# ARCHIVES OF PEDIATRICS & ADOLESCENT MEDICINE

WWW.ARCHPEDIATRICS.COM

JANUARY 2006


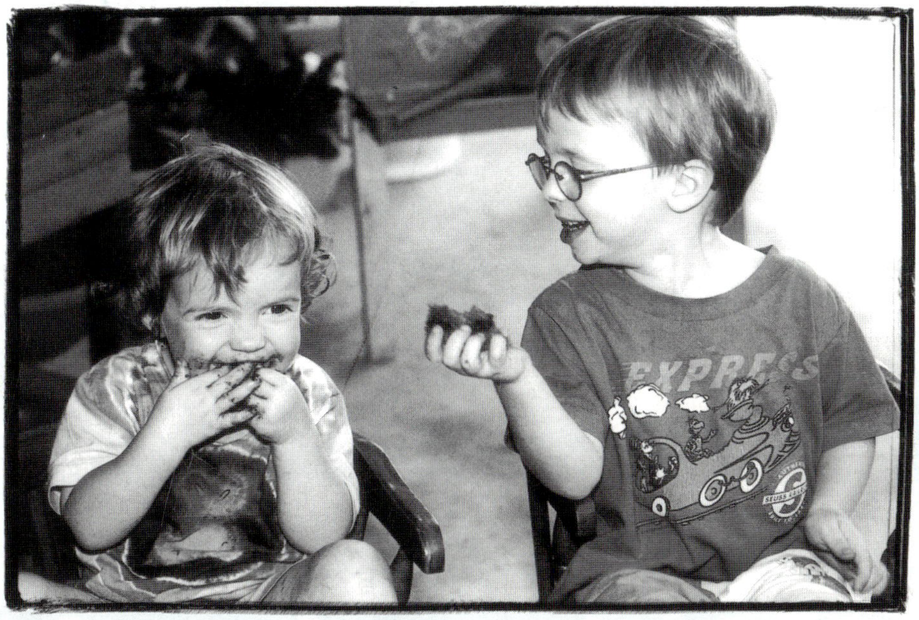


Eating cake. See page 5.


EFFECTS OF ALCOHOL ADVERTISING EXPOSURE ON DRINKING AMONG YOUTH

NEIGHBORHOOD SAFETY AND OVERWEIGHT STATUS IN CHILDREN

IMPACT OF ADOLESCENT MENTAL DISORDERS AND PHYSICAL ILLNESSES ON QUALITY OF LIFE 17 YEARS LATER

ADULTHOOD OUTCOME OF TIC AND OBSESSIVE-COMPULSIVE SYMPTOM SEVERITY IN CHILDREN WITH TOURETTE SYNDROME



COMPLETE TABLE OF CONTENTS ON PAGE 3



JAMA & ARCHIVES JOURNALS

American Medical Association

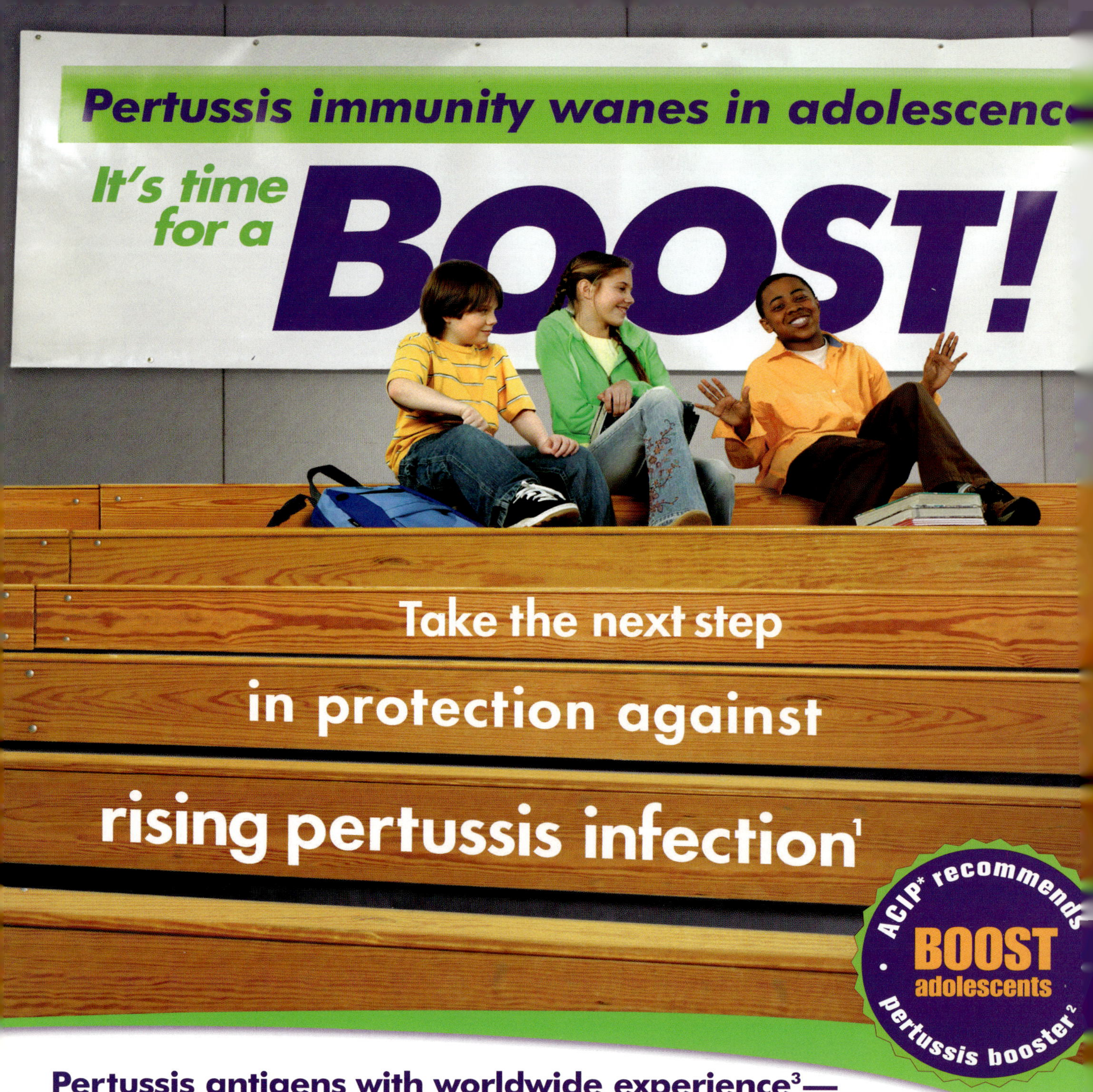

Pertussis immunity wanes in adolescenc
It's time for a BOOST!
Take the next step
in protection against
rising pertussis infection[1]
ACIP* recommends
BOOST
adolescents
pertussis booster[2]

# BOOSTRIX®

**(Tetanus Toxoid, Reduced Diphtheria Toxoid and Acellular Pertussis Vaccine, Adsorbed) (Tdap)**

The following is a brief summary only; see full prescribing information for complete product information.

**INDICATIONS AND USAGE:** BOOSTRIX is indicated for active booster immunization against tetanus, diphtheria, and pertussis as a single dose in individuals 10 through 18 years of age. The use of BOOSTRIX as a primary series or to complete the primary series has not been studied. As with any vaccine, BOOSTRIX may not protect 100% of individuals receiving the vaccine. BOOSTRIX is not recommended for treatment of actual infections.

**CONTRAINDICATIONS:** Hypersensitivity to any component of the vaccine is a contraindication (see DESCRIPTION in full prescribing information). Do not use BOOSTRIX after a serious allergic reaction (e.g., anaphylaxis) following any other tetanus toxoid, diphtheria toxoid or pertussis-containing vaccine, or any component of this vaccine (see DESCRIPTION in full prescribing information). Because of the uncertainty as to which component of the vaccine might be responsible, do not give further vaccination with any of these components; or, refer such individuals to an allergist for evaluation. The following events are contraindications to administration of BOOSTRIX: encephalopathy (e.g., coma, decreased level of consciousness, prolonged seizures) within 7 days of administration of a previous dose of a pertussis-containing vaccine that is not attributable to another identifiable cause; progressive neurologic disorder, uncontrolled epilepsy, or progressive encephalopathy. Do not vaccinate individuals with these conditions until a treatment regimen has been established and the condition has stabilized. BOOSTRIX is not contraindicated for use in individuals with HIV infection.

**WARNINGS:** The tip cap and the rubber plunger of the needleless prefilled syringes contain dry natural latex rubber that may cause allergic reactions in latex sensitive individuals. The vial stopper is latex-free. If any of the following events occurred in temporal relation to previous receipt of a Diphtheria and Tetanus Toxoids and Pertussis Vaccine Adsorbed (DTwP) vaccine or a vaccine containing an acellular pertussis component, consider carefully whether to give subsequent doses of BOOSTRIX: temperature of ≥40.5°C (105°F) within 48 hours not due to another identifiable cause; collapse or shock-like state (hypotonic-hyporesponsive episode) within 48 hours; persistent, inconsolable crying lasting ≥3 hours, occurring within 48 hours; seizures with or without fever occurring within 3 days. Persons who experienced serious Arthus-type hypersensitivity reactions following a prior dose of tetanus toxoid usually have high serum tetanus antitoxin levels and should not be given Tetanus and Diphtheria Toxoids Adsorbed For Adult Use (Td) or Tdap vaccines or even emergency doses of Td more frequently than every 10 years, even if the wound is neither clean nor minor. If Guillain-Barré syndrome has occurred within 6 weeks of receipt of prior vaccine containing tetanus toxoid, the decision to give BOOSTRIX or any vaccine containing tetanus toxoid should be based on careful consideration of the potential benefits and possible risks. The decision to administer a pertussis-containing vaccine to individuals with stable central nervous system (CNS) disorders must be made by the physician on an individual basis, with consideration of all relevant factors, and assessment of potential risks and benefits for that individual. Advise the patient, parent, or guardian of the potential increased risk involved (see PRECAUTIONS). A family history of seizures or other CNS disorders is not a contraindication to pertussis vaccine. The Advisory Committee on Immunization Practices (ACIP) has published guidelines for vaccination of persons with recent or acute illness (www.cdc.gov). Do not give BOOSTRIX to individuals with bleeding disorders such as hemophilia or thrombocytopenia, or to persons on anticoagulant therapy unless the potential benefit clearly outweighs the risk of administration. If the decision is made to administer BOOSTRIX to such persons, it should be given with caution with steps taken to avoid the risk of hematoma following the injection.

**PRECAUTIONS:** Before the injection of any biological, the physician should take all reasonable precautions to prevent allergic or other adverse reactions. Epinephrine injection (1:1,000) and other appropriate agents used for the control of immediate allergic reactions must be immediately available should an acute anaphylactic reaction occur. Immunosuppressed persons, including individuals receiving immunosuppressive therapy, may not develop the expected immune response. **Drug Interactions:** Do not mix BOOSTRIX with any other vaccine in the same syringe or vial. **Carcinogenesis, Mutagenesis, Impairment of Fertility:** BOOSTRIX has not been evaluated for carcinogenic or mutagenic potential, or for impairment of fertility. **Pregnancy:** Pregnancy Category C. Animal reproduction studies have not been conducted with BOOSTRIX. It is also not known whether BOOSTRIX can cause fetal harm when administered to a pregnant woman or can affect reproductive capacity. BOOSTRIX should be given to a pregnant woman only if clearly needed. Animal fertility studies have not been conducted with BOOSTRIX. In a developmental toxicity study, the effect of BOOSTRIX on embryo-fetal and pre-weaning development was evaluated in pregnant rats. Animals were administered INFANRIX® (Diphtheria and Tetanus Toxoids and Acellular Pertussis Vaccine Adsorbed) prior to gestation and BOOSTRIX during the period of organogenesis (gestation days 6, 8, 11) and later in pregnancy (gestation day 15), 0.1 mL/rat/occasion (a 45-fold increase compared to the human dose of BOOSTRIX on a body weight basis), by intramuscular injection. No adverse affect on pregnancy and lactation parameters, embryo-fetal or pre-weaning development was observed. There were no fetal malformations or other evidence of teratogenesis noted in this study. **Nursing Mothers:** It is not known whether BOOSTRIX is excreted in human milk. Because many drugs are excreted in human milk, caution should be exercised when BOOSTRIX is administered to a nursing woman. **Pregnancy Exposure Registry:** Healthcare providers are encouraged to register pregnant women who receive BOOSTRIX in the GlaxoSmithKline vaccination pregnancy registry by calling 1-888-825-5249. **Geriatric Use:** BOOSTRIX is not indicated for use in individuals older than 18 years. **Pediatric Use:** BOOSTRIX is not indicated for use in individuals younger than 10 years (see DOSAGE AND ADMINISTRATION in full prescribing information). For immunization of infants and children younger than 7 years against diphtheria, tetanus, and pertussis, refer to the manufacturers' package inserts for Diphtheria and Tetanus Toxoids and Acellular Pertussis Vaccine Adsorbed (DTaP) vaccines.

**ADVERSE REACTIONS:** A total of 3,289 adolescents were vaccinated with a single dose of BOOSTRIX during clinical trials. An additional 1,092 adolescents 10 to 18 years of age received a non-US formulation of BOOSTRIX (formulated to contain 0.5 mg aluminum per dose) in non-US clinical studies.

The primary safety study, conducted in the United States, was a randomized, observer-blinded, controlled study in which 3,080 adolescents 10 to 18 years of age received a single dose of BOOSTRIX and 1,034 received the control Td vaccine manufactured by Massachusetts Public Health Biologic Laboratories. There were no substantive differences in demographic characteristics between the vaccine groups. Among BOOSTRIX and control vaccine recipients approximately 75% were 10 to 14 years of age and approximately 25% were 15 to 18 years of age. Approximately 98% of participants in this study had received the recommended series of 4 or 5 doses of either DTwP or a combination of DTwP and DTaP in childhood. Data on adverse events were collected by the subjects, parents and/or guardians using standardized diaries for 15 consecutive days following the vaccine dose (i.e., day of vaccination and the next 14 days). Subjects were monitored for unsolicited adverse events that occurred within 31 days of vaccination (day 0-30) using diary cards (day 0-14) supplemented by spontaneous reports and a medical history as reported by subjects, parents, and/or guardians. Subjects were also monitored for 6 months post-vaccination for non-routine medical visits, visits to an emergency room, onset of new chronic illness, and serious adverse events. Information regarding late onset adverse events was obtained via a telephone call 6 months following vaccination. At least 97% of subjects completed the 6-month follow-up evaluation.

The adverse event information from clinical trials provides a basis for identifying adverse events that appear to be related to vaccine use and for approximating rates. However, because clinical trials are conducted under widely varying conditions, adverse event rates observed in the clinical trials of a vaccine cannot be directly compared to rates in the clinical trials of another vaccine, and may not reflect the rates observed in practice.

**Serious Adverse Events in All Safety Studies:** In the US-safety study, no serious adverse events were reported to occur within 31 days of vaccination. During the 6-month extended safety evaluation period, no serious adverse events that were of potential autoimmune origin or new onset and chronic in nature were reported to occur. In non-US studies in which serious adverse events were monitored for up to 37 days, one subject was diagnosed with insulin dependent diabetes. The association of this event with vaccination is unknown. No other serious adverse events of potential autoimmune origin or that were new onset and chronic in nature were reported to occur in these studies.

**Solicited Adverse Events in the US-Safety Study:** In a US study, the most common local adverse events following administration of BOOSTRIX were pain, redness, and swelling at the injection site. The most common general adverse events were headache and fatigue. Most of these events were reported at a similar frequency in recipients of both BOOSTRIX and Td. Any pain, grade 2 or 3 pain (but not grade 3 alone), and grade 2 or 3 headache (but not grade 3 alone) were reported at a higher rate in recipients of BOOSTRIX. The primary safety endpoint of the US study was the incidence of grade 3 pain (spontaneously painful and/or prevented normal activity) at the injection site within 15 days of vaccination. Grade 3 pain was reported in 4.6% of those who received BOOSTRIX compared with 4.0% of those who received the Td vaccine. The difference in rate of grade 3 pain was within the pre-defined clinical limit for non-inferiority (upper limit of the 95% CI for the difference ≤4%). These were the rates for solicited local and general adverse events within 15 days of vaccination with BOOSTRIX or Td vaccine for the total vaccinated cohort (all enrolled, vaccinated subjects with safety data available analyzed by vaccine received):

**Percentage of Individuals 10 to 18 Years of Age Reporting Solicited Local Adverse Events or Solicited General Adverse Events Within the 15-day* Post-Vaccination Period**

| | BOOSTRIX (N = 3,032) | Td (N = 1,013) |
|---|---|---|
| **Local** | | |
| Pain,† any | 75.3 | 71.7 |
| Pain,† grade 2 or 3 | 51.2 | 42.5 |
| Pain,‡ grade 3 | 4.6 | 4.0 |
| Redness, any | 22.5 | 19.8 |
| Redness, >20 mm | 4.1 | 3.9 |
| Redness, ≥50 mm | 1.7 | 1.6 |
| Swelling, any | 21.1 | 20.1 |
| Swelling, >20 mm | 5.3 | 4.9 |
| Swelling, ≥50 mm | 2.5 | 3.2 |
| Arm circumference increase,§ >5 mm | 28.3 | 29.5 |
| Arm circumference increase,§ >20 mm | 2.0 | 2.2 |
| Arm circumference increase,§ >40 mm | 0.5 | 0.3 |
| **General** | | |
| Fever,‖ ≥99.5°F | 13.5 | 13.1 |
| Fever,‖ >100.4°F | 5.0 | 4.7 |
| Fever,‖ >102.2°F | 1.4 | 1.0 |
| Headache, any | 43.1 | 41.5 |
| Headache,† grade 2 or 3 | 15.7 | 12.7 |
| Headache, grade 3 | 3.7 | 2.7 |
| Fatigue, any | 37.0 | 36.7 |
| Fatigue, grade 2 or 3 | 14.4 | 12.9 |
| Fatigue, grade 3 | 3.7 | 3.2 |
| Gastrointestinal symptoms,¶ any | 26.0 | 25.8 |
| Gastrointestinal symptoms,¶ grade 2 or 3 | 9.8 | 9.7 |
| Gastrointestinal symptoms,¶ grade 3 | 3.0 | 3.2 |

Td = Tetanus and Diphtheria Toxoids Adsorbed For Adult Use manufactured by Massachusetts Public Health Biologic Laboratories.

N = number of subjects in the total vaccinated cohort with local/general symptoms sheets completed.

Grade 2 = Local: painful when the limb was moved; General: interfered with normal activity.

Grade 3 = Local: spontaneously painful and/or prevented normal activity; General: prevented normal activity.

*Day of vaccination and the next 14 days.

†Statistically significantly higher (P<0.05) following BOOSTRIX as compared to Td vaccine.

‡Grade 3 injection site pain following BOOSTRIX was not inferior to Td (upper limit of two-sided 95% CI for the difference in the percentage of subjects ≤4%).

§Mid-upper region of the vaccinated arm.

‖Oral temperatures or axillary temperatures.

¶Gastrointestinal symptoms included nausea, vomiting, diarrhea and/or abdominal pain.

Mid-upper arm circumference was measured by the adolescent or their parent/guardian prior to injection and daily for 15 days following vaccination. There was no significant difference between BOOSTRIX recipients and Td recipients in the proportion of subjects reporting an increase in mid-upper arm circumference in the vaccinated arm. The incidence of unsolicited adverse events reported in the 31 days after vaccination was comparable between the 2 groups.

As with any vaccine, there is the possibility that broad use of BOOSTRIX could reveal adverse events not observed in clinical trials.

**Postmarketing Reports:** Worldwide voluntary reports of adverse events received for BOOSTRIX in persons 10 to 18 years of age since market introduction of this vaccine are listed below. This list includes serious events or events which have causal connection to components of this or other vaccines or drugs. Because these events are reported voluntarily from a population of uncertain size, it is not possible to reliably estimate their frequency or establish a causal relationship to vaccine exposure. *Blood and lymphatic system disorders:* Lymphadenitis, lymphadenopathy. *Cardiac disorders:* Myocarditis. *Injection site reactions:* Induration, inflammation, mass, nodule, warmth, local reaction. *Metabolism and nutrition disorders:* Diabetes mellitus insulin-dependent. *Musculoskeletal and connective tissue disorders:* Arthralgia, back pain, myalgia. *Nervous system disorders:* Convulsion, encephalitis, facial palsy, paraesthesia. *Skin and subcutaneous tissue disorders:* Exanthem, Henoch-Schönlein purpura, rash. In addition, extensive swelling of the injected limb has been reported following administration of BOOSTRIX.

**Reporting Adverse Events:** Report the occurrence following immunization of any event set forth in the Vaccine Injury Table from the National Childhood Vaccine Injury Act including: Anaphylaxis or anaphylactic shock within 7 days, encephalopathy or encephalitis within 7 days, brachial neuritis within 28 days, or an acute complication or sequelae (including death) of an illness, disability, injury, or condition referred to above, or any events that would contraindicate further doses of vaccine, according to this prescribing information. These events should be reported to VAERS. The VAERS toll-free number is 1-800-822-7967. Reporting forms may also be obtained at the VAERS website at www.vaers.org.

**DOSAGE AND ADMINISTRATION: Recommended Dose:** BOOSTRIX should be administered as a single 0.5 mL injection by the intramuscular route into the deltoid muscle of the upper arm in individuals 10 through 18 years of age. Do not administer this product subcutaneously or intravenously. There are no data to support repeat administration of BOOSTRIX. Five years should elapse between the subject's last dose of the recommended series of childhood DTwP and/or DTaP vaccine and the administration of BOOSTRIX. Limited data are available on the use of BOOSTRIX following Tetanus and Diphtheria Toxoids Adsorbed For Adult Use (Td) vaccine. **Additional Dosing Information:** ***Wound Management:*** Clinicians should refer to guidelines for tetanus prophylaxis in routine wound management. Adolescents 10 to 18 years of age who have completed a primary series against tetanus and who sustain wounds which are minor and uncomplicated, should receive a booster dose of a tetanus toxoid-containing vaccine only if they have not received tetanus toxoid within the preceding 10 years. In case of tetanus-prone injury (e.g., wounds contaminated with dirt, feces, soil, and saliva; puncture wounds; avulsions; and wounds resulting from missles, crushing, burns, and frostbite) in an adolescent who is in need of tetanus toxoid, BOOSTRIX can be used as an alternative to Tetanus and Diphtheria Toxoids Adsorbed For Adult Use (Td) vaccine in patients for whom the pertussis component is also indicated (see INDICATIONS AND USAGE).

Manufactured by **GlaxoSmithKline Biologicals**
Rixensart, Belgium, US License 1617
Distributed by **GlaxoSmithKline**
Research Triangle Park, NC 27709



Full prescribing information for BOOSTRIX is available at www.BOOSTRIX.com.

BRS-BO:L1

**References: 1.** Centers for Disease Control and Prevention. *Epidemiology and Prevention of Vaccine-Preventable Diseases.* Atkinson W, Hamborsky J, Wolfe S, eds. 8th ed. Washington DC: Public Health Foundation; 2004:75–88, A26–A27. **2.** ACIP recommends adolescent vaccination for tetanus, diphtheria and pertussis vaccine [press release]. Atlanta, GA: Department of Health and Human Services; Available at: www.cdc.gov/nip/pr/pr_tdap_jun2005.htm. Accessed September 27, 2005. **3.** Data on file, BOR305, GlaxoSmithKline.

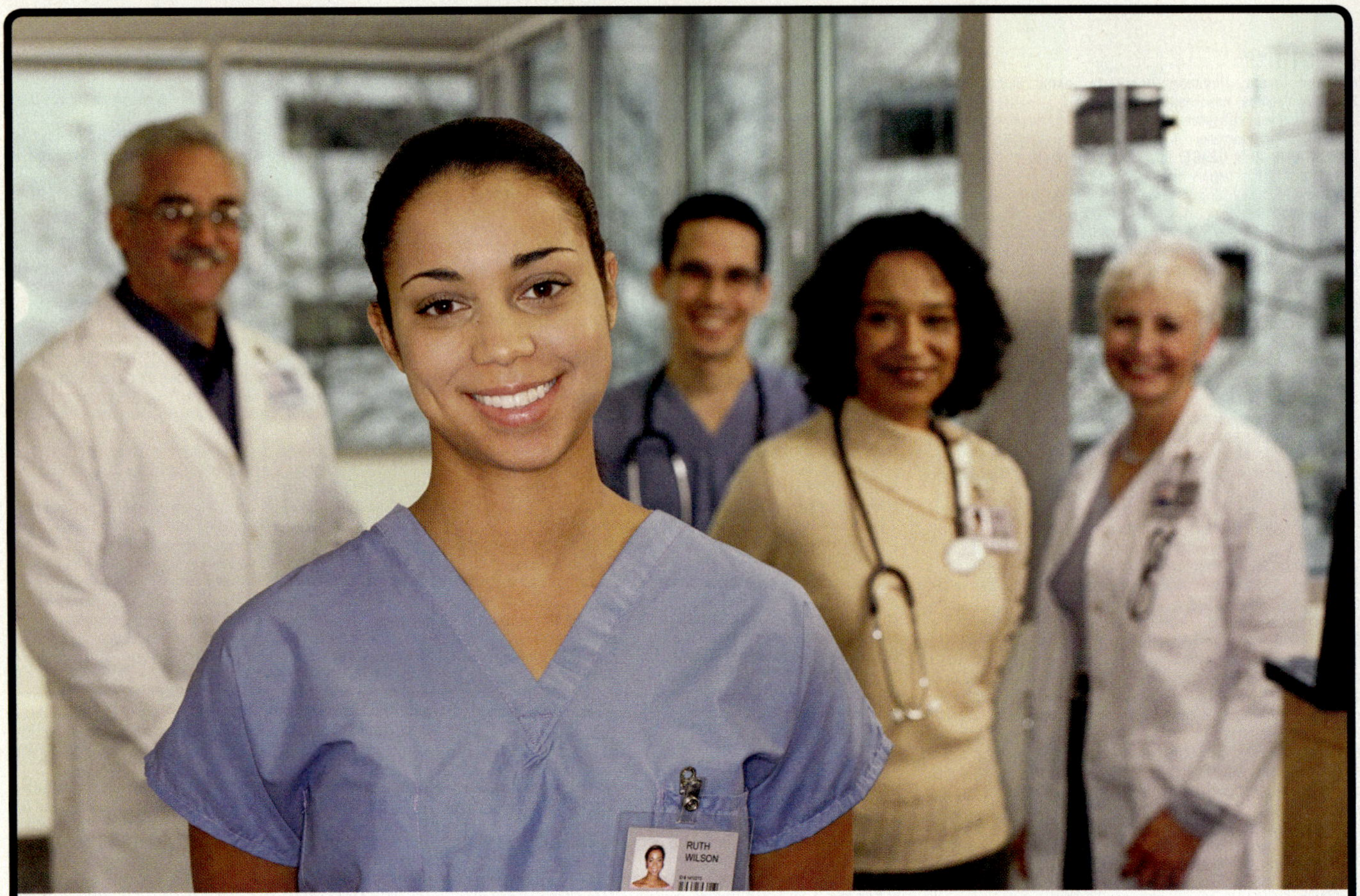
RUTH
WILSON

ARCHIVES OF PEDIATRICS & ADOLESCENT MEDICINE

JANUARY 2006 VOLUME 160, NUMBER 1 PAGES 1-112

## ON MY MIND

**Fiona** 15
*Megan A. Moreno, MD, MSEd*

## ARTICLES

**Effects of Alcohol Advertising Exposure on Drinking Among Youth** 18
*Leslie B. Snyder, PhD; Frances Fleming Milici, PhD; Michael Slater, PhD; Helen Sun, MA; Yuliya Strizhakova, PhD*

**Neighborhood Safety and Overweight Status in Children** 25
*Julie C. Lumeng, MD; Danielle Appugliese, MPH; Howard J. Cabral, PhD; Robert H. Bradley, PhD; Barry Zuckerman, MD*

**Increasing Prevalences of Overweight and Obesity in Northern Plains American Indian Children** 34
*Elenora Zephier, MPH, RD; John H. Himes, PhD, MPH; Mary Story, PhD, RD; Xia Zhou, MS*

**Weight Gain in Obese and Nonobese Adolescent Girls Initiating Depot Medroxyprogesterone Acetate, Oral Contraceptive Pills, or No Hormonal Contraceptive Method** 40
*Andrea E. Bonny, MD; Julie Ziegler, MA; Ray Harvey, MPH; Sara M. Debanne, PhD; Michelle Secic, MS; Barbara A. Cromer, MD*

## REVIEW ARTICLE

**Sedation and Analgesia for Pediatric Fracture Reduction in the Emergency Department: A Systematic Review** 46
*Russell T. Migita, MD; Eileen J. Klein, MD, MPH; Michelle M. Garrison, MPH*

## SPECIAL FEATURE

**Picture of the Month** 53
*Ismail Reisli, MD; Sevgi Keles, MD; Umit Kamis, MD; Sefika Elmas, MD; Banu Turgut Ozturk, MD*

## ARTICLES

**Enabling Parents Who Smoke to Prevent Their Children From Initiating Smoking: Results From a 3-Year Intervention Evaluation** 56
*Christine Jackson, PhD; Denise Dickinson, MPH*

**Adulthood Outcome of Tic and Obsessive-Compulsive Symptom Severity in Children With Tourette Syndrome** 65
*Michael H. Bloch, BA; Bradley S. Peterson, MD; Lawrence Scahill, MSN, PhD; Jessica Otka, BA; Lily Katsovich, MS; Heping Zhang, PhD; James F. Leckman, MD*

**Unmet Health Care Needs Among Children Evaluated for Sexual Assault** 70
*Rebecca Girardet, MD; Lauren Giacobbe; Kelly Bolton, RN; Sheela Lahoti, MD; Margaret McNeese, MD*

**Longitudinal Trends in Race/Ethnic Disparities in Leading Health Indicators From Adolescence to Young Adulthood** 74
*Kathleen Mullan Harris, PhD; Penny Gordon-Larsen, PhD; Kim Chantala, MS; J. Richard Udry, PhD*

**Multisite Controlled Study of OROS Methylphenidate in the Treatment of Adolescents With Attention-Deficit/Hyperactivity Disorder** 82
*Timothy E. Wilens, MD; Keith McBurnett, PhD; Oscar Bukstein, MD; James McGough, MD; Laurence Greenhill, MD; Marc Lerner, MD; Mark A. Stein, PhD; C. Keith Conners, PhD; John Duby, MD; Jeffrey Newcorn, MD; Charles E. Bailey, MD; Christopher J. Kratochvil, MD; Daniel Coury, MD; Charles Casat, MD; Mary Joan C. Denisco, PharmD; Patricia Halstead, MD; Leslie Bloom, BS; Brenda A. Zimmerman, MS; Joan Gu, MS; Kimberly M. Cooper, MS; Joseph M. Lynch, MD*

**Impact of Adolescent Mental Disorders and Physical Illnesses on Quality of Life 17 Years Later** 93
*Henian Chen, MD, PhD; Patricia Cohen, PhD; Stephanie Kasen, PhD; Jeffrey G. Johnson, PhD; Kathy Berenson, PhD; Kathy Gordon*

ARCHIVES OF PEDIATRICS & ADOLESCENT MEDICINE

## EDITORIALS

**Importance of Reducing Youth Exposure to Alcohol Advertising** 100
*David H. Jernigan, PhD*

**Do As I Say, Not As I Do: Does It Work for Tobacco Use Prevention?** 102
*Susan J. Curry, PhD; Robin J. Mermelstein, PhD*

**Discussing Outcome in Tourette Syndrome** 103
*Harvey S. Singer, MD*

## THE PEDIATRIC FORUM

**Can We Improve the Return Rate for Tuberculin Skin Test Readings?** 106
*Kari M. Jacono, MD; Mary Ann O'Riordan, MS; Lydia Furman, MD*

**Adult Learning** 106
*John T. Benjamin, MD*

**In Reply** 107
*Frederick P. Rivara, MD, MPH; F. Bruder Stapleton, MD*

**Potential Confounders That May Explain the Association Between Television Viewing and Poor Educational Achievement** 107
*Tracie O. Afifi, MSc; William Fleisher, MD, FRCPC; Jitender Sareen, MD, FRCPC*

**In Reply** 108
*Robert J. Hancox, MD; Richie Poulton, PhD*

**Something Else Is Missing From Research on Children's Television Viewing and Academic Performance** 109
*Jonathan M. Breslin, PhD*

**In Reply** 109
*Ariel R. Chernin, MA; Deborah L. Linebarger, PhD*

## REGULAR DEPARTMENTS

**This Month in *Archives of Pediatrics & Adolescent Medicine*** 13

**Announcements** 24, 31, 45, 55, 105

**Classified Advertising** 111

**Journal Advertiser Index** 111

**Contact Information** 112

**Instructions for authors and the author and subject indexes are available on our Web site: http://www.archpediatrics.com. If you do not have access to the Web, contact Suzanne Shuey at (206) 685-3573.**

### About the Cover

Photographer: Jan Goddard-Finegold, Houston, Tex.

# ARCHIVES OF PEDIATRICS & ADOLESCENT MEDICINE


**Mission Statement:** *The Archives of Pediatrics & Adolescent Medicine* is a monthly, peer-reviewed journal for physicians and other health care professionals who contribute to the health of children and adolescents. The *Archives* provides an open forum for dialogue on a full range of clinical, scientific, advocacy, and humanistic issues relevant to the care of pediatric patients from infancy through young adulthood. The *Archives* is a vehicle for increased attention to adolescent health, the education of pediatric health care professionals, and disease prevention and health promotion. The *Archives* publishes original studies, editorials, reviews by experts, practice commentaries, case quizzes, and updates on clinical science and practice management. The Pediatric Forum provides our readers with opportunities to express their views. *Archives* incorporates *AJDC*, the oldest journal in US pediatric literature, which originated in 1911.



JAMA & ARCHIVES JOURNALS
American Medical Association

# OMNICEF for Oral Suspension 250 mg/5 mL

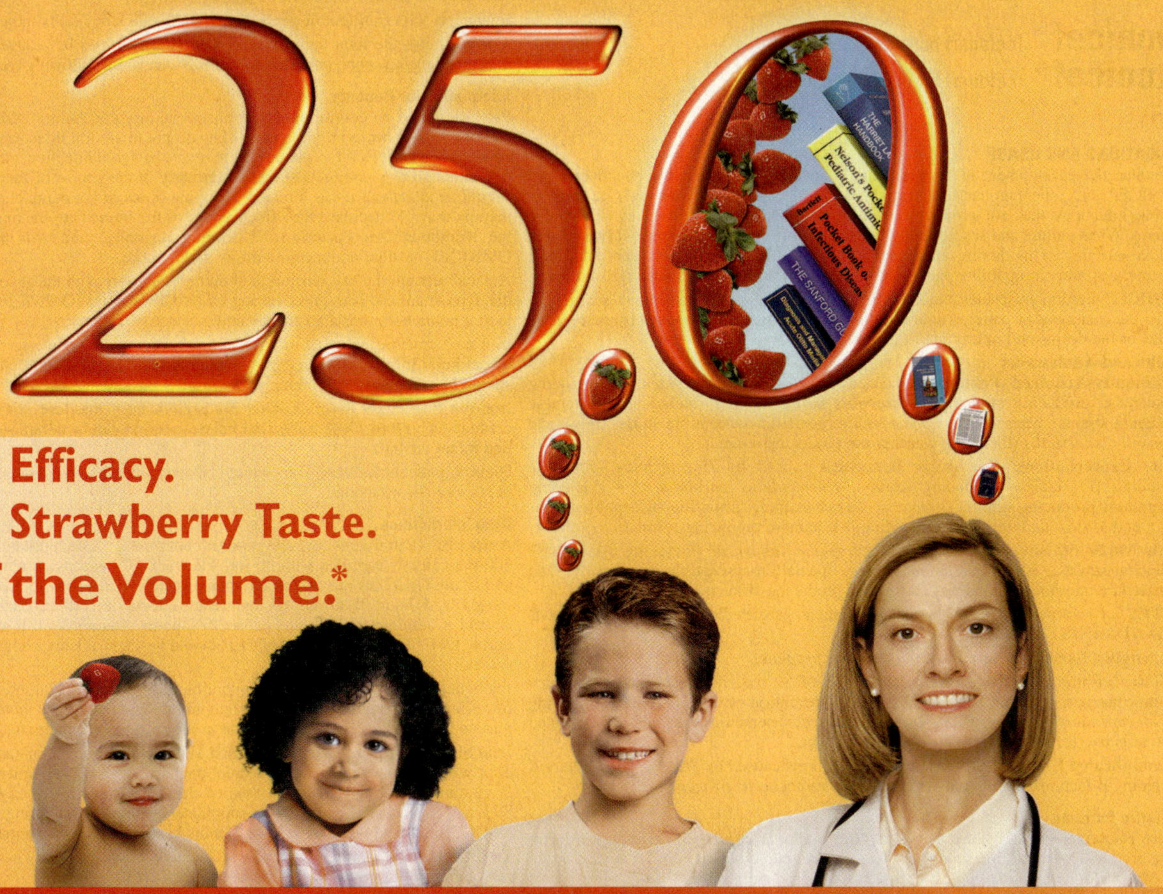


**Great Efficacy.**
**Great Strawberry Taste.**
**Half the Volume.***

## Great Minds... Concentrate on Success!

**Indications (mild to moderate infections)**[1]

**Acute Bacterial Otitis Media** and **Acute Maxillary Sinusitis** (adults and adolescents) due to *H influenzae* (including ß-lactamase producing strains), *S pneumoniae* (penicillin-susceptible strains only), and *M catarrhalis* (including ß-lactamase producing strains). Use of cefdinir in the treatment of acute maxillary sinusitis in pediatric patients is supported by evidence from adequate and well-controlled studies in adults and adolescents.

**Pharyngitis/Tonsillitis** due to *S pyogenes*. Cefdinir is effective in the eradication of *S pyogenes* from the oropharynx. Cefdinir has not, however, been studied for the prevention of rheumatic fever following *S pyogenes* pharyngitis/tonsillitis. Only intramuscular penicillin has been demonstrated to be effective for the prevention of rheumatic fever.

**Uncomplicated Skin and Skin Structure Infections** due to *S aureus* (including ß-lactamase producing strains) and *S pyogenes*.

**1/2 tsp per 20 lbs per day**††

**Important Safety Information**[1]

- To reduce the development of drug-resistant bacteria and maintain the effectiveness of OMNICEF and other antibacterial drugs, OMNICEF should be used only to treat or prevent infections that are proven or strongly suspected to be caused by bacteria
- OMNICEF is contraindicated in patients with known allergy to the cephalosporin class of antibiotics
- For patients with previous hypersensitivity reaction to penicillins, caution should be exercised because cross-hypersensitivity among ß-lactam antibiotics has been clearly documented. If an allergic reaction to cefdinir occurs, the drug should be discontinued
- Safety and efficacy in neonates and infants less than 6 months of age have not been established
- 2% of 2,289 pediatric patients discontinued medication due to adverse events in US and ex-US clinical trials. Discontinuations were primarily for gastrointestinal disturbance, usually diarrhea
- The most common reported adverse events occurring in ≥1% of pediatric patients in US clinical trials (N=1,783) were diarrhea (8%), rash (3%), and vomiting (1%)
- Maximum dose of OMNICEF for pediatric patients weighing ≥43 kg is 600 mg/day. For pediatric patients with a creatinine clearance of <30 mL/min/1.73 $m^2$ and not requiring hemodialysis, the dose of cefdinir should be 7 mg/kg (up to 300 mg) given once daily
- Antacids that contain magnesium or aluminum and iron supplements, including multivitamins that contain iron, should be taken at least 2 hours before or 2 hours after taking OMNICEF

* Compared to the 125 mg/5 mL formulation of OMNICEF.
† Calculated dose is based on 14 mg/kg/day. Dose in teaspoons is rounded to the nearest 1/4 teaspoon and is not an exact measure of calculated dose volume (mL). 1 tsp ≅ 5 mL.
‡ Once-daily dosing has not been studied in skin infections; therefore, OMNICEF for Oral Suspension should be administered twice daily in this infection (7 mg/kg BID for 10 days).


**Reference: 1.** OMNICEF® (cefdinir) for Oral Suspension Prescribing Information, Abbott Laboratories.


Please see adjacent brief summary of full prescribing information.

**OMNICEF®**
(cefdinir) for oral suspension
*125 mg/5 mL and 250 mg/5 mL*
**Expert recommended.**
**Kid preferred.**

Abbott Laboratories
Abbott Park, IL 60064

Under License of
Fujisawa Pharmaceutical Co., Ltd.
Osaka, Japan

05B-034-H712-1 • February 2005



www.OmnicefForKids.com

**BRIEF SUMMARY**
**CONSULT PACKAGE INSERT FOR FULL PRESCRIBING INFORMATION.**
03-5404-Rev. December, 2004
(Nos. 3769, 3771, 6151)

# Omnicef® (cefdinir) capsules
# Omnicef® (cefdinir) for oral suspension

℞ only

## INDICATIONS AND USAGE

To reduce the development of drug-resistant bacteria and maintain the effectiveness of OMNICEF and other antibacterial drugs, OMNICEF should be used only to treat or prevent infections that are proven or strongly suspected to be caused by susceptible bacteria. When culture and susceptibility information are available, they should be considered in selecting or modifying antibacterial therapy. In the absence of such data, local epidemiology and susceptibility patterns may contribute to the empiric selection of therapy.

OMNICEF (cefdinir) capsules and OMNICEF (cefdinir) for oral suspension are indicated for the treatment of patients with mild to moderate infections caused by susceptible strains of the designated microorganisms in the conditions listed below.

**Adults and Adolescents**

**Community-Acquired Pneumonia** caused by *Haemophilus influenzae* (including β-lactamase producing strains), *Haemophilus parainfluenzae* (including β-lactamase producing strains), *Streptococcus pneumoniae* (penicillin-susceptible strains only), and *Moraxella catarrhalis* (including β-lactamase producing strains).

**Acute Exacerbations of Chronic Bronchitis** caused by *Haemophilus influenzae* (including β-lactamase producing strains), *Haemophilus parainfluenzae* (including β-lactamase producing strains), *Streptococcus pneumoniae* (penicillin-susceptible strains only), and *Moraxella catarrhalis* (including β-lactamase producing strains).

**Acute Maxillary Sinusitis** caused by *Haemophilus influenzae* (including β-lactamase producing strains), *Streptococcus pneumoniae* (penicillin-susceptible strains only), and *Moraxella catarrhalis* (including β-lactamase producing strains).

**NOTE:** For information on use in pediatric patients, see **Pediatric Use** and **DOSAGE AND ADMINISTRATION**.

**Pharyngitis/Tonsillitis** caused by *Streptococcus pyogenes*.

**NOTE:** Cefdinir is effective in the eradication of *S. pyogenes* from the oropharynx. Cefdinir has not, however, been studied for the prevention of rheumatic fever following *S. pyogenes* pharyngitis/tonsillitis. Only intramuscular penicillin has been demonstrated to be effective for the prevention of rheumatic fever.

**Uncomplicated Skin and Skin Structure Infections** caused by *Staphylococcus aureus* (including β-lactamase producing strains) and *Streptococcus pyogenes*.

### Pediatric Patients

**Acute Bacterial Otitis Media** caused by *Haemophilus influenzae* (including β-lactamase producing strains), *Streptococcus pneumoniae* (penicillin-susceptible strains only), and *Moraxella catarrhalis* (including β-lactamase producing strains).

**Pharyngitis/Tonsillitis** caused by *Streptococcus pyogenes*.

**NOTE:** Cefdinir is effective in the eradication of *S. pyogenes* from the oropharynx. Cefdinir has not, however, been studied for the prevention of rheumatic fever following *S. pyogenes* pharyngitis/tonsillitis. Only intramuscular penicillin has been demonstrated to be effective for the prevention of rheumatic fever.

**Uncomplicated Skin and Skin Structure Infections** caused by *Staphylococcus aureus* (including β-lactamase producing strains) and *Streptococcus pyogenes*.

## CONTRAINDICATIONS

OMNICEF (cefdinir) is contraindicated in patients with known allergy to the cephalosporin class of antibiotics.

## WARNINGS

**BEFORE THERAPY WITH OMNICEF (CEFDINIR) IS INSTITUTED, CAREFUL INQUIRY SHOULD BE MADE TO DETERMINE WHETHER THE PATIENT HAS HAD PREVIOUS HYPERSENSITIVITY REACTIONS TO CEFDINIR, OTHER CEPHALOSPORINS, PENICILLINS, OR OTHER DRUGS. IF CEFDINIR IS TO BE GIVEN TO PENICILLIN-SENSITIVE PATIENTS, CAUTION SHOULD BE EXERCISED BECAUSE CROSS-HYPERSENSITIVITY AMONG β-LACTAM ANTIBIOTICS HAS BEEN CLEARLY DOCUMENTED AND MAY OCCUR IN UP TO 10% OF PATIENTS WITH A HISTORY OF PENICILLIN ALLERGY. IF AN ALLERGIC REACTION TO CEFDINIR OCCURS, THE DRUG SHOULD BE DISCONTINUED. SERIOUS ACUTE HYPERSENSITIVITY REACTIONS MAY REQUIRE TREATMENT WITH EPINEPHRINE AND OTHER EMERGENCY MEASURES, INCLUDING OXYGEN, INTRAVENOUS FLUIDS, INTRAVENOUS ANTIHISTAMINES, CORTICOSTEROIDS, PRESSOR AMINES, AND AIRWAY MANAGEMENT, AS CLINICALLY INDICATED.**

**Pseudomembranous colitis has been reported with nearly all antibacterial agents, including cefdinir, and may range in severity from mild- to life-threatening. Therefore, it is important to consider this diagnosis in patients who present with diarrhea subsequent to the administration of antibacterial agents.**

Treatment with antibacterial agents alters the normal flora of the colon and may permit overgrowth of clostridia. Studies indicate that a toxin produced by *Clostridium difficile* is a primary cause of "antibiotic-associated colitis."

After the diagnosis of pseudomembranous colitis has been established, appropriate therapeutic measures should be initiated. Mild cases of pseudomembranous colitis usually respond to drug discontinuation alone. In moderate to severe cases, consideration should be given to management with fluids and electrolytes, protein supplementation, and treatment with an antibacterial drug clinically effective against *Clostridium difficile*.

## PRECAUTIONS

### General

Prescribing OMNICEF in the absence of a proven or strongly suspected bacterial infection or a prophylactic indication is unlikely to provide benefit to the patient and increases the risk of the development of drug-resistant bacteria.

As with other broad-spectrum antibiotics, prolonged treatment may result in the possible emergence and overgrowth of resistant organisms. Careful observation of the patient is essential. If superinfection occurs during therapy, appropriate alternative therapy should be administered.

Cefdinir, as with other broad-spectrum antimicrobials (antibiotics), should be prescribed with caution in individuals with a history of colitis.

In patients with transient or persistent renal insufficiency (creatinine clearance <30 mL/min), the total daily dose of OMNICEF should be reduced because high and prolonged plasma concentrations of cefdinir can result following recommended doses.

### Information for Patients

Patients should be counseled that antibacterial drugs including OMNICEF should only be used to treat bacterial infections. They do not treat viral infections (e.g., the common cold). When OMNICEF is prescribed to treat a bacterial infection, patients should be told that although it is common to feel better early in the course of therapy, the medication should be taken exactly as directed. Skipping doses or not completing the full course of therapy may (1) decrease the effectiveness of the immediate treatment and (2) increase the likelihood that bacteria will develop resistance and will not be treatable by OMNICEF or other antibacterial drugs in the future.

Antacids containing magnesium or aluminum interfere with the absorption of cefdinir. If this type of antacid is required during OMNICEF therapy, OMNICEF should be taken at least 2 hours before or after the antacid.

Iron supplements, including multivitamins that contain iron, interfere with the absorption of cefdinir. If iron supplements are required during OMNICEF therapy, OMNICEF should be taken at least 2 hours before or after the supplement.

Iron-fortified infant formula does not significantly interfere with the absorption of cefdinir. Therefore, OMNICEF for Oral Suspension can be administered with iron-fortified infant formula.

Diabetic patients and caregivers should be aware that the oral suspension contains 2.86 g of sucrose per teaspoon.

### Drug Interactions

**Antacids:** (aluminum- or magnesium-containing): Concomitant administration of 300-mg cefdinir capsules with 30 mL Maalox® TC suspension reduces the rate ($C_{max}$) and extent (AUC) of absorption by approximately 40%. Time to reach $C_{max}$ is also prolonged by 1 hour. There are no significant effects on cefdinir pharmacokinetics if the antacid is administered 2 hours before or 2 hours after cefdinir. If antacids are required during OMNICEF therapy, OMNICEF should be taken at least 2 hours before or after the antacid.

**Probenecid:** As with other β-lactam antibiotics, probenecid inhibits the renal excretion of cefdinir, resulting in an approximate doubling in AUC, a 54% increase in peak cefdinir plasma levels, and a 50% prolongation in the apparent elimination $t_{1/2}$.

**Iron Supplements and Foods Fortified With Iron:** Concomitant administration of cefdinir with a therapeutic iron supplement containing 60 mg of elemental iron (as $FeSO4$) or vitamins supplemented with 10 mg of elemental iron reduced extent of absorption by 80% and 31%, respectively. If iron supplements are required during OMNICEF therapy, OMNICEF should be taken at least 2 hours before or after the supplement.

The effect of foods highly fortified with elemental iron (primarily iron-fortified breakfast cereals) on cefdinir absorption has not been studied.

Concomitantly administered iron-fortified infant formula (2.2 mg elemental iron/6 oz) has no significant effect on cefdinir pharmacokinetics. Therefore, OMNICEF for Oral Suspension can be administered with iron-fortified infant formula.

There have been reports of reddish stools in patients receiving cefdinir. In many cases, patients were also receiving iron-containing products. The reddish color is due to the formation of a nonabsorbable complex between cefdinir or its breakdown products and iron in the gastrointestinal tract.

### Drug/Laboratory Test Interactions

A false-positive reaction for ketones in the urine may occur with tests using nitroprusside, but not with those using nitroferricyanide. The administration of cefdinir may result in a false-positive reaction for glucose in urine using Clinitest®, Benedict's solution, or Fehling's solution. It is recommended that glucose tests based on enzymatic glucose oxidase reactions (such as Clinistix® or Tes-Tape®) be used. Cephalosporins are known to occasionally induce a positive direct Coombs' test.

### Carcinogenesis, Mutagenesis, Impairment of Fertility

The carcinogenic potential of cefdinir has not been evaluated. No mutagenic effects were seen in the bacterial reverse mutation assay (Ames) or point mutation assay at the hypoxanthine-guanine phosphoribosyltransferase locus (HGPRT) in V79 Chinese hamster lung cells. No clastogenic effects were observed *in vitro* in the structural chromosome aberration assay in V79 Chinese hamster lung cells or *in vivo* in the micronucleus assay in mouse bone marrow. In rats, fertility and reproductive performance were not affected by cefdinir at oral doses up to 1000 mg/kg/day (70 times the human dose based on mg/kg/day, 11 times based on $mg/m^2/day$).

### Pregnancy - Teratogenic Effects

**Pregnancy Category B:** Cefdinir was not teratogenic in rats at oral doses up to 1000 mg/kg/day (70 times the human dose based on mg/kg/day, 11 times based on $mg/m^2/day$) or in rabbits at oral doses up to 10 mg/kg/day (0.7 times the human dose based on mg/kg/day, 0.23 times based on $mg/m^2/day$). Maternal toxicity (decreased body weight gain) was observed in rabbits at the maximum tolerated dose of 10 mg/kg/day without adverse effects on offspring. Decreased body weight occurred in rat fetuses at $\geq$ 100 mg/kg/day, and in rat offspring at $\geq$ 32 mg/kg/day. No effects were observed on maternal reproductive parameters or offspring survival, development, behavior, or reproductive function.

There are, however, no adequate and well-controlled studies in pregnant women. Because animal reproduction studies are not always predictive of human response, this drug should be used during pregnancy only if clearly needed.

### Labor and Delivery

Cefdinir has not been studied for use during labor and delivery.

### Nursing Mothers

Following administration of single 600-mg doses, cefdinir was not detected in human breast milk.

### Pediatric Use

Safety and efficacy in neonates and infants less than 6 months of age have not been established. Use of cefdinir for the treatment of acute maxillary sinusitis in pediatric patients (age

6 months through 12 years) is supported by evidence from adequate and well-controlled studies in adults and adolescents, the similar pathophysiology of acute sinusitis in adult and pediatric patients, and comparative pharmacokinetic data in the pediatric population.

### Geriatric Use

Efficacy is comparable in geriatric patients and younger adults. While cefdinir has been well-tolerated in all age groups, in clinical trials geriatric patients experienced a lower rate of adverse events, including diarrhea, than younger adults. Dose adjustment in elderly patients is not necessary unless renal function is markedly compromised.

## ADVERSE EVENTS

### Clinical Trials - OMNICEF Capsules (Adult and Adolescent Patients):

In clinical trials, 5093 adult and adolescent patients (3841 US and 1252 non-US) were treated with the recommended dose of cefdinir capsules (600 mg/day). Most adverse events were mild and self-limiting. No deaths or permanent disabilities were attributed to cefdinir. One hundred forty-seven of 5093 (3%) patients discontinued medication due to adverse events thought by the investigators to be possibly, probably, or definitely associated with cefdinir therapy. The discontinuations were primarily for gastrointestinal disturbances, usually diarrhea or nausea. Nineteen of 5093 (0.4%) patients were discontinued due to rash thought related to cefdinir administration.

In the US, the following adverse events were thought by investigators to be possibly, probably, or definitely related to cefdinir capsules in multiple-dose clinical trials (N = 3841 cefdinir-treated patients):

**ADVERSE EVENTS ASSOCIATED WITH CEFDINIR CAPSULES US TRIALS IN ADULT AND ADOLESCENT PATIENTS (N=3841)[a]**

| | | |
|---|---|---|
| Incidence ≥ 1% | Diarrhea | 15% |
| | Vaginal moniliasis | 4% of women |
| | Nausea | 3% |
| | Headache | 2% |
| | Abdominal pain | 1% |
| | Vaginitis | 1% of women |
| Incidence <1% but >0.1% | Rash | 0.9% |
| | Dyspepsia | 0.7% |
| | Flatulence | 0.7% |
| | Vomiting | 0.7% |
| | Abnormal stools | 0.3% |
| | Anorexia | 0.3% |
| | Constipation | 0.3% |
| | Dizziness | 0.3% |
| | Dry mouth | 0.3% |
| | Asthenia | 0.2% |
| | Insomnia | 0.2% |
| | Leukorrhea | 0.2% of women |
| | Moniliasis | 0.2% |
| | Pruritus | 0.2% |
| | Somnolence | 0.2% |

[a] 1733 males, 2108 females

The following laboratory value changes of possible clinical significance, irrespective of relationship to therapy with cefdinir, were seen during clinical trials conducted in the US:

**LABORATORY VALUE CHANGES OBSERVED WITH CEFDINIR CAPSULES US TRIALS IN ADULT AND ADOLESCENT PATIENTS (N=3841)**

| | | |
|---|---|---|
| Incidence ≥ 1% | ↑Urine leukocytes | 2% |
| | ↑Urine protein | 2% |
| | ↑Gamma-glutamyltransferase[a] | 1% |
| | ↓Lymphocytes, ↑Lymphocytes | 1%, 0.2% |
| | ↑Microhematuria | 1% |
| Incidence <1% but >0.1% | ↑Glucose[a] | 0.9% |
| | ↑Urine glucose | 0.9% |
| | ↑White blood cells, ↓White blood cells | 0.9%, 0.7% |
| | ↑Alanine aminotransferase (ALT) | 0.7% |
| | ↑Eosinophils | 0.7% |
| | ↑Urine specific gravity, ↓Urine specific gravity[a] | 0.6%, 0.2% |
| | ↓Bicarbonate[a] | 0.6% |
| | ↑Phosphorus, ↓Phosphorus[a] | 0.6%, 0.3% |
| | ↑Aspartate aminotransferase (AST) | 0.4% |
| | ↑Alkaline phosphatase | 0.3% |
| | ↑Blood urea nitrogen (BUN) | 0.3% |
| | ↓Hemoglobin | 0.3% |
| | ↑Polymorphonuclear neutrophils (PMNs), ↓PMNs | 0.3%, 0.2% |
| | ↑Bilirubin | 0.2% |
| | ↑Lactate dehydrogenase[a] | 0.2% |
| | ↑Platelets | 0.2% |
| | ↑Potassium[a] | 0.2% |
| | ↑Urine pH[a] | 0.2% |

[a] N<3841 for these parameters

### Clinical Trials - OMNICEF for Oral Suspension (Pediatric Patients):

In clinical trials, 2289 pediatric patients (1783 US and 506 non-US) were treated with the recommended dose of cefdinir suspension (14 mg/kg/day). Most adverse events were mild and self-limiting. No deaths or permanent disabilities were attributed to cefdinir. Forty of 2289 (2%) patients discontinued medication due to adverse events considered by the investigators to be possibly, probably, or definitely associated with cefdinir therapy. Discontinuations were primarily for gastrointestinal disturbances, usually diarrhea. Five of 2289 (0.2%) patients were discontinued due to rash thought related to cefdinir administration.

In the US, the following adverse events were thought by investigators to be possibly, probably, or definitely related to cefdinir suspension in multiple-dose clinical trials (N=1783 cefdinir-treated patients):

**ADVERSE EVENTS ASSOCIATED WITH CEFDINIR SUSPENSION US TRIALS IN PEDIATRIC PATIENTS (N=1783)[a]**

| | | |
|---|---|---|
| Incidence ≥ 1% | Diarrhea | 8% |
| | Rash | 3% |
| | Vomiting | 1% |
| Incidence <1% but >0.1% | Cutaneous moniliasis | 0.9% |
| | Abdominal pain | 0.8% |
| | Leukopenia[b] | 0.3% |
| | Vaginal moniliasis | 0.3% of girls |
| | Vaginitis | 0.3% of girls |
| | Abnormal stools | 0.2% |
| | Dyspepsia | 0.2% |
| | Hyperkinesia | 0.2% |
| | Increased AST[b] | 0.2% |
| | Maculopapular rash | 0.2% |
| | Nausea | 0.2% |

[a] 977 males, 806 females
[b] Laboratory changes were occasionally reported as adverse events.

NOTE: In both cefdinir- and control-treated patients, rates of diarrhea and rash were higher in the youngest pediatric patients. The incidence of diarrhea in cefdinir-treated patients ≤ 2 years of age was 17% (95/557) compared with 4% (51/1226) in those >2 years old. The incidence of rash (primarily diaper rash in the younger patients) was 8% (43/557) in patients ≤ 2 years of age compared with 1% (8/1226) in those >2 years old.

The following laboratory value changes of possible clinical significance, irrespective of relationship to therapy with cefdinir, were seen during clinical trials conducted in the US:

**LABORATORY VALUE CHANGES OF POSSIBLE CLINICAL SIGNIFICANCE OBSERVED WITH CEFDINIR SUSPENSION US TRIALS IN PEDIATRIC PATIENTS (N=1783)**

| | | |
|---|---|---|
| Incidence ≥ 1% | ↑Lymphocytes, ↓Lymphocytes | 2%, 0.8% |
| | ↑Alkaline phosphatase | 1% |
| | ↓Bicarbonate[a] | 1% |
| | ↑Eosinophils | 1% |
| | ↑Lactate dehydrogenase | 1% |
| | ↑Platelets | 1% |
| | ↑PMNs, ↓PMNs | 1%, 1% |
| | ↑Urine protein | 1% |
| Incidence <1% but >0.1% | ↑Phosphorus, ↓Phosphorus | 0.9%, 0.4% |
| | ↑Urine pH | 0.8% |
| | ↓White blood cells, ↑White blood cells | 0.7%, 0.3% |
| | ↓Calcium[a] | 0.5% |
| | ↓Hemoglobin | 0.5% |
| | ↑Urine leukocytes | 0.5% |
| | ↑Monocytes | 0.4% |
| | ↑AST | 0.3% |
| | ↑Potassium[a] | 0.3% |
| | ↑Urine specific gravity, ↓Urine specific gravity | 0.3%, 0.1% |
| | ↓Hematocrit[a] | 0.2% |

[a] N=1387 for these parameters

### Postmarketing Experience

The following adverse experiences and altered laboratory tests, regardless of their relationship to cefdinir, have been reported during extensive postmarketing experience, beginning with approval in Japan in 1991: Stevens-Johnson syndrome, toxic epidermal necrolysis, exfoliative dermatitis, erythema multiforme, erythema nodosum, serum sickness, conjunctivitis, stomatitis, acute hepatitis, cholestasis, fulminant hepatitis, hepatic failure, jaundice, increased amylase, shock, anaphylaxis, facial and laryngeal edema, feeling of suffocation, acute enterocolitis, bloody diarrhea, hemorrhagic colitis, melena, pseudomembranous colitis, pancytopenia, granulocytopenia, leukopenia, thrombocytopenia, idiopathic thrombocytopenic purpura, hemolytic anemia, acute respiratory failure, asthmatic attack, drug-induced pneumonia, eosinophilic pneumonia, idiopathic interstitial pneumonia, fever, acute renal failure, nephropathy, bleeding tendency, coagulation disorder, disseminated intravascular coagulation, upper GI bleed, peptic ulcer, ileus, loss of consciousness, allergic vasculitis, possible cefdinir-diclofenac interaction, cardiac failure, chest pain, myocardial infarction, hypertension, involuntary movements, and rhabdomyolysis.

### Cephalosporin Class Adverse Events

The following adverse events and altered laboratory tests have been reported for cephalosporin-class antibiotics in general:

Allergic reactions, anaphylaxis, Stevens-Johnson syndrome, erythema multiforme, toxic epidermal necrolysis, renal dysfunction, toxic nephropathy, hepatic dysfunction including cholestasis, aplastic anemia, hemolytic anemia, hemorrhage, false-positive test for urinary glucose, neutropenia, pancytopenia, and agranulocytosis. Pseudomembranous colitis symptoms may begin during or after antibiotic treatment (see **WARNINGS**).

Several cephalosporins have been implicated in triggering seizures, particularly in patients with renal impairment when the dosage was not reduced (see **OVERDOSAGE**). If seizures associated with drug therapy occur, the drug should be discontinued. Anticonvulsant therapy can be given if clinically indicated.

## OVERDOSAGE

Information on cefdinir overdosage in humans is not available. In acute rodent toxicity studies, a single oral 5600-mg/kg dose produced no adverse effects. Toxic signs and symptoms following overdosage with other β-lactam antibiotics have included nausea, vomiting, epigastric distress, diarrhea, and convulsions. Hemodialysis removes cefdinir from the body. This may be useful in the event of a serious toxic reaction from overdosage, particularly if renal function is compromised.

**Rx only**

03-5404-Rev. December, 2004
(Nos. 3769, 3771, 6151)



Manufactured by:
**CEPH** International Corporation
Carolina, Puerto Rico 00986

For:
Abbott Laboratories
North Chicago, IL 60064

Under License of:
Fujisawa Pharmaceutical Co., Ltd.
Osaka, Japan

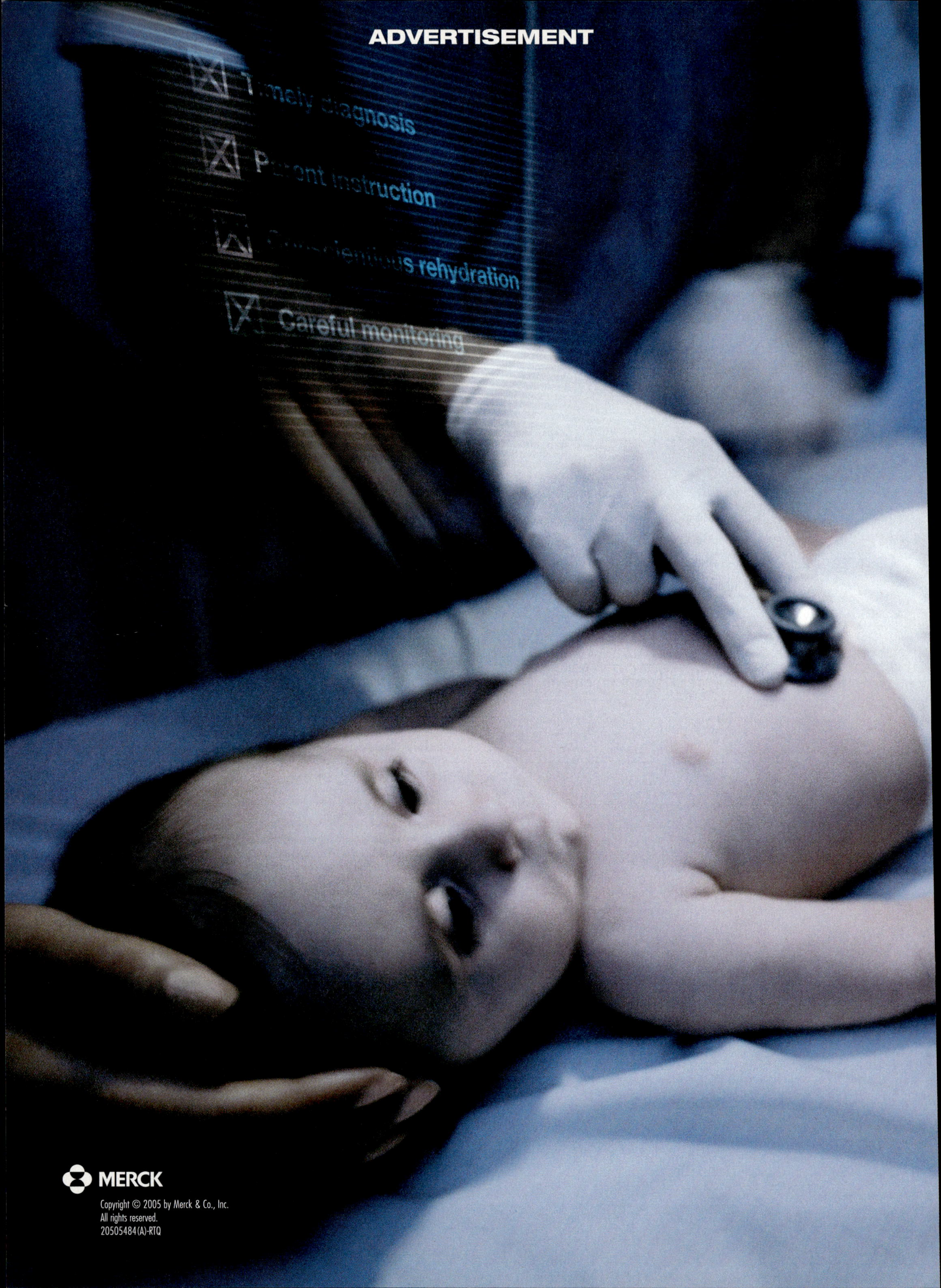
diagnosis
instruction
rehydration
Careful monitoring
MERCK

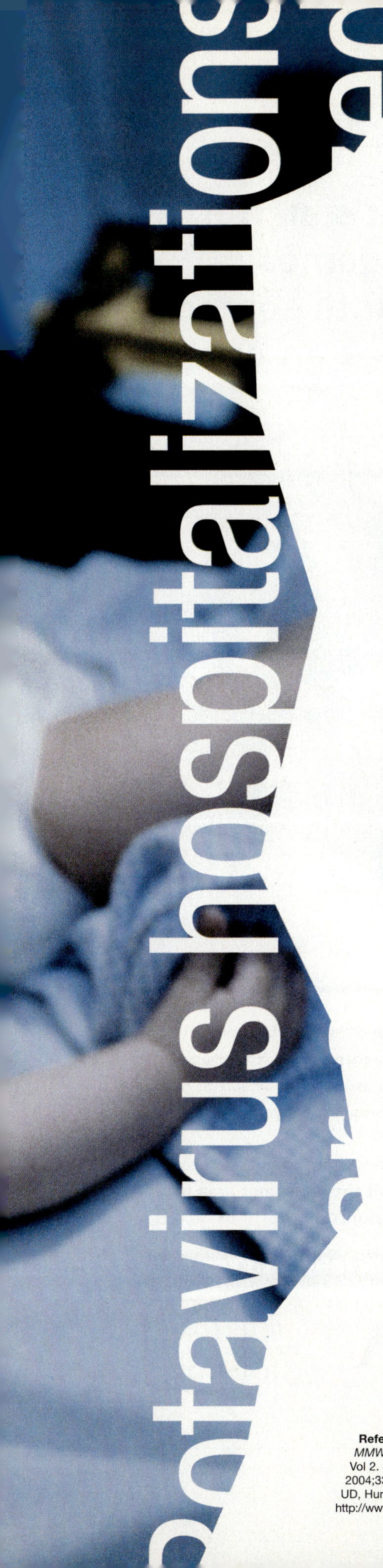


# DESPITE YOUR BEST EFFORTS, ROTAVIRUS CAUSES AN ESTIMATED 70,000 HOSPITALIZATIONS EVERY YEAR.[1]

**AN UNAVOIDABLE DISEASE...**[2]

- The most common cause of severe gastroenteritis in infants and young children in the United States[2]
- Greatest risk for severe disease occurs primarily in young children between 6 and 24 months of age.[3]

**WITH UNPREDICTABLE CONSEQUENCES**[2,4]

- No way to predict which infants will suffer severe disease[4]
- Potential for rapid deterioration in cases in which severe vomiting occurs[5]
- Responsible for an estimated 500,000 physician visits,[1] 70,000 hospitalizations,[1] and 160,000 ER visits[6] among children <5 years of age every year in the United States[1,6]
- Responsible for an estimated 100 deaths per year among children <5 years of age in the United States—an average of nearly 2 deaths per week[7]

Find out more at www.rotavirusinfo.com.

**References: 1.** Glass RI, Bresee JS, Parashar UD, et al. *Arch Pediatr.* 2005;12:844–847. **2.** Centers for Disease Control and Prevention. *MMWR.* 1999;48(RR-2):1–24. **3.** Bernstein DI, Ward RL. In: Feigin RD, Cherry JD. eds. *Textbook of Pediatric Infectious Diseases.* 4th ed. Vol 2. Philadelphia, Pa: Saunders; 1998:1901–1922. **4.** Cornell SL. *Adv Nurse Pract.* 1997;5:41–44. **5.** Clark HF, Offit PA. *Pediatr Ann.* 2004;33:537–543. **6.** Tucker AW, Haddix AC, Bresee JS, Holman MS, Parashar UD, Glass RI. *JAMA.* 1998;279:1371–1376. **7.** Parashar UD, Hummelman EG, Bresee JS, Miller MA, Glass RI. *Emerg Infect Dis.* 2003;9:565–571; Appendix B (online only.): Available at http://www.cdc.gov/ncidod/EID/vol9no5/02-0562_appB.htm. Accessed June 13, 2005.

## Effects of Alcohol Advertising Exposure on Drinking Among Youth

Youth drinking has many immediate and long-term adverse consequences including injuries, risky sexual activity, and increased risk of later alcohol abuse and dependence. This national longitudinal study examined the effects of exposure to alcohol advertising on consumption of alcohol by youth over time. The study combined a household telephone survey with data on alcohol advertising expenditures and exposure to advertisements. Youth who saw more alcohol advertisements drank more on average—every additional advertisement seen increased the number of drinks consumed by 1%. Each additional dollar spent per capita on alcohol advertising was associated with a 3% increase in the number of drinks consumed. The study clearly indicates that alcohol advertising is related to the amount of youth drinking and suggests that limiting advertisements would have a beneficial effect on drinking problems among youth.

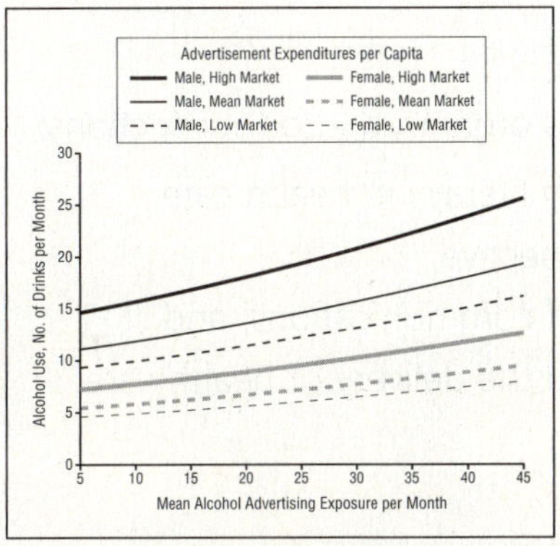


Alcohol use by mean advertising exposure, market advertising expenditures per capita, and sex.

**See page 18**

## Impact of Adolescent Mental Disorders and Physical Illnesses on Quality of Life 17 Years Later

Examining outcomes such as quality of life among patients with chronic conditions is important to better understand the impact of these illnesses on children and adolescents. This study followed a cohort of more than 600 adolescents with chronic illness at a mean age of 16 years into adulthood, at a mean age of 33 years. Adolescents with chronic physical illness had a measurably lower quality of life as adults than their healthy peers. Adolescents with Axis I psychiatric disorders had more problematic social relationships as adults, and those with personality disorders had later problems with social relationships, psychological well-being, and impaired role functioning. Mental disorders among adolescents appear to have a greater impact on adult quality of life than do chronic physical illnesses.

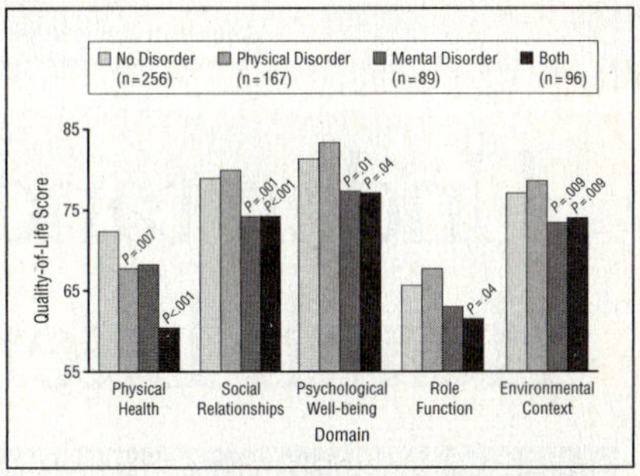


Association of mental disorders and physical illnesses at the mean age of 16 years with 5 quality-of-life domains at the mean age of 33 years.

**See page 93**

## Neighborhood Safety and Overweight Status in Children

With the marked increase in the prevalence of obesity in the United States and around the world, increased attention is being given to the physical environment in which children are raised and its effects on physical activity. This study examined 786 children in 10 urban and rural sites across the United States. Children living in the neighborhoods parents perceived as most unsafe had a 4-fold increased odds of being overweight at age 7 compared with children living in the neighborhoods perceived as being the safest. Redesign of neighborhoods has the potential to not only decrease the rates of intentional and unintentional injuries but to promote physical activity and contribute to reversing the increasing prevalence of obesity.

**See page 25**

## Adulthood Outcome of Tic and Obsessive-Compulsive Symptom Severity in Children With Tourette Syndrome

In Tourette syndrome, tics typically begin at the ages of 5 or 6 years. This study examined the clinical course of tics in patients with Tourette syndrome, as well as accompanying obsessive-compulsive (OC) symptoms. Eighty-five percent of patients observed for a mean of 7.6 years reported a reduction in tic symptoms during adolescence. The average age of worst-ever tic severity was 10.6 years. Among the 41% of patients who reported having at least moderate OC symptoms, worst-ever OC symptoms occurred about 2 years later than worst-ever tic symptoms. Obsessive-compulsive symptoms were more likely to persist than tic symptoms.

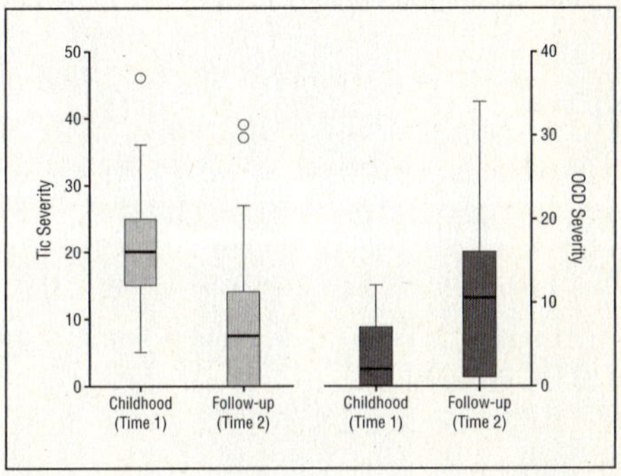


**See page 65**

# Fiona

MOTHERHOOD AND HOPE: WHAT IS THE nature of their entwined relationship? When I first learned I was pregnant, I never anticipated how much cause I would have to ponder this question—and how my answer would shape me—after the birth of my daughter.

Fiona was born at 35 weeks following a pregnancy complicated by multiple uncertain and strange findings: polyhydramnios, a single umbilical artery, a possible atrial septal defect, and a stomach bubble seen on some studies but not others—all of these were part of her ultrasound collage. My husband, Peter, and I were told, "It could be something . . . or it could be nothing."

After Fiona's birth, the diagnosis became clear: CHARGE syndrome (colobomas, heart defects, atresia choanae, retardation of growth and development, genitourinary abnormalities, and ear abnormalities). On just her third day of life, we were told that she had colobomas and would be blind. I remember coming home from the hospital that day and looking at the mural that Peter had painted in her room, knowing she would never see it. We were relieved to learn that her hearing tested normal, but we were then warned that "it could deteriorate over time." Her cognitive development? "Unlikely to be normal." There seemed to be no end to what CHARGE syndrome could affect. We were beside ourselves with sorrow and anger.

Until that point in Fiona's short life, we had received only matter-of-fact information from various subspecialists. After Fiona was transferred to another hospital for repair of her choanal atresia, we had our first encounter with hope. Our new neonatologist reviewed Fiona's case extensively with us and concluded by saying, "We have a lot to be optimistic about." I have to admit, my first thought was, "Really?"

Despite my initial skepticism, my mind kept replaying the neonatologist's words over and over throughout the remainder of the day. Peter and I began to recognize all of the positive things in front of us, most notably our beautiful little girl who interacted with us and knew us. We felt that she had a future with us, regardless of the difficulties that her syndrome might bring. The power of those 8 words—"we have a lot to be optimistic about"—far outweighed all of the bad news we had received to date.

A few days later, things took a dramatic turn for the worse when, inexplicably, Fiona became suddenly and seriously ill. We still do not know the reason. Even now, I feel a scared pain in my chest when I recall walking into the neonatal intensive care unit that day and realizing that the baby with 6 drips running into a central line, whose body had doubled in size from anasarca, was actually *my* own child.

As days passed and she did not get better, Peter and I began to understand that if improvement did not come soon, we would likely lose Fiona. We decided to make use of the time we had and offer her all that we could. We read her some of our most beloved books and played her our favorite music. Since the presidential elections were approaching, we told her about the political system and explained our own views on it. My parents asked whether they could tell Fiona about *their* political opinions, too. We had a lighthearted moment when Peter and I told them that as Fiona's parents, we reserved the right to monopolize her impressionable mind with our own ideological slants.

As difficult as those long days of waiting were, we continued to focus on the hope that the neonatologist had given us. When we began to realize that she would not recover, we put our energies into determining how to provide her with dignity while dying. We found a similar yet new kind of hope in this task in our ability to offer her honor and love, even as she passed away.

Nine days after Fiona became ill, Peter and I had gradually accumulated enough grim information about our daughter's prognosis to understand that it was time to withdraw medical support. Our favorite nurse was assigned to us the next day, and she helped us through the difficult task of extubating Fiona. Fiona's neonatologist also offered us her support and came in to be with us on her day off. After the team removed the breathing tube, the nurse placed Fiona in our arms, and we listened as she breathed softly and on her own.

Fiona lived for another 36 hours. We sat outside with her so that she could feel the light rain and the gentle breeze. All of our family members came to hold her and say goodbye. Later that day, our nurse arranged for us to have a quiet family room to spend time together privately. She brought us food, visitors, and laughter at all of the right times. Both the fellow and the resident who had been closely involved in Fiona's care visited and shared their memories of the past few weeks. As strange as it may sound, we were happy during those 2 days. Peter, Fiona, and I felt like a family, the 3 of us there together with our favorite people surrounding us. I look back on that time with immense gratitude.

After Fiona died, I entered a nebulous period that defied the boundaries of time. Days were filled with half-dreams of what might have been; nights were filled with shadowy visions of what had transpired. I occasionally awakened from sleep sweating, convinced that I had felt her familiar kicks in my belly. I sat for hours in our quiet nursery, staring at the empty crib.

I missed Fiona. I missed her as the person I had known, even if it was only for a brief time. I also missed her as the person she would have become, and I missed the dreams and expectations I had for her life.

And I missed being a mother. Who was I now? I had invested the last year of my life preparing myself for the role of a mother. Now, that responsibility had vanished. There exist no words, roles, or comfortable terms in our culture that adequately reflect the experience of a mother who has lost her only child. Simply put, I felt an overwhelming and indescribable void. I was still a pediatrician, a wife, a sister, a daughter, and a friend, but I felt that I was no longer a mother. I had lost the sense of purpose that I had cultivated with each day of Fiona's life.

I felt trapped in a paradox. I wanted to move forward with the life I had known, but I also understood that Fiona had fundamentally changed the way in which I viewed the world. I wanted to be realistic in my expectations for my life after Fiona. She was gone, and while Peter and I were brimming with grief, we were viscerally opposed to death-denying maudlin behavior; there would be no little stocking on the fireplace this Christmas. I was no longer a mom—or was I? I had become a parent—Fiona's mother—and that was something that even her death could not undo. A change had occurred; going back was impossible, but what was a truthful way forward?

My return to work finally propelled me forward. I had feared and dreaded stepping foot in the hospital again. I worried that I would not be able to find objectivity when caring for patients and that every infant would bring memories of Fiona flooding back. And for a while, every time I saw an infant, I *did* find myself thinking about Fiona. Sometimes I would have to stop in the bathroom to cry a little or just to get a grip on myself.

Thankfully, on most occasions, I could sense when my objectivity was waning, and I would ask my colleagues for help. Ever so gradually, I only cried when I saw certain infants, and then, only on certain days. Almost imperceptibly, I began to focus less on my own sense of loss and more on what I had learned from Fiona's time in the neonatal intensive care unit and from my experiences as a parent.

And so, day-by-day, I have become a slightly different pediatrician. Before Fiona, I underestimated the power that health care providers have to change attitudes, to give hope, and to offer dignity. Now, I carefully choose each word I use when talking with parents and families. Like Fiona's neonatologist, I strive to bolster realistic hopes that can be used in many ways, even in the most dire of circumstances. As I learned firsthand, when our medicines fail, families may go home with nothing but memories of their children, illuminated in part by our words, to hold in their hearts.

The other day in the hospital, I ran into one of Fiona's nurses from the neonatal intensive care unit. She looked at me and asked, "Are you Fiona's mother?" Before I had time to think—or perhaps, more aptly, overthink—I said, "Yes!" In the truth of that moment and the hug that ensued, I felt the entwining of motherhood and hope, of professional and personal, of cherishing the past while moving forward.

*Megan A. Moreno, MD, MSEd*

**Correspondence**: Dr Moreno, Adolescent Medicine, Children's Hospital and Regional Medical Center, 4800 Sand Point Way NE, M2-4, Seattle, WA 98105 (meganamoreno@hotmail.com).
**Acknowledgment**: I would like to express particular gratitude to Christine Gleason, MD, Kim Hiatt, RN, and Shannon Rojecki. I would also like to thank Chris Feutner, MD, for his valuable editing assistance with this essay.

"The best thing to spend on children is your time."
Arnold Glasow

In the treatment or prevention of bronchospasm

# What should you Expect?

# NEW XOPENEX HFA!

**In the treatment or prevention of bronchospasm**

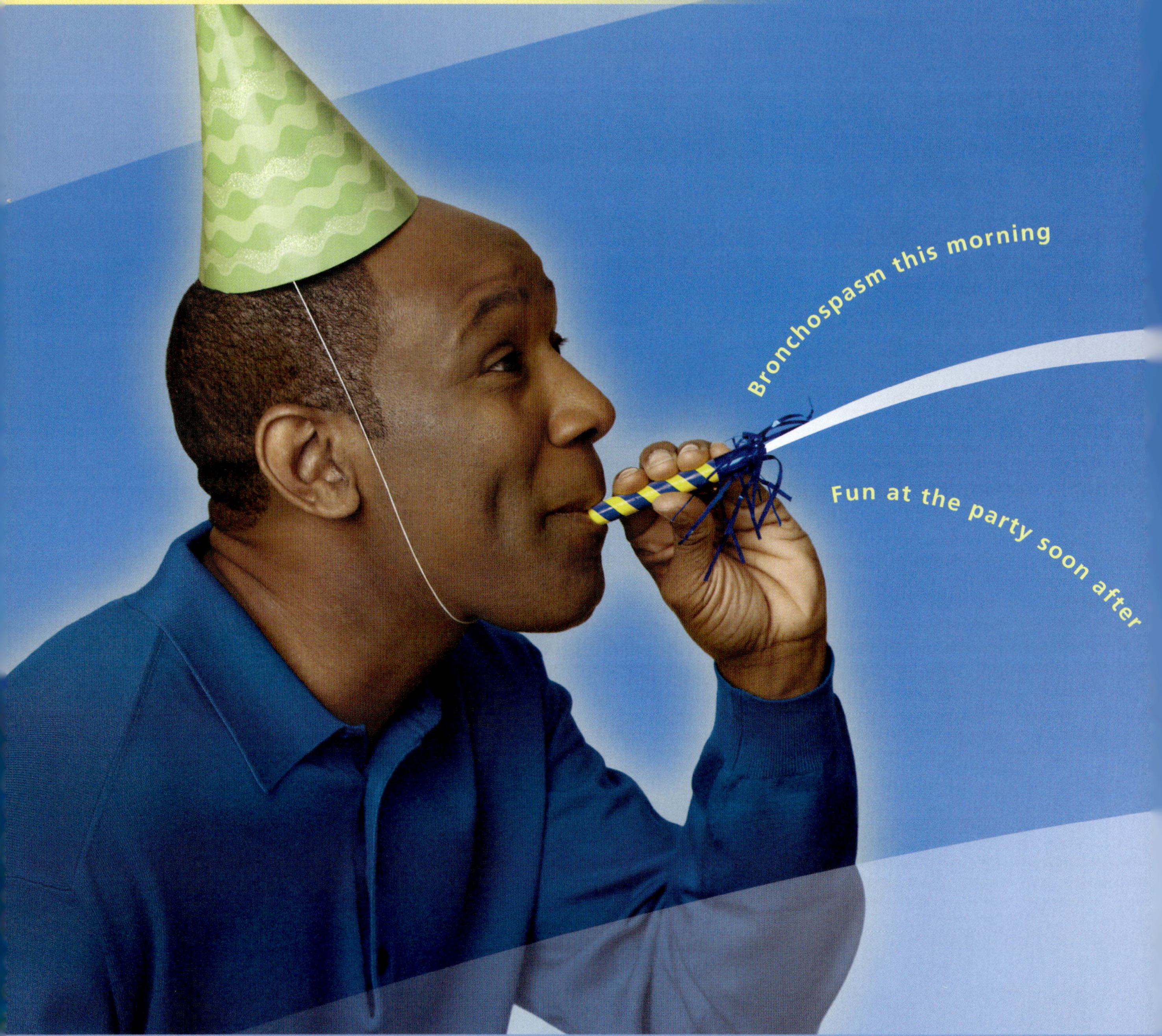


**Important Safety Information**

Xopenex HFA is contraindicated in patients with a history of hypersensitivity to levalbuterol, racemic albuterol, or any other component of Xopenex HFA. Xopenex HFA and other β-agonists can produce paradoxical bronchospasm, which may be life threatening. If additional adrenergic drugs, including other short-acting sympathomimetic bronchodilators or epinephrine, are to be administered by any route, they should be used with caution to avoid deleterious cardiovascular effects. Due to the cardiovascular side effects associated with β-agonists, caution is generally recommended for patients with cardiovascular disorders (especially coronary insufficiency, cardiac arrhythmias, and hypertension), diabetes, hyperthyroidism, or convulsive disorders. Do not exceed the recommended dose. Fatalities have been reported in association with excessive use of inhaled sympathomimetic drugs in patients with asthma. Please refer to the complete prescribing information for further information and in regard to potential drug interactions with β-blockers, diuretics, digoxin, or MAOI and tricyclic antidepressants.

# Expect Xopenex

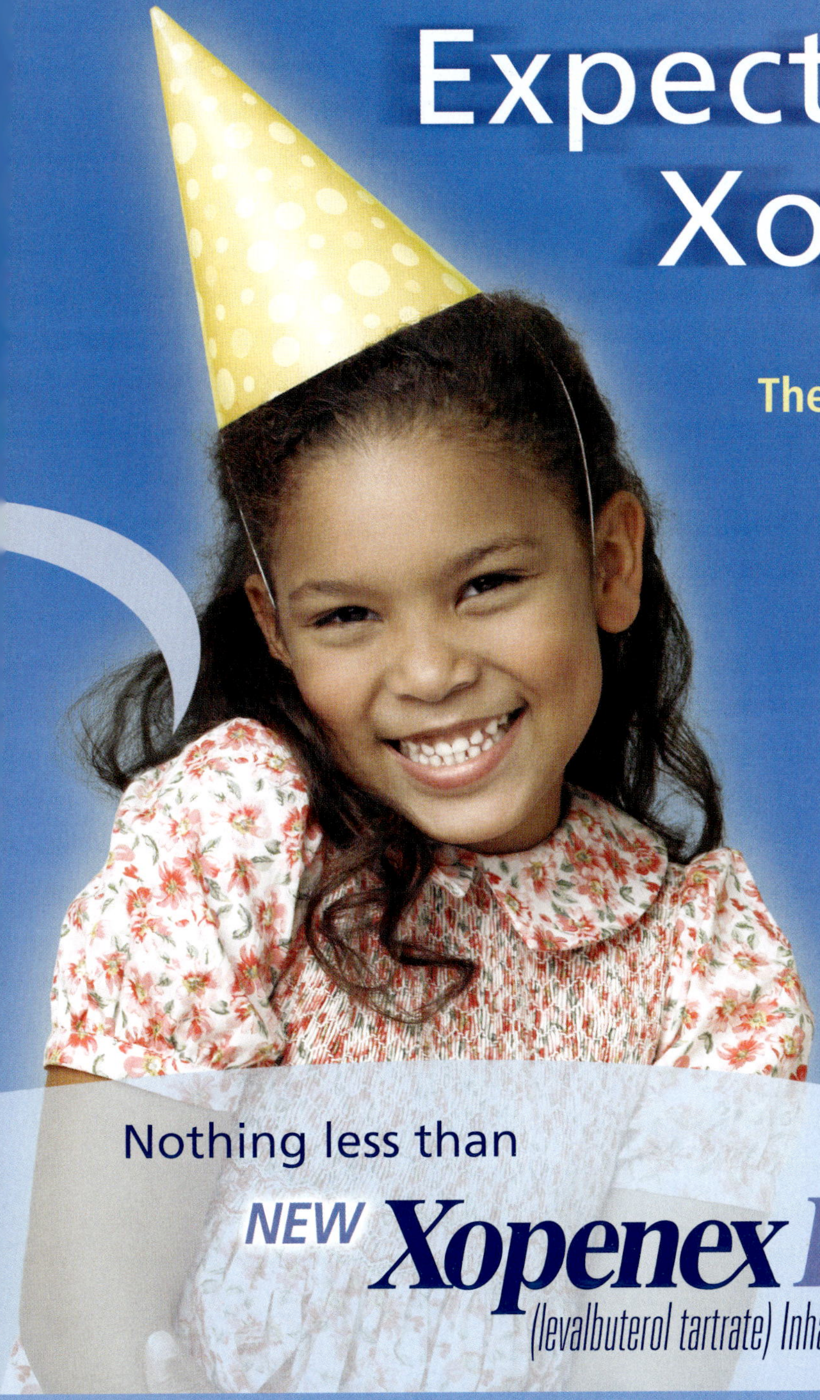

## The confidence you need, the freedom they want

- XOPENEX does not contain (S)-albuterol[1]
- Rapid onset of action for relief of bronchospasm*[1]
- Beta-adrenergic-mediated adverse events are low and comparable to placebo[1]
- Indicated for patients 4 years of age and older[1]

Nothing less than

**NEW Xopenex HFA™**
*(levalbuterol tartrate) Inhalation Aerosol*

**In patients aged 4 to 11 years,** the most common adverse events (occurring in greater than 2% of patients and more frequently than patients receiving placebo) were (90 mcg Xopenex HFA and placebo, respectively): accidental injury (9.2%; 5.7%), vomiting (10.5%; 5.7%), bronchitis (2.6%; 0%), and pharyngitis (6.6%; 5.7%).

**In patients aged 12 years and older,** the most common adverse events (occurring in greater than 2% of patients and more frequently than patients receiving placebo) were (90 mcg Xopenex HFA and placebo, respectively): pain (4.0%; 3.6%), dizziness (2.7%; 1.8%), asthma (9.4%; 6.0%), pharyngitis (7.9%; 2.4%), and rhinitis (7.4%; 3.0%).

Please see brief summary of prescribing information.

XOPENEX HFA (levalbuterol tartrate) Inhalation Aerosol is indicated for the treatment or prevention of bronchospasm in adults, adolescents, and children 4 years of age and older with reversible obstructive airway disease.

* The median onset time of a 15% increase in $FEV_1$ for XOPENEX HFA Inhalation Aerosol on Day 1 was 5.5 to 10.2 minutes for adult patients and 4.5 minutes for pediatric patients. Please refer to prescribing information.

**Reference:** 1. Xopenex HFA Prescribing Information.

# Xopenex HFA™

(levalbuterol tartrate) Inhalation Aerosol

FOR ORAL INHALATION ONLY

## BRIEF SUMMARY

### INDICATIONS AND USAGE

XOPENEX HFA (levalbuterol tartrate) Inhalation Aerosol is indicated for the treatment or prevention of bronchospasm in adults, adolescents, and children 4 years of age and older with reversible obstructive airway disease.

### CONTRAINDICATIONS

XOPENEX HFA (levalbuterol tartrate) Inhalation Aerosol is contraindicated in patients with a history of hypersensitivity to levalbuterol, racemic albuterol, or any other component of XOPENEX HFA Inhalation Aerosol.

### WARNINGS

1. Paradoxical Bronchospasm: Like other inhaled beta-adrenergic agonists, XOPENEX HFA Inhalation Aerosol can produce paradoxical bronchospasm, which may be life-threatening. If paradoxical bronchospasm occurs, XOPENEX HFA (levalbuterol tartrate) Inhalation Aerosol should be discontinued immediately and alternative therapy instituted. It should be recognized that paradoxical bronchospasm, when associated with inhaled formulations, frequently occurs with the first use of a new canister. 2. Deterioration of Asthma: Asthma may deteriorate acutely over a period of hours or chronically over several days or longer. If the patient needs more doses of XOPENEX HFA Inhalation Aerosol than usual, this may be a marker of destabilization of asthma and requires reevaluation of the patient and treatment regimen, giving special consideration to the possible need for anti-inflammatory treatment, e.g., corticosteroids.
3. Use of Anti-Inflammatory Agents: The use of a beta-adrenergic agonist alone may not be adequate to control asthma in many patients. Early consideration should be given to adding anti-inflammatory agents, e.g., corticosteroids, to the therapeutic regimen. 4. Cardiovascular Effects: XOPENEX HFA Inhalation Aerosol, like other beta-adrenergic agonists, can produce clinically significant cardiovascular effects in some patients, as measured by heart rate, blood pressure, and/or symptoms. Although such effects are uncommon after administration of XOPENEX HFA Inhalation Aerosol at recommended doses, if they occur, the drug may need to be discontinued. In addition, beta-agonists have been reported to produce electrocardiogram (ECG) changes, such as flattening of the T wave, prolongation of the QTc interval, and ST segment depression. The clinical significance of these findings is unknown. Therefore, XOPENEX HFA Inhalation Aerosol, like all sympathomimetic amines, should be used with caution in patients with cardiovascular disorders, especially coronary insufficiency, cardiac arrhythmias, and hypertension. 5. Do Not Exceed Recommended Dose: Fatalities have been reported in association with excessive use of inhaled sympathomimetic drugs in patients with asthma. The exact cause of death is unknown, but cardiac arrest following an unexpected development of a severe acute asthmatic crisis and subsequent hypoxia is suspected.
6. Immediate Hypersensitivity Reactions: Immediate hypersensitivity reactions may occur after administration of racemic albuterol, as demonstrated by rare cases of urticaria, angioedema, rash, bronchospasm, anaphylaxis, and oropharyngeal edema. The potential for hypersensitivity must be considered in the clinical evaluation of patients who experience immediate hypersensitivity reactions while receiving XOPENEX HFA Inhalation Aerosol.

### PRECAUTIONS

#### General

XOPENEX HFA (levalbuterol tartrate) Inhalation Aerosol, like all sympathomimetic amines, should be used with caution in patients with cardiovascular disorders, especially coronary insufficiency, hypertension, and cardiac arrhythmias; in patients with convulsive disorders, hyperthyroidism, or diabetes mellitus; and in patients who are unusually responsive to sympathomimetic amines. Clinically significant changes in systolic and diastolic blood pressure have been seen in individual patients and could be expected to occur in some patients after the use of any beta-adrenergic bronchodilator.

Large doses of intravenous racemic albuterol have been reported to aggravate preexisting diabetes mellitus and ketoacidosis. As with other beta-adrenergic agonist medications, XOPENEX HFA Inhalation Aerosol may produce significant hypokalemia in some patients, possibly through intracellular shunting, which has the potential to produce adverse cardiovascular effects. The decrease is usually transient, not requiring supplementation.

#### Information for Patients

The action of XOPENEX HFA Inhalation Aerosol should last for 4 to 6 hours. XOPENEX HFA Inhalation Aerosol should not be used more frequently than recommended. Do not increase the dose or frequency of doses of XOPENEX HFA Inhalation Aerosol without consulting your physician. If you find that treatment with XOPENEX HFA Inhalation Aerosol becomes less effective for symptomatic relief, your symptoms become worse, and/or you need to use the product more frequently than usual, you should seek medical attention immediately. While you are using XOPENEX HFA Inhalation Aerosol, other inhaled drugs and asthma medications should be taken only as directed by your physician.

Common adverse effects of treatment with inhaled beta-agonists include palpitations, chest pain, rapid heart rate, tremor, and nervousness. If you are pregnant or nursing, contact your physician about use of XOPENEX HFA Inhalation Aerosol. Effective and safe use of XOPENEX HFA Inhalation Aerosol includes an understanding of the way that it should be administered.

Use XOPENEX HFA Inhalation Aerosol only with the actuator supplied with the product. Discard the canister after 200 sprays have been used. Never immerse the canister in water to determine how full the canister is ("float test").

In general, the technique for administering XOPENEX HFA Inhalation Aerosol to children is similar to that for adults. Children should use XOPENEX HFA Inhalation Aerosol under adult supervision, as instructed by the patient's physician.

#### Drug Interactions

Other short-acting sympathomimetic aerosol bronchodilators or epinephrine should be used with caution with XOPENEX HFA Inhalation Aerosol. If additional adrenergic drugs are to be administered by any route, they should be used with caution to avoid deleterious cardiovascular effects.

1. Beta-blockers: Beta-adrenergic receptor-blocking agents not only block the pulmonary effect of beta-adrenergic agonists, such as XOPENEX HFA Inhalation Aerosol, but may produce severe bronchospasm in asthmatic patients. Therefore, patients with asthma should not normally be treated with beta-blockers. However, under certain circumstances, e.g., as prophylaxis after myocardial infarction, there may be no acceptable alternatives to the use of beta-adrenergic blocking agents in patients with asthma. In this setting, cardioselective beta-blockers should be considered, although they should be administered with caution. 2. Diuretics: The ECG changes and/or hypokalemia that may result from the administration of non–potassium-sparing diuretics (such as loop and thiazide diuretics) can be acutely worsened by beta-agonists, especially when the recommended dose of the beta-agonist is exceeded. Although the clinical significance of these effects is not known, caution is advised in the coadministration of beta-agonists with non–potassium-sparing diuretics. 3. Digoxin: Mean decreases of 16% to 22% in serum digoxin levels were demonstrated after single-dose intravenous and oral administration of racemic albuterol, respectively, to normal volunteers who had received digoxin for 10 days. The clinical significance of these findings for patients with obstructive airway disease who are receiving XOPENEX HFA Inhalation Aerosol and digoxin on a chronic basis is unclear. Nevertheless, it would be prudent to carefully evaluate the serum digoxin levels in patients who are currently receiving digoxin and XOPENEX HFA Inhalation Aerosol. 4. Monoamine Oxidase Inhibitors or Tricyclic Antidepressants: XOPENEX HFA Inhalation Aerosol should be administered with extreme caution to patients being treated with monoamine oxidase inhibitors or tricyclic antidepressants, or within 2 weeks of discontinuation of such agents, because the action of albuterol on the vascular system may be potentiated.

**Carcinogenesis, Mutagenesis, and Impairment of Fertility** No carcinogenesis or impairment of fertility studies have been carried out with levalbuterol tartrate. However, racemic albuterol sulfate has been evaluated for its carcinogenic potential and ability to impair fertility.

In a 2-year study in Sprague-Dawley rats, racemic albuterol sulfate caused a significant dose-related increase in the incidence of benign leiomyomas of the mesovarium at, and above, dietary doses of 2 mg/kg/day (approximately 30 times the maximum recommended daily inhalation dose of levalbuterol tartrate for adults on a $mg/m^2$ basis and approximately 15 times the maximum recommended daily inhalation dose of levalbuterol tartrate for children on a $mg/m^2$ basis). In another study, this effect was blocked by the coadministration of propranolol, a non-selective beta-adrenergic antagonist. In an 18-month study in CD-1 mice, racemic albuterol sulfate showed no evidence of tumorigenicity at dietary doses up to 500 mg/kg/day (approximately 3800 times the maximum recommended daily inhalation dose of levalbuterol tartrate for adults on a $mg/m^2$ basis and approximately 1800 times the maximum recommended daily inhalation dose of levalbuterol tartrate for children on a $mg/m^2$ basis). In a 22-month study in the Golden hamster, racemic albuterol sulfate showed no evidence of tumorigenicity at dietary doses up to 50 mg/kg/day (approximately 500 times the maximum recommended daily inhalation dose of levalbuterol tartrate for adults on a $mg/m^2$ basis and approximately 240 times the maximum recommended daily inhalation dose of levalbuterol tartrate for children on a $mg/m^2$ basis).

Levalbuterol HCl was not mutagenic in the Ames test or the CHO/HPRT Mammalian Forward Gene Mutation Assay.

Levalbuterol HCl was not clastogenic in the in vivo micronucleus test in mouse bone marrow. Racemic albuterol sulfate was negative in an in vitro chromosomal aberration assay in CHO cell cultures.

Reproduction studies in rats using racemic albuterol sulfate demonstrated no evidence of impaired fertility at oral doses up to 50 mg/kg/day (approximately 750 times the maximum recommended daily inhalation dose of levalbuterol tartrate for adults on a $mg/m^2$ basis).

**Teratogenic Effects - Pregnancy Category C** A reproduction study in New Zealand White rabbits demonstrated that levalbuterol HCl was not teratogenic when administered orally at doses up to 25 mg/kg/day (approximately 750 times the maximum recommended daily inhalation dose of levalbuterol tartrate for adults on a $mg/m^2$ basis).

However, racemic albuterol sulfate has been shown to be teratogenic in mice and rabbits. A study in CD-1 mice given racemic albuterol sulfate subcutaneously showed cleft palate formation in 5 of 111 (4.5%) fetuses at 0.25 mg/kg/day (approximately 2 times the maximum recommended daily inhalation dose of levalbuterol tartrate for adults on a $mg/m^2$ basis) and in 10 of 108 (9.3%) fetuses at 2.5 mg/kg/day (approximately 20 times the maximum recommended daily inhalation dose of levalbuterol tartrate for adults on a $mg/m^2$ basis). The drug did not induce cleft palate formation when administered subcutaneously at a dose of 0.025 mg/kg/day (less than the maximum recommended daily inhalation dose of levalbuterol tartrate for adults on a $mg/m^2$ basis). Cleft palate also occurred in 22 of 72 (30.5%) fetuses from females treated subcutaneously with 2.5 mg/kg/day of isoproterenol (positive control).

A reproduction study in Stride Dutch rabbits revealed cranioschisis in 7 of 19 (37%) fetuses when racemic albuterol sulfate was administered orally at a dose of 50 mg/kg/day (approximately 1500 times the maximum recommended daily inhalation dose of levalbuterol tartrate for adults on a $mg/m^2$ basis).

A study in which pregnant rats were dosed with radiolabeled racemic albuterol sulfate demonstrated that drug-related material is transferred from the maternal circulation to the fetus.

There are no adequate and well-controlled studies of XOPENEX HFA Inhalation Aerosol in pregnant women. Because animal reproduction studies are not always predictive of human response, XOPENEX HFA Inhalation Aerosol should be used during pregnancy only if the potential benefit justifies the potential risk to the fetus.

During marketing experience of racemic albuterol, various congenital anomalies, including cleft palate and limb defects, have been rarely reported in the offspring of patients being treated with racemic albuterol. Some of the mothers were taking multiple medications during their pregnancies. No consistent pattern of defects can be discerned, and a relationship between racemic albuterol use and congenital anomalies has not been established.

**Use in Labor and Delivery** Because of the potential for beta-adrenergic agonists to interfere with uterine contractility, the use of XOPENEX HFA Inhalation Aerosol for the treatment of bronchospasm during labor should be restricted to those patients in whom the benefits clearly outweigh the risk.

**Tocolysis** XOPENEX HFA Inhalation Aerosol has not been approved for the management of preterm labor. The benefit:risk ratio when levalbuterol tartrate is administered for tocolysis has not been established. Serious adverse reactions, including maternal pulmonary edema, have been reported during or following treatment of premature labor with beta2-agonists, including racemic albuterol.

**Nursing Mothers** Plasma concentrations of levalbuterol after inhalation of therapeutic doses are very low in humans. It is not known whether levalbuterol is excreted in human milk.

Because of the potential for tumorigenicity shown for racemic albuterol in animal studies and the lack of experience with the use of XOPENEX HFA Inhalation Aerosol by nursing mothers, a decision should be made whether to discontinue nursing or to discontinue the drug, taking into account the importance of the drug to the mother. Caution should be exercised when XOPENEX HFA Inhalation Aerosol is administered to a nursing woman.

**Pediatrics** The safety and efficacy of XOPENEX HFA Inhalation Aerosol have been established in pediatric patients 4 years of age and older in an adequate and well-controlled clinical trial. Use of XOPENEX HFA Inhalation Aerosol in children is also supported by evidence from adequate and well-controlled studies of XOPENEX HFA Inhalation Aerosol in adults, considering that the pathophysiology, systemic exposure of the drug, and clinical profile in pediatric and adult patients are substantially similar. Safety and effectiveness of XOPENEX HFA Inhalation Aerosol in pediatric patients below the age of 4 years have not been established.

**Geriatrics** Clinical studies of XOPENEX HFA Inhalation Aerosol did not include sufficient numbers of subjects aged 65 and older to determine whether they respond differently from younger subjects. Other reported clinical experience has not identified differences in responses between the elderly and younger patients. In general, dose selection for an elderly patient should be cautious, usually starting at the low end of the dosing range, reflecting the greater frequency of decreased hepatic, renal, or cardiac function, and of concomitant diseases or other drug therapy.

Albuterol is known to be substantially excreted by the kidney, and the risk of toxic reactions may be greater in patients with impaired renal function. Because elderly patients are more likely to have decreased renal function, care should be taken in dose selection, and it may be useful to monitor renal function.

**ADVERSE REACTIONS** Adverse event information concerning XOPENEX HFA (levalbuterol tartrate) Inhalation Aerosol in adults and adolescents is derived from two 8-week, multicenter, randomized, double-blind, active- and placebo-controlled trials in 748 adult and adolescent patients with asthma that compared XOPENEX HFA Inhalation Aerosol, a marketed albuterol HFA inhaler, and an HFA-134a placebo inhaler. The following lists the incidence (% XOPENEX HFA 90 mcg, marketed albuterol HFA inhaler 180 mcg, placebo, respectively) of all adverse events (whether considered by the investigator to be related or unrelated to drug) from these trials that occurred at a rate of 2% or greater in the group treated with XOPENEX HFA Inhalation Aerosol and more frequently than in the HFA-134a placebo inhaler group. Body as a whole: pain (4.0%, 3.4%, 3.6%). Central nervous system: dizziness (2.7%, 0.6%, 1.8%). Respiratory system: asthma (9.4%, 7.3%, 6.0%), pharyngitis (7.9%, 2.2%, 2.4%), rhinitis (7.4%, 2.2%, 3.0%).

Adverse events reported by less than 2% and at least 2 or more of the adolescent and adult patients receiving XOPENEX HFA Inhalation Aerosol and by a greater proportion than receiving HFA-134a placebo inhaler include cyst, flu syndrome, viral infection, constipation, gastroenteritis, myalgia, hypertension, epistaxis, lung disorder, acne, herpes simplex, conjunctivitis, ear pain, dysmenorrhea, hematuria, and vaginal moniliasis. There were no significant laboratory abnormalities observed in these studies.

Adverse event information concerning XOPENEX HFA Inhalation Aerosol in children is derived from a 4-week, randomized, double-blind trial of XOPENEX HFA Inhalation Aerosol, a marketed albuterol HFA inhaler, and an HFA-134a placebo inhaler in 150 children aged 4 to 11 years with asthma. The following lists the adverse events (% XOPENEX HFA 90 mcg, marketed albuterol HFA inhaler 180 mcg, placebo, respectively) reported for XOPENEX HFA Inhalation Aerosol in children at a rate of 2% or greater and more frequently than for placebo. Body as a whole: accidental injury (9.2%, 10.3%, 5.7%). Digestive system: vomiting (10.5%, 7.7%, 5.7%). Respiratory system: bronchitis (2.6%, 0%, 0%), pharyngitis (6.6%, 12.8%, 5.7%).

The incidence of systemic beta-adrenergic adverse effects (e.g., tremor, nervousness) was low and comparable across all treatment groups, including placebo.

**Postmarketing** In addition to the adverse events reported in clinical trials, the following adverse events have been observed in postapproval use of levalbuterol inhalation solution. These events have been chosen for inclusion due to their seriousness, their frequency of reporting, or their likely beta-mediated mechanism: angioedema, anaphylaxis, arrhythmias (including atrial fibrillation, supraventricular tachycardia, extrasystoles), asthma, chest pain, cough increased, dyspnea, nausea, nervousness, rash, tachycardia, tremor, urticaria. Because these events have been reported spontaneously from a population of unknown size, estimates of frequency cannot be made.

In addition, XOPENEX HFA Inhalation Aerosol, like other sympathomimetic agents, can cause adverse reactions such as hypertension, angina, vertigo, central nervous system stimulation, sleeplessness, headache, and drying or irritation of the oropharynx.

Rx only.

SEPRACOR 12/05

ARTICLE

# Effects of Alcohol Advertising Exposure on Drinking Among Youth

*Leslie B. Snyder, PhD; Frances Fleming Milici, PhD; Michael Slater, PhD; Helen Sun, MA; Yuliya Strizhakova, PhD*

**Objective:** To test whether alcohol advertising expenditures and the degree of exposure to alcohol advertisements affect alcohol consumption by youth.

**Design:** Longitudinal panel using telephone surveys.

**Setting:** Households in 24 US media markets, April 1999 to February 2001.

**Participants:** Individuals aged 15 to 26 years were randomly sampled within households and households within media markets. Markets were systematically selected from the top 75 media markets, representing 79% of the US population. The baseline refusal rate was 24%. Sample sizes per wave were 1872, 1173, 787, and 588. Data on alcohol advertising expenditures on television, radio, billboards, and newspapers were collected.

**Main Exposures:** Market alcohol advertising expenditures per capita and self-reported alcohol advertising exposure in the prior month.

**Main Outcome Measure:** Self-reported number of alcoholic drinks consumed in the prior month.

**Results:** Youth who saw more alcohol advertisements on average drank more (each additional advertisement seen increased the number of drinks consumed by 1% [event rate ratio, 1.01; 95% confidence interval, 1.01-1.02]). Youth in markets with greater alcohol advertising expenditures drank more (each additional dollar spent per capita raised the number of drinks consumed by 3% [event rate ratio, 1.03; 95% confidence interval, 1.01-1.05]). Examining only youth younger than the legal drinking age of 21 years, alcohol advertisement exposure and expenditures still related to drinking. Youth in markets with more alcohol advertisements showed increases in drinking levels into their late 20s, but drinking plateaued in the early 20s for youth in markets with fewer advertisements. Control variables included age, gender, ethnicity, high school or college enrollment, and alcohol sales.

**Conclusion:** Alcohol advertising contributes to increased drinking among youth.

*Arch Pediatr Adolesc Med. 2006;160:18-24*

Author Affiliations:
Department of Communications Sciences (Drs Snyder and Milici and Mss Sun and Strizhakova) and Center for Health Communication and Marketing (Dr Snyder), University of Connecticut, Storrs; and Department of Journalism and Technical Communication, Colorado State University, Ft Collins (Dr Slater). Dr Slater is currently at the School of Communication, Ohio State University, Columbus. Dr Strizhakova is currently at the Department of Communication and Journalism, Suffolk University, Boston, Mass.

THE CAUSES OF ALCOHOL USE among youth, including older children, adolescents, and young adults, are a major public health concern. Drinking among youth can result in a panoply of negative consequences, including poor grades, risky sex, alcohol addiction, and car crashes.[1-4] Drinkers younger than 21 years, who consume approximately 20% of all alcoholic drinks,[5] imbibe more heavily than adults per drinking episode[6] and are involved in twice as many fatal car crashes while drinking.[7] The problem is getting worse, with youth initiating drinking at an earlier age on average than they did in the past.[8]

There is much public policy debate about whether alcohol advertising is partially responsible for youth consumption levels. The alcohol industry is not subject to federal restrictions on their advertising practices but has voluntary advertising codes created by the major alcohol trade groups. Even when the alcohol industry adheres to a code requiring that at least 70% of the audience (50% before fall 2003) for print, radio, and television advertisements consist of adults of legal drinking age, many youth are exposed to alcohol advertisements.[9,10] There are often greater concentrations of alcohol advertisements in media aimed at youth than at adults.[10-13] However, studies of advertising content and youth exposure rates have not assessed the impact of advertising on youth. In 1997, the US Congress asked the National Institutes of Health for more scientific evidence on the relationship between advertising and alcohol use among those younger than the legal drinking age.[14]

*For editorial comment see page 100*

The most important question regarding alcohol advertising effects is whether the association between alcohol advertising and use is causal.[14] Cross-sectional surveys have found small, statistically significant, positive correlations (mean $r=0.19$) between self-reported alcohol advertising and youth drinking,[15-19] but they cannot establish causality.[20] Cumulative exposure to alcohol advertising and some effective advertising campaigns may change the way youth think about alcoholic beverages[21-27] and may increase drinking. Recently, exposure to some forms of alcohol advertising has been linked to drinking onset.[28] On the other hand, drinkers like alcohol advertisements more than nondrinkers like the advertisements,[24,26] have greater brain responses to alcohol advertisements,[29] and may remember them better.[25,30] An association between advertising exposure and drinking may therefore be due in part to drinkers reporting greater exposure than nondrinkers. It is also possible that advertisements induce drinkers to drink more. Another approach to research on alcohol advertising has shown that bans lead to a reduction in aggregate alcohol consumption,[31,32] but it is unknown how bans would affect youth.

We examined a national cohort of youth longitudinally to assess the effects of alcohol advertising on drinking amounts over time. The first hypothesis was that youth who reported greater exposure to alcohol advertising would have increased alcohol use over time. The second hypothesis concerned the effect of living in an environment with comparatively greater or fewer alcohol advertisements. By examining market-level measures of advertising expenditures per capita, we avoid the potential self-reporting bias among drinkers. We predicted that greater alcohol advertising expenditures per capita are correlated with greater youth drinking.

## METHODS

A random sample of youth aged 15 to 26 years from 24 US Nielsen media markets were interviewed 4 times during 21 months. Interviews were conducted in April through July 1999, December through January 2000, May through June 2000, and December through January 2001, using computer-aided telephone interviewing.

### SAMPLING

Twenty-four media markets were sampled to enable comparisons of advertising incidence across markets. Industry data on advertising were available for the 75 largest Nielsen media markets[33] in the United States, representing the 79% of the US population that lives in markets with populations of more than 957 000. To select markets, we conducted a cluster analysis in each of 6 US census geographic regions based on population size; population ethnic and religious composition; average income; annual state consumption of beer, wine, and liquor; state laws prohibiting sales of beer and liquor for off-premise consumption from restaurants, bars, grocery stores, gas stations, or drugstores; and percentage of households with cable television.[33-35] Markets were sampled from the identified clusters so that each geographic region in the sample was proportional to the number of top 75 markets within the region. Priority was given to markets with industry data on radio and billboard advertising, but otherwise selection was random. The selected 24 markets in the aggregate were not statistically different from the markets not selected on any of the measured criteria.

Households within markets were systematically sampled from a list of randomly selected households with telephones in the selected markets.[36] The list was purchased from Genesys Sampling Systems.[37] Within a household, the youth with the most recent birthday was selected. The mean ± SD response rate across markets at baseline was 27% ± 12%, and the refusal rate was 24% ± 7%, with many households of unknown eligibility not reached after 20 callbacks.[38] The sample sizes per wave were 1872, 1173, 787, and 588. The mobility of the 18- to 26-year-old segment of the population contributed greatly to sample attrition. Only 19% of the attrition at the second interview was due to a refusal to participate, compared with 68% due to disconnected numbers or respondent no longer in residence. Compared with youth who remained in the sample, youth who dropped out by the fourth interview were slightly older (20.2 vs 19.7 years), less likely to have been in high school (27.6% vs 42.3%), less likely to have been living at home (58.8% vs 70.7%), and drank more alcohol as of baseline (23.6 drinks per month vs14.9 drinks per month). Having greater attrition among drinkers is similar to other longitudinal youth alcohol use studies.[39] To minimize the effects of sampling and attrition, participants contributed as much data as was collected for them in the analysis (no cases were dropped), and the variables related to attrition were controlled statistically in the analyses.

The data were weighted at baseline by age, gender, and market to reflect the US population aged 15 to 26 years in the top 75 media markets. Weighting to a known population distribution adjusts for sampling fluctuations, nonresponse, and noncoverage.[36] The weighted data produced similar coefficients to the unweighted analyses.

The study received approval from the University of Connecticut institutional review board. Study participants and the parents of study participants younger than 18 years gave their oral consent before the baseline interview.

### OUTCOME MEASURE

Respondents were asked 3 questions about alcohol use: "On how many days did you drink any alcoholic beverage in the past 4 weeks" (frequency), "When you drank alcohol, how many drinks, glasses, bottles, or cans did you have per day, on average" (average quantity), and "What is the maximum number of alcoholic drinks, glasses, bottles, or cans you had on one occasion" (maximum quantity). Alcohol use was computed by multiplying drinking frequency by the mean of the average and maximum quantity of drinking. For example, if a respondent reported drinking 5 times in the past month, having 2 drinks on average, and a maximum quantity on one occasion of 4, we multiplied 5 by $(2+4)/2$ for a final score of 15. Thus, the measure estimated the number of alcoholic drinks consumed in the past month.

### ADVERTISING MEASURES

Advertising exposure was measured using 2 questions that assessed self-reported beer or liquor and premixed drink (eg, Smirnoff Ice) advertising exposure in the past month on each of 4 media (television, radio, magazines, and billboards) for a total of 8 items. The 8 items were summed to make an index. The question format was, "How many times in the past 4 weeks have you seen (media) ads for (beer/liquor or premixed drinks)?" To standardize across response formats on different surveys, "none" was coded as 0, "a few" and responses of 1 to 3 were coded as 2, "some" and responses of 4 to 6 were coded as 5, and "many" and responses of 7 or greater were coded as 10. (Ten was the modal response for the continuous response format for answers of 7 or greater.)

## MARKET ALCOHOL ADVERTISING EXPENDITURES PER CAPITA

Industry data on the amount spent on alcohol advertisements (in thousands) on television, radio, newspaper, and outdoors (mostly billboards) in each market in 1999 and 2000 were purchased from TNS Media Intelligence (formerly, Competitive Media Reporting).[40] The figure was divided by the market adult population size[33] to create an expenditures-per-capita index.

## OTHER MEASURES

Data collection took place for several months for each wave. Time of the interview per individual and per wave was measured as the number of months past the start of the study (April 1999) that the interview took place. Thus, for someone interviewed in December 1999, the time was 8 months.

## ALCOHOL SALES PER CAPITA

The total number of beer, wine, and liquor cases (in hundreds) sold per 1000 adults in each state in 2000 was purchased from an industry source.[41] It is important to control for total alcohol consumption levels because markets with greater sales may attract more alcohol advertising from brands competing to sell in markets with more heavy drinkers. In addition, adults who consume more on average may have an influence on youth drinking through tolerant attitudes and modeling. It is estimated that four fifths of all alcoholic beverages are consumed by adults.[5]

## DEMOGRAPHICS

Age was an individual's age in years beyond 15 years measured at baseline. Other demographic variables included the dummy variables of female, gender, current school status (in high school, in college, or not in school), and ethnicity (African American, Hispanic, or neither).

## STATISTICAL ANALYSIS

We used multilevel modeling to handle the complex sample and repeated-measures design.[42] There were 3 levels of analysis: (1) 4418 observations, accounting for the repeated measures within individuals, (2) 1858 individuals, and (3) 24 markets. The software used was HLM 6.01.[43] Because the outcome variable was count data (number of drinks) with many zeros (nondrinkers), we conducted nonlinear analysis using a Poisson sampling model with a log-link function.[42,44-46] The weights were applied at level 2. Analysis of the unconditional model showed that the largest share of the variance in alcohol use was within individuals (81%), reinforcing the importance of examining alcohol use within individuals.

We modeled growth in drinking over time by including month of interview in the model at level 1.[47] Since youth often increase their drinking as they age, we allowed growth to vary by age by including an interaction term between time and age.

The model examined the impact on alcohol use of alcohol advertising at the 3 levels: differences within individuals over time in advertising exposure, differences between individuals in advertising exposure, and market-level advertising expenditures. Alcohol advertising exposure at level 1 was centered on the individual's mean alcohol advertising exposure across all observations. Centering around an individual's mean is recommended when the aggregate of the level 1 predictors has a separate and distinct relationship with the outcome variable compared with variations within an individual.[42,45,47] The individual's mean advertising exposure was added as an independent variable at level 2, and market-level advertising expenditures were added at level 3. We added an interaction term between time and age and market advertising expenditures to test for differential growth in drinking over time by differences in market advertising expenditures and as youth age.

The model controlled for several potential confounders, including gender, age, ethnicity, and school status, all of which are known to vary with alcohol use.[48] Since school status could vary over time, 2 dummy variables for school status (high school, college, and no school) were entered at level 1. Another potential confounder, alcohol sales per capita, was entered at level 3. Alcohol sales, market advertising expenditures, time, and age were centered around the grand mean to aid in interpretation of the coefficients. Centering is particularly useful when dealing with interaction terms.[49] Error terms were included for all variables at level 3. Among the level 1 variables, the intercept and time were allowed to randomly vary. (If more than 2 factors were treated as randomly varying, the model would not converge.) The model tested was as follows:

$$\eta = \gamma_{000} + \gamma_{001}\text{ (Alcohol Sales per Capita)} + \gamma_{002}\text{ (Market Advertising Expenditures per Capita)} + \gamma_{010}\text{ (Female)} + \gamma_{020}\text{ (Age)} + \gamma_{030}\text{ (Black)} + \gamma_{040}\text{ (Hispanic)} + \gamma_{050}\text{ (Mean Advertising Exposure)} + \gamma_{100}\text{ (Time)} + \gamma_{110}\text{ (Time·Age)} + \gamma_{101}\text{ (Time·Age·Market Advertising Expenditures per Capita)} + \gamma_{200}\text{ (Advertising Exposure, Within Individual)} + \gamma_{300}\text{ (High School)} + \gamma_{400}\text{ (College)} + r_0 + r_1\text{ (Time)} + u_{00} + u_{01}\text{ (Female)} + u_{02}\text{ (Age)} + u_{03}\text{ (Black)} + u_{04}\text{ (Hispanic)} + u_{05}\text{ (Mean Advertising Exposure)} + u_{10}\text{ (Time)} + u_{11}\text{ (Time·Age)} + u_{20}\text{ (Advertising Exposure, Within Individual)} + u_{30}\text{ (High School)} + u_{40}\text{ (College)} + e$$

where $\eta$ is the log-link function for drinking, $\gamma$ is the estimated coefficient, $e$ is the level 1 (observation) random effect, $r$ is the level 2 (individual) random effect, and $u$ is the level 3 (market-level) random effect.

The analysis was repeated for the subset of the sample younger than 21 years because of the importance of underage drinking. The sample sizes were 2286 at level 1, 1094 at level 2, and 24 at level 3. The intercept was the only random factor among the level 1 variables. The results show the unit-specific models and the event rate ratios. The event rate ratio, which for a Poisson model is the exponential of a coefficient, can be interpreted as the percentage change in the dependent variable associated with an increase of 1 unit in the independent variable, holding other factors constant.[42]

## RESULTS

Sixty-one percent of the sample had at least 1 drink in the past month at baseline (**Table 1**). Drinkers consumed 38.5 total drinks on average in the past month at baseline (95% confidence interval [CI], 34.3-42.7), imbibing an average of 4.5 drinks per episode (95% CI, 4.3-4.8). Drinkers younger than 21 years had 29 drinks on average at baseline, with 4.5 drinks on average each drinking session (95% CI, 4.1-4.8). The market alcohol advertising spending ranged from \$78 000 (Tulsa, Okla) to \$88 750 000 (Los Angeles, Calif) during 1999 and 2000, with a mean of \$14 800 000 worth of alcohol advertising (95% CI, \$13 800 000-\$15 800 000). Per capita spending ranged from \$0.20 to \$17.3, averaging \$6.8 (95% CI, 6.6-7.0). Individuals reported seeing an average of 22.7 alcohol advertisements per month at baseline.

**Table 1. Demographics, Alcohol Advertisement Exposure, and Market Alcohol Advertisement Expenditures by Mean Alcohol Use and Changes in Alcohol Use Over Time**

| Characteristic | % of Sample | Mean Baseline Alcohol Use in Prior Month (95% CI) | Mean Change in Alcohol Use From Baseline to Time 4 (95% CI) |
|---|---|---|---|
| Total | 100.0 | 23.4 (20.7 to 26.1) | 2.4 (−1.6 to 6.4) |
| Drinkers (any drink in past month baseline) | 60.8 | 38.5 (34.3 to 42.7) | 1.2 (−6.3 to 8.7) |
| Drinkers younger than 21 y | 49.3* | 29.0 (23.9 to 34.0) | 17.5 (6.1 to −28.8) |
| Gender | | | |
| Male | 51.2 | 36.7 (37.8 to 41.5) | 1.9 (−5.8 to 9.7) |
| Female | 48.8 | 9.8 (8.0 to 11.6) | 2.7 (0.5 to 5.1) |
| Race/ethnicity | | | |
| Hispanic | 8.2 | 24.2 (21.3 to 27.1) | −.2 (−6.9 to .5) |
| Black | 11.4 | 25.6 (22.6 to 28.6) | 2.6 (−0.9 to 6.1) |
| White | 69.9 | 17.9 (13.4 to 22.4) | 3.1 (−2.1 to 8.2) |
| Education, baseline | | | |
| In high school | 28.0 | 6.5 (4.3 to 8.8) | 6.7 (3.6 to 9.9) |
| In college | 31.0 | 27.6 (22.6 to 32.5) | 13.6 (3.0 to 24.1) |
| Not in school | 41.0 | 32.9 (27.6 to 38.2) | −11.6 (−19.4 to −3.8) |
| Age, y | | | |
| 15-21, baseline | 60.0 | 14.3 (11.7 to 17.0) | 9.5 (4.7 to 14.3) |
| <18 | 27.0 | 8.5 (5.4 to 11.6) | 4.8 (1.9 to 7.7) |
| 18 (<21) | 25.0 | 20.4 (16.1 to 24.8 | 17.1 (5.7 to 28.5) |
| 21 (<23) | 16.0 | 42.1 (31.5 to 52.7) | −8.8 (−23.4 to 5.7) |
| 23-26 | 32.0 | 29.1 (24.3 to 33.8) | −6.8 (−14.3 to 0.6) |
| Television market advertising expenditures per capita | | | |
| <2 | 20.9 | 24.3 (18.0 to 30.6) | −5.4 (−13.4 to 2.7) |
| 2-5.9 | 29.0 | 24.4 (18.8 to 30.0) | −2.3 (−9.7 to 5.1) |
| 6-9.9 | 25.0 | 18.4 (14.4 to 22.4) | 5.3 (−0.3 to 11.0) |
| ≥10 | 25.1 | 26.3 (20.9 to 31.8) | 12.7 (1.7 to 23.7) |
| Advertising exposure, baseline | | | |
| <8 | 15.7 | 18.5 (11.2 to 25.9) | .7 (−8.4 to 9.9) |
| 8-29 | 55.6 | 23.3 (19.8 to 26.8) | 1.2 (−3.3 to 5.6) |
| 30-51 | 24.1 | 24.6 (19.4 to 29.8) | 8.0 (−3.5 to 19.5) |
| ≥52 | 4.6 | 34.9 (17.7 to 52.1) | −5.2 (−24.9 to 14.5) |

Abbreviation: CI, confidence interval.
*Among those younger than 21 years.

The results in **Table 2** show that advertising exposure was positively related to an increase in drinking. Holding other factors constant, individuals who saw 1 more advertisement average than other individuals had 1% more alcoholic drinks per month (event rate ratio, 1.01; 95% CI, 1.01-1.02). Within-individual variation in advertising exposure was not a statistically significant factor in drinking, so whether a youth saw more or fewer advertisements in a particular month than he or she typically saw was not as important a determinant of drinking as that person's average level of advertising exposure over time.

Market advertising expenditures per capita were related to drinking levels and to growth in drinking over time. For every additional dollar per capita spent on advertising in the market, individuals consumed 3% more alcoholic beverages per month (event rate ratio, 1.03; 95% CI, 1.01-1.05), holding constant other factors, including time. There was an interaction effect between time and age and market advertising expenditures. In markets with high levels of advertising expenditures per capita, growth in drinking over time is steepest among older youth, reaching close to 50 drinks a month for 25-year-olds (**Figure 1**). In markets with low levels of advertising expenditures per capita, the initial drinking rates were lower than in markets with high levels of advertising expenditures per capita (**Figure 2**). Younger age groups show an increase in drinking over time but at a slower rate than peers in markets with high levels of advertising expenditures per capita. Around the age of 22 years, growth flattens out, with little increase in drinking over time. Above age 23 years, drinking declines over time in the markets with low levels of advertising expenditures per capita, declining most steeply in older age groups. (The figures depict growth curves, assuming mean levels of continuous factors and zero values for dummy variables, including male, not in school, not black, and not Hispanic.)

To better illustrate the effects of the main variables of interest, **Figure 3** depicts the relationship among alcohol use, mean levels of advertising exposure, advertising expenditures per capita, and gender. We held constant the other factors in the model; therefore, the figure shows predicted drinking levels for a 20-year-old who is not currently a student, neither African American nor Hispanic, and living in a market with an average amount of alcohol sales per capita measured at the mean date of the study and who reported, in the prior month, exposure to his or her average number of advertisements. The results indicate that

**Table 2. Hierarchical Linear Modeling Parameter Estimates Predicting Alcohol Use for the Total Sample**

| | Event Rate Ratio (95% CI) |
|---|---|
| Intercept | 9.56 (7.21 to 12.67) |
| Alcohol sales per capita | 1.002 (0.999 to 1.006) |
| Market-level advertising expenditures per capita | 1.027 (1.010 to 1.045) |
| Female | 0.49 (0.41 to 0.59) |
| Age | 1.07 (1.03 to 1.12) |
| African American | 0.23 (0.12 to 0.44) |
| Hispanic | 0.47 (0.21 to 1.06) |
| Mean advertising exposure | 1.01 (1.01 to 1.04) |
| Time | 1.02 (1.01 to 1.04) |
| Time × age | 1.00 (0.99 to 1.00) |
| Time × age × market advertising expenditures per capita | 1.001 (1.000 to 1.001) |
| Advertising exposure, within individual | 1.00 (1.00 to 1.00) |
| High school student | 0.46 (0.2 to 0.73) |
| College student | 0.99 (0.86 to 1.13) |

Abbreviation: CI, confidence interval.

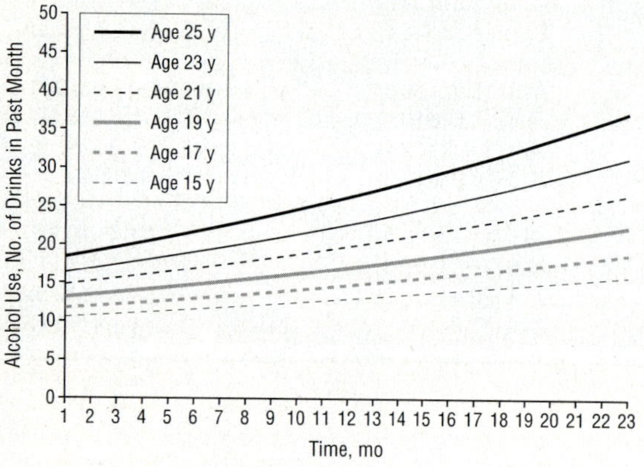


**Figure 1.** Alcohol use over time by age in markets with high alcohol advertising expenditures per capita.

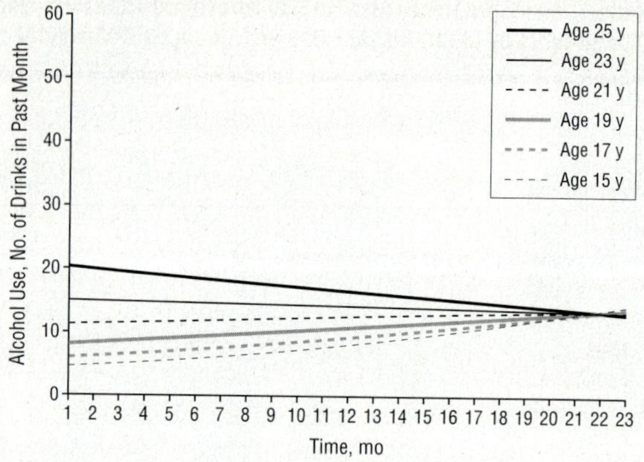


**Figure 2.** Alcohol use over time by age in markets with low alcohol advertising expenditures per capita.

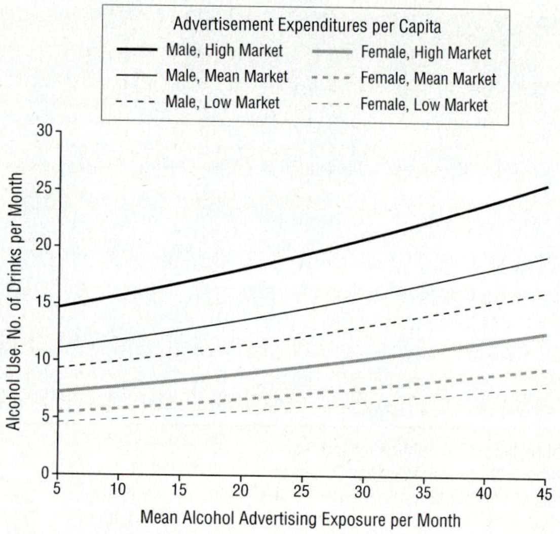


**Figure 3.** Alcohol use by mean advertising exposure, market advertising expenditures per capita, and gender.

a 20-year-old man who saw few alcohol advertisements (5) and lived in a market with minimal alcohol advertising expenditures per capita was predicted to have 9 alcoholic drinks in the past month compared with 16 drinks if he saw many advertisements (45). A man with the same profile but living in a market with the highest advertising spending per capita was predicted to have 15 drinks if he reported little advertising exposure and 26 drinks if he saw many advertisements.

We tested the same hierarchical linear model for the subset of the sample younger than the legal drinking age. The results were similar to those for the sample as a whole. Drinking was greater among underage youth who reported higher mean levels of alcohol advertising exposure (**Table 3**). Each additional average advertisement exposure was associated with an increase of 1% in drinks consumed in the past month (event rate ratio, 1.01; 95% CI, 1.001-1.021), holding constant other factors. Drinking levels were higher among underage youth living in markets with greater per capita advertising expenditures (event rate ratio, 1.03; 95% CI, 1.00-1.06), holding constant other factors. A 3-way interaction effect still occurred among time, age, and market advertising expenditures, following similar growth curves to those in Figure 1 and Figure 2.

## COMMENT

The results of the present large-scale national longitudinal study provide evidence that the amount of advertising expenditures in 15- to 26-year-olds' media environment and the amount of advertising recalled related to greater youth drinking. Youth younger than the legal drinking age displayed a similar pattern of advertising effects as the entire age range, which is important because there is often a greater policy interest in protecting underage youth from harmful communications than in protecting youth older than 21 years.

Greater alcohol advertising expenditures in a market were related to both greater levels of youth drinking and steeper increases in drinking over time. Youth who lived in markets with more alcohol advertising drank more, increased their drinking levels more over time, and continued to increase drinking levels into their late 20s. Youth who lived in markets with less alcohol advertising drank less and showed a pattern of increasing their drinking modestly until their early 20s, when their drinking levels started to decline. The results are consistent with findings from studies of advertising bans[31,32] and extend them by linking alcohol advertising expenditures per capita directly with individual youth behavior. The effect of market advertising spending on youth drinking was not attributable to differences in alcohol sales, which was controlled for statistically in the model.

The relationship between market-level advertising expenditures and youth drinking is all the more striking because it assesses the effect of the "added value" of advertising in a market, over and above national advertisements appearing in all markets. Of the more than $1 billion a year spent on alcohol advertising at the time of the study, approximately one fifth was placed on local television, radio, and billboards.[50] To the extent that additional communication produces diminishing returns, the added value of market-level advertising may underestimate the total effect of alcohol advertising.

The results are consistent with theories of cumulative effects of media exposure. Youth reporting greater amounts of exposure to alcohol advertising over the long term drank more than youth who saw fewer ads. Alcohol consumption was less sensitive to short-term differences in alcohol advertising exposure than to the long-term effects of exposure.

Given that there was an impact on drinking using an objective measure of advertising expenditures, the results are inconsistent with the hypothesis that a correlation between advertising exposure and drinking could be caused entirely by selective attention on the part of drinkers. The results also contradict claims that advertising is unrelated to youth drinking amounts: that advertising at best causes brand switching, only affects those older than the legal drinking age, or is effectively countered by current educational efforts. Alcohol advertising was a contributing factor to youth drinking quantities over time.

The strength of the study was the relatively large national sample, the use of an objective measure of advertising expenditures to complement the subjective measure of advertising exposure, and the matching of expenditure data with individual behavior. The study was limited by the industry data used to measure advertising exposure, which largely reflects the most expensive medium for advertising—television. During this period, data on outdoor advertising was spotty and may have been incomplete in some markets. It is also possible that using a measure of likely advertising exposures (such as gross rating points) would increase effects. There may also be variation in the national advertising expenditures in markets, through differences in cable systems and presence of national stations or programming, that were not measured. Note, too, that other forms of marketing were not included here (such as product placements in programming, promotions, sports sponsorships, and stadium advertising) that could affect youth drinking. Future research could examine the impact of different forms of advertising and the consumption of various alcoholic products. Other limitations of the study were the sample attrition and the fact that those who drank more at baseline were more likely to drop out of the study. Future research should also control for the effects of parent and peer influences on drinking. Finally, the study does not explain the process by which advertising affects youth.

**Table 3. Hierarchical Linear Modeling Parameter Estimates Predicting Alcohol Use Among 15- to 20-Year-Olds**

| | Event Rate Ratio (95% CI) |
|---|---|
| Intercept | 8.69 (4.01 to 18.49) |
| Alcohol sales per capita | 1.001 (0.996 to 1.006) |
| Market-level advertising expenditures per capita | 1.028 (1.002 to 1.056) |
| Female | 0.56 (0.41 to 0.76) |
| Age | 1.30 (1.16 to 1.44) |
| African American | 0.19 (0.07 to 0.53) |
| Hispanic | 0.37 (0.18 to .75) |
| Mean advertising exposure | 1.01 (1.001 to 1.021) |
| Time | 1.04 (1.01 to 1.06) |
| Time × age | 1.00 (0.99 to 1.00) |
| Time × age × market advertising expenditures per capita | 1.002 (1.001 to 1.003) |
| Advertising exposure, within individual | 1.002 (1.001 to 1.003) |
| High school student | 0.53 (0.27 to 1.02) |
| College student | 0.95 (0.56 to 1.59) |

Abbreviation: CI, confidence interval.

**Accepted for Publication:** September 12, 2005.
**Correspondence:** Leslie B. Snyder, PhD, Department of Communication Sciences, University of Connecticut, Storrs, CT 06269-1085 (leslie.snyder@uconn.edu).
**Author Contributions:** Leslie B. Snyder, PhD, had full access to all the data in the study and takes responsibility for the integrity of the data and the accuracy of the data analysis.
**Funding/Support:** This study was funded by grant 1R01AA11551 from the National Institute of Alcohol Abuse and Alcoholism, Bethesda, Md, to Dr Snyder.
**Acknowledgment:** David Kenny, PhD, Kimberly Henry, PhD, Ann O'Connell, PhD, and Cyr Emile M'Lan, PhD, reviewed the analysis and results. William Wells, PhD, Mark Hamilton, PhD, Dwayne Proctor, PhD, and Elizabeth Mitchell, PhD, contributed to the survey design. Data collection was performed by the Center for Survey Research and Analysis at the University of Connecticut.

## REFERENCES

1. Chassin L, DeLucia C. Drinking during adolescence. *Alcohol Health Res World.* 1996;20:175-180.
2. O'Malley PM, Johnston LD, Bachman JG. Alcohol use among adolescents. *Alcohol Health Res World.* 1998;22:85-94.
3. Cooper ML, Peirce RS, Huselid RF. Substance use and sexual risk taking among black adolescents and white adolescents. *Health Psychol.* 1994;13:251-262.
4. Windle M, Miller-Tutzauer C, Domenico D. Patterns of drug use from adolescence to youth adulthood, III: predictors of progression. *Am J Public Health.* 1992; 74:673-681.
5. Foster SE, Vaughan RD, Foster WH, Califano JA. Alcohol consumption and ex-

penditures for underage drinking and adult excessive drinking. *JAMA*. 2003;289:989-995.
6. Substance Abuse and Mental Health Services Administration. *National Household Survey on Drug Abuse*. Rockville, Md: Office of Applied Studies; 2001.
7. National Highway Traffic Safety Administration. *Traffic Safety Facts 2001-Alcohol*. Washington, DC: US Dept of Transportation; 2002. DOT HS 809 406.
8. Substance Abuse and Mental Health Services Administration. Alcohol Use: The National Household Survey on Drug Abuse. 2003. Available at: http://www.samhsa.gov/oas/alcohol.cfm. Accessed December 5, 2003.
9. Federal Trade Commission. Alcohol marketing and advertising. 2003. Available at: http://www.ftc.gov/os/2003/09/alcohol08report.pdf. Accessed January 24, 2004.
10. *Alcohol's Vast Adland*. Washington, DC: Georgetown University's Center on Alcohol Marketing and Youth; 2002.
11. *Overexposed: Youth a Target of Alcohol Advertising in Magazines*. Washington, DC: Georgetown University's Center on Alcohol Marketing and Youth; 2002.
12. *Radiodaze: Alcohol Ads Tune in Underage Youth*. Washington, DC: Georgetown University's Center on Alcohol Marketing and Youth; 2002.
13. Garfield CF, Chung PJ, Rathouz PJ. Alcohol advertising in magazines and adolescent readership. *JAMA*. 2003;289:2424-2426.
14. Martin SE, Snyder LB, Hamilton M, et al. Alcohol advertising and youth. *Alcohol Clin Exp Res*. 2002;26:900-906.
15. Atkin CK. Effects of media alcohol messages on adolescent audiences. *Adolesc Med*. 1993;4:527-542.
16. Adlaf EM, Kohn PM. Alcohol advertising, consumption and abuse: a covariance-structural modeling look at Strickland's data. *Br J Addict*. 1989;84:749-757.
17. Atkin CK, Neuendorf K, McDermott S. The role of alcohol advertising in excessive and hazardous drinking. *J Drug Educ*. 1983;4:313-325.
18. Atkin CK, Hocking J, Block M. Teenage drinking: does advertising make a difference? *J Commun*. 1984;28:71-80.
19. Strickland DE. Advertising exposure, alcohol consumption and misuse of alcohol. In: Grant M, Plant M, Williams A, eds. *Economics and Alcohol: Consumption and Controls*. New York, NY: Gardner Press; 1983:201-222.
20. Smart R. Does alcohol advertising affect overall consumption? a review of empirical studies. *J Stud Alcohol*. 1988;49:314-323.
21. Covell K. The appeal of image advertisements: age, gender, and product differences. *J Early Adolesc*. 1997;12:46-60.
22. Kelly KJ, Edwards RW. Image advertisements for alcohol products: is their appeal associated with adolescents' intention to consume alcohol? *Adolescence*. 1998;33:47-59.
23. Slater MD, Rouner D, Domenech-Rodriguez M, Beauvais F, Murphy K, Van Leuven JK. Adolescence responses to TV beer ads and sports content/context: gender and ethnic differences. *J Mass Commun Q*. 1997;4:108-122.
24. Waiters ED, Treno AJ, Grube JW. Alcohol advertising and youth: a focus group analysis of what young people find appealing in alcohol advertising. *Contemp Drug Probl*. 2001;28:695-715.
25. Aitken PP, Leathar DS, Scott AC. Ten- to sixteen-year-olds perceptions of advertisements for alcoholic drinks. *Alcohol Alcohol*. 1988;23:491-500.
26. Austin EW, Pinkleton BE, Fujioka Y. The role of interpretation processes and parental discussion in the media's effects on adolescents' use of alcohol. *Pediatrics*. 2000;105:343-349.
27. Grube J, Wallack L. Television beer advertising and drinking knowledge, beliefs, and intentions among schoolchildren. *Am J Public Health*. 1994;84:254-259.
28. Ellickson PL, Collins RL, Hambarsoomians K, McCaffrey DF. Does alcohol advertising promote adolescent drinking? results from a longitudinal assessment. *Addiction*. 2005;100:235-246.
29. Tapert SF, Cheung EH, Brown GG, et al. Neural response to alcohol stimuli in adolescents with alcohol use disorder. *Arch Gen Psychiatry*. 2003;60:727-735.
30. Collins RL, Schell T, Ellickson PL, McCaffrey D. Predictors of beer advertising awareness among eighth graders. *Addiction*. 2003;98:1297-1306.
31. Saffer H. Alcohol advertising bans and alcohol abuse: an international perspective. *J Health Econ*. 1991;10:65-79.
32. Saffer H, Dave D. Alcohol consumption and alcohol advertising bans. *Appl Econ*. 2002;34:1325-1334.
33. Nielsen Media Research Local Universe Estimates. Available at: http://www.nielsenmedia.com/DMAs.html..
34. US Census. 1990 Available at: http://factfinder.census.gov..
35. Adams Business Media. *Adams Liquor Handbook 1997*. New York, NY: Adams Business Media; 1998.
36. Kalton G. *Introduction to Survey Sampling*. In: Quantitative Applications in the Social Sciences Series, No. 35. Thousand Oaks, Calif: Sage; 1983.
37. Genesys Sampling Systems. Available at: http://www.m-s-g.com/genesys/genesyshme.htm.
38. American Association for Public Opinion Research Outcome Rate Calculator Version 2.1. Available at: httpp://www.aapor.org/default.asp?page=survey_methods/response _rate_calculator. Accessed March 23, 2004.
39. Adalbjarnardottir S. Adolescent psychological maturity and alcohol use: quantitative and qualitative analysis of longitudinal data. *Adolescence*. 2002;37:19-53.
40. Media Intelligence TNS . Available at: http://www.tns-mi.com.
41. Adams Business Media. *Adams Factbook 2001*. New York: Adams, 2001.
42. Raudenbush SW, Bryk AS. *Hierarchical Linear Models: Applications and Data Analysis Methods*. 2nd ed. Thousand Oaks, Calif: Sage; 2002.
43. Raudenbush SW, Bryk AS, Cheong YF, Congdon R. HLM6.01: Hierarchical Linear and Nonlinear Modeling [software]. Lincolnwood, Ill: Scientific Software International; 2005.
44. Raudenbush SW, Bryk AS, Cheong YF, Congdon R. *HLM6.01: Hierarchical Linear and Nonlinear Modeling* [manual]. Lincolnwood, Ill: Scientific Software International; 2005.
45. Hox J. *Multilevel Analysis Techniques and Applications*. Mahwah, NJ: Lawrence Erlbaum Associates; 2002.
46. Mohr CD, Armeli S, Tennen H, Carney MA, Affleck G, Hromi A. Daily interpersonal experiences, context and alcohol consumption: crying in your beer and toasting good times? *J Pers Soc Psychol*. 2001;80:489-500.
47. Singer JD, Willett JB. *Applied Longitudinal Data Analysis: Modeling Change and Event Occurrence*. New York, NY: Oxford University Press; 2003.
48. Flewelling RL, Paschall MJ, Ringwalt C. The epidemiology of underage drinking in the United States: an overview. In: Committee on Developing a Strategy to Reduce and Prevent Underage Drinking. *Reducing Underage Drinking: Issues and Interventions*. Washington DC: National Academy Press. 2004:319-350.
49. Cohen J, Cohen P, West SG, Aiken LS. *Applied Multiple Regression/Correlation Analysis for the Behavioral Sciences*. 3rd ed. Mahway, NJ: Lawrence Earlbaum Associates. 2003.
50. Snyder LB, Fleming-Milici F, Mitchell EW, Proctor D. Media, product differences, and seasonality in alcohol advertising in 1997. *J Stud Alcohol*. 2000;61:896-906.

# Neighborhood Safety and Overweight Status in Children

*Julie C. Lumeng, MD; Danielle Appugliese, MPH; Howard J. Cabral, PhD; Robert H. Bradley, PhD; Barry Zuckerman, MD*

**Objective:** To determine if there is a relationship between parental perception of neighborhood safety and overweight at the age of 7 years.

**Design:** Cross-sectional analysis of the National Institute of Child Health and Human Development Study of Early Child Care and Youth Development.

**Setting:** Ten urban and rural US sites.

**Participants:** A total of 768 children selected via conditional random sampling with complete data at follow-up.

**Main Outcome Measures:** Parents reported demographics and perception of neighborhood safety by standardized questionnaire. Child overweight status was defined as a body mass index greater than or equal to the 95th percentile for age and sex from measured anthropometrics at the age of 7 years. The base model included relationship of the safety reporter to the child, sex, and baseline body mass index *z* score at the age of 4.5 years. Covariates tested included maternal marital status, education, and depressive symptoms; child race/ethnicity; participation in structured after-school activities; Home Observation for Measurement of the Environment total score; and neighborhood social cohesiveness.

**Results:** The sample was 85% white, and 10% of the children were overweight. Neighborhood safety ratings in the lowest quartile were independently associated with a higher risk of overweight at the age of 7 years compared with safety ratings in the highest quartile (adjusted odds ratio, 4.43; 95% confidence interval, 2.03-9.65). None of the candidate covariates altered the relationship between perception of neighborhood safety and child overweight status.

**Conclusions:** Perception of the neighborhood as less safe was independently associated with an increased risk of overweight at the age of 7 years. Public health efforts may benefit from policies directed toward improving both actual and perceived neighborhood safety.

*Arch Pediatr Adolesc Med. 2006;160:25-31*

**Author Affiliations:** Center for Human Growth and Development and Department of Pediatrics and Communicable Diseases, University of Michigan, Ann Arbor (Dr Lumeng); Data Coordinating Center (Ms Appugliese) and Department of Biostatistics (Dr Cabral), Boston University School of Public Health, Boston, Mass; Center for Applied Studies in Education, University of Arkansas at Little Rock (Dr Bradley); and Department of Pediatrics, Boston University School of Medicine, Boston (Dr Zuckerman).

THE MOST RECENT US NAtional data confirm the growing obesity epidemic: 15.8% of 6- to 11-year-old children are overweight (defined as a body mass index [BMI] ≥95th percentile for age and sex)[1] and the racial disparities continue to increase.[2] Well-described risk factors for childhood overweight in the United States include African American or Hispanic race/ethnicity,[2] elevated parental BMI,[3,4] and a large amount of television viewing.[5] The most recent data suggest that lower socioeconomic status is associated with overweight in children,[4,6] but the relationship is complicated and appears to vary based on a combination of sex, age, race/ethnicity, and the degree of poverty.[7] The home environment and parenting have received significant attention in the literature,[4,8-11] but the neighborhood and built environment as independent contributors to child overweight risk have not been examined as thoroughly. The built environment, which has been associated with other health outcomes,[12-15] has been recognized by the Centers for Disease Control and Prevention as a potentially important area for public policy to address the childhood obesity epidemic[16] and an area that requires additional research.[17]

Our clinical experience in an urban pediatric clinic that serves a low-income population has been that unsafe neighborhoods significantly affect children's daily activities. Anecdotally, parents in an urban setting frequently express their reluctance to allow their children to play outside for fear of exposure to violence, crime, and illicit drug use. Prior assessments of perception of neighborhood safety have focused on physical activity levels as an outcome[18,19] or used children's (not parents') assessments of neighborhood safety.[19] However, parental perception of neighborhood safety may be more salient than the child's perception because parents of young children typically exert substantial control over where their children spend time.

We therefore sought to document our clinical impression by investigating the relationship between parental perception of neighborhood safety and overweight in children at the age of 7 years in 10 diverse regions of the United States. We focused on overweight at the age of 7 years because overweight prevalence increases most rapidly in childhood around this age,[1] and the racial/ethnic disparities in overweight prevalence also widen significantly during this same period of childhood.[1] We hypothesized that parents who perceive their neighborhood as unsafe would be more likely to have overweight children because they restrict their children's access to outdoor activities. We also hypothesized that this relationship would be attenuated by the availability of an afterschool program, a stimulating home environment, or increased social cohesiveness in the neighborhood. In examining these hypotheses, it is critical to control for potentially confounding factors known to be associated with obesity.

## METHODS

The sample was composed of children and their parents enrolled in the National Institute of Child Health and Human Development Study of Early Child Care and Youth Development (NICHD-SECCYD). The NICHD-SECCYD[20] is a longitudinal study of relationships between child behavior and development and key developmental contexts, especially child care experience. Families who participated in this study were recruited through hospital visits to mothers shortly after the birth of a child in 1991. Families lived in the areas of Little Rock, Ark; Irvine, Calif; Lawrence, Kan; Boston, Mass; Morganton, NC; Philadelphia, Pa; Pittsburgh, Pa; Charlottesville, Va; Seattle, Wash; and Madison, Wis.

Of the 8986 mothers who gave birth during the sampling period, 5416 (60%) met the eligibility criteria. Mothers were required to be healthy, to be older than 18 years, to not be planning to move within the next year, to live within an hour of the study site, and to be conversant in English with a singleton child whose birth was normal and uncomplicated. An additional inclusion criterion at the Philadelphia site was that families live in a neighborhood that was not extremely unsafe as documented by local police, given the planned home visits. One hundred thirty-one families (1.4% of the original pool of 8986 potential families) were excluded for this reason. Notably, the study protocol for the duration of the study dictated that if the neighborhood was deemed too unsafe for a home visit, the home visit would still be completed but with a security guard or police officer present.

Of the 5416 eligible families, 3015 (56%) were selected using a conditional random sampling plan that ensured that the recruited families reflected economic, educational, and ethnic diversity.[21] Of the 3015 families selected for participation, 1526 (51%) agreed to participate. Of the 1526 families who agreed to participate, 1364 (89%) completed the initial data collection.[20] This initial sample was representative of the demographics of the catchment areas from which the sample was recruited: 24% of the children were of an ethnic/racial minority, 10% of the mothers had less than a high school education, and 14% of the mothers were single at the time of the child's birth. The study involved extensive data collection at frequent intervals. Data used in this analysis were collected during assessments scheduled for children at the age of 4.5 years and in the spring and fall of the child's first grade year in school. This study was approved by the institutional review boards of all pertinent institutions.

### PERCEPTION OF NEIGHBORHOOD SAFETY

The Neighborhood Questionnaire is a 16-item measure of neighborhood characteristics that was completed during the child's first-grade year in school by the mother and another adult living in the home who acted as a caregiver (hereafter referred to as the father). More than 85% of these caregivers were fathers, 9% were the mother's partner, and the remainder were grandparents or relatives.[22] Two scales of the Neighborhood Questionnaire are the Neighborhood Safety Subscale (NSS) and the Neighborhood Social Involvement Subscale.[23]

The NSS score consists of the mean of 5 items. On the overall Neighborhood Questionnaire, the number of possible response categories (eg, items on the Likert scale) varied from 2 to 10, and on the NSS, response categories varied from 4 to 5. Responses were therefore rescaled to a 0 to 10 range and averaged to provide the overall score via the methods used in the original scale. Parents responded to the following questions: (1) "How do you feel about your neighborhood?" (2) "How satisfied are you with police protection around here?" (3) "How often are there problems with muggings, burglaries, assaults, or anything else like that around here?" (4) "How much of a problem is the selling and using of drugs around here?" and (5) "How well do the police and people in this neighborhood get along?" Higher scores represent greater perceived neighborhood safety.

All 768 children had an NSS score from at least 1 reporter; 739 had an NSS score from 2 reporters, one of whom was always the mother. The NSS scores differed significantly based on the identity of the reporter, with mothers perceiving the neighborhood as slightly safer than fathers ($\Delta = 0.16$; $P = .004$). When both parents completed the NSS questionnaire, we used the score that reflected a perception of the neighborhood as less safe based on the assumption that the parent who had the greatest concern about safety would do more to control the child's access to people and places outside the home. We therefore controlled for the identity of the neighborhood safety reporter a priori in the base model.

### OVERWEIGHT STATUS

Height and weight were measured during the laboratory visit at the age of 4.5 years and in the spring of the child's first grade year in school (when children in the United States are on average 7 years old). Trained research assistants certified for accuracy in measurement weighed the children, who were lightly clothed and without shoes, on a physician's scale (Detecto physician's scale model 437, Cardinal/Detecto, Webb City, Mo) to the nearest 100 g. Children's height was measured without shoes, using a T square, to the nearest 0.3 cm. Details of the measurement procedures are documented elsewhere.[24] The BMI was calculated as weight in kilograms divided by the square of height in meters, and child overweight was defined dichotomously as a BMI greater than or equal to the 95th percentile for age and sex based on National Center for Health Statistics norms.[25]

### INDEPENDENT VARIABLES

Demographic data consisted of the child's sex, race/ethnicity (white, black, or other), maternal marital status (single vs not), and maternal education (years of education completed). Maternal education was included as a continuous variable. We elected to use maternal education as our measure of socioeconomic status because this variable had the most complete data of the available indicators. Maternal education was correlated with income-to-needs ratio (Spearman rank correlation=0.59; $P<.001$).

Additional characteristics assumed to modify an association between perception of neighborhood safety and overweight were tested as potential covariates. These included maternal scores on the Center for Epidemiological Studies Depression Scale[26] reported during the child's first grade year, the child's participation in structured after-school activities (dichotomized as >1 hour per week vs not) reported in kindergarten, parental perception of neighborhood social cohesiveness reported on the Neighborhood Social Involvement Subscale of the Neighborhood Questionnaire during the child's first-grade year, and quality of the home environment as measured by the Home Observation for Measurement of the Environment (HOME) total score. The HOME was administered by trained observers during home visits at the child's age of 4.5 years. The HOME is an observational measure of the stimulation and support available to the child in the home.[27] The NICHD-SECCYD did not include maternal anthropometric data or child television-viewing patterns in the time frame of this analysis.

## STATISTICAL ANALYSIS

All data analysis was performed using SAS statistical software, version 8.2 (SAS Institute Inc, Cary, NC). In our analyses, we excluded children without data for NSS scores (n=337) or BMI at first grade (n=371). Children who had moved residences in the past 12 months were also excluded (n=162), since we were interested in assessing the role of the neighborhood in overweight risk. We examined the sample included in our model (n=768) vs those excluded because of missing data (n=596) and found statistically significant differences. Although the NSS scores did not differ significantly ($P=.76$), children included in the sample were more likely to be overweight (10% vs 6%; $P=.002$), slightly more likely to be female (51% vs 45%; $P=.05$), more likely to be white (85% vs 75%; $P<.001$), and had mothers who were more educated (14.7 vs 13.7 years; $P<.001$). Additional information regarding differences in the samples is available from the authors on request.

Univariate statistics were first computed to provide a description of the sample of 768 children. We dichotomized the child's BMI at the age of 7 years as overweight (BMI ≥95th percentile) vs not overweight to create a dependent variable that could be used in a multiple logistic regression model.

Then, bivariate analyses were performed to inform the development of the multivariate model. We analyzed all covariates by overweight status using *t* tests for continuous variables and cross-tabulations with $\chi^2$ tests. We analyzed associations between NSS scores and these covariates with *t* tests, analysis of variance, and correlation coefficients. To characterize the relationship among neighborhood safety, race/ethnicity, and socioeconomic status, we regressed the NSS score on race/ethnicity and socioeconomic status. We also performed a cross-tabulation of overweight status and NSS score in quartiles (with cut points at the scores 6.83, 7.67, and 8.67) to assess potential nonlinearity in their relationship. We next fit logistic regression models with overweight status as the outcome.

We accounted for clustering by site with bias-corrected generalized estimating equations based on the methods of Mancl and DeRouen.[28,29] We computed both unadjusted and adjusted odds ratios and their corresponding 95% confidence intervals from these logistic regression models. We used an $\alpha$ level of .05 (2-tailed) to determine statistical significance. A base model for estimating overweight status on the parent's perception of neighborhood safety was created including child sex and identity of the safety reporter a priori.

Each of the candidate covariates was then tested by entering them one by one into the base model. Covariates that altered the relationship of NSS scores to child overweight in these models by more than 10% were retained in the final model.[30] Although this method of modeling is not able to test for potential joint confounding, limiting the number of covariates included simultaneously in the model allowed us to maintain the stability of the model. In addition, variables found to be differentially distributed between those in the analysis sample and those not in the sample were evaluated for potential confounding effects.

## RESULTS

The sample included 768 children. The mean±SD age of the children at the time of the anthropometric measures in the spring of first grade was 7.0±0.3 years (range, 6.3-8.1 years). Approximately half of the sample were male and 10% were overweight, consistent with national data for children of this age.[31] The mean±SD NSS score was 7.69±1.5 (range, 1.3-10.0; potential range, 0.0-10.0). The NSS scores were normally distributed with a slight positive skew. Of the mothers, 42% had at least a bachelor's degree; 20% had a high school education or less (**Table 1**). Overweight children had mothers who were less educated and came from homes with lower HOME scores. However, overweight children did not differ from children who were not overweight by sex, race/ethnicity, relationship of the safety reporter to the child, maternal marital status, maternal depressive symptoms, amount of structured after-school activities, or Neighborhood Social Involvement Subscale scores (Table 1).

In bivariate analyses, lower parental neighborhood safety ratings were associated with African American race, lower maternal education, more maternal depressive symptoms, fewer structured after-school activities for the child, and a lower HOME total score. Child sex, child age (restricted to first grade), and maternal marital status were not related to parental neighborhood safety ratings (**Table 2**).

In an attempt to better characterize perception of neighborhood safety in relation to race/ethnicity and socioeconomic status, we performed regression analysis of race/ethnicity on parental neighborhood safety ratings, adjusting for maternal education as a proxy for socioeconomic status. Given the limited sample size, we categorized race/ethnicity as white and nonwhite. Race/ethnicity was significantly independently associated with parental perception of neighborhood safety. White parents were significantly more likely to perceive the neighborhood as safe (mean±SD NSS score, 7.83±1.39) than were nonwhite parents (mean±SD NSS score, 6.84±1.82), independent of socioeconomic status ($P<.001$).

### OVERWEIGHT STATUS AND NEIGHBORHOOD SAFETY

Results from the bivariate analyses showed that parents of children who were overweight in first grade perceived their neighborhoods as significantly less safe than parents of children who were not overweight ($P<.001$) (Table 1). We next evaluated the unadjusted risk of overweight in each quartile of NSS scores in a cross-

**Table 1. Characteristics of Children Who Were Overweight and Not Overweight in the Spring of First Grade**

| Characteristics | Overweight (n = 79) | Not Overweight (n = 689) | Total (n = 768) | *P* Value |
|---|---|---|---|---|
| Neighborhood Safety Subscale score, mean (SD) | 7.08 (1.6) | 7.75 (1.5) | 7.69 (1.5) | <.001 |
| Age, mean (SD), y | 7.03 (0.3) | 7.04 (0.3) | 7.04 (0.3) | .81 |
| Sex, % | | | | .63 |
| Male | 52 | 49 | 49 | |
| Female | 48 | 51 | 51 | |
| Race/ethnicity, % | | | | .84 |
| White | 85 | 85 | 85 | |
| Black | 11 | 9 | 9 | |
| Other | 4 | 6 | 6 | |
| Identity of safety reporter, % | | | | .23 |
| Mother | 57 | 64 | 63 | |
| Father or other | 43 | 36 | 37 | |
| Maternal education, mean (SD), y | 14.1 (2.3) | 14.7 (2.4) | 14.7 (2.4) | .02 |
| Maternal marital status, % | | | | .48 |
| Yes | 87 | 85 | 85 | |
| No | 13 | 15 | 15 | |
| Maternal CES-D score, mean (SD) | 9.71 (9.65) | 7.81 (7.88) | 8.01 (8.09) | .10 |
| Structured after-school activities, % | | | | .75 |
| >1 h/wk | 32 | 30 | 30 | |
| ≤1 h/wk | 68 | 70 | 70 | |
| HOME total score, mean (SD) | 45.4 (4.8) | 46.7 (4.9) | 46.6 (4.9) | .03 |
| Neighborhood Social Involvement Subscale score, mean (SD) | 5.46 (2.0) | 5.77 (1.9) | 5.74 (1.93) | .18 |

Abbreviations: CES-D, Center for Epidemiological Studies Depression Scale[26]; HOME, Home Observation for Measurement of the Environment.[27]

**Table 2. Relationship of Perceptions of Neighborhood Safety to Various Covariates**

| Covariate | Neighborhood Safety Score, Mean ± SD | Spearman Rank Correlation | *P* Value |
|---|---|---|---|
| Age | | 0.07 | .07 |
| Sex | | | .58 |
| Male | 7.65 ± 1.51 | | |
| Female | 7.71 ± 1.51 | | |
| Race | | | <.001 |
| White | 7.83 ± 1.39 | | |
| Black | 6.53 ± 1.95 | | |
| Other | 7.29 ± 1.53 | | |
| Maternal marital status | | | .05 |
| Single | 7.38 ± 1.86 | | |
| Partnered | 7.74 ± 1.43 | | |
| Maternal education | | 0.23 | <.001 |
| Maternal depressive symptoms | | −0.22 | <.001 |
| Structured after-school activities | | | .03 |
| >1 h/wk | 7.86 ± 1.40 | | |
| ≤1 h/wk | 7.60 ± 1.55 | | |
| HOME total score | | 0.24 | <.001 |
| Neighborhood social involvement | | 0.23 | <.001 |

Abbreviation: HOME, Home Observation for Measurement of the Environment.[27]

tabulation and found higher risk of overweight in quartiles 1 through 3 compared with neighborhoods perceived as most safe (NSS scores in quartile 4). We found that 17% of those in the first quartile (least perceived neighborhood safety) were overweight compared with 10% in the second quartile, 13% in the third quartile, and only 4% in the fourth quartile (highest perceived safety). We also estimated this relationship in logistic regression models that accounted for clustering by site (**Table 3**). The relationship between parental perception of neighborhood safety and a higher risk of overweight in first grade persisted in the base model, which controlled for child sex and identity of the neighborhood safety reporter (Table 3). Neither child sex nor identity of the safety reporter, variables included as confounders a priori, was significant in the model. None of the candidate covariates altered the relationship between perception of neighborhood safety and overweight in first grade by more than 10%. We tested for the presence of interactions between the covariates by adding terms to the multiple logistic regression model. We examined interactions of perception of neighborhood safety and sex, perception of neighborhood safety and identity of safety reporter, and identity of safety reporter and sex. None of these interactions were statistically significant.

## CONTROLLING FOR BMI *z* SCORE AT 4.5 YEARS

By adding BMI *z* score at the age of 4.5 years as a continuous variable into the base model (which included child sex and identity of the safety reporter) as a covariate, we were able to statistically control for variability in BMI already present at the age of 4.5 years. Statistical removal of this variability enabled us to focus on overweight that developed between the ages of 4.5 and 7 years. If adjusting for BMI *z* score at the age of 4.5 years had significantly reduced or eliminated the association between NSS scores and overweight status at the age of 7 years, it would suggest that children were overweight before parental NSS scores were obtained and therefore weaken the explanatory model. Adjusting for BMI *z* score at the age of 4.5

**Table 3. Unadjusted and Adjusted ORs for Overweight in First Grade From Logistic Regression Models Estimated via GEE and Accounting for Site as a Clustering Variable**

| | OR (95% CI) (n = 768) | | |
|---|---|---|---|
| | Unadjusted | Adjusted for Reporter and Sex | Adjusted for Reporter, Sex, and BMI *z* Score at 4.5 y |
| Neighborhood Safety Subscale score | | | |
| Quartile 1 (least safe) vs 4 (safest) | 4.55* (2.01-10.33) | 4.43* (2.03-9.65) | 3.01 (0.96-9.51) |
| Quartile 2 vs 4 | 2.64† (1.33-5.27) | 2.57† (1.21-5.47) | 2.14 (0.53-8.60) |
| Quartile 3 vs 4 | 3.58* (1.78-7.19) | 3.49* (1.62-7.53) | 3.30 (0.86-12.65) |
| Father reporter | | 1.12 (0.63-2.01) | 1.12 (0.58-2.18) |
| Male sex | | 0.94 (0.65-1.36) | 0.80 (0.41-1.54) |
| BMI z score at the age of 4.5 y | | | 9.44* (4.18-21.36) |

Abbreviations: BMI, body mass index; CI, confidence interval; GEE, generalized estimating equation; OR, odds ratio.
*$P \leq .001$.
†$P \leq .01$.

years in the base model, the relationship between parental perception of a less safe neighborhood and child overweight in first grade remained, although slightly weakened. Per our stated methods, we re-entered the same candidate covariates into the base model one by one and retained those that altered the relationship between perception of neighborhood safety and overweight in first grade by more than 10%. Again, none of the covariates altered the relationship between parental perception of neighborhood safety and overweight in first grade, and none of the interactions examined were statistically significant. The change in the odds ratio for overweight risk when controlling for BMI *z* score at 4.5 years indicates that parental perception of neighborhood safety independently increases overweight risk in the age range of 4.5 to 7 years, although the effect also operates to some degree at younger ages (Table 3).

## COMMENT

Results from a diverse sample representing 10 different sites across the United States indicate that parental perception of the neighborhood as unsafe was independently associated with an increased risk of overweight at the age of 7 years. To our knowledge, this study is the first to systematically investigate the relationship of parental perception of neighborhood safety and childhood overweight in a sample with geographic, ethnic, and socioeconomic diversity while analytically controlling for a large number of potentially confounding factors.

Previous studies in children that focused on the relationship among neighborhood safety, physical activity, and BMI have shown conflicting results. In a study[19] of Hispanic, white, and Vietnamese fourth graders of diverse socioeconomic status, children's (not parents') perceptions of a more dangerous neighborhood were associated with *increased* self-reported physical activity and *lower* BMI. Another study[18] of chronically ill 10- to 12-year-old children linked decreased activity patterns to child and parent perception of less neighborhood safety, but the generalizability of this study to healthy children is unclear. The differences in our findings and these prior studies may be partially explained by the low correlation between child and parental report of neighborhood violence[32] or the younger age of children in our study. Parental perception of neighborhood safety likely operates more strongly than that of the child in altering lifestyle because parents exert significant control over young children's activities.[33,34]

We were concerned that region of residence might mediate the relationship between neighborhood safety and overweight, but accounting for clustering based on study site did not alter the relationship. Measures of socioeconomic status also did not eliminate the observed association between perception of neighborhood safety and overweight, which would be the case if parental perception of neighborhood safety were only a proxy for socioeconomic status. In addition, potential protective factors, such as structured after-school activities, increased social cohesion in the neighborhood, or a high-quality home environment did not alter the relationship between parental perception of neighborhood safety and overweight. In effect, there may well be a relatively simple and straightforward relationship between living in a dangerous neighborhood and overweight; namely, in attempting to protect their children from harm, parents not only decrease the kind of physical activity that comes from playing outdoors in the neighborhood but inadvertently increase the likelihood of sedentary activity and snacking that comes from staying indoors.

We found significant differences in perception of neighborhood safety based on race/ethnicity. Most US neighborhoods continue to be racially segregated.[35] It is possible that one of the many contributors to the racial disparities in overweight prevalence[2] may be higher crime rates and lower perception of neighborhood safety among African Americans.[34,36] However, our study included a relatively small sample of children of minority race/ethnicity. Our inability to detect the well-documented differences in overweight prevalence by race/ethnicity, presumably because of low statistical power, suggests that these findings may not be generalizable to populations of minority race/ethnicity. The role of perceived neighborhood safety as a possible mediator between minority race/ethnicity and childhood overweight requires further investigation with a larger sample size of children of minority race/ethnicity.

## POLICY IMPLICATIONS

Although violent crime rates are lower today than they have been in 10 years, less than 10% of people report that their fear of crime has decreased.[36] It is therefore important not only to understand contributors to increased violence and crime but also to understand and address the factors that contribute to the perception that a neighborhood is unsafe. A potential area for intervention is the redesign of neighborhoods. Individuals who perceive their neighborhoods as unsafe cite open drinking and drug use as significant contributors to feeling unsafe.[36] As reviewed by Ashe et al,[37] land use planning and zoning has long been used to address endemic public health problems and could be used creatively to address the childhood obesity epidemic by improving some of the features that contribute to increased neighborhood violence and the perception of the community as unsafe. In considering neighborhood redesign, the National Institute of Health recently outlined a research agenda.[38] Of the issues that require further study, identifying factors that mediate or moderate built environment effects was of primary importance. No matter how neighborhoods are redesigned to allow children to walk to school or the neighborhood store, parents must feel safe allowing their children to do so.

## STUDY LIMITATIONS

Our study has several limitations. The findings may not be generalizable to certain populations, such as recent immigrants or the children of adolescent mothers. Our sample size of overweight children was relatively small. Therefore, the power to detect some of the differences may have been limited. We also did not have measures of actual neighborhood violence. However, prior data have indicated that poor, urban, African American mothers' ratings of their neighborhood quality correlate with actual crime rates.[39] Parents likely base their decisions on whether to send their children outside on their perception of neighborhood safety and not on statistics, which may account for a prior study[40] not showing an association of neighborhood crime statistics with overweight in preschoolers. We did not have data regarding physical activity measures or diet, which limits our ability to evaluate potential mechanisms of the association. Finally, as with many studies of this nature, the sample with complete data included in our analysis differs from the sample without complete data; therefore, our findings may not be generalizable to the reference population of the NICHD-SECCYD. Although we tested covariates that are predictors of missingness as potential covariates in the model and they did not alter the results, it remains possible that our results would have differed had complete data for the entire sample been available.

The independent effect of the neighborhood is challenging to study owing to difficulties in controlling for individual-level characteristics that may act as confounders.[41] Our data set does not include maternal weight; therefore, we were unable to control for this. However, we believe it is unlikely that maternal weight status is independently related to perception of neighborhood safety and therefore do not believe this would have acted as a significant confounder. We also did not have a measure of television viewing in our data set. An unsafe neighborhood may reduce outside activity, increase television viewing, and thereby increase the risk of overweight. However, amount of television viewing and overweight in young children has not been as strongly associated as it has been in older children.[5,42] Therefore, it seems unlikely that inclusion of television viewing would have eliminated the relationship. In addition, studies of maternal obesity or child television viewing as risk factors did not include neighborhood safety as a covariate. Understanding the independent role of each of these variables will depend on a study that is able to include all of them in predicting child overweight.

## SUMMARY

These data show a significant relationship between parental perception of an unsafe neighborhood and overweight at the age of 7 years even when many potentially confounding variables are controlled, including baseline BMI 3 years before the measures of interest. Many areas of policy development related to the built environment and neighborhood safety have not traditionally been considered relevant to child health. However, such policies may have important implications for childhood overweight. For the individual physician, these results suggest the need to understand the character of a child's neighborhood when making recommendations for lifestyle and activity changes aimed at obesity prevention and treatment.

**Accepted for Publication:** July 20, 2005.
**Correspondence:** Julie C. Lumeng, MD, 300 North Ingalls Bldg, 10th Floor, University of Michigan, Ann Arbor, MI 48109-0406 (jlumeng@umich.edu).
**Author Contributions:** Dr Lumeng had full access to all the data in the study and takes responsibility for the integrity of the data and the accuracy of the data analysis.
**Funding/Support:** This study was supported by grant 5T77 MC00015 09 from the Health Resources and Services Administration, Maternal and Child Health Bureau (Rockville, Md), and a Fellow-to-Faculty Transition Award (0275040N) to Dr Lumeng from the American Heart Association (Dallas, Tex).
**Acknowledgment:** We thank Marilyn Augustyn, MD, Michael Cabana, MD, MPH, Matthew Davis, MD, MAPP, and Robert Kahn, MD, MPH, for their thoughtful review of the manuscript.

## REFERENCES

1. Hedley A, Ogden C, Johnson C, Carroll M, Curtin L, Flegal K. Prevalence of overweight and obesity among US children, adolescents, and adults, 1999-2002. *JAMA*. 2004;291:2847-2850.
2. Strauss R, Pollack H. Epidemic increase in childhood overweight. *JAMA*. 2001; 286:2845-2848.

3. Whitaker R, Wright J, Pepe M, Seidel K, Dietz W. Predicting obesity in young adulthood from childhood and parental obesity. *N Engl J Med.* 1997;337:869-873.
4. Strauss R, Knight J. Influence of the home environment on the development of obesity in children. *Pediatrics.* 1999;103:e85.
5. Dietz W, Gortmaker S. Do we fatten our children at the television set? obesity and television viewing in children and adolescents. *Pediatrics.* 1985;75:807-812.
6. Haas J, Lee L, Kaplan C, Sonneborn D, Phillips K, Liang S. The association of race, socioeconomic status, and health insurance status with the prevalence of overweight among children and adolescents. *Am J Public Health.* 2003;93: 2105-2110.
7. Troiano R, Flegal K. Overweight children and adolescents: description, epidemiology, and demographics. *Pediatrics.* 1998;101:497-504.
8. Birch L, Davison K. Family environmental factors influencing the developing behavioral controls of food intake and childhood overweight. *Pediatr Clin North Am.* 2001;48:893-907.
9. Davison K, Cutting T, Birch L. Parents' activity-related parenting practices predict girls' physical activity. *Med Sci Sports Exerc.* 2003;35:1589-1595.
10. Birch L, Fisher J, Davison K. Learning to overeat: maternal use of restrictive feeding practices promotes girls' eating in the absence of hunger. *Am J Clin Nutr.* 2003;78:215-220.
11. Francis L, Hofer S, Birch L. Predictors of maternal child-feeding style: maternal and child characteristics. *Appetite.* 2001;37:231-243.
12. Diez Roux AV, Merkin S, Arnett D, et al. Neighborhood of residence and incidence of coronary heart disease. *N Engl J Med.* 2001;345:99-106.
13. Diez Roux AV, Merkin S, Hannan P, Jacobs D, Kiefe C. Area characteristics, individual-level socioeconomic indicators, and smoking in young adults: the coronary artery disease risk development in young adults study. *Am J Epidemiol.* 2003; 157:315-326.
14. Diez Roux AV, Jacobs D, Kiefe C. Neighborhood characteristics and components of the insulin resistance syndrome in young adults: the coronary artery risk development in young adults (CARDIA) study. *Diabetes Care.* 2002;25: 1976-1982.
15. Pearl M, Braveman P, Abrams B. The relationship of neighborhood socioeconomic characteristics to birthweight among 5 ethnic groups in California. *Am J Public Health.* 2001;91:1808-1814.
16. Koplan J, Dietz W. Caloric imbalance and public health policy. *JAMA.* 1999;282: 1579-1581.
17. Cummins S. *The Built Environment and Children's Health.* Washington, DC: National Center for Environmental Health, Centers for Disease Control and Prevention; 2004.
18. Holaday B, Swan JH, Turner-Henson A. Images of the neighborhood and activity patterns of chronically ill schoolage children. *Environ Behav.* 1997;29:348-373.
19. Romero A, Robinson T, Karemer H, et al. Are perceived neighborhood hazards a barrier to physical activity in children? *Arch Pediatr Adolesc Med.* 2001;155: 1143-1148.
20. NICHD Early Child Care Research Network. Nonmaternal care and family factors in early development: an overview of the NICHD Study of Early Child Care. *Appl Dev Psychol.* 2001;22:457-492.
21. National Institute of Child Health and Human Development. Recruitment procedures. In: *NICHD Study of Early Child Care Manual.* Bethesda, Md: National Institute of Child Health and Human Development; 1991.
22. *NICHD Study of Early Child Care and Youth Development: Phase II Instrument Document.* Research Triangle Park, NC: Research Triangle Institute; 2002:36-38.
23. Greenberg M, Lengua L, Coie J, Pinderhughes E. Predicting developmental outcomes at school entry using a multiple-risk model: four American communities. *Dev Psychol.* 1999;35:403-417.
24. *NICHD Study of Early Child Care and Youth Development Operations Manual: 54-Month Growth Measures.* Bethesda, Md: National Institute of Child Health and Human Development; 1995:1-19.
25. Kuczmarski R, Ogden C, Grummer-Strawn L, Flegal K, Guo S, Wei R. CDC growth charts. *Adv Data.* 2000;314:1-28.
26. Radloff L. The CES-D Scale: a self report depression scale for research in the general population. *J Appl Psychol.* 1977;1:385-401.
27. Caldwell B, Bradley R. *Home Observation for Measurement of the Environment.* Little Rock: University of Arkansas at Little Rock, Center for Child Development and Education; 1984.
28. Diggle P, Liang K, Zeger S. *Analysis of Longitudinal Data.* Oxford, England: Clarendon Press; 1994.
29. Mancl L, DeRouen T. A covariance estimator for GEE with improved small-sample properties. *Biometrics.* 2001;57:126-134.
30. Rothman K, Greenland S. *Modern Epidemiology.* Philadelphia, PA: Lippincott-Raven; 1998.
31. Ogden C, Flegal K, Carroll M, Johnson C. Prevalence and trends in overweight among US children and adolescents, 1999-2000. *JAMA.* 2002;288:1728-1732.
32. Thomson C, Roberts K, Curran A, Ryan L, Wright R. Caretaker-child concordance for child's exposure to violence in a preadolescent inner-city population. *Arch Pediatr Adolesc Med.* 2002;156:818-823.
33. O'Neil R, Parke R, McDowell D. Objective and subjective features of children's neighborhoods: relations to parental regulatory strategies and children's social competence. *J Appl Dev Psychol.* 2001;22:135-155.
34. Hill N, Herman-Stahl M. Neighborhood safety and social involvement: associations with parenting behaviors and depressive symptoms among African American and Euro-American mothers. *J Fam Psychol.* 2002;16:209-219.
35. Jargowsky P. *Poverty and Place: Ghettos, Barrios, and the American City.* New York, NY: Russell Sage Foundation; 1997.
36. Smith S, Steadman G, Minton T. *Criminal Victimization and Perceptions of Community Safety in 12 Cities, 1998.* Washington, DC: US Department of Justice, Bureau of Justice Statistics, Office of Community Oriented Policing Services; 1999.
37. Ashe M, Jernigan D, Kline R, Galaz R. Land use planning and the control of alcohol, tobacco, firearms, and fast food restaurants. *Am J Public Health.* 2003; 93:1404-1408.
38. Srinivasan S, O'Fallon L, Dearry A. Creating healthy communities, healthy homes, healthy people: initiating a research agenda on the built environment and public health. *Am J Public Health.* 2003;93:1446-1450.
39. Ceballo R, McLoyd V. Social support and parenting in poor, dangerous neighborhoods. *Child Dev.* 2002;73:1310-1321.
40. Burdette H, Whitaker R. Neighborhood playgrounds, fast food restaurants, and crime: relationships to overweight in low-income preschool children. *Prev Med.* 2004;38:57-63.
41. Diez Roux AV. Investigating neighborhood and area effects on health. *Am J Public Health.* 2001;91:1783-1789.
42. DuRant R, Baranowski T, Johnson M, Thompson W. The relationship among television watching, physical activity, and body composition of young children. *Pediatrics.* 1994;94:449-454.

**References: 1.** Exl BM. A review of recent developments in the use of moderately hydrolyzed whey formulae in infant nutrition. *Nutr Res* 2001;21(1–2):355–79. **2.** Cantani A. The growing genetic links and the early onset of atopic diseases in children stress the unique role of the atopic march: a meta-analysis. *J Investig Allergol Clin Immunol* 1999;9(5):314–20. **3.** Marini A, Agosti M, Motta G, Mosca F. Effects of a dietary and environmental prevention programme on the incidence of allergic symptoms in high atopic risk infants: three years follow-up. *Acta Paediatr Suppl* 1996;414:1–21. **4.** Von Berg A, Koletzko S, Grubl A, Filipiak-Pittroff B, Wichmann HE, Bauer CP, et al. The effect of hydrolyzed cow's milk formula for allergy prevention in the first year of life: the German Infant Nutritional Intervention Study, a randomized double-blind trial. *J Allergy Clin Immunol* 2003;111(3):533–40.

## All infants are potentially at risk of allergy.

- Up to 1 in 5 children develop allergy, regardless of family history.[1]

## A routine formula can increase that risk – or help reduce it.

- The intact cow's milk protein found in most routine formulas is the leading cause of food allergy in formula-fed infants.[2]
- Only GOOD START® SUPREME DHA & ARA is made with 100% whey protein, partially hydrolyzed and a patented process that breaks down intact proteins into smaller peptides.
- The result: reduced risk of food allergy vs. standard intact cow's milk formulas.[3-4,*]

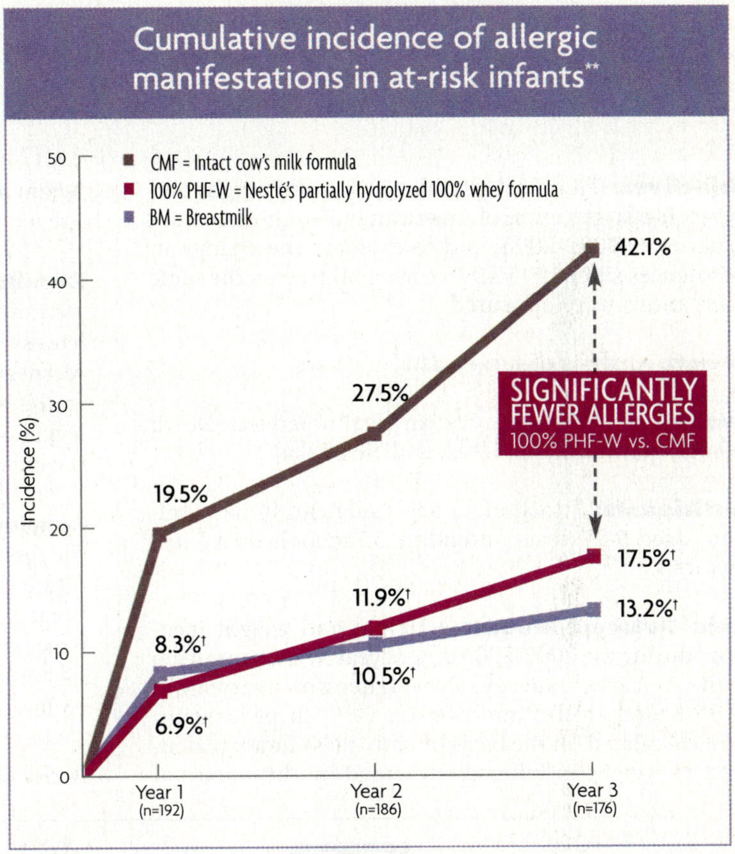


** Manifestations included atopic dermatitis, recurrent wheezing, urticaria and gastrointestinal symptoms. In infants identified as at risk based on history of atopy in both parents. Infants were exclusively fed BM or formula in Year 1. 100% PHF-W in this trial used as part of an allergy prevention program. Adapted from Marini A, et al, 1996,[3] representative of the results of 12 published clinical trials.

† $p<0.05$ vs. CMF.

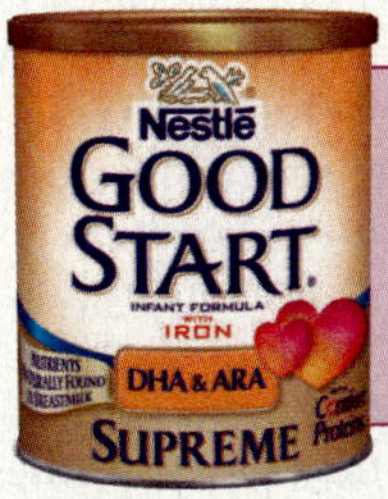


**Breastfeeding is the best allergy protection. When it isn't an option, reduce the risk with GOOD START® SUPREME DHA & ARA right from the start of formula feeding.**

**GOOD START® SUPREME DHA & ARA is a routine formula and not intended for therapeutic use.**

* No claim has yet been authorized by FDA regarding PHF-W (partially hydrolyzed whey formula). While breastfeeding is by far the best way to nourish an infant, a petition is currently under FDA review for a statement for use on label to the effect that emerging clinical research in healthy infants with family history of allergy shows that exclusive feeding of PHF-W (instead of cow's milk formula) may reduce the risk of common food allergy symptoms, particularly allergic skin rash, when used exclusively or as a supplement to breastmilk from the initiation of formula feeding. The statement would also emphasize that partially hydrolyzed whey formulas are made with cow's milk protein and are not intended to treat existing food allergy symptoms. NESTLÉ® GOOD START® SUPREME DHA & ARA is *not intended as a therapeutic formula* like extensively hydrolyzed or amino acid-based specialty formulas.

Nestlé
INFANT NUTRITION

Nestlé knows a healthy baby is where a healthy family begins.

# Increasing Prevalences of Overweight and Obesity in Northern Plains American Indian Children

*Elenora Zephier, MPH, RD; John H. Himes, PhD, MPH; Mary Story, PhD, RD; Xia Zhou, MS*

**Objectives:** To report prevalences of overweight and obesity in a large sample of American Indian children from a survey in 2002-2003, and to evaluate the change in prevalences since 1995-1996 when children on the same reservations were measured.

**Design:** Analysis of survey data.

**Setting:** Aberdeen Area Indian Health Service (North Dakota, South Dakota, Iowa, and Nebraska).

**Participants:** A total of 11 538 American Indian children (aged 5-17 years) attending 55 schools on 12 reservations.

**Main Outcome Measure:** Height and weight measured during the 2002-2003 school year by the same team as in the earlier survey. Prevalences of overweight (≥85th percentile) and obesity (≥95th percentile) were calculated on the basis of body mass index (calculated as weight in kilograms divided by the square of height in meters) and the Centers for Disease Control and Prevention growth charts.

**Results:** At 5 years of age, 47% of boys and 41% of girls were overweight, and 24% of the children were obese. Prevalences of overweight and obesity exceeded those for the most recent available data for all US children at almost every age. In the intervening 7 to 8 years between surveys, prevalences of overweight and obesity continued to increase in the children by 4.5% and 4.3%, respectively.

**Conclusions:** Prevalences of overweight and obesity in the most recent sample of American Indian children indicate that they are at even higher risk for these conditions and their health-related sequelae than the best estimates for all US children, with prevalences as high as or higher than those for any other racial or ethnic groups of children reported in the most recent national surveys.

*Arch Pediatr Adolesc Med. 2006;160:34-39*

THE HIGH LEVELS OF OVERweight and obesity among US children are a major public health concern. The National Health and Nutrition Examination Survey (NHANES) data have shown steady increases in child and adolescent overweight and obesity during the past 2 decades.[1-3] The NHANES data also indicate continuing disparities between racial and ethnic groups in the prevalence of obesity, with rates considerably higher for ethnic minority youth compared with white youth.[1-3] In NHANES data from 1999 to 2002 for youth aged 6 to 19 years, 28% of white youth, 35% of African American youth, and 40% of Mexican American youth had a body mass index (BMI) (calculated as weight in kilograms divided by the square of height in meters) greater than the 85th percentile for age and sex.[3] Recent analyses from the National Longitudinal Survey of Youth, a prospective cohort study from 1986 to 1998 among 8270 children aged 4 to 12 years, found that while overweight increased significantly and steadily among African American, Hispanic, and white children, overweight prevalence was greatest and increased most rapidly among minority children.[4]

Another group at high risk for overweight and obesity is American Indian children. Overweight and obesity rates for American Indian children, adolescents, and adults tend to be notably higher than corresponding rates for the general US population.[5,6] While several studies have examined the prevalence of overweight in American Indian children, most of these have had relatively small sample sizes and have not been population-based studies. Relatively few large studies have been conducted with American Indian youth. In 1990, a national survey on height and weight status of 9464 American Indian schoolchildren (aged 5-18 years) living on or near Indian reservations was conducted by the Indian Health Service (IHS), the Centers for Disease Control and Prevention, and tribal nutrition programs in 9 IHS service areas.[7] The overall preva-

**Author Affiliations:** Aberdeen Area Indian Health Service, Aberdeen, SD (Ms Zephier); and Division of Epidemiology and Community Health, School of Public Health, University of Minnesota, Minneapolis (Drs Himes and Story and Ms Zhou).

lence of overweight in the American Indian children (BMI, ≥85th percentile of the reference population) was 39% for age and sex according to NHANES II reference data. In 1995-1996, our group conducted a large study on overweight and obesity prevalence in American Indian school children through the Aberdeen Area IHS and involved children from 16 tribes in 4 midwestern states.[8] Height and weight were measured on 12 559 Indian children aged 5 to 17 years attending 62 schools on or near reservations in South Dakota, North Dakota, Iowa, and Nebraska. Age-adjusted prevalences of overweight (BMI, ≥85th percentile for NHANES II) were 39% for boys and 38% for girls. The age-adjusted prevalences of obesity (BMI, ≥95th percentile) for boys and girls were 22% and 18%, respectively.

These as well as other studies have all shown a high prevalence of obesity among American Indian youth.[6,9-12] Indeed, obesity has now emerged as one of the most serious public health problems facing American Indian children and adolescents. Because of the secondary health consequences of obesity, including cardiovascular disease and type 2 diabetes mellitus, there are grave implications for both the immediate and long-term health of American Indian youth.[13] Accordingly, there is a need to monitor overweight trends in American Indian children. The NHANES data have shown continuing increases in overweight among US children and youth.[1] Unfortunately, NHANES does not include American Indians living on reservations in its sampling design. The aims of this study were (1) to assess overweight and obesity in a large sample of American Indian school-aged children and adolescents living on or near reservations in the Aberdeen Area IHS area and (2) to investigate recent changes in the prevalence of overweight and obesity compared with the study conducted in 1995-1996 with children on the same reservations.

## METHODS

The analyses included data from 2 surveys of children attending primary and secondary schools at which at least 50% of enrolled children were identified as American Indian and that were located on or near the reservations included in the Aberdeen Area IHS. This IHS comprises 18 tribes in North Dakota, South Dakota, Nebraska, and Iowa.

For estimating current prevalences of overweight and obesity, data obtained during the 2002-2003 school year were used. Height and weight data were collected on 11 538 children attending 55 schools on 12 reservations (survey 2). For evaluating secular changes in prevalences, data from the most recent survey for children living on 8 of the reservations from survey 2 were compared with data from a sample of children living on the same reservations who were measured in 1995 and 1996 by the same measurement team (survey 1).[8] The samples were limited to children from 5.00 to 17.99 years of age at the time of measurement, and to children who identified themselves or who were identified by teachers as American Indian. Cases with extreme values of height or weight were excluded if measurements exceeded the median±3 times the interquartile range, calculated within whole-year, sex-specific groups.[14]

After the exclusions, the sample from survey 2 used to estimate current prevalences included data for 5508 boys and 5313 girls. For estimating secular changes in prevalences, the samples included 4763 boys and 4727 girls from survey 1 and 4835 boys and 4632 girls from survey 2. There were no significant differences between prevalences of overweight and obesity estimated from the subset of children in survey 2 used for the secular-change analyses and the complete sample in survey 2.

All children were measured by the same 7 trained individuals following the same protocols, and all measurements were standardized according to a gold-standard measurement. Weights were obtained with electronic scales (Seca Corp, Columbia, Md), which were regularly calibrated. Heights were measured with a stadiometer (Acustat; Ross Laboratories, Columbus, Ohio).[15] Informed parental consent was obtained according to individual school policies. In some schools, measurements were incorporated into regular health-screening activities. All procedures were approved by the appropriate institutional review boards for tribes and the IHS.

Overweight was defined as BMI at or above the 85th percentile for age and sex, based on the Centers for Disease Control and Prevention 2000 growth charts,[16] and obesity was defined as BMI at or above the 95th percentile according to the same reference. Exact BMI percentiles were calculated with Epi Info 2000 computer software (Centers for Disease Control and Prevention, Atlanta, Ga).

The prevalences of overweight and obesity from survey 2 calculated within single-year age groups were compared with recent national data available from NHANES 1999 to 2002[1,3] for children of all racial or ethnic groups. Prevalences for NHANES data were calculated using the case weights provided to account for the probability of sampling.

Prevalences were estimated and analyzed by coding overweight and obesity as separate dichotomous variables (0 and 1), based on the BMI percentile cutoffs specific to age and sex. This approach to estimating prevalences provides means that are unbiased estimates of prevalence for groups, and binomial distributions that approximate normality because of the large sample sizes.[17] Prevalences of overweight and obesity were calculated within whole-year age groups (eg, 10 years=10.00-10.99 years) within each sex.

For analyses of the secular changes between surveys, mixed models were fitted . The dependent variable was status as overweight or obese (0 or 1). Survey, sex, and whole-year age group were fixed categorical independent variables, and reservation was included as a random categorical variable to account for possible similarities within reservations for overweight and obesity.[18] All interactions among independent variables were evaluated. Adjusted prevalences within groups were estimated as the least squares means from the fully adjusted mixed models.

## RESULTS

The prevalences of overweight and obesity among the American Indian children measured in 2002 and 2003 are presented in **Table 1**. In general, the prevalences of overweight and obesity were slightly greater in boys than girls until the early teen years, when the trend reversed. At 5 years of age, more than 40% of the American Indian children had BMIs equal to or greater than the 85th percentile and almost one quarter of them had BMIs that equaled or exceeded the 95th percentile. At 11 years, more than half of the American Indian children were overweight.

Prevalences of overweight and obesity in the American Indian children are compared with corresponding

**Table 1. Prevalence of Overweight (≥85th Percentile of BMI) and Obesity (≥95th Percentile of BMI) in North American Indian Children by Sex and Age Group (2002-2003)**

| | Boys | | | Girls | | |
|---|---|---|---|---|---|---|
| Age, y | No. | Overweight, % | Obesity, % | No. | Overweight, % | Obesity, % |
| 5 | 302 | 47.4 | 24.2 | 311 | 40.5 | 24.1 |
| 6 | 477 | 44.7 | 22.4 | 450 | 41.6 | 18.9 |
| 7 | 510 | 43.9 | 26.1 | 483 | 42.4 | 25.5 |
| 8 | 500 | 47.0 | 27.8 | 476 | 44.3 | 28.2 |
| 9 | 581 | 48.7 | 29.8 | 525 | 46.9 | 26.1 |
| 10 | 565 | 52.7 | 35.8 | 542 | 47.1 | 25.8 |
| 11 | 530 | 57.7 | 37.2 | 538 | 51.1 | 29.9 |
| 12 | 514 | 53.9 | 35.0 | 471 | 52.2 | 29.7 |
| 13 | 459 | 48.4 | 30.5 | 484 | 49.6 | 27.5 |
| 14 | 377 | 47.5 | 29.9 | 401 | 48.1 | 25.4 |
| 15 | 283 | 39.9 | 25.1 | 264 | 46.2 | 27.3 |
| 16 | 211 | 38.4 | 23.7 | 220 | 43.6 | 22.7 |
| 17 | 199 | 36.7 | 20.1 | 148 | 40.5 | 24.3 |
| **Total*** | **5508** | 48.1 | 29.4 | **5313** | 46.3 | 26.1 |
| 95% CI | | 46.7-49.4 | 28.2-30.6 | | 44.9-47.7 | 24.9-27.3 |

Abbreviations: BMI, body mass index (calculated as weight in kilograms divided by the square of height in meters); CI, confidence interval.
*Age-adjusted.

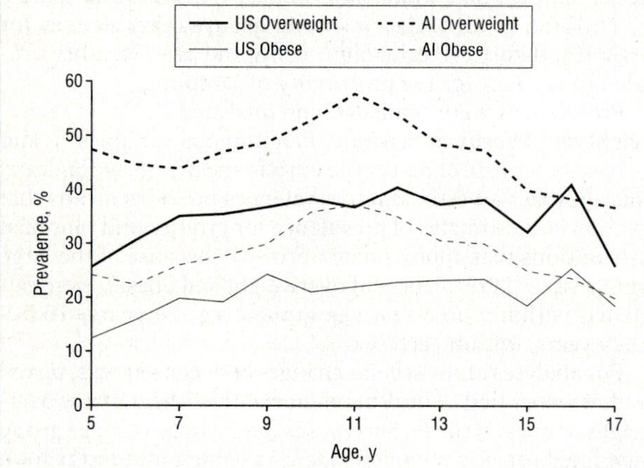


**Figure 1.** Prevalences of overweight (body mass index [calculated as weight in kilograms divided by the square of height in meters], ≥85th percentile) and obesity (body mass index, ≥95th percentile) among American Indian (AI) boys (survey 2, 2002-2003) and among all US boys (National Health and Nutrition Examination Survey, 1999-2002[1,3]) by age groups.

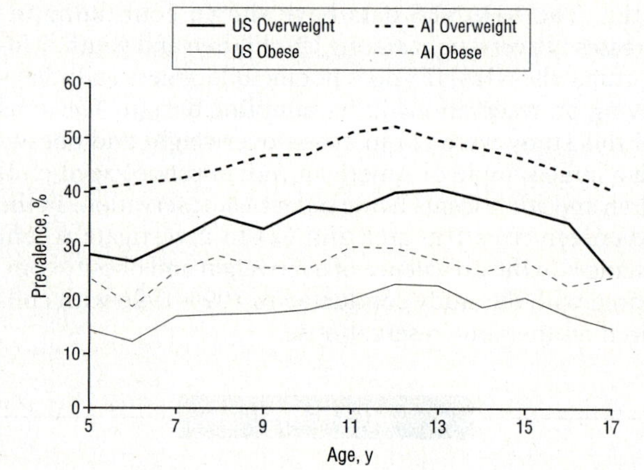


**Figure 2.** Prevalences of overweight (body mass index [calculated as weight in kilograms divided by the square of height in meters], ≥85th percentile) and obesity (body mass index, ≥95th percentile) among American Indian (AI) girls (survey 2, 2002-2003) and among all US girls (National Health and Nutrition Examination Survey, 1999-2002[1,3]) by age groups.

prevalences for all US children in **Figure 1** and **Figure 2**. At almost every age, the prevalences of both overweight and obesity among American Indian children were greater than those for their national peers at corresponding ages. At 5 years of age, the prevalence of overweight in American Indian boys was almost twice that for all US boys (47.4% vs 25.7%).

The adjusted prevalences from the mixed-model analysis of variance testing for overall changes between survey 1 (1995-1996) and survey 2 (2002-2003) for children living on the same 8 reservations are presented in **Table 2**. There were statistically significant increases in prevalences of overweight ($P<.001$) and obesity ($P<.001$) during the time between the 2 surveys (5-7 years). Also, there were significant main effects for sex (overweight, $P=.02$; obesity, $P<.001$) and age (overweight, $P<.001$; obesity, $P<.001$), but not for the interactions between survey and age (overweight, $P=.10$; obesity, $P=.58$), nor for any other interaction terms. The lack of significant interaction terms with survey indicates that there were no substantial differences between sexes or among the age groups in their patterns of secular change in prevalence of overweight and obesity. The adjusted prevalences (Table 2) indicate that the absolute changes in prevalences between surveys were 4.5% and 4.3% for overweight and obesity, respectively.

The data for boys are presented in **Figure 3** as an example of the age-related patterns in the changes in prevalences of overweight and obesity among the American Indian children between surveys. Secular increases occurred at almost all ages, and to a generally similar degree for overweight and obesity at most ages. The secular decreases in prevalences of overweight at age 7 years and obesity at age 17 years are apparent, but they are not sufficient to conclude a significant interaction between age and survey based on our analysis of variance models used to evaluate change. Similar general patterns of secular change in prevalences were seen on examination of corresponding data for girls (data not shown).

## COMMENT

The age-adjusted prevalences of overweight (BMI, ≥85th percentile) among these American Indian children aged 5 to 17 years during 2002-2003 were 48.1% in boys and 46.3% in girls. Corresponding prevalences for obesity (BMI, ≥95th percentile) were 29.4% and 26.1% for boys and girls, respectively. These levels are very high and indicate substantial health risk.[6] Although direct comparisons with previous studies in American Indians are complicated by the use of slightly different earlier BMI cutoffs, we are aware of no studies of American Indian children reporting higher prevalences of overweight and obesity.[6,19] We believe that the high prevalences among the current sample of American Indian children primarily result from the recency of the data for this cultural/ethnic group with markedly increasing prevalences over time.[19,20] The BMI and body composition data from the study by Caballero et al[21] indicate that percentage of body fat and obesity prevalences for American Indian children from the Aberdeen area in 1995-1996 did not differ appreciably from those of children in 5 other national tribal groups.

The prevalences of overweight and obesity among American Indian children in this study systematically exceeded those for the most recent data available for all US children (Figures 1 and 2). Some recent national data are available for comparisons according to sex and race or ethnicity.[1] American Indian children aged 6 to 11 years exceeded each racial or ethnic group described nationally in point prevalences for obesity (boys, 29.8%; girls, 25.7%) but were probably within the confidence intervals of the estimates for the racial or ethnic groups with the highest prevalences: Mexican American boys (27.3%) and black or African American girls (22.1%).[1] The older American Indian children (12-17 years) had prevalences of obesity (boys, 27.4%; girls, 26.8%) similar to those for Mexican American boys (27.5%) and black or African American girls (26.6%), the sex and racial-ethnic groups with the highest reported prevalences in the national survey of children aged 12 to 19 years.[1]

The age-specific data in Table 1 indicate a general trend of increasing prevalences of overweight and obesity from ages 5 until 11 years in boys and 12 years in girls, after which the prevalences generally decreased through the later adolescent years. Nevertheless, because the data are cross-sectional, any age-related changes in prevalences that might be interpreted as developmental are completely confounded by the secular changes that occurred. The data from the earlier survey 1 (1996-1997) of American Indian children[8] did not evidence such a marked age-related pattern in prevalences of overweight and obesity, nor do the data from the NHANES surveys for boys (Figures 1 and 2). We favor an interpretation of this apparent age pattern as a manifestation of the secular increases in prevalences of overweight and obesity that have become more apparent in the younger children, who, if observed longitudinally, would most likely continue their high prevalences rather than becoming less at risk as they pass through adolescence. Notably, the survey × age interaction terms in the analysis of variance models were not statistically significant, so secular changes in the age patterns of prevalences were not greater than would be expected by chance.

We restricted our analysis of secular change to children living on 8 reservations that were included in both surveys to minimize the possibility that differences between surveys might have been due to sampling issues. It is likely that some children who were younger than 10 years at the time of survey 1 were included at an older age in survey 2 as well. Because of the sampling design, we are unable to identify specific children in the 2 surveys. This likelihood of including some of the same chil-

**Table 2. Adjusted Prevalences of Overweight and Obesity From Full Model for Each Survey and Sex**

| | Adjusted Prevalences, % (95% CI) | |
|---|---|---|
| | Overweight | Obesity |
| Girls | | |
| Survey 1 | 42.0 (41.9-42.1) | 22.7 (22.6-22.8) |
| Survey 2 | 46.4 (46.3-46.5) | 27.5 (27.4-27.6) |
| Boys | | |
| Survey 1 | 42.6 (42.5-42.7) | 25.5 (25.4-25.6) |
| Survey 2 | 47.3 (47.2-47.4) | 29.2 (29.1-29.3) |
| Overall | | |
| Survey 1 | 42.3 (42.2-42.4) | 24.1 (23.9-24.2) |
| Survey 2 | 46.8 (46.7-46.9) | 28.4 (28.3-28.5) |

Abbreviation: CI, confidence interval.

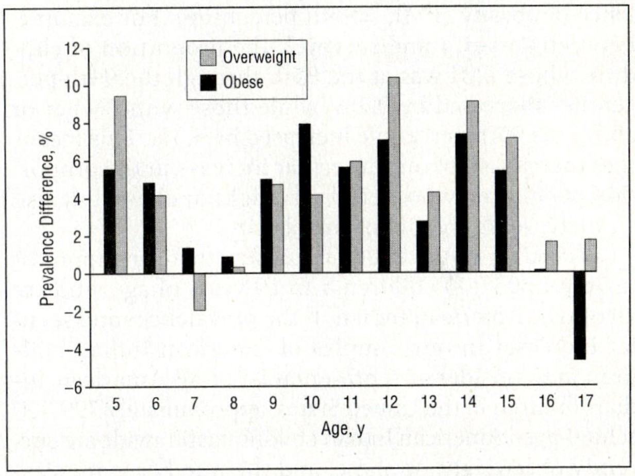


**Figure 3.** Differences in prevalences of overweight (body mass index [calculated as weight in kilograms divided by the square of height in meters], ≥85th percentile) and obesity (body mass index, ≥95th percentile) between survey 1 (1996-1997) and survey 2 (2002-2003) for American Indian boys. Differences were calculated as survey 2 minus survey 1.

dren does not invalidate any conclusions regarding secular increases in overweight and obesity. Our statistical methods allowed for such correlations between surveys in the tests of significance.

Our analyses demonstrated statistically significant increases in prevalences of overweight and obesity during the past 10 years. If the midpoint years of surveys 1 and 2 are used and both sexes are considered, the prevalences of overweight and obesity increased by approximately 4.5% and 4.3%, respectively, or approximately 7.5% to 7.2% per decade. These rates of secular increase per decade are greater than those observed for all US children aged 6 to 11 years (4.6%) and 12 to 19 years (5.9%) during a similar period before the 1999-2000 survey.[1]

Careful inspection of the results in Table 2 indicates that almost all of the secular changes in the prevalence of overweight (BMI, ≥85th percentile) were due to a shift in the portion of that group that constitutes the prevalence of obesity (BMI, ≥95th percentile). For example, between survey 1 and survey 2, the proportion of children whose BMI was at the 85th through the 94th percentiles increased by 0.2%, while those with BMI at or above the 95th percentile increased by 4.3%. This means that there was not only a secular increase in the proportion of children who were overweight or obese, but also an increase in severity of the obesity.

According to the 2000 US census, there are approximately 1 693 000 children 5 to 19 years of age who are all or part American Indian. If the prevalences and secular increases in our samples of American Indian children are considered representative of all American Indian children in the United States, approximately 799 000 school-aged American Indian children nationwide are currently overweight or obese, and the number is increasing by approximately 12 700 each year. These numbers probably underestimate the magnitude of the problem because they are based on the year 2000 and do not take into account population growth.

Our analyses indicate that American Indian children are at particularly high risk for the adverse sequelae of overweight and obesity[6,22] and that the problem continues to become more grave. Given that obesity tracks from childhood to adulthood, has adverse effects on risk factors for cardiovascular disease and other chronic diseases, and is associated with the rapid increase in type 2 diabetes mellitus, the results of our study are alarming. Recent studies have documented a 30-fold increase in type 2 diabetes in American Indian children and adolescents.[23] Obesity is highly related to the development of type 2 diabetes; up to 85% of children and adolescents with diabetes are overweight.[23-25]

Clearly, American Indian children should be identified along with Mexican American and African American children as a high-risk population, and special efforts are required to alter the progression of overweight and obesity. While the problem of overweight and obesity affects American Indian children of all ages, it appears early in life. At age 5 years, 44% of American Indian children in the present study were already overweight. A recent longitudinal study with 139 Pima Indian children found that early childhood obesity at age 5 years was the dominant predictor of obesity at age 10 years.[11] It is not clear at what age overweight and obesity begin in American Indian children, but primary prevention probably should begin at ages younger than 5 years.

Obesity is a multifactorial condition stemming from complex interactions between genetic and environmental factors. Dietary and physical activity behaviors are potentially modifiable and can be targets for change in obesity prevention and intervention efforts. Culturally tailored strategies are needed to increase physical activity and encourage healthy eating among children and their families. Efforts are also needed to produce an environment that supports healthy eating and physical activity in the community. Many reservations are economically impoverished. Poverty and living in low-income communities limit access to healthy foods.[26] To successfully combat the obesity and diabetes epidemics and help children achieve healthy weight trajectories, low-income families and communities need supportive environments with increased availability and affordability of healthier foods, such as fruits and vegetables, in grocery stores, convenience stores, commodity distribution sites, and schools. Increased play and physical activity opportunities are needed. We believe prevention of obesity in American Indian children and youth must be a public health priority. American Indian children often have been overlooked when groups at risk are identified, perhaps because they have not been adequately sampled in many surveys. Without immediate intervention, all indications are that the current generation of Indian children will face an increased burden of obesity-related chronic diseases, including type 2 diabetes and heart disease, at increasingly younger ages, which will have devastating effects on American Indian communities.

Since American Indian reservations are not included in the NHANES sampling surveys, there is a need to strengthen and develop surveillance systems to assess heights and weights in American Indian youth and monitor trends in obesity within and across reservations. Prevention and intervention efforts will be enhanced by more studies that examine the behavioral, social, genetic, and environmental factors that contribute to the development of obesity in American Indian children.

**Accepted for Publication:** July 20, 2005.
**Correspondence:** John H. Himes, PhD, MPH, Division of Epidemiology and Community Health, School of Public Health, University of Minnesota, 1300 S Second St, Suite 300, Minneapolis, MN 55454-1015 (himes@epi.umn.edu).
**Author Contributions:** Dr Himes had full access to all of the data in the study and takes responsibility for the integrity of the data and the accuracy of the data analysis.
**Funding/Support:** Data collection was supported by a grant from the Indian Health Service, Rockville, Md (Ms Zephier). Data analyses were partially supported by grant T79-MC0007-12 from the Maternal and Child Health Bureau, Rockville, Md.
**Disclaimer:** The opinions expressed herein are the private views of the authors and do not necessarily reflect the view of the IHS.

**Acknowledgment:** We gratefully acknowledge the staff for all their assistance in data collection efforts: Amy Beutler, RD; Roz Bolzer, RD; Kari Blasius, RD; Celeste Hart, RD; Margo Hoffman, RD; Mary McCormick, RD; Jody Rosedahl, RD; Valinda White, RD; and Alice Severson. We are grateful to all of the tribes, schools, and children who participated.

## REFERENCES


1. Ogden CL, Flegal KM, Carroll MD, Johnson CL. Prevalence and trends in overweight among US children and adolescents, 1999-2000. *JAMA.* 2002;288:1728-1732.
2. US Department of Health and Human Services. *The Surgeon General's Call to Action to Prevent and Decrease Overweight and Obesity.* Rockville, Md: US Dept of Health and Human Services, Office of the Surgeon General; 2001.
3. Hedley AA, Ogden CL, Johnson CL, Carroll MD, Curtin LR, Flegal KM. Prevalence of overweight and obesity among US children, adolescents, and adults, 1999-2002. *JAMA.* 2004;291:2847-2850.
4. Strauss RS, Pollack HA. Epidemic increase in childhood overweight, 1986-1998. *JAMA.* 2001;286:2845-2848.
5. Story M, Evans M, Fabsitz R, Clay T, Holy Rock B, Broussard BA. The epidemic of obesity in American Indian communities and the need for childhood obesity-prevention programs. *Am J Clin Nutr.* 1999;69(suppl):747S-754S.
6. Story M, Stevens J, Himes J, et al. Obesity in American-Indian children: prevalence, consequences, and prevention. *Prev Med.* 2003;37:S3-S12.
7. Jackson MY. Height, weight, and body mass index of American Indian schoolchildren, 1990-1991. *J Am Diet Assoc.* 1993;93:1136-1140.
8. Zephier E, Himes JH, Story M. Prevalence of overweight and obesity in American Indian school children and adolescents in the Aberdeen area: a population study. *Int J Obes Relat Metab Disord.* 1999;23(suppl):S28-S30.
9. Lindsay RS, Cook V, Hanson RL, Salbe AD, Tataranni A, Knowler WC. Early excess weight gain of children in the Pima Indian population. *Pediatrics.* 2002;109:e33.
10. Eisenmann JC, Katzmarzyk PT, Arnall DA, Kanuho V, Interpreter C, Malina RM. Growth and overweight of Navajo youth: secular changes from 1955 to 1997. *Int J Obes Relat Metab Disord.* 2000;24:211-218.
11. Salbe AD, Weyer C, Lindsay RS, Ravussin E, Tataranni PA. Assessing risk factors for obesity between childhood and adolescence, I: birth weight, childhood adiposity, parental obesity, insulin, and leptin. *Pediatrics.* 2002;110:299-306.
12. Eisenmann JC, Arnall DA, Kanuho V, McArel H. Growth status and obesity of Hopi children. *Am J Hum Biol.* 2003;15:741-745.
13. Baines DR, Welty TK, Kendrick T. Native Americans. In: Wong ND, Black HR, Gardin JM, eds. *Preventive Cardiology.* New York, NY: McGraw-Hill; 2004:473-491.
14. Tukey JW. *Exploratory Data Analysis.* Reading, Mass: Addison-Wesley Publishing Co; 1977.
15. Roche AF, Guo SM, Baumgartner RN, Falls RA. The measurement of stature [letter]. *Am J Clin Nutr.* 1988;47:922.
16. Kuczmarski RJ, Ogden CL, Guo SS, et al. 2000 CDC Growth Charts for the United States: methods and development. *Vital Health Stat 11.* 2002;(246):1-190.
17. Neter J, Kutner MH, Nachtsheim CJ, Wasserman W. *Applied Linear Statistical Models.* 4th ed. Chicago, Ill: Irwin; 1996.
18. Murray D. *Design and Analysis of Group-Randomized Trials.* New York, NY: Oxford University Press; 1998.
19. Broussard BA, Johnson A, Himes JH, et al. Prevalence of obesity in American Indians and Alaska Natives. *Am J Clin Nutr.* 1991;53(6, suppl):1535S-1542S.
20. Story M, Stevens J, Evans M, et al. Weight loss attempts and attitudes toward body size, eating, and physical activity in American Indian children: relationship to weight status and gender. *Obes Res.* 2001;9:356-363.
21. Caballero B, Himes JH, Lohman T, et al. Body composition and overweight prevalence in 1704 schoolchildren from 7 American Indian communities. *Am J Clin Nutr.* 2003;78:308-312.
22. Must A, Strauss RS. Risks and consequences of childhood and adolescent obesity. *Int J Obes Relat Metab Disord.* 1999;23(suppl 2):S2-S11.
23. Lee ET, Begum M, Wang W, et al. Type 2 diabetes and impaired fasting glucose in American Indians aged 5-40 years: the Cherokee diabetes study. *Ann Epidemiol.* 2004;14:696-704.
24. Fagot-Campagna A, Pettitt DJ, Engelgau MM, et al. Type 2 diabetes among North American children and adolescents: an epidemiologic review and a public health perspective. *J Pediatr.* 2000;136:664-672.
25. Acton KJ, Burrows NR, Moore K, Querec L, Geiss LS, Engelgau MM. Trends in diabetes prevalence among American Indian and Alaska native children, adolescents, and young adults. *Am J Public Health.* 2002;92:1485-1490.
26. Koplan JP, Liverman CT, Kraak V, eds. Preventing Childhood Obesity: Health in the Balance [prepress; excerpts available to read online at www.nap.edu]. Washington, DC: National Academies Press; 2005.


If you want to see what children can do, you must stop giving them things.
—Norman Douglas

ARTICLE

# Weight Gain in Obese and Nonobese Adolescent Girls Initiating Depot Medroxyprogesterone, Oral Contraceptive Pills, or No Hormonal Contraceptive Method

*Andrea E. Bonny, MD; Julie Ziegler, MA; Ray Harvey, MPH; Sara M. Debanne, PhD; Michelle Secic, MS; Barbara A. Cromer, MD*

**Objective:** To examine weight changes in a large cohort of obese and nonobese adolescent girls initiating depot medroxyprogesterone acetate (DMPA), an oral contraceptive (OC), or no hormonal contraceptive method (control).

**Design, Setting, and Participants:** Prospective study of 450 adolescent girls, aged 12 to 18 years, who attended 4 urban health clinics and selected DMPA, OC, or control. Data collection occurred at baseline and at 6, 12, and 18 months; consisted of structured interview and measurement of height and weight; and occurred from April 19, 2000, through September 26, 2003.

**Main Outcome Measure:** Weight was examined as mean change over 18 months and actual weight at each study visit. On the basis of preliminary analyses, we stratified the sample according to baseline obesity status (nonobese, body mass index [calculated as weight in kilograms divided by the square of height in meters] <30; obese, body mass index ≥30 ).

**Results:** Adolescent girls who were obese at initiation of DMPA gained significantly more weight than did obese girls starting OC or control ($P<.001$ for both). At 18 months, mean weight gain was 9.4, 0.2, and 3.1 kg for obese girls receiving DMPA, receiving OC, and control, respectively. Weight gain in obese girls receiving DMPA was also greater than weight gain in all nonobese categories (4.0 kg, DMPA; 2.8 kg, OC; 3.5 kg, control; $P<.001$). A significant interaction ($P=.006$) between length of time receiving DMPA and weight gain was evident for obese subjects.

**Conclusions:** Over 18 months, DMPA use was associated with increasing rates of weight gain in obese subjects. The potential contribution to severe obesity in this population is concerning.

*Arch Pediatr Adolesc Med. 2006;160:40-45*

Among adolescents receiving depot medroxyprogesterone acetate (DMPA), 41% (27/66) cite weight gain as the primary reason for discontinuing the method.[1] This clinical adverse effect contributes to low DMPA continuation rates among adolescents.[2] At 12 months of use, DMPA continuation rates as low as 27% (43/159) have been reported in this age group.[3]

Despite anecdotal reports of weight gain and documented effects of weight gain on DMPA continuation rates, weight gain has been variable in clinical studies of adolescent girls receiving DMPA.[4-6] Overweight at the time of initiation[7] and race[3,8] have been implicated as risk factors for weight gain, but current studies have been limited by either retrospective data or lack of appropriate control groups.[1,3-9] In addition, little is known about the effect of obesity status on contraceptive adverse effects, since in most controlled studies, either women of greater body weight were excluded or participants' body weight is not reported.[10]

It is important to understand better the clinical and behavioral context within which weight gain occurs with DMPA so that appropriate anticipatory guidance can be tailored to the individual user. Among adolescent girls, this could result in increased method satisfaction and prolonged use of this effective contraceptive.

The primary objective of this analysis was to examine weight changes prospectively in a large cohort of obese and nonobese adolescent girls initiating DMPA, an oral contraceptive (OC), or no hormonal contraceptive method (control).

**Author Affiliations:** Case Western Reserve University School of Medicine (Drs Bonny, Debanne, and Cromer and Mr Harvey); Department of Pediatrics, MetroHealth Medical Center (Drs Bonny and Cromer, Ms Ziegler, and Mr Harvey); and Secic Statistical Consultants (Ms Secic), Cleveland, Ohio.

## METHODS

### SUBJECTS

The study population consisted of postmenarcheal female subjects aged 12 to 18 years who attended 1 of 4 urban adolescent health clinics in a large metropolitan setting. Of the 450 subjects who enrolled in the study, 280 (62.2%) identified themselves as black, and 170 (37.8%) identified themselves as not black. Mean chronological age for the sample was 15.5 years, mean menarcheal age was 12.0 years, and mean gynecologic age (chronological age minus menarcheal age) was 3.5 years.

Adolescent girls requesting contraception, and selecting either DMPA or OC, were eligible to participate. In addition, adolescent girls attending the same health clinics, but who planned to receive no hormonal contraception, were eligible for enrollment as control subjects. The control group included adolescents who were abstinent and those using barrier contraceptive methods, although most were not sexually active. Among all 3 groups (DMPA, OC, and control), most study subjects had not received hormonal contraception before the study; 84.9% of subjects initiating DMPA, 97.4% of subjects initiating OC, and 99.3% of control subjects had not received hormonal contraception previously.

Exclusion criteria for subject participation included the following: (1) pregnancy or DMPA use within the preceding 6 months, (2) OC use within the preceding 3 months, (3) alcohol or drug dependence, (4) medical condition or medication use known to be associated with the outcomes of interest (eg, diabetes mellitus, thyroid disease, methylphenidate hydrochloride, divalproex sodium), (5) contraindications to estrogen use, and (6) need for confidential contraceptive care. After a contraceptive method was selected, eligible subjects were told about the study by their health care provider. Those who expressed interest met with a study recruiter to review the protocol. Subjects younger than 18 years gave written assent for participation, and written informed consent was obtained from a parent or legal guardian. Subjects aged 18 years provided their own written informed consent for participation. The study protocol was reviewed and approved by the institutional review board of the participating institutions.

Of the 450 girls recruited at baseline, 115 (25.6%) selected DMPA, 175 (38.9%) selected OC, and 160 (35.6%) were controls. At 18 months, study withdrawal rates according to contraceptive method were as follows: DMPA, 37.4% (43/115); OC, 46.3% (81/175); and control, 25.0% (40/160). Contraceptive continuation rates were markedly higher among study participants than that generally seen in the adolescent population, reported to be from 27% (43/159) to 34% (38/111) at 12 months.[2,3] For subjects receiving DMPA, the 3 most common reasons for study withdrawal were appointment noncompliance (46.5%), withdrawn consent (16.3%), and change of contraceptive method (9.3%). For subjects receiving OC, the major reasons for study withdrawal were appointment noncompliance (24.7%), medication noncompliance (22.2%), and positive pregnancy test (22.2%). For control subjects, the primary reasons for study withdrawal were appointment noncompliance (25.0%), change of contraceptive method (22.5%), and use of nonpermitted contraception (15.0%).

## DATA COLLECTION

The present study represents the 18-month analyses of weight data collected from April 19, 2000, through September 26, 2003, as part of a 2-year study evaluating hormonal contraception and bone mineral density.[11] A major aim of the 2-year study was to evaluate whether estrogen supplementation in subjects receiving DMPA resulted in decreased losses in bone mineral density. As such, DMPA subjects were randomly assigned to receive either monthly injections of estradiol cypionate or placebo. For the present study, subjects receiving DMPA and estradiol and subjects receiving DMPA and placebo were analyzed separately. No differences in weight gain were seen between the 2 DMPA groups, so data in DMPA subjects were combined.

Baseline data were collected on the day of enrollment and within 1 week after initiating a contraceptive method. Six-month, 12-month and 18-month data were collected on visit days scheduled for contraceptive follow-up, which coincided with time of DMPA injection for subjects using this method. At enrollment, a structured one-on-one interview was conducted to elicit information regarding current age (chronological age); age at menarche (menarcheal age); menstrual regularity; prior contraceptive use; pregnancy history; physical activity; physical and mental health problems; and use of prescription, over-the-counter, and herbal medications. Brief update interviews were conducted at 6, 12, and 18 months. At all visits, weight was measured with a calibrated digital scale, and height was measured with a calibrated stadiometer. Body mass index (BMI) was calculated as weight in kilograms divided by the square of height in meters. To reflect study participants' degree of pubertal maturation, gynecologic age was calculated by subtracting age at menarche from current chronological age.

All subjects received routine contraceptive care from their health care providers as part of their health care visits at baseline and follow-up. Routine care included counseling about potential weight gain, review of healthy eating and exercise habits, monitoring of weight changes, and referral to a registered dietitian if weight concerns arose.

## DATA ANALYSIS

The study purpose was to compare weight gain in adolescents using different contraceptive methods, with the main focus being mean group weight over time; therefore, all data points available at each study visit were eligible for analyses. Preliminary weight analyses demonstrated significant differences between subjects who were nonobese and those who were obese at baseline. The sample was thus stratified according to baseline obesity status (nonobese, BMI $<25$; overweight, BMI $\geq 25$ and $<30$; obese, BMI $\geq 30$). Further analyses demonstrated no differences in weight changes between nonobese and overweight subjects. Therefore, final analyses were performed with the stratification of nonobese and obese (nonobese, BMI $<30$ and obese, BMI $\geq 30$).

Descriptive statistics were means and standard deviations for normally distributed variables, medians and interquartile ranges for nonnormally distributed variables, and counts and percentages for categorical variables. Univariate group comparisons were completed by using $\chi^2$ tests, analyses of variance, or Kruskal-Wallis tests, as appropriate.

The main outcome measures were defined as change in weight over time and actual weight over time. We used analysis of variance modeling, stratified according to obesity status and adjusted for gynecologic age and race, to explore differences in weight changes among the 3 groups. In addition, unbalanced repeated-measures analysis of variance techniques, stratified according to obesity status and adjusted for gynecologic age and race, were used to examine the relationship between contraceptive method and weight over the 18-month study. Unbalanced repeated-measures analysis of variance techniques were used to adjust for differential withdrawal rates across treatment groups and missing data.

$P \leq .05$ was considered statistically significant. Tukey-Kramer adjustments for multiple comparisons were used as follow-up techniques in the modeling phases of the analyses. Data analyses were conducted with SAS statistical software, version 8.2 (SAS Institute Inc, Cary, NC).

**Table 1. Baseline Characteristics of Subjects According to Contraceptive Method***

| Characteristic | All Subjects (N = 450) | DMPA (n = 115) | Oral Contraceptive (n = 175) | Control (n = 160) | *P* Value† |
|---|---|---|---|---|---|
| Obese | 94 (20.9) | 15 (13.0) | 51 (29.1) | 28 (17.5) | .002 |
| Chronological age, y | 15.5 ± 1.6 | 15.8 ± 1.5 | 16.0 ± 1.4 | 14.9 ± 1.6 | <.001 |
| Menarcheal age, y | 12.1 ± 1.3 | 12.0 ± 1.5 | 12.1 ± 1.3 | 12.2 ± 1.2 | .21 |
| Gynecologic age, y | 3.5 ± 1.3 | 3.9 ± 1.5 | 3.9 ± 1.3 | 2.8 ± 1.3 | <.001 |
| Weight, kg | 65.5 ± 16.8 | 62.8 ± 14.9 | 69.3 ± 17.4 | 63.3 ± 16.8 | <.001 |
| BMI, kg/m$^2$ | 25.0 ± 5.9 | 23.8 ± 4.7 | 26.4 ± 6.4 | 24.4 ± 5.8 | <.001 |
| Race | | | | | .98 |
| Nonblack | 170 (37.8) | 43 (37.4) | 67 (38.3) | 60 (37.5) | |
| Black | 280 (62.2) | 72 (62.6) | 108 (61.7) | 100 (62.5) | |
| Regular menses | 377 (83.8) | 97 (84.3) | 139 (79.4) | 141 (88.1) | .16 |
| Previous pregnancy | 11 (2.4) | 6 (5.2) | 5 (2.9) | 0 (0.0) | <.001 |
| Physical activity‡ | | | | | .21 |
| Inactive | 40 (9.0) | 13 (11.4) | 12 (7.1) | 15 (9.4) | |
| Normal | 208 (47.2) | 58 (50.9) | 85 (50.6) | 65 (40.9) | |
| Active | 193 (43.8) | 43 (37.7) | 71 (42.3) | 79 (49.7) | |

Abbreviations: BMI, body mass index; DMPA, depot medroxyprogesterone acetate.
*Data are given as number (percentage) of subjects or mean ± SD.
†$\chi^2$ Tests or analyses of variance, as appropriate.
‡Self-description of physical activity level from a selection of 3 choices: inactive, normal, active.

**Table 2. Mean Weight Increase* From Baseline to 18 Months According to Contraceptive Method**

| Contraceptive Method | Nonobese | Obese | Tukey-Kramer Adjusted *P* Value Within Group |
|---|---|---|---|
| DMPA | 4.04 (0.44) | 9.45 (1.05) | <.001 |
| Oral contraceptive | 2.81 (0.43) | 0.16 (0.64) | .007 |
| Control | 3.50 (0.35) | 3.07 (0.75) | .99 |

Abbreviation: DMPA, depot medroxyprogesterone acetate.
*Adjusted by means of analysis of variance for race, gynecologic age, and previous pregnancy. Sample stratified according to baseline obesity status (nonobese, body mass index <30; obese, body mass index ≥30). Data are given as mean (SE) weight in kilograms.

## RESULTS

Baseline characteristics according to contraceptive method are shown in **Table 1**. There was a significantly greater percentage of obese subjects in the OC group than in the DMPA or control group. As a result, baseline weight and BMI were greater for the OC group. Stratification according to baseline obesity status resolved differences in baseline weight and BMI across contraceptive methods. The control group was significantly younger than the DMPA and OC groups at baseline according to chronological and gynecologic age. The DMPA group had a significantly higher rate of previous pregnancy compared with rates in the OC and control groups. No differences were seen across contraceptive methods in racial distribution, reported regular menses, or physical activity level.

At 18 months, study withdrawal rates according to contraceptive method were as follows: DMPA, 37.4% (43/115); OC, 46.3% (81/175); and control, 25.0% (40/160). As previously described, appointment noncompliance, medication noncompliance, withdrawn study consent, change of contraceptive method, use of nonpermitted contraception, and positive pregnancy test constituted the major reasons for study withdrawal. During the study, 17 (9.7%) of 175 subjects receiving OC, 3 (1.9%) of 160 control subjects, and 0 (0%) of 115 subjects receiving DMPA became pregnant.

Mean weight change, adjusted for race, gynecologic age, and previous pregnancy, from baseline to 18 months is demonstrated in **Table 2** according to contraceptive method and obesity status. Over the 18 months, nonobese subjects receiving DMPA, OC, or no hormonal method had mean weight changes of 4.0, 2.8, and 3.5 kg, respectively. Among obese subjects, those receiving DMPA, those receiving OC, and control had mean weight changes of 9.4, 0.2, and 3.1 kg, respectively. Weight gain in obese girls receiving DMPA was significantly greater than weight gain in obese girls receiving OC ($P<.001$) and obese girls using no hormonal method ($P<.001$). Weight gain in obese girls receiving DMPA was also greater than weight gain in all nonobese categories ($P<.001$). Nonobese subjects receiving OC gained significantly more weight than did obese subjects receiving OC ($P=.007$). In analysis of variance modeling, a significant interaction between baseline obesity status and contraceptive method ($P<.001$) was evident; adolescent girls who initiated DMPA were more likely to gain weight over time than those who initiated OC or no method, and this weight gain was accentuated by being obese at baseline.

**Table 3** shows incidence of obesity at 6, 12, and 18 months, according to contraceptive method, for subjects who were nonobese at baseline (ie, the percentage of nonobese subjects who became obese at each time point). Among nonobese subjects, 8 (19.0%) of 42 receiving DMPA, 4 (9.8%) of 41 receiving OC, and 2 (2.8%) of 71 control subjects became obese by 18 months.

Repeated-measures adjusted mean weight stratified according to baseline obesity status is shown in **Table 4**. For nonobese subjects, contraceptive method was not significantly associated with weight ($P=.31$). Predictors of weight for nonobese subjects included black race ($P=.003$), younger gynecologic age ($P=.002$), and length of time in study ($P<.001$). Conversely, perhaps because of smaller sample sizes and thus less power, race ($P=.82$) and gynecologic age ($P=.40$) were not predictive of weight for obese subjects. A significant interaction was seen, however, between contraceptive method and length of time in study ($P=.006$). This interaction effect suggests that, during the 18-month observation period, DMPA use among obese subjects was associated with an increasing rate of weight gain with longer duration of use.

**Table 3. Incidence of Obesity Among Subjects Nonobese at Baseline and at 6, 12, and 18 Months According to Contraceptive Method**

| | No. Who Became Obese/ No. Who Remained Obese, % | | |
|---|---|---|---|
| **Contraceptive Method** | **6 Months** | **12 Months** | **18 Months** |
| DMPA (100 nonobese at baseline) | 4/87 (4.6) | 6/62 (9.7) | 8/42 (19.0) |
| Oral contraceptive (124 nonobese at baseline) | 6/93 (6.5) | 7/64 (10.9) | 4/41 (9.8) |
| Control (132 nonobese at baseline) | 4/120 (3.3) | 4/97 (4.1) | 2/71 (2.8) |

Abbreviation: DMPA, depot medroxyprogesterone acetate.

## COMMENT

In this 18-month prospective study of adolescent girls initiating DMPA, OC, or no hormonal contraceptive method, we found a significant relationship between baseline obesity status and subsequent weight gain. Adolescent girls who were obese at initiation of DMPA gained significantly more weight than obese girls starting OC or no contraceptive method. In addition, obese adolescents receiving DMPA gained more weight than did nonobese adolescents using DMPA, OC, or no hormonal contraception method (control).

Among nonobese adolescents, we found no statistically significant effect of contraceptive method on weight. However, weight gain was greatest among nonobese subjects receiving DMPA, averaging 4.0 kg at 18 months. This amount of weight gain is not inconsequential and could be cause for concern in populations vulnerable to obesity.

Furthermore, weight gain in nonobese subjects receiving OC was significantly greater than in obese subjects receiving OC. Evidence suggests that hormonal steroid kinetics may contribute to differing clinical outcomes between obese and nonobese women receiving OC. A small study of ethinyl estradiol plasma concentrations in women receiving OC showed a negative correlation between ethinyl estradiol levels and body weight.[12] Women in the lowest plasma ethinyl estradiol quartile had a nonsignificant but greater mean weight than those in the highest quartile (64.0 vs 60.1 kg). However, women of extreme body weight were not included in this study. Recent evidence also demonstrates that greater body weight is associated with an increased risk of OC failure.[13,14] Among consistent OC users, the risk of pregnancy is more than 70% higher in women weighing more than 74.8 kg and nearly double in women weighing more than 86.2 kg.[14] The risk of OC failure increases among overweight women as the OC estrogen dose decreases.[13] Taken together, the results of these studies seem to suggest that lower circulating ethinyl estradiol levels may be present in obese women receiving OC compared with their nonobese peers. In the present study, less weight gain among obese subjects perhaps also reflects lower circulating contraceptive concentrations in this group.

Among adolescents who were nonobese at baseline, incidence of obesity was highest in those receiving hormonal contraception. At 18 months, incidence of obesity was 19.0% and 9.8% for nonobese subjects receiving DMPA and OC, respectively, compared with 2.8% for control subjects.

An estimated 10%, or approximately 1 million, adolescent girls aged 15 to 19 years use DMPA as their contraceptive method.[15,16] With the ever-increasing prevalence of obesity, ranging from 12.4% (28/226) to 26.6% (81/304) of adolescent girls depending on racial background,[17] the number of obese adolescents possibly choosing DMPA is potentially large. Because obese adolescents receiving OC did not gain weight, one may conclude that OC is the best contraceptive option for an obese adolescent. However, although OC use in obese adolescents was not associated with adverse effects on weight gain in this study, method discontinuation rates were markedly higher among those receiving OC compared with those receiving DMPA: 46.3% vs 37.4%, respectively. Furthermore, the pregnancy rate among adolescents receiving OC was 10%, whereas no subjects receiving DMPA became pregnant. As previously noted, new evidence also suggests that women with elevated body weight may be at greater risk for OC failure, even with good method compliance.[13,14] Unintended pregnancy in adolescence, in addition to its own effect on weight, has enormous adverse social and financial consequences. Therefore, is continued weight gain or pregnancy a larger burden for an obese adolescent?

The reasons for an interaction between obesity status and DMPA-associated weight gain are unclear. Earlier research showed a glucocorticoid agonist activity of DMPA[18] and DMPA interference with insulin action[19] and serotonin metabolism.[20] Interactions between obesity status and such DMPA mechanisms should be explored in future studies. Furthermore, interindividual variability in DMPA pharmacokinetic measures has been documented. Wide interindividual variability has been seen in serum medroxyprogesterone acetate levels at the end of the 3-month injection period[21,22] and in the time needed for resumption of ovulation after using DMPA.[23,24] Although the possible influence of weight, BMI, and race on medroxyprogesterone acetate levels has been investigated,[22,23,25] overall, few studies have done so, and the

**Table 4. Mean Weight* at Baseline and at 6, 12, and 18 Months According to Contraceptive Method**

| Contraceptive Method | Baseline | 6 Months | 12 Months | 18 Months |
|---|---|---|---|---|
| Nonobese subjects† | | | | |
| DMPA | 57.66 (1.08) | 58.07 (1.09) | 59.51 (1.15) | 62.05 (1.26) |
| Oral contraceptive | 59.40 (0.98) | 60.40 (1.01) | 61.39 (1.08) | 62.65 (1.21) |
| Control | 57.53 (0.94) | 58.94 (0.95) | 59.59 (0.98) | 60.74 (1.04) |
| Obese subjects‡ | | | | |
| DMPA | 91.61 (3.02) | 96.47 (3.09) | 99.71 (3.12) | 101.02 (3.39) |
| Oral contraceptive | 91.39 (1.75) | 91.40 (1.80) | 90.82 (1.88) | 90.10 (2.02) |
| Control | 91.44 (2.35) | 94.05 (2.39) | 94.21 (2.44) | 93.50 (2.61) |

Abbreviation: DMPA, depot medroxyprogesterone acetate.
*Adjusted by means of repeated-measures analysis of variance for race, gynecologic age, and previous pregnancy. Sample stratified according to baseline obesity status (nonobese, body mass index $<30$; obese, body mass index $\geq 30$). Data are given as mean (SE) weight in kilograms.
†Significant ($P < .001$) increases in weight, for all nonobese groups, across time. No difference according to contraceptive method.
‡Significant ($P = .006$) interaction between DMPA use and time using method in obese adolescent girls.

methodologies of some studies are unclear, suggesting a need for further investigation.

Limitations of the present study must be considered. The present study represents an analysis of secondary data from a study designed to evaluate hormonal contraception and bone mineral density in adolescents. Furthermore, subjects selected their contraceptive method rather than being randomly assigned one. Although random assignment of treatment groups would be preferable, random assignment of contraceptive method would not be ethical. In clinical practice, a variety of patient factors, including perceived ease of use, perceived adverse effects, and personal preference, affect contraceptive choice. All these variables can affect patient satisfaction and compliance with a contraceptive method. Because pregnancy is an undesirable outcome with contraception use and method compliance tends to be poor in adolescents, patient preference must dictate contraceptive choice to maximize adherence. We acknowledge that this may introduce inherent bias in the study sample as demonstrated by differences between the control subjects and adolescents receiving DMPA and OC. Although not different in racial composition and recruited from the same clinical sites as subjects receiving DMPA and OC, control subjects were significantly younger. Of note, rate of growth, and, hence, rate of weight gain, is highest in girls during the earlier phases of puberty and, hence, highest among adolescent girls of younger gynecologic age, so greater weight gain would be expected rather than lower weight gain among the younger control group.

Generalizability of the present study results also must be considered. The study sample was primarily black urban adolescents. The study findings may not be applicable to populations of other racial backgrounds or adult women.

In conclusion, to our knowledge, our study is the first to follow up and compare prospectively weight changes in a large cohort of obese and nonobese adolescent girls initiating hormonal contraception and control subjects not receiving hormonal contraception. Our study demonstrates a relationship between contraceptive weight gain and obesity; DMPA use dramatically increased rates of weight gain in obese subjects. In BMI units, the effect of the 9-kg weight gain in obese adolescents receiving DMPA is 3 in an adolescent of average height. With an estimated 150 000 obese adolescents using DMPA as a contraceptive method,[15-17] the potential contribution of DMPA to severe obesity is concerning. Significant weight gains were not observed in obese subjects receiving OC. One might conclude, therefore, that OC is the best contraceptive choice in the obese adolescent. However, with previous research documenting poor compliance and high rates of pregnancy in adolescents receiving OC, the best choice of contraception for obese teenagers is unclear, highlighting the need for further research in this area.

**Accepted for Publication:** June 23, 2005.
**Correspondence:** Andrea E. Bonny, MD, Department of Pediatrics, MetroHealth Medical Center, 2500 MetroHealth Dr, Cleveland, OH 44109 (abonny@metrohealth.org).
**Funding/Support:** This study was supported by grant M1 RR 0008012 from the US Public Health Service General Clinical Research Centers, Washington, DC, and grant R01HD39009 from the National Institutes of Health, Bethesda, Md.
**Acknowledgments:** We thank William Dietz, MD, PhD, for his critical review of the manuscript and Mary Jo Day, LPN, and Darlene Lewis, RN, for their help with subject recruitment and data collection.

## REFERENCES

1. Harel Z, Biro FM, Kollar LM, Rauh JL. Adolescents' reasons for and experience after discontinuation of the long-acting contraceptives Depo-Provera and Norplant. *J Adolesc Health.* 1996;19:118-123.
2. O'Dell CM, Forke CM, Polaneczky MM, Sondheimer SJ, Slap GB. Depot medroxyprogesterone acetate or oral contraception in postpartum adolescents. *Obstet Gynecol.* 1998;91:609-614.
3. Polaneczky M, Liblanc M. Long-term depot medroxyprogesterone acetate (Depo-Provera) use in inner-city adolescents. *J Adolesc Health.* 1998;23:81-88.
4. Moore LL, Valuck R, McDougall C, Fink W. A comparative study of one-year weight gain among users of medroxyprogesterone acetate, levonorgestrel implants, and oral contraceptives. *Contraception.* 1995;52:215-219.
5. Matson SC, Henderson KA, McGrath GJ. Physical findings and symptoms of depot medroxyprogesterone acetate use in adolescent females. *J Pediatr Adolesc Gynecol.* 1997;10:18-23.

6. Risser WL, Gefter LR, Barratt MS, Risser JM. Weight change in adolescents who used hormonal contraception. *J Adolesc Health.* 1999;24:433-436.
7. Mangan SA, Larsen PG, Hudson S. Overweight teens at increased risk for weight gain while using depot medroxyprogesterone acetate. *J Pediatr Adolesc Gynecol.* 2002;15:79-82.
8. Bonny AE, Britto MT, Huang B, Succop P, Slap GB. Weight gain, adiposity, and eating behaviors among adolescent females on depot medroxyprogesterone acetate (DMPA). *J Pediatr Adolesc Gynecol.* 2004;17:109-115.
9. Templeman C, Boyd H, Hertweck SP. Depomedroxyprogesterone acetate use and weight gain among adolescents. *J Pediatr Adolesc Gynecol.* 2000;13:45-46.
10. Speroff L, Andolsek K. Hormonal contraception and obesity. *Dialogues Contracept.* 2003;8:1-4.
11. Cromer BA, Binkovitz L, Ziegler J, Harvey R, Debanne SM. Reference values for bone mineral density in 12- to 18-year-old girls categorized by weight, race, and age. *Pediatr Radiol.* 2004;34:787-792.
12. Stadel BV, Sternthal PM, Schlesselman JJ, et al. Variation of ethinylestradiol blood levels among healthy women using oral contraceptives. *Fertil Steril.* 1980;33:257-260.
13. Holt VL, Cushing-Haugen KL, Daling JR. Body weight and risk of oral contraceptive failure. *Obstet Gynecol.* 2002;99(5 pt 1):820-827.
14. Holt VL, Scholes D, Wicklund KG, Cushing-Haugen KL, Daling JR. Body mass index, weight, and oral contraceptive failure risk. *Obstet Gynecol.* 2005;105:46-52.
15. Piccinino LJ, Mosher WD. Trends in contraceptive use in the United States: 1982-1995. *Fam Plann Perspect.* 1998;30:4-10, 46.
16. US Bureau of the Census. United States Census 2000 Summary File 1. Washington, DC: US Dept of Commerce, Economics and Statistics Administration; 2000.
17. Ogden CL, Flegal KM, Carroll MD, Johnson CL. Prevalence and trends in overweight among US children and adolescents, 1999-2000. *JAMA.* 2002;288:1728-1732.
18. Guthrie GP Jr, John WJ. The in vivo glucocorticoid and antiglucocorticoid actions of medroxyprogesterone acetate. *Endocinology.* 1980;107:1393-1396.
19. Fahmy K, Abdel-Razik M, Shaaraway M, et al. Effect of long-acting progestagen-only injectable contraceptives on carbohydrate metabolism and its hormonal profile. *Contraception.* 1991;44:419-430.
20. Ladisich W. Influence of progesterone on serotonin metabolism: a possible causal factor for mood changes. *Psychoneuroendocrinology.* 1977;2:257-266.
21. Koetsawang S, Shrimanker K, Fotherby K. Blood levels of medroxyprogesterone acetate after multiple injections of depoprovera or cycloprovera. *Contraception.* 1979;20:1-4.
22. Smit J, Botha J, McFadyen L, Beksinska M. Serum medroxyprogesterone acetate levels in new and repeat users of depot medroxyprogesterone acetate at the end of the dosing interval. *Contraception.* 2004;69:3-7.
23. Bassol S, Garza-Flores J, Cravioto MC, et al. Ovarian function following a single administration of depo-medroxyprogesterone acetate (DMPA) at different doses. *Fertil Steril.* 1984;42:216-222.
24. Ortiz A, Hirol M, Stanczyk FZ, Goebelsmann U, Mishell DR. Serum medroxyprogesterone acetate (MPA) concentrations and ovarian function following intramuscular injection of depo-MPA. *J Clin Endocrinol Metab.* 1977;44:32-38.
25. Fotherby K, Saxena BN, Shrimanker K, et al. A preliminary pharmacokinetic and pharmacodynamic evaluation of depot-medroxyprogesterone acetate and norethisterone oenanthate. *Fertil Steril.* 1980;34:131-139.

*Announcement*

**Helping the Student With Diabetes Succeed: A Guide for School Personnel Now Available From the National Diabetes Education Program.** This comprehensive guide provides school personnel, parents, and students with a framework for managing diabetes effectively in the school setting. The guide helps to ensure that students with diabetes are medically safe and have access to all educational opportunities and activities. Developed by the US Department of Health and Human Services' National Diabetes Education Program, the guide includes user-friendly tools such as a diabetes primer and glossary, sample medical management and emergency action plans, and a review of federal laws pertaining to students with diabetes. To obtain a free copy of the guide, call 1-800-438-5383 or visit the National Diabetes Education Program Web site at http://ndep.nih.gov/diabetes/youth/youth.htm.

# Sedation and Analgesia for Pediatric Fracture Reduction in the Emergency Department

## *A Systematic Review*

*Russell T. Migita, MD; Eileen J. Klein, MD, MPH; Michelle M. Garrison, MPH*

**Objective:** To assess the safety and efficacy of various forms of analgesia and sedation for fracture reduction in pediatric patients in the emergency department, as observed in randomized controlled trials in pediatric populations.

**Data Sources:** Cochrane Controlled Trials Register, CINAHL (Cumulative Index to Nursing & Allied Health Literature), and MEDLINE. The search terms "fractures," "manipulation, orthopedic," "an(a)esthetics," "analgesics," and "hypnotics and sedatives" were used.

**Study Selection:** Studies were included if they were randomized controlled trials studying sedative and/or analgesic regimens for fracture reductions in pediatric patients in the emergency department. The search yielded 915 references. From these, 8 studies inclu ding 1086 patients were selected.

**Data Extraction:** Interventions studied included intravenous regional blocks (Bier blocks), nitrous oxide, and parenteral combinations. Data on measures of effectiveness and safety were extracted.

**Data Synthesis:** Ketamine hydrochloride–midazolam hydrochloride was associated with less distress during reduction than fentanyl citrate–midazolam or propofol-fentanyl. Patients receiving ketamine-midazolam required significantly fewer airway interventions than those in whom either fentanyl-midazolam or propofol-fentanyl were used. Data comparing Bier blocks with systemic forms of sedation or analgesia were limited.

**Conclusions:** Ketamine-midazolam seems to be more effective and have fewer adverse events than fentanyl-midazolam or propofol-fentanyl. Data on other forms of analgesia or sedation are too limited to make comparisons. More research is needed to define the regimen that maximizes safety, efficacy, and efficiency for fracture reduction in pediatric patients.

*Arch Pediatr Adolesc Med. 2006;160:46-51*

LONG-BONE FRACTURES ARE one of the most common injuries treated in the emergency department (ED) setting and are also one of the most common serious injuries of childhood. Published reports of fracture rates in children range between 160 and 360 per 10 000 children.[1-3] In Singapore, 6.8% of all children require hospitalization for fracture care by age 16 years.[4] In contrast, in the United States, reimbursement policies and patient preference have led to an increasing push toward providing definitive care to patients with fractures on an outpatient basis. This care is increasingly provided in the ED rather than in the operating room.

Fracture reduction is one of the most painful procedures commonly performed in the ED, but patients and families expect the ED to be a resource for relieving a large percentage of their pain.[5] Health care providers who care for children with fractures are faced with the sometimes divergent tasks of providing effective analgesia and anxiolysis while ensuring timely, efficient, cost-effective, and safe care of the patient. The potential benefits of effective sedation during fracture reduction include diminished patient fear and discomfort; parental, provider, and patient satisfaction; decreased utilization of resources; improved outcome of the fracture reduction; and decreased reliance on general anesthesia.

Several studies have documented that children receive inadequate analgesia for fracture pain during their visit to the ED.[6-10] Furthermore, there has been a wide variation in sedation practice patterns,[11] in part because little consensus exists on the safest and most effective regimens.[12]

By systematically reviewing the literature, we hoped to answer the clinical question: What is the safest and most effective means of providing sedation and analgesia to children undergoing frac-

**Author Affiliations:** Divisions of Emergency Medicine (Drs Migita and Klein) and General Pediatrics (Ms Garrison), Department of Pediatrics, University of Washington School of Medicine; Children's Hospital and Regional Medical Center (Drs Migita and Klein); and Child Health Institute (Ms Garrison), Seattle.

ture reduction in the ED setting? In addition, we hoped to identify areas that require further research.

## METHODS

We searched several bibliographic databases, including MEDLINE (January 1, 1966, through April 30, 2005), the Cochrane Collaboration and Clinical Trials Database (as of April 30, 2005), and CINAHL (Cumulative Index to Nursing & Allied Health Literature) (as of April 30, 2005). Searches for unpublished trials were limited to the Medical Editors' Trial Amnesty. The key word search terms "fractures" or "manipulation, orthopedic" were combined with the terms "an(a)esthetics," "analgesics," or "hypnotics and sedatives." Literature searches were further restricted to studies published in the English language. Abstracts from this initial search were examined and studies were excluded if they did not study sedation for fracture reduction. We also examined articles found when viewing the bibliographies of other clinical trials or review articles as well as articles from our personal files.

We next reviewed the full text of the remaining articles identified in the search. Studies were examined by 2 of us (E.J.K. and R.T.M.); neither reviewer was blinded to journal or authors. Each reviewer independently reviewed the "Methods" section of each article to determine whether it fulfilled criteria for inclusion in the final review. A third author (M.M.G.) resolved any disagreements. Our final analysis was restricted to studies that were identified as randomized controlled trials (RCTs), exclusively included children younger than 18 years, compared pharmacological methods of sedation or analgesia for fracture reduction in the ED setting, and included clinical outcomes and/or complications. Quality was assessed by all reviewers, and studies were included if they were RCTs with adequate randomization. Because of the unique properties of the various sedation modalities, blinding was considered but was not a criterion for inclusion in this analysis. Data were extracted independently by 2 of us (E.J.K. and R.T.M.) from all studies that met inclusion criteria. The primary outcome measure selected was pain scores of individuals undergoing fracture reduction. Secondary outcomes included surrogate measures of pain such as provider, patient, or parent satisfaction; patient memory of the event; procedural success; and the need for additional medication doses. Complications such as apnea, desaturation, hypotension, vomiting, and emergence reactions as well as length of stay were tabulated when data were available.

## RESULTS

The search yielded 915 references. From these, 119 were deemed eligible for more detailed review for potential inclusion. The most common reasons for exclusion of studies from the final analysis were adult subjects, medications studied that were not for procedural pain control in the ED, not patient research (review article, letters, opinion, survey), nonorthopedic procedures, and case series. A listing of articles that were excluded from the systematic review is available on request from the corresponding author.

The final analysis included 8 studies, with some studies evaluating more than one regimen (**Table**).[13-20] Three main forms of sedation-analgesia for fracture reduction were evaluated: (1) Bier blocks, (2) parenteral medications, and (3) nitrous oxide. Bier blocks and narcotic-benzodiazepine combinations were each evaluated in 3 studies; propofol, ketamine hydrochloride, and nitrous oxide were each evaluated in 2 studies. The Bier block studies used either lidocaine hydrochloride or prilocaine hydrochloride.

### BIER BLOCKS

Three RCTs examined the effectiveness and safety of Bier block anesthesia in children undergoing fracture reduction. Bier blocks are regional nerve blocks in which an intravenous line is placed in the fractured extremity. A tourniquet is applied proximal to the injury and a local anesthetic is injected intravenously into the affected extremity. These studies compared regular-dose (3 mg/kg) and "mini-dose" (1.5 mg/kg) lidocaine hydrochloride,[13] regular-dose lidocaine with an equivalent dose of prilocaine,[14] and regular-dose lidocaine with nitrous oxide.[20]

### ARE BIER BLOCKS EFFECTIVE AT PROVIDING ANALGESIA FOR FRACTURE REDUCTION?

**Yes, but data are limited.** Only 1 RCT has compared Bier block analgesia with a systemic form of analgesia.[20] In this study, 28 children were randomized to receive either a Bier block with 3 mg/kg of lidocaine hydrochloride or self-administered 50% nitrous oxide. There were no significant differences between groups in pain scores by either child or treating physician report. However, given the small sample size, this study may be underpowered to detect a difference between the 2 regimens. Patients treated with nitrous oxide had a significantly shorter total procedure time than patients randomized to Bier block (41.1 minutes [range, 23-63 minutes] vs 61.5 minutes [range, 40-85 minutes]; $P<.001$).

### WHICH BIER BLOCK MEDICATION PROTOCOLS ARE MOST EFFECTIVE?

**Standard-dose (3-mg/kg) lidocaine hydrochloride Bier blocks seem to be more effective than either mini-dose or prilocaine Bier blocks.** Two studies have compared different drugs and doses for the Bier block. Bratt et al[13] compared standard-dose (3 mg/kg) lidocaine hydrochloride with a mini-dose Bier block (1.5 mg/kg) in a total of 283 patients. Those receiving standard-dose lidocaine reported significantly less pain than those receiving the low-dose Bier block (96% satisfactory anesthesia vs 87%; $P<.01$). This difference was even more pronounced when the fracture was completely displaced (93% vs 67%; $P<.01$). Davidson et al[14] compared 3-mg/kg doses of lidocaine hydrochloride vs prilocaine hydrochloride in a total of 249 children. In their study, children receiving lidocaine were significantly more likely to have minimal or no pain than those receiving prilocaine, per provider report (90.5% vs 78%; $P=.01$).

### ARE BIER BLOCKS SAFE?

**Probably.** The 3 RCTs that included Bier blocks observed no adverse effects among the 546 procedures.

**Table. Characteristics of Included RCTs**

| Source | Age of Subjects, y | Treatment Arm A: Intervention | n | Treatment Arm B: Intervention | n | Outcome Measures |
|---|---|---|---|---|---|---|
| Bratt et al,[13] 1996 | >3.5 | Bier block with lidocaine hydrochloride, 3 mg/kg | 140 | Bier block with lidocaine hydrochloride, 1.5 mg/kg | 143 | Faces pain score |
| Davidson et al,[14] 2002 | 3-16 | Bier block with prilocaine hydrochloride, 3 mg/kg | 116 | Bier block with lidocaine hydrochloride, 3 mg/kg | 133 | Subjective pain score; reduction success |
| Godambe et al,[15] 2003 | 3-16 | Ketamine hydrochloride, 1-2 mg/kg IV; midazolam hydrochloride, 0.05 mg/kg IV | 54 | Propofol, 1 mg/kg IV; fentanyl citrate, 1-2 μg/kg IV | 59 | OSBD-r; nurse, parent, provider satisfaction; patient recall; reduction success; sedation and recovery time |
| Kennedy et al,[16] 1998 | 5-15 | Ketamine hydrochloride, 0.5+ mg/kg IV; midazolam hydrochloride, 0.1+ mg/kg IV | 130 | Fentanyl citrate, 0.5+ μg/kg IV; midazolam hydrochloride, 0.1 mg/kg IV | 130 | OSBD-r; parent VAS; orthopedist VAS; patient recall; reduction success; recovery time |
| Havel et al,[17] 1999 | 2-18 | Propofol, 1+ mg/kg IV; morphine sulfate, 0.05-0.1+ mg/kg IV | 43 | Midazolam hydrochloride, 0.1+ mg/kg IV; morphine sulfate, 0.05-0.1+ mg/kg IV | 46 | Ramsay sedation score; patient recall; recovery time; time to discharge |
| Pierce and Fuchs,[18] 1997 | 3-18 | Ketorolac tromethamine, 1 mg/kg IV; fentanyl citrate, 1+ μg/kg IV; midazolam hydrochloride, 0.1 mg/kg IV | 17 | Fentanyl citrate, 1+ μg/kg IV; midazolam, 0.1 mg/kg IV | 17 | CHEOPS; VAS; dose required |
| Evans et al,[19] 1995 | 4-15 | Meperidine hydrochloride, 2 mg/kg IM; promethazine hydrochloride, 1 mg/kg IM | 15 | 50% Nitrous oxide | 15 | CHEOPS, reduction success |
| Gregory and Sullivan,[20] 1996 | 4-15 | Bier block with lidocaine hydrochloride, 3 mg/kg | 14 | 50% Nitrous oxide | 14 | Faces pain score, VAS, procedure time |

Abbreviations: CHEOPS, Children's Hospital of Eastern Ontario Pain Score[21]; IM, intramuscular; IV, intravenous; OSBD-r, Observational Score of Behavioral Distress, Revised[22,23]; RCTs, randomized controlled trials; VAS, visual analog scale.

## NITROUS OXIDE TREATMENT

Two RCTs examined nitrous oxide. One compared nitrous oxide with meperidine hydrochloride and promethazine hydrochloride.[19] The other compared nitrous oxide with Bier block analgesia.[20] The regimens for nitrous oxide administration were generally similar to the protocol described by Wattenmaker et al,[24] with a scavenger system used to deliver a 50:50 nitrous oxide–oxygen mixture to the patient. The anesthetic is self-administered by the patient and requires the patient to generate negative pressure to open the supply valve. After the procedure is completed, patients are administered 100% oxygen for several minutes.

### IS NITROUS OXIDE EFFECTIVE?

**Data are too limited to support this intervention's effectiveness.** The 2 RCTs that included nitrous oxide studied a total of 58 patients. Evans et al[19] compared self-administered 50% nitrous oxide vs intramuscular meperidine and promethazine. Children's Hospital of Eastern Ontario Pain Scores were not significantly different between the 2 groups (9.6 for nitrous oxide, 9.3 for meperidine-promethazine; $P>.05$). There were also no significant differences between the groups on memory or patient's reported subjective experience. Patients who were randomized to receive nitrous oxide had a significantly shorter total treatment time (30 minutes vs 83 minutes; $P<.01$).

As already described, Gregory and Sullivan[20] compared nitrous oxide vs a Bier block using lidocaine hydrochloride at 3 mg/kg. There were no significant differences between the 2 groups on either child- or provider-reported pain scales, and patients treated with nitrous oxide had a significantly shorter total procedure time than patients randomized to Bier block.

### IS NITROUS OXIDE SAFE?

**Data are too limited to make conclusions on this intervention's safety.** Drawing firm conclusions about the safety of this intervention is difficult given the few patients studied. The literature on nitrous oxide included in the study observed no adverse events.

## NARCOTIC-BENZODIAZEPINE COMBINATIONS

Three RCTs included narcotic-benzodiazepine combinations.[16-18] In addition, 1 RCT studied meperidine and promethazine, a nonselective histamine 1 antagonist with sedative and antiemetic properties.[19]

## ARE NARCOTIC-BENZODIAZEPINE COMBINATIONS EFFECTIVE?

**The evidence indicates that there are more effective drug combinations.** Kennedy et al[16] randomized a total of 260 subjects to either fentanyl citrate–midazolam hydrochloride or ketamine-midazolam. Patients randomized to receive fentanyl-midazolam had more pain and anxiety by every measure: Observational Score of Behavioral Distress, Revised (OSBD-r)[22,23] (mean±SD, 2.7±2.16 vs 1.08±1.12; *P*<.001), parental reporting of pain (5.55±3.33 vs 4.21±3.30; *P*=.05), parental reporting of anxiety (5.49±3.26 vs 4.48±3.26; *P*=.05), and orthopedists' satisfaction (8.71±2.21 vs 9.61±0.78; *P*<.001). Amnesia and depth of sedation were similar between the 2 groups. The group that received fentanyl-midazolam had shorter recovery times than the ketamine-midazolam group (113.7±36.9 minutes vs 127.6±56.2, respectively; *P*=.05).

Havel et al[17] compared midazolam–morphine sulfate with propofol-morphine. A total of 89 patients were randomized to receive either propofol-morphine or midazolam-morphine. The depth of sedation was measured by the Ramsay sedation scale at 5-minute intervals after medication administration. No pain or sedation scores were reported at the time of fracture reduction. Sedation scores at each time point and total morphine dose administered did not differ between the 2 groups. Nine (21%) of 43 patients receiving propofol-morphine had some memory of the reduction, with 1 of those patients relating detailed recall of the pain; 4 (9%) of 46 patients receiving midazolam-morphine recalled their procedure, with none recalling significant pain. Recovery time (midazolam-morphine, 48.2±45.3 minutes; propofol-morphine, 13.6±11.3 minutes) and time to discharge (midazolam-morphine, 71.9±41.9 minutes; propofol-morphine, 43.1±28.2 minutes) favored propofol-morphine.

Pierce and Fuchs[18] evaluated ketorolac tromethamine as an adjunct to fentanyl-midazolam therapy. They administered fentanyl-midazolam to all 34 patients in their study. Patients were randomized to receive ketorolac or saline placebo before fracture reduction. Patients who received ketorolac tended to receive lower doses of fentanyl citrate than those who received the saline placebo, although the difference was not statistically significant (2.26 μg/kg vs 2.85 μg/kg; *P*=.07). Pain scores were not significantly different between the 2 groups.

## ARE NARCOTIC-BENZODIAZEPINE COMBINATIONS SAFE?

**The evidence indicates that there are safer treatment regimens available.** The largest study of this combination was by Kennedy et al.[16] They found that patients receiving fentanyl-midazolam were more likely to have hypoxia (25% vs 6%; *P*<.001), need breathing cues (12% vs 1%; *P*<.01), and require oxygen (20% vs 10%; *P*<.05) than those receiving ketamine-midazolam. Vomiting was more common in the ketamine group (*P*=.05). In the study by Havel et al,[17] no difference was found in the incidence of complications when midazolam-morphine was compared with propofol-morphine therapy. Propofol-morphine therapy was associated with hypoxemia requiring supplemental oxygen, stimulation, and/or airway positioning 11.6% of the time (95% confidence interval [CI], 4.3%-26.0%) compared with 10.9% of the time (95% CI, 4.1%-24.6%) for midazolam-morphine therapy (odds ratio [OR], 1.08; 95% CI for OR, 0.24-4.76). Oversedation was noted in 32.6% of those given propofol-morphine therapy compared with 34.8% of those given midazolam-morphine therapy (OR, 0.91; 95% CI, 0.52-1.68); agitation in 4.7% vs 6.5%, respectively (OR, 0.70; 95% CI, 0.08-5.53); and injection pain in 7.0% vs 4.3%, respectively (OR, 1.65; 95% CI, 0.21-15.02). The other 2 RCTs[18,19] had small numbers (total n=64) of patients and reported that there were no adverse reactions.

## KETAMINE THERAPY

Ketamine was studied in 2 RCTs. Both of these studies combined ketamine with midazolam. One RCT compared ketamine-midazolam therapy with fentanyl-midazolam therapy,[16] while the other compared ketamine-midazolam therapy with propofol-fentanyl therapy.[15]

## IS KETAMINE-MIDAZOLAM THERAPY EFFECTIVE?

**Yes.** Kennedy et al[16] randomized 260 subjects to either fentanyl-midazolam therapy or ketamine-midazolam therapy. Observers were blinded to study purpose and design and scored the patients' distress by watching a videotape of the procedure. Compared with those who received fentanyl-midazolam, patients randomized to receive ketamine-midazolam had less pain and anxiety, less parental reporting of pain, less parental reporting of anxiety, and greater orthopedists' satisfaction. Amnesia and depth of sedation were similar between the 2 groups. The group that received ketamine-midazolam therapy had longer recovery times.

Godambe et al[15] compared ketamine-midazolam therapy with propofol-fentanyl therapy in 113 children undergoing orthopedic procedures. The primary outcome measures were behavioral distress, as measured by the OSBD-r, and recovery time. The OSBD-r was scored by independent blinded reviewers who watched videotapes of the procedures. An attempt was made to blind the observers further by placing sunglasses on the patients to hide the characteristic faces associated with ketamine and by performing mock jaw thrusts on the patients in anticipation of the greater frequency of airway positioning that would be required with propofol therapy. The OSBD-r scores during fracture reduction favored ketamine-midazolam therapy (0.084 for ketamine-midazolam vs 0.278 for propofol-fentanyl; 95% CI for the mean difference, −0.34 to −0.048). Parent visual analog scale scores, nurse satisfaction, and orthopedists' satisfaction did not differ between the 2 groups. Total sedation time (62.1 minutes vs 38.9 minutes; 95% CI for mean difference, 15.4-30.4 minutes) and recovery time (54.2 minutes vs 20.8 minutes; 95% CI for mean difference, 26.1-40.8 minutes) were significantly longer for ketamine-midazolam than for propofol-fentanyl.

### IS KETAMINE-MIDAZOLAM THERAPY SAFE?

**Ketamine-midazolam therapy is associated with fewer adverse events than other parenteral drug combinations.** Kennedy et al[16] found that ketamine-midazolam therapy was associated with fewer respiratory events, decreased need for breathing cues, and less need for supplemental oxygen than fentanyl-midazolam therapy. Vomiting was more common in the ketamine-treated group both during the ED stay (9% vs 2%; $P=.05$) and during the 7 days after the procedure (4% vs 0%; $P<.05$). Although ketamine has frequently been described as causing emergence agitation, there was no significant difference between the 2 groups in its incidence (5% vs 2%; $P=.33$). Godambe et al[15] found that patients receiving ketamine-midazolam had significantly fewer desaturation events (7% vs 31%; $P<.01$) and required fewer airway maneuvers (2% vs 25%; $P=.01$) than those who received propofol-fentanyl therapy.

### PROPOFOL THERAPY

Propofol, in combination with a narcotic analgesic, was studied in 2 RCTs. Propofol is generally combined with an analgesic, as it has no intrinsic analgesic properties. One study compared propofol-fentanyl therapy with ketamine-midazolam therapy,[15] while the other compared propofol-morphine therapy with midazolam-morphine therapy.[17]

### IS PROPOFOL THERAPY EFFECTIVE?

**Propofol therapy is not as effective as ketamine therapy. Recovery time and total sedation time are shorter with propofol than with other parenteral agents.** In the study by Godambe et al,[15] children receiving propofol-fentanyl therapy had higher OSBD-r scores (indicating greater observed distress during fracture reduction) than those receiving ketamine-midazolam therapy. Parent visual analog scale scores, nurse satisfaction, and orthopedists' satisfaction did not differ between the 2 groups. Total sedation time and recovery time were significantly shorter for propofol-fentanyl than for ketamine-midazolam.

Havel et al[17] found no differences in Ramsay sedation scores between propofol-morphine and midazolam-morphine in 89 patients. However, they did not specifically report sedation or pain scores at the time of fracture reduction. There was less recall of the event in the patients receiving midazolam-morphine therapy (9%) than in patients in the propofol-morphine group (21%). Recovery time and time to discharge favored propofol.

### IS PROPOFOL THERAPY SAFE?

**Propofol therapy is associated with more adverse events, particularly respiratory events and hypotension, than other parenteral agents.** Godambe et al[15] found that patients receiving propofol-fentanyl therapy had significantly more desaturation events (31% vs 7%; $P=.002$) and required more airway maneuvers (25% vs 2%; $P=.003$) than those who received ketamine-midazolam therapy. There was no significant difference between the 2 groups in the frequency of emergence agitation or emesis. In the study by Havel et al,[17] no difference was found in the incidence of complications when propofol-morphine therapy was compared with midazolam-morphine therapy, although the study may not have had enough power to detect a clinically important difference.

## COMMENT

There is no clear consensus on which pharmacological regimen is most effective for fracture reduction in the pediatric population.[12] In part, this is because there have been very few studies that have made direct comparisons between agents. Drawing conclusions from these studies is difficult, as many studies used different objective pain measures.

Bier blocks have been studied by many investigators and have the advantage of being associated with little risk of respiratory depression. Therefore, Bier blocks may be appropriate in centers that have less experience in managing a pediatric airway. However, Bier blocks require specialized equipment to prevent the transient neurologic sequelae associated with premature tourniquet release and do not provide anxiolysis. To date, to our knowledge, there have been no comparative studies of Bier block analgesia and parenteral sedation. The studies suggest that the most effective agent is lidocaine at a dose of 3 mg/kg.

Nitrous oxide provides the advantage of significantly shorter treatment times than other modalities. However, it is difficult to draw conclusions about the effectiveness of nitrous oxide given the very small number of patients studied in RCTs. Luhmann et al[25] recently reported results in abstract form of an RCT comparing ketamine-midazolam therapy with nitrous oxide–hematoma block. They found that patients in the nitrous oxide group had significantly less pain than those receiving ketamine, suggesting that nitrous oxide may be an excellent sedative option if combined with adequate analgesia.

Among the parenteral medications studied, the available evidence suggests that ketamine is the most effective and safest parenteral agent. However, ketamine is consistently associated with longer recovery times than other agents. Both of the RCTs in this review combined ketamine with midazolam. Other studies that have included nonorthopedic procedures in children have found that the addition of midazolam to ketamine does not reduce recovery agitation or alter the clinical effects of ketamine.[26,27] In addition, a recent practice guideline has recommended avoiding the use of coadministered benzodiazepines in most children because of the risk of additive respiratory depression.[28]

This study has several limitations. We included only studies that were written in the English language. In addition, there have been relatively few well-designed RCTs studying children who require sedation and analgesia for orthopedic procedures, including no RCTs evaluating etomidate for pediatric fracture reduction. The studies used different criteria for establishing the degree to which analgesia was achieved. Few studies used validated pain scores, and many that did were not adequately blinded. This makes it difficult to establish the relative efficacy of various interventions. It is also difficult to make firm statements about the relative safety of the different methods. Many studies reported no adverse events and did not go into detail about the mechanisms used for ascertainment of adverse events. In addition, many studies had a small enrollment. Therefore, it is difficult to make definitive statements about the safety of some of the treatment regimens. We deliberately chose to limit the reviewed studies to those that included children who required fracture reduction. Many other studies have examined the effectiveness and safety of various agents for other minor procedures; however, fracture reduction is the most painful routinely performed procedure in the pediatric population, and results gleaned from populations who were undergoing less painful procedures such as laceration repair may not be applicable to patients undergoing fracture reduction.

This systematic review identifies significant gaps in our knowledge about comparable efficacies of different sedative and analgesic modalities. Few high-quality RCTs have compared different agents, and even fewer provide validated, objective measures of pain. We were unable to perform a meta-analysis of the relative efficacies of the different treatment modalities. Future research should use a validated pain scoring system such as the Children's Hospital of Eastern Ontario Pain Score,[21] OSBD-r,[22,23] or Procedure Behavior Checklist[29] so that comparisons can be more readily made between studies. An ideal therapeutic regimen would be noninvasive, have short recovery times, and have minimal adverse effects. Although it appears from the current literature that ketamine is the superior agent for fracture reduction to date, ketamine, etomidate, propofol, and nitrous oxide all warrant further comparative study. Nitrous oxide may provide an excellent combination of attributes if combined with adequate local or regional analgesia.

**Accepted for Publication:** July 21, 2005.
**Correspondence:** Russell T. Migita, MD, Emergency Services, B-5520, Children's Hospital and Regional Medical Center, 4800 Sand Point Way NE, Seattle, WA 98105 (russ.migita@seattlechildrens.org).

## REFERENCES


1. Landin LA. Epidemiology of children's fractures. *J Pediatr Orthop B.* 1997;6:79-83.
2. Lyons RA, Sellstrom E, Delahunty AM, Loeb M, Varilo S. Incidence and cause of fractures in European districts. *Arch Dis Child.* 2000;82:452-455.
3. Stark AD, Bennet GC, Stone DH, Chishti P. Association between childhood fractures and poverty: population based study. *BMJ.* 2002;324:457.
4. Cheng JC, Ng BK, Sing SY, Lam PK. A 10-year study of the changes in the pattern and treatment of 6,493 fractures. *J Pediatr Orthop.* 1999;19:344-350.
5. Fosnocht DE, Heaps ND, Swanson ER. Patient expectations for pain relief in the ED. *Am J Emerg Med.* 2004;22:286-288.
6. Brown JC, Klein EJ, Lewis CW, Johnston BD, Cummings P. Emergency department analgesia for fracture pain. *Ann Emerg Med.* 2003;42:197-205.
7. Cimpello LB, Khine H, Avner JR. Practice patterns of pediatric versus general emergency physicians for pain management of fractures in pediatric patients. *Pediatr Emerg Care.* 2004;20:228-232.
8. Friedland LR, Kulick RM. Emergency department analgesic use in pediatric trauma victims with fractures. *Ann Emerg Med.* 1994;23:203-207.
9. Petrack EM, Christopher NC, Kriwinsky J. Pain management in the emergency department: patterns of analgesic utilization. *Pediatrics.* 1997;99:711-714.
10. Wilson JE. Oligoanalgesia in the emergency department. *Am J Emerg Med.* 1989;7:620-623.
11. Krauss B, Zurakowski D. Sedation patterns in pediatric and general community hospital emergency departments. *Pediatr Emerg Care.* 1998;14:99-103.
12. Kennedy RM, Luhmann JD, Luhmann SJ. Emergency department management of pain and anxiety related to orthopedic fracture care: a guide to analgesic techniques and procedural sedation in children. *Paediatr Drugs.* 2004;6:11-31.
13. Bratt HD, Eyres RL, Cole WG. Randomized double-blind trial of low- and moderate-dose lidocaine regional anesthesia for forearm fractures in childhood. *J Pediatr Orthop.* 1996;16:660-663.
14. Davidson AJ, Eyres RL, Cole WG. A comparison of prilocaine and lidocaine for intravenous regional anaesthesia for forearm fracture reduction in children. *Paediatr Anaesth.* 2002;12:146-150.
15. Godambe SA, Elliot V, Matheny D, Pershad J. Comparison of propofol/fentanyl versus ketamine/midazolam for brief orthopedic procedural sedation in a pediatric emergency department. *Pediatrics.* 2003;112:116-123.
16. Kennedy RM, Porter FL, Miller JP, Jaffe DM. Comparison of fentanyl/midazolam with ketamine/midazolam for pediatric orthopedic emergencies. *Pediatrics.* 1998;102:956-963.
17. Havel CJ, Strait RT, Hennes H. A clinical trial of propofol vs midazolam for procedural sedation in a pediatric emergency department. *Acad Emerg Med.* 1999;6:989-997.
18. Pierce MC, Fuchs S. Evaluation of ketorolac in children with forearm fractures. *Acad Emerg Med.* 1997;4:22-26.
19. Evans JK, Buckley SL, Alexander AH, Gilpin AT. Analgesia for the reduction of fractures in children: a comparison of nitrous oxide with intramuscular sedation. *J Pediatr Orthop.* 1995;15:73-77.
20. Gregory PR, Sullivan JA. Nitrous oxide compared with intravenous regional anesthesia in pediatric forearm fracture manipulation. *J Pediatr Orthop.* 1996;16:187-191.
21. McGrath PJ, Johnson G, Goodman JT, Schillinger J, Dunn J, Chapman JA. CHEOPS: a behavioral scale for rating postoperative pain in children. *Adv Pain Res Ther.* 1985;9:395-402.
22. Jay SM, Elliott C. Behavioral observation scales for measuring children's distress: the effects of increased methodological rigor. *J Consult Clin Psychol.* 1984;52:1106-1107.
23. Jay SM, Ozolins M, Elliott CH, Caldwell S. Assessment of children's distress during painful medical procedures. *Health Psychol.* 1983;2:133-147.
24. Wattenmaker I, Kasser JR, McGravey A. Self-administered nitrous oxide for fracture reduction in children in an emergency room setting. *J Orthop Trauma.* 1990;4:35-38.
25. Luhmann JD, Schootman M, Voytas L, Luhmann SJ, Kennedy RM. A comparison of ketamine/midazolam and nitrous oxide/hematoma block for forearm fracture reduction in children. Abstract presented at: Pediatric Academic Societies' Annual Meeting; May 1, 2004; San Francisco, Calif.
26. Sherwin TS, Green SM, Khan A, Chapman DS, Dannenberg B. Does adjunctive midazolam reduce recovery agitation after ketamine sedation for pediatric procedures? a randomized, double-blind, placebo-controlled trial. *Ann Emerg Med.* 2000;35:229-238.
27. Wathen JE, Roback MG, Mackenzie T, Bothner JP. Does midazolam alter the clinical effects of intravenous ketamine sedation in children? a double-blind, randomized, controlled emergency department trial. *Ann Emerg Med.* 2000;36:579-588.
28. Green SM, Krauss B. Clinical practice guideline for emergency department ketamine dissociative sedation in children. *Ann Emerg Med.* 2004;44:460-471.
29. LeBaron S, Zeltzer L. Assessment of acute pain and anxiety in children and adolescents by self-reports, observer reports, and a behavior checklist. *J Consult Clin Psychol.* 1984;52:729-738.

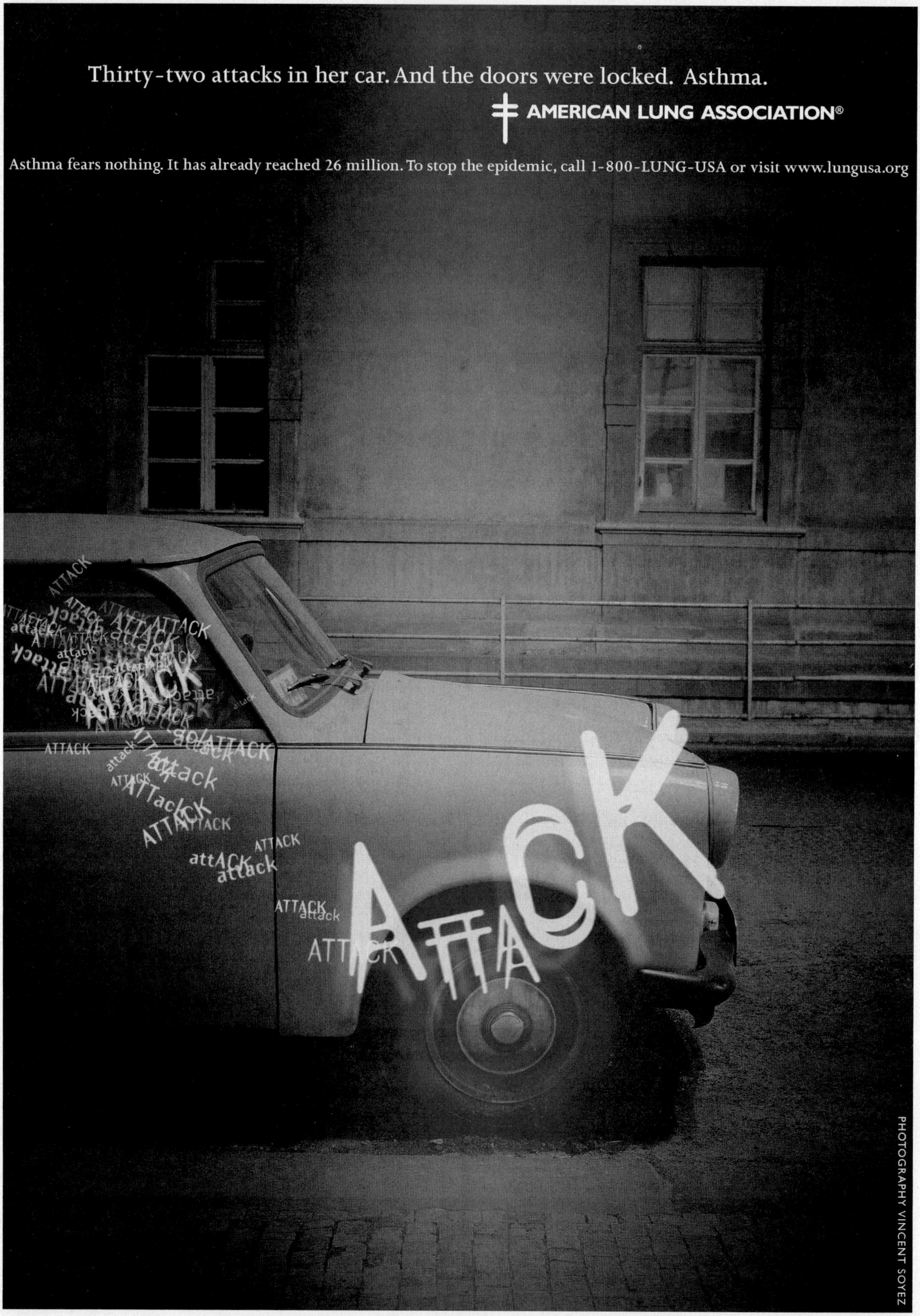
Thirty-two attacks in her car. And the doors were locked. Asthma.
AMERICAN LUNG ASSOCIATION®
Asthma fears nothing. It has already reached 26 million. To stop the epidemic, call 1-800-LUNG-USA or visit www.lungusa.org
ATTACK
PHOTOGRAPHY VINCENT SOYEZ

SECTION EDITOR: ALBERT C. YAN, MD; ASSISTANT SECTION EDITOR: SAMIR S. SHAH, MD

# Picture of the Month

*Ismail Reisli, MD; Sevgi Keles, MD; Umit Kamis, MD; Sefika Elmas, MD; Banu Turgut Ozturk, MD*

A 9-YEAR-OLD BOY WAS REFERRED TO OUR PEdiatric clinic for evaluation of inspiratory whoop, severe nocturnal coughing paroxysms of more than 2 weeks' duration, and worsening photophobia, severe bilateral eyelid ecchymosis, and red eye, despite administration of oral erythromycin (10 mg/kg, 4 times daily) for 1 week. The ophthalmologic examination revealed normal visual acuity, bilateral eyelid ecchymosis and edema, and conjunctival and corneal abnormalities (**Figure 1** and **Figure 2**). The fundus examination revealed no abnormal findings. No limitation of ocular movements was noted. Pupillary reflexes were normal. The complete blood cell count revealed an elevated white blood cell count of 30 400 cells/µL, with 60% lymphocytes. The erythrocyte sedimentation rate, platelet count, and coagulation test results were in the normal range. Orbital computed tomographic scans were negative for any malignancy. The abnormal findings at physical examination resolved over 3 weeks (**Figure 3**).

**Author Affiliations:** From the Pediatric Immunology and Allergy Division (Dr Reisli) and the Departments of Pediatrics (Drs Keles and Elmas) and Ophthalmology (Drs Kamis and Ozturk), Selçuk University Meram Medical Faculty, Konya, Turkey.

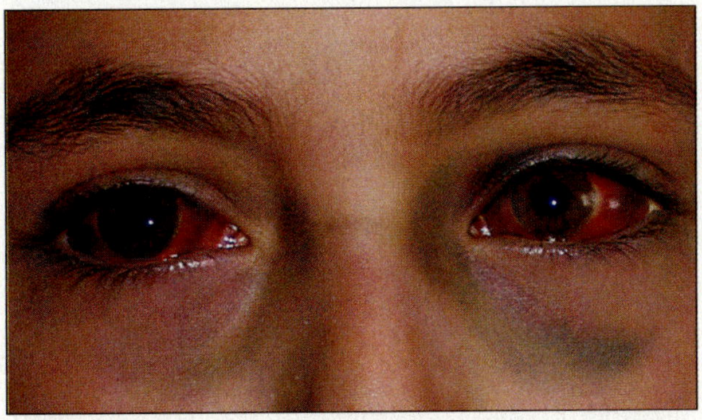

**Figure 1.** Note bilateral severe upper and lower eyelid ecchymoses, and subconjunctival hemorrhage covers the entire interpalpebral area.

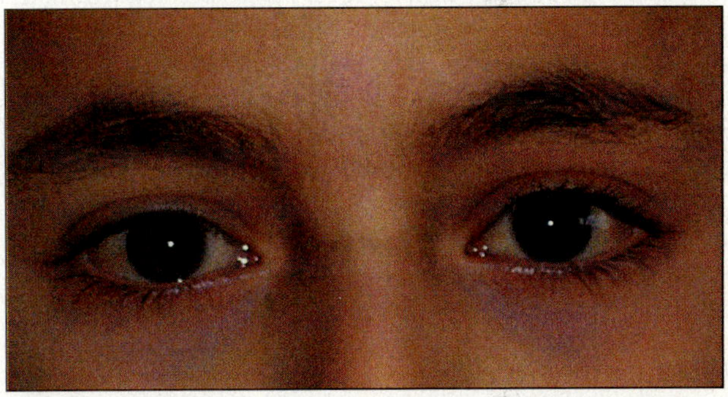

**Figure 3.** Eyelid ecchymoses and subconjunctival hemorrhages resolved over 3 weeks.

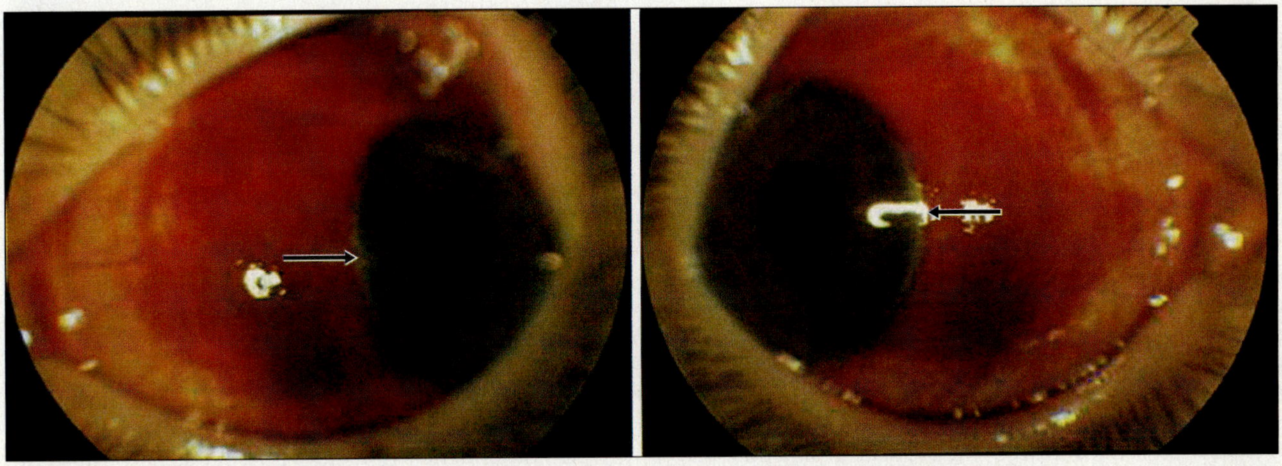

**Figure 2.** Bilateral local thinning (dellen) in the temporal peripheral cornea (arrows) is seen adjacent to the subconjunctival hemorrhages.

# Denouement and Discussion

## *Coughing Paroxysms Associated With Subconjunctival Hemorrhage and Dellen*

Subconjunctival hemorrhages are among the most frequent diagnoses in ophthalmology and commonly occur following trauma.[1] Simultaneous periorbital and subconjunctival hemorrhages are reported in a few diseases, including coagulopathic states, thrombocytopenia, trauma (occult or known), metastatic neuroblastoma, rhabdomyosarcoma, and leukemia.[2] Our patient had no history of trauma, coagulopathy, or blood dyscrasias. His only medical condition was mild persistent asthma, which was controlled with inhaled corticosteroid (400 μg/d). The coughing paroxysms suggested the cause of the subconjunctival hemorrhages and eyelid ecchymosis. Causes of coughing paroxysms are listed in **Table 1**.[3]

Although our patient had received all 4 scheduled pertussis vaccinations (diphtheria-pertussis-tetanus) and taken erythromycin for 1 week, we thought pertussis was the probable cause of the coughing paroxysms. The nasopharyngeal culture was negative for *Bordetella pertussis*; however, previously immunized patients are known to have a lower rate of positive cultures when infected. Patients previously treated with antibiotic agents may also have negative nasopharyngeal cultures for *B pertussis*. According to the clinical- and laboratory-confirmed case definitions of pertussis recently adopted by the Centers for Disease Control and Prevention in collaboration with the Council of State and Territorial Epidemiolologists (**Table 2**),[3] our patient met the criteria for diagnosis of probable pertussis.

Ophthalmologic complications of coughing paroxysms in pertussis infection include hemorrhages of the subconjunctival space, orbit, and anterior chamber, and, rarely, the retina and ocular adnexa.[2,4-6] The characteristic forceful coughing paroxysms associated with a strong Valsalva maneuver sufficiently explain all of the known associated ocular findings. The unexpected finding in our patient was the localized thinning areas in the periphery of the corneas or dellen. This is a unique case of coughing paroxysms associated with dellen secondary to subconjunctival hemorrhage.

Dellen may be observed as localized thinning in the cornea and the sclera, adjacent to corneal and conjunctival elevations such as subconjunctival hemorrhage, pterygium, limbal tumor, and postsurgical edema. They are thought to be localized in areas of dehydrations, owing to the surfacing abnormalities of the tears. In our patient, the extensive subconjunctival hemorrhage probably led to lack of wetting by the eyelids.

The diagnosis is obvious at slitlamp examination. Rapid onset, location adjacent to elevations, lack of infiltration, and coverage by intact epithelium differentiate these thinning areas from ulcerations. The diagnosis of dellen may also be confirmed during therapy. Just taping the eyelids closed may lead to improvement in 1 to 2 hours, and total disappearance will occur over 24 to 48 hours.[7] If hydration is not restored, the corneal stroma may undergo secondary degeneration leading to localized scarring and vascularization. Therefore, management should include treatment with artificial tears and lubricant supplements, eye patching, and close follow-up until the subconjunctival hemorrhage subsides. In our patient, dellen resolved in 5 days after supplemental therapy with artificial tears and lubricants. However, unilateral eye patching, with periodic alternation of which eye is patched, is recommended because bilateral eye patching is not easily tolerated. The therapy was continued for 3 weeks until the subconjunctival hemorrhages resolved. Elimination of the cause is mandatory for permanent recovery.[8]

Although dellen is usually innocuous and transient, it may be easily overlooked at penlight examination. Pediatricians should be aware of ocular complications of

**Table 1. Differential Diagnosis of Persistent Cough**

| |
|---|
| Viral infections |
| Adenovirus species |
| Influenza A and B |
| Respiratory syncytial virus |
| Rhinovirus |
| Bacterial infections |
| *Chlamydia pneumoniae* |
| *Streptococcus pneumoniae* |
| *Haemophilus influenzae* |
| Tuberculosis |
| Noninfectious causes |
| Cough variant asthma |
| Foreign body |
| Postnasal drip |
| Gastrointestinal reflux |
| Malignancy |

**Table 2. Case Definition for Pertussis***

| Variable |
|---|
| Clinical case definition |
| Cough illness lasting ≥2 weeks with one of the following: paroxysms of coughing, inspiratory whoop, or posttussive vomiting, without other apparent cause |
| Laboratory criteria for diagnosis |
| Isolation of *Bordetella pertussis* from clinical specimen or positive polymerase chain reaction for *B pertussis* |
| Case classification |
| *Probable case:* Meets the clinical case definition, is not laboratory confirmed, and is not epidemiologically linked to a laboratory-confirmed case |
| *Confirmed case:* Is laboratory confirmed or meets the clinical case definition and is either laboratory confirmed or epidemiologically linked to a laboratory-confirmed case |
| Comments |
| In outbreak settings, may be defined as cough illness lasting ≥2 weeks without other symptoms. Direct fluorescent antibody testing should not be relied on for laboratory confirmation. Serologic testing is not standardized and is not used for national reporting purposes |

*Modified from criteria developed by the Centers for Disease Control and Prevention and the Council of State and Territorial Epidemiologists.[3]

coughing paroxysm, especially if there is extensive subconjunctival hemorrhage disturbing distribution of the tear film layer.

**Accepted for Publication:** July 31, 2005.
**Correspondence:** Sevgi Keles, MD, Selçuk Üniversitesi Meram Tıp Fakültesi, Pediatri AD, 42080 Konya, Turkey (drsevgikeles@yahoo.com).

## REFERENCES


1. Fukuyama J, Hayasaka S, Yamada K, Setogawa T. Causes of subconjunctival hemorrhage. *Ophthalmologica*. 1990;200:63-67.
2. Paysse EA, Coats DK. Bilateral eyelid ecchymosis and subconjunctival hemorrhage associated with coughing paroxysms in pertussis infection. *J AAPOS*. 1998; 2:116-119.
3. Wright SW. Pertussis infections in adults. *South Med J*. 1998;91:702-708.
4. Batten FE. Complete ophthalmoplegia externa with blindness of acute onset. *BMJ*. 1903;1:249.
5. Gowring BW. A case of complete ophthalmoplegia occuring during whooping cough. *BMJ*. 1903;2:1638.
6. op de Coul ME, Budde JH. Diagnostic image (136): a boy with coughing fits and subconjunctival hemorrhage: subconjunctival hemorrhage secondary to whooping cough [in Dutch] [case report]. *Ned Tijdschr Geneeskd*. 2003;147:805.
7. Arffa RC. *Grayson's Diseases of the Cornea*. 3rd ed. St Louis, Mo: Mosby–Year Book Inc; 1991:319-321.
8. Kanski JJ. *Clinical Ophthalmology*. 4th ed. Oxford, England: Butterworth-Heinemann; 1999:117.

# Enabling Parents Who Smoke to Prevent Their Children From Initiating Smoking

## *Results From a 3-Year Intervention Evaluation*

*Christine Jackson, PhD; Denise Dickinson, MPH*

**Objective:** To evaluate effects of a home-based antismoking socialization program on the initiation of smoking among children whose parents smoke.

**Design:** Three-year randomized controlled trial.

**Participants:** Parents who were current smokers and had a child in the third grade who had not tried smoking were eligible; 873 parents-offspring pairs met these criteria, completed baseline interviews, and were randomly assigned to the intervention or control condition; 776 children (89%) completed an interview 3 years after baseline and were included in the study.

**Intervention:** During 3 months, the intervention group (n=371) received 5 printed activity guides, parenting tip sheets, child newsletters, and incentives; this group also received a booster activity guide 1 year later. The control group (n=405) received fact sheets about smoking.

**Results:** Initiation of smoking (first instance of puffing on a cigarette) was reported by 12% vs 19% of children in the intervention vs control groups. Logistic regression analysis indicated that children in the control condition had twice the odds of reporting initiation of smoking as children in the intervention condition (adjusted odds ratio, 2.16; $P<.001$), after adjusting for child sex, parent sex, parent race, parent educational achievement, child's best friends' smoking, parent smoking rate at baseline, and parent cessation status.

**Conclusion:** Children in the preinitiation phase of smoking who receive antismoking socialization from their parents are less likely to initiate smoking, even if their parents smoke.

*Arch Pediatr Adolesc Med. 2006;160:56-62*

**Author Affiliations:** Pacific Institute for Research and Evaluation, Chapel Hill Center, Chapel Hill, NC.

ALTHOUGH THE UPPER LIMIT of the age range used to define early initiation of smoking has varied across studies,[1-6] there is consensus that youth who first try smoking by age 12 years are early initiators. A comparison of prevalence estimates across studies[3-6] indicates that about 10% of 8-year-old (third grade) children, 18% to 24% of 10-year-old (fifth-grade) children, and 35% to 40% of 12-year-old (seventh-grade) children have tried smoking.

*For editorial comment see page 102*

Studies[1-3,7-11] have found strong positive associations between the initiation of smoking during childhood and habitual smoking later in life. These studies measured the age at initiation by asking adolescents[3,7-9] or young adults[1,10,11] to recall their age at first use. Despite the limitations of a retrospective assessment, the strength and consistency of the findings from these studies support the assertion that those who initiate smoking in childhood are significantly more likely to report advanced stages of smoking by late adolescence. Prospective evidence of an association between initiation during childhood and later use was obtained in a cohort study[12] of subjects who were surveyed at ages 8 through 10 years, and again at age 17 years; early cigarette use was a significant predictor of progression to advanced stages of smoking. These prospective data corroborate the results of earlier retrospective investigations of the early onset of smoking.[1-3,7-11] Together, these studies implicate the initiation of smoking in childhood as a primary risk factor for lifetime smoking.

## ANTISMOKING SOCIALIZATION

Antismoking socialization is defined as parent-child interactions that influence the development of children's cognitive and behavioral norms against smoking.[13-16] Using communication, rule setting, monitoring, guided experience, and other methods of child socialization, parents can influence children's perceptions of the prevalence of smoking, the acceptability of smoking, and the personal and social consequences of smoking. Antismoking socialization is substantially more than telling children that they should not smoke. From the child's perspective, antismoking socialization involves internalization of attitudinal and behavioral norms against initiation of smoking, acceptance of parental monitoring of access to cigarettes and affiliation with peers who have tried smoking, expectations of negative consequences for trying smoking, and expectations of positive consequences for not smoking. Antismoking socialization is a broader concept than parental attitude about smoking, which has been studied extensively.[17-19]

Few parents engage in antismoking socialization; in fact, prosmoking socialization is not uncommon.[14-16] Moreover, parental complacency is not devoid of a socializing effect; children commonly interpret parental nonresponse as tacit approval or lack of disapproval.[20] At best, the absence of antismoking socialization leaves children to perceive experimentation with smoking as an activity that lies outside the realm of overt parental concern and active parental influence.

It is reasonable to assert that parents who smoke can do little to dissuade their children from smoking. The present study, however, rested on the opposite assumption. Although smokers model smoking behavior, we reasoned that being a smoker does not preclude a parent from eliminating a child's exposure to passive smoke, talking to a child about smoking, making cigarettes inaccessible, monitoring the smoking behavior of children and their friends, and making clear the disciplinary consequences of smoking. In the present study, we evaluated whether exposure to an intervention that is designed to promote these antismoking socialization activities by parents who smoke could reduce children's likelihood of initiating smoking.

### INTERVENTION PROGRAM

Focus groups, a pilot study, and consultations with children, parents, and third-grade teachers were used to develop a home-based program called Smoke-free Kids. The program comprised 6 printed activity guides to meet the intervention objectives. Five guides were delivered in sequence after baseline data collection; the sixth guide was a booster, delivered 1 year after baseline. Examples of the intervention guides and activities can be viewed at the project's Web site (http://www.familyhealthresearch.org). The intervention also included a series of tip sheets focused on parenting skills and a series of newsletters for children. Incentives (eg, wristbands and yo-yos) were given to thank children for participating and to encourage submissions to the newsletters. Other incentives (eg, children's cameras and backpacks) were donated by local merchants and were given as prizes in program contests.

### PROGRAM EVALUATION

An earlier evaluation of the Smoke-free Kids intervention[21] showed that the intervention increased parental engagement in antismoking socialization 3 months after intervention and reduced child susceptibility to smoking 2 years after baseline. The database used for this earlier evaluation included only families for whom we had parent and child data at the 3-month and 24-month follow-ups (N=671). The database used for the present report included all children in the intervention or control condition with outcome data at 36 months (N=776). The present study used these data to test the primary hypothesis of the Smoke-free Kids intervention, namely, that children exposed to a program of antismoking socialization by parents who smoke will be significantly less likely than control subjects to initiate smoking by the sixth grade.

## METHODS

### PARTICIPANT RECRUITMENT

A volunteer sample was recruited. Administrators of 28 school districts allowed project staff to request that school principals disseminate institutional review board–approved recruitment materials. These districts were located in North Carolina, South Carolina, and Colorado, with 15, 3, and 10 districts per state, respectively. The role of these districts was limited to disseminating recruitment materials. Materials were mailed to elementary school principals with a letter that documented district cooperation. Principals were asked to distribute the materials to third-grade teachers, with the request that they send the materials home with students. Interested parents could enroll in the study with a child by mailing a signed consent form to the project office.

This voluntary recruitment method precluded obtaining an estimate of the response rate among eligible persons (ie, the self-enrolled number divided by the total number eligible). Obtaining a valid estimate of the denominator would have required a separate probability-based survey that measured the rate of smoking among parents of third-grade students in districts where recruitment occurred.

Parents who reported current smoking at baseline and who had a child in the third grade (ages 7-8 years) who had not tried smoking were eligible. The eligibility of those submitting consent forms (n=1147) was checked during telephone calls to complete the baseline interviews before randomization. During this procedure, 135 households could not be reached by telephone, and 125 (12%) of 1012 households that were reached did not meet the eligibility criteria (41 parents were nonsmokers, 2 children were not in the third grade, and 82 children reported having tried smoking), leaving 887 parents and children who completed baseline assessments and were randomized to a condition. During follow-up data collection, 14 children were found to have logic errors in their self-reported smoking status (eg, reporting abstinence at baseline and later reporting that a first puff occurred in the second grade or earlier). Because the reliability of their smoking status report was in question, these 14 children were reassigned as not eligible, leaving 873 children eligible. Of these, 776 (89%) completed a 3-year postbaseline interview and were included in the present study.

### INTERVENTION PROTOCOL

During the baseline year, participants in the intervention condition received the 5 core activity guides mailed to their homes at approximate 2-week intervals. Delivery of newsletters, tip sheets, and incentives was timed as appropriate to complement or reinforce each program guide.

Participants in the control condition received brief fact sheets with content that pertained to macrolevel variables relevant to youth smoking but not targeted by the intervention program (eg, cost of cigarettes and sales to minors). Five fact sheets were mailed to controls, one each time an activity guide was sent to participants in the intervention condition.

## SURVEY PROTOCOL

Telephone interview data were obtained from parents and children at baseline and from the children only at follow-up. At baseline, children were interviewed before their parents to avoid the possibility that the parent interview would influence parental behavior about smoking and thereby influence children's responses. Interviewers were blinded to the study condition of participants.

### Child Interview

The children's interviews were administered by staff who had at least 2 years of experience working with children and had completed 30 hours of training. The training covered ethical treatment of human subjects, reading the assent transcript, standardizing the pace of reading, and reading with a voice that did not give any hint of agreement or disagreement with responses.

Parents provided verbal consent before interviewers spoke with their children (this was in addition to the signed parental consent). This procedure included requesting that the parent "Ask your child to go sit somewhere that's quiet, let your child know that it's okay with you if he/she answers our questions about smoking, and let your child know that he/she won't have to discuss any answers after the interview ends. Please tell your child that it is okay with you if he/she sits and answers our questions privately." After providing nonbinding verbal assent, children were asked by the interviewer to move to a place that was private, comfortable, and without obvious distractions. The actual interview took about 20 minutes to complete.

### Parent Interview

Computer-assisted telephone interviews were administered to parents by a contracted survey research unit. The interviewers were jointly trained and supervised by us and by the coordinator of the research unit.

## MEASURES

### Eligibility Status at Baseline

Parents were considered eligible smokers if they had smoked at least 100 cigarettes in their lifetime and they had smoked at least 1 cigarette per week in the presence of their child (parents who said that they tried to hide their smoking from their child were not enrolled in the study). Children were considered eligible never smokers if they had never puffed on a cigarette. This widely used measure of initiation was selected based on a reliability study[22] of elementary school children's self-reported initiation of smoking. Children's consistency was evaluated by looking for logic errors between baseline and the 1-year follow-up. Almost all children (98%) provided reliable reports of "ever smoking, even one puff" during 1 year. The results of these and other analyses reported in that study[22] corroborate the results of another reliability study,[23] which found that youth are highly consistent over time in their reporting of smoking behavior.

### Dependent Variable

Initiation of smoking was defined as having ever puffed on a cigarette. Although puffing on a cigarette does not indicate regular smoking, it is the first instance of lifetime smoking. As such, it marks an important transition in children's risk of progression toward habitual smoking. Initiation of smoking at the 36-month follow-up was measured using the same method as for the assessment of initiation status at baseline.

### Covariates

Attributes of the child and of the parent smoker who enrolled the child were measured. These included child sex, relationship of the parent smoker to the child (the category of "mothers" comprised biological mothers, stepmothers, and other female guardians; and likewise for the category of "fathers"), parent race (white or nonwhite), parent educational achievement (high school or less or $\geq$1 year of college), smoking by the child's best friends (no friends initiated or $\geq$1 friend initiated), and parent smoking rate ($<$1 pack/d or $\geq$1 pack/d).

## STATISTICAL ANALYSIS

$\chi^2$ Analyses were used to test for attrition bias by comparing participants retained during 3 years (N=776) with participants who were lost to follow-up (n=97) and to evaluate the equivalence of the intervention and control groups based on demographic and smoking-specific variables. Logistic regression analyses were used to test whether the program affected initiation of smoking by the sixth grade. To develop the multivariate models, preliminary analyses were performed to determine which interaction terms should be included. We evaluated whether any of the covariates moderated the effect of program exposure on the initiation of smoking. None of these interaction terms was significant. Therefore, in the multivariate model used to estimate the intervention effect, the initiation of smoking was regressed at step 1 on the covariates and at step 2 on a dichotomous indicator of study condition. With intervention as the referent, the odds ratios (ORs) indicate the odds of initiation of smoking among control children relative to intervention children.

# RESULTS

## STUDY SAMPLE

Of the 776 children retained through follow-up, 53% were girls and all were in the second half of their sixth-grade year when the outcome data were collected (**Table 1**). Most parents (80%) who enrolled were mothers or other maternal figures, and the mean age was 36.6 years. Distributions by parent race, parent educational achievement, smoking by the child's best friends, parental smoking rate at baseline, and parental cessation status at follow-up are also given in the table.

## ATTRITION ANALYSIS

Attrition analyses compared the 97 participants lost to follow-up with the 776 participants retained during 3 years. There was no association between attrition status

**Table 1. Sample Description and Comparisons of the Intervention vs Control Groups at Baseline***

| Variable | Total Sample (N = 776) | Intervention Group (n = 371) | Control Group (n = 405) | $\chi^2$ Value | *P* Value |
|---|---|---|---|---|---|
| Child sex | | | | | |
| Female | **408** (52.6) | 206 (55.5) | 202 (49.9) | 2.5 | .12 |
| Male | **368** (47.4) | 165 (44.5) | 203 (50.1) | | |
| Parent relationship to child | | | | | |
| Father | **158** (20.4) | 75 (20.2) | 83 (20.5) | 0.009 | .92 |
| Mother | **618** (79.6) | 296 (79.8) | 322 (79.5) | | |
| Parent race | | | | | |
| White | **572** (76.3) | 265 (73.8) | 307 (78.5) | 2.3 | .13 |
| Nonwhite | **178** (23.7) | 94 (26.2) | 84 (21.5) | | |
| Parent educational achievement | | | | | |
| ≤ High school | **273** (36.1) | 145 (40.1) | 128 (32.5) | 4.7 | .03 |
| ≥1 y of College | **483** (63.9) | 217 (59.9) | 266 (67.5) | | |
| Smoking by ≥1 of child's best friends | | | | | |
| No | **611** (79.6) | 299 (81.3) | 312 (78.0) | 1.2 | .27 |
| Yes | **157** (20.4) | 69 (18.8) | 88 (22.0) | | |
| Parent smoking rate at baseline, pack/d | | | | | |
| <1 | **426** (54.9) | 208 (56.1) | 218 (53.8) | 0.4 | .53 |
| ≥1 | **350** (45.1) | 163 (43.9) | 187 (46.2) | | |
| Parent cessation status at follow-up | | | | | |
| Cessation reported | **113** (15.1) | 48 (13.3) | 65 (16.7) | 1.7 | .15 |
| No change reported | **637** (84.9) | 313 (86.7) | 324 (83.3) | | |

*Data are given as number (percentage) unless otherwise indicated. The numbers of subjects are less than the total numbers of subjects for some variables because of missing data.

and demographic attributes. The attrition rate (11.1% overall) varied only slightly (from 10.3% to 11.7%) across the categories of child sex, parent relationship to the child, parent race, and parent educational achievement. Similarly, attrition was equally likely within subgroups defined by smoking by 1 or more of the child's best friends, parent smoking rate, and parent cessation status at follow-up. The only deviation from this pattern occurred for study condition; the loss to follow-up was higher in the intervention group (12.9%) than in the control group (9.4%), although this difference was not significant ($\chi^2$=2.72, *P*=.09).

## GROUP EQUIVALENCE ANALYSIS

A preliminary analysis of data from children in the study sample (N=776) tested whether the intervention (n=371) and control (n=405) groups differed in ways that could account for differences in the study outcome. The results (Table 1) indicated that control group children were significantly more likely than intervention group children to have parents who had attended college (68% vs 60%; $\chi^2$=4.68, *P*=.03). Given the expected inverse association between parent educational achievement and child smoking, this difference would exert a conservative effect on the assessment of intervention effect on the initiation of smoking. For all other comparisons, there were no significant differences between the intervention and control groups.

## INTERVENTION EFFECT

Before the multivariate analysis, the bivariate association between each covariate and the study outcome was assessed (**Table 2**). Consistent with previous findings of risk factors for youth smoking,[24] the smoking status of the child's best friends had the strongest association with initiation of smoking. Initiation was reported by 12% of children who reported that no best friends had tried smoking vs 29% of children who had 1 or more best friends who had tried smoking. The parent smoking rate at baseline also had a significant association with the initiation of smoking at follow-up.

The bivariate association between study condition and the study outcome showed that 12% vs 19% of children in the intervention vs control groups reported initiation of smoking at follow-up ($\chi^2$=8.1, *P*<.001).

The intervention effect was estimated using the intent-to-treat model. Initiation of smoking was regressed first on the study covariates (partial model) and then on the dichotomous indicator of study condition (full model) (**Table 3**). The adjusted OR for study condition (OR, 2.16 [95% confidence interval, 1.39-3.37]; *P*<.001) indicates that children in the control condition were twice as likely as children in the intervention condition to report initiation of smoking 3 years after baseline. A comparison of the partial and full presentation of the regression model shows a significant increase in $\chi^2$ value owing to study condition (omnibus test of model coefficients, $\chi^2$=31.5, *P*<.001 for the partial model; and $\chi^2$=44.0, *P*<.001 for the full model). In addition, this comparison shows that the ORs for the control variables changed only slightly when the study condition was added to the model, indicating that the effect of the study condition on the initiation of smoking was independent of these control variables. Overall, this analysis indicates that exposure to the intervention had a significant, independent, and protective effect on the odds of the initiation of smoking at follow-up.

**Table 2. Bivariate Associations Between Predictor Variables and Initiation of Smoking***

| Variable | No. | Initiated Smoking, % | $\chi^2$ Value | *P* Value |
|---|---|---|---|---|
| Child sex | | | | |
| Female | 408 | 14.7 | 0.7 | .41 |
| Male | 368 | 16.8 | | |
| Parent relationship to child | | | | |
| Father | 158 | 12.0 | | |
| Mother | 618 | 16.7 | 2.0 | .15 |
| Parent race | | | | |
| White | 572 | 14.5 | 3.3 | .07 |
| Nonwhite | 178 | 20.2 | | |
| Parent educational achievement | | | | |
| ≤ High school | 273 | 18.7 | 3.1 | .08 |
| ≥1 y of college | 483 | 13.9 | | |
| Smoking by ≥1 of child's best friends | | | | |
| No | 611 | 12.3 | 27.3 | <.001 |
| Yes | 157 | 29.3 | | |
| Parent smoking rate at baseline, pack/d | | | | |
| <1 | 426 | 18.3 | 4.8 | .03 |
| ≥1 | 350 | 12.6 | | |
| Parent cessation status at follow-up | | | | |
| Cessation reported | 113 | 13.3 | 0.3 | .56 |
| No change reported | 637 | 15.4 | | |
| Study condition | | | | |
| Intervention group | 371 | 11.9 | 8.1 | <.001 |
| Control group | 405 | 19.3 | | |

*The numbers of subjects are less than the total numbers of subjects for some variables because of missing data.

## COMMENT

In a feasibility study, Ary et al[25] recorded conversations about avoiding tobacco use among parent-daughter dyads and found that the conversations were perceived as nonaversive and helpful by most parents and daughters. These investigators concluded that the next important research question was whether such conversations with parents can discourage young people from using tobacco. In a prospective study of naturally occurring parental antismoking socialization, Chassin et al[26] studied 182 mother-offspring pairs and found that offspring exposed to smoking-specific discussion and punishment were significantly less likely to initiate smoking. Based on this finding, Chassin et al recommended enlisting socialization by mothers as a smoking prevention strategy. The antismoking socialization program tested in the present study directly addressed the recommendations of Ary et al and Chassin et al, although the focus on parents who were smokers was unique to this investigation.

This study found that the Smoke-free Kids intervention reduced the likelihood that children of parents who smoke would initiate smoking by the sixth grade. Whereas 19% of children in the control condition had tried smoking by sixth grade, 12% of children in the intervention condition had done so. The 2.16 adjusted OR associated with this effect indicated that the control group was twice as likely to report having tried smoking. This effect was adjusted for sex of the parent who modeled smoking, child's best friends' smoking, parent smoking rate, parent cessation of smoking, and other predictors of youth smoking behavior.

That parents who smoke can be effective agents of antismoking socialization might seem counterintuitive. Indeed, one could question whether this finding is simply a research anomaly. Multiple studies of antismoking socialization interventions for parents who smoke are needed before the replicability and generalizability of this effect are known.[27] Other research studies that support the notion that parents who smoke can exert a protective antismoking effect on offspring are highlighted herein.

Investigators for nonintervention studies[13,14,26,28-31] of antismoking socialization have reported inverse associations between antismoking socialization and the risk of smoking among offspring. Some of these studies[13,14,26,30,31] found inverse associations even if the parents were smokers. In 1 study,[30] adolescents in the experimental phase of smoking who perceived strong parental disapproval of their smoking were less than half as likely to progress to established smoking as peers who did not hold that perception; the effects of parental disapproval were as strong for parents who smoked as for parents who did not smoke. More recently, an analysis of a population-based cohort of 3555 high school seniors showed that parental antismoking actions, such as restrictive rules in the home, had significant inverse associations with adolescents' odds of daily smoking, even if the parents were smokers.[31] In brief, the results of nonintervention studies[13,14,26,30,31] suggest that, if parents who smoke provide antismoking socialization, offspring will be less likely to smoke during childhood and adolescence. The results of the of the present study are consistent with this body of work.

The results of this study leave several questions unanswered: Which elements of the program accounted for the intervention effect? Could exposure to antismoking

**Table 3. Initiation of Smoking Regressed on Covariates and Study Condition***

| Variable | Partial Model | | Full Model | |
|---|---|---|---|---|
| | OR (95% CI) | *P* Value | OR (95% CI) | *P* Value |
| Child sex | | | | |
| Female | Referent | | Referent | .71 |
| Male | 1.11 (0.73-1.69) | .62 | 1.08 (0.71-1.66) | |
| Parent relationship to child | | | | |
| Father | Referent | | Referent | .04 |
| Mother | 1.94 (1.01-3.70) | .04 | 1.98 (1.03-3.81) | |
| Parent race | | | | |
| White | Referent | | Referent | .48 |
| Nonwhite | 1.12 (0.69-1.84) | .63 | 1.19 (0.73-1.97) | |
| Parent education | | | | |
| ≤ High school | Referent | | Referent | .08 |
| ≥1 y of college | 0.73 (0.48-1.13) | .16 | 0.68 (0.44-1.05) | |
| Smoking by ≥1 of child's best friends | | | | |
| No | Referent | | Referent | <.001 |
| Yes | 2.62 (1.66-4.13) | <.001 | 2.61 (1.65-4.12) | |
| Parent smoking rate at baseline, pack/d | | | | |
| <1 | Referent | | Referent | .06 |
| ≥1 | 0.65 (0.41-1.03) | .07 | 0.63 (0.40-1.01) | |
| Parent cessation status at follow-up | | | | |
| Cessation reported | Referent | | Referent | .39 |
| No change reported | 1.26 (0.67-2.35) | .46 | 1.31 (0.70-2.46) | |
| Study condition | | | | |
| Intervention group | — | — | Referent | <.001 |
| Control group | — | — | 2.16 (1.39-3.37) | |

Abbreviations: CI, 95% confidence interval; OR, odds ratio; dash, not applicable.
*Data from 750 participants were analyzed.

socialization during the elementary school years bolster the effect of middle school prevention programs, which have not had sustained effects on youth smoking?[32-34] Another issue is how to persuade parents who smoke to get involved in antismoking socialization. From our research, we know that parents who smoke are difficult to recruit. This is likely because of several factors, including low self-efficacy driven by concerns about hypocrisy and a desire to avoid experiences that could heighten feelings of guilt and worry about one's smoking. Research is needed to identify audience segments within the population of parents who smoke and to test messages designed to persuade parents in these segments that antismoking socialization is feasible for them and potentially beneficial for their children.

Limitations of the study are its design and method, which limit the external validity of the findings. By using a volunteer sample, the findings are generalizable only to adult smokers who are receptive to the opportunity to engage in antismoking socialization. With 3 years of follow-up, this study measured only the effects of antismoking socialization on children's initial experience with smoking. Longer-term follow-up with assessment of subsequent phases of smoking is needed to evaluate the duration of the effect.

## CONCLUSIONS

Children in the preinitiation phase of smoking who are exposed to antismoking socialization from their parents are less likely to try smoking, even if their parents smoke. The Smoke-free Kids intervention is a tool that parents who smoke can use to increase the range, intensity, and specificity of antismoking socialization activities to which their children are exposed.

**Accepted for Publication:** September 1, 2005.
**Correspondence:** Christine Jackson, PhD, Pacific Institute for Research and Evaluation, Chapel Hill Center, 1516 E Franklin St, Suite 200, Chapel Hill, NC 27514 (cjackson@pire.org).
**Funding/Support:** This study was supported by grant RFA CA97010 from the National Cancer Institute and the National Institute of Nursing Research, Bethesda, and the National Institute of Child Health and Human Development, Rockville, Md; and by grant R01 HD36514 from the National Institute of Child Health and Human Development.
**Acknowledgment:** We thank the many children and parents who made this study possible.

## REFERENCES

1. Breslau N, Peterson EL. Smoking cessation in young adults: age at initiation of cigarette smoking and other suspected influences. *Am J Public Health.* 1996; 86:214-220.
2. US Department of Health and Human Services. *Preventing Tobacco Use Among Young People: A Report of the Surgeon General.* Washington, DC: US Dept of Health and Human Services; 1994.
3. Johnston LD, O'Malley PM, Bachman JG. *National Survey Results on Drug Use From the Monitoring the Future Study, 1975-1992.* Rockville, Md: National Institute on Drug Abuse; 1993.
4. Jackson C, Henriksen L, Dickinson D, Levine DW. The early use of alcohol and tobacco: its relation to children's competence and parents' behavior. *Am J Public Health.* 1997;87:359-364.

5. De Moor C, Elder JP, Young RL, Wildey MB, Molgaard CA. Generic tobacco use among four ethnic groups in a school age population. *J Drug Educ.* 1989;19:257-270.
6. Cohen RY, Sattler J, Felix MR, Brownell KD. Experimentation with smokeless tobacco and cigarettes by children and adolescents: relationship to beliefs, peer use, and parental use. *Am J Public Health.* 1987;77:1454-1456.
7. Ershler J, Leventhal H, Fleming R, Glynn K. The quitting experience for smokers in sixth through twelfth grades. *Addict Behav.* 1989;14:365-378.
8. Chassin L, Presson CC, Sherman SJ, Edwards DA. The natural history of cigarette smoking: predicting young-adult smoking outcomes from adolescent smoking patterns. *Health Psychol.* 1990;9:701-716.
9. DuRant RH, Smith JA, Kreiter SR, Krowchuk DP. The relationship between early age of onset of initial substance use and engaging in multiple health risk behaviors among young adolescents. *Arch Pediatr Adolesc Med.* 1999;153:286-291.
10. Kandel DB, Yamaguchi K, Chen K. Stages of progression in drug involvement from adolescence to adulthood: further evidence for the gateway theory. *J Stud Alcohol.* 1992;53:447-457.
11. Robins LN, Przybeck TR. Age of onset of drug use as a factor in drug and other disorders. In: Jones CL, Battjes RJ, eds. *Etiology of Drug Abuse: Implications for Prevention.* Rockville, Md: National Institute on Drug Abuse; 1985:178-191. NIDA Research Monograph 56.
12. Jackson C, Dickinson D. Cigarette consumption during childhood and persistence of smoking through adolescence. *Arch Pediatr Adolesc Med.* 2004;158:1050-1056.
13. Jackson C, Henriksen L. Do as I say: parent smoking, anti-smoking socialization, and smoking onset among children. *Addict Behav.* 1997;22:107-114.
14. Henriksen L, Jackson C. Antismoking socialization: relationship to parent and child smoking status. *Health Commun.* 1998;10:87-101.
15. Fearnow M, Chassin L, Presson CC, Sherman SJ. Determinants of parental attempts to deter their children's cigarette smoking. *J Appl Dev Psychol.* 1998;19:453-468.
16. Clark PI, Scarisbrick-Hauser A, Gautam SP, Wirk SJ. Anti-tobacco socialization in homes of African-American and white parents, and smoking and nonsmoking parents. *J Adolesc Health.* 1999;24:329-339.
17. Nolte AE, Smith BJ, O'Rourke T. The relative importance of parental attitudes and behavior upon youth smoking behavior. *J Sch Health.* 1983;53:264-271.
18. Eiser JR, Morgan M, Gammage P, Gray E. Adolescent smoking: attitudes, norms and parental influence. *Br J Soc Psychol.* 1989;28(pt 3):193-202.
19. Webster RA, Hunter M, Keats JA. Peer and parental influences on adolescents' substance use: a path analysis. *Int J Addictions.* 1994;29:647-657.
20. Baumrind D, Moselle KA. A developmental perspective on adolescent drug abuse. *Adv Alcohol Subst Abuse.* 1985;4:41-67.
21. Jackson C, Dickinson D. Can parents who smoke socialize their children against smoking? results from the Smoke-free Kids intervention trial. *Tobacco Control.* 2003;12:52-59.
22. Henriksen L, Jackson C. Reliability of children's self-reported cigarette smoking. *Addict Behav.* 1999;24:271-277.
23. Brener ND, Collins JL, Kann L, Warren CW, Williams BI. Reliability of the youth risk behavior survey questionnaire. *Am J Epidemiol.* 1995;141:575-580.
24. Bauman KE, Carver K, Gleiter K. Trends in parent and friend influence during adolescence: the case of adolescent cigarette smoking. *Addict Behav.* 2001;26:349-361.
25. Ary DV, James L, Biglan A. Parent-daughter discussions to discourage tobacco use: feasibility and content. *Adolescence.* 1999;34:275-282.
26. Chassin L, Presson CC, Todd M, Rose JS, Sherman SJ. Maternal socialization of adolescent smoking: the intergenerational transmission of parenting and smoking. *Dev Psychol.* 1998;34:1189-1201.
27. Johnson BT, Eagly AH. Quantitative synthesis of social psychological research. In: Reis H, Judd C, eds. *Handbook of Research Methods in Social Psychology.* New York, NY: Cambridge University Press; 2000:496-528.
28. Distefan JM, Gilpin EA, Choi WS, Pierce JP. Parental influences predict adolescent smoking in the United States, 1989-1993. *J Adolesc Health.* 1998;22:466-474.
29. Chassin L, Presson CC, Rose JS, Sherman SJ. Maternal socialization of adolescent smoking: the intergenerational transmission of smoking-related beliefs. *Psychol Addict Behav.* 1998;12:206-216.
30. Sargent JD, Dalton M. Does parental disapproval of smoking prevent adolescents from becoming established smokers? *Pediatrics.* 2001;108:1256-1262.
31. Andersen MR, Leroux BG, Bricker JB, Kumar BJ, Peterson AV. Antismoking parenting practices are associated with reduced rates of adolescent smoking. *Arch Pediatr Adolesc Med.* 2004;158:348-352.
32. Peterson AV, Kealey KA, Mann SL, Marek PM, Sarason IG. Hutchinson Smoking Prevention Project: long-term randomized trial in school-based tobacco use prevention: results on smoking. *J Natl Cancer Inst.* 2000;92:1979-1991.
33. Rohrbach LA, Howard-Pitney B, Unger JB, et al. Independent evaluation of the California Tobacco Control Program: relationships between program exposure and outcomes, 1996-1998. *Am J Public Health.* 2002;92:975-984.
34. Wiehe S, Garrison M, Christakis D, Ebel B, Rivara F. A systematic review of school-based smoking prevention trials with long-term follow-up. *J Adolesc Health.* 2005;36:162-169.

Convulsions, infantile: alcohol has remarkable power in arresting convulsions of teething, try small doses of wine or brandy.

—From *Materia Medica Pharmacy and Therapeutics*, 1906

**PEDIARIX™ [Diphtheria and Tetanus Toxoids and Acellular Pertussis Adsorbed, Hepatitis B (Recombinant) and Inactivated Poliovirus Vaccine Combined]**

The following is a brief summary only; see full prescribing information for complete product information.

**CONTRAINDICATIONS:** Hypersensitivity to any component of the vaccine, including yeast, neomycin, and polymyxin B, is a contraindication (see DESCRIPTION in complete prescribing information). Do not use PEDIARIX after a serious allergic reaction (e.g., anaphylaxis) temporally associated with a previous dose of this vaccine or with any components of this vaccine. Because of the uncertainty as to which component of the vaccine might be responsible, do not give further vaccination with any of these components; or, refer such individuals to an allergist for evaluation. The following events are contraindications to administration of PEDIARIX: encephalopathy (e.g., coma, decreased level of consciousness, prolonged seizures) within 7 days of administration of a previous dose of a pertussis-containing vaccine that is not attributable to another identifiable cause; progressive neurologic disorder, including infantile spasms, uncontrolled epilepsy, or progressive encephalopathy. Do not vaccinate individuals with such conditions until a treatment regimen has been established and the condition has stabilized. PEDIARIX is not contraindicated for use in individuals with HIV infection.

**WARNINGS:** Administration of PEDIARIX is associated with higher rates of fever relative to separately administered vaccines. In one study that evaluated medically attended fever after the first dose of PEDIARIX or separately administered vaccines, infants who received PEDIARIX had a higher rate of medical encounters for fever within the first 4 days following vaccination. In some infants, these encounters included the performance of diagnostic studies to evaluate other causes of fever (see ADVERSE REACTIONS). The vial stopper is latex-free. The tip cap and the rubber plunger of the needleless prefilled syringes contain dry natural latex rubber that may cause allergic reactions in latex sensitive individuals. If any of the following events occur in temporal relation to receipt of whole-cell DTP or a vaccine containing an acellular pertussis component, consider carefully whether to give subsequent doses of PEDIARIX or any vaccine containing a pertussis component: temperature of ≥40.5°C (105°F) within 48 hours not due to another identifiable cause; collapse or shock-like state (hypotonic-hyporesponsive episode) within 48 hours; persistent, inconsolable crying lasting ≥3 hours, occurring within 48 hours; seizures with or without fever occurring within 3 days. If Guillain-Barré syndrome occurs within 6 weeks of receipt of prior vaccine containing tetanus toxoid, the decision to give subsequent doses of PEDIARIX or any vaccine containing tetanus toxoid should be based on careful consideration of the potential benefits and possible risks. A committee of the Institute of Medicine (IOM) has concluded that evidence is consistent with a causal relationship between whole-cell DTP vaccine and acute neurologic illness, and under special circumstances, between whole-cell DTP vaccine and chronic neurologic disease in the context of the National Childhood Encephalopathy Study (NCES) report; however, evidence was insufficient to indicate whether or not whole-cell DTP vaccine increased the overall risk of chronic neurologic disease. Acute encephalopathy and permanent neurologic damage have not been reported causally linked or in temporal association with administration of PEDIARIX, but the experience with PEDIARIX is insufficient to rule this out. Encephalopathy has been reported following INFANRIX® (Diphtheria and Tetanus Toxoids and Acellular Pertussis Vaccine Adsorbed) (see ADVERSE REACTIONS, Postmarketing Reports), but data are not sufficient to evaluate a causal relationship. The decision to administer a pertussis-containing vaccine to children with stable central nervous system (CNS) disorders must be made by the physician on an individual basis, with consideration of all relevant factors, and assessment of potential risks and benefits for that individual. Advise the parent or guardian of the potential increased risk involved (see PRECAUTIONS). A family history of seizures or other CNS disorders is not a contraindication to pertussis vaccine. For children at higher risk for seizures than the general population, an appropriate antipyretic may be administered at the time of vaccination and for the ensuing 24 hours according to the respective prescribing information recommended dosage to reduce the possibility of post-vaccination fever. Defer vaccination during the course of a moderate or severe illness with or without fever and vaccinate patients as soon as they have recovered from the acute phase of the illness. Do not give PEDIARIX to children on anticoagulant therapy or those with bleeding disorders unless the potential benefit clearly outweighs the risk of administration (see PRECAUTIONS in complete prescribing information).

**PRECAUTIONS:** Before the injection of any biological, the physician should take all reasonable precautions to prevent allergic or other adverse reactions. Epinephrine injection (1:1000) and other appropriate agents used for the control of immediate allergic reactions must be immediately available should an acute anaphylactic reaction occur. Immunosuppressed individuals, including those receiving immunosuppressive therapy, may not develop the expected immune response. **Drug Interactions:** For information regarding concomitant administration with other vaccines, refer to DOSAGE AND ADMINISTRATION in complete prescribing information. Do not mix PEDIARIX with any other vaccine in the same syringe or vial. **Carcinogenesis, Mutagenesis, Impairment of Fertility:** PEDIARIX has not been evaluated for carcinogenic or mutagenic potential, or for impairment of fertility. **Pregnancy:** Pregnancy Category C: PEDIARIX is not indicated for women of child-bearing age. Animal reproduction studies have not been conducted with PEDIARIX. It is not known whether PEDIARIX can cause fetal harm when administered to a pregnant woman or if PEDIARIX can affect reproductive capacity. **Geriatric Use:** PEDIARIX is not indicated for use in adult populations. **Pediatric Use:** Safety and effectiveness of PEDIARIX in infants younger than 6 weeks of age have not been evaluated (see DOSAGE AND ADMINISTRATION in complete prescribing information). PEDIARIX is not recommended for persons 7 years of age or older. Tetanus and Diphtheria Toxoids Adsorbed (Td) For Adult Use, inactivated poliovirus vaccine (IPV), and Hepatitis B Vaccine (Recombinant) should be used in individuals 7 years of age or older.

**ADVERSE REACTIONS:** A total of 20,739 doses of PEDIARIX have been administered to 7,028 infants as a 3-dose primary series. The most common adverse reactions observed in clinical trials were local injection site reactions (pain, redness, or swelling), fever, and fussiness. In comparative studies, administration of PEDIARIX was associated with higher rates of fever relative to separately administered vaccines (see WARNINGS). The prevalence of fever was highest on the day of vaccination and the day following vaccination. More than 98% of episodes of fever resolved within the 4-day period following vaccination (i.e., the period including the day of vaccination and the next 3 days). Rates of most other solicited adverse events following PEDIARIX were comparable to rates observed following separately administered US-licensed vaccines. The adverse event information from clinical trials provides a basis for identifying adverse events that appear to be related to vaccine use and for approximating rates. However, because clinical trials are conducted under widely varying conditions, adverse event rates observed in the clinical trials of a vaccine cannot be directly compared to rates in the clinical trials of another vaccine, and may not reflect the rates observed in practice. A total of 5,472 infants were enrolled in a German safety study that was originally designed to compare the safety and reactogenicity of PEDIARIX administered concomitantly at separate sites with 1 of 4 *Haemophilus influenzae* type b (Hib) vaccines at 3, 4, and 5 months of age. After enrollment of 1,569 infants, the study was amended to include a control group that received INFANRIX, Hib vaccine, and oral poliovirus vaccine (OPV) separately. Infants in the separate administration group received one less antigen (hepatitis B) than the infants who received PEDIARIX. Safety data were available for 4,666 infants who received PEDIARIX administered concomitantly at separate sites with 1 of 4 Hib vaccines and for 768 infants in the control group that received separate vaccines. The primary end-point of the study was the percentage of infants with any grade 3 solicited symptom (redness or swelling >20 mm, fever >103.1°F, or crying, pain, vomiting, diarrhea, loss of appetite, or restlessness that prevented normal daily activities) over the 3-dose primary series in infants who received PEDIARIX (4 groups that received PEDIARIX and Hib vaccines pooled) compared to the group that received INFANRIX and Hib vaccine separately with OPV. Analysis for the primary end-point was performed on the according-to-protocol (ATP) cohort that included only those infants who were enrolled after the protocol amendment to include a control group. Of 3,773 infants in the ATP cohort for whom safety data were available, 16.2% (95% CI: 14.9% to 17.5%) of 3,029 infants who received PEDIARIX and Hib vaccine compared to 20.3% (95% CI: 17.5% to 23.4%) of 744 infants who received separate vaccines were reported to have had at least one grade 3 solicited symptom within 4 days of vaccination (i.e., day of vaccination and the next 3 days). The difference between groups in the rate of grade 3 symptoms was 4.1% (90% CI: 1.4% to 7.1%). These were the rates for selected solicited symptoms within 4 days following each dose in a 3-dose primary series in infants who received PEDIARIX administered concomitantly with Hib vaccine and those who received separate concomitant administration of INFANRIX, Hib vaccine, and OPV for the intent-to-treat (ITT) cohort (includes all infants enrolled before and after the amendment who received the indicated vaccine and for whom at least one symptom sheet was completed):

**Percentage of German Infants With Solicited Local Reactions or Selected Systemic Adverse Events Within 4 Days of Vaccination* (ITT Cohort)**

| | PEDIARIX & Hib | | | INFANRIX, Hib, & OPV | | |
|---|---|---|---|---|---|---|
| | Dose 1 | Dose 2 | Dose 3 | Dose 1 | Dose 2 | Dose 3 |
| **N** | **4,666** | **4,619** | **4,574** | **768** | **757** | **750** |
| **Local†** | | | | | | |
| Pain, any | 14.0 | 10.2 | 9.9 | 14.2 | 9.8 | 8.1 |
| Pain, grade 2 or 3 | 2.9 | 1.2 | 1.5 | 3.6 | 1.7 | 1.1 |
| Pain, grade 3 | 0.7 | 0.3 | 0.3 | 1.3 | 0.4 | 0.1 |
| Redness, any | 18.6 | 26.6 | 25.6 | 16.1 | 21.4 | 20.8 |
| Redness, >5 mm | 6.7 | 9.9 | 9.0 | 5.9 | 8.2 | 7.7 |
| Redness, >20 mm | 1.2 | 1.0 | 1.1 | 1.8 | 0.7 | 1.1 |
| Swelling, any | 12.7 | 18.5 | 18.4 | 9.6 | 12.9 | 13.6 |
| Swelling, >5 mm | 5.6 | 7.7 | 7.8 | 3.6 | 5.2 | 4.8 |
| Swelling, >20 mm | 1.2 | 1.6 | 1.5 | 1.3 | 1.1 | 1.2 |
| **Systemic** | | | | | | |
| Restlessness, any | 41.4 | 32.0 | 26.7 | 46.4 | 35.0 | 27.6 |
| Restlessness, grade 2 or 3 | 14.4 | 10.0 | 8.9 | 20.2 | 11.5 | 8.4 |
| Restlessness, grade 3 | 3.0 | 1.5 | 1.6 | 5.7 | 3.0 | 1.7 |
| Fever‡, ≥100.4°F | 25.1 | 19.3 | 19.7 | 13.2 | 13.1 | 11.2 |
| Fever‡, >101.3°F | 5.8 | 4.1 | 4.6 | 2.2 | 2.8 | 2.1 |
| Fever‡, >103.1°F | 0.3 | 0.5 | 0.7 | 0.3 | 0.3 | 0.5 |
| Unusual cry§, any | 24.9 | 16.5 | 13.1 | 36.5 | 19.7 | 14.3 |
| Unusual cry§, grade 2 or 3 | 12.7 | 7.1 | 5.7 | 20.8 | 10.0 | 5.7 |
| Unusual cry§, grade 3 | 3.9 | 1.7 | 1.4 | 6.8 | 2.1 | 1.1 |
| Loss of appetite, any | 17.9 | 13.3 | 12.5 | 19.1 | 16.2 | 11.3 |
| Loss of appetite, grade 2 or 3 | 4.0 | 2.9 | 2.7 | 4.4 | 2.9 | 2.3 |
| Loss of appetite, grade 3 | 0.6 | 0.5 | 0.4 | 0.5 | 0.7 | 0.0 |

N = number of infants in the intent-to-treat (ITT) cohort.
Grade 2 defined as sufficiently discomforting to interfere with daily activities.
Grade 3 defined as preventing normal daily activities.
* Within 4 days of vaccination defined as day of vaccination and the next 3 days.
† Local reactions at the injection site for PEDIARIX or INFANRIX.
‡ Rectal temperatures.
§ Unusual cry lasting >1 hour.

In this study, infants were also monitored for unsolicited adverse events that occurred within 30 days following vaccination. Over the entire study period, 6 subjects in the group that received PEDIARIX reported seizures. Two of these subjects had a febrile seizure, 1 of whom also developed afebrile seizures. The remaining 4 subjects had afebrile seizures, including 2 with infantile spasms. Two subjects reported seizures within 7 days following vaccination (1 subject had both febrile and afebrile seizures, and 1 subject had afebrile seizures), corresponding to a rate of 0.22 seizures per 1,000 doses (febrile seizures 0.07 per 1,000 doses, afebrile seizures 0.14 per 1,000 doses). No subject who received concomitant INFANRIX, Hib vaccine, and OPV reported seizures. In a separate German study that evaluated the safety of INFANRIX in 22,505 infants who received 66,867 doses of INFANRIX administered as a 3-dose primary series, the rate of seizures within 7 days of vaccination with INFANRIX was 0.13 per 1,000 doses (febrile seizures 0.0 per 1,000 doses, afebrile seizures 0.13 per 1,000 doses). No cases of hypotonic-hyporesponsiveness, encephalopathy, or anaphylaxis were reported in the German study that evaluated the safety of PEDIARIX. Rates of serious adverse events that are less common than those reported in this safety study are not known at this time.

Additional safety data for PEDIARIX are available from a US study designed to evaluate lot-to-lot consistency and a bridge for a new manufacturing step. These were the rates for local reactions and selected adverse events within 4 days of vaccination with PEDIARIX administered concomitantly with a Hib vaccine at 2, 4, and 6 months of age:

**Percentage of US Infants With Solicited Local Reactions or Selected Systemic Adverse Events Within 4 Days of Vaccination* (ITT Cohort)**

| | PEDIARIX & Hib | | |
|---|---|---|---|
| | Dose 1 | Dose 2 | Dose 3 |
| **Local†** | **N = 482** | **N = 469** | **N = 466** |
| Pain, any | 30.5 | 25.4 | 23.0 |
| Pain, grade 2 or 3 | 6.2 | 5.5 | 3.6 |
| Pain, grade 3 | 1.2 | 0.6 | 0.6 |
| Redness, any | 25.3 | 32.6 | 35.6 |
| Redness, >5 mm | 9.3 | 10.4 | 8.6 |
| Redness, >20 mm | 0.6 | 1.5 | 1.3 |
| Swelling, any | 15.1 | 16.6 | 22.3 |
| Swelling, >5 mm | 6.8 | 6.2 | 6.4 |
| Swelling, >20 mm | 1.0 | 1.3 | 1.3 |
| **Systemic** | **N = 482** | **N = 469** | **N = 467** |
| Restlessness, any | 28.8 | 30.3 | 28.5 |
| Restlessness, grade 2 or 3 | 7.1 | 9.0 | 9.4 |
| Restlessness, grade 3 | 1.0 | 1.1 | 0.6 |
| Fever‡, ≥100.4°F | 26.6 | 31.3 | 25.9 |
| Fever‡, >101.3°F | 2.9 | 6.2 | 4.7 |
| Fever‡, >103.1°F | 0.0 | 0.2 | 0.6 |
| Fussiness, any | 61.8 | 63.8 | 57.0 |
| Fussiness, grade 2 or 3 | 14.9 | 21.5 | 17.1 |
| Fussiness, grade 3 | 2.7 | 3.4 | 1.7 |
| Loss of appetite, any | 21.6 | 19.8 | 18.8 |
| Loss of appetite, grade 2 or 3 | 3.1 | 3.2 | 2.4 |
| Loss of appetite, grade 3 | 0.2 | 0.4 | 0.0 |
| Sleeping more than usual, any | 46.7 | 31.8 | 28.1 |
| Sleeping more than usual, grade 2 or 3 | 10.2 | 6.0 | 4.7 |
| Sleeping more than usual, grade 3 | 1.7 | 0.4 | 0.6 |

N = number of infants in the intent-to-treat (ITT) cohort (infants who received the indicated vaccine and for whom at least one symptom sheet was completed).
Grade 2 defined as sufficiently discomforting to interfere with daily activities.
Grade 3 defined as preventing normal daily activities.
* Within 4 days of vaccination defined as day of vaccination and the next 3 days.
† Local reactions at the injection site for PEDIARIX.
‡ Rectal temperatures.

In another US study, these were the rates for fever within 4 days following dose 1 (i.e., day of vaccination and the next 3 days) at 2 months of age in infants who received PEDIARIX when administered concomitantly at separate sites with Hib and pneumococcal conjugate vaccines and those who received INFANRIX, ENGERIX-B® [Hepatitis B Vaccine (Recombinant)], IPV, Hib vaccine, and pneumococcal conjugate vaccine:

**Percentage of US Infants With Fever Within 4 Days of Dose 1* (ITT Cohort)**

| | PEDIARIX, Hib, & Pneumococcal Conjugate (N = 667) | INFANRIX, ENGERIX-B, IPV, Hib, & Pneumococcal Conjugate (N = 333) | Separate Vaccine Group Minus Combination Vaccine Group |
|---|---|---|---|
| **Fever†** | **%** | **%** | **Difference (95% CI)** |
| ≥100.4°F‡ | 27.9 | 19.8 | -8.07 (-13.54, -2.60) |
| >101.3°F | 7.0 | 4.5 | -2.54 (-5.50, 0.41) |
| >102.2°F‡ | 2.2 | 0.3 | -1.95 (-3.22, -0.68) |
| >103.1°F | 0.4 | 0.0 | -0.45 (-0.96, 0.06) |
| M.A.‡ | 1.2 | 0.0 | -1.20 (-2.03, -037) |

N = number of infants for whom at least one symptom sheet was completed, excluding 3 infants for whom temperature was not measured and 3 infants whose temperature was measured by the tympanic method.
*Within 4 days of dose 1 defined as day of vaccination and the next 3 days.
† Rectal temperatures.
‡ The group that received PEDIARIX compared to separate vaccine group p value <0.05 (2-sided Fisher Exact test) or the 95% confidence interval on the difference between groups does not include 0.
M.A. = Medically attended (a visit to or from medical personnel).

In this study, medical attention (a visit to or from medical personnel) for fever within 4 days following vaccination was sought for 8 infants who received PEDIARIX (1.2%) and no infants who received separately administered vaccines. Four infants were seen by medical personnel in an office setting; no diagnostic tests were performed in 2 of the infants and a complete blood count (CBC) was done in the other 2 infants. Of 3 infants who were seen in an emergency room, all had a CBC and a blood and urine culture performed; chest X-rays were done in 2 of the infants and a nasopharyngeal specimen was tested for Respiratory Syncytial Virus in one of the infants. One infant was hospitalized for a work-up that included a CBC, blood and urine cultures, a lumbar puncture, and a chest X-ray. All episodes of medically attended fever resolved within 4 days post-vaccination.

Limited data are available from a study conducted in Moldova in which infants received a dose of hepatitis B vaccine within 48 hours of birth followed by 3 doses of PEDIARIX at 6, 10, and 14 weeks of age. No information was collected on the HBsAg status of mothers of enrolled infants. These were the rates for local reactions and selected adverse events within 4 days of vaccination with PEDIARIX administered comcomitantly with Hib vaccine following a birth dose of hepatitis B vaccine:

**Percentage of Moldovan Infants With Solicited Local Reactions or Selected Systemic Adverse Events Within 4 Days of Vaccination* (ITT Cohort)**

| | PEDIARIX & Hib | | |
|---|---|---|---|
| | Dose 1 | Dose 2 | Dose 3 |
| **N** | **160** | **158** | **157** |
| **Local†** | | | |
| Pain, any | 25.6 | 18.4 | 14.0 |
| Pain, grade 3 | 3.1 | 0.6 | 1.9 |
| Redness, any | 41.9 | 41.8 | 47.1 |
| Redness, >20 mm | 1.9 | 2.5 | 4.5 |
| Swelling, any | 20.6 | 18.4 | 28.0 |
| Swelling, >20 mm | 4.4 | 2.5 | 7.0 |
| **Systemic** | | | |
| Restlessness, any | 13.1 | 10.8 | 8.9 |
| Restlessness, grade 3 | 1.3 | 0.6 | 0.6 |
| Fever‡, ≥100.4°F | 14.4 | 11.4 | 5.1 |
| Fever‡, >103.1°F | 0.0 | 0.6 | 0.0 |
| Fussiness, any | 25.0 | 21.5 | 17.8 |
| Fussiness, grade 3 | 2.5 | 0.6 | 0.6 |

N = number of infants in the intent-to-treat (ITT) cohort (infants who received the indicated vaccine and for whom at least one symptom sheet was completed).
Grade 3 defined as preventing normal daily activities.
*Within 4 days of vaccination defined as day of vaccination and the next 3 days.
† Local reactions at the injection site for PEDIARIX.
‡ Rectal temperatures.

Although there was no comparator group who received PEDIARIX without a birth dose of hepatitis B vaccine, available data suggest that some local adverse events may occur at a higher rate when PEDIARIX is administered after a birth dose of hepatitis B vaccine.

As with any vaccine, there is the possibility that broad use of PEDIARIX could reveal adverse events not observed in clinical trials.

**Postmarketing Reports:** Worldwide voluntary reports of adverse events received for INFANRIX and ENGERIX-B in children younger than 7 years of age since market introduction of these US-licensed vaccines are listed below. This list includes adverse events for which 20 or more reports were received with the exception of intussusception, idiopathic thrombocytopenic purpura, thrombocytopenia, anaphylactic reaction, angioedema, encephalopathy, hypotonic-hyporesponsive episode, and alopecia for which fewer than 20 reports were received. These latter events are included either because of the seriousness of the event or the strength of causal connection to components of this or other vaccines or drugs. *Body as a whole:* Asthenia[b], fever[a+b], lethargy[b], malaise[b], Sudden Infant Death Syndrome[a+b]. *Cardiovascular system:* Cyanosis[a+b], edema[b], pallor[b]. *Gastrointestinal system:* Abdominal pain[b], anorexia[b], diarrhea[a+b], intussusception[a+b], nausea[b], vomiting[a+b]. *Hematologic/lymphatic:* Idiopathic thrombocytopenic purpura[a+b], lymphadenopathy[a], thrombocytopenia[a+b]. *Hepatic:* Jaundice[b], liver function tests abnormal[b]. *Hypersensitivity:* Anaphylactic reaction[a+b], angioedema[b], hypersensitivity[a]. *Infections:* Cellulitis[a]. *Injection site reactions:* Injection site reactions[a+b]. *Musculoskeletal:* Arthralgia[b], limb swelling[a+b]. *Nervous system:* Convulsions[a+b], encephalopathy[a], headache[b], hypotonia[a+b], hypotonic-hyporesponsive episode[a], somnolence[a+b]. *Psychiatric:* Crying[a+b], irritability[a+b]. *Respiratory system:* Respiratory tract infection[a]. *Skin and appendages:* Alopecia[b], erythema[a+b], erythema multiforme[b], petechiae[b], pruritus[a+b], rash[a+b], urticaria[a+b]. *Special senses:* Ear pain[a]. [[a] Following INFANRIX; [b] Following ENGERIX-B; [a+b] Following either INFANRIX or ENGERIX-B.] These reactions were reported voluntarily from a population of uncertain size; therefore, it is not always possible to reliably estimate their frequency or establish a causal relationship to vaccination.

**Reporting Adverse Events:** Report the occurrence following immunization of any event set forth in the Vaccine Injury Table from the National Childhood Vaccine Injury Act including: Anaphylaxis or anaphylactic shock within 7 days, encephalopathy or encephalitis within 7 days, brachial neuritis within 28 days, or an acute complication or sequelae (including death) of an illness, disability, injury, or condition referred to above, or any events that would contraindicate further doses of PEDIARIX. The VAERS toll-free number is 1-800-822-7967.

Manufactured by **GlaxoSmithKline Biologicals**, Rixensart, Belgium, US License 1617

Distributed by **GlaxoSmithKline,** Research Triangle Park, NC 27709



Full prescribing information for PEDIARIX is available at www.GSKVaccines.com/Pediarix. BRS-PE:L2

 Printed in USA. PED583R0 June 2005

ARTICLE

# Adulthood Outcome of Tic and Obsessive-Compulsive Symptom Severity in Children With Tourette Syndrome

*Michael H. Bloch, BA; Bradley S. Peterson, MD; Lawrence Scahill, MSN, PhD; Jessica Otka, BA; Lily Katsovich, MS; Heping Zhang, PhD; James F. Leckman, MD*

**Background:** Tourette syndrome (TS) is a childhood-onset neuropsychiatric disorder that is characterized by both motor and phonic tics. One half to two thirds of children with TS experience a reduction or complete resolution of tic symptoms during adolescence. At least one third of adults with TS have comorbid obsessive-compulsive disorder (OCD).

**Objectives:** To clarify the clinical course of tic and OCD symptoms in children with TS and determine if baseline clinical measurements in childhood are associated with future symptom severity in late adolescence and early adulthood.

**Design:** Prospective cohort study.

**Setting:** Yale Child Study Center tic and OCD outpatient specialty clinic.

**Participants:** Forty-six children with TS who received a structured clinical evaluation prior to age 14 years.

**Main Outcome Measures:** Expert-rated tic and OCD symptom severity at follow-up interview an average of 7.6 years later (range, 3.8-12.8 years).

**Results:** Eighty-five percent of subjects reported a reduction in tic symptoms during adolescence. Only increased tic severity in childhood was associated with increased tic severity at follow-up. The average age at worst-ever tic severity was 10.6 years. Forty-one percent of patients with TS reported at one time experiencing at least moderate OCD symptoms. Worst-ever OCD symptoms occurred approximately 2 years later than worst-ever tic symptoms. Increased childhood IQ was strongly associated with increased OCD severity at follow-up.

**Conclusion:** Obsessive-compulsive disorder symptoms in children with TS became more severe at a later age and were more likely to persist than tic symptoms.

*Arch Pediatr Adolesc Med. 2006;160:65-69*

TOURETTE SYNDROME (TS) IS a childhood-onset neuropsychiatric disorder that is characterized by both motor and phonic tics. In TS, tics typically begin at age 5 or 6 years and reach their peak severity between 10 and 12 years of age.[1-3] One half to two thirds of children with TS experience a substantial decrease or complete remission of tics by the end of adolescence.[2,3] However, the continuation of tics into adulthood can have serious consequences that may include self-injurious tics and those that cause social unease, such as coprolalia.[1] Currently, no clinical measures are known to predict reliably which children will continue to express tics in adulthood.

Motor and vocal tics, the most prominent feature and diagnostic *sine qua non* of TS, are often neither the first nor the most impairing symptoms that patients with TS endure. In clinical populations, TS frequently co-occurs with obsessive-compulsive disorder (OCD), attention-deficit/hyperactivity disorder (ADHD), and other behavioral, emotional, and learning disorders. In 1 study, 65% of patients with TS in late adolescence regarded their behavioral problems (including ADHD and OCD) and learning difficulties to have had an equal or greater impact on functioning than did the tics themselves.[1]

*For editorial comment see page 103*

We conducted this study to clarify the clinical course of tic symptoms and to extend our knowledge of the course of OCD symptoms in patients with TS. We also wanted to assess prospectively whether baseline clinical measurements in children with TS were associated with adult outcome with regard to severity of tic and OCD symp-

**Author Affiliations:** Yale Child Study Center, the General Clinical Research Center, and the Departments of Pediatrics and Epidemiology and Public Health, Yale University School of Medicine, New Haven, Conn (Mr Bloch; Drs Scahill, Zhang, and Leckman; and Mss Otka and Katsovich); Division of Child and Adolescent Psychiatry and the Magnetic Resonance Imaging Unit, New York State Psychiatric Institute and Columbia University College of Physicians and Surgeons, New York (Dr Peterson).

**Table. Demographic Comparison Between Participating and Nonparticipating Patients With Tourette Syndrome***

| Characteristic | Participants | Nonparticipants | P Value |
|---|---|---|---|
| Sample size | 46 | 18 | |
| Age, y, mean ± SD | 11.42 ± 1.59 | 10.91 ± 0.97 | .21 |
| Men, No. (%) | 36 (78) | 13 (72) | .61 |
| Right handedness, No. (%) | 38 (83) | 16 (89) | .53 |
| IQ, mean ± SD | 111 ± 14.7 | 111 ± 11.3 | >.99 |
| OCD, No. (%) | 17 (37) | 3 (17) | .12 |
| ADHD, No. (%) | 9 (20) | 6 (33) | .28 |
| YGTSS[7] score, mean ± SD | 19.9 ± 8.45 | 21.5 ± 6.45 | .47 |
| CY-BOCS[8] score, mean ± SD | 2.11 ± 3.30 | 2.56 ± 5.29 | .65 |

Abbreviations: ADHD, attention-deficit/hyperactivity disorder; CY-BOCS, Children's Yale-Brown Obsessive Compulsive Scale; OCD, obsessive-compulsive disorder; YGTSS, Yale Global Tic Severity Scale.

*There were no significant differences ($P<.05$) between any of the variables examined between participating and nonparticipating subjects using $\chi^2$ or *t* tests.

toms. Our a priori hypotheses were that (1) increased severity of tic symptoms and (2) a diagnosis of ADHD in children with TS would be associated with increased tic severity at follow-up and that (3) increased severity of OCD symptoms and (4) a higher IQ in childhood would be associated with increased OCD symptom severity at follow-up.

## METHODS

### SUBJECTS

The 46 subjects included in this study were previously evaluated at the Yale Child Study Center Tic Disorder Clinic (New Haven, Conn) and had previously participated in magnetic resonance imaging studies in childhood.[4-6] Eligible subjects (1) had a previous diagnosis of TS, (2) underwent magnetic resonance imaging and a detailed evaluation prior to 14 years of age (time 1), and (3) were older than 16 years at follow-up (time 2). Exclusionary criteria in these earlier studies included a history of seizure, head trauma with loss of consciousness, ongoing or past substance abuse, or an IQ lower than 80. Parental written informed consent and subject assent were obtained at both time 1 and time 2. Compensation was provided for participation at both points under the guidelines of the Human Investigations Committee at Yale University, New Haven.

From an eligible sample of 64 subjects evaluated at time 1, 46 subjects elected to participate. Reasons for nonparticipation included subject refusal to participate in follow-up interview (n=14) or inability to locate subjects (n=4). Demographic measurements did not differ statistically significantly between participating and nonparticipating subjects as assessed during initial evaluation at time 1 (**Table**). However, there was a noticeably higher proportion of cases with comorbid OCD and a lower proportion of cases of ADHD among participating subjects compared with nonparticipating subjects at time 1.

### INTERVIEW PROCEDURE AT TIME 1

Assessment at time 1, when subjects were younger than 14 years, included current and worst-ever measures using the Yale Global Tic Severity Scale (YGTSS) and Children's Yale-Brown Obsessive Compulsive Scale (CY-BOCS).[7,8] IQ testing was performed using the Kaufman Brief Intelligence Test.[9,10] The Schedule for Tourette and Other Behavioral Syndromes, which includes the Kiddie-Schedule for Affective Disorders and Schizophrenia Epidemiologic Present and Lifetime Version for diagnosis in children and more detailed sections on TS and OCD, was used to screen for comorbid psychiatric illnesses.[11-13] Neuropsychiatric diagnoses were established using a best-estimate consensus procedure involving 2 child psychiatrists (B.S.P. and J.F.L.), who reviewed all available clinical and research data.[14]

### INTERVIEW PROCEDURE AT TIME 2

Assessments included current and worst-ever YGTSS and CY-BOCS ratings. Screening for any comorbid psychiatric conditions was conducted with the *Structured Clinical Interview for DSM-IV Axis I Disorders*.[15] Additional assessments included a thorough medication history, specific inquiry about ADHD symptoms, and ages at worst-ever tic and OCD symptoms. Overall psychosocial functioning was rated using the Global Assessment Scale after the follow-up interview.[16] Eight clinical evaluations relied solely on information provided by a parent who lived in the same home as the research subject.

### DATA ANALYSIS

All statistical procedures were performed using SPSS version 12.0.[17] Histograms were generated to examine the distribution of YGTSS and CY-BOCS scores at time 2. Because of the large number of subjects with no current tic or OCD symptoms at time 2 (YGTSS and CY-BOCS scores=0), YGTSS and CY-BOCS scores were not normally distributed. To avoid the nonnormality problem for these outcome scales, we transformed them into ordinal groupings prior to hypothesis analysis to maintain gradations in symptom severity while also maintaining ordinal groupings of roughly equal subject number. The ordinal groupings for YGTSS score (range, 0-50) at follow-up used in these analyses were 0 (n=15), 1 through 9 (n=11), 10 through 19 (n=10), and 20 or higher (n=10). These groupings roughly correspond to absence of tics (YGTSS score, 0), minimal tic symptoms (YGTSS score, 1-9), mild tic symptoms (YGTSS score, 11-19), and moderate to severe tic symptoms (YGTSS score, >20). For CY-BOCS score at follow-up (range, 0-40), groupings for ordinal logistic regression were 0 (n=24), 1 through 9 (n=10), and greater than or equal to 10 (n=9). These groupings roughly correspond to absence of OCD symptoms (CY-BOCS score, 0), subclinical OCD symptoms (CY-BOCS score, 1-9), and OCD symptoms of clinical significance (CY-BOCS score, ≥10).

The ordinal logistic regression module of SPSS 12.0 with a logit link was used for statistical analyses. This statistical package relies on the proportional odds model for ordinal logistic regression. Ordinal groupings for YGTSS and CY-BOCS ratings were used as the dependent variable in the analyses. For a priori hypothesis testing, YGTSS, CY-BOCS, and IQ scores or ADHD diagnosis at time 1 were entered as the independent variables. Each of these independent variables was then entered into individual ordinal logistic regression models. Additionally, for each ordinal logistic regression model, age at time 1 and interval between time 1 and time 2 were entered as additional covariates. Using a Bonferroni correction, the threshold for statistical significance was set at $P<.01$ to account for our 4 a priori hypotheses. All *P* values were 2 tailed.

## RESULTS

The 46 subjects were first interviewed at a mean±SD age of 11.4±1.6 years (range, 7.5-13.9 years). Demographic characteristics of subjects at time 1 are represented in the Table. At time 2, the patients with TS were at a mean±SD age of 19.0±1.8 years (range, 16.0-22.8 years). The mean±SD duration between the initial and follow-up interviews was 7.6±1.9 years (range, 3.8-12.8 years).

## CURRENT TIC STATUS

At time 2, when the patients with TS were 16 to 23 years of age, tic symptoms for the majority of patients were minimal or absent. On average, the mean±SD total tic score of the YGTSS at time 2 was 10.0±10.3 (median, 7.5; actual range, 0-39, with a possible range of 0-50). Fifteen patients (33%) reported being entirely tic free during the week before the follow-up interview, and only 10 patients (22%) were judged to have a moderate or marked level of tic severity based on their interview data (YGTSS score, ≥20 but <40). At time 1, all 46 subjects had tics of at least moderate severity (YGTSS score, ≥20). **Figure 1** demonstrates a box plot comparing tic severity between time 1 and time 2 in our study sample.

## CURRENT STATUS OF OCD SYMPTOMS

Nineteen subjects with TS reported at some point experiencing at least mild lifetime OCD symptoms (worst-ever, CY-BOCS score, ≥10). The mean±SD OCD severity score at follow-up was 10.8±9.2 (median, 13; actual range, 0-34, with a possible range of 0-40) compared with 4.1±4.2 (median, 2; actual range, 0-12) at baseline in childhood (Figure 1).

## SEVERITY AND TIMING OF TICS AND OCD SYMPTOMS DURING THE WORST-EVER PERIOD

The mean±SD worst-ever tic severity score was 31.6±7.7 (range, 15-48) at a mean±SD age of 10.6±2.6 years (range, 6-19 years). Contrary to previous reports, the level of worst-ever tic severity was not significantly associated with the patient's age during the worst-ever period (Pearson correlation coefficient, $r=0.008$; $P=.96$).[5]

In the 19 subjects who had a lifetime history of OCD symptoms, the mean±SD age at worst-ever OCD symptoms was 12.5±3.9 (range, 7-22). **Figure 2** depicts a box plot comparing age at worst-ever tic and OCD symptoms within our study sample. The mean±SD worst-ever OCD severity score reported at follow-up was 23.3±6.6 (range, 13-34).

## COMORBID CONDITIONS AND MEDICATION USE AT FOLLOW-UP

At the follow-up interview, 10 subjects had a lifetime history of ADHD symptoms. One subject had a history of ADHD symptoms but was clinically asymptomatic by the time 1 interview. Fifteen subjects (33%) had experienced a lifetime major depressive episode by the time 2 follow-up interview. Ten experienced their first depressive episode in the interval between the initial interview and the follow-up interview. Only 1 subject currently had depression. Two cases (4.3%) of bipolar disorder and 1 case of schizophrenia emerged at the follow-up interview.

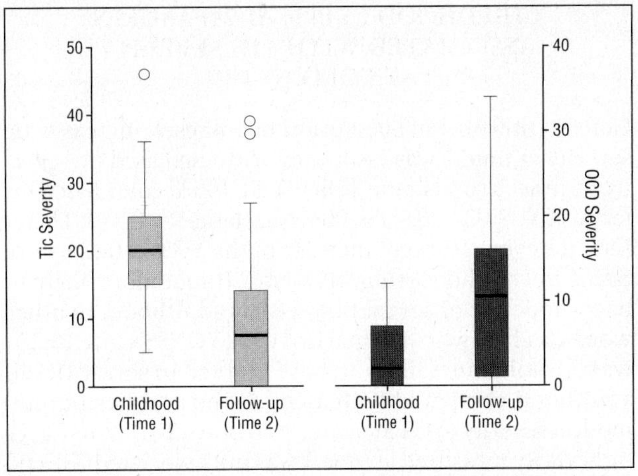


**Figure 1.** Box plots comparing tic and obsessive-compulsive disorder (OCD) symptom severity at the time of initial assessment in childhood (time 1) and follow-up in early adulthood (time 2). Tic symptom severity scores were measured by the Yale Global Tic Severity Scale[7] and are reported for all 46 subjects with Tourette syndrome. The OCD symptom severity scores were measured using the Children's Yale-Brown Obsessive Compulsive Scale[8] (CY-BOCS) and are reported for those 19 patients with Tourette syndrome with lifetime worst-ever OCD symptom severity scores that were at least in the moderate-severity range (CY-BOCS score, ≥10) as assessed at time 2.

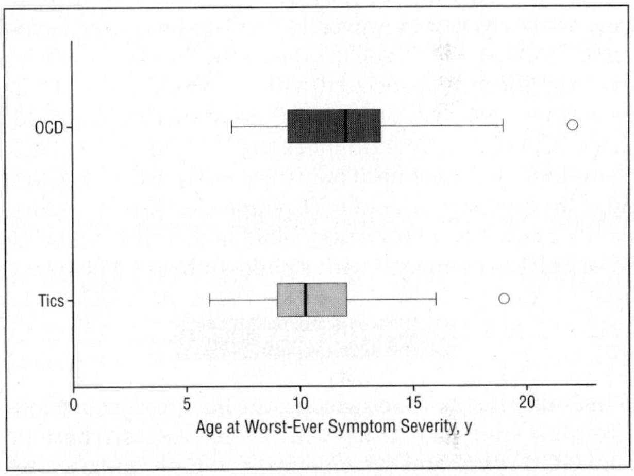


**Figure 2.** Box plot representing age when tic and obsessive-compulsive disorder (OCD) symptoms were at their worst. Age is represented for all 46 subjects with Tourette syndrome in this study sample. Age at worst-ever OCD symptoms were reported at follow-up for just those 19 patients with Tourette syndrome with lifetime worst-ever OCD symptom severity scores that were at least in the moderate-severity range (Children's Yale-Brown Obsessive Compulsive Scale score, ≥10).

At time 2, 6 subjects (13%) were using antipsychotics or $\alpha_2$-agonists (guanfacine hydrochloride or clonidine hydrochloride) (medication to treat tics), compared with 23 subjects (50%) at time 1. Five subjects (11%) were taking antipsychotics at follow-up (4 atypical antipsychotics, 1 typical) compared with 10 subjects (22%) at time 1 (9 typical antipsychotics, 1 atypical). Four subjects at both time 1 and time 2 were using selective serotonin reuptake inhibitors (fluvoxetine, sertraline hydrochloride, or clomipramine hydrochloride), although only 1 subject was taking a selective serotonin reuptake inhibitor at both times.

## CHILDHOOD CLINICAL MEASURES ASSOCIATED WITH TIC SEVERITY AT FOLLOW-UP

Consistent with 1 of our a priori hypotheses, increased tic severity at time 1 was associated with increased tic severity at time 2 (odds ratio [OR], 1.11 [95% confidence interval (CI), 1.03-1.20]; $P=.004$; Nagelerke $R^2=0.19$). Therefore, for every 10-point increase in the YGTSS tic severity rating in childhood, subjects were 2.8-fold more likely to have moderate or severe tics in early adulthood. In other words, a child who had marked tics (YGTSS score, ≥20) was 2.8-fold more likely to have marked to severe tics in adulthood compared with a child who had tics of only modest severity (YGTSS score, ≥10 but <20). Worst-ever tic severity measured at time 1 was not associated with tic severity at time 2 (OR, 1.05 [95% CI, 0.96-1.15]; $P=.32$). An ADHD diagnosis at time 1 (OR, 0.52 [95% CI, 0.14-1.95]; $P=.33$) was also not associated with follow-up tic severity.

## CHILDHOOD CLINICAL MEASURES ASSOCIATED WITH INCREASED OCD SEVERITY AT FOLLOW-UP

In contrast, OCD symptom severity at time 1 (OR, 1.04 [95% CI, 0.86-1.25]; $P=.70$) was not associated with future OCD severity. However, higher IQ score measured at time 1 (OR, 1.11 [95% CI, 1.04-1.19]; $P=.001$; $R^2=0.46$) was significantly associated with increased future OCD symptom severity. For every 10-point increase in childhood IQ, subjects were 2.8-fold more likely to express OCD symptoms at follow-up. Thus, the overall risk of developing clinically significant OCD symptoms (Y-BOCS score, ≥10) by early adulthood was 8-fold higher in a child with an IQ of 120 compared with a child with an IQ of 100.

## COMMENT

This study is, to our knowledge, the first prospective longitudinal study of patients with TS that assessed both tic and OCD symptoms systematically at both initial evaluation and follow-up in early adulthood. On average, subjects in the cohort experienced their worst-ever tics at 10 to 11 years of age, and most experienced a marked attenuation of tic severity during adolescence. Slightly less than one quarter (22%) continued to experience mild or greater tic symptoms (YGTSS scores, ≥10) at follow-up, while nearly one third were in complete remission of tic symptoms at follow-up. The only childhood clinical measure significantly associated with increased tic severity at follow-up was increased tic severity at the time of baseline assessment during childhood (<14 years). This finding stands in contrast to those of previous studies, which did not detect an association of childhood tic severity with the severity of tics later in life.[1]

The time when OCD symptoms were at their worst was approximately 2 years later than when tic symptoms were at their worst. The majority of individuals who had OCD symptoms at follow-up reported the onset of their OCD symptoms in late childhood or early adolescence, after the time of their initial evaluation. Increased childhood IQ was strongly associated with the future development of OCD symptoms in children with TS. This result is consistent with previous studies in the general population that have associated increased childhood IQ with the development of OCD in adulthood.[3]

This study has several limitations. It reports findings in a clinically referred population of children with TS whose overall illness severity and rates of comorbid illnesses are likely to be greater than in children who have TS in the general population. Furthermore, approximately one quarter of eligible subjects did not participate in the follow-up evaluation. Although participating and nonparticipating subjects did not differ significantly in any demographic or clinical characteristics at the time of initial evaluation, we cannot exclude the possibility that self-selection bias affected our findings at follow-up. In addition, because at baseline we excluded children with an IQ lower than 80, our finding that higher IQ is associated with worse future OCD symptoms in patients with TS cannot be interpreted as indicating that that those with IQs lower than 80 are not at risk of developing OCD.

Despite these limitations, we can draw 4 clinical conclusions from the findings in this study. First, tics typically diminish in severity during adolescence, even for those children who have relatively severe tic symptoms. This is welcome information for parents seeking an evaluation and treatment for TS and consistent with previous reports.[2] Given that tic symptoms are likely to decrease spontaneously during adolescence, support and tolerance from family, teachers, peers, and health care professionals may either reduce or eliminate the need for exposure to medications.[1,2] Second, the severity of tics in late childhood was associated, though only modestly so, with future tic severity in late adolescence and early adulthood. Additional work is needed to identify these high-risk individuals. Genetic studies and performance on focused neuropsychological testing as well as magnetic resonance imaging volumetric measurements may hold promise. The predictive value of perinatal risk factors also needs to be evaluated prospectively. Third, the presence of childhood ADHD symptoms was not associated with the presence or severity of adulthood tic or OCD symptoms. Fourth, OCD symptoms on average reached their peak severity 2 years later than tics. Thus, educating patients and their parents about the possibility of developing clinically significant OCD symptoms at a point later in childhood and adolescence, even if OCD symptoms are not evident at the time of initial evaluation, may be important. This may be especially important for bright children who have tics because IQ in childhood in this sample and other samples has been most predictive of increased severity of OCD symptoms in later adolescence, regardless of OCD symptoms in childhood.[11] Periodic monitoring for OCD symptoms after the initial evaluation by experts in tic disorders and OCD may be warranted, given the importance that OCD symptoms have in contributing to later psychosocial functioning.[1]

**Accepted for Publication:** June 24, 2005.
**Correspondence:** James F. Leckman, MD, Child Study Center, Yale University School of Medicine, PO Box 207900, New Haven, CT 06520-7900 (james.leckman@yale.edu).

**Author Contributions:** Dr Zhang was the statistical expert for this study. He can be reached at Department of Epidemiology and Public Health, Yale University School of Medicine, 60 College St, New Haven, CT 06520-8034 (heping.zhang@yale.edu).
**Funding/Support:** This study was supported in part by grants MH49351 (Dr Leckman), MH01232 (Dr Peterson), MH59139 (Dr Peterson), MH30929, and RR06022 from the National Institute of Mental Health, Rockville, Md; a grant from the Tourette Syndrome Association, New York, NY; the Suzanne Crosby Murphy Endowment at Columbia University, New York; the Smart Family Foundation, Wilton, Conn; Jay and Jean Kaiser; Eric Brooks; and the Chasanoff Family at the Yale University Child Study Center as well as gifts from anonymous donors.
**Acknowledgement:** We thank our many collaborators at Yale including Robert King, MD, Diane Findley, PhD, Lily Katsovich, MS, and Heidi Grantz, MSW, for their encouragement and substantial contributions in following up these families and participating in the initial assessment of these individuals. We thank Robert Schultz, PhD, for providing IQ measurements in the children of this sample. We thank Hanna Stevens, MD, PhD, and Andres Martin, MD, MPH, for their contributions toward the final manuscript of this article.

## REFERENCES

1. Erenberg G, Cruse RP, Rothner AD. The natural history of Tourette's syndrome: a follow-up study. *Ann Neurol.* 1987;22:383-385.
2. Leckman JF, Zhang H, Vitale A, et al. Course of tic severity in Tourette syndrome: the first two decades. *Pediatrics.* 1998;102:14-19.
3. Peterson BS, Pine DS, Cohen P, Brook JS. Prospective, longitudinal study of tic, obsessive-compulsive, and attention-deficit/hyperactivity disorder in an epidemiological sample. *J Am Acad Child Adolesc Psychiatry.* 2001;40:685-695.
4. Peterson BS, Skudlarski P, Anderson AW, et al. A functional magnetic resonance imaging study of tic suppression in Tourette syndrome. *Arch Gen Psychiatry.* 1998;55:326-333.
5. Peterson BS, Thomas P, Kane MJ, et al. Basal ganglia volumes in patients with Gilles de la Tourette syndrome. *Arch Gen Psychiatry.* 2003;60:415-424.
6. Peterson BS, Skudlarski P, Anderson AW, et al. Regional brain and ventricular volumes in Tourette's syndrome. *Arch Gen Psychiatry.* 2001;58:427-440.
7. Leckman JF, Riddle MA, Hardin MT, et al. The Yale Global Tic Severity Scale: initial testing of a clinician-rated scale of tic-severity. *J Am Acad Child Adolesc Psychiatry.* 1989;28:566-573.
8. Scahill L, Riddle MA, McSwiggin-Hardin M, et al. Children's Yale-Brown Obsessive Compulsive Scale: reliability and validity. *J Am Acad Child Adolesc Psychiatry.* 1997;36:844-852.
9. Grossman I, Kaufman AS, Grossman D. Correlations of scores on the Kaufman short neuropsychological assessment procedure and the Kaufman Adolescent and Adult Intelligence Test for a hospitalized depressed sample. *Percept Mot Skills.* 1993;77:1055-1058.
10. Naugle RI, Chelune GJ, Tucker GD. Validity of the Kaufman Brief Intelligence Test. *Psychol Assess.* 1993;5:182-186.
11. Ambrosini P, Metz C, Prabucki K, Lee JC. Videotape reliability of the third revised edition of the K-SADS. *J Am Acad Child Adolesc Psychiatry.* 1989;28:723-728.
12. Kaufman J, Birmaher B, Brent D, et al. Schedule for affective disorders and schizophrenia for school-age children—present and lifetime version (K-SADS-PL): initial reliability and validity data. *J Am Acad Child Adolesc Psychiatry.* 1997;36:980-988.
13. Pauls DL, Hurst CR. *Schedule for Tourette and Other Behavioral Syndromes.* New Haven, Conn: Yale University Child Study Center; 1996.
14. Leckman JF, Sholomskas D, Thompson WD, et al. Best estimate of lifetime psychiatric diagnosis. *Arch Gen Psychiatry.* 1982;39:879-883.
15. Endicott J, Spitzer RL. A diagnostic interview: the schedule for affective disorders and schizophrenia. *Arch Gen Psychiatry.* 1978;35:837-844.
16. Endicott J, Spitzer RL, Fleiss JL, Cohen J. The Global Assessment Scale. *Arch Gen Psychiatry.* 1976;33:766-771.
17. Statistical Product and Service Solutions [computer program]. Version 13.0 for Windows. Chicago, Ill: SPSS Inc; 2004.

"Better to be driven out from among men than to be disliked of children."
From *The Idle Man* by Richard Henry Dana

ARTICLE

# Unmet Health Care Needs Among Children Evaluated for Sexual Assault

*Rebecca Girardet, MD; Lauren Giacobbe; Kelly Bolton, RN; Sheela Lahoti, MD; Margaret McNeese, MD*

**Objectives:** To determine in a population of children who underwent a medical examination after alleged sexual assault the proportion who had unmet medical or psychiatric needs.

**Design:** Retrospective medical record review.

**Setting:** A referral center for alleged child victims of sexual assault in Houston, Tex, from December 1, 2003, through April 30, 2004.

**Participants:** Four hundred seventy-three children (81% girls). Nine children refused all or part of the medical evaluation.

**Main Outcome Measure:** Diagnoses that warranted intervention at the time of the medical evaluation.

**Results:** A medical or psychological diagnosis that required intervention as judged by the examiner was made in 123 children (26%) (95% confidence interval, 22%-30%). In 39 children (8% of the total study population) (95% confidence interval, 6%-11%), the diagnosis had the potential to result in significant patient morbidity if not immediately addressed. In contrast, 44 children (9%) (95% confidence interval, 7%-12%) had probable or definite physical or laboratory evidence that supported the allegation of sexual assault.

**Conclusion:** Among children undergoing a medical evaluation after an alleged sexual assault, important unmet health care needs are at least as common as forensic findings.

*Arch Pediatr Adolesc Med. 2006;160:70-73*

A REPORTED 1.2 IN 1000 children in the United States were sexually abused in 2000 through 2002.[1] Many of these children underwent a medical examination after sexual assault, with the 2-fold purpose of ensuring the health of the child and documenting any injuries or other evidence that may support the allegation. Because access to health care remains a major problem for children in the United States, with approximately 9% being uninsured in the first half of 2004,[2] many children seen for a sexual assault evaluation may have had limited prior contact with the health care system. Furthermore, children from abusive households are at potentially greater risk for inadequately addressed health needs than is the general pediatric population. While extensive literature exists concerning the incidence of forensic findings in children examined after an allegation of sexual assault, contemporary studies that examine the prevalence of unmet health care needs in this population are unavailable. The primary objective of this study was to determine in a population of children examined after alleged sexual assault the number who had other health care needs that warranted intervention at the time of the sexual assault evaluation.

The secondary objective of this study was to determine the prevalence of forensic evidence of sexual assault in our population. Many children seen for a sexual abuse evaluation are brought by parties whose primary interest is the detection and preservation of forensic evidence. The reported incidence of such findings, however, is low. In their study of 2384 children seen at a tertiary referral center for alleged sexual assault, Heger et al[3] found that less than 4% had forensic evidence and only 0.6% had a sexually transmissible disease, even though approximately two thirds reported penetration of the vagina or anus. Studies by Adams et al,[4] Kellogg et al,[5] and Bowen and Aldous[6] support these findings. The recovery of laboratory evidence in acute rape settings is also likely to be low in children, although, to our knowledge, only one published study to date has addressed this question and modern DNA amplification techniques were not used in the analysis of the samples.[7] We compared the prevalence of

**Author Affiliations:** University of Texas at Houston School of Medicine.

unmet health care needs with the prevalence of forensic findings in our population of children examined after an alleged sexual assault.

## METHODS

Institutional review board approval for this study was obtained from the University of Texas Health Sciences Center Committee for the Protection of Human Subjects. This was a retrospective review of medical records from a clinic located in a child advocacy center, which is a tertiary referral center for sexually abused children. The mission of the clinic is to provide comprehensive health care for sexually abused children; therefore, for all children seen at the clinic a complete medical history was obtained, and a physical examination was performed and the results recorded on a detailed standardized form. The medical examinations were performed by 3 board-certified pediatricians (R.G., S.L., and M.M.) specializing in sexual assault. Videocolposcopy was routinely used for the anogenital portion of the examination. Laboratory specimens for sexually transmissible infections were collected when the patient history or physical findings suggested that there was a risk for disease according to the Centers for Disease Control and Prevention 2002 sexually transmitted diseases treatment guidelines.[8] For children who had been assaulted within the previous 72 hours, additional specimens for forensic laboratory evaluation (rape evidence collection) were collected and turned over to law enforcement personnel for processing. The clinic physicians (R.G., S.L., and M.M.) conducted monthly peer review of medical records according to clinic policy.

The medical records of all sexual assault evaluations performed during the study period (December 1, 2003, through April 30, 2004) were reviewed. Three of us (R.G., L.G., and K.B.) abstracted the data for this study, with oversight of all abstraction by the lead author (R.G.). Basic demographic information, referral source, time since the alleged assault, history of prior sexual contact, anogenital findings, laboratory test results, and nonforensic diagnoses (medical and psychological) were abstracted from each medical record. Only diagnoses that were judged by the physician to require intervention at the time of the evaluation were recorded.

Both the physical findings at examination and the results of laboratory tests for sexually transmissible diseases were considered in determining the evidence for sexual abuse. The criteria published by Adams[9] in 2004 were used to categorize the children's anogenital examination findings and the likelihood of abuse. An additional category, "probable sexual contact," was also included for patients whose findings did not fall within one of the Adams categories but for whom sexual contact was considered by the authors to be the most likely cause.

## RESULTS

Four hundred seventy-three children (81% girls) were brought to the advocacy center for a sexual assault examination during the study period. The children ranged in age from 2 months to 17 years; 157 children (33%) were 13 years or older. Two hundred fifty-nine children were referred for examination by Children's Protective Services, 210 children were referred by law enforcement personnel, and the remaining 4 children were referred directly by their medical providers. Nine children received incomplete evaluations: no medical history was available and no medical evaluation was performed in 1 child with autism; a complete medical history was obtained in 2 children, but all components of the physical examination were refused; and 6 children gave a medical history but consented to only part of the medical examination or laboratory testing. A rape evidence collection kit was used in 22 children.

**Table 1. Diagnoses Warranting Intervention at Time of Examination**

| Diagnosis | No. of Children per Diagnosis* |
|---|---|
| *Candida* dermatitis/vaginitis | 16 |
| Bacterial vaginosis | 15 |
| Unprotected sexual activity | 13 |
| Suicidal ideation | 10 |
| *Chlamydia trachomatis* infection, contact/atopic dermatitis, or depression without current suicidal ideation | 7 |
| Labial adhesions | 6 |
| Dental caries, molluscum contagiosum, nonspecific vulvovaginitis, pediculosis, or urinary tract infection | 4 |
| Abnormal Papanicolaou smear, anogenital condyloma, asthma, otitis media, or pinworm infestation | 3 |
| Anemia, cerumen impaction, decreased visual acuity, hemangioma, hypoimmunization, pelvic inflammatory disease, pregnancy, suspected fistula, *Trichomonas vaginalis* or vitiligo | 2 |
| Acne, attention-deficit/hyperactivity disorder, allergic rhinitis, breast lesion, cervical cyst, conjunctivitis, encopresis, flea bites, folliculitis, gastritis, *Neisseria gonorrhoeae* infection, gynecomastia, hematochezia, hematuria, ingrown toenail, keratosis pilaris, menometrorrhagia, metrorrhagia, nongenital wart, obesity, oral thrush, perforated tympanic membrane, pharyngitis, prominent vaginal ridge, psoriasis, pustulosis, rectal prolapse, secondary amenorrhea, self-mutilation, short stature, splenomegaly, suspected anogenital streptococcal infection, suspected bipolar disorder, suspected pathologic heart murmur, suspected pseudocyesis, tinea capitus, tinea corporis, upper respiratory tract infection, urethral prolapse, or varicocele | 1 |

A medical or psychological diagnosis that warranted intervention by the examiner was made in 123 children (26% of the total who underwent at least a partial medical evaluation) (95% confidence interval, 22%-30%) (**Table 1**). Six children had medical diagnoses that could be attributed to sexual abuse, and 18 children had a psychological diagnosis. Thirty-nine children (representing 8% of the total evaluated) (95% confidence interval, 6%-11%) had a diagnosis with the potential to result in significant morbidity if not immediately addressed, including anemia, exacerbation of asthma, *Chlamydia* infection, depression without suicidal ideation, gonorrhea, menometrorrhagia, metrorrhagia, pelvic inflammatory disease, perforated tympanic membrane, pregnancy, secondary amenorrhea, self-mutilation, splenomegaly, suicidal ideation, suspected fistula, suspected pathologic heart murmur, suspected premature adrenarche, suspected pseudocyesis, and urinary tract infection. In contrast, 44 children (9% of those who underwent at least a partial anogenital examination) (95% confidence interval, 7%-

**Table 2. Evidence of Penetrating Trauma or Sexual Contact**

| Category | Physical or Laboratory Findings |
|---|---|
| Diagnostic of sexual contact | Positive urine pregnancy test results (3 patients) |
| Presence of infection | Positive vaginal culture for *Neisseria gonorrhoeae* (1 patient) |
| | *Trichomonas vaginalis* on wet mount (1 patient) |
| Probable sexual contact* | NAAT positive for *Chlamydia trachomatis* (4 patients), but vaginal culture negative (2 patients) or not performed (2 patients) |
| | NAAT positive for *N gonorrhoeae* (culture not done, 1 patient) |
| | Short curled hair at cervical os (likely pubic hair), fluid on genitalia suspicious for semen, and deep posterior hymenal notch (1 patient) |
| High specificity for abuse | Healed hymenal transection (7 patients) |
| | Absent hymen (6 patients) |
| | Hymenal laceration (3 patients) |
| | Hymenal ecchymoses and laceration (2 patients) |
| | Hymenal ecchymoses (1 patient) |
| Moderate specificity for abuse | Acute abrasion of perihymenal tissue (1 patient) |
| | Laceration and bruising of fossa navicularis (1 patient) |
| | Acute abrasion of perihymenal tissue and laceration of perineum (1 patient) |
| | Acute abrasion and laceration of fossa (1 patient) |
| | Acute abrasion of labia minora, bruising of perihymenal tissue, and acute abrasion and bruising of fossa (1 patient) |
| Indeterminate findings | Deep posterior notch (5 patients) |
| | Diminished posterior hymen (2 patients) |
| | Diminished posterior hymen and prominent anal fold vs scar (1 patient) |
| | Anal scar and dilatation, without stool in ampulla (1 patient) |

Abbreviations: NAAT, nucleic acid amplification test; UPT, urine pregnancy test.

*This category is not part of the Adams classification scale but includes patients for whom we thought the evidence indicated probable sexual contact based on the information stated. The 3 patients tested with the NAAT only for *C trachomatis* and *N gonorrhoeae* were all teenagers who had been involved in "statutory" relationships and declined definitive testing by culture.

12%) had physical or laboratory findings that potentially or definitively supported the allegation of sexual assault (**Table 2**).

Fourteen of 22 children who underwent rape evidence collection were in the group of 44 children with evidence supportive of the allegation of sexual assault. The remaining 8 children who underwent rape evidence collection had no or only nonspecific physical findings to support the allegation of sexual abuse and no diagnosis of a sexually transmissible disease. Results of forensic analyses of the evidence kits were unavailable.

## COMMENT

Medical diagnoses significantly outnumbered forensic findings in our population (26% vs 9%), and the number of children with a serious diagnosis was almost the same as the number with assault-related findings (8% vs 9%). These results indicate that sexually abused children are at high risk for unmet health care needs. This study was conducted in the southern United States, where the proportion of children with inadequate access to health care is greater than in some other parts of the United States.[10] The number of children in our study with unmet health care needs might, therefore, have been different had it been conducted in another region of the United States.

Twenty-two of the children in our study underwent rape evidence collection as part of the medical evaluation, and of these, 8 children had no physical findings or laboratory diagnosis to support the allegation of sexual abuse. Rape kits are processed by police laboratories only when requested by the judicial system. Because this process often takes months or even years in pediatric cases, an attempt to learn the outcome of these 8 kits was not made. However, even if all 8 kits contained evidence of sexual assault, the number of children with forensic evidence would have been only 11% (52 children) of the total, which is significantly lower than the number with unmet health care issues.

Our results should be of interest to medical providers, Children's Protective Services workers, foster families, and others who must be vigilant for the potential health care needs of sexually abused children. Our results also have implications for medical facilities that provide sexual assault evaluations for children. Many centers rely on nonphysician health care providers who are not independently licensed to perform sexual assault evaluations. While many of the diagnoses recorded during the study were nonemergent, that the number of children with serious diagnoses was almost the same as the number with forensic evidence indicates that this population requires comprehensive medical care in addition to having their forensic concerns addressed. Institutions that rely on extended care providers must provide careful medical oversight of sexual assault evaluations in children.

Our data also point to the need for systems that provide services to sexually abused children to carefully consider how best to meet the ongoing health care needs of this vulnerable population. We are unable to discern from our data the number of children in our population who had received inadequate medical care compared with the number who were receiving good care but happened to have an acute need on the day that we examined them. However, the high prevalence of unmet medical and psychological needs in our population suggests that at least a proportion of these children lack a "medical home." Because of their interdisciplinary design, advocacy centers that provide ongoing comprehensive medical care in addition to initial sexual assault evaluations are one solution to this problem. Ideally, the community outreach efforts of such centers can then facilitate communication with primary care physicians and, thus, provide for more permanent medical homes for these children.

Children seen for medical evaluations after alleged sexual assault are a population at risk for inadequately met health care needs, yet the systems in place to care for them are sometimes focused on the collection and documentation of potential forensic evidence rather than on medical care. To our knowledge, this study is the first to document the health care needs of this population. Unmet health care needs can be substantial in this population at high risk and should be considered in the structuring of systems designed to provide medical services for sexually abused children.

**Accepted for Publication:** June 29, 2005.
**Correspondence:** Rebecca Girardet, MD, University of Texas at Houston School of Medicine, 6431 Fannin St, MSB 3.156B, Houston, TX 77030 (Rebecca.g.girardet@uth.tmc.edu).
**Acknowledgment:** Data from the National Child Abuse and Neglect Data System Child File, 2002, were provided by the National Data Archive on Child Abuse and Neglect at Cornell University, Ithaca, NY, and are used with permission. Data were originally collected under the auspices of the Children's Bureau, Administration on Children, Youth and Families, Administration for Children and Families, US Department of Health and Human Services, Washington, DC.

## REFERENCES

1. US Department of Health and Human Services; Administration for Children and Families, Administration on Children, Youth and Families, Children's Bureau. National Child Abuse and Neglect Data System (NCANDS) Child File, 2002 [dataset]. Washington, DC; 2004. Available at: http://www.ndacan.cornell.edu. Accessed May 1, 2005.
2. Cohen RA, Martinez ME, Hao C. Health insurance coverage: estimates from the National Health Interview Survey, January-September 2004. Available at: http://www.cdc.gov/nchs/nhis.htm. Accessed May 1, 2005.
3. Heger A, Ticson L, Velasquez O, Bernier R. Children referred for possible sexual abuse: medical findings in 2384 children. *Child Abuse Negl.* 2002;26:645-659.
4. Adams JA, Harper K, Knudson S, Revilla J. Examination findings in legally confirmed child sexual abuse: it's normal to be normal. *Pediatrics.* 1994;94:310-317.
5. Kellogg ND, Parra JM, Menard S. Children with anogenital symptoms and signs referred for sexual abuse evaluations. *Arch Pediatr Adolesc Med.* 1998;152:634-641.
6. Bowen K, Aldous M. Medical evaluation of sexual abuse in children without disclosed or witnessed abuse. *Arch Pediatr Adolesc Med.* 1999;153:1160-1164.
7. Christian CW, Lavelle JM, De Jong AR, Loiselle J, Brenner L, Joffe M. Forensic evidence findings in prepubertal victims of sexual assault. *Pediatrics.* 2000;106:100-104.
8. Workowski KA, Levine WC. Centers for Disease Control and Prevention: sexually transmitted diseases treatment guidelines: 2002. *MMWR Morbid Mortal Wkly Rep.* 2002;51:69-74.
9. Adams JA. Medical evaluation of suspected child sexual abuse. *J Pediatr Adolesc Gynecol.* 2004;17:191-197.
10. CDC 2003 State Health Profiles. Available at: http://www.cdc.gov/epo/shp.index.htm. Accessed May 1, 2005.

# Longitudinal Trends in Race/Ethnic Disparities in Leading Health Indicators From Adolescence to Young Adulthood

*Kathleen Mullan Harris, PhD; Penny Gordon-Larsen, PhD; Kim Chantala, MS; J. Richard Udry, PhD*

**Objective:** To use ethnically diverse, national data to examine longitudinal trends in race/ethnic disparities in 20 leading health indicators from *Healthy People 2010* across multiple domains from adolescence to young adulthood. Much of what is known about health disparities is based on cross-sectional measures collected at a single time point.

**Design, Setting, and Participants:** Nationally representative data for more than 14 000 adolescents enrolled in wave I (1994-1995) or wave II (1996) of the National Longitudinal Study of Adolescent Health (Add Health) and followed up into adulthood (wave III; 2001-2002). We fit longitudinal regression models to assess and contrast the trend in health indicators among racial/ethnic groups of adolescents as they transition into adulthood.

**Main Outcome Measures:** Diet, inactivity, obesity, tobacco use, substance use, binge drinking, violence, sexually transmitted diseases, mental health, and health care access.

**Results:** Diet, inactivity, obesity, health care access, substance use, and reproductive health worsened with age. Perceived health, mental health, and exposure to violence improved with age. On most health indicators, white and Asian subjects were at lowest and Native American subjects at highest risk. Although white subjects had more favorable health in adolescence, they experienced greatest declines by young adulthood. No single race/ethnic group consistently leads or falters in health across all indicators.

**Conclusions:** Longitudinal data indicate that, for 15 of 20 indicators, health risk increased and access to health care decreased from the teen and adult years for most US race/ethnic groups. Relative rankings on a diverse range of health indicators (and patterns of change over time) vary by sex and race/ethnicity, causing disparities to fluctuate over time.

*Arch Pediatr Adolesc Med. 2006;160:74-81*

**Author Affiliations:** Carolina Population Center (Drs Harris, Gordon-Larsen, and Udry and Ms Chantala), Department of Sociology (Drs Harris and Udry), and Department of Nutrition, Schools of Public Health and Medicine (Dr Gordon-Larsen), The University of North Carolina at Chapel Hill.

IN THE UNITED STATES, THERE ARE large and persistent racial, ethnic, and socioeconomic disparities in health across the life course,[1-3] with increasing economic and racial inequality.[4,5] The reduction and ultimate elimination of health disparities has been identified as a major public health goal,[6,7] exemplified by *Healthy People 2010*, the nation's promotion and disease prevention strategy for the first decade of the 21st century.[8]

McGuiness and Foege[9] have described the major external (nongenetic) modifiable factors contributing to death in the United States. Tobacco use and poor diet/inactivity emerged as the 2 leading causes of preventable death in the United States, with alcohol abuse, motor vehicle crashes, sexually transmitted diseases (STDs), firearms, and illicit drug use also important.[9,10] Leading health indicators from *Healthy People 2010* with known disparities in prevalence[8] include sexually transmitted disease,[10-12] illicit drug use,[10,13-15] asthma,[16,17] lack of access to medical care,[18-20] and dental care.[21]

Health disparities research largely provides snapshots of health disparities at a single point in time or for a series of cross-sectional comparisons of different cohorts born at different times. The major contribution of our research is that we follow up the same cohort of ethnically diverse adolescents for 6 years into young adulthood to track change in disparities in health risk over time. We specifically examine 8 of 10 leading health indicators identified in *Healthy People 2010* that are particularly relevant to young people.[7,8] Measures include health indicators related to diet and inactivity, obesity, tobacco use, substance use, STDs, mental health, violence, and access to health care.

## METHODS

### SURVEY DESIGN

The National Longitudinal Study of Adolescent Health (Add Health) cohort is a nationally representative school-based study of youths (grades 7-12), followed up with multiple interview waves into young adulthood. The study used a multistage, stratified, school-based, clustered sampling design. A stratified sample of 80 high schools (and feeder middle schools) was selected with probability proportional to size. Survey procedures were approved by the Institutional Review Board of The University of North Carolina at Chapel Hill and have been previously described.[22] Wave I (1994-1995) included 20 745 adolescents (aged 12-19 years) and their parents. Wave II (1996) included 14 738 wave I adolescents (including school dropouts and excluding graduating seniors). Wave III (2001-2002) included 15 170 wave I adolescents, now aged 18 to 26 years and entering the transition to adulthood (76% response rate).[23] Total bias owing to attrition rarely exceeds 1%, which is small relative to the 20% to 80% prevalence rates for most of our measures.[23-26]

## SAMPLE

We used repeated measures of health indicators, restricting the sample to respondents interviewed at wave I or wave II and at wave III (depending on the measure) with valid data at both time points. When race/ethnic disparity in each measure is tracked from waves I through III, more than 14 000 subjects (7538 females and 6725 males) participated; from waves II through III, more than 10 000 subjects (5719 females and 5069 males) participated. In all analyses, we used wave III sampling weights and survey analysis techniques to adjust for unequal probability of selection, clustered sampling design, and attrition to ensure national representation of US teens on enrollment rosters for grades 7 through 12 in 1994-1995.[23,27,28]

## MEASURES

To provide a comprehensive picture of the major health concerns of our nation, we include a range of measures that capture 8 of 10 leading health indicators of *Healthy People 2010*[8] and that were particularly relevant to young people.

### Health Habits

Diet indicators include the number of days the respondent ate breakfast and fast foods in the past 7 days (waves II and III). Physical activity is reported using a standard physical activity behavior recall that is similar, although not identical, to other self-report questionnaires that have been used and validated in other large-scale epidemiological studies.[29,30] Wave III measures were scaled to be equivalent to those at wave II.[31] Lack of exercise is defined by self-report of no bouts of moderate to vigorous physical activity (5-8 metabolic equivalents) per week (waves II and III).

Obesity is defined using body mass index (BMI; calculated as weight in kilograms divided by the square of height in meters) from the measured height and weight at waves II and III. To deal with the discrepant obesity definitions for adolescents and adults, the International Obesity Task Force reference is used. This reference links childhood and adolescent BMI centiles to the adult BMI cut point of 30 to determine obesity prevalence at wave II.[32] For the young adult population at wave III (aged 19-26 years), we consistently use the adult BMI cut point. Measures have been described in detail elsewhere.[33]

### Health Care

The following health care measures (waves I and III) are dichotomous indicators reflecting lack of care: (1) whether the respondent had current health insurance; (2) whether the respondent needed but did not receive medical care in the last year; (3) whether the respondent needed but could not afford dental or medical care last year; (4) whether the respondent visited a dentist in the last year; and (5) whether the respondent had a physical examination within 2 years.

### General Health

Self-reported health is measured as a dichotomous indicator indicating fair or poor relative to good or excellent health. Asthma (parental report in wave I and self-reported asthma diagnosis in wave III) is measured as a dichotomous indicator.

### Substance Abuse

All measures of substance abuse are self-reported from waves I and II and reflect (1) smoking at least 1 whole cigarette daily during the last 30 days; (2) any use of marijuana in the past 30 days; (3) any use of hard drugs such as cocaine, inhalants, or injected or other illegal drugs in the past 30 days in wave I, and any use of cocaine, injected or other illegal drugs, or crystal methamphetamine in wave III; and (4) binge drinking, defined as 5 or more drinks (ie, glass of wine, can of beer, wine cooler, shot glass of liquor, or mixed drink) on 1 occasion during the past year.

### Reproductive Health

Our only measure of reproductive health is self-reported STD diagnosis (chlamydia, syphilis, gonorrhea, human immunodeficiency virus/AIDS, genital herpes, genital warts, and trichomoniasis for both sexes, and bacterial vaginosis and vaginitis for female subjects) at waves II and III.

### Mental Health

We have the following 2 indicators of mental health at waves I and III: feelings of depression (feeling depressed a lot, most, or all of the time last week) and suicide ideation (the respondent has seriously thought about suicide in the past 12 months).

### Violence

Exposure to violence in the past year is measured across the following items at waves I and III: (1) victim of violence who has been shot, stabbed, beat up, jumped, or threatened with a gun or a knife, and (2) perpetrator of a violent act who has pulled a knife or gun on someone or shot or stabbed someone.

### Race/Ethnicity

Five race and ethnic groups were used based on self-identified race and Hispanic origin at wave III. In the largest sample, tracked from waves I through III, the sample includes non-Hispanic white (n=7728), non-Hispanic black (n=3038), non-Hispanic Asian (n=1021), Hispanic (n=2340), and Native American (n=136) subjects.

## STATISTICAL ANALYSIS

We selected a marginal (or "population-average") longitudinal regression model to estimate temporal change in each health indicator; the hypotheses under investigation were best answered by examining the average experience of each race/ethnic group rather than by examining person-specific variables. Separate models were run for male and female subjects. Covariates used to predict each health indicator in the model included race/ethnic group, time, and the interaction between race/ethnic group and time. Nonsignificant interaction terms were omitted from the final model. We hypothesized that (1) each race/ethnic group experienced no change in the health indicator over time, and (2) the rate of change in the health indicator for each nonwhite race/ethnic group was equal to the rate of change in the health indicator for the white group. To determine if the significant differences in the trend in health over time could be explained by socioeconomic status (SES), median tract income and maximum parental education were included in each of the final models, but had minimal influence on estimates of variables and made no difference in the tests of the hypotheses. Hence, we report results for the models that omitted these 2 covariates.

## RESULTS

Across all sex and race/ethnic groups, there were significant increases in health risk and health disparities from adolescence into young adulthood. There were statistically significant increases over time in the proportion who get no exercise or report asthma, significant declines in breakfast consumption, and significant increases for almost every sex and race/ethnic group in the proportion of respondents who were obese, needed but could not afford medical care, used cigarettes and marijuana, had any STDs, or reported binge drinking, all indicating increasing health risk during the transition from adolescence to adulthood (**Table 1**). Reductions in risk were found in the significant declines over time across almost all sex and race/ethnic groups in the proportion who perceived their health as poor to fair, had feelings of depression or suicidal ideation, and were a victim of violence. All groups (except black and Native American male subjects) had significant declines in perpetrating violent acts.

The race/ethnic groups shift in their position as occupying the best or worst ranking across the various health indicators over time. No single race/ethnic group consistently occupies the best or worst ranking. The tendency was for Asian and non-Hispanic white subjects to generally rank best across time and across multiple domains of health risk, whereas the other minority groups ranked worst (**Table 2** and **Table 3**). However, white subjects lose their favored position more often than other groups as they age into adulthood. Native American subjects tended to appear in the worst rankings most often, followed by non-Hispanic black subjects, with Hispanic subjects in the middle range across most indicators.

Selected illustrative results are presented in **Figure 1** and **Figure 2** by category of health indicator. The full set of figures for male and female subjects in all 20 leading health indicators can be found at http://www.cpc.unc.edu/projects/addhealth/findings.

### HEALTH HABITS AND HEALTH CARE

There was a significant increase in the proportion of overweight/obese adolescents and those engaging in no weekly physical activity (female subjects shown in Figure 1A and B). The trend lines fan out, indicating increasing disparity in young adulthood, highest among black vs white subjects. The proportion of respondents with no health insurance coverage increased significantly for most groups (male subjects shown in Figure 1C). The proportion with the last physical examination more than 2 years ago (Figure 1D) also increased significantly for most male subjects, with increases for Hispanic and Native American subjects proportionately greater than those for white subjects.

### GENERAL AND MENTAL HEALTH, SUBSTANCE USE, REPRODUCTIVE HEALTH, AND VIOLENCE

Self-reports of poor health (male subjects in Figure 2A) and feelings of depression (female subjects in Figure 2B) declined significantly as adolescents aged into young adulthood, and race/ethnic disparities decreased as well. Smoking (Figure 2C) and binge drinking (Figure 2D) increased significantly for all groups, with increasing disparity over time and greatest disadvantage among white subjects. Diagnosis of STDs increased significantly in the transition to adulthood for all groups, with increasing race/ethnic disparity over time (Figure 2E). Violence declined significantly over time for all groups, with decreasing race/ethnic disparity (Figure 2F).

The overall patterns of health disparities include significantly different trends for black relative to white female subjects across almost all domains. Among male subjects, the black-white disparity in trends is significant for more than half of the indicators. For both sexes, the white-Hispanic disparity in health trends is significant for 35% of the indicators. Patterns of change in health indicators are similar for white and Asian subjects, and greater among male than female Native American compared with white subjects.

## COMMENT

To our knowledge, this research is the first to present longitudinal, nationally representative data on race/ethnic disparities in leading health indicators across the transition to adulthood. The fact that we can follow up the same individuals longitudinally to examine changes in these health risk behaviors, specifically the placement of these changes in the context of health disparities, is a major contribution of this research.

For 15 of 20 indicators, health risk increased across all race/ethnic groups during the transition to adulthood. Relative rankings on a diverse range of health indicators (and patterns of change over time) varied by sex and race/ethnicity, causing disparities to fluctuate over time. Asian and white subjects generally scored highest across the range of health indicators; Hispanic subjects scored within the moderate range; and Native American and non-Hispanic black subjects scored the lowest. Although white subjects had more favorable health risk in adolescence, they experienced the greatest decline by young adulthood.

For most of the health indicators showing increased health risk over time, race/ethnic disparities in these indicators also increased. Although the disparities increased, different race/ethnic groups occupied more and less favored positions over time, indicating that no single common approach to reduce disparities is possible given

**Table 1. Estimated Change in Sample Reporting Health Risk Factors and Health Care Access From Adolescence to Young Adulthood Within Race/Ethnicity***

| | Female Subjects | | | | |
|---|---|---|---|---|---|
| Indicator | White | Black | Native American | Asian | Hispanic |
| Breakfast, d/wk† | 0.79 (0.66 to 0.92)‡ | 0.79 (0.66 to 0.92)‡ | 0.79 (0.66 to 0.92)‡ | 0.79 (0.66 to 0.92)‡ | 0.79 (0.66 to 0.92)‡ |
| Fast food, d/wk† | −0.05 (−0.21 to 0.11) | −0.55 (−0.77 to −0.33)‡ | −0.36 (−0.97 to 0.25) | −0.23 (−0.60 to 0.13) | −0.40 (−0.62 to −0.17)‡ |
| No exercise | −0.40 (−0.42 to −0.38)‡ | −0.47 (−0.50 to −0.43)‡ | −0.34 (−0.47 to −0.22)‡ | −0.45 (−0.52 to −0.39)‡ | −0.40 (−0.43 to −0.37)‡ |
| Obese | −0.11 (−0.13 to −0.10)‡ | −0.16 (−0.19 to −0.14)‡ | −0.14 (−0.21 to −0.08)‡ | −0.05 (−0.08 to −0.02)‡ | −0.13 (−0.16 to −0.11)‡ |
| No health insurance | −0.13 (−0.15 to −0.11)‡ | −0.05 (−0.09 to −0.02)‡ | −0.17 (−0.35 to 0.00) | −0.06 (−0.13 to 0.02) | 0.03 (−0.03 to 0.09) |
| Need but did not get medical aid | −0.03 (−0.05 to −0.01) | 0.02 (−0.02 to 0.06) | 0.17 (0.08 to 0.26)‡ | −0.04 (−0.15 to 0.07) | −0.06 (−0.12 to 0.00) |
| Need but could not afford medical aid | −0.16 (−0.18 to −0.14)‡ | −0.12 (−0.14 to −0.10)‡ | −0.22 (−0.32 to −0.13)‡ | −0.11 (−0.16 to −0.06)‡ | −0.17 (−0.19 to −0.14)‡ |
| No dental examination last year | −0.39 (−0.44 to −0.35)‡ | −0.07 (−0.13 to −0.01) | −0.20 (−0.46 to 0.05) | −0.33 (−0.44 to −0.22)‡ | −0.07 (−0.15 to 0.02) |
| Last physical examination >2 y ago | −0.03 (−0.05 to −0.01)‡ | 0.05 (0.03 to 0.08)‡ | 0.04 (−0.18 to 0.26) | 0.01 (−0.08 to 0.09) | 0.04 (−0.02 to 0.10) |
| Health perceived as poor to fair | 0.02 (0.01 to 0.03)‡ | 0.03 (0.01 to 0.05)‡ | 0.03 (0.08 to 0.05)‡ | 0.02 (0.01 to 0.04)‡ | 0.03 (0.01 to 0.04)‡ |
| Asthma | −0.06 (−0.08 to −0.05)‡ | −0.06 (−0.07 to −0.04)‡ | −0.09 (−0.13 to −0.06)‡ | −0.05 (−0.07 to −0.03)‡ | −0.07 (−0.08 to −0.05)‡ |
| Daily cigarette use | −0.14 (−0.71 to −0.12)‡ | −0.07 (−0.09 to −0.05)‡ | −0.13 (−0.35 to 0.08)‡ | −0.06 (−0.10 to −0.02)‡ | −0.09 (−0.12 to −0.06)‡ |
| Marijuana use | −0.06 (−0.08 to −0.04)‡ | −0.04 (−0.06 to −0.03)‡ | −0.08 (−0.11 to −0.04)‡ | −0.03 (−0.05 to −0.01)‡ | −0.05 (−0.07 to −0.03)‡ |
| Drug use | −0.00 (−0.02 to 0.01) | −0.00 (−0.01 to 0.00) | −0.00 (−0.02 to 0.02) | −0.00 (−0.01 to 0.01) | −0.00 (−0.01 to 0.01) |
| Binge drink | −0.25 (−0.28 to −0.21)‡ | −0.02 (−0.06 to 0.01) | −0.20 (−0.43 to 0.02) | −0.11 (−0.19 to −0.06)‡ | −0.12 (−0.16 to −0.06)‡ |
| Any STD | −0.05 (−0.07 to −0.04)‡ | −0.13 (−0.16 to −0.10)‡ | −0.10 (−0.16 to −0.04)‡ | −0.04 (−0.07 to −0.02)‡ | −0.07 (−0.09 to −0.05)‡ |
| Feelings of depression | 0.05 (0.04 to 0.06)‡ | 0.06 (0.04 to 0.08)‡ | 0.06 (0.03 to 0.09)‡ | 0.04 (0.03 to 0.06)‡ | 0.06 (0.05 to 0.08)‡ |
| Suicidal thoughts | 0.10 (0.08 to 0.11)‡ | 0.08 (0.06 to 0.09)‡ | 0.17 (0.10 to 0.24)‡ | 0.09 (0.06 to 0.11)‡ | 0.09 (0.07 to 0.11)‡ |
| Attack someone | 0.01 (0.01 to 0.01)‡ | 0.04 (0.03 to 0.06)‡ | 0.05 (0.00 to 0.10) | 0.02 (0.00 to 0.04) | 0.04 (0.02 to 0.05)‡ |
| Victim of violence | 0.06 (0.05 to 0.07)‡ | 0.12 (0.09 to 0.14)‡ | 0.16 (0.07 to 0.24)‡ | 0.07 (0.04 to 0.09)‡ | 0.11 (0.09 to 0.14)‡ |

| | Male Subjects | | | | |
|---|---|---|---|---|---|
| Indicator | White | Black | Native American | Asian | Hispanic |
| Breakfast, d/wk† | 1.56 (1.41 to 1.70)‡ | 1.56 (1.41 to 1.70)‡ | 1.56 (1.41 to 1.70)‡ | 1.56 (1.41 to 1.70)‡ | 1.56 (1.41 to 1.70)‡ |
| Fast food, d/wk† | −0.35 (−0.50 to −0.20)‡ | −0.98 (−1.25 to −0.71)‡ | 0.79 (−0.18 to 1.76) | −0.17 (−0.60 to 0.27) | −0.49 (−0.79 to −0.19)‡ |
| No exercise | −0.30 (−0.32 to −0.28)‡ | −0.30 (−0.33 to −0.26)‡ | −0.27 (−0.38 to −0.17)‡ | −0.26 (−0.35 to −0.18)‡ | −0.26 (−0.30 to −0.23)‡ |
| Obese | −0.05 (−0.06 to −0.03)‡ | −0.08 (−0.12 to −0.05)‡ | −0.03 (−0.10 to 0.05)‡ | −0.12 (−0.18 to −0.06)‡ | −0.07 (−0.10 to −0.04)‡ |
| No health insurance | −0.17 (−0.19 to −0.14)‡ | −0.16 (−0.21 to −0.11)‡ | −0.19 (−0.46 to 0.09) | −0.03 (−0.13 to 0.06) | −0.11 (−0.19 to −0.04)‡ |
| Need but did not get medical aid | −0.04 (−0.06 to −0.03)‡ | −0.04 (−0.06 to −0.03)‡ | −0.06 (−0.09 to −0.03)‡ | −0.04 (−0.06 to −0.03)‡ | −0.05 (−0.06 to −0.03)‡ |
| Need but could not afford medical aid | −0.11 (−0.13 to −0.10)‡ | −0.08 (−0.10 to −0.06)‡ | −0.14 (−0.31 to 0.02) | −0.07 (−0.10 to −0.04)‡ | −0.12 (−0.14 to −0.09)‡ |
| No dental examination last year | −0.31 (−0.36 to −0.25)‡ | 0.01 (−0.06 to 0.08) | 0.30 (0.10 to 0.49)‡ | −0.32 (−0.42 to −0.22)‡ | 0.04 (−0.05 to 0.13) |
| Last physical examination >2 y ago | −0.24 (−0.27 to −0.21)‡ | −0.11 (−0.15 to −0.07)‡ | −0.08 (−0.21 to 0.04) | −0.21 (−0.29 to −0.13)‡ | −0.13 (−0.17 to −0.08)†‡ |
| Health perceived as poor to fair | 0.02 (0.01 to 0.03)‡ | 0.02 (0.01 to 0.04)‡ | 0.06 (0.03 to 0.10)‡ | 0.01 (0.00 to 0.02)‡ | 0.02 (0.01 to 0.03)‡ |
| Asthma | −0.03 (−0.04 to −0.02)‡ | −0.04 (−0.05 to −0.03)‡ | −0.03 (−0.06 to −0.01)‡ | −0.03 (−0.04 to −0.01)‡ | −0.03 (−0.05 to −0.02)‡ |
| Daily cigarette use | −0.19 (−0.21 to −0.17)‡ | −0.09 (−0.11 to −0.06)‡ | −0.15 (−0.22 to −0.07)‡ | −0.12 (−0.16 to −0.08)‡ | −0.10 (−0.13 to −0.07)‡ |
| Marijuana use | −0.16 (−0.18 to −0.13)‡ | −0.08 (−0.13 to −0.03)‡ | −0.01 (−0.18 to 0.19) | −0.03 (−0.09 to 0.03) | −0.05 (−0.10 to −0.01) |
| Drug use | −0.04 (−0.06 to −0.02)‡ | −0.02 (−0.03 to −0.01)‡ | −0.05 (−0.08 to −0.02)‡ | −0.03 (−0.04 to −0.01)‡ | −0.03 (−0.04 to −0.01)‡ |
| Binge drink | −0.35 (−0.40 to −0.32)‡ | −0.12 (−0.17 to −0.07)‡ | −0.28 (−0.42 to −0.13)‡ | −0.32 (−0.42 to −0.22)‡ | −0.23 (−0.30 to −0.16)‡ |
| Any STD | −0.02 (−0.02 to −0.01)‡ | −0.05 (−0.08 to −0.03)‡ | −0.07 (−0.13 to −0.01)‡ | −0.01 (−0.02 to 0.00) | −0.02 (−0.04 to −0.01)‡ |
| Feelings of depression | 0.02 (0.01 to 0.03)‡ | 0.03 (0.01 to 0.04)‡ | 0.03 (0.00 to 0.05) | 0.02 (0.01 to 0.04)‡ | 0.03 (0.02 to 0.05)‡ |
| Suicidal thoughts | 0.04 (0.03 to 0.06)‡ | 0.03 (0.02 to 0.04)‡ | 0.05 (0.01 to 0.09)‡ | 0.05 (0.03 to 0.07)‡ | 0.04 (0.02 to 0.05)‡ |
| Attack someone | 0.03 (0.03 to 0.04)‡ | 0.08 (0.06 to 0.10)‡ | 0.12 (0.07 to 0.18)‡ | 0.05 (0.02 to 0.07)‡ | 0.05 (0.03 to 0.06)‡ |
| Victim of violence | 0.14 (0.12 to 0.16)‡ | 0.18 (0.16 to 0.21)‡ | 0.20 (0.14 to 0.26)‡ | 0.12 (0.08 to 0.16)‡ | 0.18 (0.15 to 0.21)‡ |

Abbreviation: STD, sexually transmitted disease.

*Unless otherwise indicated, data are expressed as proportions of the sample reporting select measures at time 1 (adolescence) minus the proportion reporting select measures at time 2 (young adulthood). Numbers in parentheses are 95% confidence intervals.

†Expressed as mean number at time 1 (adolescence) minus mean number at time 2 (young adulthood) (95% confidence interval).

‡Change over time (estimated time 1 level [wave I or II] minus estimated time 2 level [wave III]) was significantly different from 0 ($P<.01$).

the race/ethnic variation in change and rankings in health risk across time. Documenting race/ethnic disparities in health indicators is essential in understanding risk and formulating preventive strategies to tackle these important behavioral/health concerns.[34-37] Furthermore, research needs to move beyond race/ethnicity to understand the underlying causes of health disparities in the United States.[38]

The extent to which socioeconomic differences may account for observed disparities in health outcomes across

**Table 2. Prevalence of Leading Health Indicators in US Females***

| Indicator | Subjects Participating in Adolescence (Waves I-II) | | | | | Subjects Participating in Young Adulthood (Wave III) | | | | |
|---|---|---|---|---|---|---|---|---|---|---|
| | White | Black | Native American | Asian | Hispanic | White | Black | Native American | Asian | Hispanic |
| Breakfast, d/wk | **4.18 (4.01 to 4.34)** | *3.41 (3.21 to 3.61)* | 3.79 (3.17 to 4.41) | 3.85 (3.33 to 4.37) | 3.89 (3.66 to 4.12) | **3.38 (3.25 to 3.52)** | *2.62 (2.42 to 2.82)* | 3.00 (2.37 to 3.63) | 3.06 (2.53 to 3.58) | 3.10 (2.89 to 3.30) |
| Fast food, d/wk | 2.04 (1.91 to 2.16) | *2.22 (2.04 to 2.39)* | **1.72 (1.29 to 2.15)** | 1.87 (1.48 to 2.25) | 1.96 (1.79 to 2.13) | 2.09 (1.95 to 2.22) | *2.77 (2.60 to 2.93)* | **2.08 (1.55 to 2.61)** | 2.10 (1.70 to 2.51) | 2.36 (2.14 to 2.57) |
| No exercise | 0.06 (0.05 to 0.07) | *0.08 (0.07 to 0.09)* | **0.04 (0.02 to 0.07)** | 0.08 (0.05 to 0.10) | 0.06 (0.05 to 0.07) | 0.46 (0.43 to 0.48) | *0.55 (0.51 to 0.59)* | **0.39 (0.23 to 0.54)** | 0.53 (0.44 to 0.62) | 0.46 (0.42 to 0.50) |
| Obese | 0.10 (0.09 to 0.12) | *0.18 (0.15 to 0.20)* | 0.14 (0.05 to 0.23) | **0.04 (0.01 to 0.06)** | 0.13 (0.10 to 0.16) | 0.21 (0.19 to 0.24) | *0.34 (0.30 to 0.38)* | 0.28 (0.13 to 0.44) | **0.09 (0.03 to 0.14)** | 0.26 (0.22 to 0.31) |
| No health insurance | 0.08 (0.07 to 0.10) | 0.15 (0.11 to 0.18) | **0.06 (0.00 to 0.11)** | 0.12 (0.04 to 0.21) | *0.33 (0.26 to 0.39)* | 0.21 (0.19 to 0.23) | 0.20 (0.17 to 0.23) | 0.23 (0.07 to 0.38) | **0.18 (0.13 to 0.23)** | *0.29 (0.25 to 0.33)* |
| Need but did not get medical aid | **0.18 (0.16 to 0.20)** | 0.25 (0.22 to 0.28) | *0.37 (0.24 to 0.49)* | 0.20 (0.13 to 0.26) | 0.24 (0.19 to 0.28) | 0.21 (0.19 to 0.22) | 0.23 (0.19 to 0.25) | **0.20 (0.09 to 0.30)** | 0.24 (0.16 to 0.31) | *0.29 (0.25 to 0.34)* |
| Need but could not afford medical aid | 0.04 (0.03 to 0.04) | 0.03 (0.02 to 0.03) | *0.06 (0.02 to 0.10)* | **0.03 (0.01 to 0.04)** | 0.04 (0.03 to 0.05) | 0.19 (0.17 to 0.21) | 0.15 (0.12 to 0.17) | *0.28 (0.15 to 0.41)* | **0.14 (0.08 to 0.20)** | 0.21 (0.17 to 0.24) |
| No dental examination last year | **0.24 (0.22 to 0.27)** | 0.43 (0.39 to 0.47) | 0.38 (0.23 to 0.52) | 0.31 (0.24 to 0.39) | *0.44 (0.39 to 0.49)* | *0.64 (0.61 to 0.66)* | **0.50 (0.46 to 0.54)** | 0.58 (0.43 to 0.73) | 0.64 (0.57 to 0.71) | 0.50 (0.45 to 0.55) |
| Last physical examination >2 y ago | **0.11 (0.09 to 0.13)** | 0.11 (0.09 to 0.14) | *0.20 (0.05 to 0.36)* | 0.17 (0.11 to 0.22) | 0.17 (0.11 to 0.22) | 0.14 (0.13 to 0.15) | **0.06 (0.04 to 0.08)** | *0.16 (0.05 to 0.27)* | 0.16 (0.10 to 0.21) | 0.12 (0.10 to 0.15) |
| Health perceived as poor to fair | **0.07 (0.06 to 0.09)** | *0.11 (0.09 to 0.13)* | 0.09 (0.04 to 0.15) | 0.09 (0.05 to 0.12) | 0.10 (0.07 to 0.12) | **0.05 (0.04 to 0.06)** | *0.08 (0.06 to 0.09)* | 0.07 (0.02 to 0.11) | 0.06 (0.03 to 0.09) | 0.07 (0.05 to 0.08) |
| Asthma | 0.12 (0.11 to 0.13) | 0.10 (0.08 to 0.13) | *0.20 (0.09 to 0.32)* | **0.09 (0.05 to 0.12)** | 0.12 (0.10 to 0.15) | 0.18 (0.17 to 0.20) | 0.16 (0.13 to 0.19) | *0.30 (0.15 to 0.44)* | **0.13 (0.09 to 0.18)** | 0.19 (0.15 to 0.22) |
| Daily cigarette use | *0.14 (0.12 to 0.16)* | **0.01 (0.01 to 0.02)** | 0.08 (−0.05 to 0.21) | 0.03 (0.00 to 0.05) | 0.05 (0.02 to 0.07) | *0.28 (0.26 to 0.31)* | **0.08 (0.06 to 0.11)** | 0.22 (0.04 to 0.39) | 0.09 (0.03 to 0.14) | 0.14 (0.09 to 0.18) |
| Use marijuana | 0.14 (0.12 to 0.16) | 0.09 (0.07 to 0.12) | *0.21 (0.13 to 0.28)* | **0.07 (0.04 to 0.10)** | 0.12 (0.10 to 0.15) | 0.20 (0.18 to 0.22) | 0.13 (0.10 to 0.16) | *0.28 (0.19 to 0.38)* | **0.11 (0.06 to 0.15)** | 0.17 (0.14 to 0.20) |
| Take hard drugs | 0.06 (0.05 to 0.07) | **0.02 (0.01 to 0.02)** | *0.08 (0.00 to 0.16)* | 0.04 (0.02 to 0.05) | 0.05 (0.03 to 0.07) | 0.06 (0.05 to 0.07) | **0.02 (0.01 to 0.02)** | *0.09 (0.00 to 0.17)* | 0.04 (0.02 to 0.06) | 0.05 (0.04 to 0.07) |
| Binge drink | 0.28 (0.25 to 0.30) | 0.13 (0.10 to 0.16) | *0.33 (0.19 to 0.47)* | **0.17 (0.09 to 0.25)** | 0.24 (0.19 to 0.29) | 0.52 (0.50 to 0.55) | **0.15 (0.12 to 0.18)** | *0.54 (0.39 to 0.68)* | 0.29 (0.21 to 0.37) | 0.35 (0.30 to 0.40) |
| Any STD | 0.03 (0.02 to 0.04) | *0.08 (0.06 to 0.10)* | 0.06 (0.02 to 0.10) | **0.02 (0.01 to 0.04)** | 0.04 (0.02 to 0.05) | 0.08 (0.07 to 0.09) | *0.21 (0.18 to 0.23)* | 0.16 (0.06 to 0.25) | **0.07 (0.02 to 0.11)** | 0.11 (0.07 to 0.14) |
| Feelings of depression | 0.12 (0.10 to 0.13) | 0.15 (0.12 to 0.17) | 0.15 (0.08 to 0.22) | **0.10 (0.06 to 0.14)** | *0.16 (0.13 to 0.18)* | 0.07 (0.06 to 0.08) | 0.09 (0.07 to 0.10) | 0.09 (0.05 to 0.14) | **0.06 (0.03 to 0.08)** | *0.09 (0.07 to 0.11)* |
| Suicidal thoughts | 0.17 (0.15 to 0.18) | **0.13 (0.11 to 0.15)** | *0.33 (0.16 to 0.51)* | 0.15 (0.11 to 0.19) | 0.16 (0.12 to 0.19) | 0.07 (0.06 to 0.08) | **0.06 (0.04 to 0.07)** | *0.16 (0.05 to 0.27)* | 0.06 (0.04 to 0.08) | 0.07 (0.05 to 0.09) |
| Attack someone | **0.01 (0.01 to 0.01)** | 0.06 (0.04 to 0.07) | *0.06 (0.00 to 0.12)* | 0.03 (0.01 to 0.05) | 0.05 (0.03 to 0.06) | **0.00 (0.00 to 0.00)** | 0.01 (0.01 to 0.02) | *0.01 (0.00 to 0.02)* | 0.01 (0.00 to 0.01) | 0.01 (0.00 to 0.01) |
| Victim of violence | **0.09 (0.08 to 0.10)** | 0.17 (0.14 to 0.21) | *0.24 (0.09 to 0.39)* | 0.09 (0.06 to 0.13) | 0.17 (0.14 to 0.19) | **0.03 (0.02 to 0.03)** | 0.06 (0.04 to 0.07) | *0.08 (0.02 to 0.15)* | 0.03 (0.02 to 0.04) | 0.05 (0.04 to 0.06) |

Abbreviation: STD, sexually transmitted disease.

*Unless otherwise indicated, data are expressed as proportions of the sample reporting select measures during adolescence (waves I and II) and young adulthood (wave III). Prevalence estimates are generated from predictions from the final interactive or main effects model for each outcome. Results were unchanged with socioeconomic status controls. Numbers in parentheses are 95% confidence intervals. Boldface indicates best and italic indicates worst ranks of health disparities.

race/ethnic groups varies across studies.[2,39] Our analytical models suggest no changes in race/ethnic disparities over time with controls for SES. Thus, factors beyond income and education may play a role in the cause of these health trends. Furthermore, SES may be related to the starting point on our health indicators in adolescence, but not to the trends in these indicators over time. It is also possible that we do not capture the complexity of the SES-health relationship across the transition from adolescence to young adulthood. For example, as teens leave their parental homes, they are likely to lose health insurance coverage owing to aging out of Medicaid coverage or leaving their parents' health insurance coverage.

The top 3 leading actual causes of death in the year 2000 were (1) tobacco use, (2) poor diet and physical inactivity, and (3) alcohol consumption.[10] We found dramatic increases in behaviors related to these 3 leading causes of death. As adolescents become young adults, they are more likely to eat fast food, get no exercise, be obese, and smoke cigarettes. Binge drinking (the most common pattern of alcohol abuse[40]) increased among male and female subjects (except black and Native American subjects). These findings underscore the importance of ongoing preventive efforts related to smoking, poor diet and physical inactivity, and alcohol consumption early in the life course.

As adolescents aged into young adulthood, an increasing proportion had no current health insurance, did not receive health care when they needed it, and did not get regular dental or physical examinations (male but not female subjects, likely due to the entrance into prime childbearing age). Race/ethnic disparities increased in the need for but inability to afford medical care, further exacerbating race/ethnic disparities in health[19,20] and potentially leading to increased mortality.[18]

**Table 3. Prevalence of Leading Health Indicators in US Male Subjects***

| Indicator | Subjects Participating in Adolescence (Wave I-II) | | | | | Subjects Participating in Young Adulthood (Wave III) | | | | |
|---|---|---|---|---|---|---|---|---|---|---|
| | White | Black | Native American | Asian | Hispanic | White | Black | Native American | Asian | Hispanic |
| Breakfast, d/wk | **4.62 (4.46 to 4.77)** | 4.37 (4.16 to 4.58) | *3.69 (3.14 to 4.24)* | 4.26 (3.81 to 4.70) | 4.60 (4.39 to 4.82) | **3.06 (2.95 to 3.16)** | 2.81 (2.61 to 3.02) | *2.13 (1.57 to 2.69)* | 2.70 (2.26 to 3.14) | 3.05 (2.83 to 3.26) |
| Fast food, d/wk | 2.27 (2.15 to 2.40) | 2.18 (2.02 to 2.34) | *3.12 (2.37 to 3.87)* | **2.03 (1.62 to 2.44)** | 2.28 (2.04 to 2.52) | 2.62 (2.49 to 2.75) | *3.16 (2.90 to 3.42)* | 2.33 (1.64 to 3.02) | **2.20 (1.86 to 2.53)** | 2.77 (2.54 to 2.99) |
| No exercise | *0.05 (0.04 to 0.06)* | 0.05 (0.04 to 0.06) | 0.04 (0.02 to 0.07) | **0.04 (0.02 to 0.06)** | 0.04 (0.03 to 0.05) | *0.35 (0.33 to 0.37)* | 0.34 (0.30 to 0.39) | 0.32 (0.18 to 0.45) | **0.31 (0.20 to 0.41)** | 0.31 (0.26 to 0.35) |
| Obese | 0.14 (0.12 to 0.16) | 0.14 (0.11 to 0.17) | *0.39 (0.11 to 0.66)* | **0.10 (0.05 to 0.14)** | 0.15 (0.11 to 0.18) | 0.19 (0.17 to 0.21) | 0.22 (0.18 to 0.26) | *0.41 (0.07 to 0.75)* | **0.21 (0.13 to 0.30)** | 0.22 (0.18 to 0.26) |
| No health insurance | 0.09 (0.08 to 0.11) | 0.13 (0.10 to 0.15) | **0.08 (0.02 to 0.14)** | 0.14 (0.06 to 0.22) | *0.27 (0.20 to 0.34)* | 0.26 (0.23 to 0.29) | 0.29 (0.24 to 0.34) | 0.27 (0.02 to 0.52) | **0.17 (0.12 to 0.22)** | *0.38 (0.33 to 0.44)* |
| Need but did not get medical aid | 0.18 (0.16 to 0.20) | 0.19 (0.16 to 0.21) | *0.30 (0.17 to 0.43)* | **0.17 (0.12 to 0.21)** | 0.19 (0.16 to 0.22) | 0.22 (0.21 to 0.24) | 0.23 (0.20 to 0.26) | 0.36 (0.21 to 0.50) | **0.21 (0.16 to 0.25)** | 0.23 (0.19 to 0.27) |
| Need but could not afford medical aid | 0.02 (0.02 to 0.03) | 0.02 (0.01 to 0.02) | *0.03 (0.01 to 0.07)* | **0.01 (0.01 to 0.02)** | 0.02 (0.02 to 0.03) | 0.13 (0.12 to 0.15) | 0.10 (0.07 to 0.12) | *0.17 (−0.03 to 0.38)* | **0.08 (0.04 to 0.12)** | 0.14 (0.11 to 0.17) |
| No dental examination last year | **0.28 (0.25 to 0.31)** | 0.47 (0.42 to 0.51) | *0.60 (0.46 to 0.74)* | 0.32 (0.23 to 0.40) | 0.47 (0.41 to 0.54) | 0.58 (0.55 to 0.61) | 0.46 (0.41 to 0.50) | **0.30 (0.18 to 0.42)** | *0.63 (0.58 to 0.69)* | 0.44 (0.40 to 0.48) |
| Last physical examination >2 y ago | 0.10 (0.08 to 0.11) | 0.09 (0.06 to 0.11) | *0.19 (0.08 to 0.30)* | **0.09 (0.04 to 0.13)** | 0.18 (0.14 to 0.22) | *0.34 (0.31 to 0.37)* | **0.20 (0.17 to 0.23)** | 0.27 (0.15 to 0.39) | 0.29 (0.21 to 0.38) | 0.31 (0.25 to 0.36) |
| Health perceived as poor to fair | 0.05 (0.04 to 0.06) | 0.08 (0.06 to 0.10) | *0.21 (0.13 to 0.30)* | **0.04 (0.02 to 0.07)** | 0.05 (0.03 to 0.07) | 0.04 (0.03 to 0.04) | 0.05 (0.04 to 0.07) | *0.15 (0.09 to 0.22)* | **0.03 (0.01 to 0.04)** | 0.04 (0.02 to 0.05) |
| Asthma | 0.12 (0.10 to 0.13) | *0.14 (0.12 to 0.17)* | 0.12 (0.03 to 0.21) | **0.10 (0.05 to 0.15)** | 0.11 (0.08 to 0.14) | 0.15 (0.14 to 0.17) | ***0.18 (0.15 to 0.22)*** | 0.16 (0.05 to 0.27) | **0.13 (0.07 to 0.19)** | 0.15 (0.11 to 0.18) |
| Daily cigarette use | *0.12 (0.10 to 0.14)* | **0.05 (0.03 to 0.06)** | 0.09 (0.02 to 0.15) | 0.06 (0.04 to 0.09) | 0.05 (0.03 to 0.07) | *0.31 (0.29 to 0.33)* | **0.13 (0.10 to 0.17)** | 0.23 (0.09 to 0.37) | 0.18 (0.13 to 0.24) | 0.56 (0.11 to 0.20) |
| Use marijuana | 0.14 (0.12 to 0.16) | 0.19 (0.15 to 0.23) | *0.28 (0.15 to 0.40)* | **0.14 (0.07 to 0.20)** | 0.15 (0.12 to 0.19) | *0.30 (0.28 to 0.32)* | 0.27 (0.23 to 0.32) | 0.27 (0.13 to 0.41) | **0.17 (0.11 to 0.22)** | 0.20 (0.16 to 0.24) |
| Use hard drugs | 0.07 (0.05 to 0.08) | **0.03 (0.02 to 0.04)** | *0.08 (0.04 to 0.13)* | 0.04 (0.02 to 0.06) | 0.05 (0.03 to 0.06) | 0.11 (0.10 to 0.12) | **0.05 (0.03 to 0.06)** | *0.14 (0.07 to 0.20)* | 0.07 (0.03 to 0.10) | 0.07 (0.05 to 0.10) |
| Binge drink | *0.32 (0.28 to 0.35)* | 0.21 (0.16 to 0.25) | 0.30 (0.18 to 0.43) | **0.17 (0.11 to 0.22)** | 0.31 (0.26 to 0.36) | *0.67 (0.64 to 0.71)* | **0.33 (0.27 to 0.38)** | 0.58 (0.44 to 0.72) | 0.49 (0.41 to 0.57) | 0.54 (0.50 to 0.58) |
| Any STD | 0.01 (0.01 to 0.02) | 0.04 (0.02 to 0.06) | *0.06 (0.01 to 0.10)* | **0.01 (0.00 to 0.01)** | 0.02 (0.01 to 0.03) | 0.03 (0.02 to 0.03) | 0.09 (0.07 to 0.11) | *0.13 (0.03 to 0.22)* | **0.01 (0.00 to 0.03)** | 0.04 (0.02 to 0.06) |
| Feelings of depression | **0.06 (0.05 to 0.07)** | 0.08 (0.06 to 0.10) | 0.07 (0.02 to 0.12) | 0.06 (0.03 to 0.10) | *0.09 (0.07 to 0.12)* | **0.04 (0.03 to 0.05)** | 0.05 (0.04 to 0.06) | 0.05 (0.01 to 0.08) | 0.04 (0.02 to 0.06) | *0.06 (0.04 to 0.08)* |
| Suicidal thoughts | 0.11 (0.10 to 0.12) | **0.08 (0.06 to 0.10)** | *0.14 (0.04 to 0.25)* | 0.12 (0.08 to 0.16) | 0.09 (0.07 to 0.11) | 0.07 (0.06 to 0.08) | **0.05 (0.03 to 0.06)** | *0.09 (0.02 to 0.16)* | 0.07 (0.05 to 0.10) | 0.06 (0.04 to 0.07) |
| Attack someone | **0.05 (0.04 to 0.06)** | 0.13 (0.11 to 0.15) | *0.21 (0.12 to 0.30)* | 0.07 (0.03 to 0.11) | 0.08 (0.05 to 0.10) | **0.02 (0.01 to 0.02)** | 0.05 (0.04 to 0.06) | *0.08 (0.04 to 0.13)* | 0.03 (0.01 to 0.04) | 0.03 (0.02 to 0.04) |
| Victim of violence | 0.25 (0.23 to 0.27) | 0.35 (0.31 to 0.38) | *0.40 (0.23 to 0.56)* | **0.21 (0.14 to 0.27)** | 0.34 (0.30 to 0.38) | 0.11 (0.10 to 0.12) | 0.16 (0.14 to 0.19) | *0.20 (0.09 to 0.30)* | **0.09 (0.06 to 0.12)** | 0.16 (0.14 to 0.19) |

Abbreviation: STD, sexually transmitted disease.

*Numbers in parentheses are 95% confidence intervals.

†Unless otherwise indicated, data are expressed as proportions of the sample reporting select measures during adolescence (waves I and II) and young adulthood (wave III). Prevalence estimates are generated from predictions from the final interactive or main effects model for each outcome. Results were unchanged with socioeconomic status controls. Boldface indicates best and italic indicates worst ranks of health disparities.

Similarly, the levels and disparities in asthma increased from adolescence to young adulthood, affecting Native American and black subjects most and confirming research that shows increasing prevalence of asthma, particularly among minorities.[16,17] Diagnosis of STDs increased over time with substantial race/ethnic disparity (highest for black subjects). Similarly, the proportion using marijuana and hard drugs (male subjects) increased over time, with increasing race/ethnic disparity in marijuana use (highest for white subjects). The trends in prevalence of STDs and illicit drug use prompts concern owing to the association of these health indicators with increased mortality risk.[9]

On the positive side, feelings of depression and suicidal ideation decreased over time (particularly for black subjects), and differences among the race/ethnic groups declined. It is possible that this co-occurrence could, as the literature shows, influence other health risk behaviors, such as a range of STD/human immunodeficiency virus–associated sexual activity,[41] substance abuse,[15] tobacco use,[42] and obesity.[43] Similarly positive was the reduction in victimization and perpetration of violence. The improvement in self-reported health indicates an interesting dichotomy as these young adults consider themselves to be in good health, despite engaging in a range of health risk behaviors with negative current (and future) health implications.

We included measures of 8 of the 10 leading health indicators highlighted in *Healthy People 2010*[8] salient for young people (not included are measures of environmental quality and immunization). Although these are admittedly a broad array of health indicators that represent several different health constructs, they are important indicators reflecting major health concerns in the United States at the beginning of the 21st century.[8] Furthermore, the meaning of health risk may change from adolescence to young adulthood (eg, sexual behavior may be considered more risky in adolescence than young adult-

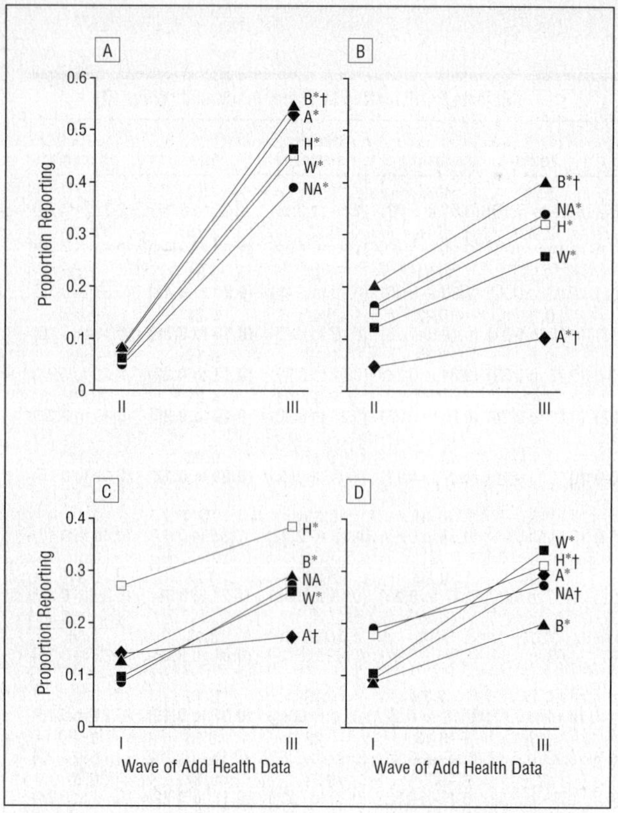

**Figure 1.** Graphs demonstrate trends over time in patterns of race/ethnic disparities in health habits and health care. A, Female subjects with no weekly exercise. B, Female subjects who are overweight or obese. C, Male subjects with no current health insurance. D, Male subjects whose last physical examination was more than 2 years ago. Asterisk indicates that the adolescent measure (wave I or II) differs significantly from the young adult measure (wave III) ($P<.05$); dagger, change over time differs significantly for the specified race/ethnic group relative to white subjects ($P<.05$); A, Asian; Add Health, National Longitudinal Study of Adolescent Health; B, black; H, Hispanic; NA, Native American; and W, white.

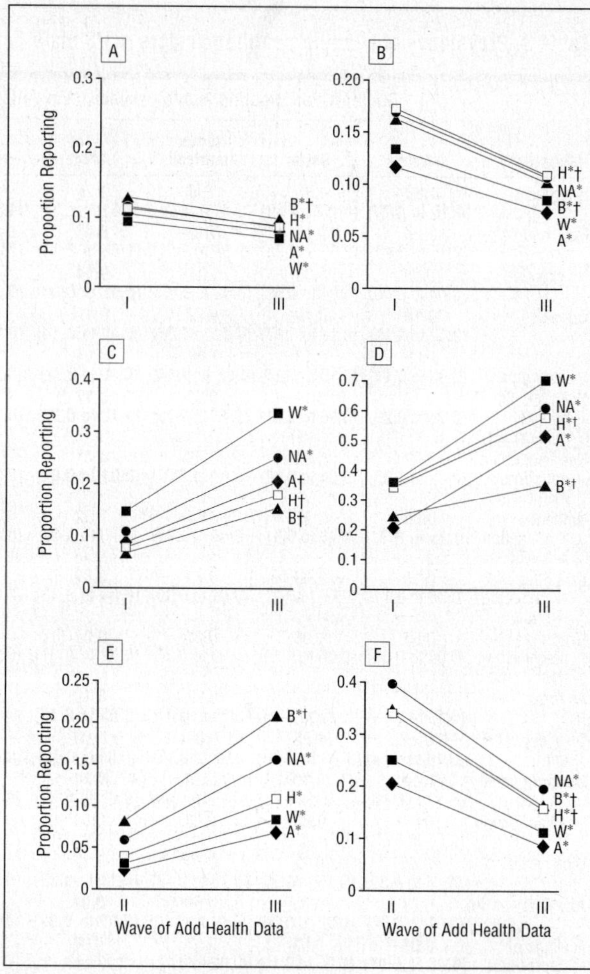

**Figure 2.** Graphs demonstrate trends over time in patterns of race/ethnic disparities in general and mental health, substance abuse, sexually transmitted disease (STD), self-reported health status, and violence. A, Female subjects with self-reported poor health. B, Female subjects with feelings of depression. C, Male subjects who smoke cigarettes daily. D, Male subjects who engage in binge drinking. E, Female subjects with a diagnosis of an STD in the past year. F, Female subjects who were victims of violence in the past year. Asterisk indicates that the adolescent measure (wave I or II) differs significantly from the young adult (wave III) measure ($P<.05$); dagger, change over time differs significantly for the specified race/ethnic group relative to white subjects ($P<.05$). Other abbreviations are described in the legend to Figure 1.

hood). Another limitation is our use of the standard race/ethnic categories, which may mask important race/ethnic heterogeneity within these groups.

Our findings indicate a strong and unprecedented decline in health during the transition to young adulthood in the current generation. Although we have no point of reference to compare these findings with those for other generations, the within-cohort trends indicate deterioration in health behaviors. As this cohort is followed up in adulthood, the assessment of morbidity and mortality outcomes associated with this increased health risk will be possible. Shifts in health profiles are part of our epidemiological history when, for example, during the demographic transition a mortality pattern of malnutrition and infectious disease shifted to one of high prevalence of chronic and degenerative diseases associated with urban-industrial lifestyles[44] and into a period of delayed degenerative diseases, a major shift in age-specific mortality patterns, and a consequent increase in life expectancy.[45] Furthermore, evidence suggests that life expectancy gains have dropped in recent decades.[46]

One finding of major concern is the fact that young US adults are engaging in a range of health risk behaviors that puts them at increased risk of future adverse health outcomes. Our findings have serious implications for the present and future health of this generation. We find substantial race/ethnic disparities in health that vary depending on the measure. Because our findings show great variability in the levels, relative rankings, and changes in race/ethnic disparities, policies to reduce race/ethnic disparities in health require completely different actions for each health indicator. Attention must be paid to national efforts to reduce and ameliorate these preventable conditions, particularly in light of national health objectives for reducing race/ethnic disparities in leading health indicators.

**Accepted for Publication:** July 8, 2005.
**Correspondence:** Penny Gordon-Larsen, PhD, The University of North Carolina at Chapel Hill, Carolina Population Center, University Square, 123 West Franklin St, Chapel Hill, NC 27516-3997 (gordon_larsen@unc.edu).
**Funding/Support:** This study was supported by grant P01

HD31921 (Drs Harris and Udry) as part of the National Longitudinal Study of Adolescent Health (Add Health) program project, grant U01 HD37558 (Dr Harris) as part of the National Institute of Child Health and Human Development (NICHD) Family and Child Well-Being Research Network, and grant K01 HD044263 (Dr Gordon-Larsen) from the NICHD, Rockville, Md.

**Additional Information:** This research uses data from Add Health, a program project designed by J. Richard Udry, PhD, Peter S. Bearman, PhD, and Kathleen Mullan Harris, PhD, with funding from the NICHD and cooperative funding from 17 other agencies. Persons interested in obtaining data files from Add Health should contact Add Health, Carolina Population Center, 123 W Franklin St, Chapel Hill, NC 27516-2524 (www.cpc.unc.edu/addhealth/contract.html).

**Acknowledgment:** We thank Carol Ford, MD, and Parker Frisbee, PhD, for their helpful comments on an earlier draft and Lani Cartier and Sally Middleton for their assistance in preparation of the manuscript. Special acknowledgment is due Ronald R. Rindfuss, PhD, and Barbara Entwisle, PhD, for assistance in the original design.

## REFERENCES

1. National Center for Health Statistics. *Health, United States, 2002.* Hyattsville, Md: National Center for Health Statistics; 2002.
2. Williams DR, Collins C. Racial residential segregation: a fundamental cause of racial disparities in health. *Public Health Rep.* 2001;116:404-416.
3. Keppel KG, Pearcy JN, Wagener DK. Trends in racial and ethnic-specific rates for the health status indicators: United States, 1990-98. Hyattsville, Md: National Center for Health Statistics; 2002. Healthy People 2000 Statistical Notes, No. 23.
4. Lenfant C. Conference on socioeconomic status and cardiovascular health and disease. *Circulation.* 1996;94:2041-2044.
5. Atkinson A-B, Bourguignon F. *Handbooks in Economics.* Vol 16. New York, NY: Elsevier Science Inc; 2000.
6. Satcher D. Eliminating racial and ethnic disparities in health: the role of the ten leading health indicators. *J Natl Med Assoc.* 2000;92:315-318.
7. US Department of Health and Human Services. National Institutes of Health strategic research plan and budget to reduce and ultimately eliminate health disparities, Vol I: fiscal years 2002-2006. Available at: http://www.ncmhd.nih.gov. Accessed June 17, 2005.
8. US Department of Health and Human Services. *Healthy People 2010: Understanding and Improving Health.* Washington, DC: US Dept of Health and Human Services, Government Printing Office; 2000.
9. McGinnis JM, Foege WH. Actual causes of death in the United States. *JAMA.* 1993;270:2207-2212.
10. Mokdad AH, Marks JS, Stroup DF, Gerberding J. Actual causes of death in the United States, 2000. *JAMA.* 2004;291:1238-1245.
11. Michaud CM, Murray CJL, Bloom BR. Burden of diseases: implications for future research. *JAMA.* 2001;285:535-539.
12. Centers for Disease Control and Prevention. *Sexually Transmitted Disease Surveillance 2000.* Atlanta, Ga: US Dept of Health and Human Services, Centers for Disease Control and Prevention; 2001.
13. Rivara FP, Mueller BA, Somes G, Mendoza CT, Rushforth NB, Kellermann AL. Alcohol and illicit drug abuse and the risk of violent death in the home. *JAMA.* 1997;278:569-575.
14. Bruner AB, Fishman M. Adolescents and illicit drug use. *JAMA.* 1998;280:597-598.
15. Regier DA, Farmer ME, Rae DS, et al. Comorbidity of mental disorders with alcohol and other drug abuse: results from the Epidemiologic Catchment Area (ECA) Study. *JAMA.* 1990;264:2511-2518.
16. Ma3ssey IT, Moore TF, Parsons VL, Tadros W. *Design and Estimation for the National Health Interview Survey, 1985-1994.* Hyattsville, Md: US Dept of Health and Human Services; 1989. Dept of Health and Human Services publication (PHS)89-1384.
17. National Center for Health Statistics. Asthma prevalence, health care use and mortality, 2000-2001. Available at: http://www.cdc.gov/nchs/products/pubs/pubd/hestats/asthma/asthma.htm. Accessed June 15, 2005.
18. Eisenberg JM, Power EJ. Transforming insurance coverage into quality health care: voltage drops from potential to delivered quality *JAMA.* 2000;284:2100-2107.
19. Schuster MA, McGlynn EA, Brook RH. How good is the quality of health care in the United States? *Milbank Q.* 1998;76:517-563.
20. Franks P, Clancy CM, Gold MR. Health insurance and mortality: evidence from a national cohort. *JAMA.* 1993;270:737-741.
21. Newacheck PW, Hughes DC, Hung YY, Wong S, Stoddard JJ. The unmet health needs of America's children. *Pediatrics.* 2000;105:989-997.
22. Harris KM, Florey F, Tabor J, Bearman PS, Jones J, Udry JR. The National Longitudinal Study of Adolescent Health: research design, 2003. Available at: http://www.cpc.unc.edu/projects/addhealth/design.html. Accessed June 17, 2005.
23. Chantala K, Kalsbeek WD, Andraca E. Non-response in wave III of the Add Health study, 2003. Available at: http://www.cpc.unc.edu/projects/addhealth/pubs/guides. Accessed June 17, 2005.
24. Chantala K, Kalsbeek WD, Andraca E. Nonresponse in wave III of the Add Health Study, 2004. Available at: http://www.cpc.unc.edu/projects/addhealth/files/W3nonres.pdf. Accessed June 17, 2005.
25. Kalsbeek WD, Yang J, Agans RP. Predictors of nonresponse in a longitudinal survey of adolescents. Paper presented at: Annual Meeting of the American Statistical Association, Joint Statistical Meetings; August 13, 2002; Alexandria, Va.
26. Kalsbeek WD, Morris CB, Vaughn BJ. Effects of nonresponse on the mean squared error of estimates from longitudinal study. Paper presented at: Annual Meeting of the American Statistical Assocation, Joint Statistical Meetings; August 5, 2001; Alexandria, Va.
27. Chantala K, Tabor T. Strategies to perform a design-based analysis using the Add Health data, 1999. Available from: http://www.cpc.unc.edu/projects/addhealth/pubs/guides. Accessed June 17, 2005.
28. Brogan D, Daniels D, Rolka D, Marsteller F, Chattopadhay M. Software for sample survey data: misuse of standard packages. In: Armitage P, Colton T, eds. *Encyclopedia of Biostatistics.* Vol 5. New York, NY: John Wiley & Sons Inc; 1998: 4167-4174.
29. Andersen RE, Crespo CH, Bartlett SJ, Cheskin LJ, Pratt M. Relationship of physical activity and television watching with body weight and level of fatness among children: results from the Third National Health and Nutrition Examination Survey. *JAMA.* 1998;279:938-942.
30. Sallis JF, Buono MJ, Roby JJ, Micale FG, Nelson JA. Seven-day recall and other physical activity self-reports in children and adolescents. *Med Sci Sports Exerc.* 1993;25:99-108.
31. Gordon-Larsen P, Nelson MC, Popkin BM. A longitudinal physical activity and sedentary behavior trends: adolescence to adulthood. *Am J Prev Med.* 2004;27:277-283.
32. Cole TJ, Bellizi MC, Flegal KM, Dietz WH. Establishing a standard definition for child overweight and obesity worldwide: international survey. *BMJ.* 2000;320: 1240-1243.
33. Gordon-Larsen P, Adair LS, Nelson MC, Popkin BM. Five-year obesity incidence in the transition period between adolescence and adulthood: the National Longitudinal Study of Adolescent Health. *Am J Clin Nutr.* 2004;80:569-575.
34. Williams DR. Race and health: basic questions, emerging directions. *Ann Epidemiol.* 1997;7:322-333.
35. Krieger N. Counting accountably: public health implications of new approaches to classifying race/ethnicity in the United States 2000 census: US and global perspectives. *Am J Public Health.* 2000;90:1687-1689.
36. Laws MB. Race and ethnicity in biomedical and health services research. *Arch Pediatr Adolesc Med.* 2001;155:972-973.
37. Flores G, Fuentes-Afflick E, Carter-Pokras O, et al. Why ethnicity and race are so important in child health services research today. *Arch Pediatr Adolesc Med.* 2001; 155:1178-1179.
38. Isaacs SL, Schroeder SA. The ignored determinant of the nation's health. *N Engl J Med.* 2004;351:1137-1142.
39. Lillie-Blanton M, Parsons PE, Gayle H, Dievler A. Racial differences in health: not just black and white, but shades of gray. *Annu Rev Public Health.* 1996;17:411-448.
40. Naimi TS, Brewer RD, Mokdad AH, Denny C, Serdula MK, Marks JS. Binge drinking among US adults. *JAMA.* 2003;289:70-75.
41. DiClemente RJ, Wingood GM, Crosby RA, Sionean C, Brown L. A prospective study of psychological distress and sexual risk behavior among black adolescent females. *Pediatrics.* 2001;108:e85. Available at: http://www.pediatrics.aapublications.org/cgi/content/full/108/5/e85. Accessed June 15, 2005.
42. Patton GC, Carlin JB, Coffey C, Wolfe R, Hibbert M, Bowes G. Depression, anxiety and smoking initiation: a prospective study over three years. *Am J Public Health.* 1998;88:1518-1522.
43. Pine DS, Goldstein RB, Wolk S, Weissman MM. The association between childhood depression and adulthood body mass index. *Pediatrics.* 2001;107:1049-1056.
44. Omran AR. The epidemiologic transition: a theory of the epidemiology of population change. *Milbank Mem Fund Q.* 1971;49:509-538.
45. Olshansky SJ, Ault AB. The fourth stage of the epidemiologic transition: the age of delayed degenerative diseases. *Milbank Q.* 1986;64:355-391.
46. Bell FC, Miller ML. *Life Tables for the United States: 1900-2050.* Baltimore, Md: Social Security Administration; 2000. Actuarial study 87.

ARTICLE

# Multisite Controlled Study of OROS Methylphenidate in the Treatment of Adolescents With Attention-Deficit/Hyperactivity Disorder

*Timothy E. Wilens, MD; Keith McBurnett, PhD; Oscar Bukstein, MD; James McGough, MD; Laurence Greenhill, MD; Marc Lerner, MD; Mark A. Stein, PhD; C. Keith Conners, PhD; John Duby, MD; Jeffrey Newcorn, MD; Charles E. Bailey, MD; Christopher J. Kratochvil, MD; Daniel Coury, MD; Charles Casat, MD; Mary Joan C. Denisco, PharmD; Patricia Halstead, MD; Leslie Bloom, BS; Brenda A. Zimmerman, MS; Joan Gu, MS; Kimberly M. Cooper, MS; Joseph M. Lynch, MD*

**Background:** Despite the persistence of attention-deficit/hyperactivity disorder (ADHD) into adolescence, little is known about the efficacy and tolerability of stimulant medications in this age group.

**Objective:** To report the results of a multisite controlled study among adolescents with ADHD evaluating the efficacy and tolerability of osmotic-release oral system (OROS) methylphenidate.

**Design:** Adolescents (N=220) having a confirmed *Diagnostic and Statistical Manual of Mental Disorders, Fourth Edition* diagnosis of ADHD underwent dose titration to identify dosages of OROS methylphenidate that improved symptoms to predefined criteria. Subjects successfully completing the dose titration phase (n=177) (ie, tolerated and responded to treatment and adhered to the protocol) were randomized to receive 2 weeks' treatment with their individualized dosage of OROS methylphenidate (18, 36, 54, or 72 mg once daily) or placebo. Treatment effectiveness was measured using investigator, parent, and adolescent assessments of ADHD.

**Results:** A significant reduction from baseline in the investigator-rated ADHD Rating Scale, the primary efficacy measure, was found with OROS methylphenidate treatment compared with placebo. Similar findings were noted with parent- and adolescent-report measures. Based on a Clinical Global Impression improvement subscale score of much or very much improved, 52% of subjects in the OROS methylphenidate group improved compared with 31% receiving placebo. Thirty-seven percent of subjects required the maximum dosage of 72 mg/d. The incidence of drug-related adverse events was similar between the 2 study groups.

**Conclusion:** In adolescents, once-daily OROS methylphenidate significantly reduced ADHD symptoms and was well tolerated using dosages up to 72 mg/d.

*Arch Pediatr Adolesc Med. 2006;160:82-90*

ATTENTION-DEFICIT/HYPERACTIVITY DISORDER (ADHD) is among the most commonly diagnosed and treated neurobehavioral disorders in children and adolescents. Studies indicate that ADHD affects approximately 8% to 10% of school-aged children,[1] and it persists into adolescence in approximately 70% of patients.[2] Children and adolescents with ADHD share many of the phenotypic characteristics of the disorder,[2,3] although adolescents may manifest more symptoms of inattention relative to hyperactivity or impulsivity.[4,5]

Stimulant medications are widely recommended among first-line therapies for ADHD,[6-8] and their safety and efficacy are well established in children with ADHD.[7,9-12] Approximately 70% of school-aged children treated with a stimulant have a positive response,[7,13,14] and this percentage increased in a trial instituted with another class of stimulant.[15] However, as noted by Smith et al[16] and by Stein and Baren,[17] few studies have investigated the use of stimulant medications or other agents in adolescents with ADHD.

This study investigates the efficacy and safety of an extended-release formulation of methylphenidate, osmotic-release oral system (OROS) methylphenidate (Concerta; ALZA Corporation, Mountain View, Calif). Osmotic-release oral system methylphenidate has been shown in short-term investigations to manage symptoms of ADHD for up to 12 hours after each single daily dose in children 6 to 12 years old,[18] with efficacy that is comparable to that of 3-times-daily methylphenidate.[18-20] In a longer-term trial, OROS methylphenidate (≤54 mg/d) showed sustained efficacy for up to 2 years without

**Author Affiliations** are listed at the end of this article.

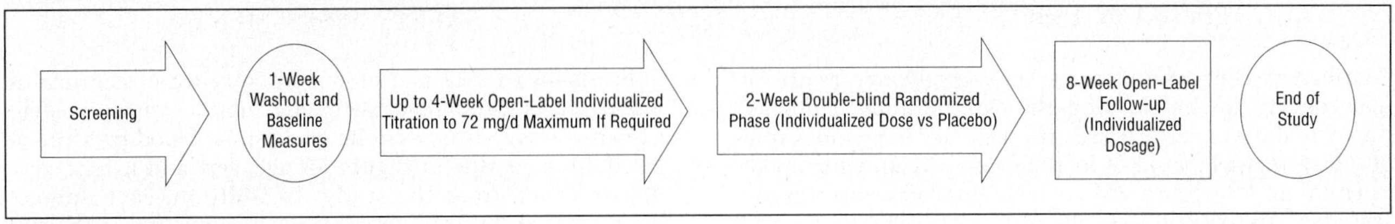


**Figure 1.** Study design.

undue adverse events.[21,22] However, anecdotal reports indicate that higher dosages of stimulants may be necessary in some adolescents.[14] In this study, a multi-informant assessment battery was used to assess responses to treatment with OROS methylphenidate (≤72 mg once daily) as reported by investigators, parents, and the adolescents. We hypothesized that OROS methylphenidate would be more efficacious than placebo in the treatment of ADHD based on investigator, parent, and adolescent rating scales.

## METHODS

### SUBJECTS

Adolescent outpatients aged 13 to 18 years having a diagnosis of ADHD (any subtype) were eligible for the study. Diagnosis of ADHD was based on a clinical evaluation using *Diagnostic and Statistical Manual of Mental Disorders, Fourth Edition* (*DSM-IV*)[23] criteria, confirmed by structured interview (using the behavior module of the Kiddie Schedule for Affective Disorders and Schizophrenia)[24] and by a Children's Global Assessment Scale[25] score of 41 to 70. Eligible subjects could be taking no medications for ADHD at the time of enrollment. Subjects using a behavioral modification program at the time of enrollment had to agree not to change the program or initiate a new program during the study period. Participants had to comply with the study visit schedule, and their parents or caregivers had to be willing to complete all assessments.

Excluded subjects included any adolescents with a history of nonresponse to methylphenidate treatment, hypersensitivity or significant intolerance to methylphenidate, clinically significant gastrointestinal tract problems, clinically important electrocardiographic or blood pressure measurement abnormalities, or coexisting medical conditions or concurrent medications likely to interfere with the safe administration of methylphenidate. Subjects requiring any of the following medications were excluded: clonidine or other $\alpha_2$-adrenergic receptor agonists, tricyclic antidepressants, selective serotonin reuptake inhibitors, theophylline, warfarin sodium, and anticonvulsant agents. Participants with psychiatric comorbidities were eligible for inclusion, except for those with Tourette syndrome or a family history of Tourette syndrome, an ongoing seizure disorder, bipolar disorder, psychotic disorder, a mood or anxiety disorder requiring drug therapy, alcohol or other drug abuse within the 6 months before study enrollment, an eating disorder, or marked anxiety, tension, or agitation.

Written approval of the study design was obtained from the institutional review boards for all participating centers before initiation of the study. For centers in California, approval was obtained from the California Research Advisory Panel. The study was conducted in accord with the Declaration of Helsinki and its amendments.

### STUDY DESIGN

This was a multisite study (15 sites) consisting of 4 phases. These included a 1-week washout phase, an open-label dose titration phase lasting up to 4 weeks, a 2-week double-blind phase consisting of a randomized comparison of an individualized once-daily dosage of OROS methylphenidate vs placebo, and an 8-week open-label follow-up safety phase assessing treatment with OROS methylphenidate at individualized dosages (data not shown) (**Figure 1**).

After a 1-week washout period during which all previous pharmacotherapies for ADHD were discontinued, eligible subjects underwent a series of baseline assessments of ADHD symptoms. Subjects then entered the open-label dose titration phase, during which an individualized dosage of OROS methylphenidate was determined for each subject based on operationalized criteria of response, defined as at least 30% improvement from baseline in the investigator-scored ADHD Rating Scale (ADHD RS)[26] and a rating of good or excellent on the global assessment of effectiveness. The ADHD RS criterion was based on the use of an ADHD RS score of at least 30% as a definition of response in several studies[27-31] of stimulant and nonstimulant therapy in adults, its approximation with a Clinical Global Impression (CGI) improvement subscale score of much or very much improved,[27-31] and its exceeding the recent inclusion and validated use of 25% reduction in ADHD symptoms as a response criterion in children.[26,32]

All subjects received OROS methylphenidate, 18 mg once daily, for a mean±SD of 7±2 days. At the end of this period, ADHD symptoms were assessed by a site investigator using the ADHD RS and the global assessment of effectiveness based on interviews with the subject and parent. If the change in ADHD symptoms from baseline met the criteria for improvement, the 18-mg/d dosage of OROS methylphenidate was defined as the individualized dosage for the subject, who then immediately entered the double-blind phase of the study. If the criteria for improvement were not met and the medication was well tolerated with no safety concerns, the subject received OROS methylphenidate, 36 mg/d, for the next mean±SD of 7±2 days. A similar procedure was followed weekly to a maximum dosage of 72 mg/d. If the criteria were not met at 72 mg/d, the subject was not permitted to continue in the study.

Subjects who successfully completed the open-label dose titration phase were assigned a randomization number within their individualized dosage level for the double-blind phase. On completion of the dose titration phase, subjects were randomized to receive placebo or their individualized dosage of OROS methylphenidate established in the dose titration phase. Investigators were supplied with packages containing the medication for each subject, identified by randomization number. Therefore, investigators and subjects were blinded as to whether a subject was receiving active medication or placebo. During the double-blind phase, ADHD symptoms, safety, and adherence were assessed at the end of each week during clinic visits, and the Child Conflict Index (CCI) was administered twice weekly by telephone interview.

Subjects were eligible to enter an 8-week open-label follow-up phase of the study and receive their individualized dosage of OROS methylphenidate after they completed the double-blind phase or discontinued the double-blind phase prematurely because of a lack of efficacy.

## EFFICACY ASSESSMENTS

Six different rating scales were used to assess the efficacy of treatment during the double-blind phase of the study. The selection of scales was partly based on scales used in previous trials of OROS methylphenidate to allow comparison with studies in children,[14-20] while a scale specific to adolescents was also included. Assessments were completed at baseline and weekly during the double-blind phase of the study. Before the start of the study, all study sites participated in an investigators' meeting at which each scale was reviewed and discussed.

### ADHD RS

The ADHD RS[26,33] is a validated instrument that has been shown to be medication sensitive among adolescents with ADHD in recent clinical trials.[34,35] It consists of an 18-item list of core ADHD symptoms corresponding to the *DSM-IV* diagnostic criteria.[33] Items are scored on a 4-point scale (from 0, never or rarely, to 3, very often). Investigator-rated and parent-rated versions of the ADHD RS were used, with changes in the investigator-rated score serving as the primary efficacy variable. Response to treatment was defined a posteriori as a decrease of at least 30% in the investigator ADHD RS score.

### Conners-Wells Adolescent Self-report of Symptoms Scale

The Conners-Wells Adolescent Self-report of Symptoms Scale[36,37] is a validated 87-item self-report assessment containing the following 9 subscales: family problems, emotional problems, conduct problems, anger control problems, hyperactivity, ADHD index, *DSM-IV* ADHD total score, *DSM-IV* ADHD inattention, and *DSM-IV* ADHD hyperactivity-impulsivity.[36,37] Items are scored on a 4-point scale (from 0, not true, to 3, very much true).

### Child Conflict Index

The CCI[38] is a validated measure of family conflicts in the home and is completed by parents. It consists of 42 items (for boys) or 36 items (for girls) reflecting attention-seeking and conflictual behavior, as well as negativity and withdrawal. Items are scored as yes (1 point) or no (0 points). The CCI has been validated in children[38] and has demonstrated clinical usefulness in detecting the effects of methylphenidate use in children.[39] The CCI was administered during telephone interviews.

### Global Assessment of Effectiveness

The investigator-rated global assessment of effectiveness uses a 4-point scale (0, poor; 1, fair; 2, good; and 3, excellent) to respond to the question: "How effective do you feel the current treatment is at the present time?" The question is answered by the investigator.

### CGI Improvement Subscale

The investigator-rated CGI improvement subscale[40] uses a 7-point scale (from 7, very much worse, to 1, very much improved) to evaluate the response of the subject to the current treatment compared with baseline. The CGI improvement subscale has been shown to be sensitive to medication effects in children[41] and in adults.[31] Based on previous studies in children,[26,32,42] the primary efficacy measure was defined as the change in the total investigator-rated ADHD RS score from baseline to the end of the 2-week double-blind period.

## SAFETY ASSESSMENT

Subjects' heart rate and blood pressure were recorded at weekly visits throughout the study. Subjects with persistent (2 consecutive visits) systolic or diastolic blood pressure at the 95th percentile or higher for age, sex, and height were discontinued from the study. In addition, each subject underwent electrocardiography at screening and at the end of the double-blind phase of the study. Spontaneous reports to the investigator of adverse events were recorded at weekly visits.

## STATISTICAL ANALYSIS

The study aimed to enroll approximately 200 subjects. Allowing for an expected 20% rate of attrition, this would ensure that the study retained at least 90% power to detect a mean difference of 7 units in the total ADHD RS score between the OROS methylphenidate–treated and placebo groups. This was based on a 2-sample, 2-sided *t* test with $\alpha = .05$ and an SD of 12.

Changes in the total scores for the ADHD RS, Conners-Wells Adolescent Self-report of Symptoms Scale, and CCI, as well as changes in heart rate and systolic and diastolic blood pressure from baseline to the end of the double-blind phase of the study, were analyzed using analysis of covariance models with treatment status (drug or placebo) and study site as factors and the corresponding baseline total score as the covariate. Possible treatment × site interactions were examined at a significance level of $\alpha = .10$. The last observation carried forward technique was used for all assessments in the double-blind phase (except for the CGI improvement subscale, which was assessed only once, at the end of the double-blind phase). Unplanned analyses of response rates at the end of the double-blind phase were conducted using the Cochran-Mantel-Haenszel correlation statistic and were stratified by study site.

# RESULTS

## SUBJECTS

The disposition of subjects in the study is shown in **Figure 2**. Two hundred twenty subjects were enrolled in the study between April 1, 2002, and October 15, 2002. Twenty-seven subjects (12%) withdrew from the dose titration phase for the following reasons: adverse events (8 subjects), withdrawal of consent (7 subjects), protocol violations (6 subjects), administrative reasons (3 subjects), lost to follow-up (2 subjects), and unable to swallow medication (1 subject). Eleven subjects (5%) did not meet defined criteria for improvement at 72 mg/d of OROS methylphenidate and were ineligible to continue in the double-blind phase. Of the 182 subjects (83%) who successfully achieved the criteria for improvement at the dose titration phase, 177 subjects were randomized into the double-blind phase; 5 subjects reached the criteria after the double-blind phase was closed and were not randomized. Of the 177 randomized subjects, one subject did not enter the double-blind phase and efficacy data were not collected for another subject. Therefore, 175 subjects were included in the efficacy analysis of the double-blind phase, but 177 subjects were included in the dosage and safety analyses.

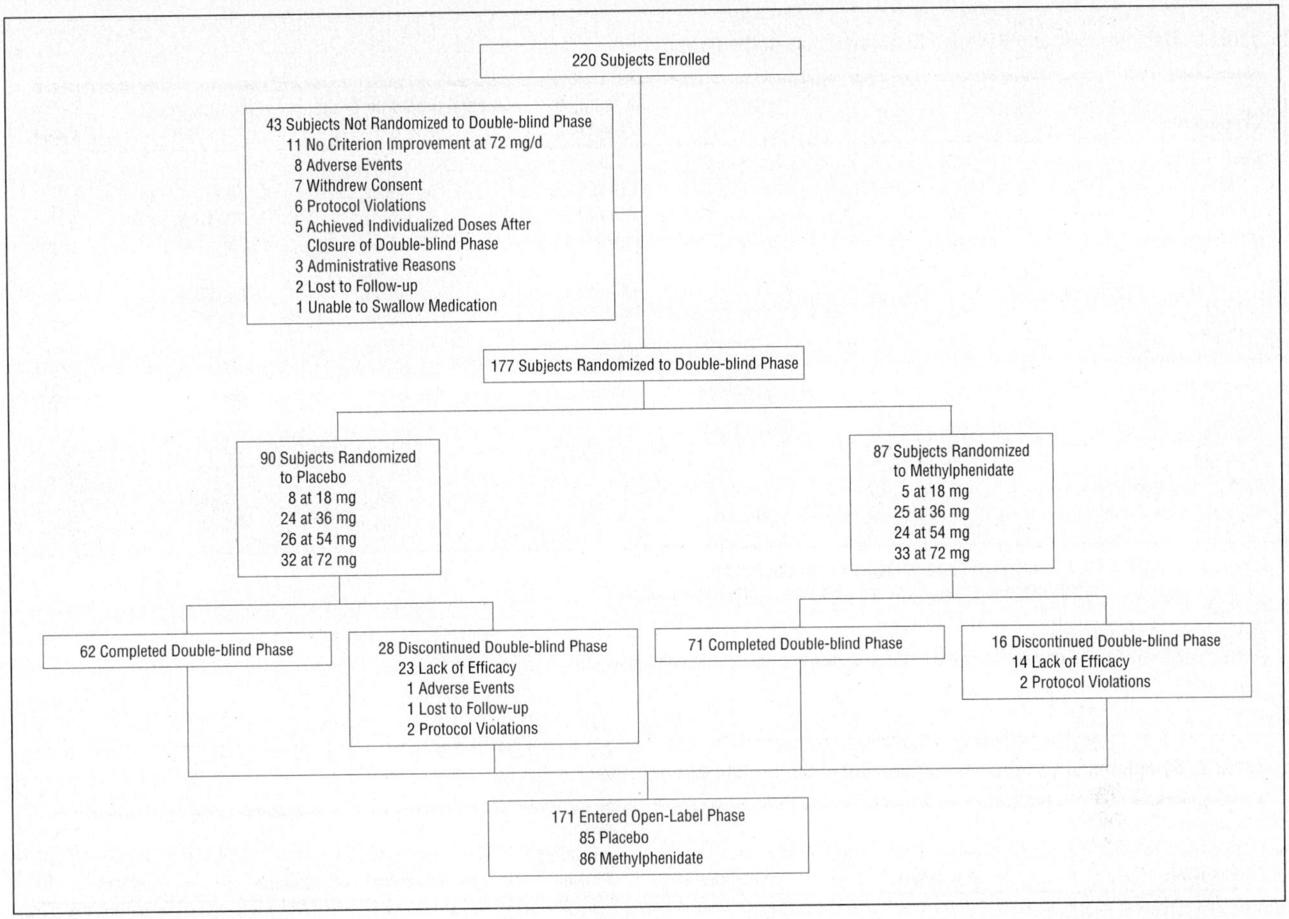


**Figure 2.** Disposition of subjects.

## DOSE TITRATION PHASE

One hundred seventy-seven subjects were assigned an individualized dosage of OROS methylphenidate (13 subjects [7.4%] at 18 mg/d; 49 subjects [28%] at 36 mg/d; 50 subjects [28%] at 54 mg/d; and 65 subjects [37%] at 72 mg/d). The mean investigator ADHD RS score for these subjects at the end of the dose titration phase was 10.64 compared with 31.26 at baseline (a change of –66%) ($t_{174}$=34.6, $P$<.001, paired $t$ test).

## DOUBLE-BLIND PHASE

The demographic and baseline characteristics of subjects for the double-blind phase are given in **Table 1**. The mean age of subjects was 14.6 years, and most subjects were white and male. Eighty-seven subjects were randomized to receive OROS methylphenidate, and 90 were randomized to receive placebo. Both groups were similarly matched for demographic characteristics and severity of ADHD at baseline, although there were significantly more male subjects in the placebo group compared with the OROS methylphenidate–treated group ($P$<.04).

Eighty-two percent (71/87) of subjects in the OROS methylphenidate–treated group completed the 2-week double-blind phase. The main reason for withdrawal was lack of efficacy (14 subjects); 8 of these subjects were receiving the highest permitted OROS methylphenidate dosage. In the placebo group, 69% (62/90) of subjects completed the double-blind phase; the main reason for withdrawal was lack of efficacy (23 subjects). Other reasons for withdrawal in the placebo group were adverse events (1 subject), lost to follow-up (2 subjects), and protocol violations (2 subjects). The difference in retention rate between treatment groups was marginally significant ($P$=.05). Of the 37 subjects who discontinued the double-blind phase early because of a lack of efficacy, all elected to enter the open-label follow-up phase, receiving their unblinded, individualized dosage of OROS methylphenidate. Of the 171 subjects who entered the open-label follow-up phase, only 3 withdrew because of a lack of efficacy.

## EFFICACY DURING THE DOUBLE-BLIND PHASE

Treatment with OROS methylphenidate was associated with clinically and statistically significant improvement from baseline compared with placebo ($F_{1,158}$=11.21, $P$=.001) for the primary efficacy variable of mean change from baseline in investigator ADHD RS score (**Table 2**). Statistically significant differences between the OROS methylphenidate–treated and placebo groups ($P$<.05) were observed for all other efficacy measures. There were no significant site × treatment interactions for the ADHD outcome measures. Post hoc responder analyses indicated that the percentages of subjects responding to treatment were significantly greater for OROS methylpheni-

**Table 1. Demographic and Baseline Characteristics of the Cohort***

| Characteristic | All Subjects (N = 177) | Methylphenidate Group (n = 87) | Placebo Group (n = 90) | *P* Value |
|---|---|---|---|---|
| Sex | | | | |
| Male | **142** (80.2) | 64 (73.6) | 78 (86.7) | .03† |
| Female | **35** (19.8) | 23 (26.4) | 12 (13.3) | |
| Age, y | 14.6 ± 1.5 | 14.8 ± 1.6 | 14.5 ± 1.4 | .16‡ |
| Race | | | | |
| White | **133** (75.1) | 65 (74.7) | 68 (75.6) | .19† |
| Black | **24** (13.6) | 9 (10.3) | 15 (16.7) | |
| Other | **20** (11.3) | 13 (14.9) | 7 (7.8) | |
| Height, mean, cm | 168.1 | 168.5 | 167.7 | .64‡ |
| Weight, mean, kg | 66.0 | 66.2 | 65.7 | .96‡ |
| ADHD RS score§ | | | | |
| Investigator | 31.26 | 31.55 | 30.99 | .70 |
| Parent | 30.82 | 30.65 | 30.99 | .93 |
| Parent Child Conflict Index | 0.272 | 0.286 | 0.259 | .30 |
| Subject Conners-Wells Adolescent Self-report of Symptoms Scale score | 91.96 | 89.81 | 94.02 | .58 |

Abbreviation: ADHD RS, Attention-Deficit/Hyperactivity Disorder Rating Scale.
*Data are given as number (percentage) or as mean ± SD unless otherwise indicated.
†$\chi^2$ Test.
‡1-Way analysis of variance.
§Baseline data are for the population in the efficacy analysis of the double-blind phase (n = 175).

**Table 2. Symptoms at Baseline and at the End of the Double-blind Phase***

| Assessment | Group | Baseline | End of the Double-blind Phase | Mean Change† | % Change | ANOVA‡ |
|---|---|---|---|---|---|---|
| ADHD RS score | | | | | | |
| Investigator | OROS methylphenidate | 31.55 ± 9.42 | 16.62 ± 11.03 | −14.93 ± 10.72 | −47 | $F_{1,158}$ = 11.21, *P* = .001 |
| | Placebo | 30.99 ± 9.64 | 21.40 ± 13.44 | −9.58 ± 9.73 | −31 | |
| Parent | OROS methylphenidate | 30.65 ± 9.81 | 16.65 ± 11.07 | −14.00 ± 10.31 | −46 | $F_{1,158}$ = 7.29, *P* = .008 |
| | Placebo | 30.99 ± 11.55 | 20.84 ± 13.58 | −10.14 ± 10.00 | −33 | |
| Parent Child Conflict Index | OROS methylphenidate | 0.286 ± 0.174 | 0.188 ± 0.145 | −0.098 ± 0.189 | −34 | $F_{1,157}$ = 8.05, *P* = .005 |
| | Placebo | 0.259 ± 0.182 | 0.247 ± 0.206 | −0.016 ± 0.150 | −6 | |
| Subject Conners-Wells Adolescent Self-report of Symptoms Scale score | OROS methylphenidate | 89.81 ± 41.44 | 57.57 ± 41.07 | −31.70 ± 28.96 | −35 | $F_{1,157}$ = 11.00, *P* = .001 |
| | Placebo | 94.02 ± 49.20 | 75.32 ± 52.20 | −18.70 ± 26.94 | −20 | |

Abbreviations: ADHD RS, Attention-Deficit/Hyperactivity Disorder Rating Scale; ANOVA, analysis of variance.
*Data are given as mean±SD unless otherwise indicated.
†From baseline to the end of the double-blind phase.
‡Comparing change from baseline for the methylphenidate vs placebo groups.

date compared with placebo for all efficacy outcome measures (**Table 3**).

## ADVERSE EVENTS DURING THE DOSE TITRATION AND DOUBLE-BLIND PHASES

The most frequently reported adverse events considered by investigators to be treatment-related during the open-label dose titration phase of the study included headache (25%), decreased appetite (21%), insomnia (15%), and abdominal pain (9%). During the double-blind phase, 16 subjects (18%) receiving OROS methylphenidate and 14 subjects (16%) receiving placebo reported at least 1 adverse event deemed by investigators to be probably or possibly related to study medication. **Table 4** gives all treatment-related adverse events in the double-blind phase that occurred in at least 2% of subjects in either study group.

Serious adverse events were reported in only 1 subject during the open-label dose titration phase of the study. While being treated with OROS methylphenidate, 18 mg/d, a 16-year-old female subject with a history of depression and suicidal ideation threatened suicide on the third day of medication use after an argument with her mother. A decision was made to discontinue study medication, and the symptoms resolved. The investigator considered the recurrence of depression to be possibly related to treatment and the suicidal ideation unlikely related to study medication. No serious adverse events were reported during the double-blind phase. No subject experienced clinically important effects on electrocardiographic indexes, heart rate, or blood pressure during the study.

**Table 3. Response Rates for Efficacy Assessments During the Double-blind Phase**

| Assessment | Criterion for Response | Response Rate, % | | P Value* |
|---|---|---|---|---|
| | | Methylphenidate Group | Placebo Group | |
| Investigator | | | | |
| ADHD RS | ≥30% Decrease from baseline | 73.3 | 56.2 | $\chi^2_1 = 4.6$, $P = .03$ |
| Global assessment of effectiveness | Subjects with good or excellent rating | 51.2 | 32.6 | $\chi^2_1 = 8.1$, $P = .004$ |
| Clinical Global Impression improvement subscale | Subjects with much improved or very much improved rating† | 51.8 | 31.0 | $\chi^2_1 = 6.4$, $P = .01$ |
| Subject Conners-Wells Adolescent Self-report of Symptoms Scale | ≥30% Decrease from baseline | 62.8 | 41.6 | $\chi^2_1 = 7.4$, $P = .007$ |

Abbreviation: ADHD RS, Attention-Deficit/Hyperactivity Disorder Rating Scale.
*Cochran-Mantel-Haenszel test comparing the methylphenidate vs placebo groups.
†Based on a 7-point scale (very much improved, much improved, minimally improved, no change, minimally worse, much worse, or very much worse).

## COMMENT

The results of this short-term multisite study involving a large group of adolescents titrated to individualized dosages of OROS methylphenidate indicate that OROS methylphenidate is associated with clinically and statistically significant improvement in ADHD compared with placebo, as measured by investigator, parent, and adolescent assessments. A large number of adolescents (37%) required 72 mg/d of OROS methylphenidate. This dosage provided effective treatment without increased risk of adverse events.

The treatment efficacy demonstrated in this trial is consistent with findings from smaller investigations among adolescent populations[16] demonstrating therapeutic benefits of methylphenidate for ADHD. A placebo-controlled crossover study[43] involving 45 adolescents with ADHD who received 1 of 3 dosages of methylphenidate 3 times daily for 6 weeks demonstrated that 78% to 91% of subjects achieved beneficial effects from methylphenidate treatment. Similarly, a review[16] of 8 controlled studies of methylphenidate use among adolescents reported a mean effect size for ADHD symptoms of 0.94 (range, 0.13-3.00), which is at the top of the range (0.47-0.96) reported in a meta-analysis[44] of studies among children. The aggregate literature involving more than 150 adolescents from 9 controlled studies thus indicates a highly significant effect of immediate-release methylphenidate on improving ADHD symptoms and functioning in adolescents. The present study extends the literature by evaluating a once-daily formulation of methylphenidate at dosages of up to 72 mg/d among a large patient population from multiple sites.

The response rate (based on the CGI improvement subscale) of 52% achieved in this study is similar to that reported in a previous multisite study[20] of OROS methylphenidate use (response rate, 47%) among school-aged children (6-12 years old),[20] as well as in the Multimodal Treatment Study of Children With Attention-Deficit/Hyperactivity Disorder,[45] in which most children received immediate-release methylphenidate 2 to 3 times daily. The consistency in response rates of these methylphenidate trials demonstrates comparable effectiveness in children and in adolescents. However, a higher placebo response was observed in our study compared with a study[20] among children (31% vs 17%). There are several possible explanations for this finding. First, as observed in the Multimodal Treatment Study of Children With Attention-Deficit/Hyperactivity Disorder,[45] subjects may have had improved ADHD symptoms or psychosocial carryover effects as a consequence of participation in our study, medication titration, and regular meetings with study personnel. Second, our study was conducted partially during the summer, and this may have resulted in less stress on the adolescents and overall improvement in both study groups. Third, it may be that more sensitive measures of attention are needed for adolescents with ADHD compared with children. Adolescents are generally less likely to display overt hyperactivity, and parents or investigators might consider this reduced hyperactivity in their evaluation of treatment effects.[46] The placebo response in our study was lower (a change of −20%) for subject-reported ratings, and there was virtually no placebo response to the CCI (a change of −6%). Fourth, in contrast to standard placebo-controlled, parallel-group trials, subjects in our study were transitioned to placebo from their lowest effective dosages, determined during open-label dose titration. It is possible that any decline in function associated with this

**Table 4. Treatment-Related Adverse Events During the Double-blind Phase Reported in at Least 2% of Subjects in Either Study Group***

| Event | Methylphenidate Group (n = 87) | Placebo Group (n = 90) |
|---|---|---|
| Headache | 3 (3.4) | 6 (6.7) |
| Decreased appetite | 2 (2.3) | 0 |
| Insomnia | 4 (4.6) | 0 |
| Abdominal pain | 1 (1.1) | 2 (2.2) |
| Nausea | 1 (1.1) | 2 (2.2) |
| Asthenia | 0 | 2 (2.2) |
| Diarrhea | 2 (2.3) | 0 |

*Data are given as number (percentage).

transition may not have been readily perceptible to investigators or parents performing the ratings.

As expected, there was a high degree of correspondence between investigator and parent ADHD RS scores because investigator ratings were based on parent ratings and on the results of interviews with parents and subjects. However, changes in parent-rated CCI scores and in subject-rated Conners-Wells Adolescent Self-report of Symptoms Scale scores also showed significant improvement over baseline for OROS methylphenidate treatment compared with placebo. The improvement in adolescent self-report measures suggests that patient self-reports may be useful for assessing treatment outcomes. The changes from baseline reported by adolescent subjects in the OROS methylphenidate–treated and placebo groups seemed lower than those recorded by investigators and parents. The implications of these response differences for the sensitivity and specificity of self-report measures need to be determined, as our results are contrary to the findings of other researchers.[47-49] The ability of adolescents to accurately report their symptoms warrants further investigation. If adolescents are able to reliably assess the effectiveness of their ADHD medication, self-reports could provide an important means of evaluating treatment outcomes as patients age and become more independent from teachers.

Teacher ratings were not included because of concerns about privacy and the difficulties of obtaining information from multiple teachers involved in an adolescent's education. Although teacher ratings are essential for assessing ADHD in studies of children up to 12 years old, they may be less critical in the evaluation of older patients because of the reduced amount of daily contact. The availability of a reliable self-report measure[37] and recent findings of the sensitivity of parent reporting in evaluating extended-release stimulant medications[20,32,41,42] suggest that adequate assessment of symptoms could be achieved without teacher ratings.

Although our study did not assess dose-response relationships with randomized dosages of OROS methylphenidate, the results of the dose titration phase of the study indicate that some adolescents benefit from higher absolute doses. This higher dosing is consistent with the greater body weight of adolescents. Bostic et al[34] demonstrated robust improvement in ADHD symptoms among adolescents who were using higher absolute doses (but similar weight-corrected doses) of pemoline relative to younger children. However, Evans et al[43] found that although some adolescents benefited from higher methylphenidate dosages, for most subjects there was little additional benefit for increasing dosages above 25 mg/d. The scarcity of data among adolescents makes it difficult to determine whether a relationship exists between weight and clinical response, or whether additional factors such as the presence of comorbidities or greater executive functioning affect dosing requirements as patients age. Regardless, the present findings suggest that adolescents may require higher absolute doses than younger children, similar to the dose-dependent variation in response to pharmacotherapy that has been observed among adults with ADHD.[50]

Dosages of OROS methylphenidate up to 72 mg administered once daily were well tolerated during our initial dose titration and the controlled study, with adverse events similar to those previously reported in controlled trials of OROS methylphenidate use among children aged 6 to 12 years.[18-20] Moreover, no subjects taking active drug discontinued treatment during the double-blind phase secondary to adverse events. There were no clinically important effects on electrocardiographic indexes, heart rate, or blood pressure, consistent with studies[18-20] of OROS methylphenidate use among children. Although spontaneous reporting may underestimate the incidence of adverse events, the adverse event profile of OROS methylphenidate use in our study is similar to that which has been well established for immediate-release methylphenidate.[51-53]

The case of suicidal ideation observed in our study was judged not likely to be related to treatment with OROS methylphenidate by an investigator. This patient had a history of depression and suicidal ideation, and it is likely that the patient's actions stemmed from an underlying idiopathic depression. Depression is a common comorbid condition associated with ADHD, with prevalence estimates for depression among patients with ADHD as high as 44%.[54,55] A modest association between ADHD and increased risk for suicide has also been reported.[56]

The findings in this study should be tempered against the methodological limitations of the study. Adolescents with unstable psychiatric and medical disorders and clinically important concurrent psychiatric comorbidity necessitating treatment were excluded from the study. Also excluded were subjects with a history of nonresponse to methylphenidate, as it was not considered ethical to enroll subjects who were unlikely to respond to treatment. Accordingly, our findings may not be generalizable to clinical practice. Moreover, data on exposure to stimulants before study entry were not collected in this study; thus, the possible effect of medication history on outcome cannot be assessed.

Two features of the study design may have biased the results toward improved efficacy and tolerability in the double-blind phase. First, a positive bias may have resulted from enrollment of only subjects who could tolerate OROS methylphenidate and experienced efficacy during the dose titration phase. However, only 11 (5%) of 220 subjects were discontinued from the study after the dose titration phase because of failure to meet the defined criteria for improvement at 72 mg/d. Second, the fact that subjects were titrated to their individualized dosage before the double-blind phase of the study may have biased the results toward a positive response in the double-blind phase. However, the upward dosing of the medication in the dose titration phase was determined by a threshold for improvement and not dosed to optimal outcome, probably biasing for a less robust outcome. Nevertheless, the substantial placebo effect observed in the double-blind phase of this study suggests that the results may have been positively biased toward improved efficacy. This placebo effect limits our ability to gauge the true extent of improvement with OROS methylphenidate therapy in the present study.

The attrition rate seen in both arms of the double-blind phase, although higher in the placebo group, may have affected the study results. In particular, discontinuation from the double-blind phase because of a perceived or real lack of efficacy, the primary reason for attrition, may have been biased by the knowledge that subjects who discontinued the study early could enter the open-label follow-up phase of the study and receive active study medication. This is supported by the fact that 97% (171/177) of subjects from the double-blind phase entered the open-label follow-up phase of the study and only 3 subjects (1.82%) of 177 withdrew from the open-label follow-up phase because of a lack of efficacy compared with 16% (14/87) of the subjects receiving OROS methylphenidate in the double-blind phase. However, in the dose titration phase, 5% (11/220) of subjects did not achieve an adequate response to OROS methylphenidate at the highest dosage tested, indicating that a small number of subjects experienced a true lack of efficacy.

The conclusions from the open-label follow-up safety analysis of this study are limited by the fact that the study was not powered to detect differences in adverse events between active treatment and placebo. The short duration of the double-blind phase also may have limited the incidence of adverse events reported and may have decreased the likelihood of detecting potential rare adverse events. In addition, the rates of adverse events reported for OROS methylphenidate use during the double-blind phase may have been underestimated, because subjects entering this study phase were already stabilized on an effective and tolerated dosage of medication and 8 subjects who could not tolerate OROS methylphenidate had been discontinued during the open-label dose titration phase.

## CONCLUSIONS

The results of this multisite controlled clinical study indicate that OROS methylphenidate treatment produces clinically and statistically significant improvement in ADHD among adolescents, as assessed by multiple raters. The study also demonstrates the efficacy and tolerability of a high OROS methylphenidate dosage, 72 mg/d, in this age group. Longer-term studies on the effectiveness and tolerability of use of stimulant medications among adolescents will increase awareness of the appropriate management of ADHD in this understudied age group.

**Accepted for Publication:** July 1, 2005.
**Author Affiliations:** Pediatric Psychopharmacology Unit, Massachusetts General Hospital, Boston (Dr Wilens); The Children's Center at Langley Porter, University of California, San Francisco (Dr McBurnett); Neuropsychiatric Institute, University of California, Los Angeles (Dr McGough); Department of Pediatrics, University of California, Irvine (Dr Lerner); Department of Psychiatry, University of Pittsburgh, Pittsburgh (Dr Bukstein), and McNeil Consumer & Specialty Pharmaceuticals, Fort Washington (Drs Denisco, Halstead, and Lynch and Mss Bloom, Zimmerman, Gu, and Cooper), Pa; New York State Psychiatric Institute (Dr Greenhill) and Department of Psychiatry, Mount Sinai School of Medicine (Dr Newcorn), New York; Department of Psychiatry, University of California, San Diego (Dr Stein); Duke University Medical Center, Durham (Dr Conners), and Behavioral Health Center, Charlotte (Dr Casat), NC; Children's Hospital Medical Center of Akron, Akron (Dr Duby), and Columbus Children's Hospital, Columbus (Dr Coury), Ohio; CNS Healthcare Orlando Research Center, Orlando, Fla (Dr Bailey); and Nebraska Medical Center, Omaha (Dr Kratochvil).
**Correspondence:** Timothy E. Wilens, MD, Massachusetts General Hospital, YAW-6-6A, 32 Fruit St, Boston, MA 02114 (twilens@partners.org).
**Financial Disclosure:** Seven of the authors were employed by McNeil Consumer & Specialty Pharmaceuticals at the time the study was conducted. These 7 authors contributed to the study design, data analysis, and preparation of the manuscript. Drs Wilens, Bukstein, Lerner, Stein, Newcorn, Kratochvil, and Coury served on the speaker's bureau for and as consultants to McNeil Consumer & Specialty Pharmaceuticals.
**Funding/Support:** This study was supported by funds from McNeil Consumer & Specialty Pharmaceuticals.
**Acknowledgment:** We acknowledge the valuable assistance of Suzanne Lamerano, MBA, BS, and Donna Votto, MMBA, BSN.

## REFERENCES

1. American Academy of Pediatrics. Clinical practice guideline: diagnosis and evaluation of the child with attention-deficit/hyperactivity disorder. *Pediatrics.* 2000; 105:1158-1170.
2. Barkley RA, Fischer M, Edelbrock CS, Smallish L. The adolescent outcome of hyperactive children diagnosed by research criteria, I: an 8-year prospective follow-up study. *J Am Acad Child Adolesc Psychiatry.* 1990;29:546-557.
3. Biederman J, Faraone SV, Taylor A, Sienna M, Williamson S, Fine C. Diagnostic continuity between child and adolescent ADHD: findings from a longitudinal clinical sample. *J Am Acad Child Adolesc Psychiatry.* 1998;37:305-313.
4. Hart EL, Lahey B, Loeber R, Applegate B, Frisk P. Developmental changes in attention-deficit hyperactivity disorder in boys: a four-year longitudinal study. *J Abnorm Child Psychol.* 1995;23:729-749.
5. Biederman J, Mick E, Faraone SV. Age-dependent decline of symptoms of attention deficit hyperactivity disorder: impact of remission definition and symptom type. *Am J Psychiatry.* 2000;157:816-818.
6. American Academy of Pediatrics Subcommittee on Attention-Deficit/Hyperactivity Disorder and Committee on Quality Improvement. Clinical practice guideline: treatment of the school-aged child with attention-deficit/hyperactivity disorder. *Pediatrics.* 2001;108:1033-1044.
7. Greenhill LL, Pliszka S, Dulcan MK, et al; American Academy of Child and Adolescent Psychiatry. Practice parameter for the use of stimulant medications in the treatment of children, adolescents, and adults. *J Am Acad Child Adolesc Psychiatry.* 2002;41(suppl):26S-49S.
8. Taylor E, Sergeant J, Doepfner M, et al; European Society for Child and Adolescent Psychiatry. Clinical guidelines for hyperkinetic disorder. *Eur Child Adolesc Psychiatry.* 1998;7:184-200.
9. Miller A, Lee S, Raina P, Klasen A, Zupanicic J, Olsen L. *A Review of Therapies for Attention-Deficit/Hyperactivity Disorder.* Ottawa, Ontario: Canadian Coordinating Office for Health Technology Assessments; 1998.
10. Lord J, Paisley S. *The Clinical Effectiveness and Cost-effectiveness of Methylphenidate for Hyperactivity in Childhood.* London, England: National Institute for Clinical Excellence; 2000.
11. National Institute for Clinical Excellence. *Guidance on the Use of Methylphenidate (Ritalin, Equasym) for Attention-Deficit/Hyperactivity Disorder (ADHD) in Childhood.* London, England: National Institute for Clinical Excellence; 2000.
12. Schachter HM, Pham B, King J, Langford S, Moher D. How efficacious and safe is short-acting methylphenidate for the treatment of attention-deficit disorder in children and adolescents? a meta-analysis. *CMAJ.* 2001;165:1475-1488.
13. Swanson JM, McBurnett K, Christian D, Wigal T. Stimulant medications in the treatment of children with ADHD. In: Ollendick TH, Prinz RJ, eds. *Advances in Clinical Child Psychology.* Vol 17. New York, NY: Plenum Press; 1995:265-322.
14. Wilens TE, Spencer TJ. The stimulants revisited. *Child Adolesc Psychiatr Clin N Am.* 2000;9:573-603 , viii.
15. Elia J, Borcherding BG, Rapoport JL, Keysor CS. Methylphenidate and dextro-

amphetamine treatments of hyperactivity: are there true nonresponders? *Psychiatry Res.* 1991;36:141-155.
16. Smith BH, Waschbusch DA, Willoughby MT, Evans S. The efficacy, safety, and practicality of treatments for adolescents with attention-deficit/hyperactivity disorder (ADHD). *Clin Child Fam Psychol Rev.* 2000;3:243-267.
17. Stein MA, Baren M. Welcome progress in the diagnosis and treatment of ADHD in adolescence. *Contemp Pediatr.* 2003;20:83.
18. Swanson J, Lerner MA, Gupta S, Shoulson I, Wigal S. Development of a new once-a-day formulation of methylphenidate for the treatment of ADHD. *Arch Gen Psychiatry.* 2003;60:204-211.
19. Pelham WE, Gnagy EM, Burrows-Maclean L, et al. Once-a-day Concerta methylphenidate versus three-times-daily methylphenidate in laboratory and natural settings. *Pediatrics.* Available at: http://pediatrics.aapublications.org/cgi/content/full/107/6/e105. 2001;107:e105. Accessed November 28, 2005.
20. Wolraich ML, Greenhill LL, Pelham W, et al. Randomized, controlled trial of OROS methylphenidate once a day in children with attention-deficit/hyperactivity disorder. *Pediatrics.* 2001;108:883-892.
21. Wilens T, Pelham W, Stein MA, et al. ADHD treatment with once-daily OROS methylphenidate: interim 12-month results from a long-term open-label study. *J Am Acad Child Adolesc Psychiatry.* 2003;42:424-433.
22. Wilens T, McBurnett K, Stein M, Lerner M, Spencer T, Wolraich M. ADHD treatment with once-daily OROS methylphenidate: final results from a long-term open-label study. *J Am Acad Child Adolesc Psychiatry.* 2005;44:1015-1023.
23. American Psychiatric Association. *Diagnostic and Statistical Manual of Mental Disorders, Fourth Edition.* Washington, DC: American Psychiatric Association; 1994.
24. Ambrosini PJ. Historical development and present status of the schedule for affective disorders and schizophrenia for school-age children. *J Am Acad Child Adolesc Psychiatry.* 2000;39:49-58.
25. Shaffer D, Gould MS, Brasic J, et al. A Children's Global Assessment Scale (CGAS). *Arch Gen Psychiatry.* 1983;40:1228-1231.
26. Faries DE, Yalcin I, Harder D, Heiligenstein JH. Validation of the ADHD Rating Scale as a clinician administered and scored instrument. *J Atten Disord.* 2001; 5:107-115.
27. Spencer T, Wilens T, Biederman J, Faraone SV, Ablon JS, Lapey K. A double-blind, crossover comparison of methylphenidate and placebo in adults with childhood-onset attention-deficit hyperactivity disorder. *Arch Gen Psychiatry.* 1995; 52:434-443.
28. Spencer T, Biederman J, Wilens TE, Johnson M, Doyle R, Parekh S. Efficacy of MPH in adults with ADHD. Scientific poster presented at: 49th Annual Meeting of the American Academy of Child and Adolescent Psychiatry; October 22-27, 2002; San Francisco, Calif.
29. Taylor FB, Russo J. Efficacy of modafinil compared to dextroamphetamine for the treatment of attention deficit hyperactivity disorder in adults. *J Child Adolesc Psychopharmacol.* 2000;10:311-320.
30. Taylor FB, Russo J. Comparing guanfacine and dextroamphetamine for the treatment of adult attention-deficit/hyperactivity disorder. *J Clin Psychopharmacol.* 2001;21:223-228.
31. Spencer T, Biederman J, Wilens T, et al. Efficacy of a mixed amphetamine salts compound in adults with attention-deficit/hyperactivity disorder. *Arch Gen Psychiatry.* 2001;58:775-782.
32. Michelson D, Allen AJ, Busner J, et al. Once-daily atomoxetine treatment for children and adolescents with attention deficit hyperactivity disorder: a randomized, placebo-controlled study. *Am J Psychiatry.* 2002;159:1896-1901.
33. DuPaul G, Power TJ, Anastopoulos AD, Reid D. *ADHD Rating Scale-IV: Checklists, Norms and Clinical Interpretations.* New York, NY: Guilford Press; 1998.
34. Bostic JQ, Biederman J, Spencer TJ, et al. Pemoline treatment of adolescents with attention deficit hyperactivity disorder: a short-term controlled trial. *J Child Adolesc Psychopharmacol.* 2000;10:205-216.
35. Prince JB, Wilens TE, Biederman J, et al. A controlled study of nortriptyline in children and adolescents with attention deficit hyperactivity disorder. *J Child Adolesc Psychopharmacol.* 2000;10:193-204.
36. Conners CK. Rating scales in attention-deficit/hyperactivity disorder: use in assessment and treatment monitoring. *J Clin Psychiatry.* 1998;59(suppl 7):24-30.
37. Conners CK, Wells KC, Parker JD, Sitarenios G, Diamond JM, Powell JW. A new self-report scale for assessment of adolescent psychopathology: factor structure, reliability, validity, and diagnostic sensitivity. *J Abnorm Child Psychol.* 1997; 25:487-497.
38. Frankel F, Weiner H. The Child Conflict Index: factor analysis, reliability, and validity for clinic-referred and nonreferred children. *J Clin Psychol.* 1990;19:239-248.
39. Stein MA, Blondis TA, Schnitzler ER, et al. Methylphenidate dosing: twice daily versus three times daily. *Pediatrics.* 1996;98:748-756.
40. National Institute of Mental Health. CGI (Clinical Global Impression) scale. *Psychopharmacol Bull.* 1985;21:839-843.
41. Biederman J, Lopez FA, Boellner SW, Chandler MC. A randomized, double-blind, placebo-controlled, parallel-group study of SLI381 (Adderall XR) in children with attention-deficit/hyperactivity disorder. *Pediatrics.* 2002;110:258-266.
42. Michelson D, Faries D, Wernicke J, et al. Atomoxetine in the treatment of children and adolescents with attention-deficit/hyperactivity disorder: a randomized, placebo-controlled, dose-response study. *Pediatrics.* 2001;108:e83.
43. Evans SW, Pelham WE, Smith BH, et al. Dose-response effects of methylphenidate on ecologically valid measures of academic performance and classroom behavior in adolescents with ADHD. *Exp Clin Psychopharmacol.* 2001;9: 163-175.
44. Lipsey MW, Wilson DB. The efficacy of psychological, educational, and behavioral treatment: confirmation from meta-analysis. *Am Psychol.* 1993;48:1181-1209.
45. MTA Cooperative Group. A 14-month randomized clinical trial of treatment strategies for attention-deficit/hyperactivity disorder. *Arch Gen Psychiatry.* 1999; 56:1073-1086.
46. Weiss M, Jain U. Clinical perspectives on the assessment of ADHD in adolescence. *ADHD Rep.* 2000;8:4-10.
47. Smith BH, Pelham WE Jr, Gnagy E, Molina B, Evans S. The reliability, validity, and unique contributions of self-report by adolescents receiving treatment for attention-deficit/hyperactivity disorder. *J Consult Clin Psychol.* 2000;68:489-499.
48. Schaughency E, McGee R, Raja SN, Feehan M, Silva PA. Self-reported inattention, impulsivity, and hyperactivity at ages 15 and 18 years in the general population. *J Am Acad Child Adolesc Psychiatry.* 1994;33:173-184.
49. Danckaerts M, Heptinstall E, Chadwick O, Taylor E. Self-report of attention deficit and hyperactivity disorder in adolescents. *Psychopathology.* 1999;32:81-92.
50. Wilens TE, Spencer TJ, Biederman J. A review of the pharmacotherapy of adults with attention-deficit/hyperactivity disorder. *J Atten Disord.* 2002;5:189-202.
51. Barkley RA, McMurray MB, Edelbrock CS, Robbins K. Side effects of methylphenidate in children with attention deficit hyperactivity disorder: a systemic, placebo-controlled evaluation. *Pediatrics.* 1990;86:184-192.
52. Greenhill LL, Osman BB. *Ritalin: Theory and Practice.* 2nd ed. Larchmont, NY: Mary Ann Liebert; 2000.
53. Klein RG, Bessler AW. Stimulant side effects in children. In: Kane JM, Lieberman JA, eds. *Adverse Effects of Psychotropic Drugs.* New York, NY: Guilford Press; 1992:470-496.
54. Anderson JC, Williams S, McGee R, Silva PA. *DSM-III* disorders in preadolescent children: prevalence in a large sample from the general population. *Arch Gen Psychiatry.* 1987;44:69-76.
55. Bird HR, Gould MS, Staghezza BM. Patterns of diagnostic comorbidity in a community sample of children aged 9 through 16 years. *J Am Acad Child Adolesc Psychiatry.* 1993;32:361-368.
56. James A, Lai FH, Dahl C. Attention deficit hyperactivity disorder and suicide: a review of possible associations. *Acta Psychiatr Scand.* 2004;110:408-415.

There's no exact time when it is important to start solid food. Fifty years ago it was begun when a baby was a year old.

—From the *Pocket Book of Baby and Child Care* by Benjamin Spock, MD, 1947

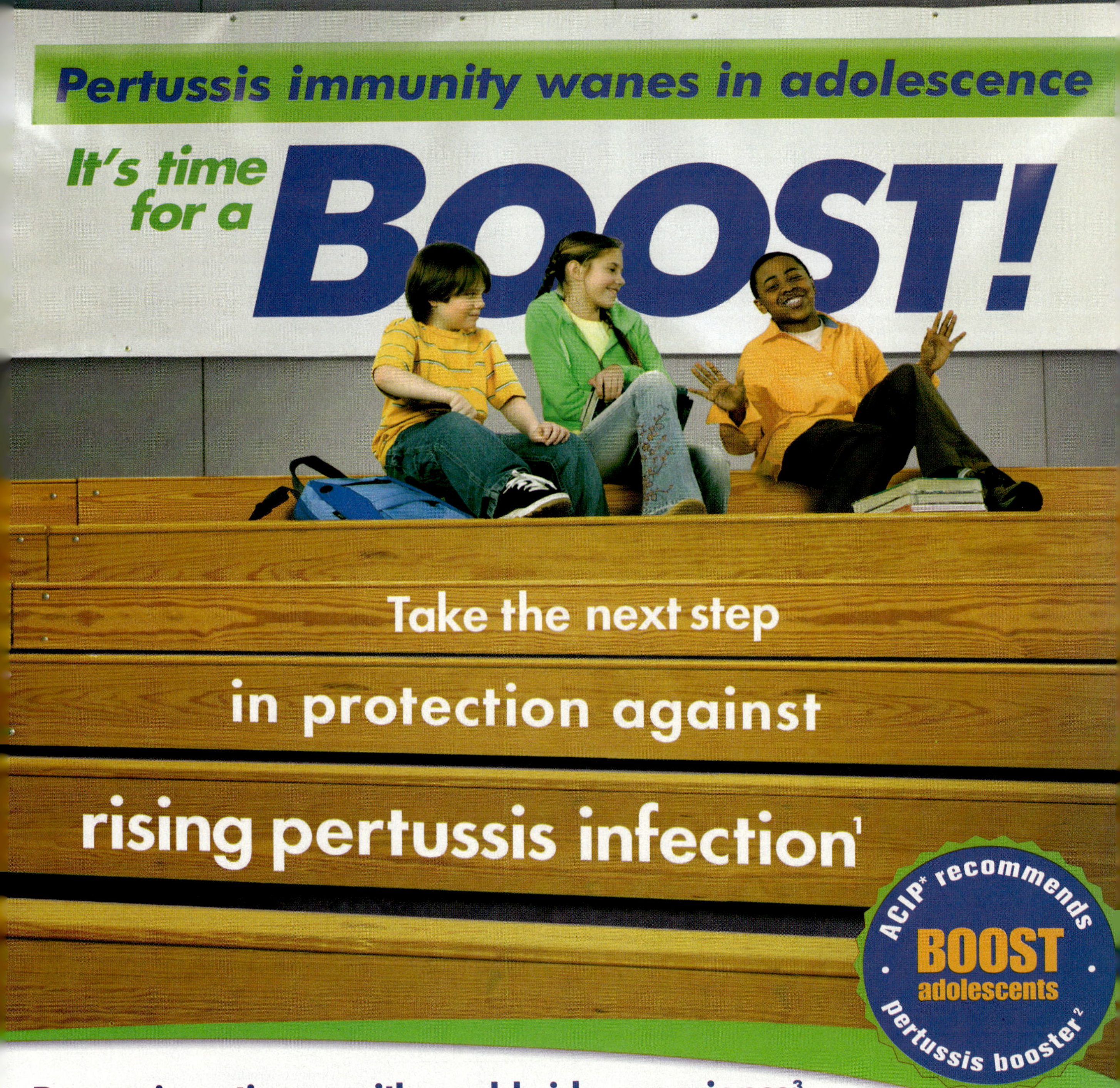
Pertussis immunity wanes in adolescence
It's time for a BOOST!
Take the next step
in protection against
rising pertussis infection[1]
ACIP* recommends
BOOST
adolescents
pertussis booster[2]

# BOOSTRIX®

**(Tetanus Toxoid, Reduced Diphtheria Toxoid and Acellular Pertussis Vaccine, Adsorbed) (Tdap)**

The following is a brief summary only; see full prescribing information for complete product information.

**INDICATIONS AND USAGE:** BOOSTRIX is indicated for active booster immunization against tetanus, diphtheria, and pertussis as a single dose in individuals 10 through 18 years of age. The use of BOOSTRIX as a primary series or to complete the primary series has not been studied. As with any vaccine, BOOSTRIX may not protect 100% of individuals receiving the vaccine. BOOSTRIX is not recommended for treatment of actual infections.

**CONTRAINDICATIONS:** Hypersensitivity to any component of the vaccine is a contraindication (see DESCRIPTION in full prescribing information). Do not use BOOSTRIX after a serious allergic reaction (e.g., anaphylaxis) following any other tetanus toxoid, diphtheria toxoid or pertussis-containing vaccine, or any component of this vaccine (see DESCRIPTION in full prescribing information). Because of the uncertainty as to which component of the vaccine might be responsible, do not give further vaccination with any of these components; or, refer such individuals to an allergist for evaluation. The following events are contraindications to administration of BOOSTRIX: encephalopathy (e.g., coma, decreased level of consciousness, prolonged seizures) within 7 days of administration of a previous dose of a pertussis-containing vaccine that is not attributable to another identifiable cause; progressive neurologic disorder, uncontrolled epilepsy, or progressive encephalopathy. Do not vaccinate individuals with these conditions until a treatment regimen has been established and the condition has stabilized. BOOSTRIX is not contraindicated for use in individuals with HIV infection.

**WARNINGS:** The tip cap and the rubber plunger of the needleless prefilled syringes contain dry natural latex rubber that may cause allergic reactions in latex sensitive individuals. The vial stopper is latex-free. If any of the following events occurred in temporal relation to previous receipt of a Diphtheria and Tetanus Toxoids and Pertussis Vaccine Adsorbed (DTwP) vaccine or a vaccine containing an acellular pertussis component, consider carefully whether to give subsequent doses of BOOSTRIX: temperature of ≥40.5°C (105°F) within 48 hours not due to another identifiable cause; collapse or shock-like state (hypotonic-hyporesponsive episode) within 48 hours; persistent, inconsolable crying lasting ≥3 hours, occurring within 48 hours; seizures with or without fever occurring within 3 days. Persons who experienced serious Arthus-type hypersensitivity reactions following a prior dose of tetanus toxoid usually have high serum tetanus antitoxin levels and should not be given Tetanus and Diphtheria Toxoids Adsorbed For Adult Use (Td) or Tdap vaccines or even emergency doses of Td more frequently than every 10 years, even if the wound is neither clean nor minor. If Guillain-Barré syndrome has occurred within 6 weeks of receipt of prior vaccine containing tetanus toxoid, the decision to give BOOSTRIX or any vaccine containing tetanus toxoid should be based on careful consideration of the potential benefits and possible risks. The decision to administer a pertussis-containing vaccine to individuals with stable central nervous system (CNS) disorders must be made by the physician on an individual basis, with consideration of all relevant factors, and assessment of potential risks and benefits for that individual. Advise the patient, parent, or guardian of the potential increased risk involved (see PRECAUTIONS). A family history of seizures or other CNS disorders is not a contraindication to pertussis vaccine. The Advisory Committee on Immunization Practices (ACIP) has published guidelines for vaccination of persons with recent or acute illness (www.cdc.gov). Do not give BOOSTRIX to individuals with bleeding disorders such as hemophilia or thrombocytopenia, or to persons on anticoagulant therapy unless the potential benefit clearly outweighs the risk of administration. If the decision is made to administer BOOSTRIX to such persons, it should be given with caution with steps taken to avoid the risk of hematoma following the injection.

**PRECAUTIONS:** Before the injection of any biological, the physician should take all reasonable precautions to prevent allergic or other adverse reactions. Epinephrine injection (1:1,000) and other appropriate agents used for the control of immediate allergic reactions must be immediately available should an acute anaphylactic reaction occur. Immunosuppressed persons, including individuals receiving immunosuppressive therapy, may not develop the expected immune response. **Drug Interactions:** Do not mix BOOSTRIX with any other vaccine in the same syringe or vial. **Carcinogenesis, Mutagenesis, Impairment of Fertility:** BOOSTRIX has not been evaluated for carcinogenic or mutagenic potential, or for impairment of fertility. **Pregnancy:** Pregnancy Category C. Animal reproduction studies have not been conducted with BOOSTRIX. It is also not known whether BOOSTRIX can cause fetal harm when administered to a pregnant woman or can affect reproductive capacity. BOOSTRIX should be given to a pregnant woman only if clearly needed. Animal fertility studies have not been conducted with BOOSTRIX. In a developmental toxicity study, the effect of BOOSTRIX on embryo-fetal and pre-weaning development was evaluated in pregnant rats. Animals were administered INFANRIX® (Diphtheria and Tetanus Toxoids and Acellular Pertussis Vaccine Adsorbed) prior to gestation and BOOSTRIX during the period of organogenesis (gestation days 6, 8, 11) and later in pregnancy (gestation day 15), 0.1 mL/rat/occasion (a 45-fold increase compared to the human dose of BOOSTRIX on a body weight basis), by intramuscular injection. No adverse affect on pregnancy and lactation parameters, embryo-fetal or pre-weaning development was observed. There were no fetal malformations or other evidence of teratogenesis noted in this study. **Nursing Mothers:** It is not known whether BOOSTRIX is excreted in human milk. Because many drugs are excreted in human milk, caution should be exercised when BOOSTRIX is administered to a nursing woman. **Pregnancy Exposure Registry:** Healthcare providers are encouraged to register pregnant women who receive BOOSTRIX in the GlaxoSmithKline vaccination pregnancy registry by calling 1-888-825-5249. **Geriatric Use:** BOOSTRIX is not indicated for use in individuals older than 18 years. **Pediatric Use:** BOOSTRIX is not indicated for use in individuals younger than 10 years (see DOSAGE AND ADMINISTRATION in full prescribing information). For immunization of infants and children younger than 7 years against diphtheria, tetanus, and pertussis, refer to the manufacturers' package inserts for Diphtheria and Tetanus Toxoids and Acellular Pertussis Vaccine Adsorbed (DTaP) vaccines.

**ADVERSE REACTIONS:** A total of 3,289 adolescents were vaccinated with a single dose of BOOSTRIX during clinical trials. An additional 1,092 adolescents 10 to 18 years of age received a non-US formulation of BOOSTRIX (formulated to contain 0.5 mg aluminum per dose) in non-US clinical studies.

The primary safety study, conducted in the United States, was a randomized, observer-blinded, controlled study in which 3,080 adolescents 10 to 18 years of age received a single dose of BOOSTRIX and 1,034 received the control Td vaccine manufactured by Massachusetts Public Health Biologic Laboratories. There were no substantive differences in demographic characteristics between the vaccine groups. Among BOOSTRIX and control vaccine recipients approximately 75% were 10 to 14 years of age and approximately 25% were 15 to 18 years of age. Approximately 98% of participants in this study had received the recommended series of 4 or 5 doses of either DTwP or a combination of DTwP and DTaP in childhood. Data on adverse events were collected by the subjects, parents and/or guardians using standardized diaries for 15 consecutive days following the vaccine dose (i.e., day of vaccination and the next 14 days). Subjects were monitored for unsolicited adverse events that occurred within 31 days of vaccination (day 0-30) using diary cards (day 0-14) supplemented by spontaneous reports and a medical history as reported by subjects, parents, and/or guardians. Subjects were also monitored for 6 months post-vaccination for non-routine medical visits, visits to an emergency room, onset of new chronic illness, and serious adverse events. Information regarding late onset adverse events was obtained via a telephone call 6 months following vaccination. At least 97% of subjects completed the 6-month follow-up evaluation.

The adverse event information from clinical trials provides a basis for identifying adverse events that appear to be related to vaccine use and for approximating rates. However, because clinical trials are conducted under widely varying conditions, adverse event rates observed in the clinical trials of a vaccine cannot be directly compared to rates in the clinical trials of another vaccine, and may not reflect the rates observed in practice.

**Serious Adverse Events in All Safety Studies:** In the US-safety study, no serious adverse events were reported to occur within 31 days of vaccination. During the 6-month extended safety evaluation period, no serious adverse events that were of potential autoimmune origin or new onset and chronic in nature were reported to occur. In non-US studies in which serious adverse events were monitored for up to 37 days, one subject was diagnosed with insulin dependent diabetes. The association of this event with vaccination is unknown. No other serious adverse events of potential autoimmune origin or that were new onset and chronic in nature were reported to occur in these studies.

**Solicited Adverse Events in the US-Safety Study:** In a US study, the most common local adverse events following administration of BOOSTRIX were pain, redness, and swelling at the injection site. The most common general adverse events were headache and fatigue. Most of these events were reported at a similar frequency in recipients of both BOOSTRIX and Td. Any pain, grade 2 or 3 pain (but not grade 3 alone), and grade 2 or 3 headache (but not grade 3 alone) were reported at a higher rate in recipients of BOOSTRIX. The primary safety endpoint of the US study was the incidence of grade 3 pain (spontaneously painful and/or prevented normal activity) at the injection site within 15 days of vaccination. Grade 3 pain was reported in 4.6% of those who received BOOSTRIX compared with 4.0% of those who received the Td vaccine. The difference in rate of grade 3 pain was within the pre-defined clinical limit for non-inferiority (upper limit of the 95% CI for the difference ≤4%). These were the rates for solicited local and general adverse events within 15 days of vaccination with BOOSTRIX or Td vaccine for the total vaccinated cohort (all enrolled, vaccinated subjects with safety data available analyzed by vaccine received):

**Percentage of Individuals 10 to 18 Years of Age Reporting Solicited Local Adverse Events or Solicited General Adverse Events Within the 15-day* Post-Vaccination Period**

| | BOOSTRIX (N = 3,032) | Td (N = 1,013) |
|---|---|---|
| **Local** | | |
| Pain,[†] any | 75.3 | 71.7 |
| Pain,[†] grade 2 or 3 | 51.2 | 42.5 |
| Pain,[‡] grade 3 | 4.6 | 4.0 |
| Redness, any | 22.5 | 19.8 |
| Redness, >20 mm | 4.1 | 3.9 |
| Redness, ≥50 mm | 1.7 | 1.6 |
| Swelling, any | 21.1 | 20.1 |
| Swelling, >20 mm | 5.3 | 4.9 |
| Swelling, ≥50 mm | 2.5 | 3.2 |
| Arm circumference increase,[§] >5 mm | 28.3 | 29.5 |
| Arm circumference increase,[§] >20 mm | 2.0 | 2.2 |
| Arm circumference increase,[§] >40 mm | 0.5 | 0.3 |
| **General** | | |
| Fever,[‖] ≥99.5°F | 13.5 | 13.1 |
| Fever,[‖] >100.4°F | 5.0 | 4.7 |
| Fever,[‖] >102.2°F | 1.4 | 1.0 |
| Headache, any | 43.1 | 41.5 |
| Headache,[†] grade 2 or 3 | 15.7 | 12.7 |
| Headache, grade 3 | 3.7 | 2.7 |
| Fatigue, any | 37.0 | 36.7 |
| Fatigue, grade 2 or 3 | 14.4 | 12.9 |
| Fatigue, grade 3 | 3.7 | 3.2 |
| Gastrointestinal symptoms,[¶] any | 26.0 | 25.8 |
| Gastrointestinal symptoms,[¶] grade 2 or 3 | 9.8 | 9.7 |
| Gastrointestinal symptoms,[¶] grade 3 | 3.0 | 3.2 |

Td = Tetanus and Diphtheria Toxoids Adsorbed For Adult Use manufactured by Massachusetts Public Health Biologic Laboratories.

N = number of subjects in the total vaccinated cohort with local/general symptoms sheets completed.

Grade 2 = Local: painful when the limb was moved; General: interfered with normal activity.

Grade 3 = Local: spontaneously painful and/or prevented normal activity; General: prevented normal activity.

*Day of vaccination and the next 14 days.

[†]Statistically significantly higher (P<0.05) following BOOSTRIX as compared to Td vaccine.

[‡]Grade 3 injection site pain following BOOSTRIX was not inferior to Td (upper limit of two-sided 95% CI for the difference in the percentage of subjects ≤4%).

[§]Mid-upper region of the vaccinated arm.

[‖]Oral temperatures or axillary temperatures.

[¶]Gastrointestinal symptoms included nausea, vomiting, diarrhea and/or abdominal pain.

Mid-upper arm circumference was measured by the adolescent or their parent/guardian prior to injection and daily for 15 days following vaccination. There was no significant difference between BOOSTRIX recipients and Td recipients in the proportion of subjects reporting an increase in mid-upper arm circumference in the vaccinated arm. The incidence of unsolicited adverse events reported in the 31 days after vaccination was comparable between the 2 groups.

As with any vaccine, there is the possibility that broad use of BOOSTRIX could reveal adverse events not observed in clinical trials.

**Postmarketing Reports:** Worldwide voluntary reports of adverse events received for BOOSTRIX in persons 10 to 18 years of age since market introduction of this vaccine are listed below. This list includes serious events or events which have causal connection to components of this or other vaccines or drugs. Because these events are reported voluntarily from a population of uncertain size, it is not possible to reliably estimate their frequency or establish a causal relationship to vaccine exposure. *Blood and lymphatic system disorders:* Lymphadenitis, lymphadenopathy. *Cardiac disorders:* Myocarditis. *Injection site reactions:* Induration, inflammation, mass, nodule, warmth, local reaction. *Metabolism and nutrition disorders:* Diabetes mellitus insulin-dependent. *Musculoskeletal and connective tissue disorders:* Arthralgia, back pain, myalgia. *Nervous system disorders:* Convulsion, encephalitis, facial palsy, paraesthesia. *Skin and subcutaneous tissue disorders:* Exanthem, Henoch-Schönlein purpura, rash. In addition, extensive swelling of the injected limb has been reported following administration of BOOSTRIX.

**Reporting Adverse Events:** Report the occurrence following immunization of any event set forth in the Vaccine Injury Table from the National Childhood Vaccine Injury Act including: Anaphylaxis or anaphylactic shock within 7 days, encephalopathy or encephalitis within 7 days, brachial neuritis within 28 days, or an acute complication or sequelae (including death) of an illness, disability, injury, or condition referred to above, or any events that would contraindicate further doses of vaccine, according to this prescribing information. These events should be reported to VAERS. The VAERS toll-free number is 1-800-822-7967. Reporting forms may also be obtained at the VAERS website at www.vaers.org.

**DOSAGE AND ADMINISTRATION: Recommended Dose:** BOOSTRIX should be administered as a single 0.5 mL injection by the intramuscular route into the deltoid muscle of the upper arm in individuals 10 through 18 years of age. Do not administer this product subcutaneously or intravenously. There are no data to support repeat administration of BOOSTRIX. Five years should elapse between the subject's last dose of the recommended series of childhood DTwP and/or DTaP vaccine and the administration of BOOSTRIX. Limited data are available on the use of BOOSTRIX following Tetanus and Diphtheria Toxoids Adsorbed For Adult Use (Td) vaccine. **Additional Dosing Information:** ***Wound Management:*** Clinicians should refer to guidelines for tetanus prophylaxis in routine wound management. Adolescents 10 to 18 years of age who have completed a primary series against tetanus and who sustain wounds which are minor and uncomplicated, should receive a booster dose of a tetanus toxoid-containing vaccine only if they have not received tetanus toxoid within the preceding 10 years. In case of tetanus-prone injury (e.g., wounds contaminated with dirt, feces, soil, and saliva; puncture wounds; avulsions; and wounds resulting from missles, crushing, burns, and frostbite) in an adolescent who is in need of tetanus toxoid, BOOSTRIX can be used as an alternative to Tetanus and Diphtheria Toxoids Adsorbed For Adult Use (Td) vaccine in patients for whom the pertussis component is also indicated (see INDICATIONS AND USAGE).

Manufactured by **GlaxoSmithKline Biologicals**
Rixensart, Belgium, US License 1617
Distributed by **GlaxoSmithKline**
Research Triangle Park, NC 27709



Full prescribing information for BOOSTRIX is available at www.BOOSTRIX.com.

BRS-BO:L1

**References: 1.** Centers for Disease Control and Prevention. *Epidemiology and Prevention of Vaccine-Preventable Diseases.* Atkinson W, Hamborsky J, Wolfe S, eds. 8th ed. Washington DC: Public Health Foundation; 2004:75–88, A26–A27. **2.** ACIP recommends adolescent vaccination for tetanus, diphtheria and pertussis vaccine [press release]. Atlanta, GA: Department of Health and Human Services; Available at: www.cdc.gov/nip/pr/pr_tdap_jun2005.htm. Accessed September 27, 2005. **3.** Data on file, BOR305, GlaxoSmithKline.

ARTICLE

# Impact of Adolescent Mental Disorders and Physical Illnesses on Quality of Life 17 Years Later

*Henian Chen, MD, PhD; Patricia Cohen, PhD; Stephanie Kasen, PhD; Jeffrey G. Johnson, PhD; Kathy Berenson, PhD; Kathy Gordon*

**Objective:** To investigate associations of mental disorders and physical illnesses during adolescence with quality of life (QOL) 17 years later.

**Design:** The Children in the Community Study, a prospective longitudinal investigation.

**Setting:** Upstate New York.

**Participants:** A community-based sample of mothers and their offspring were interviewed.

**Main Outcome Measures:** Axis I disorders and Axis II personality disorders and physical illnesses were assessed by self-report and mother report in 1985-1986. Outcome indicators of QOL were assessed in 2001-2004.

**Results:** Compared with participants without adolescent illness or disorder, those with a history of physical illness reported poorer physical health (mean difference [MD], −4.8); those with a history of an Axis I disorder reported poorer physical health (MD, −8.0) and more problematic social relationships (MD, −4.5); and those with a history of personality disorder reported poorer physical health (MD, −8.2), more problematic social relationships (MD, −5.0), lower psychological well-being (MD, −3.6), and more adversity within their environmental context (MD, −4.6) in adulthood. Comorbid physical illness and mental disorder were associated with all 5 QOL domains (MD, −3.1 to −11.9). After adjusting for all demographic variables and comorbidity, associations remained between physical illness and poor physical health (effect size [ES], −0.33); an Axis I disorder and problematic social relationships (ES, −0.37); and personality disorder and problematic social relationships (ES, −0.36), low psychological well-being (ES, −0.23), impaired role function (ES, −0.24), and an adverse environmental context (ES, −0.50).

**Conclusions:** Mental disorders may have more adverse long-term associations with QOL than do physical illnesses. Adolescent personality disorders may have a more adverse impact on adult QOL than do adolescent Axis I disorders.

*Arch Pediatr Adolesc Med. 2006;160:93-99*

QUALITY OF LIFE (QOL) has been firmly established as an important outcome in patient care and clinical research.[1-3] Improving QOL is a major goal in the treatment of individuals with chronic illnesses.[4-6] Quality of life can be viewed as a subjective, multidimensional concept, which may include self-evaluation of all aspects of life.[7,8] Data on QOL in adults and clinical samples are accumulating at a substantial rate, especially for adults in their older years; in contrast, there is minimal information about QOL during the earlier adult years. Young adults may evaluate qualitative aspects of their lives differently from older adults or patients because of variations in developmental tasks, social and work role settings, age-related expectations, and health status. Many existing QOL measures for adults focus primarily on their capacity to perform daily activities.[9] For example, the Quality of Well-Being Scale primarily covers physical problems,[10] whereas the Nottingham Health Profile is designed for people with disabilities.[11] The latter is a negative measure of health and does not include items that indicate well-being; therefore, it is more suitable as a survey tool in populations that may include people with significant disability, such as elderly people.[9] The Sickness Impact Profile assesses the impact of illness on daily activities; thus, it is best used with people who are or who perceive themselves to be ill.[9,12] Finally, certain sets of items (eg, limitations in running, moving a table, lifting groceries, climbing 1 flight of stairs, walking 1 block,

Author Affiliations: Epidemiology of Mental Disorders, New York State Psychiatric Institute (Drs Chen, Cohen, Kasen, Johnson, and Berenson and Ms Gordon), and Department of Psychiatry, College of Physicians and Surgeons (Drs Chen, Cohen, Kasen, Johnson, and Berenson), and Department of Epidemiology, Mailman School of Public Health (Drs Chen and Cohen), Columbia University, New York, NY.

bathing, washing, dressing, and preparing food) in QOL scales that tap physical functioning[13] and activities of daily life[14] are directed at older adults or disabled populations and may be less useful with a general population sample of adults. The Young Adult Quality of Life (YAQOL) instrument[9] assesses aspects of QOL related to the physical health, psychological well-being, social relationships, role function, and environmental context of young adults, thus meeting criteria for breadth of coverage of QOL. The YAQOL is the only generic measure of QOL designed specifically for young adults. A unique feature of the YAQOL, which distinguishes it from other generic QOL questionnaires for adults, is the measurement of role and residential context as well as perspective on life goals.

Research has shown that both physical illnesses[4,6,15-19] and mental disorders[2,20-26] are associated with reduced QOL. Furthermore, findings based on adult populations have indicated that the extent of impairment in QOL associated with mental disorders is comparable with the impairment associated with physical illnesses.[2,6,20,21,27-30] Previous research has focused primarily on specific illnesses or evaluated only 1 or 2 QOL domains.[16-18] Recently, researchers have begun to assess associations of physical illnesses with more comprehensive aspects of QOL[6,15-19,27,28]; however, most studies have been cross-sectional and have focused on mood and anxiety disorders in clinical samples or among older adults. To date, no community-based prospective longitudinal studies have compared associations of mental disorders and physical illnesses during adolescence with subsequent QOL during adulthood.

The purpose of the present study was to examine and compare associations between adolescent mental disorders and adult QOL and between adolescent physical illnesses and adult QOL. Indicators of QOL included 5 broad domains of physical health, social relationships, psychological well-being, role function, and the environmental context. In addition, we investigated the relative magnitudes of the associations of Axis I disorders and Axis II personality disorders (PDs) assessed in adolescence with QOL impairment during adulthood. Axis I encompasses various disorders and conditions such as mood, anxiety, disruptive, and substance-related disorders that are typically the focus of clinical attention, whereas the Axis II PDs are maladaptive, inflexible, and enduring ways of thinking, acting, and feeling that lead to distress or impairment or both.

## METHODS

### PARTICIPANTS

This study examined longitudinal data from the now-grown youths in the Children in the Community Study, an ongoing investigation of childhood behavior and development based on a sample of families randomly selected in 1975 on the basis of residence in 2 upstate New York counties.[31,32] Approximately 800 mothers and 1 randomly sampled child from each family (mean ± SD age, 5.5 ±2.8 years; in 1975) have been reinterviewed in their homes by extensively trained and supervised lay interviewers in a series of follow-up surveys during the past 30 years. These families were generally representative of the northeastern United States in terms of demographic characteristics and socioeconomic status.[32] However, the sample also reflects the relatively high proportion of Catholic (54%) and white (91%) residents living in the sampled region. Details of sampling, comparison with population, and retention rates are provided on the study Web site (www.nyspi.cpmc.columbia.edu/childcom). Earlier retention rates of 95% have dropped as the cohort became adults; this problem is shared by virtually all other recent longitudinal studies of community and clinical samples.[33]

The present study focuses on 608 (81.1%) of the 750 young adults on whom mental disorders (Axis I disorders and Axis II PDs) and physical illnesses were assessed in 1985-1986 at the mean ± SD age of 16.0 ± 2.8 years and in 2001-2004 at the mean ± SD age of 33.0 ± 2.8 years. Participants lost to attrition at the age of 33 years had higher schizotypal symptom scores at the age of 16 years and were more likely to be male than those retained in the sample. The study procedures were approved in accordance with appropriate institutional guidelines and have been approved by the institutional review board of the New York State Psychiatric Institute. A National Institutes of Health Certificate of Confidentiality has been obtained for these data. Written informed consent or assent was obtained from all participants after the interview procedures were fully explained. Assessment was performed by computer-assisted interview in participants' homes and by telephone for a small minority who moved out of the area.

### ASSESSMENT

#### Axis I Disorders

In the 1985-1986 follow-up, the parent and youth versions of the Diagnostic Interview Schedule for Children[34] were administered to assess *Diagnostic and Statistical Manual of Mental Disorders, Revised Third Edition* (*DSM-III-R*) Axis I disorders and grouped as follows: major depressive disorder, anxiety disorders (overanxious disorder, separation anxiety disorder, or social phobia), disruptive disorders (attention-deficit/hyperactivity disorder, conduct disorder, or oppositional defiant disorder), and substance abuse disorders (alcohol or marijuana or other illicit drug abuse) at the mean age of 16 years. Research has supported the reliability and validity of those psychiatric diagnoses as assessed with the Diagnostic Interview Schedule for Children and administered in the present study.[35,36]

#### Axis II PDs

No developed instruments existed for assessing PD before adulthood because recognition of the potential presence of PD in childhood or adolescence was first noted in the *DSM-III-R*. We created such an instrument by adapting items from the Personality Diagnostic Questionnaire for adults[37,38] and by selecting appropriate items from other existing scales or writing age-appropriate items when necessary.[39,40] At the mean age of 16 years, PD diagnoses based on both self-reports and mother reports were grouped at the traditional *DSM* cluster levels for analyses: cluster A (paranoid, schizoid, or schizotypal PD), cluster B (borderline, histrionic, or narcissistic PD), and cluster C (avoidant, dependent, or obsessive-compulsive PD), and at a combined "any PD" level. The PD diagnoses indicate that the individual has a specific degree of severity with regard to personality traits. The validity of those assessed PD diagnoses on an individual and a cluster level has been supported by theoretically predicted associations with risks,[40,41] correlates,[39,42] and outcomes.[43,44]

At the mean age of 33 years, those same PDs were assessed by self-reports with the Structured Clinical Interview for *Di-*

*agnostic and Statistical Manual of Mental Disorders, Fourth Edition, Axis II Personality Disorders* (SCID-II) screen. Agreement between PD diagnoses obtained at the mean age of 16 years and at the mean age of 33 years was excellent (κ=0.44) when compared with the level of agreement achieved by other instruments.[45] Moreover, we also found excellent concurrent agreement between PD symptoms obtained with our original instrument and with the SCID-II screen ($r$=0.66, 0.78, and 0.67 for cluster A, B, and C symptoms, respectively) and reasonable stability between self-reported PD symptoms from the mean age of 22 years (in an interim wave of data collection) to the mean age of 33 years ($r$=0.61, 0.64, and 0.57 for cluster A, B, and C symptoms, respectively).

### Self-reported Physical Illnesses

In interviews conducted during adolescence, physical illnesses in the past year, including allergies or asthma, musculoskeletal diseases (orthopedic problems or chronic pain), neurologic diseases (migraine or other chronic headaches or epilepsy or other neurologic problems), heart problems, mononucleosis, severe vision problems, and hearing problems, were identified and summed from both youths' and mothers' responses. For each physical illness, we asked youths, "Did you have this problem in the past year?" and "Did you go to a doctor for the problem?" Mothers were asked parallel questions: "Did s/he have this problem in the past year?" and "Did s/he see a doctor for the problem?"

### Quality of Life

The YAQOL[9] assessed 5 QOL domains in participants at the mean age of 33 years. The physical health domain was measured with an 8-item scale that assessed overall health, incapacitation due to illness, and energy level. The psychological well-being domain was measured with 3 scales that assessed expectations for the future (5 items), negative feelings (5 items), and church attendance or religious beliefs (2 items). The social relationships domain was measured with a 9-item scale that assessed the extent of contact and quality of relationships with friends and a 9-item scale that assessed the quality of relationship with a partner or close confidante. The role function domain was measured with 4 scales that assessed stress in a major productive role (employment, school, and home) due to excessive demand, conflict, safety, or health risk (6 items); degree of influence over role organization, scheduling, and decisions (5 items); role satisfaction and consistency with long-term goals (5 items); and role morale of coworkers or other students (6 items). The contextual domain was measured with 4 scales that assessed environmental factors, including residential comfort, safety, quietness, and privacy (9 items); social and service aspects of the neighborhood (8 items); ease of access to settings for work, school, shopping, leisure, and social activities (6 items); and degree of medical care access and financial support (5 items). Internal consistency reliability of the YAQOL ranged from 0.88 to 0.63 (mean, 0.73). Detailed information regarding the reliability and validity of YAQOL is available in a previous report.[9] All analyses considered indicators of QOL at the domain level. The minimum possible score for each domain was defined as 0 and the maximum possible score as 100, with higher scores indicating better QOL.

## STATISTICAL ANALYSES

Linear regression analyses were conducted to investigate the associations between adolescent physical illnesses and mental disorders, assessed at a mean age of 16 years, and adulthood QOL, assessed at a mean age of 33 years. All analyses were controlled for demographic variables (race, sex, age, family socioeconomic status, earned income, marital status, and education) because there are significant variations in aspects of QOL for those groups.[9,46,47] Unstandardized regression coefficients were interpreted as the mean difference (MD) on each QOL domain score between those with a disorder and those without any physical illnesses or mental disorders (reference group, n=256) after adjusting for all demographic variables in the equation. Regression analyses were also conducted, adjusting for all demographic variables and physical and mental disorder comorbidity to identify the independent association of each disorder with each of the QOL domains. The reference group was composed of participants without the disorder being examined. The QOL domains have different variability; thus, adjusted standardized regression coefficients are presented to make comparisons across the QOL scales. Effect sizes (ESs) of 0.20, 0.50, and 0.80 or greater were considered small, moderate, and large, respectively.[48]

# RESULTS

## SAMPLE CHARACTERISTICS AND PREVALENCE OF DISORDERS

Participants at a mean age of 33 years were 54.8% female, 91.3% white, and 8.7% black; 69.7% were married or cohabiting; 75.5% had some post–high school education; and 38.0% were from urban areas. Mean QOL domain scores were 67.8, 77.6, 80.6, 64.1, and 75.3 for physical health, social relationships, psychological well-being, role function, and environmental context, respectively. Among 5 QOL domains, correlations ranged from 0.08 to 0.50, with most in the intermediate range.

At a mean age of 16 years, 263 participants (43.3%) reported at least 1 of the physical illnesses assessed (**Table 1**). The most commonly reported illnesses were allergies or asthma (18.9%), musculoskeletal diseases (15.6%), and neurologic diseases (10.9%), whereas hearing problems, severe vision problems, heart problems, and mononucleosis each were reported by less than 6% of the participants. At this same assessment, 185 participants (30.4%) had at least 1 mental disorder, 115 (18.9%) had an Axis I disorder, 111 (18.3%) had an Axis II disorder, 41 (6.7%) had comorbid Axis I and Axis II disorders, and 96 (15.8%) had concurrent physical illnesses and mental disorders.

## ASSOCIATION OF QOL IMPAIRMENT WITH ADOLESCENT MENTAL DISORDERS AND PHYSICAL ILLNESSES

The mean QOL score for participants with a disorder was calculated and compared with a single reference group (the 256 participants without any physical illness or mental disorder). Table 1 presents the MD of QOL scores for disorders, adjusted by regression analysis for all demographic variables.

## MENTAL DISORDERS AND PHYSICAL ILLNESSES

Adolescents with a physical illness but not a mental disorder (n=167) reported poorer physical health (MD, −4.8; $P$=.007) 17 years later, whereas adolescents with a mental disorder but no physical illness (n=89) reported more

**Table 1. Mean Differences in QOL Scores in Participants With Physical Illnesses or Mental Disorders***

| | | Mean Differences in QOL Scores (N = 256) | | | | |
|---|---|---|---|---|---|---|
| **Disorder** | **No. (%) of Participants** | **Physical Health** | **Social Relationships** | **Psychological Well-being** | **Role Function** | **Environmental Context** |
| Physical illness only | 167 (27.5) | −4.8† | 0.8 | 1.8 | 1.9 | 1.3 |
| Mental disorder only | 89 (14.6) | −4.3 | −4.9† | −4.1‡ | −2.8 | −3.9† |
| Physical illness and mental disorder | 96 (15.8) | −11.9† | −4.7† | −4.2‡ | −4.1‡ | −3.1† |
| Axis I disorder only | 74 (12.2) | −8.0† | −4.5† | −1.4 | −1.2 | −0.1 |
| Axis II disorder only | 70 (11.5) | −8.2† | −5.0† | −3.6‡ | −2.3 | −4.6† |
| Axis I and Axis II disorders | 41 (6.7) | −6.2† | −5.4† | −3.7‡ | −6.3‡ | −5.1† |
| Specific disorders | | | | | | |
| Allergies or asthma | 115 (18.9) | −9.3† | −0.7 | −0.5 | −0.9 | 0.5 |
| Musculoskeletal diseases | 95 (15.6) | −11.2† | −1.4 | 0.3 | −1.3 | −1.1 |
| Neurologic diseases | 66 (10.9) | −11.8† | −4.0† | −2.9 | −1.4 | −1.3 |
| Hearing problem | 32 (5.3) | −4.7 | −1.7 | 1.7 | −3.2 | 1.3 |
| Severe vision problem | 32 (5.3) | −5.3 | 1.3 | 2.0 | −0.4 | −1.2 |
| Heart problem | 8 (1.3) | −21.8† | −3.2 | −1.8 | −0.7 | −0.9 |
| Mononucleosis | 8 (1.3) | −1.2 | 3.4 | 1.9 | −0.5 | 1.3 |
| Anxiety disorder | 62 (10.2) | −6.4‡ | −4.7† | −2.9 | −1.3 | −2.1 |
| Disruptive disorder | 39 (6.4) | −8.1‡ | −7.2† | −2.7 | −4.0 | −3.9‡ |
| Substance abuse | 24 (3.9) | −10.7† | −1.2 | 2.8 | −4.3 | 1.0 |
| Major depression | 19 (3.1) | −8.3‡ | −9.8† | −4.8 | −8.5‡ | −4.3 |
| Cluster B PD | 55 (9.0) | −7.6† | −2.7 | −2.3 | −3.8 | −4.7† |
| Cluster A PD | 48 (7.9) | −5.9‡ | −5.3† | −0.8 | −2.2 | −4.5† |
| Cluster C PD | 35 (5.8) | −9.6† | −7.8† | −9.8† | −2.0 | −7.0† |

Abbreviations: PD, personality disorder; QOL, quality of life.
*Separate regression analyses for each QOL domain score after adjusting all demographic variables. Participants were compared with a reference group of 256 people with no disorders whose QOL scores at the mean age of 33 years were as follows: physical health, 72.3; social relationships, 78.9; psychological well-being, 81.3; role function, 65.6; and environmental context, 77.1.
†$P<.01$.
‡$P<.05$.

problematic social relationships (MD, −4.9; $P=.001$), lower psychological well-being (MD, −4.1; $P=.01$), and more adversity in their environmental context (MD, −3.9; $P=.009$) 17 years later (Table 1). In addition, adolescents with comorbid physical illness and mental disorder (n=96) were more impaired in all 5 QOL domains (MDs, −3.1 to −11.9) 17 years later (**Figure 1**).

## AXIS I DISORDERS AND AXIS II PDs

Those with an Axis I disorder but no PD in adolescence (n=74) had poorer physical health (MD, −8.0; $P<.001$) and more problematic social relationships (MD, −4.5; $P=.001$) 17 years later, whereas those with a PD but no Axis I disorder in adolescence (n=70) had poorer physical health (MD, −0.82; $P=.002$), more problematic social relationships (MD, −5.0; $P=.001$), lower psychological well-being (MD, −3.6; $P=.046$), and more adversity in their environmental context (MD, −4.6; $P=.001$) (Table 1). Individuals with comorbid Axis I disorders and Axis II PDs in adolescence (n=41) were more impaired in all 5 QOL domains (MDs, −3.7 to −6.3) (**Figure 2**).

## SPECIFIC DISORDERS

Each of the 14 physical and mental disorders produced a distinctive pattern of impairment in QOL. All disorders, except mononucleosis and hearing and vision problems, were associated with impaired QOL in at least 1 and up to 4 domains (Table 1). Allergies or asthma, musculoskeletal diseases, heart problems, and substance abuse showed only an association with later poor physical health. Neurologic diseases and anxiety disorder were associated with poor physical health and problematic social relationships. Cluster B PDs (borderline, histrionic, or narcissistic PD) were associated with poor physical health and an adverse environmental context. Disruptive disorder and cluster A PDs (paranoid, schizoid, or schizotypal PD) predicted later problematic social relationships and an adverse environmental context as well as poor physical health. Major depression was associated with poor physical health, problematic social relationships, and impaired role function. Cluster C PDs (avoidant, dependent, or obsessive-compulsive PD) were associated with poor physical health, problematic social relationships, low psychological well-being, and an adverse environmental context.

## INDEPENDENT ASSOCIATION OF QOL IMPAIRMENT WITH ADOLESCENT MENTAL DISORDERS AND PHYSICAL ILLNESSES

When comorbid physical and mental disorders exist in adolescence, which contributes to impaired adult QOL? To answer this question, we tested the independent association of each type of disorder with QOL (**Table 2**). Regression analyses were adjusted for all demographic variables and comorbid disorders to identify the independent association of disorder with each of the QOL domains; the reference group was composed of participants without the disorder being examined. The ES is the

MD in QOL score between participants with and without the disorder divided by the standard deviation of the QOL score in the total sample.

## MENTAL DISORDERS AND PHYSICAL ILLNESSES

After adjusting for all demographic variables and any mental disorder, those with an adolescent history of physical illness had poorer physical health (ES, −0.33; $P<.001$) in adulthood at the mean age of 33 years. After adjusting for all demographic variables and any physical illness, those with an adolescent history of mental disorder were more impaired in all 5 QOL domains (ESs, −0.24 to −0.46) (Table 2). In our data, musculoskeletal diseases (n=95) and neurologic diseases (n=66) have been associated with high rates of mental disorders (44.2% and 42.4%, respectively). A sensitivity analyses was conducted without these 2 categories. There was an effect of physical illnesses (n=172) on the physical health QOL domain (ES, −0.25; $P=.005$); nonetheless, the effect of mental disorder was on all 5 QOL domains (ESs, −0.24 to −0.47). Those results are similar to results that considered all 7 physical illness categories assessedin our study (Table 2) but with slightly lower ESs (−0.33 to −0.25).

## AXIS I AND AXIS II DISORDERS

Table 2 gives the results of analyses adjusting for all demographic variables, any physical illness, and either any Axis I disorder or any Axis II PD. An independent adolescent Axis I disorder effect was limited to the QOL domain of social relationships (ES, −0.37; $P=.002$). In comparison, adolescent Axis II PDs had a stronger impact, with significantly more impairment in QOL domains of social relationships (ES, −0.36; $P=.006$), psychological well-being (ES, −0.23; $P=.04$), role function (ES, −0.24; $P=.04$), and environmental context (ES, −0.50; $P<.001$). To test whether these results were due to the persistence of Axis I or II disorders into adulthood, we repeated these analyses with controls for an Axis I disorder or Axis II PDs at the mean age of 33 years. The same significant effects of any adolescent Axis I disorder on QOL 17 years later were found after controlling for an adult Axis I disorder, albeit the effects were somewhat smaller. Similarly, adolescent PDs still had significant but reduced effects on social relationships, role function, and environmental context. Associations with psychological well-being were no longer significant after controlling for any PD at the mean age of 33 years.

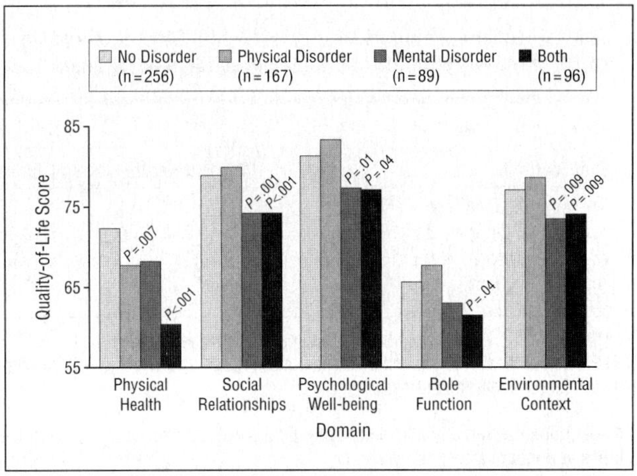


**Figure 1.** Association of mental disorders and physical illnesses at the mean age of 16 years with 5 quality-of-life domains at the mean age of 33 years.

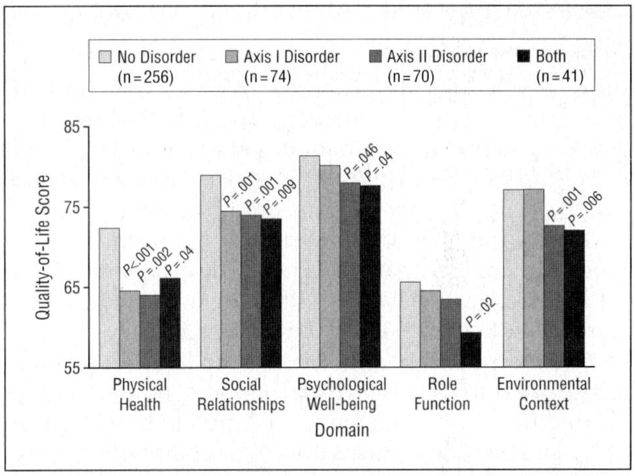


**Figure 2.** Association of Axis I and Axis II disorders at the mean age of 16 years with 5 quality-of-life domains at the mean age of 33 years.

## COMMENT

Our review of the literature indicates that these findings reported from a community-based longitudinal study provide initial support for the following: (1) mental disorders during adolescence may be more strongly associated with reduced QOL during adulthood than are adolescent physical illnesses; (2) Axis II PDs during adolescence may account for more subsequent QOL impairment than do adolescent Axis I disorders; (3) individuals with adolescent PD are at increased risk of living in a more adverse environmental context 17 years later; and (4) adolescents with comorbid physical illness and mental disorder tend to experience a particularly large reduction in QOL by adulthood.

The present findings are consistent with previous findings indicating that mental disorders are associated with considerable impairment and low QOL. Cross-sectional studies[20,23,49,50] have shown that depressive disorders are associated with QOL impairment that is comparable to the impairment associated with physical illness. Spitzer et al[2] reported findings of a cross-sectional study of 1000 adult primary care patients indicating that mental disorders tended to be associated with more impairment in QOL than were common physical illnesses. Hays et al[21] found, in a 2-year follow-up study, that depressed patients had substantial and long-lasting decrements in QOL that were equal to or greater than decrements experienced by patients with chronic medical illnesses. Our findings suggest that although physical illnesses during adolescence are likely to be associated with poor physical health outcomes, they may not be associated with poor overall functioning or low global QOL. In contrast, our findings suggest that mental disorders during adolescence tend to be associated with profound impairment in areas that include physical health, social relation-

**Table 2. Independent Association of Mental Disorders and Physical Illnesses at a Mean Age of 16 Years With Quality of Life at a Mean Age of 33 Years***

| | Effect Size | | | | |
|---|---|---|---|---|---|
| Disorder | Physical Health | Social Relationships | Psychological Well-being | Role Function | Environmental Context |
| Any physical illness (n = 263)† | −0.33‡ | 0.06 | 0.10 | 0.03 | 0.08 |
| Any mental disorder (n = 185)§ | −0.25‡ | −0.46‡ | −0.24‖ | −0.25‖ | −0.31‡ |
| Any Axis I disorder (n = 115)¶ | −0.15 | −0.37‡ | −0.12 | −0.21 | −0.04 |
| Any Axis II disorder (n = 111)# | −0.18 | −0.36‡ | −0.23‖ | −0.24‖ | −0.50‡ |

*Separate regression analyses for each quality-of-life domain.
†Participants with any physical illness at the mean age of 16 years are compared with those without physical illness, adjusted for all demographic variables and any adolescent mental disorder.
‡*P*<.01.
§Participants with any adolescent mental disorder are compared with those without mental disorder, adjusted for all demographic variables and any physical illness at a mean age of 16 years.
‖*P*<.05.
¶Participants with any adolescent Axis I disorder are compared with those without an Axis I disorder, adjusted for all demographic variables, any physical illness at a mean age of 16 years, and any adolescent Axis II disorder.
#Participants with any adolescent Axis II disorder are compared with those without an Axis II disorder, adjusted for all demographic variables, any physical illness at a mean age of 16 years, and any adolescent Axis I disorder.

ships, psychological well-being, role function, and environmental context. Furthermore, our findings suggest that mental disorders not only are associated with more impairment in adult QOL than physical illnesses but also have distinct patterns of impairment.

In addition, the present findings are of interest because they confirm that when mental disorders and physical illnesses co-occur, they often are associated with a marked reduction in QOL. Research has indicated that approximately a quarter of medical inpatients have mental disorders as well as physical illnesses, that both types of conditions contribute independently to reductions in QOL, and that these effects tend to be additive.[20,30,51] Several studies[25,52,53] also have indicated that patients with coronary disease who have symptoms of anxiety or depression are more likely than those without these symptoms to report diminished QOL.

Several limitations of the current study require discussion. First, because the present study was conducted with a sample in which a relatively high proportion was Catholic (54%) and white (91%), it is not clear whether the findings are applicable to large US populations. A second limitation of our study is that the measures of physical illnesses relied on self-report rather than medical records. We have information from both youth and mother reports and from 2 questions for each physical illness ("Did you have this problem in the past year?" and "Did you go to the doctor for the problem?"). Several studies have indicated that self-reports are fairly accurate.[54-57] However, for some diseases agreement between questionnaire data and medical record data are rather poor.[54,55] Nevertheless, these data are expected to be valid for assessing the symptom rather than the diagnosis because patients are considered to be the best experts in reporting perceived disease symptoms.[56] A third limitation is that 18.9% of this sample was lost at outcome. Participants lost to attrition at the mean age of 33 years had higher schizotypal symptom scores at the mean age of 16 years and were more likely to be male than those retained in the sample; however, there were no other significant differences in demographic variables and disorders.

**Accepted for Publication:** July 20, 2005.
**Correspondence:** Henian Chen, MD, PhD, Columbia University/NYSPI, 100 Haven Ave, 31F, New York, NY 10032 (chenhen@pi.cpmc.columbia.edu).
**Funding/Support:** This study was supported by grants MH-38914, MH-49191, and MH-60911 from the National Institute of Mental Health (Bethesda, Md).

## REFERENCES

1. Quality of life and clinical trials [editorial]. *Lancet.* 1995;346:1-2.
2. Spitzer RL, Kroenke K, Linzer M, et al. Health-related quality of life in primary care patients with mental disorders: results from the PRIME-MD 1000 study. *JAMA.* 1995;274:1511-1517.
3. Wilson IB, Cleary PD. Linking clinical variables with health-related quality of life. *JAMA.* 1995;273:59-65.
4. Guyatt GH, Feeny DH, Patrick DL. Measuring health-related quality of life. *Ann Intern Med.* 1993;118:622-629.
5. Bergner M. Quality of life, health status, and clinical research. *Med Care.* 1989; 27:S148-S156.
6. Stewart AL, Greenfield S, Hays RD, et al. The functional status and well-being of patients with chronic conditions: results from the Medical Outcomes Study. *JAMA.* 1989;262:907-913.
7. Cella DF, Bonomi AE. Measuring quality of life today: 1995 update. *Oncology (Williston Park).* 1995;9(suppl 11):47-60.
8. Bonomi AE, Patrick DL, Bushnell DM, Martin M. Validation of the United States' version of the World Health Organization Quality of Life (WHOQOL) instrument. *J Clin Epidemiol.* 2000;53:1-12.
9. Chen H, Cohen P, Kasen S, Dufur R, Smailes E, Gordon K. Construction and validation of a quality of life instrument for young adults. *Qual Life Res.* 2004; 13:747-759.
10. Kaplan RM, Bush JW, Berry CC. Health status: types of validity and the index of well-being. *Health Serv Res.* 1976;11:478-507.
11. Hunt SM, McEwen J, McKenna SP. Measuring health status: a new tool for clinicians and epidemiologists. *J R Coll Gen Pract.* 1985;35:185-188.
12. Bergner M, Bobbitt RA, Cartner WB, Gibson BS. The Sickness Impact Profile: development and final revision of a health status measure. *Med Care.* 1981; 19:787-805.
13. Ware JE, Sherbourne CD. The MOS 36-Item Short-Form Health Survey (SF-36), I: conceptual framework and item selection. *Med Care.* 1992;30:473-483.
14. The WHOQOL Group. The World Health Organization Quality of Life Assessment (WHOQOL): position paper from the World Health Organization. *Soc Sci Med.* 1995;41:1403-1409.
15. Sprangers MAG, Regt EB, Andries F, et al. Which chronic conditions are associated with better or poorer quality of life? *J Clin Epidemiol.* 2000;53:895-907.
16. Alonso J, Ferrer M, Gandek B, et al. Health-related quality of life associated with chronic conditions in eight countries: results from the International Quality of Life Assessment (IQOLA) Project. *Qual Life Res.* 2004;13:283-298.
17. Kempen G, Ormel J, Brilman EI, Relyveld J. Adaptive responses among Dutch elderly: the impact of eight chronic medical conditions on health-related quality of life. *Am J Public Health.* 1997;87:38-44.
18. Schlenk EA, Erlen JA, Dunbar-Jacob J, et al. Health-related quality of life in chronic

disorders: a comparison across studies using the MOS SF-36. *Qual Life Res.* 1998;7:57-65.
19. Singer MA, Hopman WM, MacKenzie TA. Physical functioning and mental health in patients with chronic medical conditions. *Qual Life Res.* 1999;8:687-691.
20. Wells KB, Stewart A, Hays RD, et al. The functioning and well-being of depressed patients: results from the Medical Outcomes Study. *JAMA.* 1989;262:914-919.
21. Hays RD, Wells KB, Sherbourne CD, et al. Functioning and well-being outcomes of patients with depression compared with chronic general medical illnesses. *Arch Gen Psychiatry.* 1995;52:11-19.
22. Koran LM, Thienemann ML, Davenport R. Quality of life for patients with obsessive-compulsive disorder. *Am J Psychiatry.* 1996;153:783-788.
23. Atkinson M, Zibin S, Chuang H. Characterizing quality of life among patients with chronic mental illness: a critical examination of the self-report methodology. *Am J Psychiatry.* 1997;154:99-105.
24. Ruo B, Rumsfeld JS, Hlatky MA, et al. Depressive symptoms and health-related quality of life. *JAMA.* 2003;290:215-221.
25. Huprich SK, Frisch MB. The depressive personality disorder inventory and its relationship to quality of life, hopefulness, and optimism. *J Pers Assess.* 2004;83:22-28.
26. Grant BF, Hasin DS, Stinson FS, et al. Prevalence, correlates, and disability of personality disorders in the United States: results from the national epidemiologic survey on alcohol and related conditions. *J Clin Psychiatry.* 2004;65:948-958.
27. Given CW, Given B, Azzouz F, et al. Comparison of changes in physical functioning of elderly patients with new diagnoses of cancer. *Med Care.* 2000;38:482-493.
28. Fanuele JC, Birkmeyer NJ, Abdu WA, et al. The impact of spinal problems on the health status of patients: have we underestimated the effect? *Spine.* 2000;25:1509-1514.
29. Ritsner M, Modai I, Endicott J, et al. Differences in quality of life domains and psychopathologic and psychosocial factors in psychiatric patients. *J Clin Psychiatry.* 2000;61:880-889.
30. Creed F, Morgan R, Fiddler M, et al. Depression and anxiety impair health-related quality of life and are associated with increased costs in general medical inpatients. *Psychosomatics.* 2002;43:302-309.
31. Kogan LS, Smith J, Jenkins S. Ecological validity of indicator data as predictors of survey findings. *J Soc Serv Res.* 1977;1:117-132.
32. Cohen P, Cohen J. *Adolescent Life Value and Mental Health.* Mahwah, NJ: Lawrence Erlbaum; 1996.
33. Boys A, Marsden J, Stillwell G, et al. Minimizing respondent attrition in longitudinal research: practical implications from a cohort study of adolescent drinking. *J Adolesc.* 2003;26:363-373.
34. Costello EJ, Edelbrock CS, Dulcan MK, Kalas R, Klaric SH. *Testing of the NIMH Diagnostic Interview Schedule for Children (DISC) in a Clinical Population: Final Report to the Center for Epidemiological Studies, National Institute for Mental Health.* Pittsburgh, Pa: University of Pittsburgh; 1984.
35. Cohen P, O'Connor P, Lewis SA, Malachowski B. A comparison of the agreement between DISC and K-SADS-P interviews of an epidemiological sample of children. *J Am Acad Child Psychiatry.* 1987;26:662-667.
36. Cohen P, Velez CN, Kohn M, Schwab-Stone M, Johnson J. Child psychiatric diagnosis by computer algorithm: theoretical issues and empirical tests. *J Am Acad Child Psychiatry.* 1987;26:631-638.
37. Hyler SE, Rieder R, Spitzer R, Williams J. *The Personality Diagnostic Questionnaire (PDQ).* New York: New York State Psychiatric Institute; 1982.
38. Hyler SE, Reider RO, Williams JBW, Spitzer RL, Hendler J, Lyons M. The Personality Diagnostic Questionnaire: development and preliminary results. *J Personal Disord.* 1988;2:229-237.
39. Bernstein DP, Cohen P, Velez CN, Schwab-Stone M, Siever LJ, Shinsato L. Prevalence and stability of the DSM-III-R personality disorders in a community-based survey of adolescents. *Am J Psychiatry.* 1993;150:1237-1243.
40. Bernstein D, Cohen P, Skodol A, Bezirganian S, Brook J. Childhood antecedents of adolescent personality disorders. *Am J Psychiatry.* 1996;153:907-913.
41. Cohen P. Childhood risks for young adult symptoms of personality disorder: method and substance. *Multivariate Behav Res.* 1996;31:121-148.
42. Cohen P. Personality development in childhood: old and new findings. In: Cloninger CR, ed. *Personality and Psychopathology.* Washington, DC: American Psychiatric Press; 1999:101-127.
43. Johnson JG, Cohen P, Skodol A, Oldham JM, Kasen S, Brook J. Personality disorders in adolescence and risk of major mental disorders and suicidality during adulthood. *Arch Gen Psychiatry.* 1999;56:805-811.
44. Kasen S, Cohen P, Skodol AE, Johnson JG, Smailes E, Brook JS. Childhood depression and adult personality disorder: alternative pathways of continuity. *Arch Gen Psychiatry.* 2001;58:231-236.
45. Crawford TN, Cohen P, Johnson JG, et al. Self-reported personality disorder in the Children in the Community sample: convergent and prospective validity in late adolescence and adulthood. *J Personal Disord.* 2005;19:30-52.
46. Diener E, Suh EM, Lucas RE, Smith HL. Subjective well-being: three decades of progress. *Psychol Bull.* 1999;125:276-302.
47. Hughes M, Thomas ME. The continuing significance of race revised: a study of race, class, and quality of life in America, 1972-1996. *Am Sociol Rev.* 1998;63:785-795.
48. Cohen J, Cohen P. *Applied Multiple Regression/Correlation Analysis for the Behavioral Sciences.* 3rd ed. Hillsdale, NJ: Lawrence Erlbaum; 2003.
49. Bonicatto SC, Dew MA, Zaratiegui R, Lorenzo L, Pecina P. Adult outpatients with depression: worse quality of life than in other chronic medical diseases in Argentina. *Soc Sci Med.* 2001;52:911-919.
50. Callahan CM, Kroenke K, Counsell SR, et al. Treatment of depression improves physical functioning in older adults. *J Am Geriatr Soc.* 2005;53:367-373.
51. Hemingway H, Stafford M, Stansfeld S, et al. Is the SF36 a valid measure of change in population health? results from the Whitehall II study. *BMJ.* 1997;315:1273-1279.
52. Sullivan MD, LaCroix AZ, Spertus JA, Hecht J. Five-year prospective study of the effects of anxiety and depression in patients with coronary artery disease. *Am J Cardiol.* 2000;86:1135-1138, A1136, A1139.
53. Rumsfeld JS. History of depression, angina, and quality of life following acute coronary syndromes. *Am Heart J.* 2003;145:493-499.
54. Haapanen N, Miilunpalo S, Pasanen M, Oja P, Vuori I. Agreement between questionnaire data and medical records of chronic diseases in middle-aged and elderly Finnish men and women. *Am J Epidemiol.* 1997;145:762-769.
55. Kriegsman DM, Penninx BW, van Eijk JT, Boeke AJ, Deeg DJ. Self-reports and general practitioner information on the presence of chronic diseases in community dwelling elderly: a study on the accuracy of patients' self-reports and on determinants of inaccuracy. *J Clin Epidemiol.* 1996;49:1407-1417.
56. Katz JN, Chang LC, Sangha O, Fossel AH, Bates DW. Can comorbidity be measured by questionnaire rather than medical record review? *Med Care.* 1996;34:73-84.
57. van Manen JG, Bindels PJE, Dekker FW, et al. The influence of COPD on health-related quality of life independent of the influence of comorbidity. *J Clin Epidemiol.* 2003;56:1177-1184.

**An Older but Prominent View of Child Development: Ontogeny Recapitulates Phylogeny.** This phrase expresses the 19th century idea that the development of an individual child recapitulates the history and evolutionary development of the entire race, or species. Spock's 1968 version of *Baby and Child Care* discusses this philosophical view. The idea is prominent in Freud and in the early writings of Jean Piaget. Piaget, however, sought in his later writings to explain recapitulation by appealing to general principles of structural change in cognitive development.

—From the *Stanford Encyclopedia of Philosophy*, by Edward N. Zalta, 2005

# Importance of Reducing Youth Exposure to Alcohol Advertising

Alcohol use is the leading drug problem among America's youth.[1] Every day, 7000 young people younger than 16 years take their first drink.[2] According to the National Institute on Alcohol Abuse and Alcoholism (Bethesda, Md), incidence of onset of alcohol dependence peaks in the US population at age 18 years and trails off by age 25 years.[3] The Centers for Disease Control and Prevention (Atlanta, Ga) estimate that more than 4000 persons younger than 21 years die annually as a result of excessive drinking.[4] And the drinking that young people do is excessive: more than 90% of the alcohol consumed by young people aged 12 to 20 years is drunk when the drinker is having 5 or more drinks on a single occasion, usually defined as within 2 hours.[5]

When it looked at underage drinking in the context of a 1999 report on self-regulation in the alcohol industry, the Federal Trade Commission concluded that, "While many factors may influence an underage person's drinking decisions, including among other things parents, peers and the media, there is reason to believe that advertising also plays a role."[6] As Snyder et al[7] have demonstrated in this issue of the ARCHIVES, these reasons are growing.

*See also page 18*

What is not in dispute is that young people in the United States see a lot of alcohol advertising. According to studies by the Center on Alcohol Marketing and Youth at Georgetown University (Washington, DC), in magazines in 2003, young people aged 12 to 20 years were exposed per capita to 48% more beer advertising, 20% more distilled spirits advertising, and 92% more advertising for "alcopops" (sweet, fizzy drinks such as Skyy Blue or Seagram's Smooth) than adults of the legal drinking age.[8] Regression analysis of the relationship between adolescent audiences and alcohol ad placements in 35 major US magazines that included alcohol ads found, after controlling for a variety of other factors, that beer and distilled spirits advertisements appeared more frequently in magazines with audiences with higher adolescent readerships. From 1997 through 2001, there were 1.6 times more beer advertisements for each additional 1 million readers aged 12 to 19 years, but no association between beer advertisements and each additional 1 million readers aged 20 to 24 years.[9] In the first 7 months of 2004—after the Beer Institute (Washington, DC) and the Distilled Spirits Council of the United States (Washington, DC) changed their self-regulatory codes in September 2003 to reduce the maximum youth audience threshold for alcohol advertising from 50% to 30%—73 alcohol brands exposed more youth aged 12 to 20 years per capita to their magazine advertising than adults aged 21 years and older.[10]

On television from 2001 to 2003, 12- to 20-year-olds were more likely per capita than adults of the legal drinking age to have seen close to a quarter of the more than 750 000 alcohol product advertisements placed on broadcast and cable networks and local broadcast stations.[11] Across those years, young people aged 12 to 20 years saw an average of 779 alcohol ads on television while the heaviest-watching 30% of that age group saw more than 1700 alcohol ads on television.[12,13] In the first 10 months of 2004, at least 25 alcohol brands gained half their youth exposure from ads that young people aged 12 to 20 years were more likely to see per capita than adults.[10]

On the radio, which is, after television, the second most popular medium for teenagers,[14] an analysis of audiences for a sample of 51 883 commercials for the leading 25 alcohol brands in 104 markets in the summer of 2003 found that in 14 of the 15 largest markets, young people heard more alcohol product advertising per capita than adults aged 21 years and over. In 5 of the top 15 markets, they heard more alcohol advertising than adults aged 21 to 34 years, the group sometimes identified as the actual target for alcohol advertising.[15]

Alcohol producers, like the tobacco companies in earlier years, have argued that alcohol advertising has no influence on alcohol consumption among young people. Although a number of cross-sectional studies in the United States and longitudinal studies from other countries suggested otherwise,[16] the lack of longitudinal data on alcohol advertising and youth alcohol consumption in the United States has hampered the policy debate over whether or how young people should be protected from alcohol advertising.

In 1998, the National Institute on Alcohol Abuse and Alcoholism, recognizing this deficit, funded several research groups to conduct these longitudinal studies. One group, starting with a sample of 2250 seventh-graders in Los Angeles County public schools, and using a combination of exposure and recall variables, has found that an increase in viewing television programs containing alcohol commercials was associated 1 year later with a 44% excess risk of beer use, a 34% excess risk of wine or liquor use, and a 26% excess risk of engaging in 3-drink episodes.[17] Another group followed up 3111 students in middle schools in South Dakota over 3 years and found that exposure to in-store beer displays predicted onset of drinking for nondrinkers after 2 years and that exposure to advertising in magazines and beer concession stands at sports or music events predicted greater frequency of drinking among drinkers after 2 years.[18] This group found no significant predictive effect of exposure to television advertising for either drinkers or nondrinkers.

The work of Snyder et al[7] marks the first time that a national longitudinal sample of young people in the United

States has been studied and the first time that self-reported exposure has been complemented by an objective measure of how much alcohol advertising is available in the media environment in which young people live. Their findings—that for underage drinkers, exposure to an additional alcohol ad was correlated with a 1% increase in drinking and that an additional dollar per capita spent on alcohol advertising in a local market was correlated with a 3% increase in underage alcohol consumption—calls into question the industry's argument that its roughly $1.8 billion in measured media expenditures per year have no impact on underage drinking. The fact that young people, regardless of drinking behavior at baseline, were more likely to drink more over time in environments with more alcohol advertising, even when controlling for alcohol sales in those environments, suggests that it is exposure to alcohol advertising that contributes to the drinking, rather than the reverse.

Snyder et al do not delve into the question of how alcohol advertising influences young people, but another of the research groups funded by the National Institute on Alcohol Abuse and Alcoholism has. Findings from another longitudinal study, reported at the Research Society on Alcoholism (Austin, Tex) meetings in June 2004, indicate that underage youth are drawn to elements of music, characters, story, and humor in alcohol advertising (as opposed, for example, to descriptions of product characteristics). Liking the ads was in turn correlated with the beliefs that positive outcomes from drinking were likely, that peers were likely to drink, and that peers were likely to approve of drinking. These beliefs appear to interact to produce greater intentions to drink and likelihood of drinking at later points in time.[19]

All these findings point to alcohol advertising as an important arena for interventions seeking to reduce underage drinking and its tragic consequences. Public health action on underage drinking rests on 2 key pillars: reducing the access of youth to alcohol and reducing the appeal of alcohol to young people. Policy changes, such as stricter enforcement of minimum age drinking laws; increases in alcohol prices through higher taxes or elimination of happy hours and other forms of discounting; and attention to the physical availability of alcohol, such as high concentrations of alcohol outlets near schools, have been suggested to reduce youth access to alcohol. The latter goal, reducing appeal, could be achieved, as the National Research Council (Washington, DC) and Institute of Medicine (Washington, DC) have recommended, through a national media campaign on underage drinking comparable with the existing paid media campaigns on tobacco and illegal drug use, as well as by limiting youth exposure to alcohol advertising.[1]

The Center on Alcohol Marketing and Youth has found that through the simple act of reallocating television expenditures on alcohol advertising to programming with youth audiences of less than 15% (roughly the percentage of youth aged 12 to 20 years in the general population aged 12 years and above), alcohol companies could reduce their advertising expenditures by 8% with virtually no change in their ability to reach their often-stated target audience of 21- to 34-year-olds. This change would leave 79% of television programming available for alcohol advertising and would reduce youth exposure to alcohol advertising on television by 20%.[20]

Federal surveys indicate that youth drinking stopped declining a decade ago.[2] This led the National Research Council and Institute of Medicine to conclude that further progress in reducing this problem requires "significant new intervention."[1] The research support for interventions on the "demand" side of the equation is growing. The work of Snyder et al suggests that if alcohol companies were to reduce the number of alcohol ads young people see by adopting a 15% maximum threshold for youth audiences for alcohol advertising, they could make a substantial contribution to reducing underage drinking.

*David H. Jernigan, PhD*

**Correspondence:** Dr Jernigan, Center on Alcohol Marketing and Youth, Georgetown University, Box 571444, 3300 Whitehaven St NW, Suite 5000, Washington, DC 20057 (djernigan@aol.com).
**Funding/Support:** The Center on Alcohol Marketing and Youth is supported by grants from The Pew Charitable Trusts, Philadelphia, Pa, and the Robert Wood Johnson Foundation, Princeton, NJ.
**Acknowledgment:** Thanks to Anna Haas, MA, for her research and editorial assistance.

## REFERENCES

1. Bonnie RJ, O'Connell ME, eds. *Reducing Underage Drinking: A Collective Responsibility.* Washington, DC: National Academies Press; 2004.
2. Center on Alcohol Marketing and Youth. *Underage Drinking in the United States: A Status Report, 2004.* Washington, DC: Center on Alcohol Marketing and Youth; 2005.
3. Li TK, Hewitt BG, Grant B. Alcohol use disorders and mood disorders: a National Institute on Alcohol Abuse and Alcoholism perspective. *Biol Psychiatry.* 2004;56:718-720.
4. Centers for Disease Control and Prevention. Alcohol-attributable deaths and years of potential life lost—United States, 2001. *MMWR Morb Mortal Wkly Rep.* 2004;53:866-870.
5. Pacific Institute for Research and Evaluation. *Drinking in America: Myths, Realities, and Prevention Policy.* Calverton, Md: Pacific Institute for Research and Evaluation; 2002.
6. Federal Trade Commission. *Self-Regulation in the Alcohol Industry: A Review of Industry Efforts to Avoid Promoting Alcohol to Underage Consumers.* Washington, DC: Federal Trade Commission; 1999.
7. Snyder LB, Milici FF, Slater M, Sun H, Strizhakova Y. Effects of alcohol advertising exposure on drinking among youth. *Arch Pediatr Adolesc Med.* 2006;160:18-24.
8. Center on Alcohol Marketing and Youth. *Youth Overexposed: Alcohol Advertising in Magazines, 2001 to 2003.* Washington, DC: Center on Alcohol Marketing and Youth; 2005.
9. Garfield CF, Chung PJ, Rathouz PJ. Alcohol advertising in magazines and adolescent readership. *JAMA.* 2003;289:2424-2429.
10. Center on Alcohol Marketing and Youth. *Striking a Balance: Protecting Youth From Overexposure to Alcohol Ads and Allowing Alcohol Companies to Reach the Adult Market.* Washington, DC: Center on Alcohol Marketing and Youth; 2005.
11. Center on Alcohol Marketing and Youth. *Alcohol Advertising on Television 2001 to 2003: More of the Same.* Washington, DC: Center on Alcohol Marketing and Youth; 2004.
12. Nielsen Media Research. *2001 Nielsen Persons Cume Study.* New York, NY: Nielsen Media Research; 2001.
13. Stone House Systems, Inc. T·View version 5.10.21. Kenilworth, Ill: Stone House Systems, Inc; 2004.
14. Rideout V, Roberts DF, Foehr UG. *Executive Summary, Generation M: Media in the Lives of 8–18 Year-olds.* Menlo Park, Calif: Henry J. Kaiser Family Foundation; 2005.
15. Center on Alcohol Marketing and Youth. *Youth Exposure to Radio Advertising for Alcohol—United States, Summer 2003.* Washington, DC: Center on Alcohol Marketing and Youth; 2004.

16. Hastings G, Anderson S, Cooke E, Gordon R. Alcohol marketing and young people's drinking: a review of the research. *J Public Health Policy.* 2005;26:296-311.
17. Stacy AW, Zogg JB, Unger JB, Dent CW. Exposure to televised alcohol ads and subsequent adolescent alcohol use. *Am J Health Behav.* 2004;28:498-509.
18. Ellickson PL, Collins RL, Hambarsoomians K, McCaffrey DF. Does alcohol advertising promote adolescent drinking? results from a longitudinal assessment. *Addiction.* 2005;100:235-246.
19. Chen MJ, Grube JW. Alcohol advertising and adolescent alcohol use: a latent growth analysis of the message interpretation process. Presented at: Research Society on Alcoholism; June 26, 2004; Miami, Fla.
20. Jernigan D, Ostroff J, Ross C. Alcohol advertising and youth: a measured approach. *J Public Health Policy.* 2005;26:312-325.

# Do As I Say, Not As I Do

## *Does It Work for Tobacco Use Prevention?*

TEN YEARS AGO FOOD AND DRUG ADMINISTRATION commissioner David Kessler, MD, declared tobacco use a "pediatric disease."[1] Decades of research, policy, and practice in smoking prevention make it clear that there are no magic bullets to curb this epidemic. Four and one half million children under the age of 18 currently smoke. Each day over 4000 youth try smoking for the first time and more than one third of them will become regular, daily smokers before leaving high school. Unless these trends are reversed, nearly 6.5 million children younger than age 18 who are alive today will eventually die from smoking-related disease.[2] Bold policy solutions that involve tighter governmental regulation of tobacco products have not been forthcoming.

Research on factors associated with initiation of smoking underscores the importance of multilevel smoking prevention efforts to effectively target the environmental, interpersonal, and intrapersonal factors that influence the initiation of youth smoking. Efforts to stem the influence of tobacco company marketing, easy access to tobacco through underage sales, and price affordability include advertising restrictions, mass media campaigns, strict enforcement of underage sales statutes, and price increases through tobacco taxes.[3] Consensus recommendations for schools include complete bans on smoking by anyone on school grounds and integration of tobacco use prevention programs in school curricula to reduce role modeling of smoking, teach life skills that help youth resist pressures to smoke, and reinforce antismoking attitudes and beliefs.[4]

*See also page 56*

There is more to be done. Jackson and Dickinson's study[5] in this issue of the ARCHIVES addresses head-on a potent and consistent risk factor for smoking initiation among youth—having a parent who smokes. A recent prospective study shows a dose-response relationship between the number of parents who smoke when a child is in third grade and smoking initiation by 12th grade; having 1 parent who smokes increases the risk of smoking by 64% and having 2 parents who smoke increases the risk of smoking by 105%.[6] In a continuation of their impressive program of research, the findings reported in Jackson and Dickinson's current article show that even parents who smoke can help to prevent their children from smoking. Most parents who smoke feel strongly that their children not smoke and are eager to know what they can do to lessen their child's chances of smoking. That Jackson and Dickinson successfully recruited and retained 775 families into their study attests to parents' interest in this topic.

The Jackson and Dickinson study found that third graders whose parents received a home-based intervention (Smoke-free Kids[7]) to improve communication about tobacco use were significantly less likely to try smoking by the end of sixth grade than children of parents who received fact sheets about smoking. The relatively simple intervention included 5 activity guides mailed to parents over a 3-month period, a booster guide at 1 year, tip sheets on parenting skills, and newsletters and incentives for children.

A prior publication from this study reported that by the time children reached the fifth grade introduction of the Smoke-free Kids intervention had increased a variety of factors related to antismoking socialization, such as parental self-efficacy to prevent smoking, parental reinforcement of abstinence, and parental efforts to counter prosmoking media influences.[7] Unfortunately, the current article does not examine whether the changes in parental behavior reported earlier are directly related to the observed reduction in smoking experimentation. Thus, we are left with a missing link between the intervention and the hypothesized mediators (both parental antismoking socialization and children's attitudes) and the ultimate outcome of using the Smoke-free Kids intervention on children's initiation. This pull-through is important because knowing how the intervention worked can provide more specific recommendations to parents for early approaches to preventing smoking among their children.

This understanding is particularly important given some conflicting findings in the literature about the effect that parental communications to children about smoking have on children's initiation of smoking. For example, a forthcoming paper by Huver et al[8] reports that antismoking parenting practices had their effects on adolescent tobacco use by influencing adolescent beliefs about smoking. Most important, these researchers found that, among adolescents, not all antismoking parenting practices were protective. For example, rewards for not smoking and greater frequency of talking about smoking were both associated with an *increased* likelihood of smoking. Studies by Ennett and colleagues[9] and by Engels and Willemsen[10] also found that parent-child communications about smoking may be a risk factor for smoking. Knowing more about the specific mechanisms of action in the Smoke-free Kids intervention trial may help us make sense of these conflicting findings.

Also of interest is any effect of use of the Smoke-free Kids intervention on movement from initial experimentation to more regular use of tobacco. To identify how families can protect children from smoking escalation, we need to know more about the transactional nature of parent-child communications about smoking. Simply encouraging parents to communicate to their adolescents about smoking may not be protective. Rather than focusing only on the content and frequency of communications, we may need to examine more closely the qualitative differences in how antismoking messages are delivered to youth and in the developmental appropriateness of messages and communications styles as children age. Harakeh and colleagues[11] found that both the quality and the timing of communications about smoking matter.

Jackson and Dickinson's study[5] did not directly involve pediatric practice, so one might ask what the study's implications are for frontline delivery of pediatric care. Clearly, pediatric care plays an important role in reducing the use of tobacco among our youth. The American Academy of Pediatrics outlined the role of pediatricians in tobacco use prevention and cessation in a 2001 policy statement.[12] Pediatric providers can screen all of their patients for tobacco use; encourage and reinforce youth who do not use tobacco; provide advice, assistance, and follow-up for smoking cessation to youth who do use tobacco; and screen for adult smoking in the household. There is also evidence that pediatric providers can increase smoking cessation among adults by incorporating advice and assistance to adult smokers who accompany their children to pediatric visits.[13] The results from the Jackson and Dickinson study can help pediatric providers be encouraging with parents who smoke. Even without the final analysis from this study, other work suggests that pediatricians can encourage parents to have explicit rules against smoking in the home, to talk with them about the negative aspects of smoking, to carefully monitor their children for evidence of receptivity and/or experimentation with tobacco, and to have clear disciplinary consequences for tobacco use. And, while talking about what they can do with their children, it doesn't hurt to encourage the parents to use evidence-based treatments to help themselves quit.[14]

*Susan J. Curry, PhD*
*Robin J. Mermelstein, PhD*

**Correspondence:** Dr Curry, Health Research and Policy Center, University of Illinois at Chicago, 850 W Jackson Blvd, #400, Chicago, Il 60607 (suecurry@uic.edu).

## REFERENCES

1. Gilpin B, Ballin S. Antidote for America's leading pediatric disease. *Circulation.* 1996;94:233.
2. Campaign for Tobacco-Free Kids. Tobacco use among youth. Available at: http://www.tobaccofreekids.org/ research/factsheets. Accessed October 5, 2005.
3. US Department of Health and Human Services. *Preventing Tobacco Use Among Young People: A Report of the Surgeon General*. Atlanta, Ga: US Dept of Health and Human Services, Public Health Service, Centers for Disease Control and Prevention, National Center for Chronic Disease Prevention and Health Promotion, Office on Smoking and Health, 1994.
4. Centers for Disease Control and Prevention. Guidelines for school health programs to prevent tobacco use and addiction. *MMWR Morb Mortal Wkly Rep.* 1994;43(RR-2):1-18.
5. Jackson C, Dickinson D. Enabling parents who smoke to prevent their children from initiating smoking: results from a 3-year intervention evaluation. *Arch Pediatr Adolesc Med.* 2006;160:56-62.
6. Peterson AV Jr, Leroux BG, Bricker J, Kealey KA, Marek PM, Sarason IG. Nine-year prediction of adolescent smoking by number of smoking parents [published online ahead of print June 28, 2005]. *Addict Behaviors.* http://www.sciencedirect.com. Accessed October 5, 2005.
7. Jackson C, Dickinson D. Can parents who smoke socialise their children against smoking? results from the Smoke-free Kids intervention trial. *Tob Control.* 2003; 12:52-59.
8. Huver RME, Engels RCME, deVries H. Are anti-smoking parenting practices related to adolescent smoking cognitions and behavior? *Health Educ Res.* In press.
9. Ennett ST, Bauman KE, Foshee VA, Pemberton M, Hicks KA. Parent-child communication about adolescent alcohol and tobacco use: what do parents say and does it affect youth behavior? *J Marriage Fam.* 2001;63:48-62.
10. Engels RCME, Willemsen M. Communication about smoking in Dutch families: associations between antismoking socialization and adolescent smoking-related cognitions. *Health Educ Res.* 2004;19:227-238.
11. Harakeh Z, Scholte RH, de Vries H, Engels RC. Parental rules and communication: their association with adolescent smoking. *Addiction.* 2005;100:862-870.
12. American Academy of Pediatrics, Committee on Substance Abuse. Tobacco's toll: implications for the pediatrician. *Pediatrics.* 2001;107:794-798.
13. Curry SJ, Ludman EJ, Graham E, Stout J, Grothaus L, Lozano P. Pediatric-based smoking cessation intervention for low-income women: a randomized trial. *Arch Pediatr Adolesc Med.* 2003;157:295-302.
14. Fiore MC, Bailey WC, Cohen SJ, et al. *Treating Tobacco Use and Dependence: Clinical Practice Guideline*. Rockville, Md: US Dept of Health and Human Services, Public Health Service. June 2000.

# Discussing Outcome in Tourette Syndrome

PHYSICIANS TREATING PATIENTS WITH TOURETTE syndrome (TS) should be prepared to answer several frequently asked questions posed by parents of children, or individuals, with this syndrome. Prominent in the list of inquiries are those dealing with the outcome: "Do tics get worse over time?" and "Do they ever resolve, and if so, when?" with the most focused question being "What is going to happen to my child?" Data provided in the article by Bloch et al[1] in this issue of ARCHIVES offer further insight into addressing these perplexing issues.

## GENERAL COMMENTS

Before addressing the questions regarding outcome, several general comments about TS are required as background. First, there are a myriad of different motor and

*See also page 65*

vocal tics, but their negative impact (psychosocial or physical) is typically determined by the intensity and type of movement or vocalization. For example, forceful complex motor tics or loud outbursts of profanity attract greater attention than more frequent facial grimaces or quiet throat noises. Second, tics typically wax and wane owing to unknown underlying mechanism(s), though some exacerbations may involve environmental factors such as stress, anxiety, fatigue, or infection.[2-4] Lastly, the presence of comorbid features, such as obsessive-compulsive disorder, attention-deficit/hyperactivity disorder, episodic outbursts, anxiety, and depression, is a prominent factor in the global well-being or social, educational, and functional capabilities of the individual.[5,6]

## PEAK AGE FOR TIC SEVERITY

The peak age for tic severity has been addressed in several studies. Investigators using a mathematical model to assess the course of tic severity over the first 2 decades of life have suggested that the maximum tic severity occurs between the ages of 8 and 12 years and is then followed by a steady decline in symptoms.[7] Results from the Bloch et al[1] longitudinal study are confirmatory, suggesting that the average worst-ever tic severity score occurs at a mean ± SD age of 10.6 ± 2.6 years, though the range was quite broad, from 6 to 19 years. Despite these reports, some individuals have severe, persisting tics. Although the question of exact "worst ever" tic severity was not specifically addressed, a follow-up study of 58 adults (mean age, 27.1 years [range, 21-62 years]) with TS showed that moderate to severe tics persisted in 24%.[8] A minority of tic cases may also have "catastrophic outcomes" in adulthood.[7] Lastly, patients with adult-onset tic disorder are characterized by more severe tic symptoms and a poorer response to medications as compared with patients with childhood-onset disorders.[9] In summary, in most cases of TS, motor and vocal tic severity peaks early in the second decade. One should, however, be cautious in providing parents with a specific date or else be prepared to address an irate caller when that date arrives.

## TIC OUTCOME

Tourette syndrome was originally proposed to be a lifelong disorder. Yet, as most physicians are aware, its course is actually quite variable, with some patients having a spontaneous remission or marked improvement independent of the use of tic-suppressing medication. Diminution of tics by the late teens is a relatively consistent finding.[7,10-13] In the Bloch et al[1] report, 85% of subjects reported a reduction in tic symptoms during the first 2 decades. When discussing outcome, I typically use the "rule of thirds" (one third of patients have symptoms disappear, one third of patients have symptoms get better, and one third of patients have symptoms continue).[14] This formula is, in part, derived from a study of 58 teens and young adults performed at the Cleveland Clinic (Cleveland, Ohio) in which tics virtually disappeared in 26%, diminished considerably in 46%, remained stable in 14%, and increased in 14%.[12] Furthermore, even in individuals whose tics persist, there is evidence for reduction in their impact. For example, in a 2-year follow-up of children with persistent Tourette disorder, tic impairment statistically improved, even though tic scores remained unchanged.[15] In summary, most patients show a reduction in tic severity by the late teens or early adult years.

Whether tics actually disappear completely is unclear, and results appear to be dependent on the methods used to document the presence of tics. Investigators, who have relied strictly on historical data rather than on direct observation of symptoms, have often been misled. For example, multiple recurrent tics were missed by parents in 21% of children being followed up in a longitudinal study.[16] Further, a comparison of tic assessment in adults, based on personal assessments vs videotape analysis, showed that 90% still had tics despite frequent claims of their absence.[10]

## PREDICTING OUTCOME

Whether one can predict a single individual's specific outcome is controversial. The Bloch et al[1] article suggests that an increased tic severity at the initial period of evaluation was statistically associated with an increased tic severity on repeat evaluation years later. This finding is consistent with another study in adults with TS that showed the sole predictor of adult moderate or severe tics was moderate or severe dysfunction in late adolescence.[8] One concern about each of the aforementioned observations is that they were limited to the study of young adults at mean ages of 19.0 and 27.1 years, respectively. It is therefore possible that a more extensive follow-up period could identify a different outcome pattern. Other reports have stated that early tic severity is not a good predictor of later tic severity. Tic severity at the time of initial clinical evaluation did not correlate with worst or follow-up tic severity.[7] Additionally, in the study by Goetz and colleagues,[8] the likelihood of children with moderate or severe tics improving (ie, having a mild adult condition) was approximately 75%. A prior suggestion that attention-deficit/hyperactivity disorder is more common in children with severe tic symptoms[17] was not confirmed by Bloch and colleagues.[1]

A final point is that tic outcome, even if predictable, is not synonymous with the presence or absence of obsessive-compulsive symptoms; global well-being; or social, educational, or functional capabilities. As described by Bloch et al,[1] obsessive-compulsive behaviors have a different peak age than tics and may occur after tics have subsided. Children with mild to moderate tics can also be withdrawn, aggressive, and less popular.[18] Tic severity is not a linear predictor of behavioral disturbance.[19,20] There are patients with TS without significant behavioral problems in spite of severe tics ("resilient patients") as well as those who adjust poorly despite a mild tic disorder ("vulnerable patients").[21] In summary, I believe that, to date, there are no precise clinical prognostic indicators to assist in determining tic severity outcome. It is certainly possible that additional determinants of tic outcome may be identified from genetic testing or magnetic resonance imaging volumetric measurements. In contrast, global outcome is more predictable through the use of a combination of tic ratings, neuropsychological testing, and measures of the extent of psychiatric comorbidities.

*Harvey S. Singer, MD*

**Correspondence:** Dr Singer, Division of Pediatric Neurology, Johns Hopkins Hospital, Jefferson Street Bldg 124, 600 N Wolfe St, Baltimore, MD 21287-1000 (hsinger@jhmi.edu).

## REFERENCES

1. Bloch MH, Peterson BS, Scahill L, et al. Adulthood outcome of tic and obsessive-compulsive symptom severity in children with Tourette syndrome. *Arch Pediatr Adolesc Med.* 2006;160:65-69.
2. Wood BLKK, Gbadebo O, Lichter D, Kurlan R, Miller B. Pilot study of effect of emotional stimuli on tic severity in children with Tourette's syndrome. *Mov Disord.* 2003;18:1392-1395.
3. O'Connor K, Brisebois H, Brault M, Robillard S, Loiselle J. Behavioral activity associated with onset in chronic tic and habit disorder. *Behav Res Ther.* 2003;41:241-249.
4. Hoekstra PJ, Manson WL, Steenhuis MP, Kallenberg CG, Minderaa RB. Association of common cold with exacerbations in pediatric but not adult patients with tic disorder: a prospective longitudinal study. *J Child Adolesc Psychopharmacol.* 2005;15:285-292.
5. Snider L, Seligman L, Ketchen B, et al. Tics and problem behaviors in schoolchildren: prevalence, characterization, and associations. *Pediatrics.* 2002;110:331-336.
6. Sukhodolsky DG, Scahill L, Zhang H, et al. Disruptive behavior in children with Tourette's syndrome: association with ADHD comorbidity, tic severity, and functional impairment. *J Am Acad Child Adolesc Psychiatry.* 2003;42:98-105.
7. Leckman JF, Zhang H, Vitale A, et al. Course of tic severity in Tourette syndrome: the first two decades. *Pediatrics.* 1998;102:14-19.
8. Goetz CG, Tanner CM, Stebbins GT, Leipzig G, Carr WC. Adult tics in Gilles de la Tourette's syndrome: description and risk factors. *Neurology.* 1992;42:784-788.
9. Eapen V, Lees A, Lakke J, Trimble M, Robertson M. Adult-onset tic disorders. *Mov Disord.* 2002;17:735-740.
10. Pappert EJ, Goetz CG, Louis ED, Blasucci L, Leurgans S. Objective assessments of longitudinal outcome in Gilles de la Tourette's syndrome. *Neurology.* 2003;61:936-940.
11. Bruun RD. The natural history of Tourette syndrome. In: Cohen DJ, Bruun RD, Leckman JF, eds. *Tourette Syndrome and Tic Disorders: Clinical Understanding and Treatment.* New York, NY: Wiley; 1998:21-33.
12. Erenberg G, Cruse RP, Rothner AD. The natural history of Tourette syndrome: a follow-up study. *Ann Neurol.* 1987;22:383-385.
13. Nee LE, Caine ED, Polinsky RJ, Eldridge R, Ebert MH. Gilles de la Tourette syndrome: clinical and family study of 50 cases. *Ann Neurol.* 1980;7:41-49.
14. Singer HS, Walkup JT. Tourette syndrome and other tic disorders: diagnosis, pathophysiology, and treatment. *Medicine (Baltimore).* 1991;70:15-32.
15. Coffey BJ, Biederman J, Geller D, et al. Reexamining tic persistence and tic-associated impairment in Tourette's disorder: findings from a naturalistic follow-up study. *J Nerv Ment Dis.* 2004;192:776-780.
16. McMahon WM, Carter AS, Fredine N, Pauls DL. Children at familial risk for Tourette's disorder: child and parent diagnoses. *Am J Med Genet B Neuropsychiatr Genet.* 2003;121:105-111.
17. Robertson MM, Trimble MR, Lees AJ. The psychopathology of the Gilles de la Tourette syndrome: a phenomenological analysis. *Br J Psychiatry.* 1988;152:383-390.
18. Stokes A, Bawden HN, Camfield PR, Backman JE, Dooley JM. Peer problems in Tourette's disorder. *Pediatrics.* 1991;87:936-942.
19. Hoekstra PJ, Steenhuis MP, Troost PW, Korf J, Kallenberg CG, Minderaa RB. Relative contribution of attention-deficit hyperactivity disorder, obsessive-compulsive disorder, and tic severity to social and behavioral problems in tic disorders. *J Dev Behav Pediatr.* 2004;25:272-279.
20. Singer HS, Rosenberg LA. Development of behavioral and emotional problems in Tourette syndrome. *Pediatr Neurol.* 1989;5:41-44.
21. Rosenberg LA, Brown J, Singer HS. Behavioral problems and severity of tics. *J Clin Psychol.* 1995;51:760-767.

### *Announcement*

**Submissions.** The Editors welcome contributions to Picture of the Month. Submissions should describe common problems presenting uncommonly, rather than total zebras. Cases should be of interest to practicing pediatricians, highlighting problems that they are likely to at least occasionally encounter in the office or hospital setting. High-quality clinical images (in either 35-mm slide or electronic format) along with parent or patient permission to use these images must accompany the submission. The entire discussion should comprise no more than 750 words. Articles and photographs accepted for publication will bear the contributor's name. There is no charge for reproduction and printing of color illustrations. For details regarding electronic submission, please see: http://archpedi.ama-assn.org.

## Can We Improve the Return Rate for Tuberculin Skin Test Readings?

Tuberculosis continues to cause disease in the United States despite effective treatment and a simple screening test. The Pediatric Practice of Rainbow Babies and Children's Hospital, a tertiary care children's hospital in Cleveland, Ohio, serves an inner-city population. It is located in Cuyahoga County, which had the highest number of reported tuberculosis cases in Ohio in 2003.[1] The Pediatric Practice follows American Academy of Pediatrics recommendations for targeted tuberculin skin testing by screening all children by questionnaire to identify high-risk patients.[2] Children with positive screening questionnaires have a tuberculin skin test placed, receive a reminder card, and are asked to return in 48 to 72 hours without an appointment required. The return rate is approximately 50%, lower than desired but similar to that of other studies with comparable populations.[3-5] Ozuah and colleagues[5] have shown previously that an additional telephone call increases the return rate at 72 hours.

Our objective was to determine if offering a $10 gift certificate from a local supermarket would improve the return rate for tuberculin skin test readings. This prospective intervention trial with gift certificate motivator was combined with a retrospective medical record review as the source of historical controls. The study population included all 512 children (aged 6 weeks to 18 years; 96% were African American) of 388 families who had tuberculin skin tests placed at the Pediatric Practice from November 1, 2002, through April 30, 2004. There were 113 families with 152 children in the 6-month prospective intervention arm (November 2003-April 2004) and 275 families with 360 children in the 12-month retrospective control arm (November 2002-October 2003).

There were no significant differences in age, race, sex, number of children per family, or day test was placed between the intervention and historical control groups. In the intervention group, the usual skin testing procedures were followed except that families also received verbal and written instructions that they would receive a $10 gift certificate when they returned to have the skin test read in 48 to 72 hours. Nurses were previously trained to examine for any induration and kept an ongoing patient register of skin test placements and results. Two patients had positive skin test results (induration >5 mm) during the study period, both of whom were previously known and treated.

The overall tuberculin skin test return rate for families did not change with the intervention (prospective 60 [53.1%] of 113 vs historical controls 129 [46.9%] of 275; $P=.23$). However, the intervention was associated with a significant improvement in return rate for those whose test was placed on a Thursday or Friday (19/33 [57.6%] vs 28/85 [32.9%]; $P=.02$) and for families with multiple children tested the same day (20/30 [66.7%] vs 29/75 [38.7%]; $P=.02$).

It is logistically difficult to offer the gift certificate motivator to some but not all families, and thus, our results do not support this intervention or justify this expense for general use in an urban clinic setting. Additional investigation into other interventions to improve the return rate for tuberculin skin testing is urgently needed.

*Kari M. Jacono, MD*
*Mary Ann O'Riordan, MS*
*Lydia Furman, MD*

**Correspondence:** Dr Furman, Department of Pediatrics, Division of General Academic Pediatrics, Rainbow Babies and Children's Hospital, Mather 3, MS 6019, 11100 Euclid Ave, Cleveland, OH 44106 (lmfurman@adelphia.net).

1. Ohio Department of Health tuberculosis disease data. Available at: http://www.odh.ohio.gov. Accessed January 20, 2005.
2. Pediatric Tuberculosis Collaborative Group. Targeted tuberculin skin testing and treatment of latent tuberculosis infection in children and adolescents. *Pediatrics*. 2004;114(4 pt 3):1175-1201.
3. Medchill MT. Prenatal purified protein derivative skin testing in a teaching clinic with a large Hispanic population. *Am J Obstet Gynecol*. 1999;180:1579-1583.
4. Cheng TL, Ottolini MC, Baumhaft K, Brasseux C, Wolf MD, Scheidt PC. Strategies to increase adherence with tuberculosis test reading in a high-risk population. *Pediatrics*. 1997;100:210-213.
5. Ozuah PO, Burton W, Lerro KA, Rosenstock J, Mulvihill M. Assessing the validity of tuberculin skin test readings by trained professionals and patients. *Chest*. 1999;116:104-106.

## Adult Learning

I enjoyed reading the article entitled "Closing the Quality Chasm in Health Care: The Role of Critical Reading" in the April 2005 issue of the ARCHIVES.[1] I agree with much of what was stated in that article but thought it could have gone further.

My background has been in both private practice (21 years) and, more recently, in academic medicine (11 years). My interest in understanding adult learning theory was prompted by my becoming a teacher of medical students and residents when I went into academic medicine. However, as I looked back on my practice years, I realized that, for many years, my partners and I had struggled with how to become "lifelong learners." In our practice in Charlottesville, Va, we invited speakers over the noon hour to talk to us, we attended Continuing Medical Education meetings, we published articles, some of us taught at the University of Virginia (Charlottesville) 1 day a week, and we each read up to 12 journals a month, but we were not confident that our methods promoted optimal learning.

A few years after starting my academic career, I was invited to become a member of the PediaLink (the Internet "home" for pediatricians) editorial board of the American Academy of Pediatrics (Elk Grove Village, Ill). At one of our first meetings, we were presented with the work of

Schön,[2] who described the learning cycle as "dealing with a clinical case" in which one experiences "reflection in action," which then produces "reflection on action" that through individual research and learning can lead to "improved clinical care and outcomes." In other words, it is the individual's job to ask the question, find the answer, and then use the solution to produce improved patient care. I remember the moment I first heard about this learning theory; I realized it applied totally to me—most of the knowledge I had retained from my private practice career had indeed been based on my asking myself questions, looking up answers, and then changing what I did. I realized that that knowledge did not come just from reading those 12 journals that I carefully read each month. It came from my asking a question that was answered by an article in one of those journals (or others), discussing it with my partners, and then changing (improving?) our clinical approach.

I agree with the statement that "self-directed learning involving active participation of the learner does result in changes in clinical skills and patient management,"[1(p394)] and that we need to teach residents how to learn. However, learning how to read articles properly, though important, is only one part of the solution. I think that the most important part is that those of us in academic medicine, at the American Academy of Pediatrics, and in charge of Continuing Medical Education programs all need to recognize that learning can only occur if we teach learners how to teach themselves. I would also suggest that this approach to learning needs to be applied to all levels of learning: students, residents, faculty, and practitioners.

I have been reading recently that doctors in the older age group (my age group) have a poorer knowledge base than younger doctors.[3] A commentary in the May 2005 issue of *AAP Grand Rounds*[4] theorizes that recertification may help reduce this knowledge gap in older physicians and that reading pertinent literature will help reduce this loss of knowledge. I hope this is true, but I personally don't believe it will be enough. Habits are hard to change. We sometimes don't see the need to change what we are doing when something we have done over the years has always worked. Adopting new strategies can sometimes be dangerous (eg, rotavirus vaccine) and make us hesitant to change. However, even our age group needs to be taught the importance of questioning what we do and finding our own answers.

Where do we go from here? I hope that PediaLink and its learning center will help pediatricians develop individualized learning plans and document their questions, their answers, and the resultant changes in practice. But, for many physicians, this Internet program may not be enough to change behavior by itself. There needs to be focused leadership on this subject. We need to learn much more than how to read articles; we also need to feel comfortable saying "I don't know." We need to know how to access sources of information we trust; we need to constantly rethink how we approach diagnostic problems; we need to standardize the approach we take to teaching students and residents, faculty, and practitioners; and we need to teach others that this approach is essential to improve the care of the children we treat. Learning must be interactive, it must be initiated by the learner, and it has to be a never-ending process.

We pediatricians are the luckiest people alive; we have the possibility of continuing to learn throughout our careers, and we get to do this in the context of children, their families, and our communities. It is time to focus on the process of how individuals learn and how they retain what they learn.

*John T. Benjamin, MD*

**Correspondence:** Dr Benjamin, Department of Pediatrics, University of North Carolina School of Medicine, Chapel Hill, NC 27599 (jtb@med.unc.edu).

1. Rivara FP, Stapleton FB. Closing the quality chasm in health care: the role of critical reading. *Arch Pediatr Adolesc Med*. 2005;159:394-396.
2. Schön D. *Educating the Reflective Practitioner*. San Francisco, Calif: Jossey-Bass Publishers; 1987.
3. Choudhry NK, Fletcher RH, Soumerai SB. The relationship between clinical experience and quality of health care. *Ann Intern Med*. 2005;142:260-273.
4. Robbins B. Practice may not make perfect. *AAP Grand Rounds*. 2005;13:52-53 Available at: http://aapgrandrounds.aappublications.org/cgi/content/full/13/5/52.

## *In reply*

*We appreciate the very thoughtful response of Dr Benjamin to our editorial on the role of reading in improving the quality of health care delivered by physicians. We especially appreciate his perspective as both an experienced physician and as a teacher in academic medicine. The learning cycle he describes is at the core of adult learning. We also agree that this approach to learning should be applied to all levels; this approach is central to the American Board of Pediatrics' maintenance of certification program.*

*As Dr Benjamin points out, there is a critical need for leadership in this area by our professional organizations. As has been proven repeatedly, unless professional organizations in medicine assume responsibility and leadership for important issues related to the quality of care, the federal government and/or its regulatory agencies will fill this vacuum. The resultant rules and regulations may not be to our liking. As Dr Benjamin stated, the time is now and the responsibility is ours.*

*Frederick P. Rivara, MD, MPH*
*F. Bruder Stapleton, MD*

**Correspondence:** Dr Rivara, The Child and Health Institute, University of Washington, 6200 NE 74th St, 210, Seattle, WA 98115-8160 (fpr@washington.edu).

## Potential Confounders That May Explain the Association Between Television Viewing and Poor Educational Achievement

The issue of television watching among children and adolescents, and the possible negative developmental correlates of this common childhood activity, continue to be an ongoing concern for our society and its researchers. We therefore read with interest the recent report of Hancox et al,[1] which used a powerful longitudinal epidemiologic study design to demonstrate a significant relationship between quantity of television viewing in childhood and poor educational attainment in adulthood. In their analysis, they adjusted for some of the important confounding factors that may affect educational attainment (ie, childhood IQ, gender, socioeconomic status, and behavioral problems). A surprising finding in the study was the large quantity of time children were viewing television (children aged 5-11 years: mean, 2.06 hours [SD, 0.82 hours]; adolescents aged 13-15 years: mean, 3.13 hours [SD, 1.43 hours]).

Why are children and adolescents watching so much television on weekdays? We hypothesize, based on previous literature, that excessive television watching may constitute a proxy measure for compromised parental involvement and/or an indication of a troubled home environment. Without considering the possible impact of those childhood adversities that have been already been demonstrated to be associated with diminished educational attainment, it is unclear if excessive television viewing is just an activity that occurs within households that also struggle with issues of abuse, neglect, and psychopathology. Recent literature suggests that a respondent's psychopathology,[2] experience of childhood abuse and neglect,[3,4] and parental psychopathology[5] are also significantly associated with poor educational achievement.

It is of great importance to determine if television watching remains significantly associated with poor educational achievement after adjusting for such (and other) childhood adversities. The study by Hancox et al[1] has furthered the research in this area. However, the dataset they used (The Dunedin Multidisciplinary Health and Development Study) includes variables of childhood psychopathology, childhood abuse, parental attachment, and parental psychopathology, which have been published elsewhere. We believe that their adjusting for these potential confounding variables could further our understanding of the relational complexities between television viewing and poor educational attainment.

*Tracie O. Afifi, MSc*
*William Fleisher, MD, FRCPC*
*Jitender Sareen, MD, FRCPC*

**Correspondence:** Ms Afifi, Community Health Sciences, University of Manitoba, PZ430 PsycHealth Centre, 771 Bannatyne Ave, Winnipeg, Ma R3E 3N4, Canada (toafifi@exchange.hsc.mb.ca).

1. Hancox RJ, Milne BJ, Poulton R. Association of television viewing during childhood with poor educational achievement. *Arch Pediatr Adolesc Med.* 2005;159:614-618.
2. Van Ameringen M, Mancini C, Farvolden P. The impact of anxiety disorder on educational achievement. *J Anxiety Disord.* 2003;17:561-571.
3. Kendall-Tackett KA. The effects of neglect on academic achievement and disciplinary problems: a developmental perspective. *Child Abuse Negl.* 1996;20:161-169.
4. Scher CD, Forde DR, McQuaid JR, Stein MB. Prevalence and demographic correlates of childhood maltreatment in an adult community sample. *Child Abuse Negl.* 2004;28:167-180.
5. Ensminger ME, Hanson SG, Riley AW, Juon HS. Maternal psychological distress adult sons' and daughters' mental health and educational attainment. *J Am Acad Child Adolesc Psychiatry.* 2003;42:1108-1115.

### *In reply*

*We thank Ms Afifi and colleagues for their comments. Yes, the children in our study did spend a lot of time watching television, but no more than reported for children in other countries[1] and less than children in a recent survey of children in Dunedin, New Zealand (R. McGee, PhD, written communication, August 15, 2005). We don't think that we should attribute the time spent watching television by the average child to parental neglect or a troubled home environment. Nevertheless, Afifi et al raise an important issue about potential confounding by family and environmental factors in the relationship between television viewing and educational achievement.*

*The difficulty in adjusting for putative confounders in this sort of analysis is in knowing the sequence of events. Thus, although we have information on child behavior and psychopathology in this study, much of it was collected after the children had spent several years watching television. Television appears to influence children's behavior,[2] and it is plausible that some childhood problems are a result of watching too much television rather than a cause of excessive viewing. Watching television could also be in the causal pathway between parental neglect and poor educational outcomes. Put another way, why would attentive parents restrict their children's access to television? Presumably because they believe that too much television is "bad" for children—perhaps they are right. For these reasons, we only adjusted the analyses in our report to the obvious confounders of sex, intelligence, socioeconomic status, and behavioral problems at age 5 years (ie, before we started to record viewing habits).*

*Notwithstanding these theoretical concerns, we can test whether other childhood or family and childhood factors could explain the association between television and low educational achievement using other variables from our data set as suggested by Afifi and colleagues. The* **Table** *shows the*

**Table. Results of Logistic Regression Analyses***

| | Adjustment: Sex, IQ, Socioeconomic Status | | | Adjustment: Multiple Confounders | | |
|---|---|---|---|---|---|---|
| | Sample Size | Odds Ratio | *P* Value | Sample Size | Odds Ratio | *P* Value |
| No qualifications | 943 | 1.45 | .003 | 858 | 1.54 | .004 |
| University degree | 943 | 0.64 | <.001 | 858 | 0.73 | .02 |

*Logistic regression of educational outcomes on mean weekday television viewing between ages 5 and 15 years. Odds ratios refer to change in odds of outcome per hour of viewing per day. Analyses adjusted for sex, IQ, and socioeconomic status, and after additional adjustment for multiple confounders as explained in the text.

*results of logistic regression analyses with adjustment for sex, IQ, and socioeconomic status, and after additional adjustment for mean parent and teacher Rutter scores for antisocial behavior, hyperactivity, and worry and/or fearfulness at ages 5, 7, 9, and 11 years[3]; mother's psychological malaise at ages 5, 7, and 9 years[4]; physical or sexual abuse before age 11 years[5]; an index of family cohesiveness measured at ages 7, 9, 13, and 15 years[6]; caregiver changes before age 11 years; and years spent with a single parent before age 11 years.*

*Time spent watching television during childhood and adolescence remained a significant predictor of poor educational outcomes even after adjusting for multiple potential confounders. It is always possible that some unidentified source of confounding mediates the association but the association between television and poor educational achievement appears to be remarkably robust to adjustment for the most obvious candidates. We believe that the association between childhood television and educational outcomes is unlikely to be due to confounding by a troubled home environment or compromised parental involvement.*

*Robert J. Hancox, MD*
*Richie Poulton, PhD*

**Correspondence:** Dr Hancox, Dunedin Multidisciplinary Health and Development Research Unit, Department of Preventive and Social Medicine, Dunedin School of Medicine, University of Otago, PO Box 913, Dunedin, New Zealand (bob.hancox@otago.ac.nz).

1. American Academy of Pediatrics. Children, adolescents, and television. *Pediatrics.* 2001;107:423-426.
2. Johnson JG, Cohen P, Smailes EM, Kasen S, Brook JS. Television viewing and aggressive behavior during adolescence and adulthood. *Science.* 2002;295:2468-2471.
3. McGee R, Williams S, Silva PA. Factor structure and correlates of ratings of inattention, hyperactivity, and antisocial behavior in a large sample of 9-year-old children from the general population. *J Consult Clin Psychol.* 1985;53:480-490.
4. Rodgers B, Pickles A, Power C, Collishaw S, Maughan B. Validity of the Malaise Inventory in general population samples. *Soc Psychiatry Psychiatr Epidemiol.* 1999;34:333-341.
5. Caspi A, McClay J, Moffitt TE, et al. Role of genotype in the cycle of violence in maltreated children. *Science.* 2002;297:851-854.
6. Moos RH, Moos BS. *The Family Environment Scale Manual.* Palo Alto, Calif: Consulting Psychologists Press; 1981.

## Something Else Is Missing From Research on Children's Television Viewing and Academic Performance

Chernin and Linebarger[1] do an excellent job of providing the grain of salt that should be taken with the research on children's television viewing and academic performance presented in the July 2005 issue of the ARCHIVES. Given how research on this topic has advanced from studies of total television viewing time to content-specific studies, research that focuses on total television viewing time seems to represent a regression rather than a progression in research.

However, there is one other major shortcoming of these and other studies on this topic; they focus exclusively on academic performance and skills like reading comprehension and mathematics, completely ignoring the role that television programs can play in the emotional development of children. Some of my 3-year-old daughter's favorite shows and videos over the past year have been those that would not be considered "educational"—shows like the Berenstain Bears and Madeline, for example. Although these kinds of shows don't teach academic skills, they do teach very important life lessons and opportunities to develop emotional intelligence. For example, these kinds of shows often teach children lessons about such things as empathy, fairness, kindness, honesty, sharing, safety, and so on, as well as the full range of human emotion. Even popular noneducational videos, such as *Finding Nemo*, introduce young children to emotions like fear, sadness, and joy. When used appropriately and combined with active parenting, these kinds of shows and movies can provide parents with endless teachable moments. In terms of future research opportunities, I would like to see some research on the link between content-specific television viewing and the cultivation of emotional intelligence.

*Jonathan M. Breslin, PhD*

**Correspondence:** Dr Breslin, University of Toronto Joint Centre for Bioethics, Toronto, Ontario MG5 1L4, Canada (jonathan.breslin@utoronto.ca).

1. Chernin AR, Linebarger DL. The relationship between children's television viewing and academic performance. *Arch Pediatr Adolesc Med.* 2005;159:687-689.

### In reply

*Dr Breslin is right to point out that television and film can positively impact children's social and emotional development, as evidenced by the body of research on this topic.[1-4] Our editorial addressed the cognitive benefits of appropriately designed educational television because the articles we were asked to review focused on cognitive outcomes associated with television viewing. We thank Dr Breslin for highlighting the continued need for researchers to examine the effects of various types of media content on children's emotional development.*

*Ariel R. Chernin, MA*
*Deborah L. Linebarger, PhD*

**Correspondence:** Dr Chernin, University of Pennsylvania, 3620 Walnut St, Philadelphia, PA 19104 (achernin@asc.upenn.edu).

1. Mares ML, Woodard EH. Prosocial effects on children's social interactions. In: Singer DG, Singer JD, eds. *Handbook of Children and the Media.* Thousand Oaks, Calif: Sage Publications; 2001:183-205.
2. Collins WA, Getz SK. Children's social responses following modeled reactions to provocation: prosocial effects of television drama. *J Pers.* 1976;44:488-500.
3. Friedrich L, Stein AH. Aggressive and prosocial television programs and the natural behavior of preschool children. *Monogr Soc Res Child Dev.* 1973;38:1-64.
4. Poulos RW, Rubinstein EA, Liebert RM. Positive social learning. *J Commun.* 1975;25:90-97.

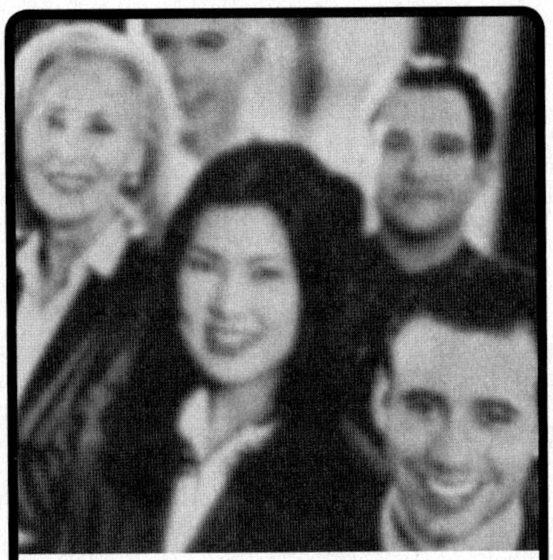

*Move* Forward.
*Move* Smart.
*Move* Now.

JAMACAREERNET
NetWorking for Physicians

*It's Your Move.*

## PEDIATRICS

PEDIATRICIAN FOR MULTI-SPECIALITY CLINIC in beautiful Southeastern Kentucky. Family oriented community with low crime rate, low cost of living. Hospital 0.5 mile from Office, Level II nursery. Call one week per month. Excellent salary and benefits. Partnership track, recent graduate, J-1, H-1 okay. Appalachian Physicians, PSC, PO Box 1477, Hazard, KY 41702. 606-487-9999.

## GROWING IN GA!

BC/BE Pediatrician needed for a growing practice in Pickens County, just 40 miles north of Atlanta. Competitive salary and benefits package. J-1 and H1-B also welcome. Please fax resume to Dr. Mahmood at **706-253-9898** or e-mail: **krazam@ellijay.com**

**"MANAGEMENT OF THE TINY BABY"**
**Conference, February 2-4, 2006**
**Disney's BoardWalk Resort**
**Orlando, Florida**

**★15 hours of Category I AMA/Credit will be awarded.★**

Distinguished faculty includes:
Dr Carl Bose, Dr Elizabeth Beierle, Dr Ronald Clyman, Dr Robert Christensen, Dr Josef Neu, Dr Seetha Shankaran, Dr Alan Spitzer, Dr Robert Urspring.

**For additional information contact: Dr Gregor Alexander, PO Box 568623, Orlando, FL 32856, 407-841-5218**

JAMACAREERNET
SEARCH LOCALLY
ACCESS GLOBALLY

**Fondation Jérôme LEJEUNE**
pour la recherche sur les maladies génétiques de l'intelligence

*The main target of the Fondation Jérôme Lejeune, a state-recommended foundation, is research into Intelligence Disability.*

"Searching, Healing, Defending"

## Grants

The Fondation Jérôme Lejeune invites interested teams and researchers to submit projects to its Scientific Committee, on fundamental or applied research programs (genetics, molecular biology, neurosciences, adult or cord blood stem cells, clinics, therapeutics, behaviour, etc.) aimed at leading to the discovery of treatments for genetic intelligence diseases, including trisomy 21 (Down syndrome), in order to improve the intelligence disease symptoms. The Fondation also considers support for congresses organization.

## Practical Information

- Please fill in the "on-line" application form on www.fondationlejeune.org
- or e-mail: conseilscientifique@fondationlejeune.org (dead-line of the return forms, 24/03/2006):

Conseil Scientifique - Fondation Jérôme Lejeune
48, rue Galande - 75005 PARIS - France

**Tel : +33 1 5310 0830    Fax : +33 1 5310 8598**

## The Penn State Children's Hospital
## Penn State College of Medicine Pediatric Hospitalist

### General Academic Pediatrician

**The PennState Children's Hospital and the Penn State College of Medicine** are seeking a full-time general pediatrician to join our existing group of four hospitalists. The group of five hospitalists will share responsibilities for general pediatric inpatient care, education of pediatric residents and medical students, and participation in clinical investigations. The General Pediatric Inpatient Service has an average daily census of 8.74 and 877 annual admissions. PennState has fully accredited pediatric and med/peds residency programs. The Department of Pediatrics has a full complement of pediatric sub-specialists, surgical sub-specialists, and excellent pediatric radiology. Applicants must be board-certified or board-eligible in general pediatrics, have exemplary clinical and teaching skills, and credentials for academic appointment to the Penn State College of Medicine. We will entertain applications at either junior or senior academic rank. Salary is competitive and commensurate with academic rank. Full benefits package.

The PennState Children's Hospital is located in Hershey, in beautiful south-central Pennsylvania, convenient to New York, Philadelphia, and Baltimore. Schools, academic community and lifestyle opportunities make Hershey an excellent family environment.

Interested candidates should send CV or contact:

**Mark Widome, MD, MPH, Interim Chief**
**General Pediatrics (Job Req #12048) PennState Children's Hospital - MC H085**
**PO Box 850**
**Hershey, PA 17033-0850**

**717-531-8006 • mdw4@psu.edu**

*The PennState Children's Hospital and the Penn State College of Medicine are equal opportunity employers. Women and minority candidates are encouraged to apply.*

## JOURNAL ADVERTISER INDEX


**ABBOTT LABS**
Omnicef OS ........ 7-9

**CLASSIFIED ADVERTISING** ........ 111
http://www.amapublications.com

**GLAXOSMITHKLINE**
Boostrix ........ 91-92, COVER 2-1
Pediarix ........ 63-64, COVER 3-4

**MERCK & COMPANY**
CORPORATE ........ 10-11

**NESTLE USA**
Good Start Supreme ........ 32-33

**SEPRACOR**
Xopenex ........ 16A-D


*Demographic and "Mini" inserts and/or ROB ad pages

While every precaution is taken to ensure accuracy, we cannot guarantee against the possibility of an occasional change or omission in the preparation of this index.

# ARCHIVES OF PEDIATRICS & ADOLESCENT MEDICINE

## CONTACT INFORMATION

### EDITORIAL OFFICE

**Editorial Office Information:** *Archives of Pediatrics & Adolescent Medicine*, Department of Pediatrics, Child Health Institute, University of Washington, 6200 NE 74th St, Suite 210, Seattle, WA 98115-8160; phone: (206) 685-3573; fax: (206) 685-3572; e-mail: archpediatrics@jama-archives.org.

**Electronic Submission:** Manuscripts should be submitted via our online manuscript submission and review system (http://manuscripts.archpediatrics.com). Manuscripts submitted through our online system should not also be submitted by mail or fax. Signed authorship forms should be sent by regular mail or fax. See the Instructions for Authors (www.archpediatrics.com) for more details.

### CONSORTIUM OF *JAMA* & *ARCHIVES* JOURNALS

The *Archives of Pediatrics & Adolescent Medicine* is a member of the consortium of AMA journals listed below.

The Journal of the American Medical Association (JAMA)
Archives of Dermatology
Archives of Facial Plastic Surgery
Archives of General Psychiatry
Archives of Internal Medicine
Archives of Neurology
Archives of Ophthalmology
Archives of Otolaryngology–Head & Neck Surgery
Archives of Pediatrics & Adolescent Medicine
Archives of Surgery

### *JAMA/ARCHIVES* MEDIA RELATIONS

Jann Ingmire; phone: (312) 464-5262; e-mail: mediarelations@jama-archives.org.

### *ARCHIVES OF PEDIATRICS* ONLINE

*Archives of Pediatrics & Adolescent Medicine* is available online at www.archpediatrics.com.

### *JAMA/ARCHIVES* REPRINTS

**Author Reprints:** Anna Goins at (312) 464-2477; fax: (312) 464-5843; e-mail: anna.goins@ama-assn.org. Minimum order: 100 reprints.

**Educational Reprints:** Rhonda Bailey Brown at (312) 464-2513; fax: (312) 464-5843; e-mail: rhonda.brown@ama-assn.org. Minimum order: 100 reprints.

**Commercial Reprints:** Phone: (312) 464-0776; fax: (312) 464-0708; e-mail: reprints@ama-assn.org. Minimum order: 500 reprints.

### PERMISSIONS

Information about obtaining permission to republish, reprint, or adapt material published in *Archives of Pediatrics & Adolescent Medicine* is available from Rhonda Bailey Brown; phone: (312) 464-2513; fax: (312) 464-5843; e-mail: permissions@ama-assn.org.

### DOCUMENT DELIVERY

Copies of individual articles are available online at www.archpediatrics.com and from the following: Infotrieve, phone: (800) 422-4633; fax: (310) 208-5971; URL: www.infotrieve.com; e-mail: orders@infotrieve.com; Institute for Scientific Information (ISI), phone: (800) 603-4367; fax: (856) 787-1679; URL: http://www.isidoc.com; e-mail: service@isidoc.com; Dialog Information Services; Proquest; Ovid Technologies, Inc; and EBSCO.

The ARCHIVES OF PEDIATRICS & ADOLESCENT MEDICINE (ISSN 01072–4710) is published monthly by the American Medical Association, 515 N State St, Chicago, IL 60610–0946, and is an official publication of the Association. The ARCHIVES OF PEDIATRICS & ADOLESCENT MEDICINE reaches more than 30 900 readers in over 83 countries each month. Periodicals postage paid at Chicago, Ill, and at additional mailing offices. GST registration number 12622 5556 RT. Canada Post International Publications Mail (Canadian Distribution) Sales Agreement No. 318728. POSTMASTER, send all address changes to *Archives of Pediatrics & Adolescent Medicine*, c/o the AMA Unified Service Center, American Medical Association, 515 N State St, Chicago, IL 60610. Printed in the USA.

### ADVERTISING

Information about advertising is available from the following sales representatives and online at www.archpediatrics.com.

**Account Manager:** Tim Melroy (nationally); phone: (973) 263-9191 ext 213.

**Manager, Marketing Services:** Nancy Bell; phone: (973) 263-9191 ext 216.

**Advertising Office:** 119 Cherry Hill Rd, Suite 330, Parsippany, NJ 07054-1114; phone: (973) 263-9191.

**Classified Advertising:** Thalia Moss, 515 N State St, Chicago, IL 60610; phone: (800) 262-2260; e-mail: classifieds@ama-assn.org.

### ADVERTISING PRINCIPLES

Advertisements in this issue have been reviewed to comply with the principles governing advertising in AMA publications. A copy of these principles is available on request and online at www.archpediatrics.com. The appearance of advertising in AMA publications is not an AMA guarantee or endorsement of the product or the claims made for the product by the manufacturer.

### ADDRESS CHANGES

Send all address changes to *Archives of Pediatrics & Adolescent Medicine*, c/o the AMA Unified Service Center, American Medical Association, 515 N State St, Chicago, IL 60610. Notification of address changes must be made at least 6 weeks in advance; include both old and new addresses and a recent mailing label if sending via mail.

### SUBSCRIPTION RATES AND SERVICE

Subscription rates are shown in the table below. For service in the US and Americas, inquiries on pricing, address changes, missing issues, subscription billing, subscription renewal, and back issues, contact the AMA Unified Service Center, 24 hours a day, 7 days a week.

**AMA members:** phone: (800) 262-3211; e-mail: msc@ama-assn.org. **Other physicians and nonphysician customers, including subscription agents:** phone: (800) 262-2350 or (312) 670-7827; fax: (312) 464-5831; e-mail: ama-subs@ama-assn.org. **Inquiries:** Unified Service Center, American Medical Association, PO Box 10946, Chicago, IL 60610-0946. For subscribers with mailing addresses outside the United States & Americas: Contact *JAMA & Archives* Journals, c/o EMD GmbH, Birkenstr.67, 10559 Berlin, Germany. Phone: +49 (30) 33099828; fax: +49 (30) 33099829; e-mail: ama@emd-germany.de.

**Annual Subscription Rates**

| | United States | Americas | UK | Rest of World |
|---|---|---|---|---|
| INDIVIDUAL | | | | |
| Print and Online | $185 | $240 | £165 | €250 |
| INSTITUTION | | | | |
| Print and Online | $375 | $485 | £315 | €470 |

In Canada, US rate plus GST. Rates for residents and medical students available at pubs.ama-assn.org, or from the AMA Unified Service Center.

**PEDIARIX™ [Diphtheria and Tetanus Toxoids and Acellular Pertussis Adsorbed, Hepatitis B (Recombinant) and Inactivated Poliovirus Vaccine Combined]**

The following is a brief summary only; see full prescribing information for complete product information.

**CONTRAINDICATIONS:** Hypersensitivity to any component of the vaccine, including yeast, neomycin, and polymyxin B, is a contraindication (see DESCRIPTION in complete prescribing information). Do not use PEDIARIX after a serious allergic reaction (e.g., anaphylaxis) temporally associated with a previous dose of this vaccine or with any components of this vaccine. Because of the uncertainty as to which component of the vaccine might be responsible, do not give further vaccination with any of these components; or, refer such individuals to an allergist for evaluation. The following events are contraindications to administration of PEDIARIX: encephalopathy (e.g., coma, decreased level of consciousness, prolonged seizures) within 7 days of administration of a previous dose of a pertussis-containing vaccine that is not attributable to another identifiable cause; progressive neurologic disorder, including infantile spasms, uncontrolled epilepsy, or progressive encephalopathy. Do not vaccinate individuals with such conditions until a treatment regimen has been established and the condition has stabilized. PEDIARIX is not contraindicated for use in individuals with HIV infection.

**WARNINGS:** Administration of PEDIARIX is associated with higher rates of fever relative to separately administered vaccines. In one study that evaluated medically attended fever after the first dose of PEDIARIX or separately administered vaccines, infants who received PEDIARIX had a higher rate of medical encounters for fever within the first 4 days following vaccination. In some infants, these encounters included the performance of diagnostic studies to evaluate other causes of fever (see ADVERSE REACTIONS). The vial stopper is latex-free. The tip cap and the rubber plunger of the needleless prefilled syringes contain dry natural latex rubber that may cause allergic reactions in latex sensitive individuals. If any of the following events occur in temporal relation to receipt of whole-cell DTP or a vaccine containing an acellular pertussis component, consider carefully whether to give subsequent doses of PEDIARIX or any vaccine containing a pertussis component: temperature of ≥40.5°C (105°F) within 48 hours not due to another identifiable cause; collapse or shock-like state (hypotonic-hyporesponsive episode) within 48 hours; persistent, inconsolable crying lasting ≥3 hours, occurring within 48 hours; seizures with or without fever occurring within 3 days. If Guillain-Barré syndrome occurs within 6 weeks of receipt of prior vaccine containing tetanus toxoid, the decision to give subsequent doses of PEDIARIX or any vaccine containing tetanus toxoid should be based on careful consideration of the potential benefits and possible risks. A committee of the Institute of Medicine (IOM) has concluded that evidence is consistent with a causal relationship between whole-cell DTP vaccine and acute neurologic illness, and under special circumstances, between whole-cell DTP vaccine and chronic neurologic disease in the context of the National Childhood Encephalopathy Study (NCES) report; however, evidence was insufficient to indicate whether or not whole-cell DTP vaccine increased the overall risk of chronic neurologic disease. Acute encephalopathy and permanent neurologic damage have not been reported causally linked or in temporal association with administration of PEDIARIX, but the experience with PEDIARIX is insufficient to rule this out. Encephalopathy has been reported following INFANRIX® (Diphtheria and Tetanus Toxoids and Acellular Pertussis Vaccine Adsorbed) (see ADVERSE REACTIONS, Postmarketing Reports), but data are not sufficient to evaluate a causal relationship. The decision to administer a pertussis-containing vaccine to children with stable central nervous system (CNS) disorders must be made by the physician on an individual basis, with consideration of all relevant factors, and assessment of potential risks and benefits for that individual. Advise the parent or guardian of the potential increased risk involved (see PRECAUTIONS). A family history of seizures or other CNS disorders is not a contraindication to pertussis vaccine. For children at higher risk for seizures than the general population, an appropriate antipyretic may be administered at the time of vaccination and for the ensuing 24 hours according to the respective prescribing information recommended dosage to reduce the possibility of post-vaccination fever. Defer vaccination during the course of a moderate or severe illness with or without fever and vaccinate patients as soon as they have recovered from the acute phase of the illness. Do not give PEDIARIX to children on anticoagulant therapy or those with bleeding disorders unless the potential benefit clearly outweighs the risk of administration (see PRECAUTIONS in complete prescribing information).

**PRECAUTIONS:** Before the injection of any biological, the physician should take all reasonable precautions to prevent allergic or other adverse reactions. Epinephrine injection (1:1000) and other appropriate agents used for the control of immediate allergic reactions must be immediately available should an acute anaphylactic reaction occur. Immunosuppressed individuals, including those receiving immunosuppressive therapy, may not develop the expected immune response. **Drug Interactions:** For information regarding concomitant administration with other vaccines, refer to DOSAGE AND ADMINISTRATION in complete prescribing information. Do not mix PEDIARIX with any other vaccine in the same syringe or vial. **Carcinogenesis, Mutagenesis, Impairment of Fertility:** PEDIARIX has not been evaluated for carcinogenic or mutagenic potential, or for impairment of fertility. **Pregnancy:** Pregnancy Category C: PEDIARIX is not indicated for women of child-bearing age. Animal reproduction studies have not been conducted with PEDIARIX. It is not known whether PEDIARIX can cause fetal harm when administered to a pregnant woman or if PEDIARIX can affect reproductive capacity. **Geriatric Use:** PEDIARIX is not indicated for use in adult populations. **Pediatric Use:** Safety and effectiveness of PEDIARIX in infants younger than 6 weeks of age have not been evaluated (see DOSAGE AND ADMINISTRATION in complete prescribing information). PEDIARIX is not recommended for persons 7 years of age or older. Tetanus and Diphtheria Toxoids Adsorbed (Td) For Adult Use, inactivated poliovirus vaccine (IPV), and Hepatitis B Vaccine (Recombinant) should be used in individuals 7 years of age or older.

**ADVERSE REACTIONS:** A total of 20,739 doses of PEDIARIX have been administered to 7,028 infants as a 3-dose primary series. The most common adverse reactions observed in clinical trials were local injection site reactions (pain, redness, or swelling), fever, and fussiness. In comparative studies, administration of PEDIARIX was associated with higher rates of fever relative to separately administered vaccines (see WARNINGS). The prevalence of fever was highest on the day of vaccination and the day following vaccination. More than 98% of episodes of fever resolved within the 4-day period following vaccination (i.e., the period including the day of vaccination and the next 3 days). Rates of most other solicited adverse events following PEDIARIX were comparable to rates observed following separately administered US-licensed vaccines. The adverse event information from clinical trials provides a basis for identifying adverse events that appear to be related to vaccine use and for approximating rates. However, because clinical trials are conducted under widely varying conditions, adverse event rates observed in the clinical trials of a vaccine cannot be directly compared to rates in the clinical trials of another vaccine, and may not reflect the rates observed in practice. A total of 5,472 infants were enrolled in a German safety study that was originally designed to compare the safety and reactogenicity of PEDIARIX administered concomitantly at separate sites with 1 of 4 *Haemophilus influenzae* type b (Hib) vaccines at 3, 4, and 5 months of age. After enrollment of 1,569 infants, the study was amended to include a control group that received INFANRIX, Hib vaccine, and oral poliovirus vaccine (OPV) separately. Infants in the separate administration group received one less antigen (hepatitis B) than the infants who received PEDIARIX. Safety data were available for 4,666 infants who received PEDIARIX administered concomitantly at separate sites with 1 of 4 Hib vaccines and for 768 infants in the control group that received separate vaccines. The primary end-point of the study was the percentage of infants with any grade 3 solicited symptom (redness or swelling >20 mm, fever >103.1°F, or crying, pain, vomiting, diarrhea, loss of appetite, or restlessness that prevented normal daily activities) over the 3-dose primary series in infants who received PEDIARIX (4 groups that received PEDIARIX and Hib vaccines pooled) compared to the group that received INFANRIX and Hib vaccine separately with OPV. Analysis for the primary end-point was performed on the according-to-protocol (ATP) cohort that included only those infants who were enrolled after the protocol amendment to include a control group. Of 3,773 infants in the ATP cohort for whom safety data were available, 16.2% (95% CI: 14.9% to 17.5%) of 3,029 infants who received PEDIARIX and Hib vaccine compared to 20.3% (95% CI: 17.5% to 23.4%) of 744 infants who received separate vaccines were reported to have had at least one grade 3 solicited symptom within 4 days of vaccination (i.e., day of vaccination and the next 3 days). The difference between groups in the rate of grade 3 symptoms was 4.1% (90% CI: 1.4% to 7.1%). These were the rates for selected solicited symptoms within 4 days following each dose in a 3-dose primary series in infants who received PEDIARIX administered concomitantly with Hib vaccine and those who received separate concomitant administration of INFANRIX, Hib vaccine, and OPV for the intent-to-treat (ITT) cohort (includes all infants enrolled before and after the amendment who received the indicated vaccine and for whom at least one symptom sheet was completed):

**Percentage of German Infants With Solicited Local Reactions or Selected Systemic Adverse Events Within 4 Days of Vaccination* (ITT Cohort)**

| | PEDIARIX & Hib | | | INFANRIX, Hib, & OPV | | |
|---|---|---|---|---|---|---|
| | **Dose 1** | **Dose 2** | **Dose 3** | **Dose 1** | **Dose 2** | **Dose 3** |
| **N** | **4,666** | **4,619** | **4,574** | **768** | **757** | **750** |
| **Local†** | | | | | | |
| Pain, any | 14.0 | 10.2 | 9.9 | 14.2 | 9.8 | 8.1 |
| Pain, grade 2 or 3 | 2.9 | 1.2 | 1.5 | 3.6 | 1.7 | 1.1 |
| Pain, grade 3 | 0.7 | 0.3 | 0.3 | 1.3 | 0.4 | 0.1 |
| Redness, any | 18.6 | 26.6 | 25.6 | 16.1 | 21.4 | 20.8 |
| Redness, >5 mm | 6.7 | 9.9 | 9.0 | 5.9 | 8.2 | 7.7 |
| Redness, >20 mm | 1.2 | 1.0 | 1.1 | 1.8 | 0.7 | 1.1 |
| Swelling, any | 12.7 | 18.5 | 18.4 | 9.6 | 12.9 | 13.6 |
| Swelling, >5 mm | 5.6 | 7.7 | 7.8 | 3.6 | 5.2 | 4.8 |
| Swelling, >20 mm | 1.2 | 1.6 | 1.5 | 1.3 | 1.1 | 1.2 |
| **Systemic** | | | | | | |
| Restlessness, any | 41.4 | 32.0 | 26.7 | 46.4 | 35.0 | 27.6 |
| Restlessness, grade 2 or 3 | 14.4 | 10.0 | 8.9 | 20.2 | 11.5 | 8.4 |
| Restlessness, grade 3 | 3.0 | 1.5 | 1.6 | 5.7 | 3.0 | 1.7 |
| Fever‡, ≥100.4ºF | 25.1 | 19.3 | 19.7 | 13.2 | 13.1 | 11.2 |
| Fever‡, >101.3ºF | 5.8 | 4.1 | 4.6 | 2.2 | 2.8 | 2.1 |
| Fever‡, >103.1ºF | 0.3 | 0.5 | 0.7 | 0.3 | 0.3 | 0.5 |
| Unusual cry§, any | 24.9 | 16.5 | 13.1 | 36.5 | 19.7 | 14.3 |
| Unusual cry§, grade 2 or 3 | 12.7 | 7.1 | 5.7 | 20.8 | 10.0 | 5.7 |
| Unusual cry§, grade 3 | 3.9 | 1.7 | 1.4 | 6.8 | 2.1 | 1.1 |
| Loss of appetite, any | 17.9 | 13.3 | 12.5 | 19.1 | 16.2 | 11.3 |
| Loss of appetite, grade 2 or 3 | 4.0 | 2.9 | 2.7 | 4.4 | 2.9 | 2.3 |
| Loss of appetite, grade 3 | 0.6 | 0.5 | 0.4 | 0.5 | 0.7 | 0.0 |

N = number of infants in the intent-to-treat (ITT) cohort.
Grade 2 defined as sufficiently discomforting to interfere with daily activities.
Grade 3 defined as preventing normal daily activities.
* Within 4 days of vaccination defined as day of vaccination and the next 3 days.
† Local reactions at the injection site for PEDIARIX or INFANRIX.
‡ Rectal temperatures.
§ Unusual cry lasting >1 hour.

In this study, infants were also monitored for unsolicited adverse events that occurred within 30 days following vaccination. Over the entire study period, 6 subjects in the group that received PEDIARIX reported seizures. Two of these subjects had a febrile seizure, 1 of whom also developed afebrile seizures. The remaining 4 subjects had afebrile seizures, including 2 with infantile spasms. Two subjects reported seizures within 7 days following vaccination (1 subject had both febrile and afebrile seizures, and 1 subject had afebrile seizures), corresponding to a rate of 0.22 seizures per 1,000 doses (febrile seizures 0.07 per 1,000 doses, afebrile seizures 0.14 per 1,000 doses). No subject who received concomitant INFANRIX, Hib vaccine, and OPV reported seizures. In a separate German study that evaluated the safety of INFANRIX in 22,505 infants who received 66,867 doses of INFANRIX administered as a 3-dose primary series, the rate of seizures within 7 days of vaccination with INFANRIX was 0.13 per 1,000 doses (febrile seizures 0.0 per 1,000 doses, afebrile seizures 0.13 per 1,000 doses). No cases of hypotonic-hyporesponsiveness, encephalopathy, or anaphylaxis were reported in the German study that evaluated the safety of PEDIARIX. Rates of serious adverse events that are less common than those reported in this safety study are not known at this time.

Additional safety data for PEDIARIX are available from a US study designed to evaluate lot-to-lot consistency and a bridge for a new manufacturing step. These were the rates for local reactions and selected adverse events within 4 days of vaccination with PEDIARIX administered concomitantly with a Hib vaccine at 2, 4, and 6 months of age:

**Percentage of US Infants With Solicited Local Reactions or Selected Systemic Adverse Events Within 4 Days of Vaccination* (ITT Cohort)**

| | PEDIARIX & Hib | | |
|---|---|---|---|
| | **Dose 1** | **Dose 2** | **Dose 3** |
| **Local†** | **N = 482** | **N = 469** | **N = 466** |
| Pain, any | 30.5 | 25.4 | 23.0 |
| Pain, grade 2 or 3 | 6.2 | 5.5 | 3.6 |
| Pain, grade 3 | 1.2 | 0.6 | 0.6 |
| Redness, any | 25.3 | 32.6 | 35.6 |
| Redness, >5 mm | 9.3 | 10.4 | 8.6 |
| Redness, >20 mm | 0.6 | 1.5 | 1.3 |
| Swelling, any | 15.1 | 16.6 | 22.3 |
| Swelling, >5 mm | 6.8 | 6.2 | 6.4 |
| Swelling, >20 mm | 1.0 | 1.3 | 1.3 |
| **Systemic** | **N = 482** | **N = 469** | **N = 467** |
| Restlessness, any | 28.8 | 30.3 | 28.5 |
| Restlessness, grade 2 or 3 | 7.1 | 9.0 | 9.4 |
| Restlessness, grade 3 | 1.0 | 1.1 | 0.6 |
| Fever‡, ≥100.4ºF | 26.6 | 31.3 | 25.9 |
| Fever‡, >101.3ºF | 2.9 | 6.2 | 4.7 |
| Fever‡, >103.1ºF | 0.0 | 0.2 | 0.6 |
| Fussiness, any | 61.8 | 63.8 | 57.0 |
| Fussiness, grade 2 or 3 | 14.9 | 21.5 | 17.1 |
| Fussiness, grade 3 | 2.7 | 3.4 | 1.7 |
| Loss of appetite, any | 21.6 | 19.8 | 18.8 |
| Loss of appetite, grade 2 or 3 | 3.1 | 3.2 | 2.4 |
| Loss of appetite, grade 3 | 0.2 | 0.4 | 0.0 |
| Sleeping more than usual, any | 46.7 | 31.8 | 28.1 |
| Sleeping more than usual, grade 2 or 3 | 10.2 | 6.0 | 4.7 |
| Sleeping more than usual, grade 3 | 1.7 | 0.4 | 0.6 |

N = number of infants in the intent-to-treat (ITT) cohort (infants who received the indicated vaccine and for whom at least one symptom sheet was completed).
Grade 2 defined as sufficiently discomforting to interfere with daily activities.
Grade 3 defined as preventing normal daily activities.
* Within 4 days of vaccination defined as day of vaccination and the next 3 days.
† Local reactions at the injection site for PEDIARIX.
‡ Rectal temperatures.

In another US study, these were the rates for fever within 4 days following dose 1 (i.e., day of vaccination and the next 3 days) at 2 months of age in infants who received PEDIARIX when administered concomitantly at separate sites with Hib and pneumococcal conjugate vaccines and those who received INFANRIX, ENGERIX-B® [Hepatitis B Vaccine (Recombinant)], IPV, Hib vaccine, and pneumococcal conjugate vaccine:

**Percentage of US Infants With Fever Within 4 Days of Dose 1* (ITT Cohort)**

| | **PEDIARIX, Hib, & Pneumococcal Conjugate (N = 667)** | **INFANRIX, ENGERIX-B, IPV, Hib, & Pneumococcal Conjugate (N = 333)** | **Separate Vaccine Group Minus Combination Vaccine Group** |
|---|---|---|---|
| **Fever†** | **%** | **%** | **Difference (95% CI)** |
| ≥100.4ºF‡ | 27.9 | 19.8 | -8.07 (-13.54, -2.60) |
| >101.3ºF | 7.0 | 4.5 | -2.54 (-5.50, 0.41) |
| >102.2ºF‡ | 2.2 | 0.3 | -1.95 (-3.22, -0.68) |
| >103.1ºF | 0.4 | 0.0 | -0.45 (-0.96, 0.06) |
| M.A.‡ | 1.2 | 0.0 | -1.20 (-2.03, -037) |

N = number of infants for whom at least one symptom sheet was completed, excluding 3 infants for whom temperature was not measured and 3 infants whose temperature was measured by the tympanic method.
*Within 4 days of dose 1 defined as day of vaccination and the next 3 days.
† Rectal temperatures.
‡ The group that received PEDIARIX compared to separate vaccine group p value <0.05 (2-sided Fisher Exact test) or the 95% confidence interval on the difference between groups does not include 0.
M.A. = Medically attended (a visit to or from medical personnel).

In this study, medical attention (a visit to or from medical personnel) for fever within 4 days following vaccination was sought for 8 infants who received PEDIARIX (1.2%) and no infants who received separately administered vaccines. Four infants were seen by medical personnel in an office setting; no diagnostic tests were performed in 2 of the infants and a complete blood count (CBC) was done in the other 2 infants. Of 3 infants who were seen in an emergency room, all had a CBC and a blood and urine culture performed; chest X-rays were done in 2 of the infants and a nasopharyngeal specimen was tested for Respiratory Syncytial Virus in one of the infants. One infant was hospitalized for a work-up that included a CBC, blood and urine cultures, a lumbar puncture, and a chest X-ray. All episodes of medically attended fever resolved within 4 days post-vaccination.

Limited data are available from a study conducted in Moldova in which infants received a dose of hepatitis B vaccine within 48 hours of birth followed by 3 doses of PEDIARIX at 6, 10, and 14 weeks of age. No information was collected on the HBsAg status of mothers of enrolled infants. These were the rates for local reactions and selected adverse events within 4 days of vaccination with PEDIARIX administered comcomitantly with Hib vaccine following a birth dose of hepatitis B vaccine:

**Percentage of Moldovan Infants With Solicited Local Reactions or Selected Systemic Adverse Events Within 4 Days of Vaccination* (ITT Cohort)**

| | PEDIARIX & Hib | | |
|---|---|---|---|
| | **Dose 1** | **Dose 2** | **Dose 3** |
| **N** | **160** | **158** | **157** |
| **Local†** | | | |
| Pain, any | 25.6 | 18.4 | 14.0 |
| Pain, grade 3 | 3.1 | 0.6 | 1.9 |
| Redness, any | 41.9 | 41.8 | 47.1 |
| Redness, >20 mm | 1.9 | 2.5 | 4.5 |
| Swelling, any | 20.6 | 18.4 | 28.0 |
| Swelling, >20 mm | 4.4 | 2.5 | 7.0 |
| **Systemic** | | | |
| Restlessness, any | 13.1 | 10.8 | 8.9 |
| Restlessness, grade 3 | 1.3 | 0.6 | 0.6 |
| Fever‡, ≥100.4ºF | 14.4 | 11.4 | 5.1 |
| Fever‡, >103.1ºF | 0.0 | 0.6 | 0.0 |
| Fussiness, any | 25.0 | 21.5 | 17.8 |
| Fussiness, grade 3 | 2.5 | 0.6 | 0.6 |

N = number of infants in the intent-to-treat (ITT) cohort (infants who received the indicated vaccine and for whom at least one symptom sheet was completed).
Grade 3 defined as preventing normal daily activities.
*Within 4 days of vaccination defined as day of vaccination and the next 3 days.
† Local reactions at the injection site for PEDIARIX.
‡ Rectal temperatures.

Although there was no comparator group who received PEDIARIX without a birth dose of hepatitis B vaccine, available data suggest that some local adverse events may occur at a higher rate when PEDIARIX is administered after a birth dose of hepatitis B vaccine.

As with any vaccine, there is the possibility that broad use of PEDIARIX could reveal adverse events not observed in clinical trials.

**Postmarketing Reports:** Worldwide voluntary reports of adverse events received for INFANRIX and ENGERIX-B in children younger than 7 years of age since market introduction of these US-licensed vaccines are listed below. This list includes adverse events for which 20 or more reports were received with the exception of intussusception, idiopathic thrombocytopenic purpura, thrombocytopenia, anaphylactic reaction, angioedema, encephalopathy, hypotonic-hyporesponsive episode, and alopecia for which fewer than 20 reports were received. These latter events are included either because of the seriousness of the event or the strength of causal connection to components of this or other vaccines or drugs. *Body as a whole:* Asthenia[b], fever[a+b], lethargy[b], malaise[b], Sudden Infant Death Syndrome[a+b]. *Cardiovascular system:* Cyanosis[a+b], edema[b], pallor[b]. *Gastrointestinal system:* Abdominal pain[b], anorexia[b], diarrhea[a+b], intussusception[a+b], nausea[b], vomiting[a+b]. *Hematologic/lymphatic:* Idiopathic thrombocytopenic purpura[a+b], lymphadenopathy[a], thrombocytopenia[a+b]. *Hepatic:* Jaundice[b], liver function tests abnormal[b]. *Hypersensitivity:* Anaphylactic reaction[a+b], angioedema[b], hypersensitivity[a]. *Infections:* Cellulitis[a]. *Injection site reactions:* Injection site reactions[a+b]. *Musculoskeletal:* Arthralgia[b], limb swelling[a+b]. *Nervous system:* Convulsions[a+b], encephalopathy[a], headache[b], hypotonia[a+b], hypotonic-hyporesponsive episode[a], somnolence[a+b]. *Psychiatric:* Crying[a+b], irritability[a+b]. *Respiratory system:* Respiratory tract infection[a]. *Skin and appendages:* Alopecia[b], erythema[a+b], erythema multiforme[b], petechiae[b], pruritus[a+b], rash[a+b], urticaria[a+b]. *Special senses:* Ear pain[a]. [[a] Following INFANRIX; [b] Following ENGERIX-B; [a+b] Following either INFANRIX or ENGERIX-B.] These reactions were reported voluntarily from a population of uncertain size; therefore, it is not always possible to reliably estimate their frequency or establish a causal relationship to vaccination.

**Reporting Adverse Events:** Report the occurrence following immunization of any event set forth in the Vaccine Injury Table from the National Childhood Vaccine Injury Act including: Anaphylaxis or anaphylactic shock within 7 days, encephalopathy or encephalitis within 7 days, brachial neuritis within 28 days, or an acute complication or sequelae (including death) of an illness, disability, injury, or condition referred to above, or any events that would contraindicate further doses of PEDIARIX. The VAERS toll-free number is 1-800-822-7967.

Manufactured by **GlaxoSmithKline Biologicals**, Rixensart, Belgium, US License 1617

Distributed by **GlaxoSmithKline,** Research Triangle Park, NC 27709



Full prescribing information for PEDIARIX is available at www.GSKVaccines.com/Pediarix. BRS-PE:L2

 Printed in USA. PED583R0 June 2005

# ARCHIVES OF PEDIATRICS & ADOLESCENT MEDICINE

WWW.ARCHPEDIATRICS.COM

FEBRUARY 2006


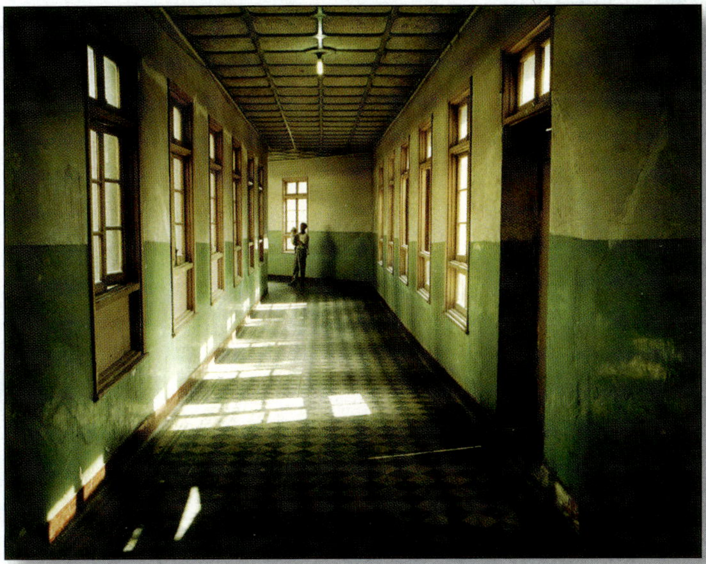

Smile China Cleft Lip Palate Mission, Provincial Children's Hospital, Lanzhou, China, July 2004. See page 119.


RANDOMIZED CONTROLLED TRIAL OF A PRIMARY CARE AND HOME-BASED INTERVENTION FOR PHYSICAL ACTIVITY AND NUTRITION BEHAVIORS

ASSOCIATION OF CONDOM USE, SEXUAL BEHAVIORS, AND SEXUALLY TRANSMITTED INFECTIONS WITH THE DURATION OF GENITAL HUMAN PAPILLOMAVIRUS INFECTION

NEONATAL ABSTINENCE SYNDROME AFTER IN UTERO EXPOSURE TO SELECTIVE SEROTONIN REUPTAKE INHIBITORS IN TERM INFANTS

SIMULATING COST-EFFECTIVENESS OF FLUORIDE VARNISH DURING WELL-CHILD VISITS FOR MEDICAID-ENROLLED CHILDREN


COMPLETE TABLE OF CONTENTS ON PAGE 117




JAMA & ARCHIVES JOURNALS
American Medical Association

**NEW XOPENEX HFA!**

**In the treatment or prevention of bronchospasm**

# Expect Xopenex

## The confidence you need, the freedom they want

- XOPENEX does not contain (S)-albuterol[1]
- Rapid onset of action for relief of bronchospasm*[1]
- Beta-adrenergic–mediated adverse events are low and comparable to placebo[1]
- Indicated for patients 4 years of age and older[1]

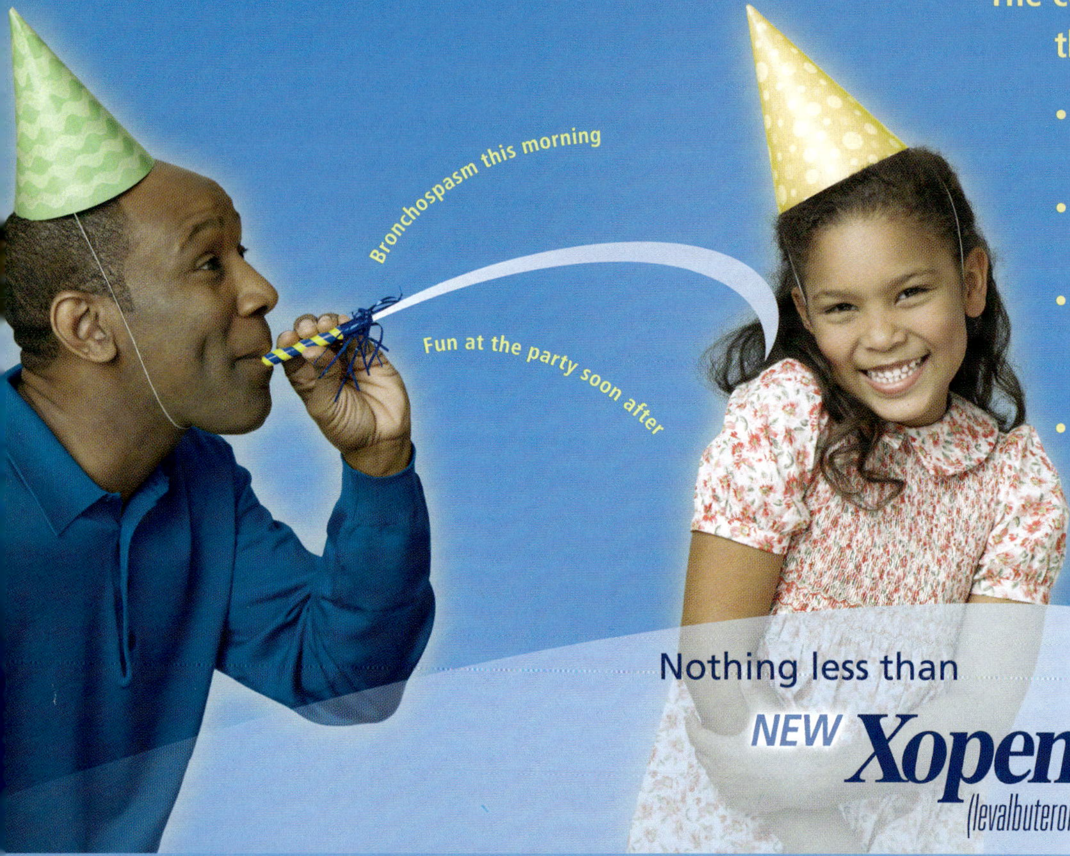


Nothing less than

**NEW Xopenex HFA™**
(levalbuterol tartrate) Inhalation Aerosol

**Important Safety Information**

Xopenex HFA is contraindicated in patients with a history of hypersensitivity to levalbuterol, racemic albuterol, or any other component of Xopenex HFA. Xopenex HFA and other β-agonists can produce paradoxical bronchospasm, which may be life threatening. If additional adrenergic drugs, including other short-acting sympathomimetic bronchodilators or epinephrine, are to be administered by any route, they should be used with caution to avoid deleterious cardiovascular effects. Due to the cardiovascular side effects associated with β-agonists, caution is generally recommended for patients with cardiovascular disorders (especially coronary insufficiency, cardiac arrhythmias, and hypertension), diabetes, hyperthyroidism, or convulsive disorders. Do not exceed the recommended dose. Fatalities have been reported in association with excessive use of inhaled sympathomimetic drugs in patients with asthma. Please refer to the complete prescribing information for further information and in regard to potential drug interactions with β-blockers, diuretics, digoxin, or MAOI and tricyclic antidepressants.

**In patients aged 4 to 11 years,** the most common adverse events (occurring in greater than 2% of patients and more frequently than patients receiving placebo) were (90 mcg Xopenex HFA and placebo, respectively): accidental injury (9.2%; 5.7%), vomiting (10.5%; 5.7%), bronchitis (2.6%; 0%), and pharyngitis (6.6%; 5.7%).

**In patients aged 12 years and older,** the most common adverse events (occurring in greater than 2% of patients and more frequently than patients receiving placebo) were (90 mcg Xopenex HFA and placebo, respectively): pain (4.0%; 3.6%), dizziness (2.7%; 1.8%), asthma (9.4%; 6.0%), pharyngitis (7.9%; 2.4%), and rhinitis (7.4%; 3.0%).

Please see brief summary of prescribing information.

XOPENEX HFA (levalbuterol tartrate) Inhalation Aerosol is indicated for the treatment or prevention of bronchospasm in adults, adolescents, and children 4 years of age and older with reversible obstructive airway disease.

* The median onset time of a 15% increase in $FEV_1$ for XOPENEX HFA Inhalation Aerosol on Day 1 was 5.5 to 10.2 minutes for adult patients and 4.5 minutes for pediatric patients. Please refer to prescribing information.



**Reference:** 1. Xopenex HFA Prescribing Information.

# Xopenex HFA™

(levalbuterol tartrate) Inhalation Aerosol

FOR ORAL INHALATION ONLY

## BRIEF SUMMARY

**INDICATIONS AND USAGE**

XOPENEX HFA (levalbuterol tartrate) Inhalation Aerosol is indicated for the treatment or prevention of bronchospasm in adults, adolescents, and children 4 years of age and older with reversible obstructive airway disease.

**CONTRAINDICATIONS**

XOPENEX HFA (levalbuterol tartrate) Inhalation Aerosol is contraindicated in patients with a history of hypersensitivity to levalbuterol, racemic albuterol, or any other component of XOPENEX HFA Inhalation Aerosol.

**WARNINGS**

1. Paradoxical Bronchospasm: Like other inhaled beta-adrenergic agonists, XOPENEX HFA Inhalation Aerosol can produce paradoxical bronchospasm, which may be life-threatening. If paradoxical bronchospasm occurs, XOPENEX HFA (levalbuterol tartrate) Inhalation Aerosol should be discontinued immediately and alternative therapy instituted. It should be recognized that paradoxical bronchospasm, when associated with inhaled formulations, frequently occurs with the first use of a new canister. 2. Deterioration of Asthma: Asthma may deteriorate acutely over a period of hours or chronically over several days or longer. If the patient needs more doses of XOPENEX HFA Inhalation Aerosol than usual, this may be a marker of destabilization of asthma and requires reevaluation of the patient and treatment regimen, giving special consideration to the possible need for anti-inflammatory treatment, e.g., corticosteroids. 3. Use of Anti-Inflammatory Agents: The use of a beta-adrenergic agonist alone may not be adequate to control asthma in many patients. Early consideration should be given to adding anti-inflammatory agents, e.g., corticosteroids, to the therapeutic regimen. 4. Cardiovascular Effects: XOPENEX HFA Inhalation Aerosol, like other beta-adrenergic agonists, can produce clinically significant cardiovascular effects in some patients, as measured by heart rate, blood pressure, and/or symptoms. Although such effects are uncommon after administration of XOPENEX HFA Inhalation Aerosol at recommended doses, if they occur, the drug may need to be discontinued. In addition, beta-agonists have been reported to produce electrocardiogram (ECG) changes, such as flattening of the T wave, prolongation of the QTc interval, and ST segment depression. The clinical significance of these findings is unknown. Therefore, XOPENEX HFA Inhalation Aerosol, like all sympathomimetic amines, should be used with caution in patients with cardiovascular disorders, especially coronary insufficiency, cardiac arrhythmias, and hypertension. 5. Do Not Exceed Recommended Dose: Fatalities have been reported in association with excessive use of inhaled sympathomimetic drugs in patients with asthma. The exact cause of death is unknown, but cardiac arrest following an unexpected development of a severe acute asthmatic crisis and subsequent hypoxia is suspected. 6. Immediate Hypersensitivity Reactions: Immediate hypersensitivity reactions may occur after administration of racemic albuterol, as demonstrated by rare cases of urticaria, angioedema, rash, bronchospasm, anaphylaxis, and oropharyngeal edema. The potential for hypersensitivity must be considered in the clinical evaluation of patients who experience immediate hypersensitivity reactions while receiving XOPENEX HFA Inhalation Aerosol.

**PRECAUTIONS**

**General**

XOPENEX HFA (levalbuterol tartrate) Inhalation Aerosol, like all sympathomimetic amines, should be used with caution in patients with cardiovascular disorders, especially coronary insufficiency, hypertension, and cardiac arrhythmias; in patients with convulsive disorders, hyperthyroidism, or diabetes mellitus; and in patients who are unusually responsive to sympathomimetic amines. Clinically significant changes in systolic and diastolic blood pressure have been seen in individual patients and could be expected to occur in some patients after the use of any beta-adrenergic bronchodilator.

Large doses of intravenous racemic albuterol have been reported to aggravate preexisting diabetes mellitus and ketoacidosis. As with other beta-adrenergic agonist medications, XOPENEX HFA Inhalation Aerosol may produce significant hypokalemia in some patients, possibly through intracellular shunting, which has the potential to produce adverse cardiovascular effects. The decrease is usually transient, not requiring supplementation.

**Information for Patients**

The action of XOPENEX HFA Inhalation Aerosol should last for 4 to 6 hours. XOPENEX HFA Inhalation Aerosol should not be used more frequently than recommended. Do not increase the dose or frequency of doses of XOPENEX HFA Inhalation Aerosol without consulting your physician. If you find that treatment with XOPENEX HFA Inhalation Aerosol becomes less effective for symptomatic relief, your symptoms become worse, and/or you need to use the product more frequently than usual, you should seek medical attention immediately. While you are using XOPENEX HFA Inhalation Aerosol, other inhaled drugs and asthma medications should be taken only as directed by your physician.

Common adverse effects of treatment with inhaled beta-agonists include palpitations, chest pain, rapid heart rate, tremor, and nervousness. If you are pregnant or nursing, contact your physician about use of XOPENEX HFA Inhalation Aerosol. Effective and safe use of XOPENEX HFA Inhalation Aerosol includes an understanding of the way that it should be administered.

Use XOPENEX HFA Inhalation Aerosol only with the actuator supplied with the product. Discard the canister after 200 sprays have been used. Never immerse the canister in water to determine how full the canister is ("float test").

In general, the technique for administering XOPENEX HFA Inhalation Aerosol to children is similar to that for adults. Children should use XOPENEX HFA Inhalation Aerosol under adult supervision, as instructed by the patient's physician.

**Drug Interactions**

Other short-acting sympathomimetic aerosol bronchodilators or epinephrine should be used with caution with XOPENEX HFA Inhalation Aerosol. If additional adrenergic drugs are to be administered by any route, they should be used with caution to avoid deleterious cardiovascular effects.

1. Beta-blockers: Beta-adrenergic receptor-blocking agents not only block the pulmonary effect of beta-adrenergic agonists, such as XOPENEX HFA Inhalation Aerosol, but may produce severe bronchospasm in asthmatic patients. Therefore, patients with asthma should not normally be treated with beta-blockers. However, under certain circumstances, e.g., as prophylaxis after myocardial infarction, there may be no acceptable alternatives to the use of beta-adrenergic blocking agents in patients with asthma. In this setting, cardioselective beta-blockers should be considered, although they should be administered with caution. 2. Diuretics: The ECG changes and/or hypokalemia that may result from the administration of non–potassium-sparing diuretics (such as loop and thiazide diuretics) can be acutely worsened by beta-agonists, especially when the recommended dose of the beta-agonist is exceeded. Although the clinical significance of these effects is not known, caution is advised in the coadministration of beta-agonists with non–potassium-sparing diuretics. 3. Digoxin: Mean decreases of 16% to 22% in serum digoxin levels were demonstrated after single-dose intravenous and oral administration of racemic albuterol, respectively, to normal volunteers who had received digoxin for 10 days. The clinical significance of these findings for patients with obstructive airway disease who are receiving XOPENEX HFA Inhalation Aerosol and digoxin on a chronic basis is unclear. Nevertheless, it would be prudent to carefully evaluate the serum digoxin levels in patients who are currently receiving digoxin and XOPENEX HFA Inhalation Aerosol. 4. Monoamine Oxidase Inhibitors or Tricyclic Antidepressants: XOPENEX HFA Inhalation Aerosol should be administered with extreme caution to patients being treated with monoamine oxidase inhibitors or tricyclic antidepressants, or within 2 weeks of discontinuation of such agents, because the action of albuterol on the vascular system may be potentiated.

**Carcinogenesis, Mutagenesis, and Impairment of Fertility** No carcinogenesis or impairment of fertility studies have been carried out with levalbuterol tartrate. However, racemic albuterol sulfate has been evaluated for its carcinogenic potential and ability to impair fertility.

In a 2-year study in Sprague-Dawley rats, racemic albuterol sulfate caused a significant dose-related increase in the incidence of benign leiomyomas of the mesovarium at, and above, dietary doses of 2 mg/kg/day (approximately 30 times the maximum recommended daily inhalation dose of levalbuterol tartrate for adults on a $mg/m^2$ basis and approximately 15 times the maximum recommended daily inhalation dose of levalbuterol tartrate for children on a $mg/m^2$ basis). In another study, this effect was blocked by the coadministration of propranolol, a nonselective beta-adrenergic antagonist. In an 18-month study in CD-1 mice, racemic albuterol sulfate showed no evidence of tumorigenicity at dietary doses up to 500 mg/kg/day (approximately 3800 times the maximum recommended daily inhalation dose of levalbuterol tartrate for adults on a $mg/m^2$ basis and approximately 1800 times the maximum recommended daily inhalation dose of levalbuterol tartrate for children on a $mg/m^2$ basis). In a 22-month study in the Golden hamster, racemic albuterol sulfate showed no evidence of tumorigenicity at dietary doses up to 50 mg/kg/day (approximately 500 times the maximum recommended daily inhalation dose of levalbuterol tartrate for adults on a $mg/m^2$ basis and approximately 240 times the maximum recommended daily inhalation dose of levalbuterol tartrate for children on a $mg/m^2$ basis).

Levalbuterol HCl was not mutagenic in the Ames test or the CHO/HPRT Mammalian Forward Gene Mutation Assay.

Levalbuterol HCl was not clastogenic in the in vivo micronucleus test in mouse bone marrow. Racemic albuterol sulfate was negative in an in vitro chromosomal aberration assay in CHO cell cultures.

Reproduction studies in rats using racemic albuterol sulfate demonstrated no evidence of impaired fertility at oral doses up to 50 mg/kg/day (approximately 750 times the maximum recommended daily inhalation dose of levalbuterol tartrate for adults on a $mg/m^2$ basis).

**Teratogenic Effects - Pregnancy Category C** A reproduction study in New Zealand White rabbits demonstrated that levalbuterol HCl was not teratogenic when administered orally at doses up to 25 mg/kg/day (approximately 750 times the maximum recommended daily inhalation dose of levalbuterol tartrate for adults on a $mg/m^2$ basis).

However, racemic albuterol sulfate has been shown to be teratogenic in mice and rabbits. A study in CD-1 mice given racemic albuterol sulfate subcutaneously showed cleft palate formation in 5 of 111 (4.5%) fetuses at 0.25 mg/kg/day (approximately 2 times the maximum recommended daily inhalation dose of levalbuterol tartrate for adults on a $mg/m^2$ basis) and in 10 of 108 (9.3%) fetuses at 2.5 mg/kg/day (approximately 20 times the maximum recommended daily inhalation dose of levalbuterol tartrate for adults on a $mg/m^2$ basis). The drug did not induce cleft palate formation when administered subcutaneously at a dose of 0.025 mg/kg/day (less than the maximum recommended daily inhalation dose of levalbuterol tartrate for adults on a $mg/m^2$ basis). Cleft palate also occurred in 22 of 72 (30.5%) fetuses from females treated subcutaneously with 2.5 mg/kg/day of isoproterenol (positive control).

A reproduction study in Stride Dutch rabbits revealed cranioschisis in 7 of 19 (37%) fetuses when racemic albuterol sulfate was administered orally at a dose of 50 mg/kg/day (approximately 1500 times the maximum recommended daily inhalation dose of levalbuterol tartrate for adults on a $mg/m^2$ basis).

A study in which pregnant rats were dosed with radiolabeled racemic albuterol sulfate demonstrated that drug-related material is transferred from the maternal circulation to the fetus.

There are no adequate and well-controlled studies of XOPENEX HFA Inhalation Aerosol in pregnant women. Because animal reproduction studies are not always predictive of human response, XOPENEX HFA Inhalation Aerosol should be used during pregnancy only if the potential benefit justifies the potential risk to the fetus.

During marketing experience of racemic albuterol, various congenital anomalies, including cleft palate and limb defects, have been rarely reported in the offspring of patients being treated with racemic albuterol. Some of the mothers were taking multiple medications during their pregnancies. No consistent pattern of defects can be discerned, and a relationship between racemic albuterol use and congenital anomalies has not been established.

**Use in Labor and Delivery** Because of the potential for beta-adrenergic agonists to interfere with uterine contractility, the use of XOPENEX HFA Inhalation Aerosol for the treatment of bronchospasm during labor should be restricted to those patients in whom the benefits clearly outweigh the risk.

**Tocolysis** XOPENEX HFA Inhalation Aerosol has not been approved for the management of preterm labor. The benefit:risk ratio when levalbuterol tartrate is administered for tocolysis has not been established. Serious adverse reactions, including maternal pulmonary edema, have been reported during or following treatment of premature labor with beta2-agonists, including racemic albuterol.

**Nursing Mothers** Plasma concentrations of levalbuterol after inhalation of therapeutic doses are very low in humans. It is not known whether levalbuterol is excreted in human milk.

Because of the potential for tumorigenicity shown for racemic albuterol in animal studies and the lack of experience with the use of XOPENEX HFA Inhalation Aerosol by nursing mothers, a decision should be made whether to discontinue nursing or to discontinue the drug, taking into account the importance of the drug to the mother. Caution should be exercised when XOPENEX HFA Inhalation Aerosol is administered to a nursing woman.

**Pediatrics** The safety and efficacy of XOPENEX HFA Inhalation Aerosol have been established in pediatric patients 4 years of age and older in an adequate and well-controlled clinical trial. Use of XOPENEX HFA Inhalation Aerosol in children is also supported by evidence from adequate and well-controlled studies of XOPENEX HFA Inhalation Aerosol in adults, considering that the pathophysiology, systemic exposure of the drug, and clinical profile in pediatric and adult patients are substantially similar. Safety and effectiveness of XOPENEX HFA Inhalation Aerosol in pediatric patients below the age of 4 years have not been established.

**Geriatrics** Clinical studies of XOPENEX HFA Inhalation Aerosol did not include sufficient numbers of subjects aged 65 and older to determine whether they respond differently from younger subjects. Other reported clinical experience has not identified differences in responses between the elderly and younger patients. In general, dose selection for an elderly patient should be cautious, usually starting at the low end of the dosing range, reflecting the greater frequency of decreased hepatic, renal, or cardiac function, and of concomitant diseases or other drug therapy.

Albuterol is known to be substantially excreted by the kidney, and the risk of toxic reactions may be greater in patients with impaired renal function. Because elderly patients are more likely to have decreased renal function, care should be taken in dose selection, and it may be useful to monitor renal function.

**ADVERSE REACTIONS** Adverse event information concerning XOPENEX HFA (levalbuterol tartrate) Inhalation Aerosol in adults and adolescents is derived from two 8-week, multicenter, randomized, double-blind, active- and placebo-controlled trials in 748 adult and adolescent patients with asthma that compared XOPENEX HFA Inhalation Aerosol, a marketed albuterol HFA inhaler, and an HFA-134a placebo inhaler. The following lists the incidence (% XOPENEX HFA 90 mcg, marketed albuterol HFA inhaler 180 mcg, placebo, respectively) of all adverse events (whether considered by the investigator to be related or unrelated to drug) from these trials that occurred at a rate of 2% or greater in the group treated with XOPENEX HFA Inhalation Aerosol and more frequently than in the HFA-134a placebo inhaler group. Body as a whole: pain (4.0%, 3.4%, 3.6%). Central nervous system: dizziness (2.7%, 0.6%, 1.8%). Respiratory system: asthma (9.4%, 7.3%, 6.0%), pharyngitis (7.9%, 2.2%, 2.4%), rhinitis (7.4%, 2.2%, 3.0%).

Adverse events reported by less than 2% and at least 2 or more of the adolescent and adult patients receiving XOPENEX HFA Inhalation Aerosol and by a greater proportion than receiving HFA-134a placebo inhaler include cyst, flu syndrome, viral infection, constipation, gastroenteritis, myalgia, hypertension, epistaxis, lung disorder, acne, herpes simplex, conjunctivitis, ear pain, dysmenorrhea, hematuria, and vaginal moniliasis. There were no significant laboratory abnormalities observed in these studies.

Adverse event information concerning XOPENEX HFA Inhalation Aerosol in children is derived from a 4-week, randomized, double-blind trial of XOPENEX HFA Inhalation Aerosol, a marketed albuterol HFA inhaler, and an HFA-134a placebo inhaler in 150 children aged 4 to 11 years with asthma. The following lists the adverse events (% XOPENEX HFA 90 mcg, marketed albuterol HFA inhaler 180 mcg, placebo, respectively) reported for XOPENEX HFA Inhalation Aerosol in children at a rate of 2% or greater and more frequently than for placebo. Body as a whole: accidental injury (9.2%, 10.3%, 5.7%). Digestive system: vomiting (10.5%, 7.7%, 5.7%). Respiratory system: bronchitis (2.6%, 0%, 0%), pharyngitis (6.6%, 12.8%, 5.7%).

The incidence of systemic beta-adrenergic adverse effects (e.g., tremor, nervousness) was low and comparable across all treatment groups, including placebo.

**Postmarketing** In addition to the adverse events reported in clinical trials, the following adverse events have been observed in postapproval use of levalbuterol inhalation solution. These events have been chosen for inclusion due to their seriousness, their frequency of reporting, or their likely beta-mediated mechanism: angioedema, anaphylaxis, arrhythmias (including atrial fibrillation, supraventricular tachycardia, extrasystoles), asthma, chest pain, cough increased, dyspnea, nausea, nervousness, rash, tachycardia, tremor, urticaria. Because these events have been reported spontaneously from a population of unknown size, estimates of frequency cannot be made.

In addition, XOPENEX HFA Inhalation Aerosol, like other sympathomimetic agents, can cause adverse reactions such as hypertension, angina, vertigo, central nervous system stimulation, sleeplessness, headache, and drying or irritation of the oropharynx.

Rx only.

SEPRACOR 12/05

**PEDIARIX™ [Diphtheria and Tetanus Toxoids and Acellular Pertussis Adsorbed, Hepatitis B (Recombinant) and Inactivated Poliovirus Vaccine Combined]**

The following is a brief summary only; see full prescribing information for complete product information.

**CONTRAINDICATIONS:** Hypersensitivity to any component of the vaccine, including yeast, neomycin, and polymyxin B, is a contraindication (see DESCRIPTION in complete prescribing information). Do not use PEDIARIX after a serious allergic reaction (e.g., anaphylaxis) temporally associated with a previous dose of this vaccine or with any components of this vaccine. Because of the uncertainty as to which component of the vaccine might be responsible, do not give further vaccination with any of these components; or, refer such individuals to an allergist for evaluation. The following events are contraindications to administration of PEDIARIX: encephalopathy (e.g., coma, decreased level of consciousness, prolonged seizures) within 7 days of administration of a previous dose of a pertussis-containing vaccine that is not attributable to another identifiable cause; progressive neurologic disorder, including infantile spasms, uncontrolled epilepsy, or progressive encephalopathy. Do not vaccinate individuals with such conditions until a treatment regimen has been established and the condition has stabilized. PEDIARIX is not contraindicated for use in individuals with HIV infection.

**WARNINGS:** Administration of PEDIARIX is associated with higher rates of fever relative to separately administered vaccines. In one study that evaluated medically attended fever after the first dose of PEDIARIX or separately administered vaccines, infants who received PEDIARIX had a higher rate of medical encounters for fever within the first 4 days following vaccination. In some infants, these encounters included the performance of diagnostic studies to evaluate other causes of fever (see ADVERSE REACTIONS). The vial stopper is latex-free. The tip cap and the rubber plunger of the needleless prefilled syringes contain dry natural latex rubber that may cause allergic reactions in latex sensitive individuals. If any of the following events occur in temporal relation to receipt of whole-cell DTP or a vaccine containing an acellular pertussis component, consider carefully whether to give subsequent doses of PEDIARIX or any vaccine containing a pertussis component: temperature of ≥40.5°C (105°F) within 48 hours not due to another identifiable cause; collapse or shock-like state (hypotonic-hyporesponsive episode) within 48 hours; persistent, inconsolable crying lasting ≥3 hours, occurring within 48 hours; seizures with or without fever occurring within 3 days. If Guillain-Barré syndrome occurs within 6 weeks of receipt of prior vaccine containing tetanus toxoid, the decision to give subsequent doses of PEDIARIX or any vaccine containing tetanus toxoid should be based on careful consideration of the potential benefits and possible risks. A committee of the Institute of Medicine (IOM) has concluded that evidence is consistent with a causal relationship between whole-cell DTP vaccine and acute neurologic illness, and under special circumstances, between whole-cell DTP vaccine and chronic neurologic disease in the context of the National Childhood Encephalopathy Study (NCES) report; however, evidence was insufficient to indicate whether or not whole-cell DTP vaccine increased the overall risk of chronic neurologic disease. Acute encephalopathy and permanent neurologic damage have not been reported causally linked or in temporal association with administration of PEDIARIX, but the experience with PEDIARIX is insufficient to rule this out. Encephalopathy has been reported following INFANRIX® (Diphtheria and Tetanus Toxoids and Acellular Pertussis Vaccine Adsorbed) (see ADVERSE REACTIONS, Postmarketing Reports), but data are not sufficient to evaluate a causal relationship. The decision to administer a pertussis-containing vaccine to children with stable central nervous system (CNS) disorders must be made by the physician on an individual basis, with consideration of all relevant factors, and assessment of potential risks and benefits for that individual. Advise the parent or guardian of the potential increased risk involved (see PRECAUTIONS). A family history of seizures or other CNS disorders is not a contraindication to pertussis vaccine. For children at higher risk for seizures than the general population, an appropriate antipyretic may be administered at the time of vaccination and for the ensuing 24 hours according to the respective prescribing information recommended dosage to reduce the possibility of post-vaccination fever. Defer vaccination during the course of a moderate or severe illness with or without fever and vaccinate patients as soon as they have recovered from the acute phase of the illness. Do not give PEDIARIX to children on anticoagulant therapy or those with bleeding disorders unless the potential benefit clearly outweighs the risk of administration (see PRECAUTIONS in complete prescribing information).

**PRECAUTIONS:** Before the injection of any biological, the physician should take all reasonable precautions to prevent allergic or other adverse reactions. Epinephrine injection (1:1000) and other appropriate agents used for the control of immediate allergic reactions must be immediately available should an acute anaphylactic reaction occur. Immunosuppressed individuals, including those receiving immunosuppressive therapy, may not develop the expected immune response. **Drug Interactions:** For information regarding concomitant administration with other vaccines, refer to DOSAGE AND ADMINISTRATION in complete prescribing information. Do not mix PEDIARIX with any other vaccine in the same syringe or vial. **Carcinogenesis, Mutagenesis, Impairment of Fertility:** PEDIARIX has not been evaluated for carcinogenic or mutagenic potential, or for impairment of fertility. **Pregnancy:** Pregnancy Category C: PEDIARIX is not indicated for women of child-bearing age. Animal reproduction studies have not been conducted with PEDIARIX. It is not known whether PEDIARIX can cause fetal harm when administered to a pregnant woman or if PEDIARIX can affect reproductive capacity. **Geriatric Use:** PEDIARIX is not indicated for use in adult populations. **Pediatric Use:** Safety and effectiveness of PEDIARIX in infants younger than 6 weeks of age have not been evaluated (see DOSAGE AND ADMINISTRATION in complete prescribing information). PEDIARIX is not recommended for persons 7 years of age or older. Tetanus and Diphtheria Toxoids Adsorbed (Td) For Adult Use, inactivated poliovirus vaccine (IPV), and Hepatitis B Vaccine (Recombinant) should be used in individuals 7 years of age or older.

**ADVERSE REACTIONS:** A total of 20,739 doses of PEDIARIX have been administered to 7,028 infants as a 3-dose primary series. The most common adverse reactions observed in clinical trials were local injection site reactions (pain, redness, or swelling), fever, and fussiness. In comparative studies, administration of PEDIARIX was associated with higher rates of fever relative to separately administered vaccines (see WARNINGS). The prevalence of fever was highest on the day of vaccination and the day following vaccination. More than 98% of episodes of fever resolved within the 4-day period following vaccination (i.e., the period including the day of vaccination and the next 3 days). Rates of most other solicited adverse events following PEDIARIX were comparable to rates observed following separately administered US-licensed vaccines. The adverse event information from clinical trials provides a basis for identifying adverse events that appear to be related to vaccine use and for approximating rates. However, because clinical trials are conducted under widely varying conditions, adverse event rates observed in the clinical trials of a vaccine cannot be directly compared to rates in the clinical trials of another vaccine, and may not reflect the rates observed in practice. A total of 5,472 infants were enrolled in a German safety study that was originally designed to compare the safety and reactogenicity of PEDIARIX administered concomitantly at separate sites with 1 of 4 *Haemophilus influenzae* type b (Hib) vaccines at 3, 4, and 5 months of age. After enrollment of 1,569 infants, the study was amended to include a control group that received INFANRIX, Hib vaccine, and oral poliovirus vaccine (OPV) separately. Infants in the separate administration group received one less antigen (hepatitis B) than the infants who received PEDIARIX. Safety data were available for 4,666 infants who received PEDIARIX administered concomitantly at separate sites with 1 of 4 Hib vaccines and for 768 infants in the control group that received separate vaccines. The primary end-point of the study was the percentage of infants with any grade 3 solicited symptom (redness or swelling >20 mm, fever >103.1°F, or crying, pain, vomiting, diarrhea, loss of appetite, or restlessness that prevented normal daily activities) over the 3-dose primary series in infants who received PEDIARIX (4 groups that received PEDIARIX and Hib vaccines pooled) compared to the group that received INFANRIX and Hib vaccine separately with OPV. Analysis for the primary end-point was performed on the according-to-protocol (ATP) cohort that included only those infants who were enrolled after the protocol amendment to include a control group. Of 3,773 infants in the ATP cohort for whom safety data were available, 16.2% (95% CI: 14.9% to 17.5%) of 3,029 infants who received PEDIARIX and Hib vaccine compared to 20.3% (95% CI: 17.5% to 23.4%) of 744 infants who received separate vaccines were reported to have had at least one grade 3 solicited symptom within 4 days of vaccination (i.e., day of vaccination and the next 3 days). The difference between groups in the rate of grade 3 symptoms was 4.1% (90% CI: 1.4% to 7.1%). These were the rates for selected solicited symptoms within 4 days following each dose in a 3-dose primary series in infants who received PEDIARIX administered concomitantly with Hib vaccine and those who received separate concomitant administration of INFANRIX, Hib vaccine, and OPV for the intent-to-treat (ITT) cohort (includes all infants enrolled before and after the amendment who received the indicated vaccine and for whom at least one symptom sheet was completed):

**Percentage of German Infants With Solicited Local Reactions or Selected Systemic Adverse Events Within 4 Days of Vaccination* (ITT Cohort)**

| | PEDIARIX & Hib | | | INFANRIX, Hib, & OPV | | |
|---|---|---|---|---|---|---|
| | Dose 1 | Dose 2 | Dose 3 | Dose 1 | Dose 2 | Dose 3 |
| **N** | **4,666** | **4,619** | **4,574** | **768** | **757** | **750** |
| **Local†** | | | | | | |
| Pain, any | 14.0 | 10.2 | 9.9 | 14.2 | 9.8 | 8.1 |
| Pain, grade 2 or 3 | 2.9 | 1.2 | 1.5 | 3.6 | 1.7 | 1.1 |
| Pain, grade 3 | 0.7 | 0.3 | 0.3 | 1.3 | 0.4 | 0.1 |
| Redness, any | 18.6 | 26.6 | 25.6 | 16.1 | 21.4 | 20.8 |
| Redness, >5 mm | 6.7 | 9.9 | 9.0 | 5.9 | 8.2 | 7.7 |
| Redness, >20 mm | 1.2 | 1.0 | 1.1 | 1.8 | 0.7 | 1.1 |
| Swelling, any | 12.7 | 18.5 | 18.4 | 9.6 | 12.9 | 13.6 |
| Swelling, >5 mm | 5.6 | 7.7 | 7.8 | 3.6 | 5.2 | 4.8 |
| Swelling, >20 mm | 1.2 | 1.6 | 1.5 | 1.3 | 1.1 | 1.2 |
| **Systemic** | | | | | | |
| Restlessness, any | 41.4 | 32.0 | 26.7 | 46.4 | 35.0 | 27.6 |
| Restlessness, grade 2 or 3 | 14.4 | 10.0 | 8.9 | 20.2 | 11.5 | 8.4 |
| Restlessness, grade 3 | 3.0 | 1.5 | 1.6 | 5.7 | 3.0 | 1.7 |
| Fever‡, ≥100.4°F | 25.1 | 19.3 | 19.7 | 13.2 | 13.1 | 11.2 |
| Fever‡, >101.3°F | 5.8 | 4.1 | 4.6 | 2.2 | 2.8 | 2.1 |
| Fever‡, >103.1°F | 0.3 | 0.5 | 0.7 | 0.3 | 0.3 | 0.5 |
| Unusual cry§, any | 24.9 | 16.5 | 13.1 | 36.5 | 19.7 | 14.3 |
| Unusual cry§, grade 2 or 3 | 12.7 | 7.1 | 5.7 | 20.8 | 10.0 | 5.7 |
| Unusual cry§, grade 3 | 3.9 | 1.7 | 1.4 | 6.8 | 2.1 | 1.1 |
| Loss of appetite, any | 17.9 | 13.3 | 12.5 | 19.1 | 16.2 | 11.3 |
| Loss of appetite, grade 2 or 3 | 4.0 | 2.9 | 2.7 | 4.4 | 2.9 | 2.3 |
| Loss of appetite, grade 3 | 0.6 | 0.5 | 0.4 | 0.5 | 0.7 | 0.0 |

N = number of infants in the intent-to-treat (ITT) cohort.
Grade 2 defined as sufficiently discomforting to interfere with daily activities.
Grade 3 defined as preventing normal daily activities.
* Within 4 days of vaccination defined as day of vaccination and the next 3 days.
† Local reactions at the injection site for PEDIARIX or INFANRIX.
‡ Rectal temperatures.
§ Unusual cry lasting >1 hour.

In this study, infants were also monitored for unsolicited adverse events that occurred within 30 days following vaccination. Over the entire study period, 6 subjects in the group that received PEDIARIX reported seizures. Two of these subjects had a febrile seizure, 1 of whom also developed afebrile seizures. The remaining 4 subjects had afebrile seizures, including 2 with infantile spasms. Two subjects reported seizures within 7 days following vaccination (1 subject had both febrile and afebrile seizures, and 1 subject had afebrile seizures), corresponding to a rate of 0.22 seizures per 1,000 doses (febrile seizures 0.07 per 1,000 doses, afebrile seizures 0.14 per 1,000 doses). No subject who received concomitant INFANRIX, Hib vaccine, and OPV reported seizures. In a separate German study that evaluated the safety of INFANRIX in 22,505 infants who received 66,867 doses of INFANRIX administered as a 3-dose primary series, the rate of seizures within 7 days of vaccination with INFANRIX was 0.13 per 1,000 doses (febrile seizures 0.0 per 1,000 doses, afebrile seizures 0.13 per 1,000 doses). No cases of hypotonic-hyporesponsiveness, encephalopathy, or anaphylaxis were reported in the German study that evaluated the safety of PEDIARIX. Rates of serious adverse events that are less common than those reported in this safety study are not known at this time.

Additional safety data for PEDIARIX are available from a US study designed to evaluate lot-to-lot consistency and a bridge for a new manufacturing step. These were the rates for local reactions and selected adverse events within 4 days of vaccination with PEDIARIX administered concomitantly with a Hib vaccine at 2, 4, and 6 months of age:

**Percentage of US Infants With Solicited Local Reactions or Selected Systemic Adverse Events Within 4 Days of Vaccination* (ITT Cohort)**

| | PEDIARIX & Hib | | |
|---|---|---|---|
| | Dose 1 | Dose 2 | Dose 3 |
| **Local†** | **N = 482** | **N = 469** | **N = 466** |
| Pain, any | 30.5 | 25.4 | 23.0 |
| Pain, grade 2 or 3 | 6.2 | 5.5 | 3.6 |
| Pain, grade 3 | 1.2 | 0.6 | 0.6 |
| Redness, any | 25.3 | 32.6 | 35.6 |
| Redness, >5 mm | 9.3 | 10.4 | 8.6 |
| Redness, >20 mm | 0.6 | 1.5 | 1.3 |
| Swelling, any | 15.1 | 16.6 | 22.3 |
| Swelling, >5 mm | 6.8 | 6.2 | 6.4 |
| Swelling, >20 mm | 1.0 | 1.3 | 1.3 |
| **Systemic** | **N = 482** | **N = 469** | **N = 467** |
| Restlessness, any | 28.8 | 30.3 | 28.5 |
| Restlessness, grade 2 or 3 | 7.1 | 9.0 | 9.4 |
| Restlessness, grade 3 | 1.0 | 1.1 | 0.6 |
| Fever‡, ≥100.4°F | 26.6 | 31.3 | 25.9 |
| Fever‡, >101.3°F | 2.9 | 6.2 | 4.7 |
| Fever‡, >103.1°F | 0.0 | 0.2 | 0.6 |
| Fussiness, any | 61.8 | 63.8 | 57.0 |
| Fussiness, grade 2 or 3 | 14.9 | 21.5 | 17.1 |
| Fussiness, grade 3 | 2.7 | 3.4 | 1.7 |
| Loss of appetite, any | 21.6 | 19.8 | 18.8 |
| Loss of appetite, grade 2 or 3 | 3.1 | 3.2 | 2.4 |
| Loss of appetite, grade 3 | 0.2 | 0.4 | 0.0 |
| Sleeping more than usual, any | 46.7 | 31.8 | 28.1 |
| Sleeping more than usual, grade 2 or 3 | 10.2 | 6.0 | 4.7 |
| Sleeping more than usual, grade 3 | 1.7 | 0.4 | 0.6 |

N = number of infants in the intent-to-treat (ITT) cohort (infants who received the indicated vaccine and for whom at least one symptom sheet was completed).
Grade 2 defined as sufficiently discomforting to interfere with daily activities.
Grade 3 defined as preventing normal daily activities.
* Within 4 days of vaccination defined as day of vaccination and the next 3 days.
† Local reactions at the injection site for PEDIARIX.
‡ Rectal temperatures.

In another US study, these were the rates for fever within 4 days following dose 1 (i.e., day of vaccination and the next 3 days) at 2 months of age in infants who received PEDIARIX when administered concomitantly at separate sites with Hib and pneumococcal conjugate vaccines and those who received INFANRIX, ENGERIX-B® [Hepatitis B Vaccine (Recombinant)], IPV, Hib vaccine, and pneumococcal conjugate vaccine:

**Percentage of US Infants With Fever Within 4 Days of Dose 1* (ITT Cohort)**

| | PEDIARIX, Hib, & Pneumococcal Conjugate (N = 667) | INFANRIX, ENGERIX-B, IPV, Hib, & Pneumococcal Conjugate (N = 333) | Separate Vaccine Group Minus Combination Vaccine Group |
|---|---|---|---|
| **Fever†** | **%** | **%** | **Difference (95% CI)** |
| ≥100.4°F‡ | 27.9 | 19.8 | -8.07 (-13.54, -2.60) |
| >101.3°F | 7.0 | 4.5 | -2.54 (-5.50, 0.41) |
| >102.2°F‡ | 2.2 | 0.3 | -1.95 (-3.22, -0.68) |
| >103.1°F | 0.4 | 0.0 | -0.45 (-0.96, 0.06) |
| M.A.‡ | 1.2 | 0.0 | -1.20 (-2.03, -037) |

N = number of infants for whom at least one symptom sheet was completed, excluding 3 infants for whom temperature was not measured and 3 infants whose temperature was measured by the tympanic method.
*Within 4 days of dose 1 defined as day of vaccination and the next 3 days.
† Rectal temperatures.
‡ The group that received PEDIARIX compared to separate vaccine group p value <0.05 (2-sided Fisher Exact test) or the 95% confidence interval on the difference between groups does not include 0.
M.A. = Medically attended (a visit to or from medical personnel).

In this study, medical attention (a visit to or from medical personnel) for fever within 4 days following vaccination was sought for 8 infants who received PEDIARIX (1.2%) and no infants who received separately administered vaccines. Four infants were seen by medical personnel in an office setting; no diagnostic tests were performed in 2 of the infants and a complete blood count (CBC) was done in the other 2 infants. Of 3 infants who were seen in an emergency room, all had a CBC and a blood and urine culture performed; chest X-rays were done in 2 of the infants and a nasopharyngeal specimen was tested for Respiratory Syncytial Virus in one of the infants. One infant was hospitalized for a work-up that included a CBC, blood and urine cultures, a lumbar puncture, and a chest X-ray. All episodes of medically attended fever resolved within 4 days post-vaccination.

Limited data are available from a study conducted in Moldova in which infants received a dose of hepatitis B vaccine within 48 hours of birth followed by 3 doses of PEDIARIX at 6, 10, and 14 weeks of age. No information was collected on the HBsAg status of mothers of enrolled infants. These were the rates for local reactions and selected adverse events within 4 days of vaccination with PEDIARIX administered comcomitantly with Hib vaccine following a birth dose of hepatitis B vaccine:

**Percentage of Moldovan Infants With Solicited Local Reactions or Selected Systemic Adverse Events Within 4 Days of Vaccination* (ITT Cohort)**

| | PEDIARIX & Hib | | |
|---|---|---|---|
| | Dose 1 | Dose 2 | Dose 3 |
| **N** | **160** | **158** | **157** |
| **Local†** | | | |
| Pain, any | 25.6 | 18.4 | 14.0 |
| Pain, grade 3 | 3.1 | 0.6 | 1.9 |
| Redness, any | 41.9 | 41.8 | 47.1 |
| Redness, >20 mm | 1.9 | 2.5 | 4.5 |
| Swelling, any | 20.6 | 18.4 | 28.0 |
| Swelling, >20 mm | 4.4 | 2.5 | 7.0 |
| **Systemic** | | | |
| Restlessness, any | 13.1 | 10.8 | 8.9 |
| Restlessness, grade 3 | 1.3 | 0.6 | 0.6 |
| Fever‡, ≥100.4°F | 14.4 | 11.4 | 5.1 |
| Fever‡, >103.1°F | 0.0 | 0.6 | 0.0 |
| Fussiness, any | 25.0 | 21.5 | 17.8 |
| Fussiness, grade 3 | 2.5 | 0.6 | 0.6 |

N = number of infants in the intent-to-treat (ITT) cohort (infants who received the indicated vaccine and for whom at least one symptom sheet was completed).
Grade 3 defined as preventing normal daily activities.
*Within 4 days of vaccination defined as day of vaccination and the next 3 days.
† Local reactions at the injection site for PEDIARIX.
‡ Rectal temperatures.

Although there was no comparator group who received PEDIARIX without a birth dose of hepatitis B vaccine, available data suggest that some local adverse events may occur at a higher rate when PEDIARIX is administered after a birth dose of hepatitis B vaccine.

As with any vaccine, there is the possibility that broad use of PEDIARIX could reveal adverse events not observed in clinical trials.

**Postmarketing Reports:** Worldwide voluntary reports of adverse events received for INFANRIX and ENGERIX-B in children younger than 7 years of age since market introduction of these US-licensed vaccines are listed below. This list includes adverse events for which 20 or more reports were received with the exception of intussusception, idiopathic thrombocytopenic purpura, thrombocytopenia, anaphylactic reaction, angioedema, encephalopathy, hypotonic-hyporesponsive episode, and alopecia for which fewer than 20 reports were received. These latter events are included either because of the seriousness of the event or the strength of causal connection to components of this or other vaccines or drugs. *Body as a whole:* Asthenia[b], fever[a+b], lethargy[b], malaise[b], Sudden Infant Death Syndrome[a+b]. *Cardiovascular system:* Cyanosis[a+b], edema[b], pallor[b]. *Gastrointestinal system:* Abdominal pain[b], anorexia[b], diarrhea[a+b], intussusception[a+b], nausea[b], vomiting[a+b]. *Hematologic/lymphatic:* Idiopathic thrombocytopenic purpura[a+b], lymphadenopathy[a], thrombocytopenia[a+b]. *Hepatic:* Jaundice[b], liver function tests abnormal[b]. *Hypersensitivity:* Anaphylactic reaction[a+b], angioedema[b], hypersensitivity[a]. *Infections:* Cellulitis[a]. *Injection site reactions:* Injection site reactions[a+b]. *Musculoskeletal:* Arthralgia[b], limb swelling[a+b]. *Nervous system:* Convulsions[a+b], encephalopathy[a], headache[b], hypotonia[a+b], hypotonic-hyporesponsive episode[a], somnolence[a+b]. *Psychiatric:* Crying[a+b], irritability[a+b]. *Respiratory system:* Respiratory tract infection[a]. *Skin and appendages:* Alopecia[b], erythema[a+b], erythema multiforme[b], petechiae[b], pruritus[a+b], rash[a+b], urticaria[a+b]. *Special senses:* Ear pain[a]. [[a] Following INFANRIX; [b] Following ENGERIX-B; [a+b] Following either INFANRIX or ENGERIX-B.] These reactions were reported voluntarily from a population of uncertain size; therefore, it is not always possible to reliably estimate their frequency or establish a causal relationship to vaccination.

**Reporting Adverse Events:** Report the occurrence following immunization of any event set forth in the Vaccine Injury Table from the National Childhood Vaccine Injury Act including: Anaphylaxis or anaphylactic shock within 7 days, encephalopathy or encephalitis within 7 days, brachial neuritis within 28 days, or an acute complication or sequelae (including death) of an illness, disability, injury, or condition referred to above, or any events that would contraindicate further doses of PEDIARIX. The VAERS toll-free number is 1-800-822-7967.

Manufactured by **GlaxoSmithKline Biologicals**, Rixensart, Belgium, US License 1617

Distributed by **GlaxoSmithKline,** Research Triangle Park, NC 27709



Full prescribing information for PEDIARIX is available at www.GSKVaccines.com/Pediarix. BRS-PE:L2

 Printed in USA. PED583R0 June 2005

# ARCHIVES OF PEDIATRICS & ADOLESCENT MEDICINE

FEBRUARY 2006 VOLUME 160, NUMBER 2 PAGES 113-224

## ARTICLES

**Randomized Controlled Trial of a Primary Care and Home-Based Intervention for Physical Activity and Nutrition Behaviors: PACE+ for Adolescents** 128
*Kevin Patrick, MD, MS; Karen J. Calfas, PhD; Gregory J. Norman, PhD; Marion F. Zabinski, PhD, MPH; James F. Sallis, PhD; Joan Rupp, MS, RD; Jennifer Covin, MPH; John Cella, MD*

**Prevalence of the Female Athlete Triad Syndrome Among High School Athletes** 137
*Jeanne F. Nichols, PhD; Mitchell J. Rauh, PhD, PT, MPH; Mandra J. Lawson, MS, RD; Ming Ji, PhD; Hava-Shoshana Barkai, MS*

**Drug Testing of Adolescents in Ambulatory Medicine: Physician Practices and Knowledge** 146
*Sharon Levy, MD, MPH; Sion Kim Harris, PhD; Lon Sherritt, MPH; Michelle Angulo, BA; John R. Knight, MD*

**Association of Condom Use, Sexual Behaviors, and Sexually Transmitted Infections With the Duration of Genital Human Papillomavirus Infection Among Adolescent Women** 151
*Marcia L. Shew, MD, MPH; J. Dennis Fortenberry, MD, MS; Wanzhu Tu, PhD; Beth E. Juliar, MA, MS; Byron E. Batteiger, MD; Brahim Qadadri, BS; Darron R. Brown, MD*

**Effect of Telephone Reminder/Recall on Adolescent Immunization and Preventive Visits: Results From a Randomized Clinical Trial** 157
*Peter G. Szilagyi, MD, MPH; Stanley Schaffer, MD, MS; Richard Barth, BS; Laura P. Shone, MSW, DrPH; Sharon G. Humiston, MD, MPH; Sandra Ambrose, MBA; Francisco Averhoff, MD, MPH*

**Simulating Cost-effectiveness of Fluoride Varnish During Well-Child Visits for Medicaid-Enrolled Children** 164
*Rocio B. Quiñonez, DMD, MS, MPH; Sally C. Stearns, PhD; Bhavna S. Talekar, BDS, MPH; R. Gary Rozier, DDS, MPH; Stephen M. Downs, MD, MPH*

**Neonatal Abstinence Syndrome After In Utero Exposure to Selective Serotonin Reuptake Inhibitors in Term Infants** 173
*Rachel Levinson-Castiel, MD; Paul Merlob, MD; Nehama Linder, MD; Lea Sirota, MD; Gil Klinger, MD*

**Access to Health Care for Young Adults With Disabling Chronic Conditions** 178
*S. Todd Callahan, MD, MPH; William O. Cooper, MD, MPH*

**Developmental Status and Service Use Among Children in the Child Welfare System: A National Survey** 183
*Michelle H. Zimmer, MD; Laura M. Panko, MD*

## SPECIAL FEATURE

**Picture of the Month** 189
*Kimberly A. Horii, MD; Amy Jo Nopper, MD; Vidya Sharma, MBBS, MPH*

## ARTICLES

**A Successful International Child Health Elective: The University of Colorado Department of Pediatrics' Experience** 191
*Steven G. Federico, MD; Pamela A. Zachar, MD; Claire M. Oravec; Tessa Mandler; Edward Goldson, MD; Jeff Brown, MD, MPH*

**Antipyretic Treatment in Young Children With Fever: Acetaminophen, Ibuprofen, or Both Alternating in a Randomized, Double-blind Study** 197
*E. Michael Sarrell, MD; Eliahu Wielunsky, MD; Herman Avner Cohen, MD*

**Variation of Cognition and Achievement With Sleep-Disordered Breathing in Full-term and Preterm Children** 203
*Judy L. Emancipator, MS; Amy Storfer-Isser, MS; H. Gerry Taylor, PhD; Carol L. Rosen, MD; H. L. Kirchner, PhD; Nathan L. Johnson, MS; Anne Marie Zambito, MPH; Susan Redline, MD, MPH*

**Effect on Hospital-Wide Sedation Practices After Implementation of the 2001 JCAHO Procedural Sedation and Analgesia Guidelines** 211
*Raymond Pitetti, MD, MPH; Peter J. Davis, MD; Robert Redlinger, RN, MSN; Jean White, RN; Eugene Wiener, MD; Karen H. Calhoun, BSN, MBA*

ARCHIVES OF PEDIATRICS & ADOLESCENT MEDICINE

## EDITORIAL

**Obesity Prevention in Primary Care** 217
*Thomas N. Robinson, MD, MPH*

## THE PEDIATRIC FORUM

**If You Don't Ask, Parents May Not Tell: Noticing Problems vs Expressing Concerns** 220
*Frances Page Glascoe, PhD*

**In Reply** 220
*Debbie Ehrmann Feldman, PT, PhD; Mélanie Couture, OT, MA; Lisa Grilli, PT, MSc; Marie-Noëlle Simard, OT, MSc; Laurent Azoulay, MSc; Julie Gosselin, OT, PhD*

## CORRECTION

**Error in E-mail Address in: Hearing Screening at Well-Child Visits** 156
*Donna R. Halloran, MD, MSPH; Terry C. Wall, MD, MPH; H. Hughes Evans, MD, PhD; J. Michael Hardin, PhD; Audie L. Woolley, MD*

## REGULAR DEPARTMENTS

**This Month in *Archives of Pediatrics & Adolescent Medicine*** 127

**Announcements** 136, 182, 188, 196

**Classified Advertising** 223

**Journal Advertiser Index** 223

**Contact Information** 224

**Instructions for authors and the author and subject indexes are available on our Web site: http://www.archpediatrics.com. If you do not have access to the Web, contact Suzanne Shuey at (206) 685-3573.**

### *About the Cover*

Photographer: Wayne Larrabee, MD, Seattle, Wash.

# ARCHIVES OF PEDIATRICS & ADOLESCENT MEDICINE


**Mission Statement:** *The Archives of Pediatrics & Adolescent Medicine* is a monthly, peer-reviewed journal for physicians and other health care professionals who contribute to the health of children and adolescents. The *Archives* provides an open forum for dialogue on a full range of clinical, scientific, advocacy, and humanistic issues relevant to the care of pediatric patients from infancy through young adulthood. The *Archives* is a vehicle for increased attention to adolescent health, the education of pediatric health care professionals, and disease prevention and health promotion. The *Archives* publishes original studies, editorials, reviews by experts, practice commentaries, case quizzes, and updates on clinical science and practice management. The Pediatric Forum provides our readers with opportunities to express their views. *Archives* incorporates *AJDC*, the oldest journal in US pediatric literature, which originated in 1911.



JAMA & ARCHIVES JOURNALS
American Medical Association

All articles published, including editorials, letters, and book reviews, represent the opinions of the authors and do not reflect the policy of the American Medical Association, the Editorial Board, or the institution with which the author is affiliated, unless this is clearly specified.

# OMNICEF (cefdinir) for Oral Suspension 250 mg/5 mL

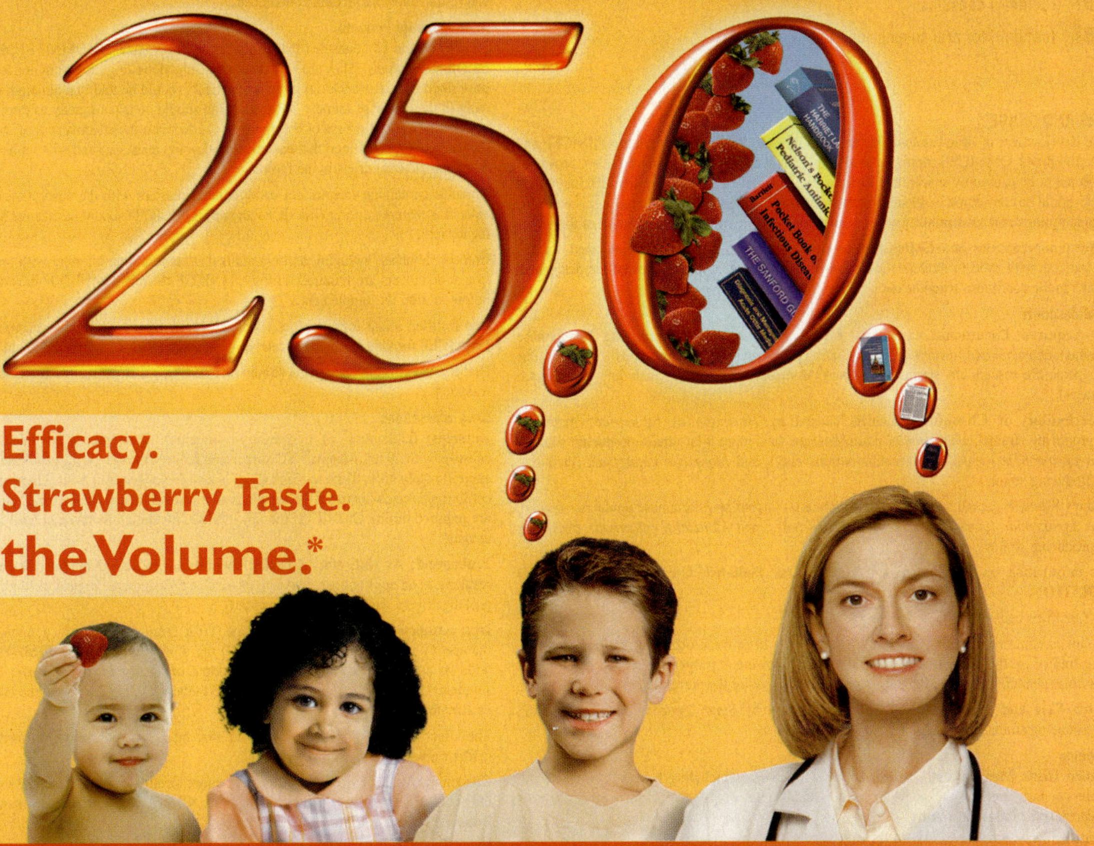


**Great Efficacy.**
**Great Strawberry Taste.**
**Half the Volume.***

## Great Minds... Concentrate on Success!

### Indications (mild to moderate infections)[1]

**Acute Bacterial Otitis Media** and **Acute Maxillary Sinusitis** (adults and adolescents) due to *H influenzae* (including ß-lactamase producing strains), *S pneumoniae* (penicillin-susceptible strains only), and *M catarrhalis* (including ß-lactamase producing strains). Use of cefdinir in the treatment of acute maxillary sinusitis in pediatric patients is supported by evidence from adequate and well-controlled studies in adults and adolescents.

**Pharyngitis/Tonsillitis** due to *S pyogenes*. Cefdinir is effective in the eradication of *S pyogenes* from the oropharynx. Cefdinir has not, however, been studied for the prevention of rheumatic fever following *S pyogenes* pharyngitis/tonsillitis. Only intramuscular penicillin has been demonstrated to be effective for the prevention of rheumatic fever.

**Uncomplicated Skin and Skin Structure Infections** due to *S aureus* (including ß-lactamase producing strains) and *S pyogenes*.

### Important Safety Information[1]

- To reduce the development of drug-resistant bacteria and maintain the effectiveness of OMNICEF and other antibacterial drugs, OMNICEF should be used only to treat or prevent infections that are proven or strongly suspected to be caused by bacteria

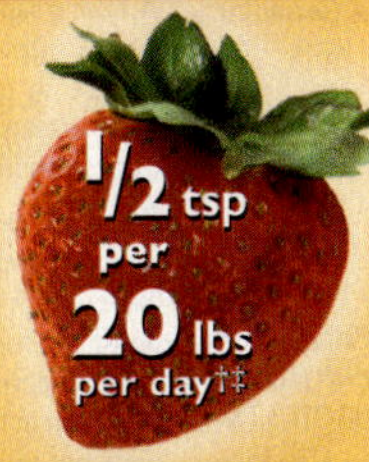


For pediatric patients weighing 20 lbs, use the 125 mg/5 mL product

- OMNICEF is contraindicated in patients with known allergy to the cephalosporin class of antibiotics
- For patients with previous hypersensitivity reaction to penicillins, caution should be exercised because cross-hypersensitivity among ß-lactam antibiotics has been clearly documented. If an allergic reaction to cefdinir occurs, the drug should be discontinued
- Safety and efficacy in neonates and infants less than 6 months of age have not been established
- 2% of 2,289 pediatric patients discontinued medication due to adverse events in US and ex-US clinical trials. Discontinuations were primarily for gastrointestinal disturbance, usually diarrhea
- The most common reported adverse events occurring in ≥1% of pediatric patients in US clinical trials (N=1,783) were diarrhea (8%), rash (3%), and vomiting (1%)
- Maximum dose of OMNICEF for pediatric patients weighing ≥43 kg is 600 mg/day. For pediatric patients with a creatinine clearance of <30 mL/min/1.73 $m^2$ and not requiring hemodialysis, the dose of cefdinir should be 7 mg/kg (up to 300 mg) given once daily
- Antacids that contain magnesium or aluminum and iron supplements, including multivitamins that contain iron, should be taken at least 2 hours before or 2 hours after taking OMNICEF

* Compared to the 125 mg/5 mL formulation of OMNICEF.
† Calculated dose is based on 14 mg/kg/day. Dose in teaspoons is rounded to the nearest 1/4 teaspoon and is not an exact measure of calculated dose volume (mL). 1 tsp ≅ 5 mL.
‡ Once-daily dosing has not been studied in skin infections; therefore, OMNICEF for Oral Suspension should be administered twice daily in this infection (7 mg/kg BID for 10 days).

**Reference: 1.** OMNICEF® (cefdinir) for Oral Suspension Prescribing Information, Abbott Laboratories.

Please see adjacent brief summary of full prescribing information.

**OMNICEF**
(cefdinir) for oral suspension
*125 mg/5 mL and 250 mg/5 mL*

**Expert recommended.**
**Kid preferred.**



astellas Under License of Astellas Pharma Inc. Japan

Abbott A Promise for Life

**PROFESSIONAL BRIEF SUMMARY-CONSULT PACKAGE INSERT FOR FULL PRESCRIBING INFORMATION.**
03-5435-Rev. July, 2005
(Nos. 3769, 3771, 6151)

# Omnicef® (cefdinir) capsules
# Omnicef® (cefdinir) for oral suspension

## Rx only

## INDICATIONS AND USAGE

To reduce the development of drug-resistant bacteria and maintain the effectiveness of OMNICEF and other antibacterial drugs, OMNICEF should be used only to treat or prevent infections that are proven or strongly suspected to be caused by susceptible bacteria. When culture and susceptibility information are available, they should be considered in selecting or modifying antibacterial therapy. In the absence of such data, local epidemiology and susceptibility patterns may contribute to the empiric selection of therapy.

OMNICEF (cefdinir) capsules and OMNICEF (cefdinir) for oral suspension are indicated for the treatment of patients with mild to moderate infections caused by susceptible strains of the designated microorganisms in the conditions listed below.

### Adults and Adolescents

**Community-Acquired Pneumonia** caused by *Haemophilus influenzae* (including β-lactamase producing strains), *Haemophilus parainfluenzae* (including β-lactamase producing strains), *Streptococcus pneumoniae* (penicillin-susceptible strains only), and *Moraxella catarrhalis* (including β-lactamase producing strains).

**Acute Exacerbations of Chronic Bronchitis** caused by *Haemophilus influenzae* (including β-lactamase producing strains), *Haemophilus parainfluenzae* (including β-lactamase producing strains), *Streptococcus pneumoniae* (penicillin-susceptible strains only), and *Moraxella catarrhalis* (including β-lactamase producing strains).

**Acute Maxillary Sinusitis** caused by *Haemophilus influenzae* (including β-lactamase producing strains), *Streptococcus pneumoniae* (penicillin-susceptible strains only), and *Moraxella catarrhalis* (including β-lactamase producing strains).

**NOTE:** For information on use in pediatric patients, see **Pediatric Use** and **DOSAGE AND ADMINISTRATION**.

**Pharyngitis/Tonsillitis** caused by *Streptococcus pyogenes*.

**NOTE:** Cefdinir is effective in the eradication of *S. pyogenes* from the oropharynx. Cefdinir has not, however, been studied for the prevention of rheumatic fever following *S. pyogenes* pharyngitis/tonsillitis. Only intramuscular penicillin has been demonstrated to be effective for the prevention of rheumatic fever.

**Uncomplicated Skin and Skin Structure Infections** caused by *Staphylococcus aureus* (including β-lactamase producing strains) and *Streptococcus pyogenes*.

### Pediatric Patients

**Acute Bacterial Otitis Media** caused by *Haemophilus influenzae* (including β-lactamase producing strains), *Streptococcus pneumoniae* (penicillin-susceptible strains only), and *Moraxella catarrhalis* (including β-lactamase producing strains).

**Pharyngitis/Tonsillitis** caused by *Streptococcus pyogenes*.

**NOTE:** Cefdinir is effective in the eradication of *S. pyogenes* from the oropharynx. Cefdinir has not, however, been studied for the prevention of rheumatic fever following *S. pyogenes* pharyngitis/tonsillitis. Only intramuscular penicillin has been demonstrated to be effective for the prevention of rheumatic fever.

**Uncomplicated Skin and Skin Structure Infections** caused by *Staphylococcus aureus* (including β-lactamase producing strains) and *Streptococcus pyogenes*.

## CONTRAINDICATIONS

OMNICEF (cefdinir) is contraindicated in patients with known allergy to the cephalosporin class of antibiotics.

## WARNINGS

**BEFORE THERAPY WITH OMNICEF (CEFDINIR) IS INSTITUTED, CAREFUL INQUIRY SHOULD BE MADE TO DETERMINE WHETHER THE PATIENT HAS HAD PREVIOUS HYPERSENSITIVITY REACTIONS TO CEFDINIR, OTHER CEPHALOSPORINS, PENICILLINS, OR OTHER DRUGS. IF CEFDINIR IS TO BE GIVEN TO PENICILLIN-SENSITIVE PATIENTS, CAUTION SHOULD BE EXERCISED BECAUSE CROSS-HYPERSENSITIVITY AMONG β-LACTAM ANTIBIOTICS HAS BEEN CLEARLY DOCUMENTED AND MAY OCCUR IN UP TO 10% OF PATIENTS WITH A HISTORY OF PENICILLIN ALLERGY. IF AN ALLERGIC REACTION TO CEFDINIR OCCURS, THE DRUG SHOULD BE DISCONTINUED. SERIOUS ACUTE HYPERSENSITIVITY REACTIONS MAY REQUIRE TREATMENT WITH EPINEPHRINE AND OTHER EMERGENCY MEASURES, INCLUDING OXYGEN, INTRAVENOUS FLUIDS, INTRAVENOUS ANTIHISTAMINES, CORTICOSTEROIDS, PRESSOR AMINES, AND AIRWAY MANAGEMENT, AS CLINICALLY INDICATED.**

**Pseudomembranous colitis has been reported with nearly all antibacterial agents, including cefdinir, and may range in severity from mild- to life-threatening. Therefore, it is important to consider this diagnosis in patients who present with diarrhea subsequent to the administration of antibacterial agents.**

Treatment with antibacterial agents alters the normal flora of the colon and may permit overgrowth of clostridia. Studies indicate that a toxin produced by *Clostridium difficile* is a primary cause of "antibiotic-associated colitis."

After the diagnosis of pseudomembranous colitis has been established, appropriate therapeutic measures should be initiated. Mild cases of pseudomembranous colitis usually respond to drug discontinuation alone. In moderate to severe cases, consideration should be given to management with fluids and electrolytes, protein supplementation, and treatment with an antibacterial drug clinically effective against *Clostridium difficile*.

## PRECAUTIONS

### General

Prescribing OMNICEF in the absence of a proven or strongly suspected bacterial infection or a prophylactic indication is unlikely to provide benefit to the patient and increases the risk of the development of drug-resistant bacteria.

As with other broad-spectrum antibiotics, prolonged treatment may result in the possible emergence and overgrowth of resistant organisms. Careful observation of the patient is essential. If superinfection occurs during therapy, appropriate alternative therapy should be administered.

Cefdinir, as with other broad-spectrum antimicrobials (antibiotics), should be prescribed with caution in individuals with a history of colitis.

In patients with transient or persistent renal insufficiency (creatinine clearance <30 mL/min), the total daily dose of OMNICEF should be reduced because high and prolonged plasma concentrations of cefdinir can result following recommended doses.

### Information for Patients

Patients should be counseled that antibacterial drugs including OMNICEF should only be used to treat bacterial infections. They do not treat viral infections (e.g., the common cold). When OMNICEF is prescribed to treat a bacterial infection, patients should be told that although it is common to feel better early in the course of therapy, the medication should be taken exactly as directed. Skipping doses or not completing the full course of therapy may (1) decrease the effectiveness of the immediate treatment and (2) increase the likelihood that bacteria will develop resistance and will not be treatable by OMNICEF or other antibacterial drugs in the future.

Antacids containing magnesium or aluminum interfere with the absorption of cefdinir. If this type of antacid is required during OMNICEF therapy, OMNICEF should be taken at least 2 hours before or after the antacid.

Iron supplements, including multivitamins that contain iron, interfere with the absorption of cefdinir. If iron supplements are required during OMNICEF therapy, OMNICEF should be taken at least 2 hours before or after the supplement.

Iron-fortified infant formula does not significantly interfere with the absorption of cefdinir. Therefore, OMNICEF for Oral Suspension can be administered with iron-fortified infant formula.

Diabetic patients and caregivers should be aware that the oral suspension contains 2.86 g of sucrose per teaspoon.

### Drug Interactions

**Antacids:** (aluminum- or magnesium-containing): Concomitant administration of 300-mg cefdinir capsules with 30 mL Maalox® TC suspension reduces the rate ($C_{max}$) and extent (AUC) of absorption by approximately 40%. Time to reach $C_{max}$ is also prolonged by 1 hour. There are no significant effects on cefdinir pharmacokinetics if the antacid is administered 2 hours before or 2 hours after cefdinir. If antacids are required during OMNICEF therapy, OMNICEF should be taken at least 2 hours before or after the antacid.

**Probenecid:** As with other β-lactam antibiotics, probenecid inhibits the renal excretion of cefdinir, resulting in an approximate doubling in AUC, a 54% increase in peak cefdinir plasma levels, and a 50% prolongation in the apparent elimination $t_{1/2}$.

**Iron Supplements and Foods Fortified With Iron:** Concomitant administration of cefdinir with a therapeutic iron supplement containing 60 mg of elemental iron (as $FeSO_4$) or vitamins supplemented with 10 mg of elemental iron reduced extent of absorption by 80% and 31%, respectively. If iron supplements are required during OMNICEF therapy, OMNICEF should be taken at least 2 hours before or after the supplement.

The effect of foods highly fortified with elemental iron (primarily iron-fortified breakfast cereals) on cefdinir absorption has not been studied.

Concomitantly administered iron-fortified infant formula (2.2 mg elemental iron/6 oz) has no significant effect on cefdinir pharmacokinetics. Therefore, OMNICEF for Oral Suspension can be administered with iron-fortified infant formula.

There have been reports of reddish stools in patients receiving cefdinir. In many cases, patients were also receiving iron-containing products. The reddish color is due to the formation of a nonabsorbable complex between cefdinir or its breakdown products and iron in the gastrointestinal tract.

### Drug/Laboratory Test Interactions

A false-positive reaction for ketones in the urine may occur with tests using nitroprusside, but not with those using nitroferricyanide. The administration of cefdinir may result in a false-positive reaction for glucose in urine using Clinitest®, Benedict's solution, or Fehling's solution. It is recommended that glucose tests based on enzymatic glucose oxidase reactions (such as Clinistix® or Tes-Tape®) be used. Cephalosporins are known to occasionally induce a positive direct Coombs' test.

### Carcinogenesis, Mutagenesis, Impairment of Fertility

The carcinogenic potential of cefdinir has not been evaluated. No mutagenic effects were seen in the bacterial reverse mutation assay (Ames) or point mutation assay at the hypoxanthine-guanine phosphoribosyltransferase locus (HGPRT) in V79 Chinese hamster lung cells. No clastogenic effects were observed *in vitro* in the structural chromosome aberration assay in V79 Chinese hamster lung cells or *in vivo* in the micronucleus assay in mouse bone marrow. In rats, fertility and reproductive performance were not affected by cefdinir at oral doses up to 1000 mg/kg/day (70 times the human dose based on mg/kg/day, 11 times based on $mg/m^2/day$).

### Pregnancy - Teratogenic Effects

**Pregnancy Category B:** Cefdinir was not teratogenic in rats at oral doses up to 1000 mg/kg/day (70 times the human dose based on mg/kg/day, 11 times based on $mg/m^2/day$) or in rabbits at oral doses up to 10 mg/kg/day (0.7 times the human dose based on mg/kg/day, 0.23 times based on $mg/m^2/day$). Maternal toxicity (decreased body weight gain) was observed in rabbits at the maximum tolerated dose of 10 mg/kg/day without adverse effects on offspring. Decreased body weight occurred in rat fetuses at $\geq$ 100 mg/kg/day, and in rat offspring at $\geq$ 32 mg/kg/day. No effects were observed on maternal reproductive parameters or offspring survival, development, behavior, or reproductive function.

There are, however, no adequate and well-controlled studies in pregnant women. Because animal reproduction studies are not always predictive of human response, this drug should be used during pregnancy only if clearly needed.

### Labor and Delivery

Cefdinir has not been studied for use during labor and delivery.

### Nursing Mothers

Following administration of single 600-mg doses, cefdinir was not detected in human breast milk.

### Pediatric Use

Safety and efficacy in neonates and infants less than 6 months of age have not been established. Use of cefdinir for the treatment of acute maxillary sinusitis in pediatric patients (age 6 months through 12 years) is supported by evidence from adequate and well-controlled studies in adults and adolescents, the similar pathophysiology of acute sinusitis in adult and pediatric patients, and comparative pharmacokinetic data in the pediatric population.

### Geriatric Use

Efficacy is comparable in geriatric patients and younger adults. While cefdinir has been well-tolerated in all age groups, in clinical trials geriatric patients experienced a lower rate of adverse events, including diarrhea, than younger adults. Dose adjustment in elderly patients is not necessary unless renal function is markedly compromised.

## ADVERSE EVENTS

**Clinical Trials - OMNICEF Capsules (Adult and Adolescent Patients):**

In clinical trials, 5093 adult and adolescent patients (3841 US and 1252 non-US) were treated with the recommended dose of cefdinir capsules (600 mg/day). Most adverse events were mild and self-limiting. No deaths or permanent disabilities were attributed to cefdinir. One hundred forty-seven of 5093 (3%) patients discontinued medication due to adverse events thought by the investigators to be possibly, probably, or definitely associated with cefdinir therapy. The discontinuations were primarily for gastrointestinal disturbances, usually diarrhea or nausea. Nineteen of 5093 (0.4%) patients were discontinued due to rash thought related to cefdinir administration.

In the US, the following adverse events were thought by investigators to be possibly, probably, or definitely related to cefdinir capsules in multiple-dose clinical trials (N = 3841 cefdinir-treated patients):

**ADVERSE EVENTS ASSOCIATED WITH CEFDINIR CAPSULES US TRIALS IN ADULT AND ADOLESCENT PATIENTS (N=3841)[a]**

| | | |
|---|---|---|
| Incidence ≥ 1% | Diarrhea | 15% |
| | Vaginal moniliasis | 4% of women |
| | Nausea | 3% |
| | Headache | 2% |
| | Abdominal pain | 1% |
| | Vaginitis | 1% of women |
| Incidence <1% but >0.1% | Rash | 0.9% |
| | Dyspepsia | 0.7% |
| | Flatulence | 0.7% |
| | Vomiting | 0.7% |
| | Abnormal stools | 0.3% |
| | Anorexia | 0.3% |
| | Constipation | 0.3% |
| | Dizziness | 0.3% |
| | Dry mouth | 0.3% |
| | Asthenia | 0.2% |
| | Insomnia | 0.2% |
| | Leukorrhea | 0.2% of women |
| | Moniliasis | 0.2% |
| | Pruritus | 0.2% |
| | Somnolence | 0.2% |

[a] 1733 males, 2108 females

The following laboratory value changes of possible clinical significance, irrespective of relationship to therapy with cefdinir, were seen during clinical trials conducted in the US:

**LABORATORY VALUE CHANGES OBSERVED WITH CEFDINIR CAPSULES US TRIALS IN ADULT AND ADOLESCENT PATIENTS (N=3841)**

| | | |
|---|---|---|
| Incidence ≥ 1% | ↑ Urine leukocytes | 2% |
| | ↑ Urine protein | 2% |
| | ↑ Gamma-glutamyltransferase[a] | 1% |
| | ↓ Lymphocytes, ↑ Lymphocytes | 1%, 0.2% |
| | ↑ Microhematuria | 1% |
| Incidence <1% but >0.1% | ↑ Glucose[a] | 0.9% |
| | ↑ Urine glucose | 0.9% |
| | ↑ White blood cells, ↓ White blood cells | 0.9%, 0.7% |
| | ↑ Alanine aminotransferase (ALT) | 0.7% |
| | ↑ Eosinophils | 0.7% |
| | ↑ Urine specific gravity, ↓ Urine specific gravity[a] | 0.6%, 0.2% |
| | ↓ Bicarbonate[a] | 0.6% |
| | ↑ Phosphorus, ↓ Phosphorus[a] | 0.6%, 0.3% |
| | ↑ Aspartate aminotransferase (AST) | 0.4% |
| | ↑ Alkaline phosphatase | 0.3% |
| | ↑ Blood urea nitrogen (BUN) | 0.3% |
| | ↓ Hemoglobin | 0.3% |
| | ↑ Polymorphonuclear neutrophils (PMNs), ↓ PMNs | 0.3%, 0.2% |
| | ↑ Bilirubin | 0.2% |
| | ↑ Lactate dehydrogenase[a] | 0.2% |
| | ↑ Platelets | 0.2% |
| | ↑ Potassium[a] | 0.2% |
| | ↑ Urine pH[a] | 0.2% |

[a] N<3841 for these parameters

**Clinical Trials - OMNICEF for Oral Suspension (Pediatric Patients):**

In clinical trials, 2289 pediatric patients (1783 US and 506 non-US) were treated with the recommended dose of cefdinir suspension (14 mg/kg/day). Most adverse events were mild and self-limiting. No deaths or permanent disabilities were attributed to cefdinir. Forty of 2289 (2%) patients discontinued medication due to adverse events considered by the investigators to be possibly, probably, or definitely associated with cefdinir therapy. Discontinuations were primarily for gastrointestinal disturbances, usually diarrhea. Five of 2289 (0.2%) patients were discontinued due to rash thought related to cefdinir administration.

In the US, the following adverse events were thought by investigators to be possibly, probably, or definitely related to cefdinir suspension in multiple-dose clinical trials (N=1783 cefdinir-treated patients):

**ADVERSE EVENTS ASSOCIATED WITH CEFDINIR SUSPENSION US TRIALS IN PEDIATRIC PATIENTS (N=1783)[a]**

| | | |
|---|---|---|
| Incidence ≥ 1% | Diarrhea | 8% |
| | Rash | 3% |
| | Vomiting | 1% |
| Incidence <1% but >0.1% | Cutaneous moniliasis | 0.9% |
| | Abdominal pain | 0.8% |
| | Leukopenia[b] | 0.3% |
| | Vaginal moniliasis | 0.3% of girls |
| | Vaginitis | 0.3% of girls |
| | Abnormal stools | 0.2% |
| | Dyspepsia | 0.2% |
| | Hyperkinesia | 0.2% |
| | Increased AST[b] | 0.2% |
| | Maculopapular rash | 0.2% |
| | Nausea | 0.2% |

[a] 977 males, 806 females

[b] Laboratory changes were occasionally reported as adverse events.

NOTE: In both cefdinir- and control-treated patients, rates of diarrhea and rash were higher in the youngest pediatric patients. The incidence of diarrhea in cefdinir-treated patients ≤2 years of age was 17% (95/557) compared with 4% (51/1226) in those >2 years old. The incidence of rash (primarily diaper rash in the younger patients) was 8% (43/557) in patients ≤2 years of age compared with 1% (8/1226) in those >2 years old.

The following laboratory value changes of possible clinical significance, irrespective of relationship to therapy with cefdinir, were seen during clinical trials conducted in the US:

**LABORATORY VALUE CHANGES OF POSSIBLE CLINICAL SIGNIFICANCE OBSERVED WITH CEFDINIR SUSPENSION US TRIALS IN PEDIATRIC PATIENTS (N=1783)**

| | | |
|---|---|---|
| Incidence ≥ 1% | ↑ Lymphocytes, ↓ Lymphocytes | 2%, 0.8% |
| | ↑ Alkaline phosphatase | 1% |
| | ↓ Bicarbonate[a] | 1% |
| | ↑ Eosinophils | 1% |
| | ↑ Lactate dehydrogenase | 1% |
| | ↑ Platelets | 1% |
| | ↑ PMNs, ↓ PMNs | 1%, 1% |
| | ↑ Urine protein | 1% |
| Incidence <1% but >0.1% | ↑ Phosphorus, ↓ Phosphorus | 0.9%, 0.4% |
| | ↑ Urine pH | 0.8% |
| | ↓ White blood cells, ↑ White blood cells | 0.7%, 0.3% |
| | ↓ Calcium[a] | 0.5% |
| | ↓ Hemoglobin | 0.5% |
| | ↑ Urine leukocytes | 0.5% |
| | ↑ Monocytes | 0.4% |
| | ↑ AST | 0.3% |
| | ↑ Potassium[a] | 0.3% |
| | ↑ Urine specific gravity, ↓ Urine specific gravity | 0.3%, 0.1% |
| | ↓ Hematocrit[a] | 0.2% |

[a] N=1387 for these parameters

**Postmarketing Experience**

The following adverse experiences and altered laboratory tests, regardless of their relationship to cefdinir, have been reported during extensive postmarketing experience, beginning with approval in Japan in 1991: Stevens-Johnson syndrome, toxic epidermal necrolysis, exfoliative dermatitis, erythema multiforme, erythema nodosum, serum sickness-like reactions, conjunctivitis, stomatitis, acute hepatitis, cholestasis, fulminant hepatitis, hepatic failure, jaundice, increased amylase, shock, anaphylaxis, facial and laryngeal edema, feeling of suffocation, acute enterocolitis, bloody diarrhea, hemorrhagic colitis, melena, pseudomembranous colitis, pancytopenia, granulocytopenia, leukopenia, thrombocytopenia, idiopathic thrombocytopenic purpura, hemolytic anemia, acute respiratory failure, asthmatic attack, drug-induced pneumonia, eosinophilic pneumonia, idiopathic interstitial pneumonia, fever, acute renal failure, nephropathy, bleeding tendency, coagulation disorder, disseminated intravascular coagulation, upper GI bleed, peptic ulcer, ileus, loss of consciousness, allergic vasculitis, possible cefdinir-diclofenac interaction, cardiac failure, chest pain, myocardial infarction, hypertension, involuntary movements, and rhabdomyolysis.

**Cephalosporin Class Adverse Events**

The following adverse events and altered laboratory tests have been reported for cephalosporin-class antibiotics in general:

Allergic reactions, anaphylaxis, Stevens-Johnson syndrome, erythema multiforme, toxic epidermal necrolysis, renal dysfunction, toxic nephropathy, hepatic dysfunction including cholestasis, aplastic anemia, hemolytic anemia, hemorrhage, false-positive test for urinary glucose, neutropenia, pancytopenia, and agranulocytosis. Pseudomembranous colitis symptoms may begin during or after antibiotic treatment (see **WARNINGS**).

Several cephalosporins have been implicated in triggering seizures, particularly in patients with renal impairment when the dosage was not reduced (see **OVERDOSAGE**). If seizures associated with drug therapy occur, the drug should be discontinued. Anticonvulsant therapy can be given if clinically indicated.

## OVERDOSAGE

Information on cefdinir overdosage in humans is not available. In acute rodent toxicity studies, a single oral 5600-mg/kg dose produced no adverse effects. Toxic signs and symptoms following overdosage with other β-lactam antibiotics have included nausea, vomiting, epigastric distress, diarrhea, and convulsions. Hemodialysis removes cefdinir from the body. This may be useful in the event of a serious toxic reaction from overdosage, particularly if renal function is compromised.

**Rx only**

Ref: 03-5435-Rev. July, 2005
(Nos. 3769, 3771, 6151)



05J-034-L150-2 **MASTER**

Manufactured by:
**CEPH** International Corporation
Carolina, Puerto Rico 00986
Under License of:
astellas Astellas Pharma Inc.
Tokyo, Japan

For:
**Abbott Laboratories**
North Chicago, IL 60064, U.S.A.

06A-034-N494-1
Printed in U.S.A.

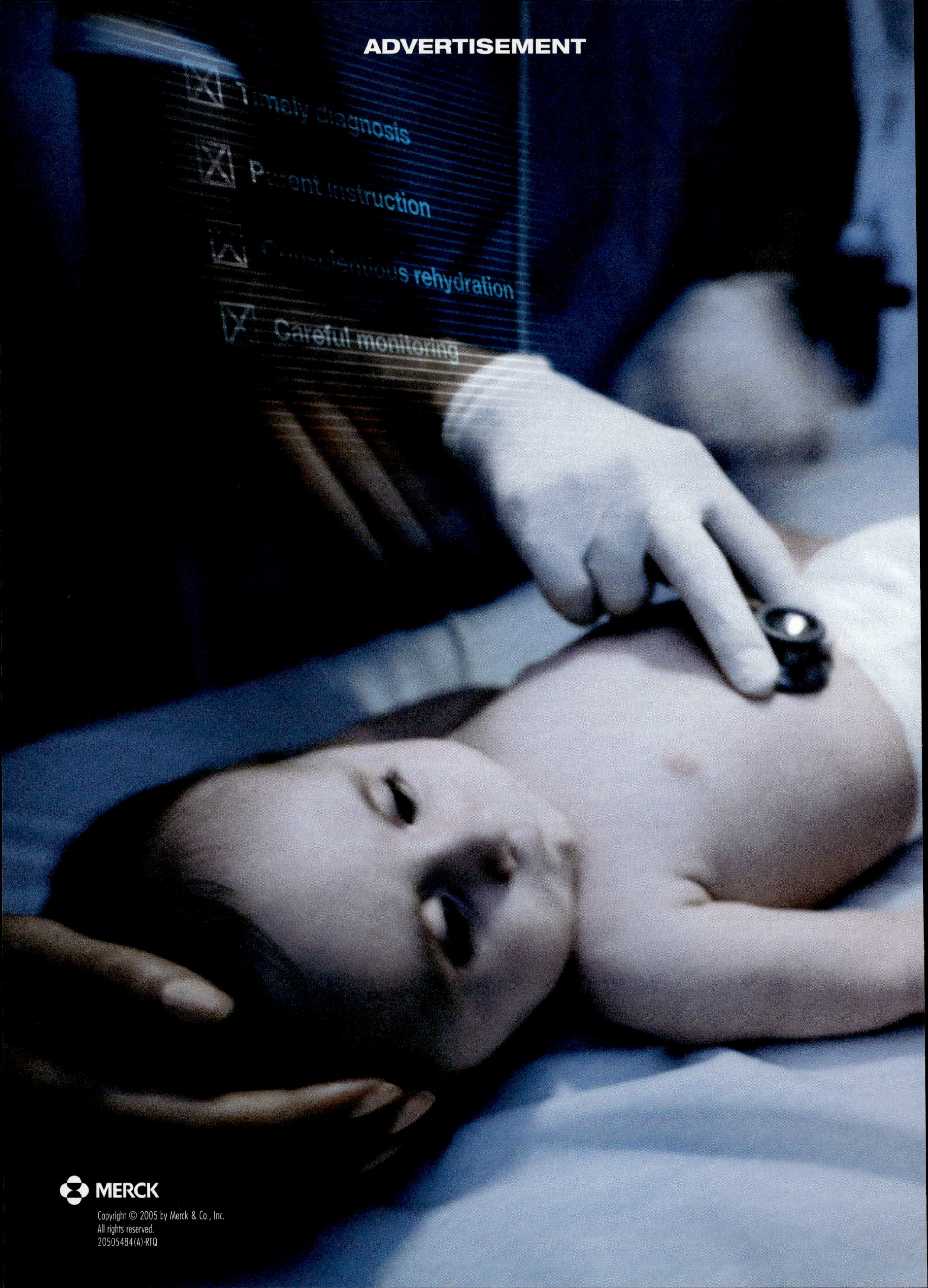
ADVERTISEMENT
Timely diagnosis
Parent instruction
rehydration
Careful monitoring
MERCK
Copyright © 2005 by Merck & Co., Inc.
All rights reserved.
20505484(A)-RTQ

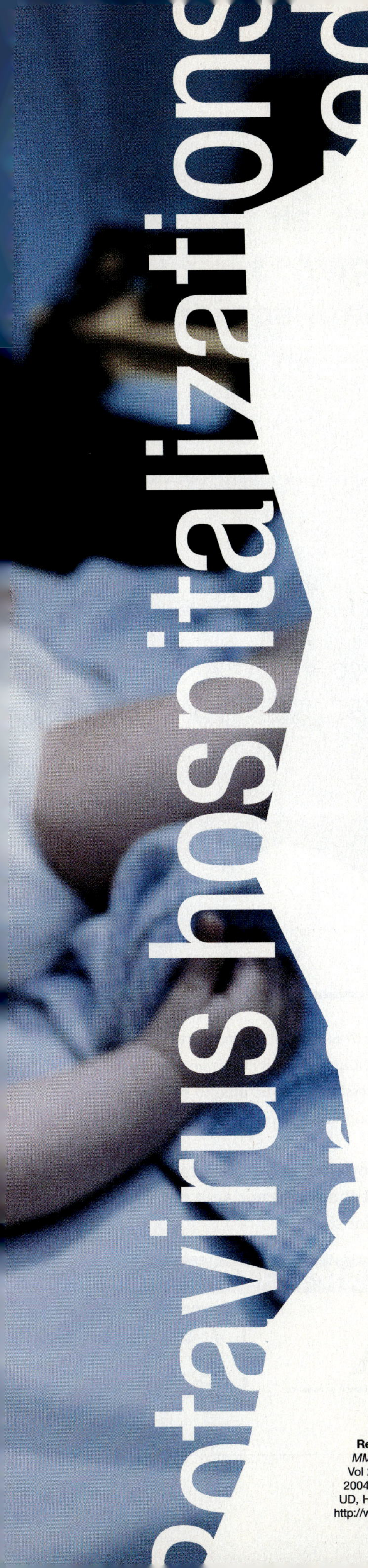


# DESPITE YOUR BEST EFFORTS, ROTAVIRUS CAUSES AN ESTIMATED 70,000 HOSPITALIZATIONS EVERY YEAR.[1]

**AN UNAVOIDABLE DISEASE...**[2]

- The most common cause of severe gastroenteritis in infants and young children in the United States[2]
- Greatest risk for severe disease occurs primarily in young children between 6 and 24 months of age.[3]

**WITH UNPREDICTABLE CONSEQUENCES**[2,4]

- No way to predict which infants will suffer severe disease[4]
- Potential for rapid deterioration in cases in which severe vomiting occurs[5]
- Responsible for an estimated 500,000 physician visits,[1] 70,000 hospitalizations,[1] and 160,000 ER visits[6] among children <5 years of age every year in the United States[1,6]
- Responsible for an estimated 100 deaths per year among children <5 years of age in the United States—an average of nearly 2 deaths per week[7]

Find out more at www.rotavirusinfo.com.

**References: 1.** Glass RI, Bresee JS, Parashar UD, et al. *Arch Pediatr.* 2005;12:844–847. **2.** Centers for Disease Control and Prevention. *MMWR.* 1999;48(RR-2):1–24. **3.** Bernstein DI, Ward RL. In: Feigin RD, Cherry JD. eds. *Textbook of Pediatric Infectious Diseases.* 4th ed. Vol 2. Philadelphia, Pa: Saunders; 1998:1901–1922. **4.** Cornell SL. *Adv Nurse Pract.* 1997;5:41–44. **5.** Clark HF, Offit PA. *Pediatr Ann.* 2004;33:537–543. **6.** Tucker AW, Haddix AC, Bresee JS, Holman MS, Parashar UD, Glass RI. *JAMA.* 1998;279:1371–1376. **7.** Parashar UD, Hummelman EG, Bresee JS, Miller MA, Glass RI. *Emerg Infect Dis.* 2003;9:565–571; Appendix B (online only.): Available at http://www.cdc.gov/ncidod/EID/vol9no5/02-0562_appB.htm. Accessed June 13, 2005.

## Randomized Controlled Trial of a Primary Care and Home-Based Intervention for Physical Activity and Nutrition Behaviors: PACE+ for Adolescents

While there has been increasing attention paid to the problem of obesity, poor nutrition, and physical inactivity among youth, few interventions have been developed that are effective in addressing these problems. Patrick and colleagues conducted a randomized controlled trial in 878 adolescents, examining the effectiveness of a multifaceted school and home-based intervention. The program significantly improved physical activity and diet although it had no effect on body mass index. Even more intensive interventions, however, may be necessary to have long-term effects on the prevalence of obesity.

See page 128

## Neonatal Abstinence Syndrome After In Utero Exposure to Selective Serotonin Reuptake Inhibitors in Term Infants

The use of selective serotonin reuptake inhibitors (SSRIs) to treat depression during pregnancy has become more common. While there is no evidence that such use is teratogenic, there have been reports of neonatal abstinence syndrome in infants born to mothers taking SSRIs. This study examined the incidence and clinical characteristics of the neonatal abstinence syndrome of 60 term infants who had prolonged in utero exposure to SSRIs. Of these infants, 1 in 7 exhibited signs of severe withdrawal and 1 in 6 had mild withdrawal symptoms. The maximum symptoms usually occurred within 2 days of birth. The long-term effects of SSRIs on infants are unknown.

See page 173

## Association of Condom Use, Sexual Behaviors, and Sexually Transmitted Infections With the Duration of Genital Human Papillomavirus Infection Among Adolescent Women

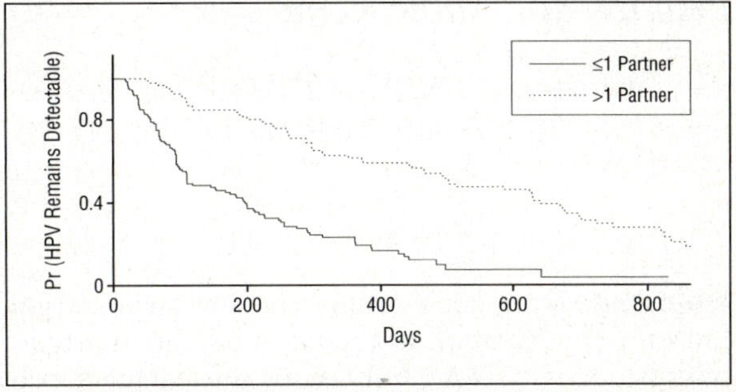


Kaplan-Meier estimates of the survival of human papillomavirus (HPV) infection (A-F). CT indicates *Chlamydia trachomatis*; TV, *Trichomonas vaginalis;* Pr, probability.

Persistent human papillomavirus (HPV) infection appears to be necessary for the development of neoplasia. Little is known about the factors associated with HPV persistence in adolescent women. The authors of this study observed adolescent women over a period of 27 months to determine the duration of persistence. The cumulative prevalence of HPV infection was 82% in this patient population, and 45% had coinfection with *Chlamydia trachomatis* and 25% with *Neisseria gonorrhoeae*. Half of all HPV infections were no longer detectable by 210 days after initial detection. Prolonged HPV infection was associated with oncogenic viral types, lower condom use, and coinfection with *C trachomatis*. Having fewer sexual partners was associated with a shorter duration of HPV infection. These findings have important public health implications.

See page 151

## Simulating Cost-effectiveness of Fluoride Varnish During Well-Child Visits for Medicaid-Enrolled Children

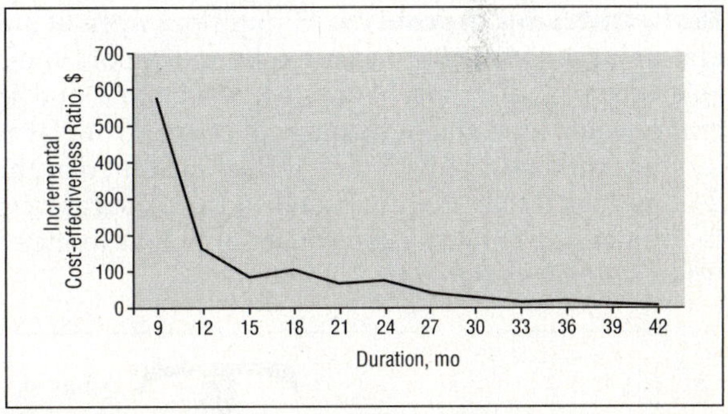


Results illustrate changing incremental cost-effectiveness ratio over simulation time by quarter discounted.

Disparities in children's oral health are large, in part owing to limited access to dental services for high-risk children. Only a minority of poor children receive regular routine prophylactic dental care. Fluoride varnish is an effective topical medication that can be applied by primary care physicians. This study examined the cost-effectiveness of routine fluoride varnish by primary care practitioners during routine well-child visits. Providing universal routine fluoride varnish at ages 9, 18, 24, and 36 months resulted in an additional 1.5 cavity-free months by 42 months of age. The net cost was $10.93 over the entire intervention period. Fluoride varnish would cost $203 per restorative treatment averted.

See page 164

ARTICLE

# Randomized Controlled Trial of a Primary Care and Home-Based Intervention for Physical Activity and Nutrition Behaviors

## *PACE+ for Adolescents*

*Kevin Patrick, MD, MS; Karen J. Calfas, PhD; Gregory J. Norman, PhD; Marion F. Zabinski, PhD, MPH; James F. Sallis, PhD; Joan Rupp, MS, RD; Jennifer Covin, MPH; John Cella, MD*

**Objective:** Many adolescents do not meet national guidelines for participation in regular moderate or vigorous physical activity (PA); limitations on sedentary behaviors; or dietary intake of fruits and vegetables, fiber, or total dietary fat. This study evaluated a health care–based intervention to improve these behaviors.

**Design:** Randomized controlled trial.

**Setting:** Primary care with follow-up at home.

**Participants:** Eight hundred seventy-eight adolescent girls and boys aged 11 to 15 years.

**Interventions:** Two experimental conditions: (1) Primary care, office-based, computer-assisted diet and PA assessment and stage-based goal setting followed by brief health care provider counseling and 12 months of monthly mail and telephone counseling and (2) a comparison condition addressing sun exposure protection.

**Main Outcome Measures:** Minutes per week of moderate plus vigorous PA measured by self-report and accelerometer; self-report of days per week of PA and sedentary behaviors; and percentage of energy from fat and servings per day of fruits and vegetables measured by three 24-hour diet recalls. Body mass index (calculated as weight in kilograms divided by the square of height in meters) was a secondary outcome.

**Results:** Compared with adolescents in the sun protection condition, girls and boys in the diet and PA intervention significantly reduced sedentary behaviors (intervention vs control change, 4.3 to 3.4 h/d vs 4.2 to 4.4 h/d for girls, respectively [$P = .001$]; 4.2 to 3.2 h/d vs 4.2 to 4.3 h/d for boys, respectively [$P = .001$]). Boys reported more active days per week (intervention vs control change: 4.1 to 4.4 d/wk vs 3.8 to 3.8 d/w, respectively [$P = .01$]), and the number of servings of fruits and vegetables for girls approached significance (intervention vs control change, 3.5 to 4.2 servings/d vs 3.5 to 3.9 servings/d, respectively [$P = .07$]). No intervention effects were seen with percentage of calories from fat or minutes of PA per week. Percentage of adolescents meeting recommended health guidelines was significantly improved for girls for consumption of saturated fat (intervention vs control change, 23.4% to 41.0% vs 18.5% to 31%, respectively [relative risk, 1.33; 95% confidence interval, 1.01-1.68]) and for boys' participation in d/wk of PA (intervention vs control change, 45.3% to 55.4% vs 41.9% to 38.0%, respectively [relative risk, 1.47; 95% confidence interval, 1.19-1.75]). No between-group differences were seen in body mass index.

**Conclusions:** Improvements in some diet, PA, and sedentary behaviors in adolescents can be enabled through the use of a 1-year, integrated intervention using the computer, health provider counseling, mail, and telephone. The amount of intervention received may contribute to its efficacy.

*Arch Pediatr Adolesc Med. 2006;160:128-136*

**Author Affiliations:** University of California, San Diego (Drs Patrick, Norman, and Zabinski and Ms Covin); San Diego State University, San Diego (Drs Calfas and Sallis and Ms Rupp); Kaiser Permanente Medical Group, San Diego (Dr Cella).

THERE IS A NEED TO IMPROVE diet, physical activity (PA), and sedentary behaviors in childhood and adolescence.[1,2] Poor dietary behaviors are a known risk factor for the development of obesity, as well as for the nation's 3 leading causes of death: coronary heart disease, cancer, and stroke. A diet rich in fruits and vegetables and low in fat is recommended for preventing these chronic diseases.[1,3-10] Energy intake has increased from the 1970s to 2000; according to the National Health and Nutrition Examination Survey,[11] children aged 6 to 11 years were consuming 133 kcal/d more in 2000 than they were just a decade earlier. Although national surveys indicate a decline in the average proportion of calories from total and saturated fat over the past several decades, the Centers for Disease Control and Prevention (Atlanta, Ga) estimated in 2000 that

*For editorial comment see page 217*

only 38% of individuals aged 2 years and older met the recommendation for total fat intake, and 41% met the recommendation for saturated fat intake.[11]

There is strong evidence of the health benefits of PA,[1,12] including improvements in longevity, cardiovascular diseases, cardiovascular disease risk factors, diabetes, obesity, osteoporosis, immune functioning, certain types of cancer, and mental health. Recent guidelines from the Dietary Guidelines for Americans[13] and an international consensus group recommend 60 minutes of daily PA for youth.[14,15] Although national survey data in the United States indicate that about two thirds of adolescent boys and one half of adolescent girls are meeting an adult-oriented recommendation for vigorous activity,[16] objective measures suggest less than 40% of teens are meeting the 60-minute guideline.[17] Girls, older adolescents, minorities, and disadvantaged youth are even less likely to be meeting this recommendation.[1]

Sedentary behaviors, particularly television viewing, are the most consistent behavioral predictor of obesity in adolescence.[18] Intervention studies show that decreasing television time is an effective method of reducing body mass index (BMI [calculated as weight in kilograms divided by the square of height in meters]) in children.[19] Substitution of PA for sedentary behaviors and increases in activity level predict 6- and 12-month reductions in BMI.[20] In addition, targeting either decreased sedentary behaviors or increased PA is associated with significant decreases in percentages of overweight people and body fat and improved aerobic fitness.[21]

Obesity in adolescence is becoming increasingly prevalent. Thirty years ago, the prevalence of obesity among adolescents aged 12 to 19 years was approximately 6%. As of the year 2002, more than 16% of adolescents were obese in the United States,[22] and this increased prevalence of childhood obesity has been universal in all age, sex, and ethnicity classifications. Childhood obesity is increasingly recognized as one of the nation's most important health issues.[2]

Interventions to improve diet, PA, and sedentary behaviors in youth can be implemented with families, in schools and communities, or in conjunction with health care. The evidence of effectiveness of most interventions is modest,[23-25] and evidence of the efficacy of health care–based interventions for these behaviors is limited to obese children and their families.[26] Based on promising feasibility and acceptability data from adolescents, their parents, and clinicians,[27,28] we conducted a randomized controlled trial of a multimodal intervention, Patient-centered Assessment and Counseling for Exercise + Nutrition (PACE+), to improve diet and PA behaviors in adolescents that could be initiated in primary care. We hypothesized that, compared with control adolescents, adolescents who completed computer-generated tailored Progress Plans addressing PA and diet behaviors, followed by brief provider counseling and 1 year of tailored telephone and mail guidance, would significantly improve PA, diet, and sedentary behaviors.

## METHODS

### PARTICIPANTS

Adolescents between the ages of 11 and 15 years were recruited through their primary care providers. A total of 45 primary care providers from 6 private clinic sites in San Diego County, California, agreed to participate in the study. A representative group of healthy adolescents seeing primary care providers was sought by contacting parents of adolescents who were already scheduled for a well child visit and by outreach to families with adolescents. Adolescents were excluded if they had health conditions that would limit the ability to comply with PA or diet recommendations. Parents gave written consent for their child to participate and each adolescent provided signed assent. Participants and parents knew the study involved randomization to either a PA and diet intervention or the comparison sun protection intervention and were not blinded to the intervention. After baseline measures but before seeing the provider, participants were randomized to either the PACE+ intervention condition or the sun protection control condition. The study was approved by the participating health care organizations and university institutional review boards for research with human subjects.

### INTERVENTION

The PACE+ intervention (**Figure 1**) was designed to promote adoption and maintenance of improved eating and PA behaviors through a computer-supported intervention initiated in primary health care settings. This was coupled with a printed manual to take home and 12 months of stage-matched telephone calls and mail contact. There was a parent intervention intended to help parents encourage behavior change attempts through praise, active support, and positive role-modeling. The intervention was based on a behavioral determinants model,[29] social cognitive theory,[30] and the Transtheoretical Model of Behavior Change.[31] The initial intervention component used a computer expert system on a kiosk in the clinical office to assess 2 nutrition target behaviors (total intake of fat, servings per day of fruits and vegetables), PA target behaviors (moderate and vigorous PA), and sedentary behaviors. A brief screening survey was used to identify patients with disordered eating, and the computer encouraged the adolescent to ask a parent or guardian for assistance with completing the assessment if needed. Stage of readiness to make a behavior change was assessed for each behavior using a simplified 3-stage model. The computer then guided the adolescent to develop stage-appropriate and tailored behavior-change Progress Plans for 1 nutrition and 1 PA behavior (either increasing minutes of PA per day or decreasing sedentary behaviors). All Progress Plans enabled the adolescent and provider to sign it as a behavioral contract.

After the adolescent completed the computer assessment, a printed Provider Summary highlighted patient-reported behaviors (both PA and nutrition), compared them with national guidelines, and displayed the behaviors the adolescent targeted for change. The Provider Summary alerted providers to areas of concern related to weight, disordered eating, or unwillingness to make changes. Providers were trained in 2-hour group sessions that included review of written materials and role-playing examples. Providers were taught to spend approximately 3 to 5 minutes counseling patients, endorse or modify the plans, and encourage full participation in the intervention.

The next component of the intervention was delivered by a 16-section printed Teen Guide, mail, and telephone using stage-based cognitive and behavioral strategies to support changes in target behaviors. The Teen Guide was provided to the adolescent after completion of the provider visit, and each section provided 2 to 3 pages of information or rationale on a specific target behavior or behavior change strategy (eg, decisional balance, self-monitoring). Most sections had worksheets to enhance the adolescent's participation in learning and applying the given strategy to each target behavior. Over the 12-month intervention, manuals were supplemented by mailed worksheets and tip sheets

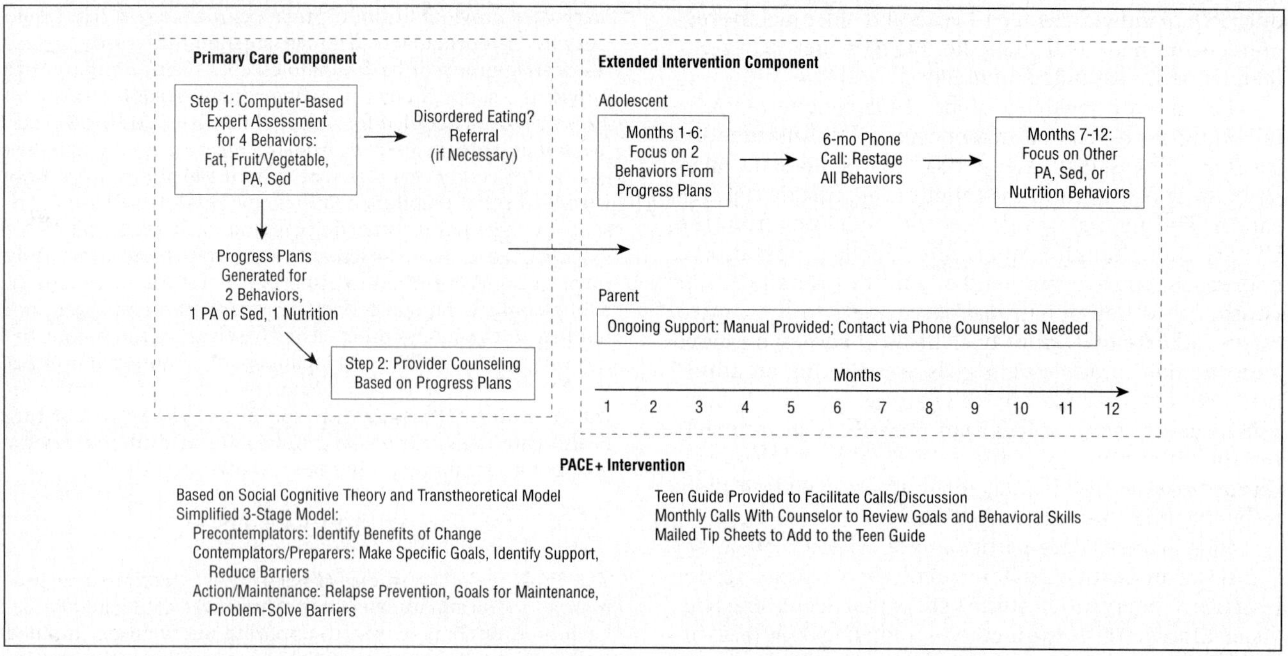


**Figure 1.** Patient-centered Assessment and Counseling for Exercise + Nutrition (PACE+) intervention overview. PA indicates physical activity; Sed, sedentary.

that allowed further tailoring by providing more guidance on change strategies, more information on foods or activities, or answers to frequently asked questions. Telephone counselors selected the most relevant tip sheets for each target behavior based on the content of each counseling call and participant questions/comments (discussed later in this article). Manuals and mailings were written at approximately a fifth-grade reading level. A companion parent manual was provided at the provider visit that supported intervention elements.

Eleven telephone counseling calls were scheduled throughout the 1-year intervention period, each lasting 10 to 15 minutes and conducted by trained research staff. During the first 6 months, 5 intervention calls were directed at the nutrition and PA behaviors that the adolescent chose to target in the initial clinical visit. A call after the 6-month measurement visit used staging data gathered in that visit to develop new Progress Plans for the remaining 2 target behaviors. Five calls were then made over the next 6 months directed primarily at the remaining 2 target behaviors. Counseling calls were structured interactions using the teen guide to help adolescents learn and apply relevant cognitive or behavioral change strategies to modify diet and PA behaviors. Up to 6 attempts were made to reach adolescents for each call. If calls were missed, the next completed call briefly addressed topic areas that would have been covered in the missed call.

Adolescents randomized to the comparison condition received an adaptation of the SunSmart sun protection behavior program developed at the University of Rhode Island, Kingston.[32] SunSmart was based on the transtheoretical model and entailed an initial primary care, office-based, computer assessment of sun protection behaviors followed by computer-generated, printed, stage-based recommendations for improvement such as wearing protective clothing and use of sunscreen. Brief counseling telephone calls were provided by the health counselor at 3 months and 6 months each, followed by a mailed feedback report and tip sheet to encourage continued sun protection behavior. Adolescents received $10 for completing the baseline measures, $15 for completing the 6-month measures, and $20 for completing the 12-month measures. On completion of scheduled measurement visits and monthly telephone calls, adolescents in both the control and intervention groups received lottery tickets for small cash prizes ($10-$50) in lotteries conducted every 6 months.

## PRIMARY OUTCOME MEASURES

Assessments were performed by trained staff at baseline before the adolescents went to the provider offices for their initial PACE+ counseling visits and at 6 and 12 months. The 7-day Physical Activity Recall is one of the most widely studied self-report measures of PA and has been evaluated with children and adolescents.[33] Subjects report hours spent in sleep and in moderate, hard, and very hard activities over the previous 7 days. The interview takes about 10 minutes to administer and focuses on salient PAs. Standardized interviewer protocol and training methods have produced same-day reliabilities across interviewers of 0.86.[34] In a sample of 102 5th-, 8th-, and 11th-grade boys and girls, the overall test retest reliability was $r = 0.77$. Reliability was not affected by obesity status or memory skills.[33] Validity of the Physical Activity Recall is strongly supported by objective measures.[35] Physical activity was calculated as the sum of reported minutes of moderate, hard, and very hard activities. The number of active days per week was calculated by summing the number of days out of 7 that an adolescent attained at least 30 minutes of vigorous activity, at least 60 minutes of moderate activity, or at least 60 minutes of a combination of vigorous and moderate activity.

Three 24-hour recalls assessed dietary intake at each assessment point. Trained data collectors conducted dietary recalls for 2 weekdays and 1 weekend day using the University of Minnesota Nutrition Data System for Research software.[36] Participants were taught how to measure food portions with 3-dimensional food models. The first interview was conducted in person and the second and third by telephone (participants were given 2-dimensional food models to use for the second and third assessments). Nutrient variables (percentage of calories from total fat and saturated fat, number of servings of fruits and vegetables, grams of fiber) were calculated by averaging values from the 3 intake records.

Participants completed a self-report measure of recent school day and non–school day time spent watching television, playing computer/video games, sitting talking on the telephone, and sitting listening to music. This survey was modified from a validated survey developed by Robinson.[19] Participants responded with an 8-point scale ranging from "none" to "6 hours or more." A composite score of sedentary behavior was calculated from a weighted sum of the school day and non–school day responses, with weights of 5 and 2, respectively.

Physical activity and dietary intake data were used to develop separate variables for direct comparison with national guidelines for number of minutes of PA per day,[15] number of hours of television per day,[37] percentage of calories from total fat and percentage of calories from saturated fat,[37] fruits and vegetables (number of servings per day), and amount of dietary fiber (grams per day).[38] Meeting the active guideline was defined as 5 or more active days per week. The television viewing guideline variable was estimated in the same way as the total sedentary variable using only the television self-report item. A cutpoint of greater than 2 hours per day defined adolescents who were not meeting the television time guideline.

## OTHER MEASURES

A wall stadiometer was used to measure standing height. Weight was measured with a calibrated digital scale. Each measure was taken twice and the average of the 2 readings calculated. Body mass index was calculated as weight in kilograms divided by the square of height in meters. Body mass index for age was determined from Centers for Disease Control and Prevention national norms using age to the nearest month and sex-specific median, standard deviation, and power of the Box-Cox transformation.[39]

Physical activity was measured with the Computer Science and Applications accelerometer (WAM 7164; Computer Science and Applications, Shalimar, Fla). This uniaxial accelerometer is small (5.1 × 3.8 × 1.5 cm), lightweight (45 g), and worn on a belt snugly around the waist. Accelerometers stored data as 1-minute averages for a 7-day period. In laboratory and field settings, Computer Science and Applications accelerometers have been shown to be a valid measure for quantifying children's activity levels.[40] Physical activity estimates of daily minutes of moderate (3-5.9 metabolic equivalents [METs]) plus vigorous PA (≥6 METs) were calculated by averaging across valid days of monitoring for each participant. Accelerometer data were considered a secondary outcome because of considerable missing data due to lost and malfunctioning monitors and compliance with participants wearing the monitor as instructed. Complete and valid data (≥3 days of 10 h/d of monitoring) from the activity monitors were available for 330 participants at baseline and 12 months. Data on numbers of calls completed to intervention participants were used to categorize adolescents into low-dose treatment and high-dose treatment groups.

## STATISTICAL ANALYSIS

All outcome analyses were conducted using the 12-month primary study end points as dependent variables. Analyses were conducted under the intent-to-treat assumption by replacing missing values at the 12-month end point with the most recent available data from either the 6-month or baseline assessment. Dependent variables with nonnormal distributions were either log or square-root transformed. The primary analyses compared differences between the PACE+ and control group on 5 outcome variables using analysis-of-covariance models controlling for the corresponding baseline outcome measure as well as age (in months), ethnicity (white non-Hispanic, all other races/ethnicities), and BMI *z* score. These covariates were selected a priori. Secondary analyses used logistic regression models to compare the proportion of PACE+ and control participants meeting 6 recommended health guidelines at 12 months. These guidelines were also tested with logistic regression models comparing low and high intervention dose levels with the control group. The logistic regression models included the corresponding baseline variable as well as age, ethnicity, and BMI *z* score as covariates. To aid interpretation of the logistic regression models, odds ratios and 95% confidence interval (CI) boundaries were corrected to risk ratios (RRs) using the method proposed by Zhang and Yu.[41] Because previous research has suggested sex differences in response to PA and diet behavior interventions,[42,43] all analyses were conducted separately for girls and boys and analyzed using SPSS version 12.0 (SPSS Inc, Chicago, Ill). *P* values were not adjusted for multiple tests. All reported *P* values are for 2-sided tests with effects considered statistically significant at $P<.05$.

## RESULTS

Recruitment occurred from May 2001 through June 2002. **Figure 2** displays the flow diagram of participants through the study. An initial letter was sent to all patients in the eligible age range from participating physicians, informing them that they may receive a telephone call in the next year about a health promotion study. Parents were given the option to send back a postcard requesting that they not be contacted about the study. A total of 1172 (7%) households returned opt-out cards. In response to the letter, some parents called to learn more about the study. After the initial mailing, adolescents were recruited in 2 ways: by calling patients of participating providers when they had an upcoming scheduled doctor's visit and by "cold-calling" patients of participating providers at random who did not return an opt-out postcard from the initial mailing. Baseline assessments were completed by 878 adolescents, 819 of whom began the intervention at the doctor's office and are included in the intent-to-treat analysis.

No differences were found between randomized participants who began the intervention and those who did not begin the intervention (n = 59) in terms of age, sex, ethnicity, provider site location, highest household education level, body weight status, or treatment group. No differences were found between intervention and comparison condition groups for sex, age, highest household education level, or body weight status at baseline. More nonwhite adolescents were randomized to the treatment group (45%) compared with the control group (38%). **Table 1** displays demographic and anthropometric characteristics of the study sample. While not fully representative of the San Diego community, in which those aged 10 to 17 years are 35% Hispanic, 7% African American, 12% Asian or other, and 45% non-Hispanic white (San Diego Association of Governments, March 7, 2003), the study sample was diverse with approximately 42% from races/ethnicities other than non-Hispanic white. Participants completing assessments at 12 months did not differ from noncompleters by treatment group, provider site location, sex, ethnicity, or highest household education level. However, completers were more likely than noncompleters to have a BMI below the 85th percentile ($P<.01$).

## EFFECT ON BEHAVIORAL OUTCOMES

The only significant ($P<.001$) between-group difference that was found for both girls and boys was im-

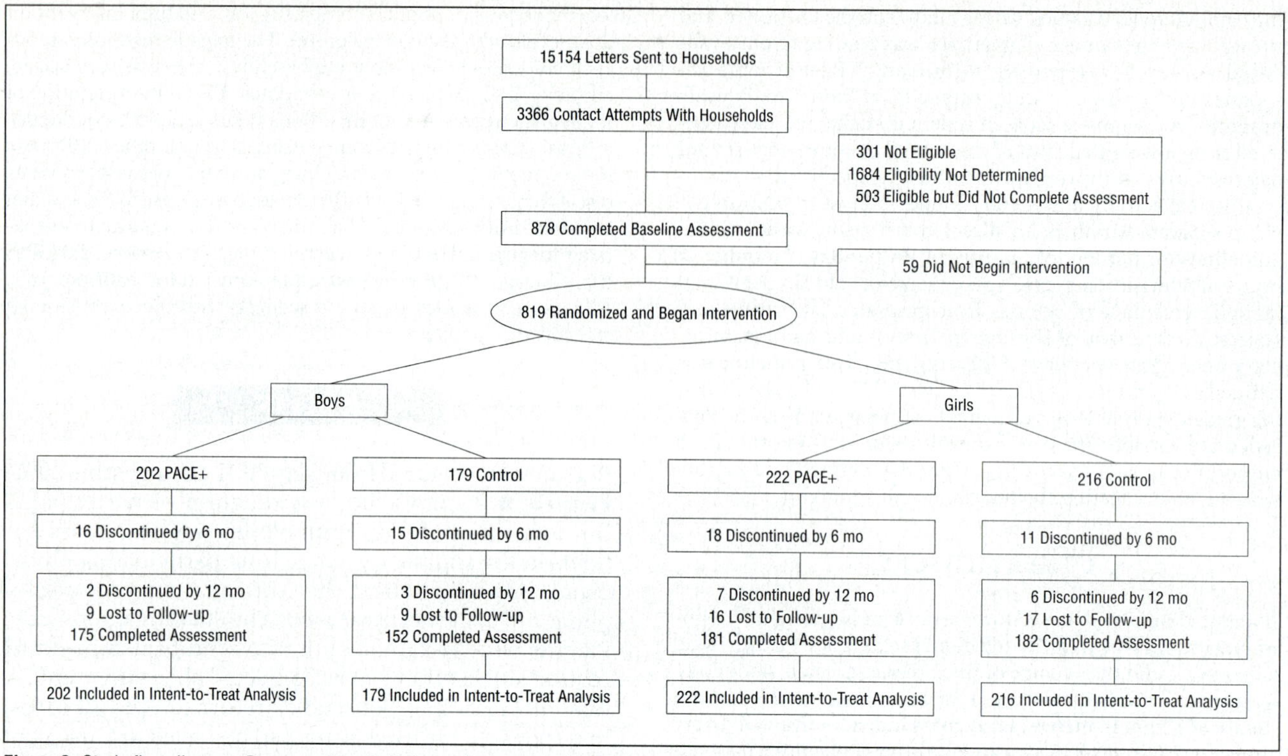


**Figure 2.** Study flow diagram. Because of the limited recruitment period (12 months), of households sent a letter (n=15 154), only 3366 had contact attempts made. Among these, eligibility could not be determined for 1684 households because of a wrong number (n=462), refusal to participate (n=892), or not reaching a household member after 8 attempts (n=330). Of the remaining eligible to participate, 503 did not complete the initial baseline assessment and 59 who completed the baseline assessment did not begin the intervention. PACE+ indicates Patient-centered Assessment and Counseling for Exercise + Nutrition.

**Table 1. PACE+ Adolescent Sample Demographic Characteristics**

| | Girls | | Boys | | |
|---|---|---|---|---|---|
| **Variable** | **PACE+** | **Control** | **PACE+** | **Control** | **Overall** |
| Participants, No. | 222 | 216 | 202 | 179 | 819 |
| Age, mean (SD), y | 12.8 (1.3) | 12.6 (1.4) | 12.6 (1.4) | 12.8 (1.3) | 12.7 (1.3) |
| Ethnicity, No. (%) | | | | | |
| Asian or Pacific Islander | 9 (4.1) | 2 (0.9) | 8 (4.0) | 7 (3.9) | 26 (3.2) |
| African American | 19 (8.6) | 6 (2.8) | 17 (8.4) | 12 (6.7) | 54 (6.6) |
| Native American | 2 (0.9) | 2 (0.9) | 1 (0.5) | 1 (0.6) | 6 (0.7) |
| Hispanic | 33 (14.9) | 28 (13.0) | 28 (13.9) | 18 (10.1) | 107 (13.1) |
| White | 121 (54.4) | 135 (62.5) | 111 (55.0) | 111 (62.0) | 478 (58.4) |
| Multiethnic or other | 38 (17.2) | 43 (19.9) | 37 (18.4) | 30 (16.7) | 148 (18.0) |
| Highest household education level, No. (%)* | | | | | |
| From no high school degree to associate's-level degree | 82 (37.8) | 80 (37.6) | 60 (30.2) | 47 (27.3) | 269 (33.6) |
| Bachelor's-level degree | 66 (30.4) | 51 (38.5) | 68 (34.2) | 53 (30.8) | 238 (29.7) |
| Graduate or professional degree | 69 (31.8) | 82 (38.5) | 71 (35.7) | 72 (41.9) | 294 (36.7) |
| Body mass index† for age, No. (%) | | | | | |
| <85th percentile | 118 (53.2) | 112 (51.9) | 116 (57.7) | 97 (54.4) | 443 (54.2) |
| ≥85th to <95th percentile | 42 (18.9) | 49 (22.7) | 29 (14.4) | 31 (17.3) | 151 (18.4) |
| ≥95th percentile | 62 (27.9) | 55 (25.5) | 56 (27.9) | 51 (28.5) | 224 (27.4) |

Abbreviations: PACE+, Patient-centered Assessment and Counseling for Exercise + Nutrition.
*n = 801.
†Calculated as weight in kilograms divided by the square of height in meters.

provement in sedentary behaviors (**Table 2**.) In addition, boys in the PACE+ group increased their number of active days per week (*P*=.01) compared with control adolescents. For the remaining behaviors, girls and boys in both the intervention and control groups improved in all behaviors, but these changes did not differ between groups.

Accelerometer data were available at baseline and 12 months on 180 girls and 150 boys. Mean±SE accelerometer estimates of average minutes per day of PA

**Table 2. Intent-to-Treat ANCOVA Analysis of Primary Outcomes for Girls and Boys***

| Outcome | Girls PACE+, Mean (SD) | Girls Control, Mean (SD) | Girls *P* Value | Boys PACE+, Mean (SD) | Boys Control, Mean (SD) | Boys *P* Value |
|---|---|---|---|---|---|---|
| Calories from fat, % | | | | | | |
| Preintervention | 32.6 (5.5) | 33.3 (7.2) | .86 | 32.6 (5.7) | 32.3 (6.2) | .31 |
| Postintervention | 31.4 (7.0) | 31.7 (6.6) | | 31.2 (6.3) | 31.6 (5.9) | |
| Change, % | −3.7 | −4.8 | | −4.3 | −2.2 | |
| Fruit and vegetable servings/d† | | | | | | |
| Preintervention | 3.5 (1.5) | 3.5 (1.8) | .07 | 3.5 (1.6) | 3.7 (1.6) | .49 |
| Postintervention | 4.2 (1.8) | 3.9 (1.7) | | 4.2 (1.7) | 4.4 (1.6) | |
| Change, % | 20.0 | 11.4 | | 20.0 | 20.0 | |
| Sedentary behaviors, h/d | | | | | | |
| Preintervention | 4.3 (3.4) | 4.2 (3.4) | .001 | 4.2 (3.7) | 4.2 (2.8) | .001 |
| Postintervention | 3.4 (2.6) | 4.4 (3.7) | | 3.2 (2.6) | 4.3 (3.5) | |
| Change, % | −21 | 4.8 | | −24 | 2.4 | |
| Physical Activity Recall mod + vig, min/wk‡ | | | | | | |
| Preintervention | 316.1 (49.2) | 284.3 (45.8) | .90 | 418.4 (54.5) | 374.0 (55.0) | .17 |
| Postintervention | 324.6 (61.5) | 313.9 (62.2) | | 486.0 (75.3) | 419.8 (79.2) | |
| Change, % | 2.7 | 10.4 | | 16.2 | 12.2 | |
| Active d/wk | | | | | | |
| Preintervention | 3.3 (2.1) | 3.1 (2.0) | .88 | 4.1 (2.0) | 3.8 (2.1) | .01 |
| Postintervention | 3.4 (2.1) | 3.3 (2.1) | | 4.4 (2.1) | 3.8 (2.1) | |
| Change, % | .03 | .06 | | 7.3 | 0.0 | |

Abbreviations: ANCOVA, analysis of covariance; mod, moderate; PACE+, Patient-centered Assessment and Counseling for Exercise + Nutrition; vig, vigorous.
*Controlling for age, ethnicity, body mass index *z* score, and baseline variable. Girls: PACE+, n = 222; control, n = 216; boys: PACE+, n = 202; control, n = 179.
†Geometric mean.
‡Square root transformed for analyses; squared means and SDs presented in this table.

(moderate + vigorous) were not found to be different between the PACE+ and the control group for girls (53.5±2.3 minutes vs 52.8±2.0 minutes , *P*=.80) or boys (72.8±3.4 minutes vs 71.3±3.3 minutes, *P*=.76).

## EFFECT ON MEETING HEALTH GUIDELINES

The proportion of adolescents meeting recommended health guidelines before and after the intervention are displayed in **Table 3**. More girls in the PACE+ group compared with the control group met the guideline for maximum percentage of daily calories from saturated fat at 12 months (RR, 1.33; 95% CI, 1.01-1.68). Changes in the proportion of girls meeting the other guidelines were not different between groups. More boys in the PACE+ group compared with the control group were meeting the PA guideline at 12 months (RR, 1.47; 95% CI, 1.19-1.75). All other changes in meeting guidelines did not differ between groups for boys.

## EFFECT OF INTERVENTION DOSE

The effect of intervention dose was tested by comparing the high and low dose levels with the control group using logistic regression analyses (**Table 4**). The number of completed counselor calls ranged from 0 to 11 out of 11 possible calls. Based on a median split, the "low dose" of 0 to 8 calls was received by 36% of adolescents, while the "high dose" of 9 to 11 calls was received by 64% of adolescents. For girls, receiving the low dose did not lead to meeting any of the health guidelines compared with control group participants while receiving the high dose was related to increased likelihood of meeting the guidelines for saturated fat (RR, 1.36; 95% CI, 1.02-1.73), fruit and vegetable consumption (RR, 1.50; 95% CI, 1.02-2.03), and sedentary behavior (RR, 1.13; 95% CI, 1.01-1.21). Compared with boys in the control group, boys who received both a low dose (RR, 1.74; 95% CI, 1.35-2.06) and high dose (RR, 1.39; 95% CI, 1.06-1.71) of the intervention were significantly more likely to meet the PA guideline.

## EFFECT ON BMI

No differences were found at 12 months between groups for BMI *z* scores, which were normed for age and sex in models controlling for baseline BMI *z* score, age, and ethnicity. In an analysis of the subgroup of adolescents with a BMI at or above the 95 percentile (n=238), mean±SE BMI *z* score estimates were 2.08±0.02 for PACE+ adolescents and 2.12±0.02 for control adolescents (*P*=.10).

## COMMENT

This is the first randomized controlled trial to evaluate the effects of a behavior change intervention for PA, diet, and sedentary behavior that integrates computer-assisted behavior assessment; health care provider counseling; and extended, tailored telephone and mail outreach. This intervention, leading to significant intervention effects on multiple behaviors, was shown to be feasible, with 64% of adolescents assigned to the intervention condition com-

**Table 3. Intent-to-Treat Logistic Regression Analyses for Meeting Recommended Health Guidelines in 438 Girls and 381 Boys***

| Guideline | Girls PACE+ | Girls Control | Girls RR (95% CI)† | Boys PACE+ | Boys Control | Boys RR (95% CI)† |
|---|---|---|---|---|---|---|
| 30% kcal from fat | | | | | | |
| Preintervention | 31.1 | 29.6 | 1.06 (0.83-1.31) | 32.2 | 34.6 | 1.10 (0.38-1.38) |
| Postintervention | 42.3 | 39.8 | | 40.6 | 38.0 | |
| Change, % | 36 | 34 | | 26 | 10 | |
| 10% kcal from saturated fat | | | | | | |
| Preintervention | 23.4 | 18.5 | 1.33 (1.01-1.68)‡ | 24.4 | 24.7 | 1.31 (0.96-1.73) |
| Postintervention | 41.0 | 31.0 | | 36.1 | 28.5 | |
| Change, % | 43 | 68 | | 48 | 15 | |
| ≥5 fruit and vegetable servings/d | | | | | | |
| Preintervention | 7.7 | 12.0 | 1.21 (0.85-1.64) | 11.9 | 13.4 | 0.80 (0.54-1.14) |
| Postintervention | 26.1 | 23.6 | | 23.3 | 28.5 | |
| Change, % | 239 | 92 | | 96 | 113 | |
| Fiber g/d | | | | | | |
| Preintervention | 12.2 | 7.9 | 0.94 (0.47-1.78) | 16.3 | 16.2 | 0.70 (0.40-1.16) |
| Postintervention | 8.6 | 7.9 | | 14.4 | 19.9 | |
| Change, % | −30 | 0 | | −12 | 23 | |
| ≤2 h/d of TV viewing | | | | | | |
| Preintervention | 71.1 | 71.8 | 1.07 (0.95-1.15) | 72.8 | 70.4 | 1.04 (0.92-1.13) |
| Postintervention | 80.6 | 76.4 | | 80.7 | 77.7 | |
| Change, % | 13 | 6 | | 11 | 10 | |
| Physical activity, d/wk | | | | | | |
| Preintervention | 37.8 | 27.8 | 0.83 (0.61-1.10) | 45.3 | 41.9 | 1.47 (1.19-1.75)‡ |
| Postintervention | 33.6 | 36.1 | | 55.4 | 38.0 | |
| Change, % | −11 | 30 | | 22 | −9 | |

Abbreviations: CI, confidence interval; PACE+, Patient-centered Assessment and Counseling for Exercise + Nutrition; RR, relative risk; TV, television.

*Girls (PACE+, n = 222; control, n = 216), boys (PACE+, n = 202; control, n = 179). Values are percentages of participants unless otherwise indicated.

†Relative risk and 95% CI estimated from corrected adjusted odds ratio controlling for age, ethnicity, body mass index (calculated as weight in kilograms divided by the square of height in meters) *z* score, and baseline status on guideline.

‡These findings differed meaningfully postintervention given that the 95% confidence intervals postintervention did not overlap.

**Table 4. Logistic Regression Analyses of the Effect of Receiving High or Low Intervention Dose Compared With the Control Condition on Meeting Recommended Health Guidelines***

| Guideline | Girls RR, (95% CI)* Low Dose (0-8 Calls) vs Control (n = 77) | Girls RR, (95% CI)* High Dose (9-11 Calls) vs Control (n = 140) | Boys RR, (95% CI)* Low Dose (0-8 Calls) vs Control (n = 73) | Boys RR, (95% CI)* High Dose (9-11 Calls) vs Control (n = 125) |
|---|---|---|---|---|
| % kcal from fat | 1.04 (0.73-1.39) | 1.06 (0.80-1.34) | 1.03 (0.70-1.13) | 1.13 (0.84-1.45) |
| % kcal from saturated fat | 1.31 (0.91-1.76) | 1.36 (1.02-1.73)† | 1.17 (0.76-1.68) | 1.34 (0.96-1.77) |
| Fruit and vegetable servings/d | 0.81 (0.44-1.39) | 1.50 (1.02-2.03)† | 0.70 (0.39-1.15) | 0.83 (0.54-1.21) |
| Fiber g/1000 kcal per day | 0.80 (0.30-2.01) | 0.82 (0.43-1.87) | 0.68 (0.31-1.34) | 0.69 (0.36-1.23) |
| Physical activity, d/wk | 0.80 (0.51-1.17) | 0.83 (0.58-1.12) | 1.74 (1.35-2.06)† | 1.39 (1.06-1.71)† |
| ≤2 h/d of TV viewing | 1.01 (0.96-1.18) | 1.13 (1.01-1.21)† | 1.02 (0.83-1.14) | 1.06 (0.92-1.16) |

Abbreviations: CI, confidence interval; RR, relative risk; TV, television.

*Relative risk and 95% CI estimated from corrected adjusted odds ratio controlling for age, ethnicity, body mass index (calculated as weight in kilograms divided by the square of height in meters) *z* score, and baseline status on guideline.

†$P<.05$.

pleting at least 9 of the 11 counseling calls. The intervention was effective in reducing sedentary time in both girls and boys, with a net change of approximately 1 hour per day. This is important given that sedentary behaviors can decrease energy intake in nonoverweight adolescents and has been suggested as an important component of interventions to prevent obesity and regulate body weight.[44] The intervention increased the number of days boys met the PA recommendation and the number of days girls met the saturated fat recommendation. These changes were documented for 12 months after the initial provider counseling, supporting the promise of ongoing telephone counseling and targeted materials to support long-term behavior changes. The results of the exploratory analysis of the effects of intervention dose suggest, at least among girls, more frequent outreach and contact can help adolescents make changes in multiple behaviors. This finding suggests the need for research on strategies to maximize participation in effective interventions that target multiple behaviors.

This study helps address the need for research on how multiple health risk behaviors can be evaluated and managed in primary care settings[45] and contributes knowledge about the efficacy of "interactive behavior change technologies" and their utility as a possible adjunct to primary care.[46] Strengths of this research include the large and diverse sample of adolescents, the involvement in the study of a range of primary care settings in San Diego, use of high-quality outcome measures, a comparison condition that controlled for many nonspecific aspects of the intervention, and long-term outcome assessment at 12 months.

There are several limitations to this study. Although we attempted to enroll a representative sample of adolescents seen in primary care, self-selection may have led to selection of adolescents and parents with a strong interest in health interventions like those tested and thus might not be generalizable to adolescents at other stages of change. Another concern is that self-report measurement of diet and PA behaviors is always an imprecise process. Although we used measures that have been validated in other studies, this does not overcome their inherent limitations. However, the accelerometer data tend to support our general findings of time spent in PA in accordance with several other studies of adolescent PA.[47]

An additional concern in interpreting results is the potential impact on our findings of measurement reactivity in which self-reported behavior is influenced by the measurement process itself. Repeated assessments of the target behaviors as well as extensive surveys on thoughts and actions used to change behaviors (not described in this article) could have motivated and even instructed adolescents in both conditions to change behaviors, and control participants reported improvements in several diet and PA behaviors. Measurement effects have been demonstrated in studies promoting PA through primary care settings,[48] and this also may occur with diet assessment. Finally, our intent-to-treat analysis used the last available value of measures for participants who dropped out. If the effect of the intervention was greater in the beginning than it was at the end, this could bias our findings.

The optimal role for health care providers in helping children and adolescents adopt and maintain healthy PA and dietary behaviors has yet to be established. This study among a group of generally healthy adolescents seen in primary care suggests limited effects of provider counseling, even when it is supported by an intervention like PACE+. More intensive interventions, perhaps using a "stepped care" approach that varies the intensity of the intervention, are showing promise in adults[49] and also may be appropriate in childhood. The increasing prevalence of problems such as childhood obesity that result from poor diet and PA, and the recognition that many childhood diseases such as diabetes and hypertension have better outcomes with improvements in these behaviors, suggest the continued need for research in this area.

**Accepted for Publication:** September 1, 2005.
**Correspondence:** Kevin Patrick, MD, MS, Department of Family and Preventive Medicine, University of California, San Diego, 9500 Gilman Dr, MC 0811 La Jolla, CA 92093-0811 (kpatrick@ucsd.edu).
**Author Contributions:** Dr Patrick had full access to all the data in the study and takes responsibility for the integrity of the data and the accuracy of the data analysis.
**Financial Disclosure:** Drs Patrick, Calfas, and Sallis are co-owners of, and receive income from, the Center for Health Interventions, LLC (San Diego, Calif), which is developing products related to the research described in this paper. The terms of this arrangement have been reviewed and approved by San Diego State University and the University of California, San Diego, in accordance with their respective conflict-of-interest policies.
**Funding/Support:** This project was supported by grants R01 CA081495 and R01 CA098861-03S1 from the National Institutes of Health National Cancer Institute, Bethesda, Md.
**Acknowledgment:** We thank the physicians at Kaiser Permanente, San Diego (La Mesa, Bonita, Clairemont Mesa, and Vandever locations); Scripps Clinic, La Jolla, Calif; and the University of California, San Diego, Perlman Ambulatory Care Center for their role in implementing the study and counseling the participants.

## REFERENCES

1. US Department of Health and Human Services. *Physical Activity and Health: A Report of the Surgeon General.* Atlanta, Ga: Centers for Disease Control and Prevention; 1996.
2. Institute of Medicine. *Preventing Childhood Obesity: Health in the Balance.* Washington, DC: National Academy of Sciences; 2004.
3. US Department of Agriculture. Nutrient database for nationwide food surveys, Release 7. Washington, DC: US Dept of Agriculture; 1991.
4. US Department of Agriculture. *The Food Guide Pyramid.* Home and Garden Bulletin No. 252. Washington, DC: US Department of Agriculture; 1992.
5. National Research Council. *Diet and Health: Implications for Reducing Chronic Disease Risk.* Washington, DC: National Academy Press; 1989.
6. National Heart, Lung, and Blood Institute. *Report of the Expert Panel on Population Strategies for Blood Cholesterol Reduction.* Bethesda, Md: US Department of Health and Human Services, Public Health Service, National Institutes of Health Publication No. 90-3046; 1990.
7. National Heart, Lung, and Blood Institute. *Report of the Expert Panel on Blood Cholesterol Levels in Children and Adolescents.* Bethesda, Md: US Department of Health and Human Services, Public Health Service, National Institutes of Health Publication No. 91-2732; 1991.
8. National Cancer Institute (NCI). *Eat More Fruits and Vegetables: 5 a Day for Better Health.* Bethesda, Md: US Department of Health and Human Services, Public Health Service, National Institutes of Health Publication No. 92-3248; 1991.
9. Weinhouse S, Bal DG, Adamson R, et al. American Cancer Society guidelines on diet, nutrition, and cancer: the work study group on diet, nutrition, and cancer. *CA Cancer J Clin.* 1991;41:334-338.
10. American Heart Association. Dietary guidelines for healthy American adults. *Circulation.* 1988;77:721A-724A.
11. Wright JD, Wang C, Kennedy-Stephenson J, Ervin RB. Dietary Intake of ten key nutrients for public health, United States:1999–2000. Advance Data from Vital and Health Statistics, Number 334. Atlanta, Ga: Centers for Disease Control and Prevention, April 17, 2003. Available at: http://www.cdc.gov/nchs/data/ad/ad334.pdf. Accessed on November 18, 2005.
12. Biddle SJH, Gorely T, Stensel DJ. Health-enhancing physical activity and sedentary behaviour in children and adolescents. *J Sports Sci.* 2004;22:679-701.
13. Dietary guidelines for Americans. US Department of Health and Human Services, US Department of Agriculture. Available at: http://www.healthierus.gov/dietaryguidelines. Accessed on May 17, 2005.
14. Biddle S, Cavill N, Sallis J. Policy framework for young people and health: enhancing physical activity. In: Biddle S, Sallis J, Cavil N, eds. *Young and Active? Young People and Health-Enhancing Physical Activity-Evidence and Implications.* London, England: Health Education Authority;1998:3-16.
15. Cavill N, Biddle S, Sallis JF. Health enhancing physical activity for young people: statement of the United Kingdom Expert Consensus Conference. *Pediatric Exercise Science.* 2001;13:12-25.
16. Pate RR, Long BJ, Heath G. Descriptive epidemiology of physical activity in adolescents. *Pediatric Exercise Science.* 1994;6:434-447.

17. Pate RR, Freedson PS, Sallis JF, et al. Compliance with physical activity guidelines: prevalence in a population of children and youth. *Ann Epidemiol.* 2002; 12:303-308.
18. Saelens BE. Helping individuals reduce sedentary behavior. In: Andersen RE, ed. *Obesity: Etiology, Assessment, Treatment, and Prevention.* Champaign, Ill: Human Kinetics; 2003:217-238.
19. Robinson TN. Reducing children's television viewing to prevent obesity: a randomized controlled trial. *JAMA.* 1999;282:1561-1567.
20. Epstein LH, Paluch RA, Kilanowski CK, Raynor HA. The effect of reinforcement of stimulus control to reduce sedentary behavior: the treatment of pediatric obesity. *Health Psychol.* 2004;23:371-380.
21. Epstein LH, Paluch RA, Gordy CC, Dorn J. Decreasing sedentary behaviors in treating pediatric obesity. *Arch Pediatr Adolesc Med.* 2000;154:220-226.
22. Ogden CL, Flegal KM, Carroll MD, Johnson CL. Prevalence and trends in overweight among US children and adolescents. *JAMA.* 2002;288:1728-1732.
23. Resnicow K, Robinson T. School-based cardiovascular disease prevention studies: review and synthesis. *Ann Epidemiol.* 1997;7(suppl):S14-S31.
24. Dishman RK, Buckworth J. Increasing physical activity: a quantitative synthesis. *Med Sci Sports Exerc.* 1996;28:706-719.
25. Contento I, Balch GI, Bronner YL, et al. The effectiveness of nutrition education and implications for nutrition education policy, programs, and research: a review of research. *J Nutr Educ.* 1995;27:275-422.
26. Epstein LH, Myers MD, Raynor HA, Saelens BE. Treatment of pediatric obesity. *Pediatrics.* 1998;101(suppl):554-570.
27. Saelens BE, Sallis J, Wilfley D, Patrick K, Cella J, Buchta R. A randomized trial of a multi-componential behavioral weight control treatment initiated in primary care versus typical care for overweight adolescents. *Obes Res.* 2002;10:22-32.
28. Patrick K, Sallis J, Lydston D, et al. Preliminary evaluation of a multi-component program for nutrition and physical activity change in primary care: PACE+ for adolescents. *Arch Pediatr Adolesc Med.* 2001;155:940-946.
29. Sallis JF, Hovell MF. Determinants of exercise behavior. *Exerc Sport Sci Rev.* 1990; 18:307-330.
30. Bandura A. *Social Foundations of Thought and Action.* Englewood Cliffs, NJ: Prentice-Hall; 1986.
31. Prochaska JO, DiClemente CC. *The Transtheoretical Approach: Crossing Traditional Boundaries of Therapy.* Homewood, Ill: Dow Jones-Irwin; 1984.
32. Weinstock MA, Rossi JS. The Rhode Island Sun Smart Project: a scientific approach to skin cancer prevention. *Clin Dermatol.* 1998;16:411-413.
33. Sallis JF, Buono MJ, Roby JJ, Micale FG, Nelson JA. Seven-day recall and other physical activity self-reports in children and adolescents. *Med Sci Sports Exerc.* 1993;25:99-108.
34. Gross LD, Sallis JF, Buono MJ, Roby JJ, Nelson JA. Reliability of interviewers using the seven-day physical activity recall. *Res Q Exerc Sport.* 1990;61:321-325.
35. Montoye HJ, Kemper HCG, Saris WHM, Washburn RA. *Measuring Physical Activity and Energy Expenditure.* Champaign, Ill: Human Kinetics; 1996.
36. Schakel SF, Sievert YA, Buzzard IM. Sources of data for developing and maintaining a nutrient database. *J Am Diet Assoc.* 1988;88:1268-1271.
37. *Healthy People 2010,* Second Edition. US Department of Health and Human Services. Available at: http://www.healthypeople.gov/Document/tableofcontents.htm#Volume2. Accessed on November 23, 2005.
38. Williams CL, Bollella M, Wynder EL. A new recommendation for dietary fiber in childhood. *Pediatrics.* 1995;96:985-988.
39. Kuczmarski RJ, Ogden CL, Grummer-Strawn LM, et al. *CDC Growth Charts: United States Advanced Data from Vital and Health Statistics.* Hyattsville, Md: National Center for Health Statistics; 2000.
40. Trost SG, Ward DS, Moorehead SM, Watson PD, Riner W, Burke JR. Validity of the computer science and applications (CSA) activity monitor in children. *Med Sci Sports Exerc.* 1998;30:629-633.
41. Zhang J, Yu KF. What's the relative risk? a method of correcting the odds ratio in cohort studies of common outcomes. *JAMA.* 1998;280:1690-1691.
42. Stone EJ, Baranowski T, Sallis JF, Cutler JA. Synthesis of behavioral research for cardiopulmonary health: emphasis on youth, gender, and ethnicity. *J Health Educ.* 1995;26:S9-17.
43. Sallis JF, McKenzie TL, Alcaraz JE, Kolody B, Faucette N, Hovell MF. The effects of a 2-year physical education program (SPARK) on physical activity and fitness in elementary school students. *Am J Public Health.* 1997;87:1328-1334.
44. Epstein LH, Roemmich JN, Paluch RA, Raynor HA. Influence of changes in sedentary behavior on energy and macronutrient intake in youth. *Am J Clin Nutr.* 2005;81:361-366.
45. Orleans TC. Addressing multiple behavioral health risks in primary care: broadening the focus of health behavior change research and practice. *Am J Prev Med.* 2004;27(suppl 2):1-3.
46. Glasgow RE, Bull SS, Piette JD, Steiner JF. Interactive behavior change technology: a partial solution to the competing demands of primary care. *Am J Prev Med.* 2004;27(2S):80-87.
47. Sirard JR, Pate RR. Physical activity assessment in children and adolescents. *Sports Med.* 2001;31:439-454.
48. van Sluijs E. *Effectiveness of Physical Activity Promotion: The Case of General Practice.* (ISBN 90-5669-088-4.) Wageningen, Netherlands: Ponsen & Looijen BV; 2004:57-70.
49. Counterweight Project Team. A new evidence-based model for weight management in primary care: the Counterweight Programme. *J Hum Nutr Diet.* 2004; 17:191-208.

ARTICLE

# Prevalence of the Female Athlete Triad Syndrome Among High School Athletes

*Jeanne F. Nichols, PhD; Mitchell J. Rauh, PhD, PT, MPH; Mandra J. Lawson, MS, RD; Ming Ji, PhD; Hava-Shoshana Barkai, MS*

**Objective:** To estimate the prevalence of the female athlete triad (disordered eating, menstrual irregularity, and low bone mass) among high school athletes.

**Design:** Observational cross-sectional study.

**Setting:** High school.

**Participants:** Female athletes (n=170) representing 8 sports were recruited from 6 high schools in southern California.

**Main Outcome Measures:** Disordered eating and menstrual status were determined by interviewer-assisted questionnaires. Bone mineral density was measured by dual-energy x-ray absorptiometry of the hip, spine (L1-L4), and total body.

**Results:** Among all athletes, 18.2%, 23.5%, and 21.8% met the criteria for disordered eating, menstrual irregularity, and low bone mass, respectively. Ten girls (5.9%) met criteria for 2 components of the triad, and 2 girls (1.2%) met criteria for all 3 components. Oligomenorrheic/amenorrheic athletes had higher mean ± SD eating restraint (1.55±1.60 vs 1.04±1.27; $P=.02$) and Eating Disorder Examination Questionnaire global scores (1.68±1.20 vs 1.33±1.14; $P=.03$) than eumenorrheic athletes. After controlling for age, age at menarche, body mass index, race/ethnicity, and sport type, athletes with oligomenorrhea/amenorrhea had significantly lower mean ± SD bone mineral densities for the trochanter (0.884±0.090 $g \cdot cm^{-2}$) than eumenorrheic athletes (0.933±0.130 $g \cdot cm^{-2}$; $P=.04$).

**Conclusions:** The prevalence of the full female athlete triad was low in our sample; however, a substantial percentage of the athletes may be at risk for long-term health consequences associated with disordered eating, menstrual irregularity, or low bone mass. Preparticipation screening to identify these components should be encouraged as a preventive approach to identify high-risk athletes.

*Arch Pediatr Adolesc Med. 2006;160:137-142*

Nearly 15 years have passed since the female athlete triad was first recognized and reported as a syndrome of 3 interrelated serious health disorders (disordered eating, menstrual dysfunction, and low bone mass).[1] Although there have been numerous reports on prevalence estimates of individual components of the triad, only 2 studies[2,3] have reported the prevalence or directly examined the interrelationships of the triad components concurrently. Lauder et al[2] examined the simultaneous occurrence of all 3 components in active-duty female soldiers and reported that no soldier exhibited the full female athlete triad. Cobb et al[3] provided evidence of the triad's existence among young adult competitive runners by demonstrating interrelationships among disordered eating, menstrual irregularity, and low bone mineral density (BMD) levels. However, they did not report whether any runner met criteria for all 3 components concurrently.

Most reports[3-8] on the individual components of the triad have been limited to collegiate, young adult, or elite athletes. The reported prevalence estimates of eating disorders or disordered eating among female collegiate and elite athletes range from 15% to 62%.[3-8] The large variation in prevalence estimates for athletes may be due to different assessment methods and criteria for classifying disordered eating, sport populations studied, training volume, or competition-level differences. In the general adolescent female population, approximately 13% to 20% have reported disordered eating attitudes and 0.4% to 4.0% have reported the practice of pathogenic behaviors, including self-induced vomiting and laxative or diuretic use.[9]

Menstrual dysfunction, including primary or secondary amenorrhea or oligomenorrhea, has been reported more often in athletes, primarily among collegiate athletes.[10,11] Menstrual dysfunction may be caused by weight fluctuations, insufficient energy availability relative to energy expenditure, and/or stress associated with intense or a high volume of training in the absence of energy imbalance.[10,12] Prevalence estimates of menstrual dysfunction among athletes have ranged from 3.4% to 66.0%.[8,10,13] The wide range in estimates may

Author Affiliations: Department of Exercise and Nutritional Sciences (Drs Nichols and Rauh and Mss Lawson and Barkai) and Graduate School of Public Health (Drs Rauh and Ji), San Diego State University, San Diego, Calif; and Graduate Program in Orthopaedic and Sports Physical Therapy, Rocky Mountain University of Health Professions, Provo, Utah (Dr Rauh).

be due in part to varying criteria used to define amenorrhea and specific sport populations sampled. To our knowledge, the prevalence of menstrual dysfunction among high school athletes has not been reported.

Data on the prevalence of low bone mass in adolescent female athletes are scarce, yet adolescence is a critical time for bone acquisition. Peak bone mass accrual in girls has been linked closely to menarche.[14] Recent literature has demonstrated the positive effect of impact exercise on bone mass in children and adolescents.[15,16] However, several studies[17-20] have demonstrated that the benefits on bone conferred by sports participation may be negated in young athletes with menstrual dysfunction. Therefore, adolescents with menstrual dysfunction may miss a key developmental period to maximize bone mineralization.

According to the National Federation of High School Associations, approximately 2.9 million girls competed in high school sports in the United States during the 2003-2004 school year, representing a 3.5-fold increase in participation since Title IX was implemented in 1972, which prohibited sex discrimination in all public education programs. Increased participation and competitiveness, greater pressure by coaches, and a preoccupation with body image that normally exists during adolescence may increase the risk of developing the triad in this population.[21,22] Currently, limited evidence exists regarding the prevalence of the female athlete triad in high school athletes in the United States. Thus, the primary objectives of our study were to estimate the prevalence of the female athlete triad as a whole and to examine the interrelationships among disordered eating, menstrual irregularity, and low bone density in female high school athletes.

## METHODS

### PARTICIPANTS

The subject sample consisted of female athletes competing on interscholastic teams from 6 high schools in southern California. Participants were 13 to 18 years old who had had initial onset of menarche or, if not menstruating, were 16 to 18 years old. Data from athletes who reported taking any medications known to affect bone mass were excluded from analysis. Subsequently, only 1 athlete was excluded because of long-term use of a steroid inhaler for asthma. A total of 589 athletes (79.6% response rate) completed questionnaires regarding menstrual history and eating behaviors and were measured, without shoes, for height and weight. One research assistant per 6 to 8 athletes reviewed the Eating Disorder Examination Questionnaire (EDE-Q)[23] response scale and questions deemed more difficult to interpret, defined terms (eg, *binge episode*), and then remained in the room to assist athletes who requested further clarification as they completed the questionnaires individually. After stratifying by eating behavior (normal vs elevated EDE-Q score) and menstrual status (eumenorrhea vs oligomenorrhea or amenorrhea), approximately 30% of the total sample was selected to receive a BMD scan. Athletes were randomly selected by sport using a weighted selection process according to the number of participants in each sport. The final sample size was 170, including track and field (n=60), cross-country running (n=33), soccer (n=21), softball (n=16), swimming (n=13), volleyball (n=11), tennis (n=10), and lacrosse (n=6). The study was approved by San Diego State University's institutional review board.

### DATA COLLECTION

#### Eating Attitudes and Behaviors

At the end of the first month of each sport season, each athlete completed the EDE-Q to identify disordered eating attitudes and behaviors.[9,23] The EDE-Q, which is a shorter version of the Eating Disorder Examination[24] and designed for self-report, is composed of 4 subscales, weight concern, shape concern, eating concern, and dietary restraint, and a global score, which is the composite mean score of the 4 subscales. Scores ranging from 0 to 6 on a Likert scale correspond to the number of days during the past 4 weeks the respondent has experienced a specific attitude, feeling, or behavior. The EDE-Q has high internal consistency[25] and moderate to high concurrent and criterion validity.[9,23,26,27] In addition to its psychometric properties, we chose the EDE-Q over other widely used questionnaires because it addresses a specific time frame and specifically assesses the frequency of eating behaviors. We evaluated EDE-Q scores as continuous and dichotomous variables. Athletes were classified as having disordered eating if they had a mean score of 4.0 or higher on the weight concern or shape concern subscales or had a mean global score of 4.0 or higher. A cutoff score of 4, which indicates that a specific attitude or behavior was reported on more than half of the past 28 days, was used to define disordered eating because it was shown to be predictive of eating disorders.[9,28] Also, scores of 4 or higher correspond to the 80th to 95th percentiles from reference norms for adolescent girls.[9] Based on this scoring rubric, athletes were divided into 2 groups: disordered eating (elevated EDE-Q score) or normal EDE-Q score.

#### Menstrual Status

Following administration of the EDE-Q, the athletes completed a menstrual status and history questionnaire, which was derived from an athletic preparticipation medical history form developed to screen for the presence of female athlete triad components.[29] The criteria for classifying athletes with menstrual irregularity were as follows: primary amenorrhea (no onset of menses by the age of 16 years), secondary amenorrhea (cessation of menstrual cycles for $\geq$3 consecutive months in the past year), or oligomenorrhea (menstrual cycles occurring at intervals >35 days after onset of menses by the age of 16 years).[22] For analyses purposes, girls who met any of these criteria were combined into a single (oligomenorrheic/amenorrheic) group and compared with girls with normal menses (eumenorrheic).

#### Bone Mineral Density

At 2 to 4 weeks after the completion of the questionnaires, bone mineral density at the spine (L1-L4), proximal femur, and total body and body composition (percentage of fat and lean tissue mass) were assessed by dual-energy x-ray absorptiometry (DXA) using a densitometer (Lunar DPX-NT; Lunar/GE Corp, Madison, Wis). Quality assurance tests were performed each morning of testing. The coefficient of variation in BMD in our laboratory was 0.6% for the total hip, 1.2% for the spine (L1-L4), and 0.99% for total body.

Currently, no consensus exists for determining osteopenia or osteoporosis in children and adolescents. Therefore, we used the World Health Organization (WHO)[30] and International Society for Clinical Densitometry (ISCD)[31] criteria to define low bone mass. Girls were categorized as having low bone mass for their age if their values for the spine or total body were 1 SD (WHO) or 2 SDs (ISCD) or more below the age-matched, sex-specific reference data from the Lunar/GE Corp pediatric database (*Z*-score of $\leq -1$ or $\leq -2$). The *Z*-scores are currently not available for the hip in children.

**Table 1. Characteristics of EDE-Q Subscales and Global Score by Eating Behavior Group and Previously Published Comparison Groups**

| | Mean (SD) | | | |
|---|---|---|---|---|
| EDE-Q Subscale | Normal EDE-Q Score (n = 139) | Elevated EDE-Q Score (Disordered Eating) (n = 31)* | EDE-Q Scores in Elite Runners With Eating Disorders or Disordered Eating† (n = 29) | Normal EDE-Q Scores for Young Adolescent Girls‡ (n = 808) |
| Weight concern | 1.26 (0.99) | 3.71 (1.48) | 3.12 (0.27) | 1.8 (1.7) |
| Shape concern | 1.59 (1.09) | 3.83 (1.49) | 3.82 (0.22) | 2.2 (1.7) |
| Eating concern | 0.47 (0.56) | 1.96 (1.31) | 2.12 (1.40) | 1.0 (1.0) |
| Dietary restraint | 0.88 (1.15) | 2.40 (1.59) | 2.98 (1.72) | 1.4 (1.5) |
| Global score | 1.06 (0.80) | 2.97 (1.23) | 3.01 (0.22) | 1.6 (1.4) |

Abbreviation: EDE-Q, Eating Disorder Examination Questionnaire.
*Disordered eating group vs normal EDE-Q score group ($P<.001$; independent *t* test).
†Data are from Hulley and Hill.[33] Mean age of the sample was 27.3 years.
‡Data are from Carter et al.[9] Mean age of the sample was 13.4 years.

## STATISTICAL ANALYSES

Outcome measures included disordered eating, menstrual status, and BMD of the spine (L1-L4), proximal femur (total hip, femoral neck, and trochanter), and total body. We reported menstrual irregularity as a dichotomous variable (eumenorrhea vs oligomenorrhea/amenorrhea), whereas eating attitudes or behaviors and BMD were reported as continuous and dichotomous variables. We used independent *t* tests to compare demographic and physical characteristics of athletes in the final sample (ie, those who received a DXA scan [n=170] compared with the girls who completed the initial study questionnaires but were not selected to receive a DXA scan [n=419]). Independent *t* tests were also used to compare physical characteristics between eumenorrheic and oligomenorrheic/amenorrheic athletes, and between athletes with normal vs elevated EDE-Q scores. We conducted $\chi^2$ analysis to determine proportions of oligomenorrheic athletes as a function of years post menarche. Univariate analysis was used to determine the relationship among menarcheal age, menstrual status, and BMD groups. Because body mass has been reported to influence scores on eating attitudes questionnaires,[32] we used analysis of covariance to control for body mass index (BMI) (calculated as weight in kilograms divided by the square of height in meters) when comparing EDE-Q scores of eumenorrheic vs oligomenorrheic/amenorrheic athletes. Analysis of covariance was also used to control for chronological age, age of menarche, BMI, ethnicity, and sport type according to mechanical loading characteristics (swimmers, runners, and high-impact sports) when comparing the BMD of eumenorrheic vs oligomenorrheic/amenorrheic athletes and athletes with disordered eating who did or did not report pathogenic behaviors.

## RESULTS

### RELIABILITY OF QUESTIONNAIRES

Test-retest intraclass correlation coefficients for the EDE-Q global score, subscales, and pathogenic behaviors, excluding binge eating, ranged from 0.84 to 0.92. The intraclass correlation coefficient for binge eating was 0.37. Interrater reliability coefficients for agreement among interviewers were 0.92 to 0.96. Test-retest reliability for the menstrual status questions ranged from 0.87 (number of consecutively missed cycles) to 1.00 (age at menarche), and the intraclass correlation coefficient for interrater reliability ranged from 0.99 to 1.00.

### PARTICIPANT CHARACTERISTICS

The athletes' self-reported race/ethnicity was as follows: 55% white, 21% Latina, 14% African American, 7% Asian, and 3% other. Athletes' age, height, weight, and BMI (mean ± SD) were 15.7 ± 1.3 years, 165.2 ± 7.0 cm, 59.4 ± 8.9 kg, and 21.8 ± 2.9 kg/m$^2$, respectively. Body fat percentage, lean tissue mass, and age of menarche were 26.6% ± 7.0%, 39.5 ± 4.6 kg, and 12.4 ± 1.2 years, respectively. No differences in ethnicity ($P=.32$), age ($P=.67$), height ($P=.92$), weight ($P=.61$), BMI ($P=.74$), or age at menarche ($P=.88$) were found between the athletes selected (n=170) and not selected (n=419). Since body composition was assessed by DXA, we do not know whether body fatness and lean tissue mass were different between the girls who received or did not receive a DXA scan.

### PREVALENCE ESTIMATES OF THE TRIAD AND ITS COMPONENTS

Of the 170 athletes in the sample, 31 (18.2%) met the criteria for disordered eating, 40 (23.5%) had menstrual irregularity (oligomenorrhea/amenorrhea), and 37 (21.8%) had low BMD for their age (WHO criteria), whereas 7 (4.1%) met the ISCD criteria for low bone mass. Ten athletes (5.9%) met criteria for any 2 triad components, whereas 2 other athletes (1.2%) met the criteria for all 3 components of the triad. Among the 419 athletes who were not selected for a BMD scan, 82 (19.6%) and 85 (20.2%) met the criteria for disordered eating and menstrual irregularity, respectively; thus, athletes within the subsample of 170 were similar to those within the larger sample.

### DISORDERED EATING

The mean EDE-Q scores on all subscales for athletes who met the criteria for disordered eating were significantly higher than those of athletes with normal EDE-Q scores (**Table 1**), thus indicating that the EDE-Q discriminated well between

**Table 2. Relationship Between Eating Behaviors and Menstrual Status Group**

| EDE-Q Subscale* | Mean (SD) Eumenorrheic (n = 130) | Mean (SD) Oligomenorrheic/ Amenorrheic† (n = 40) | P Value‡ |
|---|---|---|---|
| Weight concern | 1.63 (1.48) | 2.01 (1.30) | .06 |
| Shape concern | 1.94 (2.20) | 2.20 (1.39) | .15 |
| Dietary restraint | 1.04 (1.27) | 1.55 (1.60) | .02 |
| Global score | 1.33 (1.14) | 1.68 (1.20) | .03 |

Abbreviation: EDE-Q, Eating Disorder Examination Questionnaire.
*The EDE-Q subscales were used to classify girls with disordered eating.
†Oligomenorrhea/amenorrhea was defined as athletes who reported 3 or more consecutive missed menstrual cycles in the past year and/or cycles more than 35 days apart.
‡All comparisons were adjusted for body mass index (analysis of covariance).

**Table 3. Relationship Among Age at Menarche, Menstrual Status Group, and BMD Groups**

| Variable | Age at Menarche, Mean (SD), y | P Value |
|---|---|---|
| Eumenorrheic (n = 130) | 12.28 (1.13) | NA |
| Oligomenorrheic/amenorrheic (n = 40) | 12.81 (1.20) | .05* |
| Normal BMD (n = 127)† | 12.27 (1.17) | NA |
| BMD Z-score −1 to −2 (n = 36)‡ | 12.89 (1.17) | .004 |
| BMD Z-score ≤−2 (n = 7)§ | 13.29 (0.76) | .09∥ |

Abbreviations: BMD, bone mineral density; NA, not applicable.
*Compared with eumenorrheic athletes.
†Athletes with Z-scores greater than −1.
‡World Health Organization criteria for low bone mass.
§International Society for Clinical Densitometry criteria for low bone mass.
∥Compared with athletes with normal BMD, after adjusting for chronological age, body mass index, ethnicity, and percentage of body fat (analysis of covariance).

those with normal eating attitudes and behaviors vs disordered eating ($P<.001$). For comparison purposes, Table 1 also gives the EDE-Q scores from previously published data for elite female runners with eating disorders,[33] as well as normative data from young adolescent girls.[9]

Ten percent of the sample reported the use of pathogenic behaviors to control body weight on 2 or more of the past 28 days. The most common pathogenic behavior reported was vomiting (7%), followed by binging (6.5%), laxative use (1.8%), and diuretic use (1.2%). All athletes who reported pathogenic behaviors also met the criteria for disordered eating based on their scores for weight concern, shape concern, or global score.

## OLIGOMENORRHEA/AMENORRHEA

Menstrual irregularity was reported by 23.5% of the athletes. Of these, oligomenorrhea (17.1%) was the most common menstrual irregularity reported followed by secondary amenorrhea (5.3%) and primary amenorrhea (1.2%). Eumenorrheic and oligomenorrheic/amenorrheic athletes were similar in age, weight, BMI, and percentage of fat. Among the athletes who were less than 5 years post menarche, 17.3% reported oligomenorrhea; among those who were 5 years or more post menarche, 16.3% reported oligomenorrhea ($P=.88$). Thus, oligomenorrhea was not reported more frequently in athletes whose reproductive age was younger.

**Table 4. Bone Mineral Density and Z-Scores of Athletes by Menstrual Status Group**

| Variable | Mean (SD) Eumenorrheic (n = 130) | Mean (SD) Oligomenorrheic/ Amenorrheic* (n = 40) | P Value |
|---|---|---|---|
| Bone mineral density, g · cm$^{-2}$ | | | |
| Spine (L1-L4) | 1.175 (0.125) | 1.133 (0.133) | .21† |
| Total hip | 1.135 (0.134) | 1.091 (0.098) | .11† |
| Femoral neck | 1.114 (0.129) | 1.112 (0.010) | .28† |
| Trochanter | 0.933 (0.130) | 0.884 (0.090) | .04† |
| Total body | 1.170 (0.091) | 1.142 (0.071) | .37† |
| Z-score | | | |
| Spine | 0.169 (1.217) | −0.271 (1.131) | .10‡ |
| Total body | 0.679 (1.084) | 0.400 (0.729) | .28‡ |

*Oligomenorrhea/amenorrhea was defined as athletes who reported 3 or more consecutive missed menstrual cycles in the past year and/or cycles more than 35 days apart.
†Adjusted for chronological age, age at menarche, body mass index (calculated as weight in kilograms divided by the square of height in meters), race/ethnicity, and sport type (analysis of covariance).
‡Adjusted for age at menarche and sport type (analysis of covariance).

## ASSOCIATIONS AMONG DISORDERED EATING, MENSTRUAL IRREGULARITY, AND LOW BONE MASS

After adjusting for BMI, oligomenorrheic/amenorrheic athletes reported significantly higher dietary restraint and EDE-Q global scores than eumenorrheic athletes (**Table 2**). After adjusting for chronological age, ethnicity, BMI, and percentage of body fat, menarcheal age was significantly older in oligomenorrheic/amenorrheic athletes compared with eumenorrheic athletes and in athletes with BMD Z-scores of −1 or less (**Table 3**). After adjusting for age, age of menarche, BMI, race/ethnicity, and sport type, oligomenorrheic/amenorrheic athletes had significantly lower BMD values for the trochanter compared with eumenorrheic athletes (**Table 4**). Among athletes with disordered eating, those who reported pathogenic behaviors ($n=18$) had lower BMD for all bone sites compared with those who did not report pathogenic behaviors ($n=13$), but these differences were not statistically significant ($P=.17$ to .44).

## COMMENT

In contrast to most studies that have focused on collegiate or elite athletes, the present study included athletes from multiple high school sports. Although the percentage of athletes who met criteria for all 3 components of the triad was low, our data demonstrate its existence among high school athletes. Because 5.9% of the athletes met criteria for 2 components and approximately 20% met criteria for any 1 component of the triad, a substantial number of these young athletes may be at increased risk for the full triad over time.

Eighteen percent of the athletes were classified with disordered eating. Beals and Manore[4] found a similar percentage of athletes in multiple sports to be at risk for disordered eating (15.2%), whereas Cobb et al[3] reported elevated Eating Disorder Inventory scores in 25% of a sample of female long-distance runners. Comparisons to their findings are difficult because they studied collegiate or postcollegiate athletes and used different questionnaires to assess disordered eating. Although it is not uncommon for adolescents to report dissatisfaction with body shape and weight in the absence of pathogenic weight control behaviors, the mean scores on all EDE-Q subscales for the athletes with disordered eating were similar to those from a sample of older elite runners diagnosed as having frank eating disorders.[33] Furthermore, the EDE-Q scores of our athletes with normal eating behaviors were, on average, lower than those from a reference sample of younger adolescent girls.[9] These similarities support the scoring rubric we used to define disordered eating and demonstrate that a substantial percentage of the athletes in our study may be at risk for developing pathogenic weight control behaviors.

The percentage of athletes who reported pathogenic eating behaviors was lower than that reported previously for collegiate athletes.[4,6] Although the actual number of girls engaging in pathogenic behaviors was relatively small, 24% of those who engaged in these behaviors reported using 2 or more different pathogenic behaviors in the past 28 days. Moreover, 47% reported a frequency of 4 or more episodes in the past 28 days. Given their young age, these athletes may be at a higher risk for developing serious short- and long-term health problems associated with disordered eating, including nutrient deficiencies, cardiac disturbances, and osteoporosis.

Previous reports on the prevalence of menstrual irregularity in athletes have focused on elite athletes and/or collegiate populations. Cobb et al[3] reported menstrual dysfunction in 36% of distance runners, whereas Beals and Manore[4] reported menstrual irregularity in 31% of collegiate athletes from multiple sports. In our study, most of the athletes with menstrual irregularity reported oligomenorrhea. This finding should be interpreted cautiously because cycles more than 35 days apart may occur during the first 5 years after the onset of menarche, although 89% of girls attain normal cycles within 2 years of menarche.[34] In our sample, 75% were less than 5 years post menarche; thus, we are uncertain whether the oligomenorrheic athletes were actually experiencing menstrual dysfunction. However, the reported percentage of oligomenorrhea was similar among girls who were less than 5 or 5 or more years post menarche. The clinical significance of oligomenorrhea during the first few years post menarche needs further examination to determine whether it is predictive of low peak bone mass in young adults. Only 1.2% of our high school sample reported primary amenorrhea, whereas 7.4% of collegiate athletes have reported primary amenorrhea.[4]

Menarcheal age in our sample was similar to estimates reported for US women[35] indicating that on average, the athletes did not have delayed menarche, which had been reported previously in athletes from a variety of sports.[34,36] Consistent with previous reports,[3,20] we found a positive association between menarcheal age and menstrual irregularity. Menarcheal age of our amenorrheic athletes was approximately 6 months older than that of eumenorrheic athletes, despite no differences in chronological age, body weight, percentage of fat, or BMI. Thus, other factors predictive of late onset of menarche did not explain the differences within menstrual status groups. Moreover, the age at menarche, which was a significant predictor of BMD for all bone sites measured, was approximately 7 months older in the athletes with BMD Z-scores of −1 or less and a full year older in those with BMD Z-scores of −2 or less, although their chronological age and body fatness were similar to those of girls with normal BMD. Therefore, some young athletes may be missing a key bone development period during which participation in sports cannot compensate for other factors associated with bone mineral accrual. Clearly, adolescent athletes with persistent menstrual dysfunction are at high risk of premature osteoporosis. Moreover, bone loss or suboptimal bone mineral accrual associated with amenorrhea may not be completely reversible with the resumption of menses.[19,37]

According to WHO criteria for adult women, we found that 21.8% of the athletes had low BMD values, whereas 4.1% were classified as having low BMD using ISCD criteria. Although the WHO criteria are based on T-scores and are not directly applicable to adolescents, a BMD T-score of −1 SD corresponds to approximately 10% lower bone mass for age.[38] We support the WHO criterion to detect girls at risk earlier than when pharmacologic treatment would normally be prescribed. We believe that behavioral intervention is important for girls with Z-scores of −1 to −2. Since 98% of skeletal mass is acquired by the approximate age of 20 years, girls in their late teens are rapidly approaching their peak BMD. Thus, high school athletes with Z-scores between −1 and −2 are likely to be classified as having osteopenia or osteoporosis within a few years unless the underlying cause of their low bone mass is recognized and addressed.

Somewhat inconsistent with several reports of lower bone mass in amenorrheic vs eumenorrheic athletes,[3,18,19] BMD was significantly lower only for the trochanter in our oligomenorrheic/amenorrheic athletes. However, BMD values for all other bone sites tended to be lower in oligomenorrheic/amenorrheic compared with eumenorrheic athletes. It is possible that the younger age of our athletes and/or their relatively brief history of menstrual irregularity may have precluded results similar to those reported previously, since it has been shown that the amount of bone loss associated with amenorrhea depends on the duration of menstrual dysfunction.[39] The results of the present study underscore the need for longitudinal studies in this population.

We recognize the limitations of self-report and the ability of adolescents to accurately recall past events; however, we believe that we were able to minimize inaccurate reporting by using a semistructured interview procedure and standardizing the procedures for administering the questionnaires. The high reliability coefficients we obtained increased our confidence in the athletes' ability to recall their menstrual history and eating habits and attitudes. By explicitly discussing confidentiality issues with the athletes, we believe that we minimized underreporting of disordered eating and irregular menses, particularly by girls who feared that their results would be shared with their coach or parents. Another limitation was the lack of laboratory data on menstrual function. Assessment of reproductive hormones might have permitted better interpretation of menstrual data, especially in girls who met the criteria for oligomenorrhea/amenorrhea.

In conclusion, this study provides data to inform health care professionals and coaches of the existence of triad components among high school athletes. The prevalence estimates and relationships found between the individual components indicate a need for education and behavioral interventions in this age group. We believe that screening for disordered eating and menstrual irregularity is potentially more important for high school than for college athletes as a first step in preventing comorbidities associated with the triad, particularly because adolescence is a critical period for optimizing bone mineral accrual.

**Accepted for Publication:** August 10, 2005.
**Correspondence:** Jeanne F. Nichols, PhD, Department of Exercise and Nutritional Sciences, San Diego State University, San Diego, CA 92182-7251 (jeannebernhard@cox.net).
**Funding/Support:** This study was funded by grant 903GGP005 from the Research and Education Foundation of the National Athletic Trainers Association (Dallas, Tex) and by a grant from the Graduate Division and Research Affairs, San Diego State University, San Diego, Calif.
**Acknowledgment:** We thank the high school coaches, athletic directors, and athletes for their cooperation and enthusiasm for Project SPIRIT (Sports Injury Research in Teens), as well as the graduate student assistants associated with Project SPIRIT. We also thank Caroline A. Macera, PhD, MPH, FACSM, for reviewing the manuscript.

## REFERENCES


1. Yeager KK, Agostini R, Nattiv A, Drinkwater B. The female athlete triad: disordered eating, amenorrhea, osteoporosis. *Med Sci Sports Exerc.* 1993;25:775-777.
2. Lauder TD, Williams MV, Campbell CS, Davis G, Sherman R, Pulos E. The female athlete triad: prevalence in military women. *Mil Med.* 1999;164:630-635.
3. Cobb KL, Bachrach LK, Greendale G, et al. Disordered eating, menstrual irregularity, and bone mineral density in female runners. *Med Sci Sports Exerc.* 2003;35:711-719.
4. Beals KA, Manore MM. Disorders of the female athlete triad among collegiate athletes. *Int J Sport Nutr Exerc Metab.* 2002;12:281-293.
5. Johnson C, Powers PS, Dick R. Athletes and eating disorders: the National Collegiate Athletic Association study. *Int J Eat Disord.* 1999;26:179-188.
6. Garner DM, Rosen LW, Barry D. Eating disorders among athletes: research and recommendations. *Child Adolesc Psychiatr Clin N Am.* 1998;7:839-857.
7. Sundgot-Borgen J. Prevalence of eating disorders in elite female athletes. *Int J Sport Nutr.* 1993;3:29-40.
8. Torstveit MK, Sundgot-Borgen J. The female athlete triad: are elite athletes at increased risk? *Med Sci Sports Exerc.* 2005;37:184-193.
9. Carter JC, Stewart DA, Fairburn CG. Eating disorder examination questionnaire: norms for young adolescent girls. *Behav Res Ther.* 2001;39:625-632.
10. Loucks AB. Effects of exercise training on the menstrual cycle: existence and mechanisms. *Med Sci Sports Exerc.* 1990;22:275-280.
11. Loucks AB, Horvath SM. Athletic amenorrhea: a review. *Med Sci Sports Exerc.* 1985;17:56-72.
12. Cannavo S, Curto L, Trimarchi F. Exercise-related female reproductive dysfunction. *J Endocrinol Invest.* 2001;24:823-832.
13. Shangold M, Rebar RW, Wentz AC, Schiff I. Evaluation and management of menstrual dysfunction in athletes. *JAMA.* 1990;263:1665-1669.
14. McKay HA, Bailey DA, Mirwald RL, Davison KS, Faulkner RA. Peak bone mineral accrual and age at menarche in adolescent girls: a 6-year longitudinal study. *J Pediatr.* 1998;133:682-687.
15. McKay HA, Petit MA, Schutz RW, Prior JC, Barr SI, Khan KM. Augmented trochanteric bone mineral density after modified physical education classes: a randomized school-based exercise intervention study in prepubescent and early pubescent children. *J Pediatr.* 2000;136:156-162.
16. Fuchs RK, Bauer JJ, Snow CM. Jumping improves hip and lumbar spine bone mass in prepubescent children: a randomized controlled trial. *J Bone Miner Res.* 2001;16:148-156.
17. Bennell KL, Malcolm SA, Thomas SA, et al. Risk factors for stress fractures in track and field athletes: a twelve-month prospective study. *Am J Sports Med.* 1996;24:810-818.
18. Drinkwater BL, Bruemner B, Chesnut CH III. Menstrual history as a determinant of current bone density in young athletes. *JAMA.* 1990;263:545-548.
19. Jonnavithula S, Warren MP, Fox RP, Lazaro MI. Bone density is compromised in amenorrheic women despite return of menses: a 2-year study. *Obstet Gynecol.* 1993;81(suppl 5, pt 1):669-674.
20. Myburgh KH, Bachrach LK, Lewis B, Kent K, Marcus R. Low bone mineral density at axial and appendicular sites in amenorrheic athletes. *Med Sci Sports Exerc.* 1993;25:1197-1202.
21. Otis CL, Drinkwater B, Johnson M, Loucks A, Wilmore J. American College of Sports Medicine position stand: the Female Athlete Triad. *Med Sci Sports Exerc.* 1997;29:i-ix.
22. American Academy of Pediatrics Committee on Sports Medicine and Fitness. Medical concerns in the female athlete. *Pediatrics.* 2000;106:610-613.
23. Fairburn CG, Beglin SJ. Assessment of eating disorders: interview or self-report questionnaire? *Int J Eat Disord.* 1994;16:363-370.
24. Cooper Z, Fairburn CG. The Eating Disorder Examination: a semi-structured interview for the assessment of the specific psychopathology of eating disorders. *Int J Eat Disord.* 1987;6:1-8.
25. Luce KH, Crowther JH. The reliability of the Eating Disorder Examination-Self-Report Questionnaire Version (EDE-Q). *Int J Eat Disord.* 1999;25:349-351.
26. Mond JM, Hay PJ, Rodgers B, Owen C, Beumont PJ. Validity of the Eating Disorder Examination Questionnaire (EDE-Q) in screening for eating disorders in community samples. *Behav Res Ther.* 2004;42:551-567.
27. Binford R, Le Grange D, Jellar C. Eating Disorders Examination versus Eating Disorders Examination-Questionnaire in adolescents with full and partial-syndrome bulimia nervosa and anorexia nervosa. *Int J Eat Disord.* 2005;37:44-49.
28. Allison DB. *Handbook of Assessment Methods for Eating Behaviors and Weight Related Problems: Measures, Theory, and Research.* Thousand Oaks, Calif: Sage Publications; 1995.
29. Van de Loo DA, Johnson MD. The young female athlete. *Clin Sports Med.* 1995;14:687-707.
30. World Health Organization. Assessment of fracture risk and its application to screening for postmenopausal osteoporosis: report of a WHO Study Group. Geneva, Switzerland: World Health Organization; 1994.
31. International Society for Clinical Densitometry. Diagnosis of osteoporosis in men, premenopausal women, and children. *J Clin Densitom.* 2004;7:17-26.
32. Wilfley DE, Schwartz MB, Spurrell EB, Fairburn CG. Using the eating disorder examination to identify the specific psychopathology of binge eating disorder. *Int J Eat Disord.* 2000;27:259-269.
33. Hulley AJ, Hill AJ. Eating disorders and health in elite women distance runners. *Int J Eat Disord.* 2001;30:312-317.
34. World Health Organization. Longitudinal study of menstrual patterns in the early postmenarcheal period, duration of bleeding episodes and menstrual cycles. *J Adolesc Health Care.* 1986;7:236-244.
35. Chumlea WC, Schubert CM, Roche AF, et al. Age at menarche and racial comparisons in US girls. *Pediatrics.* 2003;111:110-113.
36. Warren MP. The effects of exercise on pubertal progression and reproductive function in girls. *J Clin Endocrinol Metab.* 1980;51:1150-1157.
37. Drinkwater BL, Nilson K, Ott S, Chesnut CH III. Bone mineral density after resumption of menses in amenorrheic athletes. *JAMA.* 1986;256:380-382.
38. Wacker W, Braden HS. Pediatric reference data for male and female total body and spine BMD and BMC. Paper presented at: Annual Meeting of the International Society of Clinical Densiometry, March 14, 2001; Dallas, Tex.
39. Davies MCHM, Jacobs HS. Bone mineral loss in young women with amenorrhea. *BMJ.* 1990;301:790-793.

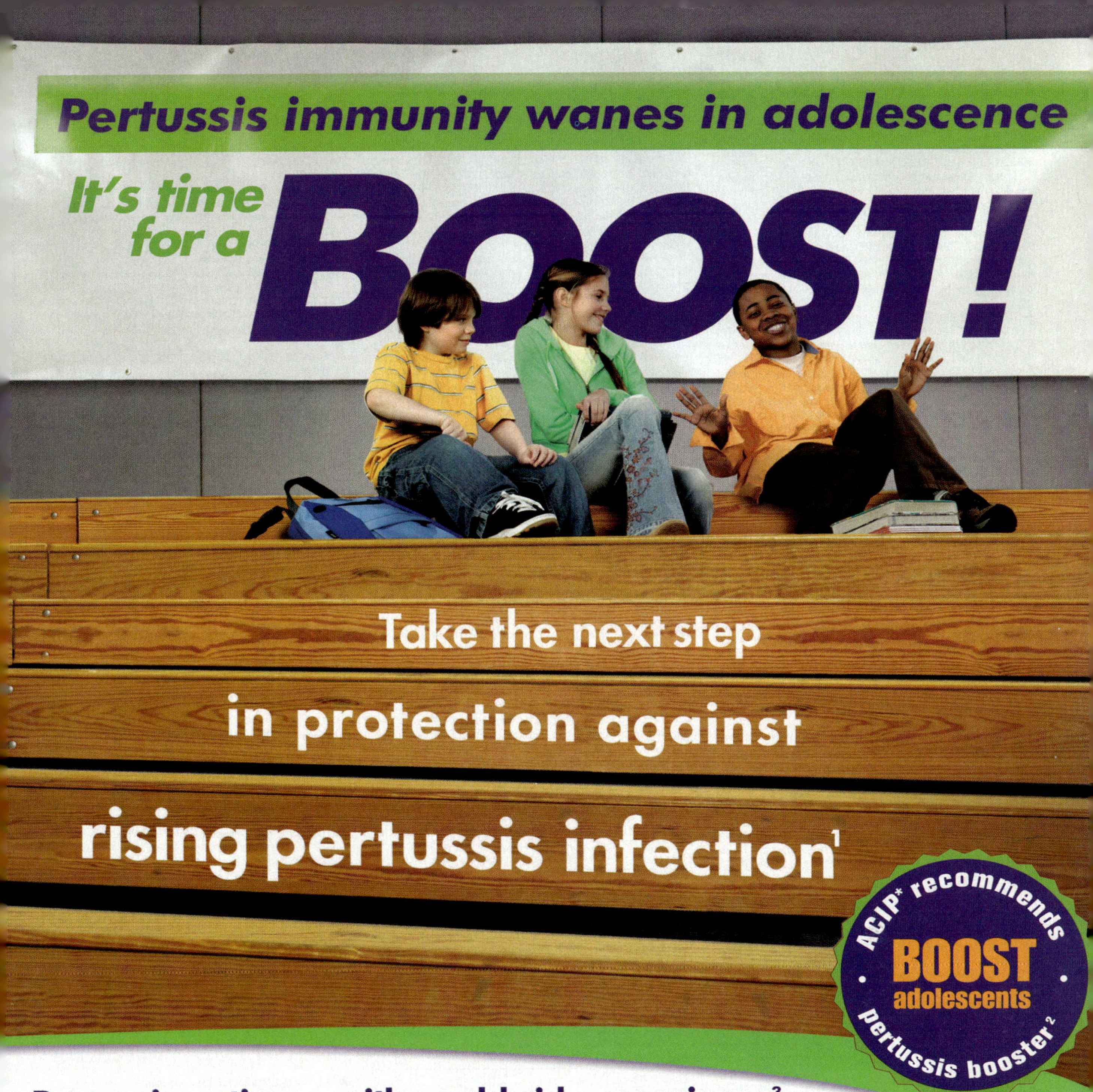


## Pertussis antigens with worldwide experience[3]—*combined* with a Td booster

### Important Safety Information

In clinical studies, adverse events included pain, redness, and swelling at the injection site, headache, fatigue, and gastrointestinal symptoms. As with other vaccines, rare adverse events may occur. As with any vaccine, vaccination with BOOSTRIX may not protect 100% of susceptible individuals. Hypersensitivity to any component of BOOSTRIX is a contraindication.

*Advisory Committee on Immunization Practices.

**BOOSTRIX®**

***Tetanus Toxoid, Reduced Diphtheria Toxoid and Acellular Pertussis Vaccine, Adsorbed***

gsk GlaxoSmithKline Vaccines

**Please see the accompanying brief summary of complete prescribing information.**


Manufactured by **GlaxoSmithKline Biologicals**, Rixensart, Belgium Distributed by **GlaxoSmithKline**, Research Triangle Park, NC 27709

# BOOSTRIX®

**(Tetanus Toxoid, Reduced Diphtheria Toxoid and Acellular Pertussis Vaccine, Adsorbed) (Tdap)**

The following is a brief summary only; see full prescribing information for complete product information.

**INDICATIONS AND USAGE:** BOOSTRIX is indicated for active booster immunization against tetanus, diphtheria, and pertussis as a single dose in individuals 10 through 18 years of age. The use of BOOSTRIX as a primary series or to complete the primary series has not been studied. As with any vaccine, BOOSTRIX may not protect 100% of individuals receiving the vaccine. BOOSTRIX is not recommended for treatment of actual infections.

**CONTRAINDICATIONS:** Hypersensitivity to any component of the vaccine is a contraindication (see DESCRIPTION in full prescribing information). Do not use BOOSTRIX after a serious allergic reaction (e.g., anaphylaxis) following any other tetanus toxoid, diphtheria toxoid or pertussis-containing vaccine, or any component of this vaccine (see DESCRIPTION in full prescribing information). Because of the uncertainty as to which component of the vaccine might be responsible, do not give further vaccination with any of these components; or, refer such individuals to an allergist for evaluation. The following events are contraindications to administration of BOOSTRIX: encephalopathy (e.g., coma, decreased level of consciousness, prolonged seizures) within 7 days of administration of a previous dose of a pertussis-containing vaccine that is not attributable to another identifiable cause; progressive neurologic disorder, uncontrolled epilepsy, or progressive encephalopathy. Do not vaccinate individuals with these conditions until a treatment regimen has been established and the condition has stabilized. BOOSTRIX is not contraindicated for use in individuals with HIV infection.

**WARNINGS:** The tip cap and the rubber plunger of the needleless prefilled syringes contain dry natural latex rubber that may cause allergic reactions in latex sensitive individuals. The vial stopper is latex-free. If any of the following events occurred in temporal relation to previous receipt of a Diphtheria and Tetanus Toxoids and Pertussis Vaccine Adsorbed (DTwP) vaccine or a vaccine containing an acellular pertussis component, consider carefully whether to give subsequent doses of BOOSTRIX: temperature of ≥40.5°C (105°F) within 48 hours not due to another identifiable cause; collapse or shock-like state (hypotonic-hyporesponsive episode) within 48 hours; persistent, inconsolable crying lasting ≥3 hours, occurring within 48 hours; seizures with or without fever occurring within 3 days. Persons who experienced serious Arthus-type hypersensitivity reactions following a prior dose of tetanus toxoid usually have high serum tetanus antitoxin levels and should not be given Tetanus and Diphtheria Toxoids Adsorbed For Adult Use (Td) or Tdap vaccines or even emergency doses of Td more frequently than every 10 years, even if the wound is neither clean nor minor. If Guillain-Barré syndrome has occurred within 6 weeks of receipt of prior vaccine containing tetanus toxoid, the decision to give BOOSTRIX or any vaccine containing tetanus toxoid should be based on careful consideration of the potential benefits and possible risks. The decision to administer a pertussis-containing vaccine to individuals with stable central nervous system (CNS) disorders must be made by the physician on an individual basis, with consideration of all relevant factors, and assessment of potential risks and benefits for that individual. Advise the patient, parent, or guardian of the potential increased risk involved (see PRECAUTIONS). A family history of seizures or other CNS disorders is not a contraindication to pertussis vaccine. The Advisory Committee on Immunization Practices (ACIP) has published guidelines for vaccination of persons with recent or acute illness (www.cdc.gov). Do not give BOOSTRIX to individuals with bleeding disorders such as hemophilia or thrombocytopenia, or to persons on anticoagulant therapy unless the potential benefit clearly outweighs the risk of administration. If the decision is made to administer BOOSTRIX to such persons, it should be given with caution with steps taken to avoid the risk of hematoma following the injection.

**PRECAUTIONS:** Before the injection of any biological, the physician should take all reasonable precautions to prevent allergic or other adverse reactions. Epinephrine injection (1:1,000) and other appropriate agents used for the control of immediate allergic reactions must be immediately available should an acute anaphylactic reaction occur. Immunosuppressed persons, including individuals receiving immunosuppressive therapy, may not develop the expected immune response. **Drug Interactions:** Do not mix BOOSTRIX with any other vaccine in the same syringe or vial. **Carcinogenesis, Mutagenesis, Impairment of Fertility:** BOOSTRIX has not been evaluated for carcinogenic or mutagenic potential, or for impairment of fertility. **Pregnancy:** Pregnancy Category C. Animal reproduction studies have not been conducted with BOOSTRIX. It is also not known whether BOOSTRIX can cause fetal harm when administered to a pregnant woman or can affect reproductive capacity. BOOSTRIX should be given to a pregnant woman only if clearly needed. Animal fertility studies have not been conducted with BOOSTRIX. In a developmental toxicity study, the effect of BOOSTRIX on embryo-fetal and pre-weaning development was evaluated in pregnant rats. Animals were administered INFANRIX® (Diphtheria and Tetanus Toxoids and Acellular Pertussis Vaccine Adsorbed) prior to gestation and BOOSTRIX during the period of organogenesis (gestation days 6, 8, 11) and later in pregnancy (gestation day 15), 0.1 mL/rat/occasion (a 45-fold increase compared to the human dose of BOOSTRIX on a body weight basis), by intramuscular injection. No adverse affect on pregnancy and lactation parameters, embryo-fetal or pre-weaning development was observed. There were no fetal malformations or other evidence of teratogenesis noted in this study. **Nursing Mothers:** It is not known whether BOOSTRIX is excreted in human milk. Because many drugs are excreted in human milk, caution should be exercised when BOOSTRIX is administered to a nursing woman. **Pregnancy Exposure Registry:** Healthcare providers are encouraged to register pregnant women who receive BOOSTRIX in the GlaxoSmithKline vaccination pregnancy registry by calling 1-888-825-5249. **Geriatric Use:** BOOSTRIX is not indicated for use in individuals older than 18 years. **Pediatric Use:** BOOSTRIX is not indicated for use in individuals younger than 10 years (see DOSAGE AND ADMINISTRATION in full prescribing information). For immunization of infants and children younger than 7 years against diphtheria, tetanus, and pertussis, refer to the manufacturers' package inserts for Diphtheria and Tetanus Toxoids and Acellular Pertussis Vaccine Adsorbed (DTaP) vaccines.

**ADVERSE REACTIONS:** A total of 3,289 adolescents were vaccinated with a single dose of BOOSTRIX during clinical trials. An additional 1,092 adolescents 10 to 18 years of age received a non-US formulation of BOOSTRIX (formulated to contain 0.5 mg aluminum per dose) in non-US clinical studies.

The primary safety study, conducted in the United States, was a randomized, observer-blinded, controlled study in which 3,080 adolescents 10 to 18 years of age received a single dose of BOOSTRIX and 1,034 received the control Td vaccine manufactured by Massachusetts Public Health Biologic Laboratories. There were no substantive differences in demographic characteristics between the vaccine groups. Among BOOSTRIX and control vaccine recipients approximately 75% were 10 to 14 years of age and approximately 25% were 15 to 18 years of age. Approximately 98% of participants in this study had received the recommended series of 4 or 5 doses of either DTwP or a combination of DTwP and DTaP in childhood. Data on adverse events were collected by the subjects, parents and/or guardians using standardized diaries for 15 consecutive days following the vaccine dose (i.e., day of vaccination and the next 14 days). Subjects were monitored for unsolicited adverse events that occurred within 31 days of vaccination (day 0-30) using diary cards (day 0-14) supplemented by spontaneous reports and a medical history as reported by subjects, parents, and/or guardians. Subjects were also monitored for 6 months post-vaccination for non-routine medical visits, visits to an emergency room, onset of new chronic illness, and serious adverse events. Information regarding late onset adverse events was obtained via a telephone call 6 months following vaccination. At least 97% of subjects completed the 6-month follow-up evaluation.

The adverse event information from clinical trials provides a basis for identifying adverse events that appear to be related to vaccine use and for approximating rates. However, because clinical trials are conducted under widely varying conditions, adverse event rates observed in the clinical trials of a vaccine cannot be directly compared to rates in the clinical trials of another vaccine, and may not reflect the rates observed in practice.

**Serious Adverse Events in All Safety Studies:** In the US-safety study, no serious adverse events were reported to occur within 31 days of vaccination. During the 6-month extended safety evaluation period, no serious adverse events that were of potential autoimmune origin or new onset and chronic in nature were reported to occur. In non-US studies in which serious adverse events were monitored for up to 37 days, one subject was diagnosed with insulin dependent diabetes. The association of this event with vaccination is unknown. No other serious adverse events of potential autoimmune origin or that were new onset and chronic in nature were reported to occur in these studies.

**Solicited Adverse Events in the US-Safety Study:** In a US study, the most common local adverse events following administration of BOOSTRIX were pain, redness, and swelling at the injection site. The most common general adverse events were headache and fatigue. Most of these events were reported at a similar frequency in recipients of both BOOSTRIX and Td. Any pain, grade 2 or 3 pain (but not grade 3 alone), and grade 2 or 3 headache (but not grade 3 alone) were reported at a higher rate in recipients of BOOSTRIX. The primary safety endpoint of the US study was the incidence of grade 3 pain (spontaneously painful and/or prevented normal activity) at the injection site within 15 days of vaccination. Grade 3 pain was reported in 4.6% of those who received BOOSTRIX compared with 4.0% of those who received the Td vaccine. The difference in rate of grade 3 pain was within the pre-defined clinical limit for non-inferiority (upper limit of the 95% CI for the difference ≤4%). These were the rates for solicited local and general adverse events within 15 days of vaccination with BOOSTRIX or Td vaccine for the total vaccinated cohort (all enrolled, vaccinated subjects with safety data available analyzed by vaccine received):

**Percentage of Individuals 10 to 18 Years of Age Reporting Solicited Local Adverse Events or Solicited General Adverse Events Within the 15-day* Post-Vaccination Period**

| | BOOSTRIX (N = 3,032) | Td (N = 1,013) |
|---|---|---|
| **Local** | | |
| Pain,[†] any | 75.3 | 71.7 |
| Pain,[†] grade 2 or 3 | 51.2 | 42.5 |
| Pain,[‡] grade 3 | 4.6 | 4.0 |
| Redness, any | 22.5 | 19.8 |
| Redness, >20 mm | 4.1 | 3.9 |
| Redness, ≥50 mm | 1.7 | 1.6 |
| Swelling, any | 21.1 | 20.1 |
| Swelling, >20 mm | 5.3 | 4.9 |
| Swelling, ≥50 mm | 2.5 | 3.2 |
| Arm circumference increase,[§] >5 mm | 28.3 | 29.5 |
| Arm circumference increase,[§] >20 mm | 2.0 | 2.2 |
| Arm circumference increase,[§] >40 mm | 0.5 | 0.3 |
| **General** | | |
| Fever,[‖] ≥99.5°F | 13.5 | 13.1 |
| Fever,[‖] >100.4°F | 5.0 | 4.7 |
| Fever,[‖] >102.2°F | 1.4 | 1.0 |
| Headache, any | 43.1 | 41.5 |
| Headache,[†] grade 2 or 3 | 15.7 | 12.7 |
| Headache, grade 3 | 3.7 | 2.7 |
| Fatigue, any | 37.0 | 36.7 |
| Fatigue, grade 2 or 3 | 14.4 | 12.9 |
| Fatigue, grade 3 | 3.7 | 3.2 |
| Gastrointestinal symptoms,[¶] any | 26.0 | 25.8 |
| Gastrointestinal symptoms,[¶] grade 2 or 3 | 9.8 | 9.7 |
| Gastrointestinal symptoms,[¶] grade 3 | 3.0 | 3.2 |

Td = Tetanus and Diphtheria Toxoids Adsorbed For Adult Use manufactured by Massachusetts Public Health Biologic Laboratories.

N = number of subjects in the total vaccinated cohort with local/general symptoms sheets completed.

Grade 2 = Local: painful when the limb was moved; General: interfered with normal activity.

Grade 3 = Local: spontaneously painful and/or prevented normal activity; General: prevented normal activity.

*Day of vaccination and the next 14 days.

[†]Statistically significantly higher (P<0.05) following BOOSTRIX as compared to Td vaccine.

[‡]Grade 3 injection site pain following BOOSTRIX was not inferior to Td (upper limit of two-sided 95% CI for the difference in the percentage of subjects ≤4%).

[§]Mid-upper region of the vaccinated arm.

[‖]Oral temperatures or axillary temperatures.

[¶]Gastrointestinal symptoms included nausea, vomiting, diarrhea and/or abdominal pain.

Mid-upper arm circumference was measured by the adolescent or their parent/guardian prior to injection and daily for 15 days following vaccination. There was no significant difference between BOOSTRIX recipients and Td recipients in the proportion of subjects reporting an increase in mid-upper arm circumference in the vaccinated arm. The incidence of unsolicited adverse events reported in the 31 days after vaccination was comparable between the 2 groups.

As with any vaccine, there is the possibility that broad use of BOOSTRIX could reveal adverse events not observed in clinical trials.

**Postmarketing Reports:** Worldwide voluntary reports of adverse events received for BOOSTRIX in persons 10 to 18 years of age since market introduction of this vaccine are listed below. This list includes serious events or events which have causal connection to components of this or other vaccines or drugs. Because these events are reported voluntarily from a population of uncertain size, it is not possible to reliably estimate their frequency or establish a causal relationship to vaccine exposure. *Blood and lymphatic system disorders:* Lymphadenitis, lymphadenopathy. *Cardiac disorders:* Myocarditis. *Injection site reactions:* Induration, inflammation, mass, nodule, warmth, local reaction. *Metabolism and nutrition disorders:* Diabetes mellitus insulin-dependent. *Musculoskeletal and connective tissue disorders:* Arthralgia, back pain, myalgia. *Nervous system disorders:* Convulsion, encephalitis, facial palsy, paraesthesia. *Skin and subcutaneous tissue disorders:* Exanthem, Henoch-Schönlein purpura, rash. In addition, extensive swelling of the injected limb has been reported following administration of BOOSTRIX.

**Reporting Adverse Events:** Report the occurrence following immunization of any event set forth in the Vaccine Injury Table from the National Childhood Vaccine Injury Act including: Anaphylaxis or anaphylactic shock within 7 days, encephalopathy or encephalitis within 7 days, brachial neuritis within 28 days, or an acute complication or sequelae (including death) of an illness, disability, injury, or condition referred to above, or any events that would contraindicate further doses of vaccine, according to this prescribing information. These events should be reported to VAERS. The VAERS toll-free number is 1-800-822-7967. Reporting forms may also be obtained at the VAERS website at www.vaers.org.

**DOSAGE AND ADMINISTRATION: Recommended Dose:** BOOSTRIX should be administered as a single 0.5 mL injection by the intramuscular route into the deltoid muscle of the upper arm in individuals 10 through 18 years of age. Do not administer this product subcutaneously or intravenously. There are no data to support repeat administration of BOOSTRIX. Five years should elapse between the subject's last dose of the recommended series of childhood DTwP and/or DTaP vaccine and the administration of BOOSTRIX. Limited data are available on the use of BOOSTRIX following Tetanus and Diphtheria Toxoids Adsorbed For Adult Use (Td) vaccine. **Additional Dosing Information:** ***Wound Management:*** Clinicians should refer to guidelines for tetanus prophylaxis in routine wound management. Adolescents 10 to 18 years of age who have completed a primary series against tetanus and who sustain wounds which are minor and uncomplicated, should receive a booster dose of a tetanus toxoid-containing vaccine only if they have not received tetanus toxoid within the preceding 10 years. In case of tetanus-prone injury (e.g., wounds contaminated with dirt, feces, soil, and saliva; puncture wounds; avulsions; and wounds resulting from missles, crushing, burns, and frostbite) in an adolescent who is in need of tetanus toxoid, BOOSTRIX can be used as an alternative to Tetanus and Diphtheria Toxoids Adsorbed For Adult Use (Td) vaccine in patients for whom the pertussis component is also indicated (see INDICATIONS AND USAGE).

Manufactured by **GlaxoSmithKline Biologicals**
Rixensart, Belgium, US License 1617
Distributed by **GlaxoSmithKline**
Research Triangle Park, NC 27709



Full prescribing information for BOOSTRIX is available at www.BOOSTRIX.com.

BRS-BO:L1

**References: 1.** Centers for Disease Control and Prevention. *Epidemiology and Prevention of Vaccine-Preventable Diseases.* Atkinson W, Hamborsky J, Wolfe S, eds. 8th ed. Washington DC: Public Health Foundation; 2004:75–88, A26–A27. **2.** ACIP recommends adolescent vaccination for tetanus, diphtheria and pertussis vaccine [press release]. Atlanta, GA: Department of Health and Human Services; Available at: www.cdc.gov/nip/pr/pr_tdap_jun2005.htm. Accessed September 27, 2005. **3.** Data on file, BOR305, GlaxoSmithKline.

# HOW COULD HUMAN PAPILLOMAVIRUS (HPV) AFFECT YOUR PATIENTS' FUTURE?

Although most **HPV** (human papillomavirus) infectio

# can be serious, an

## Cervical Cancer[1–7]

### VIRTUALLY ALL

A worldwide clinical study found virtually all cases of cervical cancer were linked to certain oncogenic types of HPV.[1]

There are 15 to 20 HPV types classified as oncogenic (high risk).[2,3]

### 10 WOMEN EVERY DAY

In the United States, an estimated 10 women **die every day from cervical cancer**— more than 3,700 women a year.[4]

## ppear to clear on their own, some HPV consequences
# thers are widely seen[1–11]

## Cervical Dysplasia[7–10]

**Case estimates of HPV-related cervical dysplasia each year in the United States[10]:**

- **330,000** new cases of high-grade cervical dysplasia (CIN 2/3)
- **1.4 million** new cases of low-grade cervical dysplasia (CIN 1)

## Genital Warts[5,9,11]

### 1 MILLION

There are an estimated 1 million new cases of genital warts each year in the United States.[11]

# Because **HPV** is often spread unknowingly,[12] **young women and adolescents** in your practice are **at risk** for HPV infection

## 80%

At least **80%** of sexually active women in the United States will have acquired a genital HPV infection by 50 years of age.[12]

## Nearly 1 out of 4

In the United States in 2000, there were almost 9.2 million sexually active young males and females **15 to 24 years of age** estimated to be infected with HPV. This translates to nearly **1 out of 4** of all the 15- to 24-year-olds in the country.[13]

## Most people are unaware of their infection[12]

- HPV infection can be **asymptomatic** or subclinical in its manifestations.[12]
- HPV is often **underdiagnosed.**[14]

**References: 1.** Walboomers JMM, Jacobs MV, Manos MM, et al. Human papillomavirus is a necessary cause of invasive cervical cancer worldwide. *J Pathol.* 1999;189:12–19. **2.** Muñoz N, Bosch FX, de Sanjose S, et al, for the International Agency for Research on Cancer Multicenter Cervical Cancer Study Group. Epidemiologic classification of human papillomavirus types associated with cervical cancer. *N Engl J Med.* 2003;348:518–527. **3.** Wiley DJ, Douglas J, Beutner K, et al. External genital warts: Diagnosis, treatment, and prevention. *Clin Infect Dis.* 2002;35(suppl 2):S210–S224. **4.** American Cancer Society. *Cancer Facts and Figures 2005.* Atlanta, Ga: American Cancer Society; 2005:20–21. **5.** National Toxicology Program. *Report on Carcinogens, Eleventh Edition.* Washington, DC: US Dept of Health and Human Services, Public Health Service, National Toxicology Program; Updated 2005. Available at: http://ntp-server.niehs.nih.gov/ntp/roc/toc11.html. Accessed November 9, 2005. **6.** Lowy DR, Kirnbauer R, Schiller JT. Genital human papillomavirus infection. *Proc Natl Acad Sci USA.* 1994;91:2436–2440. **7.** National Cancer Institute. Recent studies regarding HPV and cervical cancer: Questions and answers [fact sheet]. Available at: http://www.cancer.gov/cancertopics/factsheet/HPVCervicalQandA. Accessed August 30, 2005. **8.** Moscicki A-B, Hills N, Shiboski S, et al. Risks for incident human papillomavirus infection and low-grade squamous intraepithelial lesion development in young females. *JAMA.* 2001;285:2995–3002. **9.** Palefsky J. Abnormal Paps: An LSIL diagnosis. In: *What Your Doctor May Not Tell You About HPV and Abnormal Pap Smears.* New York, NY: Warner Books; 2002:115–128. **10.** Schiffman M, Solomon D. Findings to date from the ASCUS-LSIL triage study (ALTS). *Arch Pathol Lab Med.* 2003;127:946–949. **11.** Fleischer AB, Parrish CA, Glenn R, Feldman SR. Condylomata acuminata (genital warts): Patient demographics and treating physicians. *Sex Transm Dis.* 2001;28:643–647. **12.** Centers for Disease Control and Prevention, National Center for HIV, STD and TB Prevention, Division of Sexually Transmitted Diseases. STD prevention: Genital HPV infection [fact sheet]. Available at: http://www.cdc.gov/std/HPV/STDFact-HPV.htm. Accessed April 21, 2005. **13.** Weinstock H, Berman S, Cates W Jr. Sexually transmitted diseases among American youth: Incidence and prevalence estimates, 2000. *Perspect Sex Reprod Health.* 2004;36:6–10. **14.** Centers for Disease Control and Prevention, National Network of STD/HIV Prevention Training Centers. Core training programs: STD clinical training. Core curricular outlines for clinical training courses: HPV. June 2004. Available at: http://depts.washington.edu/nnptc/core_training/clinical/PDF/HPV%202004.pdf. Accessed August 15, 2005.

MERCK



20503284-HPV
PRINTED IN USA

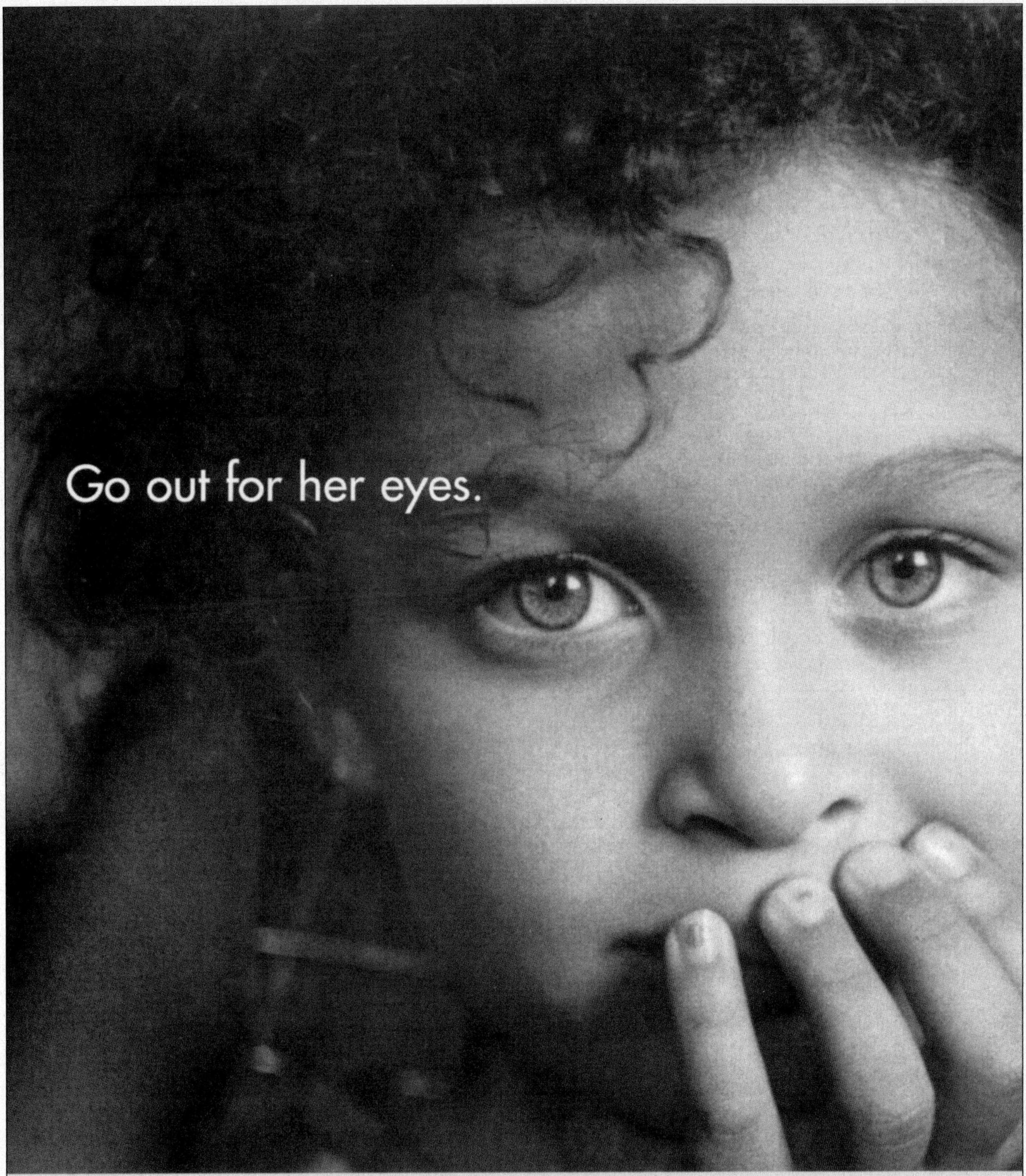


Until you can stop smoking, smoke outside for your daughter. She could get fewer earaches, be less susceptible to respiratory infections and be less likely to get asthma.

Until you can stop smoking, go out for your kids.

Take the Smoke-Free Home Pledge. Call 1 800-513-1157

American Medical Association • Environmental Protection Agency • Consumer Federation of America Foundation

ARTICLE

# Drug Testing of Adolescents in Ambulatory Medicine

## *Physician Practices and Knowledge*

*Sharon Levy, MD, MPH; Sion Kim Harris, PhD; Lon Sherritt, MPH; Michelle Angulo, BA; John R. Knight, MD*

**Objective:** To determine physicians' knowledge of urine drug testing and usual practices when performing drug testing on adolescent patients at a time when interest in drug testing of adolescents is on the rise and physicians may be consulted for advice and requests to perform tests.

**Design and Participants:** Multimodal survey conducted April to July 2004 consisting of 42 forced-choice response items. Participants were practicing physicians randomly selected from the national membership rolls of the American Academy of Pediatrics, Society of Adolescent Medicine, and American Academy of Family Physicians who provided care for 10 or more adolescents per week. We computed simple frequencies and sample design-adjusted 95% confidence intervals for each item.

**Results:** The survey was completed by 359 eligible physicians (response rate, 42%). More than 95% of respondents had ever ordered urine drug tests. Only 23% used an effective urine sample collection procedure, and only 7% used specific gravity and measurement of urine creatinine level to ensure validity of the sample, as recommended. When asked which drugs can be detected in routine panels, only 10% answered all items correctly, 47% did not know for 1 or more items, and 75% responded incorrectly for 1 or more items.

**Conclusions:** Primary care physicians do not always use proper urine sample collection and validation procedures, and they are not aware of important limitations of drug testing. The primary care workforce is not prepared to assist with drug testing programs. Physicians who order these tests need more training and access to consultation with experts.

*Arch Pediatr Adolesc Med. 2006;160:146-150*

DRUG TESTING HAS BEcome increasingly popular in American society during the past 25 years. In 1995, the US Supreme Court ruled that high schools may require student athletes to undergo drug testing, and a subsequent decision in 2002 allowed testing for any student who participates in extracurricular activities.[1] Although efficacy of drug testing by schools is unproven,[2] the Office of National Drug Control Policy encourages schools to perform drug tests for all students, claiming that urine drug testing can help identify students with drug problems and act as a deterrent for others.[3] In addition, several Internet drug-testing distributors encourage parents to perform the tests on their children at home.[4] Schools and parents need support to use drug testing effectively, and many will seek the advice of a physician. Furthermore, physicians will likely receive more requests to perform tests on adolescents as interest in this procedure continues to increase.

Improperly conducted drug tests can result in false accusation (reporting illicit drug use where none exists) or false reassurance (failing to identify actual use). The federal government has established extensive national drug testing guidelines,[5] including supervision of all federally mandated drug testing programs by a physician certified as a medical review officer by the Medical Review Officer Certification Council to protect employees and employers from the consequences of incorrect information. Adolescents, however, are far more likely to have drug testing performed by a physician who does not have medical review officer training. It is not known whether the primary care workforce is prepared to provide technical support to schools and parents or to manage an increase in drug testing requests. The objective of this study was to determine primary care physicians' drug testing practices and knowledge.

## METHODS

### SURVEY INSTRUMENT

To develop the survey instrument, the investigators conducted semistructured telephone interviews with 7 practicing physicians from different geographical regions selected at random from the membership rolls of the American Academy of Pediatrics (AAP) and the Society of Adolescent Medicine (SAM). The

**Author Affiliations:** Department of Pediatrics (Drs Levy, Harris, and Knight) and Division on Addictions (Drs Levy, Harris, and Knight, and Mss Sherritt and Angulo), Harvard Medical School, and Center for Adolescent Substance Abuse Research (Drs Levy, Harris, and Knight and Mss Sherritt and Angulo) and Divisions of General Pediatrics (Drs Levy and Knight and Ms Sherritt) and Adolescent/Young Adult Medicine (Drs Harris and Knight), Children's Hospital Boston, Boston, Mass.

interviewer presented clinical vignettes and elicited the respondents' recommendation for drug testing, which test (if any) they would order, the sample collection procedure, and what they would say to the patient and parent. We then changed details of the vignette to determine at what point the respondent would change the management plan. For example, if the respondent initially would not order a drug test, the interviewer added details indicating that the teen had more significant problems than initially indicated. Two of us (S.L. and M.A.) recorded notes, and, immediately after each interview, reviewed and tabulated results. After all of the interviews were completed, the research team met and identified themes that were used to develop the questionnaire. One of us (J.R.K.) with extensive experience in adolescent substance abuse and another (S.K.H.) with extensive experience in questionnaire development reviewed the questions for face validity. We then distributed a draft of the questionnaire to 8 physicians for pilot testing and made final revisions for clarity. In a final step, we converted the survey to an electronic format. The final tool consisted of 42 forced-choice response items measuring practice variables (n=14), knowledge (n=11), attitudes (n=10), and personal and practice demographics (n=7). This article reports results of (1) the physicians' usual urine specimen collection and validation procedures ("What special procedure, if any, do you use to collect a urine specimen for drug testing?"); (2) the physicians' knowledge of common reasons for false-positive and false-negative results ("Can the following drugs be detected by [the routine urine screen that your office orders]?"); and (3) the physicians' level of agreement with the use of drug testing in various situations ("I would recommend a teen have a drug test if a parent felt strongly that the child was using drugs and denying it.").

## PARTICIPANT SELECTION

We selected 1085 physicians (doctors of medicine or doctors of osteopathy) who were members of the AAP (n=408), the SAM (n=300), or the American Academy of Family Physicians (AAFP [n=377]). For each organization, we obtained national membership rolls sorted by state. We weighted our sample by the proportion of physicians in a given specialty listed in each state, then used a random number list to select participants. Physicians who provided primary or urgent care to an average of 10 adolescents (aged 12-18 years) per week were eligible for the study; all others were asked to return the questionnaire unanswered. We entered all available contact information (address, telephone and fax numbers, and e-mail address) into a database. We called physicians' offices and asked for a fax number if none was listed in the directory.

The study was conducted from April through July 2004 using the tailored design method.[6] All participants received a prenotification letter explaining the purpose of the study, the URL address for the Web-based questionnaire, a unique identifier that allowed access to the Web site, and a $2 bill via US mail. One week later (week 1) we sent an e-mail reminder with the URL embedded to all nonresponders with an e-mail address in our database (n=361) or a cover letter and a copy of the questionnaire via fax for those with a fax number but no e-mail address (n=293). At week 2 we sent a second reminder via the same mode. At week 3 we sent a cover letter and a copy of the survey via US mail to all nonresponders. At week 7 we sent a final reminder letter, survey, and $2 to all nonresponders. The protocol was reviewed and approved by the Children's Hospital Boston Committee on Clinical Investigations, Boston, Mass. Three hundred fifty-nine physicians (122 from the AAP, 126 from the SAM, 103 from the AAFP, and 8 who did not identify their affiliation) completed the survey, and 168 were ineligible, for a calculated response rate of 42%.[7] This is similar to response rates in other published physician surveys.[8-11]

The analytical sample was predominantly male (54%) and diverse in age (36% younger than 41 years). Thirty-four percent of our respondents were AAP members, 35% were SAM members, and 31% were AAFP members. Family physicians were more likely to be male ($P<.001$) and practice in rural settings, whereas adolescent specialists were more likely to practice in urban settings ($P<.001$).

## ANALYSIS

We used MRInterview software (SPSS Inc, Chicago, Ill) to create the online version of our survey tool, and all data from electronic surveys were exported directly into SPSS version 12.0 software (SPSS Inc) for analysis. All numerical data from surveys returned via fax or US mail were independently entered twice, compared, and reconciled by checking the original data source. Cleaned data were then imported into SPSS software for analysis.

We computed simple frequencies for all variables. All eligible physicians completed at least some answers, and we eliminated nonresponders to a particular question from the denominator for the unanswered question only. We considered physicians to be pediatricians if they belonged to the AAP, family physicians if they belonged to the AAFP, and adolescent-care providers if they belonged to SAM (whether or not they also belonged to 1 of the other 2 organizations). Eight eligible participants did not specify any affiliation but were included for group analysis. We used a $\chi^2$ statistic to determine if there were differences in knowledge (eg, substances detected by drug screens) or practice variables (eg, urine collection techniques) by specialty, sex, or age. Our sample size yielded 80% power to detect with 95% confidence differences in proportions of 10% to 15% between specialties, for base comparison proportions of 10% to 50%, respectively. We did not find differences in knowledge by physician specialty. There were differences in practice variables for SAM, AAP, and AAFP members (percentage using an effective procedure for collection being 38%, 13%, and 25%, respectively [$P=.003$], and for validation, 5%, 2%, and 15%, respectively [$P=.002$]). Although these differences are statistically significant, the low rate of effective procedures used by any specialty makes the clinical significance of this finding questionable.

# RESULTS

## DRUG TESTING PRACTICES

More than 95% of all respondents reported ever ordering a urine drug test. **Table 1** presents the procedures physicians used to collect urine samples and check validity. We considered effective procedures to include use of federal guidelines (ie, patient provides identification, empties pockets, and uses the bathroom without running water; blue dye is placed in standing water; and specimen temperature is checked immediately),[5] directly observed urination, or the presence of a staff member inside the bathroom. We considered having a staff member outside the bathroom ineffective.[12] Only 23% of respondents reported using an effective procedure.

According to the American College of Occupational and Environmental Medicine, urine creatinine level and specific gravity should be checked on every sample to prevent patients from defeating a screening test by providing diluted urine.[13] Only 7% of respondents in our sample routinely checked both, and 61% reported checking nei-

**Table 1. Procedures Used to Collect Urine Samples and Check the Validity of the Sample**

| Procedures | % of Respondents (n = 334) |
|---|---|
| Federal guidelines[5] | 10 |
| Direct observation | 7 |
| Staff member inside bathroom | 6 |
| Staff member outside bathroom | 19 |
| No procedure | 48 |
| Do not know/send out | 9 |
| Procedures to check validity of the sample | |
| Creatinine level measurement | 2 |
| Specific gravity | 29 |
| Both | 7 |
| Neither | 61 |

ther. Federal workplace testing requires a confirmatory test for any positive drug screen results,[13] yet only 26% of respondents reported doing so all or most of the time.

## KNOWLEDGE

The percentages of physicians who correctly answered items on which drugs are detectable on results of a routine urine drug test screening panel and what substances can cause false-positive screen results (ie, would result in a false-positive drug test result although a teen did not use illicit drugs) are presented in **Table 2**. Inhaled nitrous oxide can be detected in blood or urine shortly after exposure[20,21] using special techniques and precautions,[14] but it is not detected on results of routine drug screening panels. Less than two thirds of physicians answered this item correctly. Ecstasy (3,4-methylenedioxymethamphetamine) is not reliably detected by preferred assays used in drug testing laboratories.[15,22-25] Less than half of physicians answered this item correctly. Screening for oxycodone, a semisynthetic opioid whose use is rising among teens, must be specifically requested when ordering urine drug tests.[13,16] Only 12% of physicians answered this item correctly. Overall, only 10% of physicians surveyed knew that none of these 3 substances are detected by means of a standard urine panel; 47% answered that they did not know for at least 1 of the substances; and 75% answered 1 or more items incorrectly.

Almost one third of physicians did not know that alcohol used in cooking will not cause a false-positive alcohol screening result. Forty percent of respondents answered the question about whether consuming large quantities of poppy seeds can produce a positive screening test result for opioids and a positive confirmatory test result for codeine and morphine incorrectly or with "don't know."[13] Pseudoephedrine and dextromethorphan preparations, medications commonly found in over-the-counter cold preparations, can cause positive drug test results when used as directed[17,18] (dextromethorphan may cross-react with phencyclidine hydrochloride assays, but not with opioid assays[26]). When questioned about each of these items, most of the respondents answered incorrectly or with "don't know." Respondents were almost equally split when asked whether passive exposure to marijuana smoke would cause a positive drug test finding. Incidental exposure to marijuana smoke has been shown to produce a detectable concentration of $\Delta^9$-tetrahydrocannabinol metabolite in the urine, but in concentrations below the standard cutoffs.[19] In a practice known as "hot-boxing," some adolescents expose themselves to very high concentrations of passive marijuana smoke with the intention of becoming intoxicated. This may produce a positive test result,[27] although this finding would not be false positive by the definition given in our survey (positive even although a teen has not used illicit drugs). In total, less than 1% of physicians answered all of these questions regarding false-positive findings correctly; 89% answered 1 or more items incorrectly; and 74% said they did not know for at least 1 item.

When asked how long marijuana can be detected by a usual drug screening test, 330 respondents replied as follows: 8.5%, up to 48 hours; 24.5%, as long as 1 week; 31.5%, as long as 6 weeks; 7.3%, as long as 3 months; and 17.3%, as long as 6 months. The remaining 7.9% did not know.

## COMMENT

This study shows that although most primary care physicians order urine drug tests, most do not use recommended procedures for urine test collection, validation, and confirmation and lack the knowledge needed to correctly interpret positive and negative results.

False-negative test results can give physicians and parents unwarranted reassurance and delay diagnosis of a serious drug disorder. Adolescents may try to evade urine testing by drinking a large volume of water, taking a diuretic, or adding water to the collection container to intentionally dilute a urine sample below drug detection thresholds.[13] A sample can also be adulterated by adding soap or other chemicals that interfere with the assay. Proper collection and validation techniques will minimize adulteration and alert physicians to attempts at dilution.

Most of our respondents did not know that Ecstasy, oxycodone, and nitrous oxide are not detected by routine screens. Physicians and parents may be falsely reassured that their child is not using a particular drug when the child never underwent proper testing for it. Knowing which substances are tested for in a standard panel and ordering additional screening panels can prevent physicians and parents from missing a substance the adolescent is using.

Standard urine drug panels are immunoassay screens that are designed to eliminate urine specimens with negative findings from further consideration. These tests are relatively nonspecific and have the potential for false-positive results. Guidelines for federally mandated drug testing programs require a second analytical procedure using a more specific technique, such as gas chromatography/mass spectrometry, to confirm every urine drug screen with a positive finding. Misinterpretation of a false-positive finding can put adolescents at risk for false accusation of substance use and diminished trust from parents, school personnel, and counselors. In our survey, most respondents misidentified at least 1 substance that

**Table 2. Responses of 340 Respondents About Substances That Can Be Detected or Can Cause False-Positive Test Results**

| Questions | % of Respondents* | | | Reference Value |
|---|---|---|---|---|
| | Yes | No | Don't Know | |
| Detection of drugs† | | | | |
| Nitrous oxide | 1 | 59 | 36 | No[14] |
| Ecstasy (3,4-methylenedioxymethamphetamine) | 19 | 46 | 32 | No‡[15] |
| Oxycodone | 74 | 12 | 14 | No[13,16] |
| Cause false-positive results§ | | | | |
| Foods prepared with cooked alcohol | 6 | 61 | 31 | No |
| Poppy seeds | 59 | 17 | 23 | Yes[13] |
| Cold preparations containing pseudoephedrine | 48 | 27 | 25 | Yes[17] |
| Cold preparations containing dextromethorphan | 36 | 31 | 32 | Yes[18] |
| Passive exposure to marijuana smoke | 38 | 36 | 23 | No[19] |

*Percentages may not add to 100% owing to rounding.
†Indicates answers to the question "Can the following drugs be detected by the routine drug screen that your office uses?"
‡Some newer instrument–based assays can detect Ecstasy; however, preferred assays in standard drug-testing laboratories do not reliably detect it.
§Indicates answers the question: "Can the following cause false-positives on the routine drug screen that your office uses?"

can cause a false-positive finding on a drug screening test, and only one quarter order a confirmatory test all or most of the time. Physicians ordering drug tests should be familiar with causes of false-positive results, and confirmatory testing should always be performed.

A urine drug test result typically remains positive for $\Delta^9$-tetrahydrocannabinol for 1 to 3 days after a single use of marijuana.[12] However, because it is intensely lipophilic, and significant fat stores can accumulate, urine test results for $\Delta^9$-tetrahydrocannabinol can remain positive for 4 to 6 weeks in regular users.[28] In our sample, one third of respondents thought that cannabis could be detected for 1 week or less. These physicians might falsely accuse an adolescent of continued drug use if urine testing were repeated. One quarter of our respondents believed that cannabis could be detected 3 to 6 months after use. These physicians might make the opposite interpretation error and could interpret positive urine test results as continued marijuana washout longer than physiologically possible.

Previous research has demonstrated that medical school[29] and residency training[30] do not adequately prepare physicians to identify and treat drug disorders, and little has been published regarding specific training in the use of drug testing. Medical students and residents may be primarily exposed to drug testing while evaluating acutely intoxicated patients in the emergency department. In these patients, urine collection is directly observed or obtained via catheterization, and clinical signs and symptoms guide the selection of the testing panel and make confirmatory testing of lesser importance. Physicians who are interested in drug testing may seek additional training through formal medical review officer training or as part of their postgraduate medical education. The California Academy of Family Physicians produced a manual to educate family physicians on the "proper methods, uses, limitations and evaluation of urine drug testing in order to rationally employ testing in clinical practice to improve patient care, protect himself/herself, and protect the patient,"[16] but the manual is primarily intended for physicians who are treating patients receiving long-term opiate therapy for pain or addiction. Drug testing in the primary care situation, however, presents challenges and risks to the adolescent and physician. Adolescents who undergo drug testing at their parents' request may be more likely to attempt to evade testing than adults who seek medical attention of their own volition. Physicians must be well versed in the nuances of proper drug collection procedures and false-positive and false-negative findings. Drug testing requested by parents may damage the therapeutic relationship between adolescents and physicians. Adolescents are also at risk of schools or parents using drug test results punitively. Few training materials address these issues.

This study has a number of limitations. First, our sample was a national survey of physicians from the 3 specialties that provide most of the primary care to adolescents, namely, pediatricians, family physicians, and adolescent medicine providers. We used a variety of methods to contact physicians, including US mail, e-mail, and fax, to avoid the systematic exclusion of physicians who are difficult to reach by a given mode. However, we had a response rate of only 42%. Physician surveys tend to have lower response rates than surveys of the general population,[31] and our response rate is in the middle range (19%-53%) of recently reported surveys of primary care physicians.[8-11] However, we cannot exclude self-selection bias. It is possible that physicians who see fewer adolescent patients and are less familiar with laboratory testing for drugs would be less likely to complete the survey. Bias, if present, might therefore suggest that our estimates of provider proficiency and knowledge are overly optimistic. In addition, the demographic data for each professional group was similar to the demographic data of the corresponding society, making it unlikely that we systematically excluded any particular group. Furthermore, a strong demand characteristic exists in this study for physicians to present as knowledgeable, which may lead respondents to select an answer rather than select the "don't know" choice. If this is the case, some correct answers may have been guesses, further inflating our estimates of provider proficiency.

We developed a new survey instrument rather than using a previous validated tool. This was necessary because we know of no other tool designed for this purpose. It is possible that physicians found some of the questions confusing or misinterpreted them. For example, some respondents may have interpreted the question regarding whether secondhand marijuana smoke can cause false-positive drug test results as asking whether secondhand smoke contains cannabis, which it does. Physicians who interpreted the question in this way may also be misinterpreting drug test results as false positive when in fact the teenager with a positive drug test result due to secondhand marijuana smoke is exposed to the same risks as those who smoke marijuana. We pilot tested the questionnaire before the national survey and none of our pilot testers reported confusing questions or asked us to clarify any of the questions. All respondents were given the opportunity to provide feedback regarding the survey, and we did not receive any feedback regarding the clarity of questions. Few questions were skipped, and we did not identify a pattern of skipped questions that might be expected if questions were ambiguous or confusing.

## CONCLUSIONS

Overall, our findings suggest that primary care physicians are not fully aware of the limitations of drug testing and do not use recommended procedures for collecting and validating urine drug test specimens. The primary care workforce is not prepared to provide guidance to schools, parents, or patients with questions regarding drug testing. We recommend that physicians who use this procedure frequently in their office seek further training, such as that available through the Medical Review Officer Certification Council. Professional societies such as the AAP or the SAM should consider producing training materials that address the challenges of office-based urine drug testing with adolescent patients. Physicians who order drug tests infrequently should consult with a specialist such as a toxicologist or addiction specialist.

**Accepted for Publication:** August 4, 2005.
**Correspondence:** Sharon Levy, MD, MPH, Center for Adolescent Substance Abuse Research, Children's Hospital Boston, 300 Longwood Ave, Boston, MA 02115 (Sharon.Levy@childrens.harvard.edu).
**Funding/Support:** This study was supported by grant 049207 from The Robert Wood Johnson Foundation Substance Abuse Policy Research Program, Princeton, NJ, and grant K07 AA013280 from the National Institute on Alcohol Abuse and Alcoholism, Bethesda, Md (Dr Knight).
**Acknowledgment:** We thank Tai Kwong, PhD, S. Jean Emans, MD, and Shari van Hook, MPH, for reviewing this manuscript.

## REFERENCES


1. Lewin T. Schools across US await ruling on drug tests. *New York Times.* 2002§;A:26.
2. Yamaguchi R, Johnston L, O'Malley P. Relationship between student illicit drug use and school drug-testing policies. *J Sch Health.* 2003;73:159-164.
3. Office of National Drug Control Policy. *What You Need to Know About Drug Testing in Schools.* Washington, DC: White House Drug Control Policy Office; 2002.
4. Levy S, van Hook S, Knight J. A review of internet-based home drug-testing products for parents. *Pediatrics.* 2004;113:720-726.
5. Substance Abuse and Mental Health Services Administration, Department of Health and Human Services. Mandatory guidelines for federal workplace testing programs. Available at: http://www.dwp.samhsa.gov.
6. Dilman D. *Mail and Internet Surveys: The Tailored Design Method.* 2nd ed. New York, NY: John Wiley & Sons Inc; 2000.
7. American Association for Public Opinion Research. *Standard Definitions: Final Dispostions of Case Codes and Outcome Rates for Surveys.* Lenexa, Kan: American Association for Public Opinion Research; 2004.
8. Gentile DA, Oberg C, Sherwood NE, Story M, Walsh DA, Hogan M; American Academy of Pediatrics. Well-child visits in the video age: pediatricians and the American Academy of Pediatrics' guidelines for children's media use. *Pediatrics.* 2004;114:1235-1241.
9. Stille CJ, Primack WA, Savageau JA. Generalist-subspecialist communication for children with chronic conditions: a regional physician survey. *Pediatrics.* 2003;112(pt 1):1314-1320.
10. Lee A, Moretti ME, Collantes A, et al. Choice of breastfeeding and physicians' advice: a cohort study of women receiving propylthiouracil. *Pediatrics.* 2000;106:27-30.
11. Trowbridge F, Sofka D, Holt K, Barlow S. Management of child and adolescent obesity: study design and practitioner characteristics. *Pediatrics.* 2002;110:205-209.
12. Schwartz R. Testing for drugs of abuse: controversies and techniques. *Adolesc Med.* 1993;4:353-370.
13. American College of Environmental and Occupational Medicine. *Medical Review Officer Drug and Alcohol Testing Comprehensive Course Syllabus.* Elk Grove Village, Ill: American College of Environmental and Occupational Medicine; 2003.
14. Flanagan R, Streete P, Ramsey J. Volatile substance abuse. United Nations Office on Drugs and Crime Technical Series, January 1, 1997. Available at: www.unodc.org/pdf/technical_series_1997-01-01_1.pdf. Accessed December 14, 2004.
15. Hsu J, Liu C, Liu CP, et al. Performance characteristics of selected immunoassays for preliminary test of 3,4-methylenedioxymethamphetamine, methamphetamine, and related drugs in urine specimens. *J Anal Toxicol.* 2003;27:471-478.
16. Gourlay G, Heit H, Caplan Y. *Urine Drug Testing in Primary Care: Dispelling the Myths and Designing Strategies.* San Francisco: California Academy of Family Physicians; 2002.
17. Stout PR, Klette KL, Horn CK. Evaluation of ephedrine, pseudoephedrine and phenylpropanolamine concentrations in human urine samples and a comparison of the specificity of DRI amphetamines and Abuscreen online (KIMS) amphetamines screening immunoassays. *J Forensic Sci.* 2004;49:160-164.
18. Budai B, Iskandar H. Dextromethorphan can produce false positive phencyclidine testing with HPLC. *Am J Emerg Med.* 2002;20:61-62.
19. ElSohly MA. Practical challenges to positive drug tests for marijuana. *Clin Chem.* 2003;49:1037-1038.
20. Sonander H, Stenqvist O, Nilsson K. Exposure to trace amounts of nitrous oxide: evaluation of urinary gas content monitoring in anaesthetic practice. *Br J Anaesth.* 1983;55:1225-1229.
21. Sonander H, Stenqvist O, Nilsson K. Urinary $N_2O$ as a measure of biologic exposure to nitrous oxide anaesthetic contamination. *Ann Occup Hyg.* 1983;27:73-79.
22. Arria AM, Yacoubian GS Jr, Fost E, Wish ED. The pediatric forum: ecstasy use among club rave attendees. *Arch Pediatr Adolesc Med.* 2002;156:295-296.
23. Schwartz RH, Miller NS. MDMA (ecstasy) and the rave: a review. *Pediatrics.* 1997;100:705-708.
24. Stout PR, Klette KL, Wiegand R. Comparison and evaluation of DRI methamphetamine, DRI ecstasy, Abuscreen ONLINE amphetamine, and a modified Abuscreen ONLINE amphetamine screening immunoassays for the detection of amphetamine (AMP), methamphetamine (MTH), 3,4-methylenedioxyamphetamine (MDA), and 3,4-methylenedioxymethamphetamine (MDMA) in human urine. *J Anal Toxicol.* 2003;27:265-269.
25. Zhao H, Brenneisen R, Scholer A, et al. Profiles of urine samples taken from ecstasy users at rave parties: analysis by immunoassays, HPLC, and GC-MS. *J Anal Toxicol.* 2001;25:258-269.
26. Storrow AB, Magoon MR, Norton J. The dextromethorphan defense: dextromethorphan and the opioid screen. *Acad Emerg Med.* 1995;2:791-794.
27. Levy S, Knight J. Office management of substance use. Adolescent Health Update. 2003;15(3):1-8.
28. Schwartz R. Urine testing in the detection of drugs of abuse. *Arch Intern Med.* 1988;148:2407-2412.
29. Fleming M, Barry K, Davis A, Kropp S, Kahn R, Rivo M.. Medical education about substance abuse: changes in curriculum and faculty between 1976 and 1992. *Acad Med.* 1994;69:362-369.
30. Isaacson J, Fleming M, Kraus M, Kahn R, Mundt M. A national survey of training in substance use disorders in residency programs. *J Stud Alcohol.* 2000;61:912-915.
31. Asch D, Jedrziewski M, Christakis N. Response rates to mail surveys published in medical journals. *J Clin Epidemiol.* 1997;50:1129-1136.

ARTICLE

# Association of Condom Use, Sexual Behaviors, and Sexually Transmitted Infections With the Duration of Genital Human Papillomavirus Infection Among Adolescent Women

*Marcia L. Shew, MD, MPH; J. Dennis Fortenberry, MD, MS; Wanzhu Tu, PhD; Beth E. Juliar, MA, MS; Byron E. Batteiger, MD; Brahim Qadadri, BS; Darron R. Brown, MD*

**Objective:** To examine the association of potentially modifiable factors such as condom use, sexual behaviors, and concurrent sexually transmitted infections with duration of genital human papillomavirus (HPV) infections among adolescent women.

**Design:** Longitudinal observational study.

**Setting:** Study conducted at 3 inner-city clinics in Indianapolis, Ind.

**Participants:** Forty-nine HPV-positive adolescents were tested frequently for HPV infection and provided sexual behavior diaries.

**Main Exposures:** Condom use, sexual behaviors, number of partners, and concurrent infections with *Neisseria gonorrhoeae*, *Chlamydia trachomatis*, and *Trichomonas vaginalis*.

**Main Outcome Measures:** Time from onset to clearance of type-specific HPV infections was analyzed with proportional hazard models. Adjusted hazard ratios (AHRs) were used to assess the effects of risk factors on the duration of HPV infection. Because viral clearance is a preferred outcome, a variable with an AHR less than 1 was considered a risk factor (ie, associated with reduced chance of viral clearance and prolonged infection).

**Results:** Prolonged HPV infection was associated with oncogenic HPV types (AHR, 0.58 [95% confidence interval (CI), 0.39-0.84]) less than median level of condom use during an HPV infection (AHR, 0.53 [95% CI, 0.33-0.84]) and coinfection with *C trachomatis* (AHR, 0.58 [95% CI, 0.31-0.89]) or *T vaginalis* (AHR, 0.32 [95% CI, 0.16-0.64]). Not having multiple sexual partners during an HPV infection was associated with early HPV clearance (AHR, 5.52 [95% CI, 3.28-9.30]).

**Conclusions:** These findings support public health messages of reducing the number of sexual partners, promoting routine condom use, and frequent sexually transmitted infection screening that may be beneficial with HPV infections.

*Arch Pediatr Adolesc Med. 2006;160:151-156*

**Author Affiliations:** Division of Adolescent Medicine, Department of Pediatrics (Drs Shew and Fortenberry), Divisions of Biostatistics (Dr Tu and Ms Juliar) and Infectious Diseases (Drs Batteiger and Brown and Mr Qadadri), Department of Medicine, Department of Microbiology and Immunology (Drs Batteiger and Brown), and Regenstrief Institute (Dr Tu), Indiana University School of Medicine, Indianapolis.

THE PATHOGENESIS OF NEOplasia due to human papillomaviruses (HPVs) is a complex interaction of virus and host, with the ultimate incorporation of HPV DNA into the host cell genome, disruption of normal cell cycles, genomic instability, and initiation of abnormal cell clones.[1] Natural history studies show that 60% to 80% of HPV infections become undetectable over an 8- to 10-month period.[2-4] However, prolonged infection (commonly termed *HPV persistence*) appears to be a necessary but not sufficient link from initial HPV infection to subsequent neoplasia.[5,6]

Factors associated with longer HPV infections are not well defined, especially for adolescents. Infection by oncogenic viral types (ie, the approximately 20 viral types frequently identified in cancer tissue) is associated with longer HPV infection duration.[5,7,8] Other associated factors associated with longer-duration infections include older age, multiple sex partners, cigarette smoking,[9-12] immune suppression,[13] and hormonal contraception.[14] Recent studies linking genital *Chlamydia trachomatis* infections to cervical neoplasia suggest a potential role for concurrent infection in the duration of HPV infection.[15-17] Many of these earlier studies are limited by relatively infrequent follow-up intervals (ie, at 3- to 6-month intervals), inadequate assessment of concurrent sexually transmitted infections (STIs) and sexual and contraceptive behaviors, and exclusion of younger sexually active women. Given the high prevalence of sexually transmitted HPV infection among young women, additional research is needed to better define potentially modifiable factors associated with HPV persistence.

The goal of this study was to assess factors associated with the duration of HPV persistence among a cohort of middle- and late-adolescent women. Relatively shorter sampling intervals, sensitive HPV diagnostic tests, assessment of concurrent STI, and detailed measures of sexual and contraceptive behavior were used to address limitations of previous research. Quarterly and weekly self-obtained vaginal specimens were used to follow the course of HPV infection. Self-obtained specimens are well accepted by young women and of comparable accuracy to clinician-obtained specimens.[18-20]

## METHODS

### STUDY DESIGN

A description of the methods and summary of the distribution of HPV types and natural history of infection in this sample is published elsewhere.[4] Briefly, women aged 14 to 17 years, attending 1 of 3 primary care adolescent health clinics, were enrolled in a 27-month observational study of biological and behavioral factors related to STI. Study enrollment began in the spring of 1999, and the last participant in this study sample completed the observation in 2002. All eligible women were identified by clinical schedules based on age criteria, and attempts were made to recruit all eligible women at that or a subsequent clinical visit. Each participant was recruited during clinic visits by study personnel who obtained the participant's informed consent and parental permission. Prior sexual experience was not an entry criterion. No information was obtained on those who refused participation, but all eligible women were recruited equally and demographic and STI data of the cohort mirrored that of the clinic population. None of the participants had known immunodeficiency conditions at enrollment or during the follow-up period. Data analyses were limited subsequently to the 49 subjects who were infected with HPV. The research was approved by the institutional review board of Indiana University/Purdue University at Indianapolis.

At enrollment, participants received a physical examination; provided clinician-obtained vaginal and cervical specimens for STI testing; and underwent a face-to-face interview. The cycle of clinical examination, STI testing, and interview was repeated at approximately 3-month intervals for 27 months. The enrollment interview, and subsequent quarterly interviews, provided detailed information about sexual behaviors, including condom use and hormonal contraceptive use. Participants received $20 for time and effort required for each interview.

In addition, all participants completed multiple periods of daily diary completion and weekly self-obtained vaginal specimens. Each diary completion period lasted approximately 84 days (12 weeks) and was initiated and ended by a clinic visit as described earlier. Each 12-week diary collection period was followed by a 12-week rest period in which no diaries or vaginal specimens were collected. Thus, participants contributed 2 diary periods per year and up to 5 diary periods during the 27-month follow-up period.

Diaries and self-obtained specimens were collected on a weekly basis by study personnel, usually at the participants' homes. Diaries assessed whether sexual intercourse occurred on a given day and, if so, whether a condom was used. Participants received $2 for each completed diary and $5 for each vaginal specimen. During a given diary period, vaginal specimens were frozen at −20°C until the final week of diary collection. Specimens were then tested for STI as described later. All infections were treated at quarterly interviews unless the participant sought out treatment owing to concerns or symptoms.

### TYPE-SPECIFIC HPV ASSAY

All cervical and vaginal specimens were tested for HPV using a polymerase chain reaction (PCR)/reverse blot strip assay (Roche Diagnostics, Indianapolis, Ind).[21,22] This assay uses nondegenerate primer pairs to amplify 19 oncogenic HPV types (types 16, 18, 26, 31, 33, 35, 39, 45, 51, 52, 55, 56, 58, 59, 68, 73, 82, 83, and 84) and 8 nononcogenic HPV types (types 6, 11, 40, 42, 53, 54, 57, and 66).[23] To determine specimen adequacy, the GH20/PC04 human β-globin target is coamplified with HPV sequences. Reactions were amplified in a PerkinElmer TC9600 Thermal Cycler (PerkinElmer, Foster City, Calif) as previously described.[23] DNA-positive and -negative specimens were included in each assay as controls.

Reverse blot strip assays used a reference ink line and probe lines for 27 individual HPV genotypes and 2 concentrations of the β-globin control probe.[21] Bovine serum albumin–conjugated probes for each HPV type are deposited in a single line for each of the HPV types. Hybridization and visual detection of PCR products bound to immobilized probes was performed as described earlier.[4,23]

### DETECTION OF OTHER STI

Cervical and vaginal swab specimens were also evaluated for the presence of *C trachomatis*, *Neisseria gonorrhoeae*, and *Trichomonas vaginalis*. *C trachomatis* and *N gonorrhoeae* infections were identified using the Amplicor (Roche Diagnostics) *C trachomatis/N gonorrhoeae* PCR assay. Detection of *T vaginalis* DNA was performed using the Amplicor *C trachomatis/N gonorrhoeae* PCR assay with the following modifications. Samples were processed for amplification according to the manufacturer's instructions using microwell plates coated with a *T vaginalis*–specific probe.[24]

Because of the high specificity of nucleic acid amplification tests, any specimen testing positive for *C trachomatis* or *T vaginalis* was considered to represent an infection. However, a lower specificity for *N gonorrhoeae* infections is now well documented.[25,26] For this reason, all specimens positive (all women who tested positive were treated) for *N gonorrhoeae* by the Amplicor *C trachomatis/N gonorrhoeae* PCR assay were initially confirmed by 1 or more of the following tests: culture, BDProbe Tec (Becton, Dickinson, and Company, Franklin Lakes, NJ), *opa*- or *ccB*-based PCR,[27] or GENPROBE Aptima (GENPROBE, Inc, San Diego, Calif). Specimens were characterized as *N gonorrhoeae* infection only when confirmatory test results were also positive.

The STI measures assessed both prevalent (any time during the study) and concurrent infections (during an HPV infection). Prevalent measures assessed any occurrence of *C trachomatis*, *N gonorrhoeae*, or *T vaginalis* during the study period. Concurrent infections were defined as those occurring within the same period as a specific HPV infection.

### SEXUAL AND CONTRACEPTIVE BEHAVIORS

Relevant demographic, behavioral, and clinical information were obtained from interviews and diaries, including enrollment age, race (self-designated), sexual behaviors, and contraceptive and condom use behaviors.

Sexual behaviors included age at first sexual intercourse, number of sex partners, coital frequency, and condom use. The exact numbers for coital frequency and condom use were calculated from self-reports about coitus and condom use over the last

3 months using both the diaries and/or quarterly interviews depending on the time and duration of the infection. Sexual partners were the exact number of partners reported during a specific HPV infection. Initial analyses showed that number of partners was highly skewed. Therefore, number of partners was dichotomized at the sample median (as ≤1 vs ≥2 partners). Coital frequency was a continuous variable based on the number of coital events recorded during a specific HPV infection.

Condom use was defined as the proportion of condom-protected coital events during the duration of a specific HPV infection. If no coitus occurred during a specific HPV period, protection was defined as 100%. Dropping out periods of no coital activity would potentially hamper the ability to look at noncoital influences on HPV persistence. Since condom use behavior was contingent on the occurrence of coitus, assuming 100% protection for an infection period without coitus may confound the effect of condom use with that of no coitus. To ensure the validity of the analysis, we assessed the effect of condom use in both the full sample and the subsample containing only the infection periods where coitus had been reported. Because the percentage of condom-protected events had a bimodal distribution with large clusters near 0% and 100% use, condom use was dichotomized based on the sample median to "less condom use" (ie, <60% of coital events) vs "more condom use" (ie, condom use >60%). Measures of contraceptive use included self-reported use of oral contraceptive pills or depot medroxyprogesterone acetate. Participants' medical records were reviewed to verify prescription of oral contraceptive pills and injection of depot medroxyprogesterone during the period in which an HPV infection occurred.

## STATISTICAL ANALYSIS

The primary outcome variable was duration (in days) of infection by a specific HPV type. For a given infection, duration was calculated as the time between the initial onset and last detection of a specific HPV type. Prevalent infections at enrollment and incident infections were used for the analysis. Human papillomavirus infection was defined as 2 or more positive specimens for a specific HPV type. An infection with a type-specific HPV was considered to have cleared when the last positive specimen was followed by at least 2 negative specimens before the end of follow-up. When a positive specimen was obtained within 2 weeks of the end of observation, the duration of that specific infection was censored at the end of the data collection period. In other words, infection was assumed to persist at least as long as the end of the observational period if the specific HPV type was detected within 2 weeks of the end of the observation period. A single subject would contribute more than 1 infection to the analysis if she was coinfected and/or subsequently infected with a different HPV type during the observation period.

Cox regression was used to model the length of a type-specific HPV infection as a function of various sexual behaviors, hormonal contraceptive use, and infection with other STI. Since the critical event for the survival analysis is the end of a type-specific HPV infection, a hazard ratio significantly less than 1.0 implies a reduced likelihood of HPV clearance (ie, virus becomes undetectable) or longer duration of HPV infection. A hazard ratio significantly greater than 1.0, on the other hand, implies increased likelihood of HPV clearance, or shorter duration of HPV infection. Unadjusted Kaplan-Meier estimates were reported to highlight the difference in survival curves under different values of independent variables.

The analysis was performed on type-specific infections. Participants with multiple types of HPV infections, either sequentially or concurrently, would contribute multiple observations. In this research, we modeled multiple infections within the subject as unordered events. To accommodate the within-subject correlation associated with these infections, a random-subject effect with a gamma distribution was introduced into the Cox regression model (gamma frailty model).[28] For model selection, we followed a forward selection procedure with an entry criterion of $P<.05$. Data analyses were conducted using SAS version 8.2 (SAS Institute Inc, Cary, NC) and S-Plus 6.1 (Insightful Corp, Seattle, Wash).

**Table. Estimated Hazard Ratios of Viral Clearance Based on 241 Human Papillomavirus (HPV) Infections From a Cohort of 49 Adolescent Women**

| Variable | Unadjusted Hazard Ratio (95% CI) | Adjusted Hazard Ratio (95% CI) |
|---|---|---|
| Age at enrollment, y | 1.12 (0.87-1.45) | . . . |
| Race (African American vs others) | 1.19 (0.81-1.75) | . . . |
| Age at first intercourse, y | 1.26 (1.11-1.43) | . . . |
| ≤1 Partner during an HPV infection (vs ≥2 partners) | 5.45 (3.48-8.54) | 5.52 (3.28-9.30) |
| No. of coital events during an HPV infection | 0.98 (0.97-0.99) | 0.98 (0.98-0.99) |
| <60% of coital events protected by condoms during an HPV infection (vs >60% condom use)* | 0.43 (0.29-0.65) | 0.53 (0.33-0.84) |
| Oral contraceptive pill use during an HPV infection | 1.14 (0.75-1.71) | . . . |
| DMPA use during an HPV infection | 0.82 (0.53-1.25) | . . . |
| Oncogenic HPV type | 0.68 (0.48-0.97) | 0.58 (0.39-0.84) |
| *Chlamydia trachomatis* during the study† | 1.14 (0.65-2.01) | . . . |
| *Neisseria gonorrhoeae* during the study† | 1.06 (0.63-1.69) | . . . |
| *Trichomonas vaginalis* during the study† | 1.23 (0.75-2.01) | . . . |
| *C trachomatis* coinfection‡ | 0.30 (0.93-0.46) | 0.58 (0.31-0.89) |
| *N gonorrhoeae* coinfection‡ | 0.51 (0.31-0.84) | . . . |
| *T vaginalis* coinfection‡ | 0.27 (0.13-0.43) | 0.32 (0.16-0.64) |

Abbreviations: CI, confidence interval; DMPA, depot medroxyprogesterone acetate.
*Condom use was dichotomized based on sample median.
†Sexually transmitted infection was detected during study period.
‡Sexually transmitted infection was detected during the HPV infection.

## RESULTS

Participants' mean age at enrollment was 15.3 years, and 85% reported race as African American. Most participants (57 of 60) reported prior sexual experience at enrollment. Mean (SD) age at first coitus among the sexually experienced was 13.2 (1.7) years.

The mean duration of follow-up was 2.2 years (range, 2.0-2.4 years). Of the 2458 cervical or vaginal specimens collected, 353 were clinician-obtained cervical swabs (collected every 3 months at the quarterly visit) and 2105 were participants' self-obtained vaginal swabs (col-

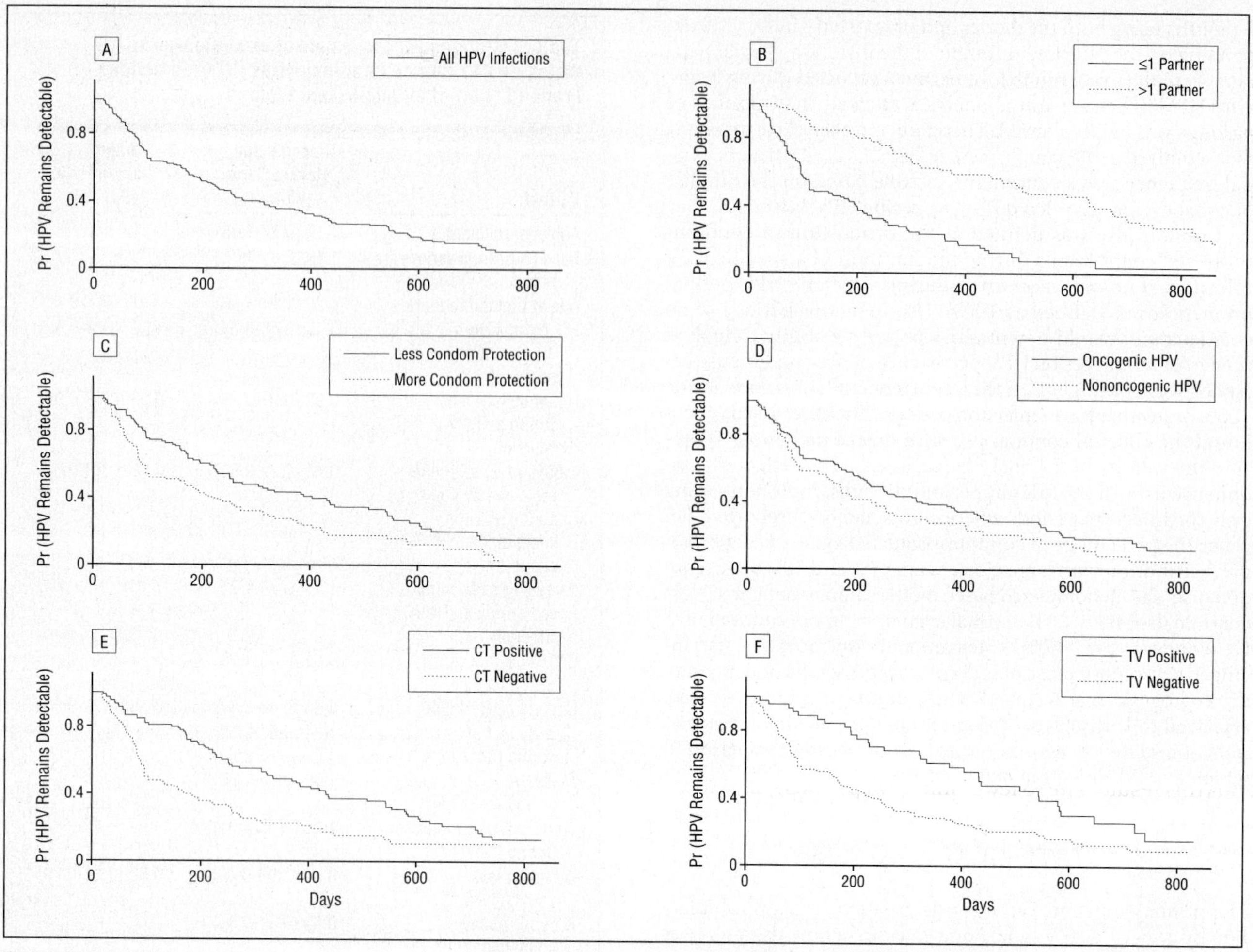


**Figure.** Kaplan-Meier estimates of the survival of human papillomavirus (HPV) infection (A-F). CT indicates *Chlamydia trachomatis*; TV, *Trichomonas vaginalis;* and Pr, probability.

lected weekly during diary collections). Overall, 2107 (85.7%) of 2458 specimens were positive for β-globin (both the low- and high-abundance bands) and were included in subsequent analyses. As previously reported, the cumulative prevalence of HPV infection was 81.7% (49/60), and those HPV-infected women were used for the survival analyses.[4]

For the 49 women who were HPV positive, the mean number of partners reported during a period associated with HPV infection was 1.7 (median, 1; range, 0-10). The mean number of coital events was 25.8. The median level of condom use was 60.4% during an HPV infection period. The STI coinfection rates during an HPV infection were as follows: 45.4% for *C trachomatis*, 25.4% for *N gonorrhoeae*, and 19.2% for *T vaginalis*. About one third of the participants reported use of oral contraceptive pills or depot medroxyprogesterone injection during the time of an HPV infection.

There were a total of 241 HPV infections with a mean duration of 232.1 days. Of these 241 infections, only 14 were prevalent at the time of enrollment. A total of 168 (70%) of 241 HPV infections were with oncogenic types. Mean duration was 251 days and 189 days for oncogenic and nononcogenic viral types, respectively. Univariate and multivariate risk ratios and 95% confidence intervals are reported in the **Table**.

Kaplan-Meier survival curves for all HPV infections are depicted in **Figure** A. Half of all infections were no longer detected by 210 days after initial detection. Depictions of the association of number of partners, condom use, HPV type, concurrent *C trachomatis* infection, and concurrent *T vaginalis* infection are seen in Figure B-F. Figure B demonstrates HPV infections associated with 1 or no partners (median infection duration, 96 days) ending earlier as compared with infections associated with multiple partners (median infection duration, 437 days). Clearance of HPV was significantly faster during infection periods associated with more frequent condom use (median duration, 58 days) compared with infections associated with less frequent condom use (median duration, 257 days) (Figure C). High-risk HPV infections were slower to clear (median duration, 228 days) than low-risk infections (median, 170 days) (Figure D). The HPV infections associated with concurrent *C trachomatis* infection cleared slower (median duration, 333 days) than those not associated with concurrent *C trachomatis* (median, 96 days) (Figure E). Finally, HPV infections associated with concurrent *T vaginalis* were slower to clear than those not associated with the infection (median time to disappearance was 436 days and 172 days, respectively) (Figure F).

In the multivariable survival analysis, women having only 1 or no sexual partners during an HPV infection were more likely to have shorter periods of HPV detection. Specifically, we estimated that the instantaneous hazard of viral clearance for women with 1 or no sexual partners during HPV infection was 5.52 times that of women with multiple partners, after controlling for the effects of other covariates (adjusted hazard ratio [AHR], 5.52 [95% confidence interval (CI), 3.28-9.30]). Clearance of HPV was less likely in women who had coitus at a higher frequency than the sample median level while infected (AHR, 0.98 [95% CI, 0.98-0.99]); women who used condoms for less than 60% of coital events while infected were less likely to have early clearance compared with women who used condoms more often (AHR, 0.53 [95% CI, 0.33-0.84]); and HPV clearance was also less likely in those women infected by an oncogenic HPV type (AHR, 0.58 [95% CI, 0.39-0.84]) and those concurrently infected with *C trachomatis* (AHR, 0.58 [95% CI, 0.31-0.89]) or *T vaginalis* (AHR, 0.32 [95% CI, 0.16-0.64]). Age at first sex and concurrent *N gonorrhoeae* infection were associated with longer periods of HPV infection in univariate but not multivariable models. Prevalent STI, concurrent oral contraceptive pill use, or concurrent depot medroxyprogesterone use were not associated with duration of the infection. When alternative analyses were performed limited to periods when sex occurred during an HPV infection (this resulted in 40 fewer infection periods), the effect of condom use remained significant in the subsample (risk ratio, 0.58 [95% CI, 0.35-0.97]).

## COMMENT

Potentially modifiable factors—sexual behaviors, less frequent condom use, and concurrent sexually transmitted infections—were associated with longer periods of detectable genital HPV infection among adolescent women. Given the importance of viral persistence in the pathogenesis of HPV-associated neoplasia, these findings may have substantial clinical and public health implications. Although persistence of HPV was not assessed directly, potential factors that influence clearance (ie, longer or shorter periods of detection) may likely also be associated with persistence. Interventions designed to influence HPV clearance—for example, to reduce number of sexual partners, increase condom use, and improve STI screening and treatment—might be similar to those already shown to be effective for reducing rates of incident STI.[29] Even with the eventual development of an HPV vaccine that protects against multiple high-risk HPV types, interventions to increase the clearance of HPV infection could influence care of women who are not immunized because of lack of vaccine access or vaccine failure or those who already had been infected with HPV.

Although mechanisms by which sexual behaviors and concurrent STI influence the clearance of HPV infection are not yet well understood, roles for local immune changes and for cervical inflammation are likely.[30] Semen in the female genital tract is associated with a marked postcoital inflammatory response in which transforming growth factor β appears to play an important role in inducing local immune hyporesponsiveness.[31] Our data linking increased levels of condom use with increased clearance of HPV infection are also consistent with observations that condom use is associated with faster regression of cervical intraepithelial neoplasia.[32]

Both *T vaginalis*[33] and *C trachomatis*[17,34] are associated with cervical cancer and its precursor, cervical dysplasia. Cervical inflammation could explain the association of concurrent *C trachomatis* or *T vaginalis* infection with duration of HPV infection.[30] Inflammation associated with these coinfections may favor a cytokine milieu compatible with prolonged HPV infection.[35]

Several limitations should be noted in considering these data. First, the sample represents a relatively small cohort of intensely studied young women. However, the sample itself was not selected on the basis of sexual activity, STI risk behaviors, contraceptive use, or HPV infection status. Thus, our results are not likely attributable to selection for specific factors that might be relevant in other populations. Second, we did not measure cigarette use, which has been linked to HPV persistence and cervical neoplasia in other studies.[12,36] Cigarette smoking is almost certainly an important risk factor for HPV persistence but it is unlikely that the range of factors identified in this study are simply surrogates for the unmeasured effect of smoking. A final limitation is the use of clearance of HPV infection as an outcome rather than a more definitive clinical outcome, such as cervical dysplasia. The incidence of higher-grade cervical dysplastic lesions is relatively low, ultimately requiring a much larger cohort to produce statistically stable estimates.[4] This does not negate the findings and impact that they could have on reducing viral infections and the potential for understanding viral persistence.

Viral clearance of HPV, and potentially persistence, appears to be a complex interaction of sexual behaviors, coexisting genital infections, and viral characteristics. This means that not only is HPV infection persistence a potentially preventable condition but HPV-related cancers may be preventable as well. Effectiveness of condoms has been questioned for some STIs, especially for HPV. The data presented suggest a strong role for condom use and strengthen the need for traditional public health approaches to reduce sexual risk behaviors and increase STI screening (and treatment) as advocated by others.[37,38]

**Accepted for Publication:** September 7, 2005.
**Correspondence:** Darron R. Brown, MD, Emerson Hall, Room 435, 545 Barnhill Dr, Indiana University School of Medicine, Indianapolis, IN 46202 (darbrow@iupui.edu)
**Funding/Support:** This study was funded by grant U19 AI43924 from the National Institutes of Health National Institute of Allergy and Infectious Diseases, Bethesda, Md. The statistical models used in this research were developed with the support of grant RO1HD42404-01 from the National Institute of Child Health and Human Development, Bethesda.
**Acknowledgment:** We thank Pat Brooks and the project staff for the Young Women's Project for their allegiance and dedication to maintenance of this cohort and data collection. We thank Timothy Breen, PhD, and the data man-

agement staff, who made this analysis and article possible. We thank William Bonnez, MD, University of Rochester School of Medicine and Dentistry, Rochester, NY, for critical review of the manuscript and helpful suggestions.

## REFERENCES


1. Burd EM. Human papillomavirus and cervical cancer. *Clin Microbiol Rev.* 2003; 16:1-17.
2. Giuliano AR, Harris R, Sedjo RL, et al. Incidence, prevalence, and clearance of type-specific human papillomavirus infections: the Young Women's Health Study. *J Infect Dis.* 2002;186:462-469.
3. Ho GYF, Bierman R, Beardsley L, et al. Natural history of cervicovaginal papillomavirus infection in young women. *N Engl J Med.* 1998;338:423-428.
4. Brown DR, Shew ML, Qadadri B, et al. A longitudinal study of genital human papillomavirus infection in a cohort of closely followed adolescent women. *J Infect Dis.* 2005;191:182-192.
5. Schlecht NF, Kulaga S, Robitaille J, et al. Persistent human papillomavirus infection as a predictor of cervical intraepithelial neoplasia. *JAMA.* 2001;286: 3106-3114.
6. Moscicki AB, Shiboski S, Broering J, et al. The natural history of human papillomavirus infection as measured by repeated DNA testing in adolescent and young women. *J Pediatr.* 1998;132:277-284.
7. Richardson H, Kelsall G, Tellier P, et al. The natural history of type-specific human papillomavirus infections in female university students. *Cancer Epidemiol Biomarkers Prev.* 2003;12:485-490.
8. Elfgren K, Kalantari M, Moberger B, Bjorn H, Dillner J. A population-based five-year follow-up study of cervical human papillomavirus infection. *Am J Obstet Gynecol.* 2000;183:561-567.
9. Castle PE, Wacholder S, Lorincz AT, et al. A prospective study of high-grade cervical neoplasia risk among human papillomavirus-infected women. *J Natl Cancer Inst.* 2002;94:1406-1414.
10. Deacon JM, Evans CD, Yule R, et al. Sexual behaviour and smoking as determinants of cervical HPV infection and of CIN3 among those infected: a case-control study nested within the Manchester cohort. *Br J Cancer.* 2000;83: 1565-1572.
11. Moscicki AB, Hills N, Shiboski S, et al. Risks for incident human papillomavirus infection and low-grade squamous intraepithelial lesion development in young females. *JAMA.* 2001;285:2995-3002.
12. Giulian AR, Sedjo RL, Roe DJ, et al. Clearance of oncogenic human papillomavirus (HPV) infection: effect of smoking (United States). *Cancer Causes Control.* 2002;13:839-846.
13. Ahdieh L, Klein RS, Burk R, et al. Prevalence, incidence, and type-specific persistence of human papillomavirus in human immunodeficiency virus (HIV)-positive and HIV-negative women. *J Infect Dis.* 2001;184:682-690.
14. Brisson J, Bairati I, Morin C, et al. Determinants of persistent detection of human papillomavirus DNA in the uterine cervix. *J Infect Dis.* 1996;173:794-799.
15. Smith JS, Munoz N, Herrero R, et al. Evidence for *Chlamydia trachomatis* as a human papillomavirus cofactor in the etiology of invasive cervical cancer in Brazil and the Philippines. *J Infect Dis.* 2002;185:324-331.
16. Anttila T, Saikku P, Koskela P, et al. Serotypes of *Chlamydia trachomatis* and risk for development of cervical squamous cell carcinoma. *JAMA.* 2001;285: 47-51.
17. Wallin KL, Wiklund F, Luostarinen T, et al. A population-based prospective study of *Chlamydia trachomatis* infection and cervical cancer. *Int J Cancer.* 2002; 101:371-374.
18. Tarkowski TA, Koumans EH, Sayer M, et al. Epidemiology of human papillomavirus infection and abnormal cytologic test results in an urban adolescent population. *J Infect Dis.* 2004;189:46-50.
19. Wright TC Jr, Denny L, Kuhn L, Pullack A, Lorizncz A. HPV DNA testing of self-collected vaginal samples compared with cytologic screening to detect cervical cancer. *JAMA.* 2000;283:81-86.
20. Gravitt PE, Lacey JV, Brinton LA, et al. Evaluation of self-collected cervicovaginal cell samples for human papillomavirus testing by polymerase chain reaction. *Cancer Epidemiol Biomarkers Prev.* 2001;10:95-100.
21. Gravitt PE, Peyton CL, Alessi TQ, et al. Improved amplification of genital human papillomaviruses. *J Clin Microbiol.* 2000;38:357-361.
22. Gravitt PE, Peyton CL, Apple RJ, Wheeler CM. Genotyping of 27 human papillomavirus types by using L1 consensus PCR products by a single hybridization, reverse line blot detection method. *J Clin Microbiol.* 1998;36:3020-3027.
23. Brown DR, Legge D, Qadadri B. Distribution of human papillomavirus types in cervicovaginal washings from women evaluated in a sexually transmitted disease clinic. *Sex Transm Dis.* 2002;29:763-768.
24. Kengne P, Veas F, Vidal N, Rey NL, Cuny G. *Trichomonas vaginalis*: repeated DNA target for highly sensitive and specific polymerase chain reaction diagnosis. *Cell Mol Biol.* 1994;40:819-831.
25. Palmer HM, Mallinson H, Woods RL, Herring AJ. Evaluation of the specificities of five DNA amplification methods for the detection of *Neisseria gonorrhoeae.* *J Clin Microbiol.* 2003;41:835-837.
26. Farrell DJ. Evaluation of AMPLICOR *Neisseria gonorrhoeae* PCR using *cppB* nested PCR and 16S rRNA PCR. *J Clin Microbiol.* 1999;37:386-390.
27. Ho BS, Feng WG, Wong BK, Egglestone SI. Polymerase chain reaction for the detection of *Neisseria gonorrhoeae* in clinical samples. *J Clin Pathol.* 1992; 45:439-442.
28. Thereau T, Grambsch P. *Modeling Survival Data: Extending the Cox Model.* New York, NY: Springer; 2002.
29. 1998 Guidelines for treatment of sexually transmitted diseases: Centers for Disease Control and Prevention. *MMWR Recomm Rep.* 1998;47:1-111.
30. Castle PE, Guiliano AR. Genital tract infections, cervical inflammation, and antioxidant nutrients—assessing their roles as human papillomavirus cofactors. *J Natl Cancer Inst Monogr.* 2003;31:29-34.
31. Robertson SA, Sharkey DJ. The role of semen in induction of maternal immune tolerance to pregnancy. *Semin Immunol.* 2001;13:243-254.
32. Hogewoning CJ, Bleeker MC, van den Brule AJ, et al. Condom use promotes regression of cervical intraepithelial neoplasia and clearance of human papillomavirus: a randomized clinical trial. *Int J Cancer.* 2003;107:811-816.
33. Zhang ZF, Graham S, Yu SZ, et al. *Trichomonas vaginalis* and cervical cancer: a prospective study in China. *Ann Epidemiol.* 1995;5:325-332.
34. Smith JS, Bosetti C, Munoz N, et al. *Chlamydia trachomatis* and invasive cervical cancer: a pooled analysis of the IARC multicentric case-control study. *Int J Cancer.* 2004;111:431-439.
35. Clerici M, Merola M, Ferrario E, et al. Cytokine production patterns in cervical intraepithelial neoplasia: association with human papillomavirus infection. *J Natl Cancer Inst.* 1997;89:245-250.
36. Castellsague X, Munoz N. Cofactors in human papillomavirus carcinogenesis—role of parity, oral contraceptives and tobacco smoking. *J Natl Cancer Inst Monogr.* 2003;31:20-28.
37. Burstein GR, Gaydos CA, Diener-West M, Howell MR, Zenilman JM, Quinn TC. Incident chlamydia trachomatis infections among inner-city adolescent females. *JAMA.* 1998;280:521-526.
38. Orr DP, Fortenberry JD, Blythe MJ. Validity of self-reported sexual behaviors in adolescent women using biomarker outcomes. *Sex Transm Dis.* 1997;24: 261-266.


## Correction

**Error in E-mail Address.** In the article "Hearing Screening at Well-Child Visits" by Halloran et al published in the October issue of the ARCHIVES (2005;159:949-955), an incorrect e-mail address was given. On page 955 in the correspondence address, the correct e-mail address for Dr Halloran is dhallor2@slu.edu.

ARTICLE

# Effect of Telephone Reminder/Recall on Adolescent Immunization and Preventive Visits

## *Results From a Randomized Clinical Trial*

*Peter G. Szilagyi, MD, MPH; Stanley Schaffer, MD, MS; Richard Barth, BS; Laura P. Shone, MSW, DrPH; Sharon G. Humiston, MD, MPH; Sandra Ambrose, MBA; Francisco Averhoff, MD, MPH*

**Objective:** To measure the effect of telephone-based reminder/recall on immunization and well-child care (WCC) visit rates among adolescents in urban practices.

**Design:** Randomized clinical trial of telephone-based reminder/recall over 18 months.

**Setting:** Four urban primary care practices.

**Participants:** Adolescents aged 11 to 14 years.

**Intervention:** Adolescents within practices were randomized to study (n=1496) or control groups (n=1510). The study group was sent audiotaped telephone reminders about a scheduled or needed immunization or WCC visit. Households were called weekly if there was no response; telephone numbers were updated weekly. Controls received standard care.

**Results:** Baseline demographics and immunization and WCC visit rates were similar for study and control groups. The intervention was largely ineffective in improving immunization or WCC visit rates. Although at the end of the study, the study group had slightly higher hepatitis B coverage (3 vaccinations)(62% vs 57.8%; $P=.02$), WCC visits were the same (53% and 54%), and impact on other vaccinations was minimal. The effect of reminder/recall was equivalent across demographic subgroups (eg, age, race/ethnicity, insurance). The major factor limiting intervention effectiveness was inaccurate telephone numbers. Seventy-one percent of study subjects with single telephone numbers throughout the study had a WCC visit vs 25% of study subjects with multiple/changed telephone numbers and 54% of controls ($P<.001$).

**Conclusions:** An intensive telephone reminder and recall system was only minimally successful in improving immunization and WCC visit rates among urban adolescents. Lack of success was largely owing to changed or inaccurate telephone numbers.

*Arch Pediatr Adolesc Med. 2006;160:157-163*

A NATIONAL HEALTH PRIORity is to improve immunization rates to reduce vaccine-preventable diseases.[1] Studies have documented effective strategies for improving childhood and adult immunization rates.[2-12]

In spite of the plethora of studies on young children and older adults, surprisingly little attention has been paid to adolescent immunizations.[13] Until recently, adolescent immunizations involved only catch-up and booster doses of tetanus vaccine and measles-containing vaccine. During the past decade, new hepatitis B,[14-16] varicella,[17] and influenza vaccination[18] guidelines heightened attention to adolescent vaccinations. Adolescent vaccinations will soon become a major public health and pediatric focus because of new policies regarding pertussis[19-21] and meningococcal[22-25] vaccines; the development of vaccines to prevent sexually transmitted infections, including human papillomavirus,[26,27] herpes simplex,[28] and chlamydia[29]; and increasing emphasis on underused vaccines such as influenza,[30,31] varicella,[32] and hepatitis A[33] and B.[34-36]

In 1997, the Advisory Committee on Immunization Practices (Atlanta, Ga), the American Academy of Pediatrics (Elk Grove Village, Ill), the American Academy of Family Physicians (Leawood, Kan), and the American Medical Association issued recommendations to improve the delivery of adolescent immunizations.[37] These guidelines highlighted barriers to adolescent immunizations: inability of health care professionals to track and recall adolescents who need vaccinations, missed opportunities for vaccinations within health care settings, and record scattering.[35,38] Additional barriers can involve parental consent, because parents are frequently absent during adolescent health visits[39]; lack of health insurance[40]; and problems with access to health care.[41-45]

Author Affiliations:
Departments of Pediatrics (Drs Szilagyi, Schaffer, and Shone, Mr Barth, and Ms Ambrose) and Emergency Medicine (Dr Humiston), University of Rochester School of Medicine and Dentistry, Strong Children's Research Center, Rochester, NY; National Immunization Program, Centers for Disease Control and Prevention, Atlanta, Ga (Dr Averhoff).

Few studies have evaluated interventions for adolescent immunizations. Studies of school-based adolescent immunization programs have noted mixed success.[46] Systematic telephone or mail reminder/recall systems, which are often,[4,5,47] but not always,[48-50] effective for increasing immunization rates among young children or adults, are recommended for adolescents but have not been evaluated for this vulnerable[33,37,39] population. A study of letter reminders to adolescents or parents noted poor response rates[51] and had no comparison group.

Our study evaluated the effectiveness of a systematic telephone-based reminder/recall system on immunization rates and well-child care (WCC) visits among adolescents attending 4 urban primary care practices that serve predominantly city residents.

## METHODS

### SETTING

The University of Rochester (Rochester, NY) Research Subjects Review Board approved this study. The study was performed at 4 urban primary care practices located in Rochester, a city with a population of 250 000 and high rates of child poverty[52] within a county of 750 000 residents. The practices included 2 pediatric group practices, a hospital-based pediatric clinic, and a family medicine–based neighborhood health center. These large practices are representative of urban primary care practices and together serve 19% of the county's children.

### ELIGIBLE POPULATION

We analyzed each practice's billing database for adolescents who had 1 or more visits at each site. From 5902 potential subjects with a birth date between June 1, 1983, and May 31, 1987 (aged 11-14 years at the start of the intervention), we excluded (1) siblings (randomly selecting 1 child per family), (2) those with no practice visits within 24 months, (3) those residing outside the county, and (4) those with no telephone number in the database. Prior power calculations to detect a 10% improvement in baseline immunization rates of 50% (power of 0.80; $\alpha = .05$) within each practice required more than 750 adolescents per practice. From 5902 potential subjects, 3006 were eligible for randomization.

### SUBJECTS

The 3006 subjects were stratified into 2 equal age groups (11-12 years and 13-14 years at the start of the study) and randomly allocated into a study group (n = 1496) or control group (n = 1510) using a random-number generator with the child as the unit of randomization. Health care professionals were unaware of group allocation for specific subjects because the intervention used research personnel and reminders from a central office.

### INTERVENTION (STUDY GROUP)

We used an automated telephone message reminder system (autodialer[53]), previously noted to improve preschool immunization rates in 2 health clinics[54,55] and a health maintenance organization setting.[56] A medical record review at the beginning of the study identified telephone numbers for the autodialers, a database tracked adolescents needing reminders, and a research assistant verified weekly upcoming appointments, recent WCC visits or immunizations, and changes in telephone numbers. The intervention mimicked an appointment-scheduling module that is linked to a telephone-reminder system. The intervention occurred between August 8, 1998, and February 29, 2000.

### ALGORITHMS FOR TELEPHONE CALLS

Adolescents were called if they were due for an annual WCC visit, a tetanus booster (>5 years since diphtheria and tetanus toxoids and pertussis vaccination), or a hepatitis B vaccination according to Advisory Committee on Immunization Practices guidelines. A variable number of calls was placed depending on the need for immunizations or WCC visits and prior response to reminder calls. The calls were voice recordings in English to request a vaccination appointment or WCC visit or to remind families of upcoming scheduled appointments. Calls were made 6 days per week during the day or early evening.

During the initial 11 months of the 18-month clinical trial, telephone calls were stopped if (1) recipients indicated from a telephone menu option that the telephone number was incorrect, the adolescent had left the practice, or the parent requested calls to be stopped or (2) 5 calls were placed within 30 days and no appointment was scheduled ("unresponsive numbers"). After 11 months, the autodialer telephone reminder calls were restarted for those subjects with "unresponsive numbers" to give families a second opportunity to respond to subsequent reminders.

### PARTICIPANT FLOW DURING THE STUDY

Based on medical record review at the end of the study, subjects who had moved or subjects for whom no medical record was found were considered "inactive" (132 study subjects and 168 controls). Because we performed an intention-to-treat analysis, these subjects were considered "behind in immunizations" or "not having a WCC visit."

### MEASURES

The key independent measure was group assignment (study vs control). Key demographic subgroups[57-59] (**Table 1**) delineated from billing files included: subject's age (11-14 years), sex, residence (inner city, rest of the city of Rochester, and suburbs), primary care practice (each of 4), insurance (6 categories), and race/ethnicity (white non-Hispanic, black non-Hispanic, Hispanic, or other/unknown). Analyses by residence, health insurance, and race/ethnicity combined subjects across practices and age groups.

Key dependent measures were obtained by blinded medical record reviews at the end of the study using a standardized medical record review form. Quality assurance checks for 5% of subjects noted more than 98% reliability.

Dependent measures were immunization-related outcomes: (1) up-to-date rates (yes/no) for hepatitis B (first, second, and third doses) and tetanus-diphtheria toxoids booster (Td); and (2) mean number of days eligible for each vaccine during the study time frame. Health care visit measures included (1) receipt (yes/no) of WCC within the prior year and (2) mean number of days eligible for WCC visits during the study time frame.

### ANALYSES

Intention-to-treat analyses were performed for the 1496 study and 1510 control subjects using $\chi^2$ tests for categorical variables and $t$ tests or analysis of variance for numeric variables.

For 2 key measures (the initial hepatitis B vaccination and a WCC visit), Kaplan-Meier survival curves were generated to determine the number of days eligible for a vaccine or WCC visit throughout the 18-month study. Results for study subjects were compared with results for control subjects using a log-rank test.

**Table 1. Baseline Demographic Characteristics of Study and Control Adolescents***

| Characteristic | Study Adolescents, % | Control Adolescents, % | P Value |
|---|---|---|---|
| No. of adolescents | 1496 | 1510 | |
| Age, y† | | | .66 |
| 11 | 23.4 | 24.3 | |
| 12 | 24.3 | 25.4 | |
| 13 | 27.0 | 26.8 | |
| 14 | 25.3 | 23.6 | |
| Male | 49.5 | 52.1 | .74 |
| Residence‡ | | | .20 |
| Inner city of Rochester, NY | 38.4 | 35.9 | |
| Rest of city of Rochester | 24.3 | 23.7 | |
| Suburbs | 37.3 | 40.4 | |
| Practice | | | .94 |
| Urban private practice 1 | 24.8 | 26.4 | |
| Urban private practice 2 | 30.7 | 31.1 | |
| Hospital-based clinic | 26.7 | 25.9 | |
| Neighborhood health center | 17.8 | 17.6 | |
| Insurance | | | .76 |
| Medicaid, fee for service | 27.1 | 25.5 | |
| Medicaid, managed care (includes SCHIP) | 9.6 | 9.6 | |
| Private, fee for service | 6.0 | 5.0 | |
| Private, managed care | 42.5 | 44.1 | |
| Uninsured | 2.6 | 3.0 | |
| Other or unknown | 9.9 | 10.5 | |
| Race/ethnicity§ | | | .24 |
| White non-Hispanic | 16.8 | 17.8 | |
| Black non-Hispanic | 36.8 | 33.9 | |
| Hispanic | 6.4 | 7.7 | |
| Other or unknown | 39.9 | 40.6 | |

Abbreviation: SCHIP, State Children's Health Insurance Program.

*Demographic characteristics were obtained from the billing files of the 4 practices.

†The study design stratified for age group (11-12 y and 13-14 y) but not for other variables.

‡The inner city of Rochester is geographically the core of the city, while the rest of the city involves other census tracts within the city boundaries. The inner city has the highest rates of poverty, the rest of the city has intermediate rates, and the suburbs have very low rates of poverty.[59]

§Race and ethnicity were not present in billing files for about 40% of subjects.

## POST HOC ANALYSIS

Because lack of telephones, incorrect telephone numbers, or changed numbers are common among impoverished families,[47,48] we anticipated that many study subjects would never receive the telephone messages. Thus, a single post hoc analysis compared results for subjects for whom only 1 telephone number was noted throughout the study vs subjects for whom multiple telephone numbers were noted throughout the study. We surmised that subjects with a single telephone number represented a less mobile[60] subgroup of families who may have had greater exposure to the intervention.

# RESULTS

## DEMOGRAPHICS

Study and control groups were similar with respect to age group, sex, practice, insurance, and race/ethnicity (Table 1). Most were from the city of Rochester, many had Medicaid coverage, and a high proportion were black or Hispanic.

**Table 2. Up-to-Date Rates of Study and Control Adolescents***

| Characteristic | Study Adolescents | Control Adolescents | Difference Between Study and Control Adolescents | P Value |
|---|---|---|---|---|
| Up-to-date at baseline | | | | |
| Hepatitis B (3 vaccinations) | 45.1 | 44.0 | 1.1 | .53 |
| Td vaccination | 24.7 | 23.8 | 0.9 | .57 |
| WCC visits (<1 y since last) | 52.3 | 54.2 | 0.1 | .30 |
| Up-to-date at end of intervention | | | | |
| Hepatitis B (3 vaccinations) | 62.0 | 57.8 | 2.2 | .02 |
| Td vaccination | 52.0 | 49.9 | 2.1 | .27 |
| WCC visits (<1 y since last) | 53.1 | 54.3 | −1.2 | .50 |
| Change in up-to-date | | | | |
| Hepatitis B (3 vaccinations) | +16.9 | +13.8 | 3.1 | .03 |
| Td vaccination | +27.3 | +26.1 | 1.2 | .50 |
| WCC visits (<1 y since last) | +0.8 | +0.1 | 0.7 | .80 |

Abbreviations: Td, tetanus-diphtheria toxoids; WCC, well-child care.

*Values are expressed as percentages unless otherwise indicated.

## IMPACT OF REMINDER/RECALL ON IMMUNIZATION AND WCC RATES

At baseline, study and control groups were similar for hepatitis B and Td coverage and WCC visit rates. At the end of the intervention, the study group had higher hepatitis B coverage (3 vaccinations)(62.0% vs 57.8%; $P = .02$), but no difference was noted in coverage for Td or WCC visit rates. Although both study and control groups experienced increases in coverage for hepatitis B and Td vaccinations, there was a statistically significant difference between study and control groups in the change in hepatitis B coverage but not in the change in Td or WCC rates (**Table 2**).

**Table 3** presents more detailed immunization and health care visit information. Since some subjects were never eligible for some immunizations, we assessed whether eligible adolescents received immunizations or WCC visits during the study. No statistically significant differences were noted between study and control groups, although there was a trend toward higher hepatitis B rates (3 vaccinations) among study subjects. The mean number of days eligible for a vaccination or a WCC visit and the mean number of WCC or other visits were also similar for study and control groups, except for slightly higher rates of Td vaccination among study subjects.

## IMPACT OF REMINDER/RECALL ON SUBGROUPS

We examined immunization and WCC visits measures for study vs control groups for the key demographic characteristics in Table 1, and no substantive differences be-

**Table 3. Immunization and Health Care Visit Status at the End of the Study**

| Outcome | Study: No. of Adolescents Eligible for Vaccination* | Study: Percentage of Eligible Adolescents Who Received Immunization or Visit† | Control: No. of Adolescents Eligible for Vaccination* | Control: Percentage of Eligible Adolescents Who Received Immunization or Visit† | Difference Between Study and Control Adolescents, % | *P* Value |
|---|---|---|---|---|---|---|
| Received during study | | | | | | |
| Hepatitis B | | | | | | |
| Vaccination 1 | 484 | 34.1 | 549 | 34.1 | 0.03 | .90 |
| Vaccination 2 | 299 | 65.2 | 294 | 61.6 | 3.7 | .30 |
| Vaccination 3 | 384 | 65.6 | 355 | 59.4 | 6.2 | .08 |
| Td vaccination | 1127 | 36.2 | 1151 | 34.3 | 1.8 | .30 |
| WCC visit | 1496 | 64.6 | 1510 | 63.8 | 0.7 | .70 |
| | **No. of Adolescents Eligible for Vaccination*** | **Mean No. of Days Eligible‡** | **No. of Adolescents Eligible for Vaccination*** | **Mean No. of Days Eligible‡** | **Difference Between Study and Control Adolescents, %** | ***P* Value** |
| Mean No. of days eligible | | | | | | |
| Hepatitis B | | | | | | |
| Vaccination 1 | 484 | 430 | 549 | 439 | −2.1 | .45 |
| Vaccination 2 | 299 | 205 | 294 | 209 | −1.7 | .84 |
| Vaccination 3 | 384 | 218 | 355 | 234 | −7.3 | .24 |
| Td vaccination | 1127 | 438 | 1151 | 454 | −3.6 | .02 |
| WCC visit | 1496 | 230 | 1510 | 242 | −5.2 | .16 |
| | **No. of Adolescents Eligible for Vaccination*** | **Mean No. of Visits** | **No. of Adolescents Eligible for Vaccination*** | **Mean No. of Visits** | **Difference Between Study and Control Adolescents, No. (%)** | ***P* Value** |
| Mean No. of visits | | | | | | |
| WCC visits | 1496 | 0.80 | 1510 | 0.77 | +0.03 (+4.1) | .20 |
| Other visits | 1496 | 2.15 | 1510 | 2.21 | −0.06 (−2.7) | .53 |
| Appointments not kept§ | 1496 | 0.56 | 1510 | 0.53 | +0.02 (+4.7) | .57 |

Abbreviations: Td, tetanus-diphtheria toxoids; WCC, well-child care.
*Number of adolescents who were eligible for the immunization at any time during the 18-month study period.
†Percentage of eligible adolescents who received the immunization or WCC visit during the intervention.
‡Mean number of days eligible among the subjects who were eligible for a vaccination or a WCC visit.
§Visits scheduled but not kept.

tween study and control groups were noted. This suggests that the reminder/recall intervention did not perform differently for subgroups that varied by these demographic characteristics.

## WANING BENEFIT OF THE INTERVENTION OVER TIME

The intervention appeared to be marginally beneficial during the first few months of the study, with benefit waning afterward. For example, during month 1, 87.8% of study and 88.4% of control subjects needed a vaccination or WCC visit, 81% of study subjects were sent a telephone reminder, and study subjects were more likely than controls to have a visit within 3 months (study subjects, 40.4%; controls, 34.4%; $P = .001$) or a vaccination (study subjects, 18.1%; controls, 11.6%; $P < .001$). For month 2, eligible study subjects again were more likely than controls to have a visit ($P < .05$) or vaccination ($P < .001$). Thereafter, benefits for WCC visits were no longer noted, and after 4 months, benefits for vaccinations were no longer noted.

The **Figure** shows Kaplan-Meier survival curves for the proportion of adolescents eligible for hepatitis B vaccination (Figure A) or WCC visit (Figure B). The y-axis shows the proportion eligible (starting with 1.0), and the x-axis shows the days during the 18-month study. As seen by comparing the "all study subjects" vs "all control subjects" groups, more control subjects than study subjects remained eligible for hepatitis B vaccination or WCC visits in the early months of the study, but the effect waned after several months.

## FACTORS LIMITING EFFECTIVENESS OF REMINDER/RECALL

Since the benefit of reminder/recall was minimal and limited to the initial months of the study, we examined factors that may have limited its effectiveness. Two factors that accounted for some reminder calls being discontinued were families (1) responding to the autodialer message that the adolescent was no longer a patient of the practice (3.4%) or (2) requesting calls to be discontinued for no stated reason (9.8%). The major group involved parents simply not responding to the reminders with no explanation (62.8%), which eventually resulted in the calls being "turned off." We cannot determine the proportion of these families that simply ignored reminders vs wrong telephone numbers.

## POST HOC ANALYSIS BY SINGLE OR MULTIPLE TELEPHONE NUMBERS

The Figure also shows Kaplan-Meier survival curves for the proportion of subjects eligible for hepatitis B vaccination (Figure A) or WCC visit (Figure B) among subjects who had 1 vs more than 1 telephone number during the study period. Fully 69% (n = 1034) of study subjects had 2 or more different telephone numbers during the 18-month study period. The one third of study subjects with a single telephone number throughout the 18-month period were far more likely ($P<.001$) to receive a hepatitis B vaccination and a WCC visit than were the study subjects who had multiple telephone numbers. Results for other outcomes followed a similar pattern.

## COMMENT

An intensive autodialer-based telephone reminder and recall system was only marginally successful in improving immunization rates and WCC visits among adolescents attending 4 urban primary care practices. An initial effect waned after several months. The small effect (4-7 percentage points) appears consistent with the small effect noted in many reminder/recall studies.[5,61] The intervention did not appear to be any more or less effective for demographic subgroups stratified by age, geographic residence, insurance status, and race/ethnicity. The major factor limiting effectiveness of reminder/recall was inaccurate telephone numbers. The initial improvements were probably owing to the reminders reaching those families with accurate telephone numbers or those who were going to respond. Continued intervention had no effect.

Patient reminder/recall can improve immunization rates[4,5,54] and preventive visit rates[62] in children or adults, but several recent studies,[47,48] including 1 autodialer-based study[63] focusing on urban infants, have failed to find benefit. The most commonly cited reason for the lack of effectiveness is difficulty in successfully contacting the patient population, a concern regarding adolescents who make few regular health care visits. In our study, lack of an accurate telephone number was the major problem. Of 1496 study subjects, 69% had at least 2 distinct telephone numbers over 18 months. The subgroup that had a single telephone number had markedly greater response to the telephone reminders than did the subgroup with 2 or more telephone numbers. Our findings confirm that the effectiveness of the patient reminder/recall is strongly associated with the accuracy of telephone numbers or addresses, which was low among this population.

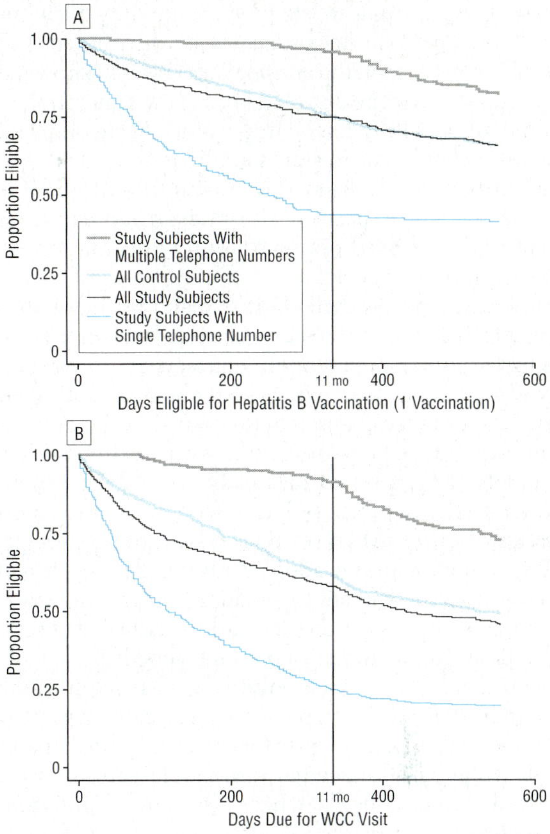


**Figure.** Kaplan-Meier survival estimates for children eligible for hepatitis B vaccination (1 vaccination) (A) and well-child care (WCC) visits (B). The study group was stratified by "single telephone number" vs "multiple telephone numbers." "Single telephone number" included subjects who had the same telephone number during the 18-month study period. "Multiple phone numbers" included subjects who had more than 1 telephone number within the 18-month study period. A, Log-rank test, all study subjects vs all control subjects, $P<.10$. Study subgroups vs each other and controls, $P<.001$. B, Log-rank test, all study subjects vs all control subjects, $P<.10$. Study subgroups vs each other and controls, $P<.001$.

Unfortunately, practices cannot discern beforehand which families are likely to change their telephone number (or addresses). Practices should update telephone numbers during all patient encounters and obtain alternate contact information such as mobile telephone numbers. Our study also suggests that new vaccines requiring multiple doses (eg, human papillomavirus vaccine) may pose a challenge for vaccinating the urban adolescent population. Given that our intervention had some initial benefit, probably because it reached those families that could be reached, health care professionals serving urban populations may consider short-term reminder/recall interventions instead of prolonged and intensive interventions.

We expect that the use of autodialers or similar technology will increase as computerized appointment scheduling modules are implemented.[58] The costs of autodialer-based reminder systems are relatively low if (1) telephone numbers are updated electronically using links with billing systems and (2) the systems are used by hospital or health systems that apply them to populations beyond adolescents.[54] As an example, 1 of the study practices has just begun using an autodialer reminder system for scheduled appointments as part of a hospitalwide autodialer reminder system. Costs to the practice are only a few hundred dollars per year because costs are distributed hospitalwide. Thus, even with very small increases in show rates, this reminder system is probably revenue generating.

Our study highlights the importance of checking adolescents' immunization status at all visits and using visits other than WCC visits as opportunities to immunize adolescents. More than half the study group had at least 1 visit with a missed opportunity for vaccination with hepatitis B or Td vaccine.

Our study has several limitations. The major threat to generalizability is the study setting—urban practices in a metropolitan area. Patient characteristics, the accuracy of telephone numbers, baseline immunization coverage, and practice characteristics may differ in other settings. Baseline vaccination rates were within the wide spectrum of rates noted nationally.[14,34,64] Demographic characteristics of our population were similar to characteristics of other urban settings. Also, although hepatitis B vaccination among adolescents will become less important (because of infant vaccination), it serves as a model for human papillomavirus vaccination because that schedule will be similar to the hepatitis B schedule.

One threat to internal validity is that we undoubtedly included adolescents who were not current patients of the practices because there was no perfect method to select eligible adolescents. Some adolescents may have received vaccinations elsewhere. The major limitation to the intervention was the inability to determine accurate telephone numbers in spite of the research assistant checking medical records and web-based directories weekly. Coordination of practice-based interventions with Medicaid managed care may improve effectiveness since the requirements to reenroll into Medicaid managed care plans provide opportunities for managed care organizations to update patient contact information.

It is possible that the autodialer was not as effective as a direct telephone call from a person would have been. Studies are lacking comparing autodialer-based reminders with person-to-person reminders. Further, we did not attempt to ascertain vaccinations received outside of the practice; however, in this community, few vaccinations are provided to adolescents in schools or public health clinics.[61] Finally, we did not perform cost analyses because we were using a labor-intensive method to update kept appointments and changes in telephone numbers.

We conclude that an intensive primary care practice-based telephone reminder/recall intervention was only marginally effective by slightly improving the receipt of adolescent immunizations visits within these urban primary care practices. The critical factor associated with success of the intervention was the accuracy of telephone numbers, which was low among our population.

An implication for health care professionals is that practices are more likely to have success with patient reminder/recall if they have accurate patient telephone numbers. In these cases, even small practices may consider using reminder systems. For practices within hospital or health systems, practice-level costs of reminder/recall systems may be low because costs would be distributed across an entire system, and large numbers of patients beyond adolescents could benefit. In these settings, an autodialer-based reminder/recall system that has only a small effect should still be considered. However, to achieve high levels of preventive care among urban adolescents, more aggressive strategies (such as outreach[13,65] or combinations of interventions) may be needed.

An implication for communities and public health is that in some settings, practice-based patient reminder/recall might be only marginally effective in improving adolescent vaccinations and preventive visits. These interventions may be more effective if combined with updated contact information from managed care organizations, immunization registries, or integrated delivery systems. With emerging new adolescent vaccines, aggressive strategies will be needed to ensure high adolescent vaccination coverage as well as receipt of preventive adolescent services.

**Accepted for Publication:** September 6, 2005.
**Correspondence:** Peter G. Szilagyi, MD, MPH, Department of Pediatrics, Strong Memorial Hospital, Box 632, Rochester, NY 14642 (peter_szilagyi@urmc.rochester.edu).
**Funding/Support:** This work was funded by the Centers for Disease Control and Prevention, Atlanta, Ga, and Cooperative Agreement TS-622 from the Association for Teachers of Preventive Medicine, Washington, DC.
**Acknowledgment:** We gratefully acknowledge the statistical consultation of Jason Roy, PhD.

## REFERENCES

1. Centers for Disease Control and Prevention (CDC). Ten great public health achievements—United States, 1900-1999. *MMWR Morb Mortal Wkly Rep.* 1999;48:241-243.
2. Gyorkos TW, Tannenbaum TN, Abrahamowicz M, et al. Evaluation of the effectiveness of immunization delivery methods. *Can J Public Health.* 1994;85(suppl 1):S14-S30.
3. Shea S, DuMouchel W, Bahamonde L. A meta-analysis of 16 randomized controlled trials to evaluate computer-based clinical reminder systems for preventive care in the ambulatory setting. *J Am Med Inform Assoc.* 1996;3:399-409.
4. Udovic S, Lieu TA. Evidence on office-based interventions to improve childhood immunization delivery. *Pediatr Ann.* 1998;27:355-361.
5. Shefer A, Briss P, Rodewald L, et al. Improving immunization coverage rates: an evidence-based review of the literature. *Epidemiol Rev.* 1999;21:96-142.
6. Szilagyi PG, Bordley C, Vann JC, et al. The effect of patient reminder/recall interventions on immunization rates: a review. *JAMA.* 2000;284:1820-1827.
7. Centers for Disease Control and Prevention. Vaccine-preventable diseases: improving vaccination coverage in children, adolescents, and adults. a report on recommendations from the Task Force on Community Preventive Services. *MMWR Morb Mortal Wkly Rep.* 1999;48(RR-8):1-15.
8. Centers for Disease Control and Prevention (CDC). National, state, and urban area vaccination levels among children aged 19-35 months—United States, 2002. *MMWR Morb Mortal Wkly Rep.* 2003;52:728-732.
9. Centers for Disease Control and Prevention (CDC). Public health and aging: influenza vaccination coverage among adults aged > or =50 years and pneumococcal vaccination coverage among adults aged > or =65 years—United States, 2002. *MMWR Morb Mortal Wkly Rep.* 2003;52:987-992.
10. Rodewald LE, Szilagyi PG, Shiuh T, et al. Is underimmunization a marker for insufficient utilization of preventive and primary care? *Arch Pediatr Adolesc Med.* 1995;149:393-397.
11. Fairbrother G, Friedman S, DuMont KA, Lobach KS. Markers for primary care: missed opportunities to immunize and screen for lead and tuberculosis by private physicians serving large numbers of inner-city Medicaid-eligible children. *Pediatrics.* 1996;97:785-790.
12. Rodewald LE, Szilagyi PG, Humiston SG, et al. A randomized study of tracking with outreach and provider prompting to improve immunization coverage and primary care. *Pediatrics.* 1999;103:31-38.
13. Schaffer SJ. The coming of age of adolescent immunization. *Pediatr Ann.* 2001;30:342-345.

14. Centers for Disease Control and Prevention (CDC). Vaccination coverage among adolescents 1 year before the institution of a seventh grade school entry vaccination requirement—San Diego, California, 1998. *MMWR Morb Mortal Wkly Rep.* 2000;49:101-102, 111.
15. Centers for Disease Control and Prevention (CDC). Hepatitis B vaccination—United States, 1982-2002. *MMWR Morb Mortal Wkly Rep.* 2002;51:549-552, 563.
16. Centers for Disease Control and Prevention. Update: recommendations to prevent hepatitis B virus transmission—United States. *JAMA.* 1999;281:790.
17. Immunization Action Coalition. Varicella prevention mandates. Available at: http://www.immunize.org/laws/varicel.htm. Accessed February 8, 2005.
18. Bridges CB, Harper SA, Fukuda K, Uyeki TM, Cox NJ, Singleton JA; Advisory Committee on Immunization Practices. Prevention and control of influenza: recommendations of the Advisory Committee on Immunization Practices (ACIP) [published correction appears in *MMWR Morb Mortal Wkly Rep.* 2003;52:526]. *MMWR Recomm Rep.* 2003;52(RR-8):1-34.
19. Vitek CR, Pascual FB, Baughman AL, Murphy TV. Increase in deaths from pertussis among young infants in the United States in the 1990s. *Pediatr Infect Dis J.* 2003;22:628-634.
20. Cherry JD. The science and fiction of the "resurgence" of pertussis. *Pediatrics.* 2003;112:405-406.
21. Edwards KM. Is pertussis a frequent cause of cough in adolescents and adults? should routine pertussis immunization be recommended? *Clin Infect Dis.* 2001;32:1698-1699.
22. Meningococcal disease and college students: recommendations of the Advisory Committee on Immunization Practices (ACIP). *MMWR Recomm Rep.* 2000;49:13-20.
23. Lingappa JR, Rosenstein N, Zell ER, Shutt KA, Schuchat A, Perkins BA. Active Bacterial Core surveillance (ABCs) team: surveillance for meningococcal disease and strategies for use of conjugate meningococcal vaccines in the United States. *Vaccine.* 2001;19:4566-4575.
24. Baker C. Meningococcal vaccine recommendation pending. *AAP News* [serial online]. December 10, 2004. Available at: http://aapnews.aappublications.org/cgi/content/full/e2004153v1. Accessed January 3, 2005.
25. FDA approves new vaccine for bacterial meningitis. WFTV.com Web site. January 18, 2005. Available at: http://www.wftv.com/health/4102986/detail.html. Accessed January 18, 2005.
26. Koutsky LA, Ault KA, Wheeler CM, et al; Proof of Principle Study Investigators. A controlled trial of a human papillomavirus type 16 vaccine. *N Engl J Med.* 2002;347:1645-1651.
27. Kulasingam SL, Myers ER. Potential health and economic impact of adding a human papillomavirus vaccine to screening programs. *JAMA.* 2003;290:781-789.
28. Skinner GR, Turyk ME, Benson CA, et al. The efficacy and safety of Skinner herpes simplex vaccine towards modulation of herpes genitalis; report of a prospective double-blind placebo-controlled trial. *Med Microbiol Immunol (Berl).* 1997;186:31-36.
29. Christiansen G, Birkelund S. Is a Chlamydia vaccine a reality? *Best Pract Res Clin Obstet Gynaecol.* 2002;16:889-900.
30. Szilagyi PG, Rodewald LE, Savageau J, et al. Improving influenza vaccination rates in children with asthma: a test of a computerized reminder system and an analysis of factors predicting vaccination compliance. *Pediatrics.* 1992;90:871-875.
31. Daley MF, Barrow J, Pearson K, et al. Identification and recall of children with chronic medical conditions for influenza vaccination. *Pediatrics.* 2004;113:e26-e33. Available at: http://pediatrics.aappublications.org/cgi/content/full/113/1/e26.
32. Vazquez M, LaRussa PS, Gershon AA, et al. Effectiveness over time of varicella vaccine. *JAMA.* 2004;291:851-855.
33. Bardenheier B, Gonzalez IM, Washington ML, et al. Parental knowledge, attitudes, and practices associated with not receiving hepatitis A vaccine in a demonstration project in Butte County, California. *Pediatrics.* 2003;112:e269. Available at: http://pediatrics.aappublications.org/cgi/content/full/112/4/e269. Accessed August 23, 2005.
34. Gonzalez IM, Averhoff FM, Massoudi MS, et al; Vaccine Safety Datalink Team. Hepatitis B vaccination among adolescents in 3 large health maintenance organizations. *Pediatrics.* 2002;110:929-934.
35. Centers for Disease Control and Prevention (CDC). Hepatitis B vaccination among high-risk adolescents and adults—San Diego, California, 1998-2001. *MMWR Morb Mortal Wkly Rep.* 2002;51:618-621.
36. Van Damme P, Van der Wielen M. Combining hepatitis A and B vaccination in children and adolescents. *Vaccine.* 2001;19:2407-2412.
37. Centers for Disease Control and Prevention. Immunization of adolescents: recommendations of the Advisory Committee on Immunization Practices, the American Academy of Pediatrics, the American Academy of Family Physicians, and the American Medical Association. *JAMA.* 1997;277:202-207.
38. Schaffer SJ, Humiston SG, Shone LP, Averhoff FM, Szilagyi PG. Adolescent immunization practices: a national survey of US physicians. *Arch Pediatr Adolesc Med.* 2001;155:566-571.
39. Gordon TE, Zook EG, Averhoff FM, Williams WW. Consent for adolescent vaccination: issues and current practices. *J Sch Health.* 1997;67:259-264.
40. Irwin CE Jr, Burg SJ, Uhler C. America's adolescents: where have we been, where are we going? *J Adolesc Health.* 2002;31:91-121.
41. Maternal and Child Health Bureau; Health Resources and Services Administration US Department of Health and Human Services. Child Health USA 2002. Available at: http://www.mchb.hrsa.gov/chusa02/main_pages/page_54.htm. Accessed May 12, 2004.
42. Klein JD, Wilson KM, McNulty M, Kapphahn C, Collins KS. Access to medical care for adolescents: results from the 1997 Commonwealth Fund Survey of the Health of Adolescent Girls. *J Adolesc Health.* 1999;25:120-130.
43. Yu SM, Bellamy HA, Schwalberg RH, Drum MA. Factors associated with use of preventive dental and health services among US adolescents. *J Adolesc Health.* 2001;29:395-405.
44. Zimmer-Gembeck MJ, Alexander T, Nystrom RJ. Adolescents report their need for and use of health care services. *J Adolesc Health.* 1997;21:388-399.
45. Marcell AV, Klein JD, Fischer I, Allan MJ, Kokotailo PK. Male adolescent use of health care services: where are the boys? *J Adolesc Health.* 2002;30:35-43.
46. Unti L, Coyle K, Woodruff BA; Demonstration Project Staff. *A Review of Adolescent School-Based Hepatitis B Vaccination Projects.* Washington, DC: US Department of Health and Human Services Public Health Service; 1996.
47. Briss PA, Rodewald LE, Hinman AR, et al. Reviews of evidence regarding interventions to improve vaccination coverage in children, adolescents, and adults: the Task Force on Community Preventive Services. *Am J Prev Med.* 2000;18:97-140.
48. Kempe A, Lowery NE, Pearson KA, et al. Immunization recall: effectiveness and barriers to success in an urban teaching clinic. *J Pediatr.* 2001;139:630-635.
49. Daley MF, Steiner JF, Kempe A, et al. Quality improvement in immunization delivery following an unsuccessful immunization recall. *Ambul Pediatr.* 2004;4:217-223.
50. Davis MM, Szilagyi PG. Can quality improvement reach into pockets of need for childhood immunizations? *Ambul Pediatr.* 2004;4:224-225.
51. Harper P, Madlon-Kay DJ. Adolescent measles vaccination: response rates to mailings addressed to patients vs parents. *Arch Fam Med.* 1994;3:619-622.
52. Monroe County Maternal/Child Health Report Card: December 2003. Health Action: Priorities for Monroe County Web site. Available at: http://www.healthaction.org/Maternal.html. Accessed January 3, 2005.
53. TeleVox Web site. Available at: http://www.televox.com/. Accessed January 3, 2005.
54. Dini EF, Linkins RW, Chaney M. Effectiveness of computer-generated telephone messages in increasing clinic visits. *Arch Pediatr Adolesc Med.* 1995;149:902-905.
55. Linkins RW, Dini EF, Watson G, Patriarca PA. A randomized trial of the effectiveness of computer-generated telephone messages in increasing immunization visits among preschool children. *Arch Pediatr Adolesc Med.* 1994;148:908-914.
56. Lieu TA, Black SB, Ray P, et al. Computer-generated recall letters for underimmunized children: how cost-effective? *Pediatr Infect Dis J.* 1997;16:28-33.
57. Klein JD. Adolescents, health services, and access to care. *J Adolesc Health.* 2000;27:293-294.
58. Newacheck PW, Hung YY, Park MJ, Brindis CD, Irwin CE Jr. Disparities in adolescent health and health care: does socioeconomic status matter? *Health Serv Res.* 2003;38:1235-1252.
59. Szilagyi PG, Schaffer S, Shone L, et al. Reducing geographic, racial, and ethnic disparities in childhood immunization rates by using reminder/recall interventions in urban primary care practices. *Pediatrics.* 2002;110:e58. Available at: http://pediatrics.aappublications.org/cgi/content/full/110/5/e58. Accessed August 23, 2005.
60. Joffe GP, Rodewald LE, Herbert T, Barth R, Szilagyi PG. Doctor-switching and utilization of health care by children on fee-for-service Medicaid. *J Urban Health.* 1999;76:322-334.
61. Jacobson Vann JC, Szilagyi PG. Patient reminder and patient recall systems to improve immunization rates. Oxford, England: Cochrane Database of Systematic Reviews. Updated May 30, 2005.
62. Campbell JR, Szilagyi PG, Rodewald LE, et al. Intent to immunize among pediatric and family medicine residents. *Arch Pediatr Adolesc Med.* 1994;148:926-929.
63. O'Brien G, Lazebnik R. Telephone call reminders and attendance in an adolescent clinic. *Pediatrics.* 1998;101:E6. Available at: http://pediatrics.aappublications.org/cgi/content/full/101/6/e6. Accessed August 23, 2005.
64. Fishbein DB. Immunization of adolescents: an update. Paper presented at: Centers for Disease Control and Prevention National Vaccine Program Office; June 2, 2005; Washington, DC.
65. Wood D, Halfon N, Donald-Sherbourne C, et al. Increasing immunization rates among inner-city, African American children: a randomized trial of case management. *JAMA.* 1998;279:29-34.

ARTICLE

# Simulating Cost-effectiveness of Fluoride Varnish During Well-Child Visits for Medicaid-Enrolled Children

*Rocio B. Quiñonez, DMD, MS, MPH; Sally C. Stearns, PhD; Bhavna S. Talekar, BDS, MPH; R. Gary Rozier, DDS, MPH; Stephen M. Downs, MD, MPH*

**Objective:** To examine the cost-effectiveness of fluoride varnish application by medical providers when implemented within a well-child periodicity schedule for Medicaid-enrolled children.

**Design:** Cost-effectiveness was analyzed using published probabilities and costs. Input parameters included the effectiveness of fluoride varnish (35.4%) applied according to the well-child periodicity schedule up to 3 years of age at $16.00 per application, annual caries increment (14%), age-specific dental care usage rates (0.2% at 9 months to 19% at 42 months), and age-related nonhospital treatment costs ($292.00-$503.00) and hospital treatment costs ($2191.00-$2940.00). Sensitivity analysis was conducted to assess the effects for varying input parameters.

**Setting:** Well-child visits during primary care.

**Participants:** Children aged 9 to 42 months.

**Intervention:** Application of universal fluoride varnish (fluoride varnish—all) at 9, 18, 24, and 36 months vs no intervention (fluoride varnish—none) was compared.

**Main Outcome Measures:** Cost per month without cavities and treatment averted during the first 42 months of life from a Medicaid payer's perspective.

**Results:** Fluoride varnish improved clinical outcomes by 1.52 cavity-free months but at a cost of $7.18 for each cavity-free month gained per child and $203 for each treatment averted. Considerable uncertainty existed for some parameters. Fluoride varnish was cost saving when dental services and nonhospital treatment costs were 1.5 to 2 times greater, respectively, than our base case estimate.

**Conclusions:** Based on these assumptions, fluoride varnish use in the medical setting is effective in reducing early childhood caries in low-income populations but is not cost saving in the first 42 months of life. Potential total cost reductions with varying parameters suggest that evaluations using a longitudinal cohort are needed.

*Arch Pediatr Adolesc Med. 2006;160:164-170*

DISPARITIES IN CHILDREN'S oral health are large, and few improvements have been reported in oral health of high-risk populations.[1] Results of the National Health and Nutrition Examination Survey suggest that the prevalence of dental caries and its treatment have become worse among children aged 2 to 4 years during the 1990s.[2] By midchildhood, more than 50% of children have detectable caries, with disproportionate prevalence and severity of disease linked to lower socioeconomic and minority group status.[3,4] These disparities arise from many complex determinants, including limited access to dental services by children at high risk.[5] Few general dentists treat children younger than 4 years and only 7% report treating patients with Medicaid coverage often or very often.[6] In 1996, the US Inspector General reported that fewer than 20% of Medicaid-enrolled children received any preventive dental care.[7]

Increasing difficulty in accessing dental services for young children at highest risk has led to innovative proposals to address this public health crisis.[8] Medical settings provide an opportunity to increase use of preventive dental services for very young children during a developmental stage when oral health routines become established. Existing guidelines encourage primary care physicians to provide a broad range of anticipatory guidance to caregivers of preschool-aged children, including preventive dental care.[9,10] The American Academy of Pediatrics and the American Academy of Pediatric Dentistry recommend that screening for early childhood caries should begin at the 1-year well-child visit.[11] Almost a dozen states have expanded preventive

**Author Affiliations:** Department of Pediatric Dentistry, School of Dentistry (Dr Quiñonez), Department of Health Policy and Administration, School of Public Health (Drs Stearns and Rozier and Talekar), and University of North Carolina at Chapel Hill; and Children's Health Services Research, Department of Pediatrics, Indiana University School of Medicine, Indianapolis (Dr Downs).

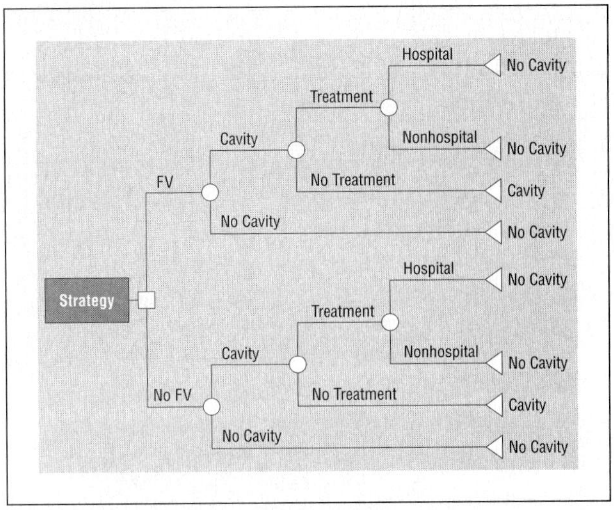


**Figure 1.** Decision tree illustrates effects of dental disease and treatment costs after fluoride varnish (FV) application in children ages 6 to 36 months in a medical setting.

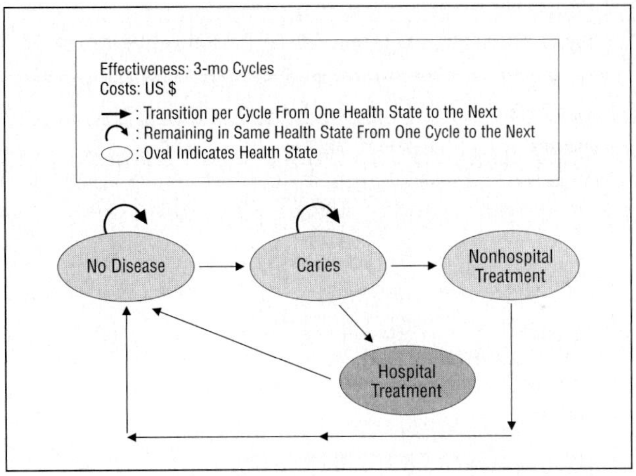


**Figure 2.** Markov model used to assess cost-effectiveness of fluoride varnish in the primary dentition.

dental services for children with public insurance to include topical fluoride application. However, the economic implications of physician-delivered interventions to prevent early childhood caries are not well understood.

Of the dental interventions available to nondental health care providers, fluoride demonstrates the strongest evidence for effectiveness in preventing dental caries.[12] Physicians have prescribed fluoride supplements and recommended fluoridated toothpaste for many years, but topical application of fluoride in medical offices is a recent innovation. Fluoride varnish (FV) is one type of topical fluoride application by physicians that is increasingly being promoted for teeth in very young children because of its ease of application, effectiveness, and safety. When applied biannually for 2 years by dental professionals, it can reduce dental caries in the primary dentition by approximately one third.[9,13,14]

The purpose of this study was to examine the cost-effectiveness of FV application by physicians using a well-child periodicity schedule (WCPS) to prevent the occurrence and progression of early-stage dental caries in a high-risk population. Because of the early stages of adoption of this intervention among public insurance programs, this analysis does not use data from any current program; rather, the analysis is based on estimates and costs from the literature. Providing universal FV applications (FV–all [FVA]) to Medicaid-enrolled children was compared with providing no such intervention (FV–none [FVN]) to Medicaid-enrolled children during the first 42 months of a child's life.

## METHODS

### MODEL DEVELOPMENT

Decision analysis was used to assess the effects of dental disease and treatment costs in children under FVA and FVN strategies in a medical setting (**Figure 1**). We developed a Markov model of the natural history of dental caries, fluoride effectiveness, and associated health states (**Figure 2**). A Markov model is a recursive decision tree and is described by the ovals in the model representing the various health states and the arrows representing the transitions from one health state to another. Each arrow is associated with a probability that represents the likelihood that a child will transition from one health state to the next in a 3-month cycle. For example, a child may enter the model with no disease and in subsequent months either remains caries free or progresses to the caries state. Once the child has experienced dental disease, he or she can either cycle within this health state if no treatment is rendered or transition to receiving dental care. Once treatment is completed, the child returns to a caries-free health state and is at risk for subsequent cavitation. In less severe circumstances, treatment may be rendered in a dental office. When the disease is severe, multiple teeth are involved, or a child is medically compromised, treatment in a hospital with the patient under general anesthesia may be required. Either of these treatment scenarios results in a return to a caries-free state after treatment completion. A cycle spent in the no-disease health state is associated with a gain in effect of 3 cavity-free months, and transitions into dental care are associated with costs representing the level of treatment. Costs of FV treatment are incurred at cycles that correspond to selected visits in the WCPS.

We derived estimates from the literature for age-specific disease incidence, fluoride effectiveness, and treatment costs. The strategies were compared by determining the cost per additional cavity-free month during the first 42 months of a child's life. The intervention consisted of FV application by the pediatric primary care provider during regular well-child visits at 9, 18, 24, and 36 months of age during the WCPS. The first cycle of the model began at 9 months, the average age at which teeth first erupt into the mouth. Although many children have a 12-month medical visit, we chose 18 months as the second time point because the 12-month visit involves multiple activities, making FV difficult to add. The 1-year interval between the 24-month and 36-month visits reflects the American Academy of Pediatrics–recommended WCPS guidelines.[15] Although the duration of treatment was the first 3 years of life, the cycles extended to 42 months to account for benefits incurred after the last FV application at the 36-month well-child visit. A half-cycle correction was applied to effectiveness. All analyses were performed using the TreeAge Pro Healthcare module (TreeAge Software Inc, Williamstown, Mass).[16]

### STUDY ASSUMPTIONS

The analysis was conducted from a Medicaid payer's perspective; thus, we assumed it would include those children en-

**Table 1. Probabilities Used to Model Cost-effectiveness of FV**

| Outcomes | Duration, mo | | | | | | | | | | | | Source |
|---|---|---|---|---|---|---|---|---|---|---|---|---|---|
| | 9 | 12 | 15 | 18 | 21 | 24 | 27 | 30 | 33 | 36 | 39 | 42 | |
| Probabilities | | | | | | | | | | | | | |
| Develop dental caries | 0.035 | 0.035 | 0.035 | 0.035 | 0.035 | 0.035 | 0.035 | 0.035 | 0.035 | 0.035 | 0.035 | 0.035 | Tang et al,[17] 1997 |
| Receive treatment | NA | 0.013 | 0.026 | 0.041 | 0.058 | 0.076 | 0.095 | 0.115 | 0.131 | 0.153 | 0.173 | 0.193 | Lee et al,[18,19] 2004; Tang et al,[17] 1997 |
| Receive treatment in hospital | NA | 0.140 | 0.140 | 0.140 | 0.140 | 0.310 | 0.310 | 0.310 | 0.310 | 0.135 | 0.135 | 0.135 | Kanellis et al,[20] 2000 |
| Effectiveness (cavity-free mo) | | | | | | | | | | | | | |
| FV effectiveness | 0.521 | 0.271 | 0.521 | 0.271 | 0.141 | 0.521 | 0.271 | 0.141 | 0.073 | 0.521 | 0.271 | 0.141 | Holm,[21] 1978; Holm,[14] 1979 |
| Cost, 2003 US $ value | | | | | | | | | | | | | |
| FV | 16 | 0 | 16 | 0 | 0 | 16 | 0 | 0 | 0 | 16 | 0 | 0 | Washington,[22] North Carolina,[23] and Iowa[24] |
| Treatment received in a hospital | NA | 2191 | 2281 | 2425 | 2568 | 2712 | 2769 | 2827 | 2884 | 2941 | 2941 | 2941 | Kanellis et al,[20] 2000 |
| Treatment received in a nonhospital | NA | 292 | 315 | 339 | 362 | 386 | 415 | 445 | 474 | 503 | 503 | 503 | Ramos-Gomez et al,[26] 1996 |

Abbreviations: FV, fluoride varnish; NA, not applicable.

rolled in Medicaid and who accessed the medical system for well-child visits. Because children enrolled in Medicaid are from a lower socioeconomic group, we assumed they would have an overall constant high risk for the development of dental caries. Our analysis did not explicitly incorporate the relationship between probability of disease and use of the medical system. However, treatment cost estimates were based on severity of disease in children who received treatment. We further assumed that FV has negligible adverse effects and that effectiveness is the same when applied by dental and medical providers at any stage of development of the primary dentition.[13] The probability of developing dental caries was constant, and dental utilization varied with child age. We assumed that once dental caries were detected, the child would be referred to a dental home for comprehensive oral health care and could continue to receive preventive dental care in a medical office.

## TRANSITION PROBABILITIES AND SOURCES

The probability estimates of various health states were derived from published data for other lower socioeconomic groups similar to the one under investigation (**Table 1**).[14,17-24,26] Values were extracted by one of us (R.B.Q.) and were reviewed by all of us.

### Probability of Cavitation

Because of the lack of longitudinal dental caries studies, the probability of cavitation was obtained from a cross-sectional, child-level caries prevalence survey of 5171 preschool-aged children recruited from mainly low-income populations.[17] Annual estimates for dental caries were available for 4 age ranges: younger than 12 months (0.5%), 12 to 23 months (6.4%), 24 to 35 months (21.6%), and 36 to 42 months (35.1%). These data were used to determine quarterly probabilities by first choosing the midpoint for each age range and subsequently deriving incidence data by linear interpolation as average 3-month rates of cavitation. These calculations resulted in a 0.035 constant probability of a child having any new dental caries in each quarter.

### Probability of a Child With Dental Caries Receiving Any Dental Treatment

The probability of a child receiving dental treatment once a carious lesion developed was determined from estimates of annual dental services use in children aged 1, 2, and 3 years enrolled in a state Medicaid program.[18,19] The number of children receiving dental treatment was divided by the total number of children with dental disease. The latter figure was estimated by multiplying the prevalence of caries at ages 1, 2, and 3 years from Tang et al[17] by the total cohort of children in the studies by Lee et al.[18,19] Annual rates were estimated and then interpolated by the quarterly time points to obtain the number of children being treated, ranging from 0.03% to 19% in each 3-month cycle, depending on age.

### Probability of Receiving Dental Treatment in a Hospital

To obtain the probability of treatment in the hospital, we used data from Kanellis et al[20] to determine the percentage of full-time-equivalent children treated in the operating room at various ages (12-23 months [0.2%], 24-35 months [1.2%], and 36-47 months [0.9%]).We assumed a constant quarterly rate of the probability of receiving treatment in the hospital and used a step function in our analysis to reflect the variation across ages.

## FV EFFECTIVENESS ESTIMATES

Three-month FV effectiveness estimates were calculated from a study that examined the caries-preventive effects of semiannual FV ap-

**Table 2. Results of Base Case Cost-effectiveness Analysis for FVN and FVA**

| Treatment | Cost, $ | Incremental Cost, $ | Effectiveness (Cavity-Free Months) | Incremental Effectiveness (Cavity-Free Months) | ICER (Cost per Cavity-Free Months) |
|---|---|---|---|---|---|
| Discounted 3% | | | | | |
| FVA, 2003 US $ | 181.66 | 10.93 | 31.49 | 1.52 | 7.18 |
| FVN, 2003 US $ | 170.73 | | 29.97 | | |

Abbreviations: FVA, fluoride varnish, all; FVN, fluoride varnish, none; ICER, incremental cost-effectiveness ratio.

plication in children beginning at 3 years of age.[14,21] This study was chosen because it was a randomized, controlled trial of FV effectiveness conducted in preschool-aged children and had the youngest subjects at enrollment of any FV study. Results indicated a preventive fraction of 35.4% per 6-month application of FV, although ranges in the literature vary from 30% to 63%.[9] Reasoning that the effectiveness of FV would undergo a constant proportional decline, we calculated effectiveness estimates for the intervals under study based on an average effectiveness of 35.4% for 6 months.[14,21] The resulting average effectiveness in the first 3 months was 57.1% and the average effectiveness in the second 3 months was 27.1%. Applying this same rate of decline, the average effectiveness of FV declined to 14.1% between 6 and 9 months and to 7.4% between 9 and 12 months from the time of FV application.

## FV AND TREATMENT COST ESTIMATES

A $16.00 FV application fee was assigned at the beginning of the 9-month, 18-month, 24-month, and 36-month cycles. This figure accounts for direct costs only and was the midpoint of the range for 2004 fees ($13.00-$19.00) that some Medicaid programs reimburse nondental providers for FV applications.[22-24] Because our analysis was conducted from a Medicaid payer's perspective, the calculated average reimbursement cost of the FV to physicians was an appropriate number to use, with no additional payment for FVA considered. Costs related to dental treatment in the hospital setting were obtained from the experience of preschool-aged children enrolled in the Iowa Medicaid Program.[20] Medicaid reimbursements per child ranged from $2100.00 to $2940.00 once adjusted for inflation using the Medical Care Component of the Consumer Price Index to reflect the 2003 US $ value.[25] Nonhospital (office-based) treatment-related costs were obtained from a retrospective study by Ramos-Gomez et al.[26] We used the 20th percentile of nonhospital costs for children experiencing decayed, extracted or missing, or filled teeth (DMFT), an epidemiologic index to describe children's oral health status (2-5 DMFT = $170-$854 and 6-10 DMFT = $394-$1373). The costs associated with 2 to 5 DMFT were used for children younger than 24 months and costs for 6 to10 DMFT were used for children older than 36 months. Interpolation of these 2 numbers was used to estimate nonhospital costs for children aged 24 to 35 months. The costs were inflated to reflect the 2003 US $ value and then deflated by 30% to reflect average Medicaid reimbursement fees as a proportion of estimated charges (Table 1).

## OUTCOMES

The primary outcomes were the average overall cost of each strategy, the number of months without cavities per child, and the incremental cost per cavity-free month gained moving from FVN to FVA. The incremental cost per cavity-free month, or the incremental cost-effectiveness ratio (ICER), was calculated as the ratio of the difference in cost between alternatives

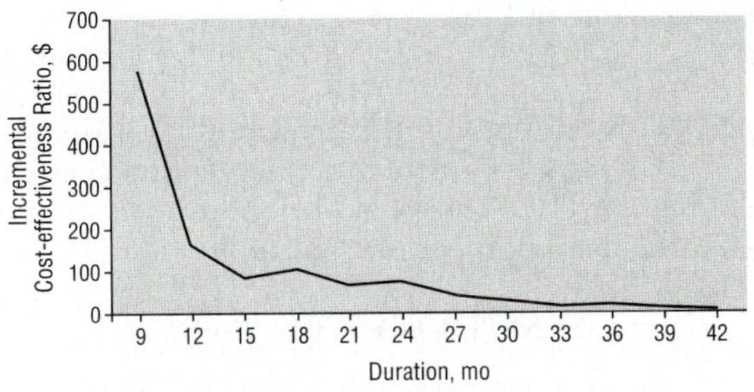


**Figure 3.** Results illustrate changing incremental cost-effectiveness ratio over simulation time by quarter discounted.

to the difference in effectiveness between the alternatives. A secondary outcome included cost per treatment averted. The FVA strategy was cost-effective if it improved outcomes and increased total costs (FV plus dental treatment), but the cost per additional unit of outcome was deemed to be worthwhile to the purchaser. The FVA strategy was cost saving if outcomes improved and total costs were less than what dental treatment costs would be in the absence of the intervention. We conducted sensitivity analyses on the effect of varying the following parameters on our primary outcomes: frequency and effectiveness of FV application, probabilities of cavitation, receiving any restorative treatment, or receiving treatment rendered in the hospital, and costs (hospital, nonhospital, and discount rate). Because some of the parameters varied with age, multipliers ranging from 0.5 to 4 were used to assess the effects of changing these parameters on the outcomes associated with the 2 strategies. Costs (dollars) and effect (cavity-free months) were discounted using an annual rate of 3%, as recommended by the panel on Cost-effectiveness in Health and Medicine.[27]

# RESULTS

## BASE CASE ANALYSIS

The results of the base case cost-effectiveness analysis (discounted) indicated that FVA was more effective than FVN, providing an additional 1.52 cavity-free months per child by 42 months of age (**Table 2**). Restorative treatment costs were reduced by $52.00 in the FVA group. However, this reduction does not offset the $64.00 cost of 4 applications. When including the direct costs associated with the FV application, the increase in cavity-free months was at an additional cost of $10.93 during the entire period, or an ICER of $7.18 per cavity-free month gained. The ICER improved as children aged, because of the increase in disease prevalence (**Figure 3**). Our analy-

**Table 3. Results of Cost per Treatment Averted (Hospital and Nonhospital)***

| Treatment | Effectiveness (Average No. of Treatments per Child up to 42 mo) | Incremental Effectiveness | ICER (Cost per Treatment Averted) |
|---|---|---|---|
| Any treatment | | | |
| FVN, 2003 US $ | 0.125 | | |
| FVA, $2003 US $ | 0.179 | −0.054 | 203 |

Abbreviations: FVA, fluoride varnish, all; FVN, fluoride varnish, none; ICER, incremental cost-effectiveness ratio.
*Incremental costs are $10.93 derived from Table 2.

sis also showed that using FVA would cost Medicaid $203.00 (beyond treatment and intervention costs) for 1 treatment averted (hospital or nonhospital) over the 42-month simulation period (**Table 3**).

## SENSITIVITY ANALYSES

Because of considerable uncertainty about some of the parameters, the base case used conservative assumptions. Therefore, sizable increases in some of these parameters may be a reasonable possibility. Because some of the parameters varied with the age of a child, the sensitivity analyses were conducted using a multiplier; for example, a multiplier of 2 for nonhospital treatment costs means that costs indicated in Table 1 are doubled. The base case values provided for all parameters were multiplied by the multiplier values indicated for each of the sensitivity analyses. Sensitivity analyses are reported using a 3% discount rate because all results were insensitive to reasonable changes for the discount rate.

### Frequency and Effectiveness of FV

The analysis demonstrated that FVA resulted in lower total costs (intervention and treatment) when FV effectiveness was 1.25 times greater than our base case assumption of 35.4% average caries reduction for 6 months. A sensitivity analysis was conducted to reflect the biannual application regimen reflected in the dental literature starting at the 9-month WCPS. Using this protocol, the total number of FV applications increased from 4 to 6 times. Results indicated effectiveness only slightly greater than the base case schedule at 1.87 cavity-free months, but with an ICER of $15.59 per cavity-free month gained, an additional $8.41 when compared with the base case results.

### Probability of Receiving Restorative Treatment in the Dental Office, Treatment in the Hospital, and Cavitation

The results were sensitive to the overall probability of receiving treatment, receiving this treatment in a hospital, and rate of cavitation. The FVA strategy became cost-saving when the probability of receiving restorative treatment was 1.5 times greater than our baseline estimates of 0.2% to 19%, depending on the child's age; the likelihood of treatment occurring in the hospital was 1.5 times greater than the baseline case, ranging from 14% to 31%; and cavitation rates were nearly doubled.

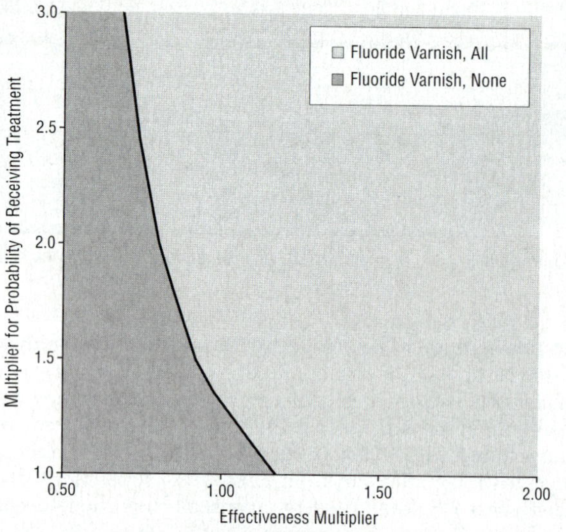


**Figure 4.** Results illustrate 2-way sensitivity analysis between fluoride varnish effectiveness and dental utilization.

### Hospital Treatment and Nonhospital Treatment Costs

Results were sensitive to costs of hospital and nonhospital treatment, with FVA becoming cost saving when nonhospital costs were doubled and hospital costs increased 1.5 times greater than for the base case.

### Two-way Sensitivity Analysis

Two-way sensitivity analysis was conducted to illustrate the joint effect of changing the probabilities of receiving treatment and nonhospital costs. Results indicated that FVA was cost saving when greater numbers of children received dental treatment and nonhospital costs doubled from the base case costs. In a second analysis, varying both the fluoride effectiveness and probability of children with caries seeking dental care, we found no evidence of cost savings at lower fluoride effectiveness levels. When fluoride effectiveness falls below two thirds of our base case effectiveness, FVA does not save money even with increased use of dental treatment (**Figure 4**).

## COMMENT

To improve access to oral health preventive services for children at risk, several Medicaid programs reimburse for FV application in the medical setting. Our analysis, from the Medicaid payer's perspective, found that FV application in a low-income population showed modest improvement in outcome of 1.52 additional months in a cavity-free state between 9 to 42 months of age but would cost Medicaid $7.18 per cavity-free month gained or $203 per restorative treatment averted.

Sensitivity analysis showed that assumptions of sometimes substantial increases in dental services utilization rates, nonhospital costs, FV effectiveness, and disease rates were required to demonstrate cost savings, with multipliers ranging from 1.25 to 2 times base case estimates. Nevertheless, the thresholds at which FVA became cost-savings fell within the range of possible values for most parameters, primarily because the absolute numbers used in our base case estimates were conservative, representing low dental services utilization and reimbursement rates among children enrolled in Medicaid reported in the literature. Since publication of these estimates, dental services in some states have increased among Medicaid populations because of the policy emphasis on access issues, often through increasing reimbursement fees to dental providers.[28] Other changes that could result in dental service utilization rates that are higher than our base case include the addition of screening and referral to any preventive oral health program in the medical home, the recent policy by the American Academy of Pediatrics[11] recommending dental referral of children at high risk at about 1 year of age rather than the traditional 3 years, and the increase in the number of pediatric dentists during the last decade.[29]

Increasing the probability of nonhospital treatment influenced the cost-effectiveness of our model and is notable because our base case estimates were selected at the 20th percentile from the only study in the literature reporting nonhospital costs in this age cohort.[26] Doubling these conservative estimates results in costs that fall slightly above the midpoint of reported ranges. Independently, hospital treatment costs reflected the highest dollar amount in the model and, thus, have an important role, given the proportion of children requiring hospitalization.

Doubling caries rates that shifted FVA to a dominant strategy in the sensitivity analysis results in a disease rate that is also plausible among certain populations that use Medicaid services, including those of Hispanic and Native American origin.[4,30] Similarly, the multiplier of 1.5 used for effectiveness of FV in our sensitivity analysis is within the range of preventive fractions observed in clinical studies.[9] Our estimates may be optimistic, because overall effectiveness levels may be attenuated when applying FV in a younger population that may be more behaviorally challenging than older children.

In summary, under these study assumptions, FV application will require that Medicaid provide additional financial resources to prevent disease in children younger than 36 months. However, assuming continued FV applications, this intervention may result in cost savings beyond 36 months of age as illustrated by the decrease in cost per cavity-free month (as measured by the ICER) over time, declining from \$578.00 initially to \$7.18 at 42 months. Cost savings may result from the effects of increasing onset of dental caries with age and the more frequent applications observed in dental offices, reflecting similar periods as those used in clinical trials of FV effectiveness. Additional benefits not examined in this study may accrue to society through improvements in the oral health status of the nation's most vulnerable children. These benefits include an increase in children's ability to learn, decreased use of dental emergency services, and increased caregiver productivity by postponing or diminishing time away from work.[30,31]

## RESEARCH AND POLICY CONSIDERATIONS

Many issues related to the cost-effectiveness of an FV Medicaid program are important when considering its implementation in a medical setting. First, research is needed to assess children's transition of care after the intervention in a medical setting to a dental setting to determine the long-term economic effect of the intervention. Second, better targeting of children at highest risk for dental caries could help improve the economic attributes of these programs for very young children. For example, holding all other assumptions constant, achieving cost savings would require the ability to identify a subset of the population with cavitation risk 2 times higher than our base case estimate. Improved caries risk assessments by primary care medical providers that go beyond identifying children of certain socioeconomic background are needed.

Third, timing and compliance issues with WCPS are important in the ability to target this high-risk population, particularly in the latter part of our simulation period. A change to annual WCPS after age 2 years creates a gap in the opportunity to apply FV at the desired 6-month interval to achieve maximum effectiveness. In addition, FV application depends on well-child visit compliance. Evidence suggests that in high-risk populations adherence to the recommended WCPS is not ideal, and some states report that only 36% of Medicaid-eligible children younger than 2 years receive all recommended visits in managed care programs.[32] Such patterns may decrease the opportunity of adequate frequency and timely application of FV. We conservatively accounted for this underuse by using only 4 of the well-child visits in our simulations. However, some of the FV application points occurred at times when the frequency of well-child care visits is decreasing and risk for caries is increasing.

## LIMITATIONS

The results of this study must be interpreted in the context of our study assumptions. Overall, limited data were available to derive our probabilities and costs. For example, even though the assumption on effectiveness of FV was made for the primary dentition, the data available for this parameter included only children older than 2 years. This limitation points to the need for longitudinal, controlled studies of the effectiveness of FV in the Medicaid population starting in the first year of life. More up-to-date information and studies of better quality and quantity could help improve some of the uncertainties around the base case estimates and refine the accuracy of our economic evaluation.

Our findings examined intermediate measures of health and were limited to the first 42 months of life; thus, effect on quality of life beyond this time frame and spending for dental services after early intervention cannot be reasonably inferred and data are not available on which to model such an effect. The denominator in the cost-effectiveness ratios was expressed as caries-free child-months rather than a standard health outcome such as quality-adjusted life-years. Efforts should be made to standardize measures that can help facilitate comparison of such programs with other medical and dental interventions. Finally, the outcomes used in our study were dichotomous, namely, the presence or absence of disease. Incremental changes in severity of caries measured by the number of teeth or surfaces affected after an FV program could produce additional benefits that were not captured in our analysis.

## CONCLUSIONS

Based on probabilities and costs derived from the literature and other secondary sources, our findings suggest that during the first 3 years of life FVA may not save money compared with FVN. However, the ICER decreased with time, approaching cost savings by 48 months of age. The sensitivity analyses also found cost savings for the intervention under higher but reasonable dental service utilization rates and nonhospital costs, which were estimated conservatively in our base case because of the traditionally poor access to dental care for children enrolled in Medicaid. The estimates in this study are based on data that are incomplete, and further research is needed to determine the benefits and costs of a dental FV program based in a primary medical care setting and how it interfaces with care in the dental home.

**Accepted for Publication:** July 8, 2005.
**Correspondence:** Rocio B. Quiñonez, DMD, MS, MPH, Department of Pediatric Dentistry, Campus Box 7450, School of Dentistry, University of North Carolina, Chapel Hill, NC 27599 (quinoner@dentistry.unc.edu).
**Funding/Support:** This study was supported by grant R01 DE 013949 from the National Institute of Dental and Craniofacial Research, National Institutes of Health, Bethesda, Md.

## REFERENCES

1. US Department of Health and Human Services. *Oral Health in America: A Report of the Surgeon General: Executive Summary.* Rockville, Md: National Institute of Dental and Craniofacial Research, National Institutes of Health. 2000:1, 5, 6. Available at: http://www.nidcr.nih.gov/sgr/sgr.htm. Accessed November 17, 2005.
2. US Department of Health and Human Services. *Healthy People 2010: With Understanding and Improving Health and Objectives for Improving Health: Oral Health.* 2nd ed. Washington, DC: US Government Printing Office; 2000. Available at: http://www.health.gov/healthypeople. Accessed November 17, 2005.
3. US Public Health Service. *Healthy People 2000 Progress Report on Oral Health.* Washington, DC: US Dept of Health and Human Services; 1995.
4. Vargas CM, Crall JJ, Schneider DA. Sociodemographic distribution of pediatric dental caries: NHANES III, 1988-1994. *J Am Dent Assoc.* 1998;129:1229-1238.
5. Mouradian WE, Wehr E, Crall JJ. Disparities in children's oral health and access to dental care. *JAMA.* 2000;284:2625-2631.
6. Seale NS, Casamassimo PS. Access to dental care for children in the United States: a survey of general practitioners. *J Am Dent Assoc.* 2003;134:1630-1640.
7. US Inspector General. *Children's Dental Services Under Medicaid: Access and Utilization.* San Francisco, Calif: US Dept of Health and Human Services; 1996. Publication OEI 09-93-00240.
8. Hegner RE. The interface between medicine and dentistry in meeting the oral health needs of young children: executive summary and white paper. *Children's Dental Health Project 2004.* Available at: http://www.cdhp.org. Accessed November 17, 2005.
9. Bader JD, Rozier RG, Lohr KN, Frame PS. Physicians' roles in preventing dental caries in preschool children: a summary of the evidence for the US Preventive Services Task Force. *Am J Prev Med.* 2004;26:315-325.
10. US Preventive Services Task Force. *Guide to Clinical Preventive Services: Counseling to Prevent Dental and Periodontal Disease.* Rockville, Md: Agency for Healthcare Research and Quality; 2005. Available at: http:odphp.osophs.dhhs.gov/pubs/guidecps/PDF/CH61.PDF. Accessed November 15, 2005.
11. Hale KJ; American Academy of Pediatrics Section on Pediatric Dentistry. Oral health risk assessment timing and establishment of the dental home. *Pediatrics.* 2003;111:1113-1116.
12. Centers for Disease Control and Prevention. Recommendations for using fluoride to prevent and control dental caries in the United States. *MMWR Morbid Mortal Wkly Rep.* 2001;50(RR-14):1-42.
13. Marinho VC, Higgins JP, Logan S, Sheiham A. Fluoride varnishes for preventing dental caries in children and adolescents. *Cochrane Database Syst Rev.* 2002;(3);CD002279.
14. Holm AK. Effect of a fluoride varnish (Duraphat) in preschool children. *Community Dent Oral Epidemiol.* 1979;7:241-245.
15. American Academy of Pediatrics Committee on Practice and Ambulatory Pediatrics. Recommendations for preventive pediatric health care. *Pediatrics.* 1995;96(2, pt 1):373-374.
16. TreeAge Pro Healthcare module. Williamstown, Mass: TreeAge Software Inc; 2004.
17. Tang JM, Altman DS, Robertson DC, O'Sullivan DM, Douglas JM, Timanoff N. Dental caries prevalence and treatment levels in Arizona preschool children. *Public Health Rep.* 1997;112:319-329.
18. Lee JY, Rozier RG, Kotch JB, Norton EC, Vann WF Jr. The Effects of the Women, Infants and Children's Program on dentally-related Medicaid expenditures. *J Public Health Dent.* 2004;64:76-81.
19. Lee JY, Rozier RG, Norton EC, Kotch JB, Vann WF Jr. Effects of WIC participation on children's use of oral health services. *Am J Public Health.* 2004;94:772-777.
20. Kanellis MJ, Damiano PC, Momany ET. Medicaid costs associated with the hospitalization of young children for restorative dental treatment under general anesthesia. *J Public Health Dent.* 2000;60:28-32.
21. Holm AK. Effect of a fluoride-containing varnish (Duraphat) in preschool children [abstract 804]. *J Dent Res.* 1978;57:275.
22. *Access to Baby and Child Dentistry Expanded.* Washington State Medicaid Reimbursement Fees 2002. Available at: http://www.smileabcd.org/images/abcde2002%20apring.pdf. Accessed November 17, 2005.
23. Into the Mouths of Babes: The NC Dental Varnish Program. Raleigh, NC; 2004. Available at: http://www.ncafp.com/imb/reimbursement.html. Accessed November 17, 2005.
24. Bureau of Oral Health, Iowa Department of Public Health; 2004. Available at: http://www.dhs.state.ia.us/medicaid/FeeSchedules2005/Physician.xls. Accessed November 17, 2005.
25. US Bureau of Labor Statistics. *Medical Consumer Index 2003.* Available at: http://www.bls.gov.cpi. Accessed November 17, 2005.
26. Ramos-Gomez FJ, Huang GF, Masouredis CM, Braham RL. Prevalence and treatment costs of infant caries in Northern California. *J Dent Child.* 1996;63:108-112.
27. Gold MR, Siegel JE, Russell LB, Weinstein MC. *Cost Effectiveness in Health and Medicine.* New York, NY: Oxford University Press; 1996.
28. North Carolina Institute of Medicine. Child Health Report Card 2004. Available at: http://www.nciom.org//docs/card2004.pdf. Accessed November 9, 2005.
29. Rutkauskas JS. Executive Director's Report. *American Academy of Pediatric Dentistry Newsletter: Pediatric Dentistry Today.* 2004;5:6.
30. Milnes AR. Description and epidemiology of nursing caries. *J Public Health Dent.* 1996;56:38-50.
31. Hollister MC, Weintraub JA. The association of oral status with systemic health, quality of life, and economic productivity. *J Dent Educ.* 1993;57:901-912.
32. Byrd RS, Hoekelman RA, Aunger P. Adherence to AAP guidelines for well-child care under managed care. *Pediatrics.* 1999;104:536-540.

**PEDIARIX™ [Diphtheria and Tetanus Toxoids and Acellular Pertussis Adsorbed, Hepatitis B (Recombinant) and Inactivated Poliovirus Vaccine Combined]**

The following is a brief summary only; see full prescribing information for complete product information.

**CONTRAINDICATIONS:** Hypersensitivity to any component of the vaccine, including yeast, neomycin, and polymyxin B, is a contraindication (see DESCRIPTION in complete prescribing information). Do not use PEDIARIX after a serious allergic reaction (e.g., anaphylaxis) temporally associated with a previous dose of this vaccine or with any components of this vaccine. Because of the uncertainty as to which component of the vaccine might be responsible, do not give further vaccination with any of these components; or, refer such individuals to an allergist for evaluation. The following events are contraindications to administration of PEDIARIX: encephalopathy (e.g., coma, decreased level of consciousness, prolonged seizures) within 7 days of administration of a previous dose of a pertussis-containing vaccine that is not attributable to another identifiable cause; progressive neurologic disorder, including infantile spasms, uncontrolled epilepsy, or progressive encephalopathy. Do not vaccinate individuals with such conditions until a treatment regimen has been established and the condition has stabilized. PEDIARIX is not contraindicated for use in individuals with HIV infection.

**WARNINGS:** Administration of PEDIARIX is associated with higher rates of fever relative to separately administered vaccines. In one study that evaluated medically attended fever after the first dose of PEDIARIX or separately administered vaccines, infants who received PEDIARIX had a higher rate of medical encounters for fever within the first 4 days following vaccination. In some infants, these encounters included the performance of diagnostic studies to evaluate other causes of fever (see ADVERSE REACTIONS). The vial stopper is latex-free. The tip cap and the rubber plunger of the needleless prefilled syringes contain dry natural latex rubber that may cause allergic reactions in latex sensitive individuals. If any of the following events occur in temporal relation to receipt of whole-cell DTP or a vaccine containing an acellular pertussis component, consider carefully whether to give subsequent doses of PEDIARIX or any vaccine containing a pertussis component: temperature of ≥40.5°C (105°F) within 48 hours not due to another identifiable cause; collapse or shock-like state (hypotonic-hyporesponsive episode) within 48 hours; persistent, inconsolable crying lasting ≥3 hours, occurring within 48 hours; seizures with or without fever occurring within 3 days. If Guillain-Barré syndrome occurs within 6 weeks of receipt of prior vaccine containing tetanus toxoid, the decision to give subsequent doses of PEDIARIX or any vaccine containing tetanus toxoid should be based on careful consideration of the potential benefits and possible risks. A committee of the Institute of Medicine (IOM) has concluded that evidence is consistent with a causal relationship between whole-cell DTP vaccine and acute neurologic illness, and under special circumstances, between whole-cell DTP vaccine and chronic neurologic disease in the context of the National Childhood Encephalopathy Study (NCES) report; however, evidence was insufficient to indicate whether or not whole-cell DTP vaccine increased the overall risk of chronic neurologic disease. Acute encephalopathy and permanent neurologic damage have not been reported causally linked or in temporal association with administration of PEDIARIX, but the experience with PEDIARIX is insufficient to rule this out. Encephalopathy has been reported following INFANRIX® (Diphtheria and Tetanus Toxoids and Acellular Pertussis Vaccine Adsorbed) (see ADVERSE REACTIONS, Postmarketing Reports), but data are not sufficient to evaluate a causal relationship. The decision to administer a pertussis-containing vaccine to children with stable central nervous system (CNS) disorders must be made by the physician on an individual basis, with consideration of all relevant factors, and assessment of potential risks and benefits for that individual. Advise the parent or guardian of the potential increased risk involved (see PRECAUTIONS). A family history of seizures or other CNS disorders is not a contraindication to pertussis vaccine. For children at higher risk for seizures than the general population, an appropriate antipyretic may be administered at the time of vaccination and for the ensuing 24 hours according to the respective prescribing information recommended dosage to reduce the possibility of post-vaccination fever. Defer vaccination during the course of a moderate or severe illness with or without fever and vaccinate patients as soon as they have recovered from the acute phase of the illness. Do not give PEDIARIX to children on anticoagulant therapy or those with bleeding disorders unless the potential benefit clearly outweighs the risk of administration (see PRECAUTIONS in complete prescribing information).

**PRECAUTIONS:** Before the injection of any biological, the physician should take all reasonable precautions to prevent allergic or other adverse reactions. Epinephrine injection (1:1000) and other appropriate agents used for the control of immediate allergic reactions must be immediately available should an acute anaphylactic reaction occur. Immunosuppressed individuals, including those receiving immunosuppressive therapy, may not develop the expected immune response. **Drug Interactions:** For information regarding concomitant administration with other vaccines, refer to DOSAGE AND ADMINISTRATION in complete prescribing information. Do not mix PEDIARIX with any other vaccine in the same syringe or vial. **Carcinogenesis, Mutagenesis, Impairment of Fertility:** PEDIARIX has not been evaluated for carcinogenic or mutagenic potential, or for impairment of fertility. **Pregnancy:** Pregnancy Category C: PEDIARIX is not indicated for women of child-bearing age. Animal reproduction studies have not been conducted with PEDIARIX. It is not known whether PEDIARIX can cause fetal harm when administered to a pregnant woman or if PEDIARIX can affect reproductive capacity. **Geriatric Use:** PEDIARIX is not indicated for use in adult populations. **Pediatric Use:** Safety and effectiveness of PEDIARIX in infants younger than 6 weeks of age have not been evaluated (see DOSAGE AND ADMINISTRATION in complete prescribing information). PEDIARIX is not recommended for persons 7 years of age or older. Tetanus and Diphtheria Toxoids Adsorbed (Td) For Adult Use, inactivated poliovirus vaccine (IPV), and Hepatitis B Vaccine (Recombinant) should be used in individuals 7 years of age or older.

**ADVERSE REACTIONS:** A total of 20,739 doses of PEDIARIX have been administered to 7,028 infants as a 3-dose primary series. The most common adverse reactions observed in clinical trials were local injection site reactions (pain, redness, or swelling), fever, and fussiness. In comparative studies, administration of PEDIARIX was associated with higher rates of fever relative to separately administered vaccines (see WARNINGS). The prevalence of fever was highest on the day of vaccination and the day following vaccination. More than 98% of episodes of fever resolved within the 4-day period following vaccination (i.e., the period including the day of vaccination and the next 3 days). Rates of most other solicited adverse events following PEDIARIX were comparable to rates observed following separately administered US-licensed vaccines. The adverse event information from clinical trials provides a basis for identifying adverse events that appear to be related to vaccine use and for approximating rates. However, because clinical trials are conducted under widely varying conditions, adverse event rates observed in the clinical trials of a vaccine cannot be directly compared to rates in the clinical trials of another vaccine, and may not reflect the rates observed in practice. A total of 5,472 infants were enrolled in a German safety study that was originally designed to compare the safety and reactogenicity of PEDIARIX administered concomitantly at separate sites with 1 of 4 *Haemophilus influenzae* type b (Hib) vaccines at 3, 4, and 5 months of age. After enrollment of 1,569 infants, the study was amended to include a control group that received INFANRIX, Hib vaccine, and oral poliovirus vaccine (OPV) separately. Infants in the separate administration group received one less antigen (hepatitis B) than the infants who received PEDIARIX. Safety data were available for 4,666 infants who received PEDIARIX administered concomitantly at separate sites with 1 of 4 Hib vaccines and for 768 infants in the control group that received separate vaccines. The primary end-point of the study was the percentage of infants with any grade 3 solicited symptom (redness or swelling >20 mm, fever >103.1°F, or crying, pain, vomiting, diarrhea, loss of appetite, or restlessness that prevented normal daily activities) over the 3-dose primary series in infants who received PEDIARIX (4 groups that received PEDIARIX and Hib vaccines pooled) compared to the group that received INFANRIX and Hib vaccine separately with OPV. Analysis for the primary end-point was performed on the according-to-protocol (ATP) cohort that included only those infants who were enrolled after the protocol amendment to include a control group. Of 3,773 infants in the ATP cohort for whom safety data were available, 16.2% (95% CI: 14.9% to 17.5%) of 3,029 infants who received PEDIARIX and Hib vaccine compared to 20.3% (95% CI: 17.5% to 23.4%) of 744 infants who received separate vaccines were reported to have had at least one grade 3 solicited symptom within 4 days of vaccination (i.e., day of vaccination and the next 3 days). The difference between groups in the rate of grade 3 symptoms was 4.1% (90% CI: 1.4% to 7.1%). These were the rates for selected solicited symptoms within 4 days following each dose in a 3-dose primary series in infants who received PEDIARIX administered concomitantly with Hib vaccine and those who received separate concomitant administration of INFANRIX, Hib vaccine, and OPV for the intent-to-treat (ITT) cohort (includes all infants enrolled before and after the amendment who received the indicated vaccine and for whom at least one symptom sheet was completed):

**Percentage of German Infants With Solicited Local Reactions or Selected Systemic Adverse Events Within 4 Days of Vaccination* (ITT Cohort)**

| | PEDIARIX & Hib | | | INFANRIX, Hib, & OPV | | |
|---|---|---|---|---|---|---|
| | Dose 1 | Dose 2 | Dose 3 | Dose 1 | Dose 2 | Dose 3 |
| **N** | **4,666** | **4,619** | **4,574** | **768** | **757** | **750** |
| **Local†** | | | | | | |
| Pain, any | 14.0 | 10.2 | 9.9 | 14.2 | 9.8 | 8.1 |
| Pain, grade 2 or 3 | 2.9 | 1.2 | 1.5 | 3.6 | 1.7 | 1.1 |
| Pain, grade 3 | 0.7 | 0.3 | 0.3 | 1.3 | 0.4 | 0.1 |
| Redness, any | 18.6 | 26.6 | 25.6 | 16.1 | 21.4 | 20.8 |
| Redness, >5 mm | 6.7 | 9.9 | 9.0 | 5.9 | 8.2 | 7.7 |
| Redness, >20 mm | 1.2 | 1.0 | 1.1 | 1.8 | 0.7 | 1.1 |
| Swelling, any | 12.7 | 18.5 | 18.4 | 9.6 | 12.9 | 13.6 |
| Swelling, >5 mm | 5.6 | 7.7 | 7.8 | 3.6 | 5.2 | 4.8 |
| Swelling, >20 mm | 1.2 | 1.6 | 1.5 | 1.3 | 1.1 | 1.2 |
| **Systemic** | | | | | | |
| Restlessness, any | 41.4 | 32.0 | 26.7 | 46.4 | 35.0 | 27.6 |
| Restlessness, grade 2 or 3 | 14.4 | 10.0 | 8.9 | 20.2 | 11.5 | 8.4 |
| Restlessness, grade 3 | 3.0 | 1.5 | 1.6 | 5.7 | 3.0 | 1.7 |
| Fever‡, ≥100.4ºF | 25.1 | 19.3 | 19.7 | 13.2 | 13.1 | 11.2 |
| Fever‡, >101.3ºF | 5.8 | 4.1 | 4.6 | 2.2 | 2.8 | 2.1 |
| Fever‡, >103.1ºF | 0.3 | 0.5 | 0.7 | 0.3 | 0.3 | 0.5 |
| Unusual cry§, any | 24.9 | 16.5 | 13.1 | 36.5 | 19.7 | 14.3 |
| Unusual cry§, grade 2 or 3 | 12.7 | 7.1 | 5.7 | 20.8 | 10.0 | 5.7 |
| Unusual cry§, grade 3 | 3.9 | 1.7 | 1.4 | 6.8 | 2.1 | 1.1 |
| Loss of appetite, any | 17.9 | 13.3 | 12.5 | 19.1 | 16.2 | 11.3 |
| Loss of appetite, grade 2 or 3 | 4.0 | 2.9 | 2.7 | 4.4 | 2.9 | 2.3 |
| Loss of appetite, grade 3 | 0.6 | 0.5 | 0.4 | 0.5 | 0.7 | 0.0 |

N = number of infants in the intent-to-treat (ITT) cohort.
Grade 2 defined as sufficiently discomforting to interfere with daily activities.
Grade 3 defined as preventing normal daily activities.
* Within 4 days of vaccination defined as day of vaccination and the next 3 days.
† Local reactions at the injection site for PEDIARIX or INFANRIX.
‡ Rectal temperatures.
§ Unusual cry lasting >1 hour.

In this study, infants were also monitored for unsolicited adverse events that occurred within 30 days following vaccination. Over the entire study period, 6 subjects in the group that received PEDIARIX reported seizures. Two of these subjects had a febrile seizure, 1 of whom also developed afebrile seizures. The remaining 4 subjects had afebrile seizures, including 2 with infantile spasms. Two subjects reported seizures within 7 days following vaccination (1 subject had both febrile and afebrile seizures, and 1 subject had afebrile seizures), corresponding to a rate of 0.22 seizures per 1,000 doses (febrile seizures 0.07 per 1,000 doses, afebrile seizures 0.14 per 1,000 doses). No subject who received concomitant INFANRIX, Hib vaccine, and OPV reported seizures. In a separate German study that evaluated the safety of INFANRIX in 22,505 infants who received 66,867 doses of INFANRIX administered as a 3-dose primary series, the rate of seizures within 7 days of vaccination with INFANRIX was 0.13 per 1,000 doses (febrile seizures 0.0 per 1,000 doses, afebrile seizures 0.13 per 1,000 doses). No cases of hypotonic-hyporesponsiveness, encephalopathy, or anaphylaxis were reported in the German study that evaluated the safety of PEDIARIX. Rates of serious adverse events that are less common than those reported in this safety study are not known at this time.

Additional safety data for PEDIARIX are available from a US study designed to evaluate lot-to-lot consistency and a bridge for a new manufacturing step. These were the rates for local reactions and selected adverse events within 4 days of vaccination with PEDIARIX administered concomitantly with a Hib vaccine at 2, 4, and 6 months of age:

**Percentage of US Infants With Solicited Local Reactions or Selected Systemic Adverse Events Within 4 Days of Vaccination* (ITT Cohort)**

| | PEDIARIX & Hib | | |
|---|---|---|---|
| | Dose 1 | Dose 2 | Dose 3 |
| **Local†** | **N = 482** | **N = 469** | **N = 466** |
| Pain, any | 30.5 | 25.4 | 23.0 |
| Pain, grade 2 or 3 | 6.2 | 5.5 | 3.6 |
| Pain, grade 3 | 1.2 | 0.6 | 0.6 |
| Redness, any | 25.3 | 32.6 | 35.6 |
| Redness, >5 mm | 9.3 | 10.4 | 8.6 |
| Redness, >20 mm | 0.6 | 1.5 | 1.3 |
| Swelling, any | 15.1 | 16.6 | 22.3 |
| Swelling, >5 mm | 6.8 | 6.2 | 6.4 |
| Swelling, >20 mm | 1.0 | 1.3 | 1.3 |
| **Systemic** | **N = 482** | **N = 469** | **N = 467** |
| Restlessness, any | 28.8 | 30.3 | 28.5 |
| Restlessness, grade 2 or 3 | 7.1 | 9.0 | 9.4 |
| Restlessness, grade 3 | 1.0 | 1.1 | 0.6 |
| Fever‡, ≥100.4ºF | 26.6 | 31.3 | 25.9 |
| Fever‡, >101.3ºF | 2.9 | 6.2 | 4.7 |
| Fever‡, >103.1ºF | 0.0 | 0.2 | 0.6 |
| Fussiness, any | 61.8 | 63.8 | 57.0 |
| Fussiness, grade 2 or 3 | 14.9 | 21.5 | 17.1 |
| Fussiness, grade 3 | 2.7 | 3.4 | 1.7 |
| Loss of appetite, any | 21.6 | 19.8 | 18.8 |
| Loss of appetite, grade 2 or 3 | 3.1 | 3.2 | 2.4 |
| Loss of appetite, grade 3 | 0.2 | 0.4 | 0.0 |
| Sleeping more than usual, any | 46.7 | 31.8 | 28.1 |
| Sleeping more than usual, grade 2 or 3 | 10.2 | 6.0 | 4.7 |
| Sleeping more than usual, grade 3 | 1.7 | 0.4 | 0.6 |

N = number of infants in the intent-to-treat (ITT) cohort (infants who received the indicated vaccine and for whom at least one symptom sheet was completed).
Grade 2 defined as sufficiently discomforting to interfere with daily activities.
Grade 3 defined as preventing normal daily activities.
* Within 4 days of vaccination defined as day of vaccination and the next 3 days.
† Local reactions at the injection site for PEDIARIX.
‡ Rectal temperatures.

In another US study, these were the rates for fever within 4 days following dose 1 (i.e., day of vaccination and the next 3 days) at 2 months of age in infants who received PEDIARIX when administered concomitantly at separate sites with Hib and pneumococcal conjugate vaccines and those who received INFANRIX, ENGERIX-B® [Hepatitis B Vaccine (Recombinant)], IPV, Hib vaccine, and pneumococcal conjugate vaccine:

**Percentage of US Infants With Fever Within 4 Days of Dose 1* (ITT Cohort)**

| | PEDIARIX, Hib, & Pneumococcal Conjugate (N = 667) | INFANRIX, ENGERIX-B, IPV, Hib, & Pneumococcal Conjugate (N = 333) | Separate Vaccine Group Minus Combination Vaccine Group |
|---|---|---|---|
| **Fever†** | **%** | **%** | **Difference (95% CI)** |
| ≥100.4ºF‡ | 27.9 | 19.8 | -8.07 (-13.54, -2.60) |
| >101.3ºF | 7.0 | 4.5 | -2.54 (-5.50, 0.41) |
| >102.2ºF‡ | 2.2 | 0.3 | -1.95 (-3.22, -0.68) |
| >103.1ºF | 0.4 | 0.0 | -0.45 (-0.96, 0.06) |
| M.A.‡ | 1.2 | 0.0 | -1.20 (-2.03, -037) |

N = number of infants for whom at least one symptom sheet was completed, excluding 3 infants for whom temperature was not measured and 3 infants whose temperature was measured by the tympanic method.
*Within 4 days of dose 1 defined as day of vaccination and the next 3 days.
† Rectal temperatures.
‡ The group that received PEDIARIX compared to separate vaccine group p value <0.05 (2-sided Fisher Exact test) or the 95% confidence interval on the difference between groups does not include 0.
M.A. = Medically attended (a visit to or from medical personnel).

In this study, medical attention (a visit to or from medical personnel) for fever within 4 days following vaccination was sought for 8 infants who received PEDIARIX (1.2%) and no infants who received separately administered vaccines. Four infants were seen by medical personnel in an office setting; no diagnostic tests were performed in 2 of the infants and a complete blood count (CBC) was done in the other 2 infants. Of 3 infants who were seen in an emergency room, all had a CBC and a blood and urine culture performed; chest X-rays were done in 2 of the infants and a nasopharyngeal specimen was tested for Respiratory Syncytial Virus in one of the infants. One infant was hospitalized for a work-up that included a CBC, blood and urine cultures, a lumbar puncture, and a chest X-ray. All episodes of medically attended fever resolved within 4 days post-vaccination.

Limited data are available from a study conducted in Moldova in which infants received a dose of hepatitis B vaccine within 48 hours of birth followed by 3 doses of PEDIARIX at 6, 10, and 14 weeks of age. No information was collected on the HBsAg status of mothers of enrolled infants. These were the rates for local reactions and selected adverse events within 4 days of vaccination with PEDIARIX administered comcomitantly with Hib vaccine following a birth dose of hepatitis B vaccine:

**Percentage of Moldovan Infants With Solicited Local Reactions or Selected Systemic Adverse Events Within 4 Days of Vaccination* (ITT Cohort)**

| | PEDIARIX & Hib | | |
|---|---|---|---|
| | Dose 1 | Dose 2 | Dose 3 |
| **N** | **160** | **158** | **157** |
| **Local†** | | | |
| Pain, any | 25.6 | 18.4 | 14.0 |
| Pain, grade 3 | 3.1 | 0.6 | 1.9 |
| Redness, any | 41.9 | 41.8 | 47.1 |
| Redness, >20 mm | 1.9 | 2.5 | 4.5 |
| Swelling, any | 20.6 | 18.4 | 28.0 |
| Swelling, >20 mm | 4.4 | 2.5 | 7.0 |
| **Systemic** | | | |
| Restlessness, any | 13.1 | 10.8 | 8.9 |
| Restlessness, grade 3 | 1.3 | 0.6 | 0.6 |
| Fever‡, ≥100.4ºF | 14.4 | 11.4 | 5.1 |
| Fever‡, >103.1ºF | 0.0 | 0.6 | 0.0 |
| Fussiness, any | 25.0 | 21.5 | 17.8 |
| Fussiness, grade 3 | 2.5 | 0.6 | 0.6 |

N = number of infants in the intent-to-treat (ITT) cohort (infants who received the indicated vaccine and for whom at least one symptom sheet was completed).
Grade 3 defined as preventing normal daily activities.
*Within 4 days of vaccination defined as day of vaccination and the next 3 days.
† Local reactions at the injection site for PEDIARIX.
‡ Rectal temperatures.

Although there was no comparator group who received PEDIARIX without a birth dose of hepatitis B vaccine, available data suggest that some local adverse events may occur at a higher rate when PEDIARIX is administered after a birth dose of hepatitis B vaccine.

As with any vaccine, there is the possibility that broad use of PEDIARIX could reveal adverse events not observed in clinical trials.

**Postmarketing Reports:** Worldwide voluntary reports of adverse events received for INFANRIX and ENGERIX-B in children younger than 7 years of age since market introduction of these US-licensed vaccines are listed below. This list includes adverse events for which 20 or more reports were received with the exception of intussusception, idiopathic thrombocytopenic purpura, thrombocytopenia, anaphylactic reaction, angioedema, encephalopathy, hypotonic-hyporesponsive episode, and alopecia for which fewer than 20 reports were received. These latter events are included either because of the seriousness of the event or the strength of causal connection to components of this or other vaccines or drugs. *Body as a whole:* Asthenia[b], fever[a+b], lethargy[b], malaise[b], Sudden Infant Death Syndrome[a+b]. *Cardiovascular system:* Cyanosis[a+b], edema[b], pallor[b]. *Gastrointestinal system:* Abdominal pain[b], anorexia[b], diarrhea[a+b], intussusception[a+b], nausea[b], vomiting[a+b]. *Hematologic/lymphatic:* Idiopathic thrombocytopenic purpura[a+b], lymphadenopathy[a], thrombocytopenia[a+b]. *Hepatic:* Jaundice[b], liver function tests abnormal[b]. *Hypersensitivity:* Anaphylactic reaction[a+b], angioedema[b], hypersensitivity[a]. *Infections:* Cellulitis[a]. *Injection site reactions:* Injection site reactions[a+b]. *Musculoskeletal:* Arthralgia[b], limb swelling[a+b]. *Nervous system:* Convulsions[a+b], encephalopathy[a], headache[b], hypotonia[a+b], hypotonic-hyporesponsive episode[a], somnolence[a+b]. *Psychiatric:* Crying[a+b], irritability[a+b]. *Respiratory system:* Respiratory tract infection[a]. *Skin and appendages:* Alopecia[b], erythema[a+b], erythema multiforme[b], petechiae[b], pruritus[a+b], rash[a+b], urticaria[a+b]. *Special senses:* Ear pain[a]. [[a] Following INFANRIX; [b] Following ENGERIX-B; [a+b] Following either INFANRIX or ENGERIX-B.] These reactions were reported voluntarily from a population of uncertain size; therefore, it is not always possible to reliably estimate their frequency or establish a causal relationship to vaccination.

**Reporting Adverse Events:** Report the occurrence following immunization of any event set forth in the Vaccine Injury Table from the National Childhood Vaccine Injury Act including: Anaphylaxis or anaphylactic shock within 7 days, encephalopathy or encephalitis within 7 days, brachial neuritis within 28 days, or an acute complication or sequelae (including death) of an illness, disability, injury, or condition referred to above, or any events that would contraindicate further doses of PEDIARIX. The VAERS toll-free number is 1-800-822-7967.

Manufactured by **GlaxoSmithKline Biologicals**, Rixensart, Belgium, US License 1617

Distributed by **GlaxoSmithKline,** Research Triangle Park, NC 27709

PEDIARIX is a trademark and TIP-LOK, INFANRIX, and ENGERIX-B are registered trademarks of GlaxoSmithKline.

Full prescribing information for PEDIARIX is available at www.GSKVaccines.com/Pediarix. BRS-PE:L2


Printed in USA. PED583R0 June 2005

ARTICLE

# Neonatal Abstinence Syndrome After In Utero Exposure to Selective Serotonin Reuptake Inhibitors in Term Infants

*Rachel Levinson-Castiel, MD; Paul Merlob, MD; Nehama Linder, MD; Lea Sirota, MD; Gil Klinger, MD*

**Objective:** To compare the prevalence and clinical characteristics of neonatal abstinence syndrome in neonates exposed and not exposed to selective serotonin reuptake inhibitors (SSRIs) in utero.

**Design:** Cohort study.

**Setting:** Tertiary care center.

**Patients:** One hundred twenty term infants, of whom 60 had prolonged in utero exposure to SSRIs, including paroxetine hydrochloride, fluoxetine, citalopram hydrobromide, sertraline hydrochloride, and venlafaxine hydrochloride.

**Main Outcome Measures:** Neonatal abstinence syndrome was assessed with the Finnegan score as follows: score of 8 or above, severe; score of 4 to 7, mild; and score of 0 to 3, normal. All infants were followed up with a standardized protocol that included repeated Finnegan score assessments and cardiorespiratory monitoring until normalization of the Finnegan score.

**Results:** Of the 60 neonates exposed to SSRIs in utero, 8 showed severe and 10 showed mild symptoms of a neonatal abstinence syndrome. All nonexposed neonates had a normal Finnegan score. In neonates who developed severe symptoms, the maximum mean daily Finnegan scores were recorded within 2 days after birth, although maximum individual scores were recorded as long as 4 days after birth.

**Conclusions:** Neonatal abstinence syndrome occurs in 30% of neonates exposed to SSRIs in utero. These neonates should be monitored for at least 48 hours after birth. The long-term effects of prolonged exposure to SSRIs, particularly in neonates who develop severe symptoms, have yet to be determined.

*Arch Pediatr Adolesc Med. 2006;160:173-176*

**Author Affiliations:** Neonatal Intensive Care Unit, Schneider Children's Medical Center of Israel, Petah Tiqwa (Drs Levinson-Castiel, Merlob, Linder, Sirota, and Klinger); Department of Neonatology, Rabin Medical Center, Petah Tiqwa (Drs Merlob, Linder, Sirota, and Klinger); and Sackler School of Medicine, Tel Aviv University, (Drs Merlob, Linder, Sirota, and Klinger), Tel Aviv, Israel.

DEPRESSION IS A COMMON disease with a lifetime risk of 10% to 25% in women.[1] Furthermore, pregnancy is a stressful state that may aggravate depression and increase the need for medical therapy. The widespread use of selective serotonin reuptake inhibitors (SSRIs), which cross the placenta,[2] has prompted investigations of the effects of maternal treatment with SSRIs on the fetus. Fetal exposure to SSRIs has not been associated with an increased incidence of major congenital malformations,[3-6] but there is growing evidence that it is associated with a neonatal abstinence syndrome (NAS).[7-12] Kallen[12] and Costei et al[13] showed increased rates of respiratory distress in exposed newborns. Zeskind and Stephens[14] observed disruptions in a wide range of neurobehavioral outcomes, and Oberlander et al[15] found that 30% of exposed infants had poor neonatal adaptation. In a recent study, 93 cases of suspected SSRI-induced neonatal withdrawal syndrome were reported.[16] However, results from large cohort studies of the symptoms of NAS in infants exposed to SSRIs in utero are not yet available. Our aim was to assess the clinical syndrome exhibited by neonates exposed to SSRIs in utero.

## METHODS

The objective of the present study was to use a standardized protocol to compare the incidence and clinical characteristics of NAS in neonates exposed and not exposed to SSRIs in utero. This cohort study was performed at Rabin Medical Center in Israel, a tertiary care facility housing a neonatology department that cares for approximately 9000 newborns per year. The study was conducted from January 1, 2002, through August 31, 2004, during which 23 254 consecutive births took place. Maternal intake of SSRIs during pregnancy, including fluoxetine, paroxetine hydrochlo-

**Table 1. Characteristics of the Study Population**

| Characteristic* | Infants Exposed to SSRIs (n = 60) | Control Infants (n = 60) | *P* Value |
|---|---|---|---|
| Maternal age, y | 32.8 ± 5.3 | 30.7 ± 5.7 | .04 |
| Mean duration of SSRI treatment, wk | 35.5 ± 8.7 | NA | NA |
| Gestational diabetes | 3 | 3 | >.99 |
| Meconium-stained amniotic fluid | 19 | 3 | <.001 |
| 5-min Apgar score <7 | 0 | 0 | NA |
| Head circumference, cm | 34.0 ± 1.2 | 34.1 ± 1.2 | .65 |
| Congenital anomalies | 3 | 1 | .60 |

Abbreviations: NA, not applicable; SSRI, selective serotonin reuptake inhibitor.

*Data are given as mean ± SD or number of patients.

ride, citalopram hydrobromide, sertraline hydrochloride, and the serotonin-noradrenaline reuptake inhibitor venlafaxine hydrochloride, was recorded in each case. All full-term infants who had had prolonged exposure to SSRIs during the entire pregnancy or at least during the third trimester were eligible for the study. The infants were identified from the delivery room records as they arrived at the nursery or from a medical history form completed by all mothers at admittance to the nursery. This form included demographic details; maternal and family illnesses; type, dosage, and duration of treatment with SSRIs or other drugs; and use of recreational drugs, tobacco, or alcohol. A control cohort of infants was similarly identified during the final 2 months of the study and included an equal number of healthy non–SSRI-exposed neonates born to healthy mothers and matched for sex, gestational age (±1 week), birth weight (±100 g), and mode of delivery.

Exclusion criteria were known or probable exposure to other medications, illicit drugs, or alcohol, which could have contributed to a NAS, congenital anomalies or conditions affecting the central nervous system. Infants who were exposed to SSRIs or who met any of the exclusion criteria were excluded from the control cohort. Preterm infants also were excluded owing to the difficulty of assessing the Finnegan score in this population.

The nurses and physicians in our center are trained to identify and record NAS symptoms. The SSRI-exposed infants in the present study were followed up after birth according to a protocol introduced in the neonatal department in 1998; it includes cardiorespiratory and temperature monitoring, assessment of the Finnegan score,[17] and blood testing. The Finnegan score is an objective method used to monitor onset, progression, and improvement of NAS symptoms in passively exposed neonates. The score rates 21 symptoms in 11 groups most commonly seen in drug-exposed neonates and is used to assess the need for pharmacologic intervention and the response to treatment. The total score is determined by adding the score assigned to each symptom group. Higher scores represent more severe NAS symptoms with a consequent risk of increased morbidity. A score of 8 or higher in 3 consecutive measurements is considered an indication for pharmacotherapy. Finnegan scores were assessed 2 hours after birth and thereafter every 8 hours after meals for 48 hours or longer if the score had not normalized in 48 hours. More frequent assessments were performed as required by the clinical situation. A severe NAS was defined as a Finnegan score of 8 or higher at 1 or more assessments, and mild NAS was defined as a score of 4 to 7 in at least 2 examinations; infants with scores of 4 or higher were assessed repeatedly until the score decreased below 4. At discharge, the medical records were reviewed, and the Finnegan scores were assessed for possible errors. In only SSRI-exposed infants, complete blood cell count, glucose level, coagulation time, and blood chemistry (urea, creatinine, electrolytes, calcium) were tested.

Findings in the exposed cohort were compared with those in the nonexposed cohort. Data are given as summary measures (mean and standard deviation). The *t* test was used to compare continuous variables and the Fisher exact test or $\chi^2$ test, as appropriate, to compare categorical values. The study was approved by the institutional research ethics board.

## RESULTS

During the study, 78 infants born to 76 women had prolonged in utero exposure to SSRIs. Eighteen were excluded from the study because of prematurity (7 infants, including 2 sets of twins), first-trimester cessation of SSRI treatment (3 infants), or concomitant maternal use of other medications that can cause withdrawal symptoms (8 infants; benzodiazepines in 6 and carbamazepine in 2). The infant of a mother who took fluoxetine until 6 days before delivery was included because of the long half-life of the drug (5-7 days). Of the 60 SSRI-exposed infants, 37 were exposed to paroxetine hydrochloride (dose range, 10-40 mg), 12 to fluoxetine (dose range, 20-60 mg), 8 to citalopram hydrobromide (dose range, 10-40 mg), 2 to venlafaxine hydrochloride (dose range, 37.5-75 mg), and 1 to sertraline hydrochloride (dose, 25 mg). In the control cohort, all families agreed to participate. The characteristics of the study population are presented in **Table 1**. Three infants exposed to SSRIs for the complete pregnancy duration had major congenital anomalies (ventricular septal defect and cleft palate, ventricular septal defect, and hydronephrosis with ureterocele). One infant in the control group had hydronephrosis. None of the infants with major congenital anomalies had any serious medical complications.

Comparison of the presence of each NAS symptom included in the Finnegan score between the SSRI-exposed infants and the control infants is presented in **Table 2**. Symptoms of NAS were present in 18 of the 60 SSRI-exposed infants (30%) vs none of the 60 control infants ($P<.001$). Of the 18 symptomatic SSRI-exposed infants, 8 (13%) had a severe NAS (Finnegan score ≥8), and 10 (17%) had a mild NAS (score, 4-7). Of the 8 infants with severe NAS, 6 neonates were exposed to paroxetine, 1 to fluoxetine, and 1 to citalopram. The characteristics of the study group infants with withdrawal symptoms are shown in **Table 3**. Maximum mean daily symptoms occurred within the first 48 hours of life, although maximum individual Finnegan scores occurred as long as 4 days after birth. No infant with symptoms required any treatment.

The relationship of SSRI dosage to NAS symptoms was assessed only in infants exposed to paroxetine hydrochloride because of subgroup sample size. Mean drug dose was 19 mg for infants with no symptoms, 23 mg for infants with mild symptoms, and 27 mg for infants with severe symptoms. Comparison of the infants with symptoms (Finnegan score >3) to those without symptoms (Finnegan score 0-3) showed a correlation between higher

**Table 2. Comparison of Finnegan Score Symptoms* in Neonates Exposed to SSRIs With Those in a Control Group**

| Symptom | SSRI-Exposed Infants (n = 60) | Control Infants (n = 60) |
|---|---|---|
| High-pitched cry | 18 | 0 |
| Sleep disturbance | 21 | 2 |
| Exaggerated Moro reflex | 3 | 0 |
| Tremor | 37 | 11 |
| Hypertonicity or myoclonus | 14 | 1 |
| Convulsions | 2 | 0 |
| Sweating | 1 | 0 |
| Fever | 3 | 0 |
| Autonomic nervous system† | 4 | 2 |
| Tachypnea | 12 | 0 |
| Gastrointestinal disturbance‡ | 34 | 2 |
| Neonatal abstinence syndrome§ | 18 | 0 |

Abbreviation: SSRI, selective serotonin reuptake inhibitor.
*Data are given as number of patients. Some patients had more than 1 symptom.
†Yawning, sneezing, sniffles.
‡Exaggerated sucking, poor feeding, regurgitation, vomiting, loose stools.
§Defined as a Finnegan score of 4 or higher.

**Table 3. Characteristics of Neonates Exposed to SSRIs Who Had Severe Neonatal Abstinence Symptoms***

| Patient No. | Maximum Mean Finnegan Score | Day of Life of Maximum Mean Finnegan Score | Duration of Hospital Stay, d |
|---|---|---|---|
| 1 | 11 | 2 | 6 |
| 2 | 8 | 1 | 7 |
| 3 | 9 | 1 | 6 |
| 4 | 10 | 2 | 5 |
| 5 | 8 | 2 | 5 |
| 6 | 8 | 2 | 5 |
| 7 | 8 | 2 | 4 |
| 8 | 9 | 2 | 4 |

Abbreviation: SSRI, selective serotonin reuptake inhibitor.
*Defined as a Finnegan score of 8 or higher.

drug dosage and NAS ($P = .01$). Examining the paroxetine hydrochloride dose used, we were unable to identify a specific cutoff point for an increased risk of NAS because most infants were exposed to a similar dose (20 mg). However, no infant exposed to a dose less than 20 mg developed any symptoms.

Laboratory test result abnormalities noted in the group exposed to SSRIs were hypoglycemia (glucose level <40 mg/dL [2.22 mmol/L]) in 3 infants, transient coagulation abnormality in 1 infant, thrombocytopenia (platelet count $<150 \times 10^3$/L; lowest count, $103 \times 10^3$/L) in 3 infants, and leukopenia (leukocyte count <10 000/μL) in 3 infants. All abnormal test results resolved within a few days.

## COMMENT

The increasing use of SSRIs during pregnancy warrants careful examination of their effects on the fetus and newborn infant. Results of the present study show that 30% of infants exposed to SSRIs in utero have symptoms of a NAS and that in 13% of these infants the symptoms are severe enough to meet the definition of a severe NAS.

Exposure to an SSRI during pregnancy has been associated with many neonatal symptoms, including respiratory distress, cyanotic events, feeding difficulties, hypoglycemia, and a wide spectrum of neurologic symptoms,[18] ranging from neurobehavioral disturbance, sleep disturbances, and increased motor activity[14] to a neonatal withdrawal syndrome.[18] A retrospective study of maternal use of fluoxetine showed that poor neonatal adaptation was more common in the SSRI-exposed infants than in controls (relative risk 8.7; 95% confidence interval, 2.9-26.6).[4] Reports of neurologic symptoms severe enough to be characterized as a withdrawal syndrome mostly have been anecdotal,[7] but recently Sanz et al[16] identified 93 cases of suspected SSRI-induced neonatal withdrawal syndrome in a large database survey. The most frequent symptoms observed in the newborns in our study were tremor, gastrointestinal or sleep disturbance, hypertonicity, and high-pitched cry. These findings are consistent with those of Sanz et al[16] who reported more neurologic and gastrointestinal than respiratory symptoms. Tachypnea, a common finding in previous studies,[12,13] was less frequently observed, probably owing to our exclusion of preterm infants. It is noteworthy that 2 of the infants in our study had seizures, but these were transient. Because of the small size of each SSRI subgroup, it was difficult to assess if there is a specific SSRI that is more likely to cause NAS symptoms. Nevertheless, in the largest subgroup of infants, those exposed to paroxetine, 6 (16%) of 37 had severe symptoms. When we compared the infants with symptoms to those without, we found a dose-response effect. Some symptoms of withdrawal, such as jitteriness, tachypnea, hypertonicity, temperature instability, and diarrhea, also can be attributed to serotoninergic hyperstimulation.[19] Laine et al[20] described such serotoninergic hyperstimulation in infants exposed to SSRIs and its correlation with drug levels. Maximum severity of symptoms would be expected to occur shortly after birth, if serotoninergic hyperstimulation is the cause of symptoms, because drug exposure does not continue after birth. However, for most infants, peak symptoms did not occur on the first day of life, so the observed symptoms were unlikely to be caused by serotoninergic hyperstimulation.

The present study is a large population-based study that includes all infants with reported prolonged exposure to SSRIs, enabling an accurate assessment of the prevalence of NAS in exposed infants. Infants were followed up prospectively from birth to identify all symptoms. The 30% rate of neonatal symptoms in our sample of SSRI-exposed infants is close to that in studies by Oberlander et al[15] (30%) and Chambers et al[4] (31.5%) but higher than the rate reported by Costei et al[13] (22%). However, in the latter study, data were not collected immediately after delivery and may underrepresent the true incidence of neonatal symptoms. Our study is the first of its kind to use the Finnegan score, which is an objective score that permits quantification of NAS symptoms, in SSRI-exposed infants. A different NAS score has been used only in case series.[21,22] Severe NAS symptoms were found in 13% of exposed neonates in our study. The study design enabled comparison of infants who were exposed with those who were not and supported the causal role of SSRIs in the observed symptoms. Prospectively following up infants until resolution of symptoms provided new information regarding the time and duration of peak symptoms. Because infants who were severely affected exhibited peak symptoms within the first 48 hours of life, this should be the minimum observation period.

Our study has some limitations. Exposure to SSRIs was determined according to maternal report. Because some mothers may elect not to report SSRI use, our study may not have captured the total exposed population. Our sample size was relatively small for each drug subgroup of exposed newborns. Because the Finnegan score routinely is used only in infants exposed to drugs, the staff was aware of exposure status, and a blinded assessment was not possible. Although the neonatal staff was well trained in the use of the Finnegan score, interobserver variability may have occurred. We tried to minimize this problem by recalculating the Finnegan score according to the symptoms noted in the medical record. Because drug levels were not measured, their correlation with symptoms was not possible.

The long-term effects of in utero exposure to SSRIs have not been demonstrated clearly.[15,23,24] Oberlander et al[15] reported symptom resolution in all infants within 48 hours of life and normal findings at 8-month follow-up. Nulman et al[23] studied 55 preschool children exposed to fluoxetine in utero and found no change in global IQ, language development, or behavioral development. However, Casper et al[24] noted subtle effects on motor development in exposed children. The long-term effects on the select group of SSRI-exposed infants who develop symptoms suggestive of a severe NAS have not been evaluated.

The high prevalence of NAS in infants exposed to SSRIs in utero should be brought to the attention of family physicians, psychiatrists, gynecologists, pediatricians, and mothers. Because maternal depression during pregnancy also entails a risk to the newborn, the risk-benefit ratio of continuing SSRI treatment should be assessed. If SSRIs are prescribed during pregnancy, use of the minimum effective dosage and avoidance of polytherapy are prudent. After birth, close monitoring is mandatory. We recommend our protocol, which includes cardiorespiratory monitoring and assessment of the Finnegan score at regular intervals. Early discharge of SSRI-exposed infants should be avoided and observation continued until symptoms subside. Breastfeeding is not contraindicated for SSRI monotherapy, but follow-up for signs of NAS after discharge is recommended.[25]

In conclusion, NAS frequently occurs after prolonged in utero exposure to SSRIs. Infants exposed to SSRIs should be closely monitored after birth by using a standardized protocol for a minimum of 48 hours. Follow-up of exposed infants, particularly those who develop severe symptoms, is needed to assess the long-term effects of prolonged exposure to SSRIs.

**Accepted for Publication:** July 20, 2005.
**Correspondence:** Gil Klinger, MD, Neonatal Intensive Care Unit, Schneider Children's Medical Center of Israel, 14 Kaplan Street, Petah Tiqwa, Israel, 49202 (gilkl@post.tau.ac.il).

## REFERENCES

1. Wisner KL, Gelenberg AJ, Leonard H, Zarin D, Frank E. Pharmacologic treatment of depression during pregnancy. *JAMA.* 1999;282:1264-1269.
2. Hendrick V, Stowe ZN, Altshuler LL, Hwang S, Lee E, Haynes D. Placental passage of antidepressant medications. *Am J Psychiatry.* 2003;160:993-996.
3. McElhatton PR, Garbis HM, Elefant E, et al. The outcome of pregnancy in 689 women exposed to therapeutic doses of antidepressants: a collaborative study of the European Network of Teratology Information Services (ENTIS). *Reprod Toxicol.* 1996;10:285-294.
4. Chambers CD, Johnson KA, Dick LM, Felix RJ, Jones KL. Birth outcomes in pregnant women taking fluoxetine. *N Engl J Med.* 1996;335:1010-1015.
5. Kulin NA, Pastuszak A, Sage SR, et al. Pregnancy outcome following maternal use of the new selective serotonin reuptake inhibitors: a prospective controlled multicenter study. *JAMA.* 1998;279:609-610.
6. Ericson A, Kallen B, Wiholm B. Delivery outcome after the use of antidepressants in early pregnancy. *Eur J Clin Pharmacol.* 1999;55:503-508.
7. Jaiswal S, Coombs RC, Isbister GK. Paroxetine withdrawal in a neonate with historical and laboratory confirmation. *Eur J Pediatr.* 2003;162:723-724.
8. Mhanna MJ, Bennet JB II, Izatt SD. Potential fluoxetine chloride (Prozac) toxicity in a newborn. *Pediatrics.* 1997;100:158-169.
9. Kent LS, Laidlaw JD. Suspected congenital sertraline dependence. *Br J Psychiatry.* 1995;167:412-413.
10. Dahl ML, Olhager E, Ahlner J. Paroxetine withdrawal syndrome in a neonate. *Br J Psychiatry.* 1997;171:391-392.
11. Spencer MJ. Fluoxetine hydrochloride (Prozac) toxicity in a neonate. *Pediatrics.* 1993;92:721-722.
12. Kallen B. Neonate characteristics after maternal use of antidepressants in late pregnancy. *Arch Pediatr Adolesc Med.* 2004;158:312-316.
13. Costei AM, Kozer E, Ho T, Ito S, Koren G. Perinatal outcome following third trimester exposure to paroxetine. *Arch Pediatr Adolesc Med.* 2002;156:1129-1132.
14. Zeskind PS, Stephens LE. Maternal selective serotonin reuptake inhibitor use during pregnancy and newborn neurobehavior. *Pediatrics.* 2004;113:368-375.
15. Oberlander TF, Misri S, Fitzgerald CE, Kostaras X, Rurak D, Riggs W. Pharmacologic factors associated with transient neonatal symptoms following prenatal psychotropic medication exposure. *J Clin Psychiatry.* 2004;65:230-237.
16. Sanz EJ, De-las-Cuevas C, Kiuru A, Bate A, Edwards R. Selective serotonin reuptake inhibitors in pregnant women and neonatal withdrawal syndrome: a database analysis. *Lancet.* 2005;365:482-487.
17. Finnegan LP. *Current Therapy in Neonatal Perinatal Medicine-2.* Neonatal abstinence syndrome. In: Nelson N, ed. Toronto, Ontario: BC Decker Inc; 1990:314-320.
18. Ruchkin V, Martin A. SSRIs and the developing brain. *Lancet.* 2005;365:451-453.
19. Isbister GK, Dawson A, Whyte IM, Prior FH, Clancy C, Smith AJ. Neonatal paroxetine withdrawal syndrome or actually serotonin syndrome? *Arch Dis Child Fetal Neonatal Ed.* 2001;85:F147-F148.
20. Laine K, Heikkinen T, Ekblad U, Kero P. Effects of exposure to selective serotonin reuptake inhibitors during pregnancy on serotonergic symptoms in newborns and cord blood monoamine and prolactin concentrations. *Arch Gen Psychiatry.* 2003;60:720-726.
21. Nordeng H, Lindemann R, Perminov KV, Reikvam A. Neonatal withdrawal syndrome after in utero exposure to selective serotonin reuptake inhibitors. *Acta Paediatr.* 2001;90:288-291.
22. Nijhuis IJ, Kok-Van Rooij GW, Bosschaart AN. Withdrawal reactions of a premature neonate after maternal use of paroxetine [letter]. *Arch Dis Child Fetal Neonatal Ed.* 2001;84:F77.
23. Nulman I, Rovet J, Stewart DE, et al. Neurodevelopment of children exposed in utero to antidepressant drugs. *N Engl J Med.* 1997;336:258-262.
24. Casper RC, Fleisher BE, Lee-Ancajas JC, et al. Follow-up of children of depressed mothers exposed or not exposed to antidepressant drugs during pregnancy. *J Pediatr.* 2003;142:402-408.
25. Merlob P, Stahl B, Sulkes J. Paroxetine during breast-feeding: infant weight gain and maternal adherence to counsel. *Eur J Pediatr.* 2004;163:135-139.

ARTICLE

# Access to Health Care for Young Adults With Disabling Chronic Conditions

*S. Todd Callahan, MD, MPH; William O. Cooper, MD, MPH*

**Objective:** To assess health insurance status and health care access of young adults with disabilities attributable to a chronic condition.

**Design and Setting:** We analyzed data from the National Health Interview Survey from 1999 to 2002. We present bivariate analysis and multiple logistic regression of reported health care access barriers in the United States stratified by health insurance status.

**Participants:** The study population included 1109 survey respondents with and 22 481 without disabling chronic conditions, aged 19 to 29 years.

**Main Outcome Measures:** Delayed or unmet health needs owing to cost, no contact with a health professional in the prior year, and no usual source of care.

**Results:** Thirty-five percent of respondents with and 15% without disabling chronic conditions reported an unmet health care need owing to cost ($P<.001$). Uninsurance rates for young adults with and without disabling chronic conditions were similar (26% vs 28%, respectively), and uninsurance was significantly associated with unmet health care needs. More than two thirds of uninsured respondents with a disabling chronic condition reported an unmet health need and 45% reported no usual source of care. After adjusting for sociodemographic factors, uninsured young adults with disabling chronic conditions had 8 times greater odds of reporting unmet health care needs and 6 times greater odds of having no usual source of care relative to insured respondents with disabling chronic conditions.

**Conclusions:** Despite increasing attention to issues of health care transition for young adults with disabling chronic conditions, this study suggests that uninsurance is as common among these young adults as nondisabled peers and is significantly associated with health care access barriers in this population.

*Arch Pediatr Adolesc Med. 2006;160:178-182*

THE POPULATION OF YOUNG adults in the United States with chronic medical and mental health conditions has more than doubled during the last 35 years, in part owing to improved diagnosis and management of conditions during childhood.[1] The provision of uninterrupted services to young adults with disabling chronic conditions as they transition from pediatric to adult health care is one of the goals of the Department of Health and Human Services as written in *Healthy People 2010*,[2] and a stated priority of many national medical organizations including the American Academy of Pediatrics and the Society for Adolescent Medicine.[3-5] The transition process places an emphasis on providing health care in a coordinated, uninterrupted manner[1]; thus continuous and affordable health insurance and a usual source of care are posited to be critically important to successful transitions.[4] The increasingly complex task of navigating changes in health care financing and delivery presents an important challenge for young adults, their families, and pediatric and adult health care providers.[6-12]

The research literature focusing on health care access for young adults with chronic health conditions is sparse. Young adults are excluded or constitute only a small proportion of the populations in studies of children or adults with disabilities, and the last comprehensive study of young adults drew on data from 1984.[13] Given the growth of this population and recent changes in health care financing and delivery, the aim of this study was to assess health insurance coverage and health care access of young adults with disabling chronic conditions using a national data source.

## METHODS

### DATA SOURCE

We analyzed responses from young adults aged 19 to 29 years who were participating in the National Health Interview Survey (NHIS) from 1999 to 2002. The NHIS is an ongoing, cross-sectional, national household survey sponsored by the National Center for Health Statistics. The purpose of the survey is to collect information about the health and health service use of the civilian noninstitutionalized population in the United States.[14] The sampling plan

**Author Affiliations:** Division of Adolescent Medicine and Behavioral Science (Dr Callahan), Division of General Pediatrics (Dr Cooper), Child and Adolescent Health Research Unit, Department of Pediatrics, Vanderbilt University Medical Center, Nashville, Tenn.

uses a multistage area probability design to yield nationally representative estimates.

The NHIS consists of a group of surveys designed to collect data on households and individuals. Data for the respondents in this study were drawn from the Person-Level file (containing sociodemographic and basic health information for each member of a household collected directly from individuals or from other adult members if the individual is unable to answer) and the Sample Adult file (containing additional health-related data obtained from 1 randomly selected adult in each household). Information in the Sample Adult file is based on self-report unless the respondent is incapable of providing the information. We calculated a response rate of 72.4% for all adults selected for the Sample Adult questionnaire during the 4 years studied.[14]

## DEFINITION OF DISABLING CHRONIC CONDITION

Young adults with disabling chronic conditions were identified by questions asking if physical, mental, or emotional problems resulted in limitation or inability to work, difficulty walking without special equipment, or limitations in activities of daily living (bathing, dressing, getting in/out of bed or a chair, using the toilet, eating, or getting around the home), instrumental activities of daily living (household chores, doing necessary business, shopping, or getting around), or any other activity. Chronic conditions were those that are not cured once acquired or that have been present for at least 3 months. Conditions related to pregnancy were not considered chronic. Young adults without disability reported none of the activity limitations. These young adults may or may not have chronic conditions. We excluded 86 participants whose limitations could not be attributed to a chronic condition.

## DESCRIPTION OF VARIABLES

### Health Care Access Variables

The dependent variables were responses to questions about unmet health needs, health professional contact, and usual source of health care. Participants were asked if they delayed or missed needed medical care or failed to fill a prescription in the last year because of cost. They were also asked when they last talked with a health professional about their health and if there was a place they usually went to when sick or in need of health advice. For this study, we categorized young adults according to whether they reported having any health professional contact during the past year. Young adults without a usual source of health care did not identify a source of care other than the emergency department.

### Health Insurance Coverage and Sociodemographic Characteristics

We used survey data to identify health insurance coverage at the time of the interview. The uninsured had no coverage through private health insurance, Medicare, Medicaid, State Children's Health Insurance Plan, or other public programs. Young adults with unknown coverage status (n = 159) were excluded from analyses.

We used NHIS-recoded variations of survey items to ascertain participants' educational attainment, marital status, household income, and major activity in the week prior to the survey. Household income was provided as a ratio of income to the US Census Bureau's poverty threshold for the survey year after considering overall family size.[15] The 20% of young adults in the study who did not provide household income data were excluded from multivariate analyses.

**Table 1. Characteristics of Young Adults With and Without Limitation***

| | Disabling Chronic Condition (n = 1101) | No Disability (n = 22 481) |
|---|---|---|
| Population estimate, No. (SE) | 1 900 000 (90 000) | 38 500 000 (512 000) |
| Male | 48.6 (1.8) | 49.5 (0.4) |
| Hispanic | 9.7 (1.0) | 15.9 (0.4) |
| White, non-Hispanic | 71.9 (1.7) | 65.0 (0.5) |
| Black, non-Hispanic | 15.3 (1.4) | 13.4 (0.4) |
| Other | 3.1 (0.6) | 5.6 (0.3) |
| Household income (ratio to poverty threshold) | | |
| 0-0.99 | 19.8 (1.5) | 12.6 (0.5) |
| 1.00-1.99 | 21.0 (1.4) | 16.0 (0.3) |
| ≥2.00 | 39.9 (1.8) | 50.7 (0.6) |
| Unknown | 19.3 (1.5) | 20.6 (0.4) |
| Marital status | | |
| Single | 61.1 (1.8) | 53.0 (0.6) |
| Married | 27.9 (1.6) | 35.2 (0.5) |
| Unmarried but living with a partner | 10.9 (1.0) | 11.6 (0.3) |
| Educational attainment | | |
| <9th grade | 4.2 (0.8) | 3.6 (0.2) |
| 9th-12th, grade no diploma | 19.8 (1.5) | 11.1 (0.3) |
| GED | 5.1 (0.8) | 2.9 (0.2) |
| High school graduate | 29.9 (1.7) | 24.0 (0.4) |
| Some college | 41.0 (1.9) | 58.4 (0.6) |
| Activity | | |
| Going to school | 9.0 (1.1) | 8.7 (0.4) |
| Working | 45.4 (1.8) | 76.2 (0.5) |
| Keeping house | 6.4 (0.8) | 7.8 (0.2) |
| Something else | 39.1 (1.8) | 7.3 (0.2) |
| Insurance coverage | | |
| Uninsured | 25.5 (1.8) | 28.0 (0.5) |
| Private insurance | 40.1 (1.9) | 64.6 (0.5) |
| Medicaid | 27.2 (1.6) | 5.3 (0.2) |
| Other insurance | 7.2 (1.0) | 2.1 (0.2) |

Abbreviation: GED, general equivalency diploma.

*Values are espressed as percentage (SE) unless otherwise indicated. Percentages are based on weighted data to represent the civilian noninstitutionalized population in the United States. Because of nonresponse, percentages may not add up to 100. Data Source: National Center for Health Statistics, National Health Interview Survey 1999 to 2002.

## STATISTICAL ANALYSES

Sociodemographic and insurance characteristics for 1101 young adults with and 22 481 without disabling chronic conditions are presented in **Table 1**. Bivariate analyses show the relationship between unmet health care needs and insurance status for young adults with and without disabling chronic conditions (**Table 2**). We used statistical weights provided by the NHIS to present population estimates, percentages, and standard errors reflecting United States population totals in the text and tables. Multivariate analyses are presented to estimate the odds of reporting unmet health care needs for the 885 young adults with and 17 903 without disabling chronic conditions who provided complete information, stratified by insurance status and adjusting for the sociodemographic variables (**Table 3**). To account for the complex sampling design employed in the NHIS, final analyses were conducted using SUDAAN statistical software (Research Triangle Institute, Research Triangle Park, NC).[16] The study protocol was approved

**Table 2. Unmet Health Care Needs of Young Adults With and Without Limitations by Insurance Status***

| | Disabling Chronic Condition | | No Disability | |
|---|---|---|---|---|
| | Uninsured | Insured | Uninsured | Insured |
| Delayed medical care owing to cost, % (SE) | 60.2 (3.6) | 14.7 (1.4) | 19.4 (0.6) | 5.4 (0.2) |
| Did not get medical care owing to cost, % (SE) | 48.3 (3.7) | 9.9 (1.0) | 16.1 (0.5) | 3.1 (0.2) |
| Could not afford to fill prescription, % (SE) | 41.4 (3.5) | 12.3 (1.3) | 14.5 (0.5) | 3.8 (0.2) |
| No contact with health professional in past year, % (SE) | 20.5 (3.1) | 7.9 (1.2) | 41.8 (0.8) | 18.6 (0.4) |
| No usual source of care, % (SE) | 45.0 (3.6) | 9.8 (1.1) | 55.8 (0.8) | 16.8 (0.4) |

*Percentages are based on weighted data to represent the civilian noninstitutionalized population in the United States. Data Source: National Center for Health Statistics, National Health Interview Survey 1999 to 2002.

**Table 3. Young Adults and Unmet Health Care Needs: AORs and 95% CIs***

| | AOR (95% CI) | | | | |
|---|---|---|---|---|---|
| Disability /Insurance Status | Delayed Medical Care Owing to Cost | Did Not Get Medical Care Owing to Cost | Could Not Afford to Fill Prescription | No Contact With Health Professional in Past Year | No Usual Source of Care |
| Disabled/uninsured | 8.40 (5.59-12.63) | 7.92 (5.17-12.14) | 4.77 (3.33-6.83) | 2.21 (1.27-3.84) | 6.38 (4.01-10.15) |
| Disabled/insured | † | † | † | † | † |
| No disability/uninsured | 1.58 (1.22-2.05) | 1.92 (1.46-2.51) | 1.32 (1.00-1.73) | 6.72 (4.68-9.65) | 10.75 (7.97-14.50) |
| No disability/insured | 0.32 (0.24-0.42) | 0.28 (0.21-0.39) | 0.32 (0.24-0.42) | 2.56 (1.78-3.67) | 2.11 (1.55-2.86) |

Abbreviations: AOR, adjusted odds ratio; CI, confidence interval.

*Also adjusted for sex, race/ethnicity, age (19-24 years or 25-29 years), marital status, major activity in the prior week, household income, and educational attainment. Data Source: National Center for Health Statistics, National Health Interview Survey 1999 to 2002.

†Reference.

by the institutional review board of Vanderbilt University (Nashville, Tenn).

## RESULTS

### DISABLING CHRONIC CONDITIONS AND UNINSURANCE

Among young adults participating in the NHIS from 1999 to 2002, 4.7% had a disabling chronic condition. Of this group, 64% reported a work limitation or inability to work. The chronic conditions most frequently leading to disability included musculoskeletal problems (33%), emotional problems including depression and anxiety (18%), and lung problems including asthma (12%).

Compared with peers without disability, young adults with disabling chronic conditions were poorer, reported lower educational attainment, and were less likely to be working (Table 1). Uninsurance rates were not significantly different for young adults with and without disabling chronic conditions (26% and 28%, respectively); however, young adults with disabling chronic conditions were more likely to have Medicaid and less likely to be privately insured.

### UNMET HEALTH CARE NEEDS/HEALTH CARE ACCESS

Uninsured young adults with disabling chronic conditions were 4 times more likely than insured young adults with disability to report unmet health care needs and no usual source of health care, and 2 times more likely to have no health professional contact in the last year (Table 2). Over two thirds of young adults with disabling chronic conditions either delayed or missed needed care owing to the high cost and 45% identified no usual source of care.

After controlling for sociodemographic characteristics, uninsured young adults with disabling chronic conditions had 8 times higher odds of delaying or missing needed care than insured young adults with disabling chronic conditions (Table 3). The uninsured with disabling chronic conditions also had twice the odds of having no health professional contact and 6 times the odds of having no usual source of health care relative to insured peers. The odds of delaying or failing to get medical care owing to cost were more than 20-fold greater for uninsured young adults with disabling chronic conditions than for insured young adults without disability.

## COMMENT

In this study, we demonstrated that uninsurance is common among young adults with disabling chronic conditions and that it is significantly associated with barriers to health care access. Five percent of young adults reported that they had a disabling chronic condition, corresponding to an estimated 2 million young adults nationally. The estimates from this study are similar to those by the US Census Bureau (5.3% of 15- to 24-year-olds).[17] In studies of children and adults, individuals with disabling chronic conditions have been shown to have higher health care use than healthy peers or those with chronic conditions or disability alone.[18,19]

Given their presumed greater need for health care services, it is troubling that 1 of every 4 young adults with a disabling chronic condition reported being uninsured. This proportion was essentially the same as that of young adults without disability. We would anticipate that young adults with disabling chronic conditions would have greater incentive to maintain health insurance coverage than peers without disability, however, the findings of this study suggest several reasons that these young adults may have particular difficulty doing so. Young adults with disabilities were significantly worse off than peers without disability in terms of poverty, educational attainment, and employment—all socioeconomic characteristics associated with uninsurance and poor health care access.[9,20-26] Most young adults obtain private insurance through employment-based coverage or dependent coverage as a full-time student. Only 54% of young adults with disabling chronic conditions were attending school or working, which may explain why only 40% of these young adults hold private health insurance coverage.

Medicaid and other public insurance programs play an important role in covering children with disabling chronic conditions, however, these public programs are frequently much more limited in size and scope for adults. For example, more stringent adult requirements mean that about one third of older adolescents who qualify for Supplemental Security Income as children will lose these benefits during a redetermination process at age 19.[27] Adult applicants for Supplemental Security Income must demonstrate an inability to work and have a monthly income of no more than $700.[28] Because many young adults with disabling chronic conditions are able to work (including 45% of the young adults in this study), meeting the requirements for Supplemental Security Income benefits as an adult may be particularly difficult.[29] State Children's Health Insurance Plan may provide coverage for some young adults with disabling chronic conditions, however, increasing budget deficits and resultant cutbacks by some states may further limit the availability of this coverage.[30]

Uninsurance was associated with health care access barriers for all young adults, but particularly for those with disabling chronic conditions. Uninsured young adults with disabling chronic conditions had 8 times greater adjusted odds of reporting unmet health care needs and 6 times greater odds of having no usual source of care relative to insured respondents with disabling chronic conditions. In this population, delayed or forgone care may represent missed opportunities to improve functioning, provide preventive services, or delay disease progression. Nearly half of uninsured young adults with disabling chronic conditions did not identify a usual source of health care. Beyond being a necessary component for transitioning young adults to developmentally appropriate care, lacking a usual source of care has been associated with poorer access to preventive services, longer hospitalizations, and increased use of emergency departments.[31-33]

The findings of this study should be considered in light of several limitations. These analyses rely on self-report and may be subject to recall or response error. Because the data are derived from a cross-sectional survey, we are limited in our ability to conclude that uninsurance resulted in the reported unmet health care needs. Finally, we would have preferred to analyze differences in unmet health care needs among those with different types of health insurance coverage (Medicaid, private, etc), but had insufficient sample size to support this level of analyses.

## CONCLUSION

Five percent of young adults in this study had a disabling chronic condition. Despite increasing attention to issues of health care transition for young adults with disabling chronic conditions, the results of this study suggest that uninsurance is as common for young adults with disabling chronic conditions as for those without disability. Moreover, the uninsured disproportionately experience health care access barriers. Improving health insurance coverage options and ensuring continuity of coverage during young adulthood may improve health care access in this population. Additional research is needed to identify barriers to maintaining health insurance coverage and the financial and health effects of barriers to health care for young adults with disabling chronic conditions.

**Accepted for Publication:** August 11, 2005.
**Correspondence:** S. Todd Callahan, MD, MPH, Division of Adolescent Medicine, Vanderbilt Children's Hospital, 11119 Doctors' Office Tower, Nashville, TN 37232 (todd.callahan@vanderbilt.edu).
**Funding/Support:** This study was supported in part by the Vanderbilt Physician-Scientist Development Program (Dr Callahan).

## REFERENCES


1. Blum RW. Transition to adult health care: setting the stage. *J Adolesc Health.* 1995;17:3-5.
2. United States Dept of Health and Human Services. *Healthy People 2010.* Available at: http://www.health.gov/healthypeople. Accessed January 25, 2005.
3. Maternal and Child Health Bureau. Achieving and measuring success: a national agenda for children with special health care needs. Available at: http://www.mchb.hrsa.gov/programs/specialneeds/measuresuccess.htm. Accessed November 9, 2005.
4. American Academy of Pediatrics; American Academy of Family Physicians; American College of Physicians-American Society of Internal Medicine. A consensus statement on health care transitions for young adults with special health care needs. *Pediatrics.* 2002;110(6 Suppl):1304-1306.
5. Rosen DS, Blum RW, Britto M, Sawyer SM, Siegel DM. Transition to adult health care for adolescents and young adults with chronic conditions: position paper of the Society for Adolescent Medicine. *J Adolesc Health.* 2003;33:309-311.
6. McManus MA, Greaney AM, Newacheck PW. Health insurance status of young adults in the United States. *Pediatrics.* 1989;84:709-716.
7. Markowitz MA, Gold M, Rice T. Determinants of health insurance status among young adults. *Med Care.* 1991;29:6-19.
8. Quinn K, Schoen C, Buatti L. *On Their Own: Young Adults Living Without Health Insurance.* New York, NY: The Commonwealth Fund; 2000.
9. Callahan ST, Cooper WO. Gender and uninsurance among young adults in the United States. *Pediatrics.* 2004;113:291-297.

10. Collins SR, Schoen C, Tenney K. *Rite of Passage? Why Young Adults Become Uninsured and How New Policies Can Help.* New York, NY: The Commonwealth Fund; 2003.
11. Callahan ST, Woods ER, Austin SB, Harris SK. Young adults in Massachusetts: who is at risk of being uninsured? *J Adolesc Health.* 2004;35:425.
12. Callahan ST, Cooper WO. Uninsurance and health care access among young adults in the US. *Pediatrics.* 2005;116:88-95.
13. McManus MA, Newacheck PW, Greaney AM. Young adults with special health care needs: prevalence, severity, and access to health services. *Pediatrics.* 1990; 86:674-682.
14. US Dept of Health and Human Services, National Center for Health Statistics. 2002 National Health Interview Survey Description. Available at: ftp://ftp.cdc.gov/pub/Health_Statistics/NCHS/Dataset_Documentation/NHIS/2000/srvydesc.pdf. Accessed August 1, 2005.
15. Proctor BD, Dalaker J. Current population reports. In: *Poverty in the United States: 2001.* Washington, DC: US Census Bureau; 2002:60-219.
16. Research Triangle Institute. *SUDAAN User's Manual, Release 8.0.* Research Triangle Park, NC: Research Triangle Institute; 2002.
17. Waldrop J, Stern SM. Disability Status: 2000. Census 2000 Brief. Available at: http://www.census.gov/prod/2003pubs/c2kbr-17.pdf. Accessed August 1, 2005.
18. Anderson G, Knickman JR. Changing the chronic care system to meet people's needs. *Health Aff (Millwood).* 2001;20:146-160.
19. Newacheck PW, Inkelas M, Kim SE. Health services use and health care expenditures for children with disabilities. *Pediatrics.* 2004;114:79-85.
20. Davidoff AJ. Insurance for children with special health care needs: patterns of coverage and burden on families to provide adequate insurance. *Pediatrics.* 2004; 114:394-403.
21. Silver EJ, Stein RE. Access to care, unmet health needs, and poverty status among children with and without chronic conditions. *Ambul Pediatr.* 2001;1:314-320.
22. Callahan ST, Cooper WO. Uninsurance and health care access among young adults in the US. *J Adolesc Health.* 2004;34:112-113.
23. Fishman E. Aging out of coverage: young adults with special health needs. *Health Aff (Millwood).* 2001;20:254-266.
24. Newacheck PW, Stoddard JJ, Hughes DC, Pearl M. Health insurance and access to primary care for children. *N Engl J Med.* 1998;338:513-519.
25. Institute of Medicine. *Coverage Matters: Insurance and Health Care.* Washington, DC: National Academy Press; 2001.
26. Institute of Medicine. *Care Without Coverage: Too Little, Too Late.* Washington, DC: National Academy Press; 2002.
27. Schulzinger R. *Youth With Disabilities in Transition: Health Insurance Options and Obstacles.* Gainesville, Fla: Institute for Child Health Policy; 2000.
28. US Social Security Administration. Red book: a summary guide to employment support for people with disabilities under the social security disability insurance and supplemental security income programs. Available at: http://purl.access.gpo.gov/GPO/LPS29365. Accessed August 1, 2005.
29. White PH. Access to health care: health insurance considerations for young adults with special health care needs/disabilities. *Pediatrics.* 2002;110:1328-1335.
30. Tobler L, Folkemer D. Rx for Medicaid: with Medicaid costs rising and revenues declining, states are looking at what to do. *State Legis.* 2003;29:16-20.
31. DeVoe JE, Fryer GE, Phillips R, Green L. Receipt of preventive care among adults: insurance status and usual source of care. *Am J Public Health.* 2003;93:786-791.
32. Hayward RA, Bernard AM, Freeman HE, Corey CR. Regular source of ambulatory care and access to health services. *Am J Public Health.* 1991;81:434-438.
33. Grumbach K, Keane D, Bindman A. Primary care and public emergency department overcrowding. *Am J Public Health.* 1993;83:372-378.

## Announcement

**Submissions.** The Editors welcome contributions to Picture of the Month. Submissions should describe common problems presenting uncommonly, rather than total zebras. Cases should be of interest to practicing pediatricians, highlighting problems that they are likely to at least occasionally encounter in the office or hospital setting. High-quality clinical images (in either 35-mm slide or electronic format) along with parent or patient permission to use these images must accompany the submission. The entire discussion should comprise no more than 750 words. Articles and photographs accepted for publication will bear the contributor's name. There is no charge for reproduction and printing of color illustrations. For details regarding electronic submission, please see: http://archpedi.ama-assn.org.

ARTICLE

# Developmental Status and Service Use Among Children in the Child Welfare System

## *A National Survey*

*Michelle H. Zimmer, MD; Laura M. Panko, MD*

**Objectives:** To estimate the prevalence of developmental delay and service use among children in the child welfare system and to identify factors that influence these outcomes.

**Design:** A descriptive study using wave 1 of the National Survey of Child and Adolescent Well-Being.

**Participants and Setting:** Children aged 0 to 10 years (n=4324) and their caregivers were interviewed within 60 days of a report being made to the child welfare system. Children's development was measured directly using standardized assessment tools. Three questions from the caregiver interviews estimated receipt of developmental services.

**Main Exposures:** Subjects were characterized as having developmental delay if any developmental measure fell more than 2 SDs below the mean. Prevalence of developmental delay and service use by age group, type of maltreatment, type of placement, race, sex, and income were reported. Odds that children aged 0 to 2, 3 to 5, and 6 to 10 years with developmental delay would receive developmental services were calculated using weighted logistic regression.

**Main Outcome Measure:** Receipt of developmental services by children with developmental delay.

**Results:** Younger children aged 0 to 2 and 3 to 5 years had higher rates, 33% and 36%, respectively, of developmental delay than school-aged children (13%) ($P<.01$). Despite their high prevalence of developmental delay, children aged 0 to 2 years were less likely to receive developmental services than preschool-aged children (odds ratio, 2.4; 95% confidence interval, 1.6-3.7) or school-aged children (odds ratio, 4.2; 95% confidence interval, 2.9-6.0).

**Conclusions:** Rates of developmental delay are high and developmental services are underused, particularly by young children in the child welfare system. Strategies for overcoming barriers to using early intervention services should be implemented.

*Arch Pediatr Adolesc Med. 2006;160:183-188*

THE LIVES OF CHILDREN IN the child welfare system are often characterized by exposure to numerous risk factors for developmental delay, including the direct effects of abuse and neglect, poverty, in utero drug exposure, parental substance abuse, and mental health disorders.[1] Studies have estimated that between 13% and 62% of children entering foster care have developmental delay.[2-5] Studies have also looked at developmental delays in clinically referred populations of maltreated children and have found higher rates of cognitive language[6] delays,[7,8] adaptive skill delays,[9] and poorer academic performance[9,10] than nonmaltreated peers.

The influence of potentially important variables such as race, sex, income, type of placement, and type of maltreatment on developmental outcomes has rarely been described for this group of children. Interpretation of the available data is limited by the use of small convenience samples, but it suggests that age group,[10] sex,[11,12] and maltreatment type[7,12,13] may be important predictors of developmental outcome. Less is known about the influence of placement type, income, and race on developmental status.

Methods used in prior studies to describe the rates of developmental delay among children in the child welfare system have serious limitations. Much of the data are based on convenience samples of patients referred to diagnostic clinics because of foster care entry, behavioral problems, or abuse itself. Convenience samples are problematic since they may have an intrinsic bias toward more severe developmental problems and may overestimate the proportion of children in the child welfare system with developmental delay. The

**Author Affiliations:** Child Development Unit (Dr Zimmer) and Department of Pediatrics (Drs Zimmer and Panko), University of Pittsburgh School of Medicine, Pittsburgh, Pa.

**Table 1. Measures Used to Assess Developmental Status of Study Subjects**

| Measure | Age, y 0-2 | 3-5 | 6-10 |
|---|---|---|---|
| Cognitive development | | | |
| Batelle Developmental Inventory cognitive subscale | * | * (3-4 y) | † |
| Kaufman Brief Intelligence Test | † | * (5 y) | * |
| Language development | | | |
| Preschool Language Scale (ages 0-5 y) | * | * | † |
| Woodcock-Johnson Tests of Achievement reading subscale (ages 6-10 y) | † | † | * |
| Adaptive skills | | | |
| Vineland Adaptive Behavior Scales daily living subscale (ages 0-10 y) | * | * | * |

*The tests were administered to the age group.
†The tests were not administered to the age group.

method of measuring development has varied considerably from study to study, with various cutoff scores between 1.0 and 2.5 SDs below the mean being used to define developmental delay. This makes it difficult to compare rates of delay from study to study.

Early intervention developmental services are important for minimizing poor developmental outcomes for children at risk.[14,15] Despite the importance of these services, there are few published data regarding the use of developmental services by children in the child welfare system. This is surprising given the fact that the federal government has mandated availability of early intervention developmental services to any child aged 0 to 5 years with an open child welfare case. One would expect that the rates of developmental service use would be very high among this population given this free federal mandate. However, our clinical experience suggests that the rate of developmental service use among this population is very low.

The National Survey of Child and Adolescent Well-Being (NSCAW) is the first publicly available data set to assess the health, development, and service use of a nationally representative sample of children and their caregivers who have come into contact with the child welfare system. This data set provides a unique opportunity to examine the prevalence of developmental delay, service use, and factors that influence developmental outcomes among this population. This data would allow appropriate care providers and policy makers to better understand the scope and severity of this problem and to design strategies to assess shortfalls in the system.

In summary, children in the child welfare system may be at risk for developmental delay, but accurate prevalence data and identification of factors that influence developmental status are lacking. Furthermore, rates of developmental service use among this high-risk population are rarely described in the literature. Therefore, the objectives of this study are to estimate the prevalence of developmental delay and developmental service use among children in the child welfare system and to identify factors that influence developmental delay and use of these services.

## METHODS

### STUDY DESIGN AND SUBJECTS

This is a descriptive study using wave 1 of the NSCAW. The NSCAW database collected information from 5504 children aged 0 to 14 years and their caregivers who were reported to the child welfare system because of a concern regarding abuse or neglect. Developmental measures and caregiver interviews were performed within 60 days of the close of the child welfare investigations. Many children remained in the home of their permanent caregivers or parents after the investigations, but if the child was living in an out-of-home placement, attempts were made to interview both the current and permanent caregivers. Since complete developmental measures were available for children aged 0 to 10 years, the analysis was constrained to children aged 0 to 10 years (n=4324).

### SURVEY DESIGN

Children were selected using a 2-stage stratified sampling design. The primary sampling units were county child welfare agencies from across the United States. The secondary sampling units were children randomly selected from lists of closed child welfare investigations from within those agencies. The sample was divided into 9 strata, 1 stratum for each of 8 key states and 1 stratum for combined data from 28 other states. Analysis weights were constructed to produce national estimates based on probability that a child would be selected from a primary sampling unit and a county within that primary sampling unit. Further details regarding the sampling design and weighting procedure are published in the NSCAW user's manual.[16] The data analysis protocol was approved by the University of Pittsburgh institutional review board.

### STUDY MEASURES

Measures used to assess cognitive, language, and adaptive skill development of the study participants are presented in **Table 1**. A subject was categorized as having developmental delay if a standard score on any developmental measure was less than 70 (2 SDs below the mean); otherwise, the subject was classified as not having developmental delay.

Three questions from the caregiver interviews were chosen to estimate receipt of developmental services: (1) Was the child ever evaluated by a medical or educational professional for a learning problem or developmental delay? (2) Is the child receiving any special education services? and (3) Does the child have an Individualized Education Plan or Individualized Family Service Plan?

Subjects were categorized by age group: 0 to 2, 3 to 5, and 6 to 10 years. These categories were chosen because they reflect the usual age cutoffs for delivery of developmental services through early intervention programs, including infant and toddler programs (ages 0-2 years), Head Start or Child Find programs (ages 3-5 years), and school-based developmental services (ages ≥6 years).

Child welfare workers were asked detailed questions about the specific nature of the alleged maltreatment. Data were coded. Then, independent raters used a modified Maltreatment Classification Scale[17] to determine maltreatment types, including physical abuse, sexual abuse, emotional abuse, neglect, and other maltreatment. This scale is used in numerous research laboratories to operationalize maltreatment types into consistent categories.[18]

Subjects were classified as living in 1 of 4 possible placements: at home, with a nonrelative foster parent, with relative foster parents (kinship care), or in a group home.

**Table 2. Sample Characteristics, Developmental Status, and Prevalence of Developmental Delay Among Children Aged 0 to 10 Years Who Were the Subjects of Child Welfare Investigations**

| | With Developmental Delay, No. (%) | | Using Developmental Services, No. (%) | |
|---|---|---|---|---|
| Characteristic | Yes | No | Yes | No |
| Total | 1118 (24) | 3206 (76) | 1326 (33) | 2998 (67) |
| Demographic characteristics | | | | |
| Age, y | | | | |
| 0-2 (n = 1998) | 564 (37) | 1434 (63) | 370 (16) | 1628 (84) |
| 3-5 (n = 834) | 280 (33) | 554 (67) | 259 (31) | 575 (69) |
| 6-10 (n = 1492) | 274 (13) | 1218 (87) | 697 (44) | 795 (56) |
| Race/ethnicity | | | | |
| African American (n = 1409) | 371 (23) | 1038 (77) | 418 (32) | 991 (68) |
| White (n = 1838) | 444 (22) | 1394 (78) | 621 (38) | 1217 (62) |
| Hispanic (n = 774) | 240 (34) | 534 (66) | 194 (22) | 580 (78) |
| Other (n = 293) | 61 (21) | 232 (79) | 88 (39) | 205 (61) |
| Sex | | | | |
| Female (n = 2089) | 485 (23) | 1604 (77) | 749 (29) | 1486 (71) |
| Male (n = 2235) | 633 (26) | 1602 (74) | 577 (38) | 1512 (62) |
| Income | | | | |
| No government assistance (n = 2656) | 687 (23) | 1969 (77) | 840 (32) | 1816 (68) |
| Government assistance (n = 1661) | 431 (26) | 1230 (74) | 483 (36) | 1178 (64) |
| Type of placement | | | | |
| Parent home (n = 3188) | 786 (24) | 2402 (76) | 907 (33) | 2281 (67) |
| Nonrelative home (n = 631) | 208 (27) | 423 (73) | 256 (35) | 375 (65) |
| Kinship care (n = 458) | 106 (27) | 352 (73) | 139 (33) | 319 (67) |
| Group home (n = 47) | 13 (64) | 18 (36) | 17 (39) | 14 (61) |
| Maltreatment type | | | | |
| Physical abuse (n = 913) | 270 (28) | 643 (72) | 299 (38) | 614 (63) |
| Sexual abuse (n = 463) | 109 (18) | 354 (82) | 141 (38) | 322 (72) |
| Emotional abuse (n = 273) | 64 (22) | 209 (78) | 77 (27) | 196 (73) |
| Neglect (n = 2015) | 516 (25) | 1499 (75) | 613 (33) | 1402 (67) |
| Other (n = 286) | 75 (28) | 211 (72) | 86 (31) | 200 (69) |

Caregivers reported the child's race. Data were collapsed into 4 categories: white, African American, Hispanic, and other races.

Caregivers were asked whether anyone in the home receives government assistance, including assistance from the Special Supplemental Nutrition Program for Women, Infants, and Children, assistance from the Temporary Assistance to Needy Families program, food stamps, housing support, or a disability check. A dichotomous variable was created to indicate whether anyone in the home receives government assistance.

## DATA ANALYSIS

Sample weights were used in all of the calculations using the survey set function of the Stata release 8 software (Stata Corp, College Station, Tex). The survey prop command was used to tabulate all of the proportions. The survey logit command was used to calculate odds ratios. To account for the complex survey design, a Wald correction was used, and statistical significance was set at $P<.01$.[19]

## RESULTS

### SUBJECT CHARACTERISTICS

Infants aged 0 to 2 years represented 46% of the sample (n=1998), preschoolers aged 3 to 5 years represented 19% (n=834), and school-aged children aged 6 to 10 years accounted for 35% (n=1492). Boys represented 52% of the study sample. Forty-two percent were white and non-Hispanic subjects, 33% were African American and non-Hispanic subjects, 18% were Hispanic subjects, and 7% were subjects of other races and ethnicities. Reasons that the youth came to the attention of the child welfare system included alleged neglect (47%), physical abuse (21%), sexual abuse (11%), emotional abuse (6%), and other types of abuse (7%). Sixty-three percent of the reports made to child welfare authorities resulted in a substantiated report of abuse or neglect. For the remaining 37% of the cases, either child welfare authorities could not gather enough information to name a perpetrator or the report was not deemed to rise to the level of abuse or neglect. Many children (74%) remained in the homes of their parents, 15% were living in foster homes, 11% were living with relative foster parents (kinship care), and 1% were living in group homes or other out-of-home facilities.

### DEVELOPMENTAL STATUS AND SERVICE USE

**Table 2** examines the prevalence of developmental delay and service use as well as whether these outcomes varied by age group, race, sex, income, type of child maltreatment, or placement status. Twenty-four percent were developmentally delayed on at least 1 measure. In the bivariate analysis, only age group was a significant predictor of developmental delay. Younger children aged 0 to

**Table 3. Odds of Developmental Service Use by Older Children Compared With Children Aged 0 to 2 Years in the Child Welfare System**

| Age, y | Any Service, OR (95% CI) | Developmental Evaluation, OR (95% CI) | IEP or IFSP, OR (95% CI) | Special Education, OR (95% CI) |
|---|---|---|---|---|
| 3-5 (n = 280; 33%) | 2.4 (1.6-3.7) | 2.5 (1.6-3.7) | 2.8 (1.4-5.8) | 3.0 (1.2-7.2) |
| 6-10 (n = 274; 13%) | 4.2 (2.9-6.0) | 4.1 (2.9-5.9) | 7.5 (4.0-14.1) | 7.2 (3.3-16.1) |

Abbreviations: CI, confidence interval; IEP, Individualized Education Plan; IFSP, Individualized Family Service Plan; OR, odds ratio.

2 and 3 to 5 years had higher rates of developmental delay, 33% and 36%, respectively, than school-aged children (13%) ($P<.01$ for both age groups). Race, sex, income, type of child maltreatment, and placement status did not have a significant impact on developmental scores or service use ($P>.05$ for all of the variables).

## USE OF DEVELOPMENTAL SERVICES AMONG CHILDREN WITH DEVELOPMENTAL DELAY

Developmental services were underused by all of the age groups. Overall, about 24% of the assessed children exhibited developmental delay, but only 38% of children with delay were using developmental services. This underuse of services appeared to be most dramatic for the youngest children, with only 20% of children aged 0 to 2 years with developmental delay, 38% of children aged 3 to 5 years with delay, and 57% of children aged 6 to 10 years with delay receiving any developmental services.

**Table 3** confirms the underuse of services by the youngest children in the sample using odds ratios, comparing service use by children aged 0 to 2 years with developmental delay vs older age groups. Children aged 3 to 5 years with delay were 2.4 times more likely to be using developmental services than children aged 0 to 2 years (95% confidence interval, 1.6-3.7). Children aged 6 to 10 years with delay were 4.2 times as likely to be using these services as compared with children aged 0 to 2 years (95% confidence interval, 2.9-6.0).

## COMMENT

Data from the NSCAW is a unique opportunity to provide national estimates of developmental status and service use among the child welfare population. Our analysis confirms the reports of high rates of developmental delay from previous studies of foster care[2-5] and maltreated children.[6-13] In our analysis, 24% of children in the child welfare system had developmental delay. The youngest children were particularly vulnerable, with 33% of infants and 36% of preschoolers having developmental delay. Developmental services were underused by all of the age groups, but children aged 0 to 2 years with delay were significantly less likely to use services than older children.

One striking finding of this study was the higher prevalence of developmental delay among the youngest children, those aged 0 to 5 years. This finding is consistent with the study by Urquiza et al[5] that measured the cognitive development of children entering protective custody. Urquiza and colleagues found higher rates of cognitive delay among children aged 0 to 2 years (45%) in comparison with older children as measured by the Bayley Scales of Infant Development.

In our analysis, factors other than age group did not account for any variability in developmental outcomes. Although our analysis failed to identify these factors, it is still likely that the reasons for the increased rate of developmental problems among this population are multifactorial. Potential factors might include the home environment and maladaptive parenting practices, including lack of exposure to age-appropriate developmental activities or poor parenting practices that do not reinforce the child's emerging developmental skills. It is possible that young children are more susceptible than older children to poor developmental outcomes because parents are often the sole caregivers for children until they enter the public school system. Other studies[20-24] highlight the importance of the home environment in promoting positive child developmental outcomes. By school age, children in abusive or neglectful homes are exposed to teachers and other caring adults who may act as protective factors, buffering the effects of maltreatment. Unfortunately, for many young children, there is no such adult in the child's life to provide the needed nurturing and developmental stimulation.

The fact that the rates of developmental delay did not vary by subtype of abuse is inconsistent with previous data suggesting that child neglect was a larger risk factor for developmental delay than other subtypes of maltreatment.[6,8,10-13] For example, Fox et al[25] compared a referred population of abused and neglected children with controls of similar socioeconomic background. Control children had the highest language scores, with all of the groups of abuse and neglect having significantly lower language scores. Severe neglect emerged as the worst prognostic language indicator. The reason for this discrepancy in findings from previous research is interesting but cannot be fully explained by this analysis. Future studies might look at a severity-of-neglect index to determine whether children with more severe degrees of neglect are more likely to experience developmental problems.

There are several potential explanations for underuse of developmental services by children aged 0 to 2 years with developmental delay in the child welfare system. One explanation is that health care and child welfare professionals are not adequately identifying the developmental needs of these young children and are not making referrals to early intervention. Furthermore, these professionals may not be aware of the federal law mandating availability of early intervention services to young children in the child welfare system. Leslie et al[26] investigated whether child welfare agencies had comprehensive policies for assessing the health and developmental status of children entering foster care, and they found that only 58% of the primary sampling units that were interviewed had policies regarding child development and only 42% provided developmental examinations. This finding suggests that child development issues are not being prioritized in many child welfare agencies. Another potential reason for underuse of services may be a reflection of the way in which the NSCAW questioned caregivers about the use of developmental services. The questions asked whether the child was evaluated by an educational or child development professional, whether the child had an Individualized Education Plan or Individualized Family Service Plan, or whether the child was receiving special education services. Although an evaluation by a child development professional and development of an Individualized Family Service Plan are typical procedures undertaken when a child is enrolled in early intervention, the NSCAW survey did not directly ask whether the child was involved in early intervention services. This line of questioning may have resulted in underreporting developmental service use by this age group. Further studies that directly assess developmental service use by parent report or linking early intervention databases to child welfare databases would help to answer this question.

The underuse of developmental services by children with clear developmental delay in the child welfare system is a travesty, particularly in light of the fact that federal legislation made these children automatically eligible for services. Our study used a very conservative cutoff for identifying developmental delay. Children were considered delayed if their developmental functioning was more than 2 SDs below average. This level of developmental delay in a child is usually not subtle and could easily be identified by persons who are regularly in contact with children.

Why are so many of these children not receiving services that are clearly needed? The answer is not completely clear, but many potential barriers to receiving early intervention services exist, including social isolation of families living in abusive homes and lack of knowledge of services available to their children. One could argue that once a child welfare professional becomes involved, the professional would identify the needs of the child and ensure that these services are put into place. With regard to developmental services, this does not appear to be happening at an acceptable rate. Children who enter foster care have another set of barriers and challenges to receiving health and developmental services. Children are often brought for health care visits by foster parents or caseworkers who are unfamiliar with the children's baseline developmental statuses. Prior health records are difficult to obtain and require consent from biological parents, making analysis of baseline developmental status challenging. In many cases, children change primary health care providers when they enter foster care. These providers are unfamiliar with the children, trying to gather basic information about the children's health statuses and visit histories rather than focusing on development.

Our findings suggest that federal laws making early intervention services available to children in the child welfare system have had little impact. Our current systems of care are failing to detect and refer this vulnerable group of children to services that provide the potential for improved developmental outcomes. This is disturbing, particularly given the growing number of children entering foster care[27] and the fact that over 1.7 million children per year are involved in the child welfare system.[28]

New strategies that might impact service use and outcomes are needed. One strategy is to empower physicians caring for children to assume a higher level of responsibility as the medical home for these vulnerable children. It may be beneficial for child health care providers to develop a system for automatically making referrals to early intervention for these children and to develop internal systems within their own practice to follow up on these referrals. Education of child welfare workers about the high prevalence of developmental delay for children in their care and the positive impact of early intervention services on outcomes is another potentially important strategy. On a systems level, child welfare agencies might examine their policies toward training caseworkers about the availability of early intervention services and begin conversations with early intervention agencies to break down communication barriers that exist between these 2 systems. Early intervention providers could develop strategies for reducing the administrative burden that prevents foster parents from enrolling children in early intervention services. Foster parents are often allowed to sign children into school but are not given the same rights to ensure that children under their care are in early intervention services.

In conclusion, this study shows that lack of service use for developmental delay is a significant problem in the child welfare population. Strategies for overcoming barriers to using early intervention services should be implemented.

**Accepted for Publication:** August 22, 2005.
**Correspondence:** Michelle H. Zimmer, MD, Division of Developmental and Behavioral Pediatrics, Cincinnati Children's Hospital Medical Center, 3333 Burnet Ave, Cincinnati, OH 45229 (michelle.zimmer@cchmc.org).
**Author Contributions:** Dr Zimmer had full access to all of the data in the study and takes responsibility for the integrity of the data and the accuracy of the data analysis.
**Acknowledgment:** This document includes data from the National Survey on Child and Adolescent Well-Being, which was developed under contract with the Administration for Children and Families, US Department of Health and Human Services, Washington, DC.

## REFERENCES

1. American Academy of Pediatrics; Committee on Early Childhood, Adoption and Dependent Care. Heath care of young children in foster care. *Pediatrics*. 2002; 109:536-540.
2. Simms MD. The foster care clinic: a community program to identify treatment needs of children in foster care. *J Dev Behav Pediatr*. 1989;10:121-128.

3. Leslie LK, Gordon JN, Ganger W, Gist K. Developmental delay in young children in child welfare by initial placement type. *Infant Ment Health J.* 2002;23:496-516.
4. Hochstadt NJ, Jaudes PK, Zimo DA, Schachter J. The medical and psychosocial needs of children entering foster care. *Child Abuse Negl.* 1987;11:53-62.
5. Urquiza AJ, Wirtz SJ, Peterson MS, Singer VA. Screening and evaluating abused and neglected children entering protective custody. *Child Welfare.* 1994;73:155-171.
6. Dietrich KN, Starr RH Jr, Weisfeld GE. Infant maltreatment: caretaker-infant interaction and developmental consequences at different levels of parenting failure. *Pediatrics.* 1983;72:532-540.
7. Allen RE, Oliver JM. The effects of child maltreatment on language development. *Child Abuse Negl.* 1982;6:299-305.
8. Eckenrode J, Laird M, Doris J. School performance and disciplinary problems among abused and neglected children. *Dev Psychol.* 1993;29:53-62.
9. Wodarski JS, Kurtz PD, Gaudin JM Jr, Howing PT. Maltreatment and the school-age child: major academic, socioemotional and adaptive outcomes. *Soc Work.* 1990;35:506-513.
10. Cicchetti D, Toth SL. A developmental psychopathology perspective on child abuse and neglect. *J Am Acad Child Adolesc Psychiatry.* 1995;34:541-565.
11. Rogeness GA, Amrung SA, Macedo CA, Harris WR, Fisher C. Psychopathology in abused and neglected children. *J Am Acad Child Psychiatry.* 1986;25:659-665.
12. Kendall-Tackett K. Timing of academic difficulties for neglected and nonmaltreated males and females. *Child Abuse Negl.* 1997;21:885-887.
13. Kendall-Tackett KA, Eckenrode J. The effects of neglect on academic achievement and disciplinary problems: a developmental perspective. *Child Abuse Negl.* 1996;20:161-169.
14. Karoly LA, Greenwood PW, Everingham SS, et al. *Investing in Our Children: What We Know and Don't Know About the Costs and Benefits of Early Childhood Interventions.* Santa Monica, Calif: Rand Corp; 1998.
15. Guralnick MJ. The effectiveness of early intervention for vulnerable children: a developmental perspective. *Am J Ment Retard.* 1998;102:319-345.
16. Dowd K, Kinsey S, Wheeless S, Suresh R; NSCAW Research Group. *National Survey of Child and Adolescent Well-Being (NSCAW): Wave 1 Data File User's Manual.* Research Triangle Park, NC: Research Triangle Institute; 2002.
17. Manly JT, Cicchetti D, Barnett D. The impact of subtype, frequency, chronicity and severity of child maltreatment on social competence and behavior problems. *Dev Psychopathol.* 1994;6:121-143.
18. Barnett D, Manly JT, Cicchetti D. Defining child maltreatment: the interface between policy and research. In: Cicchetti D, Toth SL, eds. *Child Abuse, Child Development, and Social Policy.* Norwood, NJ: Ablex Publishing Corp; 1993:7-73.
19. StataCorp. *Stata Survey Data Reference Manual: Release 8.* College Station, Tex: Stata Corp; 2003.
20. Casey PH, Bradley RH. The impact of the home environment on children's development: clinical relevance for the pediatrician. *J Dev Behav Pediatr.* 1982;3:146-152.
21. Bradley RH, Caldwell BM, Rock SL. Home environment and school performance: a ten-year follow-up and examination of three models of environmental action. *Child Dev.* 1988;59:852-867.
22. Bradley RH, Caldwell BM. The relation of infants' home environments to achievement test performance in first grade: a follow-up study. *Child Dev.* 1984;55:803-809.
23. McCulloch A, Joshi HE. Neighbourhood and family influences on the cognitive ability of children in the British National Child Development Study. *Soc Sci Med.* 2001;53:579-591.
24. Eu B, O'Neill MJ. Development of the pre-school child: the validation of a psychomotor screen, and the influence of the home environment on psychomotor development. *Aust Paediatr J.* 1983;19:78-85.
25. Fox L, Long SH, Langlois A. Patterns of language comprehension deficit in abused and neglected children. *J Speech Hear Disord.* 1988;53:239-244.
26. Leslie LK, Hurlburt MS, Landsverk J, Rolls JA, Wood PA, Kelleher KJ. Comprehensive assessments for children entering foster care: a national perspective. *Pediatrics.* 2003;112:134-142.
27. Child Welfare League of America. Family foster care fact sheet. Available at: http://cwla.org/programs/fostercare/factsheet.htm. Accessed May 2005.
28. US Dept of Health and Human Services Administration for Children Youth and Families. *Child Mistreatment.* Washington, DC: US Dept of Health and Human Services: 2000.

***Announcement***

**Topic Collections**. The *Archives* offers collections of articles in specific topic areas to make it easier for physicians to find the most recent publications in a field. These are available by subspecialty, study type, disease, or problem. In addition, you can sign up to receive a Collection E-Mail Alert when new articles on specific topics are published. Go to http://archpedi.ama-assn.org/collections to see these collections of articles.

SECTION EDITOR: ALBERT C. YAN, MD; ASSISTANT SECTION EDITOR: SAMIR S. SHAH, MD

# Picture of the Month

*Kimberly A. Horii, MD; Amy Jo Nopper, MD; Vidya Sharma, MBBS, MPH*

A RASH (**FIGURE 1** AND **FIGURE 2**) WAS noted in a 2-month-old infant who presented with a 4-week history of erythematous, annular patches and plaques concentrated on the face and periorbital areas. The cutaneous eruption appeared to be asymptomatic, and the infant was otherwise thriving.

What is your diagnosis?

**Author Affiliations:** Section of Dermatology, Children's Mercy Hospital, Kansas City, Mo.

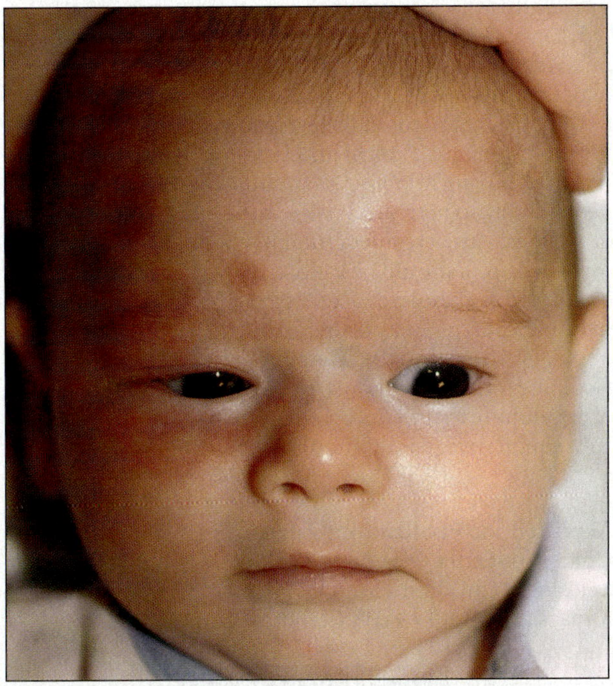

**Figure 1.** Erythematous, annular plaques concentrated around the eyes, giving the characteristic "owl's-eye" appearance.

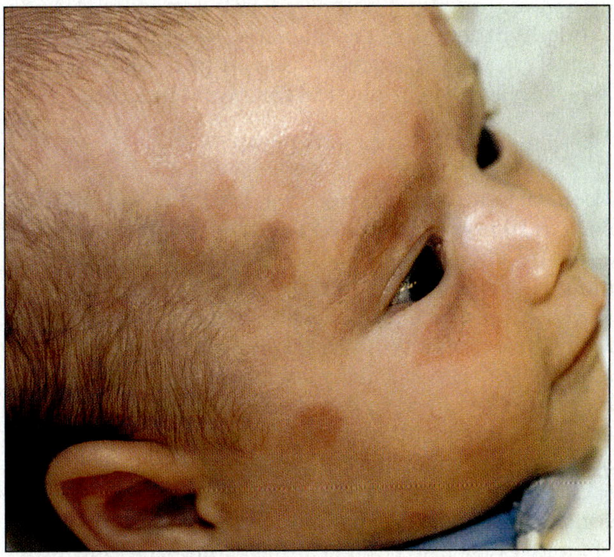

**Figure 2.** Lesions seen in profile.

# Denouement and Discussion

## *Neonatal Lupus Erythematosus*

A 2-month-old, white, male infant had a 1-month history of a rash that began on the left face and spread to involve the scalp and right lower abdomen. According to his mother, the lesions appeared to be exacerbated by sun exposure. Prenatal and medical history were unremarkable. There was no family history of rheumatologic or autoimmune disease. Aside from the skin eruption noted, the results of the remainder of the physical examination were normal with no evidence of cardiac abnormalities or hepatosplenomegaly. A complete blood cell count with differential, liver enzyme profile, and a basic chemistry panel were all normal, and a skin fungal culture was negative. Antinuclear antibody (titer of 1:320) and anti-La/SSB antibody were both positive, but surprisingly, anti-Ro/SSA antibody was negative. Complete cardiac evaluation results were normal, including a normal electrocardiogram and echocardiogram. Although his mother was clinically asymptomatic, she also had a positive antinuclear antibody and anti-La/SSB antibody but negative anti-Ro/SSA antibody and negative double-stranded DNA. By 4 months of age, all of the cutaneous lesions had resolved spontaneously with aggressive sun protection, and no new clinical symptoms or physical findings were noted.

### BACKGROUND

Neonatal lupus erythematosus was first described in a newborn in 1954 by McCuistion and Schoch,[1] and it may occur as infrequently as 1 in 20 000 births.[2] It is an uncommon, passively acquired autoimmune disease associated with the transplacental passage of maternal autoantibodies, in most cases anti-Ro/SSA and/or anti-La/SSB antibodies.[2] These transplacentally acquired maternal autoantibodies are believed to cause cell injury leading to the development of clinical disease.[2] Mothers of infants with neonatal lupus may have a known autoimmune disease such as lupus erythematosus, Sjögren syndrome, or mixed connective tissue disease; however, a sizable proportion of mothers can also be clinically asymptomatic. Owing to the subtle and varied clinical presentation of neonatal lupus, a diagnosis can be difficult to make.

### CLINICAL FEATURES AND MANAGEMENT

The clinical features of neonatal lupus can include cutaneous, cardiac, hepatic, and hematologic abnormalities. The skin eruption may be present at birth or can present during the first several weeks of life, most commonly on the head and neck, with frequent accentuation in the periorbital distribution.[3,4] Classically, the cutaneous lesions are annular erythematous plaques with scale that may be exacerbated by sun exposure.[3,4] The rash is often misdiagnosed as tinea corporis or atopic dermatitis.[4] The lesions usually resolve spontaneously over several months, but they occasionally may leave residual atrophy or telangiectasia. The most severe and life-threatening clinical manifestation of neonatal lupus is third-degree congenital heart block, which can be detected in utero during the second or third trimester.[2] Hepatobiliary and hematologic involvement may be asymptomatic and detected only through laboratory evaluation during the first several months of life.[5,6] Rarely, severe liver failure may occur in the neonatal period.[7] Although neurologic abnormalities are not a clinical feature of neonatal lupus, transient asymptomatic brain abnormalities have been detected on computed tomographic scan in several infants with neonatal lupus.[8]

Infants and their mothers will usually have positive anti-Ro/SSA antibodies, will less commonly have positive anti-La/SSB antibodies, and will rarely have a positive anti-U1RNP antibody.[2,6] Other laboratory abnormalities detected during infancy can include anemia, thrombocytopenia, neutropenia, and elevation of hepatic transaminases, $\gamma$-glutamyltransferase, or conjugated bilirubin.[5-7]

All infants with suspected neonatal lupus should receive laboratory screening for the presence of autoantibodies and hematologic or hepatic involvement as well a thorough cardiac evaluation. Neonates with congenital heart block may require pacemaker implantation. Except for those infants with congenital heart block, clinical symptoms are usually transient and resolve by age 6 to 9 months.[4,5] Often, only aggressive broad-spectrum (UV-A and UV-B) photoprotection and clinical and laboratory monitoring are required during infancy.[2] Infants and children do not appear to be at an increased risk of developing autoimmune disease as a direct result of their history of neonatal lupus; however, they should be followed up closely throughout childhood and adolescence since their overall risk of rheumatologic disease may be increased relative to the general population because of their familial predisposition.[9] Asymptomatic mothers of infants with neonatal lupus are at risk of developing rheumatologic disease in the future, and any subsequent pregnancy should be monitored closely.[4-6]

**Accepted for Publication:** August 1, 2005.
**Correspondence:** Kimberly A. Horii, MD, Section of Dermatology, Children's Mercy Hospital, 2401 Gillham Rd, Kansas City, MO 64108 (kahorii@cmh.edu).

### REFERENCES

1. McCuistion CH, Schoch EP Jr. Possible discoid lupus erythematosus in newborn infant. *AMA Arch Derm Syphilol.* 1954;70:782-785.
2. Lee LA. Neonatal lupus erythematosus. *J Investig Dermatol Symp Proc.* 2004;9:52-56.
3. Weston WL, Morelli JG, Lee LA. The clinical spectrum of anti-Ro-positive cutaneous neonatal lupus erythematosus. *J Am Acad Dermatol.* 1999;40:675-681.
4. Neiman AR, Lee LA, Weston WL, Buyon JP. Cutaneous manifestations of neonatal lupus without heart block. *J Pediatr.* 2000;137:674-680.
5. Cimaz R, Spence DL, Hornberger L, Silverman ED. Incidence and spectrum of neonatal lupus erythematosus. *J Pediatr.* 2003;142:678-683.
6. Lee LA. Neonatal lupus. *Paediatr Drugs.* 2004;6:71-78.
7. Lee LA, Sokol RJ, Buyon JP. Hepatobiliary disease in neonatal lupus. *Pediatrics.* 2002;109:e11.
8. Prendiville JS, Cabral DA, Poskitt KJ, Au S, Sargent MA. Central nervous system involvement in neonatal lupus erythematosus. *Pediatr Dermatol.* 2003;20:60-67.
9. Martin V, Lee LA, Askanase AD, Katholi M, Buyon JP. Long-term followup of children with neonatal lupus and their unaffected siblings. *Arthritis Rheum.* 2002;46:2377-2383.

ARTICLE

# A Successful International Child Health Elective

## *The University of Colorado Department of Pediatrics' Experience*

*Steven G. Federico, MD; Pamela A. Zachar, MD; Claire M. Oravec; Tessa Mandler; Edward Goldson, MD; Jeff Brown, MD, MPH*

**Objectives:** To describe the organizational features of an international child health elective (ICHE) and to document the diversity of diagnoses observed by residents.

**Design:** Faculty from the Department of Pediatrics, University of Colorado Health Sciences Center, Denver, created a steering committee in 1999 to develop and direct an ICHE, including selecting residents, selecting and organizing sites, and creating objectives and a year-long preparatory curriculum. The elective was piloted in 2000 and repeated in 2002 and 2004.

**Setting and Participants:** Residents chose from 4 ICHE sites in Peru and Guatemala, where they observed clinical care in various clinical settings during a 4-week elective.

**Main Outcome Measures:** The ICHE was evaluated via written evaluations by faculty and residents as well as written and oral reports by participating residents.

**Results:** During the 2000 and 2004 electives, residents recorded clinical cases in a data-entry log. Of the patients logged, 18% had illnesses never seen before by the residents and 5.6% had illnesses in advanced stages not previously seen by the residents. Strong reciprocal relationships were created between the department and participating international institutions. Residents reported uniformly that the elective was a valuable element of their training.

**Conclusions:** Planning and faculty involvement in ICHEs helps to ensure achievement of elective objectives. Well-organized ICHEs have the potential to augment resident education. The experience at our institution demonstrates that ICHEs can provide experience with a variety of medical systems, exposure to diverse pathophysiologic conditions, and opportunities for collaboration with international colleagues.

*Arch Pediatr Adolesc Med. 2006;160:191-196*

Author Affiliations:
Department of Pediatrics (Drs Federico, Zachar, Goldson, and Brown), University of Colorado Health Sciences Center (Mss Oravec and Mandler), Denver; and Denver Health Medical Center (Drs Federico, Zachar, and Brown).

PEDIATRIC RESIDENT INTERNATIONAL child health electives (ICHEs) in developing countries provide a unique educational experience and are an important component of pediatric residency training in the United States.[1] This type of elective provides cross-cultural medical experiences with exposure to different health care delivery systems, rarely seen diseases, and opportunities for language immersion. Previous studies have indicated that international electives may influence career decisions, leading to an increased desire to work with underserved populations and a higher likelihood of choosing a career in primary care.[2-5]

Many residency programs have developed international health electives (IHEs) with various formats. A 1995 survey of pediatric residency programs in the United States, Canada, and Puerto Rico showed that 25% of the responding programs offered formal or informal ICHEs.[1] These data suggest that ICHEs are a common component of pediatric residency training. Accordingly, the American Academy of Pediatrics has developed consensus guidelines that outline goals for pediatric residents wanting to participate in ICHEs and for programs seeking to organize ICHEs.[1]

There are several reports in the literature about the educational value of IHEs, most of which rely on survey data.[2,3,5-9] However, despite the prevalence of ICHEs in pediatric training programs and the American Academy of Pediatrics consensus guidelines, the literature reports relatively few successful pediatric ICHEs and little information about how they are organized.[6,10-12] Information about costs to residents and to the residency program, preparation of residents for travel abroad, structure of electives, site selection, and participant selection is beneficial to residency programs that seek to create successful ICHEs.

The University of Colorado Health Sciences Center Department of Pediatrics (UCDP), Denver, developed an ICHE that was piloted in April 2000. The elective has continued biannually, with the third wave of residents participating in the spring of 2004. During that period, the elective has evolved and has been successful as measured by resident and faculty evaluations, the overall safety of all participants, and the development of a reciprocal relationship with the participating institutions abroad.

The objectives of this article are to describe the organizational features of the elective, to outline the format of the elective in a way that might serve to assist other programs in the development of similar electives, and to describe the unique pathologic conditions seen in the clinical cases by the residents.

## METHODS

In 1999, a steering committee consisting of faculty members with interest and experience in international child health was formed with the intent of developing an ICHE that would be available to UCDP residents.

### PARTICIPATING RESIDENTS

The elective was specifically designed to attract residents who did not have previous experience working or traveling in developing countries, and who would otherwise be unlikely to do so. Through an organized and positive experience, we expected to foster an interest in international health in this group. Additionally, it had been noted in our institution that residents with previous international experience were successful in organizing and completing IHEs independently. Although interns may have had more time to cultivate an interest after such an experience, the committee decided to restrict the elective to second- and third-year residents for 3 main reasons: (1) there would have been logistical challenges in meeting and preparing interns in less than 12 months; (2) interns in our program are scheduled for only 1 elective month throughout their first year; and (3) more experienced residents would have more knowledge of and insight into pediatric medicine and its practices in the United States, thus maximizing the educational exchange.

### DESIGN OF ELECTIVE

Participating residents were chosen 12 months in advance to facilitate planning and schedules. Electives were arranged for the fall of the following year. Groups of residents chose one of the designated sites for a month-long rotation. The residents selected their rotations on the basis of areas of interest from a variety of services or clinics at each institution. The rotation was primarily observational, although many opportunities were provided for hands-on learning through physical examination and case discussions. The decision to make the experience observational was driven principally by UCDP's liability concerns. While abroad, residents were expected to give a collective grand rounds presentation in Spanish on the structure of pediatric training programs and the logistics of being a resident in Colorado. Clinical observations in both clinic- and hospital-based settings occurred during a 3-week period. A 1-week period was allowed at the end of each month for travel and cultural and language immersion.

At the end of the elective, residents completed a descriptive evaluation of the elective and the clinical experience obtained during the rotation. Other postrotation requirements included a formal oral presentation representing all aspects of the rotation to faculty and peers at a noon conference as well as an evening presentation open to both groups of funders. In 2002, a written report on the residents' topic of choice germane to the objectives was added. These topics were agreed on before residents left for the ICHE, to avoid redundancy.

Members of the UCDP faculty accompanied the residents during various parts of the elective months. They were assigned to solve organizational issues that could not be anticipated a priori and to provide support to ease the transition for residents who had little experience traveling outside the United States. Several opportunities for didactic teaching sessions in each of the faculty members' areas of expertise were arranged in advance. Faculty members were also asked to evaluate the elective experience and to provide feedback on their return.

### SITES

Institutions for exchange were identified on the basis of preexisting working relationships between faculty at UCDP and faculty at the proposed ICHE sites. All sites chosen were teaching institutions where residents could be incorporated into a traditional teaching structure and supervised by faculty on rounds or in clinics. A critical element in the design of the elective was reciprocity between institutions; in addition to UCDP residents rotating abroad, residents from host countries would be welcomed to rotate at UCDP. Agreements to this effect were signed between UCDP and all ICHE rotation sites on initiation of the elective.

### PROGRAM OBJECTIVES

The committee developed a written description of the elective and a set of objectives. These objectives were presented and agreed on by all participating departments (UCDP and those abroad) and were approved by the Pediatric Residency Program Committee and the chair of pediatrics from the home program:

- To gain perspective on the role of pediatrics in health care delivery in the developing and developed world
- To gain experience with common medical and public health problems in developing and developed countries
- To experience different medical systems, cultural practices, and understandings of disease causation and treatment
- To analyze residency and academic training curricula, issues, and problems in developing and developed countries
- To gain facility in medical practice and social interaction in a second language
- To share current scientific information in an area of expertise with international colleagues.

### COSTS AND PREPARATION

A comprehensive orientation program was structured for the participating UCDP residents. The orientation consisted of monthly dinner meetings where a variety of topics were covered, including aspects of tropical medicine, cultural and language competency, a general overview of Peru and Guatemala, information about travel in developing countries, and safety issues specific to the ICHE. Orientation dinners were also used as a forum for discussing organizational details of travel and the elective. Residents were asked to sign a release form created by the UCDP and agreed on by the University of Colorado Health Sciences Center legal department, copies of which are available on request from the corresponding author.

The UCDP agreed to cover the costs of resident salaries and benefits during the ICHE. This was justified by the assumption that such electives are worthwhile educational experiences and the fact that UCDP residents may choose to spend up to 2 months of their residency at sites other than UCDP-affiliated hospitals. Grant funding was received from UCDP, the Colorado Chapter of the American Academy of Pediatrics, and a private foundation (Community Child Health Foundation, Denver, Colo), which covered the cost of housing for residents while abroad as well as group ground transportation to and from the hospital. Residents received most of the recommended travel vaccines through the hospital's employee health clinic or the county immunization clinic at no or minimal charge. Residents paid for the additional travel costs, including airfare, food, local travel, and additional transportation. Residents spent approximately $1000 on ICHE expenses, not including the costs of travel on weekends or during allotted vacation time.

In addition to resident salaries, in 2004 the Department of Pediatrics began providing an administrative support person for the steering committee, as well as supporting 5% of 1 full-time faculty member as acting committee chair. Departmental support on this level can be particularly difficult to attain. The support of the department was thought to be essential to the success of an elective of this scale. All of these agreements were negotiated over time. **Table 1** gives a timeline for development and execution of the elective. This study met the exclusionary criteria from the Colorado Institutional Review Board.

**Table 1. Timeline for Elective Development and Execution**

| Time | Preparatory Activity |
|---|---|
| Months before ICHE | |
| 18 | Establish faculty steering committee |
| 18 | Develop written description and objectives for elective |
| 18 | Identify potential institutions for exchange |
| 12-15 | Create and sign letters of agreement between institutions |
| 12-15 | Select residents and faculty for ICHE participation |
| 12 | Begin orientation for residents |
| 9-12 | Create release form (legal department); residents sign form |
| 6-9 | Travel planning: air travel, housing, and ground transportation |
| 6-9 | Develop plan for clinical activities during ICHE based on participants' interests |
| 3-6 | Determine topics for faculty lectures during elective, based on interests of host institution |
| 3 | Residents receive recommended immunizations |
| 3 | Residents consider purchase of travel health insurance |
| During elective | Faculty assist with organizational issues |
| After elective | Residents and faculty complete standardized evaluation of elective; resident written and oral reports due |
| | Faculty steering committee reviews evaluations, uses feedback in planning for future ICHEs |

Abbreviation: ICHE, international child health elective.

## RESULTS

### CHARACTERISTICS OF PARTICIPATING RESIDENTS

Residents were selected for participation on the basis of their stated interest in the ICHE, availability, schedule flexibility, language abilities, and essays when necessary. All participating residents had completed more than 18 months of pediatric residency training. Although the pilot elective included 7 residents, in its current format it is limited to 3 to 4 residents in a given month because of staffing constraints within the training program.

The residents' ability to speak Spanish has been quite variable. Those who were fluent have suggested in their evaluations that their ability to follow along on rounds provided them with a more comprehensive medical experience than that of their peers. However, those with limited language skills indicated that their comprehension on medical rounds improved exponentially as the month progressed. Additionally, they reported that their conversational skills were aided tremendously by the experience.

### REPORTING ON THE EXPERIENCE

All participating groups of residents successfully completed the oral and written requirements of the elective. Residents and faculty stayed together in hotels or with families located near the hospitals. This allowed faculty to have firsthand knowledge of the daily logistics of each site. Additionally, faculty made rounds at the host institutions and gave lectures in Spanish on topics of interest to the host sites.

While abroad, each group gave a general overview of the University of Colorado Health Sciences Center training program. On their return, each group also presented an overview of their experience at a noon conference to the faculty and their peers. Since 2002, all residents fulfilled the additional requirement of submitting a written report on a variety of aspects of the residents' experiences, including pediatric training in Peru, the Peruvian health care system, infectious disease and public health issues in Peru, infectious disease–related morbidity and mortality, anatomy of a rotavirus outbreak, vaccine-preventable diseases, other infectious diseases, barriers faced by health care reform, the neonatal intensive care unit experience, an interview with Edwin Asturias, MD, infectious disease in Guatemala, overview of the pediatric residency in Guatemala, and overview of the Guatemalan health care system. These reports serve as testimony to the variety of health care issues that these residents were exposed to in their various experiences. Additionally, the reports were compiled into a yearly comprehensive overview and presented to both the faculty committee and the funders. In conjunction with the oral presentations, these reports served as a way for the department to document the fulfillment of the elective's outlined objectives.

### SITES

Originally, residents were able to choose among 3 sites located in large cities; in 2002 a regional site in Cusco, Peru, was added at the residents' request (**Table 2**). An agreement has recently been reached to add a site in Quito, Ecuador, for the 2006-2007 rotations.

In April 2000, 7 pediatric residents and 5 faculty members from UCDP participated in the pilot elective at 2 sites

**Table 2. Description of Institutions Available to ICHE Residents**

| Institution (Type) | No. of Beds | Subspecialty Clinics | Subspecialty Inpatient Services | Residents/y | Fellowships Available | Location |
|---|---|---|---|---|---|---|
| Instituto Nacional de Salud del Nino (public) | 600 Total; 600 pediatric | Full spectrum except hematology-oncology | Full spectrum except hematology-oncology | 21 | Yes | Urban area of Lima, Peru |
| Cayetano Heredia (semiprivate) | 376 Total; 47 pediatric | Full spectrum | NICU (20 beds), PICU (6 beds) | 7 | Yes | Urban area of Lima, Peru |
| Hospital Roosevelt (public) | 200 Total | Full spectrum | Full spectrum | 20 | Neonatology, oncology | Urban area of Guatemala City, Guatemala |
| Hospital Regional (public) | 26 Pediatric | None | NICU (22 beds) | None | No | Small, mountainous urban area in Cusco, Peru |

Abbreviations: ICHE, international child health elective; NICU, neonatal intensive care unit; PICU, pediatric intensive care unit.

**Table 3. Most Frequently Observed Diagnoses, Site Encountered (Inpatient vs Outpatient), and Whether Previously Seen by Residents**

| Diagnosis (Based on Code Logged by Resident) | No. of Cases Logged | No. (%) | | No. of Cases Never Seen Previously | No. of Cases Never Seen in Such an Advanced Stage of Progression |
|---|---|---|---|---|---|
| | | Inpatient Cases | Outpatient Cases | | |
| General infectious disease | 105 | 96 (17.2) | 9 (2.7) | 52 | 2 |
| General dermatology | 102 | 10 (1.8) | 92 (27.8) | 38 | 1 |
| HIV | 52 | 51 (9.1) | 1 (0.3) | 14 | 19 |
| Pneumonia | 46 | 45 (8.1) | 1 (0.3) | 1 | 0 |
| Tuberculosis | 30 | 30 (5.4) | 0 | 15 | 8 |
| Preterm infant | 30 | 28 (5.0) | 2 (0.6) | 0 | 0 |
| Bronchiolitis | 28 | 25 (4.5) | 3 (0.9) | 0 | 0 |
| Diarrhea | 27 | 11 (2.0) | 16 (4.8) | 1 | 4 |
| Warts | 25 | 0 | 25 (7.6) | 0 | 0 |
| General neurology | 24 | 14 (2.5) | 10 (3.0) | 5 | 2 |
| General respiratory | 24 | 20 (3.6) | 4 (1.2) | 1 | 2 |
| Hepatitis | 23 | 16 (2.9) | 7 (2.1) | 2 | 1 |
| Tinea infection | 22 | 1 (0.2) | 21 (6.3) | 0 | 1 |
| Asthma/RAD | 21 | 13 (2.3) | 8 (2.4) | 0 | 0 |
| FUO | 19 | 17 (3.0) | 2 (0.6) | 5 | 2 |
| Varicella | 19 | 19 (3.4) | 0 | 1 | 2 |
| Other diagnoses | 293 | 163 (29.2) | 130 (39.3) | 23 | 6 |
| **Total** | **890** | **559 (100.0)** | **331 (100.0)** | **158/890** (17.8%) | **50/890** (5.6%) |

Abbreviation: FUO, fever of unknown origin; HIV, human immunodeficiency virus; RAD, reactive airway disease.

in Lima, Peru. In 2002 and 2004, the elective sites were expanded to include the cities of Cusco and Guatemala City, Guatemala. Six residents and 6 faculty members participated in 2002, and 8 residents and 5 faculty members participated in 2004. In spring 2006, 6 residents are slated to rotate in Lima during 2 separate months and 3 will be in Guatemala City.

## PROGRAM OUTCOMES

During the 2000 and 2004 electives, a data-entry log was used to record all clinical cases seen by the residents. Recorded data included the patient's age and sex, inpatient vs outpatient setting, and a diagnostic code identifying the general category of disease. Residents also identified which of the diagnoses they had not seen previously, and which had never been seen in such an advanced state. Thirteen of 14 participating residents completed the case logs, for a participation rate of 93%. A total of 890 cases were recorded; **Table 3** gives the variety of diagnoses the residents observed during the rotation. There was a preponderance of infectious disease cases on the inpatient service, whereas in the outpatient service most cases were in the areas of dermatology and diarrhea or dehydration related to gastroenteritis. Of the cases observed, almost 18% were illnesses not previously seen by the residents and 5.6% were illnesses in advanced stages that the residents had never seen before. Many of the infectious diseases were unusual and had not been observed previously by the residents (**Table 4**).

Feedback from resident and faculty evaluations of the elective was uniformly positive. Constructive ideas were solicited each year regarding ways to improve the elective, and these ideas were implemented whenever possible. For example, language tutoring was made available at one of the sites, so that residents who were less fluent would have an increased opportunity to improve their Spanish skills. Additionally, a smaller, more regional hospital site (Cuzco) was made available per resident request; in 2002, residents spent up to 1 week in Cuzco, and in 2004 two residents spent their entire elective in Cuzco. Although this site provided more opportunities for the residents to participate actively as medical team members, the case logs disclosed that residents on the rural rotation saw fewer patients overall and fewer illnesses that were new to them or in more advanced stages than they had previously seen (**Table 5**). This led to the cancellation of Cuzco as a permanent site.

The reciprocal agreements between institutions have been successful. The UCDP has hosted approximately 4 visiting residents per year since the inception of the ICHE, mostly from the Instituto Nacional de Salud del Nino and Cayetano Heredia School of Medicine in Lima, Peru. This is consistent with the initial agreement, which specified a maximum of 1 visiting resident for every 1 sent between UCDP and the affiliated host sites. Furthermore, since the inception of the elective, UCDP has matched 3 South American graduates into its residency program, further enabling the ongoing cultural and educational exchange (eg, a primary facilitator of the development of the new site in Ecuador was a second-year resident from Quito). Finally, in December 2004, Dr Asturias, who serves as the site coordinator in Guatemala, visited Denver and the Children's Hospital as a visiting professor. The feedback from both institutions in Lima as well as Guatemala has been overwhelmingly positive. The program has been strongly encouraged to expand the elective to a yearly event to facilitate planning by both sites.

Despite these successes, the goal of reciprocity has had limitations. For instance, there have been no visiting residents to Denver from Guatemala. Most of the feedback on this limitation has centered on the expense of housing and transportation associated with a prolonged stay in the United States.

**Table 4. Infectious Disease Cases Seen**

| Diagnosis | No. of Cases (%) |
|---|---|
| Infectious disease, other | 105 (36.3) |
| Typhoid | 10 (3.5) |
| Cysticercosis | 6 (2.1) |
| *Echinococcus* species | 6 (2.1) |
| Amebiasis | 6 (2.1) |
| Tetanus | 5 (1.7) |
| Strongyloidiasis, ascariasis, toxocariasis | 4 (1.4) |
| Brucellosis | 3 (1.0) |
| Leishmaniasis | 3 (1.0) |
| Leptospirosis | 2 (0.7) |
| Other | 60 (20.8) |
| HIV | 52 (18.0) |
| Tuberculosis | 30 (10.4) |
| Hepatitis, unspecified | 23 (8.0) |
| FUO | 19 (6.6) |
| Varicella | 19 (6.6) |
| Cellulitis | 15 (5.2) |
| Upper respiratory tract infection | 9 (3.1) |
| Urinary tract infection | 6 (2.1) |
| Bacteremia | 5 (1.7) |
| Lymphadenitis | 3 (1.0) |
| Viral syndrome | 3 (1.0) |
| **Total** | **289 (100.0)** |

Abbreviations: FUO fever of unknown origin; HIV, human immunodeficiency virus.

**Table 5. Cases Logged in Large Urban Hospitals vs Regional Hospitals**

| Variable | Large Urban Hospitals | Regional Hospitals |
|---|---|---|
| No. of residents | 11 | 2 |
| No. of different diagnoses logged | 120 | 46 |
| Cases never seen previously, % per resident | 19.4 | 5.4 |
| Cases never seen in such advanced state, % per resident | 6.9 | 1.2 |

## COMMENT

The information provided about the organization, implementation, and evaluation of our elective is valuable to other pediatric training programs that are trying to create ICHEs. A significant amount of planning and faculty time, energy, and involvement is necessary to ensure that these ICHEs are a valuable learning experience and not simply an opportunity for "medical tourism." Given the detailed objectives, pretrip curriculum, pretrip and posttrip oral presentations, patient logs, language tutoring, final written reports, and evaluations, our ICHE has grown in popularity not only with the house staff but with the faculty and administration as well. We hope that these electives will gain in popularity in US pediatric training programs because of what they add to resident education and possible future international health involvement from graduating residents.

In his article on overseas electives, Northrup[9] wrote, "a two-month elective in a developing country can be a profound experience, often resembling a religious conversion, and can dramatically alter . . . perceptions of health, health care, and societal and personal responsibility." Our results support this perception. Given current restrictions on elective time and time away from the program, our experience has primarily been restricted to 1 month, but we found that 1 month can serve as an excellent beginning in international health. Northrup went on to emphasize the importance of organization in achieving an effective elective experience. We believe that the careful planning and organization that went into the development of the UCDP elective helped to ensure a positive experience for all participants.

A recent study suggested that the availability of international opportunities during residency positively affects residency program ranking by medical students.[13] Thus, IHEs may offer value as "recruiting tools" for training programs. Anecdotal evidence suggests that this is becoming true at the UCDP residency program. At a recent meeting with the intern class of 2004-2005, all of the residents reported having had some knowledge of the ICHE before their acceptance to the program. In addition, approximately 75% expressed interest in participating, and about 50% stated that it was a major factor in their ranking process. Further elucidating the effect on recruitment, the incoming intern class of 2005-2006 reported unanimous knowledge of the elective before match selection, 67% reported it as a major factor in ranking, and 96% stated an interest in participating. This level of interest has encouraged the department to expand the elective to a third country and provide it on a yearly basis.

The UCDP residents saw diverse pathologic conditions during their clinical observations in the institutions in which they were placed during the 2000 and 2004 electives. Data entry logs show that the residents observed many types of diseases that they had not encountered in the United States. This evidence of enhanced clinical experience supplements the residents' own evaluation that the elective was of value to them.

Several reports have documented that residents who have participated in an IHE are more likely to improve their knowledge of tropical medicine, to change their career plans toward areas of primary care and public health,[4] and to reduce their dependence on laboratory testing because of increased awareness of health care costs.[14] In 2003, Thompson et al[3] reviewed the literature on the topic of IHEs and discovered only 1 study that used quantitative data (National Board of Medical Examiners examination scores) rather than self-administered questionnaires to evaluate the educational effects of these programs. Our experience provides objective evidence to contribute to the pool of data supporting the benefits of IHEs.

**Accepted for Publication:** August 21, 2005.
**Correspondence:** Steven G. Federico, MD, Denver Health Medical Center, 777 Bannock St MC0132, Denver, CO 80204 (steve.federico@dhha.org).
**Author Contributions:** All authors had full access to all the data in the study and take responsibility for the integrity of the data and the accuracy of the data analysis.
**Previous Presentation:** The outcomes of this study were presented in abstract form at the annual meetings of the Pediatric Academic Societies; May 2001; Baltimore, Md; and April 2005; Washington, DC.

**Acknowledgments:** We acknowledge M. Douglas Jones, MD; Mimi Glode, MD; Adam Rosenberg, MD; and Jacinto Hernandez, MD, from the UCDP for their support of the ICHE. We also acknowledge the help of Jaime Zegarra, MD (Cayetano Heredia School of Medicine), Jorge Candela, MD (Instituto Nacional de Salud del Nino), Edwin Asturias, MD (Hospital Roosevelt), and Felix Hidalgo, MD (Hospital Regional) in creating and maintaining successful rotation sites in their home cities.

## REFERENCES

1. Torjesen K, Mandalakas A, Kahn R, Duncan B. International child health electives for pediatric residents. *Arch Pediatr Adolesc Med.* 1999;153:1297-1302.
2. Chiller TM, DeMieri P, Cohen I. International health training: the Tulane experience. *Infect Dis Clin North Am.* 1995;9:439-443.
3. Thompson MJ, Huntington MK, Hunt DD, Pinsky LE, Brodie JJ. Educational effects of international health electives on U.S. and Canadian medical students and residents: a literature review. *Acad Med.* 2003;78:342-347.
4. Miller W, Corey G, Lallinger G, Kurack D. International health and internal medicine residency training: the Duke University experience. *Am J Med.* 1995;99:291-297.
5. Gupta A, Wells C, Horwitz F, et al. The international health program: the fifteen-year experience with Yale University's Internal Medicine Residency Program. *Am J Trop Med Hyg.* 1999;61:1019-1023.
6. Nuckton T, Luther K, Weinberger M, et al. Residency training in developing nations: an international elective for U.S. physicians in training. *Teach Learn Med.* 1999;11:207-213.
7. Ulmer D. Some international efforts of medical schools to improve health care systems. *Infect Dis Clin North Am.* 1995;9:425-431.
8. Haskell A, Rovinsky D, Brown HK, Coughlin RR. The University of California at San Francisco international orthopaedic elective. *Clin Orthop Relat Res.* March 2002:12-18.
9. Northrup R. Preparing students for overseas electives [comment]. *Acad Med.* 1991;66:92.
10. Duncan B, Dalby S, Taussig L. A one-month elective in international health for senior pediatric residents. *AJDC.* 1989;143:1389-1390.
11. Torjesen H. An international health story from Case Western Reserve University. *Infect Dis Clin North Am.* 1995;9:433-437.
12. Einterz RM, Kelley CR, Mamlin JJ, Reken D. Partnerships in international health: the Indiana University-Moi experience. *Infect Dis Clin North Am.* 1995;9:453-455.
13. Dey CC, Grabowski JG, Gebreyes K, Hsu E, VanRooyen MJ. Influence of international emergency medicine opportunities on residency program selection. *Acad Emerg Med.* 2002;9:679-683.
14. Barry M, Bia F. Departments of medicine and international health. *Am J Med.* 1986;80:1019-1021.

# Antipyretic Treatment in Young Children With Fever

## *Acetaminophen, Ibuprofen, or Both Alternating in a Randomized, Double-blind Study*

*E. Michael Sarrell, MD; Eliahu Wielunsky, MD; Herman Avner Cohen, MD*

**Objective:** To compare the antipyretic benefit of acetaminophen or ibuprofen monotherapy with an alternating regimen of both drugs in young children aged 6 to 36 months.

**Design:** Randomized, double-blind, parallel-group trial.

**Setting:** Three primary pediatric community ambulatory centers in central Israel.

**Participants:** A total of 464 children aged 6 to 36 months with fever.

**Intervention:** Infants were assigned to receive either acetaminophen (12.5 mg/kg per dose every 6 hours) (n=154) or ibuprofen (5 mg/kg per dose every 8 hours) (n=155) or to receive alternating acetaminophen and ibuprofen (every 4 hours) (n=155) for 3 days after a loading dose.

**Main Outcome Measures:** Temperature, stress score, amount of antipyretic received, total days that the infant or caregiver was absent from day care or work, respectively, at the 3-day time point, recurrence of fever, and number of emergency department visits.

**Results:** The group given the alternating regimen was characterized by a lower mean temperature, more rapid reduction of fever, receiving less antipyretic medication, less stress, and less absenteeism from day care as compared with the other groups; all of the differences were statistically significant ($P<.001$). None of the regimens were associated with a significantly higher number of emergency department visits ($P=.65$) or serious long-term complications ($P=.66$). The drug used for initial loading had no effect on outcome in any of the groups.

**Conclusions:** An alternating treatment regimen of acetaminophen (12.5 mg/kg per dose) and ibuprofen (5 mg/kg per dose) every 4 hours for 3 days, regardless of the initial loading medication, is more effective than monotherapy in lowering fever in infants and children.

*Arch Pediatr Adolesc Med. 2006;160:197-202*

FEVER IS ONE OF THE MOST common presenting signs of illness in office-based primary care pediatric practice, accounting for 19% to 30% of visits.[1,2] Infants and young children are particularly susceptible to fever because of their small body size, high ratio of body surface area to weight, and low amount of subcutaneous fat. Although most experts consider fever a beneficial physiologic response to the infectious process, it can lead to patient irritability and stress as well as high parental anxiety.[3] Therefore, physicians usually prefer to prescribe antipyretic agents in addition to nonpharmacologic, physical fever-reducing modalities.[4]

Acetaminophen (paracetamol in Israel) is very widely used as an antipyretic owing to its high efficacy and good safety profile.[5] Acetaminophen is a para-aminophenol derivative that inhibits cyclooxygenase, thereby inhibiting the formation and release of prostaglandins. It is absorbed in the gastrointestinal tract, reaching peak plasma concentrations within 30 minutes. The time to maximal temperature reduction is approximately 2 hours.[6,7] The recommended dose of acetaminophen is 12 to 15 mg/kg every 6 hours.

Ibuprofen is a propionic acid derivative that, like acetaminophen, inhibits the biosynthesis of prostaglandins. It, too, is absorbed in the gastrointestinal tract, reaching peak plasma concentrations in 1 hour; the maximal temperature reduction peaks within 3 hours. The recommended dose is 5 to 10 mg/kg every 8 hours.[8,9]

Both antipyretics have been found to be equally safe in children. There are occasional descriptions of gastrointestinal bleeding or renal failure in adults using ibuprofen and of acetaminophen toxic effects in children and adults.[10]

Studies have reported that 50% or more of parents or caregivers give their children both antipyretics, but their method of alternation varies.[11] Furthermore, in about half of the cases, the dosage used is inaccurate.[12]

**Author Affiliations:** Sackler Faculty of Medicine, Tel Aviv University, Tel Aviv, Israel (Drs Sarrell, Wielunsky, and Cohen); and Pediatric Ambulatory Center General Health Services (Drs Sarrell and Cohen) and Schneider Children's Medical Center of Israel (Dr Wielunsky), Petah Tiqva, Israel.

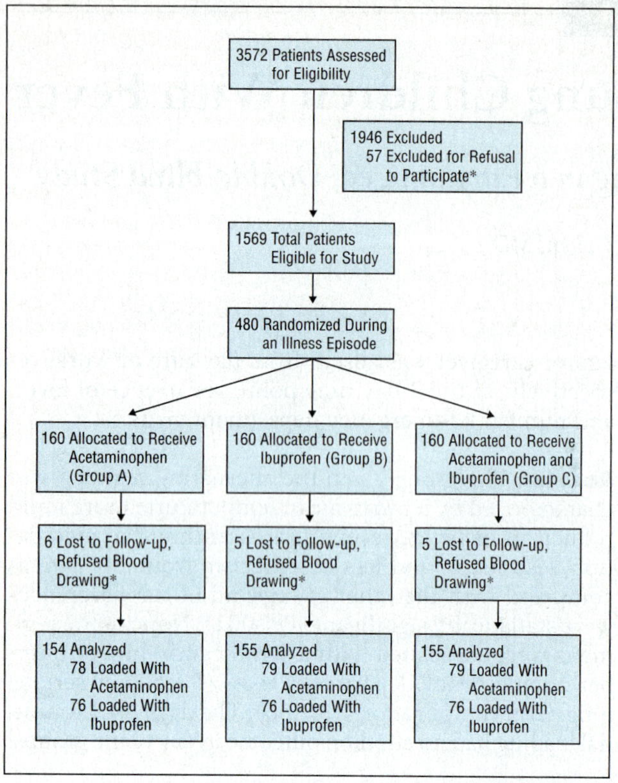


**Figure.** Flow of participants throughout the trial. Asterisk indicates that all of the children who were withdrawn from the study continued to attend the same practices.

The aim of the present study was to compare the clinical effectiveness of acetaminophen and ibuprofen alone with an alternating regimen in reducing fever and stress signs in infants and young children.

## METHODS

### SETTING

The study was approved by the local institutional human rights committee. It was conducted between September 15, 2003, and March 15, 2004, at 3 primary pediatric community centers, 2 urban and 1 rural, in central Israel.

### PATIENTS

The sample included all consecutive children aged 6 to 36 months who had a rectal temperature of at least 38.4°C. Children who were not attending day care centers or had taken any temperature-altering drugs or antibiotics within 10 days before presentation were excluded, as were children with known abnormal liver or renal laboratory values, children with medical history of any of the following: renal or hepatic impairment, gastrointestinal bleeding, known allergy to any antipyretic, congenital or acquired immunodeficiency, Reye syndrome, asthma, bronchiolitis, or malignancy, and children whose caregivers were unable to apply the Noncommunicating Children's Pain Checklist (NCCPC) to measure stress.

### DESIGN

Informed consent to participate in the study was obtained from a parent or guardian by the admitting physician (**Figure**). Thereafter, the same physician recorded the patient's background data (demographics, medical history, previous diagnosis, use of other medications, and smoking in the home). Then, the admitting nurse used a computerized random-number generator to stratify according to the center in blocks of 60 numbers so that each block comprised 20 patients randomly assigned to each treatment group, with 10 patients assigned to each loading medication. The admitting nurse also weighed the patient and obtained the initial laboratory findings along with the child's temperature (admission fever) and level of distress according to the NCCPC stress test (admission NCCPC score). She then handed the parent or guardian a sealed opaque folder holding 3 sealed envelopes: 1 containing an advice sheet explaining the physiology of fever and its nonpharmacologic management; 1 containing the prescription for the loading medication (marked "initial medication"); and 1 containing the drug prescription (marked "home prescription"), according to the assigned group and subgroup as follows:

1. Group A received acetaminophen (12.5 mg/kg per dose every 6 hours; maximum, 50 mg/kg per day). One half of the group received initial loading with acetaminophen (25 mg/kg), and the other half received initial loading with ibuprofen (10 mg/kg).
2. Group B received ibuprofen (5 mg/kg per dose every 8 hours; maximum, 20 mg/kg per day). One half of the group received initial loading with acetaminophen (25 mg/kg), and the other half received initial loading with ibuprofen (10 mg/kg).
3. Group C received acetaminophen (12.5 mg/kg per dose; maximum, 50 mg/kg per day) alternating with ibuprofen (5 mg/kg per dose; maximum, 20 mg/kg per day) every 4 hours. One half of the group received initial loading with acetaminophen (25 mg/kg), and other half received initial loading with ibuprofen (10 mg/kg).

The infant was then given the loading dose (from generic bottles marked "A" or "B") by a second nurse, who also instructed the parent or guardian in completion of a daily diary and stress questionnaire for follow-up.

The study medications were standard acetaminophen syrup (125 mg/5 mL; Acamoli; Teva Pharmaceutical Industries, Ltd, Netanya, Israel) and ibuprofen suspension (100 mg/5 mL; Nurofen Boots Healthcare International, Nottingham, England). All of the loading-dose medication bottles were outwardly identical. The medication bottles were clearly labeled by group and were distributed by the pharmacist. The doses were calculated by infant weight. The pharmacist also reinforced the physician's instructions to the parent or guardian regarding the amount and times of administration of the medication, emphasizing the importance of adhering to the prescription and not exceeding the maximal recommended daily dosage. The list of patients and medications was stored until the end of the study with the pharmacist in a sealed envelope to be opened in the event of an emergency. All of the children were evaluated and followed up by the same physician (E.M.S.), who was blinded to the group allocations (as were the parents or guardians).

### FOLLOW-UP

For each child enrolled in the study, the physician prepared a computerized questionnaire on demographic data, height of fever, days of illness, physical signs, mode of therapy, pertinent laboratory findings, new onset of illness, and emergency department visits to be completed as the study progressed.

Follow-up was conducted by a daily diary record maintained by the parent or guardian, which was accompanied by a telephone interview at 24 hours (day 1) and 48 hours (day 2) after enrollment. Parents were requested to measure the child's rectal temperature with a glass and mercury rectal thermometer at least 3 times daily during treatment, and then once daily for another 10 days. They also recorded the amount of antipyretic medication used and the number of missed work days because the child could not attend day care. In addition, they completed the NCCPC stress questionnaire.

The NCCPC stress test was designed for use in infants and young children who are unable to communicate verbally. It has been proven to be valid and reliable in the home setting.[13] Studies show that caregiver reports based on the NCCPC can predict pain behavior[14] and that caregiver pain estimates are closely related to children's self-reports.[13]

The caregiver was asked to rate how often each item in the scale occurred (not at all=0; occasionally=1; fairly often=2; and very often=3) during a 10-minute observation period in every 24-hour period in the morning before starting the day and twice more before lunch and dinner.

All of the patients were scheduled for an office visit on day 3 of the study, during which they were evaluated as they were on enrollment day, and the medication bottles were collected. Additional visits were conducted on days 5 and 10 after enrollment. Tests for renal and liver function and stool analysis for occult blood were repeated on the third and fifth days of follow-up and every 2 weeks thereafter for a total of 12 weeks. The diaries were collected on day 10 of the study.

## OUTCOME MEASURES

We evaluated body temperature, stress score, amount of antipyretic used at the 3-day time point, total days that a primary caretaker had to stay home from work because the infant could not attend day care because of his illness, recurrence of fever within 5 and 10 days after initiation of treatment, number of emergency department visits within 10 days of enrollment, hepatic and renal function, appearance of gastrointestinal symptoms or bleeding, and the appearance of Reye syndrome. Fever was evaluated according to the maximal temperature registered on any day. Children with a temperature of less than 37.8°C were considered afebrile. A score of 4 or more on the NCCPC was considered abnormal. Therapy was considered successful if the mean temperature and mean NCCPC stress score were reduced.

Renal and hepatic function were followed up by clinical symptom and appropriate laboratory investigations. Abnormal laboratory findings were defined as follows: serum creatinine level, 0.9 mg/dL or higher (≥68.6 μmol/L); blood urea nitrogen level, 18 mg/dL or higher (≥6.4 mmol/L); levels of liver enzymes serum glutamic oxaloacetic transaminase, serum glutamate pyruvate transaminase, and γ-glutamyltransferase, 20 U/L or higher; and total serum bilirubin level, 1 mg/dL or higher (≥17 μmol/L).

Gastrointestinal irritability was diagnosed by the presence of abdominal pain associated with vomiting or diarrhea as reported by the parents or caregivers. Gastrointestinal bleeding was evaluated by the presence of occult blood in stool (Cenogenics Corp, Morganville, NJ).

## SAMPLE SIZE CALCULATION

Our calculation of the minimum sample size formula for binominal proportion from an independent sample[15] was based on a double-blind clinical trial of 2 study populations of febrile children assigned at random to receive treatment A (acetaminophen) or treatment B (ibuprofen).[8] The groups were evaluated at 2 different dosages. Since the study found no significant difference between the groups in the decrease in fever, we used the variations in irritability score for the sample size calculation. The protocol required that patients be withdrawn if continuing participation could at any time be considered detrimental to their well-being.

## STATISTICAL ANALYSIS

Survey responses were analyzed using SPSS for Windows, version 12.01b (SPSS, Inc, Chicago, Ill). Between-group data were compared with a $\chi^2$ analysis to test nominal or ordinal variables of the background data. Comparison of stress, fever, and dosage according to treatment in each time was assessed with analysis of variance. Paired *t* test was used to check the differences of pain and fever between times in each group. A 2-tailed *P* value of .05 was used to define statistical significance for differences between groups and to calculate confidence intervals around differences in sample means.

## RESULTS

A total of 480 infants met the eligibility criteria, of whom 464 (96.7%) completed the study. Of the 16 infants (3.3%) who withdrew from the study, 7 (1.5%) failed to return for follow-up visits within the first 10 days, and 9 (1.9%) did not return for laboratory evaluation after symptoms were alleviated. There were no statistically significant differences ($P=.43$) between the study participants and those who dropped out in demographic data (age, sex, marital status of guardian, number of siblings in the household, neonatal or prenatal complications), diagnosis, amount of antipyretics used during the initial 3 days of treatment, other medications used, or primary outcome parameters. Although we have no long-term follow-up data for those who dropped out, all of the children in the study continued to attend the same practices, and none suffered any related illness or were lost during the study period (Figure).

Owing to the fact that the type of loading medication (acetaminophen or ibuprofen) had no statistical effect ($P=.52$), the patients were all grouped according to their maintenance medication. The groups were similar in sex, marital status of parents, number of siblings, smoking in the house, presence of prenatal or neonatal complications, and illness that caused the fever (**Table 1**).

There was no statistically significant difference among the groups in mean height of fever on the admission day ($P=.31$). Differences were significant on day 1 and continued on days 2 and 3 ($P<.001$) (**Table 2**). The mean fever of infants in group C (alternating ibuprofen and acetaminophen) was lower as the days progressed as compared with the others groups, with differences being statistically significant between groups C and A (acetaminophen) ($P<.001$) and groups C and B (ibuprofen) ($P<.001$) but not between groups A and B (Table 2).

A significant difference in the decline of stress levels (as measured with the NCCPC) was noted in all of the treatment groups ($P<.001$), but it was steeper in the infants in group C as compared with those in groups A and B. The difference was even more pronounced when we take into account that the children in group C began with a higher mean stress score ($P<.001$) (Table 2). When we

**Table 1. Background Variables of Study Sample by Group**

| Variable | Acetaminophen (Group A) (n = 154) | Ibuprofen (Group B) (n = 155) | Acetaminophen and Ibuprofen (Group C) (n = 155) | *P* Value |
|---|---|---|---|---|
| Age, mo (SD) | 18.6 (8.72) | 19.5 (9.09) | 19.3 (9.29) | .64 |
| Sex, No. (%) | | | | |
| Male | 71 (46) | 73 (40) | 62 (38) | .40 |
| Female | 83 (54) | 82 (60) | 93 (62) | |
| Parental status, No. (%) | | | | |
| 2 Parents | 128 (83) | 131 (85) | 133 (86) | .81 |
| 1 Parent | 26 (17) | 24 (15) | 22 (14) | |
| Other siblings, No. (%) | 117 (76) | 113 (73) | 114 (74) | .81 |
| Prenatal or neonatal complications, No. (%) | 22 (14) | 13 (8) | 17 (11) | .26 |
| Smoking at home, No. (%) | | | | |
| None | 135 (88) | 140 (90) | 127 (82) | .09 |
| Occasional | 19 (12) | 15 (10) | 28 (18) | |
| Initial medical illness associated with fever, No. (%) | | | | |
| URI | 66 (43) | 81 (52) | 80 (51) | .70 |
| AOM | 16 (10) | 13 (8) | 17 (11) | |
| Pharyngitis | 10 (7) | 7 (5) | 3 (2) | |
| Bronchiolitis | 8 (5) | 7 (5) | 9 (6) | |
| Gastroenteritis | 7 (5) | 7 (5) | 6 (4) | |
| Viral illness | 47 (30) | 40 (25) | 40 (26) | |

Abbreviations: AOM, acute otitis media; URI, upper respiratory tract infection.

**Table 2. Primary Outcome Measures of Treatment by Group**

| Outcome | Acetaminophen (Group A), % ± SD (95% CI) (n = 154) | Ibuprofen (Group B), % ± SD (95% CI) (n = 155) | Acetaminophen and Ibuprofen (Group C), % ± SD (95% CI) (n = 155) | *P* Value |
|---|---|---|---|---|
| Fever | | | | |
| Admission | 40.74 ± 1.01 (40.58-40.90) | 40.58 ± 1.02 (40.42-40.74) | 40.71 ± 0.93 (40.56-40.86) | .31 |
| Day 1 | 40.55 ± 1.31 (40.34-40.76) | 40.6 ± 1.46 (40.37-40.83) | 39.64 ± 1.17 (39.45-39.82) | <.001 |
| Day 2 | 39.74 ± 1.37 (39.51-39.95) | 39.66 ± 1.48 (39.42-39.89) | 38.78 ± 0.87 (38.64-38.92) | <.001 |
| Day 3 | 39.34 ± 1.19 (39.15-39.53) | 39.64 ± 1.46 (39.41-39.87) | 38.54 ± 0.74 (38.42-38.66) | <.001 |
| NCCPC | | | | |
| Admission | 18.30 ± 1.67 (18.03-18.56) | 19.00 ± 1.27 (18.80-19.20) | 19.46 ± 2.40 (19.08-19.84) | <.001 |
| NCCPC day 1 | 11.77 ± 2.64 (11.35-12.19) | 11.48 ± 2.58 (11.07-11.89) | 9.26 ± 2.49 (8.86-9.65) | <.001 |
| NCCPC day 2 | 8.87 ± 2.54 (8.47-9.27) | 8.83 ± 2.67 (8.40-9.25) | 5.09 ± 2.78 (4.65-5.53) | <.001 |
| NCCPC day 3 | 7.66 ± 2.96 (7.19-8.13) | 7.96 ± 2.71 (7.53-8.39) | 4.18 ± 2.74 (3.75-4.62) | <.001 |
| Medication | | | | |
| Day 1 | 4.33 ± 0.85 (4.20-4.47) | 2.99 ± 0.11 (2.97-3.01) | 2.57 ± 0.88 (2.43-2.71) | <.001 |
| Day 2 | 3.84 ± 0.73 (3.73-3.96) | 2.92 ± 0.27 (2.88-2.96) | 1.99 ± 0.58 (1.89-2.08) | <.001 |
| Day 3 | 2.90 ± 0.73 (2.79-3.02) | 2.84 ± 0.46 (2.77-2.92) | 1.48 ± 0.71 (1.37-1.59) | <.001 |

Abbreviations: CI, confidence interval; NCCPC, Noncommunicating Children's Pain Checklist.

calculated the percentage change through each of the days, group C showed a stress level reduction of 52.4%, 45.0%, and 17.7% from admission to day 1, from day 1 to day 2, and from day 2 to day 3, respectively, as compared with only 39.6%, 23.2%, and 9.8%, respectively, in group B and 35.7%, 24.6%, and 13.7%, respectively, in group A. Group C required significantly fewer doses of antipyretic medication per infant as compared with the other groups ($P<.001$) (Table 2). Analysis of the change in the mean rate of intake of medication by time showed that group C received a lower mean number of doses of medication per child in days 1, 2, and 3 than groups A and B; these differences were statistically significant among all of the groups on days 1 and 2, but on day 3, the difference was statistically significant only between group C and the other groups ($P<.001$)(Table 2).

Analysis over time showed that group C required 22.6% fewer doses from day 1 to day 2 and 25.7% fewer from day 2 to day 3 whereas group A required 11.2% and 24.4% fewer doses, respectively, and group B required 2.2% and 2.7% fewer doses, respectively. These changes were statistically significant ($P<.001$)(Table 2).

Recurrence of fever was evaluated 2 days after therapy ended (day 5 of the study) and 1 week after therapy (day 10 of the study). We found that alternating acetaminophen and ibuprofen maintenance therapy (group C), regardless of the type of initial loading medication, was associated with fewer fever recurrences on days 5 and 10

**Table 3. Secondary Outcome Measures and Follow-up by Group**

| Outcome | Acetaminophen (Group A) (n = 154) | Ibuprofen (Group B) (n = 155) | Acetaminophen and Ibuprofen (Group C) (n = 155) | *P* Value |
|---|---|---|---|---|
| Fever recurrence, No. (%) | | | | |
| At 5 d | 33 (21) | 27 (17) | 15 (10) | .02 |
| At 10 d | 18 (12) | 19 (12) | 14 (9) | .62 |
| Absent from day care, d, No. ± SD (95% CI) | 2.64 ± 0.58 (2.55-2.74) | 2.58 ± 0.61 (2.48-2.68) | 1.76 ± 0.69 (1.66-1.87) | <.001 |
| Patients visiting emergency department, No. (%) | 21 (14) | 20 (13) | 16 (10) | .65 |
| Patients with abnormal renal laboratory values, No. (%)* | | | | |
| Acute stage | 5 (3.3) | 4 (3.8) | 5 (3.2) | .93 |
| Follow-up | 0 | 0 | 0 | NA |
| Patients with abnormal liver laboratory values, No. (%)† | | | | |
| Acute stage | 4 (2.6) | 2 (1.3) | 2 (1.3) | .60 |
| Follow-up | 0 | 0 | 0 | NA |

Abbreviations: CI, confidence interval; NA, not applicable.
*Blood urea nitrogen level of 18 mg/dL or higher (≥6.4 mmol/L), or serum creatinine level of 0.9 mg/dL or higher (≥68.6 μmol/L).
†γ-Glutamyltransferase, serum glutamic oxaloacetic transaminase, or serum glutamate pyruvate transaminase level of 20 U/L or higher, or total serum bilirubin level of 1 mg/dL or higher (≥17 μmol/L).

as compared with acetaminophen or ibuprofen monotherapy (groups A and B, respectively). On day 5, there was a statistically significant difference among the groups ($P=.02$), but not on day 10 ($P=.62$)(**Table 3**).

The alternating group (group C) also had statistically significantly fewer day care absentees, thus requiring less work absenteeism from the parents, than the other groups (groups A and B) ($P<.001$)(Table 3).

In all of the groups, there were some cases of emergency department self-referral by the parents, but the differences were not significant by group ($P=.65$)(Table 3).

A multivariate stepwise linear regression analysis showed that the mode of therapy alone was the only significant factor influencing the result ($P=.047$).

None of the patients in any of the groups had a drug-related adverse event or serious illness. Mild elevation in levels of liver enzymes and renal findings were observed in 8 children (1.7%) and 14 children (3.0%), respectively, but none of the acute-stage laboratory abnormalities persisted to the 14-day follow-up evaluation, and there were no statistically significant differences among the groups ($P=.60$ for abnormal liver function and $P=.93$ for abnormal renal function)(Table 3).

## COMMENT

Reduction of fever in children and the maintenance of a comfortable state are important to caretakers and primary physicians. Antipyretic use therefore plays a major role in daily pediatric practice, and it must be both effective and safe.

Previous studies have described a lack of consistency among physicians, nurses, and parents with regard to the appropriate management of a febrile child.[16] The most commonly prescribed pharmacologic regimen consists of acetaminophen every 6 hours or ibuprofen every 8 hours according to the manufacturer's instructions. However, inappropriate dosing or overdosing is not uncommon. There are very few reported data on the use of an alternating regimen of acetaminophen and ibuprofen.[11,12]

In the present study, we compared the effectiveness of acetaminophen and ibuprofen alone with alternating acetaminophen and ibuprofen in reducing fever in young children. Initial loading doses of 25 mg/kg for acetaminophen or 10 mg/kg for ibuprofen were used to decrease the time to reach effective drug serum concentrations and to improve the rate of temperature decrease. Treluyer et al[17] found that without a loading dose, the time from administration of the first maintenance dose of acetaminophen to a steady-state plasma concentration is 10 to 50 hours in a febrile infant. The maintenance dose of ibuprofen (5 mg/kg per dose) was chosen on the basis of the study by Lesko and Mitchell,[10] who failed to detect a dose-response effect in children with this dose as compared with a dose of 10 mg/kg. Furthermore, doubling the maintenance dose from 5 mg/kg to 10 mg/kg increased the area under the receiver operating curve by only 1.5-fold without significant pharmacokinetic-pharmacodynamic benefit.[6] The maintenance dose of acetaminophen (12 mg/kg) was based on previous studies[4-6,12] showing that this dose is the most appropriate for fever reduction.

In a study of 27 065 children younger than 2 years, Lesko and Mitchell[10] noted that the risk of hospitalization for gastrointestinal bleeding among those receiving ibuprofen was no greater than in those receiving acetaminophen. Adverse effects of acetaminophen were mostly due to allergic reactions or inappropriate dosing because of parental failure to read or understand the label instructions, their use of an incorrect measuring device, or their use of an adult rather than pediatric preparation.[18,19] Adverse renal effects from ibuprofen have been described in adults. However, in children, the renal impairment is not significant because they use ibuprofen for only a short time.[7] In our study, none of the patients in any of the groups had serious adverse effects of the medication. The ibuprofen group had significantly more gastrointestinal irritability than the acetaminophen group because of the inflammatory action of the drug on the intestinal lining.[7] No such difference was noted in the alternating regimen group, perhaps because those patients required a lower overall dose of ibuprofen.

This study provides information only on the short-term (3-day) safety and efficacy of these drugs. We did not evaluate the repeated-dose pharmacokinetics, the biological safety, or the effect of prolonged dehydration on the likelihood of renal complications in the alternating regimen group. Acetaminophen is metabolized by the liver, but it is excreted in urine.[20] Therefore, it is important that physicians be aware that in an alternating regimen, acetaminophen may accumulate in the renal medulla—causing tubular necrosis and renal toxicity—because ibuprofen blocks the production of renal prostaglandin and inhibits the production of glutathione, which detoxifies the toxic metabolite of acetaminophen.[21]

These results cannot be extrapolated to children younger than 6 months, children with malnutrition, renal or hepatic abnormalities, metabolic, endocrine, or neoplastic disease, or peptic ulceration, or children with known adverse reactions to anti-inflammatory or antipyretic drugs. Furthermore, the small number of infants and the short time of therapy (3 days) in our sample reduces the statistical power to detect serious adverse events. It should also be noted that all of the study participants visited the physicians for treatment, so they may have been more seriously ill than most of the children who receive over-the-counter antipyretics.

These limitations notwithstanding, this study is the first randomized, double-blind, controlled clinical trial to our knowledge to assess the safety and effectiveness of an alternating regimen of acetaminophen and ibuprofen against each agent alone in children aged 6 to 36 months.

## CONCLUSIONS

Our study suggests that the alternating use of acetaminophen (12.5 mg/kg per dose) and ibuprofen (5 mg/kg per dose) every 4 hours, together with double-dose loading, reduces fever faster and for a longer duration than either agent alone with no increase in adverse events. Both dosages are easy to measure, lessening parental confusion.

**Accepted for Publication:** August 23, 2005.
**Correspondence:** E. Michael Sarrell, MD, 7 Hairis St, Moshav Gan-Haim, 44910, Israel (sarrell@netvision.net.il or michaelsar@clalit.org.il).

## REFERENCES


1. Eskerud JR, Laerum E, Fagerthun H, Lunde PK, Naess AA. Fever in general practice, I: frequency and diagnosis. *Fam Pract.* 1992;9:263-269.
2. Baucher R. Fever: approach to the febrile child. In: Green-Hernandez C, Singleton JK, Aronzon DZ, eds. *Primary Care Pediatrics.* Philadelphia, Pa: Lippincott Williams & Wilkins; 2001:343-357.
3. Guton H. *Human Physiology and Mechanisms of Disease.* 6th ed. Philadelphia, Pa: WB Saunders; 1997.
4. Baraff LJ, Bass JW, Fleisher GR, et al; Agency for Health Care Policy and Research. Practice guideline for management of infants and children 0 to 36 months of age with fever without source. *Ann Emerg Med.* 1993;22:1198-1210.
5. Vauzelle-Kervroedan F, d'Athis P, Pariente-Khayat A, Debregeas S, Olive G, Pons G. Equivalent antipyretic activity of ibuprofen and acetaminophen in febrile children. *J Pediatr.* 1997;131:683-687.
6. Brown RD, Kearns GL, Wilson JT. Integrated pharmacokinetic-pharmacodynamic model for acetaminophen, ibuprofen, and placebo antipyresis in children. *J Pharmacokinet Biopharm.* 1998;26:559-579.
7. Kelley MT, Walson PD, Edge JH, Cox S, Mortensen ME. Pharmacokinetics and pharmacodynamics of ibuprofen isomers and acetaminophen in febrile children. *Clin Pharmacol Ther.* 1992;52:181-189.
8. McIntyre J, Hull D. Comparing efficacy and tolerability of ibuprofen and acetaminophen in fever. *Arch Dis Child.* 1996;74:164-167.
9. Walson PD, Galletta G, Chomilo F, Braden NJ, Sawyer LA, Scheinbaum ML. Comparison of multidose ibuprofen and acetaminophen therapy in febrile children. *AJDC.* 1992;146:626-632.
10. Lesko SM, Mitchell AA. The safety of acetaminophen and ibuprofen among children younger than two years old. *Pediatrics.* 1999;104:e39.
11. Li SF, Lacher B, Crain EF. Acetaminophen and ibuprofen dosing by parents. *Pediatr Emerg Care.* 2000;16:394-397.
12. Mayoral CE, Marino RV, Rosenfeld W, Greensher J. Alternating antipyretics: is this an alternative? *Pediatrics.* 2000;105:1009-1012.
13. Breau LM, McGrath PJ, Camfield C, Rosmus C, Finley GA. Preliminary validation of an observational pain checklist for person with cognitive impairments and inability to communicate verbally. *Dev Med Child Neurol.* 2000;42:609-616.
14. Breau LM, Camfield C, McGrath PJ, Rosmus C, Finley GA. Measuring pain accurately in children with cognitive impairments: refinement of a caregiver scale. *J Pediatr.* 2001;138:721-727.
15. Rosner B. *Fundamentals of Biostatistics.* 4th ed. Belmont, Calif: Duxbury Press; 1995:384.
16. Sarrell M, Cohen HA, Kahan E. Physicians', nurses', and parents' attitudes to and knowledge about fever in early childhood. *Patient Educ Couns.* 2002;46:61-65.
17. Treluyer JM, Tonnelier S, d'Athis P, Leclerc B, Jolivet-Landreau I, Pons G. Antipyretic efficacy of an initial-30 mg/kg loading dose of acetaminophen vs a 15-mg/kg maintenance dose. *Pediatrics.* 2001;108:e73.
18. Lesko SM, Mitchell AA. Renal function after short-term ibuprofen use in infants and children. *Pediatrics.* 1997;100:954-957.
19. American Academy of Pediatrics; Committee on Drugs. Acetaminophen toxicity in children. *Pediatrics.* 2001;108:1020-1024.
20. Tarbell SE, Cohen IT, Marsh JL. The toddler-preschool postoperative pain scale: an observational scale for measuring postoperative pain in children aged 1-5: preliminary report. *Pain.* 1992;50:273-280.
21. McIntire SC, Rubenstein RC, Gartner JC Jr, Gilboa N, Ellis D. Acute flank pain and reversible renal dysfunction associated with nonsteroidal anti-inflammatory drug use. *Pediatrics.* 1993;92:459-460.


My mother loved children—she would have given anything if I had been one.
—Groucho Marx

ARTICLE

# Variation of Cognition and Achievement With Sleep-Disordered Breathing in Full-term and Preterm Children

*Judy L. Emancipator, MS; Amy Storfer-Isser, MS; H. Gerry Taylor, PhD; Carol L. Rosen, MD; H. L. Kirchner, PhD; Nathan L. Johnson, MS; Anne Marie Zambito, MPH; Susan Redline, MD, MPH*

**Objective:** Pediatric sleep-disordered breathing (SDB) has a disproportionately high prevalence in children who were preterm infants (preterm children) and is associated with behavioral comorbidity. Exposure to intermittent hypoxemia and sleep disruption may contribute to cognitive impairment. We quantified the association of SDB with cognition and achievement and determined whether preterm children are at a differentially increased risk for SDB-related impairments.

**Design:** Cross-sectional analyses.

**Setting:** Urban community.

**Participants:** Eight hundred thirty-five children, aged 8 to 11 years.

**Intervention(s):** None.

**Main Outcome Measures:** Scores on the Peabody Picture Vocabulary Test–Revised, Kaufman Assessment Battery for Children, and Continuous Performance Test.

**Results:** One hundred sixty-four children had SDB. In unadjusted analyses, children with SDB had poorer scores on almost all tests of cognition and achievement. Group differences were attenuated after adjusting for socioeconomic status; in these analyses, children with SDB scored lower on the Peabody Picture Vocabulary Test–Revised (mean ± SE score, 100.5 ± 1.4 vs 103.6 ± 0.7; $P = .04$), and the Kaufman Assessment Battery for Children riddles and triangles subscales. Associations were stronger in preterm than in full-term children. Of the sleep measures, snoring history was most strongly correlated with indices of cognition and achievement.

**Conclusions:** Although moderate group differences were observed for almost all cognitive measures, an attenuation of effects was observed once socioeconomic status was considered. The deficits in selective measures of academic abilities, language comprehension, and planning and organizational skills suggest a negative impact of SDB on achievement and cognition. Stronger associations in preterm children suggest the importance of screening for snoring, a good predictor of cognitive function in this population.

*Arch Pediatr Adolesc Med. 2006;160:203-210*

SLEEP-DISORDERED BREATHING (SDB), a common but underrecognized chronic health problem, is characterized by episodic periods of occlusion of the upper airway during sleep, often associated with oxygen desaturation, arousal, and impaired sleep quality. Symptoms include loud snoring, frequent awakenings, and excessive sleepiness. In adults, SDB is associated with a myriad of neurocognitive difficulties, including deficits in general intellectual function, attention, memory, and organizational abilities.[1-3]

Pediatric SDB may affect 2% to 4% of children, with a higher prevalence in certain subgroups, such as African American children and those who were preterm infants (preterm children).[4] The health impact of childhood SDB, however, is not well understood. Because learning is incremental and a strong foundation is essential during childhood, it is important to evaluate the association of SDB with children's cognitive and academic skills. Previous research has been limited by small numbers of participants,[5,6] a focus on children referred for clinical evaluation (in whom referral may have been stimulated by behavioral or cognitive concerns),[5,6] nonstandardized assessments of cognition,[7] exclusive reliance on parental observations of SDB symptoms,[8] incomplete control for confounding factors,[9] and inclusion of small numbers of children with objective evidence of sleep apnea.[10]

This study evaluates the performance of 835 children from a community-based sample on objective assessments of cognitive skills and academic achievement. We

Author Affiliations:
Department of Pediatrics, Rainbow Babies and Children's Hospital, Case Western Reserve School of Medicine, Cleveland, Ohio.

compared subgroups with and without SDB to address the following hypotheses: (1) SDB is associated with deficits in cognitive abilities and achievement; (2) preterm children, because of increased risk of neurodevelopmental disabilities related to early-life hypoxemia and ischemic injury, are at a differentially increased risk for SDB-related cognitive dysfunction; and (3) severity of overnight hypoxemia will be positively correlated with the extent of cognitive deficits.

## METHODS

### STUDY POPULATION

Methods of recruitment to the Cleveland Children's Sleep and Health Study have been previously reported.[4] In brief, the Cleveland Children's Sleep and Health Study is an urban community-based cohort of 907 children studied at 8 to 11 years of age. It was originally assembled as a stratified random sample of full-term and preterm children born at hospitals in the Cleveland, Ohio, area between January 1, 1988, and December 31, 1993. This cohort was designed to overrepresent African American and preterm children. Participants were excluded from analyses owing to inability to ascertain SDB status (n=65) or missing cognitive function data (n=7).

### STUDY PROTOCOL

Children underwent assessment at 8 to 11 years of age during a home visit, when health information was ascertained with the use of a pediatric modification of a validated questionnaire.[11] Trained research assistants (J.L.E. and A.M.Z.), blinded to the child's SDB status, administered the cognitive tests. On the night after the testing battery, children underwent an in-home sleep study. A small proportion (14%) of families and children were interviewed in a research setting rather than the home.

Institutional review boards at the participating hospitals approved the protocol. Written informed consent was obtained from the child's guardian, and assent was obtained from the child.

### SDB ASSESSMENTS

Details on the methods for the assessing SDB have been reported.[4] In brief, a 6-channel monitor recorded respiration (with rib cage and abdominal inductance plethysmography), heart rate, oxygen saturation level, and body position (SomnoStar PT-2; SensorMedics, Yorba Linda, Calif). Obstructive sleep apnea was defined as an obstructive apnea-hypopnea index (OAHI) of greater than or equal to 5 events per hour and/or an obstructive apnea index (OAI) of greater than or equal to 1 event per hour. The approach for quantifying obstructive sleep apnea has been validated by comparing the OAHI from the home study with a similar index from findings of 12-channel laboratory-based polysomnography in 55 children in whom the 2 tests were performed within 3 months (intraclass correlation coefficient, 0.85).[4] Snoring was ascertained via a questionnaire that requested the parent to report the frequency of loud snoring by the child during the past month on a 5-point scale, ranging from never to always. Habitual snoring was defined as loud snoring during the past month, occurring at least 1 to 2 times per week. Children with obstructive sleep apnea and/or who were habitual snorers were categorized as having SDB, whereas children who were not habitual snorers and did not have obstructive sleep apnea were categorized as not having SDB. For exploratory analyses, children were also classified as nonsnorers vs snorers (ie, occurring rarely or more often per week, during the past month).

### NEUROCOGNITIVE ASSESSMENTS

Cognitive skills and academic achievement were assessed with the Peabody Picture Vocabulary Test–Revised (PPVT-R),[12] Kaufman Assessment Battery for Children (K-ABC),[13] and Continuous Performance Test (CPT).[14] To administer the PPVT-R, spoken words are presented in increasing order of difficulty, and the examinee is asked to point to 1 of 4 pictures that shows the meaning of the word. The test measures comprehension of spoken words but also requires the ability to selectively attend to the response choices. The K-ABC consists of 13 subscales and 5 composite scales assessing a range of mental processing abilities and written language and mathematics skills. The K-ABC mental processing composite consists of sequential and simultaneous global mental skills. Specific subscales require memory, eye-hand coordination, spatial skills, problem solving, and executive functions that include the abilities to attend to the task and plan and organize one's approach. The CPT is a 14-minute computerized test of sustained attention and response inhibition. This test requires the child to press a key whenever an *x* appears on the screen and not to press the key when nontarget stimuli are presented. Time to respond, correct and incorrect responses, and missed targets are recorded. Raw scores on the K-ABC and PPVT-R were converted to age-adjusted standard scores based on published normative values.[13,14] Standard scores for the PPVT-R and K-ABC global measures have a mean of 100 and SD of 15, with higher scores reflecting better cognitive performance. Our primary outcome measures were standard scores from the PPVT-R, the K-ABC mental processing composite and achievement scales, the reaction time, and an index describing the child's ability to detect target stimuli while inhibiting responses to nontargets (response discrimination, D-prime) from the CPT.

### STATISTICAL ANALYSIS

Analyses were designed to obtain an unbiased estimate of the association between SDB and each measure of cognitive performance. Covariates and potential confounders, including the child's age, sex, birth weight, and indices of socioeconomic status (SES), were selected on the basis of theory and empirical research. Socioeconomic status was assessed using data on caregiver education, caregiver marital status, and census tract median income. Median income from the 2000 census was obtained by matching the child's address to the corresponding census tract. To control for prematurity and birth weight, the following 4 mutually exclusive categories were created on the basis of a combination of preterm status and birth weight: premature with extremely low birth weight (<1000 g); premature with very low birth weight (1000-1499 g); premature with low birth weight (≥1500 g), and full-term with normal birth weight (≥2500 g).

Groups were compared using 2-sample *t* tests, Wilcoxon rank sum tests, and the Pearson $\chi^2$ test for normally distributed, skewed, and categorical data, respectively (SAS software, version 9.1; SAS Institute Inc, Cary, NC). Spearman correlations were used to assess the magnitude of the association between cognitive outcomes and sleep measures. Multiple linear regression was used to assess the relationship between SDB and each cognitive outcome, adjusting for potential confounders. Graphical techniques were used to assess the relationship between continuous covariates and cognitive outcomes. Models were fit without covariate adjustment (unadjusted); adjustment for age, sex, and birth weight category (partially adjusted); and adjustment for age, sex, birth weight category, caregiver education and marital status, and median income (fully adjusted). Unless otherwise indicated, data are expressed as mean±SD.

**Table 1. Sample Characteristics***

| | Analytic Sample (n = 835) | Non-SDB (n = 671) | SDB (n = 164) | *P* Value† |
|---|---|---|---|---|
| Age, mean ± SD, y | 9.5 ± 0.8 | 9.5 ± 0.8 | 9.4 ± 0.8 | .31 |
| African American | 303 (36.3) | 218 (32.5) | 85 (51.8) | <.001 |
| Male | 419 (50.2) | 338 (50.4) | 81 (49.4) | .82 |
| Preterm | 383 (45.9) | 286 (42.6) | 97 (59.1) | <.001 |
| Prematurity by birth weight, g | | | | |
| Premature, <1000 | 75 (9.0) | 54 (8.0) | 21 (12.8) | .002 |
| Premature, 1000-1499 | 119 (14.3) | 88 (13.1) | 31 (18.9) | |
| Premature, ≥1500 | 189 (22.6) | 144 (21.5) | 45 (27.4) | |
| Full-term, ≥2500 | 452 (54.1) | 385 (57.4) | 67 (40.9) | |
| Caregiver education | | | | |
| <High school | 55 (6.6) | 40 (6.0) | 15 (9.1) | .04 |
| High school/GED | 161 (19.3) | 121 (18.0) | 40 (24.4) | |
| >High school | 619 (74.1) | 510 (76.0) | 109 (66.5) | |
| BMI, mean ± SD | 18.2 ± 3.9 | 17.9 ± 3.5 | 19.4 ± 5.0 | .005 |
| Obese (BMI ≥95th percentile) | 133 (15.9) | 88 (13.1) | 45 (27.4) | <.001 |
| History of tonsillectomy and/or adenoidectomy | 63 (7.5) | 38 (5.7) | 25 (15.2) | .002 |
| Caregiver marital status | | | | |
| Married/remarried | 585 (70.1) | 488 (72.7) | 97 (59.1) | .003 |
| Separated/widowed/divorced | 116 (13.9) | 86 (12.8) | 30 (18.3) | |
| Never married | 134 (16.0) | 97 (14.5) | 37 (22.6) | |
| Annual income, mean ± SD (median)‡† | $47 600 ± $24 000 ($46 000) | $49 600 ± $24 300 ($48 100) | $39 500 ± $20 500 ($35 900) | <.001 |
| Poverty rate, mean ± SD (median), %‡ | 13.5 ± 15.1 (6.2) | 12.5 ± 14.7 (5.3) | 17.7 ± 16.3 (12.1) | <.001 |

Abbreviations: BMI, body mass index (calculated as weight in kilograms divided by the square of height in meters); GED, general educational development test; SDB, sleep-disordered breathing.

*SDB is defined as an obstructive apnea-hypopnea index of 5 or greater, obstructive apnea index of 1 or greater, or loud snoring (1-2 times/wk or more). Unless otherwise indicated, data are expressed as number (percentage) of subjects (categorical variables).

†Compares children with and without SDB.

‡Obtained from census data (tract level).

## RESULTS

The sample was approximately 50% female and had a mean age of 9.5±0.8 years (**Table 1**). By design, approximately half of the sample (45.9%) consisted of preterm infants, including 9.0% with extremely low birth weight (<1000 g). The median income from the census tract data was $46 000 per year, and the median poverty rate was 6.2%.

One hundred sixty-four children (19.6%) children were classified as having SDB. As reported previously,[4] children with SDB were significantly more likely to be African American and to have been born prematurely. They also were more likely to live in a neighborhood with lower median income, live in a single parent household, and have a caregiver with a high school education or less. The 2 groups did not significantly differ with respect to age and sex. Tonsillectomy and/or adenoidectomy were reported more commonly among children with SDB compared with children without SDB.

Sleep characteristics of the sample are shown in **Table 2**. Overall, 21 children had an OAHI of 5 or greater, and 34 children had an OAI of 1 or greater. As expected, the percentage of sleep time at an oxygen desaturation level of less than 90% was higher among children with SDB. Approximately two thirds of parents reported that their child never snored, whereas 17.6% reported habitual snoring. Parents reported that their child slept 9.2±0.9 hours on average, with no difference for children with and without SDB.

**Table 3** shows the distribution of the unadjusted, partially adjusted, and fully adjusted PPVT-R and K-ABC scores. The unadjusted and partially adjusted (ie, not including indices of SES) results show that the SDB group scored significantly lower on the PPVT-R and K-ABC summary measures. The unadjusted analyses showed an average difference of 9 points for the PPVT-R and 5 points for the K-ABC summary scales, effect sizes that are moderate to large. There was a small attenuation of group differences once the effects of age, sex, and birth weight were considered (partially adjusted results). Further adjustment for SES, with consideration of caregiver education and marital status and median income (the latter explaining the largest proportion of variance in cognitive measures), resulted in considerable attenuation of SDB group differences. Although in fully adjusted analyses the SDB group tended to score lower on all tests and subtests, significantly lower scores were observed for the PPVT-R and the K-ABC riddles and triangles subscales only. Performance measured during the CPT showed a longer mean reaction time in children with SDB; however, this measure and response discrimination were not significantly associated with SDB after covariate adjustment. Excluding children who had had a tonsillectomy and/or adenoidectomy reduced statistical power slightly, but provided qualitatively similar results.

To address whether associations of SDB with cognitive and achievement skills may be stronger in a vulnerable group, analyses were repeated stratifying by preterm status, and the results for the preterm group are presented in **Table 4**. The fully adjusted models showed that preterm children with SDB performed significantly

**Table 2. Sleep Characteristics***

| | Analytic Sample (n = 835) | Non-SDB (n = 671) | SDB (n = 164) | *P* Value |
|---|---|---|---|---|
| OAHI, events/h | 0.7 ± 2.6 (0.2) | 0.3 ± 0.4 (0.1) | 2.4 ± 5.6 (0.5) | <.001 |
| OAHI ≥5 events/h, No. (%) | 21 (2.5) | 0 | 21 (13.1) | <.001 |
| OAI, events/h | 0.2 ± 0.9 (0.0) | 0.1 ± 0.2 (0.0) | 0.8 ± 2.0 (0.0) | <.001 |
| OAI ≥1 event/h, No. (%) | 34 (4.1) | 0 | 34 (21.3) | <.001 |
| Oxygen saturation, % | | | | |
| Minimum saturation | 84.9 ± 6.1 (86.0) | 85.0 ± 6.2 (86.0) | 84.5 ± 5.6 (86.0) | .12 |
| Mean saturation | 96.1 ± 1.4 (96.0) | 96.2 ± 1.2 (96.0) | 95.9 ± 1.9 (96.0) | .59 |
| % of time with <90% desaturation | 0.5 ± 4.9 (0.0) | 0.2 ± 1.9 (0.0) | 1.8 ± 10.4 (0.0) | <.001 |
| Frequency of loud snoring during the past mo, No. (%) | | | | |
| Never | 568 (68.0) | 553 (82.4) | 15 (9.2) | <.001 |
| <1 Time/wk (rarely) | 121 (14.5) | 118 (17.6) | 3 (1.8) | |
| 1-2 Times/wk (sometimes) | 73 (8.7) | 0 | 73 (44.5) | |
| 3-4 Times/wk (frequently) | 24 (2.9) | 0 | 24 (14.6) | |
| 5-7 Times/wk (always) | 49 (5.9) | 0 | 49 (29.9) | |
| Sleep time (parent-report), h | 9.2 ± 0.9 (9.3) | 9.2 ± 0.9 (9.3) | 9.1 ± 1.1 (9.1) | .09 |

Abbreviations: OAHI, obstructive apnea-hypopnea index; OAI, obstructive apnea index; SDB, sleep-disordered breathing.
*SDB is defined as an OAHI of 5 or greater, OAI of 1 or more, or loud snoring (1-2 times/wk or more). Unless otherwise indicated, data are expressed as mean ± SD (median) (continuous variables).

**Table 3. Distribution of Cognition and Achievement Measures by SDB***

| | Unadjusted | | | Partial Adjustment † | | | Full Adjustment‡ | | |
|---|---|---|---|---|---|---|---|---|---|
| Measure | No SDB (n = 671) | SDB (n = 164) | *P* Value | No SDB (n = 671) | SDB (n = 164) | *P* Value | No SDB (n = 671) | SDB (n = 164) | *P* Value |
| PPVT-R | 103.6 ± 0.8 | 95.0 ± 1.6 | <.001 | 103.4 ± 0.8 | 95.6 ± 1.6 | <.001 | 103.6 ± 0.7 | 100.5 ± 1.4 | .04 |
| K-ABC global scales | | | | | | | | | |
| Achievement | 102.0 ± 0.6 | 95.7 ± 1.2 | <.001 | 101.8 ± 0.6 | 96.6 ± 1.2 | .001 | 101.5 ± 0.5 | 99.7 ± 1.0 | .12 |
| Mental processing | 101.5 ± 0.5 | 96.4 ± 1.1 | <.001 | 101.2 ± 0.5 | 97.4 ± 1.0 | .001 | 100.9 ± 0.5 | 99.8 ± 1.0 | .26 |
| K-ABC subscales | | | | | | | | | |
| Riddles | 100.7 ± 0.5 | 95.2 ± 1.1 | <.001 | 100.6 ± 0.5 | 95.6 ± 1.1 | <.001 | 100.4 ± 0.5 | 98.3 ± 1.0 | .049 |
| Triangles | 10.4 ± 0.1 | 9.3 ± 0.2 | <.001 | 10.4 ± 0.1 | 9.5 ± 0.2 | <.001 | 10.3 ± 0.1 | 9.9 ± 0.2 | .045 |
| CPT | | | | | | | | | |
| Mean hit reaction time | 456.4 ± 3.1 | 471.2 ± 6.2 | .04 | 457.3 ± 2.9 | 467.8 ± 5.9 | .11 | 456.1 ± 3.2 | 460.0 ± 6.1 | .56 |
| D-prime | 1.43 ± 0.03 | 1.31 ± 0.07 | .13 | 1.42 ± 0.03 | 1.36 ± 0.06 | .37 | 1.38 ± 0.03 | 1.39 ± 0.06 | .95 |

Abbreviations: CPT, Continuous Performance Test; K-ABC, Kaufman Assessment Battery for Children; PPVT, Peabody Picture Vocabulary Test–Revised; SDB, sleep-disordered breathing.
*SDB is defined as an obstructive apnea-hypopnea index of 5 or greater, an obstructive apnea index of 1 or greater, or loud snoring (1-2 times/wk or more). Unless otherwise indicated, data are expressed as least squares mean ± SE.
†Adjusted for age, sex, and birth weight category.
‡Adjusted for age, sex, birth weight category, caregiver education, caregiver marital status, and median income (census tract, with quadratic term).

worse on the PPVT-R and the K-ABC achievement and simultaneous global scales and riddles and triangles subscales. In contrast, the differences in neurocognitive function between the full-term children with and without SDB did not achieve statistical significance after fully adjusting for covariates (data not shown).

To explore which physiological stresses associated with SDB are most closely associated with neurocognitive deficits, the strength of the associations of overnight oxygen desaturation; frequencies of apnea and hypopnea and snoring; and sleep time with each cognitive outcome were assessed. The unadjusted and fully adjusted correlations show weak associations between cognitive outcomes and the oxygen saturation measures and OAHI and OAI variables, particularly after covariate adjustment (**Table 5**). Sleep time shows a modest, positive correlation with cognitive measures in unadjusted analyses only. Frequency of snoring has the strongest association with the cognitive outcomes, which are attenuated but remain statistically significant after covariate adjustment.

Graphic techniques used to further assess the association between snoring frequency and cognitive performance showed that children who were reported to never snore in the preceding month had higher scores compared with snoring children, with no difference in those in whom snoring frequency was reported as rare compared with more frequent. Analyses that substituted snoring status as the primary predictor rather than SDB showed that the mean differences between groups were slightly greater compared with the main analysis in which SDB was the primary predictor (**Table 6**). In fully adjusted analyses, many of these group differences are statistically sig-

**Table 4. Distribution of Cognition and Achievement Measures in Preterm Children by SDB***

| Measure | Unadjusted | | | Partial Adjustment† | | | Full Adjustment‡ | | |
|---|---|---|---|---|---|---|---|---|---|
| | No SDB (n = 286) | SDB (n = 97) | *P* Value | No SDB (n = 286) | SDB (n = 97) | *P* Value | No SDB (n = 286) | SDB (n = 97) | *P* Value |
| PPVT-R | 102.0 ± 1.2 | 91.7 ± 2.0 | <.001 | 102.0 ± 1.1 | 92.0 ± 2.0 | <.001 | 102.2 ± 1.1 | 97.8 ± 1.9 | .04 |
| K-ABC global scales | | | | | | | | | |
| Achievement | 99.1 ± 0.9 | 92.0 ± 1.5 | <.001 | 99.1 ± 0.9 | 92.2 ± 1.5 | <.001 | 98.9 ± 0.9 | 95.7 ± 1.5 | .05 |
| Mental processing | 97.7 ± 0.8 | 92.2 ± 1.3 | <.001 | 97.6 ± 0.8 | 92.5 ± 1.3 | <.001 | 97.6 ± 0.8 | 95.2 ± 1.3 | .09 |
| K-ABC subscales | | | | | | | | | |
| Riddles | 99.9 ± 0.8 | 92.8 ± 1.4 | <.001 | 99.9 ± 0.8 | 93.0 ± 1.4 | <.001 | 100.0 ± 0.8 | 96.6 ± 1.4 | .03 |
| Triangles | 9.9 ± 0.2 | 8.7 ± 0.3 | <.001 | 9.9 ± 0.2 | 8.8 ± 0.3 | <.001 | 9.9 ± 0.2 | 9.3 ± 0.3 | .04 |
| CPT | | | | | | | | | |
| Mean hit reaction time | 461.0 ± 4.9 | 482.0 ± 8.5 | .03 | 461.3 ± 4.6 | 481.5 ± 7.9 | .02 | 458.5 ± 5.0 | 468.3 ± 8.5 | .29 |
| D-prime | 1.25 ± 0.05 | 1.28 ± 0.08 | .76 | 1.25 ± 0.04 | 1.27 ± 0.08 | .84 | 1.23 ± 0.05 | 1.26 ± 0.08 | .75 |

Abbreviations: See Table 3.
*SDB is defined as an obstructive apnea-hypopnea index of 5 or greater, an obstructive apnea index of 1 or greater, or loud snoring (1-2 times/wk or more). Unless otherwise indicated, data are expressed as least squares mean ± SE.
†Adjusted for age, sex, and birth weight category.
‡Adjusted for age, sex, birth weight category, caregiver education, caregiver marital status, and median income (census tract, with quadratic term).

**Table 5. Partial Spearman Correlations Relating Sleep Indices With Measures of Cognition and Achievement for the Analytic Sample***

| Measure | OAHI | OAI | Mean Saturation, % | Minimum Saturation, % | % of Time <90% Saturation | Sleep Time† | Snoring Frequency |
|---|---|---|---|---|---|---|---|
| **Unadjusted‡** | | | | | | | |
| PPVT-R | ***−0.11*** | *−0.08* | −0.04 | ***0.14*** | −0.07 | ***0.13*** | −0.18 |
| K-ABC global scales | | | | | | | |
| Achievement | ***−0.11*** | *−0.08* | −0.05 | ***0.14*** | −0.07 | ***0.15*** | ***−0.19*** |
| Mental processing | *−0.07* | *−0.07* | 0.00 | ***0.14*** | −0.04 | ***0.13*** | ***−0.16*** |
| K-ABC subscales | | | | | | | |
| Riddles | ***−0.12*** | ***−0.09*** | −0.03 | ***0.15*** | −0.05 | ***0.14*** | ***−0.19*** |
| Triangles | *−0.07* | −0.05 | −0.05 | ***0.15*** | −0.06 | ***0.12*** | ***−0.15*** |
| CPT | | | | | | | |
| Mean hit reaction time | *0.07* | *0.09* | −0.04 | −0.05 | 0.04 | 0.01 | 0.06 |
| D-prime | −0.06 | *−0.08* | 0.01 | 0.04 | −0.05 | 0.02 | −0.06 |
| **Fully Adjusted§** | | | | | | | |
| PPVT-R | −0.05 | 0.00 | 0.01 | 0.05 | −0.01 | 0.00 | ***−0.10*** |
| K-ABC global scales | | | | | | | |
| Achievement | −0.04 | −0.01 | −0.01 | 0.04 | 0.00 | 0.04 | ***−0.10*** |
| Mental processing | 0.00 | −0.01 | 0.04 | 0.04 | 0.02 | 0.03 | −0.06 |
| K-ABC subscales | | | | | | | |
| Riddles | −0.07 | −0.04 | 0.03 | *0.07* | 0.00 | 0.02 | ***−0.11*** |
| Triangles | −0.01 | 0.01 | 0.00 | *0.07* | −0.03 | 0.02 | *−0.07* |
| CPT | | | | | | | |
| Mean hit reaction time | *0.08* | 0.05 | −0.03 | −0.02 | 0.01 | 0.02 | 0.02 |
| D-prime | −0.01 | −0.02 | −0.01 | 0.01 | −0.00 | 0.02 | −0.02 |

Abbreviations: OAHI, obstructive apnea-hypopnea index; OAI, obstructive apnea index. For remaining abbreviations, see Table 3.
*Unless otherwise indicated, data are expressed as Spearman correlation. Italic values indicate *P*<.05; boldface italic, *P*<.01.
†Indicates average for weekends and weekdays (parent report).
‡Adjusted for age, sex, and birth weight category.
§Adjusted for age, sex, birth weight category, caregiver education, caregiver marital status, and median income (census tract).

nificant, with snorers demonstrating lower scores on the PPVT-R, K-ABC achievement global scale, and K-ABC subscales arithmetic (97.8±0.9 vs 100.7±0.7; *P*=.007), faces and places (100.8±0.9 vs 103.2±0.6; *P*=.01), reading/decoding (99.1±0.8 vs 101.9±0.6; *P*=.005), reading/understanding (100.8±0.8 vs 103.0±0.6; *P*=.02), and riddles and triangles (Table 6). Significant differences in the CPT measures were not observed. Results were essentially unchanged in analyses excluding children with an elevated OAHI or OAI.

## COMMENT

A major component of SDB morbidity is thought to relate to neuropsychological deficits, with concern that in

**Table 6. Distribution of Cognition and Achievement Measures by Snoring History***

| Measure | Unadjusted | | | Partial Adjustment† | | | Full Adjustment‡ | | |
|---|---|---|---|---|---|---|---|---|---|
| | Nonsnorer (n = 568) | Snorer (n = 267) | P Value | Nonsnorer (n = 568) | Snorer (n = 267) | P Value | Nonsnorer (n = 568) | Snorer (n = 267) | P Value |
| PPVT-R | 104.2 ± 0.8 | 96.9 ± 1.2 | <.001 | 104.1 ± 0.8 | 97.3 ± 1.2 | <.001 | 104.0 ± 0.8 | 100.7 ± 1.1 | .008 |
| K-ABC global scales | | | | | | | | | |
| Achievement | 102.8 ± 0.6 | 96.5 ± 0.9 | <.001 | 102.6 ± 0.6 | 97.0 ± 0.9 | <.001 | 102.1 ± 0.6 | 99.0 ± 0.8 | <.001 |
| Mental processing | 101.9 ± 0.6 | 97.4 ± 0.8 | <.001 | 101.6 ± 0.6 | 98.0 ± 0.8 | <.001 | 101.2 ± 0.5 | 99.6 ± 0.8 | .06 |
| K-ABC subscales | | | | | | | | | |
| Riddles | 101.3 ± 0.6 | 96.0 ± 0.8 | <.001 | 101.2 ± 0.6 | 96.2 ± 0.8 | <.001 | 100.9 ± 0.6 | 98.0 ± 0.8 | .002 |
| Triangles | 10.5 ± 0.1 | 9.6 ± 0.2 | <.001 | 10.5 ± 0.1 | 9.7 ± 0.2 | <.001 | 10.4 ± 0.1 | 9.9 ± 0.2 | .01 |
| CPT | | | | | | | | | |
| Mean hit reaction time | 456.9 ± 3.4 | 464.4 ± 4.9 | .21 | 457.2 ± 3.2 | 463.9 ± 4.6 | .24 | 456.4 ± 3.4 | 457.8 ± 4.9 | .80 |
| D-prime | 1.44 ± 0.04 | 1.32 ± 0.05 | .050 | 1.44 ± 0.03 | 1.33 ± 0.05 | .06 | 1.40 ± 0.04 | 1.33 ± 0.05 | .24 |

Abbreviations: See Table 3.
*Indicates parent report of loud snoring over the past month, occurring 1 to 2 times/wk or more. Unless otherwise indicated, data are expressed as least squares mean ± SE.
†Adjusted for age, sex, and birth weight category.
‡Adjusted age, sex, birth weight category, caregiver education, caregiver marital status, and median income (census tract, with quadratic term).

children, SDB may result in long-term decrements in academic achievement.[8] Although childhood SDB has been associated consistently with behavioral morbidity, including conduct problems and aggressiveness,[15-18] fewer data are available that address the association of childhood SDB and cognitive performance and achievement. This study extends previous research, addressing the association of a range of cognitive functions with SDB in a large, diverse pediatric population. The availability of several measures of SES allowed us to rigorously address potential environmental confounders. Inclusion of a large preterm group permitted assessment of low birth weight and prematurity as possible confounders while also providing an opportunity to explore differential susceptibility of a preterm population. These findings show (1) moderate to large SDB group differences for almost all cognitive measures (ie, effect sizes of 0.3-0.6), but evidence of considerable attenuation of group differences once SES (particularly neighborhood median income) was considered; (2) persistence of small to modest group differences for the PPVT-R and 2 K-ABC subscales (riddles and triangles) in adjusted analyses; (3) stronger associations of SDB with deficits in cognitive ability and academic achievement in preterm compared with full-term children; and (4) evidence that of all SDB measures (including oxygen saturation, the frequency of apneas and hypopneas, and sleep time), snoring history was most strongly associated with cognitive deficits.

Although large deficits in a broad range of neurocognitive tests were observed between SDB groups in unadjusted or partially adjusted analyses, differences were attenuated once SES was accounted for by adjusting for caregiver education and marital status and neighborhood income level. To our knowledge, this is the first time that an index of neighborhood poverty has been considered in relation to SDB. Because this measure may serve as a proxy for a wide variety of social and environmental risk factors that influence development, including quality of education and neighborhood structure, it may provide additional information over what is usually available from parent self-reported income. The findings suggest that some of the effects of childhood SDB in the literature may have been overestimated owing to incomplete consideration of confounding due to SES and premature birth or owing to other selection biases, eg, studying children at high risk for problems in behavior, cognition, and achievement.

Our findings of modest and selective cognitive deficits in children with SDB are consistent with results of previous research showing children with SDB to have poorer performances on a restricted range of neurocognitive assessments administered as part of larger test batteries.[6,9,10,19,20] In several studies, deficits were greatest for language, spatial skills, attention, and organizational skills.[10,21] In our study, the larger SDB group differences found for the PPVT-R than the K-ABC scores may reflect the relative sensitivity of the former test to accumulated verbal knowledge. This test also requires inhibition of impulsive responses—behaviors that are impaired in children with SDB.[16-18,21,22] Impairment of scores on the K-ABC riddles subscale, which requires the child to solve a verbal puzzle, is also consistent with limitations in verbal comprehension and the ability to be selective and to plan in responding to tasks. These deficits are similar to those suggested by weaknesses on the PPVT-R. The K-ABC triangles subscale scores were also impaired in children with SDB. The triangles subscale is the only timed test, and it requires children to plan and organize their responses in solving spatial puzzles, placing demands on multiple executive functions. These deficits are consistent with data from adult studies that show preferential deficits in planning and organizational skills and in efficiency of performance with SDB,[1-3] and with evidence that adults with SDB have a relatively poorer performance on timed tests, including those that make demands on spatial abilities.[23]

The pattern of deficits observed suggests that children with SDB are vulnerable to weaknesses in attending selectively to tasks and planning their responses, and these weaknesses contribute over time to more pronounced deficits in accumulated knowledge and academic skills. The latter deficits are illustrated by the SDB group's reduced scores in verbal comprehension and the reductions in academic achievement observed among snorers. Although other investigators have shown deficits in learning, memory, and general intelligence,[5,9,10] these latter studies included children referred for evaluation with high degrees of medical or psychological comorbidity[5] or did not comprehensively address confounders such as SES and prematurity.[5,9] Data from a subsample of children recruited from the Infant Practices Study[10] showed reductions in both memory and general intelligence in 5-year-old children with SDB symptoms. However, the average scores for the SDB and non-SDB groups were both higher than normative data. These findings were based on parent-reported symptoms, without evidence that deficits were specific to the small number of children with breathing pauses.[10]

Although we posited that impairments in sustained attention may underlie deficits in other cognitive functions, we did not find evidence of these deficits when a standardized continuous performance task was used. This agrees with the findings of Beebe et al[21] and Gottlieb et al,[10] who also did not find significant attentional deficits in SDB when similar measures of visual attention were used. The CPT, originally designed as a tool for evaluating attention-deficit/hyperactivity disorder, may not be sufficiently sensitive in children with mild SDB, who are not overtly somnolent. Alternatively, computer-based vigilance tasks may be less discriminating in current cohorts of children who are now regularly exposed to computer-based video games compared with the older cohorts in whom such tests were originally developed.

The pathophysiological basis for neurocognitive deficits occurring with SDB is thought to relate to exposure to intermittent hypoxemia and sleep disruption. Animal experiments have shown that intermittent hypoxemia produces apoptosis in the cerebral cortex and hippocampus,[24] which correlates with spatial learning deficits.[25] In humans, such exposures may disproportionately affect planning and organizational abilities (ie, executive functions), which are particularly dependent on the basal ganglia and frontal lobes, areas sensitive to intermittent hypoxemia. Accordingly, in several studies of adults, hypoxemia most closely predicted deficits in executive functions and psychomotor skills, whereas sleepiness predicted attentional deficits.[1,26] One study showed no threshold effect for hypoxemia or the frequency of breathing pauses, suggesting that even mild SDB may have an adverse impact on neurocognitive function.[3]

We did not observe neurocognitive deficits to be linearly associated with frequency of breathing pauses or severity of overnight desaturation. This differs from the findings from a German study of children that showed that overnight oxygen nadir was associated with selective impairment in arithmetic scores.[7] The clinical implications of this latter finding are unclear, because no other desaturation variable was associated with impairment in any academic measure, and because oxygen nadir may not provide a reliable estimate of overnight hypoxemia. In contrast, we found that reported snoring frequency was significantly correlated with cognitive and achievement scores. Even in fully adjusted analyses, significant associations were demonstrated between snoring and scores on the K-ABC achievement scale, 6 of the K-ABC subscales, and the PPVT-R. These findings are consistent with literature that has reported cognitive deficits in primary snorers[27] and in children with symptoms of SDB who have few breathing pauses.[10] The relatively small number of children with severe SDB might have limited our ability to detect dose-response relationships with indices of SDB severity. Nonetheless, these data suggest that snoring, especially assessed in general samples without high degrees of SDB severity, may provide a useful measure of chronic sleep disruption. Reported snoring at 8 to 11 years of age also may identify children who had experienced more severe SDB at earlier ages, including times of developmental susceptibility to adverse cognitive effects of hypoxemia. Although we were surprised that habitual snoring was not more strongly associated with cognitive deficits than any snoring in the preceding month, it is possible that parents of middle school children underestimate their children's snoring frequency. Regardless of the physiological basis for this observation, our data suggest that obtaining a snoring history may be useful for screening among children at risk for cognitive and achievement deficits.

A previous report from our group[4] observed a 4-fold higher prevalence of SDB in preterm children, and our present study was designed to test whether this vulnerable group experiences disproportionate morbidity associated with SDB. Preterm children have a range of learning and cognitive deficits occurring in direct proportion to their immaturity,[28,29] including deficits in language abilities, verbal learning, and spatial and organizational skills.[28] Previous research in preterm children has not considered whether unrecognized SDB may account for such deficits. Conversely, previous studies of SDB have not considered prematurity as a contributor to SDB-associated comorbidity. Our analyses identify selective cognitive deficits attributable to SDB, even after adjusting for preterm status and birth weight. Furthermore, among children with predominantly mild SDB, SDB-associated comorbidity appears more pronounced in preterm than in full-term children. Although prospective studies are required, these results suggest that children with more limited cognitive reserve and/or who have had developmental or perinatal stresses may be especially vulnerable to mild SDB in childhood. These children may be less able to compensate for SDB-related cognitive deficits, possibly because of diminished plasticity of function after early brain insults.[30-32] Alternatively, a noncausal association between SDB and cognitive dysfunction in preterm children is plausible; ie, developmental and early life stresses could increase a predisposition to SDB by adversely influencing upper airway neuromuscular control and/or airway anatomy. In either case, because some research suggests beneficial effects on cognition with treatment of childhood SDB,[15,33] there may be utility in efforts to more aggressively screen for snoring and SDB in premature children.

The strengths of our study include the large sample size with a wide range of SES and ethnicity and inclusion of sufficient numbers of preterm children to evaluate associations with birth weight and prematurity. The study used objective measures of neurocognitive function and nocturnal cardiorespiratory monitoring and contained robust measures of SES. Study weaknesses include the relatively low proportion of children with severe SDB, preventing a full evaluation of the extent to which marked hypoxemia or sleep disruption may contribute to cognitive deficits. Although validated measures for the OAHI were used that correlate excellently with full in-laboratory measures,[4] the home sleep studies did not include direct measures of sleep stages or arousal, preventing evaluation of these factors.

Our analyses suggest that some of the reported cognitive and achievement deficits attributable to mild SDB in the literature may have been overestimated owing to confounding by SES and prematurity. However, our data on a large birth cohort are consistent with an association between mild SDB, including snoring, and selective deficits in verbal comprehension and executive functions, with effects relatively greater in preterm children, who may be particularly vulnerable to stresses associated with SDB. Furthermore, our data suggest the potential utility of snoring history as a screening tool, particularly in preterm children, who appear to be at increased risk for both SDB and SDB-associated cognitive deficits.

**Accepted for Publication:** September 1, 2005.
**Correspondence:** Susan Redline, MD, MPH, 11100 Euclid Ave, Department of Pediatrics, Case Western Reserve University School of Medicine, Cleveland, OH 44106-6003 (sxr15@case.edu).
**Funding/Support:** This study was supported by grants HL HL60957, K23 HL04426, M01 RR00080, RO1 NR02707, and RO1070916 from the National Institutes of Health, Bethesda, Md.

## REFERENCES

1. Naegele B, Thouvard V, Pepin JL, et al. Deficits of cognitive executive functions in patients with sleep apnea syndrome. *Sleep.* 1995;18:43-52.
2. Bedard MA, Montplaisir J, Richer F, Rouleau I, Malo J. Obstructive sleep apnea: pathogenesis of neuropsychological deficits. *J Clin Exp Neuropsychol.* 1991; 13:950-964.
3. Adams N, Strauss M, Schluchter M, Redline S. Relation of measures of sleep-disordered breathing to neuropsychological functioning. *Am J Respir Crit Care Med.* 2001;163:1626-1631.
4. Rosen CL, Larkin EK, Kirchner HL, et al. Prevalence and risk factors for sleep-disordered breathing in 8- to 11-year-old children: association with race and prematurity. *J Pediatr.* 2003;142:383-389.
5. Rhodes SK, Shimoda KC, Waid LR, et al. Neurocognitive deficits in morbidly obese children with obstructive sleep apnea. *J Pediatr.* 1995;127:741-744.
6. Beebe DW, Groesz L, Wells C, Nichols A, McGee K. The neuropsychological effects of obstructive sleep apnea: a meta-analysis of norm-referenced and case-controlled data. *Sleep.* 2003;26:298-307.
7. Urschitz MS, Wolff J, Sokollik C, et al. Nocturnal arterial oxygen saturation and academic performance in a community sample of children. *Pediatrics.* 2005; 115:e204-e209.
8. Gozal D, Pope DW. Snoring during early childhood and academic performance at ages thirteen to fourteen years. *Pediatrics.* 2001;107:1394-1399.
9. Kaemingk KL, Pasvogel AE, Goodwin JL, et al. Learning in children and sleep disordered breathing: findings of the Tucson Children's Assessment of Sleep Apnea (tuCASA) prospective cohort study. *J Int Neuropsychol Soc.* 2003;9:1016-1026.
10. Gottlieb DJ, Chase C, Vezina RM, et al. Sleep-disordered breathing symptoms are associated with poorer cognitive function in 5-year-old children. *J Pediatr.* 2004;145:458-464.
11. Kump K, Whalen C, Tishler PV, et al. Assessment of the validity and utility of a sleep-symptom questionnaire. *Am J Respir Crit Care Med.* 1994;150:735-741.
12. Umberger FG. *Peabody Picture Vocabulary Test-Revised.* Kansas City, Mo: Test Corp America; 1985.
13. Merz WR. *Kaufman Assessment Battery for Children.* Kansas City, Mo: Test Corp America; 1984.
14. Connors CK. *Connor's Continuous Performance Test.* North Tonawanda, NY: Multi-Health System; 1995.
15. Ali NJ, Pitson D, Stradling JR. Sleep disordered breathing: effects of adenotonsillectomy on behaviour and psychological functioning. *Eur J Pediatr.* 1996; 155:56-62.
16. Chervin RD, Archbold KH, Dillon JE, et al. Inattention, hyperactivity, and symptoms of sleep-disordered breathing. *Pediatrics.* 2002;109:449-456.
17. Gottlieb DJ, Vezina RM, Chase C, et al. Symptoms of sleep-disordered breathing in 5-year-old children are associated with sleepiness and problem behaviors. *Pediatrics.* 2003;112:870-877.
18. Rosen CL, Storfer-Isser A, Taylor HG, Kirchner HL, Emancipator JL, Redline S. Increased behavioral morbidity in school-aged children with sleep-disordered breathing. *Pediatrics.* 2004;114:1640-1648.
19. Beebe DW, Gozal D. Obstructive sleep apnea and the prefrontal cortex: towards a comprehensive model linking nocturnal upper airway obstruction to daytime cognitive and behavioral deficits. *J Sleep Res.* 2002;11:1-16.
20. O'Brien LM, Mervis CB, Holbrook CR, et al. Neurobehavioral correlates of sleep-disordered breathing in children. *J Sleep Res.* 2004;13:165-172.
21. Beebe D, Wells C, Jeffries J, Chini B, Kalra M, Amin R. Neuropsychological effects of pediatric obstructive sleep apnea. *J Int Neuropsychol Soc.* 2004;10: 962-975.
22. Chervin RD, Dillon JE, Archbold KH, Ruzicka DL. Conduct problems and symptoms of sleep disorders in children. *J Am Acad Child Adolesc Psychiatry.* 2003; 42:201-208.
23. Kim HC, Young T, Matthews CG, Weber SM, Woodard AR, Palta M. Sleep-disordered breathing and neuropsychological deficits. *Am J Respir Crit Care Med.* 1997;156:1813-1819.
24. Gozal E, Row BW, Schurr A, Gozal D. Developmental differences in cortical and hippocampal vulnerability to intermittent hypoxia in the rat. *Neurosci Lett.* 2001; 305:197-201.
25. Gozal D, Daniel JM, Dohanich GP. Behavioral and anatomical correlates of chronic episodic hypoxia during sleep in the rat. *J Neurosci.* 2001;21:2442-2450.
26. Bedard MA, Montplaisir J, Malo J, Rouleau I. Persistent neuropsychological deficits and vigilance impairments in sleep apnea syndrome after treatment with continuous positive airway pressure. *J Clin Exp Neuropsychol.* 1993;15:330-341.
27. O'Brien LM, Mervis CB, Holbrook CR, et al. Neurobehavioral implications of habitual snoring in children. *Pediatrics.* 2004;114:44-49.
28. Bhutta AT, Cleves MA, Casey PH, Cradock MM, Anand KJ. Cognitive and behavioral outcomes of school-aged children who were born preterm: a meta-analysis. *JAMA.* 2002;288:728-737.
29. Taylor HG, Minich N, Bangert B, Filipek PA, Hack M. Long-term neuropsychological outcomes of very low birth weight: associations with early risks for periventricular brain insults. *J Int Neuropsychol Soc.* 2004;10:987-1004.
30. Kesler SR, Ment LR, Vohr B, et al. Volumetric analysis of regional cerebral development in preterm children. *Pediatr Neurol.* 2004;31:318-325.
31. Luciana M. Cognitive development in children born preterm: implications for theories of brain plasticity following early injury. *Dev Psychopathol.* 2003;15:1017-1047.
32. McGauhey PJ, Starfield B, Alexander C, Ensminger ME. Social environment and vulnerability of low birth weight children: a social-epidemiological perspective. *Pediatrics.* 1991;88:943-953.
33. Gozal D. Sleep-disordered breathing and school performance in children. *Pediatrics.* 1998;102:616-620.

# Effect on Hospital-Wide Sedation Practices After Implementation of the 2001 JCAHO Procedural Sedation and Analgesia Guidelines

*Raymond Pitetti, MD, MPH; Peter J. Davis, MD; Robert Redlinger, RN, MSN; Jean White, RN; Eugene Wiener, MD; Karen H. Calhoun, BSN, MBA*

**Objective:** To describe the effect of implementing the Joint Commission on Accreditation of Healthcare Organization's guidelines for procedural sedation and analgesia (PSA) on the frequency of adverse events occurring during sedation.

**Design:** Prospective, descriptive study.

**Setting:** Urban, tertiary care children's hospital.

**Participants:** Patients requiring PSA.

**Interventions:** A PSA committee and a standardized protocol for PSA were developed during a 6-month period. Institutional oversight was initiated to monitor practitioner compliance with the program. Data were abstracted from the sedation record.

**Main Outcome Measures:** The change in incidence of adverse events during PSA during the study. The strength of the association was determined by computing the Pearson product moment correlation.

**Results:** A total of 14 386 patients received PSA between July 1, 2001, and June 30, 2004. During the study, 7.6% of patients had an adverse event, with the most common being hypoxemia (39.7% of all adverse events). A trend toward a decrease in the incidence of adverse events was found during the study (Pearson product moment correlation, −0.68; $P<.001$).

**Conclusions:** Implementation of the 2001 Joint Commission on Accreditation of Healthcare Organizations guidelines for the provision of PSA appeared to lead to a decrease in the incidence of adverse events during the study. Implementation of uniform standards of monitoring and care for the provision of PSA may lead to safer conditions for pediatric patients undergoing PSA.

*Arch Pediatr Adolesc Med. 2006;160:211-216*

PROVIDING SAFE AND EFFECTIVE sedation and analgesia in children to facilitate the successful completion of a procedure or study has been a topic of concern and regulation for several years. Before the widespread use of procedural sedation and analgesia (PSA), performing a procedure in a child often required the use of restraints and distraction. However, as diagnostic imaging has advanced and invasive pediatric procedures obviating the need for surgery have become more routine, the use of sedative, hypnotic, and analgesic drugs to perform such procedures has emerged as the practice of PSA.

Pediatric sedation practices evolved to meet the various needs of the pediatric procedure. Consequently, different practice standards, different definitions, different levels of monitoring, and different requirements for documentation and patient follow-up occurred within the same institution. The Joint Commission on Accreditation of Healthcare Organizations (JCAHO) recently implemented guidelines pertaining to PSA. These guidelines were designed to ensure that accredited institutions would provide uniform standards of monitoring and care within their institutions.[1]

Before the publication of the JCAHO guidelines, different departments within our institution (Children's Hospital of Pittsburgh) provided PSA according to their standards, with the result that each department provided PSA in different ways with differing degrees of monitoring and oversight. However, the JCAHO guidelines required that each department provide sedation by following a uniform standard. We hypothesized that, as a result, the incidence of adverse events occurring dur-

**Author Affiliations:** Division of Pediatric Emergency Medicine, Departments of Pediatrics (Drs Pitetti and Davis), Anesthesiology (Dr Davis), Perioperative Services (Mr Redlinger), Quality Management (Ms White), Surgery (Dr Wiener), and Quality and Outcomes (Ms Calhoun), Children's Hospital of Pittsburgh, University of Pittsburgh School of Medicine, Pittsburgh, Pa.

ing PSA would decrease across time. In this article, we report on the implementation of the JCAHO guidelines and a prospective evaluation of 3-year quality assurance data in patients undergoing PSA at the Children's Hospital of Pittsburgh. We specifically sought to describe the incidence of adverse events that occurred during PSA, as well as changes in incidence across the study. In addition, this article details the educational process our institution went through in implementing the JCAHO guidelines. All data presented are from sedation events that occurred after implementation of the sedation program.

This study was reviewed and approved by the institutional review board of Children's Hospital of Pittsburgh.

## METHODS

### IMPLEMENTATION OF JCAHO GUIDELINES

Implementing the 2001 JCAHO guidelines at our institution required the following steps: program formation, program modifications, and program review.

### PROGRAM FORMATION

The formation of a PSA committee and the development of a standardized protocol for pediatric sedation were conducted during a 6-month period. The development and implementation of the program proceeded in 5 distinct phases. The first phase involved identifying users of PSA within the hospital and forming a steering committee to articulate a uniform hospital policy. The second phase involved identifying all areas of the hospital where PSA took place, the equipment that was available, the personnel involved, and the practice standards in use. During the third phase of the program and with the use of the American Society of Anesthesiologists (ASA) guidelines on sedation for nonanesthesiologists and the 1992 American Academy of Pediatrics guidelines for pediatric sedation, the committee developed a single, unified practice standard.[2,3] This unified sedation practice standard consisted of the following topics: defining sedation, presedation evaluation, dietary guidelines, equipment, monitoring standards, personnel and criteria for persons to be credentialed to administer sedation, documentation and development of a uniform sedation record, postrecovery standards, and discharge criteria.

The fourth step in the program involved implementing institutional oversight to monitor practitioner compliance with the program. Oversight ensured that all sedation records were completed by the physician and nursing personnel who provided sedation. The final aspect of the program involved data collection at each site that provided PSA and monthly meetings to discuss and review compliance and complications.

### PROGRAM MODIFICATIONS

Throughout the 3-year quality improvement project, the hospital's sedation committee met at monthly intervals to discuss issues pertaining to the implementation of the sedation program and to suggest modifications. Such modifications included the addition of a pain scale, the addition of provider "time-outs" (ie, break in clinical care to verify patient identity and correct patient for procedure), patient identification, surgical/procedure side-site verification (ie, verify correct site for procedure during the time-out), and providing all patients with supplemental oxygen during sedation.

### PROGRAM REVIEW

After the development of a unified practice standard and a standardized record to document the presedation assessment, sedation process, recovery, discharge appropriateness, and complications, all PSA was monitored and all sedation records were reviewed during a 3-year period. All sedation records were reviewed prospectively, and adverse events that were not initially recorded by the medical personnel providing sedation were noted during this review. Administrative review was conducted within each department that provided sedation and ensured that all sedation events were recorded. Departments that did not comply with the sedation policy were no longer allowed to provide PSA to their patients.

A nurse involved with hospital quality improvement abstracted data from the standardized record forms. For compliance purposes, process variables were recorded as being present or absent on the basis of written documentation from the sedation reviews. Variables included nil per os status, age, weight, consent, ASA physical status, identification of the persons responsible for administering the sedation, identification of the persons responsible for monitoring the patient, patient condition at discharge, level of sedation, and medications used. Adverse events were defined as the occurrence of a complication noted on the sedation record and could be secondary to the procedure or to providing PSA. The following events were defined a priori: sustained hypoxemia (pulse oximetry of $\leq$90% for $>$1 minute), apnea, aspiration (evidence of respiratory distress and a new pulmonary infiltrate at chest radiography after sedation), vomiting, hypotension (sustained systolic blood pressure less than what is considered normal at the third percentile for age), bradycardia (heart rate less than what is considered normal at the third percentile for age), prolonged recovery (requiring $>$2 hours to recover to baseline status after administration of PSA), agitation related to pain, agitation unrelated to pain (paradoxical reaction or hallucinations), change in patient's level of care (eg, hospital admission), and failed or inadequate sedation. Additional adverse events, including rash and hematoma, that occurred during sedation and were noted by health care personnel were recorded. The providers of PSA and the reviewers of the sedation records were familiar with the definitions of adverse events.

### EFFECT OF SEDATION PROGRAM ON INCIDENCE OF ADVERSE EVENTS

Our main outcome measure for the sedation program was the change in incidence of adverse events during PSA. In particular, we hypothesized that the implementation of a hospital-wide sedation policy would result in a decrease across time in the incidence of adverse events during sedation.

### STATISTICAL ANALYSIS

Clinical and demographic data are presented as means with standard deviations, medians, ranges, and proportions. The incidence of adverse events is presented as a proportion. The frequency of adverse events during each month of the study is presented graphically as a scatterplot (**Figure**). The strength of the association between the incidence of adverse events and study month was determined by computing a Pearson correlation with a 2-tailed significance of 95%. The null hypothesis was that no correlation would exist between the study month and the incidence of adverse events. The alternative hypothesis was that there would be a negative correlation between the study month and incidence of adverse events, thus suggesting that a standardized approach to sedation can reduce sedation-related adverse events.

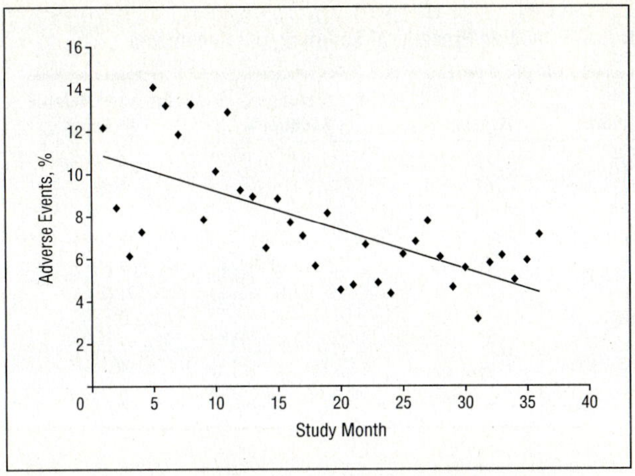


**Figure.** Scatterplot showing the percentage of adverse events during each month of the study (Pearson product moment correlation, −0.68; $P<.001$).

**Table 1. Number of Sedations Provided in Each Medical Unit Providing Procedural Sedation and Anesthesia***

| Medical Unit | Sedations Provided, No. (%) |
|---|---|
| Emergency department | 1893 (13.2) |
| Radiology | 6982 (48.5) |
| Medical ward | 452 (3.1) |
| Cardiac catheterization laboratory | 926 (6.4) |
| Dental | 923 (6.4) |
| Ear, nose, and throat/audiology | 138 (1.0) |
| Pediatric intensive care unit | 16 (0.1) |
| Gastrointestinal laboratory | 736 (5.1) |
| Interventional radiology | 2011 (14.0) |
| Special procedure room | 308 (2.1) |

*The location of sedation was not documented in 1 patient.

## RESULTS

During the 3-year study, 14 386 patients received PSA in the hospital between July 1, 2001, and June 30, 2004. The mean age of patients was 6.0 years (SD, 5.5 years; median age, 4 years; age range, 0.01-43 years). Three hundred forty-four patients (2.4%) were older than 18 years. Information pertaining to the sex and race of patients receiving PSA was not available for review. Information pertaining to ASA class was available for 10 626 patients (73.9%); 5415 (51.0%) patients were ASA class I, 4276 (40.2%) were ASA class II, 876 (8.2%) were ASA class III, and 59 (0.6%) were ASA class IV. **Table 1** depicts the number of sedations provided in each unit of the hospital that provided PSA. **Table 2** depicts the type and frequency of procedures that required PSA. The most common procedure to require PSA was magnetic resonance imaging (37.6%), followed by computed tomography (10.6%).

During the study, 1100 (7.6%) patients had an adverse event during sedation. Overall, there were 1289 adverse events, with some patients having more than 1 event. Patients who had an adverse event were significantly older than patients who did not (6.6 vs 5.9 years; $P=.001$). **Table 3** depicts the type and frequency of adverse events during PSA. The most common adverse event was hypoxemia (39.7% [512/1289] of all events). Eighty-eight patients (0.6% [6.8% {88/1289} of all adverse events]) required transfer to a higher level of medical care because of an adverse event during PSA or because of concerns about patient vital signs or level of consciousness. Of these 88 patients, 22 had hypoxemia, 1 had nausea and vomiting, 2 had bradycardia, 3 had airway obstruction, 8 had prolonged sedation, 3 had agitation, 1 had bleeding, 1 had large amounts of secretions, and 1 had hypotension. Overall, 28 patients (0.2%) required the use of a reversal agent. Three of these 28 patients required transfer to a higher level of medical care. No patient required endotracheal intubation.

**Table 2. Type and Frequency of Procedures Requiring Procedural Sedation and Anesthesia and Frequency of Adverse Events During Each Procedure**

| Procedure Type | Procedure, No. (%) | Adverse Events, No. (%)* |
|---|---|---|
| Magnetic resonance imaging | 5408 (37.6) | 396 (7.3) |
| Computed tomography | 1524 (10.6) | 104 (6.8) |
| Catheter placement | 1125 (7.8) | 83 (7.4) |
| Fracture reduction | 979 (6.8) | 98 (10.0) |
| Dental procedures | 934 (6.5) | 19 (2.0) |
| Cardiac catheterization | 925 (6.4) | 148 (16.0) |
| Laceration repair | 598 (4.2) | 74 (12.4) |
| Lumbar puncture | 565 (3.9) | 27 (4.8) |
| Esophagogastroduodenoscopy | 524 (3.6) | 24 (4.6) |
| Biopsy | 516 (3.6) | 14 (2.7) |
| Miscellaneous/other | 493 (3.4) | 39 (7.9) |
| Bone marrow aspiration | 215 (1.5) | 27 (12.6) |
| Auditory brainstem response | 154 (1.1) | 20 (13.0) |
| Colonoscopy | 107 (0.7) | 6 (5.6) |
| Angiography | 87 (0.6) | 11 (12.6) |
| Incision and drainage | 63 (0.4) | 6 (9.5) |
| Arthrocentesis | 53 (0.4) | 5 (9.4) |
| Positron emission tomography | 51 (0.4) | 2 (3.9) |
| Needle aspiration | 46 (0.3) | 6 (13.0) |
| Endoscopy | 19 (0.1) | 0 |

*Percentage of total number of procedures. More than 1 adverse event may have occurred with each procedure performed.

**Table 3. Type and Frequency of Adverse Events During Procedural Sedation and Anesthesia***

| Adverse Event | Frequency, No. (%) |
|---|---|
| Hypoxemia | 512 (3.6) |
| Prolonged sedation | 192 (1.3) |
| Agitation related to pain | 106 (0.7) |
| Transfer to higher level of care | 88 (0.6) |
| Vomiting | 85 (0.6) |
| Inability to be sedated | 92 (0.6) |
| Agitation unrelated to pain | 50 (0.3) |
| Rash | 36 (0.2) |
| Hypotension | 42 (0.3) |
| Airway obstruction | 16 (0.1) |
| Aspiration | 0 |
| Bradycardia | 10 (0.07) |
| Hematoma | 3 (0.02) |

*Some patients had more than 1 type of adverse event.

**Table 4. Frequency of Adverse Events During Sedation in Each Medical Unit Providing Procedural Sedation and Anesthesia**

| Medical Unit | No. of Sedations* | Adverse Events† | Hypoxemia‡ | Prolonged Sedation‡ | Agitation Related to Pain‡ |
|---|---|---|---|---|---|
| Cardiac catheterization laboratory | 926 | 151 (16.3) | 121 (80.1) | 3 (2.0) | 4 (2.6) |
| Emergency department | 1893 | 222 (11.7) | 88 (39.6) | 79 (35.6) | 1 (0.5) |
| Ear, nose, and throat/audiology | 138 | 15 (10.9) | 4 (26.7) | 0 | 3 (20) |
| Special procedure room | 308 | 26 (8.4) | 15 (57.7) | 1 (3.8) | 2 (7.7) |
| Radiology | 6982 | 501 (7.2) | 210 (41.9) | 101 (20.2) | 84 (16.8) |
| Interventional radiology | 2011 | 125 (6.2) | 50 (40) | 5 (4) | 11 (8.8) |
| Pediatric intensive care unit | 16 | 1 (6.2) | 1 (100) | 0 | 0 |
| Gastrointestinal laboratory | 736 | 31 (4.2) | 13 (41.9) | 1 (3.2) | 1 (3.2) |
| Medical ward | 452 | 12 (2.6) | 9 (75) | 2 (16.7) | 0 |
| Dental | 923 | 16 (1.7) | 1 (6.2) | 0 | 0 |

*The location of sedation was not documented in 1 patient.
†Data are given as number (percentage).
‡Number (percentage) of total adverse events.

**Table 5. Type and Frequency of Medications Used During Procedural Sedation and Anesthesia and the Frequency of Adverse Events Associated With Each Medication***

| Medication Type* | Medication, No. (%) | Adverse Events, No. (%)† |
|---|---|---|
| Pentobarbital‡ | 6219 (43.2) | 519 (8.3) |
| Fentanyl, midazolam | 2267 (15.8) | 219 (9.7) |
| Chloral hydrate | 2088 (14.5) | 108 (5.2) |
| Ketamine, midazolam, atropine | 1010 (7.0) | 108 (10.7) |
| Nitrous oxide‡ | 831 (5.8) | 16 (1.9) |
| Midazolam | 600 (4.2) | 0 |
| Ketamine, atropine | 532 (3.7) | 47 (8.8) |
| Meperidine, midazolam | 346 (2.4) | 16 (4.6) |
| Morphine, midazolam | 199 (1.4) | 15 (7.5) |
| Fentanyl | 114 (0.8) | 36 (31.6) |
| Meperidine, hydroxyzine | 70 (0.5) | 1 (1.4) |
| Etomidate | 21 (0.2) | 2 (9.5) |
| Propofol | 2 (0) | 0 |

*Pentobarbital was given as pentobarbital sodium; midazolam as midazolam hydrochloride; ketamine as ketamine hydrochloride; atropine as atropine sulfate; meperidine as meperidine hydrochloride; and morphine as morphine sulfate.
†Number (percentage) of total number of medications.
‡Eighty-seven (0.4%) of 14 386 patients did not have the type or amount of medications used for procedural sedation and anesthesia recorded. Pentobarbital may have been used alone or in combination with fentanyl and midazolam. Similarly, nitrous oxide may have been used in combination with meperidine and hydroxyzine or with midazolam.

Table 2 also depicts the frequency of adverse events during each procedure. The procedures with the most frequent occurrence of adverse events were cardiac catheterization (16.0%), needle aspiration (13.0%), and auditory brainstem response (13.0%). **Table 4** depicts the frequency of adverse events within each medical unit providing PSA. The medical units with the most frequent occurrence of adverse events were the cardiac catheterization laboratory (16.3%) and the emergency department (11.7%).

**Table 5** depicts the type and frequency of sedation medications used during PSA. The most common medication used for PSA was pentobarbital sodium (43.2%), alone or in combination with fentanyl citrate and midazolam hydrochloride, followed by the combination of fentanyl and midazolam (15.8%). Table 5 also depicts the frequency of adverse events according to type of sedation medication used. The medication regimens with the highest incidence of adverse events were the combination of ketamine hydrochloride, midazolam, and atropine sulfate (10.7%), followed by the combination of fentanyl and midazolam (9.7%). **Table 6** presents the frequency of adverse events reported for each sedation regimen. Seventeen of the 28 patients who required the use of a reversal agent during sedation had received pentobarbital and fentanyl, 1 had received morphine and midazolam, 3 had received meperidine hydrochloride and midazolam, and 7 had received fentanyl and midazolam. No significant association was found between the type of medication used for sedation and the use of a reversal agent.

The Figure depicts the incidence of adverse events during each month of the study. A trend toward a decrease in the incidence of adverse events was noted during the study (Pearson correlation, −0.68; $P<.001$). Correlation was significant at the 0.01 level (2-tailed).

## COMMENT

In this article, we focus on 1 institution's experience when diverse groups of physicians are mandated to develop and comply with a unified standard for PSA. Previous studies about sedation primarily focused on various groups' drug cocktails and their success and failure rates. Groups have ranged from individuals trained to provide sedation (eg, intensivists, emergency department physicians) to individuals providing sedation as an adjunct to their expertise (eg, gastroenterologists, radiologists). In this article, we view the development of a unified sedation policy from both administrative and patient safety perspectives.

Administratively, the biggest challenge for the committee was to have the physicians who were providing PSA agree to actively participate in the creation, implementation, and monitoring of the hospital-wide sedation policy. The first hurdle for the sedation committee

**Table 6. Frequency of Adverse Events According to Type of Sedation Regimen***

| Drug Group | Aspiration | Vomiting | Hypoxemia | Bradycardia | Airway Obstruction | Prolonged Sedation | Agitation Related to Pain | Agitation Unrelated to Pain | Hypotension |
|---|---|---|---|---|---|---|---|---|---|
| Chloral hydrate (n = 2088) | 0 | 16 (0.8) | 49 (2.4) | 0 | 1 (0.05) | 20 (1.0) | 1 (0.05) | 5 (0.2) | 4 (0.2) |
| Pentobarbital (n = 6219) | 0 | 26 (0.4) | 207 (3.3) | 5 (0.08) | 5 (0.08) | 90 (1.4) | 100 (1.6) | 40 (0.6) | 4 (0.06) |
| Nitrous oxide (n = 831) | 0 | 6 (0.7) | 2 (0.2) | 0 | 0 (0) | 0 | 0 | 0 | 0 |
| Ketamine, midazolam, atropine (n = 1010) | 0 | 15 (1.5) | 36 (3.6) | 0 | 1 (0.1) | 42 (4.2) | 0 | 0 | 1 (0.1) |
| Ketamine, atropine (n = 532) | 0 | 10 (1.9) | 11 (2.1) | 0 | 1 (0.2) | 19 (3.6) | 1 (0.2) | 0 | 1 (0.2) |
| Morphine, midazolam (n = 199) | 0 | 0 | 11 (5.5) | 0 | 0 | 1 (0.5) | 0 | 0 | 1 (0.5) |
| Meperidine, midazolam (n = 346) | 0 | 0 | 6 (1.7) | 0 | 0 | 0 | 1 (0.3) | 0 | 3 (0.9) |
| Fentanyl, midazolam (n = 2267) | 0 | 9 (0.4) | 162 (7.1) | 3 (0.1) | 8 (0.4) | 15 (0.7) | 2 (0.1) | 1 (0.04) | 22 (1.0) |
| Midazolam (n = 600) | 0 | 1 (0.2) | 18 (3.0) | 1 (0.2) | 0 | 4 (0.7) | 1 (0.2) | 2 (0.3) | 5 (0.8) |

*Data are given as number (percentage). Not all adverse events are included in the table. Only the most frequently used sedation regimens are included. No patient had an episode of aspiration. Pentobarbital was given as pentobarbital sodium; midazolam as midazolam hydrochloride; ketamine as ketamine hydrochloride; atropine as atropine sulfate; meperidine as meperidine hydrochloride; and morphine as morphine sulfate.

was to have them agree on definitions of what constituted PSA. Although JCAHO regulations introduced the terms *anxiolysis*, *moderate sedation/analgesia*, *deep sedation/analgesia*, and *general anesthesia*, our committee decided that PSA represented a continuum of patient responsiveness and that the individuals who administered PSA needed to have the skills to rescue patients from the deepest level of sedation. Consequently, the committee determined that we would use the term *procedural sedation* in reference to all sedation events. In addition, the committee decided that all individuals directing sedation must have completed a hospital course for sedation or be certified in pediatric advanced life support, advanced cardiac life support, or advanced trauma life support. Previously, no minimal training was required for individuals directing sedation. The requirement for certification in these courses was not intended to be a surrogate for training in providing PSA.

A second hurdle for the committee was having the various hospital departments that provided PSA actively participate in monitoring their compliance with the hospital's sedation policy. Monthly meetings of the sedation committee provided immediate feedback to each hospital department providing sedation and allowed each department to recognize deficiencies in their compliance with the hospital policy, as well as compare their department's performance with that of other departments. Having each department represented on the committee ensured that individual differences in viewpoints and concerns about the implementation of the policy were heard at the highest level of the administration, which helped ensure that the departments continued to participate actively in policy implementation. Although the decrease in incidence of adverse events noted during the study may be explained in part as a natural consequence of the increase in vigilance each unit adopted owing to increased oversight by the PSA committee, it also can be explained by interventions directed by the committee in response to trends noted during monthly program evaluations.

In addition, the committee made a conscious effort to ensure that each department completed the sedation record appropriately and documented all required information. As an example, during the study, ASA classification was documented in only 73.9% of patients. However, documentation of ASA classification improved during the study as practitioners (predominantly nonanesthesiologists) became more familiar with the concept. Similarly, practitioners became more compliant with documenting other unfamiliar items, such as side-site and procedure time-outs, as the study progressed. Items or concepts that practitioners were more familiar with, such as the documentation of adverse events, were documented appropriately from the beginning of the study. Thus, we believe that all, or nearly all, sedation events and adverse events were captured during the study.

We documented a trend toward a decrease in the incidence of adverse events during sedation provided at our institution. Reports of adverse events related to institutional sedation programs are scant. In a hospital-wide study of 1140 children sedated for a wide variety of procedures, Malviya et al[4] reported a 20% incidence of adverse events, with inadequate sedation occurring in 13.2% of patients and hypoxemia in 5.5%. In contrast to our study, in which we noted adverse events in older children, Malviya et al noted that an age younger than 1 year and an ASA class of III or IV were independent risk factors for adverse events. In a study of 1014 pediatric patients undergoing PSA in the emergency department, Agrawal et al[5] also noted that adverse events were associated with children of older age and deeper levels of sedation.

Hypoxemia and failed sedation tend to be the 2 most common adverse events in pediatric sedation. Although the incidence of hypoxemia in pediatric PSA studies varies widely, transient hypoxemia generally has no lasting sequelae.[4,6-9] Hypoxemia probably is related to the increased propensity for the pediatric airway to become obstructed. In our study, hypoxemia was a common event that generally responded to airway manipulation (jaw thrust, oral airway placement, repositioning the patient's head) and the use of supplemental oxygen.

Failed sedation probably occurs because of the difficulty of providing adequate sedation while maintaining adequate respiration. Failed sedation has financial and patient/parent satisfaction implications. In a study in which children undergoing sedation were compared with those receiving general anesthesia, Malviya et al[9] noted that the incidence of inadequate sedation was 16% and failed sedation was 7%. In a study of children sedated with pentobarbital for magnetic resonance imaging, Greenberg et al[10] noted that the failure rate was 8% and that sedation was more likely to be successful in children older than 11 years. Causes of failed sedation are multiple. Karian et al,[11] in a study of children undergoing radiological procedures, reported a 7% sedation failure rate and found that only the type of sedation medication used was a predictor of failure. In a report in which the relationship of temperament and sedation failure was evaluated for magnetic resonance imaging and computed tomography, Voepel-Lewis et al[12] noted that children whose sedation failed were less adaptable than those children whose sedation was successful.

Not surprisingly, the radiology department provided nearly half of all sedation during the study. Typically, medical procedures such as magnetic resonance imaging and computed tomography require PSA in the younger child. However, the medical unit with the highest proportion of adverse events was the cardiac catheterization laboratory, which may be related to the fact that children undergoing cardiac catheterization are more likely to have a serious medical problem, require deeper levels of sedation and analgesia, or may receive different medications than children undergoing magnetic resonance imaging or computed tomography.

This study was designed to look at all patients sedated at our institution, regardless of age. Interestingly, 2.4% of all patients sedated in the hospital were older than 18 years. Most of these patients had a history of a chronic medical condition and had received care at our institution for several years. However, they were sedated at a pediatric institution, often by physicians trained to treat children. As a result, health care personnel who provide sedation at our institution are expected to be prepared to sedate both the pediatric and the adult patient.

There are several limitations to this study. The physicians providing PSA were aware that the committee would be closely monitoring the use of PSA in the hospital. As a result, physicians may have adapted their behavior to reduce the occurrence of adverse events. Because monitoring of sedation will continue, this change in behavior would be of continued benefit. In addition, the physicians and nurses involved in PSA may have altered their recording of adverse events in an effort to decrease their department's incidence of adverse events. Finally, the level of training and clinical experience of the physicians providing PSA and the types of medications used during PSA most likely varied substantially among the medical units providing PSA, making direct comparisons difficult. In addition, patients were not randomly assigned to receive the various medications, thus limiting comparisons among sedation regimens.

## CONCLUSION

We believe that the implementation of a standardized, hospital-wide protocol for PSA, along with the establishment of a PSA committee that provides close scrutiny and evaluation of the sedation program within an institution, may lead to a marked hospital-wide decrease in the incidence of adverse events during PSA. To our knowledge, this is the first study that has looked at the potential effect of the 2001 JCAHO guidelines on providing PSA within an institution. Additional studies may confirm the potential benefit of adopting the JCAHO guidelines.

**Accepted for Publication:** August 11, 2005.
**Correspondence:** Peter J. Davis, MD, Department of Anesthesiology, Children's Hospital of Pittsburgh, 3705 Fifth Ave, Pittsburgh, PA 15213-2583 (davispj@anes.upmc.edu).

## REFERENCES


1. Joint Commission on Accreditation of Healthcare Organizations. *Revisions to Anesthesia Care Standards: Comprehensive Accreditation Manual for Hospitals*. Oakbrook Terrace, Ill: Joint Commission on Accreditation of Healthcare Organizations Department of Publications; 2001.
2. Practice guidelines for sedation and analgesia by non-anesthesiologists: a report by the American Society of Anesthesiologists Task Force on Sedation and Analgesia by Non-Anesthesiologists. *Anesthesiology*. 1996;84:459-471.
3. American Academy of Pediatrics Committee on Drugs: guidelines for monitoring and management of pediatric patients during and after sedation for diagnostic and therapeutic procedures. *Pediatrics*. 1992;89(6 pt 1):1110-1115.
4. Malviya S, Voepel-Lewis T, Tait AR. Adverse events and risk factors associated with the sedation of children by nonanesthesiologists. *Anesth Analg*. 1997;85:1207-1213.
5. Agrawal D, Manzi SF, Gupta R, Krauss B. Preprocedural fasting state and adverse events in children undergoing procedural sedation and analgesia in a pediatric emergency department. *Ann Emerg Med*. 2003;42:636-646.
6. Motas D, McDermott NB, VanSickle T, Friesen RH. Depth of consciousness and deep sedation attained in children as administered by nonanaesthesiologists in a children's hospital. *Paediatr Anaesth*. 2004;14:256-260.
7. Merola C, Albarracin C, Lebowitz P, Bienkowski RS, Barst SM. An audit of adverse events in children sedated with chloral hydrate or propofol during imaging studies. *Paediatr Anaesth*. 1995;5:375-378.
8. Lamireau T, Dubreuil M, Daconceicao M. Oxygen saturation during esophagogastroduodenoscopy in children: general anesthesia versus intravenous sedation. *J Pediatr Gastroenterol Nutr*. 1998;27:172-175.
9. Malviya S, Voepel-Lewis T, Eldevik OP, Rockwell DT, Wong JH, Tait AR. Sedation and general anaesthesia in children undergoing MRI and CT: adverse events and outcomes. *Br J Anaesth*. 2000;84:743-748.
10. Greenberg SB, Adams RC, Aspinall CL. Initial experience with intravenous pentobarbital sedation for children undergoing MRI at a tertiary care pediatric hospital: the learning curve. *Pediatr Radiol*. 2000;30:689-691.
11. Karian VE, Burrows PE, Zurakowski D, Connor L, Mason KP. Sedation for pediatric radiological procedures: analysis of potential causes of sedation failure and paradoxical reactions. *Pediatr Radiol*. 1999;29:869-873.
12. Voepel-Lewis T, Malviya S, Prochaska G, Tait AR. Sedation failures in children undergoing MRI and CT: is temperament a factor? *Paediatr Anaesth*. 2000;10:319-323.

EDITORIAL

# Obesity Prevention in Primary Care

The Institute of Medicine Committee on Prevention of Obesity in Children and Adolescents (Washington, DC) recommended that child health professionals routinely monitor and track body mass index (calculated as weight in kilograms divided by the square of height in meters) and offer relevant evidence-based counseling and guidance to improve nutrition, increase physical activity, and decrease sedentary behaviors.[1] Recent surveys indicate that child health care professionals often fail to diagnose childhood obesity, only inconsistently use body mass index and the Centers for Disease Control and Prevention (Atlanta, Ga) body mass index charts[2] and/or provide nutrition and physical activity counseling, and report low levels of confidence, proficiency, and effectiveness in evaluating and managing childhood obesity.[3-7] In addition, there is little evidence to support specific intervention strategies for primary care professionals.[1,8] It is in this context that Patrick and colleagues[9] report the results of a randomized controlled trial of Patient-centered Assessment and Counseling for Exercise + Nutrition (PACE+), a primary care–initiated intervention to improve diet, physical activity, and sedentary behaviors, in 819 11- to 15-year-olds, 438 girls and 381 boys, in this issue of the ARCHIVES. The intervention was designed to overcome many of the perceived barriers for providing obesity evaluation and counseling in the office setting by using computer-based screening and goal-setting algorithms, requiring only limited health care professional time for training (2 hours) and patient counseling, and using non–health care professional staff for continuing follow-up assessments and counseling.

*See also page 128*

The PACE+ intervention began with office-based computer-assisted screening and goal setting for nutrition, physical activity, and sedentary behaviors, the results of which were used to help guide brief health care professional counseling (designed to take 3-5 minutes). Adolescent patients and their parents were each given behavior-change manuals to take home from the visit and received a year of personalized follow-up mailings and 10- to 15-minute counseling phone calls conducted by trained research staff. Intervention implementation and participation rates were high, with nearly two thirds of adolescents completing at least 9 of the 11 scheduled follow-up counseling calls. Compared with controls, who received a sun-protection intervention including office-based computer-assisted screening followed by 2 follow-up counseling phone calls and mailings, boys and girls in the PACE+ group reported statistically significantly reducing their time spent in sedentary behaviors (mean net reductions of about an hour per day of television, computer or video games, sitting talking on the phone, and sitting listening to music), boys in the PACE+ group reported significantly more days per week of at least 30 minutes of vigorous activity or 60 minutes of moderate to vigorous activity and were more likely to report 5 or more active days per week, and girls in the PACE+ group were more likely to report eating less than 10% of daily calories from saturated fat. However, there were no significant differences between groups (boys or girls) in reported minutes per week of moderate and vigorous physical activity or objectively measured physical activity (accelerometry), the likelihood of watching 2 or fewer hours of television per day, the percentage of total calories from fat or the likelihood of consuming less than 30% of daily calories from fat, daily servings of fruit and vegetables or the likelihood of eating 5 or more fruit and vegetable servings per day, or the likelihood of eating their age-recommended grams of fiber per day. There were also no significant differences between groups in body mass index. A moderator analysis for differential effects by health care professional and/or practice site is not reported but, despite the low power of such an analysis, it is possible that effects were stronger for some health care professionals or practices than others. This may be a useful analysis to add to future studies to shed light on characteristics associated with greater effects.

Taken as a whole, the bulk of null findings and lack of confirmation of the self-reports by the available objective measures suggest that PACE+ produced only modest effects. However, that is not the whole story. While I am sure the investigators (along with myself and most readers) would have preferred to see more consistent and greater effects, we should look positively on this study. This study provides a hopeful message that a primary care–based intervention can result in some beneficial changes in adolescents' obesity-related behaviors. The statistically significant effects on reported sedentary behaviors by both boys and girls are consistent with a prior pilot study of a primary care intervention to reduce screen time in African American children,[10] possibly indicating that sedentary behaviors are an appropriate behavior-change target for the primary care setting, and screen-time reduction has been one of the most successful weight gain prevention strategies identified to date.[1,11]

The real disappointment is that there are so few other interventions that have been developed and tested for primary care settings. Experience with more intensive behavior-change interventions in other settings (eg, schools, churches, families) has taught us all that meaningful behavior changes and reducing weight gain, in particular, are very difficult to achieve. Past research and the results from PACE+, a substantial, well-designed intervention, should caution those who think that minimal office-based education is sufficient to produce meaningful effects on behavior and weight. We must not be complacent to accept and promote these simplistic approaches in the absence of supporting data, delaying efforts to push forward to find effective solutions. Instead, we need to be rigorous and systematic in our approaches to developing and testing primary care interventions to prevent and control obesity; PACE+ represents a model for this process. To my knowledge, PACE+ has been in development and testing since at least 1996, following earlier work on similar interventions for adults.[12,13] It was developed with close attention to theory and involved multiple rounds of pilot testing for feasibility and short-term efficacy[14] before being tested in this randomized clinical trial. This same process needs to be replicated over and over again with other theory-driven interventions for primary care settings.

So what can we do now? PACE+ may be a good start as we wait for intervention development and evaluation to catch up to the demand. In the meantime, child health professionals can obtain further training and practice in behavior-change counseling, linking with the experts in their own communities to increase their skills and confidence to provide counseling to patients and their families. They can also set an important example, themselves, as role models of healthful eating and physical activity. In addition, they can collaborate with fellow health care professionals and community leaders and organizations to reinforce messages and policies promoting more healthful nutrition, increased physical activity, and reduced sedentary behaviors for children and their families. Health professionals are in an influential position to help lead their communities to reduce the obesogenic environment. Managing risk factors for adult chronic disease is likely to become an even greater component of our primary care practices. To maximize our impact on child and adolescent health may require stepping beyond traditional, office-based patient care roles to actively participate in building more healthful communities. I can't think of any group with more credibility for leading this effort than child health professionals.

*Thomas N. Robinson, MD, MPH*

**Correspondence**: Dr Robinson, Division of General Pediatrics, Department of Pediatrics and Stanford Prevention Research Center, Department of Medicine, Stanford University School of Medicine, Hoover Pavilion, Room N229, 211 Quarry Rd, Mail Code 5705, Stanford, CA 94305-5705 (tom.robinson@stanford.edu).

## REFERENCES

1. Institute of Medicine Committee on Prevention of Obesity in Children and Youth. *Preventing Childhood Obesity: Health in the Balance.* Washington, DC: The National Academies Press; 2005.
2. 2000 CDC growth charts: United States. Available at: http://www.cdc.gov/growthcharts. Accessed October 30, 2005.
3. Cook S, Weitzman M, Auinger P, Barlow SE. Screening and counseling associated with obesity diagnosis in a national survey of ambulatory pediatric visits. *Pediatrics.* 2005;116:112-116.
4. Barlow SE, Dietz WH, Klish WJ, Trowbridge FL. Medical evaluation of overweight children and adolescents: reports from pediatricians, pediatric nurse practitioners, and dietitians. *Pediatrics.* 2002;110:222-228.
5. Story M, Neumark-Sztainer DR, Sherwood NE, et al. Management of child and adolescent obesity: attitudes, barriers, skills, and training needs among health care professionals. *Pediatrics.* 2002;110:210-214.
6. Perrin EM, Flower KB, Ammerman AS. Body mass index charts: useful yet underused. *J Pediatr.* 2004;144:455-460.
7. Perrin EM, Flower KB, Garrett J, Ammerman AS. Preventing and treating obesity: pediatricians' self-efficacy, barriers, resources, and advocacy. *Ambul Pediatr.* 2005;5:150-156.
8. US Preventive Services Task Force. Screening and interventions for overweight in children and adolescents: recommendation statement. *Pediatrics.* 2005;116:205-209.
9. Patrick K, Calfas KJ, Norman GJ, et al. Randomized controlled trial of a primary care and home-based intervention for physical activity and nutrition behaviors: PACE+ for adolescents. *Arch Pediatr Adolesc Med.* 2006;160:128-136.
10. Ford BS, McDonald TE, Owens AS, Robinson TN. Primary care interventions to reduce television viewing in African-American children. *Am J Prev Med.* 2002;22:106-109.
11. Robinson TN. Television viewing and childhood obesity. *Pediatr Clin North Am.* 2001;48:1017-1025.
12. Calfas KJ, Long BJ, Sallis JF, Wooten WJ, Pratt M, Patrick K. A controlled trial of physician counseling to promote the adoption of physical activity. *Prev Med.* 1996;25:225-233.
13. Calfas KJ, Sallis JF, Zabinski MF, et al. Preliminary evaluation of a multicomponent program for nutrition and physical activity change in primary care: PACE+ for adults. *Prev Med.* 2002;34:153-161.
14. Patrick K, Sallis JF, Prochaska JJ, et al. A multicomponent program for nutrition and physical activity change in primary care: PACE+ for adolescents. *Arch Pediatr Adolesc Med.* 2001;155:940-946.

I like nonsense; it wakes up the brain cells.
Fantasy is a necessary ingredient in living.
—Dr Seuss

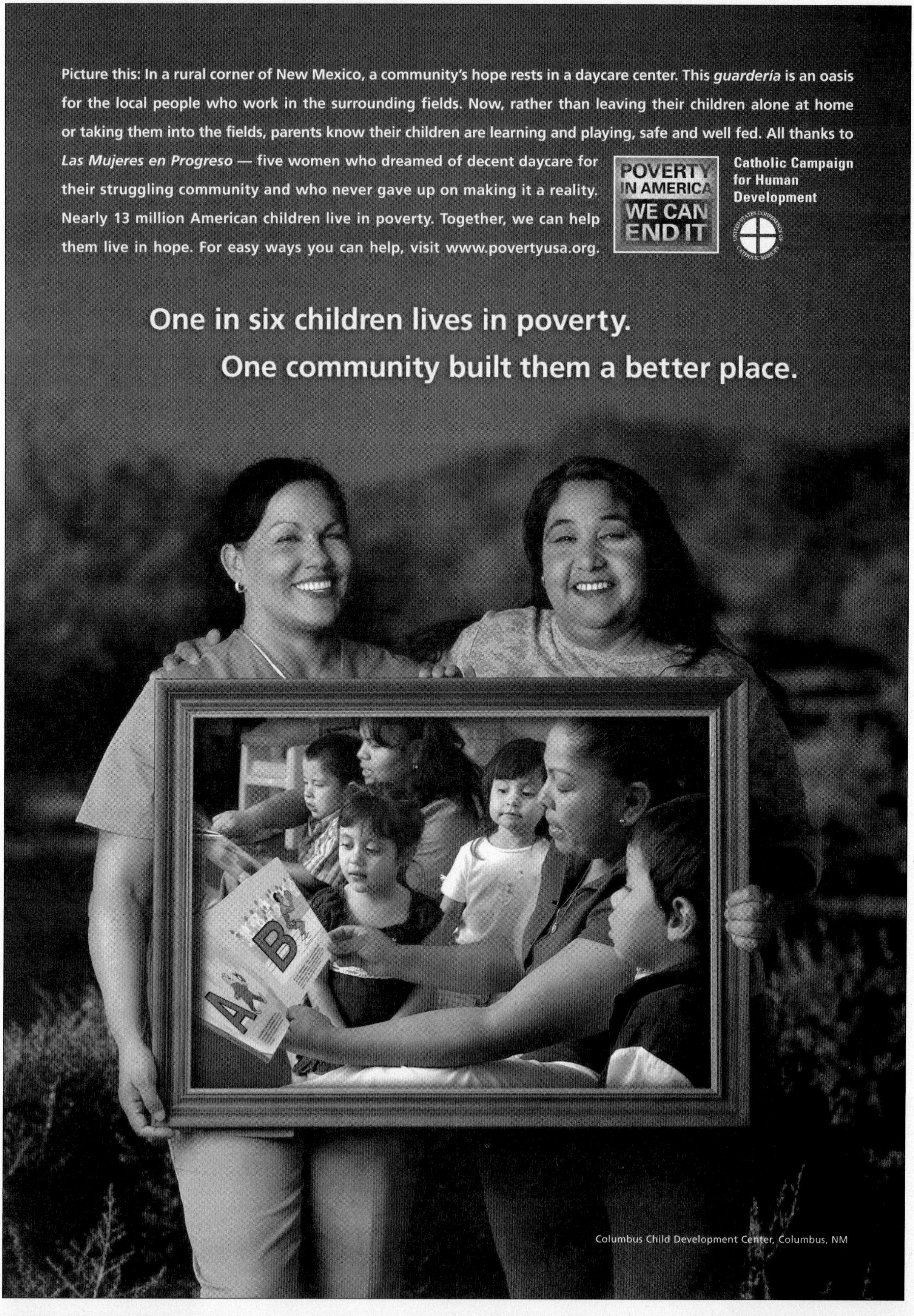
Picture this: In a rural corner of New Mexico, a community's hope rests in a daycare center. This *guarderia* is an oasis for the local people who work in the surrounding fields. Now, rather than leaving their children alone at home or taking them into the fields, parents know their children are learning and playing, safe and well fed. All thanks to *Las Mujeres en Progreso* — five women who dreamed of decent daycare for their struggling community and who never gave up on making it a reality. Nearly 13 million American children live in poverty. Together, we can help them live in hope. For easy ways you can help, visit www.povertyusa.org.
POVERTY IN AMERICA WE CAN END IT
Catholic Campaign for Human Development
UNITED STATES CONFERENCE OF CATHOLIC BISHOPS
One in six children lives in poverty.
One community built them a better place.
Columbus Child Development Center, Columbus, NM

## If You Don't Ask, Parents May Not Tell: Noticing Problems vs Expressing Concerns

I am concerned about the measurement methods and conclusions reported by Ehrmann Feldman et al[1] in "When and by Whom Is Concern First Expressed for Children With Neuromotor Problems" in the September issue of the ARCHIVES. The authors state that "parents recognized neuromotor problems in their children at older ages than did physicians,"[1(p884)] yet the research question asked of parents was not, "Who first noticed problems and when?" but instead "Who was the first person or professional who first expressed a concern regarding your child's development?" Expressing concerns and noticing potential difficulties are not synonymous. In a study I conducted on 408 families, more than one third of parents with concerns as elicited by Parents' Evaluations of Developmental Status, a brief screening and surveillance tool,[2] had spontaneously raised concerns to health care professionals.[3] Although differing levels of education and parenting experience were not associated with differences in the frequencies and types of elicited concerns, parents were more likely to have discussed concerns if they could identify a regular source of health care, were highly educated, were fathers, were worried about their child's health, and had concerns about expressive language development.

Parents with limited education are less likely to know that developmental or behavioral screening is an essential component of child health care.[4] This phenomenon may contribute to the reticence of such parents to raise concerns. Still, socioeconomic status may not account for all differences in parents' willingness to share their observations and worries. As part of my research protocols, parents were debriefed after their concerns were elicited and their children assessed with objective measures. When told about problematic performance, many parents who had not initially raised concerns reported that they had indeed held concerns but thought themselves simply anxious and overly worried and accordingly were reluctant to share their thoughts with either the research team or their child's health care professional.

What this suggests is that we should not only ask all parents about their concerns but also ask them repeatedly. In the first instance, asking about concerns establishes that developmental issues are of interest to health care professionals and prompts parents to think carefully about development as a range of domains. Asking repeatedly should help reluctant parents gain confidence in their observations and facilitate their willingness to share concerns.

Finally, parents whose children are enrolled in special services tend to have few, if any, concerns, even though their children have known difficulties.[5] This is probably a function of satisfaction with intervention, but it is also a finding that might extend to parents of children on waiting lists for services, as were the parents in the current research.

The ideal study of who first notices neurodevelopmental problems and when should be prospective, involve a general pediatric sample, and include well-crafted, effective questions for both health care professionals and parents. The value of such discussions is clear; children with disabilities are 11 times more likely to be enrolled in needed early intervention.[2]

*Frances Page Glascoe, PhD*

**Correspondence:** Dr Glascoe, Vanderbilt University, 25 Bragg Dr, East Berlin, PA 17316 (frances.p.glascoe @vanderbilt.edu).


1. Ehrmann Feldman D, Couture M, Grilli L, Simard MN, Azoulay L, Gosselin J. When and by whom is concern first expressed for children with neuromotor problems. *Arch Pediatr Adolesc Med.* 2005;159:882-886.
2. Glascoe FP. Do parents' discuss concerns about children's development with health care providers? *Ambul Child Health.* 1997;2:349-356.
3. Glascoe FP. *Parents' Evaluations of Developmental Status: A Method for Detecting and Addressing Developmental and Behavioral Problems in Children.* Nashville, Tenn: Ellsworth & Vandermeer Press Ltd; 2005.
4. Horwitz SM, Leaf PJ, Leventhal JM. Identification of psychosocial problems in pediatric primary care: do family attitudes make a difference? *Arch Pediatr Adolesc Med.* 1998;152:367-371.
5. Glascoe FP. *Collaborating With Parents: Using Parents' Evaluations of Developmental Status to Detect and Address Developmental and Behavioral Problems.* Nashville, Tenn: Ellsworth & Vandermeer Press Ltd; 1998.


### *In reply*

*Dr Glascoe is correct in stating that expressing concern to someone and noticing a problem are not synonymous. However, we did not ask about expressing concern to a professional; we asked about expressing concern in general. Moreover, the children in our study were diagnosed with neuromotor problems and not language problems or learning disabilities (although these problems may have manifested later). Delays in achieving gross motor milestones are usually recognized at an earlier age than delays in other domains of development, such as self-care and cognitive and social functioning.[1] Although parental education may affect communication between parents and a health professional,[2,3] perhaps having older children may be another important aspect related to concern about child development. We included whether having older children was associated with earlier parental awareness of potential problems, and although the result was nonsignificant, the estimated odds ratio was 1.47 (95% confidence interval, 0.53-4.03).*

*The attitude toward children with neuromotor problems may be different from that toward those with other de-*

*velopmental problems. For instance, there may be a tendency to say that the child is "lazy" and be less concerned at younger ages. (This may be true for both parents and physicians.) Even at slightly older ages, when parents mentioned their child's (motor) awkwardness to a physician, their concerns were often dismissed; physicians commonly reassure parents that children will outgrow clumsiness.[4] However, in the case of the older child who is having difficulties with language or with learning, the concern may be regarded as more urgent on the part of both the parent and physician (and possibly the teacher).*

*In our study, children were on the waiting list for services. Many expressed much concern and dissatisfaction with the long delays to receive services. Although these concerns are not addressed by our article[5] (which explored initial awareness of the problem), our experience regarding parents' ongoing concerns tends to differ from that described by Dr Glascoe.*

*Insofar as the intent of this study, it was to describe when and who was first aware of potential neuromotor problems among a cohort of children with these delays. Our study population consisted of children referred to rehabilitation from a variety of sources (not only primary care). These included general pediatrics, specialized clinics such as neonatal clinics (that follow "at risk" children [eg, those born prematurely or at very low birth weight]), orthopedics, neurology, emergency, and local community health clinics. Although we agree that a prospective study in the general pediatric population would be ideal in terms of determining the answer in the general population, it may not capture those who do not have a regular primary care physician, and there would be a need for quite a large sample, with several years of follow-up, to yield those with neuromotor problems.*

*Earlier identification of neuromotor problems led to earlier intervention for children with these problems.[5] Thus, we agree with Dr Glascoe that parents should be asked repeatedly if they have any concerns regarding their child's development so that appropriate intervention may begin early.*

*Debbie Ehrmann Feldman, PT, PhD*
*Mélanie Couture, OT, MA*
*Lisa Grilli, PT, MSc*
*Marie-Noëlle Simard, OT, MSc*
*Laurent Azoulay, MSc*
*Julie Gosselin, OT, PhD*

**Correspondence:** Dr Ehrmann Feldman, Université de Montréal, Faculté de médecine, École de Réadaptation, CP 6128 Succ Centre-ville, Montréal (QC) H3C 3J7, Canada (debbie.feldman@umontreal.ca).

1. Palfrey JS, Singer JD, Walker DK, Butler JA. Early identification of children's special needs: a study in five metropolitan communities. *J Pediatr*. 1987;111:651-659.
2. Glascoe FP. Do parents discuss concerns about children's development with health care providers? *Ambul Child Health*. 1997;2:349-356.
3. Bailey DB Jr, Hebbeler K, Scarborough A, Spiker D, Mallik S. First experiences with early intervention: a national perspective. *Pediatrics*. 2004;113:887-896.
4. Hamilton SS. Evaluation of clumsiness in children. *Am Fam Physician*. 2002;66:1435-1440.
5. Ehrmann Feldman D, Couture M, Grilli L, Simard MN, Azoulay L, Gosselin J. When and by whom is concern first expressed for children with neuromotor problems? *Arch Pediatr Adolesc Med*. 2005;159:882-886.

**Why Do We Call a Child a "Kid"?**

The Anglo-Saxon word for child is *cild*. In ancient times, just as today, people often failed to pronounce the letter *l*. The similarity of sound between this name for a child and that for a young goat, and the similarity of antics, led to the use of kid as a synonym for child.
—From *Why Do We Say It?*, Castle Books, 1985

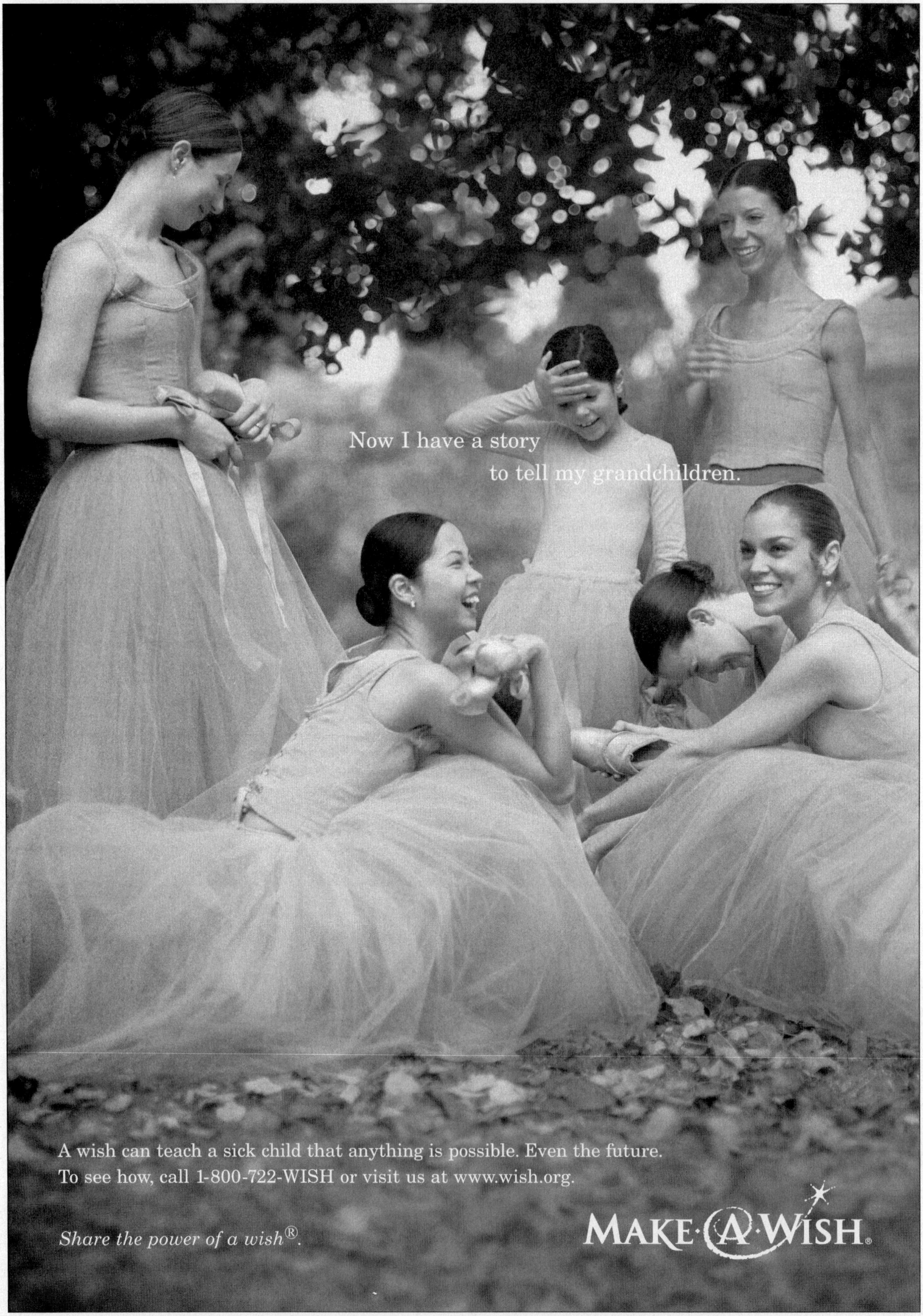

Now I have a story
to tell my grandchildren.
A wish can teach a sick child that anything is possible. Even the future.
To see how, call 1-800-722-WISH or visit us at www.wish.org.
Share the power of a wish®.
MAKE·A·WISH®

## JOURNAL ADVERTISER INDEX


**ABBOTT LABS**
Omnicef OS....121-123

**CLASSIFIED ADVERTISING**....223
http://www.amapublications.com

**GLAXOSMITHKLINE**
Boostrix....143-144, COVER 3-4
Pediarix....115-116, 171-172

**MERCK & COMPANY**
CORPORATE....124-125
CORPORATE....144A-D

**SEPRACOR**
Xopenex....COVER 2-113


*Demographic and "Mini" inserts and/or ROB ad pages

While every precaution is taken to ensure accuracy, we cannot guarantee against the possibility of an occasional change or omission in the preparation of this index.

# ARCHIVES OF PEDIATRICS & ADOLESCENT MEDICINE


## CONTACT INFORMATION

### EDITORIAL OFFICE


**Editorial Office Information:** *Archives of Pediatrics & Adolescent Medicine*, Department of Pediatrics, Child Health Institute, University of Washington, 6200 NE 74th St, Suite 210, Seattle, WA 98115-8160; phone: (206) 685-3573; fax: (206) 685-3572; e-mail: archpediatrics@jama-archives.org.


**Electronic Submission:** Manuscripts should be submitted via our online manuscript submission and review system (http://manuscripts.archpediatrics.com). Manuscripts submitted through our online system should not also be submitted by mail or fax. Signed authorship forms should be sent by regular mail or fax. See the Instructions for Authors (www.archpediatrics.com) for more details.

### CONSORTIUM OF *JAMA* & *ARCHIVES* JOURNALS

The *Archives of Pediatrics & Adolescent Medicine* is a member of the consortium of AMA journals listed below.

- The Journal of the American Medical Association (JAMA)
- Archives of Dermatology
- Archives of Facial Plastic Surgery
- Archives of General Psychiatry
- Archives of Internal Medicine
- Archives of Neurology
- Archives of Ophthalmology
- Archives of Otolaryngology–Head & Neck Surgery
- Archives of Pediatrics & Adolescent Medicine
- Archives of Surgery

### *JAMA/ARCHIVES* MEDIA RELATIONS

Jann Ingmire; phone: (312) 464-5262; e-mail: mediarelations@jama-archives.org.

### *ARCHIVES OF PEDIATRICS* ONLINE

*Archives of Pediatrics & Adolescent Medicine* is available online at www.archpediatrics.com.

### *JAMA/ARCHIVES* REPRINTS

**Author Reprints:** Anna Goins at (312) 464-2477; fax: (312) 464-5843; e-mail: anna.goins@ama-assn.org. Minimum order: 100 reprints.

**Educational Reprints:** Rhonda Bailey Brown at (312) 464-2513; fax: (312) 464-5843; e-mail: rhonda.brown@ama-assn.org. Minimum order: 100 reprints.

**Commercial Reprints:** Phone: (312) 464-0776; fax: (312) 464-0708; e-mail: reprints@ama-assn.org. Minimum order: 500 reprints.

### PERMISSIONS

Information about obtaining permission to republish, reprint, or adapt material published in *Archives of Pediatrics & Adolescent Medicine* is available from Rhonda Bailey Brown; phone: (312) 464-2513; fax: (312) 464-5843; e-mail: permissions@ama-assn.org.

### DOCUMENT DELIVERY

Copies of individual articles are available online at www.archpediatrics.com and from the following: Infotrieve, phone: (800) 422-4633; fax: (310) 208-5971; URL: www.infotrieve.com; e-mail: orders@infotrieve.com; Institute for Scientific Information (ISI), phone: (800) 603-4367; fax: (856) 787-1679; URL: http://www.isidoc.com; e-mail: service@isidoc.com; Dialog Information Services; Proquest; Ovid Technologies, Inc; and EBSCO.


The ARCHIVES OF PEDIATRICS & ADOLESCENT MEDICINE (ISSN 01072–4710) is published monthly by the American Medical Association, 515 N State St, Chicago, IL 60610–0946, and is an official publication of the Association. The ARCHIVES OF PEDIATRICS & ADOLESCENT MEDICINE reaches more than 30 900 readers in over 83 countries each month. Periodicals postage paid at Chicago, Ill, and at additional mailing offices. GST registration number 12622 5556 RT. Canada Post International Publications Mail (Canadian Distribution) Sales Agreement No. 318728. POSTMASTER, send all address changes to *Archives of Pediatrics & Adolescent Medicine,* c/o the AMA Unified Service Center, American Medical Association, 515 N State St, Chicago, IL 60610. Printed in the USA.


### ADVERTISING



### ADVERTISING PRINCIPLES

Advertisements in this issue have been reviewed to comply with the principles governing advertising in AMA publications. A copy of these principles is available on request and online at www.archpediatrics.com. The appearance of advertising in AMA publications is not an AMA guarantee or endorsement of the product or the claims made for the product by the manufacturer.

### ADDRESS CHANGES

Send all address changes to *Archives of Pediatrics & Adolescent Medicine*, c/o the AMA Unified Service Center, American Medical Association, 515 N State St, Chicago, IL 60610. Notification of address changes must be made at least 6 weeks in advance; include both old and new addresses and a recent mailing label if sending via mail.

### SUBSCRIPTION RATES AND SERVICE

Subscription rates are shown in the table below. For service in the US and Americas, inquiries on pricing, address changes, missing issues, subscription billing, subscription renewal, and back issues, contact the AMA Unified Service Center, 24 hours a day, 7 days a week.

**AMA members:** phone: (800) 262-3211; e-mail: msc@ama-assn.org. **Other physicians and nonphysician customers, including subscription agents:** phone: (800) 262-2350 or (312) 670-7827; fax: (312) 464-5831; e-mail: ama-subs@ama-assn.org. **Inquiries:** Unified Service Center, American Medical Association, PO Box 10946, Chicago, IL 60610-0946. For subscribers with mailing addresses outside the United States & Americas: Contact *JAMA* & *Archives* Journals, c/o EMD GmbH, Birkenstr.67, 10559 Berlin, Germany. Phone: +49 (30) 33099828; fax: +49 (30) 33099829; e-mail: ama@emd-germany.de.

**Annual Subscription Rates**

| | United States | Americas | UK | Rest of World |
|---|---|---|---|---|
| INDIVIDUAL | | | | |
| Print and Online | $185 | $240 | £165 | €250 |
| INSTITUTION | | | | |
| Print and Online | $375 | $485 | £315 | €470 |

In Canada, US rate plus GST. Rates for residents and medical students available at pubs.ama-assn.org, or from the AMA Unified Service Center.

## BOOSTRIX®

**(Tetanus Toxoid, Reduced Diphtheria Toxoid and Acellular Pertussis Vaccine, Adsorbed) (Tdap)**

The following is a brief summary only; see full prescribing information for complete product information.

**INDICATIONS AND USAGE:** BOOSTRIX is indicated for active booster immunization against tetanus, diphtheria, and pertussis as a single dose in individuals 10 through 18 years of age. The use of BOOSTRIX as a primary series or to complete the primary series has not been studied. As with any vaccine, BOOSTRIX may not protect 100% of individuals receiving the vaccine. BOOSTRIX is not recommended for treatment of actual infections.

**CONTRAINDICATIONS:** Hypersensitivity to any component of the vaccine is a contraindication (see DESCRIPTION in full prescribing information). Do not use BOOSTRIX after a serious allergic reaction (e.g., anaphylaxis) following any other tetanus toxoid, diphtheria toxoid or pertussis-containing vaccine, or any component of this vaccine (see DESCRIPTION in full prescribing information). Because of the uncertainty as to which component of the vaccine might be responsible, do not give further vaccination with any of these components; or, refer such individuals to an allergist for evaluation. The following events are contraindications to administration of BOOSTRIX: encephalopathy (e.g., coma, decreased level of consciousness, prolonged seizures) within 7 days of administration of a previous dose of a pertussis-containing vaccine that is not attributable to another identifiable cause; progressive neurologic disorder, uncontrolled epilepsy, or progressive encephalopathy. Do not vaccinate individuals with these conditions until a treatment regimen has been established and the condition has stabilized. BOOSTRIX is not contraindicated for use in individuals with HIV infection.

**WARNINGS:** The tip cap and the rubber plunger of the needleless prefilled syringes contain dry natural latex rubber that may cause allergic reactions in latex sensitive individuals. The vial stopper is latex-free. If any of the following events occurred in temporal relation to previous receipt of a Diphtheria and Tetanus Toxoids and Pertussis Vaccine Adsorbed (DTwP) vaccine or a vaccine containing an acellular pertussis component, consider carefully whether to give subsequent doses of BOOSTRIX: temperature of ≥40.5°C (105°F) within 48 hours not due to another identifiable cause; collapse or shock-like state (hypotonic-hyporesponsive episode) within 48 hours; persistent, inconsolable crying lasting ≥3 hours, occurring within 48 hours; seizures with or without fever occurring within 3 days. Persons who experienced serious Arthus-type hypersensitivity reactions following a prior dose of tetanus toxoid usually have high serum tetanus antitoxin levels and should not be given Tetanus and Diphtheria Toxoids Adsorbed For Adult Use (Td) or Tdap vaccines or even emergency doses of Td more frequently than every 10 years, even if the wound is neither clean nor minor. If Guillain-Barré syndrome has occurred within 6 weeks of receipt of prior vaccine containing tetanus toxoid, the decision to give BOOSTRIX or any vaccine containing tetanus toxoid should be based on careful consideration of the potential benefits and possible risks. The decision to administer a pertussis-containing vaccine to individuals with stable central nervous system (CNS) disorders must be made by the physician on an individual basis, with consideration of all relevant factors, and assessment of potential risks and benefits for that individual. Advise the patient, parent, or guardian of the potential increased risk involved (see PRECAUTIONS). A family history of seizures or other CNS disorders is not a contraindication to pertussis vaccine. The Advisory Committee on Immunization Practices (ACIP) has published guidelines for vaccination of persons with recent or acute illness (www.cdc.gov). Do not give BOOSTRIX to individuals with bleeding disorders such as hemophilia or thrombocytopenia, or to persons on anticoagulant therapy unless the potential benefit clearly outweighs the risk of administration. If the decision is made to administer BOOSTRIX to such persons, it should be given with caution with steps taken to avoid the risk of hematoma following the injection.

**PRECAUTIONS:** Before the injection of any biological, the physician should take all reasonable precautions to prevent allergic or other adverse reactions. Epinephrine injection (1:1,000) and other appropriate agents used for the control of immediate allergic reactions must be immediately available should an acute anaphylactic reaction occur. Immunosuppressed persons, including individuals receiving immunosuppressive therapy, may not develop the expected immune response. **Drug Interactions:** Do not mix BOOSTRIX with any other vaccine in the same syringe or vial. **Carcinogenesis, Mutagenesis, Impairment of Fertility:** BOOSTRIX has not been evaluated for carcinogenic or mutagenic potential, or for impairment of fertility. **Pregnancy:** Pregnancy Category C. Animal reproduction studies have not been conducted with BOOSTRIX. It is also not known whether BOOSTRIX can cause fetal harm when administered to a pregnant woman or can affect reproductive capacity. BOOSTRIX should be given to a pregnant woman only if clearly needed. Animal fertility studies have not been conducted with BOOSTRIX. In a developmental toxicity study, the effect of BOOSTRIX on embryo-fetal and pre-weaning development was evaluated in pregnant rats. Animals were administered INFANRIX® (Diphtheria and Tetanus Toxoids and Acellular Pertussis Vaccine Adsorbed) prior to gestation and BOOSTRIX during the period of organogenesis (gestation days 6, 8, 11) and later in pregnancy (gestation day 15), 0.1 mL/rat/occasion (a 45-fold increase compared to the human dose of BOOSTRIX on a body weight basis), by intramuscular injection. No adverse affect on pregnancy and lactation parameters, embryo-fetal or pre-weaning development was observed. There were no fetal malformations or other evidence of teratogenesis noted in this study. **Nursing Mothers:** It is not known whether BOOSTRIX is excreted in human milk. Because many drugs are excreted in human milk, caution should be exercised when BOOSTRIX is administered to a nursing woman. **Pregnancy Exposure Registry:** Healthcare providers are encouraged to register pregnant women who receive BOOSTRIX in the GlaxoSmithKline vaccination pregnancy registry by calling 1-888-825-5249. **Geriatric Use:** BOOSTRIX is not indicated for use in individuals older than 18 years. **Pediatric Use:** BOOSTRIX is not indicated for use in individuals younger than 10 years (see DOSAGE AND ADMINISTRATION in full prescribing information). For immunization of infants and children younger than 7 years against diphtheria, tetanus, and pertussis, refer to the manufacturers' package inserts for Diphtheria and Tetanus Toxoids and Acellular Pertussis Vaccine Adsorbed (DTaP) vaccines.

**ADVERSE REACTIONS:** A total of 3,289 adolescents were vaccinated with a single dose of BOOSTRIX during clinical trials. An additional 1,092 adolescents 10 to 18 years of age received a non-US formulation of BOOSTRIX (formulated to contain 0.5 mg aluminum per dose) in non-US clinical studies.

The primary safety study, conducted in the United States, was a randomized, observer-blinded, controlled study in which 3,080 adolescents 10 to 18 years of age received a single dose of BOOSTRIX and 1,034 received the control Td vaccine manufactured by Massachusetts Public Health Biologic Laboratories. There were no substantive differences in demographic characteristics between the vaccine groups. Among BOOSTRIX and control vaccine recipients approximately 75% were 10 to 14 years of age and approximately 25% were 15 to 18 years of age. Approximately 98% of participants in this study had received the recommended series of 4 or 5 doses of either DTwP or a combination of DTwP and DTaP in childhood. Data on adverse events were collected by the subjects, parents and/or guardians using standardized diaries for 15 consecutive days following the vaccine dose (i.e., day of vaccination and the next 14 days). Subjects were monitored for unsolicited adverse events that occurred within 31 days of vaccination (day 0-30) using diary cards (day 0-14) supplemented by spontaneous reports and a medical history as reported by subjects, parents, and/or guardians. Subjects were also monitored for 6 months post-vaccination for non-routine medical visits, visits to an emergency room, onset of new chronic illness, and serious adverse events. Information regarding late onset adverse events was obtained via a telephone call 6 months following vaccination. At least 97% of subjects completed the 6-month follow-up evaluation.

The adverse event information from clinical trials provides a basis for identifying adverse events that appear to be related to vaccine use and for approximating rates. However, because clinical trials are conducted under widely varying conditions, adverse event rates observed in the clinical trials of a vaccine cannot be directly compared to rates in the clinical trials of another vaccine, and may not reflect the rates observed in practice.

**Serious Adverse Events in All Safety Studies:** In the US-safety study, no serious adverse events were reported to occur within 31 days of vaccination. During the 6-month extended safety evaluation period, no serious adverse events that were of potential autoimmune origin or new onset and chronic in nature were reported to occur. In non-US studies in which serious adverse events were monitored for up to 37 days, one subject was diagnosed with insulin dependent diabetes. The association of this event with vaccination is unknown. No other serious adverse events of potential autoimmune origin or that were new onset and chronic in nature were reported to occur in these studies.

**Solicited Adverse Events in the US-Safety Study:** In a US study, the most common local adverse events following administration of BOOSTRIX were pain, redness, and swelling at the injection site. The most common general adverse events were headache and fatigue. Most of these events were reported at a similar frequency in recipients of both BOOSTRIX and Td. Any pain, grade 2 or 3 pain (but not grade 3 alone), and grade 2 or 3 headache (but not grade 3 alone) were reported at a higher rate in recipients of BOOSTRIX. The primary safety endpoint of the US study was the incidence of grade 3 pain (spontaneously painful and/or prevented normal activity) at the injection site within 15 days of vaccination. Grade 3 pain was reported in 4.6% of those who received BOOSTRIX compared with 4.0% of those who received the Td vaccine. The difference in rate of grade 3 pain was within the pre-defined clinical limit for non-inferiority (upper limit of the 95% CI for the difference ≤4%). These were the rates for solicited local and general adverse events within 15 days of vaccination with BOOSTRIX or Td vaccine for the total vaccinated cohort (all enrolled, vaccinated subjects with safety data available analyzed by vaccine received):

**Percentage of Individuals 10 to 18 Years of Age Reporting Solicited Local Adverse Events or Solicited General Adverse Events Within the 15-day* Post-Vaccination Period**

| | BOOSTRIX (N = 3,032) | Td (N = 1,013) |
|---|---|---|
| **Local** | | |
| Pain,† any | 75.3 | 71.7 |
| Pain,† grade 2 or 3 | 51.2 | 42.5 |
| Pain,‡ grade 3 | 4.6 | 4.0 |
| Redness, any | 22.5 | 19.8 |
| Redness, >20 mm | 4.1 | 3.9 |
| Redness, ≥50 mm | 1.7 | 1.6 |
| Swelling, any | 21.1 | 20.1 |
| Swelling, >20 mm | 5.3 | 4.9 |
| Swelling, ≥50 mm | 2.5 | 3.2 |
| Arm circumference increase,§ >5 mm | 28.3 | 29.5 |
| Arm circumference increase,§ >20 mm | 2.0 | 2.2 |
| Arm circumference increase,§ >40 mm | 0.5 | 0.3 |
| **General** | | |
| Fever,‖ ≥99.5°F | 13.5 | 13.1 |
| Fever,‖ >100.4°F | 5.0 | 4.7 |
| Fever,‖ >102.2°F | 1.4 | 1.0 |
| Headache, any | 43.1 | 41.5 |
| Headache,† grade 2 or 3 | 15.7 | 12.7 |
| Headache, grade 3 | 3.7 | 2.7 |
| Fatigue, any | 37.0 | 36.7 |
| Fatigue, grade 2 or 3 | 14.4 | 12.9 |
| Fatigue, grade 3 | 3.7 | 3.2 |
| Gastrointestinal symptoms,¶ any | 26.0 | 25.8 |
| Gastrointestinal symptoms,¶ grade 2 or 3 | 9.8 | 9.7 |
| Gastrointestinal symptoms,¶ grade 3 | 3.0 | 3.2 |

Td = Tetanus and Diphtheria Toxoids Adsorbed For Adult Use manufactured by Massachusetts Public Health Biologic Laboratories.

N = number of subjects in the total vaccinated cohort with local/general symptoms sheets completed.

Grade 2 = Local: painful when the limb was moved; General: interfered with normal activity.

Grade 3 = Local: spontaneously painful and/or prevented normal activity; General: prevented normal activity.

*Day of vaccination and the next 14 days.

†Statistically significantly higher ($P<0.05$) following BOOSTRIX as compared to Td vaccine.

‡Grade 3 injection site pain following BOOSTRIX was not inferior to Td (upper limit of two-sided 95% CI for the difference in the percentage of subjects ≤4%).

§Mid-upper region of the vaccinated arm.

‖Oral temperatures or axillary temperatures.

¶Gastrointestinal symptoms included nausea, vomiting, diarrhea and/or abdominal pain.

Mid-upper arm circumference was measured by the adolescent or their parent/guardian prior to injection and daily for 15 days following vaccination. There was no significant difference between BOOSTRIX recipients and Td recipients in the proportion of subjects reporting an increase in mid-upper arm circumference in the vaccinated arm. The incidence of unsolicited adverse events reported in the 31 days after vaccination was comparable between the 2 groups.

As with any vaccine, there is the possibility that broad use of BOOSTRIX could reveal adverse events not observed in clinical trials.

**Postmarketing Reports:** Worldwide voluntary reports of adverse events received for BOOSTRIX in persons 10 to 18 years of age since market introduction of this vaccine are listed below. This list includes serious events or events which have causal connection to components of this or other vaccines or drugs. Because these events are reported voluntarily from a population of uncertain size, it is not possible to reliably estimate their frequency or establish a causal relationship to vaccine exposure. *Blood and lymphatic system disorders:* Lymphadenitis, lymphadenopathy. *Cardiac disorders:* Myocarditis. *Injection site reactions:* Induration, inflammation, mass, nodule, warmth, local reaction. *Metabolism and nutrition disorders:* Diabetes mellitus insulin-dependent. *Musculoskeletal and connective tissue disorders:* Arthralgia, back pain, myalgia. *Nervous system disorders:* Convulsion, encephalitis, facial palsy, paraesthesia. *Skin and subcutaneous tissue disorders:* Exanthem, Henoch-Schönlein purpura, rash. In addition, extensive swelling of the injected limb has been reported following administration of BOOSTRIX.

**Reporting Adverse Events:** Report the occurrence following immunization of any event set forth in the Vaccine Injury Table from the National Childhood Vaccine Injury Act including: Anaphylaxis or anaphylactic shock within 7 days, encephalopathy or encephalitis within 7 days, brachial neuritis within 28 days, or an acute complication or sequelae (including death) of an illness, disability, injury, or condition referred to above, or any events that would contraindicate further doses of vaccine, according to this prescribing information. These events should be reported to VAERS. The VAERS toll-free number is 1-800-822-7967. Reporting forms may also be obtained at the VAERS website at www.vaers.org.

**DOSAGE AND ADMINISTRATION: Recommended Dose:** BOOSTRIX should be administered as a single 0.5 mL injection by the intramuscular route into the deltoid muscle of the upper arm in individuals 10 through 18 years of age. Do not administer this product subcutaneously or intravenously. There are no data to support repeat administration of BOOSTRIX. Five years should elapse between the subject's last dose of the recommended series of childhood DTwP and/or DTaP vaccine and the administration of BOOSTRIX. Limited data are available on the use of BOOSTRIX following Tetanus and Diphtheria Toxoids Adsorbed For Adult Use (Td) vaccine. **Additional Dosing Information: *Wound Management:*** Clinicians should refer to guidelines for tetanus prophylaxis in routine wound management. Adolescents 10 to 18 years of age who have completed a primary series against tetanus and who sustain wounds which are minor and uncomplicated, should receive a booster dose of a tetanus toxoid-containing vaccine only if they have not received tetanus toxoid within the preceding 10 years. In case of tetanus-prone injury (e.g., wounds contaminated with dirt, feces, soil, and saliva; puncture wounds; avulsions; and wounds resulting from missles, crushing, burns, and frostbite) in an adolescent who is in need of tetanus toxoid, BOOSTRIX can be used as an alternative to Tetanus and Diphtheria Toxoids Adsorbed For Adult Use (Td) vaccine in patients for whom the pertussis component is also indicated (see INDICATIONS AND USAGE).

Manufactured by **GlaxoSmithKline Biologicals**
Rixensart, Belgium, US License 1617
Distributed by **GlaxoSmithKline**
Research Triangle Park, NC 27709



Full prescribing information for BOOSTRIX is available at www.BOOSTRIX.com.

BRS-BO:L1

**References: 1.** Centers for Disease Control and Prevention. *Epidemiology and Prevention of Vaccine-Preventable Diseases.* Atkinson W, Hamborsky J, Wolfe S, eds. 8th ed. Washington DC: Public Health Foundation; 2004:75–88, A26–A27. **2.** ACIP recommends adolescent vaccination for tetanus, diphtheria and pertussis vaccine [press release]. Atlanta, GA: Department of Health and Human Services; Available at: www.cdc.gov/nip/pr/pr_tdap_jun2005.htm. Accessed September 27, 2005. **3.** Data on file, BOR305, GlaxoSmithKline.

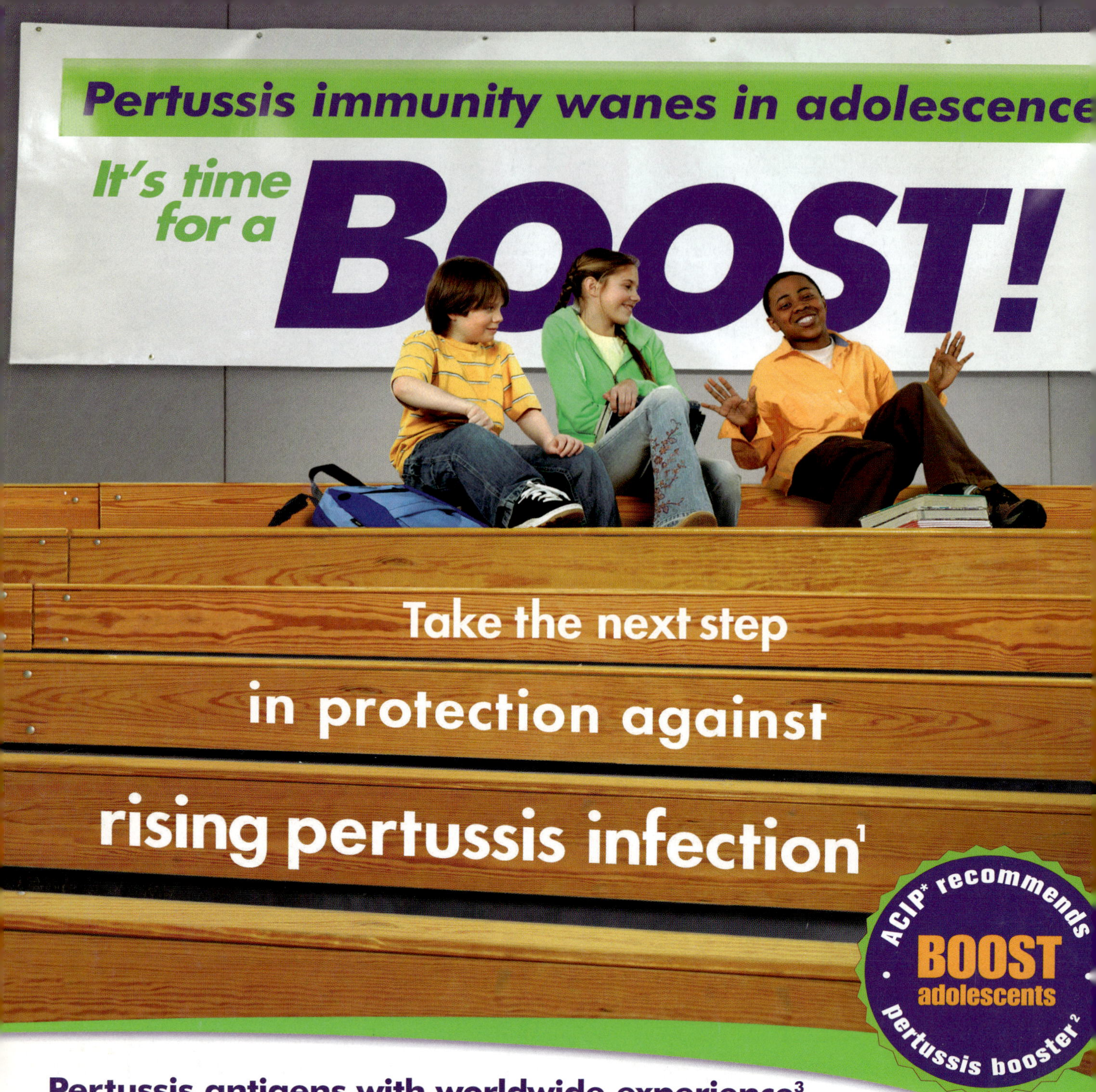


**Pertussis antigens with worldwide experience[3]—**
***combined* with a Td booster**

## Important Safety Information

In clinical studies, adverse events included pain, redness, and swelling at the injection site, headache, fatigue, and gastrointestinal symptoms. As with other vaccines, rare adverse events may occur. As with any vaccine, vaccination with BOOSTRIX may not protect 100% of susceptible individuals. Hypersensitivity to any component of BOOSTRIX is a contraindication.

*Advisory Committee on Immunization Practices.

**BOOSTRIX®**

***Tetanus Toxoid, Reduced Diphtheria Toxoid and Acellular Pertussis Vaccine, Adsorbed***

gsk GlaxoSmithKline Vaccines

**Please see the accompanying brief summary of complete prescribing information.**


Manufactured by **GlaxoSmithKline Biologicals**, Rixensart, Belgium Distributed by **GlaxoSmithKline**, Research Triangle Park, NC 27709

# ARCHIVES OF PEDIATRICS & ADOLESCENT MEDICINE

WWW.ARCHPEDIATRICS.COM

MARCH 2006

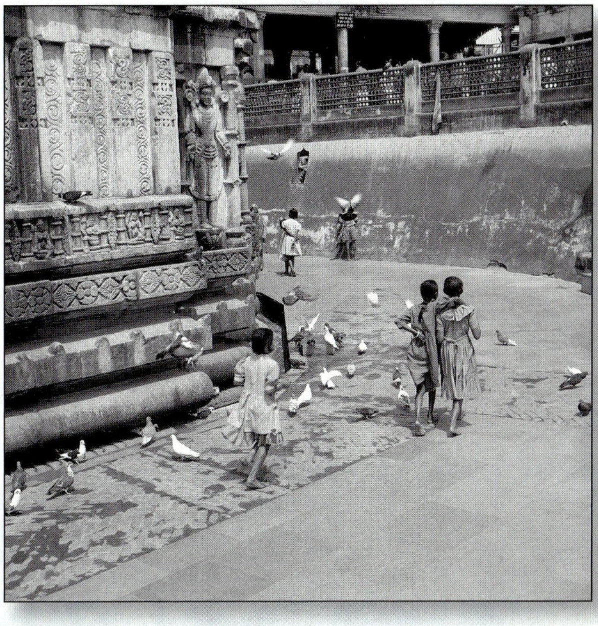

Friends. Kamakya Temple, Guwahati, Assam, India. See page 231.

RANDOMIZED PLACEBO-CONTROLLED TRIAL OF METFORMIN FOR ADOLESCENTS WITH POLYCYSTIC OVARY SYNDROME

DEPRESSIVE SYMPTOMATOLOGY AS A PREDICTOR OF EXPOSURE TO INTIMATE PARTNER VIOLENCE AMONG US FEMALE ADOLESCENTS AND YOUNG ADULTS

MATERNAL DEPRESSIVE SYMPTOMS AT 2 TO 4 MONTHS POST PARTUM AND EARLY PARENTING PRACTICES

ESTIMATED COST-EFFECTIVENESS OF GROWTH HORMONE THERAPY FOR IDIOPATHIC SHORT STATURE

COMPLETE TABLE OF CONTENTS ON PAGE 229

JAMA & ARCHIVES JOURNALS
American Medical Association

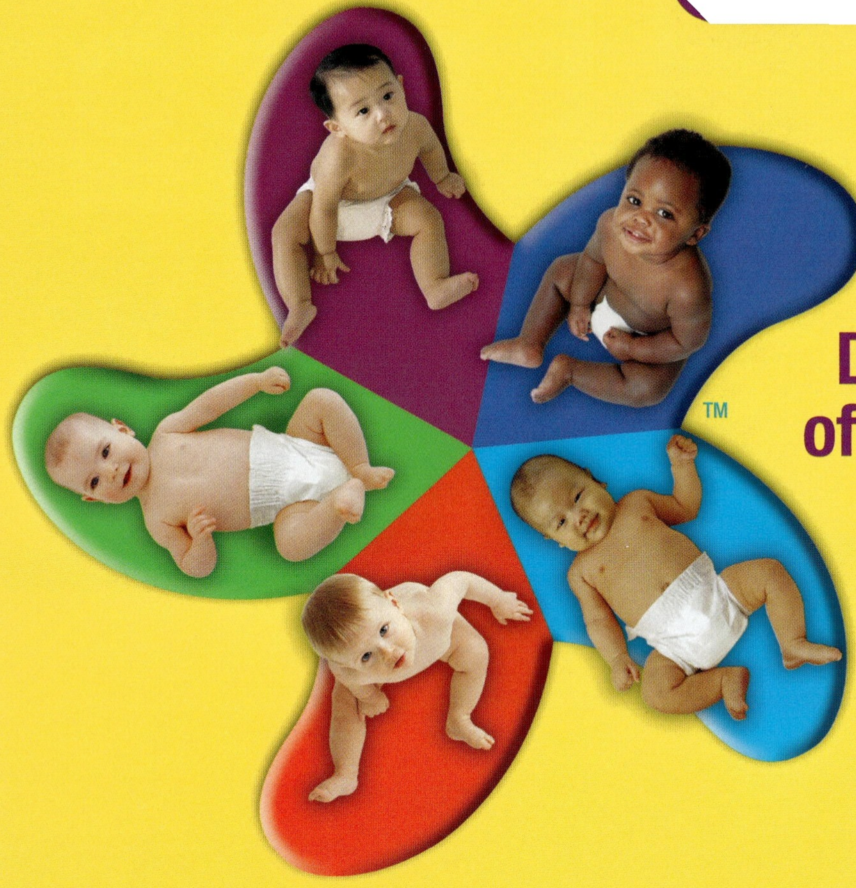


# Don't run the risk of letting one child get away

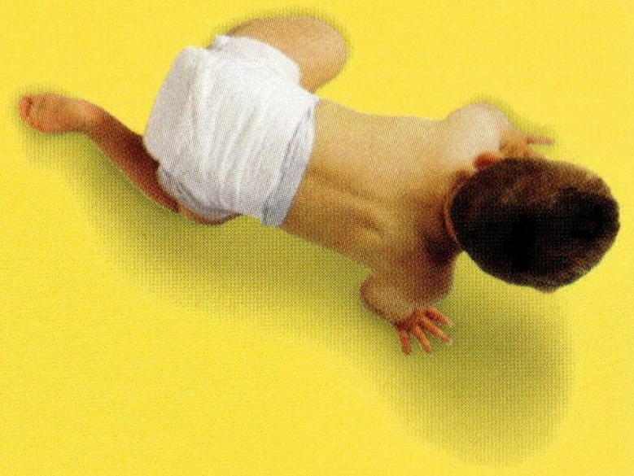

## PEDIARIX may help ensure timely vaccination with fewer injections

- With just 1 dose at 2, 4, and 6 months of age (in infants born of HBsAg-negative mothers)

*Based on analysis of the first four DTaP doses in the most recent National Immunization Survey (2003) of 21,210 children 19–35 months of age.

In clinical studies, adverse events in infants receiving PEDIARIX included injection-site reactions (pain, redness, or swelling), fever, and fussiness. Administration of PEDIARIX was associated with higher rates of fever relative to separately administered vaccines (see Adverse Reactions section of the brief summary). PEDIARIX is contraindicated in infants with known hypersensitivity to any component of the vaccine including yeast, neomycin, and polymyxin B. As with any vaccine, vaccination with PEDIARIX may not protect 100% of susceptible individuals.

**PEDIARIX™ [Diphtheria and Tetanus Toxoids and Acellular Pertussis Adsorbed, Hepatitis B (Recombinant) and Inactivated Poliovirus Vaccine Combined]**

The following is a brief summary only; see full prescribing information for complete product information.

**CONTRAINDICATIONS:** Hypersensitivity to any component of the vaccine, including yeast, neomycin, and polymyxin B, is a contraindication (see DESCRIPTION in complete prescribing information). Do not use PEDIARIX after a serious allergic reaction (e.g., anaphylaxis) temporally associated with a previous dose of this vaccine or with any components of this vaccine. Because of the uncertainty as to which component of the vaccine might be responsible, do not give further vaccination with any of these components; or, refer such individuals to an allergist for evaluation. The following events are contraindications to administration of PEDIARIX: encephalopathy (e.g., coma, decreased level of consciousness, prolonged seizures) within 7 days of administration of a previous dose of a pertussis-containing vaccine that is not attributable to another identifiable cause; progressive neurologic disorder, including infantile spasms, uncontrolled epilepsy, or progressive encephalopathy. Do not vaccinate individuals with such conditions until a treatment regimen has been established and the condition has stabilized. PEDIARIX is not contraindicated for use in individuals with HIV infection.

**WARNINGS:** Administration of PEDIARIX is associated with higher rates of fever relative to separately administered vaccines. In one study that evaluated medically attended fever after the first dose of PEDIARIX or separately administered vaccines, infants who received PEDIARIX had a higher rate of medical encounters for fever within the first 4 days following vaccination. In some infants, these encounters included the performance of diagnostic studies to evaluate other causes of fever (see ADVERSE REACTIONS). The vial stopper is latex-free. The tip cap and the rubber plunger of the needleless prefilled syringes contain dry natural latex rubber that may cause allergic reactions in latex sensitive individuals. If any of the following events occur in temporal relation to receipt of whole-cell DTP or a vaccine containing an acellular pertussis component, consider carefully whether to give subsequent doses of PEDIARIX or any vaccine containing a pertussis component: temperature of ≥40.5°C (105°F) within 48 hours not due to another identifiable cause; collapse or shock-like state (hypotonic-hyporesponsive episode) within 48 hours; persistent, inconsolable crying lasting ≥3 hours, occurring within 48 hours; seizures with or without fever occurring within 3 days. If Guillain-Barré syndrome occurs within 6 weeks of receipt of prior vaccine containing tetanus toxoid, the decision to give subsequent doses of PEDIARIX or any vaccine containing tetanus toxoid should be based on careful consideration of the potential benefits and possible risks. A committee of the Institute of Medicine (IOM) has concluded that evidence is consistent with a causal relationship between whole-cell DTP vaccine and acute neurologic illness, and under special circumstances, between whole-cell DTP vaccine and chronic neurologic disease in the context of the National Childhood Encephalopathy Study (NCES) report; however, evidence was insufficient to indicate whether or not whole-cell DTP vaccine increased the overall risk of chronic neurologic disease. Acute encephalopathy and permanent neurologic damage have not been reported causally linked or in temporal association with administration of PEDIARIX, but the experience with PEDIARIX is insufficient to rule this out. Encephalopathy has been reported following INFANRIX® (Diphtheria and Tetanus Toxoids and Acellular Pertussis Vaccine Adsorbed) (see ADVERSE REACTIONS, Postmarketing Reports), but data are not sufficient to evaluate a causal relationship. The decision to administer a pertussis-containing vaccine to children with stable central nervous system (CNS) disorders must be made by the physician on an individual basis, with consideration of all relevant factors, and assessment of potential risks and benefits for that individual. Advise the parent or guardian of the potential increased risk involved (see PRECAUTIONS). A family history of seizures or other CNS disorders is not a contraindication to pertussis vaccine. For children at higher risk for seizures than the general population, an appropriate antipyretic may be administered at the time of vaccination and for the ensuing 24 hours according to the respective prescribing information recommended dosage to reduce the possibility of post-vaccination fever. Defer vaccination during the course of a moderate or severe illness with or without fever and vaccinate patients as soon as they have recovered from the acute phase of the illness. Do not give PEDIARIX to children on anticoagulant therapy or those with bleeding disorders unless the potential benefit clearly outweighs the risk of administration (see PRECAUTIONS in complete prescribing information).

**PRECAUTIONS:** Before the injection of any biological, the physician should take all reasonable precautions to prevent allergic or other adverse reactions. Epinephrine injection (1:1000) and other appropriate agents used for the control of immediate allergic reactions must be immediately available should an acute anaphylactic reaction occur. Immunosuppressed individuals, including those receiving immunosuppressive therapy, may not develop the expected immune response. **Drug Interactions:** For information regarding concomitant administration with other vaccines, refer to DOSAGE AND ADMINISTRATION in complete prescribing information. Do not mix PEDIARIX with any other vaccine in the same syringe or vial. **Carcinogenesis, Mutagenesis, Impairment of Fertility:** PEDIARIX has not been evaluated for carcinogenic or mutagenic potential, or for impairment of fertility. **Pregnancy:** Pregnancy Category C: PEDIARIX is not indicated for women of child-bearing age. Animal reproduction studies have not been conducted with PEDIARIX. It is not known whether PEDIARIX can cause fetal harm when administered to a pregnant woman or if PEDIARIX can affect reproductive capacity. **Geriatric Use:** PEDIARIX is not indicated for use in adult populations. **Pediatric Use:** Safety and effectiveness of PEDIARIX in infants younger than 6 weeks of age have not been evaluated (see DOSAGE AND ADMINISTRATION in complete prescribing information). PEDIARIX is not recommended for persons 7 years of age or older. Tetanus and Diphtheria Toxoids Adsorbed (Td) For Adult Use, inactivated poliovirus vaccine (IPV), and Hepatitis B Vaccine (Recombinant) should be used in individuals 7 years of age or older.

**ADVERSE REACTIONS:** A total of 20,739 doses of PEDIARIX have been administered to 7,028 infants as a 3-dose primary series. The most common adverse reactions observed in clinical trials were local injection site reactions (pain, redness, or swelling), fever, and fussiness. In comparative studies, administration of PEDIARIX was associated with higher rates of fever relative to separately administered vaccines (see WARNINGS). The prevalence of fever was highest on the day of vaccination and the day following vaccination. More than 98% of episodes of fever resolved within the 4-day period following vaccination (i.e., the period including the day of vaccination and the next 3 days). Rates of most other solicited adverse events following PEDIARIX were comparable to rates observed following separately administered US-licensed vaccines. The adverse event information from clinical trials provides a basis for identifying adverse events that appear to be related to vaccine use and for approximating rates. However, because clinical trials are conducted under widely varying conditions, adverse event rates observed in the clinical trials of a vaccine cannot be directly compared to rates in the clinical trials of another vaccine, and may not reflect the rates observed in practice. A total of 5,472 infants were enrolled in a German safety study that was originally designed to compare the safety and reactogenicity of PEDIARIX administered concomitantly at separate sites with 1 of 4 *Haemophilus influenzae* type b (Hib) vaccines at 3, 4, and 5 months of age. After enrollment of 1,569 infants, the study was amended to include a control group that received INFANRIX, Hib vaccine, and oral poliovirus vaccine (OPV) separately. Infants in the separate administration group received one less antigen (hepatitis B) than the infants who received PEDIARIX. Safety data were available for 4,666 infants who received PEDIARIX administered concomitantly at separate sites with 1 of 4 Hib vaccines and for 768 infants in the control group that received separate vaccines. The primary end-point of the study was the percentage of infants with any grade 3 solicited symptom (redness or swelling >20 mm, fever >103.1°F, or crying, pain, vomiting, diarrhea, loss of appetite, or restlessness that prevented normal daily activities) over the 3-dose primary series in infants who received PEDIARIX (4 groups that received PEDIARIX and Hib vaccines pooled) compared to the group that received INFANRIX and Hib vaccine separately with OPV. Analysis for the primary end-point was performed on the according-to-protocol (ATP) cohort that included only those infants who were enrolled after the protocol amendment to include a control group. Of 3,773 infants in the ATP cohort for whom safety data were available, 16.2% (95% CI: 14.9% to 17.5%) of 3,029 infants who received PEDIARIX and Hib vaccine compared to 20.3% (95% CI: 17.5% to 23.4%) of 744 infants who received separate vaccines were reported to have had at least one grade 3 solicited symptom within 4 days of vaccination (i.e., day of vaccination and the next 3 days). The difference between groups in the rate of grade 3 symptoms was 4.1% (90% CI: 1.4% to 7.1%). These were the rates for selected solicited symptoms within 4 days following each dose in a 3-dose primary series in infants who received PEDIARIX administered concomitantly with Hib vaccine and those who received separate concomitant administration of INFANRIX, Hib vaccine, and OPV for the intent-to-treat (ITT) cohort (includes all infants enrolled before and after the amendment who received the indicated vaccine and for whom at least one symptom sheet was completed):

**Percentage of German Infants With Solicited Local Reactions or Selected Systemic Adverse Events Within 4 Days of Vaccination* (ITT Cohort)**

| | PEDIARIX & Hib | | | INFANRIX, Hib, & OPV | | |
|---|---|---|---|---|---|---|
| | **Dose 1** | **Dose 2** | **Dose 3** | **Dose 1** | **Dose 2** | **Dose 3** |
| **N** | **4,666** | **4,619** | **4,574** | **768** | **757** | **750** |
| **Local†** | | | | | | |
| Pain, any | 14.0 | 10.2 | 9.9 | 14.2 | 9.8 | 8.1 |
| Pain, grade 2 or 3 | 2.9 | 1.2 | 1.5 | 3.6 | 1.7 | 1.1 |
| Pain, grade 3 | 0.7 | 0.3 | 0.3 | 1.3 | 0.4 | 0.1 |
| Redness, any | 18.6 | 26.6 | 25.6 | 16.1 | 21.4 | 20.8 |
| Redness, >5 mm | 6.7 | 9.9 | 9.0 | 5.9 | 8.2 | 7.7 |
| Redness, >20 mm | 1.2 | 1.0 | 1.1 | 1.8 | 0.7 | 1.1 |
| Swelling, any | 12.7 | 18.5 | 18.4 | 9.6 | 12.9 | 13.6 |
| Swelling, >5 mm | 5.6 | 7.7 | 7.8 | 3.6 | 5.2 | 4.8 |
| Swelling, >20 mm | 1.2 | 1.6 | 1.5 | 1.3 | 1.1 | 1.2 |
| **Systemic** | | | | | | |
| Restlessness, any | 41.4 | 32.0 | 26.7 | 46.4 | 35.0 | 27.6 |
| Restlessness, grade 2 or 3 | 14.4 | 10.0 | 8.9 | 20.2 | 11.5 | 8.4 |
| Restlessness, grade 3 | 3.0 | 1.5 | 1.6 | 5.7 | 3.0 | 1.7 |
| Fever‡, ≥100.4°F | 25.1 | 19.3 | 19.7 | 13.2 | 13.1 | 11.2 |
| Fever‡, >101.3°F | 5.8 | 4.1 | 4.6 | 2.2 | 2.8 | 2.1 |
| Fever‡, >103.1°F | 0.3 | 0.5 | 0.7 | 0.3 | 0.3 | 0.5 |
| Unusual cry§, any | 24.9 | 16.5 | 13.1 | 36.5 | 19.7 | 14.3 |
| Unusual cry§, grade 2 or 3 | 12.7 | 7.1 | 5.7 | 20.8 | 10.0 | 5.7 |
| Unusual cry§, grade 3 | 3.9 | 1.7 | 1.4 | 6.8 | 2.1 | 1.1 |
| Loss of appetite, any | 17.9 | 13.3 | 12.5 | 19.1 | 16.2 | 11.3 |
| Loss of appetite, grade 2 or 3 | 4.0 | 2.9 | 2.7 | 4.4 | 2.9 | 2.3 |
| Loss of appetite, grade 3 | 0.6 | 0.5 | 0.4 | 0.5 | 0.7 | 0.0 |

N = number of infants in the intent-to-treat (ITT) cohort.
Grade 2 defined as sufficiently discomforting to interfere with daily activities.
Grade 3 defined as preventing normal daily activities.
* Within 4 days of vaccination defined as day of vaccination and the next 3 days.
† Local reactions at the injection site for PEDIARIX or INFANRIX.
‡ Rectal temperatures.
§ Unusual cry lasting >1 hour.

In this study, infants were also monitored for unsolicited adverse events that occurred within 30 days following vaccination. Over the entire study period, 6 subjects in the group that received PEDIARIX reported seizures. Two of these subjects had a febrile seizure, 1 of whom also developed afebrile seizures. The remaining 4 subjects had afebrile seizures, including 2 with infantile spasms. Two subjects reported seizures within 7 days following vaccination (1 subject had both febrile and afebrile seizures, and 1 subject had afebrile seizures), corresponding to a rate of 0.22 seizures per 1,000 doses (febrile seizures 0.07 per 1,000 doses, afebrile seizures 0.14 per 1,000 doses). No subject who received concomitant INFANRIX, Hib vaccine, and OPV reported seizures. In a separate German study that evaluated the safety of INFANRIX in 22,505 infants who received 66,867 doses of INFANRIX administered as a 3-dose primary series, the rate of seizures within 7 days of vaccination with INFANRIX was 0.13 per 1,000 doses (febrile seizures 0.0 per 1,000 doses, afebrile seizures 0.13 per 1,000 doses). No cases of hypotonic-hyporesponsiveness, encephalopathy, or anaphylaxis were reported in the German study that evaluated the safety of PEDIARIX. Rates of serious adverse events that are less common than those reported in this safety study are not known at this time.

Additional safety data for PEDIARIX are available from a US study designed to evaluate lot-to-lot consistency and a bridge for a new manufacturing step. These were the rates for local reactions and selected adverse events within 4 days of vaccination with PEDIARIX administered concomitantly with a Hib vaccine at 2, 4, and 6 months of age:

**Percentage of US Infants With Solicited Local Reactions or Selected Systemic Adverse Events Within 4 Days of Vaccination* (ITT Cohort)**

| | PEDIARIX & Hib | | |
|---|---|---|---|
| | **Dose 1** | **Dose 2** | **Dose 3** |
| **Local†** | **N = 482** | **N = 469** | **N = 466** |
| Pain, any | 30.5 | 25.4 | 23.0 |
| Pain, grade 2 or 3 | 6.2 | 5.5 | 3.6 |
| Pain, grade 3 | 1.2 | 0.6 | 0.6 |
| Redness, any | 25.3 | 32.6 | 35.6 |
| Redness, >5 mm | 9.3 | 10.4 | 8.6 |
| Redness, >20 mm | 0.6 | 1.5 | 1.3 |
| Swelling, any | 15.1 | 16.6 | 22.3 |
| Swelling, >5 mm | 6.8 | 6.2 | 6.4 |
| Swelling, >20 mm | 1.0 | 1.3 | 1.3 |
| **Systemic** | **N = 482** | **N = 469** | **N = 467** |
| Restlessness, any | 28.8 | 30.3 | 28.5 |
| Restlessness, grade 2 or 3 | 7.1 | 9.0 | 9.4 |
| Restlessness, grade 3 | 1.0 | 1.1 | 0.6 |
| Fever‡, ≥100.4°F | 26.6 | 31.3 | 25.9 |
| Fever‡, >101.3°F | 2.9 | 6.2 | 4.7 |
| Fever‡, >103.1°F | 0.0 | 0.2 | 0.6 |
| Fussiness, any | 61.8 | 63.8 | 57.0 |
| Fussiness, grade 2 or 3 | 14.9 | 21.5 | 17.1 |
| Fussiness, grade 3 | 2.7 | 3.4 | 1.7 |
| Loss of appetite, any | 21.6 | 19.8 | 18.8 |
| Loss of appetite, grade 2 or 3 | 3.1 | 3.2 | 2.4 |
| Loss of appetite, grade 3 | 0.2 | 0.4 | 0.0 |
| Sleeping more than usual, any | 46.7 | 31.8 | 28.1 |
| Sleeping more than usual, grade 2 or 3 | 10.2 | 6.0 | 4.7 |
| Sleeping more than usual, grade 3 | 1.7 | 0.4 | 0.6 |

N = number of infants in the intent-to-treat (ITT) cohort (infants who received the indicated vaccine and for whom at least one symptom sheet was completed).
Grade 2 defined as sufficiently discomforting to interfere with daily activities.
Grade 3 defined as preventing normal daily activities.
* Within 4 days of vaccination defined as day of vaccination and the next 3 days.
† Local reactions at the injection site for PEDIARIX.
‡ Rectal temperatures.

In another US study, these were the rates for fever within 4 days following dose 1 (i.e., day of vaccination and the next 3 days) at 2 months of age in infants who received PEDIARIX when administered concomitantly at separate sites with Hib and pneumococcal conjugate vaccines and those who received INFANRIX, ENGERIX-B® [Hepatitis B Vaccine (Recombinant)], IPV, Hib vaccine, and pneumococcal conjugate vaccine:

**Percentage of US Infants With Fever Within 4 Days of Dose 1* (ITT Cohort)**

| | PEDIARIX, Hib, & Pneumococcal Conjugate (N = 667) | INFANRIX, ENGERIX-B, IPV, Hib, & Pneumococcal Conjugate (N = 333) | Separate Vaccine Group Minus Combination Vaccine Group |
|---|---|---|---|
| **Fever†** | **%** | **%** | **Difference (95% CI)** |
| ≥100.4°F‡ | 27.9 | 19.8 | -8.07 (-13.54, -2.60) |
| >101.3°F | 7.0 | 4.5 | -2.54 (-5.50, 0.41) |
| >102.2°F‡ | 2.2 | 0.3 | -1.95 (-3.22, -0.68) |
| >103.1°F | 0.4 | 0.0 | -0.45 (-0.96, 0.06) |
| M.A.‡ | 1.2 | 0.0 | -1.20 (-2.03, -037) |

N = number of infants for whom at least one symptom sheet was completed, excluding 3 infants for whom temperature was not measured and 3 infants whose temperature was measured by the tympanic method.
*Within 4 days of dose 1 defined as day of vaccination and the next 3 days.
† Rectal temperatures.
‡ The group that received PEDIARIX compared to separate vaccine group p value <0.05 (2-sided Fisher Exact test) or the 95% confidence interval on the difference between groups does not include 0.
M.A. = Medically attended (a visit to or from medical personnel).

In this study, medical attention (a visit to or from medical personnel) for fever within 4 days following vaccination was sought for 8 infants who received PEDIARIX (1.2%) and no infants who received separately administered vaccines. Four infants were seen by medical personnel in an office setting; no diagnostic tests were performed in 2 of the infants and a complete blood count (CBC) was done in the other 2 infants. Of 3 infants who were seen in an emergency room, all had a CBC and a blood and urine culture performed; chest X-rays were done in 2 of the infants and a nasopharyngeal specimen was tested for Respiratory Syncytial Virus in one of the infants. One infant was hospitalized for a work-up that included a CBC, blood and urine cultures, a lumbar puncture, and a chest X-ray. All episodes of medically attended fever resolved within 4 days post-vaccination.

Limited data are available from a study conducted in Moldova in which infants received a dose of hepatitis B vaccine within 48 hours of birth followed by 3 doses of PEDIARIX at 6, 10, and 14 weeks of age. No information was collected on the HBsAg status of mothers of enrolled infants. These were the rates for local reactions and selected adverse events within 4 days of vaccination with PEDIARIX administered comcomitantly with Hib vaccine following a birth dose of hepatitis B vaccine:

**Percentage of Moldovan Infants With Solicited Local Reactions or Selected Systemic Adverse Events Within 4 Days of Vaccination* (ITT Cohort)**

| | PEDIARIX & Hib | | |
|---|---|---|---|
| | **Dose 1** | **Dose 2** | **Dose 3** |
| **N** | **160** | **158** | **157** |
| **Local†** | | | |
| Pain, any | 25.6 | 18.4 | 14.0 |
| Pain, grade 3 | 3.1 | 0.6 | 1.9 |
| Redness, any | 41.9 | 41.8 | 47.1 |
| Redness, >20 mm | 1.9 | 2.5 | 4.5 |
| Swelling, any | 20.6 | 18.4 | 28.0 |
| Swelling, >20 mm | 4.4 | 2.5 | 7.0 |
| **Systemic** | | | |
| Restlessness, any | 13.1 | 10.8 | 8.9 |
| Restlessness, grade 3 | 1.3 | 0.6 | 0.6 |
| Fever‡, ≥100.4°F | 14.4 | 11.4 | 5.1 |
| Fever‡, >103.1°F | 0.0 | 0.6 | 0.0 |
| Fussiness, any | 25.0 | 21.5 | 17.8 |
| Fussiness, grade 3 | 2.5 | 0.6 | 0.6 |

N = number of infants in the intent-to-treat (ITT) cohort (infants who received the indicated vaccine and for whom at least one symptom sheet was completed).
Grade 3 defined as preventing normal daily activities.
*Within 4 days of vaccination defined as day of vaccination and the next 3 days.
† Local reactions at the injection site for PEDIARIX.
‡ Rectal temperatures.

Although there was no comparator group who received PEDIARIX without a birth dose of hepatitis B vaccine, available data suggest that some local adverse events may occur at a higher rate when PEDIARIX is administered after a birth dose of hepatitis B vaccine.

As with any vaccine, there is the possibility that broad use of PEDIARIX could reveal adverse events not observed in clinical trials.

**Postmarketing Reports:** Worldwide voluntary reports of adverse events received for INFANRIX and ENGERIX-B in children younger than 7 years of age since market introduction of these US-licensed vaccines are listed below. This list includes adverse events for which 20 or more reports were received with the exception of intussusception, idiopathic thrombocytopenic purpura, thrombocytopenia, anaphylactic reaction, angioedema, encephalopathy, hypotonic-hyporesponsive episode, and alopecia for which fewer than 20 reports were received. These latter events are included either because of the seriousness of the event or the strength of causal connection to components of this or other vaccines or drugs. *Body as a whole*: Asthenia[b], fever[a+b], lethargy[b], malaise[b], Sudden Infant Death Syndrome[a+b]. *Cardiovascular system*: Cyanosis[a+b], edema[b], pallor[b]. *Gastrointestinal system*: Abdominal pain[b], anorexia[b], diarrhea[a+b], intussusception[a+b], nausea[b], vomiting[a+b]. *Hematologic/lymphatic*: Idiopathic thrombocytopenic purpura[a+b], lymphadenopathy[a], thrombocytopenia[a+b]. *Hepatic*: Jaundice[b], liver function tests abnormal[b]. *Hypersensitivity*: Anaphylactic reaction[a+b], angioedema[b], hypersensitivity[a]. *Infections*: Cellulitis[a]. *Injection site reactions*: Injection site reactions[a+b]. *Musculoskeletal*: Arthralgia[b], limb swelling[a+b]. *Nervous system*: Convulsions[a+b], encephalopathy[a], headache[b], hypotonia[a+b], hypotonic-hyporesponsive episode[a], somnolence[a+b]. *Psychiatric*: Crying[a+b], irritability[a+b]. *Respiratory system*: Respiratory tract infection[a]. *Skin and appendages*: Alopecia[b], erythema[a+b], erythema multiforme[b], petechiae[b], pruritus[a+b], rash[a+b], urticaria[a+b]. *Special senses*: Ear pain[a]. [[a] Following INFANRIX; [b] Following ENGERIX-B; [a+b] Following either INFANRIX or ENGERIX-B.] These reactions were reported voluntarily from a population of uncertain size; therefore, it is not always possible to reliably estimate their frequency or establish a causal relationship to vaccination.

**Reporting Adverse Events:** Report the occurrence following immunization of any event set forth in the Vaccine Injury Table from the National Childhood Vaccine Injury Act including: Anaphylaxis or anaphylactic shock within 7 days, encephalopathy or encephalitis within 7 days, brachial neuritis within 28 days, or an acute complication or sequelae (including death) of an illness, disability, injury, or condition referred to above, or any events that would contraindicate further doses of PEDIARIX. The VAERS toll-free number is 1-800-822-7967.

Manufactured by **GlaxoSmithKline Biologicals**, Rixensart, Belgium, US License 1617

Distributed by **GlaxoSmithKline,** Research Triangle Park, NC 27709



Full prescribing information for PEDIARIX is available at www.GSKVaccines.com/Pediarix. BRS-PE:L2

 Printed in USA. PED583R0 June 2005

# Xopenex HFA™
(levalbuterol tartrate) Inhalation Aerosol

FOR ORAL INHALATION ONLY

## BRIEF SUMMARY

**INDICATIONS AND USAGE**

XOPENEX HFA (levalbuterol tartrate) Inhalation Aerosol is indicated for the treatment or prevention of bronchospasm in adults, adolescents, and children 4 years of age and older with reversible obstructive airway disease.

**CONTRAINDICATIONS**

XOPENEX HFA (levalbuterol tartrate) Inhalation Aerosol is contraindicated in patients with a history of hypersensitivity to levalbuterol, racemic albuterol, or any other component of XOPENEX HFA Inhalation Aerosol.

**WARNINGS**

1. Paradoxical Bronchospasm: Like other inhaled beta-adrenergic agonists, XOPENEX HFA Inhalation Aerosol can produce paradoxical bronchospasm, which may be life-threatening. If paradoxical bronchospasm occurs, XOPENEX HFA (levalbuterol tartrate) Inhalation Aerosol should be discontinued immediately and alternative therapy instituted. It should be recognized that paradoxical bronchospasm, when associated with inhaled formulations, frequently occurs with the first use of a new canister. 2. Deterioration of Asthma: Asthma may deteriorate acutely over a period of hours or chronically over several days or longer. If the patient needs more doses of XOPENEX HFA Inhalation Aerosol than usual, this may be a marker of destabilization of asthma and requires reevaluation of the patient and treatment regimen, giving special consideration to the possible need for anti-inflammatory treatment, e.g., corticosteroids.
3. Use of Anti-Inflammatory Agents: The use of a beta-adrenergic agonist alone may not be adequate to control asthma in many patients. Early consideration should be given to adding anti-inflammatory agents, e.g., corticosteroids, to the therapeutic regimen. 4. Cardiovascular Effects: XOPENEX HFA Inhalation Aerosol, like other beta-adrenergic agonists, can produce clinically significant cardiovascular effects in some patients, as measured by heart rate, blood pressure, and/or symptoms. Although such effects are uncommon after administration of XOPENEX HFA Inhalation Aerosol at recommended doses, if they occur, the drug may need to be discontinued. In addition, beta-agonists have been reported to produce electrocardiogram (ECG) changes, such as flattening of the T wave, prolongation of the QTc interval, and ST segment depression. The clinical significance of these findings is unknown. Therefore, XOPENEX HFA Inhalation Aerosol, like all sympathomimetic amines, should be used with caution in patients with cardiovascular disorders, especially coronary insufficiency, cardiac arrhythmias, and hypertension. 5. Do Not Exceed Recommended Dose: Fatalities have been reported in association with excessive use of inhaled sympathomimetic drugs in patients with asthma. The exact cause of death is unknown, but cardiac arrest following an unexpected development of a severe acute asthmatic crisis and subsequent hypoxia is suspected.
6. Immediate Hypersensitivity Reactions: Immediate hypersensitivity reactions may occur after administration of racemic albuterol, as demonstrated by rare cases of urticaria, angioedema, rash, bronchospasm, anaphylaxis, and oropharyngeal edema. The potential for hypersensitivity must be considered in the clinical evaluation of patients who experience immediate hypersensitivity reactions while receiving XOPENEX HFA Inhalation Aerosol.

**PRECAUTIONS**

**General**

XOPENEX HFA (levalbuterol tartrate) Inhalation Aerosol, like all sympathomimetic amines, should be used with caution in patients with cardiovascular disorders, especially coronary insufficiency, hypertension, and cardiac arrhythmias; in patients with convulsive disorders, hyperthyroidism, or diabetes mellitus; and in patients who are unusually responsive to sympathomimetic amines. Clinically significant changes in systolic and diastolic blood pressure have been seen in individual patients and could be expected to occur in some patients after the use of any beta-adrenergic bronchodilator.

Large doses of intravenous racemic albuterol have been reported to aggravate preexisting diabetes mellitus and ketoacidosis. As with other beta-adrenergic agonist medications, XOPENEX HFA Inhalation Aerosol may produce significant hypokalemia in some patients, possibly through intracellular shunting, which has the potential to produce adverse cardiovascular effects. The decrease is usually transient, not requiring supplementation.

**Information for Patients**

The action of XOPENEX HFA Inhalation Aerosol should last for 4 to 6 hours. XOPENEX HFA Inhalation Aerosol should not be used more frequently than recommended. Do not increase the dose or frequency of doses of XOPENEX HFA Inhalation Aerosol without consulting your physician. If you find that treatment with XOPENEX HFA Inhalation Aerosol becomes less effective for symptomatic relief, your symptoms become worse, and/or you need to use the product more frequently than usual, you should seek medical attention immediately. While you are using XOPENEX HFA Inhalation Aerosol, other inhaled drugs and asthma medications should be taken only as directed by your physician.

Common adverse effects of treatment with inhaled beta-agonists include palpitations, chest pain, rapid heart rate, tremor, and nervousness. If you are pregnant or nursing, contact your physician about use of XOPENEX HFA Inhalation Aerosol. Effective and safe use of XOPENEX HFA Inhalation Aerosol includes an understanding of the way that it should be administered.

Use XOPENEX HFA Inhalation Aerosol only with the actuator supplied with the product. Discard the canister after 200 sprays have been used. Never immerse the canister in water to determine how full the canister is ("float test").

In general, the technique for administering XOPENEX HFA Inhalation Aerosol to children is similar to that for adults. Children should use XOPENEX HFA Inhalation Aerosol under adult supervision, as instructed by the patient's physician.

**Drug Interactions**

Other short-acting sympathomimetic aerosol bronchodilators or epinephrine should be used with caution with XOPENEX HFA Inhalation Aerosol. If additional adrenergic drugs are to be administered by any route, they should be used with caution to avoid deleterious cardiovascular effects.

1. Beta-blockers: Beta-adrenergic receptor-blocking agents not only block the pulmonary effect of beta-adrenergic agonists, such as XOPENEX HFA Inhalation Aerosol, but may produce severe bronchospasm in asthmatic patients. Therefore, patients with asthma should not normally be treated with beta-blockers. However, under certain circumstances, e.g., as prophylaxis after myocardial infarction, there may be no acceptable alternatives to the use of beta-adrenergic blocking agents in patients with asthma. In this setting, cardioselective beta-blockers should be considered, although they should be administered with caution. 2. Diuretics: The ECG changes and/or hypokalemia that may result from the administration of non–potassium-sparing diuretics (such as loop and thiazide diuretics) can be acutely worsened by beta-agonists, especially when the recommended dose of the beta-agonist is exceeded. Although the clinical significance of these effects is not known, caution is advised in the coadministration of beta-agonists with non–potassium-sparing diuretics. 3. Digoxin: Mean decreases of 16% to 22% in serum digoxin levels were demonstrated after single-dose intravenous and oral administration of racemic albuterol, respectively, to normal volunteers who had received digoxin for 10 days. The clinical significance of these findings for patients with obstructive airway disease who are receiving XOPENEX HFA Inhalation Aerosol and digoxin on a chronic basis is unclear. Nevertheless, it would be prudent to carefully evaluate the serum digoxin levels in patients who are currently receiving digoxin and XOPENEX HFA Inhalation Aerosol. 4. Monoamine Oxidase Inhibitors or Tricyclic Antidepressants: XOPENEX HFA Inhalation Aerosol should be administered with extreme caution to patients being treated with monoamine oxidase inhibitors or tricyclic antidepressants, or within 2 weeks of discontinuation of such agents, because the action of albuterol on the vascular system may be potentiated.

**Carcinogenesis, Mutagenesis, and Impairment of Fertility** No carcinogenesis or impairment of fertility studies have been carried out with levalbuterol tartrate. However, racemic albuterol sulfate has been evaluated for its carcinogenic potential and ability to impair fertility.

In a 2-year study in Sprague-Dawley rats, racemic albuterol sulfate caused a significant dose-related increase in the incidence of benign leiomyomas of the mesovarium at, and above, dietary doses of 2 mg/kg/day (approximately 30 times the maximum recommended daily inhalation dose of levalbuterol tartrate for adults on a mg/m$^2$ basis and approximately 15 times the maximum recommended daily inhalation dose of levalbuterol tartrate for children on a mg/m$^2$ basis). In another study, this effect was blocked by the coadministration of propranolol, a non-selective beta-adrenergic antagonist. In an 18-month study in CD-1 mice, racemic albuterol sulfate showed no evidence of tumorigenicity at dietary doses up to 500 mg/kg/day (approximately 3800 times the maximum recommended daily inhalation dose of levalbuterol tartrate for adults on a mg/m$^2$ basis and approximately 1800 times the maximum recommended daily inhalation dose of levalbuterol tartrate for children on a mg/m$^2$ basis). In a 22-month study in the Golden hamster, racemic albuterol sulfate showed no evidence of tumorigenicity at dietary doses up to 50 mg/kg/day (approximately 500 times the maximum recommended daily inhalation dose of levalbuterol tartrate for adults on a mg/m$^2$ basis and approximately 240 times the maximum recommended daily inhalation dose of levalbuterol tartrate for children on a mg/m$^2$ basis).

Levalbuterol HCl was not mutagenic in the Ames test or the CHO/HPRT Mammalian Forward Gene Mutation Assay.

Levalbuterol HCl was not clastogenic in the in vivo micronucleus test in mouse bone marrow. Racemic albuterol sulfate was negative in an in vitro chromosomal aberration assay in CHO cell cultures.

Reproduction studies in rats using racemic albuterol sulfate demonstrated no evidence of impaired fertility at oral doses up to 50 mg/kg/day (approximately 750 times the maximum recommended daily inhalation dose of levalbuterol tartrate for adults on a mg/m$^2$ basis).

**Teratogenic Effects - Pregnancy Category C** A reproduction study in New Zealand White rabbits demonstrated that levalbuterol HCl was not teratogenic when administered orally at doses up to 25 mg/kg/day (approximately 750 times the maximum recommended daily inhalation dose of levalbuterol tartrate for adults on a mg/m$^2$ basis).

However, racemic albuterol sulfate has been shown to be teratogenic in mice and rabbits. A study in CD-1 mice given racemic albuterol sulfate subcutaneously showed cleft palate formation in 5 of 111 (4.5%) fetuses at 0.25 mg/kg/day (approximately 2 times the maximum recommended daily inhalation dose of levalbuterol tartrate for adults on a mg/m$^2$ basis) and in 10 of 108 (9.3%) fetuses at 2.5 mg/kg/day (approximately 20 times the maximum recommended daily inhalation dose of levalbuterol tartrate for adults on a mg/m$^2$ basis). The drug did not induce cleft palate formation when administered subcutaneously at a dose of 0.025 mg/kg/day (less than the maximum recommended daily inhalation dose of levalbuterol tartrate for adults on a mg/m$^2$ basis). Cleft palate also occurred in 22 of 72 (30.5%) fetuses from females treated subcutaneously with 2.5 mg/kg/day of isoproterenol (positive control).

A reproduction study in Stride Dutch rabbits revealed cranioschisis in 7 of 19 (37%) fetuses when racemic albuterol sulfate was administered orally at a dose of 50 mg/kg/day (approximately 1500 times the maximum recommended daily inhalation dose of levalbuterol tartrate for adults on a mg/m$^2$ basis).

A study in which pregnant rats were dosed with radiolabeled racemic albuterol sulfate demonstrated that drug-related material is transferred from the maternal circulation to the fetus.

There are no adequate and well-controlled studies of XOPENEX HFA Inhalation Aerosol in pregnant women. Because animal reproduction studies are not always predictive of human response, XOPENEX HFA Inhalation Aerosol should be used during pregnancy only if the potential benefit justifies the potential risk to the fetus.

During marketing experience of racemic albuterol, various congenital anomalies, including cleft palate and limb defects, have been rarely reported in the offspring of patients being treated with racemic albuterol. Some of the mothers were taking multiple medications during their pregnancies. No consistent pattern of defects can be discerned, and a relationship between racemic albuterol use and congenital anomalies has not been established.

**Use in Labor and Delivery** Because of the potential for beta-adrenergic agonists to interfere with uterine contractility, the use of XOPENEX HFA Inhalation Aerosol for the treatment of bronchospasm during labor should be restricted to those patients in whom the benefits clearly outweigh the risk.

**Tocolysis** XOPENEX HFA Inhalation Aerosol has not been approved for the management of preterm labor. The benefit:risk ratio when levalbuterol tartrate is administered for tocolysis has not been established. Serious adverse reactions, including maternal pulmonary edema, have been reported during or following treatment of premature labor with beta2-agonists, including racemic albuterol.

**Nursing Mothers** Plasma concentrations of levalbuterol after inhalation of therapeutic doses are very low in humans. It is not known whether levalbuterol is excreted in human milk.

Because of the potential for tumorigenicity shown for racemic albuterol in animal studies and the lack of experience with the use of XOPENEX HFA Inhalation Aerosol by nursing mothers, a decision should be made whether to discontinue nursing or to discontinue the drug, taking into account the importance of the drug to the mother. Caution should be exercised when XOPENEX HFA Inhalation Aerosol is administered to a nursing woman.

**Pediatrics** The safety and efficacy of XOPENEX HFA Inhalation Aerosol have been established in pediatric patients 4 years of age and older in an adequate and well-controlled clinical trial. Use of XOPENEX HFA Inhalation Aerosol in children is also supported by evidence from adequate and well-controlled studies of XOPENEX HFA Inhalation Aerosol in adults, considering that the pathophysiology, systemic exposure of the drug, and clinical profile in pediatric and adult patients are substantially similar. Safety and effectiveness of XOPENEX HFA Inhalation Aerosol in pediatric patients below the age of 4 years have not been established.

**Geriatrics** Clinical studies of XOPENEX HFA Inhalation Aerosol did not include sufficient numbers of subjects aged 65 and older to determine whether they respond differently from younger subjects. Other reported clinical experience has not identified differences in responses between the elderly and younger patients. In general, dose selection for an elderly patient should be cautious, usually starting at the low end of the dosing range, reflecting the greater frequency of decreased hepatic, renal, or cardiac function, and of concomitant diseases or other drug therapy.

Albuterol is known to be substantially excreted by the kidney, and the risk of toxic reactions may be greater in patients with impaired renal function. Because elderly patients are more likely to have decreased renal function, care should be taken in dose selection, and it may be useful to monitor renal function.

**ADVERSE REACTIONS** Adverse event information concerning XOPENEX HFA (levalbuterol tartrate) Inhalation Aerosol in adults and adolescents is derived from two 8-week, multicenter, randomized, double-blind, active- and placebo-controlled trials in 748 adult and adolescent patients with asthma that compared XOPENEX HFA Inhalation Aerosol, a marketed albuterol HFA inhaler, and an HFA-134a placebo inhaler. The following lists the incidence (% XOPENEX HFA 90 mcg, marketed albuterol HFA inhaler 180 mcg, placebo, respectively) of all adverse events (whether considered by the investigator to be related or unrelated to drug) from these trials that occurred at a rate of 2% or greater in the group treated with XOPENEX HFA Inhalation Aerosol and more frequently than in the HFA-134a placebo inhaler group. Body as a whole: pain (4.0%, 3.4%, 3.6%). Central nervous system: dizziness (2.7%, 0.6%, 1.8%). Respiratory system: asthma (9.4%, 7.3%, 6.0%), pharyngitis (7.9%, 2.2%, 2.4%), rhinitis (7.4%, 2.2%, 3.0%).

Adverse events reported by less than 2% and at least 2 or more of the adolescent and adult patients receiving XOPENEX HFA Inhalation Aerosol and by a greater proportion than receiving HFA-134a placebo inhaler include cyst, flu syndrome, viral infection, constipation, gastroenteritis, myalgia, hypertension, epistaxis, lung disorder, acne, herpes simplex, conjunctivitis, ear pain, dysmenorrhea, hematuria, and vaginal moniliasis. There were no significant laboratory abnormalities observed in these studies.

Adverse event information concerning XOPENEX HFA Inhalation Aerosol in children is derived from a 4-week, randomized, double-blind trial of XOPENEX HFA Inhalation Aerosol, a marketed albuterol HFA inhaler, and an HFA-134a placebo inhaler in 150 children aged 4 to 11 years with asthma. The following lists the adverse events (% XOPENEX HFA 90 mcg, marketed albuterol HFA inhaler 180 mcg, placebo, respectively) reported for XOPENEX HFA Inhalation Aerosol in children at a rate of 2% or greater and more frequently than for placebo. Body as a whole: accidental injury (9.2%, 10.3%, 5.7%). Digestive system: vomiting (10.5%, 7.7%, 5.7%). Respiratory system: bronchitis (2.6%, 0%, 0%), pharyngitis (6.6%, 12.8%, 5.7%).

The incidence of systemic beta-adrenergic adverse effects (e.g., tremor, nervousness) was low and comparable across all treatment groups, including placebo.

**Postmarketing** In addition to the adverse events reported in clinical trials, the following adverse events have been observed in postapproval use of levalbuterol inhalation solution. These events have been chosen for inclusion due to their seriousness, their frequency of reporting, or their likely beta-mediated mechanism: angioedema, anaphylaxis, arrhythmias (including atrial fibrillation, supraventricular tachycardia, extrasystoles), asthma, chest pain, cough increased, dyspnea, nausea, nervousness, rash, tachycardia, tremor, urticaria. Because these events have been reported spontaneously from a population of unknown size, estimates of frequency cannot be made.

In addition, XOPENEX HFA Inhalation Aerosol, like other sympathomimetic agents, can cause adverse reactions such as hypertension, angina, vertigo, central nervous system stimulation, sleeplessness, headache, and drying or irritation of the oropharynx.

Rx only.

SEPRACOR 12/05

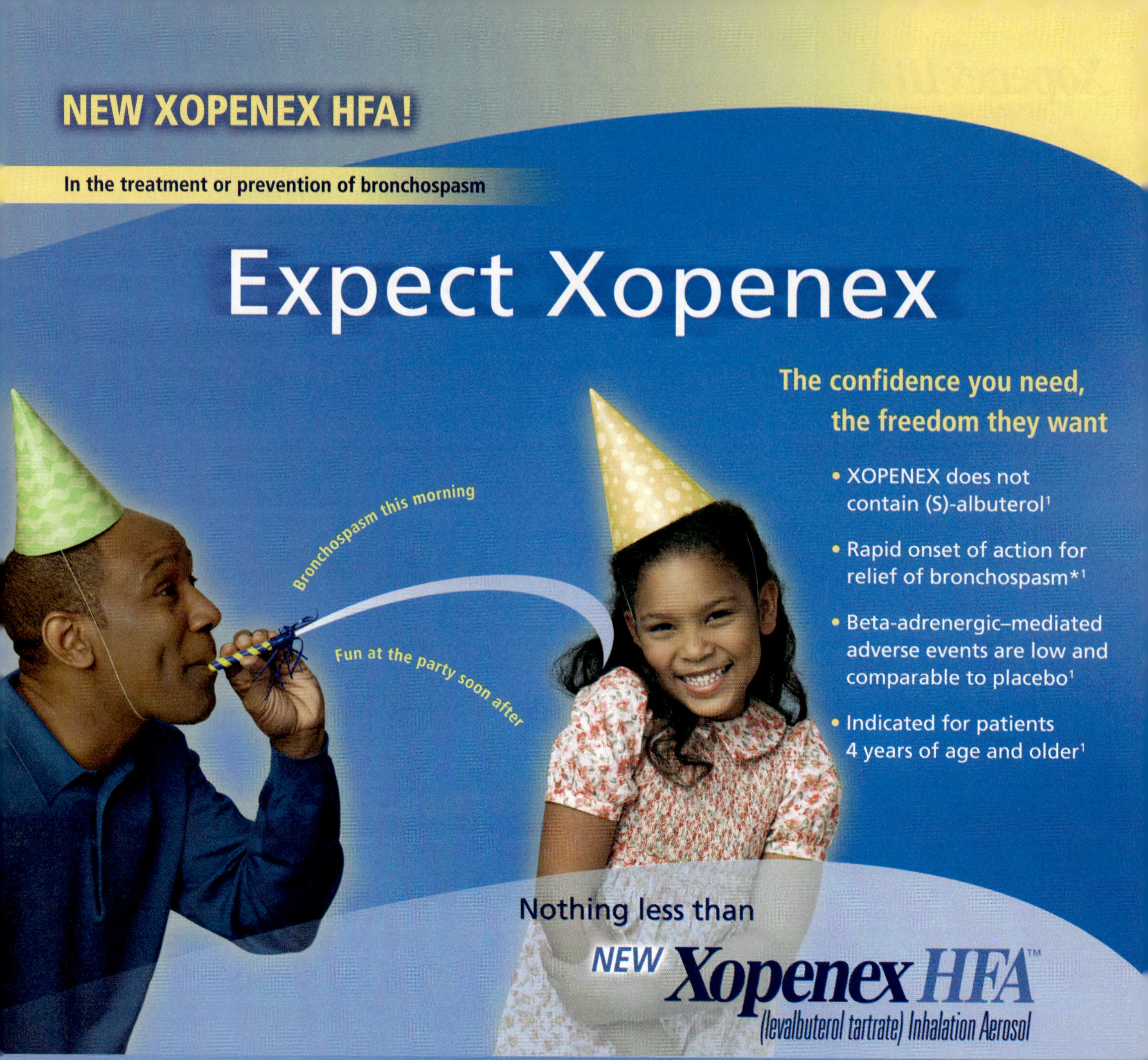


**Important Safety Information**

Xopenex HFA is contraindicated in patients with a history of hypersensitivity to levalbuterol, racemic albuterol, or any other component of Xopenex HFA. Xopenex HFA and other β-agonists can produce paradoxical bronchospasm, which may be life threatening. If additional adrenergic drugs, including other short-acting sympathomimetic bronchodilators or epinephrine, are to be administered by any route, they should be used with caution to avoid deleterious cardiovascular effects. Due to the cardiovascular side effects associated with β-agonists, caution is generally recommended for patients with cardiovascular disorders (especially coronary insufficiency, cardiac arrhythmias, and hypertension), diabetes, hyperthyroidism, or convulsive disorders. Do not exceed the recommended dose. Fatalities have been reported in association with excessive use of inhaled sympathomimetic drugs in patients with asthma. Please refer to the complete prescribing information for further information and in regard to potential drug interactions with β-blockers, diuretics, digoxin, or MAOI and tricyclic antidepressants.



**In patients aged 4 to 11 years,** the most common adverse events (occurring in greater than 2% of patients and more frequently than patients receiving placebo) were (90 mcg Xopenex HFA and placebo, respectively): accidental injury (9.2%; 5.7%), vomiting (10.5%; 5.7%), bronchitis (2.6%; 0%), and pharyngitis (6.6%; 5.7%).

**In patients aged 12 years and older,** the most common adverse events (occurring in greater than 2% of patients and more frequently than patients receiving placebo) were (90 mcg Xopenex HFA and placebo, respectively): pain (4.0%; 3.6%), dizziness (2.7%; 1.8%), asthma (9.4%; 6.0%), pharyngitis (7.9%; 2.4%), and rhinitis (7.4%; 3.0%).

Please see brief summary of prescribing information.

XOPENEX HFA (levalbuterol tartrate) Inhalation Aerosol is indicated for the treatment or prevention of bronchospasm in adults, adolescents, and children 4 years of age and older with reversible obstructive airway disease.

* The median onset time of a 15% increase in $FEV_1$ for XOPENEX HFA Inhalation Aerosol on Day 1 was 5.5 to 10.2 minutes for adult patients and 4.5 minutes for pediatric patients. Please refer to prescribing information.

**Reference:** 1. Xopenex HFA Prescribing Information.

# ARCHIVES OF PEDIATRICS & ADOLESCENT MEDICINE

MARCH 2006 VOLUME 160, NUMBER 3 PAGES 225-328



## ARTICLES

**Randomized Placebo-Controlled Trial of Metformin for Adolescents With Polycystic Ovary Syndrome** 241
*Tracey Bridger, MD, FRCPC; Suzanne MacDonald, MD, FRCPC; Franziska Baltzer, MD, FRCPC; Celia Rodd, MD, FRCPC*

**Risk of Active Tuberculosis Among Schoolchildren in Hong Kong** 247
*Chi Chiu Leung, MB; Wing Wai Yew, MB; Kwok Chiu Chang, MSc; Cheuk Ming Tam, MSc; Chi Kuen Chan, MSc; Wing Sze Law, MSc; Man Yee Wong, MPH; Shuk Nor Lee, MB; Maria Leung, MSc*

**Health-Related Quality of Life During the First Year After Traumatic Brain Injury** 252
*Melissa L. McCarthy, ScD; Ellen J. MacKenzie, PhD; Dennis R. Durbin, MD, MS; Mary E. Aitken, MD, MPH; Kenneth M. Jaffe, MD; Charles N. Paidas, MD; Beth S. Slomine, PhD; Andrea M. Dorsch, PhD; James R. Christensen, MD; Ru Ding, MS; for the Children's Health After Trauma Study Group*

**Estimated Cost-effectiveness of Growth Hormone Therapy for Idiopathic Short Stature** 263
*Joyce M. Lee, MD; Matthew M. Davis, MD, MAPP; Sarah J. Clark, MPH; Timothy P. Hofer, MD; Alex R. Kemper, MD, MPH, MS*

**Depressive Symptomatology as a Predictor of Exposure to Intimate Partner Violence Among US Female Adolescents and Young Adults** 270
*Jocelyn A. Lehrer, ScD; Stephen Buka, ScD; Steven Gortmaker, PhD; Lydia A. Shrier, MD, MPH*

**Maternal Depressive Symptoms at 2 to 4 Months Post Partum and Early Parenting Practices** 279
*Kathryn Taaffe McLearn, PhD; Cynthia S. Minkovitz, MD, MPP; Donna M. Strobino, PhD; Elisabeth Marks, MPH; William Hou, MS*

**Association of Depression and Anxiety Disorders With Weight Change in a Prospective Community-Based Study of Children Followed Up Into Adulthood** 285
*Sarah E. Anderson, MS; Patricia Cohen, PhD; Elena N. Naumova, PhD; Aviva Must, PhD*

**Development of Pediatric Comorbidity Prediction Model** 293
*Derek Tai, MSc; Paul Dick, MD, MSc; Teresa To, PhD; James G. Wright, MD, MPH*

## SPECIAL FEATURE

**Picture of the Month** 300
*Melanie Pitone, MD; Benjamin Alouf, MD*

## ARTICLES

**Impact of Specific Medical Interventions on Reducing the Prevalence of Mental Retardation** 302
*Jeffrey P. Brosco, MD, PhD; Michael Mattingly, BS; Lee M. Sanders, MD, MPH*

**Screening for Intimate Partner Violence Using an Audiotape Questionnaire: A Randomized Clinical Trial in a Pediatric Emergency Department** 311
*Megan H. Bair-Merritt, MD; Chris Feudtner, MD, PhD, MPH; Cynthia J. Mollen, MD, MSCE; Sarah Winters, MD; Mercedes Blackstone, MD; Joel A. Fein, MD, MPH*

## EDITORIALS

**Commentary on the Risk of Active Tuberculosis** 317
*John A. Jereb, MD; Lisa J. Nelson, MD, MPH; Kenneth G. Castro, MD*

**The Fog of War and the Declining Prevalence of Mental Retardation** 318
*Walton O. Schalick III, MD, PhD*

## THE PEDIATRIC FORUM

**Parent and Youth Assessments of a Handheld Wireless Device to Enhance Diabetes Mellitus Management** 321
*David A. Hanauer, MD; Katherine Wentzell, BA; Allison Tovar, BS; Jessica Zeuhlke, BS; Vikram Kumar, MD; Lori M. B. Laffel, MD, MPH*

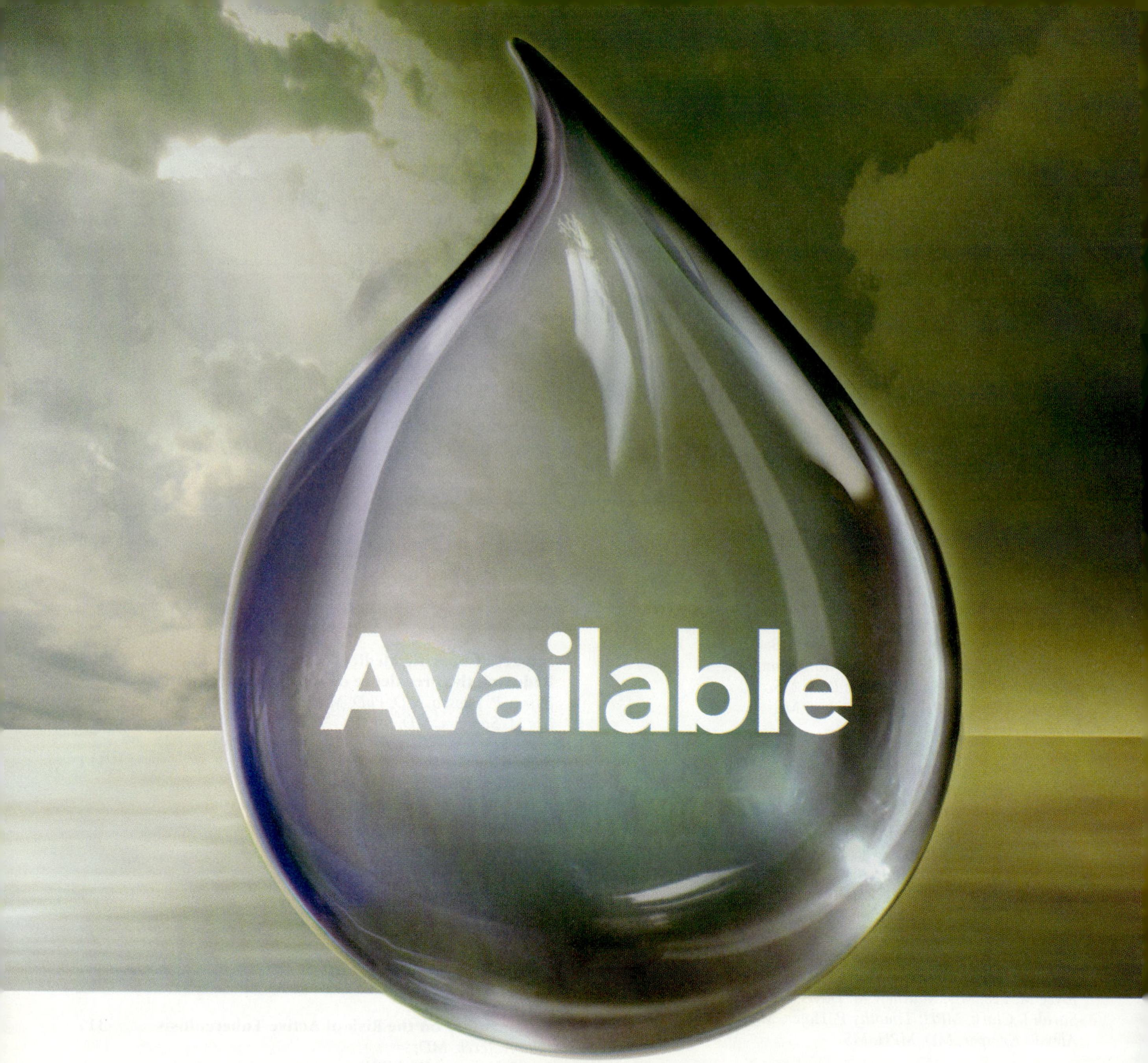
Available

ARCHIVES OF PEDIATRICS & ADOLESCENT MEDICINE

**Perfect Condom Use in a Less Than Perfect World** 321
*Mary B. Adam, MD, MA*

**In Reply** 322
*Gabriela Paz-Bailey, MD, MSc; Emilia Koumans, MD, MPH; Lauri E. Markowitz, MD*

**Increased Exclusive Breastfeeding Rates Fall Short of Proposed Healthy People 2010 Goals** 323
*Karen A. Bonuck, PhD*

**In Reply** 323
*Alex K. Anderson, PhD, MPH; Rafael Pérez-Escamilla, PhD; Donna J. Chapman, PhD, RD*

## BOOK REVIEWS AND OTHER MEDIA

**Child Abuse and Culture: Working With Diverse Families** 325
*Kristine A. Campbell, MD*

## CORRECTION

**Incorrect Author Byline and Corresponding Author Address in: Do As I Say, Not As I Do: Does It Work for Tobacco Use Prevention?** 269
*[Susan J. Curry, PhD; Robin J. Mermelstein, PhD]*

## REGULAR DEPARTMENTS

**This Month in *Archives of Pediatrics & Adolescent Medicine*** 239

**Poetry in Pediatrics** 240

**Announcements** 246, 291, 299, 324

**Classified Advertising** 327

**Journal Advertiser Index** 327

**Contact Information** 328

**Instructions for authors and the author and subject indexes are available on our Web site: http://www.archpediatrics.com. If you do not have access to the Web, contact Suzanne Shuey at (206) 685-3573.**

### About the Cover

Photographer: Kristen Imig, Seattle, Wash. Friends at Kamakya Temple, Guwahati, Assam, India, April 2000.

# ARCHIVES OF PEDIATRICS & ADOLESCENT MEDICINE

**Mission Statement:** *The Archives of Pediatrics & Adolescent Medicine* is a monthly, peer-reviewed journal for physicians and other health care professionals who contribute to the health of children and adolescents. The *Archives* provides an open forum for dialogue on a full range of clinical, scientific, advocacy, and humanistic issues relevant to the care of pediatric patients from infancy through young adulthood. The *Archives* is a vehicle for increased attention to adolescent health, the education of pediatric health care professionals, and disease prevention and health promotion. The *Archives* publishes original studies, editorials, reviews by experts, practice commentaries, case quizzes, and updates on clinical science and practice management. The Pediatric Forum provides our readers with opportunities to express their views. *Archives* incorporates *AJDC*, the oldest journal in US pediatric literature, which originated in 1911.



JAMA & ARCHIVES JOURNALS
American Medical Association

All articles published, including editorials, letters, and book reviews, represent the opinions of the authors and do not reflect the policy of the American Medical Association, the Editorial Board, or the institution with which the author is affiliated, unless this is clearly specified.

# OMNICEF (cefdinir) for Oral Suspension 250 mg/5 mL

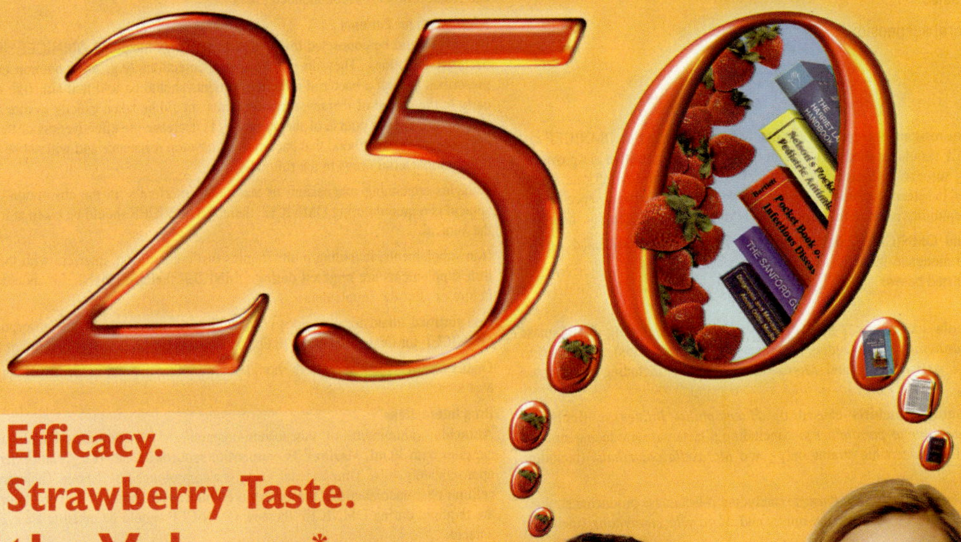


**Great Efficacy.**
**Great Strawberry Taste.**
**Half the Volume.***

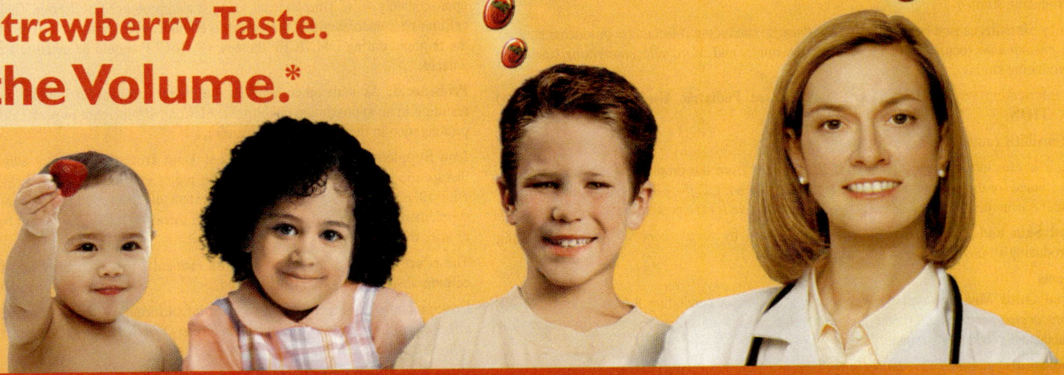

## Great Minds... Concentrate on Success!

### Indications (mild to moderate infections)[1]

**Acute Bacterial Otitis Media** and **Acute Maxillary Sinusitis** (adults and adolescents) due to *H influenzae* (including ß-lactamase producing strains), *S pneumoniae* (penicillin-susceptible strains only), and *M catarrhalis* (including ß-lactamase producing strains). Use of cefdinir in the treatment of acute maxillary sinusitis in pediatric patients is supported by evidence from adequate and well-controlled studies in adults and adolescents.

**Pharyngitis/Tonsillitis** due to *S pyogenes*. Cefdinir is effective in the eradication of *S pyogenes* from the oropharynx. Cefdinir has not, however, been studied for the prevention of rheumatic fever following *S pyogenes* pharyngitis/tonsillitis. Only intramuscular penicillin has been demonstrated to be effective for the prevention of rheumatic fever.

**Uncomplicated Skin and Skin Structure Infections** due to *S aureus* (including ß-lactamase producing strains) and *S pyogenes*.

### Important Safety Information[1]

- To reduce the development of drug-resistant bacteria and maintain the effectiveness of OMNICEF and other antibacterial drugs, OMNICEF should be used only to treat or prevent infections that are proven or strongly suspected to be caused by bacteria

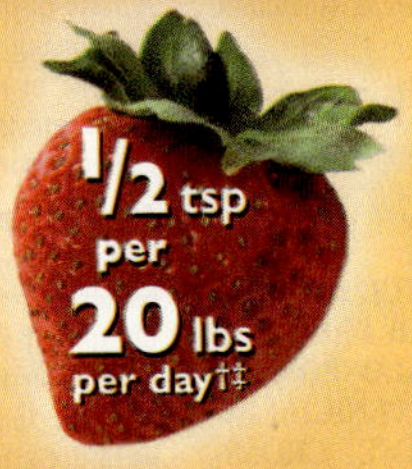


For pediatric patients weighing 20 lbs, use the 125 mg/5 mL product

- OMNICEF is contraindicated in patients with known allergy to the cephalosporin class of antibiotics
- For patients with previous hypersensitivity reaction to penicillins, caution should be exercised because cross-hypersensitivity among ß-lactam antibiotics has been clearly documented. If an allergic reaction to cefdinir occurs, the drug should be discontinued
- Safety and efficacy in neonates and infants less than 6 months of age have not been established
- 2% of 2,289 pediatric patients discontinued medication due to adverse events in US and ex-US clinical trials. Discontinuations were primarily for gastrointestinal disturbance, usually diarrhea
- The most common reported adverse events occurring in ≥1% of pediatric patients in US clinical trials (N=1,783) were diarrhea (8%), rash (3%), and vomiting (1%)
- Maximum dose of OMNICEF for pediatric patients weighing ≥43 kg is 600 mg/day. For pediatric patients with a creatinine clearance of <30 mL/min/1.73 m² and not requiring hemodialysis, the dose of cefdinir should be 7 mg/kg (up to 300 mg) given once daily
- Antacids that contain magnesium or aluminum and iron supplements, including multivitamins that contain iron, should be taken at least 2 hours before or 2 hours after taking OMNICEF

**OMNICEF**
(cefdinir) for oral suspension
*125 mg/5 mL and 250 mg/5 mL*
**Expert recommended.**
**Kid preferred.**

* Compared to the 125 mg/5 mL formulation of OMNICEF.
† Calculated dose is based on 14 mg/kg/day. Dose in teaspoons is rounded to the nearest 1/4 teaspoon and is not an exact measure of calculated dose volume (mL). 1 tsp ≅ 5 mL.
‡ Once-daily dosing has not been studied in skin infections; therefore, OMNICEF for Oral Suspension should be administered twice daily in this infection (7 mg/kg BID for 10 days).

**Reference: 1.** OMNICEF® (cefdinir) for Oral Suspension Prescribing Information, Abbott Laboratories.

Please see adjacent brief summary of full prescribing information.



astellas Under License of Astellas Pharma Inc. Japan

Abbott A Promise for Life

**PROFESSIONAL BRIEF SUMMARY-CONSULT PACKAGE INSERT FOR FULL PRESCRIBING INFORMATION.**
03-5435-Rev. July, 2005
(Nos. 3769, 3771, 6151)

# Omnicef® (cefdinir) capsules
# Omnicef® (cefdinir) for oral suspension

## Rx only

## INDICATIONS AND USAGE

To reduce the development of drug-resistant bacteria and maintain the effectiveness of OMNICEF and other antibacterial drugs, OMNICEF should be used only to treat or prevent infections that are proven or strongly suspected to be caused by susceptible bacteria. When culture and susceptibility information are available, they should be considered in selecting or modifying antibacterial therapy. In the absence of such data, local epidemiology and susceptibility patterns may contribute to the empiric selection of therapy.

OMNICEF (cefdinir) capsules and OMNICEF (cefdinir) for oral suspension are indicated for the treatment of patients with mild to moderate infections caused by susceptible strains of the designated microorganisms in the conditions listed below.

### Adults and Adolescents

**Community-Acquired Pneumonia** caused by *Haemophilus influenzae* (including β-lactamase producing strains), *Haemophilus parainfluenzae* (including β-lactamase producing strains), *Streptococcus pneumoniae* (penicillin-susceptible strains only), and *Moraxella catarrhalis* (including β-lactamase producing strains).

**Acute Exacerbations of Chronic Bronchitis** caused by *Haemophilus influenzae* (including β-lactamase producing strains), *Haemophilus parainfluenzae* (including β-lactamase producing strains), *Streptococcus pneumoniae* (penicillin-susceptible strains only), and *Moraxella catarrhalis* (including β-lactamase producing strains).

**Acute Maxillary Sinusitis** caused by *Haemophilus influenzae* (including β-lactamase producing strains), *Streptococcus pneumoniae* (penicillin-susceptible strains only), and *Moraxella catarrhalis* (including β-lactamase producing strains).

**NOTE:** For information on use in pediatric patients, see **Pediatric Use** and **DOSAGE AND ADMINISTRATION**.

**Pharyngitis/Tonsillitis** caused by *Streptococcus pyogenes.*

**NOTE:** Cefdinir is effective in the eradication of *S. pyogenes* from the oropharynx. Cefdinir has not, however, been studied for the prevention of rheumatic fever following *S. pyogenes* pharyngitis/tonsillitis. Only intramuscular penicillin has been demonstrated to be effective for the prevention of rheumatic fever.

**Uncomplicated Skin and Skin Structure Infections** caused by *Staphylococcus aureus* (including β-lactamase producing strains) and *Streptococcus pyogenes.*

### Pediatric Patients

**Acute Bacterial Otitis Media** caused by *Haemophilus influenzae* (including β-lactamase producing strains), *Streptococcus pneumoniae* (penicillin-susceptible strains only), and *Moraxella catarrhalis* (including β-lactamase producing strains).

**Pharyngitis/Tonsillitis** caused by *Streptococcus pyogenes.*

**NOTE:** Cefdinir is effective in the eradication of *S. pyogenes* from the oropharynx. Cefdinir has not, however, been studied for the prevention of rheumatic fever following *S. pyogenes* pharyngitis/tonsillitis. Only intramuscular penicillin has been demonstrated to be effective for the prevention of rheumatic fever.

**Uncomplicated Skin and Skin Structure Infections** caused by *Staphylococcus aureus* (including β-lactamase producing strains) and *Streptococcus pyogenes.*

## CONTRAINDICATIONS

OMNICEF (cefdinir) is contraindicated in patients with known allergy to the cephalosporin class of antibiotics.

## WARNINGS

**BEFORE THERAPY WITH OMNICEF (CEFDINIR) IS INSTITUTED, CAREFUL INQUIRY SHOULD BE MADE TO DETERMINE WHETHER THE PATIENT HAS HAD PREVIOUS HYPERSENSITIVITY REACTIONS TO CEFDINIR, OTHER CEPHALOSPORINS, PENICILLINS, OR OTHER DRUGS. IF CEFDINIR IS TO BE GIVEN TO PENICILLIN-SENSITIVE PATIENTS, CAUTION SHOULD BE EXERCISED BECAUSE CROSS-HYPERSENSITIVITY AMONG β-LACTAM ANTIBIOTICS HAS BEEN CLEARLY DOCUMENTED AND MAY OCCUR IN UP TO 10% OF PATIENTS WITH A HISTORY OF PENICILLIN ALLERGY. IF AN ALLERGIC REACTION TO CEFDINIR OCCURS, THE DRUG SHOULD BE DISCONTINUED. SERIOUS ACUTE HYPERSENSITIVITY REACTIONS MAY REQUIRE TREATMENT WITH EPINEPHRINE AND OTHER EMERGENCY MEASURES, INCLUDING OXYGEN, INTRAVENOUS FLUIDS, INTRAVENOUS ANTIHISTAMINES, CORTICOSTEROIDS, PRESSOR AMINES, AND AIRWAY MANAGEMENT, AS CLINICALLY INDICATED.**

**Pseudomembranous colitis has been reported with nearly all antibacterial agents, including cefdinir, and may range in severity from mild- to life-threatening. Therefore, it is important to consider this diagnosis in patients who present with diarrhea subsequent to the administration of antibacterial agents.**

Treatment with antibacterial agents alters the normal flora of the colon and may permit overgrowth of clostridia. Studies indicate that a toxin produced by *Clostridium difficile* is a primary cause of "antibiotic-associated colitis."

After the diagnosis of pseudomembranous colitis has been established, appropriate therapeutic measures should be initiated. Mild cases of pseudomembranous colitis usually respond to drug discontinuation alone. In moderate to severe cases, consideration should be given to management with fluids and electrolytes, protein supplementation, and treatment with an antibacterial drug clinically effective against *Clostridium difficile*.

## PRECAUTIONS

### General

Prescribing OMNICEF in the absence of a proven or strongly suspected bacterial infection or a prophylactic indication is unlikely to provide benefit to the patient and increases the risk of the development of drug-resistant bacteria.

As with other broad-spectrum antibiotics, prolonged treatment may result in the possible emergence and overgrowth of resistant organisms. Careful observation of the patient is essential. If superinfection occurs during therapy, appropriate alternative therapy should be administered.

Cefdinir, as with other broad-spectrum antimicrobials (antibiotics), should be prescribed with caution in individuals with a history of colitis.

In patients with transient or persistent renal insufficiency (creatinine clearance <30 mL/min), the total daily dose of OMNICEF should be reduced because high and prolonged plasma concentrations of cefdinir can result following recommended doses.

### Information for Patients

Patients should be counseled that antibacterial drugs including OMNICEF should only be used to treat bacterial infections. They do not treat viral infections (e.g., the common cold). When OMNICEF is prescribed to treat a bacterial infection, patients should be told that although it is common to feel better early in the course of therapy, the medication should be taken exactly as directed. Skipping doses or not completing the full course of therapy may (1) decrease the effectiveness of the immediate treatment and (2) increase the likelihood that bacteria will develop resistance and will not be treatable by OMNICEF or other antibacterial drugs in the future.

Antacids containing magnesium or aluminum interfere with the absorption of cefdinir. If this type of antacid is required during OMNICEF therapy, OMNICEF should be taken at least 2 hours before or after the antacid.

Iron supplements, including multivitamins that contain iron, interfere with the absorption of cefdinir. If iron supplements are required during OMNICEF therapy, OMNICEF should be taken at least 2 hours before or after the supplement.

Iron-fortified infant formula does not significantly interfere with the absorption of cefdinir. Therefore, OMNICEF for Oral Suspension can be administered with iron-fortified infant formula.

Diabetic patients and caregivers should be aware that the oral suspension contains 2.86 g of sucrose per teaspoon.

### Drug Interactions

**Antacids:** (aluminum- or magnesium-containing): Concomitant administration of 300-mg cefdinir capsules with 30 mL Maalox® TC suspension reduces the rate ($C_{max}$) and extent (AUC) of absorption by approximately 40%. Time to reach $C_{max}$ is also prolonged by 1 hour. There are no significant effects on cefdinir pharmacokinetics if the antacid is administered 2 hours before or 2 hours after cefdinir. If antacids are required during OMNICEF therapy, OMNICEF should be taken at least 2 hours before or after the antacid.

**Probenecid:** As with other β-lactam antibiotics, probenecid inhibits the renal excretion of cefdinir, resulting in an approximate doubling in AUC, a 54% increase in peak cefdinir plasma levels, and a 50% prolongation in the apparent elimination $t_{1/2}$.

**Iron Supplements and Foods Fortified With Iron:** Concomitant administration of cefdinir with a therapeutic iron supplement containing 60 mg of elemental iron (as $FeSO_4$) or vitamins supplemented with 10 mg of elemental iron reduced extent of absorption by 80% and 31%, respectively. If iron supplements are required during OMNICEF therapy, OMNICEF should be taken at least 2 hours before or after the supplement.

The effect of foods highly fortified with elemental iron (primarily iron-fortified breakfast cereals) on cefdinir absorption has not been studied.

Concomitantly administered iron-fortified infant formula (2.2 mg elemental iron/6 oz) has no significant effect on cefdinir pharmacokinetics. Therefore, OMNICEF for Oral Suspension can be administered with iron-fortified infant formula.

There have been reports of reddish stools in patients receiving cefdinir. In many cases, patients were also receiving iron-containing products. The reddish color is due to the formation of a nonabsorbable complex between cefdinir or its breakdown products and iron in the gastrointestinal tract.

### Drug/Laboratory Test Interactions

A false-positive reaction for ketones in the urine may occur with tests using nitroprusside, but not with those using nitroferricyanide. The administration of cefdinir may result in a false-positive reaction for glucose in urine using Clinitest®, Benedict's solution, or Fehling's solution. It is recommended that glucose tests based on enzymatic glucose oxidase reactions (such as Clinistix® or Tes-Tape®) be used. Cephalosporins are known to occasionally induce a positive direct Coombs' test.

### Carcinogenesis, Mutagenesis, Impairment of Fertility

The carcinogenic potential of cefdinir has not been evaluated. No mutagenic effects were seen in the bacterial reverse mutation assay (Ames) or point mutation assay at the hypoxanthine-guanine phosphoribosyltransferase locus (HGPRT) in V79 Chinese hamster lung cells. No clastogenic effects were observed *in vitro* in the structural chromosome aberration assay in V79 Chinese hamster lung cells or *in vivo* in the micronucleus assay in mouse bone marrow. In rats, fertility and reproductive performance were not affected by cefdinir at oral doses up to 1000 mg/kg/day (70 times the human dose based on mg/kg/day, 11 times based on $mg/m^2$/day).

### Pregnancy - Teratogenic Effects

**Pregnancy Category B:** Cefdinir was not teratogenic in rats at oral doses up to 1000 mg/kg/day (70 times the human dose based on mg/kg/day, 11 times based on $mg/m^2$/day) or in rabbits at oral doses up to 10 mg/kg/day (0.7 times the human dose based on mg/kg/day, 0.23 times based on $mg/m^2$/day). Maternal toxicity (decreased body weight gain) was observed in rabbits at the maximum tolerated dose of 10 mg/kg/day without adverse effects on offspring. Decreased body weight occurred in rat fetuses at ≥ 100 mg/kg/day, and in rat offspring at ≥ 32 mg/kg/day. No effects were observed on maternal reproductive parameters or offspring survival, development, behavior, or reproductive function.

There are, however, no adequate and well-controlled studies in pregnant women. Because animal reproduction studies are not always predictive of human response, this drug should be used during pregnancy only if clearly needed.

### Labor and Delivery

Cefdinir has not been studied for use during labor and delivery.

### Nursing Mothers

Following administration of single 600-mg doses, cefdinir was not detected in human breast milk.

### Pediatric Use

Safety and efficacy in neonates and infants less than 6 months of age have not been established. Use of cefdinir for the treatment of acute maxillary sinusitis in pediatric patients (age 6 months through 12 years) is supported by evidence from adequate and well-controlled studies in adults and adolescents, the similar pathophysiology of acute sinusitis in adult and pediatric patients, and comparative pharmacokinetic data in the pediatric population.

### Geriatric Use

Efficacy is comparable in geriatric patients and younger adults. While cefdinir has been well-tolerated in all age groups, in clinical trials geriatric patients experienced a lower rate of adverse events, including diarrhea, than younger adults. Dose adjustment in elderly patients is not necessary unless renal function is markedly compromised.

## ADVERSE EVENTS

**Clinical Trials - OMNICEF Capsules (Adult and Adolescent Patients):**

In clinical trials, 5093 adult and adolescent patients (3841 US and 1252 non-US) were treated with the recommended dose of cefdinir capsules (600 mg/day). Most adverse events were mild and self-limiting. No deaths or permanent disabilities were attributed to cefdinir. One hundred forty-seven of 5093 (3%) patients discontinued medication due to adverse events thought by the investigators to be possibly, probably, or definitely associated with cefdinir therapy. The discontinuations were primarily for gastrointestinal disturbances, usually diarrhea or nausea. Nineteen of 5093 (0.4%) patients were discontinued due to rash thought related to cefdinir administration.

In the US, the following adverse events were thought by investigators to be possibly, probably, or definitely related to cefdinir capsules in multiple-dose clinical trials (N = 3841 cefdinir-treated patients):

**ADVERSE EVENTS ASSOCIATED WITH CEFDINIR CAPSULES US TRIALS IN ADULT AND ADOLESCENT PATIENTS (N=3841)[a]**

| | | |
|---|---|---|
| Incidence ≥ 1% | Diarrhea | 15% |
| | Vaginal moniliasis | 4% of women |
| | Nausea | 3% |
| | Headache | 2% |
| | Abdominal pain | 1% |
| | Vaginitis | 1% of women |
| Incidence <1% but >0.1% | Rash | 0.9% |
| | Dyspepsia | 0.7% |
| | Flatulence | 0.7% |
| | Vomiting | 0.7% |
| | Abnormal stools | 0.3% |
| | Anorexia | 0.3% |
| | Constipation | 0.3% |
| | Dizziness | 0.3% |
| | Dry mouth | 0.3% |
| | Asthenia | 0.2% |
| | Insomnia | 0.2% |
| | Leukorrhea | 0.2% of women |
| | Moniliasis | 0.2% |
| | Pruritus | 0.2% |
| | Somnolence | 0.2% |

[a] 1733 males, 2108 females

The following laboratory value changes of possible clinical significance, irrespective of relationship to therapy with cefdinir, were seen during clinical trials conducted in the US:

**LABORATORY VALUE CHANGES OBSERVED WITH CEFDINIR CAPSULES US TRIALS IN ADULT AND ADOLESCENT PATIENTS (N=3841)**

| | | |
|---|---|---|
| Incidence ≥ 1% | ↑ Urine leukocytes | 2% |
| | ↑ Urine protein | 2% |
| | ↑ Gamma-glutamyltransferase[a] | 1% |
| | ↓ Lymphocytes, ↑ Lymphocytes | 1%, 0.2% |
| | ↑ Microhematuria | 1% |
| Incidence <1% but >0.1% | ↑ Glucose[a] | 0.9% |
| | ↑ Urine glucose | 0.9% |
| | ↑ White blood cells, ↓ White blood cells | 0.9%, 0.7% |
| | ↑ Alanine aminotransferase (ALT) | 0.7% |
| | ↑ Eosinophils | 0.7% |
| | ↑ Urine specific gravity, ↓ Urine specific gravity[a] | 0.6%, 0.2% |
| | ↓ Bicarbonate[a] | 0.6% |
| | ↑ Phosphorus, ↓ Phosphorus[a] | 0.6%, 0.3% |
| | ↑ Aspartate aminotransferase (AST) | 0.4% |
| | ↑ Alkaline phosphatase | 0.3% |
| | ↑ Blood urea nitrogen (BUN) | 0.3% |
| | ↓ Hemoglobin | 0.3% |
| | ↑ Polymorphonuclear neutrophils (PMNs), ↓ PMNs | 0.3%, 0.2% |
| | ↑ Bilirubin | 0.2% |
| | ↑ Lactate dehydrogenase[a] | 0.2% |
| | ↑ Platelets | 0.2% |
| | ↑ Potassium[a] | 0.2% |
| | ↑ Urine pH[a] | 0.2% |

[a] N<3841 for these parameters

**Clinical Trials - OMNICEF for Oral Suspension (Pediatric Patients):**

In clinical trials, 2289 pediatric patients (1783 US and 506 non-US) were treated with the recommended dose of cefdinir suspension (14 mg/kg/day). Most adverse events were mild and self-limiting. No deaths or permanent disabilities were attributed to cefdinir. Forty of 2289 (2%) patients discontinued medication due to adverse events considered by the investigators to be possibly, probably, or definitely associated with cefdinir therapy. Discontinuations were primarily for gastrointestinal disturbances, usually diarrhea. Five of 2289 (0.2%) patients were discontinued due to rash thought related to cefdinir administration.

In the US, the following adverse events were thought by investigators to be possibly, probably, or definitely related to cefdinir suspension in multiple-dose clinical trials (N=1783 cefdinir-treated patients):

**ADVERSE EVENTS ASSOCIATED WITH CEFDINIR SUSPENSION US TRIALS IN PEDIATRIC PATIENTS (N=1783)[a]**

| | | |
|---|---|---|
| Incidence ≥ 1% | Diarrhea | 8% |
| | Rash | 3% |
| | Vomiting | 1% |
| Incidence <1% but >0.1% | Cutaneous moniliasis | 0.9% |
| | Abdominal pain | 0.8% |
| | Leukopenia[b] | 0.3% |
| | Vaginal moniliasis | 0.3% of girls |
| | Vaginitis | 0.3% of girls |
| | Abnormal stools | 0.2% |
| | Dyspepsia | 0.2% |
| | Hyperkinesia | 0.2% |
| | Increased AST[b] | 0.2% |
| | Maculopapular rash | 0.2% |
| | Nausea | 0.2% |

[a] 977 males, 806 females

[b] Laboratory changes were occasionally reported as adverse events.

NOTE: In both cefdinir- and control-treated patients, rates of diarrhea and rash were higher in the youngest pediatric patients. The incidence of diarrhea in cefdinir-treated patients ≤2 years of age was 17% (95/557) compared with 4% (51/1226) in those >2 years old. The incidence of rash (primarily diaper rash in the younger patients) was 8% (43/557) in patients ≤2 years of age compared with 1% (8/1226) in those >2 years old.

The following laboratory value changes of possible clinical significance, irrespective of relationship to therapy with cefdinir, were seen during clinical trials conducted in the US:

**LABORATORY VALUE CHANGES OF POSSIBLE CLINICAL SIGNIFICANCE OBSERVED WITH CEFDINIR SUSPENSION US TRIALS IN PEDIATRIC PATIENTS (N=1783)**

| | | |
|---|---|---|
| Incidence ≥ 1% | ↑ Lymphocytes, ↓ Lymphocytes | 2%, 0.8% |
| | ↑ Alkaline phosphatase | 1% |
| | ↓ Bicarbonate[a] | 1% |
| | ↑ Eosinophils | 1% |
| | ↑ Lactate dehydrogenase | 1% |
| | ↑ Platelets | 1% |
| | ↑ PMNs, ↓ PMNs | 1%, 1% |
| | ↑ Urine protein | 1% |
| Incidence <1% but >0.1% | ↑ Phosphorus, ↓ Phosphorus | 0.9%, 0.4% |
| | ↑ Urine pH | 0.8% |
| | ↓ White blood cells, ↑ White blood cells | 0.7%, 0.3% |
| | ↓ Calcium[a] | 0.5% |
| | ↓ Hemoglobin | 0.5% |
| | ↑ Urine leukocytes | 0.5% |
| | ↑ Monocytes | 0.4% |
| | ↑ AST | 0.3% |
| | ↑ Potassium[a] | 0.3% |
| | ↑ Urine specific gravity, ↓ Urine specific gravity | 0.3%, 0.1% |
| | ↓ Hematocrit[a] | 0.2% |

[a] N=1387 for these parameters

**Postmarketing Experience**

The following adverse experiences and altered laboratory tests, regardless of their relationship to cefdinir, have been reported during extensive postmarketing experience, beginning with approval in Japan in 1991: Stevens-Johnson syndrome, toxic epidermal necrolysis, exfoliative dermatitis, erythema multiforme, erythema nodosum, serum sickness-like reactions, conjunctivitis, stomatitis, acute hepatitis, cholestasis, fulminant hepatitis, hepatic failure, jaundice, increased amylase, shock, anaphylaxis, facial and laryngeal edema, feeling of suffocation, acute enterocolitis, bloody diarrhea, hemorrhagic colitis, melena, pseudomembranous colitis, pancytopenia, granulocytopenia, leukopenia, thrombocytopenia, idiopathic thrombocytopenic purpura, hemolytic anemia, acute respiratory failure, asthmatic attack, drug-induced pneumonia, eosinophilic pneumonia, idiopathic interstitial pneumonia, fever, acute renal failure, nephropathy, bleeding tendency, coagulation disorder, disseminated intravascular coagulation, upper GI bleed, peptic ulcer, ileus, loss of consciousness, allergic vasculitis, possible cefdinir-diclofenac interaction, cardiac failure, chest pain, myocardial infarction, hypertension, involuntary movements, and rhabdomyolysis.

**Cephalosporin Class Adverse Events**

The following adverse events and altered laboratory tests have been reported for cephalosporin-class antibiotics in general:

Allergic reactions, anaphylaxis, Stevens-Johnson syndrome, erythema multiforme, toxic epidermal necrolysis, renal dysfunction, toxic nephropathy, hepatic dysfunction including cholestasis, aplastic anemia, hemolytic anemia, hemorrhage, false-positive test for urinary glucose, neutropenia, pancytopenia, and agranulocytosis. Pseudomembranous colitis symptoms may begin during or after antibiotic treatment (see **WARNINGS**).

Several cephalosporins have been implicated in triggering seizures, particularly in patients with renal impairment when the dosage was not reduced (see **OVERDOSAGE**). If seizures associated with drug therapy occur, the drug should be discontinued. Anticonvulsant therapy can be given if clinically indicated.

## OVERDOSAGE

Information on cefdinir overdosage in humans is not available. In acute rodent toxicity studies, a single oral 5600-mg/kg dose produced no adverse effects. Toxic signs and symptoms following overdosage with other β-lactam antibiotics have included nausea, vomiting, epigastric distress, diarrhea, and convulsions. Hemodialysis removes cefdinir from the body. This may be useful in the event of a serious toxic reaction from overdosage, particularly if renal function is compromised.

**Rx only**

Ref: 03-5435-Rev. July, 2005
(Nos. 3769, 3771, 6151)

TM – Trademark



05J-034-L150-2 **MASTER**

Manufactured by:
**CEPH** International Corporation
Carolina, Puerto Rico 00986

Under License of:
astellas Astellas Pharma Inc.
Tokyo, Japan

For:
**Abbott Laboratories**
North Chicago, IL 60064, U.S.A.

06A-034-N494-1
Printed in U.S.A.

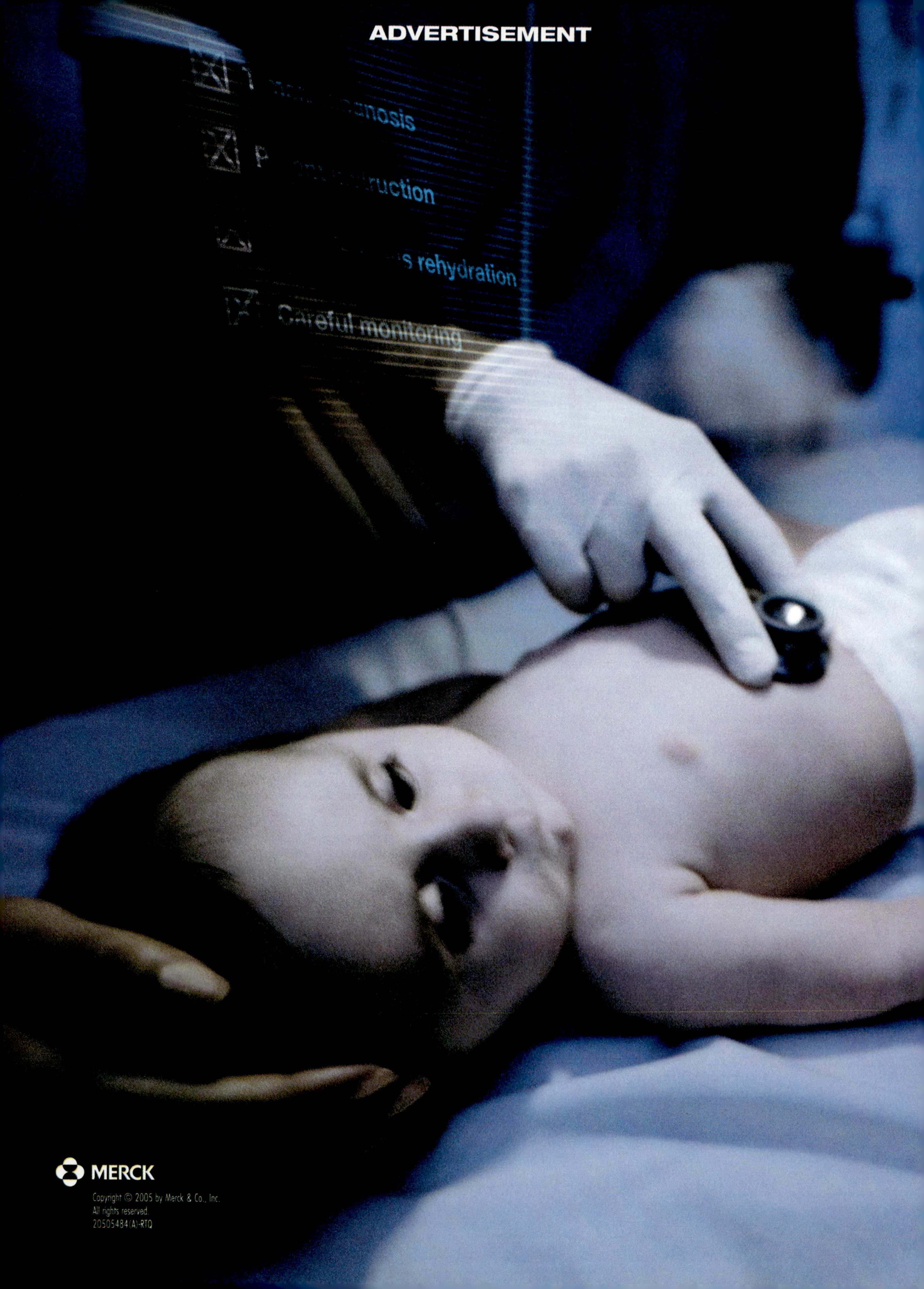
ADVERTISEMENT
rehydration
Careful monitoring
MERCK
Copyright © 2005 by Merck & Co., Inc.
All rights reserved.
20505484(A)-RTQ

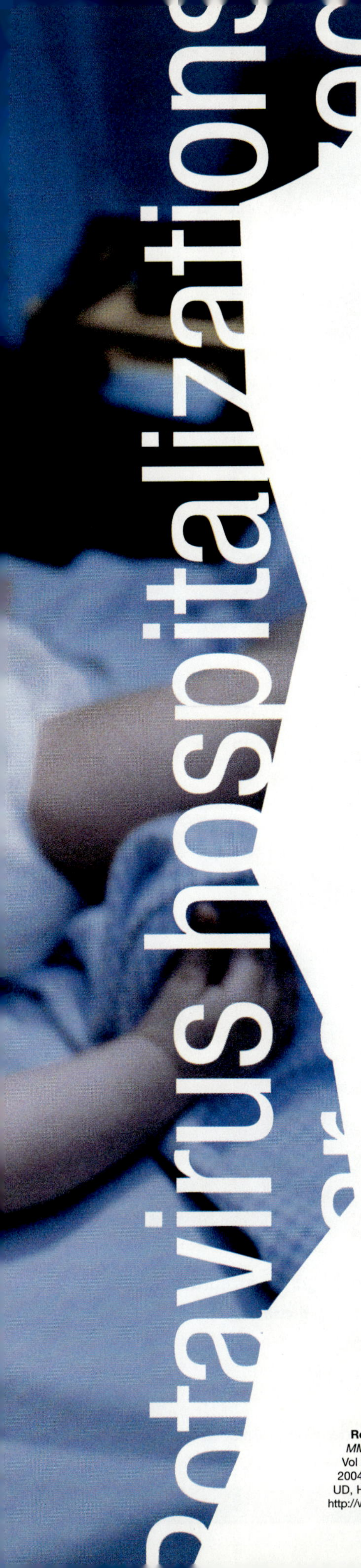


# DESPITE YOUR BEST EFFORTS, ROTAVIRUS CAUSES AN ESTIMATED 70,000 HOSPITALIZATIONS EVERY YEAR.[1]

**AN UNAVOIDABLE DISEASE...**[2]

- The most common cause of severe gastroenteritis in infants and young children in the United States[2]
- Greatest risk for severe disease occurs primarily in young children between 6 and 24 months of age.[3]

**WITH UNPREDICTABLE CONSEQUENCES**[2,4]

- No way to predict which infants will suffer severe disease[4]
- Potential for rapid deterioration in cases in which severe vomiting occurs[5]
- Responsible for an estimated 500,000 physician visits,[1] 70,000 hospitalizations,[1] and 160,000 ER visits[6] among children <5 years of age every year in the United States[1,6]
- Responsible for an estimated 100 deaths per year among children <5 years of age in the United States—an average of nearly 2 deaths per week[7]

Find out more at www.rotavirusinfo.com.

**References: 1.** Glass RI, Bresee JS, Parashar UD, et al. *Arch Pediatr*. 2005;12:844–847. **2.** Centers for Disease Control and Prevention. *MMWR*. 1999;48(RR-2):1–24. **3.** Bernstein DI, Ward RL. In: Feigin RD, Cherry JD. eds. *Textbook of Pediatric Infectious Diseases*. 4th ed. Vol 2. Philadelphia, Pa: Saunders; 1998:1901–1922. **4.** Cornell SL. *Adv Nurse Pract*. 1997;5:41–44. **5.** Clark HF, Offit PA. *Pediatr Ann*. 2004;33:537–543. **6.** Tucker AW, Haddix AC, Bresee JS, Holman MS, Parashar UD, Glass RI. *JAMA*. 1998;279:1371–1376. **7.** Parashar UD, Hummelman EG, Bresee JS, Miller MA, Glass RI. *Emerg Infect Dis*. 2003;9:565–571; Appendix B (online only.): Available at http://www.cdc.gov/ncidod/EID/vol9no5/02-0562_appB.htm. Accessed June 13, 2005.

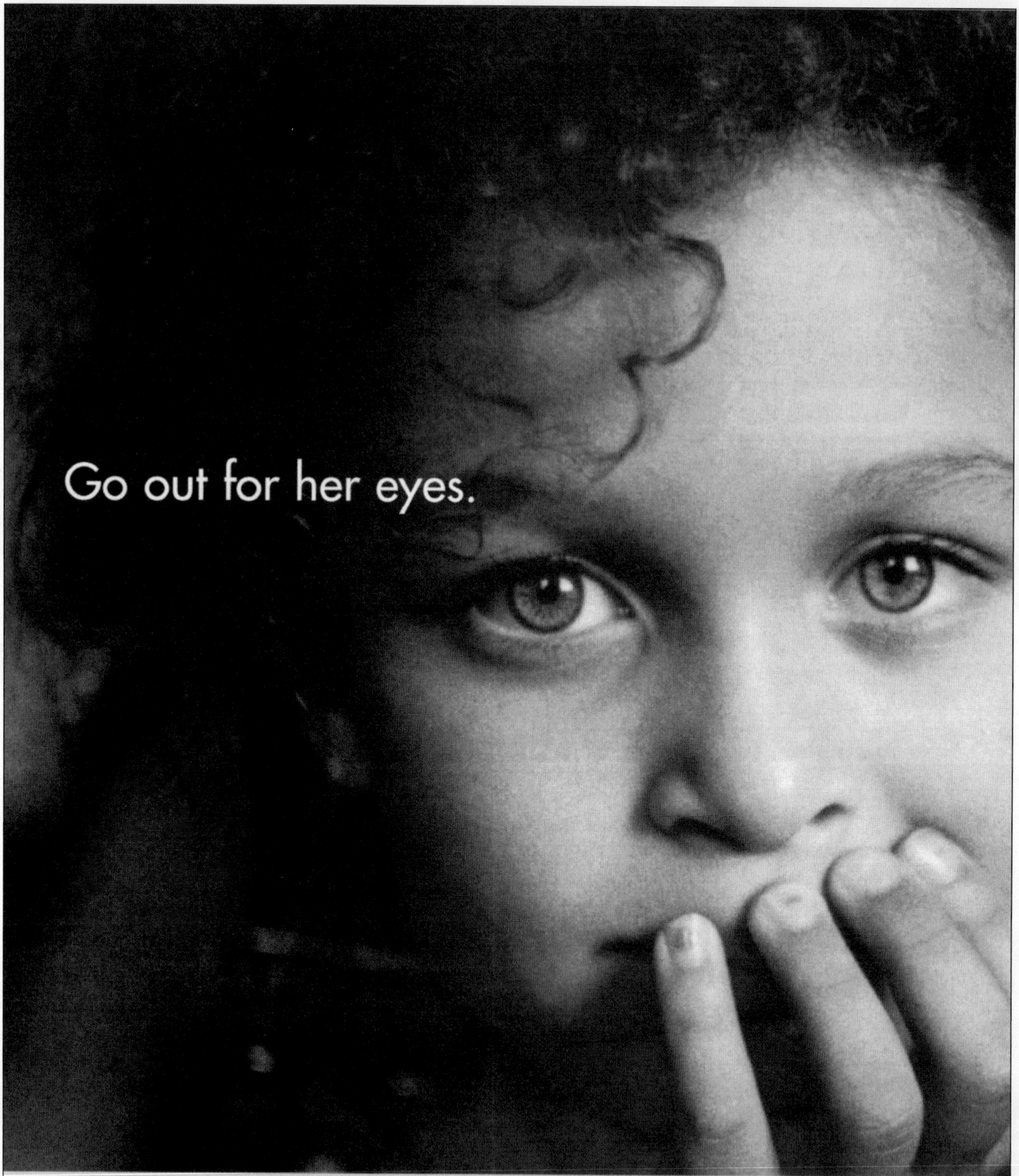
Go out for her eyes.

## A Randomized Placebo-Controlled Trial of Metformin for Adolescents With Polycystic Ovary Syndrome

Polycystic ovary syndrome is characterized by menstrual dysfunction and evidence of hyperandrogenism, and occurs in 5% to 10% of women between adolescence and menopause. Insulin resistance and hyperinsulinemia appear to play a key role in the pathophysiology of the disorder. This randomized controlled trial sought to determine if metformin would reduce serum testosterone levels in hyperandrogenic, hyperinsulinemic adolescents with the disorder. At 12 weeks of treatment, metformin lowered serum testosterone, increased the likelihood of menses 2.5-fold, and improved high-density lipoprotein cholesterol without affecting body weight. Longer follow-up studies are needed to determine the overall benefit of metformin treatment.

See page 241

## Maternal Depressive Symptoms at 2 to 4 Months Post Partum and Early Parenting Practices

Increased attention has been paid to the effects of maternal depression on infants and young children because as many as a quarter of mothers of young children have depressive symptoms. McLearn and colleagues studied nearly 5000 mothers 2 to 4 months post partum. Mothers with depressive symptoms were 27% less likely to breastfeed, 30% less likely to play with their baby, and 26% less likely to talk with their infants than mothers without depressive symptoms. Maternal depressive symptoms appear to be common in the postpartum period and adversely affect parenting practices. This study emphasizes the need for links between adult and pediatric systems of care.

See page 279

## Depressive Symptomatology as a Predictor of Exposure to Intimate Partner Violence Among US Female Adolescents and Young Adults

While many studies have shown that intimate partner violence increases the risk of subsequent depression, little is known about whether depressive symptoms are a risk factor for intimate partner violence in adolescents or adults. Lehrer and colleagues used data from the Add Health study to examine whether depressive symptomatology was associated with an increased risk of subsequent physical abuse. A total of 1659 adolescent women who were in a relationship with the opposite sex at a mean age of 15.9 years were observed for 5 years to a mean age of 21.3 years. Ten percent of women at baseline had high levels of depressive symptoms; their risk of subsequent moderate to severe intimate partner violence was nearly double that of women with the lowest level of depressive symptoms. Each 1-point increase in depressive symptomatology was associated with a 3% increase in the odds of violence.

See page 270

## Estimated Cost-effectiveness of Growth Hormone for Idiopathic Short Stature

In July 2003, the US Food and Drug Administration approved the use of recombinant growth hormone for the long-term treatment of idiopathic short stature. With this indication, it is estimated that 400 000 children in the United States now qualify for growth hormone treatment. The authors sought to estimate the cost-effectiveness of growth hormone therapy for idiopathic short stature based on the efficacy data used by the Food and Drug Administration for approval of this indication. The estimated incremental cost-effectiveness ratio of growth hormone therapy for idiopathic short stature, compared with no therapy, is $52 634 per inch or $100 000 per child, which reflects an incremental growth of 1.9 in. Alternate treatment strategies such as increased duration of growth hormone therapy and high pubertal dosing of growth hormone did not substantially improve the cost-effectiveness ratio. The significance of a cost of more than $50 000 per inch gained is difficult to judge without a better understanding of the benefits associated with height gain after growth hormone treatment.

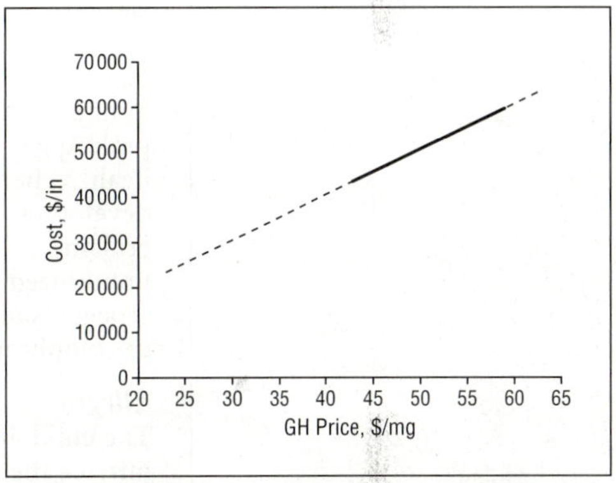


**Figure.** Estimated incremental cost per inch of growth (dashed line) based on the drug price of growth hormone (GH). The solid line represents the current range of GH prices.

See page 263

## Poetry in Pediatrics

### Trio in A Minor for Pediatrician, Mother, and Child

Chief Complaint taps his baton
and they break the sterile hush—
the fussy child with chords of sobs,
as healer asks Mom of febrile nights

*Moderato*
Asks melodic queries of
the present's past
nature of stool:
blood or mucus?
nature of vomitus:
blood or bile?
asks of syncopated functions,
do ins and outs go on?
suckled breasts, how long the child has fed
soiled diapers, how many the child has wet
asks of cough staccatos,
coryza legatos,
ear tugging, nasal flaring,
breathing, wheezing, grunting, eating,
peeing, teething, walking, grieving?
queries: a healer's seeds to sow.

*Adagio*
Her solo, Mother delivers with pride
gravidas and paras hold pain and bliss
her lone voice sounds a tremolo of joy for her
bundle of 7 pounds, 13 ounces of
pink Apgar-9 perfection
healthy, home from the hospital,
developing, mama-dada babbling
cruising, mimicking, grasping
immunized from lyrical exanthems,
arpeggios of rubella rubeola varicella
uncomplicated child

*Allegro*
The child whose uvula
mirrors the metronome,
now history taking
hastens.
contact to illness,
smoking exposure,
pets in the house,
poisons.
His tympanic cave
boiling with rage,
the child's wail
crescendos.
His cries of coda
mean the fat healer has sung,
and now is the time for
the healer's forte, his fortissimo:
his serpentine stethoscope lies in wait, soon to be
heavy on the heart of the sick child
The third musician heeds not the score,
and the song, now his alone, plays on
unrelentingly, unconductibly,
inconsolably.

*Victoria S. S. Wong, MS-3*

ARTICLE

# Randomized Placebo-Controlled Trial of Metformin for Adolescents With Polycystic Ovary Syndrome

*Tracey Bridger, MD, FRCPC; Suzanne MacDonald, MD, FRCPC; Franziska Baltzer, MD, FRCPC; Celia Rodd, MD, FRCPC*

**Objective:** To determine whether metformin or placebo could, in conjunction with healthy lifestyle counseling, decrease serum testosterone levels and related aberrations in adolescents with hyperandrogenism, hyperinsulinemia, and polycystic ovarian syndrome.

**Design:** Randomized, placebo-controlled, double-blind trial.

**Setting:** Pediatric university teaching hospital.

**Participants:** Twenty-two adolescents aged 13 to 18 years with hyperinsulinemia and polycystic ovarian syndrome.

**Intervention:** Participants were randomly assigned to take a 12-week course of either metformin or placebo.

**Main Outcome Measures:** Pretreatment and posttreatment oral glucose tolerance tests, fasting lipid profiles, and clinical measurements.

**Results:** There was a significant decline in mean serum testosterone concentration with metformin (−38.3 ng/dL) compared with placebo (−0.86 ng/dL) (95% confidence interval, −∞ to −0.29 for the mean difference between groups). At completion, the relative risk of menses was 2.50 times higher in the metformin group compared with the placebo (95% confidence interval, 1.12 to 5.58). Measures of insulin sensitivity, including insulin area under the curve and HOMA (homeostasis model assessment), demonstrated improvement only with metformin, but these did not reach statistical significance. High-density lipoprotein cholesterol levels increased by 6.98 mg/dL with metformin vs a decrease of −2.33 mg/dL with placebo (95% confidence interval, 0.78 to 18.23 for the mean difference between groups). There were no significant changes in body mass index, hirsutism, triglyceride levels, or total and low-density lipoprotein cholesterol levels.

**Conclusion:** Metformin significantly lowered total testosterone concentrations, increased the likelihood of menses, and improved high-density lipoprotein cholesterol levels without affecting measures of insulin sensitivity or body weight.

*Arch Pediatr Adolesc Med. 2006;160:241-246*

POLYCYSTIC OVARY SYNDROME (PCOS) is a common disorder in women, characterized by menstrual dysfunction and evidence of hyperandrogenism (clinical or biochemical).[1,2] It is diagnosed in at least 5% to 10% of women between adolescence and menopause, making it one of the most prevalent hormonal disorders in this population.[3-6] Once thought to be purely a cosmetic and fertility problem, it is now known that women with PCOS have increased risk factors for cardiovascular disease and are at risk of developing diabetes.[7-9]

Although the pathogenesis is not fully understood, evidence suggests insulin resistance and hyperinsulinemia play a key pathophysiologic role by promoting excess androgen production from both the ovaries and adrenal glands.[10,11] Many studies have demonstrated improvement of hyperinsulinemia, hyperandrogenemia, and clinical status in women by weight loss or treatment with insulin-sensitizing agents (such as metformin or troglitazone).[12,13]

Polycystic ovary syndrome is increasingly recognized in adolescent girls and is one of the most frequent causes of androgen excess in this age group.[14] The metabolic features seen in adult women with PCOS have also been reported in adolescents with the disorder, including hyperinsulinemia.[15-17] From these data, we infer that the pathogenesis is likely similar to that in adult women, which suggests a therapeutic role for reducing insulin levels or increasing insulin sensitivity in adolescents with PCOS.

There are currently very few studies of metformin in adolescent girls, and its use in this population remains controversial. Moreover, there are no randomized, pla-

Author Affiliations: Department of Pediatrics, Memorial University of Newfoundland, St John's (Dr Bridger); Department of Pediatrics, McGill University, Montreal, Quebec (Drs MacDonald, Baltzer, and Rodd).

cebo-controlled studies of metformin in adolescents with PCOS.[1,14,18]

The primary objective of this study was to determine whether metformin or placebo, in conjunction with healthy lifestyle counseling, could reduce serum testosterone levels in adolescents with hyperandrogenism, hyperinsulinemia, and PCOS. Secondary objectives centered on the efficacy of metformin in restoring menses, attenuating insulin resistance, and/or improving lipid profiles in adolescents with this disorder.

## METHODS

### STUDY PARTICIPANTS

We enrolled 22 adolescents with PCOS and concomitant hyperinsulinemia from the Endocrinology and Adolescent Medicine clinics of the Montreal Children's Hospital (Montreal, Quebec) between 1999 and 2002. Participants were at least 12 years old and had a history of menarche at least 2 years prior to enrollment. Diagnosis of PCOS was based on previously reported criteria.[7] All subjects had chronic oligomenorrhea ($\leq$6 menses in the preceding year) and clinical or biochemical evidence of hyperandrogenism. We excluded subjects with other causes of hyperandrogenism, such as hyperprolactinemia, androgen-secreting tumors, or late-onset congenital adrenal hyperplasia. Congenital adrenal hyperplasia was specifically ruled out by measuring 17 hydroxyprogesterone levels using an adrenocorticotropin (ACTH) stimulation test.

Sample size was based on power calculations and the published effects of metformin treatment in adult women. We approached eligible candidates sequentially until this goal was achieved, and baseline demographic features did not differ between participants and nonparticipants (not shown). Exclusion criteria included diabetes mellitus, renal or hepatic disease, pregnancy, allergies to metformin, taking oral contraceptives in the 6 months prior to enrollment, or taking medications that could influence the effects of insulin or androgens.

The study was approved by the research ethics board of the Montreal Children's Hospital. Each young woman gave informed consent and/or assent, and informed consent was obtained from their parents.

### STUDY PROTOCOL

After a 12-hour overnight fast, the adolescents came to the study center and underwent a standard 75-g oral glucose tolerance test (OGTT). At baseline, serum was collected to measure total testosterone level, progesterone level, and lipid profile. At 0-, 30-, 60-, 90-, and 120-minute intervals after the glucose load, glucose and insulin levels were drawn. Glucose tolerance was assessed by criteria from the American Diabetes Association (Alexandria, Va).[19] Progesterone was measured to determine the phase of the menstrual cycle for accurate assessment of the serum lipids.

We performed a complete physical examination for all participants, including measuring height and weight, determining blood pressure, and assessing hirsutism using the Ferriman and Gallwey scoring system.[20] This scoring system ranges from 0 to 36, with values greater or equal to 8 considered moderately hirsute.

All participants were provided with healthy eating and physical activity counseling according to the Health Canada and Fitness Vitality healthy lifestyle program. A copy of this information was provided with a 3-month calendar to document medication adverse events, menses, and lifestyle changes. Patients were then randomized by draw sequential sampling, without replacement, to receive either metformin at the final dose of 750 mg or identically appearing placebo tablets twice per day. They were advised to increase the medications over a 4-week period to minimize adverse effects. Telephone contact was made after 4 to 6 weeks to discuss their progress.

After 12 weeks, the adolescents returned for a second OGTT, baseline blood samples, and an interview as during the first visit. Unused pills were returned to estimate compliance.

### ASSAYS

Blood samples were centrifuged immediately, and serum for hormones and high-density lipoprotein (HDL) cholesterol was stored at −20° C until assayed. Glucose, triglyceride, and total cholesterol levels were immediately analyzed on the Vitros (Ortho-Clinical, Johnson and Johnson, New Brunswick, NJ). High-density lipoprotein cholesterol was analyzed on the Cobas Miros platform (Roche Diagnostics, Hoffman La Roche Ltd, Basel, Switzerland). Progesterone was assayed by Centaur chemiluminescence platform (Chiron Corp, Emeryville, Calif). Insulin, dehydroepiandrosterone sulfate, and prolactin were analyzed by the chemiluminescent Immulite platform (Diagnostic Systems, Webster, Tex). Serum was analyzed by radio immunoassay kits for total testosterone (Pantax, Santa Monica, Calif), 17 beta estradiol, 17 hydroxyprogesterone (Diagnostic Systems) and luteinizing hormone and follicle-stimulating hormone (Diagnostic Products Corp, Los Angeles, Calif).

Insulin sensitivity was estimated by calculating the insulin area under the curve (AUC), a measure that has been validated in women with PCOS against the hyperglycemic-euglycemic clamp.[21] We also calculated the homeostasis model assessment (HOMA = [fasting insulin result × fasting glucose result]/22.5) and quantitative insulin sensitivity check index (QUICKI = 1/[logarithm of fasting insulin result + logarithm of fasting glucose result]), both previously validated using the hyperglycemic-euglycemic clamp.[22-24]

### DATA ANALYSIS

Statistical analysis was performed with R, version 2.1.1. For continuous variables, the difference between posttreatment and baseline values were calculated for each subject and the groups compared for equality of variance by F test. When variances were equal, the mean difference in each group and 95% confidence interval (CI) for the difference between the 2 means were tested for equality by a standard Welch *t* test procedure. The Satterthwaite method was invoked for unequal variances (null hypothesis, $H_O$; mean difference, 0). Categorical data (eg, return of menses) were compared by Fisher exact test and expressed as a relative risk with associated 95% confidence interval ($H_O$ relative risk, 1). In both cases, failure of the 95% confidence interval to cross the $H_O$ value reflects $P<.05$.

## RESULTS

Of 22 subjects recruited (n = 11 in each group), only 1 subject did not complete the study. One adolescent in the placebo arm was able to provide information about her compliance and clinical well-being at the end of the study period but was unable to present for the OGTT and physical examination.

### PREINTERVENTION CHARACTERISTICS

The clinical characteristics of the 2 groups of adolescent girls at baseline are depicted in **Table 1**. They ranged

**Table 1. Clinical Characteristics and Serum Hormone Concentrations in Adolescents With PCOS at Baseline**

| Characteristic | Metformin Group | Placebo Group |
|---|---|---|
| Age, mean ± SD, y | 16.07 ± 0.97 | 16.08 ± 1.39 |
| Body mass index, mean ± SD* | 33.6 ± 5.6 | 30.81 ± 3.0 |
| Ferriman and Gallwey score, mean ± SD | 5.3 ± 5.0 | 7.2 ± 7.6 |
| Total testosterone, mean ± SD, ng/dL (nmol/L) | 174.3 ± 54.0 (6.03 ± 1.88) | 167.3 ± 46.0 (5.80 ± 1.58) |
| Insulin AUC, mean ± SD, µU/mL · min (pmol/L · min) | 15 246 ± 10 097 (109 374 ± 72 433) | 15 460 ± 12 377 (110 905 ± 88 788) |
| Fasting glucose, mean ± SD, mg/dL (mmol/L) | 77.9 ± 7.2 (4.33 ± 0.4) | 80.6 ± 8.3 (4.48 ± 0.46) |
| HOMA, mean ± SD | 5.75 ± 10.08 | 2.79 ± 1.45 |
| QUICKI, mean ± SD | 0.34 ± 0.07 | 0.36 ± 0.05 |
| Total cholesterol, mean ± SD, mg/dL (mmol/L) | 164.9 ± 27.5 (4.25 ± 0.71) | 171.1 ± 48.9 (4.41 ± 1.26) |
| LDL cholesterol, mean ± SD, mg/dL (mmol/L) | 88.5 ± 19.8 (2.28 ± 0.51) | 93.5 ± 41.9 (2.41 ± 1.08) |
| HDL cholesterol, mean ± SD, mg/dL (mmol/L) | 45.8 ± 18.6 (1.18 ± 0.48) | 42.3 ± 10.9 (1.09 ± 0.28) |
| Triglycerides, mean ± SD, mg/dL (mmol/L) | 133.9 ± 55.1 (1.53 ± 0.63) | 168 ± 77.9 (1.92 ± 0.89) |
| Ethnicity, No. | | |
| White, non-Hispanic | 7 | 10 |
| Black, non-Hispanic | 2 | 0 |
| Hispanic | 1 | 0 |
| Asian | 1 | 1 |
| Menses in 6 months before enrollment, No. | 2 | 3 |
| Girls with menses during 6 months before enrollment, No. | 2 | 3 |

Abbreviations: AUC, area under the curve; HDL, high-density lipoprotein; HOMA, homeostasis model assessment; LDL, low-density lipoprotein; PCOS, polycystic ovarian syndrome; QUICKI, quantitative insulin sensitivity check index.

*Body mass index is calculated as weight in kilograms divided by the square of height in meters.

in age from 13 to 18 years with an average age of 16.0 years at the start of the study period. All were overweight or obese with body mass index (BMI), calculated as weight in kilograms divided by the square of height in meters, ranging from 26.0 to 44.7. By definition, all were hyperandrogenemic with significantly elevated levels of total testosterone. Subjects in both groups came from similar ethnic backgrounds. All participants had had fewer than 6 menses in the year preceding the study with no significant difference in the 2 proportions at baseline.

## POSTINTERVENTION CHARACTERISTICS

At completion, the weights and BMI had not significantly changed. Total testosterone levels dropped significantly in the cohort treated with metformin (mean difference, −38.3 ng/dL) compared with placebo (mean difference, −0.86 ng/dL) (95% CI, −∞ to −0.29 for the difference between group means). In neither group was there a change in the Ferriman and Gallwey scores or acanthosis nigricans (**Table 2**). Ten of 11 adolescents in the metformin group experienced menses, compared with only 4 of 11 adolescents in the placebo group. The relative risk of menses was statistically significant at 2.50 (95% CI, 1.12 to 5.58).

## GLUCOSE AND INSULIN PROFILES

Fasting blood glucose levels were all normal at baseline and remained this way at the end of the study regardless of the treatment prescribed. None of the study recruits were diabetic based on the American Diabetes Association interpretation of the OGTT, a requirement for participation. The baseline OGTTs revealed that 1 adolescent in the metformin arm had impaired glucose tolerance. At the end of the study, her results demonstrated persistent impaired glucose tolerance. None of the girls in the placebo arm had any glucose intolerance at baseline, but 1 developed this at the end of the 12-week interval.

The areas under the insulin response curve were elevated and were not significantly different in the 2 arms at baseline. With metformin, there was a suggestive trend toward lower insulin AUC with treatment, but this was not statistically significant (with metformin, insulin AUC declined by −3662 µU/mL·minute, compared with +2093 µU/mL·minute for placebo; 95% CI, −17 531 to 6024 for the mean difference between groups). Homeostasis model assessment calculations also showed a trend toward improved insulin sensitivity with metformin treatment, but again these were not statistically significant (HOMA: metformin therapy [mean difference, −1.06] compared with placebo [mean difference, 0.86] [95% CI, −9.26 to 5.42 for the difference between group means]; QUICKI: metformin therapy [mean difference, 0.00] compared with placebo [mean difference, −0.01] [95% CI, −0.03 to 0.05 for the difference between group means]).

## LIPID PROFILE

On average, the baseline levels of total, low-density lipoprotein and HDL cholesterol were normal for all participants (Table 1). At the end of the trial, metformin had significantly improved HDL cholesterol concentrations compared with placebo. The increase with treatment was +6.98 mg/dL vs −2.33 mg/dL for placebo (95% CI, 0.78 to 18.23 for the mean difference between groups). Other cholesterol parameters were not significantly different (Table 2). Triglycerides were elevated in both baseline cohorts and fell with metformin treatment, but this did not reach statistical significance. No decline was noted with placebo. All young women were in the follicular phase of their menstrual cycle at baseline; 1 participant

**Table 2. Change From Baseline in Clinical Characteristics and Blood Tests After Administration of Metformin or Placebo for 12 Weeks**

| Characteristic | Mean Difference: Metformin Group | Mean Difference: Placebo Group | 95% Confidence Interval for the Mean Difference Between Groups |
|---|---|---|---|
| Body mass index* | −0.16 | −0.19 | −1.01 to 0.32 |
| Ferriman and Gallwey score | 0 | 0 | NA |
| Total testosterone, ng/dL | −38.3 | −0.86 | −∞ to −0.29 |
| Insulin AUC, μU/mL · min | −3662 | 2093 | −17 531 to 6024 |
| Fasting glucose, mg/dL | 0.31 | 0.36 | −3.42 to 5.22 |
| HOMA | −1.06 | 0.86 | −9.26 to 5.42 |
| QUICKI | 0.00 | −0.01 | −0.03 to 0.05 |
| Total cholesterol, mg/dL | −0.78 | −8.15 | −17.07 to 31.82 |
| LDL cholesterol, mg/dL | −3.10 | −7.76 | −12.80 to 20.56 |
| HDL cholesterol, mg/dL | 6.98 | −2.33 | 0.78 to 18.23 |
| Triglycerides, mg/dL | −13.13 | 7.00 | −70.00 to 29.75 |
| Girls with restored menses, No. | 10/11 | 4/11 | 1.12 to 5.58 (relative risk, 2.50) |

Abbreviations: AUC, area under the curve; HDL, high-density lipoprotein; HOMA, homeostasis model assessment; LDL, low-density lipoprotein; NA, not applicable; QUICKI, quantitative insulin sensitivity check index.

*Body mass index is calculated as weight in kilograms divided by the square of height in meters.

in the placebo group was excluded from the comparisons because she was in the luteal phase at completion of the study.

## COMPLIANCE

Pill counts were performed at the end of the trial. Two adolescents in the placebo arm admitted to not taking all the required tablets. One of them stated that they caused gastrointestinal adverse effects and discontinued the pills after taking about 45% of them. The second participant did not return for the second OGTT and stated that she only took about 50% of the pills. In the metformin treatment arm, 5 of 11 admitted to poor compliance (defined as <70% of pills taken), citing gastrointestinal disturbances. Based on pill counts, 8% to 60% of the metformin tablets were not consumed. Of note, in the metformin group, all of the noncompliant subjects and 6 of 7 compliant subjects had least 1 menses during the study period; therefore, metformin treatment was associated with restoration of menses in 10 of 11 treated subjects.

## COMMENT

To our knowledge, this is the first study to evaluate the effect of metformin and lifestyle counseling on insulin levels, testosterone levels, and menstrual patterns in adolescent girls with hyperinsulinemia and PCOS in a randomized, double-blind, placebo-controlled study. We found that metformin resulted in a clinically significant impact on menses, significantly reduced serum testosterone levels, and significantly increased HDL cholesterol levels.

All of our study subjects were overweight or obese at baseline and did not achieve a significant reduction in BMI with lifestyle intervention and metformin or placebo. In the 2 published pediatric, unrandomized, and uncontrolled studies using metformin for PCOS, a moderate reduction in weight was noted. Both studies by Glueck et al[25] and Arslanian et al[26] were small in sample size, and in the latter, the BMI was significantly lowered because of a significant increase in height. Two small, randomized, double-blind, placebo-controlled trials by Kay et al[27] and Freemark and Bursey[28] evaluated metformin in obese adolescents (not with PCOS) and showed that those treated with metformin had a significantly greater weight loss compared with the placebo groups, although the differences were modest. Of note, the subjects in the Kay et al[27] and Freemark and Bursey[28] studies were also prescribed weight-reduction diets. The adult literature is equally inconclusive with regard to weight reduction, which suggests that metformin may not contribute to weight loss directly.

Metformin did, however, result in a significant reduction in total testosterone levels compared with placebo. Our study design could not determine whether reduced androgen levels were a consequence of the downward trend in insulin levels or some other biologic effects of metformin. Given the duration of the study, it comes as little surprise that this did not necessarily translate into a change in degree of hirsutism. Two earlier studies in overweight adolescents with PCOS demonstrated conflicting results; Arslanian et al[26] described significant reductions in both free and total testosterone levels with metformin, and Glueck et al[25] noted a nonsignificant downward trend in testosterone levels. In both studies, moderate weight loss was noted and only in the former study were insulin levels measured, which were decreased with metformin. The small (n=10) study by Ibanez et al[29] in nonobese adolescent girls with PCOS observed a decrease in both androgen levels and hirsutism with metformin, associated with a concomitant decrease in insulin concentrations and without any weight loss.

We found a significant rise in HDL cholesterol levels in the metformin group compared with the placebo group by the end of the study period. We did not find significant changes in other lipid parameters. The mean triglyceride concentrations were elevated in both study groups at the start of the study, with a nonsignificant reduction in triglyceride levels observed in the metformin-treated group alone. Again, the impact of metformin in adolescents has been inconsistent. Glueck et al[25] observed a significant reduction in total cholesterol levels in a nonrandomized study while Arslanian et al[26] saw no significant change in cholesterol or triglyceride levels. In the randomized double-blind placebo-controlled trial by Kay et al[27] of obese adolescents (not with PCOS), a significant improvement in the lipid profile was seen with metformin treatment (decreased total cholesterol and triglyceride levels). In all 3 of these studies, metformin treatment was associated with weight loss. In 2 of these studies, insulin levels were assessed and found to be reduced with metformin.

Most importantly, menses was 2.5 times more likely to occur in the metformin group compared with the placebo group. Metformin has been deemed to be beneficial in the restoration of menses in other studies, from 40% to 100% (40%, Glueck et al[25]; 91%, Arslanian et al[26]; and 100%, Ibanez et al[29]). Indeed, Ibanez et al confirmed that menses returned, and the majority of these cycles were ovulatory.[30,31]

We noted an improvement in measures of insulin sensitivity, including the insulin AUC and HOMA, in the adolescents treated with metformin, but not in the control group. However, this trend failed to achieve statistical significance, possibly reflecting sample size and inherent variability of the measure. Because some clinical benefits were noted, we postulate that this reduction may have had biologic effects. Earlier studies by Arslanian et al[26] and Ibanez et al[30,31] in adolescents with PCOS have demonstrated a significant decline in insulin levels assessed by both fasting insulin-glucose ratios and formal pharmacokinetic AUC. However, most studies in female and male adolescents have also demonstrated a decrease in BMI or body weight with metformin treatment, which could conceivably alter insulin sensitivity.[25-28]

Poor compliance in nearly half (5/11) of the adolescents randomized to metformin and/or our small sample size may have limited the ability to detect statistically significant differences in insulin concentrations despite the clinical impact on menses and testosterone levels. Comparing our results with the other trials carried out in adolescents suggests that important biologic effects can occur without weight loss and without statistically significant improvements in measures of insulin sensitivity. This raises the question as to whether metformin has additional biologic actions besides that of an insulin sensitizer or whether the impact of metformin is noted with very small decreases in insulin concentrations.

The use of insulin-sensitizing agents, especially metformin, has generally been accepted in adult women with PCOS although not all studies have demonstrated consistent benefits.[13] In adolescents with PCOS, there have been fewer studies of metformin, and controversy remains with regards to its benefits and mechanisms of action. It is difficult to directly compare our study with those previously published because of the inherent differences in study design, although most appear to demonstrate that metformin treatment leads to clinical improvement. The goal of this therapy in the adolescent is more likely to focus on the reduction of hirsutism and acne with return of menses as a less important outcome. Fertility and long-term cardiovascular health appear more remote concerns for these young adults.

Our randomized placebo-controlled study, albeit small in sample size, demonstrated a significant decrease in testosterone levels and an increase in the frequency of menses in adolescents with oligomenorrhea or amenorrhea. Measures of insulin sensitivity improved, although not significantly. Poor compliance with metformin and/or sample size were major limitations as was the short duration of the study.

Despite other adolescent preoccupations, the increased frequency of menses observed with a combination of metformin and lifestyle therapy may benefit uterine health. In addition, the significant increase in HDL cholesterol levels may benefit overall health in the future, as might the trend toward improvement in insulin AUC, although longer term follow-up studies will be needed to explore these questions.

**Accepted for Publication:** September 13, 2005.
**Corresponding Author:** Tracey Bridger, MD, FRCPC, Paediatric Endocrinology, Janeway Child Health and Rehabilitation Centre, 300 Prince Philip Dr, St John's, Newfoundland and Labrador, Canada A1B 3V6 (traceybridger@hotmail.com).
**Funding/Support:** Montreal Children's Hospital Research Institute, Montreal, Quebec, and Aventis Pharmaceutical, Laval, Quebec, supplied metformin and an identical appearing placebo.

## REFERENCES

1. Pfeifer SM, Dayal M. Treatment of the adolescent patient with polycystic ovary syndrome. *Obstet Gynecol Clin North Am.* 2003;30:337-352.
2. Zawadzki JK, Dunaif A. Diagnostic criteria for polycystic ovary syndrome: towards a rational approach. In: Dunaif A, Givens JR, Haseltine FP, Merriam GR, eds. *Current Issues in Endocrinology and Metabolism: Polycystic Ovary Syndrome.* Boston, Mass: Blackwell Scientific; 1992:377-384.
3. Knochenhauer ES, Key TJ, Kahsar-Miller M, Waggoner W, Boots LR, Azziz R. Prevalence of the polycystic ovary syndrome in unselected black and white women of the southeastern United States: a prospective study. *J Clin Endocrinol Metab.* 1998;83:3078-3082.
4. Asuncion M, Calvo RM, San Millan JL, et al. A prospective study of the prevalence of the polycystic ovary syndrome in unselected Caucasian women from Spain. *J Clin Endocrinol Metab.* 2000;85:2434-2438.
5. Diamanti-Kandarakis E, Kouli CR, Bergiele AT, et al. A survey of the polycystic ovary syndrome in the Greek island of Lesbos: hormonal and metabolic profile. *J Clin Endocrinol Metab.* 1999;84:4006-4011.
6. Azziz R, Woods KS, Reyna R, Key TJ, Knochenhauer ES, Yildiz BO. The prevalence and features of the polycystic ovary syndrome in an unselected population. *J Clin Endocrinol Metab.* 2004;89:2745-2749.
7. Legro RS, Kunselman AR, Dodson WC, Dunaif A. Prevalence and predictors of risk for type 2 diabetes mellitus and impaired glucose tolerance in polycystic ovary syndrome: a prospective, controlled study in 254 affected women. *J Clin Endocrinol Metab.* 1999;84:165-169.
8. Ehrmann DA, Barnes RB, Rosenfield RL, Cavaghan MK, Imperial J. Prevalence of impaired glucose tolerance and diabetes in women with polycystic ovary syndrome. *Diabetes Care.* 1999;22:141-146.
9. Wild S, Pierpoint T, McKeigue P, Jacobs H. Cardiovascular disease in women with polycystic ovary syndrome at long-term follow-up: a retrospective cohort study. *Clin Endocrinol (Oxf).* 2000;52:595-600.
10. Barbieri RL, Smith S, Ryan KJ. The role of hyperinsulinemia in the pathogenesis of ovarian hyperandrogenism. *Fertil Steril.* 1988;50:197-212.
11. Dunaif A, Segal KR, Futterweit W, Dobrjansky A. Profound peripheral insulin resistance, independent of obesity, in polycystic ovary syndrome. *Diabetes.* 1989;38:1165-1174.
12. Huber-Buchholz MM, Carey DGP, Norman RJ. Restoration of reproductive po-

tential by lifestyle modification in obese polycystic ovary syndrome: role of insulin sensitivity and luteinizing hormone. *J Clin Endocrinol Metab.* 1999;84:1470-1474.
13. Taylor AE. Insulin lowering medications in polycystic ovary syndrome. *Obstet Gynecol Clin North Am.* 2000;27:583-595.
14. Kent SC, Legro RS. Polycystic ovary syndrome in adolescents. *Adolesc Med.* 2002;13:73-88.
15. Apter D. Endocrine and metabolic abnormalities in adolescents with a PCOS-like condition: consequences for adult reproduction. *Trends Endocrinol Metab.* 1998;9:58-61.
16. Lewy VD, Danadian K, Witchel SF, Arslanian S. Early metabolic abnormalities in adolescent girls with polycystic ovarian syndrome. *J Pediatr.* 2001;138:38-44.
17. Silfen ME. Early endocrine, metabolic, and sonographic characteristics of polycystic ovary syndrome (PCOS): comparison between nonobese and obese adolescents. *J Clin Endocrinol Metab.* 2003;88:4682-4688.
18. Dean H. Metformin use in adolescent with PCOS: an invited editorial from the pediatric endocrinology perspective. *J Pediatr Adolesc Gynecol.* 2003;16:109-111.
19. Expert Committee on the Diagnosis and Classification of Diabetes Mellitus. Report of the Expert Committee on the Diagnosis and Classification of Diabetes Mellitus. *Diabetes Care.* 2000;23:S5-S19.
20. Ferriman D, Gallwey JD. Clinical assessment of body hair growth in women. *J Clin Endocrinol Metab.* 1961;21:1440-1447.
21. Ciampelli M. Assessment of insulin sensitivity from measurements in the fasting state and during an oral glucose tolerance test in polycystic ovary syndrome and menopausal patients. *J Clin Endocrinol Metab.* 2005;90:1398-1406.
22. Skrha J, Haas T, Sindelka G, et al. Comparison of the insulin action parameters from hyperinsulinemic clamps with homeostasis model assessment and QUICKI indexes in subjects with different endocrine disorders. *J Clin Endocrinol Metab.* 2004;89:135-141.
23. Katz A, Nambi SS, Mather K, et al. Quantitative insulin sensitivity check index: a simple, accurate method for assessing insulin sensitivity in humans. *J Clin Endocrinol Metab.* 2000;85:2402-2410.
24. Matthews DR, Hosker JP, Rudenski AS, Naylor BA, Treacher DF, Turner RC. Homeostasis model assessment: insulin resistance and beta-cell function from fasting plasma glucose and insulin concentrations in man. *Diabetologia.* 1985;28:412-419.
25. Glueck CJ, Wang P, Fontaine R, Tracy T, Sieve-Smith L. Metformin to restore normal menses in oligo-amenorrheic teenage girls with polycystic ovary syndrome (PCOS). *J Adolesc Health.* 2001;29:160-169.
26. Arslanian SA, Lewy V, Danadian K, Saad R. Metformin therapy in obese adolescents with polycystic ovary syndrome and impaired glucose intolerance: amelioration of exaggerated adrenal response to adrenocorticotropin with reduction of insulinemia/insulin resistance. *J Clin Endocrinol Metab.* 2002;87:1555-1559.
27. Kay JP, Alemzadeh R, Langley G, D'Angelo L, Smith P, Holshouser S. Beneficial effects of metformin in normoglycemic morbidly obese adolescents. *Metabolism.* 2001;50:1457-1461.
28. Freemark M, Bursey D. The effects of metformin on body mass index and glucose tolerance in obese adolescents with fasting hyperinsulinemia and a family history of type 2 diabetes. *Pediatrics.* 2001;107:E55.
29. Ibanez L, Valls C, Potau N, Marcos MV, de Zegher F. Sensitization to insulin in adolescent girls to normalize hirsutism, hyperandrogenism, oligomenorrhea, dyslipidemia, and hyperinsulinism after precocious pubarche. *J Clin Endocrinol Metab.* 2000;85:3526-3530.
30. Ibanez L, Valls C, Ferrer A, Marcos MV, Rodriguez-Hierro F, de Zegher F. Sensitization to insulin induces ovulation in nonobese adolescents with anovulatory hyperandrogenism. *J Clin Endocrinol Metab.* 2001;86:3595-3598.
31. Ibanez L, Potau N, Ferrer A, Rodriguez-Hierro F, Marcos MV, de Zegher F. Anovulation in eumenorrheic, nonobese adolescent girls born small for gestational age: insulin sensitization induces ovulation, increases lean body mass, and reduces abdominal fat excess, dyslipidemia, and subclinical hyperandrogenism. *J Clin Endocrinol Metab.* 2002;87:5702-5705.

## Announcement

**Submissions.** The Editors welcome contributions to Picture of the Month. Submissions should describe common problems presenting uncommonly, rather than total zebras. Cases should be of interest to practicing pediatricians, highlighting problems that they are likely to at least occasionally encounter in the office or hospital setting. High-quality clinical images (in either 35-mm slide or electronic format) along with parent or patient permission to use these images must accompany the submission. The entire discussion should comprise no more than 750 words. Articles and photographs accepted for publication will bear the contributor's name. There is no charge for reproduction and printing of color illustrations. For details regarding electronic submission, please see: http://archpedi.ama-assn.org.

# Risk of Active Tuberculosis Among Schoolchildren in Hong Kong

*Chi Chiu Leung, MB; Wing Wai Yew, MB; Kwok Chiu Chang, MSc; Cheuk Ming Tam, MSc; Chi Kuen Chan, MSc; Wing Sze Law, MSc; Man Yee Wong, MPH; Shuk Nor Lee, MB; Maria Leung, MSc*

**Objective:** To estimate the risk of active tuberculosis (TB) and its implication on preventive treatment among BCG-vaccinated schoolchildren.

**Design:** Cohort and case-control designs.

**Setting:** Community settings in a high-prevalence area.

**Participants:** Children in primary school. The main exposure was their tuberculin response.

**Main Outcome Measures:** Of 94 928 primary schoolchildren tuberculin tested during a routine school revaccination program in 1999, 656 with a tuberculin response at 20 mm or more were followed up prospectively through the territory-wide TB registry up to December 31, 2003, for the development of TB. In a separate case-control analysis, the tuberculin responses of children who subsequently had active TB (at the age of 10-15 years) were compared with those of their sex- and age-matched classmates to ascertain the relative risks of TB for different tuberculin reaction categories. The absolute and relative risks were applied to the 1999 cohort for estimating the incidence of TB among different tuberculin reactors.

**Results:** The annual incidence (95% confidence interval) of active TB was estimated to be 13.4 (5.6-40.6) per 100 000 for the entire cohort and 7.5 (2.4-24.5), 7.5 (1.7-32.0), 16.0 (4.4-57.2), 92.6 (26.6-320.2), and 340.6 (163.3-626.4) per 100 000 for children with a tuberculin reaction at 0 to 4, 5 to 9, 10 to 14, 15 to 19, and 20 mm or more, respectively. By using 10 mm as the cutoff, 482 (95% confidence interval, 163-1391) children have to be treated to prevent a single case of active TB within 5 years. Treatment will cover 17.5% of the cohort, but prevent only 54.1% of all active TB cases.

**Conclusion:** It is desirable to reexamine the existing screening method for BCG-vaccinated children from high-prevalence countries.

*Arch Pediatr Adolesc Med. 2006;160:247-251*

Tuberculin skin testing has been used for a long time as a diagnostic test for latent tuberculosis (TB) infection. Tuberculin-positive children from high-prevalence countries are regularly given treatment for latent TB infection in the United States,[1] while such treatment is seldom recommended in the absence of other risk factors like recent contact or human immunodeficiency virus infection in their home countries. It would be desirable to quantify the actual risk of TB among these children, so that the appropriateness of the recommendation can be examined in light of better scientific evidence. While a prospective cohort might be the ideal approach to tackle this issue, the relatively low incidence of disease[2] among children poses a significant problem in relation to sample size and follow-up.

In many countries with a high prevalence of TB, neonatal BCG vaccination is regularly performed.[3] For the past 30 years, BCG (Glaxo strain) has been given to all newborns in Hong Kong, with a coverage rate of about 99%.[4] BCG revaccination was also practiced among primary schoolchildren (aged mainly from 6-12 years) until its cessation in 2000. All primary schools in Hong Kong were covered. The BCG team (a group of well-experienced inoculators) of the Tuberculosis and Chest Service used to visit each primary school once every 4 years in rotation to conduct tuberculin skin testing with 1 U of purified protein derivative (PPD) RT-23. Schoolchildren with a tuberculin reaction of 9 mm or less were of-

*For editorial comment see page 317*

Author Affiliations:
Tuberculosis and Chest Service, Department of Health (Drs Leung, Chang, Tam, Chan, Law, Wong, and Lee, and Ms Leung), and Tuberculosis and Chest Unit, Grantham Hospital (Dr Yew), Hong Kong.

fered revaccination. In general, treatment for latent TB infection was not offered. The revaccination program was stopped in 2000 on the advice of the local Advisory Committee on Immunization. A postcessation surveillance program was launched from January 1, 2001, to June 30, 2003, to record the BCG revaccination history of all TB patients aged 10 to 15 years on notification. With data available from these regular services, we engaged in a 2-part study, combining the benefits of cohort and case-control design, to quantify the risk of active TB among schoolchildren in Hong Kong.

## METHODS

### PART 1: COHORT STUDY

From the paper records of the School Revaccination Program, all schoolchildren with a tuberculin response at 20 mm or more in 1999 were retrieved, and cross matched with the computerized statutory TB notification registry in Hong Kong every 6 months until December 31, 2003, using name (in English), sex, and date of birth as identifiers. The medical and public health records of all identified TB cases were retrieved from relevant chest clinics or hospitals for verification of identity and confirmation of the diagnosis. An active case of TB was defined as disease proved by isolation of *Mycobacterium tuberculosis* or, in the absence of bacteriological confirmation, disease diagnosed on clinical, radiological, and/or histological grounds together with an appropriate response to treatment. The incidence of active TB was quantified, with the 95% confidence interval estimated by assuming a Poisson distribution in the occurrence of the cases.

### PART 2: MATCHED CASE-CONTROL STUDY

The school BCG records of active TB patients aged 10 to 15 years, from January 1, 2001, to June 30, 2003, were retrieved together with those of their classmates. Each case was matched to 8 controls by class, sex, and age to control for the potential confounding effects of these variables, and to maximize the statistical power to detect any significant differences among multiple tuberculin reaction categories. All students who had not been tested with a tuberculin skin test during the school BCG revaccination were excluded. Univariate conditional logistic regression analysis was used because of the matched design to estimate the odds ratios for active TB among different tuberculin reaction categories.[5] A commercially available software program (SPSS version 10; SPSS Inc, Chicago, Ill) was used for analysis. $P<.05$ was considered statistically significant.

The odds ratios obtained in part 2 were multiplied to the absolute incidence derived for the strongest reactors in part 1 to obtain the annual risks of active TB for other tuberculin reaction categories. These were then applied to the 1999 cohort to estimate the numbers needed to treat to prevent a single case of active TB. For simplicity, only those active TB cases occurring within the first 5 years were considered, and the protective efficacy of treatment was assumed to be 100%.

The study has been approved by the Ethics Committee of the Department of Health of Hong Kong.

## RESULTS

In 1999, a total of 94 928 primary school students were successfully tested for tuberculin response in the School Revaccination Program. The distribution of tuberculin skin test results is summarized in the **Figure**. Of those with a tuberculin test reaction of less than 10 mm, 99.7% were given a BCG revaccination. Of 662 students (0.7%) with a tuberculin reaction at 20 mm or more, 6 with missing data on date of birth were excluded, leaving 656 students for analysis. All except 6 (0.9%) were Chinese. Approximately 54% were females. The mean (SD) age was 9.80 (2.13) years. The mean (SD) duration of follow-up was 4.48 (0.26) years.

Up to December 31, 2003, 10 active TB patients (7 pulmonary, 1 extrapulmonary, and 2 combined) were identified. Four cases were confirmed by culture, including one with a positive sputum smear result. The diagnosis of the rest was verified by their clinicoradiological picture and subsequent response to treatment. There were 7 female and 3 male patients (Fisher exact test, 2-tailed; $P=.36$). The median age at disease onset was 12.5 (range, 9.5-13.6) years. The median interval from tuberculin skin testing to the development of disease was 286.5 (range, 20-1649) days. All of them had received a BCG vaccination at birth. Three reported a history of TB contact (2 household and 1 nonhousehold) within 5 years. All enjoyed good health in the past, except for one with Down syndrome. The incidence rate of active TB was 340.6 (95% confidence interval, 163.3-626.4) per 100 000 person-years among schoolchildren with a tuberculin reaction at 20 mm or more.

From January 1, 2001, to June 30, 2003, a total of 103 active TB patients aged 10 to 15 years were reported to the Department of Health. Fourteen had not met the school BCG team because of recent immigration or cessation of the School Revaccination Program. Five students missed the tuberculin skin testing because of parental refusal or absence from school, and the school BCG records of 1 student could not be retrieved, leaving 83 patients with complete tuberculin skin testing records (from December 8, 1992, to March 27, 2000) for analysis. The mean (SD) age of these 83 patients at notification of disease was 14.18 (1.54) years, and the mean (SD) interval from tuberculin skin testing to disease was 5.21 (2.00) years. All 83 patients (59 pulmonary, 20 extrapulmonary, and 4 both) were new cases. Only 16 (19.3%) were positive for TB by sputum smear result, and 30 (36.1%) were confirmed to have TB by culture result. The rest met the definition for active TB by their clinicoradiological picture and subsequent response to treatment. The neonatal BCG vaccination history was available for only 75 patients. Seventy-four reported BCG vaccination and 1 did not. BCG scars were checked in 76 patients, with 16 showing 0 scars, 45 showing 1 scar, and 15 showing 2 scars. Matching the 83 patients by class identified 2505 classmates in 79 different schools. Eighty-four students did not participate in the regular revaccination program, leaving 2421 with tuberculin skin testing results.

The proportions of males were 39.8% and 49.1% among patients and their classmates, respectively ($P=.10$). The mean (SD) age at tuberculin skin testing was 8.97 (1.88) years for patients and 8.90 (1.79) years for their classmates (unpaired *t* test, $P=.72$). The mean (SD) tuberculin test response was 9.64 (7.95) mm for patients and 4.09 (5.13) mm for their classmates (unpaired *t* test, $P<.001$). All students with a tuberculin response at 9 mm or less had been revaccinated.

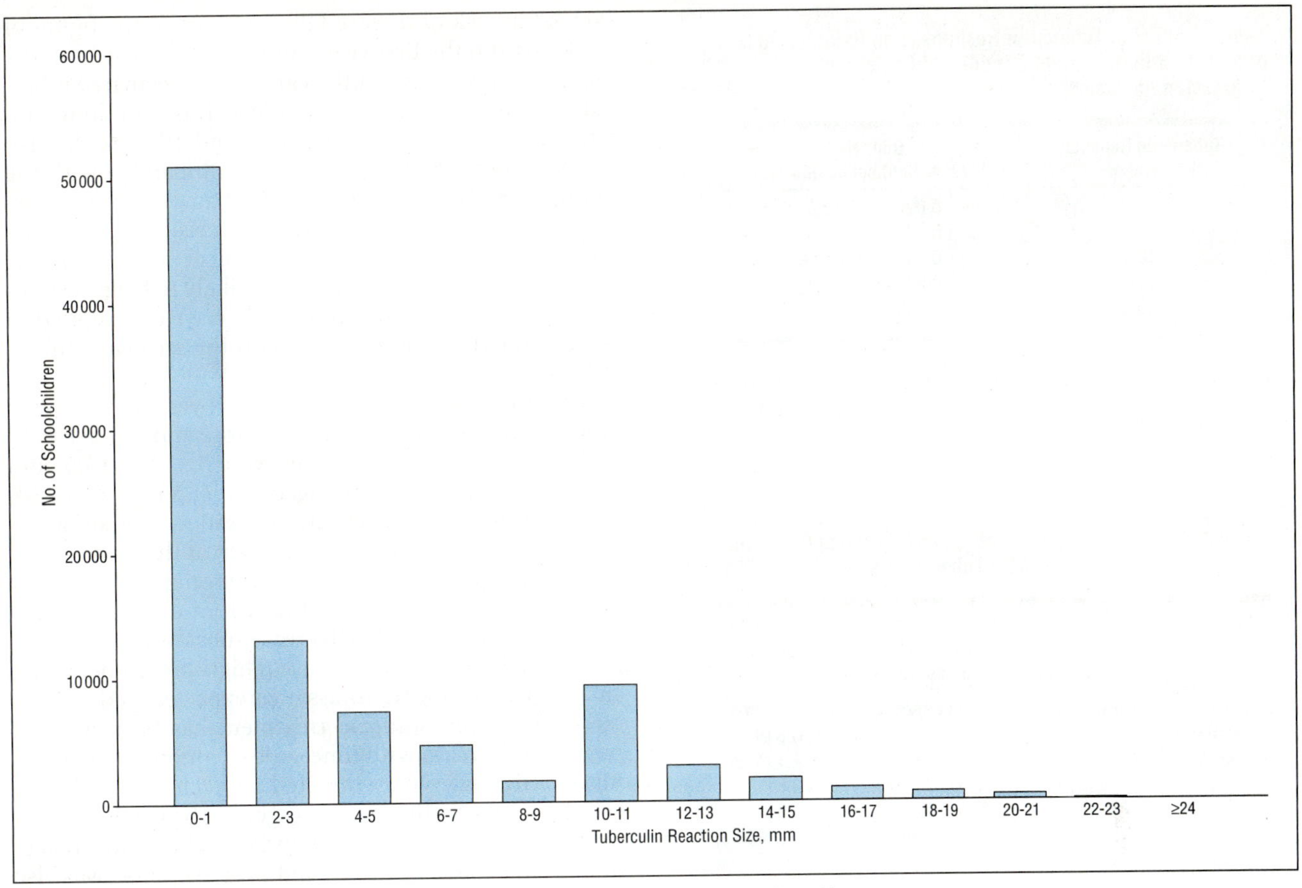


**Figure.** Distribution of tuberculin response among 94 928 children in primary schoolchildren in Hong Kong.

A total of 649 sex-, age-, and class-matched controls were successfully matched to the 83 patients in a ratio of 8:1, except for 4 patients in special classes (for whom 2, 4, 5, and 6 controls were matched, respectively). The selected controls differed significantly from those disease-free classmates not chosen as controls by sex (39.4% vs 52.6% males; $\chi^2$ test, $P<.001$) and age (mean±SD, 9.05±1.95 vs 8.85±1.74 years; unpaired $t$ test, $P=.02$), but there was no significant difference in their distribution of tuberculin response ($\chi^2$ test, $P=.17$).

The cases and matched controls were comparable by sex (39.8% vs 39.4% males; $\chi^2$ test, $P=.96$) and age (mean±SD, 8.97±1.88 vs 9.05±1.95 years; paired $t$ test, $P=.75$). The distribution of tuberculin responses between cases and controls is summarized in **Table 1**. **Table 2** shows the results of univariate conditional logistic regression analysis of the tuberculin responses for all identified active TB cases and their controls. Similar results were obtained when analysis was restricted to the 30 culture-confirmed cases and their matched controls.

On applying the incidence rate derived in part 1 and the odds ratios of Table 2 to the 94 928 primary schoolchildren tuberculin tested in 1999, the respective incidences of active TB among different tuberculin reactors are summarized in **Table 3**. **Table 4** lists the proportions of the student population to be covered and the number of active TB cases preventable within 5 years by using different cutoffs, based on the estimations shown in Table 3.

**Table 1. Comparison of Tuberculin Responses Between Active TB Patients and Their Sex-, Age-, and Class-Matched Controls During the School BCG Revaccination Program***

| Tuberculin Reaction, mm | Patients (n = 83) | Classmates (n = 649) |
|---|---|---|
| 0-4 | 33 (39.8) | 454 (70.0) |
| 5-9 | 5 (6.0) | 64 (9.9) |
| 10-14 | 13 (15.7) | 94 (14.5) |
| 15-19 | 18 (21.7) | 30 (4.6) |
| ≥20 | 14 (16.9) | 7 (1.1) |

Abbreviation: TB, tuberculosis.
*Data are given as number (percentage) of each group. $P<.001$ ($\chi^2$ test) for the difference between groups.

## COMMENT

In this study, tuberculin reaction size was a strong predictor of active TB. The overall pattern was similar to the J-shaped pattern reported in northern Malawi, apart from the absence of a definite trough among those with low-grade sensitivity.[6] The risk started to increase for the 10- to 14-mm group, and increased sharply for a reaction size of 15 mm or more, supporting previous studies[7] that the latter is more indicative of infection among subjects with a previous BCG vaccination. By using 10 mm as the cutoff, 482 children have to be treated to prevent a single case of active TB within 5 years (Table 4). Treatment will

**Table 2. Effect of Tuberculin Responses on Relative Odds of Active TB in Univariate Conditional Logistic Regression Analysis***

| Tuberculin Reaction Category, mm | Odds Ratio (95% Confidence Interval) |
|---|---|
| 0-4 | 0.022 (0.007-0.072) |
| 5-9 | 0.022 (0.005-0.094) |
| 10-14 | 0.047 (0.013-0.168) |
| 15-19 | 0.272 (0.078-0.940) |
| ≥20 | 1.000 |

Abbreviation: TB, tuberculosis.

*The case-control ratio was 1:8; cases and controls were matched for sex, age, and class (83 classes in total). The model coefficients were as follows: −2 log likelihood = 280.49 and $\chi^2$ = 117.24 ($P$<.001).

**Table 3. Estimated Incidence of Active TB Among Children in Primary School Tested With Tuberculin Skin Test in 1999**

| Tuberculin Reaction, mm | No. (%) of Schoolchildren | Active TB Rate per 100 000 Person-Years* | No. (%) of Cases per Year† |
|---|---|---|---|
| 0-4 | 68 099 (71.7) | 7.5 (2.4-24.5) | 5.1 (39.8) |
| 5-9 | 10 195 (10.7) | 7.5 (1.7-32.0) | 0.8 (6.2) |
| 10-14 | 13 250 (14.0) | 16.0 (4.4-57.2) | 2.1 (16.4) |
| 15-19 | 2722 (2.9) | 92.6 (26.6-320.2) | 2.5 (19.5) |
| ≥20 | 662 (0.7) | 340.6 (163.3-626.4) | 2.3 (18.0) |
| Overall | 94 928 (100.0) | 13.4 (5.6-40.6) | 12.8 (100.0) |

Abbreviation: TB, tuberculosis.

*The 95% confidence intervals are given in parentheses, and those for tuberculin reaction categories other than 20 mm or more were estimated by keeping the TB incidence for the latter at the mean level.

†Individual percentages may not total 100 because of rounding.

**Table 4. Effect of Using Different Cutoffs in Tuberculin Skin Testing on Proportions of Schoolchildren Eligible for Treatment of Latent TB Infection and Potential TB Cases Preventable Within 5 Years**

| Cutoff, mm | No. (%) of Schoolchildren Eligible | No. (%) of TB Cases Prevented in 5 y* | No. of Children Needed to Treat to Prevent 1 Case† |
|---|---|---|---|
| ≥0 | 94 928 (100.0) | 63.8 (100.0) | 1487 (469-4533) |
| ≥5 | 26 829 (28.3) | 38.3 (60.0) | 700 (226-2092) |
| ≥10 | 16 634 (17.5) | 34.5 (54.1) | 482 (163-1391) |
| ≥15 | 3384 (3.6) | 23.9 (37.5) | 141 (53-375) |
| ≥20 | 662 (0.7) | 11.3 (17.7) | 59 (32-122) |

Abbreviation: TB, tuberculosis.

*Assuming 100% efficacy of treatment of latent TB infection.

†Data in parentheses are 95% confidence intervals.

cover 17.5% of the cohort, but prevent only 54.1% of all active TB cases. If the cutoff is increased to 15 mm, only 141 children need treatment to prevent a case of active TB. Only 3.6% of children will be subjected to treatment, but an additional 16.6% of cases will be missed.

Among schoolchildren incidentally found to have a tuberculin reaction at 20 mm or more, the annual incidence of active TB was as high as 341 per 100 000. However, their risk of disease falls far short of the figure of 12.9% within the first year,[8] and 1.6% per year from the second year to the seventh year[1] for unvaccinated tuberculin-positive TB contacts. Among those children with a tuberculin reaction between 15 and 19 mm, the risk was 92.6 per 100 000, which was comparable with the figure of 90.4 per 100 000 reported among similar vaccinated children in Singapore.[9] Such risk is just a quarter of those with a tuberculin reaction at 20 mm or more. Because most of both groups were likely to have been infected, more recent infection might have contributed to the greater risk among those with the strongest tuberculin reaction.

Children from birth to the age of 14 years have a lower risk of active TB compared with those at other ages.[2] In 2001, the TB notification rates were 5.4, 3.5, 13.5, and 52.5 per 100 000 for those aged 0 to 4, 5 to 9, 10 to 14, and 15 to 19 years, respectively. A question naturally arises whether tuberculin-positive children at the mean age of 9 years may have a higher risk of developing active TB in the late teens. However, the risk of developing disease has been reported to decrease substantially with the passage of time after infection.[8] In high-prevalence areas, substantial ongoing transmission is expected, and the protective effect of isoniazid treatment has been well reported to decrease with time, at least among human immunodeficiency virus–infected subjects.[10,11] Among a cohort of tuberculin reactors (aged 1-18 years) detected during a BCG trial from 1949 to 1951, the annual risk of developing active TB (averaged over 20 years) was also lowest among those aged 7 to 12 years at recruitment.[12] Even in low-prevalence areas, 55% of immigrants with TB had the condition diagnosed within the first 5 years of arrival.[13] Considering the less than 100% protective efficacy of the recommended treatment, compounded by often poor adherence and sometimes isoniazid resistance, in field conditions,[14,15] the numbers needed to treat to prevent an active TB case are unlikely to deviate excessively from those previously estimated.

One unit of PPD RT23 was used in this study, not the 5 U of PPD standard commonly used in the United States. Stronger reactions might be expected if 2 U of PPD RT23 (the equivalent of 5 U of PPD standard[16,17]) were used. This would increase the percentage of children to be covered with each cutoff, and the number of children to be treated to prevent a single case of active TB. Because children with a tuberculin reaction at 10 mm or more were not revaccinated, BCG revaccination would not confound the results for any cutoffs more than 9 mm, even if there was any protective effect.

Undernotification is always a point of concern for all notifiable diseases.[18] In a local audit of TB notifications by reviewing discharge codes, microbiological reports, or hospital reports in 1995, the undernotification rates were 3.0%, 27.6%, and 31.4% for chest clinics, chest hospitals, and general hospitals, respectively.[19] After a series of improvement measures, notifications from sources other than chest clinics increased drastically,[20] in line with what was previously observed in 2 London, England, hospitals.[21,22] With incomplete notification, some degree of underestimation is likely, but it would be expected to affect all tuberculin reactor categories. Because tuberculin testing was done during primary school age, the bulk of the 1999 cohort should be in the age range of 10 to 14 years from the time of tuberculin testing to the end of 2003. The estimated incidence of active TB for the study cohort was 13.4 per 100 000 person-years (Table 3), while the reported incidences from the territory-wide TB notification registry were 13.5, 8.5, and 10.3 per 100 000 person-years for children aged 10 to 14 years in 2001,[2] 2002,[23] and 2003,[24] respectively. Even if we apply the relative risks derived from part 2 directly to the notification figures for the same years, there will not be any substantial changes in the various estimates in Table 3 and 4.

Considering the sharp contrast in disease risk between those with a tuberculin reaction of less than 15 mm and those with a reaction of 15 mm or more (Table 2), it might be worthwhile to reexamine the existing tuberculin test screening criterion in children with clear documentation of BCG vaccination, at least outside the contact settings. A tuberculin reaction is known to wane rapidly after neonatal BCG vaccination.[25,26] However, in a study[27] on 2588 randomly selected Saudi children, while the tuberculin-positive rate was not significantly different between vaccinated and unvaccinated children at the age of 5 years, the tuberculin sensitivity increased more steeply with age in the BCG-vaccinated than in the unvaccinated children, so that the difference between the 2 groups became statistically significant in those aged 12 and 13 years. Because booster phenomenon is also well reported in BCG-vaccinated children,[28] the possibility of interaction with ongoing environmental antigenic stimulation cannot be completely excluded. An interferon $\gamma$ assay measuring the production of interferon $\gamma$ in T lymphocytes on stimulation with PPD is not expected to differentiate false-positive cross-reactors from those with genuine infection.[29] However, a modified version of that test using ESAT-6 and CFP-10, antigens not present in BCG, has recently been reported to show a high degree of sensitivity and specificity for culture-confirmed TB, which is unaffected by previous BCG vaccination.[30,31] The modified test also showed a better correlation with the degree of exposure than the tuberculin test in a mass contact screening exercise.[32] It is conceivable that an adapted version of the test may help to sort out the truly infected children among BCG-vaccinated immigrants from high-prevalence areas. More systematic studies are, therefore, warranted in this direction.

**Accepted for Publication:** September 14, 2005.
**Correspondence:** Chi Chiu Leung, MB, Wanchai Chest Clinic, 99 Kennedy Rd, Wanchai, Hong Kong (cc_leung@dh.gov.hk).
**Author Contributions:** Dr Leung had full access to all the data in the study and takes responsibility for the integrity of the data and the accuracy of the data analysis.
**Financial Disclosure:** None.

## REFERENCES

1. American Thoracic Society. Targeted tuberculin testing and treatment of latent tuberculosis infection. *MMWR Recomm Rep.* 2000;49(RR-6):1-51.
2. Hong Kong Tuberculosis and Chest Service. *Annual Report of Tuberculosis and Chest Service for 2001.* Hong Kong: Dept of Health; 2002.
3. WHO. Expanded Program on Immunization: immunization schedules in the WHO Western Pacific region, 1995. *WHO Wkly Epidemic Rec.* 1996;71:133-138.
4. Leung CC, Tam CM, Chan SL, et al. Efficacy of the BCG revaccination program in a cohort given BCG vaccination at birth in Hong Kong. *Int J Tuberc Lung Dis.* 2001;5:717-723.
5. Campbell MJ. *Statistics at Square Two: Understanding Modern Statistical Applications in Medicine.* London, England: BMJ Books; 2001:51-55.
6. Fine PE, Sterne JA, Ponnighaus JM, Rees RJ. Delayed-type hypersensitivity, mycobacterial vaccines and protective immunity. *Lancet.* 1994;344:1245-1249.
7. American Thoracic Society. Diagnostic standards and classification of tuberculosis in adults and children. *Am J Respir Crit Care Med.* 2000;161:1376-1395.
8. Ferebee SH. Controlled chemoprophylaxis trials in tuberculosis: a general review. *Bibl Tuberc.* 1970;26:28-106.
9. Chee CB, Soh CH, Boudville IC, et al. Interpretation of the tuberculin skin test in *Mycobacterium bovis* BCG-vaccinated Singaporean schoolchildren. *Am J Respir Crit Care Med.* 2001;164:958-961.
10. Quigley MA, Mwinga A, Hosp M, et al. Long-term effect of preventive therapy for tuberculosis in a cohort of HIV-infected Zambian adults. *AIDS.* 2001;15:215-222.
11. Woldehanna S, Volmink J. Treatment of latent tuberculosis infection in HIV infected persons. *Cochrane Database Syst Rev.* 2004;(1):CD000171.
12. Comstock GW, Livesay VT, Woolpert SF. The prognosis of a positive tuberculin reaction in childhood and adolescence. *Am J Epidemiol.* 1974;99:131-138.
13. McKenna MT, McCray E, Onorato I. The epidemiology of tuberculosis among foreign-born persons in the United States, 1986-1993. *N Engl J Med.* 1995;332:1071-1076.
14. International Union Against Tuberculosis. Committee on Prophylaxis Efficacy of various durations of isoniazid preventive therapy for tuberculosis. *Bull World Health Organ.* 1982;60:555-564.
15. Ferebee SH, Mount FW. Tuberculosis morbidity in a controlled trial of the prophylactic use of isoniazid among household contacts. *Am Rev Respir Dis.* 1962;85:490-510.
16. Teixeira L, Maciel E, Dutra ME, Perkins MD, Johnson JL, do Valle Dettoni V. Simultaneous comparison of reactivity to purified protein derivative RT-23 and Tubersol in health care workers in Vitoria, Brazil. *Int J Tuberc Lung Dis.* 2000;4:1074-1077.
17. Munoz-Barret JM, Macias-Hernandez AE, Hernandez-Ramos I, et al. Comparative tuberculin reactivity to two protein derivatives. *Rev Invest Clin.* 1996;48:377-381.
18. Jenkinson D. Whooping cough: what proportion of cases is notified in an epidemic? *BMJ.* 1983;287:185-186.
19. Health Services Research Group, Department of Community Medicine, University of Hong Kong. *Services for the Treatment of Patients With Tuberculosis in Hong Kong: Final Report to the Project Steering Group.* Hong Kong: University of Hong Kong; 2000.
20. Hong Kong Tuberculosis and Chest Service. *Annual Report of the Tuberculosis and Chest Service for 1999.* Hong Kong: Dept of Health; 2000.
21. Sheldon CD, King K, Cock H, Wilkinson P, Barnes NC. Notification of tuberculosis: how many cases are never reported? *Thorax.* 1992;47:1015-1018.
22. Brown JS, Wells F, Duckworth G, Paul EA, Barnes NC. Improving notification rates for tuberculosis. *BMJ.* 1995;310:974.
23. Hong Kong Tuberculosis and Chest Service. *Annual Report of Tuberculosis and Chest Service for 2002.* Hong Kong: Dept of Health; 2003.
24. Hong Kong Tuberculosis and Chest Service. *Annual Report of Tuberculosis and Chest Service for 2003.* Hong Kong: Dept of Health; 2004.
25. Bozaykut A, Ipek IO, Ozkars MY, et al. Effect of BCG vaccine on tuberculin skin tests in 1-6-year-old children. *Acta Paediatr.* 2002;91:235-238.
26. Karalliedde S, Katugaha LP, Uragoda CG. Tuberculin response of Sri Lankan children after BCG vaccination at birth. *Tubercle.* 1987;68:33-38.
27. Al-Kassimi FA, Abdullah AK, al-Orainey IO, et al. The significance of positive Mantoux reactions in BCG-vaccinated children. *Tubercle.* 1991;72:101-104.
28. Sepulveda RL, Burr C, Ferrer X, et al. Booster effect of tuberculin testing in healthy 6-year-old school children vaccinated with Bacillus Calmette-Guerin at birth in Santiago, Chile. *Pediatr Infect Dis J.* 1988;7:578-581.
29. Mazurek GH, LoBue PA, Daley CL, et al. Comparison of a whole-blood interferon $\gamma$ assay with tuberculin skin testing for detecting latent *Mycobacterium tuberculosis* infection. *JAMA.* 2001;286:1740-1747.
30. Lalvani A, Pathan AA, Durkan H, et al. Enhanced contact tracing and spatial tracking of *Mycobacterium tuberculosis* infection by enumeration of antigen-specific T cells. *Lancet.* 2001;357:2017-2021.
31. Mori T, Sakatani M, Yamagishi F, et al. Specific detection of tuberculosis infection: an interferon-$\gamma$–based assay using new antigens. *Am J Respir Crit Care Med.* 2004;170:59-64.
32. Ewer K, Deeks J, Alvarez L, et al. Comparison of T-cell–based assay with tuberculin skin test for diagnosis of *Mycobacterium tuberculosis* infection in a school tuberculosis outbreak. *Lancet.* 2003;361:1168-1173.

# Health-Related Quality of Life During the First Year After Traumatic Brain Injury

*Melissa L. McCarthy, ScD; Ellen J. MacKenzie, PhD; Dennis R. Durbin, MD, MS; Mary E. Aitken, MD, MPH; Kenneth M. Jaffe, MD; Charles N. Paidas, MD; Beth S. Slomine, PhD; Andrea M. Dorsch, PhD; James R. Christensen, MD; Ru Ding, MS; for the Children's Health After Trauma Study Group*

**Objectives:** To document health-related quality of life (HRQOL) of children with traumatic brain injury (TBI) and to examine the relationship between TBI severity and HRQOL during the first year after injury.

**Design:** Prospective cohort study.

**Setting:** Four pediatric level I trauma centers.

**Patients:** Children with TBI (n=330).

**Main Exposure:** Traumatic brain injury.

**Main Outcome Measures:** A primary caregiver completed telephone interviews at baseline, 3 months, and 12 months to measure the child's HRQOL using the Pediatric Quality of Life Inventory. The HRQOL outcomes were modeled as a function of injury, patient characteristics, and family characteristics using longitudinal, multivariable regression.

**Results:** A considerable proportion of children had impaired HRQOL at 3 months (42% of children) and 12 months (40% of children) after injury. Multiple dimensions of HRQOL were negatively affected among children with moderate or severe TBI (decrease of 3.7 to 17.6) ($P<.05$) and did not improve significantly over time. Concomitant lower extremity fractures and spinal injuries resulted in large declines in overall HRQOL, particularly at 3 months after injury (decrease of 12.9 and 8.1, respectively) ($P<.05$). The HRQOL scores were also reduced by preexisting psychosocial conditions (decrease of 2.9 to 12.3), impaired family functioning (decrease of 5.1 to 6.8), having Medicaid coverage or being uninsured (decrease of 3.1 to 5.5), and single-parent households (decrease of 3.2 to 3.4) ($P<.05$).

**Conclusions:** Moderate or severe TBI resulted in measurable declines in children's HRQOL after injury. Injury-related factors impacted HRQOL more compared with patient and family characteristics during the first year after injury.

*Arch Pediatr Adolesc Med. 2006;160:252-260*

DURING THE PAST DECADE, a number of instruments have been developed to measure children's health-related quality of life (HRQOL).[1-9] These instruments have 3 distinguishing features: (1) they measure function at the level of the person (as opposed to the organ or organ system); (2) they measure outcome from the child's or parent's perspective (as opposed to the clinician's); and (3) they measure health as a multidimensional construct that includes physical, social, and emotional well-being. Furthermore, they can be self-administered or administered over the phone, making them practical for clinical and research applications.[10,11]

Although numerous studies have documented the neurobehavioral consequences following traumatic brain injury (TBI) in children,[12-26] only 2 have focused primarily on children's HRQOL.[27,28] Interestingly, neither found a significant relationship between the severity of TBI and HRQOL.[27,28] Stancin et al[27] used the Child Health Questionnaire to measure HRQOL at 4 years after injury among 84 subjects with moderate to severe TBI and 50 children with an orthopedic injury. Although the psychosocial health of children with severe TBI was poorer compared with those with an orthopedic injury when examined alone, no significant differences remained after controlling for socioeconomic and premorbid problems. Coster et al[28] also did not find a significant relationship between TBI severity and HRQOL using the Pediatric Evaluation of Disability Inventory among 57 young children with TBI at 6 months after injury. The findings from these 2 studies are surprising given that previous research that has

**Author Affiliations** are listed at the end of this article.
**Group Information:** The Children's Health After Trauma Study Group investigators are listed at the end of the article.

measured neuropsychological and behavioral outcomes among children with moderate to severe TBI has noted significant and persistent deficits in this patient population long after the acute injury.[13,15,17,20,24,29,30] It could be that the HRQOL instruments used in the studies by Stancin and colleagues and Coster and colleagues were not sensitive enough to discriminate among different levels of TBI severity, or it could be that HRQOL is more affected by premorbid and family characteristics than injury-related factors.

The purpose of this article is to document HRQOL among children hospitalized with TBI during the first year after injury and to examine the relationship between severity of injury and HRQOL after adjusting for premorbid, socioeconomic, and family characteristics. To do this, we compared the outcomes of children hospitalized with TBI of varying severity using the Pediatric Quality of Life Inventory (PedsQL), an instrument that we previously demonstrated to be a reliable and valid measure of HRQOL among children with TBI.[31]

## METHODS

### STUDY POPULATION

Children aged 5 to 15 years who were discharged alive after being hospitalized 1 or more nights at 1 of 4 level I pediatric trauma center hospitals (Johns Hopkins Hospital, Baltimore, Md; Children's Hospital of Philadelphia, Philadelphia, Pa; Harborview Medical Center, Seattle, Wash; and Arkansas Children's Hospital, Little Rock) for treatment of TBI with an Abbreviated Injury Scale (AIS) severity score of 2 or greater were eligible for the study.[32]

Children were excluded for the following reasons: (1) they or their parents were non-English speaking; (2) they had a preexisting medical condition that seriously impacted preinjury physical (eg, amputation), psychological (eg, schizophrenia or bipolar disorder), or cognitive (eg, mental retardation or prior TBI-related hospitalization) function; or (3) they were part of a suspected child abuse case. To increase the generalizability of the study and to evaluate the effects of preinjury risk factors on HRQOL, children with preinjury learning disabilities or behavioral problems were eligible.

The sample was stratified by AIS severity to enroll adequate numbers of children with more severe TBI. Consecutive children within each study group were enrolled until there were approximately 95 children with head injuries with AIS scores of 2, 3, and 4. The target number for children with head injuries with AIS scores of 5 was 50 because they are less frequent.

### PROCEDURES

The institutional review boards of all of the 4 participating sites approved the study. Between January 15, 2002, and July 31, 2003, the study coordinators identified 536 children with an eligible injury. However, 98 (18%) of the children were deemed ineligible on full review of all of the demographic and injury characteristics. The study coordinators approached all of the eligible children and their families. Those who consented agreed to complete 3 telephone interviews over a 1-year period and to allow pertinent injury and treatment information to be abstracted from the child's medical record.

All of the interviews were conducted by a professional survey research firm with a primary caregiver of the injured child. The first, or baseline, interview conducted within 3 weeks of the initial hospitalization (median, 16 days) was designed to measure the child's preinjury HRQOL and to obtain background information on the child and his or her family. During the baseline interview, the respondent was instructed to think of the child 1 month prior to the injury when answering the HRQOL questions. During the follow-up interviews, the respondent was asked to rate the child's HRQOL during the previous month.

### MEASUREMENT

Health-related quality of life was measured with the PedsQL.[1,33] The PedsQL was selected over other pediatric HRQOL instruments primarily because it advocates a modular assessment strategy that allows for the integration of generic and disease-specific scales. For this study, the PedsQL generic instrument was supplemented with a cognitive function scale since cognitive dysfunction is a common and serious impairment following TBI.[34] Numerous studies[31,35-42] have confirmed the PedsQL to be a reliable and valid instrument for measuring HRQOL among children with different types of illnesses or injuries, including TBI.

The PedsQL generic core comprises 23 items that measure 4 health domains: (1) physical functioning, (2) emotional functioning, (3) social functioning, and (4) school functioning. The scales can be aggregated into summary scales of physical health (same as the physical functioning scale), psychosocial health (emotional, social, and school functioning scales), and total health (all of the 4 scales). The PedsQL cognitive function scale comprises 6 items. All of the PedsQL scales have a possible range from 0 (poor health) to 100 (excellent health). Scale scores more than 1 SD below the healthy sample mean are considered impaired.[34,40]

The child's age, race, health insurance coverage, and the presence of preexisting physical or psychosocial health conditions were obtained from the respondent during the baseline interview. The most prevalent preexisting physical conditions were asthma (18%) and allergies (17%) whereas the most common psychosocial conditions were an attentional problem (12%), a learning disability (11%), and a behavioral problem (7%). The respondent was also queried about his or her age, race, marital status, highest grade in school completed, total annual income of the household, and relationship to the child. Finally, the general functioning scale of the Family Assessment Device was administered to the respondents.[43,44] This 12-item scale is a self-reported measure of overall family functioning.[43-45] The scale has a possible range of 1 to 4, and scores of 2 and higher are considered unhealthy family functioning.

The nature and severity of all of the injuries sustained were characterized according to the AIS.[32,46] This scale classifies more than 2000 injuries according to the body region of injury (eg, head, chest, lower extremity), type of structure involved (eg, nerve, vessel, bone), location of injury within the body region (eg, femur, tibia), and nature of injury (eg, abrasion, crush). The AIS grades each injury according to its associated threat to life on an ordinal scale from 1 (minor) to 6 (unsurvivable). Typical head injuries sustained by the study sample included a closed vault fracture (AIS score=2), comminuted vault fracture or subarachnoid hemorrhage (AIS score=3), epidural or subdural hematoma (AIS score=4), or a diffuse axonal injury (AIS score=5). To reflect overall injury severity, the New Injury Severity Scale score was computed. The New Injury Severity Scale score is the sum of the squares of the 3 most severe injuries sustained.[47] The New Injury Severity Scale score ranges from 0 to 75, and higher scores reflect greater severity. Finally, the mechanism of injury, hospital length of stay, and disposition were recorded for all of the subjects.

**Table 1. Percentage Distribution of Patient Characteristics of Subjects by Traumatic Brain Injury Severity**

| Patient Characteristic | Overall, % (n = 330) | Mild TBI, % (n = 185) | Moderate TBI, % (n = 103) | Severe TBI, % (n = 42) |
|---|---|---|---|---|
| Age, y | | | | |
| 5-7 | 28.4 | 27.0 | 35.9 | 16.7 |
| 8-10 | 26.4 | 28.7 | 26.2 | 16.7 |
| 11-12 | 20.3 | 20.5 | 15.5 | 30.9 |
| 13-15 | 24.9 | 23.8 | 22.4 | 35.7 |
| Sex, male | 69.4 | 69.2 | 68.9 | 71.4 |
| Race | | | | |
| White | 68.5 | 65.4 | 68.9 | 81.0 |
| Nonwhite | 31.5 | 34.6 | 31.1 | 19.0 |
| Health insurance | | | | |
| Uninsured | 0.3 | 0.5 | 0.0 | 0.0 |
| Commercial | 73.3 | 71.9 | 77.7 | 69.1 |
| Medicaid | 26.4 | 27.6 | 22.3 | 30.9 |
| Preexisting physical condition | 37.9 | 35.1 | 41.7 | 40.5 |
| Preexisting psychosocial condition | 25.1 | 22.7 | 27.2 | 30.9 |
| Normal total PedsQL score at baseline | 89.1 | 88.1 | 89.3 | 92.9 |

Abbreviations: PedsQL, Pediatric Quality of Life Inventory; TBI, traumatic brain injury.

## DATA ANALYSIS

First, we compared those who enrolled with those who did not by different patient and injury characteristics using a $\chi^2$ test of homogeneity. We also compared the distribution of different patient, respondent, and family characteristics by the severity of TBI sustained among those who enrolled. Second, we compared the mean PedsQL scale scores among the TBI severity groups by analysis of variance, and we examined the percentage of subjects with HRQOL outcomes that were 1 and 2 SDs lower than general population norms.[1,40] Because the PedsQL scale scores of children who sustained head injuries with AIS scores of 2 and 3 were similar, these 2 groups were combined. Throughout this article, head injuries with AIS scores of 2 and 3 are referred to as mild TBI, head injuries with AIS scores of 4 as moderate TBI, and head injuries with AIS scores of 5 as severe TBI.

Finally, to examine the impact of TBI on HRQOL over time controlling for the influence of other factors, generalized estimating equation modeling was used.[48] Selected PedsQL scale scores of all of the enrolled subjects were modeled separately as a function of time, head injury severity (maximum AIS score of the head-body region), the presence of an injury with an AIS score of 2 or higher to each other body region, mechanism of injury, Glasgow Coma Scale score, patient characteristics (ie, age, race, sex, preexisting conditions), respondent characteristics (ie, age, race, sex, relationship to child, education), and family characteristics (ie, family functioning, marital status, total household income, health insurance coverage). All of the independent variables were initially forced into the models and dropped sequentially based on their association with the outcomes. Possible interactions were tested and regression diagnostics were examined to evaluate multicollinearity and goodness of fit. Variables were considered statistically significant at $P \leq .05$ and were noted as borderline significant at $.05 < P \leq .10$. Only variables that were significant at $P \leq .10$ were included in the final models.

## RESULTS

Of the 438 children eligible for the study, 381 (87%) consented and 330 (75%) enrolled. Children who did not enroll were more likely to lack health insurance (10%) than those who enrolled (<1%) ($P < .05$). In addition, children who did not enroll were hospitalized longer than those who enrolled (8.3 vs 5.3 days, respectively) ($P \leq .01$). Of the 330 who enrolled, 302 (92%) completed the interview at 3 months and 288 (87%) completed the interview at 12 months. Seventeen subjects (5%) did not complete either follow-up interview. Those who were not followed up were more likely to be younger, nonwhite, and part of a single-parent household compared with those who were followed up ($P \leq .05$) (data not shown).

**Table 1** and **Table 2** display the patient, respondent, and family characteristics of the sample by the severity of TBI sustained. The mean age of all of the enrolled subjects was 10.4 years (range, 5.1-15.9 years). Subjects were more likely to be male (69%), white (69%), and in good health prior to the injury (89%). There were no significant differences in patient characteristics by the severity of TBI sustained (all $P > .10$). The respondents for children with severe TBI were more likely to be the father (31%) compared with respondents for children with mild (12%) or moderate (13%) TBI ($P \leq .05$). A greater proportion of respondents for children with mild TBI had not completed high school (24%) than respondents for children with moderate (11%) or severe (10%) TBI ($P = .001$). Finally, the respondents for children with moderate and severe TBI reported better preinjury family functioning (94% and 93%, respectively) than respondents for children with mild TBI (79%) ($P < .05$) (Table 2).

Traffic-related injuries (39%) and falls (36%) were the most common injuries (**Table 3**). The mean New Injury Severity Scale score was 21 (range, 4-66). Subjects with severe TBI were significantly more likely to sustain a thoracic (33%), abdominal (17%), spinal (17%), or upper extremity (26%) fracture than subjects with mild TBI (AIS score=2) (4%, 3%, 3%, and 9%, respectively) ($P < .01$).

Children with severe TBI had significantly poorer HRQOL scores after injury ($P \leq .05$) than children with mild TBI, except for social functioning (not significantly different at 3 months only [$P = .15$]) and emotional functioning (not significantly different at 3 or 12 months [$P = .51$ and $P = .15$, respectively]) (**Table 4**).

**Table 2. Percentage Distribution of Respondent and Family Characteristics of Subjects by Traumatic Brain Injury Severity**

| Respondent or Family Characteristic | Overall, % (n = 330) | Mild TBI, % (n = 185) | Moderate TBI, % (n = 103) | Severe TBI, % (n = 42) |
|---|---|---|---|---|
| Respondent* | | | | |
| Mother | 80.3 | 81.1 | 83.5 | 69.0 |
| Father | 14.6 | 11.9 | 12.6 | 31.0 |
| Other | 5.1 | 7.0 | 3.9 | 0.0 |
| Respondent age, y | | | | |
| 21-34 | 33.3 | 36.2 | 31.1 | 26.2 |
| 35-40 | 30.9 | 30.8 | 32.0 | 28.6 |
| ≥41 | 35.8 | 33.0 | 36.9 | 45.2 |
| Educational level of respondent* | | | | |
| <High school graduate | 18.2 | 24.3 | 10.7 | 9.5 |
| High school graduate | 33.3 | 31.9 | 36.9 | 31.0 |
| Some college | 26.7 | 22.2 | 32.0 | 33.3 |
| College graduate | 21.8 | 21.6 | 20.4 | 26.2 |
| Marital status of respondent | | | | |
| Married or partner | 63.6 | 66.0 | 62.1 | 57.1 |
| Not married or no partner | 36.4 | 34.0 | 37.9 | 42.9 |
| Total household income, $† | | | | |
| <20 000 | 18.3 | 18.8 | 16.7 | 20.0 |
| 20 000-49 999 | 36.0 | 35.9 | 38.5 | 30.0 |
| 50 000-99 999 | 34.0 | 34.3 | 36.5 | 27.5 |
| ≥100 000 | 11.7 | 11.0 | 8.3 | 22.5 |
| Healthy family functioning before injury* | 85.5 | 78.9 | 94.2 | 92.9 |

Abbreviation: TBI, traumatic brain injury.
*Difference is significant between study groups ($P \leq .05$).
†Data were missing for 10 subjects.

**Table 3. Percentage Distribution of Injury Characteristics of Subjects by Traumatic Brain Injury Severity**

| Injury Characteristic | Overall, % (n = 330) | Mild TBI, % (n = 185) | Moderate TBI, % (n = 103) | Severe TBI, % (n = 42) |
|---|---|---|---|---|
| Mechanism of injury* | | | | |
| Traffic related | 38.8 | 33.0 | 35.0 | 73.8 |
| Fall | 36.1 | 36.8 | 42.7 | 16.7 |
| Other | 25.1 | 30.2 | 22.3 | 9.5 |
| New Injury Severity Scale score* | | | | |
| 4 | 13.6 | 24.3 | 0.0 | 0.0 |
| 5-9 | 26.4 | 47.0 | 0.0 | 0.0 |
| 10-24 | 23.0 | 21.1 | 35.9 | 0.0 |
| ≥25 | 37.0 | 7.6 | 64.1 | 100.0 |
| Hospital length of stay, d* | | | | |
| 1-2 | 31.8 | 47.0 | 17.5 | 0.0 |
| 3 | 20.9 | 22.2 | 25.2 | 4.7 |
| 4-7 | 24.9 | 21.1 | 35.0 | 16.7 |
| ≥8 | 22.4 | 9.7 | 22.3 | 78.6 |
| Disposition* | | | | |
| Home | 84.2 | 94.6 | 84.5 | 19.1 |
| Rehabilitation hospital | 15.8 | 5.4 | 5.5 | 80.9 |
| Location of injury with AIS score ≥2 | | | | |
| Face | 12.7 | 11.9 | 9.7 | 3.8 |
| Thorax* | 8.2 | 3.8 | 5.8 | 33.3 |
| Abdomen* | 5.5 | 3.2 | 4.8 | 16.7 |
| Spine* | 5.2 | 3.2 | 3.9 | 16.7 |
| Upper extremity* | 11.2 | 8.6 | 9.7 | 26.2 |
| Lower extremity* | 16.1 | 15.1 | 12.6 | 28.6 |

Abbreviations: AIS, Abbreviated Injury Scale; TBI, traumatic brain injury.
*Difference is significant between study groups ($P \leq .05$).

When comparing children with severe TBI with those with moderate TBI, physical functioning was the only significant difference at both 3 and 12 months after injury ($P \leq .05$).

Using the total PedsQL score as an overall measure of HRQOL, **Figure 1** displays the proportion of children with impaired HRQOL by TBI severity. Overall, a considerable proportion of children had impaired HRQOL at 3 months

**Table 4. Mean Pediatric Quality of Life Inventory Scores by Traumatic Brain Injury Severity***

| PedsQL Scale | PedsQL Score Overall, Mean (n = 330) | PedsQL Score for Mild TBI, Mean (n = 185) | PedsQL Score for Moderate TBI, Mean (n = 103) | PedsQL Score for Severe TBI, Mean (n = 42) |
|---|---|---|---|---|
| Total | | | | |
| At baseline | 88.9 | 88.3 | 89.1 | 90.8 |
| At 3 mo† | 74.8 | 77.4 | 73.4 | 67.4 |
| At 12 mo† | 77.7 | 80.0 | 76.4 | 70.3 |
| Physical function | | | | |
| At baseline | 95.0 | 94.3 | 95.4 | 96.7 |
| At 3 mo† | 78.1 | 81.5 | 77.8 | 65.2 |
| At 12 mo† | 84.7 | 87.3 | 83.4 | 75.5 |
| Emotional function | | | | |
| At baseline | 86.0 | 85.4 | 86.7 | 87.0 |
| At 3 mo | 71.0 | 72.0 | 69.8 | 69.6 |
| At 12 mo | 73.1 | 74.9 | 70.9 | 70.1 |
| Social function | | | | |
| At baseline | 90.4 | 90.0 | 90.0 | 93.6 |
| At 3 mo | 78.7 | 80.3 | 77.5 | 75.4 |
| At 12 mo‡ | 80.9 | 83.2 | 79.1 | 75.1 |
| School function | | | | |
| At baseline | 84.1 | 83.6 | 84.1 | 86.0 |
| At 3 mo† | 71.2 | 75.4 | 68.7 | 59.1 |
| At 12 mo† | 72.2 | 74.2 | 72.3 | 62.9 |
| Psychosocial function | | | | |
| At baseline | 86.8 | 86.3 | 87.0 | 88.9 |
| At 3 mo | 73.7 | 76.0 | 72.0 | 68.2 |
| At 12 mo | 75.3 | 77.4 | 74.1 | 68.8 |
| Cognitive function | | | | |
| At baseline | 86.2 | 85.6 | 85.7 | 90.0 |
| At 3 mo† | 68.2 | 72.3 | 66.1 | 56.4 |
| At 12 mo† | 68.4 | 71.2 | 66.0 | 61.4 |

Abbreviations: PedsQL, Pediatric Quality of Life Inventory; TBI, traumatic brain injury.

*There were 433 subjects at baseline, 391 at 3 months after injury, and 377 at 12 months after injury.

†Difference is significant between at least 2 of the study groups ($P \leq .05$).

‡Difference is borderline significant between at least 2 of the study groups ($.05 < P < .10$).

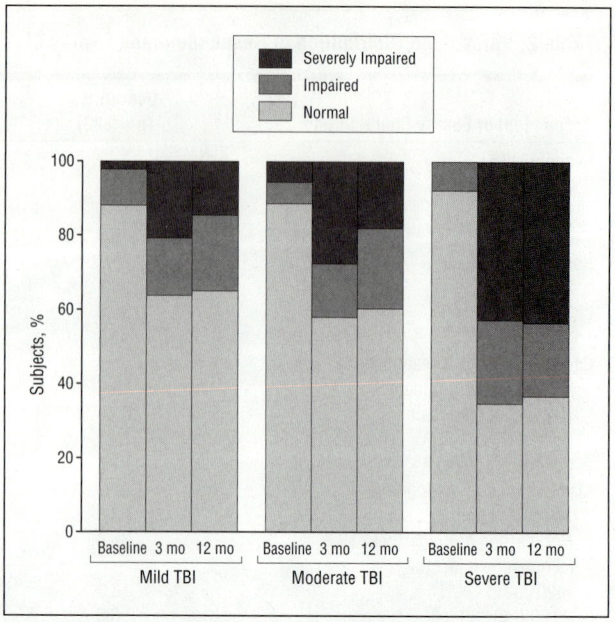


**Figure 1.** Percentage of subjects with impaired health-related quality of life by traumatic brain injury (TBI) severity at baseline, 3 months after injury, and 12 months after injury. The health-related quality of life is measured by the total Pediatric Quality of Life Inventory score. Severely impaired indicates 2 SDs below the general population norm; impaired, 1 SD below the general population norm.

(42%) and 12 months (40%) after injury. At 3 months after injury, more children with mild TBI (64%; relative risk=1.3; 95% confidence interval, 1.1-1.5) or moderate TBI (58%; relative risk=1.3; 95% confidence interval, 1.1-1.7) had normal HRQOL compared with children with severe TBI (35%). Similarly, at 12 months after injury, HRQOL of a relatively small proportion of children with severe TBI was normal (37%) compared with the other TBI groups (relative risk=0.4; 95% confidence interval, 0.2-0.7).

**Figure 2** compares the mean total PedsQL scores of the different study groups at 12 months after injury with scores for children with different medical conditions.[1,34-38,40-42,49,50] Health-related quality of life of children with mild TBI is similar to that of children with type 1 diabetes mellitus.[49] Health-related quality of life of children with moderate TBI is most similar to that of children who survived acute lymphoblastic leukemia whereas HRQOL of children with severe TBI most resembled that of children who were seen at a rheumatology or oncology clinic.[34,42,50]

**Table 5** displays the changes in HRQOL scores associated with different risk factors. Of note, the type and severity of injuries sustained are associated with the greatest reductions in HRQOL at 3 and 12 months after injury. Children with moderate or severe TBI had significantly poorer physical, cognitive, psychosocial, and overall HRQOL scores compared with children with mild TBI (all $P < .10$). Furthermore, there is a significant interaction effect between type and severity of injury and time. At 3 and 12 months after injury, the presence of a concomitant lower extremity fracture (decrease of 24.1 and 7.3, respectively), upper extremity fracture (decrease of 8.9 and 7.8, respectively), concomitant spinal injury (decrease of 13.2 and 7.7, respectively), or severe TBI (decrease of 11.7 and 9.6, respectively) ($P < .05$) was associated with the largest decrements in physical function. Although the impact of a concomitant lower extremity fracture and a concomitant spinal injury (ie, spinal fracture or dislocation) on physical function lessened over time, the impact of a concomitant upper extremity fracture or severe TBI did not. A similar pattern was noted for psychosocial function and overall HRQOL; however, the magnitude of the impact was not as strong (except for TBI), and only the impact of the concomitant lower extremity fracture lessened over time. None of the associated injuries to other body regions significantly influenced HRQOL (all $P > .10$). There was also a strong dose-response relationship noted between the severity of TBI and cognitive function (**Figure 3**).

The only patient characteristic to demonstrate a significant relationship to HRQOL was the presence of a preexisting psychosocial condition, which was associated with a significant reduction in all of the dimensions of HRQOL (range of decrease, 2.9-12.3) ($P \leq .05$).

Although none of the respondent characteristics significantly influenced HRQOL, several family character-

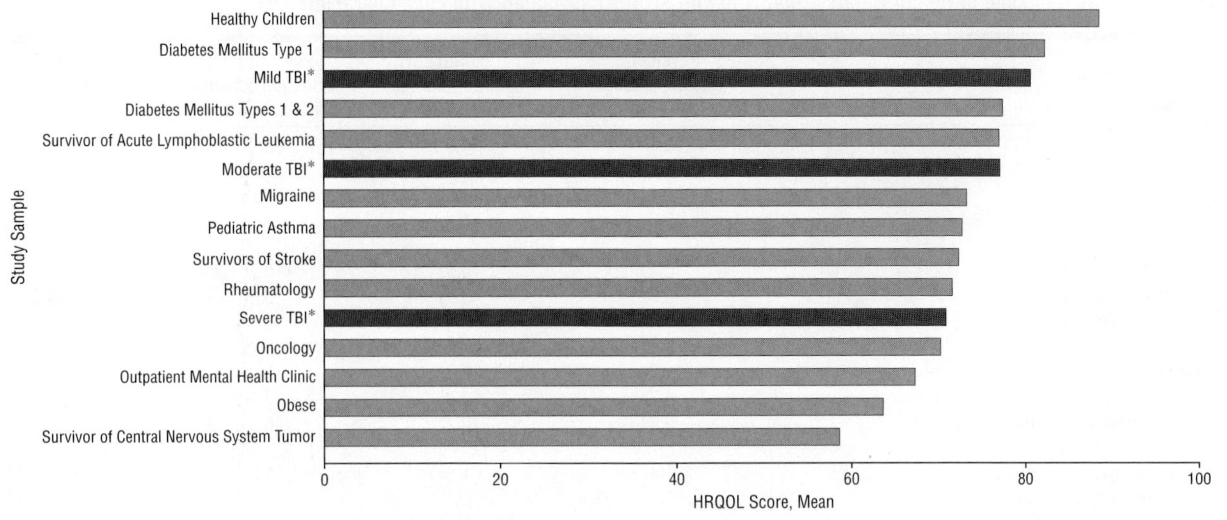


**Figure 2.** Mean health-related quality of life (HRQOL) scores among different study samples. The HRQOL is measured by the total Pediatric Quality of Life Inventory score. TBI indicates traumatic brain injury; asterisk, the HRQOL was measured at 12 months after injury.

istics did. The HRQOL scores of children who came from single-parent households were significantly lower than those of children who lived with both parents or 1 parent and a partner (range of decrease, 3.2-3.4) ($P \leq .05$). Similarly, unhealthy family functioning was associated with a significant reduction in HRQOL (range of decrease, 5.1-6.8) ($P \leq .05$). Finally, children who were covered by Medicaid or were uninsured had poorer HRQOL outcomes compared with children with private health insurance (range of decrease, 3.1-5.5) ($P \leq .05$). Family income was significantly related to HRQOL when examined alone (subjects with lower family income had poorer HRQOL outcomes compared with subjects from higher income households), but because of its strong correlation to health insurance coverage and marital status, it did not remain significant in the multivariable model (all $P > .10$; data not shown).

## COMMENT

This is the first study to our knowledge to document the HRQOL outcomes during the first year after injury of a cohort of children who sustained TBI severe enough to warrant hospitalization, and we found that the severity of injury significantly impacted HRQOL. Our findings are consistent with other studies[12-20,22-26] that have examined neuropsychological and behavioral outcomes following TBI. All of the dimensions of HRQOL measurably declined among children who sustained severe TBI and did not improve over time. With the exception of physical function, multiple dimensions of HRQOL were also negatively impacted among children who sustained moderate TBI.

Our results suggest that there is a strong relationship between the severity of TBI and HRQOL during the first year after injury. Coster et al[28] may not have found a significant association between TBI severity and HRQOL during the first 6 months after injury because the majority of their patients sustained mild TBI. In a multivariable analysis, Stancin et al[27] also did not find a relationship between TBI severity and HRQOL as measured by the Child Health Questionnaire. Although it could be that the Child Health Questionnaire is not sufficiently sensitive for children with TBI, it seems more likely that the relationship between TBI severity and HRQOL weakens over time. Since numerous studies[16,17,20,22-24] have demonstrated that children with severe TBI have persistent long-term deficits that should negatively impact HRQOL, it will be important in future research to measure HRQOL outcomes multiple times over a long follow-up period to determine how HRQOL and the factors that influence it change over time.

The results of this study demonstrate the importance of measuring the impact of associated injuries on children's health. The poorest HRQOL outcomes were among children who sustained TBI and an associated extremity fracture or spinal injury (ie, spinal fractures or dislocations). These results concur with earlier studies[51,52] that noted that a significant proportion of children who sustained an extremity injury had physical and role limitations 1 year later. We also found that a small but significant proportion of children with extremity fractures, particularly lower extremity fractures, had impaired HRQOL at 1 year after injury.[53] MacKenzie et al[54] also found that among adult trauma patients, injuries to the head, spine, or extremities (particularly lower extremities) were more frequently associated with functional limitations after injury compared with injuries to other body regions.

Children with moderate or severe TBI had worse physical and psychosocial functioning during the first year after injury compared with children with mild TBI. Evidence that children who sustain moderate to severe TBI are at higher risk of developing a psychiatric disorder after injury is beginning to accumulate.[55,56] Other researchers[13,15,29,57,58] have also found that children who sustain moderate to severe TBI exhibit more depressive symptoms, behavioral problems, and difficulties at school compared with children with an orthopedic injury.

**Table 5. Estimated Change in Health-Related Quality of Life Scores Associated With Each Characteristic***

| Characteristic† | Physical Function, Change in Scale Score | Cognitive Function, Change in Scale Score | Psychosocial Function, Change in Scale Score | Total PedsQL, Change in Scale Score |
|---|---|---|---|---|
| Intercept | 99.2 | 91.9 | 92.9 | 94.4 |
| Time | | | | |
| 3 mo (baseline) | −7.9‡ | −11.6‡ | −8.2‡ | −8.1‡ |
| 12 mo (baseline) | −5.5‡ | −13.2‡ | −8.2‡ | −7.5‡ |
| Head injury severity | | | | |
| Moderate TBI (mild TBI) | 0.4 | −0.3 | 0.2 | 0.2 |
| Severe TBI (mild TBI) | 2.7‡ | 5.4‡ | 3.3§ | 3.2‡ |
| Head injury severity and time | | | | |
| Moderate TBI at 3 mo (mild TBI at 3 mo) | −5.8‡ | −7.1‡ | −5.2‡ | −5.3‡ |
| Severe TBI at 3 mo (mild TBI at 3 mo) | −11.7‡ | −17.6‡ | −7.2§ | −8.2‡ |
| Moderate TBI at 12 mo (mild TBI at 12 mo) | −4.7‡ | −4.7§ | −3.3§ | −3.7‡ |
| Severe TBI at 12 mo (mild TBI at 12 mo) | −9.6‡ | −10.7‡ | −6.5‡ | −7.3‡ |
| Concomitant LE fracture | | | | |
| LE fracture (no LE fracture) | 1.4 | 1.9 | 2.5 | 2.2 |
| Concomitant LE fracture and time | | | | |
| LE fracture at 3 mo (no LE fracture at 3 mo) | −24.1‡ | −5.9 | −9.2‡ | −12.9‡ |
| LE fracture at 12 mo (no LE fracture at 12 mo) | −7.3§ | −0.9 | −2.0 | −3.3 |
| Concomitant UE fracture | | | | |
| UE fracture (no UE fracture) | 1.9 | 4.0 | 0.2 | 0.7 |
| Concomitant UE fracture and time | | | | |
| UE fracture at 3 mo (no UE fracture at 3 mo) | −8.9§ | −6.3 | −5.2 | −6.1§ |
| UE fracture at 12 mo (no UE fracture at 12 mo) | 7.8‡ | −11.1‡ | −9.0‡ | −8.7‡ |
| Concomitant spinal injury | | | | |
| Spinal injury at baseline (no spinal injury at baseline) | 0.3 | 0.5 | 0.8 | 0.7 |
| Concomitant spinal injury and time | | | | |
| Spinal injury at 3 mo (no spinal injury at 3 mo) | −13.2§ | −5.2 | −6.3§ | −8.1‡ |
| Spinal injury at 12 mo (no spinal injury at 12 mo) | −7.7 | −9.8§ | −6.3§ | −6.5§ |
| Mechanism of injury | | | | |
| Traffic-related (fall) | −2.7§ | −3.6§ | −2.7§ | −2.5§ |
| Other (fall) | −1.1 | −0.4 | −0.2 | −0.2 |
| Patient characteristics | | | | |
| Preexisting psychosocial condition (no preexisting psychosocial condition) | −2.9‡ | −12.3‡ | −8.0‡ | −6.7‡ |
| Preexisting physical condition (no preexisting physical condition) | −1.0 | 0.7 | −2.0§ | −1.9§ |
| Family characteristics | | | | |
| Single or no partner (married or partner) | −3.4‡ | −1.6 | −3.2‡ | −3.2‡ |
| Poor family functioning (good family functioning) | −5.1‡ | −4.8§ | −6.8‡ | −6.5‡ |
| Medicaid or uninsured (commercial insurance) | −3.1‡ | −5.5‡ | −3.7‡ | −3.6‡ |

Abbreviations: LE, lower extremity; PedsQL, Pediatric Quality of Life Inventory; TBI, traumatic brain injury; UE, upper extremity.
*These estimates reflect the increase or decrease in the PedsQL scale scores associated with a given characteristic compared with the reference group adjusted for all of the other covariates in the tables.
†Reference group is in parentheses for each parameter.
‡Parameters are significant ($P \leq .05$).
§Parameters are borderline significant ($.05 < P < .10$).

With increasing TBI severity, parents reported more cognitive dysfunction. Moreover, the cognitive dysfunction persisted over time. Our results concur with numerous other studies[14,16,20,30,59,60] that have described cognitive deficits at 1 year after injury among children who sustain moderate to severe TBI.

The presence of a preexisting psychosocial condition was associated with a reduction in many domains of HRQOL, even after adjusting for preinjury function. Other studies[19,61,62] involving trauma patients have also noted the importance of controlling for the presence of comorbidities when examining the impact of an injury on HRQOL.

During the first year after injury, unhealthy family functioning, single-parent households, and being uninsured or covered by Medicaid all had a small but negative impact on children's HRQOL. These results are consistent with those of other studies[15,18] that have also found that preinjury family functioning influences different health outcomes after TBI. It could be that single-parent households have fewer resources (ie, financial and/or social) available to devote to a child's recovery compared with 2-parent households. Similarly, financial resources could also explain why the HRQOL outcomes were poorer among children covered by Medicaid or who were uninsured. Stancin et al[27] noted a significant association between socioeconomic status and HRQOL. Contrary to the results of other studies,[15,29,63] we did not find a significant interaction effect between family characteristics and the severity of TBI sustained.

The results of this study must be considered in the context of several limitations. First, preinjury HRQOL scores were obtained shortly after injury, which could have bi-

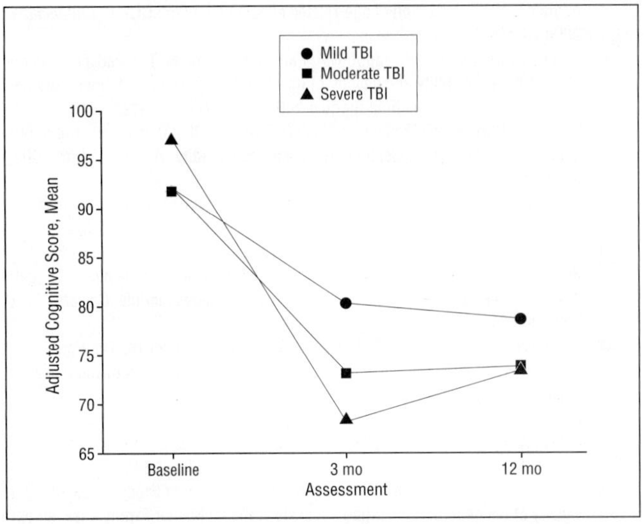


**Figure 3.** Adjusted mean cognitive score by traumatic brain injury (TBI) severity. Scores were adjusted for associated injury, mechanism of injury, patient characteristics, and family characteristics.

ased the respondent's perceptions. Although the preinjury HRQOL scores were not significantly different among the study groups when examined alone, the multivariable regression results showed that the parents of children with severe TBI reported better preinjury HRQOL compared with that which the parents of the children with an extremity fracture reported. While this may reflect a small overestimation of preinjury function, an estimate is important to have when evaluating injury sequelae.[15] Second, HRQOL was based on a primary caregiver's perspective; future research should incorporate the child's perceptions of his or her HRQOL. Finally, we may have underestimated the reduction in HRQOL as a result of severe TBI or a lack of health insurance since children with either of these characteristics were less likely to participate.

Despite these limitations, this study illustrates that it is possible to use a brief instrument to assess a child's physical and psychosocial health following TBI. While it is not feasible to conduct in-depth follow-up assessments on all children who sustain TBI severe enough to warrant hospitalization, it may be that an instrument such as the PedsQL can help clinicians to monitor the recovery of children following different types of injuries and to systematically identify those in need of further evaluation and services.

**Accepted for Publication:** September 15, 2005.
**Author Affiliations:** Departments of Emergency Medicine (Dr McCarthy and Ms Ding), Surgery (Dr Paidas), Psychiatry (Dr Slomine), Physical Medicine and Rehabilitation (Dr Christensen), and Pediatrics (Dr Christensen), School of Medicine, and Center for Injury Research and Policy, Bloomberg School of Public Health (Dr MacKenzie), Johns Hopkins University, Baltimore, Md; Department of Pediatrics, School of Medicine, University of Pennsylvania, Philadelphia (Dr Durbin); Department of Pediatrics, College of Medicine, University of Arkansas for Medical Sciences, Little Rock (Dr Aitken); Departments of Rehabilitation Medicine (Dr Jaffe) and Pediatrics (Dr Jaffe) and Division of Rehabilitation Psychology (Dr Dorsch), Children's Hospital and Regional Medical Center, School of Medicine, University of Washington, Seattle; and Departments of Neuropsychology (Dr Slomine) and Pediatric Rehabilitation Medicine (Dr Christensen), Kennedy Krieger Institute, Baltimore.
**Correspondence:** Melissa L. McCarthy, ScD, 5802 Smith Ave, Davis Bldg, Room 220, Baltimore, MD 21209 (mmccarth@jhmi.edu).
**Author Contributions:** Dr McCarthy had full access to all of the data in the study and takes responsibility for the integrity of the data and the accuracy of the data analysis.
**Children's Health After Trauma (CHAT) Study Group Institutions and Investigators:** Johns Hopkins University, Baltimore, Md, Melissa McCarthy, ScD; Ellen MacKenzie, PhD; Charles Paidas, MD; Beth Slomine, PhD; James Christensen, MD; Ronald Berk, PhD; Susan Ziegfeld, MSN, CRNP; Vinita Misra Knight, MPH, CSTR; University of Pennsylvania, Philadelphia, Dennis Durbin, MD, MS; University of Arkansas for Medical Sciences, Little Rock, Mary Aitken, MD, MPH; Patricia Korehbandi, RN, MS, CHES; University of Washington, Seattle, Kenneth Jaffe, MD; Patricia Klotz, RN, BSN; Andrea Dorsch, PhD; Kennedy Krieger Institute, Baltimore, Beth Slomine; James Christensen; Children's Hospital of Philadelphia, Philadelphia, Eileen Houseknecht, RN, BSN; Arkansas Children's Hospital, Little Rock, Donna Parnell, RN, MNSc.
**Funding/Support:** This study was funded by grant R49/CCR319701 from the National Center for Injury Prevention and Control, Centers for Disease Control and Prevention, Atlanta, Ga.
**Acknowledgment:** We would like to express our appreciation to the study coordinators who worked hard to successfully recruit all of the injured children and families involved. They are Mss Eileen Houseknecht, Patricia Klotz, Patricia Korehbandi, Vinita Misra Knight, Donna Parnell, and Susan Ziegfeld.

## REFERENCES

1. Varni JW, Seid M, Kurtin PS. PedsQL 4.0: reliability and validity of the Pediatric Quality of Life Inventory version 4.0 generic core scales in healthy and patient populations. *Med Care.* 2001;39:800-812.
2. Daltroy LH, Liang MH, Fossel AH, Goldberg MJ; Pediatric Outcomes Instrument Development Group. The POSNA pediatric musculoskeletal functional health questionnaire: report on reliability, validity, and sensitivity to change. *J Pediatr Orthop.* 1998;18:561-571.
3. Landgraf JM, Abetz LA, Ware JE. *The CHQ User's Manual.* 1st ed. Boston, Mass: Health Institute, New England Medical Center; 1996.
4. Torrance GW, Feeny DH, Furlong WJ, Barr RD, Zhang Y, Wang Q. Multiattribute utility function for a comprehensive health status classification system: Health Utilities Index Mark 2. *Med Care.* 1996;34:702-722.
5. Msall ME, DiGaudio K, Rogers BT, et al. The Functional Independence Measure for Children (WeeFIM): conceptual basis and pilot use in children with developmental disabilities. *Clin Pediatr (Phila).* 1994;33:421-430.
6. Starfield B, Bergner M, Ensminger M, et al. Adolescent health status measurement: development of the Child and Health Illness Profile. *Pediatrics.* 1993;91:430-435.
7. Haley SM, Coster WJ, Ludlow LH, Haltiwanger JT, Andrellos PJ. *Pediatric Evaluation and Disability Inventory (PEDI): Development, Standardization and Administration Manual.* 1st ed. Boston, Mass: New England Medical Center Hospitals Inc, PEDI Research Group; 1992.
8. Stein RE, Jessop DJ. Functional status II(R): a measure of child health status. *Med Care.* 1990;28:1041-1055.
9. Kaplan RM, Anderson JP, Wu AW, Mathews WC, Kozin F, Orenstein D. The Quality of Well-being Scale: applications in AIDS, cystic fibrosis, and arthritis. *Med Care.* 1989;27:S27-S43.

10. Ware JE. Conceptualization and measurement of health-related quality of life: comments on an evolving field. *Arch Phys Med Rehabil.* 2003; 84(suppl 2):S43-S51.
11. Andresen EM, Meyers AR. Health-related quality of life outcomes. *Arch Phys Med Rehabil.* 2000;81(suppl 2):S30-S45.
12. Ewing-Cobbs L, Barnes M, Fletcher JM, Levin HS, Swank PR, Song J. Modeling of longitudinal academic achievement scores after pediatric traumatic brain injury. *Dev Neuropsychol.* 2004;25:107-133.
13. Schwartz L, Taylor HG, Drotar D, Yeates KO, Wade SL, Stancin T. Long-term behavior problems following pediatric traumatic brain injury: prevalence, predictors and correlates. *J Pediatr Psychol.* 2003;28:251-263.
14. Yeates KO, Taylor HG, Wade SL, Drotar D, Stancin T, Minich N. A prospective study of short- and long-term neuropsychological outcomes after traumatic brain injury in children. *Neuropsychology.* 2002;16:514-523.
15. Taylor HG, Yeates KO, Wade SL, Drotar D, Klein SK, Stancin T. Influences on first-year recovery from traumatic brain injury in children. *Neuropsychology.* 1999; 13:76-89.
16. Broman SH, Michel ME. *Traumatic Head Injury in Children.* New York, NY: Oxford University Press; 1995.
17. Fay GC, Jaffe KM, Polissar NL, Liao S, Rivara JB, Martin KM. Outcome of pediatric traumatic brain injury at three years: a cohort study. *Arch Phys Med Rehabil.* 1994;75:733-741.
18. Rivara JB, Jaffe KM, Polissar NL, et al. Family functioning and children's academic performance and behavior problems in the year following traumatic brain injury. *Arch Phys Med Rehabil.* 1994;75:369-379.
19. Greenspan AI, MacKenzie EJ. Functional outcome after pediatric head injury. *Pediatrics.* 1994;94:425-432.
20. Jaffe KM, Fay GC, Polissar NL, et al. Severity of pediatric traumatic brain injury and neurobehavioral recovery at one year: a cohort study. *Arch Phys Med Rehabil.* 1993;74:587-595.
21. Kraus JF, Fife D, Conroy C. Pediatric brain injuries: the nature, clinical course, and early outcomes in a defined United States' population. *Pediatrics.* 1987; 79:501-507.
22. Levin HS, Eisenberg HM, Wigg NR, Kobayashi K. Memory and intellectual ability after head injury in children and adolescents. *Neurosurgery.* 1982;11: 668-673.
23. Brink JD, Imbus C, Woo-Sam J. Physical recovery after severe closed head trauma in children and adolescents. *J Pediatr.* 1980;97:721-727.
24. Rutter M, Chadwick O, Shaffer D, Brown G. A prospective study of children with head injuries, I: design and methods. *Psychol Med.* 1980;10:633-645.
25. Levin HS, Eisenberg HM. Neuropsychological outcome of closed head injury in children and adolescents. *Childs Brain.* 1979;5:281-292.
26. Fuld PA, Fisher P. Recovery of intellectual ability after closed head-injury. *Dev Med Child Neurol.* 1977;19:495-502.
27. Stancin T, Drotar D, Taylor HG, Yeates KO, Wade SL, Minich NM. Health-related quality of life of children and adolescents after traumatic brain injury. *Pediatrics.* 2002;109:E34.
28. Coster WJ, Haley S, Baryza MJ. Functional performance of young children after traumatic brain injury: a 6-month follow-up study. *Am J Occup Ther.* 1994; 48:211-218.
29. Taylor HG, Yeates KO, Wade SL, Drotar D, Stancin T, Minich N. A prospective study of short- and long-term outcomes after traumatic brain injury in children: behavior and achievement. *Neuropsychology.* 2002;16:15-27.
30. Jaffe KM, Polissar NL, Fay GC, Liao S. Recovery trends over three years following pediatric traumatic brain injury. *Arch Phys Med Rehabil.* 1995;76:17-26.
31. McCarthy ML, MacKenzie EJ, Durbin DR, et al. The Pediatric Quality of Life Inventory: an evaluation of its reliability and validity for children with traumatic brain injury. *Arch Phys Med Rehabil.* 2005;86:1901-1909.
32. Association for the Advancement of Automotive Medicine; Committee on Injury Scaling. *The Abbreviated Injury Scale: 1990 Revision.* Des Plaines, Ill: Association for the Advancement of Automotive Medicine; 1990.
33. Varni JW, Seid M, Rode CA. The PedsQL: measurement model for the pediatric quality of life inventory. *Med Care.* 1999;37:126-139.
34. Varni JW, Burwinkle TM, Katz ER, Meeske K, Dickinson P. The PedsQL in pediatric cancer: reliability and validity of the pediatric quality of life inventory generic core scales, multidimensional fatigue scale, and cancer module. *Cancer.* 2002;94:2090-2106.
35. Bastiaansen D, Koot HM, Bongers IL, Varni JW, Verhulst FC. Measuring quality of life in children referred for psychiatric problems: psychometric properties of the PedsQL 4.0 generic core scales. *Qual Life Res.* 2004;13:489-495.
36. Friefeld S, Yeboah O, Jones JE, deVeber G. Health-related quality of life and its relationship to neurological outcome in child survivors of stroke. *CNS Spectr.* 2004;9:465-475.
37. Powers SW, Patton SR, Hommel KA, Hershey AD. Quality of life in paediatric migraine: characterization of age-related effects using PedsQL 4.0. *Cephalalgia.* 2004;24:120-127.
38. Varni JW, Burwinkle TM, Rapoff MA, Kamps JL, Olson N. The PedsQL in pediatric asthma: reliability and validity of the Pediatric Quality of Life Inventory generic core scales and asthma module. *J Behav Med.* 2004;27:297-318.
39. Varni JW, Burwinkle TM, Seid M, Skarr D. The PedsQL 4.0 as a pediatric population health measure: feasibility, reliability, and validity. *Ambul Pediatr.* 2003; 3:329-341.
40. Schwimmer JB, Burwinkle TM, Varni JW. Health-related quality of life of severely obese children and adolescents. *JAMA.* 2003;289:1813-1819.
41. Varni JW, Burwinkle TM, Jacobs JR, Gottschalk M, Kaufman F, Jones KL. The PedsQL in type 1 and type 2 diabetes: reliability and validity of the pediatric quality of life inventory generic core scales and type 1 diabetes module. *Diabetes Care.* 2003;26:631-637.
42. Varni JW, Seid M, Knight TS, Burwinkle TM, Brown J, Szer IS. The PedsQL in pediatric rheumatology: reliability, validity and responsiveness of the pediatric quality of life inventory generic core scales and rheumatology module. *Arthritis Rheum.* 2002;46:714-725.
43. Miller IW, Epstein NB, Bishop DS, Keitner GI. The McMaster Family Assessment Device: reliability and validity. *J Marital Fam Ther.* 1985;11:345-356.
44. Byles J, Byrne C, Boyle M, Offord D. Ontario Child Health Study: reliability and validity of the general functioning subscale of the McMaster Family Assessment Device. *Fam Process.* 1988;27:97-104.
45. Epstein NB, Baldwin LM, Bishop DS. The McMaster Family Assessment Device. *J Marital Fam Ther.* 1983;9:171-180.
46. MacKenzie EJ. Injury severity scales: overview and directions for future research. *J Emerg Med.* 1984;2:537-549.
47. Osler T, Baker SP, Long W. A modification of the injury severity score that both improves accuracy and simplifies scoring. *J Trauma.* 1997;43:922-926.
48. Diggle PJ, Liang K, Zeger SL. *Analysis of Longitudinal Data.* 1st ed. New York, NY: Oxford University Press; 1994.
49. Laffel LM, Connell A, Vangess L, Goebel-Fabri A, Mansfield A, Anderson BJ. Relationship to patient management and diabetes-specific family conflict. *Diabetes Care.* 2003;26:3067-3073.
50. Eiser C, Vance YH, Horne B, Glaser A, Galvin H. The value of the PedsQL in assessing quality of life in survivors of childhood cancer. *Child Care Health Dev.* 2003;29:95-102.
51. Wesson DE, Williams JI, Spence LJ, Filler RM, Armstrong PF, Pearl RH. Functional outcome in pediatric trauma. *J Trauma.* 1989;29:589-592.
52. Hu X, Wesson DE, Logsetty S, Spence LJ. Functional limitations and recovery in children with severe trauma: a one-year follow-up. *J Trauma.* 1994;37:209-213.
53. Ding R, McCarthy ML, Houseknecht E, et al. The health-related quality of life of children with an extremity fracture: a one year follow-up study. *J Pediatr Orthop.* In press.
54. MacKenzie EJ, Siegel JH, Shapiro S, Moody M, Smith RT. Functional recovery and medical costs of trauma: an analysis by type and severity of injury. *J Trauma.* 1988;28:281-297.
55. Max JE, Lansing AE, Koele SL, Castillo CS, Bokura H, Schachar R. Attention deficit hyperactivity disorder in children and adolescents following traumatic brain injury. *Dev Neuropsychol.* 2004;25:159-177.
56. Gerring JP, Brady KD, Chen A, et al. Premorbid prevalence of ADHD and development of secondary ADHD after closed head injury. *J Am Acad Child Adolesc Psychiatry.* 1998;37:647-654.
57. Kirkwood M, Janusz J, Yeates KO, et al. Prevalence and correlates of depressive symptoms following traumatic brain injuries in children. *Neuropsychol Dev Cogn C Child Neuropsychol.* 2000;6:195-208.
58. Janusz JA, Kirkwood MW, Yeates KO, Taylor HG. Social problem-solving skills in children with traumatic brain injury: long-term outcomes and prediction of social competence. *Neuropsychol Dev Cogn C Child Neuropsychol.* 2002; 8:179-194.
59. Roncadin C, Guger S, Archibald J, Barnes M, Dennis M. Working memory after mild, moderate, or severe childhood closed head injury. *Dev Neuropsychol.* 2004; 25:21-36.
60. Jaffe KM, Fay GC, Polissar NL, et al. Severity of pediatric traumatic brain injury and neurobehavioral outcome: a cohort study. *Arch Phys Med Rehabil.* 1993; 74:587-595.
61. Pollak AN, McCarthy ML, Bess RS, Agel J, Swiontkowski MF. Outcomes after treatment of high-energy tibial plafond fractures. *J Bone Joint Surg Am.* 2003; 85-A:1893-1900.
62. McCarthy ML, MacKenzie EJ, Bosse MJ, Copeland CE, Hash CS, Burgess AR. Functional status following orthopedic trauma in young women. *J Trauma.* 1995; 39:828-837.
63. Yeates KO, Taylor HG, Drotar D, et al. Preinjury family environment as a determinant of recovery from traumatic brain injuries in school-age children. *J Int Neuropsychol Soc.* 1997;3:617-630.

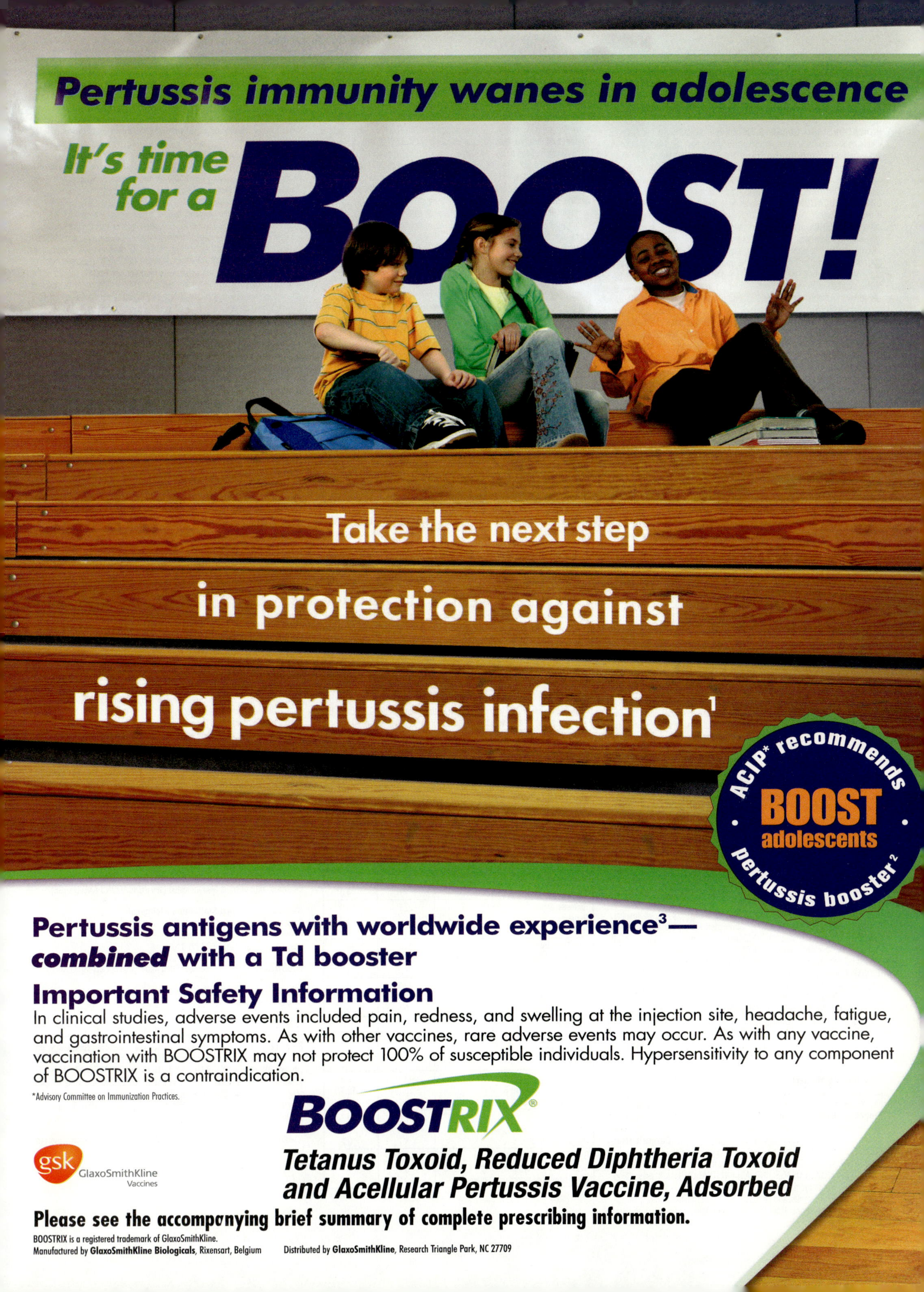

Pertussis immunity wanes in adolescence
It's time for a BOOST!
Take the next step in protection against rising pertussis infection[1]
ACIP* recommends BOOST adolescents pertussis booster[2]
Pertussis antigens with worldwide experience[3]— combined with a Td booster
Important Safety Information
In clinical studies, adverse events included pain, redness, and swelling at the injection site, headache, fatigue, and gastrointestinal symptoms. As with other vaccines, rare adverse events may occur. As with any vaccine, vaccination with BOOSTRIX may not protect 100% of susceptible individuals. Hypersensitivity to any component of BOOSTRIX is a contraindication.
*Advisory Committee on Immunization Practices.
BOOSTRIX®
Tetanus Toxoid, Reduced Diphtheria Toxoid and Acellular Pertussis Vaccine, Adsorbed
gsk GlaxoSmithKline Vaccines
Please see the accompanying brief summary of complete prescribing information.
BOOSTRIX is a registered trademark of GlaxoSmithKline.
Manufactured by GlaxoSmithKline Biologicals, Rixensart, Belgium
Distributed by GlaxoSmithKline, Research Triangle Park, NC 27709

## BOOSTRIX®

**(Tetanus Toxoid, Reduced Diphtheria Toxoid and Acellular Pertussis Vaccine, Adsorbed) (Tdap)**

The following is a brief summary only; see full prescribing information for complete product information.

**INDICATIONS AND USAGE:** BOOSTRIX is indicated for active booster immunization against tetanus, diphtheria, and pertussis as a single dose in individuals 10 through 18 years of age. The use of BOOSTRIX as a primary series or to complete the primary series has not been studied. As with any vaccine, BOOSTRIX may not protect 100% of individuals receiving the vaccine. BOOSTRIX is not recommended for treatment of actual infections.

**CONTRAINDICATIONS:** Hypersensitivity to any component of the vaccine is a contraindication (see DESCRIPTION in full prescribing information). Do not use BOOSTRIX after a serious allergic reaction (e.g., anaphylaxis) following any other tetanus toxoid, diphtheria toxoid or pertussis-containing vaccine, or any component of this vaccine (see DESCRIPTION in full prescribing information). Because of the uncertainty as to which component of the vaccine might be responsible, do not give further vaccination with any of these components; or, refer such individuals to an allergist for evaluation. The following events are contraindications to administration of BOOSTRIX: encephalopathy (e.g., coma, decreased level of consciousness, prolonged seizures) within 7 days of administration of a previous dose of a pertussis-containing vaccine that is not attributable to another identifiable cause; progressive neurologic disorder, uncontrolled epilepsy, or progressive encephalopathy. Do not vaccinate individuals with these conditions until a treatment regimen has been established and the condition has stabilized. BOOSTRIX is not contraindicated for use in individuals with HIV infection.

**WARNINGS:** The tip cap and the rubber plunger of the needleless prefilled syringes contain dry natural latex rubber that may cause allergic reactions in latex sensitive individuals. The vial stopper is latex-free. If any of the following events occurred in temporal relation to previous receipt of a Diphtheria and Tetanus Toxoids and Pertussis Vaccine Adsorbed (DTwP) vaccine or a vaccine containing an acellular pertussis component, consider carefully whether to give subsequent doses of BOOSTRIX: temperature of ≥40.5°C (105°F) within 48 hours not due to another identifiable cause; collapse or shock-like state (hypotonic-hyporesponsive episode) within 48 hours; persistent, inconsolable crying lasting ≥3 hours, occurring within 48 hours; seizures with or without fever occurring within 3 days. Persons who experienced serious Arthus-type hypersensitivity reactions following a prior dose of tetanus toxoid usually have high serum tetanus antitoxin levels and should not be given Tetanus and Diphtheria Toxoids Adsorbed For Adult Use (Td) or Tdap vaccines or even emergency doses of Td more frequently than every 10 years, even if the wound is neither clean nor minor. If Guillain-Barré syndrome has occurred within 6 weeks of receipt of prior vaccine containing tetanus toxoid, the decision to give BOOSTRIX or any vaccine containing tetanus toxoid should be based on careful consideration of the potential benefits and possible risks. The decision to administer a pertussis-containing vaccine to individuals with stable central nervous system (CNS) disorders must be made by the physician on an individual basis, with consideration of all relevant factors, and assessment of potential risks and benefits for that individual. Advise the patient, parent, or guardian of the potential increased risk involved (see PRECAUTIONS). A family history of seizures or other CNS disorders is not a contraindication to pertussis vaccine. The Advisory Committee on Immunization Practices (ACIP) has published guidelines for vaccination of persons with recent or acute illness (www.cdc.gov). Do not give BOOSTRIX to individuals with bleeding disorders such as hemophilia or thrombocytopenia, or to persons on anticoagulant therapy unless the potential benefit clearly outweighs the risk of administration. If the decision is made to administer BOOSTRIX to such persons, it should be given with caution with steps taken to avoid the risk of hematoma following the injection.

**PRECAUTIONS:** Before the injection of any biological, the physician should take all reasonable precautions to prevent allergic or other adverse reactions. Epinephrine injection (1:1,000) and other appropriate agents used for the control of immediate allergic reactions must be immediately available should an acute anaphylactic reaction occur. Immunosuppressed persons, including individuals receiving immunosuppressive therapy, may not develop the expected immune response. **Drug Interactions:** Do not mix BOOSTRIX with any other vaccine in the same syringe or vial. **Carcinogenesis, Mutagenesis, Impairment of Fertility:** BOOSTRIX has not been evaluated for carcinogenic or mutagenic potential, or for impairment of fertility. **Pregnancy:** Pregnancy Category C. Animal reproduction studies have not been conducted with BOOSTRIX. It is also not known whether BOOSTRIX can cause fetal harm when administered to a pregnant woman or can affect reproductive capacity. BOOSTRIX should be given to a pregnant woman only if clearly needed. Animal fertility studies have not been conducted with BOOSTRIX. In a developmental toxicity study, the effect of BOOSTRIX on embryo-fetal and pre-weaning development was evaluated in pregnant rats. Animals were administered INFANRIX® (Diphtheria and Tetanus Toxoids and Acellular Pertussis Vaccine Adsorbed) prior to gestation and BOOSTRIX during the period of organogenesis (gestation days 6, 8, 11) and later in pregnancy (gestation day 15), 0.1 mL/rat/occasion (a 45-fold increase compared to the human dose of BOOSTRIX on a body weight basis), by intramuscular injection. No adverse affect on pregnancy and lactation parameters, embryo-fetal or pre-weaning development was observed. There were no fetal malformations or other evidence of teratogenesis noted in this study. **Nursing Mothers:** It is not known whether BOOSTRIX is excreted in human milk. Because many drugs are excreted in human milk, caution should be exercised when BOOSTRIX is administered to a nursing woman. **Pregnancy Exposure Registry:** Healthcare providers are encouraged to register pregnant women who receive BOOSTRIX in the GlaxoSmithKline vaccination pregnancy registry by calling 1-888-825-5249. **Geriatric Use:** BOOSTRIX is not indicated for use in individuals older than 18 years. **Pediatric Use:** BOOSTRIX is not indicated for use in individuals younger than 10 years (see DOSAGE AND ADMINISTRATION in full prescribing information). For immunization of infants and children younger than 7 years against diphtheria, tetanus, and pertussis, refer to the manufacturers' package inserts for Diphtheria and Tetanus Toxoids and Acellular Pertussis Vaccine Adsorbed (DTaP) vaccines.

**ADVERSE REACTIONS:** A total of 3,289 adolescents were vaccinated with a single dose of BOOSTRIX during clinical trials. An additional 1,092 adolescents 10 to 18 years of age received a non-US formulation of BOOSTRIX (formulated to contain 0.5 mg aluminum per dose) in non-US clinical studies.

The primary safety study, conducted in the United States, was a randomized, observer-blinded, controlled study in which 3,080 adolescents 10 to 18 years of age received a single dose of BOOSTRIX and 1,034 received the control Td vaccine manufactured by Massachusetts Public Health Biologic Laboratories. There were no substantive differences in demographic characteristics between the vaccine groups. Among BOOSTRIX and control vaccine recipients approximately 75% were 10 to 14 years of age and approximately 25% were 15 to 18 years of age. Approximately 98% of participants in this study had received the recommended series of 4 or 5 doses of either DTwP or a combination of DTwP and DTaP in childhood. Data on adverse events were collected by the subjects, parents and/or guardians using standardized diaries for 15 consecutive days following the vaccine dose (i.e., day of vaccination and the next 14 days). Subjects were monitored for unsolicited adverse events that occurred within 31 days of vaccination (day 0-30) using diary cards (day 0-14) supplemented by spontaneous reports and a medical history as reported by subjects, parents, and/or guardians. Subjects were also monitored for 6 months post-vaccination for non-routine medical visits, visits to an emergency room, onset of new chronic illness, and serious adverse events. Information regarding late onset adverse events was obtained via a telephone call 6 months following vaccination. At least 97% of subjects completed the 6-month follow-up evaluation.

The adverse event information from clinical trials provides a basis for identifying adverse events that appear to be related to vaccine use and for approximating rates. However, because clinical trials are conducted under widely varying conditions, adverse event rates observed in the clinical trials of a vaccine cannot be directly compared to rates in the clinical trials of another vaccine, and may not reflect the rates observed in practice.

**Serious Adverse Events in All Safety Studies:** In the US-safety study, no serious adverse events were reported to occur within 31 days of vaccination. During the 6-month extended safety evaluation period, no serious adverse events that were of potential autoimmune origin or new onset and chronic in nature were reported to occur. In non-US studies in which serious adverse events were monitored for up to 37 days, one subject was diagnosed with insulin dependent diabetes. The association of this event with vaccination is unknown. No other serious adverse events of potential autoimmune origin or that were new onset and chronic in nature were reported to occur in these studies.

**Solicited Adverse Events in the US-Safety Study:** In a US study, the most common local adverse events following administration of BOOSTRIX were pain, redness, and swelling at the injection site. The most common general adverse events were headache and fatigue. Most of these events were reported at a similar frequency in recipients of both BOOSTRIX and Td. Any pain, grade 2 or 3 pain (but not grade 3 alone), and grade 2 or 3 headache (but not grade 3 alone) were reported at a higher rate in recipients of BOOSTRIX. The primary safety endpoint of the US study was the incidence of grade 3 pain (spontaneously painful and/or prevented normal activity) at the injection site within 15 days of vaccination. Grade 3 pain was reported in 4.6% of those who received BOOSTRIX compared with 4.0% of those who received the Td vaccine. The difference in rate of grade 3 pain was within the pre-defined clinical limit for non-inferiority (upper limit of the 95% CI for the difference ≤4%). These were the rates for solicited local and general adverse events within 15 days of vaccination with BOOSTRIX or Td vaccine for the total vaccinated cohort (all enrolled, vaccinated subjects with safety data available analyzed by vaccine received):

**Percentage of Individuals 10 to 18 Years of Age Reporting Solicited Local Adverse Events or Solicited General Adverse Events Within the 15-day* Post-Vaccination Period**

| | BOOSTRIX (N = 3,032) | Td (N = 1,013) |
|---|---|---|
| **Local** | | |
| Pain,† any | 75.3 | 71.7 |
| Pain,† grade 2 or 3 | 51.2 | 42.5 |
| Pain,‡ grade 3 | 4.6 | 4.0 |
| Redness, any | 22.5 | 19.8 |
| Redness, >20 mm | 4.1 | 3.9 |
| Redness, ≥50 mm | 1.7 | 1.6 |
| Swelling, any | 21.1 | 20.1 |
| Swelling, >20 mm | 5.3 | 4.9 |
| Swelling, ≥50 mm | 2.5 | 3.2 |
| Arm circumference increase,§ >5 mm | 28.3 | 29.5 |
| Arm circumference increase,§ >20 mm | 2.0 | 2.2 |
| Arm circumference increase,§ >40 mm | 0.5 | 0.3 |
| **General** | | |
| Fever,‖ ≥99.5°F | 13.5 | 13.1 |
| Fever,‖ >100.4°F | 5.0 | 4.7 |
| Fever,‖ >102.2°F | 1.4 | 1.0 |
| Headache, any | 43.1 | 41.5 |
| Headache,† grade 2 or 3 | 15.7 | 12.7 |
| Headache, grade 3 | 3.7 | 2.7 |
| Fatigue, any | 37.0 | 36.7 |
| Fatigue, grade 2 or 3 | 14.4 | 12.9 |
| Fatigue, grade 3 | 3.7 | 3.2 |
| Gastrointestinal symptoms,¶ any | 26.0 | 25.8 |
| Gastrointestinal symptoms,¶ grade 2 or 3 | 9.8 | 9.7 |
| Gastrointestinal symptoms,¶ grade 3 | 3.0 | 3.2 |

Td = Tetanus and Diphtheria Toxoids Adsorbed For Adult Use manufactured by Massachusetts Public Health Biologic Laboratories.

N = number of subjects in the total vaccinated cohort with local/general symptoms sheets completed.

Grade 2 = Local: painful when the limb was moved; General: interfered with normal activity.

Grade 3 = Local: spontaneously painful and/or prevented normal activity; General: prevented normal activity.

*Day of vaccination and the next 14 days.

†Statistically significantly higher ($P<0.05$) following BOOSTRIX as compared to Td vaccine.

‡Grade 3 injection site pain following BOOSTRIX was not inferior to Td (upper limit of two-sided 95% CI for the difference in the percentage of subjects ≤4%).

§Mid-upper region of the vaccinated arm.

‖Oral temperatures or axillary temperatures.

¶Gastrointestinal symptoms included nausea, vomiting, diarrhea and/or abdominal pain.

Mid-upper arm circumference was measured by the adolescent or their parent/guardian prior to injection and daily for 15 days following vaccination. There was no significant difference between BOOSTRIX recipients and Td recipients in the proportion of subjects reporting an increase in mid-upper arm circumference in the vaccinated arm. The incidence of unsolicited adverse events reported in the 31 days after vaccination was comparable between the 2 groups.

As with any vaccine, there is the possibility that broad use of BOOSTRIX could reveal adverse events not observed in clinical trials.

**Postmarketing Reports:** Worldwide voluntary reports of adverse events received for BOOSTRIX in persons 10 to 18 years of age since market introduction of this vaccine are listed below. This list includes serious events or events which have causal connection to components of this or other vaccines or drugs. Because these events are reported voluntarily from a population of uncertain size, it is not possible to reliably estimate their frequency or establish a causal relationship to vaccine exposure. *Blood and lymphatic system disorders:* Lymphadenitis, lymphadenopathy. *Cardiac disorders:* Myocarditis. *Injection site reactions:* Induration, inflammation, mass, nodule, warmth, local reaction. *Metabolism and nutrition disorders:* Diabetes mellitus insulin-dependent. *Musculoskeletal and connective tissue disorders:* Arthralgia, back pain, myalgia. *Nervous system disorders:* Convulsion, encephalitis, facial palsy, paraesthesia. *Skin and subcutaneous tissue disorders:* Exanthem, Henoch-Schönlein purpura, rash. In addition, extensive swelling of the injected limb has been reported following administration of BOOSTRIX.

**Reporting Adverse Events:** Report the occurrence following immunization of any event set forth in the Vaccine Injury Table from the National Childhood Vaccine Injury Act including: Anaphylaxis or anaphylactic shock within 7 days, encephalopathy or encephalitis within 7 days, brachial neuritis within 28 days, or an acute complication or sequelae (including death) of an illness, disability, injury, or condition referred to above, or any events that would contraindicate further doses of vaccine, according to this prescribing information. These events should be reported to VAERS. The VAERS toll-free number is 1-800-822-7967. Reporting forms may also be obtained at the VAERS website at www.vaers.org.

**DOSAGE AND ADMINISTRATION: Recommended Dose:** BOOSTRIX should be administered as a single 0.5 mL injection by the intramuscular route into the deltoid muscle of the upper arm in individuals 10 through 18 years of age. Do not administer this product subcutaneously or intravenously. There are no data to support repeat administration of BOOSTRIX. Five years should elapse between the subject's last dose of the recommended series of childhood DTwP and/or DTaP vaccine and the administration of BOOSTRIX. Limited data are available on the use of BOOSTRIX following Tetanus and Diphtheria Toxoids Adsorbed For Adult Use (Td) vaccine. **Additional Dosing Information:** ***Wound Management:*** Clinicians should refer to guidelines for tetanus prophylaxis in routine wound management. Adolescents 10 to 18 years of age who have completed a primary series against tetanus and who sustain wounds which are minor and uncomplicated, should receive a booster dose of a tetanus toxoid-containing vaccine only if they have not received tetanus toxoid within the preceding 10 years. In case of tetanus-prone injury (e.g., wounds contaminated with dirt, feces, soil, and saliva; puncture wounds; avulsions; and wounds resulting from missles, crushing, burns, and frostbite) in an adolescent who is in need of tetanus toxoid, BOOSTRIX can be used as an alternative to Tetanus and Diphtheria Toxoids Adsorbed For Adult Use (Td) vaccine in patients for whom the pertussis component is also indicated (see INDICATIONS AND USAGE).

Manufactured by **GlaxoSmithKline Biologicals**
Rixensart, Belgium, US License 1617
Distributed by **GlaxoSmithKline**
Research Triangle Park, NC 27709

BOOSTRIX and INFANRIX are registered trademarks of GlaxoSmithKline.

Full prescribing information for BOOSTRIX is available at www.BOOSTRIX.com.

BRS-BO:L1

**References: 1.** Centers for Disease Control and Prevention. *Epidemiology and Prevention of Vaccine-Preventable Diseases.* Atkinson W, Hamborsky J, Wolfe S, eds. 8th ed. Washington DC: Public Health Foundation; 2004:75–88, A26–A27. **2.** ACIP recommends adolescent vaccination for tetanus, diphtheria and pertussis vaccine [press release]. Atlanta, GA: Department of Health and Human Services; Available at: www.cdc.gov/nip/pr/pr_tdap_jun2005.htm. Accessed September 27, 2005. **3.** Data on file, BOR305, GlaxoSmithKline.

# Estimated Cost-effectiveness of Growth Hormone Therapy for Idiopathic Short Stature

*Joyce M. Lee, MD; Matthew M. Davis, MD, MAPP; Sarah J. Clark, MPH; Timothy P. Hofer, MD; Alex R. Kemper, MD, MPH, MS*

**Objective:** To estimate the cost-effectiveness of growth hormone (GH) therapy for idiopathic short stature (ISS).

**Design:** Cost-effectiveness analysis.

**Setting:** Decision model.

**Patients:** A cohort of 10-year-old prepubertal boys with ISS treated with GH.

**Interventions:** Comparison of children treated for 5 years with GH therapy vs children receiving no intervention.

**Main Outcome Measures:** Incremental cost per child, incremental growth per child, and incremental cost per inch of final height gain.

**Results:** The estimated incremental cost-effectiveness ratio of GH therapy for ISS in the base case analysis compared with no therapy was $52 634 per inch (per 2.54 cm), or $99 959 per child, reflecting an incremental growth of 1.9 in (4.8 cm). Alternate treatment strategies such as increased duration of GH treatment and high pubertal dosing of GH did not substantially improve the cost-effectiveness ratio. Probabilistic sensitivity analyses showed that growth variability in response to GH had the greatest impact on the cost-effectiveness of GH therapy.

**Conclusions:** Targeted treatment of children with ISS with the greatest potential for growth appears critical for maximizing cost-effectiveness of GH treatment. However, the significance of the cost per inch is difficult to judge until the utility gains associated with height gain after GH therapy for ISS can be ascertained.

*Arch Pediatr Adolesc Med. 2006;160:263-269*

IN JULY 2003, THE US FOOD AND Drug Administration (FDA) approved the use of recombinant growth hormone (GH) for the long-term treatment of idiopathic short stature (ISS)—also called non-growth hormone-deficient short stature—defined by height SDs ≤ −2.25 and associated with growth rates unlikely to permit attainment of adult height in the normal range, in pediatric patients whose epiphyses are not closed and for whom diagnostic evaluation excludes other causes associated with short stature that should be observed or treated by other means.[1]

With this indication, it is estimated that 400 000 children in the United States now qualify for GH therapy.[2] While endocrinologists are the most likely prescribers of GH, general pediatricians will likely encounter patients with this new indication for GH and may be asked by parents for guidance about its effectiveness and cost.

The FDA approval was based on evidence from 2 clinical trials: the only randomized, double-blind, placebo-controlled study to final height conducted at the National Institutes of Health (NIH),[3] Bethesda, Md, and an uncontrolled European dose-response study.[4] In the placebo study, children treated with GH had a final adult height approximately 3.7 cm (1.5 in) taller than that of the placebo group.[3] The dose-response study suggested that the amount of height gained is dose dependent, with higher doses leading to increased growth.[4]

Considerable debate exists about the benefits of a 1- to 2-in (2.5- to 5.1-cm) height gain from GH therapy in otherwise healthy short children. Although some studies suggest that ISS can be associated with psychosocial impairment, it is not associated with physical disability.[5] In addition, GH therapy has not been shown to improve quality of life in children with short stature.[6] Furthermore, GH therapy is expensive: at current prices, it may cost $20 000 or more per year for a 30-kg child,[2] and because GH therapy is usually continued until final adult height is reached, treatment can last 5 years or more.

Rising pharmaceutical costs are a prominent concern for the US health care system.[7] Cost-effectiveness studies of pharmaceutical interventions can serve as a useful decision-making tool for both clinicians and payers. Two studies published in 2002 evaluated the cost-effectiveness of GH therapy for ISS, but both were performed before the availability of the most recent GH efficacy data.[8,9] Given that a much larger cohort of children is now eligible for GH

Author Affiliations: Divisions of Pediatric Endocrinology (Dr Lee) and General Pediatrics (Drs Lee, Davis, and Kemper and Ms Clark), Child Health Evaluation and Research Unit (Drs Lee, Davis, and Kemper and Ms Clark), Gerald R. Ford School of Public Policy (Dr Davis), and Veterans Affairs Health Services Research and Development (Dr Hofer), University of Michigan, Ann Arbor.

**Table 1. Base Case Scenario of the Hypothetical Cohort With Idiopathic Short Stature***

| Variable | Assumption | References |
|---|---|---|
| Age at initiation | 10 y | 9, 10 |
| Sex | Male | 3, 4, 10 |
| Duration of treatment | 5 y | 3, 4 |
| Drug dosage | 0.37 mg/kg per wk† | 4, 11 |
| Weight | 5th Percentile adjusted for chronologic age | 12 |
| Discontinuation rate | 30% in first year of treatment | 13 |
| Health care events associated with height monitoring | Annual visit with pediatric endocrinologist<br>Annual bone-age radiograph | |
| Health care events associated with GH treatment | GH therapy<br>3 Visits/y with pediatric endocrinologist<br>Annual bone-age radiograph<br>Annual thyroid function tests<br>Annual insulin-like growth factor I level measurement | 14 |
| Height gain for height monitoring | 0 in | 3 |
| Height gain for standard GH treatment (0.37 mg/kg per wk) | 2.8 in | 4 |

Abbreviation: GH, growth hormone.
Conversion factor: To convert inches to centimeters, multiply by 2.54.
*Height 2.25 SDs below the mean, no evidence of GH deficiency based on GH stimulation tests, and no comorbid conditions that compromise growth.
†Drug dosage for the baseline case was derived from the dosing approved by the US Food and Drug Administration for GH treatment of idiopathic short stature.

therapy, a reassessment of its cost-effectiveness with respect to the recent efficacy data is warranted.

The objectives of this study were to estimate the cost-effectiveness of GH therapy for ISS based on the efficacy data used for FDA approval of this indication, and to evaluate the cost-effectiveness of alternate GH treatment strategies for ISS.

## METHODS

### DECISION ANALYSIS MODEL

We constructed a deterministic decision tree to compare GH treatment of ISS with the strategy of height monitoring for ISS, given the lack of alternate treatment options for ISS. Growth hormone efficacy was measured in terms of final adult height gain (final adult height minus baseline predicted adult height at the start of treatment). Given that GH treatment has not yet been proven to improve psychosocial adjustment or quality of life in children with ISS,[6] this aspect of GH therapy was not considered in the model. The analysis was conducted from the perspective of the health care payer.

### ASSUMPTIONS FOR THE BASE CASE SCENARIO

Because most GH trials for ISS predominantly enrolled male children, our base case scenario consisted of a hypothetical cohort of 10-year-old prepubertal male children with ISS (height 2.25 SD below the mean, no evidence of GH deficiency on the basis of GH stimulation tests, and no comorbid conditions that compromise growth). Assumptions regarding duration of treatment, drug dosing, patient weight, treatment dropout, and GH efficacy were based on the 2 clinical trials used for FDA approval (a randomized, double-blind, placebo-controlled NIH study[3] and an uncontrolled European dose-response study[4]) and other published studies where appropriate (**Table 1**).[9-14]

### FINAL HEIGHT GAIN

Final height gain for the no-intervention group was derived from the placebo-treated group of the NIH randomized controlled trial.[3] Although mean final height gain for this group was approximately −0.3 in (−0.8 cm), the 95% confidence interval for this figure overlapped 0 in. Therefore, we assumed a height gain of 0 in for the no-intervention group. Final height gain for the GH intervention cohort was assumed to be 2.8 in (7.1 cm), which was the mean adult height gain of children in the arm of the dose-response study that used 0.37 mg/kg per week.[4]

Given that a number of clinical trials of GH for ISS have shown that growth velocity in the first year of treatment is double the pretreatment growth velocity and declines with each successive year of treatment,[4,15,16] the model assumed a height gain for each year that was proportional to the increase in growth velocity for each successive year of treatment.

An overall discontinuation rate of 30% in the first year of treatment was assumed, based on rates from observational studies.[13] Given that one recent study of children with ISS showed that children who discontinued treatment had growth rates similar to those of children who continued with treatment,[10] children with early discontinuation of GH treatment were assumed to accumulate a height gain calculated pro rata for the number of years of treatment. Finally, GH was not assumed to accelerate puberty in this model, as recent studies have shown that GH treatment does not appear to accelerate bone age or induce an earlier onset of puberty in children.[4,17]

### COSTS

Direct medical costs, including pharmacy costs, physician costs, and laboratory and radiologic costs, for both the GH-treated group and the no-intervention group, were estimated as follows (in 2004 US dollars): GH cost per milligram, $52; cost of physician visit, $58; bone-age radiograph, $17; free thyroxine and thyrotropin measurement, $74; and insulin-like growth factor I determination, $27. Indirect costs such as transportation costs and parental wages lost because of physicians' visits were not included.

Regardless of the potential for GH treatment, an initial evaluation is necessary for all children to identify possible organic causes of poor growth. Therefore, the costs associated with the initial evaluation for short stature, including possible laboratory studies, GH stimulation testing, and imaging studies, were not included in this model, because they would be identical for children in the GH treatment and no-intervention groups.

Growth hormone is regarded as a safe medication with infrequent and rare adverse events.[18] Given that studies of GH

**Table 2. Growth Assumptions for Sensitivity Analyses***

| Sensitivity Analysis | Height Gain, in | References |
|---|---|---|
| Deterministic, mean | | |
| Lower efficacy | 1.8 | 4 |
| Higher efficacy | 3.9 | 4 |
| Low-dosage GH (0.24 mg/kg per wk) | 2.1 | 4 |
| Standard-dosage GH (0.37 mg/kg per wk) × 2 y followed by high-pubertal-dosage GH (0.7 mg/kg per wk) × 3 y | 4.6 | 23 |
| Standard-dosage GH (0.37 mg/kg per wk) × 1 y followed by high-pubertal-dosage GH (0.7 mg/kg per wk) × 4 y | 5.0 | 23 |
| 7-y Treatment duration (ages 8-15 y) | 3.8 | 15, 16 |
| 10-y Treatment duration (ages 5-15 y) | 5.2 | 15, 16 |
| Probabilistic, mean ± SD | | |
| % of variance due to growth variability | | |
| 50 | 2.8 ± 1.64 | 3, 4 |
| 30 | 2.8 ± 1.28 | |
| 10 | 2.8 ± 0.73 | |

Abbreviation: GH, growth hormone.
Conversion factor: To convert inches to centimeters, multiply by 2.54.
*Estimates of height gain for the sensitivity analyses of discontinuation rate and age at initiation were the same as the base case analysis.

side effects in ISS are currently underpowered to assess the frequency of more serious rare adverse events,[19] the costs of side effects of GH therapy were not considered in the model.

Charge data from our hospital were converted to costs by multiplying charges by 0.5.[20] Retail GH prices obtained from a query of several US pharmacies were averaged and then verified with another drug reference publication.[21] Costs are expressed in 2004 US dollars.

All modeling was conducted with @RISK software (version 4.5; Palisade Corp, Newfield, NY). We applied a 3% yearly discount rate to both costs and height gain on the basis of consensus guidelines for conducting cost-effectiveness analyses published by the Panel on Cost-effectiveness in Health and Medicine.[22]

## COST-EFFECTIVENESS CALCULATIONS

The incremental cost-effectiveness ratio for GH treatment of ISS was defined as the incremental cost of GH treatment divided by its incremental clinical benefit in dollars per inch.

## DETERMINISTIC SENSITIVITY ANALYSES

Key assumptions were varied over plausible ranges to examine several parameter effects on the model estimates of GH cost-effectiveness. One-way sensitivity analyses were performed, including (1) final height gain ranging from 1.8 to 3.9 in (4.6-9.9 cm), based on the confidence intervals from the dose-response study[4]; (2) a discontinuation rate ranging from 10% to 40%; (3) age at initiation of 8 or 12 years, with 5 years of treatment; (4) the use of a low dosage (0.24 mg/kg per week) or high dosing of GH at puberty (0.7 mg/kg per week for the last 3 or 4 years of therapy); and (5) a prolonged treatment duration of 7 years (from ages 8-15 years) and 10 years (from ages 5-15 years).

Growth assumptions for the sensitivity analyses are shown in **Table 2**. Assumptions of height gain for the sensitivity analyses of discontinuation rate and age of initiation were the same as in the base case analysis. Assumptions for low-dosage GH were based on the 0.24–mg/kg per week arm of the dose-response study.[4] Assumptions for high pubertal GH dosing (0.7 mg/kg per week during the last 3 or 4 years of a 5-year treatment duration) were based on a randomized trial of GH-deficient children treated with high doses for 3 or 4 years, who were 1.8 (4.6 in) and 2.2 in (5.6 cm) taller than children treated with standard-dose GH.[23] This additional growth with high-dose therapy was added to the baseline estimate of 2.8 in (7.1 cm).

An increased duration of treatment has been shown to be positively associated with height gain and growth velocity plateaus at a stable rate into the fifth and sixth years of treatment.[15,16] Therefore, the model assumed total baseline growth for the first 5 years of treatment (2.8 in), and for years 6 to 10 of treatment, incremental growth was assumed to be similar to that in the fifth year of treatment.

## PROBABILISTIC SENSITIVITY ANALYSES

We also performed probabilistic sensitivity analyses to assess the impact of growth variability on the cost-effectiveness of this therapy. Rather than using fixed estimates of height gain, we constructed a probabilistic Monte Carlo simulation for the base case analysis. Mean height gain was varied over a normal distribution using variance estimates from the dose-response study.

Variance in height gain with GH has 2 determinants: growth variability and error in estimating the predicted adult height. The relative contribution of these 2 determinants to the variance in height gain is unknown. However, one plausible estimate is that growth variability represents 50% of the variance, as the variance of height gain of the 0.37–mg/kg per week arm of the dose-response study was 5.43, compared with the variance of height gain of the placebo group in the placebo-controlled trial, which was 2.57.[3,4] Therefore, we modeled scenarios in which growth variability represented 50%, 30%, and 10% of the variance of height gain from the dose-response study (Table 2) and limited the distribution to a minimum height gain of 0 in and a maximum height gain of 12 in (30.5 cm). Cost-effectiveness ratios were calculated for 10 000 iterations and the distributions of the ratios were examined.

## RESULTS

The estimated incremental cost-effectiveness ratio of GH treatment for the base case analysis compared with no treatment was $52 634 per inch (per 2.54 cm), with an incremental height gain of 1.9 in (4.8 cm) during 5 years and an incremental cost per child of $99 959 (**Table 3**). Although mean growth per child was assumed to be 2.8 in (7.1 cm) for children who completed 5 years of GH treatment, the mean incremental height gain for the entire cohort was lower (1.9 in) because of early discontinuation of GH treatment in 30% of the cohort, who accumulated a

**Table 3. Estimated Incremental Cost per Child and Incremental Growth per Child for the Base Case**

| | Average Cost per Child, $ | Average Growth per Child, in | Incremental Cost per Child, $ | Incremental Growth per Child, in | Incremental Cost per Inch, $ |
|---|---|---|---|---|---|
| Height monitoring | 248 | 0 | ... | ... | ... |
| Standard GH treatment (0.37 mg/kg per wk) | 100 207 | 1.9 | 99 959 | 1.9 | 52 634 |

Abbreviation: GH, growth hormones; ellipses, not applicable.
Conversion factor: To convert inches to centimeters, multiply by 2.54.

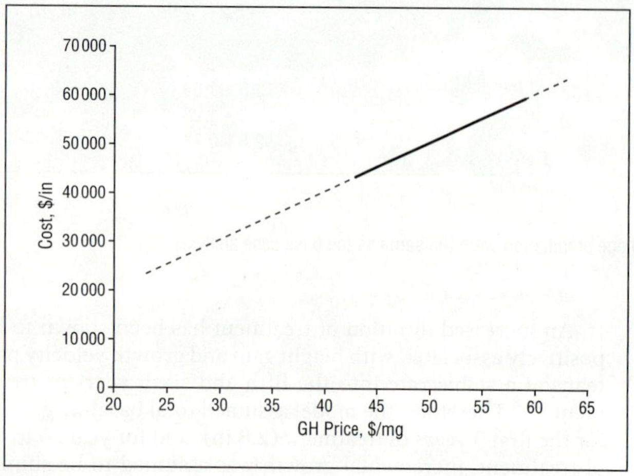


**Figure.** Estimated incremental cost per inch of growth (dashed line) based on the drug price of growth hormone (GH). The solid line represents the current range of GH prices. To convert inches to centimeters, multiply by 2.54.

height gain calculated pro rata for the number of years of treatment. The **Figure** illustrates the effect of GH price per milligram on the cost-effectiveness ratio.

## DETERMINISTIC SENSITIVITY ANALYSES

The results of the deterministic sensitivity analyses are shown in **Table 4**. The incremental cost-effectiveness of GH for ISS was most sensitive to estimates of drug efficacy. With higher estimates of efficacy, the incremental cost per inch was more favorable ($38 783), and with lower estimates of efficacy, the incremental cost per inch was less favorable ($81 875).

Because of weight-based dosing and increases in weight with increasing age, GH cost per inch was somewhat sensitive to the age at initiation ($42 792 for earlier initiation by 2 years; $66 411 for later initiation by 2 years). The discontinuation rate did not appreciably affect the cost per inch.

Alternate treatment strategies, including high-dosage GH at puberty and increased duration of treatment, resulted in increases in the incremental growth per child, but also resulted in marked increases in the incremental cost per child because of the use of more drug overall. There were no substantive improvements in the cost per inch, even when generous assumptions of GH efficacy were used.

Analyses using hospital charge rather than cost data were also conducted, with no appreciable differences in the incremental cost per inch (data not shown).

## PROBABILISTIC SENSITIVITY ANALYSES

When plausible estimates of growth variability in response to GH were used in our model, the mean incremental cost-effectiveness ratio was significantly higher in the probabilistic analyses compared with our deterministic analyses, with wide 95% confidence intervals (**Table 5**). Only when growth variability represented 10% of the variance of height gain did the cost per inch approximate the figure calculated from the base case analysis, with a significant narrowing of the confidence intervals.

## COMMENT

This study found that the estimated incremental cost-effectiveness of GH therapy for ISS is approximately $52 000 per inch (per 2.54 cm). This is substantially higher than a previously cited cost estimate of $35 000 per inch, which was not generated by formal economic analysis and was developed before the availability of the recent efficacy data.[9] To our knowledge, this study is the first formal analysis of the cost-effectiveness of GH therapy for ISS that used data from the clinical trials that were the basis for the FDA approval. In addition, our study is unique in that it assessed the cost-effectiveness of alternate GH treatment strategies.

We found that an earlier age at initiation of GH therapy did lead to an improved cost per inch, but it is unclear whether this represents a viable treatment strategy. Some studies have shown growth deceleration in children who discontinue GH treatment before reaching final adult height,[24] so earlier onset of treatment with premature discontinuation of GH therapy may not lead to sustained gains in final adult height. Other treatment strategies to improve GH efficacy, such as high-dose GH therapy during the pubertal years or an increased duration of treatment, did not lead to substantive changes in the cost per inch but did lead to considerable increases in the cost per child, despite generous assumptions regarding efficacy.

Through our probabilistic sensitivity analyses, we found that growth variability in response to GH had the greatest impact on the incremental cost-effectiveness of GH therapy for ISS, as plausible estimates of growth variability led to a mean incremental cost per inch of approximately $125 000. When we modeled a smaller variance in drug response attributable to growth variability (vs errors in predicting adult height), the cost per inch estimates improved dramatically and the confidence intervals narrowed considerably. Therefore, targeting of GH therapy to children with ISS who are most likely to re-

**Table 4. Estimated Incremental Cost per Child, Incremental Growth per Child, and Cost per Inch for Deterministic Sensitivity Analyses**

| Sensitivity Analyses | Incremental Cost per Child, $ | Incremental Growth per Child, in | Cost per Inch, $ |
|---|---|---|---|
| Efficacy | | | |
| Lower (1.8 in) | 99 959 | 1.2 | 81 875 |
| Higher (3.9 in) | 99 959 | 2.6 | 38 783 |
| Age at initiation | | | |
| Treatment from ages 8-13 y | 81 268 | 1.9 | 42 792 |
| Treatment from ages 12-16 y | 126 123 | 1.9 | 66 411 |
| Discontinuation rate, % | | | |
| 0 | 137 779 | 2.6 | 53 531 |
| 40 | 87 352 | 1.7 | 52 174 |
| Dosing | | | |
| Low-dosage GH (0.24 mg/kg per wk) | 65 092 | 1.4 | 45 700 |
| Standard-dosage GH (0.37 mg/kg per wk) × 2 y followed by high-dosage GH at puberty (0.7 mg/kg per wk) × 3 y | 155 440 | 3.1 | 49 821 |
| Standard-dosage GH (0.37 mg/kg per wk) × 1 y followed by high-dosage GH at puberty (0.7 mg/kg per wk) × 4 y | 170 866 | 3.4 | 50 384 |
| Treatment duration, y | | | |
| 7 (Ages 8-15 y) | 122 513 | 2.5 | 49 396 |
| 10 (Ages 5-15 y) | 145 550 | 3.2 | 45 156 |

Abbreviation: GH, growth hormone.
Conversion factor: To convert inches to centimeters, multiply by 2.54.

spond to GH, rather than universal treatment of all eligible children, represents an important treatment strategy for improving the cost-effectiveness of this therapy.

The chief challenge in implementing such a strategy, however, is that ISS represents a heterogeneous group of children with short stature of various causes. Diagnoses such as insulin-like growth factor I deficiency, partial GH insensitivity, genetic short stature, familial short stature, and constitutional delay of puberty all fit the classification of ISS,[25] no doubt contributing to significant growth variability among children with ISS. Further studies are needed to determine which subsets of children with ISS will have the greatest therapeutic response; the subset of patients who have insulin-like growth factor I deficiency may be one such candidate group.[26]

The impact of GH therapy on quality of life is uncertain, and quality-adjusted life-years or other utility measures for incremental height gains have not been formally generated from primary data.[8] Therefore, future studies to assess the quality-adjusted life-years gained with additional height gain due to GH therapy are required to understand the significance of a cost per inch of $52 000. One threshold for cost-effectiveness frequently cited in the literature is $50 000 to $100 000 per quality-adjusted life-year gained, but whether such a range is appropriate for judging gains in height is not known.[27]

## LIMITATIONS

A limitation of this analysis is that it was based largely on 2 clinical trials,[3,4] each with a small number of enrolled patients. Assumptions from the studies may not be entirely generalizable because of the small sample sizes. However, to date they represent the best available data and were the basis for FDA approval and for determination of the FDA-approved GH dosing for ISS. Although

**Table 5. Estimated Incremental Cost per Inch for Probabilistic Sensitivity Analyses**

| % of Variance Due to Growth Variability | Cost-effectiveness Ratio (95% CI), $ |
|---|---|
| 50 | 125 416 (24 369-417 154) |
| 30 | 93 820 (27 716-270 616) |
| 10 | 57 482 (34 830-107 518) |

Abbreviation: CI, confidence interval.

we did not perform a systematic review of the literature, we are unaware of other data that would change these assumptions.

Growth assumptions for the base case analysis were based on an open-label dose-response study, which did not include an untreated group and was not blinded. Ideally, cost-effectiveness studies are based on the results of randomized controlled trials; the NIH trial[3] was the first and only randomized, double-blind, placebo-controlled trial of GH therapy for ISS, and it included intent-to-treat analyses. However, in that study GH was administered at a dose and dosing frequency now considered suboptimal (0.22 mg/kg per week given subcutaneously 3 times per week).[3,28]

Because of the lack of definitive GH trials for ISS regarding alternate treatment strategies, height gains associated with a longer duration and high-pubertal-dose treatment had to be extrapolated on the basis of studies in the literature. However, we used growth assumptions that favored GH therapy. For example, one study[15] of GH-treated children with ISS showed that GH treatment in patients treated for anywhere from 2 to 10 years led to a height gain of greater than 5 cm (1.9 in) above their predicted height, which is substantially lower than our assumptions for a longer duration of treatment. Furthermore, growth assumptions for high pubertal dosing were derived from studies performed on GH-deficient children and not children with ISS. Studies have shown that children with GH deficiency tend to have better catch-up growth and a greater final height gain than children with ISS.[23,29,30] Therefore, our high-dose growth assumptions were likely generous estimates of growth for children with ISS.

Growth assumptions may also be optimistic in that we assumed 100% adherence until discontinuation or completion. Nonadherent children will likely have less overall growth as they discontinue taking their shots, but they may continue to incur standard GH drug costs if their nonadherence is unrecognized, resulting in a higher incremental cost per inch.

Our model was based on charge data from our institution, so it may not be generalizable to other health care settings. Our model may also underestimate the costs of GH therapy, as it does not account for mild potential side effects associated with GH therapy or rare complications. Safety studies of GH-treated patients with ISS thus far have not shown a significant rate of adverse effects, but longer-term safety data are currently unavailable.[19] Given that growth assumptions favored GH therapy and costs may have been underestimated, our estimate of the incremental cost per inch is likely a conservative figure.

Finally, this study was performed from the health care payer perspective. Further studies looking at the cost-effectiveness from a societal perspective may yield different results, as some studies have shown in males that greater heights in adolescence are associated with greater financial and career success.[31]

## IMPLICATIONS

With the ISS indication, it has been estimated that more than 400 000 children aged 4 to 15 years are now eligible for GH therapy. At an average incremental cost per child of approximately $100 000, the potential cost of treating all eligible children with ISS is approximately $40 billion dollars. Not all patients with ISS will be treated with GH, but if just one tenth of all eligible children are treated, the cost will still be considerable.

Since the licensure of GH therapy for ISS, a number of commentaries have highlighted the cost of GH therapy as an important issue for the health care system and society.[2,32] There is debate about whether GH for ISS constitutes a medical treatment or an enhancement therapy. Some authors have referred to GH as a "lifestyle drug," a drug that improves quality of life rather than alleviates illness.[33] Certainly lifestyle drugs and their costs have been a frequent topic of interest in the adult literature, but to our knowledge GH therapy represents the first costly lifestyle medication to emerge in the field of pediatrics. Given that the rising cost of prescription drug therapies is a prominent issue for our health care system,[7] GH therapy for ISS represents one of its major challenges.

**Accepted for Publication:** September 20, 2005.
**Correspondence:** Joyce M. Lee, MD, Division of Pediatric Endocrinology, University of Michigan, 300 NIB, Room 6E08, Campus Box 0456, Ann Arbor, MI 48109-0456 (joyclee@umich.edu).
**Funding/Support:** Dr Lee is supported by Pediatric Health Services Research Training Grant T32 HD07534-05 from the National Institute of Child Health and Human Development, Bethesda, Md.

## REFERENCES


1. Orloff DG. FDA approval letter for Humatrope. Available at: http://www.fda.gov/cder/foi/appletter/2003/19640se1-033ltr.pdf. Accessed February 15, 2005.
2. Cuttler L, Silvers JB. Growth hormone treatment for idiopathic short stature: implications for practice and policy. *Arch Pediatr Adolesc Med.* 2004;158:108-110.
3. Leschek EW, Rose SR, Yanovski JA, et al. Effect of growth hormone treatment on adult height in peripubertal children with idiopathic short stature: a randomized, double-blind, placebo-controlled trial. *J Clin Endocrinol Metab.* 2004;89:3140-3148.
4. Wit JM, Rekers-Mombarg LT, Cutler GB, et al. Growth hormone (GH) treatment to final height in children with idiopathic short stature: evidence for a dose effect. *J Pediatr.* 2005;146:45-53.
5. Wheeler PG, Bresnahan K, Shephard BA, Lau J, Balk EM. Short stature and functional impairment: a systematic review. *Arch Pediatr Adolesc Med.* 2004;158:236-243.
6. Ross JL, Sandberg DE, Rose SR, et al. Psychological adaptation in children with idiopathic short stature treated with growth hormone or placebo. *J Clin Endocrinol Metab.* 2004;89:4873-4878.
7. Levit K, Smith C, Cowan C, Lazenby H, Sensenig A, Catlin A. Trends in U.S. health care spending, 2001. *Health Aff (Millwood).* 2003;22:154-164.
8. Bryant J, Cave C, Mihaylova B, et al. Clinical effectiveness and cost-effectiveness of growth hormone in children: a systematic review and economic evaluation. *Health Technol Assess.* 2002;6(18):1-168.
9. Finkelstein BS, Imperiale TF, Speroff T, Marrero U, Radcliffe DJ, Cuttler L. Effect of growth hormone therapy on height in children with idiopathic short stature: a meta-analysis. *Arch Pediatr Adolesc Med.* 2002;156:230-240.
10. Kemp SF, Kuntze J, Attie KM, et al. Efficacy and safety results of long-term growth hormone treatment of idiopathic short stature. *J Clin Endocrinol Metab.* 2005;90:5247-5253.
11. Humatrope prescribing information. Available at: http://pi.lilly.com/us/humatrope-pi.pdf. Accessed November 1, 2004.
12. Hogler W, Briody J, Moore B, Lu PW, Cowell CT. Effect of growth hormone therapy and puberty on bone and body composition in children with idiopathic short stature and growth hormone deficiency. *Bone.* 2005;37:642-650.
13. Coste J, Letrait M, Carel JC, et al. Long-term results of growth hormone treatment in France in children of short stature: population, register based study. *BMJ.* 1997;315:708-713.
14. Gharib H, Cook DM, Saenger PH, et al. American Association of Clinical Endocrinologists medical guidelines for clinical practice for growth hormone use in adults and children—2003 update. *Endocr Pract.* 2003;9:64-76.
15. Hintz RL, Attie KM, Baptista J, Roche A; Genentech Collaborative Group. Effect of growth hormone treatment on adult height of children with idiopathic short stature. *N Engl J Med.* 1999;340:502-507.
16. Ranke MB, Wilton P, eds. *GH Therapy in KIGS: 10 Years' Experience.* Heidelberg, Germany: Barth; 1999.
17. Leschek EW, Troendle JF, Yanovski JA, et al. Effect of growth hormone treatment on testicular function, puberty, and adrenarche in boys with non–growth hormone–deficient short stature: a randomized, double-blind, placebo-controlled trial. *J Pediatr.* 2001;138:406-410.
18. Wyatt D. Lessons from the National Cooperative Growth Study. *Eur J Endocrinol.* 2004;151(suppl 1):S55-S59.
19. Quigley CA, Gill AM, Crowe BJ, et al. Safety of growth hormone treatment in pediatric patients with idiopathic short stature. *J Clin Endocrinol Metab.* 2005;90:5188-5196.
20. Centers for Medicare and Medicaid Services. Statewide average operating cost-to-charge ratios—July 2004 [Table 8A]. Acute inpatient prospective payment system: federal regulations and notices: CMS-1428-F. Available at: http://www.cms.hhs.gov/AcuteInpatientPPS/Downloads/cms1428f_v.pdf. Accessed July 7, 2005.
21. Growth hormone for normal short children. *Med Lett Drugs Ther.* 2003;45:89-90.
22. Gold MRSJ, Russell LB, Weinstein MC, eds. *Cost-effectiveness in Health and Medicine.* New York, NY: Oxford University Press; 1996.
23. Mauras N, Attie KM, Reiter EO, Saenger P, Baptista J; Genentech, Inc, Cooperative Study Group. High dose recombinant human growth hormone (GH) treat-

ment of GH-deficient patients in puberty increases near-final height: a randomized, multicenter trial. *J Clin Endocrinol Metab.* 2000;85:3653-3660.
24. Fjellestad-Paulsen A, Simon D, Czernichow P. Short children born small for gestational age and treated with growth hormone for three years have an important catch-down five years after discontinuation of treatment. *J Clin Endocrinol Metab.* 2004;89:1234-1239.
25. Rosenfeld R, Allen DB, MacGillivray MH, et al. Growth hormone use in pediatric growth hormone deficiency and other pediatric growth disorders. *Am J Manag Care.* 2000;6(15, suppl):S805-S816.
26. Rosenfeld RG, Hwa V. Toward a molecular basis for idiopathic short stature. *J Clin Endocrinol Metab.* 2004;89:1066-1067.
27. Ubel PA, Hirth RA, Chernew ME, Fendrick AM. What is the price of life and why doesn't it increase at the rate of inflation? *Arch Intern Med.* 2003;163:1637-1641.
28. Hopwood NJ, Hintz RL, Gertner JM, et al. Growth response of children with non–growth-hormone deficiency and marked short stature during three years of growth hormone therapy. *J Pediatr.* 1993;123:215-222.
29. Coutant R, Rouleau S, Despert F, Magontier N, Loisel D, Limal JM. Growth and adult height in GH-treated children with nonacquired GH deficiency and idiopathic short stature: the influence of pituitary magnetic resonance imaging findings. *J Clin Endocrinol Metab.* 2001;86:4649-4654.
30. Guyda HJ. Four decades of growth hormone therapy for short children: what have we achieved? *J Clin Endocrinol Metab.* 1999;84:4307-4316.
31. Persico N, Postlewaite A, Silverman D. The effect of adolescent experience on labor market outcomes: the case of height. *J Polit Econ.* 2004;112:1019-1053.
32. Freemark M. Growth hormone treatment of "idiopathic short stature": not so fast. *J Clin Endocrinol Metab.* 2004;89:3138-3139.
33. Ashworth M, Clement S, Wright M. Demand, appropriateness and prescribing of "lifestyle drugs": a consultation survey in general practice. *Fam Pract.* 2002; 19:236-241.

## Correction

**Incorrect Author Byline and Corresponding Author Address:** In the online version only of the January issue of the ARCHIVES, the editorial by Curry and Mermelstein entitled, "Do As I Say, Not As I Do: Does It Work for Tobacco Use Prevention?" (2006;160:102-103) had the wrong author listed at the end of the editorial and in the Table of Contents. The authors should have been Susan J. Curry, PhD, and Robin J. Mermelstein, PhD. The ARCHIVES regrets the error. This correction was made previously to online versions of this article. In addition, the address for the corresponding author changed and should read: Dr Curry, Health Policy and Administration, Institute for Health Research and Policy, University of Illinois at Chicago, 1747 W Roosevelt Rd, Room 558, M/C 275, Chicago, IL 60608 (suecurry@uic.edu).

# Depressive Symptomatology as a Predictor of Exposure to Intimate Partner Violence Among US Female Adolescents and Young Adults

*Jocelyn A. Lehrer, ScD; Stephen Buka, ScD; Steven Gortmaker, PhD; Lydia A. Shrier, MD, MPH*

**Objective:** To examine whether depressive symptomatology is predictive of subsequent intimate partner violence victimization among a national prospective sample of female adolescents and young adults.

**Design:** Home interview data from 2 waves of the school-based National Longitudinal Study of Adolescent Health were used to examine whether baseline depressive symptomatology was associated with increased risk of past-year exposure to physical abuse by a current partner at 5-year follow-up, controlling for age, race/ethnicity, parental education, retrospective childhood physical and sexual abuse, and baseline dating violence and forced sex.

**Setting:** A stratified random sample of 80 US high schools and 52 middle schools.

**Participants:** All young women (n=1659) were in a current opposite-sex relationship at follow-up.

**Main Exposure:** Baseline past-week depressive symptomatology, measured as both a dichotomous and continuous variable.

**Main Outcome Measures:** Past-year exposure to mild and moderate to severe physical abuse by a current intimate partner.

**Results:** In adjusted models with dichotomous depressive symptoms, high baseline symptom levels were associated with 1.86 times the odds of subsequent exposure to moderate to severe partner violence (95% confidence interval, 1.05-3.29). In adjusted models with continuous depressive symptoms, an increase of 1 SD in baseline symptom levels was associated with a 24% increase in odds of exposure to mild partner violence and a 24% increase in the odds of exposure to moderate to severe partner violence.

**Conclusions:** The findings of this study suggest that depressive symptomatology among girls during adolescence is associated with increased risk of subsequent exposure to physical partner violence. Prevention, identification, and treatment of depressive symptomatology among adolescent girls may help to reduce the likelihood of subsequent victimization.

*Arch Pediatr Adolesc Med. 2006;160:270-276*

**Author Affiliations:** Center for Reproductive Health Research and Policy, University of California, San Francisco (Dr Lehrer); Department of Society, Human Development, and Health, Harvard School of Public Health (Drs Buka and Gortmaker) and Harvard Medical School (Dr Shrier) and Division of Adolescent Medicine, Boston Children's Hospital (Dr Shrier), Boston, Mass.

WHILE DEPRESSION IS understood to be a common outcome of exposure to intimate partner violence (IPV) among female adolescents and young adults,[1] little research has examined the reverse relationship—the extent to which depressive symptomatology in adolescence may be associated with risk of exposure to future abuse by an intimate partner, independent of factors such as prior dating violence or childhood abuse. Increased understanding of the depression-IPV relationship may contribute to prevention efforts by helping to identify girls at risk of future IPV exposure.

Lifetime prevalence of major depressive disorder and minor depression among girls aged 15 to 24 years have been estimated to be 21% and 10%, respectively.[2] The time of transition from adolescence to adulthood is a time of peak depression onset.[3] At the same time, 8.8% of female high school students in the national 2003 Youth Risk Behavior Surveillance System survey reported past-year experience of physical abuse by a dating partner.[4] Estimates of dating violence victimization among girls in smaller studies range from 8% to 57%; studies vary in the period assessed.[5] Nationally, 22% of women 18 years and older report experiencing physical IPV at some point in their lifetime.[6]

Depressive symptomatology, dysthymia, and major depression during adolescence have been found to be associated with a broad range of functional impairments and adverse outcomes in later adolescence and young adulthood, including diminished self-esteem, self-mastery and life satisfaction, internalizing behavior problems, interpersonal difficulties, increased need for social support, career dissatisfaction,[7] divorce,[8-11] impaired work and social functioning, lower social class, increased work absence, unemployment,[12] diminished educational attainment,[9,11,12] female teenage childbearing,[10] and decreased likelihood of on-time marriage.[13] In addition to predicting adverse social outcomes, diagnosed depression in adolescence is associated with subsequent substance abuse[14] and is a strong and specific predictor of depression in early adulthood[7,12,15-18] as well as suicide and suicide attempts.[12,19] One study found that depression at age 18 years was associated with impaired psychological and social functioning at age 21 years regardless of depression status at age 21 years, suggesting that depression during the time of transition to adulthood is associated with continued psychosocial vulnerability and poorer functioning in young adulthood regardless of depression status in young adulthood[19]; other studies support the finding of vulnerability beyond the duration of the depressive episode.[14]

Few prospective studies have examined IPV exposure as a potential outcome related to adolescent depressive symptomatology, and findings among these studies have been mixed. A 3-year study of a high-risk sample found that women's baseline depressive symptomatology was predictive of their male partners' subsequent perpetration of psychological but not physical abuse.[20] A 6-year study of male and female high school students found that depressive symptomatology in adolescence was not associated with subsequent physical aggression in dating relationships or marriage (perpetration and victimization were not distinguished).[21] A retrospective national study of married or cohabiting adults found that premarital depression was not associated with subsequent IPV victimization among women.[22] A 5-year study of female high school students found that the proportion of days spent in depressive episodes was positively associated with psychological and physical abuse by boyfriends over the follow-up period; temporal order of depressive episodes and abuse could not be ascertained.[16]

Given the high prevalence of depressive symptomatology and IPV exposure among female youth in the United States, as well as research demonstrating many adverse psychosocial outcomes for adolescents with depressive symptomatology, this study examined whether depressive symptomatology among adolescent girls is predictive of subsequent IPV exposure in late adolescence and young adulthood. Analyses were conducted with prospective, population-based data from the National Longitudinal Study of Adolescent Health (Add Health).[23]

## METHODS

### DESIGN

The Add Health study is a longitudinal study of the determinants and contexts of youth health and risk behaviors. In summary, a stratified random sample of 80 US high schools and 52 middle schools was selected with probability of selection proportional to school size. Stratification was with respect to region of country, urbanicity, school size, school type, and race/ethnic composition. Wave 1 structured, closed-ended home interviews were conducted with youth in grades 7 through 12 in 1995; 82% of wave 1 home interview subjects with sampling weights had a parental figure who participated in a wave 1 parent interview. Wave 2 home interview data were collected in 1996 (n with sampling weights = 13 570) and wave 3 data were collected in 2001 and 2002 (n with sampling weights = 10 828). Written informed consent was provided by youth participants as well as a parental figure at waves 1 and 2 and by youth participants at wave 3. Approval for the full Add Health study was granted by the institutional review board of the University of North Carolina at Chapel Hill School of Public Health; approval for the present data analysis was granted by the Human Subjects Committee of the Harvard School of Public Health (Boston, Mass).

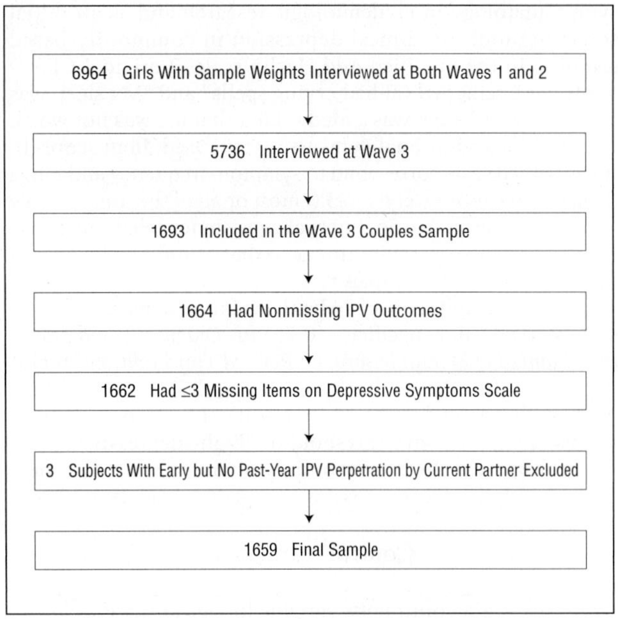


**Figure.** Sample selection flowchart. IPV indicates intimate partner violence.

### SAMPLE

The study sample was restricted to the 1659 girls in the contractual use data set[24] who participated in home interviews at waves 1, 2, and 3; had sample weights; and were selected for the couples sample of the Add Health study. One half of all wave 3–eligible subjects were randomly selected to be considered for the wave 3 couples sample. By design, the couples sample includes one-third dating couples, one-third cohabiting couples, and one-third married couples. Criteria for inclusion in the couples sample were (1) involvement in a current relationship; (2) relationship duration of 3 months or more; (3) opposite-sex relationship; and (4) partner 18 years or older. The sample for the present study was also restricted to subjects who had nonmissing data regarding IPV outcomes and who had 3 or fewer missing items on the wave 2 depressive symptoms scale. Three subjects who reported that their partner had physically abused them more than 1 year prior to the wave 3 interview, but not within the past year, were also excluded so as to maintain temporal clarity between wave 2 depressive symptoms and IPV exposure (**Figure**).

### MEASURES

#### Baseline Depressive Symptomatology

Self-reported past-week depressive symptomatology was assessed both as a dichotomous and continuous variable at wave 2, with a 19-item, modified Center for Epidemiologic Studies Scale (CES-D) used in the Add Health survey.[25] The original 20-item scale has been widely used as a measure of depressive symptomatology in epidemiologic research and as an initial screening tool for clinical depression in community-based samples. In the modified Add Health scale, 2 original CES-D items were removed ("I had crying spells" and "My sleep was restless") and 1 item was added ("I felt that life was not worth living"). Two additional items were rephrased. Item scores in the modified scale correspond to symptom frequency and range from 0 ("never or rarely") to 3 ("most or all of the time"); scale scores range from 0 to 56. Internal consistency reliability in the present sample was 0.89, similar to that found for the CES-D in other adolescent samples.[26-28]

A CES-D cutoff score of 24 has been found to maximize sensitivity (0.84) and specificity (0.75) for *Diagnostic and Statistical Manual of Mental Disorders, Revised Third Edition*[29] major depressive disorder or dysthymia for adolescent girls.[27] Proportionally adapted to the 19-item scale, the cutoff score used in this study for above-threshold or "high" depressive symptomatology was 23.[30,31] Secondary analyses were also performed with the continuous scale for greater statistical power.

### Control Variables

**Age.** This was a continuous variable for age at wave 2.

**Race/Ethnicity.** Four categories were used: non-Hispanic white, non-Hispanic black, Hispanic, and other. Youth reporting more than 1 race/ethnicity were assigned to the category with which they indicated they most identify.

**Wave 1 Parental Education.** This was a dichotomous variable indicating whether the highest educational attainment among resident parental figures at wave 1 was less than high school. Data were obtained from the parent interview.

### Covariates

**Childhood Experience of Physical and/or Sexual Abuse.** At wave 3, subjects were asked 2 self-administered questions regarding the time before they entered the sixth grade: (1) "How often had your parents or other adult caregivers slapped, hit, or kicked you?" and (2) "How often had one of your parents or other adult caregivers touched you in a sexual way, forced you to touch him or her in a sexual way, or forced you to have sexual relations?" A dichotomous variable was created reflecting subject report of being slapped, hit, or kicked more than 5 times and/or report of any occurrence of sexual abuse.

**Dating Violence and/or Forced Sex Between Waves 1 and 2.** At wave 2, subjects were asked whether any partner they had had since wave 1 ever threatened them with violence, pushed or shoved them, or thrown something at them that could hurt. Subjects who indicated at wave 2 that they had ever had sexual intercourse were also asked whether they were ever physically forced to have sexual intercourse against their will since the wave 1 interview. These data were collected with audio computer-assisted self-interview.[32,33] A dichotomous variable was created reflecting 1 or more affirmative responses to these items.

### Outcome Variables

**Mild Violence.** At wave 3, subjects were asked 1 self-administered question regarding how often in the past year their current partner had threatened them with violence, pushed or shoved them, or thrown something at them that could hurt. A dichotomous variable was created reflecting any past-year experience of this outcome.

**Moderate to Severe Physical Violence.** At wave 3, subjects were asked 1 self-administered question regarding how often in the past year their current partner had slapped, hit, or kicked them and another question regarding how often in the past year they had had an "injury, such as a sprain, bruise, or cut" because of a fight with their current partner. A dichotomous variable was created reflecting experience of either or both of these outcomes.

## STATISTICAL ANALYSIS

All analyses were conducted with SAS version 8 (SAS Institute Inc, Cary, NC). Logistic regression models were estimated using the 2 dichotomous violence variables as dependent variables. The SAS proc GENMOD function (generalized estimating equations) was used for all regressions, with specification of an independent working correlation structure. The use of generalized estimating equations accounts for data clustering to provide robust standard error estimation.

Multivariate models first adjusted for control variables of age, race/ethnicity, and parental education (model 1) and then additionally adjusted for covariates of childhood physical/sexual abuse and dating violence/forced sex (model 2). All baseline data for these analyses were collected at wave 2, except for wave 1 parental education and wave 3 retrospective childhood abuse.

Potential interactions between depressive symptomatology and each of the 2 prior abuse covariates were examined separately in unadjusted and adjusted models predicting mild and moderate to severe abuse outcomes, with both the dichotomous and continuous depressive symptoms variables. These interaction terms were insignificant in all model specifications and were not included in final models.

In addition, 2 variables reflecting wave 2 alcohol abuse comorbidity (frequent drinking and heavy drinking) were considered for inclusion as covariates; neither variable was included in final models because they were not associated in bivariate or multivariate models with either IPV outcome, and their addition to the adjusted models did not alter the effect size or significance of depressive symptoms. This may have been owing to insufficient statistical power.

Variables reflecting subjects' relationship status were also not included in final models because relationship status was viewed as a potential mediator between depressive symptoms and IPV exposure. Inclusion of relationship status variables in preliminary analyses, however, produced no difference in the effect size or significance level of depressive symptomatology with regard to either IPV outcome.

All analyses used adjusted grand sample weights to account for wave 3 nonresponse and subgroup oversampling. For analyses examining the outcome of mild IPV, a subsample of 1632 subjects was used; 27 subjects who reported exposure to moderate to severe but not mild violence at wave 3 were excluded. For analyses examining moderate to severe IPV, a subsample of 1525 subjects was used; 134 subjects who experienced mild but not moderate to severe violence were excluded. For the 15 subjects who were missing 3 or fewer items on the wave 2 depressive symptoms scale, the mean of the remaining items was imputed for each missing item.

# RESULTS

## SAMPLE CHARACTERISTICS

The sample of girls was 68.5% non-Hispanic white, 15.6% non-Hispanic black, 10.6% Hispanic, and 5.3% other race/ethnicities (**Table 1**). The mean ages at baseline and follow-up were 15.9 years and 21.3 years, respectively; the wave 3 age range was 18 to 27 years. Ten percent of sub-

**Table 1. Sample Characteristics of 1659 Subjects***

| Characteristic | Percentage† |
|---|---|
| Wave 2 age, y, mean (SD) | 15.9 (1.6) |
| Wave 3 age, y, mean (SD) | 21.3 (1.6) |
| Race/ethnicity | |
| Non-Hispanic white | 68.5 |
| Non-Hispanic black | 15.6 |
| Hispanic | 10.6 |
| Other | 5.3 |
| Parent education <12 y | 10.1 |
| Parent education missing | 10.5 |
| Wave 3 marital status | |
| Married | 25.7 |
| Cohabiting | 24.9 |
| Dating/other | 49.4 |
| Wave 2 depressive symptom score, mean (SD) | 11.4 (8.1) |
| Childhood sexual and/or physical abuse | 10.2 |
| Baseline dating violence and/or forced sex | 12.4 |
| Wave 3 partner violence | |
| Threatened, pushed, or threw object | 17.0 |
| Hit, slapped, or kicked | 9.6 |
| Injury | 4.8 |
| Any violence or injury | 18.6 |
| Years between waves 2 and 3, mean (SD) | 5.4 (0.2) |

*Number of subjects is unweighted.
†Unless otherwise noted. Percentages and means are weighted.

jects came from homes where the highest parental education level was less than 12th grade. The mean baseline depressive symptoms scale score was 11.4, and 10.2% of subjects had above-threshold symptom scores. At wave 3, 25.7% of subjects were married, 24.9% were cohabiting, and 49.4% were considered to be dating. The mean number of years between wave 2 and 3 interviews was 5.4. One percent of subjects were married at both waves 2 and 3.

## DEPRESSIVE SYMPTOMATOLOGY AND SUBSEQUENT IPV EXPOSURE

Twenty-eight percent of subjects with high depressive symptom levels at baseline reported any IPV or injury at follow-up as compared with 17.5% of subjects with lower symptom levels (odds ratio [OR], 1.84 [95% confidence interval (CI), 1.20-2.84]) (**Table 2**).

In bivariate analyses with the dichotomous depressive symptoms variable, girls with high baseline symptom levels had 1.66 times the odds of subsequent exposure to mild IPV and 2.46 times the odds of exposure to moderate to severe IPV as compared with girls with lower baseline symptom levels (results not shown). In fully adjusted analyses, high depressive symptomatology was not significantly associated with likelihood of exposure to mild IPV ($P=.11$) (**Table 3**); girls with high depressive symptoms had 1.86 times the odds of subsequent exposure to moderate to severe IPV (95% CI, 1.05-3.29) (**Table 4**).

In bivariate analyses with continuous depressive symptomatology, a 1-point increase in baseline symptoms was associated with a 3% increase in the odds of subsequent exposure to mild IPV (95% CI, 1.01-1.05) and a 4% increase in the odds of exposure to moderate to severe IPV (95% CI, 1.02-1.06). In fully adjusted analyses, each

**Table 2. Percentage of 1659 Subjects Who Reported Past-Year Intimate Partner Violence at Wave 3, by Wave 2 Depressive Symptom Level***

| | Subjects With High Wave 2 Depressive Symptoms, % | Subjects Without High Wave 2 Depressive Symptoms, % |
|---|---|---|
| Threatened, pushed, or threw object | 23.5 | 16.3 |
| Hit, slapped, or kicked | 20.0 | 8.5 |
| Injury | 6.7 | 4.6 |
| Any violence or injury | 28.1 | 17.5 |

*Number of subjects is unweighted. Percentages are weighted.

**Table 3. Association Between Dichotomous Wave 2 Depressive Symptomatology and Wave 3 Mild Intimate Partner Violence in 1632 Subjects***

| | Model 1† | Model 2‡ |
|---|---|---|
| Wave 2 dichotomous depressive symptoms | 1.64 (1.01-2.68)§ | 1.49 (0.91-2.45) |
| Wave 2 age | 0.98 (0.89-1.08) | 0.98 (0.89-1.08) |
| Race/ethnicity | | |
| Non-Hispanic white | 1.00 | 1.00 |
| Non-Hispanic black | 1.67 (1.03-2.71)§ | 1.70 (1.06-2.74)§ |
| Hispanic | 0.95 (0.53-1.72) | 0.97 (0.53-1.77) |
| Other | 0.96 (0.46-1.99) | 0.92 (0.45-1.89) |
| Parent education <12 y | 1.30 (0.73-2.33) | 1.33 (0.74-2.39) |
| Parent education missing | 0.88 (0.52-1.46) | 0.91 (0.54-1.52) |
| Childhood sexual and/or physical abuse | | 1.39 (0.83-2.33) |
| Baseline dating violence and/or forced sex | | 1.40 (0.84-2.30) |

*Number of subjects is unweighted. Values are expressed as adjusted odds ratio (95% confidence interval).
†Model 1 includes depressive symptoms, age, race/ethnicity, parental education, and indicator for parental education missing.
‡Model 2 includes all variables of model 1 and adds childhood sexual/physical abuse and baseline dating violence/forced sex.
§$P<.05$.

1-point increase in depressive symptomatology was associated with a 3% increase in the odds of exposure to mild IPV (95% CI, 1.01-1.05) and a 3% increase in the odds of exposure to moderate to severe IPV (95% CI, 1.01-1.05) (tables available on request).

Regarding covariates and controls, adjusted analyses demonstrated that childhood physical/sexual abuse and baseline dating violence/forced sex were each associated with approximately 2 times the odds of exposure to moderate to severe IPV (Table 4). Additional analyses found that the lack of association observed between the abuse covariates and mild IPV in the fully adjusted model did not seem to be due to a mediating effect of depressive symptomatology.[34]

## COMMENT

Findings from this prospective study suggest that depressive symptomatology among adolescent girls is as-

**Table 4. Association Between Dichotomous Wave 2 Depressive Symptomatology and Wave 3 Moderate to Severe Intimate Partner Violence in 1525 Subjects***

| | Model 1† | Model 2‡ |
|---|---|---|
| Wave 2 dichotomous depressive symptoms | 2.26 (1.32-3.87)§ | 1.86 (1.05-3.29)‖ |
| Wave 2 age | 1.04 (0.93-1.17) | 1.03 (0.91-1.16) |
| Race/ethnicity | | |
| Non-Hispanic white | 1.00 | 1.00 |
| Non-Hispanic black | 1.21 (0.64-2.26) | 1.22 (0.65-2.29) |
| Hispanic | 1.10 (0.57-2.12) | 1.15 (0.57-2.31) |
| Other | 1.10 (0.53-2.31) | 1.02 (0.51-2.04) |
| Parent education <12 y | 1.61 (0.84-3.08) | 1.70 (0.88-3.28) |
| Parent education missing | 1.00 (0.55-1.82) | 1.11 (0.61-2.02) |
| Childhood sexual and/or physical abuse | | 1.99 (1.11-3.57)‖ |
| Baseline dating violence and/or forced sex | | 2.05 (1.18-3.53)§ |

*Number of subjects is unweighted. Values are expressed as adjusted odds ratio (95% confidence interval).

†Model 1 includes depressive symptoms, age, race/ethnicity, parental education, and indicator for parental education missing.

‡Model 2 includes all variables of model 1 and adds childhood sexual/physical abuse and baseline dating violence/forced sex.

§$P<.01$.

‖$P<.05$.

sociated with increased risk of subsequent physical abuse by an intimate partner in late adolescence and young adulthood, independent of childhood physical or sexual abuse as well as prior experience of dating violence or forced sex. Twenty-eight percent of girls with high levels of baseline depressive symptomatology, corresponding to an elevated likelihood of mood disorder, reported some form of past-year physical IPV victimization 5 years later. Girls with high baseline depressive symptoms had 1.86 times the odds of girls with lower symptom levels of subsequent exposure to moderate to severe IPV, and victimization risk was also found to increase with increasing levels of continuous depressive symptomatology. The finding that childhood abuse and dating violence/forced sex were associated with subsequent IPV risk also provides prospective evidence that prior abuse is predictive of revictimization among young women.

The time of transition from adolescence to adulthood is one of increasing independence from parents, strengthening self-concept, and critical decision making regarding education, occupation, and intimate relationships, all of which have a salient impact on the long-term social trajectory of the individual.[16,19] Depression that occurs during this time of transition may have a particularly significant impact on maturational processes and choices made, generating a trajectory of risk for continued psychosocial impairment and psychopathology.[11,15,16,35,36]

Regarding social pathways that may be affected by depression in adolescence, studies of peer group homophily and assortative mating have found that adolescents and adults with depressive symptoms or disorders often associate, in friendship,[37,38] dating,[20] and marriage,[39] with others who have similar levels of symptomatology. In turn, depressive symptoms and disorders among men have been found to be positively associated with subsequent psychological[20] and/or physical[22] aggression toward an intimate partner.

Depressive symptomatology is also associated with a range of adolescent risk behaviors including substance use and abuse,[40-42] and depressed youth are more likely to associate with deviant or risky peer groups[18] from which partner selection is likely to occur. Alcohol and drug use, in turn, have been associated in some studies with males' physical abuse perpetration toward their dating partners,[43] cohabiting partners, and wives.[44] Depressive symptomatology has also been associated with antisocial behavior among young men[20,45]; delinquency[46] and antisocial behavior[20,21] among male adolescents are associated with increased likelihood of physical IPV perpetration. In sum, depressive symptomatology may elevate girls' risk of future IPV exposure by way of its contribution to risky peer group affiliations and assortative partnering with high-risk mates.

In addition to differential selection into abusive relationships, young women with a history of depressive symptomatology may be less likely to leave abusive relationships (or take a longer time to leave) for various reasons. First, insofar as depression in adolescence is predictive of outcomes such as teenage childbearing, diminished educational attainment, and unemployment, it may be associated with increased economic dependency on future partners and thus decreased likelihood of relationship exit.[47,48] Second, increasing social isolation of the woman from family and friends is a common feature of abusive relationships, and diminished social support is another obstacle to relationship exit.[49,50] Depressed youth often have impaired social relationships and diminished support from family members and peers,[11,35,51] such that young women with former or current depression may enter intimate relationships from a starting point of greater isolation than those with no former or current depression. This diminished potential pool of external support may contribute to an increased likelihood of not leaving, or returning to, an abusive partner. Girls with a history of depression and diminished social support may also place an elevated premium on intimacy and maintenance of a relationship with a romantic partner and be more willing to tolerate acts of violence from an otherwise seemingly secure partner.[48]

Third, depression is a primary psychological response to abuse, and Barnett[48] notes that depression or other mental health difficulties due to IPV may impair women's ability to mobilize to exit their relationships. Women who have a history of vulnerability to depression may have an increased likelihood of responding to the stressor of IPV with depression or other debilitation, contributing to a decreased likelihood of relationship exit. Further research should examine these and other potential mechanisms.

This study has several limitations. First, the adapted CES-D scale is not a diagnostic instrument. The wave 2 measurement of past-week depressive symptomatology may also not fully reflect the severity, chronicity, or recurrence of symptomatology over the period between waves 2 and 3, which may be relevant to likelihood of future IPV exposure. However, depressive symptoms and disorders in adolescence are predictive of subsequent disorder in young adulthood, and a number of studies have noted the stability of depressed mood among adolescents, although a consistent pattern of findings has not yet emerged for girls.[11,52-54] Second, incomplete measurement of confounding factors may have contributed to the observation of an association between depressive symptomatology and IPV exposure. The childhood abuse, dating violence, and sexual coercion covariates do not account for all relevant time in respondents' lives, and the wave 2 sexual coercion item focuses only on forced intercourse. The Add Health study also does not include a measure of exposure to interparental violence, which has been found to be predictive of women's subsequent depressive symptomatology[55] and abuse by an intimate partner.[56] Third, IPV is frequently underreported by survivors,[57,58] which may have led to bias in results. Fourth, this study did not address perpetration; this relationship should be examined with surveys that distinguish between violence committed in self-defense or retaliation and self-initiated acts.[59] Finally, the generalizability of the study findings is limited, given the specific nature of the sample.

Overall, this study provides evidence that elevated levels of depressive symptomatology among adolescent girls are associated with an increased vulnerability to subsequent IPV exposure in late adolescence and young adulthood. However, the question of whether depressive symptomatology plays an independent role in shaping the trajectory toward future IPV exposure among young women, or whether it is simply a marker for IPV risk, is not fully resolved with the present study and warrants further investigation. If depressive symptomatology among adolescent girls becomes recognized as an independent predictor of subsequent IPV exposure, this will be one more reason to increase efforts in the prevention, identification, and treatment of depressive symptomatology among adolescent girls. If depressive symptomatology comes to be understood as a marker for risk of IPV exposure, it may be helpful in identifying high-risk girls for targeted intervention efforts.

**Accepted for Publication:** September 21, 2005.
**Correspondence:** Jocelyn A. Lehrer, ScD, 4601 25th St, 7, San Francisco, CA 94114 (jlehrer1@gmail.com).
**Funding/Support:** This research uses data from Add Health, a program project designed by J. Richard Udry, PhD, Peter S. Bearman, PhD, and Kathleen Mullan Harris, PhD, and funded by grant P01-HD31921 from the National Institute of Child Health and Human Development, Rockville, Md, with cooperative funding from 17 other agencies. Partial funding for research came from the National Institute of Mental Health Academic Fellowship on Mental Health and Developmental Disorders.
**Role of the Sponsor:** The funders were not involved in the design, conduct, analysis, or interpretation of the data or in preparation, review, or approval of the manuscript.
**Additional Information:** Persons interested in obtaining data files from Add Health should contact Add Health, Carolina Population Center, 123 W Franklin St, Chapel Hill, NC 27516-2524 (addhealth@unc.edu).
**Acknowledgment:** Special acknowledgment is due Ronald R. Rindfuss, PhD, and Barbara Entwisle, PhD, for assistance in the Add Health Study original design.

## REFERENCES

1. Campbell JC. Health consequences of intimate partner violence. *Lancet*. 2002;359:1331-1336.
2. Kessler RC, Walters E. Epidemiology of *DSM-III-R* major depression and minor depression among adolescents and young adults in the National Comorbidity Survey. *Depress Anxiety*. 1998;7:3-14.
3. Hankin BL, Abramson LY, Moffitt TE, et al. Development of depression from preadolescence to young adulthood: emerging gender differences in a 10-year longitudinal study. *J Abnorm Psychol*. 1998;107:128-140.
4. Grunbaum JA, Kann L, Kinchen SA, et al. Youth Risk Behavior Surveillance—United States, 2003 [published correction appears in *MMWR Morb Mortal Wkly Rep*. 2004;53:536. *MMWR Morb Mortal Wkly Rep*. 2005;54:608]. *MMWR Surveill Summ*. 2004;53:1-96.
5. Hickman LJ, Jaycox LH, Aronoff J. Dating violence among adolescents: prevalence, gender distribution, and prevention program effectiveness. *Trauma Violence Abuse*. 2004;5:123-142.
6. Tjaden P, Thoennes N. *Extent, Nature and Consequences of Intimate Partner Violence: Findings From the National Violence Against Women Survey*. Washington, DC: US Dept of Justice; 2000.
7. Giaconia RM, Reinherz HZ, Paradis AD, et al. Major depression and drug disorders in adolescence: general and specific impairments in early adulthood. *J Am Acad Child Adolesc Psychiatry*. 2001;40:1426-1433.
8. Kessler RC, Walters EE, Forthofer MS. The social consequences of psychiatric disorders, III: probability of marital stability. *Am J Psychiatry*. 1998;155:1092-1096.
9. Kessler RC, Foster CL, Saunders WB, et al. Social consequences of psychiatric disorders, I: educational attainment. *Am J Psychiatry*. 1995;152:1026-1032.
10. Kessler RC, Berglund PA, Foster CL, et al. Social consequences of psychiatric disorders, II: teenage parenthood. *Am J Psychiatry*. 1997;154:1405-1411.
11. Kandel DB, Davies M. Adult sequelae of adolescent depressive symptoms. *Arch Gen Psychiatry*. 1986;43:255-262.
12. Weissman MM, Wolk S, Goldstein RB, et al. Depressed adolescents grown up. *JAMA*. 1999;281:1707-1713.
13. Forthofer MS, Kessler RC, Story AL, et al. The effects of psychiatric disorders on the probability and timing of first marriage. *J Health Soc Behav*. 1996;37:121-132.
14. Birmaher B, Ryan N, Williamson D, et al. Childhood and adolescent depression: a review of the past 10 years, part I. *J Am Acad Child Adolesc Psychiatry*. 1996;35:1427-1439.
15. Rao U, Ryan ND, Birmaher B, et al. Unipolar depression in adolescents: clinical outcome in adulthood. *J Am Acad Child Adolesc Psychiatry*. 1995;34:566-578.
16. Rao U, Hammen C, Daley S. Continuity of depression during the transition to adulthood: a 5-year longitudinal study of young women. *J Am Acad Child Adolesc Psychiatry*. 1999;38:908-915.
17. Lewinsohn PM, Rohde P, Klein DN, et al. Natural course of adolescent major depressive disorder I: continuity into young adulthood. *J Am Acad Child Adolesc Psychiatry*. 1999;38:56-63.
18. Fergusson DM, Woodward LJ. Mental health, educational and social role outcomes of adolescents with depression. *Arch Gen Psychiatry*. 2002;59:225-231.
19. Reinherz HZ, Giaconia RM, Carmola Hauf AM, et al. Major depression in the transition to adulthood: risks and impairments. *J Abnorm Psychol*. 1999;108:500-510.
20. Kim HK, Capaldi DM. The association of antisocial behavior and depressive symptoms between partners and risk for aggression in romantic relationships. *J Fam Psychol*. 2004;18:82-96.
21. Andrews JA, Capaldi D, Foster SL, et al. Adolescent and family predictors of physical aggression, communication, and satisfaction in young adult couples: a prospective analysis. *J Consult Clin Psychol*. 2000;68:195-208.
22. Kessler RC, Molnar BE, Feurer ID, et al. Patterns and mental health predictors of domestic violence in the United States: results from the National Comorbidity Survey. *Int J Law Psychiatry*. 2001;24:487-508.
23. Harris KM, Florey F, Tabor J, Bearman PS, Jones J, Udry JR. The National Longitudinal Study of Adolescent Health: research design. Available at: http://www.cpcunc.edu/projects/addhealth/design. Accessed July 15, 2004.
24. Udry JR. *The National Longitudinal Study of Adolescent Health (Add Health), Waves I & II, 1994–1996; Wave III, 2001–2002*. Chapel Hill: Carolina Population Center, University of North Carolina at Chapel Hill; 2003.
25. Radloff L. The CES-D Scale: a self-report depression scale for research in the general population. *Appl Psychol Meas*. 1977;1:385-401.

26. Roberts RE, Andrews JA, Lewinsohn PM, et al. Assessment of depression in adolescents using the Center for Epidemiologic Studies Depression Scale. *Psychol Assess.* 1990;2:122-128.
27. Roberts RE, Lewinsohn P, Seeley J. Screening for adolescent depression: a comparison of depression scales. *J Am Acad Child Adolesc Psychiatry.* 1991;30:58-66.
28. Garrison CZ, Addy CL, Jackson KL, et al. The CES-D as a screen for depression and other psychiatric disorders in adolescents. *J Am Acad Child Adolesc Psychiatry.* 1991;30:636-641.
29. American Psychiatric Association. *Diagnostic and Statistical Manual of Mental Disorders, Revised, Third Edition.* Washington, DC: American Psychiatric Association; 1987.
30. Shrier LA, Harris S, Beardslee W. Temporal associations between depressive symptoms and self-reported sexually transmitted disease among adolescents. *Arch Pediatr Adolesc Med.* 2002;156:599-606.
31. Goodman E, Capitman J. Depressive symptoms and cigarette smoking in teens. *Pediatrics.* 2000;106:748-755.
32. Des Jarlais DC, Paone D, Milliken J, et al. Audio-computer interviewing to measure risk behavior for HIV among injecting drug users: a quasi-randomized trial. *Lancet.* 1999;353:1657-1661.
33. Supple AJ, Aquilino WS, Wright DL. Collecting sensitive self-report data with laptop computers: impact on the response tendencies of adolescents in a home interview. *J Res Adolesc.* 1999;9:467-488.
34. Baron RM, Kenny DA. The mediator-moderator variable distinction in social psychological research: conceptual, strategic and statistical considerations. *J Pers Soc Psychol.* 1986;51:1173-1182.
35. Merikangas K, Angst J. The challenge of depressive disorders in adolescence. In: Rutter MJ, ed. *Psychosocial Disturbances in Young People: Challenges for Prevention.* Victoria, Australia: Cambridge University Press; 1995:131-165.
36. Reinherz HZ, Paradis AD, Giaconia RM, et al. Childhood and adolescent predictors of major depression in the transition to adulthood. *Am J Psychiatry.* 2003;160:2141-2147.
37. Hogue A, Steinberg L. Homophily of internalized distress in adolescent peer groups. *Dev Psychol.* 1995;31:897-906.
38. Rosenblatt A, Greenberg J. Examining the world of the depressed: do depressed people prefer others who are depressed? *J Pers Soc Psychol.* 1991;60:620-629.
39. Lindeman S, Kaprio J, Isometsa E, et al. Spousal resemblance for history of major depressive episode in the previous year. *Psychol Med.* 2002;32:363-367.
40. Lewinsohn PM, Gotlib IH, Seeley JR. Adolescent psychopathology, IV: specificity of psychosocial risk factors for depression and substance abuse in older adolescents. *J Am Acad Child Adolesc Psychiatry.* 1995;34:1221-1229.
41. Deykin EY, Levy JC, Wells V. Adolescent depression, alcohol and drug abuse. *Am J Public Health.* 1987;77:178-182.
42. Kelder SH, Murray NG, Orpinas P, et al. Depression and substance use in minority middle-school students. *Am J Public Health.* 2001;91:761-766.
43. O'Keefe M. Predictors of dating violence among high school students. *J Interpers Violence.* 1997;12:546-568.
44. Pan HS, Neidig PH, OLeary KD. Predicting mild and severe husband-to-wife physical aggression. *J Consult Clin Psychol.* 1994;62:975-981.
45. Zoccolillo M. Co-occurrence of conduct disorder and its adult outcomes with depressive and anxiety disorders: a review. *J Am Acad Child Adolesc Psychiatry.* 1992;31:547-556.
46. Malamuth NM, Sockloskie RJ, Koss MP, et al. Characteristics of aggressors against women: testing a model using a national sample of college students. *J Consult Clin Psychol.* 1991;59:670-681.
47. Anderson DK, Saunders DG. Leaving an abusive partner: an empirical review of predictors, the process of leaving, and psychological well-being. *Trauma Violence Abuse.* 2003;4:163-191.
48. Barnett OW. Why battered women do not leave, part 1: external inhibiting factors within society. *Trauma Violence Abuse.* 2000;1:343-372.
49. Walker L. Assessment of abusive spousal relationships. In: Beach SR, ed. *Marital and Family Processes in Depression.* Washington, DC: American Psychological Association; 1996:338-356.
50. Barnett OW. Why battered women do not leave, part 2: external inhibiting factors—social support and internal inhibiting factors. *Trauma Violence Abuse.* 2001;2:3-35.
51. Lewinsohn PM, Gotlib IH, Seeley JR. Depression-related psychosocial variables: are they specific to depression in adolescents? *J Abnorm Psychol.* 1997;106:365-375.
52. Holsen I, Kraft P, Vitterso J. Stability in depressed mood in adolescence: results from a 6-year longitudinal panel study. *J Youth Adolesc.* 2000;29:61-78.
53. Patten CA, Choi WS, Vickers KS, et al. Persistence of depressive symptoms in adolescents. *Neuropsychopharmacology.* 2001;25(suppl 5):S89-S91.
54. Charman T. The stability of depressed mood in young adolescents: a school-based survey. *J Affect Disord.* 1994;30:109-116.
55. Maker AH, Kemmelmeier M, Peterson C. Long-term psychological consequences in women of witnessing parental physical conflict and experiencing abuse in childhood. *J Interpers Violence.* 1998;13:574-589.
56. Hotaling GT, Sugarman DB. An analysis of risk markers in husband to wife violence: the current state of knowledge. *Violence Vict.* 1986;1:101-124.
57. Sugarman DB, Hotaling GT. Intimate violence and social desirability: a meta-analytic review. *J Interpers Violence.* 1997;12:275-290.
58. Koss MP, Goodman LA, Browne A, et al. *No Safe Haven: Male Violence Against Women at Home, at Work and In the Community.* Washington, DC: American Psychological Association; 1994.
59. Lewis SF, Fremouw W. Dating violence: a critical review of the literature. *Clin Psychol Rev.* 2001;21:105-127.

"Look there,
look in the eyes,
and look in the hearts,
of those who watch while a baby sleeps,
who will come at a call if he wakes and weeps,
who forget the diapers and broken toys,
who remember the tears and fears and joys,
and the catch in the throat, and the heart's clutch,
when small hands fumble, and reach, and touch—
Yes, look in their hearts, and the signs are clear . . .
A baby lives here."
—Anonymous

**PEDIARIX™ [Diphtheria and Tetanus Toxoids and Acellular Pertussis Adsorbed, Hepatitis B (Recombinant) and Inactivated Poliovirus Vaccine Combined]**

The following is a brief summary only; see full prescribing information for complete product information.

**CONTRAINDICATIONS:** Hypersensitivity to any component of the vaccine, including yeast, neomycin, and polymyxin B, is a contraindication (see DESCRIPTION in complete prescribing information). Do not use PEDIARIX after a serious allergic reaction (e.g., anaphylaxis) temporally associated with a previous dose of this vaccine or with any components of this vaccine. Because of the uncertainty as to which component of the vaccine might be responsible, do not give further vaccination with any of these components; or, refer such individuals to an allergist for evaluation. The following events are contraindications to administration of PEDIARIX: encephalopathy (e.g., coma, decreased level of consciousness, prolonged seizures) within 7 days of administration of a previous dose of a pertussis-containing vaccine that is not attributable to another identifiable cause; progressive neurologic disorder, including infantile spasms, uncontrolled epilepsy, or progressive encephalopathy. Do not vaccinate individuals with such conditions until a treatment regimen has been established and the condition has stabilized. PEDIARIX is not contraindicated for use in individuals with HIV infection.

**WARNINGS:** Administration of PEDIARIX is associated with higher rates of fever relative to separately administered vaccines. In one study that evaluated medically attended fever after the first dose of PEDIARIX or separately administered vaccines, infants who received PEDIARIX had a higher rate of medical encounters for fever within the first 4 days following vaccination. In some infants, these encounters included the performance of diagnostic studies to evaluate other causes of fever (see ADVERSE REACTIONS). The vial stopper is latex-free. The tip cap and the rubber plunger of the needleless prefilled syringes contain dry natural latex rubber that may cause allergic reactions in latex sensitive individuals. If any of the following events occur in temporal relation to receipt of whole-cell DTP or a vaccine containing an acellular pertussis component, consider carefully whether to give subsequent doses of PEDIARIX or any vaccine containing a pertussis component: temperature of ≥40.5°C (105°F) within 48 hours not due to another identifiable cause; collapse or shock-like state (hypotonic-hyporesponsive episode) within 48 hours; persistent, inconsolable crying lasting ≥3 hours, occurring within 48 hours; seizures with or without fever occurring within 3 days. If Guillain-Barré syndrome occurs within 6 weeks of receipt of prior vaccine containing tetanus toxoid, the decision to give subsequent doses of PEDIARIX or any vaccine containing tetanus toxoid should be based on careful consideration of the potential benefits and possible risks. A committee of the Institute of Medicine (IOM) has concluded that evidence is consistent with a causal relationship between whole-cell DTP vaccine and acute neurologic illness, and under special circumstances, between whole-cell DTP vaccine and chronic neurologic disease in the context of the National Childhood Encephalopathy Study (NCES) report; however, evidence was insufficient to indicate whether or not whole-cell DTP vaccine increased the overall risk of chronic neurologic disease. Acute encephalopathy and permanent neurologic damage have not been reported causally linked or in temporal association with administration of PEDIARIX, but the experience with PEDIARIX is insufficient to rule this out. Encephalopathy has been reported following INFANRIX® (Diphtheria and Tetanus Toxoids and Acellular Pertussis Vaccine Adsorbed) (see ADVERSE REACTIONS, Postmarketing Reports), but data are not sufficient to evaluate a causal relationship. The decision to administer a pertussis-containing vaccine to children with stable central nervous system (CNS) disorders must be made by the physician on an individual basis, with consideration of all relevant factors, and assessment of potential risks and benefits for that individual. Advise the parent or guardian of the potential increased risk involved (see PRECAUTIONS). A family history of seizures or other CNS disorders is not a contraindication to pertussis vaccine. For children at higher risk for seizures than the general population, an appropriate antipyretic may be administered at the time of vaccination and for the ensuing 24 hours according to the respective prescribing information recommended dosage to reduce the possibility of post-vaccination fever. Defer vaccination during the course of a moderate or severe illness with or without fever and vaccinate patients as soon as they have recovered from the acute phase of the illness. Do not give PEDIARIX to children on anticoagulant therapy or those with bleeding disorders unless the potential benefit clearly outweighs the risk of administration (see PRECAUTIONS in complete prescribing information).

**PRECAUTIONS:** Before the injection of any biological, the physician should take all reasonable precautions to prevent allergic or other adverse reactions. Epinephrine injection (1:1000) and other appropriate agents used for the control of immediate allergic reactions must be immediately available should an acute anaphylactic reaction occur. Immunosuppressed individuals, including those receiving immunosuppressive therapy, may not develop the expected immune response. **Drug Interactions:** For information regarding concomitant administration with other vaccines, refer to DOSAGE AND ADMINISTRATION in complete prescribing information. Do not mix PEDIARIX with any other vaccine in the same syringe or vial. **Carcinogenesis, Mutagenesis, Impairment of Fertility:** PEDIARIX has not been evaluated for carcinogenic or mutagenic potential, or for impairment of fertility. **Pregnancy:** Pregnancy Category C: PEDIARIX is not indicated for women of child-bearing age. Animal reproduction studies have not been conducted with PEDIARIX. It is not known whether PEDIARIX can cause fetal harm when administered to a pregnant woman or if PEDIARIX can affect reproductive capacity. **Geriatric Use:** PEDIARIX is not indicated for use in adult populations. **Pediatric Use:** Safety and effectiveness of PEDIARIX in infants younger than 6 weeks of age have not been evaluated (see DOSAGE AND ADMINISTRATION in complete prescribing information). PEDIARIX is not recommended for persons 7 years of age or older. Tetanus and Diphtheria Toxoids Adsorbed (Td) For Adult Use, inactivated poliovirus vaccine (IPV), and Hepatitis B Vaccine (Recombinant) should be used in individuals 7 years of age or older.

**ADVERSE REACTIONS:** A total of 20,739 doses of PEDIARIX have been administered to 7,028 infants as a 3-dose primary series. The most common adverse reactions observed in clinical trials were local injection site reactions (pain, redness, or swelling), fever, and fussiness. In comparative studies, administration of PEDIARIX was associated with higher rates of fever relative to separately administered vaccines (see WARNINGS). The prevalence of fever was highest on the day of vaccination and the day following vaccination. More than 98% of episodes of fever resolved within the 4-day period following vaccination (i.e., the period including the day of vaccination and the next 3 days). Rates of most other solicited adverse events following PEDIARIX were comparable to rates observed following separately administered US-licensed vaccines. The adverse event information from clinical trials provides a basis for identifying adverse events that appear to be related to vaccine use and for approximating rates. However, because clinical trials are conducted under widely varying conditions, adverse event rates observed in the clinical trials of a vaccine cannot be directly compared to rates in the clinical trials of another vaccine, and may not reflect the rates observed in practice. A total of 5,472 infants were enrolled in a German safety study that was originally designed to compare the safety and reactogenicity of PEDIARIX administered concomitantly at separate sites with 1 of 4 *Haemophilus influenzae* type b (Hib) vaccines at 3, 4, and 5 months of age. After enrollment of 1,569 infants, the study was amended to include a control group that received INFANRIX, Hib vaccine, and oral poliovirus vaccine (OPV) separately. Infants in the separate administration group received one less antigen (hepatitis B) than the infants who received PEDIARIX. Safety data were available for 4,666 infants who received PEDIARIX administered concomitantly at separate sites with 1 of 4 Hib vaccines and for 768 infants in the control group that received separate vaccines. The primary end-point of the study was the percentage of infants with any grade 3 solicited symptom (redness or swelling >20 mm, fever >103.1°F, or crying, pain, vomiting, diarrhea, loss of appetite, or restlessness that prevented normal daily activities) over the 3-dose primary series in infants who received PEDIARIX (4 groups that received PEDIARIX and Hib vaccines pooled) compared to the group that received INFANRIX and Hib vaccine separately with OPV. Analysis for the primary end-point was performed on the according-to-protocol (ATP) cohort that included only those infants who were enrolled after the protocol amendment to include a control group. Of 3,773 infants in the ATP cohort for whom safety data were available, 16.2% (95% CI: 14.9% to 17.5%) of 3,029 infants who received PEDIARIX and Hib vaccine compared to 20.3% (95% CI: 17.5% to 23.4%) of 744 infants who received separate vaccines were reported to have had at least one grade 3 solicited symptom within 4 days of vaccination (i.e., day of vaccination and the next 3 days). The difference between groups in the rate of grade 3 symptoms was 4.1% (90% CI: 1.4% to 7.1%). These were the rates for selected solicited symptoms within 4 days following each dose in a 3-dose primary series in infants who received PEDIARIX administered concomitantly with Hib vaccine and those who received separate concomitant administration of INFANRIX, Hib vaccine, and OPV for the intent-to-treat (ITT) cohort (includes all infants enrolled before and after the amendment who received the indicated vaccine and for whom at least one symptom sheet was completed):

**Percentage of German Infants With Solicited Local Reactions or Selected Systemic Adverse Events Within 4 Days of Vaccination* (ITT Cohort)**

| | PEDIARIX & Hib | | | INFANRIX, Hib, & OPV | | |
|---|---|---|---|---|---|---|
| | Dose 1 | Dose 2 | Dose 3 | Dose 1 | Dose 2 | Dose 3 |
| **N** | **4,666** | **4,619** | **4,574** | **768** | **757** | **750** |
| **Local[†]** | | | | | | |
| Pain, any | 14.0 | 10.2 | 9.9 | 14.2 | 9.8 | 8.1 |
| Pain, grade 2 or 3 | 2.9 | 1.2 | 1.5 | 3.6 | 1.7 | 1.1 |
| Pain, grade 3 | 0.7 | 0.3 | 0.3 | 1.3 | 0.4 | 0.1 |
| Redness, any | 18.6 | 26.6 | 25.6 | 16.1 | 21.4 | 20.8 |
| Redness, >5 mm | 6.7 | 9.9 | 9.0 | 5.9 | 8.2 | 7.7 |
| Redness, >20 mm | 1.2 | 1.0 | 1.1 | 1.8 | 0.7 | 1.1 |
| Swelling, any | 12.7 | 18.5 | 18.4 | 9.6 | 12.9 | 13.6 |
| Swelling, >5 mm | 5.6 | 7.7 | 7.8 | 3.6 | 5.2 | 4.8 |
| Swelling, >20 mm | 1.2 | 1.6 | 1.5 | 1.3 | 1.1 | 1.2 |
| **Systemic** | | | | | | |
| Restlessness, any | 41.4 | 32.0 | 26.7 | 46.4 | 35.0 | 27.6 |
| Restlessness, grade 2 or 3 | 14.4 | 10.0 | 8.9 | 20.2 | 11.5 | 8.4 |
| Restlessness, grade 3 | 3.0 | 1.5 | 1.6 | 5.7 | 3.0 | 1.7 |
| Fever[‡], ≥100.4°F | 25.1 | 19.3 | 19.7 | 13.2 | 13.1 | 11.2 |
| Fever[‡], >101.3°F | 5.8 | 4.1 | 4.6 | 2.2 | 2.8 | 2.1 |
| Fever[‡], >103.1°F | 0.3 | 0.5 | 0.7 | 0.3 | 0.3 | 0.5 |
| Unusual cry[§], any | 24.9 | 16.5 | 13.1 | 36.5 | 19.7 | 14.3 |
| Unusual cry[§], grade 2 or 3 | 12.7 | 7.1 | 5.7 | 20.8 | 10.0 | 5.7 |
| Unusual cry[§], grade 3 | 3.9 | 1.7 | 1.4 | 6.8 | 2.1 | 1.1 |
| Loss of appetite, any | 17.9 | 13.3 | 12.5 | 19.1 | 16.2 | 11.3 |
| Loss of appetite, grade 2 or 3 | 4.0 | 2.9 | 2.7 | 4.4 | 2.9 | 2.3 |
| Loss of appetite, grade 3 | 0.6 | 0.5 | 0.4 | 0.5 | 0.7 | 0.0 |

N = number of infants in the intent-to-treat (ITT) cohort.
Grade 2 defined as sufficiently discomforting to interfere with daily activities.
Grade 3 defined as preventing normal daily activities.
* Within 4 days of vaccination defined as day of vaccination and the next 3 days.
† Local reactions at the injection site for PEDIARIX or INFANRIX.
‡ Rectal temperatures.
§ Unusual cry lasting >1 hour.

In this study, infants were also monitored for unsolicited adverse events that occurred within 30 days following vaccination. Over the entire study period, 6 subjects in the group that received PEDIARIX reported seizures. Two of these subjects had a febrile seizure, 1 of whom also developed afebrile seizures. The remaining 4 subjects had afebrile seizures, including 2 with infantile spasms. Two subjects reported seizures within 7 days following vaccination (1 subject had both febrile and afebrile seizures, and 1 subject had afebrile seizures), corresponding to a rate of 0.22 seizures per 1,000 doses (febrile seizures 0.07 per 1,000 doses, afebrile seizures 0.14 per 1,000 doses). No subject who received concomitant INFANRIX, Hib vaccine, and OPV reported seizures. In a separate German study that evaluated the safety of INFANRIX in 22,505 infants who received 66,867 doses of INFANRIX administered as a 3-dose primary series, the rate of seizures within 7 days of vaccination with INFANRIX was 0.13 per 1,000 doses (febrile seizures 0.0 per 1,000 doses, afebrile seizures 0.13 per 1,000 doses). No cases of hypotonic-hyporesponsiveness, encephalopathy, or anaphylaxis were reported in the German study that evaluated the safety of PEDIARIX. Rates of serious adverse events that are less common than those reported in this safety study are not known at this time.

Additional safety data for PEDIARIX are available from a US study designed to evaluate lot-to-lot consistency and a bridge for a new manufacturing step. These were the rates for local reactions and selected adverse events within 4 days of vaccination with PEDIARIX administered concomitantly with a Hib vaccine at 2, 4, and 6 months of age:

**Percentage of US Infants With Solicited Local Reactions or Selected Systemic Adverse Events Within 4 Days of Vaccination* (ITT Cohort)**

| | PEDIARIX & Hib | | |
|---|---|---|---|
| | Dose 1 | Dose 2 | Dose 3 |
| **Local[†]** | **N = 482** | **N = 469** | **N = 466** |
| Pain, any | 30.5 | 25.4 | 23.0 |
| Pain, grade 2 or 3 | 6.2 | 5.5 | 3.6 |
| Pain, grade 3 | 1.2 | 0.6 | 0.6 |
| Redness, any | 25.3 | 32.6 | 35.6 |
| Redness, >5 mm | 9.3 | 10.4 | 8.6 |
| Redness, >20 mm | 0.6 | 1.5 | 1.3 |
| Swelling, any | 15.1 | 16.6 | 22.3 |
| Swelling, >5 mm | 6.8 | 6.2 | 6.4 |
| Swelling, >20 mm | 1.0 | 1.3 | 1.3 |
| **Systemic** | **N = 482** | **N = 469** | **N = 467** |
| Restlessness, any | 28.8 | 30.3 | 28.5 |
| Restlessness, grade 2 or 3 | 7.1 | 9.0 | 9.4 |
| Restlessness, grade 3 | 1.0 | 1.1 | 0.6 |
| Fever[‡], ≥100.4°F | 26.6 | 31.3 | 25.9 |
| Fever[‡], >101.3°F | 2.9 | 6.2 | 4.7 |
| Fever[‡], >103.1°F | 0.0 | 0.2 | 0.6 |
| Fussiness, any | 61.8 | 63.8 | 57.0 |
| Fussiness, grade 2 or 3 | 14.9 | 21.5 | 17.1 |
| Fussiness, grade 3 | 2.7 | 3.4 | 1.7 |
| Loss of appetite, any | 21.6 | 19.8 | 18.8 |
| Loss of appetite, grade 2 or 3 | 3.1 | 3.2 | 2.4 |
| Loss of appetite, grade 3 | 0.2 | 0.4 | 0.0 |
| Sleeping more than usual, any | 46.7 | 31.8 | 28.1 |
| Sleeping more than usual, grade 2 or 3 | 10.2 | 6.0 | 4.7 |
| Sleeping more than usual, grade 3 | 1.7 | 0.4 | 0.6 |

N = number of infants in the intent-to-treat (ITT) cohort (infants who received the indicated vaccine and for whom at least one symptom sheet was completed).
Grade 2 defined as sufficiently discomforting to interfere with daily activities.
Grade 3 defined as preventing normal daily activities.
* Within 4 days of vaccination defined as day of vaccination and the next 3 days.
† Local reactions at the injection site for PEDIARIX.
‡ Rectal temperatures.

In another US study, these were the rates for fever within 4 days following dose 1 (i.e., day of vaccination and the next 3 days) at 2 months of age in infants who received PEDIARIX when administered concomitantly at separate sites with Hib and pneumococcal conjugate vaccines and those who received INFANRIX, ENGERIX-B® [Hepatitis B Vaccine (Recombinant)], IPV, Hib vaccine, and pneumococcal conjugate vaccine:

**Percentage of US Infants With Fever Within 4 Days of Dose 1* (ITT Cohort)**

| | PEDIARIX, Hib, & Pneumococcal Conjugate (N = 667) | INFANRIX, ENGERIX-B, IPV, Hib, & Pneumococcal Conjugate (N = 333) | Separate Vaccine Group Minus Combination Vaccine Group |
|---|---|---|---|
| **Fever[†]** | **%** | **%** | **Difference (95% CI)** |
| ≥100.4°F[‡] | 27.9 | 19.8 | -8.07 (-13.54, -2.60) |
| >101.3°F | 7.0 | 4.5 | -2.54 (-5.50, 0.41) |
| >102.2°F[‡] | 2.2 | 0.3 | -1.95 (-3.22, -0.68) |
| >103.1°F | 0.4 | 0.0 | -0.45 (-0.96, 0.06) |
| M.A.[‡] | 1.2 | 0.0 | -1.20 (-2.03, -037) |

N = number of infants for whom at least one symptom sheet was completed, excluding 3 infants for whom temperature was not measured and 3 infants whose temperature was measured by the tympanic method.
*Within 4 days of dose 1 defined as day of vaccination and the next 3 days.
† Rectal temperatures.
‡ The group that received PEDIARIX compared to separate vaccine group p value <0.05 (2-sided Fisher Exact test) or the 95% confidence interval on the difference between groups does not include 0.
M.A. = Medically attended (a visit to or from medical personnel).

In this study, medical attention (a visit to or from medical personnel) for fever within 4 days following vaccination was sought for 8 infants who received PEDIARIX (1.2%) and no infants who received separately administered vaccines. Four infants were seen by medical personnel in an office setting; no diagnostic tests were performed in 2 of the infants and a complete blood count (CBC) was done in the other 2 infants. Of 3 infants who were seen in an emergency room, all had a CBC and a blood and urine culture performed; chest X-rays were done in 2 of the infants and a nasopharyngeal specimen was tested for Respiratory Syncytial Virus in one of the infants. One infant was hospitalized for a work-up that included a CBC, blood and urine cultures, a lumbar puncture, and a chest X-ray. All episodes of medically attended fever resolved within 4 days post-vaccination.

Limited data are available from a study conducted in Moldova in which infants received a dose of hepatitis B vaccine within 48 hours of birth followed by 3 doses of PEDIARIX at 6, 10, and 14 weeks of age. No information was collected on the HBsAg status of mothers of enrolled infants. These were the rates for local reactions and selected adverse events within 4 days of vaccination with PEDIARIX administered comcomitantly with Hib vaccine following a birth dose of hepatitis B vaccine:

**Percentage of Moldovan Infants With Solicited Local Reactions or Selected Systemic Adverse Events Within 4 Days of Vaccination* (ITT Cohort)**

| | PEDIARIX & Hib | | |
|---|---|---|---|
| | Dose 1 | Dose 2 | Dose 3 |
| **N** | **160** | **158** | **157** |
| **Local[†]** | | | |
| Pain, any | 25.6 | 18.4 | 14.0 |
| Pain, grade 3 | 3.1 | 0.6 | 1.9 |
| Redness, any | 41.9 | 41.8 | 47.1 |
| Redness, >20 mm | 1.9 | 2.5 | 4.5 |
| Swelling, any | 20.6 | 18.4 | 28.0 |
| Swelling, >20 mm | 4.4 | 2.5 | 7.0 |
| **Systemic** | | | |
| Restlessness, any | 13.1 | 10.8 | 8.9 |
| Restlessness, grade 3 | 1.3 | 0.6 | 0.6 |
| Fever[‡], ≥100.4°F | 14.4 | 11.4 | 5.1 |
| Fever[‡], >103.1°F | 0.0 | 0.6 | 0.0 |
| Fussiness, any | 25.0 | 21.5 | 17.8 |
| Fussiness, grade 3 | 2.5 | 0.6 | 0.6 |

N = number of infants in the intent-to-treat (ITT) cohort (infants who received the indicated vaccine and for whom at least one symptom sheet was completed).
Grade 3 defined as preventing normal daily activities.
*Within 4 days of vaccination defined as day of vaccination and the next 3 days.
† Local reactions at the injection site for PEDIARIX.
‡ Rectal temperatures.

Although there was no comparator group who received PEDIARIX without a birth dose of hepatitis B vaccine, available data suggest that some local adverse events may occur at a higher rate when PEDIARIX is administered after a birth dose of hepatitis B vaccine.

As with any vaccine, there is the possibility that broad use of PEDIARIX could reveal adverse events not observed in clinical trials.

**Postmarketing Reports:** Worldwide voluntary reports of adverse events received for INFANRIX and ENGERIX-B in children younger than 7 years of age since market introduction of these US-licensed vaccines are listed below. This list includes adverse events for which 20 or more reports were received with the exception of intussusception, idiopathic thrombocytopenic purpura, thrombocytopenia, anaphylactic reaction, angioedema, encephalopathy, hypotonic-hyporesponsive episode, and alopecia for which fewer than 20 reports were received. These latter events are included either because of the seriousness of the event or the strength of causal connection to components of this or other vaccines or drugs. *Body as a whole*: Asthenia[b], fever[a+b], lethargy[b], malaise[b], Sudden Infant Death Syndrome[a+b]. *Cardiovascular system*: Cyanosis[a+b], edema[b], pallor[b]. *Gastrointestinal system*: Abdominal pain[b], anorexia[b], diarrhea[a+b], intussusception[a+b], nausea[b], vomiting[a+b]. *Hematologic/lymphatic*: Idiopathic thrombocytopenic purpura[a+b], lymphadenopathy[a], thrombocytopenia[a+b]. *Hepatic*: Jaundice[b], liver function tests abnormal[b]. *Hypersensitivity*: Anaphylactic reaction[a+b], angioedema[b], hypersensitivity[a]. *Infections*: Cellulitis[a]. *Injection site reactions*: Injection site reactions[a+b]. *Musculoskeletal*: Arthralgia[b], limb swelling[a+b]. *Nervous system*: Convulsions[a+b], encephalopathy[a], headache[b], hypotonia[a+b], hypotonic-hyporesponsive episode[a], somnolence[a+b]. *Psychiatric*: Crying[a+b], irritability[a+b]. *Respiratory system*: Respiratory tract infection[a]. *Skin and appendages*: Alopecia[b], erythema[a+b], erythema multiforme[b], petechiae[b], pruritus[a+b], rash[a+b], urticaria[a+b]. *Special senses*: Ear pain[a]. [[a] Following INFANRIX; [b] Following ENGERIX-B; [a+b] Following either INFANRIX or ENGERIX-B.] These reactions were reported voluntarily from a population of uncertain size; therefore, it is not always possible to reliably estimate their frequency or establish a causal relationship to vaccination.

**Reporting Adverse Events:** Report the occurrence following immunization of any event set forth in the Vaccine Injury Table from the National Childhood Vaccine Injury Act including: Anaphylaxis or anaphylactic shock within 7 days, encephalopathy or encephalitis within 7 days, brachial neuritis within 28 days, or an acute complication or sequelae (including death) of an illness, disability, injury, or condition referred to above, or any events that would contraindicate further doses of PEDIARIX. The VAERS toll-free number is 1-800-822-7967.

Manufactured by **GlaxoSmithKline Biologicals**, Rixensart, Belgium, US License 1617

Distributed by **GlaxoSmithKline,** Research Triangle Park, NC 27709



Full prescribing information for PEDIARIX is available at www.GSKVaccines.com/Pediarix. BRS-PE:L2

 Printed in USA. PED583R0 June 2005

# Maternal Depressive Symptoms at 2 to 4 Months Post Partum and Early Parenting Practices

*Kathryn Taaffe McLearn, PhD; Cynthia S. Minkovitz, MD, MPP; Donna M. Strobino, PhD; Elisabeth Marks, MPH; William Hou, MS*

**Objective:** To determine whether maternal depressive symptoms, reported when infants are 2 to 4 months old, are associated with mothers' early parenting practices.

**Design:** Secondary data analyses collected from the National Evaluation of Healthy Steps for Young Children. Data sources included newborn enrollment questionnaires and parent interviews when infants were 2 to 4 months old. Maternal depressive symptoms were assessed using the Center for Epidemiological Studies Depression Scale.

**Setting:** Twenty-four pediatric practices across the United States.

**Participants:** A total of 5565 families enrolled in Healthy Steps; 4874 mothers (88%) completed 2- to 4-month interviews and provided Center for Epidemiologic Studies Depression Scale data; 17.8% of mothers reported having depressive symptoms.

**Main Outcome Measures:** Ten parenting practices assessed in 3 domains: safety (sleep position and lowering water temperature), feeding (cereal, water, or juice; continuing breastfeeding), and practices to promote child development (showing books, playing with infant, talking to infant, and following 2 or more routines).

**Results:** Mothers with and without depressive symptoms reported similar uses of safety and feeding practices. Mothers with depressive symptoms had reduced odds of continuing breastfeeding (adjusted odds ratio [AOR], 0.73; 95% confidence interval [CI], 0.61-0.88), showing books (AOR, 0.81; 95% CI, 0.68-0.97), playing with the infant (AOR, 0.70; 95% CI, 0.54-0.90), talking to the infant (AOR, 0.74; 95% CI, 0.63-0.86), and following routines (AOR, 0.61; 95% CI, 0.52-0.72).

**Conclusion:** Maternal depressive symptoms are common in early infancy and contribute to unfavorable parenting practices.

*Arch Pediatr Adolesc Med. 2006;160:279-284*

DEPRESSION IS A PREVALENT health problem among women of childbearing age, with mothers of infants and young children being at particular risk in part because of the routine demands of parenting.[1] Prevalence rates vary depending on the population being studied. The prevalence of depressive symptoms among mothers of children younger than 3 years ranged from 19% to 24% in 2 nationally representative US samples.[1,2] For low-income mothers with young children, depressive symptoms are more prevalent,[3-5] whereas longitudinal studies of pregnant and postpartum women consistently find that 9% to 12% of mothers have depressive symptoms.[6-8]

Many investigators, using both observational and interview methods, have demonstrated that maternal depressive symptoms are related to adverse caregiving and health-related behaviors, which in turn influence children's health and development.[9-12] A meta-analysis[13] of small direct-observation studies found associations between maternal depression and impaired parenting, especially among mothers of infants. Depressed mothers were less likely to engage in positive behaviors during play and feeding opportunities and were more likely to be disengaged and display higher levels of hostile behaviors.

In large national samples, investigators reported that mothers with depressive symptoms engaged in poorer preventive health practices with their toddlers, such as decreased use of car seats and electrical outlet covers.[2,14] Maternal depressive symptoms have been associated with lower levels of positive parent-child interactive behaviors, such as playing, reading, following routines, and cuddling, and higher levels of negative behaviors, such as being irritable, yelling or spanking in the first 3 years of life, and decreased use of health care seeking for their young children.[1,2,5,15]

Only a few large studies have focused on maternal depressive symptoms in the postpartum period and their association with

**Author Affiliations:** National Center for Children in Poverty, Mailman School of Public Health, Columbia University, New York, NY (Dr McLearn and Ms Marks); and Department of Population and Family Health Sciences, Bloomberg School of Public Health, Johns Hopkins University, Baltimore, Md (Drs Minkovitz and Strobino and Mr Hou). Dr McLearn is currently with Center for Children's Healthcare Improvement, Department of Pediatrics, University of North Carolina, Chapel Hill. Ms Marks is currently with Population Health Division, Research Centre of the University of Montreal Hospital Centre, Montreal, Quebec.

early parenting behaviors. Using a community sample of low-income women, the presence of postpartum depressive symptoms was associated with decreased odds of having a smoke detector or placing the infant on his or her back to sleep and increased odds of using corporal punishment during the first year of life.[5] Smaller direct-observation studies have found that depressed mothers were less likely to engage in positive developmental behaviors during early interactions, such as talking, playing, or being affectionate with their newborns, and were more likely to display anger and disengagement.[16-18]

The science of early development is clear about the importance of parenting and early caregiving relationships, especially during infancy, when there is total dependency for safety, health, protection, nurturing, and stability.[9,11] Infants' early development also depends on the health and well-being of their parents. When a mother is coping with postpartum depressive symptoms, it places a burden on the caregiving relationship at a time when early patterns of parenting are established.[9,11,19] Despite this fact, we are unaware of any studies that have used a diverse, large nationwide sample to determine whether the presence of depressive symptoms in mothers is associated with a broad array of caregiving practices related to health and development in the postpartum period.

In this study, we examined whether maternal depressive symptoms at 2 to 4 months post partum are associated with parenting practices in a large nationwide sample of mothers and infants. We posited that depressive symptoms exhibited in the early months of caring for an infant were associated with lower levels of engagement in positive parenting behaviors to promote child health and development. The diversity and size of our sample allowed us to address limitations of smaller studies and adjust for possible confounders of the relationship between maternal depressive symptoms and parenting practices. We examined 10 parenting practices that fall into 3 domains: safety practices, feeding practices, and behaviors that promote early development. Extensive evidence, professional guidelines, and the American Academy of Pediatrics (AAP) policy statements highlight the importance of these practices.[11,20-27]

## METHODS

### SAMPLE

Data for this study were obtained from a sample of intervention and control group families at 15 sites across the United States that participated in the National Evaluation of Healthy Steps for Young Children.[28] Healthy Steps is a new model of pediatric care that incorporates child development specialists and enhanced developmental services into pediatric practices that serve families with young children. The design was a randomization trial at 6 sites (up to 400 enrolled) and quasi-experimental at 9 sites (up to 200 enrolled at the intervention site and 200 at the comparison site). Sites began staggered enrollment in September 1996 with completion at the last site in November 1998.

Newborns whose families intended to use the Healthy Steps sites for their care were enrolled consecutively in the hospital at birth or at the first office visit within the first 4 weeks of life. Newborns were ineligible if they did not complete an office visit within the first 4 weeks, they were to be adopted or placed in foster care, their mother did not speak English or Spanish, or their parents expected to move within 6 months. The eligible sample for the analyses reported in this article included mothers who completed forms at enrollment and a telephone interview at 2 to 4 months and who provided self-reported data of depressive symptoms using a 14-item modified Center for Epidemiologic Studies Depression Scale (CES-D) at 2 to 4 months.

### DATA SOURCES

Two data sources, available in English and Spanish, were used. The first was a short questionnaire completed by parents at the time of entry into Healthy Steps; this questionnaire provided maternal and family demographic characteristics. The second was a computer-assisted Healthy Steps telephone interview conducted with the mother (virtually all respondents) when the child was 2 to 4 months of age. The structured interview included questions about the presence of depressive symptoms, early parenting practices, and additional demographic characteristics.[29]

The 10 early parenting practices included in this study were selected from 17 parenting practices included in the Healthy Steps interview. They were selected based on evidence of their importance for child health and development, near complete data, and variability at 2 to 4 months. Two dichotomous variables were chosen to assess infant safety practices: using the prone sleep position at both naptime and bedtime and lowering the temperature of the hot water heater in the home. Placing an infant to sleep in the supine or stomach position is associated with sudden infant death syndrome, the leading cause of postneonatal mortality in the United States.[30] Since 1992, the AAP has recommended that newborns be placed on their backs to sleep.[21] Lowering the hot water temperature is an important preventive safety measure to decrease tap water scald burns, especially among infants and young children.[25,31,32]

The 4 infant feeding practices included continuation of breastfeeding at 2 to 4 months among mothers who had ever put the infant to the breast and whether or not the infant had been given water, juice, or cereal during the last week. The AAP advises that breast milk or infant formula provides sufficient nutrients in the first 4 to 6 months. Breastfeeding is associated with decreased infectious and chronic diseases and has shown a modest positive influence on infant cognitive development.[24,33] The early use of juice in the diet can result in insufficient nutrition, dental caries, and short stature[34]; early water use is associated with electrolyte imbalance and can lead to water intoxication and even death[35]; and there is no nutritional indication to introduce cereal before the age of 4 months.[36] Four practices to foster healthy development included showing books daily to the infant, playing daily with the infant, talking daily to the infant while working in the home, and following 2 or more routines at meals, naptime, and bedtime. To promote development, showing books from infancy onward has been positively associated with subsequent language acquisition and school achievement.[37,38] The 3 other parenting practices—talking to, playing with, and establishing predictable routines for infants—provide important opportunities to stimulate cognitive, social, physical, and emotional development.[37,39]

The presence of maternal depressive symptoms was measured in the 2- to 4-month interview using a modified version of the CES-D. The CES-D is a 20-item self-report scale designed to measure the frequency of depressive symptoms experienced in the previous week.[40] Using the modified 14-item CES-D, scores of 11 or higher indicated the presence of maternal depressive symptoms; this value was calibrated against the cutoff of 16 used for the 20-item scale. Correlation of the reduced-item version with the full 20-item scale exceeded 0.95 in a sample of high-risk pregnant women.[41] The α coefficient for the 14-item CES-D for Healthy Steps mothers was .85, similar to that for the total scale for the general population.[40]

## STATISTICAL ANALYSIS

We used $\chi^2$ statistics to compare parenting practices among mothers with and without depressive symptoms at 2 to 4 months post partum. Multiple logistic regression models were used to estimate the overall unadjusted and adjusted relations of the presence of maternal depressive symptoms with parenting practices. These models assessed whether differences by depressive symptoms were due to covariates that may potentially be associated with both depressive symptoms and parenting practices. These covariates were mother's age, race, ethnicity, marital or partner status, level of education, and employment status; whether she was a first-time mother; father's employment status; household income; whether the family owned their home; and child's age (**Table 1**).

In addition, because of a possible correlation of observations among families receiving pediatric care at the same site, multiple logistic regression analyses were also adjusted for the site of health care and enrollment in the Healthy Steps intervention group. Analyses were conducted using SAS statistical software, version 8.2 (SAS Institute Inc, Cary, NC).

The Committee on Human Subjects Research of the Johns Hopkins Bloomberg School of Public Health and the institutional review board of Columbia University College of Physicians and Surgeons granted study approval. For participants in this study, written informed consent was obtained at the time of enrollment, and oral consent was obtained before the 2- to 4-month interview.

# RESULTS

## STUDY SAMPLE

A total of 5565 families completed enrollment forms; 4891 mothers (87.9%) completed the 2- to 4-month survey, and 4874 (87.6%) also provided depressive symptom data. When compared with nonresponders, mothers in the sample were more likely to be older than 20 years, white, non-Hispanic, married, and high school graduates and to report that the infant's father was employed.

Table 1 shows the percentage of women with depressive symptoms by demographic characteristics and the distribution of the demographic characteristics for the total sample. At 2 to 4 months post partum, 17.8% of mothers reported depressive symptoms. Mothers who were younger than 20 years, from a minority background, Hispanic, and not living with the biological father of the child, who had low incomes, and who had less than a high school education were more likely to report depressive symptoms than mothers without these characteristics (Table 1). Depressive symptoms were not associated with mothers being employed or parity.

## SAFETY PRACTICES

Significantly fewer mothers with depressive symptoms than mothers without depressive symptoms lowered the temperature on water heaters (24.3% vs 31.0%) (**Table 2**). Comparable percentages used the wrong sleep position (14.3% vs 11.9%). The unadjusted odds ratios for lowering temperature on the water heater indicated decreased odds for mothers with depressive symptoms; however, it was not significant when adjusted for covariates (**Table 3**).

## FEEDING PRACTICES

The frequencies of less-than-optimal newborn feeding practices at 2 to 4 months (giving cereal, water, or juice) differed between mothers with and without depressive symptoms, ranging from 11.9% to 40.0% in mothers without depressive symptoms and 16.8% to 50.5% in mothers with depressive symptoms (Table 2). Although the unadjusted regression model indicated that mothers with depressive symptoms had increased odds of engaging in

**Table 1. Mothers With Depressive Symptoms and All Mothers by Parent and Family Characteristics at 2 to 4 Months Post Partum**

| Demographic Characteristic | Mothers With Depressive Symptoms, No. (%) (n = 867) | Mothers With Specific Characteristic,* No. (%) (n = 4874) | P Value |
|---|---|---|---|
| Mother's age at child's birth, y | | | |
| <20 | 172 (26.6) | 646 (13.3) | <.001 |
| 20-29 | 455 (18.5) | 2460 (50.6) | |
| ≥30 | 239 (13.6) | 1760 (36.2) | |
| Mother's race | | | |
| African American | 285 (24.6) | 1158 (24.1) | <.001 |
| Non–African American | 570 (15.6) | 3650 (75.9) | |
| Mother's ethnicity | | | |
| Hispanic | 190 (20.4) | 930 (19.8) | .02 |
| Non-Hispanic | 651 (17.3) | 3771 (80.2) | |
| Mother's marital status at 2-4 months | | | |
| Married, living with child's biological father | 393 (13.0) | 3027 (64.6) | <.001 |
| Not married, living with child's biological father | 149 (23.8) | 627 (13.4) | |
| Other | 294 (28.5) | 1033 (22.0) | |
| Mother's educational level at 2-4 months | | | |
| <High school graduate | 219 (28.0) | 781 (16.1) | <.001 |
| High school graduate | 267 (20.9) | 1276 (26.3) | |
| Some college or vocational school | 227 (15.9) | 1424 (29.3) | |
| College graduate or beyond | 152 (11.0) | 1376 (28.3) | |
| Mother's employment status at 2-4 months | | | |
| Employed | 288 (16.4) | 1754 (36.0) | .06 |
| Not employed | 579 (18.6) | 3120 (64.0) | |
| Maternal parity | | | |
| First-time mother | 424 (17.9) | 2370 (48.6) | .86 |
| Not first-time mother | 443 (17.7) | 2504 (51.4) | |
| Household income at 2-4 months, $ | | | |
| <20 000 | 444 (27.6) | 1607 (33.0) | <.001 |
| 20 000-44 999 | 274 (16.2) | 1695 (34.8) | |
| ≥45 000 | 149 (9.5) | 1572 (32.2) | |
| Home ownership at 2 to 4 months | | | |
| Owns home | 368 (14.6) | 2529 (51.9) | <.001 |
| Rents home | 499 (21.3) | 2345 (48.1) | |

*Less than 2% missing data except for mother's ethnicity (3.6%) and marital status (3.8%).

**Table 2. Percentages and Unadjusted Odds Ratios of Mothers With and Without Depressive Symptoms Reporting Parenting Practices at 2 to 4 Months Post Partum**

| Parenting Practices | With Depressive Symptoms, % (n = 867) | Without Depressive Symptoms, % (n = 4007) | Total Sample, % (n = 4874) | Unadjusted Odds Ratio (95% CI) | *P* Value |
|---|---|---|---|---|---|
| Safety | | | | | |
| Used wrong sleep position | 14.3 | 11.9 | 12.3 | 1.24 (1.00-1.53) | .05 |
| Lowered water temperature* | 24.3 | 31.0 | 29.8 | 0.72 (0.60-0.85) | <.001 |
| Feeding | | | | | |
| Gave cereal | 34.6 | 27.0 | 28.4 | 1.43 (1.22-1.67) | <.001 |
| Gave water | 50.5 | 40.0 | 41.8 | 1.53 (1.32-1.78) | <.001 |
| Gave juice | 16.8 | 11.9 | 12.8 | 1.50 (1.22-1.83) | <.001 |
| Continued to breastfeed* | 43.8 | 56.9 | 54.7 | 0.59 (0.50-0.70) | <.001 |
| Developmental | | | | | |
| Showed book to infant at least once a day | 22.4 | 28.2 | 27.1 | 0.74 (0.62-0.87) | <.001 |
| Played with infant at least once a day | 87.4 | 91.9 | 91.1 | 0.61 (0.49-0.77) | <.001 |
| Always talked to infant while working | 59.6 | 64.1 | 63.3 | 0.83 (0.71-0.96) | .01 |
| Followed 2 or more routines | 59.6 | 66.9 | 65.6 | 0.66 (0.57-0.78) | <.001 |

Abbreviation: CI, confidence interval.
*Among the 3670 mothers who ever breastfed.

**Table 3. Odds Ratios for Parenting Practices Among Mothers With Depressive Symptoms Compared With Those With No Symptoms, Adjusted Models**

| Parenting Practices | Odds Ratio (95% CI)* | *P* Value |
|---|---|---|
| Safety | | |
| Used wrong sleep position | 1.13 (0.91-1.42) | .24 |
| Lowered water temperature | 0.93 (0.78-1.22) | .46 |
| Feeding | | |
| Gave cereal | 1.11 (0.94-1.32) | .13 |
| Gave water | 1.05 (0.90-1.25) | .47 |
| Gave juice | 1.09 (0.88-1.35) | .37 |
| Continued to breastfeed | 0.73 (0.61-0.88) | <.001 |
| Developmental | | |
| Showed book to infant at least once a day | 0.81 (0.68-0.97) | .02 |
| Played with infant at least once a day | 0.70 (0.54-0.90) | .004 |
| Always talked to infant while working | 0.74 (0.63-0.86) | <.001 |
| Followed 2 or more routines | 0.61 (0.52-0.72) | <.001 |

Abbreviation: CI, confidence interval.
*Adjusted for the following covariates: parity, maternal age, race, ethnicity, marital status, maternal educational level, maternal employment income, home ownership, child's age, site, and intervention status.

these practices, the adjusted odds ratios for these variables were not significant (Table 3). Among mothers who had ever breastfed (76% for women without depressive symptoms and 71% for women with depressive symptoms), mothers with depressive symptoms had more than one-quarter reduced odds of continuing to breastfeed at 2 to 4 months compared with mothers without depressive symptoms (Tables 2 and 3).

## DEVELOPMENTAL PRACTICES

Smaller percentages of mothers with depressive symptoms reported positive developmental parenting practices than mothers without symptoms; the odds of each practice also differed significantly in both the unadjusted and adjusted logistic regression models. Playing with the infant was the most frequent developmental practice, with 87.4% of mothers with depressive symptoms and 91.9% of mothers without depressive symptoms reporting they played with their infant at least once a day (Table 2). Frequencies of the 3 other developmental practices ranged from 28.2% to 66.9% in mothers without depressive symptoms and from 22.4% to 59.6% in mothers with depressive symptoms (Table 2). After adjusting for covariates, mothers with depressive symptoms had 19% reduced odds of showing a book to their infants at least once a day, one-quarter reduced odds of playing with their infant at least once a day and talking to their infants while working in the home, and one-third reduced odds of following 2 or more daily routines (Table 3).

## COMMENT

The findings from this study provide a snapshot of early parenting practices among mothers with depressive symptoms in the critical first months post partum. Although we posited that there would be a significant relation between each of the parenting practices and the presence of maternal depressive symptoms, we found that the safety and feeding practices did not vary by depressive symptoms, after adjustment for covariates, with 1 exception. After controlling for covariates, we found that mothers with depressive symptoms had decreased odds of continuing breastfeeding. Our breastfeeding findings are different from those reported by Chung et al,[5] who found no difference in breastfeeding duration for longer than 1 month. Their study used a smaller, community-based low-income sample, whereas this study used a larger, diverse national sample.

After adjusting for covariates, we also found that mothers with depressive symptoms had decreased odds of showing picture books, playing and talking with their infants, and following daily routines. These findings suggest that parenting practices that require more active interaction with infants, such as continuing breastfeeding and playing or talking with the infant, were reduced. Similar results have been found in direct-observation studies of mothers.[13,16] As other experts have noted, the presence of elevated maternal depressive symptoms often results in the increased feelings of hopelessness and helplessness that can discourage mothers from engaging in parenting practices that have less concrete tangible outcomes.[42]

In this study, although depressive symptoms did not appear to influence several preventive parenting practices for mothers with newborns after adjustment for covariates, other studies[2] with mothers of toddlers found differences in practices such as car seat use and covering electrical outlets. This may be due to the more demanding nature of parenting toddlers. In both studies, however, the presence of depressive symptoms resulted in reduced odds of mothers showing books or reading to their children on a daily basis, a parenting behavior that requires more sustained interaction from the mother.

Several limitations to this study should be noted. First, self-report measures of parenting may lead to overreporting of behaviors that are socially desirable among mothers who do not have depressive symptoms. In this study, which used a broad array of parenting practices, we have no evidence of overstating for mothers with or without depressive symptoms. Among mothers with depressive symptoms, the bias may be in the opposite direction, with the depressive symptoms leading to underestimates of actual parenting practices as a result of feelings of decreased self-efficacy about parenting ability.[2] However, the review by Richters[43] of 22 studies suggests that depressed mothers do not have distorted perceptions of their children. In addition, D'Souza-Vazirani et al[44] found no difference in the validity of maternal report for children's short-term health care use based on the presence of maternal depressive symptoms. Our study findings suggest that it is possible to identify reduced positive parenting practices among mothers with depressive symptoms without having to use expensive direct-observation measures. Although a recent study[45] suggests variability in the validity of self-reported home safety practices, lowering water temperature was among the more reliable measures and sleep position was not assessed.

Second, we used a self-report measure for depressive symptoms as opposed to a structured diagnostic instrument. Nevertheless, prior studies[2] have found significant relationships between diminished parenting and self-reported depressive symptoms and suggest that the nondiagnostic CES-D may be more appropriate and preferable for pediatric practice and policy.

The findings from this study offer important implications for pediatric health care professionals and practice. The first is the need to screen for maternal depressive symptoms among all mothers during the postpartum period, when parenting practices are being established and when pediatric practices have frequent contact with families to provide guidance. Experts have stated that the scope of professional responsibility for pediatric physicians includes universal screening, guidance, and referrals for maternal depression.[2,20,46,47] The US Preventive Services Task Force has recommended 2-item screeners by primary care professionals to detect depressive symptoms.[48] A recent study[49] in a busy urban pediatric practice found a significant increase in the detection of depressive symptoms among mothers during the first postpartum year following implementation of a universal postpartum depression screening during well-child care visits. Second, the challenge and opportunity for pediatricians when providing anticipatory guidance to mothers with depressive symptoms are to discuss the mother's engagement in parenting practices that require more ongoing interactions, such as continuing breastfeeding, playing, talking, providing routines, and showing books.

The results of this study add to the burgeoning evidence that highlights the importance of screening for maternal depressive symptoms in the postpartum period. Once depressive symptoms are identified, pediatric health care professionals have an important role in providing ongoing counseling and anticipatory guidance to enhance parental efficacy, as well as in referring mothers to appropriate health care professionals to assist with their depressive symptoms.[4,50] To maximize pediatric physician interactions with mothers with depressive symptoms, further efforts are needed to ensure that linkages exist between adult and pediatric systems of care and that communities have adequate mental health resources. Such an approach has the potential to foster positive parenting, child health and development, and family well-being.

**Accepted for Publication:** October 21, 2005.
**Correspondence:** Cynthia S. Minkovitz, MD, MPP, Department of Population and Family Health Sciences, Johns Hopkins Bloomberg School of Public Health, 615 N Wolfe St, E4636, Baltimore, MD 21205 (cminkovi@jhsph.edu).
**Author Contributions:** Dr McLearn had full access to all the data in the study and takes responsibility for the integrity of the data and the accuracy of the data analysis.
**Funding/Support:** This study received funding from The Commonwealth Fund, New York, NY.
**Disclaimer:** The views presented herein are those of the authors and not necessarily those of the funders, their directors, officers, or staff.
**Previous Presentation:** Presented at the Pediatric Academic Society Meeting; San Francisco, Calif; May 3, 2004.

## REFERENCES

1. Lyons-Ruth K, Wolfe R, Lyubchik A, Steingard R. Depressive symptoms in parents of children under age 3: sociodemographic predictors, current correlates, and associated parenting behaviors. In: Halfon N, McLearn KT, Schuster MA, eds. *Child Rearing in America: Challenges Facing Parents With Young Children.* New York, NY: Cambridge University Press; 2002:217-259.
2. McLennan JD, Kotelchuck M. Parental prevention practices for young children in the context of maternal depression. *Pediatrics.* 2000;105:1090-1095.
3. Hall LA, Williams CA, Greenberg RS. Supports, stressors, and depressive symptoms in low-income mothers of young children. *Am J Public Health.* 1985; 75:518-522.
4. Lanzi RG, Pascoe JM, Keltner B, Ramey SL. Correlates of maternal depressive symptoms in a national Head Start program sample. *Arch Pediatr Adolesc Med.* 1999;153:801-807.
5. Chung EK, McCollum KF, Elo IT, Lee HJ, Calhane JF. Maternal depressive symptoms and infant health practices among low-income women. *Pediatrics.* 2004; 113:e523-e529.
6. O'Hara MW, Neunaber DJ, Zekoski EM. Prospective study of postpartum depression: prevalence, course, and predictive factors. *J Abnorm Psychol.* 1984; 93:158-171.
7. Evans J, Heron J, Francomb H, Oke S, Golding J. Cohort study of depressed mood during pregnancy and after childbirth. *BMJ.* 2001;323:257-259.

8. Luoma I, Tamminen T, Kaukonem P, et al. Longitudinal study of maternal depressive symptoms and child well-being. *J Am Acad Child Adolesc Psychiatry.* 2001;40:1367-1374.
9. Bornstein MH. Parenting infants. In: Bornstein MH, ed. *Handbook of Parenting, Volume 1: Children and Parenting.* Mahwah, NJ: Erlbaum; 1995:3-39.
10. Zeanah CH, Boris NW, Larrieu JA. Infant development and developmental risk: a review of the past 10 years. *J Am Acad Child Adolesc Psychiatry.* 1997;36:165-178.
11. Shonkoff JP, Phillips DA, eds. *From Neurons to Neighborhoods: The Science of Early Childhood Development.* Washington, DC: Institute of Medicine, National Research Council, Board on Children, Youth, and Families; 2000.
12. Downey G, Coyne JC. Children of depressed parents: an integrative review. *Psychol Bull.* 1990;108:50-76.
13. Lovejoy MC, Graczyk PA, O'Hare E, Neuman G. Maternal depression and parenting behavior: a meta-analytic review. *Clin Psychol Rev.* 2000;20:561-592.
14. Leiferman J. The effect of maternal depressive symptomology on maternal behaviors associated with child health. *Health Educ Behav.* 2002;29:596-607.
15. Minkovitz CS, Strobino D, Scharfstein D, et al. Maternal depressive symptoms and children's receipt of health care in the first three years of life. *Pediatrics.* 2005; 115:306-314.
16. Field T. Psychologically depressed parents. In: Bornstein MH, ed. *Handbook of Parenting. Volume 4: Applied and Practical Parenting.* Mahwah, NJ: Lawrence Erlbaum Associates; 1995:85-99.
17. Field T, Healy BT, Goldstein S, Guthertz M. Behavior-state matching and synchrony in mother-infant interactions of nondepressed versus depressed dyads. *Dev Psychol.* 1990;26:7-14.
18. Fleming AS, Ruble DN, Flett GL, Van Wagner V. Adjustment in first-time mothers: changes in mood and mood content during the early postpartum months. *Dev Psychol.* 1990;26:137-143.
19. American Academy of Pediatrics, Task Force on the Family. Family pediatrics. *Pediatrics.* 2003;111:1541-1571.
20. Green M, Palfrey JS, eds. *Bright Futures: Guidelines for Health Supervision of Infants, Children, and Adolescents.* 2nd ed. Arlington, Va: National Center for Education in Maternal and Child Health; 2000.
21. American Academy of Pediatrics, Task Force on Infant Sleep Position and Sudden Infant Death Syndrome. Changing concepts of sudden infant death syndrome: implications for infant sleeping environment and sleep position. *Pediatrics.* 2000;105:650-656.
22. American Academy of Pediatrics, Committee on Injury and Poison Prevention. Office-based counseling for injury prevention. *Pediatrics.* 1994;94:566-567.
23. US Department of Health and Human Services. *Healthy People 2010: Understanding and Improving Health.* 2nd ed. Washngton, DC: US Dept of Health and Human Services; November 2000.
24. American Academy of Pediatrics, Work Group on Breastfeeding. Breastfeeding and the use of human milk. *Pediatrics.* 1997;100:1035-1039.
25. Gielen AC, McDonald E, Wilson MEH, et al. Effects of improved access to safety counseling, products, and home visits on parents' safety practices: results of a randomized trial. *Arch Pediatr Adolesc Med.* 2002;156:33-40.
26. Debaryshe BD. Joint picture-book reading correlates of early oral language skill. *J Child Lang.* 1993;20:455-461.
27. Halfon N, McLearn KT. Families with children under 3: what we know and implications for results and policy. In: Halfon N, McLearn KT, Schuster MA, eds. *Child Rearing in America: Challenges Facing Parents With Young Children.* New York, NY: Cambridge University Press; 2002:367-412.
28. Minkovitz CS, Hughart N, Strobino D, et al. A practice-based intervention to enhance quality of care in the first three years of life: results from the Healthy Steps for Young Children Program. *JAMA.* 2003;290:3081-3091.
29. Minkovitz C, Strobino DM, Hughart N, Scharfstein D, Guyer B. Early effects of the Healthy Steps for Young Children Program. *Arch Pediatr Adolesc Med.* 2001; 155:470-479.
30. Gibson E, Cullen JA, Spinner S, Rankin K, Spitzer AR. Infant sleep position following new AAP guidelines. *Pediatrics.* 1995;96:69-72.
31. American Academy of Pediatrics. *The Injury Prevention Program (TIPP).* Chicago, Ill: American Academy of Pediatrics; 1994.
32. Katcher ML. Scald burns from hot tap water. *JAMA.* 1981;246:1219-1222.
33. Slusser WM, Lange L. Breastfeeding in the United States today: are families prepared? In: Halfon N, McLearn KT, Schuster MA, eds. *Child Rearing in America: Challenges Facing Parents With Young Children.* New York, NY: Cambridge University Press; 2002:178-216.
34. AAP Committee on Nutrition. The use and misuse of fruit juice in pediatrics. *Pediatrics.* 2001;107:1210-1213.
35. Keating JP, Schears GJ, Dodge PR. Oral water intoxication in infants: an American epidemic. *AJDC.* 1991;145:985-990.
36. American Academy of Pediatrics, Committee on Nutrition. *Pediatric Nutrition Handbook.* 5th ed. Elk Grove Village, Ill: American Academy of Pediatrics; 2004.
37. Britto PB, Fuligni AS, Brooks-Gunn J. Reading, rhymes, and routines: American parents and their young children. In: Halfon N, McLearn KT, Schuster MA, eds. *Child Rearing in America: Challenges Facing Parents With Young Children.* New York, NY: Cambridge University Press; 2002:117-145.
38. Bus AG, van Ijzendoorn MH, Pellegrini AD. Joint book reading makes success in learning to read: a meta-analysis on intergenerational transmission of literacy. *Rev Educ Res.* 1995;65:1-21.
39. Bradley RH. Environment and parenting. In: Bronstein M, ed. *Handbook of Parenting, Volume 2.* Hillsdale, NJ: Erlbaum; 1995.
40. Radloff LS. The CES-D scale: a self-report depression scale for research in the general population. *Appl Psychol Meas.* 1977;1:385-401.
41. Strobino D. *Utilization of Health Care by Drug Using Pregnant Women: Final Report.* Bethesda, Md: National Institute on Drug Abuse; 2000. Publication R01:DA07621-03.
42. Akisal H. Mood disorders: clinical features. In: Kaplan H, Sadock B, eds. *Comprehensive Textbook of Psychiatry.* 6th ed. Baltimore, Md: Williams & Wilkins; 1995:1123-1151.
43. Richters JE. Depressed mothers as informants about their children: a critical review of the evidence for distortion. *Psychol Bull.* 1992;112:485-499.
44. D'Souza-Vazirani D, Minkovitz CS, Strobino DM. Validity of maternal report of acute health care use for children younger than 3 years. *Arch Pediatr Adolesc Med.* 2005;159:167-172.
45. Robertson AS, Rivara FP, Ebel BE, Lymp JF, Christakis DA. Validation of parent self reported home safety practices. *Inj Prev.* 2005;11:209-212.
46. Zuckerman BS, Beardslee WR. Maternal depression: a concern for pediatricians. *Pediatrics.* 1987;79:110-117.
47. Olson AL, Kemper KJ, Kelleher KJ, Hammond CS, Zuckerman BS, Dietrich AJ. Primary care pediatricians' roles and perceived responsibilities in the identification and management of maternal depression. *Pediatrics.* 2002;110:1169-1176.
48. US Preventive Services Task Force. Screening for depression: recommendations and rationale. *Ann Intern Med.* 2002;136:760-764.
49. Chaudron LH, Szilagyi PG, Kitzman HJ, Wadkins HI, Cornwell Y. Detection of postpartum depressive symptoms by screening at well-child visits. *Pediatrics.* 2004; 113:551-558.
50. Carter AS, Garrity-Rokous FE, Chazan-Cohen R, Little C, Briggs-Gowan MJ. Maternal depression and comorbidity: predicting early parenting, attachment security, and toddler social-emotional problems and competencies. *J Am Acad Child Adolesc Psychiatry.* 2001;40:18-26.

"You can be a warm father and a real man at the same time."
—From *Handbook on Baby and Child Care*, by Dr Benjamin Spock, 1947

# Association of Depression and Anxiety Disorders With Weight Change in a Prospective Community-Based Study of Children Followed Up Into Adulthood

*Sarah E. Anderson, MS; Patricia Cohen, PhD; Elena N. Naumova, PhD; Aviva Must, PhD*

**Objective:** To investigate childhood to adulthood weight change associated with anxiety and depression.

**Design:** The Children in the Community Study. A prospective longitudinal investigation.

**Setting:** Albany and Saratoga Counties, New York.

**Participants:** Eight hundred twenty individuals (403 females and 417 males) assessed at 4 time points: in 1983 when they were 9 to 18 years old (n=776), in 1985 to 1986 when they were 11 to 22 years old (n=775), in 1991 to 1994 when they were 17 to 28 years old (n=776), and in 2001 to 2003 when they were 28 to 40 years old (n=661).

**Main Exposures:** Anxiety disorders and depression assessed by structured diagnostic interview.

**Main Outcome Measures:** Centers for Disease Control and Prevention body mass index *z* score (BMI*z*), a measure of weight status; and association of anxiety and depression with BMI*z* level and annual change.

**Results:** In females, anxiety disorders were associated with higher weight status, a BMI*z* of 0.13 (95% confidence interval, 0.01-0.25) units higher compared with females without anxiety disorders. Female depression was associated with a gain in BMI*z* of 0.09 units/y (95% confidence interval, 0.03-0.15 units/y), modified by the age when depression was first observed, such that early depression onset was associated with a higher subsequent BMI*z* than depression onset at older ages. In males, childhood depression was associated with a lower BMI*z* (−0.46; 95% confidence interval, −0.93 to 0.02 units lower at the age of 9 years), but BMI*z* trajectories for males with or without depression converged in adulthood; male anxiety disorders were not substantively associated with weight status.

**Conclusions:** Anxiety disorders and depression were associated with a higher BMI*z* in females, whereas these disorders in males were not associated with a higher BMI*z*. These results, if causal and confirmed in other prospective studies, support treating female anxiety and depression as part of comprehensive obesity prevention efforts.

*Arch Pediatr Adolesc Med. 2006;160:285-291*

Author Affiliations: Gerald J. and Dorothy R. Friedman School of Nutrition Science and Policy, Tufts University (Ms Anderson and Dr Must), and Department of Public Health and Family Medicine, Tufts University School of Medicine (Drs Naumova and Must), Boston, Mass; and Department of Psychiatry, College of Physicians and Surgeons, Columbia University, and Department of Epidemiology, New York State Psychiatric Institute, New York, NY (Dr Cohen).

THE PREVALENCE OF OBESITY among US children, adolescents, and adults represents a public health crisis.[1] Obesity often has roots early in life, and if present in adolescence is likely to persist into adulthood.[2] Understanding the predictive factors associated with weight gain is important for obesity prevention; obesity treatment will be most effective when targeted, and informed by understanding of etiologic pathways and correlates.

Evidence suggests that a child's social and psychological environment contributes to obesity risk. Psychosocial difficulty during childhood is associated with increased risk for adult obesity,[3] and with rapid weight gain in children.[4] Physical or verbal abuse,[5] and parental neglect,[6] are associated with a higher obesity risk, as is poor quality of a child's home environment.[7] Thus, childhood adversity can increase risk for later obesity; these associations may be mediated by negative psychological symptoms.

That psychopathological dysfunction and obesity are associated has long been hypothesized, but studies have yielded conflicting results. Some cross-sectional population-based studies[8-17] show associations between poorer psychological functioning and obesity, while others[18-24] do not. Similar variability exists among studies[19,21,24-26] of pediatric populations.

Evidence from the few prospective studies[27-34] conducted suggests that psychological disorders are associated with weight gain. Limitations of these studies include having observations at only 2 time points,[27-32] relatively short periods of follow-up,[27,30,33,34] and clinical rather than population-based samples.[28]

Our objectives were to evaluate the association of anxiety disorders and major depressive disorder (depression), defined based on *Diagnostic and Statistical*

*Manual of Mental Disorders (DSM)* diagnostic criteria, with weight trajectory in a community-based cohort of children followed up into adulthood.

## METHODS

### STUDY POPULATION

The Children in the Community Study is a prospective cohort study of determinants and correlates of psychological health. In these analyses, we have examined the influence of depression and anxiety disorders on childhood to adulthood weight trajectory. Children in the Community Study design and operations have been described previously.[35,36] Briefly, 976 families with children born between 1965 and 1974, residing in Albany and Saratoga Counties in Upstate New York, were sampled in 1975. The sample was demographically representative of the area, and was primarily of white race/ethnicity (91.5%). Participants were assessed in 1983 (wave 1, n=776) when they were 9 to 18 years old, in 1985 to 1986 (wave 2, n=775) when they were 11 to 22 years old, in 1991 to 1994 (wave 3, n=776) when they were 17 to 28 years old, and in 2001 to 2003 (wave 4, n=661) when they were 28 to 40 years old. Trained interviewers conducted in-home interviews with participants at waves 1 to 4, and a parent (usually the mother) at waves 1 to 3. Informed consent (or assent for children) was obtained at each wave. The institutional review boards of the New York State Psychiatric Institute and Tufts–New England Medical Center, Boston, approved this study. Eight hundred twenty individuals (403 females and 417 males) contributed data to these analyses: 593 (72.3%) with data for 4 waves, 176 (21.5%) with data for 3 waves, 37 (4.5%) with data for 2 waves, and 14 (1.7%) with data for 1 wave.

### MAIN EXPOSURES

Depression and anxiety disorders were assessed using structured diagnostic interviews for *DSM* disorders. The Diagnostic Interview Schedule for Children[37] was administered, separately, to a parent and the participant at waves 1 and 2. Parents and children provide unique nonoverlapping information,[38] and in accordance with current practice, disorders were identified if either reported a minimum number of items meeting *DSM-III* criteria and the combined parent-child symptom score was at least 1 SD above the mean. At wave 3, the Diagnostic Interview Schedule for Children, with minor adjustments made for age appropriateness and comparability across *DSM* revisions,[35] was administered to participants. At wave 4, disorders were assessed using the Structured Clinical Interview for *DSM-IV*. The Diagnostic Interview Schedule for Children and the Structured Clinical Interview for *DSM-IV* assessed whether an individual had symptoms consistent with a *DSM* disorder at any point during the year leading up to the interview. In addition, during the wave 2 assessment, disorders were identified if they occurred at any point between waves 1 and 2.

For each participant, we determined if the participant was observed to have met the diagnostic criteria for an anxiety disorder or depression at any of the 4 interviews. If the diagnostic criteria were met, the age of the participant at the interview during which the disorder was first identified was designated as the age of observed onset. For example, if a participant did not meet the diagnostic criteria for depression at wave 1 or 2, and did meet the diagnostic criteria for depression at wave 3, we defined the age we first observed depression in this individual as his or her age at wave 3.

The specific disorders that could be considered "anxiety" were not identical across waves. We defined *anxiety* as follows: at waves 1 and 2, separation anxiety, social phobia, or overanxious disorder; and at waves 3 and 4 (when participants were adults), social phobia, generalized anxiety disorder, obsessive-compulsive disorder, panic disorder, or agoraphobia.

Depression is often accompanied by symptoms of anxiety, some of which may be severe enough to meet the diagnostic criteria for an anxiety disorder. Thus, we do not attempt to separate depression from comorbid anxiety.

### MAIN OUTCOMES

Body mass index (BMI) was calculated as weight in kilograms divided by the square of height in meters, from height and weight reported at each wave. At wave 1, a parent reported the participant's height and weight. At wave 2, a parent and the participant reported the participant's height and weight. At waves 3 and 4, participants self-reported their height and weight. Agreement between participant- and parent-reported height and weight at wave 2 was high (intraclass correlation coefficient for height, 0.92; and for weight, 0.95). At wave 2, we used the participant's report of height and weight if the participant was older than 13 years; otherwise, we used the parent report. Reported height for individuals across waves was examined for consistency and implausible values, such as decreases in height over time. Approximately 30% of individuals reported a decrease in height; however, in all except 64 individuals, the difference was 1 inch or less (≤2.54 cm). Height decreases were adjusted by substituting a "stable adult height" if the participant reported 2 or more identical heights; otherwise, the mean of reported adult heights was used. *Adult* was defined herein as follows: for males, those older than 17 years; and for females, those older than 15 years. Similar methods were used to stabilize height for 18 individuals reporting growth of greater than 1 inch (>2.54 cm) between 2 waves after the age of 20 years. Observations (<1%) were not included in analyses if implausible and not accompanied by stable estimates.

Participants were observed during childhood and adulthood, necessitating a measure of weight status comparable throughout this period. Body mass index is commonly used to assess weight status in adults, but BMI is not a good measure for comparison of relative weight status among children of different ages because it increases with age, independent of adiposity, during childhood. Instead, in children, it is recommended that weight status be determined relative to age- and sex-specific reference data.[39,40] Therefore, we used the Centers for Disease Control and Prevention BMI-for-age reference data,[41] which are available for children and adolescents aged 2 to 20 years, to calculate a BMI *z* score (BMI*z*) for each participant at each wave. The BMI*z* scores correspond with growth chart percentiles and allow for tracking a child's relative weight through childhood and adolescence. A BMI*z* of 0 equals the 50th percentile; 1.04, the 85th percentile; and 1.65, the 95th percentile. To provide continuity from childhood to adulthood, we used the age 20 reference to calculate BMI*z* when individuals were 20 years or older, as have others.[42] Because BMI*z* is a continuous measure of relative weight adjusted for age and sex, we were able to assess the association of depression and anxiety disorders on weight trajectory over an age range spanning childhood, adolescence, and adulthood.

### COVARIATES

Socioeconomic status was defined by an index (mean, 10; SD, 1) of family income, parental education, work status, occupation, and receipt of public assistance.[36] Potential confounding variables included whether medications were taken for emotional or behavioral problems before the age of 21 years, assessed by self-report at wave 4, and whether the participant reported being a

**Table 1. Age, Weight Status, Anxiety, and Depression of Participants Studied in 1983, 1985 to 1986, 1991 to 1994, and 2001 to 2003***

| | Females (n = 403) | | | | Males (n = 417) | | | |
|---|---|---|---|---|---|---|---|---|
| Characteristic | 1983 (n = 388) | 1985-1986 (n = 374) | 1991-1994 (n = 382) | 2001-2003 (n = 351) | 1983 (n = 388) | 1985-1986 (n = 401) | 1991-1994 (n = 394) | 2001-2003 (n = 310) |
| Age, y | | | | | | | | |
| Mean | 13.9 | 16.2 | 22.1 | 33.1 | 13.7 | 16.2 | 22.1 | 33.2 |
| Range | 9.1-18.5 | 11.1-21.6 | 16.6-27.9 | 27.8-39.0 | 9.2-18.6 | 11.2-22.7 | 16.7-28.2 | 27.8-40.1 |
| BMI, mean (SD) | 20.3 (3.3) | 21.1 (3.2) | 23.1 (4.4) | 26.3 (6.1) | 21.1 (4.5) | 22.1 (3.8) | 24.6 (4.2) | 27.5 (5.0) |
| BMI *z* score | | | | | | | | |
| Mean (SD) | 0.2 (0.9) | 0.1 (0.9) | 0.1 (0.9) | 0.7 (0.9) | 0.4 (1.1) | 0.3 (1.0) | 0.3 (1.0) | 0.9 (0.9) |
| >85th Percentile | 66 (17.0) | 44 (11.8) | 67 (17.5) | 134 (38.2)† | 88 (22.7) | 72 (18.0) | 77 (19.5) | 138 (44.5)† |
| >95th Percentile | 12 (3.1) | 8 (2.1) | 18 (4.7) | 59 (16.8)‡ | 34 (8.8) | 26 (6.5) | 35 (8.9) | 56 (18.1)‡ |
| Anxiety§ | 105 (27.1) | 129 (34.5) | 163 (42.7) | 172 (49.0) | 71 (18.3) | 92 (22.9) | 89 (22.6) | 95 (30.6) |
| Depression§ | 16 (4.1) | 30 (8.0) | 63 (16.5) | 89 (25.4) | 9 (2.3) | 15 (3.7) | 28 (7.1) | 45 (14.5) |

Abbreviation: BMI, body mass index (calculated as weight in kilograms divided by the square of height in meters).

*Data are given as number (percentage) of each group unless otherwise indicated. The BMI *z* score was obtained from the Centers for Disease Control and Prevention BMI-for-age growth reference.[41] Anxiety disorders and depression were based on *Diagnostic and Statistical Manual of Mental Disorders* diagnostic criteria, as assessed by structured diagnostic interview. Wave 1 was in 1983; 2, 1985 to 1986; 3, 1991 to 1994; and 4, 2001 to 2003.

†The 85th percentile BMI *z* score corresponds to a BMI of 26.5 in women and 27.0 in men at 20 years or older. At the 2001 to 2003 wave, 155 (44.2%) of the women and 211 (68.1%) of the men had a BMI of 25 or greater.

‡The 95th percentile BMI *z* score corresponds to a BMI of 31.8 in women and 30.6 in men at 20 years or older. At the 2001 to 2003 wave, 76 (21.7%) of the women and 68 (21.9%) of the men had a BMI of 30 or greater.

§Data are given for individuals observed at each wave who met the diagnostic criteria for an anxiety disorder or depression at that wave or a previous wave.

current smoker, assessed by self-report at each wave. Analyses were conducted separately for males and females because we hypothesized that the association between anxiety or depression and weight status would depend on sex.

## STATISTICAL ANALYSIS

We used linear mixed models[43] to estimate differences in BMI*z* level and annual change in BMI*z* associated with observed onset of anxiety disorder or depression, compared with participants who were never observed as having an anxiety disorder or depression. We used age (in years) as the measure of time in these models.

Our model-building strategy was established a priori and used to assess whether observed onset of female anxiety, male anxiety, female depression, or male depression was associated with BMI*z* level or annual change in BMI*z*; we used the term *trajectory* when referring simultaneously to BMI*z* level and annual change. We controlled for socioeconomic status in all models. The BMI*z* trajectory was defined as a cubic function of age. We determined the effect of anxiety disorders and depression on BMI*z* level and annual change in BMI*z*, and assessed whether the participant's age at the wave in which anxiety or depression was first recognized modified these associations. We assessed potential confounding variables (current smoking and early medication use) by determining whether their inclusion changed model estimates. We identified those individuals with an anxiety disorder who did not meet criteria (at any point in the study) for depression, and evaluated the result of using this more restricted definition of anxiety.

## RESULTS

### CHARACTERISTICS OF STUDY PARTICIPANTS

The mean BMI*z* for males and females increased by greater than 0.5 units between waves 3 and 4 (**Table 1**). During the study, 310 individuals (119 males and 191 females) met the diagnostic criteria for an anxiety disorder; of these individuals, 86 males and 116 females did not also meet the criteria for depression. The mean age at the wave in which an anxiety disorder was first recognized was 17.5 years in females (range, 9.4-38.0 years) and 16.8 years in males (range, 9.3-39.4 years). One hundred forty-eight individuals (50 males and 98 females) met the diagnostic criteria for depression during the study. The mean age at the wave in which depression was first identified was 23.8 years in females (range, 9.7-38.4 years) and 23.5 years in males (range, 10.1-37.5 years).

### ANXIETY DISORDERS: ASSOCIATION WITH BMI*z*

In females, anxiety disorders were associated with higher weight status; our model estimated that the mean BMI*z* for females observed as having had an anxiety disorder was 0.13 units higher compared with females of the same age and socioeconomic status who were not observed as having had an anxiety disorder (**Table 2**). This difference of 0.13 units, comparing females with an anxiety disorder with females without an anxiety disorder, was unrelated to the number of years elapsed since observed anxiety disorder onset (ie, annual change in BMI*z* was estimated to be essentially the same, a difference in annual BMI*z* change of −0.0002 units/y, regardless of whether the participant had been recognized as having an anxiety disorder). In males, anxiety disorders were not associated with a substantive or statistically significant difference in BMI*z* level or annual change in BMI*z* compared with males without an anxiety disorder (Table 2). We found no evidence that the association of BMI*z* with anxiety disorders in either females or males was related to age at first recognition of anxiety. Controlling for cigarette smoking or early medication use did not substantively change results.

Using a definition of anxiety disorder restricted to females who had never met the diagnostic criteria for de-

**Table 2. Estimated Difference in BMI*z* Trajectory (Level and Annual Change) Associated With Anxiety Disorder and Depression***

| | Model Estimate of Mean Difference in BMI*z* | | | | | |
|---|---|---|---|---|---|---|
| | Anxiety Disorders | | Anxiety Disorders Not Comorbid With Depression† | | Depression | |
| BMI*z* Variable | Females | Males | Females | Males | Females | Males |
| Level | 0.13 (0.01 to 0.25)‡ | 0.004 (−0.16 to 0.17) | 0.18 (0.03 to 0.33)‡ | −0.01 (−0.20 to 0.18) | −0.07 (−0.21 to 0.07) | −0.46 (−0.93 to 0.02) |
| Change (per year) | −0.0002 (−0.01 to 0.01) | 0.01 (−0.004 to 0.02) | −0.003 (−0.01 to 0.01) | 0.01 (−0.01 to 0.02) | 0.09 (0.03 to 0.15)‡ | −0.005 (−0.03 to 0.02) |
| Level × age (in years) interaction | § | § | § | § | § | 0.02 (−0.01 to 0.05) |
| Change (per year) × age (in years) interaction | ‖ | ‖ | ‖ | ‖ | −0.003 (−0.005 to −0.001)‡ | ‖ |

Abbreviation: BMI*z*, body mass index *z* score.
*Data are given as mean difference in BMI*z* (95% confidence interval). The BMI*z* scores were obtained from the Centers for Disease Control and Prevention BMI-for-age growth reference.[41] Anxiety disorders and depression were based on *Diagnostic and Statistical Manual of Mental Disorders* diagnostic criteria, as assessed by structured diagnostic interview. Estimates from linear mixed-effects models of BMI*z* assessed at 4 waves; all models were adjusted for age, age$^2$, age$^3$, and socioeconomic status. We subtracted 9 (age of the youngest individual at wave 1) from age to maximize the interpretability of variable estimates.[44]
†Individuals who met the criteria for an anxiety disorder and did not meet the criteria for depression during the study.
‡Statistically significant estimates ($\alpha$ = .05).
§Addition of term for interaction between age and BMI*z* level did not improve model fit.
‖Addition of term for interaction between age and BMI*z* annual change did not improve model fit.

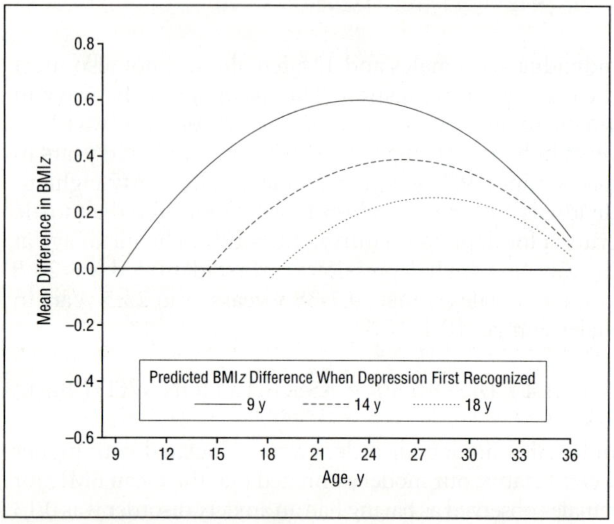


**Figure 1.** Mean difference calculated from model estimates of body mass index *z* score (BMI*z*) with age for females with depression first recognized at the ages of 9, 14, or 18 years compared with females without depression (reference line at 0). The linear mixed-effects model was as follows: BMI*z*=1.77−[0.14(Age−9)]+{0.01[(Age−9)$^2$]}−{0.0002[(Age−9)$^3$]}−[0.12 (Socioeconomic Status)]−[0.07(Depression)]+[0.09(Years of Depression)]−{0.003[(Age−9) (Years of Depression)]}.

pression increased the estimated mean difference in BMI*z* associated with anxiety to 0.18 units higher compared with other females (Table 2). Our results for males with anxiety disorders that were not comorbid with depression were virtually the same as those for male anxiety disorders overall (Table 2).

## DEPRESSION: ASSOCIATION WITH BMI*z*

For females, a history of depression was associated with greater yearly gains in BMI*z* compared with females without a history of depression; the annual change in BMI*z* for females observed as having had depression was greater by 0.09 units/y than the annual change in BMI*z* for females who had never been identified as having had depression. The magnitude of this annual BMI*z* change was modified by age at first recognition of depression and by the number of years elapsed since depression was recognized; the estimated yearly gain in BMI*z* was reduced by 0.003 units for each additional year of age a female was when depression was first recognized and each year elapsed since then (Table 2 and **Figure 1**). In males, the first recognition of depression was of borderline statistical significance (*P*=.06) and predicted a lower BMI*z* compared with males without depression. Childhood depression was associated with the greatest estimated difference in BMI*z* (a 9-year-old boy with depression would be estimated to have a BMI*z* of 0.46 units lower than a boy of the same age without depression). The BMI*z* trajectories converged with increasing age for males with and without a history of depression; each additional year of age reduced the difference between estimated BMI*z* for males with depression compared with males without depression by 0.02 units (Table 2 and **Figure 2**). Controlling for cigarette smoking or early medication use did not substantively change results.

## COMMENT

We found that *DSM* disorders of anxiety or depression were associated in females with a higher BMI*z*. The BMI*z* was predicted to be 0.13 or 0.18 units higher, depending on depression comorbidity, for females recognized as having had an anxiety disorder compared with the BMI*z* level of similar females without an anxiety disorder. The estimated annual change in BMI*z* was essentially the same for females irrespective of whether they had been observed as having had an anxiety disorder and, thus,

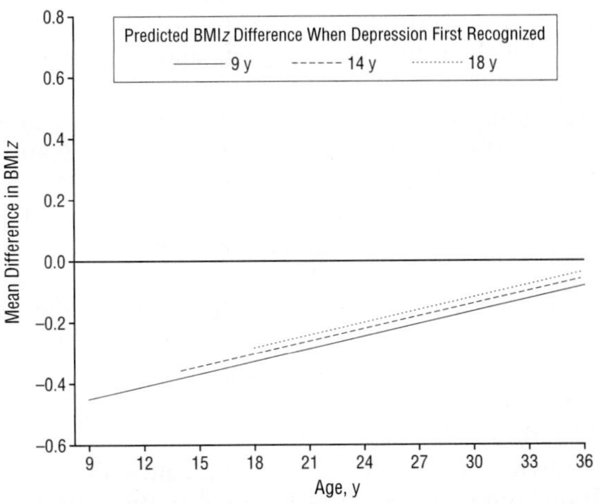


**Figure 2.** Mean difference calculated from model estimates of body mass index *z* score (BMI*z*) with age for males with depression first recognized at the ages of 9, 14, or 18 years compared with males without depression (reference line at 0). The linear mixed-effects model was as follows: BMI*z*=1.78−[0.13(Age−9)]+{0.01[(Age−9)$^2$]}−{0.0002[(Age−9)$^3$]}−[0.11 (Socioeconomic Status)]−[0.46(Depression)]−[0.005(Years of Depression)]+{0.02[(Age−9) (Depression)]}.

the estimated mean difference of 0.13 or 0.18 units was maintained over time. A 0.18-unit difference in BMI*z* would translate, depending on initial BMI, to a difference in adult BMI of, for example, approximately 25 to 26, 28 to 30, or 30 to 32. For a woman with a height of 64 inches (163 cm) (the average height of US women aged 20-40 years),[45] these BMI changes correspond to 2.7-, 4.2-, and 5.3-kg weight differences, respectively. Although these average weight differences are not large, obesity results from incremental increases in weight, and successful prevention is likely to require interventions targeted toward many factors, no one of which, alone, is sufficient to prevent obesity.

The association of female depression with BMI*z* depended on age at first recognition of depression and the number of years since elapsed. Our model predicted that a 30-year-old woman first recognized with depression at the age of 14 years would have a BMI*z* that was 0.34 units higher than a similar woman without depression; if depression were first recognized at the age of 18 years, the estimated difference in BMI*z* at the age of 30 years would be reduced to 0.23 units. A 0.34-unit difference in BMI*z* translates to a difference in BMI of approximately 24 to 26, 25 to 27, or 27 to 30; for a woman of average height, these values represent weight differences of 4.8, 5.3, and 7.4 kg, respectively. Our model estimated that differences in BMI*z* were largest for adolescents and young adults when depression was present at an early age (Figure 1); irrespective of the age of depression recognition, differences between BMI*z* trajectories for women with and without a history of depression lessened as women approached their 30s. However, statistical power at later ages was not as great as at younger ages.

In males, the association of anxiety disorders with BMI*z* trajectory was small and not statistically significant. Thus, our results suggest that anxiety disorders do not greatly influence weight status in males. Childhood depression for males was associated with lower weight; the magnitude of the difference was inversely related to age. Our results for male depression were of borderline statistical significance. Our model predicted that a 14-year-old male with depression would have a BMI*z* 0.36 units lower than a similar male without depression; however, by the age of 30 years, the BMI*z* difference between these men would be reduced to 0.12 units, and by the age of 35 years, to less than 0.05 units. In adult males, a 0.12-unit difference in BMI*z* translates to a difference in BMI of approximately 25 to 24.5 or 29 to 28; for a man with a height of 69 inches (176 cm) (the average height of US men aged 20-40 years),[45] these BMI differences represent weight differences of 1.5 and 2.2 kg, respectively.

The literature describing associations between obesity and psychological disorders is replete with cross-sectional and clinical studies,[46,47] but contains fewer prospective studies.[27-34] Several of these studies[27,30,31] use symptom scales that are not directly comparable to *DSM* criteria, and others[27-32] are limited to observations at 2 time points. Our analyses of the association of anxiety and depression with weight are unique in using structured diagnostic interviews to assess *DSM* disorders in a community-based cohort studied at 4 occasions spanning childhood and early adulthood.

Our results are broadly consistent with other prospective studies[28,30] in finding that psychological distress, especially when present in childhood, predicts higher weight. The study[33] most methodologically comparable to ours found that adolescent depression increased risk for later obesity in girls, but not boys. However, anxiety disorders were not studied, and the study outcome was obesity at the age of 26 years. In an earlier analysis[29] that used data from the 1983 and 1991 to 1994 waves of the Children in the Community Study, young adulthood BMI was associated with symptoms of conduct disorder and depression.

The relationship of depression to BMI*z* we observed in males was fundamentally different from that observed in females. Our results are consistent with those of other investigators[9,10,14,16,17,33] in reporting null or inverse associations between depressive symptoms and weight in males. Differences in results in these mainly cross-sectional studies could be due to influences of age on the association of depression with weight.

Longitudinal studies of anxiety and weight are rare. Mustillo et al[34] observed no association between children's weight trajectory and *DSM* anxiety disorders; however, comparability to our results is limited by differences in objective and approach. Cross-sectional studies of anxiety and weight provide inconsistent results; in 2 studies,[9,18] anxiety symptoms were inversely associated with weight. Like ours, more recent studies[13,16] observed positive associations between obesity and anxiety, particularly in women.

Depression and anxiety are often comorbid disorders.[48,49] An estimated 60% of adults with depression have had an anxiety disorder,[49] and up to 40% of adults with anxiety disorders have had depression.[50] In our study, 66.0% of males and 76.5% of females with depression also met the diagnostic criteria for an anxiety disorder. Attempting to separate the influence of depression on weight from the influence of anxiety on weight is counterproductive because "pure" depression is not common. In contrast, only 27.7% of males and 39.3% of females with an anxiety disorder met the diagnostic criteria for depression; that results of our female anxiety model were strengthened in this subset counters the potential argument that our observed association between anxiety and BMI*z* was due primarily to depression.

By early adulthood, females with depression outnumber males by approximately 2:1.[51] Atypical depression, characterized by increased appetite, hypersomnia, and decreased activity level, is more common in women than men,[52] suggesting a potential mechanism for the association we observed.

Our analyses provide evidence that anxiety disorders and depression are associated with higher weight in females. A strength of our study is assessment of depression and anxiety disorders consistent with *DSM* criteria. In contrast to symptom scales, use of *DSM* diagnostic criteria facilitates interpretability and generalizability of results.

There were several limitations of our analyses. First, we modeled the association of first recognition of anxiety or depression with BMI*z*, but it is unlikely that we captured true disorder onset, and some individuals with depression or anxiety were likely not identified (eg, if a disorder began after wave 3 and remitted well before wave 4). Also, because we did not continuously assess weight and do not know the true age of disorder onset, we cannot decisively establish whether weight change preceded or followed anxiety or depression onset. Second, height and weight were self-reported; self-reported height and weight have been shown to be accurate in adults and older teenagers.[53,54] In younger adolescents (aged 12-16 years), accuracy is related to age, with values for younger youth more likely to be inaccurate.[55] Third, it is possible that missing data biased our results. However, we assessed 94.6% of participants at waves 1, 2, and 3 and 80.6% of participants at wave 4; participants missing data at wave 4 did not differ substantively in age or BMI*z* at waves 1, 2, or 3. Finally, although we controlled for socioeconomic status, smoking, and medication use, it is possible that our results are biased by residual confounding due to imperfect measurement of these variables or the lack of measurement of other unknown confounders.

In conclusion, our analysis of a community-based cohort studied from childhood until adulthood provides evidence that, in females, anxiety disorders and depression are associated with higher weight. The potential for sex and age to influence whether an association between weight and anxiety disorders or depression is seen cross-sectionally or in short-term studies underscores the necessity of applying a life-course approach. Our results suggest that efforts to improve mental health in populations may also help prevent female obesity; consideration of the potential for psychological antecedents and correlates of obesity could improve prevention and treatment.

**Accepted for Publication:** October 20, 2005.
**Correspondence:** Sarah E. Anderson, MS, Tufts University, 136 Harrison Ave, Boston, MA 02111 (sarah.anderson@tufts.edu).
**Author Contributions:** Ms Anderson and Dr Must had full access to all the data in the study and take responsibility for the integrity of the data and the accuracy of the data analysis.
**Funding/Support:** This study was supported by grants T32 DK62032-11 and R21 DK64254 from the National Institute of Diabetes and Digestive and Kidney Diseases, Bethesda, Md; grant HD-40685 from the National Institute of Child Health and Human Development, Bethesda; and grants MH-36971, MH-38916, and MH-49191 from the National Institute of Mental Health, Rockville, Md.
**Role of the Sponsor:** The funding bodies had no role in data extraction and analyses, in the writing of the manuscript, or in the decision to submit the manuscript for publication.
**Acknowledgment:** We thank Paul Jacques, PhD, for his helpful comments on an earlier draft of the manuscript.

## REFERENCES

1. Hedley AA, Ogden CL, Johnson CL, Carroll MD, Curtin LR, Flegal KM. Prevalence of overweight and obesity among US children, adolescents, and adults, 1999-2002. *JAMA*. 2004;291:2847-2850.
2. Guo S, Wu W, Chumlea WC, Roche AF. Predicting overweight and obesity in adulthood from body mass index values in childhood and adolescence. *Am J Clin Nutr*. 2002;76:653-658.
3. Johnson J, Cohen P, Kasen S, Brook J. Childhood adversities associated with risk for eating disorders or weight problems during adolescence or early adulthood. *Am J Psychiatry*. 2002;159:394-400.
4. Mellbin T, Vuille JC. Rapidly developing overweight in school children as an indicator of psychosocial stress. *Acta Paediatr Scand*. 1989;78:568-575.
5. Williamson DF, Thompson TJ, Anda RF, Dietz WH, Felitti VJ. Body weight and obesity in adults and self-reported abuse in childhood. *Int J Obes Relat Metab Disord*. 2002;26:1075-1082.
6. Lissau I, Sorensen TI. Parental neglect during childhood and increased risk of obesity in young adulthood. *Lancet*. 1994;343:324-327.
7. Strauss RS, Knight J. Influence of the home environment on the development of obesity in children. *Pediatrics*. 1999;103:e85. Available at: http://pediatrics.aappublications.org/cgi/content/full/103/6/e85. Accessed August 12, 2004.
8. Moore ME, Stunkard A, Srole L. Obesity, social class, and mental illness. *JAMA*. 1962;181:962-966.
9. Crisp AH, McGuiness B. Jolly fat: relation between obesity and psychoneurosis in general population. *BMJ*. 1976;1:7-9.
10. Istvan J, Zavela K, Weidner G. Body weight and psychological distress in NHANES I. *Int J Obes Relat Metab Disord*. 1992;16:999-1003.
11. Carpenter KM, Hasin DS, Allison DB, Faith MS. Relationships between obesity and *DSM-IV* major depressive disorder, suicide ideation, and suicide attempts: results from a general population study. *Am J Public Health*. 2000;90:251-257.
12. Onyike CU, Crum RM, Lee HB, Lyketsos CG, Eaton WW. Is obesity associated with major depression? results from the Third National Health and Nutrition Examination Survey. *Am J Epidemiol*. 2003;158:1139-1147.
13. Becker ES, Margraf J, Turke V, Soeder U, Neumer S. Obesity and mental illness in a representative sample of young women. *Int J Obes Relat Metab Disord*. 2001;25(suppl 1):S5-S9.
14. Kawada T, Suzuki S. Obesity has an inverse relationship with a depressive state. *J Occup Health*. 2001;43:371-374.
15. Dong C, Sanchez LE, Price RA. Relationship of obesity to depression: a family-based study. *Int J Obes Relat Metab Disord*. 2004;28:790-795.
16. Jorm AF, Korten AE, Christensen H, Jacomb PA, Rodgers B, Parslow RA. Association of obesity with anxiety, depression and emotional well-being: a community survey. *Aust N Z J Public Health*. 2003;27:434-440.
17. Palinkas LA, Wingard DL, Barrett-Connor E. Depressive symptoms in overweight and obese older adults: a test of the "jolly fat" hypothesis. *J Psychosom Res*. 1996;40:59-66.
18. Stewart A, Brook R. Effects of being overweight. *Am J Public Health*. 1983;73:171-178.
19. Sallade J. A comparison of the psychological adjustment of obese vs non-obese children. *J Psychosom Res*. 1973;17:89-96.

20. Hallstrom T, Noppa H. Obesity in women in relation to mental illness, social factors and personality traits. *J Psychosom Res.* 1981;25:75-82.
21. Renman C, Engstrom I, Silfverdal SA, Aman J. Mental health and psychosocial characteristics in adolescent obesity: a population-based case-control study. *Acta Paediatr.* 1999;88:998-1003.
22. Hayes D, Ross CE. Body and mind: the effect of exercise, overweight, and physical health on psychological well-being. *J Health Soc Behav.* 1986;27:387-400.
23. Han TS, Tijhuis MAR, Lean MEJ, Seidell JC. Quality of life in relation to overweight and body fat distribution. *Am J Public Health.* 1998;88:1814-1820.
24. Lamertz CM, Jacobi C, Yassouridis A, Arnold K, Henkel AW. Are obese adolescents and young adults at higher risk for mental disorders? a community survey. *Obes Res.* 2002;10:1152-1160.
25. Erickson SJ, Robinson TN, Haydel KF, Killen JD. Are overweight children unhappy? body mass index, depressive symptoms, and overweight concerns in elementary school children. *Arch Pediatr Adolesc Med.* 2000;154:931-935.
26. Braet C, Mervielde I, Vandereycken W. Psychological aspects of childhood obesity: a controlled study in a clinical and nonclinical sample. *J Pediatr Psychol.* 1997;22:59-71.
27. Lumeng JC, Gannon K, Cabral HJ, Frank DA, Zucherman B. Association between clinically meaningful behavior problems and overweight in children. *Pediatrics.* 2003;112:1138-1145.
28. Pine DS, Goldstein RB, Wolk S, Weissman MM. The association between childhood depression and adulthood body mass index. *Pediatrics.* 2001;107:1049-1056.
29. Pine DS, Cohen P, Brook J, Coplan JD. Psychiatric symptoms in adolescence as predictors of obesity in early adulthood: a longitudinal study. *Am J Public Health.* 1997;87:1303-1310.
30. Goodman E, Whitaker RC. A prospective study of the role of depression in the development and persistence of adolescent obesity. *Pediatrics.* 2002;110:497-504.
31. DiPietro L, Anda RF, Williamson DF, Stunkard AJ. Depressive symptoms and weight change in a national cohort of adults. *Int J Obes Relat Metab Disord.* 1992;16:745-753.
32. Barefoot JC, Heitmann BL, Helms MJ, Williams RB, Surwit RS, Siegler IC. Symptoms of depression and changes in body weight from adolescence to mid-life. *Int J Obes Relat Metab Disord.* 1998;22:688-694.
33. Richardson LP, Davis R, Poulton R, et al. A longitudinal evaluation of adolescent depression and adult obesity. *Arch Pediatr Adolesc Med.* 2003;157:739-745.
34. Mustillo S, Worthman C, Erkanli A, Keeler G, Angold A, Costello EJ. Obesity and psychiatric disorder: developmental trajectories. *Pediatrics.* 2003;111:851-859.
35. Cohen P, Cohen J, Kasen S, et al. An epidemiological study of disorders in late childhood and adolescence–I: age- and gender-specific prevalence. *J Child Psychol Psychiatry.* 1993;34:851-867.
36. Cohen P, Cohen J. *Life Values and Adolescent Mental Health.* Mahwah, NJ: Lawrence A Erlbaum Associates; 1996.
37. Costello EJ, Edelbrock CS, Duncan MK, Kalas R. *Testing of the NIMH Diagnostic Interview Schedule for Children (DISC) in a Clinical Population: Final Report to the Center for Epidemiological Studies, NIHM.* Pittsburgh, Pa: University of Pittsburgh; 1984.
38. Costello EJ, Edelbrock CS, Costello AJ. Validity of the NIMH Diagnostic Interview Schedule for Children: a comparison between psychiatric and pediatric referrals. *J Abnorm Child Psychol.* 1985;13:579-595.
39. American Academy of Pediatrics' Committee on Nutrition. Prevention of pediatric overweight and obesity. *Pediatrics.* 2003;112:424-430.
40. Barlow SE, Dietz WH. Obesity evaluation and treatment: Expert Committee recommendations: the Maternal and Child Health Bureau, Health Resources and Services Administration and the Department of Health and Human Services. *Pediatrics.* 1998;102:e29. Available at: http://pediatrics.org/cgi/content/full/102/3/e29. Accessed. July 22, 2004.
41. Ogden CL, Kuczmarski RL, Flegal KM, et al. Centers for Disease Control and Prevention 2000 growth charts for the United States: improvements to the 1977 National Center for Health Statistics version. *Pediatrics.* 2002;109:45-60.
42. Wright CM, Parker L, Lamont D, Craft AW. Implications of childhood obesity for adult health: findings from thousand families cohort study. *BMJ.* 2001;323:1280-1284.
43. Singer JD, Willett JB. Modeling discontinuous and nonlinear change. In: Singer JD, Willett JB, eds. *Applied Longitudinal Data Analysis: Modeling Change and Event Occurrence.* New York, NY: Oxford University Press Inc; 2003:189-242.
44. Singer JD, Willett JB. Doing data analysis with the multilevel model for change. In: Singer JD, Willett JB, eds. *Applied Longitudinal Data Analysis: Modeling Change and Event Occurrence.* New York, NY: Oxford University Press Inc; 2003:113-116.
45. McDowell MA, Fryar CD, Hirsch R, Ogden CL. *Anthropometric Reference Data for Children and Adults: US Population, 1999-2002.* Atlanta, Ga: Centers for Disease Control and Prevention, US Dept of Health and Human Services; 2005. Advance Data From Vital and Health Statistics, No. 361.
46. Friedman MA, Brownell KD. Psychological correlates of obesity: moving to the next research generation. *Psychol Bull.* 1995;117:3-20.
47. Faith MS, Matz PE, Jorge MA. Obesity-depression associations in the population. *J Psychosom Res.* 2002;53:935-942.
48. Kessler RC, Chiu WT, Demler O, Walters EE. Prevalence, severity, and comorbidity of 12-month *DSM-IV* disorders in the National Comorbidity Survey Replication. *Arch Gen Psychiatry.* 2005;62:617-627.
49. Kessler RC, Nelson CB, McGonagle KA, Liu J, Swartz M, Blazer DG. Comorbidity of *DSM-III-R* major depressive disorder in the general population: results from the US National Comorbidity Survey. *Br J Psychiatry Suppl.* 1996;(30):17-30.
50. Overbeek T, Griez EJL. At the interface of depression and anxiety: comorbidity and concepts. In: Griez EJL, Faravelli C, Nutt DJ, Zohar J, eds. *Mood Disorders: Clinical Management and Research Issues.* Hoboken, NJ: John Wiley & Sons; 2005:503-526.
51. Saluja G, Iachan R, Scheidt P, Overpeck MD, Sun W, Giedd J. Prevalence of and risk factors for depressive symptoms among young adolescents. *Arch Pediatr Adolesc Med.* 2004;158:760-765.
52. American Psychiatric Association. *Diagnostic and Statistical Manual of Mental Disorders, Fourth Edition.* Washington, DC: American Psychiatric Association; 1994.
53. Stewart AL. The reliability and validity of self-reported weight and height. *J Chronic Dis.* 1982;35:295-309.
54. Brener ND, McManus T, Galuska DA, Lowry R, Wechsler H. Reliability and validity of self-reported height and weight among high school students. *J Adolesc Health.* 2003;32:281-287.
55. Strauss RS. Comparison of measured and self-reported weight and height in a cross-sectional sample of young adolescents. *Int J Obes Relat Metab Disord.* 1999;23:904-908.

# Development of Pediatric Comorbidity Prediction Model

*Derek Tai, MSc; Paul Dick, MD, MSc; Teresa To, PhD; James G. Wright, MD, MPH*

**Objective:** To develop a comorbidity model for children that can be used with hospital discharge administrative databases.

**Design:** Retrospective study using administrative data obtained from the Canadian Institute for Health Information Discharge Abstract Database and the Deaths File to develop a logistic regression model. Hosmer-Lemeshow $\chi^2$ test was used to examine model fit. The C statistic was used to assess model discrimination. Bootstrapping was used to determine the stability of regression coefficients.

**Setting:** We used linked administrative databases to compile 339 077 hospital discharge abstracts from April 1, 1991, through March 31, 2002.

**Participants:** Children between ages 1 and 14 years in Ontario, Canada.

**Main Outcome Measure:** Death within 1 year of hospital discharge.

**Results:** The 27-variable pediatric comorbidity model predicted 1-year mortality with a C statistic of 0.83 in the Ontario data set from which it was derived. The presence of brain cancer (odds ratio, 76.38 [95% confidence interval, 53.40-109.27]) at hospital admission was the strongest predictor, followed by diabetes insipidus (odds ratio, 39.23 [95% confidence interval, 20.75-74.17]).

**Conclusion:** Using clinical judgment and empirical modeling strategies, we were able to identify 27 diagnoses highly predictive of death for children between 1 and 14 years of age within 1 year of hospital discharge.

*Arch Pediatr Adolesc Med. 2006;160:293-299*

**Author Affiliations:** Department of Surgery (Dr Wright), University of Toronto (Mr Tai), and the Population Health Sciences Program (Drs Wright and To and Mr Tai) and Department of Paediatrics (Dr Dick) The Hospital for Sick Children, Toronto, Ontario.

COMPARISON OF HEALTH care outcomes across treatments, institutions, or health care professionals requires adjustment for risks, such as comorbidity, that inherently increase or decrease the likelihood of poor health outcomes, thereby allowing more valid comparisons. Comorbidities are defined as acute or chronic conditions unrelated to the principal diagnosis responsible for hospital admission.[1-3] Patients with comorbidities have higher risks of complications and death, are less responsive and tolerant to conventional therapies, and have longer hospital stays and higher resources use.[1-6] Although studied extensively in adults, comorbidity has received little attention in children. Because low proportions of children require long-term care,[4,7,8] pediatric risk adjustments have focused mainly on acute care settings that use physiologic indicators, such as the Pediatric Risk of Mortality Score,[9] the Clinical Risk Index for Babies,[10] and Score for Neonatal Acute Physiology,[11] to predict imminent in-hospital death of gravely ill patients. While acute clinical factors are central to evaluating risk for imminent (ie, 30 days) deaths and complications, their usefulness for predicting long-term outcomes (ie, 1 year) is probably limited. The purpose of this study was to identify comorbid conditions related to death within 1 year of hospital discharge for children and adolescents between ages 1 and 14 years. Infants younger than 1 year were omitted because mortality and morbidity in this age group are mostly due to congenital conditions. Children 14 years and older were excluded because beyond this age disease epidemiology is more akin to young adults.

## METHODS

### SOURCES OF ADMINISTRATIVE DATA

Hospital discharges for children between ages 1 and 14 years in Ontario, Canada, from April 1, 1991, through March 31, 2002, were compiled from the Canadian Institute for Health Information (CIHI) Discharge Abstract Data-

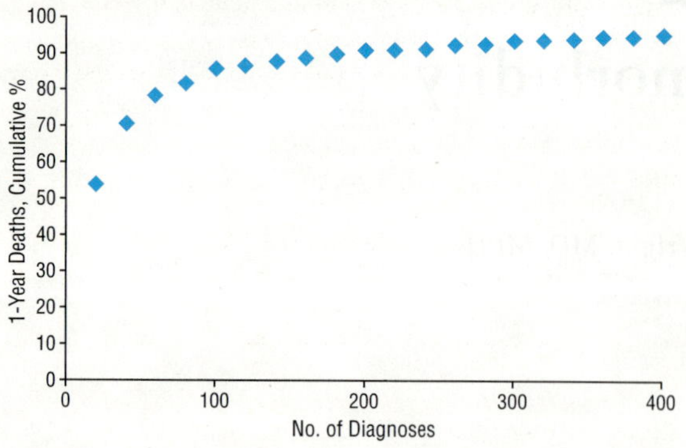


**Figure.** Cumulative percentage of 1-year deaths represented by the top 400 of 1294 most frequently recorded *International Classification of Diseases, Ninth Revision*[12] codes for the cohort of inpatients (n=1988) who died following their index hospital discharges.

base. The CIHI is a federally chartered institution established to provide health information pertinent for health services research. Abstracts are completed by hospital-based coders after patients leave the hospital, recording diagnoses noted during the entire hospital admission. The Ontario discharge data contain 16 diagnoses and 10 surgical procedures coded using the *International Classification of Diseases, Ninth Revision*[12] (*ICD-9*) codes. Corresponding diagnosis-type indicators specify whether it is a preexisting comorbidity or a complication. Only diagnoses coded as comorbidities were used to develop our prediction model. In addition, demographic (eg, sex and date of birth) and administrative (eg, hospital admission and discharge dates) information were obtained. According to the Institute for Clinical Evaluative Sciences Practice Atlas[13] chapter entitled "A Summary of Studies on the Quality of Health Care in Administrative Databases in Canada," the documentation of patient demographic variables in the health administrative databases is complete and reliable. Recording of comorbid condition is accurate but may be incomplete. Undercoding is an inherent limitation of all administrative databases.

To determine patient status, we used the Deaths File created by the Institute for Clinical Evaluative Sciences in North York, Ontario. The Deaths File has 1 observation for every resident in Ontario with a valid health card number who is registered dead in either the Registered Persons Database or CIHI record of in-hospital deaths. The Registered Persons Database is an administrative database maintained by the Ministry of Health and Long-Term Care to keep track of all Ontario Health Insurance Plan users. The Registered Persons Database records patient information including birth date, sex, postal code, and death date. The Deaths File is updated whenever new Registered Persons Database or CIHI data become available. Each year between 2% and 3% of deaths are reported only in CIHI. In case of discrepancy, the CIHI death date supersedes.

## OUTCOMES

Using the Institute for Clinical Evaluative Sciences key number, an encrypted form of health card number (a unique patient identifier), we linked the CIHI Discharge Abstract Database with the Deaths File to identify patients' vital status (ie, alive or dead) at 1 year from the date of hospital discharge. Twenty-seven records with death dates preceding those of hospital discharge were deleted. Our decision to study mortality at 1 year was based on the need to extend our observation window to capture more deaths because childhood mortality is a rare outcome. Although factors other than comorbidities may affect vital status in a longer window, we chose 1 year so that our model would have greater utility than one predicting 30- or 60-day mortality.

From this linked database, we identified 541 825 first and recurring hospital discharges from Ontario hospitals for children between 1 and 14 years of age within the 8-year accrual window, from April 1, 1993, to April 1, 2001. To make certain that we included only 1 abstract per inpatient, we used only the index or first hospital discharge in 2 years, enumerating backward from the date of hospital discharge. Based on this criterion, there were 339 077 index hospital discharges. Comparing the numbers of total and index hospital discharges, the volume of readmissions was low.

## POTENTIAL RISK FACTORS FOR THE PEDIATRIC COMORBIDITY PREDICTION MODEL

The 16 diagnosis fields in the linked database were collapsed, yielding 1294 distinct *ICD-9* codes recorded for those who died subsequent to their index hospital discharge. Codes were ranked from most to least frequent. The top 200 represented 90.8% of 1-year deaths, whereas the next 200 represented only an additional 4.4% (**Figure**). If we compiled diagnoses irrespective of the outcome, we would have identified prevalent conditions, such as common cold, that are almost certainly not associated with mortality. Including such diagnoses would render the model with low or no discriminative power.

We aimed to include the fewest number of variables that would still adjust for risks of 1-year mortality adequately, not only because the model is easier to use but also because it prevents the potential peril of overfitting when the ratio of risk factors to outcomes is greater than 10:1.[14,15] Both empirical modeling strategies and clinical judgment were used to develop our prediction model. First, a panel of 2 pediatric clinicians (ie, a surgeon and a pediatrician) independently aggregated the 200 *ICD-9* codes into homogenous diagnostic categories (eg, seizures and epilepsy). The clinicians convened to reconcile the minor differences between diagnostic groupings. Second, we used the Pearson $\chi^2$ test to examine associations between each diagnostic group and death within 1 year of index hospital discharge using a $P$ value $<.20$. This threshold was chosen because a more lenient cutoff would include too many variables whereas a more stringent one would fail to pick up important ones. Third, we omitted procedure codes that were not diagnoses (eg, kidney donor, V594). Fourth, we deleted diagnosis codes that were not clinically plausible predictors of 1-year mortality (eg, cardiac arrest, 4275). Fifth, diagnostic groups associated with fewer than 15 deaths were removed from further analysis because our aim was to capture diagnoses both relatively frequent and having significant associations with 1-year mortality. The remaining variables were entered into a multivariable logistic regression model, and forward stepwise regression was used to eliminate variables until only those significant at $P<.20$ were left in the final model. A more stringent $P$ value, such as $P=.05$, is not recommended because of the risk of excluding important variables from the prediction model.[16]

The goodness of fit of the final model was examined using the Hosmer-Lemeshow $\chi^2$ test. The Hosmer-Lemeshow test measures deviations between the observed and predicted number of cases who were alive or dead within subgroups of similar risks. Under the null hypothesis that prediction within each subgroup is correct, the model is calibrated to the data if the $P$ value is large. The discrimination of the model was calculated by measuring the area under the receiver operating characteristic curve, which is equivalent to the C statistic, ranging from 0 to 1 with 1 indicating a perfect prediction. A prediction model with excellent discrimination generally has a C statistic between 0.8 and 0.9.[16] If the model has no ability to discriminate patients who died less than 1 year after hospital discharge from those who did not, the expected value of the C statistic is 0.5.

Bootstrap estimates of standard errors, a technique developed by Efron[17] in 1979, were calculated to assess the accuracy of parameter estimates of diagnostic groups included in the final model. Bootstrapping relies on drawing a large number of independent bootstrap samples.[17] Each bootstrap replicate is obtained by randomly sampling *n* times, with replacement, from the original database of size *n*. Because a bootstrap replicate is drawn with replacement, each replicate might contain multiple copies of an observation or none at all. Our bootstrap algorithm generated 150 replicates. Parameter estimates were calculated for each, and the standard deviation of these point estimates was the bootstrap estimate of standard errors. The standard errors were used to compute 95% bootstrap confidence intervals (CIs) for parameter estimates, which were exponentiated to yield 95% bootstrap CIs of odds ratios (ORs). SAS statistical software (SAS Institute Inc, Cary, NC) was used to conduct all statistical analyses in this study.

## RESULTS

In total, 595 905 *ICD-9* codes were compiled for 339 077 index hospital discharges, identified by unique Institute for Clinical Evaluative Sciences key numbers. Each hospital discharge was associated with 1 or more diagnosis codes. The minimum, maximum, and median number of *ICD-9* codes for index hospital discharges were 1.0, 16.0, and 3.0, respectively. One thousand nine hundred eighty-eight deaths were identified subsequent to index hospital discharges, in which 880 died within 1 year or less and 1108 died after 1 year. Descriptive statistics for age and length of stay for index hospital discharges are presented in **Table 1**.

A list of the 37 diagnostic groups entered into multivariable logistic regression is presented in **Table 2** along with the *ICD-9* codes used to generate them. The frequency of each group was recorded during index hospital admission, along with the number of inpatients who had the diagnosis and died within 1 year of the date of hospital discharge. **Table 3** presents the results of the logistic regression along with the bootstrap results. Six diagnostic groups did not enter the model based on the preset *P* value of .20: cerebral palsy, urinary tract infection, pleural effusion, anemia, esophagitis, and acute renal failure. Four diagnostic groups (ie, gastroenteritis, otitis media, dehydration, and asthma) that had negative associations with 1-year mortality were excluded. Hence, the final list of the pediatric comorbidity prediction model consists of 27 variables. Table 3 presents the logistic regression coefficients and associated ORs with 95% CIs. The presence of brain cancer at hospital admission was the strongest predictor of 1-year post–hospital discharge mortality (OR, 76.38 [95%CI, 53.40-109.27]), followed by diabetes insipidus (OR, 39.23 [95% CI, 20.75-74.17]).

The Hosmer-Lemeshow $\chi^2$ test was performed to examine goodness of fit. Based on the large sample size, the model was poorly calibrated ($P<.001$). However, the model's predictive validity was excellent with a C statistic of

**Table 1. Descriptive Analyses of Age and Length of Stay for 339 077 Index Hospital Discharges**

| Statistic | Age, y | Length of Stay, d |
|---|---|---|
| Mean | 5.86 | 2.69 |
| Median | 5.00 | 2.00 |
| Mode | 1.00 | 1.00 |
| Standard deviation | 4.31 | 9.76 |
| Maximum | 14 | 2434 |
| Minimum | 1 | 1 |

0.83. A bootstrap algorithm was executed to draw 150 replicates with replacement from the database to estimate bootstrap standard errors, which in turn were used to generate 95% bootstrap CIs. Table 3 lists the adjusted ORs, in descending order, with their respective 95% bootstrap CIs.

## COMMENT

Sicker patients, even with optimal care, are likely to experience worse outcomes than their healthier counterparts. The ability to make valid comparison and thereby draw unbiased conclusions about quality of care hinges on the availability of appropriate risk-adjustment models to account for differences in patients' characteristics. Our goal was to create a statistical model that can be generated from an administrative hospital discharge database. Although clinical data are the gold standard for risk adjustment, administrative data are less expensive to acquire and less cumbersome to use because the data are already collected and computer readable. For these reasons, it is likely that administrative data will be used more regularly in the future for risk adjustment purposes. Administrative data have been used successfully in adults to identify potential comorbidity risk factors for outcomes, such as death.[18-25] The CIHI database used in our study encompassed an entire population, the province of Ontario (with negligible care provided to residents outside the province), permitting stable estimates of rare events, such as childhood mortality.

Validity is a crucial attribute that encompasses both clinical and statistical considerations. For health care professionals to accept and ultimately use our mortality prediction rule, it must be clinically valid. Health care professionals appraise the validity of a model by examining whether it includes the major variables that they judge to be important. To reduce the model to a working number of diagnoses and not rely exclusively on statistical modeling, in our first step we used clinicians to cluster homogenous codes into independent diagnostic groups. This was performed in part recognizing that *ICD-9* codes lack diagnostic criteria and many diagnostic labels are used interchangeably. The 2 clinicians involved are experienced health services researchers who have solid understanding of the health administrative databases used in this study and the use of *ICD-9* and *International Statistical Classification of Diseases, 10th Revision*[26] codes in documenting diagnoses. Instead of relying solely on their own clinical experience to prognosticate mortality, their

**Table 2. Potential Risk Factors of 1-Year Mortality Derived From Clinical and Statistical Criteria**

| Diagnostic Groups | Descriptions (*ICD-9*[12] codes) | No. of Times This Diagnostic Group Was Recorded During Index Hospital Admission | No. (%) of Inpatients Who Had Condition(s) That Belong to This Diagnostic Group and Had Died Within 1 Year |
|---|---|---|---|
| Seizure | Convulsions (7803); grand mal status (3453); generalized convulsive epilepsy (3451); epilepsy, unspecified (3459); partial epilepsy, without impairment of consciousness (3455) | 14 073 | 93 (0.66) |
| Feeding problem | Gastrostomy status (V441), feeding problem (7833) | 879 | 54 (6.1) |
| Pyrexia | Pyrexia unknown origin (8786) | 8786 | 66 (0.75) |
| Pneumonia | Pneumonia, organism NOS (486); bronchopneumonia, organism NOS (485); pneumonia, organism NOS (4860) | 21 425 | 69 (0.32) |
| Leukemia | Acute lymphoid leukemia (2040), acute lymphoid leukemia of unspecified cell type (2080), acute myeloid leukemia (2050) | 692 | 45 (6.5) |
| Septicemia | *Staphylococcus* infection NOS (411), other specified bacterial infections (418), *Streptococcus* infection NOS (410), *Escherichia coli* infection NOS (414), septicemia NOS (389), *Staphylococcus* septicemia (381), *Pseudomonas* infection NOS (417), *Klebsiella* infection NOS (413), *Haemophilus influenzae* infection NOS (415), *streptococcal* septicemia (380), infection and inflammatory reaction due to internal prosthetic device, implant, and graft (9966) | 9316 | 115 (1.2) |
| Dehydration | Volume depletion (2765), hyperosmolality (2760) | 26 460 | 29 (0.11) |
| Asthma | Asthma NOS (4939), extrinsic asthma (4930) | 38 104 | 30 (0.079) |
| Agranulocytosis | Agranulocytosis (2880) | 709 | 29 (4.1) |
| Respiratory failure | Respiratory failure (7991), dyspnea and respiratory abnormalities (7860) | 5923 | 86 (1.5) |
| Asphyxia | Anoxic brain damage (3481), cerebral edema (3485), coma and stupor (7800), drowning and nonfatal submersion (9941), asphyxia (7990) | 1031 | 138 (13) |
| Pneumonitis | Pneumonitis due to inhalation of food or vomitus (5070) | 364 | 39 (11) |
| Cerebral palsy | Cerebral palsy NOS (3439), congenital quadriplegia (3432), hemiplegia NOS (3429), lack of coordination (7813) | 1770 | 35 (2.0) |
| Esophagitis | Esophagitis (5301) | 669 | 25 (3.7) |
| Gastroenteritis | Enteritis due to specified virus (86), other and unspecified noninfectious gastroenteritis and colitis (558/5580) | 29 698 | 35 (0.12) |
| Otitis media | Otitis media NOS (3829) | 16 438 | 17 (0.10) |
| Urinary tract infection | Urinary tract infection NOS (5990) | 4819 | 26 (0.54) |
| Hydrocephalus | Obstructive hydrocephalus (3314), ventricular shunt status (V452), congenital hydrocephalus (7423) | 936 | 46 (4.9) |
| Diabetes insipidus | Diabetes insipidus (2535) | 93 | 37 (40) |
| Ventricular septal defect | Ventricular septal defect (7454) | 735 | 21 (2.9) |
| Congenital subaortic stenosis | Congenital subaortic stenosis (7468) | 535 | 15 (2.8) |
| Brain cancer | Malig neoplasm of the brainstem (1917), malig neoplasm of the cerebellum (1916), malig neoplasm of the ventricles (1915), malig neoplasm of other parts of the brain (1918), malig neoplasm of the brain, unspecified (1919), malig neoplasm of the cerebrum, except lobes and ventricles (1910), brain neoplasm NOS (2396), secondary malig neoplasm of other parts of the nervous system (meninges) (1984), secondary malig neoplasm of the brain and spinal cord (1983), neoplasm of uncertain behavior of endocrine glands and nervous system (brain and spinal cord) (2375) | 429 | 69 (16) |
| Head injury | Closed skull fractures with cerebral laceration and contusion (8001), closed skull base fractures with cerebral laceration and contusion (8011), subarachnoid hemorrhage following injury without mention of open intracranial wound (8520), other conditions of brain (3488), intracranial injury without mention of open intracranial wound (8540), traumatic brain hemorrhage (8530), cerebral cortex contusion without mention of open intracranial wound (8510), closed skull vault fracture with other and unspecified intracranial hemorrhage (8003), compression of brain (3483), abrasion head (9100) | 7301 | 141 (1.9) |
| Lung contusion | Closed fracture of rib(s) (8070); abrasion or friction burn without mention of infection (9110); lung injury without mention of open wound into thorax (8612); posttraumatic pulmonary insufficiency (5185); traumatic pneumothorax, closed (8600); pulmonary collapse (5180) | 1889 | 83 (4.4) |

*(continued)*

**Table 2. Potential Risk Factors of 1-Year Mortality Derived From Clinical and Statistical Criteria (cont)**

| Diagnostic Groups | Descriptions (*ICD-9*[12] codes) | No. of Times This Diagnostic Group Was Recorded During Index Hospital Admission | No. (%) of Inpatients Who Had Condition(s) That Belong to This Diagnostic Group and Had Died Within 1 Year |
|---|---|---|---|
| Pleural effusion | Pleural effusion NOS (5119) | 573 | 18 (3.1) |
| Heart failure | Congestive heart failure (4280), heart failure NOS (4289), acute edema of lung, unspecified (5184), other primary cardiomyopathies (4254) | 273 | 41 (15) |
| Developmental delay | Development delay NOS (3159), mental retardation NOS (319), other specified delays in development (3158), severe mental retardation (3181), lack of expected normal physiological development in childhood (7834) | 2872 | 79 (2.8) |
| Anemia | Anemia NOS (2859), anemia secondary to blood loss (chronic) (2800), other specified aplastic anemias (2848), acute posthemorrhagic anemia (2851) | 5434 | 34 (0.63) |
| Hypertension | Essential hypertension, unspecified (4019) | 351 | 16 (4.6) |
| Shock | Hypotension NOS (4589), shock NOS (7855), traumatic shock (9584) | 225 | 53 (24) |
| Arrhythmia | Sinoatrial node dysfunction (4278), cardiac dysrhythmia NOS (4279) | 628 | 22 (3.5) |
| Stroke | Cerebral artery occlusion NOS (4349), intracerebral hemorrhage (431), cerebrovascular anomaly (7478) | 246 | 35 (14) |
| Femur fracture | Fracture femur NOS, closed (8210); abrasion hip leg (9160) | 2491 | 23 (0.92) |
| Coagulopathy | Thrombocytopenia NOS (2875), primary thrombocytopenia (2873), other and unspecified coagulation defects (2869) | 1232 | 24 (1.9) |
| Candidiasis | Candidiasis site NOS (1129) | 92 | 16 (17) |
| Acute renal failure | Acute renal failure NOS (5849), acute renal failure (584), acute glomerulonephritis (5809) | 188 | 15 (8.0) |
| Acidosis | Acidosis (2762) | 576 | 27 (4.7) |

Abbreviations: *ICD-9, International Classification of Diseases, Ninth Revision;* malig, malignant; NOS, not otherwise specified.

judgments on grouping were guided by data. Each diagnostic group almost certainly has differing mortality risk. Even within each diagnosis, severity of disease affects outcome. However, the purpose of this study was to develop a model that provided the ability to adjust for risk of mortality, not to determine mortality risk for every diagnosis. Other extensively used comorbidity indexes have been constructed using similar principles. For example, the Charlson Index,[27] the most commonly used comorbidity risk adjustment tool for adults, lumps all cancer into 1 group, although different cancers have strikingly different mortality rates.

## MODEL PERFORMANCE

One standard model-performance indicator is how well risk-adjusted predictions fit the actual outcomes. A small *P* value suggests poor fit. In this study, because the sample size was large, even small discrepancies between the model's prediction and observed counts were anticipated to be significant. The C statistic was calculated to evaluate the model's predictive performance. In absolute terms, the ability of our model to predict 1-year mortality was excellent, as indicated by a C statistic of 0.83. In relative terms, Wang and colleagues[22] adapted the Charlson Index[27] to a Medicare claims database to predict 1-year mortality and reported a C statistic of 0.72.

In theory, it would be optimal to establish a model that handles more diagnostic details as well as being thoroughly calibrated. However, a tool that is too detailed may be too laborious to use. While we might be able to produce a better-calibrated model by including more diagnostic information, it could be difficult to validate such a model with other data sets. Moreover, we could be calibrating for many rare diagnoses that have limited usefulness.

Discrimination is more important than calibration because the objective is to create a general risk-adjustment model with the intent to adjust for baseline differences in average background comorbidity. If the study population has specific high-risk comorbidities, the investigator should identify the specific and relevant covariates to be incorporated in the adjustment model. For example, when studying a specific population of children with airway obstruction who underwent 2 different modalities of tracheostomy, additional clinical comorbidities associated with tracheostomy, such as congenital airway anomalies, should be included in the risk-adjustment model. We believe it is not possible to produce a parsimonious general risk-adjustment tool that is well calibrated for all conceivable pediatric populations.

## MODEL VALIDATION

Bleeker et al[28] suggested that both internal and external validations be used to ascertain performance of a new regression model. In our study, rather than using the split-half method, we used the entire data set to develop the model and performed bootstrapping as the measure of

**Table 3. Logistic Regression and Bootstrapping Models for Predicting 1-Year Mortality After Index Hospital Discharge in Ontario, 1993-2001**

| | Multivariable Logistic Regression | | | |
|---|---|---|---|---|
| **Diagnostic Groups** | **Regression Parameter Estimates** | **SE** | **OR (95% CI)** | **Bootstrap (95% BootCI)** |
| Brain cancer | 4.34 | 0.18 | 76.38 (53.40-109.27) | (46.47-125.56) |
| Diabetes insipidus | 3.67 | 0.33 | 39.23 (20.75-74.17) | (17.13-89.84) |
| Asphyxia | 3.24 | 0.13 | 25.49 (19.74-32.91) | (17.88-36.33) |
| Shock | 3.17 | 0.25 | 23.69 (14.61-38.42) | (12.04-46.63) |
| Leukemia | 3.060 | 0.22 | 21.34 (13.77-33.065) | (11.09-41.04) |
| Heart failure | 3.039 | 0.25 | 20.89 (12.92-33.78) | (10.46-41.72) |
| Feeding problem | 2.16 | 0.19 | 8.67 (5.94-12.66) | (5.18-14.50) |
| Pneumonitis | 2.080 | 0.24 | 8.003 (4.99-12.85) | (4.31-14.85) |
| Stroke | 2.055 | 0.29 | 7.81 (4.39-13.87) | (3.40-17.90) |
| Candidiasis | 1.97 | 0.39 | 7.16 (3.36-15.28) | (2.61-19.63) |
| Head injury | 1.91 | 0.12 | 6.76 (5.36-8.54) | (5.35-8.85) |
| Acidosis | 1.85 | 0.32 | 6.33 (3.41-11.74) | (3.03-13.24) |
| Hypertension | 1.84 | 0.37 | 6.29 (3.016-13.11) | (2.25-17.58) |
| Developmental delay | 1.54 | 0.16 | 4.67 (3.39-6.42) | (3.05-7.14) |
| Respiratory failure | 1.35 | 0.15 | 3.85 (2.90-5.13) | (2.76-5.38) |
| Lung contusion | 1.24 | 0.17 | 3.46 (2.49-4.80) | (2.30-5.19) |
| Ventricular septal defect | 1.23 | 0.31 | 3.41 (1.85-6.28) | (1.48-7.88) |
| Congenital subaortic stenosis | 1.22 | 0.37 | 3.38 (1.63-7.00) | (1.37-8.31) |
| Arrhythmia | 0.78 | 0.34 | 2.19 (1.13-4.23) | (0.89-5.37) |
| Septicemia | 0.75 | 0.13 | 2.11 (1.63-2.75) | (1.56-2.86) |
| Coagulopathy | 0.67 | 0.31 | 1.96 (1.065-3.59) | (0.80-4.76) |
| Agranulocytosis | 0.62 | 0.30 | 1.86 (1.031-3.35) | (0.79-4.38) |
| Pyrexia | 0.59 | 0.17 | 1.80 (1.30-2.50) | (1.31-2.47) |
| Hydrocephalus | 0.47 | 0.24 | 1.60 (1.01-2.56) | (0.79-3.24) |
| Pneumonia | 0.47 | 0.14 | 1.59 (1.22-2.083) | (1.19-2.12) |
| Femur fracture | 0.40 | 0.27 | 1.49 (0.87-2.55) | (0.77-2.90) |
| Seizure | 0.38 | 0.14 | 1.46 (1.12-1.91) | (1.08-1.97) |

Abbreviations: BootCI, bootstrap confidence interval; CI, confidence interval; OR, odds ratio.

internal validation. Bootstrapping to look at the stability of the individual coefficients is sensitive in capturing the destabilizing effect of a few highly influential observations within a diagnostic group.

Because our model was developed using an entire population, external validation might not be as critical. However, to evaluate whether we developed a model of pediatric comorbidity that predicts well in diverse settings, retesting of the model in an independent database to evaluate the coefficients derived in an Ontario population is important. We expect that slight differences in patterns of care and coding practices could affect the type of clinical data available for risk adjustment and could potentially change the relationship between the risk factors and outcomes. Future studies should also examine whether the pediatric comorbidity model has utility in predicting other outcomes, such as length of hospital stay.

## STRENGTHS AND LIMITATIONS OF THE PEDIATRIC COMORBIDITY PREDICTION MODEL

The model has several strengths. First, the model has a relatively small number of variables that can be easily generated and replicated in other administrative databases using *ICD-9* codes. Second, to our knowledge, it was the first population study that used administrative data to quantify the relationship between individual pediatric comorbidities and 1-year mortality. Third, the variables in the model are clinically sensible because pediatric clinicians were involved at all stages of model building.

The study has 2 potential limitations. First, we were not able to compare the model's performance against that derived from health records. Second, the model needs to be externally validated. Nonetheless, our research offers the first Charlson-like tool for pediatrics to adjust for comorbidity using administrative data. We anticipate the pediatric comorbidity risk-adjustment model will prove to be useful to outcome researchers working with administrative data in assessing the existence and direction of confounding by comorbidity.

**Accepted for Publication:** October 13, 2005.
**Correspondence:** Derek Tai, MSc, University of Toronto, 133 Wild Orchid Crescent, Markham, Ontario L6C 1V6, Canada (derek.tai@utoronto.ca).
**Funding/Support:** This study was supported by the Research Institute, The Hospital for Sick Children, Toronto, Ontario.
**Additional Information:** Dr Wright is the RB Salter Chair of Pediatric Surgical Research at The Hospital for Sick Children.
**Acknowledgment:** We thank all biostatisticians at the Institute for Clinical Evaluative Sciences (North York, Ontario) for help with SAS programming.

## REFERENCES


1. Guralnik JM. Assessing the impact of comorbidity in the older population. *Ann Epidemiol.* 1996;6:376-380.
2. Rozzini R, Frisoni GB, Ferrucci L, et al. Geriatric Index of Comorbidity: validation and comparison with other measures of comorbidity. *Age Ageing.* 2002;31:277-285.
3. Yates JW. Comorbidity considerations in geriatric oncology research. *CA Cancer J Clin.* 2001;51:329-336.
4. Iezzoni LI. *Risk Adjustment for Measuring Healthcare Outcomes.* 3rd ed. Chicago, Ill: Health Administration Press; 2003.
5. Iezzoni LI. The risks of risk adjustment. *JAMA.* 1997;278:1600-1607.
6. Rochon PA, Katz JN, Morrow LA, et al. Comorbid illness is associated with survival and length of hospital stay in patients with chronic disability: a prospective comparison of three comorbid indices. *Med Care.* 1996;34:1093-1101.
7. Kuhlthau K, Ferris TGG, Iezzoni LI. Risk adjustment for pediatric quality indicators. *Pediatrics.* 2004;113:210-216.
8. Beal AC, Patrick J, Dougherty D, et al. Quality measures for children's health care. *Pediatrics.* 2004;113:199-209.
9. Pollack MM, Ruttimann UE, Getson PR. Pediatric Risk of Mortality (PRISM) Score. *Crit Care Med.* 1988;16:1110-1116.
10. The CRIB (Clinical Risk Index for Babies) score: a tool for assessing initial neonatal risk and comparing performance of neonatal intensive care units. The International Neonatal Network [published correction appears in *Lancet.* 1993;342:626]. *Lancet.* 1993;342:193-198.
11. Richardson DK, Gray JE, McCormick MC, et al. Score for Neonatal Acute Physiology (SNAP): a physiologic severity index for neonatal intensive care. *Pediatrics.* 1993;91:617-623.
12. World Health Organization. *International Classification of Diseases, Ninth Revision (ICD-9).* Geneva, Switzerland: World Health Organization; 1977.
13. Goel V, Williams JI, Anderson GM, et al. *Patterns of Health Care in Ontario. The ICES Practice Atlas.* 2nd ed. Ottawa, Ontario: Canadian Medical Association; 1996:54-64.
14. Concato J, Feinstein AR, Holford TR. The risk of determining risk with multivariable models. *Ann Intern Med.* 1993;118:201-210.
15. Iezzoni LI. Statistically derived predictive models: caveat emptor. *J Gen Intern Med.* 1999;14:388-389.
16. Hosmer DW, Lemeshow S. *Applied Logistic Regression.* 2nd ed. Toronto, Ontario: John Wiley & Sons; 2000.
17. Efron B, Tibshirani RJ. *An Introduction to the Bootstrap.* New York, NY: Chapman & Hall; 1993.
18. Deyo RA, Cherkin DC, Ciol MA. Adapting a clinical comorbidity index for use with *ICD-9-CM* administrative databases. *J Clin Epidemiol.* 1992;45:613-619.
19. Romano PS, Roos LL, Jollis JG. Adapting a clinical comorbidity index for use with *ICD-9-CM* administrative data: differing perspectives. *J Clin Epidemiol.* 1993;46:1075-1079.
20. D'Hoore W, Bouchaert A, Tilquin C. Practical considerations on the use of the Charlson Comorbidity Index with administrative databases. *J Clin Epidemiol.* 1996;49:1429-1433.
21. Schneeweiss S, Malcolm M. Use of comorbidity scores for control of confounding in studies using administrative databases. *Int J Epidemiol.* 2000;29:891-898.
22. Wang PS, Walker A, Tsuang M, et al. Strategies for improving comorbidity measures based on Medicare and Medicaid claims data. *J Clin Epidemiol.* 2000;53:571-578.
23. Quan H, Parsons GA, Ghali WA. Validity of information on comorbidity derived from *ICD-9-CM* administrative data. *Med Care.* 2002;40:675-685.
24. Klabunde CN, Potosky AL, Legler JM, et al. Development of a comorbidity index using physician claims data. *J Clin Epidemiol.* 2000;53:1258-1267.
25. Klabunde CN, Warren JL, Legler JM. Assessing comorbidity using claims data: an overview. *Med Care.* 2002;40(8)(suppl):IV-26-35.
26. World Health Organization. *International Statistical Classification of Diseases, 10th Revision (ICD-10).* Geneva, Switzerland: World Health Organization; 1992.
27. Charlson ME, Pompei P, Ales KL, et al. A new method of classifying prognostic comorbidity in longitudinal studies: development and validation. *J Chronic Dis.* 1987;40:373-383.
28. Bleeker SE, Moll HA, Steyerberg EW, et al. External validation is necessary in prediction research: a clinical example. *J Clin Epidemiol.* 2003;56:826-832.

SECTION EDITOR: ALBERT C. YAN, MD; ASSISTANT SECTION EDITOR: SAMIR S. SHAH, MD

# Picture of the Month

*Melanie Pitone, MD; Benjamin Alouf, MD*

AN OTHERWISE HEALTHY 3-MONTH-OLD male infant had umbilical erythema and watery stools. He had been slightly fussy and cried during feeding. His parents reported intermittent emesis and diarrhea over the last several weeks, with body temperature to 38.8°C. During this illness, he developed redness of the umbilicus that, after resolving spontaneously, recurred over the last 2 days.

On examination, his weight was 7.1 kg (75th percentile); temperature, 38.1°C; heart rate, 153/min; respiratory rate, 40/min; blood pressure, 62/47 mm Hg; and oxygen saturation, 98% on room air. He appeared mildly ill, pale, and quiet. His lips were dry, he had a 2/6 flow murmur heard best at the left sternal border, his skin was mottled, and his feet were cool. The abdomen was soft without apparent tenderness. Periumbilical erythema and induration extended a distance of 0.5 cm around the umbilicus.

Initial laboratory testing revealed a white blood cell count of 34 800/μL, with a differential of 60% neutrophils and 26% lymphocytes. The hemoglobin level was 10.3 g/dL, the platelet count was $1.103 \times 10^6$/μL, and the C-reactive protein level was 2.9 mg/dL. Abdominal radiography revealed a single dilated loop of bowel in the midabdomen with adjacent thickening of the anterior abdominal wall. Isotonic saline improved his perfusion and color. The patient began receiving intravenous piperacillin and tazobactam for broad-spectrum bowel and skin flora coverage.

The following day, the surrounding erythema had improved. However, spontaneous purulent drainage was noted at the umbilicus (**Figure 1**), so an ultrasound was performed (**Figure 2**).

What is your diagnosis?

**Author Affiliations:** Division of Pediatric Emergency Medicine (Dr Pitone) and Department of Pediatrics (Dr Alouf), Alfred I. duPont Hospital for Children, Wilmington, Del.

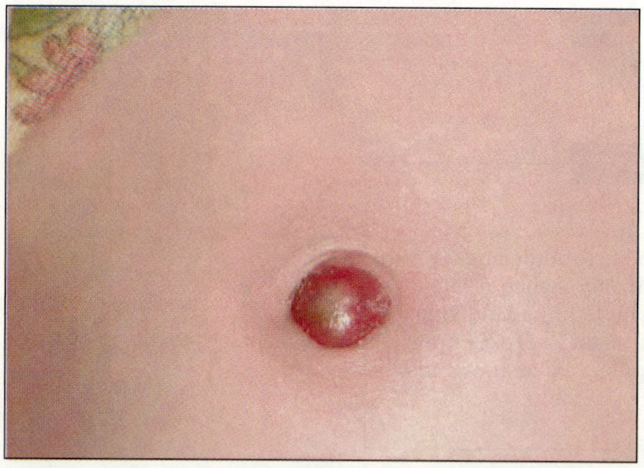

**Figure 1.** Erythema and purulent collection at the umbilicus. Methicillin sodium–sensitive *Staphylococcus aureus* was isolated from a culture of drainage fluid.

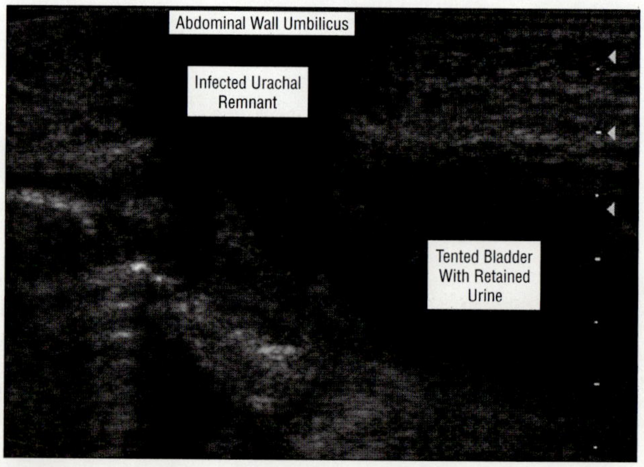


**Figure 2.** The ultrasound revealed an infected urachal remnant associated with urinary retention.

# Denouement and Discussion

## *Infected Urachal Cyst*

The lesion was surgically excised, and histopathologic analysis revealed an infected urachal cyst with an umbilical artery remnant.

The urachus is a fibrous structure derived from the embryonic communication that extends from the bladder to the umbilicus.[1] In the newborn period, it becomes a fibrous structure known as the medial umbilical ligament. It is normally obliterated, but urachal abnormalities result from a failure of this structure to regress. Four types of urachal abnormalities are recognized, including patent urachus, urachal sinus, urachal diverticulum, and urachal cyst. The patent urachus is the most severe and is usually diagnosed early in the newborn period because of its more obvious presentation of urinary drainage from the umbilicus. It is a direct connection between the bladder and the umbilicus due to complete persistence of the urachus. The urachal sinus and diverticulum, by contrast, represent partial urachal remnants. The urachal sinus communicates with the umbilicus but is closed to the bladder. The urachal (or vesicourachal) diverticulum is open to the bladder but closed to the umbilicus. The final and most common type is the urachal cyst—a partial remnant, but with no direct connection to either the umbilicus or the bladder.[2] Data derived from autopsies indicate an incidence of urachal cysts of 1 in 5000 births and a 3:1 male-female ratio.[3]

Urachal anomalies can have diverse presentations because the size of the defect and extent of the communication can vary significantly. Clinical presentations include palpable masses, umbilical drainage, and vesicular obstruction due to bladder compression. They are occasionally diagnosed at autopsy. Urachal cysts can rupture and cause symptoms of an acute intraperitoneal process. If a cyst becomes infected, umbilical erythema or drainage, dysuria, abdominal pain, or peritonitis may occur.[4,5] The route of infection may occur via direct extension from the skin, umbilicus, or bladder, or via hematogenous or lymphatic means.[6]

The differential diagnosis of umbilical abnormalities is broad, and it can include cellulitis, omphalitis, urinary tract infection, pelvic inflammatory disease, appendicitis with or without rupture, inflammatory bowel disease, Meckel diverticulum, strangulated umbilical hernia, bowel perforation, and intra-abdominal abscesses.[4,6]

The urachal cyst represents a diagnostic challenge. Retrospective studies have documented the sensitivity of ultrasound to be between 75% and 100% for urachal cysts.[7,8] Alternative imaging studies include the use of contrast fistulography if drainage is present or computed tomography if a malignant process is suspected.[7] In addition, the high rate of associated urinary tract abnormalities warrants routine intravenous pyelography and/or retrograde cystourethrography.[7]

Simple incision and drainage of an infected urachal cyst may address the acute infection, but it is not curative, as the rate of reinfection is approximately 30%.[9] Additionally, any remaining urachal tissue is at risk for adenocarcinomatous transformation.[9] Therefore, optimal treatment of urachal cysts requires surgical excision. If no infection or limited infection is present, primary excision is possible.[3,9] Primary excision of an acutely infected cyst creates the risk of perioperative complications, including wound infection and bladder injury. Secondary excision after antibiotic therapy reduces the risk of complications and allows for faster healing and resolution of inflammation.[3,9,10]

In adult patients, laparoscopy has been successfully used for the removal of urachal remnants. However, its use in younger patients requires further investigation.[2,11-13]

Patients with infected urachal cysts have varied clinical presentations. Clinicians should maintain an index of suspicion for this process in young patients with acute intra-abdominal processes marked by abdominal distention or rigidity or by apparent cellulitis of the abdominal wall.[9] Antibiotic therapy and primary or secondary excision will be required for complete treatment.

**Accepted for Publication:** September 14, 2005.
**Correspondence:** Melanie Pitone, MD, Division of Pediatric Emergency, Alfred I. duPont Hospital for Children, 1600 Rockland Rd, Wilmington, DE 19899 (mpitone@nemours.org).

## REFERENCES


1. Pomeranz A. Anomalies, abnormalities, and care of the umbilicus. *Pediatr Clin North Am.* 2004;51:819-827.
2. Allen JW, Song J, Velcek FT. Acute presentation of infected urachal cysts: case report and review of diagnosis and therapeutic interventions. *Pediatr Emerg Care.* 2004;20:108-111.
3. Minevich E, Wacksman J, Lewis AG, et al. The infected urachal cyst: primary excision versus a staged approach. *J Urol.* 1997;157:1869-1872.
4. Goldberg R, Pritchard B, Gelbard M. Umbilical inflammatory conditions: case report and differential diagnosis. *J Emerg Med.* 1992;10:151-156.
5. Mesrobian HG, Zacharias A, Balcom AH, Cohen RD. Ten years experience with isolated urachal anomalies in children. *J Urol.* 1997;158:1316-1318.
6. Ogbevoen JO, Jaffe DM, Langer JC. Intraperitoneal rupture of an infected cyst: a rare cause of peritonitis in children. *Pediatr Emerg Care.* 1996;12:41-43.
7. Nagasaki A, Handa N, Kawanami T. Diagnosis of urachal anomalies in infancy and childhood by contrast fistulography, ultrasound and CT. *Pediatr Radiol.* 1991;21:321-323.
8. Cilento BG, Bauer SB, Retik AB, et al. Urachal anomalies: defining the best diagnostic modality. *Urology.* 1998;52:120-122.
9. Goldman IL, Caldamone AA, Gauderer M, et al. Infected urachal cysts: a review of 10 cases. *J Urol.* 1988;140:375-378.
10. McCollum MO, Macneily AE, Blair GK. Surgical implications of urachal remnants: presentation and management. *J Pediatr Surg.* 2003;38:798-803.
11. Stone NN, Garden RJ, Weber H. Laparoscopic excision of a urachal cyst. *Urology.* 1995;45:161-164.
12. Jorion JL. Laparoscopic removal of a urachal cyst. *J Urol.* 1994;151:1006-1007.
13. Siegel JF, Winfield HN, Valderrama E, et al. Laparoscopic excision of urachal cyst. *J Urol.* 1994;151:1631-1633.

# Impact of Specific Medical Interventions on Reducing the Prevalence of Mental Retardation

*Jeffrey P. Brosco, MD, PhD; Michael Mattingly, BS; Lee M. Sanders, MD, MPH*

**Objective:** To explore the impact of medical interventions on reducing the prevalence of mental retardation (MR) in the United States over the last 50 years.

**Design:** We reviewed the medical literature and other data from 1950 to 2000 to construct estimates of the general and condition-specific prevalence of MR in the United States over time. We further explored the existing literature to document historically important influences on condition-specific prevalence, including the year that an effective intervention was introduced, the likelihood of success of the intervention, and the availability of such interventions nationwide. Specific conditions included congenital syphilis, Rh hemolytic disease of the newborn, measles, *Haemophilus influenzae* type B meningitis, congenital hypothyroidism, phenylketonuria, and congenital rubella syndrome.

**Setting:** Twentieth-century North America.

**Participants:** Children with MR or 1 of the 7 specific conditions listed earlier.

**Main Outcome Measures:** Case-specific and general prevalence of MR from 1950 to 2000.

**Results:** The prevalence of MR caused by a number of specific medical conditions has decreased sharply over the last 50 years. However, the incidence of each of these conditions is relatively low, and cases of MR due to these conditions represent, at most, 16.5% of the total number of cases of MR in 1950.

**Conclusion:** Although specific medical interventions have prevented thousands of cases of MR, their contribution to the overall prevalence of MR is relatively small.

*Arch Pediatr Adolesc Med. 2006;160:302-309*

IN 1962, PRESIDENT JOHN F. Kennedy announced a bold new initiative: the federal government would conduct "a comprehensive and coordinated attack on the problem of mental retardation [MR]."[1] Kennedy was inspired by his sister Rose, who had a developmental disability, and counseled by his sister Eunice Shriver, a dynamic and forceful advocate for persons with MR. He convened an expert panel that recommended investing in scientific research, improving health care, and training a special education workforce. Unlike the work of many similar governmental task forces, most of their recommendations were implemented—largely through the efforts of Eunice Shriver, her spouse R. Sargent Shriver, and pediatrician Robert Cooke, MD.[2] Since 1960, the number of federal programs for persons with developmental disabilities has grown from 15 to more than 50, with overall spending topping $40 billion per year.[3,4]

*For editorial comment see page 318*

The Kennedy administration was not the first US governmental body to use scientific medicine to try to reduce the burden of MR, although it was the first large-scale federal investment in MR. In the early 1800s, state governments began opening institutions where persons with MR could live if their families were unable to care for them. Based on expert medical opinion, hundreds of these large institutions were built in the 19th century with the hope that MR could be alleviated with the proper environmental treatment. Simple cures were elusive, however, and with chronic underfunding, most of these institutions became warehouses where persons unable to care for themselves were neglected and maltreated. Descriptions of deplorable conditions in large state-funded institutions began to appear in the 1880s and continued through the 1970s, although most of these institutions have since closed.[5]

In the early 20th century, eugenics provided hope that science could eliminate the need for large state institutions. Although today the word *eugenics* brings horrific images of science and policy gone mad, at one stage in US history it was promoted by respectable scientists and lead-

**Author Affiliations:**
Department of Pediatrics, Miller School of Medicine, University of Miami, Miami, Fla.

ers across the political spectrum.[6] By combining Darwin's theory of evolution with an emerging understanding of genetics, advocates of eugenics hoped to eliminate pain from disease and inequity in US society in a single generation. They understood human behavior in simple genetic terms: characteristics such as intelligence, honesty, and sobriety were passed on according to mendelian genetics. The future therefore lay in encouraging "fit" couples to marry and discouraging others from parenthood. Because persons with MR could not be trusted to understand the wisdom of eugenics, many states passed laws that led to the involuntary sterilization of adults with MR. Although rarely explicit in their eugenic beliefs, physicians routinely withheld care from children with MR, such as infants born with Down syndrome, to reduce the burden to families and society.[7]

The Kennedy panel's recommendations departed sharply from the science of eugenics, but they continued the historical trend of increasing government commitment to biomedical research. Through the 1930s and especially during World War II, Americans began to accept a larger role for the federal government in national affairs, and the birth of the National Institutes of Health, Bethesda, Md, in the 1940s is 1 small example. Although not specifically related to the newly opened National Institutes of Health, the spectacular success of the Salk and Sabin vaccines in the 1950s seemed to confirm that faith in biomedical research was well placed. It seemed only natural for the Kennedy panel to call for expanded biomedical research as a key to reducing the burden of MR. Indeed, the National Institute for Child Health and Human Development, Rockville, Md, was established in 1962 in part to stimulate research on MR.[2]

The Kennedy panel's focus on applying knowledge gained from the laboratory to the individual doctor-patient interaction characterizes 20th-century medicine in the United States. Although there have been successful public health programs that have reduced the burden of MR, such as lead abatement and infant nutrition, modern medicine has grown increasingly focused on applying technological solutions to individual patient problems.[8-10] As part of a larger study on the epidemiology of MR, this study focuses on a single question: what has been the impact of our federal government's commitment to biomedical solutions to prevent new cases of MR? We hypothesized that, contrary to policymaker expectations, specific medical interventions have had a relatively small impact on the prevalence of MR in the United States over the last 50 years. To test this hypothesis, we identified selected conditions with successful medical interventions that once routinely caused MR. We then compared the prevalence of the selected conditions with the overall prevalence of MR in the United States.

## METHODS

We used existing epidemiologic data to create a 50-year, retrospective description of the general and condition-specific prevalence of MR in the United States. To collect this data, we reviewed the medical literature and other existing data from 1900 to 2000, with a focus on the last 50 years. Our search included the electronic databases MEDLINE (1967 to present), Histline, and CALLCAT (the database associated with Calder Library, University of Miami, Miami, Fla), as well as relevant Web sites such as those of the Centers for Disease Control and Prevention (CDC) (keywords are available on request). We also searched reference lists from each of these sources to locate other articles, books, and historical works that were not present in electronic databases.

**Table 1. Causes of Mental Retardation With Specific Medical Interventions**

| Cause | Medical Intervention |
|---|---|
| Congenital syphilis | Screening and antimicrobial therapy |
| Measles encephalitis | Vaccination |
| Kernicterus | Maternal treatment for Rh incompatibility |
| Bacterial meningitis | Vaccination or antibiotics |
| Congenital hypothyroidism | Newborn screening and treatment |
| Phenylketonuria | Newborn screening and treatment |
| Congenital rubella syndrome | Vaccination |
| Galactosemia | Newborn screening and treatment |
| Tuberculosis meningitis | Nutrition and antibiotics |
| Whooping cough | Vaccination |
| Fetal hydantoin syndrome | No phenytoin during pregnancy |
| Pelvic irradiation | Limited x-ray exposure during pregnancy |
| HIV encephalitis | Reduced perinatal transmission |
| Stroke in sickle cell disease | Transfusion therapy |
| Brain tumors | Reduced radiation therapy |
| Metabolic disorders | Transplantation or gene therapy |

Abbreviation: HIV, human immunodeficiency virus.

## SPECIFIC MEDICAL CONDITIONS

Our previous research had identified more than a dozen medical conditions for which specific medical intervention can prevent MR, including newborn screening programs, vaccines, and advances in nutritional and pharmacologic treatments (**Table 1**).[11] Not all of these interventions had their origins in federal research funding, but all of them benefited from the national decision to focus on biomedical research as the primary means of reducing the burden of MR.[12]

We selected 7 conditions to study in detail: congenital syphilis (CS), Rh hemolytic disease of the newborn (Rh disease), measles, *Haemophilus influenzae* type b (Hib) meningitis, congenital hypothyroidism (CH), phenylketonuria (PKU), and congenital rubella syndrome (CRS). We chose these 7 conditions for several reasons: (1) all of them were recognized in the 1950s as specific causes of MR with a high probability of finding or implementing a cure[12-15]; (2) they account for all of the relatively high-incidence conditions noted in Table 1; (3) they are the commonly discussed "success" stories in the prevention of MR[12,16-23]; and (4) interventions for these conditions depend largely on care provided through the individual doctor-patient relationship, ie, they exemplify the traditional biomedical approach to preventing disease or complications in each individual patient.

## CONDITION-SPECIFIC PREVALENCE OF MR

We used a common set of variables to construct estimates of the condition-specific prevalence of MR over the last 50 years: (1) the incidence of the condition; (2) the number of cases of MR likely to arise from that condition (natural history); (3) the efficacy of the intervention to cure the condition; and (4) the population-wide availability of the intervention.

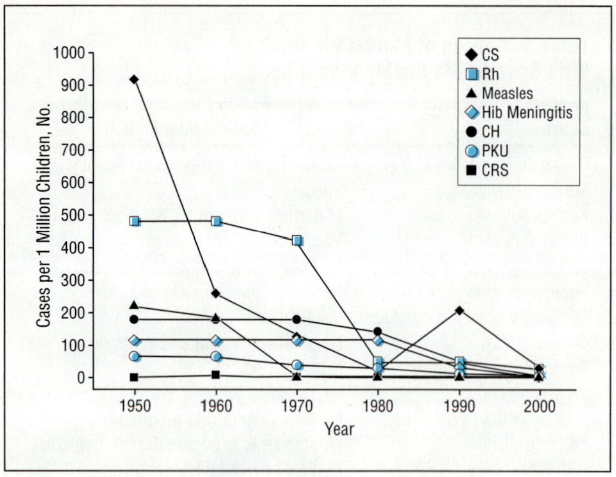


**Figure 1.** Estimated prevalence of mental retardation by selected causes. CS indicates congenital syphilis; Rh, Rh hemolytic disease of the newborn; Hib, *Haemophilus influenzae* type b; CH, congenital hypothyroidism; PKU, phenylketonuria; and CRS, congenital rubella syndrome.

In an effort to bias toward the null hypothesis, we chose assumptions that would maximize the efficacy and availability of each specific medical intervention. For the 2 genetic conditions, we estimated the incidence as birth prevalence; for the 5 other conditions, we used the prevalence estimates from longitudinal studies. For all 7 of the conditions, we calculated the number of cases of MR likely to arise from the condition by using published reports of the natural history of the condition, ie, the likelihood that a condition would lead to MR before age 10 years. For each condition, we then used the randomized studies of specific interventions to estimate the efficacy of preventing MR. For the 2 genetic conditions, we assumed that population-wide availability of the intervention occurred as universal screening was available for that condition. This was estimated by noting the year in which screening programs were introduced state by state, and we generally assumed 100% sensitivity and 100% specificity. For the other 5 conditions, we noted the date that effective interventions were available and assumed that the reductions in prevalence were related to the newly introduced interventions.

## GENERAL PREVALENCE OF MR

Because the diagnosis of MR is usually not made before age 5 years, we searched for estimates of the general prevalence of MR in persons who were school-aged and older. When prevalence was reported by age, we chose the cohort closest to age 10 years.

## RESULTS

## CONDITION-SPECIFIC PREVALENCE OF MR

Regarding data sources, we were unable to locate research programs that tracked condition-specific prevalence of MR over time in the United States. However, there were longitudinal studies of the prevalence of 5 of the 7 specific conditions. For the other 2 conditions (CH and PKU), we assumed that the incidence has been relatively constant over the last 50 years, and we used the reported incidence from a recent large study, the 2000 National Newborn Screening Report.[24] We recognize that this reported incidence does not take into account fetal loss, but it does provide a good estimate of the number of births with each condition per 1 million live births (birth prevalence). Furthermore, published studies of the natural history, efficacy of treatment, and availability of treatment for the 7 conditions led to the following condition-specific estimates of the impact of specific medical interventions (**Figure 1**).

### Congenital Syphilis

We calculated the incidence of CS by dividing the number of reported CS cases by the total number of births in that year; the incidence ranged from 1 case of CS per 272 births in 1950 to 1 case of CS per 13 000 births in 1980.[25] In general, the epidemiology of CS has followed the pattern of syphilis more generally. Dramatic decreases in CS followed public health efforts to screen and treat the general population in the late 1940s and 1950s. Rates reached a low in the 1950s and have since become cyclic with a generally increasing trend. A rise in the number of cases in the late 1980s and the peak in 1991 have many causes, including the epidemic of crack/cocaine use and changes in the public health approach to syphilis.[25,26] In 1988, the CDC adopted a new case definition of CS that included stillbirths and asymptomatic infants of untreated or inadequately treated mothers.[27] Since 1991, rates of CS in the general population have continued to decrease amid continuing preventive efforts, such as the CDC's National Syphilis Elimination Plan.[28]

With regard to the natural history, CS is the result of placental transmission of *Treponema pallidum* from an infected mother to the fetus, causing multiple organ system damage. Mental retardation is associated with approximately 25% of CS cases that are detected clinically.[29] We assumed that MR occurs in the same percentage of cases under the revised 1988 definition (25%), although we did exclude a presumed 5% of cases that represent stillbirths and 1% that result in neonatal death.[30]

Efforts to eradicate CS have focused on elimination of adult disease as well as screening pregnant women. Prenatal detection and treatment with antibiotics prevent clinical CS in 98% of cases.[31] Penicillin has been widely available since the late 1940s.[32] Public health efforts to reach all of the affected persons have varied as described earlier.

### Rh Disease

Before 1970, Rh disease of the newborn, or erythroblastosis fetalis, was a relatively common occurrence in approximately 10% of the mothers who did not have the blood group antigen rhesus (Rh).[12] Rh disease has declined over the last 3 decades and is relatively rare today, but there are no longitudinal studies of the incidence of Rh disease in the United States. We assumed that the incidence in the United States would have followed roughly the same pattern as that in Canada over the last 50 years.[33]

In 1950, Gerver and Day[34] found that 9% of children who were treated with transfusion and recovered from Rh disease had IQ scores in the range of 61 to 80; among healthy controls, only 3% had IQ scores in that range. Using an IQ score of 70 as the criterion for MR and assuming that scores were evenly distributed between 61 and 80, we calculated that Rh disease would lead to excess cases of MR in 3% of children who required transfusion.

In the late 1960s, a group of investigators[35] demonstrated that human anti-D globulin could eliminate potentially antigenic fetal cells in a mother who was Rh negative and could thus prevent severe hemolysis for subsequent babies who were Rh positive. Treatment with RhoGAM reduces the risk of initial sensitization from 20% to less than 1%.[12,33,36] By the 1980s, the number of cases of Rh disease decreased dramatically owing to the use of anti-Rh immunoglobulin and to changing family fertility patterns.[12,33]

### Measles

As part of the National Immunization Program, the CDC posts the number of reported cases of measles from 1950 through 1998.[37] However, widespread underreporting was likely before 1963, when nearly every child in the United States had contracted measles. Therefore, we assumed that every child in the birth cohorts of 1950 and 1960 had measles before age 10 years[38]; for 1970 through 1998, we used the CDC reports of the incidence of measles.

Approximately 1 in 1000 children with clinical measles develops encephalitis.[36,39] Although most children with encephalitis recover without sequelae, approximately 15% die and 25% of survivors develop complications such as MR.[39] We assumed that approximately 1 in 5000 cases of measles leads to MR.

Several effective vaccines against measles were licensed in 1963, and by 1968, the Moraten strain emerged as the live-attenuated vaccine of choice.[12,40] The vaccines were widely available almost immediately after licensing in 1963, and reported cases of measles dropped 10-fold within 5 years.[12] Measles continued its downward trend when the CDC organized a nationwide measles eradication campaign from 1967 to 1969.[40] A resurgence of measles in the 1990s was associated with decreased vaccination rates in children younger than 2 years and with primary vaccine failure leading to waning immunity in adolescents.[39]

### Hib Meningitis

Between 1980 and 1990, the incidence of invasive Hib meningitis in the United States was 40 to 100 cases per 100 000 children for children younger than 5 years in the United States. With routine use of the Hib conjugate vaccine, the incidence of invasive Hib meningitis decreased to 1 case per 100 000 children in the last several years.[41] We assumed that the incidence from 1950 to 1980 was approximately 70 cases per 100 000 children.

With regard to natural history, Hib meningitis was once the leading cause of acquired MR in the United States. Slightly more than half of the Hib meningitis invasive cases presented as meningitis, and one third of children with Hib meningitis went on to have MR. Approximately 1 in 10 children died from Hib meningitis.[12,39]

Effective conjugate vaccines were licensed for use in the United States for children aged at least 18 months in December 1987 and for infants aged at least 2 months in October 1990.[42] Widespread use of each vaccine quickly followed licensure, and by 1993, there was evidence of a dramatic decrease in the number of cases of Hib meningitis.[42]

### Congenital Hypothyroidism

The reported incidence of CH has varied little in different populations over the last 50 years. We used the incidence as determined by the 2000 National Newborn Screening Report[24] and adjusted for a 25% false-positive rate and 27 false negatives per million cases screened[43] to arrive at an incidence of 1 case per 2700 live births as the basis for our estimates over the past 50 years.

In the United States, most cases of CH result from thyroid dysgenesis, inborn errors of thyroxine synthesis, and transplacental maternal thyrotropin receptor–blocking antibody. In 1972, Klein et al[44] found that 48% of children clinically diagnosed with hypothyroidism had childhood IQs of less than 70.

Sporadic hypothyroidism was described as early as the middle of the 19th century, and the efficacy of thyroid replacement therapy was described by Osler in the 1890s.[45] Although recipients of replacement therapy often returned to normal skeletal growth patterns, they retained the central nervous system abnormalities associated with the condition, including MR. In contrast, children detected by neonatal screening and treated early tend to have much higher IQs, with only about 4% having scores under 70.[46,47] Indeed, as early as 1957, Smith et al[48] noted that infants treated before age 6 months had improved intellectual outcomes.

Unfortunately, clinical signs of CH are often not obvious until a later age; therefore, very few children were treated early enough to prevent MR. Early detection through infant screening programs began with pilot studies in Quebec in 1972, and a universal screening program was in place by 1974 in that province. Universal screening and treatment of CH began in Pittsburgh, Pa, New England, and Oregon soon after, and by 1996, all of the US states required universal infant screening and treatment.[49]

We assumed that from 1950 through 1970, clinical diagnosis rarely resulted in treatment early enough to improve IQ outcomes and that 48% of cases thus developed MR. Based on the number of state screening programs at the beginning of each decade and the effectiveness of newborn screening in detecting CH, we estimated that by 1980, almost 20% of infants in the United States would have been detected by neonatal screening and adequately treated.[50] As of 2000, we calculated that there were approximately 27 cases of MR caused by CH in the United States, half as a result of missed cases.

### Phenylketonuria

According to the 2000 National Newborn Screening Report, the incidence of PKU is approximately 1 case per 15 500 live births.[24]

**Table 2. Estimated Prevalence of Mental Retardation by All Causes**

| Year | Cases of MR per 1 Million Children, No. | Source |
|---|---|---|
| 1942 | 12 000 | Lemkau et al[72] |
| 1956 | 34 000 | Goodman et al[73] |
| 1957 | 20 000 | Jastak and Whiteman[74] |
| 1969 | 74 000 | Lemkau and Imre[75] |
| 1980 | 37 000 | McDermott[76] |
| 1991 | 12 000 | Boyle et al[77] |
| 1995 | 20 000 | Larson et al[78] |

Phenylalanine hydroxylase deficiency results in toxic levels of serum phenylalanine and is the metabolic cause of classic PKU. About 94% of untreated or late-treated cases of classic PKU are associated with IQ scores of less than 70.[51]

It was postulated in 1953 that restricting the phenylalanine intake of affected individuals could prevent the severe MR that almost always accompanies the condition.[52] When treatment of the disorder is initiated in the first weeks of life after detection by neonatal screening, virtually no children score below 70 on standard measures of IQ.[51,53-55]

Before 1963, early phenylalanine testing was only feasible in younger siblings of affected individuals. However, the introduction in 1963 of the Guthrie Test, a semiquantitative phenylalanine assay that could be applied to a drop of dried blood, made universal infant screening practical.[56] Most US states quickly adopted the test, and today, all of the states have mandatory universal screening programs. We assumed that 94% of false-negative cases result in MR and that 3% of screened and treated cases will result in MR.

### Congenital Rubella Syndrome

In the United States, epidemics of rubella occurred every 8 to 11 years through the 20th century. The last major epidemic was in 1964 to 1965, when there were approximately 20 000 cases of CRS.[57] For the period between 1969 and 2004, we used the estimated incidence of CRS as reported by the CDC.[58]

Infection with the rubella virus during pregnancy may lead to CRS. The association between maternal infection and fetal disease was first detected by Gregg[59] in 1941, and 2 years later, Swan et al[60] confirmed the occurrence of central nervous system abnormalities in affected infants. When maternal infection occurs during the first month of pregnancy, 50% of children will later be diagnosed with MR; overall, 10% of all of the cases of CRS result in MR.[61] Because neonatal mortality in CRS is approximately 10%,[62] we assumed that 9% of children born with CRS would later be diagnosed with MR.

The rubella virus was isolated in 1960, and an effective vaccine was soon developed.[63-65] In 1969, a vaccination program concentrating on young children began in the United States. The maturation of this cohort and efforts beginning in 1977 to inoculate postpubertal females led to dramatic decreases in CRS by the 1980s. Although epidemics of rubella have not recurred, rubella has not been eradicated. In response to an increase in cases in 1990 and 1991, the Childhood Immunization Initiative in 1993 intensified efforts to ensure a universally immunized population.[66] Rubella and CRS now occur exclusively among immigrant populations from countries without vaccination programs.[57,67]

## PREVALENCE OF MR BY SELECTED CAUSES

For each condition, we estimated the number of cases of MR likely to arise by age 10 years for each decade from 1950 to 2000 (Figure 1). Over this time period, CS and Rh disease were the most significant acquired causes of MR. Although the trends for CS, measles, and CRS have been cyclical, the prevalence of MR due to these infections has fallen dramatically over the past 50 years. The peak number of cases of MR due to CRS was 450 cases per million persons in the epidemic years of 1964 to 1965. Also, Rh disease, Hib meningitis, CH, and PKU cause much fewer cases of MR than they did in the 1950s. The net effect of medical interventions in these 7 conditions is a significant decrease in the number of cases of MR.

## PREVALENCE OF MR BY ALL OF THE CAUSES

There have been no longitudinal studies of the prevalence of MR in the United States, and cross-sectional estimates of prevalence have varied dramatically over the last 100 years.[13,18,21,68-71] **Table 2** includes representative estimates for each decade since 1940. Although the variation is partly owing to differences in case ascertainment and the population studied, changes in case definition are, by far, the most important factor.[11] For example, the 1961 definition proposed by the American Association on Mental Retardation[79] considered MR likely in anyone with general intellectual functioning 1 SD below the mean, which implies that as many as 16% of the population would qualify. By 1973, the criterion was changed to 2 SDs below the mean, or approximately 3% of the general population.[79] Based on more recent definitions, estimates of the prevalence of MR in the 1990s have ranged between 1% and 3% for the US school-aged population.[71,77,78]

To gauge the impact of medical interventions on the prevalence of MR over the last 50 years, we compared the combined prevalence of the 7 condition-specific causes of MR with the estimates of the general prevalence of MR (**Figure 2**). Using the lowest estimated prevalence of MR, 1.2%, the condition-specific causes of MR accounted for approximately 16.5% of the total number of cases of MR in 1950 and for 0.005% of the total number of cases of MR in 2000.

## COMMENT

In 1962, President Kennedy's Panel on Mental Retardation[80] announced their hope to reduce the prevalence of MR by 50% by the year 2000. This bold, long-term goal reflected national optimism in the power of science to cure disease and improve quality of life. Our analysis suggests that there have been sharp decreases in the case-specific prevalence of MR due to 7 specific medical conditions in the last 50 years, but there are limitations inherent in historical epidemiology. Data from an ongoing surveillance program do not exist, as the only such program in the United States began too recently to reflect trends that began 4 or 5 decades ago.[77] In using cross-sectional data, we tried to err on the side of proving the null hypothesis. For example, we compared the reduction in MR cases from specific causes with the lowest estimate of the general prevalence of MR. If we had chosen 3% as the point of comparison, the condition-specific causes of MR would have accounted for only 7% of the total number of cases of MR in 1950. Furthermore, to maximize our estimates of the effectiveness of medical interventions, we did not account for factors that likely would have lowered the effectiveness of screening and treatment (eg, local variations from standard medical practice, poor adherence to treatment, screening tests for genetic conditions with sensitivity less than 100%[81]). Lastly, we attributed the entire decrease in cases of MR to specific medical interventions, although other factors may have been important.[33,82] Despite such limitations in our analysis, there is ample evidence that the number of cases of MR due to these specific conditions has decreased over the last 50 years. Our figures represent 1 estimate of that decline, and we suggest that although different assumptions may change the shape of the graphs documenting the decline, the overall trend would persist.

These case-specific rates can be combined to provide 1 estimate of the impact of medical interventions on the prevalence of MR. At first glance, the impact seems to be small but significant. There are more factors to be investigated, however, before reaching conclusions about the general impact of medical interventions. As suggested by Table 1, there are other conditions that cause MR that may be approached through specific medical interventions. These remaining conditions have such a low incidence, however, that they are unlikely to substantially alter our finding. In this study, we also did not consider causes of MR for which prenatal or preconceptional screening is available (**Table 3**). Down syndrome, for example, accounts for approximately 5% of all of the cases of MR,[83] and widespread screening and termination of pregnancy might have some impact on the overall prevalence of MR.[84] We chose not to consider conditions such as Down syndrome in this initial study in part because there is a difference between the unambiguous good of a medical intervention that prevents MR in an otherwise healthy individual and the more controversial intervention that prevents the birth of an individual likely to have MR. Furthermore, our initial data review did not suggest substantial changes in the incidence of Down syndrome over the last 50 years.

Medical interventions over the last 50 years may also have contributed to a rise in the prevalence of MR. The increased life span of persons with MR, for example, increases the prevalence of MR: children with Down syndrome now live well into adulthood.[85] Furthermore, the clinical success of neonatalogists and cardiothoracic surgeons, among other clinicians, means that many children who would have died in infancy 1 or 2 generations ago now survive to be school-aged and are frequently diagnosed with MR and other neurodevelopmental disabilities.[86,87] Our ongoing research will help quantify more precisely whether modern medicine has contributed significantly to the prevalence of MR.

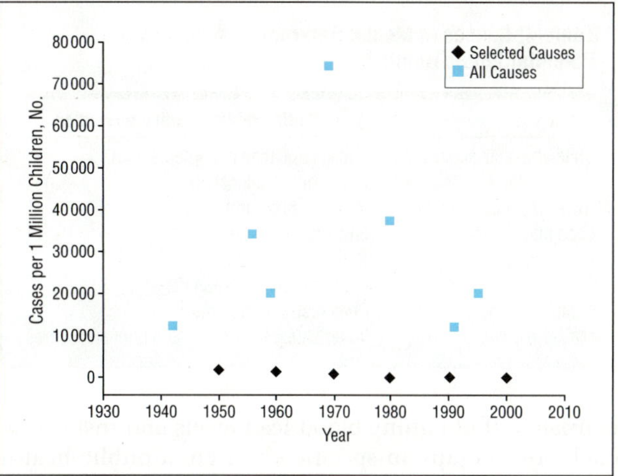


**Figure 2.** Estimated prevalence of mental retardation from all of the causes and selected causes.

**Table 3. Causes of Mental Retardation With Available Prenatal or Preconceptional Screening**

| Cause |
|---|
| Down syndrome |
| Neurofibromatosis |
| Tuberous sclerosis |
| Fragile X syndrome |
| Tay-Sachs disease |
| Maple syrup urine disease |
| Duchenne muscular dystrophy |
| Other genetic abnormalities |

Our study's focus was to test the assumptions of the 1963 Kennedy panel's primary prevention approach to MR, which proposed biomedical models to treat specific conditions that cause MR.[1] Although the panel's approach was successful for a number of conditions, our data suggest that the overall impact has been relatively small because specific medical conditions account for a relatively small fraction of the total cases of MR. This is not to say that the nation's optimism in science was misplaced—thousands of lives have been saved because of specific medical interventions, and the astonishing complexity of neurodevelopment is slowly being revealed. It is only through understanding the causes of MR and other conditions that appropriate prevention and treatment can be implemented.

Future research may reveal, however, that broad-based public health interventions may have had a larger impact on the prevalence of MR than specific medical interventions (**Table 4**). For example, lead poisoning leading to encephalitis caused relatively few cases of MR, but the vast numbers of subclinical cases of lead poisoning likely shifted the mean IQ to the left, thus resulting in diagnoses of MR among children who would otherwise have had low-average cognitive functioning. Whereas the Kennedy panel's approach to lead poisoning might have

**Table 4. Causes of Mental Retardation With Potential Public Health Interventions**

| Cause | Potential Public Health Intervention |
|---|---|
| Child abuse or neglect | Public education and intervention |
| Fetal alcohol effects | Public health education |
| Iron-deficiency anemia | Nutrition programs |
| Lead intoxication | Environmental intervention |
| Malnutrition | Nutrition programs |
| Neural tube abnormalities | Folic acid before pregnancy |
| Traumatic brain injury | Child restraint systems |
| Near-drowning | Water safety instruction and pool enclosures |

consisted of obtaining blood lead levels and instituting chelation therapy in specific children, a public health approach that eliminates lead from paint and gasoline protects all children from subclinical poisoning.[88] Similarly, infant nutrition programs that provided supplemental iron may have shifted the distribution of IQ scores to the right, thus dramatically reducing the prevalence of MR.[12] Indeed, the so-called Flynn effect provides some evidence of rising IQ scores and a lower prevalence of MR over the past 5 decades.[89,90]

This study does not consider the effectiveness, and indeed the greater importance, of other nonmedical approaches to improving the lives of persons with disabilities. Although it may be difficult to measure the cognitive impact of deinstitutionalization and special education programs, individuals with disabilities and their advocates have convinced the nation of the fundamental soundness of the disability rights movement. The late 20th century is characterized by a spectacular change in attitudes toward persons with disabilities,[91] and surely this is the most salient feature in understanding MR in the United States over the last 50 years.

**Accepted for Publication:** October 19, 2005.
**Correspondence:** Jeffrey P. Brosco, MD, PhD, Department of Pediatrics, University of Miami, PO Box 016820 (D-820), Miami, FL 33101 (jbrosco@miami.edu).
**Funding/Support:** This study was supported by a Generalist Scholar Award (Dr Brosco) from the Robert Wood Johnson Foundation, Princeton, NJ.
**Previous Presentations:** This work was presented at the Annual Meeting of the Pediatric Academic Societies; May 3, 2003; Seattle, Wash; and at the Comparative and Interdisciplinary Approaches to Child Health in the 20th Century Colloquium; October 29, 2004; Montreal, Quebec.
**Acknowledgment:** We thank Michael Weitzman, MD, Louis Elsas, MD, Charles Mitchell, MD, Lee Worley, MD, and the anonymous reviewers of the ARCHIVES for their comments on the manuscript.

## REFERENCES

1. President's Panel on Mental Retardation. *Mental Retardation: A National Plan for a National Problem.* Washington, DC: US Dept of Health, Education, and Welfare; 1963.
2. Shorter E. *The Kennedy Family and the Story of Mental Retardation.* Philadelphia, Pa: Temple University Press; 2000.
3. Braddock D. *Federal Policy Toward Mental Retardation and Developmental Disabilities.* Baltimore, Md: Brookes; 1987.
4. Brosco JP. How the history of children with disabilities affects current policy in the US. Paper presented at: 11th World Congress of the International Association for the Scientific Study of Intellectual Disabilities; August 5, 2000; Seattle, Wash.
5. Trent JW. *Inventing the Feeble Mind: A History of Mental Retardation in the United States.* Berkeley, Calif: University of California Press; 1994.
6. Kevles DJ. *In the Name of Eugenics: Genetics and the Uses of Human Heredity.* Cambridge, Mass: Harvard University Press; 1995.
7. Pernick MS. *The Black Stork: Eugenics and the Death of "Defective" Babies in American Medicine and Motion Pictures Since 1915.* New York, NY: Oxford University Press; 1996.
8. Starr P. *The Social Transformation of American Medicine: The Rise of a Sovereign Profession and the Making of a Vast Industry.* New York, NY: Basic Books; 1983.
9. Rosenberg CE. *The Care of Strangers: The Rise of America's Hospital System.* New York, NY: Basic Books; 1987.
10. Rothman DJ. *Beginnings Count: The Technological Imperative in American Health Care.* New York, NY: Oxford University Press; 1997.
11. Brosco JP. More than the names have changed: the prevalence of mental retardation in the United States. Paper presented at: Annual Meeting of the American Association for the History of Medicine; May 3, 2003; Boston, Mass.
12. Alexander D. Prevention of mental retardation: four decades of research. *Ment Retard Dev Disabil Res Rev.* 1998;4:50-58.
13. Heber RF. *Epidemiology of Mental Retardation.* Springfield, Ill: Thomas; 1970.
14. Stern EM. Mental retardation. In: Fishman H, ed. *The Encyclopedia of Mental Health.* Vol 4. New York, NY: Franklin Watts Inc; 1963:1180-1193.
15. Levinson A, Bigler J. *Mental Retardation in Infants and Children.* Chicago, Ill: Year Book Medical Publishers Inc; 1960.
16. Sells CJ, Bennett FC. Prevention of mental retardation: the role of medicine. *Am J Ment Defic.* 1977;82:117-129.
17. Crocker AC. Prevention of mental retardation: 1985. *Ann N Y Acad Sci.* 1986;477:329-338.
18. Stein ZA. Strategies for the prevention of mental retardation. *Bull N Y Acad Med.* 1975;51:130-142.
19. Brockley JA. History of mental retardation: an essay review. *Hist Psychol.* 1999;2:25-36.
20. Centerwall SA, Centerwall WR. The discovery of phenylketonuria: the story of a young couple, two retarded children, and a scientist. *Pediatrics.* 2000;105:89-103.
21. Lakin KC, Braddock D, Smith G. Trends and milestones. *Ment Retard.* 1994;32:248.
22. Moser HW. Prevention of mental retardation (genetics). In: Rowitz L, ed. *Mental Retardation in the Year 2000.* New York, NY: Springer-Verlag; 1992:140-148.
23. Scheerenberger RC. *A History of Mental Retardation: A Quarter Century of Promise.* Baltimore, Md: Brookes; 1987.
24. National Newborn Screening and Genetics Resource Center. *National Newborn Screening Report: 2000.* Austin, Tex: National Newborn Screening and Genetics Resource Center; 2003.
25. Nakashima A, Rolfs R, Flock M, Kilmarx P, Greenspan J. Epidemiology of syphilis in the United States, 1941-1993. *Sex Transm Dis.* 1996;23:16-23.
26. Brandt AM. AIDS in historical perspective: four lessons from the history of sexually transmitted diseases. *Am J Public Health.* 1988;78:367-371.
27. Centers for Disease Control and Prevention. Guidelines for the prevention and control of congenital syphilis. *MMWR Morb Mortal Wkly Rep.* 1988;37(suppl 1):1-13.
28. Centers for Disease Control and Prevention. Congenital syphilis: United States, 2000. *MMWR Morb Mortal Wkly Rep.* 2001;50:573-577.
29. Stokes JHB, Ingraham NR. *Modern Clinical Syphilology: Diagnosis, Treatment, Case Study.* Vol 1. 3rd ed. Philadelphia, Pa: WB Saunders; 1944.
30. Gust DA, Levine WC, St Louis ME, Braxton J, Berman SM. Mortality associated with congenital syphilis in the United States, 1992-1998. *Pediatrics.* 2002;109:E79.
31. Alexander JM, Sheffield JS, Sanchez PJ, Mayfield J, Wendel GD Jr. Efficacy of treatment for syphilis in pregnancy. *Obstet Gynecol.* 1999;93:5-8.
32. Parascandola J. The introduction of antibiotics into therapeutics. In: Numbers RL, ed. *Sickness and Health in America.* 3rd ed. Madison, Wis: University of Wisconsin Press; 1997:102-112.
33. Joseph KS, Kramer MS. The decline in Rh hemolytic disease: should Rh prophylaxis get all the credit? *Am J Public Health.* 1998;88:209-215.
34. Gerver J, Day RW. Intelligence quotient of children who have recovered from erythroblastosis fetalis. *J Pediatr.* 1950;36:342-348.
35. Freda VJ. Recent advances in the Rh problem. *Trans N Engl Obstet Gynecol Soc.* 1964;18:91-104.
36. Behrman RE, Kliegman RM, Jenson HB. *Nelson Textbook of Pediatrics.* 17th ed. Philadelphia, Pa: WB Saunders; 2003.

37. Centers for Disease Control and Prevention. Measles history: US disease and vaccination coverage: reported measles cases, 1950-1998. Available at: http://www.cdc.gov/nip/diseases/measles/history.htm. Accessed June 15, 2005.
38. National Center for Health Statistics. Vital statistics of the United States, 1999, volume I, natality: live births, birth rates, and fertility rates, by race: United States, 1909-99. Available at: http://www.cdc.gov/nchs. Accessed June 15, 2005.
39. Long SS, Pickering LK, Prober CG, eds. *Principles and Practice of Pediatric Infectious Diseases.* 2nd ed. New York, NY: Churchill Livingstone; 2003.
40. Baker JP. Immunization and the American way: 4 childhood vaccines. *Am J Public Health.* 2000;90:199-207.
41. Centers for Disease Control and Prevention. Haemophilus influenzae serotype b (Hib) disease. Available at: http://www.cdc.gov/nip/publications/pink/hib.pdf. Accessed September 4, 2005.
42. Adams WG, Deaver KA, Cochi SL, et al. Decline of childhood Haemophilus influenzae type b (Hib) disease in the Hib vaccine era. *JAMA.* 1993;269:221-226.
43. Fisher DA. Effectiveness of newborn screening programs for congenital hypothyroidism: prevalence of missed cases. *Pediatr Clin North Am.* 1987;34:881-890.
44. Klein AH, Meltzer S, Kenny FM. Improved prognosis in congenital hypothyroidism treated before age three months. *J Pediatr.* 1972;81:912-915.
45. Klein RZ. Infantile hypothyroidism then and now: the results of neonatal screening. *Curr Probl Pediatr.* 1985;15:1-58.
46. New England Congenital Hypothyroidism Collaborative. Effects of neonatal screening for hypothyroidism: prevention of mental retardation by treatment before clinical manifestations. *Lancet.* 1981;2:1095-1098.
47. New England Congenital Hypothyroidism Collaborative. Neonatal hypothyroidism screening: status of patients at 6 years of age. *J Pediatr.* 1985;107:915-919.
48. Smith DW, Blizzard RM, Wilkins L. The mental prognosis in hypothyroidism of infancy and childhood. *Pediatrics.* 1957;19:1011-1022.
49. Gruters A, Jenner A, Krude H. Long-term consequences of congenital hypothyroidism in the era of screening programmes. *Best Pract Res Clin Endocrinol Metab.* 2002;16:369-382.
50. Fisher DA, Dussault J, Foley TP, Klein AH. Screening for congenital hypothyroidism: results of screening one million North American infants. *J Pediatr.* 1979;94:700-705.
51. Pitt D. The natural history of untreated phenylketonuria. *Med J Aust.* 1971;1:378-383.
52. Bickel H, Gerrard J, Hickmans EM. Influence of phenylalanine intake on phenylketonuria. *Lancet.* 1953;2:812-813.
53. Smith I, Wolff OH. Natural history of phenylketonuria and influence of early treatment. *Lancet.* 1974;2:540-544.
54. Berry HK, O'Grady DJ, Perlmutter LJ, Bofinger MK. Intellectual development and academic achievement of children treated early for phenylketonuria. *Dev Med Child Neurol.* 1979;21:311-320.
55. Pietz J, Benninger C, Schmidt H, Scheffner D, Bickel H. Long-term development of intelligence (IQ) and EEG in 34 children with phenylketonuria treated early. *Eur J Pediatr.* 1988;147:361-367.
56. Guthrie R, Susi A. A simple phenylalanine method for detecting phenylketonuria in large populations of newborn infants. *Pediatrics.* 1963;32:338-343.
57. Centers for Disease Control and Prevention. Vaccines timeline. Available at: http://www.cdc.gov/nip/vaccine/vacc-timeline.htm#2000. Accessed October 2, 2005.
58. Centers for Disease Control and Prevention. Achievements in public health: elimination of rubella and congenital rubella syndrome: United States, 1969-2004. *MMWR Morb Mortal Wkly Rep.* 2005;54:279-282.
59. Gregg NM. Congenital cataract following German measles in the mother. *Trans Ophthalmol Soc Aust.* 1941;3:35-46.
60. Swan C, Tostevin AL, Moore B, Mayo H, Glack GHB. Congenital defects in infants following infectious disease during pregnancy. *Med J Aust.* 1943;2:201-210.
61. South MA, Sever JL. Teratogen update: the congenital rubella syndrome. *Teratology.* 1985;31:297-307.
62. Centers for Disease Control and Prevention. *Rubella Surveillance Report No. 1.* Atlanta, Ga: Centers for Disease Control and Prevention; 1969.
63. Meyer HM Jr. The control of rubella and other virus infections in the prevention of mental retardation. *Ment Retard.* 1969;7:17-18.
64. Meyer HM Jr, Parkman PD, Hopps HE. The control of rubella. *Pediatrics.* 1969;44:5-20.
65. Meyer HM Jr, Parkman PD. Rubella vaccination: a review of practical experience. *JAMA.* 1971;215:613-619.
66. Centers for Disease Control and Prevention. Reported vaccine-preventable diseases: United States, 1993, and the Childhood Immunization Initiative. *MMWR Morb Mortal Wkly Rep.* 1994;43:57-60.
67. Reef SE, Frey TK, Theall K, et al. The changing epidemiology of rubella in the 1990s: on the verge of elimination and new challenges for control and prevention. *JAMA.* 2002;287:464-472.
68. Scott KG. Theoretical epidemiology: environment and lifestyle. In: Kavanagh JF, ed. *Understanding Mental Retardation.* Baltimore, Md: Paul H. Brookes; 1988:23-33.
69. Rumeau-Rouquette C, Grandjean H, Cans C, du Mazaubrun C, Verrier A. Prevalence and time trends of disabilities in school-age children. *Int J Epidemiol.* 1997;26:137-145.
70. Crocker AC. Current strategies in prevention of mental retardation. *Pediatr Ann.* 1982;11:450-454, 457.
71. Roeleveld N, Zielhuis GA, Gabreels F. The prevalence of mental retardation: a critical review of recent literature. *Dev Med Child Neurol.* 1997;39:125-132.
72. Lemkau P, Tietze C, Cooper M. Mental hygiene problems in an urban district, third paper. *Ment Hyg.* 1942;26:275-288.
73. Goodman MB, Gruenberg EM, Downing JJ, Rogot E. A prevalence study of mental retardation in a metropolitan area. *Am J Public Health.* 1956;46:702-707.
74. Jastak JF, Whiteman M. The prevalence of mental retardation in Delaware: preliminary report on a state-wide survey. In: Fund MM, ed. *Nature and Transmission of the Genetic and Cultural Characteristics of Human Populations.* New York, NY: Milbank; 1957:143.
75. Lemkau PV, Imre PD. Results of a field epidemiologic study. *Am J Ment Defic.* 1969;73:858-863.
76. McDermott S. Explanatory model to describe school district prevalence rates for mental retardation and learning disabilities. *Am J Ment Retard.* 1994;99:175-185.
77. Boyle CA, Yeargin-Allsopp M, Doernberg NS, Holmgreen P, Murphy CC, Schendel DE. Prevalence of selected developmental disabilities in children 3-10 years of age: the Metropolitan Atlanta Developmental Disabilities Surveillance Program, 1991. *MMWR CDC Surveill Summ.* 1996;45:1-14.
78. Larson S, Lakin C, Anderson L, Kwak N, Lee JH, Anderson D. Prevalence of mental retardation and/or developmental disabilities: analysis of the 1994/1995 NHIS-D. *MR/DD Data Brief.* 2000;2:1-11.
79. American Association on Mental Retardation. *Mental Retardation: Definition, Classification, and Systems of Supports.* 10th ed. Washington, DC: American Association on Mental Retardation; 2002.
80. President's Panel on Mental Retardation. *National Action to Combat Mental Retardation.* Washington, DC: US Government Printing Office; 1962.
81. Kwon C, Farrell PM. The magnitude and challenge of false-positive newborn screening test results. *Arch Pediatr Adolesc Med.* 2000;154:714-718.
82. McKeown T. *The Role of Medicine: Dream, Mirage, or Nemesis?* Princeton, NJ: Princeton University Press; 1979.
83. Yeargin-Allsopp M, Murphy CC, Cordero JF, Decoufle P, Hollowell JG. Reported biomedical causes and associated medical conditions for mental retardation among 10-year-old children, metropolitan Atlanta, 1985 to 1987. *Dev Med Child Neurol.* 1997;39:142-149.
84. Liu S, Joseph KS, Wen SW, et al. Secular trends in congenital anomaly-related fetal and infant mortality in Canada, 1985-1996. *Am J Med Genet.* 2001;104:7-13.
85. Yang Q, Rasmussen SA, Friedman JM. Mortality associated with Down's syndrome in the USA from 1983 to 1997: a population-based study. *Lancet.* 2002;359:1019-1025.
86. Aylward GP. Cognitive and neuropsychological outcomes: more than IQ scores. *Ment Retard Dev Disabil Res Rev.* 2002;8:234-240.
87. Wernovsky G, Shillingford AJ, Gaynor JW. Central nervous system outcomes in children with complex congenital heart disease. *Curr Opin Cardiol.* 2005;20:94-99.
88. Warren C. *Brush with Death: A Social History of Lead Poisoning.* Baltimore, Md: Johns Hopkins University Press; 2000.
89. Kanaya T. The Flynn effect and U.S. policies: the impact of rising IQ scores on American society via mental retardation diagnoses. *Am Psychol.* 2003;58:778-790.
90. Neisser U. *The Rising Curve: Long-term Gains in IQ and Related Measures.* 1st ed. Washington, DC: American Psychological Association; 1998.
91. Shapiro JP. *No Pity: People With Disabilities Forging a New Civil Rights Movement.* New York, NY: Times Books; 1994.

# Screening for Intimate Partner Violence Using an Audiotape Questionnaire

## *A Randomized Clinical Trial in a Pediatric Emergency Department*

*Megan H. Bair-Merritt, MD; Chris Feudtner, MD, PhD, MPH; Cynthia J. Mollen, MD, MSCE; Sarah Winters, MD; Mercedes Blackstone, MD; Joel A. Fein, MD, MPH*

**Objective:** To compare women's acceptability ratings of 2 different intimate partner violence screening methods, an audiotape questionnaire and a written questionnaire, in a pediatric emergency department.

**Design:** Randomized clinical trial.

**Setting:** An urban, pediatric, tertiary care center emergency department.

**Participants:** Female caregivers of children.

**Main Exposure:** Intimate partner violence screening by either an audiotape or written questionnaire method.

**Main Outcome Measures:** Perceptions of each screening method's safety, acceptability, and ease of use.

**Results:** Fifty (10%) of 497 participants reported intimate partner violence, 30 (11%) of 266 in the audiotape group and 20 (9%) of 231 in the written questionnaire group ($P = .30$). Women in the audiotape group were significantly more likely to report that the audiotape method did not put them at risk and was private. Women in both groups were satisfied with their screening method and were willing to use it again. Women in both groups preferred their given method over the idea of direct emergency department provider screening.

**Conclusions:** Screening for intimate partner violence with an audiotape method appears to have several advantages compared with screening by a written questionnaire, and the audiotape method may be associated with slightly higher rates of disclosing intimate partner violence.

**Trial Registration:** http://clinicaltrials.gov/show/NCT00122395

*Arch Pediatr Adolesc Med. 2006;160:311-316*

**Author Affiliations:** Pediatric Generalist Research Group, Division of General Pediatrics (Drs Bair-Merritt, Feudtner, and Winters) and Division of Emergency Medicine (Drs Blackstone and Fein), Children's Hospital of Philadelphia, Philadelphia, Pa; and Leonard Davis Institute of Health Economics (Dr Feudtner) and Center for Clinical Epidemiology and Biostatistics, School of Medicine (Drs Feudtner and Mollen), University of Pennsylvania, Philadelphia.

INTIMATE PARTNER VIOLENCE (IPV) affects 2 to 4 million women each year, with an estimated 3.3 to 10 million children exposed to this violence.[1] In response to this national endemic, many professional organizations have developed policies recommending routine screening for IPV in health care environments, including emergency departments (EDs)[2,3] and pediatric office settings.[4]

Though no specific guidelines exist regarding IPV screening in a pediatric ED, this setting could provide an important site at which to identify abused women, as the prevalence of IPV is believed to be higher in families who seek care in this environment than in the general population.[5] Screening for IPV in pediatric EDs, however, may be hindered by multiple factors. Among these, ED providers are reluctant to screen secondary to time constraints.[6-9] Also, research has suggested that physicians should not ask IPV questions when children older than 3 years are present secondary to concerns that the child might later disclose the details of the conversation to the perpetrator.[10]

Self-administered IPV screening methods may offer solutions to limited provider time and issues of privacy. Three different styles of self-administered methods include written, computer-based, and audiotape-based questionnaires. While women state that they are comfortable with a written (pen-and-paper) method of screening for IPV, illiteracy (affecting 28% of ED patients in 1 study[11]) could hinder the effectiveness of this method. Additionally, women involved in abusive relationships express concerns that a written questionnaire will become part of their child's medical record, potentially placing them at increased risk.[12] Computer-based screening questionnaires have been found to be acceptable to ED patients and to be effective in eliciting personal information.[13] This technology, however, may be lim-

Every year, thousands of children are injured in their own homes. In order for us to figure out how to best provide home safety programs for our families in the future, we'd like to ask you some questions about your home.

1. Do you have a working smoke alarm in your house?
2. Do you have working batteries in your smoke alarm?
3. Do you practice a family fire escape route?
4. Do you store cleaning supplies and poisonous items out of children's reach?
5. Do you have a latch or lock to prevent your child from getting into the space where you store cleaning supplies and poisonous items?
6. Do you have the poison control center's phone number near your phone?

Every year, millions of women are abused by a partner. And, the safety of moms can affect the health and safety of children. So, in order for us to figure out how to best provide women with help if they are in a violent relationship with a partner, we would like to ask you some personal safety questions.

7. Do you feel safe in your current relationship with your partner?
8. Have you been hit, kicked, punched, or otherwise hurt by a partner within the past year?
9. Is there a partner from a previous relationship who is making you feel unsafe now?
10. Within the past year, has a partner repeatedly used words, yelled, or screamed at you in a way that frightened you, threatened you, put you down, or made you feel rejected?

**Figure 1.** Safety questionnaire.

ited owing to the expense and technological complexity associated with its implementation.

The audiotape screening method, with lower associated costs and the potential for improved privacy, involves the use of a personal audiotape and headset with a prerecorded screening questionnaire that prompts the respondent to circle "yes" or "no" answers on a sheet of paper without listing the corresponding question (which is only heard by the respondent via the audiotape). When compared with face-to-face screening by an adult emergency medicine physician, this technique had comparable rates of disclosure and was found to be logistically feasible.[14] To our knowledge, however, the perceived safety, ease, and acceptability of this method have not been examined and this method of screening has not been studied in a pediatric ED environment in which the dynamics of screening, including the presence of older children, may be different than in an adult setting.

We therefore conducted a randomized clinical trial examining female caregivers' perceptions of the safety, acceptability, and ease of use of an audiotape-based method for IPV screening in a pediatric ED. We compared this method with a written questionnaire, hypothesizing that women would find the audiotape method safer and more acceptable and that its use would not be unduly cumbersome.

## METHODS

### STUDY DESIGN AND SITE

We conducted a randomized clinical trial in the ED of an urban, academic, tertiary care children's hospital that serves as both a local and national referral center. At the time of the study, more than 70 000 children were seen in this ED annually. The patient population of this ED is predominantly African American. Just more than half of the patients at this ED are insured through Medicaid-based health maintenance organizations. The study was approved by the institution's Committee for the Protection of Human Subjects.

### SCREENING QUESTIONNAIRE DEVELOPMENT

The safety screening questionnaire comprised 10 questions, including 6 general safety questions about fire safety and poisoning prevention and 4 IPV questions (**Figure 1**). The questionnaire required dichotomous yes or no responses for all of the questions except 1 (question 7) in which a "not applicable" option was also offered. The IPV questions were asked after the 6 general safety questions, with the consideration that respondents are more likely to answer more intrusive questions honestly if they are placed in a context and at a later point in a questionnaire.[15] Representatives (Jill Posner, MD, MSCE, and Linda Hawkins, MSEd) from the Injury Free Coalition for Kids recommended the content of the general safety questions. The IPV questions were based on the Feldhaus Partner Violence Screen, a validated IPV screening tool for use in the ED.[16] One additional question assessing emotional abuse, taken from an IPV instrument validated in an ED population of low-income African American women, was asked as the last question.[17]

After women completed the screening questionnaire, trained research assistants (RAs) asked 10 questions created by us to assess the perceived safety, acceptability, and ease of administration of the survey method. Responses to these questions were rated on a 5-point Likert scale ranging from "strongly agree" to "strongly disagree." Respondent demographic information was collected at the end of the survey.

Prior to enrolling subjects, we assessed the understandability of the questionnaire using cognitive interviewing techniques with 15 women in the pediatric ED. The measure was then modified based on the interview responses. The 4 IPV questions were easily understood and were not modified. A certified translator created a Spanish-language version of the questionnaire, and we piloted this version with 3 native Spanish speakers.

To further pilot test the audiotape method, we asked an additional 10 women to complete the questionnaire using the audiotape, and we then repeated the survey verbally to assure that, when using the audiotape, they had recorded their answers as they had intended even though the answer sheet contained only yes and no choices without written questions. None of the 10 women had gotten off track.

### STUDY STAFF AND MEDICAL STAFF PREPARATION

Prior to beginning the study, 3 of us (M.H.B.-M., S.W., and J.F.), along with a representative (Ana Lisa Yoder, LSW) from a local IPV resource and advocacy organization, provided information about this project and about management of IPV with or without concurrent child abuse for the ED attending and fellow physicians, nurses, and social workers. During these sessions, participants were taught to affirm the woman's experiences, emphasize that the abuse was not her fault and that help was available, assess current safety, and offer the assistance of a social worker. Social workers are available 24 hours per day, 7 days per week in this ED.

### PARTICIPANTS

All of the English- and Spanish-speaking women who brought a child to our pediatric ED between January 17, 2005, and March 24, 2005, were eligible to participate if they met the following requirements: (1) they were not accompanied by another adult (thereby establishing a setting in which subjects could answer questions in a safe and confidential manner); (2) the child was not undergoing acute resuscitation; and (3) they were aged 18 years or older or were an emancipated minor.

## ENROLLMENT

Trained RAs who staff this ED between 8 AM and midnight 7 days per week approached potential subjects for consent. During the consent, women were told that the investigators were interested in conducting a study about safety in the home, including smoke alarms, poisoning prevention, and IPV, and they were informed that if they disclosed either IPV or concern about the safety of their children, the RA would inform the attending physician, who may seek the help of the hospital social worker.

## RANDOMIZATION METHOD

We prepared identical, sealed, opaque packets containing either the audiotape answer sheet or the written questionnaire. Using a computer-based random number generator, the 2 types of packets were compiled in a random order and sequentially numbered by a work-study student who was not associated with data collection. As each participant consented and enrolled, the RA provided her with the next packet in the random sequence.

## INTERVENTION

Subjects randomized to the audiotape group were provided with an audiotape player with a headset and the answer sheet, which was blank other than listing numbers 1 through 10 with yes and no written next to each number. The RA instructed the participant to press the play button and to circle yes or no on the answer sheet in response to each question. The RA did not offer further assistance but remained present for questions.

Subjects randomized to the written questionnaire group were given a written copy of the survey and were asked to complete the items. As with the audiotape method, the RA did not provide help but remained in the room in case the woman had questions.

After completion of the 10 safety screening questions by either method, the RA verbally administered the 10 Likert scale questions assessing the primary study outcomes—the perceived safety, acceptability, and ease of use of the method.

The RAs were instructed to stop the interview if, at any point, another non–medical-providing adult entered the room. After completion of all of the instruments, participants received a packet of information about fire safety and poisoning prevention. If a subject stated that she did not have a smoke alarm, batteries, or latches, she received these items. If a subject responded that she was in a violent relationship, the RA provided her with a hotline card and informed the attending or fellow physician of this issue.

## STATISTICAL ANALYSES

All of the data were entered twice into a database program; the 2 copies were then compared for discrepancies. Dichotomous variables were compared using a $\chi^2$ test of binomial proportions. For the principal test for differences in our primary outcomes, the Likert-scaled method acceptability questions, we conducted bivariate analyses using the Wilcoxon rank sum test. The Wilcoxon rank sum test was selected based on the nonnormal distribution of the responses. In addition to these bivariate analyses, we also conducted a multivariable analysis using ordinal logistic regression. This enabled us to look for confounding by IPV disclosure through determining whether the regression coefficients changed more than 10% with and without adjustment for this variable. Through multivariable analysis, we also reported a summary odds ratio measure and assured the stability of our findings across statistical methods.[18]

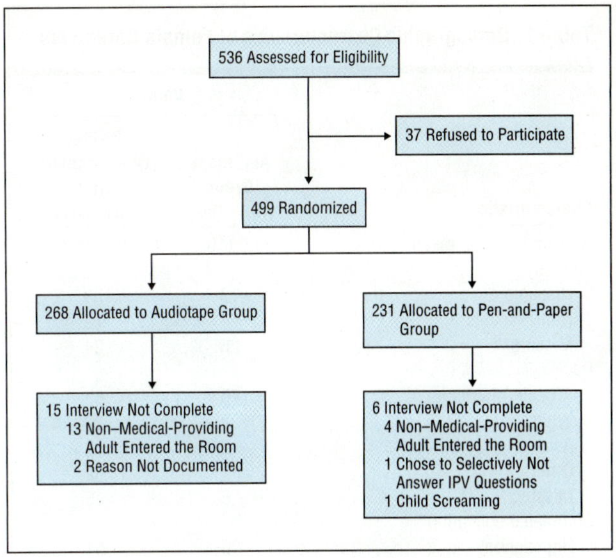


**Figure 2.** Flow diagram of study enrollment. IPV indicates intimate partner violence.

## RESULTS

We enrolled 499 subjects, and the randomization procedure assigned 231 of them to the written questionnaire group and 268 of them to the audiotape group (**Figure 2**). Ninety-four percent of the women who were approached for the study participated. Characteristics of participants in the audiotape and written questionnaire groups were comparable with most women having a high school education and identifying themselves as non-Hispanic African American (**Table 1**).

More than half of the women in both groups had a child older than 3 years in the room. Overall, 10% of the women reported IPV in the past 12 months, defined as either responding no to the question about feeling safe with their current partner or answering yes to any of the remaining 3 IPV questions (**Table 2**). Disclosure rates of IPV were minimally higher in the audiotape group than in the written questionnaire group (11% vs 9%, respectively, equal to a 2% absolute difference or an approximately 20% relative difference), though this difference was not statistically significant ($P$=.30). Regarding the IPV questions, emotional abuse was reported most commonly in both groups. Of the 50 women disclosing abuse in the past year, most (32 women) answered affirmatively to only 1 of the IPV questions, with fewer respondents answering affirmatively to 2 (13 women), 3 (4 women), or 4 (3 women) of the IPV questions.

No statistically significant differences existed between methods with regard to the women's responses to the 6 general safety questions about fire safety and poisoning prevention (results not shown; all $P$>.05). The majority of female caregivers answered that they had a working smoke alarm (audiotape group, 96% of the wom-

**Table 1. Demographic Characteristics of Female Caregivers**

| Characteristic | Value* Audiotape Group (n = 268) | Written Questionnaire Group (n = 231) |
|---|---|---|
| Respondent age, mean (SD), y | 34.0 (10.2) | 32.4 (8.8) |
| Ethnicity | | |
| Hispanic | 3 | 3 |
| Non-Hispanic | 71 | 73 |
| Missing | 26 | 24 |
| Race | | |
| African American | 70 | 63 |
| White | 22 | 27 |
| Asian | 2 | 3 |
| Other | 1 | 2 |
| Missing | 5 | 5 |
| Completed education | | |
| High school | 56 | 51 |
| College | 21 | 25 |
| Graduate school | 6 | 9 |
| Technical school | 6 | 5 |
| Other | 5 | 7 |
| Missing | 6 | 3 |
| Age of primary child in room, mean (SD), y | 6.2 (5.4) | 6.1 (5.2) |
| Presence of child older than 3 y in room | 62 | 61 |

*Values are expressed as percentages unless otherwise indicated.

**Table 2. Intimate Partner Violence Disclosure***

| Disclosure | Audiotape Group, No./Total No. (%) | Written Questionnaire Group, No./Total No. (%) | RR (95% CI) |
|---|---|---|---|
| Any IPV | 30/266 (11) | 20/231 (9) | 1.2 (0.8-1.7) |
| Unsafe in current relationship | 2/222 (1) | 3/181 (2) | 0.5 (0.1-3.2) |
| Physical abuse | 10/265 (4) | 9/230 (4) | 1.0 (0.4-2.3) |
| Past partner making participant feel unsafe now | 8/265 (3) | 3/230 (1) | 2.3 (0.6-8.6) |
| Emotional abuse | 24/265 (9) | 15/230 (7) | 1.4 (0.8-2.6) |

Abbreviations: CI, confidence interval; IPV, intimate partner violence; RR, relative risk.

*If answers to all of the 4 questions were missing, IPV data were considered missing. To provide a conservative estimate, if women answered at least 1 IPV question, their data were included in "Any IPV," with the remaining questions considered no evidence of abuse.

en; written group, 98% of the women), had working batteries in the smoke alarm (audiotape group, 95% of the women; written group, 97% of the women), and stored cleaning supplies and poisons out of children's reach (audiotape group, 90% of the women; written group, 89% of the women). In comparison, results were mixed regarding affirmative answers for practicing a fire escape route (audiotape group, 40% of the women; written group, 45% of the women), having a latch for poisonous items (audiotape group, 53% of the women; written group, 58% of the women), and having the telephone number to the poison control center (audiotape group, 59% of the women; written group, 60% of the women).

Women in the audiotape group were less likely to display concern that this method puts a woman in a violent relationship at risk ($P<.001$) and were more likely to consider the method private ($P=.001$) (**Table 3**). In contrast, there was no difference between the audiotape and written groups regarding the perceived privacy of the method for screening for fire safety and poisoning prevention ($P=.30$). Only 16% of women in the audiotape group and 21% of women in the written questionnaire group agreed or strongly agreed that they would prefer that an ED physician or nurse ask the question directly rather than being screened using the method to which they were randomly assigned.

The majority of women in both groups responded that they were satisfied with using the method to answer IPV questions, that they would be willing to use the method again to answer IPV questions, and that the method was a safe way for women to disclose IPV. The majority of women in both groups either disagreed or strongly disagreed that the method was hard to use, and no difference existed between the numbers of women who requested assistance from the RA in the audiotape group (6%) and the written questionnaire group (8%) (relative risk, 0.8; 95% confidence interval, 0.4-1.5).

Intimate partner violence disclosure had the potential to act as a confounder because disclosure differed somewhat between groups, and it also may be related to responses regarding the method acceptability questions. Estimates of subjects' assessments of the 2 screening methods, however, changed by less than 5% in ordinal logistic regression models with and without IPV disclosure as a covariate, providing evidence that the findings regarding the safety, acceptability, and ease of use are not confounded by self-reported IPV. We show the odds ratios and 95% confidence intervals for each question with no covariate adjustment in **Figure 3**, with the same pattern of responses as observed in Table 3.

A subanalysis of women reporting IPV reflected a pattern of responses similar to that of the larger group (Table 3). Like the larger sample, abused women in the audiotape group were significantly more likely to view the method as private ($P=.03$) and to prefer their method to the idea of direct provider screening ($P=.02$). Questions comparing the methods' safety and whether it put women at risk were not statistically significant ($P=.11$ and .22, respectively), though both questions had a mean difference of 0.5, with abused women more likely to agree that the method was safe and more likely to disagree that the method placed women at risk.

## COMMENT

This randomized clinical trial comparing the safety, acceptability, and ease of use of an audiotape vs written questionnaire for IPV screening in a pediatric ED demon-

**Table 3. Perceptions Regarding Screening Method**

| Perception | All Women, Degree of Agreement* (n = 499) Mean (SD) | P Value† | Women Who Disclosed IPV, Degree of Agreement* (n = 50) Mean (SD) | P Value† |
|---|---|---|---|---|
| Puts women at risk | | | | |
| AT | 4.2 (0.7) | <.001 | 4.1 (0.7) | .22 |
| WQ | 3.8 (0.9) | | 3.6 (1.3) | |
| Private | | | | |
| AT | 1.6 (0.7) | .001 | 1.6 (0.9) | .03 |
| WQ | 1.9 (0.9) | | 2.4 (1.3) | |
| Difficult to use | | | | |
| AT | 4.5 (0.7) | .06 | 4.6 (0.6) | .44 |
| WQ | 4.6 (0.6) | | 4.7 (0.5) | |
| Prefer physician or nurse to ask | | | | |
| AT | 3.6 (1.1) | .07 | 3.9 (1.1) | .02 |
| WQ | 3.4 (1.1) | | 3.0 (1.4) | |
| Safe way to disclose IPV | | | | |
| AT | 1.7 (0.8) | .26 | 1.4 (0.6) | .11 |
| WQ | 1.8 (0.9) | | 1.9 (1.1) | |
| Willing to use again | | | | |
| AT | 1.7 (0.8) | .30 | 1.6 (0.6) | .93 |
| WQ | 1.6 (0.7) | | 1.8 (1.1) | |
| Satisfied | | | | |
| AT | 1.6 (0.6) | .46 | 1.6 (0.6) | .52 |
| WQ | 1.6 (0.7) | | 1.7 (0.8) | |

Abbreviations: AT, audiotape; IPV, intimate partner violence; WQ, written questionnaire.

*The degree of agreement is rated on a Likert scale of 1 through 5. A score of 1 indicates that the participant strongly agrees; 5, the participant strongly disagrees.

†*P* values are from the Wilcoxon rank sum test.

strated that female caregivers considered the audiotape method to be at least equivalent to the written questionnaire, with the suggestion that screening by audiotape may have some important advantages. Specifically, women found the audiotape method more private and less likely to put an abused woman at risk. Neither group felt that the use of the method was cumbersome, and there was no difference in the need for assistance between groups. Both groups appeared to prefer their given method over the concept of direct provider screening.

The findings of this study should be interpreted in light of several methodological limitations. First, the study did not have sufficient power to detect a modest difference in the rates of disclosing IPV. Second, implementation of our study was aided by RAs who provided the audiotapes, looked at the women's responses, and informed physicians of IPV disclosure. Whether an audiotape-based screening could be effectively integrated into another pediatric ED with fewer resources is unclear. Third, we excluded women who were with another adult during this initial study; whether the level of privacy offered by the audiotape screening method circumvents this barrier to more universal screening is an important question for future research. Finally, this study sought to assess the perceptions that all female caregivers had of the 2 methods as opposed to solely examining the opinions of abused women. Future research might better elucidate abused women's views about an audiotape-based screening.

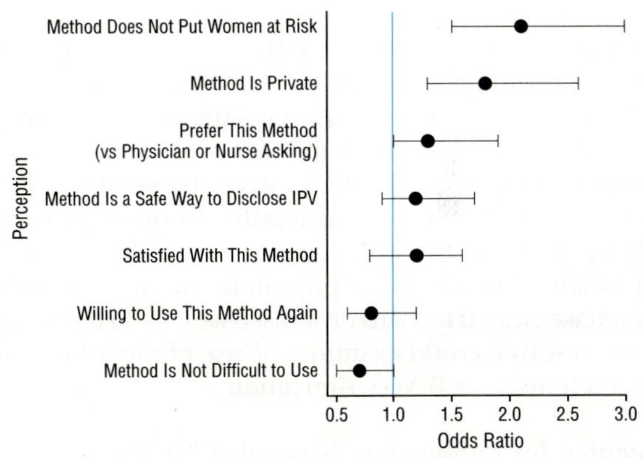


**Figure 3.** Comparison of perceptions specific to screening methods (audiotape or written questionnaire) among participants. The written questionnaire group is the referent group. Error bars indicate 95% confidence intervals; IPV, intimate partner violence.

Women's perceptions of the privacy associated with IPV screening have important implications in a pediatric setting because the screening dynamics differ from an adult setting. In a pediatric environment, the caregiver is not the practitioner's patient; furthermore, older children often are present in the room. When interviewed, abused women express concerns about disclosing IPV information in the presence of older children, leading some authorities to recommend that pediatric providers attempt to ask about IPV when caregivers are alone.[12] Implementing a self-administered method that is viewed as private may alleviate this obstacle.

Women reported apparently disparate findings regarding the perceptions of risk and safety. Although female caregivers believed that the audiotape method was less likely to put women at risk, there was no significant difference between the audiotape and written groups regarding their overall perceptions of safety. Without formal psychometric testing, we do not know whether these 2 questions are measuring the same construct. Clarifying how safety and risk are distinguishable may have important implications for screening and intervention design.

Considering safety and risk with IPV screening is essential. The 2004 US Preventive Services Task Force stated that insufficient evidence exists to recommend either for or against routine IPV screening and that "no studies have directly addressed the harms of screening . . . [for IPV]. Possible harms of screening may include loss of contact with established support systems, psychological distress, and an escalation of abuse."[19] Though this study suggests that the audiotape method engenders less perceived risk for screening, exploration of the actual risks would best be assessed using other indicators such as police reports or women's self-reports of violence after screening.

We also note that the majority of women preferred their self-administered screening method compared with the prospect of provider-based screening. To our knowledge, preferences for provider- vs self-administered IPV instruments have not been previously studied in a pediatric environment.

Intimate partner violence affects the lives of pediatric patients and their caregivers, and pediatricians as a group are recognizing the importance of routine screening. The results of this study suggest that an audiotape with a headset is an option for pediatric ED IPV screening, as it may have some advantages over a written questionnaire. Future work should examine whether these results are reproducible and feasible in other pediatric EDs and whether the audiotape method is deemed to be safe when other adults are present in the room. Finally, though we elected to focus on abused women in this study, future research could examine the use of these methods to screen men for IPV victimization.

**Accepted for Publication:** November 10, 2005.
**Correspondence:** Megan H. Bair-Merritt, MD, Children's Hospital of Philadelphia, 3535 Market St, Room 1550, Philadelphia, PA 19104 (merritt@email.chop.edu).
**Author Contributions:** Dr Bair-Merritt had full access to all of the data in the study and takes responsibility for the integrity of the data and the accuracy of the data analysis.
**Funding/Support:** The drawer safety latches, smoke alarm batteries, audiotape players, and audiotapes were provided by the Dyson Foundation, Millbrook, NY. Safety information and smoke alarms were donated by local fire departments, fire safety groups, and poison safety control centers.
**Role of the Sponsor:** The Dyson Foundation had no role in the study design or conduct, collection, management, analysis or interpretation of the data, or preparation or review of the manuscript.

## REFERENCES


1. Novello A, Rosenberg M, Saltzman L, Shosky J. From the Surgeon General, US Public Health Service. *JAMA*. 1992;267:3132.
2. Joint Commission on Accreditation of Healthcare Organizations. *Comprehensive Accreditation Manual for Hospitals: The Official Handbook.* Oakbrook Terrace, Ill: Joint Commission on Accreditation of Healthcare Organizations; 1998.
3. American College of Emergency Physicians. Emergency medicine and domestic violence: policy No. 400163. Available at: http://www.acep.org.
4. American Academy of Pediatrics Committee on Child Abuse and Neglect. The role of the pediatrician in recognizing and intervening on behalf of abused women. *Pediatrics*. 1998;101:1091-1092.
5. Duffy SJ, McGrath ME, Becker BM, Linakis JG. Mothers with histories of domestic violence in a pediatric emergency department. *Pediatrics*. 1999;103:1007-1013.
6. Ernst AA, Weiss SJ. Intimate partner violence from the emergency medicine perspective. *Women Health*. 2002;35:71-81.
7. McGrath ME, Bettacchi A, Duffy SJ, Peipert JF, Becker BM, St Angelo L. Violence against women: provider barriers to intervention in emergency departments. *Acad Emerg Med*. 1997;4:297-300.
8. Ellis JM. Barriers to effective screening for domestic violence by registered nurses in the emergency department. *Crit Care Nurs Q*. 1999;22:27-41.
9. Dowd MD, Kennedy C, Knapp JF, Stallbaumer-Rouyer J. Mothers' and health care providers' perspectives on screening for intimate partner violence in a pediatric emergency department. *Arch Pediatr Adolesc Med*. 2002;156:794-799.
10. Zink T, Jacobson J. Screening for intimate partner violence when children are present: the victim's perspective. *J Interpers Violence*. 2003;18:872-890.
11. Logan P, Schwab R, Salomone J, Watson W. Patient understanding of emergency department discharge instructions. *South Med J*. 1996;89:770-774.
12. Zink T. Should children be in the room when the mother is screened for partner violence? *J Fam Pract*. 2000;49:130-136.
13. Rhodes KV, Lauderdale DS, He T, Howes DS, Levinson W. "Between me and the computer": increased detection of intimate partner violence using a computer questionnaire. *Ann Emerg Med*. 2002;40:476-484.
14. Furbee PM, Sikora R, Williams JM, Derk SJ. Comparison of domestic violence screening methods: a pilot study. *Ann Emerg Med*. 1998;31:495-501.
15. Bradburn N, Sudman S, Wansink B. *Asking Questions: The Definitive Guide to Questionnaire Design: For Market Research, Political Polls, and Social and Health Questionnaires*. San Francisco, Calif: Jossey-Bass; 2004:79-115.
16. Feldhaus KM, Koziol-McLain J, Amsbury HL, Norton IM, Lowenstein SR, Abbott JT. Accuracy of 3 brief screening questions for detecting partner violence in the emergency department. *JAMA*. 1997;277:1357-1361.
17. Heron SL, Thompson M, Jackson E, Kaslow N. Do responses to an intimate partner violence screen predict scores on a comprehensive measure of intimate partner violence in low-income black women? *Ann Emerg Med*. 2003;42:483-491.
18. Rosenbaum P. *Observational Studies*. 2nd ed. New York, NY: Springer-Verlag; 2002:333-360.
19. US Preventive Services Task Force. Screening for family and intimate partner violence: recommendation statement. *Ann Intern Med*. 2004;140:382-386.

# Commentary on the Risk of Active Tuberculosis

One of the fundamental questions in tuberculosis (TB) control is the optimal interpretation of the tuberculin skin test (TST) when it is administered to apparently healthy persons. The answer has far-reaching consequences: for the individual patient, a diagnosis and a treatment plan; and for public health, guidance about who should be tested and treated for asymptomatic infection with *Mycobacterium tuberculosis*, or latent TB infection (LTBI). If vaccination with BCG is known or presumed, then the solution is complicated by the inconsistent BCG influence on TST results and the unpredictable but generally poor efficacy of this vaccine. In this issue of ARCHIVES, Leung et al add to our knowledge with their longitudinal study linking TST results to subsequent TB disease in schoolchildren in Hong Kong.[1]

Their study derived from the discontinuation of routine school-age revaccination with BCG. In Hong Kong, children still are vaccinated at birth, and until recently they were revaccinated if they had induration of less than 10 mm after receiving 1 tuberculin unit (TU) of RT-23.[1] As a consequence, the authors had a rich data set of TST results, with a study cohort of almost 95 000 children.

*See also page 247*

This type of research, although simple in concept, rarely is attempted because it is so intricate in the implementation and analysis. The requirements include a large, stable cohort with graded TST results obtained through standard methods, a uniform case definition for TB disease, complete case ascertainment (ie, both detection and confirmation), and accurate linkage between the data about the cases and the study cohort. The relatively low prevalence rate of LTBI and low incidence rate of TB disease after infection (we assume generally intact immunity in the study subjects) dictate the large cohort. Studying school-age children allows some convenience because of stability of the population and access to data, but it compounds the problems of the case definition and ascertainment because of the vagaries of diagnosing TB disease in children.[2]

Leung et al streamlined their follow-up tasks by tracing the cohort subset of 656 children who had reactions of at least 20 mm of induration to the TST and who thus (by circular argument, we note) probably would have the greatest rate of TB disease. The incidence rate from this subset established the anchor for estimating the rates for the other cohort subsets via case-control comparisons. Even in the greatest-risk subset, only 10 TB cases were found, which calculated to an incidence rate of 340.6 per 100 000 person-years. Finding or missing a case could have shifted the rate by 10%, which is a study limitation that is reflected in broad statistical confidence intervals throughout the study. Also, we suspect misclassification of the TST reaction sizes because of digit-preference, as seen in the modal spike of 10- to 11-mm readings (the Figure of the current report).[1] We wonder whether health care workers could have avoided revaccinating children with BCG by scoring the TST reactions that were almost 10 mm as 10 mm. This type of systematic bias could lead to errors in this study, especially for the cohort subsets with reaction sizes bordering on 10 mm.

The authors confirmed previous findings that the TST induration size predicts the likelihood of subsequent TB disease.[3] We were impressed that the Hong Kong children who had TST indurations of 5 mm or less still had a TB incidence rate of 7.5 per 100 000 person-years, more than 8 times the reported rate of 0.9 per 100 000 for US children aged 10 to 14 years in 2001.[4] A major factor explaining this difference between Hong Kong and US incidence rates must have been infections with *Mycobacterium tuberculosis* subsequent to skin testing. A conservative measurement of the annual risk of infection in Hong Kong is 0.5%,[5] which is 25 to 50 times greater than the estimated risk for the United States.[6,7] Other factors that could explain cases in the tuberculin nonreactors are a decrease in the test sensitivity caused by the low dose of RT-23 tuberculin used in this study (1 U, instead of the 2 U recommended by the World Health Organization), inevitable mistakes in skin testing, the imperfect sensitivity of the TST, and possibly incorrect matching between the TB case registry and the TST results.

The US Centers for Disease Control and Prevention recommends that recent immigrants from countries with large TB burdens be skin tested and offered treatment for LTBI. We welcome the authors' challenge to this recommendation. They concluded that 482 school-aged children from Hong Kong who have TST induration of at least 10 mm would have to be treated for preventing a single TB case within 5 years. We suspect even poorer efficiency than they suggested, because they used a small tuberculin dose and because they assumed perfect rates for completion and efficacy of treatment. A more realistic idea of treatment completion among children is 70%.[8] The efficacy of isoniazid treatment for preventing TB disease is 90% or less.[9] However, we believe that the finding of Leung et al that only 54.1% of cases could be prevented was a byproduct of the large risk of incident infection in Hong Kong. For the United States, with its much lower probability of new infections or re-infections, we predict that a comprehensive program for finding and treating LTBI in immigrants could prevent much more than half of the subsequent cases.

The majority of TB cases reported in the United States are in persons born outside the United States, mostly in high-burden countries.[10] The disparity is growing, which reflects a stagnant incidence rate in the immigrant populations and a declining rate for the US-born population. Increasingly, the success of TB control in the United States will depend on fighting the global TB epidemic, finding prevalent disease among emigrants in their countries of origin, and preventing future cases in immigrants by treating LTBI. The Institute of Medicine, in its report *Ending Neglect*, strongly advocated these strategies, and the returns that would be accrued from investing in global TB control have been demonstrated.[11,12]

We agree with Leung et al that a study of school-age children, who are in the "golden age" of relative resistance to TB disease,[13] probably understates the impact of finding and treating LTBI in immigrants from high-burden countries. Nonetheless, we need to improve our programmatic practices, test methods, and medical treatments so that we prevent TB disease more efficiently. Indiscriminant skin testing wastes resources. We must focus on the groups with the greatest prevalence of infection and on the infected individuals who are most likely to have subsequent TB disease.[9] Ongoing advances in blood tests that might someday replace the TST, a fickle and archaic test, offer prospects for improving efficiency. The new tests have greater positive predictive value than the TST for *M tuberculosis* infection, because BCG and most other mycobacterial infections apparently do not cause positive results.[14] Thus, these tests should improve the selection of patients for treatment. However, their ability to predict subsequent disease has yet to be studied as in the manner presented by Leung et al, and their capabilities for diagnosing LTBI and TB disease in children have not been determined sufficiently.[15] Last, the inherent problems of isoniazid treatment of LTBI—the long treatment duration, which hampers treatment completion, and apprehension over adverse effects—need to be overcome either with advances in treatment supervision or with replacement of the regimen by one that is safer, briefer, and equally as effective. The study presented by Leung et al, even with its limitations, provides an up-to-date building block for understanding tuberculin testing in a high-burden country and encourages us all to improve our methods for TB prevention in the United States.

*John A. Jereb, MD*
*Lisa J. Nelson, MD, MPH*
*Kenneth G. Castro, MD*

**Correspondence:** Dr Jereb, Mail Stop E-10, 1600 Clifton Rd, Atlanta, GA 30333 (jxj4@cdc.gov).

**REFERENCES**

1. Leung CC, Yew WW, Chang KC, et al. Risk of active tuberculosis among schoolchildren in Hong Kong. *Arch Pediatr Adolesc Med.* 2006;160:247-251.
2. Hesseling AC, Schaaf HS, Gie RP, Starke JR, Beyers N. A critical review of diagnostic approaches used in the diagnosis of childhood tuberculosis. *Int J Tuberc Lung Dis.* 2002;6:1038-1045.
3. Fine PE, Sterne JA, Ponninghaus JM, Rees RJ. Delayed-type hypersensitivity, mycobacterial vaccines and protective immunity. *Lancet.* 1994;344:1245-1249.
4. Nelson LJ, Schneider E, Wells CD, Moore M. Epidemiology of childhood tuberculosis in the United States, 1993-2001: the need for continued vigilance. *Pediatrics.* 2004;114:333-341.
5. Leung CC, Yew WW, Tam CM, et al. Tuberculin response in BCG vaccinated schoolchildren and the estimation of annual risk of infection in Hong Kong. *Thorax.* 2005; 60:124-129.
6. Jereb J, Albalak R, Castro KG. The Arden House Conference on Tuberculosis, revisited: perspectives for tuberculosis elimination in the United States. *Semin Respir Crit Care Med.* 2004;25:255-269.
7. Daniel TM, Debanne SM. Estimation of the annual risk of tuberculosis infection for white men in the United States. *J Infect Dis.* 1997;175:1535-1537.
8. Alperstein G, Morgan KR, Mills K, Daniels L. Compliance with anti-tuberculosis preventive therapy among 6-year-old children. *Aust N Z J Public Health.* 1998; 22:210-213.
9. Centers for Disease Control and Prevention. Targeted tuberculin testing and treatment of latent tuberculosis infection. *MMWR Recomm Rep.* 2000;49:1-51.
10. Centers for Disease Control and Prevention. *Reported Tuberculosis in the United States, 2004.* Atlanta, Ga: US Dept of Health and Human Services; 2005.
11. Institute of Medicine. *Ending Neglect: The Elimination of Tuberculosis in the United States.* Washington, DC: National Academy Press; 2000.
12. Schwartzman K, Oxlade O, Barr RG, et al. Domestic returns from investment in the control of tuberculosis in other countries. *N Engl J Med.* 2005;353:1008-1020.
13. Marais BJ, Gie RP, Schaaf HS, et al. The natural history of childhood intrathoracic tuberculosis: a critical review of literature from the pre-chemotherapy era. *Int J Tuberc Lung Dis.* 2004;8:392-402.
14. Pai M, Riley LW, Colford JM Jr. Interferon-γ assays in the immunodiagnosis of tuberculosis: a systematic review. *Lancet Infect Dis.* 2004;4:761-776.
15. Mazurek GH, Jereb J, Lobue P, Iademarco MF, Metchock B, Vernon A. Division of Tuberculosis Elimination, National Center for HIV, STD, and TB Prevention, Centers for Disease Control and Prevention (CDC). Guidelines for using the QuantiFERON-TB Gold test for detecting *Mycobacterium tuberculosis* infection, United States. *MMWR Recomm Rep.* 2005;54:49-55.

# The Fog of War and the Declining Prevalence of Mental Retardation

According to legend, Canute the Great, the 11th century king of England, Norway, and Denmark, ordered his throne brought to the seashore at low tide. Ruler of an extensive realm, he commanded the incoming tide not wet the hem of his gown. The tide paid no attention. The moistened Canute reputedly chastened his followers, how empty is the authority of kings in comparison with a higher power which alone controls nature.[1]

*See also page 302*

We need to be reminded of our limitations. In the face of great strides in medical research, legislators, scientists, and the public are often seduced into unbridled optimism by medical breakthroughs—the hope of cure. Such optimism is impelled by revolutionary therapies and dramatic leaps in understanding, the basis of Nobel Prizes. Similarly, the power of clean water, safe food production, and general sanitation stand as modern accomplishments. But our perception is also driven by publicly waged wars on cancer, drugs, and AIDS, for these wars are backed by presidential prestige and congressional allocations, high-profile stuff.

In the early 1960s, President Kennedy invoked one such war against a condition his own family had experienced—mental retardation (MR). Kennedy and Eunice Shriver, in particular, helped establish a mandate to take on this "major national health problem," which struck 10 times more people than diabetes mellitus and 600 more than polio.[2] They assembled a presidential panel of experts to generate a report and a battle plan to take on MR.

In this issue, Brosco and colleagues[3] use a blend of historical and epidemiological analysis to chasten us once again. Beginning with Kennedy's declaration, they follow the war's impact on 5 infectious and 2 genetic conditions to assess the overall effect on MR's prevalence. By comparing contemporary estimates of MR from 1950 to 2000 and the imputed impact of condition-specific preventions, they identify both a general downward trend in MR and relative declines for each of the 7 conditions. The battle plan seemingly had an impact on those diseases preventable by conventional means, optimistically cutting their proportion of the total number of cases from 16.5% to 0.005%. The problem is the condition-specific effects are a small percentage of the general trend.

As cogent as this study is, it demands a measure of the economist's *ceteris paribus*. All things weren't equal over the 50 years studied. Not the least static among them was the growth of neonatology and its professionalizing imperatives for "rescuing" increasingly premature infants.[4] Concomitantly, care for children with Down syndrome altered with the growth of pediatric cardiac surgery, multidisciplinary clinics, and antibiotics. Nor can the legalization of abortion be underestimated in its impact of bringing to term children with a variety of disabilities.[5,6] The authors intentionally avoided such conditions and interventions. This is, of course, the matter of heated, protracted debate in the United States, particularly around disabilities.[7] Finally, the very racial makeup of America has changed over the last 50 years, providing different genetic bases to their already heavily inflected denominators. The *ceteris* were not *paribus*.

Certainly, the impact of broad-based initiatives from folate to iron supplementation and from welfare-based nutrition programs, like Women, Infants, and Children, to fluctuating funding for special education all played a part in the changing milieu of MR epidemiology. So too did the quagmire in 50 years of changing definitions of MR and their variable application in interventions like Head Start. The authors appropriately target the role of such wider efforts for future campaigns.

Health care professionals don't often agree on the "success" of disease wars, but scientists invariably see the benefits to basic research.[8] Like the program to take man to the moon, with its resulting Tang, intensive care unit cardiorespiratory sensors, and myriad other devices, these wars have unanticipated benefits. A significant one is educating the general public about disabilities.

In the early to mid-1960s, for example, the "right to treatment" movement synergized with Kennedy's mandates, coinciding in the landmark 1966 *Rouse v Cameron* case in Washington, DC. The case validated the right of those involuntarily committed to institutions to receive treatment rather than merely confinement, the so-called quid pro quo for loss of liberty.[9] Social welfare programs for the mentally disabled helped alter their civil rights, blending into the incipient disability rights movement, akin to the Civil Rights and Women's Rights movements of the 1960s.

Nor was the Kennedy push aimed only at prevention. It also targeted education and general care. Indeed the presidential panel made 95 recommendations, many taken up in legislation. When enacted in Public Laws 88-156[10] and 88-164[11] in 1963, the collective acts doubled the spending ceiling for the Maternal and Child Health Bureau's state grant program and, in an unprecedented move, required all 50 states to generate comprehensive blueprints of services for those with MR. Funding came for centers for research, yes, but also for clinics and treatment centers. In 1963, Kennedy signed the Community Mental Health Centers Act, creating many such centers across the country.[12] The bills also funded training centers for students and residents and 3 sets of education grants to teach teachers who worked with those with disabilities.[13]

These changes came against a backdrop of swelling interest nationally in finding ways to adapt to MR and childhood disability more broadly.[14] Such interest extended from researchers, including the work of Ivar Asbjørn Følling, MD, and Robert Guthrie, PhD, MD, with phenylketonuria, and psychologists' behavioral adaptation scales as well as family groups, such as the 1950s National Association for Retarded Children, coalescing around the identity of MR as a condition.[15] Likewise, the March of Dimes, polio's old nemesis, reacted to its initial successes and shifted its resources toward birth defects.

On the other hand, medical social scientists like Thomas McKeown, PhD, Ivan Illich, PhD, and Archibald Cochrane, MB, BCh, criticized our emphasis on scientific and clinical discoveries for improving public health and clinical care.[16-19] One may interpret the present study as a late extension of that American *crise du coeur* over the value of science to health.[20] While McKeown's thesis about a rising standard of living improving longevity more than science or public health has been effectively overturned, there is an ongoing debate over the health returns from economic investment in scientific medicine.[21,22] Nevertheless, the questions raised by McKeown and others about the relative value of socioeconomic development, public health interventions, and condition-specific therapy remain a critical subject for today's policy makers.

A previous war, of a sort, was declared on childhood disabilities by a US president. Responding to a variety of motivations, not the least his own experience with polio, Franklin D. Roosevelt included funding for disabled children in the Social Security Act of 1935.[23] The US Children's Bureau, the funding's administrator, began by trying to count America's disabled children. One may wonder that those on Kennedy's panel did not start in a similar fashion, thus filling in the data gaps, with which Brosco and his colleagues[3] are struggling. After all, this is lesson 6 from Errol Morris' 2003 movie *The Fog of War*, chronicling Robert S. McNamara's reflections on the Vietnam War: "get the data." However in this war, data are not enough.

As one US Department of Health and Human Services document noted in 1988, "We have heard a good deal about a war on drugs and a war on AIDS. If we are waging a war on mental retardation and related disabilities, it is increasingly being waged by a handful of troops being provided with pea-shooters for scientific weapons."[24(p713)] Whether investment in genomics and molecular biology, for example, will really offer stronger weapons remains to be seen; we can only hope to have the wisdom to use them appropriately.

In the fog of war, wisdom is especially difficult to divine. The belated perspective of history is often the only arbiter. But then, wise King Canute probably knew that almost a thousand years ago.

*Walton O. Schalick III, MD, PhD*

**Correspondence:** Dr Schalick, Division of Newborn Medicine, One Children's Place, Box 8116, St Louis, MO 63110 (schalick_w@kids.wustl.edu).

## REFERENCES


1. Henry of Huntingdon. *Historia Anglorum: The History of the English People.* Greenway D, trans-ed. Oxford, England: Clarendon Press; 1996.
2. US House of Representatives. *Supplemental Appropriations to Combat Mental Retardation.* Washington, DC: Government Printing Office; 1963:5.
3. Brosco JP, Mattingly M, Sanders LM. Impact of specific medical interventions on reducing the prevalence of mental retardation. *Arch Pediatr Adolesc Med.* 2006; 160:302-309.
4. Baker JP. Technology in the nursery: incubators, ventilators, and the rescue of premature infants. In: Stern AM, Markel H, eds. *Formative Years: Children's Health in The United States, 1880-2000.* Ann Arbor: University of Michigan Press; 2004: 66-90.
5. Reagan LJ. *When Abortion Was a Crime: Women, Medicine and Law in the United States, 1867-1973.* Berkeley: University of California Press; 1997.
6. Finer LB, Henshaw SK. Estimates of US abortion incidence in 2001 and 2002. Available at: http://www.guttmacher.org/pubs/2005/05/18/ab_incidence.pdf. Accessed December 17, 2005.
7. Parens E, Asch A, eds. *Prenatal Testing and Disability Rights.* Washington, DC: Georgetown University Press; 2000.
8. Berkowitz ED. *To Improve Human Health: A History of the Institute of Medicine.* Washington, DC: Institute of Medicine; 1998:219.
9. Braddock DL, Parish SL. An institutional history of disability. In: Albrecht GL, Seelman KD, Bury M, eds. *Handbook of Disability Studies.* Thousand Oaks, Calif: Sage Press; 2001:11-68.
10. Maternal and Child Health and Mental Retardation Planning Amendments of 1963, Pub L No. 88-156 (1963).
11. Mental Retardation Facilities and Community Mental Health Centers Construction Act of 1963, Pub L No. 88-164 (1963).
12. Grob G. *The Mad Among Us: A History of the Care of America's Mentally Ill.* New York, NY: Free Press; 1994.
13. Berkowitz ED. Social welfare and the American state. In: Critchlow DT, Hawley W, Hawley EW, eds. *Federal Social Policy: The Historical Dimension.* State College: Penn State Press. 1984:171-200.
14. Schalick WO. Children, youth and adolescence. In: Albrecht GL, ed. *Encyclopedia of Disability.* Thousand Oaks, Calif: Sage Press; 2005:245-254.
15. Ainsworth P, Baker PC. *Understanding Mental Retardation: A Resource for Parents, Caregivers and Counselors.* Jackson: University Press of Mississippi; 2004.
16. McKeown T. *The Modern Rise of Population.* New York, NY: Academic Press; 1976.
17. McKeown T. *The Role of Medicine: Dream, Mirage, or Nemesis?* London, England: Nuffield Provincial Hospitals Trust; 1976.
18. Illich I. *Limits to Medicine: Medical Nemesis: The Expropriation of Health.* New York, NY: Pantheon; 1982.
19. Cochrane AL. *Effectiveness and Efficiency: Random Reflections on Health Service.* London, England: Nuffield Provincial Hospitals Trust; 1972.
20. Alvarez-Dardet C, Ruiz MT. Thomas McKeown and Archibald Cochrane: a journey through the diffusion of their ideas. *BMJ.* 1993;306:1252-1254.
21. Cutler DM. *Your Money or Your Life: Strong Medicine for America's Health Care System.* New York, NY: Oxford University Press; 2004.
22. Colgrove J. The McKeown Thesis: a historical controversy and its enduring legacy. *Am J Public Health.* 2002;92:725-729.
23. Lindenmeyer K. *A Right to Childhood: The US Children's Bureau and Child Welfare, 1912-46.* Urbana: University of Illinois Press; 1997.
24. Departments of Health and Human Services, Education, and Related Agencies of the United States and the US Congress. *Departments of Labor, Health and Human Services, Education, and Related Agencies Appropriations for 1989.* Washington, DC: Government Printing Office; 1988:713.


"American physicians at the turn of the century in country districts were not remarkable for the thoroughness of their physical examinations. . . . [one] story tells of a large family in which all the boys were sewn into their clothes in the fall when the cold weather approached. At bedtime blankets were thrown on the floor and the youngsters lay down on them, clothes and all. In the spring the clothes were ripped off and the children saw themselves for the first time in months."

—*The Illustrated Treasury of Medical Curiosa*, by Art Newman, 1988

## Parent and Youth Assessments of a Handheld Wireless Device to Enhance Diabetes Mellitus Management

Diabetes mellitus is a complex disease that requires both the patient and the family to focus on many medical management tasks such as checking blood glucose (BG) levels and administering insulin. Careful adherence to these tasks can often result in better outcomes.[1] Several studies have shown that the use of emerging technologies by adolescents and youths can have a positive impact on diabetes care[2] and reduce healthcare utilization without adversely affecting outcomes.[3] It is becoming increasingly important to explore both interest in and usability of patient-centered implementations using new tools to determine how best to engage hard-to-reach populations such as youths, especially with the proliferation of wireless transmission technologies.

Personal digital assistants (PDAs) are considered to be promising tools for diabetes management.[4] Successful implementation of a diabetes mellitus management tool on PDAs has been difficult; a recent study using PDAs in children with diabetes mellitus had to be stopped early secondary to usability issues resulting from both human factors and technical limitations.[5]

We assessed the acceptability of an experimental, handheld, wireless PDA system among youths with diabetes mellitus and their parents. We administered surveys separately to 40 children with diabetes mellitus (aged 8-18 years) and their parents both before and after a 1-month pilot trial[6] using a BG meter enabled with an infrared port for uploading data to a PDA. The PDA was capable of transmitting the data to a central, secure server via a wireless modem.

At baseline, only 1 family maintained a computer log of BG levels while 39 of 40 families had home computers. Only 3 youths and 6 parents reported owning a PDA at the time of study entry, yet most participants (92%) successfully used the PDA and wirelessly transmitted data at least once. About 80% of parents and 90% of children reported that having the BG values automatically downloaded to the PDA made it easier to keep track of their numbers. Slightly more than 70% of parents and 66% of children reported beaming BG results once each day, whereas only 9% of parents and 14% of children reported beaming results every time their BG level was checked. The low frequency of beaming every time demonstrates that it is important to maintain realistic expectations for new technology use by busy families.

Nevertheless, more than half of participants (61% of parents and 58% of children) reported that they would want to send data to their health care team via this modality. Additionally, 90% of parents and children reported that they liked knowing that the daily BG values could potentially be available for others to view, including members of the health care team.

Our results show that parents and youths will accept a PDA to aid with BG level monitoring at least in the short-term. More advanced and widely accepted technologies will likely continue to emerge, and it will be important to assess what gains might be achieved by introducing new tools to an age group that generally adopts new technology with enthusiasm.

*David A. Hanauer, MD*
*Katherine Wentzell, BA*
*Allison Tovar, BS*
*Jessica Zeuhlke, BS*
*Vikram Kumar, MD*
*Lori M. B. Laffel, MD, MPH*

**Correspondence:** Dr Laffel, Pediatric and Adolescent Section, Joslin Diabetes Center, One Joslin Place, Boston, MA 02215 (lori.laffel@joslin.harvard.edu).
**Funding/Support:** This investigator-initiated clinical trial was supported by Roche Diagnostics Corporation, Indianapolis, Ind. Dr Kumar was supported by the Paul and Daisy Soros Fellowship for New Americans, New York, NY. Additional support for Dr Laffel came from the Charles H. Hood Foundation and the Katherine Adler Astrove Youth Education Fund, Boston.

1. Evans JM, Newton RW, Ruta DA, MacDonald TM, Stevenson RJ, Morris AD. Frequency of blood glucose monitoring in relation to glycaemic control: observational study with diabetes database. *BMJ*. 1999;319:83-86.
2. Marrero DG, Kronz KK, Golden MP, Wright JC, Orr DP, Fineberg NS. Clinical evaluation of computer-assisted self-monitoring of blood glucose system. *Diabetes Care*. 1989;12:345-350.
3. Chase HP, Pearson JA, Wightman C, Roberts MD, Oderberg AD, Garg SK. Modem transmission of glucose values reduces the costs and need for clinic visits. *Diabetes Care*. 2003;26:1475-1479.
4. Kerkenbush NL, Lasome CE. The emerging role of electronic diaries in the management of diabetes mellitus. *AACN Clin Issues*. 2003;14:371-378.
5. Keshavjee K, Lawson ML, Malloy M, Hubbard S, Grass M. Technology failure analysis: understanding why a diabetes management tool developed for a Personal Digital Assistant (PDA) didn't work in a randomized controlled trial. *AMIA Annu Symp Proc*. 2003:889.
6. Kumar VS, Wentzell KJ, Mikkelsen T, Pentland A, Laffel LM. The DAILY (Daily Automated Intensive Log for Youth) trial: a wireless, portable system to improve adherence and glycemic control in youth with diabetes. *Diabetes Technol Ther*. 2004;6:445-453.

## Perfect Condom Use in a Less Than Perfect World

Dr Paz-Bailey and colleagues[1] are to be applauded for their careful assessment of perfect condom use and its impact on risk reduction for gonococcal and chlamydial infections in young women. In their study, they have clearly used important methodological advances in assessing proper condom use like examining how the condom is used in each act of intercourse. In defining variables for analysis, they state, "Consistent and correct use included those with consistent condom use who reported none of the 5 assessed condom errors; consistent but not correct use included those who used condoms for every act of vaginal intercourse but reported 1 or more condom errors; and inconsistent use of condoms was defined as no use or some use but less than 100%."[1(p537)]

This delineation of the variable for "correct and consistent" makes one important error. The use of this variable does not acceptably identify the difference between user and method failure. It would be incorrect to attribute all episodes of slippage and breakage to "user failure." When used consistently and correctly, condoms will substantially reduce but not eliminate one's risk of acquiring gonorrhea or chlamydia infection because some slippage and breakage will occur even in experienced individuals, which is the result of method failure, not user failure.

This study offers hope because it demonstrates risk reduction for women, but it also highlights the challenge of the need for perfect use to obtain this degree of risk reduction. This challenge will confront physicians as they seek to teach patients about correct condom use and condom effectiveness in clear terms. Physicians and public health professionals will need to take the time to explain what patients might expect with typical use of condoms (occasional user errors and method failure) as well as perfect use with a perfectly performing product. Unfortunately, the risk reduction from less than perfect use is underwhelming. We all wish we lived in a perfect world, one without sexually transmitted diseases. In reality, requiring adolescents and adults to perform perfectly to obtain risk reduction is unlikely to provide the reduction in sexually transmitted diseases we hope for on a population level. However, physicians can and should aggressively advocate for the good of the patient, and risk reduction can take multiple forms in addition to condoms. A fully orbed approach includes encouraging abstinence in adolescents, routine testing and treatment of sexually transmitted infections, and counseling sexually active patients to decrease their lifetime number of partners.

*Mary B. Adam, MD, MA*

**Correspondence:** Dr Adam, Department of Pediatrics, University of Arizona College of Medicine, 3961 N Hillwood Pl, Tucson, AZ 85750 (adammb@pol.net).

1. Paz-Bailey G, Koumans EH, Sternberg M, et al. The effect of correct and consistent condom use on chlamydial and gonococcal infection among urban adolescents. *Arch Pediatr Adolesc Med.* 2005;159:536-542.

### *In reply*

*We appreciate Dr Adam raising the issue of possible limitations in the definition of correct condom use described in our article. We included in our definition of correct condom use both episodes of user and method failure. Although we agree that method failure such as breakage or slippage cannot always be controlled by the user, it is likely that incorrect use can lead to these events and its frequency could be reduced through patient education.*

*The most prevalent condom error reported by adolescents in our study was starting sex without a condom. As summarized by a Centers for Disease Control and Prevention report, proper use of a condom requires: (1) using a new condom for each act of vaginal, oral, and anal intercourse; (2) putting the condom on correctly before any genital contact; (3) withdrawing while the penis is still erect and holding the condom firmly to keep it from slipping off; and (4) using only water-based lubricants, not those that are petroleum based.*[1]

*Previous studies have evaluated correlates of condom failure. Some of the factors that have been identified with an increased risk of breakage or slippage include opening condoms with sharp objects, infrequent condom use, having less lifetime condom experience, never receiving instruction on correct condom use, young age, and low partner motivation to use condoms.*[2] *Condom breakage or slippage may be especially likely among those who have never been taught how to use condoms correctly, and increased experience with condoms and sex education may reduce the likelihood of condom breakage. Discussing the issue of condom errors and potential problems and encouraging consistent use may improve condom effectiveness, even if product failure may occasionally happen.*

*The use of condoms is beneficial not only because of the protection it provides against some sexually transmitted diseases but also because of its effectiveness in preventing human immunodeficiency virus and unwanted pregnancies. With approximately half of all 15- to 19-year-old adolescents in the United States being sexually active,*[3] *rates of adolescent pregnancies and sexually transmitted diseases remain a significant concern.*

*Abstaining from intercourse should be encouraged for adolescents because it is the surest way to prevent sexually transmitted diseases, including human immunodeficiency virus infection, and pregnancy. Adolescents who are sexually active should also be counseled regarding the benefits of postponing future sexual relationships. In addition, we recommend that health care professionals actively support and encourage the correct and consistent use of reliable contraception and condoms by adolescents who are sexually active or contemplating sexual activity. More research is needed to identify methods to increase correct and consistent condom use by sexually active adolescents and to evaluate the effectiveness of strategies to promote condom use, including condom education and availability.*

*Gabriela Paz-Bailey, MD, MSc*
*Emilia Koumans, MD, MPH*
*Lauri E. Markowitz, MD*

**Correspondence:** Dr Paz-Bailey, Centers for Disease Control and Prevention, Unit 3321, APO AA, Miami, FL 34024-3321 (gpbz@cdc.gov).

1. Centers for Disease Control and Prevention. Update: barrier protection against HIV infection and other sexually transmitted diseases. *MMWR Morb Mortal Wkly Rep.* 1993;42:589-597.
2. Crosby RA, Sanders SA, Yarber WL, Graham CA, Dodge B. Condom use errors and problems among college men. *Sex Transm Dis.* 2002;29:552-557.
3. Kaplan DW, Feinstein RA, Fisher MM, et al; Committee on Adolescence. Condom use by adolescents. *Pediatrics.* 2001;107:1463-1469.

## Increased Exclusive Breastfeeding Rates Fall Short of Proposed Healthy People 2010 Goals

The Anderson et al article[1] on a peer counseling intervention to increase exclusive breastfeeding (EBF) is timely, given proposed Healthy People 2010 revised goals of 60% of mothers EBF at 3 months and 25% at 6 months.[2] Currently, just 46% of US mothers EBF at hospital discharge, while 17% do so at 6 months.[3] The Anderson et al study involved several elements of "best practice" education and support, including prenatal home visits (n=3), daily hospital visits, and postpartum home visits (n=9), designed to boost EBF.

Anderson et al found dramatic differences in EBF rates through 3 months in this low-income Latina community. Results, reported as risks of non-EBF, suggest that 59% of intervention group women vs 44% of controls were EBF at hospital discharge. (Though unstated, one assumes this is a dichotomous variable and that all other mothers weren't EBF.) By 3 months, EBF rates fell but were still significantly higher in the intervention group, 20.6% vs 1.4% of controls. The study hospital is 1 of only 42 (as of 2004) Baby-Friendly hospitals in the United States (ie, certified as implementing the 10 Steps to Successful Breastfeeding).

Additional implementation details would help determine the acceptability of this resource-intensive intervention. That is, the reference to peer counselor coverage being 89% for the prenatal home visits leaves unclear how many women received 0, 1, 2, or 3 prenatal home visits. Similarly, the number of women receiving hospital and home visits during the first through sixth weeks is unclear. Authors state that the cost-effectiveness of EBF peer counseling should be further studied. Any such work must incorporate the considerable time required for travel and supervision, as opposed to clinical contact time alone.

The intrapartum experience is key. Thus, it is discouraging that EBF rates in both groups were not higher, given the study hospital's Baby-Friendly status. At Baby-Friendly hospitals, 78.4% of mothers EBF at hospital discharge (median, 86% [range, 25%-100%])[4] vs 59% in the Anderson et al treatment group. Neither Hispanic ethnicity nor low-income status is associated with decreased EBF in Baby-Friendly hospitals.[4] Therefore, the sample's characteristics are unlikely to explain the low EBF rates relative to other Baby-Friendly hospitals. Variation in EBF assessment undoubtedly accounts for some, but not all, of the discrepancy.

The difficulty of sustaining EBF is clear. Just 21% of women receiving this intensive intervention and delivering in a Baby-Friendly hospital were EBF at 3 months. Considerable effort will be required to reach the proposed Healthy People 2010 goal of 60% EBF at 3 months.

*Karen A. Bonuck, PhD*

**Correspondence:** Dr Bonuck, Department of Epidemiology and Population Health, Montefiore Medical Center/Albert Einstein College of Medicine, 111 E 210th St, Bronx, NY 10467 (kbonuck@montefiore.org).

1. Anderson AK, Damio G, Young S, Chapman DJ, Perez-Escamilla R. A randomized trial assessing the efficacy of peer counseling on exclusive breastfeeding in a predominantly Latina low-income community. *Arch Pediatr Adolesc Med.* 2005;159:836-841.
2. Healthy People 2010 midcourse review: revised objectives for 16-19—breastfeeding. Available at: http://www.healthypeople.gov. Accessed September 22, 2005.
3. Ryan AS, Wnejun Z, Acosta A. Breastfeeding continues to increase into the new millennium. *Pediatrics.* 2002;110:1103-1109.
4. Merewood A, Mehta SD, Chamberlain LB, et al. Breastfeeding rates in US Baby-Friendly hospitals: results of a national survey. *Pediatrics.* 2005;116:628-634.

### *In reply*

*We recently reported the efficacy of peer counseling on EBF in a predominantly Latina, low-income community in Hartford, Conn.[1] Our study, to our knowledge, the first of its kind in the United States, assessed the efficacy of peer counseling on EBF and showed a significant impact with an effect size similar to or stronger than the one found in other countries.[2]*

*Dr Bonuck seems impressed with the findings from our study but unclear with the EBF definition used. As reported in the article,[1] we used the strictest definition of EBF (ie, no other food or fluid other than breast milk) as proposed by Labbok and Krasovec.[3] While in the hospital and soon before hospital discharge, mothers were directly asked by the interviewer to respond to these questions: (1) How are you feeding your newborn (exclusive breastfeeding; breast and formula feeding; exclusive formula feeding), and (2) Has your newborn received anything besides breast milk (yes or no). At each follow-up contact, the question was asked in relation to the previous week, the previous 24 hours, and since the baby was born.*

*Dr Bonuck also requests additional implementation details of our intervention. The 89% prenatal peer counselor coverage reported reflects participants who received all 3 prenatal home visits. The remaining 11% of participants were not seen at all points either because they stated not needing any support or because the peer counselors were unable to establish contact. With regard to the in-hospital breastfeeding support, 17% of mother-infant pairs were missed by the peer counselors because the delivery took place at a time when the peer counselor was not able to be in the hospital before the mother was fdischarged. The percentage of mothers who did not receive all the scheduled home visits from the assigned peer counselors ranged from 23.8% to 36.5% at different points and included mothers who opted not to receive peer counselor support and those who had stopped breastfeeding or missed an appointment. We did collect data on peer counselors' time for travel and cost of supervision, which are yet to be analyzed, to estimate the potential cost-effectiveness of our EBF peer counseling model.*

*As Dr Bonuck rightly points out, the variation across hospitals in EBF assessment in the study by Merewood et al[4] is likely to account for some of the differences observed in hospital EBF rates when compared with our study. Whereas we used a standardized and rigorous definition of EBF, Merewood et al based their assessment on data routinely collected by the hospitals. What is more worrisome is that those data were based on at least 3 different definitions for EBF across institutions. Thus, we strongly recommend caution in attempting to compare in-hospital EBF rates between the 2 studies. Contrary to the findings by Merewood et al, we did find strong differences in EBF behaviors across ethnic groups in our study.*[5]

*Alex K. Anderson, PhD, MPH*
*Rafael Pérez-Escamilla, PhD*
*Donna J. Chapman, PhD, RD*

**Correspondence:** Dr Anderson, Department of Foods and Nutrition, University of Georgia, Athens, GA 30602 (anderson@fcs.uga.edu).

1. Anderson AK, Damio G, Young S, Chapman DJ, Perez-Escamilla R. A randomized trial assessing the efficacy of peer counseling on exclusive breastfeeding in a predominantly Latina low-income community. *Arch Pediatr Adolesc Med.* 2005;159:836-841.
2. Perez-Escamilla R, Guerrero ML. Epidemiology of breastfeeding: advances and multidisciplinary applications. *Adv Exp Med Biol.* 2004;554:45-59.
3. Labbok M, Krasovec K. Toward consistency in breastfeeding definitions. *Stud Fam Plann.* 1990;21:226-230.
4. Merewood A, Mehta SD, Chamberlain LB, et al. Breastfeeding rates in US Baby-Friendly hospitals: results of a national survey. *Pediatrics.* 2005;116:628-634.
5. Anderson AK. *Determinant of Exclusive Breastfeeding Among Low-Income Inner-City Women* [master's thesis]. Farmington, Conn: School of Public Health, University of Connecticut; 2005.

## *Announcement*

**Trial Registration Required.** In concert with the International Committee of Medical Journal Editors (ICMJE), *Archives of Pediatrics and Adolescent Medicine* will require, as a condition of consideration for publication, registration of all trials in a public trials registry (such as http://ClinicalTrials.gov). Trials must be registered at or before the onset of patient enrollment. This policy applies to any clinical trial starting enrollment after July 1, 2005. For trials that began enrollment before this date, registration will be required by September 13, 2005, before considering the trial for publication. The trial registration number should be supplied at the time of submission.

For details about this new policy, and for information on how the ICMJE defines a clinical trial, see the editorials by DeAngelis et al in the September 8, 2004 (2004;292:1363-1364) and June 15, 2005 (2005;293: 2927-2929) issues of *JAMA*. Also see the Instructions to Authors on our Web site: www.archpediatrics.com.

SECTION EDITOR: ABRAHAM BERGMAN, MD

## Child Abuse and Culture: Working With Diverse Families

*by Lisa Aronson Fontes, 239 pages, $30, ISBN, 1-59385-130-8, New York, NY, The Guilford Press, 2005.*

After finishing Lisa Aronson Fontes' *Child Abuse and Culture: Working With Diverse Families*, I found myself rereading *The Spirit Catches You and You Fall Down*,[1] Anne Fadiman's story of a Hmong family and the medical, social, and legal systems of central California caring for Lia, a young girl with a severe seizure disorder. The book alternates the perspective of Lia's well-meaning American pediatricians with the perspective of her well-meaning immigrant parents, pulling the reader along the tumbling downhill course of 1 child caught between 2 cultures. In the end, Lia does poorly, her parents are grieving, and her pediatricians are saddened and frustrated by the outcome.

Granted an omniscient perspective through Fadiman's graceful narrative, the reader gains the uncomfortable sense that Lia would have done better if everyone involved had merely understood one another. In *Child Abuse and Culture: Working With Diverse Families*, Fontes constructs solutions to the many challenges presented through the experiences of Lia and her caretakers. Where Fadiman's book leaves us doubting our ability to work effectively in cross-cultural circumstances, Fontes' well-referenced text pushes ahead, offering concrete guidance to professionals providing care to children in communities distinguished by language, culture, race, religion, or socioeconomic status.

Fontes' primary audience is the multidisciplinary child protection team, with a chapter structure that approximates the course of an investigation into a report of child maltreatment. Fontes presents the impact of culture at each stage, from initial suspicion of abuse through family assessment and child interview. A cross-disciplinary bibliography supports her recommendations. Anecdotes from her own experience as a social worker, therapist, and mother keep the reader engaged. Questions at the end of each chapter feel pedantic to the casual reader but provide structure for a multidisciplinary team interested in improving the quality of services provided to minority families.

There is an important unintended audience for this book. *Child Abuse and Culture: Working With Diverse Families* provides pediatricians with a unique perspective on the daily interactions that we have with children and families. The chapter on sexual abuse is a guide for the HEADSS (home, education/employment, activities, drugs, sexuality, and suicide/depression) evaluation of a Latino teen. A segment on immigration sheds light on why a 15-year-old Somali refugee looks and acts more like a young woman in her 20s. Tucked into a discussion of physical abuse is a culturally specific argument against the use of corporal punishment in an African American family.

The first pages of Fontes' work led me to expect a dry dissertation on cultural competency and a compendium of traditional practices often confused with abuse (eg, coining, moxibustion). Instead, the book develops rapidly into an accessible and thoughtful discussion of how we can improve the protection of children and their families despite challenging cultural barriers. There are no perfect answers to cross-cultural understanding, but Fontes has created a strong structure from which we can begin our work. We can hope that Lia's story would have unfolded quite differently with the benefit of such understanding between her family and her pediatricians.

*Kristine A. Campbell, MD*

**Correspondence:** Dr Campbell, General Academic Pediatrics, Children's Hospital of Pittsburgh, 3705 Fifth Ave, CHOB Third Floor, Pittsburgh, PA 15213 (kristinea.campbell@chp.edu).

1. Fadiman A. *The Spirit Catches You and You Fall Down*. New York, NY: The Noonday Press; 1997:341.

## Director of the Children's Evaluation and Rehabilitation Center (CERC)

The Albert Einstein College of Medicine (AECOM) is searching for The Director for its Children's Evaluation and Rehabilitation Center (CERC). The successful candidate must have expertise in developmental medicine, demonstrated skill in clinical care and/or research, and a collaborative vision. Major expectations of the Director will be to facilitate the growth of clinical and related basic and translational research programs, and to play a leadership role in a new initiative in autism arising from collaboration between Developmental Pediatrics, Child Neurology and Neuroscience.

CERC is an integral part of AECOM's Rose F. Kennedy Center for Research in Mental Retardation and Developmental Disabilities, which provides a base for basic and clinical Neuroscience, Pediatric and cognitive research at AECOM. CERC also is one of the largest clinical centers of its kind in the United States providing a broad spectrum of services for infants, children, adolescents and adults with physical, developmental, language and learning disabilities. A multidisciplinary professional staff of more than 130 individuals provides over 58,000 diagnostic, therapeutic and related service visits, and trains close to 1,000 professionals annually.

Nominations and/or CV's should be sent electronically to: **CERC Search Committee, c/o Michael Reichgott, M.D., Ph.D., Associate Dean for Clinical Affairs and GME; reichgot@aecom.yu.edu**

We welcome applicants who will add diversity to our academic leadership and faculty. EOE

**ALBERT EINSTEIN COLLEGE OF MEDICINE**
*Advancing science, building careers*



### JOURNAL ADVERTISER INDEX


**ABBOTT LABS**

Omnicef OS ............ 233-235

**CLASSIFIED ADVERTISING** ............ 327
http://www.amapublications.com

**GLAXOSMITHKLINE**

Boostrix ............ 261-262, COVER 3-4

Pediarix ............ 277-278, COVER 2-225

**MERCK & COMPANY**

CORPORATE ............ 236-237

Gardasil ............ 240A-B

Rotateq ............ 230

**SEPRACOR**

Xopenex ............ 227-228


*Demographic and "Mini" inserts and/or ROB ad pages

While every precaution is taken to ensure accuracy, we cannot guarantee against the possibility of an occasional change or omission in the preparation of this index.

ARCHIVES OF PEDIATRICS & ADOLESCENT MEDICINE

# CONTACT INFORMATION

## EDITORIAL OFFICE

**Editorial Office Information:** *Archives of Pediatrics & Adolescent Medicine*, Department of Pediatrics, Child Health Institute, University of Washington, 6200 NE 74th St, Suite 210, Seattle, WA 98115-8160; phone: (206) 685-3573; fax: (206) 685-3572; e-mail: archpediatrics@jama-archives.org.

**Electronic Submission:** Manuscripts should be submitted via our online manuscript submission and review system (http://manuscripts.archpediatrics.com). Manuscripts submitted through our online system should not also be submitted by mail or fax. Signed authorship forms should be sent by regular mail or fax. See the Instructions for Authors (www.archpediatrics.com) for more details.

## CONSORTIUM OF *JAMA* & *ARCHIVES* JOURNALS

The *Archives of Pediatrics & Adolescent Medicine* is a member of the consortium of AMA journals listed below.

The Journal of the American Medical Association (JAMA)
Archives of Dermatology
Archives of Facial Plastic Surgery
Archives of General Psychiatry
Archives of Internal Medicine
Archives of Neurology
Archives of Ophthalmology
Archives of Otolaryngology–Head & Neck Surgery
Archives of Pediatrics & Adolescent Medicine
Archives of Surgery

## *JAMA/ARCHIVES* MEDIA RELATIONS

Jann Ingmire; phone: (312) 464-5262; e-mail: mediarelations@jama-archives.org.

## *ARCHIVES OF PEDIATRICS* ONLINE

*Archives of Pediatrics & Adolescent Medicine* is available online at www.archpediatrics.com.

## *JAMA/ARCHIVES* REPRINTS

**Author Reprints:** Anna Goins at (312) 464-2477; fax: (312) 464-5843; e-mail: anna.goins@ama-assn.org. Minimum order: 100 reprints.

**Educational Reprints:** Rhonda Bailey Brown at (312) 464-2513; fax: (312) 464-5843; e-mail: rhonda.brown@ama-assn.org. Minimum order: 100 reprints.

**Commercial Reprints:** Phone: (312) 464-0776; fax: (312) 464-0708; e-mail: reprints@ama-assn.org. Minimum order: 500 reprints.

## PERMISSIONS

Information about obtaining permission to republish, reprint, or adapt material published in *Archives of Pediatrics & Adolescent Medicine* is available from Rhonda Bailey Brown; phone: (312) 464-2513; fax: (312) 464-5843; e-mail: permissions@ama-assn.org.

## DOCUMENT DELIVERY

Copies of individual articles are available online at www.archpediatrics.com and from the following: Infotrieve, phone: (800) 422-4633; fax: (310) 208-5971; URL: www.infotrieve.com; e-mail: orders@infotrieve.com; Institute for Scientific Information (ISI), phone: (800) 603-4367; fax: (856) 787-1679; URL: http://www.isidoc.com; e-mail: service@isidoc.com; Dialog Information Services; Proquest; Ovid Technologies, Inc; and EBSCO.

The ARCHIVES OF PEDIATRICS & ADOLESCENT MEDICINE (ISSN 01072–4710) is published monthly by the American Medical Association, 515 N State St, Chicago, IL 60610–0946, and is an official publication of the Association. The ARCHIVES OF PEDIATRICS & ADOLESCENT MEDICINE reaches more than 30 900 readers in over 83 countries each month. Periodicals postage paid at Chicago, Ill, and at additional mailing offices. GST registration number 12622 5556 RT. Canada Post International Publications Mail (Canadian Distribution) Sales Agreement No. 318728. POSTMASTER, send all address changes to *Archives of Pediatrics & Adolescent Medicine,* c/o the AMA Unified Service Center, American Medical Association, 515 N State St, Chicago, IL 60610. Printed in the USA.

## ADVERTISING

Information about advertising is available from the following sales representatives and online at www.archpediatrics.com.

**Account Manager:** Tim Melroy (nationally); phone: (973) 263-9191 ext 213.

**Manager, Marketing Services:** Nancy Bell; phone: (973) 263-9191 ext 216.

**Advertising Office:** 119 Cherry Hill Rd, Suite 330, Parsippany, NJ 07054-1114; phone: (973) 263-9191.

**Classified Advertising:** Thalia Moss, 515 N State St, Chicago, IL 60610; phone: (800) 262-2260; e-mail: classifieds@ama-assn.org.

## ADVERTISING PRINCIPLES

Advertisements in this issue have been reviewed to comply with the principles governing advertising in AMA publications. A copy of these principles is available on request and online at www.archpediatrics.com. The appearance of advertising in AMA publications is not an AMA guarantee or endorsement of the product or the claims made for the product by the manufacturer.

## ADDRESS CHANGES

Send all address changes to *Archives of Pediatrics & Adolescent Medicine*, c/o the AMA Unified Service Center, American Medical Association, 515 N State St, Chicago, IL 60610. Notification of address changes must be made at least 6 weeks in advance; include both old and new addresses and a recent mailing label if sending via mail.

## SUBSCRIPTION RATES AND SERVICE

Subscription rates are shown in the table below. For service in the US and Americas, inquiries on pricing, address changes, missing issues, subscription billing, subscription renewal, and back issues, contact the AMA Unified Service Center, 24 hours a day, 7 days a week.

**AMA members:** phone: (800) 262-3211; e-mail: msc@ama-assn.org. **Other physicians and nonphysician customers, including subscription agents:** phone: (800) 262-2350 or (312) 670-7827; fax: (312) 464-5831; e-mail: ama-subs@ama-assn.org. **Inquiries:** Unified Service Center, American Medical Association, PO Box 10946, Chicago, IL 60610-0946. For subscribers with mailing addresses outside the United States & Americas: Contact *JAMA & Archives* Journals, c/o EMD GmbH, Birkenstr.67, 10559 Berlin, Germany. Phone: +49 (30) 33099828; fax: +49 (30) 33099829; e-mail: ama@emd-germany.de.

**Annual Subscription Rates**

| | United States | Americas | UK | Rest of World |
|---|---|---|---|---|
| INDIVIDUAL | | | | |
| Print and Online | $185 | $240 | £165 | €250 |
| INSTITUTION | | | | |
| Print and Online | $375 | $485 | £315 | €470 |

In Canada, US rate plus GST. Rates for residents and medical students available at pubs.ama-assn.org, or from the AMA Unified Service Center.

# BOOSTRIX®

**(Tetanus Toxoid, Reduced Diphtheria Toxoid and Acellular Pertussis Vaccine, Adsorbed) (Tdap)**

The following is a brief summary only; see full prescribing information for complete product information.

**INDICATIONS AND USAGE:** BOOSTRIX is indicated for active booster immunization against tetanus, diphtheria, and pertussis as a single dose in individuals 10 through 18 years of age. The use of BOOSTRIX as a primary series or to complete the primary series has not been studied. As with any vaccine, BOOSTRIX may not protect 100% of individuals receiving the vaccine. BOOSTRIX is not recommended for treatment of actual infections.

**CONTRAINDICATIONS:** Hypersensitivity to any component of the vaccine is a contraindication (see DESCRIPTION in full prescribing information). Do not use BOOSTRIX after a serious allergic reaction (e.g., anaphylaxis) following any other tetanus toxoid, diphtheria toxoid or pertussis-containing vaccine, or any component of this vaccine (see DESCRIPTION in full prescribing information). Because of the uncertainty as to which component of the vaccine might be responsible, do not give further vaccination with any of these components; or, refer such individuals to an allergist for evaluation. The following events are contraindications to administration of BOOSTRIX: encephalopathy (e.g., coma, decreased level of consciousness, prolonged seizures) within 7 days of administration of a previous dose of a pertussis-containing vaccine that is not attributable to another identifiable cause; progressive neurologic disorder, uncontrolled epilepsy, or progressive encephalopathy. Do not vaccinate individuals with these conditions until a treatment regimen has been established and the condition has stabilized. BOOSTRIX is not contraindicated for use in individuals with HIV infection.

**WARNINGS:** The tip cap and the rubber plunger of the needleless prefilled syringes contain dry natural latex rubber that may cause allergic reactions in latex sensitive individuals. The vial stopper is latex-free. If any of the following events occurred in temporal relation to previous receipt of a Diphtheria and Tetanus Toxoids and Pertussis Vaccine Adsorbed (DTwP) vaccine or a vaccine containing an acellular pertussis component, consider carefully whether to give subsequent doses of BOOSTRIX: temperature of ≥40.5°C (105°F) within 48 hours not due to another identifiable cause; collapse or shock-like state (hypotonic-hyporesponsive episode) within 48 hours; persistent, inconsolable crying lasting ≥3 hours, occurring within 48 hours; seizures with or without fever occurring within 3 days. Persons who experienced serious Arthus-type hypersensitivity reactions following a prior dose of tetanus toxoid usually have high serum tetanus antitoxin levels and should not be given Tetanus and Diphtheria Toxoids Adsorbed For Adult Use (Td) or Tdap vaccines or even emergency doses of Td more frequently than every 10 years, even if the wound is neither clean nor minor. If Guillain-Barré syndrome has occurred within 6 weeks of receipt of prior vaccine containing tetanus toxoid, the decision to give BOOSTRIX or any vaccine containing tetanus toxoid should be based on careful consideration of the potential benefits and possible risks. The decision to administer a pertussis-containing vaccine to individuals with stable central nervous system (CNS) disorders must be made by the physician on an individual basis, with consideration of all relevant factors, and assessment of potential risks and benefits for that individual. Advise the patient, parent, or guardian of the potential increased risk involved (see PRECAUTIONS). A family history of seizures or other CNS disorders is not a contraindication to pertussis vaccine. The Advisory Committee on Immunization Practices (ACIP) has published guidelines for vaccination of persons with recent or acute illness (www.cdc.gov). Do not give BOOSTRIX to individuals with bleeding disorders such as hemophilia or thrombocytopenia, or to persons on anticoagulant therapy unless the potential benefit clearly outweighs the risk of administration. If the decision is made to administer BOOSTRIX to such persons, it should be given with caution with steps taken to avoid the risk of hematoma following the injection.

**PRECAUTIONS:** Before the injection of any biological, the physician should take all reasonable precautions to prevent allergic or other adverse reactions. Epinephrine injection (1:1,000) and other appropriate agents used for the control of immediate allergic reactions must be immediately available should an acute anaphylactic reaction occur. Immunosuppressed persons, including individuals receiving immunosuppressive therapy, may not develop the expected immune response. **Drug Interactions:** Do not mix BOOSTRIX with any other vaccine in the same syringe or vial. **Carcinogenesis, Mutagenesis, Impairment of Fertility:** BOOSTRIX has not been evaluated for carcinogenic or mutagenic potential, or for impairment of fertility. **Pregnancy:** Pregnancy Category C. Animal reproduction studies have not been conducted with BOOSTRIX. It is also not known whether BOOSTRIX can cause fetal harm when administered to a pregnant woman or can affect reproductive capacity. BOOSTRIX should be given to a pregnant woman only if clearly needed. Animal fertility studies have not been conducted with BOOSTRIX. In a developmental toxicity study, the effect of BOOSTRIX on embryo-fetal and pre-weaning development was evaluated in pregnant rats. Animals were administered INFANRIX® (Diphtheria and Tetanus Toxoids and Acellular Pertussis Vaccine Adsorbed) prior to gestation and BOOSTRIX during the period of organogenesis (gestation days 6, 8, 11) and later in pregnancy (gestation day 15), 0.1 mL/rat/occasion (a 45-fold increase compared to the human dose of BOOSTRIX on a body weight basis), by intramuscular injection. No adverse affect on pregnancy and lactation parameters, embryo-fetal or pre-weaning development was observed. There were no fetal malformations or other evidence of teratogenesis noted in this study. **Nursing Mothers:** It is not known whether BOOSTRIX is excreted in human milk. Because many drugs are excreted in human milk, caution should be exercised when BOOSTRIX is administered to a nursing woman. **Pregnancy Exposure Registry:** Healthcare providers are encouraged to register pregnant women who receive BOOSTRIX in the GlaxoSmithKline vaccination pregnancy registry by calling 1-888-825-5249. **Geriatric Use:** BOOSTRIX is not indicated for use in individuals older than 18 years. **Pediatric Use:** BOOSTRIX is not indicated for use in individuals younger than 10 years (see DOSAGE AND ADMINISTRATION in full prescribing information). For immunization of infants and children younger than 7 years against diphtheria, tetanus, and pertussis, refer to the manufacturers' package inserts for Diphtheria and Tetanus Toxoids and Acellular Pertussis Vaccine Adsorbed (DTaP) vaccines.

**ADVERSE REACTIONS:** A total of 3,289 adolescents were vaccinated with a single dose of BOOSTRIX during clinical trials. An additional 1,092 adolescents 10 to 18 years of age received a non-US formulation of BOOSTRIX (formulated to contain 0.5 mg aluminum per dose) in non-US clinical studies.

The primary safety study, conducted in the United States, was a randomized, observer-blinded, controlled study in which 3,080 adolescents 10 to 18 years of age received a single dose of BOOSTRIX and 1,034 received the control Td vaccine manufactured by Massachusetts Public Health Biologic Laboratories. There were no substantive differences in demographic characteristics between the vaccine groups. Among BOOSTRIX and control vaccine recipients approximately 75% were 10 to 14 years of age and approximately 25% were 15 to 18 years of age. Approximately 98% of participants in this study had received the recommended series of 4 or 5 doses of either DTwP or a combination of DTwP and DTaP in childhood. Data on adverse events were collected by the subjects, parents and/or guardians using standardized diaries for 15 consecutive days following the vaccine dose (i.e., day of vaccination and the next 14 days). Subjects were monitored for unsolicited adverse events that occurred within 31 days of vaccination (day 0-30) using diary cards (day 0-14) supplemented by spontaneous reports and a medical history as reported by subjects, parents, and/or guardians. Subjects were also monitored for 6 months post-vaccination for non-routine medical visits, visits to an emergency room, onset of new chronic illness, and serious adverse events. Information regarding late onset adverse events was obtained via a telephone call 6 months following vaccination. At least 97% of subjects completed the 6-month follow-up evaluation.

The adverse event information from clinical trials provides a basis for identifying adverse events that appear to be related to vaccine use and for approximating rates. However, because clinical trials are conducted under widely varying conditions, adverse event rates observed in the clinical trials of a vaccine cannot be directly compared to rates in the clinical trials of another vaccine, and may not reflect the rates observed in practice.

**Serious Adverse Events in All Safety Studies:** In the US-safety study, no serious adverse events were reported to occur within 31 days of vaccination. During the 6-month extended safety evaluation period, no serious adverse events that were of potential autoimmune origin or new onset and chronic in nature were reported to occur. In non-US studies in which serious adverse events were monitored for up to 37 days, one subject was diagnosed with insulin dependent diabetes. The association of this event with vaccination is unknown. No other serious adverse events of potential autoimmune origin or that were new onset and chronic in nature were reported to occur in these studies.

**Solicited Adverse Events in the US-Safety Study:** In a US study, the most common local adverse events following administration of BOOSTRIX were pain, redness, and swelling at the injection site. The most common general adverse events were headache and fatigue. Most of these events were reported at a similar frequency in recipients of both BOOSTRIX and Td. Any pain, grade 2 or 3 pain (but not grade 3 alone), and grade 2 or 3 headache (but not grade 3 alone) were reported at a higher rate in recipients of BOOSTRIX. The primary safety endpoint of the US study was the incidence of grade 3 pain (spontaneously painful and/or prevented normal activity) at the injection site within 15 days of vaccination. Grade 3 pain was reported in 4.6% of those who received BOOSTRIX compared with 4.0% of those who received the Td vaccine. The difference in rate of grade 3 pain was within the pre-defined clinical limit for non-inferiority (upper limit of the 95% CI for the difference ≤4%). These were the rates for solicited local and general adverse events within 15 days of vaccination with BOOSTRIX or Td vaccine for the total vaccinated cohort (all enrolled, vaccinated subjects with safety data available analyzed by vaccine received):

**Percentage of Individuals 10 to 18 Years of Age Reporting Solicited Local Adverse Events or Solicited General Adverse Events Within the 15-day* Post-Vaccination Period**

| | BOOSTRIX (N = 3,032) | Td (N = 1,013) |
|---|---|---|
| **Local** | | |
| Pain,† any | 75.3 | 71.7 |
| Pain,† grade 2 or 3 | 51.2 | 42.5 |
| Pain,‡ grade 3 | 4.6 | 4.0 |
| Redness, any | 22.5 | 19.8 |
| Redness, >20 mm | 4.1 | 3.9 |
| Redness, ≥50 mm | 1.7 | 1.6 |
| Swelling, any | 21.1 | 20.1 |
| Swelling, >20 mm | 5.3 | 4.9 |
| Swelling, ≥50 mm | 2.5 | 3.2 |
| Arm circumference increase,§ >5 mm | 28.3 | 29.5 |
| Arm circumference increase,§ >20 mm | 2.0 | 2.2 |
| Arm circumference increase,§ >40 mm | 0.5 | 0.3 |
| **General** | | |
| Fever,‖ ≥99.5°F | 13.5 | 13.1 |
| Fever,‖ >100.4°F | 5.0 | 4.7 |
| Fever,‖ >102.2°F | 1.4 | 1.0 |
| Headache, any | 43.1 | 41.5 |
| Headache,† grade 2 or 3 | 15.7 | 12.7 |
| Headache, grade 3 | 3.7 | 2.7 |
| Fatigue, any | 37.0 | 36.7 |
| Fatigue, grade 2 or 3 | 14.4 | 12.9 |
| Fatigue, grade 3 | 3.7 | 3.2 |
| Gastrointestinal symptoms,¶ any | 26.0 | 25.8 |
| Gastrointestinal symptoms,¶ grade 2 or 3 | 9.8 | 9.7 |
| Gastrointestinal symptoms,¶ grade 3 | 3.0 | 3.2 |

Td = Tetanus and Diphtheria Toxoids Adsorbed For Adult Use manufactured by Massachusetts Public Health Biologic Laboratories.

N = number of subjects in the total vaccinated cohort with local/general symptoms sheets completed.

Grade 2 = Local: painful when the limb was moved; General: interfered with normal activity.

Grade 3 = Local: spontaneously painful and/or prevented normal activity; General: prevented normal activity.

*Day of vaccination and the next 14 days.

†Statistically significantly higher (P<0.05) following BOOSTRIX as compared to Td vaccine.

‡Grade 3 injection site pain following BOOSTRIX was not inferior to Td (upper limit of two-sided 95% CI for the difference in the percentage of subjects ≤4%).

§Mid-upper region of the vaccinated arm.

‖Oral temperatures or axillary temperatures.

¶Gastrointestinal symptoms included nausea, vomiting, diarrhea and/or abdominal pain.

Mid-upper arm circumference was measured by the adolescent or their parent/guardian prior to injection and daily for 15 days following vaccination. There was no significant difference between BOOSTRIX recipients and Td recipients in the proportion of subjects reporting an increase in mid-upper arm circumference in the vaccinated arm. The incidence of unsolicited adverse events reported in the 31 days after vaccination was comparable between the 2 groups.

As with any vaccine, there is the possibility that broad use of BOOSTRIX could reveal adverse events not observed in clinical trials.

**Postmarketing Reports:** Worldwide voluntary reports of adverse events received for BOOSTRIX in persons 10 to 18 years of age since market introduction of this vaccine are listed below. This list includes serious events or events which have causal connection to components of this or other vaccines or drugs. Because these events are reported voluntarily from a population of uncertain size, it is not possible to reliably estimate their frequency or establish a causal relationship to vaccine exposure. *Blood and lymphatic system disorders:* Lymphadenitis, lymphadenopathy. *Cardiac disorders:* Myocarditis. *Injection site reactions:* Induration, inflammation, mass, nodule, warmth, local reaction. *Metabolism and nutrition disorders:* Diabetes mellitus insulin-dependent. *Musculoskeletal and connective tissue disorders:* Arthralgia, back pain, myalgia. *Nervous system disorders:* Convulsion, encephalitis, facial palsy, paraesthesia. *Skin and subcutaneous tissue disorders:* Exanthem, Henoch-Schönlein purpura, rash. In addition, extensive swelling of the injected limb has been reported following administration of BOOSTRIX.

**Reporting Adverse Events:** Report the occurrence following immunization of any event set forth in the Vaccine Injury Table from the National Childhood Vaccine Injury Act including: Anaphylaxis or anaphylactic shock within 7 days, encephalopathy or encephalitis within 7 days, brachial neuritis within 28 days, or an acute complication or sequelae (including death) of an illness, disability, injury, or condition referred to above, or any events that would contraindicate further doses of vaccine, according to this prescribing information. These events should be reported to VAERS. The VAERS toll-free number is 1-800-822-7967. Reporting forms may also be obtained at the VAERS website at www.vaers.org.

**DOSAGE AND ADMINISTRATION: Recommended Dose:** BOOSTRIX should be administered as a single 0.5 mL injection by the intramuscular route into the deltoid muscle of the upper arm in individuals 10 through 18 years of age. Do not administer this product subcutaneously or intravenously. There are no data to support repeat administration of BOOSTRIX. Five years should elapse between the subject's last dose of the recommended series of childhood DTwP and/or DTaP vaccine and the administration of BOOSTRIX. Limited data are available on the use of BOOSTRIX following Tetanus and Diphtheria Toxoids Adsorbed For Adult Use (Td) vaccine. **Additional Dosing Information:** ***Wound Management:*** Clinicians should refer to guidelines for tetanus prophylaxis in routine wound management. Adolescents 10 to 18 years of age who have completed a primary series against tetanus and who sustain wounds which are minor and uncomplicated, should receive a booster dose of a tetanus toxoid-containing vaccine only if they have not received tetanus toxoid within the preceding 10 years. In case of tetanus-prone injury (e.g., wounds contaminated with dirt, feces, soil, and saliva; puncture wounds; avulsions; and wounds resulting from missles, crushing, burns, and frostbite) in an adolescent who is in need of tetanus toxoid, BOOSTRIX can be used as an alternative to Tetanus and Diphtheria Toxoids Adsorbed For Adult Use (Td) vaccine in patients for whom the pertussis component is also indicated (see INDICATIONS AND USAGE).

Manufactured by **GlaxoSmithKline Biologicals**
Rixensart, Belgium, US License 1617
Distributed by **GlaxoSmithKline**
Research Triangle Park, NC 27709

BOOSTRIX and INFANRIX are registered trademarks of GlaxoSmithKline.

Full prescribing information for BOOSTRIX is available at www.BOOSTRIX.com.

BRS-BO:L1

**References: 1.** Centers for Disease Control and Prevention. *Epidemiology and Prevention of Vaccine-Preventable Diseases.* Atkinson W, Hamborsky J, Wolfe S, eds. 8th ed. Washington DC: Public Health Foundation; 2004:75–88, A26–A27. **2.** ACIP recommends adolescent vaccination for tetanus, diphtheria and pertussis vaccine [press release]. Atlanta, GA: Department of Health and Human Services; Available at: www.cdc.gov/nip/pr/pr_tdap_jun2005.htm. Accessed September 27, 2005. **3.** Data on file, BOR305, GlaxoSmithKline.

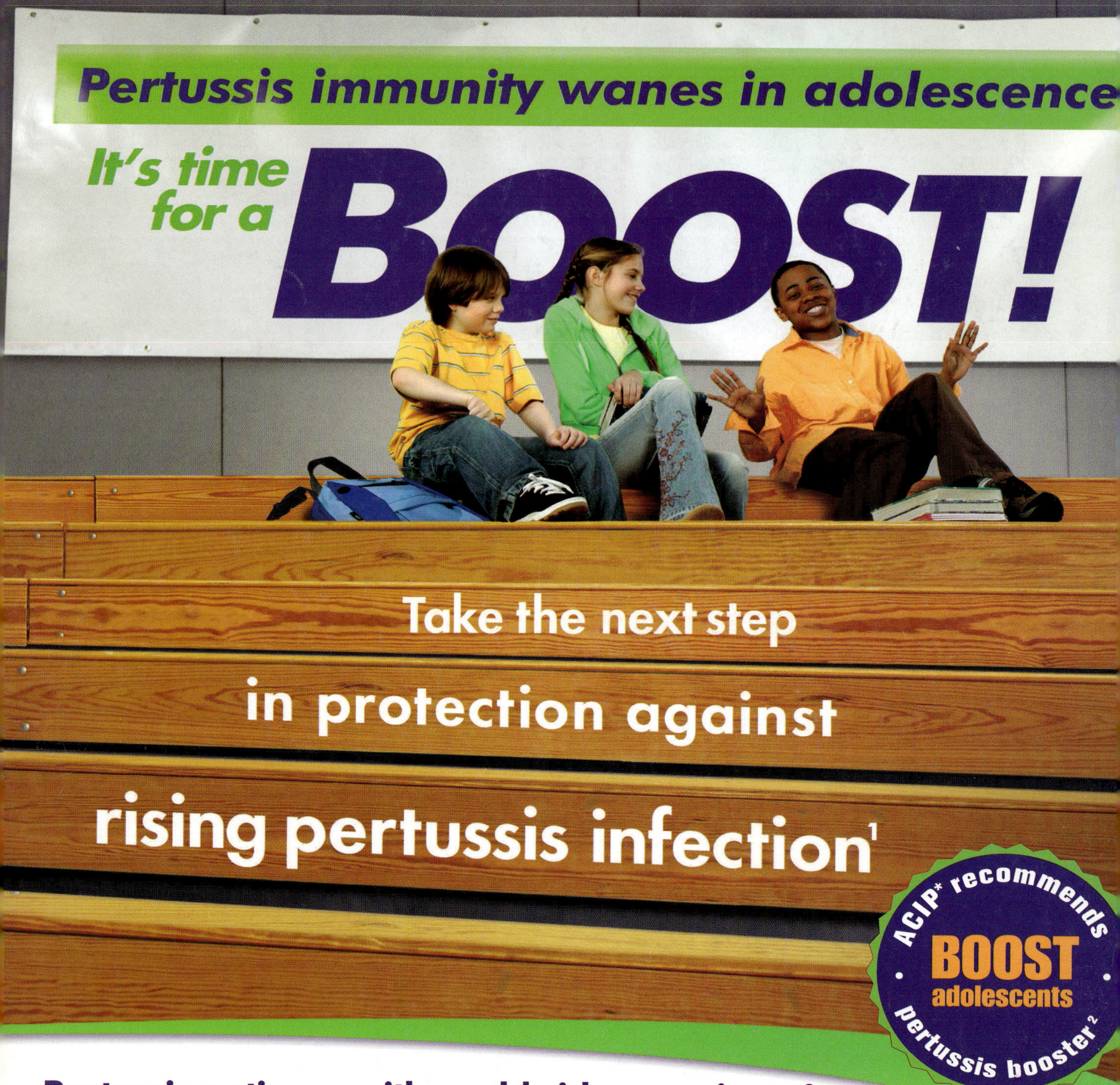
Pertussis immunity wanes in adolescence
It's time for a BOOST!
Take the next step
in protection against
rising pertussis infection[1]
ACIP* recommends
BOOST
adolescents
pertussis booster[2]

# ARCHIVES OF PEDIATRICS & ADOLESCENT MEDICINE

WWW.ARCHPEDIATRICS.COM

APRIL 2006


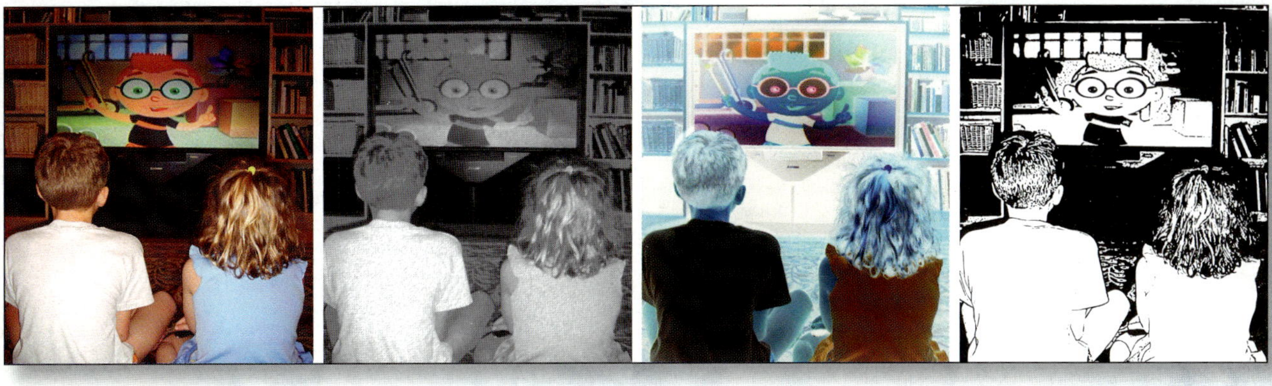

Little Einsteins. See page 335.


DOES CHILDREN'S SCREEN TIME PREDICT REQUESTS FOR ADVERTISED PRODUCTS?

CONTENT AND RATINGS OF MATURE-RATED VIDEO GAMES

TELEVISION EXPOSURE AND OVERWEIGHT RISK IN PRESCHOOLERS

WHEN CHILDREN EAT WHAT THEY WATCH

SHORT-TERM AND LONG-TERM EFFECTS OF VIOLENT MEDIA ON AGGRESSION IN CHILDREN AND ADULTS

TELEVISION VIEWING AND RISK OF SEXUAL INITIATION BY YOUNG ADOLESCENTS

EFFECTS OF MEDIA VIOLENCE ON HEALTH RELATED OUTCOMES AMONG YOUNG MEN

CONTENT ANALYSIS OF HEALTH AND PHYSICAL ACTIVITY MESSAGES MARKETED DURING AFTER-SCHOOL TV PROGRAMMING



COMPLETE TABLE OF CONTENTS ON PAGE 333





JAMA & ARCHIVES JOURNALS
American Medical Association

**In the treatment or prevention of bronchospasm**

**New**

# Expect Xopenex

## ...To Go

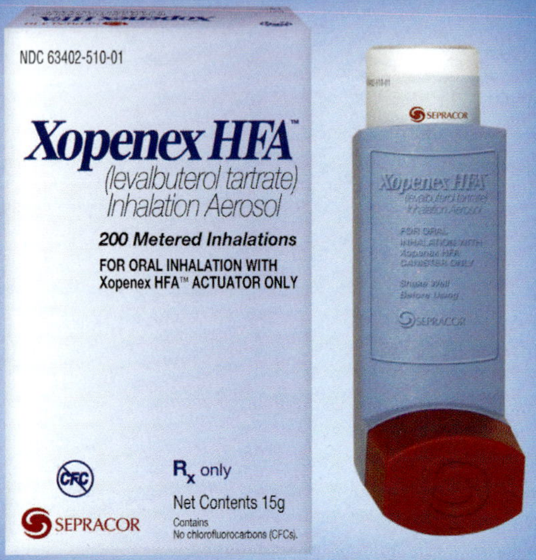


## Now in an MDI

**Same trusted single-isomer technology**

**Does not contain (S)-albuterol[1]**

Nothing less than

**NEW Xopenex HFA™**
(levalbuterol tartrate) Inhalation Aerosol

XOPENEX HFA (levalbuterol tartrate) Inhalation Aerosol is indicated for the treatment or prevention of bronchospasm in adults, adolescents, and children 4 years of age and older with reversible obstructive airway disease.

**Important Safety Information**

Xopenex HFA is contraindicated in patients with a history of hypersensitivity to levalbuterol, racemic albuterol, or any other component of Xopenex HFA. Xopenex HFA and other β-agonists can produce paradoxical bronchospasm, which may be life threatening. If additional adrenergic drugs, including other short-acting sympathomimetic bronchodilators or epinephrine, are to be administered by any route, they should be used with caution to avoid deleterious cardiovascular effects. Due to the cardiovascular side effects associated with β-agonists, caution is generally recommended for patients with cardiovascular disorders (especially coronary insufficiency, cardiac arrhythmias, and hypertension), diabetes, hyperthyroidism, or convulsive disorders. Do not exceed the recommended dose. Fatalities have been reported in association with excessive use of inhaled sympathomimetic drugs in patients with asthma. Please refer to the complete prescribing information for further information and in regard to potential drug interactions with β-blockers, diuretics, digoxin, or MAOI and tricyclic antidepressants.

**In patients aged 4 to 11 years,** the most common adverse events (occurring in greater than 2% of patients and more frequently than patients receiving placebo) were (90 mcg Xopenex HFA and placebo, respectively): accidental injury (9.2%; 5.7%), vomiting (10.5%; 5.7%), bronchitis (2.6%; 0%), and pharyngitis (6.6%; 5.7%).

**In patients aged 12 years and older,** the most common adverse events (occurring in greater than 2% of patients and more frequently than patients receiving placebo) were (90 mcg Xopenex HFA and placebo, respectively): pain (4.0%; 3.6%), dizziness (2.7%; 1.8%), asthma (9.4%; 6.0%), pharyngitis (7.9%; 2.4%), and rhinitis (7.4%; 3.0%).

**Reference:** 1. Xopenex HFA Prescribing Information.

Please see brief summary of prescribing information.

# Xopenex HFA™
## (levalbuterol tartrate) Inhalation Aerosol

FOR ORAL INHALATION ONLY

## BRIEF SUMMARY

**INDICATIONS AND USAGE**

XOPENEX HFA (levalbuterol tartrate) Inhalation Aerosol is indicated for the treatment or prevention of bronchospasm in adults, adolescents, and children 4 years of age and older with reversible obstructive airway disease.

**CONTRAINDICATIONS**

XOPENEX HFA (levalbuterol tartrate) Inhalation Aerosol is contraindicated in patients with a history of hypersensitivity to levalbuterol, racemic albuterol, or any other component of XOPENEX HFA Inhalation Aerosol.

**WARNINGS**

1. Paradoxical Bronchospasm: Like other inhaled beta-adrenergic agonists, XOPENEX HFA Inhalation Aerosol can produce paradoxical bronchospasm, which may be life-threatening. If paradoxical bronchospasm occurs, XOPENEX HFA (levalbuterol tartrate) Inhalation Aerosol should be discontinued immediately and alternative therapy instituted. It should be recognized that paradoxical bronchospasm, when associated with inhaled formulations, frequently occurs with the first use of a new canister. 2. Deterioration of Asthma: Asthma may deteriorate acutely over a period of hours or chronically over several days or longer. If the patient needs more doses of XOPENEX HFA Inhalation Aerosol than usual, this may be a marker of destabilization of asthma and requires reevaluation of the patient and treatment regimen, giving special consideration to the possible need for anti-inflammatory treatment, e.g., corticosteroids.
3. Use of Anti-Inflammatory Agents: The use of a beta-adrenergic agonist alone may not be adequate to control asthma in many patients. Early consideration should be given to adding anti-inflammatory agents, e.g., corticosteroids, to the therapeutic regimen. 4. Cardiovascular Effects: XOPENEX HFA Inhalation Aerosol, like other beta-adrenergic agonists, can produce clinically significant cardiovascular effects in some patients, as measured by heart rate, blood pressure, and/or symptoms. Although such effects are uncommon after administration of XOPENEX HFA Inhalation Aerosol at recommended doses, if they occur, the drug may need to be discontinued. In addition, beta-agonists have been reported to produce electrocardiogram (ECG) changes, such as flattening of the T wave, prolongation of the QTc interval, and ST segment depression. The clinical significance of these findings is unknown. Therefore, XOPENEX HFA Inhalation Aerosol, like all sympathomimetic amines, should be used with caution in patients with cardiovascular disorders, especially coronary insufficiency, cardiac arrhythmias, and hypertension. 5. Do Not Exceed Recommended Dose: Fatalities have been reported in association with excessive use of inhaled sympathomimetic drugs in patients with asthma. The exact cause of death is unknown, but cardiac arrest following an unexpected development of a severe acute asthmatic crisis and subsequent hypoxia is suspected.
6. Immediate Hypersensitivity Reactions: Immediate hypersensitivity reactions may occur after administration of racemic albuterol, as demonstrated by rare cases of urticaria, angioedema, rash, bronchospasm, anaphylaxis, and oropharyngeal edema. The potential for hypersensitivity must be considered in the clinical evaluation of patients who experience immediate hypersensitivity reactions while receiving XOPENEX HFA Inhalation Aerosol.

**PRECAUTIONS**

**General**

XOPENEX HFA (levalbuterol tartrate) Inhalation Aerosol, like all sympathomimetic amines, should be used with caution in patients with cardiovascular disorders, especially coronary insufficiency, hypertension, and cardiac arrhythmias; in patients with convulsive disorders, hyperthyroidism, or diabetes mellitus; and in patients who are unusually responsive to sympathomimetic amines. Clinically significant changes in systolic and diastolic blood pressure have been seen in individual patients and could be expected to occur in some patients after the use of any beta-adrenergic bronchodilator.

Large doses of intravenous racemic albuterol have been reported to aggravate preexisting diabetes mellitus and ketoacidosis. As with other beta-adrenergic agonist medications, XOPENEX HFA Inhalation Aerosol may produce significant hypokalemia in some patients, possibly through intracellular shunting, which has the potential to produce adverse cardiovascular effects. The decrease is usually transient, not requiring supplementation.

**Information for Patients**

The action of XOPENEX HFA Inhalation Aerosol should last for 4 to 6 hours. XOPENEX HFA Inhalation Aerosol should not be used more frequently than recommended. Do not increase the dose or frequency of doses of XOPENEX HFA Inhalation Aerosol without consulting your physician. If you find that treatment with XOPENEX HFA Inhalation Aerosol becomes less effective for symptomatic relief, your symptoms become worse, and/or you need to use the product more frequently than usual, you should seek medical attention immediately. While you are using XOPENEX HFA Inhalation Aerosol, other inhaled drugs and asthma medications should be taken only as directed by your physician.

Common adverse effects of treatment with inhaled beta-agonists include palpitations, chest pain, rapid heart rate, tremor, and nervousness. If you are pregnant or nursing, contact your physician about use of XOPENEX HFA Inhalation Aerosol. Effective and safe use of XOPENEX HFA Inhalation Aerosol includes an understanding of the way that it should be administered.

Use XOPENEX HFA Inhalation Aerosol only with the actuator supplied with the product. Discard the canister after 200 sprays have been used. Never immerse the canister in water to determine how full the canister is ("float test").

In general, the technique for administering XOPENEX HFA Inhalation Aerosol to children is similar to that for adults. Children should use XOPENEX HFA Inhalation Aerosol under adult supervision, as instructed by the patient's physician.

**Drug Interactions**

Other short-acting sympathomimetic aerosol bronchodilators or epinephrine should be used with caution with XOPENEX HFA Inhalation Aerosol. If additional adrenergic drugs are to be administered by any route, they should be used with caution to avoid deleterious cardiovascular effects.

1. Beta-blockers: Beta-adrenergic receptor-blocking agents not only block the pulmonary effect of beta-adrenergic agonists, such as XOPENEX HFA Inhalation Aerosol, but may produce severe bronchospasm in asthmatic patients. Therefore, patients with asthma should not normally be treated with beta-blockers. However, under certain circumstances, e.g., as prophylaxis after myocardial infarction, there may be no acceptable alternatives to the use of beta-adrenergic blocking agents in patients with asthma. In this setting, cardioselective beta-blockers should be considered, although they should be administered with caution. 2. Diuretics: The ECG changes and/or hypokalemia that may result from the administration of non–potassium-sparing diuretics (such as loop and thiazide diuretics) can be acutely worsened by beta-agonists, especially when the recommended dose of the beta-agonist is exceeded. Although the clinical significance of these effects is not known, caution is advised in the coadministration of beta-agonists with non–potassium-sparing diuretics. 3. Digoxin: Mean decreases of 16% to 22% in serum digoxin levels were demonstrated after single-dose intravenous and oral administration of racemic albuterol, respectively, to normal volunteers who had received digoxin for 10 days. The clinical significance of these findings for patients with obstructive airway disease who are receiving XOPENEX HFA Inhalation Aerosol and digoxin on a chronic basis is unclear. Nevertheless, it would be prudent to carefully evaluate the serum digoxin levels in patients who are currently receiving digoxin and XOPENEX HFA Inhalation Aerosol. 4. Monoamine Oxidase Inhibitors or Tricyclic Antidepressants: XOPENEX HFA Inhalation Aerosol should be administered with extreme caution to patients being treated with monoamine oxidase inhibitors or tricyclic antidepressants, or within 2 weeks of discontinuation of such agents, because the action of albuterol on the vascular system may be potentiated.

**Carcinogenesis, Mutagenesis, and Impairment of Fertility** No carcinogenesis or impairment of fertility studies have been carried out with levalbuterol tartrate. However, racemic albuterol sulfate has been evaluated for its carcinogenic potential and ability to impair fertility.

In a 2-year study in Sprague-Dawley rats, racemic albuterol sulfate caused a significant dose-related increase in the incidence of benign leiomyomas of the mesovarium at, and above, dietary doses of 2 mg/kg/day (approximately 30 times the maximum recommended daily inhalation dose of levalbuterol tartrate for adults on a mg/m² basis and approximately 15 times the maximum recommended daily inhalation dose of levalbuterol tartrate for children on a mg/m² basis). In another study, this effect was blocked by the coadministration of propranolol, a non-selective beta-adrenergic antagonist. In an 18-month study in CD-1 mice, racemic albuterol sulfate showed no evidence of tumorigenicity at dietary doses up to 500 mg/kg/day (approximately 3800 times the maximum recommended daily inhalation dose of levalbuterol tartrate for adults on a mg/m² basis and approximately 1800 times the maximum recommended daily inhalation dose of levalbuterol tartrate for children on a mg/m² basis). In a 22-month study in the Golden hamster, racemic albuterol sulfate showed no evidence of tumorigenicity at dietary doses up to 50 mg/kg/day (approximately 500 times the maximum recommended daily inhalation dose of levalbuterol tartrate for adults on a mg/m² basis and approximately 240 times the maximum recommended daily inhalation dose of levalbuterol tartrate for children on a mg/m² basis).

Levalbuterol HCl was not mutagenic in the Ames test or the CHO/HPRT Mammalian Forward Gene Mutation Assay.

Levalbuterol HCl was not clastogenic in the in vivo micronucleus test in mouse bone marrow. Racemic albuterol sulfate was negative in an in vitro chromosomal aberration assay in CHO cell cultures.

Reproduction studies in rats using racemic albuterol sulfate demonstrated no evidence of impaired fertility at oral doses up to 50 mg/kg/day (approximately 750 times the maximum recommended daily inhalation dose of levalbuterol tartrate for adults on a mg/m² basis).

**Teratogenic Effects - Pregnancy Category C** A reproduction study in New Zealand White rabbits demonstrated that levalbuterol HCl was not teratogenic when administered orally at doses up to 25 mg/kg/day (approximately 750 times the maximum recommended daily inhalation dose of levalbuterol tartrate for adults on a mg/m² basis).

However, racemic albuterol sulfate has been shown to be teratogenic in mice and rabbits. A study in CD-1 mice given racemic albuterol sulfate subcutaneously showed cleft palate formation in 5 of 111 (4.5%) fetuses at 0.25 mg/kg/day (approximately 2 times the maximum recommended daily inhalation dose of levalbuterol tartrate for adults on a mg/m² basis) and in 10 of 108 (9.3%) fetuses at 2.5 mg/kg/day (approximately 20 times the maximum recommended daily inhalation dose of levalbuterol tartrate for adults on a mg/m² basis). The drug did not induce cleft palate formation when administered subcutaneously at a dose of 0.025 mg/kg/day (less than the maximum recommended daily inhalation dose of levalbuterol tartrate for adults on a mg/m² basis). Cleft palate also occurred in 22 of 72 (30.5%) fetuses from females treated subcutaneously with 2.5 mg/kg/day of isoproterenol (positive control).

A reproduction study in Stride Dutch rabbits revealed cranioschisis in 7 of 19 (37%) fetuses when racemic albuterol sulfate was administered orally at a dose of 50 mg/kg/day (approximately 1500 times the maximum recommended daily inhalation dose of levalbuterol tartrate for adults on a mg/m² basis).

A study in which pregnant rats were dosed with radiolabeled racemic albuterol sulfate demonstrated that drug-related material is transferred from the maternal circulation to the fetus.

There are no adequate and well-controlled studies of XOPENEX HFA Inhalation Aerosol in pregnant women. Because animal reproduction studies are not always predictive of human response, XOPENEX HFA Inhalation Aerosol should be used during pregnancy only if the potential benefit justifies the potential risk to the fetus.

During marketing experience of racemic albuterol, various congenital anomalies, including cleft palate and limb defects, have been rarely reported in the offspring of patients being treated with racemic albuterol. Some of the mothers were taking multiple medications during their pregnancies. No consistent pattern of defects can be discerned, and a relationship between racemic albuterol use and congenital anomalies has not been established.

**Use in Labor and Delivery** Because of the potential for beta-adrenergic agonists to interfere with uterine contractility, the use of XOPENEX HFA Inhalation Aerosol for the treatment of bronchospasm during labor should be restricted to those patients in whom the benefits clearly outweigh the risk.

**Tocolysis** XOPENEX HFA Inhalation Aerosol has not been approved for the management of preterm labor. The benefit:risk ratio when levalbuterol tartrate is administered for tocolysis has not been established. Serious adverse reactions, including maternal pulmonary edema, have been reported during or following treatment of premature labor with beta2-agonists, including racemic albuterol.

**Nursing Mothers** Plasma concentrations of levalbuterol after inhalation of therapeutic doses are very low in humans. It is not known whether levalbuterol is excreted in human milk.

Because of the potential for tumorigenicity shown for racemic albuterol in animal studies and the lack of experience with the use of XOPENEX HFA Inhalation Aerosol by nursing mothers, a decision should be made whether to discontinue nursing or to discontinue the drug, taking into account the importance of the drug to the mother. Caution should be exercised when XOPENEX HFA Inhalation Aerosol is administered to a nursing woman.

**Pediatrics** The safety and efficacy of XOPENEX HFA Inhalation Aerosol have been established in pediatric patients 4 years of age and older in an adequate and well-controlled clinical trial. Use of XOPENEX HFA Inhalation Aerosol in children is also supported by evidence from adequate and well-controlled studies of XOPENEX HFA Inhalation Aerosol in adults, considering that the pathophysiology, systemic exposure of the drug, and clinical profile in pediatric and adult patients are substantially similar. Safety and effectiveness of XOPENEX HFA Inhalation Aerosol in pediatric patients below the age of 4 years have not been established.

**Geriatrics** Clinical studies of XOPENEX HFA Inhalation Aerosol did not include sufficient numbers of subjects aged 65 and older to determine whether they respond differently from younger subjects. Other reported clinical experience has not identified differences in responses between the elderly and younger patients. In general, dose selection for an elderly patient should be cautious, usually starting at the low end of the dosing range, reflecting the greater frequency of decreased hepatic, renal, or cardiac function, and of concomitant diseases or other drug therapy.

Albuterol is known to be substantially excreted by the kidney, and the risk of toxic reactions may be greater in patients with impaired renal function. Because elderly patients are more likely to have decreased renal function, care should be taken in dose selection, and it may be useful to monitor renal function.

**ADVERSE REACTIONS** Adverse event information concerning XOPENEX HFA (levalbuterol tartrate) Inhalation Aerosol in adults and adolescents is derived from two 8-week, multicenter, randomized, double-blind, active- and placebo-controlled trials in 748 adult and adolescent patients with asthma that compared XOPENEX HFA Inhalation Aerosol, a marketed albuterol HFA inhaler, and an HFA-134a placebo inhaler. The following lists the incidence (% XOPENEX HFA 90 mcg, marketed albuterol HFA inhaler 180 mcg, placebo, respectively) of all adverse events (whether considered by the investigator to be related or unrelated to drug) from these trials that occurred at a rate of 2% or greater in the group treated with XOPENEX HFA Inhalation Aerosol and more frequently than in the HFA-134a placebo inhaler group. Body as a whole: pain (4.0%, 3.4%, 3.6%). Central nervous system: dizziness (2.7%, 0.6%, 1.8%). Respiratory system: asthma (9.4%, 7.3%, 6.0%), pharyngitis (7.9%, 2.2%, 2.4%), rhinitis (7.4%, 2.2%, 3.0%).

Adverse events reported by less than 2% and at least 2 or more of the adolescent and adult patients receiving XOPENEX HFA Inhalation Aerosol and by a greater proportion than receiving HFA-134a placebo inhaler include cyst, flu syndrome, viral infection, constipation, gastroenteritis, myalgia, hypertension, epistaxis, lung disorder, acne, herpes simplex, conjunctivitis, ear pain, dysmenorrhea, hematuria, and vaginal moniliasis. There were no significant laboratory abnormalities observed in these studies.

Adverse event information concerning XOPENEX HFA Inhalation Aerosol in children is derived from a 4-week, randomized, double-blind trial of XOPENEX HFA Inhalation Aerosol, a marketed albuterol HFA inhaler, and an HFA-134a placebo inhaler in 150 children aged 4 to 11 years with asthma. The following lists the adverse events (% XOPENEX HFA 90 mcg, marketed albuterol HFA inhaler 180 mcg, placebo, respectively) reported for XOPENEX HFA Inhalation Aerosol in children at a rate of 2% or greater and more frequently than for placebo. Body as a whole: accidental injury (9.2%, 10.3%, 5.7%). Digestive system: vomiting (10.5%, 7.7%, 5.7%). Respiratory system: bronchitis (2.6%, 0%, 0%), pharyngitis (6.6%, 12.8%, 5.7%).

The incidence of systemic beta-adrenergic adverse effects (e.g., tremor, nervousness) was low and comparable across all treatment groups, including placebo.

**Postmarketing** In addition to the adverse events reported in clinical trials, the following adverse events have been observed in postapproval use of levalbuterol inhalation solution. These events have been chosen for inclusion due to their seriousness, their frequency of reporting, or their likely beta-mediated mechanism: angioedema, anaphylaxis, arrhythmias (including atrial fibrillation, supraventricular tachycardia, extrasystoles), asthma, chest pain, cough increased, dyspnea, nausea, nervousness, rash, tachycardia, tremor, urticaria. Because these events have been reported spontaneously from a population of unknown size, estimates of frequency cannot be made.

In addition, XOPENEX HFA Inhalation Aerosol, like other sympathomimetic agents, can cause adverse reactions such as hypertension, angina, vertigo, central nervous system stimulation, sleeplessness, headache, and drying or irritation of the oropharynx.

Rx only.

## HAVRIX®
## (Hepatitis A Vaccine, Inactivated)

The following is a brief summary only; see full prescribing information for complete product information.

**INDICATIONS AND USAGE:** HAVRIX is indicated for active immunization of persons ≥12 months of age against disease caused by hepatitis A virus (HAV). Primary immunization should be administered at least 2 weeks prior to expected exposure to HAV. When passive protection against hepatitis A is required either following exposure to hepatitis A virus or in persons requiring both immediate and long-term protection, HAVRIX may be administered concomitantly with immune globulin (IG) with different syringes and at different injection sites. Duration of immunity following a complete vaccination schedule has not been established.

**CONTRAINDICATIONS:** Hypersensitivity to any component of the vaccine, including neomycin, is a contraindication (see DESCRIPTION in full prescribing information). This vaccine is contraindicated in patients with previous hypersensitivity to any hepatitis A-containing vaccine.

**WARNINGS:** There have been rare reports of anaphylaxis/anaphylactoid reactions following commercial use of the vaccine. The tip cap and the rubber plunger of the needleless prefilled syringes contain dry natural latex rubber that may cause allergic reactions in latex sensitive individuals. The vial stopper is latex-free. Hepatitis A has a relatively long incubation period. Hepatitis A vaccine may not prevent hepatitis A infection in those who have an unrecognized hepatitis A infection at the time of vaccination. Additionally, it may not prevent infection in those who do not achieve protective antibody titers (although the lowest titer needed to confer protection has not been determined).

**PRECAUTIONS: General:** Prior to immunization with HAVRIX, the patient's current health status and medical history should be reviewed. The physician should review the patient's immunization history for possible vaccine sensitivity, previous vaccination-related adverse reactions and occurrence of any adverse–event-related symptoms and/or signs, in order to determine the existence of any contraindication to immunization with HAVRIX and to allow an assessment of benefits and risks. Appropriate medical treatment and supervision should be readily available for immediate use in case of a rare anaphylactic reaction following the administration of the vaccine. Epinephrine injection (1:1,000) and other appropriate agents used for the control of immediate allergic reactions must be immediately available. A separate, sterile syringe and needle or a sterile disposable unit should be used for each patient to prevent the transmission of other infectious agents from person to person. Needles should be disposed of properly and should not be recapped. As with any vaccine, if administered to immunosuppressed persons, including those receiving immunosuppressive therapy, the expected immune response may not be obtained. **Drug Interactions:** HAVRIX may be given concurrently with Hib conjugate vaccines in children 15 to 18 months of age (see CLINICAL PHARMACOLOGY in full prescribing information and ADVERSE REACTIONS). The safety of HAVRIX given concomitantly with INFANRIX has been evaluated (see ADVERSE REACTIONS). Insufficient data are available to assess the immune response of a fourth dose of DTaP vaccine when administered with HAVRIX. There are limited data to assess the concomitant use of HAVRIX with other vaccines. (See Immune Response to Concomitantly Administered Vaccines in full prescribing information.)

**Carcinogenesis, Mutagenesis, Impairment of Fertility:** HAVRIX has not been evaluated for its carcinogenic potential, mutagenic potential, or potential for impairment of fertility. **Pregnancy:** Pregnancy Category C. Animal reproduction studies have not been conducted with HAVRIX. It is also not known whether HAVRIX can cause fetal harm when administered to a pregnant woman or can affect reproduction capacity. Give HAVRIX to a pregnant woman only if clearly needed. **Nursing Mothers:** It is not known whether HAVRIX is excreted in human milk. Because many drugs are excreted in human milk, use caution when administering HAVRIX to a nursing woman. **Pediatric Use:** The safety and effectiveness of HAVRIX have been evaluated in 20,436 subjects 1 year to 18 years of age. (See CLINICAL PHARMACOLOGY and DOSAGE AND ADMINISTRATION in full prescribing information.) The safety and effectiveness of HAVRIX have not been established in subjects less than 12 months of age. **Geriatric Use:** Clinical studies of HAVRIX did not include sufficient numbers of subjects 65 years of age and older to determine whether they respond differently from younger subjects. Other reported clinical experience has not identified differences in overall safety between these subjects and younger adult subjects.

**ADVERSE REACTIONS:** As with all pharmaceuticals, however, it is possible that expanded commercial use of the vaccine could reveal rare adverse events. The adverse events most frequently reported by volunteers in clinical trials were injection-site soreness (56% of adults; 21% of children); headache (14% of adults; less than 9% of children). Other solicited and unsolicited events are listed below:

**Incidence 1% to 10% of Injections:** ***Local Reactions at Injection Site:*** Induration, redness, swelling; ***Body as a Whole:*** Fatigue, fever (>37.5°C), malaise; ***Gastrointestinal:*** Anorexia, nausea.

**Incidence <1% of Injections:** ***Local Reaction at Injection Site:*** Hematoma; ***Dermatologic:*** Pruritus, rash, urticaria; ***Respiratory:*** Pharyngitis, other upper respiratory tract infections; ***Gastrointestinal:*** Abdominal pain, diarrhea, dysgeusia, vomiting; ***Musculoskeletal:*** Arthralgia, elevation of creatine phosphokinase, myalgia; ***Hematologic:*** Lymphadenopathy; ***Central Nervous System:*** Hypertonic episode, insomnia, photophobia, vertigo.

**Additional safety data:** Safety data were obtained from 2 additional sources in which large populations were vaccinated. In an outbreak setting in which 4,930 individuals were immunized with a single dose of either 720 EL.U. or 1440 EL.U. of HAVRIX, the vaccine was well tolerated and no serious adverse events due to vaccination were reported. Overall, less than 10% of vaccinees reported solicited general adverse events following the vaccine. The most common solicited local adverse event was pain at the injection site, reported in 22.3% of subjects at 24 hours and decreasing to 2.4% by 72 hours.

In a field efficacy trial, 19,037 children received the 360 EL.U. dose of HAVRIX. The most commonly reported adverse events were injection-site pain (9.5%) and tenderness (8.1%), reported following first doses of HAVRIX. Other adverse events were infrequent and comparable to the control vaccine ENGERIX-B® [Hepatitis B Vaccine (Recombinant)].

In subjects with chronic liver disease, HAVRIX was safe and well tolerated. Local injection site reactions were similar among all 4 groups, and no serious adverse reactions attributed to the vaccine were reported in subjects with chronic liver disease.

***Safety Data for HAVRIX 720 EL.U./0.5 mL Beginning at 11 Months of Age:*** In the multicenter study described under CLINICAL PHARMACOLOGY in full prescribing information, parents/guardians recorded local and general symptoms on diary cards for 4 days (Days 0 to 3) after vaccination. In the 3 groups of children who received HAVRIX alone, safety data were available for 723 children who received 1,396 documented doses of HAVRIX. Additional safety data were available for 181 children who received HAVRIX coadministered with INFANRIX and Hib conjugate vaccine. Most adverse events were mild and transient. The frequencies of solicited local and systemic reactions following receipt of HAVRIX were monitored during the 4-day observation period.

The following rates of solicited adverse events in children who received their first dose of HAVRIX alone at between 11 and 25 months of age were observed. Among local reactions: pain was reported in 15-21% of subjects, redness in 16-21%, swelling in 8% of subjects. Among general reactions, irritability was reported in 24-36% of subjects, loss of appetite in 16-19% of subjects, drowsiness in 15-17% of subjects and fever >39.5°C in ≤2% of subjects. Following the booster dose of HAVRIX, among local reactions: pain was reported in 16-21% of subjects, redness in 17-22%, swelling in 8-10% of subjects. Following the booster dose of HAVRIX, among general reactions, irritability was reported in 19-29% of subjects, loss of appetite in 14-18% of subjects, drowsiness in 13-16% of subjects and fever >39.5°C in ≤1% of subjects.

Drowsiness and loss of appetite occurred at statistically significantly higher rates in subjects 15 to 18 months of age who received Hib conjugate vaccine (PRP-T) and INFANRIX concomitantly with HAVRIX as compared to subjects 15 to 18 months of age who received Hib conjugate vaccine (PRP-T) and INFANRIX (drowsiness 34% and 22% and loss of appetite 29% and 19%, respectively). With the exception of fever (>39.5°C), the solicited general symptoms occurred at statistically significantly higher rates in subjects 15 to 18 months of age who received Hib conjugate vaccine (PRP-T) and INFANRIX concomitantly with HAVRIX as compared to subjects 15 to 18 months of age who received HAVRIX alone (irritability 46% and 30%, drowsiness 34% and 17%, and loss of appetite 29% and 17%, respectively).

A febrile seizure was reported in an 18-month old subject two days after receiving the first dose of HAVRIX. Other serious adverse events reported during the course of this study included a single case each of hepatitis ~5 months post dose 1, insulin-dependent diabetes ~4 months post dose 1, and Kawasaki's disease ~3 1/2 months post dose 1. The association of these events with vaccination is unknown.

**Postmarketing Reports:** Rare voluntary reports of adverse events in people receiving HAVRIX since market introduction include the following: ***Local:*** Localized edema; ***Body as a Whole:*** Anaphylaxis/anaphylactoid reactions, somnolence; ***Cardiovascular:*** Syncope; ***Hepatobiliary:*** Jaundice, hepatitis; ***Dermatologic:*** Erythema multiforme, hyperhydrosis, angioedema; ***Respiratory:*** Dyspnea; ***Hematologic:*** Lymphadenopathy, thrombocytopenia; ***Central Nervous System:*** Convulsions, encephalopathy, dizziness, neuropathy, myelitis, paresthesia, Guillain-Barré syndrome, multiple sclerosis; ***Other:*** Congenital abnormality.

The US Department of Health and Human Services has established the Vaccine Adverse Events Reporting System (VAERS) to accept reports of suspected adverse events after the administration of any vaccine, including, but not limited to, the reporting of events required by the National Childhood Vaccine Injury Act of 1986. The toll-free number for VAERS forms and information is 1-800-822-7967. Reporting forms may also be obtained at the VAERS website at www.vaers.org.

Manufactured by **GlaxoSmithKline Biologicals**, Rixensart, Belgium

Distributed by **GlaxoSmithKline**, Research Triangle Park, NC 27709



BRS-HA:L20

**References: 1.** Centers for Disease Control and Prevention. Recommended childhood and adolescent immunization schedule—United States, 2006. *MMWR.* 2006;54(51&52):Q1–Q4. **2.** Bell BP, Shapiro CN. Hepatitis A virus. In: Long SS, Pickering LK, Prober CG, eds. *Principles and Practice of Pediatric Infectious Diseases.* 2nd ed. Philadelphia, Pa: Churchill Livingstone; 2003:1188–1192. **3.** Armstrong GL, Bell BP. Hepatitis A virus infection in the United States: model-based estimates and implication for childhood immunizations. *Pediatrics.* 2002;109:839–845.



Printed in USA. HAP283R0 February 2006

**ACIP *recommends vaccination of children against hepatitis A**[1]**

# *Hepatitis A spreads FAST... especially among children*[2,3]

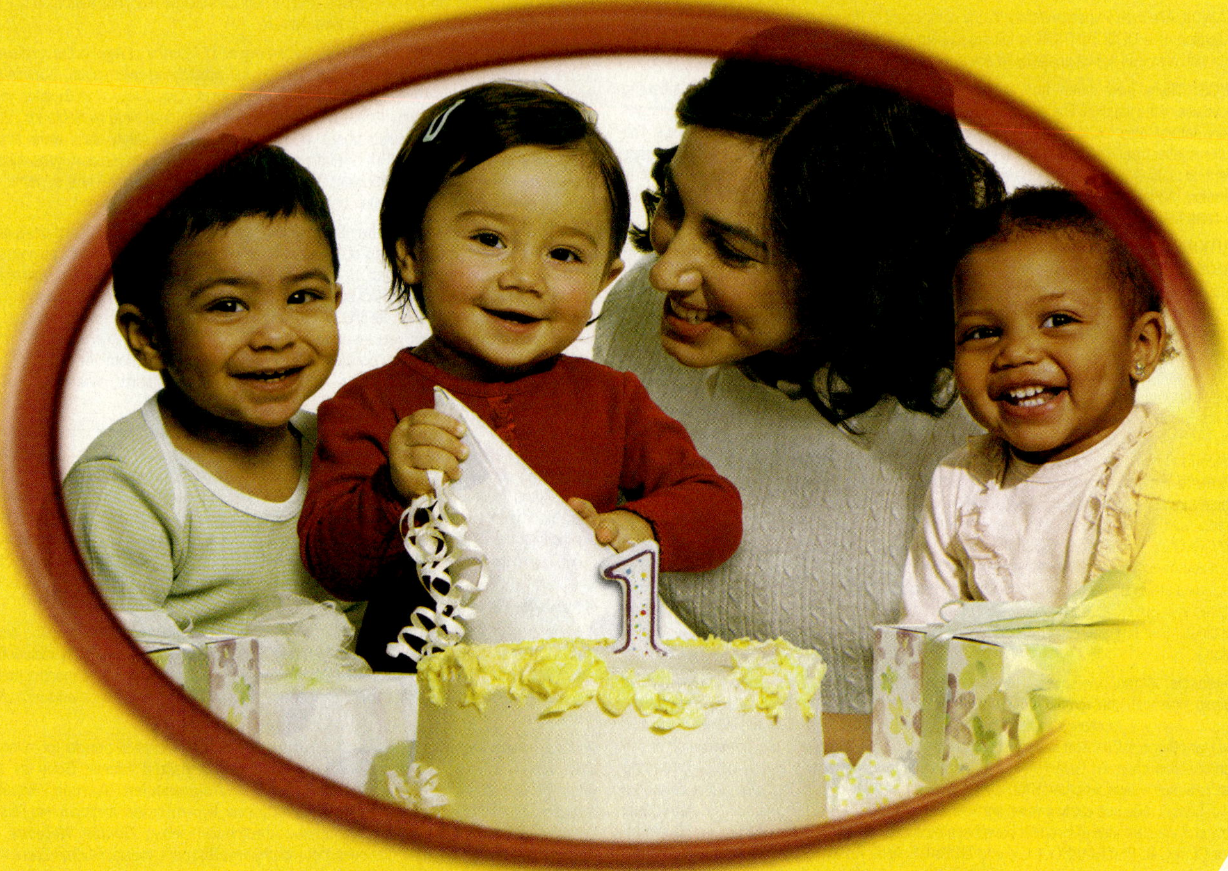

## *HAVRIX provides excellent protection*

HAVRIX is indicated for active immunization against hepatitis A virus in children 12 months of age and older.

## Important Safety Information

In clinical trials, the most common solicited adverse events were injection-site soreness and headache.

Greater incidences of general adverse events were observed in subjects who received HAVRIX at the same time as Hib conjugate and DTaP vaccines. As with any vaccine, rare adverse events may occur. (See Adverse Reactions section of the Prescribing Information for HAVRIX for potential side effects.) HAVRIX is contraindicated in people with hypersensitivity to any component of the vaccine, including neomycin.

* Advisory Committee on Immunization Practices recommends routine nationwide vaccination against hepatitis A in all children 1–2 years of age.

**Please see references and brief summary of complete prescribing information for HAVRIX on adjacent page.**

HAVRIX is a registered trademark of GlaxoSmithKline.

Manufactured by **GlaxoSmithKline Biologicals**, Rixensart, Belgium
Distributed by **GlaxoSmithKline**, Research Triangle Park, NC 27709

gsk GlaxoSmithKline Vaccines

**Havrix®**
**Hepatitis A Vaccine, Inactivated**

# ARCHIVES OF PEDIATRICS & ADOLESCENT MEDICINE

APRIL 2006 VOLUME 160, NUMBER 4 PAGES 329-456


## ARTICLES


**Effects of Media Violence on Health-Related Outcomes Among Young Men** 341
*Sonya S. Brady, PhD; Karen A. Matthews, PhD*

**Short-term and Long-term Effects of Violent Media on Aggression in Children and Adults** 348
*Brad J. Bushman, PhD; L. Rowell Huesmann, PhD*

**Disentangling the Relation Between Television Viewing and Cognitive Processes in Children With Attention-Deficit/Hyperactivity Disorder and Comparison Children** 354
*Ignacio David Acevedo-Polakovich, MS; Elizabeth Pugzles Lorch, PhD; Richard Milich, PhD; Rebecca D. Ashby, BA*

**Does Children's Screen Time Predict Requests for Advertised Products? Cross-sectional and Prospective Analyses** 363
*Lisa J. Chamberlain, MD, MPH; Yun Wang, MS; Thomas N. Robinson, MD, MPH*

**Development and Validation of a Smoking Media Literacy Scale for Adolescents** 369
*Brian A. Primack, MD, EdM; Melanie A. Gold, DO; Galen E. Switzer, PhD; Renee Hobbs, EdD; Stephanie R. Land, PhD; Michael J. Fine, MD, MSc*

**Television Viewing and Risk of Sexual Initiation by Young Adolescents** 375
*Sarah L. Ashby, MD, MS; Christine M. Arcari, PhD, MPH; M. Bruce Edmonson, MD, MPH*

**Social Interactions in Adolescent Television Viewing** 383
*Jason Fletcher, MS*

**Is Television Viewing Associated With Social Isolation? Roles of Exposure Time, Viewing Context, and Violent Content** 387
*David S. Bickham, PhD; Michael Rich, MD, MPH*

**Parental Media Mediation Styles for Children Aged 2 to 11 Years** 395
*Shari Barkin, MD; Edward Ip, PhD; Irma Richardson, MHA; Sara Klinepeter; Stacia Finch, MA; Marina Krcmar, PhD*

**Content and Ratings of Mature-Rated Video Games** 402
*Kimberly M. Thompson, ScD; Karen Tepichin, BS; Kevin Haninger, AB*

**Metabolic and Physiologic Responses to Video Game Play in 7- to 10-Year-Old Boys** 411
*Xuewen Wang, MSEd; Arlette C. Perry, PhD*

**Television Exposure and Overweight Risk in Preschoolers** 417
*Julie C. Lumeng, MD; Sahand Rahnama, BS; Danielle Appugliese, MPH; Niko Kaciroti, PhD; Robert H. Bradley, PhD*

**Parental Weight Status as a Moderator of the Relationship Between Television Viewing and Childhood Overweight** 425
*Elizabeth A. Vandewater, PhD; Xuan Huang, MA*

**A Content Analysis of Health and Physical Activity Messages Marketed to African American Children During After-School Television Programming** 432
*Corliss Wilson Outley, PhD; Abdissa Taddese*

**When Children Eat What They Watch: Impact of Television Viewing on Dietary Intake in Youth** 436
*Jean L. Wiecha, PhD; Karen E. Peterson, ScD, RD; David S. Ludwig, MD, PhD; Juhee Kim, ScD; Arthur Sobol, MA; Steven L. Gortmaker, PhD*


## EDITORIALS


**Media as a Public Health Issue** 445
*Dimitri A. Christakis, MD, MPH; Frederick J. Zimmerman, PhD*

**Exploring the Impact of Media on Children: The Challenges That Remain** 446
*Amy B. Jordan, PhD*

**The Effect of Media on Children and Adolescents: It's About Time** 448
*Donald Shifrin, MD*

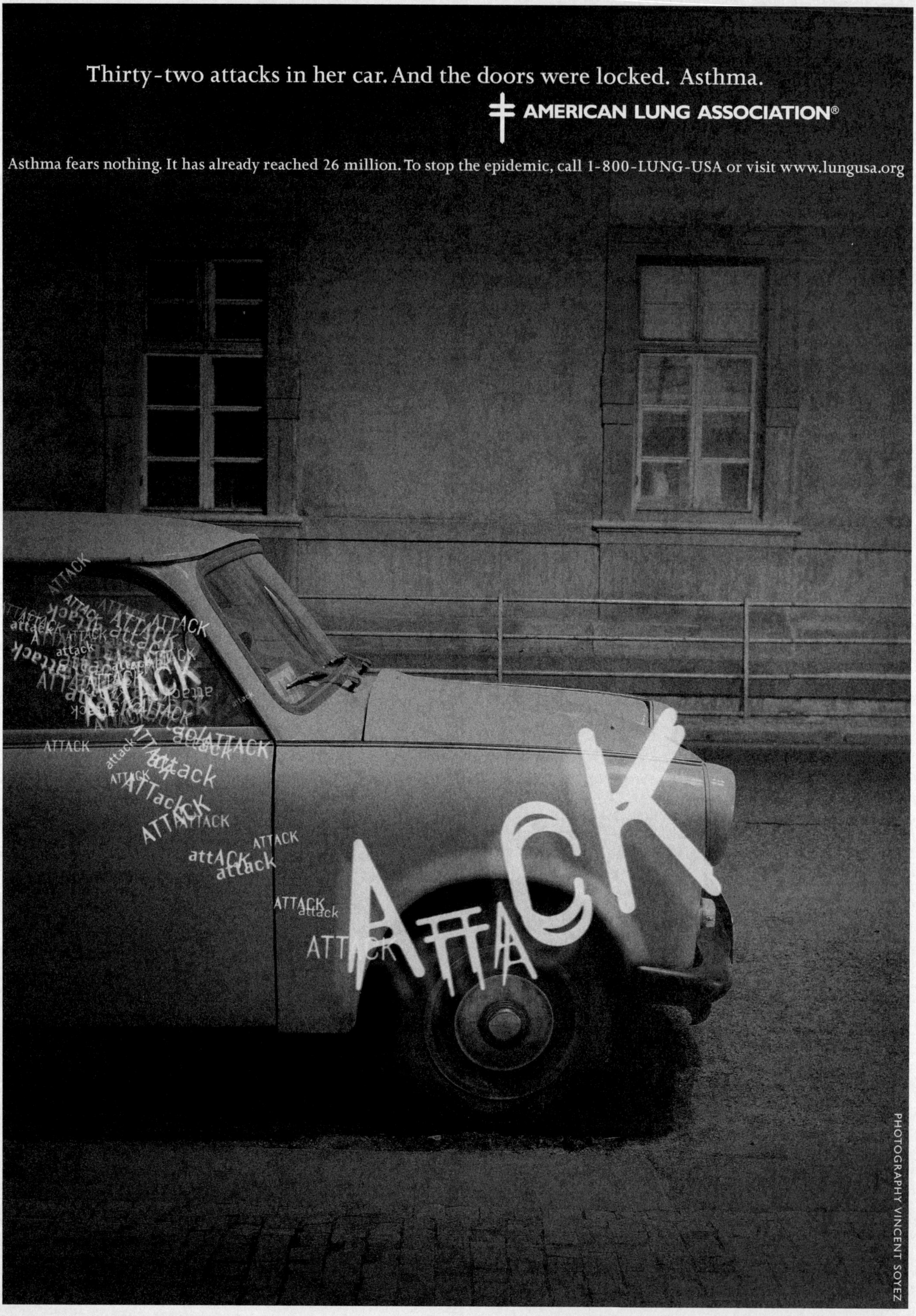
Thirty-two attacks in her car. And the doors were locked. Asthma.
AMERICAN LUNG ASSOCIATION®
Asthma fears nothing. It has already reached 26 million. To stop the epidemic, call 1-800-LUNG-USA or visit www.lungusa.org
ATTACK
PHOTOGRAPHY VINCENT SOYEZ

ARCHIVES OF PEDIATRICS & ADOLESCENT MEDICINE

## THE PEDIATRIC FORUM

**Needle Aspiration and Intramuscular Vaccination** 451
*Moshe Ipp, MD; Jonathan Sam, BSc; Patricia C. Parkin, MD*

**Cranberry Therapy for Children's Urinary Tract Infections** 451
*Kathi J. Kemper, MD, MPH*

**Dismissing Families: A Slippery Slope** 452
*Kathi J. Kemper, MD, MPH; Caryl J. Guth, MD*

**Dismissing Families: A Critical Issue** 452
*Michael P. Elston, MD, MS*

**In Reply** 452
*Erin Flanagan-Klygis, MD; Joel Frader, MD; Lisa Sharp, PhD*

**Advocacy by Any Other Name Would Smell as Sweet** 453
*Lisa J. Chamberlain, MD, MPH; Lee M. Sanders, MD, MPH; John I. Takayama, MD, MPH*

## REGULAR DEPARTMENTS

**This Month in *Archives of Pediatrics & Adolescent Medicine*** 340

**Announcements** 347, 352, 360, 401

**Classified Advertising** 455

**Journal Advertiser Index** 455

**Contact Information** 456

**Instructions for authors and the author and subject indexes are available on our Web site: http://www.archpediatrics.com. If you do not have access to the Web, contact Suzanne Shuey at (206) 685-3573.**

### About the Cover

Photographer: Danielle Zerr, MD, Seattle, Wash.

# ARCHIVES OF PEDIATRICS & ADOLESCENT MEDICINE


**Mission Statement:** *The Archives of Pediatrics & Adolescent Medicine* is a monthly, peer-reviewed journal for physicians and other health care professionals who contribute to the health of children and adolescents. The *Archives* provides an open forum for dialogue on a full range of clinical, scientific, advocacy, and humanistic issues relevant to the care of pediatric patients from infancy through young adulthood. The *Archives* is a vehicle for increased attention to adolescent health, the education of pediatric health care professionals, and disease prevention and health promotion. The *Archives* publishes original studies, editorials, reviews by experts, practice commentaries, case quizzes, and updates on clinical science and practice management. The Pediatric Forum provides our readers with opportunities to express their views. *Archives* incorporates *AJDC*, the oldest journal in US pediatric literature, which originated in 1911.



JAMA & ARCHIVES JOURNALS
American Medical Association

All articles published, including editorials, letters, and book reviews, represent the opinions of the authors and do not reflect the policy of the American Medical Association, the Editorial Board, or the institution with which the author is affiliated, unless this is clearly specified.

**PROFESSIONAL BRIEF SUMMARY-CONSULT PACKAGE INSERT FOR FULL PRESCRIBING INFORMATION.**
03-5435-Rev. July, 2005
(Nos. 3769, 3771, 6151)

# Omnicef® (cefdinir) capsules
# Omnicef® (cefdinir) for oral suspension

**Rx only**

## INDICATIONS AND USAGE

To reduce the development of drug-resistant bacteria and maintain the effectiveness of OMNICEF and other antibacterial drugs, OMNICEF should be used only to treat or prevent infections that are proven or strongly suspected to be caused by susceptible bacteria. When culture and susceptibility information are available, they should be considered in selecting or modifying antibacterial therapy. In the absence of such data, local epidemiology and susceptibility patterns may contribute to the empiric selection of therapy.

OMNICEF (cefdinir) capsules and OMNICEF (cefdinir) for oral suspension are indicated for the treatment of patients with mild to moderate infections caused by susceptible strains of the designated microorganisms in the conditions listed below.

### Adults and Adolescents

**Community-Acquired Pneumonia** caused by *Haemophilus influenzae* (including β-lactamase producing strains), *Haemophilus parainfluenzae* (including β-lactamase producing strains), *Streptococcus pneumoniae* (penicillin-susceptible strains only), and *Moraxella catarrhalis* (including β-lactamase producing strains).

**Acute Exacerbations of Chronic Bronchitis** caused by *Haemophilus influenzae* (including β-lactamase producing strains), *Haemophilus parainfluenzae* (including β-lactamase producing strains), *Streptococcus pneumoniae* (penicillin-susceptible strains only), and *Moraxella catarrhalis* (including β-lactamase producing strains).

**Acute Maxillary Sinusitis** caused by *Haemophilus influenzae* (including β-lactamase producing strains), *Streptococcus pneumoniae* (penicillin-susceptible strains only), and *Moraxella catarrhalis* (including β-lactamase producing strains).

**NOTE:** For information on use in pediatric patients, see **Pediatric Use** and **DOSAGE AND ADMINISTRATION**.

**Pharyngitis/Tonsillitis** caused by *Streptococcus pyogenes*.

**NOTE:** Cefdinir is effective in the eradication of *S. pyogenes* from the oropharynx. Cefdinir has not, however, been studied for the prevention of rheumatic fever following *S. pyogenes* pharyngitis/tonsillitis. Only intramuscular penicillin has been demonstrated to be effective for the prevention of rheumatic fever.

**Uncomplicated Skin and Skin Structure Infections** caused by *Staphylococcus aureus* (including β-lactamase producing strains) and *Streptococcus pyogenes*.

### Pediatric Patients

**Acute Bacterial Otitis Media** caused by *Haemophilus influenzae* (including β-lactamase producing strains), *Streptococcus pneumoniae* (penicillin-susceptible strains only), and *Moraxella catarrhalis* (including β-lactamase producing strains).

**Pharyngitis/Tonsillitis** caused by *Streptococcus pyogenes*.

**NOTE:** Cefdinir is effective in the eradication of *S. pyogenes* from the oropharynx. Cefdinir has not, however, been studied for the prevention of rheumatic fever following *S. pyogenes* pharyngitis/tonsillitis. Only intramuscular penicillin has been demonstrated to be effective for the prevention of rheumatic fever.

**Uncomplicated Skin and Skin Structure Infections** caused by *Staphylococcus aureus* (including β-lactamase producing strains) and *Streptococcus pyogenes*.

## CONTRAINDICATIONS

OMNICEF (cefdinir) is contraindicated in patients with known allergy to the cephalosporin class of antibiotics.

## WARNINGS

**BEFORE THERAPY WITH OMNICEF (CEFDINIR) IS INSTITUTED, CAREFUL INQUIRY SHOULD BE MADE TO DETERMINE WHETHER THE PATIENT HAS HAD PREVIOUS HYPERSENSITIVITY REACTIONS TO CEFDINIR, OTHER CEPHALOSPORINS, PENICILLINS, OR OTHER DRUGS. IF CEFDINIR IS TO BE GIVEN TO PENICILLIN-SENSITIVE PATIENTS, CAUTION SHOULD BE EXERCISED BECAUSE CROSS-HYPERSENSITIVITY AMONG β-LACTAM ANTIBIOTICS HAS BEEN CLEARLY DOCUMENTED AND MAY OCCUR IN UP TO 10% OF PATIENTS WITH A HISTORY OF PENICILLIN ALLERGY. IF AN ALLERGIC REACTION TO CEFDINIR OCCURS, THE DRUG SHOULD BE DISCONTINUED. SERIOUS ACUTE HYPERSENSITIVITY REACTIONS MAY REQUIRE TREATMENT WITH EPINEPHRINE AND OTHER EMERGENCY MEASURES, INCLUDING OXYGEN, INTRAVENOUS FLUIDS, INTRAVENOUS ANTIHISTAMINES, CORTICOSTEROIDS, PRESSOR AMINES, AND AIRWAY MANAGEMENT, AS CLINICALLY INDICATED.**

**Pseudomembranous colitis has been reported with nearly all antibacterial agents, including cefdinir, and may range in severity from mild- to life-threatening. Therefore, it is important to consider this diagnosis in patients who present with diarrhea subsequent to the administration of antibacterial agents.**

Treatment with antibacterial agents alters the normal flora of the colon and may permit overgrowth of clostridia. Studies indicate that a toxin produced by *Clostridium difficile* is a primary cause of "antibiotic-associated colitis."

After the diagnosis of pseudomembranous colitis has been established, appropriate therapeutic measures should be initiated. Mild cases of pseudomembranous colitis usually respond to drug discontinuation alone. In moderate to severe cases, consideration should be given to management with fluids and electrolytes, protein supplementation, and treatment with an antibacterial drug clinically effective against *Clostridium difficile*.

## PRECAUTIONS

### General

Prescribing OMNICEF in the absence of a proven or strongly suspected bacterial infection or a prophylactic indication is unlikely to provide benefit to the patient and increases the risk of the development of drug-resistant bacteria.

As with other broad-spectrum antibiotics, prolonged treatment may result in the possible emergence and overgrowth of resistant organisms. Careful observation of the patient is essential. If superinfection occurs during therapy, appropriate alternative therapy should be administered.

Cefdinir, as with other broad-spectrum antimicrobials (antibiotics), should be prescribed with caution in individuals with a history of colitis.

In patients with transient or persistent renal insufficiency (creatinine clearance <30 mL/min), the total daily dose of OMNICEF should be reduced because high and prolonged plasma concentrations of cefdinir can result following recommended doses.

### Information for Patients

Patients should be counseled that antibacterial drugs including OMNICEF should only be used to treat bacterial infections. They do not treat viral infections (e.g., the common cold). When OMNICEF is prescribed to treat a bacterial infection, patients should be told that although it is common to feel better early in the course of therapy, the medication should be taken exactly as directed. Skipping doses or not completing the full course of therapy may (1) decrease the effectiveness of the immediate treatment and (2) increase the likelihood that bacteria will develop resistance and will not be treatable by OMNICEF or other antibacterial drugs in the future.

Antacids containing magnesium or aluminum interfere with the absorption of cefdinir. If this type of antacid is required during OMNICEF therapy, OMNICEF should be taken at least 2 hours before or after the antacid.

Iron supplements, including multivitamins that contain iron, interfere with the absorption of cefdinir. If iron supplements are required during OMNICEF therapy, OMNICEF should be taken at least 2 hours before or after the supplement.

Iron-fortified infant formula does not significantly interfere with the absorption of cefdinir. Therefore, OMNICEF for Oral Suspension can be administered with iron-fortified infant formula.

Diabetic patients and caregivers should be aware that the oral suspension contains 2.86 g of sucrose per teaspoon.

### Drug Interactions

**Antacids:** (aluminum- or magnesium-containing): Concomitant administration of 300-mg cefdinir capsules with 30 mL Maalox® TC suspension reduces the rate ($C_{max}$) and extent (AUC) of absorption by approximately 40%. Time to reach $C_{max}$ is also prolonged by 1 hour. There are no significant effects on cefdinir pharmacokinetics if the antacid is administered 2 hours before or 2 hours after cefdinir. If antacids are required during OMNICEF therapy, OMNICEF should be taken at least 2 hours before or after the antacid.

**Probenecid:** As with other β-lactam antibiotics, probenecid inhibits the renal excretion of cefdinir, resulting in an approximate doubling in AUC, a 54% increase in peak cefdinir plasma levels, and a 50% prolongation in the apparent elimination $t_{1/2}$.

**Iron Supplements and Foods Fortified With Iron:** Concomitant administration of cefdinir with a therapeutic iron supplement containing 60 mg of elemental iron (as $FeSO_4$) or vitamins supplemented with 10 mg of elemental iron reduced extent of absorption by 80% and 31%, respectively. If iron supplements are required during OMNICEF therapy, OMNICEF should be taken at least 2 hours before or after the supplement.

The effect of foods highly fortified with elemental iron (primarily iron-fortified breakfast cereals) on cefdinir absorption has not been studied.

Concomitantly administered iron-fortified infant formula (2.2 mg elemental iron/6 oz) has no significant effect on cefdinir pharmacokinetics. Therefore, OMNICEF for Oral Suspension can be administered with iron-fortified infant formula.

There have been reports of reddish stools in patients receiving cefdinir. In many cases, patients were also receiving iron-containing products. The reddish color is due to the formation of a nonabsorbable complex between cefdinir or its breakdown products and iron in the gastrointestinal tract.

### Drug/Laboratory Test Interactions

A false-positive reaction for ketones in the urine may occur with tests using nitroprusside, but not with those using nitroferricyanide. The administration of cefdinir may result in a false-positive reaction for glucose in urine using Clinitest®, Benedict's solution, or Fehling's solution. It is recommended that glucose tests based on enzymatic glucose oxidase reactions (such as Clinistix® or Tes-Tape®) be used. Cephalosporins are known to occasionally induce a positive direct Coombs' test.

### Carcinogenesis, Mutagenesis, Impairment of Fertility

The carcinogenic potential of cefdinir has not been evaluated. No mutagenic effects were seen in the bacterial reverse mutation assay (Ames) or point mutation assay at the hypoxanthine-guanine phosphoribosyltransferase locus (HGPRT) in V79 Chinese hamster lung cells. No clastogenic effects were observed *in vitro* in the structural chromosome aberration assay in V79 Chinese hamster lung cells or *in vivo* in the micronucleus assay in mouse bone marrow. In rats, fertility and reproductive performance were not affected by cefdinir at oral doses up to 1000 mg/kg/day (70 times the human dose based on mg/kg/day, 11 times based on $mg/m^2$/day).

### Pregnancy - Teratogenic Effects

**Pregnancy Category B:** Cefdinir was not teratogenic in rats at oral doses up to 1000 mg/kg/day (70 times the human dose based on mg/kg/day, 11 times based on $mg/m^2$/day) or in rabbits at oral doses up to 10 mg/kg/day (0.7 times the human dose based on mg/kg/day, 0.23 times based on $mg/m^2$/day). Maternal toxicity (decreased body weight gain) was observed in rabbits at the maximum tolerated dose of 10 mg/kg/day without adverse effects on offspring. Decreased body weight occurred in rat fetuses at $\geq$ 100 mg/kg/day, and in rat offspring at $\geq$ 32 mg/kg/day. No effects were observed on maternal reproductive parameters or offspring survival, development, behavior, or reproductive function.

There are, however, no adequate and well-controlled studies in pregnant women. Because animal reproduction studies are not always predictive of human response, this drug should be used during pregnancy only if clearly needed.

### Labor and Delivery

Cefdinir has not been studied for use during labor and delivery.

### Nursing Mothers

Following administration of single 600-mg doses, cefdinir was not detected in human breast milk.

### Pediatric Use

Safety and efficacy in neonates and infants less than 6 months of age have not been established. Use of cefdinir for the treatment of acute maxillary sinusitis in pediatric patients (age 6 months through 12 years) is supported by evidence from adequate and well-controlled studies in adults and adolescents, the similar pathophysiology of acute sinusitis in adult and pediatric patients, and comparative pharmacokinetic data in the pediatric population.

### Geriatric Use

Efficacy is comparable in geriatric patients and younger adults. While cefdinir has been well-tolerated in all age groups, in clinical trials geriatric patients experienced a lower rate of adverse events, including diarrhea, than younger adults. Dose adjustment in elderly patients is not necessary unless renal function is markedly compromised.

## ADVERSE EVENTS

**Clinical Trials - OMNICEF Capsules (Adult and Adolescent Patients):**

In clinical trials, 5093 adult and adolescent patients (3841 US and 1252 non-US) were treated with the recommended dose of cefdinir capsules (600 mg/day). Most adverse events were mild and self-limiting. No deaths or permanent disabilities were attributed to cefdinir. One hundred forty-seven of 5093 (3%) patients discontinued medication due to adverse events thought by the investigators to be possibly, probably, or definitely associated with cefdinir therapy. The discontinuations were primarily for gastrointestinal disturbances, usually diarrhea or nausea. Nineteen of 5093 (0.4%) patients were discontinued due to rash thought related to cefdinir administration.

In the US, the following adverse events were thought by investigators to be possibly, probably, or definitely related to cefdinir capsules in multiple-dose clinical trials (N = 3841 cefdinir-treated patients):

**ADVERSE EVENTS ASSOCIATED WITH CEFDINIR CAPSULES US TRIALS IN ADULT AND ADOLESCENT PATIENTS (N=3841)[a]**

| | | |
|---|---|---|
| Incidence ≥ 1% | Diarrhea | 15% |
| | Vaginal moniliasis | 4% of women |
| | Nausea | 3% |
| | Headache | 2% |
| | Abdominal pain | 1% |
| | Vaginitis | 1% of women |
| Incidence <1% but >0.1% | Rash | 0.9% |
| | Dyspepsia | 0.7% |
| | Flatulence | 0.7% |
| | Vomiting | 0.7% |
| | Abnormal stools | 0.3% |
| | Anorexia | 0.3% |
| | Constipation | 0.3% |
| | Dizziness | 0.3% |
| | Dry mouth | 0.3% |
| | Asthenia | 0.2% |
| | Insomnia | 0.2% |
| | Leukorrhea | 0.2% of women |
| | Moniliasis | 0.2% |
| | Pruritus | 0.2% |
| | Somnolence | 0.2% |

[a] 1733 males, 2108 females

The following laboratory value changes of possible clinical significance, irrespective of relationship to therapy with cefdinir, were seen during clinical trials conducted in the US:

**LABORATORY VALUE CHANGES OBSERVED WITH CEFDINIR CAPSULES US TRIALS IN ADULT AND ADOLESCENT PATIENTS (N=3841)**

| | | |
|---|---|---|
| Incidence ≥ 1% | ↑ Urine leukocytes | 2% |
| | ↑ Urine protein | 2% |
| | ↑ Gamma-glutamyltransferase[a] | 1% |
| | ↓ Lymphocytes, ↑ Lymphocytes | 1%, 0.2% |
| | ↑ Microhematuria | 1% |
| Incidence <1% but >0.1% | ↑ Glucose[a] | 0.9% |
| | ↑ Urine glucose | 0.9% |
| | ↑ White blood cells, ↓ White blood cells | 0.9%, 0.7% |
| | ↑ Alanine aminotransferase (ALT) | 0.7% |
| | ↑ Eosinophils | 0.7% |
| | ↑ Urine specific gravity, ↓ Urine specific gravity[a] | 0.6%, 0.2% |
| | ↓ Bicarbonate[a] | 0.6% |
| | ↑ Phosphorus, ↓ Phosphorus[a] | 0.6%, 0.3% |
| | ↑ Aspartate aminotransferase (AST) | 0.4% |
| | ↑ Alkaline phosphatase | 0.3% |
| | ↑ Blood urea nitrogen (BUN) | 0.3% |
| | ↓ Hemoglobin | 0.3% |
| | ↑ Polymorphonuclear neutrophils (PMNs), ↓ PMNs | 0.3%, 0.2% |
| | ↑ Bilirubin | 0.2% |
| | ↑ Lactate dehydrogenase[a] | 0.2% |
| | ↑ Platelets | 0.2% |
| | ↑ Potassium[a] | 0.2% |
| | ↑ Urine pH[a] | 0.2% |

[a] N<3841 for these parameters

**Clinical Trials - OMNICEF for Oral Suspension (Pediatric Patients):**

In clinical trials, 2289 pediatric patients (1783 US and 506 non-US) were treated with the recommended dose of cefdinir suspension (14 mg/kg/day). Most adverse events were mild and self-limiting. No deaths or permanent disabilities were attributed to cefdinir. Forty of 2289 (2%) patients discontinued medication due to adverse events considered by the investigators to be possibly, probably, or definitely associated with cefdinir therapy. Discontinuations were primarily for gastrointestinal disturbances, usually diarrhea. Five of 2289 (0.2%) patients were discontinued due to rash thought related to cefdinir administration.

In the US, the following adverse events were thought by investigators to be possibly, probably, or definitely related to cefdinir suspension in multiple-dose clinical trials (N=1783 cefdinir-treated patients):

**ADVERSE EVENTS ASSOCIATED WITH CEFDINIR SUSPENSION US TRIALS IN PEDIATRIC PATIENTS (N=1783)[a]**

| | | |
|---|---|---|
| Incidence ≥ 1% | Diarrhea | 8% |
| | Rash | 3% |
| | Vomiting | 1% |
| Incidence <1% but >0.1% | Cutaneous moniliasis | 0.9% |
| | Abdominal pain | 0.8% |
| | Leukopenia[b] | 0.3% |
| | Vaginal moniliasis | 0.3% of girls |
| | Vaginitis | 0.3% of girls |
| | Abnormal stools | 0.2% |
| | Dyspepsia | 0.2% |
| | Hyperkinesia | 0.2% |
| | Increased AST[b] | 0.2% |
| | Maculopapular rash | 0.2% |
| | Nausea | 0.2% |

[a] 977 males, 806 females

[b] Laboratory changes were occasionally reported as adverse events.

NOTE: In both cefdinir- and control-treated patients, rates of diarrhea and rash were higher in the youngest pediatric patients. The incidence of diarrhea in cefdinir-treated patients ≤2 years of age was 17% (95/557) compared with 4% (51/1226) in those >2 years old. The incidence of rash (primarily diaper rash in the younger patients) was 8% (43/557) in patients ≤2 years of age compared with 1% (8/1226) in those >2 years old.

The following laboratory value changes of possible clinical significance, irrespective of relationship to therapy with cefdinir, were seen during clinical trials conducted in the US:

**LABORATORY VALUE CHANGES OF POSSIBLE CLINICAL SIGNIFICANCE OBSERVED WITH CEFDINIR SUSPENSION US TRIALS IN PEDIATRIC PATIENTS (N=1783)**

| | | |
|---|---|---|
| Incidence ≥ 1% | ↑ Lymphocytes, ↓ Lymphocytes | 2%, 0.8% |
| | ↑ Alkaline phosphatase | 1% |
| | ↓ Bicarbonate[a] | 1% |
| | ↑ Eosinophils | 1% |
| | ↑ Lactate dehydrogenase | 1% |
| | ↑ Platelets | 1% |
| | ↑ PMNs, ↓ PMNs | 1%, 1% |
| | ↑ Urine protein | 1% |
| Incidence <1% but >0.1% | ↑ Phosphorus, ↓ Phosphorus | 0.9%, 0.4% |
| | ↑ Urine pH | 0.8% |
| | ↓ White blood cells, ↑ White blood cells | 0.7%, 0.3% |
| | ↓ Calcium[a] | 0.5% |
| | ↓ Hemoglobin | 0.5% |
| | ↑ Urine leukocytes | 0.5% |
| | ↑ Monocytes | 0.4% |
| | ↑ AST | 0.3% |
| | ↑ Potassium[a] | 0.3% |
| | ↑ Urine specific gravity, ↓ Urine specific gravity | 0.3%, 0.1% |
| | ↓ Hematocrit[a] | 0.2% |

[a] N=1387 for these parameters

**Postmarketing Experience**

The following adverse experiences and altered laboratory tests, regardless of their relationship to cefdinir, have been reported during extensive postmarketing experience, beginning with approval in Japan in 1991: Stevens-Johnson syndrome, toxic epidermal necrolysis, exfoliative dermatitis, erythema multiforme, erythema nodosum, serum sickness-like reactions, conjunctivitis, stomatitis, acute hepatitis, cholestasis, fulminant hepatitis, hepatic failure, jaundice, increased amylase, shock, anaphylaxis, facial and laryngeal edema, feeling of suffocation, acute enterocolitis, bloody diarrhea, hemorrhagic colitis, melena, pseudomembranous colitis, pancytopenia, granulocytopenia, leukopenia, thrombocytopenia, idiopathic thrombocytopenic purpura, hemolytic anemia, acute respiratory failure, asthmatic attack, drug-induced pneumonia, eosinophilic pneumonia, idiopathic interstitial pneumonia, fever, acute renal failure, nephropathy, bleeding tendency, coagulation disorder, disseminated intravascular coagulation, upper GI bleed, peptic ulcer, ileus, loss of consciousness, allergic vasculitis, possible cefdinir-diclofenac interaction, cardiac failure, chest pain, myocardial infarction, hypertension, involuntary movements, and rhabdomyolysis.

**Cephalosporin Class Adverse Events**

The following adverse events and altered laboratory tests have been reported for cephalosporin-class antibiotics in general:

Allergic reactions, anaphylaxis, Stevens-Johnson syndrome, erythema multiforme, toxic epidermal necrolysis, renal dysfunction, toxic nephropathy, hepatic dysfunction including cholestasis, aplastic anemia, hemolytic anemia, hemorrhage, false-positive test for urinary glucose, neutropenia, pancytopenia, and agranulocytosis. Pseudomembranous colitis symptoms may begin during or after antibiotic treatment (see **WARNINGS**).

Several cephalosporins have been implicated in triggering seizures, particularly in patients with renal impairment when the dosage was not reduced (see **OVERDOSAGE**). If seizures associated with drug therapy occur, the drug should be discontinued. Anticonvulsant therapy can be given if clinically indicated.

## OVERDOSAGE

Information on cefdinir overdosage in humans is not available. In acute rodent toxicity studies, a single oral 5600-mg/kg dose produced no adverse effects. Toxic signs and symptoms following overdosage with other β-lactam antibiotics have included nausea, vomiting, epigastric distress, diarrhea, and convulsions. Hemodialysis removes cefdinir from the body. This may be useful in the event of a serious toxic reaction from overdosage, particularly if renal function is compromised.

**Rx only**

Ref: 03-5435-Rev. July, 2005
(Nos. 3769, 3771, 6151)



05J-034-L150-2 **MASTER**

Manufactured by:
**CEPH** International Corporation
Carolina, Puerto Rico 00986

Under License of:
astellas
Astellas Pharma Inc.
Tokyo, Japan

For:
**Abbott Laboratories**
North Chicago, IL 60064, U.S.A.

06A-034-N494-1
Printed in U.S.A.

## Does Children's Screen Time Predict Requests for Advertised Products?

The average child will see more than 40 000 television commercials each year, in addition to frequent product placements in television shows and movies. In a diverse sample of third- and fourth-grade students, Chamberlain and colleagues found that children who report more screen media exposure at the beginning of the third grade would report more requests for advertised toys, food, and drinks through the end of the fourth grade than those with less screen time. Third-graders had nearly 23 hours of reported screen media use per week. This study supports efforts to limit the exposure of children to product advertisements.

See page 363

## When Children Eat What They Watch

Wiecha and colleagues studied 548 students (mean age, 11.7 years) from 5 schools in Massachusetts and observed them for nearly 2 years. Each additional hour of television viewing was associated with 167 additional calories per day, with increases in consumption of foods commonly advertised on television. Although children and youth are encouraged to watch what they eat, many youth appear to eat what they watch and in the process increase their risk for excessive energy intake.

See page 436

## Content and Ratings of Mature-Rated Video Games

During the last 5 years, the average time spent playing video games by 8- to 18-year-olds nearly doubled. While the mature (M) rating of video games should lead to restrictions on children's exposure to the content in these games, the limited existing data suggest that many children younger than 17 years play M-rated games. In a random sample of M-rated video games available in 2004, all involved intentional acts of violence, which accounted for more than one third of game play time. All of the games rewarded or required the player to injure human characters. An average of 145 characters died per hour of game play. One third of the games had sexual themes and two thirds used profanity an average of 17 times per hour. Nearly all of the teen-rated games depicted violence as well. Children's exposure to violence from these games is potentially enormous.

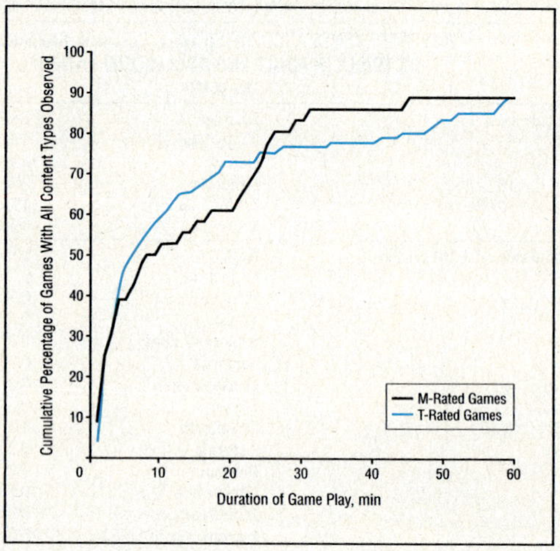


Cumulative percentage of video games with all content types observed by duration of game play.

See page 402

## Television Exposure and Overweight Risk in Preschoolers

The relationship between television viewing and risk of being overweight has been most thoroughly described for school-aged children. Lumeng and colleagues studied a national sample of 1016 children in preschool. Six percent of the children were overweight by 36 months of age and 10% by 54 months. More than two thirds of the children were exposed to 2 or more hours of television per day. Television exposure predicted overweight status at 36 months but not at 54 months.

See page 417

# Effects of Media Violence on Health-Related Outcomes Among Young Men

*Sonya S. Brady, PhD; Karen A. Matthews, PhD*

**Objective:** To test the effects of media violence exposure on blood pressure, negative affect, hostile social information processing, uncooperative behavior, and attitudes toward health risk behaviors among young men varying in lifetime violence exposure within the home and community.

**Design:** Experimental laboratory study.

**Setting:** University campus situated within an urban environment.

**Participants:** One hundred male undergraduates aged 18 to 21 years.

**Intervention:** Men who had previously reported differing amounts of lifetime home and community violence were randomly assigned to play *The Simpsons: Hit and Run* (low-violence condition) or *Grand Theft Auto III* (high-violence condition).

**Main Outcome Measures:** Systolic and diastolic blood pressure; negative affect; hostile social information processing; uncooperative behavior; and permissive attitudes toward violence, alcohol use, marijuana use, and sexual activity without condom use.

**Results:** Men randomly assigned to play *Grand Theft Auto III* exhibited greater increases in diastolic blood pressure from a baseline rest period to game play, greater negative affect, more permissive attitudes toward using alcohol and marijuana, and more uncooperative behavior in comparison with men randomly assigned to play *The Simpsons*. Only among participants with greater exposure to home and community violence, play of *Grand Theft Auto III* led to elevated systolic blood pressure in comparison with play of *The Simpsons* (mean, 13 vs 5 mm Hg).

**Conclusions:** Media violence exposure may play a role in the development of negative attitudes and behaviors related to health. Although youth growing up in violent homes and communities may become more physiologically aroused by media violence exposure, all youth appear to be at risk for potentially negative outcomes.

*Arch Pediatr Adolesc Med. 2006;160:341-347*

EXPERIMENTAL STUDIES CONSISTENTLY show that media violence increases blood pressure, negative emotions, and aggressive behavior in the immediate aftermath of exposure, including physical assault (hitting, kicking, choking, wrestling), in samples of children and younger adolescents and willingness to inflict electric shock or loud aversive noises on a peer in samples of older adolescents and young adults.[1] Results from the few existing longitudinal survey studies suggest that greater exposure to television and media violence in childhood increases the occurrence of meaningful aggression-related outcomes and criminality well into young adulthood,[2-5] even after statistically controlling for potential confounds, such as early aggressive behavior, family socioeconomic status, parenting characteristics, and community safety.[4,5]

Anderson and Bushman[6] have integrated previous influential theories of aggression[7-9] into a comprehensive framework for understanding human aggression. Their General Aggression Model posits that characteristics of the situation (eg, media violence exposure) influence the internal state of an individual, including cognitions (eg, proviolent attitudes), affect (eg, anger), and arousal (eg, increased blood pressure). Internal states in turn influence appraisals (eg, interpreting others' actions as hostile) and decision processes (eg, choosing to aggress). Repeated violence exposure may lead to the development of a hostile, aggressive personality.

One less understood issue is whether media violence exposure influences risky health behaviors and social interactions more broadly than aggression-related outcomes. In addition to modeling aggression, violence models general risk taking and disregard for the well-being of others. The General Aggression Model suggests that media violence exposure may increase the likelihood that individuals engage in impulsive rather than thoughtful courses of action.[6] Although a consistent body of research links real-world violence exposure to adolescent substance use and sexual risk tak-

**Author Affiliations:** University of Pittsburgh (Drs Brady and Matthews), Pittsburgh, Pa. Dr Brady is now a postdoctoral fellow in the Health Psychology Program at the University of California, San Francisco.

ing,[10-16] to our knowledge, only 1 study has examined the association between media violence exposure and such behaviors, and this study yielded mixed results. Male youth aged 11 to 25 years who watched television programs involving contact sports and realistic crime (eg, *COPS*) reported higher levels of risk behaviors (eg, alcohol and other drug use), while those who watched violent drama (eg, *NYPD Blue*) reported lower levels.[17] Real-world violence exposure[18,19] and media violence exposure[1,20,21] are linked with hostile appraisals and aggressive behavior, but research has not addressed whether violence exposure influences social behaviors in ways that do not directly involve aggression, such as the decision whether to cooperate or compete with a peer.

A second less understood issue is whether some youth are at particular risk for experiencing adverse outcomes when exposed to media violence. Huesmann and colleagues[22] have conceptualized societal "cultures of violence" as a potentially important moderator of media violence effects. Acute exposure to media violence may activate aggressive patterns of thought, affect, and behavior more strongly among individuals who are accustomed to aggressive styles of interaction and who have potentially developed more aggressive attitudes, appraisals of others' actions, and behavioral scripts as a result. In a comprehensive review of children's adjustment to real-world violence, Margolin and Gordis[23] highlighted the need to examine the cumulative effects of different types of violence exposure (eg, family, community) as well as unique effects. Previous studies have not tested whether exposure to violence within the home and/or community interacts with media violence exposure to influence outcomes.

The present study examines the effects of acute media violence exposure and lifetime home and community violence exposure on cognitive-behavioral, affective, and physiological health outcomes within the context of a quasi-experimental study design. Young men exposed to differing amounts of lifetime violence were randomly assigned to play a video game high or low in violent content. Consistent with the General Aggression Model,[6] we hypothesized that both home and community and media violence exposure would be associated with greater increases in blood pressure during game play, greater negative affect and more permissive attitudes toward violence immediately after game play, and more hostile social information processing during a laboratory task subsequent to game play. Because violence models general risk taking and disregard for the well-being of others, we also hypothesized that home and community and media violence exposure would be associated with more permissive attitudes toward health risk behavior and with greater uncooperative behavior. Finally, we hypothesized that effects of the media violence condition would be greater among those young men high in lifetime home and community violence exposure.

## METHODS

### STUDY DESIGN

We recruited 100 participants from a pool of 180 undergraduate men aged 18 to 21 years who completed a survey of violence exposure and engagement in harmful health behaviors. We decided to conduct the present laboratory experiment on men because young men are known to have greater exposure to violent media in comparison with young women.[24]

Participants identified their ethnicity as white/Caucasian (n=83), black/African American (n=10), Asian/Asian American (n=4), and Hispanic/Latino (n=2). One participant declined to identify his ethnicity. In some studies, individuals of black ethnicity have exhibited greater stress-related increases in blood pressure in comparison with individuals of white ethnicity.[25-27] All but 1 of the black participants were in the highest tertile for home and community violence exposure, raising the possibility that effects of lifetime violence exposure would be confounded with ethnicity. We thus included a dichotomous ethnicity variable (white/Caucasian or minority) as a covariate in supplemental analyses.

The university institutional review board approved all parts of the study protocol and participants provided their informed consent. We matched pairs of men on ethnicity and lifetime home and community violence exposure tertile and randomly assigned them to the high- or low-violence video game. All participants began their laboratory visit by watching a relaxing video about Hawaii for 10 minutes. They then viewed 4 minutes of videotaped game play demonstrating the "mission" they would be asked to complete, followed by 10 minutes of video game play. We made blood pressure readings at minutes 5, 3, and 1 of the 10-minute resting baseline period and minutes 10, 7.5, 5, and 2.5 during game play. After game play, participants completed an affect checklist and a measure of attitudes toward harmful health behaviors and violence. In 2 subsequent tasks administered in counterbalanced order, participants watched a videotaped social scenario and responded to a structured clinical interview and then engaged in a game during which they could cooperate or compete with a confederate. At the end of the study, participants completed a paper-and-pencil measure asking them to rate features of the video game. We reimbursed participants for their time.

## MEASURES

### Previous Violence Exposure

Participants completed the Community Experiences Questionnaire[18] during the survey, prior to their laboratory visit. The Community Experiences Questionnaire contains items assessing direct victimization (11 items [eg, hit/punched/slapped; coerced through violence/threats]) and witnessed victimization (14 items [eg, robbery; gunshots]). Participants indicated whether each item had occurred never (0), once (1), a few times (2), or lots of times (3) and indicated whether they had experienced each item within the home and within their community (including school and work). Violence exposure scores were summed to create total overall violence ($\alpha = .90$), total community violence ($\alpha = .89$), and total home violence ($\alpha = .82$) scales. Because of slight positive skew, home violence exposure was transformed by taking the square root of the original variable.

During the survey, participants estimated the typical number of hours per week they spent playing video games during grades 7 through 9 (mean [SD], 11.0 [11.9] hours per week ), grades 10 through 12 (mean [SD], 10.1 [10.1] hours per week), and college (mean [SD], 6.6 [7.3] hours per week). We created a composite score by weighting each estimation according to recency of period (1, 2, or 3) and summing across scores. Because of positive skew, this composite score was transformed by taking the square root of the original variable. The resulting variable was examined as a covariate in supplemental analyses.

### Video Games and Manipulation Check

We randomly assigned participants to play a video game high in violence, *Grand Theft Auto III*, or a video game comparatively low in violence, *The Simpsons: Hit and Run*. Both games involve driving through a virtual city to complete various missions. Participants randomly assigned to play *Grand Theft Auto III* played the role of a criminal and were instructed by a member of the mafia to "introduce a bat" to the face of a drug dealer who was supplying drugs to prostitutes employed by the mafia. Participants randomly assigned to play *The Simpsons: Hit and Run* played the role of Homer Simpson and were instructed by Homer's wife, Marge, to deliver daughter Lisa's science project to school before Principal Skinner arrived and Lisa's science project would be marked late.

All participants began their mission in the same game location as that shown in the videotape prior to game play. Participants were instructed to complete the mission they had just viewed and to play the game "however you would like" in any remaining time after completing the mission. The percentage of participants able to complete the *Grand Theft Auto III* and *Simpsons* missions in the allotted 10-minute period was 78% and 96%, respectively. Only 1 person appeared not to attempt any part of his mission. The mean (SD) time spent engaging in mission-related game play was 5 minutes, 24 seconds (2 minutes, 34 seconds) for *Grand Theft Auto III* and 4 minutes, 42 seconds (1 minute, 21 seconds) for *The Simpsons*. Thus, virtually all participants completed the mission or spent a substantial amount of time attempting to complete the mission as instructed.

As a manipulation check, participants completed a paper-and-pencil Video Game Rating Sheet allowing them to rate features of the game on a 7-point Likert scale (1, "not at all" to 7, "very").[28,29] Participants perceived *Grand Theft Auto III* to be more violent in content (mean, 6.0 vs 3.1; $t=10.8$; $P<.001$) and graphics (mean, 5.6 vs 2.4; $t=12.8$; $P<.001$) in comparison with *The Simpsons: Hit and Run*. Ratings of difficulty, enjoyability, and frustration did not significantly differ between games. Participants perceived *Grand Theft Auto III* to be slightly more exciting and faster in action than *The Simpsons: Hit and Run* (mean differences were <1 scale point). Within-game correlations between ratings of excitement and fast action were both 0.50. We summed ratings of excitement and fast action to create a composite score and included the score as a covariate in supplemental analyses.

### Physiological Measures

We monitored systolic (SBP) and diastolic blood pressure using an IBS Model SD-700A automated blood pressure monitor (IBS Corp, Waltham, Mass) with a standard occluding cuff placed on the participant's left arm. We averaged all measures taken during a particular period. Participants' resting SBP ranged from 96 to 136 mm Hg (mean [SD], 113 [9] mm Hg), while resting diastolic blood pressure ranged between 41 to 84 mm Hg (mean [SD] 61 [9] mm Hg). Increases in physiological parameters from the baseline rest period to playing the video game were all significantly different from zero (**Table 1**). Change scores from the baseline rest period to playing the video game were regressed on the baseline rest measure to control for potential "ceiling effects" among individuals with greater resting blood pressures. These residualized change scores were analyzed in subsequent analyses.

### Laboratory-Assessed Negative Affect

Immediately after video game play, we measured negative affect with the Reduced Profile of Mood States.[30] The 9-item negative affect score ($\alpha=.79$) is the sum of 3 affective subscores (anxiety, depression, and anger). Because of slight positive skew, scores were transformed by computing the square root of the original variable.

### Permissive Attitudes Toward Violence and Other Harmful Health Behaviors

After video game play, participants completed the Funk et al[31] 15-item Attitudes Towards Violence Scale ($\alpha=.76$). Participants used a 7-point Likert scale (−3, "very harmful to my health to +3, "very helpful to my health") to indicate the perceived health benefit or risk of engaging in alcohol use, marijuana use, and sex without use of a condom. Attitudes with greater negative values indicate greater perception of harm.

### Hostile Social Information Processing

Participants watched a videotaped social scenario and responded to a structured clinical interview designed to measure hostile cognitive bias in evaluating the scenario.[32] In the scenario, a teacher alerts his class to his suspicion that some students have cheated and dwells at length on his disappointment in students who have cheated and his pride in students who have earned their test scores. The teacher hands back a high test score to Billy and asks to speak with him at the end of class. Participants imagined that they were Billy and rated the likelihood that the teacher would accuse them of cheating on a 5-point Likert scale (1, "not at all likely" to 5, "very likely").

### Uncooperative Behavior

Participants engaged in a "mixed-motive" game with a confederate, during which they could cooperate or compete to earn points exchangeable for money at the completion of the study (all participants were later given \$5).[33] On each of 30 trials, the participant chose to divide points worth money with his "partner" (in actuality, a preprogrammed computer), either equally by clicking on the "cooperate" box on the computer screen or unequally by clicking on the "compete" box. The "partner" cooperated only 30% of the time, creating a situation that could be construed by the participant as provocation, while also providing an economical incentive for the participant to cooperate (if both the participant and partner chose to compete, both lost the maximum number of points). "Compete" responses were tallied across 30 trials.

### Parental Socioeconomic Status—Covariate

When completing the survey, participants reported the maximum years of education achieved by any parent in their primary household (mean [SD], 16.6 [3.1] years [range, 11-24 years]).

### Association With Deviant Peers—Covariate

During the survey, participants completed a 13-item questionnaire to indicate their association with deviant peers,[34] both for current ($\alpha=.83$) and high school ($\alpha=.84$) friends. The 2 scores ($r=0.65$; $P<.001$) were summed to create an overall composite for association with deviant peers (mean [SD], 35.6 [14.0]). Low scores indicated that few of a participant's friends had ever engaged in any deviant behavior (eg, smoking cigarettes, hitting other people, cheating on tests).

## STATISTICAL ANALYSIS

For each outcome separately, we tested main effects of the media violence condition (dichotomous) and real-world violence exposure (continuous) by including both variables in the first step of a univariate general linear model. When main ef-

**Table 1. Violence Exposure and Outcome Variable Distributions and Correlations***

| | Mean (SD) | Violence Exposure: Total | Violence Exposure: Community | Violence Exposure: Home | Laboratory Video Game Condition (*Grand Theft Auto III* = 1) | Change in Blood Pressure to Game Play: SBP | Change in Blood Pressure to Game Play: DBP | Negative Affect After Game | Permissive Attitudes Toward: Violence | Permissive Attitudes Toward: Alcohol | Permissive Attitudes Toward: Marijuana | Permissive Attitudes Toward: Sexual Activity Without Condom | Hostile Social Information Processing |
|---|---|---|---|---|---|---|---|---|---|---|---|---|---|
| Violence exposure | | | | | | | | | | | | | |
| Total | 26.2 (14.8) | | | | | | | | | | | | |
| Community | 19.2 (10.6) | 0.89† | | | | | | | | | | | |
| Home | 7.1 (7.1) | 0.72† | 0.38† | | | | | | | | | | |
| Laboratory video game condition (*Grand Theft Auto III* = 1) | | −0.01 | −0.02 | −0.03 | | | | | | | | | |
| Change in blood pressure to game play | | | | | | | | | | | | | |
| SBP | 7.4 (8.4) | 0.22‡ | 0.20‡ | 0.13 | 0.22‡ | | | | | | | | |
| DBP | 5.0 (7.6) | 0.02 | 0.03 | −0.06 | 0.22‡ | 0.26§ | | | | | | | |
| Negative affect after game play | 12.9 (3.9) | 0.02 | 0.03 | 0.04 | 0.24‡ | 0.09 | 0.01 | | | | | | |
| Permissive attitudes toward | | | | | | | | | | | | | |
| Violence | 2.0 (0.45) | 0.33§ | 0.33§ | 0.22‡ | −0.01 | 0.02 | −0.03 | 0.22‡ | | | | | |
| Alcohol | −1.1 (0.95) | 0.24‡ | 0.19 | 0.20‡ | 0.24‡ | 0.08 | −0.02 | 0.03 | 0.43† | | | | |
| Marijuana | −1.6 (1.2) | 0.08 | 0.08 | 0.02 | 0.27§ | 0.18 | 0.15 | 0.02 | 0.25‡ | 0.41† | | | |
| Sexual activity without condom | −1.8 (1.0) | 0.08 | 0.17 | −0.07 | 0.08 | −0.14 | 0.02 | −0.08 | 0.21‡ | 0.17 | 0.02 | | |
| Hostile social information processing | 3.5 (1.0) | 0.10 | −0.03 | 0.25‡ | 0.05 | −0.03 | 0.07 | 0.04 | −0.01 | 0.09 | 0.10 | −0.09 | |
| Competitive responses with confederate | 13.6 (4.4) | −0.02 | 0.04 | −0.12 | 0.21‡ | 0.16 | 0.12 | −0.07 | 0.12 | 0.24‡ | 0.15 | 0.20‡ | −0.06 |

Abbreviations: DBP, diastolic blood pressure; SBP, systolic blood pressure.
*Means and standard deviations are based on untransformed variables.
†$P<.001$.
‡$P<.05$.
§$P<.01$.

fects were significant, we calculated 95% confidence intervals (CIs) for mean differences between violence exposure groups based on a median split for the continuous lifetime violence exposure variables. When interaction terms (tested in a second univariate model) were significant, we conducted simple effects tests to determine whether the media violence condition was associated with an outcome within high– and low–home and community violence exposure groups and compared effect sizes within each group using partial $\eta^2$. For all significant main effects and interactions, analyses were performed again with inclusion of covariates (composite rating of video game excitement and fast action, prior experience playing video games, ethnicity, parental socioeconomic status, association with deviant peers). We conducted separate analyses to test the effects of home, community, and total real-world violence exposure. *P* values $\leq .05$ (2-tailed) were considered statistically significant.

## RESULTS

Table 1 presents means and standard deviations of violence exposure and laboratory outcome measures and their intercorrelations. **Table 2** presents correlations between these measures and covariates.

As hypothesized, young men randomly assigned to play *Grand Theft Auto III* exhibited greater changes in SBP (mean difference, 3.58 [95% CI, 0.41-6.75]) and diastolic blood pressure (mean difference, 2.84 [95% CI, 0.29-5.39]), greater negative affect (mean difference, 1.86 [95% CI, 0.34-3.38]), more permissive attitudes toward using alcohol (mean difference, 0.46 [95% CI, 0.09-0.83]) and marijuana (mean difference, 0.62 [95% CI, 0.18-1.06]), and greater uncooperative behavior (mean difference, 1.89 [95% CI, 0.13-3.65]) in comparison with young adults randomly assigned to play *The Simpsons: Hit and Run* (**Table 3**). Contrary to hypothesis, the violent video game condition was not associated with hostile social information processing, permissive attitudes toward violence, and attitudes toward sexual activity without condom use.

Consistent with our hypothesis, greater total home and community violence exposure was associated with greater changes in SBP (mean difference, 3.52 [95% CI, 0.26-6.78]) (Table 3). Domain-specific analyses (Table 1) suggested that community violence exposure, in particular, was associated with greater changes in SBP. Greater total home and community violence exposure was associated with more permissive attitudes toward violence (mean difference, 0.30 [95% CI, 0.13-0.47]) and drinking alcohol (mean difference, 0.42 [95% CI, 0.05-0.79] (Table 3). Associations remained when home and com-

**Table 2. Correlations Between Covariates and Violence Exposure and Outcome Variables**

| | Video Game Excitement/ Fast Action | Ethnic Minority Status (1 = Minority) | Parent Education, y | Prior Experience Playing Video Games | Association With Deviant Peers |
|---|---|---|---|---|---|
| Violence exposure | | | | | |
| Total | 0.06 | 0.22* | −0.09 | 0 | 0.49† |
| Community | 0.08 | 0.18 | 0.10 | −0.03 | 0.48† |
| Home | 0.02 | 0.22* | −0.20* | 0.07 | 0.32‡ |
| Laboratory video game condition (*Grand Theft Auto III* = 1) | 0.28‡ | −0.03 | −0.10 | 0 | 0.06 |
| Change in blood pressure to game play | | | | | |
| SBP | −0.05 | 0.16 | −0.20* | 0.05 | 0.18 |
| DBP | 0.08 | 0 | −0.03 | 0.17 | −0.06 |
| Negative affect after game play | 0.25* | −0.15 | −0.16 | −0.15 | 0.12 |
| Permissive attitudes toward | | | | | |
| Violence | 0.05 | −0.02 | 0.12 | −0.13 | 0.30‡ |
| Alcohol | 0.03 | 0 | 0.10 | −0.06 | 0.29‡ |
| Marijuana | 0 | −0.08 | −0.12 | 0.20* | 0.38† |
| Sexual activity without condom | −0.06 | −0.04 | 0.30‡ | −0.01 | 0.08 |
| Hostile social information processing | 0.14 | −0.05 | 0.01 | −0.12 | 0.08 |
| Competitive responses with confederate | −0.01 | −0.14 | −0.02 | −0.15 | 0.24* |

Abbreviations: See Table 1.
*$P<.05$.
†$P<.001$.
‡$P<.01$.

**Table 3. Means and Standard Deviations of Outcome Variables by Laboratory Media Violence Condition and Total Lifetime Violence Exposure**

| | Low Lifetime Violence, Mean (SD) | | High Lifetime Violence, Mean (SD) | | *F* Test (*P* Value)* | | |
|---|---|---|---|---|---|---|---|
| | GTA III | Simpsons | GTA III | Simpsons | Life Violence | Video Game | Interaction |
| Change in blood pressure to game play† | | | | | | | |
| SBP | 5.0 (6.5) | 6.3 (7.7) | 13.3 (9.6) | 5.4 (7.3) | 5.2 (.02) | 5.4 (.02)‡ | 11.3 (.001)‡ |
| DBP | 6.5 (7.1) | 3.2 (7.2) | 6.2 (8.6) | 4.2 (7.7) | 0.03 (.86) | 4.9 (.03)‡ | 0.46 (.50) |
| Total negative affect after game play§ | 13.4 (3.6) | 11.8 (3.6) | 14.3 (5.2) | 12.2 (2.7) | 0.06 (.80) | 5.7 (.02) | 0.001 (.97) |
| Permissive attitudes toward | | | | | | | |
| Violence | 1.8 (0.33) | 2.0 (0.50) | 2.3 (0.48) | 2.1 (0.38) | 11.5 (.001)‡ | 0.01 (.92) | 2.4 (.12) |
| Alcohol | −1.1 (0.74) | −1.5 (0.93) | −0.58 (1.1) | −1.1 (0.86) | 6.5 (.01) | 6.7 (.01)‡ | 0.01 (.94) |
| Marijuana | −1.4 (1.1) | −2.0 (1.2) | −1.2 (1.0) | −1.8 (1.2) | 0.77 (.38) | 7.7 (.01)‡ | 0.24 (.63) |
| Sexual activity without condom | −1.6 (1.2) | −2.2 (0.87) | −1.8 (1.1) | −1.6 (0.90) | 0.71 (.40) | 0.62 (.43) | 1.97 (.16) |
| Hostile social information processing | 3.3 (1.2) | 3.5 (0.88) | 3.8 (0.85) | 3.4 (1.0) | 0.98 (.32) | 0.26 (.61) | 1.2 (.28) |
| Competitive responses with confederate | 15.2 (3.8) | 11.4 (4.2) | 14.0 (4.6) | 13.8 (4.5) | 0.03 (.87) | 4.5 (.04)‡ | 3.2 (.08) |

Abbreviations: DBP, diastolic blood pressure; GTA III, *Grand Theft Auto III*; SBP, systolic blood pressure; Simpsons, *The Simpsons: Hit and Run*.
**F* test and *P* values for main effects were obtained from analyses without inclusion of the interaction term.
†Residualized change scores from the initial rest period to game play are used in analyses.
‡Finding remained significant after inclusion of covariates: composite rating of video game excitement/fast action, ethnic minority status, parental socioeconomic status, prior experience playing video games, and association with deviant peers.
§Means and standard deviations are presented using the original mood rating scale, ranging from 0 to 45 for total negative affect. The square root of the total negative affect score was used in analyses.

munity violence exposure were examined separately. Domain-specific analyses revealed that greater home violence exposure was associated with more hostile attributions during the social scenario (mean difference, 0.50 [95% CI, 0.11-0.88]). Contrary to hypothesis, real-world violence exposure variables were not associated with negative affect and uncooperative behavior.

Two interactions between lifetime violence exposure variables and media violence condition emerged (Table 3). Within the low–total violence exposure group, the video game condition was not associated with change in SBP, while within the high–total violence exposure group, play of *Grand Theft Auto III* predicted greater changes in SBP than play of *The Simpsons: Hit and Run*. The violent video game condition explained roughly 21% of the variance in SBP change within the high–total violence exposure group and virtually none of the variance in SBP change within the low–total violence exposure group. Interactions between the video game condition and both community and home violence exposure yielded identical patterns to that described for total violence exposure.

Violence exposure within the community interacted with the video game condition to predict hostile attributions during the social scenario ($F=4.0$; $P<.05$). The video game condition was not associated with hostile attributions within the low–community violence exposure group ($F=0.96$; partial $\eta^2=0.02$) but was associated with more hostile attributions within the high–community violence exposure group ($F=3.0$; $P<.10$; partial $\eta^2=0.06$).

Analyses controlling for covariates showed the same pattern of results with few exceptions: the violent video game condition was no longer associated with negative affect; lifetime violence exposure was no longer associated with SBP and alcohol use.

## COMMENT

In response to playing a very popular video game, *Grand Theft Auto III*, young men exhibited increased blood pressure, more negative affect, and more hostile social information processing, consistent with the results of other experimental studies and the General Aggression Model.[1,6] Participants randomly assigned to play *Grand Theft Auto III* also expressed more permissive attitudes toward using alcohol and marijuana and were less cooperative during a subsequent task than participants randomly assigned to play a less violent video game. To our knowledge, the present study is the first experimental study to show that media violence is associated with permissive attitudes toward health risk behaviors that do not directly involve hostility or aggression.

Young men with higher levels of home and community violence exposure may be more susceptible to certain outcomes as a result of media violence exposure. In the present study, media violence exposure was associated with greater SBP and hostile social information processing among participants with greater lifetime violence exposure. The act in *Grand Theft Auto III* that participants were asked to commit (ie, striking another person with a baseball bat) may have appeared more realistic to those who had witnessed or been victimized by violence within the home or community, thus resulting in greater physiological response. Perhaps owing to learning experiences, individuals from violent communities may have greater difficulty imagining a nonhostile interpretation for the ambiguous actions of others after playing a video game that "primes" hostile thought patterns. Main effects of media violence exposure on negative affect, uncooperative behavior, and permissive attitudes toward health risk behavior were also observed in the present study. These findings demonstrate that all young adults, regardless of background, are potentially affected by media violence exposure.

Strengths of the present study include the use of random assignment and the selection of commonly played games, which are likely to increase the generalizability of results. Limitations include the inability to generalize findings beyond young men who were sufficiently advantaged to attend a major public university. In addition, selected video games may have differed in ways other than violence; these differences, rather than violent content, may have influenced outcomes. The finding most vulnerable to this possibility is the link observed between play of *Grand Theft Auto III* and permissive attitudes toward using alcohol and marijuana. Because *Grand Theft Auto III* includes characters who are drug dealers, it is possible that observation of a drug dealer may have relaxed players' attitudes toward alcohol and marijuana use. However, participants randomly assigned to play *Grand Theft Auto III* took a punitive stance against drugs during their "mission" (ie, striking a drug dealer with a baseball bat), raising the possibility that other mechanisms may have been responsible for the relaxing of attitudes toward alcohol and marijuana use (eg, violent content may not only appear to condone aggression but also general risk-taking and law-breaking behavior). The General Aggression Model also suggests that media violence exposure may increase the likelihood that individuals engage in impulsive rather than thoughtful courses of action.[6]

School-based research on young children shows that negative effects of media violence exposure are reduced when use of television and video games are reduced,[35] when attitude-change interventions emphasize the unrealistic nature of media,[36,37] and when parents coview and comment on violent TV programs.[38] Results of the present study suggest that media violence exposure may predispose adolescents and young adults toward greater engagement in general health risk behaviors and toward tension and conflict in social interactions with others. Adolescents and their parents may benefit from media education campaigns.

**Accepted for Publication:** December 22, 2005.
**Correspondence:** Sonya S. Brady, PhD, Health Psychology Program, University of California, San Francisco, 3333 California St, Suite 465, Box 0848, San Francisco, CA 94143-0848 (sonya.brady@ucsf.edu).
**Funding/Support:** This research was supported by Ruth L. Kirschstein National Research Service Award T32 MH019391 and grants HL07852, HL07858, and HL25767 and a professional development award through the University of Pittsburgh Provost's Office, Pittsburgh, Pa.
**Acknowledgment:** We thank Sabrina DellaMea, BS, Heather Koston, BS, Diana Buck, BA, Leslie Mitrik, BS, and Karen Kenyon, BS, for assistance during data collection, entry, and coding. We also thank Adam Rixey, BA, for his skill in playing the 4-minute video game segments that were recorded and shown to participants.

## REFERENCES

1. Anderson CA, Berkowitz L, Donnerstein E, et al. The influence of media violence on youth. *Psychological Sci Public Interest.* 2003;4:81-110.
2. Eron LD, Lefkowitz MM, Huesmann LR, Walder LO. Does television violence cause aggression? *Am Psychol.* 1972;27:253-263.
3. Huesmann LR. Psychological processes promoting the relation between exposure to media violence and aggressive behavior by the viewer. *J Soc Issues.* 1986;42:125-139.
4. Huesmann LR, Moise-Titus J, Podolski C, Eron LD. Longitudinal relations between children's exposure to TV violence and their aggressive and violent behavior in young adulthood: 1977-1992. *Dev Psychol.* 2003;39:201-221.

5. Johnson JG, Cohen P, Smailes EM, Kasen S, Brook JS. Television viewing and aggressive behavior during adolescence and adulthood. *Science*. 2002;295: 2468-2471.
6. Anderson CA, Bushman BJ. Human aggression. *Annu Rev Psychol*. 2002;53: 27-51.
7. Berkowitz L. On the formation and regulation of anger and aggression: a cognitive-neoassociationistic analysis. *Am Psychol*. 1990;45:494-503.
8. Bandura A. Social cognitive theory: an agentic perspective. *Annu Rev Psychol*. 2001;52:1-26.
9. Huesmann LR. The role of social information processing and cognitive schema in the acquisition and maintenance of habitual aggressive behavior. In: Geen RG, Donnerstein E, eds. *Human Aggression: Theories, Research and Implications for Policy*. New York, NY: Academic Press; 1998:73-109.
10. Acierno R, Kilpatrick DG, Resnick H, Saunders B, De Arellano M, Best C. Assault, PTSD, family substance use, and depression as risk factors for cigarette use in youth: findings from the National Survey of Adolescents. *J Trauma Stress*. 2000;13:381-396.
11. Albus KE, Weist MD, Perez-Smith AM. Associations between youth risk behavior and exposure to violence: implications for the provision of mental health services in urban schools. *Behav Modif*. 2004;28:548-564.
12. Berenson AB, Wiemann CM, McCombs S. Exposure to violence and associated health-risk behaviors among adolescent girls. *Arch Pediatr Adolesc Med*. 2001; 155:1238-1242.
13. Kilpatrick DG, Acierno R, Saunders B, Resnick H, Best CL, Schnurr PP. Risk factors for adolescent substance abuse and dependence: data from a national sample. *J Consult Clin Psychol*. 2000;68:19-30.
14. Schwab-Stone ME, Ayers TS, Kasprow W, et al. No safe haven: a study of violence exposure in an urban community. *J Am Acad Child Adolesc Psychiatry*. 1995;34:1343-1352.
15. Silverman JG, Raj A, Mucci LA, Hathaway JE. Dating violence against adolescent girls and associated substance use, unhealthy weight control, sexual risk behavior, pregnancy, and suicidality. *JAMA*. 2001;286:572-579.
16. Sullivan TN, Kung EM, Farrell AD. Relation between witnessing violence and drug use initiation among rural adolescents: parental monitoring and family support as protective factors. *J Clin Child Adolesc Psychol*. 2004;33:488-498.
17. Krcmar M, Greene K. Connections between violent television exposure and adolescent risk taking. *Media Psychology*. 2000;2:195-217.
18. Schwartz D, Proctor LJ. Community violence exposure and children's social adjustment in the school peer group: the mediating roles of emotion regulation and social cognition. *J Consult Clin Psychol*. 2000;68:670-683.
19. Shahinfar A, Kupersmidt JB, Matza LS. The relation between exposure to violence and social information processing among incarcerated adolescents. *J Abnorm Psychol*. 2001;110:136-141.
20. Kirsh SJ, Olczak PV. Violent comic books and perceptions of ambiguous provocation situations. *Media Psychology*. 2000;2:47-62.
21. Bushman BJ, Anderson CA. Violent video games and hostile expectations: a test of the General Aggression Model. *Pers Soc Psychol Bull*. 2002;28:1679-1686.
22. Huesmann LR, Moise JF, Podolski C. The effects of media violence on the development of antisocial behavior. In: Stoff DM, Breiling J, Maser JD, eds. *Handbook of Antisocial Behavior*. New York, NY: John Wiley & Sons, Inc; 1997:181-193.
23. Margolin G, Gordis EB. The effects of family and community violence on children. *Annu Rev Psychol*. 2000;51:445-479.
24. Funk JB. Reevaluating the impact of video games. *Clin Pediatr (Phila)*. 1993;32: 86-90.
25. Dysart JM, Treiber FA, Pflieger K, Davis H, Strong WB. Ethnic differences in the myocardial and vascular reactivity to stress in normotensive girls. *Am J Hypertens*. 1994;7:15-22.
26. Murphy JK, Alpert BS, Moes D, Somes G. Race and cardiovascular reactivity: a neglected relationship. *Hypertension*. 1986;8:1075-1083.
27. Treiber FA, Davis H, Musante L, et al. Ethnicity, gender, family history of myocardial infarction, and hemodynamic responses to laboratory stressors in children. *Health Psychol*. 1993;12:6-15.
28. Anderson CA, Dill KE. Video games and aggressive thoughts, feelings, and behavior in the laboratory and life. *J Pers Soc Psychol*. 2000;78:772-790.
29. Anderson CA, Ford CM. Affect of the game player: short-term effects of highly and mildly aggressive video games. *Pers Soc Psychol Bull*. 1986;12:390-402.
30. Usala PD, Hertog C. Measurement of affective states in adults: evaluation of an adjective rating scale instrument. *Res Aging*. 1989;11:403-426.
31. Funk JB, Elliott R, Urman ML, Flores GT, Mock RM. The Attitudes Towards Violence Scale: a measure for adolescents. *J Interpers Violence*. 1999;14:1123-1136.
32. Chen E, Matthews KA. Development of the Cognitive Appraisal and Understanding of Social Events (CAUSE) videos. *Health Psychol*. 2003;22:106-110.
33. Van Egeren LF, Fabrega H, Thornton DW. Electrocardiographic effects of social stress on coronary-prone (type A) individuals. *Psychosom Med*. 1983;45:195-203.
34. Metzler CW, Noell J, Biglan A, Ary D, Smolkowski K. The social context for risky sexual behavior among adolescents. *J Behav Med*. 1994;17:419-438.
35. Robinson TN, Wilde ML, Navracruz LC, Haydel KF, Varady A. Effects of reducing children's television and video game use on aggressive behavior: a randomized controlled trial. *Arch Pediatr Adolesc Med*. 2001;155:17-23.
36. Huesmann LR, Eron LD, Klein R, Brice P, Fischer P. Mitigating the imitation of aggressive behaviors by children's attitudes about media violence. *J Pers Soc Psychol*. 1983;44:899-910.
37. Rosenkoetter LI, Rosenkoetter SE, Ozretich RA, Acock AC. Mitigating the harmful effects of violent television. *J Appl Dev Psychol*. 2004;25:25-47.
38. Nathanson AI. Identifying and explaining the relationship between parental mediation and children's aggression. *Communic Res*. 1999;26:124-143.

ARTICLE

# Short-term and Long-term Effects of Violent Media on Aggression in Children and Adults

*Brad J. Bushman, PhD; L. Rowell Huesmann, PhD*

**Objectives:** To test whether the results of the accumulated studies on media violence and aggressive behavior are consistent with the theories that have evolved to explain the effects. We tested for the existence of both short-term and long-term effects for aggressive behavior. We also tested the theory-driven hypothesis that short-term effects should be greater for adults and long-term effects should be greater for children.

**Design:** Meta-analysis.

**Participants:** Children younger than 18 years and adults.

**Main Exposures:** Violent media, including TV, movies, video games, music, and comic books.

**Main Outcome Measures:** Measures of aggressive behavior, aggressive thoughts, angry feelings, physiological arousal (eg, heart rate, blood pressure), and helping behavior.

**Results:** Effect size estimates were combined using meta-analytic procedures. As expected, the short-term effects of violent media were greater for adults than for children whereas the long-term effects were greater for children than for adults. The results also showed that there were overall modest but significant effect sizes for exposure to media violence on aggressive behaviors, aggressive thoughts, angry feelings, arousal levels, and helping behavior.

**Conclusions:** The results are consistent with the theory that short-term effects are mostly due to the priming of existing well-encoded scripts, schemas, or beliefs, which adults have had more time to encode. In contrast, long-term effects require the learning (encoding) of scripts, schemas, or beliefs. Children can encode new scripts, schemas, and beliefs via observational learning with less interference and effort than adults.

*Arch Pediatr Adolesc Med. 2006;160:348-352*

THE BODY OF EMPIRICAL RESEARCH linking children's exposure to media violence with subsequent increases in their aggressive and violent behavior was already substantial by the 1970s. The 1972 Surgeon General's Scientific Advisory Committee on Television and Social Behavior report[1] and the National Institute of Mental Health 10-year follow-up report[2] provided widely accessible summaries of this growing body of research. By the 1980s, most child development scholars had accepted the theory that exposure to media violence, at least during some periods of a child's development, increased their risk for aggression.[3] However, it has only been in the 1990s and more recently that meta-analyses have provided systematic summaries of the entire body of research.[4,5] Similarly, it has been during this time that the attention of researchers has turned more toward investigating the processes producing the effects and developing a more coherent theoretical understanding of the effects.[6]

In this article, we describe what we believe are the major psychological processes that account for the relationship between children's exposure to different kinds of violence in their world and the increase in the risk for violence and aggression that this exposure produces. We then use meta-analyses to show that, on the whole, the available empirical data show the patterns one would expect from this theory. Although the focus of this article is on exposure to media violence, the theoretical premise is that the same processes operate when children are exposed to media violence as when they are exposed to violence on the street, in the home, or among their peers.

The psychological processes that link children's exposure to violence with subsequent increases in children's aggressive behaviors can be divided into those that produce more immediate but transient short-term changes in behavior and those that produce more delayed but enduring long-term changes in behavior. Long-term increases in children's aggressive behavior are now generally agreed to be a consequence of the child's learning scripts for aggressive behavior, cognitions supporting aggression, and aggression-promoting emotions through the observation of others behaving violently. This observational learning generally requires the repeated observation of violence. On the other hand, short-term increases in children's aggressive behavior following

**Author Affiliations:** Vrije Universiteit, Amsterdam, the Netherlands (Dr Bushman); and Institute for Social Research, University of Michigan, Ann Arbor (Drs Bushman and Huesmann).

the observation of violence are owing to 3 other quite different psychological processes: (1) the priming of already existing aggressive behavioral scripts, aggressive cognitions, or angry emotional reactions; (2) simple mimicking of aggressive scripts; and (3) changes in emotional arousal stimulated by the observation of violence.

Neuroscientists and cognitive psychologists posit that the human mind acts as an associative network in which ideas are partially activated, or primed, by stimuli that they are associated with.[7] The activation produced by an observed stimulus spreads in the network and moves even remotely related concepts closer to a threshold of influence. Thus, an encounter with an event or object can prime related concepts, ideas, and emotions in a person's memory, even without the person being aware of it.[8] For example, the mere presence of a weapon in a person's visual field can increase aggressive thoughts or behaviors.[9] Seeing people fight activates scripts for behavior related to fighting and other aggressive ideas. Any cognitions, behaviors, or emotions that have ever been linked to an observed violent scene will be activated within milliseconds when that scene is observed.

Human and primate young have an innate tendency to imitate whomever they observe.[10,11] Neuroscientists have discovered "mirror neurons" in primates that seem to promote such processing.[12] Consequently, children who observe (in the media or in the environment around them) others exhibiting a specific aggressive behavior, eg, hitting, are more likely to perform the same aggressive behavior immediately.[11,13,14] Theoretically, the more similar that children think they and the observed model are, the more readily imitation will take place, but the imitation mechanism is so powerful that even fantasy characters are imitated by young children.

Observed violence often consists of high-action sequences that are very arousing for youth as measured by increased heart rate, blood pressure, skin conductance of electricity, and other physiological indices of arousal. To the extent that media violence highly arouses the observer, aggressive behaviors may become more likely in the short run for 2 possible reasons. First, high arousal generated by exposure to violence makes any dominant response tendency more likely to be carried out in the short term. Consequently, the child with aggressive tendencies behaves even more aggressively.[15,16] Second, when a child is highly aroused (eg, by viewing violence), a mild specific emotion (eg, mild anger) experienced some time later may be felt more severely (eg, intense anger) than otherwise because some of the emotional response stimulated by the violent media presentation is misattributed as being due to the provocation. This process is called excitation transfer.[17,18]

By observational learning, we mean the process through which behavioral scripts, world schemas, and normative beliefs become encoded in a child's mind simply as a consequence of the child observing others. Observational learning is a powerful extension of imitation in which logical induction and abstraction are used to encode complex representations. For example, extensive observation of violence biases children's world schemas toward hostility, and they then attribute more hostility to others' actions,[19,20] which in turn increases the likelihood of children behaving aggressively themselves.[21] Similarly, through repeated observation of real-life aggressive models and aggressive models portrayed in the media, children develop normative beliefs that aggression is appropriate, and they acquire social scripts for how to behave aggressively. Whereas short-term mimicry requires only 1 exposure to an observed behavior, long-term observational learning usually (but not always) requires repeated exposures. The more that the child's attention is riveted on the observed behavior, the fewer are the number of repetitions needed. However, numerous other factors besides attention affect the extent of the learning. The current conceptions of this process have grown out of the convergence of social learning theory[13] with more recent theories of social information processing.[19,22-25] The more that the child identifies with the observed people and the more that the observed scripts for behavior are rewarded and portrayed as appropriate, the more firmly will the scripts be encoded and the more likely it is that more general beliefs about such behaviors will be extracted and encoded.[13,26]

This observational learning interacts with conditioning by family and peers to build behavioral scripts and social cognitions that are highly resistant to change. The reinforcements that a child receives from imitating a positive or negative behavior strongly influence the likelihood of that behavior persisting.[15,26] Similarly, if the world schemas and normative beliefs that a child acquires through observing others (again, in real life and in the media) lead to valuable outcomes for the child, they will become more firmly encoded and more resistant to change.[27]

The long-term effects that exposure to violence has on children also involve the vicarious conditioning of emotional reactions. Through classical conditioning, fear or anger can become linked with specific stimuli after only a few exposures.[28-30] These emotions influence behavior in social settings away from the media source through stimulus generalization. A child may then react with inappropriate fear or anger in a novel situation that is similar to one that the child has observed in the media. Repeated exposure to emotionally arousing media can also lead to habituation of certain natural emotional reactions. This process is often called *desensitization*, and it has been used to explain a reduction in distress-related physiological reactivity to media portrayals of violence. Indeed, violent scenes do become less arousing over time,[31] and brief exposure to media violence can reduce physiological reactions to real-world violence.[32] Behaviors that might seem unusual to the child viewer at first will begin to seem more normative after repeated presentations. For example, most persons seem to have an innate negative emotional response to observing blood and violence as evidenced by increased heart rates, perspiration, and self-reports of discomfort that often accompany such exposure. However, with repeated exposure, this negative emotional response habituates, and the child becomes desensitized. The child can then think about and plan proactive aggressive acts without experiencing negative affect.

For both adults and children, we expect that there will be positive relationships between their degree of exposure to media violence and their subsequent short-term displays of aggressive behaviors, emotions, and ideas. Priming, imitation, and excitation transfer would all contribute to these effects.

These short-term effects should be more pronounced for adults than for children because priming depends on the prior

**Table. Effects of Media Violence on Aggressive and Helpful Behavior, Aggressive Thoughts, Angry Feelings, and Physiological Arousal Levels for All of the Studies Combined***

| Measure | Average Correlation (95% CI) | Studies, No. | Participants, No. | Fail-Safe N |
|---|---|---|---|---|
| Aggressive behavior | 0.19 (0.19 to 0.20) | 262 | 48 430 | 151 984 |
| Helpful behavior | −0.08 (−0.11 to −0.04) | 59 | 3243 | 157 |
| Aggressive thoughts | 0.18 (0.17 to 0.19) | 140 | 22 967 | 34 447 |
| Angry feelings | 0.27 (0.24 to 0.30) | 50 | 4838 | 8654 |
| Physiological arousal | 0.26 (0.20 to 0.31) | 27 | 1356 | 927 |

Abbreviation: CI, confidence interval.
*Physiological arousal includes, for example, increased heart rate and blood pressure.

existence of a well-encoded network of aggressive scripts, beliefs, and schemas. The development and elaboration of such networks require time and repeated learning experiences, so adults are more likely to possess well-elaborated, rich networks of associations involving aggressive scripts, beliefs, and schemas. Consequently, observations of violence by adults will prime a set of related aggressive constructs larger than that for children and will prime them more rapidly.

There should be positive relationships for both adults and children between their degree of exposure to media violence earlier in life and their subsequent long-term displays of aggressive scripts, beliefs, and schemas. Observational learning of scripts, schemas, and beliefs and the desensitization of negative emotional reactions to violence are the 2 processes that contribute to these effects.

These long-term effects should be more pronounced for children than for adults because observational learning and desensitization both depend on the observer having a mind that is readily modifiable. The younger the children are, the more susceptible they should be to encoding aggressive scripts, schemas, or beliefs through observational learning; also, the younger the children are, the more quickly their emotional responses to observing violence should habituate. For adults, learning new scripts, schemas, and beliefs requires replacing old ones, and the process is likely to take longer and require the observation of more powerful scenes. In the rest of this article, we examine whether meta-analyses of the accumulated empirical data on media violence are consistent with these predictions.

## METHODS

### DATA SOURCES

To retrieve relevant studies, we searched the PsychINFO database from 1887 (starting date) to 2000 using the terms *violen** or *aggress** as well as the terms *TV*, *televis**, *film*, *movie*, *screen*, *music*, *radio*, *video*, *video game*, *computer game*, *cartoon*, *comic*, *pornograph**, *erotic**, *news*, *book*, *magazine*, or *sport*. The asterisk is a wild card that gives all of the possible forms of the word (eg, *aggress** searches for the terms *aggress*, *aggressed*, *aggression*, *aggressive*, *aggressively*, and *aggressor*). We restricted the search to empirical studies involving human participants. We also searched the reference sections of previous meta-analyses of violent media and aggression.[4,33-35]

### STUDY SELECTION

Two inclusion criteria were used. First, the study needed to include a measure or manipulation of violent media exposure (eg, TV programs, films, video games, music, and comic books). Second, the study needed to include a measure of aggressive behavior, aggressive cognition, aggressive affect, physiological arousal, or helping behavior. A total of 431 studies involving 68 463 participants met these criteria. There were 264 studies involving 50 312 children and 167 studies involving 18 151 adults.

### CODED CHARACTERISTICS

The following characteristics were coded for each study: (1) type of study (ie, longitudinal study, laboratory experiment, field experiment, correlational study); (2) participant age (ie, children aged <18 years, adults); and (3) type of dependent variable (ie, aggressive behavior, aggressive thoughts, angry feelings, physiological arousal, helping behavior).

Each article was coded by one of us (B.J.B.). To assess coding reliability, an additional 3 judges each coded a random sample of 50 articles. A different random sample (with replacement) was selected for each judge. There was perfect agreement among judges on coded variables.

### META-ANALYTIC APPROACH

The effect size index was the correlation coefficient. Because the distribution of the correlation coefficient is not normal unless the population correlation coefficient equals 0, we applied Fisher $z$ transformation to each correlation coefficient before pooling them. Each $z$ score was weighted by the inverse of its variance (ie, N–3). Thus, larger studies had more weight computing the average correlation. Then, we transformed $z$ scores back to correlations. We also computed a 95% confidence interval for the average correlation. If the 95% confidence interval excludes the value 0, the correlation is significantly different from 0.

We used both fixed- and random-effects analyses, although the 2 approaches yielded the same pattern of results. Thus, we report only the fixed-effects analyses in this article.

In a meta-analysis, it is difficult to find unpublished studies. Studies with nonsignificant effects are often not published; they end up in file drawers rather than in peer-reviewed journals. If studies in file drawers had been published, the average correlation would be smaller. "Fail-safe N" is the number of studies with nonsignificant correlations that are needed to reduce the average correlation to 0.[36] If the fail-safe N is large, then the results are probably not affected by publication bias.

## RESULTS

### OVERALL EFFECTS OF MEDIA VIOLENCE

As shown in the **Table**, there were significant, if modest, overall positive effect sizes showing that exposure to media violence was positively related to subsequent aggressive behavior, aggressive ideas, arousal, and anger. Additionally, there was a significant negative effect of exposure to violence on subsequent helping behavior. Because the confidence intervals exclude the value 0, the average correlations were all significantly different from 0. Also, the fail-safe N values are quite large, indicating that the file drawer problem is not that serious.

## AGE DIFFERENCES IN SHORT-TERM AND LONG-TERM VIOLENT MEDIA EFFECTS

We expected the short-term effects of violent media on aggression to be larger for adults than for children. In contrast, we expected the long-term effects of violent media on aggression to be larger for children than for adults. This pattern of results would be supported by a significant interaction between the type of study and age on violent media–related effect size estimates. We tested this hypothesis using the Statistical Analysis System (SAS Institute, Inc, Cary, NC) general linear model procedure.[37] Age was a dichotomous variable in the model (ie, child vs adult). Study type was also dichotomous (laboratory experiment vs longitudinal study). The analysis revealed no main effect for age ($\chi^2=0.21$, N=166, $P>.05$). There was a main effect for type of study ($\chi^2=14.25$, N=166, $P<.001$), but it was qualified by the predicted interaction between age and study type ($\chi^2=6.87$, N=166, $P<.009$). As can be seen in the **Figure**, media-related aggression was greater for adults than for children in laboratory studies, but it was greater for children than for adults in longitudinal studies.

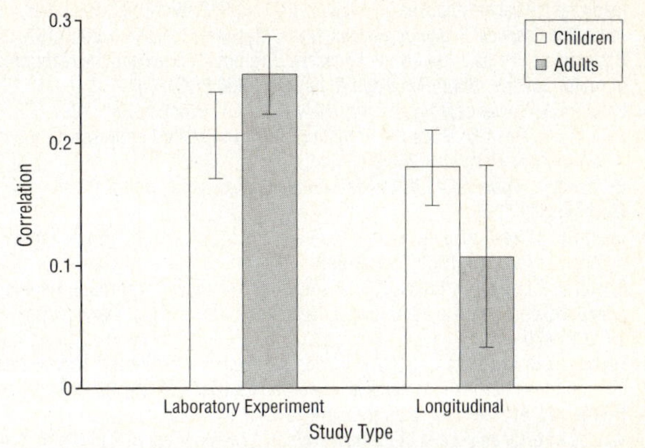


**Figure.** Interactive effects of age and study type on media-related aggression. Error bars indicate 95% confidence intervals.

## COMMENT

In summary, none of our theoretical predictions about the relationship between exposure to media violence and subsequent aggression were contradicted by the meta-analytic data. As predicted, adults displayed larger effect sizes than children in short-term studies whereas children displayed larger effect sizes than adults in long-term studies. This is consistent with the theory that short-term effects are mostly due to the priming of existing well-encoded scripts, schemas, or beliefs whereas long-term effects require the learning (encoding) of scripts, schemas, or beliefs. Young minds with fewer existing encoded cognitions can encode new scripts, schemas, and beliefs via observational learning with less interference and effort than adults. Additionally, we showed that there were overall modest but significant effect sizes for exposure to media violence on aggressive behaviors, emotions, and cognitions.

There are important implications to be drawn from these conclusions for clinical practice. Although observing violence may increase aggression in the short term for adults and children, long-term effects are most likely to occur for children. Consequently, children need the most protection from repeated exposures to violence. Infrequent exposure is not likely to produce lasting consequences, but parents particularly need to be urged to protect their children against the kinds of repeated exposures that heavy play with violent video games or immersion in violent TV programs is likely to produce.

Parents also need to realize that the size of the long-term effect that such exposure has on children will depend on the extent to which the child perceives the violence as realistic, justified, and rewarded as well as on the extent to which the child identifies with the perpetrator. Action heroes are more dangerous teachers of violent behavior than villains. Finally, parents need to be as concerned about the beliefs and attitudes that are being conveyed in violent shows as they are about their child mimicking the behaviors shown. The changes in how the child perceives the world from viewing violence and the beliefs about aggression that the child acquires from viewing violence are likely to influence the child's behavior in the long term as much as the specific scripts for aggression that the child learns from viewing violence.

**Accepted for Publication:** November 30, 2005.
**Correspondence:** Brad J. Bushman, PhD, Institute for Social Research, University of Michigan, 426 Thompson St, Ann Arbor, MI 48106 (bbushman@umich.edu).

## REFERENCES


1. Surgeon General's Scientific Advisory Committee on Television and Social Behavior. *Television and Growing Up: The Impact of Televised Violence.* Rockville, Md: National Institute of Mental Health; 1972.
2. Pearl D, Bouthilet L, Lazar J, eds. *Television and Behavior: Ten Years of Scientific Progress and Implications for the Eighties.* Rockville, Md: US Dept of Health and Human Services, Public Health Service, Alcohol, Drug Abuse, and Mental Health Administration, National Institute of Mental Health; 1982.
3. Murray JP. Results of an informal poll of knowledgeable persons concerning the impact of television violence. *Newsl Am Psychol Assoc Div Child Youth Fam Serv.* 1984;7:2-3.
4. Paik H, Comstock G. The effects of television violence on antisocial behavior: a meta-analysis. *Communic Res.* 1994;21:516-546.
5. Anderson CA, Bushman BJ. Media violence and societal violence. *Science.* 2002; 295:2377-2378.
6. Huesmann LR, Moise-Titus J, Podolski C, Eron L. Longitudinal relations between children's exposure to TV violence and their aggressive and violent behavior in young adulthood: 1977-1992. *Dev Psychol.* 2003;39:201-221.
7. Fiske ST, Taylor SE. *Social Cognition.* Reading, Mass: Addison-Wesley; 1984.
8. Bargh JA, Pietromonaco P. Automatic information processing and social perception: the influence of trait information presented outside of conscious awareness on impression formation. *J Pers Soc Psychol.* 1982;43:437-449.
9. Berkowitz L, LePage A. Weapons as aggression-eliciting stimuli. *J Pers Soc Psychol.* 1967;7:202-207.
10. Hurley S, Chatter N. *Perspectives on Imitation: From Cognitive Neuroscience to Social Science.* Cambridge, Mass: MIT Press; 2004.

11. Meltzoff AN, Moore MK. Imitation of facial and manual gestures by human neonates: resolving the debate about early imitation. In: Muir D, Slater A, eds. *Infant Development: The Essential Readings.* Malden, Mass: Blackwell Publishers; 2000:167-181.
12. Rizzolatti G, Fadiga L, Gallese V, Fogassi L. Premotor cortex and the recognition of motor actions. *Brain Res Cogn Brain Res.* 1996;3:131-141.
13. Bandura A. *Social Learning Theory.* New York, NY: Prentice-Hall; 1997.
14. Bandura A, Ross D, Ross SA. Imitation of film-mediated aggressive models. *J Abnorm Soc Psychol.* 1963;66:3-11.
15. Berkowitz L. *Aggression: Its Causes, Consequences, and Control.* Boston, Mass: McGraw-Hill; 1993.
16. Geen RG, O'Neal EC. Activation of cue-elicited aggression by general arousal. *J Pers Soc Psychol.* 1969;11:289-292.
17. Bryant J, Zillmann D. Effect of intensification of annoyance through unrelated residual excitation on substantially delayed hostile behavior. *J Exp Soc Psychol.* 1979;15:470-480.
18. Zillmann D, Bryant J, Comisky PW. Excitation and hedonic valence in the effect of erotica on motivated inter-male aggression. *Eur J Soc Psychol.* 1981;11:233-252.
19. Dodge KA. Attributional bias in aggressive children. In: Kendall PC, ed. *Advances in Cognitive-Behavioral Research and Therapy.* Vol 4. San Diego, Calif: Academic Press; 1985:73-110.
20. Gerbner G, Gross L, Morgan M, Signorielli N. Growing up with television: the cultivation perspective. In: Bryant J, Zillmann D, eds. *Media Effects.* Hillsdale, NJ: Erlbaum; 1994:17-41.
21. Dodge KA, Pettit GS, Bates JE. Social information-processing patterns partially mediate the effect of early physical abuse on later conduct problems. *J Abnorm Psychol.* 1995;104:632-643.
22. Anderson CA, Huesmann LR. Human aggression: a social-cognitive view. In: Hogg MA, Cooper J, eds. *Sage Handbook of Social Psychology.* London, England: Sage; 2003:296-323.
23. Anderson CA, Bushman BJ. Human aggression. *Annu Rev Psychol.* 2002;53:27-51.
24. Huesmann LR. An information processing model for the development of aggression. *Aggress Behav.* 1988;14:13-24.
25. Huesmann LR. The role of social information processing and cognitive schema in the acquisition and maintenance of habitual aggressive behavior. In: Geen RG, Donnerstein E, eds. *Human Aggression: Theories, Research, and Implications for Social Policy.* San Diego, Calif: Academic Press; 1998:73-109.
26. Bandura A. *Social Foundations of Thought and Action: A Social Cognitive Theory.* Upper Saddle River, NJ: Prentice-Hall; 1986.
27. Huesmann LR, Guerra N. Children's normative beliefs about aggression and aggressive behavior. *J Pers Soc Psychol.* 1997;72:408-419.
28. Cantor J. Confronting children's fright responses to mass media. In: Zillmann D, Bryant J, eds. *Media, Children, and the Family: Social Scientific, Psychodynamic, and Clinical Perspectives.* Hillsdale, NJ: Lawrence Erlbaum Associates; 1994:139-150.
29. Cantor J, Reilly S. Adolescents' fright reactions to television and films. *J Commun.* 1982;32:87-89.
30. Harrison K, Cantor J. Tales from the screen: enduring fright reactions to scary media. *Media Psychol.* 1999;1:97-116.
31. Cline VB, Croft RG, Courrier S. Desensitization of children to television violence. *J Pers Soc Psychol.* 1973;27:360-365.
32. Thomas MH, Horton RW, Lippincott EC, Drabman RS. Desensitization to portrayals of real life aggression as a function of television violence. *J Pers Soc Psychol.* 1977;35:450-458.
33. Hearold S. A synthesis of 1043 effects of television on social behavior. In: Comstock G, ed. *Public Communication and Behavior.* Vol 1. New York, NY: Academic Press; 1986:65-133.
34. Hogben M. Factors moderating the effect of television aggression on viewer behavior. *Communic Res.* 1998;25:220-247.
35. Wood W, Wong FY, Chachere JG. Effects of media violence on viewers' aggression in unconstrained social interaction. *Psychol Bull.* 1991;109:371-383.
36. Rosenthal R. *Meta-analytic Procedures for Social Research.* Newbury Park, Calif: Sage; 1991.
37. Wang MC, Bushman BJ. *Integrating Results Through Meta-analytic Review Using SAS Software.* Cary, NC: SAS Institute Inc; 1999.

## Announcement

**Submissions.** The Editors welcome contributions to Picture of the Month. Submissions should describe common problems presenting uncommonly, rather than total zebras. Cases should be of interest to practicing pediatricians, highlighting problems that they are likely to at least occasionally encounter in the office or hospital setting. High-quality clinical images (in either 35-mm slide or electronic format) along with parent or patient permission to use these images must accompany the submission. The entire discussion should comprise no more than 750 words. Articles and photographs accepted for publication will bear the contributor's name. There is no charge for reproduction and printing of color illustrations. For details regarding electronic submission, please see: http://archpedi.ama-assn.org.

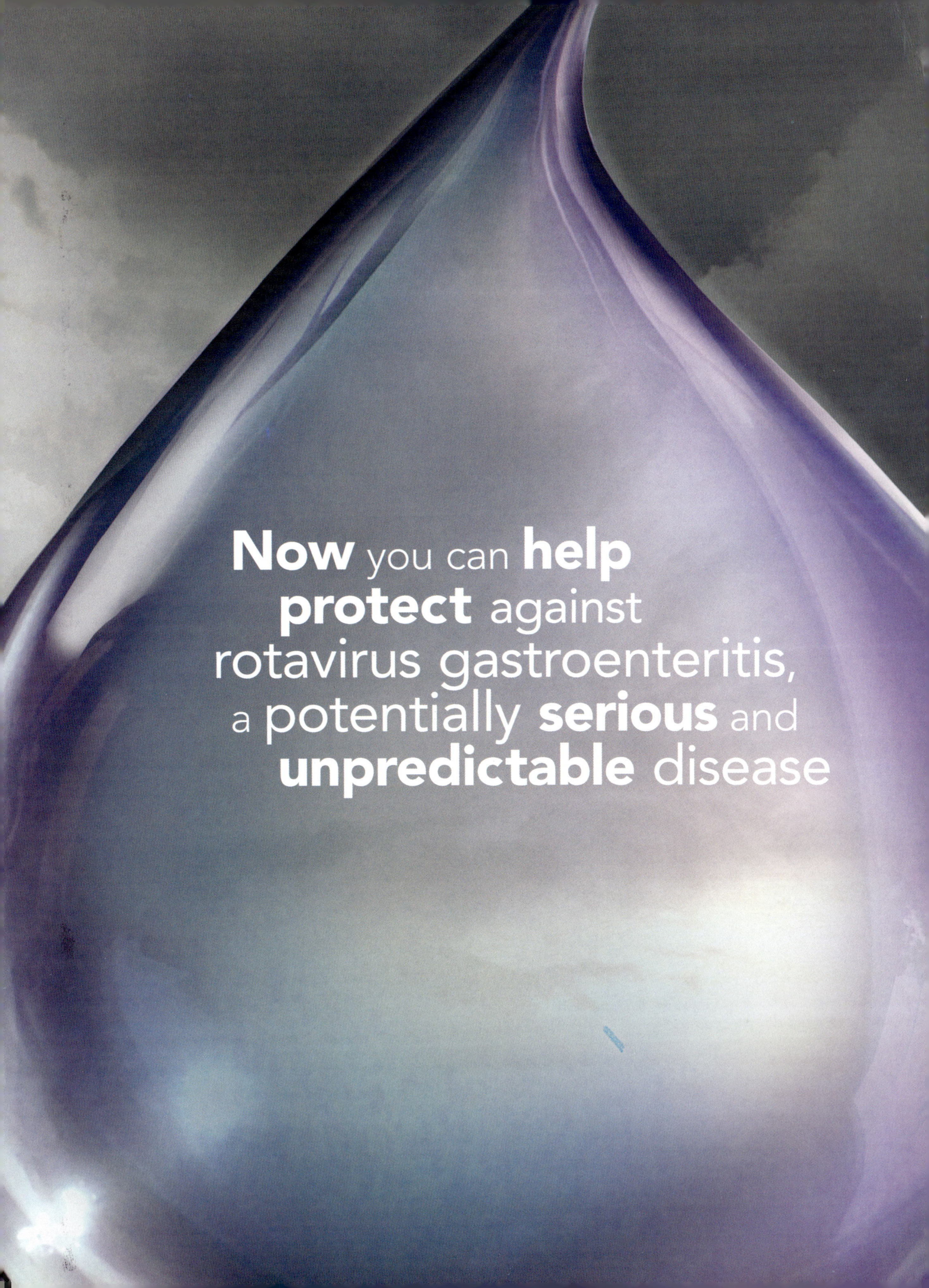
**Now** you can **help**
**protect** against
rotavirus gastroenteritis,
a potentially **serious** and
**unpredictable** disease

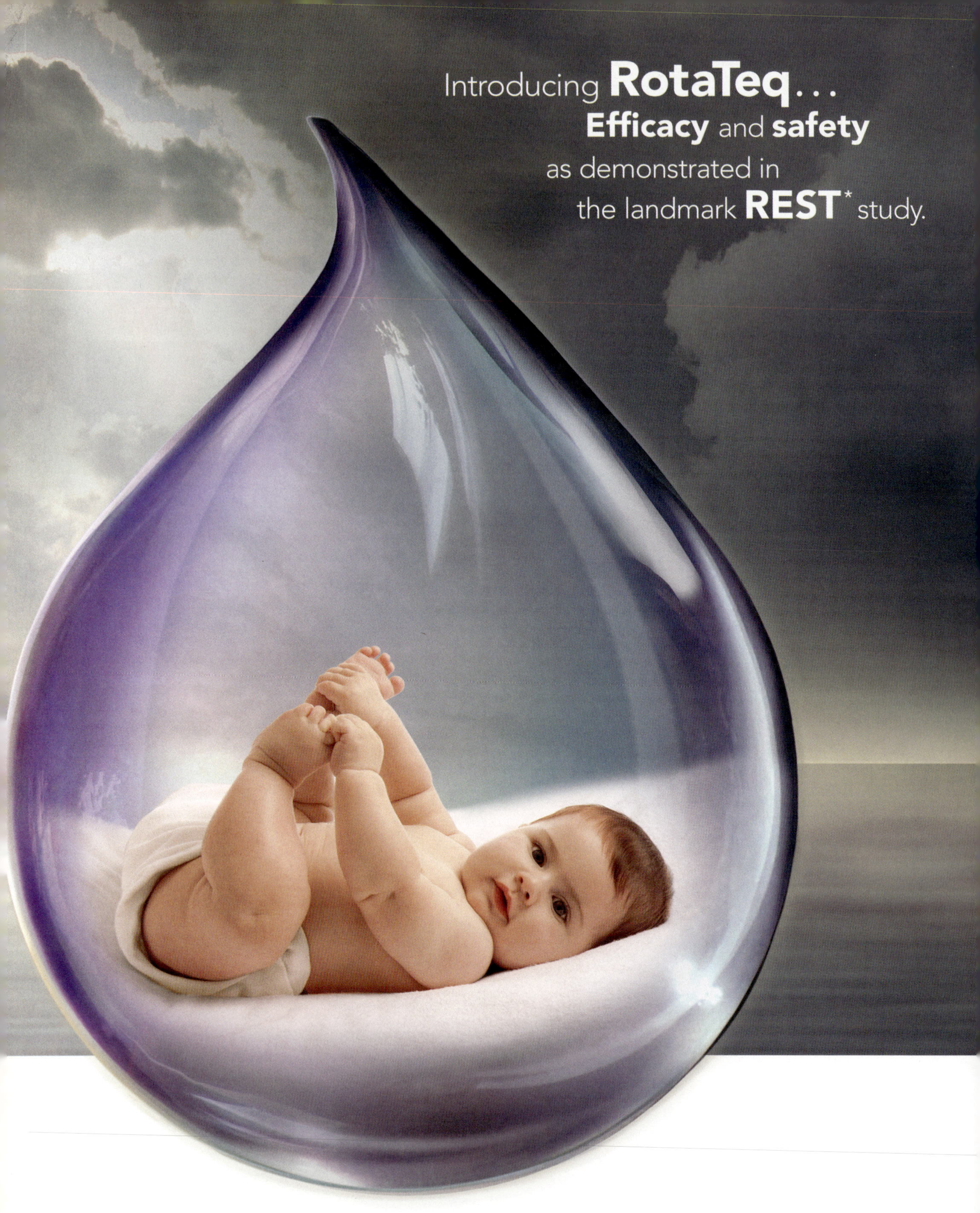
Introducing RotaTeq...
Efficacy and safety
as demonstrated in
the landmark REST* study.

ARTICLE

# Disentangling the Relation Between Television Viewing and Cognitive Processes in Children With Attention-Deficit/Hyperactivity Disorder and Comparison Children

*Ignacio David Acevedo-Polakovich, MS; Elizabeth Pugzles Lorch, PhD; Richard Milich, PhD; Rebecca D. Ashby, BA*

**Objectives:** To develop causal hypotheses regarding the effects of television viewing on cognitive processes in children and to examine the proposition that deleterious effects of television may be stronger among children with attention-deficit/hyperactivity disorder.

**Design:** Longitudinal study involving 2 phases occurring 18 months apart.

**Setting:** University research facilities in Lexington.

**Participants:** Fifty-nine children with attention-deficit/hyperactivity disorder and 106 comparison children. The children's mean age was 7.18 years at phase 1 and 8.74 years at phase 2.

**Main Outcome Measures:** Laboratory measures of visual attention to television, cognitive engagement to televised stories, factual recall of televised stories, and causal recall of televised stories. Parental reports of a child's weekly television viewing.

**Results:** Among comparison children, phase 1 television viewing negatively predicted phase 2 visual attention and phase 2 cognitive engagement (after accounting for phase 1 levels of the outcome variables and any relevant demographic variables). Also among comparison children, phase 1 attention negatively predicted phase 2 television viewing, even after accounting for phase 1 levels of television viewing and relevant demographic variables. These patterns were not observed among children with attention-deficit/hyperactivity disorder.

**Conclusions:** Contrary to recent arguments, television viewing was associated with cognitive abilities in comparison children but not children with attention-deficit/hyperactivity disorder, a finding that suggests more careful examinations of the relation between television viewing and children's cognitive abilities are in order. Future studies should consider the possibility that any effects of television may be limited to certain developmental periods.

*Arch Pediatr Adolesc Med. 2006;160:354-360*

THE AVERAGE US CHILD SPENDS almost 27 hours per week watching television, a figure that has remained constant over the past 5 years.[1] Not surprisingly, the potential effects of television on children's cognitive abilities have received much attention in popular and professional discourse.[2-4] Commentary on this issue ranges from omnibus indictments of television as a deleterious influence on children's cognitive development[2] to encouraging endorsements of the current television landscape as supportive of increased cognitive complexity and improved problem solving.[3] Unfortunately, much of this commentary does not rise above speculation because little research has actually examined the effects of media exposure on children's cognitive abilities.[4]

Among the emerging research in this area, a handful of studies have examined the relation between television viewing and processes such as attention and comprehension. Findings suggest that television viewing is negatively correlated with later performance in both of these areas,[5,6] and have led some scholars to speculate that television viewing may play an exacerbating, if not causal, role in the development of attention-deficit/hyperactivity disorder (ADHD).[6] This hypothesis is consistent with evidence indicating that children with ADHD watch more television than their peers[7] and experience significant impairments in comprehending stories, a crucial skill in achieving academic success.[8]

There is some debate surrounding the suggestion that the existing correlational evidence supports the contention that television has deleterious effects on children's cognitive abilities.[9,10] Some scholars[9] have argued that because individual variation in attentional styles is evident even during infancy, this evidence could also be given the interpretation that chil-

Author Affiliations:
Departments of Psychology, University of Kentucky, Lexington (Mr Acevedo-Polakovich and Drs Lorch and Milich), and Auburn University, Auburn, Ala (Ms Ashby).

dren with a predisposition for attention problems are more likely to watch television at an early age. In response to this argument, it has been suggested that the negative effects of television viewing on cognitive processes may be particularly salient in children predisposed for ADHD.[10] Accordingly, research is needed that helps clarify the causal direction of the relations between television viewing and cognitive abilities and addresses the issue of whether, as recently suggested, these differ in children with ADHD and comparison children.

Lorch and colleagues[8,11] have used a television viewing method to understand the attention and story comprehension abilities of children with ADHD and comparison children. In this approach, children watch 2 television programs, 1 in the presence of toys and 1 in the absence of toys. Visual attention to the television is recorded throughout each program. At the end of each program, children are asked questions assessing their recall of specific factual information (ie, "what" questions assessing a child's understanding and recall of specific factual information from the show) and causal relations (ie, "why" questions assessing a child's ability to link earlier information in the story with later information to understand why an event occurred). The television viewing method has the advantage of directly assessing the cognitive processes involved in story comprehension, and is especially appropriate for research involving children with ADHD because it does not involve reading, a skill in which children with ADHD are frequently impaired.[12]

The results of studies using this method consistently reveal that in the absence of toys there are no significant differences in visual attention or story recall between children with ADHD and comparison children. However, when toys are present, children with ADHD show a steeper decrease in visual attention than do comparison children, and exhibit significantly poorer performance on questions testing causal relations.[8] In addition, the amount of time that children spend in long looks at the television (ie, ≥15 seconds) accounts for the recall differences between children with ADHD and comparison children.[8,11] This finding is important because long looks are considered an overt indicator of deeper cognitive processing.[13]

While the television viewing method has allowed for an increased understanding of the manner in which the attention problems of children with ADHD may impact their story comprehension, to our knowledge, no research has used data gathered using this approach to examine the relation between television viewing and cognitive abilities in a longitudinal study. Accordingly, the present study uses longitudinal data that include variables obtained through the use of the television viewing method to develop more careful hypotheses about the causal relation between television viewing and cognitive processing, and to examine whether—as suggested by other researchers[10]—this relation differs between children with ADHD and comparison children.

## METHODS

### PARTICIPANTS

Data for this study were provided by 165 children participating in a longitudinal research project, approved by the University of Kentucky institutional review board, examining the comprehension of televised stories in children with ADHD and a comparison sample. Participants with ADHD (n=59) were recruited from clinical settings. Comparison children (n=106) were recruited through newspaper advertisements. Before their children's enrollment in this study, parents provided written informed consent and completed a semistructured interview and several standardized assessment instruments to verify their children's diagnostic status. Children accepted into the ADHD group averaged more than 12.24 symptoms of ADHD (SD, 3.44 symptoms). Children accepted into the comparison sample averaged less than 1 symptom of ADHD (SD, 0.72 symptoms). Data were collected in 2 phases spaced approximately 18 months apart, with children being a mean age of 7.18 years (SD, 1.71 years) at phase 1 and 8.74 years (SD, 1.76 years) at phase 2.

### PROCEDURE

During each of the phases, children visited university research facilities to complete several experimental tasks related to story processing, including those used in this study and described later. While the children completed these tasks, surveys and standardized questionnaires regarding their behavior, social environment, media use, and media environment were completed by their parents.

### MEASURES

#### Television Viewing

Parents were asked to report the number of hours that their children spent watching television, excluding VCR use, during specific periods on weekdays (eg, "Monday through Thursday, 6 AM–noon") and during these same periods on each specific weekend days (eg, "Friday, 6:00 AM–noon"). Collectively, these periods spanned the entire week. Parent reports were then combined to form a total weekly television viewing composite. Existing evidence suggests that data gathered using this approach to the assessment of television viewing approximate actual behavior better than global questions focused on estimates of daily or weekly television viewing.[14]

#### Visual Attention to and Comprehension of Televised Stories

The television viewing method was used to assess children's comprehension of and attention to televised stories. Because the toys present condition most closely simulates the home viewing environment and allows for the assessment of children's allocation of attention to the programs vs the toys, only data from this viewing condition are included in the present study. During the 2 phases of the study, the children viewed different episodes of the cartoon show, *Rugrats*. This show was chosen because it appeals to children across a wide age range and maintains a strong narrative structure that facilitates story comprehension assessment. The children were videotaped while the program was presented, and the videotapes were later coded for moment-to-moment visual attention. After the program was finished, all children viewing a given program were asked the same series of questions involving factual and causal information. Four variables obtained during each of the 2 phases are included in the present study: (1) *attention*, operationalized as the total percentage of time that a child's gaze was fixed on the television screen; (2) *cognitive engagement*, operationalized as the total amount of time that a child spent in looks at the television lasting 15 or more seconds; (3) *factual recall*, operationalized as the percentage of factual questions a child answered correctly;

**Table 1. Data for the Effects of Diagnosis on Variables Included in This Study**

| | Control Group | | ADHD Group | | 1-Way ANOVA Results | |
|---|---|---|---|---|---|---|
| Variable | Mean | SD | Mean | SD | F Value | $\eta^2$ |
| Age, y | 7.86 | 1.73 | 8.21 | 1.77 | 1.34 | 0.01 |
| Male sex* | 55 | 50 | 78 | 41 | 7.98 | 0.05† |
| Mother's education, y | 15.93 | 2.15 | 14.67 | 2.41 | 10.26 | 0.07† |
| Weekly television viewing, h | | | | | | |
| Phase 1 | 14.55 | 10.23 | 18.82 | 7.96 | 6.60 | 0.05‡ |
| Phase 2 | 14.92 | 8.14 | 19.41 | 9.08 | 9.07 | 0.06† |
| Attention* | | | | | | |
| Phase 1 | 43.04 | 30.01 | 23.90 | 20.50 | 16.35 | 0.11§ |
| Phase 2 | 54.19 | 31.08 | 32.25 | 24.50 | 18.71 | 0.12§ |
| Cognitive engagement score | | | | | | |
| Phase 1 | 211.52 | 205.23 | 68.05 | 108.42 | 21.45 | 0.13§ |
| Phase 2 | 282.03 | 234.24 | 118.31 | 145.00 | 20.40 | 0.13§ |
| Factual recall score | | | | | | |
| Phase 1 | 52.24 | 25.44 | 45.37 | 22.72 | 2.55 | 0.02 |
| Phase 2 | 65.33 | 19.68 | 52.21 | 22.09 | 13.16 | 0.09§ |
| Causal recall score | | | | | | |
| Phase 1 | 41.24 | 24.62 | 33.88 | 22.02 | 3.12 | 0.02§ |
| Phase 2 | 53.99 | 21.05 | 43.76 | 17.95 | 8.49 | 0.06† |

Abbreviations: ADHD, attention-deficit/hyperactivity disorder; ANOVA, analysis of variance.
*Data are given as percentage.
†$P<.01$.
‡$P<.05$.
§$P<.001$.

and (4) *causal recall*, operationalized as the percentage of causal questions a child answered correctly.

## RESULTS

### DESCRIPTIVE INFORMATION

Means and SDs for all variables included in this study are presented separately by diagnostic group in **Table 1**, along with 1-way analysis of variance results. For demographic variables, there were no differences between groups in the mean age across both data collection times; however, children with ADHD were significantly more likely to be male and had mothers who reported significantly fewer years of education. For the principal variables of interest in this study, the children with ADHD were described by their parents as watching significantly more weekly television than the comparison children at both phases, and performed more poorly on laboratory tasks assessing visual attention, cognitive engagement, and recall of causal information at both phases of the study. Children with ADHD also performed more poorly than comparison children on factual recall at phase 2 but not phase 1.

### CORRELATIONS AMONG VARIABLES

The correlations among all variables examined in this study are reported in **Table 2**. Correlations calculated from data provided by children with ADHD are reported above the diagonal line formed by the NA (not applicable) results, and correlations calculated from data provided by comparison children are reported below this diagonal line. As can be observed, among comparison children, most longitudinal correlations between television viewing and laboratory measures collected at a different phase were significant, suggesting the possibility of bidirectional causal effects. By comparison, these correlations were not significant and most approached 0 among children with ADHD, suggesting the possibility that the relations between television viewing and the laboratory measures differ in children with ADHD and comparison children.

Fisher *r*-to-*z* comparisons were used to test the differences between samples in the longitudinal relation between television viewing and laboratory measures. There were significant (2-tailed) differences between diagnostic groups in the correlations between phase 1 television viewing and phase 2 attention ($z=2.16$, $P=.03$), between phase 1 television viewing and phase 2 cognitive engagement ($z=2.22$, $P=.03$), and between phase 1 television viewing and phase 2 factual recall ($z=1.80$, $P=.07$). In each case, the correlation obtained in the comparison group was significantly greater than that obtained in the ADHD sample. No other group differences in correlations were significant.

Cross-lagged hierarchical regression analyses were then conducted to develop causal hypotheses about significant longitudinal correlations involving television viewing and the laboratory measures obtained through the television viewing method. Cross-lagged comparisons estimate the linear relation between a predictor variable measured at an early point (eg, phase 1 television viewing) and a criterion variable measured at a later point (eg, phase 2 attention to television) after accounting for levels of the criterion variable at the time the predictor variable was assessed (eg, phase 1 attention to television).[15] Although not a definitive demonstration of causality, the identification of a significant relation between the pre-

**Table 2. Correlations Among Variables Considered in This Study***

| Variable | Age | Male Sex | Mother's Education | Phase 1 Weekly Television Viewing | Phase 1 % of Attention | Phase 1 Cognitive Engagement | Phase 1 Factual Recall | Phase 1 Causal Recall | Phase 2 Weekly Television Viewing | Phase 2 % of Attention | Phase 2 Cognitive Engagement | Phase 2 Factual Recall | Phase 2 Causal Recall |
|---|---|---|---|---|---|---|---|---|---|---|---|---|---|
| Age | NA | 0.02 | −0.30† | 0.03 | −0.03 | −0.11 | 0.40‡ | 0.51§ | 0.06 | 0.20 | 0.15 | 0.42‡ | 0.41‡ |
| Male sex | 0.07 | NA | 0.02 | 0.20 | −0.09 | −0.13 | 0.01 | 0.13 | 0.14 | 0.05 | 0.00 | 0.18 | 0.04 |
| Mother's education | 0.05 | −0.05 | NA | −0.13 | 0.03 | 0.09 | 0.04 | −0.22 | −0.20 | 0.02 | −0.03 | −0.01 | −0.04 |
| Phase 1 | | | | | | | | | | | | | |
| Weekly television viewing | −0.14 | 0.02 | −0.34§ | NA | −0.18 | −0.09 | 0.02 | −0.05 | 0.60§ | −0.07 | 0.01 | 0.10 | 0.02 |
| % of Attention | 0.14 | −0.20† | 0.27‡ | −0.48§ | NA | 0.85§ | 0.15 | 0.16 | −0.22 | 0.49§ | 0.43‡ | 0.03 | 0.01 |
| Cognitive engagement | 0.14 | −0.18† | 0.24† | −0.43§ | 0.93§ | NA | 0.03 | 0.00 | −0.14 | 0.38§ | 0.30* | −0.11 | −0.26* |
| Factual recall | 0.74§ | 0.01 | 0.27‡ | −0.16 | 0.30‡ | 0.27‡ | NA | 0.78§ | −0.02 | 0.20 | 0.24‖ | 0.60§ | 0.46§ |
| Causal recall | 0.76§ | 0.05 | 0.19† | −0.21† | 0.22† | 0.23† | 0.77§ | NA | −0.01 | 0.25‖ | 0.27† | 0.66§ | 0.48§ |
| Phase 2 | | | | | | | | | | | | | |
| Weekly television viewing | −0.10 | 0.02 | −0.40§ | 0.66§ | −0.46§ | −0.40§ | −0.07 | −0.14 | NA | −0.25‖ | −0.25‖ | 0.03 | −0.02 |
| % of Attention | 0.22† | −0.12 | 0.33‡ | −0.41§ | 0.51§ | 0.45§ | 0.20† | 0.35§ | −0.53§ | NA | 0.85§ | 0.34‡ | 0.35‡ |
| Cognitive engagement | 0.15 | −0.13 | 0.24† | −0.35§ | 0.48§ | 0.43§ | 0.17‖ | 0.30‡ | −0.48§ | 0.92§ | NA | 0.39‡ | 0.39‡ |
| Factual recall | 0.60§ | 0.04 | 0.13 | −0.20† | 0.15 | 0.12 | 0.68§ | 0.68§ | −0.05 | 0.28‡ | 0.26‡ | NA | 0.73§ |
| Causal recall | 0.65§ | 0.02 | 0.19‖ | −0.19‖ | 0.19‖ | 0.14 | 0.68§ | 0.71§ | −0.10 | 0.35§ | 0.29‡ | 0.77§ | NA |

Abbreviation: NA, data not applicable.

*Correlations obtained from data provided by children with attention-deficit/hyperactivity disorder are reported above the diagonal line formed by the NA results, and correlations obtained from data provided by comparison children are reported below this diagonal line.

†$P<.05$.

‡$P<.01$.

§$P<.001$.

‖$P<.10$.

dictor and criterion variables using this approach provides stronger evidence for a possible causal mechanism than other correlational approaches.[16] Where indicated by significantly different correlations (ie, phase 1 television viewing to phase 2 cognitive engagement, phase 2 attention, and phase 2 factual recall), separate analyses were calculated in each diagnostic group. Because the sex distribution and the amount of education received by the mother differed between diagnostic groups, these predictors were statistically controlled for whenever they evinced a significant correlation with an outcome to avoid confounding the effects of these predictors with those of diagnostic status.

## TELEVISION VIEWING AS A PREDICTOR OF SUBSEQUENT ATTENTION AND COMPREHENSION

### Attention

As summarized in **Table 3**, among comparison children, phase 1 television viewing negatively predicted phase 2 attention, even after accounting for a participant's age and phase 1 attention. This effect was not observed among children with ADHD (Table 3).

### Cognitive Engagement

As summarized in Table 3, among comparison children, phase 1 television viewing negatively predicted phase 2 cognitive engagement, even after accounting for phase 1 cognitive engagement. The significant effect of phase 1 television viewing on phase 2 cognitive engagement was not observed among children with ADHD (Table 3).

### Factual and Causal Recall

As summarized in Table 3, phase 1 television viewing did not predict phase 2 factual recall after accounting for the effects of phase 1 factual recall in either sample of children. As suggested by the *r*-to-*z* comparisons previously described, the effect of phase 1 television viewing on phase 2 causal recall was examined in a sample including all children regardless of diagnostic status. These results are summarized in **Table 4**. As can be observed, phase 1 television viewing did not predict phase 2 causal recall after accounting for the effects of phase 1 causal recall and mother's education.

## ATTENTION AND COMPREHENSION AS PREDICTORS OF SUBSEQUENT TELEVISION VIEWING

Analyses examining the relation between phase 2 television viewing and phase 1 performance on laboratory measures of attention, cognitive engagement, factual recall, and causal recall (after accounting for phase 1 amounts of television viewing and the effects of significant covariates) are summarized in **Table 5**. As can be observed, among phase 1 laboratory measures, only phase 1 visual attention acted as a significant (negative) predictor of phase 2 television viewing. Post hoc analyses, reported in Table 3, suggest that the effect of phase 1 attention on phase 2 television viewing may be limited to comparison children.

**Table 3. Summary of Hierarchical Regression Results Conducted Separately by Diagnostic Group**

| | Comparison Sample | | ADHD Sample | |
|---|---|---|---|---|
| Phase 2 Outcome Variable | β Value | Change in $R^2$ | β Value* | Change in $R^2$ |
| Visual attention | | | | |
| Step 1 predictors | | | | |
| Mother's education | .21† | 0.30‡ | NA | 0.24‡ |
| Phase 1 % of attention | .46‡ | | .49‡ | |
| Step 2 predictors | | | | |
| Mother's education | .17§ | 0.02§ | NA | 0 |
| Phase 1 % of attention | .39‡ | | .49‡ | |
| Phase 1 weekly television viewing | −.17§ | | .02 | |
| Cognitive engagement | | | | |
| Step 1 predictors | | | | |
| Phase 1 % of cognitive engagement | .43‡ | 0.18‡ | .30† | 0.09† |
| Step 2 predictors | | | | |
| Phase 1 % of cognitive engagement | .34‖ | 0.03† | .30† | 0 |
| Phase 1 weekly television viewing | −.20† | | .04 | |
| Factual recall | | | | |
| Step 1 predictors | | | | |
| Phase 1 % of factual recall | .68‡ | 0.46‡ | .60‡ | 0.36‡ |
| Step 2 predictors | | | | |
| Phase 1 % of factual recall | .66‡ | 0.01 | .60‡ | 0.01 |
| Phase 1 weekly television viewing | −.09 | | .09 | |
| Television use | | | | |
| Step 1 predictors | | | | |
| Mother's education | −.19† | 0.47‡ | NA | 0.36‡ |
| Phase 1 weekly television viewing | .60‡ | | .60‡ | |
| Step 2 predictors | | | | |
| Mother's education | −.17† | 0.02§ | NA | 0.01 |
| Phase 1 weekly television viewing | .53‡ | | −.58‡ | |
| Phase 1 % of attention | −.16§ | | −.11 | |

Abbreviations: ADHD, attention-deficit/hyperactivity disorder; NA, data not applicable.
*Results are being reported without mother's education as a predictor because this variable was not significantly related to phase 2 cognitive engagement when included in the regression equation (β = .10, $P = .32$).
†$P < .05$.
‡$P < .001$.
§$P < .10$.
‖$P < .01$.

**Table 4. Hierarchical Regression Results Using Phase 1 Television Viewing to Predict Phase 2 Causal Recall in a Sample Including Comparison Children and Children With ADHD**

| Predictor Variable | β Value | Change in $R^2$ |
|---|---|---|
| Step 1 predictors | | |
| Mother's education | .12* | 0.44† |
| Phase 1 causal recall | .64† | |
| Step 2 predictors | | |
| Mother's education | .11‡ | 0 |
| Phase 1 causal recall | .64† | |
| Phase 1 weekly television | −.03 | |

Abbreviation: See Table 1.
*$P < .05$.
†$P < .001$.
‡$P < .10$.

## COMMENT

This study sought to further develop causal hypotheses about the relation between television viewing and 2 important cognitive abilities: attention and comprehension. An additional goal was to examine the recent proposition that these relations may differ between children with ADHD and comparison children. Results suggest that, among comparison children, increased levels of television viewing at phase 1 were associated with decreased performance on phase 2 measures of visual attention and cognitive engagement, a finding that is consistent with previous literature in this area.[5,6] However, the relation between television viewing and visual attention among comparison children seems to have a bidirectional component because reduced performance on phase 1 visual attention measures was associated with increased television viewing at phase 2. This last finding is consistent with arguments suggesting that children who have difficulty paying attention may favor television and other electronic media to a greater extent than the media environment of children without attention problems.[9] More important, contrary to recent suggestions that any deleterious longitudinal relation between television and cognitive outcomes may be more salient among children with ADHD,[10] no effects of television viewing were observed among children with this diagnosis. Indeed, Fisher *r*-to-*z* comparisons indicated that the longitudinal relations between television viewing and laboratory measures of attention, cognitive engagement, and factual recall were in fact smaller in children with ADHD than in comparison children. Findings are of particular interest because they are based on an approach that directly assesses the cognitive processes that are hypothesized to affect story comprehension rather than rely on parent or child reports of symptoms or imputations about cognitive performance based on standardized achievement tests.

One possible explanation for the finding that television viewing may have an effect on attention and cognitive engagement only among comparison children is that the cognitive processing deficits associated with ADHD are so strongly rooted in biological predisposition that, among children with this diagnosis, environmental characteristics such as television viewing have a negligible effect on these cognitive processing areas.[9] Alternatively, characteristics of the current sample may limit the ability of this study to identify any effects of television viewing among children with ADHD. For instance, the effects of television viewing on attention and cognitive engagement may occur at younger ages and, thus, have taken hold by the time children are of elementary school age. Another possibility is that, among children with ADHD in the age group being considered in this study, a longer period is required to observe effects of television viewing on the cognitive processes being measured in the laboratory. While this alternative would still run counter to the speculation that the effects of television are strongest among children with ADHD, it does allow for the possibility of added environmental contributions to the cognitive deficits exhibited by these children. Finally, it is possible that the direct laboratory assessment of visual attention used in this study examines a different spectrum of attentional abilities than those assessed by the rating forms or clinical impressions used in other studies and, therefore, influences the results.

Contrary to prior literature in this area,[5] current results showed no effect of television viewing on subsequent story comprehension in either group. The same developmental and measurement considerations as discussed previously may apply to this finding. In addition, it should be considered that in the present study, comprehension was assessed via recall of televised content. It may be the case that television exposure may affect comprehension of information presented through other media (eg, orally or in print), but not televised content.

A first limitation that should be considered when evaluating this study's findings is associated with the cross-lagged approach used. As stated previously, results obtained from this approach provide stronger evidence for a possible causal mechanism than other correlational approaches, but are not a definitive demonstration of causality. As discussed previously, findings also are limited by the age range of the children sampled. The possibility that findings are influenced by the television viewing method being used has already been discussed in this paper. An additional methodological limitation involves the use of a weekly composite of television viewing to assess television viewing, an approach that fails to capture possible differences associated with the content of the programming viewed by children. Existing research[17] using comparison samples suggests that educational and prosocial programming can foster the development of academic and social skills in children. As such, current results can only be generalized to quantitative increments in television viewing, but leave open the possibility that different types of programming content can differentially affect children's cognitive abilities. Finally, particularly among children with ADHD, current sample sizes may have prevented the identification of additional effects. For instance, it was noted earlier that many of the longitudinal correlations involving weekly television viewing and laboratory measures obtained through the television viewing method seemed to have greater magnitude among comparison children than children with ADHD; however, in the present study, not all of these diagnostic group differences were significant. Research involving larger samples of children with ADHD could be more sensitive to smaller effect sizes.

Overall, the pattern of results obtained in the present study suggests that by elementary school age, television viewing may have an effect on the attention and cognitive engagement abilities of comparison children but not of those children with ADHD. While limited to the age

**Table 5. Hierarchical Regression Results Predicting Phase 2 Television Viewing With Phase 1 Laboratory Measures of Attention and Comprehension in a Sample Including Comparison Children and Children With ADHD**

| Phase 1 Predictor Variable | β Value | Change in $R^2$ |
|---|---|---|
| Visual attention | | |
| Step 1 predictors | | |
| Mother's education | −.17* | 0.46† |
| Phase 1 weekly television viewing | .61† | |
| Step 2 predictors | | |
| Mother's education | −.15‡ | 0.02‡ |
| Phase 1 weekly television viewing | .55† | |
| Phase 1 visual attention | −.15‡ | |
| Cognitive engagement | | |
| Step 1 predictors | | |
| Mother's education | −.17* | 0.46† |
| Phase 1 weekly television viewing | .61† | |
| Step 2 predictors | | |
| Mother's education | −.15‡ | 0.01 |
| Phase 1 weekly television viewing | .57† | |
| Phase 1 cognitive engagement | −.11 | |
| Factual recall | | |
| Step 1 predictors | | |
| Mother's education | −.17* | 0.46† |
| Phase 1 weekly television viewing | .61† | |
| Step 2 predictors | | |
| Mother's education | −.18* | 0 |
| Phase 1 weekly television viewing | .61† | |
| Phase 1 factual recall | .03 | |
| Causal recall | | |
| Step 1 predictors | | |
| Mother's education | −.17* | 0.46† |
| Phase 1 weekly television viewing | .61† | |
| Step 2 predictors | | |
| Mother's education | −.17* | 0 |
| Phase 1 weekly television viewing | .61† | |
| Phase 1 causal recall | 0 | |

Abbreviation: See Table 1.
*$P<.01$.
†$P<.001$.
‡$P<.10$.

group under study, this finding contradicts recent speculation that children with ADHD may be most at risk for any deleterious effects of television viewing[10] and raises the interesting possibility that, at certain developmental periods, it may be comparison children who are most at risk for these effects. Certainly, future research should continue to examine this question using approaches that overcome the limitations of the present study. Studies contrasting children with ADHD and comparison children at younger ages, and research using children of the same age sampled in the present study but allowing for greater time for any effects of television viewing on children with ADHD to take place, seem particularly indicated. Television and ADHD are inexorable realities of the current developmental landscape facing children in the United States; it is to these children's benefit that scholarly discussion about the possible relation between television and attention problems move away from speculation and toward an empirically informed understanding.

**Accepted for Publication:** December 21, 2005.
**Correspondence:** Ignacio David Acevedo-Polakovich, MS, Department of Psychology, University of Kentucky, Lexington, KY 40506-0044 (Acevedo@uky.edu).
**Funding/Support:** This study was supported by grant MH47386 from the National Institute of Mental Health, Bethesda, Md; and by National Institutes of Health National Research Service Award DA07304 from the National Institute on Drug Abuse, Bethesda.
**Role of the Sponsor:** The funding bodies had no role in data extraction and analyses, in the writing of the manuscript, or in the decision to submit the manuscript for publication.
**Acknowledgment:** We thank the 2 anonymous reviewers for their helpful comments, which vastly improved the direction and presentation of this article.

## REFERENCES

1. Rideout V, Roberts DF, Foehr UG. *Generation M: Media in the Lives of 8-18 Year-Olds.* Menlo Park, Calif: Henry J. Kaiser Family Foundation; 2005.
2. Winn M. *The Plug-in Drug: Television, Computers, and Family Life.* 2nd rev ed. New York, NY: Penguin Putnam Books; 2002.
3. Johnson S. *Everything Bad Is Good for You: How Today's Popular Culture Is Actually Making Us Smarter.* New York, NY: Riverhead Books; 2005.
4. Christakis DA. The effect of media on children and adolescents [editorial]. *Arch Pediatr Adolesc Med.* 2005;159:595.
5. Zimmerman FJ, Christakis DA. Children's television viewing and cognitive outcomes: a longitudinal analysis of national data. *Arch Pediatr Adolesc Med.* 2005; 159:619-625.
6. Christakis DA, Zimmerman FJ, DiGiuseppe DL, McCarthy CA. Early television exposure and subsequent attentional problems in children. *Pediatrics.* 2004;113: 708-713.
7. Acevedo-Polakovich ID, Lorch EP, Milich R. TV or not TV: questions and answers regarding television and ADHD. *ADHD Rep.* 2005;13:6-11.
8. Lorch EP, Berthiaume K, Milich R, van den Broek P. Story comprehension impairments in children with ADHD. In: Cain K, Oakhill J, eds. *Cognitive Bases of Children's Language Comprehension Difficulties.* New York, NY: Guilford Publications. In press.
9. Barkley RA. ADHD and television exposure: correlation as cause. *ADHD Rep.* 2004; 12:1-4.
10. Zimmerman FJ, Christakis DA. ADHD and television: a reply to Barkley. *ADHD Rep.* 2004;12:5-6.
11. Pugzles Lorch E, Eastham D, Milich R, et al. Difficulties in comprehending causal relations among children with ADHD: the role of cognitive engagement. *J Abnorm Psychol.* 2004;113:56-63.
12. Tannock R. Language, reading, and motor control problems in ADHD: a potential behavioral phenotype. In: Greenhill L, ed. *Learning Disabilities: Implications for Psychiatric Treatment.* Washington, DC: American Psychiatric Association Publishing; 2000:129-167.
13. Richards JE, Anderson DR. Attentional inertia in children's extended looking at television. In: Kail RV, ed. *Advances in Child Development and Behavior.* Amsterdam, the Netherlands: Academic Press; 2004:163-212.
14. Anderson DR, Field DE, Collins PA, Lorch EP, Nathan JG. Estimates of young children's time with television: a methodological comparison of parent reports with time-lapse video home observation. *Child Dev.* 1985;56:1345-1357.
15. Horvath LS, Milich R, Lynam D, Leukefled C, Clayton R. Personality and substance use: a cross-lagged panel design. *Individual Differences Res.* 2004; 2:175-183.
16. Cohen J, Cohen P. *Applied Multiple Regression/Correlation for the Behavioral Sciences.* 2nd ed. Hillsdale, NJ: Lawrence Erlbaum Associates; 1983.
17. Chernin AR, Linebarger DL. The relationship between children's television viewing and academic performance. *Arch Pediatr Adolesc Med.* 2005;159:687-689.

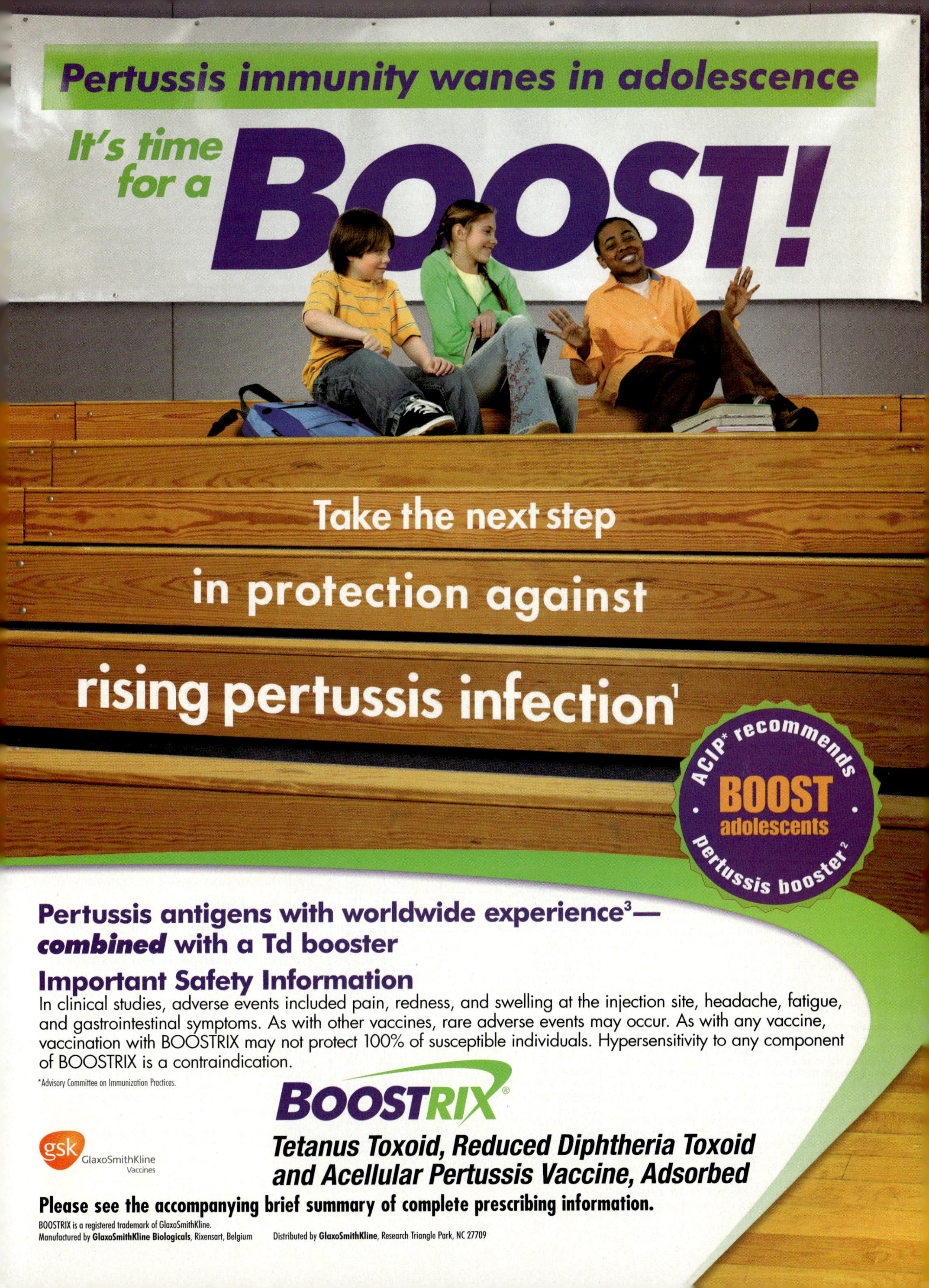
Pertussis immunity wanes in adolescence
It's time for a BOOST!
Take the next step
in protection against
rising pertussis infection[1]
ACIP* recommends
BOOST
adolescents
pertussis booster[2]
Pertussis antigens with worldwide experience[3]—
combined with a Td booster
Important Safety Information
In clinical studies, adverse events included pain, redness, and swelling at the injection site, headache, fatigue, and gastrointestinal symptoms. As with other vaccines, rare adverse events may occur. As with any vaccine, vaccination with BOOSTRIX may not protect 100% of susceptible individuals. Hypersensitivity to any component of BOOSTRIX is a contraindication.
*Advisory Committee on Immunization Practices.
BOOSTRIX®
Tetanus Toxoid, Reduced Diphtheria Toxoid and Acellular Pertussis Vaccine, Adsorbed
gsk GlaxoSmithKline Vaccines
Please see the accompanying brief summary of complete prescribing information.
BOOSTRIX is a registered trademark of GlaxoSmithKline.
Manufactured by GlaxoSmithKline Biologicals, Rixensart, Belgium
Distributed by GlaxoSmithKline, Research Triangle Park, NC 27709

# BOOSTRIX®

**(Tetanus Toxoid, Reduced Diphtheria Toxoid and Acellular Pertussis Vaccine, Adsorbed) (Tdap)**

The following is a brief summary only; see full prescribing information for complete product information.

**INDICATIONS AND USAGE:** BOOSTRIX is indicated for active booster immunization against tetanus, diphtheria, and pertussis as a single dose in individuals 10 through 18 years of age. The use of BOOSTRIX as a primary series or to complete the primary series has not been studied. As with any vaccine, BOOSTRIX may not protect 100% of individuals receiving the vaccine. BOOSTRIX is not recommended for treatment of actual infections.

**CONTRAINDICATIONS:** Hypersensitivity to any component of the vaccine is a contraindication (see DESCRIPTION in full prescribing information). Do not use BOOSTRIX after a serious allergic reaction (e.g., anaphylaxis) following any other tetanus toxoid, diphtheria toxoid or pertussis-containing vaccine, or any component of this vaccine (see DESCRIPTION in full prescribing information). Because of the uncertainty as to which component of the vaccine might be responsible, do not give further vaccination with any of these components; or, refer such individuals to an allergist for evaluation. The following events are contraindications to administration of BOOSTRIX: encephalopathy (e.g., coma, decreased level of consciousness, prolonged seizures) within 7 days of administration of a previous dose of a pertussis-containing vaccine that is not attributable to another identifiable cause; progressive neurologic disorder, uncontrolled epilepsy, or progressive encephalopathy. Do not vaccinate individuals with these conditions until a treatment regimen has been established and the condition has stabilized. BOOSTRIX is not contraindicated for use in individuals with HIV infection.

**WARNINGS:** The tip cap and the rubber plunger of the needleless prefilled syringes contain dry natural latex rubber that may cause allergic reactions in latex sensitive individuals. The vial stopper is latex-free. If any of the following events occurred in temporal relation to previous receipt of a Diphtheria and Tetanus Toxoids and Pertussis Vaccine Adsorbed (DTwP) vaccine or a vaccine containing an acellular pertussis component, consider carefully whether to give subsequent doses of BOOSTRIX: temperature of ≥40.5°C (105°F) within 48 hours not due to another identifiable cause; collapse or shock-like state (hypotonic-hyporesponsive episode) within 48 hours; persistent, inconsolable crying lasting ≥3 hours, occurring within 48 hours; seizures with or without fever occurring within 3 days. Persons who experienced serious Arthus-type hypersensitivity reactions following a prior dose of tetanus toxoid usually have high serum tetanus antitoxin levels and should not be given Tetanus and Diphtheria Toxoids Adsorbed For Adult Use (Td) or Tdap vaccines or even emergency doses of Td more frequently than every 10 years, even if the wound is neither clean nor minor. If Guillain-Barré syndrome has occurred within 6 weeks of receipt of prior vaccine containing tetanus toxoid, the decision to give BOOSTRIX or any vaccine containing tetanus toxoid should be based on careful consideration of the potential benefits and possible risks. The decision to administer a pertussis-containing vaccine to individuals with stable central nervous system (CNS) disorders must be made by the physician on an individual basis, with consideration of all relevant factors, and assessment of potential risks and benefits for that individual. Advise the patient, parent, or guardian of the potential increased risk involved (see PRECAUTIONS). A family history of seizures or other CNS disorders is not a contraindication to pertussis vaccine. The Advisory Committee on Immunization Practices (ACIP) has published guidelines for vaccination of persons with recent or acute illness (www.cdc.gov). Do not give BOOSTRIX to individuals with bleeding disorders such as hemophilia or thrombocytopenia, or to persons on anticoagulant therapy unless the potential benefit clearly outweighs the risk of administration. If the decision is made to administer BOOSTRIX to such persons, it should be given with caution with steps taken to avoid the risk of hematoma following the injection.

**PRECAUTIONS:** Before the injection of any biological, the physician should take all reasonable precautions to prevent allergic or other adverse reactions. Epinephrine injection (1:1,000) and other appropriate agents used for the control of immediate allergic reactions must be immediately available should an acute anaphylactic reaction occur. Immunosuppressed persons, including individuals receiving immunosuppressive therapy, may not develop the expected immune response. **Drug Interactions:** Do not mix BOOSTRIX with any other vaccine in the same syringe or vial. **Carcinogenesis, Mutagenesis, Impairment of Fertility:** BOOSTRIX has not been evaluated for carcinogenic or mutagenic potential, or for impairment of fertility. **Pregnancy:** Pregnancy Category C. Animal reproduction studies have not been conducted with BOOSTRIX. It is also not known whether BOOSTRIX can cause fetal harm when administered to a pregnant woman or can affect reproductive capacity. BOOSTRIX should be given to a pregnant woman only if clearly needed. Animal fertility studies have not been conducted with BOOSTRIX. In a developmental toxicity study, the effect of BOOSTRIX on embryo-fetal and pre-weaning development was evaluated in pregnant rats. Animals were administered INFANRIX® (Diphtheria and Tetanus Toxoids and Acellular Pertussis Vaccine Adsorbed) prior to gestation and BOOSTRIX during the period of organogenesis (gestation days 6, 8, 11) and later in pregnancy (gestation day 15), 0.1 mL/rat/occasion (a 45-fold increase compared to the human dose of BOOSTRIX on a body weight basis), by intramuscular injection. No adverse affect on pregnancy and lactation parameters, embryo-fetal or pre-weaning development was observed. There were no fetal malformations or other evidence of teratogenesis noted in this study. **Nursing Mothers:** It is not known whether BOOSTRIX is excreted in human milk. Because many drugs are excreted in human milk, caution should be exercised when BOOSTRIX is administered to a nursing woman. **Pregnancy Exposure Registry:** Healthcare providers are encouraged to register pregnant women who receive BOOSTRIX in the GlaxoSmithKline vaccination pregnancy registry by calling 1-888-825-5249. **Geriatric Use:** BOOSTRIX is not indicated for use in individuals older than 18 years. **Pediatric Use:** BOOSTRIX is not indicated for use in individuals younger than 10 years (see DOSAGE AND ADMINISTRATION in full prescribing information). For immunization of infants and children younger than 7 years against diphtheria, tetanus, and pertussis, refer to the manufacturers' package inserts for Diphtheria and Tetanus Toxoids and Acellular Pertussis Vaccine Adsorbed (DTaP) vaccines.

**ADVERSE REACTIONS:** A total of 3,289 adolescents were vaccinated with a single dose of BOOSTRIX during clinical trials. An additional 1,092 adolescents 10 to 18 years of age received a non-US formulation of BOOSTRIX (formulated to contain 0.5 mg aluminum per dose) in non-US clinical studies.

The primary safety study, conducted in the United States, was a randomized, observer-blinded, controlled study in which 3,080 adolescents 10 to 18 years of age received a single dose of BOOSTRIX and 1,034 received the control Td vaccine manufactured by Massachusetts Public Health Biologic Laboratories. There were no substantive differences in demographic characteristics between the vaccine groups. Among BOOSTRIX and control vaccine recipients approximately 75% were 10 to 14 years of age and approximately 25% were 15 to 18 years of age. Approximately 98% of participants in this study had received the recommended series of 4 or 5 doses of either DTwP or a combination of DTwP and DTaP in childhood. Data on adverse events were collected by the subjects, parents and/or guardians using standardized diaries for 15 consecutive days following the vaccine dose (i.e., day of vaccination and the next 14 days). Subjects were monitored for unsolicited adverse events that occurred within 31 days of vaccination (day 0-30) using diary cards (day 0-14) supplemented by spontaneous reports and a medical history as reported by subjects, parents, and/or guardians. Subjects were also monitored for 6 months post-vaccination for non-routine medical visits, visits to an emergency room, onset of new chronic illness, and serious adverse events. Information regarding late onset adverse events was obtained via a telephone call 6 months following vaccination. At least 97% of subjects completed the 6-month follow-up evaluation.

The adverse event information from clinical trials provides a basis for identifying adverse events that appear to be related to vaccine use and for approximating rates. However, because clinical trials are conducted under widely varying conditions, adverse event rates observed in the clinical trials of a vaccine cannot be directly compared to rates in the clinical trials of another vaccine, and may not reflect the rates observed in practice.

**Serious Adverse Events in All Safety Studies:** In the US-safety study, no serious adverse events were reported to occur within 31 days of vaccination. During the 6-month extended safety evaluation period, no serious adverse events that were of potential autoimmune origin or new onset and chronic in nature were reported to occur. In non-US studies in which serious adverse events were monitored for up to 37 days, one subject was diagnosed with insulin dependent diabetes. The association of this event with vaccination is unknown. No other serious adverse events of potential autoimmune origin or that were new onset and chronic in nature were reported to occur in these studies.

**Solicited Adverse Events in the US-Safety Study:** In a US study, the most common local adverse events following administration of BOOSTRIX were pain, redness, and swelling at the injection site. The most common general adverse events were headache and fatigue. Most of these events were reported at a similar frequency in recipients of both BOOSTRIX and Td. Any pain, grade 2 or 3 pain (but not grade 3 alone), and grade 2 or 3 headache (but not grade 3 alone) were reported at a higher rate in recipients of BOOSTRIX. The primary safety endpoint of the US study was the incidence of grade 3 pain (spontaneously painful and/or prevented normal activity) at the injection site within 15 days of vaccination. Grade 3 pain was reported in 4.6% of those who received BOOSTRIX compared with 4.0% of those who received the Td vaccine. The difference in rate of grade 3 pain was within the pre-defined clinical limit for non-inferiority (upper limit of the 95% CI for the difference ≤4%). These were the rates for solicited local and general adverse events within 15 days of vaccination with BOOSTRIX or Td vaccine for the total vaccinated cohort (all enrolled, vaccinated subjects with safety data available analyzed by vaccine received):

**Percentage of Individuals 10 to 18 Years of Age Reporting Solicited Local Adverse Events or Solicited General Adverse Events Within the 15-day* Post-Vaccination Period**

| | BOOSTRIX (N = 3,032) | Td (N = 1,013) |
|---|---|---|
| **Local** | | |
| Pain,† any | 75.3 | 71.7 |
| Pain,† grade 2 or 3 | 51.2 | 42.5 |
| Pain,‡ grade 3 | 4.6 | 4.0 |
| Redness, any | 22.5 | 19.8 |
| Redness, >20 mm | 4.1 | 3.9 |
| Redness, ≥50 mm | 1.7 | 1.6 |
| Swelling, any | 21.1 | 20.1 |
| Swelling, >20 mm | 5.3 | 4.9 |
| Swelling, ≥50 mm | 2.5 | 3.2 |
| Arm circumference increase,§ >5 mm | 28.3 | 29.5 |
| Arm circumference increase,§ >20 mm | 2.0 | 2.2 |
| Arm circumference increase,§ >40 mm | 0.5 | 0.3 |
| **General** | | |
| Fever,‖ ≥99.5°F | 13.5 | 13.1 |
| Fever,‖ >100.4°F | 5.0 | 4.7 |
| Fever,‖ >102.2°F | 1.4 | 1.0 |
| Headache, any | 43.1 | 41.5 |
| Headache,† grade 2 or 3 | 15.7 | 12.7 |
| Headache, grade 3 | 3.7 | 2.7 |
| Fatigue, any | 37.0 | 36.7 |
| Fatigue, grade 2 or 3 | 14.4 | 12.9 |
| Fatigue, grade 3 | 3.7 | 3.2 |
| Gastrointestinal symptoms,¶ any | 26.0 | 25.8 |
| Gastrointestinal symptoms,¶ grade 2 or 3 | 9.8 | 9.7 |
| Gastrointestinal symptoms,¶ grade 3 | 3.0 | 3.2 |

Td = Tetanus and Diphtheria Toxoids Adsorbed For Adult Use manufactured by Massachusetts Public Health Biologic Laboratories.

N = number of subjects in the total vaccinated cohort with local/general symptoms sheets completed.

Grade 2 = Local: painful when the limb was moved; General: interfered with normal activity.

Grade 3 = Local: spontaneously painful and/or prevented normal activity; General: prevented normal activity.

*Day of vaccination and the next 14 days.

†Statistically significantly higher (P<0.05) following BOOSTRIX as compared to Td vaccine.

‡Grade 3 injection site pain following BOOSTRIX was not inferior to Td (upper limit of two-sided 95% CI for the difference in the percentage of subjects ≤4%).

§Mid-upper region of the vaccinated arm.

‖Oral temperatures or axillary temperatures.

¶Gastrointestinal symptoms included nausea, vomiting, diarrhea and/or abdominal pain.

Mid-upper arm circumference was measured by the adolescent or their parent/guardian prior to injection and daily for 15 days following vaccination. There was no significant difference between BOOSTRIX recipients and Td recipients in the proportion of subjects reporting an increase in mid-upper arm circumference in the vaccinated arm. The incidence of unsolicited adverse events reported in the 31 days after vaccination was comparable between the 2 groups.

As with any vaccine, there is the possibility that broad use of BOOSTRIX could reveal adverse events not observed in clinical trials.

**Postmarketing Reports:** Worldwide voluntary reports of adverse events received for BOOSTRIX in persons 10 to 18 years of age since market introduction of this vaccine are listed below. This list includes serious events or events which have causal connection to components of this or other vaccines or drugs. Because these events are reported voluntarily from a population of uncertain size, it is not possible to reliably estimate their frequency or establish a causal relationship to vaccine exposure. *Blood and lymphatic system disorders:* Lymphadenitis, lymphadenopathy. *Cardiac disorders:* Myocarditis. *Injection site reactions:* Induration, inflammation, mass, nodule, warmth, local reaction. *Metabolism and nutrition disorders:* Diabetes mellitus insulin-dependent. *Musculoskeletal and connective tissue disorders:* Arthralgia, back pain, myalgia. *Nervous system disorders:* Convulsion, encephalitis, facial palsy, paraesthesia. *Skin and subcutaneous tissue disorders:* Exanthem, Henoch-Schönlein purpura, rash. In addition, extensive swelling of the injected limb has been reported following administration of BOOSTRIX.

**Reporting Adverse Events:** Report the occurrence following immunization of any event set forth in the Vaccine Injury Table from the National Childhood Vaccine Injury Act including: Anaphylaxis or anaphylactic shock within 7 days, encephalopathy or encephalitis within 7 days, brachial neuritis within 28 days, or an acute complication or sequelae (including death) of an illness, disability, injury, or condition referred to above, or any events that would contraindicate further doses of vaccine, according to this prescribing information. These events should be reported to VAERS. The VAERS toll-free number is 1-800-822-7967. Reporting forms may also be obtained at the VAERS website at www.vaers.org.

**DOSAGE AND ADMINISTRATION: Recommended Dose:** BOOSTRIX should be administered as a single 0.5 mL injection by the intramuscular route into the deltoid muscle of the upper arm in individuals 10 through 18 years of age. Do not administer this product subcutaneously or intravenously. There are no data to support repeat administration of BOOSTRIX. Five years should elapse between the subject's last dose of the recommended series of childhood DTwP and/or DTaP vaccine and the administration of BOOSTRIX. Limited data are available on the use of BOOSTRIX following Tetanus and Diphtheria Toxoids Adsorbed For Adult Use (Td) vaccine. **Additional Dosing Information:** ***Wound Management:*** Clinicians should refer to guidelines for tetanus prophylaxis in routine wound management. Adolescents 10 to 18 years of age who have completed a primary series against tetanus and who sustain wounds which are minor and uncomplicated, should receive a booster dose of a tetanus toxoid-containing vaccine only if they have not received tetanus toxoid within the preceding 10 years. In case of tetanus-prone injury (e.g., wounds contaminated with dirt, feces, soil, and saliva; puncture wounds; avulsions; and wounds resulting from missles, crushing, burns, and frostbite) in an adolescent who is in need of tetanus toxoid, BOOSTRIX can be used as an alternative to Tetanus and Diphtheria Toxoids Adsorbed For Adult Use (Td) vaccine in patients for whom the pertussis component is also indicated (see INDICATIONS AND USAGE).

Manufactured by **GlaxoSmithKline Biologicals**
Rixensart, Belgium, US License 1617
Distributed by **GlaxoSmithKline**
Research Triangle Park, NC 27709



Full prescribing information for BOOSTRIX is available at www.BOOSTRIX.com.

BRS-BO:L1

**References: 1.** Centers for Disease Control and Prevention. *Epidemiology and Prevention of Vaccine-Preventable Diseases.* Atkinson W, Hamborsky J, Wolfe S, eds. 8th ed. Washington DC: Public Health Foundation; 2004:75–88, A26–A27. **2.** ACIP recommends adolescent vaccination for tetanus, diphtheria and pertussis vaccine [press release]. Atlanta, GA: Department of Health and Human Services; Available at: www.cdc.gov/nip/pr/pr_tdap_jun2005.htm. Accessed September 27, 2005. **3.** Data on file, BOR305, GlaxoSmithKline.

ARTICLE

# Does Children's Screen Time Predict Requests for Advertised Products?

## *Cross-sectional and Prospective Analyses*

*Lisa J. Chamberlain, MD, MPH; Yun Wang, MS; Thomas N. Robinson, MD, MPH*

**Objective:** To examine children's screen media exposure and requests for advertised toys and food/drinks.

**Design:** Prospective cohort study.

**Setting:** Twelve elementary schools in northern California.

**Participants:** Eight hundred twenty-seven third grade children participated at baseline; 386 students in 6 schools were followed up for 20 months.

**Intervention:** None.

**Main Outcome Measures:** Child self-reported requests for advertised toys and foods/drinks.

**Results:** At baseline, children's screen media time was significantly associated with concurrent requests for advertised toys (Spearman $r=0.15$ [TV viewing] and $r=0.20$ [total screen time]; both $P<.001$) and foods/drinks (Spearman $r=0.16$ [TV viewing] and $r=0.18$ [total screen time]; both $P<.001$). In prospective analysis, children's screen media time at baseline was significantly associated with their mean number of toy requests 7 to 20 months later (Spearman $r=0.21$ [TV viewing] and r=0.24 [total screen time]; both $P<.001$) and foods/drinks requests (Spearman $r=0.14$ [TV viewing] and r=0.16 [total screen time]; both $P<.01$). After adjusting for baseline requests and sociodemographic variables, the relationship between screen media exposure and future requests for advertised foods/drinks remained significant for total TV viewing and total screen media exposure. The relationship with future requests for toys remained significant for total screen media exposure.

**Conclusions:** Screen media exposure is a prospective risk factor for children's requests for advertised products. Future experimental studies on children's health- and consumer-related outcomes are warranted.

*Arch Pediatr Adolesc Med. 2006;160:363-368*

CHILDREN ARE IMMERSED IN advertising in media. A recent national survey found that the average child in the United States spends 6 and a half hours a day using media, more than any other waking-time activity, and the majority of media time is spent watching television.[1] In the new era of expanded media channel options, niche programming and advertising have singled out children as a targeted audience.[2] The average US child will see more than 40 000 television commercials a year[3] in addition to frequent product placements in television programs and movies.

Advertising to children is used to change their preferences for advertised products and to change their requests to parents for such items. Consistently, studies have shown that advertising influences children's preferences, choices, and requests for advertised products.[2,4-15] These influences start very young. In 1 experimental trial, preschool children demonstrated preferences for foods seen in ads only briefly.[12] In another study, 63% of Latino preschoolers had asked for a toy seen on TV in the previous 2 weeks and 55% had made a request for advertised food or drinks.[4] Since parents control family budgets, child requests are important forces for family spending and may negatively impact interactions between parents and children.[2,4,10] In addition, in a small-scale randomized controlled trial, a screen media reduction curriculum for third and fourth graders resulted in children making fewer toy purchase requests compared with controls.[16]

Much of the past research exploring the effects of television advertising on children was conducted in the 1970s. Recently, this area of research has become more relevant to children's health, with evi-

Author Affiliations: Division of General Pediatrics, Department of Pediatrics (Drs Chamberlain and Robinson) and Stanford Prevention Research Center, Department of Medicine (Ms Wang and Dr Robinson), Stanford University School of Medicine, Palo Alto, Calif.

dence that food advertising is playing a role in the childhood obesity epidemic.[14,17] As the home screen media environment, children's media use, and advertising have changed, new data are needed to explore the role of advertising in today's children's health and behaviors. Prospective studies are also needed to examine the temporal relationships between screen media exposure and potential outcomes to establish media as a risk factor for purchase requests. Therefore, in a large, ethnically and socioeconomically diverse sample, we conducted a prospective study of preadolescents' screen media exposures and their concurrent and future requests for advertised toys and foods/drinks. We hypothesized that children who reported more screen media exposure at the beginning of third grade would report more requests for advertised toys and food and drinks, both then and during the subsequent 20 months. Establishing screen media exposure as a risk factor for purchase requests would provide stronger support for further efforts to reduce screen time and/or advertising exposure as potential clinical and public health intervention strategies.

## METHODS

All third grade students from 12 public elementary schools in northern California and their parents were eligible to participate in a randomized controlled trial of obesity prevention (6 schools) and smoking prevention (6 schools). Assessments were performed by trained research staff at baseline (September-October 1999), in the spring of third grade (April-May 2000), in the fall of fourth grade (September-October, 2000), and in the spring of fourth grade, approximately 20 months after baseline (April-May 2001). At each point, children completed self-report questionnaires on 2 non-Monday weekdays. A research staff member read each question out loud. Classroom teachers did not participate in the assessments. Parents were interviewed by telephone at baseline by trained interviewers following a standardized protocol.

Tracking and confidentiality were maintained by using unique identification numbers. Parents or guardians provided passive informed consent for their children to participate in each assessment. During classroom assessments, research assistants acquired verbal assent for participation from each child. Children who declined to participate did another nonpunitive activity with their classroom teacher. Parents gave active verbal consent for their own participation in telephone interviews. The study was approved by the participating school districts and the Stanford University Panel for the Protection of Human Subjects in Medical Research (Stanford, Calif).

### MEASURES

#### Demographics

Children reported their date of birth and sex. Ethnicity was obtained from school district records. Parents reported the main language spoken at home, their marital status, and the highest level of education completed by parents or guardians.

#### Media Use and Home Media Environment

Children reported the time they spent "watching television," "watching movies or videos on a VCR," and "playing video games" separately for before school and after school "yesterday" and "last Saturday" on the first assessment day and "yesterday" on the second assessment day. Prior to reading these items, the research staff led children through several participatory time-estimating exercises.[18] This instrument was adapted from a similar instrument previously used in young adolescents with high test-retest reliability ($r=0.94$).[19] For purposes of this analysis, children's screen media use reports derived 4 variables: average weekday television viewing; average Saturday television viewing; total weekly TV viewing (the sum of $5\times$ the average weekday viewing and $2\times$ Saturday viewing); and weekly total screen time (the sum of $5\times$ average weekday TV, movies or videos, and video games use and $2\times$ Saturday TV, movies or videos, and video games use). Children also reported if there was a TV set in the room where they regularly slept.

#### Purchase Requests

Children were asked, "In the past week, have you asked someone to buy you any foods or drinks that you have seen on TV?" and "In the past week, have you asked someone to buy you any toys that you have seen on TV?" For each question, those who responded yes were asked to write the names of up to 4 specific items they had requested and the responses were scored from 0 to 4 for analysis.

### STATISTICAL ANALYSIS

The baseline sample for cross-sectional analysis included children from all 12 schools. Because the obesity-prevention intervention included screen time reduction, only participants from the 6 schools randomly assigned to smoking prevention were included in the prospective analysis sample.

To test our hypothesis, we used nonparametric Spearman rank correlations. First, we examined baseline (fall, third grade) screen exposure variables and baseline requests first for toys and then baseline requests for foods/drinks. Then we examined the prospective sample for correlations between baseline screen exposure and the mean number of requests for toys and foods/drinks over the subsequent assessments (mean of spring third grade, fall fourth grade, and spring of fourth grade).

We performed multivariate linear regression to further examine these relationships, adjusting for covariates. First, all variables were centered[20] (for example, boys were coded $+0.5$ and girls were coded $-0.5$). In model 1, we regressed follow-up requests on screen media exposure, baseline requests, and their interaction. In model 2, we additionally adjusted for sex and ethnicity and all first-order, 2-way interactions. In model 3, using the subset of participants with parent interviews, we further adjusted for parent education, marital status, and language spoken at home and all first-order, 2-way interactions. Statistical significance was defined at a 2-tailed $\alpha=0.05$. Analysis was performed with SAS for Windows, version 9.1 (SAS Institute Inc, Cary, NC).

## RESULTS

Of 860 children enrolled in the 12 elementary schools at baseline, 836 (97%) completed surveys. Nonparticipants included 22 parent refusals, 1 child unable to participate owing to cognitive difficulties, and 1 child who was absent on all assessment days. We randomly chose 1 child for analysis from each of 9 sibling sets to avoid violating the assumption of independence, leaving a final baseline analysis sample of 827 children. Of the 827 students, 410 were enrolled in 1 of the 6 smoking-

**Table 1. Participant Characteristics at Baseline**

| | Baseline Sample (12 Schools) | Prospective Sample (6 Schools) |
|---|---|---|
| Sample size | 827 | 392 |
| Boys, % | 48 | 47 |
| Age, y, mean (SD) | 8.45 (0.38) | 8.45 (0.39) |
| Race/ethnicity, % | | |
| Hispanic/Latino | 35 | 39 |
| Filipino | 27 | 25 |
| White | 17 | 15 |
| Asian/Pacific Islander | 15 | 13 |
| African American | 4 | 4 |
| Other | 2 | 4 |
| Primary language spoken at home, %* | | |
| English | 72 | 66 |
| Spanish | 20 | 25 |
| Other | 8 | 9 |
| Marital status, %* | | |
| Married | 74 | 71 |
| Separated/divorced | 17 | 20 |
| Single, never married | 8 | 9 |
| Widowed | <1 | <1 |
| Maximum parent education level, %* | | |
| <High school | 8 | 10 |
| High school graduate or GED | 23 | 23 |
| Some college/technical school | 33 | 31 |
| 4-year college graduate | 28 | 29 |
| Some/graduate degree | 8 | 7 |
| Screen media use, h, mean (SD) | | |
| Weekly TV exposure | 10.8 (10.8) | 11.3 (11.2) |
| Average weekday TV exposure | 1.6 (1.7) | 1.7 (1.8) |
| Saturday TV exposure | 1.4 (1.8) | 1.4 (1.8) |
| Weekly total screen time | 22.8 (24.7) | 24 (26) |
| TV in child's bedroom, % | 70 | 70 |
| Children's purchase requests, mean (SD) | | |
| No. of toy requests per week | 0.95 (1.29) | 1.15 (1.41) |
| No. of food requests per week | 0.61 (1.14) | 0.77 (1.29) |

Abbreviation: GED, general equivalency diploma; TV, television.
*From parent survey data, N = 684 to 691 (baseline sample), N = 315 to 320 owing to missing data.

**Table 2. Cross-sectional Association Between Screen Media Exposure and Requests for Toys and Food/Drinks***

| | Toy Requests | Food/Drink Requests |
|---|---|---|
| Weekly TV exposure | 0.15† | 0.16† |
| Weekday TV exposure | 0.16† | 0.17† |
| Saturday TV exposure | 0.10‡ | 0.09§ |
| Weekly total screen time | 0.20† | 0.18† |

*Values are expressed as nonparametric Spearman rank correlation coefficients.
†$P<.001$.
‡$P<.01$.
§$P<.05$.

**Table 3. Prospective Association Between Baseline Screen Media Exposure and Subsequent Requests for Toys and Foods/Drinks***

| | Toy Requests | Food/Drink Requests |
|---|---|---|
| Weekly TV exposure | 0.21† | 0.13‡ |
| Weekday TV exposure | 0.19† | 0.15§ |
| Saturday TV exposure | 0.19† | 0.06 |
| Weekly total screen time | 0.22† | 0.16§ |

*Values are expressed as nonparametric Spearman rank correlation coefficients.
†$P<.001$.
‡$P<.05$.
§$P<.01$.

prevention schools. Of the 410 students, there were 14 parent refusals, 2 child refusals, 2 children were unable to complete the surveys, 1 child was absent, and 5 children from sibling sets were removed, which resulted in a potential prospective sample of 386 students. There were an additional 39 children with no follow-up data: 22 children had moved and 17 parents refused participation, leaving 347. Overall, 347 (85%) of 410 students in the 6 smoking-prevention schools participated in at least 1 follow-up assessment and were included in the final prospective analysis sample. Two hundred ninety (84%) of these children also had complete parent interview data for parent education, marital status, and the language spoken at home and were included in the model 3 analysis sample.

Characteristics of the baseline and prospective analysis samples are presented in **Table 1**. The sample was ethnically and sociodemographically diverse. Children reported watching more than 10 hours of TV and more than 22 hours of total screen time per week. Children reported making nearly 1 request per week for toys and more than 1 request every 2 weeks for food/drinks. The smaller prospective sample with complete parent data for model 3 was nearly identical to the full prospective sample for all variables.

Spearman rank correlation coefficients between baseline screen exposure variables and baseline requests for toys and food/drinks are reported in **Table 2**. All correlations were statistically significant (range, 0.09-0.20), confirming the hypothesis that screen exposure is cross-sectionally related to children's requests for advertised products.

To test whether the amount of screen media exposure is a prospective risk factor for future requests for toys or food/drinks, we examined Spearman correlations between baseline screen media exposure and the average toy and food/drink requests at 7, 12, and 20 months (**Table 3**). All screen media exposure variables were significantly associated with the mean of future requests for toys ($r$=0.19-0.24) and weekly TV viewing; weekday TV viewing and weekly total screen viewing time were significantly associated with the frequency of future requests for food/drinks ($r$=0.14-0.16), confirming the hypothesis that screen exposure is related to subsequent requests for advertised products. Having a TV in the bedroom was not significantly correlated with requests for advertised products cross-sectionally at baseline or prospectively ($r$=0.5-0.6).

As a secondary analysis, we further examined these prospective relationships, adjusting for demographic factors using multivariate linear regression (**Table 4**). After adjusting for baseline requests for toys (model 1),

**Table 4. Relationships of Baseline Media Exposure and Future Requests for Advertised Toys and Foods and Drinks Adjusting for Demographic Variables***

| | No. of Toy Requests | | No. of Food/Drink Requests | |
|---|---|---|---|---|
| | Parameter (SE) | *P* Value | Parameter (SE) | *P* Value |
| Model 1 | | | | |
| Weekly TV exposure | 0.005 (0.031) | .88 | 0.011 (0.004) | .005 |
| Weekday TV exposure | 0.048 (0.031) | .12 | 0.066 (0.024) | .006 |
| Saturday TV exposure | 0.006 (0.005) | .20 | 0.044 (0.023) | .053 |
| Weekly total screen time | 0.008 (0.002) | .001 | 0.006 (0.002) | <.001 |
| Model 2 | | | | |
| Weekly TV exposure | 0.009 (0.036) | .80 | 0.019 (0.005) | <.001 |
| Weekday TV exposure | 0.074 (0.047) | .06 | 0.103 (0.030) | <.001 |
| Saturday TV exposure | 0.010 (0.006) | .11 | 0.079 (0.026) | .002 |
| Weekly total screen time | 0.010 (0.003) | .002 | 0.011 (0.002) | <.001 |
| Model 3 | | | | |
| Weekly TV exposure | 0.008 (0.063) | .90 | 0.022 (0.007) | .001 |
| Weekday TV exposure | 0.068 (0.056) | .22 | 0.134 (0.042) | .002 |
| Saturday TV exposure | 0.008 (0.009) | .40 | 0.100 (0.046) | .03 |
| Weekly total screen time | 0.012 (0.004) | .004 | 0.010 (0.003) | .003 |

*Model 1 adjusts for baseline level of requests made for toys and foods/drinks and their interaction with media exposure. Model 2 adjusts for baseline level of requests made for toys and foods/drinks, sex, ethnicity, and all first-order, 2-way interactions between variables. Model 3 adjusts for baseline level of requests made for toys and foods/rinks, parental education (ordinal), marital status (married/not married), language spoken in the home (English/other), and all first-order, 2-way interactions between variables.

weekly total screen time was significantly associated with future toy requests. This result was consistent when further adjusting for ethnicity/race and sex (model 2) and parent education, marital status, and language spoken at home (model 3).

Television viewing exposure variables alone were not statistically significantly related to future requests for toys. For food/drink requests, baseline hours of weekly TV viewing, weekday TV viewing, and weekly total screen time remained significantly associated with future food/drink requests after adjusting for baseline food requests (model 1), and all screen time exposure variables were significantly related to future food/drink requests after adjusting for ethnicity/race and sex (model 2) and parent education, marital status, and language spoken at home (model 3). As in the bivariate analyses, a TV in the bedroom was not significantly correlated with requests for advertised products.

## COMMENT

We hypothesized that in a racially/ethnically and sociodemographically diverse sample of third and fourth grade public school children those who report more screen media exposure at the beginning of third grade would report more requests for advertised toys and food and drinks, both concurrently at baseline and subsequently, through the end of fourth grade. Our findings confirmed our hypothesis. Past research provided evidence that advertising exposure influences children's concurrent or immediate preferences, choices, and requests.[4-9,11-13,15,16,21] Our findings confirm those past findings, using contemporary data from a more diverse sample, and extend them by following up children prospectively. Our prospective findings demonstrate that baseline screen media exposure predicts future requests for advertised toys and foods/drinks. In this prospective study, the screen media exposure was antecedent to the outcome of requests; therefore, we are able to define media exposure as a true risk factor[22,23] for future requests for toys and food/drinks.

In our sociodemographically diverse sample, we found that third graders reported an average of nearly 11 hours per week of TV watching and nearly 23 hours per week of total screen media use. The media consumption was similar[24] to less[25] than other reports in the literature. They also reported requesting an average of about 1 advertised toy per week and 2 foods or drinks every 3 weeks, which is consistent with the literature.[4] Our primary prospective analysis demonstrated that TV and other screen media exposure are true risk factors for future requests for advertised products. In multivariate analysis, we also explored these relationships adjusted for baseline requests and sociodemographic factors. Only the relationship between the hours of Saturday TV viewing and requests for advertised foods or drinks became nonsignificant in prospective analysis, although the magnitude of the correlation was about the same. The relationships between screen media exposure and future food/drink requests remained statistically significant in the multivariate analysis. These results indicated that, even after adjustment for baseline product requests and demographic variables, an extra 1 hour per day in total weekly TV viewing at baseline was associated with an average extra request for an advertised food/drink about every 6 to 13 weeks (0.08-0.15 requests per week) 7 to 20 weeks later, and an extra 1 hour per day of total screen media exposure was associated with an average extra request for an advertised food/drink about every 13 to 24 weeks (0.08-0.04 requests per week) 7 to 20 months later. Because our media time self-reports are slightly lower than other reported samples, it is possible that these effects would be even larger if examined in other samples reporting greater exposure, making these results even more compelling.

When adjusting for baseline toy requests and demographic variables, however, only baseline total screen media exposure continued to be statistically significantly related to future toy requests. An extra hour per day of total screen media exposure at baseline was associated with an average extra request for an advertised toy about every 12 to 18 weeks (0.06-0.08 requests per week) 7 to 20 months later.

For both the toy and food/drink multivariate analysis, we did not find any consistent evidence of significant differences by sex, race/ethnicity, parent education, marital status, or language spoken in the home. In addition, we found no evidence for baseline requests or demographic variables as significant moderators of the associations between baseline screen exposure and subsequent requests for toys.

Although both toy and food/drink requests were significantly predicted by TV viewing and total screen media exposure more than 6 months earlier, it is interesting to speculate on potential reasons for the difference between toy and food/drink requests in the multivariate analysis. First, it is possible that excessive power was lost because of the addition of variables that may not have sufficiently added to the fit of the models. Additional power was sacrificed by using a smaller sample in model 3 because it required complete parent survey data. It is also possible that advertising trends and preferences for toys are more transient or seasonal than those for food/drinks. If individual toy popularity and toy advertising change more frequently with time and age, the link between TV exposure at 1 point and requests for toys more than 6 months later may be weaker. The media variable that did remain statistically significant, total screen media exposure, included video game, movie, videotape, and DVD use in addition to TV. More total screen media time might also produce greater overall exposure to marketing for toy products, thus creating a more durable and sustained level of requests. Alternatively, this group of children who use greater amounts of multiple forms of screen media may represent a subset within our population more heavily geared to consumerism and/or whose families are more likely to respond positively to such requests, themselves leading to additional subsequent requests.

It is always possible that the lack of association in toy requests could be influenced by biased sampling, in which there was a differential in sampling between those predisposed to the effects of toy advertising vs food/drink advertising. However, we had data for 85% of the eligible population-based sample and there were no significant differences in age, sex, marital status, language spoken at home, or educational level of parents for those with and without complete data. Therefore, we believe that sample bias is an unlikely explanation.

A limitation of our study is that we assessed screen media exposure as a proxy for advertising exposure and not advertising directly. It would be methodologically difficult to measure actual exposure and attention to advertising in a population-based study. In a study where consumerism is the outcome of interest, it would be ideal to assess and catalog advertising as direct or product placement on TV, video games, movie, videotape, and DVD in movies. However, from a practical standpoint and in the current policy environment, the easiest way for parents to reduce exposure to screen advertising is to reduce screen time. Therefore, we believe that assessing total screen time was the most reasonable method for drawing relevant practical and policy conclusions. In addition, this study does not take into consideration that new requests may have displaced requests for similar products; however, in analyzing requests over time it is clear that overall requests increased. Despite its limitations, the current study does document that screen media exposure is a true prospective risk factor for subsequent consumeristic behavior, adding to the evidence supporting behavioral and policy interventions to reduce children's exposure to screen media and advertising, whether implemented at the individual family level, institutional level, or the population level through legislation and changes in social norms.

One compelling reason to study the effects of media and advertising on children is to further explore their role in the current obesity epidemic.[14] Advertising and consumerism have been identified as potential targets for both individual and population-based strategies to prevent obesity.[2,26] A causal relationship has been established between children's exposure to food advertisements and food choice[15] and a school-based intervention to reduce screen time resulted in reduced toy requests.[16] Investigators in Australia found that overweight children were more susceptible to food advertising than their lean counterparts.[11] Our study contributes support that reducing children's exposure to screen media may reduce their requests for advertised foods and drinks, which are predominantly high in calories and low in nutritional density.[14]

Potential policy actions should be grounded in empirically derived evidence. Further prospective studies could be designed to further establish advertising directed at children as a risk factor for obesity and consumerism and help identify biological, psychological, and/or social factors that may moderate an individual's susceptibility to advertising and marketing messages and/or mediate their effects on behavioral and physiological outcomes. The finding that screen media exposure is a true risk factor for subsequent requests for advertised products provides rationale for studies examining the effects of individual- and population-level interventions to reduce screen media exposure in general, and advertising in particular, for their impacts on child health.

**Accepted for Publication:** December 15, 2005.
**Correspondence:** Lisa J. Chamberlain, MD, MPH, Division of General Pediatrics, Stanford University School of Medicine, 750 Welch Rd, Suite 325, Palo Alto, CA 94304 (lchamberlain@stanford.edu).
**Author Contributions:** Dr Robinson had full access to all the data in the study and takes responsibility for the integrity of the data and the accuracy of the data analysis.
**Funding/Support:** The study was supported in part by grant R01 HL62224 from the National Heart, Lung, and Blood Institute, National Institutes of Health, Bethesda, Md.

**Acknowledgment:** We would like to acknowledge Helena C. Kraemer, PhD, for statistical guidance and K. Farish Haydel, BA, Michelle Fujimoto, RD, Sally McCarthy, BA, Connie Watanabe, MS, Janine Bishop, MPH, and the participating children, parents, teachers, and schools for their support, guidance, and participation.

## REFERENCES


1. Roberts D, Foehr U, Rideout V. *Generation M: Media in the Lives of 8-18 Year Olds.* Menlo Park, Calif: The Henry J. Kaiser Family Foundation; 2005. Available at: http://www.kff.org/entmedia/upload/Executive-Summary-Generation-M-Media-in-the-Lives-of-8-18-Year-olds.pdf.
2. Kunkel D, Wilcox B, Cantor J, Palmer E, Linn S, Dowrick P. Report of the APA Task Force on advertising and children. Section: psychological issues in the increasing commercialization of childhood. February 20, 2004. Available at: http://www.apa.org/releases/childrenads.pdf.
3. Kunkel D. *Children and Television Advertising.* Thousand Oaks, Calif: Sage Publications; 2001.
4. Borzekowski DL, Poussaint AF. Latino American Preschoolers and the Media. Philadelphia, Pa: Annenberg Public Policy Center; 1998. Annenberg Public Policy Center Report Series 24.
5. Goldberg ME, Gorn GJ. Children's reactions to television advertising: an experimental approach. *J Consum Res.* 1974;1:69-75.
6. Galst J, White M. The unhealthy persuader: the reinforcing value of television and children's purchase-influencing attempts at the supermarket. *Child Dev.* 1976;47:1089-1096.
7. Isler L, Popper E, Ward S. Children's purchase requests and parental responses: results from a diary study. *J Advert Res.* 1987;27:28-39.
8. Goldberg M. A quasi-experiment assessing the effectiveness of TV advertising directed to children. *J Mark Res.* 1990;27:445-454.
9. Gorn G, Florsheim R. The effects of commercials for adult products on children. *J Consum Res.* 1985;11:962-967.
10. Goldberg ME, Gorn GJ. Some unintended consequences of TV advertising to children. *J Consum Res.* 1978;5:22-29.
11. Halford JC, Gillespie J, Brown V, Pontin EE, Dovey TM. Effect of television advertisements for foods on food consumption in children. *Appetite.* 2004;42:221-225.
12. Borzekowski DL, Robinson TN. The 30-second effect: an experiment revealing the impact of television commercials on food preferences of preschoolers. *J Am Diet Assoc.* 2001;101:42-46.
13. Jeffrey DB, McLellarn RW, Fox DT. The development of children's eating habits: the role of television commercials. *Health Educ Q.* 1982;9:174-189.
14. Story M, French S. Food advertising and marketing directed at children and adolescents in the US. *Int J Behav Nutr Phys Act.* 2004;1:3.
15. Gorn GJ, Goldberg ME. Behavioral evidence of the effects of televised food messages on children. *J Consum Res.* 1982;9:200-205.
16. Robinson TN, Saphir MN, Kraemer HC, Varady A, Haydel KF. Effects of reducing television viewing on children's requests for toys: a randomized controlled trial. *J Dev Behav Pediatr.* 2001;22:179-184.
17. Henry J. Kaiser Family Foundation. The role of media in childhood obesity. February 2004. Available at: http://www.kff.org/entmedia/upload/The-Role-Of-Media-in-Childhood-Obesity.pdf. Accessed January 21, 2006.
18. Robinson TN. Reducing children's television viewing to prevent obesity: a randomized controlled trial. *JAMA.* 1999;282:1561-1567.
19. Robinson TN, Killen JD. Ethnic and gender differences in the relationships between television viewing and obesity, physical activity and dietary fat intake. *J Health Educ.* 1995;26:S91-S98.
20. Kraemer HC, Blasey CM. Centring in regression analyses: a strategy to prevent errors in statistical inference. *Int J Methods Psychiatr Res.* 2004;13:141-151.
21. Coon KA, Tucker KL. Television and children's consumption patterns: a review of the literature. *Minerva Pediatr.* 2002;54:423-436.
22. Kraemer HC, Kazdin AE, Offord DR, Kessler RC, Jensen PS, Kupfer DJ. Coming to terms with the terms of risk. *Arch Gen Psychiatry.* 1997;54:337-343.
23. Kazdin AE, Kraemer HC, Kazdin AE, Kessler RC, Kupfer DJ, Offord DR. Contributions of risk-factor research to developmental psychopathology. *Clin Psychol Rev.* 1997;17:375-406.
24. Wiecha JL, Sobol AM, Peterson KE, Gortmaker SL. Household television access: associations with screen time, reading, and homework among youth. *Ambul Pediatr.* 2001;1:244-251.
25. Roberts D, Foehr U, Rideout V, Brodie M. *Kids & Media: the New Millennium.* Menlo Park, Calif: Kaiser Family Foundation; 1999. Report 1536.
26. Koplan J, Liverman C, Kraak V. *Preventing Childhood Obesity: Health in the Balance.* Washington, DC: Institute of Medicine; 2005.


"When is the ideal time for us to have another baby?" a mother will ask.

"Ideal for whom?" I generally reply.

"Well, I'd like him to want the baby—and to see it as his."

This is wishful thinking. No first child ever wants the invasion of a second child. Parents should decide for themselves when they feel they can handle another.

—From *Touchpoints* by T. Berry Brazelton, 2004

# Development and Validation of a Smoking Media Literacy Scale for Adolescents

*Brian A. Primack, MD, EdM; Melanie A. Gold, DO; Galen E. Switzer, PhD; Renee Hobbs, EdD; Stephanie R. Land, PhD; Michael J. Fine, MD, MSc*

**Objectives:** To develop a smoking media literacy (SML) scale by using empiric survey data from a large sample of high school students and to assess reliability and criterion validity of the scale.

**Design:** On the basis of an established theoretical framework, 120 potential items were generated, and items were eliminated or altered on the basis of input from experts and students. Cross-sectional responses to scale items, demographics, smoking-related variables, and multiple covariates were obtained to refine the scale and determine its reliability and validity.

**Setting:** One large Pittsburgh, Pa, high school.

**Participants:** A total of 1211 high school students aged 14 to 18 years.

**Main Outcome Measures:** Current smoking, susceptibility to smoking, attitudes toward smoking, and smoking norms.

**Results:** Factor analysis demonstrated a strong 1-factor scale with 18 items ($\alpha = 0.87$). After controlling for all covariate data, SML had a statistically significant and independent association with current smoking ($P = .01$), susceptibility ($P < .001$), and attitudes ($P < .001$), but not norms ($P = .42$). Controlling for all covariates, an increase of 1 point on the 10-point SML scale was associated with a 22% decrease in the odds of being a smoker and a 31% decrease in the odds of being susceptible to smoking.

**Conclusions:** Smoking media literacy can be measured with excellent reliability and concurrent criterion validity. Given the independent association between SML and smoking, media literacy may be a promising tool for future tobacco control interventions.

*Arch Pediatr Adolesc Med. 2006;160:369-374*

**Author Affiliations:** Center for Research on Health Care (Drs Primack, Gold, Switzer, and Fine), Division of General Internal Medicine, Department of Medicine (Drs Primack, Switzer, and Fine), and Division of Adolescent Medicine, Department of Pediatrics (Dr Gold), University of Pittsburgh School of Medicine, Pittsburgh, Pa; Temple University School of Communications and Theater, Philadelphia, Pa (Dr Hobbs); Graduate School of Public Health, University of Pittsburgh (Dr Land); and Center for Health Equity Research and Promotion, Veterans Affairs Pittsburgh Health Care System (Dr Fine).

CIGARETTE SMOKING IS THE leading cause of preventable death and disease in the United States,[1] and about 90% of those who die from smoking began during adolescence.[2] However, traditional school-based smoking prevention programs have not been successful in affecting clinically relevant smoking behaviors.[3-6]

Youth aged 8 to 18 years are exposed to 8 hours 33 minutes of mass media content daily,[7] including a substantial number of positive portrayals of cigarette smoking.[8-10] Research has demonstrated a strong association between exposure to certain mass media messages and smoking in adolescents. For instance, more than half of adolescent smoking initiation has been linked to watching smoking in movies.[11-13] Exposure to mass media messages such as promotions and advertisements also significantly increases the risk of smoking initiation by adolescents.[2,14-17]

Media literacy therefore represents a promising framework for development of innovative school-based tobacco control programs.[18] Acknowledging the effects of mass media on attitudes and behavior, media literacy teaches youth to understand, analyze, and evaluate advertising and other mass media messages, enabling them to actively process media messages rather than passively remain message targets.[19,20] Media literacy has been shown to be both feasible and teachable,[20,21] making it attractive as an intervention.

Recognizing its potential, the American Academy of Pediatrics,[18] the Centers for Disease Control and Prevention,[22] and the US Office of National Drug Control Policy[23] have called for the use of media literacy to reduce harmful health behaviors such as smoking. One consistent limitation of smoking media literacy (SML) evaluations, however, is the lack of a reliable, validated scale measuring this construct in youth. Development of such a

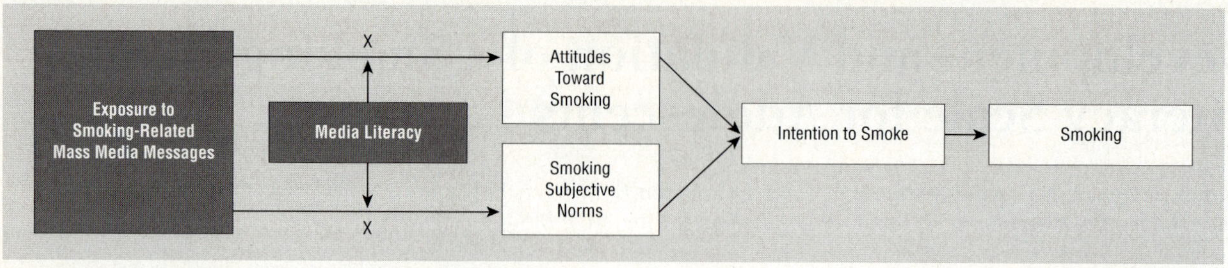


**Figure 1.** The theory of reasoned action, applied to mass media and smoking. Media literacy interventions, which examine the manipulative construction of tobacco industry messages and the salient omissions of those messages, would be expected to decrease positive attitudes toward smoking. Media literacy would also be expected to correct misperceptions regarding the normality of smoking by (1) exposing the industry techniques used to make behaviors seem more normative and (2) emphasizing the difference between "television reality" and "real reality."

**Table 1. Media Literacy Framework***

| Media Literacy Domain | Related Media Literacy Core Concepts |
|---|---|
| Authors and audiences (AA) | AA1: authors create media messages for profit and/or influence |
| | AA2: authors target specific audiences |
| Messages and meanings (MM) | MM1: messages contain values and specific points of view |
| | MM2: different people interpret messages differently |
| | MM3: messages affect attitudes and behaviors |
| | MM4: multiple production techniques are used |
| Representation and reality (RR) | RR1: messages filter reality |
| | RR2: messages omit information |

*Core concepts from 2 major theories of media literacy[28,29] were integrated into this model.

psychometrically appropriate scale is necessary to evaluate the effectiveness of media literacy interventions designed to reduce adolescent smoking.

To validate a measure of SML, it is necessary to apply an appropriate theory of health behavior. The theory of reasoned action has been used to accurately predict adolescent smoking.[24-27] According to this theory, an individual's behavior is determined by his or her intention to perform the behavior, which is in turn predicted by his or her attitude toward the behavior and perception of norms regarding it.[24] Media literacy theoretically affects both attitudes and norms involving smoking (**Figure 1**).

The aims of this study were (1) to develop a scale measuring SML in adolescents, using empiric survey data from a large sample of high school students, and (2) to assess internal consistency (ie, reliability) and concurrent criterion validity of the SML scale.

## METHODS

Our study was conducted in 3 distinct phases, in which we (1) rigorously developed a pool of potential SML scale items, (2) collected empiric cross-sectional data from adolescents, and (3) refined the scale and assessed its reliability and validity.

### PHASE 1: ITEM DEVELOPMENT

Two major accepted theoretical models exist describing media literacy[28,29]; although the models overlap substantially, there are differences in emphasis. A British model emphasizes understanding (1) the purposes of media producers and characteristics of target audiences, (2) the multiple complex production techniques used to convey meaning, and (3) the ability to distinguish media representations from reality.[28] A US model emphasizes that (1) media messages are carefully constructed with the use of their own complex language, (2) different individuals interpret messages differently, (3) messages contain inherent values and perspectives, and (4) media messages are usually created for profit and/or power.[29] To maximize content validity of the scale, we combined the 2 models into a comprehensive framework integrating core concepts from each model (**Table 1**). We then developed 120 Likert-type scale items (strongly disagree, disagree, agree, strongly agree), with 15 items representing each of the 8 core concepts. We developed items related to both persuasive media (such as promotions and advertisements) and narrative media (such as episodes of smoking in films and on television) because of the important role each genre plays in media literacy.[30] We also included both general and smoking-specific items.

We distributed this pool of items for review to a convenience sample of 8 leading national experts in media literacy, tobacco control, and public health. We also held 2 hour-long focus groups with 9th- to 11th-grade adolescents. One was held at a primarily white high school in a middle-income neighborhood (8 students) and the second at a predominantly African American high school in a low-income neighborhood (11 students). Items were eliminated or altered on the basis of consensus of both experts and students, resulting in a 51-item pool, with several items representing each of the 8 core concepts of media literacy.

### PHASE 2: DATA COLLECTION IN A DEVELOPMENT SAMPLE

We administered this refined item pool to a sample of all students aged 14 to 18 years at a large Pittsburgh, Pa, public high school (enrollment, 1690). In addition to media literacy items, we asked students to provide demographic information, smoking-related data, and covariate information. Demographic information included age, sex, parental education (as a surrogate for socioeconomic status), race, and ethnicity. Smoking-related data obtained measured 4 smoking-related variables defined by the theory of reasoned action: (1) current smoking, defined as having smoked in the past 30 days; (2) intention to smoke, assessed with Pierce and coworkers' reliable and valid susceptibility scale[31]; (3) attitudes toward smoking, assessed with 18 items based on Buller and coworkers' reliable and valid scale[32]; and (4) smoking subjective norms, assessed with 3 items based on the Fishbein-Ajzen-Hansen question-

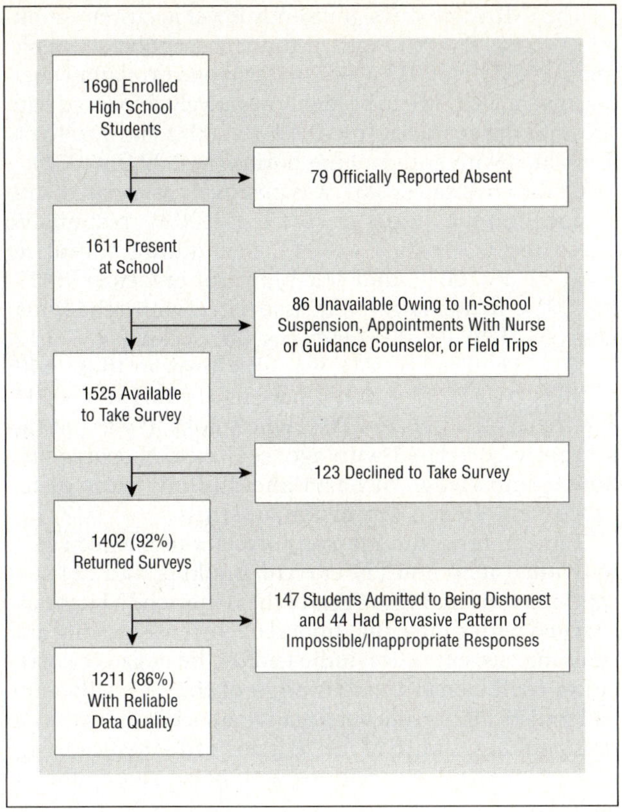


**Figure 2.** Study population and response rate.

naire.[33] A high score on this norms scale (stronger "antismoking norms") indicates that the individual feels that those close to him or her do not approve of smoking. Covariates obtained included media use habits, parent smoking, friend smoking, sibling smoking, stress, depression, self-report of grades, knowledge of the effects and addictiveness of tobacco, demanding parenting, responsive parenting, sensation seeking, and rebellious behavior. Covariates were measured with previously validated and/or commonly used scales.[11,31,32]

The vast majority (1402) of the 1525 students eligible to complete the survey participated (**Figure 2**). Before data analysis, we defined specific criteria to detect and eliminate questionnaires with poor data quality. If 3 or more responses were deemed impossible or extremely improbable (such as claims to have smoked an average of 120 cigarettes per day), that respondent's data were eliminated from the analysis. By this process, data from 44 students (3%) were eliminated. In addition, students were asked in a final survey item to appraise their honesty with the survey. Those who admitted having been dishonest (147 students) were eliminated from the analysis, resulting in a final sample size of 1211 (86% of returned surveys). The unpaired, 2-tailed *t* test, an exact linear rank test for comparing 2 ordered multinomial proportions (using a Wilcoxon statistic), and a $\chi^2$ test confirmed that those eliminated from the analysis were no different in terms of age, race, or reported parental education, respectively. Those eliminated were, however, more likely to be male (71% vs 48%; $P<.001$).

Approval for the project was granted by both the superintendent of the school district and the institutional review board of the University of Pittsburgh. Both bodies agreed to a waiver of parental informed consent, since students did not place their names or any other unique personal identifiers on the questionnaires. All students completed the questionnaire during social studies classes, and those who completed the questionnaire were given a packet of trail mix.

**Table 2. Scale Item Core Concepts, Factor Loadings, and Correlations With Smoking Outcomes***

| Item No. | Related Core Concept† | Factor Loading | Pearson *r* Between Item and Current Smoking | Pearson *r* Between Item and Susceptibility to Smoking |
|---|---|---|---|---|
| 1 | AA1 | 0.47 | −0.10 | −0.10 |
| 2 | AA1 | 0.58 | −0.01 | **−0.14** |
| 3 | AA1 | 0.62 | −0.10 | **−0.19** |
| 4 | AA2 | 0.54 | −0.05 | −0.10 |
| 5 | MM1 | 0.54 | −0.09 | **−0.20** |
| 6 | MM1 | 0.58 | **−0.12** | **−0.13** |
| 7 | MM2 | 0.51 | −0.03 | **−0.11** |
| 8 | MM2 | 0.55 | −0.02 | **−0.14** |
| 9 | MM2 | 0.52 | −0.06 | **−0.15** |
| 10 | MM3 | 0.54 | **−0.12** | **−0.13** |
| 11 | MM3 | 0.60 | **−0.12** | **−0.15** |
| 12 | MM4 | 0.48 | −0.08 | **−0.20** |
| 13 | MM4 | 0.48 | **−0.15** | **−0.15** |
| 14 | RR1 | 0.47 | **−0.12** | **−0.12** |
| 15 | RR1 | 0.62 | **−0.17** | **−0.17** |
| 16 | RR1 | 0.55 | **−0.19** | **−0.24** |
| 17 | RR2 | 0.56 | **−0.17** | **−0.22** |
| 18 | RR2 | 0.66 | **−0.20** | **−0.22** |

*All items were tested on a 4-point Likert scale: strongly disagree, disagree, agree, or strongly agree. Wording of actual items is available from the authors. For boldface entries, $P<.05$ by the Dunn-Sidak method of correction.

†See Table 1 for explanation.

## PHASE 3: SCALE REFINEMENT AND DETERMINATION OF RELIABILITY AND VALIDITY

We performed iterative principal components analysis (PCA) using varimax rotation with the 51 media literacy items to determine the underlying factor structure produced by these items.[34] The first iteration of PCA showed 1 strong factor with an eigenvalue of 8.2 explaining 53% of the variance, a much weaker but possible second factor, and a scree plot indicating a likely 1-factor solution. We conducted a second PCA on the 23 items that maintained a loading of at least 0.45 on 1 of the first 2 factors. This PCA resulted in a conclusive 1-factor solution with an eigenvalue of 6.0 explaining 87% of the variance (the second factor's eigenvalue was 0.9). Eighteen of the 23 items were related to this primary factor with a loading of greater than 0.45, and all were retained in the scale (**Table 2**). We used a cutoff factor loading of 0.45 to ensure that the scale did not contain too many or too few items and to ensure that the selected items were highly correlated with the underlying construct of media literacy. Qualitative analysis of the final 18 items confirmed that the scale did seem to measure SML and not other competing constructs. For instance, the items appropriately represented each of the theoretical domains of the framework (Table 2). In addition, retained items related to both narrative (items 7, 10, 12, and 14) and persuasive media, and some items were general (items 7, 10, 11, 12, and 18) while others were smoking-specific. Finally, some items (items 3 and 5) had strong cynical sentiment, whereas other items (items 7, 8, 9, and 12) were neutral in tone. This is consistent with the theoretical construct of media literacy: cynicism and anti-industry attitudes can result from critical appraisal of media messages, but it is only one aspect of media literacy. The final 18-item scale has excellent internal consistency, with a Cronbach $\alpha=0.87$. For ease of intuitive interpretation and potential future application, the resulting 54-point SML scale was con-

**Table 3. Baseline Respondent Characteristics**

| Characteristic | Finding |
|---|---|
| Age, mean (SD), y | 15.9 (1.2) |
| Sex, No. (%) M | 572 (47.7) |
| Race, No. (%) | |
| White | 1092 (91.7) |
| Black | 49 (4.1) |
| Other | 50 (4.2) |
| Hispanic ethnicity, No. (%) | 11 (0.9) |
| Parental education, No. (%)* | |
| ≥1 Parent did not graduate from high school | 58 (5.2) |
| Both parents graduated from high school, neither from college | 365 (32.9) |
| 1 Parent graduated from college, 1 from high school | 320 (28.9) |
| Both parents graduated from college | 365 (32.9) |
| Current smoker, No. (%)† | 216 (19.0) |
| Susceptible to smoking, No. (%)‡ | 575 (50.0) |
| Prosmoking attitude score, mean (SD) (range, 18-72) | 36.2 (9.1) |
| Antismoking norms score, mean (SD) (range, 3-12) | 8.7 (1.9) |
| Household member smokes, No. (%) | 468 (38.9) |
| Close friend smokes, No. (%) | 628 (56.9) |
| Sibling smokes, No. (%) | 267 (22.7) |
| Smoking media literacy score, mean (SD) (range, 0-10) | 6.9 (1.3) |

*Parental education was used as a surrogate for socioeconomic status.
†Current smoking was defined as smoking at least once in the past 30 days.
‡Susceptibility to smoking was defined by at least 1 positive response on the reliable and valid 3-item scale of Pierce et al.[31]

verted to a 10-point scale by dividing the raw 54-point score by 5.4.

We then assessed concurrent criterion validity by examining associations between students' SML scale values and smoking-related variables and covariates in the theory of reasoned action. We first computed pairwise Pearson correlation coefficients between SML and all smoking measures and covariates. We also computed Pearson correlation coefficients between the major clinically significant smoking measures (current smoking and susceptibility) and each of the individual SML items. Significance was defined with a $P<.05$ but was corrected by the Dunn-Sidak method to reduce the likelihood of false-positive significant results.[35] When variables were dichotomous, 2-group $t$ tests of the SML scores were used instead. Regression techniques were then used to determine whether associations between SML and each of the 4 theory of reasoned action variables remained after controlling for major factors known to predict smoking: sex, age, socioeconomic status, media use habits, parent smoking, friend smoking, sibling smoking, stress, depression, self-report of grades, knowledge of the effects and addictiveness of tobacco, demanding parenting, responsive parenting, sensation seeking, and rebellious behavior. Multiple linear regression was used for continuous outcome variables and logistic regression was used for binary outcome variables. Race and Hispanic ethnicity were not included in the regression model because of the extremely low proportions of nonwhite and Hispanic participants.

## RESULTS

The sample had a nearly equal sex distribution, and mean age was 15.9 years (**Table 3**). The sample was predominantly white, with few African Americans and Latinos. Of the sample, 19% reported smoking in the past 30 days and 50% were classified as susceptible to smoking.

The SML score was significantly lower in current smokers ($t=6.60$, $P<.001$) and in those susceptible to smoking ($t=9.60$, $P<.001$). Pairwise Pearson correlation coefficients showed SML to be highly negatively associated with prosmoking attitudes ($r=-0.49$, $P<.001$) and positively associated with antismoking norms ($r=0.22$, $P<.001$).

Of the covariates, SML was positively associated with socioeconomic status ($r=0.13$, $P=.003$), responsive parenting ($r=0.18$, $P<.001$), demanding parenting ($r=0.22$, $P<.001$), and self-report of grades ($r=0.27$, $P<.001$). It was negatively associated with rebelliousness ($r=-0.26$, $P<.001$) and sensation seeking ($r=-0.12$, $P=.01$). The level of SML was also lower in those with siblings ($t=3.62$, $P<.001$), parents ($t=3.61$, $P<.001$), and friends ($t=7.26$, $P<.001$) who smoke. It was not significantly correlated with age, sex, race, Hispanic ethnicity, knowledge of harm and addictiveness of tobacco, self-esteem, depression, or stress.

Table 2 shows the Pearson correlations between each individual item and (1) current smoking and (2) susceptibility to smoking. Each of the items tended to be associated with a lower likelihood of current smoking and smoking susceptibility, indicated by the negative correlation coefficients. In addition, 9 of the 18 coefficients had statistically significant negative associations with current smoking, and 16 of the 18 items had statistically significant negative associations with being susceptible to smoking.

Multivariate regression analyses (**Table 4**) showed that, after controlling for all covariates, the SML score was independently associated with current smoking ($P=.01$), susceptibility to smoking ($P<.001$), and antismoking attitudes ($P<.001$). After controlling for all of these cofactors, however, the SML score was not independently associated with smoking norms ($P=.42$). Logistic regression was used for binary outcomes (smoking and susceptibility), so we report odds ratios with 95% confidence intervals. Multiple linear regression was used for the continuous outcomes (attitude and norms), so for these outcomes we report the regression coefficients, standard errors, and $P$ values. These $P$ values help determine whether the regression coefficients are significantly greater than zero, indicating that the variable being tested is an independent predictor of the outcome.

## COMMENT

This study shows that SML is a construct that can be adequately measured with a Likert-type scale with promising reliability and validity. Internal consistency of the developed scale is excellent (Cronbach $\alpha=0.87$). Content validity appears strong because scale items were based on a carefully developed framework integrating the most accepted models of media literacy and because the resultant scale contains items representing each of the framework's core concepts. In addition, the associations noted in this study seem to support the scale's concurrent criterion validity. As would be expected, those with higher media literacy were less likely to smoke, less susceptible to smoking, less likely to have positive attitudes toward smoking, and more likely to have antismoking norms.

**Table 4. Multivariate Associations Between SML and Smoking***

| | Odds Ratio (95% CI) | | Positive Attitude Toward Smoking | | Antismoking Norms | |
|---|---|---|---|---|---|---|
| | Current Smoking† | Susceptibility to Smoking‡ | Coefficient (SE) | *P* Value | Coefficient (SE) | *P* Value |
| SML (1 point on 10-point scale) | **0.78 (0.65-0.95)** | **0.69 (0.59-0.80)** | **−2.26 (0.20)** | **<.001** | 0.04 (0.05) | .42 |
| Age (1 yr) | **1.32 (1.06-1.64)** | 0.92 (0.79-1.08) | −0.04 (0.22) | .84 | **−0.13 (0.05)** | **.02** |
| Sex (M vs F) | 1.21 (0.74-1.98) | 0.99 (0.69-1.43) | −0.62 (0.51) | .23 | −0.17 (0.13) | .18 |
| SES (1 point on 5-point scale based on parental education) | 1.12 (0.86-1.46) | 1.13 (0.93-1.37) | 0.05 (0.27) | .86 | 0.00 (0.07) | .97 |
| Smoking knowledge (1 point on 5-point scale) | **0.76 (0.60-0.96)** | 0.99 (0.84-1.18) | **−0.60 (0.24)** | **.01** | **0.20 (0.06)** | **.001** |
| Electronic media use (1 h/d) | 1.02 (0.98-1.07) | 0.98 (0.95-1.02) | −0.05 (0.05) | .33 | 0.01 (0.01) | .31 |
| Responsive parenting (1 point on 7-point scale) | 0.96 (0.77-1.21) | 0.99 (0.82-1.20) | −0.26 (0.26) | .32 | **0.15 (0.06)** | **.02** |
| Authoritative parenting (1 point on 7-point scale) | 1.04 (0.84-1.29) | 0.93 (0.78-1.10) | **−0.64 (0.24)** | **.01** | **0.25 (0.06)** | **<.001** |
| Sensation seeking (1 point on 7-point scale) | **1.27 (1.01-1.59)** | **1.38 (1.17-1.63)** | **0.71 (0.22)** | **.001** | −0.02 (0.05) | .67 |
| Rebelliousness (1 point on 7-point scale) | **1.63 (1.28-2.07)** | **1.47 (1.21-1.78)** | **1.04 (0.27)** | **<.001** | **−0.28 (0.06)** | **<.001** |
| Depression (1 point on 7-point scale based on PRIME-MD) | 1.21 (0.97-1.50) | 1.10 (0.93-1.29) | 2.28 (0.22) | <.001 | −0.03 (0.06) | .54 |
| Self-esteem (1 point on 7-point scale) | 0.97 (0.78-1.20) | **0.81 (0.69-0.95)** | −0.04 (0.22) | .87 | −0.02 (0.05) | .77 |
| Stress (1 point on 4-point scale) | 1.18 (0.86-1.63) | 1.07 (0.85-1.34) | −0.12 (0.32) | .71 | −0.05 (0.08) | .49 |
| Grades (1 point on self-reported 4-point scale) | **0.59 (0.39-0.88)** | 0.90 (0.65-1.23) | −0.26 (0.46) | .56 | 0.14 (0.11) | .21 |
| Sibling smoking (yes vs no) | **1.73 (1.03-2.89)** | 1.20 (0.75-1.91) | −0.79 (0.66) | .23 | −0.28 (0.16) | .07 |
| Parent smoking (yes vs no) | **2.01 (1.24-3.26)** | 1.09 (0.75-1.60) | **1.10 (0.54)** | **.04** | **−0.52 (0.13)** | **<.001** |
| Friend smoking (yes vs no) | **15.18 (5.84-39.41)** | **4.02 (2.75-5.88)** | **3.26 (0.57)** | **<.001** | **−0.84 (0.14)** | **<.001** |

Abbreviations: CI, confidence interval; PRIME-MD, Primary Care Evaluation of Mental Disorders questionnaire; SES, socioeconomic status; SML, smoking media literacy.

*Boldface values are statistically significant at $P<.05$.

†Defined as smoking at least once in the past 30 days.

‡Defined by at least 1 positive response on the reliable and valid 3-item scale of Pierce et al.[31]

Nearly all of the individual SML items were significantly associated with reduced susceptibility to smoking, and 9 of 18 were significantly associated with reduced current smoking, even attitudinally neutral statements such as "People are influenced by advertising."

After controlling for major known covariates of smoking, SML retained its significant relationship with smoking, intention to smoke, and attitudes, but not smoking norms. There are several potential reasons for this finding. First, media literacy may indeed have less of an association with smoking-related norms than has been hypothesized. Second, this may signify a weakness in the SML scale's ability to fully capture the intended construct of media literacy. Third, the mean for the antismoking norms was relatively high, so an association might be lacking because the distribution was limited or skewed. Finally, it is possible that our measurement of smoking norms was not ideal. Although we selected relevant items from a scale shown to have acceptable reliability and validity,[33] we did not include all items from the original scale. It is also possible that even the full Fishbein-Ajzen-Hansen questionnaire does not completely assess the construct of "smoking norms" because it includes items assessing the subject's sense of approval of smoking solely by parents (father and mother) and peers (best friend, friends, romantic partner). Because youth behavior is likely to be influenced not only by parents and peers but also by coaches, mentors, teachers, actors, sports stars, and other important public figures, it may be necessary to develop a more comprehensive smoking norms scale based on the model of the successful Fishbein-Ajzen-Hansen questionnaire.

These findings suggest that media literacy may be a useful intervention with regard to tobacco control. In this adolescent population, an increase of 1 point on the 10-point SML scale was associated with a 22% decrease in the odds of being a smoker and a 31% decrease in the odds of being susceptible to smoking, even after controlling for multiple known smoking covariates. Indeed, as shown by logistic regression, the association of smoking with media literacy was stronger than the association of smoking with many other factors thought to be important predictors of smoking, such as knowledge of the harm and addictiveness of smoking, depression, self-esteem, socioeconomic status, responsive parenting, demanding parenting, and stress level. This would imply that SML may be an important part of comprehensive tobacco control interventions, especially since it is feasible and teachable.

This research had several limitations. First, the study population was drawn from a single large high school and was largely homogeneous in terms of its racial and ethnic background. This scale should therefore be tested and these results confirmed in more diverse populations. Baseline values for smoking and susceptibility approximate previously reported values, however.[31,32] For instance, the Monitoring the Future study[36] recently reported that 16% of 10th-grade students and 25% of 12th-grade students reported current (30-day) smoking. These values are similar to the overall 19% rate we found among all 9th through 12th graders. Also, our study addressed only content (face) and concurrent criterion validity, so it will be particularly important to assess construct validity of the scale in the future. Although there is currently no gold standard for measuring an individual's media literacy, there are accepted scales used in educational settings that could be adapted for smoking-specific media.[37] Students' scores on these measures could be compared with SML scores to support or weaken this scale's construct validity. It will also be important to confirm these findings in a longitudinal setting. Although a cross-sectional study can show concurrent associations between SML and smoking, the more clinically relevant question remains to be answered: whether individuals with different levels of media literacy take up smoking at different rates. This question could ideally be answered with a prospective cohort study.

Given the substantial exposure of adolescents to mass media messages, many of which have been shown to successfully promote smoking, it is not surprising that organizations such as the American Academy of Pediatrics and the Centers for Disease Control and Prevention recommend media literacy—the systematic assessment and evaluation of mass media messages—to buffer the impact of mass media messages on adolescent smoking.[18,22] To evaluate such programs with appropriate rigor, however, it was necessary to develop a scale measuring the construct of SML in adolescents. This scale seems to have strong psychometric properties, and its association with theoretically derived markers of smoking suggests the potential utility of SML as an intervention in this population.

**Accepted for Publication:** December 15, 2005.
**Correspondence:** Brian A. Primack, MD, EdM, Center for Research on Health Care, 230 McKee Pl, Suite 600, Room 4, Pittsburgh, PA 15213 (bprimack@pitt.edu).
**Author Contributions:** Dr Primack had full access to all the data in the study and takes responsibility for the integrity of the data and the accuracy of the data analysis.
**Funding/Support:** This study was supported by the Maurice Falk Foundation and Tobacco-Free Allegheny, Pittsburgh.
**Role of the Sponsor:** The funding agencies were not involved in the design and conduct of the study; collection, management, analysis, and interpretation of the data; or preparation, review, or approval of the manuscript.
**Acknowledgment:** We acknowledge the active participation and support of Baldwin High School, Pittsburgh, including the students, teachers, principal Stephen Puskar, and social services director Annette Giovanazzi, PhD. We thank Katie Steinkamp, MHPE, CHES, and Jessica Viglione for their assistance with data management.

## REFERENCES

1. Mokdad AH, Marks JS, Stroup DF, Gerberding JL. Actual causes of death in the United States, 2000. *JAMA*. 2004;291:1238-1245.
2. Centers for Disease Control and Prevention. *Preventing Tobacco Use Among Young People: A Report of the Surgeon General*. Atlanta, Ga: US Dept of Health and Human Services; 1994.
3. Peterson AV Jr, Kealey KA, Mann SL, Marek PM, Sarason IG. Hutchinson Smoking Prevention Project: long-term randomized trial in school-based tobacco use prevention—results on smoking. *J Natl Cancer Inst*. 2000;92:1979-1991.
4. Ellickson PL, Bell RM, McGuigan K. Preventing adolescent drug use: long-term results of a junior high program. *Am J Public Health*. 1993;83:856-861.
5. Flay BR, Koepke D, Thomson SJ, Santi S, Best JA, Brown KS. Six-year follow-up of the first Waterloo school smoking prevention trial. *Am J Public Health*. 1989; 79:1371-1376.
6. Luepker RV, Pallonen UE, Murray DM, Pirie PL. Validity of telephone surveys in assessing cigarette smoking in young adults. *Am J Public Health*. 1989;79: 202-204.
7. Rideout V, Roberts D, Foehr U. *Generation M: Media in the Lives of 8-18 Year-Olds*. Menlo Park, Calif: Kaiser Family Foundation; 2005.
8. Dozier DM, Lauzen M, Day C, Payne S, Tafoya M. Leaders and elites: portrayals of smoking in popular films. *Tob Control*. 2005;14:7-9.
9. Fischer PM, Schwartz MP, Richards JW Jr, Goldstein AO, Rojas TH. Brand logo recognition by children aged 3 to 6 years: Mickey Mouse and Old Joe the Camel. *JAMA*. 1991;266:3145-3148.
10. Long JA, O'Connor PG, Gerbner G, Concato J. Use of alcohol, illicit drugs, and tobacco among characters on prime-time television. *Subst Abus*. 2002;23: 95-103.
11. Dalton MA, Sargent JD, Beach ML, et al. Effect of viewing smoking in movies on adolescent smoking initiation: a cohort study. *Lancet*. 2003;362:281-285.
12. Sargent JD, Beach ML, Adachi-Mejia AM, et al. Exposure to movie smoking: its relation to smoking initiation among US adolescents. *Pediatrics*. 2005;116: 1183-1191.
13. Sargent JD, Beach ML, Dalton MA, et al. Effect of seeing tobacco use in films on trying smoking among adolescents: cross sectional study. *BMJ*. 2001;323: 1394-1397.
14. Pierce JP, Choi WS, Gilpin EA, Farkas AJ, Berry CC. Tobacco industry promotion of cigarettes and adolescent smoking. *JAMA*. 1998;279:511-515.
15. Gilpin EA, Pierce JP, Rosbrook B. Are adolescents receptive to current sales promotion practices of the tobacco industry? *Prev Med*. 1997;26:14-21.
16. Altman DG, Levine DW, Coeytaux R, Slade J, Jaffe R. Tobacco promotion and susceptibility to tobacco use among adolescents aged 12 through 17 years in a nationally representative sample. *Am J Public Health*. 1996;86:1590-1593.
17. Wakefield MA, Ruel EE, Chaloupka FJ, Slater SJ, Kaufman NJ. Association of point-of-purchase tobacco advertising and promotions with choice of usual brand among teenage smokers. *J Health Commun*. 2002;7:113-121.
18. Committee on Public Education. Media education: American Academy of Pediatrics, Committee on Public Education. *Pediatrics*. 1999;104:341-343.
19. Buckingham D. *Media Education: Literacy, Learning, and Contemporary Culture*. Malden, Mass: Blackwell Publishing; 2003.
20. Hobbs R, Frost R. Measuring the acquisition of media-literacy skills. *Reading Res Q*. 2003;38:330-355.
21. Aufderheide P, Firestone C. *Media Literacy: A Report of the National Leadership Conference on Media Literacy*. Queenstown, Md: Aspen Institute; 1993.
22. Centers for Disease Control and Prevention. *MediaSharp: Analyzing Tobacco and Alcohol Messages*. Atlanta, Ga: Centers for Disease Control and Prevention; 1999.
23. Office of National Drug Control Policy. *Helping Youth Navigate the Media Age: A New Approach to Drug Prevention*. Washington, DC: Office of National Drug Control Policy; 2001.
24. Ajzen I, Fishbein M. *Understanding Attitudes and Predicting Social Behavior*. Englewood Cliffs, NJ: Prentice-Hall; 1980.
25. O'Callaghan FV, Callan VJ, Baglioni A. Cigarette use by adolescents: attitude-behavior relationships. *Subst Use Misuse*. 1999;34:455-468.
26. McGahee TW, Kemp V, Tingen M. A theoretical model for smoking prevention studies in preteen children. *Pediatr Nurs*. 2000;26:135-138.
27. Unger JB, Rohrbach LA, Howard KA, Boley Cruz T, Johnson CA, Chen X. Attitudes toward anti-tobacco policy among California youth: associations with smoking status, psychosocial variables and advocacy actions. *Health Educ Res*. 1999; 14:751-763.
28. Bazalgette C. Key aspects of media education. In: Alvarado M, Boyd-Barrett O, eds. *Media Education: An Introduction*. London, England: British Film Institute; 1992:198-219.
29. Thoman E. *Skills and Strategies for Media Education*. Santa Monica, Calif: Center for Media Literacy; 2003.
30. Hobbs R. The seven great debates in the media literacy movement. *J Commun*. 1998;48:16-32.
31. Pierce JP, Choi WS, Gilpin EA, Farkas AJ, Merritt RK. Validation of susceptibility as a predictor of which adolescents take up smoking in the United States. *Health Psychol*. 1996;15:355-361.
32. Buller DB, Borland R, Woodall WG, Hall JR, Burris-Woodall P, Voeks JH. Understanding factors that influence smoking uptake. *Tob Control*. 2003;12(suppl 4):IV16-IV25.
33. Hanson MJ. The theory of planned behavior applied to cigarette smoking in African-American, Puerto Rican, and non-Hispanic white teenage females in the journal. *Nurs Res*. 1997;46:155-161.
34. DeVellis R. *Scale Development: Theory and Applications*. Vol 26. 2nd ed. Thousand Oaks, Calif: Sage Publishing; 2003.
35. Rosner B. *Fundamentals of Biostatistics*. 5th ed. Pacific Grove, Calif: Duxbury Press; 1999.
36. Johnston LD, O'Malley PM, Bachman JG, Schulenberg JE. *Monitoring the Future National Survey Results on Drug Use, 1975-2004: Volume 1, Secondary School Students*. Bethesda, Md: National Institute on Drug Abuse; 2005. NIH Publication No. 05-5727.
37. Hobbs R. Does media literacy work? an empirical study of learning how to analyze advertisements. *Advertising Soc Rev*. 2004;5:1-28.

ARTICLE

# Television Viewing and Risk of Sexual Initiation by Young Adolescents

*Sarah L. Ashby, MD, MS; Christine M. Arcari, PhD, MPH; M. Bruce Edmonson, MD, MPH*

**Objective:** To determine if television viewing is associated with the risk of initiating sexual intercourse in young adolescents.

**Design:** Secondary analysis of data obtained from 1994 through 1996.

**Setting:** The National Longitudinal Study of Adolescent Health.

**Participants:** The 4808 students younger than 16 years who had not initiated intercourse before baseline interview.

**Exposures:** Primary exposure was self-reported daily television watching, categorized as low (<2 hours) or high (≥2 hours) use. Secondary exposure was parental regulation of television programming watched.

**Main Outcome Measure:** Odds ratio for initiating intercourse by 1-year follow-up, adjusted for potential confounders.

**Results:** At baseline, 2414 (48.8%) subjects watched television 2 or more hours per day. By 1-year follow-up, 791 (15.6%) subjects had initiated intercourse. Sexual initiation was associated with high television use (adjusted odds ratio, 1.35; 95% confidence interval, 1.01-1.79) and lack of parental regulation of television programming (adjusted odds ratio, 1.35; 95% confidence interval, 1.01-1.80). Most subjects (73.8%) reported strong parental disapproval of sex; their overall rate of initiation was 12.5%, and their risk was independently associated with high television use (adjusted odds ratio, 1.72; 95% confidence interval, 1.24-2.40) and lack of parental regulation of television programming (adjusted odds ratio, 1.35; 95% confidence interval, 1.01-1.81). Among adolescents who did not report strong parental disapproval, the rate of sexual initiation was higher (24.1%) but unrelated to television use.

**Conclusion:** Among young adolescents who reported strong parental disapproval of sex, watching television 2 or more hours per day and lack of parental regulation of television programming were each associated with increased risk of initiating sexual intercourse within a year.

*Arch Pediatr Adolesc Med. 2006;160:375-380*

Initiation of sexual intercourse by younger adolescents is associated with risky sexual behaviors and increases the risk of multiple partners, unwanted pregnancy, sexually transmitted infections, and pelvic inflammatory disease.[1-5] Several predictors of sexual intercourse during early adolescent years have been identified. These predictors include early puberty, poor self-esteem, depression, poor academic performance, being less religious, low parental education, lack of attentive and nurturing parents, and cultural and family patterns of early sexual experience.[6-12] Exposure to television is another proposed factor.[13,14] Although television watching appears to be useful in predicting certain behaviors, most notably violent behavior,[15] it is less clear whether television watching is linked to sexual behavior.

Survey research results demonstrate that television programming watched by adolescents contains high levels of sexual content, includes little information about sexual risks, and is an important source of information about sex for adolescents.[16-18] Results of a 2005 Kaiser Family Foundation survey showed that the mean amount of television watched per day was more than 3 hours for teens aged 11 to 14 years and about 2.5 hours for those aged 15 to 18 years.[19] Content analysis demonstrates that 70% of the programs favored by teenagers include sexual content.[18] Moreover, adolescents aged 13 to 15 years rank entertainment media as their leading source of information about sexuality and sexual health.[16] Almost 75% of 15- to 17-year-olds believe that sexual content on television influences the behavior of their peers "somewhat" or "a lot."[17]

As recently reviewed by Escobar-Chaves et al,[14] few studies have directly addressed the question of whether adolescent exposure to television affects sexual

**Author Affiliations:** Division of General Pediatrics and Adolescent Medicine, Department of Pediatrics (Drs Ashby and Edmonson), and Department of Population Health Sciences (Dr Arcari), University of Wisconsin School of Medicine and Public Health, Madison.

behavior, and only 2 have been based on longitudinal data.[20,21] Peterson et al[21] found some evidence for a relationship between amount of television viewed and sexual experience in certain subgroups of adolescents. In the other study, Collins et al[20] found that viewing more sexual content on television was associated with an increased 1-year risk of sexual initiation.

We performed a secondary analysis of longitudinal data from a large nationally representative sample of adolescents to determine whether self-reported hours of television viewed was associated with initiation of sexual intercourse in young adolescents (aged <16 years) during the subsequent year. We also studied whether parental regulation of television programming was associated with risk of initiation. We hypothesized that adolescents would be more likely to initiate intercourse within 1 year if they (1) watched more television or (2) lacked a parental rule about television programming.

## METHODS

### SAMPLE

We used data from waves 1 and 2 of the National Longitudinal Study of Adolescent Health (Add Health).[22] The sampling frame was all high schools in the United States that had an 11th grade and at least 30 students. A systematic, random sample of 80 high schools and 52 associated feeder schools from across the United States was then selected, stratified according to region, urbanicity, school type, ethnic composition, and school size. Subjects were weighted on the basis of the complex sampling design to establish a representative cohort of all 7th through 12th grade students in the United States.[23] In Add Health, 20 745 of the original in-school sample were randomly selected for in-home interviews, conducted in 1995, which included questions about more sensitive health behaviors. Of these, 16 706 were selected for a second interview approximately 1 year later, and 13 568 completed the interview and received a weight. Median interval between baseline and follow-up interviews was 11 months (interquartile range, 10-12 months). Adolescents who were younger than 16 years at baseline interview and completed 2 interviews (n=7063) were included in our study if they reported at baseline interview that they had never had sexual intercourse (n=5518), if they provided information about the primary exposure of interest (hours of television per week, n=5497), and if covariate data were complete (n=5178). Because of small sample sizes of other races/ethnicities, we further restricted our analysis to subjects who reported their race/ethnicity as non-Hispanic white, non-Hispanic black, or Hispanic (n=4808).

### MEASURES

#### Exposure Variables

Hours of television watched per day at baseline interview was the primary exposure of interest and was calculated from self-reported hours (0-99) of television watched per week. We chose to categorize television use as low (<2 h/d) or high (≥2 h/d). A cutoff of 2 h/d was selected to correspond to the American Academy of Pediatrics[24] recommended limit for children's television exposure. Two hours per day was also the median daily television exposure for subjects in our sample. In our final models, we explored television hours parameterized as a continuous variable and used an alternate categorization scheme to look for a dose-response effect by using the following categories of hours of television watched: 0 to less than the 25th percentile, 25th to less than the 50th percentile, 50th to less than the 75th percentile, 75th to less than the 90th percentile, and 90th percentile or greater.

Parental monitoring was a secondary exposure of interest. At baseline interview, subjects were asked if their parents allow them to make their own decisions about which television programs they watch. We refer to adolescents as having a *content rule* if they answered no to this question. Subjects were also asked if they made their own decisions about how much television they watch, but we excluded this *amount rule* variable from our final models because of the concern that it may be highly correlated with hours of television viewed.

#### Outcome Variable

Initiation of sexual intercourse (defined as penile-vaginal intercourse) was the primary outcome of interest and was reported (yes/no) at follow-up interview. Answers to this and other sensitive questions were obtained by using a confidential computer-assisted self-interviewing system and were entered into a laptop computer.

#### Covariates

Sociodemographic variables included in this analysis were age (years/months) at baseline interview, sex, race/ethnicity, and maternal education. Race/ethnicity was self-reported and categorized as non-Hispanic white, non-Hispanic black, or Hispanic. Maternal education was reported by the resident mother or mother figure for most subjects or, otherwise, by the subject; responses were classified as less than high school, high school graduate, more than high school, or college or more. Parental presence was assessed by asking each respondent how frequently his/her mother or father was present before school, after school, and at bedtime. We created a dichotomous variable that defined *decreased parental presence at home* as occurring when a parent was *sometimes*, *almost never*, or *never* present at any of these times. Perceived parental tolerance of intercourse was measured by asking subjects at baseline interview if mother and/or father would approve of them having sex at this time of life. If subjects reported anything other than *strong disapproval* they were placed in the category of *does not perceive strong parental disapproval of sex.* Depression was assessed using the sum of responses to 19 items selected from the Center for Epidemiologic Studies Depression Scale, which measures depressive symptoms in the community and has been validated in junior and senior high school students.[25,26] Higher scores indicated more depressive symptoms. For the purposes of our study, we defined depression as scoring in the top quartile on this scale. Self-esteem was assessed by summing 6 of 10 items modified from the Rosenberg Self-Esteem Inventory, which has good reliability (Cronbach $\alpha = .86$).[7] We defined low self-esteem as a score below the median. Subjects were asked to assess the importance of religion by using a 5-point scale. We recoded these answers and created a dichotomous variable that classified as *less religious* all who did not respond that religion was *very important.* Educational aspirations were measured with a question asking subjects to rank on a scale of 1 to 5 how likely it is that they will go to college. We recoded answers dichotomously and placed subjects who did not answer *highly likely* in the category of *less likely to attend college.* Other potential covariates that were explored in the univariate analyses but excluded from multivariate models were taking a virginity pledge (yes/no), intelligence as measured by means of the Add Health Picture Vocabulary Test, and pubertal status.

## DATA ANALYSIS

Data were weighted by using commercially available software (Stata version 9.0; Stata Corp, College Station, Tex) according to Add Health recommendations to account for complex sampling design.[27] We performed univariate and multivariate logistic regression analyses to examine the relationship between baseline television viewing and 1-year initiation of sexual intercourse. Preliminary analysis demonstrated that this relationship varied according to parental attitude toward adolescent engagement in sexual intercourse; therefore, we stratified subsequent analyses according to this variable. We chose to include only covariates that appeared to be related to primary exposure and outcome in univariate analysis or that had been included in previous literature on this subject. We tested for 2-way multiplicative interactions between amount of television watched and all other covariates at the $P<.01$ level.

# RESULTS

Our final study sample (n=4808) included approximately equal numbers of male and female subjects and had significantly more whites than blacks or Hispanics. Subjects in the final sample watched television a mean of 2.5 h/d and a median of 2.0 h/d. **Table 1** shows selected characteristics of subjects. We stratified analyses according to parental attitude toward sex (strong disapproval vs all others) on the basis of differences between the 2 groups in the relationship between television watching and sexual initiation (**Table 2**).

**Table 1. Characteristics of 4808 Study Subjects at Baseline Interview**

| Subject Characteristics* | Unweighted No. of Subjects (Weighted %) |
|---|---|
| Sex | |
| Female | 2682 (53.5) |
| Male | 2126 (46.5) |
| Race/ethnicity | |
| Non-Hispanic white | 3178 (77.1) |
| Non-Hispanic black | 912 (11.2) |
| Hispanic | 718 (11.7) |
| Maternal education | |
| College or more | 1266 (23.3) |
| More than high school | 1410 (29.7) |
| High school | 1400 (31.2) |
| Less than high school | 732 (15.8) |
| Does not perceive strong parental disapproval of sex | 1292 (26.2) |
| Decreased parental presence at home | 2159 (44.1) |
| Depressed | 1097 (22.4) |
| Less religious | 2510 (54.1) |
| Low self-esteem | 2211 (45.9) |
| Less likely to attend college | 1982 (42.6) |
| Watches television ≥2 h/d | 2414 (48.8) |
| Makes own decisions about television programming watched (no content rule) | 3234 (67.2) |
| Makes own decision about amount of television watched (no amount rule) | 3667 (75.2) |

*See Methods section for variable description and categorization.

## HOURS OF TELEVISION WATCHED

Overall, subjects who watched television 2 or more hours per day were more likely to initiate sex within 1 year (adjusted odds ratio [aOR], 1.35; 95% confidence interval [CI], 1.01-1.79). **Table 3** shows that this relationship was even stronger (aOR, 1.72; 95% CI, 1.24-2.40) for subjects who reported strong parental disapproval of sex. We failed to find a statistically significant relationship between watching television 2 or more hours per day and 1-year sexual initiation for subjects who did not report strong parental disapproval (Table 3).

We looked for evidence of a stepwise relationship between television hours and risk of sexual initiation among subjects who reported strong parental disapproval of sex. Compared with adolescents in the first quartile of television watching (<0.9 h/d), those in the second quartile (0.9-1.9 h/d) were not more likely to initiate intercourse (aOR, 1.05; 95% CI, 0.70-1.57). For adolescents in the third quartile of television watching (2.0-2.9 h/d), the risk was higher (aOR, 2.14; 95% CI, 1.40-3.26). For adolescents in the 75th to 90th percentile (3.0-4.9 h/d), the aOR was 2.24 (95% CI, 1.46-3.42). For subjects in the top decile of television viewing (≥5 h/d), however, the risk of sexual initiation (aOR, 1.02; 95% CI, 0.62-1.66) was not increased compared with those in the lowest quartile of television watching.

## PARENTAL REGULATION OF TELEVISION PROGRAMMING (CONTENT RULE)

Lack of parental regulation of television programming was significantly associated with 1-year sexual initiation in subjects who reported strong parental disapproval of sex, and the relationship persisted after controlling for multiple possible confounders (Table 3).

## INTERACTION BETWEEN HOURS OF TELEVISION WATCHED AND PARENTAL REGULATION

We failed to find evidence of statistically significant multiplicative or additive interaction between television viewing and a content rule on the risk of sexual initiation. However, despite a lower overall rate of intercourse among subjects who reported strong parental disapproval of sex, adolescents who watched television 2 or more hours per day and reported no content rule had the highest rate of sexual initiation (17.1%; 95% CI, 14.5%-20.1%), approximately twice the risk (aOR, 2.48; 95% CI, 1.66-3.70) observed in subjects who watched fewer than 2 h/d and reported a content rule (initiation rate, 6.9%; 95% CI, 5.0%-9.5%).

## OTHER COVARIATES

For subjects who reported strong parental disapproval of sex, 1-year initiation of sexual intercourse was independently associated ($P<.05$) with increased age at baseline interview, being black, maternal education of high school or less, being less religious, and being more depressed. For subjects who reported anything other than strong parental disapproval of sex, 1-year initiation of sexual intercourse was independently associated ($P<.05$) with increased age at baseline interview and being black.

**Table 2. Risk of Initiating Sexual Intercourse Within 1 Year According to Amount of Television Watched and Perceived Parental Attitude Toward Sexual Initiation**

| | Amount of Television Watched | | | | | | |
|---|---|---|---|---|---|---|---|
| | <2 h/d | | | ≥2 h/d | | | |
| Perceives Strong Disapproval of Sex | No. of Subjects | No. Who Initiated Sex | Initiation Rate (%)* | No. of Subjects | No. Who Initiated Sex | Initiation Rate (%)* | *P* Value |
| Yes (n = 3516) | 1768 | 203 | 9.5 | 1748 | 276 | 15.8 | <.001 |
| No (n = 1292) | 626 | 162 | 25.0 | 666 | 150 | 23.2 | .61 |
| **All (N = 4808)** | **2394** | **365** | 13.5 | **2414** | **426** | 17.8 | .02 |

*Weighted to account for sample design.

**Table 3. Odds Ratios for 1-Year Initiation of Sexual Intercourse Stratified According to Adolescent Perception of Parental Attitude Toward Sexual Initiation**

| | Perceives Strong Disapproval of Sex (n = 3516) | | Does Not Perceive Strong Disapproval of Sex (n = 1292) | |
|---|---|---|---|---|
| Subject Characteristics | OR (95% CI) | aOR* (95% CI) | OR (95% CI) | aOR* (95% CI) |
| Watches television ≥2 h/d | 1.78 (1.29-2.47) | 1.72 (1.24-2.40) | 0.91 (0.62-1.32) | 0.89 (0.60-1.33) |
| Makes own decisions about television programming watched | 1.51 (1.15-1.99) | 1.35 (1.01-1.81) | 1.45 (0.85-2.47) | 1.38 (0.76-2.49) |
| Age (in years) at baseline interview | 1.53 (1.32-1.77) | 1.53 (1.32-1.77) | 1.35 (1.11-1.64) | 1.31 (1.08-1.59) |
| Sex | | | | |
| Female | 1.22 (0.91-1.63) | 1.20 (0.88-1.64) | 1.37 (1.00-1.88) | 1.18 (0.85-1.62) |
| Male | 1.00 | | | |
| Maternal education | | | | |
| College or more | 1.00 | | | |
| More than high school | 1.42 (0.94-2.15) | 1.23 (0.79-1.91) | 1.16 (0.74-1.81) | 1.19 (0.74-1.92) |
| High school | 1.95 (1.35-2.83) | 1.61 (1.08-2.40) | 1.34 (0.85-2.12) | 1.30 (0.81-2.09) |
| Less than high school | 2.53 (1.62-3.93) | 1.85 (1.08-3.17) | 1.39 (0.84-2.30) | 1.39 (0.80-2.41) |
| Race | | | | |
| Non-Hispanic white | 1.00 | | | |
| Non-Hispanic black | 1.89 (1.31-2.73) | 1.77 (1.26-2.47) | 1.56 (1.10-2.21) | 1.65 (1.09-2.50) |
| Hispanic | 1.39 (0.93-2.08) | 1.01 (0.63-1.62) | 1.12 (0.57-2.20) | 1.01 (0.51-1.97) |
| Decreased parental presence at home | 1.15 (0.91-1.47) | 1.08 (0.83-1.40) | 1.28 (0.92-1.78) | 1.31 (0.94-1.84) |
| Depressed | 2.21 (1.69-2.90) | 1.72 (1.27-2.33) | 1.06 (0.78-1.45) | 0.88 (0.63-1.23) |
| Less religious | 1.59 (1.20-2.11) | 1.63 (1.25-2.12) | 0.99 (0.70-1.45) | 0.99 (0.68-1.45) |
| Low self-esteem | 1.48 (1.15-1.91) | 1.11 (0.83-1.48) | 1.64 (1.07-2.50) | 1.51 (0.98-2.32) |
| Less likely to attend college | 1.61 (1.23-2.10) | 1.29 (0.96-1.73) | 1.28 (0.88-1.89) | 1.27 (0.84-1.91) |

Abbreviations: aOR, adjusted odds ratio; CI, confidence interval; OR, odds ratio.
*Adjusted for all variables listed.

## COMMENT

We used longitudinal data to examine the relationships between amount (hours per day) of television viewing and parental regulation of content on sexual initiation. Studying data in a large, nationally representative sample of young adolescents, we found a positive association between viewing television 2 or more hours per day and the subsequent 1-year risk of initiation of sexual intercourse in adolescents who report strong parental disapproval of sex. We also found that lack of parental regulation of television programming was associated with increased 1-year risk of sexual initiation in these adolescents. The magnitude of these associations remained constant after controlling for multiple potential confounders. Although we failed to find any statistically significant interaction between the amount of television watched and parental regulation of content, we found that among subjects who reported strong parental disapproval of sex, the rate of initiation was highest among those who watched television 2 or more hours per day and had no content rule and that the risk of sexual initiation was approximately twice that observed in subjects who watched less television and reported a content rule.

Our finding that hours of television viewed is associated with 1-year sexual initiation differs somewhat from results of the 2 other longitudinal studies available on this subject.[20,21] Peterson et al[21] found a positive, but inconsistent, relationship between hours of television watched and sexual initiation for boys; however, this study was based on television viewing data from the 1970s, which may not reflect more recent programming. Collins et al[20] reported that the amount of sexual content viewed, but not hours of television watched, was a significant risk factor for sexual initiation. This finding was based on a multivariate model that, by design, retained separate variables for amount of television watched and amount of sexual content watched.[20] Because we did not have any data available on the sexual content of programs watched by the subjects in our study, it is difficult to compare our results directly with those of Collins et al.[20]

Previous research results showed that adolescent perception of parental attitude toward sex is related to sexual initiation.[28,29] On the basis of our results, we hypothesize that for adolescents who do not perceive strong parental disapproval of sex and are already at higher risk for sexual initiation, television may not have affected their behavior. However, for adolescents who perceive strong parental disapproval of sex and are at lower risk for sexual initiation, contradictory messages, such as those seen on television, may be more influential.

Although results of our study and those of Collins et al[20] provide evidence that television watching increases the risk of sexual initiation by adolescents, neither study's results resolve the question of whether attempting to control content or limit amount of television watched would be most likely to reduce this risk. Limiting amount of television may be easier and more effective than limiting content, given the pervasiveness of sexual content in television programming.[18] In addition, unlike limiting content, limiting the amount of television children watch may have collateral benefits such as prevention of obesity[30] and reduction in aggressive behavior.[31]

We found that adolescents in the top 10th percentile of television viewing (≥5 h/d) were not at increased risk of sexual initiation. This result provides support for a theoretical *babysitter effect*[20] or *displacement effect* in which certain adolescents may spend extraordinary amounts of time viewing television and are therefore less likely to participate in other activities or to initiate sexual activity. Failure to account for such an effect may distort attempts to understand the true effect of increased television watching, especially if amount of television is modeled as a continuous variable.

We found that lack of a content rule was associated with 1-year sexual initiation only among adolescents who reported strong parental disapproval of sex, a result related to that of Peterson et al,[21] who found that coviewing television and discussing television with parents were related to decreased sexual initiation in certain adolescents. These results support the hypothesis that parental regulation of television viewing may affect television-related outcomes in some adolescents.

Effects of parental regulation have been studied previously. Although results of some studies showed that certain types of regulation are associated with differences in television-related behavior,[32-34] additional research is needed to understand whether mediation of television use by parents might influence television-related sexual behavior.

Strengths of this study include use of a data set that is longitudinal, provides a nationally representative sample, and has good measures of individual and family characteristics that are important control variables. Using longitudinal data eliminates the potential for reverse causality, a possible problem in cross-sectional studies.[35,36] The generalizability of our study results is strengthened by the comparability of mean hours of television watched in our sample to that in other large nationally representative samples.[19]

Our study has several limitations. First, the available measure of television exposure, a self-reported global estimate, was crude and may be less accurate than a viewing diary or other format that includes more than 1 measure across time. We recommend that future surveys designed to explore determinants of adolescent health include more extensive questions to establish the quantity and quality of adolescent exposure to multiple types of media. Second, although we adjusted for many potential confounders, our results still may be subject to residual confounding due to unmeasured social or environmental factors. In particular, rules about television content may be a proxy measure for parental willingness to monitor other behaviors that may be associated with the risk of sexual initiation. Third, available data provided no direct measure of the content of television programming watched. Although this is an important limitation given the diversity of programming that different adolescents are likely to select, it is still reasonable to assume that those who watch more television will see more sexual content given the high level of sexual content in shows that adolescents watch. Fourth, our outcome measure was limited to sexual intercourse defined as vaginal/penile intercourse, and we had no information on oral sex or other types of sexual behavior that are increasingly prevalent among teens. Future surveys should include questions about other types of sexual behavior. Fifth, because we excluded those who had already initiated intercourse, we necessarily selected for subjects who were slightly younger, included somewhat more female and white subjects, included fewer black subjects, and had a higher maternal educational status (data not shown). Finally, the data used for the study were almost 10 years old, and the sexual content of television programming has changed over that time.[18] In addition, as adolescents have increasing sources of media available to them, such as the Internet, the amount of television they watch and its role in their lives may be changing.[19]

The American Academy of Pediatrics recommends that children and adolescents view television no more than 2 hours each day and that parents take an active role in guiding television use.[24,37] Although there is limited evidence about the effectiveness of these recommendations, our results suggest that successful implementation of these guidelines may diminish the risk of early sexual initiation by young adolescents. Further research is needed to understand how families might effectively minimize the potential harms to children and adolescents associated with television exposure, whether by limiting total amount of television watched or by limiting access to specific types of programming. Interventions, including clinic-based interventions, designed to alter television use and improve parental mediation of television use should continue to be developed and tested to determine if they are feasible and effective in changing television use and its behavioral effects.

**Accepted for Publication:** December 15, 2005.
**Correspondence:** Sarah L. Ashby, MD, MS, 2870 University Ave, Madison, WI 53705 (slashby@aap.net).
**Funding/Support:** This research uses data from Add Health, a program project designed by J. Richard Udry, PhD, Peter S. Bearman, MA, PhD, and Kathleen Mullan Harris, PhD, and funded by grant P01-HD31921 from the National Institute of Child Health and Human Development, with cooperative funding from 17 other agencies. Special acknowledgment is due to Ronald R. Rindfuss, PhD, and Barbara Entwisle, PhD, for assistance in the original design. Persons interested in obtaining data files from Add Health should contact Add Health, Carolina Population Center, 123 W Franklin St, Chapel Hill, NC 27516-2524 (addhealth@unc.edu).
**Acknowledgment:** This research was performed while Dr Ashby was a National Institutes of Health National Research Service Award fellow at the University of Wisconsin-Madison.

## REFERENCES


1. Edgardh K. Sexual behavior and early coitarche in a national sample of 17-year-old Swedish girls. *Sex Transm Infect.* 2000;76:98-102.
2. Suss AL, Homel P, Hammerschlag M, Bromberg K. Risk factors for pelvic inflammatory disease in inner-city adolescents. *Sex Transm Dis.* 2000;27:289-291.
3. Coker AL, Richter DL, Valois RF, McKeown RE, Garrison CZ, Vincent ML. Correlates and consequences of early initiation of sexual intercourse. *J Sch Health.* 1994;64:372-377.
4. O'Donnell BL, O'Donnell CR, Stueve A. Early sexual initiation and subsequent sex-related risks among urban minority youth: the Reach for Health Study. *Fam Plann Perspect.* 2001;33:268-275.
5. Kaestle CE, Halpern CT, Miller WC, Ford CA. Young age at first sexual intercourse and sexually transmitted infections in adolescents and young adults. *Am J Epidemiol.* 2005;161:774-780.
6. Rosenthal SL, Von Ranson KM, Cotton S, Biro FM, Mills L, Succop PA. Sexual initiation: predictors and developmental trends. *Sex Transm Dis.* 2001;28:527-532.
7. Resnick MD, Bearman PS, Blum RW, et al. Protecting adolescents from harm: findings from the National Longitudinal Study of Adolescent Health. *JAMA.* 1997;278:823-832.
8. Santelli JS, DiClemente RJ, Miller KS, Kirby D. Sexually transmitted diseases, unintended pregnancy, and adolescent health promotion. *Adolesc Med.* 1999;10:87-108.
9. Lammers C, Ireland M, Resnick M, Blum R. Influences on adolescents' decision to postpone onset of sexual intercourse: a survival analysis of virginity among youths aged 13 to 18 years. *J Adolesc Health.* 2000;26:42-48.
10. Santelli JS, Beilenson P. Risk factors for adolescent sexual behavior, fertility, and sexually transmitted diseases. *J Sch Health.* 1992;62:271-279.
11. Hofferth S. Factors affecting initiation of sexual intercourse. In: Hayes C, ed. *Risking the Future: Adolescent Sexuality, Pregnancy and Childbearing.* Vol 2. Washington, DC: National Academy Press; 1987:7-35.
12. Mott FL, Fondell MM, Hu PN, Kaleski-Jones L, Menaghan EG. The determinants of first sex by age 14 in a high-risk adolescent population. *Fam Plann Perspect.* 1996;28:13-18.
13. Ashby SL, Rich M. Video killed the radio star: the effect of music videos on adolescent health. *Adolesc Med Clin.* 2005;16:371-394.
14. Escobar-Chaves SL, Tortolero SR, Markham CM, Low BJ, Eitel P, Thickstun P. Impact of the media on adolescent sexual attitudes and behaviors. *Pediatrics.* 2005;116:303-326.
15. Hogan MJ. Adolescents and media violence: six crucial issues for practitioners. *Adolesc Med Clin.* 2005;16:249-268.
16. Henry J. Kaiser Family Foundation. *Kaiser Family Foundation and Children Now National Surveys: Talking With Kids About Tough Issues.* Menlo Park, Calif: Henry J. Kaiser Family Foundation; 1997.
17. Henry J. Kaiser Family Foundation. *Teens, Sex and TV.* Menlo Park, Calif: Henry J. Kaiser Family Foundation; 2002.
18. Kunkel D, Eyal K, Finnerty K, Biely E, Donnerstein E. *Sex on TV4: A Biennial Report to the Kaiser Family Foundation.* Santa Barbara, Calif: Henry J. Kaiser Family Foundation; 2005.
19. Roberts DF, Foehr U, Rideout V. *Generation M: Media in the Lives of 8-18 Year-Olds.* Menlo Park, Calif: Henry J. Kaiser Family Foundation; 2005.
20. Collins RL, Elliott MN, Berry SH, et al. Watching sex on television predicts adolescent initiation of sexual behavior. *Pediatrics.* 2004;114:e280-e289. Available at: http://www.pediatrics.aappublications.org/cgi/content/full/114/3/e280. Accessed January 19, 2006.
21. Peterson JL, Moore KA, Furstenberg FF Jr. Television viewing and early initiation of sexual intercourse: is there a link? *J Homosex.* 1991;21:93-118.
22. Udry JR. *The National Longitudinal Study of Adolescent Health (Add Health), Waves I & II, 1994–1996; Wave III, 2001–2002.* Chapel Hill: Population Center, University of North Carolina at Chapel Hill; 2003.
23. Harris KM, Florey F, Tabor J, Bearman PS, Jones J, Udry JR. The National Longitudinal Study of Adolescent Health: research design. Available at: http://www.cpc.unc.edu/projects/addhealth/design. Accessed January 16, 2006.
24. American Academy of Pediatrics. Committee on Public Education: children, adolescents, and television. *Pediatrics.* 2001;107:423-426.
25. Radloff LS. The use of the Center for Epidemiologic Studies Depression scale in adolescents and young adults. *J Youth Adolesc.* 1991;20:149-166.
26. Roberts RE, Lewinsohn PM, Seeley JR. Screening for adolescent depression: a comparison of depression scales. *J Am Acad Child Adolesc Psychiatry.* 1991;30:58-66.
27. Chantala K, Tabor J. Strategies to perform a design-based analysis using the Add Health data. Available at: http://www.cpc.unc.edu/projects/addhealth/files/weight1.pdf. Accessed August 1, 2005.
28. Miller B. *Families Matter.* Washington, DC: National Campaign to Prevent Teen Pregnancy; 1998.
29. Jaccard J, Dittus P, Gordon V. Maternal correlates of adolescent sexual and contraceptive behaviors. *Fam Plann Perspect.* 1996;28:159-165.
30. Robinson TN. Reducing children's television viewing to prevent obesity: a randomized controlled trial. *JAMA.* 1999;282:1561-1567.
31. Robinson TN, Wilde ML, Navracruz LC, Haydel KF, Varady A. Effects of reducing children's television and video game use on aggressive behavior: a randomized controlled trial. *Arch Pediatr Adolesc Med.* 2001;155:17-23.
32. Vandewater EA, Park SE, Huang X, Wartella EA. "No - you can't watch that" parental rules and young children's media use. *Am Behav Sci.* 2005;48:608-623.
33. Desmond RJ, Singer JL, Singer DG, Calam R, Colimore K. Family mediation patterns and television viewing: young children's use and grasp of the medium. *Hum Commun Res.* 1985;11:461-480.
34. Nathanson AI. Identifying and explaining the relationship between parental mediation and children's aggression. *Commun Res.* 1999;26:124-143.
35. Brown JD, Newcomer SF. Television viewing and adolescents' sexual behavior. *J Homosex.* 1991;21:77-91.
36. Klein JD, Brown JD, Childers KW, Oliveri J, Porter C, Dykers C. Adolescents' risky behavior and mass media use. *Pediatrics.* 1993;92:24-31.
37. American Academy of Pediatrics. Sexuality, contraception, and the media. *Pediatrics.* 2001;107:191-194.

**PEDIARIX™ [Diphtheria and Tetanus Toxoids and Acellular Pertussis Adsorbed, Hepatitis B (Recombinant) and Inactivated Poliovirus Vaccine Combined]**

The following is a brief summary only; see full prescribing information for complete product information.

**CONTRAINDICATIONS:** Hypersensitivity to any component of the vaccine, including yeast, neomycin, and polymyxin B, is a contraindication (see DESCRIPTION in complete prescribing information). Do not use PEDIARIX after a serious allergic reaction (e.g., anaphylaxis) temporally associated with a previous dose of this vaccine or with any components of this vaccine. Because of the uncertainty as to which component of the vaccine might be responsible, do not give further vaccination with any of these components; or, refer such individuals to an allergist for evaluation. The following events are contraindications to administration of PEDIARIX: encephalopathy (e.g., coma, decreased level of consciousness, prolonged seizures) within 7 days of administration of a previous dose of a pertussis-containing vaccine that is not attributable to another identifiable cause; progressive neurologic disorder, including infantile spasms, uncontrolled epilepsy, or progressive encephalopathy. Do not vaccinate individuals with such conditions until a treatment regimen has been established and the condition has stabilized. PEDIARIX is not contraindicated for use in individuals with HIV infection.

**WARNINGS:** Administration of PEDIARIX is associated with higher rates of fever relative to separately administered vaccines. In one study that evaluated medically attended fever after the first dose of PEDIARIX or separately administered vaccines, infants who received PEDIARIX had a higher rate of medical encounters for fever within the first 4 days following vaccination. In some infants, these encounters included the performance of diagnostic studies to evaluate other causes of fever (see ADVERSE REACTIONS). The vial stopper is latex-free. The tip cap and the rubber plunger of the needleless prefilled syringes contain dry natural latex rubber that may cause allergic reactions in latex sensitive individuals. If any of the following events occur in temporal relation to receipt of whole-cell DTP or a vaccine containing an acellular pertussis component, consider carefully whether to give subsequent doses of PEDIARIX or any vaccine containing a pertussis component: temperature of ≥40.5°C (105°F) within 48 hours not due to another identifiable cause; collapse or shock-like state (hypotonic-hyporesponsive episode) within 48 hours; persistent, inconsolable crying lasting ≥3 hours, occurring within 48 hours; seizures with or without fever occurring within 3 days. If Guillain-Barré syndrome occurs within 6 weeks of receipt of prior vaccine containing tetanus toxoid, the decision to give subsequent doses of PEDIARIX or any vaccine containing tetanus toxoid should be based on careful consideration of the potential benefits and possible risks. A committee of the Institute of Medicine (IOM) has concluded that evidence is consistent with a causal relationship between whole-cell DTP vaccine and acute neurologic illness, and under special circumstances, between whole-cell DTP vaccine and chronic neurologic disease in the context of the National Childhood Encephalopathy Study (NCES) report; however, evidence was insufficient to indicate whether or not whole-cell DTP vaccine increased the overall risk of chronic neurologic disease. Acute encephalopathy and permanent neurologic damage have not been reported causally linked or in temporal association with administration of PEDIARIX, but the experience with PEDIARIX is insufficient to rule this out. Encephalopathy has been reported following INFANRIX® (Diphtheria and Tetanus Toxoids and Acellular Pertussis Vaccine Adsorbed) (see ADVERSE REACTIONS, Postmarketing Reports), but data are not sufficient to evaluate a causal relationship. The decision to administer a pertussis-containing vaccine to children with stable central nervous system (CNS) disorders must be made by the physician on an individual basis, with consideration of all relevant factors, and assessment of potential risks and benefits for that individual. Advise the parent or guardian of the potential increased risk involved (see PRECAUTIONS). A family history of seizures or other CNS disorders is not a contraindication to pertussis vaccine. For children at higher risk for seizures than the general population, an appropriate antipyretic may be administered at the time of vaccination and for the ensuing 24 hours according to the respective prescribing information recommended dosage to reduce the possibility of post-vaccination fever. Defer vaccination during the course of a moderate or severe illness with or without fever and vaccinate patients as soon as they have recovered from the acute phase of the illness. Do not give PEDIARIX to children on anticoagulant therapy or those with bleeding disorders unless the potential benefit clearly outweighs the risk of administration (see PRECAUTIONS in complete prescribing information).

**PRECAUTIONS:** Before the injection of any biological, the physician should take all reasonable precautions to prevent allergic or other adverse reactions. Epinephrine injection (1:1000) and other appropriate agents used for the control of immediate allergic reactions must be immediately available should an acute anaphylactic reaction occur. Immunosuppressed individuals, including those receiving immunosuppressive therapy, may not develop the expected immune response. **Drug Interactions:** For information regarding concomitant administration with other vaccines, refer to DOSAGE AND ADMINISTRATION in complete prescribing information. Do not mix PEDIARIX with any other vaccine in the same syringe or vial. **Carcinogenesis, Mutagenesis, Impairment of Fertility:** PEDIARIX has not been evaluated for carcinogenic or mutagenic potential, or for impairment of fertility. **Pregnancy:** Pregnancy Category C: PEDIARIX is not indicated for women of child-bearing age. Animal reproduction studies have not been conducted with PEDIARIX. It is not known whether PEDIARIX can cause fetal harm when administered to a pregnant woman or if PEDIARIX can affect reproductive capacity. **Geriatric Use:** PEDIARIX is not indicated for use in adult populations. **Pediatric Use:** Safety and effectiveness of PEDIARIX in infants younger than 6 weeks of age have not been evaluated (see DOSAGE AND ADMINISTRATION in complete prescribing information). PEDIARIX is not recommended for persons 7 years of age or older. Tetanus and Diphtheria Toxoids Adsorbed (Td) For Adult Use, inactivated poliovirus vaccine (IPV), and Hepatitis B Vaccine (Recombinant) should be used in individuals 7 years of age or older.

**ADVERSE REACTIONS:** A total of 20,739 doses of PEDIARIX have been administered to 7,028 infants as a 3-dose primary series. The most common adverse reactions observed in clinical trials were local injection site reactions (pain, redness, or swelling), fever, and fussiness. In comparative studies, administration of PEDIARIX was associated with higher rates of fever relative to separately administered vaccines (see WARNINGS). The prevalence of fever was highest on the day of vaccination and the day following vaccination. More than 98% of episodes of fever resolved within the 4-day period following vaccination (i.e., the period including the day of vaccination and the next 3 days). Rates of most other solicited adverse events following PEDIARIX were comparable to rates observed following separately administered US-licensed vaccines. The adverse event information from clinical trials provides a basis for identifying adverse events that appear to be related to vaccine use and for approximating rates. However, because clinical trials are conducted under widely varying conditions, adverse event rates observed in the clinical trials of a vaccine cannot be directly compared to rates in the clinical trials of another vaccine, and may not reflect the rates observed in practice. A total of 5,472 infants were enrolled in a German safety study that was originally designed to compare the safety and reactogenicity of PEDIARIX administered concomitantly at separate sites with 1 of 4 *Haemophilus influenzae* type b (Hib) vaccines at 3, 4, and 5 months of age. After enrollment of 1,569 infants, the study was amended to include a control group that received INFANRIX, Hib vaccine, and oral poliovirus vaccine (OPV) separately. Infants in the separate administration group received one less antigen (hepatitis B) than the infants who received PEDIARIX. Safety data were available for 4,666 infants who received PEDIARIX administered concomitantly at separate sites with 1 of 4 Hib vaccines and for 768 infants in the control group that received separate vaccines. The primary end-point of the study was the percentage of infants with any grade 3 solicited symptom (redness or swelling >20 mm, fever >103.1°F, or crying, pain, vomiting, diarrhea, loss of appetite, or restlessness that prevented normal daily activities) over the 3-dose primary series in infants who received PEDIARIX (4 groups that received PEDIARIX and Hib vaccines pooled) compared to the group that received INFANRIX and Hib vaccine separately with OPV. Analysis for the primary end-point was performed on the according-to-protocol (ATP) cohort that included only those infants who were enrolled after the protocol amendment to include a control group. Of 3,773 infants in the ATP cohort for whom safety data were available, 16.2% (95% CI: 14.9% to 17.5%) of 3,029 infants who received PEDIARIX and Hib vaccine compared to 20.3% (95% CI: 17.5% to 23.4%) of 744 infants who received separate vaccines were reported to have had at least one grade 3 solicited symptom within 4 days of vaccination (i.e., day of vaccination and the next 3 days). The difference between groups in the rate of grade 3 symptoms was 4.1% (90% CI: 1.4% to 7.1%). These were the rates for selected solicited symptoms within 4 days following each dose in a 3-dose primary series in infants who received PEDIARIX administered concomitantly with Hib vaccine and those who received separate concomitant administration of INFANRIX, Hib vaccine, and OPV for the intent-to-treat (ITT) cohort (includes all infants enrolled before and after the amendment who received the indicated vaccine and for whom at least one symptom sheet was completed):

**Percentage of German Infants With Solicited Local Reactions or Selected Systemic Adverse Events Within 4 Days of Vaccination* (ITT Cohort)**

| | PEDIARIX & Hib | | | INFANRIX, Hib, & OPV | | |
|---|---|---|---|---|---|---|
| | **Dose 1** | **Dose 2** | **Dose 3** | **Dose 1** | **Dose 2** | **Dose 3** |
| **N** | **4,666** | **4,619** | **4,574** | **768** | **757** | **750** |
| **Local†** | | | | | | |
| Pain, any | 14.0 | 10.2 | 9.9 | 14.2 | 9.8 | 8.1 |
| Pain, grade 2 or 3 | 2.9 | 1.2 | 1.5 | 3.6 | 1.7 | 1.1 |
| Pain, grade 3 | 0.7 | 0.3 | 0.3 | 1.3 | 0.4 | 0.1 |
| Redness, any | 18.6 | 26.6 | 25.6 | 16.1 | 21.4 | 20.8 |
| Redness, >5 mm | 6.7 | 9.9 | 9.0 | 5.9 | 8.2 | 7.7 |
| Redness, >20 mm | 1.2 | 1.0 | 1.1 | 1.8 | 0.7 | 1.1 |
| Swelling, any | 12.7 | 18.5 | 18.4 | 9.6 | 12.9 | 13.6 |
| Swelling, >5 mm | 5.6 | 7.7 | 7.8 | 3.6 | 5.2 | 4.8 |
| Swelling, >20 mm | 1.2 | 1.6 | 1.5 | 1.3 | 1.1 | 1.2 |
| **Systemic** | | | | | | |
| Restlessness, any | 41.4 | 32.0 | 26.7 | 46.4 | 35.0 | 27.6 |
| Restlessness, grade 2 or 3 | 14.4 | 10.0 | 8.9 | 20.2 | 11.5 | 8.4 |
| Restlessness, grade 3 | 3.0 | 1.5 | 1.6 | 5.7 | 3.0 | 1.7 |
| Fever‡, ≥100.4ºF | 25.1 | 19.3 | 19.7 | 13.2 | 13.1 | 11.2 |
| Fever‡, >101.3ºF | 5.8 | 4.1 | 4.6 | 2.2 | 2.8 | 2.1 |
| Fever‡, >103.1ºF | 0.3 | 0.5 | 0.7 | 0.3 | 0.3 | 0.5 |
| Unusual cry§, any | 24.9 | 16.5 | 13.1 | 36.5 | 19.7 | 14.3 |
| Unusual cry§, grade 2 or 3 | 12.7 | 7.1 | 5.7 | 20.8 | 10.0 | 5.7 |
| Unusual cry§, grade 3 | 3.9 | 1.7 | 1.4 | 6.8 | 2.1 | 1.1 |
| Loss of appetite, any | 17.9 | 13.3 | 12.5 | 19.1 | 16.2 | 11.3 |
| Loss of appetite, grade 2 or 3 | 4.0 | 2.9 | 2.7 | 4.4 | 2.9 | 2.3 |
| Loss of appetite, grade 3 | 0.6 | 0.5 | 0.4 | 0.5 | 0.7 | 0.0 |

N = number of infants in the intent-to-treat (ITT) cohort.
Grade 2 defined as sufficiently discomforting to interfere with daily activities.
Grade 3 defined as preventing normal daily activities.
* Within 4 days of vaccination defined as day of vaccination and the next 3 days.
† Local reactions at the injection site for PEDIARIX or INFANRIX.
‡ Rectal temperatures.
§ Unusual cry lasting >1 hour.

In this study, infants were also monitored for unsolicited adverse events that occurred within 30 days following vaccination. Over the entire study period, 6 subjects in the group that received PEDIARIX reported seizures. Two of these subjects had a febrile seizure, 1 of whom also developed afebrile seizures. The remaining 4 subjects had afebrile seizures, including 2 with infantile spasms. Two subjects reported seizures within 7 days following vaccination (1 subject had both febrile and afebrile seizures, and 1 subject had afebrile seizures), corresponding to a rate of 0.22 seizures per 1,000 doses (febrile seizures 0.07 per 1,000 doses, afebrile seizures 0.14 per 1,000 doses). No subject who received concomitant INFANRIX, Hib vaccine, and OPV reported seizures. In a separate German study that evaluated the safety of INFANRIX in 22,505 infants who received 66,867 doses of INFANRIX administered as a 3-dose primary series, the rate of seizures within 7 days of vaccination with INFANRIX was 0.13 per 1,000 doses (febrile seizures 0.0 per 1,000 doses, afebrile seizures 0.13 per 1,000 doses). No cases of hypotonic-hyporesponsiveness, encephalopathy, or anaphylaxis were reported in the German study that evaluated the safety of PEDIARIX. Rates of serious adverse events that are less common than those reported in this safety study are not known at this time.

Additional safety data for PEDIARIX are available from a US study designed to evaluate lot-to-lot consistency and a bridge for a new manufacturing step. These were the rates for local reactions and selected adverse events within 4 days of vaccination with PEDIARIX administered concomitantly with a Hib vaccine at 2, 4, and 6 months of age:

**Percentage of US Infants With Solicited Local Reactions or Selected Systemic Adverse Events Within 4 Days of Vaccination* (ITT Cohort)**

| | PEDIARIX & Hib | | |
|---|---|---|---|
| | **Dose 1** | **Dose 2** | **Dose 3** |
| **Local†** | **N = 482** | **N = 469** | **N = 466** |
| Pain, any | 30.5 | 25.4 | 23.0 |
| Pain, grade 2 or 3 | 6.2 | 5.5 | 3.6 |
| Pain, grade 3 | 1.2 | 0.6 | 0.6 |
| Redness, any | 25.3 | 32.6 | 35.6 |
| Redness, >5 mm | 9.3 | 10.4 | 8.6 |
| Redness, >20 mm | 0.6 | 1.5 | 1.3 |
| Swelling, any | 15.1 | 16.6 | 22.3 |
| Swelling, >5 mm | 6.8 | 6.2 | 6.4 |
| Swelling, >20 mm | 1.0 | 1.3 | 1.3 |
| **Systemic** | **N = 482** | **N = 469** | **N = 467** |
| Restlessness, any | 28.8 | 30.3 | 28.5 |
| Restlessness, grade 2 or 3 | 7.1 | 9.0 | 9.4 |
| Restlessness, grade 3 | 1.0 | 1.1 | 0.6 |
| Fever‡, ≥100.4ºF | 26.6 | 31.3 | 25.9 |
| Fever‡, >101.3ºF | 2.9 | 6.2 | 4.7 |
| Fever‡, >103.1ºF | 0.0 | 0.2 | 0.6 |
| Fussiness, any | 61.8 | 63.8 | 57.0 |
| Fussiness, grade 2 or 3 | 14.9 | 21.5 | 17.1 |
| Fussiness, grade 3 | 2.7 | 3.4 | 1.7 |
| Loss of appetite, any | 21.6 | 19.8 | 18.8 |
| Loss of appetite, grade 2 or 3 | 3.1 | 3.2 | 2.4 |
| Loss of appetite, grade 3 | 0.2 | 0.4 | 0.0 |
| Sleeping more than usual, any | 46.7 | 31.8 | 28.1 |
| Sleeping more than usual, grade 2 or 3 | 10.2 | 6.0 | 4.7 |
| Sleeping more than usual, grade 3 | 1.7 | 0.4 | 0.6 |

N = number of infants in the intent-to-treat (ITT) cohort (infants who received the indicated vaccine and for whom at least one symptom sheet was completed).
Grade 2 defined as sufficiently discomforting to interfere with daily activities.
Grade 3 defined as preventing normal daily activities.
* Within 4 days of vaccination defined as day of vaccination and the next 3 days.
† Local reactions at the injection site for PEDIARIX.
‡ Rectal temperatures.

In another US study, these were the rates for fever within 4 days following dose 1 (i.e., day of vaccination and the next 3 days) at 2 months of age in infants who received PEDIARIX when administered concomitantly at separate sites with Hib and pneumococcal conjugate vaccines and those who received INFANRIX, ENGERIX-B® [Hepatitis B Vaccine (Recombinant)], IPV, Hib vaccine, and pneumococcal conjugate vaccine:

**Percentage of US Infants With Fever Within 4 Days of Dose 1* (ITT Cohort)**

| | **PEDIARIX, Hib, & Pneumococcal Conjugate (N = 667)** | **INFANRIX, ENGERIX-B, IPV, Hib, & Pneumococcal Conjugate (N = 333)** | **Separate Vaccine Group Minus Combination Vaccine Group** |
|---|---|---|---|
| **Fever†** | **%** | **%** | **Difference (95% CI)** |
| ≥100.4ºF‡ | 27.9 | 19.8 | -8.07 (-13.54, -2.60) |
| >101.3ºF | 7.0 | 4.5 | -2.54 (-5.50, 0.41) |
| >102.2ºF‡ | 2.2 | 0.3 | -1.95 (-3.22, -0.68) |
| >103.1ºF | 0.4 | 0.0 | -0.45 (-0.96, 0.06) |
| M.A.‡ | 1.2 | 0.0 | -1.20 (-2.03, -037) |

N = number of infants for whom at least one symptom sheet was completed, excluding 3 infants for whom temperature was not measured and 3 infants whose temperature was measured by the tympanic method.
*Within 4 days of dose 1 defined as day of vaccination and the next 3 days.
† Rectal temperatures.
‡ The group that received PEDIARIX compared to separate vaccine group p value <0.05 (2-sided Fisher Exact test) or the 95% confidence interval on the difference between groups does not include 0.
M.A. = Medically attended (a visit to or from medical personnel).

In this study, medical attention (a visit to or from medical personnel) for fever within 4 days following vaccination was sought for 8 infants who received PEDIARIX (1.2%) and no infants who received separately administered vaccines. Four infants were seen by medical personnel in an office setting; no diagnostic tests were performed in 2 of the infants and a complete blood count (CBC) was done in the other 2 infants. Of 3 infants who were seen in an emergency room, all had a CBC and a blood and urine culture performed; chest X-rays were done in 2 of the infants and a nasopharyngeal specimen was tested for Respiratory Syncytial Virus in one of the infants. One infant was hospitalized for a work-up that included a CBC, blood and urine cultures, a lumbar puncture, and a chest X-ray. All episodes of medically attended fever resolved within 4 days post-vaccination.

Limited data are available from a study conducted in Moldova in which infants received a dose of hepatitis B vaccine within 48 hours of birth followed by 3 doses of PEDIARIX at 6, 10, and 14 weeks of age. No information was collected on the HBsAg status of mothers of enrolled infants. These were the rates for local reactions and selected adverse events within 4 days of vaccination with PEDIARIX administered comcomitantly with Hib vaccine following a birth dose of hepatitis B vaccine:

**Percentage of Moldovan Infants With Solicited Local Reactions or Selected Systemic Adverse Events Within 4 Days of Vaccination* (ITT Cohort)**

| | PEDIARIX & Hib | | |
|---|---|---|---|
| | **Dose 1** | **Dose 2** | **Dose 3** |
| **N** | **160** | **158** | **157** |
| **Local†** | | | |
| Pain, any | 25.6 | 18.4 | 14.0 |
| Pain, grade 3 | 3.1 | 0.6 | 1.9 |
| Redness, any | 41.9 | 41.8 | 47.1 |
| Redness, >20 mm | 1.9 | 2.5 | 4.5 |
| Swelling, any | 20.6 | 18.4 | 28.0 |
| Swelling, >20 mm | 4.4 | 2.5 | 7.0 |
| **Systemic** | | | |
| Restlessness, any | 13.1 | 10.8 | 8.9 |
| Restlessness, grade 3 | 1.3 | 0.6 | 0.6 |
| Fever‡, ≥100.4ºF | 14.4 | 11.4 | 5.1 |
| Fever‡, >103.1ºF | 0.0 | 0.6 | 0.0 |
| Fussiness, any | 25.0 | 21.5 | 17.8 |
| Fussiness, grade 3 | 2.5 | 0.6 | 0.6 |

N = number of infants in the intent-to-treat (ITT) cohort (infants who received the indicated vaccine and for whom at least one symptom sheet was completed).
Grade 3 defined as preventing normal daily activities.
*Within 4 days of vaccination defined as day of vaccination and the next 3 days.
† Local reactions at the injection site for PEDIARIX.
‡ Rectal temperatures.

Although there was no comparator group who received PEDIARIX without a birth dose of hepatitis B vaccine, available data suggest that some local adverse events may occur at a higher rate when PEDIARIX is administered after a birth dose of hepatitis B vaccine.

As with any vaccine, there is the possibility that broad use of PEDIARIX could reveal adverse events not observed in clinical trials.

**Postmarketing Reports:** Worldwide voluntary reports of adverse events received for INFANRIX and ENGERIX-B in children younger than 7 years of age since market introduction of these US-licensed vaccines are listed below. This list includes adverse events for which 20 or more reports were received with the exception of intussusception, idiopathic thrombocytopenic purpura, thrombocytopenia, anaphylactic reaction, angioedema, encephalopathy, hypotonic-hyporesponsive episode, and alopecia for which fewer than 20 reports were received. These latter events are included either because of the seriousness of the event or the strength of causal connection to components of this or other vaccines or drugs. *Body as a whole*: Asthenia[b], fever[a+b], lethargy[b], malaise[b], Sudden Infant Death Syndrome[a+b]. *Cardiovascular system*: Cyanosis[a+b], edema[b], pallor[b]. *Gastrointestinal system*: Abdominal pain[b], anorexia[b], diarrhea[a+b], intussusception[a+b], nausea[b], vomiting[a+b]. *Hematologic/lymphatic*: Idiopathic thrombocytopenic purpura[a+b], lymphadenopathy[a], thrombocytopenia[a+b]. *Hepatic*: Jaundice[b], liver function tests abnormal[b]. *Hypersensitivity*: Anaphylactic reaction[a+b], angioedema[b], hypersensitivity[a]. *Infections*: Cellulitis[a]. *Injection site reactions*: Injection site reactions[a+b]. *Musculoskeletal*: Arthralgia[b], limb swelling[a+b]. *Nervous system*: Convulsions[a+b], encephalopathy[a], headache[b], hypotonia[a+b], hypotonic-hyporesponsive episode[a], somnolence[a+b]. *Psychiatric*: Crying[a+b], irritability[a+b]. *Respiratory system*: Respiratory tract infection[a]. *Skin and appendages*: Alopecia[b], erythema[a+b], erythema multiforme[b], petechiae[b], pruritus[a+b], rash[a+b], urticaria[a+b]. *Special senses*: Ear pain[a]. [[a] Following INFANRIX; [b] Following ENGERIX-B; [a+b] Following either INFANRIX or ENGERIX-B.] These reactions were reported voluntarily from a population of uncertain size; therefore, it is not always possible to reliably estimate their frequency or establish a causal relationship to vaccination.

**Reporting Adverse Events:** Report the occurrence following immunization of any event set forth in the Vaccine Injury Table from the National Childhood Vaccine Injury Act including: Anaphylaxis or anaphylactic shock within 7 days, encephalopathy or encephalitis within 7 days, brachial neuritis within 28 days, or an acute complication or sequelae (including death) of an illness, disability, injury, or condition referred to above, or any events that would contraindicate further doses of PEDIARIX. The VAERS toll-free number is 1-800-822-7967.

Manufactured by **GlaxoSmithKline Biologicals**, Rixensart, Belgium, US License 1617

Distributed by **GlaxoSmithKline,** Research Triangle Park, NC 27709



Full prescribing information for PEDIARIX is available at www.GSKVaccines.com/Pediarix. BRS-PE:L2

 Printed in USA. PED583R0 June 2005

ARTICLE

# Social Interactions in Adolescent Television Viewing

*Jason Fletcher, MS*

**Objective:** To examine whether social interactions influence the television viewing choices of adolescents in grades 7 through 12.

**Design:** Data from a nationally representative cross-sectional survey were used to examine the association between individual-level and school-level television choices. An instrumental variables approach was used to solve the simultaneity problem found in models that examine the association between individual and aggregate choices.

**Setting:** In-home interviews in the United States collected in 1996.

**Participants:** A sample of 4532 students in grades 7 through 12 in 132 US public and private schools who participated in the National Longitudinal Study of Adolescent Health (Add Health).

**Main Exposure:** The reported television viewing choices of an individual's schoolmates.

**Main Outcome Measure:** The number of hours of television individuals reported viewing in a week.

**Results:** The number of hours of television that adolescents report viewing per week was associated with their peers' reported hours of television viewing. Adjusted for other covariates, a 1-hour increase in average school-level television viewing was associated with an increase in almost half an hour of television viewing at the individual level.

**Conclusions:** Evidence suggests that social interactions within schools influence the hours of television that adolescents report viewing. This finding is important for both future attempts at modeling the determinants of adolescent television viewing and suggestions for future policy interventions. The presence of social interactions implies that interventions that affect the social norms of television viewing within schools could also change individual television viewing. In reducing the number of hours of television watched, these interventions could also positively affect adolescent obesity, emotional problems, and academic achievement.

*Arch Pediatr Adolesc Med. 2006;160:383-386*

TELEVISION IS A UBIQUITOUS part of adolescents' lives, and its effects are controversial. Many studies have reported several negative consequences of television viewing, including increases in obesity, attentional problems and aggression, and decreases in several measures of academic achievement.[1-4] In contrast, other studies have shown that some types of programming are associated with positive developmental outcomes.[5] There have also been several randomized interventions aimed at reducing television as a means of decreasing negative outcomes.[3,6] This article examines the importance of social interactions in adolescent television choices. Social interactions follow the conceptual idea of the establishment of a social norm of television viewing within peer groups. The idea of interdependent choices, or social interactions, across individuals, where individual choices are affected by the choices of peers, is becoming established in the social sciences as an important aspect of individual decision making. Current research examines potential social interactions in crime, school attendance, and unemployment.[7-9] For example, a student might choose to attend school on a particular day based on whether his or her friends will attend school. The intuitive reason for this interdependence in choices is that friends want to be involved in activities together whether the activities are pleasant (eg, skipping school to go to the mall) or unpleasant (eg, attending school).

This study tested whether social norms created by schoolmates influence individual choices in television viewing. In addition to contributing to conceptual models of the determinants of television viewing among adolescents, the results of

**Author Affiliation:** Department of Agricultural and Applied Economics, University of Wisconsin–Madison.

this study can be used to inform policies that seek to change television viewing choices. Evidence of social interactions suggests several new directions for potential interventions. If social norms are an important determinant of individual television viewing, interventions that seek to shape these norms within schools could be a valuable future direction for research. Some forms of social interactions also imply that interventions on a subset of individuals within a school will have a spillover effect on students who did not receive the intervention. Both implications of finding social interactions in television viewing choices represent new and interesting directions for future policy suggestions.

## METHODS

### DATA

Data for this study were drawn from the National Longitudinal Study of Adolescent Health (Add Health). Add Health is a nationally representative study of adolescents in grades 7 through 12 and their outcomes in young adulthood, and was begun in 1994 under a grant from the National Institute of Child Health and Human Development, with co-funding from 17 other federal agencies. Data at the individual, family, school, and community levels were collected in 2 waves between 1994 and 1996. More information about the Add Health data are provided elsewhere.[10,11] The sample used in this study consists of all adolescents in grades 7 through 12 in the wave II public-use data collected in 1996. Of the 4532 observations available in wave II, 3594 adolescents have valid school identification codes, which are necessary to calculate school-level variables and place individuals in their school environments. The sample of students with valid school identification codes is similar to those students with missing codes across many of the covariates examined in this study, but they are slightly more likely to be white (0.72 vs 0.68) and have married parents (0.65 vs 0.54), less likely to be male (0.46 vs 0.55), and on average have a higher family income ($48 300 vs $43 500). Of the remaining sample, 3583 had valid television hours data and 3141 had complete covariate data after family income was imputed using single imputation techniques for 600 individuals. The use of this data set was preapproved by the University of Wisconsin Institutional Review Board, Madison.

### MEASURES

#### Outcome Variables

The primary outcome measure was self-reported hours of television viewing per week at the individual level.

#### Independent Variables

The primary predictor of interest was the mean reported hours of television viewing of an individual's school. For each individual, this measure was the sample average of all individuals in the same school (except the individual). Several important covariates were also included in the analysis. The individual's sex was included because it is well documented that male students watch more television than female students do.[12] Likewise, race (white, black, or Hispanic) was included to capture known differences in television viewing across these groups.[13] Overweight status was included because it has consistently been shown to be highly correlated with television viewing.[1,13] An individual's grade in school and grade point average were included because television viewing decreases as students age and academic achievement is likely to be negatively correlated with television viewing. Family income, rural status, and employment were included to control for availability of activities for adolescents that are substitutes for television. Finally, school-level characteristics (eg, racial composition and income) were included to capture differences in the school environment across individuals. Since geographic identifiers are unavailable in the data set, no variables that directly measure community access to television programming can be used in the analysis.

### STATISTICAL ANALYSIS

The analytical approaches included multivariate linear regression and 2-stage least squares regression using the Huber-White estimator of variance to account for the fact that more than 1 child was assessed in each school.[14] Wave II sample weights were also used to adjust for the complex sampling design in the data. The estimated regression model was of the following form:

$$Y_{is} = \beta \bar{X}_{is} + \delta \bar{X}_{-is} + \alpha \bar{Y}_{is} + \epsilon_{is}$$

where individual $i$ in school $s$ chooses television viewing level $Y_{is}$ and has individual characteristics $X$. School-level variables are included in $\bar{X}$ (with individual $i$ omitted), and school-level television choices are included in $\bar{Y}$ (with individual $i$ omitted). The main parameter of interest is $\alpha$, which is the estimate of the importance of social interaction in individual television choices. Two-stage least squares regression is necessary in the empirical analysis because group behavior affects individual behavior and vice versa. This simultaneity in choices leads to the reflection problem first discussed by Manski[15,16] in the economics literature. The reflection problem occurs in most empirical research that attempts to demonstrate an association between individual-level and group-level behavior. Manski proved that most estimates of $\alpha$ are not identified without using instrumental variables or other methods.[16] The instrumental variables approach solves the reflection problem by finding a variable that is related to the individual outcome at the individual level but not at the group level.[17,18] For this analysis, employment status was used to identify the relationship between group television viewing and individual television viewing. Intuitively, the assumption is that an individual's employment status is related (negatively) to the individual's television viewing, because individuals who are employed have less available time to watch television, but the proportion of employed students in an individual's school is not associated with the individual's choice of how much television to watch. The proportion of employed students is assumed to affect the individual's television viewing only through its affect on the school-level television viewing measure.

## RESULTS

**Table 1** gives descriptive statistics of the variables used in the study. The mean number of hours per week of television viewing was almost 15. The average number of children in the 131 schools in the sample was nearly 40. Students are exposed to a wide variety of school-level employment; the school-level proportion of students working varies from 0% to 95% of the sampled student body. Finally, the school-level average number of hours of television viewing varies between 2 and 32 hours per week.

**Table 2** gives the results of the regressions of the determinants of individual hours of television viewing. Before examining potential social interactions, ordinary least squares results showing the individual, family, and school-

**Table 1. Descriptive Statistics Wave II of the Add Health Data Set, 3189 Observations**

| Variable | Mean (SD) | Minimum | Maximum |
|---|---|---|---|
| Outcome | | | |
| Television viewing, h/wk | 14.63 (14.91) | 0 | 160 |
| Individual and family characteristics | | | |
| Male sex | 0.49 (0.50) | 0 | 1 |
| White | 0.65 (0.48) | 0 | 1 |
| Black | 0.21 (0.41) | 0 | 1 |
| Hispanic | 0.11 (0.31) | 0 | 1 |
| Grade point average | 2.82 (0.76) | 1 | 4 |
| School grade | 9.92 (1.45) | 7 | 13 |
| Rural | 0.27 (0.44) | 0 | 1 |
| Urban | 0.30 (0.46) | 0 | 1 |
| Overweight | 0.23 (0.42) | 0 | 1 |
| Employed | 0.58 (0.49) | 0 | 1 |
| Family income ($10 000-$10 999) | 4.55 (4.36) | 0 | 90 |
| Married household | 0.66 (0.47) | 0 | 1 |
| School-level characteristics | | | |
| No. of students per school | 39.15 (17.14) | 11 | 99 |
| Overweight | 23.02 (11.56) | 0 | 58 |
| Income | 45.21 (18.62) | 14 | 136 |
| Hispanic | 11.05 (19.12) | 0 | 92 |
| Black | 20.42 (28.06) | 0 | 100 |
| Employed | 57.94 (18.02) | 9 | 95 |
| Television viewing, h/wk | 14.82 (5.28) | 2 | 32 |

Abbreviation: Add Health, National Longitudinal Study of Adolescent Health.

level correlates of individual television hours are listed in column 1. Robust standard errors that allow for correlated errors at the school level are shown under the coefficients, and wave II sample weights are used. Male students report watching 2 hours of television per week more than female students. While black students report 5 more hours of television viewing than do white students, there was little difference between white and Hispanic students in television viewing time. As students age, they report watching less television. Employed students report watching television almost 2 hours less than unemployed students do. Students with higher grade point averages also report watching fewer hours of television. Finally, while family income had a small and statistically insignificant relationship with television viewing, students who attended schools with wealthier classmates report less television viewing.

Column 2 lists results for 2-stage least squares analysis. To estimate this empirical model, an instrumental variable must be chosen. Without an instrumental variable, the coefficient of interest ($\alpha$ in the equation) is not identified. The instrumental variable must meet 2 criteria for the estimation results to be valid. First, the variable must be strongly related to the school-level average of television hours. This criterion was met because the (unreported) first-stage relationship between school-level employment and school-level television hours had a *t* statistic of almost 17. Second, the variable must be uncorrelated with the unobserved error term. Because it was impossible to document that this criterion is satisfied, in practice it must be assumed. Suggestive evidence that school-level employment was uncorrelated with the unobserved error can be found in the result from column 1 that school-level employment was uncorrelated with the individual choice of television hours.

**Table 2. Television Regression Results***

| Dependent Variable | Television Hours: Ordinary Least Squares Analysis | Television Hours: 2-Staged Least Squares Analysis |
|---|---|---|
| Individual and family characteristics | | |
| Male sex | 2.001 (0.644-3.357)† | 2.027 (0.653 to 3.401)† |
| Black | 5.317 (3.339-7.295)† | 4.634 (2.060 to 7.208)† |
| Hispanic | 0.138 (−1.924-2.200) | 0.755 (−1.002 to 2.512) |
| Grade point average | −1.394 (−2.130-−0.657)† | −1.227 (−1.982 to −0.472)† |
| Married household | −0.865 (−2.161-0.431) | −0.804 (−2.077 to 0.469) |
| Family income | 0.008 (−0.107-0.124) | 0.014 (−0.100 to 0.29) |
| Rural | −0.502 (−1.813-0.810) | −0.451 (−1.711 to 0.810) |
| Urban | −0.321 (−1.822-1.180) | −0.317 (−1.793 to 1.160) |
| Overweight | 0.584 (−0.650-1.819) | 0.531 (−0.715 to 1.778) |
| School grade | −0.667 (−1.152-−0.182)† | −0.545 (−0.904 to −0.186) |
| Employed | −1.939 (−3.236-0.643)† | −1.969 (−3.283 to −0.654)† |
| School-level variables | | |
| Income | −0.092 (−0.133-−0.052)† | −0.045 (−0.101 to 0.010) |
| White | −0.021 (−0.059-0.017) | |
| Employment | −0.022 (−0.077-0.032) | |
| Television viewing, h | | 0.441 (0.064 to 0.817)‡ |
| Constant | 31.782 (25.467-38.097)† | 18.680 (8.487 to 28.874)† |
| No. of observations | 3141 | 3141 |
| $R^2$ | 0.105 | 0.106 |

*Unless otherwise specified, values indicate number, with robust 95% confidence interval in parentheses.
†Significant at 1%.
‡Significant at 5%.

The results in column 2 for individual and family variables change little from the results in column 1. The main result was that the level of school television viewing was positively related to individual hours. The results suggest that a 1-hour increase in school-level hours increases the individual's television viewing by almost half an hour per week (95% confidence interval, 0.06-0.82).

## COMMENT

This analysis has produced evidence that individual choices of how many hours to watch television are determined, in part, by choices by schoolmates. The inclusion of potential confounding variables and the use of instrumental variables suggest that these associations may be causal; not only are television choices correlated within school, but decisions by peers of how much television to watch affects television choices at the individual level. However, since this framework can only show the existence of social influences on individual decisions and not the mechanism underlying the process, why and how the social influences affect individual decisions are unclear. It could be that individuals in the same school watch similar amounts of television so that they can discuss television during school. The data set contained information only on hours of television watched and not specific content, which does not allow the hypothesized mechanism to be tested explicitly.[19] Further examinations of the mechanism through which social interactions shape individuals' television choices are an important area for future research.

Several important limitations of this research require elaboration. It is possible that the ability of parents to choose schools for their children account for some portion of the relationship. If parents who do not actively monitor their children's television viewing send their children to similar schools, a portion of the results could be spurious. This unobserved parental trait would have to be inadequately controlled for in the covariates for this to be a substantive concern. Including a variable that measures the frequency of parental participation in parent-teacher association events was not significant when included in the regression analyses. While this variable was not available for all students, it does allow some confidence that the results are likely not significantly affected by unobserved parental characteristics.

An additional potential weakness of this research has been the reliance on measures of self-reported television viewing rather than actual viewing.[20-23] This problem is not unique to this research but might be particularly concerning if self-reported measures of television viewing are affected by social norms within schools. Examination of this issue would require additional data that are unavailable.

With these caveats in mind, overall the results suggest the presence of social interactions in adolescents' television choices. The importance of this finding for policy makers is that social interactions imply that policies that shape social norms in schools could be an effective direction for interventions to reduce television viewing. In addition, interventions on a subset of students within schools are likely to have a spillover effect on students in the same school who did not receive the intervention. Both types of interventions represent interesting areas for future efforts to decrease television viewing among adolescents.

**Accepted for Publication:** November 22, 2005.
**Correspondence:** Jason Fletcher, MS, Department of Agricultural and Applied Economics, 427 Lorch St, University of Wisconsin-Madison, Madison, WI 53706 (jmfletcher@wisc.edu).
**Funding/Support:** This study was supported by the Ruth L. Kirschstein National Research Service Award T32 MH18029-19 from the National Institute of Mental Health, Bethesda, Md (Mr Fletcher).
**Acknowledgment:** This research used data from Add Health, a program project designed by J. Richard Udry, Peter S. Bearman, and Kathleen Mullan Harris and funded by grant P01-HD31921 from the National Institute of Child Health and Human Development with cooperative funding from 17 other agencies. Persons interested in obtaining data files from Add Health may contact Add Health, Carolina Population Center, 123 W Franklin St, Chapel Hill, NC 27516-2524 (addhealth@unc.edu). Special acknowledgment is due Ronald R. Rindfuss and Barbara Entwisle for assistance in the original design.

## REFERENCES

1. Christakis DA, Zimmerman FJ, DiGiuseppe DL, McCarty CA. Early television exposure and subsequent attentional problems in children. *Pediatrics.* 2004;113:708-713.
2. Anderson DR, Huston AC, Schmitt KL, Linebarger DL, Wright JC. Early childhood television viewing and adolescent behavior. *Monogr Soc Res Child Dev.* 2001;66:I-VIII, 1-147.
3. Robinson TN, Wilde ML, Navracruz LC, Haydel KF, Varady A. Effects of reducing children's television and video game use on aggressive behavior: a randomized controlled trial. *Arch Pediatr Adolesc Med.* 2001;155:17-23.
4. Zimmerman FJ, Christakis DA. Children's television viewing and cognitive outcomes: a longitudinal analysis of national data. *Arch Pediatr Adolesc Med.* 2005;159:619-625.
5. Wright JC, Huston AC, Murphy KC, et al. The relations of early television viewing to school readiness and vocabulary of children from low-income families: the early window project. *Child Dev.* 2001;72:1347-1366.
6. Robinson TN. Reducing children's television viewing to prevent obesity: a randomized controlled trial. *JAMA.* 1999;282:1561-1567.
7. Glaeser EL, Sacerdote BE, Scheinkman JA. Crime and social interactions. *Q J Econ.* 1996;111:507-548.
8. Lalive R, Cattaneo A. *Social Interactions and Schooling Decisions.* Zurich, Switzerland: University of Zurich; October 2004. Working Paper.
9. Lalive R. *Social Interactions in Unemployment.* Zurich, Switzerland: University of Zurich; 2003. IZA Discussion Paper 803.
10. Bearman PS, Jones J, Udry JR. The National Longitudinal Study of Adolescent Health: research design. Carolina Population Center, University of North Carolina at Chapel Hill; 1997. Available at: http://www.cpc.unc.edu/projects/addhealth/design.html. Accessed August 19, 2005.
11. Udry JR. *The National Longitudinal Study of Adolescent Health (Add Health), Waves I & II, 1994–1996; Wave III, 2001–2002* [machine-readable data file and documentation]. Carolina Population Center, University of North Carolina at Chapel Hill; 2003.
12. Crespo CJ, Smit E, Troiano RP, Bartlett SJ, Macera CA, Andersen RE. Television watching, energy intake, and obesity in US children: results from the Third National Health and Nutrition Examination Survey, 1988-1994. *Arch Pediatr Adolesc Med.* 2001;155:360-365.
13. Flores G, Tomany-Korman SC, Olson L. Does disadvantage start at home? racial and ethnic disparities in health-related early childhood home routines and safety practices. *Arch Pediatr Adolesc Med.* 2005;159:158-165.
14. Deaton A. *The Analysis of Household Surveys.* Baltimore, Md: Johns Hopkins University Press; 1997.
15. Manski CF. Economic analysis of social interactions. *J Econ Perspect.* 2000;14:115-136.
16. Manski CF. Identification of endogenous social effects: the reflection problem. *Rev Econ Stud.* 1993;60:531-542.
17. Durlauf SN. Neighborhood effects. In: Henderson V, Thisse JF, eds. *Handbook of Regional and Urban Economics.* Vol 4. New York, NY: North-Holland; 2004.
18. Blume LE, Durlauf SN. Identifying social interactions: a review. University of Wisconsin-Madison; 2005. SSRI Working Paper 2005-12.
19. Chernin AR, Linebarger DL. The relationship between children's television viewing and academic performance. *Arch Pediatr Adolesc Med.* 2005;159:687-689.
20. Wiecha JL, Sobol AM, Peterson KE, Gortmaker SL. Household television access: associations with screen time, reading, and homework among youth. *Ambul Pediatr.* 2001;1:244-251.
21. Anderson DR, Field DE, Collins PA, Lorch EP, Nathan JG. Estimates of young children's time with television: a methodological comparison of parent reports with time-lapse video home observation. *Child Dev.* 1985;56:1345-1357.
22. Strasburger VC, Donnerstein E. Children, adolescents, and the media: issues and solutions. *Pediatrics.* 1999;103:129-139.
23. Borzekowski DL, Robinson T. Viewing the viewers: ten video cases of children's television viewing behaviors. *J Broadcasting Electronic Media.* 1999;43:506-528.

# Is Television Viewing Associated With Social Isolation?

## *Roles of Exposure Time, Viewing Context, and Violent Content*

*David S. Bickham, PhD; Michael Rich, MD, MPH*

**Objective:** To estimate associations between children's peer integration and amount of time they spend (1) watching television, (2) watching violent television, and (3) coviewing television with friends.

**Design:** Survey using nationally representative data from the Panel Study of Income Dynamics–Child Development Supplement Wave 1.

**Setting:** Nationwide survey of families with young children performed in 1997.

**Participants:** Of 3562 children, 1356 had sufficient data for inclusion in analyses (563 children aged 6 to 8 years and 793 children aged 9 to 12 years).

**Main Exposure:** Total time viewing television, with and without friends present, and time viewing violent and nonviolent television content.

**Main Outcome Measure:** Amount of time children spent with friends as reported in two 24-hour activity diaries.

**Results:** Viewing violent programs (but not nonviolent programs) was negatively related to time children spent with friends (aged 6-8 years, unstandardized regression coefficient [$\beta$] = −0.34, 95% confidence interval [CI], −0.59 to −0.08; aged 9-12 years, $\beta$ = −0.41, 95% CI, −0.65 to −0.18). More time viewing television with friends was associated with more time engaging in other activities with friends (aged 6-8 years, $\beta$ = 0.98, 95% CI, 0.61 to 1.36; aged 9-12 years, $\beta$ = 1.03, 95% CI, 0.72 to 1.34).

**Conclusions:** The more time that children spent viewing violent programs, the less time they spent with their friends. While this study cannot determine the direction of effects for this relationship, a cyclical process between violent media and peer integration best explains the findings. To optimize social development and mental health, children's access to violent media should be limited.

*Arch Pediatr Adolesc Med. 2006;160:387-392*

CHILDREN'S SUCCESS WITH peer relationships has substantial, long-lasting effects on their social adjustment and overall mental health. Failing in these relationships increases the risk for social isolation, anxiety disorder, agoraphobia, and antisocial behavior, including aggression and gang involvement.[1-6] Peer rejection during childhood is linked to serious disorders and behavioral consequences in adolescence and adulthood, including dropping out of school, criminal behavior, and psychoses.[1] To help children succeed socially, parents and pediatricians must understand and guide behaviors and activities that affect peer integration and social development. Television viewing, while frequently cited as a cause of social isolation,[7] is often overlooked as a potential contributor to problems with peer relationships. This study uses a nationally representative data set to investigate the complex relationship between television viewing and children's peer relationships.

It is a widely held belief that the time children spend with media displaces more valuable pursuits.[7-9] Once activities such as eating, sleeping, and self-care are accounted for, children have roughly 51 hours of discretionary time each week.[10] Recent studies have found that on average, school-aged American children spend approximately 27 hours a week watching television.[11] It is easy to understand, therefore, how television viewing is seen as interfering with children's important developmental activities.

Peer interaction allows children the opportunity to develop social skills and build relationships.[12] Research on the relationship between television and social interactions is limited and findings are mixed. Some studies have found no relationship between television viewing and social time,[13] while others have found that television displaces participation in some social activities.[14] Still others have found that the more time children spent watching television, the less time they spent with their families.[15]

**Author Affiliations:** Center on Media and Child Health, Harvard Medical School, Harvard School of Public Health, Boston, Mass.

**Table 1. Mean Television (TV) Viewing Time and Time Spent With Friends**

| Independent Variables | Mean (SD) | |
|---|---|---|
| | Children Aged 6-8 y (n = 563) | Children Aged 9-12 y (n = 793) |
| Time watching TV, min/48 h* | 289.67 (182.37) | 290.34 (200.47) |
| Time watching TV with no friends, min/48 h | 272.27 (178.99) | 263.36 (189.92) |
| Time with friends (no TV), min/48 h | 168.69 (214.82) | 251.44 (266.64) |
| Time watching TV with friends, min/48 h | 17.40 (55.84) | 26.99 (79.62) |
| Time watching violent TV programs,† min/48 h | 85.21 (82.76) | 82.65 (105.76) |
| Time watching nonviolent TV programs,† min/48 h | 128.24 (108.24) | 139.83 (123.48) |

*Values for time-use variables represent minutes of viewing during both diary days (weekday and weekend combined). All values are weighted to represent national estimates.

†For violent and nonviolent TV programs, n = 411 for children aged 6 to 8 years; n = 604 for children aged 9 to 12 years.

Assuming television simply displaces peer interactions underestimates the complex role it has in children's lives. Television is a rich medium that can teach a variety of social behaviors. Meta-analyses conclude that viewing violent television increases children's antisocial behaviors and decreases their positive social behaviors.[16-18] Such negative social behaviors can lead to social isolation, while positive social behaviors can lead to successful peer relationships.[19-22] The content of television, therefore, may be at least as important to children's social integration as the time they spend with the medium.[23]

The context in which television is viewed may also influence children's social interactions. While television viewing is often perceived as an isolating activity, it frequently occurs in the company of friends.[24] Because socializing builds interpersonal skills,[12] television viewing with friends may provide a venue for these skills to develop.

While television may isolate children, the reverse causal direction is also plausible—lonely children may turn to television for entertainment and companionship. Children who are marginalized by their peers use television to escape the stresses of their lives and meet their social needs.[25] Conversely, children who are socially integrated spend less time watching television.[26-29] In this model, it is social isolation that motivates media use. Overall, it is most likely that both effects occur—children who watch more television become more socially isolated, which leads them to spend more time watching television.

The purpose of this study is to investigate the extent to which television viewing is associated with children's peer integration. It tests the hypothesis that the more time children watch television, the less time they spend with their friends. Additionally, children's exposure to violent and nonviolent programs will be distinguished to determine the independent relationship of these 2 types of content with peer integration. Finally, this study investigates whether coviewing television is linked to the amount of time children spend with friends not watching television.

## METHOD

### DATA

Data for this study were drawn from the Panel Study of Income Dynamics–Child Development Supplement (PSID-CDS) Wave 1 collected in 1997.[30] Since 1968, the PSID has been an ongoing, nationally representative panel study of adults conducted by the Survey Research Center at the Institute for Social Research, University of Michigan, Ann Arbor. In 1997, the CDS was added and included a battery of questionnaires for families with children aged 6 months to 12 years. It resulted in data representing 3562 children.

Data collection procedures for the PSID-CDS were approved by the University of Michigan institutional review board, and the analytical protocol was approved by the University of Texas at Austin institutional review board.

Time-use diaries were used to collect detailed information about children's activities. This method yields the most complete, valid, and reliable data possible without an extraordinary commitment of time or money.[10,31] It is less costly and intrusive than observational methods and less likely to be socially biased than summative self-reports.[32] Time-use diary reports of children's television viewing have been validated by comparison with observational data from videotapes made of the child's home.[33]

On 2 randomly chosen days (1 weekend and 1 weekday), primary caregivers completed comprehensive time-use diaries. The primary caregiver, with help from the child when appropriate, accounted for every minute of activity performed by their child for 24-hour periods from midnight to 11:59 PM the next night. Along with duration of activities, parents reported location, other people who were present, and any secondary concurrent activity. When television was the primary activity reported, the title of the program or movie viewed was also requested.

Two coders used their own knowledge and information gained from Web sites to determine the presence of violence in each show reported by the participants. News, sports, and other nonfiction programs contained widely variable content and were not coded. Programs were considered violent if violence was a central theme to the program. These programs generally depicted considerably more violence than normally exists in most children's lives and often included main characters whose profession included responding to or participating in violence. The coders reached an appropriate level of interrater reliability ($\kappa$=0.81).

The number of minutes each child watched television as a primary or secondary activity was computed by summing every instance of viewing broadcast, cable, or videos reported in the time-use diaries for both days. Viewing of violent and nonviolent content was similarly calculated. Mean values for viewing are presented in **Table 1**.

### SUBSAMPLES

Only children 6 years and older were included in this study because it is at this age, around school entry, when children begin shifting their social focus from family to peers.[34,35] Analyses were performed separately for 6- to 8-year-olds and 9- to 12-year-olds.

This study used 2 subsamples from the PSID-CDS. The television viewing subsample contained 1356 children of the total sample (n = 3562) who returned 2 time-use diaries and had complete data on variables in the models. This subsample was used in analyses that considered total television viewing and viewing context. The television viewing subsample included 563 children aged 6 to 8 years and 793 children aged 9 to 12 years.

The violent content viewing subsample consisted of 1015 children from the television viewing subsample whose diaries contained 70% or more codeable data. This subsample included 411 children aged 6 to 8 years and 604 children aged 9 to 12 years.

### MEASURING TIME SPENT WITH FRIENDS

Peer integration was operationalized as the amount of time children spent with their friends. Because the time-use diaries included a report of people present during activities, it was possible to determine the total amount of time each child spent with his or her friends during the 2 days. The time children watched television with their friends was also calculated and subtracted from the total amount of time they spent with their friends to prevent overlap between the independent variable (ie, television viewing) and dependent variable (ie, time with friends). The mean and standard deviation of time with friends (no television) and time watching television with friends are provided in Table 1.

### COVARIATES

The PSID-CDS contains multiple family and child level variables that may contribute to children's television exposure and/or peer integration. The following were included in analyses as control variables: (1) age in years was included to control for age differences within each age group (overall mean [SD] age, 9.05 [2.04] years); (2) sex was coded with girls as 1 and boys as 0 (girls, n=683, boys, n=673); (3) parental education was determined by the number of years of education completed by the head of each child's household (mean [SD], 12.67 [2.73] years); (4) the primary caregiver's report of total family income in 1996 was divided by the Census Bureau poverty threshold for that size family to determine the income-to-needs ratio[36] (mean [SD], 2.92 [3.74]); (5) children who were reported to have a race/ethnicity of black, Hispanic, Asian, Native American, or other were considered to be minorities (minority, n=706; nonminority, n=650); (6) the Home Observation for Measurement of the Environment short form[37] combines observational items completed by the researcher and self-report questions completed by the participant to measure emotional support and cognitive stimulation parents provide their children (scores were standardized within age groups); (7) the 6-item, 5-point Parental Warmth Scale developed by Child Trends was used to measure warmth of the relationship between child and parent[38] (mean [SD], 4.33 [0.62]).

### ANALYSIS PLAN AND DETAILS

Ordinary least squares regression was performed using STATA 8.0 statistical software (Stata Corp, College Station, Tex) to test the relationships between television viewing and the amount of time children spent with their friends while controlling for the variables listed previously. Sampling weights were applied to all analyses to represent national estimates and commands were used to help correct for nonindependent, sibling data. Unstandardized regression coefficients are reported to allow for the translation of results into meaningful time-use differences.

**Table 2. Regression Analysis for Television Viewing and Control Variables Predicting Non-Television Time With Friends**

| Independent Variables | β* (95% CI) Children Aged 6-8 y (n = 563) | β* (95% CI) Children Aged 9-12 y (n = 793) |
|---|---|---|
| Television (no friends) | −0.20† (−0.32 to −0.08) | −.31‡ (−0.43 to −0.19) |
| Age, y | 34.38§ (8.12 to 60.64) | 6.70 (−14.38 to 27.79) |
| Parental education | 12.67† (4.69 to 20.65) | 3.07 (−6.68 to 12.82) |
| Income-needs ratio | −1.81 (−10.24 to 6.63) | −3.13§ (−6.17 to −0.08) |
| Minority status | 17.71 (−36.92 to 72.34) | −56.93§ (−113.35 to −0.51) |
| Sex | 1.16 (−41.21 to 43.53) | −17.24 (−66.01 to 31.52) |
| Home‖ score | 4.25 (−19.14 to 27.63) | 1.16 (−26.20 to 28.51) |
| Parental warmth | 12.90 (−35.55 to 61.36) | −19.85 (−61.58 to 21.88) |
| $R^2$ | .09‡ | .07‡ |

Abbreviation: CI, confidence interval.
*Regression coefficients (β) are unstandardized and weighted to represent national estimates.
†$P<.01$.
‡$P<.001$.
§$P<.05$.
‖The Home Observation for Measurement of the Environment short form measures emotional support and cognitive stimulation parents provide their children.

## RESULTS

### TOTAL TELEVISION VIEWING AND TIME WITH FRIENDS

The more time children spent watching television without friends present, the less time they spent with their friends engaging in other activities (**Table 2**). For 6- to 8-year-olds, the unstandardized coefficient of −0.21 can be interpreted to indicate that a difference of 1 hour more of television watched corresponded to a difference of about 13 minutes or, on average, 7.5% less time with friends. For 9- to 12-year-olds, 1 hour more television watched corresponded to about 19 fewer minutes (7.4%) spent with friends.

### VIOLENT/NONVIOLENT TELEVISION AND TIME WITH FRIENDS

**Table 3** presents the regression results for viewing each of the 2 categories (violent and nonviolent) of television programming. These 2 types of viewing were moderately correlated with one another in each of the age groups (children aged 6-8 years, $r=0.36$, $P<.001$; 9-12 years, $r=0.32$, $P<.001$).

The more time children spent watching violent television without friends, the less non-television time they spent with their friends. Among 6- to 8-year-olds, an additional 1 hour of violent television viewing corresponded to about 20 minutes (12.1%) less time spent with friends. For 9- to 12-year-olds, viewing 1 additional hour of violent television corresponded to 25 minutes (9.8%)

**Table 3. Regression Analysis for Violent and Nonviolent Television Program Viewing and Control Variables Predicting Non-Television Time With Friends**

| Independent Variables | β* (95% CI) Children Aged 6-8 y (n = 411) | β* (95% CI) Children Aged 9-12 y (n = 604) |
|---|---|---|
| Violent television programs (without friends present) | −0.34† (−0.59 to −0.08) | −0.41† (−0.65 to −0.18) |
| Nonviolent television programs (without friends present) | −0.00 (−0.25 to 0.25) | −0.18 (−0.44 to 0.09) |
| Age, y | 45.18† (15.15 to 75.21) | 0.39 (−23.26 to 24.04) |
| Parental education | 10.01‡ (.34 to 19.67) | 5.51 (−6.71 to 17.73) |
| Income-needs ratio | −2.39 (−11.00 to 6.22) | −3.50‡ (−6.73 to −0.27) |
| Minority status | 37.92 (−29.59 to 105.42) | −21.04 (−87.24 to 45.16) |
| Sex | 26.31 (−23.84 to 76.47) | −13.16 (−65.10 to 38.77) |
| Home§ score | 19.79 (−5.47 to 45.04) | 7.89 (−24.10 to 39.88) |
| Parental warmth | 2.02 (−58.36 to 62.40) | −38.51 (−87.42 to 10.40) |
| $R^2$ | .09‖ | .04‖ |

Abbreviation: CI, confidence interval.
*Regression coefficients (β) are unstandardized and weighted to represent national estimates.
†$P<.01$.
‡$P<.05$.
§The Home Observation for Measurement of the Environment short form measures emotional support and cognitive stimulation parents provide their children.
‖$P<.001$.

**Table 4. Regression Analysis for Television Viewing With Friends and Control Variables Predicting Non-Television Time With Friends**

| Independent Variables | β* (95% CI) Children Aged 6-8 y (n = 563) | β* (95% CI) Children Aged 9-12 y (n = 793) |
|---|---|---|
| Television with friends | 0.98† (0.61 to 1.36) | 1.03† (0.72 to 1.34) |
| Age, y | 28.77‡ (3.10 to 54.44) | −4.19 (−24.17 to 15.78) |
| Parental education | 12.18§ (4.35 to 20.02) | 2.59 (−7.34 to 12.51) |
| Income-needs ratio | −0.37 (−8.83 to 8.10) | −2.18 (−5.02 to 0.66) |
| Minority status | 16.68 (−33.68 to 67.04) | −64.24‡ (−115.99 to −12.49) |
| Sex | 9.36 (−31.28 to 50.00) | −41.47 (−88.95 to 6.00) |
| Home‖ score | 13.37 (−9.10 to 35.84) | 9.25 (−16.25 to 34.74) |
| Parental warmth | 18.70 (−28.66 to 66.06) | −28.06 (−68.05 to 11.93) |
| $R^2$ | .13† | .12† |

Abbreviation: CI, confidence interval.
*Regression coefficients (β) are unstandardized and weighted to represent national estimates.
†$P<.001$.
‡$P<.05$.
§$P<.01$.
‖The Home Observation for Measurement of the Environment short form measures emotional support and cognitive stimulation parents provide their children.

less time spent with their friends. Viewing nonviolent television programming was not significantly related to the amount of time children spent with their friends.

## COVIEWING TELEVISION WITH FRIENDS AND OTHER TIME WITH FRIENDS

The more time children of either age group spent coviewing television with their friends, the more time they spent with their friends engaging in non-television activities (**Table 4**). For 6- to 8-year-olds, 1 more hour of watching television with friends corresponded to 59 minutes more time with their friends not watching television. For 9- to 12-year-old children, each hour of television viewing with friends corresponded to about 62 minutes more non-television time spent with friends.

## COMMENT

This study used nationally representative data and time-use diaries to investigate the relationship between television viewing time, content, context, and peer integration. As children spent more total time watching television, they spent a small but significantly shorter amount of time with friends not viewing television. The more violent television programs that children watched, the less non-television time they spent with friends. Viewing nonviolent television programs had no effect on time spent with friends. More time coviewing television with friends was associated with more non-television time with friends. These findings indicate that displacement is not a sufficient explanation for observed relationships between children's television viewing and social activities.

## A PROCESS MODEL

There is strong evidence from many previous studies that violent media contributes to children's antisocial behaviors, suggesting a plausible link between children's violent television exposure and peer integration. As children watch more violent television, they become more aggressive and exhibit fewer positive social behaviors.[16-18] Aggressive behaviors have been associated with peer rejection and less popularity.[20,21,39] Increased aggression influenced by viewing violent television may prompt peers to reject and socially isolate the aggressive child.

These data are correlational and cannot test causality or the directions of relationships. An alternative explanation for the results is that social isolation precedes increased violent media use. As aggressive children become more isolated from their peers, they have more discretionary time that they then fill by watching television. Because they are aggressive, these children may be attracted to violent content.[40,41]

The model that may most accurately represent real-world effects of violent television is one that synthesizes both directions of influence into a cyclical process, a downward spiral from violent television viewing to aggressive behavior to social isolation to viewing more violent television.[41,42] Exposure to violent television could, therefore, be the catalyst for a cyclical system leading toward an aggressive, socially isolated lifestyle.

## COVIEWING WITH FRIENDS

The more time children spent coviewing television with friends, the more time they spent with their friends engaging in other activities. Again, it is important to consider both directions of influence in the interpretation of this result. Children may forge stronger relationships with their friends around television and thus be more likely to continue their interactions away from the medium. Alternatively, children who regularly spend time with their friends may engage in a variety of activities with them. Viewing television together may be one activity in the repertoire of a rich childhood friendship. Regardless of the direction of influence, this finding does not support the hypothesis that viewing television with friends interferes with relationships or replaces other shared activities.

## LIMITATIONS

The large number of television programs reported by the participants of the PSID-CDS necessitated a limited violence coding procedure. Differing depictions of violence on television can influence the viewer in different ways[43]; the binary, violent vs nonviolent coding used in this study does not capture important yet subtle differences in content. Further research using more precise and objective coding strategies is necessary to understand more fully the relationship between violent television viewing and social isolation.

Although time-use diaries are a valid and accurate method of measuring television viewing, they may be limited by recall bias because they are filled out for the previous day. Additionally, because diaries were collected for 2 sample days, activities that occur rarely are likely to be underrepresented. While 80% of children watch television every day,[11] viewing with friends is a much less common activity and may be underreported in these data. There was not enough coviewing reported to permit analyses examining differences in viewing violent vs nonviolent television programs with friends. Finally, the cross-sectional nature of these data does not permit analyses of the direction of influence between television viewing and peer integration. Longitudinal research is necessary to further examine the direction and strength of this relationship.

## CONCLUSIONS

The more time that children between the ages of 6 and 12 years spent watching violent television, the less time they spent with their friends. This content-specific relationship indicates that television may not simply displace peer interactions. At the time our study data were collected, the National Television Violence Study found this type of content was readily available to children—61% of all television programs and 66% of children's programming contained violence.[44,45]

These results demonstrate that it is important to consider television content whenever investigating the relationships between media use and behaviors. Other research has reached similar conclusions with different behavioral outcomes. Educational television viewing among children in preschool has been shown to have long-term positive effects on children's academic success,[46] while early viewing of violence predicts aggression and violent crime in adulthood.[47]

These findings expand and enrich our understanding of the effects of television exposure on the healthy social development of children. Violent television viewing may influence younger children to be more antisocial, resulting in their becoming socially isolated which, in turn, attracts them to more violent media. To optimize children's social development and long-term mental health, parents, teachers, and pediatricians should discourage the viewing of violent television programs.

In response to these and other findings indicating the potential effects of violent media, pediatricians should incorporate media use histories in children's health maintenance visits to determine how much time children view television or play video games, what content they are exposed to, and with whom they view or play. Special attention should be given to a child's media exposure when there are indications of social isolation, declining school performance, or aggressive, anxious, or withdrawn behavior. Parents should be urged to remove televisions, video games, and Internet access from children's bedrooms and to budget media use for school-aged children to time after all homework, sports, and social obligations have been completed. Parents should be encouraged to make themselves aware of their children's media use, watching television or using other media with them, and discussing problematic content. Finally, pediatricians should encourage the development of media literacy, the ability to use media critically and to protect oneself, for both children and parents. Aware of the potential risks to their children's mental health and social development, parents should model and enforce healthy and safe media use habits in their homes.

**Accepted for Publication:** December 7, 2005.
**Correspondence:** David S. Bickham, PhD, Center on Media and Child Health, Children's Hospital Boston/Harvard Medical School, 300 Longwood Ave, Boston, MA 02115 (david.bickham@childrens.harvard.edu).
**Funding/Support:** The Panel Study of Income Dynamics Child Development Supplement is funded by grant R01-HD33474 from the National Institute of Child Health and Human Development, Bethesda, Md. This research was supported by the Center for Research on Interactive Technology, Television and Children at the University of Texas at Austin and the Center on Media and Child Health at Children's Hospital, Boston.
**Acknowledgment:** The authors would like to thank Elizabeth Vandewater, PhD, Aletha Huston, PhD, Ellen Wartella, PhD, Joanne Cantor, PhD, and Edward Anderson, PhD, for their comments on earlier versions of this research and Brandy King, MLIS, for her contributions.

## REFERENCES


1. Parker JG, Asher SR. Peer relations and later personal adjustment: are low-accepted children at risk? *Psychol Bull.* 1987;102:357-389.
2. Cowen EL, Pederson A, Babigian M, Izzo LD, Trost MR. Long-term follow-up of early detected vulnerable children. *J Consult Clin Psychol.* 1973;41:438-446.
3. Coie JD, Lochman RT, Hymna C. Predicting early adolescent disorder from childhood aggression and peer rejection. *J Consult Clin Psychol.* 1992;60:783-792.
4. Dishion TJ, Nelson SE, Yasui M. Predicting early adolescent gang involvement from middle school adaptation. *J Clin Child Adolesc Psychol.* 2005;34:62-73.
5. Laird RD, Pettit GS, Dodge KA, Bates JE. Peer relationship antecedents of delinquent behavior in late adolescence: is there evidence of demographic group differences in developmental processes? *Dev Psychopathol.* 2005;17:127-144.
6. Werner NE, Crick NR. Maladaptive peer relationships and the development of relational and physical aggression during middle childhood. *Soc Dev.* 2004;13:495-514.
7. Winn M. *The Plug-In Drug: Television, Computers, and Family Life.* New York, NY: Penguin Books; 2002.
8. Healy JM. *Failure to Connect: How Computers Affect Our Children's Minds–and What We Can Do About It.* New York, NY: Touchstone; 1998.
9. Pawlowski C. *Glued to the Tube: The Threat of Television Addiction to Today's Family.* Naperville, Ill: Sourcebooks; 2000.
10. Hofferth SL, Sandberg JF. How American children spend their time. *J Marriage Fam.* 2001;63:295-308.
11. Roberts DF, Foehr UG, Rideout VJ. *Generation M: Media in the Lives of 8-18 Year-Olds.* Menlo Park, Calif: Kaiser Family Foundation; 2005.
12. Berndt TJ, Ladd GW. *Contributions of Peer Relationships to Children's Development.* New York, NY: Wiley; 1989.
13. Neuman SB. The displacement effect: assessing the relation between television viewing and reading performance. *Reading Research Quarterly.* 1988;23:414-440 .
14. Williams TM. *The Impact of Television: A Natural Experiment in Three Communities.* New York, NY: Academic Press; 1986.
15. Vandewater EA, Bickham DS, Lee JH. Time well spent? Relating television use to children's free-time activities. *Pediatrics.* 2006;117:181-191.
16. Paik HJ, Comstock GA. The effects of television violence on antisocial behavior: a meta-analysis. *Communic Res.* 1994;21:516-546.
17. Hearold S. A synthesis of l043 effects of television on social behavior. In: Comstock G, ed. *Public Communication and Behavior.* Vol 1. San Diego, Calif: Academic Press; 1986:65-133.
18. Bushman BJ, Anderson CA. Media violence and the American public: scientific facts versus media misinformation. *Am Psychol.* 2001;56:477-489.
19. Coie JD, Dodge KA, Kupersmidt JB. Group behavior and social status. In: Asher SR, Coie JD, eds. *Peer Rejection in Childhood.* New York, NY: Cambridge University Press; 1990:17-59.
20. Dodge KA. Behavioral antecedents of peer social status. *Child Dev.* 1983;54:1386-1399.
21. Ladd GW, Price JM. Play styles of peer-accepted and peer-rejected children on the playground. In: Hart CH, ed. *Children on Playgrounds: Research Perspectives and Applications.* Albany: State University of New York Press; 1993:130-161.
22. Mize J, Ladd GW. A cognitive-social learning approach to social skill training with low-status preschool children. *Dev Psychol.* 1990;26:388-397.
23. Huston AC, Wright JC, Marquis J, Green SB. How young children spend their time: television and other activities. *Dev Psychol.* 1999;35:912-925.
24. Livingstone S, Lemish D. Doing comparative research with children and young people. In: Livingstone S, Bovill M, eds. *Children and Their Changing Media Environment.* Hillsdale, NJ: Lawrence Erlbaum Associates; 2001:31-50.
25. Kubey RW. Television use in everyday life: coping with unstructured time. *J Commun.* 1986;36:108-123.
26. Edgar P. *Children and Screen Violence.* St Lucia: University of Queensland Press; 1977.
27. Johnstone J. Social integration and mass media use among adolescents: a case study. In: Blumler JG, Katz E, eds. *The Uses of Mass Communication: Current Perspectives on Gratification Research.* Beverly Hills, Calif: Sage Publications; 1974.
28. Krosnick JA, Anand SN, Hartl SP. Psychosocial predictors of heavy television viewing among preadolescents and adolescents. *Basic Appl Soc Psych.* 2003;25:87-110.
29. Kubey R, Csikszentmihalyi M. *Television and the Quality of Life: How Viewing Shapes Everyday Experience.* Hillsdale, NJ: Lawrence Erlbaum Associates; 1990.
30. Brown C, Duncan GJ, Stafford F. Data watch: the panel study of income dynamics. *J Econ Perspect.* 1996;10:155-168.
31. Juster FT, Stafford FP. The allocation of time: empirical findings, behavior models, and problems of measurement. *J Econ Lit.* 1991;29:471-522.
32. Hofferth S. Family reading to young children: social desirability and cultural biases in reporting. Paper presented at: National Research Council Workshop on Measurement of and Research on Time Use; May 1999; Washington, DC.
33. Anderson DR, Field DE, Collins PA, Lorch EP, Nathan JG. Estimates of young children's time with television: a methodological comparison of parent reports with time-lapse video home observation. *Child Dev.* 1985;56:1345-1357.
34. Hazan C, Shaver PR. Attachment as an organizational framework for research on close relationships. *Psychol Inq.* 1994;5:1-22.
35. Hazan C, Zeifman D. Sex and the psychological tether. In: Bartholomew K, Perlman D, eds. *Attachment Processes in Adulthood: Advances in Personal Relationships.* Vol 5. London, England: Jessica Kingsley; 1994:151-177.
36. US Census Bureau. Poverty thresholds. Available at: http://www.census.gov/hhes/poverty/threshld/thresh96.html. Accessed August 1, 2005.
37. Caldwell BM, Bradley RH. *Home Observation for Measurement of the Environment.* Little Rock, Ark: University of Arkansas Press; 1984.
38. *Parental warmth scale: JOBS In-Home Baseline Survey.* Child Trends Inc. Washington, DC: Child Trends; 1992.
39. Coie JD, Kupersmidt J. A behavioral analysis of emerging social status in boys' groups. *Child Dev.* 1983;54:1400-1416.
40. Bushman BJ. Moderating role of trait aggressiveness in the effects of violent media on aggression. *J Pers Soc Psychol.* 1995;69:950-960.
41. Slater MD, Henry KL, Swaim RC, Anderson LI. Violent media content and aggressiveness in adolescents: a downward spiral model. *Communic Res.* 2003;30:713-736.
42. Huesmann LR, Lagerspetz K, Eron LD. Intervening variables in the TV violence-aggression relation: evidence from two countries. *Dev Psychol.* 1984;20:746-775.
43. Kunkel D, Wilson BJ, Linz D, et al. Violence in television programming overall: University of California, Santa Barbara study. In: *National Television Violence Study.* Vol 1. Studio City, Calif: Mediascope; 1996:1-172.
44. Federman J, ed. *National Television Violence Study, Volume 3: Executive Summary.* Santa Barbara, Calif: Center for Communication and Social Policy; 1998.
45. *Executive Summary, National Television Violence Study, Volume 1.* Studio City, Calif: Mediascope; 1996.
46. Anderson DR, Huston AC, Schmitt KL, Linebarger DL, Wright JC. Early childhood television viewing and adolescent behavior: the recontact study. *Monogr Soc Res Child Dev.* 2001;66:1-147.
47. Huesmann LR, Miller LS. Long-term effects of repeated exposure to media violence in childhood. In: Huesmann LR, ed. *Aggressive Behavior: Current Perspectives.* New York, NY: Plenum Press; 1994:153-186.

**ACIP recommends vaccination of children against hepatitis A*[1]**

# Hepatitis A spreads FAST... especially among children[2,3]

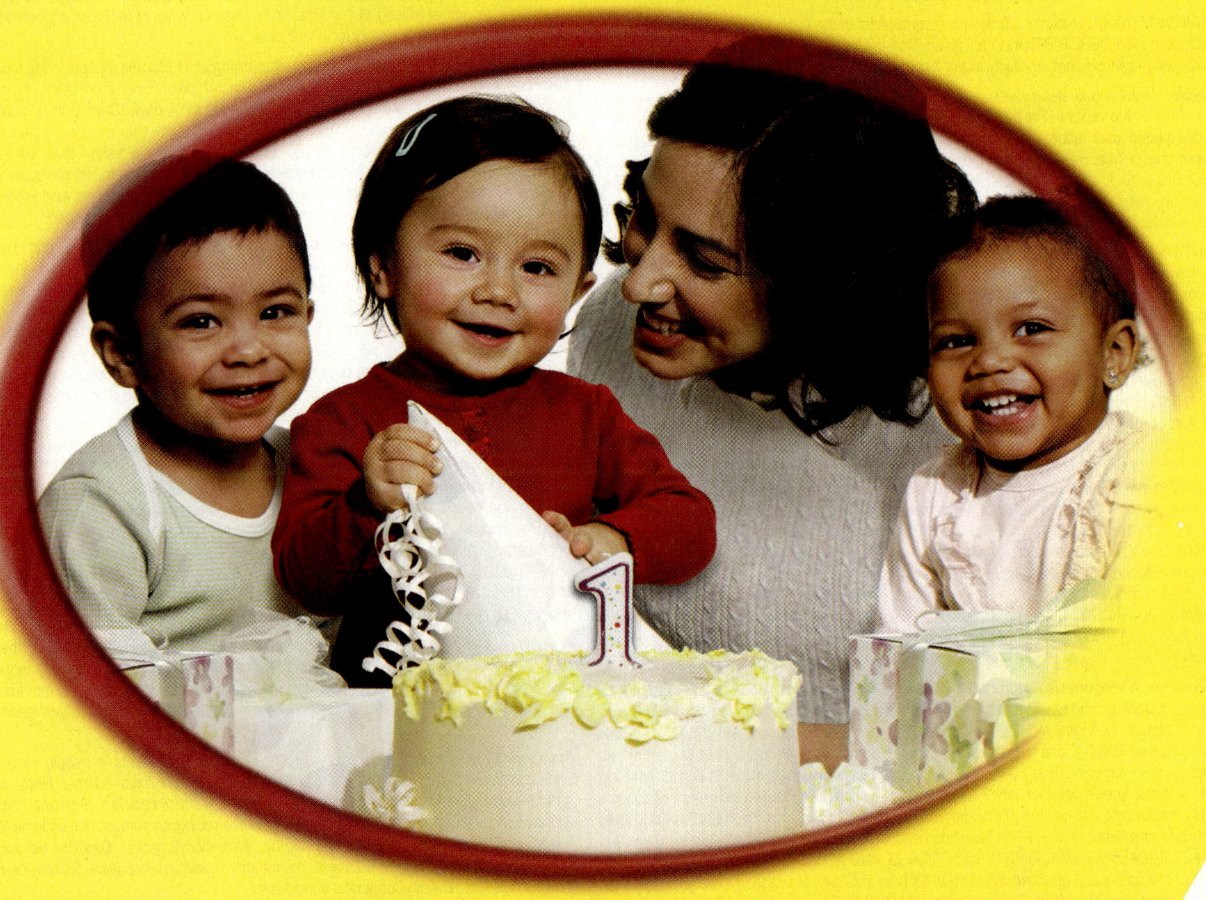

## HAVRIX provides excellent protection

HAVRIX is indicated for active immunization against hepatitis A virus in children 12 months of age and older.

## Important Safety Information

In clinical trials, the most common solicited adverse events were injection-site soreness and headache.

Greater incidences of general adverse events were observed in subjects who received HAVRIX at the same time as Hib conjugate and DTaP vaccines. As with any vaccine, rare adverse events may occur. (See Adverse Reactions section of the Prescribing Information for HAVRIX for potential side effects.) HAVRIX is contraindicated in people with hypersensitivity to any component of the vaccine, including neomycin.

*Advisory Committee on Immunization Practices recommends routine nationwide vaccination against hepatitis A in all children 1–2 years of age.

**Please see references and brief summary of complete prescribing information for HAVRIX on adjacent page.**



Manufactured by **GlaxoSmithKline Biologicals**, Rixensart, Belgium
Distributed by **GlaxoSmithKline**, Research Triangle Park, NC 27709

gsk GlaxoSmithKline Vaccines

**Havrix®**
**Hepatitis A Vaccine, Inactivated**

# HAVRIX®
# (Hepatitis A Vaccine, Inactivated)

The following is a brief summary only; see full prescribing information for complete product information.

**INDICATIONS AND USAGE:** HAVRIX is indicated for active immunization of persons ≥12 months of age against disease caused by hepatitis A virus (HAV). Primary immunization should be administered at least 2 weeks prior to expected exposure to HAV. When passive protection against hepatitis A is required either following exposure to hepatitis A virus or in persons requiring both immediate and long-term protection, HAVRIX may be administered concomitantly with immune globulin (IG) with different syringes and at different injection sites. Duration of immunity following a complete vaccination schedule has not been established.

**CONTRAINDICATIONS:** Hypersensitivity to any component of the vaccine, including neomycin, is a contraindication (see DESCRIPTION in full prescribing information). This vaccine is contraindicated in patients with previous hypersensitivity to any hepatitis A-containing vaccine.

**WARNINGS:** There have been rare reports of anaphylaxis/anaphylactoid reactions following commercial use of the vaccine. The tip cap and the rubber plunger of the needleless prefilled syringes contain dry natural latex rubber that may cause allergic reactions in latex sensitive individuals. The vial stopper is latex-free. Hepatitis A has a relatively long incubation period. Hepatitis A vaccine may not prevent hepatitis A infection in those who have an unrecognized hepatitis A infection at the time of vaccination. Additionally, it may not prevent infection in those who do not achieve protective antibody titers (although the lowest titer needed to confer protection has not been determined).

**PRECAUTIONS: General:** Prior to immunization with HAVRIX, the patient's current health status and medical history should be reviewed. The physician should review the patient's immunization history for possible vaccine sensitivity, previous vaccination-related adverse reactions and occurrence of any adverse–event-related symptoms and/or signs, in order to determine the existence of any contraindication to immunization with HAVRIX and to allow an assessment of benefits and risks. Appropriate medical treatment and supervision should be readily available for immediate use in case of a rare anaphylactic reaction following the administration of the vaccine. Epinephrine injection (1:1,000) and other appropriate agents used for the control of immediate allergic reactions must be immediately available. A separate, sterile syringe and needle or a sterile disposable unit should be used for each patient to prevent the transmission of other infectious agents from person to person. Needles should be disposed of properly and should not be recapped. As with any vaccine, if administered to immunosuppressed persons, including those receiving immunosuppressive therapy, the expected immune response may not be obtained. **Drug Interactions:** HAVRIX may be given concurrently with Hib conjugate vaccines in children 15 to 18 months of age (see CLINICAL PHARMACOLOGY in full prescribing information and ADVERSE REACTIONS). The safety of HAVRIX given concomitantly with INFANRIX has been evaluated (see ADVERSE REACTIONS). Insufficient data are available to assess the immune response of a fourth dose of DTaP vaccine when administered with HAVRIX. There are limited data to assess the concomitant use of HAVRIX with other vaccines. (See Immune Response to Concomitantly Administered Vaccines in full prescribing information.)

**Carcinogenesis, Mutagenesis, Impairment of Fertility:** HAVRIX has not been evaluated for its carcinogenic potential, mutagenic potential, or potential for impairment of fertility. **Pregnancy:** Pregnancy Category C. Animal reproduction studies have not been conducted with HAVRIX. It is also not known whether HAVRIX can cause fetal harm when administered to a pregnant woman or can affect reproduction capacity. Give HAVRIX to a pregnant woman only if clearly needed. **Nursing Mothers:** It is not known whether HAVRIX is excreted in human milk. Because many drugs are excreted in human milk, use caution when administering HAVRIX to a nursing woman. **Pediatric Use:** The safety and effectiveness of HAVRIX have been evaluated in 20,436 subjects 1 year to 18 years of age. (See CLINICAL PHARMACOLOGY and DOSAGE AND ADMINISTRATION in full prescribing information.) The safety and effectiveness of HAVRIX have not been established in subjects less than 12 months of age. **Geriatric Use:** Clinical studies of HAVRIX did not include sufficient numbers of subjects 65 years of age and older to determine whether they respond differently from younger subjects. Other reported clinical experience has not identified differences in overall safety between these subjects and younger adult subjects.

**ADVERSE REACTIONS:** As with all pharmaceuticals, however, it is possible that expanded commercial use of the vaccine could reveal rare adverse events. The adverse events most frequently reported by volunteers in clinical trials were injection-site soreness (56% of adults; 21% of children); headache (14% of adults; less than 9% of children). Other solicited and unsolicited events are listed below:

**Incidence 1% to 10% of Injections:** ***Local Reactions at Injection Site:*** Induration, redness, swelling; ***Body as a Whole:*** Fatigue, fever (>37.5°C), malaise; ***Gastrointestinal:*** Anorexia, nausea.

**Incidence <1% of Injections:** ***Local Reaction at Injection Site:*** Hematoma; ***Dermatologic:*** Pruritus, rash, urticaria; ***Respiratory:*** Pharyngitis, other upper respiratory tract infections; ***Gastrointestinal:*** Abdominal pain, diarrhea, dysgeusia, vomiting; ***Musculoskeletal:*** Arthralgia, elevation of creatine phosphokinase, myalgia; ***Hematologic:*** Lymphadenopathy; ***Central Nervous System:*** Hypertonic episode, insomnia, photophobia, vertigo.

**Additional safety data:** Safety data were obtained from 2 additional sources in which large populations were vaccinated. In an outbreak setting in which 4,930 individuals were immunized with a single dose of either 720 EL.U. or 1440 EL.U. of HAVRIX, the vaccine was well tolerated and no serious adverse events due to vaccination were reported. Overall, less than 10% of vaccinees reported solicited general adverse events following the vaccine. The most common solicited local adverse event was pain at the injection site, reported in 22.3% of subjects at 24 hours and decreasing to 2.4% by 72 hours.

In a field efficacy trial, 19,037 children received the 360 EL.U. dose of HAVRIX. The most commonly reported adverse events were injection-site pain (9.5%) and tenderness (8.1%), reported following first doses of HAVRIX. Other adverse events were infrequent and comparable to the control vaccine ENGERIX-B® [Hepatitis B Vaccine (Recombinant)].

In subjects with chronic liver disease, HAVRIX was safe and well tolerated. Local injection site reactions were similar among all 4 groups, and no serious adverse reactions attributed to the vaccine were reported in subjects with chronic liver disease.

***Safety Data for HAVRIX 720 EL.U./0.5 mL Beginning at 11 Months of Age:*** In the multicenter study described under CLINICAL PHARMACOLOGY in full prescribing information, parents/guardians recorded local and general symptoms on diary cards for 4 days (Days 0 to 3) after vaccination. In the 3 groups of children who received HAVRIX alone, safety data were available for 723 children who received 1,396 documented doses of HAVRIX. Additional safety data were available for 181 children who received HAVRIX coadministered with INFANRIX and Hib conjugate vaccine. Most adverse events were mild and transient. The frequencies of solicited local and systemic reactions following receipt of HAVRIX were monitored during the 4-day observation period.

The following rates of solicited adverse events in children who received their first dose of HAVRIX alone at between 11 and 25 months of age were observed. Among local reactions: pain was reported in 15-21% of subjects, redness in 16-21%, swelling in 8% of subjects. Among general reactions, irritability was reported in 24-36% of subjects, loss of appetite in 16-19% of subjects, drowsiness in 15-17% of subjects and fever >39.5°C in ≤2% of subjects. Following the booster dose of HAVRIX, among local reactions: pain was reported in 16-21% of subjects, redness in 17-22%, swelling in 8-10% of subjects. Following the booster dose of HAVRIX, among general reactions, irritability was reported in 19-29% of subjects, loss of appetite in 14-18% of subjects, drowsiness in 13-16% of subjects and fever >39.5°C in ≤1% of subjects.

Drowsiness and loss of appetite occurred at statistically significantly higher rates in subjects 15 to 18 months of age who received Hib conjugate vaccine (PRP-T) and INFANRIX concomitantly with HAVRIX as compared to subjects 15 to 18 months of age who received Hib conjugate vaccine (PRP-T) and INFANRIX (drowsiness 34% and 22% and loss of appetite 29% and 19%, respectively). With the exception of fever (>39.5°C), the solicited general symptoms occurred at statistically significantly higher rates in subjects 15 to 18 months of age who received Hib conjugate vaccine (PRP-T) and INFANRIX concomitantly with HAVRIX as compared to subjects 15 to 18 months of age who received HAVRIX alone (irritability 46% and 30%, drowsiness 34% and 17%, and loss of appetite 29% and 17%, respectively).

A febrile seizure was reported in an 18-month old subject two days after receiving the first dose of HAVRIX. Other serious adverse events reported during the course of this study included a single case each of hepatitis ~5 months post dose 1, insulin-dependent diabetes ~4 months post dose 1, and Kawasaki's disease ~3 1/2 months post dose 1. The association of these events with vaccination is unknown.

**Postmarketing Reports:** Rare voluntary reports of adverse events in people receiving HAVRIX since market introduction include the following: ***Local:*** Localized edema; ***Body as a Whole:*** Anaphylaxis/anaphylactoid reactions, somnolence; ***Cardiovascular:*** Syncope; ***Hepatobiliary:*** Jaundice, hepatitis; ***Dermatologic:*** Erythema multiforme, hyperhydrosis, angioedema; ***Respiratory:*** Dyspnea; ***Hematologic:*** Lymphadenopathy, thrombocytopenia; ***Central Nervous System:*** Convulsions, encephalopathy, dizziness, neuropathy, myelitis, paresthesia, Guillain-Barré syndrome, multiple sclerosis; ***Other:*** Congenital abnormality.

The US Department of Health and Human Services has established the Vaccine Adverse Events Reporting System (VAERS) to accept reports of suspected adverse events after the administration of any vaccine, including, but not limited to, the reporting of events required by the National Childhood Vaccine Injury Act of 1986. The toll-free number for VAERS forms and information is 1-800-822-7967. Reporting forms may also be obtained at the VAERS website at www.vaers.org.

Manufactured by **GlaxoSmithKline Biologicals**, Rixensart, Belgium

Distributed by **GlaxoSmithKline**, Research Triangle Park, NC 27709



BRS-HA:L20

**References: 1.** Centers for Disease Control and Prevention. Recommended childhood and adolescent immunization schedule—United States, 2006. *MMWR.* 2006;54(51&52):Q1–Q4. **2.** Bell BP, Shapiro CN. Hepatitis A virus. In: Long SS, Pickering LK, Prober CG, eds. *Principles and Practice of Pediatric Infectious Diseases.* 2nd ed. Philadelphia, Pa: Churchill Livingstone; 2003:1188–1192. **3.** Armstrong GL, Bell BP. Hepatitis A virus infection in the United States: model-based estimates and implication for childhood immunizations. *Pediatrics.* 2002;109:839–845.


Printed in USA. HAP283R0 February 2006

ARTICLE

# Parental Media Mediation Styles for Children Aged 2 to 11 Years

*Shari Barkin, MD; Edward Ip, PhD; Irma Richardson, MHA; Sara Klinepeter; Stacia Finch, MA; Marina Krcmar, PhD*

**Background:** Studies indicate that children use media (television, video, and computer) more than the recommended limit of 2 h/d, but little is known about parents' role in mediating their children's media use.

**Design:** Office-based survey. Data were collected on demographics, reported media behaviors, parental awareness about media effects, television in the bedroom, and parental concern. We developed logistic regression models to examine factors associated with the following 3 mediation approaches: restrictive, instructive, and unlimited.

**Setting:** Pediatric Research in Office Settings practices.

**Participants:** Parents with children aged 2 to 11 years (n=1831) presenting for a well-child visit.

**Results:** Almost half of parents reported a single mediation approach, including restrictive for 23%, instructive for 11%, and unlimited for 7%, with 59% reporting the use of multiple strategies. Restrictive (odds ratio [OR], 1.16; *P*<.001) and instructive (OR, 1.06; *P*=.02) approaches were associated with increased awareness about negative media effects, whereas a decreased awareness existed for those who used an unlimited approach (OR, 0.87; *P*<.001). A restrictive strategy also occurred with increased parental concern (OR, 1.77; *P*<.001) and 2 adults in the home (OR, 1.64; *P*<.01). The only strategy associated with the child's age was instructive mediation, noted more often with younger children (OR, 1.41; *P*<.001). Allowing unlimited media use occurred when parents permitted a television in the child's bedroom (OR, 2.13; *P*<.001) and were Latino (OR, 2.03; *P*<.01) or African American (OR, 2.20; *P*<.001). Mother as primary decision maker and maternal education were not statistically significant.

**Conclusions:** Pediatric health care providers should identify parental practices and reinforce active media mediation strategies.

*Arch Pediatr Adolesc Med. 2006;160:395-401*

**Author Affiliations:** Departments of Pediatrics (Dr Barkin and Ms Richardson) and Public Health Sciences (Dr Ip), Wake Forest University Baptist Medical Center, and Department of Communication, Wake Forest University (Dr Krcmar), Winston-Salem, NC; University of Virginia (Ms Klinepeter), Charlottesville; and Pediatric Research in Office Settings, Department of Practice and Research, Center for Child Health Research, American Academy of Pediatrics, Elk Grove Village, Ill (Ms Finch).

According to the American Academy of Pediatrics (AAP), American children and adolescents aged 2 to 18 years spend an average of more than 4 hours using electronic media daily, more than they spend on any other single activity except sleep.[1] Media exposure has been associated with aggressive behavior,[2-5] poor moral reasoning,[6] desensitization,[7] the conception of the world as a mean and scary place,[8] obesity,[9,10] and decreased attention span.[11] Conversely, it has also been associated with positive social interactions,[12] improved intelligence scores,[13] improved problem-solving skills,[14] accelerated language acquisition,[15,16] and enhanced school performance.[17] The difference exists in the content of the programming and the time spent engaged in media use.[9,11-15,18]

Owing to these facts, the AAP recommends limiting media exposure to no more than 1 to 2 hours per day of educational, quality programs for children older than 2 years. In addition, the AAP recommends that parents use the media's influence in a positive manner by helping their children to be intelligent media viewers, restricting their media exposure, watching with their children, explaining what the child sees, and creating an electronic media–free environment in children's rooms.[19,20] To have this effect, however, it is necessary that parents engage in some form of mediation, by setting limits on media exposure and discussing content with children. These behaviors have been found to mitigate some of the negative effects of media exposure on children.[21,22]

Research on mediation suggests that various types exist,[23] including (1) restrictive mediation, in which parents set rules or prohibit exposure to certain content, (2) instructive mediation, in which parents discuss certain portions of the programming they view together, and (3) social coviewing, in which the programming is watched together. Social coviewing is associated with overall heavier viewing patterns for parents and their children.[1] It is unlimited viewing that is perhaps most problematic and may require the greatest intervention.

Active mediation, such as restrictive and instructive approaches, has positive associations with younger children,[15,18-22] mothers as media decision makers,[21] increased parental education,[24] and increased socioeconomic levels.[23,25] Several family variables still remain largely unexplored. For example, positive parent-child relationships have an association with increased effective rule setting in contexts such as eating and sleeping[26]; therefore the quality of the parent-child relationship might also have a potential association with increased media mediation. The influence of ethnicity or family structure on media mediation is not known. It is possible that in homes where 2 parents reside, mediation is more likely simply because 2 parents are available to provide mediation. It is clear that in parenting areas such as discipline, one's own experiences as a child influence current strategies.[26] Likewise, past media experience as a child could influence tendencies to provide mediation as a parent. It is important, therefore, to discern the effects of all these potential contributors on parental mediation strategies.

In a world where media burgeons and children's exposure is likely to grow, understanding how parents mediate their children's media use and the attendant associations becomes necessary. Information is needed to shape interventions suitable for the pediatric provider's office, a venue that children and their families routinely use.

Most surveys that purport to estimate the percentage of parents who use mediation[21-24] are limited by small sample sizes. In 1 of the larger samples, Cheng et al[27] reported a convenience sample of almost 700 parents. That study was limited in its assessment of various mediation styles. These authors found that female parents and younger children were more likely to be associated with limits on violent television viewing.[21-24,27]

Conducting a study with a national scope allows an assessment of an expanded model of potential influences on media mediation. The purpose of the present analysis was to explore how often parents mediate media, what strategies they use, and what variables predict active media mediation to inform the development of potential interventions based in the pediatric provider's office.

## METHODS

This study was conducted by Pediatric Research in Office Settings, the practice-based research network of the AAP. Institutional review board approval was obtained from the Wake Forest University School of Medicine, Winston-Salem, NC, and the AAP. Parents participated in an office-based survey before the visit for the well-child examination of children aged 2 to 11 years. We limited enrollment to 1 child per family with English- or Spanish-speaking parents. A list of participating practices is given in the box at the end of the article.

### SURVEY INSTRUMENT

Parents/legal guardians answered questions regarding demographics (age of child, number of children in the home, self-identified race/ethnicity of the child, parental home structure, maternal education), reported media behaviors, television in the bedroom, parental awareness about negative violent media effects, parental media concern, primary decision maker about media use, parent-child relationship, and parental history of television use as a child.

Media-related behavior questions included "When this child is at home, how many hours per day does he or she watch television/videos? play computer games/Gameboy?" This was broken down by hours on an average weekday and average weekend day. For the purposes of our analysis, we collapsed these data to reflect hours of average media use (inclusive of television, video, computer games, and electronic handheld devices) per day. Our survey presented 3 survey items assessing parental strategies for their child's media use. These questions asked, in the past month, how often the parent restricted use, explained content, or allowed unlimited media use. The response scale for each question ranged from "never" to "always" on a 4-point scale. Three media-related questions assessed parental awareness about the potential negative outcomes of watching violent media, including "Watching violent television programs makes children more afraid," "Children's behavior is not influenced by what they see on television," and "Children who watch violent television think real-life violence is normal behavior." These responses were rated on a 5-point scale from "strongly disagree" to "strongly agree." We developed an awareness scale (range, 3-15; Cronbach $\alpha = 0.6$) from these 3 questions. A higher value on the awareness scale indicated better understanding of the effects of exposure to violent media.

To gauge parental concern about media use, parents responded yes or no to the question, "I'm concerned about what this child sees in the media." Also, we assessed parents' perception of their relationship with their child with the statement, "My relationship with this child is poor, fair, good, very good, or excellent." Respondents chose 1 response.

Questions were also asked about the primary caregiver's own childhood experience with media. The following 3 statements make up the Family History Scale: "My family watched a lot of television," "My family allowed children to watch as much television as they wanted," and "My family monitored the programs that children watched on television." Each question was answered on a 3-point scale; the range of the Family History Scale was 3 to 9 points, with a mean of 5.1 (SD, 2.1) and Cronbach $\alpha$ of 0.60. Higher numbers indicated more exposure to television.

### STATISTICAL ANALYSIS

We examined descriptive statistics and bivariate associations with the outcomes of interest including use of restrictive, instructive, or unlimited media mediation. Each outcome was dichotomized as never/sometimes vs often/always. We chose this cut point owing to response variation and the underlying concept that parents are more likely to be similar in these identified categories. We assessed bivariate associations with those variables determined from our literature search or clinical judgment to have a potential contribution to parental media behaviors. These included age of the child, awareness that violent media exposure can influence children's behavior, parental concern about media exposure, maternal education level, ethnicity, relationship between parent and child, mother as primary decision maker, number of children in the home, family history, and a 1- vs 2-parent home structure. To create a parsimonious model, we included those variables that had a statistically significant bivariate association (odds ratio or $\chi^2$ for categorical variables; correlation for continuous variables) with the outcomes of interest at the .05 level in logistic regression models to examine factors associated with the 3 mediation styles.

## RESULTS

### STUDY SAMPLE

Participants included 1831 families with children aged 2 to 11 years attending their well-child visit. They represented families from 64 community-based pediatric practices in 27 states, Canada, and Puerto Rico. **Table 1** includes the sample description. Most caregivers completing the survey were mothers (89.6%), with 24.3% of the respondents indicating that they run a single-parent home. About half of the patients were aged 2 to 5 years. Most (70.0%) of the patients were white, 11.4% were Latino, and 11.7% were African American. Most of the caregivers reported that the mother's education was less than a college degree, with more than one third of respondents indicating that the mothers were college graduates or beyond. Almost half of the sample reported that the mother was the primary decision maker for their child's media use. Close to three fourths of respondents indicated that they were concerned about their child's media use. Almost three fourths of caregivers reported that when they were children, their family allowed unlimited television use or watched a lot of television. Of the respondents, 74.9% indicated that children who watch violent media (1) are more afraid, (2) are influenced by what they see, and (3) think real-life violence is normal. For the 1775 parents who completed the questions on awareness of violent media effects, the mean (SD) score was 12.0 (2.4); for the 1782 who completed the Family History Scale, the mean (SD) score was 5.2 (2.1).

### REPORTED MEDIA USE AND PARENTAL MEDIA MEDIATION STYLES

Parents reported mutiple mediation styles, including restrictive (restricting content or time of viewing), instructive (parent/guardian explaining media to the child as they watch together), and/or unlimited viewing (allowing the child to decide the period of time to engage in media activities). Respondents reported mean (SD) media exposure in general as 2.7(1.5) h/d. The amount of media exposure time varied depending on reported media mediation style, with means of 2.4 (1.3) hours for restrictive, 2.9 (1.5) hours for instructive, and 4.1 (1.6) hours for unlimited mediation styles. In our sample, 36% of children had televisions in their bedrooms. The likelihood of having a television in a child's bedroom was twice as high if the child was aged 6 to 11 vs 2 to 5 years (odds ratio [OR], 2.24; 95% confidence interval [CI], 1.86-2.71). Moreover, parents who reported a television in their child's bedroom indicated increased exposure to media (mean [SD] of 3.6 [2] hours vs 2.5 [1.7] hours; $P<.001$).

**Table 1. Description of Study Sample**

| Variable | No. (%) of Respondents* |
|---|---|
| Relationship to child | |
| Mother | 1639 (89.7) |
| Father | 144 (7.9) |
| Other | 45 (2.5) |
| Age of child, y | |
| 2-5 | 968 (54.3) |
| 6-11 | 816 (45.7) |
| Ethnicity/race | |
| White | 1176 (70.0) |
| African American | 197 (11.7) |
| Latino | 191 (11.4) |
| Multirace | 63 (3.8) |
| Other | 52 (3.1) |
| Maternal education | |
| <High school | 123 (6.9) |
| ≥High school, <college graduate | 1008 (56.2) |
| ≥College graduate | 662 (36.9) |
| No. of children in the home | |
| 1 | 342 (20.1) |
| >1 | 1361 (79.9) |
| Relationship with child | |
| Poor-fair | 96 (5.3) |
| Very good | 1699 (94.7) |
| Mother as primary decision maker for media use | |
| Yes | 808 (45.6) |
| No | 962 (54.4) |
| Parental concern about media use | |
| Yes | 1269 (72.1) |
| No | 492 (27.9) |
| No. of parents in the home | |
| 1 | 436 (24.3) |
| 2 | 1359 (75.7) |

*Includes 1831 parents who participated in an office-based survey before the visit for a well-child examination of children aged 2 to 11 years. Numbers vary owing to missing data.

A little more than half of respondents (59%) indicated that they used multiple media mediation strategies. The remaining 41% of respondents indicated that they used a single approach, including restrictive for 23.4%, instructive for 11.2%, and unlimited for 6.9%.

Media mediation strategies did not differ in a statistically significant way for younger children (aged 2-5 years) compared with older children (6-11 years) (**Figure 1**). Once we examined the logistic regression models controlling for other variables, however, an instructive mediation strategy was positively associated with younger children (**Table 2**).

Logistic regression models (Table 2) indicated that restrictive and instructive approaches had positive associations with increased awareness about negative media effects, whereas a decreased awareness existed for those who used an unlimited approach. Those respondents who indicated parental concern about their child's media exposure and who had 2 adults in the home were more likely to use a restrictive media strategy (**Figure 2**). Allowing unlimited media use occurred more often when parents permitted a television in the child's bedroom. Conversely, the absence of a television in the child's bedroom was associated with a restrictive strategy. Latino and African American ethnicities were associated with allowing unlimited media use more than was white ethnicity in our sample (**Figure 3**). The number of children in the home (1 vs >1) and mother as the primary decision maker for media use did not have statistically significant bivariate relationships and, therefore, were not included in the logistic regression models.

## COMMENT

Parents play a key role in shaping how their children use the media.[23,27,28] In the present large-scale national sample, a majority (59%) of parents reported using a variety of mediation strategies. It is reassuring that only 7% allowed unlimited media use and engaged in no mediation. A third of the sample reported using a single active media strategy, including 11% who used instructive mediation and 23% who used restrictive mediation. In this sample with a national scope, unlike other studies, we did not see that mother as a primary decision maker or younger children were associated with a restrictive media mediation strategy.[21] However, we noted that parents reported using an instructive strategy more often with younger children. Each media strategy demonstrated varying degrees of reported media exposure, with a restrictive approach associated with the least amount of exposure (mean [SD], 2.4 [1.3] hours) and an unlimited approach associated with the greatest amount of exposure (4.1 [1.6] hours). If we take the average, our findings are consistent with previous studies.[29,30] Our data emphasize that exposure to media has an important influential factor, ie, parents.

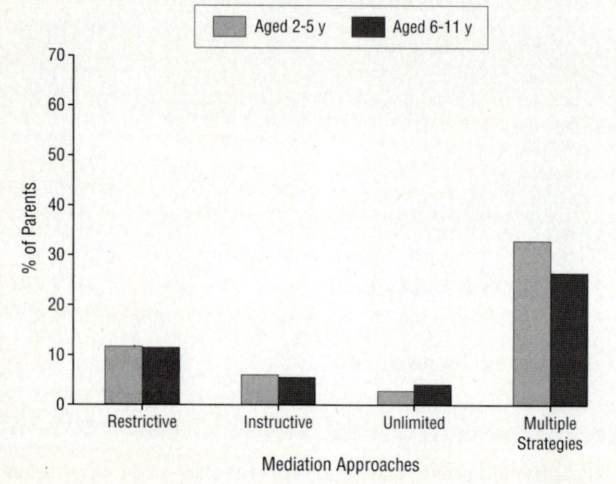


**Figure 1.** Parental media mediation approaches for children aged 2 to 5 vs 6 to 11 years. Mediation approaches are described in the "Reported Media Use and Parental Media Mediation Styles" subsection of the "Results" section.

Our research identified some other factors associated with increased active parental mediation. Our data identified demographic factors, such as single-parent homes and children of African American and Latino ethnicites, associated with less active mediation. This fact may be further compounded because African American and Latino families watch more television on average.[1] Therefore, more overall viewing combined with less active mediation may put African American and Latino children at greater risk for the problematic effects of media content. These populations may benefit most from promotion of active media mediation strategies by practitioners.

Moreover, our data suggest that parents who understand that media can have harmful effects and who express concern about those effects are more likely to mediate actively. Therefore, 1 strategy to increase mediation is to provide information to parents about the negative effects of media. Given that a higher level of parental concern increases restrictive mediation, encouraging a healthy

**Table 2. Logistic Regression Model of Parental Mediation Approaches***

| | Mediation Approach | | | | | |
|---|---|---|---|---|---|---|
| | Restrictive | | Instructive | | Unlimited | |
| Variable | OR (95% CI) | *P* Value | OR (95% CI) | *P* Value | OR (95% CI) | *P* Value |
| Child's age | 0.96 (0.74-1.25) | .75 | 1.41 (1.13-1.77) | .00 | 0.91 (0.69-1.19) | .47 |
| Maternal education | | | | | | |
| <High school | 0.79 (0.47-1.35) | .31 | 1.75 (1.02-2.98) | .09 | 1.71 (1.00-2.91) | .08 |
| High school/college | 1.04 (0.78-1.39) | .31 | 1.25 (0.98-1.60) | .72 | 1.22 (0.90-1.65) | .64 |
| Race/ethnicity | | | | | | |
| African American | 0.71 (0.48-1.07) | .40 | 1.06 (0.72-1.56) | .77 | 2.20 (1.49-3.26) | .00 |
| Latino | 0.53 (0.36-0.78) | .01 | 0.98 (0.67-1.43) | .44 | 2.03 (1.36-3.01) | .01 |
| Parental concern | 1.77 (1.35-2.33) | <.001 | 0.93 (0.73-1.20) | .59 | 0.79 (0.59-1.05) | .10 |
| Relationship with child | 1.43 (0.84-2.44) | .19 | 1.90 (1.19-3.04) | .01 | 0.71 (0.42-1.22) | .22 |
| 2 Parents in the home | 1.64 (1.15-2.35) | .01 | 0.78 (0.55-1.11) | .17 | 0.72 (0.50-1.04) | .08 |
| Awareness of violent media effects | 1.16 (1.09-1.22) | <.001 | 1.06 (1.01-1.12) | .02 | 0.87 (0.82-0.92) | <.001 |
| Family history of media use | 0.96 (0.91-1.02) | .22 | 0.97 (0.92-1.02) | .21 | 1.16 (1.09-1.24) | <.001 |
| Television in bedroom | 0.71 (0.53-0.94) | .02 | 1.03 (0.79-1.33) | .85 | 2.13 (1.61-2.82) | <.001 |

Abbreviations: CI, confidence interval; OR, odds ratio.

*Higher ORs indicate increased use of individual media strategy. Reference groups include children aged 6 to 11 years, maternal college attainment or beyond, white race/ethnicity, no parental concern, poor to fair relationship between the parent and child, and 1 parent in the home. Model includes 1831 parents who participated in an office-based survey before the visit for a well-child examination of children aged 2 to 11 years. Mediation approaches are described in the "Reported Media Use and Parental Media Mediation Styles" subsection of the "Results" section.

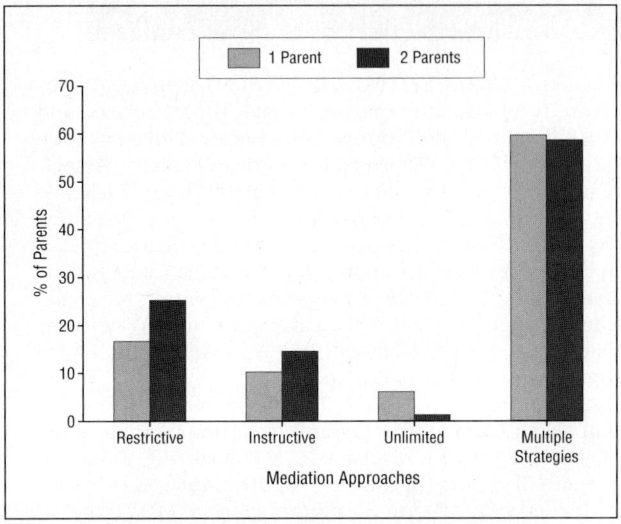


**Figure 2.** Number of parents in the home and use of mediation approaches. Mediation approaches are described in the "Reported Media Use and Parental Media Mediation Styles" subsection of the "Results" section.

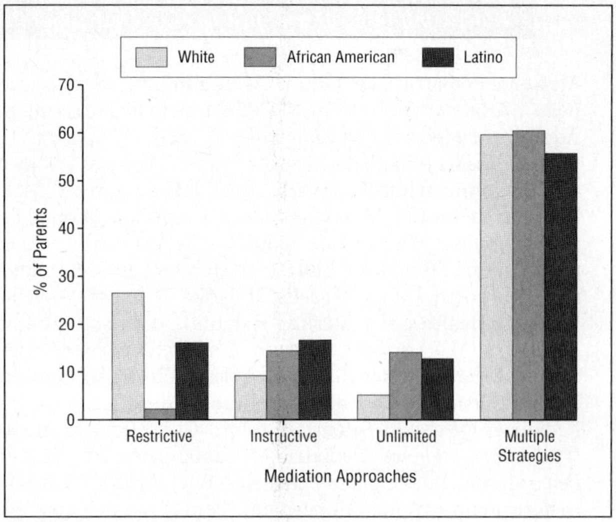


**Figure 3.** Mediation approaches across different ethnicities. Mediation approaches are described in the "Reported Media Use and Parental Media Mediation Styles" subsection of the "Results" section.

level of concern about media exposure among parents may influence their willingness to try active mediation strategies. Conversely, we could provide information about positive educational programming available to children.[14,31] The data are limited, however, in that they focus primarily on young children's programming (≤5 years of age). Research is needed to assess what programs exist with strong educational, positive effects for children older than 5 years.

The negative effects of exposure to media,[3] especially when parents do not play an active role in mediating that exposure,[32] make it critical to minimize the barriers to parental mediation. In this sample we found that 36% of parents allowed children to have a television set in their bedroom. Many of the parents of childen with a television in their bedroom allowed unlimited viewing, regardless of the child's age. A growing body of evidence links excessive media exposure (>2 h/d) to poorer cognitive outcomes.[33,34] In a recent study, third graders found to have a television in their bedroom had a significant negative association with their cognitive test scores.[33] Televisions in the bedroom not only might be detrimental to an elementary school-aged child's health, it also might create an opportunity for unsupervised media exposure. It is not clear what drives parents' decisions to allow children to have a television in their bedroom. Entering into a dialogue with families about this topic could provide an important starting point for making active parental mediation possible.

During the course of the study, the concept of media has continued to expand. We asked families to report on use of television, videos, computer games, and electronic handheld devices. We cannot make an association between this use and the now even fuller gamut of media use in our society, such as instant messaging, or multiple uses of the computer simultaneously, such as doing one's homework while watching a movie in the corner of the screen. Although self-reported information on media exposure is commonly presented in studies, evidence suggests that this method can lead to overestimation.[35] Conversely, it could lead to underestimation, because parents could be unaware of their child's exposure if a television is in the bedroom. In this study, we focused on parental perceptions of their child's media use and did not gather data on parental use. In future work, gathering these data would be useful because it is family behaviors that often guide children's exposure to media.[36]

We asked 1 yes/no question to gauge parental media concern. This does not allow us to investigate the complexity of parental concern but mirrors how clinicians usually ask the question during a routine office visit. From this question, we cannot infer whether families are unconcerned because they control the media use to their satisfaction or because they are unconcerned about the problem regardless of their family behaviors. However, nearly 75% of parents indicated concern, regardless of their reported media mediation strategies.

Although proportions of African American and Latino children in our sample were substantial and approach the national population percentages, it is possible that our findings do not accurately represent these populations. In addition, all data were derived from a self-administered survey of parents' reports that can be associated with socially desirable reporting. Nevertheless, we identified statistically significant and clinically meaningful information to help direct our next steps as pediatric health care providers working with families. Finally, we asked families to report behaviors that occurred in their home; therefore, we cannot make statements or implications related to other environments such as schools and the homes of friends or other family members. It will be important for future researchers to describe mediation strategies that occur in these environments as well.

Children use television and computers at younger and younger ages,[24] making mediation increasingly important. The pediatric health care provider interacts with families of young children, educating them on healthy behaviors routinely. Our study indicates that

## Participating Pediatric Practices or Individual Practitioners by American Academy of Pediatrics Chapter

*Alabama*: Pediatric Care Group (Montgomery); *Alaska*: Anchorage Pediatric Group, LLC (Anchorage), Joy Neyhart, MD (Juneau); *Arizona*: Orange Grove Pediatrics (Tucson); *California 1*: Palo Alto Medical Foundation (Palo Alto), Pediatric and Adolescent Medical Associates of the Pacific Coast, Inc (Salinas); *California 3*: East County Community Clinic–Lakeside (Lakeside), La Jolla Pediatrics (La Jolla); *Colorado*: Rocky Mountain Health Center (Denver); *Connecticut*: Pediatric Associates of Connecticut, PC (Waterbury), Jeff Cersonsky, MD (Southbury); *Florida*: Atlantic Coast Pediatrics (Merritt Island); *Georgia*: Victor Lui, MD (Chamblee), Snapfinger Woods Pediatric Associates, PC (Decatur); *Indiana*: Georgetown Pediatrics (Indianapolis), Jeffersonville Pediatrics (Jeffersonville); *Kansas*: Ashley Clinic (Chanute); *Louisiana*: Carousel Pediatrics (Metairie), Shalom Clinic for Children (Natchitoches); *Maryland*: Steven E. Caplan, MD (Baltimore); *Maine*: Maine Coast Pediatrics (Ellsworth); *Massachusetts*: Holyoke Pediatric Associates (Holyoke), Mary Lane Pediatric Associates (Ware); *Michigan*: Pediatric Health Care (Sterling Heights); *Minnesota*: Brainerd Medical Center, PA (Brainerd), Lakeview Clinic–Watertown Pediatrics (Watertown); *Missouri*: Children's Mercy Hospital Pediatric Care Center (Kansas City); *New Hampshire*: Foundation Pediatrics (Nashna); *New York 1*: Elmwood Pediatric Group (Rochester), Lewis Pediatrics (Rochester); *New York 3*: Pediatric Primary Care at Montefiore Medical Center (Bronx); *North Carolina*: Aegis Family Health Center–Winston East Pediatrics (Winston-Salem), Guilford Child Health, Inc–High Point (High Point); *Ohio*: Oxford Pediatrics & Adolescents (Oxford); *Oklahoma*: Pediatric & Adolescent Care, LLP (Tulsa); *Ontario*: Richard J. MacDonald, MD (Oakville, Ontario); *Pennsylvania*: Buckingham Pediatrics (Buckingham), Laurel Health Center–Blossburg (Blossburg), Pediatric Practices of Northeastern Pennsylvania (Honesdale), Pennridge Pediatric Associates (Sellersville); *Puerto Rico*: Ethel Lamela, MD (Isabela); *Quebec*: Clinique Enfant-Medic (Dollard des Ormeaux); *South Carolina*: Palmetto Pediatrics & Adolescent Clinic, PA (Columbia); *Tennessee*: East Tennessee State University Physicians & Associates (Johnson City); *Texas*: The Pediatric Clinic (Greenville), Su Clinica Familiar (Harlingen), Winnsboro Pediatrics (Winnsboro); *Utah*: Utah Valley Pediatrics, LC (American Fork), Willow Creek Pediatrics–Draper (Draper); *Vermont*: Brattleboro Pediatrics (Brattleboro), Rebecca Collman, MD (Colchester), Springfield Pediatric Network (Springfield), University Pediatrics, UHC Campus (Burlington), University Pediatrics (Williston); *Washington*: Central Washington Family Medicine (Yakima); *West Virginia*: Grant Memorial Pediatrics (Petersburg); *Wisconsin*: Gundersen Clinic–Whitehall (Whitehall); *Wyoming*: Jackson Pediatrics (Jackson).

when providers discuss media use, they need to identify parental media concerns, share information about potential negative media effects, and encourage active media mediation approaches, such as restriction and instruction, with parents of children aged 2 to 11 years. For many families, this discussion could begin with ascertaining the presence of a television in the child's bedroom.

**Accepted for Publication:** July 12, 2005.
**Correspondence:** Shari Barkin, MD, Department of Pediatrics, Wake Forest University Baptist Medical Center, 1 Medical Center Blvd, Winston-Salem, NC 27157 (sbarkin@wfubmc.edu).
**Financial Disclosure:** None.
**Funding/Support:** This study was supported by grant HD 42260 from the National Institute of Child Health and Human Development, Rockville, Md; the Agency for Healthcare Research and Quality, Rockville; the Robert Wood Johnson Generalist Faculty Scholars Program, San Antonio, Tex; and the Friends of Children Fund, American Academy of Pediatrics, Elk Grove Village, Ill.
**Acknowledgment:** We especially appreciate the efforts of the Pediatric Research in Office Settings practices and practitioners. A list of the participating practices appears in a box on this page.

## REFERENCES


1. Roberts DF, Foehr UG, Rideout VJ, Brodie M. Kids & media @ the new millennium. Available at: http://www.kff.org/entmedia/loader.cfm?url=/commonspot/security/getfile.cfm&PageID=1326. Accessed February 6, 2005.
2. Donnerstein E, Slaby R, Eron LD, eds. *Violence and Youth: Psychology's Response*. Vol 2. Washington, DC: American Psychological Association; 1994.
3. Paik H, Comstock G. The effects of television violence on antisocial behavior: a meta-analysis. *Communic Res.* 1994;21:516-546.
4. Boyatzis J, Matillo GM, Nesbitt KM. Effects of the "Mighty Morphin Power Rangers" on children's aggression with peers. *Child Study J.* 1995;25:45-55.
5. Wilson BJ, Kunkel D, Lintz D, et al. *Television Violence and Its Context: National Television Violence Study.* Vol 1. Newbury Park, Calif: Sage Publications; 1997.
6. Krcmar M, Curtis S. Mental models: understanding the effect of fantasy violence on children's moral reasoning. *J Commun.* 2003;53:460-468.
7. Thomas MH, Horton RW, Lippincott EC, Drabman RS. Desensitization to portrayals of real-life aggression as a function of exposure to television violence. *J Pers Soc Psychol.* 1977;35:450-458.
8. Gerbner G, Gross L, Morgan M, Signorielli N. Growing up with television: the cultivation perspective. In: Bryant J, Zillman D, eds. *Media Effects.* Hillsdale, NJ: Lawrence A Erlbaum Associates; 1994. .
9. Dennison BA, Erb TA, Jenkins PL. Television viewing and television in bedroom associated with overweight risk among low-income preschool children. *Pediatrics.* 2002;109:1028-1035.
10. Reilly JJ, Armstrong J, Dorosty AR, et al. Early life risk factors for obesity in childhood: cohort study [published online ahead of print May 20, 2005]. *BMJ.* 2005; 330:1357.
11. Christakis DA, Zimmerman FJ, DiGiuseppe DL, McCarty CA. Early television exposure and subsequent attentional problems in children. *Pediatrics.* 2004;113: 708-713.
12. Friedrich-Cofer LK, Huston-Stein A, Kipnis DM, Susman EJ, Clewett AS. Environmental enhancement of prosocial television content: effects on interpersonal behavior, imaginative play, and self-regulation in a natural setting. *Dev Psychol.* 1979;15:637-646.
13. Haugland SW. The effect of computer software on preschool children's developmental gains. *J Comput Childhood Educ.* 1992;3:15-30.
14. Anderson DR, Bryant J, Wilder A, Santomero A, Williams MV, Crawley AM. Researching Blue's Clues: viewing behavior and impact. *Media Psychology.* 2000; 2:179-194.
15. Linebarger DL, Walker D. Infants' and toddlers' television viewing and language outcomes. *Am Behav Sci.* 2005;48:624-645.
16. Wright JC. The relations of early television viewing to school readiness and vocabulary of children from low-income families: the Early Window Project. *Child Dev.* 2001;72:1347-1366.
17. Anderson DR, Huston AC, Schmitt KL, Linebarger DL, Wright JC. Early childhood television viewing and adolescent behavior: the recontact study. *Monogr Soc Res Child Dev.* 2001;66:I-VII, 1-147.
18. Gentile DA, Lynch PJ, Linder JR, Walsh DA. The effects of violent video game habits on adolescent hostility, aggressive behaviors, and school performance. *J Adolesc.* 2004;27:5-22.

19. Television and the family. Available at:http://www.aap.org/family/tv1.htm. Accessed July 30, 2004.
20. American Academy of Pediatrics, Committee on Public Education. Media violence. *Pediatrics.* 2001;108:1222-1226.
21. Nathanson AI, Yang M. The effects of mediation content and form on children's responses to violent television. *Hum Commun Res.* 2003;21:516-546.
22. Nathanson AI. Identifying and explaining the relationship between parental mediation and children's aggression. *Communic Res.* 1999;26:124-143.
23. Valkenburg PM, Krcmar M, Peeters AL, Marseille NM. Developing a scale to assess three styles of television mediation: "instructive mediation," "restrictive mediation," and "social coviewing". *J Broadcast Electron Media.* 1999;43:52-66.
24. Desmond RJ, Singer SL, Singer DG. *Family Mediation: Parental Communication Patterns and the Influence of Television on Children.* Hillsdale, NJ: Lawrence Earlbaum Associates; 1990.
25. Salomon G. Effects of encouraging Israeli mothers to co-view Sesame Street with their 5-year-old. *Child Dev.* 1977;48:1146-1151.
26. Noller P, Fitzpatrick MA. *Communication in Family Relationships.* Englewood Cliffs, NJ: Prentice Hall; 1993.
27. Cheng TL, Brenner RA, Wright JL, Sachs HC, Moyer P, Rao MR. Children's violent television viewing: are parents monitoring? *Pediatrics.* 2004;114:94-99.
28. Bernard-Bonnin AC, Gilbert S, Rousseau E, Masson P, Maheux B. Television and the 3- to 10-year-old child. *Pediatrics.* 1991;88:48-54.
29. Roberts DR, Foehr UG. Generation M: media in the lives of 8-18 year olds. Available at:http://www.kff.org/entmedia/7251.cfm. Accessed July 10, 2005.
30. Zimmerman FJ, Christakis DA. Children's television viewing and cognitive outcomes: a longitudinal analysis of national data. *Arch Pediatr Adolesc Med.* 2005;159:619-625.
31. Fisch SM, Truglio RT, Cole CF. The impact of Sesame Street on preschool children: a review and synthesis of 30 years' research. *Media Psychol.* 1999;1:165-190.
32. Cantor J, Wilson B. Media and violence: intervention strategies for reducing aggression. *Media Psychol.* 2003;5:363-403.
33. Borzekowski DL, Robinson TN. The remote, the mouse, and the No. 2 pencil: the household media environment and academic achievement among third grade students. *Arch Pediatr Adolesc Med.* 2005;159:607-613.
34. Hancox RJ, Milne BJ, Poulton R. Association of television viewing during childhood with poor educational achievement. *Arch Pediatr Adolesc Med.* 2005;159:614-618.
35. Anderson DR, Field DE, Collins PA, Lorch EP, Nathan JG. Estimates of young children's time with television: a methodological comparison of parent reports with time-lapse video home observation. *Child Dev.* 1985;56:1345-1357.
36. Taras HL, Sallis JF, Nader PR, Nelson J. Children's television-viewing habits and the family environment. *AJDC.* 1990;144:357-359.

## *Trial Registration Required*

In concert with the International Committee of Medical Journal Editors (ICMJE), *Archives of Pediatrics and Adolescent Medicine* will require, as a condition of consideration for publication, registration of all trials in a public trials registry (such as http://ClinicalTrials.gov). Trials must be registered at or before the onset of patient enrollment. This policy applies to any clinical trial starting enrollment after July 1, 2005. For trials that began enrollment before this date, registration will be required by September 13, 2005, before considering the trial for publication. The trial registration number should be supplied at the time of submission.

For details about this new policy, and for information on how the ICMJE defines a clinical trial, see the editorials by DeAngelis et al in the September 8, 2004 (2004;292:1363-1364) and June 15, 2005 (2005;293:2927-2929) issues of *JAMA*. Also see the Instructions to Authors on our Web site: www.archpediatrics.com.

ARTICLE

# Content and Ratings of Mature-Rated Video Games

*Kimberly M. Thompson, ScD; Karen Tepichin, BS; Kevin Haninger, AB*

**Objectives:** To quantify the depiction of violence, blood, sexual themes, profanity, substances, and gambling in video games rated M (for "mature") and to measure agreement between the content observed and the rating information provided to consumers on the game box by the Entertainment Software Rating Board.

**Design:** We created a database of M-rated video game titles, selected a random sample, recorded at least 1 hour of game play, quantitatively assessed the content, performed statistical analyses to describe the content, and compared our observations with the Entertainment Software Rating Board content descriptors and results of our prior studies.

**Setting:** Harvard University, Boston, Mass.

**Participants:** Authors and 1 hired game player.

**Main Exposure:** M-rated video games.

**Main Outcome Measures:** Percentages of game play depicting violence, blood, sexual themes, gambling, alcohol, tobacco, or other drugs; use of profanity in dialogue, song lyrics, or gestures.

**Results:** Although the Entertainment Software Rating Board content descriptors for violence and blood provide a good indication of such content in the game, we identified 45 observations of content that could warrant a content descriptor in 29 games (81%) that lacked these content descriptors. M-rated video games are significantly more likely to contain blood, profanity, and substances; depict more severe injuries to human and nonhuman characters; and have a higher rate of human deaths than video games rated T (for "teen").

**Conclusion:** Parents and physicians should recognize that popular M-rated video games contain a wide range of unlabeled content and may expose children and adolescents to messages that may negatively influence their perceptions, attitudes, and behaviors.

*Arch Pediatr Adolesc Med. 2006;160:402-410*

The Entertainment Software Rating Board (ESRB) assigns age-based rating symbols and content descriptors that appear on video game boxes to inform consumers about game content.[1] To receive a rating, game manufacturers submit videotaped footage and other information to the ESRB for review by 3 independent raters. We previously quantified the content of video games rated E (for "everyone") and T (for "teen") and observed content that could warrant ESRB content descriptors in games lacking such content descriptors.[2-4] Although video games rated M (for "mature") continue to raise concerns and attract media attention, to our knowledge, no study to date quantifies the content of potential concern to physicians,[5,6] parents, and others[7] or the correspondence between game content and the ESRB content descriptors displayed on the game box.

Recent studies document the increasing popularity of video games among children and adolescents, with 91% of 8- to 18-year-olds reporting that they played a console video game at least once.[8] In the last 5 years, the average time spent playing video games by 8- to 18-year-olds nearly doubled from 26 to 49 minutes per day.[8,9] The results indicate an average of 2.1 video game consoles per home, with 31% of children and adolescents surveyed reporting 3 or more consoles.[9] Children and adolescents with video game consoles in their rooms reported significantly more time spent playing video games, while parental rules restricting TV and video game use appear to reduce reported video game play time.[9] Unfortunately, the same survey did not ask about M-rated video games played. However, 27% and 65% of respondents reported they had played *Duke Nukem* or *Grand Theft Auto*, respectively; 12% reported playing a game of which their parents would disapprove; and only 17% indicated that their parents check the ratings on games.[9]

In addition, the most recent Federal Trade Commission report on marketing violent entertainment to children cited industry data showing that in 2002 consumers purchased nearly 40% of M-rated video games for children younger than 17 years.[10] The Federal Trade Commission also reported that 69% of unaccompanied chil-

**Author Affiliations:** Kids Risk Project, Harvard School of Public Health, Harvard University, Boston, Mass.

**Violence:** Intentional acts in which the aggressor causes or attempts to cause physical injury or death to another character. We exclude actions that lead to unintentional physical harm, the effects of natural disasters, or the presence of dangerous obstacles not attributed to another character. Note that characters include humans and nonhumans (eg, monsters, ghosts, animals, and personified robots) that attack the player or other characters.

**Planning Violence:** Precursor acts in which a character selects, modifies, or acquires a weapon; acquires ammunition; aims prior to committing violence; or discusses detailed plans for killing or injuring other characters.

**Depictions of Injury:** An injured or dead character lying on the ground or remnants of blood from a known violent act.

**Portrayal of Violence:**

**Mild:** The most severe depiction of violence in the game involves minor auditory or visual representations of injury and pain that primarily serve to notify the player that a character is injured (eg, characters grunt or turn red when injured but do not scream or bleed).

**Moderate:** The most severe depiction of violence involves more realistic representations of injury and pain (eg, characters scream, fall over, or bleed when injured).

**Strong:** The most severe depiction of violence involves graphic representations of injury and pain that exaggerate or focus attention on suffering (eg, characters scream in agony or bleed excessively when injured or when otherwise physically tortured).

**Blood:** A red fluid originating from an injured human or any colored fluid originating from an injured creature.

**Sexual Themes:** Behaviors (eg, provocative touching or moaning) or dialogue related to sex and prostitution, as well as depictions of exposed breasts, buttocks, or genitals. We otherwise exclude pronounced cleavage, large breasts, and provocative clothing as sexual material given the vague ESRB definition of "suggestive themes" (ie, "mild provocative references or materials").

**Profanity:** Use of abusive and vulgar language, anatomical references without the use of such words, and obscene gestures involving the middle finger or its full-arm equivalent. We include use of "God," "Jesus," and "hell" only when characters use these words abusively, but we otherwise exclude taunts, mean language, or words censored by bleeps.

**Substances:** Use of alcohol, tobacco, or illicit drugs; scenes in which the player views images related to at least 1 substance; or scenes in which characters discuss drug deals or using substances. We exclude medicinal herbs, tonics, or ambiguous "potions."

**Gambling:** Characters betting money for prizes.

**Figure 1.** Definitions of content used in the study. ESRB indicates Entertainment Software Rating Board.

dren aged 13 to 16 years participating in its mystery shopper survey successfully purchased M-rated video games.[10] Industry data also identified M-rated *Grand Theft Auto: San Andreas* and *Halo 2* as the best-selling video games of 2004.[11] A national study of 5756 students in Canada found that approximately 22% of boys in grades 3 through 6 and 50% of boys in grades 7 through 10 identified 1 or more M-rated video games among their 3 favorite games.[12] Thus, while the M-rating should theoretically lead to restrictions on children's exposure to the content in these games, the limited existing data suggest that many children younger than 17 years currently play M-rated video games.

Legislative efforts to restrict the sale of violent video games to minors[13] and lawsuits covered in the popular media demonstrate the public concern about the potential health impacts of video games on children.[5,6] With respect to video games, a meta-analysis of experimental and nonexperimental studies found that playing violent video games increased aggression in children and young adults.[14] A recent experimental study of mostly adults, designed to detect only moderate or large effects, did not find an increase in aggressive thoughts or behaviors after 1 month of playing an M-rated online fantasy game.[15] Given the very limited evidence, understanding the effects of video games on brain processing, learning, attitudes, and behaviors requires additional research, and currently, health care professionals must offer advice to parents in the absence of good data from rigorous longitudinal studies. To our knowledge, this study provides the first set of quantitative data available to physicians and parents to help them better understand the content of M-rated video games and the accuracy of the rating information provided.

**Table 1. ESRB Content Descriptors Assigned to Game Titles**

| ESRB Content Descriptor | No. (%) of Game Titles* Random Sample (n = 36) | All M-Rated (N = 147) |
|---|---|---|
| Violence | | |
| Intense violence | 3 (8.3) | 22 (15.0) |
| Sexual violence | 0 | 0 |
| Violence | 30 (83.3) | 112 (76.2) |
| Animated violence† | 2 (5.6) | 8 (5.4) |
| Fantasy violence | 0 | 0 |
| Cartoon violence | 0 | 0 |
| Mild violence | 0 | 2 (1.4) |
| Mild animated violence† | 0 | 0 |
| Mild fantasy violence | 0 | 0 |
| Mild cartoon violence | 0 | 0 |
| Blood | | |
| Blood and gore | 20 (55.6) | 81 (55.1) |
| Blood | 13 (36.1) | 49 (33.3) |
| Animated blood and gore† | 1 (2.8) | 3 (2.0) |
| Animated blood | 1 (2.8) | 5 (3.4) |
| Sexual themes | | |
| Strong sexual content | 3 (8.3) | 8 (5.4) |
| Mature sexual themes‡ | 1 (2.8) | 8 (5.4) |
| Suggestive themes | 1 (2.8) | 3 (2.0) |
| Nudity | 0 | 2 (1.4) |
| Partial nudity | 1 (2.8) | 3 (2.0) |
| Profanity | | |
| Strong language | 9 (25.0) | 32 (21.8) |
| Strong lyrics | 1 (2.8) | 1 (0.7) |
| Language | 0 | 0 |
| Lyrics | 0 | 0 |
| Mild language | 1 (2.8) | 3 (2.0) |
| Mild lyrics | 0 | 0 |
| Substances | | |
| Use of alcohol | 0 | 0 |
| Use of tobacco | 0 | 0 |
| Use of drugs | 1 (2.8) | 5 (3.4) |
| Alcohol reference | 0 | 0 |
| Tobacco reference | 0 | 0 |
| Drug reference | 0 | 1 (0.7) |
| Humor | | |
| Mature humor | 0 | 2 (1.4) |
| Crude humor | 0 | 0 |
| Comic mischief | 1 (2.8) | 2 (1.4) |
| Gambling | 0 | 1 (0.7) |

Abbreviations: ESRB, Entertainment Software Rating Board; M, mature.
*Columns sum to 89 and 353, respectively, because some game titles received more than 1 content descriptor.
†The ESRB no longer uses the word "animated" in this content descriptor.
‡The ESRB no longer uses the word "mature" in this content descriptor.

## METHODS

We created a database of all 147 M-rated video game titles scheduled for release on the major video game consoles (Xbox [Microsoft Corporation, Redmond], GameCube [Nintendo of

**Table 2. ESRB Content Descriptors Assigned to Games in Sample Compared With Observed Content**

| Game Title | Console | Year Released | ESRB Content Descriptor | Observed Content: Violence | Blood | Sexual Themes | Profanity | Substances |
|---|---|---|---|---|---|---|---|---|
| Action | | | | | | | | |
| *Brute Force* | Xbox (Microsoft Corp, Redmond) | 2003 | Blood, violence | Yes | Yes | No | Yes | No |
| *Drakengard* | PS2 (Sony Computer Entertainment America, Foster City, Calif) | 2004 | Blood and gore, violence | Yes | Yes | No | Yes | No |
| *Gungrave* | PS2 | 2002 | Blood, violence | Yes | Yes | No | Yes | Yes |
| *Hitman: Contracts* | Xbox | 2004 | Blood and gore, intense violence, strong language, strong sexual content, use of drugs | Yes | Yes | Yes | No | Yes |
| *Max Payne* | PS2 | 2001 | Blood, violence | Yes | Yes | Yes | Yes | Yes |
| *McFarlane's Evil Prophecy* | PS2 | 2004 | Blood and gore, violence | Yes | Yes | No | Yes | No |
| *Nightshade* | PS2 | 2004 | Blood, violence | Yes | Yes | No | No | No |
| *Ninja Gaiden* | Xbox | 2004 | Blood and gore, violence | Yes | Yes | No | No | No |
| *Rune: Viking Warlord* | PS2 | 2001 | Animated blood and gore, animated violence | Yes | Yes | No | No | Yes |
| *Syphon Filter: The Omega Strain* | PS2 | 2004 | Blood, strong language, violence | Yes | Yes | No | Yes | Yes |
| *The Chronicles of Riddick: Escape From Butcher Bay* | Xbox | 2004 | Blood, intense violence, strong language | Yes | Yes | Yes | Yes | Yes |
| *Twisted Metal: Black* | PS2 | 2001 | Blood and gore, violence | Yes | Yes | No | Yes | No |
| Action adventure | | | | | | | | |
| *Genma Onimusha* | Xbox | 2002 | Blood and gore, violence | Yes | Yes | No | No | No |
| *Grand Theft Auto: Vice City* | PS2 | 2002 | Blood and gore, strong language, strong sexual content, violence | Yes | Yes | Yes | Yes | Yes |
| *Metal Gear Solid: The Twin Snakes* | GCN (Nintendo of America, Redmond) | 2004 | Blood and gore, suggestive themes, violence | Yes | Yes | Yes | Yes | Yes |
| *Onimusha 2: Samurai's Destiny* | PS2 | 2002 | Blood and gore, violence | Yes | Yes | Yes | Yes | Yes |
| *Resident Evil 3: Nemesis* | GCN | 2003 | Blood and gore, violence | Yes | Yes | No | No | Yes* |
| *Rogue Ops* | Xbox | 2003 | Blood, mild language, violence | Yes | Yes | No | Yes | Yes |
| *Run Like Hell* | PS2 | 2002 | Blood and gore, strong language, violence | Yes | Yes | Yes | Yes | Yes* |
| *The Thing* | Xbox | 2002 | Blood and gore, violence | Yes | Yes | No | Yes | No |
| Shooting | | | | | | | | |
| *Cold Winter* | PS2 | 2005 | Blood and gore, intense violence, strong language | Yes | Yes | No | Yes | Yes |
| *Red Faction II* | Xbox | 2003 | Blood and gore, violence | Yes | Yes | No | Yes | No |
| *Resident Evil Dead Aim* | PS2 | 2003 | Blood and gore, violence | Yes | Yes | No | No | Yes |
| *Robocop* | Xbox | 2003 | Blood, violence | Yes | Yes | No | No | Yes |
| *Silent Scope Complete* | Xbox | 2004 | Blood, violence | Yes | Yes | No | Yes | No |
| *Soldier of Fortune II: Double Helix* | Xbox | 2003 | Blood, violence | Yes | Yes | No | Yes | Yes |
| *Unreal II: The Awakening* | Xbox | 2004 | Blood and gore, violence | Yes | Yes | Yes | Yes | Yes |

(*continued*)

America, Redmond], and PlayStation 2 [Sony Computer Entertainment America, Foster City, Calif]) in the United States by April 1, 2004. Using data from the ESRB[1] and several video game Web sites,[16-18] we verified the release of each game title, recorded the ESRB-assigned content descriptors, and classified each game title by 1 of 10 primary genres.

We randomly selected 25% (n = 37) of the 147 M-rated video game titles to play. However, given the postponed release of *Painkiller* until 2006, we played only 36 games. All of the games played remain available for sale or rental. When possible, we purchased or rented the games with their original game manuals intact. For consistency, a research assistant with considerable video-gaming experience played the entire random sample of video games and recorded all game play on DVD for later coding. The player first read the manual and played the game to become familiar with the game features, then restarted the video game from the beginning and recorded at least 1 hour of game play, including any required game introductions and setup.

One of us with considerable video-gaming experience (K.T.) reviewed and manually coded all of the recorded game play us-

**Table 2. ESRB Content Descriptors Assigned to Games in Sample Compared With Observed Content (cont)**

| Game Title | Console | Year Released | ESRB Content Descriptor | Observed Content: Violence | Blood | Sexual Themes | Profanity | Substances |
|---|---|---|---|---|---|---|---|---|
| Adventure | | | | | | | | |
| *Eternal Darkness: Sanity's Requiem* | GCN | 2002 | Blood and gore, violence | Yes | Yes | No | Yes | No |
| *Fatal Frame II: Crimson Butterfly* | PS2 | 2003 | Blood, violence | Yes | No | No | No | No |
| *Shadow Man: 2econd Coming* | PS2 | 2002 | Blood and gore, strong language, violence | Yes | Yes | No | Yes | Yes* |
| *Silent Hill 2* | PS2 | 2001 | Blood and gore, violence | Yes | Yes | Yes | Yes | No |
| Fighting | | | | | | | | |
| *Kengo: Master of Bushido* | PS2 | 2000 | Animated blood, animated violence | Yes | No | Yes | No | No |
| *Pride FC* | PS2 | 2003 | Blood, strong lyrics, violence | Yes | Yes | No | No | No |
| Role-Playing | | | | | | | | |
| *Fallout: Brotherhood of Steel* | Xbox | 2004 | Blood and gore, mature sexual themes, strong language, violence | Yes | Yes | Yes | Yes | Yes |
| Sports | | | | | | | | |
| *BMX XXX* | PS2 | 2002 | Comic mischief, partial nudity, strong language, strong sexual content | Yes | No | Yes | Yes† | Yes* |
| Strategy | | | | | | | | |
| *Legion: The Legend of Excalibur* | PS2 | 2002 | Blood, violence | Yes | Yes | Yes | No | Yes |

Abbreviations: GCN, Nintendo GameCube; ESRB, Entertainment Software Rating Board; PS2, Sony PlayStation 2.
*Game contains alcohol, tobacco, or drug references but was released before the ESRB began assigning these content descriptors.
†Game contains explicit language and song lyrics.

ing standard coding instruments (available on request) and then 2 of us (K.T. and K.H.) entered the data into Microsoft Access (Version 2002; Microsoft Corporation). We used the same coding methods as in our earlier studies in which we obtained excellent agreement between coders ($\kappa = 0.93$).[2-4] In addition, to assess the consistency of our method in this study, 1 of us (K.M.T.) independently coded all 36 games for evidence of each specific type of content for comparison with a κ statistic.

**Figure 1** provides the definitions of content we used.[2-4] To quantify the amount of violence in each game, we divided the recorded game play into 1-second intervals and noted whether each second of game play contained acts of violence. For each second of game play not already coded as "committing violence," we coded the second as "planning violence" if it showed a character planning acts of violence, as "depicting injuries" if it depicted injuries from violence, or as "not violent" if it failed to meet either of these criteria. To further characterize the overall portrayal of violence, we used the 3 categories defined in Figure 1 to separately code the highest (and most severe) portrayal of injuries depicted to human and nonhuman characters using a method previously shown to provide good agreement between independent coders.[4] We also noted the types of weapons used for violence, whether the player could select or modify these weapons, whether violence resulted in injury or death, the number of human and nonhuman deaths from violence, whether injuring or killing human and nonhuman characters was rewarded or was required to advance in the game, and whether destroying objects was rewarded or required to advance in the game, although we did not code the destruction of objects as violence. To quantify the amount of blood, we noted whether each second of game play depicted blood and further identified whether each second depicted human or nonhuman blood. We did not code blood as a depiction of injury unless the blood came from a known act of violence. We also noted whether the game depicted the mutilation or severing of body parts. To quantify the amount of sexual themes, we noted whether each second of game play depicted sexual behaviors, sexual dialogue, and/or nudity. We also noted the sex of the characters involved and whether the player could play each game as a male or female character. To quantify profanity, we counted each occurrence and noted the specific gesture or word(s) used. We noted whether the profanity occurred in the game as dialogue, written text, or song lyrics. To quantify the amount of alcohol, tobacco, and drugs in the game, we noted whether each second of game play depicted any type of substance, and we separately noted whether each second involved substance use. Finally, we counted the number of seconds of game play that depicted gambling.

We performed statistical tests using SAS statistical software (Version 9.0 for Windows; SAS Institute Inc, Cary, NC).

## RESULTS

**Table 1** lists ESRB content descriptors by type and compares the 89 content descriptors assigned to the 36 video game titles in the random sample with the 353 content descriptors assigned to all 147 M-rated video game titles. No statistically significant difference exists between the 2 distributions of content descriptors. The range of content descriptors reflects continued changes to the ESRB rating system. For example, in 2003, the ESRB added new content descriptors for violence (intense violence, sexual violence, fantasy violence, and cartoon violence) and for substances (alcohol reference, tobacco reference, and drug reference). Overall, 98% of game titles rated M received content descriptors for violence (ie, descriptors under that

**Table 3. ESRB Content Descriptors for Violence and Blood Compared With Observations of Violence and Blood**

| Game Title | Violence, % | | Blood, % | | Deaths per Hour | | Depiction of Injuries From Violence | | Rewards | Weapons |
|---|---|---|---|---|---|---|---|---|---|---|
| | Acts | All | Human | All | Human | All | Human | Nonhuman | | |
| Action | | | | | | | | | | |
| *Brute Force* | 28.4 | 39.5 | 2.8 | 10.1 | 33 | 132 | Strong | Strong | RD,RI,RK | B,E,G,K,P* |
| *Drakengard* | 61.6 | 74.7 | 29.7 | 36.6 | 1140 | 1142 | Strong | Strong | RD,RI,RK | E,F,G,K,M,P* |
| *Gungrave* | 50.2 | 60.3 | 14.4 | 14.5 | 618 | 702 | Strong | Moderate | RD,RI,RK | B,E,F,G,K,P,O* |
| *Hitman: Contracts* | 8.7 | 44.4 | 21.5 | 33.4† | 109 | 133 | Strong | Strong | RI,RK | B,G,T,O* |
| *Max Payne* | 7.3 | 22.4 | 15.9 | 15.9 | 62 | 62 | Strong | . . . | RD,RI,RK | G,P,O* |
| *McFarlane's Evil Prophecy* | 42.5 | 50.9 | 0.9 | 43.0† | 3 | 514 | Strong | Strong | RD,RI,RK | B,E,F,G,K,M,P* |
| *Nightshade* | 37.6 | 46.2 | 2.6 | 9.1† | 39 | 266 | Moderate | Strong | RD,RI,RK | B,E,K,M,P* |
| *Ninja Gaiden* | 30.1 | 38.5 | 17.1 | 18.1† | 118 | 126 | Strong | Strong | RD,RI,RK | B,F,G,K,M,P* |
| *Rune: Viking Warlord* | 8.1 | 34.2 | 27.7 | 31.2 | 28 | 72 | Strong | Moderate | RD,RI,RK | B,F,K,M,P,O* |
| *Syphon Filter: The Omega Strain* | 28.4 | 45.6 | 15.1 | 15.1 | 119 | 119 | Strong | . . . | RD,RI,RK | B,E,G,K,P* |
| *The Chronicles of Riddick: Escape from Butcher Bay* | 10.7 | 31.7 | 20.7 | 21.1 | 34 | 35 | Strong | Strong | RD,RI,RK | B,G,K* |
| *Twisted Metal: Black* | 53.1 | 60.9 | 3.7 | 3.7† | 60 | 60 | Strong | . . . | RD,RI,RK | E,F,G,P,O* |
| Action adventure | | | | | | | | | | |
| *Genma Onimusha* | 40.9 | 55.4 | 10.9 | 27.7 | 61 | 132 | Strong | Strong | RD,RI,RK | B,K,M,P* |
| *Grand Theft Auto: Vice City* | 6.3 | 10.4 | 3.3 | 3.3 | 32 | 32 | Strong | . . . | RD,RI,RK | B,E,G,K,O* |
| *Metal Gear Solid: The Twin Snakes* | 7.6 | 15.3 | 5.5 | 5.5 | 5 | 5 | Strong | . . . | RI | B,G,O* |
| *Onimusha 2: Samurai's Destiny* | 14.7 | 22.5 | 6.5 | 9.7 | 67 | 95 | Strong | Strong | RD,RI,RK | B,G,K,P* |
| *Resident Evil 3: Nemesis* | 14.0 | 36.8 | 31.9 | 33.6† | 78 | 79 | Strong | Strong | RD,RI,RK | E,G,K,P* |
| *Rogue Ops* | 5.9 | 24.5 | 8.0 | 8.0 | 26 | 26 | Strong | . . . | RD,RI,RK | B,E,G,P* |
| *Run Like Hell* | 6.4 | 11.7 | 1.7 | 10.6† | 6 | 36 | Strong | Moderate | RD,RI,RK | B,E,G* |
| *The Thing* | 4.7 | 21.3 | 4.5 | 17.6† | 12 | 57 | Strong | Strong | RD,RI,RK | E,F,G,P* |
| Shooting | | | | | | | | | | |
| *Cold Winter* | 15.5 | 37.8 | 27.9 | 28.2† | 59 | 68 | Strong | Moderate | RD,RI,RK | E,F,G,P,O* |
| *Red Faction II* | 39.7 | 50.5 | 23.7 | 23.7† | 200 | 200 | Strong | . . . | RI,RK | E,G,P* |
| *Resident Evil Dead Aim* | 11.1 | 29.7 | 13.5 | 13.7 | 58 | 58 | Strong | . . . | RI,RK | B,G* |
| *Robocop* | 26.2 | 33.3 | 6.0 | 6.0 | 103 | 108 | Strong | Moderate | RD,RI,RK | B,E,F,G,P* |
| *Silent Scope Complete* | 48.1 | 54.4 | 1.9 | 1.9 | 339 | 339 | Moderate | . . . | RD,RI,RK | E,G,P |
| *Soldier of Fortune II: Double Helix* | 19.0 | 33.1 | 14.1 | 14.1 | 98 | 98 | Strong | . . . | RD,RI,RK | E,G,K,P* |
| *Unreal II: The Awakening* | 22.2 | 31.4 | 4.0 | 6.6† | 12 | 109 | Strong | Strong | RI,RK | B,E,G,P* |
| Adventure | | | | | | | | | | |
| *Eternal Darkness: Sanity's Requiem* | 6.4 | 13.3 | 0.5 | 4.2† | 1 | 31 | Strong | Strong | RD,RI,RK | B,K,M* |
| *Fatal Frame II: Crimson Butterfly* | 11.7 | 20.7 | 0 | 0 | 10 | 23 | Moderate | Moderate | RI,RK | O* |
| *Shadow Man: 2econd Coming* | 10.8 | 53.9 | 2.9 | 41.9† | 29 | 50 | Strong | Strong | RD,RI,RK | B,G,K,M* |
| *Silent Hill 2* | 4.7 | 13.4 | 1.0 | 12.5† | 2 | 14 | Strong | Strong | RI,RK | B,G,O* |
| Fighting | | | | | | | | | | |
| *Kengo: Master of Bushido* | 48.4 | 58.8 | 0 | 0 | 0 | 1 | Moderate | Moderate | RD,RI,RK | K,M* |
| *Pride FC* | 18.1 | 20.5 | 8.0 | 8.0 | 0 | 0 | Strong | . . . | RI | B |
| Role-Playing | | | | | | | | | | |
| *Fallout: Brotherhood of Steel* | 17.0 | 38.8 | 9.6 | 30.8† | 17 | 155 | Moderate | Strong | RD,RI,RK | B,G,T,O* |
| Sports | | | | | | | | | | |
| *BMX XXX* | 0.8 | 1.3 | 0 | 0 | 0 | 0 | Moderate | Moderate | RD,RI | O |
| Strategy | | | | | | | | | | |
| *Legion: The Legend of Excalibur* | 35.1 | 43.6 | 25.5 | 25.5† | 149 | 154 | Strong | Moderate | RD,RI,RK | B,F,K,M,P,O* |

Abbreviations: B, body as weapon; E, explosive as weapon; ESRB, Entertainment Software Rating Board; F, fire as weapon; G, gun as weapon; K, knife or sword as weapon; M, magic as weapon; O, other weapon; P, projectile as weapon; RD, game rewards destruction of objects; RI, game rewards injuring characters; RK, game rewards killing characters; T, toxic substance as weapon.

*Player can select weapons.

†Game depicts the mutilation of body parts.

heading in Figure 1); 94%, for blood; 14%, for sexual themes; 24%, for profanity; 4%, for substances; 3%, for humor; and 1%, for gambling.

**Table 2** lists game titles in the random sample by genre, along with their console and release year, and compares the content we observed with the ESRB-assigned content descriptors. Overall, we identified 45 observations of content that could warrant a content descriptor in 29 games (81%) that did not receive these content descriptors from the ESRB. This statistic excludes images and dialogue related to alcohol, tobacco, and illicit drugs in games released before 2003 when the ESRB assigned content descriptors for only the use of these substances. We did not observe content indicated by 4 ESRB-assigned content descriptors in 4 games (11%) within 1 hour of game play, although we note that this content occurs later in these games. We also know from extended play of some games that content for which the ESRB did not assign a content descriptor sometimes occurs after 1 hour of game play (eg, a sexually provoca-

**Table 4. ESRB Content Descriptors for Sexual Themes Compared With Observed Sexual Themes**

| | Duration of Game Play, s | Duration of Observed Sexual Themes, s (% of Game Play) | | | |
|---|---|---|---|---|---|
| | | Total | Dialogue or Writing | Behavior | Partial Nudity |
| Strong sexual content and partial nudity | | | | | |
| *BMX XXX* | 4193 | 1739 (41.5)* | 653 (15.6)†‡ | 344 (8.2)†‡ | 1211 (28.9)† |
| Strong sexual content | | | | | |
| *Grand Theft Auto: Vice City* | 4228 | 203 (4.8)* | 83 (2.0)†‡ | 121 (2.9)†‡ | 21 (0.5)† |
| *Hitman: Contracts* | 4121 | 75 (1.8)* | 0 | 75 (1.8)†‡ | 0 |
| Mature sexual themes | | | | | |
| *Fallout: Brotherhood of Steel* | 4209 | 177 (4.2)* | 133 (3.2)† | 138 (3.3)† | 39 (0.9)† |
| Suggestive themes | | | | | |
| *Metal Gear Solid: The Twin Snakes* | 4700 | 8 (0.2) | 8 (0.2)† | 0 | 0 |
| No descriptors | | | | | |
| *Kengo: Master of Bushido* | 4407 | 5 (0.1) | 0 | 0 | 5 (0.1)‡ |
| *Legion: The Legend of Excalibur* | 4055 | 12 (0.3) | 0 | 0 | 12 (0.3)† |
| *Max Payne* | 3741 | 77 (2.1)* | 77 (2.1)‡ | 0 | 0 |
| *Onimusha 2: Samurai's Destiny* | 4647 | 214 (4.6)* | 77 (1.7)†‡ | 200 (4.3)†‡ | 7 (0.2)† |
| *Run Like Hell* | 4047 | 108 (2.7) | 2 (0)† | 11 (0.3)†‡ | 97 (2.4)† |
| *Silent Hill 2* | 4127 | 8 (0.2) | 0 | 8 (0.2)§ | 0 |
| *The Chronicles of Riddick: Escape From Butcher Bay* | 3911 | 6 (0.2) | 6 (0.2)‡ | 0 | 0 |
| *Unreal II: The Awakening* | 4153 | 59 (1.4) | 0 | 0 | 59 (1.4)† |

Abbreviation: ESRB, Entertainment Software Rating Board.
*Game depicts prostitution.
†Female characters engage in this activity.
‡Male characters engage in this activity.
§Nonhuman characters engage in this activity.

tive female character in *Ninja Gaiden* and tobacco use in *Soldier of Fortune II: Double Helix*). We found excellent agreement between the 2 of us (K.M.T. and K.T.) who coded all of the games for each type of content ($\kappa = 0.97$).

**Table 3** summarizes our observations of violence and blood. All 36 games involved intentional acts of violence (100%), with 35 games (97%) receiving content descriptors for violence. We observed wide variation in the amounts of violence in the games, with games containing an average of 22% violent game play time (range, 0.8%-62%). Including the additional game play associated with planning violence and depiction of injuries increases the average to 36% of game play time directly related to violence (range, 1.3%-75%). We also observed 28 games (78%) that rewarded or required the player to destroy objects.

Overall, 35 games (97%) received content descriptors for blood and we observed blood in 33 (92%) of 36 games, with 18% of game play time depicting blood (range, 1.9%-43%) and 12% of game play time depicting human blood (range, 0.5%-32%). We did not observe blood within 1 hour of game play in 2 games (6%) that received content descriptors for blood. These results indicate that ESRB content descriptors for violence and blood provide a good indication that an M-rated video game contains such content.

We observed 6011 character deaths from violence in approximately 42 hours of game play, occurring at an average rate of 145 character deaths per hour (range, 0-1142). This included 4268 human deaths, occurring at an average rate of 104 human deaths per hour (range, 0-1140). Overall, we identified 24 games (67%) that depicted deaths from violence of nonhuman characters, including the player, and 33 games (92%) that depicted deaths from violence of human characters, including the player. All 36 games (100%) rewarded or required the player to injure characters, while 33 games (92%) rewarded or required the player to kill.

Analysis of the overall portrayal of violence shows that all 36 games (100%) depicted injuries to human characters and 25 (69%) of 36 games depicted injuries to nonhuman characters, including injuries to the player. Examining the portrayal of violence to human characters, we found that 6 (17%) of 36 games portrayed violence characterized as "moderate" and 30 games (83%) portrayed violence characterized as "strong." Examining the portrayal of violence to nonhuman characters, we found that 9 (25%) of 36 games portrayed "moderate" violence and 16 games (44%) portrayed "strong" violence.

Table 3 also shows that games depicted an average of 4 types of weapons (range, 1-7), with players able to select weapons in 33 games (92%), and that 35 games (97%) depicted weapons other than the body. A total of 24 games (67%) used the body as a weapon, 27 (75%) used guns, 22 (61%) used projectiles, 18 (50%) used knives or swords, 18 (50%) used explosives, 10 (28%) used fire, 10 (28%) used magic, 2 (6%) used toxic substances, and 13 (36%) used other weapons (eg, automobile, club, broken bottle). These findings represent a subset given our limited game play time.[2-4]

**Table 4** lists game titles by ESRB content descriptor for sexual themes and shows our observations of characters engaging in dialogue or behaviors related to sex or showing exposed breasts, buttocks, or genitals. We observed sexual themes in 13 (36%) of 36 games, with 5 games (14%) receiving content descriptors for sexual themes. On average, the 13 games in which we observed sexual themes depicted sexual themes for 4.9% of game play time (range, 0.1%-42%). Expanding our definition of sexual themes to

**Table 5. ESRB Content Descriptors for Profanity Compared With Observed Profanity**

| | No. of Observed Uses of Profanity per Hour | | | |
|---|---|---|---|---|
| Game Title | Total | Dialogue or Writing | Song Lyrics | Gestures |
| Strong language | | | | |
| *BMX XXX* | 201 | 166 | 35 | |
| *Cold Winter* | 3 | 3 | | |
| *Fallout: Brotherhood of Steel* | 13 | 13 | | |
| *Grand Theft Auto: Vice City* | 23 | 23 | | |
| *Hitman: Contracts* | 0 | 0 | | |
| *Run Like Hell* | 16 | 16 | | |
| *Shadow Man: 2econd Coming* | 17 | 17 | | |
| *Syphon Filter: The Omega Strain* | 3 | 3 | | |
| *The Chronicles of Riddick: Escape From Butcher Bay* | 57 | 56 | | 1 |
| Strong lyrics* | | | | |
| *Pride FC* | 0 | 0 | | |
| Mild language | | | | |
| *Rogue Ops* | 5 | 5 | | |
| No descriptors | | | | |
| *Brute Force* | 3 | 3 | | |
| *Drakengard* | 2 | 2 | | |
| *Eternal Darkness: Sanity's Requiem* | 1 | 1 | | |
| *Gungrave* | 7 | 7 | | |
| *Max Payne* | 9 | 9 | | |
| *McFarlane's Evil Prophecy* | 3 | 3 | | |
| *Metal Gear Solid: The Twin Snakes* | 1 | 1 | | |
| *Onimusha 2: Samurai's Destiny* | 1 | 1 | | |
| *Red Faction II* | 9 | 9 | | |
| *Silent Hill 2* | 3 | 3 | | |
| *Silent Scope Complete* | 1 | 1 | | |
| *Soldier of Fortune II: Double Helix* | 1 | 1 | | |
| *The Thing* | 21 | 21 | | |
| *Twisted Metal: Black* | 4 | 4 | | |
| *Unreal II: The Awakening* | 7 | 7 | | |

Abbreviation: See Table 5.
*The ESRB content descriptor for "strong lyrics" is not limited to profanity ("profanity and explicit references to sexuality, violence, alcohol, or drug use in music.")

include pronounced cleavage, large breasts, or provocative clothing would imply sexual themes in 17 games (47%). We observed the depiction of prostitution in 6 (17%) of 36 games. Overall, 32 games (89%) contained playable male characters, 12 games (33%) contained playable female characters, and 10 games (28%) allowed the player to select among a list of characters or personalize characters. Games were significantly more likely to depict female characters partially nude than male characters ($P<.007$), based on a 2-sided binomial exact test.

**Table 5** lists game titles by ESRB content descriptor for profanity and presents the observed uses of profanity per hour in dialogue, writing, lyrics, or gestures. We observed the use of profanity in 24 games (67%), with 11 games (31%) receiving content descriptors for profanity. The sample included 15 games (42%) that did not receive content descriptors for profanity when we observed such content and 2 games (6%) that received content descriptors for profanity for which we did not observe within 1 hour of game play. On average, the 24 games in which we observed profanity contained 17 uses of profanity per hour (range, 0.8-201). These observations include a game (*Twisted Metal: Black*) that did not receive a content descriptor for profanity despite containing use of the words "motherfucker," "bitch," and "piss." The game that received a content descriptor for mild language (*Rogue Ops*) contained the same words and number of uses per hour as the group of 15 games with unlabeled profanity.

**Table 6** lists game titles by ESRB content descriptor for substances and shows the percentage of game play depicting substances. We observed the depiction or use of substances in 21 (58%) of 36 games, with only 1 game (3%) receiving a content descriptor for substances. We found 17 games (47%) depicted alcohol, 8 games (22%) depicted tobacco, and 5 games (14%) depicted illicit drugs, with 12 (33%) of 36 games depicting characters using substances. On average, the 21 games in which we observed substances depicted substances for 3.4% of game play time, with 1.1% of game play time depicting substance use.

We did not observe gambling for money in any of the games, with no games receiving a content descriptor for gambling.

Compared with our prior analyses, this study suggests that nearly all M-rated (100%) and T-rated (98%) video games contain violence. Remarkably, M-rated video games contained a significantly smaller percentage of violent game play than did T-rated video games (22% for M-rated video games vs 36% for T-rated video games) based on a 2-sided Wilcoxon rank sum exact test ($P<.008$). However, game players are significantly more likely to encounter blood in M-rated video games than in T-rated video games (2-sided Fisher exact test, $P<.001$). Partly because of the increased presence of blood, M-rated video games depict more severe injuries to human ($P<.001$) and nonhuman characters ($P<.001$) than do T-rated video games, based on 2-sided Wilcoxon rank sum exact tests. We also observed a higher rate of human deaths in M-rated video games than in T-rated video games (2-sided Wilcoxon rank sum exact tests, $P<.001$), a result driven by the 23% of T-rated video games that do not depict deaths. Conditioning on the subset of M-rated and T-rated games that depict human deaths, we did not observe different rates.

In terms of other content, M-rated video games are significantly more likely than T-rated video games to contain profanity ($P<.001$) and substances ($P<.001$) but not sexual themes, based on 2-sided Fisher exact tests. Overall, M-rated video games are significantly more likely to contain unlabeled content than are T-rated video games (81% for M-rated video games vs 48% for T-rated video games), based on a 2-sided Fischer exact test ($P<.001$).

Because most video games contain more than 1 hour of game play, we emphasize that our method means that we miss some content. **Figure 2** shows the cumulative percentage of the different types of content found as a function of game play time for this sample, which demonstrates that by playing each game for approximately

**Table 6. ESRB Content Descriptors for Substances Compared With Observed Substances**

| Game Title | Duration of Game Play, s | Duration of Observed Substances, s (% of Game Play) | | | |
|---|---|---|---|---|---|
| | | Total | Alcohol | Tobacco | Drugs |
| Use of drugs | | | | | |
| *Hitman: Contracts* | 4121 | 43 (1.0) | 6 (0.1) | 0 | 43 (1.0) |
| No descriptors | | | | | |
| *BMX XXX** | 4193 | 27 (0.6) | 13 (0.3) | 0 | 14 (0.3) |
| *Cold Winter* | 4115 | 111 (2.7) | 39 (0.9) | 72 (1.7)† | 0 |
| *Fallout: Brotherhood of Steel* | 4209 | 466 (11.1) | 466 (11.1)† | 0 | 0 |
| *Grand Theft Auto: Vice City* | 4228 | 224 (5.3) | 149 (3.5)† | 0 | 114 (2.7) |
| *Gungrave* | 3896 | 347 (8.9) | 47 (1.2)† | 300 (7.7)† | 0 |
| *Legion: The Legend of Excalibur* | 4055 | 133 (3.3) | 133 (3.3)† | 0 | 0 |
| *Max Payne* | 3741 | 215 (5.7) | 86 (2.3) | 29 (0.8)† | 100 (2.7) |
| *Metal Gear Solid: The Twin Snakes* | 4700 | 90 (1.9) | 0 | 90 (1.9) | 0 |
| *Onimusha 2: Samurai's Destiny* | 4647 | 476 (10.2) | 342 (7.4)* | 181 (3.9) | 0 |
| *Resident Evil 3: Nemesis* | 4082 | 207 (5.1) | 207 (5.1) | 0 | 0 |
| *Resident Evil Dead Aim* | 4063 | 69 (1.7) | 69 (1.7) | 0 | 0 |
| *Robocop* | 4062 | 153 (3.8) | 39 (1.0) | 0 | 114 (2.8) |
| *Rogue Ops* | 3936 | 33 (0.8) | 0 | 33 (0.8)† | 0 |
| *Run Like Hell* | 4047 | 30 (0.7) | 30 (0.7) | 0 | 0 |
| *Rune: Viking Warlord* | 5781 | 76 (1.3) | 76 (1.3)† | 0 | 0 |
| *Shadow Man: 2econd Coming* | 4125 | 66 (1.6) | 66 (1.6) | 0 | 0 |
| *Soldier of Fortune II: Double Helix*‡ | 4212 | 18 (0.4) | 18 (0.4)† | 0 | 0 |
| *Syphon Filter: The Omega Strain* | 4071 | 35 (0.9) | 35 (0.9)† | 0 | 0 |
| *The Chronicles of Riddick: Escape From Butcher Bay* | 3911 | 124 (3.2) | 0 | 124 (3.2) | 0 |
| *Unreal II: The Awakening* | 4153 | 83 (2.0) | 0 | 83 (2.0)† | 0 |

Abbreviation: See Table 5.
*Game contains alcohol and drug references in song lyrics but did not receive an ESRB content descriptor for "mild lyrics" ("mild references to profanity, sexuality, violence, alcohol, or drug use in music").
†Game depicts use of this substance.
‡Game depicts use of tobacco during an optional training sequence that was excluded from analysis.

1 hour, we observed approximately 90% of content indicated by the ESRB content descriptors. These findings are consistent with our prior sample of T-rated video games[2] as also shown.

## COMMENT

The results of our study suggest that parents and physicians should pay careful attention to the actual content of any M-rated video game that their children might play, particularly since the M-rating indicates that the intended audience is for ages 17 years and older. Compared with our studies of T-rated video games, we found significantly more blood, severe injuries, and human deaths in M-rated games, although we also found a significantly smaller percentage of violent game play in M-rated video games. We believe that current discussions about restricting children's access to violent games may miss the reality that both T-rated and M-rated games contain significant amounts of violence.

These results confirm that the presence of an ESRB content descriptor means that game players likely will find the indicated content in the game but that parents should not interpret the absence of a content descriptor to mean the absence of content. Parents should recognize that the content descriptors on M-rated video games usually do not provide information about all types of content in the game, notably the depiction of substances. Our observation that 20 (56%) of 36 games depicted substances while only 1 game (3%) received a content descriptor for substances should motivate consideration of children's exposure to substances in video games (and more broadly in all media[19]). While some might argue

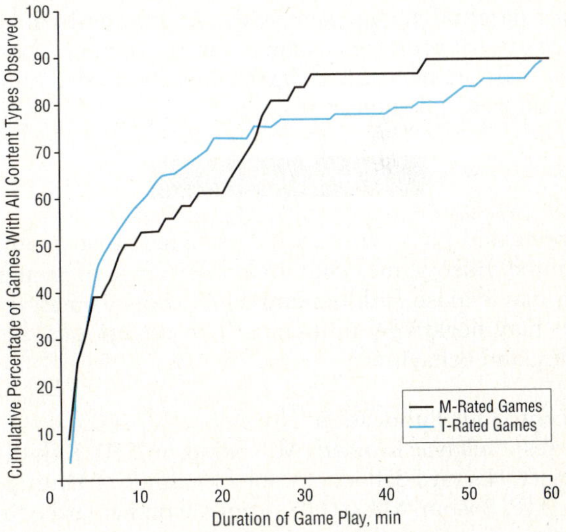


**Figure 2.** Cumulative percentage of video games with all content types observed by duration of game play.

about the need to provide content descriptors for M-rated video games given the intended audience of ages 17 years and older, we note that the ESRB does not provide specific criteria for assigning content descriptors. Even within a rating category, the ESRB assigns content descriptors to some games but not others with the same content, which creates confusion for parents who seek accurate and consistent rating information. We emphasize that the ESRB should provide greater clarity about its content descriptors and rating standards. In addition, since our studies consistently found content for which the ESRB did not assign content descriptors, we continue to believe that the ESRB should play the video games before assigning its ratings and provide assurance to parents and to the public about the quality of the rating information.

This study relies on the same methods and consequently implies the same methodological limitations as our other studies of video games.[2-4] In this study, our random sample represented only 25% of M-rated video games with 1 game in the sample not reaching the market prior to completion of the study. In the context of evolving games and ratings, this sample represents a cross-section of M-rated video games. We did not unlock additional material in games by entering codes (eg, from Web sites[16-18]), but parents should know that codes can alter game play. The ESRB's recent decision to change the rating of *Grand Theft Auto: San Andreas* from M to AO (for "adults only") resulted from the ability of players to unlock sexually explicit content.[20] Parents should look for the ESRB warning "Game Experience May Change During Online Play" and recognize that online game play may not reflect the game's original rating and content descriptors.

We emphasize that no study or rating system can replace parental engagement with children and adolescents experiencing video games and that more research is needed to understand the health impacts of video games on children and adolescents.

## CONCLUSIONS

Parents and physicians should recognize that popular M-rated video games contain a wide range of content and may expose children and adolescents to messages that may negatively influence their perceptions, attitudes, and behaviors.

**Accepted for Publication:** November 30, 2005.
**Correspondence:** Kimberly M. Thompson, ScD, Kids Risk Project, Harvard School of Public Health, 677 Huntington Ave, Boston, MA 02115 (kimt@hsph.harvard.edu).
**Funding/Support:** This research received support from gifts to the Kids Risk Project, Harvard School of Public Health.
**Acknowledgment:** We thank Roberto Tepichin, BS, JD, for playing the video games.

## REFERENCES

1. Entertainment Software Rating Board Web site. Available at: http://www.esrb.org. Accessed April 1, 2004.
2. Haninger K, Thompson KM. Content and ratings of teen-rated video games. *JAMA*. 2004;291:856-865.
3. Thompson KM, Haninger K. Violence in E-rated video games. *JAMA*. 2001;286:591-598.
4. Haninger K, Ryan MS, Thompson KM. Violence in teen-rated video games. *MedGenMed*. 2004 March 11;6:1.
5. Cook DE, Kestenbaum C, Honaker LM, Anderson ER Jr; American Academy of Family Physicians; American Psychiatric Association. Joint statement on the impact of entertainment violence on children, congressional public health summit, July 26, 2000. Available at: http://www.aap.org/advocacy/releases/jstmtevc.htm. Accessed August 1, 2003.
6. American Academy of Pediatrics Committee on Communications. Media violence. *Pediatrics*. 1995;95:949-951.
7. Grossman D, Degaetano G. *Stop Teaching Our Kids to Kill: A Call to Action Against TV, Movie and Video Game Violence*. New York, NY: Crown; 1999.
8. Roberts DF, Foehr UG, Rideout VJ, Brodie M. *Kids & Media @ the New Millennium: A Comprehensive Analysis of Children's Media Use*. Menlo Park, Calif: Kaiser Family Foundation; 1999.
9. Roberts DF, Foehr UG, Rideout VJ. *Generation M: Media in the Lives of 8-18 Year-Olds*. Menlo Park, Calif: Kaiser Family Foundation; 2005.
10. Federal Trade Commission. Marketing violent entertainment to children: a fourth follow-up review of industry practices in the motion picture, music recording & electronic game industries. July 2004. Available at: http://www.ftc.gov/os/2004/07/040708kidsviolencerpt.pdf. Accessed May 4, 2005.
11. The NPD Group. Top 10 video game titles ranked by total US units sold in 2004. Available at: http://www.npdfunworld.com/funServlet?nextpage=trend_body.html&content_id=2079. Accessed August 29, 2005.
12. Canadian Teachers' Federation. Kids' take on media. Available at: http://www.ctf-fce.ca/bilingual/pubs/ctfreport/kidsenglish.pdf. Accessed November 4, 2005.
13. Saunders KW. Regulating youth access to violent video games: three responses to first amendment concerns. Michigan State-DCL Law Review, p 51, 2003. Available at: http://papers.ssrn.com/sol3/papers.cfm?abstract_id=443140.
14. Anderson CA, Bushman BJ. Effects of violent video games on aggressive behavior, aggressive cognition, aggressive affect, physiological arousal, and prosocial behavior: a meta-analytic review of the scientific literature. *Psychol Sci*. 2001;12:353-359.
15. Williams D, Skoric D. Internet fantasy violence: a test of aggression in an online game. *Commun Monogr*. 2005;72:217-233. Available at: http://www.ingentaconnect.com/content/routledg/rcmm/2005/00000072/00000002/art00005.
16. IGN games. Available at: http://games.ign.com. Accessed April 1, 2004.
17. GameSpot Web site. Available at: http://www.gamespot.com. Accessed April 1, 2004.
18. Game FAQs. GameSpot Web site. Available at: http://www.gamespot.com. Accessed April 1, 2004.
19. Thompson KM. Addicted media: substances on screen. *Child Adolesc Psychiatr Clin N Am*. 2005;14:473-489.
20. Entertainment Software Rating Board Web site. ESRB concludes investigation into *Grand Theft Auto: San Andreas*; revokes M (mature) rating (July 20, 2005). Available at: http://www.esrb.org/about_updates.asp#7-20-05. Accessed November 4, 2005.

ARTICLE

# Metabolic and Physiologic Responses to Video Game Play in 7- to 10-Year-Old Boys

*Xuewen Wang, MSEd; Arlette C. Perry, PhD*

**Objective:** To examine the metabolic, physiologic, and hemostatic responses to action video game play in a group of young boys.

**Design:** Comparison study.

**Setting:** Laboratory of Clinical and Applied Physiology, University of Miami.

**Participants:** Twenty-one boys aged 7 to 10 years.

**Main Outcome Measures:** Blood pressure monitored before and during game play and blood glucose and lactate levels measured before and immediately after game play. Measurements were continuously recorded throughout game play. Dependent *t* tests were used to compare measurements recorded at baseline and during or after game play. Effect sizes using the Cohen *d* were examined for comparisons.

**Results:** Significant increases from baseline were found for heart rate (18.8%; $P<.001$), systolic (22.3%; $P<.001$) and diastolic (5.8%; $P=.006$) blood pressure, ventilation (51.9%; $P<.001$), respiratory rate (54.8%; $P<.001$), oxygen consumption (49.0%; $P<.001$), and energy expenditure (52.9%; $P<.001$). Effect sizes for these comparisons were medium or large. No significant changes were found from baseline to after video game play for lactate (18.2% increase; $P=.07$) and glucose (0.9% decrease; $P=.59$) levels.

**Conclusions:** Video game play results in significant increases in various metabolic and physiologic variables in young children. Thus, it should not be combined with television viewing for the evaluation of sedentary activities. The magnitude of change, however, was lower than that observed during standard physical exercise and below national health recommendations. As such, video game play should not be considered a substitute for regular physical activities that significantly stress the metabolic pathways required for the promotion of cardiovascular conditioning.

*Arch Pediatr Adolesc Med. 2006;160:411-415*

THE PREVALENCE OF OBESITY and overweight is increasing in adults and children throughout the world.[1] For example, in children aged 6 to 11 years, the prevalence of obesity has increased from 6.5% (NHANES II [second National Health and Nutrition Examination Survey]) to 11.3% (NHANES III) to 15.3% (NHANES 1999-2000).[2] Although the rising prevalence of obesity is multifactorial, insufficient physical activity is suspected to play a primary role.[3] Television viewing is considered a sedentary behavior that has gained much attention recently. Children and adolescents have been reported to watch television for 2.77 to 3.54[4,5] hours per day, averaging 19.39 to 24.78 hours of television viewing per week. Dietz and Gortmaker[6] reported that each additional hour of television viewing per week increased the risk of obesity by 2%. The experimental study by Robinson[7] found strong evidence of a causal link between television viewing and children's overweight.

Television viewing and video game play may be combined for the purpose of evaluating sedentary behaviors.[8] Playing video games, however, may not be a passive activity and may not have the same impact on the prevalence of overweight as watching television. Watching television expends the same energy as sitting quietly.[9] Unlike television viewing, however, studies have shown increases in oxygen consumption ($VO_2$), blood pressure (BP), heart rate (HR), and energy cost in response to video game play. For example, Segal and Dietz[10] found that video game play significantly increased HR, systolic BP (SBP), diastolic BP (DBP), and $VO_2$ in 16- to 25-year-old young adults. Ridley and Olds[11] found that the magnitude of energy expenditure (EE) is related to the amount of body movement associated with video game play in 11- to 12-year-old children. However, there is a lack of research

**Author Affiliations:** Exercise and Sport Sciences Department, School of Education, University of Miami, Coral Gables, Fla.

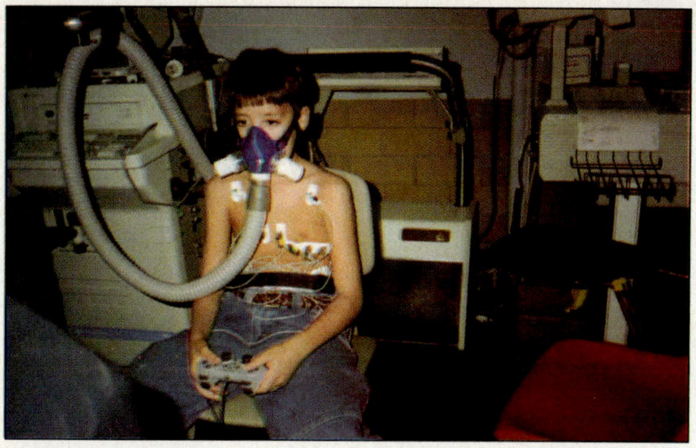

**Figure 1.** Video game data collection using a metabolic cart and an electrocardiograph.

in young children, who constitute a large video game consumer population.

Given the rising rates of childhood obesity and the implications of sedentary behaviors contributing to this problem, it is important to determine the calorie expenditure of video game play in young children. It is also important to examine additional metabolic responses to video game play, including glucose and lactate levels, to determine their comparability with values typically observed during exercise. Thus, the purpose of this study is to examine the metabolic and physiologic responses to action video game play in a group of 7- to 10-year-old boys.

## METHODS

### PARTCIPANTS

Volunteers were recruited through direct communication with local public school officials in after-school programs, parks and recreation departments, and youth centers. Volunteers enjoyed playing video games and considered themselves very experienced at playing all video games. All the participants were boys aged 7 to 10 years (10 were white, 9 were Hispanic, and 2 were African American). Testing was conducted at the Laboratory of Clinical and Applied Physiology, University of Miami. An informed consent form was signed by the participants and their parents in accordance with the guidelines of the institutional review board for the use of human subjects at the University of Miami. Before testing began, an orientation was given to all the parents and children to discuss the procedures and protocol requirements during testing.

### PROCEDURES

Height was measured in shoeless boys using a stadiometer (Detecto Scale Inc, Brooklyn, NY) and was recorded to the nearest 0.1 cm. Weight was measured to the nearest 0.1 kg using a balance scale (Detecto Scale Inc), with calibration procedures performed before data collection. Body mass index (BMI) was calculated as weight in kilograms divided by the square of height in meters.

After the participants maintained a seated position for 5 minutes, BP was measured twice by a trained investigator (A.C.P.) using standard procedures,[12] with 5 minutes of rest between the 2 measurements. The mean of the 2 measures was recorded to the nearest 2.0 mm Hg. If the 2 measurements were more than 4 mm Hg apart, a third measurement was taken after 5 minutes, and the mean of the 3 measurements was recorded. Blood pressure was measured by the same investigator halfway through game play.

Before video game play, all the participants underwent a familiarization period using the mask and electrodes required for testing. A simulated testing session without blood analysis and video game play was provided at this time so that participants felt more comfortable during actual testing.

A metabolic cart (model 2900; SensorMedics, Yorba Linda, Calif) was used to measure physiologic responses (including ventilation [VE], tidal volume, and respiratory rate) and metabolic responses (including $VO_2$ per kilogram, EE, and respiratory quotient) during video game play. Data were continuously monitored and recorded throughout the testing session. A small-sized 3-valve mask (Hans-Rudolph Inc, Kansas City, Mo) was fitted to the participant's face. The mask covered the boy's nose and mouth and was customized for each individual to ensure a tight seal around the edges. This was achieved by adding gauze to the nasal bridge area and petroleum jelly to the area on the perimeter of the mask. Both HR and 12-lead electrocardiography were continuously monitored using an electrocardiograph (MAX-1; SensorMedics) (**Figure 1**).

### HEMOSTATIC VARIABLES

Approximately 200 µL of blood was obtained from the tip of the middle finger of the nondominant hand as part of baseline data collection and before video game play. Blood samples were also obtained again from the top of the middle finger of the dominant hand immediately after completion of game play. Samples were immediately analyzed for lactate and glucose concentrations according to the user instructions of the VITROS DT60 II Analyzer (Johnson & Johnson Clinical Diagnostics Inc, Rochester, NY). Calibration was conducted in accordance with methods described by the manufacturer.

### VIDEO GAME

The video game *Tekken 3* (Namco Hometek Inc, San Jose, Calif), an action video game played on a Sony Playstation (Sony Computer Entertainment America, Foster City, Calif), was selected. Players controlled their character against the computer-controlled character in a mock martial arts contest. Buttons on the video game controller included "move left," "move right," "jump," "duck," "high punch," "low punch," "high kick," and "low kick." The participants started from the "Arcade Mode" and had identical game variables, including game time, opponent level, and game rules, throughout the study. Instructions regarding how to operate the video game were given to participants during the familiarization period and again immediately before video game play. The participants were allowed to pick their own character and to change this character at any time during the game. They were encouraged to do their best and were told that they were competing against other players in the study. The Playstation and video game console were turned on after 5 minutes of baseline data collection of metabolic and physiologic measurements. The Playstation and video game were turned off after 15 minutes of game play, and blood samples were obtained again. The mask was subsequently removed for the comfort of the child.

### ANALYTIC METHODS

All the statistical analyses were completed using a software program (SPSS version 10.1; SPSS Inc, Chicago, Ill). Mean ± SD are reported for all the variables. For each participant, mean values of measurements obtained by continuous monitoring us-

**Table 1. Comparison of Physiologic and Metabolic Measurements at Baseline vs During Video Game Play and of Hemostatic Measurements at Baseline vs After Game Play Using Dependent *t* Tests in 21 Boys**

| Measurement | Baseline, Mean ± SD | During or After Game Play, Mean ± SD | Change, % (95% CI) | *P* Value | Cohen *d* |
|---|---|---|---|---|---|
| Physiologic variables | | | | | |
| HR, beats · $min^{-1}$ | 86.9 ± 10.9 | 103.2 ± 7.0 | 18.8 (−21.52 to −10.99) | <.001 | 1.41* |
| SBP, mm Hg | 106.0 ± 16.8 | 129.6 ± 13.3 | 22.3 (−34.42 to −12.95) | <.001 | 1.00* |
| DBP, mm Hg | 67.0 ± 7.1 | 70.9 ± 6.2 | 5.8 (−6.57 to −1.24) | .006 | 0.67† |
| VE, L · $min^{-1}$ | 5.2 ± 1.6 | 7.9 ± 2.1 | 51.9 (−3.56 to −1.97) | <.001 | 1.59* |
| Tidal volume, L | 0.32 ± 0.08 | 0.31 ± 0.07 | −3.1 (−0.03 to 0.05) | .69 | 0.15 |
| Respiratory rate, per minute | 16.6 ± 4.6 | 25.7 ± 5.1 | 54.8 (−11.00 to −7.16) | <.001 | 2.16* |
| Metabolic variables | | | | | |
| $VO_2$, mL · $min^{-1}$ · $kg^{-1}$ | 4.90 ± 1.3 | 7.30 ± 1.6 | 49.0 (−3.06 to −1.64) | <.001 | 1.52* |
| RQ | 0.85 ± 0.04 | 0.84 ± 0.04 | −1.2 (−0.017 to 0.022) | .79 | 0.17 |
| Energy expenditure, kcal · $hr^{-1}$ · $kg^{-1}$ | 1.36 ± 0.44 | 2.08 ± 0.47 | 52.9 (−31.11 to −15.16) | <.001 | 1.49* |
| Hemostatic variables | | | | | |
| Glucose, mg · $dL^{-1}$ | 109.95 ± 7.93 | 108.95 ± 9.39 | −0.9 (−2.82 to 4.82) | .59 | 0.13 |
| Lactate, mmol · $L^{-1}$ | 1.92 ± 0.52 | 2.27 ± 0.68 | 18.2 (−0.73 to 0.036) | .07 | 0.41 |

Abbreviations: CI, confidence interval; DBP, diastolic blood pressure; HR, heart rate; RQ, respiratory quotient (calculated as carbon dioxide production/$VO_2$); SBP, systolic blood pressure; VE, ventilation; $VO_2$, oxygen consumption.

*A Cohen *d* value of 0.8 or greater indicates a large effect size.

†A Cohen *d* value of 0.50 to 0.8 indicates a medium effect size.

ing a metabolic cart and an electrocardiograph were calculated for the 5-minute baseline period, the 15 minutes of game play, and the most active 3 minutes of game play. Dependent *t* tests were used to compare measurements at baseline with those during video game play, including all the physiologic and metabolic variables. Mean values of measurements for the most active 3 minutes were also compared with their corresponding baseline values using dependent *t* tests. The most active minutes were simply those with the highest metabolic values. We chose to use the average of the most active 3 minutes rather than 1 minute to avoid any single aberrant or unusual value produced during a single minute of video game play. Thus, we used the most active 3 minutes rather than 1 minute against which to compare baseline values. Hemostatic measurements before game play were compared with those immediately after game play. $P \leq .05$ was considered statistically significant.

Effect sizes for the dependent *t* tests were examined using the Cohen *d*. A *d* value of 0.8 or greater refers to a large effect size, and a value of 0.5 to 0.8 refers to a medium effect size. Both large and medium effect sizes have been used to indicate a substantial difference between means. A Cohen *d* value less than 0.5 refers to a small effect size, which indicates a trivial difference between mean values.

## RESULTS

Twenty-one boys volunteered for the study (age, 8.8±1.1 years; height, 139.5±7.4 cm; weight, 31.8±7.6 kg; and BMI, 16.2±3.0). The height, weight, and BMI of the participants were at the 90th, 75th, and 25th percentile, respectively, for their age and sex.[13,14]

**Table 1** includes comparisons of metabolic and physiologic measurements at baseline and during game play and comparison of hemostatic variables at baseline and immediately after game play. Values during game play were significantly higher than their respective baseline values for HR, SBP, DBP, VE, respiratory rate, $VO_2$, and EE. Specifically, $VO_2$ showed a 49.0% increase, from 4.90 to 7.30 mL·$min^{-1}$·$kg^{-1}$, and EE showed a 52.9% increase, from 1.36 to 2.08 kcal·$hr^{-1}$·$kg^{-1}$. Of the aforementioned variables, HR, SBP, VE, respiratory rate, $VO_2$, and EE had Cohen *d* values much greater than 0.8, thereby reflecting large effect sizes. Diastolic BP showed an increase in medium effect size. In contrast, tidal volume, respiratory quotient, and glucose concentration showed numerical decreases; however, their *t* test values were not significant, and their effect sizes were small. Lactate level showed a nonsignificant increase and a small effect size.

**Table 2** provides the significant results from dependent *t* tests comparing metabolic and physiologic measurements during baseline with those during the most active 3 minutes of video game play. Significantly greater values were observed for the most active 3 minutes compared with baseline for HR, VE, respiratory rate, $VO_2$, and EE. Cohen *d* values for these comparisons substantially exceeded 0.8, thereby reflecting large effect sizes. The $VO_2$ showed a 75.5% increase, from 4.90 to 8.60 mL·$min^{-1}$·$kg^{-1}$, and EE showed an 86.0% increase, from 1.36 to 2.53 kcal·$hr^{-1}$·$kg^{-1}$. In summary, most metabolic and physiologic variables examined during video game play showed significant increases from baseline. Furthermore, VE, respiratory rate, $VO_2$, and EE showed a 75% or greater increase from baseline to the most active 3 minutes of video game play. Hemostatic variables did not show significant changes after video game play.

## COMMENT

The present study evaluated the metabolic and physiologic effects of video game play in young children. Participants included white, Hispanic, and African American boys averaging 8.8 years of age with above-average height and weight and a low BMI. Their mean resting SBP and DBP were 106.0 and 67.0 mm Hg, respectively, which are considered average for their age and sex. To our knowl-

**Table 2. Significant Results From Dependent *t* Tests Comparing Physiologic and Metabolic Measurements at Baseline and During the Most Active 3 Minutes of Video Game Play in 21 Boys**

| Measurement | Baseline, Mean ± SD | Most Active 3 Minutes, Mean ± SD | Change, % (95% CI) | Cohen *d** |
|---|---|---|---|---|
| Physiologic variables | | | | |
| HR, beats · $min^{-1}$ | 86.9 ± 10.9 | 116.0 ± 12.2 | 33.5 (−36.35 to −11.43) | 1.63 |
| VE, L · $min^{-1}$ | 5.2 ± 1.6 | 9.5 ± 2.3 | 82.7 (−5.50 to −3.26) | 1.78 |
| Respiratory rate, per minute | 16.6 ± 4.6 | 30.3 ± 6.1 | 82.5 (−16.77 to −10.64) | 2.04 |
| Metabolic variables | | | | |
| $VO_2$, mL · $min^{-1}$ · $kg^{-1}$ | 4.90 ± 1.3 | 8.60 ± 2.0 | 75.5 (−151.29 to −82.27) | 1.60 |
| Energy expenditure, kcal · $hr^{-1}$ · $kg^{-1}$ | 1.36 ± 0.44 | 2.53 ± 0.58 | 86.0 (−45.94 to −26.74) | 1.79 |

Abbreviations: CI, confidence interval; HR, heart rate; VE, ventilation; $VO_2$, oxygen consumption.
*A Cohen *d* value of 0.8 or greater indicates a large effect size. $P<.001$ for all.

edge, this is the first study to examine the metabolic and physiologic responses to video game play in children younger than 10 years. It is also the first study to measure serum glucose and lactate levels before and after video game play.

These findings show that during action video game play there was a significant increase in EE. The values rose to levels similar to those reported by Ridley and Olds,[11] whose participants played driving simulation games and were older (mean age, 12.5 years). Because our average EE during game play was 2.08 kcal · $h^{-1}$ · $kg^{-1}$ body weight and the reported average time children spend playing video games is 20 to 39 minutes a day,[4,5,15] a 9-year-old child at 28.5 kg (50th percentile for body weight[13]) may expend an extra 19.76 to 38.53 kcal daily by playing video games. Although this value seems small, after many years, it translates into weight loss of approximately 1.8 kg per year and 9.0 kg in 5 years.

In addition, physiologic changes elicited by video game play included a 22.3% increase in SBP and a 5.8% increase in DBP, which are in accordance with changes seen for adults during video game play.[10,16,17] Our results show that the mean BP was 129.6/70.9 mm Hg and that the mean HR was 103.2 beats · $min^{-1}$ during game play. Although the highest SBP during game play was 150 mm Hg for 1 participant, the increases in BP or HR generally did not represent a clinically significant or unsafe situation for participants during video game play (Table 1).

We found that respiratory rate and VE increased statistically significantly during game play. Denot-Ledunois and colleagues[18] concluded that video game play may increase arousal and elicit a strong emotional response, both of which would lead to the observed increase in breathing frequency and VE in our study. On the other hand, the act of focusing attention on game play may actually prompt children to inhibit any movement and, in particular, breathing. According to the previous investigators,[18] the increases in breathing rate and VE found in our study were most likely due to a stronger arousal and emotional component during game play than to attention load.

We also measured serum glucose and lactate levels before and after video game play. The purpose of examining these measures was to compare metabolic responses with those typically observed during regular exercise. Lactate levels, which typically increase during exercise, increased 18.2% from baseline to after game play; however, the change was not statistically significant. Because many video games involve hand movements, which constitute activation of a small amount of body mass, one would expect video games that invoke larger body mass movements to result in greater accumulation of lactate. Glucose levels barely changed during video game play, which is in contrast to what has been observed in response to physical exercise.[19] Therefore, video game play did not elicit the same metabolic responses as exercise, which may be because of the smaller amount of muscle mass involved.

Investigators often use metabolic equivalents (METs) to quantify the intensity of exercise, thereby enabling comparison of intensity across different exercises. One MET is equivalent to 3.5 mL $O_2$ · $kg^{-1}$ · $min^{-1}$, which represents the energy expended at rest. In the present study, the mean $VO_2$ at baseline was 4.9 mL · $kg^{-1}$ · $min^{-1}$, corresponding to 1.4 METs. It was somewhat higher than expected, indicating that our children may have some level of excitation or arousal in anticipation of game play. The mean $VO_2$ during video game play was 7.30 mL · $kg^{-1}$ · $min^{-1}$ and during the most active 3 minutes was 8.60 mL · $kg^{-1}$ · $min^{-1}$, corresponding to 2.1 and 2.5 METs, respectively. The calculated energy cost during video game play was approximately equivalent to walking 2.0 mph,[9] which is similar to that reported by Segal and Dietz[10] for adults. In addition, SBP, DBP, and HR in the present study increased to approximately the same level shown for cycling at a work rate of 60 W or walking at 3 mph in boys of similar age and body composition.[20] In contrast, the $VO_2$ values observed in this study were much lower than those for cycling at 60 W or walking at 3 mph. Based on $VO_2$ and MET levels, the intensity of video game play is less than moderate. Public health officials have suggested that 20 to 30 minutes of moderate to vigorous activity per day is recommended for children. In fact, up to 60 or more minutes of moderate-intensity activity daily has been recommended by several health organizations.[21] Therefore, video game play is insufficient for children to meet these guidelines, although metabolic variables were significantly higher than those observed at baseline.

Recent studies[22,23] have also shown a significant association between electronic game use and obesity, with nearly a 2-fold increased risk of obesity for every hour spent playing electronic games daily.[22] An inverse relationship between time spent using video games and daily physical activity has also been observed.[24] Thus, if video game play is used as a substitute for regular physical activity, the positive association between game play and obesity is certainly plausible; however, if it is used to replace time spent watching television or simply resting, video game play can serve to more positively affect EE. The volunteers in our study considered themselves to be very experienced at video game play, yet they were very slender for their age.

There are several limitations that should be noted regarding this study. First, the sample size was small, and the participants were all relatively lean. Children with large BMIs may manifest different EE levels during video game play than lean children. Therefore, we could not generalize our results to larger samples in practice. Second, no girls were included in this study. Because in adults there are reported sex differences in free fatty acid, glycogen, and glucose use during exercise,[25] we believed that combining boys and girls might confound the results of metabolic variables during video game play. Third, the data were collected in a laboratory. Although the children were familiarized with the equipment and testing procedures before actual data collection, it still was not a natural setting in which children typically play video games. This was observed because the baseline MET level was higher than 1 and thereby might have resulted in a smaller increase during game play.

In summary, the present study demonstrates that video game play is not a passive activity in young children because it results in significant increases in various physiologic and metabolic responses. As such, we recommend not combining it with television viewing for the purpose of evaluating sedentary activities. In contrast, the intensity of video game play is insufficient for the enhancement of cardiovascular conditioning. Despite similarities between video game play and cycling or walking with respect to physiologic variables, such as HR and BP, metabolic variables, such as $VO_2$, glucose, and lactate levels, were lower than those associated with physical exercise. These differences may have been due to the smaller amount of muscle mass actually used during video game play. Thus, although video game play should not be considered a sedentary activity, it should in no way be considered a substitute for regular physical activities that significantly stress the metabolic pathways required for the enhancement of cardiovascular conditioning.

**Accepted for Publication:** June 3, 2005.
**Correspondence:** Arlette C. Perry, PhD, Exercise and Sport Sciences Department, School of Education, University of Miami, PO Box 248065, Coral Gables, FL 33124 (aperry@miami.edu).

## REFERENCES

1. World Health Organization. *Obesity, Preventing and Managing the Global Epidemic: Report of the WHO Consultation of Obesity.* Geneva, Switzerland: World Health Organization; 1997.
2. Ogden CL, Carroll MD, Flegal KM. Epidemiologic trends in overweight and obesity. *Endocrinol Metab Clin North Am.* 2003;32:741-760.
3. Boreham C, Riddoch C. The physical activity, fitness and health of children. *J Sports Sci.* 2001;19:915-929.
4. Roberts DF, Foehr UG, Rideout VJ, Brodie M. *Kids & Media @ the New Millennium: A Comprehensive National Analysis of Children's Media Use.* Menlo Park, Calif: Henry J. Kaiser Family Foundation; 1999.
5. Woodard E, Gridina N. *Media in the Home 2000: The Fifth Annual Survey of Parents and Children.* Philadelphia: Annenberg Public Center, University of Pennsylvania; 2000.
6. Dietz WH Jr, Gortmaker SL. Do we fatten our children at the television set? obesity and television viewing in children and adolescents. *Pediatrics.* 1985;75:807-812.
7. Robinson TN. Television viewing and childhood obesity. *Pediatr Clin North Am.* 2001;48:1017-1025.
8. von Kries R, Toschke AM, Koletzko B, Slikker W Jr. Maternal smoking during pregnancy and childhood obesity. *Am J Epidemiol.* 2002;156:954-961.
9. Ainsworth BE, Haskell WL, Leon AS, et al. Compendium of physical activities: classification of energy costs of human physical activities. *Med Sci Sports Exerc.* 1993;25:71-80.
10. Segal KR, Dietz WH. Physiologic resoponses to playing a video game. *AJDC.* 1991;145:1034-1036.
11. Ridley K, Olds T. Video center games: energy cost and children's behaviors. *Pediatr Exerc Sci.* 2001;13:413-421.
12. Kirkendall WM, Burton AC, Epstein FH, Freis ED. Recommendations for human blood pressure determination by sphygmomanometers. *Circulation.* 1967;36:980-988.
13. National Center for Health Statistics. Birth to 36 months: boys: length-for-age and weight-for-age percentiles. Available at: http://www.cdc.gov/nchs/data/nhanes/growthcharts/set2clinical/cj41l067.pdf. Accessed November 21, 2000.
14. National Center for Health Statistics. 2 to 20 years: boys: body mass index-for-age percentiles. Available at: http://www.cdc.gov/nchs/data/nhanes/growthcharts/set2clinical/cj41l073.pdf. Accessed October 16, 2000.
15. Stanger J, Gridina N. *Media in the Home 1999: The Fourth Annual Survey of Parents and Children.* Philadelphia: Annenberg Public Center, University of Pennsylvania; 1999.
16. Gwinup G, Haw T, Elias A. Cardiovascular changes in video-game players: cause for concern? *Postgrad Med.* 1983;74:245-248.
17. Turner JR, Carroll D. Heart rate and oxygen consumption during mental arithmetic, a video game, and graded exercise: further evidence of metabolically-exaggerated cardiac adjustments? *Psychophysiology.* 1985;22:261-267.
18. Denot-Ledunois S, Vardon G, Perruchet P, Gallego J. The effect of attentional load on the breathing pattern in children. *Int J Psychophysiol.* 1998;29:13-21.
19. Coggan AR. Plasma glucose metabolism during exercise in humans. *Sports Med.* 1991;11:102-124.
20. Turley KR, Wilmore JH. Cardiovascular responses to submaximal exercise in 7- to 9-yr-old boys and girls. *Med Sci Sports Exerc.* 1997;29:824-832.
21. Fulton JE, Garg M, Galuska DA, Rattay KT, Caspersen CJ. Public health and clinical recommendations for physical activity and physical fitness: special focus on overweight youth. *Sports Med.* 2004;34:581-599.
22. Stettler N, Signer TM, Suter PM. Electronic games and environmental factors associated with childhood obesity in Switzerland. *Obes Res.* 2004;12:896-903.
23. Tremblay MS, Willms JD. Is the Canadian childhood obesity epidemic related to physical inactivity? *Int J Obes Relat Metab Disord.* 2003;27:1100-1105.
24. Janz KF, Mahoney LT. Maturation, gender, and video game playing are related to physical activity intensity in adolescents: the Muscation Study. *Pediatr Exerc Sci.* 1997;9:353-363.
25. Tarnopolsky MA, Ruby BC. Sex differences in carbohydrate metabolism. *Curr Opin Clin Nutr Metab Care.* 2001;4:521-526.

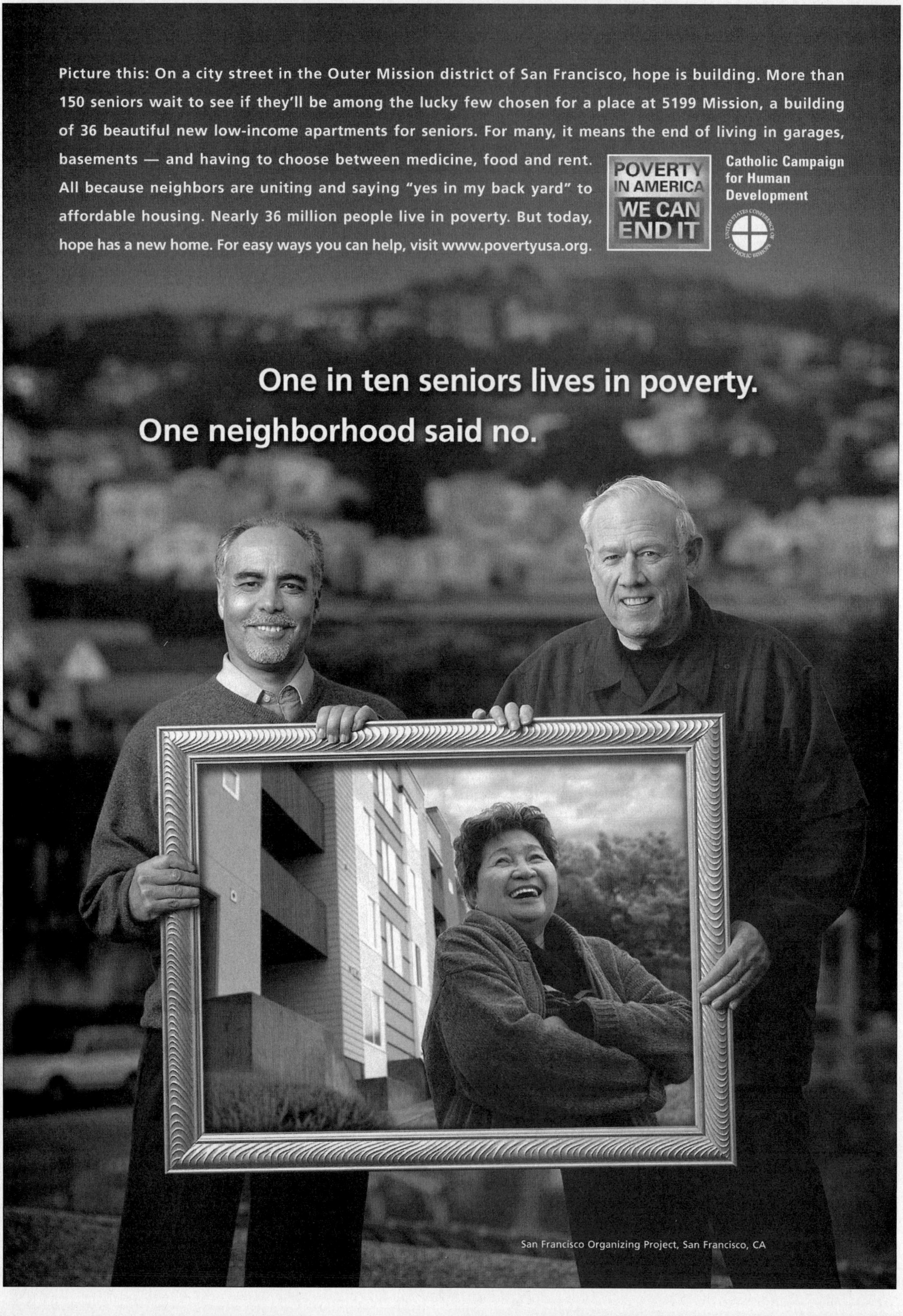
Picture this: On a city street in the Outer Mission district of San Francisco, hope is building. More than 150 seniors wait to see if they'll be among the lucky few chosen for a place at 5199 Mission, a building of 36 beautiful new low-income apartments for seniors. For many, it means the end of living in garages, basements — and having to choose between medicine, food and rent. All because neighbors are uniting and saying "yes in my back yard" to affordable housing. Nearly 36 million people live in poverty. But today, hope has a new home. For easy ways you can help, visit www.povertyusa.org.
POVERTY IN AMERICA
WE CAN END IT
Catholic Campaign for Human Development
UNITED STATES CONFERENCE OF CATHOLIC BISHOPS
One in ten seniors lives in poverty.
One neighborhood said no.
San Francisco Organizing Project, San Francisco, CA

# Television Exposure and Overweight Risk in Preschoolers

*Julie C. Lumeng, MD; Sahand Rahnama, BS; Danielle Appugliese, MPH; Niko Kaciroti, PhD; Robert H. Bradley, PhD*

**Objective:** To test the independent effect of television exposure in preschool-aged children on overweight risk.

**Design:** Cross-sectional and longitudinal analysis of the National Institute of Child Health and Human Development Study of Early Child Care and Youth Development.

**Setting:** Ten US sites.

**Participants:** One thousand sixteen children selected via conditional random sampling.

**Main Exposure:** Being awake in the room with the television on for 2 hours or more per day, by maternal report at age 36 months.

**Main Outcome Measures:** Child overweight (body mass index [calculated as weight in kilograms divided by the square of height in meters] ≥95th percentile) calculated from measured anthropometrics at ages 36 and 54 months. Covariates tested included child sex and race; maternal marital status, education, age, and depressive symptoms; income-needs ratio, child behavior problems; Home Observation for Measurement of the Environment total score; hours per week in nonparental care; and proportion of television exposure that was educational.

**Results:** At age 36 months, 5.8% of children were overweight; at age 54 months, 10.0% were overweight. Exposure to 2 or more hours of television per day was associated with an increased risk of overweight at both age 36 months (odds ratio, 2.92; 95% confidence interval, 1.36-6.24) and age 54 months (odds ratio, 1.71; 95% confidence interval, 1.03-2.83) in unadjusted analyses. Only maternal age altered the concurrent relationship, and the effect of television remained significant (odds ratio, 2.61; 95% confidence interval, 1.21-5.62). Television exposure at age 36 months was no longer a significant predictor of overweight at age 54 months when controlling for covariates.

**Conclusion:** Excessive television exposure is a risk factor for overweight in preschoolers independent of a number of potential confounders associated with the quality of the home environment.

*Arch Pediatr Adolesc Med. 2006;160:417-422*

**Author Affiliations:** Center for Human Growth and Development (Drs Lumeng and Kaciroti and Mr Rahnama) and Department of Pediatrics and Communicable Diseases (Dr Lumeng), University of Michigan, Ann Arbor; Data Coordinating Center, Boston University, Boston, Mass (Ms Appugliese); and Center for Applied Studies in Education, University of Arkansas at Little Rock (Dr Bradley).

EXCESSIVE TELEVISION (TV) viewing has been linked to a variety of adverse outcomes in children.[1,2] The relationship between TV viewing and overweight risk has been more thoroughly described in school-aged[3-10] than in preschool-aged[11-17] children, and only 2 studies in preschoolers control for important potential confounders.[12,13] The American Academy of Pediatrics recommends that total media time be limited to less than 2 hours per day in children aged 2 years and older.[2] Helping families achieve this goal requires more information, including whether the relationship is confounded by family characteristics that have not been previously controlled, such as overall quality of the home environment or maternal depressive symptoms. In addition, the relationship in US children has been evaluated only in low-income groups,[13] who watch significantly more television.[18] It is possible that the relationship may be stronger in low-income populations or that important confounders of the relationship are present to a greater degree in low-income families. Excessive television viewing in preschoolers may also simply be a marker for an understimulating home environment, which has been independently linked to overweight risk.[19]

The present study seeks to address these gaps in the current literature. We investigate the relationship between television exposure and overweight risk in an age range in which there are limited data and in socioeconomic strata of the United States in which it has not previously been studied in large samples. We control for a number of covariates that have not previously been available and examine both the cross-sectional and longitudinal relationships between television exposure and overweight risk. We hypothesized that a relationship between excessive television exposure and overweight risk would be present both cross-sectionally and longitudinally, but that it would be confounded by markers of quality of the home environment.

## METHODS

The sample was composed of children and their parents enrolled in the National Institute of Child Health and Human Development Study of Early Child Care and Youth Development.[20] This is a longitudinal study of relations between child behavior and development, particularly in relation to child care experience. Families were recruited shortly after the birth of a child in 1991 from 10 areas of the United States, both urban and rural. Details of the recruitment methods and sampling plan are available elsewhere.[21] The initial sample included 1364 children and was representative of the demographics of the catchment areas from which the sample was recruited.[20] We examined the cross-sectional relationship between television exposure and overweight risk with data collected at age 36 months and the longitudinal relationship with data collected at ages 36 and 54 months. This study was approved by the institutional review boards of all pertinent institutions.

Our outcome measure in the cross-sectional analysis was overweight status at age 36 months. We evaluated 3 outcome measures in the longitudinal analysis: overweight status at age 54 months; incidence of new cases of overweight between the ages of 36 and 54 months; and change in body mass index (BMI), calculated as weight in kilograms divided by the square of height in meters, between the ages of 36 and 54 months.[22] Height and weight were measured during the laboratory visits at ages 36 and 54 months by trained research assistants.[23] Body mass index was calculated and child overweight defined dichotomously as a BMI greater than or equal to the 95th percentile for age and sex based on National Center for Health Statistics norms.[24]

Mothers reported hours of TV exposure by questionnaire when the child was aged 36 months, describing 2 weekdays (Tuesday and Wednesday) and 2 weekend days for each of the three 6-hour time blocks between 6 AM and midnight in 15-minute increments. Television exposure was defined as "being awake in the room when the television is on" and included both broadcast and cable television as well as videos.[25] The mean±SD television exposure on weekdays (3.61±2.53 hours) and on weekends (3.58±2.67 hours) were correlated ($r$=0.75, $P$<.001). We indexed average daily TV exposure by multiplying mean weekday exposure by 5, summing this with mean weekend exposure, and dividing by 7. Given that the American Academy of Pediatrics recommends less than 2 hours of media exposure per day,[1,2] we dichotomized our predictor to "less than 2 hours of television per day" vs "greater than or equal to 2 hours of television per day" to simplify interpretation of the results.

Demographic data consisted of the child's sex, the child's race/ethnicity ("white" or "not white"), maternal marital status ("single" vs "not"), years of maternal education, and maternal age. Additional characteristics hypothesized to modify an association between TV exposure and overweight were often available only for a subset of subjects and were therefore tested as potential covariates separately from the main analysis. Parents reported average hours per day in nonparental care via telephone interview every 3 months, and we calculated average hours per day in nonparental care between the ages of 24 and 36 months (n=1016). Maternal depressive symptoms were indexed with the Center for Epidemiologic Studies Depression scale (n=928), one of the most widely used and validated measures of depressive symptomatology, which asks respondents to self-report the frequency of 20 depressive symptoms. Potential scores range from 0 to 60, with higher scores reflecting more depressive symptoms and scores greater than 16 reflecting a high risk for a clinical diagnosis of depression.[26]

The income-to-needs ratio (n=912) is the ratio of total family income relative to the poverty line for a family of a particular size. A family with an income-to-needs ratio less than 1 is considered "poor." Child behavioral problems were indexed with the Child Behavior Checklist (n=1014), a 99-item rating scale that is the most widely used assessment of behavioral problems in young children.[27] Scores are presented as T scores that have a mean of 50 with a standard deviation of 15. A cut-off of 70 is frequently used to denote clinically significant behavioral problems. The quality of the home environment was measured by the Home Observation for Measurement of the Environment (HOME) (n=996), one of the most widely used indices of the quality and quantity of stimulation and support available to a child in the home. Information is obtained during a home visit via observation and interview. It is composed of 55 items, each of which is scored in a binary fashion (yes/no), with scores therefore ranging from 0 to 55 and higher scores indicating higher-quality home environments. The HOME has consistently been correlated with cognitive, language, achievement, and social-emotional outcomes.[28]

We included an index of educational TV exposure based on the hypothesis that educational programming is higher quality and would therefore potentially promote healthier eating habits and exercise or, at a minimum, limit exposure to unhealthy advertising messages. Parents reported, in the same format described earlier, exposure to 6 programs comprising a significant proportion of children's programming on the Public Broadcasting Service in the early 1990s.[25] Mean±SD daily educational TV exposure (1.70±1.68 hours) was correlated with average daily total TV exposure (3.59±2.50 hours) ($r$=0.64, $P$<.001). We calculated the proportion of total daily TV exposure that was educational (n=917).

All data analysis was performed using SAS 8.2 (SAS Institute Inc, Cary, NC). We excluded children without data for television exposure (n=267) or BMI at age 36 months (n=273). We examined the sample included in our model (n=1016) vs those excluded because of missing data (n=348) and found significant differences. Neither average daily TV exposure nor overweight prevalence at age 36 months differed significantly in those with and without complete data ($P$=.51 and $P$=.67, respectively). Children included in the sample compared with those excluded were more likely to be white (82.8% vs 73.6%, $P$<.001) and had mothers who were more educated (14.4 vs 13.7 years, $P$<.001). We tested the location of data collection (each of the 10 sites) as a variable in the final model, as well as its interaction term, and found these to be nonsignificant.

Univariate statistics were first computed to provide a description of the sample of 1016 children. Then, bivariate analyses were performed to inform the development of the multiple logistic regression models. We analyzed all covariates by TV exposure (<2 hours per day vs ≥2 hours per day) using $t$ tests for continuous variables and cross tabulations with $\chi^2$ tests for categorical variables. We sought to confirm the utility of the American Academy of Pediatrics–defined cut point of fewer than 2 hours of television per day and therefore performed a logistic regression analysis evaluating the relationship between TV exposure and overweight risk at age 36 months by quartile of average daily TV exposure (with cut points at 1.75, 3.00, and 4.90 hours per day). All remaining analyses use TV exposure (<2 hours per day vs ≥2 hours per day) as the primary predictor.

To evaluate the cross-sectional relationship between TV exposure and overweight risk at age 36 months, we first created a logistic regression model adjusting for the demographic covariates sex; race/ethnicity; and maternal marital status, education, and age simultaneously. Second, a base model was created using maximum likelihood ratios to derive the most parsimonious model with the best fit for the demographic covariates (sex; race/ethnicity; and maternal marital status, education, and age). Doing so allowed us to limit the number of covariates included simultaneously in the model, thereby maintaining the stability of the model when the additional covariates of interest were tested. After this base model was identified, we tested additional covariates, most of which were only available for a subset of the sample, each individually in the model as potential confounders. These were hours per day in nonparental care, Center for Epidemiologic Studies Depression scale score, income-needs ratio, Child Behavior Checklist total score, HOME score, and proportion of TV exposure that was educational.

To evaluate the longitudinal relationship between TV exposure at age 36 months and overweight risk at age 54 months, we repeated the analysis described earlier but with overweight status at age 54 months as the outcome (both with and without BMI $z$ score at age 36 months as a covariate in the model). We also evaluated incidence (new cases of overweight emerging between the ages 36 and 54 months) as an outcome. We evaluated change in BMI between the ages 36 and 54 months using multiple linear regression and the Mallows Cp criterion[29] to identify the most parsimonious model for this continuous outcome.

We computed both unadjusted and adjusted odds ratios (ORs) and their corresponding 95% confidence intervals (CIs) from the logistic regression models. We used a $P$ value of less than .05 (2-tailed) to determine statistical significance.

**Table 1. Characteristics of Children by Amount of Television Exposure Per Day**

| Characteristic | <2 Hours TV per Day (n = 322) | ≥2 Hours TV per Day (n = 694) | P Value |
|---|---|---|---|
| Child overweight at age 36 m, % | | | .004 |
| Yes | 2.5 | 6.9 | |
| No | 97.5 | 93.1 | |
| Sex, % | | | .23 |
| Male | 53.7 | 49.7 | |
| Female | 46.3 | 50.3 | |
| Race, % | | | <.001 |
| White | 89.4 | 79.7 | |
| Not white | 10.6 | 20.3 | |
| Maternal marital status, % | | | .004 |
| Single | 8.4 | 14.8 | |
| Not single | 91.6 | 85.2 | |
| Maternal education, mean (SD), y | 15.4 (2.7) | 14.0 (2.3) | <.001 |
| Maternal age, mean (SD), y | 29.8 (5.1) | 27.8 (5.6) | <.001 |
| Income-needs ratio, mean (SD) | 4.5 (4.2) | 3.2 (2.6) | <.001 |
| Child Behavior Checklist total score, mean (SD) | 31.7 (17.2) | 38.6 (18.2) | <.001 |
| Center for Epidemiologic Studies Depression scale score, mean (SD) | 8.2 (7.2) | 10.4 (8.6) | <.001 |
| HOME total score, mean (SD) | 43.5 (7.2) | 41.0 (7.2) | <.001 |
| Time in nonparental care, mean (SD), h/wk | 22.0 (15.8) | 22.6 (17.2) | .58 |
| Proportion of TV exposure that was educational, mean (SD) | 0.60 (0.30) | 0.50 (0.30) | <.001 |

Abbreviations: HOME, Home Observation for Measurement of the Environment; TV, television.

## RESULTS

The sample included 1016 children. About half of the sample was male and 5.5% were overweight (BMI ≥95th percentile).[30,31] Fewer than one third (31.7%) of children were exposed to less than 2 hours of TV per day. In bivariate analyses, 2 or more hours of television exposure per day was associated with families who were less likely to be white; were more likely to be headed by single mothers; had lower income-needs ratios, lower HOME scores, and a lower proportion of television exposure that was educational; and had less educated, younger mothers with more depressive symptoms. Children exposed to 2 or more hours of TV per day had more reported behavior problems. Child sex and hours in nonparental care were not related to TV exposure (**Table 1**).

### TELEVISION EXPOSURE AT AGE 36 MONTHS AND CONCURRENT OVERWEIGHT STATUS

Bivariate analyses showed that children who were exposed to 2 or more hours of TV per day were significantly more likely to be overweight than children exposed to less than 2 hours of TV per day ($P$=.004) (Table 1). We first evaluated the unadjusted risk of overweight in each quartile of TV exposure in a cross-tabulation and found higher risk of overweight in quartiles 2 through 4 in comparison with children watching 1.75 or fewer hours of TV per day (TV exposure in quartile 1). We found that 2.0% of those in the first quartile (least TV exposure) were overweight, compared with 5.6% in the second quartile, 5.8% in the third quartile, and 8.8% in the fourth quartile (greatest amount of TV exposure). We estimated this relationship in logistic regression models. Using quartile 1 as a reference, each of the 3 other quartiles conferred additional obesity risk in the unadjusted analysis ($P$=.02): quartile 2, OR, 2.98, 95% CI, 1.06-8.40; quartile 3, OR, 3.06, 95% CI, 1.10-8.55; and quartile 4, OR, 4.87, 95% CI, 1.81-13.06. Overweight risk did not differ significantly between quartiles 2, 3, and 4. In summary, results of the quartile analysis supported dichotomizing TV exposure by the American Academy of Pediatrics guidelines, and we proceeded with additional analyses using this dichotomous variable as the predictor in our models.

A relationship between 2 or more hours of TV exposure per day and overweight at age 36 months was present in the unadjusted analysis (OR, 2.92; 95% CI, 1.36-6.24). In the unadjusted analyses, both maternal age and income-needs ratio were found to be associated with overweight while maternal education and marital status approached statistical significance (**Table 2**). In the adjusted analysis controlling for all demographic covariates (sex; race; and maternal education, marital status, and age) simultaneously, a relationship between TV exposure and overweight at age 36 months persisted (Table 2).

In the analysis resulting from using the maximum likelihood ratio to derive the most parsimonious model, both watching 2 or more hours of TV per day (OR, 2.61; 95% CI, 1.21-5.62) and maternal age (OR, 0.95; 95% CI, 0.90-0.995) predicted overweight at age 36 months. We tested for the presence of an interaction between TV exposure and maternal age and it was not statistically significant,

**Table 2. Unadjusted and Adjusted Odds Ratios for Concurrent Overweight at Age 36 Months for 1016 Children**

| Covariate | Unadjusted | | Adjusted* | |
|---|---|---|---|---|
| | OR (95% CI) | *P* Value | OR (95% CI) | *P* Value |
| ≥2 h TV exposure per day | 2.92 (1.36-6.24) | .006 | 2.64 (1.21-5.76) | .01 |
| Sex | | | | .68 |
| Male | 1.12 (0.65-1.92) | .69 | 1.12 (0.65-1.94) | |
| Female | 1.00 | | 1.00 | |
| Race | | | | .25 |
| White | 0.96 (0.47-1.93) | .90 | 1.58 (0.72-3.47) | |
| Not white | 1.00 | | 1.00 | |
| Maternal education | 0.89 (0.80-1.00) | .05 | 0.99 (0.86-1.14) | .93 |
| Maternal age | 0.94 (0.89-0.98) | .009 | 0.95 (0.89-1.01) | .11 |
| Mother single | 1.94 (1.00-3.79) | .05 | 1.64 (0.75-3.55) | .21 |
| Income-needs ratio | 0.84 (0.74-0.96) | .01 | NA | NA |
| Child Behavior Checklist total score | 1.01 (1.00-1.03) | .09 | NA | NA |
| Center for Epidemiologic Studies Depression scale score | 1.01 (0.98-1.05) | .42 | NA | NA |
| HOME total score | 0.97 (0.94-1.00) | .08 | NA | NA |
| Time in nonparental care | 1.00 (0.98-1.01) | .72 | NA | NA |
| Proportion of TV exposure that was educational | 0.92 (0.33-2.49) | .86 | NA | NA |

Abbreviations: CI, confidence interval; HOME, Home Observation for Measurement of the Environment; NA, not applicable; OR, odds ratio; TV, television.
*Adjusted for demographic covariates.

indicating that the relationship between TV exposure and overweight did not differ based on maternal age. Per our analytic plan, we next tested each additional covariate (hours per day in nonparental care, maternal depressive symptoms, income-needs ratio, child behavior problems, quality of the home environment, and proportion of TV exposure that was educational) individually in the model with TV exposure and maternal age. None of these covariates were statistically significant in these models, nor did they significantly alter the relationship between TV exposure and overweight risk at age 36 months.

### TELEVISION EXPOSURE AT AGE 36 MONTHS AND FUTURE OVERWEIGHT STATUS AT AGE 54 MONTHS

Data regarding TV exposure at age 36 months and anthropometric data at age 54 months were available for 946 of 1016 subjects. Of these 946, 10% were overweight at age 54 months. In the unadjusted analysis, 2 or more hours of TV exposure per day predicted overweight status at age 54 months (OR, 1.71; 95% CI, 1.03-2.83). After adjusting for demographic covariates (sex; race; and maternal education, marital status, and age), however, the main effect of TV exposure became nonsignificant. The most parsimonious model predicting overweight at age 54 months created using maximum likelihood ratios included only maternal education. Television exposure was not statistically significant in the model.

Anthropometric data were available at both ages 36 and 54 months for 893 children. Of the 852 children who were not overweight at age 36 months, 62 became overweight by age 54 months. Watching 2 or more hours of TV per day did not predict the new onset of overweight at age 54 months in the unadjusted analysis (OR, 0.74; 95% CI, 0.42-1.32), nor did it predict the change in BMI from ages 36 to 54 months in the unadjusted analysis ($P = .39$).

## COMMENT

Results indicated that being awake in a room with a television on for 2 or more hours per day at age 36 months was independently associated with an increased concurrent risk of overweight. To our knowledge, this study is the first to investigate the relationship between excessive TV exposure and childhood overweight in a preschool-aged sample with geographic, ethnic, and socioeconomic diversity while analytically controlling for a large number of potentially confounding factors. Children who watched 2 or more hours of TV per day had more behavior problems and mothers with more depressive symptoms as well as significantly less stimulating home environments. Excessive TV exposure was not simply a marker for these factors but was a significant independent risk factor for childhood overweight during the preschool age range. Neither spending time outside of parental care nor watching educational TV muted the effect of excessive TV exposure on overweight.

Television exposure at age 36 months did not predict overweight risk at age 54 months. Given prior data that TV exposure increases throughout childhood,[18] it is unlikely that TV exposure in our sample decreased over time, although we do not have these data and cannot confirm this supposition. Given that maternal education was the most powerful predictor of overweight risk at age 54 months, we hypothesize that other risk factors connected to socioeconomic status or maternal cognitive functioning may overwhelm the contributing effect of TV exposure. Some of these factors presumably have a cumulative effect over childhood and may only begin to overwhelm the robust effect of TV exposure as children age. These may include maternal feeding behaviors,[32] maternal weight status,[33] family dietary choices,[34] and exercise patterns.[35] Studies that have detected a longitudinal relationship between TV exposure and overweight risk have also had larger sample sizes with longer follow-up than our study had.[12]

Our findings on correlates of excessive TV exposure mirror prior work[12,13,18] in that children from disadvantaged environments watch more television. Despite the previously documented associations between behavior problems, TV exposure, and overweight risk,[36-38] the relationship between TV exposure and overweight risk was not accounted for by child behavior problems. Although depression is associated with increased TV exposure[39] and obesity[40] in adults, and maternal depression is associated with increased TV exposure in preschool-aged children,[41] the relationship between excessive TV exposure and overweight risk was not accounted for by maternal depressive symptoms. Overweight risk has been associated with understimulating home environments in older children,[19] but TV exposure is an independent risk factor for overweight in preschool children, regardless of the overall quality of the home environment.

The mechanism of effect of TV exposure on overweight risk is undoubtedly multifactorial. Prior studies indicate that it appears to operate independently from reduced physical activity.[15] Excessive TV exposure may instead operate through the extensive advertising messages for unhealthy foods targeted at very young children[42] or from a tendency of children to snack while watching TV. Although educational TV exposure did not mute the effect of excessive total TV exposure on overweight risk, this may be because educational television in the United States does not equate with the absence of advertising for unhealthy foods.[43] Therefore, it remains possible that even the limited advertising on public educational television for children may be 1 mechanism of effect. Finally, our measure of TV exposure deserves comment. Being awake in the room with the television on is a broadly defined measure as compared with "watching television." Such an index is developmentally appropriate for children in this age range, given that children this age rarely actually sit watching the television with no other activity for prolonged periods of time. Our findings suggest that exposing children to TV even as "background noise" while they engage in other activities may increase overweight risk. It may be equally relevant in clinical practice to ask parents how often the child is in the presence of a TV that is "on" as it is to ask how much time the child spends "watching TV."

Our study has several limitations. Our sample size of overweight children was relatively small; therefore, the power to detect some effects may have been limited. Data regarding physical activity, diet, or maternal obesity were not available, which limits our ability to evaluate potential mechanisms of association. In addition, the cross-sectional nature of our analysis at age 36 months limits the ability to infer causation. Finally, as with many studies of this nature, the sample with complete data included in our analysis differed from the sample without complete data and therefore our findings may not be valid to generalize to the reference population of the National Institute of Child Health and Human Development Study of Early Child Care and Youth Development. Although we tested covariates that are predictors of missingness in the model and they did not alter the results, it remains possible that our results would have differed had complete data for the entire sample been available.

These data show a significant relationship between exposure to 2 or more hours of television per day at age 36 months and concurrent overweight, independent of a variety of demographic factors, child behavior problems, maternal depressive symptoms, amount of time spent in nonparental care, and proportion of TV exposure that is educational. These results provide further support for the utility of discussing television exposure during the well-child examination in the preschool years and before. The longitudinal results support the need to evaluate how low maternal educational level may shape the preschooler's environment to increase overweight risk. Although reduced TV exposure is a message that should be provided to all families, broadly based prevention and intervention efforts may best be placed in disadvantaged populations. School-based intervention programs have effectively reduced TV exposure and BMI in older children,[44,45] but to our knowledge, there are no randomized controlled trials assessing such interventions in preschoolers. The most effective method of reaching these parents is a public health challenge where additional work is needed.

**Accepted for Publication:** December 9, 2005.
**Correspondence:** Julie C. Lumeng, MD, 300 North Ingalls Building, 10th Floor, University of Michigan, Ann Arbor, MI 48109-0406 (jlumeng@umich.edu).
**Funding/Support:** This study was supported by the Fellow-to-Faculty Transition Award 0275040N and the Midwest Affiliate Grant-in-Aid 0455563Z (J.C.L.), both from the American Heart Association, Dallas, Tex.
**Author Contributions:** Dr Lumeng had full access to all the data in the study and takes responsibility for the integrity of the data and the accuracy of the data analysis.
**Acknowledgment:** We thank Kay Rhee, MD; Tiffany Cardinal, BS; and Jacinta Sitto, BA, for their thoughtful review of the manuscript.

## REFERENCES

1. Committee on Public Education. Media education. *Pediatrics.* 1999;104:341-342.
2. Committee on Public Education. Children, adolescents, and television. *Pediatrics.* 2001;107:423-426.
3. Dietz WH, Gortmaker SL. Do we fatten our children at the television set? Obesity and television viewing in children and adolescents. *Pediatrics.* 1985;75:807-812.
4. Obarzanek E, Schreiber GB, Crawford PB, et al. Energy intake and physical activity in relation to indexes of body fat: the National Heart, Lung, and Blood Institute Growth and Health Study. *Am J Clin Nutr.* 1994;60:15-22.
5. Gortmaker SL, Must A, Sobol AM, Peterson K, Colditz GA, Dietz WH. Television viewing as a cause of increasing obesity among children in the United States, 1986-1990. *Arch Pediatr Adolesc Med.* 1996;150:356-362.
6. Kimm SY, Obarzanek E, Barton BA, et al. Race, socioeconomic status, and obesity in 9- to 10-year-old girls: the NHLBI Growth and Health Study. *Ann Epidemiol.* 1996;6:266-275.
7. Guillaume M, Lapidus L, Bjorntorp P, Lambert A. Physical activity, obesity, and cardiovascular risk factors in children: the Belgian Luxembourg Child Study II. *Obes Res.* 1997;5:549-556.
8. Hancox RJ, Milne BJ, Poulton R. Association between child and adolescent television viewing and adult health: a longitudinal birth cohort. *Lancet.* 2004;364:257-262.
9. Crespo CJ, Smit E, Troiano RP, Bartlett SJ, Macera CA, Andersen RE. Television watching, energy intake, and obesity in US children: results from the third National Health and Nutrition Examination Survey, 1988-1994. *Arch Pediatr Adolesc Med.* 2001;155:360-365.

10. Dowda M, Ainsworth BE, Addy CL, Saunders R, Riner W. Environmental influences, physical activity, and weight status in 8- to 16-year-olds. *Arch Pediatr Adolesc Med.* 2001;155:711-717.
11. Locard E, Mamelle N, Billette A, Miginiac M, Munoz F, Rey S. Risk factors for obesity in a five year old population: parental versus environmental factors. *Int J Obes Relat Metab Disord.* 1992;16:721-729.
12. Reilly JJ, Armstrong J, Dorosty AR, et al. Early life risk factors for obesity in childhood: cohort study. *BMJ.* 2005;330:1357.
13. Dennison BA, Erb TA, Jenkins PL. Television viewing and television in bedroom associated with overweight risk among low-income preschool children. *Pediatrics.* 2002;109:1028-1035.
14. Durant RH, Baranowski T, Johnson M, Thompson WO. The relationship among television watching, physical activity, and body composition of young children. *Pediatrics.* 1994;94:449-455.
15. Moore LL, Nguyen US, Rothman KJ, Cupples LA, Ellison RC. Preschool physical activity level and change in body fatness in young children: the Framingham Children's Study. *Am J Epidemiol.* 1995;142:982-988.
16. Janz KF, Levy SM, Burns TL, Torner JC, Willing MC, Warren JJ. Fatness, physical activity, and television viewing in children during the adiposity rebound period: the Iowa Bone Development Study. *Prev Med.* 2002;35:563-571.
17. Sugimori H, Yoshida K, Izuno T, et al. Analysis of factors that influence body mass index from ages 3 to 6 years: a study based on the Toyama cohort study. *Pediatr Int.* 2004;46:302-310.
18. Certain LK, Kahn RS. Prevalence, correlates and trajectory of television viewing among infants and toddlers. *Pediatrics.* 2002;109:634-642.
19. Strauss RS, Knight J. Influence of the home environment on the development of obesity in children. *Pediatrics.* 1999;103:e85.
20. NICHD Early Child Care Research Network. Nonmaternal care and family factors in early development: an overview of the NICHD Study of Early Child Care. *J App Dev Psychol.* 2001;22:457-492.
21. Recruitment procedures. *NICHD Study of Early Child Care Manual.* Available at: http://secc.rti.org/. Accessed February 2, 2006.
22. Cole TJ, Faith MS, Pietrobelli A, Heo M. What is the best measure of adiposity change in growing children: BMI, BMI %, BMI z-score or BMI centile? *Eur J Clin Nutr.* 2005;59:419-425.
23. 54-month growth measures. *NICHD Study of Early Child Care and Youth Development Operations Manual.* Available at: http://secc.rti.org/. Accessed February 2, 2006.
24. Kuczmarski RJ, Ogden CL, Grummer-Strawn LM, Flegal KM, Guo SS, Wei R. CDC growth charts. *Adv Data.* 2000;314:1-28.
25. NICHD Study of Early Child Care and Youth Development Television Viewing Questionnaire, Form 38V. Available at: http://secc.rti.org/. Accessed February 2, 2006.
26. Radloff LS. The CES-D scale: a self-report depression scale for research in the general population. *Applied Psychol Measurement.* 1977;1:385-401.
27. Achenbach TM. *Manual for the Child Behavior Checklist/2-3 and 1992 Profile.* Burlington, Vt: University of Vermont Department of Psychiatry; 1992.
28. Caldwell BM, Bradley RH. *Home Observation for Measurement of the Environment.* Little Rock, Ark: University of Arkansas at Little Rock, Center for Child Development and Education; 1984.
29. Neter J, Kutner MH, Wasserman W, Nachtsheim CJ. *Applied Linear Statistical Models,* 4th ed. Columbus, Ohio: McGraw-Hill/Irwin; 1996.
30. Hedley AA, Ogden CL, Johnson CL, Carroll MD, Curtin LR, Flegal KM. Prevalence of overweight and obesity among US children, adolescents, and adults, 1999-2002. *JAMA.* 2004;291:2847-2850.
31. Mei Z, Scanlon KS, Grummer-Strawn LM, Freedman DS, Yip R, Trowbridge FL. Increasing prevalence of overweight among US low-income preschool children: the Centers for Disease Control and Prevention Pediatric Nutrition Surveillance, 1983 to 1995. *Pediatrics.* 1998;101:e12.
32. Baughcum AE, Powers SW, Johnson SB, et al. Maternal feeding practices and beliefs and their relationships to overweight in early childhood. *J Dev Behav Pediatr.* 2001;22:391-408.
33. Ball K, Crawford D. Socioeconomic status and weight change in adults: a review. *Soc Sci Med.* 2005;60:1987-2010.
34. Drewnowski A, Specter SE. Poverty and obesity: the role of energy density and energy costs. *Am J Clin Nutr.* 2004;79:6-16.
35. Crespo CJ, Ainsworth BE, Keteyian SJ, Heath GW, Smit E. Prevalence of physical inactivity and its relation to social class in US adults: results from the Third National Health and Nutrition Examination Survey, 1988-1994. *Med Sci Sports Exerc.* 1999;31:1821-1827.
36. Lumeng JC, Gannon K, Cabral HJ, Frank DA, Zuckerman B. Association between clinically meaningful behavior problems and overweight in children. *Pediatrics.* 2003;112:1138-1145.
37. Christakis DA, Zimmerman FJ, DiGiuseppe DL, McCarty CA. Early television exposure and subsequent attentional problems in children. *Pediatrics.* 2004;113:708-713.
38. Singer MI, Slovak K, Frierson T, York P. Viewing preferences, symptoms of psychological trauma, and violent behaviors among children who watch television. *J Am Acad Child Adolesc Psychiatry.* 1998;37:1041-1048.
39. Sidney S, Sternfeld B, Haskell WL, Jacobs DR, Chesney MA, Hulley SB. Television viewing and cardiovascular risk factors in young adults: the CARDIA study. *Ann Epidemiol.* 1996;6:154-159.
40. Carpenter KM, Hasin DS, Allison DB, Faith MS. Relationships between obesity and DSM-IV major depressive disorder, suicide ideation, and suicide attempts: results from a general population study. *Am J Public Health.* 2000;90:251-257.
41. Burdette HL, Whitaker RC, Kahn RS, Havery-Berino J. Association of maternal obesity and depressive symptoms with television-viewing time in low-income preschool children. *Arch Pediatr Adolesc Med.* 2003;157:894-899.
42. Lewis MK, Hill AJ. Food advertising on British children's television: a content analysis and experimental study with nine-year olds. *Int J Obes Relat Metab Disord.* 1998;22:206-214.
43. About PBS Sponsorship. Available at: http://www.pbs.org/aboutpbs/aboutpbs_sponsorship.html. Accessed August 25, 2005.
44. Gortmaker SL, Peterson K, Wiecha J, et al. Reducing obesity via a school-based interdisciplinary intervention among youth: Planet Health. *Arch Pediatr Adolesc Med.* 1999;153:409-418.
45. Robinson TN. Reducing children's television viewing to prevent obesity: a randomized controlled trial. *JAMA.* 1999;282:1561-1567.

The Walt Disney Internet Group announced in early July that it is teaming up with Sprint to develop a line of mobile phones, due out next year, aimed squarely at preteen children.

—From *Time*, "Young and Wireless" by Michele Oreckli, August 1, 2005

In the treatment or prevention of bronchospasm

**New**

# Expect Xopenex

## ...To Go

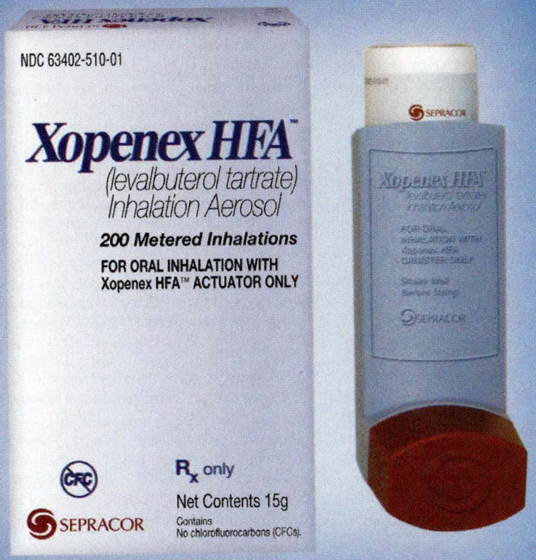


## Now in an MDI

**Same trusted single-isomer technology**

**Does not contain (S)-albuterol[1]**

Nothing less than

**NEW Xopenex HFA™**
(levalbuterol tartrate) Inhalation Aerosol

XOPENEX HFA (levalbuterol tartrate) Inhalation Aerosol is indicated for the treatment or prevention of bronchospasm in adults, adolescents, and children 4 years of age and older with reversible obstructive airway disease.

**Important Safety Information**

Xopenex HFA is contraindicated in patients with a history of hypersensitivity to levalbuterol, racemic albuterol, or any other component of Xopenex HFA. Xopenex HFA and other β-agonists can produce paradoxical bronchospasm, which may be life threatening. If additional adrenergic drugs, including other short-acting sympathomimetic bronchodilators or epinephrine, are to be administered by any route, they should be used with caution to avoid deleterious cardiovascular effects. Due to the cardiovascular side effects associated with β-agonists, caution is generally recommended for patients with cardiovascular disorders (especially coronary insufficiency, cardiac arrhythmias, and hypertension), diabetes, hyperthyroidism, or convulsive disorders. Do not exceed the recommended dose. Fatalities have been reported in association with excessive use of inhaled sympathomimetic drugs in patients with asthma. Please refer to the complete prescribing information for further information and in regard to potential drug interactions with β-blockers, diuretics, digoxin, or MAOI and tricyclic antidepressants.

**In patients aged 4 to 11 years,** the most common adverse events (occurring in greater than 2% of patients and more frequently than patients receiving placebo) were (90 mcg Xopenex HFA and placebo, respectively): accidental injury (9.2%; 5.7%), vomiting (10.5%; 5.7%), bronchitis (2.6%; 0%), and pharyngitis (6.6%; 5.7%).

**In patients aged 12 years and older,** the most common adverse events (occurring in greater than 2% of patients and more frequently than patients receiving placebo) were (90 mcg Xopenex HFA and placebo, respectively): pain (4.0%; 3.6%), dizziness (2.7%; 1.8%), asthma (9.4%; 6.0%), pharyngitis (7.9%; 2.4%), and rhinitis (7.4%; 3.0%).

**Reference:** 1. Xopenex HFA Prescribing Information.

Please see brief summary of prescribing information.

# Xopenex HFA™

(levalbuterol tartrate) Inhalation Aerosol

FOR ORAL INHALATION ONLY

## BRIEF SUMMARY

### INDICATIONS AND USAGE

XOPENEX HFA (levalbuterol tartrate) Inhalation Aerosol is indicated for the treatment or prevention of bronchospasm in adults, adolescents, and children 4 years of age and older with reversible obstructive airway disease.

### CONTRAINDICATIONS

XOPENEX HFA (levalbuterol tartrate) Inhalation Aerosol is contraindicated in patients with a history of hypersensitivity to levalbuterol, racemic albuterol, or any other component of XOPENEX HFA Inhalation Aerosol.

### WARNINGS

1. Paradoxical Bronchospasm: Like other inhaled beta-adrenergic agonists, XOPENEX HFA Inhalation Aerosol can produce paradoxical bronchospasm, which may be life-threatening. If paradoxical bronchospasm occurs, XOPENEX HFA (levalbuterol tartrate) Inhalation Aerosol should be discontinued immediately and alternative therapy instituted. It should be recognized that paradoxical bronchospasm, when associated with inhaled formulations, frequently occurs with the first use of a new canister. 2. Deterioration of Asthma: Asthma may deteriorate acutely over a period of hours or chronically over several days or longer. If the patient needs more doses of XOPENEX HFA Inhalation Aerosol than usual, this may be a marker of destabilization of asthma and requires reevaluation of the patient and treatment regimen, giving special consideration to the possible need for anti-inflammatory treatment, e.g., corticosteroids.
3. Use of Anti-Inflammatory Agents: The use of a beta-adrenergic agonist alone may not be adequate to control asthma in many patients. Early consideration should be given to adding anti-inflammatory agents, e.g., corticosteroids, to the therapeutic regimen. 4. Cardiovascular Effects: XOPENEX HFA Inhalation Aerosol, like other beta-adrenergic agonists, can produce clinically significant cardiovascular effects in some patients, as measured by heart rate, blood pressure, and/or symptoms. Although such effects are uncommon after administration of XOPENEX HFA Inhalation Aerosol at recommended doses, if they occur, the drug may need to be discontinued. In addition, beta-agonists have been reported to produce electrocardiogram (ECG) changes, such as flattening of the T wave, prolongation of the QTc interval, and ST segment depression. The clinical significance of these findings is unknown. Therefore, XOPENEX HFA Inhalation Aerosol, like all sympathomimetic amines, should be used with caution in patients with cardiovascular disorders, especially coronary insufficiency, cardiac arrhythmias, and hypertension. 5. Do Not Exceed Recommended Dose: Fatalities have been reported in association with excessive use of inhaled sympathomimetic drugs in patients with asthma. The exact cause of death is unknown, but cardiac arrest following an unexpected development of a severe acute asthmatic crisis and subsequent hypoxia is suspected.
6. Immediate Hypersensitivity Reactions: Immediate hypersensitivity reactions may occur after administration of racemic albuterol, as demonstrated by rare cases of urticaria, angioedema, rash, bronchospasm, anaphylaxis, and oropharyngeal edema. The potential for hypersensitivity must be considered in the clinical evaluation of patients who experience immediate hypersensitivity reactions while receiving XOPENEX HFA Inhalation Aerosol.

### PRECAUTIONS

#### General

XOPENEX HFA (levalbuterol tartrate) Inhalation Aerosol, like all sympathomimetic amines, should be used with caution in patients with cardiovascular disorders, especially coronary insufficiency, hypertension, and cardiac arrhythmias; in patients with convulsive disorders, hyperthyroidism, or diabetes mellitus; and in patients who are unusually responsive to sympathomimetic amines. Clinically significant changes in systolic and diastolic blood pressure have been seen in individual patients and could be expected to occur in some patients after the use of any beta-adrenergic bronchodilator.

Large doses of intravenous racemic albuterol have been reported to aggravate preexisting diabetes mellitus and ketoacidosis. As with other beta-adrenergic agonist medications, XOPENEX HFA Inhalation Aerosol may produce significant hypokalemia in some patients, possibly through intracellular shunting, which has the potential to produce adverse cardiovascular effects. The decrease is usually transient, not requiring supplementation.

#### Information for Patients

The action of XOPENEX HFA Inhalation Aerosol should last for 4 to 6 hours. XOPENEX HFA Inhalation Aerosol should not be used more frequently than recommended. Do not increase the dose or frequency of doses of XOPENEX HFA Inhalation Aerosol without consulting your physician. If you find that treatment with XOPENEX HFA Inhalation Aerosol becomes less effective for symptomatic relief, your symptoms become worse, and/or you need to use the product more frequently than usual, you should seek medical attention immediately. While you are using XOPENEX HFA Inhalation Aerosol, other inhaled drugs and asthma medications should be taken only as directed by your physician.

Common adverse effects of treatment with inhaled beta-agonists include palpitations, chest pain, rapid heart rate, tremor, and nervousness. If you are pregnant or nursing, contact your physician about use of XOPENEX HFA Inhalation Aerosol. Effective and safe use of XOPENEX HFA Inhalation Aerosol includes an understanding of the way that it should be administered.

Use XOPENEX HFA Inhalation Aerosol only with the actuator supplied with the product. Discard the canister after 200 sprays have been used. Never immerse the canister in water to determine how full the canister is ("float test").

In general, the technique for administering XOPENEX HFA Inhalation Aerosol to children is similar to that for adults. Children should use XOPENEX HFA Inhalation Aerosol under adult supervision, as instructed by the patient's physician.

#### Drug Interactions

Other short-acting sympathomimetic aerosol bronchodilators or epinephrine should be used with caution with XOPENEX HFA Inhalation Aerosol. If additional adrenergic drugs are to be administered by any route, they should be used with caution to avoid deleterious cardiovascular effects.

1. Beta-blockers: Beta-adrenergic receptor-blocking agents not only block the pulmonary effect of beta-adrenergic agonists, such as XOPENEX HFA Inhalation Aerosol, but may produce severe bronchospasm in asthmatic patients. Therefore, patients with asthma should not normally be treated with beta-blockers. However, under certain circumstances, e.g., as prophylaxis after myocardial infarction, there may be no acceptable alternatives to the use of beta-adrenergic blocking agents in patients with asthma. In this setting, cardioselective beta-blockers should be considered, although they should be administered with caution. 2. Diuretics: The ECG changes and/or hypokalemia that may result from the administration of non–potassium-sparing diuretics (such as loop and thiazide diuretics) can be acutely worsened by beta-agonists, especially when the recommended dose of the beta-agonist is exceeded. Although the clinical significance of these effects is not known, caution is advised in the coadministration of beta-agonists with non–potassium-sparing diuretics. 3. Digoxin: Mean decreases of 16% to 22% in serum digoxin levels were demonstrated after single-dose intravenous and oral administration of racemic albuterol, respectively, to normal volunteers who had received digoxin for 10 days. The clinical significance of these findings for patients with obstructive airway disease who are receiving XOPENEX HFA Inhalation Aerosol and digoxin on a chronic basis is unclear. Nevertheless, it would be prudent to carefully evaluate the serum digoxin levels in patients who are currently receiving digoxin and XOPENEX HFA Inhalation Aerosol. 4. Monoamine Oxidase Inhibitors or Tricyclic Antidepressants: XOPENEX HFA Inhalation Aerosol should be administered with extreme caution to patients being treated with monoamine oxidase inhibitors or tricyclic antidepressants, or within 2 weeks of discontinuation of such agents, because the action of albuterol on the vascular system may be potentiated.

**Carcinogenesis, Mutagenesis, and Impairment of Fertility** No carcinogenesis or impairment of fertility studies have been carried out with levalbuterol tartrate. However, racemic albuterol sulfate has been evaluated for its carcinogenic potential and ability to impair fertility.

In a 2-year study in Sprague-Dawley rats, racemic albuterol sulfate caused a significant dose-related increase in the incidence of benign leiomyomas of the mesovarium at, and above, dietary doses of 2 mg/kg/day (approximately 30 times the maximum recommended daily inhalation dose of levalbuterol tartrate for adults on a mg/m² basis and approximately 15 times the maximum recommended daily inhalation dose of levalbuterol tartrate for children on a mg/m² basis). In another study, this effect was blocked by the coadministration of propranolol, a non-selective beta-adrenergic antagonist. In an 18-month study in CD-1 mice, racemic albuterol sulfate showed no evidence of tumorigenicity at dietary doses up to 500 mg/kg/day (approximately 3800 times the maximum recommended daily inhalation dose of levalbuterol tartrate for adults on a mg/m² basis and approximately 1800 times the maximum recommended daily inhalation dose of levalbuterol tartrate for children on a mg/m² basis). In a 22-month study in the Golden hamster, racemic albuterol sulfate showed no evidence of tumorigenicity at dietary doses up to 50 mg/kg/day (approximately 500 times the maximum recommended daily inhalation dose of levalbuterol tartrate for adults on a mg/m² basis and approximately 240 times the maximum recommended daily inhalation dose of levalbuterol tartrate for children on a mg/m² basis).

Levalbuterol HCl was not mutagenic in the Ames test or the CHO/HPRT Mammalian Forward Gene Mutation Assay.

Levalbuterol HCl was not clastogenic in the in vivo micronucleus test in mouse bone marrow. Racemic albuterol sulfate was negative in an in vitro chromosomal aberration assay in CHO cell cultures.

Reproduction studies in rats using racemic albuterol sulfate demonstrated no evidence of impaired fertility at oral doses up to 50 mg/kg/day (approximately 750 times the maximum recommended daily inhalation dose of levalbuterol tartrate for adults on a mg/m² basis).

**Teratogenic Effects - Pregnancy Category C** A reproduction study in New Zealand White rabbits demonstrated that levalbuterol HCl was not teratogenic when administered orally at doses up to 25 mg/kg/day (approximately 750 times the maximum recommended daily inhalation dose of levalbuterol tartrate for adults on a mg/m² basis).

However, racemic albuterol sulfate has been shown to be teratogenic in mice and rabbits. A study in CD-1 mice given racemic albuterol sulfate subcutaneously showed cleft palate formation in 5 of 111 (4.5%) fetuses at 0.25 mg/kg/day (approximately 2 times the maximum recommended daily inhalation dose of levalbuterol tartrate for adults on a mg/m² basis) and in 10 of 108 (9.3%) fetuses at 2.5 mg/kg/day (approximately 20 times the maximum recommended daily inhalation dose of levalbuterol tartrate for adults on a mg/m² basis). The drug did not induce cleft palate formation when administered subcutaneously at a dose of 0.025 mg/kg/day (less than the maximum recommended daily inhalation dose of levalbuterol tartrate for adults on a mg/m² basis). Cleft palate also occurred in 22 of 72 (30.5%) fetuses from females treated subcutaneously with 2.5 mg/kg/day of isoproterenol (positive control).

A reproduction study in Stride Dutch rabbits revealed cranioschisis in 7 of 19 (37%) fetuses when racemic albuterol sulfate was administered orally at a dose of 50 mg/kg/day (approximately 1500 times the maximum recommended daily inhalation dose of levalbuterol tartrate for adults on a mg/m² basis).

A study in which pregnant rats were dosed with radiolabeled racemic albuterol sulfate demonstrated that drug-related material is transferred from the maternal circulation to the fetus.

There are no adequate and well-controlled studies of XOPENEX HFA Inhalation Aerosol in pregnant women. Because animal reproduction studies are not always predictive of human response, XOPENEX HFA Inhalation Aerosol should be used during pregnancy only if the potential benefit justifies the potential risk to the fetus.

During marketing experience of racemic albuterol, various congenital anomalies, including cleft palate and limb defects, have been rarely reported in the offspring of patients being treated with racemic albuterol. Some of the mothers were taking multiple medications during their pregnancies. No consistent pattern of defects can be discerned, and a relationship between racemic albuterol use and congenital anomalies has not been established.

**Use in Labor and Delivery** Because of the potential for beta-adrenergic agonists to interfere with uterine contractility, the use of XOPENEX HFA Inhalation Aerosol for the treatment of bronchospasm during labor should be restricted to those patients in whom the benefits clearly outweigh the risk.

**Tocolysis** XOPENEX HFA Inhalation Aerosol has not been approved for the management of preterm labor. The benefit:risk ratio when levalbuterol tartrate is administered for tocolysis has not been established. Serious adverse reactions, including maternal pulmonary edema, have been reported during or following treatment of premature labor with beta2-agonists, including racemic albuterol.

**Nursing Mothers** Plasma concentrations of levalbuterol after inhalation of therapeutic doses are very low in humans. It is not known whether levalbuterol is excreted in human milk.

Because of the potential for tumorigenicity shown for racemic albuterol in animal studies and the lack of experience with the use of XOPENEX HFA Inhalation Aerosol by nursing mothers, a decision should be made whether to discontinue nursing or to discontinue the drug, taking into account the importance of the drug to the mother. Caution should be exercised when XOPENEX HFA Inhalation Aerosol is administered to a nursing woman.

**Pediatrics** The safety and efficacy of XOPENEX HFA Inhalation Aerosol have been established in pediatric patients 4 years of age and older in an adequate and well-controlled clinical trial. Use of XOPENEX HFA Inhalation Aerosol in children is also supported by evidence from adequate and well-controlled studies of XOPENEX HFA Inhalation Aerosol in adults, considering that the pathophysiology, systemic exposure of the drug, and clinical profile in pediatric and adult patients are substantially similar. Safety and effectiveness of XOPENEX HFA Inhalation Aerosol in pediatric patients below the age of 4 years have not been established.

**Geriatrics** Clinical studies of XOPENEX HFA Inhalation Aerosol did not include sufficient numbers of subjects aged 65 and older to determine whether they respond differently from younger subjects. Other reported clinical experience has not identified differences in responses between the elderly and younger patients. In general, dose selection for an elderly patient should be cautious, usually starting at the low end of the dosing range, reflecting the greater frequency of decreased hepatic, renal, or cardiac function, and of concomitant diseases or other drug therapy.

Albuterol is known to be substantially excreted by the kidney, and the risk of toxic reactions may be greater in patients with impaired renal function. Because elderly patients are more likely to have decreased renal function, care should be taken in dose selection, and it may be useful to monitor renal function.

**ADVERSE REACTIONS** Adverse event information concerning XOPENEX HFA (levalbuterol tartrate) Inhalation Aerosol in adults and adolescents is derived from two 8-week, multicenter, randomized, double-blind, active- and placebo-controlled trials in 748 adult and adolescent patients with asthma that compared XOPENEX HFA Inhalation Aerosol, a marketed albuterol HFA inhaler, and an HFA-134a placebo inhaler. The following lists the incidence (% XOPENEX HFA 90 mcg, marketed albuterol HFA inhaler 180 mcg, placebo, respectively) of all adverse events (whether considered by the investigator to be related or unrelated to drug) from these trials that occurred at a rate of 2% or greater in the group treated with XOPENEX HFA Inhalation Aerosol and more frequently than in the HFA-134a placebo inhaler group. Body as a whole: pain (4.0%, 3.4%, 3.6%). Central nervous system: dizziness (2.7%, 0.6%, 1.8%). Respiratory system: asthma (9.4%, 7.3%, 6.0%), pharyngitis (7.9%, 2.2%, 2.4%), rhinitis (7.4%, 2.2%, 3.0%).

Adverse events reported by less than 2% and at least 2 or more of the adolescent and adult patients receiving XOPENEX HFA Inhalation Aerosol and by a greater proportion than receiving HFA-134a placebo inhaler include cyst, flu syndrome, viral infection, constipation, gastroenteritis, myalgia, hypertension, epistaxis, lung disorder, acne, herpes simplex, conjunctivitis, ear pain, dysmenorrhea, hematuria, and vaginal moniliasis. There were no significant laboratory abnormalities observed in these studies.

Adverse event information concerning XOPENEX HFA Inhalation Aerosol in children is derived from a 4-week, randomized, double-blind trial of XOPENEX HFA Inhalation Aerosol, a marketed albuterol HFA inhaler, and an HFA-134a placebo inhaler in 150 children aged 4 to 11 years with asthma. The following lists the adverse events (% XOPENEX HFA 90 mcg, marketed albuterol HFA inhaler 180 mcg, placebo, respectively) reported for XOPENEX HFA Inhalation Aerosol in children at a rate of 2% or greater and more frequently than for placebo. Body as a whole: accidental injury (9.2%, 10.3%, 5.7%). Digestive system: vomiting (10.5%, 7.7%, 5.7%). Respiratory system: bronchitis (2.6%, 0%, 0%), pharyngitis (6.6%, 12.8%, 5.7%).

The incidence of systemic beta-adrenergic adverse effects (e.g., tremor, nervousness) was low and comparable across all treatment groups, including placebo.

**Postmarketing** In addition to the adverse events reported in clinical trials, the following adverse events have been observed in postapproval use of levalbuterol inhalation solution. These events have been chosen for inclusion due to their seriousness, their frequency of reporting, or their likely beta-mediated mechanism: angioedema, anaphylaxis, arrhythmias (including atrial fibrillation, supraventricular tachycardia, extrasystoles), asthma, chest pain, cough increased, dyspnea, nausea, nervousness, rash, tachycardia, tremor, urticaria. Because these events have been reported spontaneously from a population of unknown size, estimates of frequency cannot be made.

In addition, XOPENEX HFA Inhalation Aerosol, like other sympathomimetic agents, can cause adverse reactions such as hypertension, angina, vertigo, central nervous system stimulation, sleeplessness, headache, and drying or irritation of the oropharynx.

Rx only.

SEPRACOR 12/05

# Parental Weight Status as a Moderator of the Relationship Between Television Viewing and Childhood Overweight

*Elizabeth A. Vandewater, PhD; Xuan Huang, MA*

**Objective:** To examine whether and to what extent the relationship between television viewing and children's weight status differs according to parental weight status.

**Design:** Population-level survey including in-home and telephone interview components.

**Setting:** United States.

**Participants:** Representative sample of children aged 6 to 19 years in 2002 (n=1483).

**Main Exposure:** Hours of television viewing.

**Main Outcome Measures:** Child weight status (normal weight, at risk for overweight, overweight) as defined by current Centers for Disease Control and Prevention standards.

**Results:** Parental obesity increased the risk of child overweight for all of the children except boys aged 6 to 9 years. There were significant interactions between television viewing hours and parental obesity among boys aged 14 to 19 years and girls aged 10 to 13 years. For these 2 groups, the odds of overweight status increased with viewing hours for children with at least 1 obese parent but not at all for children of normal-weight parents.

**Conclusions:** Results indicate that when parental obesity is taken into account, television viewing hours do not significantly relate to increased odds of childhood overweight, and parental body mass index may serve to moderate the relationship between television viewing and child weight status among adolescents (but not among younger children). Further examination of the moderating effect of parental body mass index on the relationship between television viewing and child weight status is warranted.

*Arch Pediatr Adolesc Med. 2006;160:425-431*

**Author Affiliations:** Population Research Center (Dr Vandewater), Human Development and Family Sciences (Drs Vandewater and Huang), Center for Research on Interactive Technology, Television, and Children (Drs Vandewater and Huang), and Children's Digital Media Center (Drs Vandewater and Huang), University of Texas, Austin.

THE PREVALENCE OF OBESITY in American youth has reached alarming levels. The proportion of overweight children and adolescents, defined as a body mass index (BMI) exceeding the 95th percentile for age- and sex-based norms, has tripled in the past 3 decades.[1] Current estimates indicate that among children aged 6 through 19 years, approximately 31% are at risk for overweight and 16% are overweight.[2,3] Many believe that time spent watching television is at least partly to blame for obesity in the nation's youth. Children spend 3 to 5 hours per day watching television, more time than in any other single free-time activity except sleep.[4,5] Perhaps because of this, the notion that television use must somehow be responsible for the increased prevalence of obesity in American children and adolescents in recent years is dearly held by the lay public and scholars alike.[6-9]

In their seminal study, Dietz and Gortmaker[10] found that the prevalence of obesity in a large epidemiologic sample of adolescents aged 12 to 17 years increased 2% for each additional hour of television watched. It is this study that is widely cited as evidence that television causes obesity in children and adolescents. However, this finding has been surprisingly difficult to replicate. Robinson and Killen[11] found that television viewing was only weakly associated with BMI among white boys in a large sample (n=1912) of ninth-graders. Robinson et al[12] found that baseline hours of television viewing were not associated with either baseline or longitudinal changes in BMI in a large sample (n=971) of sixth- and seventh-grade girls. McMurray et al[13] found no relationship between television or video game use and BMI in a sample of 2389 adolescents aged 10 to 17 years once the influence of socioeconomic status and ethnicity were controlled. Finally, DuRant et al[14] also found no relationship between BMI and television watching in a longitudinal sample of young children (aged 3-4 years).

However, it is worth noting that interventions with random controlled trial designs have found a causal relationship between reduction of television viewing and reduction of children's BMI. Gortmaker et al[15] designed a school-based intervention to reduce obesity in middle school youth (grades 6-8) by altering key physical activity and dietary risk factors, including reductions in television viewing. They found reductions in the prevalence of obesity related to reduced television viewing for girls (although not for boys). Robinson[16] found that elementary school children (third- and fourth-graders) who received classroom curriculum designed to reduce television use over 1 school year showed significant decreases in BMI.

The general discrepancy between findings from epidemiologic and intervention studies (although they are somewhat more limited in number) is puzzling. We believe that the answer may lie in the influence of moderating variables. That is, the generally weak relationship found between children's television use and their weight status in epidemiologic samples may be owing to the fact that the strength of this relationship differs for different groups of children, thus diluting the linear relationships in heterogeneous samples. Identification of moderating influences would be an important step for both epidemiologic researchers as well as those interested in designing targeted interventions. However, examination of moderators of the relationship between television viewing and child weight status is surprisingly lacking.

In this article, we focus on 1 possible moderator of the relationship between children's television viewing and their weight status—parental weight status. Parental (especially maternal) BMI has been found to explain as much as 70% of the variance in children's BMI.[17-21] Thus, parental weight status represents both environmental and genetic risk factors that may importantly moderate the relationship between media use and obesity. Two mechanisms for this moderating effect seem readily apparent. First, the inactivity accompanying television viewing may be more consequential for the weight status of children at familial risk of overweight than for those without such risk. Second, children with familial risk of obesity may be more susceptible to televised food advertising—the vast majority of which is for nutrient-poor, high-fat foods.[22,23] This may be either because their parents themselves are more likely to buy and consume such foods[24] or because of evidence indicating that overweight children eat more in response to food advertising than normal-weight children.[25] Although we cannot discern the various mechanisms with these data, both scenarios suggest that television viewing might be related to increased risk of overweight or obesity more so among children at familial risk of overweight than among those without such risk.

However, to the extent that parental weight status has been included in studies at all (and often it is not), it has been treated as a covariate. Although this approach has its utility, controlling for its effects obviates the researcher's ability to assess how relationships among variables of interest might differ at different levels of the covariate (ie, moderator effects). If the relationship between television viewing and child weight status operates differently for children with different levels of familial risk for overweight, then this might at least partly explain some of the lack of findings in studies using heterogeneous samples of children that fail to take parental BMI into account. This study examines the question of whether the relationship between television use and weight status differs for children at different levels of familial risk for obesity as indicated by parental weight status.

## METHODS

### SAMPLE

The sample was drawn from cross-sectional data collected as a part of the Child Development Supplement (CDS) to the Panel Study of Income Dynamics in 2002 to 2003. Since 1968, the Panel Study of Income Dynamics has been an ongoing, nationally representative panel study focusing primarily on the transfer of social and economic capital within families. As its name implies, the CDS to the Panel Study of Income Dynamics focuses on children and provides additional information about parents' and children's education, health, cognitive and behavioral development, and time use. In 2002 to 2003, the CDS contacted families who remained active in the Panel Study of Income Dynamics as of 2001. The CDS successfully reinterviewed 2017 families (91%) who provided data on 2908 children and adolescents aged 6 to 19 years. For a complete description of sampling and data collection procedures, see the CDS user guide.[26]

The sample used for the present study comprised 1483 children aged 6 to 19 years (736 boys and 747 girls) for whom complete data on all of the variables of interest were available. The median income of the families was $53 375, with 16.1% of the families falling below poverty level. Twenty percent of the parents had not graduated high school, 31% had a high school diploma, 23% had some college, and 26% had attained a bachelor degree or higher. Fifty-six percent were European American and 44% were African American. The study was approved by the institutional review boards of the University of Michigan, Ann Arbor, where the data were collected, and the University of Texas, Austin, where analyses for this study were conducted.

### MEASURES

#### Child BMI

Weight and height information was collected via strain-gauge lithium bath scales[27] and measurement tape, respectively, during the home interview. Children were measured in stocking feet and, in the case of weight, in light clothing with pockets emptied. Body mass index was calculated from height and weight by using the formula from the National Center for Chronic Disease Prevention and Health Promotion (weight in kilograms divided by the height in meters squared). Because BMI varies by age and sex, BMI was converted to a BMI *z* score using the Centers for Disease Control and Prevention's BMI growth reference to determine an age- and sex-specific BMI *z* score for subjects aged 2 to 20 years.[28]

The definition of overweight among children is a statistical definition based on the 2000 Centers for Disease Control and Prevention growth reference for the United States.[28] Overweight is defined as being at or above the 95th percentile of BMI for age. Being at risk for overweight is defined as being at or above the 85th percentile but less than the 95th percentile of BMI for age. (Descriptive statistics for this and all of the other measures are presented in **Table 1**.)

**Table 1. Sample Characteristics**

| Characteristic | Boys | | | Girls | | |
|---|---|---|---|---|---|---|
| | Aged 6-9 y (n = 135) | Aged 10-13 y (n = 281) | Aged 14-19 y (n = 320) | Aged 6-9 y (n = 134) | Aged 10-13 y (n = 248) | Aged 14-19 y (n = 365) |
| Child weight status, % | | | | | | |
| Child of normal weight | 62 | 61 | 66 | 64 | 58 | 68 |
| Child at risk for overweight | 17 | 12 | 14 | 13 | 17 | 15 |
| Child overweight | 21 | 27 | 20 | 23 | 25 | 17 |
| Predictors | | | | | | |
| Parental weight status, % | | | | | | |
| Both parents of normal weight | 16 | 20 | 21 | 23 | 18 | 20 |
| ≥1 Parent overweight | 52 | 43 | 42 | 35 | 46 | 39 |
| ≥1 Parent obese | 32 | 37 | 37 | 42 | 36 | 41 |
| Television viewing, mean (SD), h | 5.55 (3.07) | 5.61 (3.68) | 5.64 (3.83) | 4.25 (2.77) | 5.36 (3.36) | 5.26 (3.70) |
| Covariates | | | | | | |
| Family income-needs ratio, mean (SD) | 3.38 (2.26) | 4.46 (4.67) | 4.65 (5.15) | 3.62 (2.20) | 4.73 (6.68) | 5.32 (7.73) |
| Household head education, mean (SD), y | 13.16 (2.24) | 13.74 (2.20) | 13.63 (2.25) | 13.65 (1.99) | 13.75 (2.12) | 13.70 (2.48) |
| Child race, % | | | | | | |
| White | 56 | 55 | 51 | 57 | 61 | 59 |
| African American | 44 | 45 | 49 | 43 | 39 | 41 |
| Child maturational status, mean (SD) | 70.93 (2.30) | 80.47 (5.40) | 96.46 (3.75) | 71.82 (2.49) | 84.10 (5.37) | 97.29 (2.42) |

### Biological Parent BMI

Parents' weight and height information was collected via self-report in 1999 and 2001. Data collected in 2001 were used to calculate parental BMI. However, in a small number of cases where 2001 data were unavailable, 1999 data were used (for father's weight status, n=36; for mother's weight status, n=42). Parental BMI was used to categorize the weight status of parents using the Centers for Disease Control and Prevention recommended cutoff points for overweight (BMI >25) and obesity (BMI >30).[29] Parental obesity was considered present when 1 or both parents had a BMI greater than 30. Parental overweight was considered present when 1 or both parents had a BMI greater than 25 but no more than 30.

### Amount of Children's Television Viewing

Information on children's television viewing was assessed via two 24-hour time-use diaries providing detailed accounts of type, number, duration, and location of activities that children engaged in during each 24-hour period.[5,30,31] On 1 randomly chosen weekday and 1 randomly chosen weekend day, all of the activities that the child engaged in were reported. Children aged 10 years and older were encouraged to complete their own time-use diaries; younger children were aided by primary caregivers. A primary activity and its duration were recorded to account for every minute of the two 24-hour diaries, and, if appropriate, a secondary activity was also noted. The measure was created by summing the minutes children spent watching television as a primary or secondary activity across both days. This sum was then divided by 60 to express television viewing in hours.

### Validity of Time-Use Diaries

A fairly extensive body of research has demonstrated the validity and reliability of time-use diaries as representations of the ways both children and adults spend their time.[32-35] When direct observation techniques are compared with time-use dairies, the mean values for time allocated to different activities are very close and the correlations are quite high, on the order of 0.70 to 0.80.[34,35] Of particular relevance to this study, Anderson et al[36] specifically examined the accuracy of parent report of young (aged 5 years on average) children's media use. Using video cameras, they recorded all of the children's viewing in approximately 100 families for a 10-day period while the children's parents also completed a viewing diary. The correlation between the 2 methods was quite high (0.84), indicating that time-use diaries filled out by parents provided fairly accurate representations of children's weekly viewing. Thus, time-use diaries have been shown to be a highly reliable and valid method of recording the way individuals spend their time in large-scale survey samples, such as that used here, where observing individuals over 24-hour periods is neither logistically nor financially feasible.

## COVARIATES

### Sociodemographic Characteristics

Based on demonstrated relationships with television viewing, weight status, or both, a number of sociodemographic characteristics were treated as covariates in the analyses. These included the following: (1) family income-to-needs ratio, which was a proportion of the family's income by the poverty threshold for that family, with higher income-to-needs ratios reflecting more disposable income in a family; (2) education of the household head, denoting the number of years of education completed by the household head; and (3) child race.

### Child Maturational Status

Because maturation-related misclassification may result in overestimations of overweight prevalence rates among early-maturing adolescents and underestimations among later-maturing adolescents,[37,38] we controlled for child maturational status. This was assessed using the Khamis-Roche method for predicting the percentage of adult stature.[39] The method is applicable to children aged 4 to 17 years and thus was not applied to children in the sample who were aged 18 or 19 years. Percentage of adult stature has been shown to be significantly correlated with maturational status (range, $r$=0.50-0.70) and thus a good proxy for maturational status when other, more invasive measures are not available.[40-42] It is calculated using current stature (meters), current weight (kilograms), and mid–

**Table 2. Multinomial Logistic Regression Models Predicting Child Weight Status From Child's Television Use and Parental Weight Status***

| | Boys | | | Girls | | |
|---|---|---|---|---|---|---|
| Variable | Aged 6-9 y (n = 135) | Aged 10-13 y (n = 281) | Aged 14-19 y (n = 320) | Aged 6-9 y (n = 134) | Aged 10-13 y (n = 248) | Aged 14-19 y (n = 365) |
| **Child at Risk for Overweight Compared With Child of Normal Weight** | | | | | | |
| Parental weight status | | | | | | |
| ≥1 Parent overweight | 1.27 (0.26-6.15) | 0.53 (0.18-1.59) | 1.46 (0.42-5.10) | 0.67 (0.12-3.82) | 1.84 (0.56-6.03) | 5.18 (1.40-19.15)† |
| ≥1 Parent obese | 1.95 (0.37-10.21) | 0.81 (0.21-3.05) | 2.39 (0.75-7.59) | 1.45 (0.17-12.44) | 2.25 (0.66-7.70) | 8.98 (2.47-32.68)‡ |
| Television viewing, h | 1.11 (0.94-1.31) | 0.94 (0.77-1.13) | 0.86 (0.68-1.07) | 1.22 (0.99-1.50)§ | 1.08 (0.86-1.37) | 1.27 (0.95-1.70) |
| Parent overweight × television viewing, h | ... | 0.99 (0.78-1.25) | 1.15 (0.86-1.54) | ... | 0.93 (0.71-1.23) | 0.82 (0.60-1.12) |
| Parent obese × television viewing, h | ... | 0.87 (0.62-1.23) | 1.21 (0.92-1.61) | ... | 0.95 (0.67-1.34) | 0.86 (0.62-1.19) |
| **Child Overweight Compared With Child of Normal Weight** | | | | | | |
| Parental weight status | | | | | | |
| ≥1 Parent overweight | 0.42 (0.08-2.12) | 0.95 (0.30-3.00) | 3.56 (0.89-14.16)§ | 1.11 (0.21-6.01) | 2.10 (0.47-9.40) | 8.35 (1.49-46.80)† |
| ≥1 Parent obese | 0.28 (0.04-1.79) | 6.77 (2.31-19.82)‡ | 6.89 (1.61-29.45)‖ | 7.42 (1.42-38.88)† | 4.79 (1.06-21.63)† | 7.20 (1.52-34.12)‡ |
| Television viewing, h | 1.42 (1.15-1.74)‡ | 1.28 (1.01-1.62)† | 0.84 (0.69-1.02)§ | 1.18 (0.97-1.44) | 0.91 (0.67-1.23) | 1.24 (1.03-1.49)† |
| Parent overweight × television viewing, h | ... | 0.79 (0.59-1.05) | 1.28 (1.01-1.62)† | ... | 0.97 (0.64-1.47) | 0.87 (0.68-1.11) |
| Parent obese × television viewing, h | ... | 0.76 (0.58-1.01)§ | 1.16 (0.89-1.50) | ... | 1.48 (1.01-2.17)† | 0.82 (0.66-1.02)§ |

*Values are expressed as odds ratio (95% confidence interval). All of the values control for family income-needs ratio, education of the household head, child race (white, n = 0; African American, n = 1), and child maturational status. Ellipses indicate nonsignificant interaction terms, with only main effects reported.

†$P<.05$.

‡$P<.001$.

§$P<.10$.

‖$P<.01$.

parent stature (meters), where mid–parent stature represents the average height of both parents. The regression equation for predicting adult stature takes the following form: predicted adult stature $= \beta_0 + \beta_1(\text{stature}) + \beta_2(\text{weight}) + \beta_3(\text{mid–parent stature})$, where $\beta_1$, $\beta_2$, and $\beta_3$ are the coefficients by which stature, weight, and mid–parent stature, respectively, should be multiplied. Percentage of adult stature at a given age is then predicted by dividing adult stature by current stature. The β weights used in the equation differ for boys and girls at individual ages, respectively, and are specified by Khamis and Roche.[39]

## STATISTICAL ANALYSIS

Multinomial logistic regressions predicting child weight status were used to examine the possibility that the relationship between television use and weight status differs for children at different levels of familial risk for obesity. The odds of a child being at risk for overweight (BMI, 85th-94th percentile) and of being overweight (BMI, ≥95th percentile) were each compared with the odds of a child being of normal weight for the following: (1) each hour of television viewed; (2) familial risk of obesity (both parents of normal weight, at least 1 parent overweight, or at least 1 parent obese); and (3) the interaction between television viewing hours and familial risk of obesity for these factors. Children were stratified by age and sex for a variety of reasons. Because there are known differences in both children's television viewing[5] and risk for overweight and obesity,[2] the sample was stratified by age and sex to examine the models separately (ie, for boys aged 6-9, 10-13, and 14-19 years and girls aged 6-9, 10-13, and 14-19 years). All of the models included the following covariates: family income-needs ratio, years of education of the household head, child race, and child maturational status.

The regression models for each sex × age group predicted the odds of a child being at risk for overweight or being overweight compared with the odds of a child being of normal weight based on television viewing (in hours), parental weight status, and the interaction of television viewing and parental weight status. We first conducted analyses without interaction terms (the product of parent's weight status and centered television viewing in hours) and then analyses including interaction terms. Interaction terms were centered to protect against collinearity issues that arise when nonindependent terms (in this case, the interaction terms and the main effect) are included in the same model.[43] If interaction terms were not statistically significant at $P<.05$, the model without interaction terms was presented in this article. Otherwise, the model with interaction terms was interpreted.

Stata version 8.0 (StataCorp, College Station, Tex) was used for all of the analyses. Because of the existence of sibling pairs in the data, standard errors were corrected for nonindependence. Stata version 8.0 provides options for correcting possible deflation of standard errors due to nonindependence in the data (such as when siblings each provide data) by means of using a robust estimator of variance that does not assume independence of observations.

# RESULTS

Table 1 displays descriptive statistics for the variables of interest. Results of multinomial logistic regression models for each sex and age group are presented in **Table 2**. The odds ratios shown in Table 2 represent the odds of a child being either at risk for overweight (compared with children of normal weight) or overweight (compared with children of normal weight). Odds ratios of 1.0 represent exactly even odds. Odds ratios above 1.0 indicate increased odds, and odds ratios below 1.0 indicate decreased odds. Interactions between television viewing hours and parental weight status, which significantly predicted child weight status at $P<.05$, are plotted in **Figure 1** and **Figure 2**.

## DESCRIPTIVE STATISTICS

Of the children included in this study, more than one third either were at risk of overweight or were overweight. Many children had parents who were overweight or obese. About four fifths of all of the children had at least 1 overweight or obese parent. Only one fifth of the children had both parents of normal weight. Children in this sample watched an average of 4 to 6 hours of television across 2 days (1 randomly selected weekday and 1 randomly selected weekend day).

## PARENTAL WEIGHT STATUS

Having at least 1 obese parent presented an increased risk of child overweight for most of the age × sex groups. The 1 exception to these findings was among boys aged 6 to 9 years for whom parental weight status was unrelated to child weight status. Having at least 1 overweight parent was generally unrelated to risk of being at risk for overweight or being overweight. The 1 exception to this finding was among girls aged 14 to 19 years for whom at least 1 overweight parent as well as at least 1 obese parent dramatically increased the odds of being either at risk for overweight or overweight compared with being of normal weight (Table 2).

## TELEVISION VIEWING HOURS

Hours of television viewing were related to increased odds of child overweight relative to normal weight among 3 groups: boys aged 6 to 9 years, boys aged 10 to 13 years, and girls aged 14 to 19 years. Television viewing hours were generally unrelated to odds of being at risk for overweight compared with normal weight.

## INTERACTION OF PARENTAL WEIGHT STATUS AND TELEVISION VIEWING

There were significant interactions between parental weight status and television viewing for 2 of the 6 age and sex groups: older adolescent boys (aged 14-19 years) and younger adolescent girls (aged 10-13 years) (Table 2). These interactions are plotted in Figure 1 and Figure 2, respectively. As shown in Figure 1, the risk of overweight increased with television viewing hours for boys with at least 1 overweight parent but not for boys with normal-weight parents. For boys with normal-weight parents, by contrast, television viewing hours and risk of overweight were unrelated. This same pattern is evident, but much more so, among girls aged 10 to 13 years. Among girls aged 10 to 13 years with at least 1 obese parent, the probability of overweight status dramatically increased as television viewing increased. For younger adolescent girls with normal-weight parents, increases in television viewing were unrelated to increased risk of overweight.

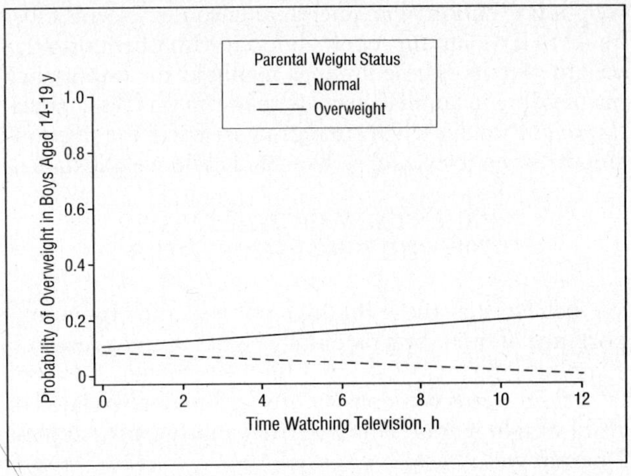


**Figure 1.** The interaction of parental weight status and television viewing on the probability of child overweight for boys aged 14 to 19 years. The time spent watching television is a 2-day total.

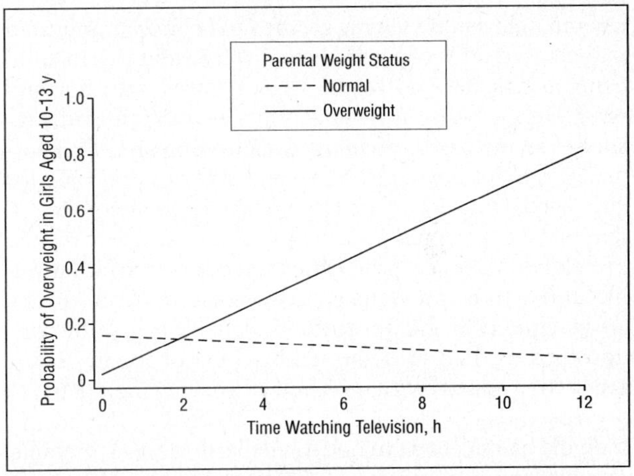


**Figure 2.** The interaction of parental weight status and television viewing on the probability of child overweight for girls aged 10 to 13 years. The time spent watching television is a 2-day total.

## COMMENT

We began this study with the premise that the relationship between television viewing hours and child weight status would be moderated by parental weight status. Specifically, we speculated that for children who were at risk of familial obesity, the relationship between television viewing and a status of child at risk for overweight or overweight would be strongly positive. Though reasonable, this hypothesis received only moderate support. Results indicated that this was the case for 2 of the 6 sex × age groups that we examined—girls aged 10 to 13 years and boys aged 14 to 19 years.

For these 2 groups, the probability of elevated weight status increased with television viewing only among children whose parents were obese. This was particularly true for younger adolescent girls (aged 10-13 years), but it was also evident among older adolescent boys (aged 14-19 years). Among these sex and age groups, children with normal-weight parents could seemingly watch television with impunity—at least with regard to risk of elevated weight status.

These findings may be owing to developmental changes with respect to the relationship between parental weight status and child weight status or between television viewing and weight status. Whatever the case, they certainly have implications for intervention designs. It seems that among younger children (particularly those with normal-weight parents), decreasing television viewing may be an important component of prevention of a status of childhood at risk for overweight or overweight. For older children, however, decreasing television viewing as either an overweight prevention or an intervention strategy seems most likely to have an impact on children with obese or overweight parents. These findings highlight the importance of attending to familial characteristics (in this case, parental weight status) when attempting to assess the relationship between television viewing and child weight status.

### PARENTAL WEIGHT STATUS AND CHILD WEIGHT STATUS

We believe that these findings point to the crucial importance of including parental weight status in research examining factors related to child weight status. Parental weight status was consistently and strongly related to child weight status. This was particularly true if at least 1 parent was obese.

### TELEVISION VIEWING AND CHILD WEIGHT STATUS

Overall, television viewing seemed to be more implicated in increased odds of a child being overweight than a child being at risk for overweight. Looking across the age and sex groups, television viewing hours were significantly related to an increased risk of overweight compared with normal weight for boys aged 6 to 9 and 10 to 13 years and for girls aged 14 to 19 years. Despite the general conviction that television viewing is strongly and consistently related to childhood obesity,[6-8] this pattern of results is, in fact, much like those from previous epidemiologic research in this area—equivocal and not particularly strong.[11,12] The relationships are there for some children but not others, or they are even reversed (with more television viewing related to decreased risk of elevated weight). Moreover, the magnitude of the effects were not particularly large—the highest positive odds ratio was 1.42 (the lowest, 1.24).

### LIMITATIONS AND FUTURE DIRECTIONS

In these analyses, we examined age and sex groups, controlling for ethnicity. It is quite possible (and indeed probable) that the relationship between television viewing and child weight status varies importantly by ethnicity as well as age and sex. Unfortunately, the sample size limited our ability to examine associations among different age and sex groups also defined by ethnicity. Examining the extent to which ethnicity plays a role in the relationships among parental weight status, television viewing, and child weight status will be an important area for future research.

Although a number of studies indicate that self-reported height and weight are highly correlated with observed measures (on the order of $r=0.90$),[44-46] there is also evidence that a systematic bias exists such that adults tend to overestimate their height and underestimate their weight.[47,48] Thus, to the extent that parents in this study underestimated their BMI, the findings would be biased toward the null hypothesis.

Another important limitation is the lack of information regarding parents' viewing habits. That is, it seems likely that parental media use itself would be a strong moderator of the relationship between childhood media use and BMI. Our ability to examine this possibility in these data was hampered by the fact that information regarding parents' own viewing habits was not collected. The connection between parents' and children's viewing habits and the intersection of these viewing habits with both parental and child obesity is a crucial area of further investigation.

Parental weight status represents both genetic and environmental influences on children's weight status. Although we cannot separate these influences in these data, doing so is an important component to furthering the understanding of the nature of familial influences on childhood obesity. Similarly, although we had theoretical reasons for focusing on parental weight status, other familial factors (such as parents' own activity levels, media use, family eating habits) clearly merit further investigation.

## CONCLUSIONS

We believe that the varied nature of these results highlights the notion that the relationship between television viewing and child weight status is neither simple nor the same across children of differing sexes and ages. These findings may help to explain the generally weak association between television viewing and child weight status often found in existing research based on heterogeneous populations. These findings may also have important implications for prevention and intervention designs. Our findings suggest that reductions in BMI with concomitant reductions in television viewing will be evident in some groups of children but not others. Specifically, television viewing hours alone seemed importantly related to risk of overweight among younger groups of boys (between the ages of 6 and 13 years) but not for other groups of children. However, for other children, especially adolescent boys and girls, the relationship between television viewing and overweight was only evident among children at familial risk of obesity (those with at least 1 obese parent). Thus, these findings suggest that researchers interested in designing childhood weight status interventions should certainly consider parental obesity in their project designs.

We understand that this message is somewhat at odds with both popular and scholarly convictions that television viewing—alone—is largely to blame for the current epidemic of being at risk for overweight and being overweight among American children. Although it is not an unreasonable hypothesis, empirical evidence for it is, to date, surprisingly equivocal.[11,12,14] The findings of this study suggest that parental weight status is an important moderator of the relationship between television viewing and child weight status and that researchers interested in understanding and intervening in childhood obesity would do well to collect information from parents as well as children. As noted, in this study, we focused exclusively on parental weight status as a moderator of the relationship between television viewing and child weight status. It seems reasonable to assume that there may be other important familial moderators (or mediators) as well. To date, however, surprisingly few studies, either epidemiologic or experimental in nature, include parental or familial contextual information in their data collection schemes. Thus, we know little about the contextual factors affecting relationships between television viewing and childhood overweight.[49,50]

Our view is that it behooves us to understand the true nature of the role that media use plays in the development of obesity. To do this, we would argue that research agendas must move beyond a focus on single linkages between television viewing and childhood overweight so that we may arrive at a more nuanced and complex understanding of the ways in which (and for whom) they are related and unrelated. As a very real threat to public health, it is crucial to identify central contributing factors to the development of obesity so that we may appropriately target prevention and intervention efforts. It seems safe to say that technology is here to stay, and it is virtually guaranteed to play an ever-increasing role in our daily lives. Thus, a thorough understanding of the nature of its impact on health and well-being is a vital component of the public health agenda in the United States.

**Accepted for Publication:** December 16, 2005.
**Correspondence:** Elizabeth A. Vandewater, PhD, Human Development and Family Sciences, University of Texas at Austin, 1 University Station, A2700, Austin, TX 78712-1097 (evandewater@mail.utexas.edu).
**Funding/Support:** This study was supported by grant R01-HD40851-01 and Population Research Center grant 5-R24-HD42849 from the National Institute of Child Health and Human Development, Rockville, Md. The Children's Digital Media Center at the University of Texas, Austin, is funded by grant BCS-0126127 from the National Science Foundation, Arlington, Va. The Panel Study of Income Dynamics Child Development Supplement is funded by grants R01-HD33474 and R01-HD044027 from the National Institute of Child Health and Human Development.

## REFERENCES


1. Troiano RP, Flegal KM. Overweight children and adolescents: description, epidemiology, and demographics. *Pediatrics.* 1998;101:497-504.
2. Ogden CL, Flegal K, Carrol MD, Johnson CL. Prevalence and trends in the overweight among US children and adolescents, 1999-2000. *JAMA.* 2002;288:1728-1732.
3. Hedley AA, Ogden CL, Johnson CL, Carrol MD, Curtin LR, Flegal KM. Prevalence of overweight and obesity among US children, adolescents, and adults, 1999-2002. *JAMA.* 2004;291:2847-2850.
4. Huston AC, Wright JC, Marquis J, Green SB. How young children spend their time: television and other activities. *Dev Psychol.* 1999;35:912-925.
5. Wright JC, Huston AC, Vandewater EA, et al. American children's use of electronic media in 1997: a national survey. *J Appl Dev Psychol.* 2001;22:31-47.
6. Gortmaker SL, Dietz WH, Sobol AM, Wehler CA. Increasing pediatric obesity in the United States. *AJDC.* 1987;141:535-540.
7. Chen JL, Kennedy CM. Television viewing and children's health. *J Soc Pediatr Nurs.* 2001;6:35-38.
8. Dietz WH. The obesity epidemic in young children: reduce television viewing and promote playing. *BMJ.* 2001;322:313-314.
9. Gortmaker SL, Must A, Perrin JM, Sobol AM, Dietz WH. Social and economic consequences of overweight in adolescence and young adulthood. *N Engl J Med.* 1993;329:1008-1012.
10. Dietz WH, Gortmaker SL. Do we fatten our children at the television set? obesity and television viewing in children and adolescents. *Pediatrics.* 1985;75:807-812.
11. Robinson TN, Killen JD. Ethnic and gender differences in the relationships between television viewing and obesity, physical activity, and dietary fat intake. *J Health Educ.* 1995;26(suppl 2):S91-S98.
12. Robinson TN, Hammer LD, Killen JD, et al. Does television viewing increase obesity and reduce physical activity? cross-sectional and longitudinal analyses among adolescent girls. *Pediatrics.* 1993;91:273-280.
13. McMurray RG, Harrell JS, Deng S, Bradley CB, Cox LM, Bangdiwala SI. The influence of physical activity, socioeconomic status, and ethnicity on the weight status of adolescents. *Obes Res.* 2000;8:130-139.
14. DuRant RH, Baranowski T, Johnson M, Thompson WO. The relationship among television watching, physical activity, and body composition of young children. *Pediatrics.* 1994;94:449-455.
15. Gortmaker SL, Peterson K, Wiecha J, et al. Reducing obesity via a school-based interdisciplinary intervention among youth: Planet Health. *Arch Pediatr Adolesc Med.* 1999;153:409-418.
16. Robinson TN. Reducing children's television viewing to prevent obesity: a randomized controlled trial. *JAMA.* 1999;282:1561-1567.
17. Garn SM, Sullivan TV, Hawthorne VM. Fatness and obesity of the parents of obese individuals. *Am J Clin Nutr.* 1989;50:1308-1313.
18. Locard E, Mamelle N, Billette A, Miginiac M, Munoz F, Rey S. Risk factors of obesity in a five year old population: parental vs environmental factors. *Int J Obes Relat Metab Disord.* 1992;16:721-729.
19. Mossberg HO. 40-year follow-up of overweight children. *Lancet.* 1989;2:491-493.
20. Stunkard AJ, Harris JR, Pedersen NL, McClearn GE. The body mass index of twins who have been reared apart. *N Engl J Med.* 1990;322:1483-1487.
21. Whitaker RC, Wright JA, Pepe MS, Seidel KD, Dietz WH. Predicting obesity in young adulthood from childhood and parental obesity. *N Engl J Med.* 1997;337:869-873.
22. Kotz K, Story M. Food advertisements during children's Saturday morning television programming: are they consistent with dietary recommendations? *J Am Diet Assoc.* 1994;94:1296-1301.
23. Harrison K, Marske AL. Nutritional content of foods advertised during the television programs children watch most. *Am J Public Health.* 2005;95:1568-1574.
24. Coon KA, Tucker K. Television and children's consumption patterns: a review of the literature. *Minerva Pediatr.* 2002;54:423-436.
25. Halford JCG, Gillespie J, Brown V, Pontin EE, Dowling H. Effect of television advertisements for foods on food consumption in children. *Appetite.* 2004;42:221-225.
26. Panel Study of Income Dynamics. Child Development Supplement documentation. Available at: http://psidonline.isr.umich.edu/CDS/wavesdoc.html. Accessed November 1, 2004.
27. Measurement Specialities Inc. Thinner MS-7 model. Available at: http://www.msiusa.com/default/index.asp. Accessed May 20, 2005.
28. Kuczmarski RJ, Ogden C, Guo SS, et al. 2000 CDC growth charts for the United States: methods and development. *Vital Health Stat 11.* 2002;(246):1-190.
29. National Heart, Lung, and Blood Institute; North American Association for the Study of Obesity. *The Practical Guide: Identification, Evaluation, and Treatment of Overweight and Obesity in Adults.* Bethesda, Md: National Institutes of Health; 2000. NIH publication 00-4084.
30. Hofferth SL, Sandberg JF. How American children spend their time. *J Marriage Fam.* 2001;63:295-308.
31. Yeung WJ, Sandberg JF, Davis-Kean PE. Children's time with fathers in intact families. *J Marriage Fam.* 2001;63:136-154.
32. Robinson JP. *How Americans Use Time: A Social-Psychological Analysis of Everyday Behavior.* New York, NY: Praeger; 1977.
33. Juster FT. Response errors in the measurement of time use. *J Am Stat Assoc.* 1986;81:390-402.
34. Juster FT, Stafford FP. The allocation of time: empirical findings, behavioral models, and problems of measurement. *J Econ Lit.* 1991;29:471-522.
35. Juster FT, Stafford FP, eds. *Time, Goods, and Well-being.* Ann Arbor, Mich: Institute for Social Research, University of Michigan; 1985.
36. Anderson DR, Field DE, Collins PA, Lorch EP, Natham JG. Estimates of young children's time with television: a methodological comparison of parent reports with time-lapse video home observation. *Child Dev.* 1985;56:1345-1357.
37. Himes JH. Maturation-related deviations and misclassification of stature and weight in adolescence. *Am J Hum Biol.* 1999;11:499-504.
38. Wang Y. Is obesity associated with early sexual maturation? a comparison of the association in American boys vs girls. *Pediatrics.* 2002;110:903-910.
39. Khamis HJ, Roche AF. Predicting adult stature without using skeletal age: the Khamis-Roche method. *Pediatrics.* 1994;94:504-507.
40. Beunen GP, Malina RM, Lefevre J, Claessens AL, Renson R, Simons J. Prediction of adult stature and noninvasive assessment of biological maturation. *Med Sci Sports Exerc.* 1997;29:225-230.
41. Himes JH, Obarzanek E, Baranowski T, Wilson DM, Rochon J, McClanahan BS. Early sexual maturation, body composition, and obesity in African-American girls. *Obes Res.* 2004;12(suppl):64S-72S.
42. Roche AF, Tyleshevski F, Rogers E. Non-invasive measurement of physical maturity in children. *Res Q Exerc Sport.* 1983;54:364-371.
43. Aiken LS, West SG. *Multiple Regression: Testing and Interpreting Interactions.* Thousand Oaks, Calif: Sage; 1991.
44. Goodman E, Hinden BR, Khandelwal S. Accuracy of teen and parental reports of obesity and body mass index. *Pediatrics.* 2000;106:52-58.
45. Jeffery RW. Bias in reported body weight as a function of education, occupation, health and weight concern. *Addict Behav.* 1996;21:217-222.
46. Wang Z, Patterson CM, Hills AP. A comparison of self-reported and measured height, weight, and BMI in Australian adolescents. *Aust N Z J Public Health.* 2002;26:473-478.
47. Palta M, Prineas RJ, Berman R, Hannan PJ. Comparison of self-reported and measured height and weight. *Am J Epidemiol.* 1982;115:223-230.
48. Rowland ML. Self-reported weight and height. *Am J Clin Nutr.* 1990;52:1125-1133.
49. Gorely T, Marshall SJ, Biddle SJH. Couch kids: correlates of television viewing among youth. *Int J Behav Med.* 2004;11:152-163.
50. Koplan JP, Liverman CT, Kraak VA, eds. *Preventing Childhood Obesity: Health in the Balance.* Washington, DC: National Academies Press; 2005.

# A Content Analysis of Health and Physical Activity Messages Marketed to African American Children During After-School Television Programming

*Corliss Wilson Outley, PhD; Abdissa Taddese*

**Objective:** To examine the number of food advertisements African American children are exposed to during children's television programming aired on predominantly African American and general television stations.

**Design:** A content analysis was conducted to identify and analyze the health-related content (HRC) and physical activity–related content (PARC) of food advertisements shown during children's television programming.

**Setting:** Three sets of television advertisements from 3 stations (Black Entertainment Television, The WB [Warner Bros], and Disney Channel) served as the sample during a 1-week period in July 2005 (July 11-15), from 3 PM to 9 PM.

**Results:** In total, 1098 advertisements were recorded, with 256 food and beverage commercials used for this study. Results indicate that 36.3% of all commercials were based on fast food restaurants, 31.3% were for drinks, 16.8% were for candy, 13.7% were for cereals, and 2.0% were for snacks (percentages do not total 100 because of rounding). Compared with The WB and Disney Channel, Black Entertainment Television had significantly ($P$=.001) more food and beverage advertisements. Few HRC or PARC advertisements were shown. Of 256 food and beverage commercials, only 8.2% contained HRC and 9.4% had PARC. Also, the HRC and PARC scenes contained messages that were implied vs explicitly talking about the health or physical benefits of the product.

**Conclusions:** African American children are overexposed to numerous types of food and beverage advertisements. These advertisements do not provide an adequate level of positive HRC and PARC messages. Consequently, the messages that are portrayed may undermine efforts to teach African American children about the importance of healthy living and physical activity.

*Arch Pediatr Adolesc Med. 2006;160:432-435*

**Author Affiliation:** School of Kinesiology, University of Minnesota, Minneapolis.

OBESITY IS BECOMING A MAjor public health concern, affecting 1 of 5 children in the United States.[1-4] Studies have shown an alarming increase in obesity among children in the United States during the past decade. Between 10% and 20% of children and teenagers in the United States are obese.[4,5] The prevalence of obesity in US children varies by racial and ethnic group as well. Estimates indicate that 13% of African American children are overweight or obese.[6] Consequently, more African Americans are experiencing health problems due to obesity, such as high cholesterol, stroke, asthma, sleep apnea, and diabetes mellitus. Limited access to high-quality foods, poor dietary choices, sedentary lifestyles, cultural norms, and low socioeconomic status contribute to the high prevalence of obesity among African American children. Despite these influences, researchers have begun to investigate the role of the media and its influences on obesity.

Television viewing in America starts at an early age. Children as young as 2 to 6 years are viewing approximately 2 hours of television each day.[4,6,7] According to a recent study,[7] children in the United States between the ages of 6 and 11 years watch an average of more than 23 hours of television a week, while children between the ages of 12 and 17 years watch an average of more than 21 hours per week. Furthermore, it is estimated that the average child views more than 40 000 advertisements each year.[7] Television viewership also differs by racial and ethnic groups. Previous studies[8-10] indicate that African American children watch significantly more television than white children. Studies[5] have documented that African American prime-time television shows contain 60% more food commercials (fast food, candy and sweets, and unhealthy foods) compared with general prime-time market shows. To our knowledge, the effect of television viewing and obesity risk among African Americans is an area that has received little attention, despite the fact that much television viewing is taking place in African American households.

There are 4 main propositions to explain the relationship between television viewing and obesity: (1) television displaces participation in exercise and other active leisure behaviors, (2) increased food consumption occurs during viewing, (3) advertisement exposure leads to increased consumption of advertised foods, and (4) there are subsequent attempts by children to influence parental food purchases after repeated advertisement exposure.[5,10,11] Each of these propositions illustrates the vulnerability of children to the food messages that are portrayed during television advertisements. Although many believe there is a link between television watching, decreased physical activity, and obesity, what children watch and the messages they are receiving from the advertisements may be more important. This is significant given that most food advertised during children's programming is fast foods, soft drinks, sweets, and sugar-sweetened cereal, all of which has been linked to children's misconceptions about the health benefits of the advertised foods and increased consumption of high-caloric high-fat foods.[12-14]

In recent years, the food and beverage industry has viewed children and adolescents as major consumers. As a result, children and adolescents are targeted aggressively by food advertisers, and are exposed to a growing and unprecedented amount of advertising through television. There have been few studies focused on the after-school hours, from 3 PM to 9 PM. Thus, the present study represents an attempt to examine the health- and physical activity–related messages presented during after-school children's television programs on a predominately African American network and those airing on general programming networks.

## METHODS

### SAMPLE

Nielsen Media Research[15] indicates that 72% of African American children (aged 2-11 years) and 65% of teenagers (aged 12-17 years) watch network and advertisement-supported cable stations. The selected television stations for this study include Black Entertainment Television (BET), The WB (Warner Bros), and Disney Channel. Each channel represents a different television segment. The WB is the fifth largest television network in the nation, BET is an advertisement-supported cable station, and Disney Channel is a cable station supported by private and nonprofit advertisements. BET is the first television network devoted to programming for African American viewers between the ages of 18 and 34 years, and reaches more than 80 million households (78% African American). Historically, The WB has featured African American shows that have drawn an African American audience. Although few prime-time shows exist with predominately African American casts, their Kids' WB children's programming is rated number 1 among all US children. Finally, Nielsen Media Research points out that although Disney Channel is not an advertiser-supported channel (some programming is underwritten via select sponsorship advertisement), several shows (eg, *That's So Raven*) are among the top rated for African American children. Each of these was selected based on these findings and for being among the top-ranked stations for African American viewers younger than 18 years.[16]

The stations were broadcast in the Midwest region of the United States for a 1-week period, July 11-15, 2005. The commercials broadcast on each network were recorded between 3 PM and 9 PM. All of the commercials that aired during the recorded period were included. A total of 35 hours of after-school television programs were analyzed.

### CODING PROCEDURE

The coding scheme was based on earlier studies[12-14] and included new categories. The final instrument was pilot tested by having 3 upper-level recreation students independently analyze 3 hours of televised after-school programs. The results of the pilot test were used to revise the instrument. The final instrument used for this study contained 2 sections. Section 1 focused on basic television station information (program type, commercial length, presence of models, and type of product advertised). Section 2 described the health-related content (HRC) or physical activity–related content (PARC) of the advertisement. For this study, HRC was defined as any scene that provided visual and verbal information related to mental or physical health, medical treatments (eg, medications), and food/nutrition. In contrast, PARC was defined as any scene that provided verbal or visual information related to leisure-related physical activities. Although previous studies have looked at these 2 categories collectively, research warrants having an accurate examination of HRC and PARC separately because both are viewed as predictors of obesity.

This section also looked at (1) the level of accuracy (accurate, accurate but misleading, or inaccurate) for the HRC and PARC and (2) their implicit or explicit assertions. The level of accuracy was measured by examining the amount of information the HRC and PARC provided that was free from errors and did not mislead the viewer. An advertisement that illustrates its cereal product as "no preservatives" and "no additives" (and the statements are true based on US nutritional guidelines) is a good example of an accurate advertisement. An accurate but misleading message was defined as one that provides information without errors but withholds or deletes additional information that can counter the primary target message (eg, a commercial that flaunts a cereal product's low-sugar content but does not reveal the high level of carbohydrates, calories, and fat that equal the regular cereal version). Inaccurate messages were those that provided information on a product that was erroneous or left out, that could possibly assist viewers in their decision making. For example, this can occur when a product is advertised as having the ingredients to increase children's running capacity to that of a jaguar or to mimic a cartoon inanimate superstrength (eg, Popeye's can of spinach).

Implicit messages were those that implied a link between the advertised product and the HRC or PARC message but relied on the viewer to make the connection. Explicit HRC is when the commercial message regarding health outcomes is directly linked to the advertised product. For example, a commercial that implied eating a particular food was linked to health by describing the food product ingredients (eg, whole wheat) or unique quality (eg, low in sugar) was deemed implicit. Likewise, a commercial that overtly stated that the featured product could lower cholesterol was coded as explicit.

### DATA COLLECTION

Two researchers (A.T. and an undergraduate student) were trained to conduct the content analysis. This training included a review of the instrument and definitions before beginning analysis. In addition, the examiners jointly viewed and coded 3 hours of after-school programming to become familiar with the procedures. For the actual study, each researcher independently viewed and coded all of the commercials in a private computer/media laboratory. To ensure that the data were recorded accurately, the examiners were encouraged to stop,

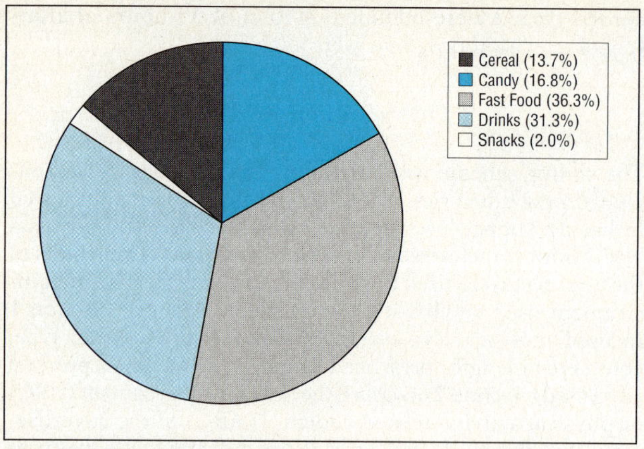


**Figure.** Type of food advertised during after-school programming. Percentages do not total 100 because of rounding.

restart, and rewind the videotape, and to use slow motion as needed. At the end of their coding, the researchers compared and discussed any differences to reach an agreed on decision.

## RESULTS

The 36 hours of after-school programming analyzed included a total of 1098 commercials. Food and beverage advertisements accounted for 256 (23.3%) of the total advertisements broadcast during the study period. A total of 174 minutes, or 2 hours 54 minutes, of the 36 hours sampled was commercial time. The number of commercials per half hour ranges from 15 to 20 (average, 18). The commercial length ranges from 25 to 55 seconds. On average, more than 7 in 10 of the food commercials presented were repeated several times throughout the day. Of the advertisements, 63.3% aired on BET, 32.4% aired on The WB, and only 4.3% aired on Disney Channel.

### TYPE OF PRODUCTS ADVERTISED

The food and beverage products advertised were grouped into the following categories: fast food restaurants, drinks, candy, cereal, and snacks. According to our findings (**Figure**), fast food represented most advertisements, followed by drinks, candy, cereal, and snacks. We investigated whether there were differences in the type of products being advertised by the varying stations (**Table 1**). The top 3 fast food advertisements were for McDonald's (30.1%), SONIC (16.0%), and Domino's Pizza (15.1%). Fast food advertisements were aired more often on BET compared with the other 2 stations. There was a significant difference in the drink products that were advertised, with all of the Kool-Aid advertisements (25.0%) being aired on BET ($P = .001$). The next leading drink product was Coke and Gatorade (16.3% each). There were no significant differences in the type of snacks advertised on the varying stations. Cinnamon Toast Crunch represented 34.3% of the total cereal products that were recorded. This was followed by Cheerios, which represented 20.0% of the cereal advertisements aired. The third largest advertised cereal product was Frosted Flakes (17.1%). Candy products were advertised mainly on The WB compared with BET or Disney Channel. The major advertised candy product was Air Heads (41.9%). This was followed by M&M's (27.9%) and various gum products (14.0%).

**Table 1.** $\chi^2$ **Analysis Between Type of Food Advertised and Television Stations***

| Product Type | BET | The WB | Disney Channel |
|---|---|---|---|
| Fast food† | 65.6 | 34.4 | 0 |
| Drinks† | 82.5 | 11.3 | 6.3 |
| Snacks | 60.0 | 0 | 40.0 |
| Cereal† | 42.9 | 45.7 | 11.4 |
| Candy† | 39.5 | 60.5 | 0 |

Abbreviations: BET, Black Entertainment Television; WB, Warner Bros.
*Data are given as percentage of food advertised on each station. Percentages may not total 100 because of rounding.
†The difference between stations is significant ($P = .001$).

**Table 2.** $\chi^2$ **Test of Television Stations Containing Health-Related Content**

| | Health-Related Content* | |
|---|---|---|
| Television Station | Yes | No |
| BET (n = 162)† | 21 (13.0) | 141 (87.0) |
| The WB (n = 83)† | 0 | 83 (100.0) |
| Disney Channel (n = 11)† | 0 | 11 (100.0) |
| **Total** (N = 256) | **21** (8.2) | **235** (91.8) |

Abbreviations: See Table 1.
*Data are given as number (percentage) of each station.
†The difference between stations is significant ($P = .001$).

### HEALTH-RELATED CONTENT

Of 256 food and beverage commercials viewed, only 8.2% contained HRC information (**Table 2**). The HRC advertisements all promoted health or nutritional factors (eg, showed that the product contains no or low sugar, the product has low fat, or "the product is good"). Most of the health-related commercials aired were implicit (90.5%), with few being explicit (9.5%). Few commercials explicitly illustrated positive health-related information to sell their products to young viewers. Many focused on taste, color, and smell to market the food products.

Next, we determined the accuracy of the claims regarding the HRC information aired in each advertisement. Of the commercials, 47.6% provided accurate information. In comparison, 28.6% were accurate but misleading and 23.8% were inaccurate and misleading. There was a significant difference in the amount of HRC information provided in the advertisements between the 3 stations, with more HRC advertisements on BET.

### PHYSICAL ACTIVITY–RELATED CONTENT

Much like the HRC advertisements, the PARC advertisement sample was small. Only 9.4% of the food and beverage commercials contained PARC (**Table 3**). When it comes to PARC, Disney Channel aired the most advertisements, followed by The WB and BET. Again, rarely did advertisers attempt to make a direct link between their product and physical activity messages. Few models that were portrayed in the commercials were shown explicitly using products while participating in physical activity (34.6%). There were no significant ($P$=.19) differences between the stations in the total number of commercials that were implicit or explicit in their message form. Approximately 38.5% of the commercials were accurate, 38.5% were accurate but misleading, and 23.1% were inaccurate and misleading (percentages do not total 100 because of rounding).

## COMMENT

In summary, our results indicate that African American children are being exposed to numerous types of food and beverage advertisements being aired during after-school programming. In the past, much research focused on the links between children being exposed to an unprecedented volume of televised food and beverage advertisements and the unprecedented rates of childhood obesity. Many of these researchers have indicated that most children who are at a high risk of becoming overweight are African American children who come from low-income families. It is argued that these children watch significantly more hours of television. The more children watch television, the greater the chance of them being exposed to advertisements for foods that are high in fat and sugar. In addition, these children are exposed to HRC and PARC that does not reflect nutritional and physical activity guidelines. Although this study does not look at the relationship between television watching and obesity, it does provide a bird's-eye view into the type of advertisements shown during the after-school hours and the information they convey. Unfortunately, many of the products being advertised can be considered unhealthy and not conforming to the health recommendations set by the US government.

This study illustrates this is especially true for children watching the predominant African American television network, BET. BET had the most advertisements that are deemed unhealthy compared with those that the general television stations aired during after-school programming. This study supports previous findings[5,17,18] that suggest African American television shows have a disproportionate number of unhealthy food images and may influence the eating behavior and knowledge of vulnerable African American children.

This study is one of the first to examine the effects of media on children during the after-school programming hours. Past studies have more often focused on Saturday morning and weekday prime-time television programming. Yet, the out-of-school time hours have become a leading focus of researchers investigating positive youth development. Data suggest that there are approximately 8 million children between the ages of 5 and 14 years who spend the after-school hours without adult supervision.[19] Research[19] has shown that, during these hours, children without adult supervision are at significantly greater risk of nonattendance from school, stress, receiving poor grades, risk-taking behavior, and substance abuse. Those who spend more hours on their own and begin self-care at younger ages are at increased risk of poor development outcomes. We hope that these findings will be used to further research that will examine the inequitable advertising that African American children are exposed to and its effect on their health. Given the increase in the number of African American children who are overweight and obese, their cultural predisposition to watch television programs that feature African American characters,[5,17,18] and the lack of obesity prevention programs designed to address disproportionate target marketing, research on the effect of media on African American children in the United States must become a priority.

**Table 3. $\chi^2$ Test of Television Stations Containing Physical Activity–Related Content**

| Television Station | Physical Activity–Related Content* | |
|---|---|---|
| | Yes | No |
| BET (n = 162)† | 7 (4.3) | 155 (95.7) |
| The WB (n = 83)† | 12 (14.5) | 71 (85.5) |
| Disney Channel (n = 11)† | 5 (45.5) | 6 (54.5) |
| **Total** (N = 256) | **24** (9.4) | **232** (90.6) |

Abbreviations: See Table 1.
*Data are given as number (percentage) of each station.
†The difference between stations is significant ($P$ = .001).

**Accepted for Publication:** December 21, 2005.
**Correspondence:** Corliss Wilson Outley, PhD, School of Kinesiology, University of Minnesota, 1900 University Ave SE, Minneapolis, MN 55443 (coutley@umn.edu).

## REFERENCES


1. Micic D. Obesity in children and adolescents—a new epidemic? consequences in adult life. *J Pediatr Endocrinol.* 2001;14(suppl 5):1345-1352; discussion, 1365.
2. Kimm SYS, Obarzanek E. Childhood obesity. *Pediatrics.* 2002;110:1003-1007.
3. Ogden CL, Flegal KM, Carroll MD, Johnson CL. Prevalence and trends in overweight among US children and adolescents, 1999-2000. *JAMA.* 2002;288: 1728-1732.
4. Kaiser JH. The role of media in childhood obesity [Kaiser Family Foundation Web site]. Available at: http://www.kff.org/entmedia/upload/The-Role-Of-Media-in-Childhood-Obesity.pdf. Accessed June 23, 2005.
5. Henderson VR, Kelly B. Food advertising in the age of obesity. *J Nutr Educ Behav.* 2005;37:191-196.
6. Crawford PB, Story M, Wang MC, Ritchie LD, Sabry ZI. Ethnic issues in the epidemiology of childhood obesity. *Pediatr Clin North Am.* 2001;48:855-878.
7. Story M, French S. Food advertising and marketing directed at children and adolescents in the US. Available at: http://www.ijbnpa.org/content/1/1/3. Accessed July 9, 2005.
8. Stroman CA. Television's role in the socialization of African American children and adolescents. *J Negro Educ.* 2001;60:314-327.
9. Larson RW, Richards MH, Sims B, Dworkin J. How urban African American young adolescents spend their time. *Am J Community Psychol.* 2001;29:565-597.
10. Tirodkar MA, Jain A. Food messages on African American television shows. *Am J Public Health.* 2003;93:439-441.
11. Robinson TN, Hammer LD, Killen JD, et al. Does television viewing increase obesity and reduce physical activity? *Pediatrics.* 1993;91:273-280.
12. Taras HL, Gage M. Advertised foods on children's television. *Arch Pediatr Adolesc Med.* 1995;149:649-652.
13. Story M, Faulkner P. The prime time diet. *Am J Public Health.* 1990;80:738-740.
14. Byrd-Bredbenner C, Grassos D. Prime-time health. *Int Electronic J Health Educ.* 1999;2:159-169.
15. Nielsen Media Research. TV audience special study: African American audience: 2005. Available at: http://www.nielsenmedia.com/ethnicmeasure/african-american/indexAA.html. Accessed September 3, 2005.
16. Byrd-Bredbenner C, Grasso D, Finckenor M. Nutrition-related content in prime-time television programming. *Top Clin Nutr.* 2001;16:61-72.
17. Brown JD, Pardun CJ. Little in common: racial and gender differences in adolescent's television diets. *J Broadcasting Electronic Media.* 2004;48:266-278.
18. Li-Vollmer M. Race representation in child-targeted television commercials. *Mass Commun Sociol.* 2002;5:207-228.
19. The future of children: when school is out, executive summary [The Future of Children Web site]. Available at: http://www.futureofchildren.org/usr_doc/vol9no2ES.pdf. Accessed July 28, 2005.

ARTICLE

# When Children Eat What They Watch

## *Impact of Television Viewing on Dietary Intake in Youth*

*Jean L. Wiecha, PhD; Karen E. Peterson, ScD, RD; David S. Ludwig, MD, PhD; Juhee Kim, ScD; Arthur Sobol, MA; Steven L. Gortmaker, PhD*

**Objectives:** To test whether increased television viewing is associated with increased total energy intake and with increased consumption of foods commonly advertised on television, and to test whether increased consumption of these foods mediates the relationship between television viewing and total energy intake.

**Design:** Prospective observational study with baseline (fall 1995) and follow-up (spring 1997) measures of youth diet, physical activity, and television viewing. We used food advertising data to identify 6 food groups for study (sweet baked snacks, candy, fried potatoes, main courses commonly served as fast food, salty snacks, and sugar-sweetened beverages).

**Setting and Participants:** Five public schools in 4 communities near Boston. The sample included 548 students (mean age at baseline, 11.70 years; 48.4% female; and 63.5% white).

**Main Outcome Measures:** Change in total energy intake and intake of foods commonly advertised on television from baseline to follow-up.

**Results:** After adjusting for baseline covariates, each hour increase in television viewing was associated with an additional 167 kcal/d (95% confidence interval, 136-198 kcal/d; $P<.001$) and with increases in the consumption of foods commonly advertised on television. Including changes in intakes of these foods in regression models provided evidence of their mediating role, diminishing or rendering nonsignificant the associations between change in television viewing and change in total energy intake.

**Conclusions:** Increases in television viewing are associated with increased calorie intake among youth. This association is mediated by increasing consumption of calorie-dense low-nutrient foods frequently advertised on television.

*Arch Pediatr Adolesc Med. 2006;160:436-442*

OVERWEIGHT PREVALENCE has increased sharply among all sex and racial/ethnic groups in the United States. Among 12- to 19-year old individuals, overweight (body mass index [BMI] [calculated as weight in kilograms divided by the square of height in meters] ≥95th age- and sex-specific percentile) prevalence increased from 4.6% in the mid 1960s to 15.5% in 2000.[1] In many cross-sectional[2-4] and longitudinal[5-10] studies, a positive association exists between hours of television viewing and measures of obesity and overweight in youth. Television viewing time also predicts obesity, development of type 2 diabetes mellitus,[11,12] and poor lipid profiles[13,14] in adults. In randomized controlled trials[10,15-17] among youth, changes in television viewing have been instrumental in reducing overweight.

While published studies are consistent with a causal relationship between television viewing and overweight, the mechanisms driving this are not well understood. Television viewing could influence energy balance by reducing energy expenditure relative to other uses of leisure time, by increasing energy intake (eg, through snacking and exposure to food marketing), or by a combination of these. Although television viewing itself is a sedentary activity, contributing little to nonbasal energy expenditure, studies[18-20] show only a weak or modest negative correlation between time spent on television viewing and time spent in moderate and vigorous physical activity. A randomized controlled trial[21] found that increasing screen time resulted in reduced energy expenditure and increased energy intake.

Television's potential role in increasing energy intake must be considered in the context of the extraordinary amount of television-based food advertising that occurs annually. Television advertisements account for roughly 75% of food manufacturers' and 95% of fast food restaurants' advertising expenditures.[22] In

Author Affiliations:
Departments of Society, Human Development, and Health (Drs Wiecha, Peterson, and Gortmaker and Mr Sobol) and Nutrition (Drs Peterson and Kim), Harvard School of Public Health, and Department of Medicine, Children's Hospital (Dr Ludwig), Boston, Mass.

1997, when data collection for this study ended, food industries spent $11 billion on advertising.[22] Food manufacturers, responsible for most ($7 billion) of this, spent 25% of their advertising dollars promoting candy, cookies, salty snacks, and soft drinks—and 5% promoting fruits, vegetables, grains, beans, meat, poultry, and fish.[22] Fast food restaurants spent more than $1 billion on advertising in 1999.[23]

Studies[22,24-28] suggest these dollars are spent effectively—food advertising works. For example, several studies show associations between exposure to advertisements and children's requests for specific foods, food purchasing, and food consumption. Television viewing, a major venue for advertising exposure, is directly associated with calorie intake among adults[11] and youth[29,30] in cross-sectional studies, and with intake of foods commonly advertised on television (FCAT)—soft drinks, fried foods, and snacks—among youth.[3] These types of foods pose risks for overeating and weight gain. Fast food restaurant use, which is heavily promoted on television, is positively associated with calorie intake in youth[31] and with BMI among adults.[32] In a recent study,[30] on days when children ate fast food, they consumed more calories, fat, added sugars, and sugar-sweetened beverages and fewer servings of milk, fruits, and nonstarchy vegetables than on days when they did not eat fast food. Prospective studies[33] among children have indicated a positive relationship between intake of sugar-sweetened soft drinks and obesity incidence.

The present study examines whether increases in adolescents' television viewing time are associated with increases in total energy intake (TEI), and whether viewing increases are also associated with increases in intake of FCAT (candy, fast foods, fried potatoes, sweet baked snacks, salty snacks, and sugar-sweetened beverages). We also examine whether changes in intakes of these foods mediate the relationship between change in viewing time and change in TEI.

## METHODS

### THEORETICAL FRAMEWORK

In light of the literature, we hypothesize that increases in television viewing time will result in increases in TEI. One causal pathway will consist of increased consumption of FCAT. To test this hypothesis, we examine a longitudinal observational cohort in which we collected measures of television viewing and food consumption at 2 time points. Statistical models in which change in an independent variable predicts change in a dependent variable may provide stronger evidence for causality than predictions involving the independent variable measured at just 1 point in time (eg, baseline).[34] Attenuation of the association between an independent and a dependent variable by the addition of a second independent variable in the causal pathway can provide evidence for mediation in the context of a plausible theoretical framework.[35] In addition, a mediator variable is also independently associated with exposure and outcome. Therefore, in our analyses of the relationship of change in television viewing time to change in TEI, we evaluate evidence for the mediating effects of FCAT by examining the associations between television and FCAT; FCAT and TEI; and television, FCAT, and TEI. In our models, we control for other characteristics of respondents that could potentially influence energy intake at follow-up, including baseline BMI, age, sex, indicator variables for race/ethnicity, baseline physical activity of 3.5 metabolic equivalents (METs) or more, change in physical activity of 3.5 METs or more, and school.

### SUBJECTS

Data were collected as part of the Planet Health intervention and evaluation, a group randomized controlled trial that took place in 10 schools in 4 communities in the Boston metropolitan area between fall 1995 and spring 1997. Schools were matched and then randomized to the control and intervention conditions, and no differences were observed between these groups on baseline measures, including age, BMI, TEI, television viewing, or physical activity levels. The 548 students composing the analytic sample attended the 5 randomly assigned control schools that did not take part in the intervention designed to reduce obesity prevalence.[16] The median annual household income of ZIP code areas where the control schools were located averaged $34 200, according to 1990 census data, lower than that for all households in Massachusetts in 1990 ($41 000), but similar to the US figure ($33 952).[36] A total of 780 subjects (64.5% of those eligible) completed the baseline evaluation in fall 1995 at the control schools after excluding individuals who transferred schools at baseline, were in special education classes, were in grades other than sixth or seventh, or did not complete the English-language version of the questionnaire. Follow-up data were collected in spring 1997 for 655 subjects (84.0% of the baseline group), reflecting loss to follow-up of 18.0% for girls and 14.0% for boys. The main reason for lack of follow-up data was school transfer (half of those not followed up) and school absence (one quarter). Of the 571 subjects with complete data on all variables, 548 were included in these analyses after excluding 23 with implausible daily energy intakes (≤500 or ≥7000 kcal). Further details on sampling and exclusions are available elsewhere.[16] The study was approved by the Committee on Human Subjects at the Harvard School of Public Health.

The 548 subjects were a mean ± SD age of 11.70 ± 0.75 years at baseline, and 48.4% were female. Of the subjects, 63.5% were white, 15.3% were Hispanic, 13.9% were African American, 7.7% were Asian, 0.9% were American Indian, and 7.7% were another ethnicity (this totals >100% because respondents could select multiple descriptors). Anthropometric data and student surveys were collected in fall 1995, when subjects were in either grade 6 or grade 7, and follow-up measurements were collected approximately 19 months later, in spring 1997 (when subjects were in grade 7 or 8).

### ANTHROPOMETRIC DATA

For BMI, height without shoes was measured to the nearest 0.1 cm using a stadiometer (Irwin Shorr, Olney, Md) and weight in light clothes was measured to the nearest 0.1 kg on a portable electronic scale (model 770; Seca, Hanover, Md), calibrated using a standard weights "step-up" test (Seca).

### ASSESSMENT OF DIET, PHYSICAL ACTIVITY LEVEL, AND TELEVISION VIEWING

Measures of dietary intake, physical activity level, and television viewing were obtained via an optically scannable student food and activity survey, used with permission of the Brigham and Women's Hospital, Boston. Students completed the food and activity survey independently in class under the supervision of teachers who participated in a 1-hour training session before administration.

**Table 1. Groups of Foods Advertised on Television and Measured on the Food Frequency Questionnaire**

| Group | Item (Serving Type Where Specified)* | Response Categories |
|---|---|---|
| Sugar-sweetened beverages | Soda (can) | Never or less than one can per month, 1-3 cans per month, 1 can per week, 2-6 cans per week, 1 can per day, 2 or more cans per day |
| | Hawaiian punch, lemonade, Kool-Aid, or other sweetened fruit drink (glass) | Never or less than 1 glass per month, 1-3 glasses per month, 1 glass per week, 2-4 glasses per week, 5-6 glasses per week, 1 glass per day, 2 or more glasses per day |
| | Iced tea, not diet (glass) | Never or less than 1 glass per month, 1-3 glasses per month, 1-4 glasses per week, 5 or more glasses per week |
| Salty snacks | Crackers, potato chips (small bag), corn chips (small bag, including Doritos and Fritos, etc), pretzels | Never or less than once per month, 1-3 times per month, 1-4 times per week, or 5 or more times per week |
| Fried potatoes | Fried potatoes (eg, tater tots or French fries) | Less than 1 order per month, 1-3 orders per month, 1 order per week, 2-4 orders per week, 5 or more orders per week |
| Sweet snacks | Cookies (one) | Never or less than one per month, 1-3 per month, 1 per week, 2 to 6 per week, 1 to 3 per day, 4 or more per day |
| | Brownies (one) | Never or less than one per month, 1-3 per month, 1 per week, 2-4 per week, 5 or more per week |
| | Pie (one slice) | Never or less than one per month, 1-3 per month, 1 per week, 2 to 6 per week, 1 or more per day |
| | Pop-Tarts or turnovers (one) | Never or less than one per month, 1-3 per month, 1-6 per week, 1 or more per day |
| | Cake (one slice) | Never or less than one per month, 1-3 per month, 1 per week, or 2 or more per week |
| | Snack cakes (eg, Twinkies, one package) or donuts (one) | Never or less than one per month, 1-3 per month, 1 per week, 2-6 per week, 1 or more per day |
| Candy | Chocolate (one bar or packet) | Never or less than 1 per month, 1-3 per month, 1 per week, 2-6 per week, 1 or more per day |
| | Candy without chocolate (eg, Life Savers, one pack) | Never or less than one per month, 1-3 per month, 1 per week, 2-4 per week, 5 or more per week |
| | Fruit leathers (one pack) | Never or less than 1 per month, 1-3 per month, 1-4 per week, 5 or more per week |
| Fast food–type main courses | Fried chicken (one serving), cheeseburger (one burger), hamburger (one burger), pizza (one slice), tacos or burritos (one), chicken nuggets (six nuggets), and hot dog (one) | Never or less than once per month, 1-3 per month, 1 per week, 2-4 per week, 5 or more per week |

*Manufacturers: Kool-Aid and Life Savers (Kraft Foods, Northfield, Ill); Doritos and Fritos (Frito-Lay, Division of Pepsico, Purchase, NY); Pop-Tarts (Kellogg's, Battle Creek, Mich); Twinkies (Interstate Bakeries Corp, Kansas City, Mo).

## DIETARY INTAKE

The FCAT were identified from the data of Gallo.[22] Comparable foods were identified from the youth food frequency questionnaire component of the food and activity survey, an instrument adapted and validated for use in ethnically and socioeconomically diverse populations.[37-39] Six FCAT groups were created to best match the available youth food frequency questionnaire data with information on food advertising[22,23]: sugar-sweetened beverages, salty snacks, fried potatoes, sweet baked snacks, candy, and main courses commonly served at fast food restaurants.

The youth food frequency questionnaire asked how often in the past 30 days food items were consumed. There were 4 to 6 response categories typically offered. For example, response categories for soda (1 of 3 items composing sugar-sweetened beverages) were never or less than 1 can per month, 1 to 3 cans per month, 1 can per week, 2 to 6 cans per week, 1 can per day, or 2 cans or more per day. For each item, the uppermost category was truncated at the highest value (eg, ≥2 glasses per day was assigned a value of 2) and the lowest category was coded as 0.5 per month. If a food item was left blank, it was recoded as a 0. **Table 1** describes the food groups and the response categories for each item.

Total energy intake was estimated from all foods on the youth food frequency questionnaire by the Channing Laboratory, Boston, using calorie values assigned to standard portion sizes from releases 10 and 11 of the US Department of Agriculture Nutrient Database for Standard Reference. In a separate study,[37] the Pearson product moment correlation coefficient for TEI estimated by comparing 2 food frequency questionnaires with three 24-hour recalls was 0.49.

## PHYSICAL ACTIVITY

Physical activity level was assessed with the youth activity questionnaire component of the food and activity survey. The youth activity questionnaire included 16 items that estimate hours per day spent in moderate and vigorous activities (≥3.5 METs)[40] over the past month. Walking was excluded because of low agreement among measures in other studies.[36] The youth activity questionnaire is based on a 14-item physical activity questionnaire demonstrated to have good reproducibility and validity in adults[41,42] and high school youth.[36] In a validation study among 53 participants in Planet Health, using repeat 24-hour physical activity recalls 1 month apart, the 16 youth activity questionnaire items for activity of 3.5 METs or more had a deattenuated correlation[43] with the 24-hour recall of $r=0.80$, with equivalent means.[16]

## TELEVISION

Time spent watching television was measured with the 11-item television and video measure.[16] Seven of these questions asked about hours of television typically viewed during each day of the week. The midpoint of each response category was used to estimate total viewing, and the uppermost category (eg, "5 or more hours per day") was assigned a value of 5. Items were appropriately weighted and summed to obtain a television viewing hour-per-day estimate. Other items in the television and video measure assessed video and computer game use and were not included in this analysis. In the validation sample (n=53), we found a deattenuated[43] correlation of television viewing via the television and video measure and the 24-hour recall of $r=0.54$, with equivalent means.[16] Television data were imputed among 7 students missing 1 or more days of television data in 1995 and among 3 students in 1997. When weekdays were missing, the imputed value was equal to the mean of the other weekdays for that student. When weekend days were missing, the imputed value was equal to the value for the available weekend day or, for 4 students missing both weekend days in 1995, the mean value for the sample was used. Sample means for television viewing were unchanged by imputation.

## DEMOGRAPHIC VARIABLES

Age was calculated from birth date and date of anthropometric examinations. Sex was classified at the time of examination by measurers or from school list data. Racial/ethnic categories were derived from the question, "How do you describe yourself?," to which students could select multiple responses from the following list: white, black, Hispanic, Asian or Pacific Islander, American Indian or Alaskan Native, or other. Participants indicating black were classified as African American. Indicator variables were used to classify the 5 schools, with the largest school omitted as the referent. The distribution of subjects from each of the 5 schools was as follows: 261 (47.6%), 122 (22.3%), 79 (14.4%), 48 (8.8%), and 38 (6.9%).

## STATISTICAL ANALYSES

SAS statistical software, version 8.2 (SAS Institute Inc, Cary, NC), was used for all analyses. For adjusted analyses, we used PROC SURVEYREG to estimate regressions because these take into account clustering at the school level. PROC SURVEYREG uses an implicit Taylor linearization estimation method. Change variables were calculated as the 1997 value minus the 1995 value to obtain continuous measures.

We estimated adjusted associations of change in television viewing with change in TEI in a series of regression models. Predictor variables in each model included baseline television viewing and change in viewing, baseline BMI, TEI, age, sex, indicator variables for race/ethnicity, baseline physical activity of 3.5 METs or more, change in physical activity of 3.5 METs or more, and indicator variables for schools.

In the first set of models, the outcome was change in TEI. We evaluated the mediating role of intake of FCAT by adding baseline and change variables for the 6 food groups individually and then simultaneously to create 7 regressions in addition to the basic model for TEI. Foods were considered potential mediating, and not confounding, variables because in our theoretical model, we posit that increases in FCAT intake follow increases in television viewing in a temporal manner and, therefore, are part of the causal pathway. Empirically, this suggests that changes in television viewing predict changes in FCAT intake, and that FCAT intake predicts TEI. Two analyses were undertaken to examine evidence for the hypothesized mediation. First, we assessed evidence for independent associations between changes in intakes of the food groups and change in TEI (all models were significant at $P<.05$; data not shown). Second, we estimated an additional set of regression models (shown later) to assess whether changes in television viewing predicted change in number of servings per day of each food group.

**Table 2. Baseline (Fall 1995) and Follow-up (Spring 1997) Dietary and Activity Characteristics of the Cohort (N = 548)***

| Characteristic | Baseline Value | Follow-up Value | Crude Change |
|---|---|---|---|
| Dietary | | | |
| Total daily intake, kcal | 2141 ± 1076 | 2299 ± 1128 | 158 ± 1199 |
| Baked sweet snacks† | 1.18 ± 1.53 | 1.43 ± 1.56 | 0.25 ± 1.75 |
| Candy† | 0.42 ± 0.44 | 0.51 ± 0.49 | 0.10 ± 0.52 |
| Fast food–type main courses† | 0.70 ± 0.63 | 0.74 ± 0.60 | 0.04 ± 0.65 |
| Fried potatoes† | 0.12 ± 0.15 | 0.16 ± 0.17 | 0.05 ± 0.20 |
| Salty snacks† | 0.64 ± 0.59 | 0.72 ± 0.58 | 0.09 ± 0.68 |
| Sugar-sweetened beverages† | 1.21 ± 1.10 | 1.43 ± 1.09 | 0.22 ± 1.14 |
| All foods commonly advertised on television† | 4.27 ± 3.19 | 5.00 ± 3.27 | 0.74 ± 3.29 |
| Physical activity and inactivity | | | |
| Television viewing, h/d | 2.44 ± 1.41 | 2.29 ± 1.38 | −0.16 ± 1.30 |
| Reported activity ≥3.5 METs, h/d | 1.34 ± 1.09 | 1.28 ± 1.03 | −0.06 ± 0.97 |

Abbreviation: MET, metabolic equivalent.
*Data are given as mean ± SD.
†All food values are in servings per day.

## RESULTS

Dietary and activity data are summarized in **Table 2**. The mean±SD BMI at baseline was 20.73±3.99. The TEI increased from baseline to follow-up. Although the average hours of television viewing changed little, 152 subjects (27.7%) increased television viewing by 1 h/d or less and 83 (15.1%) increased viewing by more than 1 h/d (data not shown). All mean FCAT intakes increased during the study period. The highest daily number of servings at follow-up were reported for baked sweet snacks, sugar-sweetened beverages, and fast food–type main courses, and the combined category indicated roughly 5 servings of FCAT per day, or 35 per week.

In adjusted analyses, baseline viewing and change in television viewing predicted change in daily TEI (**Table 3**). With no foods in the model, each hour of increase in television viewing was associated with a 167-kcal increment. Baseline television viewing time was also independently associated with change in TEI. The FCAT mediated these associations; coefficients for television viewing time (baseline and change) were greatly reduced, and some were rendered insignificant when foods were added into the models. For example, adjusting for sugar-sweetened beverages reduced the kilocalories associated with a 1-hour increase in television viewing from 167 to 123, a 26% reduction; and adjusting for fast food–type main courses or all FCAT combined rendered the association between television increasing and TEI nonsignificant. Baseline television viewing predicted change in calorie intake when no foods were in the model, but was no longer a predictor in models controlling for change in baked sweet snacks, candy, fast food–type main courses, sugar-sweetened beverages, or all foods combined.

In support of the hypothesis of mediation, **Table 4** shows that increased television viewing time was also associated with increased intake of FCAT. These relation-

**Table 3. Adjusted Change in Daily Caloric Intake Associated With Baseline and Each 1-h/d Increase in Television Viewing and Evidence for Mediation of This Relationship by Change in Intake of Foods Commonly Advertised on Television (N = 548)**

| | Additional Kilocalories at Follow-up Associated With Each Hour of Television Viewing at Baseline | | Additional Kilocalories at Follow-up Associated With Each Hour Increase in Television Viewing | |
|---|---|---|---|---|
| Variable | Mean (95% Confidence Interval) | *P* Value | Mean (95% Confidence Interval) | *P* Value |
| Basic model (no foods in model)* | 127.0 (27.7 to 226.2) | .02 | 167.0 (135.9 to 197.9) | <.001 |
| Baked sweet snacks† | 33.5 (−31.0 to 98.1) | .22 | 74.5 (17.7 to 131.3) | .02 |
| Candy | 50.3 (−69.1 to 169.6) | .31 | 70.7 (9.9 to 131.5) | .03 |
| Fast food–type main courses | 44.8 (−47.4 to 36.9) | .25 | 42.1 (−16.9 to 101.1) | .12 |
| Fried potatoes | 77.9 (18.9 to 136.9) | .02 | 99.3 (71.0 to 127.6) | .001 |
| Salty snacks | 67.7 (10.9 to 124.4) | .03 | 87.8 (33.4 to 142.2) | .01 |
| Sugar-sweetened beverages | 66.6 (−26.6 to 159.8) | .12 | 122.8 (68.2 to 177.5) | .003 |
| All foods | −36.1 (−103.3 to 31.2) | .21 | −5.1 (−81.7 to 71.5) | .86 |

*Estimated from a regression equation controlling for baseline body mass index, total energy intake, physical activity duration of 3.5 metabolic equivalents or more, and age; change in physical activity duration of 3.5 metabolic equivalents or more; and sex, race/ethnicity, and school indicator variables. All change values are the 1997 value minus the 1995 value.

†Coefficients in subsequent models were estimated from separate regression equations controlling for variables as in the basic model, with the addition of change in daily servings of the food group shown controlling for baseline servings per day of the food group.

**Table 4. Adjusted Change in Servings per Day of Foods Commonly Advertised on Television Associated With Baseline and 1-h/d Increase in Television Viewing (N = 548)***

| | Additional Servings per Day at Follow-up Associated With Each Hour of Baseline Television Viewing | | Additional Servings per Day at Follow-up Associated With Each Hour Increase in Television Viewing | |
|---|---|---|---|---|
| Type of Food† | Mean (95% Confidence Interval) | *P* Value | Mean (95% Confidence Interval) | *P* Value |
| Baked sweet snacks | 0.21 (0.08 to 0.33) | .01 | 0.21 (0.14 to 0.29) | .002 |
| Candy | 0.06 (0.03 to 0.10) | .006 | 0.08 (0.02 to 0.14) | .02 |
| Fast food–type main courses | 0.06 (0.04 to 0.08) | .001 | 0.09 (0.06 to 0.12) | .001 |
| Fried potatoes | 0.02 (−0.004 to 0.04) | .08 | 0.03 (0.01 to 0.04) | .004 |
| Salty snacks | 0.06 (0.01 to 0.12) | .04 | 0.09 (0.04 to 0.14) | .009 |
| Sugar-sweetened beverages | 0.14 (0.12 to 0.16) | <.001 | 0.11 (0.01 to 0.22) | .04 |
| All foods | 0.54 (0.37 to 0.72) | .001 | 0.60 (0.41 to 0.78) | .001 |

*Estimated from a regression equation controlling for baseline intake of the test food group, body mass index, total energy intake, physical activity of 3.5 metabolic equivalents or more, and age; change in physical activity of 3.5 metabolic equivalents or more; and sex, race/ethnicity, and school indicator variables.

†Baked sweet snacks include brownies, cake, cookies, donuts, pies, Pop-Tarts (Kellogg's, Battle Creek, Mich), and snack cakes; candy: candy other than chocolate, chocolate, and fruit leathers; fast food–type main courses: cheeseburgers, chicken nuggets, fried chicken, hamburgers, hot dogs, pizza, and tacos/burritos; fried potatoes: French fries and potato puffs; salty snacks: corn chips, crackers, potato chips, and pretzels; and sugar-sweetened beverages: fruit drinks, nondiet iced tea, and nondiet soda.

ships are necessary to demonstrate that intakes of these foods can mediate television's effect on TEI. The table shows the coefficients for change in servings per day of these foods associated with baseline and change in television viewing. With the exception of fried potatoes, higher intakes of all foods at follow-up were significantly positively associated with baseline television viewing level. Moreover, change in television viewing was significantly associated with change in consumption of each food group. With each 1-hour increment in television viewing, increases in servings per day ranged from 0.03 (fried potatoes) to 0.21 (baked sweet snacks) across food groups, or 0.2 to 1.4 servings per week.

## COMMENT

Identifying the mechanisms by which television increases risk of obesity through its influence on energy balance is important in providing evidence for causality for this well-documented observation. We show that, among youth, increases in television viewing predict increases in TEI, and that increasing intakes of FCAT mediate this relationship.

These results build on other recent research. Epstein et al[21] found that in experimental manipulations, increasing screen time by 50% was associated with a 250-kcal/d increase in energy intake among youth. Increasing consumption of non–nutrient-dense foods high in added sugars and fats, a pattern typical of fast food meals that include a burger, French fries, and soda, may compromise diet quality by increasing energy intake,[29-32] displacing more healthful food options,[30] and promoting weight gain.[33] The growth in fast food consumption in the US population is, therefore, of great concern. While fast food meals accounted for 3% of eating occasions and 3% of daily calorie intake in 1977, in 1995 they accounted for 9% of eating occasions and 12% of calories.[44] Concurrent evidence[45,46] suggests that total average daily energy intakes among youth have increased, reflecting in part increased intake of added sugars.[47] Among adolescents, about 40% of added sugars derive from soda,[48] consumption of which increased by 131% between the late 1970s and the mid 1990s.[49] Our analyses support a link between television viewing and these unhealthy dietary changes, suggesting that television advertising for food has a powerful influence on diets. Indeed, studies show that television viewing is inversely associated with intake of fruits and vegetables,[31,50] which receive little air time[22] despite their potential to promote health in various ways and protect against weight gain.[51]

Several limitations of the analysis relate to measurement error and its attendant effect on regression analyses. The validity of the television measure is limited by recall bias and instrument design, although prior studies indicate modest validity. Dietary intake is typically measured with a large component of random measurement error. In linear regression models with random error in the dependent variable (such as total energy or food intake), regression coefficients will be unbiased, although the $R^2$ value for the model will be reduced; conversely, random measurement errors in independent variables will attenuate regression coefficients and reduce their ability to function effectively as mediating or control variables.[52] In using dietary intake, television viewing time, and physical activity measures as independent variables, random error due to questionnaire design, recall error, and within-person variability not captured by the instrument may, therefore, attenuate regression coefficients. When food servings are converted to energy intake, additional errors are introduced because of assumptions about serving size and food composition. Another potential source of error is in the use of television viewing time as a proxy for exposure to advertising. Although we assumed that, on average, youth who watched more television were exposed to more advertisements, we did not assess what programs or channels subjects were exposed to, both of which could affect the total "dose" of advertising. We also had limited ability to control for other potential confounding variables, such as baseline levels of moderate and vigorous physical activity and body composition, which may also have contributed to bias in estimates of association.

Causality is suggested but not proved by our findings, which are observational and not experimental. Generalizability may be limited because of the nature of our sample. Further research could address these limitations through a randomized trial to reduce television viewing in a broader population of youth using survey instruments that collected data on sources of food.

In conclusion, although children and youth are encouraged to watch what they eat, many youth seem to eat what they watch, and in the process increase their risk for increasing their energy intake. In the absence of regulations restricting food advertising aimed at children, reduction in television viewing is a promising approach to reducing excess energy intake. Although a threshold of safe exposure to television and food marketing has not been empirically demonstrated, the American Academy of Pediatrics has long advocated limiting children to no more than 2 hours of television per day to decrease sedentary time and to decrease exposure to content that may encourage a range of negative behaviors.[53] This study adds more evidence in support of this recommendation.

**Accepted for Publication:** July 25, 2005.
**Correspondence:** Jean L. Wiecha, PhD, Harvard School of Public Health, 677 Huntington Ave, Seventh Floor, Boston, MA 02115 (jwiecha@hsph.harvard.edu).
**Author Contributions:** Dr Wiecha had full access to all the data in the study and takes responsibility for the integrity of the data and the accuracy of the data analysis.
**Funding/Support:** This study was supported by grant HD-30780 from the National Institute of Child Health and Human Development, Rockville, Md; Prevention Research Centers grants U48/CCU115807 and U48/DP00064-00S1 from the Centers for Disease Control and Prevention, Atlanta, Ga; grant R01DK59240 from the National Institute of Diabetes and Digestive and Kidney Diseases, Bethesda, Md; and the Charles H. Hood Foundation, Boston.
**Role of the Sponsor:** The funding bodies had no role in data extraction and analyses, in the writing of the manuscript, or in the decision to submit the manuscript for publication.
**Disclaimer:** This work is solely the responsibility of the authors and does not represent official views of the Centers for Disease Control and Prevention or other granting institutions.
**Acknowledgment:** We thank Alice Colby for her assistance with manuscript preparation.

## REFERENCES

1. Ogden CL, Flegal KM, Carroll MD, Johnson CL. Prevalence and trends in overweight among US children and adolescents, 1999-2000. *JAMA*. 2002;288:1728-1732.
2. Obarzanek E, Schreiber GB, Crawford PB, et al. Energy intake and physical activity in relation to indexes of body fat: the National Heart, Lung, and Blood Institute Growth and Health Study. *Am J Clin Nutr*. 1994;60:15-22.
3. Utter J, Neumark-Sztainer D, Jeffery R, Story M. Couch potatoes or French fries: are sedentary behaviors associated with body mass index, physical activity, and dietary behaviors among adolescents? *J Am Diet Assoc*. 2003;103:1298-1305.
4. Andersen RE, Crespo CJ, Bartlett SJ, Cheskin LJ, Pratt M. Relationship of physical activity and television watching with body weight and level of fatness among children: results from the Third National Health and Nutrition Examination Survey. *JAMA*. 1998;279:938-942.
5. Dietz WH Jr, Gortmaker SL. Do we fatten our children at the television set? obesity and television viewing in children and adolescents. *Pediatrics*. 1985;75:807-812.
6. Dietz WH, Gortmaker SL. TV or not TV: fat is the question. *Pediatrics*. 1993;91:499-501.
7. Proctor MH, Moore LL, Gao D, et al. Television viewing and change in body fat from preschool to early adolescence: the Framingham Children's Study. *Int J Obes Relat Metab Disord*. 2003;27:827-833.
8. Gortmaker SL, Must A, Sobol AM, Peterson K, Colditz GA, Dietz WH. Television viewing as a cause of increasing obesity among children in the United States, 1986-1990. *Arch Pediatr Adolesc Med*. 1996;150:356-362.
9. Berkey CS, Rockett HR, Field AE, et al. Activity, dietary intake, and weight changes in a longitudinal study of preadolescent and adolescent boys and girls. *Pediatrics*. 2000;105:e56. Available at: http://pediatrics.aappublications.org/cgi/content/full/105/4/e56. Accessed January 23, 2006.
10. Ludwig DS, Gortmaker SL. Programming obesity in childhood. *Lancet*. 2004;364:226-227.

11. Hu FB, Leitzmann MF, Stampfer MJ, Colditz GA, Willett WC, Rimm EB. Physical activity and television watching in relation to risk for type 2 diabetes mellitus in men. *Arch Intern Med.* 2001;161:1542-1548.
12. Hu FB, Li TY, Colditz GA, Willett WC, Manson JE. Television watching and other sedentary behaviors in relation to risk of obesity and type 2 diabetes mellitus in women. *JAMA.* 2003;289:1785-1791.
13. Fung TT, Hu FB, Yu J, et al. Leisure-time physical activity, television watching, and plasma biomarkers of obesity and cardiovascular disease risk. *Am J Epidemiol.* 2000;152:1171-1178.
14. Fung TT, Rimm EB, Spiegelman D, et al. Association between dietary patterns and plasma biomarkers of obesity and cardiovascular disease risk. *Am J Clin Nutr.* 2001;73:61-67.
15. Epstein LH, Valoski AM, Vara LS, et al. Effects of decreasing sedentary behavior and increasing activity on weight change in obese children. *Health Psychol.* 1995; 14:109-115.
16. Gortmaker SL, Peterson K, Wiecha J, et al. Reducing obesity via a school-based interdisciplinary intervention among youth: Planet Health. *Arch Pediatr Adolesc Med.* 1999;153:409-418.
17. Robinson TN. Reducing children's television viewing to prevent obesity: a randomized controlled trial. *JAMA.* 1999;282:1561-1567.
18. Pate RR, Heath GW, Dowda M, Trost SG. Associations between physical activity and other health behaviors in a representative sample of US adolescents. *Am J Public Health.* 1996;86:1577-1581.
19. Lowry R, Wechsler H, Galuska DA, Fulton JE, Kann L. Television viewing and its associations with overweight, sedentary lifestyle, and insufficient consumption of fruits and vegetables among US high school students: differences by race, ethnicity, and gender. *J Sch Health.* 2002;72:413-421.
20. Marshall SJ, Biddle SJ, Gorely T, Cameron N, Murdey I. Relationships between media use, body fatness and physical activity in children and youth: a meta-analysis. *Int J Obes Relat Metab Disord.* 2004;28:1238-1246.
21. Epstein LH, Paluch RA, Consalvi A, Riordan K, Scholl T. Effects of manipulating sedentary behavior on physical activity and food intake. *J Pediatr.* 2002;140: 334-339.
22. Gallo A. Food advertising in the United States. In: Frazao E, ed. *America's Eating Habits: Changes and Consequences.* Washington, DC: Economic Research Service, US Dept of Agriculture; 1999:173-180. Agriculture Information Bulletin 750.
23. Nestle M. *Food Politics: How the Food Industry Influences Nutrition and Health.* Berkeley: University of California Press; 2002.
24. Taras HL, Sallis JF, Patterson TL, Nader PR, Nelson JA. Television's influence on children's diet and physical activity. *J Dev Behav Pediatr.* 1989;10:176-180.
25. Borzekowski DL, Robinson TN. The 30-second effect: an experiment revealing the impact of television commercials on food preferences of preschoolers. *J Am Diet Assoc.* 2001;101:42-46.
26. Galst J, White M. The unhealthy persuader: the reinforcing value of television and children's purchase influence attempts at the supermarket. *Child Dev.* 1976; 47:1089-1096.
27. Goldberg M, Gorn G, Gibson W. TV messages for snacks and breakfast foods: do they influence children's preferences? *J Consum Res.* 1978;5:73-81.
28. Gorn GJ, Goldberg ME. Behavioral evidence of the effects of televised food messages on children. *J Consum Res.* 1982;9:200-205.
29. McNutt SW, Hu Y, Schreiber GB, Crawford PB, Obarzanek E, Mellin L. A longitudinal study of the dietary practices of black and white girls 9 and 10 years old at enrollment: the NHLBI Growth and Health Study. *J Adolesc Health.* 1997; 20:27-37.
30. Bowman SA, Gortmaker SL, Ebbeling CB, Pereira MA, Ludwig DS. Effects of fast-food consumption on energy intake and diet quality among children in a national household survey. *Pediatrics.* 2004;113(pt 1):112-118.
31. French SA, Story M, Neumark-Sztainer D, Fulkerson JA, Hannan P. Fast food restaurant use among adolescents: associations with nutrient intake, food choices and behavioral and psychosocial variables. *Int J Obes Relat Metab Disord.* 2001; 25:1823-1833.
32. Binkley JK, Eales J, Jekanowski M. The relation between dietary change and rising US obesity. *Int J Obes Relat Metab Disord.* 2000;24:1032-1039.
33. Ludwig DS, Peterson KE, Gortmaker SL. Relation between consumption of sugar-sweetened drinks and childhood obesity: a prospective, observational analysis. *Lancet.* 2001;357:505-508.
34. Shadish WR, Cook TD, Campbell DT. *Experimental and Quasi-experimental Designs for Generalized Causal Inference.* Boston, Mass: Houghton Mifflin Co; 2002.
35. Baron RM, Kenny DA. The moderator-mediator variable distinction in social psychological research: conceptual, strategic, and statistical considerations. *J Pers Soc Psychol.* 1986;51:1173-1182.
36. Peterson KE, Field AE, Fox MK. *Validation of YRBSS Questions on Dietary Behaviors and Physical Activity Among Adolescents in Grades 9-12.* Atlanta, Ga: Division of Adolescent and School Health, Centers for Disease Control and Prevention; 1996.
37. Rockett HR, Breitenbach M, Frazier AL, et al. Validation of a youth/adolescent food frequency questionnaire. *Prev Med.* 1997;26:808-816.
38. Rockett HR, Wolf AM, Colditz GA. Development and reproducibility of a food frequency questionnaire to assess diets of older children and adolescents. *J Am Diet Assoc.* 1995;95:336-340.
39. Field AE, Peterson KE, Gortmaker SL, et al. Reproducibility and validity of a food frequency questionnaire among fourth to seventh grade inner-city school children: implications of age and day-to-day variation in dietary intake. *Public Health Nutr.* 1999;2:293-300.
40. Ainsworth BE, Haskell WL, Leon AS, et al. Compendium of physical activities: classification of energy costs of human physical activities. *Med Sci Sports Exerc.* 1993;25:71-80.
41. Wolf AM, Hunter DJ, Colditz GA, et al. Reproducibility and validity of a self-administered physical activity questionnaire. *Int J Epidemiol.* 1994;23:991-999.
42. Chasan-Taber S, Rimm EB, Stampfer MJ, et al. Reproducibility and validity of a self-administered physical activity questionnaire for male health professionals. *Epidemiology.* 1996;7:81-86.
43. Rosner B, Willett WC. Interval estimates for correlation coefficients corrected for within-person variation: implications for study design and hypothesis testing. *Am J Epidemiol.* 1988;127:377-386.
44. Lin B, Guthrie J, Frazao E. Nutrient contribution of food away from home. In: Frazao E, ed. *America's Eating Habits: Changes and Consequences.* Washington, DC: Economic Research Service, US Dept of Agriculture; 1999:213-239. Agriculture Information Bulletin 750.
45. Dixon LB, Ernst ND. Choose a diet that is low in saturated fat and cholesterol and moderate in total fat: subtle changes to a familiar message. *J Nutr.* 2001; 131(suppl):510S-526S.
46. Cavadini C, Siega-Riz AM, Popkin BM. US adolescent food intake trends from 1965 to 1996. *Arch Dis Child.* 2000;83:18-24.
47. Krebs-Smith SM. Choose beverages and foods to moderate your intake of sugars: measurement requires quantification. *J Nutr.* 2001;131(suppl):527S-535S.
48. Guthrie JF, Morton JF. Food sources of added sweeteners in the diets of Americans. *J Am Diet Assoc.* 2000;100:43-51.
49. Tippett K, Cleveland L. How current diets stack up: comparison with dietary guidelines. In: Frazao E, ed. *America's Eating Habits: Changes and Consequences.* Washington, DC: Economic Research Service, US Dept of Agriculture; 1999:51-70. Agriculture Information Bulletin 750.
50. Boynton-Jarrett R, Thomas TN, Peterson KE, Wiecha J, Sobol AM, Gortmaker SL. Impact of television viewing patterns on fruit and vegetable consumption among adolescents. *Pediatrics.* 2003;112:1321-1326.
51. Ludwig DS, Pereira MA, Kroenke CH, et al. Dietary fiber, weight gain, and cardiovascular disease risk factors in young adults. *JAMA.* 1999;282:1539-1546.
52. Fox J. *Applied Regression Analysis, Linear Models and Related Methods.* Thousand Oaks, Calif: Sage Publications; 1997.
53. Committee on Communications, American Academy of Pediatrics. Children, adolescents, and television. *Pediatrics.* 1995;96:786-787.

## BOOSTRIX®

**(Tetanus Toxoid, Reduced Diphtheria Toxoid and Acellular Pertussis Vaccine, Adsorbed) (Tdap)**

The following is a brief summary only; see full prescribing information for complete product information.

**INDICATIONS AND USAGE:** BOOSTRIX is indicated for active booster immunization against tetanus, diphtheria, and pertussis as a single dose in individuals 10 through 18 years of age. The use of BOOSTRIX as a primary series or to complete the primary series has not been studied. As with any vaccine, BOOSTRIX may not protect 100% of individuals receiving the vaccine. BOOSTRIX is not recommended for treatment of actual infections.

**CONTRAINDICATIONS:** Hypersensitivity to any component of the vaccine is a contraindication (see DESCRIPTION in full prescribing information). Do not use BOOSTRIX after a serious allergic reaction (e.g., anaphylaxis) following any other tetanus toxoid, diphtheria toxoid or pertussis-containing vaccine, or any component of this vaccine (see DESCRIPTION in full prescribing information). Because of the uncertainty as to which component of the vaccine might be responsible, do not give further vaccination with any of these components; or, refer such individuals to an allergist for evaluation. The following events are contraindications to administration of BOOSTRIX: encephalopathy (e.g., coma, decreased level of consciousness, prolonged seizures) within 7 days of administration of a previous dose of a pertussis-containing vaccine that is not attributable to another identifiable cause; progressive neurologic disorder, uncontrolled epilepsy, or progressive encephalopathy. Do not vaccinate individuals with these conditions until a treatment regimen has been established and the condition has stabilized. BOOSTRIX is not contraindicated for use in individuals with HIV infection.

**WARNINGS:** The tip cap and the rubber plunger of the needleless prefilled syringes contain dry natural latex rubber that may cause allergic reactions in latex sensitive individuals. The vial stopper is latex-free. If any of the following events occurred in temporal relation to previous receipt of a Diphtheria and Tetanus Toxoids and Pertussis Vaccine Adsorbed (DTwP) vaccine or a vaccine containing an acellular pertussis component, consider carefully whether to give subsequent doses of BOOSTRIX: temperature of ≥40.5°C (105°F) within 48 hours not due to another identifiable cause; collapse or shock-like state (hypotonic-hyporesponsive episode) within 48 hours; persistent, inconsolable crying lasting ≥3 hours, occurring within 48 hours; seizures with or without fever occurring within 3 days. Persons who experienced serious Arthus-type hypersensitivity reactions following a prior dose of tetanus toxoid usually have high serum tetanus antitoxin levels and should not be given Tetanus and Diphtheria Toxoids Adsorbed For Adult Use (Td) or Tdap vaccines or even emergency doses of Td more frequently than every 10 years, even if the wound is neither clean nor minor. If Guillain-Barré syndrome has occurred within 6 weeks of receipt of prior vaccine containing tetanus toxoid, the decision to give BOOSTRIX or any vaccine containing tetanus toxoid should be based on careful consideration of the potential benefits and possible risks. The decision to administer a pertussis-containing vaccine to individuals with stable central nervous system (CNS) disorders must be made by the physician on an individual basis, with consideration of all relevant factors, and assessment of potential risks and benefits for that individual. Advise the patient, parent, or guardian of the potential increased risk involved (see PRECAUTIONS). A family history of seizures or other CNS disorders is not a contraindication to pertussis vaccine. The Advisory Committee on Immunization Practices (ACIP) has published guidelines for vaccination of persons with recent or acute illness (www.cdc.gov). Do not give BOOSTRIX to individuals with bleeding disorders such as hemophilia or thrombocytopenia, or to persons on anticoagulant therapy unless the potential benefit clearly outweighs the risk of administration. If the decision is made to administer BOOSTRIX to such persons, it should be given with caution with steps taken to avoid the risk of hematoma following the injection.

**PRECAUTIONS:** Before the injection of any biological, the physician should take all reasonable precautions to prevent allergic or other adverse reactions. Epinephrine injection (1:1,000) and other appropriate agents used for the control of immediate allergic reactions must be immediately available should an acute anaphylactic reaction occur. Immunosuppressed persons, including individuals receiving immunosuppressive therapy, may not develop the expected immune response. **Drug Interactions:** Do not mix BOOSTRIX with any other vaccine in the same syringe or vial. **Carcinogenesis, Mutagenesis, Impairment of Fertility:** BOOSTRIX has not been evaluated for carcinogenic or mutagenic potential, or for impairment of fertility. **Pregnancy:** Pregnancy Category C. Animal reproduction studies have not been conducted with BOOSTRIX. It is also not known whether BOOSTRIX can cause fetal harm when administered to a pregnant woman or can affect reproductive capacity. BOOSTRIX should be given to a pregnant woman only if clearly needed. Animal fertility studies have not been conducted with BOOSTRIX. In a developmental toxicity study, the effect of BOOSTRIX on embryo-fetal and pre-weaning development was evaluated in pregnant rats. Animals were administered INFANRIX® (Diphtheria and Tetanus Toxoids and Acellular Pertussis Vaccine Adsorbed) prior to gestation and BOOSTRIX during the period of organogenesis (gestation days 6, 8, 11) and later in pregnancy (gestation day 15), 0.1 mL/rat/occasion (a 45-fold increase compared to the human dose of BOOSTRIX on a body weight basis), by intramuscular injection. No adverse affect on pregnancy and lactation parameters, embryo-fetal or pre-weaning development was observed. There were no fetal malformations or other evidence of teratogenesis noted in this study. **Nursing Mothers:** It is not known whether BOOSTRIX is excreted in human milk. Because many drugs are excreted in human milk, caution should be exercised when BOOSTRIX is administered to a nursing woman. **Pregnancy Exposure Registry:** Healthcare providers are encouraged to register pregnant women who receive BOOSTRIX in the GlaxoSmithKline vaccination pregnancy registry by calling 1-888-825-5249. **Geriatric Use:** BOOSTRIX is not indicated for use in individuals older than 18 years. **Pediatric Use:** BOOSTRIX is not indicated for use in individuals younger than 10 years (see DOSAGE AND ADMINISTRATION in full prescribing information). For immunization of infants and children younger than 7 years against diphtheria, tetanus, and pertussis, refer to the manufacturers' package inserts for Diphtheria and Tetanus Toxoids and Acellular Pertussis Vaccine Adsorbed (DTaP) vaccines.

**ADVERSE REACTIONS:** A total of 3,289 adolescents were vaccinated with a single dose of BOOSTRIX during clinical trials. An additional 1,092 adolescents 10 to 18 years of age received a non-US formulation of BOOSTRIX (formulated to contain 0.5 mg aluminum per dose) in non-US clinical studies.

The primary safety study, conducted in the United States, was a randomized, observer-blinded, controlled study in which 3,080 adolescents 10 to 18 years of age received a single dose of BOOSTRIX and 1,034 received the control Td vaccine manufactured by Massachusetts Public Health Biologic Laboratories. There were no substantive differences in demographic characteristics between the vaccine groups. Among BOOSTRIX and control vaccine recipients approximately 75% were 10 to 14 years of age and approximately 25% were 15 to 18 years of age. Approximately 98% of participants in this study had received the recommended series of 4 or 5 doses of either DTwP or a combination of DTwP and DTaP in childhood. Data on adverse events were collected by the subjects, parents and/or guardians using standardized diaries for 15 consecutive days following the vaccine dose (i.e., day of vaccination and the next 14 days). Subjects were monitored for unsolicited adverse events that occurred within 31 days of vaccination (day 0-30) using diary cards (day 0-14) supplemented by spontaneous reports and a medical history as reported by subjects, parents, and/or guardians. Subjects were also monitored for 6 months post-vaccination for non-routine medical visits, visits to an emergency room, onset of new chronic illness, and serious adverse events. Information regarding late onset adverse events was obtained via a telephone call 6 months following vaccination. At least 97% of subjects completed the 6-month follow-up evaluation.

The adverse event information from clinical trials provides a basis for identifying adverse events that appear to be related to vaccine use and for approximating rates. However, because clinical trials are conducted under widely varying conditions, adverse event rates observed in the clinical trials of a vaccine cannot be directly compared to rates in the clinical trials of another vaccine, and may not reflect the rates observed in practice.

**Serious Adverse Events in All Safety Studies:** In the US-safety study, no serious adverse events were reported to occur within 31 days of vaccination. During the 6-month extended safety evaluation period, no serious adverse events that were of potential autoimmune origin or new onset and chronic in nature were reported to occur. In non-US studies in which serious adverse events were monitored for up to 37 days, one subject was diagnosed with insulin dependent diabetes. The association of this event with vaccination is unknown. No other serious adverse events of potential autoimmune origin or that were new onset and chronic in nature were reported to occur in these studies.

**Solicited Adverse Events in the US-Safety Study:** In a US study, the most common local adverse events following administration of BOOSTRIX were pain, redness, and swelling at the injection site. The most common general adverse events were headache and fatigue. Most of these events were reported at a similar frequency in recipients of both BOOSTRIX and Td. Any pain, grade 2 or 3 pain (but not grade 3 alone), and grade 2 or 3 headache (but not grade 3 alone) were reported at a higher rate in recipients of BOOSTRIX. The primary safety endpoint of the US study was the incidence of grade 3 pain (spontaneously painful and/or prevented normal activity) at the injection site within 15 days of vaccination. Grade 3 pain was reported in 4.6% of those who received BOOSTRIX compared with 4.0% of those who received the Td vaccine. The difference in rate of grade 3 pain was within the pre-defined clinical limit for non-inferiority (upper limit of the 95% CI for the difference ≤4%). These were the rates for solicited local and general adverse events within 15 days of vaccination with BOOSTRIX or Td vaccine for the total vaccinated cohort (all enrolled, vaccinated subjects with safety data available analyzed by vaccine received):

**Percentage of Individuals 10 to 18 Years of Age Reporting Solicited Local Adverse Events or Solicited General Adverse Events Within the 15-day* Post-Vaccination Period**

| | BOOSTRIX (N = 3,032) | Td (N = 1,013) |
|---|---|---|
| **Local** | | |
| Pain,† any | 75.3 | 71.7 |
| Pain,† grade 2 or 3 | 51.2 | 42.5 |
| Pain,‡ grade 3 | 4.6 | 4.0 |
| Redness, any | 22.5 | 19.8 |
| Redness, >20 mm | 4.1 | 3.9 |
| Redness, ≥50 mm | 1.7 | 1.6 |
| Swelling, any | 21.1 | 20.1 |
| Swelling, >20 mm | 5.3 | 4.9 |
| Swelling, ≥50 mm | 2.5 | 3.2 |
| Arm circumference increase,§ >5 mm | 28.3 | 29.5 |
| Arm circumference increase,§ >20 mm | 2.0 | 2.2 |
| Arm circumference increase,§ >40 mm | 0.5 | 0.3 |
| **General** | | |
| Fever,‖ ≥99.5°F | 13.5 | 13.1 |
| Fever,‖ >100.4°F | 5.0 | 4.7 |
| Fever,‖ >102.2°F | 1.4 | 1.0 |
| Headache, any | 43.1 | 41.5 |
| Headache,† grade 2 or 3 | 15.7 | 12.7 |
| Headache, grade 3 | 3.7 | 2.7 |
| Fatigue, any | 37.0 | 36.7 |
| Fatigue, grade 2 or 3 | 14.4 | 12.9 |
| Fatigue, grade 3 | 3.7 | 3.2 |
| Gastrointestinal symptoms,¶ any | 26.0 | 25.8 |
| Gastrointestinal symptoms,¶ grade 2 or 3 | 9.8 | 9.7 |
| Gastrointestinal symptoms,¶ grade 3 | 3.0 | 3.2 |

Td = Tetanus and Diphtheria Toxoids Adsorbed For Adult Use manufactured by Massachusetts Public Health Biologic Laboratories.

N = number of subjects in the total vaccinated cohort with local/general symptoms sheets completed.

Grade 2 = Local: painful when the limb was moved; General: interfered with normal activity.

Grade 3 = Local: spontaneously painful and/or prevented normal activity; General: prevented normal activity.

*Day of vaccination and the next 14 days.

†Statistically significantly higher (P<0.05) following BOOSTRIX as compared to Td vaccine.

‡Grade 3 injection site pain following BOOSTRIX was not inferior to Td (upper limit of two-sided 95% CI for the difference in the percentage of subjects ≤4%).

§Mid-upper region of the vaccinated arm.

‖Oral temperatures or axillary temperatures.

¶Gastrointestinal symptoms included nausea, vomiting, diarrhea and/or abdominal pain.

Mid-upper arm circumference was measured by the adolescent or their parent/guardian prior to injection and daily for 15 days following vaccination. There was no significant difference between BOOSTRIX recipients and Td recipients in the proportion of subjects reporting an increase in mid-upper arm circumference in the vaccinated arm. The incidence of unsolicited adverse events reported in the 31 days after vaccination was comparable between the 2 groups.

As with any vaccine, there is the possibility that broad use of BOOSTRIX could reveal adverse events not observed in clinical trials.

**Postmarketing Reports:** Worldwide voluntary reports of adverse events received for BOOSTRIX in persons 10 to 18 years of age since market introduction of this vaccine are listed below. This list includes serious events or events which have causal connection to components of this or other vaccines or drugs. Because these events are reported voluntarily from a population of uncertain size, it is not possible to reliably estimate their frequency or establish a causal relationship to vaccine exposure. *Blood and lymphatic system disorders:* Lymphadenitis, lymphadenopathy. *Cardiac disorders:* Myocarditis. *Injection site reactions:* Induration, inflammation, mass, nodule, warmth, local reaction. *Metabolism and nutrition disorders:* Diabetes mellitus insulin-dependent. *Musculoskeletal and connective tissue disorders:* Arthralgia, back pain, myalgia. *Nervous system disorders:* Convulsion, encephalitis, facial palsy, paraesthesia. *Skin and subcutaneous tissue disorders:* Exanthem, Henoch-Schönlein purpura, rash. In addition, extensive swelling of the injected limb has been reported following administration of BOOSTRIX.

**Reporting Adverse Events:** Report the occurrence following immunization of any event set forth in the Vaccine Injury Table from the National Childhood Vaccine Injury Act including: Anaphylaxis or anaphylactic shock within 7 days, encephalopathy or encephalitis within 7 days, brachial neuritis within 28 days, or an acute complication or sequelae (including death) of an illness, disability, injury, or condition referred to above, or any events that would contraindicate further doses of vaccine, according to this prescribing information. These events should be reported to VAERS. The VAERS toll-free number is 1-800-822-7967. Reporting forms may also be obtained at the VAERS website at www.vaers.org.

**DOSAGE AND ADMINISTRATION: Recommended Dose:** BOOSTRIX should be administered as a single 0.5 mL injection by the intramuscular route into the deltoid muscle of the upper arm in individuals 10 through 18 years of age. Do not administer this product subcutaneously or intravenously. There are no data to support repeat administration of BOOSTRIX. Five years should elapse between the subject's last dose of the recommended series of childhood DTwP and/or DTaP vaccine and the administration of BOOSTRIX. Limited data are available on the use of BOOSTRIX following Tetanus and Diphtheria Toxoids Adsorbed For Adult Use (Td) vaccine. **Additional Dosing Information: *Wound Management:*** Clinicians should refer to guidelines for tetanus prophylaxis in routine wound management. Adolescents 10 to 18 years of age who have completed a primary series against tetanus and who sustain wounds which are minor and uncomplicated, should receive a booster dose of a tetanus toxoid-containing vaccine only if they have not received tetanus toxoid within the preceding 10 years. In case of tetanus-prone injury (e.g., wounds contaminated with dirt, feces, soil, and saliva; puncture wounds; avulsions; and wounds resulting from missles, crushing, burns, and frostbite) in an adolescent who is in need of tetanus toxoid, BOOSTRIX can be used as an alternative to Tetanus and Diphtheria Toxoids Adsorbed For Adult Use (Td) vaccine in patients for whom the pertussis component is also indicated (see INDICATIONS AND USAGE).

Manufactured by **GlaxoSmithKline Biologicals**
Rixensart, Belgium, US License 1617
Distributed by **GlaxoSmithKline**
Research Triangle Park, NC 27709



Full prescribing information for BOOSTRIX is available at www.BOOSTRIX.com.

BRS-BO:L1

**References: 1.** Centers for Disease Control and Prevention. *Epidemiology and Prevention of Vaccine-Preventable Diseases.* Atkinson W, Hamborsky J, Wolfe S, eds. 8th ed. Washington DC: Public Health Foundation; 2004:75–88, A26–A27. **2.** ACIP recommends adolescent vaccination for tetanus, diphtheria and pertussis vaccine [press release]. Atlanta, GA: Department of Health and Human Services; Available at: www.cdc.gov/nip/pr/pr_tdap_jun2005.htm. Accessed September 27, 2005. **3.** Data on file, BOR305, GlaxoSmithKline.

# Media as a Public Health Issue

GIVEN THE ENORMOUS INFLUENCE THAT electronic media in all of their forms exerts on the lives of children, it is astonishing how little parents, researchers, and policymakers have been spurred to action. This is not to say that there have not been episodic public outcries about violence and sex on television and even some modicum of congressional action regarding them. However, these efforts have lacked consistency, thoughtfulness, and staying power. Most of what has been done to date to understand, curtail, or regulate the negative effects of media on children can be viewed as failure. Every single children's G-rated movie released in US theaters from 1937 to 1999 contained at least 1 act of violence.[1] The quantity of advertising has increased to more than 16 minutes per hour of programming, and to 21 minutes per hour during daytime television.[2] The amount of sex on television has doubled since 1998.[3] The majority of video games rated E (for "Everyone") contain intentional violence.[4] The V-chip, mandated amidst great fanfare in 2000, has produced no tangible benefits. The ratings systems used for television and video games have not proven helpful to parents.[5,6]

Much of what we know about media's effects on children is based on studies of television that, since television's creation some 60 years ago, have left an increasingly large footprint in American households. Those studies have demonstrated potentially profound effects—both positive and negative—on children's cognitive, social, and behavioral development.[7-18]

However, too much of the data on television and children are dated. They are dated because the content of television has changed dramatically over the past 20 years. They are dated because the way in which it has been used has changed as well, with more and more children watching alone. They are dated because the age at which children start watching has steadily and dramatically declined so that today, many children begin their viewing careers as infants.[15] They are dated because as a medium, television is quickly being overtaken by other technologies in the competition for children's screen time.[15,16] Children's use of the internet, video games, instant messaging, and podcasts are largely unexplored. Furthermore, existing technology will soon make every cellular phone a miniature television. It was alarming enough (to some) that two thirds of teenagers have televisions in their bedrooms. Soon, they will all have them in their pockets.

Why is it that something that is widely recognized as being so influential and potentially dangerous has resulted in so little effective action? To be sure, there has been some lack of political will to take on the enormously powerful and influential entertainment industry. In part, however, the disconnect between consensus and action can be explained by what has been called the "third person effect."[17] We all agree that media can be bad, but not for our children—only for other people's. The third person effect has its roots in a misguided and insular naïveté, a sense that one's own child's vulnerabilities are fundamentally different from society's as a whole. However, it also owes much to the fact that media are enormously popular not only with children but also with adults. We are concerned about its pervasiveness, but we do not want to relinquish the purchase it has on our lives. There are more televisions than toilets in the United States. Adults who grew up prior to the media explosion and purport to limit their usage have themselves become addicted to their iPods, BlackBerries, laptops, and TiVo. Is updating one's to-do list every 15 minutes really better than idly playing *Pokémon Emerald*? Is checking e-mail at every free moment functionally different from instant messaging one's adolescent friends?

Given that it will prove impossible to stem the rising tide of media usage, we must ask ourselves what is needed to advance research and inform public policy. First, media need to be recognized as a major public health issue rather than as a series of commercial endeavors in need of regulation, as they are among the most profound influences on children in this country; this intersects with many other issues that are critically important to child health, including violence, obesity, tobacco and alcohol use, and risky sexual behaviors. Declaring violence a public health issue as opposed to solely a criminal justice one has been instrumental in curtailing it.[18] Similarly, understanding children's media use as a component of public health may help to cut the Gordian knot of adult defensiveness that surrounds the issue. Second, a more nuanced approach to the role of media is in order. The current debate is too adversarial and often poorly informed. Television and other media must be viewed as more than sources of evil or mere idle pleasures; their potential to enrich the lives of our children are, in fact, enormous, and that potential needs to be explored and actualized. We need to find ways to optimize the role of media in our society, taking advantage of their positive attributes and minimizing their negative ones. Finally, a better evidence base is needed. Too much research is descriptive, cross-sectional, or, when interventional, is based on small, select populations with short-term follow-up. Robust, prospective, experimental, population-based effectiveness trials are needed. These studies should include pragmatic strategies for optimizing usage. Pragmatism is key. No more studies demonstrating how much children watch or how many exceed the American Academy of Pediatrics guidelines are needed. Better studies of *how* they watch and how viewing habits can be improved are necessary. Such solution-oriented research is the key to advancing public health.[19] Can appropriate use of educational video games increase language acquisition and reading in preschool-aged children? Can computers in classrooms improve children's long-term academic achievement? Can modeling appropriate eating and sexual practices reduce obesity and risky sexual behaviors? Such studies are expensive to conduct and difficult to manage, but given their importance, they should be a priority. Pending congressional legislation, particularly the Children and Media Research Act (CAMRA) that would help establish a research agenda and earmark dollars to the National Institute of Child Health and Human Development, Rockville, Md, for research on the effects of media on children should be passed.

Finally, the industry should be put to task for making unchecked and outlandish claims about products' abilities to make children geniuses in music, art, science, and math.[20] Such scrutiny will do more than protect the public from false advertisements; it will motivate the industry to collaborate with academia so that high-quality products can be developed, tested, and marketed.

Representing the current state of the science in a wide variety of disciplines on the effects of media on children, this issue of the ARCHIVES is an important start in furthering this research. We hope that it is just that, a start, outlining the important questions that must be addressed. The potential impact of media on our children and our society mandates that these studies lead to a rapid expansion of rigorous controlled trials and long-term follow-up studies to better understand how to reverse the scales and make the effects of media more positive than negative.

*Dimitri A. Christakis, MD, MPH*
*Frederick J. Zimmerman, PhD*

**Correspondence:** Dr Christakis, Child Health Institute, University of Washington, 6200 NE 74th St, Suite 210, Seattle, WA 98115 (dachris@u.washington.edu).

## REFERENCES

1. Yokota F, Thompson KM. Violence in G-rated animated films. *JAMA*. 2000;283:2716-2720.
2. American Association of Advertising Agencies; Association of National Advertisers. *2001 Television Commercial Monitoring Report*. New York, NY: American Association of Advertising Agencies; 2002.
3. Kunkel D, Eyal K, Finnerty K, Biely E, Donnerstein E. *Sex on TV 4*. Menlo Park, Calif: Kaiser Family Foundation; 2005.
4. Thompson KM, Haninger K. Violence in E-rated video games. *JAMA*. 2001;286:591-598.
5. Jordan A, Woodard E. *Parents' Use of the V-Chip to Supervise Children's Television Use*. Philadelphia, Pa: Annenberg Public Policy Center; 2003.
6. Walsh DA, Gentile DA. A validity test of movie, television, and video-game ratings. *Pediatrics*. 2001;107:1302-1308.
7. Christakis DA, Zimmerman FJ, DiGiuseppe DL, McCarty CA. Early television exposure and subsequent attentional problems in children. *Pediatrics*. 2004;113:708-713.
8. Friedrich LK, Stein AH. Prosocial television and young children: the effects of verbal labeling and role playing on learning and behavior. *Child Dev*. 1975;46:27-38.
9. Gadberry S. Effects of restricting first graders' TV-viewing on leisure time use, IQ change, and cognitive style. *J Appl Dev Psychol*. 1980;1:45-57.
10. MacBeth TM, ed. *Tuning In to Young Viewers: Social Science Perspectives on Television*. Thousand Oaks, Calif: Sage Publications; 1996.
11. Robinson TN. Reducing children's television viewing to prevent obesity: a randomized controlled trial. *JAMA*. 1999;282:1561-1567.
12. Rice ML, Huston AC, Truglio R, Wright JA. Words from "Sesame Street": learning vocabulary while viewing. *Dev Psychol*. 1990;26:421-438.
13. Lesser GS. *Children and Television: Lessons from Sesame Street*. New York, NY: Random House; 1974.
14. Anderson DR, Huston AC, Schmitt KL, Linebarger DL, Wright JC. Early childhood television viewing and adolescent behavior: the recontact study. *Monogr Soc Res Child Dev*. 2001;66:I-VIII, 1-47.
15. Rideout VJ, Vandewater EA, Wartella EA. *Zero to Six: Electronic Media in the Lives of Infants, Toddlers, and Preschoolers*. Menlo Park, Calif: Kaiser Family Foundation; 2003.
16. Christakis DA, Ebel BE, Rivara FP, Zimmerman FJ. Television, video, and computer game usage in children under 11 years of age. *J Pediatr*. 2004;145:652-656.
17. Perloff RM. The third person effect. In: Bryant J, Zillmann D, eds. *Media Effects: Advances in Theory and Research*. Mahwah, NJ: Lawrence Erlbaum Associates; 2002:489-506.
18. Mercy JA, Rosenberg ML, Powell KE, Broome CV, Roper WL. Public health policy for preventing violence. *Health Aff*. 1993;12:7-29.
19. Robinson TN, Sirard JR. Preventing childhood obesity: a solution-oriented research paradigm. *Am J Prev Med*. 2005;28(suppl 2):194-201.
20. Garrison M, Christakis DA. *A Teacher in the Living Room? Educational Media for Babies, Toddlers, and Preschoolers*. Menlo Park, Calif: Kaiser Family Foundation; 2005.

# Exploring the Impact of Media on Children

## *The Challenges That Remain*

THE RESEARCH PRESENTED IN THIS SPECIAL ISsue of *Archives of Pediatrics and Adolescent Medicine* clearly illustrates that the media have disturbing potential to negatively affect many aspects of children's healthy development, including weight status (Vandewater and Huang,[1] Weicha et al,[2] Outley and Taddese,[3] and Lumeng et al[4]), sexual initiation (Ashby et al[5]), aggressive feelings and beliefs (Brady and Matthews[6] and Bushman and Huesmann[7]), consumerism (Chamberlain et al[8]), and social isolation (Bickham and Rich[9]). Such evidence offers increasing support for the American Academy of Pediatrics' recommendation that children older than 2 years spend no more than 2 hours per day with screen media, preferably educational screen media.[10]

The empirical studies that make up this collection reflect the variety of methods that are now used in this field: content analysis, laboratory and field experiments, cross-sectional and longitudinal surveys, and meta-analysis. We are clearly becoming more creative and sophisticated in how we study the problem and more nuanced in the ways we think about audiences. Despite these advances, those who work in this field must continue to grapple with difficult issues.

First, there is no gold standard for a measure of media exposure that is thoroughly tested and widely accepted.[11] A critical cornerstone of media effects research is the ability to tie the amount of time children spend with a specific medium or a constellation of media to attitudes, beliefs, and behaviors. However, consider the variety of ways in which media exposure is operationalized by the research in this special issue alone. Barkin et al[12] asked parents in pediatric office settings, "When this child is at home, how many hours per day does he or she watch television/videos? play computer games/Gameboy?" The National Institute of Child Health and Human Development Study of Early Child Care interview data used by Lumeng et al[4] defined toddlers' television exposure as "being awake in the room when the television is on," and asked mothers to describe 2 weekdays and 2 weekend days for each of the three 6-hour time blocks between 6 AM and midnight in 15-minute increments. Bickham and Rich[9] and Vandewater and Huang,[1] using data from the Panel Study of Income Dynamics–Child Development Supplement, derive their exposure measure from the number of minutes of television viewing reported in two 24-hour time use diaries filled out by parents and children. Parents' recall is triggered in very different ways depending on the measure.

Self-report measures of media use by children are similarly inconsistent. Chamberlain et al[8] provided third-grade children in-school time-estimating exercises and subsequently had the children report time spent "watching television" separately for before school and after school "yesterday" and "last Saturday." The National Longitudinal Study of Adolescent Health data used by Ashby et al[5] and Fletcher[13] simply asked adolescents how many hours of television they viewed per week, whereas the subjects in Weicha et al's Planet Health study[2] reported the average number of hours viewed on each of 7 days of the week.

The use of different media exposure measures makes it impossible to know whether contradictory findings are an artifact of different measurement instruments. Vandewater and Huang,[1] for example, did not find a consistent correlation between children's heavy television viewing and child weight status, although field experiments[14] and correlational[15] and longitudinal surveys[16] have. The differences may be partially explained by their reliance on time use diaries, which may or may not offer a superior measurement of children's time with television.

A second important challenge facing the field is the changing landscape of the media environment. A plethora of studies are now available that offer snapshots of the kinds of messages to which children are routinely exposed, including 2 in this issue (Outley and Taddese[3] and Thompson et al[17]). Once upon a time such snapshots would be a good assessment of media exposure, and one could argue that children who watched more television would receive more of the messages in those snapshots than children who watched less television.[18] Today's media environment, however, is not quite so monolithic. Children have dozens of channels, hundreds of programs, and a variety of media from which to choose. The rise of niche audiences means that children's media use is quite idiosyncratic, both within media and across media. As a consequence, media time cannot be a proxy for message exposure. Moroever, researchers must take caution not to overextend the findings of their content analyses. Outley and Taddese[3] found that the dominant African American television network, BET, had more advertising for unhealthy foods than the WB network or the Disney Channel. This important finding suggests one consequence of niche programming for different audiences. The authors write, "This study is one of the first to examine the effects of media on children during the after-school programming hours." However, content analysis is not effects research unless it actually examines the reception of messages by audiences. Although this study is an ambitious undertaking, future researchers should focus on assessing time spent with media as well as exposure to particular messages to more convincingly directly tie exposure to effects.

Finally, for decades we have known that excessive media use and exposure to problematic content are detrimental to children's healthy development. Despite this fact, we have been slow to develop interventions that are evaluated and replicated across a variety of settings. Several authors in this issue write that parents need to be educated about the negative effects of media (eg, Bushman and Huesmann[7]), but it is not clear how to target messages in such a way that parents will feel that they have the power to make changes within the home. Studies are needed that explore mediation strategies in the home, such as that provided by Barkin et al,[12] and how the American Academy of Pediatrics' recommendation is received by those who would have the most influence over children's media use—namely, parents. Other authors (eg, Bickham and Rich[9]) suggest that pediatricians encourage the development of media literacy, but studies indicate that few primary care physicians have the time or the inclination to address such matters in office visits because their time is limited and they believe that their efforts in this realm would be futile.[19,20] That said, effective school-[21,22] and clinic-based[23] interventions have been developed and evaluated, offering a window into potential strategies for influencing children's media use behaviors. Rigorously evaluated interventions are few in number, however. Funding must be made available, and efforts must be undertaken to create targeted campaigns that both raise parental awareness and provide simple strategies for reducing media time and limiting exposure to negative content.

*Amy B. Jordan, PhD*

**Correspondence:** Dr Jordan, The Annenberg Public Policy Center, University of Pennsylvania, 3620 Walnut St, Philadelphia, PA 19104-6220 (Ajordan@asc.upenn.edu).

## REFERENCES

1. Vandewater EA, Huang X. Parental weight status as a moderator of the relationship between television viewing and childhood overweight. *Arch Pediatr Adolesc Med.* 2006;160:425-431.
2. Weicha JL, Peterson KE, Ludwig DS, Kim J, Sobol A, Gortmaker SL. When children eat what they watch: impact of television viewing on dietary intake in youth. *Arch Pediatr Adolesc Med.* 2006;160:436-442.
3. Outley CW, Taddese A. A content analysis of health and physical activity messages marketed to African American children during after-school television programming. *Arch Pediatr Adolesc Med.* 2006;160:432-435.

4. Lumeng JC, Rahnama S, Appugliese D, Kaciroti N, Bradley RH. Television exposure and overweight risk in preschoolers. *Arch Pediatr Adolesc Med.* 2006;160:417-422.
5. Ashby SL, Arcari CM, Edmonson MB. Television viewing and risk of sexual initiation by young adolescents. *Arch Pediatr Adolesc Med.* 2006;160:375-380.
6. Brady SS, Matthews KA. Effects of media violence on health-related outcomes among young men. *Arch Pediatr Adolesc Med.* 2006;160:341-347.
7. Bushman BJ, Huesmann LR. Short-term and long-term effects of violent media on aggression in children and adults. *Arch Pediatr Adolesc Med.* 2006;160:348-352.
8. Chamberlain LJ, Wang Y, Robinson TN. Does children's screen time predict requests for advertised products? cross-sectional and prospective analyses. *Arch Pediatr Adolesc Med.* 2006;160:363-368.
9. Bickham DS, Rich M. Is television viewing associated with social isolation? roles of exposure time, viewing context, and violent content. *Arch Pediatr Adolesc Med.* 2006;160:387-392.
10. American Academy of Pediatrics, Committee on Public Education. American Academy of Pediatrics: children, adolescents, and television. *Pediatrics.* 2001;107:423-426.
11. Jordan A, Trentacoste N, Manganello J, Henderson V, Fishbein M. Measuring the time teens spend with media: challenges and opportunities. *Media Psychol.* In press.
12. Barkin S, Ip E, Richardson I, Klinepeter S, Finch S, Krcmar M. Parental media mediation styles for children aged 2 to 11 years. *Arch Pediatr Adolesc Med.* 2006;160:395-401.
13. Fletcher J. Social interactions in adolescent television viewing. *Arch Pediatr Adolesc Med.* 2006;160:383-386.
14. Robinson TN. Reducing children's television viewing to prevent obesity: a randomized controlled trial. *JAMA.* 1999;282:1561-1567.
15. Armstrong CA, Sallis JF, Alcaraz JE, Kolody B, McKenzie TL, Hovell MF. Children's television viewing, body fat, and physical fitness. *Am J Health Promot.* 1998;2:363-368.
16. Gortmaker SL, Must A, Sobol AM, Peterson K, Colditz GA, Dietz WH. Television viewing as a cause of increasing obesity among children in the United States, 1986-1990. *Arch Pediatr Adolesc Med.* 1996;150:356-362.
17. Thompson KM, Tepichin K, Haninger K. Content and ratings of mature-rated video games. *Arch Pediatr Adolesc Med.* 2006;160:402-410.
18. Gerbner G, Gross L, Morgan M, Signorielli N. Growing up with television: the cultivation perspective. In: Bryant J, Zillmann D, eds. *Media Effects: Advances in Theory and Research.* Hillsdale, NJ: Lawrence Erlbaum; 1994:17-41.
19. Strasburger VC. Adolescents and the media: why don't paediatricians and parents "get it"? *Med J Aust.* 2005;183:425-426.
20. Gentile DA, Oberg C, Sherwood N, Story M, Walsh D. Hogan. Well-child visits in the video age: pediatricians and the American Academy of Pediatrics' guidelines for children's media use. *Pediatrics.* 2004;114:1235-1241.
21. Robinson TN. Can a school-based intervention to reduce television use decrease adiposity in children in grades 3 and 4? *West J Med.* 2000;173:40.
22. Gortmaker SL, Peterson K, Wiecha J, et al. Reducing obesity via a school-based interdisciplinary intervention among youth. *Arch Pediatr Adolesc Med.* 1999;153:409-418.
23. Epstein LH, Paluch RA, Consalvi A, Riordan K, School T. Effects of manipulating sedentary behavior on physical activity and food intake. *J Pediatr.* 2002;140:334-339.

# Effect of Media on Children and Adolescents

## *It's About Time*

IN THE OCTOBER 2004 ISSUE OF *NATIONAL GEOGRAPHIC*, Joel Bourne[1] postulated about the circumstances that would occur if a category 3 or 4 storm changed into a category 5 storm before it hit the Louisiana coast and New Orleans, La. The ensuing calamity and damage to the city and its citizens if the levies were breached was exactingly detailed as the worst natural disaster in the history of the United States. Foreshadowing the event, geologist Shea Penland stated, "It's not if it will happen. It's when."

In this issue of the ARCHIVES, we read about a different storm: research articles that reveal more evidence of the power of electronic media exposure to breach the protections of our children's cognitive, social, behavioral, and physical health. Does ongoing exposure to media erode children's behaviors and attitudes enough to compare with an impending disaster? These and newer studies may reveal whether that is not an inappropriate hyperbole.

Media immersion begins early. A study[1] from almost 3 years ago showed that 50% of households with children aged 0 to 6 years had more than 3 TVs. Thirty percent of children aged 0 to 3 years and 43% of those aged 3 to 6 years had TVs in their bedrooms. Seventy-five percent of these children watched DVDs daily, and 72% of parents who were surveyed believed that computers "mostly helped." Fifty-eight percent of the parents said that educational videos were "very important," and 25% owned *Baby Einstein* videos. Ninety percent of parents said that they had TV rules, but 58% would let children watch alone.

Children's educational DVDs and interactive games for infants and toddlers are a $100 million business fueled by marketing strategies that tout or intimate cognitive and social development. This is despite the fact that, to my knowledge, there are no scientific studies on outcomes from any DVDs, programs, or games that are currently available except for *Sesame Street*. Companies market primarily to parental anxieties to give their children every academic advantage. Most companies realize that money spent doing research would not change the reality that parents rely more on other parents' experience with these products than on studies or "expert advice."[3]

The market continues to flourish in the face of the 1999 recommendation by the American Academy of Pediatrics (AAP) that urges parents to "avoid television for less than 2 years, secondary to early brain development showing babies and toddlers have a critical need for direct interactions with parents."[4]

Research needs to continue on the context and content of parental strategies regarding media exposure in the face of the recommendations by the AAP.[4] Are parents aware and/or concerned about media exposure time? Is media exposure a family affair? Will discussing these kinds of published results impact the parents' decisions?

Do the media usage habits of young children carry on to older ages? A study by the Kaiser Family Foundation[5] found that children aged 8 to 18 years had an average media usage time of 6 hours and 21 minutes. Sixty-eight percent of these children had TVs in their rooms, and 31%

had computers. Fifty percent of the children lived in households with no TV rules, and of the other 50% with rules, only 1 in 5 reported that the rules are enforced. Total media exposure time for most of the children exceeded the time spent in all other activities except sleep. Also noted was that the total average time spent using media was much greater (more than 9 hours) in certain categories, such as low contentedness (18%), heavy video gaming (13%), and for children with poorer academic grades (10% who had received grades of *C*s and *D*s).

The research by Bickham and Rich[6] is certainly of interest within these subgroups of preteens and teens. They structured their study to describe the effect of television and violent television viewing on peer relationships. They postulated that "lonely children may turn to television for entertainment and companionship."[6] Is more media or specific media exposure a predictor of social isolation? When aggressive behaviors or poor academic grades are noted, attention should be given to documenting specific and total media exposure time.

"Generation Speed," a study of 1000 children aged 12 to 17 years that was performed by Johns Hopkins University, Baltimore, Md, and reported in *Seventeen* magazine,[7] revealed that 97% of the children multitasked, using several electronic appliances simultaneously. Although not described in this issue of the ARCHIVES, this is an area of media use that has leapfrogged to the forefront of concern related to the potential effect of partial and simultaneous attention on learning capability and cognitive function. New technology will continue to extend this trend to younger children. Future research will have to create new testing that may reveal perhaps both the positive and negative outcomes of media multitasking.

Although there are no articles in this issue of the ARCHIVES specifically detailing Internet exposure, teens are living and playing online. A study by Lenhart et al[8] showed that 87% (21 million) of children aged 12 to 17 years use the Internet. Of these children, 17 million play games online, 31% get health information, 50% have a cellular phone, and 51% have broadband access. Teens look at the Internet now as a place for communication, social networking, and personal expression. However, with expected expansion of broadband and wireless services as well as cellular video content delivery, we could see significantly more portable connectivity and media use.

Remember that all media imply an economic imperative: they are there to make money. Toddler "edutainment," video games, movies, Internet portals, social networking sites, music, electronic devices, phones, and TV are all positioning the young consumer to purchase products.[9]

This media-oriented generation is targeted from birth. Branding has become ubiquitous for and among the youngest children. Children and teens are divided into demographic niches exposing them to specific marketing strategies and product placements from home to school, malls, and sports arenas. Media exposure carries the specter of advertising with it, even with TiVo and digital video recorders promising to allow less advertising exposure. Every brand covets children's and teens' eyes. Combined, children and teens spend more than $200 billion yearly. Because children younger than age 8 years are unable to decipher advertising cognitively, popular children's television characters are selling low-nutrition, high-calorie foods. More than $10 billion per year is spent on marketing foods and beverages that kids buy and eat.[10] The study by Wiecha et al[11] regarding the impact of viewing on dietary intake again reiterates that "television advertising for food has a powerful influence on diets."[11] More research must be done on the direct viewing of advertisements to separate out the protective factors allowing children and teens to resist the urge to drink, smoke, or eat.

It is about time we concluded that we cannot outspend the media. Media researchers may often censure but rarely censor the media. Media exposure is inevitable, and most media have eroded the dividing line that separated childhood from adulthood. Even with the plethora of (mostly unused) rating systems for parents, there are latch-key children, children with dangerous community environments, and children who may need more media secondary to psychosocial issues. The media exposure for these children and teens will bypass parental guidance, as will that for children with TVs, computers, and gaming systems in their bedrooms.

We are conducting an ongoing, uncontrolled experiment on this generation in terms of media exposure and potential future behavioral and physical consequences, and it seems unopposed by the media industry and most parents. This issue of the ARCHIVES illuminates only some of those consequences.

What of risks that are not apparent or foreshadowed? Cognitive risks from this flood with imagery. Does TV viewing lead to poor educational outcomes? There are many confounding factors that allow media scholars only to speculate. However, for every 100 ninth-graders, only 67 graduate from high school, 38 go to college, and 18 obtain a college degree within 6 years.[12] Of the 1.2 million high school seniors taking the ACT college admission test, only 51% were found to have the reading skills needed to succeed in college.[13] Within the many factors involved in this outcome, is the amount of time spent using media significant?

In reviewing the data from the study by Zimmerman and Christakis[14] on cognitive outcomes related to television viewing, Chernin and Linebarger[15] stated that because there were no reliable and valid estimates of content-based measures, the results put forth were "not sufficient to substantiate the American Academy of Pediatrics' recommendations."[15]

For almost 40 years, the AAP has been concerned about TV's power to be the "other parent."[16] Since the early 1990s, the AAP has been engaged in an educational campaign that recognizes the risks and benefits of media exposure. The AAP policy statements provided for parents, pediatricians, and policy makers give recommendations to guide but not isolate children and adolescents from the media. Acknowledging that the mechanisms of some risks have multiple factors, researchers with studies included in this issue of the ARCHIVES have continued to emphasize the usefulness of the AAP's recommendations, which include the following guidelines: (1) not allowing the bedroom to be a media center with TV, video games, and Internet access; (2)

limiting media time to 1 to 2 hours of quality programming; (3) discouraging TV viewing for children younger than 2 years (believing that at this age, there is more to be learned from a 3-dimensional world than a 2-dimensional one regardless of content); (4) viewing and discussing content together; (5) turning off the TV when no one is watching and during meals; and (6) being a good media role model. These are noncomplex, salable actions that can be implemented by most parents or caregivers and reinforced by pediatricians. Because the topography of media exposure has evolved from 10 feet (TV) to 2 feet (computers) to 10 inches (cellular telephones), these actions (with the exception of being a good role model) are important but may only achieve short-term interventions. Technology will continue to present new media opportunities to all children.

The AAP will continue to advocate for specific content as opposed to the amount of media research from earlier ages. Also, researchers will need to devise newer techniques to test the hypothesis that interactive media may have positive cognitive and physical outcomes.

As research becomes available, the AAP's continuing advocacy position promoting media education and literacy will still be of utmost urgency.[17] It has been shown that media messages target and affect behaviors and attitudes. Parents and schools should be natural allies in producing media-literate children. This implies that children will comprehend that all media messages are constructed and will then develop the ability to decipher the purpose and actual meaning of that message rather than integrate it into their value system. Additionally, media literacy should allow for positive and prosocial media messages to be appreciated.

Like the 30-year, $10 billion plan that could have protected the Louisiana wetlands and New Orleans, media literacy curricula will be difficult to accept and implement. There is always hope that politicians and the industry could be a significant part of the solution. However, President Clinton once said, "Governments don't raise children, parents do." Because our government rejected that plan, Louisiana waited unprepared for the storm that could and did come. It is about time we validate this research on the behavioral, cognitive, social, and physical outcomes of media exposure rather than wait for more evidence of possible adverse effects. Increased awareness by physicians, ongoing innovative research beginning at earlier ages, and soliciting active partnerships to teach media literacy should allow us to protect our most precious resource. It's about time.

*Donald Shifrin, MD*

**Correspondence:** Dr Shifrin, Pediatric Associates, 2700 Northrup Way, Bellevue, WA 98004-1461 (peddoc07@aol.com).

**Additional Information:** Dr Shifrin is chair of the Committee on Communications, American Academy of Pediatrics.

## REFERENCES

1. Bourne Jr JK. Gone With the Water. *National Geographic.* October 2004;92.
2. Kaiser Family Foundation. Zero to six: electronic media in the lives of infants, toddlers, and preschoolers. Available at: http://www.kff.org/entmedia/entmedia102803pkg.cfm. Accessed January 25, 2006.
3. Kaiser Family Foundation. A teacher in the living room? educational media for babies, toddlers, and preschoolers. Available at: http://www.kff.org/entmedia/entmedia121405pkg.cfm Accessed January 25, 2006.
4. American Academy of Pediatrics; Committee on Public Education. Media violence. *Pediatrics.* 2001;108:1222-1226.
5. Kaiser Family Foundation. Generation M: media in the lives of 8-18 year-olds. Available at: http://www.kff.org/entmedia/entmedia030905pkg.cfm. Accessed January 25, 2006.
6. Bickham DS, Rich M. Is television viewing associated with social isolation? roles of exposure time, viewing context, and violent content. *Arch Pediatr Adolesc Med.* 2006;160:387-392.
7. Joiner W. Generation Speed. *Seventeen Magazine.* November 2005:147-149.
8. Lenhart A, Madden M, Hitlin P. Teens and technology: youth are leading the transition to a fully wired and mobile nation. Available at: http://www.pewinternet.org/PPF/r/162/report_display.asp. Accessed January 26, 2006.
9. Leonhardt D, Kerwin K. Hey kid, buy this. *Bus Week.* June 30, 1997:62.
10. Institute of Medicine. Food marketing to children and youth: threat or opportunity? Available at: http://www.iom.edu/CMS/3788/21939/31330.aspx. Accessed January 26, 2006.
11. Wiecha JL, Peterson KE, Ludwig DS, Kim J, Sobol A, Gortmaker SL. When children eat what they watch: impact of television viewing on dietary intake in youth. *Arch Pediatr Adolesc Med.* 2006;160:436-442.
12. National High School Alliance. Conversations about the American high school. Available at: http://www.hsalliance.org. Accessed January 26, 2006.
13. Levin T. Many who plan on college aren't ready, report finds. *NY Times.* August 17, 2005:15.
14. Zimmerman FJ, Christakis DA. Children's television viewing and cognitive outcomes: a longitudinal analysis of national data. *Arch Pediatr Adolesc Med.* 2005;159:619-625.
15. Chernin AR, Linebarger DL. The relationship between children's television viewing and academic performance. *Arch Pediatr Adolesc Med.* 2005;159:687-689.
16. Steyer J. *The Other Parent: The Inside Story of the Media's Effect on Our Children.* New York, NY: Atria; 2002.
17. American Academy of Pediatrics. Media education. Available at: http://www.aap.org/visit/cmte11.htm. Accessed January 30, 2006.

## Needle Aspiration and Intramuscular Vaccination

Needle aspiration is the process of pulling back on the syringe plunger prior to injection. Its purported importance is to prevent accidental entry of the needle into a blood vessel, but there is no scientific evidence to support its need. The most recent guidelines published by the American Academy of Pediatrics (Elk Grove Village, Ill) recommend that aspiration prior to intramuscular vaccination may not be necessary,[1] while the Canadian guidelines continue to recommend aspiration.[2] It is not surprising therefore that both techniques are currently being used by vaccinators. The objective of this survey was to determine which technique vaccinators are currently using.

A 22-item categorical questionnaire was sent to all community pediatric offices registered with the Continuing Medical Education Department, Hospital for Sick Children, Toronto, Ontario (n=248). The Hospital for Sick Children Research Ethics Board granted ethical approval for the study. The primary outcome was whether community pediatricians and nurses aspirate prior to intramuscular vaccine injection. The $\chi^2$ test was used for comparison of categorical variables, with a $P$ value $<.05$ considered significant.

Of the 248 offices mailed questionnaires, 40 were excluded because they did not routinely administer vaccinations and 123 responded with valid data, for an overall office response rate of 59% (123/208). A total of 167 completed questionnaires were returned by individual vaccinators: 135 (81%) from pediatricians and 32 (19%) from nurses. Of the 167 respondents, 123 (74%) aspirated prior to intramuscular vaccination. Of aspirators, 45% (55/123) reported at least 1 major complication (eg, crying for > 3 hours, seizures, or other) following vaccination, compared with 48% (21/44) of nonaspirators ($P=.70$). Of those who did aspirate, 3% (4/119) did so for the recommended 5 to 10 seconds, while the remainder aspirated for less than 5 seconds. Of nonaspirators, 43% (18/42) reported that they thought aspiration increased pain response compared with 11% (13 of 121) of aspirators ($P<.001$).

A review of the literature indicates a paucity of scientific data for the optimal method to administer intramuscular vaccine injections, and there is no scientific data to support aspiration prior to injection, only expert opinion.[3] Slow aspiration and slow injection time have been recommended to avoid damage to local tissues, which might cause pain, but also without scientific validation.[3,4] In this survey, only 3% of respondents aspirated for the recommended 5 to 10 seconds. The remainder aspirated far too quickly for the procedure to be effective and would not have accomplished the safety objective for which it had been designed.

This survey of vaccinators demonstrates that the majority of respondents still aspirate prior to intramuscular vaccination but most do it too rapidly to be effective. Aspiration is time-consuming if done properly, and the current recommendation to aspirate prior to intramuscular vaccination may need to be reconsidered.

*Moshe Ipp, MD*
*Jonathan Sam, BSc*
*Patricia C. Parkin, MD*

**Correspondence:** Dr Ipp, Division of Pediatric Medicine, The Hospital for Sick Children, 155 University Ave, Toronto, Ontario M5G 1X8, Canada (mm.ipp@utoronto.ca).
**Funding/Support:** This study was supported by unrestricted research grant from GlaxoSmithKline.

1. American Academy of Pediatrics. Red book. In: Pickering LK, ed. *Active and Passive Immunization: Report of the Committee on Infectious Diseases.* 26th ed. Elk Grove Village, Ill: American Academy of Pediatrics; 2003:1-93.
2. National Advisory Committee on Immunization. Immunization technique. In: *Canadian Immunization Guide.* 6th ed. Ottawa, Ontario: Health Canada; 2002:38-40. Cat H49-8/2002E.
3. Beyea SC, Nicholl LH. Administration of medications via the intramuscular route: an integrative review of the literature and research-based protocol for the procedure. *Appl Nurs Res.* 1995;8:23-33.
4. Zelman S. Notes on techniques of intramuscular injection: the avoidance of needless pain and morbidity. *Am J Med Sci.* 1961;241:563-574.

## Cranberry Therapy for Children's Urinary Tract Infections

In "Reevaluating Antibiotic Therapy for Urinary Tract Infections [UTIs] in Children" Yared and Edwards suggest that "pediatricians should thoughtfully reexamine their practice of prescribing prophylactic antibiotics; this practice further contributes to antibiotic pressure and resistance."[1(p993)] I concur. So do many families. In fact, many families turn to home remedies such as cranberry juice to prevent recurrent UTIs, often without discussing this therapy with their physician.[2]

Although cranberry juice and capsules have proven effective in adult women with recurrent UTIs, they have only been studied in pediatric populations at very high risk for recurrent UTIs and not in the typical population receiving prophylactic antibiotics. Many questions need to be addressed: pharmacokinetics of different cranberry products (juice vs fresh berries vs dried fruit vs dried in capsules; organic, pure juice vs corn syrup–sweetened juice diluted with water or other juices); the effectiveness of cranberry vs other members of its botanical family, such as blueberry; safety; optimal dose; frequency; duration; synergy with medications; impact on use of other medications; and short- and long-term economic impact, for example.

I wonder if the authors would agree that it is high time for a thoughtful series of studies of cranberry therapy in children to learn if, in select cases, we can use fruit juice instead of "bug juice" to prevent recurrent UTIs, thereby decreasing antibiotic pressure and resistance.

*Kathi J. Kemper, MD, MPH*

**Correspondence:** Dr Kemper, Departments of Pediatrics, Public Health Sciences, and Family and Community Medicine, Wake Forest University School of Medicine, Medical Center Boulevard, Winston-Salem, NC 27157 (kkemper@wfubmc.edu).

1. Yared A, Edwards KM. Reevaluating antibiotic therapy for urinary tract infections in children. *Arch Pediatr Adolesc Med.* 2005;159:992-993.
2. Kemper KJ, Super E, Woods C, Nagaraj S. Cranberry use among pediatric nephrology patients. *Ambul Pediatr.* 2005;5:249-252.

## Dismissing Families: A Slippery Slope

After reading "Dismissing the Family Who Refuses Vaccines: A Study of Pediatrician Attitudes" by Flanagan-Klygis et al,[1] I spent a sleepless night feeling sad, ashamed, and angry. How can physicians dedicated to patient-centered care "fire" families who make independent health decisions? We are not generals demanding obedience; we are servants of life, of free human beings. They come to us for help, not demands to do it "our way or the highway."

What's next? Will we fire families who let their children watch more than the "maximum" of 2 hours of television daily? Fire parents who let their children ride in the back of pick-up trucks? Fire parents who do not feed their children at least 5 servings of fruits and vegetables daily? Or just those who serve less than 3? Or those who overfeed their children and allow them to become obese? Or those who don't have sufficient funds to buy food or shelter and have hungry, homeless children? Or those of different religious or cultural or racial backgrounds?

On just what part of the Hippocratic oath or conventional medical ethics are we relying when we make such decisions or are they based purely on a sense of self-righteousness?

Many patients are voting with their feet and have already started firing this kind of rigid pediatrician, turning instead to humanistic clinicians from other disciplines such as family medicine, chiropractic, and naturopathy. We have not just started on this slippery slope; we are well on our way. It is time to turn around and head back to the high ground of true service before we hit the depths of petty tyranny.

*Kathi J. Kemper, MD, MPH*
*Caryl J. Guth, MD*

**Correspondence:** Dr Kemper, Departments of Pediatrics, Public Health Sciences, and Family and Community Medicine, Wake Forest University School of Medicine, Medical Center Boulevard, Winston-Salem, NC 27157 (kkemper@wfubmc.edu).

1. Flanagan-Klygis EA, Sharp L, Frader JE. Dismissing the family who refuses vaccines: a study of pediatrician attitudes. *Arch Pediatr Adolesc Med.* 2005;159:929-934.

## Dismissing Families: A Critical Issue

As a former practicing family physician providing care to pediatric and adolescent patients, I applaud the ARCHIVES' efforts to bring attention to this critical issue.

In my former practice I, too, dismissed families from my practice for refusing childhood immunizations. Following the lead of a pediatrician mentor of mine, I would exhaust all efforts to provide cogent arguments to support the proven safety and effectiveness of these most successful preventive regimens. When these arguments failed, I advised these well-meaning but misguided parents that they were asking me to "voluntarily contribute to the death of their child from a disease we could prevent"; an ethical breach they could not ask of me. Most understood, and although it seldom changed their preconceptions, it at least provided a conceptual basis to interpret the decision to terminate the patient-physician relationship.

I believe it is essential that practicing physicians be given the support of their college or academy and their academic colleagues and be provided sound scientific and ethical bases on which to render care in the face of this pernicious public health threat. Drs Flanagan-Klygis, Sharp, and Frader[1] bring voice to the ever-present need for physicians to advocate for the highest-quality care for their patients.

*Michael P. Elston, MD, MS*

**Correspondence:** Dr Elston, Medical Management, Western Health, 529 Kansas City St, 200, Rapid City, SD 57701 (melston@rcrh.org).

1. Flanagan-Klygis EA, Sharp L, Frader JE. Dismissing the family who refuses vaccines: a study of pediatrician attitudes. *Arch Pediatr Adolesc Med.* 2005;159:929-934.

### *In reply*

*We appreciate the recent letters to the editor regarding our study entitled "Dismissing the Family Who Refuses Vaccines: a Study of Pediatrician Attitudes" published in October.[1] We intended to stimulate a thoughtful discussion about the pros and cons of family dismissal for vaccine refusal, not demonize physicians who choose to sever their professional relationships with patients. Those who dismiss families have reasonable concerns; a more scholarly editorial could have added to the discussion about this very important issue. Unfortunately, in his editorial,[2] Dr Hendricks minimized the significance of prevalent acceptance of dismissal and emphasized the use of a formal, somewhat legalistic documentation of parental vaccine refusal. Just as a signed informed consent document cannot take the place of face-to-face discussions with patients about risks and benefits of purposed treatments, paper memorialization should never take the place of substantive discussions and education with families about vaccination risks and benefits.*

*We hope that pediatricians will take note of our findings and readdress the issue of family dismissal for themselves and their colleagues. We think all will agree we should put our patients first when encountering parents who refuse vaccines and find a balance between maintaining access to and continuity of all pediatric care and ensuring the importance of immunization's part in preventive medicine.*

*Erin Flanagan-Klygis, MD*
*Joel Frader, MD*
*Lisa Sharp, PhD*

**Correspondence:** Dr Flanagan-Klygis, Rush Medical College, 1645 W Jackson St, Suite 200, Chicago, IL 60612 (erin_flanagan-klygis@rush.edu).

1. Flanagan-Klygis EA, Frader J, Sharp L. Dismissing the family who refuses vaccines: a study of pediatrician attitudes. *Arch Pediatr Adolesc Med*. 2005;159:929-934.
2. Hendricks JW. Does immunization refusal warrant discontinuing the physician-patient relationship? *Arch Pediatr Adolesc Med*. 2005;159:994.

## Advocacy by Any Other Name Would Smell as Sweet

We are responding to the thoughtful editorial by Dr Bergman[1] to our study "Child Advocacy Training: Curriculum Outcomes and Resident Satisfaction."[2] We could discuss many of the details of advocacy training that Dr Bergman mentions, but the real issue is how to create and disseminate educational experiences that will serve all physicians, not only future pediatricians.

It is important to determine what is meant by advocacy both in terms of its historical roots and dynamic boundaries. We would suggest that this is a dynamic conversation involving pediatrics and beyond. We believe that the term *advocacy* incorporates a broad range of physician engagement. To advocate is when one "defends, maintains, publicly recommends, or raises his voice in behalf of a proposal or tenet."[3] The venue is not inherent in the definition. This personal calling to "publicly defend" can manifest at the individual level in the clinic or hospital[1]; at the system level, for example, in hospital administrative meetings[4]; in the community[5]; or in the policy arena.[6]

A consensus definition of advocacy is important because it allows pediatricians to participate beyond pediatric circles in a conversation occurring throughout medicine[7] and medical education.[8,9] This is a dynamic conversation about greater civic engagement by physicians. In this broader arena, advocacy is often used to describe such engagement in simple terms: "Advocacy only means taking the problems that one faces day to day and pursuing their resolution outside their usual place of presentation"[10(p458)] and working "informally with others to solve a health problem in the community."[5(p97)]

The content and requirements for advocacy training will depend on the changing environment and vulnerability of medical practice to political decision making. We need vibrant training now because so much of pediatric illness is dependent on the interaction among a variety of changing communities: regional, neighborhood, school, family, and health care, as examples. All pediatricians, regardless of specialty, should be trained in and share a collective foundation of skills that include child advocacy. We agree that advocacy is not a pediatric specialty. Along with professionalism, interpersonal communication, and other competencies, advocacy may best be considered a cross-cutting theme for physician education. The Pediatric Residency Review Committee's move to require "structured educational experiences that prepare residents for the role of advocate"[11] is a first step for this recognition—but it is just the first step.

Dr Bergman articulates where the current challenges lie. Continued guidance from those who have dedicated their lives to advocacy, more national discussions such as this, and the hard work of organizations such as the Resident Advocacy Special Interest Group of the Ambulatory Pediatrics Association and the Community Pediatrics Training Initiative of the American Academy of Pediatrics will ensure that the role of the pediatrician will evolve in way that benefits children the most.

*Lisa J. Chamberlain, MD, MPH*
*Lee M. Sanders, MD, MPH*
*John I. Takayama, MD, MPH*

**Correspondence:** Dr Chamberlain, Stanford University School of Medicine, General Pediatrics, 750 Welch Rd, Suite 325, Palo Alto, CA 94304 (lchamberlain@stanford.edu).

1. Bergman AB. Advocacy is not a specialty. *Arch Pediatr Adolesc Med*. 2005;159:892.
2. Chamberlain LJ, Sanders LM, Takayama JI. Child advocacy training: curriculum outcomes and resident satisfaction. *Arch Pediatr Adolesc Med*. 2005;159:842-847.
3. Oxford English Dictionary. Available at: http://dictionary.oed.com. Accessed February 6, 2006.
4. Rivara FP. Sustaining optimism. *Arch Pediatr Adolesc Med*. 2004;158:414-415.
5. Gruen RL, Pearson SD, Brennan TA. Physician-citizens—public roles and professional obligations. *JAMA*. 2004;291:94-98.
6. Bergman AB. The practice of political medicine. *Pediatr Ann*. 1995;24:405-408.
7. ABIM Foundation; American Board of Internal Medicine; ACP-ASIM Foundation; American College of Physicians-American Society of Internal Medicine; European Federation of Internal Medicine. Medical professionalism in the new millennium: a physician charter. *Ann Intern Med*. 2002;136:243-246.
8. Calleson DC, Jordan C, Seifer SD. Community-engaged scholarship: is faculty work in communities a true academic enterprise? *Acad Med*. 2005;80:317-321.
9. Oandasan IF, Barker KK. Educating for advocacy: exploring the source and substance of community-responsive physicians. *Acad Med*. 2003;78(10 suppl):S16-S19.
10. Horton R. The doctor's role in advocacy. *Lancet*. 2002;359:458.
11. Residency Review Committee for Pediatrics. Program requirements for resident training in pediatrics. Available at: http://www.acgme.org. Accessed February 7, 2006.

## JOURNAL ADVERTISER INDEX

**ABBOTT LABS**
Omnicef OS .......... 337-339

**CLASSIFIED ADVERTISING**
http://www.amapublications.com .......... 455

**GLAXOSMITHKLINE**
Boostrix .......... 361-362, 443-444
Havrix .......... 331-332, 393-394
Pediarix .......... 381-382, COVER 3-4

**MERCK & COMPANY**
Gardasil .......... 368A-D
Rotateq .......... 352A-E

**SEPRACOR**
Xopenex .......... 423-424, COVER 2-329

*Demographic and "Mini" inserts and/or ROB ad pages

While every precaution is taken to ensure accuracy, we cannot guarantee against the possibility of an occasional change or omission in the preparation of this index.

ARCHIVES OF PEDIATRICS & ADOLESCENT MEDICINE

# CONTACT INFORMATION

## EDITORIAL OFFICE

**Editorial Office Information:** *Archives of Pediatrics & Adolescent Medicine*, Department of Pediatrics, Child Health Institute, University of Washington, 6200 NE 74th St, Suite 210, Seattle, WA 98115-8160; phone: (206) 685-3573; fax: (206) 685-3572; e-mail: archpediatrics@jama-archives.org.

**Electronic Submission:** Manuscripts should be submitted via our online manuscript submission and review system (http://manuscripts.archpediatrics.com). Manuscripts submitted through our online system should not also be submitted by mail or fax. Signed authorship forms should be sent by regular mail or fax. See the Instructions for Authors (www.archpediatrics.com) for more details.

## CONSORTIUM OF *JAMA* & *ARCHIVES* JOURNALS

The *Archives of Pediatrics & Adolescent Medicine* is a member of the consortium of AMA journals listed below.

The Journal of the American Medical Association (JAMA)
Archives of Dermatology
Archives of Facial Plastic Surgery
Archives of General Psychiatry
Archives of Internal Medicine
Archives of Neurology
Archives of Ophthalmology
Archives of Otolaryngology–Head & Neck Surgery
Archives of Pediatrics & Adolescent Medicine
Archives of Surgery

## *JAMA/ARCHIVES* MEDIA RELATIONS

Jann Ingmire; phone: (312) 464-5262; e-mail: mediarelations@jama-archives.org.

## *ARCHIVES OF PEDIATRICS* ONLINE

*Archives of Pediatrics & Adolescent Medicine* is available online at www.archpediatrics.com.

## *JAMA/ARCHIVES* REPRINTS

**Author Reprints:** Anna Goins at (312) 464-2477; fax: (312) 464-5843; e-mail: anna.goins@ama-assn.org. Minimum order: 100 reprints.

**Educational Reprints:** Rhonda Bailey Brown at (312) 464-2513; fax: (312) 464-5843; e-mail: rhonda.brown@ama-assn.org. Minimum order: 100 reprints.

**Commercial Reprints:** Phone: (312) 464-0776; fax: (312) 464-0708; e-mail: reprints@ama-assn.org. Minimum order: 500 reprints.

## PERMISSIONS

Information about obtaining permission to republish, reprint, or adapt material published in *Archives of Pediatrics & Adolescent Medicine* is available from Rhonda Bailey Brown; phone: (312) 464-2513; fax: (312) 464-5843; e-mail: permissions@ama-assn.org.

## DOCUMENT DELIVERY

Copies of individual articles are available online at www.archpediatrics.com and from the following: Infotrieve, phone: (800) 422-4633; fax: (310) 208-5971; URL: www.infotrieve.com; e-mail: orders@infotrieve.com; Institute for Scientific Information (ISI), phone: (800) 603-4367; fax: (856) 787-1679; URL: http://www.isidoc.com; e-mail: service@isidoc.com; Dialog Information Services; Proquest; Ovid Technologies, Inc; and EBSCO.

The ARCHIVES OF PEDIATRICS & ADOLESCENT MEDICINE (ISSN 01072–4710) is published monthly by the American Medical Association, 515 N State St, Chicago, IL 60610–0946, and is an official publication of the Association. The ARCHIVES OF PEDIATRICS & ADOLESCENT MEDICINE reaches more than 30 900 readers in over 83 countries each month. Periodicals postage paid at Chicago, Ill, and at additional mailing offices. GST registration number 12622 5556 RT. Canada Post International Publications Mail (Canadian Distribution) Sales Agreement No. 318728. POSTMASTER, send all address changes to *Archives of Pediatrics & Adolescent Medicine,* c/o the AMA Unified Service Center, American Medical Association, 515 N State St, Chicago, IL 60610. Printed in the USA.

## ADVERTISING

Information about advertising is available from the following sales representatives and online at www.archpediatrics.com.

**Account Manager:** Tim Melroy (nationally); phone: (973) 263-9191 ext 213.

**Manager, Marketing Services:** Nancy Bell; phone: (973) 263-9191 ext 216.

**Advertising Office:** 119 Cherry Hill Rd, Suite 330, Parsippany, NJ 07054-1114; phone: (973) 263-9191.

**Classified Advertising:** Thalia Moss, 515 N State St, Chicago, IL 60610; phone: (800) 262-2260; e-mail: classifieds@ama-assn.org.

## ADVERTISING PRINCIPLES

Advertisements in this issue have been reviewed to comply with the principles governing advertising in AMA publications. A copy of these principles is available on request and online at www.archpediatrics.com. The appearance of advertising in AMA publications is not an AMA guarantee or endorsement of the product or the claims made for the product by the manufacturer.

## ADDRESS CHANGES

Send all address changes to *Archives of Pediatrics & Adolescent Medicine*, c/o the AMA Unified Service Center, American Medical Association, 515 N State St, Chicago, IL 60610. Notification of address changes must be made at least 6 weeks in advance; include both old and new addresses and a recent mailing label if sending via mail.

## SUBSCRIPTION RATES AND SERVICE

Subscription rates are shown in the table below. For service in the US and Americas, inquiries on pricing, address changes, missing issues, subscription billing, subscription renewal, and back issues, contact the AMA Unified Service Center, 24 hours a day, 7 days a week.

**AMA members:** phone: (800) 262-3211; e-mail: msc@ama-assn.org. **Other physicians and nonphysician customers, including subscription agents:** phone: (800) 262-2350 or (312) 670-7827; fax: (312) 464-5831; e-mail: ama-subs@ama-assn.org. **Inquiries:** Unified Service Center, American Medical Association, PO Box 10946, Chicago, IL 60610-0946. For subscribers with mailing addresses outside the United States & Americas: Contact *JAMA & Archives* Journals, c/o EMD GmbH, Birkenstr.67, 10559 Berlin, Germany. Phone: +49 (30) 33099828; fax: +49 (30) 33099829; e-mail: ama@emd-germany.de.

**Annual Subscription Rates**

| | United States | Americas | UK | Rest of World |
|---|---|---|---|---|
| INDIVIDUAL | | | | |
| Print and Online | $185 | $240 | £165 | €250 |
| INSTITUTION | | | | |
| Print and Online | $375 | $485 | £315 | €470 |

In Canada, US rate plus GST. Rates for residents and medical students available at pubs.ama-assn.org, or from the AMA Unified Service Center.

**PEDIARIX™ [Diphtheria and Tetanus Toxoids and Acellular Pertussis Adsorbed, Hepatitis B (Recombinant) and Inactivated Poliovirus Vaccine Combined]**

The following is a brief summary only; see full prescribing information for complete product information.

**CONTRAINDICATIONS:** Hypersensitivity to any component of the vaccine, including yeast, neomycin, and polymyxin B, is a contraindication (see DESCRIPTION in complete prescribing information). Do not use PEDIARIX after a serious allergic reaction (e.g., anaphylaxis) temporally associated with a previous dose of this vaccine or with any components of this vaccine. Because of the uncertainty as to which component of the vaccine might be responsible, do not give further vaccination with any of these components; or, refer such individuals to an allergist for evaluation. The following events are contraindications to administration of PEDIARIX: encephalopathy (e.g., coma, decreased level of consciousness, prolonged seizures) within 7 days of administration of a previous dose of a pertussis-containing vaccine that is not attributable to another identifiable cause; progressive neurologic disorder, including infantile spasms, uncontrolled epilepsy, or progressive encephalopathy. Do not vaccinate individuals with such conditions until a treatment regimen has been established and the condition has stabilized. PEDIARIX is not contraindicated for use in individuals with HIV infection.

**WARNINGS:** Administration of PEDIARIX is associated with higher rates of fever relative to separately administered vaccines. In one study that evaluated medically attended fever after the first dose of PEDIARIX or separately administered vaccines, infants who received PEDIARIX had a higher rate of medical encounters for fever within the first 4 days following vaccination. In some infants, these encounters included the performance of diagnostic studies to evaluate other causes of fever (see ADVERSE REACTIONS). The vial stopper is latex-free. The tip cap and the rubber plunger of the needleless prefilled syringes contain dry natural latex rubber that may cause allergic reactions in latex sensitive individuals. If any of the following events occur in temporal relation to receipt of whole-cell DTP or a vaccine containing an acellular pertussis component, consider carefully whether to give subsequent doses of PEDIARIX or any vaccine containing a pertussis component: temperature of ≥40.5°C (105°F) within 48 hours not due to another identifiable cause; collapse or shock-like state (hypotonic-hyporesponsive episode) within 48 hours; persistent, inconsolable crying lasting ≥3 hours, occurring within 48 hours; seizures with or without fever occurring within 3 days. If Guillain-Barré syndrome occurs within 6 weeks of receipt of prior vaccine containing tetanus toxoid, the decision to give subsequent doses of PEDIARIX or any vaccine containing tetanus toxoid should be based on careful consideration of the potential benefits and possible risks. A committee of the Institute of Medicine (IOM) has concluded that evidence is consistent with a causal relationship between whole-cell DTP vaccine and acute neurologic illness, and under special circumstances, between whole-cell DTP vaccine and chronic neurologic disease in the context of the National Childhood Encephalopathy Study (NCES) report; however, evidence was insufficient to indicate whether or not whole-cell DTP vaccine increased the overall risk of chronic neurologic disease. Acute encephalopathy and permanent neurologic damage have not been reported causally linked or in temporal association with administration of PEDIARIX, but the experience with PEDIARIX is insufficient to rule this out. Encephalopathy has been reported following INFANRIX® (Diphtheria and Tetanus Toxoids and Acellular Pertussis Vaccine Adsorbed) (see ADVERSE REACTIONS, Postmarketing Reports), but data are not sufficient to evaluate a causal relationship. The decision to administer a pertussis-containing vaccine to children with stable central nervous system (CNS) disorders must be made by the physician on an individual basis, with consideration of all relevant factors, and assessment of potential risks and benefits for that individual. Advise the parent or guardian of the potential increased risk involved (see PRECAUTIONS). A family history of seizures or other CNS disorders is not a contraindication to pertussis vaccine. For children at higher risk for seizures than the general population, an appropriate antipyretic may be administered at the time of vaccination and for the ensuing 24 hours according to the respective prescribing information recommended dosage to reduce the possibility of post-vaccination fever. Defer vaccination during the course of a moderate or severe illness with or without fever and vaccinate patients as soon as they have recovered from the acute phase of the illness. Do not give PEDIARIX to children on anticoagulant therapy or those with bleeding disorders unless the potential benefit clearly outweighs the risk of administration (see PRECAUTIONS in complete prescribing information).

**PRECAUTIONS:** Before the injection of any biological, the physician should take all reasonable precautions to prevent allergic or other adverse reactions. Epinephrine injection (1:1000) and other appropriate agents used for the control of immediate allergic reactions must be immediately available should an acute anaphylactic reaction occur. Immunosuppressed individuals, including those receiving immunosuppressive therapy, may not develop the expected immune response. **Drug Interactions:** For information regarding concomitant administration with other vaccines, refer to DOSAGE AND ADMINISTRATION in complete prescribing information. Do not mix PEDIARIX with any other vaccine in the same syringe or vial. **Carcinogenesis, Mutagenesis, Impairment of Fertility:** PEDIARIX has not been evaluated for carcinogenic or mutagenic potential, or for impairment of fertility. **Pregnancy:** Pregnancy Category C: PEDIARIX is not indicated for women of child-bearing age. Animal reproduction studies have not been conducted with PEDIARIX. It is not known whether PEDIARIX can cause fetal harm when administered to a pregnant woman or if PEDIARIX can affect reproductive capacity. **Geriatric Use:** PEDIARIX is not indicated for use in adult populations. **Pediatric Use:** Safety and effectiveness of PEDIARIX in infants younger than 6 weeks of age have not been evaluated (see DOSAGE AND ADMINISTRATION in complete prescribing information). PEDIARIX is not recommended for persons 7 years of age or older. Tetanus and Diphtheria Toxoids Adsorbed (Td) For Adult Use, inactivated poliovirus vaccine (IPV), and Hepatitis B Vaccine (Recombinant) should be used in individuals 7 years of age or older.

**ADVERSE REACTIONS:** A total of 20,739 doses of PEDIARIX have been administered to 7,028 infants as a 3-dose primary series. The most common adverse reactions observed in clinical trials were local injection site reactions (pain, redness, or swelling), fever, and fussiness. In comparative studies, administration of PEDIARIX was associated with higher rates of fever relative to separately administered vaccines (see WARNINGS). The prevalence of fever was highest on the day of vaccination and the day following vaccination. More than 98% of episodes of fever resolved within the 4-day period following vaccination (i.e., the period including the day of vaccination and the next 3 days). Rates of most other solicited adverse events following PEDIARIX were comparable to rates observed following separately administered US-licensed vaccines. The adverse event information from clinical trials provides a basis for identifying adverse events that appear to be related to vaccine use and for approximating rates. However, because clinical trials are conducted under widely varying conditions, adverse event rates observed in the clinical trials of a vaccine cannot be directly compared to rates in the clinical trials of another vaccine, and may not reflect the rates observed in practice. A total of 5,472 infants were enrolled in a German safety study that was originally designed to compare the safety and reactogenicity of PEDIARIX administered concomitantly at separate sites with 1 of 4 *Haemophilus influenzae* type b (Hib) vaccines at 3, 4, and 5 months of age. After enrollment of 1,569 infants, the study was amended to include a control group that received INFANRIX, Hib vaccine, and oral poliovirus vaccine (OPV) separately. Infants in the separate administration group received one less antigen (hepatitis B) than the infants who received PEDIARIX. Safety data were available for 4,666 infants who received PEDIARIX administered concomitantly at separate sites with 1 of 4 Hib vaccines and for 768 infants in the control group that received separate vaccines. The primary end-point of the study was the percentage of infants with any grade 3 solicited symptom (redness or swelling >20 mm, fever >103.1°F, or crying, pain, vomiting, diarrhea, loss of appetite, or restlessness that prevented normal daily activities) over the 3-dose primary series in infants who received PEDIARIX (4 groups that received PEDIARIX and Hib vaccines pooled) compared to the group that received INFANRIX and Hib vaccine separately with OPV. Analysis for the primary end-point was performed on the according-to-protocol (ATP) cohort that included only those infants who were enrolled after the protocol amendment to include a control group. Of 3,773 infants in the ATP cohort for whom safety data were available, 16.2% (95% CI: 14.9% to 17.5%) of 3,029 infants who received PEDIARIX and Hib vaccine compared to 20.3% (95% CI: 17.5% to 23.4%) of 744 infants who received separate vaccines were reported to have had at least one grade 3 solicited symptom within 4 days of vaccination (i.e., day of vaccination and the next 3 days). The difference between groups in the rate of grade 3 symptoms was 4.1% (90% CI: 1.4% to 7.1%). These were the rates for selected solicited symptoms within 4 days following each dose in a 3-dose primary series in infants who received PEDIARIX administered concomitantly with Hib vaccine and those who received separate concomitant administration of INFANRIX, Hib vaccine, and OPV for the intent-to-treat (ITT) cohort (includes all infants enrolled before and after the amendment who received the indicated vaccine and for whom at least one symptom sheet was completed):

**Percentage of German Infants With Solicited Local Reactions or Selected Systemic Adverse Events Within 4 Days of Vaccination* (ITT Cohort)**

| | PEDIARIX & Hib | | | INFANRIX, Hib, & OPV | | |
|---|---|---|---|---|---|---|
| | **Dose 1** | **Dose 2** | **Dose 3** | **Dose 1** | **Dose 2** | **Dose 3** |
| **N** | **4,666** | **4,619** | **4,574** | **768** | **757** | **750** |
| **Local†** | | | | | | |
| Pain, any | 14.0 | 10.2 | 9.9 | 14.2 | 9.8 | 8.1 |
| Pain, grade 2 or 3 | 2.9 | 1.2 | 1.5 | 3.6 | 1.7 | 1.1 |
| Pain, grade 3 | 0.7 | 0.3 | 0.3 | 1.3 | 0.4 | 0.1 |
| Redness, any | 18.6 | 26.6 | 25.6 | 16.1 | 21.4 | 20.8 |
| Redness, >5 mm | 6.7 | 9.9 | 9.0 | 5.9 | 8.2 | 7.7 |
| Redness, >20 mm | 1.2 | 1.0 | 1.1 | 1.8 | 0.7 | 1.1 |
| Swelling, any | 12.7 | 18.5 | 18.4 | 9.6 | 12.9 | 13.6 |
| Swelling, >5 mm | 5.6 | 7.7 | 7.8 | 3.6 | 5.2 | 4.8 |
| Swelling, >20 mm | 1.2 | 1.6 | 1.5 | 1.3 | 1.1 | 1.2 |
| **Systemic** | | | | | | |
| Restlessness, any | 41.4 | 32.0 | 26.7 | 46.4 | 35.0 | 27.6 |
| Restlessness, grade 2 or 3 | 14.4 | 10.0 | 8.9 | 20.2 | 11.5 | 8.4 |
| Restlessness, grade 3 | 3.0 | 1.5 | 1.6 | 5.7 | 3.0 | 1.7 |
| Fever‡, ≥100.4°F | 25.1 | 19.3 | 19.7 | 13.2 | 13.1 | 11.2 |
| Fever‡, >101.3°F | 5.8 | 4.1 | 4.6 | 2.2 | 2.8 | 2.1 |
| Fever‡, >103.1°F | 0.3 | 0.5 | 0.7 | 0.3 | 0.3 | 0.5 |
| Unusual cry§, any | 24.9 | 16.5 | 13.1 | 36.5 | 19.7 | 14.3 |
| Unusual cry§, grade 2 or 3 | 12.7 | 7.1 | 5.7 | 20.8 | 10.0 | 5.7 |
| Unusual cry§, grade 3 | 3.9 | 1.7 | 1.4 | 6.8 | 2.1 | 1.1 |
| Loss of appetite, any | 17.9 | 13.3 | 12.5 | 19.1 | 16.2 | 11.3 |
| Loss of appetite, grade 2 or 3 | 4.0 | 2.9 | 2.7 | 4.4 | 2.9 | 2.3 |
| Loss of appetite, grade 3 | 0.6 | 0.5 | 0.4 | 0.5 | 0.7 | 0.0 |

N = number of infants in the intent-to-treat (ITT) cohort.
Grade 2 defined as sufficiently discomforting to interfere with daily activities.
Grade 3 defined as preventing normal daily activities.
* Within 4 days of vaccination defined as day of vaccination and the next 3 days.
† Local reactions at the injection site for PEDIARIX or INFANRIX.
‡ Rectal temperatures.
§ Unusual cry lasting >1 hour.

In this study, infants were also monitored for unsolicited adverse events that occurred within 30 days following vaccination. Over the entire study period, 6 subjects in the group that received PEDIARIX reported seizures. Two of these subjects had a febrile seizure, 1 of whom also developed afebrile seizures. The remaining 4 subjects had afebrile seizures, including 2 with infantile spasms. Two subjects reported seizures within 7 days following vaccination (1 subject had both febrile and afebrile seizures, and 1 subject had afebrile seizures), corresponding to a rate of 0.22 seizures per 1,000 doses (febrile seizures 0.07 per 1,000 doses, afebrile seizures 0.14 per 1,000 doses). No subject who received concomitant INFANRIX, Hib vaccine, and OPV reported seizures. In a separate German study that evaluated the safety of INFANRIX in 22,505 infants who received 66,867 doses of INFANRIX administered as a 3-dose primary series, the rate of seizures within 7 days of vaccination with INFANRIX was 0.13 per 1,000 doses (febrile seizures 0.0 per 1,000 doses, afebrile seizures 0.13 per 1,000 doses). No cases of hypotonic-hyporesponsiveness, encephalopathy, or anaphylaxis were reported in the German study that evaluated the safety of PEDIARIX. Rates of serious adverse events that are less common than those reported in this safety study are not known at this time.

Additional safety data for PEDIARIX are available from a US study designed to evaluate lot-to-lot consistency and a bridge for a new manufacturing step. These were the rates for local reactions and selected adverse events within 4 days of vaccination with PEDIARIX administered concomitantly with a Hib vaccine at 2, 4, and 6 months of age:

**Percentage of US Infants With Solicited Local Reactions or Selected Systemic Adverse Events Within 4 Days of Vaccination* (ITT Cohort)**

| | PEDIARIX & Hib | | |
|---|---|---|---|
| | **Dose 1** | **Dose 2** | **Dose 3** |
| **Local†** | **N = 482** | **N = 469** | **N = 466** |
| Pain, any | 30.5 | 25.4 | 23.0 |
| Pain, grade 2 or 3 | 6.2 | 5.5 | 3.6 |
| Pain, grade 3 | 1.2 | 0.6 | 0.6 |
| Redness, any | 25.3 | 32.6 | 35.6 |
| Redness, >5 mm | 9.3 | 10.4 | 8.6 |
| Redness, >20 mm | 0.6 | 1.5 | 1.3 |
| Swelling, any | 15.1 | 16.6 | 22.3 |
| Swelling, >5 mm | 6.8 | 6.2 | 6.4 |
| Swelling, >20 mm | 1.0 | 1.3 | 1.3 |
| **Systemic** | **N = 482** | **N = 469** | **N = 467** |
| Restlessness, any | 28.8 | 30.3 | 28.5 |
| Restlessness, grade 2 or 3 | 7.1 | 9.0 | 9.4 |
| Restlessness, grade 3 | 1.0 | 1.1 | 0.6 |
| Fever‡, ≥100.4°F | 26.6 | 31.3 | 25.9 |
| Fever‡, >101.3°F | 2.9 | 6.2 | 4.7 |
| Fever‡, >103.1°F | 0.0 | 0.2 | 0.6 |
| Fussiness, any | 61.8 | 63.8 | 57.0 |
| Fussiness, grade 2 or 3 | 14.9 | 21.5 | 17.1 |
| Fussiness, grade 3 | 2.7 | 3.4 | 1.7 |
| Loss of appetite, any | 21.6 | 19.8 | 18.8 |
| Loss of appetite, grade 2 or 3 | 3.1 | 3.2 | 2.4 |
| Loss of appetite, grade 3 | 0.2 | 0.4 | 0.0 |
| Sleeping more than usual, any | 46.7 | 31.8 | 28.1 |
| Sleeping more than usual, grade 2 or 3 | 10.2 | 6.0 | 4.7 |
| Sleeping more than usual, grade 3 | 1.7 | 0.4 | 0.6 |

N = number of infants in the intent-to-treat (ITT) cohort (infants who received the indicated vaccine and for whom at least one symptom sheet was completed).
Grade 2 defined as sufficiently discomforting to interfere with daily activities.
Grade 3 defined as preventing normal daily activities.
* Within 4 days of vaccination defined as day of vaccination and the next 3 days.
† Local reactions at the injection site for PEDIARIX.
‡ Rectal temperatures.

In another US study, these were the rates for fever within 4 days following dose 1 (i.e., day of vaccination and the next 3 days) at 2 months of age in infants who received PEDIARIX when administered concomitantly at separate sites with Hib and pneumococcal conjugate vaccines and those who received INFANRIX, ENGERIX-B® [Hepatitis B Vaccine (Recombinant)], IPV, Hib vaccine, and pneumococcal conjugate vaccine:

**Percentage of US Infants With Fever Within 4 Days of Dose 1* (ITT Cohort)**

| | PEDIARIX, Hib, & Pneumococcal Conjugate (N = 667) | INFANRIX, ENGERIX-B, IPV, Hib, & Pneumococcal Conjugate (N = 333) | Separate Vaccine Group Minus Combination Vaccine Group |
|---|---|---|---|
| **Fever†** | **%** | **%** | **Difference (95% CI)** |
| ≥100.4°F‡ | 27.9 | 19.8 | -8.07 (-13.54, -2.60) |
| >101.3°F | 7.0 | 4.5 | -2.54 (-5.50, 0.41) |
| >102.2°F‡ | 2.2 | 0.3 | -1.95 (-3.22, -0.68) |
| >103.1°F | 0.4 | 0.0 | -0.45 (-0.96, 0.06) |
| M.A.‡ | 1.2 | 0.0 | -1.20 (-2.03, -037) |

N = number of infants for whom at least one symptom sheet was completed, excluding 3 infants for whom temperature was not measured and 3 infants whose temperature was measured by the tympanic method.
*Within 4 days of dose 1 defined as day of vaccination and the next 3 days.
† Rectal temperatures.
‡ The group that received PEDIARIX compared to separate vaccine group p value <0.05 (2-sided Fisher Exact test) or the 95% confidence interval on the difference between groups does not include 0.
M.A. = Medically attended (a visit to or from medical personnel).

In this study, medical attention (a visit to or from medical personnel) for fever within 4 days following vaccination was sought for 8 infants who received PEDIARIX (1.2%) and no infants who received separately administered vaccines. Four infants were seen by medical personnel in an office setting; no diagnostic tests were performed in 2 of the infants and a complete blood count (CBC) was done in the other 2 infants. Of 3 infants who were seen in an emergency room, all had a CBC and a blood and urine culture performed; chest X-rays were done in 2 of the infants and a nasopharyngeal specimen was tested for Respiratory Syncytial Virus in one of the infants. One infant was hospitalized for a work-up that included a CBC, blood and urine cultures, a lumbar puncture, and a chest X-ray. All episodes of medically attended fever resolved within 4 days post-vaccination.

Limited data are available from a study conducted in Moldova in which infants received a dose of hepatitis B vaccine within 48 hours of birth followed by 3 doses of PEDIARIX at 6, 10, and 14 weeks of age. No information was collected on the HBsAg status of mothers of enrolled infants. These were the rates for local reactions and selected adverse events within 4 days of vaccination with PEDIARIX administered comcomitantly with Hib vaccine following a birth dose of hepatitis B vaccine:

**Percentage of Moldovan Infants With Solicited Local Reactions or Selected Systemic Adverse Events Within 4 Days of Vaccination* (ITT Cohort)**

| | PEDIARIX & Hib | | |
|---|---|---|---|
| | **Dose 1** | **Dose 2** | **Dose 3** |
| **N** | **160** | **158** | **157** |
| **Local†** | | | |
| Pain, any | 25.6 | 18.4 | 14.0 |
| Pain, grade 3 | 3.1 | 0.6 | 1.9 |
| Redness, any | 41.9 | 41.8 | 47.1 |
| Redness, >20 mm | 1.9 | 2.5 | 4.5 |
| Swelling, any | 20.6 | 18.4 | 28.0 |
| Swelling, >20 mm | 4.4 | 2.5 | 7.0 |
| **Systemic** | | | |
| Restlessness, any | 13.1 | 10.8 | 8.9 |
| Restlessness, grade 3 | 1.3 | 0.6 | 0.6 |
| Fever‡, ≥100.4°F | 14.4 | 11.4 | 5.1 |
| Fever‡, >103.1°F | 0.0 | 0.6 | 0.0 |
| Fussiness, any | 25.0 | 21.5 | 17.8 |
| Fussiness, grade 3 | 2.5 | 0.6 | 0.6 |

N = number of infants in the intent-to-treat (ITT) cohort (infants who received the indicated vaccine and for whom at least one symptom sheet was completed).
Grade 3 defined as preventing normal daily activities.
*Within 4 days of vaccination defined as day of vaccination and the next 3 days.
† Local reactions at the injection site for PEDIARIX.
‡ Rectal temperatures.

Although there was no comparator group who received PEDIARIX without a birth dose of hepatitis B vaccine, available data suggest that some local adverse events may occur at a higher rate when PEDIARIX is administered after a birth dose of hepatitis B vaccine.

As with any vaccine, there is the possibility that broad use of PEDIARIX could reveal adverse events not observed in clinical trials.

**Postmarketing Reports:** Worldwide voluntary reports of adverse events received for INFANRIX and ENGERIX-B in children younger than 7 years of age since market introduction of these US-licensed vaccines are listed below. This list includes adverse events for which 20 or more reports were received with the exception of intussusception, idiopathic thrombocytopenic purpura, thrombocytopenia, anaphylactic reaction, angioedema, encephalopathy, hypotonic-hyporesponsive episode, and alopecia for which fewer than 20 reports were received. These latter events are included either because of the seriousness of the event or the strength of causal connection to components of this or other vaccines or drugs. *Body as a whole:* Asthenia[b], fever[a+b], lethargy[b], malaise[b], Sudden Infant Death Syndrome[a+b]. *Cardiovascular system:* Cyanosis[a+b], edema[b], pallor[b]. *Gastrointestinal system:* Abdominal pain[b], anorexia[b], diarrhea[a+b], intussusception[a+b], nausea[b], vomiting[a+b]. *Hematologic/lymphatic:* Idiopathic thrombocytopenic purpura[a+b], lymphadenopathy[a], thrombocytopenia[a+b]. *Hepatic:* Jaundice[b], liver function tests abnormal[b]. *Hypersensitivity:* Anaphylactic reaction[a+b], angioedema[b], hypersensitivity[a]. *Infections:* Cellulitis[a]. *Injection site reactions:* Injection site reactions[a+b]. *Musculoskeletal:* Arthralgia[b], limb swelling[a+b]. *Nervous system:* Convulsions[a+b], encephalopathy[a], headache[b], hypotonia[a+b], hypotonic-hyporesponsive episode[a], somnolence[a+b]. *Psychiatric:* Crying[a+b], irritability[a+b]. *Respiratory system:* Respiratory tract infection[a]. *Skin and appendages:* Alopecia[b], erythema[a+b], erythema multiforme[b], petechiae[b], pruritus[a+b], rash[a+b], urticaria[a+b]. *Special senses:* Ear pain[a]. [[a] Following INFANRIX; [b] Following ENGERIX-B; [a+b] Following either INFANRIX or ENGERIX-B.] These reactions were reported voluntarily from a population of uncertain size; therefore, it is not always possible to reliably estimate their frequency or establish a causal relationship to vaccination.

**Reporting Adverse Events:** Report the occurrence following immunization of any event set forth in the Vaccine Injury Table from the National Childhood Vaccine Injury Act including: Anaphylaxis or anaphylactic shock within 7 days, encephalopathy or encephalitis within 7 days, brachial neuritis within 28 days, or an acute complication or sequelae (including death) of an illness, disability, injury, or condition referred to above, or any events that would contraindicate further doses of PEDIARIX. The VAERS toll-free number is 1-800-822-7967.

Manufactured by **GlaxoSmithKline Biologicals**, Rixensart, Belgium, US License 1617

Distributed by **GlaxoSmithKline,** Research Triangle Park, NC 27709



Full prescribing information for PEDIARIX is available at www.GSKVaccines.com/Pediarix. BRS-PE:L2

 Printed in USA. PED583R0 June 2005

**Nearly 1 in 6 children did not receive all recommended DTaP doses*[1]**

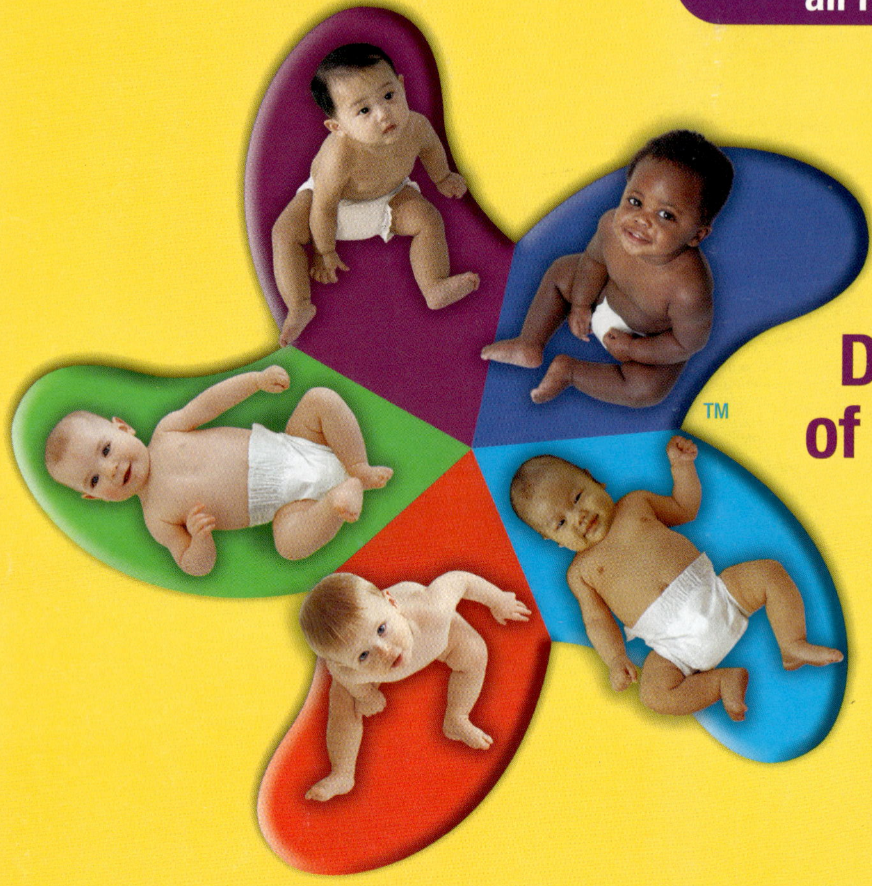


# Don't run the risk of letting one child get away

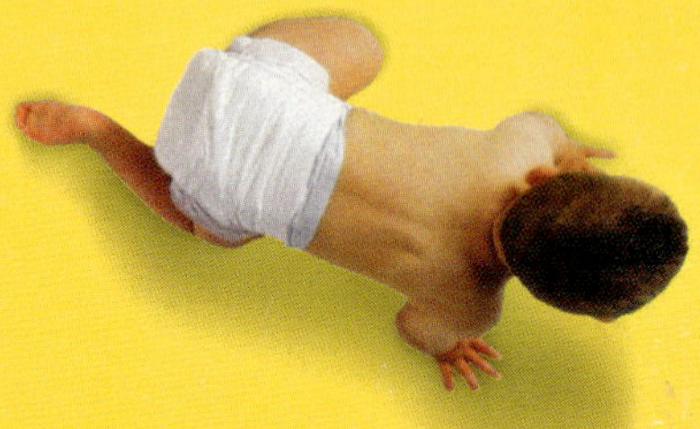

## PEDIARIX may help ensure timely vaccination with fewer injections

- With just 1 dose at 2, 4, and 6 months of age (in infants born of HBsAg-negative mothers)

*Based on analysis of the first four DTaP doses in the most recent National Immunization Survey (2003) of 21,210 children 19–35 months of age.

In clinical studies, adverse events in infants receiving PEDIARIX included injection-site reactions (pain, redness, or swelling), fever, and fussiness. Administration of PEDIARIX was associated with higher rates of fever relative to separately administered vaccines (see Adverse Reactions section of the brief summary). PEDIARIX is contraindicated in infants with known hypersensitivity to any component of the vaccine including yeast, neomycin, and polymyxin B. As with any vaccine, vaccination with PEDIARIX may not protect 100% of susceptible individuals.

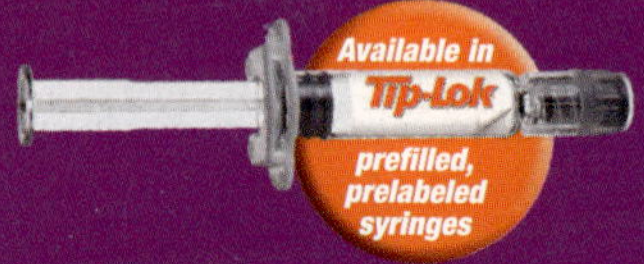


**Please see brief summary for PEDIARIX on the following page.**

**References: 1.** Centers for Disease Control and Prevention. National, state, and urban area vaccination coverage among children aged 19–35 months—United States, 2003. *MMWR.* 2004;53(29):658–661.



Pediarix®

**Diphtheria and Tetanus Toxoids and Acellular Pertussis Adsorbed, Hepatitis B (Recombinant) and Inactivated Poliovirus Vaccine Combined**

gsk GlaxoSmithKline Vaccines

# ARCHIVES OF PEDIATRICS & ADOLESCENT MEDICINE

WWW.ARCHPEDIATRICS.COM

MAY 2006


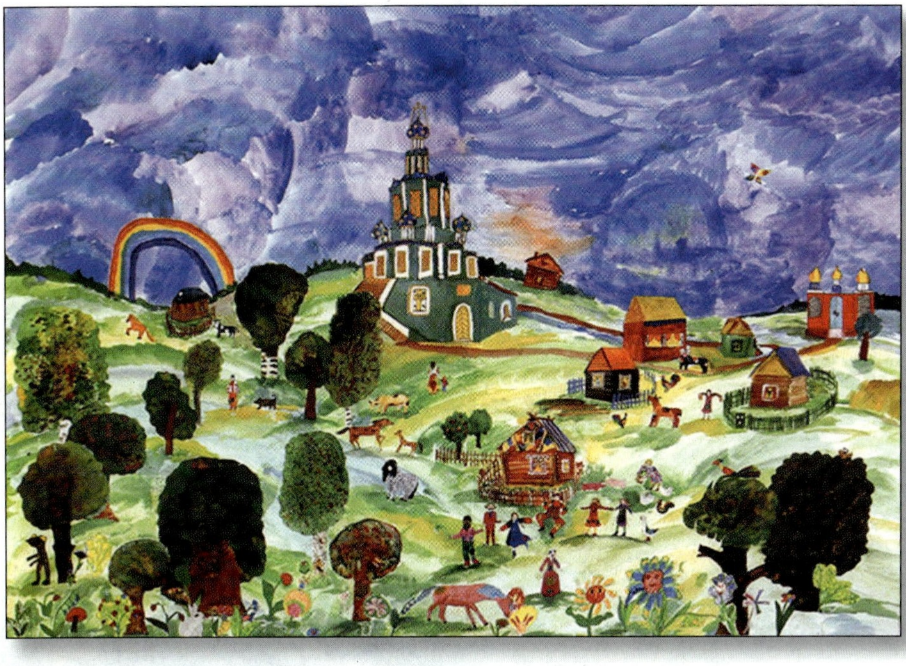

*Land of Russia.* A collaborative mural by the orphans of Maria's Children, Moscow, Russia, 1996.
See page 464.

COMMERCIAL VALUE OF UNDERAGE DRINKING AND ADULT ABUSIVE AND DEPENDENT DRINKING TO THE ALCOHOL INDUSTRY

EMERGENCY DEPARTMENT–BASED RANDOMIZED CLINICAL TRIAL TO IMPROVE ASTHMA OUTCOMES

PREVALENCE OF DIABETES AND IMPAIRED FASTING GLUCOSE AMONG US ADOLESCENTS

RELATIONSHIP BETWEEN EARLY INTRODUCTION OF SOLID FOODS AND THE DEVELOPMENT OF ALLERGIC DISEASE

COMPLETE TABLE OF CONTENTS ON PAGE 459




JAMA & ARCHIVES JOURNALS
American Medical Association

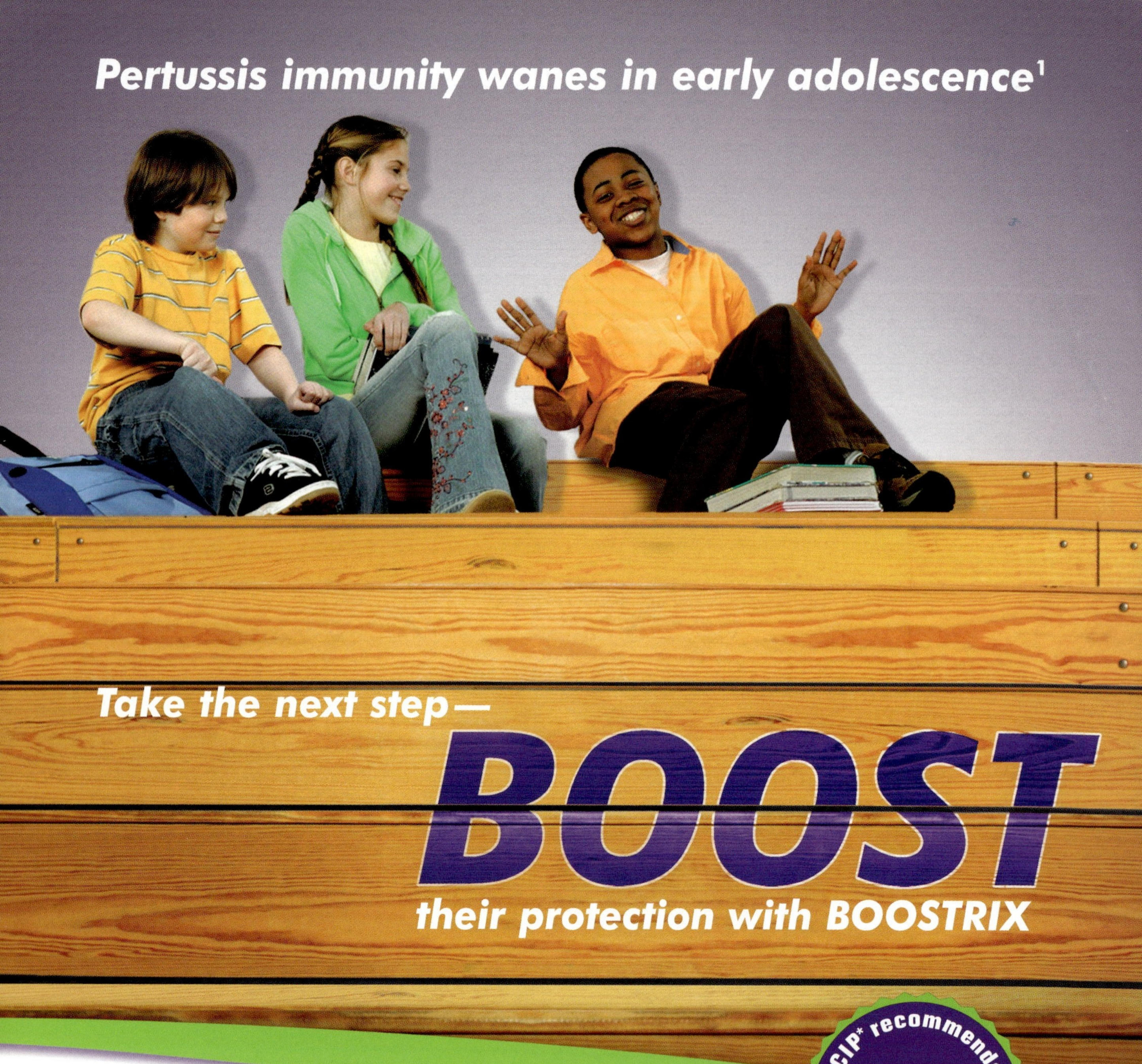


## Important Safety Information

In clinical studies, adverse events included pain, redness, and swelling at the injection site, headache, fatigue, and gastrointestinal symptoms. As with other vaccines, rare adverse events may occur. As with any vaccine, vaccination with BOOSTRIX may not protect 100% of susceptible individuals. Hypersensitivity to any component of BOOSTRIX is a contraindication.

*Advisory Committee on Immunization Practices.

BOOSTRIX®

gsk GlaxoSmithKline Vaccines

*Tetanus Toxoid, Reduced Diphtheria Toxoid and Acellular Pertussis Vaccine, Adsorbed*

**Please see references and brief summary of complete prescribing information on the adjacent page.**

# BOOSTRIX®

## (Tetanus Toxoid, Reduced Diphtheria Toxoid and Acellular Pertussis Vaccine, Adsorbed) (Tdap)

The following is a brief summary only; see full prescribing information for complete product information.

**INDICATIONS AND USAGE:** BOOSTRIX is indicated for active booster immunization against tetanus, diphtheria, and pertussis as a single dose in individuals 10 through 18 years of age. The use of BOOSTRIX as a primary series or to complete the primary series has not been studied. As with any vaccine, BOOSTRIX may not protect 100% of individuals receiving the vaccine.

**CONTRAINDICATIONS:** Hypersensitivity to any component of the vaccine is a contraindication (see DESCRIPTION in full prescribing information). Do not use BOOSTRIX after a serious allergic reaction (e.g., anaphylaxis) following any other tetanus toxoid, diphtheria toxoid or pertussis-containing vaccine, or any component of this vaccine (see DESCRIPTION in full prescribing information). Because of the uncertainty as to which component of the vaccine might be responsible, do not give further vaccination with any of these components; or, refer such individuals to an allergist for evaluation. The following events are contraindications to administration of BOOSTRIX: encephalopathy (e.g., coma, decreased level of consciousness, prolonged seizures) within 7 days of administration of a previous dose of a pertussis-containing vaccine that is not attributable to another identifiable cause; progressive neurologic disorder, uncontrolled epilepsy, or progressive encephalopathy. Do not vaccinate individuals with these conditions until a treatment regimen has been established and the condition has stabilized.

**WARNINGS:** The tip cap and the rubber plunger of the needleless prefilled syringes contain dry natural latex rubber that may cause allergic reactions in latex sensitive individuals. The vial stopper is latex-free. If any of the following events occurred in temporal relation to previous receipt of a Diphtheria and Tetanus Toxoids and Pertussis Vaccine Adsorbed (DTwP) vaccine or a vaccine containing an acellular pertussis component, consider carefully whether to give subsequent doses of BOOSTRIX: temperature of ≥40.5°C (105°F) within 48 hours not due to another identifiable cause; collapse or shock-like state (hypotonic-hyporesponsive episode) within 48 hours; persistent, inconsolable crying lasting ≥3 hours, occurring within 48 hours; seizures with or without fever occurring within 3 days. Persons who experienced serious Arthus-type hypersensitivity reactions following a prior dose of tetanus toxoid usually have high serum tetanus antitoxin levels and should not be given Tetanus and Diphtheria Toxoids Adsorbed For Adult Use (Td) or Tdap vaccines or even emergency doses of Td more frequently than every 10 years, even if the wound is neither clean nor minor. If Guillain-Barré syndrome has occurred within 6 weeks of receipt of prior vaccine containing tetanus toxoid, the decision to give BOOSTRIX or any vaccine containing tetanus toxoid should be based on careful consideration of the potential benefits and possible risks. The decision to administer a pertussis-containing vaccine to individuals with stable central nervous system (CNS) disorders must be made by the physician on an individual basis, with consideration of all relevant factors, and assessment of potential risks and benefits for that individual. Advise the patient, parent, or guardian of the potential increased risk involved (see PRECAUTIONS). A family history of seizures or other CNS disorders is not a contraindication to pertussis vaccine. The Advisory Committee on Immunization Practices (ACIP) has published guidelines for vaccination of persons with recent or acute illness (www.cdc.gov). Do not give BOOSTRIX to individuals with bleeding disorders such as hemophilia or thrombocytopenia, or to persons on anticoagulant therapy unless the potential benefit clearly outweighs the risk of administration. If the decision is made to administer BOOSTRIX to such persons, it should be given with caution with steps taken to avoid the risk of hematoma following the injection.

**PRECAUTIONS: General:** Before the injection of any biological, the physician should take all reasonable precautions to prevent allergic or other adverse reactions. Epinephrine injection (1:1,000) and other appropriate agents used for the control of immediate allergic reactions must be immediately available should an acute anaphylactic reaction occur. Immunosuppressed persons, including individuals receiving immunosuppressive therapy, may not develop the expected immune response. **Drug Interactions:** Do not mix BOOSTRIX with any other vaccine in the same syringe or vial. **Carcinogenesis, Mutagenesis, Impairment of Fertility:** BOOSTRIX has not been evaluated for carcinogenic or mutagenic potential, or for impairment of fertility. **Pregnancy:** Pregnancy Category C. Animal reproduction studies have not been conducted with BOOSTRIX. It is also not known whether BOOSTRIX can cause fetal harm when administered to a pregnant woman or can affect reproductive capacity. BOOSTRIX should be given to a pregnant woman only if clearly needed. Animal fertility studies have not been conducted with BOOSTRIX. In a developmental toxicity study, the effect of BOOSTRIX on embryo-fetal and pre-weaning development was evaluated in pregnant rats. Animals were administered INFANRIX® (Diphtheria and Tetanus Toxoids and Acellular Pertussis Vaccine Adsorbed) prior to gestation and BOOSTRIX during the period of organogenesis (gestation days 6, 8, 11) and later in pregnancy (gestation day 15), 0.1 mL/rat/occasion (a 45-fold increase compared to the human dose of BOOSTRIX on a body weight basis), by intramuscular injection. No adverse affect on pregnancy and lactation parameters, embryo-fetal or pre-weaning development was observed. There were no fetal malformations or other evidence of teratogenesis noted in this study. **Nursing Mothers:** It is not known whether BOOSTRIX is excreted in human milk. Because many drugs are excreted in human milk, caution should be exercised when BOOSTRIX is administered to a nursing woman. **Pregnancy Exposure Registry:** Healthcare providers are encouraged to register pregnant women who receive BOOSTRIX in the GlaxoSmithKline vaccination pregnancy registry by calling 1-888-825-5249. **Geriatric Use:** BOOSTRIX is not indicated for use in individuals older than 18 years. **Pediatric Use:** BOOSTRIX is not indicated for use in individuals younger than 10 years (see DOSAGE AND ADMINISTRATION in full prescribing information). For immunization of infants and children younger than 7 years against diphtheria, tetanus, and pertussis, refer to the manufacturers' package inserts for Diphtheria and Tetanus Toxoids and Acellular Pertussis Vaccine Adsorbed (DTaP) vaccines.

**ADVERSE REACTIONS:** A total of 3,608 adolescents were vaccinated with a single dose of BOOSTRIX during clinical trials. An additional 1,092 adolescents 10 to 18 years of age received a non-US formulation of BOOSTRIX (formulated to contain 0.5 mg aluminum per dose) in non-US clinical studies.

The primary safety study, conducted in the United States, was a randomized, observer-blinded, controlled study in which 3,080 adolescents 10 to 18 years of age received a single dose of BOOSTRIX and 1,034 received the control Td vaccine manufactured by Massachusetts Public Health Biologic Laboratories. There were no substantive differences in demographic characteristics between the vaccine groups. Among BOOSTRIX and control vaccine recipients approximately 75% were 10 to 14 years of age and approximately 25% were 15 to 18 years of age. Approximately 98% of participants in this study had received the recommended series of 4 or 5 doses of either DTwP or a combination of DTwP and DTaP in childhood. Data on adverse events were collected by the subjects, parents and/or guardians using standardized diaries for 15 consecutive days following the vaccine dose (i.e., day of vaccination and the next 14 days). Subjects were monitored for unsolicited adverse events that occurred within 31 days of vaccination (day 0-30) using diary cards (day 0-14) supplemented by spontaneous reports and a medical history as reported by subjects, parents, and/or guardians. Subjects were also monitored for 6 months post-vaccination for non-routine medical visits, visits to an emergency room, onset of new chronic illness, and serious adverse events. Information regarding late onset adverse events was obtained via a telephone call 6 months following vaccination. At least 97% of subjects completed the 6-month follow-up evaluation.

In a study conducted in Germany, BOOSTRIX was administered to 319 children 10 to 12 years of age previously vaccinated with 5 doses of acellular pertussis-containing vaccines, 193 of these subjects had previously received 5 doses of INFANRIX. Adverse events were recorded on diary cards during the 15 days following vaccination. Unsolicited adverse events that occurred within 31 days of vaccination (day 0-30) were recorded on the diary card or verbally reported to the investigator. Subjects were monitored for 6 months post-vaccination for physician office visits, emergency room visits, onset of new chronic illness, and serious adverse events. The 6-month follow-up evaluation, conducted via telephone interview, was completed by 90% of subjects.

The adverse event information from clinical trials provides a basis for identifying adverse events that appear to be related to vaccine use and for approximating rates. However, because clinical trials are conducted under widely varying conditions, adverse event rates observed in the clinical trials of a vaccine cannot be directly compared to rates in the clinical trials of another vaccine, and may not reflect the rates observed in practice.

**Serious Adverse Events in All Safety Studies:** In the US-safety study and German-safety study, no serious adverse events were reported to occur within 31 days of vaccination. During the 6-month extended safety evaluation period, no serious adverse events that were of potential autoimmune origin or new onset and chronic in nature were reported to occur. In non-US studies in which serious adverse events were monitored for up to 37 days, one subject was diagnosed with insulin dependent diabetes 20 days following administration of BOOSTRIX. No other serious adverse events of potential autoimmune origin or that were new onset and chronic in nature were reported to occur in these studies.

**Solicited Adverse Events in the US-Safety Study:** In a US study, the most common local adverse events following administration of BOOSTRIX were pain, redness, and swelling at the injection site. The most common general adverse events were headache and fatigue. Most of these events were reported at a similar frequency in recipients of both BOOSTRIX and Td. Any pain, grade 2 or 3 pain (but not grade 3 alone), and grade 2 or 3 headache (but not grade 3 alone) were reported at a higher rate in recipients of BOOSTRIX. The primary safety endpoint of the US study was the incidence of grade 3 pain (spontaneously painful and/or prevented normal activity) at the injection site within 15 days of vaccination. Grade 3 pain was reported in 4.6% of those who received BOOSTRIX compared with 4.0% of those who received the Td vaccine. The difference in rate of grade 3 pain was within the pre-defined clinical limit for non-inferiority (upper limit of the 95% CI for the difference ≤4%). These were the rates for solicited local and general adverse events within 15 days of vaccination with BOOSTRIX or Td vaccine for the total vaccinated cohort (all enrolled, vaccinated subjects with safety data available analyzed by vaccine received):

**Percentage of Individuals 10 to 18 Years of Age Reporting Solicited Local Adverse Events or Solicited General Adverse Events Within the 15-day* Post-Vaccination Period**

| | BOOSTRIX (N = 3,032) % | Td (N =1,013) % |
|---|---|---|
| **Local** | | |
| Pain,† any | 75.3 | 71.7 |
| Pain,† grade 2 or 3 | 51.2 | 42.5 |
| Pain,‡ grade 3 | 4.6 | 4.0 |
| Redness, any | 22.5 | 19.8 |
| Redness, >20 mm | 4.1 | 3.9 |
| Redness, ≥50 mm | 1.7 | 1.6 |
| Swelling, any | 21.1 | 20.1 |
| Swelling, >20 mm | 5.3 | 4.9 |
| Swelling, ≥50 mm | 2.5 | 3.2 |
| Arm circumference increase,§ >5 mm | 28.3 | 29.5 |
| Arm circumference increase,§ >20 mm | 2.0 | 2.2 |
| Arm circumference increase,§ >40 mm | 0.5 | 0.3 |
| **General** | | |
| Fever,‖ ≥99.5°F | 13.5 | 13.1 |
| Fever,‖ >100.4°F | 5.0 | 4.7 |
| Fever,‖ >102.2°F | 1.4 | 1.0 |
| Headache, any | 43.1 | 41.5 |
| Headache,† grade 2 or 3 | 15.7 | 12.7 |
| Headache, grade 3 | 3.7 | 2.7 |
| Fatigue, any | 37.0 | 36.7 |
| Fatigue, grade 2 or 3 | 14.4 | 12.9 |
| Fatigue, grade 3 | 3.7 | 3.2 |
| Gastrointestinal symptoms,¶ any | 26.0 | 25.8 |
| Gastrointestinal symptoms,¶ grade 2 or 3 | 9.8 | 9.7 |
| Gastrointestinal symptoms,¶ grade 3 | 3.0 | 3.2 |

Td = Tetanus and Diphtheria Toxoids Adsorbed For Adult Use manufactured by Massachusetts Public Health Biologic Laboratories.
N = number of subjects in the total vaccinated cohort with local/general symptoms sheets completed.
Grade 2 = Local: painful when the limb was moved; General: interfered with normal activity.
Grade 3 = Local: spontaneously painful and/or prevented normal activity; General: prevented normal activity.
*Day of vaccination and the next 14 days.
†Statistically significantly higher (P<0.05) following BOOSTRIX as compared to Td vaccine.
‡Grade 3 injection site pain following BOOSTRIX was not inferior to Td (upper limit of two-sided 95% CI for the difference in the percentage of subjects ≤4%).
§Mid-upper region of the vaccinated arm.
‖Oral temperatures or axillary temperatures.
¶Gastrointestinal symptoms included nausea, vomiting, diarrhea and/or abdominal pain.

Mid-upper arm circumference was measured by the adolescent or their parent/guardian prior to injection and daily for 15 days following vaccination. There was no significant difference between BOOSTRIX recipients and Td recipients in the proportion of subjects reporting an increase in mid-upper arm circumference in the vaccinated arm. The incidence of unsolicited adverse events reported in the 31 days after vaccination was comparable between the 2 groups.

**Solicited Adverse Events in the German Safety Study:** No cases of whole arm swelling were spontaneously reported. Two individuals (2/193) reported large injection site swelling (range 110 to 200 mm diameter), in one case associated with grade 3 pain. Neither individual sought medical attention. These episodes were reported to resolve without sequelae within 5 days. These were the rates of solicited local adverse events and fever within 15 days of vaccination for those subjects who had previously been vaccinated with 5 doses of INFANRIX:

**Rates of Solicited Adverse Events Reported Within the 15-day* Post-Vaccination Period Following Administration of BOOSTRIX in Individuals 10 to 12 Years of Age Who Had Previously Received 5 Doses of INFANRIX**

| Adverse Event | BOOSTRIX (N = 193) % (95% CI) |
|---|---|
| Pain, any | 62.2 (54.9-69.0) |
| Pain, grade 2 or 3 | 33.2 (26.6-40.3) |
| Pain, grade 3 | 5.7 (2.9-10.0) |
| Redness, any | 47.7 (40.4-55.0) |
| Redness, >20 mm | 15.0 (10.3-20.9) |
| Redness, ≥50 mm | 10.9 (6.9-16.2) |
| Swelling, any | 38.9 (31.9-46.1) |
| Swelling, >20 mm | 17.6 (12.5-23.7) |
| Swelling, ≥50 mm | 14.0 (9.4-19.7) |
| Fever, ≥99.5 | 8.8 (5.2-13.7) |
| Fever, >100.4 | 4.1 (1.8-8.0) |
| Fever, >102.2 | 1.0 (0.1-3.7) |

N = number of subjects with local/general symptoms sheets completed.
Grade 2 = Painful when the limb was moved.
Grade 3 = Spontaneously painful and/or prevented normal activity.
*Day of vaccination and the next 14 days.

As with any vaccine, there is the possibility that broad use of BOOSTRIX could reveal adverse events not observed in clinical trials.

**Postmarketing Reports:** Worldwide voluntary reports of adverse events received for BOOSTRIX in persons 10 to 18 years of age since market introduction of this vaccine are listed below. This list includes serious events or events which have causal connection to components of this or other vaccines or drugs. Because these events are reported voluntarily from a population of uncertain size, it is not possible to reliably estimate their frequency or establish a causal relationship to vaccine exposure. *Blood and lymphatic system disorders:* Lymphadenitis, lymphadenopathy. *Cardiac disorders:* Myocarditis. *Injection site reactions:* Induration, inflammation, mass, nodule, warmth, local reaction. *Metabolism and nutrition disorders:* Diabetes mellitus insulin-dependent. *Musculoskeletal and connective tissue disorders:* Arthralgia, back pain, myalgia. *Nervous system disorders:* Convulsion, encephalitis, facial palsy, paraesthesia. *Skin and subcutaneous tissue disorders:* Exanthem, Henoch-Schönlein purpura, rash. In addition, extensive swelling of the injected limb has been reported following administration of BOOSTRIX.

**Reporting Adverse Events:** Report the occurrence following immunization of any event set forth in the Vaccine Injury Table from the National Childhood Vaccine Injury Act including: Anaphylaxis or anaphylactic shock within 7 days, encephalopathy or encephalitis within 7 days, brachial neuritis within 28 days, or an acute complication or sequelae (including death) of an illness, disability, injury, or condition referred to above, or any events that would contraindicate further doses of vaccine, according to this prescribing information. These events should be reported to VAERS. The VAERS toll-free number is 1-800-822-7967. Reporting forms may also be obtained at the VAERS website at www.vaers.hhs.gov.

**DOSAGE AND ADMINISTRATION: Recommended Dose:** BOOSTRIX should be administered as a single 0.5 mL injection by the intramuscular route into the deltoid muscle of the upper arm in individuals 10 through 18 years of age. Do not administer this product subcutaneously or intravenously. There are no data to support repeat administration of BOOSTRIX. Five years should elapse between the subject's last dose of the recommended series of childhood DTwP and/or DTaP vaccine and the administration of BOOSTRIX. Limited data are available on the use of BOOSTRIX following Tetanus and Diphtheria Toxoids Adsorbed For Adult Use (Td) vaccine. **Additional Dosing Information: *Wound Management:*** Clinicians should refer to guidelines for tetanus prophylaxis in routine wound management. Adolescents 10 to 18 years of age who have completed a primary series against tetanus and who sustain wounds which are minor and uncomplicated, should receive a booster dose of a tetanus toxoid-containing vaccine only if they have not received tetanus toxoid within the preceding 10 years. In case of tetanus-prone injury (e.g., wounds contaminated with dirt, feces, soil, and saliva; puncture wounds; avulsions; and wounds resulting from missles, crushing, burns, and frostbite) in an adolescent who is in need of tetanus toxoid, BOOSTRIX can be used as an alternative to Tetanus and Diphtheria Toxoids Adsorbed For Adult Use (Td) vaccine in patients for whom the pertussis component is also indicated (see INDICATIONS AND USAGE).

Manufactured by **GlaxoSmithKline Biologicals**
Rixensart, Belgium, US License 1617
Distributed by **GlaxoSmithKline**
Research Triangle Park, NC 27709



Full prescribing information for BOOSTRIX is available at www.BOOSTRIX.com.
BRS-BO:L3

**References: 1.** Centers for Disease Control and Prevention. Preventing tetanus, diphtheria, and pertussis among adolescents: use of tetanus toxoid, reduced diphtheria toxoid and acellular pertussis vaccines: recommendations of the Advisory Committee on Immunization Practices (ACIP). Early Release 2006;55(February 23, 2006):1–43. **2.** Centers for Disease Control and Prevention. Recommended childhood and adolescent immunization schedule—United States, 2006. *MMWR.* 2006;54(51&52):Q1–Q4.

# ARCHIVES OF PEDIATRICS & ADOLESCENT MEDICINE

MAY 2006 VOLUME 160, NUMBER 5 PAGES 457-560


## COVER ART


**Maria's Children** 464
*Jan Adams, MD*


## ON MY MIND


**986 Grams** 465
*Jorge E. Gomez, MD*


## COMMENTARIES


**Returning to the Basics: A New Era in Pediatric Education** 466
*Aaron Friedman, MD; Edward Schor, MD; Bonita Stanton, MD; Bruder Stapleton, MD; Barry Zuckermann, MD*

**Pediatric Organ Transplantation Needs: Organ Donation Best Practices** 468
*Susan L. Bratton, MD, MPH; Nikoleta S. Kolovos, MD; Elizabeth S. Roach, RN, BSN; Virginia McBride, MPH, RN; Judy L. Geiger, RN, BSN; Rebecka L. Meyers, MD*


## ARTICLES


**Estimate of the Commercial Value of Underage Drinking and Adult Abusive and Dependent Drinking to the Alcohol Industry** 473
*Susan E. Foster, MSW; Roger D. Vaughan, DrPH; William H. Foster, PhD; Joseph A. Califano, Jr, LLB*

**Patterns and Knowledge of Nonmedical Use of Stimulants Among College Students** 481
*Bronwen C. Carroll, MD; Thomas J. McLaughlin, ScD; Diane R. Blake, MD*

**Pediatricians' Clinical Decision Making: Results of 2 Randomized Controlled Trials of Test Performance Characteristics** 487
*Colin M. Sox, MD, MS; Thomas D. Koepsell, MD, MPH; Jason N. Doctor, PhD; Dimitri A. Christakis, MD, MPH*

**Error Reduction in Pediatric Chemotherapy: Computerized Order Entry and Failure Modes and Effects Analysis** 495
*George R. Kim, MD; Allen R. Chen, MD, PhD; Robert J. Arceci, MD, PhD; Sandra H. Mitchell, RPh, MSIS; K. Michelle Kokoszka, RN; Denise Daniel, RN; Christoph U. Lehmann, MD*


## SPECIAL FEATURE


**Picture of the Month** 499
*Kathryn S. Moffett, MD; Jon E. Welch, MD*


## REVIEW ARTICLE


**Systematic Review of the Relationship Between Early Introduction of Solid Foods to Infants and the Development of Allergic Disease** 502
*Beth A. Tarini, MD; Aaron E. Carroll, MD, MS; Colin M. Sox, MD, MS; Dimitri A. Christakis, MD, MPH*


## ARTICLES


**Excessive Crying Beyond 3 Months May Herald Other Features of Multiple Regulatory Problems** 508
*Rüdiger von Kries, MD, MSc; Helen Kalies, MSc, MPH; Mechthild Papoušek, MD*

**Maternal Infant-Feeding Style and Children's Adiposity at 5 Years of Age** 513
*Hillary L. Burdette, MD, MS; Robert C. Whitaker, MD, MPH; Waynitra C. Hall, MS; Stephen R. Daniels, MD, PhD*

**Prevalence of Diabetes and Impaired Fasting Glucose Levels Among US Adolescents: National Health and Nutrition Examination Survey, 1999-2002** 523
*Glen E. Duncan, PhD, RCEPSM*

**Genetic Testing of Minors for Alpha$_1$-Antitrypsin Deficiency** 531
*Charlie Strange, MD; Mary Allison Moseley; Yonge Jones; Laura Schwarz; Lianqi Xie; Mark L. Brantly, MD*

**Improved Asthma Outcomes in a High-Morbidity Pediatric Population: Results of an Emergency Department–Based Randomized Clinical Trial** 535
*Stephen J. Teach, MD, MPH; Ellen F. Crain, MD, PhD; Deborah M. Quint, BA; Michelle L. Hylan, BA; Jill G. Joseph, MD, PhD*

**Parental Misperceptions About Children and Firearms** 542
*Frances Baxley, MD; Matthew Miller, MD, ScD*

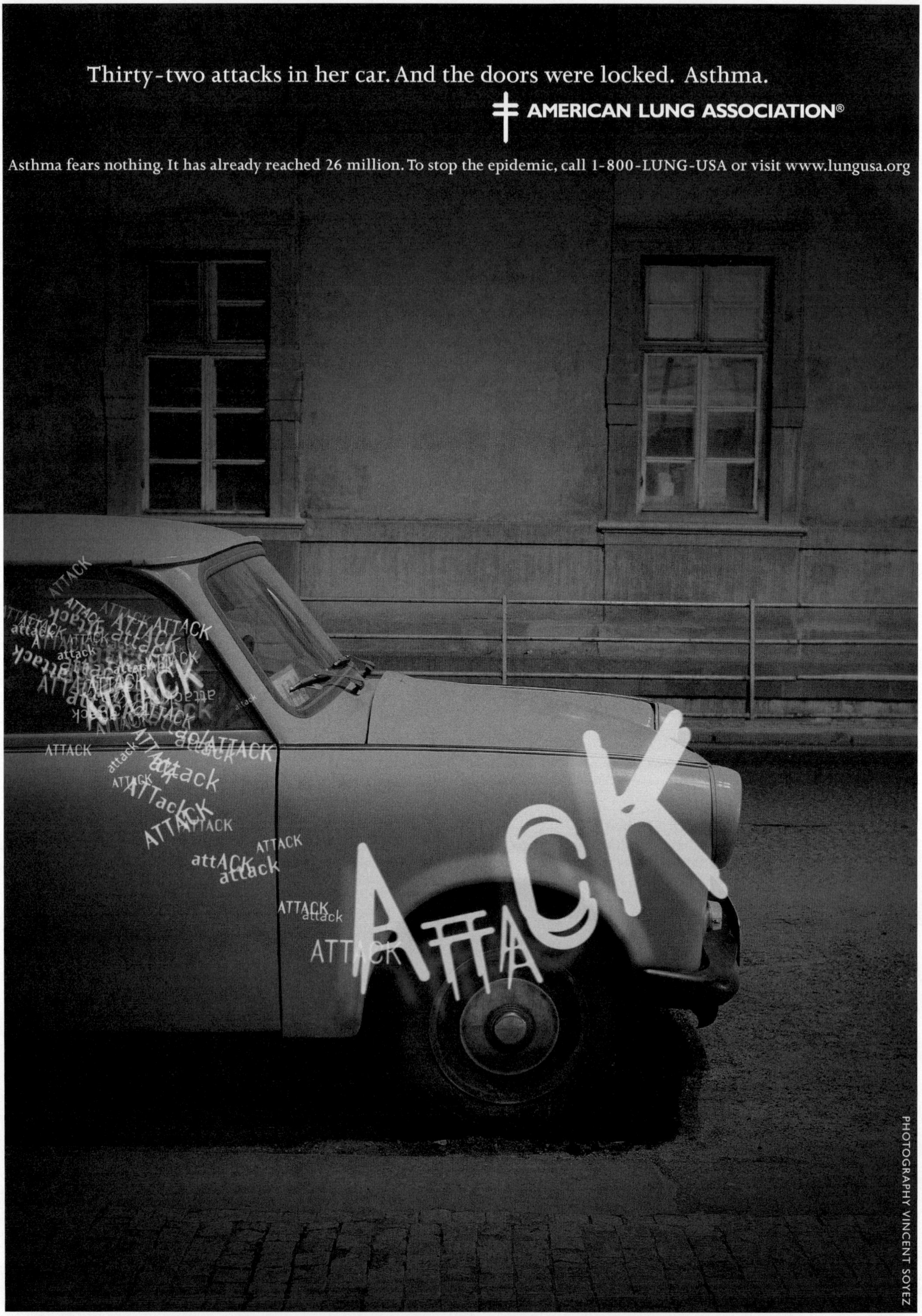
Thirty-two attacks in her car. And the doors were locked. Asthma.
AMERICAN LUNG ASSOCIATION®
Asthma fears nothing. It has already reached 26 million. To stop the epidemic, call 1-800-LUNG-USA or visit www.lungusa.org
ATTACK
PHOTOGRAPHY VINCENT SOYEZ

ARCHIVES
OF
PEDIATRICS &
ADOLESCENT MEDICINE

EDITORIALS

**Autism and Autism Spectrum Disorders** 548
*Frederick P. Rivara, MD, MPH*

**Meeting the Need for Transplantable Organs Through the US Donation System** 548
*Marc I. Lorber, MD*

**Implications for Primary Care of Diabetes and Impaired Fasting Glucose Prevalence in Adolescents** 550
*Arlan L. Rosenbloom, MD*

**Prospects for the Prevention of Allergy: A Losing Battle or a Battle Still Worth Fighting?** 552
*Robert A. Wood, MD*

BOOK REVIEWS AND OTHER MEDIA

**A Young Mind in a Growing Brain** 557
*Esther H. Wender, MD*

REGULAR DEPARTMENTS

**This Month in *Archives of Pediatrics & Adolescent Medicine*** 463

**Announcements** 467, 492, 534, 554

**Poetry in Pediatrics** 556

**Classified Advertising** 559

**Journal Advertiser Index** 559

**Contact Information** 560

**Instructions for authors and the author and subject indexes are available on our Web site: http://www.archpediatrics.com. If you do not have access to the Web, contact Suzanne Shuey at (206) 685-3573.**

***About the Cover***

*Land of Russia*, a collaborative mural by the orphans of Maria's Children, Moscow, Russia, 1996.

# ARCHIVES OF PEDIATRICS & ADOLESCENT MEDICINE


**Mission Statement:** *The Archives of Pediatrics & Adolescent Medicine* is a monthly, peer-reviewed journal for physicians and other health care professionals who contribute to the health of children and adolescents. The *Archives* provides an open forum for dialogue on a full range of clinical, scientific, advocacy, and humanistic issues relevant to the care of pediatric patients from infancy through young adulthood. The *Archives* is a vehicle for increased attention to adolescent health, the education of pediatric health care professionals, and disease prevention and health promotion. The *Archives* publishes original studies, editorials, reviews by experts, practice commentaries, case quizzes, and updates on clinical science and practice management. The Pediatric Forum provides our readers with opportunities to express their views. *Archives* incorporates *AJDC*, the oldest journal in US pediatric literature, which originated in 1911.




JAMA & ARCHIVES JOURNALS
American Medical Association

## Estimate of the Commercial Value of Underage Drinking and Adult Abusive and Dependent Drinking to the Alcohol Industry

Individuals who begin drinking before the age of 15 years are 4 times more likely to become alcohol dependent than those who do not drink before the age of 21 years. Foster et al examined underage drinking, the amount of drinking, and the cash value from this consumption to the alcohol industry. Forty-seven percent of underage youth are current drinkers and 25% met the criteria for alcohol abuse and dependence. The total cash value of underage drinking was $22.5 billion in 2001, accounting for 17.5% of total consumer expenditures for alcohol. Early initiation of alcohol use provides substantial financial value to the alcohol industry. Restricting alcohol advertising can have a substantial effect on this problem.

See page 473

## Systematic Review of the Relationship Between Early Introduction of Solid Foods to Infants and the Development of Allergic Disease

Current recommendations advise the introduction of solid foods to infants after the age of 4 to 6 months. This systematic review sought to examine the evidence that early solid feeding before the age of 4 months increases the risk of allergic disease. Of the 13 studies that met inclusion criteria, only 1 study was a controlled trial. Five studies found an association between early solid feeding and eczema, while 4 studies found no association. There was a lack of strong evidence that early solid feeding increases the risk of persistent asthma, persistent food allergy, allergic rhinitis, or dander allergy.

See page 502

## Prevalence of Diabetes and Impaired Fasting Glucose Levels Among US Adolescents: National Health and Nutrition Examination Survey, 1999-2002

Because the prevalence of being overweight among youth has dramatically increased in the United States during the last decade, a corresponding increase in the prevalence of diabetes is expected. In this national sample, 0.5% of adolescents reported having been diagnosed with diabetes, 71% of whom had type 1 diabetes and 29% had type 2. Among nondiabetic youth, 11% had impaired fasting blood glucose levels, 42% of whom were overweight or at risk for being overweight. Based on this sample, 39 000 adolescents in the United States have type 2 diabetes, and 2.8 million have impaired fasting glucose levels. These data have important implications for public health because of the high rate of conversion from impaired fasting glucose levels to type 2 diabetes.

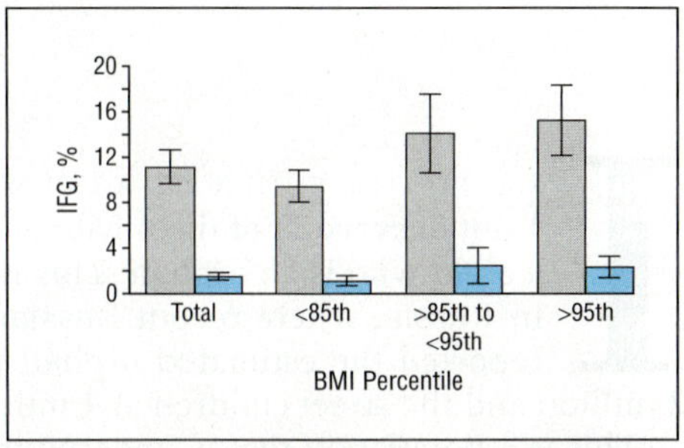


**Figure 1.** Prevalence of impaired fasting glucose (IFG) level as a function of body mass index (BMI) percentile among 1496 US adolescents. Gray-shaded bars indicate prevalence estimates using a fasting plasma glucose cut-point value of 5.6 mmol/L (100 mg/dL) to define impaired fasting glucose level, and blue-shaded bars indicate prevalence estimates using a cut-point value of 6.1 mmol/L (110 mg/dL).

See page 523

## Improved Asthma Outcomes in a High-Morbidity Pediatric Population: Results of an Emergency Department–Based Randomized Clinical Trial

Appropriate care of children with asthma continues to be problematic. This study took a different approach by randomizing emergency department patients with asthma to usual care or to a scheduled visit 2 to 15 days after emergency department discharge to a specialized asthma clinic located in the emergency department. Of those randomized to the intervention, 70% attended. In the subsequent 6-month follow-up period, the intervention patients had significantly fewer unscheduled visits, although there was no impact on the number of hospitalizations. There was significant improvement in asthma symptoms. This study may have important implications for the future role of the urban emergency department in asthma care.

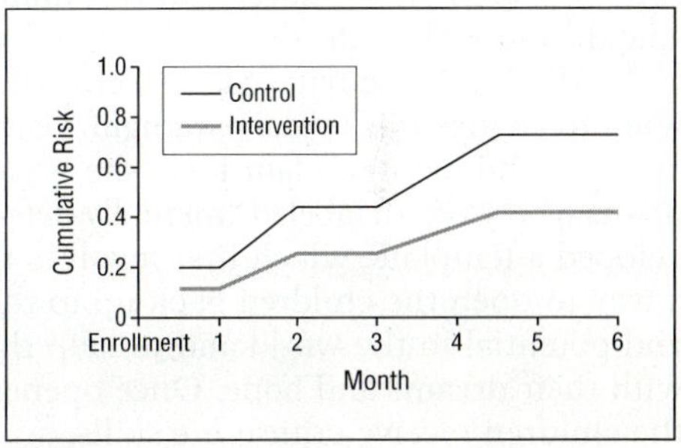


**Figure 2.** Cox proportional hazards regression of cumulative risk of having 1 or more emergency department visits during the 6-month follow-up period.

See page 535

# Maria's Children

IMAGINE THE FUTURE OF A COUNTRY IN WHICH 1 out of every 21 of the inhabitants is currently a child who is an orphan. This is the situation in Russia, where recent Russian media have reported the estimated orphan population at 2 million and the street children at 4 million.

This is a population that is undernourished, understimulated, underbonded, undereducated (both academically and in life skills), and abused in nearly every physical, sexual, and psychological way imaginable. There are exceptions of course, but the average government orphanage is a grim place indeed, understaffed with underpaid and overworked employees.

The result of this hopeless situation for these forgotten children who are anathema in their own country is a nearly 25% suicide rate and, without intervention, a life span that averages 25 years. The children, unprepared in any way for the challenging Russian life, are dumped out of the orphanages at age 16 years. They are offered few options in life—cannon fodder for the army, various criminal occupations such as drug trafficking and prostitution, or work in paint or shoe factories (which are highly toxic). They are lost to disease, drug and alcohol addiction, white slavery, and the military along with suicide and violent death.

In 1993, a Moscovite, Maria Yeliseyeva, decided to work to change this brutal paradigm. Using her skills as an artist and her abundant love, she began with 12 orphans who were all labeled "mentally defective." She developed a template, which first involves teaching art as a way to open the children back up to their own value and potential in the world and to help them reconnect with their dreams and hope. Once opened to their joy, the children receive critical life skills.

Maria's project, Maria's Children, Moscow, Russia, now involves nearly 400 orphans, refugees, street kids, and children from cerebral palsy schools. Besides creating their joyous art, the kids at her studio learn to cook and prepare a meal each day and they learn computer skills, English language skills, music, sewing, money management, and a variety of other skills. The project stays with the youth into adulthood until they are on their feet. The statistics for the lucky ones from this project are very good—no suicides or early deaths, no youth lost to prostitution, no out-of-wedlock pregnancies, and so on.

As a Minnesota family practitioner, I was clowning in Moscow with Patch Adams, MD, when I met Maria in 1995. I decided to find a way to fund Maria's efforts. The American foundation, Maria's Children International, continues to fund Maria's project and has funded 2 additional projects in Russia using the same template. Chuezhik Puezhik is the St Petersburg, Russia, project, and it involves children from 2 orphanages (one of which involves orphans who are all human immunodeficiency virus positive). Dmitrov, Russia, is the location of the most recent project, and a new studio is currently being built from funds raised by Maria's Children International.

If you visit our Web sites (http://www.mariaschildren.com and http://www.mariaschildren.org), you will be stunned by the pure joy expressed by these kids whose lives have been opened in this way.

*Jan Adams, MD*

**Correspondence**: Dr Adams, Maria's Children International, 4321 W Highway 13, Savage, MN 55378 (info@mariaschildren.com).

The more you read, the more things you will know. The more that you learn, the more places you'll go.
—Dr Seuss

# 986 Grams

THERE IS NOTHING MORE TO BE DONE.
I take this little being,
Who without will, without malice,
Has devastated a family,
Into a warm blanket and
To a room where a couple awaits
The unthinkable.

I hand the bundle to a terrified mother
Who knows she will have to wait
To hand her back.
A father sits just out of reach,
Pressing his hands into the sofa
Unsure of anything anymore except that
His tears will come soon.

I could save myself this agony.
Orders, laboratories, and adjustments
Await me.
I stay,
Until I have to tell them
There is no more waiting,
And they collapse into wretched sobs
Against a background of
Ventilators cycling and alarms sounding
For those that go on.

I go back to the tedious work,
Haunted by a vision of their
Lonely walk to the parking lot,
In the blazing light of this
Most unbearable of all days,
Suffocating in their thoughts,
And finding no comfort.

*Jorge E. Gomez, MD*

**Correspondence**: Dr Gomez, Department of Pediatrics, University of Texas Health Science Center, 7703 Floyd Curl Dr, MSC7808, San Antonio, TX 78229-3900 (gomezje@uthscsa.edu).

COMMENTARY

# Returning to the Basics

## *A New Era in Pediatric Education*

It is axiomatic that the care of children should reflect our knowledge of the dynamic interaction of genes, environment, and time on human biology. Pediatricians have long been concerned with issues in development as they relate to normal/abnormal behavioral and cognitive and somatic growth. Advances in molecular biology, imaging technologies, and the human genome project have greatly accelerated our understanding of the significance of the timing of these interactions. The Institute of Medicine's publication *Children's Health, the Nation's Wealth* proposes a new conceptualization of child health as a developmental model. It emphasizes the effect of each period of life and the interactions that occur at that period on subsequent periods. The explosion of evidence through functional imaging and genetic and behavioral studies regarding the unique importance of specific developmental stages on subsequent health and function stands in marked contrast to the paucity of information on those topics in current training for medical students and pediatric/family medicine residents. Pediatric chairs and educators around the country are challenged by this gap, leaving some to suggest that much current pediatric training may be unhinged from both significant advances in knowledge in the basic sciences and to emerging clinical realities.

What is wrong with the way we are teaching and learning now? Why is change needed? Despite substantial increases in investment in health (including child health), disparities in outcomes are increasing both within and between nations. Our increasing basic science knowledge should be used to reduce these disparities not by reducing improvements to the healthiest but rather by increasing the improvements in those with the poorest health. This developmental approach is especially important for the chronically ill child and for the child whose illness is sufficiently complex to require an understanding of basic pathophysiology.

The breadth and range of new and critical knowledge acquired in the last decade but not yet fully integrated into teaching or practice are extensive. Examples of quantum leaps in "basic" knowledge that should be integrated into clinical practice include the following:

- Genomic (single and multiple genes) contributions to complex diseases
- Sensitive and critical periods in development
- Effects of the physical and social environment and the role of physician as advocate
- Importance of tailoring therapy to the individual rather than on the basis of group/aggregate data (the public health model)
- Understanding and motivating behavior and behavioral change, especially regarding compliance with health care instructions
- Information about cultural/world health

Some of these concepts are relatively new, and only recently has associated genetic, biologic, physiologic, and behavioral evidence become compelling. In many cases, medical school and residency curricula contain only anecdotal references to these concepts. It is time to develop a systematic approach to their inclusion in the education of the next generation of pediatricians. The implications cross traditional subspecialty lines within pediatrics and child health. Determination of the information needed by child health care workers and the manner in which it should be taught is beyond the purview of any single group or discipline. As chairs and educators dedicated to child health, we are concerned that our profession lacks a systematic approach to the delivery of this emerging and vitally important transdisciplinary body of knowledge.

The effective integration of this vast array of new knowledge into clinical practice will require a structured educational experience based on a defined curriculum. One workable and familiar format might be through a case-based approach. Certain themes might be considered in each case analysis:

- Why did this happen to this child at this particular time? (requiring an understanding of genetics, development, and the environment)
- What could have been done to prevent it?
- Does the illness change the risk for subsequent generations?
- How will the family be able to cope with the illness?
- What skills does the pediatrician need to help the parents and patients in this process?
- Does it change what the pediatrician does in the future care of the child and family?

The audience for pediatric teaching is vast. At a minimum it includes medical students, residents, faculty, practitioners, and—given the increasing access of the general population to medical advances—the family and children as well as the health sections of popular press. Although there would be similarities in the manner in which the material would be presented to the different audiences, there would be differences as well.

Most faculty will need to learn how to think in this manner before they can become effective teachers. The skills necessary for such a teaching approach are generally not ones employed in the daily teaching activities of clinicians. We would anticipate that the Federation of Pediatric Organizations might sponsor a faculty development program in this regard. For interested faculty unable to attend a national meeting, the Federation of Pediatric Organizations might make other materials available, including videos on its web site demonstrating case presentations using this approach. As new scientific information emerges, it can be incorporated into case studies for teaching faculty and others.

For premedical students, we should consider revamping premedical school requirements, including genetics and developmental biology, perhaps in lieu of calculus and/or 2 years of chemistry. Courses relevant to culture, psychology, and education should be encouraged.

For medical students during their third year pediatric clerkship, a standardized format incorporating the points addressed in questions listed earlier could be required for student presentations (and encouraged for faculty presentations). Early exposure to this thinking will be important. Consideration might be given to a longitudinal or fourth-year elective refocusing on basic sciences as they apply to pediatrics. Such a course might be web-based, perhaps building on web-based case studies that already exist at the Council on Medical Student Education in Pediatrics.

For residents, the format of "morning report" could be altered to accommodate this emphasis, although modeling of expectations would need to be provided perhaps through videos of successful approaches. Department chairs could poll their faculties about teaching cases that have a developmental approach, and the basic sciences might need to be better represented on the American Board of Pediatrics certifying examination.

Fellows represent a unique opportunity. Their training represents a hybrid of in-depth clinical and basic science training emphasizing new scientific knowledge. If the integrated case formats were emphasized during fellowship training, tomorrow's faculty would become well versed in this approach.

For pediatricians already in practice, we might emphasize the interconnectedness of basic science and practice through practical discussions in clinical journals and pediatric newsletters. This might be similar to the series of articles published in the *New England Journal of Medicine* with an evidence-based developmental focus. For example, practitioners with little understanding of sleep physiology and its developmental changes, of behavioral development (separation vs autonomy), or of the role of social environment, especially stress, may overlook beneficial management strategies. Similar examples can be developed for other problems, such as age-related vulnerability and different morbidities of urinary tract infections. Addressing questions in a format that uses all available and relevant information will result in better care.

We are not describing trivial changes in pediatric medical education because we are not seeking trivial changes in pediatric practice and child health outcomes. We want every pediatrician to have the information needed to maximize the developmental trajectory of each patient—in much the same manner that pediatricians plot the growth of their patients and assess their trajectory on a growth chart. Every therapy and every action or inaction should take into account the implications for the whole child, now and in the future.

*Aaron Friedman, MD*
*Edward Schor, MD*
*Bonita Stanton, MD*
*Bruder Stapleton, MD*
*Barry Zuckermann, MD*

**Correspondence**: Dr Stanton, Carman and Ann Adams Department of Pediatrics, Children's Hospital of Michigan, Wayne State University School of Medicine, 3901 Beaubien Blvd, Detroit, MI 48201 (bstanton@dmc.org).
**Acknowledgment**: We thank Doug Jones, MD, who has been an inspiration and thought leader in the evolution of this educational innovation.

# Pediatric Organ Transplantation Needs

## *Organ Donation Best Practices*

According to the national Organ Procurement and Transplantation Network, of the more than 87 000 people currently awaiting organ transplantation in the United States, more than 6000 will die annually before receiving an

*See also page 548*

organ. Two hundred sixty of those who will die are children.[1,2] Another 40 children per year will be removed from the list when their medical conditions deteriorate so badly that transplantation is no longer possible.[1] The number of adult and child candidates for transplantation has risen over the past decade with adult candidate numbers increasing by 19% annually. Over the same time, pediatric candidates also increased in number but less dramatically (16% over the decade) (**Figure 1**). However, increased numbers of adult candidates compete for organs previously available to children. Among children, the greatest increased organ needs are for small bowel (increased from 70 in 1995 to 155 in 2004) and kidney transplants (increased from 585 in 1995 to 875 in 2004).

All pediatric transplants have size limitations that are met in different ways for different organs. Size match is least important for kidneys where a 1-year-old infant can accommodate an adult kidney. At the other extreme, heart organ donors must be between 80% and 200% of the recipient's weight. Liver donors must be between 50% and 200% of the recipient's weight. Split livers have the potential to increase the donor liver supply but for many reasons are often not used as widely as was predicted when the technique was developed.

### LIMITED AVAILABILITY

In 2004, 14 138 deceased and live organ donors donated a total of 27 025 organs, only a third of the number needed for the 87 000 candidates waiting for "the gift of life."[1] Obviously, this is a dramatic shortage and a serious medical problem for the many waiting patients.

#### Live Donors

Live donors are sometimes an option for pediatric candidates, and **Figure 2** illustrates recent trends in live donations of kidneys and livers for children. Live kidney donors now exceed deceased donors for pediatric kidney recipients; conversely, the number of living liver donations remains a small fraction of actual liver transplantations.

#### Deceased Donors

National studies estimate that there are between 12 000 and 14 000 eligible potential deceased donors each year.[3] This same study found that 39% of families declined consent for organ donation; however, another 16% were never asked, thus depriving them of the opportunity to make an informed decision consistent with their values.

Barriers to donation include failure of hospitals to identify potential donors and notify the organ procurement organizations (OPOs), failure to discuss donation with families, use of requestors not knowledgeable about

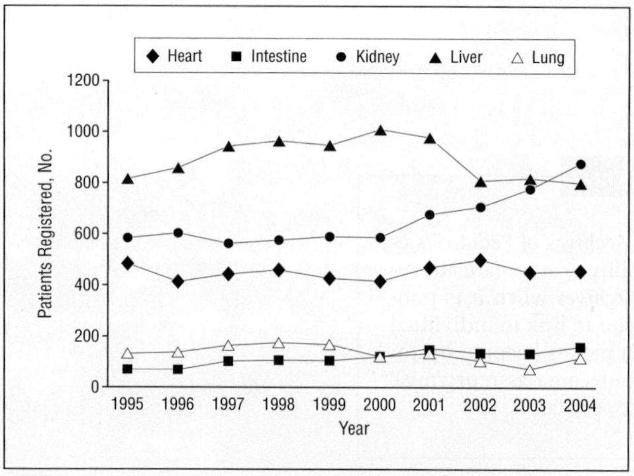


**Figure 1.** Patients younger than 18 years listed for organ transplantation during 1995 through 2004. The greatest increases are for kidney and small-bowel transplantations.

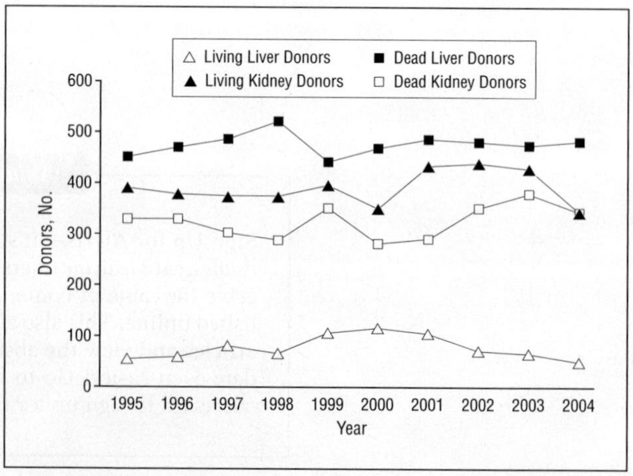


**Figure 2.** Pediatric kidney and liver transplant recipients from living and deceased donors, 1995 through 2004.

the donation process, and cultural barriers between potential donor families and medical staff discussing donation. Increased focus to identify potential donors and to improve consent processes is needed in all hospitals so that families wanting to donate have that opportunity and the request for donation is delivered in the most culturally sensitive and efficacious manner.

It is believed that if best practices were used, the rate of organ donation would increase nationally. Therefore, the Health Resources and Services Administration in the US Department of Health and Human Services launched the Organ Donation Breakthrough Collaborative in April 2003 to identify and promote best practices in organ donation for adoption by hospitals and OPOs.[4,5] The goal of the initiative was to raise the overall rate of average donor conversion (potential donors who become actual donors) to 75% among the participating hospitals and OPOs and to ultimately implement similar practices and success across all hospitals with significant donor potential.

In the first phase of the collaborative, 95 large hospitals participated; however, no children's hospitals were included. Success was achieved on a variety of organ donation outcome measures, such as timely notifications to the OPO of potential donors, use of appropriate requestors for donation consent, increased numbers of referred donors, and higher organ donation conversion rates. A second collaborative was launched in 2004 and included 11 children's hospitals. One goal of including children's hospitals was to help focus on special donation needs of pediatric patients and their families because the number of pediatric donors has been declining slightly over the past decade (**Figure 3**).

## ORGAN DONATION BEST PRACTICES

### Organizational Structure

A strong culture of hospital accountability is encouraged with emphasis on hospital leadership participation at all levels, including doctors, nurses, and administrators. Integrated relationships between transplantation centers, hospital physicians, and medical examiners support continuing communication for all individuals who participate in the donation process and family-centered end-of-life care. Close monitoring with frequent comparisons of donation performance against both local and national benchmarks is used to motivate change, and real-time feedback for the hospital and clinical leaders is encouraged.

### Consent Process

**Early Referral and Linkage.** One of the first priorities is early referral and linkage between the OPO and hospital so potential donors are identified well before brain death is pronounced. Although notification of imminent brain death to the local OPO is mandated by the Centers for Medicare & Medicaid Services[6] and is a focus of the Joint Commission of Accreditation of Health Care Organizations,[7] late or no contact clearly limits potential donation.[8,9] Development of "trigger tools" for physicians and nurses to identify patients at risk of progression to brain death is useful to enhance the process. A typical trigger for OPO notification would be for a patient with a Glasgow Coma Score of 4 or 5 or less in a brain-injured, mechanically ventilated patient. However, centers are encouraged to develop triggers that are appropriate for the local patient population and practice. A focus on timely referral for hospitals participating in both collaboratives improved the early notification rate from just over 50% in 2002 to greater than 90% in 2004 (Virginia McBride, RN, MPH; written communication; March 2005).

Early notification gives the OPO coordinator time to determine donor suitability and provides time for the family to acknowledge the patient's medical condition—critical elements for a stepwise approach to organ donation consent. At 2 large trauma centers in Missouri, a stepwise approach is initiated immediately upon referral to the OPO. Following the referral, the procurement coordinator notifies an on-call, in-house chaplain to introduce himself or herself to the family. The chaplains are experienced in both grief counseling and the donation process, and the early notification allows for family assessment up to 90 minutes prior to the arrival of OPO staff (Ron Gegg, RN, BSN CPTC; written communication; March 2005).[10,11] If the topic of organ donation has been broached prematurely before the family has accepted the terminal condition of their loved one, a second approach by a skilled requestor from the OPO often leads to donation consent even after an initial decline. Mid-America Transplant Services tracked this process between July 2004 and January 2005. It reviewed 86 referrals to evaluate the stepwise approach. When it was followed, 87% of individuals consented to organ donation compared with 57% when the process was not followed.[12]

**Cultural Competence.** The medical team and OPOs must strive to offer information regarding donation in a culturally appropriate manner. Hospitals and OPOs often offer training in organ donation to social workers and chaplains, who can focus on the family's spiritual and cultural needs. Historically, nonwhite Americans have donated organs at lower rates compared with whites.[13,14] A team member of the same background as the donor family can enhance cultural understanding and avoid language barriers.[15,16] Although Ben Taub Hospital in Houston, Tex, has a large minority population in which one might expect lower donation rates, a program using "like" requestors has been associated with dramatic improvement in donation rates among both Hispanic and African American individuals. Community education regarding the need for organ donation among minorities is very important because of increased transplantation need among minority candidates[17] and because improved renal graft survival is seen when the donor and recipients are of the same ethnicity.[18]

**Scripted Consent Process.** Use of an appropriate script by trained requestors appears to improve the experi-

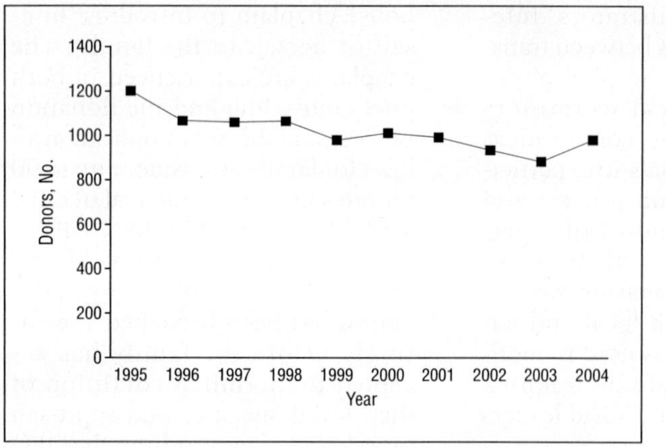


**Figure 3.** Pediatric donors (<18 years of age) during 1995 through 2004.

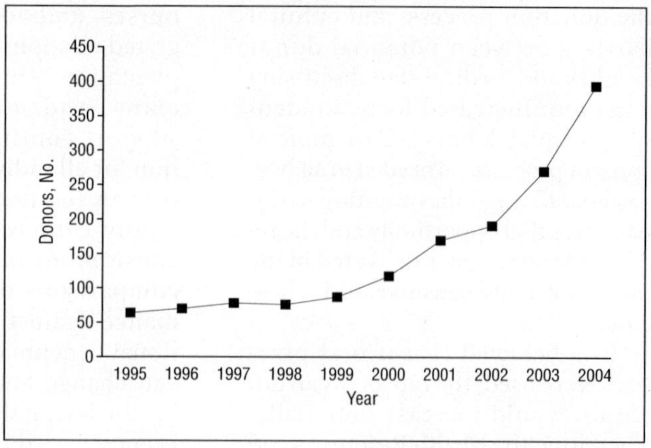


**Figure 4.** Trends in donors after cardiac death during 1995 through 2004.

ence for families. Trained hospital and OPO requestors must assess and reassess the effectiveness of approach techniques. Typically, this assessment is done with case reviews after each donor case.

**Presumptive Approach.** In years past, requestors have been reluctant to discuss the great unmet need for donor organs with families of potential donors despite a 1993 Gallup poll demonstrating that over 85% of respondents favor organ transplantation.[19] Many believe that the majority of families and patients will choose to donate if they are educated about the need for organ donation. Families are approached with the assumption that they want to help others and will donate. This includes giving information on needs of candidates on the transplant waiting list who may be helped by the donation. The University of Pennsylvania Center for Bioethics is studying this presumptive approach to consent for organ donation and offers online information and onsite training to hospitals and OPOs.[20]

**In-House Coordinators.** Placement of OPO in-house coordinators at large trauma centers has been associated with substantial improvement in referral rates of potential donors and higher consent and donation conversion rates.[7,21] The in-house coordinator serves as both a member of the acute care team and the OPO, ensuring good communication, enhancing use of audits and standards, and serving as a bridge between the teams to meet the needs of potential donor families. Clearly this strategy is not possible in smaller hospitals or OPOs but is used with success in large trauma systems.[21]

**Physician's Role in Discussing Organ Donation.** In 1998, the US Health Care Financing Administration changed the federal Conditions of Participation for organ and tissue donation to include the use of trained "designated" requestors.[22] This caused some unintended tension between staff of the OPO and hospital physicians based on the misconception that only OPO staff may approach the family and that physicians were excluded from counseling families regarding donation. This is not accurate; however, physicians who participate in donation consent need to be aware of important issues regarding brain death as well as organ donation and should participate in training to work effectively with OPO coordinators.[23]

Physicians need to initiate discussions of donation separately after conversations regarding the child's grave prognosis and explanations of brain death have occurred. In some hospitals, the OPO staff make all requests for organ donation. The physician would organize the approach for consent with the OPO staff.

Typically families who consent to organ donation have a good understanding of brain death, feel that they had sufficient time and privacy to make their decision regarding donation, and feel that the person requesting donation was sensitive to their needs.[23] A collaborative approach between OPOs, physicians, and other hospital staff (social workers, chaplains, and nurses) is often ideal for such a detailed and sometimes lengthy process.

## Other Strategies

**Donation After Cardiac Death.** Organ donation in the early 1960s was from non–heart-beating patients and led to the understanding of the dead donor rule, the concept that it is unethical to cause death by procuring organs and unethical for cadaveric organ procurement to precede death.[24] French physicians developed and implemented a concept of brain death in 1966, which facilitated organ donation among patients without neurological function. The United States and other countries quickly developed brain death criteria,[25,26] and the number of non–heart-beating donors virtually disappeared because organ preservation and graft function from non–heart-beating donors was poor. Forty years ago, organ procurement and preservation techniques were relatively primitive, and the physiologic function of organs from brain-dead, heart-beating donors was superior. Given today's environment of critical organ shortage and improved preservation techniques, the potential for donation by non–heart-beating donors has re-emerged and is now known as donation after cardiac death (DCD).[27]

Donation after cardiac death may be considered in a patient with a terminal condition, where additional aggressive therapy will only prolong the dying process, and cardiac death is expected to occur rapidly (typically within 1 hour) after withdrawal of support. After the decision to withdraw support has been made, the option for donation can be addressed.

The ethical principles for DCD were reviewed by the Institute of Medicine in 1997 and again in 2000. The Institute of Medicine recommended that all US OPOs explore the option of DCD in cooperation with local hospitals, health care professionals, and communities.[28] They also recommended that decisions to withdraw life-sustaining treatment be made independently of and prior to any staff-initiated discussion of organ or tissue donation, and finally, like all end-of-life care, the donation process should be patient- and family-centered. The American Medical Association offers professional resources regarding DCD, which state that consent must be voluntary, that the health care team must not be compromised by conflict of interest, and that providers making end-of-life decisions must be separate from the transplantation team. The American Medical Association recommends that recipients of the organs be informed of the source and approve their acceptance.[29]

Over the past decade, 1514 people have donated organs after cardiac death in the United States with a dramatic increase in the last 2 years (**Figure 4**). Two hundred one donors younger than 18 years old were donors after cardiac death during the years 1995 through 2004. This included 35 children younger than 6 years (Virginia McBride, RN, MPH; written communication; March 2005). Several reports show that renal and liver grafts from DCD donors have graft function and recipient survival rates comparable with donations from brain-dead donors.[30-33]

Currently DCD programs for children are evolving with gradual acceptance by providers. A recent report from the University of Chicago showed that families of pediatric patients support the concept of DCD and want to be approached if their children were in a situation where withdrawal of life support was considered.[34]

**Care of Potential Donors.** Another way to improve donation rates is providing meticulous care to potential donors so that cardiovascular instability does not either preclude the diagnosis of brain death or occur prior to successful recovery of organs. Optimal care of the potential donor requires a sound grasp of the physiologic derangement unique to brain death, including hemodynamic instability, diabetes insipidus, disseminated intravascular coagulation due to release of thromboplastin from the injured brain tissue, and neurogenic pulmonary edema. Uncontrolled progression from brain death to cardiac death results in loss of 10% to 20% of potential donors.[35]

Overwhelming untreated infection generally precludes donation; however, bacteremia is not an absolute contraindication to donation,[36] and outcomes for recipients do not differ between selected infected and noninfected donors,[37] making aggressive treatment of infection critical.

The goals of cardiovascular support are to achieve normovolemia, maintain blood pressure, and optimize cardiac output.[38] Many OPOs routinely administer steroids and thyroid hormone to potential donors who require either vasopressor support or high-dose inotropes. Case series suggest that hormone replacement therapies tend to lower the need for vasopressors.[39-41] Cardiac function may improve in young potential donors, and if the initial echocardiogram shows poor function, a repeat examination after a period of stability may be indicated.

Respiratory management includes avoidance of high static airway pressures and normalization of $PaCO_2$ and $PaO_2$. Early bronchoscopy has been advocated for adult and larger pediatric patients to evaluate anatomy, remove secretions, and optimize lung expansion.[38,41] Reported lung procurement rates have historically been low (20%).[42]

Organ procurement organizations are evaluating the number of organs used from each donor to determine care pathways associated with greater organ yield per donor.[43,44] Many OPOs rely on input from pediatric critical care providers for donor care because the OPO coordinators typically have less pediatric experience and a team approach remains critical in donor management.

### Prioritizing the Needs of Children

Policy makers recognize that children not only often have size limitations for potential organs, but also stand to gain considerable medical and personal quality-of-life benefit from transplantation. Children are given priority allocation of kidneys from all deceased donors younger than 35 years to achieve transplantation within specifically identified time goals. Pediatric liver transplant candidates are also preferentially offered grafts from donors younger than 18 years.[45] Finally, children younger than age 17 years are now given priority to lungs recovered from pediatric donors.[46]

### Current Status

Organ donation processes are complex. Recognizing the complexity, establishing standards of care, and working in a collaborative fashion may help families choose donation. Compared with 2003, there were 10.8% more deceased donors in 2004.[47] More than 184 of the nation's largest hospitals have sustained donation rates of 75% or greater for at least 12 of the last 18 months owing to renewed focus on donation practices. The 11 pediatric hospitals also showed improvement. Compared with a year ago, conversion rates among the 11 centers increased to 64% from 48% (November through March 2004-2005 vs 2003-2004) and 5 of the centers achieved conversion rates of 75% or greater (Ron Gegg, RN, BSN CPTC; written communication; March 2005).

A sustained focus on the donation process is required for all hospitals to realize these goals. Pediatricians can educate their patients and parents about donation and work with their community hospital and OPO to ensure that families of potential pediatric donors are offered compassionate end-of-life care, including information about donation. Intensive care providers must work with OPOs to manage potential donors and develop DCD programs to decrease the number of children who die or have diminished quality of life while awaiting transplantation.

*Susan L. Bratton, MD, MPH*
*Nikoleta S. Kolovos, MD*
*Elizabeth S. Roach, RN, BSN*
*Virginia McBride, MPH, RN*
*Judy L. Geiger, RN, BSN*
*Rebecka L. Meyers, MD*

**Correspondence:** Dr Bratton, 295 Chipeta Way, PO Box 581289, Salt Lake City, UT 84158-0289 (susan.bratton@hsc.utah.edu).
**Funding/Support:** This work was supported in part by the Health Resources and Services Administration.
**Disclaimer:** The content is the responsibility of the authors alone and does not necessarily reflect the views or policies of the Department of Health and Human Services, nor does mention of trade names, commercial products, or organizations imply endorsement by the US Government.

## REFERENCES

1. Organ Procurement and Transplantation Network. Available at: http://www.optn.org/data. Accessed January 26, 2005 and March 22, 2005.
2. Fast facts about transplants, July 1, 2003, to June 30, 2004. Scientific registry of transplant recipients. Available at: http://www.ustransplant.org. Accessed January 26, 2005.
3. Sheehy E, Conrad SL, Brigham LE, et al. Estimating the potential number of organ donors in the United States. *N Engl J Med.* 2003;349:667-674.
4. Secretary Thompson's organ donation initiative. Available at: http://www.organdonor.gov/SecInitiative.htm. Accessed January 26, 2005.
5. The Organ Donation Breakthrough Collaborative: best practices final report (September 2003). Available at: http://organdonor.gov/bestpractice.htm. Accessed March 8, 2005.
6. Centers for Medicare & Medicaid Services. Conditions of participation: conditions for coverage identification of potential organ, tissue, and eye donors. Available at: http://new.cms.hhs.gov/apps/media/press/release.asp?counter=40. Accessed March 9, 2004.
7. Health care at the crossroads: strategies for narrowing the organ donation gap and protecting patients. Available at: http://www.jcaho.org/about+us/public+policy+initiatives/organ+donation.htm. Accessed February 23, 2005.
8. Tsai E, Shemie SD, Cox PN, Furst S, McCarthy L, Hebert D. Organ donation in children: role of the pediatric intensive care unit. *Pediatr Crit Care Med.* 2000;1:156-160.
9. Opdam HI, Silverster W. Identifying the potential organ donor: an audit of hospital deaths. *Intensive Care Med.* 2004;30:1390-1397.
10. Schweiger M, Wasler A, Prenner A, et al. Improving the rate of organ donation. *Transplant Proc.* 2004;36:2543-2545.
11. Bardell T, Hunter DJ, Kent WD, Jain MK. Do medical students have the knowledge needed to maximize organ donation rates? *Can J Surg.* 2003;46:453-457.
12. Mid-America Transplant Services Leadership meeting. St Louis, Mo; March 10, 2005.
13. Siminoff LA, Lawrence RH, Arnold RM. Comparison of black and white families' experiences and perceptions regarding organ donation requests. *Crit Care Med.* 2003;31:146-151.
14. Perez LM, Schulman B, Davis F, et al. Organ donation in three major American cities with large Latino and black populations. *Transplantation.* 1988;46:553-557.
15. Minniefield WJ, Muti P. Organ donation survey results of a Buffalo, New York, African-American community. *J Natl Med Assoc.* 2002;94:979-986.
16. Pietz CA, Mayes T, Naclerio A, Taylor R. Pediatric organ transplantation and the Hispanic population: approaching families and obtaining their consent. *Transplant Proc.* 2004;36:1237-1240.
17. Center for Reducing Health Disparities. The net transfer of transplant organs across race, sex and income. *Am J Med.* 2004;117:670-675.
18. Weller JM, Wu SC, Ferguson CW, et al. Influence of race on cadaveric kidney donor and recipient graft survival: a multifactorial analysis. *Am J Kidney Dis.* 1987;9:191-199.
19. The Gallup Organization. *The American Public's Attitudes Toward Organ Donation and Transplantation.* Boston, Mass: The Partnership for Organ Donation Inc; 1993.
20. The Program for Transplant Policy and Ethics. Presumptive Approach to Consent. Available at: http://www.bioethics.upenn.edu/bioethics/?pageID=4. Accessed April 4, 2005.
21. Shafer TJ, Ehrle RN, Davis KD, et al. Increasing organ recovery from a level I trauma center: inhouse coordinator intervention. *Prog Transplant.* 2004;14:250-263.
22. Medicare and Medicaid programs; hospital conditions of participation; identification of potential organ, tissue, and eye donors and transplant hospitals' provision of transplant-related data: HCFA. Final rule. *Fed Regist.* 1998;63:33856-33875.
23. Williams MA, Lipsett PA, Rushton CH, et al. The physician's role in discussing organ donation with families. *Crit Care Med.* 2003;31:1568-1572.
24. Ethics Committee, American College of Critical Care Medicine, Society of Critical Care Medicine. Recommendation for nonheartbeating donation. *Crit Care Med.* 2001;29:1826-1831.
25. American Academy of Pediatrics Task Force on Brain Death in Children. Report of special task force: guidelines for the determination of brain death in children. *Pediatrics.* 1987;80:298-300.
26. Wijdicks EF. The diagnosis of brain death. *N Engl J Med.* 2001;344:1215-1221.
27. Koogler T, Costarino AT Jr. The potential benefits of pediatric nonheartbeating organ donor. *Pediatrics.* 1998;101:1049-1052.
28. Institute of Medicine. *Non-Heart-Beating Organ Transplantation: Medical and Ethical Issues in Procurement.* Washington, DC: National Academies Press; 1997.
29. Organ procurement following cardiac death. Available at: http://www.ama-assn.org/ama/pub/category/8447.html. Accessed September 28, 3005.
30. D'Alessandro AM, Fernandez LA, Chin LT, et al. Donation after cardiac death: the University of Wisconsin experience. *Ann Transplant.* 2004;9:68-71.
31. Manzarbeitia CY, Ortiz JA, Rothstein KD, et al. Long-term outcome of controlled, non-heart-beating donor liver transplantation. *Transplantation.* 2004;78:211-215.
32. Cooper JT, Chin LT, Krieger NR, et al. Donation after cardiac death: the University of Wisconsin experience with renal transplantation. *Am J Transplant.* 2004;4:1490-1494.
33. Rudich SM, Kaplan B, Magee JC, et al. Renal transplantations performed using non-heart-beating organ donors: going back to the future? *Transplantation.* 2002;74:1715-1720.
34. Koogler TK, Stark A, Kaplan B, Myers GR. Parents'/guardians' views on donation after cardiac death. *Crit Care Med.* 2006;33:A105.
35. Lopez-Navidad A, Domingo P, Viedma MA. Professional characteristics of the transplantation coordinator. *Transplant Proc.* 1997;29:1607-1613.
36. Angelis M, Cooper JT, Freeman RB. Impact of donor infections on outcome of orthotopic liver transplantation. *Liver Transpl.* 2003;9:451-462.
37. Freeman RB, Giatras I, Falagas ME, et al. Outcome of transplantation of organs procured from bacteremic donors. *Transplantation.* 1999;68:1107-1111.
38. Wood KE, Becker BN, McCartney JG, D'Alessandro AM, Coursin DB. Care of the potential organ donor. *N Engl J Med.* 2004;351:2730-2739.
39. Zuppa AF, Nadkarni V, Davis L, et al. The effect of thyroid hormone infusion on vasopressor support in critically ill children with cessation of neurologic function. *Crit Care Med.* 2004;32:2318-2322.
40. Salim A, Vassiliu P, Velmahos GC, et al. The role of thyroid hormone in potential organ donors. *Arch Surg.* 2001;136:1377-1380.
41. Perrot M, Snell GI, Babcock WD, et al. Strategies to optimize the use of currently available lung donors. *J Heart Lung Transplant.* 2004;23:1127-1134.
42. Reilly PM, Morgan L, Grossman MD, et al. Lung procurement from solid organ donors: role of fluid resuscitation in procurement failures. Available at: http://www.ispub.com/ostia/index.php?xmlFilePath=journals/ijeicm/vol3n2/organ.xml. Accessed on March 3, 2006.
43. Rosendale JD, Chabalewski FL, McBride M, et al. Increased transplanted organs from the use of a standardized donor management protocol. *Am J Transplant.* 2002;2:761-768.
44. Donkin M, Daher N, Kolovos NS, et al. The effect of specialized pediatric management on organ recovery from potential pediatric transplant donors. *Crit Care Med.* 2004;32(suppl):A82.
45. OPTN/UNOS board approves policies to benefit children needing livers, kidneys. Organ Procurement and Transplantation Network. Available at: http://www.optn.org/news/newsDetail.asp?id=373. Accessed March 8, 2004.
46. OPTN/UNOS board approves lung allocation policy based on transplant benefit. Organ Procurement and Transplantation Network. Available at: http://www.optn.org/SharedContentDocuments/Lung_Policy_Release.doc. Accessed March 30, 2005.
47. Transplants by donor type. Organ Procurement and Transplantation Network. Available at: http://www.optn.org/latestData/step2.asp. Accessed March 8, 2005.

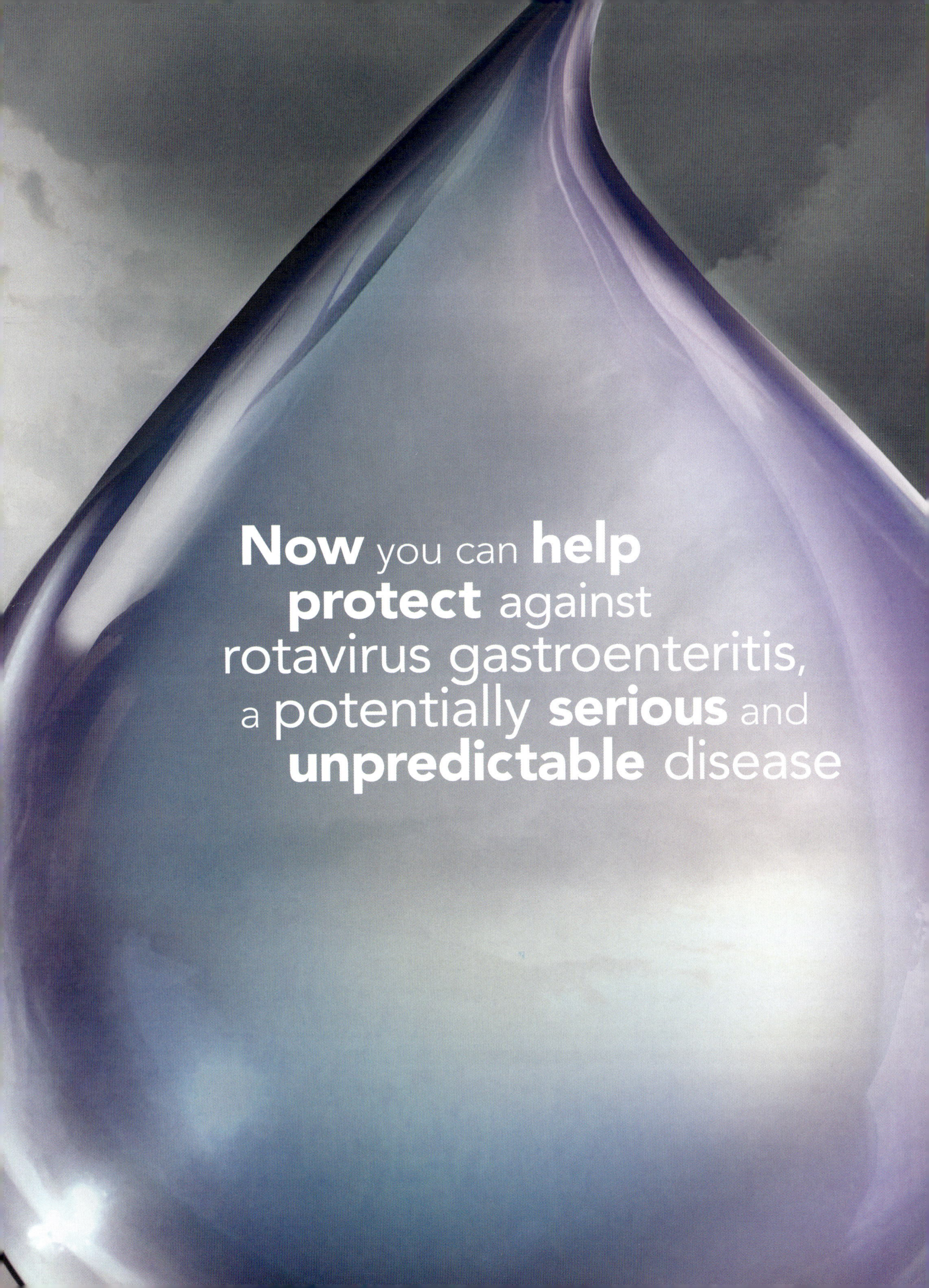
Now you can help protect against rotavirus gastroenteritis, a potentially serious and unpredictable disease

ARTICLE

# Estimate of the Commercial Value of Underage Drinking and Adult Abusive and Dependent Drinking to the Alcohol Industry

*Susan E. Foster, MSW; Roger D. Vaughan, DrPH; William H. Foster, PhD; Joseph A. Califano, Jr, LLB*

**Objectives:** To document quantity and cash value of underage and adult *Diagnostic and Statistical Manual of Mental Disorders, Fourth Edition* (*DSM-IV*)–defined abusive and dependent drinking as well as underage drinking and adult *DSM-IV*–defined abusive and dependent drinking combined to the alcohol industry.

**Design:** Analysis of multiple cross-sectional national data sets.

**Setting:** The 2001 National Household Survey on Drug Abuse, the 2001 Youth Risk Behavior Survey, the 2001 Behavioral Risk Factor Surveillance Survey, the 2000 US Census, the 2000 to 2001 National Epidemiological Survey on Alcohol and Related Conditions, and the 2001 Adams Business Research.

**Participants:** A total of 260 580 persons aged 12 years and older across 4 data sources.

**Main Exposure:** Underage drinking or pathological drinking defined as meeting the *DSM-IV* criteria for abusive or dependent drinking.

**Main Outcome Measures:** Total amount of alcohol consumed and the cash value for alcohol consumed among underage and adult drinkers with *DSM-IV*–defined alcohol abuse and dependence as well as all underage drinkers combined with adult drinkers with *DSM-IV*–defined alcohol abuse and dependence.

**Results:** The short-term cash value of underage drinking to the alcohol industry was $22.5 billion in 2001—17.5% of total consumer expenditures for alcohol. The long-term commercial value of underage drinking is the contribution of underage drinking to maintaining consumption among adult drinkers with alcohol abuse and dependence, which was equal to at least $25.8 billion in 2001.

**Conclusions:** The combined value of illegal underage drinking and adult pathological drinking to the industry was at least $48.3 billion, or 37.5% of consumer expenditures for alcohol, in 2001. Alternative estimates suggest that these costs may be closer to $62.9 billion, or 48.8% of consumer expenditures for alcohol.

*Arch Pediatr Adolesc Med. 2006;160:473-478*

An important national health objective in the United States is to prevent and reduce the incidence of pathological drinking among Americans.[1] Federal dietary guidelines recognize that "higher levels of alcohol intake raise the risk for high blood pressure, stroke, heart disease, certain cancers, accidents, violence, suicides, birth defects, and overall mortality. Too much alcohol may cause cirrhosis of the liver, inflammation of the pancreas, and damage to the brain and heart."[2] Abusive and dependent drinking is recognized clinically as a pathological condition in the *Diagnostic and Statistical Manual of Mental Disorders, Fourth Edition (DSM-IV)*.[3] Alcohol abuse and alcoholism cost the nation $184 billion in 1998,[4] more than cancer ($107 billion) or obesity ($100 billion).[5]

Research suggests that an effective way to prevent pathological drinking is to delay the onset of regular drinking.[6-14] For example, Grant and Dawson[6] found that individuals who begin drinking before age 15 years are 4 times likelier to become alcohol dependent than those who do not drink before age 21 years, and they also found that the odds of lifetime alcohol dependence were reduced by 14% with each increasing year of age at first use. Expanding on these findings, DeWit et al[12] found that the incidence of lifetime alcohol abuse and dependence is greatest for those who begin drinking between the ages of 11 and 14 years. Despite knowledge of this relationship between early onset of drinking and later abuse and dependence, more than 13 000 teens younger than age 21 years take their first drink each day.[15] Slightly more than 6000 of these beginning drinkers are younger than age 16 years.[15] In 2001, 47% of 12- to 20-year-olds reported that they were current drinkers; 30% of them admitted to binge drinking in the past month.[15]

Author Affiliations: The National Center on Addiction and Substance Abuse (Ms S. E. Foster, Drs Vaughan and W. H. Foster, and Mr Califano) and Department of Biostatistics, Mailman School of Public Health (Dr Vaughan), Columbia University, New York, NY.

Not only are younger drinkers likelier to become pathological drinkers, but pathological drinkers—young and old—consume a disproportionate share of the alcohol. For example, in 1981, Gerstein[16] estimated that 10% of the drinkers drank 57% of the alcohol. Greenfield and Rogers[17] found that 2.5% of drinkers aged 18 years and older—the heaviest drinkers—drink 27% of the alcohol. Foster et al[18] confirmed and expanded on the findings by Greenfield and Rogers. However, to our knowledge, no research has determined the share of the nation's alcohol consumption that is attributable to pathological drinking. Foster and colleagues have documented the commercial value of underage drinking and adult excessive drinking to the alcohol industry, but no research has documented the combined commercial value of underage drinking and adult pathological drinking to the industry.

In this article, we close this gap in research. First, we reexamine the incidence of underage and adult drinking. Next, we consider the proportion of underage and adult drinking that can be clinically characterized as abusive and dependent drinking as well as the percentage of alcohol consumed by such drinkers. Finally, we document the commercial value of underage and adult abusive and dependent drinking to the alcohol industry as well as the combined commercial value of underage drinking and adult abusive and dependent drinking to the industry.

## METHODS

### DATA SOURCES AND MEASURES

We relied on several national data sets to help define the following: (1) the number and proportion of underage and adult drinkers; (2) alcohol consumption by underage and adult drinkers as well as by underage and adult drinkers with alcohol abuse and dependence; and (3) the cash value of underage drinking as well as of underage and adult abusive and dependent drinking to the alcohol industry.

### NUMBER AND PROPORTION OF UNDERAGE AND ADULT DRINKERS

To compute alcohol consumption by age group, we first used the 2000 US Census[19] to estimate the number of people in the United States aged 12 to 20 years and 21 years and older.

To estimate the proportion of people aged 12 to 20 years who drank in the past month (ie, current drinkers), we considered several data sets, including the 2001 National Household Survey of Drug Abuse (NHSDA)[20] and the 2001 Youth Risk Behavior Survey (YRBS).[21] The NHSDA, administered by the Substance Abuse and Mental Health Services Administration, Rockville, Md, used a nationally representative sample of 55 561 persons, including 24 264 persons aged 12 to 20 years and 31 297 persons aged 21 years and older. The YRBS, administered by the Centers for Disease Control and Prevention, Atlanta, Ga, used a nationally representative sample of 13 601 persons in grades 9 through 12, with observed ages from 12 to 18 years (if the participating high school students were older than 18 years, they were recoded as 18-year-olds). We concluded that the YRBS data are the most accurate for purposes of estimating the proportion of underage individuals (aged 12-20 years) who drank in the past 30 days. Several studies[22-27] have demonstrated that the NHSDA data tend to underestimate the proportion of underage drinkers who consume alcohol and the amounts they consume since it is based on personal interviews performed in a household and because children are only interviewed when a parent is in the home. The YRBS provides more accurate estimates because it is administered in schools, with the added benefit of anonymity, and because of the order and content of the survey questions.[22-27]

To estimate the proportion of persons aged 21 years and older who drank in the past month, we used the 2001 Behavioral Risk Factor Surveillance Survey,[28] which was also administered by the Centers for Disease Control and Prevention. The 2001 Behavioral Risk Factor Surveillance Survey is a telephone survey of 212 510 respondents, including 148 325 persons aged 21 years or older.

### ALCOHOL CONSUMPTION BY UNDERAGE AND ADULT DRINKERS AND BY UNDERAGE AND ADULT DRINKERS WITH ALCOHOL ABUSE AND DEPENDENCE

We used the 2001 NHSDA to compute the amount of alcohol consumed by underage and adult drinkers, the prevalence of abusive and dependent drinking as defined by *DSM-IV* criteria, and the amount of alcohol consumed by underage and adult drinkers with alcohol abuse and dependence. The NHSDA asked the following questions about alcohol consumption: "Think specifically about the past 30 days—that is, since (fill in date), up to and including today. During the past 30 days, on how many days did you drink 1 or more drinks of an alcoholic beverage?" and "On the days when you drank during the past 30 days, how many drinks did you usually have? Count as a drink a can or bottle of beer; a wine cooler or a glass of wine, champagne, or sherry; a shot of liquor; or a mixed drink or cocktail." The NHSDA also included the items necessary for a *DSM-IV* diagnosis of alcohol abuse or dependence.

We defined pathological drinking according to the *DSM-IV* criteria for alcohol abuse and dependence. The NHSDA asked respondents about the 4 domains related to alcohol abuse, defined by the *DSM-IV* as "a maladaptive pattern of substance use manifested by recurrent and significant adverse consequences,"[3] and the 7 domains related to alcohol dependence, defined by the *DSM-IV* as "a maladaptive pattern of substance use leading to clinically significant impairment or distress."[3]

A respondent was labeled as abusing alcohol if he or she exhibited any 1 of 4 conditions in the previous year. The respondent was labeled as substance dependent by the *DSM-IV* criteria if the respondent exhibited 3 or more of 7 conditions at any time in the previous year.[3]

### CASH VALUE OF UNDERAGE DRINKING AND UNDERAGE AND ADULT ABUSIVE AND DEPENDENT DRINKING TO THE ALCOHOL INDUSTRY

To estimate consumer expenditures linked to underage drinking and to underage and adult drinkers who met or did not meet the *DSM-IV* criteria for abusive or dependent drinking, the total amount (in gallons and liters) of beer, distilled spirits, and wine consumed by each group in 2001 was calculated using data on consumer expenditures for alcohol reported by the alcohol industry and published by Adams Business Research.[29-31]

Estimating the cash value of underage and adult drinkers also requires information on the proportion of the type of drink (beer vs distilled spirits vs wine) consumed by underage and adult drinkers and by those who met vs did not meet the *DSM-IV* criteria for alcohol abuse or dependence. To our knowledge, no data documenting the proportions by type of alcoholic beverages consumed by underage drinkers aged 12 to 18 years are available. However, Foster et al[18] found that the pattern of drinking among underage drinkers aged 12 to 20 years closely resembles the pattern of drinking among adult excessive drinkers.

We estimated patterns of alcohol consumption using the 2001 to 2002 National Epidemiological Survey on Alcohol and Related Conditions (NESARC).[32] This nationally representative survey of those aged 18 and older, administered by the National Institute on Alcohol Abuse and Alcoholism, asked participants to identify type of drink by the categories of beer, distilled spirits, wine, and "coolers" of all types. Because the price of coolers is typically similar to that of beer,[33-35] we redistributed the percentage of cooler consumption into the beer category, producing consumption estimates for adults who met the *DSM-IV* criteria for abuse or dependence of 70.8% beer, 18.3% distilled spirits, and 10.9% wine whereas other adult drinkers consumed 56.1% beer, 16.7% distilled spirits, and 27.2% wine. Using this same data set, we found that underage drinkers (aged 18-20 years) who met the *DSM-IV* criteria for abuse or dependence consumed 79.6% beer, 17.5% distilled spirits, and 2.9% wine whereas other underage drinkers consumed 71.5% beer, 20.8% distilled spirits, and 7.7% wine. We applied the estimated beverage type computed among those aged 18 to 20 years to all of the underage drinkers.

To present a range of estimates of the cash value of underage and pathological drinking, we also used the NESARC to compute alternative estimates of drinking rates, consumption, and pathological drinking rates among adults aged 21 years and older.

## STATISTICAL ANALYSIS

To calculate the amount of alcohol consumed by underage and adult drinkers who met and did not meet the *DSM-IV* criteria for alcohol abuse and dependence, we followed a basic formula: $T_i = P_i \times A_i \times C_i$, where $T_i$ is the total estimated number of drinks consumed in the past 30 days by those in the $i^{th}$ age category, $P_i$ is the estimated proportion of the population in the $i^{th}$ age category who drank in the past 30 days, $A_i$ is the mean number of drinks consumed by drinkers in the $i^{th}$ age category in the past 30 days, $C_i$ is the number of people in the population in the $i^{th}$ age category, and i refers to those who are aged either 12 to 20 years or 21 years and older. To compute these equations, we estimated the number of persons aged 12 to 20 years as well as 21 years and older (ie, $C_i$) using the 2000 US Census data, and we multiplied that by the proportion of those who drank in the past 30 days (ie, $P_i$) using the 2001 YRBS data for those aged 12 to 20 years and the 2001 Behavioral Risk Factor Surveillance Survey data for adults. We then multiplied the resulting numbers of people aged 12 to 20 years and those aged 21 years and older who drank in the past 30 days by the estimated mean amount of alcohol consumed among drinkers within the age category (ie, $A_i$) using the 2001 NHSDA data. We annualized the results to compute the total number of drinks consumed by persons aged 12 years and older. To determine the number of people who met the *DSM-IV* criteria for alcohol abuse or dependence, we multiplied the estimated proportion of drinkers in each category who met the *DSM-IV* criteria for alcohol abuse or dependence by the number of drinkers in each age category.

To calculate the cash value of each age and *DSM-IV* group, we multiplied the total amount of alcohol (in the form of beer, wine, and distilled spirits) consumed in the United States in 2001, as reported in the 2003 Adams Beverage Group handbooks,[29-31] by the percentage of total alcohol consumed by each age and *DSM-IV* group. The cost per drink was then calculated by taking the total consumer expenditures for beer, distilled spirits, and wine as reported by the Adams Beverage Group and dividing each amount by the total number of drinks of beer, distilled spirits, and wine, respectively. Consumer expenditures were calculated by multiplying the overall proportion of drinks that each group consumed by the proportion of that amount that was estimated to be beer, distilled spirits, or wine and finally by the average computed price per drink for beer, distilled spirits, and wine ($1.05, $1.34, and $1.30, respectively[29-31]).

**Table 1. Summary of National Data Sets Used in Estimations**

| Data Source | Sample Size, No. | Year | Application |
|---|---|---|---|
| US Census | US population | 2000 | Estimation of the number of people in each age category |
| Youth Risk Behavior Survey | 13 601 persons aged 12-18 y | 2001 | Estimation of the proportion of persons aged <21 y who drank alcohol in the past month |
| Behavior Risk Factor Surveillance Survey | 212 510 persons, including 148 325 persons aged ≥21 y | 2001 | Estimation of the proportion of persons aged ≥21 y who drank alcohol in the past month |
| National Household Survey of Drug Abuse | 55 561 persons aged ≥12 y | 2001 | Estimation of alcohol consumption and proportion of persons aged ≥12 y who met *DSM-IV* criteria for alcohol abuse or dependence |
| National Epidemiological Survey on Alcohol and Related Conditions | 43 093 persons aged ≥18 y | 2001-2002 | Estimation of proportion of drink type consumed (alternative estimation of alcohol consumption and proportion of persons who met *DSM-IV* criteria for alcohol abuse or dependence) |

Abbreviation: *DSM-IV, Diagnostic and Statistical Manual of Mental Disorders, Fourth Edition.*

Although we have accounted for the fact that underage and adult drinkers with alcohol abuse and dependence consume lower-cost beverages (ie, more beer), they also may consume lower-cost products within each beverage type. If so, our results will be marginally overestimated since, in the absence of empirical data, we were unable to calculate the impact that such behavior would have on consumer expenditures among these groups.

Using these procedures, we accounted for all but 0.3% of consumer expenditures. We reallocated this small remainder of the $128.6 billion reported by Adams Beverage Group[29-31] across the age and drinking categories according to their computed percentages of all alcohol expenditures. All of the analyses using nationally representative data sets incorporated the appropriate weighting variables provided with each data set.

## RESULTS

### CASH VALUE OF UNDERAGE DRINKING AND ABUSIVE AND DEPENDENT DRINKING TO THE ALCOHOL INDUSTRY

A summary of the data sets and how they were used is presented in **Table 1**. We calculated the proportion of people in each age group who drank in the past 30 days in 2001 and the percentage of each category who met the *DSM-IV* criteria for alcohol abuse or dependence. Among youth aged 12 to 20 years, 47.1% were current drinkers. The percentages of drinkers who met the *DSM-IV* crite-

**Table 2. Distribution of Drinkers and Those Meeting *Diagnostic and Statistical Manual of Mental Disorders, Fourth Edition* Criteria for Alcohol Abuse or Dependence**

| Age, y | Population Aged ≥12 y, %* | Persons Who Drank Alcohol in the Past 30 d, % (95% CI)† | Persons Within Age Category Meeting *DSM-IV* Criteria for Alcohol Abuse or Dependence, % (95% CI)‡ | Drinkers Within Age Category Meeting *DSM-IV* Criteria for Alcohol Abuse or Dependence, % (95% CI)§ | All Persons Who Met *DSM-IV* Criteria for Alcohol Abuse or Dependence, %‡ |
|---|---|---|---|---|---|
| 12-20 | 15.4 | 47.1 (44.8-49.3) | 12.2 (11.5-12.8) | 25.9 (24.5-27.3) | 30.1 |
| ≥21 | 84.6 | 53.8 (53.5-54.3) | 5.1 (4.8-5.5) | 9.6 (8.9-10.2) | 69.9 |
| **Total** | **100.0** | **52.8 (52.1-53.5)** | **6.2 (5.9-6.6)** | **11.8 (11.1-12.5)** | **100.0** |

Abbreviations: CI, confidence interval; *DSM-IV, Diagnostic and Statistical Manual of Mental Disorders, Fourth Edition.*
*Data are from the 2000 US Census.
†For the age category of 12 to 20 years, data are from the 2001 Youth Risk Behavior Survey. For the age category of 21 years and older, data are from the 2001 Behavior Risk Factor Surveillance Survey.
‡Calculated values.
§Data are from the 2001 National Household Survey of Drug Abuse.

**Table 3. Consumption of Alcohol Among Those Who Drank Alcohol in the Past 30 Days by Age Category and *Diagnostic and Statistical Manual of Mental Disorders, Fourth Edition* Criteria for Alcohol Abuse or Dependence**

| Age, y | No. of Drinks/mo, Mean (95% CI)* | Drinks/y, No. in Millions (95% CI)† | Drinks Consumed Within Age Category, % (95% CI)† | All Drinks Consumed, % (95% CI)† |
|---|---|---|---|---|
| 12-20 | 35.2 (32.9-37.5) | 20 104.0 (17 650.1-22 817.7) | 100.0 (NA) | 18.1 (17.3-18.8) |
| Met *DSM-IV* criteria | 64.3 (58.9-69.7) | 9509.9 (8864.9-10 126.9) | 47.3 (46.1-48.3) | 8.5 (8.0-9.1) |
| Did not meet *DSM-IV* criteria | 25.0 (22.7-27.4) | 10 594.1 (8785.2-12 690.8) | 52.7 (51.7-53.9) | 9.5 (7.9-11.4) |
| ≥21 | 25.4 (24.0-26.8) | 91 226.8 (80 285.9-113 484.5) | 100.0 (NA) | 81.9 (81.2-82.7) |
| Met *DSM-IV* criteria | 66.4 (60.3-72.5) | 22 791.1 (20 856.2-34 788.8) | 25.0 (22.6-27.3) | 20.5 (18.7-22.2) |
| Did not meet *DSM-IV* criteria | 21.0 (19.7-22.4) | 68 435.7 (59 429.7-78 695.7) | 75.0 (72.7-77.4) | 61.5 (53.4-70.1) |
| Total | 26.7 (25.2-28.3) | 111 330.8 (97 935.3-136 302.2) | 100.0 (NA) | 100.0 (NA) |
| Met *DSM-IV* criteria | 65.8 (59.9-71.6) | 32 301.0 (29 721.1-44 915.7) | 29.0 (NA) | 29.0 (NA) |
| Did not meet *DSM-IV* criteria | 21.5 (20.1-22.9) | 79 029.9 (68 214.9-91 386.5) | 71.0 (NA) | 71.0 (NA) |

Abbreviations: CI, confidence interval; *DSM-IV, Diagnostic and Statistical Manual of Mental Disorders, Fourth Edition*; NA, not applicable.
*Data are from the 2001 National Household Survey of Drug Abuse.
†Calculated values.

ria for alcohol abuse and dependence were 25.9% among those aged 12 to 20 years and 9.6% among those aged 21 years and older. Whereas people aged 12 to 20 years composed 15.4% of the population aged 12 years and older, they composed 30.1% of those meeting the *DSM-IV* criteria for alcohol abuse or dependence. Underage drinkers were 2.7 times likelier to meet the *DSM-IV* criteria for alcohol abuse or dependence as compared with adult drinkers. These results are presented in **Table 2**.

The mean number of drinks, the total number of drinks, and the percentage of drinks consumed by age and *DSM-IV* categories are presented in **Table 3**. Those who met the *DSM-IV* criteria for alcohol abuse or dependence drank, on average, 3 times as much per month as those who did not meet the criteria. Underage drinkers (aged 12 to 20 years) who met the *DSM-IV* criteria represent one quarter (25.9%) of drinkers in that age group, but they consumed nearly half of all drinks (47.3%) in that age category. Adult drinkers (aged 21 years and older) who met the *DSM-IV* criteria represent 9.6% of drinkers in that age group, but they consumed 25.0% of all drinks in that age category.

The cash value of alcohol consumption is presented in **Table 4**. An estimated $128.6 billion was spent on alcohol in the United States in 2001.[29-31] Of this amount, 28.3%, or $36.3 billion, was attributable to abusive or dependent drinking. Underage abusive and dependent drinking alone accounted for 8.2% of total consumer expenditures for alcohol; adult abusive and dependent drinking accounted for 20.1% of all of the expenditures.

The total cash value of underage drinking was $22.5 billion in 2001, or 17.5% of total consumer expenditures for alcohol. Adult drinkers who met the *DSM-IV* criteria for alcohol abuse and dependence accounted for another $25.8 billion in consumer expenditures for alcohol. Underage drinkers and adults who met the *DSM-IV* criteria for alcohol abuse or dependence together were responsible for 37.5% ($48.3 billion) of all of the consumer expenditures for alcohol.

## CASH VALUE OF UNDERAGE DRINKING AND ABUSIVE AND DEPENDENT DRINKING TO THE ALCOHOL INDUSTRY USING AN ALTERNATIVE ESTIMATE

We used the NESARC data instead of the NHSDA and Behavioral Risk Factor Surveillance Survey data to compute alternative estimates of drinking rates, consumption, and pathological drinking rates for adults aged 21 years and older. Because the NESARC did not include persons aged 12 to 17 years, we continued to use the YRBS data to estimate drinking rates and the NHSDA data to estimate drinking amounts and pathological drinking rates among underage drinkers. In this alternative analysis, we found that underage drinkers and adults who met the *DSM-IV* criteria for alcohol abuse or dependence together were responsible for nearly half (48.8%, or $62.9 billion) of all of the consumer expenditures for alcohol.

## COMMENT

There are several limitations of our research. First, several data sets were used to derive various estimates for youth and adults. Although it would have been preferable to have 1 source of data, thereby controlling for possible moderating factors such as item construction, method of administration, and time, no such single data source exists. Therefore, as in other research of this nature, we used the data sources that provided valid estimates of all of the quantities of interest and provided a conservative and alternative estimate. All of the data that we used were publicly available national data sources.

We also made several assumptions about the proportion of each type of alcoholic beverage consumed by the various age and drinking groups. More research is clearly necessary, especially among underage drinkers, to obtain direct estimates of consumption amount by type and cost. The operational definition of the term *drink* also needs further exploration. The estimates produced by the NHSDA[20] were based on the number of drinks of wine, beer, or distilled spirits whereas alternative approaches (the 2001-2002 NESARC,[32] the study by Kaskutas and Graves,[36] and the study by Dawson[37]) were based on the actual size of the beverage consumed rather than on the number of drinks.

For the alcohol industry, increases in alcohol consumption come either from new customers or from increased drinking among existing customers. This analysis demonstrates that early initiation of alcohol use provides substantial financial value to the alcohol industry in both areas. The short-term cash value is the immediate return of at least $22.5 billion in consumer expenditures linked to alcohol consumed by minors—ie, new customers. Because these underage drinkers are likelier to become adult drinkers with alcohol abuse and dependence, the longer-term cash value of early initiation is their significant contribution to the $25.8 billion per year in consumer expenditures for alcohol consumed by adult drinkers with alcohol abuse and dependence—ie, increased drinking among existing customers. Almost all (96.8%) of the adult drinkers with alcohol abuse and dependence began drinking prior to the age of 21 years.[20] The combined annual worth of all underage drinking (including abusive and dependent drinking) and all adult abusive and dependent drinking to the industry is at least $48.3 billion, or 37.5% of total consumer expenditures for alcohol, with alternative estimates suggesting that these costs may be closer to $62.9 billion, or 48.8% of total consumer expenditures for alcohol. Projected into the future, this present pattern of illegal underage drinking and adult abusive and dependent drinking will realize at least one-half trillion dollars in cash revenues for the alcohol industry over the next decade—an extraordinary commercial motive to insure that such consumer behavior continues unabated.

**Table 4. Expenditures on Alcohol by Age Category and *Diagnostic and Statistical Manual of Mental Disorders, Fourth Edition* Criteria for Alcohol Abuse or Dependence Using Total Sales Reported by Industry**

| Age, y | Drinks, No. in Billions | Total Dollars in Billions | Total Dollars, % |
|---|---|---|---|
| 12-20 | | | |
| Met *DSM-IV* criteria | 9.5 | 10.5 | 8.2 |
| Did not meet *DSM-IV* criteria | 10.6 | 12.0 | 9.3 |
| ≥21 | | | |
| Met *DSM-IV* criteria | 22.8 | 25.8 | 20.1 |
| Did not meet *DSM-IV* criteria | 68.4 | 80.3 | 62.4 |
| **Total** | **111.3** | **128.6** | **100.0** |

Abbreviation: *DSM-IV, Diagnostic and Statistical Manual of Mental Disorders, Fourth Edition.*

The drinking behavior of 25.9% of the underage drinkers already met clinical criteria for alcohol abuse and dependence. Although youth aged 12 to 20 years composed 15.4% of the population aged 12 years and older, they made up 30.1% of all of the drinkers in the United States who met the *DSM-IV* criteria for abusive and dependent drinking. Of the $128.6 billion in consumer expenditures for alcohol in the United States in 2001, $36.3 billion, or 28.3% of market sales, came from drinking on the part of adults and children who met the *DSM-IV* criteria for alcohol abuse and dependence in the past year. A drinker with alcohol abuse and dependence is 3 times more valuable to the alcohol industry since such drinkers consume 3 times the amount of alcohol that other drinkers consume.

With at least 37.5% of sales linked to underage drinking and adult abusive and dependent drinking, the alcohol industry has a compelling financial motive to attempt to maintain or increase rates of underage drinking. Alcohol advertisements in magazines, for example, expose youth aged 12 to 20 years to 45% more beer advertisements and 27% more advertisements for distilled spirits than adults of legal drinking age.[38-40] The same pattern of overexposure of children relative to adults with advertisements for beer and distilled spirits also can be seen in radio and television advertising.[41,42] Furthermore, exposure of children and teens to magazine and television alcohol advertisements has increased, even more so for girls than boys, despite national reports[43-45] calling for limits on advertising by the alcohol industry to children and teens younger than 21 years. Allegations that the alcohol industry profits from unfair and deceptive marketing practices aimed at underage drinkers to assure this flow of profits is the subject of several lawsuits filed against the alcohol industry.[46-48]

The financial interests of the alcohol industry appear to be antithetic to the public health interests of the nation in preventing and limiting pathological drinking. The public health implications of this research are two-fold. First, because of this apparent conflict of interest, the alcohol industry is not a good candidate to regulate its own marketing and sales practices, particularly as they relate to underage drinking. Second, the fact that 25.9% of underage drinkers (12.2% of youth aged 12-20 years) already met *DSM-IV* criteria for abusive and dependent drinking underscores the critical importance of comprehensive prevention strategies and treatment options tailored to the needs of teens.

**Accepted for Publication:** October 26, 2005.
**Correspondence:** Susan E. Foster, The National Center on Addiction and Substance Abuse at Columbia University, 633 Third Ave, New York, NY 10017 (sfoster@casacolumbia.org)
**Acknowledgment:** We thank Elizabeth Peters for her expert assistance with the data analysis, David Man, PhD, who provided library assistance, and Jane Carlson, BS, for her help with manuscript preparation.

## REFERENCES


1. US Department of Health and Human Services. *Healthy People 2010: With Understanding and Improving Health and Objectives for Improving Health.* 2nd ed. Washington, DC: US Government Printing Office; 2000. Available at: http://www.healthypeople.gov/Document/pdf/uih/2010uih.pdf. Accessed February 7, 2005.
2. US Department of Agriculture; US Department of Health and Human Services. *Nutrition and Your Health: Dietary Guidelines for Americans.* Washington, DC: US Dept of Health and Human Services; 2000.
3. American Psychiatric Association. *Diagnostic and Statistical Manual of Mental Disorders, Fourth Edition.* Washington, DC: American Psychiatric Association; 1994.
4. Harwood H. *Updating Estimates of the Economic Costs of Alcohol Abuse in the United States: Estimates, Update Methods, and Data.* Falls Church, Va: The Lewin Group for the National Institute on Alcohol Abuse and Alcoholism; 2000.
5. National Heart, Lung, and Blood Institute; National Institute of Diabetes and Digestive and Kidney Diseases; National Institutes of Health. *Clinical Guidelines on the Identification, Evaluation, and Treatment of Overweight and Obesity in Adults: The Evidence Report.* Bethesda, Md: National Institutes of Health; 1998. Available at: http://www.nhlbi.nih.gov/guidelines/obesity/ob_home.htm. Accessed February 22, 2005.
6. Grant BF, Dawson DA. Age of onset of drug use and its association with DSM-IV drug abuse and dependence: results from the National Longitudinal Alcohol Epidemiologic Survey. *J Subst Abuse.* 1998;10:163-173.
7. Grant BF, Stinson FS, Hartford TC. Age at onset of alcohol use and DSM-IV alcohol abuse and dependence: a 12-year follow-up. *J Subst Abuse.* 2001;13:493-504.
8. Grant BF. The impact of a family history of alcoholism on the relationship between age at onset of alcohol use and DSM-IV alcohol dependence: results from the National Longitudinal Alcohol Epidemiologic Survey. *Alcohol Health Res World.* 1998;22:144-147.
9. Brook DW, Brook JS, Zhang C, Cohen P, Whiteman M. Drug use and the risk of major depressive disorder, alcohol dependence, and substance use disorders. *Arch Gen Psychiatry.* 2002;59:1039-1044.
10. Hasin DS, Glick H. Severity of DSM-III-R alcohol dependence: United States, 1988. *Br J Addict.* 1992;87:1725-1730.
11. Windle M. Alcohol use and abuse: some findings from the National Adolescent Student Health Survey. *Alcohol Health Res World.* 1991;15:5-10.
12. DeWit DJ, Adlaf EM, Offord DR, Ogborne AC. Age at first alcohol use: a risk factor for the development of alcohol disorders. *Am J Psychiatry.* 2000;157:745-750.
13. Barnes GM, Welte JW. Patterns and predictors of alcohol use among 7-12th grade students in New York State. *J Stud Alcohol.* 1986;47:53-62.
14. Chou SP, Pickering RP. Early onset of drinking as a risk factor for lifetime alcohol-related problems. *Br J Addict.* 1992;87:1199-1204.
15. Centers for Disease Control and Prevention. *Youth Risk Behavior Surveillance System.* Atlanta, Ga: US Dept of Health and Human Services; 2001.
16. Gerstein DR. Alcohol use and consequences. In: Moore MH, Gerstein DR, eds. *Alcohol and Public Policy: Beyond the Shadow of Prohibition.* Washington, DC: National Academy Press; 1981:182-224.
17. Greenfield TK, Rogers JD. Who drinks most of the alcohol in the US? the policy implications. *J Stud Alcohol.* 1999;60:78-89.
18. Foster SE, Vaughan RD, Foster WH, Califano JA. Alcohol consumption and expenditures for underage drinking and adult excessive drinking. *JAMA.* 2003;289:989-995.
19. US Department of Commerce; US Census Bureau. Profiles of general demographic characteristics, 2002. Available at: http://landview.census.gov/prod/cen2000/dp1/2kh00.pdf. Accessed January 23, 2003.
20. Office of Applied Studies, Substance Abuse and Mental Health Services Administration, US Department of Health and Human Services. *National Household Survey on Drug Abuse, 2001* [computer file]. ICPSR version. Research Triangle Park, NC: Research Triangle Institute [producer], 2002. Ann Arbor, Mich: Inter-university Consortium for Political and Social Research [distributor], 2003.
21. Centers for Disease Control and Prevention. *Youth Risk Behavioral Surveillance.* Atlanta, Ga: US Dept of Health and Human Services; 1999.
22. Cowan CD. Coverage, sample design, and weighting in three federal surveys. *J Drug Issues.* 2001;31:599-614.
23. Fendrich M, Johnson TP. Examining prevalence differences in three national surveys of youth: impact of consent procedures, mode, and editing rules. *J Drug Issues.* 2001;31:615-642.
24. Fowler FJ Jr, Stringfellow VL. Learning from experience: estimating teen use of alcohol, cigarettes, and marijuana from three survey protocols. *J Drug Issues.* 2001;31:643-664.
25. Gfroerer J, Wright D, Kopstein A. Prevalence of youth substance use: the impact of methodological differences between two national surveys. *Drug Alcohol Depend.* 1997;47:19-30.
26. Schuman H, Presser S. *Questions and Answers in Attitude Surveys: Experiments on Form, Wording and Content.* New York, NY: Sage; 1981.
27. Harrison LD. Understanding the differences in youth drug prevalence rates produced by the MTF, NHSDA, and YRBS studies. *J Drug Issues.* 2001;31:665-694.
28. Centers for Disease Control and Prevention. *Behavioral Risk Factor Surveillance System Survey Data.* Atlanta, Ga: US Dept of Health and Human Services; 2001.
29. Adams Beverage Group. *Adams Beer Handbook.* Norwalk, Ct: Adams Business Research; 2002.
30. Adams Beverage Group. *Adams Liquor Handbook.* Norwalk, Ct: Adams Business Research; 2002.
31. Adams Beverage Group. *Adams Wine Handbook.* Norwalk, Ct: Adams Business Research; 2002.
32. National Institute on Alcohol Abuse and Alcoholism. *2001-2002 National Epidemiologic Survey on Alcohol and Related Conditions.* Bethesda, Md: National Institute on Alcohol Abuse and Alcoholism; 2002.
33. Roberts M. Hard beverages tap into America's thirst for something different, 2002. Available at: http://www.restaurant.org/rusa/magArticle. Accessed July 21, 2005.
34. Grapefinds. Beer. Available at: http://www.grapefinds.net/db/Beer. Accessed July 21, 2005.
35. Beverages & More! Product list.Available at: http://www.bevmo.com/productlist. Accessed July 21, 2005.
36. Kaskutas LA, Graves K. An alternative to standard drinks as a measure of alcohol consumption. *J Subst Abuse.* 2000;12:67-78.
37. Dawson DA. Volume of ethanol consumption: effects of different approaches to measurement. *J Stud Alcohol.* 1998;59:191-197.
38. Center on Alcohol Marketing and Youth. *Overexposed: Youth a Target of Alcohol Advertising in Magazines.* Washington, DC: Center on Alcohol Marketing and Youth; 2002.
39. Garfield CF, Chung PJ, Rathouz PJ. Alcohol advertising in magazines and adolescent readership. *JAMA.* 2003;289:2424-2429.
40. Center on Alcohol Marketing and Youth. *Radio Daze: Alcohol Ads Tune in Underage Youth.* Washington, DC: Center on Alcohol Marketing and Youth; 2003.
41. Center on Alcohol Marketing and Youth. *Television: Alcohol's Vast Adland.* Washington, DC: Center on Alcohol Marketing and Youth; 2002.
42. Jernigan DH, Ostroff J, Ross C, O'Hara JA III. Sex differences in adolescent exposure to alcohol advertising in magazines. *Arch Pediatr Adolesc Med.* 2004;158:629-634.
43. Committee on Developing a Strategy to Reduce and Prevent Underage Drinking. *Reducing Underage Drinking: A Collective Responsibility.* Bonnie RJ, O'Connell ME, eds; Washington, DC: Board on Children, Youth and Families, Division of Behavioral and Social Sciences and Education, Research Council and Institute of Medicine; 2004.
44. American Medical Association. Underage drinkers at higher risk of brain damage than adults, American Medical Association report reveals. Available at: http://www.alcoholpolicysolutions.net/pdf/RUDC_dec_nr.pdf. Accessed December 9, 2002.
45. National Center on Addiction and Substance Abuse. *Teen Tipplers: America's Underage Drinking Epidemic.* New York, NY: National Center on Addiction and Substance Abuse, Columbia University; 2002.
46. *Hakki v Zima Co et al,* Superior Court of the District of Columbia, Case No. 03-cv-2621-GK (2003).
47. *Kreft v Zima Beverage Co et al,* District Court and County of Denver, Colo, Case No. 03-cv-9229 (2003).
48. *Wilson v Zima Co et al,* Superior Court Division, General Court of Justice, Mecklenburg County, NC, Case No. 04-cvs-626 (2004).

**PEDIARIX™ [Diphtheria and Tetanus Toxoids and Acellular Pertussis Adsorbed, Hepatitis B (Recombinant) and Inactivated Poliovirus Vaccine Combined]**

The following is a brief summary only; see full prescribing information for complete product information.

**CONTRAINDICATIONS:** Hypersensitivity to any component of the vaccine, including yeast, neomycin, and polymyxin B, is a contraindication (see DESCRIPTION in complete prescribing information). Do not use PEDIARIX after a serious allergic reaction (e.g., anaphylaxis) temporally associated with a previous dose of this vaccine or with any components of this vaccine. Because of the uncertainty as to which component of the vaccine might be responsible, do not give further vaccination with any of these components; or, refer such individuals to an allergist for evaluation. The following events are contraindications to administration of PEDIARIX: encephalopathy (e.g., coma, decreased level of consciousness, prolonged seizures) within 7 days of administration of a previous dose of a pertussis-containing vaccine that is not attributable to another identifiable cause; progressive neurologic disorder, including infantile spasms, uncontrolled epilepsy, or progressive encephalopathy. Do not vaccinate individuals with such conditions until a treatment regimen has been established and the condition has stabilized. PEDIARIX is not contraindicated for use in individuals with HIV infection.

**WARNINGS:** Administration of PEDIARIX is associated with higher rates of fever relative to separately administered vaccines. In one study that evaluated medically attended fever after the first dose of PEDIARIX or separately administered vaccines, infants who received PEDIARIX had a higher rate of medical encounters for fever within the first 4 days following vaccination. In some infants, these encounters included the performance of diagnostic studies to evaluate other causes of fever (see ADVERSE REACTIONS). The vial stopper is latex-free. The tip cap and the rubber plunger of the needleless prefilled syringes contain dry natural latex rubber that may cause allergic reactions in latex sensitive individuals. If any of the following events occur in temporal relation to receipt of whole-cell DTP or a vaccine containing an acellular pertussis component, consider carefully whether to give subsequent doses of PEDIARIX or any vaccine containing a pertussis component: temperature of ≥40.5°C (105°F) within 48 hours not due to another identifiable cause; collapse or shock-like state (hypotonic-hyporesponsive episode) within 48 hours; persistent, inconsolable crying lasting ≥3 hours, occurring within 48 hours; seizures with or without fever occurring within 3 days. If Guillain-Barré syndrome occurs within 6 weeks of receipt of prior vaccine containing tetanus toxoid, the decision to give subsequent doses of PEDIARIX or any vaccine containing tetanus toxoid should be based on careful consideration of the potential benefits and possible risks. A committee of the Institute of Medicine (IOM) has concluded that evidence is consistent with a causal relationship between whole-cell DTP vaccine and acute neurologic illness, and under special circumstances, between whole-cell DTP vaccine and chronic neurologic disease in the context of the National Childhood Encephalopathy Study (NCES) report; however, evidence was insufficient to indicate whether or not whole-cell DTP vaccine increased the overall risk of chronic neurologic disease. Acute encephalopathy and permanent neurologic damage have not been reported causally linked or in temporal association with administration of PEDIARIX, but the experience with PEDIARIX is insufficient to rule this out. Encephalopathy has been reported following INFANRIX® (Diphtheria and Tetanus Toxoids and Acellular Pertussis Vaccine Adsorbed) (see ADVERSE REACTIONS, Postmarketing Reports), but data are not sufficient to evaluate a causal relationship. The decision to administer a pertussis-containing vaccine to children with stable central nervous system (CNS) disorders must be made by the physician on an individual basis, with consideration of all relevant factors, and assessment of potential risks and benefits for that individual. Advise the parent or guardian of the potential increased risk involved (see PRECAUTIONS). A family history of seizures or other CNS disorders is not a contraindication to pertussis vaccine. For children at higher risk for seizures than the general population, an appropriate antipyretic may be administered at the time of vaccination and for the ensuing 24 hours according to the respective prescribing information recommended dosage to reduce the possibility of post-vaccination fever. Defer vaccination during the course of a moderate or severe illness with or without fever and vaccinate patients as soon as they have recovered from the acute phase of the illness. Do not give PEDIARIX to children on anticoagulant therapy or those with bleeding disorders unless the potential benefit clearly outweighs the risk of administration (see PRECAUTIONS in complete prescribing information).

**PRECAUTIONS:** Before the injection of any biological, the physician should take all reasonable precautions to prevent allergic or other adverse reactions. Epinephrine injection (1:1000) and other appropriate agents used for the control of immediate allergic reactions must be immediately available should an acute anaphylactic reaction occur. Immunosuppressed individuals, including those receiving immunosuppressive therapy, may not develop the expected immune response. **Drug Interactions:** For information regarding concomitant administration with other vaccines, refer to DOSAGE AND ADMINISTRATION in complete prescribing information. Do not mix PEDIARIX with any other vaccine in the same syringe or vial. **Carcinogenesis, Mutagenesis, Impairment of Fertility:** PEDIARIX has not been evaluated for carcinogenic or mutagenic potential, or for impairment of fertility. **Pregnancy:** Pregnancy Category C: PEDIARIX is not indicated for women of child-bearing age. Animal reproduction studies have not been conducted with PEDIARIX. It is not known whether PEDIARIX can cause fetal harm when administered to a pregnant woman or if PEDIARIX can affect reproductive capacity. **Geriatric Use:** PEDIARIX is not indicated for use in adult populations. **Pediatric Use:** Safety and effectiveness of PEDIARIX in infants younger than 6 weeks of age have not been evaluated (see DOSAGE AND ADMINISTRATION in complete prescribing information). PEDIARIX is not recommended for persons 7 years of age or older. Tetanus and Diphtheria Toxoids Adsorbed (Td) For Adult Use, inactivated poliovirus vaccine (IPV), and Hepatitis B Vaccine (Recombinant) should be used in individuals 7 years of age or older.

**ADVERSE REACTIONS:** A total of 20,739 doses of PEDIARIX have been administered to 7,028 infants as a 3-dose primary series. The most common adverse reactions observed in clinical trials were local injection site reactions (pain, redness, or swelling), fever, and fussiness. In comparative studies, administration of PEDIARIX was associated with higher rates of fever relative to separately administered vaccines (see WARNINGS). The prevalence of fever was highest on the day of vaccination and the day following vaccination. More than 98% of episodes of fever resolved within the 4-day period following vaccination (i.e., the period including the day of vaccination and the next 3 days). Rates of most other solicited adverse events following PEDIARIX were comparable to rates observed following separately administered US-licensed vaccines. The adverse event information from clinical trials provides a basis for identifying adverse events that appear to be related to vaccine use and for approximating rates. However, because clinical trials are conducted under widely varying conditions, adverse event rates observed in the clinical trials of a vaccine cannot be directly compared to rates in the clinical trials of another vaccine, and may not reflect the rates observed in practice. A total of 5,472 infants were enrolled in a German safety study that was originally designed to compare the safety and reactogenicity of PEDIARIX administered concomitantly at separate sites with 1 of 4 *Haemophilus influenzae* type b (Hib) vaccines at 3, 4, and 5 months of age. After enrollment of 1,569 infants, the study was amended to include a control group that received INFANRIX, Hib vaccine, and oral poliovirus vaccine (OPV) separately. Infants in the separate administration group received one less antigen (hepatitis B) than the infants who received PEDIARIX. Safety data were available for 4,666 infants who received PEDIARIX administered concomitantly at separate sites with 1 of 4 Hib vaccines and for 768 infants in the control group that received separate vaccines. The primary end-point of the study was the percentage of infants with any grade 3 solicited symptom (redness or swelling >20 mm, fever >103.1°F, or crying, pain, vomiting, diarrhea, loss of appetite, or restlessness that prevented normal daily activities) over the 3-dose primary series in infants who received PEDIARIX (4 groups that received PEDIARIX and Hib vaccines pooled) compared to the group that received INFANRIX and Hib vaccine separately with OPV. Analysis for the primary end-point was performed on the according-to-protocol (ATP) cohort that included only those infants who were enrolled after the protocol amendment to include a control group. Of 3,773 infants in the ATP cohort for whom safety data were available, 16.2% (95% CI: 14.9% to 17.5%) of 3,029 infants who received PEDIARIX and Hib vaccine compared to 20.3% (95% CI: 17.5% to 23.4%) of 744 infants who received separate vaccines were reported to have had at least one grade 3 solicited symptom within 4 days of vaccination (i.e., day of vaccination and the next 3 days). The difference between groups in the rate of grade 3 symptoms was 4.1% (90% CI: 1.4% to 7.1%). These were the rates for selected solicited symptoms within 4 days following each dose in a 3-dose primary series in infants who received PEDIARIX administered concomitantly with Hib vaccine and those who received separate concomitant administration of INFANRIX, Hib vaccine, and OPV for the intent-to-treat (ITT) cohort (includes all infants enrolled before and after the amendment who received the indicated vaccine and for whom at least one symptom sheet was completed):

**Percentage of German Infants With Solicited Local Reactions or Selected Systemic Adverse Events Within 4 Days of Vaccination* (ITT Cohort)**

| | PEDIARIX & Hib | | | INFANRIX, Hib, & OPV | | |
|---|---|---|---|---|---|---|
| | Dose 1 | Dose 2 | Dose 3 | Dose 1 | Dose 2 | Dose 3 |
| **N** | **4,666** | **4,619** | **4,574** | **768** | **757** | **750** |
| **Local[†]** | | | | | | |
| Pain, any | 14.0 | 10.2 | 9.9 | 14.2 | 9.8 | 8.1 |
| Pain, grade 2 or 3 | 2.9 | 1.2 | 1.5 | 3.6 | 1.7 | 1.1 |
| Pain, grade 3 | 0.7 | 0.3 | 0.3 | 1.3 | 0.4 | 0.1 |
| Redness, any | 18.6 | 26.6 | 25.6 | 16.1 | 21.4 | 20.8 |
| Redness, >5 mm | 6.7 | 9.9 | 9.0 | 5.9 | 8.2 | 7.7 |
| Redness, >20 mm | 1.2 | 1.0 | 1.1 | 1.8 | 0.7 | 1.1 |
| Swelling, any | 12.7 | 18.5 | 18.4 | 9.6 | 12.9 | 13.6 |
| Swelling, >5 mm | 5.6 | 7.7 | 7.8 | 3.6 | 5.2 | 4.8 |
| Swelling, >20 mm | 1.2 | 1.6 | 1.5 | 1.3 | 1.1 | 1.2 |
| **Systemic** | | | | | | |
| Restlessness, any | 41.4 | 32.0 | 26.7 | 46.4 | 35.0 | 27.6 |
| Restlessness, grade 2 or 3 | 14.4 | 10.0 | 8.9 | 20.2 | 11.5 | 8.4 |
| Restlessness, grade 3 | 3.0 | 1.5 | 1.6 | 5.7 | 3.0 | 1.7 |
| Fever[‡], ≥100.4°F | 25.1 | 19.3 | 19.7 | 13.2 | 13.1 | 11.2 |
| Fever[‡], >101.3°F | 5.8 | 4.1 | 4.6 | 2.2 | 2.8 | 2.1 |
| Fever[‡], >103.1°F | 0.3 | 0.5 | 0.7 | 0.3 | 0.3 | 0.5 |
| Unusual cry[§], any | 24.9 | 16.5 | 13.1 | 36.5 | 19.7 | 14.3 |
| Unusual cry[§], grade 2 or 3 | 12.7 | 7.1 | 5.7 | 20.8 | 10.0 | 5.7 |
| Unusual cry[§], grade 3 | 3.9 | 1.7 | 1.4 | 6.8 | 2.1 | 1.1 |
| Loss of appetite, any | 17.9 | 13.3 | 12.5 | 19.1 | 16.2 | 11.3 |
| Loss of appetite, grade 2 or 3 | 4.0 | 2.9 | 2.7 | 4.4 | 2.9 | 2.3 |
| Loss of appetite, grade 3 | 0.6 | 0.5 | 0.4 | 0.5 | 0.7 | 0.0 |

N = number of infants in the intent-to-treat (ITT) cohort.
Grade 2 defined as sufficiently discomforting to interfere with daily activities.
Grade 3 defined as preventing normal daily activities.
* Within 4 days of vaccination defined as day of vaccination and the next 3 days.
† Local reactions at the injection site for PEDIARIX or INFANRIX.
‡ Rectal temperatures.
§ Unusual cry lasting >1 hour.

In this study, infants were also monitored for unsolicited adverse events that occurred within 30 days following vaccination. Over the entire study period, 6 subjects in the group that received PEDIARIX reported seizures. Two of these subjects had a febrile seizure, 1 of whom also developed afebrile seizures. The remaining 4 subjects had afebrile seizures, including 2 with infantile spasms. Two subjects reported seizures within 7 days following vaccination (1 subject had both febrile and afebrile seizures, and 1 subject had afebrile seizures), corresponding to a rate of 0.22 seizures per 1,000 doses (febrile seizures 0.07 per 1,000 doses, afebrile seizures 0.14 per 1,000 doses). No subject who received concomitant INFANRIX, Hib vaccine, and OPV reported seizures. In a separate German study that evaluated the safety of INFANRIX in 22,505 infants who received 66,867 doses of INFANRIX administered as a 3-dose primary series, the rate of seizures within 7 days of vaccination with INFANRIX was 0.13 per 1,000 doses (febrile seizures 0.0 per 1,000 doses, afebrile seizures 0.13 per 1,000 doses). No cases of hypotonic-hyporesponsiveness, encephalopathy, or anaphylaxis were reported in the German study that evaluated the safety of PEDIARIX. Rates of serious adverse events that are less common than those reported in this safety study are not known at this time.

Additional safety data for PEDIARIX are available from a US study designed to evaluate lot-to-lot consistency and a bridge for a new manufacturing step. These were the rates for local reactions and selected adverse events within 4 days of vaccination with PEDIARIX administered concomitantly with a Hib vaccine at 2, 4, and 6 months of age:

**Percentage of US Infants With Solicited Local Reactions or Selected Systemic Adverse Events Within 4 Days of Vaccination* (ITT Cohort)**

| | PEDIARIX & Hib | | |
|---|---|---|---|
| | Dose 1 | Dose 2 | Dose 3 |
| **Local[†]** | **N = 482** | **N = 469** | **N = 466** |
| Pain, any | 30.5 | 25.4 | 23.0 |
| Pain, grade 2 or 3 | 6.2 | 5.5 | 3.6 |
| Pain, grade 3 | 1.2 | 0.6 | 0.6 |
| Redness, any | 25.3 | 32.6 | 35.6 |
| Redness, >5 mm | 9.3 | 10.4 | 8.6 |
| Redness, >20 mm | 0.6 | 1.5 | 1.3 |
| Swelling, any | 15.1 | 16.6 | 22.3 |
| Swelling, >5 mm | 6.8 | 6.2 | 6.4 |
| Swelling, >20 mm | 1.0 | 1.3 | 1.3 |
| **Systemic** | **N = 482** | **N = 469** | **N = 467** |
| Restlessness, any | 28.8 | 30.3 | 28.5 |
| Restlessness, grade 2 or 3 | 7.1 | 9.0 | 9.4 |
| Restlessness, grade 3 | 1.0 | 1.1 | 0.6 |
| Fever[‡], ≥100.4°F | 26.6 | 31.3 | 25.9 |
| Fever[‡], >101.3°F | 2.9 | 6.2 | 4.7 |
| Fever[‡], >103.1°F | 0.0 | 0.2 | 0.6 |
| Fussiness, any | 61.8 | 63.8 | 57.0 |
| Fussiness, grade 2 or 3 | 14.9 | 21.5 | 17.1 |
| Fussiness, grade 3 | 2.7 | 3.4 | 1.7 |
| Loss of appetite, any | 21.6 | 19.8 | 18.8 |
| Loss of appetite, grade 2 or 3 | 3.1 | 3.2 | 2.4 |
| Loss of appetite, grade 3 | 0.2 | 0.4 | 0.0 |
| Sleeping more than usual, any | 46.7 | 31.8 | 28.1 |
| Sleeping more than usual, grade 2 or 3 | 10.2 | 6.0 | 4.7 |
| Sleeping more than usual, grade 3 | 1.7 | 0.4 | 0.6 |

N = number of infants in the intent-to-treat (ITT) cohort (infants who received the indicated vaccine and for whom at least one symptom sheet was completed).
Grade 2 defined as sufficiently discomforting to interfere with daily activities.
Grade 3 defined as preventing normal daily activities.
* Within 4 days of vaccination defined as day of vaccination and the next 3 days.
† Local reactions at the injection site for PEDIARIX.
‡ Rectal temperatures.

In another US study, these were the rates for fever within 4 days following dose 1 (i.e., day of vaccination and the next 3 days) at 2 months of age in infants who received PEDIARIX when administered concomitantly at separate sites with Hib and pneumococcal conjugate vaccines and those who received INFANRIX, ENGERIX-B® [Hepatitis B Vaccine (Recombinant)], IPV, Hib vaccine, and pneumococcal conjugate vaccine:

**Percentage of US Infants With Fever Within 4 Days of Dose 1* (ITT Cohort)**

| | PEDIARIX, Hib, & Pneumococcal Conjugate (N = 667) | INFANRIX, ENGERIX-B, IPV, Hib, & Pneumococcal Conjugate (N = 333) | Separate Vaccine Group Minus Combination Vaccine Group |
|---|---|---|---|
| **Fever[†]** | **%** | **%** | **Difference (95% CI)** |
| ≥100.4°F[‡] | 27.9 | 19.8 | -8.07 (-13.54, -2.60) |
| >101.3°F | 7.0 | 4.5 | -2.54 (-5.50, 0.41) |
| >102.2°F[‡] | 2.2 | 0.3 | -1.95 (-3.22, -0.68) |
| >103.1°F | 0.4 | 0.0 | -0.45 (-0.96, 0.06) |
| M.A.[‡] | 1.2 | 0.0 | -1.20 (-2.03, -037) |

N = number of infants for whom at least one symptom sheet was completed, excluding 3 infants for whom temperature was not measured and 3 infants whose temperature was measured by the tympanic method.
*Within 4 days of dose 1 defined as day of vaccination and the next 3 days.
† Rectal temperatures.
‡ The group that received PEDIARIX compared to separate vaccine group p value <0.05 (2-sided Fisher Exact test) or the 95% confidence interval on the difference between groups does not include 0.
M.A. = Medically attended (a visit to or from medical personnel).

In this study, medical attention (a visit to or from medical personnel) for fever within 4 days following vaccination was sought for 8 infants who received PEDIARIX (1.2%) and no infants who received separately administered vaccines. Four infants were seen by medical personnel in an office setting; no diagnostic tests were performed in 2 of the infants and a complete blood count (CBC) was done in the other 2 infants. Of 3 infants who were seen in an emergency room, all had a CBC and a blood and urine culture performed; chest X-rays were done in 2 of the infants and a nasopharyngeal specimen was tested for Respiratory Syncytial Virus in one of the infants. One infant was hospitalized for a work-up that included a CBC, blood and urine cultures, a lumbar puncture, and a chest X-ray. All episodes of medically attended fever resolved within 4 days post-vaccination.

Limited data are available from a study conducted in Moldova in which infants received a dose of hepatitis B vaccine within 48 hours of birth followed by 3 doses of PEDIARIX at 6, 10, and 14 weeks of age. No information was collected on the HBsAg status of mothers of enrolled infants. These were the rates for local reactions and selected adverse events within 4 days of vaccination with PEDIARIX administered comcomitantly with Hib vaccine following a birth dose of hepatitis B vaccine:

**Percentage of Moldovan Infants With Solicited Local Reactions or Selected Systemic Adverse Events Within 4 Days of Vaccination* (ITT Cohort)**

| | PEDIARIX & Hib | | |
|---|---|---|---|
| | Dose 1 | Dose 2 | Dose 3 |
| **N** | **160** | **158** | **157** |
| **Local[†]** | | | |
| Pain, any | 25.6 | 18.4 | 14.0 |
| Pain, grade 3 | 3.1 | 0.6 | 1.9 |
| Redness, any | 41.9 | 41.8 | 47.1 |
| Redness, >20 mm | 1.9 | 2.5 | 4.5 |
| Swelling, any | 20.6 | 18.4 | 28.0 |
| Swelling, >20 mm | 4.4 | 2.5 | 7.0 |
| **Systemic** | | | |
| Restlessness, any | 13.1 | 10.8 | 8.9 |
| Restlessness, grade 3 | 1.3 | 0.6 | 0.6 |
| Fever[‡], ≥100.4°F | 14.4 | 11.4 | 5.1 |
| Fever[‡], >103.1°F | 0.0 | 0.6 | 0.0 |
| Fussiness, any | 25.0 | 21.5 | 17.8 |
| Fussiness, grade 3 | 2.5 | 0.6 | 0.6 |

N = number of infants in the intent-to-treat (ITT) cohort (infants who received the indicated vaccine and for whom at least one symptom sheet was completed).
Grade 3 defined as preventing normal daily activities.
*Within 4 days of vaccination defined as day of vaccination and the next 3 days.
† Local reactions at the injection site for PEDIARIX.
‡ Rectal temperatures.

Although there was no comparator group who received PEDIARIX without a birth dose of hepatitis B vaccine, available data suggest that some local adverse events may occur at a higher rate when PEDIARIX is administered after a birth dose of hepatitis B vaccine.

As with any vaccine, there is the possibility that broad use of PEDIARIX could reveal adverse events not observed in clinical trials.

**Postmarketing Reports:** Worldwide voluntary reports of adverse events received for INFANRIX and ENGERIX-B in children younger than 7 years of age since market introduction of these US-licensed vaccines are listed below. This list includes adverse events for which 20 or more reports were received with the exception of intussusception, idiopathic thrombocytopenic purpura, thrombocytopenia, anaphylactic reaction, angioedema, encephalopathy, hypotonic-hyporesponsive episode, and alopecia for which fewer than 20 reports were received. These latter events are included either because of the seriousness of the event or the strength of causal connection to components of this or other vaccines or drugs. *Body as a whole*: Asthenia[b], fever[a+b], lethargy[b], malaise[b], Sudden Infant Death Syndrome[a+b]. *Cardiovascular system*: Cyanosis[a+b], edema[b], pallor[b]. *Gastrointestinal system*: Abdominal pain[b], anorexia[b], diarrhea[a+b], intussusception[a+b], nausea[b], vomiting[a+b]. *Hematologic/lymphatic*: Idiopathic thrombocytopenic purpura[a+b], lymphadenopathy[a], thrombocytopenia[a+b]. *Hepatic*: Jaundice[b], liver function tests abnormal[b]. *Hypersensitivity*: Anaphylactic reaction[a+b], angioedema[b], hypersensitivity[a]. *Infections*: Cellulitis[a]. *Injection site reactions*: Injection site reactions[a+b]. *Musculoskeletal*: Arthralgia[b], limb swelling[a+b]. *Nervous system*: Convulsions[a+b], encephalopathy[a], headache[b], hypotonia[a+b], hypotonic-hyporesponsive episode[a], somnolence[a+b]. *Psychiatric*: Crying[a+b], irritability[a+b]. *Respiratory system*: Respiratory tract infection[a]. *Skin and appendages*: Alopecia[b], erythema[a+b], erythema multiforme[b], petechiae[b], pruritus[a+b], rash[a+b], urticaria[a+b]. *Special senses*: Ear pain[a]. [[a] Following INFANRIX; [b] Following ENGERIX-B; [a+b] Following either INFANRIX or ENGERIX-B.] These reactions were reported voluntarily from a population of uncertain size; therefore, it is not always possible to reliably estimate their frequency or establish a causal relationship to vaccination.

**Reporting Adverse Events:** Report the occurrence following immunization of any event set forth in the Vaccine Injury Table from the National Childhood Vaccine Injury Act including: Anaphylaxis or anaphylactic shock within 7 days, encephalopathy or encephalitis within 7 days, brachial neuritis within 28 days, or an acute complication or sequelae (including death) of an illness, disability, injury, or condition referred to above, or any events that would contraindicate further doses of PEDIARIX. The VAERS toll-free number is 1-800-822-7967.

Manufactured by **GlaxoSmithKline Biologicals**, Rixensart, Belgium, US License 1617

Distributed by **GlaxoSmithKline,** Research Triangle Park, NC 27709



Full prescribing information for PEDIARIX is available at www.GSKVaccines.com/Pediarix. BRS-PE:L2

 Printed in USA. PED583R0 June 2005

# Patterns and Knowledge of Nonmedical Use of Stimulants Among College Students

*Bronwen C. Carroll, MD; Thomas J. McLaughlin, ScD; Diane R. Blake, MD*

**Objective:** To determine patterns and knowledge of nonmedical use of stimulants among a sample of college students.

**Design:** Completion of an anonymous survey consisting of 23 questions designed to explore college student use of medications intended to treat attention-deficit/hyperactivity disorder.

**Setting:** A private liberal arts college in New England.

**Participants:** Three hundred forty-seven undergraduate students.

**Main Outcome Measure:** Nonmedical use of stimulants.

**Results:** Thirty-one students (9.2%) reported nonmedical stimulant use. Two hundred forty students (71.4%) had peers who used nonprescribed stimulants, 149 (44.3%) knew of peers who made stimulant medication–seeking visits to a physician although they did not believe that they had attention-deficit/hyperactivity disorder, and 178 (53.0%) knew of people who sold stimulants to students. Nonprescription users were significantly more knowledgeable about the effects of stimulants than nonusers, and nonusers whose peers used nonprescribed stimulants were more knowledgeable about the effects of stimulants than nonusers whose peers did not use nonprescribed stimulants. After controlling for age, race, and sex, the variables that predicted nonmedical use of stimulants were beliefs that stimulants help individuals study better, stay awake, and lose weight.

**Conclusions:** A substantial proportion of college students in this sample were using nonprescribed stimulants. Among nonusers, those whose peers use nonprescribed stimulants were much more knowledgeable about the effects of stimulant use than those whose peers do not use stimulants. This knowledge may confer an increased risk of future nonmedical stimulant use if students become tempted to seek the beneficial effects experienced by their peers.

*Arch Pediatr Adolesc Med. 2006;160:481-485*

Attention-deficit/hyperactivity disorder (ADHD) is characterized by symptoms of inattention and/or hyperactivity-impulsivity that cause impairments in executive function and learning ability that generally persist into adult life.[1] The effectiveness of stimulants on the behavior of hyperactive children was first observed in the 1930s, and use of these medications has been well established for the treatment of ADHD.[2-4] Between 1990 and 1995, there was a 9-fold increase in the population-adjusted rate of ADHD-related stimulant medication prescriptions.[5] During the same period, increased nonmedical use of stimulant medications was also noted. The Monitoring the Future Survey[6] found that the annual prevalence of nonmedical use of Ritalin (methylphenidate hydrochloride) among nationally representative samples of high school seniors increased substantially from 0.1% in 1992 to 2.8% in 1998, and then declined slightly to 2.3% in 2003. However, responses to a new question using a different format to ask about Ritalin use on the 2003 version of the Monitoring the Future Survey documented a higher annual prevalence of 4.0%.[6] The biological mechanism associated with methylphenidate abuse was established in a review of 60 studies showing that methylphenidate functions in a manner similar to dextroamphetamine or cocaine. Both methylphenidate and cocaine block the dopamine transporter, producing comparable increases in synaptic dopamine levels.[7] However, stimulant medications are noteworthy in that individuals without ADHD may experience beneficial effects similar to those of individuals with ADHD.[8]

Both the abuse and misuse of stimulant medications by normal college students have received a considerable amount of attention in the lay press. Increasing numbers of reports have chronicled student use of stimulants as study aids[9-16] and for recreational purposes.[9,11-14,17] The trend of students giving away and/or selling their prescribed stimulant medications to other

**Author Affiliations:**
Departments of Pediatrics (Drs Carroll, McLaughlin, and Blake) and Psychiatry (Dr McLaughlin), University of Massachusetts Medical School, Worcester.

**Table 1. Characteristics of Sample***

| Characteristic (N = 347) | No. (%) |
|---|---|
| Age, mean (SD), y | 19.2 (1.1) |
| Female | 206 (59) |
| Race/ethnicity† | |
| White | 281 (81) |
| African American or black | 16 (5) |
| Asian | 32 (9) |
| Hispanic | 22 (6) |
| Other | 9 (3) |
| ADHD diagnosis | 11 (3) |
| No ADHD diagnosis, No. (%) (n = 336) | |
| Personal nonmedical use | 31 (9) |
| No personal nonmedical use/nonmedical use among peers | 210 (62) |
| No personal nonmedical use/no nonmedical use among peers | 95 (28) |

Abbreviation: ADHD, attention-deficit/hyperactivity disorder.
*Data are presented as number (percentage) unless otherwise indicated.
†Numbers do not add up to total because participants were allowed to choose more than 1 category.

students has recently been noted.[11-14,16] College students seeking stimulants inappropriately from college health services has been reported as well.[16]

The issue of nonmedical use of stimulants has not received as much attention in the medical literature as might be expected. Nevertheless, several reports have documented a problem. Nationally representative samples of 6th through 12th-grade students have shown annual prevalence rates of 4% and 4.5% for nonmedical use of methylphenidate.[18,19] Nonmedical use of stimulants among college students has also been demonstrated. More than 16% of students at a public liberal arts college reported trying methylphenidate recreationally,[20] and 3% of students surveyed at a large public university admitted to past-year nonmedical use of methylphenidate.[21] A recently published study of students at a midwestern university revealed that 17% of men and 11% of women reported nonmedical use of stimulants.[22] Student distribution of stimulant medications has been described as well. Samples of students in grade school and high school have demonstrated rates of 16% and 23% for being approached to sell, give, or trade their prescription stimulant medications.[19,23] Furthermore, not only are students approached, but some actually engage in the distribution of stimulant medication, with 14.7% reporting having given away medication and an additional 7.3% having sold their medication.[24]

Such reports are concerning and suggest that further research is needed to examine and address the nonmedical use of stimulant medications among children and young adults. The present study was undertaken to further explore nonmedical use of stimulant medication among college students. This study goes beyond existing work in that it investigates students' beliefs about the effects of stimulant medications and analyzes trends within peer groups.

## METHODS

A survey consisting of 23 questions about college student use of medications intended to treat ADHD was developed and a pilot survey conducted on 15 young people. Face validity was checked during the administration pilot to ensure that the questions were interpreted with the same meanings as we intended. The survey was administered at a private liberal arts college with a student enrollment of approximately 6000. A cover sheet emphasized that participation was voluntary and that the surveys were completely anonymous and could not be traced back to the student. Students were offered candy to thank them for participating.

Participants were recruited from large lecture hall classes. Once the professor concluded the lecture, a brief announcement was made asking for volunteers to complete a survey. Surveys were then distributed to the entire class; 347 surveys were collected. The manner in which the surveys were distributed precluded the calculation of an exact response rate. A stack of surveys was handed to the person seated at the end of each row and passed along the row. Students who did not want to participate could pass the stack without taking a survey. The response rate is estimated at approximately 80%. Both the University of Massachusetts institutional review board and the institutional review board at the participating college approved the protocol for this study.

Demographic questions included age, sex, and race/ethnicity. Students were then asked if they had ever been diagnosed as having ADHD. The next set of questions asked if they had ever visited a physician because they believed that they might have ADHD, to obtain a prescription for ADHD medication because they believed that they had ADHD, or to obtain a prescription for ADHD medication to help them study or for reasons other than believing that they had ADHD. The questions on ADHD medications listed examples including Adderall (amphetamine and dextroamphetamine) and Ritalin and Concerta (methylphenidate). The survey went on to determine if students had ever used ADHD medications without a prescription, if they had knowledge of peers who used ADHD medications to help them study despite not having ADHD or who had visited a physician to obtain a prescription for ADHD medication despite not believing that they had ADHD, and if they had knowledge of individuals selling ADHD medications to students. Finally, students were then asked to indicate if each of 10 statements about ADHD medications was true or false.

Descriptive analyses included frequencies, means, and standard deviations. Bivariate analyses included the Fisher exact test to compare responses among various groups and the Spearman rank correlation. Binary logistic regression models, in which the outcome was coded as nonmedical use vs nonuse, were used to identify predictors associated with nonmedical use of stimulants.

## RESULTS

General characteristics of the sample are described in **Table 1**. Eleven (3%) of the survey respondents reported receiving an actual ADHD diagnosis, and 10 (2.9%) had received a prescription for stimulants. The remaining analyses were performed for the 336 students who did not report having been given an ADHD diagnosis. Thirty-one (9.2%) reported using nonprescribed stimulants. Three students acknowledged visiting a physician seeking ADHD medications although they believed that they did not have ADHD, 240 (71.6%) knew of peers who used nonprescribed stimulants, 149 (44.3%) knew of peers who had visited a physician to get a prescription for ADHD medication despite not believing that they had ADHD, and 178 (53.0%) knew of people selling ADHD medications to students.

Students who identified themselves as white were significantly more likely than students of other back-

**Table 2. Association of Nonmedical Use With Other Characteristics**

| Variable | Nonmedical Use No. (%) (n = 31) | No Nonmedical Use No. (%) (n = 305) | Fisher Exact Test, *P* Value |
|---|---|---|---|
| Visited physician for ADHD evaluation | 4 (12.9) | 7 (2.3) | .01 |
| Sought medication because thought had ADHD | 3 (9.7) | 0 (0) | .001 |
| Sought medication but did not think had ADHD | 2 (6.5) | 1 (.03) | .02 |
| Knew peers who used ADHD medications nonmedically | 30 (96.8) | 210 (68.9) | <.001 |
| Knew peers who sought medication but did not think had ADHD | 21 (67.7) | 128 (42.0) | .007 |
| Knew of people selling ADHD medications | 24 (77.4) | 154 (50.5) | .004 |

Abbreviation: ADHD, attention-deficit/hyperactivity disorder.

**Table 3. Correlations Between Endorsement of Stimulant Effects and Degree of Exposure to Nonmedical Use**

| Medication Effect (n = 326)* | Nonmedical Users (n = 31), % | Nonusers With Nonmedical Use Among Peers (n = 207), % | Nonusers Without Nonmedical Use Among Peers (n = 88), % | Spearman ρ | *P* Value |
|---|---|---|---|---|---|
| Study longer | 96.8 | 78.8 | 54.5 | .29 | <.001 |
| Study better | 83.9 | 64.7 | 40.9 | .26 | <.001 |
| Relax | 10.0 | 27.5 | 46.6 | −.23 | <.001 |
| Remember more | 27.6 | 28.5 | 28.4 | −.003 | .96 |
| Perform better in sports | 10.3 | 6.8 | 10.2 | −.03 | .60 |
| Good mood | 22.6 | 12.6 | 23.0 | −.06 | .24 |
| Stay awake | 96.8 | 73.4 | 44.3 | .34 | <.001 |
| Maintain better complexion | 0.0 | 4.4 | 5.7 | −.06 | .27 |
| Lose weight | 51.7 | 24.9 | 12.5 | .22 | <.001 |
| Build muscle | 0.0 | 2.5 | 3.4 | −.05 | .36 |

*Ten students did not complete this section of the survey.

**Table 4. Stepwise Logistic Regression for Nonmedical Use (Yes/No)***

| Predictor Variable | Regression Coefficient | *P* Value | Odds Ratio | 95% CI |
|---|---|---|---|---|
| Study better | 1.15 | .04 | 3.17 | 1.05-9.60 |
| Stay awake | 2.20 | .03 | 9.04 | 1.17-69.60 |
| Lose weight | 0.90 | .03 | 2.45 | 1.08-5.56 |

Abbreviation: CI, confidence interval.
*Age, sex, and race were forced into the model, although they had no significant effect.

grounds to know peers who used nonprescribed stimulants (Fisher exact test; $P=.001$) and to know peers who visited physicians seeking stimulants despite not believing that they had ADHD ($P\leq.001$). There were no significant differences between men's and women's responses to any of the questions, with 1 exception. Women were more likely than men to agree that stimulant medications help people lose weight ($P=.004$).

**Table 2** describes associations between nonmedical use of stimulants and other characteristics. When nonusers were further subdivided into those whose peers used nonprescribed stimulants and those whose peers did not use nonprescribed stimulants, members of the former group were more likely to know peers who sought stimulants from physicians for nontherapeutic uses ($P<.001$) and to know of people who sold ADHD medications to students ($P=.004$).

**Table 3** includes the 10 statements used in the survey, and participants were divided into 3 subgroups: (1) nonprescription users, (2) nonusers with nonprescription use among peers, and (3) nonusers without nonprescription use among peers. As demonstrated in Table 3, the efficacy of stimulants in helping one study longer, study better, stay awake, and lose weight was endorsed most strongly by nonprescription users, followed by nonusers whose peers used nonprescribed stimulants. Nonusers whose peers did not use nonprescription stimulants provided the weakest endorsement for these statements. The same trend in the reverse direction was found for beliefs regarding stimulant use and relaxation. Nonprescription users were least likely to agree that stimulants promote relaxation, whereas nonusers whose peers did not use nonprescribed stimulants were the most likely to believe that these agents promoted relaxation. No significant trends were found among groups for the endorsement of false statements about stimulant effects, such as stimulants promoting improved sports performance, complexion, or muscle growth.

**Table 4** indicates that in the multivariate logistic regression model, after controlling for age, race, and sex, nonprescribed stimulant use was independently predicted by the endorsement of 3 statements about stimulants: that they help one study better, help one stay awake, and help one lose weight. The regression accounted for 8% of the variability in response to nonprescribed stimulant use. The *C* statistic of 0.771 demonstrated reasonable goodness of fit.

## COMMENT

The results of this study demonstrate that nonmedical use of stimulants is occurring among some groups of college students. It is concerning not only that nearly 10% of students reported nonmedical use of stimulants, but also that 71.7% reported nonmedical use of stimulants among their peers and 53.3% knew of people selling ADHD medications to students. These estimates suggest that nonmedical use of stimulants has become a relatively common aspect of student life on this college campus. Although the anonymity of the survey was emphasized to participants, students may have felt more comfortable reporting nonprescription stimulant use by "peers" rather than their own use, so the true percentage of students using nonprescribed stimulants may be even higher than reported.

We were surprised that only 3% of our sample reported having an ADHD diagnosis. Possible explanations for this finding include that surveys were collected in large lecture halls, and perhaps students with ADHD are less likely to attend class or perhaps those who do attend are less likely to stay to complete a survey. It has been reported that young adults with ADHD are less likely to graduate from college,[25] which could be due to lower rates of class attendance. Additionally, the public setting in which surveys were filled out may have made students with ADHD self-conscious about acknowledging their diagnosis.

The low rate of reported ADHD diagnoses also raises the possibility that ADHD has been underdiagnosed among this sample of college students. A recent study by Faraone et al[26] found that only 25% of adults diagnosed as having ADHD received the diagnosis during childhood or adolescence.

To our knowledge, this is the first study that describes the phenomenon of students seeking stimulant medications from health care professionals for nontherapeutic purposes. Only 1.2% of students acknowledged engaging in this behavior themselves, yet almost half of the students (44.7%) knew of peers who had done so. These figures underscore the importance of health care professionals seeking corroborating data from parents, teachers, and previous health care professionals if at all possible when college students schedule an appointment to discuss symptoms of ADHD. Of course, students must be willing to provide consent to allow disclosure of relevant information to prevent any breach of patient confidentiality.

Our findings also demonstrate that nonprescription users were more likely than nonusers to have visited a physician to obtain stimulant medications for nonmedical uses. However, some of the nonprescription users endorsed a belief that they had ADHD. Therefore, it is possible that a subgroup of the nonprescription users had undiagnosed ADHD. In their study, Faraone et al[26] found that more than half of the sample they studied with undiagnosed ADHD had previously discussed their symptoms with health care professionals; furthermore, 7 of their top 10 reasons for self-referral were signs or symptoms of ADHD. This suggests that the nonprescription users in our study may be a heterogeneous group composed of students with untreated ADHD as well as students seeking an unfair advantage. Medical encounters with these students could offer health care professionals the opportunity for education and intervention for both types of students. Given that undiagnosed ADHD and inappropriate stimulant-seeking behavior are potential problems on college campuses that require considerably different treatment responses, the results of this study highlight the need for increased awareness of this issue by college health care professionals.

This study demonstrates that nonmedical use of stimulants clusters within peer groups. Nonprescription stimulant users were more likely than nonusers to know peers with nonprescription use, to know peers who visited a physician to obtain stimulants, and to know people who sell ADHD medications to students. Likewise, nonusers whose peers used nonprescribed stimulants were more likely than nonusers whose peers did not use nonprescribed stimulants to know of peers visiting physicians to seek stimulants inappropriately and to know of people selling ADHD medications to students.

To our knowledge, this is also the first study to examine the beliefs of college students regarding the effects of ADHD medications. Although it may not be surprising that nonprescription users were significantly more knowledgeable about stimulant effects than nonusers, it is interesting that nonusers whose peers use nonprescribed stimulants were significantly more knowledgeable about stimulant effects than nonusers whose peers did not use nonprescribed stimulants. It appears that nonusers whose peers use nonprescribed stimulants are more likely to hold beliefs that may increase their risk for future nonprescribed stimulant use. They may be learning about the effects of stimulants from their peers, either through report or through direct observation. These nonusing students may be at higher risk themselves if they become tempted to try stimulants based on the benefits reported by their peers.

The recent findings of Hall et al[22] support our contention that students whose peers use nonprescription stimulants may be at heightened risk for future nonmedical use themselves. Their analysis revealed that for both men and women, knowing peers who used nonprescribed stimulants predicted nonprescription use. Additionally, knowing how to acquire stimulants easily was a factor predicting men's use, and being offered stimulants by another student was a factor predicting women's use.[22] Our finding that students whose peers use nonprescribed stimulants were more likely to know of individuals selling ADHD medications to students extends the findings of Hall and colleagues. It is plausible that having peers who use nonprescribed stimulants might increase the likelihood of being offered stimulants by another student.

There are several limitations to this study. The disproportionate recruitment of female respondents (61.3%) suggests that there may have been a sex selection bias. Since other groups have reported higher rates of nonmedical use of stimulants among men than women,[22] the disproportionate number of female respondents in this study may have resulted in lower overall rates of students endorsing nonmedical use of stimulants, and it may also explain why we did not find differing rates of stimulant use among men and women.

Although our results may not be generalizable to other colleges or geographic regions, they do complement the results of studies conducted on other college campuses. A study undertaken at another Eastern liberal arts college reported higher rates of recreational methylphenidate use,[20] whereas a survey at a midwestern public university found lower rates of nonmedical use of methylphenidate.[21] On the other hand, a study from another midwestern university found higher rates of nonmedical use of stimulants but lower rates of students whose peers used nonprescribed stimulants when compared with the results of this study.[22] Geographic variation in prescription stimulant use has been recognized[27] and may parallel geographic variation in nonmedical use of stimulants given that the latter has been associated with increased numbers of students giving away or selling their prescription stimulant medication.[24]

Additionally, this study did not address duration or frequency of use. Thus, it is not known whether the nonprescription users in this study were taking stimulants regularly or only on occasion. Also, the circumstances of how students began nonmedical use of stimulants and the sources students used to procure stimulants were not examined.

Finally, the method of survey distribution created some limitations. It would have been preferable to approach students in such a manner that a precise response rate could be calculated. However, the practicalities of distributing surveys in lecture halls quickly enough to encourage participation precluded gathering the necessary data. In addition, as with any study in which potential subjects are offered an incentive to encourage participation, the possibility exists that we inadvertently created bias by offering students candy. Candy was chosen as an incentive because it is inexpensive, portable to lecture halls, and unlikely to be considered coercive. A bowl of candy was placed at the lecture hall exit and was not monitored. Since taking candy was not contingent on completing a survey, and eating candy was not required to participate, it is unlikely that the offer of candy biased our results.

Additional research is needed to better understand the scope of nonmedical use of stimulants among college students nationally and to determine geographic variation. More detailed information from nonprescription stimulant users regarding their decisions to begin using stimulants, their interactions with the medical community, and their sources of stimulants will be helpful in designing interventions to combat this problem. College health services should also consider initiating campaigns to educate undergraduates regarding the potential dangers of inappropriate stimulant use, including the possibility of nonmedical use of stimulants serving as a gateway to other illicit drug use. Such efforts could potentially be helpful in reaching students at heightened risk for nonmedical use of stimulants, such as those whose peers use nonprescribed stimulants, before nonmedical use of stimulants is initiated.

**Accepted for Publication:** October 9, 2005.

**Correspondence:** Diane R. Blake, MD, University of Massachusetts Medical School, Department of Pediatrics, 55 Lake Ave N, Worcester, MA 01655 (Diane.Blake@umassmed.edu).

## REFERENCES


1. First MB, Frances A, Pincus HA. *DSM-IV-TR Handbook of Differential Diagnosis.* Washington, DC: American Psychiatric Publishing; 2002.
2. Greenhill LL, Pliszka S, Dulcan MK, et al. Practice parameters for the use of stimulant medications in the treatment of children, adolescents, and adults. *J Am Acad Child Adolesc Psychiatry.* 2002;41(suppl 2):26S-49S.
3. Spencer T, Biederman J, Wilens T, Harding M, O'Donnell D, Griffin S. Pharmacotherapy of attention-deficit hyperactivity disorder across the life cycle. *J Am Acad Child Adolesc Psychiatry.* 1996;35:409-432.
4. Biederman J, Spencer T, Wilens T. Evidence-based pharmacotherapy for attention-deficit hyperactivity disorder. *Int J Neuropsychopharmacol.* 2004;7:77-97.
5. Robison LM, Sclar DA, Skaer TL, Galin RS. National trends in the prevalence of attention-deficit/hyperactivity disorder and the prescribing of methylphenidate among school-age children: 1990-1995. *Clin Pediatr (Phila).* 1999;38:209-217.
6. Johnston LD, O'Malley PM, Bachman JG, Schulenberg JE. *Monitoring the Future National Survey Results on Drug Use, 1975-2003: Vol I: Secondary School Students.* Bethesda, Md: National Institute on Drug Abuse; 2004. NIH publication 04-5507.
7. Kollins SH, MacDonald EK, Rush CR. Assessing the abuse potential of methylphenidate in nonhuman and human subjects: a review. *Pharmacol Biochem Behav.* 2001;68:611-627.
8. Rapoport JL, Buchsbaum MS, Zahn TP, Weingartner H, Ludlow C, Mikkelsen EJ. Dextroamphetamine: cognitive and behavioral effects in normal prepubertal boys. *Science.* 1978;199:560-563.
9. Cho A. Making the grade. *Berkeley Medical Journal.* Fall 2000. Available at: www.ocf.berkeley.edu/~issues/fall00/Allison.html. Accessed December 12, 2005.
10. CNN.com. Ritalin abuse scoring high on college illegal drug circuit. Available at: http://archives.cnn.com/2001/HEALTH/children/01/08/college.ritalin/. Accessed March 18, 2005.
11. Medill News Service. Ritalin on rise in the region. Available at: http://mesh.medill.northwestern.edu/mnschicago/archives/2001/01/ritalin_on_rise.html. Accessed March 18, 2005.
12. Scruggs J. Students turn to prescription drugs for new highs. *Daily Helmsman.* March 4, 2005. Available at: www.dailyhelmsman.com. Accessed December 12, 2005.
13. Shulas G. Adderall misuse up in schools. *Connecticut Post.* February 13, 2005:A1.
14. Sprang J. Students turn to "study drugs" too often when facing academic pressures. *Daily Cardinal.* March 14, 2005. Available at: www.dailycardinal.com/article.php?storyid=893405. Accessed December 12, 2005.
15. Zamiska N. Pressed to do well on admissions tests, students take drugs: stimulants prescribed for attention disorders find new unapproved use. *Wall Street Journal.* November 8, 2004:A1.
16. Nadler M. Pharmaceutical U. *Boston Magazine.* May 2004. Available at: www.bostonmagazine.com/index.cfm/fuseaction/article.view/articleID/63b1ecf4-3324-4dcf-8188-defc1ab04440. Accessed December 12, 2005.
17. Mertl M. Running on Ritalin. *Psychology Today.* September/October 2000. Available at: www.findarticles.com/p/articles/mi_m1175/is_5_33/ai_66380389. Accessed December 12, 2005.
18. McCabe SE, Teter CJ, Boyd CJ, et al. Prevalence and correlates of illicit methylphenidate use among 8th, 10th, and 12th grade students in the United States, 2001. *J Adolesc Health.* 2004;35:501-504.
19. McCabe SE, Teter CJ, Boyd CJ. The use, misuse and diversion of prescription stimulants among middle and high school students. *Subst Use Misuse.* 2004;39:1095-1116.
20. Babcock Q, Byrne T. Student perceptions of methylphenidate abuse at a public liberal arts college. *J Am Coll Health.* 2000;49:143-145.
21. Teter CJ, McCabe SE, Boyd CJ, Guthrie SK. Illicit methylphenidate use in an undergraduate student sample: prevalence and risk factors. *Pharmacotherapy.* 2003;23:609-617.
22. Hall KM, Irwin MM, Bowman KA, Frankenberger W, Jewett DC. Illicit use of prescribed stimulant medication among college students. *J Am Coll Health.* 2005;53:167-174.
23. Musser CJ, Ahmann PA, Theye FW, Mundt P, Broste SK, Mueller-Rizner N. Stimulant use and the potential for abuse in Wisconsin as reported by school administrators and longitudinally followed children. *J Dev Behav Pediatr.* 1998;19:187-192.
24. Poulin C. Medical and nonmedical stimulant use among adolescents: from sanctioned to unsanctioned use. *CMAJ.* 2001;165:1039-1044.
25. Murphy KR, Barkley RA, Bush T. Young adults with attention deficit hyperactivity disorder: subtype differences in comorbidity, educational and clinical history. *J Nerv Ment Dis.* 2002;190:147-157.
26. Faraone SV, Spencer TJ, Montano CB, Biederman J. Attention-deficit/hyperactivity disorder in adults: a survey of current practice in psychiatry and primary care. *Arch Intern Med.* 2004;164:1221-1226.
27. Cox ER, Motheral BR, Henderson RR, Mager D. Geographic variation in the prevalence of stimulant medication use among children 5 to 14 years old: results from a commercially insured US sample. *Pediatrics.* 2003;111:237-243.

# Pediatricians' Clinical Decision Making

## *Results of 2 Randomized Controlled Trials of Test Performance Characteristics*

*Colin M. Sox, MD, MS; Thomas D. Koepsell, MD, MPH; Jason N. Doctor, PhD; Dimitri A. Christakis, MD, MPH*

**Objective:** To determine whether presenting test performance characteristics influences clinical management.

**Design:** Two questionnaire-based, randomized controlled trials.

**Setting:** Mailed surveys with 2 clinical vignettes.

**Participants:** Randomly selected US pediatricians (N=1502).

**Intervention:** Vignette-specific, randomly assigned test information: no additional information (control), test characteristics (TC), or TC defined. In the pertussis vignette, the TC group received the direct fluorescent antibody test's sensitivity and specificity, and the TC defined group received the same information with definitions. In the urinalysis vignette, the TC group received the false-positive rate of persistent microhematuria in predicting renal disease, and the TC defined group received a definition of this information.

**Main Outcome Measures:** In the pertussis vignette, diagnostic test choice and management of erythromycin therapy and hospital discharge plans. In the urinalysis vignette, serum laboratory testing and nephrology referral plans.

**Results:** Six hundred fifty-three participants (49.5% of those eligible) returned completed surveys. In the pertussis vignette, significantly more of the TC (73%) and TC defined (71%) groups ordered the best-performing test than did controls (21%) ($P<.001$ for both comparisons). Receiving test characteristics did not significantly affect erythromycin therapy or hospital discharge plans ($P\geq.40$). In the urinalysis vignette, the TC defined group referred to nephrology (30%) and checked laboratory tests (88%) significantly more often than did controls (19%, $P=.01$; 78%, $P=.01$, respectively), but the TC and control groups' testing and referral plans did not differ significantly (22% vs 19%, $P=.36$; 75% vs 78%, $P=.48$, respectively).

**Conclusion:** Providing test performance characteristics influenced certain clinical decisions, sometimes in unexpected ways.

*Arch Pediatr Adolesc Med. 2006;160:487-492*

**Author Affiliations:** Center for Child Health Care Studies, Department of Ambulatory Care and Prevention, Harvard Medical School, and Harvard Pilgrim Healthcare, Boston, Mass (Dr Sox); Departments of Epidemiology (Dr Koepsell), Medical Education (Dr Doctor), and Health Services (Dr Koepsell), and Pediatrics (Dr Christakis), University of Washington, and Child Health Institute and Children's Hospital and Regional Medical Center (Dr Christakis), Seattle.

THE INSTITUTE OF MEDICINE'S report *To Err Is Human*[1,2] prioritized improvement in the quality of health care and increased awareness of its importance. Although improving care can be difficult,[3] advances in information technology, such as electronic medical records and computerized provider order entry, have provided useful tools for this task.[4,5] Decision support linked to computer provider order entry has been shown to improve many types of care,[6] including medication prescribing,[7,8] guideline compliance, and diagnostic test ordering.[9-11] The health information technology revolution under way in the United States has been influenced by requirements to report quality, incentives to improve billing efficiencies, and financial support from the Department of Health and Human Services.[15] It is only a matter of time before health information technology tools become more widely available.[16]

As outlined in *Medical Decision Making*,[17] physicians approach clinical problems in a stepwise fashion. A list of hypotheses (differential diagnosis) is generated, the hypotheses are tested, the test results evaluated and interpreted, and a course of action is chosen. During the hypothesis-testing phase of medical decision making, appropriate diagnostic test ordering is important, as excessive use of diagnostic tests is an expensive problem in medicine.[18] Physicians' discomfort with uncertainty sometimes motivates them to order tests for defensive reasons.[19] Interventions targeting physician behavioral factors[20] and using quality improvement strategies[21] have had some success at improving test ordering.

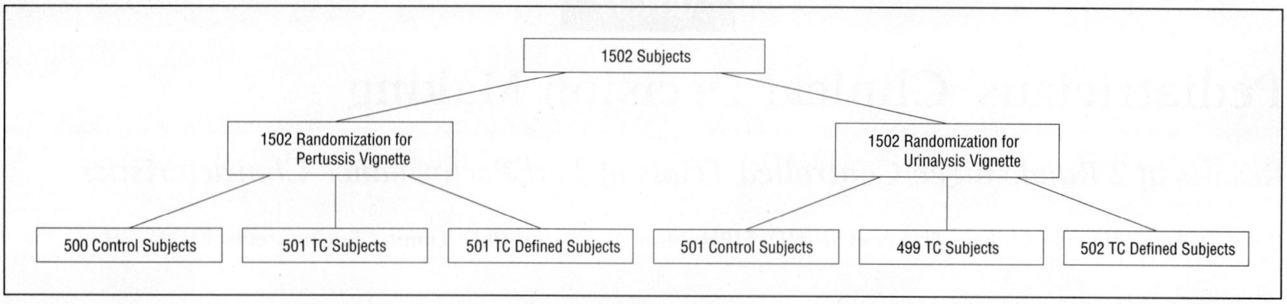


**Figure 1.** Randomization of subjects. TC indicates pediatricians who received test characteristics alone; TC defined, pediatricians who received test characteristics defined.

The format used to present test information can independently influence the hypothesis-testing phase. In a randomized controlled trial,[22] general practitioners were given a clinical vignette with test results presented in 1 of 3 ways (test result only, test result and test sensitivity and specificity, or test result and the positive likelihood ratio presented in plain language). Physicians who received the test result and the positive likelihood ratio in plain language more accurately estimated the patient's posttest probability of disease.[22] Although this study evaluated the hypothesis-testing phase of medical decision making, the influence of the format of presentation of test characteristics on physicians' choice of tests or patient management has not been rigorously tested, to our knowledge. While decision support linked to computerized provider order entry has reduced unnecessary serologic and radiologic tests ordered among adult patients,[10,11,14] the influence of providing test performance with test results on pediatricians' subsequent clinical management has not been studied.

Our study examined 2 sets of research questions to address our hypothesis that presenting general pediatricians with information about test accuracy would influence patient management. Our first research question sought to determine whether presenting pediatricians with the sensitivity and specificity of direct fluorescent antibody (DFA) testing for pertussis would influence their initial choice of a diagnostic test and subsequent patient management. We hypothesized that pediatricians receiving test performance characteristics would choose the test with the highest sensitivity and specificity and would choose an appropriate management plan. Our second research question sought to determine whether presenting pediatricians with the high false-positive rate of persistent microhematuria detected on screening urinalysis (96%) would influence their subsequent patient evaluation. We hypothesized that subjects receiving test performance information would be less likely to evaluate the patient further.

## METHODS

### STUDY DESIGN

We implemented 2 questionnaire-based, randomized controlled trials in a mailed survey that asked pediatricians to manage 2 clinical vignettes. The questionnaire required approximately 7 minutes to complete. For each of 2 vignettes, we randomized subjects in a factorial design into 1 of 3 vignette-specific test characteristics groups (**Figure 1**). Therefore, each subject received 1 of 9 versions of the questionnaire. We randomized subjects using a computerized random-number generator. Subjects were blinded to randomization, and allocation was concealed.

In February 2002, we mailed potential subjects a 4-page questionnaire, a prepaid return envelope, a dollar bill as a token of appreciation, and a letter stating that participation was voluntary and that responses would be kept confidential. Subjects were given the opportunity to decline to participate. We sent nonresponders a replacement survey at 4-week intervals, for a maximum of 4 mailings per subject, and sent a reminder postcard after the second mailing. We contacted the institutions of nonresponders to confirm that the mailing addresses were correct. The University of Washington Institutional Review Board approved this study.

### SUBJECTS

Our target study population was a random selection of pediatricians practicing general pediatrics in the United States. We recruited our sample from the 2002 American Medical Association Masterfile of licensed physicians in the United States. Compiled for the US Department of Defense, this list is considered a complete collection of physicians' names, addresses, specialty, age, and sex and is not limited to members of the American Medical Association. From among 44 561 pediatricians without listed secondary specialties, 1502 were randomly selected for participation. To power the study to detect a 15% difference in management choices between test performance information groups and assuming a 50% response rate, we chose our sample size to ensure at least 175 participants in each group.

### QUESTIONNAIRE VIGNETTES

We developed the questionnaire and pilot tested it among 22 nonstudy pediatricians. We will refer to the questionnaire's 2 clinical vignettes as "the pertussis vignette" and "the urinalysis vignette." For each vignette, subjects were presented with a diagnostic test result followed by their randomly assigned, vignette-specific information about test performance. Both vignettes had a control group, a TC group, and a TC defined group. The TC groups were presented information that included the scientific terms *sensitivity*, *specificity*, or *false-positive rate*, with the corresponding numerical values as frequencies (because medical students understand probabilities easier when they are presented as frequencies[23]). The TC defined groups received the same information defined using nonscientific terminology.

After being provided with test information, subjects were asked to make management decisions about the case. We assumed that subjects would estimate the posttest probability of disease during the hypothesis-testing phase of medical decision-making, before making management decisions. We hypothesized that providing test performance information would aid subjects in their disease probability estimations, because they are needed to make Bayesian calculations of the posttest probability of disease.[17]

The pertussis vignette presented a 5-month-old girl with perioral cyanosis and a hacking cough; subjects were instructed to assume that the likelihood she had pertussis was 30% (vignette details are available in an appendix from the corresponding author). Subjects were asked to choose one of several diagnostic tests to evaluate her nasopharyngeal secretions for pertussis, including culture, DFA testing, or polymerase chain reaction. Subjects in the control group were presented with no further information and were asked if they "happened to know the sensitivity and specificity" of the 3 tests. The other 2 groups were given the sensitivity and specificity of culture (35% and 100%, respectively), DFA testing (50% and 95%, respectively), and polymerase chain reaction (95% and 99%, respectively) for *Bordetella pertussis*.[24,25] The vignette continued with information that the patient was hospitalized, DFA testing of her sputum was ordered, and treatment with erythromycin was started. Three days later, her symptoms were somewhat improved, and results of the DFA testing were negative for pertussis. Controls received no additional information about this test result, the TC group was presented the sensitivity and specificity of DFA testing (50% and 95%, respectively), while the TC defined group was given the following information: "The pertussis DFA has a sensitivity of 50%, meaning that if 100 patients infected with pertussis were tested with the pertussis DFA, 50 would test positive and 50 would test negative by DFA. Similarly, the pertussis DFA has a specificity of 95%, meaning that if 100 patients who are not infected with pertussis were tested with the DFA for pertussis, 5 would test positive and 95 would test negative." We then asked subjects to decide whether to continue the patient's treatment with erythromycin and whether to discharge the patient from the hospital.

The urinalysis vignette presented a healthy 5-year-old boy with persistent microhematuria detected by routine screening urinalysis (vignette details are available in an appendix from the corresponding author). Using data obtained from the literature,[26-31] we calculated the false-positive rate of persistent microscopic hematuria detected by screening urinalysis to be 96%. The control group received the test result only, with no additional information. The TC group was given the following information: "When screening asymptomatic patients with urinalysis for diseases whose clinical outcome might be improved with early treatment, persistent microscopic hematuria has an estimated false-positive rate of 96%." The TC defined group was given the following nontechnical explanation of this information: "The literature suggests that, of 100 asymptomatic children who have persistent microscopic hematuria detected by routine urinalysis, 96 will not have significant nephrologic renal disease for which early treatment might improve clinical outcome." We then asked subjects if they would refer the patient to a pediatric nephrologist or check his serum electrolyte, urea nitrogen, and creatinine levels.

## ADDITIONAL DEMOGRAPHIC DATA

To collect information about subjects' training, we asked if they were board certified in pediatrics, a US medical school graduate, and currently in a pediatric residency program. We defined *foreign medical school graduate* as a graduate of a medical school located outside of the United States.

To collect information about clinical practice, we asked subjects to report the percentage of clinical time spent in general pediatrics and whether they worked in a practice that had 1 or 2 pediatricians, or more. We defined general pediatrician as one

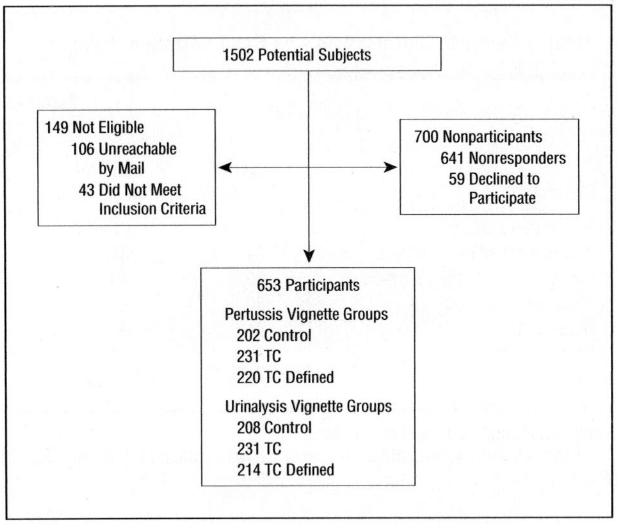


**Figure 2.** Response to survey. TC indicates pediatricians who received test characteristics alone; TC defined, pediatricians who received test characteristics defined.

who reported spending more than 80% of clinical time in general pediatrics. We defined small primary practice as a primary practice that included 1 or 2 pediatricians.

## MAIN OUTCOME MEASURES

In the pertussis vignette, we assessed subjects' choice of an initial pertussis diagnostic test and whether they continued the patient's treatment with erythromycin and discharged the patient from the hospital. In the urinalysis vignette, we assessed whether subjects referred the patient to a pediatric nephrologist and/or checked the patient's serum electrolyte, urea nitrogen, and creatinine levels.

## STATISTICAL ANALYSIS

For each outcome, we performed comparisons between the vignette-specific control group and its TC or TC defined group. We conducted $\chi^2$ tests to examine the effect of receiving test characteristics on the 5 dichotomous outcomes. If we found statistically significant differences between groups using a subject characteristic, we conducted logistic regression analyses controlling for that characteristic. All analyses were conducted using STATA 8.0 (StataCorp LP, College Station, Tex).

# RESULTS

## STUDY PARTICIPATION

We mailed questionnaires to 1502 physicians identified in the American Medical Association Masterfile as pediatricians without subspecialization. Of these, 106 questionnaires (7%) were returned by the post office without forwarding addresses, and 43 physicians (3%) did not meet inclusion criteria. Of the 1353 potentially eligible subjects, 59 (4%) declined to participate and 653 returned completed surveys, leaving 641 potentially eligible nonresponders (**Figure 2**), for an estimated response rate[32] of 49.75% (653/1313). There were no statistically significant differences by age, sex, or test characteristics group between participants and nonresponders.

**Table 1. Subject Characteristics by Randomization Groups***

| Characteristic | Overall (n = 653) | Pertussis Vignette (n = 643): Control (n = 202) | Pertussis Vignette (n = 643): TC Group (n = 231) | Pertussis Vignette (n = 643): TC Defined Group (n = 220) | Urinalysis Vignette (n = 643): Control (n = 208) | Urinalysis Vignette (n = 643): TC Group (n = 231) | Urinalysis Vignette (n = 643): TC Defined Group (n = 214) |
|---|---|---|---|---|---|---|---|
| Age, mean ± SD, y | 43 ± 11 | 43 ± 11 | 43 ± 11 | 44 ± 11 | 43 ± 11 | 43 ± 11 | 44 ± 11 |
| Board certified in pediatrics | 81 | 81 | 82 | 79 | 80 | 79 | 84 |
| Foreign medical school graduate | 20 | 19 | 22 | 19 | 20 | 21 | 19 |
| General pediatrician | 80 | 81 | 82 | 76 | 80 | 77 | 84 |
| Male sex | 44 | 40 | 43 | 50 | 31 | 45 | 37 |
| Small primary practice | 22 | 13 | 17 | 17 | 15 | 17 | 14 |
| Resident | 16 | 22 | 21 | 23 | 22 | 23 | 22 |

Abbreviations: TC, test characteristics.

*Data are given as percentages unless otherwise indicated. The only significant difference between randomization groups was by sex for the urinalysis vignette ($P = .02$).

**Table 2. Effect of Providing Sensitivity and Specificity of the *Bordetella pertussis* DFA on Pediatricians' Patient Management**

| Outcome | Randomization Groups for the Pertussis DFA Vignette, %: Control (n = 202) | TC Group* (n = 231) | TC Defined Group* (n = 220) | *P* Value |
|---|---|---|---|---|
| Continued erythromycin | 92 | 90 | | .55 |
| therapy | 92 | | 94 | .40 |
| Discharged patient | 87 | 86 | | .79 |
| from the hospital | 87 | | 87 | .99 |

Abbreviations: DFA, direct fluorescent antibody (DFA); TC, test characteristics.

*The TC group received the DFA's sensitivity and specificity; the TC defined group received the same information with nontechnical definitions of these terms.

**Table 3. Effect of Providing False-Positive Rate of Persistent Microhematuria Found on Screening Urinalysis on Pediatricians' Subsequent Patient Evaluation**

| Outcome | Randomization Groups for the Screening Urinalysis Vignette, %: Control (n = 208) | TC Group* (n = 231) | TC Defined Group* (n = 214) | *P* Value |
|---|---|---|---|---|
| Referred to pediatric | 19 | 22 | | .36 |
| nephrology | 19 | | 30 | .01 |
| Checked serum electrolyte, | 78 | 75 | | .48 |
| urea nitrogen, and creatinine levels | 78 | | 88 | .01 |

Abbreviations: DFA, direct fluorescent antibody (DFA); TC, test characteristics.

*The TC group received the false-positive rate of persistent microhematuria in predicting renal disease; the TC defined group received a nontechnical definition of this information.

For the pertussis vignette, 202 participants were in the control group, 231 in the TC group, and 220 in the TC defined group. For the urinalysis vignette, 208 participants were in the control group, 231 in the TC group, and 214 in the TC defined group (**Table 1**). The only significant difference in participant characteristics by randomization groups was by sex for the urinalysis vignette ($P = .02$) (Table 1).

## PERTUSSIS VIGNETTE

Providing participants with the sensitivity and specificity of the 3 tests influenced which test they chose, as significantly more of the TC (73%) and TC defined (71%) groups chose the polymerase chain reaction test (the only test for which sensitivity and specificity were ≥95%) than did controls (21%, $P < .001$ in both comparisons) (**Table 2**). Among the controls, 45% reported that they knew the sensitivity and specificity of pertussis culture, 34% knew the values for DFA testing, and 18% knew the values for polymerase chain reaction.

The vast majority of participants chose to continue the patient's erythromycin therapy, and receiving test characteristics had no significant influence on these decisions (90% of the TC group vs 92% of controls, $P = .55$; and 94% of the TC defined group vs 92% of controls, $P = .40$). Similarly, most participants chose to discharge the patient from the hospital, and receiving test characteristics had no significant influence on these decisions (86% of the TC group vs 87% of controls, $P = .79$; and 87% of the TC defined group vs 87% of controls, $P = .99$) (Table 2).

## URINALYSIS VIGNETTE

Significantly more participants in the TC defined group than controls chose to refer the patient to a nephrologist (30% vs 19%, $P = .01$), while there was no significant difference in referral between the TC group and the controls (22% vs 19%, $P = .36$). Significantly more subjects in the TC defined group than controls decided to check the patient's serum electrolyte, urea nitrogen, and creatinine levels (88% vs 78%, $P = .01$), while there was no significant difference in laboratory test ordering between the TC group and the controls (75% vs 78%, $P = .48$) (**Table 3**). Controlling for sex in logistic regression analyses had little effect on any of these results.

## COMMENT

Providing laboratory test performance characteristics influenced pediatricians' clinical decision making, but to different degrees. In the pertussis vignette, few participants reported familiarity with the performance characteristics of commonly used tests. Providing the sensitivity and specificity of diagnostic tests for pertussis dramatically increased the proportion of participants who chose the best-performing test, but it did not influence their clinical management decisions. The subjects' posttest probability of pertussis was perhaps higher than their treatment threshold. On the other hand, it is possible that their decisions to continue erythromycin therapy were primarily influenced by its low cost or favorable adverse effect profile. In the urinalysis vignette, receiving test characteristics alone did not significantly influence participants' decisions to refer the patient or to conduct serum laboratory tests, but receiving test characteristics defined increased the frequency of both evaluations. The direction of this effect contradicted our hypothesis, as we expected that presenting pediatricians with the high false-positive rate of persistent microhematuria would decrease their subsequent workup of the patient's hematuria. The increased evaluation of microhematuria may have been in part due to the "certainty effect,"[33] as presenting the nonzero probability of renal disease may have instilled concern. This result supports others' findings that false-positive laboratory results lead to increased resource use.[34]

The format of the test performance information influenced practice to different degrees, as patient management after receiving test characteristics defined differed significantly from that controls for 3 of the 5 measures, while receiving the test characteristics alone significantly affected only 1 measure. Perhaps participants in the TC group did not understand the scientific terminology that was used; the TC defined group was given the same information described without using scientific language. Presenting the test characteristics defined might be difficult to implement using computerized provider order entry, because the time required to read lengthy decision support might limit the influence of the intervention. The test characteristics alone information was more concise, but it did not significantly influence most management decisions.

Several limitations to this study warrant comment. First, physicians who returned completed surveys may be different from those who did not. However, there were no significant differences in age or sex between responders and nonresponders, and our response rate was similar to the mean response rates in published studies[35,36] of physicians. Second, decisions made by participants in our vignettes may not represent their actual clinical practice. However, vignettes have been shown to be a valid tool for measuring the quality of clinical practice,[37] and our primary comparison was between randomized groups. Third, in retrospect it might have been preferable to avoid the use of the term *false-positive rate* presented to the TC group in the urinalysis vignette. Although some have used this term to refer to 1 minus predictive value positive (as our survey did),[38] it also has been used to refer to 1 minus specificity.[17,39] A false-positive rate would be termed a *false-alarm rate* in other disciplines.[40] An occasional participant may have been confused by the potential ambiguity of this term. However, we believe that an interpretation of a false-positive rate of 96% as 1 minus specificity would be implausible because it would imply a specificity of 4%, a value that would essentially render any such test useless for clinical diagnostic purposes.

Providing diagnostic test performance characteristics sometimes influenced pediatricians' patient management in unexpected ways. Presenting a representative sample of US pediatricians with the same information in different formats influenced their clinical decisions to different degrees. Future research should determine the format for presenting test characteristics that maximally influences physicians' clinical decision making. In addition, interviews should be performed among pediatricians who do not respond to decision support as expected in an effort to understand why sometimes this information is not influential. In light of the substantial investment that the Department of Health and Human Services recently made to promote the use of health information technology in the United States,[15] our findings reinforce the importance of verifying that point-of-care decision support has the desired effect.

**Accepted for Publication:** October 27, 2005.
**Correspondence:** Colin M. Sox, MD, MS, Center for Child Health Care Studies, Department of Ambulatory Care and Prevention, Harvard Medical School, and Harvard Pilgrim Health Care, Inc, 133 Brookline Ave, Sixth Floor, Boston, MA 02215 (colin_sox@hms.harvard.edu).
**Funding/Support:** This study was supported in part by the Nesholm Family Foundation, Seattle, and by the Clinical Scholars Program (Dr Sox) and the Generalist Physician Faculty Scholars Program (Dr Christakis) of The Robert Wood Johnson Foundation, Princeton, NJ.
**Disclaimer:** The opinions are those of the authors and do not necessarily represent the views of The Robert Wood Johnson Foundation.
**Acknowledgment:** We acknowledge the helpful feedback received on this project from Alison Galbraith, MD, MPH, and from Hal Sox, MD. We also acknowledge the assistance of the Clinical Scholars Program work-in-progress seminar at the University of Washington.

## REFERENCES

1. Kohn LT, Corrigan JM, Donaldson MS. *To Err Is Human: Building a Safer Health System.* eds. Washington, DC: National Academy Press; 1999.
2. Leape LL, Berwick DM, Bates DW. What practices will most improve safety? *JAMA.* 2002;288:501-507.
3. Chassin MR. Improving the quality of care. *N Engl J Med.* 1996;335:1060-1064.
4. Bates DW, Gawande AA. Improving safety with information technology. *N Engl J Med.* 2003;348:2526-2534.
5. Bates DW. The quality case for information technology in healthcare. *BMC Med Inform Decis Mak.* 2002;2:e7.
6. Bates DW, Kuperman GJ, Wang S, et al. Ten commandments for effective clinical decision support: making the practice of evidence-based medicine a reality. *J Am Med Inform Assoc.* 2003;10:523-530.
7. Chertow GM, Lee J, Kupermann GJ, et al. Guided medication dosing for inpatients with renal insufficiency. *JAMA.* 2001;286:2839-2844.
8. Christakis DA, Zimmerman FJ, Wright JA, Garrison MM, Rivara FP, Davis RL.

A randomized controlled trial of point-of-care evidence to improve the antibiotic prescribing practices for otitis media in children. *Pediatrics.* 2001;107:e15 Accessed June 1, 2005.
9. Tierney WM, McDonald CJ, Martin DK, Rogers MP. Computerized display of past test results: effect on outpatient testing. *Ann Intern Med.* 1987;107:569-574.
10. Harpole LH, Khorasani R, Fiskio J, Kuperman GJ, Bates DW. Automated evidence-based critiquing of orders for abdominal radiographs: impact on utilization and appropriateness. *J Am Med Inform Assoc.* 1997;4:511-521.
11. Solomon DH, Shmerling RH, Schur PH, Lew R, Fiskio J, Bates DW. A computer based intervention to reduce unnecessary serologic testing. *J Rheumatol.* 1999; 26:2578-2584.
12. Tierney WM, McDonald CJ, Hui SL, Martin DK. Computer predictions of abnormal test results: effects on outpatient testing. *JAMA.* 1988;259:1194-1198.
13. Tierney WM, Miller ME, McDonald CJ. The effect on test ordering of informing physicians of the charges of outpatient diagnostic tests. *N Engl J Med.* 1990; 322:1499-1504.
14. Chen P, Tanasijevic MJ, Schoenenberger RA, Fiskio J, Kuperman GJ, Bates DW. A computer-based intervention for improving the appropriateness of antiepileptic drug level monitoring. *Am J Clin Pathol.* 2003;119:432-438.
15. Agency for Healthcare Research and Quality. HHS awards $139 million to drive adoption of health information technology [press release]. October 13, 2004. Available at: http://www.ahrq.gov/news/press/pr2004/hhshitpr.htm. Accessed January 4, 2005.
16. Committee on Quality of Health Care in AmericaInstitute of Medicine. *Using Information Technology: Crossing the Quality Chasm: A New Health System for the 21st Century.* Washington, DC: National Academy Press; 2001:164-180.
17. Sox HC, Blatt MA, Higgins MC, Marton KI. Differential diagnosis. In: Sox HC, ed. *Medical Decision Making.* Stoneham, Mass: Butterworth Publishers; 1988:9-26.
18. Bates DW, Boyle DL, Rittenberg E, et al. What proportion of common diagnostic tests appear redundant? *Am J Med.* 1998;104:361-368.
19. DeKay ML, Asch DA. Is the defensive use of diagnostic tests good for patients, or bad? *Med Decis Making.* 1998;18:19-28.
20. Solomon DH, Hashimoto H, Daltroy L, Liang MH. Techniques to improve physicians' use of diagnostic tests: a new conceptual framework. *JAMA.* 1998; 280:2020-2027.
21. Verstappen WH, van der Weijden T, Sijbrandij J, et al. Effect of a practice-based strategy on test ordering performance of primary care physicians: a randomized trial. *JAMA.* 2003;289:2407-2412.
22. Steurer J, Fischer JE, Bachmann LM, Koller M, Riet GT. Communicating accuracy of tests to general practitioners: a controlled trial. *BMJ.* 2002;324:824-826.
23. Kurzenhauser S, Hoffrage U. Teaching Bayesian reasoning: an evaluation of a classroom tutorial for medical students. *Med Teach.* 2002;24:516-521.
24. Tilley PA, Kanchana MV, Knight I, Blondeau J, Antonishyn N, Deneer H. Detection of *Bordetella pertussis* in a clinical laboratory by culture, polymerase chain reaction, and direct fluorescent antibody staining; accuracy, and cost. *Diagn Microbiol Infect Dis.* 2000;37:17-23.
25. Loeffelholz MJ, Thompson CJ, Long KS, Gilchrist MJ. Comparison of PCR, culture, and direct fluorescent-antibody testing for detection of *Bordetella pertussis. J Clin Microbiol.* 1999;37:2872-2876.
26. Vehaskari VM, Rapola J, Koskimies O, Savilahti E, Vilska J, Hallman N. Microscopic hematuria in school children: epidemiology and clinicopathologic evaluation. *J Pediatr.* 1979;95:676-684.
27. Feld LG, Meyers KE, Kaplan BS, Stapleton FB. Limited evaluation of microscopic hematuria in pediatrics. *Pediatrics.* 1998;102:e42.
28. Hisano S, Kwano M, Hatae K, et al. Asymptomatic isolated microhaematuria: natural history of 136 children. *Pediatr Nephrol.* 1991;5:578-581.
29. Ito K, Kawaguchi H, Hattori M. Screening for proteinuria and hematuria in school children: is it possible to reduce the incidence of chronic renal failure in children and adolescents? *Acta Paediatr Jpn.* 1990;32:710-715.
30. Murakami M, Yamamoto H, Ueda Y, Murakani D, Yamauchi K. Urinary screening of elementary and junior high-school children over a 13-year period in Tokyo. *Pediatr Nephrol.* 1991;5:50-53.
31. Gauthier B, Trachtman H, Frank R, Valderrama E. Familial thin basement membrane nephropathy in children with asymptomatic microhematuria. *Nephron.* 1989; 51:502-508.
32. Council of American Survey Research Organizations. *On the Definition of Response Rates: A Special Report From the CASRO Task Force on Completion Rates.* Port Jefferson, NY: Council of American Survey Research Organizations; 1982.
33. Kahneman D, Tversky A. Choices, values and frames. In: Kahneman D, Slovic P, Tversky A, eds. *Choices, Values and Frames.* 3rd ed. Cambridge, England: Cambridge University Press; 2000:1-16.
34. Bates DW, Goldman L, Lee TH. Contaminate blood cultures and resource utilization: the true consequences of false-positive results. *JAMA.* 1991;265:365-369.
35. Asch DA, Jedrzeiwski MK, Christakis NA. Response rates to mail surveys published in medical journals. *J Clin Epidemiol.* 1997;50:1129-1136.
36. Cummings SM, Savitz LA, Konrad TR. Reporting response rates to mailed physician questionnaires. *Health Serv Res.* 2001;35:1347-1355.
37. Peabody JW, Luck J, Glassman P, et al. Measuring the quality of physician practice by using clinical vignettes: a prospective validation study. *Ann Intern Med.* 2004;141:771-780.
38. Fleiss JL. *Statistical Methods for Rates and Proportions.* 2nd ed. New York, NY: John Wiley & Sons Inc; 1981.
39. Rembold CM, Watson D. Posttest probability calculation by weights: a simple form of Bayes' theorem. *Ann Intern Med.* 1988;108:115-120.
40. Olson RH. On the use of Bayes' theorem in estimating false alarm rate. *Mon Weather Rev.* 1965;19:557-558.

*Announcement*

**Submissions.** The Editors welcome contributions to Picture of the Month. Submissions should describe common problems presenting uncommonly, rather than total zebras. Cases should be of interest to practicing pediatricians, highlighting problems that they are likely to at least occasionally encounter in the office or hospital setting. High-quality clinical images (in either 35-mm slide or electronic format) along with parent or patient permission to use these images must accompany the submission. The entire discussion should comprise no more than 750 words. Articles and photographs accepted for publication will bear the contributor's name. There is no charge for reproduction and printing of color illustrations. For details regarding electronic submission, please see: http://archpedi.ama-assn.org.

**ACIP recommends vaccination of children against hepatitis A*[1]**

## Hepatitis A spreads FAST... especially among children[2,3]

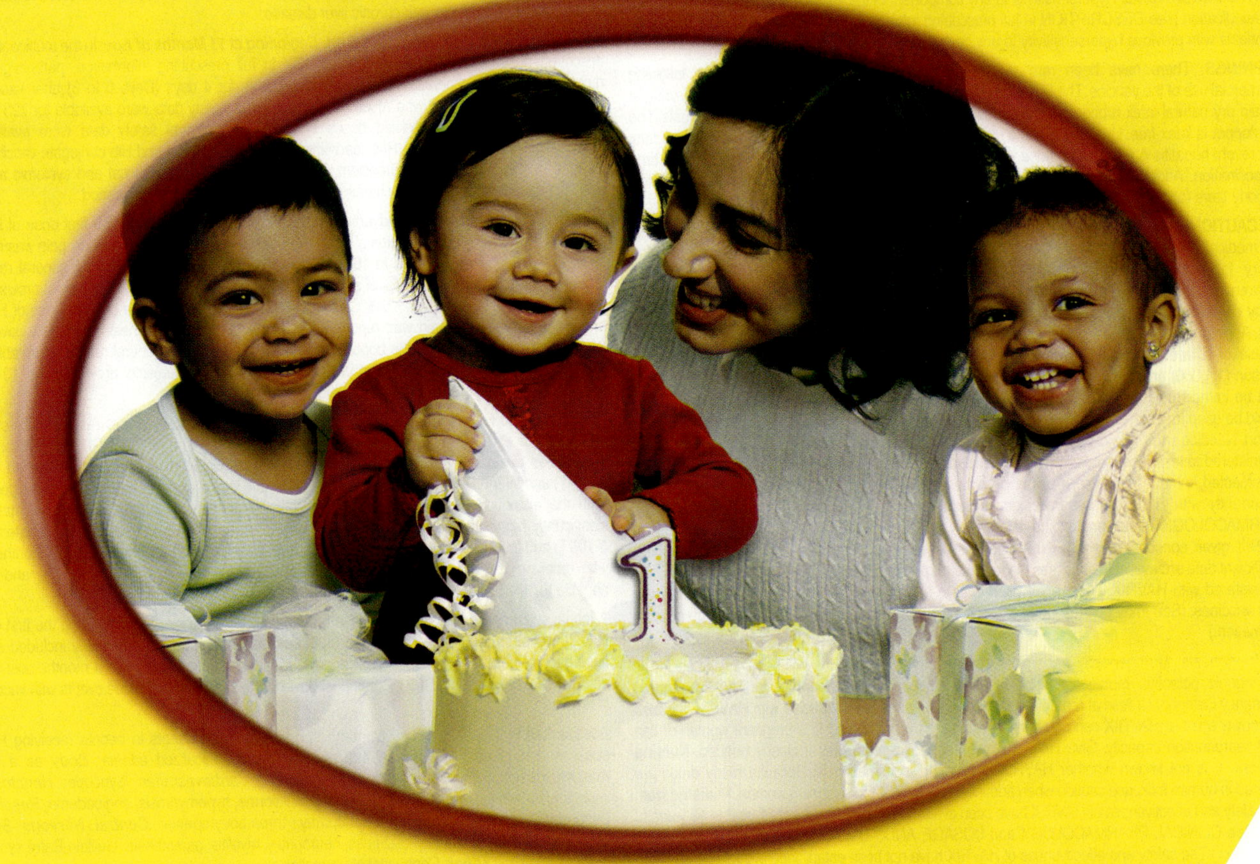

## HAVRIX provides excellent protection

HAVRIX is indicated for active immunization against hepatitis A virus in children 12 months of age and older.

### Important Safety Information

In clinical trials, the most common solicited adverse events were injection-site soreness and headache.

Greater incidences of general adverse events were observed in subjects who received HAVRIX at the same time as Hib conjugate and DTaP vaccines. As with any vaccine, rare adverse events may occur. (See Adverse Reactions section of the Prescribing Information for HAVRIX for potential side effects.) HAVRIX is contraindicated in people with hypersensitivity to any component of the vaccine, including neomycin.

* Advisory Committee on Immunization Practices recommends routine nationwide vaccination against hepatitis A in all children 1–2 years of age.

**Please see references and brief summary of complete prescribing information for HAVRIX on adjacent page.**

HAVRIX is a registered trademark of GlaxoSmithKline.

Manufactured by **GlaxoSmithKline Biologicals**, Rixensart, Belgium
Distributed by **GlaxoSmithKline**, Research Triangle Park, NC 27709

gsk GlaxoSmithKline Vaccines

**Havrix®**
**Hepatitis A Vaccine, Inactivated**

# HAVRIX®
# (Hepatitis A Vaccine, Inactivated)

The following is a brief summary only; see full prescribing information for complete product information.

**INDICATIONS AND USAGE:** HAVRIX is indicated for active immunization of persons ≥12 months of age against disease caused by hepatitis A virus (HAV). Primary immunization should be administered at least 2 weeks prior to expected exposure to HAV. When passive protection against hepatitis A is required either following exposure to hepatitis A virus or in persons requiring both immediate and long-term protection, HAVRIX may be administered concomitantly with immune globulin (IG) with different syringes and at different injection sites. Duration of immunity following a complete vaccination schedule has not been established.

**CONTRAINDICATIONS:** Hypersensitivity to any component of the vaccine, including neomycin, is a contraindication (see DESCRIPTION in full prescribing information). This vaccine is contraindicated in patients with previous hypersensitivity to any hepatitis A-containing vaccine.

**WARNINGS:** There have been rare reports of anaphylaxis/anaphylactoid reactions following commercial use of the vaccine. The tip cap and the rubber plunger of the needleless prefilled syringes contain dry natural latex rubber that may cause allergic reactions in latex sensitive individuals. The vial stopper is latex-free. Hepatitis A has a relatively long incubation period. Hepatitis A vaccine may not prevent hepatitis A infection in those who have an unrecognized hepatitis A infection at the time of vaccination. Additionally, it may not prevent infection in those who do not achieve protective antibody titers (although the lowest titer needed to confer protection has not been determined).

**PRECAUTIONS: General:** Prior to immunization with HAVRIX, the patient's current health status and medical history should be reviewed. The physician should review the patient's immunization history for possible vaccine sensitivity, previous vaccination-related adverse reactions and occurrence of any adverse–event-related symptoms and/or signs, in order to determine the existence of any contraindication to immunization with HAVRIX and to allow an assessment of benefits and risks. Appropriate medical treatment and supervision should be readily available for immediate use in case of a rare anaphylactic reaction following the administration of the vaccine. Epinephrine injection (1:1,000) and other appropriate agents used for the control of immediate allergic reactions must be immediately available. A separate, sterile syringe and needle or a sterile disposable unit should be used for each patient to prevent the transmission of other infectious agents from person to person. Needles should be disposed of properly and should not be recapped. As with any vaccine, if administered to immunosuppressed persons, including those receiving immunosuppressive therapy, the expected immune response may not be obtained. **Drug Interactions:** HAVRIX may be given concurrently with Hib conjugate vaccines in children 15 to 18 months of age (see CLINICAL PHARMACOLOGY in full prescribing information and ADVERSE REACTIONS). The safety of HAVRIX given concomitantly with INFANRIX has been evaluated (see ADVERSE REACTIONS). Insufficient data are available to assess the immune response of a fourth dose of DTaP vaccine when administered with HAVRIX. There are limited data to assess the concomitant use of HAVRIX with other vaccines. (See Immune Response to Concomitantly Administered Vaccines in full prescribing information.)

**Carcinogenesis, Mutagenesis, Impairment of Fertility:** HAVRIX has not been evaluated for its carcinogenic potential, mutagenic potential, or potential for impairment of fertility. **Pregnancy:** Pregnancy Category C. Animal reproduction studies have not been conducted with HAVRIX. It is also not known whether HAVRIX can cause fetal harm when administered to a pregnant woman or can affect reproduction capacity. Give HAVRIX to a pregnant woman only if clearly needed. **Nursing Mothers:** It is not known whether HAVRIX is excreted in human milk. Because many drugs are excreted in human milk, use caution when administering HAVRIX to a nursing woman. **Pediatric Use:** The safety and effectiveness of HAVRIX have been evaluated in 20,436 subjects 1 year to 18 years of age. (See CLINICAL PHARMACOLOGY and DOSAGE AND ADMINISTRATION in full prescribing information.) The safety and effectiveness of HAVRIX have not been established in subjects less than 12 months of age. **Geriatric Use:** Clinical studies of HAVRIX did not include sufficient numbers of subjects 65 years of age and older to determine whether they respond differently from younger subjects. Other reported clinical experience has not identified differences in overall safety between these subjects and younger adult subjects.

**ADVERSE REACTIONS:** As with all pharmaceuticals, however, it is possible that expanded commercial use of the vaccine could reveal rare adverse events. The adverse events most frequently reported by volunteers in clinical trials were injection-site soreness (56% of adults; 21% of children); headache (14% of adults; less than 9% of children). Other solicited and unsolicited events are listed below:

**Incidence 1% to 10% of Injections:** ***Local Reactions at Injection Site:*** Induration, redness, swelling; ***Body as a Whole:*** Fatigue, fever (>37.5°C), malaise; ***Gastrointestinal:*** Anorexia, nausea.

**Incidence <1% of Injections:** ***Local Reaction at Injection Site:*** Hematoma; ***Dermatologic:*** Pruritus, rash, urticaria; ***Respiratory:*** Pharyngitis, other upper respiratory tract infections; ***Gastrointestinal:*** Abdominal pain, diarrhea, dysgeusia, vomiting; ***Musculoskeletal:*** Arthralgia, elevation of creatine phosphokinase, myalgia; ***Hematologic:*** Lymphadenopathy; ***Central Nervous System:*** Hypertonic episode, insomnia, photophobia, vertigo.

**Additional safety data:** Safety data were obtained from 2 additional sources in which large populations were vaccinated. In an outbreak setting in which 4,930 individuals were immunized with a single dose of either 720 EL.U. or 1440 EL.U. of HAVRIX, the vaccine was well tolerated and no serious adverse events due to vaccination were reported. Overall, less than 10% of vaccinees reported solicited general adverse events following the vaccine. The most common solicited local adverse event was pain at the injection site, reported in 22.3% of subjects at 24 hours and decreasing to 2.4% by 72 hours.

In a field efficacy trial, 19,037 children received the 360 EL.U. dose of HAVRIX. The most commonly reported adverse events were injection-site pain (9.5%) and tenderness (8.1%), reported following first doses of HAVRIX. Other adverse events were infrequent and comparable to the control vaccine ENGERIX-B® [Hepatitis B Vaccine (Recombinant)].

In subjects with chronic liver disease, HAVRIX was safe and well tolerated. Local injection site reactions were similar among all 4 groups, and no serious adverse reactions attributed to the vaccine were reported in subjects with chronic liver disease.

***Safety Data for HAVRIX 720 EL.U./0.5 mL Beginning at 11 Months of Age:*** In the multicenter study described under CLINICAL PHARMACOLOGY in full prescribing information, parents/guardians recorded local and general symptoms on diary cards for 4 days (Days 0 to 3) after vaccination. In the 3 groups of children who received HAVRIX alone, safety data were available for 723 children who received 1,396 documented doses of HAVRIX. Additional safety data were available for 181 children who received HAVRIX coadministered with INFANRIX and Hib conjugate vaccine. Most adverse events were mild and transient. The frequencies of solicited local and systemic reactions following receipt of HAVRIX were monitored during the 4-day observation period.

The following rates of solicited adverse events in children who received their first dose of HAVRIX alone at between 11 and 25 months of age were observed. Among local reactions: pain was reported in 15-21% of subjects, redness in 16-21%, swelling in 8% of subjects. Among general reactions, irritability was reported in 24-36% of subjects, loss of appetite in 16-19% of subjects, drowsiness in 15-17% of subjects and fever >39.5°C in ≤2% of subjects. Following the booster dose of HAVRIX, among local reactions: pain was reported in 16-21% of subjects, redness in 17-22%, swelling in 8-10% of subjects. Following the booster dose of HAVRIX, among general reactions, irritability was reported in 19-29% of subjects, loss of appetite in 14-18% of subjects, drowsiness in 13-16% of subjects and fever >39.5°C in ≤1% of subjects.

Drowsiness and loss of appetite occurred at statistically significantly higher rates in subjects 15 to 18 months of age who received Hib conjugate vaccine (PRP-T) and INFANRIX concomitantly with HAVRIX as compared to subjects 15 to 18 months of age who received Hib conjugate vaccine (PRP-T) and INFANRIX (drowsiness 34% and 22% and loss of appetite 29% and 19%, respectively). With the exception of fever (>39.5°C), the solicited general symptoms occurred at statistically significantly higher rates in subjects 15 to 18 months of age who received Hib conjugate vaccine (PRP-T) and INFANRIX concomitantly with HAVRIX as compared to subjects 15 to 18 months of age who received HAVRIX alone (irritability 46% and 30%, drowsiness 34% and 17%, and loss of appetite 29% and 17%, respectively).

A febrile seizure was reported in an 18-month old subject two days after receiving the first dose of HAVRIX. Other serious adverse events reported during the course of this study included a single case each of hepatitis ~5 months post dose 1, insulin-dependent diabetes ~4 months post dose 1, and Kawasaki's disease ~3 1/2 months post dose 1. The association of these events with vaccination is unknown.

**Postmarketing Reports:** Rare voluntary reports of adverse events in people receiving HAVRIX since market introduction include the following: ***Local:*** Localized edema; ***Body as a Whole:*** Anaphylaxis/anaphylactoid reactions, somnolence; ***Cardiovascular:*** Syncope; ***Hepatobiliary:*** Jaundice, hepatitis; ***Dermatologic:*** Erythema multiforme, hyperhydrosis, angioedema; ***Respiratory:*** Dyspnea; ***Hematologic:*** Lymphadenopathy, thrombocytopenia; ***Central Nervous System:*** Convulsions, encephalopathy, dizziness, neuropathy, myelitis, paresthesia, Guillain-Barré syndrome, multiple sclerosis; ***Other:*** Congenital abnormality.

The US Department of Health and Human Services has established the Vaccine Adverse Events Reporting System (VAERS) to accept reports of suspected adverse events after the administration of any vaccine, including, but not limited to, the reporting of events required by the National Childhood Vaccine Injury Act of 1986. The toll-free number for VAERS forms and information is 1-800-822-7967. Reporting forms may also be obtained at the VAERS website at www.vaers.org.

Manufactured by **GlaxoSmithKline Biologicals**, Rixensart, Belgium

Distributed by **GlaxoSmithKline**, Research Triangle Park, NC 27709



BRS-HA:L20

**References: 1.** Centers for Disease Control and Prevention. Recommended childhood and adolescent immunization schedule—United States, 2006. *MMWR.* 2006;54(51&52):Q1–Q4. **2.** Bell BP, Shapiro CN. Hepatitis A virus. In: Long SS, Pickering LK, Prober CG, eds. *Principles and Practice of Pediatric Infectious Diseases.* 2nd ed. Philadelphia, Pa: Churchill Livingstone; 2003:1188–1192. **3.** Armstrong GL, Bell BP. Hepatitis A virus infection in the United States: model-based estimates and implication for childhood immunizations. *Pediatrics.* 2002;109:839–845.



Printed in USA. HAP283R0 February 2006

# Error Reduction in Pediatric Chemotherapy

## *Computerized Order Entry and Failure Modes and Effects Analysis*

*George R. Kim, MD; Allen R. Chen, MD, PhD; Robert J. Arceci, MD, PhD; Sandra H. Mitchell, RPh, MSIS; K. Michelle Kokoszka, RN; Denise Daniel, RN; Christoph U. Lehmann, MD*

**Objective:** To implement and evaluate the impact of computerized provider order entry (CPOE) on reducing ordering errors in pediatric chemotherapy.

**Design:** Before-and-after study from 2001 to 2004.

**Setting:** Pediatric Oncology in an academic medical center.

**Intervention:** Implementation of a CPOE system guided by multidisciplinary failure modes and effects analysis into pediatric chemotherapy.

**Main Outcome Measures:** Completion data on chemotherapy steps of high morbidity/mortality potential if missed (as determined by attending oncologists) from 1259 pre-CPOE paper and 1116 post-CPOE pediatric chemotherapy orders.

**Results:** After CPOE deployment, daily chemotherapy orders were less likely to have improper dosing (relative risk [RR], 0.26; 95% confidence interval [CI], 0.11-0.61), incorrect dosing calculations (RR, 0.09; 95% CI, 0.03-0.34), missing cumulative dose calculations (RR, 0.32; 95% CI, 0.14-0.77), and incomplete nursing checklists (RR, 0.51; 95% CI, 0.33-0.80). There was no difference in the likelihood of improper dosing on treatment plans and a higher likelihood of not matching medication orders to treatment plans (RR, 5.4; 95% CI, 3.1-9.5).

**Conclusion:** Failure modes and effects analysis–guided CPOE reduced ordering errors in pediatric chemotherapy and provided data for further improvements.

*Arch Pediatr Adolesc Med. 2006;160:495-498*

THE COMPLEXITY OF PEDIATRIC chemotherapy makes it vulnerable to errors.[1] As a specialized medication process, it combines the risks for errors in pediatric drug dosage calculation (which is dependent on age, weight, and body surface area) and the risks associated with the narrow therapeutic profile and high potential for acute and cumulative toxicities of antineoplastic agents.[2] Those risks, combined with potential interruptions in the execution of detailed protocols (due to the labile physiological conditions of patients), create a higher probability and impact of errors and worse outcomes[3] in an already vulnerable population.

Because of these inherent vulnerabilities, error reduction and prevention in pediatric chemotherapy is also complex and requires a systematic approach, strong leadership, and multidisciplinary cooperation for success.[4,5] Error management in this domain requires global and specific consideration of the medication process and the information that controls it and coordination and communication among physicians, nurses, pharmacists, and allied health professionals. In addition, there must be ongoing surveillance and data collection and analysis to evaluate the effect of interventions[6] on the medication process[7] and to identify the introduction of new types of errors.[8]

One approach to reduce and prevent errors in medicating patients is to model the process as a series of steps performed by individuals (physicians, nurses, clerks, and pharmacists) who pass information from one to another.[9] With such a model, domain experts may be able to assess failure modes (mechanisms, likelihood, and impacts of the failure of individual steps)[10] for the process. With this assessment, interventions may be planned to reduce variation in the human performance (of repetitive or complex tasks) that leads to errors.[11] For medication processes, one highly promoted information technology (IT) application advocated by health care industry leaders to reduce errors is computerized provider order entry (CPOE)[12] because of its ability to reduce variability through automation and clinical decision support.

We herein describe the incorporation of CPOE into the pediatric chemotherapy process and its impact on process errors at an academic medical center.

**Author Affiliations:** Divisions of Health Sciences Informatics (Drs Kim and Lehmann) and Pediatric Oncology (Drs Chen and Arceci and Mss Kokoszka and Daniel), The Johns Hopkins School of Medicine, and Department of Pharmacy, The Johns Hopkins Hospital (Ms Mitchell), Baltimore, Md.

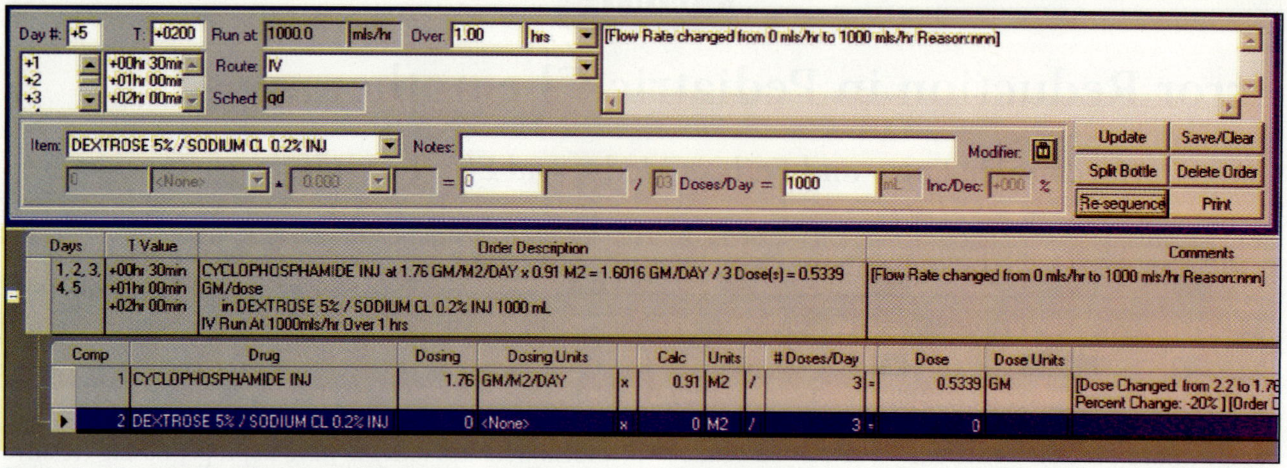


**Figure.** Sample screen shot of the pediatric chemotherapy computerized provider order entry interface.

## METHODS

This study was conducted in Pediatric Oncology of the Johns Hopkins Children's Center/Sidney Kimmel Comprehensive Cancer Center, Baltimore, Md, which provides chemotherapy to more than 200 children with a variety of neoplastic disorders. In response to a sentinel event, and as part of a safety and quality improvement program (the Quality Improvement Initiative) in pediatric oncology, paper-based order entry of pediatric chemotherapy was converted to CPOE.

### FAILURE MODES AND EFFECTS ANALYSIS

As part of a hospital leadership–driven initiative to reduce errors in chemotherapy, a multidisciplinary team consisting of staff from pediatric oncology (physicians, nurses, and physician assistants), pharmacy, and hospital information systems conducted a failure modes and effects analysis (FMEA) of the pediatric chemotherapy process and made recommendations to guide the implementation of functions for CPOE.

### IMPLEMENTATION OF CPOE

Recommendations of the multidisciplinary team, based on the FMEA findings and a pre-CPOE audit (described in "Data Collection"), were used to guide the modification of an available pharmacy system (RxTFC Pharmacy Information System; GE Medical Systems Information Technologies, BDM Information Systems Ltd, Saskatoon, Saskatchewan) to meet the needs of pediatric chemotherapy and to address the identified failure modes. A sample of the interface is shown in the **Figure**.

### DATA COLLECTION

To evaluate the impact of the introduction of CPOE into the pediatric chemotherapy process and to create a benchmark for further improvements, a 2-phase daily audit of pediatric chemotherapy treatments was administered before and after CPOE deployment. Before CPOE deployment, audit data were collected from July 31 to August 1, 2001, and August 14, 2001, to August 22, 2002 (241 days) using a paper-based survey tool from 1259 sequential chemotherapy orders (representing 176 patients). After CPOE deployment, audit data were collected from February 3, 2003, to February 12, 2004 (296 days) using a Web-based direct-entry tool (part of the CPOE application) from 1116 orders (representing 167 patients). Use of these data was approved by the Quality Assurance committee and the Division Chair at The Johns Hopkins University School of Medicine.

### DATA ANALYSIS

Using all chemotherapy orders for an individual patient in 1 day as the unit of analysis, we captured successful correct completion rates of specific steps of "high importance" (as determined by attending oncologists according to their potential for morbidity and mortality if not correctly completed) from the pre- and post-CPOE periods. The specific steps measured and compared were correct order format on the treatment plan (proper medication dose on the associated chemotherapy protocol/treatment plan), correct order format on the order (proper medication dose on an individual order), order and treatment plan match (proper match of a medication dose to its associated protocol), cumulative dose on the treatment plan (verification of the cumulative dose of a medication on a protocol), correct calculation (verification of the medication dose calculation), and nursing checklist (documentation of the nurse review).

## RESULTS

### FMEA RECOMMENDATIONS

Medication process steps, their failure modes (the potential severity and probability of occurrence), and the consensus recommendation to reduce errors are summarized in **Table 1**.

Of the different medication steps (prescription, ordering, transcription, dispensing, and administration), failure modes of high severity were identified in the ordering and administration steps. Of those, error types of medium to medium-high probability involved the misidentification of patients, patient variables (height and weight), and medications. Consensus recommendations to reduce these error types were to (1) limit choices (by predefined menus instead of free-text entry), (2) enforce entry of required data (height and weight), and (3) provide alerts for abnormal values. Failure modes of low to medium-high probability involved dosing errors due to mismatch of drug orders to chemotherapy protocols or miscalculation. Consensus recommendations to reduce error probability were to (1) enforce protocol specification and (2) automate calculations.

**Table 1. Abbreviated Failure Modes and Effects Analysis Matrix for Steps of High Importance**

| Step/Failure Mode | Probability of Occurrence | Action by CPOE to Reduce Occurrence |
|---|---|---|
| Wrong patient/parameter | Medium to medium high | Limited menu |
| Wrong medication | Medium to medium high | Order sets, limited formulary |
| Wrong dose/protocol | Low to medium high | Forced entry |
| Wrong dose/calculation | Low to medium high | Autocalculation |
| Missed check | Medium to medium high | Autocheck |

Abbreviation: CPOE, computerized provider order entry.

**Table 2. Audit Data Analysis of High Importance Steps**

| | Errors on Paper, No. (%) | Errors on CPOE, No. (%) | RR With CPOE (95% CI) |
|---|---|---|---|
| Correct order format (treatment plan) | 50/1255 (4.0) | 28/1063 (2.6) | 0.66 (0.42-1.04) |
| Correct order format (order) | 26/1153 (2.3) | 6/1028 (0.06) | 0.26 (0.11-0.61) |
| Order and treatment plan match | 14/1253 (1.1) | 67/1112 (6.0) | 5.4 (3.1-9.5) |
| Cumulative dose on treatment plan | 5/28 (18) | 29/512 (5.7) | 0.32 (0.14-0.77) |
| Correct calculation | 3/52 (5.8) | 6/1102 (0.54) | 0.09 (0.03-0.34) |
| Nursing checklist present | 59/1237 (4.8) | 27/1101 (2.5) | 0.51 (0.33-0.80) |

Abbreviations: CI, confidence interval; CPOE, computerized provider order entry; RR, relative risk.

## AUDIT DATA ANALYSIS

Completion rates of oncologist-identified steps of high importance from the pre- and post-CPOE periods are summarized in **Table 2**.

After CPOE deployment, daily chemotherapy orders were less likely to have improper dosing on orders (relative risk [RR], 0.26; 95% confidence interval [CI], 0.11-0.61), incorrect dosing calculations (RR, 0.09; 95% CI, 0.03-0.34), missing cumulative dose calculations (RR, 0.32; 95% CI, 0.14-0.77), and incomplete nursing checklists (RR, 0.51; 95% CI, 0.33-0.80). There was no difference in the likelihood of improper dosing on treatment plans and a higher likelihood of not matching medication orders to treatment plans (RR, 5.4; 95% CI, 3.1-9.5).

## COMMENT

The risks to patients posed by potential errors in the pediatric chemotherapy process are multidimensional, owing to inherent toxicities of the sometimes experimental drugs used, complexities of the protocols followed, and clinical lability of the patients' disease processes. In addition, children, possibly owing to the additional need for individualized dosing based on weight and body surface area, are at higher risk for medication errors (approximately 3 times that of adults[13]) in general.[7]

For these reasons, the maxim *primum non nocere*[14] mandates systematic error management in the pediatric chemotherapy process as an essential part of improving pediatric oncology outcomes.[15] Such management includes an informed and iterative approach to (1) model the clinical process in which errors occur; (2) identify the errors, their mechanisms, probabilities of occurrence, and impacts; (3) modify the process to eliminate or reduce the errors; (4) evaluate the effect of modifications on the process (and outcomes); and (5) update clinical process models on the basis of evaluation data.[16] Systematic error management is vital to good clinical care in complex processes (such as patient medication) and complex settings (such as hospitals).

Other proactive and reactive approaches to error management in pediatric chemotherapy include (manual) multidisciplinary check of order sets,[17] integrated incident and error reporting,[18] knowledge acquisition and computer-aided planning of therapy with decision support for individualized therapy,[19] standardization of the terminology used,[20] and education of caregivers,[21] in addition to standard approaches such as root cause analysis[22] (mandated by the Joint Commission on Accreditation of Healthcare Organizations for the investigation of sentinel events in accredited hospitals) of errors when they occur.

Failure modes effects analysis is a methodology adapted from the military[23] and recommended by the Joint Commission on Accreditation of Healthcare Organizations for redesigning health care processes[24] as a proactive, systematic approach for identifying "the ways that a process or design can fail, why it might fail, and how it can be made safer."[25] Failure modes effects analysis is directly applicable to the incorporation of IT such as CPOE into a complex process such as pediatric chemotherapy. Using domain and IT expertise, the assessment identifies and prioritizes specific process errors (failure modes) and suggests ways that IT (in this case CPOE) can help to mitigate them. The collection of data (also determined by domain expertise, in this case attending oncologists) provides evidence and benchmarks for further improvement efforts.

According to literature and to the experience of the team, most medication process errors (in general) and pediatric chemotherapy errors (in particular) occur at the prescribing/ordering step,[26] to which the team recommendations were directed to (1) automate calculations (via embedded calculators), (2) reduce free-text and handwritten entry (via drop-down medication lists), (3) reduce prescriber memory load (via autocompletion of specific data fields), and (4) enforce prescriber completion of essential data fields (via pop-up alerts). These functions were incorporated into the design and implementation of the application and its interface.

Incorporation of CPOE has been advocated as an effective way to reduce medication errors,[27,28] but its implementation and deployment must be tailored to the needs of specific clinical processes. In pediatrics and neonatology, CPOE has been demonstrated to mitigate errors in specialized medication processes (such as total parenteral nutrition[29] and continuous intravenous infusions[30]), and these deployments have succeeded through guidance by domain and IT experts who are familiar with the processes.

Error management must consist of continued surveillance for persistence of old errors and anticipation of the introduction of new ones. In the first iteration of CPOE error, there was an unanticipated but statistically significant decrease in the matching of orders (chemotherapy drug doses) to specific protocols. A review of the data suggested several reasons for this:

- No automated drug-protocol linkage. At the time of this study, this feature was not included.
- User interface problem. New or experimental drugs did not appear on the predefined menu after CPOE deployment, requiring users to enter them manually, resulting in drug-protocol nonmatch. Before CPOE deployment, all orders were handwritten, which may have also resulted in underreporting of drug-protocol nonmatches.
- Human transcription failure. After CPOE deployment, protocols were still paper based, forcing prescribers to switch back and forth between electronic and print interfaces.

These considerations provide a basis for the next iteration of the CPOE application, which will include automated linkage of chemotherapy order sets to specific protocols at the Johns Hopkins Children's Center (planned for 2006).

A strength of this study was the inclusion of audit data from all patient encounters in the pre- and post-CPOE time frames. A limitation was the focus on process and not outcomes. Inclusion of outcome measures is projected for a future iteration.

In conclusion, pediatric chemotherapy is a complex medication process that is vulnerable to human error. Computerized provider order entry is a recognized IT intervention that can reduce errors, but its incorporation into the process must be guided by domain and IT expertise. We have described an FMEA-guided implementation of CPOE in pediatric chemotherapy at an academic medical center with data that demonstrate its impact on reducing process errors.

**Accepted for Publication:** November 22, 2005.
**Correspondence:** George R. Kim, MD, The Johns Hopkins School of Medicine, 600 N Wolfe St, Nelson 2-133, Baltimore, MD 21287-3200 (grkim@jhmi.edu).
**Author Contributions:** All of the authors had full access to all the data in the study and take responsibility for the integrity of the data and the accuracy of the data analysis.
**Funding/Support:** This study was supported by the Center for Innovation and Quality Patient Care at The Johns Hopkins Hospital.

## REFERENCES

1. Scavuzzo J, Gamba N. Bridging the gap: the virtual chemotherapy unit. *J Pediatr Oncol Nurs.* 2004;21:27-32.
2. Womer RB, Tracy E, Soo-Hoo W, Bickert B, DiTaranto S, Barnsteiner JH. Multidisciplinary systems approach to chemotherapy safety: rebuilding processes and holding the gains. *J Clin Oncol.* 2002;20:4705-4712.
3. Taylor RE, Bailey CC, Robinson K, et al; International Society of Paediatric Oncology; United Kingdom Children's Cancer Study Group. Results of a randomized study of preradiation chemotherapy versus radiotherapy alone for nonmetastatic medulloblastoma: the International Society of Paediatric Oncology/United Kingdom Children's Cancer Study Group PNET-3 Study. *J Clin Oncol.* 2003;21:1581-1591.
4. Branowicki P, O'Neill JB, Dwyer JL, Marino BL, Houlahan K, Billett A. Improving complex medication systems: an interdisciplinary approach. *J Nurs Adm.* 2003; 33:199-200.
5. Dinning C, Branowicki P, O'Neill JB, Marino BL, Billett A. Chemotherapy error reduction: a multidisciplinary approach to create templated order sets. *J Pediatr Oncol Nurs.* 2005;22:20-30.
6. Apkon M, Mattera JA, Lin Z, et al. A randomized outpatient trial of a decision-support information technology tool. *Arch Intern Med.* 2005;165:2388-2394.
7. Lehmann CU, Kim GR. Prevention of medication errors. *Clin Perinatol.* 2005;32: 107-123.
8. Ash JS, Berg M, Coiera E. Some unintended consequences of information technology in health care: the nature of patient care information system–related errors. *J Am Med Inform Assoc.* 2004;11:104-112.
9. Coiera E. Four rules for the reinvention of health care. *BMJ.* 2004;328:1197-1199.
10. Bonnabry P, Cingria L, Ackermann M, Sadeghipour F, Bigler L, Mach N. Use of a prospective risk analysis method to improve the safety of the cancer chemotherapy process. *Int J Qual Health Care.* 2006;18:9-16.
11. Norman DA. Design rules based on analyses of human error. *Commun ACM.* 1983;26:254-258.
12. Computer physician order entry. Leapfrog Group Web site. Washington, DC: Leapfrog Group; 2005. Available at: http://www.leapfroggroup.org/for_hospitals/leapfrog_safety_practices/cpoe. Updated 2005. Accessed November 16, 2005 .
13. Kaushal R, Bates DW, Landrigan C, et al. Medication errors and adverse drug events in pediatric inpatients. *JAMA.* 2001;285:2114-2120.
14. Smith CM. Origin and uses of *primum non nocere*—above all, do no harm! *J Clin Pharmacol.* 2005;45:371-377.
15. Kaushal R, Shojania KG, Bates DW. Effects of computerized physician order entry and clinical decision support systems on medication safety: a systematic review. *Arch Intern Med.* 2003;163:1409-1416.
16. Pape TM, Guerra DM, Muzquiz M, et al. Innovative approaches to reducing nurses' distractions during medication administration. *J Contin Educ Nurs.* 2005;36: 108-116.
17. Marino BL, Branowicki P, Bennett JA, et al. Evaluating process changes in a pediatric hospital medication system. *Outcomes Manag.* 2002;6:10-15.
18. France DJ, Miles P, Cartwright J, et al. A chemotherapy incident reporting and improvement system. *Jt Comm J Qual Saf.* 2003;29:171-180.
19. Garde S, Baumgarten B, Basu O, et al. A meta-model of chemotherapy planning in the multi-hospital/multi-trial-center–environment of pediatric oncology. *Methods Inf Med.* 2004;43:171-183.
20. Merzweiler A, Ehlerding H, Creutzig U, et al. Standardizing terminology in pediatric oncology: the basic data set [in German]. *Klin Padiatr.* 2002;214:212-217.
21. Kline NE. Promoting patient safety through the development of a pediatric chemotherapy and biotherapy provider program [editorial]. *J Pediatr Oncol Nurs.* 2004;21:65-66.
22. Wald H, Shojania KG. Root cause analysis. In: Shojania KG, Duncan BW, McDonald KM, et al, eds. Making Health Care Safer: A Critical Analysis of Patient Safety Practices. Rockville, Md: Agency for Healthcare Research and Quality; July 2001. Evidence Report/Technology Assessment No. 43. AHRQ Publication No. 01-E058. Available at: http://www.ahrq.gov/clinic/ptsafety/. Accessed November 18, 2005.
23. Haapenen P, Helminen A. Failure mode and effects analysis of software-based automation systems. STUK-YTO- TR 190. Helsinki, Finland; 2002. Available at: http://www.fmeainfocentre.com/download/softwarefmea.pdf. Accessed November 18, 2005.
24. O'Leary D. Reducing medical errors: a review of innovative strategies to improve patient safety. Testimony before the House Committee on Energy and Commerce Subcommittee on Health, May 8, 2002. Available at: http://www.jcaho.org/news+room/on+capitol+hill/oleary_test.htm. Accessed November 16, 2005.
25. Joint Commission on Accreditation of Healthcare Organizations. Team identifies ways to mitigate risks in new accreditation process. *Jt Comm Perspect.* 2004; 24:15-16.
26. Barber N, Rawlins M, Dean Franklin B. Reducing prescribing error: competence, control, and culture. *Qual Saf Health Care.* 2003;12(suppl 1):i29-i32.
27. Kohn L, Corrigan J, Donaldson M, eds. *To Err is Human: Building a Safer Health System: Institute of Medicine.* Washington, DC: National Academy Press; 1999.
28. Patient safety. Leapfrog Group Web site. Available at: http://www.leapfroggroup.org/safety1.htm. Accessed July 26, 2004.
29. Lehmann CU, Conner KG, Cox JM. Preventing provider errors: online total parenteral nutrition calculator. *Pediatrics.* 2004;113:748-753.
30. Giannone G. Computer-supported weight-based drug infusion concentrations in the neonatal intensive care unit. *Comput Inform Nurs.* 2005;23:100-105.

SECTION EDITOR: ALBERT C. YAN, MD; ASSISTANT SECTION EDITOR: SAMIR S. SHAH, MD

# Picture of the Month

*Kathryn S. Moffett, MD; Jon E. Welch, MD*

A 7-YEAR-OLD GIRL PRESENTED WITH 6 DAYS of vomiting and abdominal pain in addition to a 3.5-kg weight loss over the past 6 months. On examination, she was pale and thin. Her weight was 16.9 kg (<5th percentile for age), and her height was 116 cm (10th percentile). Abdominal examination revealed a well-defined, firm, mobile, nontender, and nonpulsatile 8 × 8-cm mass in the left upper quadrant extending into the epigastric region. Laboratory studies showed a microcytic anemia with a hemoglobin concentration of 9.0 g/dL; the hematocrit was 26.8%. Amylase and lipase levels were normal. Hemoccult test results for stool and emesis were positive for blood. Abdominal radiography was performed (see **Figure 1** and **Figure 2**).

What is your diagnosis?

**Author Affiliations:** Department of Pediatrics, West Virginia University, Morgantown.

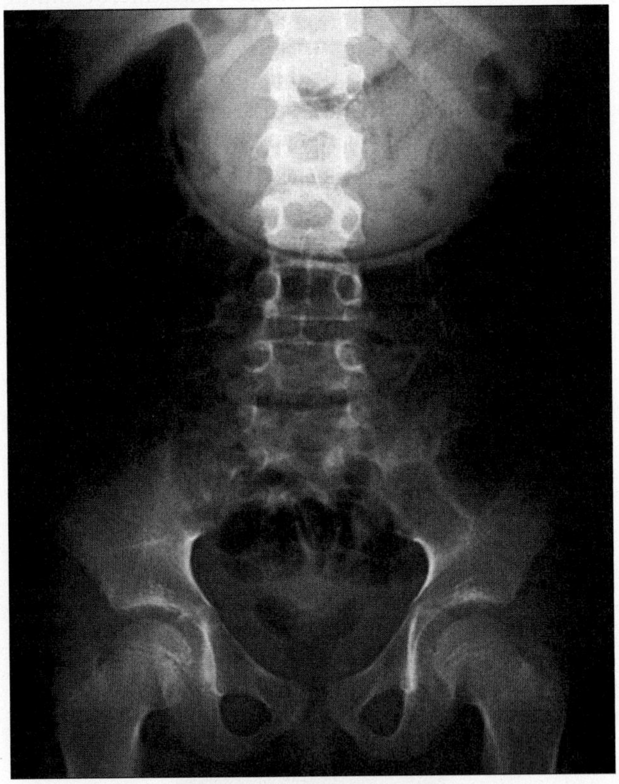

**Figure 1.** Upright radiograph of the abdomen.

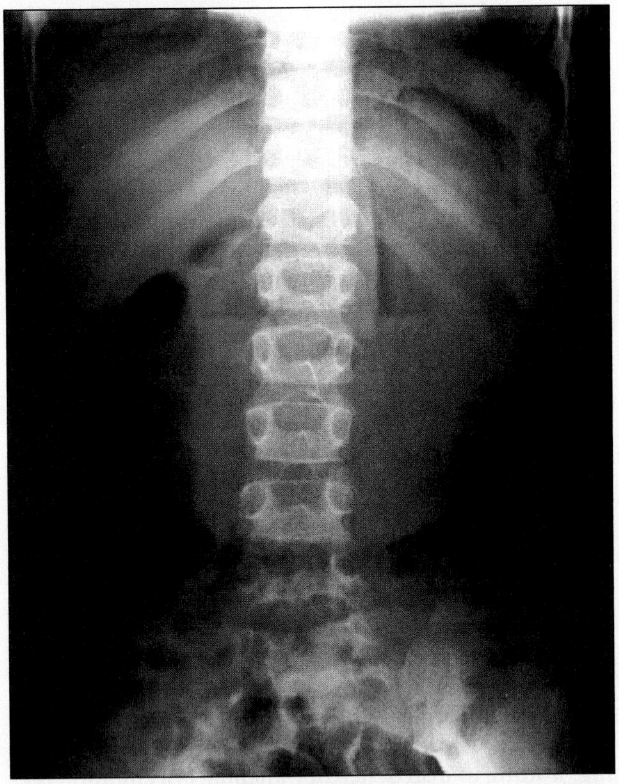

**Figure 2.** Kidneys, ureters, and bladder (KUB) radiograph.

# Denouement and Discussion

## Trichobezoar

Abdominal radiography revealed a mass in the stomach (see Figure 1 and Figure 2). Open surgical resection of the stomach revealed a trichobezoar (hair bezoar) (see **Figure 3**) and evidence of gastritis. Upon further inquiry with the family, we learned that the child had had a history of trichotillomania since 2 years of age; however, at the time, she had no signs of alopecia. Within days of the surgical removal of the bezoar, the child's appetite improved and she quickly gained weight. Her anemia was attributed to iron deficiency from chronic blood loss associated with gastritis as well as poor oral intake. Following surgery, outpatient child psychiatry consultation was arranged.

The accumulation of foreign ingested material in the form of masses or concretions may result in a gastric bezoar.[1] Bezoars are classified according to their composition: phytobezoars, trichobezoars, and pharmacobezoars. Phytobezoars, composed of vegetable matter, are the most common type with the persimmon fruit (diospyrobezoar) accounting for the majority of cases. Banana seeds have also been reported.[2] Trichobezoars, composed of hair, typically occur in young women and girls with psychiatric disorders such as trichotillomania (hair pulling) and trichophagia (hair eating), which usually precede trichobezoar formation. Pharmacobezoars, composed of ingested medications, have become increasingly recognized from such medications as iron, antacids, theophylline, enteric-coated aspirin, nifedipine, sodium alginate, and sucralfate. Bezoars composed of a variety of other substances, such as shellac, fungus, milk curd, tissue paper, cement, vinyl gloves, and Styrofoam cups, have been described.[3]

Trichobezoars form in patients with trichotillomania and trichophagia. They begin as retained hairs between the gastric folds; the hair is then denatured by gastric acid, becomes black (regardless of hair color), and combines with food to form an enmeshed mass. Trichobezoars become colonized by bacteria, resulting in a foul smell. A small number of patients have been reported in whom the gastric trichobezoar has a long tail and extends throughout the small bowel to the cecum. This condition, known as the Rapunzel syndrome, occurs almost exclusively in young girls.[4-6]

Many affected patients remain asymptomatic for many years and develop symptoms insidiously. Common complaints include abdominal pain, nausea, vomiting, early satiety, anorexia, and weight loss. Gastrointestinal bleeding, leading to iron deficiency anemia, is a common presentation because there is a high association of gastric ulcers or gastritis in patients with bezoars. The ulcers may be due to peptic ulcer disease or pressure necrosis. Although many bezoars become quite large, gastric outlet obstruction is an uncommon presentation.

Bezoars have rarely been associated with a vast array of other gastrointestinal complications. These include gastrointestinal perforation, peritonitis, protein-losing enteropathy, steatorrhea, pancreatitis, intussusception, dysphagia, obstructive jaundice, appendicitis, constipation, and pneumatosis intestinalis. These other gastrointestinal complications may occur either when "the Rapunzel," or the string of a long tail of hair, extends into the small intestine or when an embolus of hair lodges in the small intestine, becoming the lead point for obstruction or intussusception.[6,7]

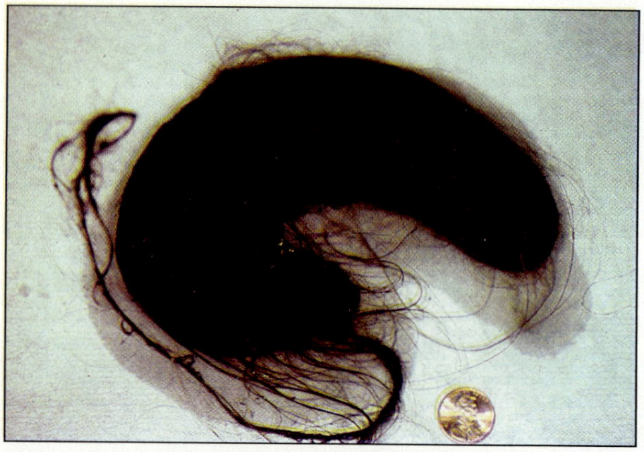

**Figure 3.** Hair bezoar.

On physical examination, most patients with a gastric bezoar may have minimal findings except for an occasional painless abdominal mass or halitosis. Pallor may accompany anemia. Parents may report that the child eats frequent small meals with early satiety. Patients with trichobezoars may have patchy areas of alopecia, a result of the accompanying trichotillomania.

Bezoars are usually discovered as an incidental finding in a patient with nonspecific symptoms. Abdominal radiograph with or without barium, abdominal ultrasound, or computed tomographic scan may show the bezoar as mass or a filling defect. Therapy for bezoars should be tailored to the composition of the concretion and to the underlying pathophysiologic features. Removal of the bezoar does not alleviate the underlying process that precipitated the bezoar. Preventive therapy should be implemented to avoid a reported 14% recurrence rate. Patients should be encouraged to seek psychiatric evaluation, especially in children with trichobezoars.

**Accepted for Publication:** September 14, 2005.
**Correspondence:** Kathryn S. Moffett, MD, Department of Pediatrics, West Virginia University, HSC-9214, Morgantown, WV 26506-9214 (kmoffett@hsc.wvu.edu).

## REFERENCES

1. De Bakey M, Ochsner A. Bezoars and concretions. *Surgery.* 1938;4:934-936.
2. Schoeffl V, Varatorn R, Blinnikov O, Vidamaly V. Intestinal obstruction due to phytobezoars of banana seeds: a case report. *Asian J Surg.* 2004;27:348-351.
3. Zamir D, Goldblum C, Linova L, Polychuck I, Reitblat T, Yoffe B. Phytobezoars and trichobezoars: a 10-year experience. *J Clin Gastroenterol.* 2004;38:873-876.
4. Balik E, Ulman I, Taneli C, Demircan M. The Rapunzel syndrome: a case report and review of the literature. *Eur J Pediatr Surg.* 1993;3:171-173.
5. Pul N, Pul M. The Rapunzel syndrome (trichobezoar) causing gastric perforation in a child: a case report. *Eur J Pediatr.* 1996;155:18-19.
6. Singla SL, Rattan KN, Kaushik N, Pandit SK. Rapunzel syndrome: a case report. *Am J Gastroenterol.* 1999;94:1970-1971.
7. Frey AS, McKee M, King RA, Martin A. Hair apparent: Rapunzel syndrome. *Am J Psychiatry.* 2005;162:242-248.

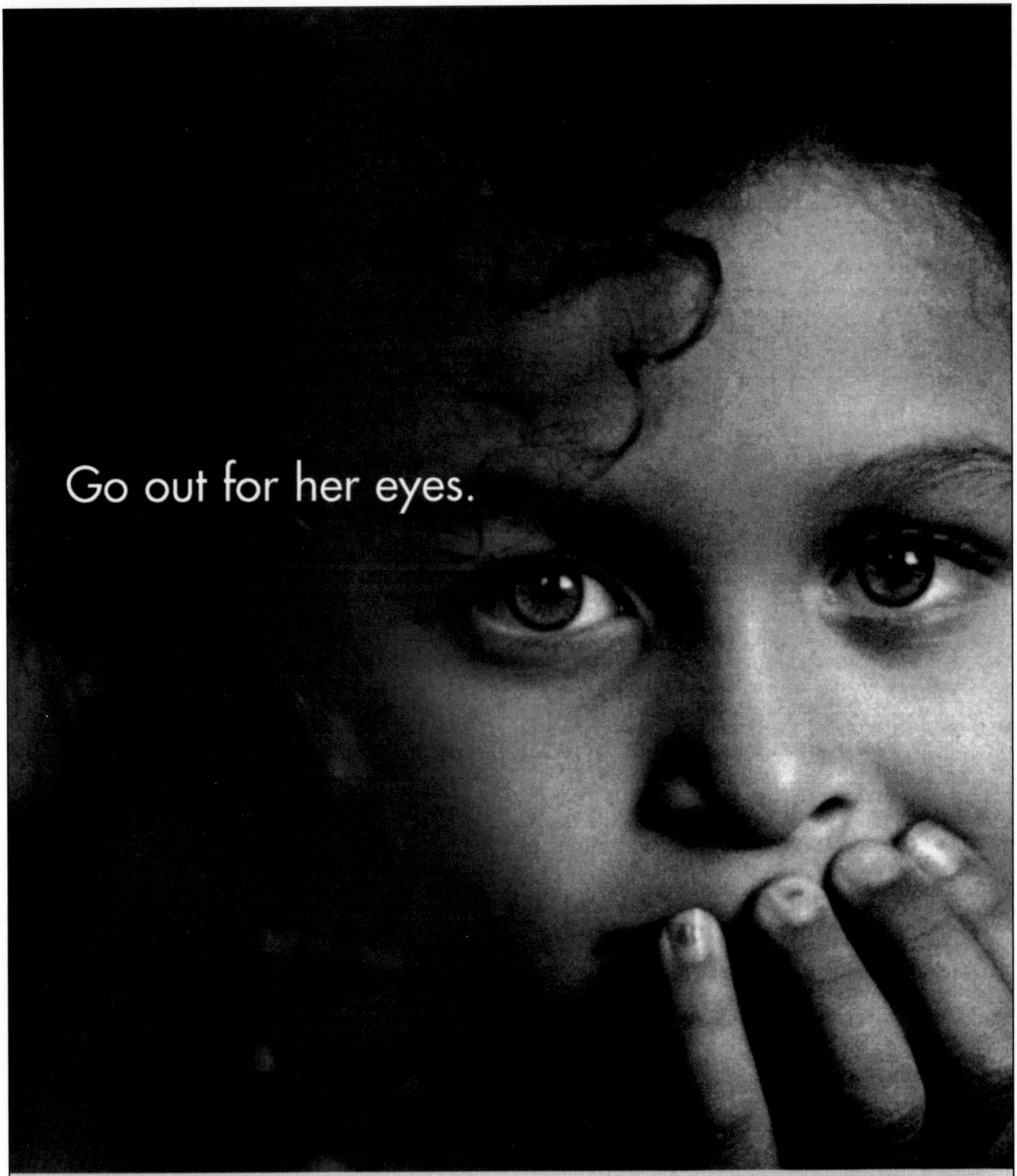


Until you can stop smoking, smoke outside for your daughter. She could get fewer earaches, be less susceptible to respiratory infections and be less likely to get asthma.

Until you can stop smoking, go out for your kids.

Take the Smoke-Free Home Pledge. Call 1 800-513-1157

American Medical Association • Environmental Protection Agency • Consumer Federation of America Foundation

# Systematic Review of the Relationship Between Early Introduction of Solid Foods to Infants and the Development of Allergic Disease

*Beth A. Tarini, MD; Aaron E. Carroll, MD, MS; Colin M. Sox, MD, MS; Dimitri A. Christakis, MD, MPH*

**Objective:** To assess the evidence that early solid feeding (before age 4 months) increases the risk of allergic disease.

**Data Sources:** MEDLINE, the Cochrane Library, and the Drugs and Pharmacology section of EMBASE with key words "infant," "food," and "allergy."

**Study Selection:** We found 2719 article citations and reviewed references of relevant articles. We critically evaluated the methods and results of articles that met inclusion criteria. We identified 13 studies that met inclusion criteria. There was only 1 controlled trial.

**Data Extraction:** Allergic disease.

**Data Synthesis:** Five studies found a positive association between early solid feeding and eczema, with a persistence of the association for 10 years in 1 study. Four studies found no association. One study found an association between early solid feeding and pollen allergy. We found no strong evidence to support the association between early solid feeding and the development of persistent asthma, persistent food allergy, allergic rhinitis, or animal dander allergy.

**Conclusions:** Systematic review of available evidence suggests that early solid feeding may increase the risk of eczema. However, there are little data supporting an association between early solid feeding and other allergic conditions. Since many studies had problematic methods, additional controlled trials are needed to help guide physicians as they advise parents about the allergic risks of early introduction of solids.

*Arch Pediatr Adolesc Med. 2006;160:502-507*

**Author Affiliations:** Robert Wood Johnson Clinical Scholars Program (Drs Tarini and Christakis); Department of Pediatrics, University of Washington (Drs Tarini and Christakis), and Child Health Institute and Children's Hospital and Regional Medical Center (Dr Christakis), Seattle; Children's Health Services Research, Indiana University School of Medicine, and Regenstrief Institute for Health Care, Indianapolis (Dr Carroll); Center for Child Health Care Studies, Department of Ambulatory Care and Prevention, Harvard Medical School and Harvard Pilgrim Healthcare, Boston, Mass (Dr Sox).

THE AGE WHEN INFANTS ARE introduced to solid foods has varied greatly during the last century, from 1 year of age in the 1900s to a few weeks of age in the 1950s.[1] Currently, the American Academy of Pediatrics,[2] the World Health Organization,[3] and the European Academy of Allergology and Clinical Immunology[4] recommend avoidance of solid feeding for at least the first 4 months of life, citing studies that have suggested an increased risk of allergy associated with earlier introduction of solids. However, there has been no systematic review of the evidence that early solid feeding increases an infant's risk of allergic disease.

*For editorial comment see page 552*

The timing of introduction of solids to infants is an important issue that physicians frequently confront while caring for infants. Counseling parents is further complicated by the fact that, despite recommendations to the contrary, many parents continue to feed their infants solids before the age of 4 months.[5,6] The 1988-1994 National Health and Nutrition Examination Survey reported that 52% of nonbreastfed infants and 29% of breastfed infants were introduced to infant cereal at 2 to 3 months of age.[2]

Given that pediatricians are frequently asked for advice on when to start infants on solid foods and, to our knowledge, no systematic synthesis of the literature has been performed, we conducted a systematic review to evaluate the evidence of the effect of early solid feeding of infants on the risk of allergic disease.

## METHODS

We searched MEDLINE (from January 1, 1966, through March 1, 2005), the Cochrane Library (as of March 1, 2005), and the Drugs and Pharmacology section of EMBASE (1991 through March 1, 2005) using the key words "infant" and "food" and "allergy" and restricted our search to human studies and English-language publications. We also reviewed the bibliographies of relevant articles to identify additional studies. We used a keyword search because it was more robust than alternative literature searches using MeSH headings or key words of specific allergic conditions.

We designed this systematic review to follow a number of inclusion and exclusion criteria. We included randomized controlled trials and case-control and cohort studies. We chose to include cohort studies because some, but not all, of these cohort studies have been cited in feeding recommendations.[2,4] Therefore, given the clinical influence that these cohort studies exert, we felt that they merited evaluation in our review.

We immediately eliminated articles that did not examine the relationship between the introduction of solid foods to infants and the development of any of the following allergic diseases: asthma, eczema, food allergy, pollen allergy, allergic rhinitis, and animal dander allergy. We did not include outcomes that frequently are due to nonallergic causes (such as cough, respiratory illness, or vomiting) in order to avoid type II error. We defined "solid foods" as any food other than breast milk, cow's milk, or formula.

Therefore, studies were included only if they met all of the following criteria: (1) explicit mention of early (at < 4 months of age) introduction of solids, (2) presence of a comparison group for early feeders, (3) absence of additional and simultaneous allergy reduction interventions (such as prenatal maternal diet restriction, environmental allergen avoidance, or additional infant hypoallergenic dietary restrictions), (4) measurement of 1 of the aforementioned clinically defined allergic diseases, and (5) English-language publication.

If a citation could not be excluded based on the title or abstract, then the entire article was reviewed. After articles that clearly did not meet the inclusion criteria were excluded, 2 of us (B.A.T. and C.M.S.) independently evaluated all remaining articles to determine if they met inclusion criteria; another of us (A.E.C) resolved discrepancies. We did not blind authors to the titles, authors, or journal publication of the articles. We defined duplicate publications as multiple original articles that reported identical outcomes measured on the same population during the same period. For duplicate publications, we included the first published article unless minor differences between publications existed. In this latter case, we included the publication that provided the most information.

## RESULTS

### LITERATURE SEARCH

Our literature search identified 2719 article titles. Thirty-nine articles required joint review by 3 of us (B.A.T, C.M.S., and A.E.C.). None of these 39 articles was a randomized controlled trial. We found 2 sets (4 articles) of duplicate publications.[7-10]

Thirteen studies met inclusion criteria (**Table**). Major reasons for exclusion were (1) no information regarding timing of solid food introduction, (2) multiple simultaneous interventions in addition to timing of solids, (3) attempts to compare groups with confounding differences at baseline, (4) delay of only a select group of solids, (5) comparison groups were not "early" and "late" feeders, and (6) allergic disease was not clinically defined. The references for these excluded articles are available on request.

We also excluded studies in which the intervention consisted of a combined prenatal and postnatal dietary intervention because the methods (control group had neither maternal nor infant dietary restriction) did not permit evaluation of the individual contribution of infant diet to the outcomes.[22-24] Additionally, these studies evaluated the effect of delayed, not early, introduction of solid feeding.[22-24]

We present the studies according to the allergic outcomes reported; as a result, some studies appear multiple times. Furthermore, cohorts are followed up longitudinally and so some have been described in multiple publications. For simplicity, we refer to each follow-up publication for a cohort as a different study.

### ECZEMA

#### Summary

Nine cohort studies evaluated the relationship between solids before the age of 3 to 4 months and eczema.[7,9,11-17] Five of these studies found a positive association,[7,11-14] while 4 studies found no association.[9,15-17] Of these 9 studies, 5 were based on 2 cohorts followed up longitudinally.[7,9,11,12,14]

#### Studies Finding a Positive Association Between Early Introduction of Solid Foods and Eczema

Two studies followed up the same birth cohort of 135 Finnish infants of atopic parent(s), evaluating them for eczema at 1 and 5 years of age.[9,14] Sixty-five mothers initiated solid foods at 3 months of age (against protocol), but none introduced cow's milk before 6 months of age. An unreported, but "similar," number of infants in each group avoided fish, citrus fruit, and eggs by their mothers' initiative. Criteria for eczema were either (1) previous diagnosis by a physician and eczema noted during an examination by the author (a physician) or (2) eczema on examination at the 1- and 5-year study evaluations. No information on the blinding of the examining author was provided.

By 1 year of age, 24% of these Finnish infants were diagnosed with eczema: 14% of breastfed infants vs 35% of solid-fed infants ($P<.01$).[14] However, by 5 years of age, 24% of both feeding groups had eczema.[9] Although these cohort studies suggest that the association between early feeding of solids to infants of atopic parent(s) and eczema wanes by 5 years of age, these results merit cautious interpretation because 17% of participants were lost to follow-up.

Forsyth et al[13] examined whether introduction of solid foods at a specific time before 3 months of age was associated with eczema in a birth cohort of 671 Scottish infants. The rate of eczema (adjusted for maternal age, social class, type of milk feed, and maternal history of allergic disease) during 1 to 2 years of age was significantly higher among infants introduced to solids at 8 to 12 weeks of age compared with other ages (<8 weeks, 5.4%; 8-12 weeks, 17%; >12 weeks, 8.3%; $P<.05$).

Three studies followed up a birth cohort during the Christchurch Child Development Study in New Zealand[7,11,12] for 10 years. Since compliance with maternal diaries was only 61% by age 2 years, maternal recall and physicians' records provided the missing information. At age 2 years, eczema rates were significantly higher in infants fed solids before 4 months of age: before 4 months

**Table. Characteristics of Included Studies***

| Disease | No. of Subjects | Exclusive to Subjects With Atopic Family History | Age at Study Conclusion | Disease Risk |
|---|---|---|---|---|
| Eczema | | | | |
| Fergusson et al[7] | 1265 | No | 10 y | Increased |
| Fergusson et al[11] | 1265 | No | 2 y | Increased |
| Fergusson et al[12] | 1265 | No | 3 y | Increased |
| Forsyth et al[13] | 671 | No | 2 y | Increased |
| Kajosaari and Saarinen[14] | 135 | Yes | 1 y | Increased |
| Kajosaari[9] | 135 | Yes | 5 y | No difference |
| Moore et al[15] | 525† | Yes | 1 y | No difference |
| Van Asperen et al[16] | 79 | Yes | 16-20 mo | No difference |
| Zutavern et al[17] | 642 | No | 5.5 y | No difference |
| Asthma | | | | |
| Armentia et al[18] | 500‡ | No | 41.5 y ± 18.5§ | Increased |
| Fergusson et al[19] | 1265 | No | 4 y | No difference |
| Kajosaari[9] | 135 | Yes | 5 y | No difference |
| Wheezing | | | | |
| Forsyth et al[13] | 671 | No | 2 y | No difference |
| Van Asperen et al[16] | 79 | Yes | 16-20 mo | No difference |
| Wilson et al[20] | 545 | No | 7.3 y (6.1-9.9)‖ | Increased |
| Zutavern et al[17] | 642 | No | 5.5 y | No difference |
| Food allergy | | | | |
| Kajosaari and Saarinen[14] | 135 | Yes | 1 y | Increased |
| Kajosaari[9] | 135 | Yes | 5 y | No difference |
| Allergic rhinitis | | | | |
| Van Asperen et al[16] | 79 | Yes | 16-20 mo | No difference |
| Pollen allergy | | | | |
| Kajosaari[9] | 135 | Yes | 5 y | Increased |
| Animal dander allergy | | | | |
| Kajosaari[9] | 135 | Yes | 5 y | No difference |
| Allergic disease | | | | |
| Parihar et al[21] | 425¶ | No | 0-2 y | Increased |

*All studies are cohort design unless otherwise noted.
†Designed as randomized-controlled trial, analyzed as a cohort.
‡Case-control design.
§Mean age ± SD.
‖Mean age (range).
¶Cross-sectional design.

of age, 17.8% vs after 4 months of age, 12.6% ($P<.05$).[11] Furthermore, the association was found to be dose dependent; rates of eczema increased with the number of different food types given: 0 foods, 13.4% had eczema; 1 to 2 types of foods, 17%; 3 to 4 types, 17.4%; and more than 5 types, 33.3% ($P<.05$).[11] However, this study found no association between eczema and either the specific types of foods or the estimated mean volume of solids. Parental history of atopy had an independent and stronger influence on rates of childhood eczema than early solid feeding (23.7% of children with atopic parents vs 13.0% of those without; $P<.001$).[11] No significant interaction was found between parental history, early solid feeding, and rate of eczema.

At 3 years of age, the positive association between early solid feeding and eczema persisted in the Christchurch cohort.[12] After adjusting for parental history and type of milk diet, the cumulative rates of eczema were found to be 16.6% for those offered no solids before 4 months, 20.5% for those offered 1 to 3 types of solid foods, and 25% for those offered 4 or more types ($P<.01$).[12]

At 10 years of age, the authors found a positive effect of early solids on recurrent eczema in the Christchurch cohort.[7] The authors defined recurrent eczema as having 3 previous physician visits for eczema, having at least 3 years of eczema symptoms, and receiving regular medications for eczema.[7] Eighty-four percent of the original cohort was followed up for 10 years. Although the overall prevalence of recurrent eczema decreased, the adjusted prevalence increased significantly with increasing types of solid foods introduced: 5.4% for no solids, 7.5% for 1 to 3 solids, and 12.7% for 4 or more solids ($P<.05$).[7] However, no particular food type was significantly associated with eczema.[7] In summary, the strengths of the Christchurch cohort's findings are the length of follow-up and the dose-dependent nature of the relationship.

### Studies Finding No Association Between Early Introduction of Solid Foods and Eczema

In addition to the 5-year follow-up study of the Finnish infant cohort,[9] 3 studies found no association between early solid feeding and eczema.[15-17] After studying 475 of 525 infants in a British birth cohort with a parental history of eczema or asthma, Moore et al[15] found no significant association between introduction of solids before 3 months of age and eczema (diagnosed through interval physical examinations) by 3, 6, or 12 months of age. Although initially designed as a randomized controlled trial to promote exclusive breastfeeding, poor compliance led to analysis of the study as a cohort. Multivariate analysis controlling for type of milk, early introduction of solids, social class, and family history of atopy found that only severity of atopic family history and type of milk independently predicted eczema at age 3 months (both $P<.01$) and severity of family history alone significantly predicted eczema at 6 and 12 months of age ($P<.02$). However, problematic study design warrants cautious interpretation of these results.

Van Asperen et al[16] studied a birth cohort of 79 Australian infants with a parental history of atopic disease (confirmed by skin prick tests) and found no significant association between eczema and solid feeding before 4 months of age (<4 months of age, 48.5%; >4 months of age, 47.8%). However, this study had the following problems: (1) incomplete follow-up (100% retention at 16 months, 75% at 20 months), (2) small sample size, (3) no indication of a blinded determination of eczema status, and (4) no indication that results were adjusted for cow's milk intake.

Zutavern et al[17] evaluated 604 of a birth cohort of 642 British children at 5.5 years of age and, in a multivariate analysis, found none of the early feeding exposures (rice by 3 months of age; fruits, vegetables, and cereals by 4 months of age; or any solid food by 3 months of age) to be significantly associated with development of eczema at 5.5 years of life. Unlike the previous study by Fergusson et al,[11] this study found no significant association between the numbers of food types introduced before age 4 months and eczema.

## ASTHMA OR WHEEZING

### Summary

One case-control and 6 cohort studies examined the association between early solid feeding and the development of asthma and/or wheezing.[9,13,16-20] The case-control study found a positive association with asthma.[18] Three cohort studies found no significant association with asthma by 4,[19] 5,[9] or 7[20] years of life, respectively. Three cohort studies found no significant association with episodes of wheezing,[13,16,17] while 1 found a positive association.[20]

### Studies Finding a Positive Association Between Early Introduction of Solid Foods and Asthma

The case-control study compared 250 cases of grass-pollen asthma (identified by allergy and pulmonary testing) with 250 asthma-free controls from an allergy clinic.[18] Grass pollen was the major aeroallergen responsible for allergic asthma in the geographic area; patients not native to the area were excluded. Cases and controls were not age matched (Table). Recall of exposure to cereals before 3 months of age was associated with grass-pollen asthma in an adjusted model (adjusted for mite asthma, animal asthma, food asthma, sex, and urban origin of patients; odds ratio, 6.24; $P=.71$). However, these findings should be interpreted cautiously because it is unclear whether the results were adjusted for family history and the exposure status is susceptible to recall bias.

### Studies Finding No Association Between Early Introduction of Solid Foods and Asthma

A longitudinal evaluation of the Christchurch cohort found that introduction to solids before 4 months of age was not associated with the cumulative rate of asthma or "wheezy bronchitis" by 4 years of age (solid fed, 7.2% vs nonsolid fed, 6.2%) and parental asthma was the only factor significantly related to variation in asthma rates.[19] Authors included "wheezy bronchitis" because it accounted for only 10 of the 77 "asthmatic" children[19] and differentiating it from asthma is difficult at a young age.

Among the 135 Finnish infants of atopic parent(s), Kajosaari[9] found no association between solid feeding at 3 months of age and asthma at 5 years of age. At 5 years of age, only 51 of 65 exclusively breastfed children and 62 of 70 children fed early solids were available for follow-up.[9]

### Study Finding No Association Between Early Introduction of Solid Foods and Asthma But a Positive Association With Wheezing

Wilson et al[20] retrospectively evaluated a subset (81%) of the birth cohort of Scottish infants at a mean age of 7.3 years (range, 6.1-9.9 years) and found an increased risk of wheezing, but not asthma, with introduction of solids before age 15 weeks. The outcome of wheeze required either a history of persistent wheeze since birth or during the previous 12 months. The outcome of asthma required either a previous physician diagnosis or current treatment with asthma medications. After adjustment for parental history of atopy, sex, and social class, the estimated probability of ever wheezing was significantly higher for those introduced to solids before 15 weeks of age (21.0% [95% confidence interval, 19.9%-21.1%]) compared with after (9.7% [95% confidence interval, 8.6%-10.8%]; $P<.01$). Using the cutoff of 15 weeks of age, the probability of ever having asthma was not significantly associated with the timing of solid feeding.

### Studies Finding No Association Between Early Introduction of Solid Foods and Wheezing

Forsyth et al[13] studied the same Scottish birth cohort until 2 years of age and found no relationship between the timing of solid foods introduction and episodes of wheezing during various age intervals (adjusted for maternal age, social class, type of milk feed, and maternal history of allergic disease).

In the birth cohort of 79 British infants of atopic parent(s), Van Asperen et al[16] found no significant association between introduction of solids before 4 months of age and wheezing (unadjusted for parental smoking or introduction of cow's milk).

Zutavern et al[17] evaluated about 600 of 642 children in a British birth cohort and found no association between early solid feeding and "transient" and "preschool wheezing." The authors defined "transient wheezing" as wheezing in the first 2 years of life only and "preschool wheezing" as either wheezing from age 1 to 4 years or wheezing during the fifth year of life with a history of at least 1 previous wheezing episode. Multivariate analysis revealed (1) no association between timing of solids (rice before age 3 months; fruits, vegetables, and cereals by 4 months of age; and any solid food by 3 months of age) and transient or preschool wheezing[17] and (2) no significant association between the number of food types introduced before 4 months of age and wheezing.

## FOOD ALLERGY

Longitudinal follow-up of the birth cohort of 135 Finnish infants of atopic parent(s) found early solid feeding to be significantly associated with food allergy by 1 year of age.[14] Food allergy was defined as a "history of skin rash or heavy vomiting after ingestion of a food." Allergy to fish, eggs, or citrus fruit prompted additional evaluation with an "elimination/challenge/rechallenge" protocol. At 1 year of age, infants who had received solids at 3 months of age were significantly more likely to have a history of food allergy compared with exclusively breastfed infants (37% vs 7%; $P<.001$).[14] Even when considering a history of food allergy to either fish, eggs, or citrus fruit individually, solid-fed infants were still more likely to have a positive history of allergy (26% vs 7%; $P<.01$).[14] However, evaluation of these food allergies with an elimination/challenge/rechallenge protocol decreased the proportion of food allergies in the solid-fed group to about 12%, and differences between the groups were no longer statistically significant.[14] This finding raises the concern that some nonallergic children were misclassified as allergic. When the criteria for food allergy were modified to include a positive clinical history and positive skin prick tests (fish, milk, wheat), at 5 years of age, there was no difference in allergy to any food between the 2 feeding groups.[9]

## ALLERGIC RHINITIS

In the birth cohort of 79 British infants of atopic parent(s), Van Asperen et al[16] found no association between early solid feeding (<4 months of age) and rhinitis by 16 to 20 months of age (no solids, 51.5%; solids, 58.6%; $P>.05$). Rhinitis was defined as "any history of nasal discharge and/or blockage occurring continuously for at least 4 weeks and excluding obvious infective rhinitis."[16(p526)]

## POLLEN ALLERGY

In the study of 135 Finnish infants of atopic parent(s), Kajosaari[9] found that exclusively breastfed infants were significantly less likely to have pollen allergy at 5 years of age than infants introduced to solid foods at 3 months of age (no solids, 20%; solids <3 months of age, 37%; $P=.04$). The investigators defined pollen allergy as positive skin prick test results to birch, elm, timothy, or ragweed that matched a clinical history of pollen allergy.

## ANIMAL DANDER ALLERGY

Kajosaari[9] found no association between cumulative incidence of animal dander allergy and solid feeding at 3 months of age. Animal dander allergy was determined by clinical history and positive skin prick test results to dog or cat epithelium.

## ANY ALLERGIC DISEASE

Using a cross-sectional study design, Parihar et al[21] found introduction of solids before the age of 3 months to be significantly associated with "allergic disease" in children before the age of 2 years at a pediatric clinic in Chandigarh, India. A child with 1 or more major allergic conditions (allergic asthma, rhinitis, atopic dermatitis, and urticaria) was categorized as allergic. No mean age of the study population was provided, although the 2 groups (with and without allergic disease) were reportedly "well-matched" for age. However, the 2 groups differed with respect to family history of allergy and age of introduction of cow's milk.

Parihar et al found that more children with allergic disease had been given semisolids before 3 months of age: 9.4% of children with allergies vs 1.4% of children without ($P<.01$). Significantly more children with allergies than those without had been fed cereals before 4 months of age and had received more solids during 4 to 6 months of life, although the authors didn't provide confidence intervals. However, study results should be interpreted cautiously since it is unclear whether the results were adjusted for family history of allergy and age at introduction of cow's milk.

## COMMENT

The evidence that introduction of solid food to infants before 4 months of age increases the risk of allergic disease is conflicting and inconsistent. In general, there is insufficient evidence to suggest that, on its own, the early introduction of solids to infants is associated with an increased risk of asthma, food allergy, allergic rhinitis, or animal allergies. However, based on the current literature, we can make limited and cautious conclusions. There is a consistent association between the persistence of eczema and the introduction of solid foods before age 4 months that is supported by long-term follow-up studies and the dose-dependent nature of the association. The results of 1 cohort study suggest a relationship between pollen allergy and early solid feeding in children with an atopic family history.

Unfortunately, many of the reviewed studies lacked a rigorous design and so were susceptible to multiple biases. For example, there was only 1 controlled trial (nonrandomized). While it is understandably difficult to evaluate the relationship of interest with a randomized controlled design, such a design would account for unmeasured and unknown confounders associated with early solid feeding. Moreover, some of the studies presented in this review failed to adjust for important known confounders, such as milk type used or parental history of atopy.

Exposure ascertainment was another important source of bias in identified studies. For example, some studies introduced recall bias by retrospectively collecting data on feeding. Most studies failed to systematically define the quality and quantity of solid foods that were introduced. This latter issue is important given the finding of Fergusson et al[11] of a dose-response relationship between number of food types and eczema.

Some study results may have been influenced by outcome misclassification. For example, incidence of some clinical outcomes may vary substantially depending on definitions used. In the study of 135 Finnish infants, when food allergy was evaluated by history in combination with a food challenge protocol instead of by history alone, the proportion of children with food allergy decreased.[14] Finally, lack of blinding to feeding history during study examinations may have led to a biased evaluation of outcome status.

There are a number of limitations to this systematic review that warrant consideration. We only evaluated articles in the English language and perhaps missed relevant studies published in other languages. We did not include studies that evaluated vomiting and/or diarrhea as outcomes because we felt that these were nonspecific symptoms of allergy. As a result, we may have missed a portion of children who had allergic gastrointestinal disorders. Additionally, some studies were based on the same ethnically homogeneous cohort of children[9,14] and some populations may have different genetic tendencies toward allergy as well as variable local prevalence of certain health outcomes. Finally, the potential for delayed timing of solid food introduction to affect the risk of allergic disease either alone, in concert with additional hypoallergenic interventions (such as prenatal or environmental), or in certain susceptible subgroups are valid concerns. However, evaluation of these factors is beyond the scope of this article.

In summary, we found that the evidence linking early solid feeding of infants and allergic disease is inconsistent and conflicting. We propose that organizations modify their recommendations regarding the relationship between the timing of introduction of solid feeding of infants and allergic disease risk to reflect the evidence presented in this review. Physicians who counsel parents on infant feeding issues should both educate parents that early solids do not confer a nutritional advantage and temper strong parental concerns that feeding small amounts of solids before 4 months of age will inevitably cause their child to a develop an allergic condition.

**Accepted for Publication:** September 6, 2005.
**Correspondence:** Beth A. Tarini, MD, Robert Wood Johnson Clinical Scholars Program, University of Washington, Health Sciences H-220, Box 357183, Seattle, WA 98195-7183 (btarini@u.washington.edu).
**Author Contributions:** Dr Tarini had full access to all the data in the study and takes responsibility for the integrity of the data and the accuracy of the data analysis.
**Funding/Support:** This study was supported by The Robert Wood Johnson Foundation Clinical Scholars Program. Dr Christakis is supported by the Robert Wood Johnson Generalist Physician Faculty Scholars Program. This study was also supported in part by the Nesholm Family Foundation.
**Disclaimer:** The views expressed in this article are those of the authors and do not necessarily represent the views of the Robert Wood Johnson Foundation or the University of Washington.
**Acknowledgment:** We acknowledge the helpful feedback on this project from Tom Koepsell, MD, MPH.

## REFERENCES

1. American Academy of Pediatrics Committee on Nutrition. On the feeding of solid foods to infants. *Pediatrics.* 1958;21:685-692.
2. American Academy of Pediatrics Committee on Nutrition. *Pediatric Nutrition Handbook.* 5th ed. Elk Grove, Ill: AAP; 2004.
3. World Health Organization. Prevention of allergy and allergic asthma. Paper presented at: WHO/WAO Meeting on the Prevention of Allergy and Allergic Asthma; January 8-9, 2002; Geneva, Switzerland.
4. Muraro A, Dreborg S, Halken S, et al. Dietary prevention of allergic diseases in infants and small children, part III: critical review of published peer-reviewed observational and interventional studies and final recommendations. *Pediatr Allergy Immunol.* 2004;15:291-307.
5. Skinner JD, Carruth BR, Houck K, et al. Transitions in infant feeding during the first year of life. *J Am Coll Nutr.* 1997;16:209-215.
6. Crocetti M, Dudas R, Krugman S. Parental beliefs and practices regarding early introduction of solid foods to their children. *Clin Pediatr (Phila).* 2004;43:541-547.
7. Fergusson DM, Horwood LJ, Shannon FT. Early solid feeding and recurrent childhood eczema: a 10-year longitudinal study. *Pediatrics.* 1990;86:541-546.
8. Fergusson DM, Horwood LJ. Early solid food diet and eczema in childhood: a 10-year longitudinal study. *Pediatr Allergy Immunol.* 1994;5(suppl 1):44-47.
9. Kajosaari M. Atopy prophylaxis in high-risk infants. *Adv Exp Med Biol.* 1991;310:453-458.
10. Kajosaari M. Atopy prevention in childhood: the role of diet. Prospective 5-year follow-up of high-risk infants with six months exclusive breastfeeding and solid food elimination. *Pediatr Allergy Immunol.* 1994;5(suppl 1):26-28.
11. Fergusson DM, Horwood LJ, Beautrais AL, Shannon FT, Taylor B. Eczema and infant diet. *Clin Allergy.* 1981;11:325-331.
12. Fergusson DM, Horwood LJ, Shannon FT. Risk factors in childhood eczema. *J Epidemiol Community Health.* 1982;36:118-122.
13. Forsyth JS, Ogston SA, Clark A, Florey CD, Howie PW. Relation between early introduction of solid food to infants and their weight and illnesses during the first two years of life. *BMJ.* 1993;306:1572-1576.
14. Kajosaari M, Saarinen UM. Prophylaxis of atopic disease by six months' total solid food elimination: evaluation of 135 exclusively breast-fed infants of atopic families. *Acta Paediatr Scand.* 1983;72:411-414.
15. Moore WJ, Midwinter RE, Morris AF, Colley JR, Soothill JF. Infant feeding and subsequent risk of atopic eczema. *Arch Dis Child.* 1985;60:722-726.
16. Van Asperen PP, Kemp AS, Mellis CM. Relationship of diet in the development of atopy in infancy. *Clin Allergy.* 1984;14:525-532.
17. Zutavern A, von Mutius E, Harris J, et al. The introduction of solids in relation to asthma and eczema. *Arch Dis Child.* 2004;89:303-308.
18. Armentia A, Banuelos C, Arranz ML, et al. Early introduction of cereals into children's diets as a risk-factor for grass pollen asthma. *Clin Exp Allergy.* 2001;31:1250-1255.
19. Fergusson DM, Horwood LJ, Shannon FT. Asthma and infant diet. *Arch Dis Child.* 1983;58:48-51.
20. Wilson AC, Forsyth JS, Greene SA, Irvine L, Hau C, Howie PW. Relation of infant diet to childhood health: seven year follow up of cohort of children in Dundee infant feeding study. *BMJ.* 1998;316:21-25.
21. Parihar H, Kumar L, Puri R, Kumar V. The incidence of allergic diseases and feeding patterns in children up to 2 years of age. *Indian J Pediatr.* 1984;51:7-12.
22. Zeiger RS, Heller S, Mellon MH, et al. Effect of combined maternal and infant food-allergen avoidance on development of atopy in early infancy: a randomized study. *J Allergy Clin Immunol.* 1989;84:72-89.
23. Zeiger RS, Heller S, Mellon MH, Halsey JF, Hamburger RN, Sampson HA. Genetic and environmental factors affecting the development of atopy through age 4 in children of atopic parents: a prospective randomized study of food allergen avoidance. *Pediatr Allergy Immunol.* 1992;3:110-127.
24. Zeiger RS, Heller S. The development and prediction of atopy in high-risk children: follow-up at age seven years in a prospective randomized study of combined maternal and infant food allergen avoidance. *J Allergy Clin Immunol.* 1995;95:1179-1190.

ARTICLE

# Excessive Crying Beyond 3 Months May Herald Other Features of Multiple Regulatory Problems

*Rüdiger von Kries, MD, MSc; Helen Kalies, MSc, MPH; Mechthild Papoušek, MD*

**Objective:** To assess duration of excessive crying and its relation to sleep and eating disturbances in a population sample of infants.

**Design:** Cross-sectional study.

**Setting:** Random digit-dialing survey, enrolling birth cohorts between 1999 and 2003, in Germany.

**Participants:** Children aged 4 years and younger.

**Main Exposures:** Excessive crying, retrospectively ascertained according to modified Wessel's criteria, and duration of excessive crying.

**Main Outcome Measures:** Severe eating or sleeping problems at interview.

**Results:** The participation rate in the random digit-dialing survey was 62%. The analysis was confined to 1865 children with complete data. The observed prevalence for excessive crying ever was 16.3% (95% confidence interval [CI], 14.7-18.1), beyond 3 months 5.8% (95% CI, 4.8-6.9), and beyond 6 months 2.5% (95% CI, 1.9-3.3). Excessive crying only in the first 3 months did not increase the prevalence of sleep or eating disturbances whereas crying beyond 6 months did; prevalence of eating disorders was 19.1% (95% CI, 9.1- 33.3) and prevalence of sleeping disorders was 12.8% (95% CI, 4.8-25.7) compared with 2.7% (95% CI, 1.9–3.6) and 3.6% (95% CI, 2.7-4.6), respectively, in children without excessive crying.

**Conclusions:** Persistence of crying beyond the first 6 months heralded a higher prevalence of eating or sleeping difficulties in children with excessive crying than in children without excessive crying. These parents should be offered support and counseling over a broader spectrum of features related to multiple regulatory problems.

*Arch Pediatr Adolesc Med. 2006;160:508-511*

EXCESSIVE CRYING IS A COMmon condition in infants which may interfere with the mother-infant, father-infant, and mother-father interaction[1] and may increase the risk of child abuse.[2] Prevalence estimates vary depending on the case definition used.[3] Most articles use modifications of Wessel's "rule of three" (excessive crying for 3 hours per day, 3 days per week, for 3 weeks) to define excessive crying.[4] Although excessive crying is often limited to the first 3 months of life, there is a substantial proportion of children in whom excessive crying persists beyond the third month.[3,5] In clinical settings, persistent crying may be associated with other features of multiple regulatory problems and constitute a severe threat to the developing mother-child relationship,[6] and some articles point to interdependencies between prolonged excessive crying and other behavioral and mental problems later in life.[7-9] However, little is known about the association between typical or prolonged excessive crying and sleeping or eating disturbances in population samples.[10]

In a cross-sectional study, the interdependencies between excessive crying and sleeping or eating disturbances were assessed in a representative sample of 1865 children aged 6 to 47 months at interview.

## METHODS

Questions on behavioral problems like excessive crying, sleeping disturbances, and feeding difficulties in children were added to the nationwide, random digit-dialing telephone interview to assess vaccination. This survey on children born between July 1, 1999, and June 30, 2003, was conducted between July 2002, and January 2004 by computer-assisted telephone interviews.[11]

Informed consent was obtained from all participating parents. The response rate to the telephone survey was 62%. A total of 2827 interviews were completed. The analyses were confined to interviews carried out for chil-

**Author Affiliations:** Division of Pediatric Epidemiology at the Institute of Social Pediatrics and Adolescent Medicine, Ludwig-Maximilians-University, Munich, Germany.

**Table 1. Demographics of the Study Population Compared With German Reference Data (Microcensus)[12]**

| | Study Population, % | Microcensus, % |
|---|---|---|
| Sex | | |
| Male | 52.1 | 50.9 |
| Female | 47.9 | 49.1 |
| Nationality | | |
| German | 93.0 | 90.4 |
| Non-German | 7.0 | 9.6 |
| No. of siblings | | |
| None | 35.3 | 40.5 |
| 1 | 42.9 | 40.1 |
| 2 | 15.0 | 13.6 |
| 3 | 4.9 | 3.7 |
| ≥4 | 1.9 | 2.1 |
| Net household income, € | | |
| <1500 | 13.2 | 24.4 |
| 1500-3000 | 55.8 | 60.1 |
| 3000-5000 | 19.1 | 12.5 |
| ≥5000 | 4.6 | 2.9 |
| Mean age of mother at birth, y | 29.9 | 30.3 |

dren aged 6 months to 4 years. This accounted for a reduction of sample size from 2827 to 2349. For 1865 of these interviews, complete data for all relevant questions were available. The proportion of valid questionnaires, therefore, was reduced to 49%. The median age at interview was 25 months (minimum, 6 months; maximum, 47 months).

The validity of the survey was assessed by comparing data on geographic distribution, demographic, and social components with official data provided by the Federal Statistical Office, Wiesbaden, Germany.[12]

Excessive crying was retrospectively ascertained with a modification of Wessel's criteria by asking the parents to remember the child's first 3 months and answer the following questions: "Did your child cry or fuss for more than 3 hours per day?", "Did this condition occur on at least 3 days per week?", "Did this condition persist for longer than 3 weeks?" All 3 questions had to be answered with yes for the diagnosis of excessive crying in the first 3 months.

The duration of excessive crying was ascertained by asking "Did your child also cry or fuss for at least 3 hours per day on at least 3 days a week after the first 3 months?" If yes, the parents were asked for how long this condition persisted (age in weeks/months or until interview). In the latter case, the age at interview was used to define the duration of excessive crying. Duration of crying was categorized as never, beyond 3 months, and beyond 6 months.

Eating difficulties at the time of interview were defined by the questions "Does your child fuss around during regular meals?" and "Does your child need distraction to keep eating?" For each question, the parents were asked to answer on a scale from 1 to 5 (never, rarely, occasionally, mostly, and always, respectively). A child was categorized as having eating difficulties if they scored 4 points or higher on both scales.

Poor sleeping at the time of interview was defined from answers to the question "On how many nights per week does your child wake up on average?" A poor sleeper was defined as a child with at least 5 wake-ups per week who stayed awake an average of 15 minutes.[7]

The statistical analyses were carried out using SAS statistical software (version 8.0; SAS Institute, Cary, NC). We used the Clopper-Pearson exact method to calculate 95% confidence intervals (CIs).[13]

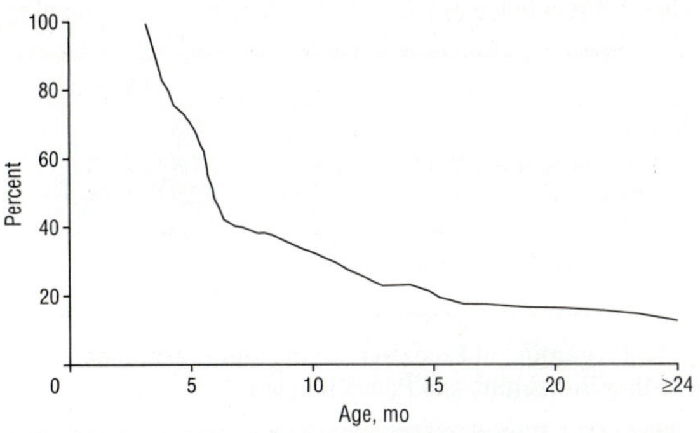


**Figure.** Children with excessive crying beyond the first 3 months of life (n=108); percentage of children with persistent crying at different ages.

## RESULTS

The response rate to the telephone survey was 62% for both surveys. Comparison with official data provided by the Federal Statistical Office revealed that data from telephone interviews were representative for families with age-eligible children in Germany with regard to geographic (Bundesland) and demographic factors (number of siblings, nationality, maternal age). Children from households with higher incomes were overrepresented (**Table 1**).

For 304 of 1865 children, the mothers reported crying or fussing for more than 3 hours a day on at least 3 days per week for more than 3 weeks, which accounts for a prevalence of excessive crying in the first 3 months of 16.3% (95% CI, 14.7-18.1).

Excessive crying was observed beyond the third month in 108 children. The duration of excessive crying was reported by the parents of 94 of these children. Excessive crying persisted at the time of interview in 14 of these children (observation period truncated at 24-42 months). Excessive crying waned during the first 6 months in most of the 108 children with excessive crying beyond the third month. However, persistence of crying for more than 6 months was reported in 47 (44%) of these children (**Figure**). The prevalence for excessive crying was 5.8% (95% CI, 4.8-6.9) beyond 3 months and 2.5% (95% CI; 1.9-3.3) beyond 6 months.

The prevalence of eating disorders was constant around 3% in the second, third, and fourth years of life compared with 1.4% in the first year. The prevalence of sleeping disorders, in contrast, decreased from the first to the fourth year of life (**Table 2**). In children with excessive crying limited to the first 3 months of life and in those with prolonged excessive crying up to 6 months, the prevalence of poor sleeping and eating difficulties was not significantly higher than in children without any excessive crying. In children with excessive crying beyond 6 months, however, the prevalence of eating and sleeping difficulties increased dramatically (**Table 3**). Children with excessive crying beyond the first 6 months were 8.9 times more likely to have eating difficulties and 6.6 times more likely to have sleeping difficulties than those without excessive crying (**Table 4**).

**Table 2. Prevalence of Eating Difficulties and Poor Sleeping by Age**

| | 1 y | 2 y | 3 y | 4 y |
|---|---|---|---|---|
| Interviews, No. | 70 | 618 | 829 | 348 |
| Eating difficulties, No. (95% CI) | 1.4 (0-7.7) | 3.6 (2.2-5.3) | 3.4 (2.3-4.8) | 3.2 (1.6-5.6) |
| Poor sleeping, No. (95% CI) | 12.9 (6.1-23.0) | 5.5 (3.8-7.6) | 2.5 (1.6-3.8) | 1.4 (0.5-3.3) |

Abbreviation: CI, confidence interval.

**Table 3. Duration of Excessive Crying and Prevalence of Eating Difficulties and Poor Sleeping**

| Duration of Excessive Crying | Difficulty Eating, No. (95% CI) | Poor Sleeping, No. (95% CI) |
|---|---|---|
| Never (n = 1561) | 2.7 (1.9-3.6) | 3.6 (2.7-4.6) |
| First 3 mo only (n = 196) | 4.6 (2.1-8.5) | 3.1 (1.1-6.5) |
| ≤6 mo (n = 61) | 3.3 (0.4-11.3) | 1.6 (0.0-8.8) |
| >6 mo (n = 47) | 19.1 (9.1-33.3) | 12.8 (4.8-25.7) |

Abbreviation: CI, confidence interval.

**Table 4. Association Between Duration of Excessive Crying and Prevalence of Eating Difficulties and Poor Sleeping***

| Duration of Excessive Crying | Difficulty Eating, No. (95% CI) | Poor Sleeping, No. (95% CI) |
|---|---|---|
| Never (n = 1561) | 1 (Baseline) | 1 (Baseline) |
| First 3 mo only (n = 196) | 1.7 (0.8-3.6) | 0.9 (0.4-2.2) |
| ≤6 mo (n = 61) | 1.2 (0.3-5.2) | 0.6 (0.1-4.1) |
| >6 mo (n = 47) | 8.9 (4.0-20.0) | 6.6 (2.5-17.0) |

Abbreviation: CI, confidence interval.
*Odds ratios with adjustment for age; reference, no excessive crying.

## COMMENT

This study is an extension of previous work and demonstrates that excessive crying does not always stop after the first 3 months of life.[5] Among those with excessive crying beyond the first 3 months, 56% stopped crying within the first 6 months, but 44% continued to cry excessively. A significantly increased prevalence of eating and sleeping difficulties was observed only in children with excessive crying beyond the sixth month of life.

These findings are relevant for counseling parents and with respect to the interpretation of studies on long-term effects of excessive crying. However, these studies have given contradictory results; some studies have not found a relationtionship between excessive crying and sleep problems and other indicators of multiple regulatory problems,[14-16] while others have found either sleeping or other regulatory problems.[7,17-19] Some of these discrepancies may be owing to the studying of different groups of children, including children with typical colic only or those with colic and prolonged excessive crying. A recent study further underlined the differences in the prognostic value of classic excessive crying vs prolonged crying; children with prolonged crying (but not those with colic only) had an adjusted mean IQ that was 9 points lower than the control group.[9]

The fact that our survey was taken by a representative population sample strengthened our data. The response rates in this survey were similar to response rates in other telephone surveys conducted in Germany and the United States.[20-22] The overrepresentation of children from households with higher incomes might potentially influence the observed association between excessive crying and sleeping or eating disturbances. In our data, however, income was not associated with crying, sleeping, or eating disturbances (data not shown).

The size of the study allowed us to look at the more severe spectrum of eating and sleeping disorders, although the numbers in the final categories were small and accounted for wide CIs. Since our main interest was to assess the relationship between these conditions and classic infantile colic, we focused on crying in the first 3 months and its extension beyond. A possible link to excessive crying starting after the first 3 months would be missed. Nine children with excessive crying beyond 6 months who fussed around at most or all meals additionally required distraction to be fed at all or most meals. Six children with excessive crying beyond 6 months who woke up on 5 or more days per week for at least 15 minutes were between the ages of 24 and 47 months at interview, which is an age when such poor sleeping is quite unusual. Identifying children with excessive crying in the first 3 months of life who may proceed to severe behavioral problems is one of the challenges in counseling parents of children with excessive crying.

Although some risk factors for excessive crying have been identified, such as maternal smoking during pregnancy[12,23] and cow's milk allergy,[24,25] the etiology of excessive infant crying is still poorly understood. The absence of a dose effect related to the duration of excessive crying was surprising. The few children with excessive crying and either severe sleeping or eating disorders might constitute a group of children with multiple regulatory problems outside the continuous spectrum of normal behavior.

The prevalence of any excessive crying was a bit higher in our study than in other retrospective studies. Prevalence estimates vary with the case definition used.[3] The higher prevalence may have resulted from a slight modification of Wessel's rule of three.[3] We asked for crying or fussing longer than 3 hours per day, at least for 3 days per week, and for more than 3 weeks. Since there is no generally accepted case definition, any definition is acceptable as long as it is clearly stated.[3] To test whether recall bias might affect the categorization of excessive crying, we checked the prevalence estimates for different categories of excessive crying by age at interview. The number of parents interviewed at children's ages of 2, 3, and 4 years (618, 829, and 348, respectively) was sufficient to allow for meaningful comparisons. There was no significant difference in the prevalence of crying within the first 3 months or up to 6 months by age at interview, whereas the proportion of children with excessive crying beyond 6 months increased significantly by age at interview (5 of 618, 21 of 829, and 20 of 348 at the ages of 2, 3, and 4 years, respectively). However, the associations of excessive crying with sleeping or eating difficulties did not vary by age at interview (data not shown).

A further limitation of this study is its design; a cohort study might allow for a more valid estimation of the prevalence of excessive crying. We asked parents to remember the first 3 months first and then to report whether excessive crying extended beyond the first 3 months. Recall bias related to a selective recall of crying in the first 3 months in parents of children with multiple regulatory disorders would result in on overestimation of the proportion of children's excessive crying in the first 3 months. However, eating difficulties and poor sleeping were not more common in children with excessive crying limited to the first 3 months of life.

There are 2 further observations suggesting that the parents' recall about crying in the first 3 months was not grossly wrong. The onset of excessive crying stated by parents (interquartile range, week 1-3) matched the typical pattern.[26] The parents might remember their child's crying in the first months of life less well when interviewed in later years of life (year 3-4 vs year 1-2). The remembered prevalence of crying, however, did not decrease with age at interview (data not shown).

We therefore feel that these limitations of the study design do not invalidate our findings. If excessive crying extends beyond the sixth month, the affected children have an increased risk for relevant eating and sleeping difficulties. Their parents should be offered support and counseling over a broader spectrum of features related to multiple regulatory problems.

**Accepted for Publication:** October 27, 2005.
**Correspondence:** Rüdiger von Kries, MD, MSc, Department of Epidemiology, Institute for Social Pediatrics and Adolescent Medicine, Ludwig-Maximilians-University, Munich, Heiglhofstr 63, D–81377 Munich, Germany (prof.von.kries@gmx.de).
**Funding/Support:** This study is a spin-off from a vaccination coverage study. The questions on behavioral issues were added to ask the parents something that might worry them more than vaccination coverage. The vaccination coverage study was funded by GlaxoSmithKline and Sanofi Pasteur MSD.

## REFERENCES


1. Raiha H, Lehtonen L, Huhtala V, Saleva K, Korvenranta H. Excessively crying infant in the family: mother-infant, father-infant and mother-father interaction. *Child Care Health Dev.* 2002;28:419-429.
2. Reijneveld SA, van-der-Wal MF, Brugman E, Sing RA, Verloove-Vanhorick SP. Infant crying and abuse. *Lancet.* 2004;364:1340-1342.
3. Reijneveld SA, Brugman E, Hirasing RA. Excessive infant crying: the impact of varying definitions. *Pediatrics.* 2001;108:893-897.
4. Wessel MA, Cobb JC, Jackson EB, Harris GS Jr, Detwiler AC. Paroxysmal fussing in infancy, sometimes called colic. *Pediatrics.* 1954;14:421-435.
5. Wurmser H, Laubereau B, Hermann M, Papousek M, von-Kries R. Excessive infant crying: often not confined to the first 3 months of age. *Early Hum Dev.* 2001;64:1-6.
6. Papousek M, von Hofacker N. Persistent crying in early infancy: a non-trivial condition of risk for the developing mother-infant relationship. *Child Care Health Dev.* 1998;24:395-424.
7. Wolke D, Meyer R, Ohrt B, Riegel K. Co-morbidity of crying and feeding problems with sleeping problems in infancy: concurrent and predictive associations. *Early Devel Parenting.* 1995;4:191-207.
8. Wolke D, Rizzo P, Woods S. Persistent infant crying and hyperactivity problems in middle childhood. *Pediatrics.* 2002;109:1054-1060.
9. Rao MR, Brenner RA, Schisterman EF, Vik T, Mills JL. Long term cognitive development in children with prolonged crying. *Arch Dis Child.* 2004;89:989-992.
10. Barr RG. Colic and crying syndromes in infants. *Pediatrics.* 1998;102(Suppl E):1282-1286.
11. Kalies H, Grote V, Schmitt H-J, von Kries R. Immunisation status of children in Germany: temporal trend and regional differences. *Eur J Pediatr.* 2005 In press.
12. Fachserie 1, Reihe 3, Bevölkerung und Erwerbstätigkeit, Haushalte und Familien. German Federal Statistical Office. Wiesbaden, Germany: Federal Statistical Office; 2002.
13. Clopper C, Pearson E. The use of confidence of fiducial limits illustrated in the case of the binomial. *Biometrics.* 1934;26:404-408.
14. Kirjavainen J, Kirjavainen T, Huhtala V, Lehtonen L, Korvenranta H, Kero P. Infants with colic have a normal sleep structure at 2 and 7 months of age. *J Pediatr.* 2001;138:218-223.
15. Lehtonen L, Korhonen T, Korvenranta H. Temperament and sleeping patterns in colicky infants during the first year of life. *J Dev Behav Pediatr.* 1994;15:416-420.
16. Raiha H, Lehtonen L, Korhonen T, Korvenranta H. Family functioning 3 years after infantile colic. *J Dev Behav Pediatr.* 1997;18:290-294.
17. Stahlberg MR. Infantile colic: occurrence and risk factors. *Eur J Pediatr.* 1984;143:108-111.
18. Rautava P, Lehtonen L, Helenius H, Sillanpaa M. Infantile colic: child and family three years later. *Pediatrics.* 1995;96:43-47.
19. Canivet C, Jakobsson I, Hagander B. Infantile colic—follow-up at four years of age: still more "emotional." *Acta Paediatr.* 2000;89:13-17.
20. Centers for Disease Control and Prevention (CDC). National, state, and urban area vaccination coverage among children aged 19-35 months—United States, 2003. *MMWR Morb Mortal Wkly Rep.* 2004;53:658-661.
21. Meyer N, Fischer R, Weitkunat R, et al. Evalutation of health monitoring in Bavaria by computer-assisted telephone interviews (CATI) in comparison to the German National Health Examination Survey conducted in 1998 by the Robert Koch Institute. *Gesundheitswesen.* 2002;64:329-336.
22. Rehmet S, Ammon A, Pfaff G, Bocter N, Petersen LR. Cross-sectional study on influenza vaccination, Germany, 1999-2000. *Emerg Infect Dis.* 2002;8:1442-1447.
23. Shenassa ED, Brown MJ. Maternal smoking and infantile gastrointestinal dysregulation: the case of colic. *Pediatrics.* 2004;114:e497-e505.
24. Lothe L, Lindberg T. Cow's milk whey protein elicits symptoms of infantile colic in colicky formula-fed infants: a double-blind crossover study. *Pediatrics.* 1989;83:262-266.
25. Lothe L, Lindberg T, Jakobsson I. Cow's milk formula as a cause of infantile colic: a double-blind study. *Pediatrics.* 1982;70:7-10.
26. Crowcroft NS, Strachan DP. The social origins of infantile colic: questionnaire study covering 76,747 infants. *BMJ.* 1997;314:1325-1328.

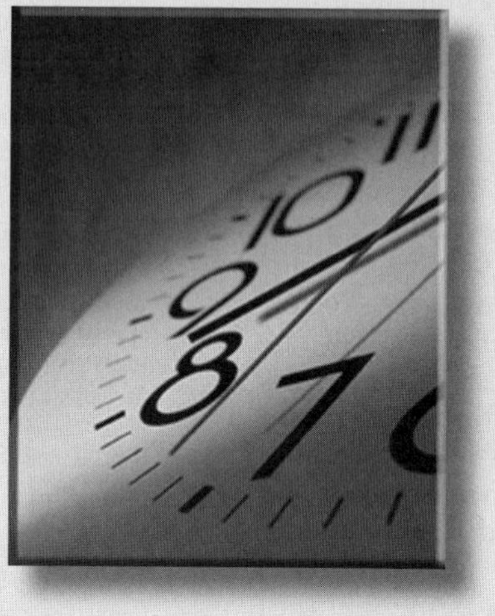

ARTICLE

# Maternal Infant-Feeding Style and Children's Adiposity at 5 Years of Age

*Hillary L. Burdette, MD, MS; Robert C. Whitaker, MD, MPH; Waynitra C. Hall, MS; Stephen R. Daniels, MD, PhD*

**Objectives:** To examine the relationship between maternal infant-feeding style and adiposity in childhood and to determine whether feeding style explains any of the association between maternal obesity and childhood adiposity.

**Design:** Prospective cohort study.

**Setting:** Cincinnati metropolitan area.

**Participants:** A total of 313 preschool children; 80% were white and 20% were black.

**Main Outcome Measures:** Seven factors describing maternal infant-feeding style derived from the Infant Feeding Questionnaire administered at age 3 years; maternal obesity, defined as a body mass index of 30 or higher before pregnancy; and adiposity at 5 years of age as assessed by dual-energy x-ray absorptiometry.

**Results:** The mean ± SD fat mass was 4.55 ± 1.64 kg. Seventeen percent of the mothers were obese before pregnancy. Children whose mothers had high concern about the infant overeating or becoming overweight (the highest tertile of the "overeating" factor) had 0.67 kg (95% confidence interval, 0.31-1.03 kg) higher fat mass than children whose mothers did not have high concern (the other 2 tertiles). None of the other 6 feeding factors were related to childhood adiposity. Children of obese mothers had 0.54 kg (95% confidence interval, 0.10-0.98 kg) higher fat mass than children of nonobese mothers. High concern about the infant overeating, which was more common in obese mothers, accounted for 15% of this 0.54-kg difference.

**Conclusion:** High maternal concern about an infant overeating or becoming overweight was associated with higher adiposity at 5 years of age and explained some of the association between maternal obesity and child adiposity.

*Arch Pediatr Adolesc Med. 2006;160:513-520*

AMIDST THE CURRENT EPIDEMIC of childhood obesity, more consideration is being given to starting obesity prevention efforts early in life, even during gestation or at birth.[1] One potential target for these prevention efforts is infant feeding. Although there has been much research on the association between later obesity and what infants eat, such as breast milk, infant formula, and other complementary foods,[2,3] there has been far less research on contextual factors in infant feeding. Many of these contextual factors are related to the parental feeding style, particularly the feeding style of the mother, who is often the primary infant feeder.

The term *maternal infant-feeding style* is used herein to describe a mother's practices and beliefs about feeding her infant, such as whether the mother controls feeding with a regular schedule, uses food to soothe her infant, is aware of her infant's hunger cues, or worries about her infant eating too much or too little. To the extent that the mother's infant-feeding style has an enduring impact on the child's developing system of appetite regulation and is associated with the child's later adiposity, this maternal feeding style, and not just what the infant eats, may be an appropriate focus in obesity prevention.

Although maternal obesity has been identified as the strongest risk factor for the early development of obesity in children,[4] this risk factor can operate through many potential mechanisms.[5] One of the modifiable mechanisms may be the mother's style of feeding her infant. If obese and nonobese mothers have different feeding styles and these styles are also associated with childhood obesity, it is possible that altering these feeding styles might be a way to help obese parents prevent obesity in their children.

Some maternal feeding practices, such as pushing children to eat or restricting children from certain snack foods, are thought to be related to the development of later obesity, but those studies have focused on feeding preschool children and not on feeding infants.[6,7] To our knowledge, there are only 2 validated instruments that ask mothers about aspects of their infant feeding style hypothesized to

**Author Affiliations:** Division of Gastroenterology and Nutrition, Children's Hospital of Philadelphia, Philadelphia, Pa (Dr Burdette and Ms Hall); Department of Pediatrics, University of Pennsylvania School of Medicine, Philadelphia (Dr Burdette); Mathematica Policy Research Inc, Princeton, NJ (Dr Whitaker); and Division of Cardiology, Cincinnati Children's Hospital Medical Center, and Department of Pediatrics, University of Cincinnati College of Medicine, Cincinnati, Ohio (Dr Daniels).

affect later adiposity.[8,9] The developers of these instruments examined the association of maternal infant-feeding style with children's later height and weight, but there were no direct measures of children's adiposity in these studies, and all anthropometric measurements were made at younger than 24 months.[9,10] To our knowledge, there have been no other studies relating maternal infant-feeding style to children's later weight or adiposity.

In this study, we attempted to address 2 research questions. (1) Are there any aspects of the mother's feeding style during infancy that are associated with the child's adiposity at 5 years of age? (2) How much, if any, of the association between maternal obesity before pregnancy and childhood adiposity is explained by maternal infant-feeding style?

## METHODS

### STUDY DESIGN AND PARTICIPANTS

This study involves data collected on preschool children participating in a prospective cohort study describing normal changes in body fatness during early childhood. In 2001 and 2002 we recruited 372 children aged 3 years for this study from the Cincinnati metropolitan area by placing brochures in pediatric offices and day care centers and by placing advertisements in community newspapers. All the children met the following eligibility criteria: full-term gestation (≥37 weeks), no chronic health conditions affecting growth and development, and parents who were either both black or both white. Parental race was reported by the child's mother. The institutional review board at Cincinnati Children's Hospital Medical Center approved the study. Informed written consent was obtained from the parents.

### CHILD ADIPOSITY AND BODY MASS INDEX

Dual-energy x-ray absorptiometry (DXA) is considered the most accurate measure of adiposity in children,[11] and it was used to measure children's body composition at a mean age of 5.0 years (range, 4.8-5.2 years). The entire body was scanned in the array-fan beam mode using a Hologic 4500 instrument (Hologic Inc, Bedford, Mass) and pediatric software (version 12.3, Hologic Inc). Body composition measures derived from DXA included lean body mass, total fat mass, and percentage of body fat (total fat mass divided by total body mass). The DXA measurements at 5 years of age were available for 313 children (84% of the original cohort).

Height and weight were measured at the initial study visit and at the time of DXA. Heights were measured using a wall-mounted stadiometer, and weights were measured using a digital scale. Height and weight were measured twice, and, for each measure, the average value was calculated. These height and weight values were then used to calculate body mass index (BMI) (calculated as weight in kilograms divided by the square of height in meters), and the BMI percentile and *z* score for each BMI value were established using the 2000 Centers for Disease Control and Prevention growth reference.[12] For the DXA and anthropometric measurements, the child was lightly dressed in a T-shirt and in shorts or pants with an elastic waist.

### MATERNAL INFANT-FEEDING STYLE

At the time of the initial study visit (mean ± SD child age, 3.3 ± 0.3 years), each mother was asked to complete the Infant Feeding Questionnaire (IFQ),[9] a self-administered instrument containing 20 questions about different aspects of maternal infant-feeding style during the child's first year of life that are hypothesized to be related to the risk of childhood obesity. The IFQ has 12 items about the context of a mother's feeding practices, such as how, when, and why she fed her infant, and 8 questions about a mother's beliefs concerning infant feeding (**Table 1**). Each item has 5 response options ranging from "never" to "always" for questions about practices and from "disagree a lot" to "agree a lot" for questions about beliefs.

The IFQ measures the following 7 factors: (1) concern about infant undereating or becoming underweight (undereating), (2) concern about infant's hunger (hunger), (3) awareness of infant's hunger and satiety cues (infant cues), (4) concern about infant overeating or becoming overweight (overeating), (5) feeding infant on schedule (schedule), (6) using food to calm infant's fussiness (food to calm), and (7) social interaction with the infant during feeding (social) (Table 1). The 5 response options for each question were assigned the values 0 (never/disagree a lot) through 4 (always/agree a lot). Answers were averaged across the items for each factor to give a possible score for each factor ranging from 0 to 4. This is the same scoring method used in a previous study.[9]

### MATERNAL OBESITY

The mother's BMI was calculated from maternal report of height and weight before pregnancy (data collected at the first study visit). Maternal obesity was defined as having a BMI of 30 or higher.

### COVARIATES

At the first study visit, the mothers provided information about the children's sex, birth weight, and breastfeeding history. The duration of breastfeeding was categorized as follows: never and less than 3, 3 to 5, 6 to 12, and more than 12 months. Mothers also reported information to allow construction of the following maternal variables: age (years), race (white vs black), marital status (single vs married), education (high school or less vs some college vs college or more), current smoking status (smoker vs nonsmoker), household income (<$50 000 vs $50 000-$74 999 vs ≥$75 000), and whether the mother enrolled the child in WIC (Special Supplemental Nutrition Program for Women, Infants, and Children) during infancy (yes vs no).

### DATA ANALYSIS

#### Variable Construction

We created continuous and binary outcome measures from the DXA data and from the BMI data (4 total outcome variables). From DXA, the continuous outcome measure was fat mass, which was adjusted for lean body mass and sex, as has been previously described.[13,14] These adjustments in fat mass were made to account for normal variation in fat mass related to body size and sex, and they allowed us to pool data across the sexes. Fat mass was selected a priori as the primary outcome variable because it is a direct measure of adiposity and, as a continuous measure, was likely to be more sensitive than a binary measure to any differences in maternal infant-feeding style.

To facilitate clinical interpretation of the DXA results, we also classified children as having either "high" or "normal" adiposity, creating a secondary (binary) outcome measure. Because there are no established reference data to determine a cutoff point for overweight/obesity in children based on body composition data from DXA, children were categorized as having high adiposity if they had a percentage of body fat in the sex-specific upper quartile for the cohort. In this cohort, this value was greater than 29% for females and greater than 24% for males, cutoff points that are

**Table 1. Descriptive Statistics for the 7 Maternal Feeding Factors From the Infant Feeding Questionnaire**

| Factor and Item | Score, Median (Range) | "Outlier" Tertile |
|---|---|---|
| Undereating | 0.75 (0-4.00) | High concern (high values) |
| Worried infant was not eating enough | | |
| Struggled to get infant to eat | | |
| Worried infant would become underweight | | |
| Infant needed encouragement to eat enough | | |
| Hunger | 0.33 (0-4.00) | High concern (high values) |
| Cereal in bottle so infant would stay full longer | | |
| Cereal in bottle so infant would sleep longer at night | | |
| Before age 4 mo, infant wanted more than just formula and/or breast milk | | |
| Infant cues | 3.75 (0.75-4.00) | Low awareness (low values) |
| Infant knew when hungry | | |
| Infant knew when full | | |
| I knew when infant was full | | |
| I knew when infant was hungry | | |
| Overeating | 0.33 (0-2.67) | High concern (high values) |
| Worried that infant was eating too much | | |
| Worried that infant would become overweight | | |
| Upset if infant ate too much | | |
| Schedule | 1.00 (0-4.00) | High control (high values) |
| Allowed infant to eat whenever wanted* | | |
| Only allowed infant to eat at set times | | |
| Food to calm | 1.50 (0-3.50) | High use (high values) |
| Feeding infant was the best way to stop fussiness | | |
| When fussy, feeding infant was first thing you would do | | |
| Social | 3.50 (0-4.00) | Low contact (low values) |
| Talked or sang to infant while feeding | | |
| Held infant while giving bottle | | |

*The score for this item was reverse coded.

consistent with previous studies[15,16] investigating cutoff points for obesity in children based on the relationship between percentage of body fat and cardiovascular risk factors.

Because most other studies of childhood obesity risk factors are based on BMI, we also analyzed 2 other secondary outcome measures—BMI $z$ score (continuous) and BMI at the 85th percentile or higher (binary). These 2 measures are analogous to our DXA measures of fat mass and high adiposity, respectively.

The 7 feeding factor scores from the IFQ were not normally distributed (the median value was close to either 0 or 4) (Table 1), and not all the scores ranged from 0 to 4, so we converted each factor into a binary variable using the following method. For each factor, we divided the sample into 3 groups of approximately equal size, breaking the group as close as possible to the tertile cutoff points for the factor score. Given the skew of the data, 1 tertile contained the values in the "outlier" tail of the distribution. We further divided the children into 2 groups—a group with values in this outlier tertile and a group with values in the other 2 tertiles (Table 1). In all the analyses using the 7 IFQ factors, we made comparisons between these 2 groups. For 6 of the 7 factors, the children in the outlier tertile were those we hypothesized would have increased adiposity at 5 years of age. We hypothesized that the outlier tertile of the factor "high concern about the child undereating or being underweight" would be associated with lower fat mass.

### Bivariate and Multivariate Analyses

Multivariate linear regression was used to compare the mean fat mass, adjusted for lean body mass and sex, between the 2 levels of each feeding factor (Table 1) and between obese and nonobese mothers. $\chi^2$ Tests and $t$ tests were used to evaluate the bivariate relationship between the 3 other outcome measures (high adiposity, BMI $z$ score, and overweight) and (1) the 7 feeding factors and (2) maternal obesity.

After examining these bivariate relationships among child adiposity, maternal infant-feeding style (7 feeding factors), and maternal obesity, we used regression models to evaluate the extent to which the relationship between maternal obesity before pregnancy and child adiposity at age 5 years was mediated by maternal infant-feeding style. Using fat mass as the dependent variable, linear regression models were run with the base model containing lean body mass and sex and with 5 subsequent models, each adding variables to the previous model as follows: model 1, maternal obesity; model 2, birth weight; model 3, maternal covariates (race, age, marital status, smoking status, education, household income, and enrolled child in WIC); model 4, breastfeeding duration; and model 5, the maternal infant-feeding factors that were significantly associated, in bivariate analysis, with child fat mass and maternal obesity. We then assessed the change in the regression coefficient for maternal obesity between models 4 and 5 to determine the extent to which these feeding factors mediated the relationship between maternal obesity and child adiposity.[17] Similar linear regression models were used with BMI $z$ score as the dependent variable, and similar logistic models were used for the binary dependent variables of high adiposity and overweight. None of these models, however, contained lean body mass or sex.

## RESULTS

### DESCRIPTION OF SAMPLE

Of the 313 children in this analysis, 166 (53%) were boys; 80% of the mothers were white and 20% were black. The

**Table 2. Fat Mass by Construct of Maternal Infant-Feeding Style From the Infant Feeding Questionnaire**

| | DXA | | Anthropometrics | |
|---|---|---|---|---|
| | Total Fat, Mean ± SE, kg* | High Adiposity, %† | BMI $z$ Score, Mean ± SE | Overweight, %‡ |
| Undereating | | | | |
| High concern | 4.42 ± 0.14 | 28.7 | 0.12 ± 0.09 | 15.7 |
| Normal | 4.62 ± 0.10 | 22.9 | 0.60 ± 0.07 | 30.7 |
| *P* value§ | .25 | .26 | <.001 | .004 |
| Hunger | | | | |
| High concern | 4.42 ± 0.15 | 18.7 | 0.52 ± 0.11 | 31.9 |
| Normal | 4.60 ± 0.10 | 27.5 | 0.40 ± 0.07 | 23.0 |
| *P* value§ | .29 | .10 | .33 | .10 |
| Infant cues | | | | |
| Low awareness | 4.54 ± 0.13 | 25.9 | 0.38 ± 0.10 | 22.3 |
| Normal | 4.55 ± 0.10 | 24.4 | 0.47 ± 0.07 | 27.4 |
| *P* value§ | .94 | .77 | .44 | .33 |
| Overeating | | | | |
| High concern | 5.05 ± 0.16 | 33.3 | 0.84 ± 0.11 | 38.5 |
| Normal | 4.38 ± 0.09 | 22.1 | 0.30 ± 0.06 | 21.3 |
| *P* value§ | <.001 | .05 | <.001 | .003 |
| Schedule | | | | |
| High control | 4.30 ± 0.16 | 17.5 | 0.42 ± 0.11 | 25.0 |
| Normal | 4.64 ± 0.09 | 27.5 | 0.44 ± 0.06 | 25.8 |
| *P* value§ | .07 | .08 | .84 | .89 |
| Food to calm | | | | |
| High use | 4.48 ± 0.13 | 24.8 | 0.36 ± 0.08 | 24.0 |
| Normal | 4.60 ± 0.10 | 25.0 | 0.48 ± 0.07 | 26.6 |
| *P* value§ | .47 | .97 | .30 | .61 |
| Social | | | | |
| Low contact | 4.47 ± 0.13 | 24.6 | 0.49 ± 0.09 | 31.0 |
| Normal | 4.60 ± 0.10 | 25.1 | 0.40 ± 0.07 | 21.9 |
| *P* value§ | .44 | .92 | .40 | .07 |

Abbreviations: BMI, body mass index (calculated as weight in kilograms divided by the square of height in meters); DXA, dual-energy x-ray absorptiometry.
*Adjusted for the child's lean body mass and sex.
†Upper quartile of percentage of body fat for sex.
‡Defined as a BMI at the 85th percentile or higher for age and sex.
§*P* value for *t* test or $\chi^2$ test.

mean ± SD birth weight of the children was 3388 ± 554 g, with 12% of the newborns weighing 4000 g or more. Sixty-eight mothers (22%) enrolled their infants in WIC, and 231 children (74%) were breastfed. At the time of the child's birth, the mean ± SD age of the mothers was 30 ± 5.0 years. Half of the mothers had completed college, 86% were married, and 7% were smokers.

The mean ± SD maternal BMI before pregnancy was 24.9 ± 5.6, and 17% of the mothers (n=52) were obese before becoming pregnant. At 5 years of age, the percentages of children with BMI at the 85th percentile or higher and at the 95th percentile or higher were 26% and 10%, respectively. Total fat mass and BMI $z$ score were significantly correlated ($r$=0.735; $P$<.001), as were percentage of body fat and BMI $z$ score ($r$=0.552; $P$<.001). The mean ± SD fat mass (unadjusted), lean body mass, and percentage body fat were 4.55 ± 1.64 kg, 14.05 ± 1.93 kg, and 23% ± 5.43%, respectively. After adjusting for lean body mass, girls had significantly higher fat mass than boys (5.18 vs 3.99 kg; $P$<.001). Mean fat mass is, hereafter, reported after adjustment for lean body mass and sex.

Comparing the 313 children who underwent DXA at 5 years of age with the 59 children in the original cohort who did not undergo DXA, there was no significant difference between the 2 groups in BMI $z$ score at 3 years of age (0.34 vs 0.37; $P$=.86) or in the percentage with BMI at the 85th percentile or higher (22% vs 25%; $P$=.67) or at the 95th percentile or higher (6.7% vs 7.1%; $P$=.91).

## MATERNAL INFANT-FEEDING STYLE AND CHILD ADIPOSITY

The only maternal infant-feeding factor that was significantly related to fat mass at 5 years of age was high concern about the infant overeating or becoming overweight (**Table 2**). Compared with children whose mothers had lower levels of concern (lowest 2 tertiles), the children whose mothers had high concern had a 0.67 kg (95% confidence interval, 0.31-1.03 kg) greater fat mass at 5 years of age. Because the standard deviation in fat mass was 1.64 kg, this 0.67-kg difference represents an effect size of 0.41 SD unit (0.67/1.64). These children were also more likely to have high adiposity. Mothers who reported high control over their infant feeding schedules tended to have children with lower rather than higher fat mass at age 5 years.

Mothers who were concerned about their infant overeating or becoming overweight also had children with higher BMI $z$ scores and prevalence of overweight (Table 2). In the opposite direction, mothers with high concern about their infant undereating or becoming underweight had children with lower BMI $z$ scores and prevalence of overweight.

## MATERNAL OBESITY

At 5 years of age, children born to mothers who were obese before pregnancy were more likely to have higher fat mass and BMI $z$ scores and to be overweight (**Table 3**). Mothers who were obese before pregnancy were significantly more concerned about their infant overeating or becoming overweight. Although none of the other differences in maternal infant-feeding style between obese and nonobese mothers were statistically significant, obese mothers also tended to exert less control over the infant feeding schedule, to have lower social contact during feeding, and to have less concern about the infant being underweight.

## MULTIVARIATE MODELS

Because "overeating" was the only factor significantly related to adiposity at age 5 years and maternal obesity before pregnancy, this was the only feeding factor included in the regression analyses. Based on the regression models, children born to obese mothers had a 0.54-kg greater fat mass (95% confidence interval, 0.10-0.98 kg) than children born to nonobese mothers, even after controlling for the child's lean body mass, sex, birth weight, a variety of maternal covariates (race, age, marital status, smoking status, education, household income, and WIC enrollment), and breastfeeding status (model 4 under "fat mass" in **Table 4**). This is a difference in fat mass of one third of a standard deviation.

This difference was reduced to 0.46 kg (a 15% reduction) by the addition of the "overeating" feeding factor in the final model (model 5 under "fat mass" in Table 4). In this final model, the unstandardized regression coefficient on the "overeating" factor was 0.60 (95% confidence interval, 0.23-0.98), which means that after controlling for all the covariates, including birth weight, maternal obesity, and breastfeeding duration, children whose mothers had high concern about their overeating or becoming overweight during infancy had a 0.60-kg higher fat mass at 5 years of age. Maternal obesity, birth weight, maternal covariates, breastfeeding duration, and the "overeating" feeding factor together explained 36% of the variance in child fat mass.

The regression models using the 2 BMI-derived dependent variables produced results similar to those using fat mass as the dependent variable. When BMI $z$ score was used, there was a 13% reduction in the regression coefficient on maternal obesity (from 0.53 SD of BMI to 0.46 SD of BMI) between model 4 and model 5 (Table 4). The addition of the "overeating" infant feeding factor to the logistic model for overweight reduced the odds ratio for maternal obesity by 8% (**Table 5**).

**Table 3. Relationship of Maternal Obesity* Before Pregnancy to Child Fat Mass and BMI at 5 Years of Age and to Maternal Infant-Feeding Style**

| | Mother Obese (n = 52) | Mother Not Obese (n = 256) | $P$ Value† |
|---|---|---|---|
| DXA | | | |
| Fat mass, mean ± SD, kg‡ | 5.03 ± 0.20 | 4.45 ± 0.09 | .008 |
| High adiposity, %§ | 30.8 | 23.4 | .26 |
| Anthropometric | | | |
| BMI $z$ score, mean ± SD | 1.00 ± 0.15 | 0.33 ± 0.06 | <.001 |
| Overweight, %‖ | 50.0 | 20.7 | <.001 |
| Maternal infant-feeding style, % | | | |
| High concern about undereating | 25 | 37 | .11 |
| High concern about hunger | 35 | 27 | .29 |
| Low awareness of infant cues | 31 | 36 | .45 |
| High concern about overeating | 37 | 23 | .04 |
| High control of schedule | 15 | 27 | .08 |
| High use of food to calm | 35 | 40 | .48 |
| Low social contact | 50 | 38 | .12 |

Abbreviations: BMI, body mass index (calculated as weight in kilograms divided by the square of height in meters); DXA, dual-energy x-ray absorptiometry.

*Defined as a BMI of 30 or higher; 5 mothers were missing data on BMI before pregnancy.

†$P$ value for $\chi^2$ test.

‡Adjusted for the child's lean body mass and sex.

§Upper quartile of percentage of body fat.

‖Defined as a BMI at the 85th percentile or higher for age and sex.

# COMMENT

## SUMMARY OF MAIN FINDINGS

The IFQ described maternal infant-feeding style in terms of 7 factors, but only a single factor—concern about the infant overeating or becoming overweight—was significantly associated with fat mass at 5 years of age, as measured directly using DXA. This factor was also associated with high adiposity (percentage of body fat in the upper quartile of study participants), BMI $z$ score, and overweight (BMI ≥85th percentile). Low awareness of infant satiety cues, high use of food to calm infant fussiness, and low social contact with the infant during feeding were not significantly related to childhood adiposity. High control over the infant feeding schedule tended to be associated with lower, rather than higher, childhood adiposity.

Mothers who were obese (BMI ≥30) before pregnancy had children with significantly higher fat mass, BMI $z$ scores, and prevalence of overweight at 5 years of age. This relationship between maternal obesity and the child's later adiposity/BMI was explained, in part, by maternal concern that the infant was overeating or would become overweight. This finding was independent of birth weight, breastfeeding, and maternal covariates, such as race, education, and income.

## LIMITATIONS

This study was limited by the fact that the mothers completed the IFQ when the child was 3 years of age rather than at the end of infancy. This could have led to poorer recall of the infant feeding style or could have biased that recall because of the child's weight at the time the IFQ was completed. Controlling for BMI at age 3 years would not necessarily overcome this potential limitation, and

**Table 4. Linear Regression Models Predicting Child Fat Mass and BMI *z* Score**

| | Maternal Obesity b (95% CI)* | F Change Statistic (*df*)† | *P* Value† | Model $R^2$‡ |
|---|---|---|---|---|
| Fat mass§ | | | | |
| Model 1: maternal obesity | 0.58 (0.16-1.00) | 7.22 (1) | .008 | 0.27 |
| Model 2: maternal obesity + BW | 0.53 (0.10-0.95) | 4.80 (1) | .03 | 0.29 |
| Model 3: maternal obesity + BW + maternal covariates‖ | 0.57 (0.14-1.01) | 1.58 (9) | .12 | 0.32 |
| Model 4: maternal obesity + BW + maternal covariates‖ + BF duration | 0.54 (0.10-0.98) | 1.52 (4) | .20 | 0.33 |
| Model 5: maternal obesity + BW + maternal covariates‖ + BF duration + "overeating"¶ | 0.46 (0.02-0.89) | 10.15 (1) | .002 | 0.36 |
| BMI *z* score | | | | |
| Model 1: maternal obesity | 0.68 (0.39-0.96) | 21.85 (1) | <.001 | 0.07 |
| Model 2: maternal obesity + BW | 0.57 (0.30-0.85) | 23.21 (1) | <.001 | 0.13 |
| Model 3: maternal obesity + BW + maternal covariates‖ | 0.54 (0.25-0.82) | 2.71 (9) | .005 | 0.20 |
| Model 4: maternal obesity + BW + maternal covariates‖ + BF duration | 0.53 (0.24-0.81) | 1.85 (4) | .12 | 0.22 |
| Model 5: maternal obesity + BW + maternal covariates‖ + BF duration + "overeating"¶ | 0.46 (0.18-0.73) | 15.82 (1) | <.001 | 0.26 |

Abbreviations: BF, breastfeeding; BMI, body mass index (calculated as weight in kilograms divided by the square of height in meters); BW, birth weight; CI, confidence interval.

*The unstandardized regression coefficient (b) (and its 95% CI) for maternal obesity represents the kilogram difference in fat mass (or SD units of BMI) at 5 years of age between children whose mothers were obese (BMI ≥30) before pregnancy and children whose mothers were not obese before pregnancy.

†F change statistic and degrees of freedom are for the comparison of the specified model to the previous model, and the *P* value is for the F change statistic.

‡Proportion of variance in fat mass (or BMI *z* score) explained by the model.

§All models for fat mass are also adjusted for lean body mass and sex.

‖Maternal covariates include race, age, marital status, smoking status, education, household income, and enrollment of child in WIC (Special Supplemental Nutrition Program for Women, Infants, and Children).

¶"Overeating" indicates a high concern about infant overeating or becoming overweight.

**Table 5. Logistic Regression Models Predicting Child High Adiposity and Overweight***

| | Maternal Obesity Odds Ratio (95% CI)† | Likelihood Ratio Statistic (*df*)‡ | *P* Value§ |
|---|---|---|---|
| High adiposity | | | |
| Model 1: maternal obesity | 1.45 (0.75-2.80) | 1.20 (1) | .27 |
| Model 2: maternal obesity + BW | 1.30 (0.66-2.53) | 4.59 (1) | .03 |
| Model 3: maternal obesity + BW + maternal covariates‖ | 1.09 (0.52-2.30) | 22.52 (9) | .007 |
| Model 4: maternal obesity + BW + maternal covariates‖ + BF duration | 1.03 (0.48-2.21) | 6.55 (4) | .16 |
| Model 5: maternal obesity + BW + maternal covariates‖ + BF duration + "overeating"¶ | 0.95 (0.44-2.05) | 2.33 (1) | .13 |
| Overweight | | | |
| Model 1: maternal obesity | 3.83 (2.06-7.13) | 17.52 (1) | <.001 |
| Model 2: maternal obesity + BW | 3.46 (1.84-6.52) | 5.16 (1) | .02 |
| Model 3: maternal obesity + BW + maternal covariates‖ | 3.70 (1.82-7.53) | 22.02 (9) | .009 |
| Model 4: maternal obesity + BW + maternal covariates‖ + BF duration | 3.69 (1.80-7.59) | 3.48 (4) | .48 |
| Model 5: maternal obesity + BW + maternal covariates‖ + "overeating"¶ | 3.39 (1.62-7.10) | 7.72 (1) | .005 |

Abbreviations: BF, breastfeeding; BMI, body mass index (calculated as weight in kilograms divided by the square of height in meters); BW, birth weight; CI, confidence interval.

*High adiposity is defined as the upper quartile of percentage of body fat, and overweight is defined as a BMI at the 85th percentile or higher.

†Odds ratio and 95% CI of high adiposity or overweight associated with maternal obesity before pregnancy (BMI ≥30).

‡The likelihood ratio statistic and degrees of freedom comparing the specified model with the previous model.

§*P* value is for the likelihood ratio statistic.

‖Maternal covariates include race, age, marital status, smoking status, education, household income, and enrollment of child in WIC (Special Supplemental Nutrition Program for Women, Infants, and Children).

¶"Overeating" indicates high concern about infant overeating or becoming overweight.

doing so would inappropriately control for a factor on the causal pathway between infant-feeding style and adiposity at age 5 years.[18]

In addition to this limitation, IFQ scores were not normally distributed and could have failed to detect meaningful clinical variation in some of the 7 factors. The present study may have also lacked power to detect some differences in maternal infant-feeding style that are of potential clinical significance. For example, there was a tendency for children to have lower fat mass if their mothers exerted high control over the infant feeding schedule, and there was also a tendency for obese mothers to report being less likely to exert high control over the infant feeding schedule. These findings warrant further study because they have implications for advising parents about infant feeding.

## RELATIONSHIP TO PREVIOUS STUDIES

Kramer and colleagues[8] administered the 10-item Maternal Feeding Attitudes Questionnaire to mothers at delivery. This instrument asked mothers about how they planned to feed their children. It was designed to assess a mother's tendency to "push" food into her child (eg, by trying to feed a fussy infant even if the infant had just been fed), with higher scores indicating a "pushier" feeding style. Scores were not significantly associated with BMI at 12 (n=382) or 24 (n=347) months of age.[10] The IFQ was previously administered to 453 mothers of varying sociodemographic backgrounds with children 11 to 23 months of age.[9] Consistent with the present study, maternal concern about the infant overeating or becoming overweight was the only infant-feeding factor that was associated with an increased relative weight (weight-for-height ≥90th percentile) in the children.

A strong and graded relationship between maternal BMI before pregnancy and childhood obesity (BMI ≥95th percentile) has previously been demonstrated,[4] suggesting that maternal obesity is the primary clinical risk factor, available at birth, for predicting preschooler obesity. To our knowledge, only 1 other study[19] has demonstrated the relationship between maternal obesity before pregnancy and childhood adiposity using DXA, a direct measure of adiposity.

## INTERPRETATION OF THE RESULTS

Maternal concern about her infant overeating or becoming overweight explained some of the relationship between maternal obesity and childhood adiposity. However, this feeding factor was associated with later fatness, independent of maternal obesity, suggesting that this feeding factor represents more than a mother's concern about transmitting to the child any of her own genetic susceptibility to obesity. Maternal concern about the infant overeating may be a marker for a behavioral eating pattern in the child that promotes obesity. Others have shown that an infant's eating style, as measured by the vigor of nipple sucking, is associated with later body weight.[20-22]

We do not have data on weight during infancy, but the present study suggests that mothers have some concern about their infant's appetite and weight, independent of birth weight, that predicts adiposity at age 5 years. Mothers may begin to alter feeding strategies in response to their infant's appetite and weight. Several studies indicate that higher levels of maternal control, manifested as restriction over a child's intake of snack foods, are associated with higher BMI levels in the children,[23,24] especially in children of obese mothers.[25] However, it is not clear whether this restriction is a response to the child's weight or the cause of it. Our findings suggest that mothers are concerned about their child's weight before the preschool years.

Our finding that maternal concern about the infant becoming overweight is associated with later adiposity seems to contradict other studies[26,27] suggesting that parents do not accurately perceive when their preschool children are overweight. One possible explanation for these different findings is that many parents may consider it unreasonable to label infants or young children as "overweight" or that such a label may be a reflection of poor parenting. However, asking parents whether they are concerned that their child "will become overweight" may reveal parents' more latent concerns about their infant's weight.

## CLINICAL IMPLICATIONS

Interactions during feeding are an important part of establishing attachment between mother and child.[28] Therefore, absent any clearer evidence that specific maternal infant-feeding styles are related to later adiposity, practitioners should avoid overzealous recommendations that might interfere with feeding interactions.

Because obesity is partly a heritable disorder and because feeding and infant growth contribute to parents' sense of competence in their ability to nurture their children, the topic of overeating or overweight can be sensitive. Clinicians may find it useful, however, to ask parents during their child's infancy whether they are "concerned about their infant eating too much or becoming overweight." These questions could also be paired with questions about the infant "not eating enough or becoming underweight."

Such questions may serve to open an early and constructive dialogue with parents about weight-related issues. For all parents, certain household behaviors can be encouraged that may prevent obesity[29] while providing health benefits unrelated to obesity.[30] For parents who express concern about obesity in their children, there are constructive ways to expand the dialogue.[31] Useful areas for open-ended inquiry include asking about the family history of obesity, which members of the family share a concern about the child's obesity risk, what specifically is causing the concern, what household interventions have already been tried, and what are the perceived barriers and facilitators to those efforts. Responses to these questions can help form an action plan that is based on the family's input.

**Accepted for Publication:** November 15, 2005.
**Correspondence:** Hillary L. Burdette, MD, MS, Division of Gastroenterology and Nutrition, Children's Hospital of Philadelphia, 34th Street and Civic Center Boulevard, Philadelphia, PA 19104 (burdette@email.chop.edu).
**Author Contributions:** Dr Burdette had full access to all the data in the study and takes responsibility for the integrity of the data and the accuracy of the data analysis.
**Funding/Support:** This work was supported by grant R01HL/DK64022 from the National Institutes of Health (Drs Whitaker and Daniels).
**Role of the Sponsor:** The sponsor had no role in the design and conduct of the study; the collection, management, analysis, and interpretation of the data; or the preparation, review, and approval of the manuscript.
**Acknowledgment:** We thank Karen Munson, RN, for her role in managing the data collection.

## REFERENCES

1. Institute of Medicine. *Preventing Childhood Obesity: Health in the Balance.* Washington, DC: National Academies Press; 2005.
2. Owen CG, Martin RM, Whincup PH, Smith GD, Cook DG. Effect of infant feeding on the risk of obesity across the life course: a quantitative review of published evidence. *Pediatrics.* 2005;115:1367-1377.
3. Mehta KC, Specker BL, Bartholmey S, Giddens J, Ho ML. Trial on timing of introduction to solids and food type on infant growth. *Pediatrics.* 1998;102:569-573.
4. Whitaker RC. Predicting preschooler obesity at birth: the role of maternal obesity in early pregnancy. *Pediatrics.* 2004;114:e29-e36.

5. Whitaker RC, Dietz WH. Role of the prenatal environment in the development of obesity. *J Pediatr.* 1998;132:768-776.
6. Faith MS, Scanlon KS, Birch LL, Francis LA, Sherry B. Parent-child feeding strategies and their relationships to child eating and weight status. *Obes Res.* 2004; 12:1711-1722.
7. Birch LL, Fisher JO. Development of eating behaviors among children and adolescents. *Pediatrics.* 1998;101:539-549.
8. Kramer MS, Barr RG, Leduc DG, Boisjoly C, Pless IB. Maternal psychological determinants of infant obesity: development and testing of two new instruments. *J Chronic Dis.* 1983;36:329-335.
9. Baughcum AE, Powers SW, Johnson SB, et al. Maternal feeding practices and beliefs and their relationships to overweight in early childhood. *J Dev Behav Pediatr.* 2001;22:391-408.
10. Kramer MS, Barr RG, Leduc DG, Boisjoly C, Pless IB. Infant determinants of childhood weight and adiposity. *J Pediatr.* 1985;107:104-107.
11. Chan GM. Performance of dual-energy x-ray absorptiometry in evaluating bone, lean body mass, and fat in pediatric subjects. *J Bone Miner Res.* 1992;7:369-374.
12. Kuczmarski RJ, Ogden CL, Guo SS, et al. 2000 CDC Growth Charts for the United States: methods and development. *Vital Health Stat 11.* 2002;(246):1-190.
13. Allison DB, Paultre F, Goran MI, Poehlman ET, Heymsfield SB. Statistical considerations regarding the use of ratios to adjust data. *Int J Obes Relat Metab Disord.* 1995;19:644-652.
14. Spruijt-Metz D, Lindquist CH, Birch LL, Fisher JO, Goran MI. Relation between mothers' child-feeding practices and children's adiposity. *Am J Clin Nutr.* 2002; 75:581-586.
15. Dwyer T, Blizzard CL. Defining obesity in children by biological endpoint rather than population distribution. *Int J Obes Relat Metab Disord.* 1996;20:472-480.
16. Williams DP, Going SB, Lohman TG, et al. Body fatness and risk for elevated blood pressure, total cholesterol, and serum lipoprotein ratios in children and adolescents. *Am J Public Health.* 1992;82:358-363.
17. Baron RM, Kenny DA. The moderator-mediator variable distinction in social psychological research: conceptual, strategic, and statistical considerations. *J Pers Soc Psychol.* 1986;51:1173-1182.
18. Tu YK, West R, Ellison GT, Gilthorpe MS. Why evidence for the fetal origins of adult disease might be a statistical artifact: the "reversal paradox" for the relation between birth weight and blood pressure in later life. *Am J Epidemiol.* 2005;161:27-32.
19. Berkowitz RI, Stallings VA, Maislin G, Stunkard AJ. Growth of children at high risk of obesity during the first 6 y of life: implications for prevention. *Am J Clin Nutr.* 2005;81:140-146.
20. Stunkard AJ, Berkowitz RI, Stallings VA, Schoeller DA. Energy intake, not energy output, is a determinant of body size in infants. *Am J Clin Nutr.* 1999; 69:524-530.
21. Agras WS, Kraemer HC, Berkowitz RI, Korner AF, Hammer LD. Does a vigorous feeding style influence early development of adiposity? *J Pediatr.* 1987;110: 799-804.
22. Agras WS, Kraemer HC, Berkowitz RI, Hammer LD. Influence of early feeding style on adiposity at 6 years of age. *J Pediatr.* 1990;116:805-809.
23. Birch LL, Fisher JO. Mothers' child-feeding practices influence daughters' eating and weight. *Am J Clin Nutr.* 2000;71:1054-1061.
24. Lee Y, Mitchell DC, Smiciklas-Wright H, Birch LL. Diet quality, nutrient intake, weight status, and feeding environments of girls meeting or exceeding recommendations for total dietary fat of the American Academy of Pediatrics. *Pediatrics.* 2001;107:E95.
25. Faith MS, Berkowitz RI, Stallings VA, Kerns J, Storey M, Stunkard AJ. Parental feeding attitudes and styles and child body mass index: prospective analysis of a gene-environment interaction. *Pediatrics.* 2004;114:e429-e436.
26. Baughcum AE, Chamberlin LA, Deeks CM, Powers SW, Whitaker RC. Maternal perceptions of overweight preschool children. *Pediatrics.* 2000;106:1380-1386.
27. Carnell S, Edwards C, Croker H, Boniface D, Wardle J. Parental perceptions of overweight in 3-5 y olds. *Int J Obes (Lond).* 2005;29:353-355.
28. Slaughter CW, Bryant AH. Hungry for love: the feeding relationship in the psychological development of young children. *Permanente J.* 2004;8:23-29.
29. Whitaker RC. Obesity prevention in pediatric primary care: four behaviors to target. *Arch Pediatr Adolesc Med.* 2003;157:725-727.
30. Burdette HL, Whitaker RC. Resurrecting free play in young children: looking beyond fitness and fatness to attention, affiliation, and affect. *Arch Pediatr Adolesc Med.* 2005;159:46-50.
31. Whitaker RC. Mental health and obesity in pediatric primary care: a gap between importance and action. *Arch Pediatr Adolesc Med.* 2004;158:826-828.

## IN OTHER ARCHIVES JOURNALS

### ARCHIVES OF GENERAL PSYCHIATRY

**Suicidality in Pediatric Patients Treated With Antidepressant Drugs**

*Tarek A. Hammad, MD, PhD, MSc, MS; Thomas Laughren, MD; Judith Racoosin, MD, MPH*

**Context:** There has been concern that widely used antidepressant agents might be associated with an increased risk of suicidal ideation and behavior (suicidality) in pediatric patients.
**Objective:** To investigate the relationship between antidepressant drugs and suicidality in pediatric patients participating in randomized, placebo-controlled trials.
**Data Sources:** Data were derived from 23 trials conducted in 9 drug company–supported programs evaluating the effectiveness of antidepressants in pediatric patients and 1 multicenter trial (the Treatment for Adolescents With Depression Study) that evaluated fluoxetine hydrochloride.
**Study Selection:** All placebo-controlled trials submitted to the Food and Drug Administration were eligible for inclusion. Evaluable data were derived from 4582 patients in 24 trials. Sixteen trials studied patients with major depressive disorder, and the remaining 8 studied obsessive-compulsive disorder (n=4), generalized anxiety disorder (n=2), attention-deficit/hyperactivity disorder (n=1), and social anxiety disorder (n=1). Only 20 trials were included in the risk ratio analysis of suicidality because 4 trials had no events in the drug or placebo groups.
**Data Extraction:** Individual patient data were available for all the trials.
**Data Synthesis:** A meta-analysis was conducted to obtain overall suicidality risk estimates for each drug individually, for selective serotonin reuptake inhibitors in depression trials as a group, and for all evaluable trials combined. There were no completed suicides in any of these trials. The multicenter trial was the only individual trial to show a statistically significant risk ratio (4.62; 95% confidence interval [CI], 1.02-20.92). The overall risk ratio for selective serotonin reuptake inhibitors in depression trials was 1.66 (95% CI, 1.02-2.68) and for all drugs across all indications was 1.95 (95% CI, 1.28-2.98). The overall risk difference for all drugs across all indications was 0.02 (95% CI, 0.01-0.03).
**Conclusion:** Use of antidepressant drugs in pediatric patients is associated with a modestly increased risk of suicidality. *(2006;63:332-339)*

**Correspondence:** *Thomas Laughren, MD, Division of Neuropharmacological Drug Products, HFD-120, 5600 Fishers Ln, Rockville, MD 20857 (laughren@cder.fda.gov).*

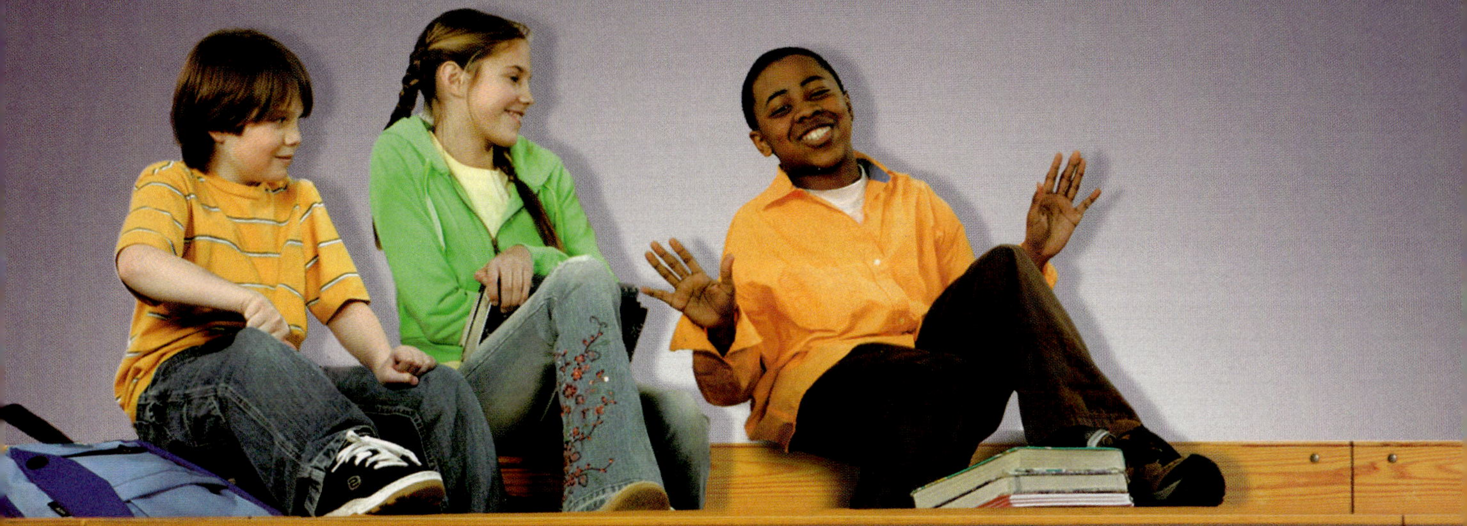

# BOOSTRIX®

## (Tetanus Toxoid, Reduced Diphtheria Toxoid and Acellular Pertussis Vaccine, Adsorbed) (Tdap)

The following is a brief summary only; see full prescribing information for complete product information.

**INDICATIONS AND USAGE:** BOOSTRIX is indicated for active booster immunization against tetanus, diphtheria, and pertussis as a single dose in individuals 10 through 18 years of age. The use of BOOSTRIX as a primary series or to complete the primary series has not been studied. As with any vaccine, BOOSTRIX may not protect 100% of individuals receiving the vaccine.

**CONTRAINDICATIONS:** Hypersensitivity to any component of the vaccine is a contraindication (see DESCRIPTION in full prescribing information). Do not use BOOSTRIX after a serious allergic reaction (e.g., anaphylaxis) following any other tetanus toxoid, diphtheria toxoid or pertussis-containing vaccine, or any component of this vaccine (see DESCRIPTION in full prescribing information). Because of the uncertainty as to which component of the vaccine might be responsible, do not give further vaccination with any of these components; or, refer such individuals to an allergist for evaluation. The following events are contraindications to administration of BOOSTRIX: encephalopathy (e.g., coma, decreased level of consciousness, prolonged seizures) within 7 days of administration of a previous dose of a pertussis-containing vaccine that is not attributable to another identifiable cause; progressive neurologic disorder, uncontrolled epilepsy, or progressive encephalopathy. Do not vaccinate individuals with these conditions until a treatment regimen has been established and the condition has stabilized.

**WARNINGS:** The tip cap and the rubber plunger of the needleless prefilled syringes contain dry natural latex rubber that may cause allergic reactions in latex sensitive individuals. The vial stopper is latex-free. If any of the following events occurred in temporal relation to previous receipt of a Diphtheria and Tetanus Toxoids and Pertussis Vaccine Adsorbed (DTwP) vaccine or a vaccine containing an acellular pertussis component, consider carefully whether to give subsequent doses of BOOSTRIX: temperature of ≥40.5°C (105°F) within 48 hours not due to another identifiable cause; collapse or shock-like state (hypotonic-hyporesponsive episode) within 48 hours; persistent, inconsolable crying lasting ≥3 hours, occurring within 48 hours; seizures with or without fever occurring within 3 days. Persons who experienced serious Arthus-type hypersensitivity reactions following a prior dose of tetanus toxoid usually have high serum tetanus antitoxin levels and should not be given Tetanus and Diphtheria Toxoids Adsorbed For Adult Use (Td) or Tdap vaccines or even emergency doses of Td more frequently than every 10 years, even if the wound is neither clean nor minor. If Guillain-Barré syndrome has occurred within 6 weeks of receipt of prior vaccine containing tetanus toxoid, the decision to give BOOSTRIX or any vaccine containing tetanus toxoid should be based on careful consideration of the potential benefits and possible risks. The decision to administer a pertussis-containing vaccine to individuals with stable central nervous system (CNS) disorders must be made by the physician on an individual basis, with consideration of all relevant factors, and assessment of potential risks and benefits for that individual. Advise the patient, parent, or guardian of the potential increased risk involved (see PRECAUTIONS). A family history of seizures or other CNS disorders is not a contraindication to pertussis vaccine. The Advisory Committee on Immunization Practices (ACIP) has published guidelines for vaccination of persons with recent or acute illness (www.cdc.gov). Do not give BOOSTRIX to individuals with bleeding disorders such as hemophilia or thrombocytopenia, or to persons on anticoagulant therapy unless the potential benefit clearly outweighs the risk of administration. If the decision is made to administer BOOSTRIX to such persons, it should be given with caution with steps taken to avoid the risk of hematoma following the injection.

**PRECAUTIONS: General:** Before the injection of any biological, the physician should take all reasonable precautions to prevent allergic or other adverse reactions. Epinephrine injection (1:1,000) and other appropriate agents used for the control of immediate allergic reactions must be immediately available should an acute anaphylactic reaction occur. Immunosuppressed persons, including individuals receiving immunosuppressive therapy, may not develop the expected immune response. **Drug Interactions:** Do not mix BOOSTRIX with any other vaccine in the same syringe or vial. **Carcinogenesis, Mutagenesis, Impairment of Fertility:** BOOSTRIX has not been evaluated for carcinogenic or mutagenic potential, or for impairment of fertility. **Pregnancy:** Pregnancy Category C. Animal reproduction studies have not been conducted with BOOSTRIX. It is also not known whether BOOSTRIX can cause fetal harm when administered to a pregnant woman or can affect reproductive capacity. BOOSTRIX should be given to a pregnant woman only if clearly needed. Animal fertility studies have not been conducted with BOOSTRIX. In a developmental toxicity study, the effect of BOOSTRIX on embryo-fetal and pre-weaning development was evaluated in pregnant rats. Animals were administered INFANRIX® (Diphtheria and Tetanus Toxoids and Acellular Pertussis Vaccine Adsorbed) prior to gestation and BOOSTRIX during the period of organogenesis (gestation days 6, 8, 11) and later in pregnancy (gestation day 15), 0.1 mL/rat/occasion (a 45-fold increase compared to the human dose of BOOSTRIX on a body weight basis), by intramuscular injection. No adverse affect on pregnancy and lactation parameters, embryo-fetal or pre-weaning development was observed. There were no fetal malformations or other evidence of teratogenesis noted in this study. **Nursing Mothers:** It is not known whether BOOSTRIX is excreted in human milk. Because many drugs are excreted in human milk, caution should be exercised when BOOSTRIX is administered to a nursing woman. **Pregnancy Exposure Registry:** Healthcare providers are encouraged to register pregnant women who receive BOOSTRIX in the GlaxoSmithKline vaccination pregnancy registry by calling 1-888-825-5249. **Geriatric Use:** BOOSTRIX is not indicated for use in individuals older than 18 years. **Pediatric Use:** BOOSTRIX is not indicated for use in individuals younger than 10 years (see DOSAGE AND ADMINISTRATION in full prescribing information). For immunization of infants and children younger than 7 years against diphtheria, tetanus, and pertussis, refer to the manufacturers' package inserts for Diphtheria and Tetanus Toxoids and Acellular Pertussis Vaccine Adsorbed (DTaP) vaccines.

**ADVERSE REACTIONS:** A total of 3,608 adolescents were vaccinated with a single dose of BOOSTRIX during clinical trials. An additional 1,092 adolescents 10 to 18 years of age received a non-US formulation of BOOSTRIX (formulated to contain 0.5 mg aluminum per dose) in non-US clinical studies.

The primary safety study, conducted in the United States, was a randomized, observer-blinded, controlled study in which 3,080 adolescents 10 to 18 years of age received a single dose of BOOSTRIX and 1,034 received the control Td vaccine manufactured by Massachusetts Public Health Biologic Laboratories. There were no substantive differences in demographic characteristics between the vaccine groups. Among BOOSTRIX and control vaccine recipients approximately 75% were 10 to 14 years of age and approximately 25% were 15 to 18 years of age. Approximately 98% of participants in this study had received the recommended series of 4 or 5 doses of either DTwP or a combination of DTwP and DTaP in childhood. Data on adverse events were collected by the subjects, parents and/or guardians using standardized diaries for 15 consecutive days following the vaccine dose (i.e., day of vaccination and the next 14 days). Subjects were monitored for unsolicited adverse events that occurred within 31 days of vaccination (day 0-30) using diary cards (day 0-14) supplemented by spontaneous reports and a medical history as reported by subjects, parents, and/or guardians. Subjects were also monitored for 6 months post-vaccination for non-routine medical visits, visits to an emergency room, onset of new chronic illness, and serious adverse events. Information regarding late onset adverse events was obtained via a telephone call 6 months following vaccination. At least 97% of subjects completed the 6-month follow-up evaluation.

In a study conducted in Germany, BOOSTRIX was administered to 319 children 10 to 12 years of age previously vaccinated with 5 doses of acellular pertussis-containing vaccines, 193 of these subjects had previously received 5 doses of INFANRIX. Adverse events were recorded on diary cards during the 15 days following vaccination. Unsolicited adverse events that occurred within 31 days of vaccination (day 0-30) were recorded on the diary card or verbally reported to the investigator. Subjects were monitored for 6 months post-vaccination for physician office visits, emergency room visits, onset of new chronic illness, and serious adverse events. The 6-month follow-up evaluation, conducted via telephone interview, was completed by 90% of subjects.

The adverse event information from clinical trials provides a basis for identifying adverse events that appear to be related to vaccine use and for approximating rates. However, because clinical trials are conducted under widely varying conditions, adverse event rates observed in the clinical trials of a vaccine cannot be directly compared to rates in the clinical trials of another vaccine, and may not reflect the rates observed in practice.

**Serious Adverse Events in All Safety Studies:** In the US-safety study and German-safety study, no serious adverse events were reported to occur within 31 days of vaccination. During the 6-month extended safety evaluation period, no serious adverse events that were of potential autoimmune origin or new onset and chronic in nature were reported to occur. In non-US studies in which serious adverse events were monitored for up to 37 days, one subject was diagnosed with insulin dependent diabetes 20 days following administration of BOOSTRIX. No other serious adverse events of potential autoimmune origin or that were new onset and chronic in nature were reported to occur in these studies.

**Solicited Adverse Events in the US-Safety Study:** In a US study, the most common local adverse events following administration of BOOSTRIX were pain, redness, and swelling at the injection site. The most common general adverse events were headache and fatigue. Most of these events were reported at a similar frequency in recipients of both BOOSTRIX and Td. Any pain, grade 2 or 3 pain (but not grade 3 alone), and grade 2 or 3 headache (but not grade 3 alone) were reported at a higher rate in recipients of BOOSTRIX. The primary safety endpoint of the US study was the incidence of grade 3 pain (spontaneously painful and/or prevented normal activity) at the injection site within 15 days of vaccination. Grade 3 pain was reported in 4.6% of those who received BOOSTRIX compared with 4.0% of those who received the Td vaccine. The difference in rate of grade 3 pain was within the pre-defined clinical limit for non-inferiority (upper limit of the 95% CI for the difference ≤4%). These were the rates for solicited local and general adverse events within 15 days of vaccination with BOOSTRIX or Td vaccine for the total vaccinated cohort (all enrolled, vaccinated subjects with safety data available analyzed by vaccine received):

**Percentage of Individuals 10 to 18 Years of Age Reporting Solicited Local Adverse Events or Solicited General Adverse Events Within the 15-day* Post-Vaccination Period**

| | BOOSTRIX (N = 3,032) % | Td (N =1,013) % |
|---|---|---|
| **Local** | | |
| Pain,† any | 75.3 | 71.7 |
| Pain,† grade 2 or 3 | 51.2 | 42.5 |
| Pain,‡ grade 3 | 4.6 | 4.0 |
| Redness, any | 22.5 | 19.8 |
| Redness, >20 mm | 4.1 | 3.9 |
| Redness, ≥50 mm | 1.7 | 1.6 |
| Swelling, any | 21.1 | 20.1 |
| Swelling, >20 mm | 5.3 | 4.9 |
| Swelling, ≥50 mm | 2.5 | 3.2 |
| Arm circumference increase,§ >5 mm | 28.3 | 29.5 |
| Arm circumference increase,§ >20 mm | 2.0 | 2.2 |
| Arm circumference increase,§ >40 mm | 0.5 | 0.3 |
| **General** | | |
| Fever,‖ ≥99.5°F | 13.5 | 13.1 |
| Fever,‖ >100.4°F | 5.0 | 4.7 |
| Fever,‖ >102.2°F | 1.4 | 1.0 |
| Headache, any | 43.1 | 41.5 |
| Headache,† grade 2 or 3 | 15.7 | 12.7 |
| Headache, grade 3 | 3.7 | 2.7 |
| Fatigue, any | 37.0 | 36.7 |
| Fatigue, grade 2 or 3 | 14.4 | 12.9 |
| Fatigue, grade 3 | 3.7 | 3.2 |
| Gastrointestinal symptoms,¶ any | 26.0 | 25.8 |
| Gastrointestinal symptoms,¶ grade 2 or 3 | 9.8 | 9.7 |
| Gastrointestinal symptoms,¶ grade 3 | 3.0 | 3.2 |

Td = Tetanus and Diphtheria Toxoids Adsorbed For Adult Use manufactured by Massachusetts Public Health Biologic Laboratories.
N = number of subjects in the total vaccinated cohort with local/general symptoms sheets completed.
Grade 2 = Local: painful when the limb was moved; General: interfered with normal activity.
Grade 3 = Local: spontaneously painful and/or prevented normal activity; General: prevented normal activity.
*Day of vaccination and the next 14 days.
†Statistically significantly higher (P<0.05) following BOOSTRIX as compared to Td vaccine.
‡Grade 3 injection site pain following BOOSTRIX was not inferior to Td (upper limit of two-sided 95% CI for the difference in the percentage of subjects ≤4%).
§Mid-upper region of the vaccinated arm.
‖Oral temperatures or axillary temperatures.
¶Gastrointestinal symptoms included nausea, vomiting, diarrhea and/or abdominal pain.

Mid-upper arm circumference was measured by the adolescent or their parent/guardian prior to injection and daily for 15 days following vaccination. There was no significant difference between BOOSTRIX recipients and Td recipients in the proportion of subjects reporting an increase in mid-upper arm circumference in the vaccinated arm. The incidence of unsolicited adverse events reported in the 31 days after vaccination was comparable between the 2 groups.

**Solicited Adverse Events in the German Safety Study:** No cases of whole arm swelling were spontaneously reported. Two individuals (2/193) reported large injection site swelling (range 110 to 200 mm diameter), in one case associated with grade 3 pain. Neither individual sought medical attention. These episodes were reported to resolve without sequelae within 5 days. These were the rates of solicited local adverse events and fever within 15 days of vaccination for those subjects who had previously been vaccinated with 5 doses of INFANRIX:

**Rates of Solicited Adverse Events Reported Within the 15-day* Post-Vaccination Period Following Administration of BOOSTRIX in Individuals 10 to 12 Years of Age Who Had Previously Received 5 Doses of INFANRIX**

| Adverse Event | BOOSTRIX (N = 193) % (95% CI) |
|---|---|
| Pain, any | 62.2 (54.9-69.0) |
| Pain, grade 2 or 3 | 33.2 (26.6-40.3) |
| Pain, grade 3 | 5.7 (2.9-10.0) |
| Redness, any | 47.7 (40.4-55.0) |
| Redness, >20 mm | 15.0 (10.3-20.9) |
| Redness, ≥50 mm | 10.9 (6.9-16.2) |
| Swelling, any | 38.9 (31.9-46.1) |
| Swelling, >20 mm | 17.6 (12.5-23.7) |
| Swelling, ≥50 mm | 14.0 (9.4-19.7) |
| Fever, ≥99.5 | 8.8 (5.2-13.7) |
| Fever, >100.4 | 4.1 (1.8-8.0) |
| Fever, >102.2 | 1.0 (0.1-3.7) |

N = number of subjects with local/general symptoms sheets completed.
Grade 2 = Painful when the limb was moved.
Grade 3 = Spontaneously painful and/or prevented normal activity.
*Day of vaccination and the next 14 days.

As with any vaccine, there is the possibility that broad use of BOOSTRIX could reveal adverse events not observed in clinical trials.

**Postmarketing Reports:** Worldwide voluntary reports of adverse events received for BOOSTRIX in persons 10 to 18 years of age since market introduction of this vaccine are listed below. This list includes serious events or events which have causal connection to components of this or other vaccines or drugs. Because these events are reported voluntarily from a population of uncertain size, it is not possible to reliably estimate their frequency or establish a causal relationship to vaccine exposure. *Blood and lymphatic system disorders:* Lymphadenitis, lymphadenopathy. *Cardiac disorders:* Myocarditis. *Injection site reactions:* Induration, inflammation, mass, nodule, warmth, local reaction. *Metabolism and nutrition disorders:* Diabetes mellitus insulin-dependent. *Musculoskeletal and connective tissue disorders:* Arthralgia, back pain, myalgia. *Nervous system disorders:* Convulsion, encephalitis, facial palsy, paraesthesia. *Skin and subcutaneous tissue disorders:* Exanthem, Henoch-Schönlein purpura, rash. In addition, extensive swelling of the injected limb has been reported following administration of BOOSTRIX.

**Reporting Adverse Events:** Report the occurrence following immunization of any event set forth in the Vaccine Injury Table from the National Childhood Vaccine Injury Act including: Anaphylaxis or anaphylactic shock within 7 days, encephalopathy or encephalitis within 7 days, brachial neuritis within 28 days, or an acute complication or sequelae (including death) of an illness, disability, injury, or condition referred to above, or any events that would contraindicate further doses of vaccine, according to this prescribing information. These events should be reported to VAERS. The VAERS toll-free number is 1-800-822-7967. Reporting forms may also be obtained at the VAERS website at www.vaers.hhs.gov.

**DOSAGE AND ADMINISTRATION: Recommended Dose:** BOOSTRIX should be administered as a single 0.5 mL injection by the intramuscular route into the deltoid muscle of the upper arm in individuals 10 through 18 years of age. Do not administer this product subcutaneously or intravenously. There are no data to support repeat administration of BOOSTRIX. Five years should elapse between the subject's last dose of the recommended series of childhood DTwP and/or DTaP vaccine and the administration of BOOSTRIX. Limited data are available on the use of BOOSTRIX following Tetanus and Diphtheria Toxoids Adsorbed For Adult Use (Td) vaccine. **Additional Dosing Information:** ***Wound Management:*** Clinicians should refer to guidelines for tetanus prophylaxis in routine wound management. Adolescents 10 to 18 years of age who have completed a primary series against tetanus and who sustain wounds which are minor and uncomplicated, should receive a booster dose of a tetanus toxoid-containing vaccine only if they have not received tetanus toxoid within the preceding 10 years. In case of tetanus-prone injury (e.g., wounds contaminated with dirt, feces, soil, and saliva; puncture wounds; avulsions; and wounds resulting from missles, crushing, burns, and frostbite) in an adolescent who is in need of tetanus toxoid, BOOSTRIX can be used as an alternative to Tetanus and Diphtheria Toxoids Adsorbed For Adult Use (Td) vaccine in patients for whom the pertussis component is also indicated (see INDICATIONS AND USAGE).

Manufactured by **GlaxoSmithKline Biologicals**
Rixensart, Belgium, US License 1617

Distributed by **GlaxoSmithKline**
Research Triangle Park, NC 27709



Full prescribing information for BOOSTRIX is available at www.BOOSTRIX.com.
BRS-BO:L3

**References:** **1.** Centers for Disease Control and Prevention. Preventing tetanus, diphtheria, and pertussis among adolescents: use of tetanus toxoid, reduced diphtheria toxoid and acellular pertussis vaccines: recommendations of the Advisory Committee on Immunization Practices (ACIP). Early Release 2006;55(February 23, 2006):1–43. **2.** Centers for Disease Control and Prevention. Recommended childhood and adolescent immunization schedule—United States, 2006. *MMWR.* 2006;54(51&52):Q1–Q4.

ARTICLE

# Prevalence of Diabetes and Impaired Fasting Glucose Levels Among US Adolescents

## *National Health and Nutrition Examination Survey, 1999-2002*

*Glen E. Duncan, PhD, RCEPSM*

**Objective:** To determine the current prevalence of self-reported diabetes and impaired fasting glucose levels among US adolescents.

**Design and Setting:** Cross-sectional, National Health and Nutrition Examination Survey (1999-2002).

**Participants:** A sample of 4370 adolescents (aged 12-19 years) with self-reported diabetes and a subsample of 1496 adolescents without self-reported diabetes who had fasted for at least 8 hours. Subjects who reported having diabetes and using insulin were further categorized as having type 1 diabetes, those reporting having diabetes and not using insulin as having type 2 diabetes, and those with a fasting plasma glucose level greater than or equal to 5.6 mmol/L (100 mg/dL) as having impaired fasting glucose levels.

**Main Outcome Measures:** Prevalence of self-reported diabetes, type 1 and type 2 diabetes, and impaired fasting glucose levels among US adolescents.

**Results:** In the full sample, 0.5% (95% confidence interval [CI], 0.24%-0.76%) of adolescents reported having diabetes. Of those reporting diabetes, roughly 71% (95% CI, 56%-86%) were categorized as having type 1 and 29% (95% CI, 14%-44%) as having type 2 diabetes. In the subsample, roughly 11% (95% CI, 8%-14%) had impaired fasting glucose levels. Using population-based sample weights, these proportions were equivalent to 39 005 US adolescents with type 2 diabetes and 2 769 736 with impaired fasting glucose levels.

**Conclusions:** The prevalence of type 2 diabetes and impaired fasting glucose levels is substantial among US adolescents. These estimates have important implications for public health because of the high rate of conversion from impaired fasting glucose level to type 2 diabetes in adults and the increased risk of cardiovascular disease in individuals with type 2 diabetes.

*Arch Pediatr Adolesc Med. 2006;160:523-528*

THE CURRENT ESTIMATE OF the number of people in the United States with diabetes is 18.2 million, or 6.3% of the population.[1] This figure includes 13 million people with diagnosed diabetes and 5.2 million with undiagnosed diabetes. About 210 000 people younger than 20 years have diabetes, and approximately 1 in every 400 to 500 children and adolescents has type 1 diabetes.[1] Although type 2 diabetes is an emerging problem among youth,[2-5] nationally representative data to monitor diabetes trends in this age group are not available.

*For editorial comment see page 550*

In the only population-based study of diabetes among US adolescents (aged 12-19 years) to date,[6] the prevalence of diabetes was estimated at 0.41% between 1988 and 1994. Although the presence of type 2 diabetes was reported, the survey sample size was not large enough to obtain precise prevalence estimates because of the relatively low prevalence at the time of the survey. More recent reports indicate that impaired glucose tolerance is highly prevalent among overweight youth,[7] and that prediabetes in youth is associated with altered fat partitioning in muscle and intra-abdominal regions and the development of severe peripheral insulin resistance.[8] Similarly, the metabolic syndrome is common among US adolescents[9-11] and has increased significantly over the past decade.[10]

Because the prevalence of being overweight has continued to increase substantially over the past several decades among US children and adolescents,[12,13] it is also likely that the prevalence of diabetes has increased among these youths. Further

**Author Affiliation:** Nutritional Sciences Program, Department of Epidemiology, University of Washington, Seattle.

supporting this contention, a recent report indicates that the lifetime probability of being diagnosed with diabetes is substantial for individuals born in the United States in the year 2000.[14] The objective of this article is to present the most recent national estimates for the prevalence of diabetes and impaired fasting glucose levels among US adolescents, based on data from the 1999-2000 and 2001-2002 National Health and Nutrition Examination Surveys (NHANES).

## METHODS

The NHANES design is a stratified, multistage probability sample of the civilian noninstitutionalized US population. Approximately 9965 persons aged 2 months to 85 years were studied in the NHANES 1999-2000 survey period, and 11 039 in the 2001-2002 survey period. A subsample of more than 3000 individuals from each survey was invited to attend a morning examination after fasting overnight. Fully informed consent and assent were obtained from all participants and these documents were approved by the National Center for Health Statistic's Institutional Review Board.

Details of the NHANES protocol are available elsewhere.[15] Briefly, blood specimens were stored frozen until they were shipped to a central laboratory for analysis. Plasma glucose levels were measured with an enzymatic technique using the hexokinase/glucose-6-phospate dehydrogenase reaction. Whole-blood hemoglobin $A_{1c}$ levels were measured using fully automated glycohemoglobin analyzers (CLC330 and CLC385; Primus Corp, Kansas City, Mo) and boromate affinity high-performance liquid chromatography, serum insulin levels were measured using a double-antibody radioimmunoassay technique, and serum C-peptide levels were measured using a polyethylene glycol–accelerated double-antibody technique. Height was measured in an upright position with a stadiometer and weight was also measured in a standing position on a self-zeroing scale. The poverty-to-income ratio, a ratio of family income to poverty thresholds established by the US Census Bureau, was used as a measure of socioeconomic status.

Data from each survey were linked using a unique survey participant identifier. The full sample consisted of 4370 adolescents (aged 12-19 years) who were given a personal interview on diabetes, including use of medications and symptoms associated with diabetes. All subjects were asked the lead-in question pertaining to history of diabetes: "Have you ever been told by a doctor or health professional that you have diabetes or sugar diabetes?" Subjects with a missing response (n=1) or those who responded "borderline" (n=1) were excluded from the analyses. Thus, the only possible responses were "yes" or "no." Pregnant women (n=101) and subjects categorized as "other Hispanics" (n=231) and "other races, including multiracial" (n=202) were also excluded from the analyses, the latter because of inadequate sample sizes for these groups. The subsample consisted of 1496 adolescents with a fasting (≥ 8 hours) glucose value recorded and who responded "no" to the lead-in question on diabetes history. Only subjects who had complete data were included in the subsample analyses.

### DEFINITIONS

In the full sample, subjects who responded "yes" to the lead-in question were further categorized by specific diabetes type. Those who reported using insulin were categorized as having type 1 diabetes, and those who reported not using insulin as having type 2 diabetes. Subjects in the subsample with a fasting glucose level of less than 5.6 mmol/L (100 mg/dL) were categorized as having normal fasting glucose levels, and those with a value greater than or equal to 5.6 mmol/L (100 mg/dL) as having impaired fasting glucose levels.[16] Using the Centers for Disease Control and Prevention growth charts for the United States in the year 2000, being overweight among adolescents was defined as having a body mass index (BMI) (calculated as weight in kilograms divided by the square of height in meters) of greater than or equal to the 95th percentile for age and sex; at risk for being overweight was defined as having a BMI value greater than or equal to the 85th percentile but less than the 95th percentile for age and sex; and normal weight was defined as having a BMI of less than the 85th percentile for age and sex.[17]

### STATISTICAL ANALYSIS

Data were analyzed using SAS statistical software (version 9.1; SAS Institute Inc, Cary, NC). The full sample was analyzed using the 4-year full sample interview weights to estimate means and 95% confidence intervals (CIs), and the masked variance units (pseudoprimary and pseudostratum sampling units) to estimate the standard error of those means. The subsample was analyzed using the 4-year fasting weights and the masked variance units. Continuous variables are presented as mean±SE. Categorical variables are presented as frequency, weighted frequency (based on sampling weights), and proportion with 95% CI. All proportions are based on a percentage of the weighted frequencies. Differences in continuous variables were tested univariately using *t* tests for independent samples, and prevalence values for categorical variables were compared using $\chi^2$ tests for proportions. Statistical significance was established at $\alpha=.05$ a priori.

## RESULTS

The full sample included 4370 subjects, equivalent to a weighted sample of 26 649 401 adolescents, with mean age of 15.4±0.1 years. The sex distribution was roughly 48% female and 52% male, and the race distribution was 12.8% Mexican American, 16.6% non-Hispanic black, and 70.6% non-Hispanic white. The percentage of self-reported diabetes in the total sample and self-reported diabetes by sex and race are presented in **Table 1**. There was no difference (*P*=.94) in age among subjects reporting "yes" for having diabetes (15.4±0.6 years) or "no" to the lead-in question on diabetes history (15.4±0.1 years). There was a significant association between self-reported diabetes and sex, and between self-reported diabetes and race (*P*<.001).

The percentage of diabetes type in the overall sample and the percentage of diabetes by sex and race are presented in **Table 2**. There was no difference (*P*=.34) in age among subjects categorized as having type 1 (15.8±0.6 years) or type 2 (14.5±0.0 years) diabetes. Among subjects categorized as having type 1 diabetes (n=10; estimate=95 066), 5.9% also reported taking oral agents (n=2; estimate=5635). Among subjects categorized as having type 2 diabetes (n=8; estimate=39 005), 31.3% reported taking oral agents (n=1; estimate=12 205). There was a significant association between diabetes type and sex, and between diabetes type and race (*P*<.001).

The subsample included 1496 subjects, equivalent to a weighted sample of 24 885 638 adolescents, with a mean age of 15.4±0.1 years. The sex distribution was roughly 49% female and 51% male and the race distribution was 11.6% Mexican American, 15.3% non-Hispanic black, and

**Table 1. Percentage of Self-reported Diabetes Among 4370 US Adolescents*†**

| | Total (N = 4370) | Weighted Frequency (Percentage [95% CI]) Diabetes (n = 18) | No Diabetes (n = 4352) |
|---|---|---|---|
| Total population | 26 649 401 | 134 071 (0.50 [0.24-0.76]) | 26 515 330 (99.50 [99.24-99.76]) |
| By sex‡ and race‡ | | | |
| Female | 12 755 217 | 61 060 (45.54 [11.23-79.86]) | 12 694 157 (47.87 [45.70-50.05]) |
| Male | 13 894 184 | 73 011 (54.46 [20.14-88.77]) | 13 821 173 (52.13 [49.95-54.30]) |
| Mexican American | 3 409 373 | 10 437 (7.78 [0.00-16.14]) | 3 398 936 (12.82 [9.49-16.14]) |
| Non-Hispanic, black | 4 434 147 | 18 727 (13.97 [1.80-26.14]) | 4 415 420 (16.65 [13.02-20.29]) |
| Non-Hispanic, white | 18 805 881 | 104 907 (78.25 [62.21-94.29]) | 18 700 974 (70.53 [67.10-73.95]) |

Abbreviation: CI, confidence interval.

*Respondents (aged 12-19 years) were asked "Have you ever been told by a doctor or health professional that you have diabetes or sugar diabetes?" to determine diabetes status.

†Data are from the 1999-2000 and 2001-2002 National Health and Nutrition Examination Surveys. Values are expressed as frequency, weighted frequency (based on sample weights), and percentage with 95% CI.

‡Indicates significant association between row and column variables by $\chi^2$ test ($P<.001$).

**Table 2. Diabetes Type Among 18 US Adolescents With Self-reported Diabetes*†**

| | Total (N = 18) | Weighted Frequency (Percentage [95% CI]) Type 1 (n = 10) | Type 2 (n = 8) |
|---|---|---|---|
| Total population | 134 071 | 95 066 (70.91 [55.99-85.82]) | 39 005 (29.09 [14.18-44.01]) |
| By sex‡ and race‡ | | | |
| Female | 61 060 | 38 322 (40.31 [0.00-96.80]) | 22 737 (58.29 [52.78-63.80]) |
| Male | 73 011 | 56 743 (59.69 [3.20-100]) | 16 268 (41.71 [36.20-47.22]) |
| Mexican American | 10 437 | 3912 (4.11 [0.00-12.64]) | 6525 (16.73 [8.84-24.62]) |
| Non-Hispanic, black | 18 727 | 11 677 (12.28 [2.51-22.06]) | 7051 (18.08 [16.36-19.79]) |
| Non-Hispanic, white | 104 907 | 79 477 (83.60 [68.53-98.68]) | 25 430 (65.20 [59.02-71.37]) |

Abbreviation: CI, confidence interval.

*Respondents (aged 12-19 years) were asked "Have you ever been told by a doctor or health professional that you have diabetes or sugar diabetes?" Subjects who responded "yes" and reported using insulin were categorized as having type 1 diabetes and those who reported not using insulin as having type 2 diabetes.

†Data are from the 1999-2000 and 2001-2002 National Health and Nutrition Examination Surveys. Values are expressed as frequency, weighted frequency (based on sample weights), and percentage with 95% CI.

‡Indicates significant association between row and column variables by $\chi^2$ test ($P<.001$).

**Table 3. Percentage of Impaired Fasting Glucose Levels Among 1496 US Adolescents***

| | Total (N = 1496) | Weighted Frequency (Percentage [95% CI]) NFG (n = 1318) | IFG (n = 178) |
|---|---|---|---|
| Total population | 24 885 638 | 22 115 903 (88.87 [85.83-91.92]) | 2 769 736 (11.13 [8.09-14.17]) |
| By sex† and race† | | | |
| Female | 12 079 241 | 11 201 134 (50.65 [46.63-54.67]) | 878 107 (31.70 [21.09-42.32]) |
| Male | 12 806 397 | 10 914 769 (49.35 [45.33-53.37]) | 1 891 628 (68.30 [57.68-78.91]) |
| Mexican American | 2 877 893 | 2 438 858 (15.93 [11.33-20.52]) | 439 035 (15.85 [9.08-22.62]) |
| Non-Hispanic, black | 3 803 133 | 3 522 359 (11.03 [7.92-14.14]) | 280 773 (10.14 [5.52-14.76]) |
| Non-Hispanic, white | 18 204 612 | 16 154 685 (73.05 [68.64-77.45]) | 2 049 927 (74.01 [65.36-82.66]) |

Abbreviations: CI, confidence interval; IFG, impaired fasting glucose level; NFG, normal fasting glucose level.

*Respondents were aged 12 to 19 years. Data are from the 1999-2000 and 2001-2002 National Health and Nutrition Examination Surveys. Values are expressed as frequency, weighted frequency (based on sample weights), and percentage with 95% CI.

†Indicates significant association between row and column variables by $\chi^2$ test ($P<.001$).

73.1% non-Hispanic white. The proportion of subjects in the subsample (by fasting glucose level group and by sex and race) is presented in **Table 3**. Age was not different ($P=.83$) among subjects having normal (15.4±0.1 years) and impaired (15.4±0.3 years) fasting glucose levels. There was a significant association between fasting glucose group and sex, and between fasting glucose group and race ($P<.001$).

**Table 4. Clinical Measures for 1496 US Adolescents by Fasting Glucose Level Status***

| | Total (N = 1496) | NFG (n = 1318) | IFG (n = 178) |
|---|---|---|---|
| Weighted frequency | 24 885 638 | 22 115 903 | 2 769 736 |
| Age ± SE, y | 15.4 ± 0.1 | 15.4 ± 0.1 | 15.4 ± 0.3 |
| Glucose ± SE, mmol/L (mg/dL) | 5.1 ± 0.02 (91.5 ± 0.3) | 5.0 ± 0.02 (89.9 ± 0.3)† | 5.8 ± 0.03 (104.7 ± 0.6) |
| Percent hemoglobin $A_{1c}$ ± SE | 5.10 ± 0.02 | 5.09 ± 0.02† | 5.24 ± 0.03 |
| Insulin ± SE, U/mL | 12.4 ± 0.3 | 11.8 ± 0.3† | 17.6 ± 1.5 |
| C-peptide ± SE, nmol/L | 0.68 ± 0.01 | 0.66 ± 0.01† | 0.83 ± 0.05 |
| PIR ± SE | 2.7 ± 0.1 | 2.7 ± 0.1 | 2.7 ± 0.1 |
| BMI ± SE, kg/m$^2$ | 23.0 ± 0.2 | 22.8 ± 0.2 | 23.9 ± 0.6 |
| | | Weighted Frequency (Percentage [95% CI]) | |
| **BMI status‡** | | | |
| Normal (<85th percentile) | 16 937 629 | 15 337 016 (69.35 [66.37-72.33]) | 1 600 614 (57.79 [45.76-69.82]) |
| At risk (≥85th to <95th percentile) | 3 605 267 | 3 098 036 (14.01 [11.31-16.71]) | 507 231 (18.31 [9.83-26.79]) |
| Overweight (≥95th percentile) | 4 342 742 | 3 680 851 (16.64 [14.39-18.90]) | 661 891 (23.90 [15.88-31.91]) |

Abbreviations: BMI, body mass index (calculated as weight in kilograms divided by the square of height in meters); CI, confidence interval; IFG, impaired fasting glucose; NFG, normal fasting glucose; PIR, poverty-to-income ratio.

*Respondents were aged 12 to 19 years. Data are from the 1999-2000 and 2001-2002 National Health and Nutrition Examination Surveys. Values are expressed as mean ± SE, except for Centers for Disease Control–defined BMI percentiles which are expressed as frequency, weighted frequency (based on sample weights), and percentage with 95% CIs.

†Indicates significant difference between groups at $P<.01$.

‡Indicates significant association between row and column variables by $\chi^2$ test ($P<.001$).

Demographic and clinical measures for the subjects in the subsample are presented in **Table 4**. Fasting glucose, hemoglobin $A_{1c}$, insulin, and C-peptide levels were significantly different ($P<.01$) between groups, whereas BMI and the poverty-to-income ratio were not different between groups ($P>.05$). There was a significant association ($P<.001$) between the fasting glucose group and BMI status, expressed as a percentile for age and sex.

## CONCLUSIONS

This study provides the most recent national estimates of the prevalence of diabetes and impaired fasting glucose levels among US adolescents. Eighteen subjects in the full sample had self-reported diabetes. Using population-based sample weights, this was equivalent to 134 071 US adolescents aged 12 to 19 years with self-reported diabetes, or 0.5% of all people in this age group. This estimate is reasonable and consistent with the estimate that 206 000 (0.25%) people younger than 20 years have diagnosed diabetes, as reported elsewhere.[1]

The absolute percentage of self-reported diabetes was higher among boys than girls (eg, 54% vs 46%, respectively), and among non-Hispanic white youth than non-Hispanic black and Mexican American youth. This pattern was consistent when self-reported diabetes was expressed as a function of the number of individuals in a given sex or race with diabetes by the total number of individuals of that sex or race in the population. For example, about 0.53% of all adolescent boys in the population had self-reported diabetes (73 011 cases of self-reported diabetes among boys divided by 13 894 184 boys in the population), compared with about 0.48% of all adolescent girls in the population. Similarly, about 0.56% of all non-Hispanic white youth in the population had self-reported diabetes (104 907 cases of self-reported diabetes among non-Hispanic white youth divided by 18 805 881 non-Hispanic white youth in the population) compared with 0.42% of all non-Hispanic black and 0.31% of all Mexican American adolescents in the population. These percentages are different among adults (≥20 years), where the total prevalence of diabetes by race/ethnicity is highest among non-Hispanic black adults (11.4%), followed by non-Hispanic white (8.4%) and Hispanic/Latino adults (8.2%).[1]

By examining information on self-reported diabetes and medication use, subjects were further categorized as having type 1 or type 2 diabetes. In this analysis, 10 subjects with self-reported diabetes were categorized as having type 1 diabetes, whereas 8 subjects were categorized as having type 2 diabetes. Using population-based sample weights, this was equivalent to 95 066 adolescents with type 1 diabetes and 39 005 adolescents with type 2 diabetes. Thus, among the US adolescents in the population who have diabetes, 71% have type 1 diabetes and 29% have type 2 diabetes. Type 2 diabetes was once a condition only seen in adults, but this study provides evidence to support recent clinic-based reports and regional studies[2,3,5,18] that point to an emerging problem of type 2 diabetes among US youth.

The absolute percentage of type 1 diabetes was higher among boys than girls, while the absolute percentage of type 2 diabetes was higher among girls than boys. About 78% of all adolescent boys in the population with self-reported diabetes had type 1 diabetes (56 743 cases of type 1 diabetes among boys divided by 73 011 boys in the population with self-reported diabetes), and 22% of all adolescent boys in the population with self-reported diabetes had type 2 diabetes. On the other hand, 63% of all adolescent girls in the population with self-reported diabetes had type 1 diabetes and 37% had type 2 diabetes. The absolute percentage of type 1 and type 2 diabetes was higher among non-Hispanic white than non-Hispanic black and Mexican American youth. About 76% of all non-Hispanic white youth in the population with self-reported diabetes had type 1 diabetes (79 477 cases of type 1 diabetes among non-Hispanic white youth divided by 104 907 non-Hispanic youth in the population with self-reported diabetes), and 24% of all non-Hispanic white adolescents in the population with self-reported diabetes had type 2 diabetes. This is in contrast to 62% of all non-Hispanic black youth in the population with self-reported diabetes having type 1 diabetes and 38% having type 2 diabetes, and 37% of all Mexican American youth in the population with self-reported diabetes having type 1 diabetes and 63% having type 2 diabetes. Thus, the relative percentage of type 2 diabetes is highest among Mexican American adolescents, followed by non-Hispanic black and non-Hispanic white adolescents.

There were 178 subjects in the subsample who had impaired fasting glucose levels. Using population-based sample weights, this was equivalent to 2 769 736 US adolescents with impaired fasting glucose levels, or about 11% of all people in this age group. The number of adolescents with impaired fasting glucose levels in this study is about 9 percentage points higher than previously reported (1.76%).[6] However, at the time of that report the cut-point value for defining impaired fasting glucose levels was 6.1 mmol/L (110 mg/dL). The much higher prevalence of impaired fasting glucose levels in this study was entirely a result of the lowered cut-point value. There were only 24 subjects in the subsample who had impaired fasting glucose levels when using a value of 6.1 mmol/L (110 mg/dL). This was equivalent to 379 729 US adolescents with impaired fasting glucose levels, or about 1.5% (95% CI, 0.82-2.23) of all people in this age group. Sinha et al[7] found that 21% of overweight adolescents aged 11 to 18 years had impaired glucose tolerance. However, it is important to note that their subjects were at high risk for diabetes, impaired fasting glucose levels, and/or impaired glucose tolerance as the entire sample had a BMI at or above the 95th percentile for age and sex. Although BMI was not different between the normal and impaired fasting glucose level groups in the present study when expressed on an absolute basis (ie, 22.8 vs 23.9, respectively), more than 15% of all adolescents with impaired fasting glucose levels were overweight (661 891 cases of impaired fasting glucose levels among overweight adolescents divided by 4 342 742 overweight adolescents in the population) compared with 14.1% who were at risk for being overweight and 9.5% who were normal weight. This was also the case when a cut-point value of 6.1 mmol/L (110 mg/dL) was used; roughly 2.4% of overweight or at risk for being overweight adolescents had impaired fasting glucose levels compared with 1.1% of normal-weight youth. Thus, impaired fasting glucose levels were more common among overweight youth on a relative basis in the present study, regardless of the cut-point value used. The distribution of impaired fasting glucose levels as a function of BMI percentile is shown in the **Figure**.

Impaired fasting glucose levels were more common in boys than girls (14.8% of all boys in the population vs 7.3% of all girls in the population). In contrast, Fagot-Campagna et al[6] reported that slightly more girls than boys had impaired fasting glucose levels. Impaired fasting glucose levels were more common among Mexican American adolescents at 15.3% (439 035 cases of impaired fasting glucose levels among Mexican American adolescents divided by 2 877 893 Mexican American adolescents in the population) compared with 11.3% of all non-Hispanic white and 7.4% of all non-Hispanic black adolescents. These data are consistent with a previous report[1] demonstrating large differences in the prevalence of impaired fasting glucose levels among the major race groups.

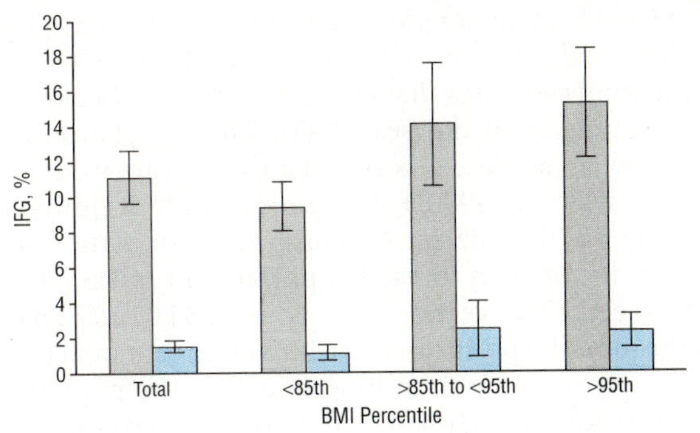


**Figure.** Prevalence of impaired fasting glucose (IFG) level as a function of body mass index (BMI) (calculated as weight in kilograms divided by the square of height in meters) percentile among 1496 US adolescents (aged 12-19 years). Gray-shaded bars indicate prevalence estimates using a fasting plasma glucose cut-point value of 5.6 mmol/L (100 mg/dL) to define impaired fasting glucose level, and blue-shaded bars indicate prevalence estimates using a cut-point value of 6.1 mmol/L (110 mg/dL). Data are presented as percent ± SE.

As expected, there were differences in several physiologic measures of glucose metabolism between adolescents categorized as having normal or impaired fasting glucose levels. By definition (as previously mentioned in the "Methods" section), fasting plasma glucose would have to be different between groups; levels were about 5.0 mmol/L (90 mg/dL) in those with normal fasting glucose levels and 5.8 mmol/L (105 mg/dL) in those with impaired fasting glucose levels. Fasting plasma insulin levels were also higher in subjects with impaired vs normal fasting glucose levels. This is consistent with the findings of Weiss et al[8] who found significantly higher fasting insulin levels in young subjects with impaired glucose tolerance compared with matched youth with normal glucose tolerance. The impaired glucose tolerance group in that study also exhibited marked insulin resistance (measured by the glucose clamp technique) and higher fasting C-peptide levels. Similarly in this study, C-peptide levels were higher in the impaired vs normal fasting glucose group. Together these findings suggest that abnormalities in glucose metabolism (that manifest as impaired fasting glucose levels and/or impaired glucose tolerance) in adolescents are primarily owing to insulin resistance and not an absolute reduction in β-cell function.

A few limitations of this study are worth noting. First, the population estimate of diabetes prevalence among US adolescents aged 12 to 19 years was based on a self-reported history of diabetes in a small number of subjects (n = 18). The sample weights used to calculate population totals in the current NHANES are based on population estimates that incorporate the US Census Bureau counts from the year 2000. The population estimate for US adolescents aged 12 to 19 years in the full sample was 26 649 401 based on sample weights applied to 4370 subjects. Although this population estimate is lower than the actual population of US adolescents (aged 12-19 years), which is about 32 012 573 based on the monthly postcensal civilian noninstitutional population (April 1, 2000, to June 1, 2000), the population in this study was estimated after applying several exclusion criteria. Using all subjects (aged 12-19 years) in the current NHANES without applying the exclusion criteria gives a sample of 4902 adolescents, equivalent to a population of 32 113 578. Thus, the population of US adolescents in this study is quite reasonable and consistent with US Census data. Likewise, the population estimate of diabetes prevalence among US adolescents provided in this study (134 071 or 0.5% of all people in this age group) also appears quite reasonable, as evidenced by the report discussed previously[1] where it was estimated that 206 000 (0.25%) people younger than 20 years have diagnosed diabetes.

Similar to this limitation, the classification of subjects into a specific type of diabetes was also based on self-reported use (or nonuse) of insulin, which was not optimal. However, this was the best method of doing so based on the available data in the current NHANES. It has been proposed that approximately 1 in every 400 to 500 children and adolescents younger than 20 years has type 1 diabetes.[1] Based on the results of the present study, approximately 1 in every 338 adolescents aged 12 to 19 years has type 1 diabetes and 1 in every 823 has type 2 diabetes. Thus, type 1 diabetes remains the major contributor to the diagnosis of diabetes in a pediatric population. Finally, the classification of and prevalence estimate for impaired fasting glucose levels were determined from one measurement. Although only subjects who had fasted for at least 8 hours were included in this analysis, confirmation of these findings may require an additional fasting blood draw and/or an oral glucose tolerance test. Despite these limitations, this study does provide evidence that the prevalence of type 2 diabetes and impaired fasting glucose level is substantial among US adolescents. These findings have important implications for public health because of the high rate of conversion from impaired fasting glucose level to type 2 diabetes in adults, and the increased risk of cardiovascular disease among adults with type 2 diabetes. These data provide a compelling rationale for prevention of diabetes and impaired fasting glucose levels among adolescents in the US population.

**Accepted for Publication:** October 9, 2005.
**Correspondence:** Glen E. Duncan, PhD, RCEPSM, Department of Epidemiology, 305 Raitt Hall, Box 353410, University of Washington, Seattle, WA 98195 (duncag@u.washington.edu).
**Funding/Support:** This study was funded by a career development award from the National Institutes of Health (K01 DK61999).
**Author Contribution:** The author had full access to all the data in the study and takes responsibility for the integrity of the data and the accuracy of the data analysis.

## REFERENCES

1. Centers for Disease Control and Prevention. *National Diabetes Fact Sheet: General Information and National Estimates on Diabetes in the United States, 2003.* Atlanta, Ga: US Dept of Health and Human Services, Centers for Disease Control and Prevention; 2004.
2. Rosenbloom AL, Joe JR, Young RS, Winter WE. Emerging epidemic of type 2 diabetes in youth. *Diabetes Care.* 1999;22:345-354.
3. Fagot-Campagna A. Emergence of type 2 diabetes mellitus in children: epidemiological evidence. *J Pediatr Endocrinol Metab.* 2000;13(Suppl 6):1395-1402.
4. American Diabetes Association. Type 2 diabetes in children and adolescents. *Diabetes Care.* 2000;23:381-389.
5. Fagot-Campagna A, Pettitt DJ, Engelgau MM, et al. Type 2 diabetes among North American children and adolescents: an epidemiologic review and a public health perspective. *J Pediatr.* 2000;136:664-672.
6. Fagot-Campagna A, Saaddine JB, Flegal KM, Beckles GL. Diabetes, impaired fasting glucose, and elevated HbA1c in US adolescents: the Third National Health and Nutrition Examination Survey. *Diabetes Care.* 2001;24:834-837.
7. Sinha R, Fisch G, Teague B, et al. Prevalence of impaired glucose tolerance among children and adolescents with marked obesity. *N Engl J Med.* 2002;346:802-810.
8. Weiss R, Dufour S, Taksali SE, et al. Prediabetes in obese youth: a syndrome of impaired glucose tolerance, severe insulin resistance, and altered myocellular and abdominal fat partitioning. *Lancet.* 2003;362:951-957.
9. Cook S, Weitzman M, Auinger P, Nguyen M, Dietz WH. Prevalence of a metabolic syndrome phenotype in adolescents: findings from the third National Health and Nutrition Examination Survey, 1988-1994. *Arch Pediatr Adolesc Med.* 2003;157:821-827.
10. Duncan GE, Li SM, Zhou XH. Prevalence and trends of a metabolic syndrome phenotype among US adolescents, 1999-2000. *Diabetes Care.* 2004;27:2438-2443.
11. Weiss R, Dziura J, Burgert TS, et al. Obesity and the metabolic syndrome in children and adolescents. *N Engl J Med.* 2004;350:2362-2374.
12. Ogden CL, Flegal KM, Carroll MD, Johnson CL. Prevalence and trends in overweight among US children and adolescents, 1999-2000. *JAMA.* 2002;288:1728-1732.
13. Hedley AA, Ogden CL, Johnson CL, Carroll MD, Curtin LR, Flegal KM. Prevalence of overweight and obesity among US children, adolescents, and adults, 1999-2002. *JAMA.* 2004;291:2847-2850.
14. Narayan KM, Boyle JP, Thompson TJ, Sorensen SW, Williamson DF. Lifetime risk for diabetes mellitus in the United States. *JAMA.* 2003;290:1884-1890.
15. The National Health and Nutrition Examination Survey page. National Center for Health Statistics Web site. Available at: http://www.cdc.gov/nchs/about/major/nhanes/datalink.htm#1999%20NHANES. Accessed February 17, 2006.
16. American Diabetes Association. Clinical Practice Recommendations 2005. *Diabetes Care.* 2005;28(Suppl 1):S1-79.
17. Kuczmarski RJ, Ogden CL, Guo SS, et al. 2000 CDC growth charts for the United States: methods and development. *Vital Health Stat 11.* 2002:1-190.
18. Fagot-Campagna A, Burrows NR, Williamson DF. The public health epidemiology of type 2 diabetes in children and adolescents: a case study of American Indian adolescents in the Southwestern United States. *Clin Chim Acta.* 1999;286:81-95.

**PEDIARIX™ [Diphtheria and Tetanus Toxoids and Acellular Pertussis Adsorbed, Hepatitis B (Recombinant) and Inactivated Poliovirus Vaccine Combined]**

The following is a brief summary only; see full prescribing information for complete product information.

**CONTRAINDICATIONS:** Hypersensitivity to any component of the vaccine, including yeast, neomycin, and polymyxin B, is a contraindication (see DESCRIPTION in complete prescribing information). Do not use PEDIARIX after a serious allergic reaction (e.g., anaphylaxis) temporally associated with a previous dose of this vaccine or with any components of this vaccine. Because of the uncertainty as to which component of the vaccine might be responsible, do not give further vaccination with any of these components; or, refer such individuals to an allergist for evaluation. The following events are contraindications to administration of PEDIARIX: encephalopathy (e.g., coma, decreased level of consciousness, prolonged seizures) within 7 days of administration of a previous dose of a pertussis-containing vaccine that is not attributable to another identifiable cause; progressive neurologic disorder, including infantile spasms, uncontrolled epilepsy, or progressive encephalopathy. Do not vaccinate individuals with such conditions until a treatment regimen has been established and the condition has stabilized. PEDIARIX is not contraindicated for use in individuals with HIV infection.

**WARNINGS:** Administration of PEDIARIX is associated with higher rates of fever relative to separately administered vaccines. In one study that evaluated medically attended fever after the first dose of PEDIARIX or separately administered vaccines, infants who received PEDIARIX had a higher rate of medical encounters for fever within the first 4 days following vaccination. In some infants, these encounters included the performance of diagnostic studies to evaluate other causes of fever (see ADVERSE REACTIONS). The vial stopper is latex-free. The tip cap and the rubber plunger of the needleless prefilled syringes contain dry natural latex rubber that may cause allergic reactions in latex sensitive individuals. If any of the following events occur in temporal relation to receipt of whole-cell DTP or a vaccine containing an acellular pertussis component, consider carefully whether to give subsequent doses of PEDIARIX or any vaccine containing a pertussis component: temperature of ≥40.5°C (105°F) within 48 hours not due to another identifiable cause; collapse or shock-like state (hypotonic-hyporesponsive episode) within 48 hours; persistent, inconsolable crying lasting ≥3 hours, occurring within 48 hours; seizures with or without fever occurring within 3 days. If Guillain-Barré syndrome occurs within 6 weeks of receipt of prior vaccine containing tetanus toxoid, the decision to give subsequent doses of PEDIARIX or any vaccine containing tetanus toxoid should be based on careful consideration of the potential benefits and possible risks. A committee of the Institute of Medicine (IOM) has concluded that evidence is consistent with a causal relationship between whole-cell DTP vaccine and acute neurologic illness, and under special circumstances, between whole-cell DTP vaccine and chronic neurologic disease in the context of the National Childhood Encephalopathy Study (NCES) report; however, evidence was insufficient to indicate whether or not whole-cell DTP vaccine increased the overall risk of chronic neurologic disease. Acute encephalopathy and permanent neurologic damage have not been reported causally linked or in temporal association with administration of PEDIARIX, but the experience with PEDIARIX is insufficient to rule this out. Encephalopathy has been reported following INFANRIX® (Diphtheria and Tetanus Toxoids and Acellular Pertussis Vaccine Adsorbed) (see ADVERSE REACTIONS, Postmarketing Reports), but data are not sufficient to evaluate a causal relationship. The decision to administer a pertussis-containing vaccine to children with stable central nervous system (CNS) disorders must be made by the physician on an individual basis, with consideration of all relevant factors, and assessment of potential risks and benefits for that individual. Advise the parent or guardian of the potential increased risk involved (see PRECAUTIONS). A family history of seizures or other CNS disorders is not a contraindication to pertussis vaccine. For children at higher risk for seizures than the general population, an appropriate antipyretic may be administered at the time of vaccination and for the ensuing 24 hours according to the respective prescribing information recommended dosage to reduce the possibility of post-vaccination fever. Defer vaccination during the course of a moderate or severe illness with or without fever and vaccinate patients as soon as they have recovered from the acute phase of the illness. Do not give PEDIARIX to children on anticoagulant therapy or those with bleeding disorders unless the potential benefit clearly outweighs the risk of administration (see PRECAUTIONS in complete prescribing information).

**PRECAUTIONS:** Before the injection of any biological, the physician should take all reasonable precautions to prevent allergic or other adverse reactions. Epinephrine injection (1:1000) and other appropriate agents used for the control of immediate allergic reactions must be immediately available should an acute anaphylactic reaction occur. Immunosuppressed Individuals, including those receiving immunosuppressive therapy, may not develop the expected immune response. **Drug Interactions:** For information regarding concomitant administration with other vaccines, refer to DOSAGE AND ADMINISTRATION in complete prescribing information. Do not mix PEDIARIX with any other vaccine in the same syringe or vial. **Carcinogenesis, Mutagenesis, Impairment of Fertility:** PEDIARIX has not been evaluated for carcinogenic or mutagenic potential, or for impairment of fertility. **Pregnancy:** Pregnancy Category C: PEDIARIX is not indicated for women of child-bearing age. Animal reproduction studies have not been conducted with PEDIARIX. It is not known whether PEDIARIX can cause fetal harm when administered to a pregnant woman or if PEDIARIX can affect reproductive capacity. **Geriatric Use:** PEDIARIX is not indicated for use in adult populations. **Pediatric Use:** Safety and effectiveness of PEDIARIX in infants younger than 6 weeks of age have not been evaluated (see DOSAGE AND ADMINISTRATION in complete prescribing information). PEDIARIX is not recommended for persons 7 years of age or older. Tetanus and Diphtheria Toxoids Adsorbed (Td) For Adult Use, inactivated poliovirus vaccine (IPV), and Hepatitis B Vaccine (Recombinant) should be used in individuals 7 years of age or older.

**ADVERSE REACTIONS:** A total of 20,739 doses of PEDIARIX have been administered to 7,028 infants as a 3-dose primary series. The most common adverse reactions observed in clinical trials were local injection site reactions (pain, redness, or swelling), fever, and fussiness. In comparative studies, administration of PEDIARIX was associated with higher rates of fever relative to separately administered vaccines (see WARNINGS). The prevalence of fever was highest on the day of vaccination and the day following vaccination. More than 98% of episodes of fever resolved within the 4-day period following vaccination (i.e., the period including the day of vaccination and the next 3 days). Rates of most other solicited adverse events following PEDIARIX were comparable to rates observed following separately administered US-licensed vaccines. The adverse event information from clinical trials provides a basis for identifying adverse events that appear to be related to vaccine use and for approximating rates. However, because clinical trials are conducted under widely varying conditions, adverse event rates observed in the clinical trials of a vaccine cannot be directly compared to rates in the clinical trials of another vaccine, and may not reflect the rates observed in practice. A total of 5,472 infants were enrolled in a German safety study that was originally designed to compare the safety and reactogenicity of PEDIARIX administered concomitantly at separate sites with 1 of 4 *Haemophilus influenzae* type b (Hib) vaccines at 3, 4, and 5 months of age. After enrollment of 1,569 infants, the study was amended to include a control group that received INFANRIX, Hib vaccine, and oral poliovirus vaccine (OPV) separately. Infants in the separate administration group received one less antigen (hepatitis B) than the infants who received PEDIARIX. Safety data were available for 4,666 infants who received PEDIARIX administered concomitantly at separate sites with 1 of 4 Hib vaccines and for 768 infants in the control group that received separate vaccines. The primary end-point of the study was the percentage of infants with any grade 3 solicited symptom (redness or swelling >20 mm, fever >103.1°F, or crying, pain, vomiting, diarrhea, loss of appetite, or restlessness that prevented normal daily activities) over the 3-dose primary series in infants who received PEDIARIX (4 groups that received PEDIARIX and Hib vaccines pooled) compared to the group that received INFANRIX and Hib vaccine separately with OPV. Analysis for the primary end-point was performed on the according-to-protocol (ATP) cohort that included only those infants who were enrolled after the protocol amendment to include a control group. Of 3,773 infants in the ATP cohort for whom safety data were available, 16.2% (95% CI: 14.9% to 17.5%) of 3,029 infants who received PEDIARIX and Hib vaccine compared to 20.3% (95% CI: 17.5% to 23.4%) of 744 infants who received separate vaccines were reported to have had at least one grade 3 solicited symptom within 4 days of vaccination (i.e., day of vaccination and the next 3 days). The difference between groups in the rate of grade 3 symptoms was 4.1% (90% CI: 1.4% to 7.1%). These were the rates for selected solicited symptoms within 4 days following each dose in a 3-dose primary series in infants who received PEDIARIX administered concomitantly with Hib vaccine and those who received separate concomitant administration of INFANRIX, Hib vaccine, and OPV for the intent-to-treat (ITT) cohort (includes all infants enrolled before and after the amendment who received the indicated vaccine and for whom at least one symptom sheet was completed):

**Percentage of German Infants With Solicited Local Reactions or Selected Systemic Adverse Events Within 4 Days of Vaccination* (ITT Cohort)**

| | PEDIARIX & Hib | | | INFANRIX, Hib, & OPV | | |
|---|---|---|---|---|---|---|
| | Dose 1 | Dose 2 | Dose 3 | Dose 1 | Dose 2 | Dose 3 |
| **N** | **4,666** | **4,619** | **4,574** | **768** | **757** | **750** |
| **Local[†]** | | | | | | |
| Pain, any | 14.0 | 10.2 | 9.9 | 14.2 | 9.8 | 8.1 |
| Pain, grade 2 or 3 | 2.9 | 1.2 | 1.5 | 3.6 | 1.7 | 1.1 |
| Pain, grade 3 | 0.7 | 0.3 | 0.3 | 1.3 | 0.4 | 0.1 |
| Redness, any | 18.6 | 26.6 | 25.6 | 16.1 | 21.4 | 20.8 |
| Redness, >5 mm | 6.7 | 9.9 | 9.0 | 5.9 | 8.2 | 7.7 |
| Redness, >20 mm | 1.2 | 1.0 | 1.1 | 1.8 | 0.7 | 1.1 |
| Swelling, any | 12.7 | 18.5 | 18.4 | 9.6 | 12.9 | 13.6 |
| Swelling, >5 mm | 5.6 | 7.7 | 7.8 | 3.6 | 5.2 | 4.8 |
| Swelling, >20 mm | 1.2 | 1.6 | 1.5 | 1.3 | 1.1 | 1.2 |
| **Systemic** | | | | | | |
| Restlessness, any | 41.4 | 32.0 | 26.7 | 46.4 | 35.0 | 27.6 |
| Restlessness, grade 2 or 3 | 14.4 | 10.0 | 8.9 | 20.2 | 11.5 | 8.4 |
| Restlessness, grade 3 | 3.0 | 1.5 | 1.6 | 5.7 | 3.0 | 1.7 |
| Fever[‡], ≥100.4°F | 25.1 | 19.3 | 19.7 | 13.2 | 13.1 | 11.2 |
| Fever[‡], >101.3°F | 5.8 | 4.1 | 4.6 | 2.2 | 2.8 | 2.1 |
| Fever[‡], >103.1°F | 0.3 | 0.5 | 0.7 | 0.3 | 0.3 | 0.5 |
| Unusual cry[§], any | 24.9 | 16.5 | 13.1 | 36.5 | 19.7 | 14.3 |
| Unusual cry[§], grade 2 or 3 | 12.7 | 7.1 | 5.7 | 20.8 | 10.0 | 5.7 |
| Unusual cry[§], grade 3 | 3.9 | 1.7 | 1.4 | 6.8 | 2.1 | 1.1 |
| Loss of appetite, any | 17.9 | 13.3 | 12.5 | 19.1 | 16.2 | 11.3 |
| Loss of appetite, grade 2 or 3 | 4.0 | 2.9 | 2.7 | 4.4 | 2.9 | 2.3 |
| Loss of appetite, grade 3 | 0.6 | 0.5 | 0.4 | 0.5 | 0.7 | 0.0 |

N = number of infants in the intent-to-treat (ITT) cohort.
Grade 2 defined as sufficiently discomforting to interfere with daily activities.
Grade 3 defined as preventing normal daily activities.
* Within 4 days of vaccination defined as day of vaccination and the next 3 days.
† Local reactions at the injection site for PEDIARIX or INFANRIX.
‡ Rectal temperatures.
§ Unusual cry lasting >1 hour.

In this study, infants were also monitored for unsolicited adverse events that occurred within 30 days following vaccination. Over the entire study period, 6 subjects in the group that received PEDIARIX reported seizures. Two of these subjects had a febrile seizure, 1 of whom also developed afebrile seizures. The remaining 4 subjects had afebrile seizures, including 2 with infantile spasms. Two subjects reported seizures within 7 days following vaccination (1 subject had both febrile and afebrile seizures, and 1 subject had afebrile seizures), corresponding to a rate of 0.22 seizures per 1,000 doses (febrile seizures 0.07 per 1,000 doses, afebrile seizures 0.14 per 1,000 doses). No subject who received concomitant INFANRIX, Hib vaccine, and OPV reported seizures. In a separate German study that evaluated the safety of INFANRIX in 22,505 infants who received 66,867 doses of INFANRIX administered as a 3-dose primary series, the rate of seizures within 7 days of vaccination with INFANRIX was 0.13 per 1,000 doses (febrile seizures 0.0 per 1,000 doses, afebrile seizures 0.13 per 1,000 doses). No cases of hypotonic-hyporesponsiveness, encephalopathy, or anaphylaxis were reported in the German study that evaluated the safety of PEDIARIX. Rates of serious adverse events that are less common than those reported in this safety study are not known at this time.

Additional safety data for PEDIARIX are available from a US study designed to evaluate lot-to-lot consistency and a bridge for a new manufacturing step. These were the rates for local reactions and selected adverse events within 4 days of vaccination with PEDIARIX administered concomitantly with a Hib vaccine at 2, 4, and 6 months of age:

**Percentage of US Infants With Solicited Local Reactions or Selected Systemic Adverse Events Within 4 Days of Vaccination* (ITT Cohort)**

| | PEDIARIX & Hib | | |
|---|---|---|---|
| | Dose 1 | Dose 2 | Dose 3 |
| **Local[†]** | **N = 482** | **N = 469** | **N = 466** |
| Pain, any | 30.5 | 25.4 | 23.0 |
| Pain, grade 2 or 3 | 6.2 | 5.5 | 3.6 |
| Pain, grade 3 | 1.2 | 0.6 | 0.6 |
| Redness, any | 25.3 | 32.6 | 35.6 |
| Redness, >5 mm | 9.3 | 10.4 | 8.6 |
| Redness, >20 mm | 0.6 | 1.5 | 1.3 |
| Swelling, any | 15.1 | 16.6 | 22.3 |
| Swelling, >5 mm | 6.8 | 6.2 | 6.4 |
| Swelling, >20 mm | 1.0 | 1.3 | 1.3 |
| **Systemic** | **N = 482** | **N = 469** | **N = 467** |
| Restlessness, any | 28.8 | 30.3 | 28.5 |
| Restlessness, grade 2 or 3 | 7.1 | 9.0 | 9.4 |
| Restlessness, grade 3 | 1.0 | 1.1 | 0.6 |
| Fever[‡], ≥100.4°F | 26.6 | 31.3 | 25.9 |
| Fever[‡], >101.3°F | 2.9 | 6.2 | 4.7 |
| Fever[‡], >103.1°F | 0.0 | 0.2 | 0.6 |
| Fussiness, any | 61.8 | 63.8 | 57.0 |
| Fussiness, grade 2 or 3 | 14.9 | 21.5 | 17.1 |
| Fussiness, grade 3 | 2.7 | 3.4 | 1.7 |
| Loss of appetite, any | 21.6 | 19.8 | 18.8 |
| Loss of appetite, grade 2 or 3 | 3.1 | 3.2 | 2.4 |
| Loss of appetite, grade 3 | 0.2 | 0.4 | 0.0 |
| Sleeping more than usual, any | 46.7 | 31.8 | 28.1 |
| Sleeping more than usual, grade 2 or 3 | 10.2 | 6.0 | 4.7 |
| Sleeping more than usual, grade 3 | 1.7 | 0.4 | 0.6 |

N = number of infants in the intent-to-treat (ITT) cohort (infants who received the indicated vaccine and for whom at least one symptom sheet was completed).
Grade 2 defined as sufficiently discomforting to interfere with daily activities.
Grade 3 defined as preventing normal daily activities.
* Within 4 days of vaccination defined as day of vaccination and the next 3 days.
† Local reactions at the injection site for PEDIARIX.
‡ Rectal temperatures.

In another US study, these were the rates for fever within 4 days following dose 1 (i.e., day of vaccination and the next 3 days) at 2 months of age in infants who received PEDIARIX when administered concomitantly at separate sites with Hib and pneumococcal conjugate vaccines and those who received INFANRIX, ENGERIX-B® [Hepatitis B Vaccine (Recombinant)], IPV, Hib vaccine, and pneumococcal conjugate vaccine:

**Percentage of US Infants With Fever Within 4 Days of Dose 1* (ITT Cohort)**

| | PEDIARIX, Hib, & Pneumococcal Conjugate (N = 667) | INFANRIX, ENGERIX-B, IPV, Hib, & Pneumococcal Conjugate (N = 333) | Separate Vaccine Group Minus Combination Vaccine Group |
|---|---|---|---|
| **Fever[†]** | **%** | **%** | **Difference (95% CI)** |
| ≥100.4°F[‡] | 27.9 | 19.8 | -8.07 (-13.54, -2.60) |
| >101.3°F | 7.0 | 4.5 | -2.54 (-5.50, 0.41) |
| >102.2°F[‡] | 2.2 | 0.3 | -1.95 (-3.22, -0.68) |
| >103.1°F | 0.4 | 0.0 | -0.45 (-0.96, 0.06) |
| M.A.[‡] | 1.2 | 0.0 | -1.20 (-2.03, -037) |

N = number of infants for whom at least one symptom sheet was completed, excluding 3 infants for whom temperature was not measured and 3 infants whose temperature was measured by the tympanic method.
*Within 4 days of dose 1 defined as day of vaccination and the next 3 days.
† Rectal temperatures.
‡ The group that received PEDIARIX compared to separate vaccine group p value <0.05 (2-sided Fisher Exact test) or the 95% confidence interval on the difference between groups does not include 0.
M.A. = Medically attended (a visit to or from medical personnel).

In this study, medical attention (a visit to or from medical personnel) for fever within 4 days following vaccination was sought for 8 infants who received PEDIARIX (1.2%) and no infants who received separately administered vaccines. Four infants were seen by medical personnel in an office setting; no diagnostic tests were performed in 2 of the infants and a complete blood count (CBC) was done in the other 2 infants. Of 3 infants who were seen in an emergency room, all had a CBC and a blood and urine culture performed; chest X-rays were done in 2 of the infants and a nasopharyngeal specimen was tested for Respiratory Syncytial Virus in one of the infants. One infant was hospitalized for a work-up that included a CBC, blood and urine cultures, a lumbar puncture, and a chest X-ray. All episodes of medically attended fever resolved within 4 days post-vaccination.

Limited data are available from a study conducted in Moldova in which infants received a dose of hepatitis B vaccine within 48 hours of birth followed by 3 doses of PEDIARIX at 6, 10, and 14 weeks of age. No information was collected on the HBsAg status of mothers of enrolled infants. These were the rates for local reactions and selected adverse events within 4 days of vaccination with PEDIARIX administered comcomitantly with Hib vaccine following a birth dose of hepatitis B vaccine:

**Percentage of Moldovan Infants With Solicited Local Reactions or Selected Systemic Adverse Events Within 4 Days of Vaccination* (ITT Cohort)**

| | PEDIARIX & Hib | | |
|---|---|---|---|
| | Dose 1 | Dose 2 | Dose 3 |
| **N** | **160** | **158** | **157** |
| **Local[†]** | | | |
| Pain, any | 25.6 | 18.4 | 14.0 |
| Pain, grade 3 | 3.1 | 0.6 | 1.9 |
| Redness, any | 41.9 | 41.8 | 47.1 |
| Redness, >20 mm | 1.9 | 2.5 | 4.5 |
| Swelling, any | 20.6 | 18.4 | 28.0 |
| Swelling, >20 mm | 4.4 | 2.5 | 7.0 |
| **Systemic** | | | |
| Restlessness, any | 13.1 | 10.8 | 8.9 |
| Restlessness, grade 3 | 1.3 | 0.6 | 0.6 |
| Fever[‡], ≥100.4°F | 14.4 | 11.4 | 5.1 |
| Fever[‡], >103.1°F | 0.0 | 0.6 | 0.0 |
| Fussiness, any | 25.0 | 21.5 | 17.8 |
| Fussiness, grade 3 | 2.5 | 0.6 | 0.6 |

N = number of infants in the intent-to-treat (ITT) cohort (infants who received the indicated vaccine and for whom at least one symptom sheet was completed).
Grade 3 defined as preventing normal daily activities.
*Within 4 days of vaccination defined as day of vaccination and the next 3 days.
† Local reactions at the injection site for PEDIARIX.
‡ Rectal temperatures.

Although there was no comparator group who received PEDIARIX without a birth dose of hepatitis B vaccine, available data suggest that some local adverse events may occur at a higher rate when PEDIARIX is administered after a birth dose of hepatitis B vaccine.

As with any vaccine, there is the possibility that broad use of PEDIARIX could reveal adverse events not observed in clinical trials.

**Postmarketing Reports:** Worldwide voluntary reports of adverse events received for INFANRIX and ENGERIX-B in children younger than 7 years of age since market introduction of these US-licensed vaccines are listed below. This list includes adverse events for which 20 or more reports were received with the exception of intussusception, idiopathic thrombocytopenic purpura, thrombocytopenia, anaphylactic reaction, angioedema, encephalopathy, hypotonic-hyporesponsive episode, and alopecia for which fewer than 20 reports were received. These latter events are included either because of the seriousness of the event or the strength of causal connection to components of this or other vaccines or drugs. *Body as a whole*: Asthenia[b], fever[a+b], lethargy[b], malaise[b], Sudden Infant Death Syndrome[a+b]. *Cardiovascular system*: Cyanosis[a+b], edema[b], pallor[b]. *Gastrointestinal system*: Abdominal pain[b], anorexia[b], diarrhea[a+b], intussusception[a+b], nausea[b], vomiting[a+b]. *Hematologic/lymphatic*: Idiopathic thrombocytopenic purpura[a+b], lymphadenopathy[a], thrombocytopenia[a+b]. *Hepatic*: Jaundice[b], liver function tests abnormal[b]. *Hypersensitivity*: Anaphylactic reaction[a+b], angioedema[b], hypersensitivity[a]. *Infections*: Cellulitis[a]. *Injection site reactions*: Injection site reactions[a+b]. *Musculoskeletal*: Arthralgia[b], limb swelling[a+b]. *Nervous system*: Convulsions[a+b], encephalopathy[a], headache[b], hypotonia[a+b], hypotonic-hyporesponsive episode[a], somnolence[a+b]. *Psychiatric*: Crying[a+b], irritability[a+b]. *Respiratory system*: Respiratory tract infection[a]. *Skin and appendages*: Alopecia[b], erythema[a+b], erythema multiforme[b], petechiae[b], pruritus[a+b], rash[a+b], urticaria[a+b]. *Special senses*: Ear pain[a]. [[a] Following INFANRIX; [b] Following ENGERIX-B; [a+b] Following either INFANRIX or ENGERIX-B.] These reactions were reported voluntarily from a population of uncertain size; therefore, it is not always possible to reliably estimate their frequency or establish a causal relationship to vaccination.

**Reporting Adverse Events:** Report the occurrence following immunization of any event set forth in the Vaccine Injury Table from the National Childhood Vaccine Injury Act including: Anaphylaxis or anaphylactic shock within 7 days, encephalopathy or encephalitis within 7 days, brachial neuritis within 28 days, or an acute complication or sequelae (including death) of an illness, disability, injury, or condition referred to above, or any events that would contraindicate further doses of PEDIARIX. The VAERS toll-free number is 1-800-822-7967.

Manufactured by **GlaxoSmithKline Biologicals**, Rixensart, Belgium, US License 1617

Distributed by **GlaxoSmithKline,** Research Triangle Park, NC 27709



Full prescribing information for PEDIARIX is available at www.GSKVaccines.com/Pediarix.

BRS-PE:L2

 Printed in USA. PED583R0 June 2005

# Genetic Testing of Minors for Alpha$_1$-Antitrypsin Deficiency

*Charlie Strange, MD; Mary Allison Moseley; Yonge Jones; Laura Schwarz; Lianqi Xie; Mark L. Brantly, MD*

**Background:** Alpha$_1$-antitrypsin deficiency (AATD) is a genetic disorder primarily affecting the lungs and liver of affected individuals, causing severe panlobular emphysema and cirrhosis.

**Objective:** To describe the demographics and feasibility of a home test for AATD in children and adolescents.

**Design:** Case series of parents who test their children for AATD.

**Setting:** Nonprofit supported program in which participants telephoned or e-mailed requests for alpha$_1$-antitrypsin testing.

**Participants:** All persons younger than 18 years whose parents or guardians chose to test for AATD from January 1, 2002, to October 1, 2004.

**Interventions:** Home-administered finger-stick blood spot test for alpha$_1$-antitrypsin genotype and questionnaire.

**Main Outcome Measures:** The alpha$_1$-antitrypsin genotypes and questionnaire responses.

**Results:** The Alpha Coded Testing Study tested 422 children and adolescents with a confidential test for AATD. Testing was suggested by a family member in most (76.7%) of the cases and was responsible for the many carrier (*PIMZ* and *PIMS*) genotypes (51.9%) in the study. Interest in testing was equally distributed among all ages. Test confidentiality was seen as an important reason to test (64.1% with a Likert scale score of 4-5 on a 5-point scale). Parents and guardians of the minors suggested that testing benefits (mean [SD] Likert score, 3.5 [1.4] on a 5-point scale) were higher than risks (mean [SD] Likert score, 1.7 [1.2]) ($P$=.001).

**Conclusion:** Parents value genetic testing of their children at risk for AATD when testing can be done in a confidential setting.

*Arch Pediatr Adolesc Med. 2006;160:531-534*

Alpha$_1$-antitrypsin (AAT) is an abundant plasma glycoprotein that inhibits neutrophil elastase. Individuals who inherited *AAT* genes associated with deficiency are at high risk for the development of chronic obstructive pulmonary disease and cirrhosis. The prevalence of AAT deficiency (AATD) in the United States is between 1 in 2857 and 1 in 5097, occurring mainly in white populations of European lineage, with an incidence similar to that of cystic fibrosis.[1-4] Cigarette smoking substantially decreases the age of onset of chronic obstructive pulmonary disease in individuals with AATD.

Early identification of AATD allows affected individuals to learn about their condition, make educated decisions regarding lifestyle choices, anticipate insurance and medical needs, and assess career choice options. However, the most important decision may concern smoking behavior. Because tobacco smoking often begins during adolescence, genetic testing of children at risk for AATD has the potential to affect lung health.

From November 1972 to September 1974, 200 000 Swedish newborns were screened for AATD; 183 children had a severe deficiency.[4] When studied in late adolescence, only 3% of those identified smoked cigarettes.[5] However, in targeted studies[6] of the parents, objective measures of psychological stress were encountered. When added to the potential for genetic information misuse in the absence of symptoms by employers or insurance companies, the 2003 American Thoracic Society/European Respiratory Society statement concluded that testing of minors should not be performed in the absence of a family history of AATD.[7]

The goal of this article is to report the demographics of children and adolescents, and the perceptions of their parents, testing for AATD through the Alpha Coded Testing (ACT) Study.

## METHODS

The ACT Study began January 16, 2001, to query issues surrounding genetic testing for AATD. The study and all questionnaires were

Author Affiliations: Division of Pulmonary and Critical Care Medicine (Dr Strange, Mss Moseley and Schwarz, and Mr Jones) and Department of Biometry (Ms Xie), Medical University of South Carolina, Charleston; and Division of Pulmonary and Critical Care Medicine, University of Florida Health Sciences Center at Gainesville (Dr Brantly).

**Table 1. Age Distribution and Genotypes of Tested Individuals**

| | Age, y | | | | | | |
|---|---|---|---|---|---|---|---|
| Genotype* | 0-3 (n = 79) | 4-6 (n = 70) | 7-9 (n = 71) | 10-12 (n = 66) | 13-15 (n = 83) | 16-18 (n = 153) | Total (N = 422)† |
| *PIMM* | 33 | 32 | 28 | 36 | 39 | 20 | **188** (44.5) |
| *PIMS* | 6 | 4 | 6 | 6 | 7 | 4 | **33** (7.8) |
| *PIMZ* | 36 | 31 | 35 | 19 | 36 | 29 | **186** (44.1) |
| *PISS* | 1 | 1 | 0 | 2 | 0 | 0 | **4** (0.9) |
| *PISZ* | 0 | 1 | 2 | 3 | 0 | 0 | **6** (1.4) |
| *PIZZ* | 3 | 1 | 0 | 0 | 1 | 0 | **5** (1.2) |

*The *PIMM* genotype is present in approximately 92% of the US population and produces a normal serum level of alpha$_1$-antitrypsin (AAT). The *PIMS* (5.7%) and *PIMZ* (2.3%) genotypes carry 1 deficient gene and serum levels are intermediate between *PIMM* and the genotypes *PISZ* (0.1%) and *PIZZ* (0.02%), which have severe reductions in serum AAT concentrations.[9]

†Data are given as number (percentage).

approved by the Medical University of South Carolina Institutional Review Board for Research with Human Subjects, and a Certificate of Confidentiality was obtained from the National Institutes of Health. Study participation was advertised as an option for AAT testing by the Alpha-1 Foundation and the Alpha-1 Association, 2 nonprofit organizations dedicated to AAT detection. Participants were required to telephone, e-mail, or visit a study booth at an Alpha-1 Education Day for study materials. Individuals wanting an *AAT* genotype for themselves or their minor children administered a home finger-stick test for blood spot analysis.[8] Consent forms, informational brochures, and a study questionnaire accompanied all mailings. Results of testing were returned only to the requesting individual, who then had the option of telling others about the test results. Participants had the option of having their name and contact information deleted from the study 3 weeks after receiving results. The other option was to maintain consent for further study of testing outcomes for 5 years. Results were mailed with genotype-specific support information. For the first 20 months of the study, a posttest questionnaire and postage-paid envelope were mailed.

Summary statistics were performed using SAS statistical software (SAS Institute Inc, Cary, NC). Mean risk and mean benefit scores were calculated from mean Likert responses for participants who gave answers to all questions. A *t* test was used to compare continuous variables. $P<.05$ was considered significant.

## RESULTS

Between January 1, 2002, and October 1, 2004, the ACT Study enrolled 2831 persons who requested a confidential, self-administered, finger-stick test kit, including 422 younger than 18 years. Participation for the 422 minors in the ACT Study was dependent on the following: (1) parent or legal guardian signed consent and (2) return of a completed pretest research questionnaire. **Table 1** shows the age distribution and genotypes of the participants. Of the 422 respondents, 212 (50.2%) were male, 208 (49.3%) were female, and 2 (0.5%) did not respond. Testing for the first time was reported by 386 (91.5%) participants. Individuals in the study requested removal of contact information after results returned in 174 (41.2%) cases.

Respondent race was as follows (data available for 421 respondents): 375 (89.1%) were white, 7 (1.7%) were Hispanic, 2 (0.5%) were Native American, and 1 (0.2%) was Asian; 35 (8.3%) responded as having more than 1 race, and 1 (0.2%) did not state race. As expected for minor testing, the test was recommended most often by a family member (319 [76.7%] of 416 subjects with this information). Recommendations for testing also came from physicians for 24 subjects (5.8%), the participants alone for 11 subjects (2.6%), the media or Internet for 6 subjects (1.4%), other sources for 25 subjects (6.0%), and a combination of sources for 31 subjects (7.5%).

The distribution of responses to a Likert scale query on whether confidentiality was a reason for participation were also obtained. The query answered by 220 participants was as follows: "I enrolled because the test was confidential and results cannot be traced." Test confidentiality was measured on a scale from 0 (not a reason) to 5 (a very important reason). Of the 220 participants, 34 (15.5%) answered 0; 17 (7.7%), 1; 13 (5.9%), 2; 15 (6.8%), 3; 26 (11.8%), 4; and 115 (52.3%), 5. Of the 250 responses to smoking status, 227 (90.8%) were never smokers, 17 (6.8%) reported current smoking, and 6 (2.4%) reported an ex-smoking status. Of the 17 smokers, 10 (58.8%) reported they were very likely (Likert scale score, 4-5) to quit if they received results of being severely deficient in AAT.

Likert responses from 1 to 5 were collected (1 indicates no risk; and 5, high risk) for a series of potential testing risks that included the loss of insurance or increased insurance cost, discovery of true paternity, and encountering religious issues associated with testing. Participants who answered all risk questions (n=162) had a mean (SD) Likert response of 1.7 (1.2). Likert responses for selected questions of benefits of testing were graded from a score of 1 (no benefit) to a score of 5 (important benefit). A mean (SD) score of 3.5 (1.4) was recorded from participants who answered all benefit questions (n=173) for questions including the benefits of establishing diagnosis, screening for other manifestations of disease, finding individuals without abnormal genes, and better understanding family genetics. Participants reported receiving more benefits than risks from AATD testing ($P$=.001) (**Table 2**).

## COMMENT

Testing of children and adolescents for genetic conditions that clinically present later in life is termed *predispositional testing*. In AATD, however, there is a unique gene × environment interaction that is responsible for the most common associated disease: emphysema. The environmental determinants of emphysema include cigarette smoking and dusty environments, both of which are amenable to prevention before the age of 18 years.[10,11] Although most children and adolescents being tested are asymptomatic, the genetic information being provided has the potential to be life changing.

One critical issue addressed by this article is whether genetic testing for AATD is likely harmful or helpful to minors or the family. In the absence of long-term outcomes, the attitudes of the parents were sampled in this large genetic testing study. The only other large study of AATD testing in which parental questionnaires were obtained remains the experience of the Swedish studies[4] of early identification of AATD.

Sveger and Thelin[12] described the attitudes of parents of 4-year-old children with AATD that had been detected in the Swedish birth-testing cohort. They found that 92% of the parents believed the knowledge of AATD did not have a negative effect on their own self-image. Of the parents, 50% had positive attitudes about testing their child, 80% thought the test should be offered to all children, and 94% wanted to test their remaining or future children.[12]

Some negative effects of testing were recorded in the Swedish experience. Although most parents experienced initial concern, poor emotional adjustment was found in 8% of mothers and 6% of fathers at 5 to 7 years after diagnosis. In general, parents of AAT-deficient children had a higher frequency of poor physical and/or mental health compared with control parents. However, by the time the children were 16 years old, the only difference noted was a higher incidence of anxiety in mothers, but not in fathers, of AAT-deficient children.[6]

Parents' smoking habits were examined because of concerns about secondary smoke inhalation. Although parents were advised to stop smoking, it was extremely difficult for them to quit completely.[5] In fact, fathers of the children were smoking at twice the frequency of the control cohorts.

Adolescents in the Swedish cohort (N=50) supported general screening for AATD, with 94% supporting testing during the neonatal period.[13] Of this cohort, 50% reported that knowledge of the results had affected their lives, especially regarding air pollution and smoking, and 88% recognized the importance of avoiding cigarette smoke for optimal lung protection. They found no early adult negative psychosocial consequences from their neonatal screening of AATD, with all participants (N=50) recommending AATD screening. In a separate questionnaire survey, 3% of adolescents from the Swedish cohort (N=150) were smoking compared with 12% of an age-matched nondeficient cohort (N=50).[5]

The American Thoracic Society/European Respiratory Society standards for the diagnosis and management of individuals with AATD recommend testing for newborns, children, and adolescents with unexplained liver disease.[7] The standards' document recommends predispositional testing for siblings of known deficient individuals who would have a 1 in 4 chance or more of being severely deficient and recommends testing if the genetic testing outcome serves as a motivator for the individual to quit cigarette smoking.[7] However, the document recommends against testing of minors independent of these circumstances.

**Table 2. The Risks and Benefits of AATD Testing**

| Category | No. of Participants* | Likert Scale Score, Mean (SD) |
|---|---|---|
| Risks | | |
| Losing health insurance | 171 | 2.3 (1.6) |
| Higher health insurance | 169 | 2.2 (1.5) |
| Losing your job | 170 | 1.5 (1.1) |
| Psychological risks associated with genetic knowledge | 173 | 2.1 (1.3) |
| Religious issues associated with genetic knowledge | 169 | 1.4 (0.9) |
| Knowledge concerning children's true parents | 166 | 1.4 (1.0) |
| Increased stress knowing that I have normal genes while a family member has abnormal *AAT* genes | 172 | 1.9 (1.3) |
| Benefits | | |
| Establishing a diagnosis | 181 | 3.8 (1.5) |
| Benefit of drug treatment not available without a diagnosis | 179 | 3.6 (1.6) |
| Genetic knowledge that may be helpful for family members | 183 | 3.8 (1.5) |
| Networking with others who have the genetic condition | 177 | 3.0 (1.6) |
| Screening for other manifestations of AATD | 181 | 3.5 (1.5) |
| Peace of mind if the genetic test result is normal | 182 | 4.0 (1.4) |

Abbreviation: AATD, $alpha_1$-antitrypsin deficiency.
*There were differing numbers of responses because of missing data.

One reason that predispositional testing of minors remains controversial for AATD and other genetic conditions is the absence of protective legislation at the federal level to prevent genetic discrimination, particularly regarding health and life insurance costs. Consistent with previous studies in AATD, we found that confidentiality in genetic testing remains a high concern. One of the reasons for high study enrollment is likely the confidentiality protection afforded by the study and its Certificate of Confidentiality. The ACT Study was designed to protect the confidentiality of participants by only disclosing test results to the individual or, in the case of minors, to the parent or guardian. We do not know the extent that parents shared genetic information or its implications with their children, an important determinant of whether models such as this should be advanced. Furthermore, long-term health outcomes of testing remain unknown.

The present study does not reflect the current practice of AAT testing in a community practice setting.[14,15]

One alternative for community testing is a model that has been used in other genetic diseases.[16] If a parent is severely deficient, with a *PIZZ* genotype, test results of the spouse have a high chance of being normal, with a genotype of *PIMM*. In this case, testing of children is unnecessary because all with parental genes will be genotype *PIMZ*. This pattern undoubtedly plays a major role in the many *PIMZ* carriers in this study. Advocates of testing both parents argue that the practice is more cost-effective than testing all children. However, if either parent is not homozygous, the testing model does not provide the genotypes of children and adolescents.

There are several limitations to the study. Because questionnaires were completed at participants' homes, there is a significant amount of missing data, as reflected in the data tables. In addition, we do not know the extent of influence from adolescents on the parental response to these questions. Finally, because of the few severely deficient (*PISZ* and *PIZZ*) responses, and the failure to query after test results were returned, we cannot define differences in responses between genotypes.

Because cigarette smoking and environmental dust exposure can have a significantly negative effect on the health of individuals with AATD and these exposures begin in adolescence, we believe that genetic testing should be accessible to all families in which AATD has been detected. Our study demonstrates that parents and guardians value genetic testing of minors for AATD.

**Accepted for Publication:** November 15, 2005.
**Correspondence:** Charlie Strange, MD, Division of Pulmonary and Critical Care Medicine, Medical University of South Carolina, 96 Jonathan Lucas St, Suite 812-CSB, Charleston, SC 29425 (strangec@musc.edu).
**Financial Disclosure:** Drs Strange and Brantly received grants from the Alpha-1 Foundation, a nonprofit corporation that funds the current testing program, and from ZLB Behring and Talecris Biotherapeutics. Dr Strange is on the speakers bureau for Baxter and ZLB Behring, manufacturers of AAT augmentation products. Dr Brantly has received grants from Baxter, the National Institutes of Health, Ono Pharmaceuticals, the State of Florida Health and Human Service, the American Red Cross, Bayer Biologics, and PPL Therapeutics.

## REFERENCES


1. O'Brien ML, Buist NR, Murphey WH. Neonatal screening for alpha$_1$-antitrypsin deficiency. *J Pediatr.* 1978;92:1006-1010.
2. Silverman EK, Miletich JP, Pierce JA, et al. Alpha-$_1$-antitrypsin deficiency: high prevalence in the St Louis area determined by direct population screening. *Am Rev Respir Dis.* 1989;140:961-966.
3. Spence WC, Morris JE, Pass K, Murphy PD. Molecular confirmation of alpha$_1$-antitrypsin genotypes in newborn dried blood specimens. *Biochem Med Metab Biol.* 1993;50:233-240.
4. Sveger T. Liver disease in alpha$_1$-antitrypsin deficiency detected by screening of 200,000 infants. *N Engl J Med.* 1976;294:1316-1321.
5. Sveger T, Piitulainen E, Arborelius M Jr. Lung function in adolescents with $\alpha_1$-antitrypsin deficiency. *Acta Paediatr.* 1994;83:1170-1173.
6. Sveger T, Thelin T, McNeil TF. Neonatal $\alpha$-$_1$-antitrypsin screening: parents' views and reactions 20 years after the identification of the deficiency state. *Acta Paediatr.* 1999;88:315-318.
7. American Thoracic Society/European Respiratory Society. American Thoracic Society/European Respiratory Society Statement: standards for the diagnosis and management of individuals with alpha-$_1$ antitrypsin deficiency. *Am J Respir Crit Care Med.* 2003;168:818-900.
8. Strange C, Dickson R, Carter C, et al. Genetic testing for alpha$_1$-antitrypsin deficiency. *Genet Med.* 2004;6:204-210.
9. de Serres FJ. Worldwide racial and ethnic distribution of alpha$_1$-antitrypsin deficiency: summary of an analysis of published genetic epidemiologic surveys. *Chest.* 2002;122:1818-1829.
10. Piitulainen E, Eriksson S. Decline in FEV$_1$ related to smoking status in individuals with severe $\alpha_1$-antitrypsin deficiency (PiZZ). *Eur Respir J.* 1999;13:247-251.
11. Mayer AS, Stoller JK, Bartelson BB, Ruttenber AJ, Sandhaus RA, Newman LS. Occupational exposure risks in individuals with PI*Z $\alpha_1$-antitrypsin deficiency. *Am J Respir Crit Care Med.* 2000;162:553-558.
12. Sveger T, Thelin T. Four-year-old children with $\alpha_1$-antitrypsin deficiency: clinical follow-up and parental attitudes towards neonatal screening. *Acta Paediatr Scand.* 1981;70:171-177.
13. Sveger T, Thelin T, McNeil TF. Young adults with $\alpha_1$-antitrypsin deficiency identified neonatally: their health, knowledge about and adaptation to the high-risk condition. *Acta Paediatr.* 1997;86:37-40.
14. American Society of Human Genetics, American College of Medical Genetics. Points to consider: ethical, legal, and psychosocial implications of genetic testing in children and adolescents. *Am J Hum Genet.* 1995;57:1233-1241.
15. Committee on Bioethics, American Academy of Pediatrics. Ethical issues with genetic testing in pediatrics. *Pediatrics.* 2001;107:1451-1455.
16. El-Serag HB, Inadomi JM, Kowdley KV. Screening for hereditary hemochromatosis in siblings and children of affected patients: a cost-effectiveness analysis. *Ann Intern Med.* 2000;132:261-269.

ARTICLE

# Improved Asthma Outcomes in a High-Morbidity Pediatric Population

## *Results of an Emergency Department–Based Randomized Clinical Trial*

*Stephen J. Teach, MD, MPH; Ellen F. Crain, MD, PhD; Deborah M. Quint, BA; Michelle L. Hylan, BA; Jill G. Joseph, MD, PhD*

**Objective:** To determine if an emergency department–based asthma follow-up clinic could improve outcomes within a high-morbidity pediatric population.

**Design:** Prospective, randomized clinical trial with 6 months of follow-up.

**Setting:** Emergency department of an urban pediatric medical center.

**Participants:** Convenience sample of 488 patients aged 12 months to 17 years, inclusive, with prior physician-diagnosed asthma and 1 or more other unscheduled visits in the previous 6 months and/or 1 or more hospitalizations in the prior 12 months.

**Intervention:** Single follow-up clinic visit focusing on 3 domains: asthma self-monitoring and management, environmental modification and trigger control, and linkages and referrals to ongoing care.

**Main Outcome Measures:** The primary outcome measure was unscheduled visits for acute asthma care. Secondary outcomes included compliance with a medical plan and asthma quality of life. Analysis was by intention to treat with adjustment for baseline differences.

**Results:** Of those randomized to the clinic visit, 172 (70.5%) of 244 attended. The intervention group had significantly fewer mean unscheduled visits for asthma care during follow-up (1.39 vs 2.34; relative risk [RR] = 0.60 [95% confidence interval (CI), 0.46-0.77]). At 6 months, significantly more patients in the intervention group reported use of inhaled corticosteroids in the prior 2 days (49.3% vs 26.5%; RR = 2.03 [95% CI, 1.57-2.62]), no limitation in daytime quality of life (43.8% vs 34.4%; RR = 1.36 [95% CI, 1.06-1.73]), and no functional limitations in quality of life (49.8% vs 40.8%; RR = 1.33 [95% CI, 1.08-1.63]).

**Conclusion:** Attendance in the follow-up clinic was high. The intervention decreased subsequent unscheduled health care use while improving compliance and quality of life.

*Arch Pediatr Adolesc Med. 2006;160:535-541*

**Author Affiliations:** Division of Emergency Medicine (Dr Teach) and Center for Health Services and Community Research, Children's Research Institute, Children's National Medical Center (Drs Teach and Joseph and Mss Quint and Hylan), George Washington University School of Medicine and Health Sciences (Drs Teach and Joseph), Washington, DC; Division of Emergency Medicine, Department of Pediatrics, Jacobi Medical Center, Albert Einstein College of Medicine, Bronx, NY (Dr Crain). Ms Hylan is now with the Genzyme Corporation, Cambridge, Mass. Dr Joseph is now with the University of California at Davis School of Medicine.

DESPITE THE INTRODUCTION of standardized care guidelines,[1] emergency department (ED) visits for pediatric asthma have not declined.[2] These visits are concentrated disproportionately among minority, disadvantaged, and urban children,[2-4] and this population's ED recidivism rate is high.[5,6] In fact, many urban children with asthma and their families view EDs as their primary source of asthma care.[7,8] A specific objective of Healthy People 2010 is a nearly 50% reduction in the rate of ED visits for asthma in children younger than 5 years.[9]

Recent systematic reviews[10,11] have confirmed the efficacy of structured education and controller medications in improving asthma outcomes among pediatric patients, including decreasing ED use. Little is known, however, about how ED-based programs can apply these measures to decrease asthma morbidity after ED discharge. One approach has been to attempt to improve primary care follow-up rates after ED visits, previously reported to range from 6% to 46%.[12-16] Some ED studies have shown that facilitated follow-up can modestly increase primary care visits in the short-term but that these efforts have not decreased unscheduled visits for acute care in the long-term.[12,13,17] Other studies have provided asthma education and improved care during ED visits[18] or after ED visits by telephone[19] or have encouraged specific behaviors by ED professionals at the point of discharge.[15] None of them has reduced subsequent unscheduled health care use for asthma.

The current study took a different approach by delivering a novel intervention in which the ED itself became the site of highly individualized, comprehensive follow-up asthma care. The intervention, known as Improving Pediatric Asthma Care in the District of Columbia (IMPACT DC), targeted frequent users of an urban pediatric ED. It consisted of a single visit scheduled for 2 to 15 days after ED discharge to a specialized asthma clinic located in the ED. The clinic provided education and clinical care, focusing on 3 distinct domains: asthma self-monitoring and management, environmental modification and trigger control, and linkages and referrals to ongoing primary care.

Our primary hypothesis was that this intervention would decrease subsequent unscheduled visits (to both EDs and other sources of urgent care) for acute asthma care during a 6-month follow-up period. We further hypothesized that the intervention would decrease hospitalizations for asthma, improve compliance with an individualized medical plan and with trigger control, increase scheduled primary care practitioner (PCP) visits for routine asthma care, and decrease asthma symptoms while improving asthma quality of life (QOL).

## METHODS

We enrolled patients in a prospective, randomized clinical trial in the ED at Children's National Medical Center in Washington, DC, from April 2002 until January 2004. Children's National Medical Center is an urban tertiary care pediatric medical center with an ED volume of 72 778 visits in 2003. Of these visits, 4482 (6.1%) included a primary discharge diagnosis of asthma among patients aged 12 months to 17 years, inclusive. Trained research assistants recruited subjects among those with respiratory complaints. Inclusion criteria included: (1) age between 12 months and 17 years, inclusive; (2) prior physician-diagnosed asthma; (3) 1 or more other unscheduled visits for acute asthma care (to an ED or other health care source) in the previous 6 months and/or 1 or more hospitalizations for asthma in the prior 12 months; (4) a parent or guardian available for interview; (5) residence in Washington, DC, or a contiguous Maryland county; and (6) requirement for 3 or more doses of nebulized albuterol in the ED at the time of enrollment.

Exclusion criteria included: (1) significant medical comorbidities affecting the cardiorespiratory system; (2) a visit to an allergist or a pulmonologist in the prior 6 months; (3) 2 or more of the following: a current written asthma medical action plan, current use of more than 1 controller medication, or a scheduled visit for asthma care with their PCP in the prior 2 weeks; (4) enrollment in another asthma research study; (5) unavailability for telephone follow-up; or (6) primary language other than English or Spanish.

Acute asthma therapy while the patient was in the ED at the enrollment visit was at the discretion of the treating ED physicians. This care was largely guided by an existing clinical pathway for acute asthma exacerbation that suggested a 5-day course of oral prednisolone or prednisone be initiated in the ED.

### BASELINE DATA COLLECTION AND RANDOMIZATION

After obtaining informed consent and assent and while the patient was still in the ED, the research assistants obtained baseline data from the parent or guardian that assessed demographics, asthma history, medication use, asthma classification by the criteria of the National Heart, Lung, and Blood Institute (NHLBI),[1] asthma symptoms and QOL, linkages to primary and specialty sources of care, and triggers in the home. Race and ethnicity were self-described by parents and guardians and were collected because they are independent predictors of asthma severity.[20] Symptom questions were drawn from the National Cooperative Inner-City Asthma Study (NCICAS).[21,22] Quality of life was assessed through the use of a measure developed and validated for pediatric asthma.[23,24]

Randomization was then accomplished in blocks of 30 participants. To accomplish this, the project director prepared batches of 30 opaque, sealed envelopes, 15 containing a folded slip of paper specifying randomization to the control group and 15 specifying randomization to the intervention group. Each batch of 30 envelopes was then exhaustively shuffled and numbered with participant identification numbers. During enrollment, the research assistants opened each sequential envelope after informed consent and assent was obtained and after the baseline interview was conducted.

The intervention consisted of a single visit to the IMPACT DC asthma clinic where each family met with an asthma educator and a physician. This clinic was physically located in the ED, using space available on weekday mornings. The control group received an asthma educational booklet but no specialized follow-up.

### INTERVENTION

All clinical activities of the intervention were based on a shared dialogue with the families and development of a tailored treatment plan. In common with the NCICAS,[22] these family-centered principles were theoretically grounded in the Health Belief Model and promotion of self-efficacy.[25] Following a fully specified protocol requiring 60 to 90 minutes, education and care were provided in 3 domains.

#### Asthma Self-monitoring and Management

Educators first reviewed the basic physiology of asthma with emphasis on its chronicity. After evaluating asthma severity and treatment history, the physician completed an individualized medical action plan and provided any necessary device teaching (metered-dose inhaler, spacer, diskus, compressor, nebulizer). Controller medications were prescribed for a total of 3 months. Self-monitoring was taught by symptoms and/or by peak flow measurement.

#### Environmental Modification and Trigger Control

After evaluation of potential environmental triggers in the home, each family was educated on their control. The protocol emphasized an "asthma-safe sleep zone" for the child. Each child was provided hypoallergenic bed encasings.

#### Linkages and Referrals to Ongoing Primary Care

Clinic staff stressed the importance of longitudinal asthma care by a PCP. A full report of the clinic visit, together with a digital photograph of the child and a copy of the medical action plan, was mailed to each child's PCP, insurance asthma case manager, and school nurse. In addition, the asthma educator scheduled a follow-up appointment with the PCP within 4 weeks. Any child with severe, persistent asthma was instructed to pursue further ongoing care with an asthma specialist.

### FOLLOW-UP

Research assistants blinded to randomization status performed follow-up telephone interviews with each child's parent or guardian at 1, 3, and 6 months after enrollment. The primary outcome measure was the rate of unscheduled visits (to EDs and other sources of urgent care) for acute asthma care during the 6-month period following randomization. Other utilization outcomes included hospital admissions for acute asthma and routine (scheduled >24 hours in advance) PCP visits for nonacute asthma care. Other secondary outcomes included asthma medication and device use, efforts to control asthma triggers in the home, linkages to care providers (PCPs, asthma specialists, asthma case managers, and school nurses), asthma classification by NHLBI criteria, current asthma symptoms, and asthma QOL.

## VALIDATION STUDY

To validate parental recall of ED visits, a random subset of 30 participants each from the intervention and control groups were recontacted after completion of the 6-month interview and asked to recall visits made to the ED at Children's National Medical Center during the prior 2 months. Their responses were compared with hospital records.

## STATISTICAL CONSIDERATIONS

All outcomes were analyzed among those completing follow-up for the relevant period using an intention-to-treat paradigm. Initially, baseline sociodemographic and clinical characteristics in the intervention and control groups were compared using means and frequencies. All subsequent estimates of relative risk (RR) were adjusted for age, sex, race/ethnicity, insurance type, household income, environmental tobacco smoke exposure, and the corresponding baseline variable. All estimates of RR are reported with 95% confidence intervals (CIs).

All models included a specific dependent variable and a binary indicator of the randomly assigned study group. Process measures (elements of medical management, environmental modification, and care coordination) were compared between groups at the 1-month follow-up using multiple logistic regression models. For the primary outcome measure (unscheduled visits for asthma care) and for other measures of health care use, the analysis compared adjusted 6-month rates and RRs. Depending on the degree of dispersion in the rates, these models were based on either Poisson or negative binomial regression models. The latter were used whenever the degree of dispersion exceeded that accommodated by the Poisson model. Similar to the approach used with the process measures, multiple logistic regression models were also used to compare symptom and QOL measures between the 2 study groups at the 1-, 3-, and 6-month follow-ups. Finally, a Cox proportional hazards time-to-event model was developed to estimate and compare the cumulative probability of 1 or more ED visits during the 6-month follow-up period. All analyses were conducted using procedures in STATA version 8[26] and SAS version 9.[27]

## HUMAN SUBJECTS

The institutional review board at Children's National Medical Center approved this study. Legal guardians provided written informed consent. Participants 6 years and older provided written assent.

## RESULTS

The research assistants screened 2791 patients during the 22-month enrollment period (**Figure 1**). Of these, 2270 (81.3%) were ineligible. The main reasons for ineligibility were no prior physician-diagnosed asthma (30.8%), no other unscheduled visits for asthma in prior 6 months and no hospitalization in prior 12 months (19.3%), acute asthma exacerbation not the primary reason for ED visit (18.6%), and significant medical comorbidities (8.6%). Of the 521 eligible patients identified, 490 (94.0%) were enrolled and randomized. Two were subsequently excluded because of enrollment violations, leaving 488 participants available for analysis. Follow-up through 6 months was available for 437 (89.5%) of these participants.

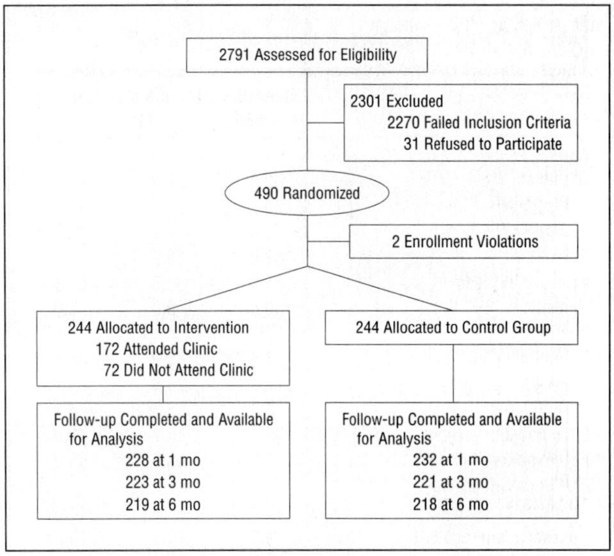


**Figure 1.** Progress of participants through trial.

Baseline demographics of all participants are described in **Table 1**. The intervention and control groups were similar except for the proportions of each reporting environmental tobacco smoke exposure in the home and in the distribution of hospital admissions for asthma and scheduled asthma care visits in the prior 12 months.

Of those randomized to the intervention, 172 (70.5%) of 244 attended. The intervention was implemented with high uniformity. All patients left the clinic with a completed medical action plan, a mattress pad and pillow cover, and a spacer (if prescribed inhaled medicines). Of the 172 patients attending the clinic, 167 (97.1%) were prescribed inhaled corticosteroids (via inhaler or nebulizer), and 69 (40.1%) were prescribed leukotriene antagonists.

Process measures at 1 month after enrollment are reported in **Table 2**. There were significantly more families in the intervention group reporting use of a written medical action plan, use of inhaled corticosteroids and leukotriene antagonists in the prior 2 days, and use of a spacer whenever using metered-dose inhalers. In addition, significantly more families in the intervention group reported use of bed encasings and no daily smoking within the home. There were no significant differences between the groups in the proportion of families who identified the PCP as their usual source of asthma care, had contact with the school nurse regarding asthma care, or had contact with an asthma case manager from their insurance company.

Improvements in certain process measures continued for the full 6 months of follow-up. Reported use of inhaled corticosteroids in the prior 2 days was significantly greater in the intervention group compared with the con-

**Table 1. Participant Characteristics at Enrollment***

| | Overall (n = 488) | Intervention (n = 244) | Control (n = 244) |
|---|---|---|---|
| Age, y | | | |
| 1-5 | 60.0 | 59.4 | 60.7 |
| 6-10 | 26.2 | 28.7 | 23.8 |
| ≥11 | 13.8 | 11.9 | 15.6 |
| Male | 63.9 | 65.2 | 62.7 |
| African American | 85.9 | 86.5 | 85.3 |
| Hispanic | 9.4 | 9.8 | 9.0 |
| Insurance type | | | |
| Public | 68.4 | 70.0 | 66.8 |
| Private | 27.9 | 26.8 | 29.1 |
| Uninsured | 3.7 | 3.3 | 4.1 |
| Total household income ≤$30,000 | 42.9 | 42.2 | 43.6 |
| ETS exposure in home | 63.5 | 68.9 | 58.2 |
| NHLBI classification | | | |
| Severe persistent | 16.0 | 17.6 | 14.3 |
| Moderate persistent | 14.3 | 14.8 | 13.9 |
| Mild persistent | 29.1 | 29.5 | 28.7 |
| Mild intermittent | 40.6 | 38.1 | 43.0 |
| ED visits in prior 12 mo | | | |
| 0 | 8.0 | 9.4 | 6.6 |
| 1-2 | 40.2 | 35.7 | 44.7 |
| 3-4 | 25.0 | 28.3 | 21.7 |
| ≥5 | 26.8 | 26.6 | 27.1 |
| Other urgent visits in prior 12 mo | | | |
| 0 | 39.9 | 41.6 | 38.3 |
| 1-2 | 26.8 | 23.5 | 30.0 |
| 3-4 | 17.3 | 17.7 | 16.9 |
| ≥5 | 16.1 | 17.3 | 14.8 |
| Admissions in prior 12 mo | | | |
| 0 | 69.7 | 74.2 | 65.2 |
| 1-2 | 25.8 | 21.7 | 29.9 |
| 3-4 | 3.7 | 3.7 | 3.7 |
| ≥5 | 0.8 | 0.4 | 1.2 |
| Scheduled visits in prior 12 mo | | | |
| 0 | 23.9 | 26.3 | 21.5 |
| 1-2 | 50.8 | 52.5 | 49.2 |
| 3-4 | 14.5 | 12.5 | 16.5 |
| ≥5 | 10.8 | 8.8 | 12.8 |
| Identifiable PCP | 94.3 | 94.7 | 93.9 |
| Primary source of asthma care | | | |
| ED | 61.7 | 63.5 | 59.8 |
| PCP | 34.6 | 33.2 | 36.1 |
| Other | 3.7 | 3.3 | 4.1 |
| Has written MAP | 20.5 | 21.0 | 20.1 |
| ICS use in prior month | 24.2 | 19.7 | 28.7 |
| LTRA use in prior month | 10.5 | 11.6 | 9.4 |

Abbreviations: ED, emergency department; ETS, environmental tobacco smoke; ICS, inhaled corticosteroids; LTRA, leukotriene antagonists; MAP, medical action plan; NHLBI, National Heart, Lung, and Blood Institute; PCP, primary care practitioner.

*Values are expressed as percentage of participants. The following variables have missing data: insurance type (n = 1), other urgent visits (n = 2), scheduled visits (n = 6), written MAP (n = 1), and LTRA use in prior 1 month (n = 2).

**Table 2. Selected Process Measures at 1-Month Follow-up, With Relative Risks Adjusted for Covariates***

| | Unadjusted Proportion, % | | |
|---|---|---|---|
| | Intervention (n = 228) | Control (n = 232) | Adjusted Relative Risk (95% CI) |
| Asthma self-monitoring and management | | | |
| Written asthma plan used in prior month | 61.8 | 40.1 | 1.53 (1.26-1.86) |
| ICS use in prior 2 d | 64.0 | 32.6 | 2.09 (1.70-2.56) |
| LTRA use in prior 2 d | 27.6 | 14.4 | 1.73 (1.20-2.49) |
| Using spacer whenever using MDI | 48.7 | 26.5 | 1.96 (1.44-2.66) |
| Used peak flow meter in prior month if older than 5 y | 77.8 | 75.0 | 1.05 (0.89-1.25) |
| Influenza vaccination in prior month | 17.0 | 10.2 | 1.52 (0.92-2.52) |
| Environmental modification and trigger control | | | |
| Mattress pad or pillow cover on child's bed or pillow | 74.6 | 23.3 | 3.00 (2.38-3.78) |
| Damp dusting in bedroom | 85.5 | 79.7 | 1.08 (0.99-1.17) |
| Daily smoking inside home | 4.4 | 9.9 | 0.35 (0.16-0.76) |
| Linkages and referrals to ongoing primary care | | | |
| PCP identified as usual source of asthma care | 48.7 | 49.1 | 1.02 (0.87-1.21) |
| Discussed asthma care with PCP in prior month | 54.3 | 59.8 | 0.95 (0.80-1.13) |
| Contact with school nurse in prior month (if in school) | 23.1 | 24.1 | 0.91 (0.58-1.41) |
| Contact with asthma case manager in prior month | 18.9 | 11.3 | 1.42 (0.89-2.28) |

Abbreviations: CI, confidence interval; ICS, inhaled corticosteroids; LTRA, leukotriene antagonists; MDI, metered-dose inhaler; PCP, primary care practitioner.

*Adjustments made for age, sex, race/ethnicity, insurance type, household income, environmental tobacco smoke exposure, and corresponding baseline variable.

trol group at both 3 months (54.3% vs 25.6%; adjusted RR=2.37 [95% CI, 1.83-3.04]) and 6 months (49.3% vs 26.5%; adjusted RR=2.03 [95% CI, 1.57-2.62]).

Utilization outcomes during the 6-month follow-up period are reported in **Table 3**. There were significantly fewer total mean unscheduled visits among children randomized to the intervention (1.39 vs 2.34; RR=0.60 [95% CI, 0.46-0.77]). This benefit of the intervention was also observed when ED visits and other unscheduled visits were considered separately. In addition, as depicted in **Figure 2**, there was a significantly higher cumulative risk in the control group of making 1 or more ED visits during the 6-month follow-up period (RR=1.74 [95% CI, 1.31-2.31]). There were no significant differences in the number of hospital admissions or scheduled PCP visits between the 2 groups. Of the 219 intervention patients with a complete 6-month follow-up, 32 (14.6%) had 1 or more visits to an asthma specialist outside of our intervention compared with 38 (17.4%) of 218 control patients (*P*=.42).

As presented in **Table 4**, data reporting asthma symptoms, NHLBI classification, and QOL during the follow-up period are skewed, with large proportions reporting being symptom free. We therefore analyzed them as the proportions in each group reporting no symptoms, no persistent asthma criteria, and no compromise in QOL. The intervention improved asthma symptoms and QOL in the first month after randomization, with selected improvements persisting to the 6-month follow-up. Significantly more children in the intervention group, for example, were free of both diurnal and nocturnal symptoms and sleep disturbance at 1 month after enrollment. Similarly, persistent asthma symptoms were less common at 1 month among those randomized to the intervention, and QOL was significantly improved, whether assessed with respect to daytime, nighttime, or functional limitations. At 3 and 6 months, diminished but still significant benefits in QOL remained.

Validation of 1 of the primary outcomes (ED use) showed good agreement (unweighted $\kappa = 0.67$) between caregiver report and hospital records for 2-month recall of ED visits. In addition, there was no difference between the intervention and control groups in the proportion of caregivers with accurate 2-month recall of ED visits (27 [90.0%] of 30 in both groups; $P > .99$).

**Table 3. Rates of Health Care Use During 6-Month Follow-up Period, Adjusted for Covariates***

| | Adjusted Mean Rate of Visits During 6 Months | | |
|---|---|---|---|
| | Intervention (n = 219) | Control (n = 218) | Adjusted Relative Risk (95% CI) |
| Total unscheduled visits for asthma (ED and elsewhere) | 1.39 | 2.34 | 0.60 (0.46-0.77) |
| ED visits for asthma | 0.64 | 1.19 | 0.54 (0.40-0.72) |
| Unscheduled visits for asthma to source other than ED | 0.68 | 1.13 | 0.60 (0.44-0.84) |
| Hospital admissions for asthma | 0.10 | 0.18 | 0.56 (0.33-1.08) |
| Scheduled visits with PCP for asthma | 2.05 | 2.04 | 1.00 (0.85-1.18) |

Abbreviations: CI, confidence interval; ED, emergency department; PCP, primary care practitioner.

*Adjustments made for age, sex, race/ethnicity, insurance type, household income, environmental tobacco smoke exposure, and corresponding baseline variable.

## COMMENT

Using a rigorous randomized design with blinded interviews and intention-to-treat analysis, we demonstrated that a single comprehensive follow-up visit after ED discharge improved asthma care and outcomes in a high-morbidity population of urban, largely disadvantaged, and minority children. The intervention was unique in at least 3 important respects. First, it was an entirely ED-based effort that did not rely on facilitated follow-up with either primary care services or a specialized asthma center. Second, it achieved rates of follow-up after ED care for asthma far in excess of those reported in similar urban pediatric populations.[12-16] Finally, unlike prior ED-based efforts, the intervention improved multiple measures of asthma treatment adherence, symptom control, QOL, and health care use. Perhaps most importantly, it decreased the rate of unscheduled visits for asthma during the entire 6-month follow-up period.

Expert published guidelines[1,28] stress that asthma care should occur through a longitudinal relationship with a PCP, and evidence exists that application of these guidelines in primary care improves asthma outcomes.[29,30] Nonetheless, EDs remain a primary source of asthma care for many inner-city families. Rand et al,[7] for example, documented that more than 40% of an unselected group of 392 inner-city children with asthma in Baltimore, Md, had visited an ED in the prior 6 months, and Dinkevich et al[8] found that just more than half of 308 inner-city families of children with asthma in New York, NY, identified the ED as their usual source of asthma care. In our series, 61.7% of the patients identified the ED as their primary source of asthma care.

Unfortunately, while EDs often provide quality episodic care, they rarely address nonacute issues in asthma care. Few ED physicians, for example, prescribe inhaled corticosteroids after an acute asthma exacerbation.[31] For this reason, NHLBI guidelines[1] recommend a primary care follow-up after all acute exacerbations. Motivated at least

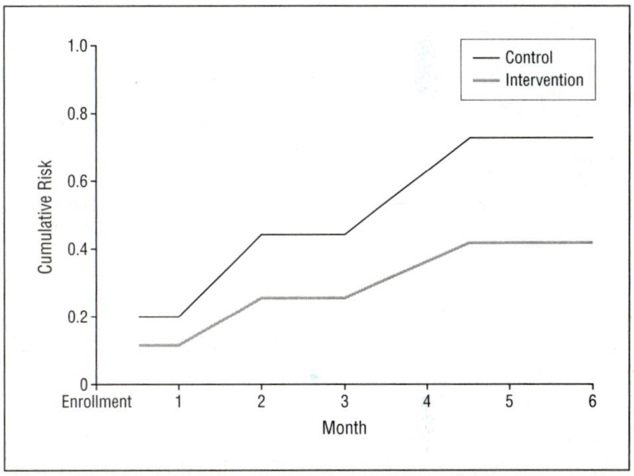


**Figure 2.** Cox proportional hazards regression of cumulative risk of having 1 or more emergency department visits during the 6-month follow-up period, adjusted for age, sex, race/ethnicity, insurance type, household income, environmental tobacco smoke exposure, baseline National Heart, Lung, and Blood Institute classification, and reported emergency department visits at baseline. There were 219 patients in the intervention group and 218 in the control group. Adjusted relative risk = 1.74 (95% confidence interval, 1.31-2.31).

in part by these guidelines, prior ED-based interventions have focused on improving rates of primary care follow-up. Zorc et al[12] and Smith et al[13] have recently reported randomized trials of facilitated follow-up after acute ED visits for pediatric asthma care. Although these interventions successfully increased follow-up visits, they did not reduce subsequent ED visits or hospital admissions. Other evidence outside of randomized trials also suggests that primary care follow-up after acute exacerbations is not associated with a decrease in subsequent ED visits.[14]

There are several factors that may explain the success of the intervention described herein. First, it was designed to exploit the "teachable moment," an approach

**Table 4. Participants Reporting No Asthma Symptoms in Prior 14 Days, No Persistent Asthma Criteria, and No Compromise in Quality of Life (QOL) in Prior 4 Weeks***

| | 1 Month (n = 421) | | | 3 Months (n = 419) | | | 6 Months (n = 437) | | |
|---|---|---|---|---|---|---|---|---|---|
| | Unadjusted % | | | Unadjusted % | | | Unadjusted % | | |
| | Intervention (n = 210) | Control (n = 211) | Adjusted RR (95% CI) | Intervention (n = 210) | Control (n = 209) | Adjusted RR (95% CI) | Intervention (n = 219) | Control (n = 218) | Adjusted RR (95% CI) |
| No days of symptoms in prior 14 d | 51.4 | 32.7 | 1.67 (1.31-2.15) | 48.6 | 42.1 | 1.18 (0.94-1.46) | 46.6 | 43.6 | 1.11 (0.90-1.37) |
| No nights of symptoms in prior 14 nights | 69.1 | 56.4 | 1.23 (1.05-1.43) | 66.7 | 57.4 | 1.15 (0.99-1.35) | 56.4 | 59.6 | 0.95 (0.81-1.13) |
| No nights of sleep disturbance in prior 14 nights | 66.7 | 53.6 | 1.28 (1.09-1.51) | 65.2 | 56.5 | 1.15 (0.98-1.34) | 59.4 | 61.9 | 0.98 (0.84-1.15) |
| No days of slowed activities in prior 14 d | 60.0 | 46.5 | 1.37 (1.13-1.67) | 57.6 | 50.7 | 1.16 (0.97-1.40) | 53.9 | 52.3 | 1.07 (0.89-1.29) |
| No days of missed school in prior 14 d (if in school) | 81.5 | 70.1 | 1.14 (0.98-1.34) | 77.7 | 73.0 | 1.13 (0.97-1.31) | 71.8 | 65.7 | 1.16 (0.96-1.39) |
| No persistent asthma criteria | 69.3 | 58.6 | 1.25 (1.09-1.44) | 73.0 | 65.6 | 1.12 (0.99-1.27) | 69.9 | 64.7 | 1.03 (0.90-1.18) |
| No compromise in daytime QOL in prior 4 wk | 44.3 | 31.3 | 1.53 (1.18-1.97) | 44.8 | 35.9 | 1.27 (0.99-1.63) | 43.8 | 34.4 | 1.36 (1.06-1.73) |
| No compromise in nighttime QOL in prior 4 wk | 42.4 | 26.1 | 1.70 (1.28-2.26) | 41.9 | 29.7 | 1.40 (1.07-1.84) | 35.6 | 34.9 | 1.06 (0.82-1.38) |
| No functional limitations in QOL in prior 4 wk | 49.5 | 29.9 | 1.74 (1.35-2.23) | 51.4 | 35.9 | 1.46 (1.16-1.85) | 49.8 | 40.8 | 1.33 (1.08-1.63) |

Abbreviations: CI, confidence interval; RR, relative risk.

*Data reported for those 437 patients completing all 6 months of follow-up. Relative risks adjusted for age, sex, race/ethnicity, insurance type, household income, environmental tobacco smoke exposure, and corresponding baseline variable.

documented to improve outcomes in injury prevention,[32] drug and alcohol abuse,[33,34] smoking,[35] and weight loss.[36] The high rate of clinic attendance (70.5% of those randomized to the intervention) suggests that participants were highly motivated under these circumstances to seek education and improved care. Second, the intervention was comprehensive, addressing environmental change, medical care, and care coordination, and it was highly family- and patient-centered. Several studies have identified this individualized approach to asthma care as especially important to inner-city families.[37,38] Third, we obtained very high levels of self-reported adherence with inhaled corticosteroids, use of which has been independently associated with improved asthma outcomes.[11,30] Finally, we provided access to follow-up care within the familiar context of the ED. Based on their prior pattern of frequent ED use for asthma, it may not be surprising that families were comfortable returning to the ED. We do not know whether this comprehensive intervention would be as successful if applied in venues other than the ED.

The intervention was also designed to strengthen each family's relationship to their child's PCP, but it did not achieve this objective. It is possible that the intervention might even have negatively impacted the role of the PCPs by establishing an effective ED-based system for short-term asthma management. In any case, the intervention did not increase PCP contact for scheduled asthma care, and this may be an important limitation to its sustained effect.

Despite its successes, the intervention has other limitations. First, participants were recruited in a single large, urban pediatric ED, and results may not be generalizable to other geographic areas. Emergency departments with populations similar to the one studied herein clearly exist in other cities; however, and as noted earlier, patients and families see them as important sources of their asthma care.[7,8] Second, participants were deliberately selected based on high prior rates of health care use for asthma, and the effect of the intervention on patients with less frequent prior ED visits is uncertain. Previous work has shown, however, that a relatively small group of inner-city children contributes disproportionately to overall pediatric ED visits for asthma. Data from Pittsburgh, Pa, and Milwaukee, Wis, for example, demonstrated that 16% to 20% of ED patients with asthma made 36% to 50% of all ED visits.[5,6] Third, all of the outcomes were based on caregiver recall for periods of 1 to 3 months, and they are therefore subject to recall bias. However, numerous other studies have relied on the same methods, including the NCICAS, which asked participants to recall use during the prior 2 to 3 months.[2,3,21,22,39] We also validated one of the most important outcomes, ED use, and we found no evidence of selectively biased recall between the 2 study groups. Fourth, we only followed up participants for 6 months after enrollment. It is possible that the effect of the intervention diminished thereafter. Fifth, we performed no cost-benefit analysis of the intervention. This was beyond the budgeted scope of the project. Finally, a single physician provided all the medical care for the intervention, and therefore, the results may be due in part to a practitioner effect.

In conclusion, we found that a single follow-up visit to a comprehensive ED-based asthma clinic resulted in significant and clinically relevant improvements in care and outcomes in a high-morbidity pediatric population. We believe that this finding may have implications for the future role of the urban ED in asthma care and potentially in other chronic pediatric conditions with acute exacerbations. At the least, these methods may serve as a useful model in similar urban EDs with a high volume of inner-city children with asthma.

**Accepted for Publication:** October 19, 2005.
**Corresponding Author:** Stephen J. Teach, MD, MPH, Division of Emergency Medicine, Children's National Medical Center, 111 Michigan Ave NW, Washington, DC 20010 (steach@cnmc.org).
**Author Contributions:** Ms Quint had full access to all the data in the study and takes responsibility for the integrity of the data and the accuracy of the data analysis.
**Financial Disclosure:** Dr Teach serves on the Speakers' Bureau for the AstraZeneca Corporation.
**Funding/Support:** We would like to acknowledge the financial support of the Robert Wood Johnson Foundation (RWJF). This study was also supported by grant M01-RR020359 from the General Clinical Research Center Program of the National Center for Research Resources, National Institutes of Health, US Department of Health and Human Services.
**Role of the Sponsor:** The RWJF was not involved in the design and conduct of the study; collection, management, analysis, or interpretation of the data; or preparation, review, or approval of the manuscript. Material donations were provided by the AstraZeneca, GlaxoSmithKline, Merck, and Monaghan Medical corporations.
**Acknowledgment:** We would like to acknowledge the statistical support of Robert McCarter, ScD, and Cheng Shao, MPH, and the database support of Bruce M. Sprague, BS.

## REFERENCES

1. National Heart, Lung, and Blood Institute. *National Asthma Education and Prevention Program.Expert Panel Report 2: Guidelines for the Diagnosis and Management of Asthma.* Bethesda, Md: National Institutes of Health; 1997. NIH publication 97-4051.
2. Mannino DM, Homa DM, Akinbami LJ, et al. Surveillance for asthma—United States, 1980-1999. *MMWR Surveill Summ.* 2002;51:1-13.
3. Kattan M, Mitchell H, Eggleston P, et al. Characteristics of inner-city children with asthma: the National Cooperative Inner-City Asthma Study. *Pediatr Pulmonol.* 1997;24:253-262.
4. Shields AE, Comstock C, Weiss KB. Variations in asthma care by race/ethnicity among children enrolled in a state Medicaid program. *Pediatrics.* 2004;113:496-504.
5. Friday GA Jr, Khine H, Lin MS, Caliguri LA. Profile of children requiring emergency treatment for asthma. *Ann Allergy Asthma Immunol.* 1997;78:221-224.
6. Morris RD, Naumova EN, Goldring J, Hersch M, Munasinghe RL, Anderson H. Childhood asthma surveillance using computerized billing records: a pilot study. *Public Health Rep.* 1997;112:506-512.
7. Rand CS, Butz AM, Kolodner K, Huss K, Eggleston P, Malveaux F. Emergency department visits by urban African American children with asthma. *J Allergy Clin Immunol.* 2001;105(pt 1):83-90.
8. Dinkevich EI, Cunningham SJ, Crain EF. Parental perceptions of access to care and quality of care for inner-city children with asthma. *J Asthma.* 1998;35:63-71.
9. US Department of Health and Human Services. Respiratory diseases. In: *Healthy People 2010: Objectives for Improving Health.* Vol 2. McLean, Va: International Medical Publishing, Inc; 2000:24-16.
10. Wolf FM, Guevara JP, Grum CM, Clark NM, Cates CJ. Educational interventions for asthma in children. *Cochrane Database Syst Rev.* 2003;(1):CD000326.
11. Adams NP, Bestall JC, Lasserson TJ, Jones PW. Inhaled fluticasone versus placebo for chronic asthma in adults and children. *Cochrane Database Syst Rev.* 2005;(2):CD003135.
12. Zorc JJ, Scarfone RJ, Li Y, et al. Scheduled follow-up after a pediatric emergency department visit for asthma: a randomized trial. *Pediatrics.* 2003;111:495-502.
13. Smith SR, Jaffe DM, Fisher EB, Trinkaus KM, Highstein G, Strunk RC. Improving follow-up for children with asthma after an acute emergency department visit. *J Pediatr.* 2004;145:772-777.
14. Cabana MD, Bruckman D, Bratton SL, Kemper AR, Clark NM. Association between outpatient follow-up and pediatric emergency department asthma visits. *J Asthma.* 2003;40:741-749.
15. Petersen DL, Murphy DE, Jaffe DM, et al. A tool to organize instructions at discharge after treatment of asthmatic children in an emergency department. *J Asthma.* 1999;36:597-603.
16. Stevens MW, Gorelick MH. Short-term outcomes after acute treatment of pediatric asthma. *Pediatrics.* 2001;107:1357-1362.
17. Komoroski EM, Graham CJ, Kirby RS. A comparison of interventions to improve clinic follow-up compliance after a pediatric emergency department visit. *Pediatr Emerg Care.* 1996;12:87-90.
18. Cunningham SJ, Crain EF. Reduction of morbidity in asthmatic children given a spacer device. *Chest.* 1994;106:753-757.
19. Khan MS, O'Meara M, Stevermuer TL, Henry RL. Randomized controlled trial of asthma education after discharge from an emergency department. *J Paediatr Child Health.* 2004;40:674-677.
20. Boudreaux ED, Emond SD, Clark S, Carmago CA. Race/ethnicity and asthma among children presenting to the emergency department: differences in disease severity and management. *Pediatrics.* 2003;111:e615-e621. Available at: http://pediatrics.aappublications.org/cgi/content/full/111/5/e615.
21. Mitchell H, Senturia Y, Gergen P, et al. Design and methods of the National Cooperative Inner-City Asthma Study. *Pediatr Pulmonol.* 1997;24:237-252.
22. Evans R III, Gergen PJ, Mitchell H, et al. A randomized clinical trial to reduce asthma morbidity among inner-city children: results of the National Cooperative Inner-City Asthma Study. *J Pediatr.* 1999;135:332-338.
23. Bukstein DA, McGrath MM, Buchner DA, Landgraf J, Goss TF. Evaluation of a short form for measuring health-related quality of life among pediatric asthma patients. *J Allergy Clin Immunol.* 2000;105:245-251.
24. Gorelick MH, Brousseau DC, Stevens MW. Validity and responsiveness of a brief, asthma-specific quality-of-life instrument in children with acute asthma. *Ann Allergy Asthma Immunol.* 2004;92:47-51.
25. Rosenstock IM, Strecher VJ, Becker MH. Social learning theory and the Health Belief Model. *Health Educ Q.* 1988;15:175-183.
26. StataCorp. *Statistical Software: Release 8.0.* College Station, Tex: Stata Corporation; 2003.
27. SAS Institute Inc. *Statistical Software version 9.1.3.* Cary, NC: SAS Institute Inc; 2004.
28. American Academy of Allergy, Asthma, and Immunology. *Pediatric Asthma: Promoting Best Practice.* Milwaukee, Wis: American Academy of Allergy, Asthma, and Immunology; 1999:40-48.
29. Lieu TA, Quesenberry CP Jr, Capra AM, Sorel ME, Martin KE, Mendoza GR. Outpatient management practices associated with reduced risk of pediatric asthma hospitalization and emergency department visits. *Pediatrics.* 1997;100:334-341.
30. Adams RJ, Fuhlbrigge A, Finkelstein JA, et al. Impact of inhaled anti-inflammatory therapy on hospitalization and emergency department visits for children with asthma. *Pediatrics.* 2001;107:706-711.
31. Thomas JA, Potter MW, Counselman FL, Smith DG. Emergency physician practice and steroid use in the management of acute exacerbations of asthma. *Am J Emerg Med.* 2001;19:465-468.
32. Posner JC, Hawkins LA, Garcia-Espana F, Durbin DR. A randomized, clinical trial of a home safety intervention based in an emergency department setting. *Pediatrics.* 2004;113:1603-1608.
33. Dill PL, Wells-Parker E, Soderstrom CA. The emergency care setting for screening and intervention for alcohol use problems among injured and high-risk drivers: a review. *Traffic Inj Prev.* 2004;5:278-291.
34. Gentilello LM, Rivara FP, Donovan DM, et al. Alcohol interventions in a trauma center as a means of reducing the risk of injury recurrence. *Ann Surg.* 1999;230:473-480.
35. McBride CM, Emmons KM, Lipkus IM. Understanding the potential of teachable moments: the case of smoking cessation. *Health Educ Res.* 2003;18:156-170.
36. Gorin AA, Phelan S, Hill JO, Wing RR. Medical triggers are associated with better short- and long-term weight loss outcomes. *Prev Med.* 2004;39:612-616.
37. Mansour ME, Lanphear BP, DeWitt TG. Barriers to asthma care in urban children: parent perspectives. *Pediatrics.* 2000;106:512-519.
38. Wissow LS, Roter D, Bauman LJ, et al. Patient-provider communication during the emergency department care of children with asthma. *Med Care.* 1998;36:1439-1450.
39. Joseph CL, Havstad S, Anderson EW, Brown R, Johnson CC, Clark NM. Effect of asthma intervention on children with undiagnosed asthma. *J Pediatr.* 2005;146:96-104.

# Parental Misperceptions About Children and Firearms

*Frances Baxley, MD; Matthew Miller, MD, ScD*

**Objective:** To assess the accuracy of parental predictions about their children's self-reported behavior around household guns.

**Design:** Survey.

**Setting:** Family practice clinic in rural Alabama.

**Participants:** Convenience sample of parents and their children aged 5 to 14 years.

**Intervention:** Questionnaires about firearms administered separately to children and their parents.

**Main Outcome Measures:** Rates of concordance and discordance between parents and their children living in homes with guns about whether the children knew the storage location of household firearms and had ever handled firearms in the home.

**Results:** Of 420 parent-child dyads, 314 agreed to participate; 201 of the 314 homes contained guns. Children younger than 10 years were as likely as older children to report knowing the storage location (73% vs 79%, respectively) and to report having handled a household gun (36% vs 36%, respectively). Thirty-nine percent of parents who reported that their children did not know the storage location of household guns and 22% of parents who reported that their children had never handled a household gun were contradicted by their children's reports. Such discordance between parent and child reports was unrelated to whether parents stored their firearms locked away or had ever discussed firearm safety with their children.

**Conclusions:** Many parents who were living in homes with firearms and who reported that their children had never handled firearms in their homes were contradicted by their children's self-reports. Parents who locked their guns away and discussed gun safety with their children were as likely to be contradicted as parents who did not take such safety measures.

*Arch Pediatr Adolesc Med. 2006;160:542-547*

In the United States, firearm injury accounts for 10% of all deaths among children aged 5 to 14 years, surpassed only by malignant neoplasms and motor vehicle crashes.[1] For every firearm-related child death in this age group, 3 children are injured by nonfatal gunshots,[2] and 25% of those children have permanent physical sequelae.[3] Many of these injuries occur when a child gains access to household firearms that are stored loaded and/or in unlocked locations.[4-13]

Several medical associations advise parents who decide to keep firearms in the home to store all of the household guns locked away and to separate ammunition from the gun.[14-18] Despite these recommendations, firearms are as likely to be present in US homes with children as in homes without children, and they are often stored in unlocked locations and/or loaded.[19]

To our knowledge, our study is the first to examine how well parents' perceptions about their children's access to household guns coincide with their children's self-reports. We surveyed parents and their children (aged 5-14 years) attending a pediatric and family practice clinic in rural Alabama to assess how accurately parents could predict whether their children reported knowing where household firearms were stored and reported ever handling firearms in their homes.

Author Affiliations:
Department of Family and Community Medicine, San Francisco General Hospital, San Francisco, Calif (Dr Baxley); and Department of Health Policy and Management, Harvard School of Public Health, Boston, Mass (Dr Miller).

## METHODS

During the summer of 2002, research assistants in a pediatric ambulatory and family practice clinic located in rural Alabama approached all of the parents of children aged 5 to 14 years who were attending well-child or sick appointments and asked them to participate in this study. Parents and their children who agreed to participate were separated and given questionnaires about firearm ownership; neither heard the responses of the other. Parents completed questionnaires in the waiting area; in a separate room, children were read the questionnaires aloud and their responses were recorded. During each week of enrollment, at least three fourths of all of the parent-child pairs agreed to participate in the study. If a parent accompanied 2 children, the younger child's questionnaire was selected for inclusion in the study. Each parent and child questionnaire was coded with a unique alphanumeric identifier used to match parent-child pairs without the use of names. Written informed consent was obtained from parents, and verbal informed consent was obtained from children.

## PARENTS' SURVEYS

Parents' surveys comprised 20 items. Sixteen items were about firearms. After an initial set of demographic questions to determine the age and sex of their children, parents were asked a series of questions to elicit information about family firearm ownership and storage practices, including questions about whether household firearms were stored loaded and/or locked away when not in use (as distinguished from having child-safety locks). Specifically, parents were asked the following questions: (1) Are any firearms in your home stored loaded? (2) Is the firearm(s) in your home stored locked up when not in use? (3) Does your child know where the firearm(s) in your home is stored? (4) Has your child ever handled the firearm(s) in your home? and (5) Have you discussed firearm safety with your child?

## CHILDREN'S SURVEYS

Children's surveys comprised 18 items. Children were asked the following questions (in order): (1) Are there any toy guns in your house? (2) What kind of toy guns (including BB guns)? (3) Are there any real guns in your house? (4) Do you know where the real gun(s) in your house is stored? and (5) Have you ever held or played with the real gun(s) in your house? Completed questionnaires were placed in a box for data entry at a later time. To determine the rate of participation, data collectors tallied the number of families approached and the number who consented each day. Children who reported ever handling a firearm in their home were asked, "Was this done with your parents' knowledge and permission?" During the informed consent process, children were told that their answers would be kept confidential unless there was concern that they might be putting themselves at risk of harm.

Only households with firearms were included in the study. Data on firearm storage practices among all of the households with firearms are based on parent responses. Concordance and discordance rates between parental perceptions and children's self-report are based on parent-child dyads for which the parent reported at least 1 firearm in the home and for whom we have complementary responses regarding knowledge of where household firearms were stored and whether the child had ever handled a household firearm.

Concordance between parents' perceptions and the self-reported behavior of their children is summarized as the sensitivity of the parent's report relative to the child's behavior. For example, with respect to whether parents accurately identified children who had handled firearms in their homes, the sensitivity is the percentage of children who reported having handled firearms in the home who were correctly identified by their parents as having handled them (true positives divided by the sum of true positives plus false negatives). Discordance is expressed using another metric commonly used in screening literature: 1 minus the negative predictive value (1–NPV). The complement of the NPV (1–NPV) is the percentage of parents who reported that their children are naïve with respect to guns who were contradicted by their children's reports. Bivariate relationships between categorical variables were evaluated using Pearson $\chi^2$ statistic.

**Table 1. Characteristics of 201 Households With Children and Guns**

| Characteristic | Prevalence, No. (%) |
|---|---|
| Child's sex | |
| Boy | 100 (50) |
| Girl | 101 (50) |
| Child's age, y | |
| <10 | 93 (46) |
| 10-14 | 108 (54) |
| Purpose of gun(s) | |
| Protection only | 53 (26) |
| Recreation only | 90 (45) |
| Both protection and recreation | 58 (29) |
| Parent's report of child | |
| Knows gun storage location | 141 (70) |
| Does not know gun storage location | 60 (30) |
| Has handled gun in home | 61 (30) |
| Never handled gun in home | 140 (70) |
| Knows gun storage location and/or has handled gun in home | 147 (73) |
| Does not know gun storage location and has never handled gun in home | 54 (27) |
| Parent report | |
| Discussed gun safety with child | 183 (91) |
| Never discussed gun safety with child | 18 (9) |

## RESULTS

Of the 314 parents, 201 (64%) reported the presence of at least 1 gun in the home (**Table 1**). Approximately half of all of the children in homes with guns were boys (n=100); slightly more than half were aged 10 to 14 years (n=108). Forty-five percent of the homes contained guns for recreational purposes only, 26% for protection only, and 29% for both purposes. Ninety-one percent of parents in homes with guns discussed gun safety with their children. Nine in 10 parents were female.

Among the 196 parents who reported household guns and provided full information about how those guns were stored, 110 (56%) stored all of the household guns unloaded and locked away, 61 (31%) stored at least 1 firearm unloaded and unlocked, and 25 (13%) stored at least 1 gun loaded (**Table 2**). Gun storage practices were not significantly associated with the sex or age of the child, but they were associated with the reason parents gave for keeping a gun. Seventy percent of households with firearms used only for recreational purposes stored their firearms unloaded and locked away compared with 52% of households with firearms kept solely for protection (rate ratio [RR], 1.35; 95% confidence interval [CI], 1.00-1.83). Parents who reported that their children either knew the storage location of household firearms or had ever handled firearms in their homes were more likely to store all of the household firearms locked up and unloaded (RR, 1.53; 95% CI, 1.07-2.18).

One hundred ninety children and their parents living in homes with guns reported definitively whether they

**Table 2. Unadjusted Associations Between Household Firearm Storage Practices and Parental Responses to Questions About Children and Guns in 196 Homes**

| | Gun(s) Unloaded and Locked Away (n = 110) | | Gun(s) Unloaded and Unlocked (n = 61) | | Gun(s) Loaded (Locked or Unlocked) (n = 25) | |
|---|---|---|---|---|---|---|
| **Characteristic** | % | RR (95% CI) | % | RR (95% CI) | % | RR (95% CI) |
| Child's sex | | | | | | |
| Boy | 54 | 0.92 (0.71-1.17) | 36 | 1.37 (0.90-2.10) | 10 | 0.68 (0.32-1.44) |
| Girl | 59 | | 26 | | 15 | |
| Child's age, y | | | | | | |
| <10 | 55 | 0.97 (0.75-1.24) | 36 | 1.33 (0.87-2.01) | 9 | 0.57 (0.26-1.25) |
| 10-14 | 57 | | 27 | | 16 | |
| Purpose of gun(s) | | | | | | |
| Protection only | 52 | Reference | 36 | Reference | 12 | Reference |
| Recreation only | 70 | 1.35 (1.00-1.83)* | 24 | 0.66 (0.39-1.12) | 6 | 0.47 (0.15-1.48) |
| Both protection and recreation | 38 | 0.73 (0.48-1.12) | 38 | 1.05 (0.64-1.73) | 24 | 2.01 (0.83-4.86) |
| Parent's report of child | | | | | | |
| Knows gun storage location | 61 | 1.35 (0.99-1.86) | 26 | 0.61 (0.40-0.91)* | 13 | 1.08 (0.48-2.45) |
| Does not know gun storage location | 45 | | 41 | | 12 | |
| Has handled gun in home | 63 | 1.20 (0.93-1.54) | 23 | 0.67 (0.40-1.12) | 13 | 1.06 (0.48-2.32) |
| Never handled gun in home | 53 | | 35 | | 12 | |
| Knows gun storage location and/or has handled gun in home | 62 | 1.53 (1.07-2.18)* | 26 | 0.56 (0.37-0.83)† | 12 | 0.93 (0.41-2.09) |
| Does not know gun storage location and never handled gun in home | 40 | | 46 | | 13 | |
| Parent report | | | | | | |
| Discussed gun safety with child | 58 | 1.49 (0.82-2.70) | 29 | 0.58 (0.35-0.98) | 13 | 1.16 (0.30-4.54) |
| Never discussed gun safety with child | 39 | | 50 | | 11 | |

Abbreviations: CI, confidence interval; RR, rate ratio.
*$P<.05$.
†$P<.10$.

**Table 3. Unadjusted Correlates of Parent and Child Responses to Questions About Whether Children Know Where Firearms Are Stored or Ever Handled Firearms in the Home***

| | Parent Reported Child Knows Location (n = 141) | | Child Reported Knowing Location (n = 145) | | Parent Reported Child Has Handled Firearm (n = 61) | | Child Reported Having Handled Firearm (n = 63) | |
|---|---|---|---|---|---|---|---|---|
| **Characteristic** | % | RR (95% CI) | % | RR (95% CI) | % | RR (95% CI) | % | RR (95% CI) |
| Child's sex | | | | | | | | |
| Boy | 75 | 1.02 (0.86-1.21) | 79 | 1.08 (0.92-1.27) | 48 | 2.31 (1.45-3.68) | 52 | 2.84 (1.75-4.61) |
| Girl | 73 | | 73 | | 21 | | 18 | |
| Child's age, y | | | | | | | | |
| <10 | 67 | 0.84 (0.71-1.00) | 73 | 0.92 (0.78-1.08) | 36 | 1.06 (0.70-1.59) | 36 | 1.00 (0.67-1.49) |
| 10-14 | 80 | | 79 | | 34 | | 36 | |
| Household firearms | | | | | | | | |
| All locked | 79 | 1.19 (0.98-1.44) | 79 | 1.16 (0.97-1.39) | 37 | 1.25 (0.80-1.96) | 34 | 0.86 (0.58-1.29) |
| Some unlocked | 66 | | 71 | | 30 | | 39 | |
| Purpose of firearms | | | | | | | | |
| Protection only | 49 | Reference | 55 | Reference | 16 | Reference | 27 | Reference |
| Recreation only | 84 | 1.72 (1.27-2.34) | 88 | 1.58 (1.21-2.07) | 49 | 3.14 (1.53-6.43) | 42 | 1.56 (0.90-2.70) |
| Both protection and recreation | 80 | 1.63 (1.18-2.25) | 76 | 1.37 (1.02-1.85) | 27 | 1.74 (0.76-3.98) | 33 | 1.25 (0.67-2.35) |
| Parent report | | | | | | | | |
| Discussed gun safety with child | 78 | 2.07 (1.09-3.92) | 78 | 1.16 (0.83-1.63) | 38 | Undefined | 36 | 1.27 (0.54-2.98) |
| Never discussed gun safety with child | 38 | | 67 | | 0 | | 29 | |

Abbreviations: CI, confidence interval; RR, rate ratio.
*One hundred seventy-seven parents and their children reported definitively whether they thought their children had ever handled a firearm in their homes and had ever handled a firearm in their homes, respectively. One hundred ninety parents and their children reported definitively whether they thought their children knew where household firearms were stored and knew where household firearms were stored, respectively.

knew and thought their children knew, respectively, the storage location of the guns in their homes. One hundred forty-one of these parents (74%) reported that they thought their children knew where household firearms were stored (**Table 3**). Parents accompanying girls were as likely as parents accompanying boys to report that their children knew where household guns were stored. Parents were less likely, however, to expect their children

**Table 4. Concordance and Discordance Between Parent and Child Responses to Questions About Household Firearms***

| Characteristic | Child Reported Knowing Firearm Storage Location | | | | Child Reported Handling Firearms in the Home | | | |
|---|---|---|---|---|---|---|---|---|
| | Sensitivity, % | *P* Value | 1−NPV, % | *P* Value | Sensitivity, % | *P* Value | 1−NPV, % | *P* Value |
| All children | 87 | NA | 39 | NA | 60 | NA | 22 | NA |
| Child's sex | | | | | | | | |
| Boy | 84 | .31 | 50 | .11 | 64 | .33 | 36 | .002 |
| Girl | 90 | | 28 | | 50 | | 12 | |
| Child's age, y | | | | | | | | |
| <10 | 83 | .22 | 38 | .88 | 56 | .50 | 24 | .51 |
| 10-14 | 90 | | 40 | | 64 | | 19 | |
| Household firearms | | | | | | | | |
| All locked | 88 | .66 | 46 | .26 | 68 | .10 | 17 | .13 |
| Some unlocked | 85 | | 30 | | 48 | | 29 | |
| Purpose of firearms | | | | | | | | |
| Protection only | 69 | Reference | 33 | Reference | 25 | Reference | 24 | Reference |
| Recreation only | 87 | .10 | 71 | .02 | 71 | .04 | 23 | .96 |
| Both protection and recreation | 98 | .01 | 9 | .20 | 63 | .09 | 17 | .495 |
| Parent report | | | | | | | | |
| Discussed gun safety with child | 89 | .009 | 40 | .93 | 64 | .01 | 21 | .496 |
| Never discussed gun safety with child | 60 | | 39 | | 0 | | 29 | |

Abbreviations: NA, not applicable; NPV, negative predictive value.

*Concordance is the sensitivity of parents' responses to their children's responses and is equal to the percentage of children who reported ever handling a firearm in their homes who are identified by their parents as having handled a firearm in their homes (ie, true positives divided by the sum of true positives plus false negatives). Discordance is the complement of the NPV (1−NPV) and is equal to the percentage of parents who reported that their children have never handled a firearm in their homes and are contradicted by their children's reports.

to know the storage location if the children they accompanied were younger than 10 years (RR, 0.84; 95% CI, 0.71-1.00). Parents were more likely to report that their children knew where household firearms were stored if firearms were owned for recreation only (RR, 1.72; 95% CI, 1.27-2.34) or for both recreation and protection (RR, 1.63; 95% CI, 1.18-2.25) as compared with owning them for protection only. In contrast to parents' expectations, children younger than 10 years were as likely as older children to report that they knew the storage location of household firearms (RR, 0.92; 95% CI, 0.78-1.08). Children were also as likely to report knowing the storage location in homes where all of the household firearms were locked away as in homes with at least 1 unlocked firearm (RR, 1.16; 95% CI, 0.97-1.39).

One hundred seventy-seven children and their parents living in homes with guns reported definitively whether they had ever and thought their children had ever, respectively, handled a firearm in their homes. Sixty-one parents (34%) in gun-owning households reported that they thought their children had handled a firearm in the home (Table 3). Sixty-three children (36%) in homes with firearms reported that they had handled a firearm in the home. Parents accompanying boys were more likely than parents accompanying girls to expect their children to have handled a household gun (RR=2.31; 95% CI, 1.45-3.68). Compared with parents who kept guns solely for protection, parents who kept guns solely for recreational purposes were significantly more likely to report that their children had handled a gun in the home (RR, 3.14; 95% CI, 1.53-6.43). Consistent with parents' expectations, boys were more likely than girls to report having handled a gun in the home (RR, 2.84; 95% CI, 1.75-4.61); children younger than 10 years were as likely as children aged 10 to 14 years to have handled a firearm in the home (RR, 1.00; 95% CI, 0.67-1.29); children in homes where all of the guns were locked away were as likely as children in homes where firearms were unlocked to have handled firearms in the home (RR, 0.86; 95% CI, 0.58-1.29). Among the 63 children who reported ever handling a firearm in the home, 18 reported that they jointly owned the gun with a parent or grandparent; 1 child reported that the gun was his own (not shown). Sixty-two of 63 children who reported handling a firearm also reported that they had parental permission to do so.

The vast majority of children who reported knowing where firearms were stored in their homes were identified by their parents as knowing so (sensitivity, 87%) (**Table 4**). Significantly fewer parents who kept firearms solely for protection or who never discussed firearm safety with their children were able to identify whether their children knew the storage location (sensitivity, 69% and 60%, respectively, compared with all of the other parents). Overall, 39% of parents who reported that their children were unaware of the storage location of the guns were contradicted by their children's reports (1−NPV=39%). Among parents in households in which firearms were kept for protection, half reported that their children did not know where the household firearms were stored; 1 in 3 parents were contradicted by their children's reports (1−NPV=33%).

Of the children who reported that they had handled firearms in the home, 60% were identified by their parents as ever having handled firearms (sensitivity, 60%) (Table 4). Parents who kept firearms solely for protection were significantly less likely to accurately predict that their children reported having handled firearms in the home. Of the 27% of children living in homes where firearms were kept solely for protection who reported having handled firearms in their homes, only 1 in 4 were identified by their parents as ever having handled firearms (sensitivity, 25%) (Table 4). Among the 66% of all of the parents living in homes with firearms who reported that their children had not handled a household gun, 22% were contradicted by their children's reports (1–NPV=22%). Parents accompanying boys were significantly more likely than parents accompanying girls to be contradicted (36% vs 12%, respectively; $P<.05$).

## COMMENT

To our knowledge, this is the first study to explore whether a child's access to household firearms is associated with the age or sex of children in the home, the firearm counseling parents give children about gun safety, or the manner in which household firearms are stored. In contrast to previous studies[20,21] that found a greater tendency to store firearms unloaded and locked away if at least 1 child in the home was younger than 13 years, we found no statistically significant association between the child's age and household firearm storage practices. Although it is possible that parents in rural Alabama do not consider their children's age relevant to their decision about how to store household firearms, it is also possible that they factor age into storage decisions but distinguish between teenagers and younger children rather than between the ages of children included in our study, ie, between ages 5 and 14 years. It is also possible that we found no association between storage practices and the child's age because we only knew the age of the child accompanying the parent on the day of the survey rather than the age and sex distribution of all of the children living in each home.

In our study, children younger than 10 years were as likely as older children to report knowing where household firearms were stored as well as handling firearms in the home. Furthermore, children in homes where all of the guns were stored locked away were as likely as children in homes with firearms stored unlocked to report having handled a gun in the home. Because we do not know whether a child who reported ever handling firearms in his or her home had in fact handled firearms under storage conditions reflected by his or her parent's response to questions about current storage practices, we cannot say that locking firearms away had no effect on the ease with which children could gain access to household firearms. In addition, because we asked only whether the child knew where firearms were stored or had *ever* handled a household firearm rather than the frequency or ease with which the child could gain access to the gun (eg, in a moment of crisis), our findings do not necessarily mean that storage practices are ineffective in retarding children's access to guns in the home.

Parents' beliefs about their children's broader experience with guns were associated with storage practices. Parents who reported that their children either knew the storage location of household guns or had, at some point, handled a gun in the home were more likely than those who did not report these details to store all of the household firearms locked up and unloaded (62% vs 40%, respectively). This finding suggests that addressing the disconnect between parental perceptions and children's reported knowledge of and behavior around household firearms might induce some parents to alter their storage practices.

Although the vast majority of children (87%) who reported knowing where firearms were stored in their homes were correctly identified by their parents as knowing so, fewer children (60%) who reported ever handling firearms in their homes were correctly identified by their parents as having handled firearms. Findings from other studies[22,23] also suggest that parental misperceptions about their ability to predict their own children's likelihood of handling firearms are common. For example, in a survey of parents in metropolitan Atlanta, Ga, three quarters of parents believed that their children could tell the difference between toy and real guns and trusted that if their children encountered a real gun, they would tell an adult rather than handle it.[23] A later study[24] among different subjects demonstrated that 63% of boys between the ages of 8 and 12 years who found a real gun handled it (approximately half of whom thought it was a toy or were unsure whether it was a real gun), and 30% actually pulled the trigger with enough force to fire the gun had it not been disabled. More than 90% of these children said they had previously received gun safety instructions.

Ninety-one percent of parents in our study who lived in gun-owning households said they had discussed gun safety with their children; 64% reported storing guns locked away. Previous work[25] has shown that discussing gun safety and locking household guns away are the 2 measures most commonly relied on by parents to ensure their children's safety around guns in the home. Indeed, the American Academy of Pediatrics,[14] the American Academy of Family Practice,[15] and the American Medical Association[16] encourage these measures as effective means of decreasing pediatric firearm morbidity. Parents in our study who had taken such safety measures, however, were no less likely to be contradicted by their children's reports about knowing where household guns were stored or about handling household guns. This finding suggests that common preventative measures for ensuring children's safety around household guns often fail to prevent children from gaining unacknowledged access to household guns and may, in fact, lead parents to have misplaced confidence in their ability to accurately predict their children's broader experience with guns in the home.

Our study has various limitations. It is set in rural Alabama, limiting generalizability. Results are based on self-report and thus are subject to potential inaccuracies attributable to social desirability responses, recall bias, intentional distortions, or noncandid responses.[26] For example, parents might be reluctant to admit that their children know where firearms are stored (or that their children have handled firearms in the home) if they feel that researchers will not approve of this practice. Children may be reluctant to report handling firearms in the home for fear of being discovered to have broken house rules, or they may report having had permission when they did not.

Our finding that 62 of 63 children who reported having handling firearms in the home said they did so with parental knowledge may be an example of noncandid response since two fifths of parents accompanying these children reported that their children never handled a firearm in their homes. Alternatively, this apparent contradiction could result if fathers had accurate information about their children's activities around guns but mothers did not (as 90% of our parents were female). Nevertheless, although this discrepancy highlights a limitation to our study, our findings still suggest that in a region where gun ownership is prevalent and where children are frequently included in gun-related activities, many mothers appear to be misinformed about the extent of their children's potential access and exposure to household guns.

Despite these limitations, the picture that emerges from our study is that parental predictions, most of which are maternal predictions, tend to be more sensitive than specific with regard to their children's behavior around household guns. Two fifths of the parents in our study who reported that their children did not know the storage location of guns in their homes and one fifth who reported that their children never handled a firearm in their homes were contradicted by their children's reports.

**Accepted for Publication:** October 31, 2005.
**Correspondence:** Matthew Miller, MD, ScD, Harvard School of Public Health, 677 Huntington Ave, Room 305, Boston, MA 02115 (mmiller@hsph.harvard.edu).
**Author Contributions:** Drs Baxley and Miller had full access to all of the data in the study and take full responsibility for the integrity of the data and the accuracy of the data analysis.
**Acknowledgment:** We acknowledge the helpful comments provided by Deborah Azrael, PhD, David Hemenway, PhD, and Renee M. Johnson, PhD, and the support of Nath Camp, MD, and the entire staff of the family and pediatric practice at which this survey took place.

## REFERENCES


1. Centers for Disease Control and Prevention. Web-based Injury Statistics Query and Reporting System (WISQARS). Available at: http://www.cdc.gov/ncipc/wisqars. Accessed August 1, 2005.
2. Eber GB, Annest JL, Mercy JA, Ryan GW. Nonfatal and fatal firearm-related injuries among children aged 14 years and younger: United States, 1993-2000. *Pediatrics.* 2004;113:1686-1692.
3. Rivara FP, Mueller BA. The epidemiology and causes of childhood injuries. *J Soc Issues.* 1987;43:13-31.
4. Coyne-Beasley T, Schoenbach VJ, Johnson RM. "Love our kids, lock your guns": a community-based firearm safety counseling and gun lock distribution program. *Arch Pediatr Adolesc Med.* 2001;155:659-664.
5. Grossman DC, Reay DT, Baker SA. Self-inflicted and unintentional firearm injuries among children and adolescents: the source of the firearm. *Arch Pediatr Adolesc Med.* 1999;153:875-878.
6. Wintemute GJ, Teret SP, Kraus JF, Wright MA, Bradfield G. When children shoot children: 88 unintended deaths in California. *JAMA.* 1987;257:3107-3109.
7. Grossman DC, Mueller BA, Riedy C, et al. Gun storage practices and risk of youth suicide and unintentional firearm injuries. *JAMA.* 2005;293:707-714.
8. Miller M, Azrael D, Hemenway D, Vriniotis M. Firearm storage practices and rates of unintentional firearm deaths in the United States. *Accid Anal Prev.* 2005;37:661-667.
9. Martin JR, Sklar DP, McFeeley P. Accidental firearm fatalities among New Mexico children. *Ann Emerg Med.* 1991;20:58-61.
10. Beaver BL, Moore VL, Peclet M, Haller JA, Smialek J, Hill JL. Characteristics of pediatric firearm fatalities. *J Pediatr Surg.* 1990;25:97-100.
11. Powell EC, Jovtis E, Tanz RR. Incidence and circumstances of nonfatal firearm-related injuries among children and adolescents. *Arch Pediatr Adolesc Med.* 2001;155:1364-1368.
12. Brent DA, Perper JA, Moritz G, Baugher M, Schweers J, Roth C. Firearms and adolescent suicide: a community case-control study. *AJDC.* 1993;147:1066-1071.
13. Kellermann AL, Rivara FP, Somes G, et al. Suicide in the home in relation to gun ownership. *N Engl J Med.* 1992;327:467-472.
14. American Academy of Pediatrics. Firearms injury prevention. Available at: http://www.aap.org/family/tipp-firearms.htm. Accessed August 1, 2005.
15. American Academy of Family Physicians. Firearms/handgun firearms, handguns, and assault weapons. Available at: http://www.aafp.org/x6823.xml. Accessed August 1, 2005.
16. American Medical Association. Policy No. H-145.990: prevention of firearm accidents in children. Available at: http://www.ama-assn.org/apps/pf_new/pf_online?f_n=browse&doc=policyfiles/HnE/H-145.990.HTM. Accessed August 1, 2005.
17. Committee on Injury and Poison Prevention; American Academy of Pediatrics. Firearm-related injuries affecting the pediatric population. *Pediatrics.* 2000;105:888-895.
18. Society for Adolescent Medicine. Adolescents and firearms: position paper of the Society for Adolescent Medicine. *J Adolesc Health.* 1998;23:117-118.
19. Johnson RM, Coyne-Beasley T, Runyan CW. Firearm ownership and storage practices, US households, 1992-2002: a systematic review. *Am J Prev Med.* 2004;27:173-182.
20. Schuster MA, Franke TM, Bastian AM, Sor S, Halfon N. Firearm storage patterns in US homes with children. *Am J Public Health.* 2000;90:588-594.
21. Azrael D, Miller M, Hemenway D. Are household firearms stored safely? it depends on whom you ask. *Pediatrics.* 2000;106:E31.
22. Hardy MS, Armstrong FD, Martin BL, Strawn KN. A firearm safety program for children: they just can't say no. *J Dev Behav Pediatr.* 1996;17:216-221.
23. Farah MM, Simon HK, Kellermann AL. Firearms in the home: parental perceptions. *Pediatrics.* 1999;104:1059-1063.
24. Jackman GA, Farah MM, Kellermann AL, Simon HK. Seeing is believing: what do boys do when they find a real gun? *Pediatrics.* 2001;107:1247-1250.
25. Knight-Bohnhoff K, Harris MB. Parents' behaviors, knowledge, and beliefs related to unintentional firearm injuries among children and youth in the southwest. *J Pediatr Health Care.* 1998;12:139-146.
26. Aday L. *Designing and Conducting Health Surveys.* San Francisco, Calif: Jossey-Bass Publishers; 1989.


In 1943 an editor of Pocket Books asked me to write a book and said, half jokingly, "It doesn't have to be a very good book because at 25 cents a copy we can sell ten thousand every year."

—From *A Better World for Our Children*, by Benjamin Spock, 1994

# Autism and Autism Spectrum Disorders

FEW PROBLEMS IN CHILD HEALTH HAVE GARnered as much attention in the last few years as autism. There are a number of reasons for this. First, a new category of disease termed "autism spectrum disorders" has been created that encompasses not only autism but disorders such as pervasive developmental disorder, Asperger disorder, and Rett syndrome. Second, the reported prevalence of the problem has increased markedly in recent years from as few as 4 per 10 000 children in the 1980s to as many as 50 per 10 000 today. It is unclear how much of this increased prevalence is because of better identification of affected children, increased services for children with autism, or broadened case definitions. Finally, at least some of the attention given to autism is concern that it might be induced by toxins in the environment affecting children before or after birth. Parents are concerned about these issues and turn to child experts—pediatricians—for advice.

The mission of *Archives of Pediatrics & Adolescent Medicine* is to advance child health by publishing carefully reviewed science on important health issues. The ARCHIVES will therefore publish a special theme issue in April 2007 on autism spectrum disorder that includes autism so as to foster a better understanding of the environmental and genetic risk (and protective) factors for autism; efficient and sensitive methods to screen for autism, especially in the primary care physician's office; confirmatory tools to accurately diagnose autism and autism spectrum disorders; and information on the natural history of autism. We are especially interested in rigorously conducted studies on interventions for children with autism, as well as for their families. We will be happy to consider articles that consider policy implications of diagnosis and treatment of children with autism from the point of view of their families, communities, schools, and society as a whole. The common theme of articles we seek is that they be rigorous work that advances the field and contributes ultimately to improve the health of these children. In our experience, articles in these theme issues, taken as a whole, have made important contributions to advancing the field.

Papers submitted by September 1, 2006, will have the best chance for inclusion in this issue. Please consult our Web site at www.archpediatrics.com for submission information.

*Frederick P. Rivara, MD, MPH*

**Correspondence**: Dr Rivara, *Archives of Pediatrics & Adolescent Medicine*, Department of Pediatrics, Child Health Institute, University of Washington, 6200 NE 74th St, Suite 210, Seattle, WA 98115-8160 (archpediatrics @jama-archives.org).

# Meeting the Need for Transplantable Organs Through the US Donation System

BRATTON ET AL[1] REPORT SOME OF THE recent approaches being used to improve donor organ availability. Although their focus was pediatric patients, they point out that the problem has risen to crisis proportions for children and adults alike. Certainly, the donor shortage has become one of the most pressing problems facing the field of transplantation on many levels. Improved results have established transplantation as the preferred treatment for many forms of organ failure, leading to the tremendous growth in transplant waiting lists. This growth contrasts dramatically with only modest increases in the number of available transplantable organs.[2] This frustrating reality challenges patients, their families, and caregivers alike as the promise of transplantation cannot be delivered with increasing frequency. Instead of transplantation, candidates must endure long waiting times, often leading to medical deterioration and sometimes death, never having had the opportunity to receive a needed organ.

*See also page 468*

The Organ Donation Best Practices resulted from a recent initiative of the US Department of Health and Human Services called the Organ Donation Breakthrough Collaborative.[3] This initiative sought to identify successful approaches used in the best organ procurement organizations as an educational template. Thought leaders representing the organ donation and transplantation communities worked with government officials to examine attributes of those organizations where donation rates appeared high, setting goals to increase the average conversion rate of eligible donors from 43% to 75%

in the nation's largest 200 hospitals, to increase donations by up to 1900 per year, and to increase the number of transplantation procedures by 6000 per year.[3] A qualitative case study approach identified and described best practices associated with higher organ donation rates. Acknowledged limitations of the study included a relatively small sample size, the use of nonvalidated assumptions regarding "high performers," and the absence of a control group. Nevertheless, a series of principles were developed into a list of 15 best practices. These were then applied in a pilot study that sought to determine whether the approach might improve organ donation rates.

The Breakthrough Collaborative has been successful in bringing government officials together with the organ donation and transplant community to conduct a successful project, and the Department of Health and Human Services has been quite proactive in its support of organ donation during recent years. However, the US transplant waiting list presently exceeds 90 000 people in need of transplants, yet, as the authors observed, 14 138 people donated 27 025 organs for transplantation (deceased and living donors) in 2004.[2] During that same time, more than 45 000 new transplant candidates were added to the United Network for Organ Sharing transplant waiting lists.[2] The modest gains in donation activity have been inadequate, and efforts have not yet impacted significantly on the magnitude of the donor organ shortage. Conversion rates (percentage of the total potential organ donors who become actual donors) for deceased donors have been estimated in the 40% to 50% range nationally from a total pool approximating 13 000 potential donors.[4] Assuming the Breakthrough Collaborative approaches are successful over time and conversion rates can be increased to the 75% range nationally, one might anticipate approximately 10 000 deceased donors annually from individuals meeting traditional brain death criteria.

Recovery of organs from individuals who become donors after cardiac death represents another approach with potential for increasing the number of transplantable organs. Although concern that organs from such donors may present technical and management challenges, it appears that donors after cardiac death could add substantially to the number of deceased donor organs.[5,6] This approach has been used with varying success; again, commonly cited barriers have included concern that donor organ quality will be inferior (resulting from longer warm ischemia time) and added expense (resulting from delayed or poor graft function after transplantation). Although analyses to date have been somewhat anecdotal, reports have been encouraging. A detailed, systematic evaluation of transplant outcomes from donors after cardiac death should be undertaken because demonstration of similar results to more standard donor organs would almost certainly lead to widespread acceptance of this approach.

The consent process represents another area where some have argued for change. Our system, based on altruism and volunteerism, has been the subject of ethical and legal debate since the very early applications of clinical transplantation. Individuals must specify their willingness to be an organ donor, either by advanced directive or after death through consent from surviving family members. The most common advanced directive has been the driver's license, where people may "opt in" to become an organ donor at the time of initial receipt or renewal. Unfortunately, this depends on the interest of the employees at state motor vehicle offices, who are often inadequately trained to discharge this important responsibility. Additionally, there has been a widespread reluctance among hospital personnel to override objections of surviving family members (even in the presence of a signed donor card), especially because discussion about organ donation usually has not occurred prior to the tragic death of a loved one.

"Mandated choice" or "required request" represents one alternative to our traditional opt-in system. This method forces consideration of the donation question because individuals (or surviving family members) must specify their wish to donate or not. This approach has been used, but in practice, the actual request usually comes at the time of tragedy, and it does not appear to have had significant impact on donation rates. The most evident advantage of mandated choice is that individual wishes become known, but the most obvious downside is that people are forced to make a decision about a subject about which they have been inadequately informed and usually at a very inopportune time.

Another alternative has been called "presumed consent." This assumes that a deceased individual is presumed to consent for organ donation unless she or he has registered a prior refusal. The individual's rights are protected because each person must be offered an advanced opportunity to register a written refusal. This approach would spare people the emotional stress of the organ donation process, especially the "bad timing" effects associated with the present system. It has also been suggested that this is a more psychologically acceptable approach vs the present opt-in system. On the other hand, like the current system, a sophisticated infrastructure must be in place to register and track each person's decision. Also, some have argued that the assumption of consent inherent to this approach undermines the altruism and volunteerism of the present system, that it would negatively impact individual rights, and that the approach would increase the potential for abuse through conscription of organs.

Presumed consent has been operational in several European countries, including Belgium and Spain, for some years. The Spanish approach uses a modification whereby relatives of a potential donor must be approached to determine the deceased person's wishes. This so-called soft presumed consent approach, combined with a very effective donation advocacy system, has been credited among the reasons leading to the remarkable improvement in organ donation rates in Spain during recent years.[7] A similar soft presumed consent is used in Belgium, where the transplant surgeon must search for any opposition to donation as well as search the national registry prior to proceeding. Despite the inherent problems, many have advocated in favor of such an approach in the United States; the Advisory Committee on Transplantation of the US Department of Health and Human Services recently recommended that demonstration projects should be undertaken to test the feasibility of adopting a presumed consent model.[8]

Finally, living donation has also received considerable recent attention. The practice of living donor transplantation has evolved from one associated with considerable reluctance to become a common activity in most major medical centers. Recognizing that living donation is a complicated subject, the severe shortage of organs from deceased donors, reports indicating superior outcomes using live donor organs, and the widespread societal acceptance of live donation as a "good thing to do," physicians have become increasingly more vigorous advocates.

Live donation represents the only setting in medicine where healthy people undergo major operative intervention without medical need (that is, their own need), and this activity must be considered as a special category. Many ethical considerations have been topics of concern, especially as live donation has become increasingly more common.[9-11] The unique relationship between the transplant surgeon and the live donor, the specific information that should be disclosed to organ donors, medical considerations making donation acceptable, determination of acceptable risk (and who decides), and compensation for donation represent a few important and controversial subjects. Growing international concerns with a "black market" for donor organs and the potential for exploitation represent additional concerns.[12-14]

As transplantation has transitioned from a promising clinical research activity to a remarkably successful treatment for end-stage organ failure, the serious shortage of suitable organs has generated considerable tension. Efforts such as the Breakthrough Collaborative and others have focused attention on the problem. However, progress has been very slow. The serious mismatch between demand for organs and inadequate supply requires continuing work to identify durable and meaningful solutions. Much debate lies ahead as ongoing efforts strive to deliver the promise of this remarkable therapy for all who might benefit.

*Marc I. Lorber, MD*

**Correspondence:** Dr Lorber, Surgery Section of Organ Transplantation, Yale University School of Medicine, 333 Cedar St, FMB 112, New Haven, CT 06520 (marc.lorber@yale.edu).

## REFERENCES

1. Bratton SL, Kolovos NS, Roach ES, McBride V, Geiger JL, Meyers RL. Pediatric organ transplantation needs: organ donation best practices. *Arch Pediatrics.* 2006; 160:468-472.
2. United Network for Organ Sharing data. Available at: http://www.unos.org/data. Accessed March 10, 2006.
3. The Organ Donation Breakthrough Collaborative: best practices final report (September 2003). Available at: http://organdonor.gov/bestpractice.htm. Accessed March 8, 2005.
4. Sheehy E, Conrad SL, Brigham LE, et al. Estimating the number of potential organ donors in the United States. *N Engl J Med.* 2003;349:667-674.
5. D'Alessandro AM, Fernandez LA, Chin LT, et al. Donation after cardiac death: the University of Wisconsin experience. *Ann Transplant.* 2004;9:68-71.
6. Howard RJ, Schold JD, Cornell DL. A 10-year analysis of organ donation after cardiac death in the United States. *Transplantation.* 2005;80:564-568.
7. Miranda B, Vilardell J, Grinyo JM. Optimizing cadaveric organ procurement: the Catalan and Spanish experience. *Am J Transpl.* 2003;3:1189-1196.
8. Recommendations to the HHS secretary: recommendation 37. Available at: http://www.organdonor.gov/acot.html. Accessed March 10, 2006.
9. Abecassis M, Adams M, Adams P, et al. Consensus statement on the live organ donor. *JAMA.* 2000;284:2919-2926.
10. Morris PJ, Monaco AP. The living donor. *Transplantation.* 2003;76:1242.
11. US Department of Health and Human Services Advisory Committee on Organ Transplantation. Available at: http://www.organdonor.gov/acot.html. Accessed March 10, 2006.
12. Rothman DJ. Ethical and social consequences of selling a kidney. *JAMA.* 2002; 288:1640-1641.
13. Goyal M, Mehta RL, Schneiderman LJ, Sehgal AR. Economic and health consequences of selling a kidney in India. *JAMA.* 2002;288:1589-1593.
14. Eighth Plenary Meeting of the Fifty-Seventh World Health Assembly in Geneva. Human organ and tissue transplantation. *Transplantation.* 2005;79:635.

# Implications for Primary Care of Diabetes and Impaired Fasting Glucose Prevalence in Adolescents

IN HIS ARTICLE IN THIS ISSUE, DUNCAN[1] ESTIMATES the prevalence for type 1 diabetes mellitus (T1DM) and type 2 diabetes mellitus (T2DM) from self-reports by 4370 adolescents aged 12 to 19 years in the National Health and Nutrition Examination Survey, and frequency of impaired fasting glucose in a tested subsample of subjects. A fundamental problem in

*See also page 523*

interpreting the diabetes prevalence data is the case definition of T1DM and of T2DM. During the past several decades, we have gone from classifying the main forms of diabetes by age group (juvenile onset vs maturity onset) to differentiating by treatment (insulin-dependent vs non-insulin-dependent) to the contemporary separation by etiology.[2] Type 1 diabetes mellitus is a disease predominantly of autoimmune-mediated insulin deficiency, whereas T2DM results from a combination of insulin resistance and inadequate islet cell capacity to meet the increased insulin demands. The case definition in this study, which lacks validation from medical records, harks back to classification by treatment; those who reported using insulin were considered to have T1DM and those who reported that they were not using insulin were considered to have T2DM. The concern about case definition based on insulin use is exemplified by the recognition that pediatric endocrinologists treat approximately 50% of their patients who have T2DM with insulin, either as monotherapy or in conjunction with oral hypoglycemic agents. Two of 10 subjects in

Duncan's study were taking insulin and thus classified as having T1DM, but they were also taking oral agents, making it likely that they had T2DM. Only 1 of the 8 subjects who self-reported diabetes and that they were not taking insulin reported that they were taking an oral hypoglycemic agent. The diagnosis of diabetes is therefore questionable in 7 of these subjects because only about 10% of pediatric patients with T2DM can control their disease for more than a brief period with lifestyle change alone.[3,4] These concerns are magnified when the small numbers of purported subjects with diabetes are stratified by ethnicity for each diabetes type, resulting in wide 95% confidence intervals for the estimates.[1]

Despite these shortcomings, the percentage estimates for total diabetes represented by T1DM and T2DM in this age group are reasonably consistent with contemporary clinic-based data that varies by ethnic mix, with T2DM accounting for 15% to 45% of all diabetes cases.[3-5] Furthermore, the total number of individuals in this age group with each type of diabetes is consistent with other estimates.

What is particularly relevant to the practitioner in this article is the examination of fasting glucose, hemoglobin $A_{1c}$, and C-peptide levels in a subsample of 1496 subjects who answered "no" to the question of whether they had diabetes. Applying the contemporary criterion for impaired fasting glucose of 5.6 mmol/L (100 mg/dL), 11% were abnormal, with fairly tight 95% confidence intervals of 8% to 14%. As would be expected, there was a significant association between glucose levels and body mass index percentile for age and sex, hemoglobin $A_{1c}$, insulin, and C-peptide levels. This is a substantial percentage of young people with impaired fasting glucose, especially considering that in the evolution of T2DM, fasting serum glucose increases following the rise in postprandial glycemia.

Many practitioners may be surprised by the low glucose level that serves as the criterion for impaired fasting glucose. Twenty-five years ago, the National Diabetes Data Group recommended a fasting plasma glucose concentration greater than 7.8 mmol/L (140 mg/dL) for the diagnosis of diabetes.[6] An international expert committee lowered this limit to 7 mmol/L (126 mg/dL) in 1997 based on epidemiologic evidence of complications such as retinopathy at lower levels.[7] This report also introduced the concept of impaired fasting glucose for individuals with fasting glucose levels of 6.1 to 6.9 mmol/L (110-125 mg/dL). When this committee reconvened only a few years later, it analyzed data from 4 diverse populations to ascertain a level of fasting glucose predictive of the development of diabetes and concluded that 6.1 mmol/L (110 mg/dL) was inappropriately high, recommending that impaired fasting glucose be considered at levels of 5.6 to 6.9 mmol/L (100-125 mg/dL).[8] Rather than being arbitrary consensus, these changes reflect increasing sophistication of epidemiologic analysis. They also reflect the appreciation that such measurements exist on a continuum from absolutely normal to absolutely abnormal, with predictive value for the eventual development of disease increasing as one moves more toward the abnormal. This has also been the experience with blood pressure and lipid measurements, for which "normal" cutoff values have continuously been lowered as more long-term data accumulate. A further indication of this phenomenon has been the recent report of a long-term follow-up of 13 163 Israeli Defense Forces recruits aged 26 to 45 years. Those with normal fasting plasma glucose levels of less than 5.6 mmol/L (<100 mg/dL) in the upper range of 5.1 to 5.5 mmol/L (91-99 mg/dL) were at much greater risk of developing T2DM during the years of follow-up than those with lower levels. This risk was heightened by greater body mass index and serum triglyceride levels above 1.69 mmol/L (150 mg/dL).[9]

What are the implications for primary care practice with regard to the high frequency of impaired fasting glucose in youth and the recognition that normal fasting glucose in the upper range is a risk factor? Impaired fasting glucose has been associated with progression to diabetes in adults, but the natural history has not been defined for adolescents. Whether weight loss will prevent or slow the progression to diabetes in this age group is also unknown, although studies in adults with impaired glucose tolerance indicate that lifestyle change (weight loss and increased physical activity) is effective in decreasing progression to T2DM over a period of 5 to 6 years.[10-13] Furthermore, the tracking of cardiovascular risk factors from childhood into adulthood is well documented and emphasizes the importance of testing and intervention for those who treat children and adolescents.[14]

The American Diabetes Association published a consensus statement on T2DM in children in 2000 which recommended fasting plasma glucose measurement in children older than 10 years who have a body mass index greater than the 85th percentile for age and sex and have 2 other risk factors, including first- or second-degree relatives with T2DM, high-risk ethnicity, and signs of insulin resistance such as acanthosis nigricans, hypertension, dyslipidemia, or polycystic ovarian syndrome. These recommendations were not evidence-based, and included the option that clinical judgment may be used to test high-risk patients who might not meet these criteria.[15] It now seems appropriate to focus on the clinical judgment criterion for glucose as well as lipid testing for any child or adolescent who is overweight, or who has a family history of T2DM, hypertension, early cardiovascular disease, or dyslipidemia. Abnormal test results need to be verified on more than one occasion and, because postprandial blood glucose rises earlier in the evolution of T2DM than does fasting glucose concentration, a 2-hour postprandial or postglucose load value should be obtained. Adolescents who have been considered sufficiently at risk for testing for impaired fasting glucose should be retested every couple of years if normal according to the American Diabetes Association guidelines. More frequent testing should be motivated by indications of increasing insulin resistance such as weight gain, appearance or worsening of acanthosis nigricans, hypertension, or polycystic ovarian syndrome. These developments should also motivate lipid testing. Not only do abnormal glucose values need to be treated, but upper-range normal values can be cited to motivate lifestyle changes.

A substantial number of pediatric patients, those with body mass index greater than 85th percentile for age and sex, are going to require the kind of monitoring for cardiovascular risk factors that has been considered standard of care for older adults. The costs of this monitoring are insignificant in comparison to the potential for prevention of early cardiovascular disease, but only if there are individual and community resources to effect lifestyle change, and if necessary, maintain compliance with medications for hyperglycemia, hypertension, and dyslipidemia. The obstacles are enormous in contemporary society where daily physical activity opportunities are limited for many youngsters, entertainment is sedentary, and high-fat, high-energy foods are cheap, ubiquitous, convenient, and heavily promoted. It is to be hoped that the recognition of the public health time bomb reflected in the report by Duncan[1] will lead to a pervasive societal effort to prevent obesity, a daunting task of such magnitude that enormous community and governmental commitments will be required.[16]

*Arlan L. Rosenbloom, MD*

**Correspondence:** Dr Rosenbloom, Children's Medical Services Center, 1701 SW 16th Ave, Gainesville, FL 32608 (rosenal@peds.ufl.edu).

## REFERENCES

1. Duncan GE. Prevalence of diabetes and impaired fasting glucose levels among US adolescents: National Health and Nutrition Examination Survey, 1999-2002. *Arch Pediatr Adolesc Med.* 2006;160:523-528.
2. American Diabetes Association. Diagnosis and classification of diabetes mellitus. *Diabetes Care.* 2005;28(suppl 1):S37-S42.
3. Rapaport R, Silverstein JH, Garzarella L, Rosenbloom AL. Type 1 and type 2 diabetes mellitus in childhood in the United States: practice patterns by pediatric endocrinologists. *J Pediatr Endocrinol Metab.* 2004;17:871-877.
4. Macaluso CJ, Bauer UE, Deeb LC, et al. Type 2 diabetes mellitus among Florida children and adolescents, 1994 through 1998. *Public Health Rep.* 2002;117:373-379.
5. Rosenbloom AL, Silverstein JH. *Type 2 Diabetes in Children and Adolescents: A Clinician's Guide to Diagnosis, Epidemiology, Pathogenesis, Prevention, and Treatment.* Alexandria, Va: American Diabetes Association; 2003:17-24.
6. National Diabetes Data Group. Classification and diagnosis of diabetes mellitus and other categories of glucose intolerance. *Diabetes.* 1979;28:1039-1057.
7. Report of the Expert Committee on the Diagnosis and Classification of Diabetes Mellitus. *Diabetes Care.* 1997;20:1183-1197.
8. Expert Committee on the Diagnosis and Classification of Diabetes Mellitus. Report of the Expert Committee on the Diagnosis and Classification of Diabetes Mellitus. *Diabetes Care.* 2003;26(suppl 1):S5-S20.
9. Tirosh A, Shai I, Tekes-Manova D, et al; Israeli Diabetes Research Group. Normal fasting plasma glucose levels and type 2 diabetes in young men. *N Engl J Med.* 2005;353:1454-1462.
10. Pan XR, Li GW, Hu YH, et al. Effects of diet and exercise in preventing NIDDM in people with impaired glucose tolerance: the Da Qing IGT and Diabetes Study. *Diabetes Care.* 1997;20:537-544.
11. Tuomilehto J, Lindstrom J, Eriksson JG, et al. Prevention of type 2 diabetes mellitus by changes in lifestyle among subjects with impaired glucose tolerance. *N Engl J Med.* 2001;344:1343-1350.
12. Swinburn BA, Metcalf PA, Ley SJ. Long-term (5-year) effects of a reduced-fat diet intervention in individuals with glucose intolerance. *Diabetes Care.* 2001;24:619-624.
13. Diabetes Prevention Program Research Group. Reduction in the incidence of type 2 diabetes with lifestyle intervention or metformin. *N Engl J Med.* 2002;346:393-403.
14. Freedman DS, Kahn LK, Dietz WH, Srinivasan SR, Berenson GS. Relationship of childhood obesity to coronary heart disease risk factors in adulthood: the Bogalusa Heart Study. *Pediatrics.* 2001;108:712-718.
15. American Diabetes Association. Type 2 diabetes in children. *Diabetes Care.* 2000;23:381-389.
16. Rosenbloom AL, Silverstein JH. Primary and secondary prevention and treatment of type 2 diabetes in children. *Ann Nestle.* 2005;63:23-37.

# Prospects for the Prevention of Allergy

## *A Losing Battle or a Battle Still Worth Fighting?*

ONE OF THE GREAT CONTROVERSIES IN PEdiatric allergy during the past 2 decades has been and remains the potential to prevent the development of allergy and asthma. The controversy stems largely from the lack of quality studies and conflicting data from the few studies that have been done; some studies have demonstrated significant protection and most others have shown little or no effect.

*See also page 502*

Possible approaches to allergy prevention include maternal dietary restrictions during pregnancy, breastfeeding, dietary restrictions while breastfeeding, the use of hypoallergenic infant formulas, and delays in the introduction of foods into the infant's diet, both in general and specifically in regard to more allergenic foods.[1] In addition, the use of probiotics or other immunomodulatory agents and the avoidance of environmental allergens and irritants, such as tobacco smoke, have been suggested as possible approaches to allergy prevention.

The apparently rapid increase in the prevalence of allergic disease during the past few decades compels us to consider anything that might stem this rising tide, although it should be equally compelling to avoid recommendations that are not grounded in science. The hesitancy to make unfounded recommendations is particularly important because all of these suggested approaches require substantial education and motivation on the part of the family; most are inconvenient, many are costly, and some may place infants and mothers at significant nutritional risk.

Among these possible approaches, delaying the introduction of solid foods into the infant's diet is one of the most commonly recommended. As with most of these recommendations, this one was based on a few studies that suggested benefit without questioning their validity, and based on largely ignoring other negative studies. We are therefore indebted to Tarini and colleagues[2] for their excellent review of this topic in this issue of the ARCHIVES.

In the review by Tarini et al, a total of 13 studies were identified that met their inclusion criteria, only one of which was a controlled trial. Five of these 13 studies found a positive association between early solid feeding and eczema, while 4 found no such association. None of the studies provided strong evidence to support the association between early solid feeding and the development of persistent food allergy, persistent asthma, or allergic rhinitis. Therefore, they concluded that early solid feeding may increase the risk of eczema but that there is little data supporting an association. As with most studies regarding allergy prevention, they recommended that additional controlled trials be performed to provide sound advice to physicians and families regarding the timing of solid food introduction.

Given this degree of uncertainty, what then should we be recommending to our patients? The first decision is whether a recommendation should be made globally, that is, to all families regardless of their atopic predisposition or whether it should be reserved for those with a higher risk of developing allergies. Although asthma and allergies commonly occur in children from families without any history of allergic disease,[3,4] a careful family history remains the most simple and effective tool to screen for atopic risk.

At this point, most prevention strategies are best reserved for children at higher risk of developing allergies, at least until more definitive strategies can be recommended. There are probably only 2 measures that should be universally recommended, breastfeeding and the avoidance of environmental tobacco smoke. Environmental tobacco smoke exposure, especially during pregnancy and infancy, clearly increases the risk of childhood allergy and asthma.[5-7] Although no study has proven that environmental tobacco smoke avoidance is beneficial, it is still logical to advise avoidance of environmental tobacco smoke exposure.

With regard to dietary measures, exclusive breastfeeding should be recommended first and foremost. However, this is not meant to imply that breastfeeding has been conclusively shown to prevent allergy. While some studies have demonstrated protection,[8,9] others have failed to do so.[10,11] Two meta-analyses on this subject concluded that exclusive breastfeeding does seem to have some protective effect on the development of allergy,[12,13] and given the other benefits of breastfeeding, there is little doubt about this recommendation.

As for other dietary measures, the recommendations are less clear. Maternal avoidance of allergenic foods during pregnancy has not been shown to be helpful,[14] although there is evidence that sensitization may begin in utero and many experts still recommend that at least peanut and tree nuts be avoided in the maternal diet during pregnancy. Maternal avoidance of allergenic foods during lactation, particularly milk, egg, and peanut, has been studied extensively without conclusive results, but a general notion that while there may be a preventative effect in the first 1 to 2 years of life, there is not likely to be any longer-term benefit.[15,16] In addition, these avoidance diets during pregnancy and lactation may put mothers and infants at nutritional risk and should only be considered for highly motivated families with a high risk of allergy.

The use of hydrolyzed infant formulas as a preventative measure has also been studied extensively. Most studies have shown that extensively hydrolyzed formulas are clearly superior to cow's-milk formulas and some have shown that partially hydrolyzed formulas might be as or even more effective than extensively hydrolyzed products.[17-20] This approach has not been shown to be superior to exclusive breastfeeding, but may make sense as a supplement to breast milk in high-risk infants.

The final dietary strategies involve the delay in food introduction to the infant and toddler. As noted previously, convincing proof for the preventive effects of the delayed introduction of solid foods is lacking. It has also been suggested that certain allergenic foods, such as milk, egg, and peanut, be withheld from the diet of at-risk children. In fact, a current position statement from the American Academy of Pediatrics recommends withholding milk until age of 1 year, egg until age of 2 years, and peanut, tree nuts, and fish until age of 3 years in high-risk infants.[21] It should also be noted, however, that there is little evidence to support these recommendations and a similar position statement from the European Societies for Paediatric Allergology and Clinical Immunology and Paediatric Gastroenterology, Hepatology, and Nutrition makes no such recommendation.[22]

Other potential approaches that have been studied with mixed results include the avoidance of house dust mites and other environmental allergens,[23-25] the use of probiotics and other immunomodulatory agents,[26-29] and certain medications.[30] There is some evidence that each of these approaches might have some effect, but none appear to be long lasting. For example, probiotics have been shown to potentially reduce early atopic dermatitis, but convincing data on the prevention of food and other allergies is currently lacking. This is an area of active research, however, that we will be hearing more about in the next few years.

Given these limited and often conflicting data, how should we proceed? Is this really a losing battle or a battle still worth fighting? Families with affected children are often intensely committed to reduce allergy in subsequent children and should certainly be provided with this information. We need to be careful when providing information, however, without being dogmatic given the current state of knowledge. In the long run, I remain extremely optimistic that some combination of these, and potentially other new strategies, will have a significant impact on the rising tide of allergic disease.

*Robert A. Wood, MD*

**Correspondence:** Dr Wood, Johns Hopkins University, 600 N Wolfe St, Baltimore, MD 21287 (rwood@jhmi.edu).

## REFERENCES

1. Arshad SH. Primary prevention of asthma and allergy. *J Allergy Clin Immunol.* 2005;116:3-14.
2. Tarini BA, Carroll AE, Sox CM, Christakis DA. Systematic review of the relationship between early introduction of solid foods to infants and the development of allergic disease. *Arch Pediatr Adolesc Med.* 2006;160:502-507.
3. Bergmann RL, Edenharter G, Bergmann KE, et al. Predictability of early atopy by cord blood-IgE and parental history. *Clin Exp Allergy.* 1997;27:752-760.
4. Bergmann R, Woodcock A. Whole population or high-risk group? Childhood asthma. *Eur Respir J Suppl.* 1998;27:9s-12s.
5. Jaakkola JJ, Gissler M. Maternal smoking in pregnancy, fetal development, and childhood asthma. *Am J Public Health.* 2004;94:136-140.

6. Gilliland FD, Berhane K, Li YF, Rappaport EB, Peters JM. Effects of early onset asthma and in utero exposure to maternal smoking on childhood lung function. *Am J Respir Crit Care Med.* 2003;167:917-924.
7. Lodrup Carlsen KC, Carlsen KH. Effects of maternal and early tobacco exposure on the development of asthma and airway hyperreactivity. *Curr Opin Allergy Clin Immunol.* 2001;1:139-143.
8. Schoetzau A, Filipiak-Pittroff B, Franke K, et al. Effect of exclusive breast-feeding and early solid food avoidance on the incidence of atopic dermatitis in high-risk infants at 1 year of age. *Pediatr Allergy Immunol.* 2002;13:234-242.
9. Gruskay FL. Comparison of breast, cow, and soy feedings in the prevention of onset of allergic disease: a 15-year prospective study. *Clin Pediatr (Phila).* 1982; 21:486-491.
10. Wright AL, Holberg CJ, Taussig LM, Martinez FD. Factors influencing the relation of infant feeding to asthma and recurrent wheeze in childhood. *Thorax.* 2001; 56:192-197.
11. Sears MR, Greene JM, Willan AR, et al. Long term relation between breast feeding and development of atopy and asthma in children and young adults: a longitudinal study. *Lancet.* 2002;360:901-907.
12. Gdalevich M, Mimouni D, Mimouni M. Breast-feeding and the risk of bronchial asthma in childhood: a systematic review with meta-analysis of prospective studies. *J Pediatr.* 2001;139:261-266.
13. Mimouni Bloch A, Mimouni D, Mimouni M, Gdalevich M. Does breastfeeding protect against allergic rhinitis during childhood: a metaanalysis of prospective studies. *Acta Paediatr.* 2002;91:275-279.
14. Falth-Magnusson K, Kjellman NI. Allergy prevention by maternal elimination diet during late pregnancy: a 5-year follow-up of a randomized study. *J Allergy Clin Immunol.* 1992;89:709-713.
15. Zeiger RS, Heller S, Mellon MH, et al. Effect of combined maternal and infant food-allergen avoidance on development of atopy in early infancy: a randomized study. *J Allergy Clin Immunol.* 1989;84:72-89.
16. Zeiger RS, Heller S. The development and prediction of atopy in high risk children: follow-up at age seven years in a prospective randomized study of combined maternal and infant food allergen avoidance. *J Allergy Clin Immunol.* 1995; 95:1179-1190.
17. von Berg A, Koletzko S, Grubl A, et al. The effect of hydrolyzed cow's milk formula for allergy prevention in the first year of life: the German Infant Nutritional Intervention Study, a randomized double-blind trial. *J Allergy Clin Immunol.* 2003; 111:533-540.
18. Halken S, Hansen KS, Jacobsen HP, et al. Comparison of a partially hydrolyzed infant formula with two extensively hydrolyzed formulas for allergy prevention: a prospective, randomized study. *Pediatr Allergy Immunol.* 2000;11:149-161.
19. Ram FS, Ducharme FM, Scarlett J. Cow's milk protein avoidance and development of childhood wheeze in children with a family history of atopy. *Cochrane Database Syst Rev.* 2002;3:CD003795.
20. Hays T, Wood RA. A systematic review of the role of hydrolyzed infant formulas in allergy prevention. *Arch Pediatr Adolesc Med.* 2005;159:810-816.
21. American Academy of Pediatrics, Committee on Nutrition: hypoallergenic infant formulas. *Pediatrics.* 2000;106:346-349.
22. Host A, Koletzko B, Dreborg S, et al. Dietary products used in infants for treatment and prevention of food allergy. Joint Statement of the European Society for Paediatric Allergology and Clinical Immunology (ESPACI) Committee on Hypoallergenic Formulas and the European Society for Paediatric Gastroenterology, Hepatology and Nutrition (ESPGHAN) Committee on Nutrition. *Arch Dis Child.* 1999;81:80-84.
23. Arshad SH, Bojarskas J, Tsitoura S, et al. Prevention of sensitization to house dust mite by allergen avoidance in school age children: a randomized controlled study. *Clin Exp Allergy.* 2002;32:843-849.
24. Simpson A, Simpson B, Custovic A, Craven M, Woodcock A. Stringent environmental control in pregnancy and early life: the long term effects on mite, cat and dog allergen. *Clin Exp Allergy.* 2003;33:1183-1189.
25. van Strien RT, Koopman LP, Kerkhof M, et al. Mattress encasings and mite al lergen levels in the Prevention and Incidence of Asthma and Mite Allergy study. *Clin Exp Allergy.* 2003;33:490-495.
26. Kalliomaki M, Salminen S, Arvilommi H, Kero P, Koskinen P, Isolauri E. Probiotics in primary prevention of atopic disease: a randomized placebo-controlled trial. *Lancet.* 2001;357:1076-1079.
27. Kalliomaki M, Salminen S, Poussa T, Arvilommi H, Isolauri E. Probiotics and prevention of atopic disease: 4-year follow-up of a randomised placebo-controlled trial. *Lancet.* 2003;361:1869-1871.
28. Rautava S, Kalliomaki M, Isolauri E. New therapeutic strategy for combating the increasing burden of allergic disease: probiotics—a Nutrition, Allergy, Mucosal Immunology and Intestinal Microbiota (NAMI) Research Group report. *J Allergy Clin Immunol.* 2005;116:31-37.
29. Peat JK, Mihrshahi S, Kemp AS, et al. Three-year outcomes of dietary fatty acid modification and house dust mite reduction in the Childhood Asthma Prevention Study. *J Allergy Clin Immunol.* 2004;114:807-813.
30. Allergic factors associated with the development of asthma and the influence of cetirizine in a double-blind, randomised, placebo-controlled trial: first results of ETAC. Early Treatment of the Atopic Child. *Pediatr Allergy Immunol.* 1998;9:116-124.

# Attending

SO SLEEP
small and feral, scurries
about the floor of a dark kitchen,
eludes me, as the buses
roar by on the avenue
along the light rails
of their head lamps
and I wait
for the release of sleep.

As a young man
I could not sleep
when it was the night on call
or the night after that night or
the night immediately before. Babies
fled to the far side
of their steel-barred cribs
when I approached

out of the dark with a white tray
of sharps, intent on settling with them
and returning to sleep. Their parents
watched, thin-lipped, or left the room.
But on this night I cannot sleep

I prowl gray stairs
from ward to ward.
The parents cradling their babes
continue rocking
as I approach their chairs

as I crouch, silver-haired
to introduce myself. They relax
their shoulders; they smile,
as they should. They seem relieved
to see me here.
I am astonished. It is good.

*Ted McMahon, MD*

## A Young Mind in a Growing Brain

*by Jerome Kagan and Norbert Herschkowitz, 257 pages, ISBN 0-8058-5425-8, Mahwah, NJ, Lawrence Erlbaum Associates, 2005.*

This book is written by a psychologist, well known through his illustrious career in the research of normal child development, and a pediatrician with an expertise in neuroscience. Its focus is on the "simultaneous examination of the psychological milestones of human development . . . and what has been learned about brain growth,"(pix) during the first 8 years of life. They repeatedly point to the limitations of our current knowledge, both in developmental behavior and the neuroscience of development. They take great pains to say that correlations in timing between changes in the brain and psychological competence do not prove that one is the cause of the other. Despite these limitations, their motivation in writing this book is their belief that simultaneous descriptions of the behavioral and biological features of a developmental stage will generate fruitful questions for further research in both psychology and neuroscience.

As someone who specializes in the field of developmental and behavioral pediatrics, I was especially interested in the summary of research findings in the psychology of development. The importance of this topic to pediatricians was stressed by Julius B. Richmond, MD, a scholar in our field, who said that child development is a basic science for pediatrics.[1] Much of the research in child development is recent and was unknown to me. The findings that relate to the early development of language were fascinating. Pediatricians, either with general or subspecialty interests, will find these reviews of the emergence of behavioral competencies to be of great interest.

Each chapter is devoted to a specific period in development, beginning with a review of psychological competencies that emerge during that period and then moving to what is known about neurodevelopment during that same age span. Preceding this sequence of topics, the authors present an overview entitled "Brain and Behavioral Development" where they introduce themes that are repeated throughout the book. They point out that the simultaneous emergence of a psychological competence and a brain structure does not mean, necessarily, a causal connection between the 2, although they also assert that a psychological competence cannot emerge before the neurological structures are in place. Thus, specific aspects of psychological development are at least partially dependent on the maturation of neuronal circuits. Again, there is new information about the development of neural connections, and the correlations between this and psychological development are interesting and provocative.

The chapter on prenatal development contains a well-written and interesting review of fetal brain development that is of special relevance in recognizing the potential impact of factors that may have a deleterious effect on that process.

I was especially fascinated by chapter 5, "The Second Year," and its review of research on the development of speech. Chapter 4, called "The Second Transition: 7 to 12 Months," contains a thought-provoking review of the concept of temperament, a topic that Jerome Kagan has studied extensively. In that section, the authors review the psychological research and also discuss temperament in the context of research on attachment. They argue convincingly that interpretation of infants' reaction to the "strange situation" is probably due more to the infants' temperaments than to the qualities of their caregiver relationships.

I found some of the neuroscience difficult to follow without a more extensive background in the field, and I do not have the background to comment on the accuracy of the science contained in these chapters. Also, the summarizing chapter, called "Reflections," was repetitive and overly wordy.

This book will, I believe, be of great interest to pediatricians, especially those whose interests include development and behavior. The book provides a fascinating review of what is known about child development during the early years. As the authors hoped, the description of brain structures and connections that arise during definable periods of psychological development provokes many interesting questions about their connection. This book should, therefore, also be read by those interested in research in these areas.

*Esther H. Wender, MD*

**Correspondence:** Dr Wender, Department of Pediatrics, University of Washington School of Medicine, 5880 NE Twin Spits Rd, Hansville, WA 98340 (wenfried@earthlink.net).

1. Richmond JB. Child development: a basic science for pediatrics. *Pediatrics*. 1967;39:649.

## PEDIATRICS

WESTERN NEW YORK: Expanding practice seeking additional Pediatrician. Board Certified/Board Eligible. Send CV to Rajiv C. Parikh, MD, 1134 Central Ave, Dunkirk, NY 14048.

PEDIATRIC OPPORTUNITIES AVAILABLE: NORTH SEATTLE Metro Area, Suburban Los Angeles, South Eastern Idaho. Single and multi specialty groups, very attractive compensation and benefits, partnership. Call Chris Warner 206-782-1277, E-mail: panther@seanet.com

## ACKNOWLEDGMENT SERVICE

Acknowledgments in confirmation of advertising orders are sent each week. Upon receipt, please verify that your ad will be running under the appropriate heading and that your scheduling is correct. Changes to the schedule, cancellations or corrections must be communicated in writing by fax, e-mail, or regular mail prior to the published closing date of the scheduled issue.

## JOURNAL ADVERTISER INDEX

**CLASSIFIED ADVERTISING** .................. 559
http://www.amapublications.com

**GLAXOSMITHKLINE**
Boostrix .................. 521-522, COVER 2-457
Havrix .................. 493-494, COVER 3-4
Pediarix .................. 479-480, 529-530

**MERCK & COMPANY**
Gardasil .................. 464A-C
Rotateq .................. 472A-E

*Demographic and "Mini" inserts and/or ROB ad pages
While every precaution is taken to ensure accuracy, we cannot guarantee against the possibility of an occasional change or omission in the preparation of this index.

ARCHIVES OF PEDIATRICS & ADOLESCENT MEDICINE

# CONTACT INFORMATION

## EDITORIAL OFFICE

**Editorial Office Information:** *Archives of Pediatrics & Adolescent Medicine*, Department of Pediatrics, Child Health Institute, University of Washington, 6200 NE 74th St, Suite 210, Seattle, WA 98115-8160; phone: (206) 685-3573; fax: (206) 685-3572; e-mail: archpediatrics@jama-archives.org.

**Electronic Submission:** Manuscripts should be submitted via our online manuscript submission and review system (http://manuscripts.archpediatrics.com). Manuscripts submitted through our online system should not also be submitted by mail or fax. Signed authorship forms should be sent by regular mail or fax. See the Instructions for Authors (www.archpediatrics.com) for more details.

## CONSORTIUM OF *JAMA* & *ARCHIVES* JOURNALS

The *Archives of Pediatrics & Adolescent Medicine* is a member of the consortium of AMA journals listed below.

- The Journal of the American Medical Association (JAMA)
- Archives of Dermatology
- Archives of Facial Plastic Surgery
- Archives of General Psychiatry
- Archives of Internal Medicine
- Archives of Neurology
- Archives of Ophthalmology
- Archives of Otolaryngology–Head & Neck Surgery
- Archives of Pediatrics & Adolescent Medicine
- Archives of Surgery

## *JAMA/ARCHIVES* MEDIA RELATIONS

Jann Ingmire; phone: (312) 464-5262; e-mail: mediarelations@jama-archives.org.

## *ARCHIVES OF PEDIATRICS* ONLINE

*Archives of Pediatrics & Adolescent Medicine* is available online at www.archpediatrics.com.

## *JAMA/ARCHIVES* REPRINTS

**Author Reprints:** Anna Goins at (312) 464-2477; fax: (312) 464-5843; e-mail: anna.goins@ama-assn.org. Minimum order: 100 reprints.

**Educational Reprints:** Rhonda Bailey Brown at (312) 464-2513; fax: (312) 464-5843; e-mail: rhonda.brown@ama-assn.org. Minimum order: 100 reprints.

**Commercial Reprints:** Phone: (312) 464-0776; fax: (312) 464-0708; e-mail: reprints@ama-assn.org. Minimum order: 500 reprints.

## PERMISSIONS

Information about obtaining permission to republish, reprint, or adapt material published in *Archives of Pediatrics & Adolescent Medicine* is available from Rhonda Bailey Brown; phone: (312) 464-2513; fax: (312) 464-5843; e-mail: permissions@ama-assn.org.

## DOCUMENT DELIVERY

Copies of individual articles are available online at www.archpediatrics.com and from the following: Infotrieve, phone: (800) 422-4633; fax: (310) 208-5971; URL: www.infotrieve.com; e-mail: orders@infotrieve.com; Institute for Scientific Information (ISI), phone: (800) 603-4367; fax: (856) 787-1679; URL: http://www.isidoc.com; e-mail: service@isidoc.com; Dialog Information Services; Proquest; Ovid Technologies, Inc; and EBSCO.

The ARCHIVES OF PEDIATRICS & ADOLESCENT MEDICINE (ISSN 01072–4710) is published monthly by the American Medical Association, 515 N State St, Chicago, IL 60610–0946, and is an official publication of the Association. The ARCHIVES OF PEDIATRICS & ADOLESCENT MEDICINE reaches more than 30 900 readers in over 83 countries each month. Periodicals postage paid at Chicago, Ill, and at additional mailing offices. GST registration number 12622 5556 RT. Canada Post International Publications Mail (Canadian Distribution) Sales Agreement No. 318728. POSTMASTER, send all address changes to *Archives of Pediatrics & Adolescent Medicine,* c/o the AMA Unified Service Center, American Medical Association, 515 N State St, Chicago, IL 60610. Printed in the USA.

## ADVERTISING

Information about advertising is available from the following sales representatives and online at www.archpediatrics.com.

**Account Manager:** Tim Melroy (nationally); phone: (973) 263-9191 ext 213.

**Manager, Marketing Services:** Nancy Bell; phone: (973) 263-9191 ext 216.

**Advertising Office:** 119 Cherry Hill Rd, Suite 330, Parsippany, NJ 07054-1114; phone: (973) 263-9191.

**Classified Advertising:** Thalia Moss, 515 N State St, Chicago, IL 60610; phone: (800) 262-2260; e-mail: classifieds@jama-archives.org.

## ADVERTISING PRINCIPLES

Advertisements in this issue have been reviewed to comply with the principles governing advertising in AMA publications. A copy of these principles is available on request and online at www.archpediatrics.com. The appearance of advertising in AMA publications is not an AMA guarantee or endorsement of the product or the claims made for the product by the manufacturer.

## ADDRESS CHANGES

Send all address changes to *Archives of Pediatrics & Adolescent Medicine*, c/o the AMA Unified Service Center, American Medical Association, 515 N State St, Chicago, IL 60610. Notification of address changes must be made at least 6 weeks in advance; include both old and new addresses and a recent mailing label if sending via mail.

## SUBSCRIPTION RATES AND SERVICE

Subscription rates are shown in the table below. For service in the US and Americas, inquiries on pricing, address changes, missing issues, subscription billing, subscription renewal, and back issues, contact the AMA Unified Service Center, 24 hours a day, 7 days a week.

**AMA members:** phone: (800) 262-3211; e-mail: msc@ama-assn.org. **Other physicians and nonphysician customers, including subscription agents:** phone: (800) 262-2350 or (312) 670-7827; fax: (312) 464-5831; e-mail: ama-subs@ama-assn.org. **Inquiries:** Unified Service Center, American Medical Association, PO Box 10946, Chicago, IL 60610-0946. For subscribers with mailing addresses outside the United States & Americas: Contact *JAMA & Archives* Journals, c/o EMD GmbH, Birkenstr.67, 10559 Berlin, Germany. Phone: +49 (30) 33099828; fax: +49 (30) 33099829; e-mail: ama@emd-germany.de.

**Annual Subscription Rates**

| | United States | Americas | UK | Rest of World |
|---|---|---|---|---|
| INDIVIDUAL | | | | |
| Print and Online | $185 | $240 | £165 | €250 |
| INSTITUTION | | | | |
| Print and Online | $375 | $485 | £315 | €470 |

In Canada, US rate plus GST. Rates for residents and medical students available at pubs.ama-assn.org, or from the AMA Unified Service Center.

## HAVRIX®
## (Hepatitis A Vaccine, Inactivated)

The following is a brief summary only; see full prescribing information for complete product information.

**INDICATIONS AND USAGE:** HAVRIX is indicated for active immunization of persons ≥12 months of age against disease caused by hepatitis A virus (HAV). Primary immunization should be administered at least 2 weeks prior to expected exposure to HAV. When passive protection against hepatitis A is required either following exposure to hepatitis A virus or in persons requiring both immediate and long-term protection, HAVRIX may be administered concomitantly with immune globulin (IG) with different syringes and at different injection sites. Duration of immunity following a complete vaccination schedule has not been established.

**CONTRAINDICATIONS:** Hypersensitivity to any component of the vaccine, including neomycin, is a contraindication (see DESCRIPTION in full prescribing information). This vaccine is contraindicated in patients with previous hypersensitivity to any hepatitis A-containing vaccine.

**WARNINGS:** There have been rare reports of anaphylaxis/anaphylactoid reactions following commercial use of the vaccine. The tip cap and the rubber plunger of the needleless prefilled syringes contain dry natural latex rubber that may cause allergic reactions in latex sensitive individuals. The vial stopper is latex-free. Hepatitis A has a relatively long incubation period. Hepatitis A vaccine may not prevent hepatitis A infection in those who have an unrecognized hepatitis A infection at the time of vaccination. Additionally, it may not prevent infection in those who do not achieve protective antibody titers (although the lowest titer needed to confer protection has not been determined).

**PRECAUTIONS: General:** Prior to immunization with HAVRIX, the patient's current health status and medical history should be reviewed. The physician should review the patient's immunization history for possible vaccine sensitivity, previous vaccination-related adverse reactions and occurrence of any adverse–event-related symptoms and/or signs, in order to determine the existence of any contraindication to immunization with HAVRIX and to allow an assessment of benefits and risks. Appropriate medical treatment and supervision should be readily available for immediate use in case of a rare anaphylactic reaction following the administration of the vaccine. Epinephrine injection (1:1,000) and other appropriate agents used for the control of immediate allergic reactions must be immediately available. A separate, sterile syringe and needle or a sterile disposable unit should be used for each patient to prevent the transmission of other infectious agents from person to person. Needles should be disposed of properly and should not be recapped. As with any vaccine, if administered to immunosuppressed persons, including those receiving immunosuppressive therapy, the expected immune response may not be obtained. **Drug Interactions:** HAVRIX may be given concurrently with Hib conjugate vaccines in children 15 to 18 months of age (see CLINICAL PHARMACOLOGY in full prescribing information and ADVERSE REACTIONS). The safety of HAVRIX given concomitantly with INFANRIX has been evaluated (see ADVERSE REACTIONS). Insufficient data are available to assess the immune response of a fourth dose of DTaP vaccine when administered with HAVRIX. There are limited data to assess the concomitant use of HAVRIX with other vaccines. (See Immune Response to Concomitantly Administered Vaccines in full prescribing information.)

**Carcinogenesis, Mutagenesis, Impairment of Fertility:** HAVRIX has not been evaluated for its carcinogenic potential, mutagenic potential, or potential for impairment of fertility. **Pregnancy:** Pregnancy Category C. Animal reproduction studies have not been conducted with HAVRIX. It is also not known whether HAVRIX can cause fetal harm when administered to a pregnant woman or can affect reproduction capacity. Give HAVRIX to a pregnant woman only if clearly needed. **Nursing Mothers:** It is not known whether HAVRIX is excreted in human milk. Because many drugs are excreted in human milk, use caution when administering HAVRIX to a nursing woman. **Pediatric Use:** The safety and effectiveness of HAVRIX have been evaluated in 20,436 subjects 1 year to 18 years of age. (See CLINICAL PHARMACOLOGY and DOSAGE AND ADMINISTRATION in full prescribing information.) The safety and effectiveness of HAVRIX have not been established in subjects less than 12 months of age. **Geriatric Use:** Clinical studies of HAVRIX did not include sufficient numbers of subjects 65 years of age and older to determine whether they respond differently from younger subjects. Other reported clinical experience has not identified differences in overall safety between these subjects and younger adult subjects.

**ADVERSE REACTIONS:** As with all pharmaceuticals, however, it is possible that expanded commercial use of the vaccine could reveal rare adverse events. The adverse events most frequently reported by volunteers in clinical trials were injection-site soreness (56% of adults; 21% of children); headache (14% of adults; less than 9% of children). Other solicited and unsolicited events are listed below:

**Incidence 1% to 10% of Injections:** ***Local Reactions at Injection Site:*** Induration, redness, swelling; ***Body as a Whole:*** Fatigue, fever (>37.5°C), malaise; ***Gastrointestinal:*** Anorexia, nausea.

**Incidence <1% of Injections:** ***Local Reaction at Injection Site:*** Hematoma; ***Dermatologic:*** Pruritus, rash, urticaria; ***Respiratory:*** Pharyngitis, other upper respiratory tract infections; ***Gastrointestinal:*** Abdominal pain, diarrhea, dysgeusia, vomiting; ***Musculoskeletal:*** Arthralgia, elevation of creatine phosphokinase, myalgia; ***Hematologic:*** Lymphadenopathy; ***Central Nervous System:*** Hypertonic episode, insomnia, photophobia, vertigo.

**Additional safety data:** Safety data were obtained from 2 additional sources in which large populations were vaccinated. In an outbreak setting in which 4,930 individuals were immunized with a single dose of either 720 EL.U. or 1440 EL.U. of HAVRIX, the vaccine was well tolerated and no serious adverse events due to vaccination were reported. Overall, less than 10% of vaccinees reported solicited general adverse events following the vaccine. The most common solicited local adverse event was pain at the injection site, reported in 22.3% of subjects at 24 hours and decreasing to 2.4% by 72 hours.

In a field efficacy trial, 19,037 children received the 360 EL.U. dose of HAVRIX. The most commonly reported adverse events were injection-site pain (9.5%) and tenderness (8.1%), reported following first doses of HAVRIX. Other adverse events were infrequent and comparable to the control vaccine ENGERIX-B® [Hepatitis B Vaccine (Recombinant)].

In subjects with chronic liver disease, HAVRIX was safe and well tolerated. Local injection site reactions were similar among all 4 groups, and no serious adverse reactions attributed to the vaccine were reported in subjects with chronic liver disease.

***Safety Data for HAVRIX 720 EL.U./0.5 mL Beginning at 11 Months of Age:*** In the multicenter study described under CLINICAL PHARMACOLOGY in full prescribing information, parents/guardians recorded local and general symptoms on diary cards for 4 days (Days 0 to 3) after vaccination. In the 3 groups of children who received HAVRIX alone, safety data were available for 723 children who received 1,396 documented doses of HAVRIX. Additional safety data were available for 181 children who received HAVRIX coadministered with INFANRIX and Hib conjugate vaccine. Most adverse events were mild and transient. The frequencies of solicited local and systemic reactions following receipt of HAVRIX were monitored during the 4-day observation period.

The following rates of solicited adverse events in children who received their first dose of HAVRIX alone at between 11 and 25 months of age were observed. Among local reactions: pain was reported in 15-21% of subjects, redness in 16-21%, swelling in 8% of subjects. Among general reactions, irritability was reported in 24-36% of subjects, loss of appetite in 16-19% of subjects, drowsiness in 15-17% of subjects and fever >39.5°C in ≤2% of subjects. Following the booster dose of HAVRIX, among local reactions: pain was reported in 16-21% of subjects, redness in 17-22%, swelling in 8-10% of subjects. Following the booster dose of HAVRIX, among general reactions, irritability was reported in 19-29% of subjects, loss of appetite in 14-18% of subjects, drowsiness in 13-16% of subjects and fever >39.5°C in ≤1% of subjects.

Drowsiness and loss of appetite occurred at statistically significantly higher rates in subjects 15 to 18 months of age who received Hib conjugate vaccine (PRP-T) and INFANRIX concomitantly with HAVRIX as compared to subjects 15 to 18 months of age who received Hib conjugate vaccine (PRP-T) and INFANRIX (drowsiness 34% and 22% and loss of appetite 29% and 19%, respectively). With the exception of fever (>39.5°C), the solicited general symptoms occurred at statistically significantly higher rates in subjects 15 to 18 months of age who received Hib conjugate vaccine (PRP-T) and INFANRIX concomitantly with HAVRIX as compared to subjects 15 to 18 months of age who received HAVRIX alone (irritability 46% and 30%, drowsiness 34% and 17%, and loss of appetite 29% and 17%, respectively).

A febrile seizure was reported in an 18-month old subject two days after receiving the first dose of HAVRIX. Other serious adverse events reported during the course of this study included a single case each of hepatitis ~5 months post dose 1, insulin-dependent diabetes ~4 months post dose 1, and Kawasaki's disease ~3 1/2 months post dose 1. The association of these events with vaccination is unknown.

**Postmarketing Reports:** Rare voluntary reports of adverse events in people receiving HAVRIX since market introduction include the following: ***Local:*** Localized edema; ***Body as a Whole:*** Anaphylaxis/anaphylactoid reactions, somnolence; ***Cardiovascular:*** Syncope; ***Hepatobiliary:*** Jaundice, hepatitis; ***Dermatologic:*** Erythema multiforme, hyperhydrosis, angioedema; ***Respiratory:*** Dyspnea; ***Hematologic:*** Lymphadenopathy, thrombocytopenia; ***Central Nervous System:*** Convulsions, encephalopathy, dizziness, neuropathy, myelitis, paresthesia, Guillain-Barré syndrome, multiple sclerosis; ***Other:*** Congenital abnormality.

The US Department of Health and Human Services has established the Vaccine Adverse Events Reporting System (VAERS) to accept reports of suspected adverse events after the administration of any vaccine, including, but not limited to, the reporting of events required by the National Childhood Vaccine Injury Act of 1986. The toll-free number for VAERS forms and information is 1-800-822-7967. Reporting forms may also be obtained at the VAERS website at www.vaers.org.

Manufactured by **GlaxoSmithKline Biologicals**, Rixensart, Belgium

Distributed by **GlaxoSmithKline**, Research Triangle Park, NC 27709



BRS-HA:L20

---

**References: 1.** Centers for Disease Control and Prevention. Recommended childhood and adolescent immunization schedule—United States, 2006. *MMWR.* 2006;54(51&52):Q1–Q4. **2.** Bell BP, Shapiro CN. Hepatitis A virus. In: Long SS, Pickering LK, Prober CG, eds. *Principles and Practice of Pediatric Infectious Diseases.* 2nd ed. Philadelphia, Pa: Churchill Livingstone; 2003:1188–1192. **3.** Armstrong GL, Bell BP. Hepatitis A virus infection in the United States: model-based estimates and implication for childhood immunizations. *Pediatrics.* 2002;109:839–845.



Printed in USA. HAP283R0 February 2006

# ARCHIVES OF PEDIATRICS & ADOLESCENT MEDICINE

WWW.ARCHPEDIATRICS.COM

JUNE 2006


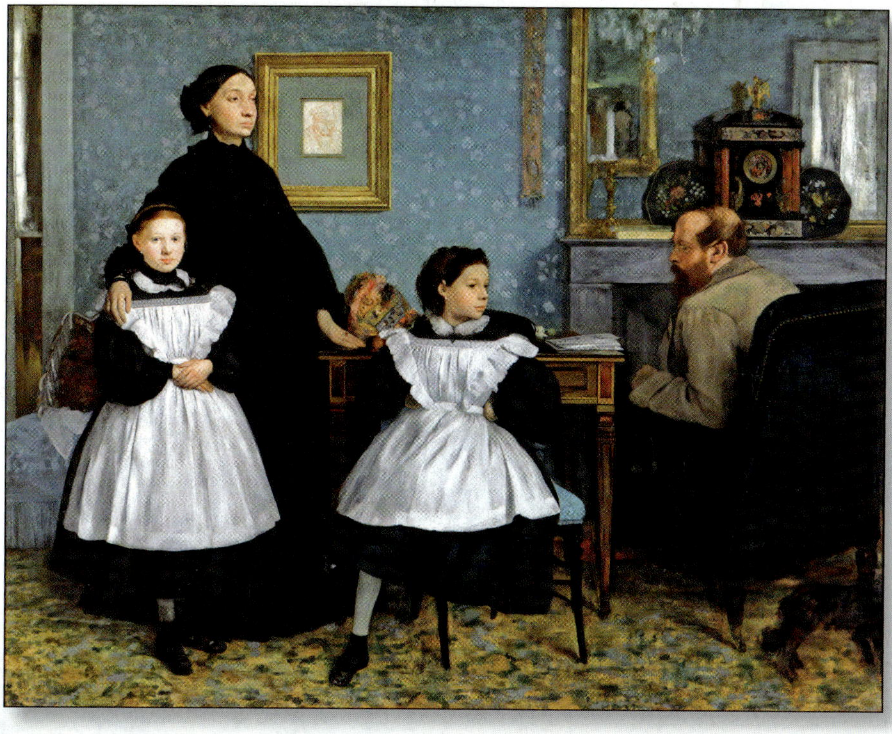

Edgar Degas (1834-1917), *The Bellelli Family* (1859-1867). See page 568.

RACE, ETHNICITY, SOCIOECONOMIC STATUS, AND OBESITY

EFFECTS OF REGULAR PHYSICAL ACTIVITY ON GLYCEMIC CONTROL

NEBULIZER-TARGETED ASTHMA EDUCATION

A WEB-BASED PEDIATRIC ADVANCED LIFE SUPPORT COURSE

COMPLETE TABLE OF CONTENTS ON PAGE 561

JAMA & ARCHIVES JOURNALS
American Medical Association

# ARCHIVES OF PEDIATRICS & ADOLESCENT MEDICINE

JUNE 2006 VOLUME 160, NUMBER 6 PAGES 561-664


## COVER ART


**Edgar Degas (1834-1917): *The Bellelli Family*, 1859-1867** 568
*Thomas D. Koepsell, MD, MPH*


## COMMENTARY


**International Exchanges: A Missed Opportunity in Pediatric Graduate Education** 570
*Joel J. Alpert, MD; Samuel L. Katz, MD; Tom Lissauer, MD*


## ARTICLES


**Effects of Regular Physical Activity on Control of Glycemia in Pediatric Patients With Type 1 Diabetes Mellitus** 573
*Antje Herbst, MD; Rainer Bachran, MD; Thomas Kapellen, MD; Reinhard W. Holl, PhD; for the DPV Science Initiative*

**Obesity Among US Urban Preschool Children: Relationships to Race, Ethnicity, and Socioeconomic Status** 578
*Robert C. Whitaker, MD, MPH; Sean M. Orzol, MPH*

**Forensic Laboratory Evidence in Sexually Abused Children and Adolescents** 585
*Karen L. Young, MD; Jerry G. Jones, MD; Toss Worthington, RNP; Pippa Simpson, PhD; Patrick H. Casey, MD*

**Incidence and Correlates of Unwanted Sex in Relationships of Middle and Late Adolescent Women** 591
*Margaret J. Blythe, MD; J. Dennis Fortenberry, MD, MS; M'Hamed Temkit, MS; Wanzhu Tu, PhD; Donald P. Orr, MD*

**Symptomatic Children With Hereditary Hemorrhagic Telangiectasia: A Pediatric Center Experience** 596
*Meir Mei-Zahav, MD; Michelle Letarte, PhD; Marie E. Faughnan, MD; Salma A. Abdalla, PhD; Ursula Cymerman, MS; Ian B. MacLusky, MD*

**The Clinical and Demographic Characteristics of Nonneuronopathic Gaucher Disease in 887 Children at Diagnosis** 603
*Paige Kaplan, MBBCh; Hans C. Andersson, MD; Katherine A. Kacena, PhD; John D. Yee, MD, MPH*

**Risk-Compensation Behavior in Children: Myth or Reality?** 610
*I. Barry Pless, MD; Helen Magdalinos, BA, CCLS; Brent Hagel, PhD*

**Effectiveness of Child Safety Seats vs Seat Belts in Reducing Risk for Death in Children in Passenger Vehicle Crashes** 617
*Michael R. Elliott, PhD; Michael J. Kallan, MS; Dennis R. Durbin, MD, MSCE; Flaura K. Winston, MD, PhD*

**Effectiveness of Nebulizer Use–Targeted Asthma Education on Underserved Children With Asthma** 622
*Arlene M. Butz, RN, CRNP, ScD; Mona G. Tsoukleris, PharmD, BCPS; Michele Donithan, MHS; Van Doren Hsu, PharmD; Ilene Zuckerman, PharmD, PhD; Kim Elizabeth Mudd, MSN; Richard E. Thompson, PhD; Cindy Rand, PhD; Mary Elizabeth Bollinger, DO*

**Racial and Ethnic Disparities in Pediatric Tuberculosis in North Carolina** 631
*Jason E. Stout, MD, MHS; Kapil K. Saharia, MD, MPH; Savithri Nageswaran, MD; Amina Ahmed, MD; Carol Dukes Hamilton, MD*

**Effects of Antibullying School Program on Bullying and Health Complaints** 638
*Minne Fekkes, MSc, PhD; Frans I. M. Pijpers, MD, PhD; S. Pauline Verloove-Vanhorick, MD, PhD*


## SPECIAL FEATURE


**Picture of the Month** 645
*Sabrina J. Braham, BA; Amy E. Gilliam, MD*


## ARTICLE


**Evaluation of a Novel Web-Based Pediatric Advanced Life Support Course** 649
*James M. Gerard, MD; Anthony J. Scalzo, MD; Steven P. Laffey, MD; Glen Sinks, RN, MSN, CS, FNP, EMT-P; Diana Fendya, RN, MSN; Patrice Seratti, BS*

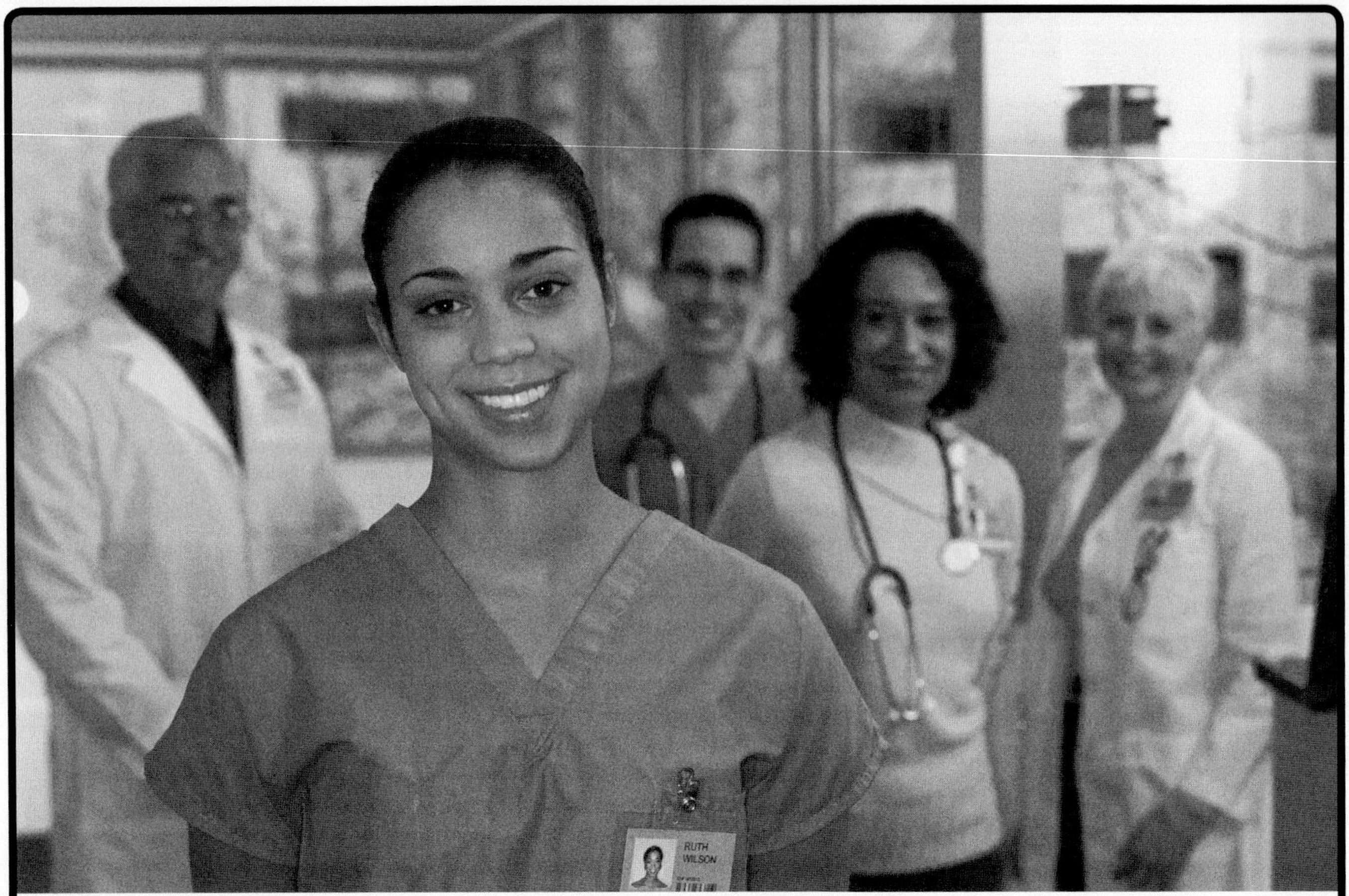

ARCHIVES OF PEDIATRICS & ADOLESCENT MEDICINE

## EDITORIALS

**Obesity Among Latino Preschoolers: Do Children Outgrow the "Epidemiologic Paradox"?** 656
*Elena Fuentes-Afflick, MD, MPH*

**Pediatric Advanced Life Support Your Way** 658
*Jane F. Knapp, MD; Robert D. Schremmer, MD*

## BOOK REVIEWS AND OTHER MEDIA

**"I'm, Like, SO Fat!": Helping Your Teen Make Healthy Choices About Eating and Exercise in a Weight-Obsessed World** 660
*Lenna L. Liu, MD, MPH*

## CORRECTIONS

**Error in Abstract in: Hearing Thresholds and Tympanic Membrane Sequelae in Children Managed Medically or Surgically for Otitis Media With Effusion** 588
*Robert Stenstrom, MD, PhD; I. Barry Pless, MD; Philippe Bernard, MD, PhD*

**Error in Text in: Schoolwide Food Practices Are Associated With Body Mass Index in Middle School Students** 614
*Martha Y. Kubik, PhD, RN; Leslie A. Lytle, PhD, RD; Mary Story, PhD*

## REGULAR DEPARTMENTS

**This Month in *Archives of Pediatrics & Adolescent Medicine*** 567

**Announcements** 577, 601, 628, 655

**Call for Papers** 637

**Classified Advertising** 663

**Journal Advertiser Index** 663

**Contact Information** 664

**Instructions for authors and the author and subject indexes are available on our Web site: http://www.archpediatrics.com. If you do not have access to the Web, contact Suzanne Shuey at (206) 685-3573.**

### About the Cover

Edgar Degas (1834-1917), French. *The Bellelli Family*, 1859-1867. Oil on canvas. Musée d'Orsay, Paris, France. Photo credit: Réunion des Musées Nationaux/Art Resource, New York, NY.

# ARCHIVES OF PEDIATRICS & ADOLESCENT MEDICINE


**Mission Statement:** *The Archives of Pediatrics & Adolescent Medicine* is a monthly, peer-reviewed journal for physicians and other health care professionals who contribute to the health of children and adolescents. The *Archives* provides an open forum for dialogue on a full range of clinical, scientific, advocacy, and humanistic issues relevant to the care of pediatric patients from infancy through young adulthood. The *Archives* is a vehicle for increased attention to adolescent health, the education of pediatric health care professionals, and disease prevention and health promotion. The *Archives* publishes original studies, editorials, reviews by experts, practice commentaries, case quizzes, and updates on clinical science and practice management. The Pediatric Forum provides our readers with opportunities to express their views. *Archives* incorporates *AJDC*, the oldest journal in US pediatric literature, which originated in 1911.



JAMA & ARCHIVES JOURNALS
American Medical Association

All articles published, including editorials, letters, and book reviews, represent the opinions of the authors and do not reflect the policy of the American Medical Association, the Editorial Board, or the institution with which the author is affiliated, unless this is clearly specified.

**PEDIARIX™ [Diphtheria and Tetanus Toxoids and Acellular Pertussis Adsorbed, Hepatitis B (Recombinant) and Inactivated Poliovirus Vaccine Combined]**

The following is a brief summary only; see full prescribing information for complete product information.

**CONTRAINDICATIONS:** Hypersensitivity to any component of the vaccine, including yeast, neomycin, and polymyxin B, is a contraindication (see DESCRIPTION in complete prescribing information). Do not use PEDIARIX after a serious allergic reaction (e.g., anaphylaxis) temporally associated with a previous dose of this vaccine or with any components of this vaccine. Because of the uncertainty as to which component of the vaccine might be responsible, do not give further vaccination with any of these components; or, refer such individuals to an allergist for evaluation. The following events are contraindications to administration of PEDIARIX: encephalopathy (e.g., coma, decreased level of consciousness, prolonged seizures) within 7 days of administration of a previous dose of a pertussis-containing vaccine that is not attributable to another identifiable cause; progressive neurologic disorder, including infantile spasms, uncontrolled epilepsy, or progressive encephalopathy. Do not vaccinate individuals with such conditions until a treatment regimen has been established and the condition has stabilized. PEDIARIX is not contraindicated for use in individuals with HIV infection.

**WARNINGS:** Administration of PEDIARIX is associated with higher rates of fever relative to separately administered vaccines. In one study that evaluated medically attended fever after the first dose of PEDIARIX or separately administered vaccines, infants who received PEDIARIX had a higher rate of medical encounters for fever within the first 4 days following vaccination. In some infants, these encounters included the performance of diagnostic studies to evaluate other causes of fever (see ADVERSE REACTIONS). The vial stopper is latex-free. The tip cap and the rubber plunger of the needleless prefilled syringes contain dry natural latex rubber that may cause allergic reactions in latex sensitive individuals. If any of the following events occur in temporal relation to receipt of whole-cell DTP or a vaccine containing an acellular pertussis component, consider carefully whether to give subsequent doses of PEDIARIX or any vaccine containing a pertussis component: temperature of ≥40.5°C (105°F) within 48 hours not due to another identifiable cause; collapse or shock-like state (hypotonic-hyporesponsive episode) within 48 hours; persistent, inconsolable crying lasting ≥3 hours, occurring within 48 hours; seizures with or without fever occurring within 3 days. If Guillain-Barré syndrome occurs within 6 weeks of receipt of prior vaccine containing tetanus toxoid, the decision to give subsequent doses of PEDIARIX or any vaccine containing tetanus toxoid should be based on careful consideration of the potential benefits and possible risks. A committee of the Institute of Medicine (IOM) has concluded that evidence is consistent with a causal relationship between whole-cell DTP vaccine and acute neurologic illness, and under special circumstances, between whole-cell DTP vaccine and chronic neurologic disease in the context of the National Childhood Encephalopathy Study (NCES) report; however, evidence was insufficient to evaluate whether or not whole-cell DTP vaccine increased the overall risk of chronic neurologic disease. Acute encephalopathy and permanent neurologic damage have not been reported causally linked or in temporal association with administration of PEDIARIX, but the experience with PEDIARIX is insufficient to rule this out. Encephalopathy has been reported following INFANRIX® (Diphtheria and Tetanus Toxoids and Acellular Pertussis Vaccine Adsorbed) (see ADVERSE REACTIONS, Postmarketing Reports), but data are not sufficient to evaluate a causal relationship. The decision to administer a pertussis-containing vaccine to children with stable central nervous system (CNS) disorders must be made by the physician on an individual basis, with consideration of all relevant factors, and assessment of potential risks and benefits for that individual. Advise the parent or guardian of the potential increased risk involved (see PRECAUTIONS). A family history of seizures or other CNS disorders is not a contraindication to pertussis vaccine. For children at higher risk for seizures than the general population, an appropriate antipyretic may be administered at the time of vaccination and for the ensuing 24 hours according to the respective prescribing information recommended dosage to reduce the possibility of post-vaccination fever. Defer vaccination during the course of a moderate or severe illness with or without fever and vaccinate patients as soon as they have recovered from the acute phase of the illness. Do not give PEDIARIX to children on anticoagulant therapy or those with bleeding disorders unless the potential benefit clearly outweighs the risk of administration (see PRECAUTIONS in complete prescribing information).

**PRECAUTIONS:** Before the injection of any biological, the physician should take all reasonable precautions to prevent allergic or other adverse reactions. Epinephrine injection (1:1000) and other appropriate agents used for the control of immediate allergic reactions must be immediately available should an acute anaphylactic reaction occur. Immunosuppressed individuals, including those receiving immunosuppressive therapy, may not develop the expected immune response. **Drug Interactions:** For information regarding concomitant administration with other vaccines, refer to DOSAGE AND ADMINISTRATION in complete prescribing information. Do not mix PEDIARIX with any other vaccine in the same syringe or vial. **Carcinogenesis, Mutagenesis, Impairment of Fertility:** PEDIARIX has not been evaluated for carcinogenic or mutagenic potential, or for impairment of fertility. **Pregnancy:** Pregnancy Category C: PEDIARIX is not indicated for women of child-bearing age. Animal reproduction studies have not been conducted with PEDIARIX. It is not known whether PEDIARIX can cause fetal harm when administered to a pregnant woman or if PEDIARIX can affect reproductive capacity. **Geriatric Use:** PEDIARIX is not indicated for use in adult populations. **Pediatric Use:** Safety and effectiveness of PEDIARIX in infants younger than 6 weeks of age have not been evaluated (see DOSAGE AND ADMINISTRATION in complete prescribing information). PEDIARIX is not recommended for persons 7 years of age or older. Tetanus and Diphtheria Toxoids Adsorbed (Td) For Adult Use, inactivated poliovirus vaccine (IPV), and Hepatitis B Vaccine (Recombinant) should be used in individuals 7 years of age or older.

**ADVERSE REACTIONS:** A total of 20,739 doses of PEDIARIX have been administered to 7,028 infants as a 3-dose primary series. The most common adverse reactions observed in clinical trials were local injection site reactions (pain, redness, or swelling), fever, and fussiness. In comparative studies, administration of PEDIARIX was associated with higher rates of fever relative to separately administered vaccines (see WARNINGS). The prevalence of fever was highest on the day of vaccination and the day following vaccination. More than 98% of episodes of fever resolved within the 4-day period following vaccination (i.e., the period including the day of vaccination and the next 3 days). Rates of most other solicited adverse events following PEDIARIX were comparable to rates observed following separately administered US-licensed vaccines. The adverse event information from clinical trials provides a basis for identifying adverse events that appear to be related to vaccine use and for approximating rates. However, because clinical trials are conducted under widely varying conditions, adverse event rates observed in the clinical trials of a vaccine cannot be directly compared to rates in the clinical trials of another vaccine, and may not reflect the rates observed in practice. A total of 5,472 infants were enrolled in a German safety study that was originally designed to compare the safety and reactogenicity of PEDIARIX administered concomitantly at separate sites with 1 of 4 *Haemophilus influenzae* type b (Hib) vaccines at 3, 4, and 5 months of age. After enrollment of 1,569 infants, the study was amended to include a control group that received INFANRIX, Hib vaccine, and oral poliovirus vaccine (OPV) separately. Infants in the separate administration group received one less antigen (hepatitis B) than the infants who received PEDIARIX. Safety data were available for 4,666 infants who received PEDIARIX administered concomitantly at separate sites with 1 of 4 Hib vaccines and for 768 infants in the control group that received separate vaccines. The primary end-point of the study was the percentage of infants with any grade 3 solicited symptom (redness or swelling >20 mm, fever >103.1°F, or crying, pain, vomiting, diarrhea, loss of appetite, or restlessness that prevented normal daily activities) over the 3-dose primary series in infants who received PEDIARIX (4 groups that received PEDIARIX and Hib vaccines pooled) compared to the group that received INFANRIX and Hib vaccine separately with OPV. Analysis for the primary end-point was performed on the according-to-protocol (ATP) cohort that included only those infants who were enrolled after the protocol amendment to include a control group. Of 3,773 infants in the ATP cohort for whom safety data were available, 16.2% (95% CI: 14.9% to 17.5%) of 3,029 infants who received PEDIARIX and Hib vaccine compared to 20.3% (95% CI: 17.5% to 23.4%) of 744 infants who received separate vaccines were reported to have had at least one grade 3 solicited symptom within 4 days of vaccination (i.e., day of vaccination and the next 3 days). The difference between groups in the rate of grade 3 symptoms was 4.1% (90% CI: 1.4% to 7.1%). These were the rates for selected solicited symptoms within 4 days following each dose in a 3-dose primary series in infants who received PEDIARIX administered concomitantly with Hib vaccine and those who received separate concomitant administration of INFANRIX, Hib vaccine, and OPV for the intent-to-treat (ITT) cohort (includes all infants enrolled before and after the amendment who received the indicated vaccine and for whom at least one symptom sheet was completed):

**Percentage of German Infants With Solicited Local Reactions or Selected Systemic Adverse Events Within 4 Days of Vaccination* (ITT Cohort)**

| | PEDIARIX & Hib | | | INFANRIX, Hib, & OPV | | |
|---|---|---|---|---|---|---|
| | Dose 1 | Dose 2 | Dose 3 | Dose 1 | Dose 2 | Dose 3 |
| **N** | **4,666** | **4,619** | **4,574** | **768** | **757** | **750** |
| **Local†** | | | | | | |
| Pain, any | 14.0 | 10.2 | 9.9 | 14.2 | 9.8 | 8.1 |
| Pain, grade 2 or 3 | 2.9 | 1.2 | 1.5 | 3.6 | 1.7 | 1.1 |
| Pain, grade 3 | 0.7 | 0.3 | 0.3 | 1.3 | 0.4 | 0.1 |
| Redness, any | 18.6 | 26.6 | 25.6 | 16.1 | 21.4 | 20.8 |
| Redness, >5 mm | 6.7 | 9.9 | 9.0 | 5.9 | 8.2 | 7.7 |
| Redness, >20 mm | 1.2 | 1.0 | 1.1 | 1.8 | 0.7 | 1.1 |
| Swelling, any | 12.7 | 18.5 | 18.4 | 9.6 | 12.9 | 13.6 |
| Swelling, >5 mm | 5.6 | 7.7 | 7.8 | 3.6 | 5.2 | 4.8 |
| Swelling, >20 mm | 1.2 | 1.6 | 1.5 | 1.3 | 1.1 | 1.2 |
| **Systemic** | | | | | | |
| Restlessness, any | 41.4 | 32.0 | 26.7 | 46.4 | 35.0 | 27.6 |
| Restlessness, grade 2 or 3 | 14.4 | 10.0 | 8.9 | 20.2 | 11.5 | 8.4 |
| Restlessness, grade 3 | 3.0 | 1.5 | 1.6 | 5.7 | 3.0 | 1.7 |
| Fever‡, ≥100.4°F | 25.1 | 19.3 | 19.7 | 13.2 | 13.1 | 11.2 |
| Fever‡, >101.3°F | 5.8 | 4.1 | 4.6 | 2.2 | 2.8 | 2.1 |
| Fever‡, >103.1°F | 0.3 | 0.5 | 0.7 | 0.3 | 0.3 | 0.5 |
| Unusual cry§, any | 24.9 | 16.5 | 13.1 | 36.5 | 19.7 | 14.3 |
| Unusual cry§, grade 2 or 3 | 12.7 | 7.1 | 5.7 | 20.8 | 10.0 | 5.7 |
| Unusual cry§, grade 3 | 3.9 | 1.7 | 1.4 | 6.8 | 2.1 | 1.1 |
| Loss of appetite, any | 17.9 | 13.3 | 12.5 | 19.1 | 16.2 | 11.3 |
| Loss of appetite, grade 2 or 3 | 4.0 | 2.9 | 2.7 | 4.4 | 2.9 | 2.3 |
| Loss of appetite, grade 3 | 0.6 | 0.5 | 0.4 | 0.5 | 0.7 | 0.0 |

N = number of infants in the intent-to-treat (ITT) cohort.
Grade 2 defined as sufficiently discomforting to interfere with daily activities.
Grade 3 defined as preventing normal daily activities.
* Within 4 days of vaccination defined as day of vaccination and the next 3 days.
† Local reactions at the injection site for PEDIARIX or INFANRIX.
‡ Rectal temperatures.
§ Unusual cry lasting >1 hour.

In this study, infants were also monitored for unsolicited adverse events that occurred within 30 days following vaccination. Over the entire study period, 6 subjects in the group that received PEDIARIX reported seizures. Two of these subjects had a febrile seizure, 1 of whom also developed afebrile seizures. The remaining 4 subjects had afebrile seizures, including 2 with infantile spasms. Two subjects reported seizures within 7 days following vaccination (1 subject had both febrile and afebrile seizures, and 1 subject had afebrile seizures), corresponding to a rate of 0.22 seizures per 1,000 doses (febrile seizures 0.07 per 1,000 doses, afebrile seizures 0.14 per 1,000 doses). No subject who received concomitant INFANRIX, Hib vaccine, and OPV reported seizures. In a separate German study that evaluated the safety of INFANRIX in 22,505 infants who received 66,867 doses of INFANRIX administered as a 3-dose primary series, the rate of seizures within 7 days of vaccination with INFANRIX was 0.13 per 1,000 doses (febrile seizures 0.0 per 1,000 doses, afebrile seizures 0.13 per 1,000 doses). No cases of hypotonic-hyporesponsiveness, encephalopathy, or anaphylaxis were reported in the German study that evaluated the safety of PEDIARIX. Rates of serious adverse events that are less common than those reported in this safety study are not known at this time.

Additional safety data for PEDIARIX are available from a US study designed to evaluate lot-to-lot consistency and a bridge for a new manufacturing step. These were the rates for local reactions and selected adverse events within 4 days of vaccination with PEDIARIX administered concomitantly with a Hib vaccine at 2, 4, and 6 months of age:

**Percentage of US Infants With Solicited Local Reactions or Selected Systemic Adverse Events Within 4 Days of Vaccination* (ITT Cohort)**

| | PEDIARIX & Hib | | |
|---|---|---|---|
| | Dose 1 | Dose 2 | Dose 3 |
| **Local†** | **N = 482** | **N = 469** | **N = 466** |
| Pain, any | 30.5 | 25.4 | 23.0 |
| Pain, grade 2 or 3 | 6.2 | 5.5 | 3.6 |
| Pain, grade 3 | 1.2 | 0.6 | 0.6 |
| Redness, any | 25.3 | 32.6 | 35.6 |
| Redness, >5 mm | 9.3 | 10.4 | 8.6 |
| Redness, >20 mm | 0.6 | 1.5 | 1.3 |
| Swelling, any | 15.1 | 16.6 | 22.3 |
| Swelling, >5 mm | 6.8 | 6.2 | 6.4 |
| Swelling, >20 mm | 1.0 | 1.3 | 1.3 |
| **Systemic** | **N = 482** | **N = 469** | **N = 467** |
| Restlessness, any | 28.8 | 30.3 | 28.5 |
| Restlessness, grade 2 or 3 | 7.1 | 9.0 | 9.4 |
| Restlessness, grade 3 | 1.0 | 1.1 | 0.6 |
| Fever‡, ≥100.4°F | 26.6 | 31.3 | 25.9 |
| Fever‡, >101.3°F | 2.9 | 6.2 | 4.7 |
| Fever‡, >103.1°F | 0.0 | 0.2 | 0.6 |
| Fussiness, any | 61.8 | 63.8 | 57.0 |
| Fussiness, grade 2 or 3 | 14.9 | 21.5 | 17.1 |
| Fussiness, grade 3 | 2.7 | 3.4 | 1.7 |
| Loss of appetite, any | 21.6 | 19.8 | 18.8 |
| Loss of appetite, grade 2 or 3 | 3.1 | 3.2 | 2.4 |
| Loss of appetite, grade 3 | 0.2 | 0.4 | 0.0 |
| Sleeping more than usual, any | 46.7 | 31.8 | 28.1 |
| Sleeping more than usual, grade 2 or 3 | 10.2 | 6.0 | 4.7 |
| Sleeping more than usual, grade 3 | 1.7 | 0.4 | 0.6 |

N = number of infants in the intent-to-treat (ITT) cohort (infants who received the indicated vaccine and for whom at least one symptom sheet was completed).
Grade 2 defined as sufficiently discomforting to interfere with daily activities.
Grade 3 defined as preventing normal daily activities.
* Within 4 days of vaccination defined as day of vaccination and the next 3 days.
† Local reactions at the injection site for PEDIARIX.
‡ Rectal temperatures.

In another US study, these were the rates for fever within 4 days following dose 1 (i.e., day of vaccination and the next 3 days) at 2 months of age in infants who received PEDIARIX when administered concomitantly at separate sites with Hib and pneumococcal conjugate vaccines and those who received INFANRIX, ENGERIX-B® [Hepatitis B Vaccine (Recombinant)], IPV, Hib vaccine, and pneumococcal conjugate vaccine:

**Percentage of US Infants With Fever Within 4 Days of Dose 1* (ITT Cohort)**

| | PEDIARIX, Hib, & Pneumococcal Conjugate (N = 667) | INFANRIX, ENGERIX-B, IPV, Hib, & Pneumococcal Conjugate (N = 333) | Separate Vaccine Group Minus Combination Vaccine Group |
|---|---|---|---|
| **Fever†** | **%** | **%** | **Difference (95% CI)** |
| ≥100.4°F‡ | 27.9 | 19.8 | -8.07 (-13.54, -2.60) |
| >101.3°F | 7.0 | 4.5 | -2.54 (-5.50, 0.41) |
| >102.2°F‡ | 2.2 | 0.3 | -1.95 (-3.22, -0.68) |
| >103.1°F | 0.4 | 0.0 | -0.45 (-0.96, 0.06) |
| M.A.‡ | 1.2 | 0.0 | -1.20 (-2.03, -037) |

N = number of infants for whom at least one symptom sheet was completed, excluding 3 infants for whom temperature was not measured and 3 infants whose temperature was measured by the tympanic method.
*Within 4 days of dose 1 defined as day of vaccination and the next 3 days.
† Rectal temperatures.
‡ The group that received PEDIARIX compared to separate vaccine group p value <0.05 (2-sided Fisher Exact test) or the 95% confidence interval on the difference between groups does not include 0.
M.A. = Medically attended (a visit to or from medical personnel).

In this study, medical attention (a visit to or from medical personnel) for fever within 4 days following vaccination was sought for 8 infants who received PEDIARIX (1.2%) and no infants who received separately administered vaccines. Four infants were seen by medical personnel in an office setting; no diagnostic tests were performed in 2 of the infants and a complete blood count (CBC) was done in the other 2 infants. Of 3 infants who were seen in an emergency room, all had a CBC and a blood and urine culture performed; chest X-rays were done in 2 of the infants and a nasopharyngeal specimen was tested for Respiratory Syncytial Virus in one of the infants. One infant was hospitalized for a work-up that included a CBC, blood and urine cultures, a lumbar puncture, and a chest X-ray. All episodes of medically attended fever resolved within 4 days post-vaccination.

Limited data are available from a study conducted in Moldova in which infants received a dose of hepatitis B vaccine within 48 hours of birth followed by 3 doses of PEDIARIX at 6, 10, and 14 weeks of age. No information was collected on the HBsAg status of mothers of enrolled infants. These were the rates for local reactions and selected adverse events within 4 days of vaccination with PEDIARIX administered comcomitantly with Hib vaccine following a birth dose of hepatitis B vaccine:

**Percentage of Moldovan Infants With Solicited Local Reactions or Selected Systemic Adverse Events Within 4 Days of Vaccination* (ITT Cohort)**

| | PEDIARIX & Hib | | |
|---|---|---|---|
| | Dose 1 | Dose 2 | Dose 3 |
| **N** | **160** | **158** | **157** |
| **Local†** | | | |
| Pain, any | 25.6 | 18.4 | 14.0 |
| Pain, grade 3 | 3.1 | 0.6 | 1.9 |
| Redness, any | 41.9 | 41.8 | 47.1 |
| Redness, >20 mm | 1.9 | 2.5 | 4.5 |
| Swelling, any | 20.6 | 18.4 | 28.0 |
| Swelling, >20 mm | 4.4 | 2.5 | 7.0 |
| **Systemic** | | | |
| Restlessness, any | 13.1 | 10.8 | 8.9 |
| Restlessness, grade 3 | 1.3 | 0.6 | 0.6 |
| Fever‡, ≥100.4°F | 14.4 | 11.4 | 5.1 |
| Fever‡, >103.1°F | 0.0 | 0.6 | 0.0 |
| Fussiness, any | 25.0 | 21.5 | 17.8 |
| Fussiness, grade 3 | 2.5 | 0.6 | 0.6 |

N = number of infants in the intent-to-treat (ITT) cohort (infants who received the indicated vaccine and for whom at least one symptom sheet was completed).
Grade 3 defined as preventing normal daily activities.
*Within 4 days of vaccination defined as day of vaccination and the next 3 days.
† Local reactions at the injection site for PEDIARIX.
‡ Rectal temperatures.

Although there was no comparator group who received PEDIARIX without a birth dose of hepatitis B vaccine, available data suggest that some local adverse events may occur at a higher rate when PEDIARIX is administered after a birth dose of hepatitis B vaccine.

As with any vaccine, there is the possibility that broad use of PEDIARIX could reveal adverse events not observed in clinical trials.

**Postmarketing Reports:** Worldwide voluntary reports of adverse events received for INFANRIX and ENGERIX-B in children younger than 7 years of age since market introduction of these US-licensed vaccines are listed below. This list includes adverse events for which 20 or more reports were received with the exception of intussusception, idiopathic thrombocytopenic purpura, thrombocytopenia, anaphylactic reaction, angioedema, encephalopathy, hypotonic-hyporesponsive episode, and alopecia for which fewer than 20 reports were received. These latter events are included either because of the seriousness of the event or the strength of causal connection to components of this or other vaccines or drugs. *Body as a whole:* Asthenia[b], fever[a+b], lethargy[b], malaise[b], Sudden Infant Death Syndrome[a+b]. *Cardiovascular system:* Cyanosis[a+b], edema[b], pallor[a]. *Gastrointestinal system:* Abdominal pain[b], anorexia[b], diarrhea[a+b], intussusception[a+b], nausea[b], vomiting[a+b]. *Hematologic/lymphatic:* Idiopathic thrombocytopenic purpura[a+b], lymphadenopathy[a], thrombocytopenia[a+b]. *Hepatic:* Jaundice[b], liver function tests abnormal[b]. *Hypersensitivity:* Anaphylactic reaction[a+b], angioedema[b], hypersensitivity[a]. *Infections:* Cellulitis[a]. *Injection site reactions:* Injection site reactions[a+b]. *Musculoskeletal:* Arthralgia[b], limb swelling[a+b]. *Nervous system:* Convulsions[a+b], encephalopathy[a], headache[b], hypotonia[a+b], hypotonic-hyporesponsive episode[a], somnolence[a+b]. *Psychiatric:* Crying[a+b], irritability[a+b]. *Respiratory system:* Respiratory tract infection[a]. *Skin and appendages:* Alopecia[b], erythema[a+b], erythema multiforme[b], petechiae[b], pruritus[a+b], rash[a+b], urticaria[a+b]. *Special senses:* Ear pain[a]. [[a] Following INFANRIX;[b] Following ENGERIX-B;[a+b] Following either INFANRIX or ENGERIX-B.] These reactions were reported voluntarily from a population of uncertain size; therefore, it is not always possible to reliably estimate their frequency or establish a causal relationship to vaccination.

**Reporting Adverse Events:** Report the occurrence following immunization of any event set forth in the Vaccine Injury Table from the National Childhood Vaccine Injury Act including: Anaphylaxis or anaphylactic shock within 7 days, encephalopathy or encephalitis within 7 days, brachial neuritis within 28 days, or an acute complication or sequelae (including death) of an illness, disability, injury, or condition referred to above, or any events that would contraindicate further doses of PEDIARIX. The VAERS toll-free number is 1-800-822-7967.

Manufactured by **GlaxoSmithKline Biologicals**, Rixensart, Belgium, US License 1617
Distributed by **GlaxoSmithKline,** Research Triangle Park, NC 27709



Full prescribing information for PEDIARIX is available at www.GSKVaccines.com/Pediarix. BRS-PE:L2

## Obesity Among US Urban Preschool Children: Relationships to Race, Ethnicity, and Socioeconomic Status

In the United States, one of the great concerns in the obesity epidemic is the disparity among racial and ethnic groups in the prevalence of obesity. Data from the Fragile Families and Child Well-being Study represent a birth cohort from 75 hospitals across 20 large cities in 15 states. At 3 years of age, 26% of Hispanic children were obese compared with 16% of black children and 15% of white children. This higher prevalence of obesity in Hispanic children was not explained by maternal education, household income, or children's food security status. Other yet unidentified factors must be explored to explain these differences, particularly since they occur so early in life.

See page 578

## Evaluation of a Novel Web-Based Pediatric Advanced Life Support Course

A basic component of quality health care is that it be current, which requires continued lifelong learning by physicians. Unfortunately, most continuing medical education has been found to be ineffective in either changing behavior or improving care. Few studies have examined the efficacy of Web-based learning compared with traditional styles of continuing medical education. Gerard and colleagues conducted a randomized controlled trial to compare a traditional pediatric advanced life support course with a Web-based version. Students taking the Web-based pediatric advanced life support course performed very similarly to those taking the traditional course on follow-up evaluation, and all indicated that they would recommend it to a colleague. The findings in this study support the continued development and promotion of the Web-based pediatric advanced life support course.

See page 649

## Incidence and Correlates of Unwanted Sex in Relationships of Middle and Late Adolescent Women

Unwanted sex is a common element of the sexual experiences of many young women and is associated with harm to both physical and mental health. In this study of 279 females with a mean age of 16 years, 41% reported unwanted sex at least once. The most common type was owing to fear that the partner would get angry if denied sex; 10% reported being forced to have sex. Risk factors for unwanted sex were the woman having a baby with the partner, lack of sexual control with a partner, lower condom use, and partner's use of marijuana. These same behaviors can put women at risk of sexually transmitted infections and unwanted pregnancies.

See page 591

## Effects of Regular Physical Activity on Control of Glycemia in Pediatric Patients With Type 1 Diabetes Mellitus

The effect of physical activity training on glycemic control of children with diabetes remains controversial. In this large cohort of 18 392 children with type 1 diabetes from 179 sites in Germany and Austria, regular physical activity was assessed. Glycemic control (as measured by hemoglobin $A_{1c}$) was better at all ages in patients with more regular physical activity; in girls, this was also accompanied by a lower body mass index (calculated as weight in kilograms divided by the square of height in meters). Physical activity did not increase the chance of symptomatic hypoglycemia. Regular physical activity should be recommended in all patients with diabetes.

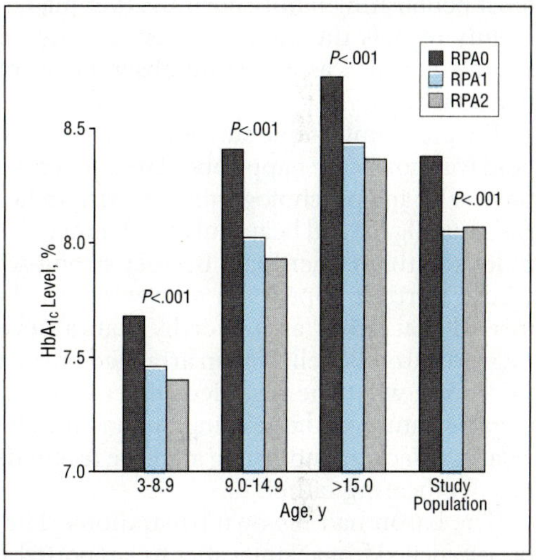


Glycosylated hemoglobin $A_{1c}$ ($HbA_{1c}$) level in age groups stratified by frequency of regular physical activity (RPA) per week. RPA0 indicates none; RPA1, 1 or 2 times per week; and RPA2, 3 or more times per week.

See page 573

## Effectiveness of Nebulizer Use–Targeted Asthma Education on Underserved Children With Asthma

Despite the availability of effective medication, many children with asthma have inadequate control of their symptoms, which results in frequent emergency department visits and hospital admissions. The objective of this randomized trial was to examine the effectiveness of a home-based educational intervention targeting symptom recognition and nebulizer use in young children with persistent asthma. Although most children in the study received appropriate nonurgent asthma care, the nebulizer education intervention had no impact on home nebulizer practice, asthma morbidity, or health care use. This study found a high rate of undertreatment and asthma mortality in young inner-city children.

See page 622

COVER ART

# Edgar Degas (1834-1917)

## The Bellelli Family, *1859-1867*

IN 1856, THE ASPIRING YOUNG FRENCH ARTIST Edgar Degas traveled to Italy to study the work of the Renaissance masters and to visit members of his extended family. After stops in Naples and Rome, he stayed for several months in Florence with his aunt Laura; her husband, Baron Gennaro Bellelli; and their daughters, Giovanna and Giulia. Following his return to Paris in 1859, he spent much of the next year turning his many drawings of his cousins and their parents into what is now regarded as one of the most penetrating family portraits ever made. *The Bellelli Family* reveals the young Degas's talents not only as a painter but also as an astute observer of interpersonal relationships.

Despite comfortable surroundings, the Bellelli household was not a very happy one. The 2 parents appear both physically and psychologically far apart. In her youth, Degas's intelligent and beautiful aunt Laura had been deeply in love with another man. But her strong-willed father, whose portrait appears in a drawing on the wall, dismissed that suitor as unworthy. Laura's eventual marriage to Baron Bellelli was an arranged one, and she came to despise what she regarded as her husband's idle and irritable nature. In the painting, she and the girls are shown wearing black, in mourning after the recent death of Laura's overbearing father.

The baron had his own frustrations. The family had been expelled from Naples after he supported a failed revolution there, and they were living in exile in Florence. In the painting, he sits apart, disengaged from the rest of the family and preoccupied with his own affairs. With his back turned to us, he barely deigns to take part in the family portrait at all.

The 2 young girls are a source of warmth in this chilly scene. Degas was fond of his 2 cousins, writing in a letter: "The older one [Giovanna, age 10 years] is really a little beauty; the younger one [Giulia, age 7 years] has the wit of a devil and the goodness of a little angel. . . ."[1(p71)] Giovanna was the obedient one, a mama's girl. In the picture, she stands primly in front of her mother, with Laura's protective right arm on her shoulder. Giulia was the restless one, tied to her mother but also seeking the attention of her distracted father. She sits perched on a chair in the middle of the picture, one leg curled up under her. On one side, she is at Laura's fingertips; on the other, she looks toward her father across the gap between them, forming a child-bridge between her 2 estranged parents.

Tension in the Bellelli household was relieved permanently when the baron died 5 years later. The next time Degas visited Florence, Giovanna and Giulia were teenagers. He made few drawings of them. Perhaps they had become less interesting to him as adolescents, and perhaps he to them. Laura Bellelli kept the love letters from her youthful paramour until she died at age 83 years. Degas, who later became a founding member of the Impressionists, never married. At his death, also at age 83 years, *The Bellelli Family* was found neglected and dusty among his possessions. It now hangs in the Musée d'Orsay in Paris, showing in ways that no photograph could ever reveal what it was like to be part of the troubled Bellelli family.

*Thomas D. Koepsell, MD, MPH*

**Correspondence**: Dr Koepsell, Department of Epidemiology, University of Washington, F-261F, Health Sciences, Box 357236, Seattle, WA 98195-7236 (koepsell@u.washington.edu).

REFERENCES

1. McMullen R. *Degas: His Life, Times, and Work.* Boston, Mass: Houghton Mifflin; 1984.

# International Exchanges

## *A Missed Opportunity in Pediatric Graduate Education*

IN APRIL 2002, MORE THAN 100 pediatricians from the United Kingdom, United States, and Australia convened in London, England, to commemorate the 50th anniversary of the inception of the exchange program between St Mary's Hospital in London and the Children's Hospital Medical Center in Boston, Mass. The attendees were former US pediatric residents or UK registrars who participated in either the London/Boston exchange that existed from 1952 through 1978 or the exchange between Oxford University (Oxford, England) and the Duke University Department of Pediatrics (Durham, NC), which began in 1986 and continued unchanged through 2005. These 2 bilateral exchanges produced a generation of trainees who made important contributions both to their home and visited countries. That and the profound influence of the experience on their careers and personal lives as described by the attendees prompted us to reflect on the importance of structured pediatric training programs for residents between countries, the additional opportunities exchanges provide, and the practical difficulties in achieving them. (The reunion report is available from the authors.)

### BACKGROUND

Going abroad holds a distinguished place in the history of medical education. For centuries, physicians have traveled widely to advance their clinical skills and knowledge, seeking out renowned centers of medical education and research. William Halsted, professor of surgery at The Johns Hopkins University (Baltimore, Md), initiated an exchange in the 1890s of surgical residents in different lands and wrote the first recorded manuscript on resident international exchange programs.[1]

The Children's Hospital Medical Center/St Mary's exchange was conceived by Reginald Lightwood, consultant pediatrician at St Mary's, and Charles A. Janeway, pediatrician-in-chief at the Boston Children's Hospital. Janeway had been pivotal in rejuvenating the International Pediatric Association. Janeway was an internationalist who believed his residents would benefit by studying medicine in the United Kingdom, with its emphasis on clinical medicine; out-of-hospital care, including outpatient and home services; and exposure to the National Health Service. Lightwood believed coming to the United States would provide his registrars with exposure to US scientific and technological accomplishments. Both believed exchanges would enhance career opportunities for their trainees.

The Oxford/Duke resident exchange was established by Samuel Katz, professor and chair of pediatrics at Duke, and Richard Moxon, professor and chair of pediatrics at Oxford. Katz and Moxon had studied at The Johns Hopkins University and Boston Children's, respectively, and became committed to establishing a US/UK exchange program.

### CURRENT EXCHANGES

To ascertain the status of past and present international exchanges, we surveyed 199 US-approved civilian pediatric residencies. We obtained 121 (60.8%) responses, which included 76.5% (101/132) of university-affiliated programs and 29.8% (20/67) of nonuniversity programs. Ten (9.9%) university-affiliated programs reported a bilateral resident exchange program, and 1 (5.0%) nonuniversity program reported a bilateral exchange. The university-affiliated exchanges were with the United Kingdom, Africa,[1] Asia,[1] and Latin America. The nonuniversity exchange was with Latin America. The 2 additional US/UK exchanges were between the Children's Hospital of Philadelphia, Pennsylvania, and the Hospital for Sick Children, London (1956-1985) and between the Boston City/Boston University and Princess Alexandra Children's Hospital, Brighton, England, and Westminster Hospital, London (1974-1978).

A similar survey was conducted of UK training programs in 2001.[2] Most of the UK programs were unilateral electives, with UK registrars going largely to Africa and Asia. A number of UK programs also had Commonwealth physicians, especially from Australia and New Zealand, coming to the United Kingdom. We completed a literature search for the years 1966 through 2002 regarding bilateral exchanges and found only limited reference to pediatric electives.[3]

### OBSTACLES

There are currently formidable obstacles to overcome for a bilateral exchange program to succeed, especially between developed countries. The first obstacle is that any exchange must conform to each country's training and specialty requirements in content and duration. The residency training regulations of the American Board of Pediatrics now allow only a maximum of 6 months away time; the time allowed for UK trainees is similarly restricted. In 2006, the Oxford/Duke program is under review because of further decreases in UK registrar work hours.

Another major set of hurdles to US/UK exchanges has been the requirement for examinations to meet each country's medical licensure qualifications. American residents in the recent past needed to make 2 advance trips to the United Kingdom to take examinations. Current changes in UK regulations now enable US pediatric residents with 2 years of postgraduate training to become registrars without taking further examinations. The UK registrars still must pass the US written and clinical examinations; the latter can be taken only in the United States.

Obtaining the necessary finances is another hurdle. Beginning with modest costs, the exchange has become an expensive arrangement, and the Oxford/Duke exchange now costs approximately $35 000 annually per participant. Costs include not only travel but also health insurance and malpractice insurance (currently more than $4000 for the 6 months) for the British resident. Car rental, car insurance, and document fees add another $4300. The resident and registrar each receives the other's salary, and salaries are generally similar in purchasing power.

## LESSONS LEARNED

A number of lessons have been learned from the US/UK exchanges. To succeed, both programs must have resident numbers large enough to ensure a steady flow of quality candidates from each program. The reason for the short life of the Boston City Hospital US/UK exchange program was that the pool of residents was too small. Family circumstances such as schooling and housing need to be organized. In some circumstances, participants have exchanged homes and cars.

Finally, the commitment of program leadership is essential. The department heads and faculty must be prepared to devote time and energy and to identify the necessary resources.

## CONCLUSIONS

Exchanges offer considerable opportunity for learning in an increasingly complex world. Medical students and residents participate in international electives, often in developing countries, and are able to develop their clinical skills and learn about providing health care when resources are limited. The type of bilateral exchange we describe is different. Like residency, the training is structured and overseen by experienced faculty.

In graduate medical education, we believe bilateral exchanges between the United States and other countries have been underused and represent a missed educational opportunity. Not all resident programs have the will or resources to conduct a successful exchange, but we urge those who can to commit to developing international exchanges, choosing countries most appropriate for their particular program goals. Sustained exchanges between the United States and other developed countries can succeed only with careful planning. We believe the institutional and personal benefits far outweigh the efforts and resources required.

*Joel J. Alpert, MD*
*Samuel L. Katz, MD*
*Tom Lissauer, MD*

**Correspondence:** Dr Albert, Department of Pediatrics, Boston University School of Medicine, 91 E Concord St, Boston, MA 02118 (e-mail: Joel.Alpert@bmc.org).
**Acknowledgment:** We are grateful to Donna Staton, MD, MPH, and Howard Bauchner, MD, for helpful reading of this article; to the participants in the St Mary's/Boston and Duke/Oxford bilateral exchange programs; and to Enriqueta Bond, PhD, president of the Burroughs Wellcome Fund (Research Triangle Park, NC), for supporting the London reunion.

## REFERENCES

1. Rutkow IM, Hempel K. An experiment in surgical education—the first international exchange of residents: the letters of Halsted, Kuttner, Heuer, and Landois. *Arch Surg.* 1988;123:115-121.
2. Nicoll A, Carter E, Golden B, Robson J, Southall D, Williams T. Developing sustainable international partnerships in child health and paediatric care. *Arch Dis Child.* 2001;84:315-319.
3. Torjesen K, Mandalakas A, Kahn R, Duncan B. International child health electives for pediatric residents. *Arch Pediatr Adolesc Med.* 1999;153:1297-1302.

"Medicine would be the ideal profession if it did not involve giving pain."
—Samuel Hopkins Adams

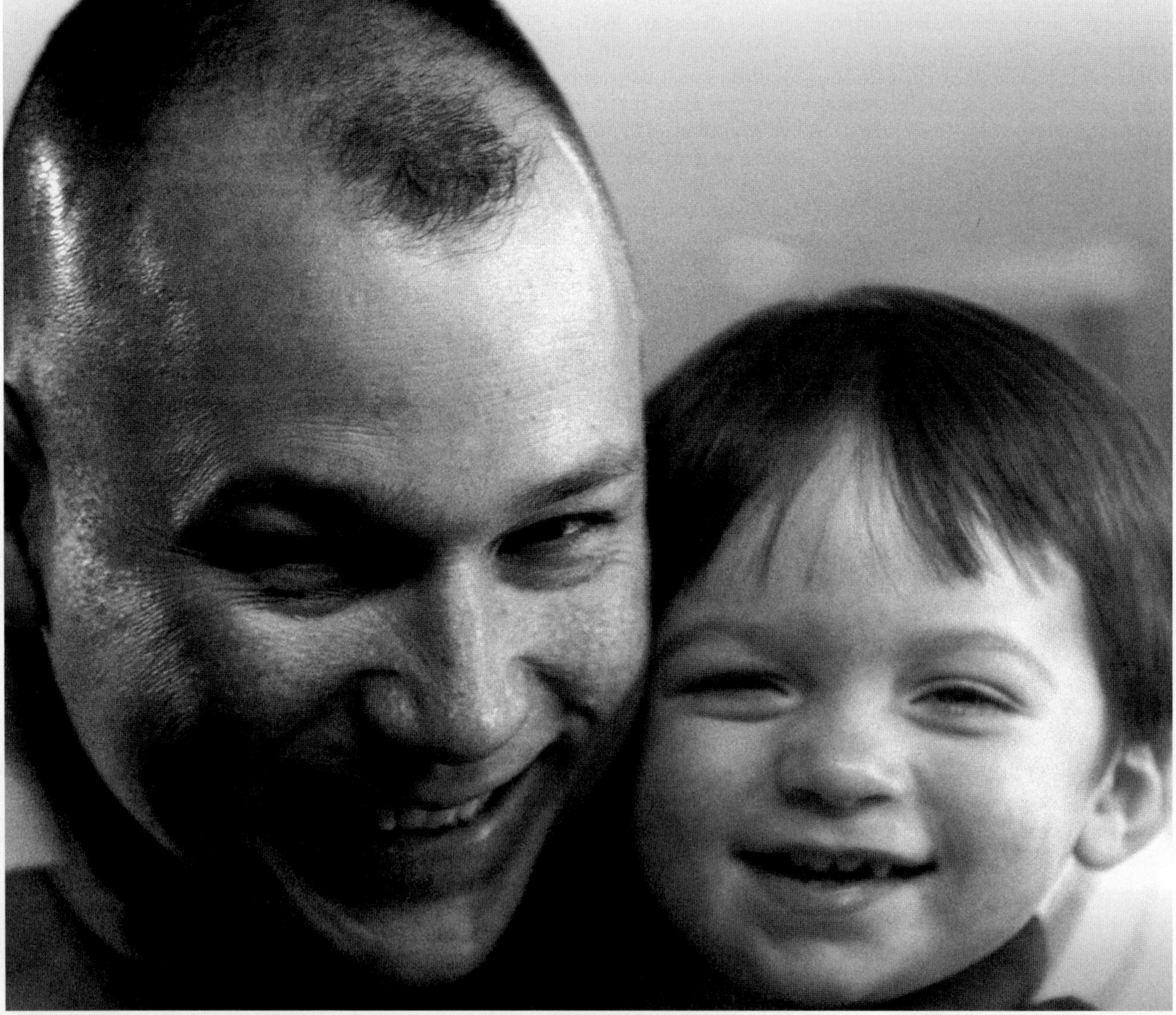

ARTICLE

# Effects of Regular Physical Activity on Control of Glycemia in Pediatric Patients With Type 1 Diabetes Mellitus

*Antje Herbst, MD; Rainer Bachran, MD; Thomas Kapellen, MD; Reinhard W. Holl, PhD; for the DPV Science Initiative*

**Objective:** To evaluate the effect of regular physical activity (RPA) on the control of glycemia (glycosylated hemoglobin $A_{1c}$ level) and the frequency of severe hypoglycemia in a large cohort of patients with type 1 diabetes mellitus.

**Design:** Cross-sectional analysis of data for 19 143 patients, comparing control of glycemia and rate of hypoglycemia by frequency of RPA.

**Setting:** One hundred seventy-nine pediatric diabetes clinics in Germany and Austria.

**Participants:** Patients aged 3 to 20 years with type 1 diabetes mellitus.

**Main Exposure:** Patients were grouped by the frequency of RPA per week as follows: RPA0, none; RPA1, 1 or 2 times per week; and RPA2, 3 or more times per week.

**Main Outcome Measures:** Glycosylated hemoglobin $A_{1c}$ level, body mass index (calculated as weight in kilograms divided by the square of height in meters) *z* score, and frequency of severe hypoglycemia.

**Results:** Glycosylated hemoglobin $A_{1c}$ level was higher in the groups with less frequent RPA (8.4% in group RPA0 vs 8.1% in group RPA2; $P<.001$). This effect was found in both sexes and in all age groups ($P<.001$). In female patients but not in male patients, the body mass index *z* score decreased from 0.60 in group RPA0 to 0.51 in group RPA2 ($P<.001$). Multiple regression analysis revealed that RPA was one of the most important factors influencing the glycosylated hemoglobin level. No association was noted between frequency of RPA and frequency of severe hypoglycemia or hypoglycemia with loss of consciousness or seizure.

**Conclusions:** In pediatric patients with type 1 diabetes mellitus, frequency of RPA is a major factor influencing the control of glycemia without increasing the risk for severe hypoglycemia. Regular physical activity should be recommended in pediatric patients with type 1 diabetes mellitus.

*Arch Pediatr Adolesc Med. 2006;160:573-577*

**Author Affiliations:** Department of Paediatrics, University of Bonn, Bonn (Dr Herbst); Hospital for Children and Adolescents, University of Leipzig, Leipzig (Dr Kapellen); and Institute for Biomedical Engineering, University of Ulm, Ulm (Dr Holl), Germany. Dr Bachran is in private practice in Oberhausen, Germany.
**Group Information:** For a current listing of the members of the DPV Science Initiative see http://dpv.mathematik.uni-ulm.de.

PHYSICAL ACTIVITY IS KNOWN to acutely reduce the blood glucose level and to increase insulin sensitivity in human beings with[1-3] and without[4,5] diabetes mellitus (DM). Furthermore, exercise increases insulin-stimulated glucose uptake in muscle, and this effect is higher in trained muscle than in untrained muscle.[6,7] It has been shown that exercise reduces the counterregulatory responses of epinephrine and the muscle sympathetic nerve activity during hypoglycemia the day after exercise.[8,9] Fewer hypoglycemic symptoms have been reported in groups that exercise compared with control groups.[8]

As a consequence, exercise might be a risk factor for hypoglycemia or severe hypoglycemia in patients with type 1 diabetes mellitus (T1DM) and, thus, endanger the patient. Regular physical activity (RPA) can improve the lipoprotein profile, lower blood pressure, and improve cardiovascular fitness and quality of life in patients with T1DM.[1,10] The effect of physical activity training on the control of glycemia remains controversial, as some studies[1,10] have shown, and some studies[2,11-14] have failed to show, an independent effect of physical activity training on the control of glycemia as measured by the glycosylated hemoglobin ($HbA_{1c}$) level in patients with T1DM. The present study evaluates the influence of RPA on the frequency of severe hypoglycemia and on metabolic control ($HbA_{1c}$ level) in a large cohort of 18 392 pediatric patients in a multicenter survey in Germany and Austria.

## METHODS

Data were provided by the Pediatric Quality Initiative[15] and included anonymized longitudi-

**Table 1. Characteristics of Study Population Stratified by Frequency of Regular Physical Activity***

| Variable | Age, y | T1DM Duration, y | $HbA_{1c}$, % | Insulin Dosage, IU/kg per d | BMI z Score | Per 100 Patient-Years: Severe Hypoglycemia | Per 100 Patient-Years: Hypoglycemia With Loss of Consciousness |
|---|---|---|---|---|---|---|---|
| RPA0 | 12.9 | 4.8 ± 3.9 | 8.4 ± 1.9 | 0.85 ± 0.3 | 0.48 ± 0.9 | 23.5 ± 14.3 | 4.7 ± 31.9 |
| RPA1 | 12.7 | 4.8 ± 3.8 | 8.0 ± 1.6 | 0.84 ± 0.3 | 0.44 ± 0.9 | 21.8 ± 8.2 | 5.1 ± 30.8 |
| RPA2 | 14.0 | 5.2 ± 3.8 | 8.1 ± 1.6 | 0.84 ± 0.3 | 0.44 ± 0.8 | 23.6 ± 8.0 | 5.1 ± 28.3 |
| *P* value† | <.001 | <.001 | <.001 | <.005 | <.05 | <.01 | .70 |

Abbreviations: BMI, body mass index (calculated as weight in kilograms divided by the square of height in meters); $HbA_{1c}$, glycosylated hemoglobin $A_{1c}$; NS, not significant; RPA, frequency of regular physical activity per week; RPA0, none (n = 8589); RPA1, 1 or 2 times per week (n = 7056); RPA2, 3 or more times per week (n = 3498); T1DM, type 1 diabetes mellitus.

*Data are given as mean ± SD.

†Statistical comparison by Kruskal-Wallis test followed by Bonferroni correction.

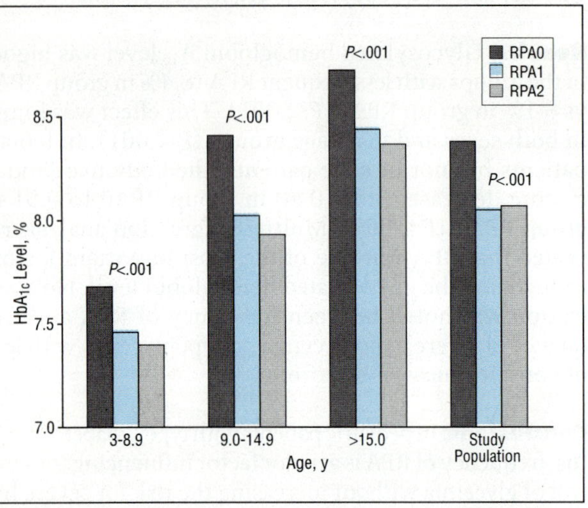


**Figure 1.** Glycosylated hemoglobin $A_{1c}$ ($HbA_{1c}$) level in age groups stratified by frequency of regular physical activity (RPA) per week. RPA0 indicates none; RPA1, 1 or 2 times per week; and RPA2, 3 or more times per week.

nal data for 19 143 patients aged 3 to 20 years (mean age, 12.8 years; 9140 female patients) with T1DM from 179 centers in Germany and Austria. Data are generated locally in an ongoing process by the participating centers using Diabetessoftware zur Prospektiven Verlaufsdokumentation (DPV) software (Diabetes Software for Prospective Documentation)[16] and transmitted in an anonymized form to the Pediatric Quality Initiative for central analysis. Twice a year the plausibility of these data is reviewed and inconsistent data are reconfirmed with the centers.

At every visit to the diabetologist, the DPV software requires information about the frequency of the patient's RPA. The patient or the parents of young children are asked about the patient's RPA and its frequency. Regular physical activity is defined as physical activity performed regularly at least once a week for at least 30 minutes. School sports are excluded. We included only patients for whom information on the frequency of RPA was available continuously for at least 1 year and evaluated the most recent year of complete documentation for each patient. Data obtained between January 1997 and December 2004 were included in this cross-sectional study. The study protocol was approved by the local human subjects committee of the University of Ulm, Ulm, Germany, and the study was carried out in accord with the Declaration of Helsinki.

Patients were grouped by the frequency of RPA per week as follows: RPA0, none (n=8589), RPA1, 1 or 2 times per week (n=7056), and RPA2, 3 or more times per week (n=3498). We divided the total analyzed population into the following 3 age groups: 3 to 8.9 years (n=3530), 9 to 14.9 years (n=8458), and 15 years or older (n=7155). We excluded children younger than 3 years from the study because the extensive physical activity in this age group is performed spontaneously and cannot be defined as regular.

For the occurrence of hypoglycemic episodes, we differentiated between severe hypoglycemia requiring help from another person and hypoglycemia with occurrence of seizure or loss of consciousness. For purposes of comparison, body mass index (BMI) (calculated as weight in kilograms divided by the square of height in meters) was expressed as BMI *z* score[17] and $HbA_{1c}$ values were transformed to Diabetes Control and Complications Trial normal values[18] using the LMS transformation of Cole.[19]

## STATISTICAL ANALYSES

The incidence of severe hypoglycemia or hypoglycemia with seizure or loss of consciousness is expressed as frequency per hundred patient-years. Data about insulin dosage are given as the mean daily dose per kilogram of body weight.

Data were evaluated statistically using the Kruskal-Wallis test for comparison between groups followed by the Bonferroni step-down correction in cases of multiple comparison, using SAS for Windows software (SAS Institute Inc, Cary, NC). Multiple linear regression analysis was performed to extract possible explanatory variables affecting the frequency of hypoglycemia and the $HbA_{1c}$ level. $P<.05$ was considered statistically significant.

## RESULTS

The frequency of RPA ranged from 0 to 9 (mean, 1.3) times per week. The general characteristics of the RPA groups are given in **Table 1**. The mean duration of DM was 4.9 years; the mean $HbA_{1c}$ level was 8.2%. In group RPA2, the mean age of patients was higher and the mean duration of DM was longer than in groups RPA0 and RPA1.

### $HbA_{1c}$ LEVEL

The $HbA_{1c}$ level differed among the RPA groups ($P<.001$) and was lower in the groups with more frequent RPA. This difference was present in all age groups ($P<.001$ in each age group) (**Figure 1**) and in both sexes ($P<.001$ in female and male patients).

A multivariate model with $HbA_{1c}$ level as the dependent variable and with age, BMI *z* score, sex, RPA, insulin dosage, and duration of T1DM as independent variables revealed that RPA was one of the most important factors influencing the $HbA_{1c}$ level. Other factors influencing $HbA_{1c}$ level were age, sex, and insulin dosage (**Table 2**). Thus, the $HbA_{1c}$ level was lower in patients with more frequent RPA, in male patients, in younger patients, and in patients receiving a higher insulin dosage. Body mass index had no influence on $HbA_{1c}$ level. After statistical control of all of these factors, the $HbA_{1c}$ level decreased by 30% from RPA0 to RPA1 and by 37% from RPA1 to RPA2.

## BODY MASS INDEX

In female patients but not in male patients, the BMI *z* score was lower in the groups with more frequent RPA ($P<.001$) (**Figure 2**). The main difference in BMI *z* score in female patients was found between the RPA0 group (0.60) and the RPA1 group (0.50). In the RPA2 group, the mean BMI *z* score (0.51) was not lower than in the RPA1 group.

## INSULIN DOSAGE

In male patients but not in female patients, the insulin dosage differed among the RPA groups ($P<.01$). Insulin dosage was higher in the groups with less frequent RPA. For male patients, the mean daily insulin dosage in the RPA0 group was 0.02 IU/kg higher than in the RPA1 group and was 0.02 IU/kg higher in the RPA1 group than in the RPA2 group. Analysis of the different age groups confirmed this effect in patients aged 9 to 15 years ($P<.001$) or 14.9 years or older ($P<.001$) but not in patients aged 3 to 8.9 years, the youngest age group.

## HYPOGLYCEMIA

The mean frequency of severe hypoglycemia was 22.9 per hundred patient-years in the analyzed population, and the mean frequency of hypoglycemia with occurrence of seizure or loss of consciousness was 4.9 per hundred patient-years. Multiple regression analysis (Poisson distribution) with frequency of severe hypoglycemia as the dependent factor and RPA, age, sex, BMI *z* score, $HbA_{1c}$ level, mean insulin dosage, and T1DM duration as independent factors revealed no influence of any of these factors on severe hypoglycemia. The same results were found for the frequency of hypoglycemia with occurrence of seizure or loss of consciousness. Thus, the frequency of RPA had no significant influence on the frequency of severe hypoglycemia or hypoglycemia with occurrence of seizure or loss of consciousness.

**Table 2. Results of Multiple Regression Analysis With Glycosylated Hemoglobin Level as the Dependent Variable**

| Variable | Regression Coefficient β | 95% CI for exp(β) | *P* Value |
|---|---|---|---|
| RPA | −0.302 | −0.434 to −0.247 | <.001 |
| Age, y | 0.074 | 0.067 to 0.081 | <.001 |
| Sex | −0.097 | −0.145 to −0.049 | <.001 |
| Insulin dosage | 0.990 | 0.904 to 1.077 | .001 |

Abbreviations: CI, confidence interval; RPA, frequency of regular physical activity per week.

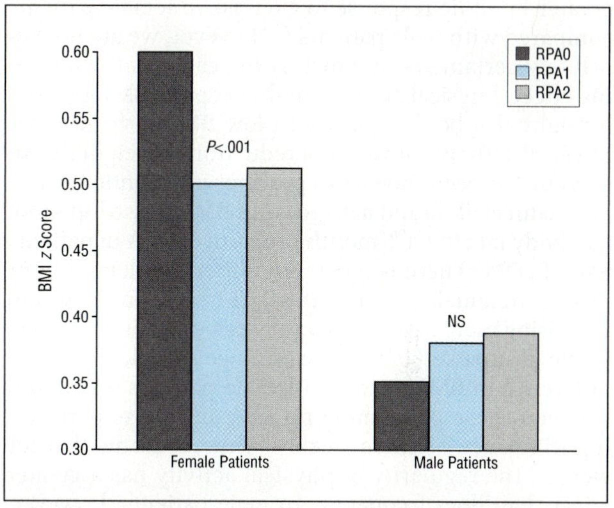


**Figure 2.** Body mass index (BMI) (calculated as weight in kilograms divided by the square of height in meters) *z* score in female and male patients stratified by frequency of regular physical activity (RPA) per week. NS indicates not significant; RPA0, none; RPA1, 1 or 2 times per week, and RPA2, 3 or more times per week.

## COMMENT

This study evaluated the influence of the frequency of RPA on metabolic control ($HbA_{1c}$ level), frequency of severe hypoglycemia, insulin dosage, and BMI in a large cohort of 19 143 patients with T1DM.

### $HbA_{1c}$ LEVEL

Our results show that the frequency of RPA is one of the most important factors influencing the $HbA_{1c}$ level. The $HbA_{1c}$ level was lower in the groups with greater RPA frequency. This effect was found in both sexes and in all age groups. Previous publications revealed controversial results; some studies[1,10,20,21] have shown an independent effect of physical activity training on the control of glycemia as measured by the $HbA_{1c}$ level in patients with T1DM, whereas other studies[2,11-14,22,23] have failed to show this effect. Most of the previous studies were designed as intervention studies and assessed the effect of an exercise program on $HbA_{1c}$ level during a defined period. The controversial results might be because of the different methodological approaches or because of few patients.[1,2,10,13,20-23] The FinnDiane Study[24] included a larger cohort of patients with T1DM (1030 adults) and assessed leisure time physical activity during 12 months. A lower $HbA_{1c}$ level was found in physically more active women but not in men. In another study,[14] 142 children and adolescents with T1DM were interviewed about their physical activity using a structured questionnaire. Performing intensive sports activity or taking part in competitive sports was not associated with better or worse metabolic control. Our study includes a large cohort of patients. However, the definition of the physical activity used in our study is based on the DPV questionnaire. This definition is not specific because it includes the patient's self-reported frequency of physical activity but does not consider the individual kind or intensity of the activity. This might limit our results and affect the strength of the association of the analyzed parameters.

## BODY MASS INDEX

Our study revealed a positive effect of RPA on BMI in female patients but not in male patients. This is important because, during puberty, adolescents with T1DM tend to become overweight[25] and girls with T1DM have a higher risk for gaining weight than are boys with T1DM.[26] Our data suggest that for weight normalization, girls benefit from RPA more than boys do. This might be caused by a greater lipolytic response to exercise in female patients compared with male patients.[27] However, we are not absolutely certain about which is the cause and which is the effect. Physical activity might keep the BMI low, but it might also be that girls with low BMI perform more physical activity. However, a reduction in weight due to exercise has been shown in a previous intervention study: Lehmann et al[1] found a decrease in BMI, waist-hip ratio, and body fat after a 3-month program of RPA in patients with T1DM. There is one more important detail in our results: in female patients, the BMI *z* score in the group exercising more than 3 times per week was not lower than in the group exercising once or twice a week. The main difference in BMI *z* score in female patients was found between those performing no RPA and those performing RPA once or twice weekly. Thus, it seems that for weight, the regularity of physical activity has a greater effect than does frequency. In male patients, however, we found a slight (not significant) weight gain in the group with more frequent RPA. We suggest that this higher BMI is not due to greater body fat mass but to greater muscle mass.

## INSULIN DOSAGE

An effect of exercise on insulin dosage has been shown.[14,28] Our data confirm that RPA is associated with a lower insulin dosage as a long-term effect. However, we found this effect only in male patients and only in those 9 years and older. The FinnDiane Study[24] found the same sex difference and revealed an association between greater physical activity and lower use of exogenous insulin in men but not in women. The authors speculated that men tend to reduce their insulin dosage to prevent exercise-induced hypoglycemia more than women do. We believe this issue should be followed up in further studies.

In our study, in the younger age group (<9 years), we found no difference in insulin dosage among the RPA groups. One reason might be that in this age group a higher proportion of patients still are in remission and, therefore, factors other than physical activity exert a major influence on insulin dosage.

## HYPOGLYCEMIA

Better control of glycemia (lower $HbA_{1c}$ level) is related to more frequent mild and severe hypoglycemia.[29,30] Thus, one might argue that RPA, by lowering the $HbA_{1c}$ level, indirectly bears the risk for a higher incidence of hypoglycemia in patients with T1DM. We analyzed the influence of RPA on the occurrence of severe hypoglycemia and of hypoglycemia with loss of consciousness or seizure. Mild hypoglycemia was not assessed in our study. Our data show that the frequency of RPA does not constitute an independent risk factor for severe hypoglycemia or hypoglycemia with loss of consciousness. One reason might be that RPA enables the patient to implement management strategies to prevent exercise-induced hypoglycemia. It has been shown that the intrasubject blood glucose response to moderate exercise is reliable and repeatable when preexisting meal, exercise, and insulin regimens are kept constant.[31] Thus, the well-educated patient with T1DM is able to learn about his or her individual glucose response to RPA and can establish an individual strategy (ie, intake of carbohydrates or reduction of insulin dosage before exercise) to prevent exercise-induced hypoglycemia.

Our results are influenced by the educational status of the analyzed patients concerning glucose management before exercise. However, preventing exercise-induced hypoglycemia is only possible in cases of planned exercise by a reasonable patient. This is not the case in very young children, who exert physical activity spontaneously and often unexpectedly by the parents. These children were not the subject of our study and might be at higher risk for hypoglycemia due to physical activity.

## CONCLUSIONS

Regular physical activity should be recommended in patients with T1DM. Regular physical activity results in better control of glycemia, including a lower $HbA_{1c}$ level and, in female patients, lower BMI. The risk for severe hypoglycemia or hypoglycemia with loss of consciousness or seizure is not elevated in pediatric patients with a high frequency of RPA.

**Accepted for Publication:** November 23, 2005.
**Correspondence:** Antje Herbst, MD, Department of Paediatrics, University of Bonn, Adenaueralle 119, 53113 Bonn, Germany (herbstantje@web.de).
**Funding/Support:** The DPV Science Initiative was supported by the German Federal Ministry of Health, Novo Nordisk Germany, the Dr Bürger-Büsing Foundation, and the German Diabetes Foundation.
**Acknowledgment:** We thank the pediatric diabetes centers who have joined the DPV Science Initiative and collaborated in this investigation: In Germany: Aachen, Ahlen, Aue, Augsburg, Aurich, Bad Driburg, Bad Hersfeld, Bad Kösen, Bad Lauterberg, Bad Oeynhausen, Berlin, Bielefeld, Bocholt, Bonn, Bottrop, Bremen, Bremerhaven, Bruckmühl, Celle, Chemnitz, Coesfeld, Darmstadt, Datteln, Deggendorf, Delmenhorst, Detmold, Dortmund, Dresden, Düren-Birkesdorf, Düsseldorf, Erfurt, Erlangen, Essen, Esslingen, Eutin, Freiburg, Friedrichshafen, Fulda, Fürth, Gaissach, Garmisch-Partenkirchen, Gelnhausen, Gelsenkirchen, Gießen, Göppingen, Görlitz, Göttingen, Hachenburg, Hagen, Halle, Hamburg, Hamm, Hanau, Hannover, Heidelberg, Heidenheim, Heilbronn, Herdecke, Herford, Heringsdorf, Hermeskeil,

Herten, Hildesheim, Hinrichsegen, Homburg, Itzehoe, Jena, Kaiserslautern, Karlsburg, Karlsruhe, Kassel, Kaufbeuren, Kempen, Kiel, Koblenz, Köln, Konstanz, Krefeld, Landshut, Leipzig, Lingen, Lippstadt, Ludwigsburg, Ludwigshafen, Lübeck, Lüdenscheid, Magdeburg, Mannheim, Marburg, Mechernich, Memmingen, Minden, Moers, Mönchengladbach, München, Münster, Mutterstadt, Neuburg, Neunkirchen, Neuss, Neuwied, Nürnberg, Oberhausen, Offenbach, Oldenburg, Osnabrück, Paderborn, Passau, Pforzheim, Rastatt, Ravensburg, Recklinghausen, Regensburg, Remscheid, Rendsburg, Rheine, Rosenheim, Rostock, Rotenburg/Wümme, Saaldorf-Surheim, Saalfeld, Saarbrücken, Saarlouis, Scheidegg, Schw. Gemünd, Schweinfurt, Schwerin, Siegen, Singen, Sinsheim, Stade, Stolberg, Stuttgart, Suhl, Sylt, Trier, Tübingen, Ulm, Vechta, Viersen, Waiblingen, Waldshut, Weiden, Weingarten, Wetzlar, Wiesbaden, Worms, and Wuppertal; and in Austria, Innsbruck and Wien.

## REFERENCES


1. Lehmann R, Kaplan V, Bingisser R, Bloch KE, Spinas GA. Impact of physical activity on cardiovascular risk factors in IDDM. *Diabetes Care.* 1997;20:1603-1611.
2. Wallberg-Henriksson H, Gunnarsson R, Henriksson J, et al. Increased peripheral insulin sensitivity and muscle mitochondrial enzymes but unchanged blood glucose control in type I diabetics after physical training. *Diabetes.* 1982;31:1044-1050.
3. Yki-Jarvinen H, DeFronzo RA, Koivisto VA. Normalization of insulin sensitivity in type I diabetic subjects by physical training during insulin pump therapy. *Diabetes Care.* 1984;7:520-527.
4. Schmitz KH, Jacobs DR Jr, Hong CP, Steinberger J, Moran A, Sinaiko AR. Association of physical activity with insulin sensitivity in children. *Int J Obes Relat Metab Disord.* 2002;26:1310-1316.
5. Mikines KJ, Sonne B, Farrell PA, Tronier B, Galbo H. Effect of physical exercise on sensitivity and responsiveness to insulin in humans. *Am J Physiol.* 1988;254:E248-E259.
6. Dela F, Mikines KJ, von Linstow M, Secher NH, Galbo H. Effect of training on insulin-mediated glucose uptake in human muscle. *Am J Physiol.* 1992;263:E1134-E1143.
7. Kristiansen S, Gade J, Wojtaszewski JF, Kiens B, Richter EA. Glucose uptake is increased in trained vs. untrained muscle during heavy exercise. *J Appl Physiol.* 2000;89:1151-1158.
8. Sandoval DA, Guy DL, Richardson MA, Ertl AC, Davis SN. Effects of low and moderate antecedent exercise on counterregulatory responses to subsequent hypoglycemia in type 1 diabetes. *Diabetes.* 2004;53:1798-1806.
9. Galassetti P, Tate D, Neill RA, Morrey S, Wasserman DH, Davis SN. Effect of sex on counterregulatory responses to exercise after antecedent hypoglycemia in type 1 diabetes. *Am J Physiol Endocrinol Metab.* 2004;287:E16-E24.
10. Zoppini G, Carlini M, Muggeo M. Self-reported exercise and quality of life in young type 1 diabetic subjects. *Diabetes Nutr Metab.* 2003;16:77-80.
11. Zinman B, Ruderman N, Campaigne BN, Devlin JT, Schneider SH; American Diabetes Association. Physical activity/exercise and diabetes. *Diabetes Care.* 2004;27:S58-S62.
12. Wasserman DH, Zinman B. Exercise in individuals with IDDM. *Diabetes Care.* 1994;17:924-937.
13. Roberts L, Jones TW, Fournier PA. Exercise training and glycemic control in adolescents with poorly controlled type 1 diabetes mellitus. *J Pediatr Endocrinol Metab.* 2002;15:621-627.
14. Raile K, Kapellen T, Schweiger A, et al. Physical activity and competitive sports in children and adolescents with type 1 diabetes. *Diabetes Care.* 1999;22:1904-1905.
15. Hecker W, Grabert M, Holl RW; German Paediatric Diabetology Group. Quality of paediatric IDDM care in Germany: a multicentre analysis. *J Pediatr Endocrinol Metab.* 1999;12:31-38.
16. Grabert M, Schweiggert F, Holl RW. A framework for diabetes documentation and quality management in Germany: 10 years of experience with DPV. *Comput Methods Programs Biomed.* 2002;69:115-121.
17. Kromeyer-Hauschild K, Wabitsch M, Kunze D, et al. Percentiles of body mass index in children and adolescents evaluated from different regional German studies [in German]. *Monatsschr Kinderheilkd.* 2001;149:807-818.
18. DCCT Research Group. Feasibility of centralized measurements of glycated hemoglobin in the Diabetes Control and Complications Trial: a multicenter study. *Clin Chem.* 1987;33:2267-2271.
19. Cole TJ. The LMS method for constructing normalized growth standards. *Eur J Clin Nutr.* 1990;44:45-60.
20. Mosher PE, Nash MS, Perry AC, LaPerriere AR, Goldberg RB. Aerobic circuit exercise training: effect on adolescents with well-controlled insulin-dependent diabetes mellitus. *Arch Phys Med Rehabil.* 1998;79:652-657.
21. Marrero DG, Fremion AS, Golden MP. Improving compliance with exercise in adolescents with insulin-dependent diabetes mellitus: results of a self-motivated home exercise program. *Pediatrics.* 1988;81:519-525.
22. Landt KW, Campaigne BN, James FW, Sperling MA. Effects of exercise training on insulin sensitivity in adolescents with type I diabetes. *Diabetes Care.* 1985;8:461-465.
23. Huttunen NP, Lankela SL, Knip M, et al. Effect of once-a-week training program on physical fitness and metabolic control in children with IDDM. *Diabetes Care.* 1989;12:737-740.
24. Wadén J, Tikkanen H, Forsblom C, et al; FinnDiane Study Group. Leisure time physical activity is associated with poor glycemic control in type 1 diabetic women: the FinnDiane study. *Diabetes Care.* 2005;28:777-782.
25. Holl RW, Grabert M, Sorgo W, Heinze E, Debatin KM. Contributions of age, gender and insulin administration to weight gain in subjects with IDDM. *Diabetologia.* 1998;41:542-547.
26. Mortensen HB, Robertson KJ, Aanstoot HJ, et al; Hvidore Study Group on Childhood Diabetes. Insulin management and metabolic control of type 1 diabetes mellitus in childhood and adolescence in 18 countries. *Diabet Med.* 1998;15:752-759.
27. Galassetti P, Tate D, Neill RA, Morrey S, Davis SN. Effect of gender on counterregulatory responses to euglycemic exercise in type 1 diabetes. *J Clin Endocrinol Metab.* 2002;87:5144-5150.
28. Mauvais-Jarvis F, Sobngwi E, Porcher R, et al. Glucose response to intense aerobic exercise in type 1 diabetes: maintenance of near euglycemia despite a drastic decrease in insulin dose. *Diabetes Care.* 2003;26:1316-1317.
29. DCCT Research Group. Epidemiology of severe hypoglycemia in the Diabetes Control and Complications Trial. *Am J Med.* 1991;90:450-459.
30. Allen C, LeCaire T, Palta M, Daniels K, Meredith M, D'Alessio DJ; Wisconsin Diabetes Registry Project. Risk factors for frequent and severe hypoglycemia in type 1 diabetes. *Diabetes Care.* 2001;24:1878-1881.
31. Temple MY, Bar-Or O, Riddell MC. The reliability and repeatability of the blood glucose response to prolonged exercise in adolescent boys with IDDM. *Diabetes Care.* 1995;18:326-332.

# Obesity Among US Urban Preschool Children

## *Relationships to Race, Ethnicity, and Socioeconomic Status*

*Robert C. Whitaker, MD, MPH; Sean M. Orzol, MPH*

**Objectives:** To determine whether there are racial/ethnic differences in the prevalence of obesity among preschool children and to determine whether these differences are explained by socioeconomic factors.

**Design:** Cross-sectional assessment.

**Setting:** Twenty large US cities, from 2001 to 2003.

**Participants:** Of the 4898 children enrolled at birth in the Fragile Families and Child Well-being Study, we analyzed data for the 2452 who, at the age of 3 years, had their height and weight measured during a maternal survey.

**Main Exposures:** Three socioeconomic indicators were the main exposures—maternal education, household income, and children's food security status, as assessed by the US Household Food Security Survey Module.

**Main Outcome Measure:** Obesity, defined as a body mass index at the 95th percentile or higher for age and sex.

**Results:** Of the mothers, 41.0% had education beyond high school, 52.9% of households had an income above the federal poverty threshold, and 79.5% of the children were food secure. The prevalence of obesity was 25.8% among Hispanics (any race), 16.2% among blacks, and 14.8% among whites. Compared with whites, the odds of obesity were significantly higher in Hispanics (odds ratio, 2.00; 95% confidence interval, 1.46-2.73), but not in blacks (odds ratio, 1.10; 95% confidence interval, 0.82-1.48). Neither of these odds ratios changed meaningfully after adjusting for all 3 socioeconomic indicators (Hispanics: odds ratio, 1.86 [95% confidence interval, 1.33-2.60]; and blacks: odds ratio, 1.07 [95% confidence interval, 0.78-1.47]).

**Conclusion:** In a sample of preschool children drawn from 20 large US cities, the high prevalence of obesity among Hispanics relative to blacks or whites was not explained by racial/ethnic differences in maternal education, household income, or food security.

*Arch Pediatr Adolesc Med. 2006;160:578-584*

IN THE UNITED STATES, A DISPARity among racial/ethnic groups in the prevalence of obesity[1] is one of the great concerns and enigmas in the obesity epidemic.[2,3] Addressing this disparity is important because it may underlie similar disparities in obesity-related health conditions, such as diabetes mellitus and hypertension.[4,5] However, to address this racial/ethnic disparity in obesity, we need to understand more about its modifiable root causes.

*For editorial comment see page 656*

It is not known, for example, at what age the disparity emerges, even though it seems to be established by adolescence.[6-8] The origin of this disparity may lie in the preschool years, because maternal obesity might influence the risk of childhood obesity by altering the prenatal and the early postnatal environments[9-11] and because the behaviors affecting energy balance begin to develop early in life.

Even if a racial/ethnic disparity in obesity prevalence exists in early childhood, it is not clear that it reflects varying socioeconomic conditions across racial/ethnic groups. Few studies have compared the prevalence of obesity in preschool children across racial/ethnic groups, and, to our knowledge, none has explored whether these differences are related to measures of socioeconomic status. The 1999-2002 National Health and Nutrition Examination Survey provided data on obesity prevalence among 2- to 5-year-old children by racial/ethnic group,[12,13] but the sample size of preschool children in the National Health and Nutrition Examination Survey limits the analysis of the relationship between socioeconomic factors and obesity within racial/ethnic groups. Other prevalence studies in preschool children were conducted in a specific geographic location[14] or were restricted to low-income children.[15]

Although there is no single measure of socioeconomic status for children,[16] parental education and household income are commonly used and have independently explained variability in childhood obesity in

Author Affiliations:
Mathematica Policy Research, Inc, Princeton, NJ.

prior studies.[17,18] However, among children in economically disadvantaged households, specific measures of material resources may be better than reports of annual household income at capturing meaningful short-term variability in economic well-being. Household food insecurity—a limited or uncertain availability of nutritionally adequate and safe food because of constraints in economic resources[19]—may be a specific form of material deprivation that is associated with childhood obesity. Food insecurity has been associated with an increased prevalence of obesity in women.[20-25] However, the relationship between food insecurity and obesity in children is less clear.[26-31] Food insecurity is an important factor to identify insofar as it can potentially be addressed by food assistance programs.

We used data on 3-year-old children in the Fragile Families and Child Well-being Study,[32,33] a birth cohort study of children from 20 large US cities, to address the following questions: (1) Are there differences in the prevalence of obesity among preschoolers across 3 major racial/ethnic groups—non-Hispanic whites, non-Hispanic blacks, and Hispanics (any race)? and (2) To what extent is any difference in obesity prevalence between these racial/ethnic groups explained by 3 socioeconomic indicators—household income, maternal education, and food security?

## METHODS

### STUDY DESIGN AND SAMPLE

The Fragile Families and Child Well-being Study is an ongoing birth cohort study whose sampling design is described elsewhere in detail.[32,33] The cohort was drawn from births occurring from 1998 to 2000 in 75 hospitals across 20 large (population, >200 000) US cities in 15 states. Nonmarital births, so-called fragile families, were oversampled relative to marital births (3:1).

Families were ineligible (<5% of sampled births) if the child was being placed for adoption, if the mother did not speak either English or Spanish well enough to understand the survey questions, or if the mother was too ill after delivery to participate in an interview. Most hospitals did not allow mothers younger than 18 years to participate. Among eligible mothers, 81.8% of those married and 87.1% of those unmarried agreed to participate. The institutional review boards at all 75 birth hospitals, and those at Princeton University, Princeton, and Columbia University, New York, NY, approved the data collection procedures. All mothers gave informed written consent.

After a survey of mothers in the birth hospital, follow-up surveys of the mothers were conducted approximately 1 and 3 years after delivery. At 3 years, 2452 (50.1%) of the original 4898 mothers in the birth cohort agreed to complete the survey as an in-home interview, during which their child's height and weight were measured. This report involves these 2452 children who, during the in-home survey, were a mean ± SD age of 38.6 ± 3.3 months.

### CHILDHOOD OBESITY

Interviewers were trained to measure the children's height and weight using a protocol modeled after the one established by the Centers for Disease Control and Prevention.[34] Children were measured while wearing light clothing and no shoes. Weight was obtained with an electronic scale (Bella Digital Scale, model 840; SECA, Hanover, Md). Stature was obtained with a portable stadiometer (Road Rod Stadiometer, model 214; SECA). Measurements were taken once and recorded to the nearest pound and to the nearest 0.1 cm. From these measurements, we calculated body mass index (BMI) (calculated as weight in kilograms divided by the square of height in meters) and computed BMI percentiles for age and sex using the Centers for Disease Control and Prevention 2000 growth reference.[35] We classified all children with a BMI at the 95th percentile or higher as obese.[36]

### RACE/ETHNICITY AND SOCIOECONOMIC INDICATORS

#### Race/Ethnicity

The mother was asked separately about her own race and ethnicity (Hispanic origin) and that of the child's father. We created 4 mutually exclusive race/ethnicity categories—non-Hispanic white, non-Hispanic black, Hispanic (any race), and other race (non-Hispanic)—that are hereafter referred to as white, black, Hispanic, and other. For 86.3% of the children, the race/ethnicity category of the 2 parents was the same and was used as the child's category. In the cases in which the race/ethnicity of the 2 parents differed, we based the child's race/ethnicity on the mother's race/ethnicity.

#### Maternal Education

This variable was based on the mother's report of her educational status 3 years after delivery, and children were placed in 1 of 4 maternal education categories: less than high school, high school degree or equivalent, some college, and college graduate (bachelor's degree) or more.

#### Household Income

Income data were not available from the 3-year survey. However, on the birth and 1-year surveys, the mother was asked to report the pretax income of the entire household during the prior 12 months. She was instructed to include her own income plus the income of all those living with her and to consider income from all sources, including public assistance. On both surveys, when the mother did not report household income, income was imputed using a regression model that contained other variables available in the survey, such as marital status, age, immigrant status, number of other adults in the household, whether the mother worked in the past year, and whether she received welfare in the past year. In our analysis, we used the income data reported on the 1-year survey, because these data were missing for fewer respondents than on the birth survey. In the 90 cases (3.7% of the sample) in which the mother did not participate in the 1-year survey, household income data were obtained from the birth survey. Altogether, income data were imputed for 142 (5.8%) of the cases in our study sample.

We calculated the income-to-poverty ratio by dividing the household income by the income at the US poverty threshold for a given household size for the year of the survey (data available at: http://www.census.gov/hhes/poverty/threshld.html). By using this ratio, we then placed children into 1 of 5 income categories: less than 0.50, 0.50 to 0.99, 1.00 to 1.85, 1.86 to 1.99, 2.00 to 2.99, and 3.00 or greater. We selected these categories because they divided the study population into groups of similar size while also using the cut point of 1.85, the criterion for determining income eligibility for the Special Supplemental Nutrition Program for Women, Infants, and Children.

#### Food Security

Households are considered "food secure" when all members have "access at all times to enough food for an active healthy life."[19(p1575)] The standard for measuring food security is the 18-

| Item | Positive Response |
|---|---|
| We relied on only a few kinds of low-cost food to feed the children because we were running out of money to buy food. Was that often, sometimes, or never true for you in the last 12 months? | Often or sometimes |
| We couldn't feed the children a balanced meal because we couldn't afford that. Was that often, sometimes, or never true for you in the last 12 months? | Often or sometimes |
| The children were not eating enough because we just couldn't afford enough food. Was that often, sometimes, or never true for you in the last 12 months? | Often or sometimes |
| In the last 12 months, did you ever cut the size of any of the children's meals because there wasn't enough money for food? | Yes |
| In the last 12 months, did any of the children ever skip meals because there wasn't enough money for food? | Yes |
| How often did this [item above] happen–almost every month, some months but not every month, or in only 1 or 2 months? | Almost every month or some months but not every month |
| In the last 12 months, were the children ever hungry but you just couldn't afford more food? | Yes |
| In the last 12 months, did any of the children ever not eat for a whole day because there wasn't enough money for food? | Yes |

**Figure.** Items on the Children's Food Security Scale. The first 2 items were preceded by the following: "Now I'm going to read you several statements that people have made about their food situation."

item US Household Food Security Survey Module,[37,38] which mothers completed as part of the 3-year survey. The items assess food security along a continuum by asking about a range of conditions and behaviors families experience when, because of lack of money or other resources, the quality or amount of available food is constrained.

The Children's Food Security Scale consists of the 8 questions in the module that reference the children in the household (**Figure**).[37] The scale score is based on the total number of food-insecure conditions reported.[39] We used previously described procedures to score item responses as positive and to code any missing responses.[37] Categorical designations of food security status based on the children's scale are not well established.[39] We used 3 mutually exclusive categories: "fully food secure" (0 positive items), "reduced diet quality" (1 or 2 positive responses), and "reduced food intake" (≥3 positive responses). In doing so, we tried to distinguish positive responses on the first 2 items ("relied on a few kinds of low-cost food for children" and "couldn't feed the children a balanced meal"), which might have indicated reduced diet quality, from positive responses on later items, which indicated reduced food intake.

## DATA ANALYSES

We conducted all our analyses using categorical variables to facilitate interpretation of our results. We used $\chi^2$ tests to examine the bivariate relationship of childhood obesity to race/ethnicity and to the 3 socioeconomic indicators (maternal education, household income, and children's food security). $\chi^2$ Tests were also used to compare the levels of the 3 socioeconomic indicators within each of the 3 major racial/ethnic groups (whites, blacks, and Hispanics). In these and other analyses in which we examined subject characteristics by race/ethnicity, we excluded the "other" group, because it contained too few subjects (n=75) to permit stable estimates for that group.

We used logistic regression models, with childhood obesity as the dependent variable, to determine to what extent, if any, the socioeconomic indicators mediated the relationship between race/ethnicity and obesity. We focused on the extent to which the odds ratios for the racial/ethnic groups changed between the base model (race/ethnicity as the only independent variable) and the models containing the socioeconomic indicators (entered individually and as a group). A small change from the base-model odds ratios for race/ethnicity or the lack of any significant bivariate association between the socioeconomic indicator and obesity would suggest that the socioeconomic indicator did not mediate the relationship between race/ethnicity and obesity.[40]

Because studies[7,17,41] of older children have suggested that race/ethnicity may modify the relationship between socioeconomic indicators and obesity, we also examined the bivariate association between each socioeconomic indicator and obesity after stratifying by race/ethnicity. We then developed logistic regression models to assess the statistical significance of any apparent interaction. By using the likelihood ratio statistic, we compared 2 logistic models: (1) a "reduced model" that contained only race/ethnicity plus the socioeconomic indicator and (2) a "full model" that also contained the variables for the interaction between race/ethnicity and the socioeconomic indicator. Because of the few children in the other race category, we excluded this group from these regression analyses. In the regression models, race/ethnicity was entered as 2 dummy variables (black and Hispanic). To limit the number of terms needed to model each interaction (and the degrees of freedom for statistical testing), each socioeconomic indicator was added to the model as a single linearly ordered variable—values of 1 through 5 for the income categories, 1 through 4 for the education categories, and 1 through 3 for the food security categories. Each interaction was modeled as 2 variables (black × socioeconomic indicator and Hispanic × socioeconomic indicator).

## RESULTS

In comparing the 2452 children in the initial birth cohort who had height and weight measurements (those in the study sample) with the 2446 children who did not (those not in the study sample), we found the mean household income to be lower (income-to-poverty ratio at the child's birth, 1.70 vs 1.99; $P<.001$) and the racial/ethnic composition different (white, 19.3% vs 22.8%; black, 52.2% vs 43.0%; Hispanic, 25.4% vs 29.3%; and other race/ethnicity, 3.1% vs 4.9%; $P<.001$). However, there was no significant difference ($P=.10$) between these 2 groups in the mothers' education level at delivery.

In the study sample, 41.0% of mothers had some education beyond high school and 52.9% of children lived in households with incomes above the federal poverty threshold (**Table 1**). Based on the Children's Food Security Scale, 16.5% of children had reduced diet quality and another 4.0% had reduced food intake. Of the 116 children who had reduced food intake, 22 met the criteria for "food insecurity with hunger" (≥5 positive items on the children's scale).[39]

The prevalence of obesity (BMI, ≥95th percentile) was 18.4%, and the prevalence of BMI at the 90th percentile or higher, the 85th percentile or higher, and less than the 5th percentile was 27.2%, 35.6%, and 4.2%, respectively. There was no significant difference in the prevalence of obesity between boys and girls (18.9% vs 17.8%; $P=.47$), nor was there a significant difference by sex within racial/ethnic group (data not shown).

The prevalence of obesity was not significantly different between black and white children. However, among Hispanic children, one fourth of whom were obese (Table 1), the prevalence of obesity was significantly higher than in either black or white children. There was a significant in-

**Table 1. Prevalence of Preschooler Obesity by Level of Socioeconomic Indicator***

| Indicator | Prevalence of Factor (N = 2452)† | Prevalence of Obesity |
|---|---|---|
| Race/ethnicity | | |
| White, non-Hispanic | 474 (19.3) | 70/474 (14.8) |
| Black, non-Hispanic | 1280 (52.2) | 207/1280 (16.2) |
| Hispanic (any race) | 623 (25.4) | 161/623 (25.8) |
| Other race, non-Hispanic | 75 (3.1) | 12/75 (16.0) |
| *P* value‡ | ... | <.001 |
| Maternal education | | |
| Less than high school | 731 (29.8) | 157/731 (21.5) |
| High school degree or equivalent | 713 (29.1) | 125/713 (17.5) |
| Some college | 745 (30.4) | 129/745 (17.3) |
| College graduate or more | 260 (10.6) | 38/260 (14.6) |
| *P* value§ | ... | .008 |
| Household income-poverty ratio | | |
| <0.50 | 670 (27.3) | 113/670 (16.9) |
| 0.50-0.99 | 485 (19.8) | 107/485 (22.1) |
| 1.00-1.85 | 562 (22.9) | 109/562 (19.4) |
| 1.86-2.99 | 360 (14.7) | 59/360 (16.4) |
| ≥3.00 | 375 (15.3) | 62/375 (16.5) |
| *P* value§ | ... | .48 |
| Children's food security‖ | | |
| Fully food secure | 1939 (79.5) | 361/1939 (18.6) |
| Reduced diet quality | 402 (16.5) | 71/402 (17.7) |
| Reduced food intake | 97 (4.0) | 13/97 (13.4) |
| *P* value§ | ... | .23 |

*Obesity was defined as a body mass index at the 95th percentile or higher.

†Data signify the number (percentage) of subjects at each level of the indicator. Percentages may not total 100 because of rounding. For the 2452 subjects, data were missing on maternal education for 3 subjects and on the food security measures for 14 subjects.

‡*P* value for the $\chi^2$ test (Pearson). *P* values for specific comparisons between non-Hispanic blacks (B), non-Hispanic whites (W), and Hispanics (H) are as follows: B vs W, *P*=.47; B vs H, *P*<.001; and W vs H, *P*<.001.

§*P* value for the $\chi^2$ test (Cochran-Armitage trend test).

‖Categories are based on the Children's Food Security Scale: fully food secure (0 positive responses), reduced diet quality (1 or 2 positive responses), and reduced food intake (≥3 positive responses).

verse relationship between maternal education and obesity prevalence, but there was no significant relationship between household income and obesity or between children's food security level and obesity. These findings on the bivariate relationship with the 3 socioeconomic indicators also held true when we used the 90th or 85th percentile as a BMI cut point. When all 18 items on the US Household Food Security Survey Module, including the 10 adult-referenced items, were scored to establish a single measure of household food security,[37] this measure was also not significantly related to childhood obesity. The prevalence of obesity was 18.4%, 18.0%, and 15.2% in the categories of food secure, food insecure without hunger, and food insecure with hunger, respectively (*P*=.47).

Hispanics and blacks had similar levels of food security and income, but Hispanics had lower levels of maternal education than blacks (**Table 2**). Whites had significantly higher levels of food security, income, and education than either Hispanics or blacks. Despite the differences between the racial/ethnic groups on socioeconomic indicators, there was no evidence that these indicators were important mediators of the risk of obesity in Hispanic children (**Table 3**). In re-

**Table 2. Comparison Between Racial/Ethnic Groups in the Prevalence of Socioeconomic Indicators***

| Indicator | Whites (Non-Hispanic) | Blacks (Non-Hispanic) | Hispanics (Any Race) |
|---|---|---|---|
| Maternal education | | | |
| Less than high school | 69 (14.6) | 350 (27.4) | 298 (47.9) |
| High school degree or equivalent | 113 (23.8) | 429 (33.5) | 156 (25.1) |
| Some college | 151 (31.9) | 433 (33.9) | 138 (22.2) |
| College graduate or more | 141 (29.7) | 67 (5.2) | 30 (4.8) |
| Income-to-poverty ratio | | | |
| <0.50 | 34 (7.2) | 431 (33.7) | 191 (30.7) |
| 0.50-0.99 | 53 (11.2) | 267 (20.9) | 149 (23.9) |
| 1.00-1.85 | 101 (21.3) | 290 (22.7) | 159 (25.5) |
| 1.86-2.99 | 107 (22.6) | 179 (14.0) | 63 (10.1) |
| ≥3.00 | 179 (37.8) | 113 (8.8) | 61 (9.8) |
| Children's food security | | | |
| Fully food secure | 405 (85.6) | 1002 (78.8) | 471 (76.2) |
| Reduced diet quality | 60 (12.7) | 216 (17.0) | 116 (18.8) |
| Reduced food intake | 8 (1.7) | 54 (4.2) | 31 (5.0) |

*Data are given as number (percentage) of each group. Percentages are based on the total for each indicator and may not total 100 because of rounding. All *P* values for the $\chi^2$ test comparing the difference in the prevalence of a given socioeconomic indicator between 2 racial/ethnic groups were significant at *P*<.001, except as follows: children's food security, blacks vs whites, *P*=.002, and blacks vs Hispanics, *P*=.44; and household income-to-poverty ratio, blacks vs Hispanics, *P*=.04.

gression models that controlled for maternal education, household income, and children's food security (as single indicators or together), the odds of obesity were still 84% to 104% higher for Hispanic children compared with white children (Table 3). Maternal education, for example, reduced the odds ratio for Hispanic race/ethnicity only 8.0%, from 2.00 to 1.84. In both models that contained income (models 2 and 4 in Table 3), the odds of obesity were approximately 40% higher in those children with household incomes between 50% and 99% of the poverty threshold than in those below 50% of the poverty threshold, but there was no evidence that income differences accounted for the increased risk of obesity in Hispanic children.

We conducted several sensitivity tests of the regression models shown in Table 3. By using blacks rather than whites as the referent racial/ethnic group, the odds of obesity in each model were still significantly higher for Hispanic children compared with black children, with the odds ratios ranging from 1.74 to 1.83 in the models. Our findings in all the models were not significantly changed when we (1) made the cut point for the binary dependent variable either at a BMI at the 85th percentile or higher or at a BMI at the 90th percentile or higher, (2) excluded those cases in which income data were imputed, (3) used the 18-item household food security measure rather than the children's measure, (4) used the father's race/ethnicity rather than the mother's race/ethnicity for those children whose parents differed in their race/ethnicity, (5) excluded children whose parents differed in race/ethnicity, or (6) examined models for boys and girls separately.

Stratified analyses (**Table 4**) showed an inverse bivariate relationship between maternal education and child obesity in whites and Hispanics, but not in blacks. Although income was not significantly related to obesity

**Table 3. Odds of Preschooler Obesity From Multivariate Logistic Regression Models***

| | Model | | | | |
|---|---|---|---|---|---|
| **Variable†** | **Base** | **1** | **2** | **3** | **4** |
| Race/ethnicity | | | | | |
| White, non-Hispanic | 1.00 | 1.00 | 1.00 | 1.00 | 1.00 |
| Black, non-Hispanic | 1.10 (0.82-1.48) | 1.04 (0.76-1.42) | 1.09 (0.80-1.50) | 1.12 (0.83-1.50) | 1.07 (0.78-1.47) |
| Hispanic (any race) | 2.00 (1.46-2.73) | 1.84 (1.32-2.55) | 1.96 (1.41-2.73) | 2.04 (1.49-2.79) | 1.86 (1.33-2.60) |
| Other race, non-Hispanic | 1.00 (0.50-2.00) | 1.00 (0.50-1.99) | 0.99 (0.50-1.98) | 1.02 (0.51-2.03) | 1.01 (0.51-2.02) |
| Maternal education | | | | | |
| <High school degree | . . . | 1.00 | . . . | . . . | 1.00 |
| High school degree | NA | 0.86 (0.66-1.13) | NA | NA | 0.83 (0.63-1.09) |
| Some college | NA | 0.87 (0.66-1.14) | NA | NA | 0.83 (0.62-1.10) |
| College degree or more | NA | 0.74 (0.49-1.12) | NA | NA | 0.69 (0.43-1.11) |
| Income-to-poverty ratio | | | | | |
| <0.50 | . . . | . . . | 1.00 | . . . | 1.00 |
| 0.50-0.99 | NA | NA | 1.37 (1.02-1.85) | NA | 1.38 (1.02-1.87) |
| 1.00-1.85 | NA | NA | 1.18 (0.88-1.58) | NA | 1.22 (0.90-1.65) |
| 1.86-2.99 | NA | NA | 1.06 (0.74-1.50) | NA | 1.11 (0.77-1.61) |
| ≥3.00 | NA | NA | 1.08 (0.75-1.56) | NA | 1.20 (0.80-1.81) |
| Children's food security | | | | | |
| Fully food secure | . . . | . . . | . . . | 1.00 | 1.00 |
| Reduced diet quality | NA | NA | NA | 0.91 (0.69-1.21) | 0.90 (0.67-1.20) |
| Reduced food intake | NA | NA | NA | 0.64 (0.35-1.16) | 0.63 (0.34-1.15) |
| *P* value‡ | NA | .47 | .32 | .26 | .31 |

Abbreviation: NA, not applicable (ie, the variable was not included in the regression model).

*Data are given as odds ratio (95% confidence interval). Obesity indicates a body mass index (calculated as the weight in kilograms divided by the square of height in meters) at the 95th percentile or higher.

†The referents were as follows: for race/ethnicity, non-Hispanic white; for maternal education, less than a high school degree; for income-to-poverty ratio, less than 0.50; and for children's food security, fully food secure.

‡Values are for the likelihood ratio statistic comparing the base model with the specified model.

**Table 4. Prevalence of Preschooler Obesity by Level of Socioeconomic Indicator and by Race/Ethnicity***

| Variable | Whites (Non-Hispanic) | Blacks (Non-Hispanic) | Hispanics (Any Race) |
|---|---|---|---|
| Maternal education | | | |
| Less than high school | 14/69 (20.3) | 52/350 (14.9) | 90/298 (30.2) |
| High school degree or equivalent | 16/113 (14.2) | 70/429 (16.3) | 37/156 (23.7) |
| Some college | 24/151 (15.9) | 73/433 (16.9) | 28/138 (20.3) |
| College graduate or more | 16/141 (11.3) | 12/67 (17.9) | 6/30 (20.0) |
| *P* value† | .14 | .40 | .02 |
| Income-to-poverty ratio | | | |
| <0.50 | 6/34 (17.6) | 55/431 (12.8) | 50/191 (26.2) |
| 0.50-0.99 | 10/53 (18.9) | 49/267 (18.4) | 44/149 (29.5) |
| 1.00-1.85 | 16/101 (15.8) | 53/290 (18.3) | 38/159 (23.9) |
| 1.86-2.99 | 16/107 (15.0) | 29/179 (16.2) | 13/63 (20.6) |
| ≥3.00 | 22/179 (12.3) | 21/113 (18.6) | 16/61 (26.2) |
| *P* value† | .19 | .09 | .50 |
| Children's food security | | | |
| Fully food secure | 57/405 (14.1) | 175/1002 (17.5) | 119/471 (25.3) |
| Reduced diet quality | 11/60 (18.3) | 25/216 (11.6) | 33/116 (28.4) |
| Reduced food intake | 2/8 (25.0) | 4/54 (7.4) | 7/31 (22.6) |
| *P* value† | .24 | .006 | .84 |

*Data are given as number/total (percentage) of subjects in each group. Obesity indicates a body mass index (calculated as the weight in kilograms divided by the square of height in meters) at the 95th percentile or higher.

†Values are for the $\chi^2$ test (Cochran-Armitage trend test).

in any of the racial/ethnic groups, it was only among white children that those in the highest income stratum had the lowest prevalence of obesity. Only among blacks was the prevalence of obesity significantly higher in children who were fully food secure. Based on regression models to test the statistical significance of the interaction between race/ethnicity and each of the 3 socioeconomic indicators, the *P* values for the likelihood ratio statistics were as follows: education ($P=.04$), income ($P=.09$), and children's food security ($P=.02$).

## COMMENT

### SUMMARY OF MAIN FINDINGS

Based on heights and weights measured between 2001 and 2003 for more than 2400 three-year-old children living in 20 large US cities, we found that the prevalence of obesity was significantly higher in Hispanics than in either whites or blacks, but that it did not differ significantly between whites and blacks. This elevated risk for obesity in Hispanic children was not explained by racial/ethnic differences in 3 socioeconomic indicators (maternal education, household income, and children's food security).

### COMPARISON WITH PRIOR STUDIES

The differences we found in obesity prevalence by race/ethnicity are consistent with those of 2 other large national studies. In the 1999-2002 National Health and Nutrition Examination Survey, the estimated prevalence of obesity among the 739 two- to five-year-old non-Hispanic white, non-Hispanic black, and Mexican American children was 8.6%, 8.8%, and 13.1%, respectively.[13] A similar pattern by race/ethnicity was also seen in 2000 data from the Special

Supplemental Nutrition Program for Women, Infants, and Children for more than 2 million 2- to 4-year-old white, African American, and Hispanic children in whom the prevalence of obesity was 11.4%, 11.7%, and 17.9%, respectively.[15] Both studies, like ours, showed that the prevalence of obesity in Hispanics was approximately 50% higher than in either blacks or whites. Our data were collected more recently, and the higher prevalence of obesity that we found in each racial/ethnic group could partly reflect continuing increases in the prevalence of obesity in US preschool children.

We found no overall association between the level of food security and childhood obesity. This finding is consistent with those of several other studies,[26-31] despite the differences between them in the age of the children studied, the specific measure of food security, and the cut point for obesity or overweight. To our knowledge, no other studies have examined whether the association between food security and childhood obesity differs by race/ethnicity. The significant interaction between food security and race/ethnicity, suggested by our findings, should be explored in future studies, as should the application of the Children's Food Security Scale, which, to our knowledge, has not been used in prior studies of childhood obesity.

Our data suggest that the association of maternal education and household income with childhood obesity also differs by race/ethnicity. Interaction between socioeconomic status and race/ethnicity has been shown in other studies[7,17,41] of obesity in older children or adolescents. In these studies, an inverse relationship between socioeconomic status and obesity was seen primarily in white children but not in nonwhite children, a finding that was particularly true among females. This interaction between socioeconomic status and race/ethnicity may be one reason for the inconsistent findings across studies that have focused on the overall relationship between obesity and socioeconomic status in children.[42]

## LIMITATIONS

Although this sample was drawn from 15 states, all the children were living in large metropolitan areas and many were born to unwed parents. The findings are not meant to apply to all US 3-year-old children, especially those living outside large cities. Less emphasis should be placed on the specific prevalence of obesity that we found within subgroups, as defined by race/ethnicity and socioeconomic factors, and more emphasis should be placed on how the prevalence differed across these subgroups.

Overall, the sample contained a broad range of household income and maternal education levels, but when our analyses were stratified by race, some sample sizes were small. The study involved only half the original birth cohort. Those who had height and weight measurements had a different racial/ethnic composition and lower income levels than those who did not have these measurements. We cannot determine how these differences might have influenced our findings about the relationship between childhood obesity and the socioeconomic factors we examined. For example, it is possible that the Hispanic children who had anthropometric measurements were less likely to be obese than the Hispanic children who did not have these measurements. However, even if the prevalence of obesity were 40% lower in the measured Hispanic children than in the unmeasured Hispanic children, the prevalence of obesity among all Hispanic children in the birth cohort would still have been 20%.

Socioeconomic status is a complex construct that is only partly captured by the indicators we studied. Income was not measured at the same time as maternal education and food security. Furthermore, among those at the lower end of the income distribution, actual income levels may fluctuate greatly. Income also does not reflect wealth or the possession of assets, economic or social, which may be more strongly associated with childhood obesity. Despite these limitations in measuring income, we found no association between childhood obesity and food insecurity, a specific form of material deprivation that might influence diet quality and thereby obesity.

## IMPLICATIONS

Although there is great concern about a racial/ethnic disparity in childhood obesity,[2] we found that obesity in preschoolers was highly prevalent in all 3 major racial/ethnic groups and that the principal disparity between these groups was for Hispanic children. We found no evidence that this disparity was related to household income, maternal education, or children's food security. This suggests that other unidentified factors, including genes conferring susceptibility to obesity, are the more likely explanation. Thus far, studies in young children have failed to identify possible environmental or behavioral factors to explain this disparity, but measuring such factors in young children is challenging. In this cohort, we have previously shown that perceived neighborhood safety, outdoor play time, and television viewing are all unrelated to childhood obesity,[43] and further analyses (Hillary L. Burdette, MD, MS, and R.C.W., unpublished data, 2005) have shown that these negative findings apply to all 3 racial/ethnic groups. Other studies[44-46] have not found significant differences in the diet of Hispanic children that could explain their higher prevalence of obesity.

Qualitative research[47,48] among low-income Hispanic children has suggested some potentially obesity-promoting factors in how mothers approach feeding their young children. However, it is not clear that these practices and beliefs about feeding are different from those among low-income black or white mothers[49-52] or are strongly related to child weight.[53] Less is known from qualitative research about how physical activity patterns in preschool children may differ by race/ethnicity.

This disparity in obesity between Hispanic and non-Hispanic children seems to develop early in life, so future research into modifiable determinants of this disparity should focus on the period from conception to school entry. This research might benefit from more emphasis on qualitative studies across racial/ethnic groups of those cultural factors that can influence energy balance, such as how young children are nourished and spend their time. Such studies might better detect the differences that underlie this disparity and that may not be easily understood through large epidemiologic studies.

**Accepted for Publication:** November 22, 2005.
**Correspondence:** Robert C. Whitaker, MD, MPH, Mathematica Policy Research, Inc, PO Box 2393, Princeton, NJ 08543-2393 (rwhitaker@mathematica-mpr.com).

**Author Contributions:** Dr Whitaker had full access to all the data in the study and takes responsibility for the integrity of the data and the accuracy of the data analysis.
**Funding/Support:** This study was supported by grant 43-3AEM-4-80086 from the Economic Research Service, US Department of Agriculture; grants R01-HD41141 and R01-HD36916 from the National Institutes of Health; and a consortium of private foundations.
**Role of the Sponsor:** The funding bodies had no role in data extraction and analyses, in the writing of the manuscript, or in the decision to submit the manuscript for publication.
**Acknowledgment:** We thank Shannon M. Phillips for her technical assistance and Ronette R. Briefel, DrPH, Thomas D. Koepsell, MD, MPH, Elizabeth Goodman, MD, Mark Nord, PhD, and Ram Chandran, PhD, for their critical review of earlier drafts of this article and for their helpful suggestions.

## REFERENCES

1. Flegal KM, Carroll MD, Ogden CL, Johnson CL. Prevalence and trends in obesity among US adults, 1999-2000. *JAMA.* 2002;288:1723-1727.
2. US Department of Health and Human Services. *The Surgeon General's Call to Action to Prevent and Decrease Overweight and Obesity.* Rockville, Md: Office of the Surgeon General, Public Health Service, US Dept of Health and Human Services; 2001.
3. US Department of Health and Human Services. *Healthy People 2010: Understanding and Improving Health.* 2nd ed. Washington, DC: US Government Printing Office; 2000.
4. Must A, Spadano J, Coakley EH, Field AE, Colditz G, Dietz WH. The disease burden associated with overweight and obesity. *JAMA.* 1999;282:1523-1529.
5. Winkleby MA, Robinson TN, Sundquist J, Kraemer HC. Ethnic variation in cardiovascular disease risk factors among children and young adults. *JAMA.* 1999; 281:1006-1013.
6. Kimm SY, Barton BA, Obarzanek E, et al. Racial divergence in adiposity during adolescence: the NHLBI Growth and Health Study. *Pediatrics.* 2001;107:e34. http://www.pediatrics.aappublications.org/cgi/content/full/107/3/e34. Accessed November 15, 2005.
7. Gordon-Larsen P, Adair LS, Popkin BM. The relationship of ethnicity, socioeconomic factors, and overweight in US adolescents. *Obes Res.* 2003;11:121-129.
8. Goodman E. The role of socioeconomic status gradients in explaining differences in US adolescents' health. *Am J Public Health.* 1999;89:1522-1528.
9. Whitaker RC. Predicting preschooler obesity at birth: the role of maternal obesity in early pregnancy. *Pediatrics.* 2004;114:e29-e36. http://www.pediatrics.aappublications.org/cgi/content/full/114/1/e29. Accessed November 15, 2005.
10. Whitaker RC, Dietz WH. Role of the prenatal environment in the development of obesity. *J Pediatr.* 1998;132:768-776.
11. Berkowitz RI, Stallings VA, Maislin G, Stunkard AJ. Growth of children at high risk of obesity during the first 6 y of life: implications for prevention. *Am J Clin Nutr.* 2005;81:140-146.
12. Ogden CL, Flegal KM, Carroll MD, Johnson CL. Prevalence and trends in overweight among US children and adolescents, 1999-2000. *JAMA.* 2002;288:1728-1732.
13. Hedley AA, Ogden CL, Johnson CL, Carroll MD, Curtin LR, Flegal KM. Prevalence of overweight and obesity among US children, adolescents, and adults, 1999-2002. *JAMA.* 2004;291:2847-2850.
14. Nelson JA, Chiasson MA, Ford V. Childhood overweight in a New York City WIC population. *Am J Public Health.* 2004;94:458-462.
15. Sherry B, Mei Z, Scanlon KS, Mokdad AH, Grummer-Strawn LM. Trends in state-specific prevalence of overweight and underweight in 2- through 4-year-old children from low-income families from 1989 through 2000. *Arch Pediatr Adolesc Med.* 2004;158:1116-1124.
16. Krieger N, Williams DR, Moss NE. Measuring social class in US public health research. *Annu Rev Public Health.* 1997;18:341-378.
17. Goodman E, Adler NE, Daniels SR, Morrison JA, Slap GB, Dolan LM. Impact of objective and subjective social status on obesity in a biracial cohort of adolescents. *Obes Res.* 2003;11:1018-1026.
18. Goodman E, Slap GB, Huang B. The public health impact of socioeconomic status on adolescent depression and obesity. *Am J Public Health.* 2003;93:1844-1850.
19. Life Sciences Research Office, Federation of American Societies for Experimental Biology. Core indicators of nutritional state for difficult-to-sample populations. *J Nutr.* 1990;120(suppl 11):1559-1600.
20. Centers for Disease Control and Prevention (CDC). Self-reported concern about food security associated with obesity: Washington, 1995-1999. *MMWR Morb Mortal Wkly Rep.* 2003;52:840-842.
21. Adams EJ, Grummer-Strawn L, Chavez G. Food insecurity is associated with increased risk of obesity in California women. *J Nutr.* 2003;133:1070-1074.
22. Laraia BA, Siega-Riz AM, Evenson KR. Self-reported overweight and obesity are not associated with concern about enough food among adults in New York and Louisiana. *Prev Med.* 2004;38:175-181.
23. Olson CM. Nutrition and health outcomes associated with food insecurity and hunger. *J Nutr.* 1999;129(suppl):521S-524S.
24. Townsend MS, Peerson J, Love B, Achterberg C, Murphy SP. Food insecurity is positively related to overweight in women. *J Nutr.* 2001;131:1738-1745.
25. Kaiser LL, Townsend MS, Melgar-Quinonez HR, Fujii ML, Crawford PB. Choice of instrument influences relations between food insecurity and obesity in Latino women. *Am J Clin Nutr.* 2004;80:1372-1378.
26. Alaimo K, Olson CM, Frongillo EA Jr. Low family income and food insufficiency in relation to overweight in US children: is there a paradox? *Arch Pediatr Adolesc Med.* 2001;155:1161-1167.
27. Casey PH, Szeto K, Lensing S, Bogle M, Weber J. Children in food-insufficient, low-income families. *Arch Pediatr Adolesc Med.* 2001;155:508-514.
28. Cutts DB, Pheley AM, Geppert JS. Hunger in midwestern inner-city young children. *Arch Pediatr Adolesc Med.* 1998;152:489-493.
29. Jones SJ, Jahns L, Laraia BA, Haughton B. Lower risk of overweight in school-aged food insecure girls who participate in food assistance. *Arch Pediatr Adolesc Med.* 2003;157:780-784.
30. Kaiser LL, Melgar-Quinonez HR, Lamp CL, Johns MC, Sutherlin JM, Harwood JO. Food security and nutritional outcomes of preschool-age Mexican-American children. *J Am Diet Assoc.* 2002;102:924-929.
31. Matheson DM, Varady J, Varady A, Killen JD. Household food security and nutritional status of Hispanic children in the fifth grade. *Am J Clin Nutr.* 2002; 76:210-217.
32. Reichman NE, Teitler JO, Garfinkel I, McLanahan SS. Fragile families: sample and design. *Child Youth Serv Rev.* 2001;23:303-326.
33. Carlson M, McLanahan S, England P. Union formation in fragile families. *Demography.* 2004;41:237-261.
34. Centers for Disease Control and Prevention. *Enhanced Pediatric Nutrition Surveillance System (PedNSS) Manual.* Atlanta, Ga: Centers for Disease Control and Prevention; 1994.
35. Kuczmarski RJ, Ogden CL, Guo SS, et al. 2000 CDC Growth Charts for the United States: methods and development. *Vital Health Stat 11.* 2002;No. 246:1-190.
36. Institute of Medicine. *Preventing Childhood Obesity: Health in the Balance.* Washington, DC: National Academies Press; 2005.
37. Bickel G, Nord M, Price C, Hamilton W, Cook J. *Guide to Measuring Household Food Security, Revised 2000.* Alexandria, Va: Food and Nutrition Service, US Dept of Agriculture; 2000.
38. Carlson SJ, Andrews MS, Bickel GW. Measuring food insecurity and hunger in the United States. *J Nutr.* 1999;129(suppl):510S-516S.
39. Nord M, Bickel G. *Measuring Children's Food Security in US Households, 1995-99: Food Assistance and Nutrition Research Report No. 25.* Alexandria, Va: Food and Rural Economics Division, Economic Research Service, US Dept of Agriculture; 2002.
40. Baron RM, Kenny DA. The moderator-mediator variable distinction in social psychological research. *J Pers Soc Psychol.* 1986;51:1173-1182.
41. Kimm SY, Obarzanek E, Barton BA, et al. Race, socioeconomic status, and obesity in 9- to 10-year-old girls: the NHLBI Growth and Health Study. *Ann Epidemiol.* 1996;6:266-275.
42. Sobal J, Stunkard AJ. Socioeconomic status and obesity: a review of the literature. *Psychol Bull.* 1989;105:260-275.
43. Burdette HL, Whitaker RC. A national study of neighborhood safety, outdoor play, television viewing, and obesity in preschool children. *Pediatrics.* 2005;116: 657-662.
44. Cullen KW, Baranowski T, Owens E, et al. Ethnic differences in social correlates of diet. *Health Educ Res.* 2002;17:7-18.
45. Grummer-Strawn LM, Mei Z. Does breastfeeding protect against pediatric overweight? analysis of longitudinal data from the Centers for Disease Control and Prevention Pediatric Nutrition Surveillance System. *Pediatrics.* 2004;113:e81-e86. http://www.pediatrics.aappublications.org/cgi/content/full/113/2/e81. Accessed November 15, 2005.
46. Bowman SA, Gortmaker SL, Ebbeling CB, Pereira MA, Ludwig DS. Effects of fast-food consumption on energy intake and diet quality among children in a national household survey. *Pediatrics.* 2004;113:112-118.
47. Kaiser LL, Martinez NA, Harwood JO, Garcia LC. Child feeding strategies in low-income Latino households. *J Am Diet Assoc.* 1999;99:601-603.
48. Crawford PB, Gosliner W, Anderson C, et al. Counseling Latina mothers of preschool children about weight issues. *J Am Diet Assoc.* 2004;104:387-394.
49. Baughcum AE, Burklow KA, Deeks CM, Powers SW, Whitaker RC. Maternal feeding practices and childhood obesity: a focus group study of low-income mothers. *Arch Pediatr Adolesc Med.* 1998;152:1010-1014.
50. Jain A, Sherman SN, Chamberlin LA, Carter Y, Powers SW, Whitaker RC. Why don't low-income mothers worry about their preschoolers being overweight? *Pediatrics.* 2001;107:1138-1146.
51. Sherry B, McDivitt J, Birch LL, et al. Attitudes, practices, and concerns about child feeding and child weight status among socioeconomically diverse white, Hispanic, and African-American mothers. *J Am Diet Assoc.* 2004;104:215-221.
52. Bentley M, Gavin L, Black MM, Teti L. Infant feeding practices of low-income, African-American, adolescent mothers: an ecological, multigenerational perspective. *Soc Sci Med.* 1999;49:1085-1100.
53. Baughcum AE, Powers SW, Johnson SB, et al. Maternal feeding practices and beliefs and their relationships to overweight in early childhood. *J Dev Behav Pediatr.* 2001;22:391-408.

ARTICLE

# Forensic Laboratory Evidence in Sexually Abused Children and Adolescents

*Karen L. Young, MD; Jerry G. Jones, MD; Toss Worthington, RNP; Pippa Simpson, PhD; Patrick H. Casey, MD*

**Objectives:** To determine if forensic laboratory evidence could be recovered from alleged sexual abuse victims more than 24 hours after the event and to determine if age or historical factors could be used to determine the need for forensic evidence collections.

**Design:** Retrospective study of hospital records matched with forensic evidence reports from the Arkansas State Crime Laboratory, Little Rock.

**Setting:** The emergency department at Arkansas Children's Hospital, Little Rock.

**Participants:** Eighty children (aged <12 years) and adolescents (aged ≥12 years) who presented to the emergency department within 72 hours of an alleged event of sexual abuse or assault with genital contact.

**Main Outcome Measures:** Cases positive for semen were correlated with age of the victim and postevent length of time to presentation to the emergency department.

**Results:** Of the 80 subjects, 16 had positive findings for semen. All 16 subjects who tested positive for semen presented to the emergency department less than 24 hours after the alleged abuse or assault event ($P<.001$). Of the 16 subjects who tested positive, 13 (81%) were adolescents. None of the prepubertal children had semen recovered from any body site; semen was recovered only from clothing or linen in those 3 children.

**Conclusions:** Forensic evidence collections from body sites in child and adolescent rape patients are unlikely to yield positive results for semen (1) more than 24 hours after the event and (2) when taken from prepubertal patients. Consideration should be given to amending guidelines regarding forensic evidence collections in child and adolescent sexual abuse or assault victims.

*Arch Pediatr Adolesc Med. 2006;160:585-588*

When an allegation of sexual abuse is reported within 72 hours after the event, the American Academy of Pediatrics[1] recommends that children and adolescents be taken immediately to a medical facility so that a physical examination can be performed and forensic evidence collected when appropriate. However, when the likelihood of forensic evidence contributing positively to the diagnosis of sexual abuse is low, the potential emotional harm to the child by evidence collection may be greater than the likelihood of benefit.[2] The child can perceive the evidence collection as uncomfortable,[2] frightening, and reminiscent of the abuse. Sedation, when required, also has attendant risks.

The goals of this study were to determine the usefulness of forensic collections for semen in child (aged <12 years) and adolescent (aged ≥12 years) sexual assault victims more than 24 hours after the event and to find other factors that may be reliably associated with the presence or absence of semen.

The standard of care is to perform forensic evidence collections if the event occurred less than 72 hours before presentation or if bleeding or recent injury is present. This "72-hour rule" is based on adult data and may not hold true for children.[2] Some adult data suggest that sperm could be found inside the adult cervix after this period if there was significant trauma, pain, or bleeding, so physician judgment should always be used.[3-5]

Most published studies involving evidence collection kits in children provide little information as to how often these kits are actually positive for semen, and whether some circumstances warrant omission of forensic specimen collection with confidence that the likelihood of missing evidence is low. Dahlke et al,[6] in 1977, reported sperm detection in 3% of children younger than 11 years who were raped, compared with 36% of 11- to 14-year-old subjects who were raped.

Author Affiliations:
Department of Pediatrics, College of Medicine (Drs Young, Jones, Simpson, and Casey and Ms Worthington), Center for Children at Risk (Dr Jones and Ms Worthington), Biostatistics Section (Dr Simpson), and Center for Applied Research and Evaluation (Dr Casey), University of Arkansas for Medical Sciences, Little Rock.

**Table 1. Characteristics of the 16 Patients Positive for Semen**

| Patient No./ Sex/Age, y | Time to Emergency Department, h* | Genital-to-Genital Contact | Bathed or Wiped | Location of Semen | Method Used† |
|---|---|---|---|---|---|
| 1/F/6 | Immediate | Yes | Unknown | Underwear | p30 |
| 2/F/8 | Immediate | Yes | Unknown | Underwear and washcloth | p30 |
| 3/M/11 | Immediate | No | Unknown | Underwear | p30 |
| 4/F/12 | <24 | Yes | Wiped | Vaginal and underwear | Cell |
| 5/F/13 | Immediate | Yes | Unknown | Unknown | Unknown |
| 6/F/13 | Immediate | Yes | Unknown | Vaginal | Cell |
| 7/F/13 | <24 | Yes | Wiped | Vaginal | Cell |
| 8/F/14 | Immediate | Yes | No | Vaginal, pants, and underwear | Cell |
| 9/F/14 | <24 | Yes | Unknown | Vaginal | Cell |
| 10/F/14 | <24 | Yes | Unknown | Vaginal, rectal, and underwear | Cell |
| 11/F/14 | <24 | Yes | Bathed and wiped | Vaginal, rectal, and underwear | Cell |
| 12/F/14 | Immediate | Yes | Wiped | Vaginal, shorts, and underwear | Cell |
| 13/F/14 | <24 | Yes | No | Vaginal, pants, and underwear | p30 |
| 14/F/14 | Immediate | Yes | Wiped | Vaginal and shorts | Cell |
| 15/F/16 | Immediate | Yes | Unknown | Vaginal | Cell |
| 16/F/16 | Immediate | Yes | No | Vaginal and underwear | Cell |

*Immediate indicates less than 6 hours.
†These methods are described in the "Laboratory Analyses" subsection of the "Methods" section.

## METHODS

### SETTING

This study was a retrospective review of records of suspected victims of sexual abuse or sexual assault who were examined and had forensic evidence collected in the emergency department of Arkansas Children's Hospital, Little Rock. The University of Arkansas for Medical Sciences Hospital institutional review board approved this study.

### SUBJECTS AND RECORD ABSTRACTION

We reviewed the medical records of 110 patients aged 16 years and younger who had forensic evidence processed by the Arkansas State Crime Laboratory, Little Rock, over a 30-month period from October 25, 1992, to April 4, 1995. Adequate medical records for 80 of 110 of those patients were obtained and were included in the study. The forensic semen analysis results for all subjects obtained from the Arkansas State Crime Laboratory were matched to the subjects' emergency department visit when the forensic evidence was collected. Specific information was then extracted from that visit and included in this study.

### PROCEDURES

The sexual abuse examinations and forensic laboratory collections were performed primarily by pediatric residents who were supervised by pediatric faculty physicians. Forensic collections were obtained when the sexual abuse or assault occurred within the previous 72 hours. Speculum examination with attempted cervical specimen collection was done for adolescents.

The forensic evidence kits contained swabs, slides, and containers and bags for collecting oral, vaginal, and rectal samples, linens, skin scrapings, clothing, or other particulate matter that could aid law enforcement investigators and prosecuting attorneys in confirming the sexual abuse and/or identification of a perpetrator. Kits contained printed instructions for collecting the forensic evidence. Nurses trained in forensic evidence collection assisted in the collections, and the protocols were followed in a standardized fashion. The kits were then submitted to the Arkansas State Crime Laboratory for analysis.

### LABORATORY ANALYSES

Investigators at the Arkansas State Crime Laboratory who tested the 80 kits used 2 possible methods to identify the presence of sperm in the forensic collections: (1) direct microscopic identification of sperm (designated "cell" in **Table 1**) or (2) crossover electrophoresis, which identifies a prostate-specific antigen by causing a union with a matching antibody using an electrical accelerant to process the results (designated "p30" in Table 1). Prostate-specific antigen, also referred to as p30, is a seminal plasma protein found only in adult male urine and seminal fluid.[3,7]

The p30 antigen can be detected in vaginal fluid only if semen were present[7] and only up to a maximum of 48 hours. Usually, p30 is nondetectable in the vagina after 48 hours.[3] Cell microscopy, or direct visualization, was the other method of laboratory analysis. Both highly sensitive methods detected and identified spermatozoa collected on oral, vaginal, or rectal swabs from the victim or from stains on clothing or linens.

### STATISTICAL ANALYSES

The association between forensic examination results and the time from the alleged event to presentation at the emergency department was investigated using an exact Cochran-Armitage trend test with computer software (StatXact 4.01, StatXact Software; Cytel, Cambridge, Mass).

## RESULTS

Of the 80 children and adolescents in this study, 49 (61%) were younger than 12 years and 31 (39%) were 12 years or older. The median age of the 80 children and adolescents in the study was 9 years (mean, 8.5 years). The age range was 4 months to 16 years. Of the subjects, 8 (10%) were male, of whom 6 (75%) were younger than 12 years.

**Table 2. Forensic Evidence Results by Age***

| Forensic Evidence Result | Subjects Aged <12 y | Subjects Aged ≥12 y | Total |
|---|---|---|---|
| Positive | 3 (6) | 13 (42) | **16** (20) |
| Negative | 46 (94) | 18 (58) | **64** (80) |
| **Total** | **49** (**100**) | **31** (**100**) | **80** (**100**) |

*Data are given as number (percentage) of each group.

**Table 3. Time to Emergency Department Presentation for the 80 Subjects***

| Result of Collections Processed | Total No. of Subjects | Immediate† | ≤24 h† | >24 h† |
|---|---|---|---|---|
| Negative | 64 | 3 (5) | 22 (34) | 39 (61) |
| Positive | 16 | 10 (62) | 6 (38) | 0 |

*$P < .001$ for the difference between times using an exact Cochran-Armitage trend test.
†Data are given as number (percentage) of each group.

Of the 80 subjects, 64 had a negative semen test result, while 16 had a positive result when their kits were analyzed at the Arkansas State Crime Laboratory (**Table 2**).

The findings of our study are presented in relation to historical findings, victims' ages, and site of semen recovery.

## HISTORICAL FINDINGS

All 16 subjects who tested positive for semen from body sites and/or linens presented to the emergency department less than 24 hours after the alleged abuse or assault event, and 10 (62%) arrived at the emergency department immediately after the alleged event. Table 1 details the characteristics noted in the 16 subjects who tested positive. **Table 3** shows the length of time between the event and presentation to the emergency department for all 80 patients. Of the semen-positive patients, 1 was known to have bathed and washed the genital area before the visit and 4 had wiped; 3 patients had not wiped or bathed; and in 8 patients, the bathing history was unknown. All 15 semen-positive girls reported genital-to-genital contact; the only semen-positive boy disclosed penile-leg contact.

## AGES OF VICTIMS

Positive test results for semen were present in 3 (6%) of the 49 children younger than 12 years, whereas results were positive in 15 (48%) of the 31 adolescents. The 3 youngest children with positive collections for semen were aged 6, 8, and 11 years, and presented to the emergency department promptly after the alleged sexual assault. Of the 16 patients who tested positive for semen, 13 (81%) were adolescents.

## SITE OF POSITIVE TEST RESULT FOR SEMEN

None of the prepubertal children had semen recovered from any body site; semen was recovered only from clothing or linen in those instances. Four adolescents had semen found in the vagina only. The remaining 8 adolescents with known sites of recovery had seminal fluid in specimens from multiple body sites and/or clothing (Table 1).

# COMMENT

Many findings on investigation of suspected child sexual abuse and assault influence the decisions of law enforcement to arrest a suspected offender and a social agency to take steps to protect a victim. When forensic laboratory evidence plays a role, it can be invaluable. The collections are not necessarily emotionally benign procedures, however, especially for prepubertal children. Establishment of medical evidence that justifies the guidelines for forensic collections in the pediatric population is imperative, because extrapolation from adult data may not be reliable when applied to children or adolescents.

Christian et al[2] report that more than 90% of 67 children younger than 10 years with positive forensic evidence findings were seen within 24 hours of their sexual abuse or assault. All evidence recovered after 24 hours was found on clothing and linens, except for 1 child, on whom a pubic hair was identified 44 hours after the assault.[2] Our findings are consistent with those in the report of Christian et al. All of the patients in our study who tested positive for semen arrived in the emergency department within 24 hours of the event. Christian et al reported some form of forensic evidence recovered from 24.9% of their collections, although only 11% of that was from body sites. Our yield was only 6%. This difference can likely be explained by the fact that Christian et al reported findings that included blood, semen, hair, sperm, and others (grease stain and synthetic fibers), whereas our findings were limited to semen and sperm. We would like to emphasize the critical role that early forensic evidence collections have in the recovery of semen from body sites for all age groups, while allowing for the importance of physician judgment to deviate from the standard on a case-by-case basis. We also agree with Christian et al that recovery and analysis of unwashed clothing and linens should be vigorously pursued because seminal fluid and blood can remain stable for long periods on cloth. In the study by Christian et al,[2] most of the evidence positive for semen was found on linens and clothing. In our study, this was exclusively the case for the 3 prepubertal children.

The prepubertal age group of victims seems to be predictive of the absence of semen. No child younger than 12 years had semen recovered from any body site in this study. Christian et al,[2] in, to our knowledge, the only other published study regarding forensic evidence collections in childhood, found that 11% of children younger than 10 years were positive for forensic findings from body sites, including blood, semen, hair, and other. Our study was limited to semen. One possible explanation for the low detection rates of sperm in children younger than 12 years may be that the sexual abuse of prepubertal children is less likely to involve vaginal intercourse because of the relatively small size of the hymen and vagina. The likelihood of identification of seminal fluids in the vagina is, thus, diminished. The collection technique for prepubertal children is also different from that of adolescents and adults. For vaginal swabs in young children, a blind swab is the preferred collection method, and there is no anticipation of collecting cervical fluids. In the adolescent and adult collections, a vaginal speculum is used, thus ensuring that deep vaginal, cervical, and other noticeable fluids can be obtained, which would likely increase the positive yield. One study[8] reports that it is possible that sperm can be found in the adult endocervix up to 6 days after intercourse. In vaginal samples, motile sperm commonly are not found after a few hours.[9] In a study[10] that looked at 1007 adult rape survivors, 919 vaginal specimens were collected and 344 (37.4%) were positive for sperm; 37% of the total number of cases were examined within 20 hours of the assault.

This study had limitations. It was a retrospective review, and many patient medical records had incomplete data. In addition, the number of semen-positive subjects was small.

In conclusion, our findings support those of the study by Christian et al[2] that forensic evidence collections from child or adolescent patients are unlikely to yield positive results more than 24 hours after the event. No child younger than 12 years in our study was positive for semen from body sites; if semen is present in children younger than 12 years, it is likely to be on linens and clothing. Evaluation of these findings by experts in the field is recommended so that guidelines can be amended to reflect the latest medical evidence.

**Accepted for Publication:** December 9, 2005.
**Correspondence:** Karen L. Young, MD, University of Arkansas for Medical Sciences, Arkansas Children's Hospital, 800 Marshall St, Slot 512-24A, Little Rock, AK 72202 (youngkaren@uams.edu).
**Acknowledgments:** We thank Cherise Martini, BS, for her significant contribution to this study as a research assistant; the Arkansas State Crime Laboratory for providing the results of the forensic evidence collections; retired Arkansas State Police Lieutenant Mary Margaret Kesterson for providing assistance in obtaining some of the data in this study; and Suzanne Speaker, MS, medical writer for the Department of Pediatrics, University of Arkansas for Medical Sciences, for contributing to this article.

## REFERENCES

1. Committee on Child Abuse and Neglect, American Academy of Pediatrics. Guidelines for the evaluation of sexual abuse of children: subject review. *Pediatrics.* 1999;103:186-191.
2. Christian CW, Lavelle JM, De Jong AR, Loiselle J, Brenner L, Joffe M. Forensic evidence findings in prepubertal victims of sexual assault. *Pediatrics.* 2000; 106(pt 1):100-104.
3. Finkel MA, Giardino AP, eds. *Medical Evaluation of Child Sexual Abuse: A Practical Guide.* 2nd ed. Thousand Oaks, Calif: Sage Publications; 2002.
4. Heger AS, Emans SJ, Muram D, eds. *Evaluation of the Sexually Abused Child.* 2nd ed. New York, NY: Oxford University Press; 2000.
5. *A National Protocol for Sexual Assault Medical Forensic Examination: Adults/Adolescents: President's DNA Initiative.* Washington, DC: Office on Violence Against Women, US Dept of Justice; 2004. Report NCJ 206554.
6. Dahlke MB, Cooke C, Cunnane M, Chawla J, Lau P. Identification of semen in 500 patients seen because of rape. *Am J Clin Pathol.* 1977;68:740-746.
7. Sensabaugh GF. Isolation and characterization of a semen-specific protein from human seminal plasma: a potential new marker for semen identification. *J Forensic Sci.* 1978;23:106-115.
8. Nicholson R. Vitality of spermatozoa in the endocervical canal. *Fertil Steril.* 1965; 16:758-764.
9. Soules MR, Pollard AA, Brown KM, Verma M. The forensic laboratory evaluation of evidence in alleged rape. *Am J Obstet Gynecol.* 1978;130:142-147.
10. Tucker S, Claire E, Ledray LE, Werner JS. Sexual assault evidence collection. *Wis Med J.* 1990;89:407-411.

## *Correction*

**Error in Abstract.** The article "Hearing Thresholds and Tympanic Membrane Sequelae in Children Managed Medically or Surgically for Otitis Media With Effusion," by Stenstrom et al in the December issue of the ARCHIVES (2005;159:1151-1156), contained 2 incorrect numbers in the abstract. The sentence in the methods paragraph of the abstract on page 1151 should read as follows: "Thirty of 57 medical subjects received ventilation tubes and 18 of 56 VT subjects received more than 1 set of tubes."

# HAVRIX®
# (Hepatitis A Vaccine, Inactivated)

The following is a brief summary only; see full prescribing information for complete product information.

**INDICATIONS AND USAGE:** HAVRIX is indicated for active immunization of persons ≥12 months of age against disease caused by hepatitis A virus (HAV). Primary immunization should be administered at least 2 weeks prior to expected exposure to HAV. When passive protection against hepatitis A is required either following exposure to hepatitis A virus or in persons requiring both immediate and long-term protection, HAVRIX may be administered concomitantly with immune globulin (IG) with different syringes and at different injection sites. Duration of immunity following a complete vaccination schedule has not been established.

**CONTRAINDICATIONS:** Hypersensitivity to any component of the vaccine, including neomycin, is a contraindication (see DESCRIPTION in full prescribing information). This vaccine is contraindicated in patients with previous hypersensitivity to any hepatitis A-containing vaccine.

**WARNINGS:** There have been rare reports of anaphylaxis/anaphylactoid reactions following commercial use of the vaccine. The tip cap and the rubber plunger of the needleless prefilled syringes contain dry natural latex rubber that may cause allergic reactions in latex sensitive individuals. The vial stopper is latex-free. Hepatitis A has a relatively long incubation period. Hepatitis A vaccine may not prevent hepatitis A infection in those who have an unrecognized hepatitis A infection at the time of vaccination. Additionally, it may not prevent infection in those who do not achieve protective antibody titers (although the lowest titer needed to confer protection has not been determined).

**PRECAUTIONS: General:** Prior to immunization with HAVRIX, the patient's current health status and medical history should be reviewed. The physician should review the patient's immunization history for possible vaccine sensitivity, previous vaccination-related adverse reactions and occurrence of any adverse–event-related symptoms and/or signs, in order to determine the existence of any contraindication to immunization with HAVRIX and to allow an assessment of benefits and risks. Appropriate medical treatment and supervision should be readily available for immediate use in case of a rare anaphylactic reaction following the administration of the vaccine. Epinephrine injection (1:1,000) and other appropriate agents used for the control of immediate allergic reactions must be immediately available. A separate, sterile syringe and needle or a sterile disposable unit should be used for each patient to prevent the transmission of other infectious agents from person to person. Needles should be disposed of properly and should not be recapped. As with any vaccine, if administered to immunosuppressed persons, including those receiving immunosuppressive therapy, the expected immune response may not be obtained. **Drug Interactions:** HAVRIX may be given concurrently with Hib conjugate vaccines in children 15 to 18 months of age (see CLINICAL PHARMACOLOGY in full prescribing information and ADVERSE REACTIONS). The safety of HAVRIX given concomitantly with INFANRIX has been evaluated (see ADVERSE REACTIONS). Insufficient data are available to assess the immune response of a fourth dose of DTaP vaccine when administered with HAVRIX. There are limited data to assess the concomitant use of HAVRIX with other vaccines. (See Immune Response to Concomitantly Administered Vaccines in full prescribing information.)

**Carcinogenesis, Mutagenesis, Impairment of Fertility:** HAVRIX has not been evaluated for its carcinogenic potential, mutagenic potential, or potential for impairment of fertility. **Pregnancy:** Pregnancy Category C. Animal reproduction studies have not been conducted with HAVRIX. It is also not known whether HAVRIX can cause fetal harm when administered to a pregnant woman or can affect reproduction capacity. Give HAVRIX to a pregnant woman only if clearly needed. **Nursing Mothers:** It is not known whether HAVRIX is excreted in human milk. Because many drugs are excreted in human milk, use caution when administering HAVRIX to a nursing woman. **Pediatric Use:** The safety and effectiveness of HAVRIX have been evaluated in 20,436 subjects 1 year to 18 years of age. (See CLINICAL PHARMACOLOGY and DOSAGE AND ADMINISTRATION in full prescribing information.) The safety and effectiveness of HAVRIX have not been established in subjects less than 12 months of age. **Geriatric Use:** Clinical studies of HAVRIX did not include sufficient numbers of subjects 65 years of age and older to determine whether they respond differently from younger subjects. Other reported clinical experience has not identified differences in overall safety between these subjects and younger adult subjects.

**ADVERSE REACTIONS:** As with all pharmaceuticals, however, it is possible that expanded commercial use of the vaccine could reveal rare adverse events. The adverse events most frequently reported by volunteers in clinical trials were injection-site soreness (56% of adults; 21% of children); headache (14% of adults; less than 9% of children). Other solicited and unsolicited events are listed below:

**Incidence 1% to 10% of Injections:** ***Local Reactions at Injection Site:*** Induration, redness, swelling; ***Body as a Whole:*** Fatigue, fever (>37.5°C), malaise; ***Gastrointestinal:*** Anorexia, nausea.

**Incidence <1% of Injections:** ***Local Reaction at Injection Site:*** Hematoma; ***Dermatologic:*** Pruritus, rash, urticaria; ***Respiratory:*** Pharyngitis, other upper respiratory tract infections; ***Gastrointestinal:*** Abdominal pain, diarrhea, dysgeusia, vomiting; ***Musculoskeletal:*** Arthralgia, elevation of creatine phosphokinase, myalgia; ***Hematologic:*** Lymphadenopathy; ***Central Nervous System:*** Hypertonic episode, insomnia, photophobia, vertigo.

**Additional safety data:** Safety data were obtained from 2 additional sources in which large populations were vaccinated. In an outbreak setting in which 4,930 individuals were immunized with a single dose of either 720 EL.U. or 1440 EL.U. of HAVRIX, the vaccine was well tolerated and no serious adverse events due to vaccination were reported. Overall, less than 10% of vaccinees reported solicited general adverse events following the vaccine. The most common solicited local adverse event was pain at the injection site, reported in 22.3% of subjects at 24 hours and decreasing to 2.4% by 72 hours.

In a field efficacy trial, 19,037 children received the 360 EL.U. dose of HAVRIX. The most commonly reported adverse events were injection-site pain (9.5%) and tenderness (8.1%), reported following first doses of HAVRIX. Other adverse events were infrequent and comparable to the control vaccine ENGERIX-B® [Hepatitis B Vaccine (Recombinant)].

In subjects with chronic liver disease, HAVRIX was safe and well tolerated. Local injection site reactions were similar among all 4 groups, and no serious adverse reactions attributed to the vaccine were reported in subjects with chronic liver disease.

***Safety Data for HAVRIX 720 EL.U./0.5 mL Beginning at 11 Months of Age:*** In the multicenter study described under CLINICAL PHARMACOLOGY in full prescribing information, parents/guardians recorded local and general symptoms on diary cards for 4 days (Days 0 to 3) after vaccination. In the 3 groups of children who received HAVRIX alone, safety data were available for 723 children who received 1,396 documented doses of HAVRIX. Additional safety data were available for 181 children who received HAVRIX coadministered with INFANRIX and Hib conjugate vaccine. Most adverse events were mild and transient. The frequencies of solicited local and systemic reactions following receipt of HAVRIX were monitored during the 4-day observation period.

The following rates of solicited adverse events in children who received their first dose of HAVRIX alone at between 11 and 25 months of age were observed. Among local reactions: pain was reported in 15-21% of subjects, redness in 16-21%, swelling in 8% of subjects. Among general reactions, irritability was reported in 24-36% of subjects, loss of appetite in 16-19% of subjects, drowsiness in 15-17% of subjects and fever >39.5°C in ≤2% of subjects. Following the booster dose of HAVRIX, among local reactions: pain was reported in 16-21% of subjects, redness in 17-22%, swelling in 8-10% of subjects. Following the booster dose of HAVRIX, among general reactions, irritability was reported in 19-29% of subjects, loss of appetite in 14-18% of subjects, drowsiness in 13-16% of subjects and fever >39.5°C in ≤1% of subjects.

Drowsiness and loss of appetite occurred at statistically significantly higher rates in subjects 15 to 18 months of age who received Hib conjugate vaccine (PRP-T) and INFANRIX concomitantly with HAVRIX as compared to subjects 15 to 18 months of age who received Hib conjugate vaccine (PRP-T) and INFANRIX (drowsiness 34% and 22% and loss of appetite 29% and 19%, respectively). With the exception of fever (>39.5°C), the solicited general symptoms occurred at statistically significantly higher rates in subjects 15 to 18 months of age who received Hib conjugate vaccine (PRP-T) and INFANRIX concomitantly with HAVRIX as compared to subjects 15 to 18 months of age who received HAVRIX alone (irritability 46% and 30%, drowsiness 34% and 17%, and loss of appetite 29% and 17%, respectively).

A febrile seizure was reported in an 18-month old subject two days after receiving the first dose of HAVRIX. Other serious adverse events reported during the course of this study included a single case each of hepatitis ~5 months post dose 1, insulin-dependent diabetes ~4 months post dose 1, and Kawasaki's disease ~3 1/2 months post dose 1. The association of these events with vaccination is unknown.

**Postmarketing Reports:** Rare voluntary reports of adverse events in people receiving HAVRIX since market introduction include the following: ***Local:*** Localized edema; ***Body as a Whole:*** Anaphylaxis/anaphylactoid reactions, somnolence; ***Cardiovascular:*** Syncope; ***Hepatobiliary:*** Jaundice, hepatitis; ***Dermatologic:*** Erythema multiforme, hyperhydrosis, angioedema; ***Respiratory:*** Dyspnea; ***Hematologic:*** Lymphadenopathy, thrombocytopenia; ***Central Nervous System:*** Convulsions, encephalopathy, dizziness, neuropathy, myelitis, paresthesia, Guillain-Barré syndrome, multiple sclerosis; ***Other:*** Congenital abnormality.

The US Department of Health and Human Services has established the Vaccine Adverse Events Reporting System (VAERS) to accept reports of suspected adverse events after the administration of any vaccine, including, but not limited to, the reporting of events required by the National Childhood Vaccine Injury Act of 1986. The toll-free number for VAERS forms and information is 1-800-822-7967. Reporting forms may also be obtained at the VAERS website at www.vaers.org.

Manufactured by **GlaxoSmithKline Biologicals**, Rixensart, Belgium

Distributed by **GlaxoSmithKline**, Research Triangle Park, NC 27709



BRS-HA:L20

**References: 1.** Centers for Disease Control and Prevention. Recommended childhood and adolescent immunization schedule—United States, 2006. *MMWR.* 2006;54(51&52):Q1–Q4. **2.** Bell BP, Shapiro CN. Hepatitis A virus. In: Long SS, Pickering LK, Prober CG, eds. *Principles and Practice of Pediatric Infectious Diseases.* 2nd ed. Philadelphia, Pa: Churchill Livingstone; 2003:1188–1192. **3.** Armstrong GL, Bell BP. Hepatitis A virus infection in the United States: model-based estimates and implication for childhood immunizations. *Pediatrics.* 2002;109:839–845.

 Printed in USA. HAP283R0 February 2006

# Incidence and Correlates of Unwanted Sex in Relationships of Middle and Late Adolescent Women

*Margaret J. Blythe, MD; J. Dennis Fortenberry, MD, MS; M'Hamed Temkit, MS; Wanzhu Tu, PhD; Donald P. Orr, MD*

**Objectives:** To determine the 3-month incidence of unwanted sex and to examine relationship factors and health-risk behaviors associated with incident unwanted sex.

**Design:** Data collected from face-to-face interviews every 3 months in a longitudinal study with a minimum of 2 interviews and maximum of 10 across 27 months.

**Setting:** Primary health care clinics for teens in an urban setting.

**Participants:** Adolescent women aged 14 through 17 years.

**Main Outcome Measures:** At each 3-month visit, cervical and vaginal specimens were obtained for the evaluation of *Chlamydia trachomatis*, *Neisseria gonorrhoeae*, and *Trichomonas vaginalis* infection; for each partner, relationship characteristics and sexual behaviors were assessed, as well as the occurrence of unwanted sex. A logistic model was used to account for within-subject variability to model the probability of unwanted sex as a function of predictor variables.

**Results:** A total of 279 participants with a mean age of 15.9 years were enrolled, and most were African American (88.5% [247/279]). Unwanted sex was reported by 40.9% (n=114) of participants and in 15.5% (292/1880) of partner-visits. The most prevalent type of unwanted sex was due to fear that the partner would get angry if denied sex (37.6%, or 105 participants). Factors associated with unwanted sex included having a baby with the partner, lower relationship quality, lack of sexual control, less condom use, and partner marijuana use.

**Conclusions:** Unwanted sex occurs often within the sexual relationships of teens. These unwanted sexual experiences result in risk for sexually transmitted infections and pregnancies. Sexual health counseling to reduce risk should focus on both the patient's and the partner's behaviors.

*Arch Pediatr Adolesc Med. 2006;160:591-595*

Unwanted sex is a common element of many young women's sexual experiences, often within the context of established romantic and sexual relationships.[1-4] Unwanted sex refers to increasing degrees of incentive, pressure, or threat used by one partner to obtain sex that is unwanted by the other partner.[4,5]

Unwanted sex, especially in more extreme forms of sexual coercion or rape, is associated with harm to mental and physical health. Depression, anxiety disorders, and posttraumatic stress disorder are all more common among women with a history of sexual coercion.[6] Sexual coercion also is linked to younger age at sexual initiation, more lifetime sexual partners, unplanned pregnancy, and sexually transmitted infections (STIs), including human immunodeficiency virus.[7-10] Unwanted sex occurs in a wide range of partnerships, from those in which the partner is barely known (eg, on a first date) to those in which the young woman has been sexually involved for months or years.

In addition to relationship characteristics, other factors may increase the health risks of unwanted sex. For example, condom use may be difficult to negotiate in circumstances associated with unwanted sex.[10] Substance use also may increase the risk of unwanted sex; approximately half of unwanted sexual events involve alcohol.[2,11] Risk of unwanted sex may be increased when a partner is drinking but the young woman is not.[12,13] Marijuana use is associated with unwanted sex, but in few studies is overall marijuana use distinguished from use within the context of a specific relationship.[13]

Research related to unwanted sex among adolescent women has at least 3 limitations. First, most research addresses only relatively extreme experi-

Author Affiliations: Departments of Pediatrics (Drs Blythe, Fortenberry, and Orr) and Medicine (Mr Temkit and Dr Tu), and Regenstrief Institute (Dr Tu), Indiana University Medical Center, Indianapolis.

ences of unwanted sex involving high levels of threat, coercion, or violence.[1,2,6,13] In these studies, more subtle and more subjective forms of unwanted sex that may be common in ongoing sexual relationships are not evaluated.[14] Nonetheless, these apparently less traumatic forms of unwanted sex still may be associated with adverse outcomes. Second, much of the research about unwanted sex is not relationship specific.[15] Unwanted sex occurs in the context of changes within relationships as well as change from one relationship to another. Romantic ideals and still-developing gender-role expectations about sexual relationships may influence the occurrence of unwanted sex as relationships change.[16] Third, much of the research addresses the prevalence rather than the incidence of unwanted sex. Prevalence measures are appropriate for less common forms of unwanted sex and sexual violence (eg, date rape) but are less relevant for assessing more subtle forms that may occur in many relationships, as well as when relatively short-term relationship and behavioral correlates are investigated.[17] Thus, the purposes of this study were 4-fold: (1) to determine the 3-month incidence of unwanted sex among adolescent women; (2) to evaluate relationship factors associated with incident unwanted sex; (3) to examine health-risk behaviors such as condom nonuse, alcohol use, and marijuana use in association with incident unwanted sex; and (4) to investigate associations of unwanted sex with incident STIs.

## METHODS

### STUDY DESIGN AND PROCEDURES

Data were collected as part of a longitudinal study of risk and protective factors associated with STIs among young women in middle and late adolescence. Data were obtained from face-to-face interviews performed at enrollment and quarterly clinic visits and from STI testing of clinical specimens obtained at each visit. Each participant provided at least 2 and as many as 10 interviews across 27 months. Interviews required between 25 and 40 minutes, and participants received $20 for each interview as compensation for time and effort. At each visit, cervical and vaginal specimens were obtained for diagnosis of *Neisseria gonorrhoeae*, *Chlamydia trachomatis*, and *Trichomonas vaginalis* infections. Diagnostic testing was performed using polymerase chain reaction for each organism. Informed consent was obtained from each participant, and written permission was obtained from a parent or legal guardian. This research was approved by the institutional review board of Indiana University/Purdue University at Indianapolis-Clarian. As part of the protocol for ensuring participant safety, disclosed cases of neglect, abuse, or sexual violence were referred to clinic staff and social workers for evaluation.

### PARTICIPANTS

Participants were adolescent women receiving health care in 1 of 3 primary health care clinics in Indianapolis. These clinics serve primarily lower- and middle-income residents from areas with high rates of teen pregnancy and sexually transmitted diseases. Clinic patients were eligible if they were aged 14 through 17 years at enrollment, spoke English, and were not pregnant at the time of enrollment. However, participants who became pregnant continued in the study.

### MEASURES

Measures were chosen to represent demographic, relationship, and behavioral characteristics thought to be associated with unwanted sex. Self-reported race was recorded as nonblack or black because of the substantial racial homogeneity of the sample. Age was calculated as the age on the day of the interview.

Relationship characteristics were assessed for each partner (as many as 5 partners) within the past 3 months. Because unwanted sex may occur in relationships in which coitus has not occurred previously, participants identified partners on the basis of noncoital sexual behaviors (oral-genital contact, genital touching, sexual kissing) if vaginal or anal sexual contact had not occurred. For each identified partner, the following items assessed relationship characteristics and sexual behaviors. *Duration of relationship* reflected the time (in months) since the first sexual contact (if any) with a specific partner. Participants were asked if they had a baby with the specific partner (no/yes). Relationship-specific substance use was assessed by means of 4 items reflecting frequency of alcohol and marijuana use (by participant herself or by a specific partner) before sex. Response options were "never," "some," and "a lot." *Coital frequency* was measured as the number of sex acts reported with a specific partner. Retrospective reports of partner-specific coital frequency show good correlation to prospective diary records, except at high coital frequencies.[18] *Condom nonuse* was calculated as the proportion of sex acts with a specific partner not protected by condoms.

Other relationship-specific measures included *sexual lack of control* and *relationship quality*. *Sexual lack of control* (2 items: $\alpha = .72$) addressed the degree to which the participant felt unable to manage sexual situations with a specific partner at a specific visit. Items were "Sometimes things just get out of control with him" and "It's easy for him to take advantage of me." Four response options were "strongly disagree," "disagree," "agree," and "strongly agree." Higher scores indicated less perceived sexual control with a specific partner at a specific visit. *Relationship quality* (5 items: $\alpha = .92$) reflects affiliation and comfort with a partner. An example item is: "We enjoy spending time together." Response options were "strongly disagree," "disagree," "agree," and "strongly agree." Score ranges were from 5 to 20, with higher scores indicating higher relationship quality. Prior research results show that relationship quality is an important correlate of STI-related behaviors such as condom use.[19]

Sexually transmitted infection was measured by the absence or presence of any of 3 STIs (*N gonorrhoeae*, *C trachomatis*, or *T vaginalis*) at any given visit.

The outcome measure was derived from 4 items related to partner-specific, visit-specific unwanted sex. These items were designed to assess the occurrence of unwanted sex in the previous 3 months. Formative research with this sample shows that *sex* is used to refer to penile-vaginal intercourse (Dr Fortenberry, oral communication, March 2005). Therefore, the term *unwanted sex* refers to unwanted penile-vaginal intercourse rather than other forms of sexual contact. Specific items included: "Would he break up with you unless you would have sex?"; "Does he ever make you have any kind of sex when you don't want to?"; "Would he get mad if you didn't want to have sex?"; and, "Does he give you money or gifts for any kind of sex?" Response options for each item were "definitely no," "maybe," and "definitely yes." These items were chosen to assess subtle power and relational imbalances that may be more common in sexual decision making than overt threats and use of force.[20] For the purposes of this research, unwanted sex by a specific partner at a specific 3-month visit was considered present if there was any positive response ("maybe" or "definitely yes") to any

**Table 1. Prevalence and Incidence of Unwanted Sex According to Type of Unwanted Sex**

| | No. (%) of Participants or Partner-Visits | |
|---|---|---|
| Type of Unwanted Sex | Prevalence* | Incidence† |
| Partner angry if denied sex | 105 (37.6) | 251 (13.4) |
| Sex that was not wanted | 26 (9.3) | 51 (2.7) |
| Fear of relationship termination | 27 (9.7) | 53 (2.8) |
| Exchange of money/gifts | 13 (4.7) | 27 (1.4) |
| Any | 114 (40.9) | 292 (15.5) |

*Prevalence refers to any report of unwanted sex (N = 279 participants).
†Incidence refers to any report of unwanted sex with a specific partner during the previous 3 months (N = 1880 partner-visits).

of the 4 items. The outcome measure was therefore dichotomous (no/yes) partner- and visit-specific unwanted sex.

## STATISTICAL ANALYSES

A logistic model with a random intercept to account for within-subject variability was used to model the probability of unwanted sex as a function of predictor variables. In this analysis, the random intercept reflected the subject-specific propensity of giving a "yes" response in an outcome variable. The model was fitted using the procedure PROC NLMIXED from the statistical software package SAS version 8.2 (SAS Institute Inc, Cary, NC); the initial values used in the model-fitting procedure were obtained from PROC GENMOD. For model selection, we first screened all independent variables through a series of bivariate logistic models with a random intercept. Independent variables with bivariate $P<.30$ were included in a full multivariable model so the effect of each variable could be reassessed after adjustment for the effects of other potentially important covariates. A final model was obtained through backward elimination of variables with $P>.05$.

## RESULTS

A total of 279 participants were enrolled, with a mean age at enrollment of 15.9 years. Most participants (88.5% [n=247]) reported race as African American, while 0.7% (n=2) reported Hispanic/Latino ethnicity, and 10.8% (n=30) reported race as white. The mean number of interviews for each participant was 5.4, and the mean number of partners identified at each visit was 1.3. Thus, participants identified 1502 partners for a total of 1883 partner-visits. Missing data on unwanted sex reduced the final sample to 1880 partner-visits.

Unwanted sex was reported at least once (ie, prevalence) by 40.9% (114/279) of the participants and in 15.5% (292/1880) of partner-visits (ie, incidence) (**Table 1**). The most prevalent type of unwanted sex (37.6% [105/279] of participants) was due to fear that the partner would get angry if denied sex. About 10% of participants reported being forced to have sex (Table 1).

Demographic, relationship, and behavioral characteristics of the partner-visits without and with unwanted sex are shown in **Table 2**. These bivariate associations, unadjusted for multiple within-subject observations, suggest that recent unwanted sex with a given partner is more likely in relationships of longer duration, if the woman has a baby with a partner, when less sexual control is perceived with the partner, when coital frequency and condom nonuse are higher, and when marijuana or alcohol are used by either partner (**Table 3**).

**Table 2. Unwanted Sex During the Past 3 Months According to Demographic, Relationship, and Behavioral Correlates**

| | Unwanted Sex, Past 3 Months* | |
|---|---|---|
| Demographic, Relationship, or Behavioral Correlate | No (n = 1588) | Yes (n = 292) |
| African American | 1432 (90.2) | 244 (83.6) |
| Age, y | 16.8 ± 1.3 | 17.0 ± 1.3 |
| Relationship duration, y | 0.9 ± 1.2 | 1.4 ± 1.7 |
| Baby with partner | 110 (6.9) | 55 (18.8) |
| Relationship quality | 15.9 ± 3.5 | 15.0 ± 4.1 |
| Sexual lack of control | 2.8 ± 1.0 | 3.6 ± 1.5 |
| Coital frequency | 8.1 ± 16.4 | 13.6 ± 21.3 |
| Condom nonuse, % | 5.6 ± 15.7 | 10.7 ± 19.2 |
| Coital events without condom, % | 38 ± 40 | 54 ± 40 |
| Sexually transmitted infections | 321 (20.2) | 71 (24.3) |
| Marijuana use before sex | 313 (19.7) | 95 (32.5) |
| Partner's marijuana use | 548 (34.5) | 162 (55.5) |
| Alcohol use before sex | 182 (11.5) | 68 (23.3) |
| Partner's alcohol use | 464 (29.2) | 143 (49.0) |

*Data are given as number (percentage) or mean±SD.

Demographic, relationship, and behavioral characteristics of the partner-visits associated with unwanted sex are shown in Table 3. These analyses are adjusted for multiple within-subject observations (column 2, univariate), for other predictors (column 3, full model), and including only significant correlates of unwanted sex (column 4, final model). After backward elimination of nonsignificant predictors, factors associated in the final model with unwanted sex during the past 3 months included having a baby with a specific partner (odds ratio [OR], 4.4; 95% confidence interval [CI], 2.48-7.90]), lesser relationship quality (OR, 0.92; 95% CI, 0.88-0.97), lack of sexual control with a partner (OR, 1.80; 95% CI, 1.52-2.13), higher proportion of coital events without condom use (OR, 2.30; 95% CI, 1.49-3.55), and partner marijuana use before sex (OR, 1.80; 95% CI, 1.25-2.59). Variables not associated with unwanted sex were race, age, duration of relationship, STI, participant's marijuana use before sex, participant's alcohol use before sex, and partner's alcohol use before sex.

## COMMENT

Unwanted sex is a common aspect of sexual relationships of adolescent women, even when reported across a relatively short 3-month interval. Moreover, the data show that relationship factors (such as relationship quality, relationship duration, and having a baby with a partner) and behavioral factors (such as condom nonuse and marijuana use) are characteristics of relationships in which incident unwanted sex is more likely to occur. The data cannot be used to assess causal associations of unwanted sex; rather, they point to the complex interpersonal and behavioral contexts that may link unwanted

**Table 3. Demographic, Relationship, and Behavioral Correlates Associated With Unwanted Sex in the Past 3 Months**

| Demographic, Relationship, or Behavioral Correlate | Univariate* OR (95% CI) | Full Model OR (95% CI)† | Final Model OR (95% CI)‡ |
|---|---|---|---|
| African American, % | 0.38 (0.17-0.84) | 0.47 (0.20-1.09) | ... |
| Age, y | 1.09 (0.93-1.27) | 0.84 (0.70-1.01) | ... |
| Relationship duration, y | 1.37 (1.21-1.55) | 1.18 (1.01-1.37) | ... |
| Baby with partner, % | 4.79 (2.77-8.26) | 3.61 (1.93-6.77) | 4.42 (2.48-7.90) |
| Relationship quality§ | 0.92 (0.88-0.96) | 0.92 (0.88-0.98) | 0.92 (0.88-0.97) |
| Sexual lack of control | 2.01 (1.72-2.35) | 1.76 (1.48-2.09) | 1.80 (1.52-2.13) |
| Condom nonuse, % | 2.84 (1.89-4.24) | 2.19 (1.39-3.46) | 2.30 (1.49-3.55) |
| Sexually transmitted infections, % | 1.39 (0.96-2.03) | 1.44 (0.95-2.20) | ... |
| Marijuana use before sex | 1.86 (1.25-2.78) | 1.16 (0.70-1.91) | ... |
| Partner's marijuana use | 2.29 (1.65-3.18) | 1.62 (1.08-3.42) | 1.80 (1.25-2.59) |
| Alcohol use before sex | 1.75 (1.13-2.71) | 1.13 (0.66-1.93) | ... |
| Partner's alcohol use | 1.93 (1.38-2.68) | 1.07 (0.70-1.63) | ... |

Abbreviations: CI, confidence interval; OR, odds ratio.
*Adjusted for multiple observations within each subject by random subject effect.
†Variables with $P<.30$ in bivariate analyses are included in the full model.
‡Variables with $P<.05$ in the full model are included in the final model.
§Scale with possible total of 5 to 20 when 4 items are summed.

sex to other health risks. Clinically, these data suggest a reasonably high yield of screening for occurrence of unwanted sex at almost any routine health care visit, even if these visits occur at relatively frequent intervals (eg, at quarterly visits for contraceptives).

The data also point to the importance of attention to relationship issues as part of understanding risks associated with unwanted sex.[14] Results of some studies suggest that young women perceive unwanted sex as part of normal heterosexual relationships.[14,21] If sexual negotiation (including sexual refusal) is a skill learned during adolescence, then some degree of trial-and-error learning might be expected as experience, both positive and negative, accumulates. However, association of unwanted sex with lower perceived relationship quality, as well as condom nonuse, suggests the possibility of more serious consequences. Although the unwanted sex addressed in our study resembles the unwanted but consensual sex defined as *sexual compliance*, more extreme forms of sexual coercion and violence also may be characteristic of some sexually compliant relationships.[22,23]

The distinction of types of unwanted sex is important because our data do not directly address sex associated with violence, physical intimidation, or force. However, about 10% of the participants in our study responded affirmatively to an item ("Does he ever make you have any kind of sex when you don't want to?") that is similar to an item in the 2003 Youth Risk Behavior Surveillance Study. In that study, approximately 11.9% of high school students indicated forced sexual intercourse had occurred.[24] However, in our study, this type of sex in the past 3 months was addressed, whereas the Youth Risk Behavior Survey was used to assess lifetime prevalence. Other research documents an even higher prevalence of unwanted sex (as high as 44%), although using a variety of definitions of unwanted sex and diverse samples from which the data were drawn.[1,10,13,25]

Unwanted sex associated with relationship factors appears to be a relatively common phenomenon. Fear of relationship termination is often a component of the psychological pressure associated with unwanted sex. This type of unwanted sex usually is discussed in the context of verbal coercion in which sexual activity may occur in efforts to enhance the relationship, please a partner, or avoid conflict.[2,22,26] A study of junior and senior high school students indicated that one third of unwanted sexual experiences were often efforts to please the partner.[9] Other influences on sexual decision making also may be relevant to adolescents. Sex for money or gifts was described by 4.7% of the participants in our study and occurred in 1.4% of partner-visits. From one perspective, this measure cannot be used to assess unwanted sex directly because the participant's evaluation of the sex as wanted or unwanted was not assessed. However, inclusion of this measure is justified because of substantial research interest in social and economic power differentials in adolescent sexual relationships.[27] To our knowledge, only 1 study of youth in South America studied sex for money in a teen population, and researchers found it was not associated with sexual coercion at the initiation of sexual activity.[25]

Our findings are consistent with other research findings linking various health-risk behaviors with unwanted sex.[4,28-30] Condom nonuse was associated independently with unwanted sex, which is consistent with other research linking sexual coercion and sexual violence to risk of STIs.[8-10] According to a survey of junior and high school students, 25% of unwanted sexual experiences occur around use of alcohol and other drugs.[9] Data from the National Longitudinal Study of Adolescent Health indicate the use of alcohol and other drugs was twice as likely to be reported at last sex for those teens who had ever experienced forced sex compared with those who had not.[10] Alcohol and marijuana use were common within sexual relationships of teens in this study. Our finding that a partner's marijuana use rather than the young woman's use was associated with unwanted sex emphasizes the importance of focusing on both the individual and the partner's behaviors when counseling on avoidance of risk.

To reduce the number of unwanted sexual encounters between young people, one must clarify the meaning of pressure, and one must teach young people to be more effective communicators.[31] There is limited understanding of the negotiation strategies that facilitate or diminish sexually coercive behaviors. In episodes of sexual activity with the partners under the influence of substances, the lines between consensual and nonconsensual activity easily might be blurred.[14] Consent to sex has to be viewed in the context of the communication and perception of consent. Women may not clearly say no in response to unwanted sexual activity but may try to communicate their unwillingness in nonverbal and nonassertive ways. Alternatively, substance use by the partner may result in his being less sensitive to the young woman's unwillingness.[18,21,32]

Limitations of our study include the use of a clinic-based sample of relatively homogeneous racial and socioeconomic composition. The history of sexual coercion is based on self-report; self-reports of unwanted sex appear to be reasonably valid and reliable but may vary as individuals reevaluate experiences across time.[33] We also measured the occurrence of unwanted sex in generic terms, without specifically addressing the types of unwanted sexual contact. Thus, incidence rates of unwanted sex may be somewhat lower than would have been identified if specific unwanted sexual acts were assessed.

In summary, the experience of unwanted sex is common among adolescent women and is related to engaging in sexual behaviors that put them at risk of STIs and pregnancies.

**Accepted for Publication:** December 11, 2005.
**Correspondence:** Margaret J. Blythe, MD, Indiana University School of Medicine, 1001 W 10th St, Bryce Building B-2006, Indianapolis, IN 46202 (e-mail: mblythe@iupui.edu).
**Author Contributions:** Dr Fortenberry had full access to all the data in the study and takes responsibility for the integrity of the data and the accuracy of the data analysis.
**Funding/Support:** This research was supported by grant U19 AI43924 from the National Institute of Allergy and Infectious Diseases and grant RO1 HD 042404 from the National Institute of Child Health and Human Development.

## REFERENCES

1. Biglan A, Noell J, Ochs L, Smolkowski K, Metsler C. Does sexual coercion pay a role in the high-risk sexual behavior of adolescent and young adult women? *J Behav Med.* 1995;18:549-568.
2. Koss MP, Gidycz CA, Wisniewski N. The scope of rape: incidence and prevalence of sexual aggression and victimization in a national sample of higher education students. *J Consult Clin Psychol.* 1987;55:162-170.
3. Spitzberg BH. An analysis of empirical estimates of sexual aggression victimization and perpetration. *Violence Vict.* 1999;14:241-260.
4. Pacifici C, Stoolmiller M, Nelson C. Evaluating a prevention program for teenagers on sexual coercion: a differential effectiveness approach. *J Consult Clin Psychol.* 2001;69:552-559.
5. O'Sullivan LF, Byers ES, Finkelman L. The context and aftermath of sexual coercion: a comparison of male and female college students' experiences of sexual coercion. *Psychol Women Q.* 1998;22:177-196.
6. Miller BC, Monson BH, Norton MC. The effects of forced sexual intercourse on white female adolescents. *Child Abuse Negl.* 1995;19:1289-1301.
7. Abma J, Driscoll A, Moore K. Young women's degree of control over first intercourse: an exploratory analysis. *Fam Plann Perspect.* 1998;30:12-18.
8. Noell J, Rohde P, Seeley J, Ochs L. Childhood sexual abuse, adolescent sexual coercion and sexually transmitted infection acquisition among homeless female adolescents. *Child Abuse Negl.* 2001;25:137-148.
9. Erickson PI, Rapkin AJ. Unwanted sexual experiences among middle and high school youth. *J Adolesc Health.* 1991;12:319-325.
10. Upchurch DM, Kusunlik Y. Associations between forced sex, sexual and protective practices and sexually transmitted diseases among a national sample of adolescent girls. *Womens Health Issues.* 2004;14:75-84.
11. Abbey A, Ross LT, McDuffie D, McAuslan P. Alcohol and dating risk factors for sexual assault among college women. *Psychol Women Q.* 1996;20:147-169.
12. Abbey A. Alcohol-related sexual assault: a common problem among college students. *J Stud Alcohol Suppl.* 2002;(14):118-128.
13. Rickert VI, Wiemann CM, Vaughan RD, White JW. Rates and risk factors for sexual violence among an ethnically diverse sample of adolescents. *Arch Pediatr Adolesc Med.* 2004;158:1132-1139.
14. Adams-Curtis LE, Forbes GB. College women's experiences of sexual coercion: a review of cultural, perpetrator, victim, and situational variables. *Trauma Violence Abuse.* 2004;5:91-122.
15. Irwin CE Jr, Rickert VI. Coercive sexual experiences during adolescence and young adulthood: a public health problem. *J Adolesc Health.* 2005;36:359-361.
16. Lichtenstein B. Domestic violence, sexual ownership, and HIV risk in women in the American deep south. *Soc Sci Med.* 2005;60:701-714.
17. Marston C. What is heterosexual coercion? Interpreting narratives from young people in Mexico City. *Sociol Health Illn.* 2005;27:68-91.
18. Fortenberry JD, Cecil H, Zimet GD, Orr DP. Concordance between self-report questionnaires and coital diaries for sexual behaviors of adolescent women with sexually transmitted diseases. In: Bancroft J, ed. *Researching Sexual Behavior.* Bloomington: Indiana University Press; 1997:237-249.
19. Katz BP, Fortenberry JD, Zimet GD, Blythe MJ, Orr DP. Partner-specific relationship characteristics and condom use among young people with sexually transmitted infections. *J Sex Res.* 2000;37:69-75.
20. Struckman-Johnson C, Struckman-Johnson D, Anderson PB. Tactics of sexual coercion: when men and women won't take no for an answer. *J Sex Res.* 2003;40:76-86.
21. Frith H, Kitzinger C. Reformulating sexual script theory: developing a discursive psychology of sexual negotiation. *Theory Psychol.* 2001;11:209-232.
22. O'Sullivan LF, Allgeier ER. Feigning sexual desire: consenting to unwanted sexual activity in heterosexual dating relationships. *J Sex Res.* 1998;35:234-244.
23. Impett EA, Peplau LA. Sexual compliance: gender, motivational, and relationship perspectives. *J Sex Res.* 2003;40:87-100.
24. Grunbaum JA, Kann L, Kinchen S, et al. Youth Risk Behavior Surveillance—United States, 2003. *MMWR Surveill Summ.* 2004;53(No. SS-2):1-96. Available at http://iier.isciii.es/mmwr/preview/mmwrhtml/ss5302al.htm. Accessed March 16, 2006.
25. Caceres CF, Vanoss Marin B, Sid Hudes E. Sexual coercion among youth and young adults in Lima, Peru. *J Adolesc Health.* 2000;27:361-367.
26. Livingston JA, Buddie AM, Testa M, VanZile-Tamsen C. The role of sexual precedence in verbal coercion. *Psychol Women Q.* 2004;28:287-297.
27. Tschann JM, Adler NE, Millstein SG, Gurvey JE, Ellen JM. Relative power between sexual partners and condom use among adolescents. *J Adolesc Health.* 2002;31:17-25.
28. Muehlenhard CL, Linton MA. Date rape and sexual aggression in dating situations: incidence and risk factors. *J Counsel Psychol.* 1987;34:186-196.
29. Malamuth NM, Sockloskie RJ, Koss MP, Tanaka JS. Characteristics of aggressors against women: testing a model using a national sample of college students. *J Consult Clin Psychol.* 1991;59:670-681.
30. Jordan TR, Price JH, Telljohann SK, Chesney BK. Junior high school students' perceptions regarding nonconsensual sexual behavior. *J Sch Health.* 1998;68:289-296.
31. Rosenthal DA. Understanding sexual coercion among young adolescents: communicative clarity, pressure, and acceptance. *Arch Sex Behav.* 1997;26:481-493.
32. Kitzinger C, Frith H. Just say no? The use of conversation analysis in developing a feminist perspective on sexual refusal. *Discourse Soc.* 1999;10:293-316.
33. Aalsma MC, Zimet GD, Fortenberry JD, Blythe M, Orr DP. Reports of childhood sexual abuse by adolescents: stability over time. *J Sex Res.* 2002;39:259-263.

ARTICLE

# Symptomatic Children With Hereditary Hemorrhagic Telangiectasia

## *A Pediatric Center Experience*

*Meir Mei-Zahav, MD; Michelle Letarte, PhD; Marie E. Faughnan, MD; Salma A. Abdalla, PhD; Ursula Cymerman, MS; Ian B. MacLusky, MD*

**Objective:** To assess the clinical and genetic characteristics of symptomatic children with hereditary hemorrhagic telangiectasia (HHT).

**Design:** Cross-sectional study.

**Setting:** The HHT clinics in Toronto.

**Participants:** All children with symptomatic HHT treated from April 1, 1996, through December 31, 2002.

**Interventions:** Participants were screened for visceral arteriovenous malformations (AVMs). Molecular testing was performed in the children or their affected family members.

**Main Outcome Measures:** Prevalence of epistaxis, telangiectases, pulmonary and cerebral AVMs, and genetic characteristics.

**Results:** Fourteen children presented with manifestations of HHT. Seven had cardiorespiratory symptoms related to pulmonary AVMs. Three had neurological symptoms secondary to bleeding from spinal or cerebral AVMs. Two were referred because of skin telangiectases and 2, because of multiple episodes of epistaxis. Screening results revealed a cerebral AVM in 1 of 11 neurologically asymptomatic children. Of the children without respiratory symptoms, 1 was diagnosed as having definite and 1, suspected pulmonary AVMs. Four children with pulmonary AVMs carried an endoglin gene mutation (HHT type 1), and 1 carried an activin receptor–like kinase 1 gene mutation (HHT type 2). The 2 children with spinal AVMs belong to the same HHT type 2 family. No mutation was found in 1 child with pulmonary and 1 with cerebral AVMs.

**Conclusions:** Visceral AVMs and mucosal telangiectases are present in children with HHT and can lead to life-threatening events. Failure to identify a disease-associated mutation for each child suggests complex mutations or novel HHT genes.

*Arch Pediatr Adolesc Med. 2006;160:596-601*

**Author Affiliations:** Division of Respiratory Medicine, Department of Pediatrics (Drs Mei-Zahav and MacLusky), and Cancer Research Program (Drs Letarte and Abdalla and Ms Cymerman), The Hospital for Sick Children Toronto, Division of Respiratory Medicine, St Michael's Hospital (Dr Faughnan), Heart and Stroke Richard Lewar Center of Excellence (Dr Letarte), and Department of Immunology (Drs Letarte and Abdalla), Division of Respirology (Drs Mei-Zahav, Faughnan, and MacLusky), University of Toronto, Toronto, Ontario.

HEREDITARY HEMORRHAGIC telangiectasia (HHT), or Rendu-Osler-Weber syndrome, is an autosomal dominant vascular dysplasia. Although initially thought to be rare, recent reports suggest a prevalence of 1:5000 to 1:10 000.[1,2] Hereditary hemorrhagic telangiectasia is characterized by mucocutaneous telangiectatic lesions, resulting in epistaxis in 90% of patients[3] and gastrointestinal tract bleeding in 20% to 30%.[4] Visceral arteriovenous malformations (AVMs) are predominantly found in the pulmonary, cerebral, and hepatic circulations.[5,6]

The clinical characteristics of HHT in children are not well described. Symptoms and signs tend to develop in late childhood and early adulthood,[2,5,6] and many children do not experience epistaxis or develop skin telangiectases in the first decade of life.[6] Multiple reports[7-12] of cerebral and pulmonary AVMs in children have been published; however, prevalence of such AVMs has not been established, and there are no published series describing the clinical presentations and genetics of HHT in childhood.

We aimed to characterize the clinical presentation, presence of asymptomatic visceral AVMs, and genotype in children symptomatic for HHT.

## METHODS

Pediatric and adult HHT clinics were established at The Hospital for Sick Children and St Michael's Hospital, respectively, in Toronto in 1996. Both are tertiary care referral centers affiliated with the University of Toronto. All children and adolescents (aged 0-18 years) presenting with symptoms of HHT from April 1,

1996, through December 31, 2002, were included in the current study. Children referred because of a family history and found to have HHT were not included.

The children were examined carefully for skin and mucosal telangiectases. Thorough examinations of the oral and conjunctival mucous membranes and anterior rhinoscopy for nasal telangiectases were also performed.

The children were screened for visceral AVMs. Pulmonary AVMs were diagnosed by means of echocardiography with agitated saline contrast and enhanced chest computed tomography followed by pulmonary angiography when indicated. Cerebral AVMs were diagnosed by means of head magnetic resonance imaging, followed by cerebral angiography when indicated.

Clinical diagnosis of HHT was based on the established clinical diagnostic criteria for HHT. These criteria include recurrent epistaxis, multiple skin telangiectases, visceral AVMs or telangiectases, and a first-degree family member with HHT.[13] Having 3 criteria confirms the diagnosis, whereas having 2 criteria leads to a diagnosis of suspected HHT.[13]

Molecular testing for HHT mutations was performed as part of a research project aimed at developing a clinically applicable diagnostic test and at understanding basic mechanisms of the disease. Informed consent was obtained from participating patients and/or their parents, as appropriate, and the research protocols were approved by the Ethics Committee of the Research Institute at the Hospital for Sick Children.

Genomic DNA was extracted from blood lymphocytes using commercially available DNA extraction kits (DNAzol [Gibco BRL, Gaithersburg, Md] or Puregene DNA isolation kit [Gentra Systems Inc, Minneapolis, Minn]). Mutation analysis for the endoglin gene (*ENG*; for HHT type 1 [HHT1]) was performed by means of quantitative multiplex polymerase chain reaction and exon sequencing as described previously.[14,15] Mutation analysis for activin receptor–like kinase 1 (*ACVRL1*; for HHT type 2 [HHT2]) was performed by exon sequencing according to published procedures.[16,17]

## RESULTS

We examined 127 children in the Toronto HHT clinics from April 1, 1996, through December 31, 2002. One hundred thirteen were referred because of a family history of HHT, and 14 (age range, 0-15 years; median age, 9 years) because of symptoms or signs of HHT. This report describes these 14 children. Their clinical presentation, disease characteristics, and results of molecular analysis are summarized in the **Table**. Nine (64%) had a family history of HHT, and mutations were found in 8.

Seven children (50%) presented with pulmonary AVMs; 3 (21%), with cerebral or spinal AVMs; and 4 (29%), with mucocutaneous telangiectases. Epistaxis was common, being observed in 12 children (86%), but usually mild; severe nosebleeds were described in only 3 children.

### CLINICAL PRESENTATION OF PULMONARY AVMs

Of the 7 children with pulmonary AVMs, 5 had a prolonged history of dyspnea and cyanosis that started years before the diagnosis, 1 presented with congestive heart failure, and 1 presented with hemoptysis. The pulmonary presentation and outcome of patients 1 through 5, 7, and 10 were reported in a large series summarizing the outcome of transcatheter embolotherapy for pulmonary AVMs[18] and diffuse pulmonary AVMs.[19] However, complete screening for other AVMs and HHT mutation analysis were not described previously.

Patient 1 was diagnosed at 11 months of age as having lactic acidosis and mitochondrial myopathy, probably unrelated to HHT. The diagnosis of HHT was established 3 years later, after referral because of epistaxis, dyspnea, and cyanosis. A large pulmonary AVM was found in the left lower lobe and required embolization. After 5 years of follow-up, the child is well, with no evidence of pulmonary AVMs. This child was the first in the family to show signs of HHT. Molecular analysis revealed an *ENG* splice-site mutation (g.IVS3+1G>A), which leads to an exon 3 skip and expression of an in-frame smaller and unstable *ENG*-mutant protein. The child's asymptomatic mother was subsequently shown to have pulmonary and hepatic AVMs. She had passed on the mutation to her child but had not inherited it from her parents, who did not carry the mutation and showed no signs of HHT. Results of DNA fingerprinting with 8 different markers confirmed that the child and his mother share the expected alleles with their respective parents.[15] This mutation was thus occurring de novo in the mother. This same splice-site variant has also been reported in an unrelated family with several generations of HHT,[20] confirming that the same mutation can arise in distinct families.

Patient 2 had a very complicated course characterized by multiple-organ involvement. She was diagnosed in early childhood as having hypothyroidism and developmental delay. She was noted to have long-standing cyanosis and multiple mucocutaneous telangiectases. However, the diagnosis of HHT was only established at 12 years of age, when she manifested diffuse pulmonary AVMs and an occipital cerebral AVM. She also had liver disease, with elevated transaminase levels and with coagulopathy that remained enigmatic even after a liver biopsy. Transcatheter embolotherapies resulted in only transient improvement. Lung transplantation was offered but refused. Epistaxis appeared at 17 years of age. The patient continued to have severe cyanosis and died at 18 years of age. A novel *ENG* exon 5 substitution (c.640G>A), which converts glycine to serine at codon 214, was identified. The patient did not have a family history of HHT. The same sequence variant was found in her asymptomatic mother and is likely disease associated because it was not identified in more than 200 individuals who underwent testing. However, confirmation of this sequence variant as disease associated requires further study.

Patient 3 presented at 7 years of age with multiple telangiectases and prolonged cyanosis. During 13 years of follow-up, multiple pulmonary AVMs were embolized on 3 occasions (**Figure**, second embolotherapy), with symptomatic improvement and resolution of hypoxemia. A previously unreported *ENG* mutation was found in the patient and 2 affected relatives: a 4-base insertion c.982_983insGCCT in exon 7, which causes a frame shift.

Patients 4 and 5 presented with severe cyanosis. Diffuse pulmonary AVMs required multiple transcatheter embolizations (and right lower lobectomy in patient 4), with only transient improvement.

Patient 6 presented with severe respiratory distress soon after birth. A large pulmonary AVM, causing congestive heart failure, was found in the left upper lobe, and lo-

**Table. Clinical and Molecular Characteristics of Children Presenting With HHT**

| Patient No./Sex/Age at Diagnosis, y | Presenting Symptom | Treatment | Outcome | Other Clinical Characteristics at Presentation and Follow-up | | | | Family History | Mutation | Follow-up, y |
|---|---|---|---|---|---|---|---|---|---|---|
| | | | | PAVM Screening | CAVM Screening | Epi* | Tel | | | |
| **Pulmonary AVMs** | | | | | | | | | | |
| 1/M/4 | Cyanosis | Embolotherapy | Well | † | Normal | Y (4) | Y | Y | *ENG* splice site, g.IVS3 + 1G>A | 5 |
| 2/F/12 | Cyanosis | Embolotherapy ×2 | Dead | † | CAVM observed | Y (17) | Y | N | *ENG* exon 5, missense, c.640G>A | 6 |
| 3/F/7 | Cyanosis | Embolotherapy ×3 | Well | † | Normal | Y (10) | Y | Y | *ENG* exon 7, insertion, c.982_983insGCCT | 12 |
| 4/F/9 | Cyanosis | Lobectomy, multiple embolotherapies | Mild cyanosis | † | Normal | Y | Y | Y | Not performed | 12 |
| 5/M/15 | Cyanosis | Multiple embolotherapies | Mild cyanosis | † | Normal | Y | Y | N | No *ENG* or *ACVRL1* mutation found in patient | 7 |
| 6/F/0‡ | Congestive heart failure | Lobectomy | Well | † | Normal | N | Y | Y | *ACVRL1* exon 4, missense, c.383C>A | 14 |
| 7/F/11 | Hemoptysis | Embolotherapy ×2, laser ablation of airways Tel | Well | † | Normal | N | Y | Y | *ENG*, duplication of exons 3-8, c.1134_1135ins220-1134 | 13 |
| **Spinal and Cerebral AVMs** | | | | | | | | | | |
| 8/M/5 | Paraplegia, urinary retention | Ligation of feeding artery | Prolonged rehabilitation, new AVM embolized | Normal | Normal | Y (6) | N | Y | *ACVRL1* exon 8, missense, c.1232G>A | 8 |
| 9/M/9 | Loss of consciousness, seizures | Embolotherapy | Well | Normal, only chest radiography performed | Normal | Y (7) | N | Y | *ACVRL1* exon 8, missense, c.1232G>A | 11 |
| 10/F/15 | Right hemiparesis, seizures | Embolotherapy | Prolonged rehabilitation | PAVM embolized | † | Y | Y | Y | No *ENG* or *ACVRL1* mutation found in family | 7 |
| **Skin Tel and Epi** | | | | | | | | | | |
| 11/F/8 | Skin Tel, Epi, TIA | No treatment | Well | Normal | Normal | Y (6) | Y | N | No *ENG* or *ACVRL1* mutation found in patient | 2 |
| 12/M/8 | Skin Tel, Epi | No treatment | Well | Normal | Normal | Y (3) | Y | Tel in family | No *ENG* or *ACVRL1* mutation found in family | 2 |
| 13/M/10 | Epi | Cauterization | Well | Normal | Normal | Y (10) | Y | Epi and Tel in family | No *ENG* or *ACVRL1* mutation found in patient | 5 |
| 14/M/11 | Epi | Laser ablation | Well | Suspected PAVMs | Normal | Y (4) | Y | Y | *ACVRL1* exon 8, missense, c.1232G>A | 3 |

Abbreviations: *ACVRL1*, activin receptor–like kinase 1 gene; AVM, arteriovenous malformation; CAVM, cerebral AVM; *ENG*, endoglin gene; Epi, epistaxis; HHT, hereditary hemorrhagic telangiectasia; N, no; PAVM, pulmonary AVM; Tel, telangiectases; TIA, transient ischemic attack, Y, yes.

*Numbers in parentheses indicate years of follow-up since the patient first presented with symptoms.

†Arteriovenous malformation was diagnosed and treated as part of the clinical course.

‡Diagnosis was neonatal.

bectomy was performed. After 14 years of follow-up, except for a few cutaneous telangiectases that appeared during follow-up, she is asymptomatic with no evidence of pulmonary AVMs. A missense mutation in exon 4 of *ACVRL1* (c.383C>A), which changes alanine to aspartic acid at codon 128, was found in this child and her affected parent.[21]

Patient 7 presented at 11 years of age with recurrent hemoptysis. Chest imaging revealed multiple pulmonary AVMs, which were embolized with significant improvement. Recurrent hemoptysis due to laryngeal and tracheal telangiectases responded well to laser ablation. Six years later, she required transcatheter embolotherapy of bilateral pulmonary AVMs causing hypoxia, with resolution of symptoms. Skin telangiectases were noticed at 15 years of age. A duplication of *ENG* exons 3 through 8 was found in this patient and her affected parent, and a large unstable intracellular protein could be observed, as previously reported for an unrelated family.[12]

## CLINICAL PRESENTATION OF CEREBRAL AND SPINAL AVMs

Three children presented with neurological symptoms. Patients 8 and 9, first cousins, were diagnosed as having spinal AVMs, and their initial course was described elsewhere.[22] Patient 8 experienced new neurological symptoms 3 years after the feeding artery to the AVM was ligated. A new spinal AVM was found and embolized. These 2 children belong to the same family with HHT2, characterized by an *ACVRL1* missense mutation (c.1232G>A), which converts arginine to glutamine at codon 411, and was reported as a disease-causing mutation in seemingly unrelated families.[23]

Patient 10 presented with right hemiparesis, headache, and seizures. Two cerebral AVMs were found and embolized. Complete sequencing of *ENG* and *ACVRL1* genes failed to identify a mutation in her clinically affected relatives.

All 3 patients required rehabilitation, with resolution of most symptoms.

## MUCOCUTANEOUS TELANGIECTASES AND EPISTAXIS

Only 4 children were referred because of mucocutaneous telangiectases and epistaxis; however, all children presented with mucocutaneous telangiectases and/or epistaxis during follow-up. Epistaxis appeared as early as 3 years of age (mean±SD age of first episode, 7.5±4.0 years).

Patient 11 was referred because of multiple skin telangiectases, epistaxis, and an episode of a transient ischemic attack, with no family history of HHT. Results of a physical examination revealed multiple skin telangiectases on her palms and nasal mucosa. Echocardiography with agitated saline injection and chest computed tomography failed to demonstrate pulmonary AVMs. Pulmonary angiography was not performed because the probability of finding an AVM large enough to be embolized was very low. Head magnetic resonance imaging did not display any ischemic or hemorrhagic changes. No cerebral AVMs were seen. The cause of the transient ischemic attack could not be determined, and migraine remains a probable diagnosis. However, the presence of minute pulmonary AVMs cannot be ruled out. Molecular analysis failed to reveal a mutation in the *ENG* or the *ACVRL1* gene.

Patient 12 presented with multiple telangiectases on his face and extremities and epistaxis that started at 3 years of age and tended to be frequent (up to few times a week) and difficult to control (each episode lasting up to 1 hour). However, epistaxis was not treated before referral to our clinic. Patients 13 and 14 presented with epistaxis and were both treated successfully with cauterization or laser ablation. Patient 14 was found to carry the previously reported familial *ACVRL1* missense mutation (c.1232G>A) and is unrelated to patients 8 and 9.[17]

## ASYMPTOMATIC AVMs DETECTED ON SCREENING

Thirteen children were screened for pulmonary and cerebral AVMs. Of the 11 neurologically asymptomatic children, patient 2 was found to have a cerebral AVM. Of the children with no respiratory symptoms, patient 10 was found to have pulmonary AVMs and underwent transcatheter embolotherapy. Patient 14, with genetically proven HHT2, had echocardiographic and computed tomographic findings suggestive of small pulmonary AVMs. He is being followed up conservatively.

## CLINICAL DIAGNOSTIC CRITERIA FOR HHT

Eleven of the 14 children currently meet the established diagnostic criteria for definite HHT. However, because

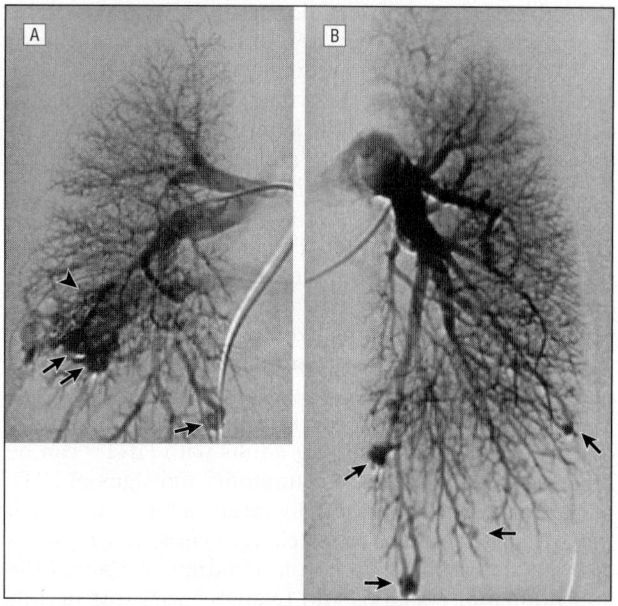


**Figure.** Pulmonary angiography revealing multiple pulmonary arteriovenous malformations (arrows) in the right (A) and left (B) lungs of patient 3 and coils in the right lung (arrowhead).

epistaxis or telangiectases appeared in 5 children after their first presentation, 4 of them did not meet these criteria at presentation. As of this writing, 3 children still did not have sufficient criteria for a definite diagnosis of HHT. The transient ischemic attack in patient 11 raises a major concern that she has pulmonary AVMs; however, extensive workup failed to demonstrate any. Thus, according to the diagnostic criteria, she is suspected of having HHT. Patients 12 and 13 have telangiectases and severe epistaxis with no evidence of visceral AVMs and no family history of HHT. However, telangiectases and/or epistaxis exist in these families, and screening for visceral AVMs was not performed in family members.

## COMMENT

A pediatric HHT clinic was established in Toronto for treating children with HHT. In a recent series[24] describing 15 children with HHT, epistaxis was common, appearing as early as 4 years of age. However, symptoms of visceral AVMs were rare, and screening for visceral AVMs was performed in only 6 children.

Five of the symptomatic children in our series presented with acute life-threatening events, including stroke, hemoptysis, and congestive heart failure. Five presented with chronic hypoxia. Previous reports[2,25-28] have established the prevalence of cerebral and pulmonary AVMs at 5% to 10% and 15% to 33%, respectively, in adults with HHT. Much less attention has been given to children with this disease. It was also shown that most pulmonary AVMs grow during life,[26] but it is not known whether all pulmonary AVMs are present at birth or some develop later. Multiple cases of fatal complications of cerebral AVMs have been reported in children with HHT.[7,10-12] We examined 127 children, 113 of them because of a family history and 14 because of symptoms. Ten children presented with symptomatic visceral AVMs.

Considering the autosomal dominant inheritance of the disease, we estimate that 50% of the children do have HHT. A prevalence of symptomatic visceral AVMs of 16% (10/63) is suggested by these data. In our series, we also demonstrated that the first symptom of HHT in children can be life threatening and can occur at any time from birth onward. A family history of HHT was known for at least 9 children, and screening might have revealed these lesions earlier. The favorable reported outcomes of transcatheter embolotherapy in adults and children[8,18] suggest that early intervention could have prevented life-threatening events.

Although epistaxis was common in our series, it was usually mild, in contrast to that found in adults.

The application to children of the clinical diagnostic criteria established mostly for adults with HHT[13] can be misleading. As mentioned, symptoms and signs of HHT generally develop during childhood and adolescence, such that the absence of epistaxis, telangiectases, or symptoms of visceral AVMs is common in children. We noted the appearance of epistaxis and telangiectases during follow-up in 5 patients. We also demonstrated the presence of asymptomatic visceral AVMs diagnosed on the basis of screening results in 3 children (patients 2, 10, and 14). Folz et al[24] concluded that findings in 15 children referred because of symptoms and signs suggestive of HHT could establish the diagnosis in only 2 children. Therefore, the clinical diagnostic criteria should be used cautiously in children, and the diagnosis of HHT and screening for visceral AVMs should be considered in all children with a family history of HHT regardless of symptoms.

Genetic analysis was helpful in establishing the diagnosis of HHT in children. We confirmed 8 cases by identifying the disease-causing mutation. However, we were unable to find *ENG* or *ACVRL1* mutations in 5 cases with a clinical diagnosis. For patients 11 through 13, in whom family history was minimal and no mutation was found, one could argue that the diagnosis is questionable and remains to be confirmed by additional criteria. In patients 5 and 10, in whom clinical diagnosis was definite, the mutation might be complex and require techniques other than quantitative multiplex polymerase chain reaction and exon sequencing. It can also be postulated that these patients have a different type of HHT. A possible HHT type 3, now linked to chromosome 5, was suggested in a family with a high frequency of pulmonary AVMs.[29,30] Mutations in the *MADH4* gene, which encodes Smad4, were recently described in patients with a combined syndrome of juvenile polyposis and HHT.[31] Another method shown to be valuable in the diagnosis of HHT is capillary microscopy,[32] which can help in establishing the diagnosis of HHT in future studies.

Our study also shows that AVMs occur in children with different types of *ENG* mutations, including a single base-pair substitution, a large and a small insertion, and a splice variant, in agreement with haploinsufficiency as the underlying model of HHT1.[14,15,20,33] Furthermore, one child with HHT2 had a pulmonary AVM (patient 6), and another had suspected pulmonary AVMs (patient 14). Although pulmonary AVMs are less frequent than in HHT1,[29] they do occur in HHT2.[17] We also observed the appearance of spinal AVMs in 2 children from a family with HHT2. Spinal AVMs have rarely been described in patients with HHT2.[34] Mutation analysis thus provides an important tool in the diagnosis of HHT, particularly in children because of variation in the age at onset and clinical manifestations even within a single family.

This study illustrates the heterogeneity of presentation of severe cases of HHT in children at a tertiary specialized pediatric center. However, there are limitations to this study. First, the study group is too small to represent the full clinical spectrum of HHT in childhood. Second, these children probably represent the more severe cases because only children presenting with symptoms were included. To ascertain the whole spectrum of pediatric HHT, a disorder with an autosomal mode of inheritance, large prospective studies should be conducted. The inclusion of mutation analysis in the diagnostic criteria will increase the probability of detecting children early in life and determine the prevalence of AVMs in children with both types of HHT.

In summary, pulmonary and cerebral AVMs are found in children with HHT and can lead to life-threatening complications, often as the first presentation of HHT. The clinical diagnostic criteria for HHT likely underestimate the presence of this disease in children. Screening for visceral AVMs in asymptomatic children with a family history of HHT is under way in our centers to evaluate their prevalence and to determine whether screening can prevent serious complications associated with pulmonary and cerebral AVMs.

**Accepted for Publication:** December 18, 2005.
**Correspondence:** Meir Mei-Zahav, MD, Division of Respiratory Medicine, Department of Pediatrics, The Hospital for Sick Children, 555 University Ave, Toronto, Ontario, Canada M5G 1X8 (meirmeizahav@hotmail.com).
**Funding/Support:** This study was supported by grants HHT-FY-02-226 from the March of Dimes (Dr Letarte) and POP-PPP-62030 from the Canadian Institutes of Health Research (Drs Letarte and Faughnan).
**Acknowledgment:** We thank HHT Solutions and Diane Rushlow for their contributions in the mutation analysis and Victoria Snell for her assistance in preparing the manuscript.

## REFERENCES

1. Kjeldsen AD, Vase P, Green A. Hereditary haemorrhagic telangiectasia: a population-based study of prevalence and mortality in Danish patients. *J Intern Med.* 1999;245:31-39.
2. Plauchu H, de Chadarevian JP, Bideau A, Robert JM. Age-related clinical profile of hereditary hemorrhagic telangiectasia in an epidemiologically recruited population. *Am J Med Genet.* 1989;32:291-297.
3. AAssar OS, Friedman CM, White RI Jr. The natural history of epistaxis in hereditary hemorrhagic telangiectasia. *Laryngoscope.* 1991;101:977-980.
4. Vase P, Grove O. Gastrointestinal lesions in hereditary hemorrhagic telangiectasia. *Gastroenterology.* 1986;91:1079-1083.
5. Shovlin CL, Letarte M. Hereditary haemorrhagic telangiectasia and pulmonary arteriovenous malformations: issues in clinical management and review of pathogenic mechanisms. *Thorax.* 1999;54:714-729.
6. Guttmacher AE, Marchuk DA, White RI Jr. Hereditary hemorrhagic telangiectasia. *N Engl J Med.* 1995;333:918-924.
7. Morgan T, McDonald J, Anderson C, et al. Intracranial hemorrhage in infants and children with hereditary hemorrhagic telangiectasia (Osler-Weber-Rendu syndrome). *Pediatrics.* 2002;109:E12.

8. Lee DW, White RI Jr, Egglin TK, et al. Embolotherapy of large pulmonary arteriovenous malformations: long-term results. *Ann Thorac Surg.* 1997;64:930-939.
9. Bennhagen RG, Holje G, Laurin S, Pesonen E. Coil embolization of a neonatal pulmonary arteriovenous malformation. *Pediatr Cardiol.* 2002;23:235-238.
10. Garcia-Monaco R, Taylor W, Rodesch G, et al. Pial arteriovenous fistula in children as presenting manifestation of Rendu-Osler-Weber disease. *Neuroradiology.* 1995;37:60-64.
11. Jessurun GA, Kamphuis DJ, van der Zande FH, Nossent JC. Arteriovenous malformations in the Netherlands Antilles: high prevalence of hereditary hemorrhagic telangiectasia-related single and multiple cerebral arteriovenous malformations. *Clin Neurol Neurosurg.* 1993;95:193-198.
12. Bourdeau A, Cymerman U, Paquet ME, et al. Endoglin expression is reduced in normal vessels but still detectable in arteriovenous malformations of patients with hereditary hemorrhagic telangiectasia type 1. *Am J Pathol.* 2000;156:911-923.
13. Shovlin CL, Guttmacher AE, Buscarini E, et al. Diagnostic criteria for hereditary hemorrhagic telangiectasia (Rendu-Osler-Weber syndrome). *Am J Med Genet.* 2000;91:66-67.
14. Cymerman U, Vera S, Pece-Barbara N, et al. Identification of hereditary hemorrhagic telangiectasia type 1 in newborns by protein expression and mutation analysis of endoglin. *Pediatr Res.* 2000;47:24-35.
15. Cymerman U, Vera S, Karabegovic A, Abdalla S, Letarte M. Characterization of several novel endoglin mutations associated with hereditary hemorrhagic telangiectasia. *Hum Mutat.* 2003;21:482-492.
16. Abdalla SA, Pece-Barbara N, Vera S, et al. Analysis of ALK-1 and endoglin in newborns from families with hereditary hemorrhagic telangiectasia type 2. *Hum Mol Genet.* 2000;9:1227-1237.
17. Abdalla SA, Cymerman U, Johnson RM, Deber CM, Letarte M. Disease-associated mutations in conserved residues of ALK-1 kinase domain. *Eur J Hum Genet.* 2003;11:279-287.
18. Faughnan ME, Thabet A, Mei-Zahav M, et al. Pulmonary arteriovenous malformations in children: outcomes of transcatheter embolotherapy. *J Pediatr.* 2004;145:826-831.
19. Faughnan ME, Lui YW, Wirth JA, et al. Diffuse pulmonary arteriovenous malformations: characteristics and prognosis. *Chest.* 2000;117:31-38.
20. Pece N, Vera S, Cymerman U, White RI Jr, Wrana JL, Letarte M. Mutant endoglin in hereditary hemorrhagic telangiectasia type 1 is transiently expressed intracellularly and is not a dominant negative. *J Clin Invest.* 1997;100:2568-2579.
21. Abdalla SA, Cymerman U, Rushlow D, et al. Novel mutations and polymorphisms in genes causing hereditary hemorrhagic telangiectasia. *Hum Mutat.* 2005;25:320-321.
22. Mandzia JL, terBrugge KG, Faughnan ME, Hyland RH. Spinal cord arteriovenous malformations in two patients with hereditary hemorrhagic telangiectasia. *Childs Nerv Syst.* 1999;15:80-83.
23. Bayrak-Toydemir P, Mao R, Lewin S, McDonald J. Hereditary hemorrhagic telangiectasia: an overview of diagnosis and management in the molecular era for clinicians. *Genet Med.* 2004;6:175-191.
24. Folz BJ, Zoll B, Alfke H, Toussaint A, Maier RF, Werner JA. Manifestations of hereditary hemorrhagic telangiectasia in children and adolescents. *Eur Arch Otorhinolaryngol.* 2006;263:53-61.
25. Haitjema T, Westermann CJ, Overtoom TT, et al. Hereditary hemorrhagic telangiectasia (Osler-Weber-Rendu disease): new insights in pathogenesis, complications, and treatment. *Arch Intern Med.* 1996;156:714-719.
26. Vase P, Holm M, Arendrup H. Pulmonary arteriovenous fistulas in hereditary hemorrhagic telangiectasia. *Acta Med Scand.* 1985;218:105-109.
27. Haitjema T, Disch F, Overtoom TT, Westermann CJ, Lammers JW. Screening family members of patients with hereditary hemorrhagic telangiectasia. *Am J Med.* 1995;99:519-524.
28. Nanthakumar K, Graham AT, Robinson TI, et al. Contrast echocardiography for detection of pulmonary arteriovenous malformations. *Am Heart J.* 2001;141:243-246.
29. Wallace GM, Shovlin CL. A hereditary hemorrhagic telangiectasia family with pulmonary involvement is unlinked to the known HHT genes, endoglin and ALK-1. *Thorax.* 2000;55:685-690.
30. Cole SG, Begbie MF, Wallace GM, Shovlin CL. A new locus for hereditary haemorrhagic telangiectasia (HHT3) maps to chromosome 5. *J Med Genet.* 2005;42:577-582.
31. Gallione CJ, Repetto GM, Legius E, et al. A combined syndrome of juvenile polyposis and hereditary haemorrhagic telangiectasia associated with mutations in *MADH4* (*SMAD4*). *Lancet.* 2004;363:852-859.
32. Mager JJ, Westermann CJ. Value of capillary microscopy in the diagnosis of hereditary hemorrhagic telangiectasia. *Arch Dermatol.* 2000;136:732-734.
33. Shovlin CL, Hughes JM, Scott J, Seidman CE, Seidman JG. Characterization of endoglin and identification of novel mutations in hereditary hemorrhagic telangiectasia. *Am J Hum Genet.* 1997;61:68-79.
34. McDonald JE, Miller FJ, Hallam SE, Nelson L, Marchuk DA, Ward KJ. Clinical manifestations in a large hereditary hemorrhagic telangiectasia (HHT) type 2 kindred. *Am J Med Genet.* 2000;93:320-327.

## *Announcement*

**Submissions.** The Editors welcome contributions to Picture of the Month. Submissions should describe common problems presenting uncommonly, rather than total zebras. Cases should be of interest to practicing pediatricians, highlighting problems that they are likely to at least occasionally encounter in the office or hospital setting. High-quality clinical images (in either 35-mm slide or electronic format) along with parent or patient permission to use these images must accompany the submission. The entire discussion should comprise no more than 750 words. Articles and photographs accepted for publication will bear the contributor's name. There is no charge for reproduction and printing of color illustrations. For details regarding electronic submission, please see: http://archpedi.ama-assn.org.

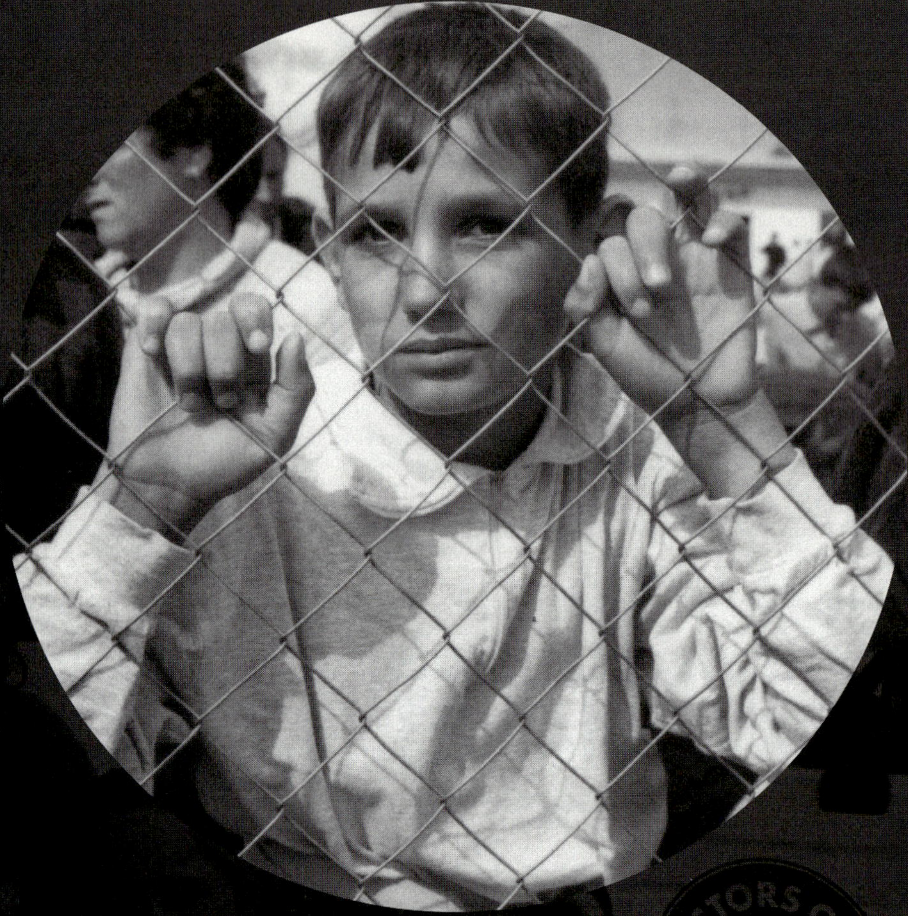

ARTICLE

# The Clinical and Demographic Characteristics of Nonneuronopathic Gaucher Disease in 887 Children at Diagnosis

*Paige Kaplan, MBBCh; Hans C. Andersson, MD; Katherine A. Kacena, PhD; John D. Yee, MD, MPH*

**Objective:** To describe the clinical and demographic characteristics of nonneuronopathic Gaucher disease (GD) in children at the time of diagnosis.

**Design:** Longitudinal observational database of the International Collaborative Gaucher Group Gaucher Registry.

**Setting:** Data reported to the Registry from January 1, 1989, to June 3, 2005, were included in this report.

**Patients/Participants:** All 887 patients were diagnosed as having nonneuronopathic GD from birth to younger than 18 years and did not receive enzyme replacement therapy.

**Main Outcome Measures:** Eight measures of the clinical manifestations and demographics of nonneuronopathic GD.

**Results:** The most common signs and symptoms noted were splenomegaly (95%), hepatomegaly (87%), radiologic bone disease (81%), thrombocytopenia (50%), anemia (40%), growth retardation (34%), bone pain (27%), and bone crisis (9%). Anemia and more severe splenomegaly and hepatomegaly were observed more frequently in younger patients. Skeletal manifestations were found more often in older children. Only 23% were identified as Ashkenazi Jews.

**Conclusions:** Nonneuronopathic GD commonly manifests in childhood and affects many ethnic groups. The high prevalence of rare mutations may be associated with earlier onset and/or more severe disease. Increased awareness of the clinical and demographic characteristics of nonneuronopathic GD in children may improve early recognition of this treatable lysosomal storage disorder, decrease morbidity, and prevent irreversible sequelae.

*Arch Pediatr Adolesc Med. 2006;160:603-608*

GAUCHER DISEASE (GD), the most common lysosomal storage disorder, is caused by a deficiency of the lysosomal enzyme glucocerebrosidase, leading to the accumulation of glucocerebroside within tissue macrophages in multiple organs.[1] Gaucher disease is almost always attributable to mutations in the glucocerebrosidase gene located on the long arm of chromosome 1 and is inherited in an autosomal recessive manner. Clinically, there are 3 subtypes of GD: nonneuronopathic (type 1), acute neuronopathic (type 2), and chronic neuronopathic (type 3).

Nonneuronopathic GD is the most prevalent form (94%) and is differentiated from the acute neuronopathic (1%) and chronic neuronopathic (5%) forms by the absence of central nervous system involvement.[2] The manifestations of nonneuronopathic GD include splenomegaly, hepatomegaly, anemia, thrombocytopenia, bone disease (ie, bone marrow infiltration, Erlenmeyer flask deformity of the distal femur, osteopenia, osteoporosis, infarction, avascular necrosis, and pathologic fractures), and growth retardation.[2-4] Bone pain is common, manifesting as mild to moderate intermittent pain or more severe acute "bone crises" accompanied by periosteal elevation, leukocytosis, and fever, which may cause debilitation for several days and require narcotic analgesics. Clinical expression of GD is highly variable among patients,[2] but, particularly when manifested during childhood, the natural history of GD is that of a progressive, multisystemic, and debilitating disorder.

Because GD has typically been described as an adult disorder affecting mainly Ashkenazi Jews, many physicians do not consider this diagnosis when evaluating signs and symptoms of the disorder in children. Early recognition of GD by physicians caring for children is important because safe and effective treatment with enzyme replacement is available, and early intervention can decrease morbidity and reduce the risk of later complications.[5,6] Enzyme replacement therapy has

**Author Affiliations:** Section of Metabolic Diseases, Department of Pediatrics, The Children's Hospital of Philadelphia, University of Pennsylvania School of Medicine, Philadelphia (Dr Kaplan); Hayward Genetics Center, Tulane University Medical Center, New Orleans, La (Dr Andersson); and Genzyme Corporation, Cambridge, Mass (Drs Kacena and Yee).

been shown to prevent progressive manifestations of GD and ameliorate GD-associated anemia, thrombocytopenia, organomegaly, bone pain, and bone crises.[6] Because GD is relatively uncommon in non-Ashkenazi populations (estimated incidence, 1:57 000 live births),[7] no large study of the pediatric manifestations of GD has been reported. Although a previous report of the International Collaborative Gaucher Group (ICGG) Gaucher Registry data noted that most affected people manifest GD in childhood, the clinical and demographic data for childhood GD were not separately analyzed.[8]

This study analyzes data from the ICGG Gaucher Registry to characterize the manifestations at the time of diagnosis of a large population of children and adolescents with nonneuronopathic GD. This description of pediatric nonneuronopathic GD should increase the recognition and earlier diagnosis of this condition in childhood, allowing for the initiation of treatment before the development of severe morbidity or irreversible disease complications.

## METHODS

The ICGG Gaucher Registry is an observational database of clinical, biochemical, and therapeutic characteristics of patients with GD (hereafter referred to as GD patients), regardless of disease severity and treatment status.[8] The ICGG Gaucher Registry, initiated in 1991 and supported by Genzyme Corporation, Cambridge, Mass, is governed by a collaborative group of international physician experts in GD (the ICGG). With appropriate institutional review board or ethics committee approvals, more than 700 physicians from 52 countries have voluntarily submitted data on their patients to the ICGG Gaucher Registry.

All nonneuronopathic GD patients included in this report were diagnosed from January 1, 1989, to June 3, 2005, ranged in age from birth to younger than 18 years at diagnosis, and had not received enzyme replacement therapy. A definitive diagnosis was based on results of enzyme analysis of glucocerebrosidase activity and/or DNA analysis of the glucocerebrosidase gene. To avoid inclusion of children who did not manifest signs or symptoms of GD, patients with a prenatal diagnosis were excluded from this study.

Patients were categorized into the following 3 groups according to age at diagnosis: birth to younger than 6 years, 6 to younger than 12 years, and 12 to younger than 18 years. For each clinical variable studied, the data closest to the diagnosis date were analyzed within an interval of ±2 years from diagnosis and before initiation of enzyme replacement therapy. Genotype frequency distributions for common, rare, and unknown mutations were determined. Hemoglobin level was analyzed as a binary variable, with anemia defined as below the reference age- and sex-adjusted value as follows: less than 10.1 g/dL for infants younger than 6 months; less than 9.5 g/dL for children 6 months to younger than 2 years; less than 10.5 g/dL for children 2 to younger than 12 years; less than 12 g/dL for boys 12 years and older; and less than 11 g/dL for girls 12 years and older. Platelet counts were analyzed in patients with intact spleens. Patients with partial or total splenectomy underwent separate analysis. Platelet counts were used to classify thrombocytopenia into the following groups: severe ($<60 \times 10^3/\mu L$), moderate ($60 \times 10^3/\mu L$ to $120 \times 10^3/\mu L$), and mild/normal ($>120 \times 10^3/\mu L$). Liver and spleen volumes were measured by means of magnetic resonance imaging, computed tomography, or ultrasonography and reported as multiples of normal size predicted for body weight (MN).[9] Ultrasound measurements were converted to volumetric equivalents using the formula developed by Elstein et al.[10] Splenomegaly was classified into the following groups: severe (>15 MN), moderate (>5 to 15 MN), and mild/normal (<5 MN). Hepatomegaly was divided into the following groups: severe (>2.5 MN), moderate (>1.25 to 2.5 MN), and mild/normal (≤1.25 MN).

The following 3 skeletal parameters were examined: bone pain, bone crisis, and radiologic evidence of bone disease. Bone pain was defined as being present if the patient or the parents reported this event as occurring within 1 month (30 days) before the diagnosis visit. Bone crisis was defined as present if the patient or the parents reported this event any time before diagnosis. Bone crisis was defined as pain with acute onset that requires immobilization of the affected area and narcotics for the relief of pain and that may be accompanied by periosteal elevation, elevated white blood cell count, fever, or debilitation that lasts longer than 3 days. Radiologic evidence of bone disease was tabulated.

Growth was assessed using height *z* scores, calculated for age and sex using the December 2000 Centers for Disease Control and Prevention growth charts[11] because data on midparental heights were not available. Growth was divided into the following 3 groups: less than the 5th percentile, 5th to 25th percentile, and greater than the 25th percentile.

Data analysis was conducted using SAS software, version 8.2 (SAS Institute Inc, Cary, NC). Age group at diagnosis, sex, ethnicity, and geographic region were tabulated. Median age at diagnosis was studied across common genotype groupings. The *P* value test for trend in severity across age groups was calculated (Jonckheere-Terpstra 2-sided tests).[12,13] We used the Jonckheere-Terpstra test to test the null hypothesis that the distribution of disease severity is the same across the 3 age groups vs the alternative hypothesis that there are significant differences among the age groups in their respective ordering for each clinical variable studied.[12,13]

## RESULTS

On June 21, 2005, the ICGG Gaucher Registry contained data for 887 nonneuronopathic GD patients who had been diagnosed between birth and age younger than 18 years. Hemoglobin and platelet data from the time of diagnosis were reported for 68% and 64% of the patients, respectively; 27% of patients had data for spleen and liver volumes; and 34% had radiologic examination data. Genotype data were available for 72% of the patients.

Of the 887 total study patients, the 2 largest ethnic groups were non-Jewish white subjects (30%) and Ashkenazi Jews (23%) (**Table 1**). The largest groups of pediatric patients participating in the ICGG Gaucher Registry were from the United States (29%) and Latin America (25%). Europe and Israel contributed 19% and 15% of participating patients, respectively.

Genotype data for this population indicate that 4 common mutations constitute 72% of all GD alleles: *N370S*, *L444P*, *IVS2+1*, and *84GG* (**Table 2**). (The mutations are notated according to standard nomenclature.[14]) Two hundred twenty-five (18%) of all 1270 reported alleles were rare, and 132 (10%) were unknown. Forty-seven percent of patients had at least 1 rare or unknown allele. Patients with the *N370S/N370S* genotype had a median age at diagnosis of 10 years. Patients with the *L444P/L444P* genotype had a median age at diagnosis of 1 year. All other allele groupings had a median diagnosis age ranging from 3 to 7 years.

For hemoglobin levels and spleen and liver volumes, younger patients tended to have significantly

**Table 1. Patient Demographics at Diagnosis***

| Demographic Variables | No. (%) of Patients (N = 887) |
|---|---|
| Age at diagnosis, y | |
| 0 to <6 | 425 (48) |
| 6 to <12 | 274 (31) |
| 12 to <18 | 188 (21) |
| Sex | |
| Male | 454 (51) |
| Female | 433 (49) |
| Ethnicity | |
| White, non-Jewish | 262 (30) |
| Jewish, Ashkenazi | 207 (23) |
| Unknown | 118 (13) |
| African American/Caribbean | 102 (11) |
| Hispanic | 91 (10) |
| Other† | 57 (6) |
| Arab | 50 (6) |
| Geographic region | |
| United States | 253 (29) |
| Latin America | 222 (25) |
| Europe | 165 (19) |
| Israel | 130 (15) |
| Asian Pacific‡ | 46 (5) |
| Middle East§ | 38 (4) |
| Canada | 33 (4) |

*Total percentages may be higher than 100% owing to rounding.
†Includes 3% or less each of Asian, multiethnic, American Indian, and Jewish Sephardic.
‡Includes Australia, Japan, New Zealand, South Africa.
§Excludes Israel and includes Egypt, Jordan, Saudi Arabia, Lebanon, and the Palestinian Authority.

**Table 2. Comparison of Age at Diagnosis for Different Genotype Groups**

| Genotype* | No. (%) of Patients (n = 635) | Median Age at Diagnosis (25th-75th Percentile), y† |
|---|---|---|
| *N370S*/rare allele‡ | 184 (29) | 7 (5-11) |
| *N370S*/*L444P* | 128 (20) | 7 (4-11) |
| *N370S*/*N370S* | 121 (19) | 10 (5-14) |
| Other§ | 58 (9) | 4 (2-7) |
| *L444P*/rare allele‡ | 57 (9) | 4 (2-9) |
| *N370S*/*84GG* | 43 (7) | 4 (2-6) |
| *L444P*/*L444P* | 29 (5) | 1 (1-1) |
| *N370S*/*IVS2+1* | 15 (2) | 3 (2-6) |

*Genotype information was not available for 252 patients. For those patients, median (25th-75th percentile) age at diagnosis was 6 (3-10) years.
†Age at diagnosis indicates severity of disease.
‡Rare allele is defined as a known allele that is not *N370S*, *L444P*, *IVS2+1*, or *84GG*, or as an unknown allele (results do not match any known allele).
§Includes patients who have any combination of rare or unknown alleles.

more severe abnormalities at the time of diagnosis (**Table 3**). Across all age groups, 40% of patients had anemia; 50% had platelet counts less than $120 \times 10^3$/μL; 95% had spleen volumes greater than 5 MN; and 87% had liver volumes greater than 1.25 MN. Twenty-seven (5%) of the 570 patients submitting platelet count information reported partial or total splenectomy at the time of diagnosis, with 93% and 7% of these patients presenting with mild/normal and moderate thrombocytopenia, respectively; none had platelet counts less than $60 \times 10^3$/μL.

Overall, most children (81%) had at least 1 radiologic skeletal abnormality at the time of diagnosis (**Table 4**). The 2 most common radiologic manifestations were Erlenmeyer flask deformity (49%) and bone marrow infiltration (38%). Bone pain was reported in 27% and a history of bone crisis, in 9%. Older children had significantly ($P<.001$) more severe skeletal disease (Table 4). Growth was less than the 5th percentile of height for sex and age at diagnosis (**Figure 1**) in 34% of children (Table 4); in 28%, from the 5th to 25th percentiles; and 39%, greater than the 25th percentile.

## COMMENT

Without definitive and uninterrupted treatment, nonneuronopathic (type 1) GD, particularly when diagnosed in childhood, is a progressive multisystemic disorder with substantial morbidity, potential for disability, reduced quality of life, and even reduced life expectancy.[15] Fortunately, the underlying enzyme deficiency and resulting pathology can be treated effectively with enzyme replacement therapy (with recombinant glucocerebrosidase or imiglucerase for injection [Cerezyme]).[4-6] However, there is reason to believe that there are children with GD that is unrecognized and undiagnosed and who may experience unnecessary morbidity and irreversible disease sequelae if treatment is not initiated at the earliest signs and symptoms. In part, this may be because nonneuronopathic GD is often thought to be an adult disorder primarily affecting or even restricted to Ashkenazi Jews.

The data described in this report clearly indicate that many patients with nonneuronopathic GD are symptomatic when they are children. Furthermore, in this international population, 77% of children who manifested nonneuronopathic GD were not Ashkenazi Jews. In fact, nonneuronopathic GD is prevalent across all ethnic groups, and many physicians caring for children can expect to encounter 1 or more children with nonneuronopathic GD in their practice.

The hematologic and organ volume factors indicate that symptoms and signs that manifest at a younger age may indicate more severe disease. Statistically significant differences in disease severity were noted among the 3 age groups. Anemia and hepatosplenomegaly at the time of diagnosis were greatest in the youngest group (birth to <6 years). Thrombocytopenia was prevalent in all age groups. This finding supports our clinical experience that the hematologic and visceral manifestations tend to appear first in the natural history of GD.

The skeletal manifestations of GD may progress slowly and only become apparent in the teenage years, although growth failure is often obvious much earlier. Exemplifying the progressive nature of skeletal pathology in GD, bone pain and bone crisis increased with the age at diagnosis. Children with GD who manifest evidence of bone pain are often incorrectly characterized as having normal growing pains. In this study, 27% of children diagnosed as having GD presented with bone pain

**Table 3. Patient Hematologic and Organ Volume Characteristics at Diagnosis***

| | Age at Diagnosis, y | | | | |
|---|---|---|---|---|---|
| | 0 to <6 | 6 to <12 | 12 to <18 | All Ages | *P* Value† |
| Hemoglobin, patient population | n = 287 | n = 184 | n = 131 | n = 602 | <.05 |
| Anemic‡ | 128 (45) | 62 (34) | 49 (37) | 239 (40) | |
| Not anemic | 159 (55) | 122 (66) | 82 (63) | 363 (60) | |
| Thrombocytopenia with spleen intact (platelet count, $\times 10^3/\mu L$),§ patient population | n = 277 | n = 176 | n = 117 | n = 570 | .003 |
| Severe (<60) | 24 (9) | 12 (7) | 15 (13) | 51 (9) | |
| Moderate (60 to <120) | 98 (35) | 75 (43) | 58 (50) | 231 (41) | |
| Mild/normal (≥120) | 155 (56) | 89 (51) | 44 (38) | 288 (51) | |
| Splenomegaly (spleen volume, MN),‖ patient population | n = 115 | n = 72 | n = 54 | n = 241 | <.001 |
| Severe (>15) | 84 (73) | 26 (36) | 14 (26) | 124 (51) | |
| Moderate (>5-15) | 30 (26) | 42 (58) | 34 (63) | 106 (44) | |
| Mild/normal (≤5) | 1 (1) | 4 (6) | 6 (11) | 11 (5) | |
| Hepatomegaly (liver volume, MN),‖ patient population | n = 111 | n = 68 | n = 58 | n = 237 | <.001 |
| Severe (>2.5) | 32 (29) | 4 (6) | 1 (2) | 37 (16) | |
| Moderate (>1.25 to 2.5) | 74 (67) | 56 (82) | 38 (66) | 168 (71) | |
| Mild/normal (≤1.25) | 5 (5) | 8 (12) | 19 (33) | 32 (14) | |

Abbreviation: MN, multiples of normal size predicted for body weight.

*Diagnosis is defined as the data point closest to the diagnosis date but no more than ±2 years from diagnosis. Unless otherwise indicated, data are expressed as number (percentage) of patients. Total percentages may be greater than 100% owing to rounding.

†Indicates *P* value test for trend and severity across age groups (Jonckheere-Terpstra 2-sided tests).[12,13]

‡Anemia is defined according to age and sex norms for hemoglobin concentrations as follows: less than 11 g/dL for boys 12 years and older; less than 10 g/dL for girls 12 years and older; less than 9.5 g/dL for children aged 2 to younger than 12 years; less than 8.5 for children aged 6 months to younger than 2 years; and less than 9.1 g/dL for infants younger than 6 months.

§Among the 27 patients with partial or total splenectomy, 25 (93%) were classified as mild/normal, and 2 (7%) were classified as moderate.

‖Normal organ volumes, measured by magnetic resonance imaging, computed tomography, or ultrasonography, are approximately 2.5% for the liver and 0.2% for the spleen (described in Ludwig[9]).

**Table 4. Patient Skeletal Manifestations at Diagnosis***

| | Age, y | | | | |
|---|---|---|---|---|---|
| Skeletal Manifestations | 0 to <6 | 6 to <12 | 12 to <18 | All Ages | *P* Value† |
| Bone pain, patient population | n = 214 | n = 144 | n = 102 | n = 460 | <.001 |
| Patients reporting | 33 (15) | 51 (35) | 40 (39) | 124 (27) | |
| Bone crisis, patient population | n = 207 | n = 143 | n = 99 | n = 449 | <.001 |
| Patients reporting | 8 (4) | 16 (11) | 15 (15) | 39 (9) | |
| Radiologic evidence of bone disease, patient population | n = 134 | n = 95 | n = 75 | n = 304 | <.001 |
| Any evidence of radiologic bone disease‡ | 97 (72) | 80 (84) | 69 (92) | 246 (81) | .06 |
| Erlenmeyer flask deformity | 59 (44) | 48 (51) | 43 (57) | 150 (49) | .009 |
| Marrow infiltration | 40 (30) | 41 (43) | 35 (47) | 116 (38) | .04 |
| Osteopenia | 21 (16) | 20 (21) | 21 (28) | 62 (20) | .16 |
| Avascular necrosis | 8 (6) | 6 (6) | 9 (12) | 23 (8) | .11 |
| Infarction | 6 (5) | 11 (12) | 7 (9) | 24 (8) | .50 |
| Lytic lesions | 7 (5) | 9 (9) | 5 (7) | 21 (7) | .87 |
| New fractures | 2 (1) | 3 (3) | 1 (1) | 6 (2) | |
| Height, percentile, patient population | n = 245 | n = 150 | n = 101 | n = 496 | .50 |
| <5th | 79 (32) | 62 (41) | 26 (26) | 167 (34) | |
| 5th-25th | 77 (31) | 34 (23) | 27 (27) | 138 (28) | |
| >25th | 89 (36) | 54 (36) | 48 (48) | 191 (39) | |

*Diagnosis is defined as the data point closest to the diagnosis date but no more than ±2 years from diagnosis. Unless otherwise indicated, data are expressed as number (percentage) of patients. Total percentages may be greater than 100% owing to rounding.

†Indicates *P* value test for trend and severity across age groups (Jonckheere-Terpstra 2-sided tests).[12,13]

‡Some patients demonstrated more than 1 indicator of bone disease.

at the time of diagnosis. Older children were more likely to have more severe radiologic manifestations of GD, with evidence of bone disease in 72% of the group diagnosed between birth and age younger than 6 years; 84%, between ages 6 and younger than 12 years; and 92%, between ages 12 and younger than 18 years.

The high prevalence of bone disease (81%) reported in children with nonneuronopathic GD at the time of diagnosis has several implications. First, evidence of early and potentially reversible bone disease is rarely evident on physical examination and may not correlate with the degree of visceral and hematologic involvement. Appropriate radio-

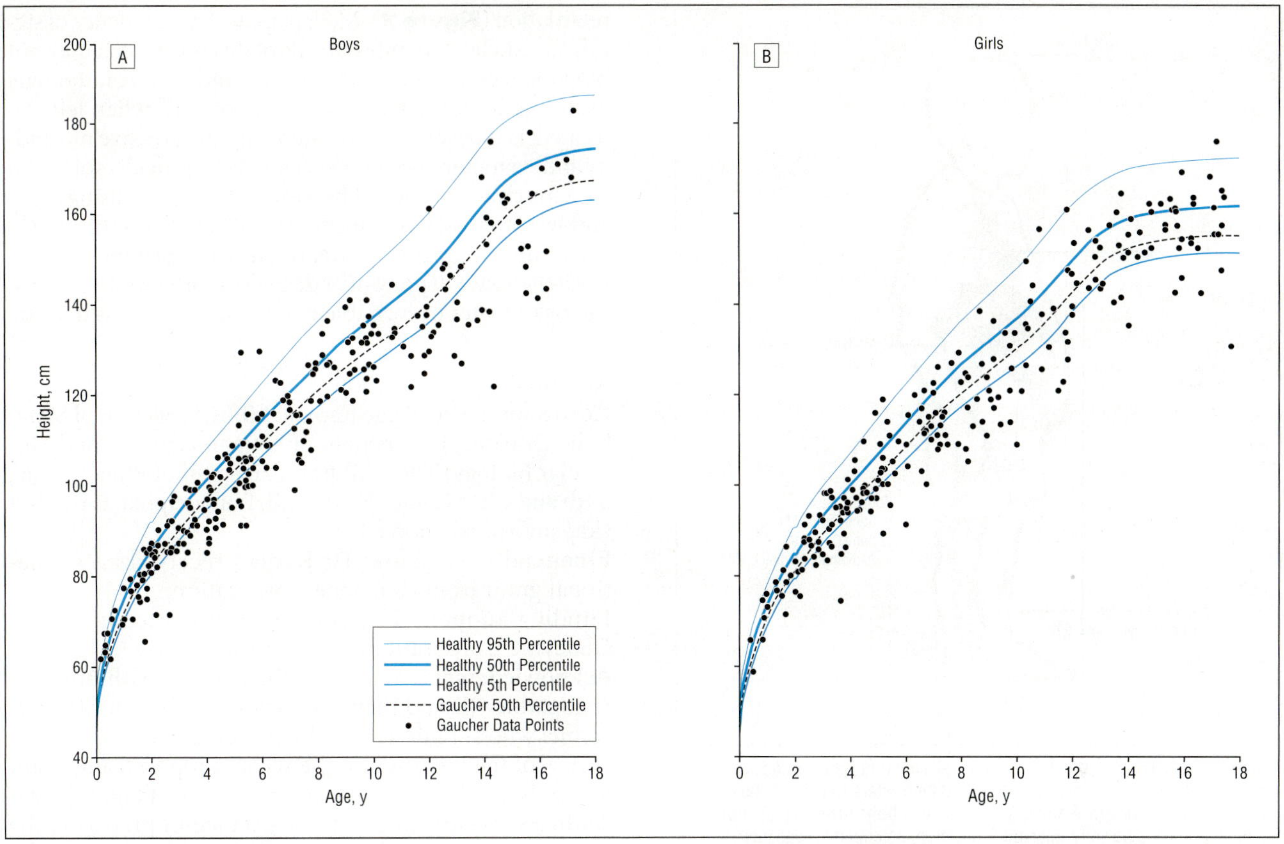


**Figure 1.** Height at diagnosis for 256 boys (A) and 240 girls (B) with the 5th, 50th, and 95th percentiles of the healthy population and 50th percentile reference curves for the population with Gaucher disease.

graphic studies are required and must be evaluated by a radiologist familiar with the bone changes of GD. Second, the presence of severe manifestations, particularly avascular necrosis, fractures, and lytic lesions, indicates a clinically aggressive form of GD, a fact that is often unrecognized by physicians whose focus is restricted to the hematologic and visceral manifestations of GD. For many nonneuronopathic GD patients, the morbidity of bone disease has the greatest long-term impact on quality of life. Untreated bone disease can lead to severe acute and chronic pain sometimes requiring even opioid analgesia; decreased bone mass, density, and strength; and increased risk of pathologic fractures. Avascular necrosis and joint collapse may affect linear growth and require joint replacement, ambulation with crutches, and/or the use of a wheelchair. Finally, the increasing prevalence of bone disease at diagnosis among older children with GD may indicate a need for earlier diagnosis and initiation of enzyme replacement therapy to prevent or reduce the risk of irreversible bone complications.[6,16]

Linear growth retardation is common in the pediatric nonneuronopathic GD population, with more than 30% of all children below the fifth percentile for height at the time of diagnosis. For all 3 age groups, the median height was below the expected height based on population standards. Because most patients (66%) in our population were American, Canadian, European, or Israeli, the National Center for Health Statistics 2000 growth data[11] were used for comparison. One possible explanation for the poorer growth seen in the group younger than 6 years may be more severe and earlier disease manifestations. Previous literature suggests that enzyme replacement therapy significantly improves growth in children with GD.[4] The goal of treatment is to normalize growth and achieve normal peak skeletal mass within 3 years of initiating enzyme replacement therapy.[17]

Nonneuronopathic GD in children can be caused by a wide range of glucocerebrosidase mutations. The 4 most common mutations (*N370S*, *L444P*, *84GG*, and *IVS2+1*) accounted for 72% of all mutated alleles in our nonneuronopathic GD population, and the remaining 28% of alleles were rare, unique, or unknown. The method of genotyping is not recorded in the ICGG Gaucher Registry, and it is possible that only common mutations were analyzed.

The manifestation of GD in childhood may indicate more severe disease than GD found in patients who present in adulthood. Childhood presentation represents an earlier accumulation of pathologic amounts of undegraded substrate in viscera and bone, which results in clinical signs and symptoms and indicates more severe disease.[16] This finding agrees with our clinical experience. We believe that all children should undergo regular evaluation.

The GD in patients with the *L444P/L444P* genotype in this study was classified as nonneuronopathic. However, these patients are at risk for development of neuronopathic disease (type 3) in later childhood and should undergo regular evaluation for central nervous system manifestations of GD.

Although the ICGG Gaucher Registry is the largest longitudinal database of the GD population, registry data are

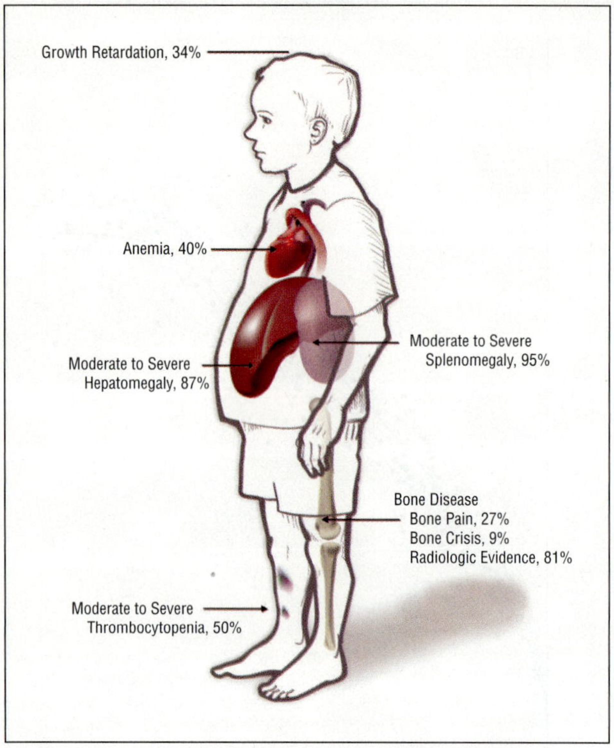


**Figure 2.** Prevalence of affected organ involvement in Gaucher disease among children at diagnosis. Growth retardation refers to patients below the fifth percentile for height. Radiologic evidence of bone disease may indicate Erlenmeyer flask deformity, marrow infiltration, osteopenia, avascular necrosis, infarction, and/or new fractures. Anemia is defined according to age and sex references for hemoglobin concentrations as follows: less than 11 g/dL for boys 12 years and older; less than 10 g/dL for girls 12 years and older; less than 9.5 g/dL for children aged 2 to younger than 12 years; less than 8.5 for children aged 6 months to younger than 2 years; and less than 9.1 g/dL for infants younger than 6 months. Hepatomegaly (liver volume in multiples of normal size predicted for body weight [MN]) is defined as moderate (>1.25 to 2.5 MN) to severe (>2.5 MN). Splenomegaly (spleen volume in multiples of normal) is defined as moderate (>5 to 15 MN) to severe (>15 MN). Thrombocytopenia is defined as moderate (platelet count, $60 \times 10^3/\mu L$ to $>120 \times 10^3/\mu L$) to severe (platelet count, $<60 \times 10^3/\mu L$).

voluntarily reported by physicians caring for GD patients and are not subject to independent verification. Therefore, the data may have limitations. First, the subjects may not represent the full spectrum of disease severity. Second, the prevalence of signs and symptoms could be biased by the identification of siblings of index cases. Third, differing testing modalities may have been used (as occurs for organ volume measurements and genotyping). Fourth, there may be variable quantities of data submitted by different physicians.

Nevertheless, the ICGG Gaucher Registry offers the largest cohort available with longitudinal data, making statistical analysis of clinical characteristics possible for a disorder in which its rarity essentially obviates the ability to conduct large-scale clinical trials.

In summary, nonneuronopathic GD is a treatable lysosomal storage disorder that most commonly manifests during childhood. A definitive diagnosis requires an enzyme assay demonstrating deficient or absent activity of glucocerebrosidase supplemented by mutational analysis of the glucocerebrosidase gene. Common disease manifestations in children include splenomegaly, hepatomegaly, anemia, thrombocytopenia, easy bruising, and significant growth retardation (**Figure 2**). Most patients have evidence of significant skeletal manifestations of disease, which may not be evident on physical examination and require radiologic examination for detection.[16] Pediatric GD, when left untreated, is most often associated with progressive morbidity and even shortened life expectancy. All providers of health care for children should be aware of the presenting signs and symptoms of nonneuronopathic GD because the timely initiation of appropriate treatment with enzyme replacement therapy will prevent or decrease morbidity and reduce the risk of later irreversible complications of this disease.

**Accepted for Publication:** December 22, 2005.
**Correspondence:** Paige Kaplan, MBBCh, Section of Metabolic Diseases, Department of Human Genetics and Molecular Biology, The Children's Hospital of Philadelphia, 34th and Civic Center Boulevard, Philadelphia, PA 19104 (kaplan@email.chop.edu).
**Financial Disclosure:** Dr Kaplan received an educational grant from Genzyme Corporation.
**Funding/Support:** This study was supported in part by Genzyme Corporation.
**Acknowledgment:** We thank the patients with nonneuronopathic GD and their physicians and health care personnel who submit data to the ICGG; the ICGG for their review of the manuscript; the ICGG support team; Trent Richardson, MAMS, for the graphic design of Figure 2; and Andrea Gwosdow, PhD, for assistance in preparing the manuscript.

## REFERENCES

1. Brady RO, Kanfer J, Shapiro D. Metabolism of glucocerebrosides. *J Biol Chem.* 1965;240:39-42.
2. Beutler E, Grabowski GA. Gaucher disease. In: Scriver CR, Beaudet AL, Sly WS, et al, eds. *The Metabolic and Molecular Bases of Inherited Disease.* 8th ed. New York, NY: McGraw-Hill Co; 2001:3635-3668.
3. Zevin S, Abrahamov A, Hadas-Halpern I, et al. Adult-type Gaucher disease in children. *Q J Med.* 1993;86:565-573.
4. Kaplan P, Mazur A, Manor O, et al. Acceleration of retarded growth in children with Gaucher disease after treatment with alglucerase. *J Pediatr.* 1996;129:149-153.
5. Barton NW, Brady RO, Dambrosia JM, et al. Replacement therapy for inherited enzyme deficiency. *N Engl J Med.* 1991;324:1464-1470.
6. Weinreb NJ, Charrow J, Andersson HC, et al. Effectiveness of enzyme replacement therapy in 1028 patients with non-neuronopathic Gaucher disease after 2 to 5 years of treatment. *Am J Med.* 2002;113:112-119.
7. Meikle PJ, Hopwood JJ, Clague AE, Carey WF. Prevalence of lysosomal storage disorders. *JAMA.* 1999;281:249-254.
8. Charrow J, Andersson HC, Kaplan P, et al. The Gaucher Registry. *Arch Intern Med.* 2000;160:2835-2843.
9. Ludwig J. *Current Methods of Autopsy Practice.* Philadelphia, Pa: WB Saunders Co; 1979.
10. Elstein D, Hadas-Halpern I, Azuri Y, Abrahamov A, Bar-Ziv Y, Zimran A. Accuracy of ultrasonography in assessing spleen and liver size in patients with Gaucher disease. *J Ultrasound Med.* 1997;16:209-211.
11. Kuczmarski RJ, Ogden CL, Grummer-Strawn LM, et al. CDC growth charts: United States. *Adv Data.* 2000;(314):1-27.
12. Hollander M, Wolfe DA. *Nonparametric Statistical Methods.* 2nd ed. New York, NY: John Wiley & Sons Inc; 1999.
13. Stokes ME, Davis CS, Koch GG. *Categorical Data Analysis Using the SAS System.* 2nd ed. Cary, NC: SAS Institute Inc; 2000.
14. Wain HM, Bruford EA, Lovering RC, Lush MJ, Wright MW, Povey S. Guidelines for human gene nomenclature. *Genomics.* 2002;79:464-470.
15. Weinreb N, Deegan P, Kacena K, Mistry P, Pastores GM, vom Dahl S. Life expectancy in type 1 (non-neuronopathic) Gaucher disease. http://www.ashg.org/cgi-bin/ashg05s/ashg05. Accessed December 9, 2005.
16. Charrow J, Andersson HC, Kaplan P, et al. Enzyme replacement therapy and monitoring for children with non-neuronopathic Gaucher disease: consensus recommendations. *J Pediatr.* 2004;144:112-120.
17. Pastores GM, Weinreb NJ, Aerts H, et al. Therapeutic goals in the treatment of Gaucher disease. *Semin Hematol.* 2004;41(4)(suppl 5):4-14.

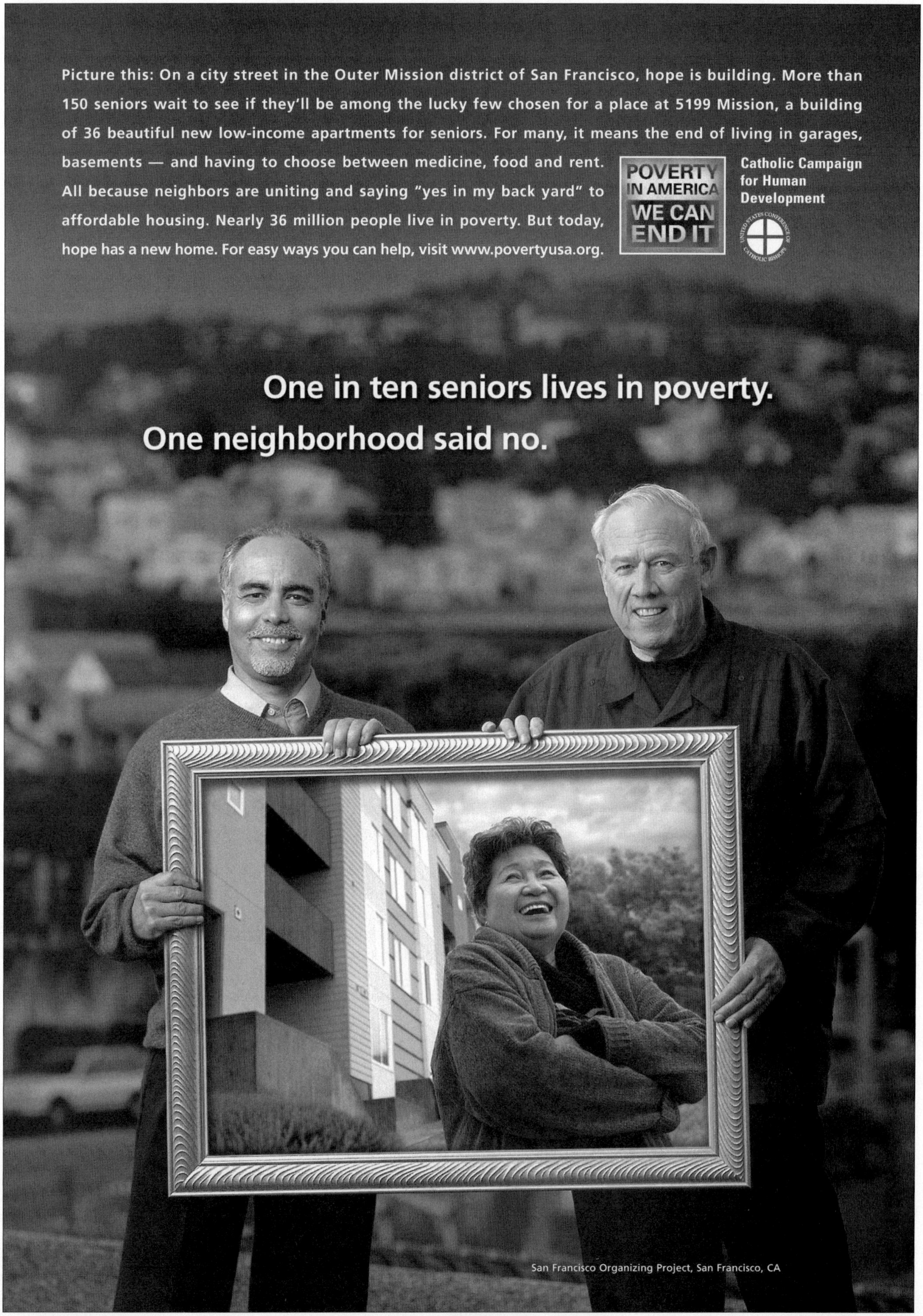
Picture this: On a city street in the Outer Mission district of San Francisco, hope is building. More than 150 seniors wait to see if they'll be among the lucky few chosen for a place at 5199 Mission, a building of 36 beautiful new low-income apartments for seniors. For many, it means the end of living in garages, basements — and having to choose between medicine, food and rent. All because neighbors are uniting and saying "yes in my back yard" to affordable housing. Nearly 36 million people live in poverty. But today, hope has a new home. For easy ways you can help, visit www.povertyusa.org.
POVERTY IN AMERICA
WE CAN END IT
Catholic Campaign for Human Development
UNITED STATES CONFERENCE OF CATHOLIC BISHOPS
One in ten seniors lives in poverty.
One neighborhood said no.
San Francisco Organizing Project, San Francisco, CA

ARTICLE

# Risk-Compensation Behavior in Children

## Myth or Reality?

*I. Barry Pless, MD; Helen Magdalinos, BA, CCLS; Brent Hagel, PhD*

**Objective:** To assess risk compensation and risk homeostasis theory in children.

**Design:** We used a case-control study design in children aged 8 to 18 years who had an injury while participating in an activity that did or could entail the use of protective equipment (PE).

**Setting:** Montreal Children's Hospital emergency department from December 1, 2001, to November 30, 2002.

**Participants:** We interviewed consenting children and compared the reports of risk-taking behaviors in those who did and those who did not report using PE.

**Main Outcome Measures:** Indicators of risk-taking behavior and injury severity.

**Results:** A total of 674 children presented with injuries during the study, and 394 were interviewed (235 PE users and 159 nonusers). There was no evidence of an association between indicators of risk-taking behavior and PE use after adjusting for age, sex, personality, and type of activity and no relationship between injury severity and PE use.

**Conclusions:** Results of this study provide no support for hypotheses about risk homeostasis theory among children using PE. The validity of the theory appears highly doubtful for children in this age range.

*Arch Pediatr Adolesc Med. 2006;160:610-614*

RISK HOMEOSTASIS THEORY (RHT) has perplexed the injury-prevention field for the past quarter century. The theory can be understood by analogy with a thermostat that adjusts the heat depending on the temperature of the surrounding area, which results in homeostasis—"resistance to change or maintaining an equilibrium." With respect to injuries, RHT asserts that everyone has an acceptable preset level of risk taking, such that when a safety measure is applied, thus decreasing risk, the preventive benefit of the measure will be offset by more dangerous or risky behavior.

The theory was popularized by Wilde[1] in 1984 and has been the topic of much heated debate that continues to the present.[2-7] The debate is fueled in part by the many important implications of the theory for several aspects of injury prevention.

These aspects range from the formulation of public health policies or programs to research strategies. For example, if RHT were proved and as widely applicable as its adherents contend, preventing injuries would require fostering changes in the risk tolerance of entire populations—a daunting, if not impossible, task. For researchers determined to find new strategies for prevention, it would suggest that most such efforts are futile.

Before struggling with these issues, we need first to assess the strength of the evidence in support of RHT. Several investigators have attempted to do so and have identified a number of critical deficiencies[8,9] to which Wilde and his colleagues have offered rebuttals.[6,10,11] The main criticism is that convincing empirical evidence is lacking. Most supposedly supportive studies are based on secondary analyses, almost exclusively in the domain of driving and motor vehicle crashes. These analyses have been dismissed as flawed or superseded by stronger evidence.

Several related issues also have been largely overlooked. One such is whether the theory, if true, applies equally to all subgroups in the population. In particular, it is not known whether children are affected in the same way as adults. There is virtually no mention of children in Wil-

Author Affiliations:
Departments of Pediatrics and Epidemiology and Biostatistics, Faculty of Medicine, McGill University (Dr Pless), and Montreal Children's Hospital (Dr Pless and Ms Magdalinos), Montreal, Quebec; and Departments of Paediatrics and Community Health Sciences, Alberta Children's Hospital, Faculty of Medicine, University of Calgary, Alberta (Dr Hagel).

de's text, and only 2 possibly pertinent articles have been published. Morrongiello and Major[12] found that parents appear to permit their children to engage in riskier behaviors when safety devices, such as bicycle helmets, are used. This premise, however, is an example of adult behavior and does not address the child question directly. In another study, Mok et al[13] provided pilot study data from interviews with 6- to 14-year-old children that offer modest support for RHT.

This article presents the results of an extension of that pilot study. It differs with respect to the larger number of children involved and the manner in which the data are analyzed. As in the pilot study, it is based on self-reported risk-taking behaviors of injured children who did and did not use protective equipment (PE) during sports and recreational activities. The sample is large enough to permit us to detect a 2-fold or greater difference in risk-compensatory behavior between the groups.[13]

## METHODS

In Canada, the parents of all children attending a children's hospital emergency department (ED) for an injury are asked to provide details of the event. This information is recorded on a form used by the Canadian Hospitals Injury Reporting and Prevention Program (CHIRPP).[14] From these reports at the Montreal Children's Hospital from December 1, 2001, through November 30, 2002, we selected children aged 8 to 18 years who had an injury while participating in an activity that did or could entail the use of PE. We then interviewed these children and compared reports of behaviors from those who did and those who did not report using any such equipment. The research ethics board of the Montreal Children's Hospital approved this study.

An interviewer (H.M.) blinded to PE use status contacted families by telephone shortly after the ED visit, explained the purpose of the study, and sought verbal consent from parents. She then asked the child a series of questions about PE (eg, helmet) use, actual behavior (eg, whether, at the time of injury, the child judged that he or she was cycling or skating faster than usual), and severity (eg, equipment damage). Type of activity was taken from the CHIRPP form and confirmed during the telephone interview. Ages and categories were obtained from the CHIRPP form and confirmed by telephone interviews (**Table 1** and **Table 2**). For the regression models, we classified age as younger than 11 years, 11 to 14 years, and 15 to 18 years; personality as careful or one who takes chances (on the basis of the Zuckerman scale[15]), and activity into 5 groups: hockey, ski/snowboard, football, bicycle, or scooter.

The questions used focused on actual behavior and were intended to provide more compelling information than the hypothetical questions used in the pilot study. Because the previous form of the question could lead to bias, the new questions were based on a specified event (eg, when you were injured bicycling, were you taking more chances than usual). The interview included administration of the Zuckerman thrill- and adventure-seeking subscale.[15] An individual could obtain a score between 0 and 10, with 10 indicating high thrill and adventure seeking, a proxy for risk taking. These scores were divided into 3 risk categories: 0-4, low; 5-8, medium; and 9-10, high.

We calculated that with a sample of 400 children there would be 80% power to detect a 50% reported change in behavior, assuming a PE use rate of about 50% (ie, to 25% or 75%). The number of respondents we sought was based on estimates of anticipated nonresponses, refusals, and those who could not be traced.

**Table 1. Sociodemographic and Clinical Characteristics: Completed vs Not-Completed Interviews**

| Characteristic | Respondents, No. (%) Completed Interviews (n = 394) | Not-Completed Interviews (n = 280) |
|---|---|---|
| Sex | | |
| Male | 277 (70.3) | 215 (76.8) |
| Female | 117 (29.7) | 65 (23.2) |
| Age, y | | |
| <11 | 57 (14.5) | 45 (16.1) |
| 11-14 | 184 (47.7) | 148 (52.9) |
| 15-18 | 153 (38.8) | 87 (31.1) |
| Type of injury | | |
| Bruise, sprain, laceration | 204 (51.8) | 149 (53.2) |
| Fracture, dislocation | 158 (40.1) | 102 (36.4) |
| Head: minor injury or concussion | 32 (8.1) | 29 (10.4) |
| Body part | | |
| Upper extremity | 205 (52.0) | 147 (52.5) |
| Lower extremity | 92 (23.4) | 68 (24.3) |
| Trunk | 32 (8.1) | 15 (5.4) |
| Head and neck | 65 (16.5) | 50 (17.9) |
| Where injury occurred | | |
| Arena | 92 (23.4) | 57 (20.4) |
| Ski hill | 121 (30.7) | 30 (10.7) |
| Park | 43 (10.9) | 44 (15.7) |
| Rink | 42 (10.7) | 16 (5.7) |
| Street | 75 (19.0) | 109 (38.9) |
| School | 15 (3.8) | 20 (7.1) |
| Home | 6 (1.5) | 4 (1.4) |
| Activity | | |
| Skate, hockey (street, field, or ice) | 144 (36.5) | 71 (25.4) |
| Ski, snowboard | 120 (30.5) | 30 (10.7) |
| Football | 17 (4.3) | 30 (10.7) |
| Bicycle | 62 (15.7) | 83 (29.6) |
| Scooter, in-line skates, skateboard | 51 (12.9) | 66 (23.6) |
| Disposition | | |
| Left or advice only | 83 (21.1) | 53 (18.9) |
| Treated, follow-up | 289 (73.4) | 214 (76.4) |
| Short stay in emergency department or admission | 22 (5.6) | 13 (4.6) |
| Protective equipment* | | |
| Users | 188 (47.7) | 137 (48.9) |
| Nonusers | 76 (19.3) | 64 (22.8) |
| Missing | 130 (33.0) | 79 (28.2) |

*On the basis of Canadian Hospitals Injury Reporting and Prevention Program data.

## RESULTS

Using CHIRPP reports for the 10 months from December 2001 through November 2002, we identified 674 children meeting the selection criteria and successfully interviewed 394 (58.5%). The average time between the ED visit and initial follow-up was 27 days, with a maximum of 49 days. Messages were left but not returned by 169 families; 15 were wrong numbers, and 90 did not answer after 3 attempts at different times of day. Only 4 were outright refusals, and 2 were missed for other reasons. Table 1 shows that those who completed the interview differed importantly from those who did not only by where the injury occurred, activity at the time of injury, and PE use.

**Table 2. Sociodemographic and Clinical Characteristics in Protective Equipment Users vs Nonusers**

| Characteristic | Protective Equipment Users, No. (%) (n = 235) | Protective Equipment Nonusers, No. (%) (n = 159) | Odds Ratio (95% Confidence Interval) |
|---|---|---|---|
| Sex | | | |
| Male | 183 (77.8) | 94 (59.1) | 2.43 (1.57-3.78) |
| Female | 52 (22.1) | 65 (40.9) | 1.00 |
| Age, y | | | |
| <11 | 42 (17.9) | 15 (9.4) | 2.07 (1.06-4.05) |
| 11-14 | 105 (44.7) | 79 (49.7) | 0.98 (0.64-1.52) |
| 15-18 | 88 (37.4) | 65 (40.9) | 1.00 |
| Type of injury | | | |
| Bruise, sprain, laceration | 120 (51.1) | 84 (52.8) | 1.00 |
| Fracture, dislocation | 97 (41.3) | 61 (38.4) | 1.11 (0.52-2.35) |
| Head: minor injury or concussion | 18 (7.7) | 14 (8.8) | 1.24 (0.57-2.67) |
| Body part | | | |
| Head and neck | 38 (16.2) | 27 (17.0) | 0.47 (0.18-1.20) |
| Upper extremity | 126 (53.6) | 79 (49.7) | 0.53 (0.23-1.24) |
| Lower extremity | 47 (20.0) | 45 (28.3) | 0.34 (0.14-0.86) |
| Trunk | 24 (10.2) | 8 (5.0) | 1.00 |
| Where injury occurred | | | |
| Arena | 83 (35.3) | 9 (5.7) | 12.30 (4.07-37.11) |
| Ski hill | 71 (30.2) | 50 (31.4) | 1.89 (0.74-4.83) |
| Park | 23 (9.8) | 20 (12.6) | 1.52 (0.54-4.39) |
| Rink | 16 (6.8) | 26 (16.4) | 0.82 (0.28-2.38) |
| Street | 33 (14.0) | 42 (26.4) | 1.04 (0.39-2.78) |
| Home or school | 9 (3.8) | 12 (7.5) | 1.00 |
| Activity | | | |
| Skate, hockey (street, field, or ice) | 101 (43.0) | 43 (27.0) | 1.00 |
| Ski, snowboard | 69 (29.4) | 51 (32.1) | 4.69 (2.37-9.30) |
| Football | 12 (5.1) | 5 (3.1) | 2.70 (1.36-5.37) |
| Bicycle | 36 (15.3) | 26 (16.4) | 4.80 (1.45-15.85) |
| Scooter, in-line skates, skateboard | 17 (7.2) | 34 (21.4) | 2.77 (1.28-5.98) |
| Disposition | | | |
| Left or advice only | 53 (22.6) | 30 (18.9) | 1.00 |
| Treated, follow-up | 172 (73.2) | 117 (73.6) | 2.12 (0.82-5.49) |
| Short stay in emergency department or admission | 10 (4.2) | 12 (7.5) | 1.18 (0.74-4.22) |

Initial information obtained from the CHIRPP form revealed that 325 children used PE. However, at the interview, only 234 claimed to have done so (55% used a helmet, 23% used knee pads, <1% used wrist guards, and <1% used other PE). All analyses that follow are based on the number interviewed. As shown in Table 1, 70.3% were boys, and 86.5% were 11 years or older. Nearly one third were injured while skating or playing hockey, 30.5% while skiing or snowboarding, and 15.7% while bicycling. Only 5.6% were admitted to the hospital or kept for observation in the ED; 40.1% had a fracture or dislocation, and 16.5% involved a head-neck injury. The most commonly injured body parts were the upper and lower extremities (52.0% and 23.4%, respectively). About one third of the injuries occurred on a ski hill (30.7%) or in an arena (23.4%), 19.0% on the street, and 10.9% in a park.

Table 2 provides a comparison of sociodemographic and clinical characteristics between PE users and nonusers on the basis of the completed interview sample. A significantly higher percentage of PE users were boys; they were injured in an arena or while skiing, snowboarding, skating, or playing hockey. The PE users were also more likely to be younger children. Use of PE was not, however, related to type of injury or severity (using treatment provided in the ED as a proxy for severity).

**Table 3. Risk Taking, Past Injury, and Injury Severity in Protective Equipment Users vs Nonusers**

| Question | Protective Equipment Users, No. (%) (n = 235) | Protective Equipment Nonusers, No. (%) (n = 159) | Odds Ratio (95% Confidence Interval) |
|---|---|---|---|
| Type of person | | | |
| Careful | 138 (58.7) | 77 (48.4) | 1.00 |
| Risk taker | 97 (41.3) | 82 (51.6) | 1.51 (1.01-2.27) |
| Zuckerman score | | | |
| Low risk | 70 (29.8) | 49 (30.8) | 1.00 |
| Medium risk | 118 (50.5) | 80 (50.3) | 0.91 (0.51-1.64) |
| High risk | 47 (20.0) | 30 (18.9) | 0.94 (0.55-1.61) |
| Damage to helmet | | | |
| No | 208 (88.5) | NA | NA |
| Yes | 8 (3.4) | NA | NA |
| Missing | 19 (8.1) | 159 (100) | NA |
| Equipment damage | | | |
| No | 120 (51.1) | NA | NA |
| Yes | 6 (2.6) | NA | NA |
| NA | 109 (46.4) | 159 (100) | NA |
| Previous helmet use | | | |
| No | 11 (4.7) | 20 (12.6) | 1.00 |
| Yes | 57 (24.3) | 6 (3.8) | 0.06 (0.02-0.17) |
| NA (first use) | 167 (71.1) | 133 (83.6) | NA |
| Past injury same activity | | | |
| No | 159 (67.7) | 125 (78.6) | 1.00 |
| Yes | 68 (28.9) | 23 (14.5) | 0.06 (0.02-0.18) |
| NA (first use) | 8 (3.4) | 11 (6.9) | NA |

Abbreviation: NA, not applicable.

In **Table 3**, we compare PE users and nonusers with respect to measures of risk taking, past injuries, and proxies for injury severity. Significantly more of the PE nonusers described themselves as risk takers, but there were no differences in the Zuckerman thrill-seeking scores. The PE users were more likely to report having used a helmet previously and to have been injured previously in the same activity, although in neither case did the odds ratio exclude the null.

In **Table 4**, we directly test the RHT by asking PE users and nonusers specific questions about risky behavior. Both the unadjusted and adjusted odds ratios indicate no evidence of a relationship between these indicators of risk-taking behavior and PE use after adjusting for age, sex, personality, and type of activity.

In **Table 5** we examined the relationship between non–PE-related injury severity and PE use. The RHT would predict that, for example, as arm injury severity in an individual wearing a helmet increases, the proportion wearing a helmet should increase (ie, with RHT we would expect more severe arm injuries as the result of helmeted riders taking more chances). Using disposition in the ED as a proxy for severity, we found no evidence to suggest such a relationship ($P=.56$).

## COMMENT

Taken together, our findings provide little support for the existence of risk compensation among children in this age group. This study is one of the first attempts to test the RHT directly in children. To our knowledge, there are no other studies in the literature in which this question is addressed in a similar manner. Thus, until such time as other study results are reported, these findings are the best indication of how RHT affects children.

With a much larger sample, we may have been able to search for, and possibly find, what might be regarded as an example of effect modification. This possibility arises because we previously postulated that there might be important subgroups in any population, including children. These subgroups might consist of inherent risk takers or thrill seekers at one extreme or the exceptionally cautious at the other. If RHT were to operate, it would be most evident among a middle group, but it is uncertain how large this group might be. However, as some data in Table 3 suggest, PE users may be different from non-PE users with respect to risk-taking behavior.

We acknowledge that these findings depend heavily on the ability of children in this age group to provide reasoned responses. Conclusions also depend on the assumption that those responses are not biased. Both assumptions seem reasonable but cannot be proved with the data at hand. The question of bias is important in this context only if it operates in what is, in effect, the null direction (ie, so that children who actually take more risks when using PE report not doing so perhaps because this response is more socially acceptable).

Despite the number of respondents involved, whether the number is sufficient to fully test the hypothesis is uncertain. We estimated that the sample was large enough to detect a 25% difference in responses, assuming a base rate (ie, for non-PE users) of 50%. That estimate was remarkably accurate, and although none of the differences approached 25%, the order of magnitude was so small that we believe the conclusion is well supported.

Among the limitations that also must be considered are the statistical requirements for the logistic regression on which the results rest heavily. To the extent that we were able to do so, these requirements appear to have been met. Another statistical issue is that of multiple testing. We did not deem it necessary to adjust for repeated tests using the same data, and not doing so made it more likely for us to find a difference. Hence, we are being conservative in our interpretation of a null result.

The use of CHIRPP data poses other limitations, especially with respect to the generalizability of the results. If there were solid reasons for believing that children seen at this hospital differ in some important ways from others and that those differences might influence their responses, this must be taken into account. However, we think it highly unlikely that the children in our sample were so unusual, but it is also possible that having chosen to test the hypothesis in children who have

**Table 4. Risk Taking and Protective Equipment Use: Unadjusted and Adjusted Odds Ratios**

| Protective Equipment Use | Risk-Taking Behavior, No. (%) | | Odds Ratio (95% Confidence Interval) Unadjusted | Adjusted* |
|---|---|---|---|---|
| **Going Fast** | | | | |
| Yes | 112 (59.6) | 123 (59.7) | 0.99 (0.65-1.50) | 1.16 (0.73-1.84) |
| No | 76 (40.4) | 83 (40.3) | 1.00 | 1.00 |
| **Speed Faster Than Usual** | | | | |
| Yes | 51 (60.7) | 184 (59.4) | 1.06 (0.63-1.79) | 0.96 (0.53-1.73) |
| No | 33 (39.3) | 126 (40.6) | 1.00 | 1.00 |
| **Taking Chances** | | | | |
| Yes | 73 (62.9) | 162 (58.3) | 1.22 (0.76-1.95) | 0.71 (0.42-1.21) |
| No | 43 (37.1) | 116 (41.7) | 1.00 | 1.00 |
| **More Chances Than Usual** | | | | |
| Yes | 34 (52.3) | 201 (61.1) | 0.70 (0.40-1.23) | 1.45 (0.77-2.74) |
| No | 31 (47.7) | 128 (38.9) | 1.00 | 1.00 |
| **Dangerous Activity** | | | | |
| Yes | 49 (53.8) | 186 (61.4) | 0.73 (0.45-1.21) | 1.41 (0.82-2.43) |
| No | 42 (46.2) | 117 (38.6) | 1.00 | 1.00 |
| **More Dangerous Than Usual** | | | | |
| Yes | 44 (56.4) | 191 (60.4) | 0.85 (0.50-1.44) | 1.40 (0.79-2.51) |
| No | 34 (43.6) | 125 (39.6) | 1.00 | 1.00 |

*Adjusted for age, sex, risk tolerance (Zuckerman score), and type of activity.

**Table 5. Protective Equipment Use According to Severity* Among Those With Injuries to an Unprotected Body Part**

| Protective Equipment Use | Mild (Advice Only) | Intermediate (Treated) | Severe (Admitted) | Total |
|---|---|---|---|---|
| Yes | 10 (16.9) | 38 (15.6) | 1 (6.2) | **49** (15.4) |
| No | 49 (83.1) | 205 (84.4) | 15 (93.8) | **269** (84.6) |
| **Total** | **59 (100.0)** | **243 (100.0)** | **16 (100.0)** | **318 (100.0)** |

*Disposition in the emergency department as proxy for severity; $P=.56$ (determined by $\chi^2$ analysis).

been injured might constitute a bias. Nevertheless, it is difficult to imagine that asking these questions of children who have not been injured would result in anything more than speculation because they would not have a memory cueing/anchoring event on which to base their responses.

There were large differences in PE use when we compared CHIRPP forms with follow-up interviews. On the basis of the CHIRPP form, those missed were less likely to wear PE. If they were also less likely to take additional risks when they were injured, their inclusion would have increased the association between PE use and risk taking. On the other hand, if these individuals were more likely to take additional risks when they were injured, their inclusion would have reduced the association between PE use and risk taking.

Our 58.5% response rate raises the possibility of a selection bias. However, we conducted a sensitivity analysis by including nonresponders in the examination of the relation between PE use and injury severity and found almost identical results (ie, no statistically significant relationships).

On the basis of these results, there appears to be little, if any, basis for believing that risk compensation is a phenomenon that influences the behavior of children using PE. Although this finding does not necessarily relegate RHT to the realm of myth, at least for children it does not seem to be a significant reality. The practical and important public health implication of this conclusion is that efforts must continue to persuade children to protect themselves by whatever means possible. Our results indicate that doing so will not result in greater risk taking and more injuries.[16]

**Accepted for Publication:** December 21, 2005.
**Correspondence:** I. Barry Pless, MD, Montreal Children's Hospital, 2300 Tupper St, Room F-259, Montreal, Quebec, Canada H3H 1P3 (barry.pless@mcgill.ca).
**Author Contributions:** Barry Pless had full access to all the data in the study and takes full responsibility for the integrity of the data and the accuracy of the data analysis.
**Funding/Support:** Dr Hagel is supported through a Professorship in Child Health and Wellness, funded by an anonymous donor to the Alberta Children's Hospital Foundation.
**Acknowledgment:** We thank Sofia Bamboulas, Sébastien Dubé, MSc, and Xun Zhang, PhD, for invaluable assistance.

## REFERENCES

1. Wilde GJS. *Target Risk.* Toronto, Ontario: PDE Publishing; 1984.
2. Evans WN, Graham JD. Risk reduction or risk compensation: the case of mandatory safety-belt use laws. *J Risk Uncertain.* 1991;4:61-73.
3. McKenna FP. Evidence and assumptions relevant to risk homeostasis. *Ergonomics.* 1985;28:1539-1541.
4. Robertson LS, Pless IB. Does risk homoeostasis theory have implications for road safety: against. *BMJ.* 2002;324:1149-1152.
5. Wilde GJS. Accident countermeasures and behavioral compensation: the position of risk homeostasis theory. *J Occup Accid.* 1989;10:267-292.
6. Wilde GJS. Risk homeostasis theory: an overview. *Inj Prev.* 1998;4:89-91.
7. Wilde GJ. Does risk homoeostasis theory have implications for road safety: for. *BMJ.* 2002;324:1149-1152.
8. O'Neill B, Williams A. Risk homeostasis hypothesis: a rebuttal. *Inj Prev.* 1998;4:92-93.
9. Shannon HS, Szatmari P. Seat-belt legislation and risk homeostasis: further analysis of the British data. *Accid Anal Prev.* 1994;26:803-805.
10. Adams J, Hillman M. The risk compensation theory and bicycle helmets. *Inj Prev.* 2001;7:89-90.
11. Adams J, Hillman M. Bicycle helmets: risk taking is influenced by people's perception of safety and danger. *BMJ.* 2001;322:1063-1064.
12. Morrongiello BA, Major K. Influence of safety gear on parental perceptions of injury risk and tolerance or children's risk taking. *Inj Prev.* 2002;8:27-31.
13. Mok D, Gore G, Hagel B, Mok E, Magdalinos H, Pless B. Risk compensation in children's activities: a pilot study. *Paediatr Child Health.* 2004;9:327-330.
14. Mackenzie SG, Pless IB. CHIRPP: Canada's principal injury surveillance program: Canadian Hospitals Injury Reporting and Prevention Program. *Inj Prev.* 1999;5:208-213.
15. Zuckerman M, Link K. Construct validity for the sensation-seeking scale. *J Consult Clin Psychol.* 1968;32:420-426.
16. Pless B. Taking risks with injury prevention. *CMAJ.* 2002;167:767-768.

## *Correction*

**Error in Text.** In the article titled "Schoolwide Food Practices Are Associated With Body Mass Index in Middle School Students," by Kubik et al published in the December 2005 issue of the ARCHIVES (2005;159:1111-1114) the estimated regression coefficient in the model was incorrectly interpreted as representing a 10% increase in body mass index (BMI) for every additional food practice permitted in a school. As described in the article, the dependent variable in the model was specified as BMI, calculated as weight in kilograms divided by the square of height in meters. Therefore, the estimated regression coefficient of $\beta=0.10$ would be correctly interpreted as a 0.10 BMI unit increase for every additional food practice a school permitted. In the abstract on page 1111, right-hand column, "Results" section, the third sentence should have read as follows: "Body mass index (BMI) of the students increased a 0.10 BMI unit for every additional food practice permitted in their school ($P<.03$)." On page 1113, left-hand column, "Results" section, paragraph 2, the last sentence should have read as follows: "Results indicated that for every additional food practice allowed by a school, student BMI increased by a 0.10 BMI unit ($P<.03$)." Also on page 1113, bottom left-hand column and upper right-hand column, "Comment" section, first paragraph, the fifth sentence should have read as follows: "However, the most important study finding was the positive association between these school food practices and student BMI, with BMI increasing a 0.10 BMI unit for every additional food practice allowed."

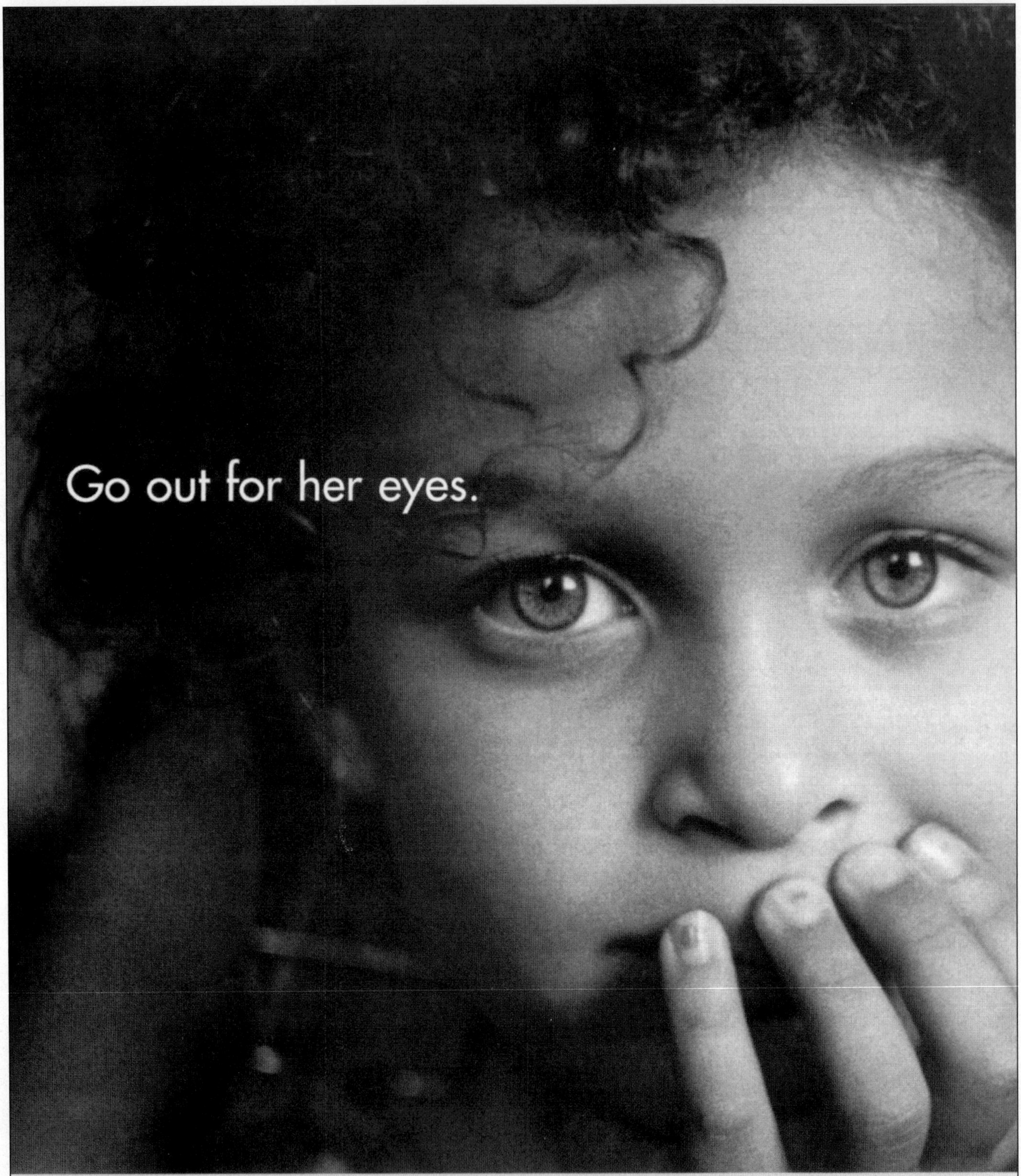


Until you can stop smoking, smoke outside for your daughter. She could get fewer earaches, be less susceptible to respiratory infections and be less likely to get asthma.

Until you can stop smoking, go out for your kids.

Take the Smoke-Free Home Pledge. Call 1 800-513-1157

American Medical Association • Environmental Protection Agency • Consumer Federation of America Foundation

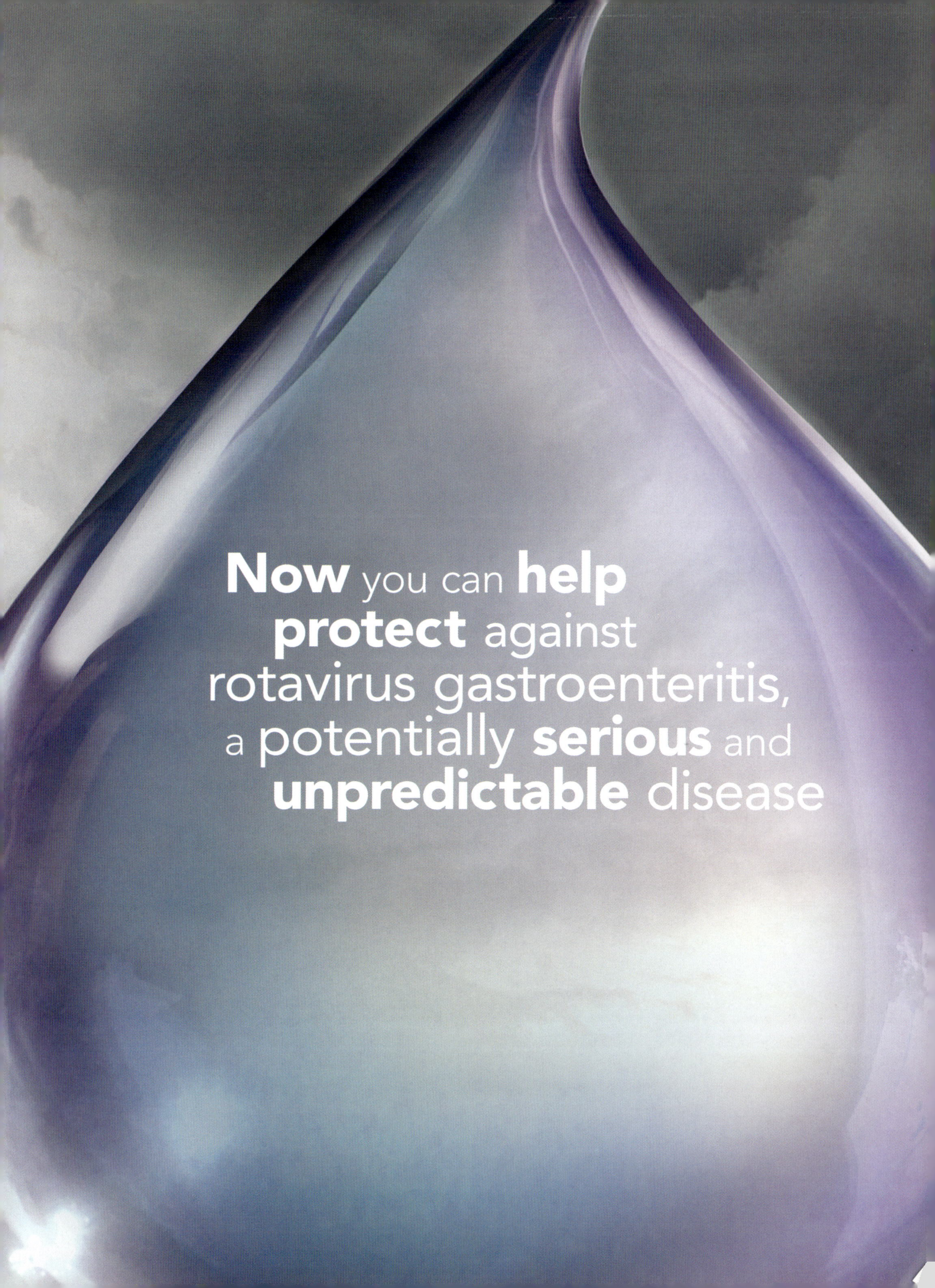
Now you can help protect against rotavirus gastroenteritis, a potentially serious and unpredictable disease

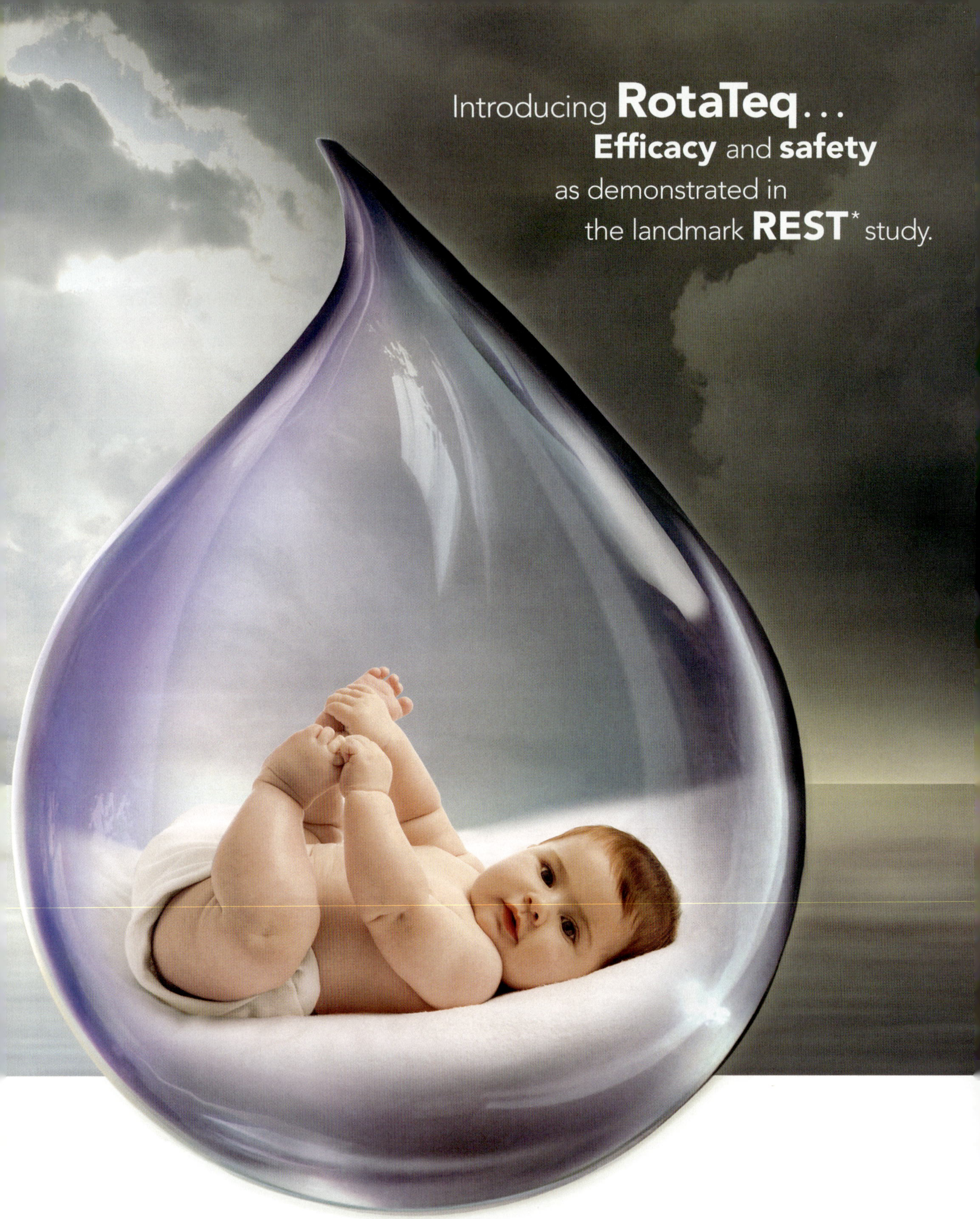
Introducing RotaTeq...
Efficacy and safety
as demonstrated in
the landmark REST* study.

ARTICLE

# Effectiveness of Child Safety Seats vs Seat Belts in Reducing Risk for Death in Children in Passenger Vehicle Crashes

*Michael R. Elliott, PhD; Michael J. Kallan, MS; Dennis R. Durbin, MD, MSCE; Flaura K. Winston, MD, PhD*

**Objective:** To provide an estimate of benefit, if any, of child restraint systems over seat belts alone for children aged from 2 through 6 years.

**Design:** Cohort study.

**Setting:** A sample of children in US passenger vehicle crashes was obtained from the National Highway Transportation Safety Administration by combining cases involving a fatality from the US Department of Transportation Fatality Analysis Reporting System with a probability sample of cases without a fatality from the National Automotive Sampling System.

**Participants:** Children in two-way crashes occurring between 1998 and 2003.

**Main Exposure:** Use of child restraint systems (rear-facing and forward-facing car seats, and shield and belt-positioning booster seats) vs seat belts. Potentially confounding variables included seating position, vehicle type, model year, driver and passenger ages, and driver survival status.

**Main Outcomes Measure:** Death of child passengers from injuries incurred during the crash.

**Results:** Compared with seat belts, child restraints, when not seriously misused (eg, unattached restraint, child restraint system harness not used, 2 children restrained with 1 seat belt) were associated with a 28% reduction in risk for death (relative risk, 0.72; 95% confidence interval, 0.54-0.97) in children aged 2 through 6 years after adjusting for seating position, vehicle type, model year, driver and passenger ages, and driver survival status. When including cases of serious misuse, the effectiveness estimate was slightly lower (21%) (relative risk, 0.79; 95% confidence interval, 0.59-1.05).

**Conclusion:** Based on these findings as well as previous epidemiological and biomechanical evidence for child restraint system effectiveness in reducing nonfatal injury risk, efforts should continue to promote use of child restraint systems through improved laws and with education and disbursement programs.

*Arch Pediatr Adolesc Med. 2006;160:617-621*

Author Affiliations:
Department of Biostatistics, University of Michigan School of Public Health, and Institute for Social Research, University of Michigan, Ann Arbor (Dr Elliott); Center for Clinical Epidemiology and Biostatistics (Mr Kallan and Dr Durbin) and Divisions of Pediatric Emergency Medicine (Dr Durbin) and General Pediatrics (Dr Winston), University of Pennsylvania School of Medicine, Leonard Davis Institute of Health Economics, University of Pennsylvania, (Dr Winston), Philadelphia; and TraumaLink Injury Research Center, Children's Hospital of Philadelphia (Drs Durbin and Winston).

CHILD RESTRAINT POLICY, including the passage of state child restraint laws, relies on evaluation of the risks of nonuse of child restraint systems and the benefits of their use in protecting children in crashes, most notably in the form of effectiveness estimates. However, previous estimates of real-world child restraint effectiveness have varied based on the analytical method chosen (most notably, the crash database chosen for analysis) and factors under study, including the outcome (nonfatal injury vs death) and the comparison group (children restrained with seat belts vs unrestrained children).[1-6]

Estimating effectiveness of child restraint systems through analysis of crash databases is potentially problematic because of the association between how passengers are restrained in a given crash and whether that crash will be in the given database. Analyses estimating the effectiveness of restraints are often conducted using the US Department of Transportation Fatality Analysis Reporting System (FARS), a census of crashes in the United States in which at least 1 person died. FARS has a sufficient number of outcomes of fatal child injuries for analysis but has a potentially biased selection of crashes in that inclusion of crashes is associated with the outcome of interest, fatalities. Using only data from FARS to assess child restraint system effectiveness in reducing risk for death in passenger vehicle crashes implicitly assumes that surviving children in fatal accidents have restraint practices that are similar to those of children in other serious crashes that do not result in fatalities. If child restraint systems are highly effective in reducing risk for death relative to seat belts, children in crashes who survived because they were restrained in a child restraint system rather than a seat belt will not be included in the FARS database unless someone else in the crash died. This will lead to a potential underrepresentation of child restraint system use among surviving children and a consequent underestimation of the effectiveness of child restraint systems in reducing risk for fatal injury if only FARS data are used.

One method for dealing with selection bias inherent in a FARS-only analysis would be a matched case-control or double-sampling method[7] that compares outcomes in children using different restraint types within a vehicle. Such analyses face limitations in this setting owing to small sample sizes, especially if other factors such as age or seating position are also matched for. We pursue an alternative analytical approach, that of combining the FARS database with the National Automotive Sampling System Crashworthiness Data System (NASS CDS), which includes a national probability sample of 2-way crashes. The NASS CDS provides a cross-section of crashes without regard to injury outcome but includes relatively few crashes with fatal child outcomes. By combining data from FARS and NASS CDS, we can obtain a sample of the entire cohort of children involved in 2-way crashes in the United States during a given period, with an identification of all of the fatally injured children during that time. Such analysis need not rely on assumptions about the representativeness of fatal crashes in the entire crash population.

Using sled tests, Kahane[1] previously estimated a mortality risk reduction of 46% for children in child restraints compared with unrestrained children. Using the double-sampling method applied to FARS data, Partyka[5] and Hertz[6] found reductions of 47% to 59% in fatality risk for children aged 1 to 4 years in child restraint systems compared with unrestrained children. In more recent years, child restraint and seat belt use rates have increased dramatically.[8] This study builds on the work of Kahane,[1] Partyka,[5] and Hertz[6] by providing a current estimate of restraint effectiveness based on newer model year vehicles and restraints and by providing an estimate of the incremental benefit, if present, of child restraint systems over seat belts alone for young children.

## METHODS

### DATA SOURCES

A census of children involved in crashes in the 50 states, the District of Columbia, and Puerto Rico, in which at least 1 passenger in 1 of the vehicles involved in the crash died, was obtained from the National Highway Traffic Safety Administration FARS database.[9] To be included in FARS, a crash must involve a motor vehicle traveling on a traffic way customarily open to the public and result in the death of a person (occupant of a vehicle or a nonoccupant such as a pedestrian) within 30 days of the crash. We restricted our analyses to the 92% of vehicles that were nondrivable (could not be driven from the crash scene) for compatibility with the NASS CDS. Further, to focus on the effectiveness of current child restraint systems, only crashes between 1998 and 2003 were analyzed. A few crashes in which only nonoccupants died were also excluded. Because all US state laws require child restraints for children younger than 2 years but some states still allow seat belt restraints for children aged 2 years or older, this study was limited to children from the ages of 2 through 6 years. Within FARS, we identified 7813 children aged 2 through 6 years who were vehicle occupants restrained in a child restraint system or a seat belt in a nondrivable passenger car, van, pickup truck, or sport-utility vehicle that was involved in a crash with at least 1 passenger fatality between 1998 and 2003. Of these 7813 children involved in fatal crashes, 1096 children (14%) were killed.

A sample of children involved in nonfatal crashes was obtained from NASS CDS.[10] The NASS CDS is a representative 3-stage probability sample selected annually from all police-reported crashes that resulted in at least 1 vehicle having to be towed from the scene because of damage. Approximately 5000 vehicles per year were sampled as part of the NASS CDS. Both vehicles in a NASS CDS–investigated crash were not necessarily nondrivable; therefore, we restricted our analyses to the 83% of vehicles that were nondrivable. Within NASS CDS, we identified 1433 children aged 2 through 6 years who were restrained in a child restraint system or seat belt in a passenger car, van, pickup truck, or sport-utility vehicle involved in a nonfatal crash sampled between 1998 and 2003. Because of the complex sample design of NASS CDS, these 1433 children represent 956 820 children meeting our inclusion criteria.

### VARIABLE DEFINITIONS

Our exposure variable of interest was child restraint system use vs seat belt use. Child restraint systems included rear-facing and forward-facing car seats, and shield and belt-positioning booster seats. Our primary analysis included all children 2 through 6 years old classified as either child restraint system or seat belt users, regardless of how the restraint was used. Our secondary analysis excluded the small fraction of children in FARS when the restraints were seriously misused. These included seat belt users who used a shoulder belt without a lap belt or improperly used the seat belt, for example, by restraining multiple children with a single seat belt, and also included child restraint users who did not attach the restraint to the vehicle seat or did not use the harness straps. Such misuse would usually be classified as nonuse in the NASS CDS; thus, a similar restriction was not necessary for the sample from NASS CDS. We also included driver, child, and vehicle characteristics of seating position (front seat vs rear seat), vehicle type (passenger car, pickup truck, van or minivan, and sport utility vehicle), model year (before 1990, 1990-1993, 1994-1997, after 1997), driver age (<20 years vs ≥20 years), passenger age (dummy variables for years 2-6), and driver survival status (as a marker of crash severity) as potential confounders. Direction of impact was not ascertained consistently in the 2 databases and was excluded from the analysis.

### STATISTICAL ANALYSES

Bivariate analyses comparing fatalities and nonfatalities and restraint type with respect to crash characteristics (seating position, vehicle type, model year, driver and passenger ages, and driver survival status) were conducted. Robust $\chi^2$ tests were performed to assess the differences in distributions in the bivariate analyses. Logistic regression modeling was used to compute the relative risk (RR) for death in children in child restraint systems vs seat belts. To estimate adjusted RRs, we used odds ratios from logistic regression; odds ratios will approximate RRs when the outcome is uncommon, as it was in this study. Because child restraint system users may differ from seat belt users in other crash characteristics, both unadjusted and adjusted analyses were conducted.

**Table 1. Child Occupant and Crash Characteristics, Overall and by Restraint Use*†**

| Characteristic | Overall | CRS‡ | Seat Belt§ | *P* Value |
|---|---|---|---|---|
| Fatality status | | | | |
| Fatal | 0.11 (1096) | 0.12 (508) | 0.11 (588) | .88 |
| Nonfatal | 99.89 (8150) | 99.88 (3795) | 99.89 (4355) | |
| Age, y | | | | |
| 2 | 21.2 (2243) | 42.8 (1875) | 2.9 (368) | <.001 |
| 3 | 17.3 (1981) | 29.3 (1338) | 7.3 (643) | |
| 4 | 19.2 (1875) | 17.8 (718) | 20.4 (1157) | |
| 5 | 15.0 (1615) | 7.6 (278) | 21.2 (1337) | |
| 6 | 27.3 (1532) | 2.5 (94) | 48.2 (1438) | |
| Seating position | | | | |
| Front seat | 15.7 (1549) | 13.4 (360) | 17.6 (1189) | .47 |
| Rear seat | 84.3 (7697) | 86.6 (3943) | 82.4 (3754) | |
| Vehicle type | | | | |
| Passenger car | 67.7 (5003) | 71.4 (2271) | 64.5 (2732) | .46 |
| Pickup truck | 5.6 (941) | 3.1 (367) | 7.7 (574) | |
| Van/minivan | 17.2 (1688) | 16.0 (861) | 18.3 (827) | |
| Sport-utility vehicle | 9.5 (1614) | 9.6 (804) | 9.4 (810) | |
| Model year | | | | |
| Before 1990 | 15.6 (1749) | 13.0 (734) | 17.7 (1015) | .73 |
| 1990-1993 | 23.4 (1953) | 23.4 (893) | 23.3 (1060) | |
| 1994-1997 | 33.8 (2692) | 37.2 (1259) | 31.0 (1433) | |
| 1998-2004 | 27.2 (2852) | 26.4 (1417) | 28.0 (1435) | |
| Driver age, y | | | | |
| <20 | 4.0 (603) | 3.4 (268) | 4.5 (335) | .71 |
| ≥20 | 96.0 (8643) | 96.6 (4035) | 95.5 (4608) | |
| Driver fatality | | | | |
| Yes | 0.28 (2744) | 0.29 (1299) | 0.28 (1445) | .70 |
| No | 99.72 (6502) | 99.71 (3004) | 99.72 (3498) | |
| Total | | 45.7 (4303) | 54.3 (4943) | |

Abbreviations: CRS, child restraint system; FARS, Fatality Analysis Reporting System (US Department of Transportation); NASS CDS, National Automotive Sampling System Crashworthiness Data System.

*Data are based on combined FARS/NASS CDS data set for crashes occurring between 1998 and 2003. Data are weighted according to their probability of selection: FARS cases with weights of 1; NASS cases with weights proportional to the inverse of their probability of selection.

†Data indicate weighted percent (unweighted number).

‡Includes 162 subjects with serious CRS misuse.

§Includes 89 subjects with serious seat belt misuse.

Because sampling in NASS CDS was based on model year and the severity of injury (including hospitalization status), subjects in less serious crashes were underrepresented in the study sample in a manner potentially associated with the predictors of interest. To account for this potential bias, case weights equal to the inverse of the probability of selection and adjusted to known crash totals were used to account for the oversampling of serious crashes in NASS CDS. (Case weights in FARS were set to 1, consistent with FARS being a census of all fatalities.) To adjust inference to account for the disproportional probability of selection of subjects and stratification and clustering of subjects by geographic region and vehicle, robust $\chi^2$ tests of association and Taylor series linearization estimates of the logistic regression parameter variances were calculated using SAS-callable SUDAAN: Software for the Statistical Analysis of Correlated Data, version 9.1 (Research Triangle Institute, Research Triangle Park, NC).

## RESULTS

Data in the cohort (constructed as described earlier) included 9246 children, weighted to represent 964 633 children in nondrivable vehicles in crashes between 1998 and 2003. **Table 1** gives the distribution of the variables used in the analysis, overall and by type of restraint used. Approximately 1 (0.11%) of 1000 children in a 2-way crash died. Somewhat fewer than half (45%) of all children were in child restraint systems, although younger children were much more likely to be restrained in child restraint systems. One (15.7%) of 6 children were in the front seat, two thirds (67.7%) were in passenger cars, one (15.6%) of 6 were in pre-1990 model year vehicles, and relatively few (4.0%) were driven by teenaged drivers; none of these factors were significantly associated with restraint type in bivariate analyses.

**Table 2. Relative Risk for Death, Child Restraint System Use vs Seat Belt Use, Unadjusted and Adjusted for Seating Position, Vehicle Type, Model Year, Driver and Passenger Age, and Driver Death**

| Variable | Unadjusted RR (95% CI) | Adjusted RR (95% CI) |
|---|---|---|
| All restrained | 1.03 (0.72-1.46) | 0.79 (0.59-1.05) |
| Excluding serious misuse of restraint | 0.93 (0.65-1.32) | 0.72 (0.54-0.97) |

Abbreviations: CI, confidence interval, RR, relative risk.

**Table 2** summarizes little difference in the unadjusted risk for death between users of child restraint systems and users of seat belts (RR, 1.03; 95% confidence interval, 0.72-1.46). After adjusting for seating position, vehicle type, model year, driver and passenger ages, and driver survival status, children in child restraint systems had a 21% reduction in risk for death compared with children in seat belts, although this difference was only marginally significant (RR, 0.79; 95% confidence interval, 0.59-1.05). After excluding the cases of serious child restraint system and seat belt misuse from FARS, children in child restraint systems had a 28% reduction in risk for death compared with children in seat belts (RR, 0.72; 95% confidence interval, 0.54-0.97).

## COMMENT

Our analysis indicated that children aged 2 through 6 years in child restraint systems had a 21% reduction in mortality risk compared with children in seat belts. When cases of serious misuse of child restraint systems and seat belts are excluded, mortality risk was reduced by 28%. This effectiveness estimate is less than that reported by Kahane,[1] Partyka,[5] and Hertz,[6] all of whom compared mortality risk in children in child restraint systems with those who were not restrained. Hertz[6] conducted the most recent National Highway Transportation Safety Administration effectiveness analyses based on crashes between 1988 and 1994. Using a matched-pairs analysis, he found that, among children aged 1 to 4 years in passenger cars, those in child restraint systems experienced a 54% reduction in deaths compared with unrestrained children. In the same analysis, Hertz[6] found that children in seat belts experienced a 47% reduction in deaths compared with unrestrained children. The crude relative effectiveness of child restraint systems vs seat belts based on this analysis would be 0.54 divided by 0.47, or 1.149, a 14.9% improvement in mortality reduction afforded by child restraint systems over seat belts.

In a more recent series of analyses, Levitt[4] and Dubner and Levitt[11] used FARS data from 1975 to 2003 and, by various methods, directly compared the mortality with child restraint systems vs seat belts in children aged 2 to 6 years and could not demonstrate a difference in effectiveness. Levitt and Porter[12] restricted the FARS data set to 2-vehicle crashes in which someone in the other vehicle (ie, the vehicle without the index child occupant) died, under the assumption that the distribution of restraint use among children in potentially fatal crashes is independent of whether someone in the other vehicle dies, after adjusting for various crash-related characteristics.

The precision of these previous effectiveness estimates and their relevance to today's fleet were limited by their reliance on FARS (the limits of which were presented in the introduction), by the inclusion of older vehicles and restraints, and by failing to control for the severity (potential unsurvivability) of the crashes. Our analysis based on a modern cohort of children involved in crashes in which the car was rendered undrivable addressed many of the limitations of these previous analyses and found effectiveness estimates for child restraint systems to be greater than that for seat belts alone, with estimates greater than those of both Levitt[4] and Hertz.[6]

Child restraint systems offer a considerable safety advantage over seat belts alone for biomechanical reasons. Child restraint systems are designed to reduce risk for ejection during a crash, better distribute the load of the crash through structurally stronger bones rather than soft tissues, limit the crash forces experienced by the vehicle occupant by prolonging the time of deceleration, and potentially limit the contact of the occupant with intruding vehicle structures. Optimal performance of restraint systems depends on an adequate fit between the restraint system and the occupant at the time of the crash. Increased risk for injury in young children restrained in seat belts as a result of improper loading of deceleration forces has been documented for nearly 50 years.[13-15] Child restraint systems offer improved fit of restraints for children who are too small for the adult-sized seat belt, thereby affording a mechanical protection advantage over seat belts. If restraint systems are seriously misused, however, their safety performance would be expected to be diminished. We adjusted for serious seat belt and child restraint system misuse (as defined in the "Methods" section) and found a slight increase in the relative effectiveness of child restraint systems compared with seat belts. In addition, previous in-depth analyses have demonstrated that most crashes in which children in child restraint systems die were of such severity that survival of the child was unlikely.[16,17] Considering this, we included a variable for driver death (as a proxy for a potentially nonsurvivable crash) in our multivariate analyses.

Previous assessments of child restraint system effectiveness using nonfatal injury as an outcome have demonstrated the safety benefits of child restraint systems over seat belts alone for young children.[2,3,17] The current study extends this evidence to include increased effectiveness of child restraint systems over seat belts alone in preventing death.

Our analysis was not without limitations. Restraint status information was missing for approximately 6% of children aged 2 through 6 years in the FARS data set and 9% of such children in the NASS CDS data set. Systematic differences between these subjects and those with restraint status provided may bias results, although the effect of such bias is likely to be small, given the relatively small amount of missing data. (Among restrained children aged 2 through 6 years, seating position was missing in 4% of FARS cases and less than 1% of NASS CDS cases, and less than 1% in both data sets were missing driver survival status, driver age, vehicle type, or model year.) In addition, the possibility of differential misclassification bias exists. Thus, if police misclassified fatally injured children in restraint systems as being in seat belts or unrestrained less often than NASS CDS crash investigators did for survivors of passenger vehicle crashes, the resulting RR for children in child restraint systems vs seat belts would be biased upward (ie, toward 1). Previous work suggests that, when a crash involves a fatality, the validity of police-reported restraint use improves.[18] Therefore, to the extent that misclassification in restraint use exists in our sources of data, it is more likely that it may result in an underestimate of child restraint system effectiveness. Finally, while we have argued that using only the FARS data set puts one at risk for selection bias, use of the NASS CDS to obtain a representative sample of the full two-way crash population may suffer from confounding between child restraint system use and crash severity, leading to either upward or downward bias in the estimate of child restraint system effectiveness. For example, if drivers who restrain their children in child restraint systems are less likely to be involved in potentially fatal crashes (ie, those fatal with the child in either a child restraint system or a seat belt, in a child restraint system only, or in a seat belt only), use of the NASS CDS population may overstate the effectiveness of child restraint systems vs seat belts by confounding child restraint use with safer driving behavior. The restriction of NASS CDS to two-way crashes and use of adjustment factors such as vehicle type, model year, age of driver, and, especially, survival status of the driver should reduce this confounding.

## IMPLICATIONS

Our analysis, which considered key predictors other than restraint use that are associated with injury severity and addressed selection bias problems inherent in a FARS-only analysis by combing FARS and NASS CDS data into a single cohort, provides evidence that using child restraint systems rather than seat belts reduces mortality in children aged 2 through 6 years. Based on our current findings as well as the long-standing biomechanical evidence for child restraint effectiveness and previous demonstrations of the importance of child restraint systems in reducing nonfatal injury risk,[3,19] efforts should continue to promote child restraint use through improved child restraint laws and with education and disbursement programs. Further research is needed, however, to further refine restraint effectiveness estimation procedures and to ensure that the results are applicable to the current fleet, because this information is needed for evidence-based policy and product design.

**Accepted for Publication:** November 23, 2005.
**Correspondence:** Flaura K. Winston, MD, PhD, 3535 TraumaLink Injury Research Center, 10th Floor, Children's Hospital of Philadelphia, 34th St and Civic Center Blvd, Philadelphia, PA 19104 (flaura@mail.med.upenn.edu).
**Funding/Support:** We acknowledge the commitment, partnership, and financial support of State Farm Mutual Automobile Insurance Company for the conduct of this research study.

**Disclaimer:** The results presented in this report are the interpretation solely of the authors and are not necessarily the views of State Farm Mutual Automobile Insurance Company.

## REFERENCES

1. Kahane CJ. *An Evaluation of Child Passenger Safety: The Effectiveness and Benefits of Safety Seats.* Washington, DC: US Dept of Transportation; 1986. DOT-HS-806-890.
2. Arbogast KB, Durbin DR, Cornejo RA, Kallan MJ, Winston FK. An evaluation of the effectiveness of forward facing child restraint systems. *Accid Anal Prev.* 2004;36:585-589.
3. Durbin DR, Elliott MR, Winston FK. Belt-positioning booster seats and reduction in risk of injury among children in vehicle crashes. *JAMA.* 2003;289:2835-2840.
4. Levitt SD. Evidence that child safety seats are no more effective than seat belts in reducing fatalities for children aged two and up. Available at: http://www.freakonomics.com/LevittAcademicPaper.pdf. Accessed July 25, 2005.
5. Partyka S. *Lives Saved by Child Restraints from 1982 through 1987.* Washington, DC: US Dept of Transportation; 1986. DOT-HS-807-371.
6. Hertz E. Revised estimates of child restraint effectiveness. Available at http://www-nrd.nhtsa.dot.gov/pdf/nrd-30/NCSA/RNotes/1996/childest.pdf. Accessed October 24, 2005.
7. Evans L. Double pair comparison: a new method to determine how occupant characteristics affect fatality risk in traffic crashes. *Accid Anal Prev.* 1986;18:217-227.
8. Winston FK, Chen IG, Elliott MR, Arbogast KB, Durbin DR. Recent trends in child restraint practices in the United States. *Pediatrics.* 2004;113:458-464.
9. National Highway Traffic Safety Administration. *FARS Analytic Reference Guide, 1975-2002.* Washington, DC: US Dept of Transportation; 2005. Available at ftp://ftp.nhtsa.dot.gov/FARS/FARS-DOC/USERGUIDE-2002.pdf. Accessed July 25, 2005.
10. National Highway Traffic Safety Administration. National Automotive Sampling System (NASS) Crashworthiness Data System. Washington, DC: US Dept of Transportation; 1997. Available at http://www-nass.nhtsa.dot.gov/NASS/cds/AnalyticalManuals/aman1997.pdf. Accessed July 25, 2005.
11. Dubner SJ, Levitt SD. Freakonomics: the seat-belt solution. *New York Times Magazine.* July 10, 2005:20.
12. Levitt S, Porter J. Sample selection in the estimation of air bag and seat belt effectiveness. *Rev Econ Stat.* 2001;83:603-615.
13. Kulowski K, Rost W. Intra-abdominal injury from safety belts in auto accidents. *Arch Surg.* 1956;73:970-971.
14. Garrett JW, Braunstein PW. The seat belt syndrome. *J Trauma.* 1962;2:220-238.
15. Agran PF, Dunkle DE, Winn DG. Injuries to a sample of seat belted children evaluated and treated in a hospital emergency room. *J Trauma.* 1987;27:58-64.
16. Sherwood CP, Ferguson SA, Crandall JR. *Factors Leading to Crash Fatalities to Child in Child Restraints: Proceedings of the 47th Conference of the Association for the Advancement of Automotive Medicine, September 22-24, 2003.* Arlington: Virginia University, Center for Applied Biomechanics, Charlottesville/Insurance Institute for Highway Safety; 2003.
17. Huelke DF, Sherman HW, Murphy MJ, Kaplan RJ, Flora JD. *Effectiveness of Current and Future Restraint Systems in Fatal and Serious Injury Automobile Crashes.* Warrendale, PA: Society of Automotive Engineers; 1979. SAE Paper 790323.
18. Schiff MA, Cummings P. Comparison of reporting of seat belt use by police and crash investigators: variation in agreement by injury severity. *Accid Anal Prev.* 2004;36:961-965.
19. Winston FK, Durbin DR, Kallan MJ, Moll EK. The danger of premature graduation to seat belts for young children. *Pediatrics.* 2000;105:1179-1183.

"I just can't get over how much babies cry. I really had no idea what I was getting into. To tell you the truth, I thought it would be more like getting a cat."

—From *Operating Instructions* by Anne Lamott, 1993

# Effectiveness of Nebulizer Use–Targeted Asthma Education on Underserved Children With Asthma

*Arlene M. Butz, RN, CRNP, ScD; Mona G. Tsoukleris, PharmD, BCPS; Michele Donithan, MHS; Van Doren Hsu, PharmD; Ilene Zuckerman, PharmD, PhD; Kim Elizabeth Mudd, MSN; Richard E. Thompson, PhD; Cindy Rand, PhD; Mary Elizabeth Bollinger, DO*

**Objective:** To determine the effectiveness of a home-based asthma education intervention in increasing appropriate nebulizer use and reducing symptom frequency, emergency department (ED) visits, and hospitalizations over 12 months.

**Design:** A randomized clinical trial.

**Settings:** Pediatric primary care, pulmonary/allergy, and ED practices associated with the University of Maryland Medical System and The Johns Hopkins Hospital, Baltimore.

**Participants:** Children with persistent asthma, aged 2 to 9 years, with regular nebulizer use and an ED visit or hospitalization within the past 12 months. Children were randomized into the intervention (n = 110) or control (n = 111) group. Follow-up data were available for 95 intervention and 86 control children.

**Intervention:** Home-based asthma education, including symptom recognition, home treatment of acute symptoms, appropriate asthma medication, and nebulizer practice.

**Main Outcome Measures:** Estimates of mean differences in asthma symptom frequency, number of ED visits and hospitalizations and appropriate quick relief, controller medication, and nebulizer practice over 12 months.

**Results:** Of the 221 children, 181 (81.9%) completed the study. There were no significant differences in home nebulizer practice, asthma morbidity, ED visits, or hospitalizations between groups (*P* range, .11-.79). Although most children received appropriate nonurgent asthma care (mean, 2 visits per 6 months), more than one third of all children received at least 6 quick-relief medication prescriptions during 12 months, with no difference by group.

**Conclusions:** A nebulizer education intervention had no effect on asthma severity or health care use. Of concern is the high quick-relief and low controller medication use in young children with asthma seen nearly every 3 months for nonurgent care.

*Arch Pediatr Adolesc Med. 2006;160:622-628*

**Author Affiliations:** Divisions of General Pediatrics (Dr Butz) and Pediatric Allergy and Immunology (Ms Mudd), Department of Pulmonary and Critical Care (Dr Rand), The Johns Hopkins University Medical Institutions; University of Maryland School of Pharmacy (Drs Tsoukleris, Hsu, and Zuckerman); Departments of Epidemiology (Ms Donithan) and Biostatistics (Dr Thompson), The Johns Hopkins University Bloomberg School of Public Health; and The University of Maryland School of Medicine (Dr Bollinger), Baltimore, Md.

ASTHMA, THE LEADING chronic illness among US children, affects approximately 6.2 million children younger than 18 years,[1] with the highest prevalence in African American boys from birth to the age of 4 years.[2,3] Management of acute asthma symptoms in children begins at home. Decisions of when and how to treat home acute asthma episodes rely on the parent's and child's ability to accurately identify symptoms and to implement timely and appropriate medication therapy. Yet, one third of caregivers make significant errors in accurately perceiving their child's asthma symptom severity[4] that may result in overuse or underuse of short-acting β-agonist or quick-relief asthma medications. In young children, nebulizers are used to deliver quick-relief medications for symptom relief and to provide some controller medications, but are only effective if properly administered. However, many families fail to properly use nebulizers.[5,6] Nebulizer use in young children is common, ranging from 33% to 71% in children younger than 12 years.[5-7] Although metered-dose inhalers (MDIs) are as effective as nebulized medications for asthma in young children,[8-11] many families prefer nebulizers to dispense medication to their child because of the parental lack of confidence in administering MDIs to young children and the difficulty of some children in coordinating respiration with MDIs.[12] Physician preference for nebulizer administration of asthma medications is low, but those who favor nebulizer delivery usually do so because of the perceived direct aerosolization of medication into the respiratory system vs MDIs.[13]

Most asthma educational programs and national guidelines[14,15] lack specific content addressing appropriate nebulizer practice and warnings of overdependence on quick-relief medications for asthma control. Furthermore, overuse of short-acting β-agonist medications delivered via MDI or nebulizer has been associated with fatal asthma.[16,17] The present study determines the effectiveness of a home-based asthma educational intervention (INT) targeting symptom recognition and nebulizer use in young children with persistent asthma in reducing symptoms and health care use and in increasing appropriate home asthma medication use. We hypothesized that children receiving the intervention would demonstrate a decrease in asthma symptoms, improvement in appropriate nebulizer and asthma medication use, and a decrease in emergency department (ED) visits and hospitalizations.

## METHODS

### STUDY DESIGN

This was a 2-group randomized clinical trial conducted to evaluate the effectiveness of a home-based INT vs basic or standard asthma education (CON) on symptom frequency, appropriate nebulizer and asthma medication use, and ED visits and hospitalizations in children aged 2 to 9 years who had persistent asthma. The institutional review boards of The Johns Hopkins University Medical Institutions and the University of Maryland School of Medicine, Baltimore, approved the study protocols. We obtained informed consent from all participating parents, including consent for electronic monitoring of the child's nebulizer and collection of the child's pharmacy records. Assent was obtained from children 7 years and older. Data collection included telephone-administered questionnaires, pharmacy records, and electronic monitoring of home nebulizer use.

### STUDY SUBJECTS

Children were recruited from pediatric practices affiliated with 2 large urban university hospitals, including pediatric primary care (29.9%), pulmonary/allergy specialty (50.2%), and ED (19.9%) practices between October 1, 2001, and December 31, 2003, and were followed up for 12 months. Eligibility criteria were as follows: aged 2 to 9 years, previous medical diagnosis of asthma, daytime asthma symptom frequency at least 2 or more times a week within the past 30 days, nighttime asthma symptom frequency at least 2 or more times a month for the past 30 days, use of a nebulizer to administer asthma medication within the past 30 days, resident of Baltimore, and 1 or more ED visits for asthma within the past 12 months or hospitalization for asthma in the past 12 months. A total of 513 children were recruited, of whom 254 (49.5%) were eligible; 221 (85.3%) provided consent and were randomized into the 2 study groups (INT or CON) (**Figure**). Ineligibility was primarily due to low or no nebulizer use in the prior 30 days and to children newly diagnosed as having asthma. At the 12-month follow-up, 181 (81.9%) of the children had complete interview and pharmacy record data to be included in the analysis (Figure). Incomplete pharmacy record data (n=30) were the primary reason for exclusion in final analysis. Three children died of asthma complications during the follow-up study, as described later. Children excluded from follow-up (n=40) did not significantly differ from children with complete data (n=181)

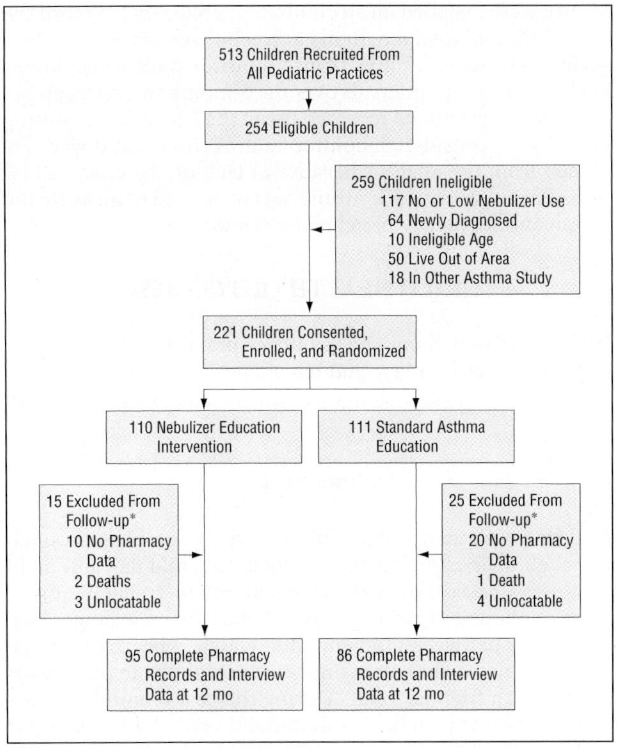


**Figure.** Flow diagram of subject progress through a randomized trial. The asterisk indicates that $P=.09$ for the differences by group for those excluded from follow-up.

by group status, age, sex, race/ethnicity, parental educational level, specialty care, days of nebulizer use in the past 30 days, or baseline asthma severity.

### INT PROGRAM

The 6-month home-based asthma/nebulizer educational intervention was based on the Wee Wheezers Program,[18] the A+ Asthma Club Program,[19] an asthma symptom identification program, or children[4,20] and nebulizer therapy recommendations.[12,13] Parents of children in the INT group received 6 home visits of 1-hour sessions. The intervention curricula are detailed elsewhere.[21]

Parents of children randomized into the CON group received basic asthma education comparable to asthma education received during nonurgent care visits, during 3 home visits addressing dose and frequency of current asthma medications in the home, use of a peak flow meter, importance of an asthma action plan, and importance of regular asthma care. Specific quick-relief and controller medication use, symptom identification, and nebulizer use technique were not included in the educational content for CON families.

All home education visits were delivered by 3 community health nurses with pediatric asthma training and were supervised monthly by a pediatric nurse asthma specialist (A.M.B.). Families of both groups were randomly assigned to each nurse to ensure equal exposure to any differences in nurse teaching style. Most families completed all assigned educational home visits (CON group, mean [SD] of 2.9 (0.5) of 3 assigned visits; and INT group, mean [SD] of 5.6 (1.2) of 6 assigned visits).[21]

### ELECTRONIC MONITOR OF NEBULIZER USE

Electronic nebulizer monitors, fitting all brands of nebulizer devices and developed by Hill-Rom Company, Inc (St Paul,

Minn), were installed on all children's nebulizers to record the date, time, and total length of each nebulizer use event, as described elsewhere.[22] Electronic monitor data were downloaded at 3-month intervals over the 6-month intervention period. Monitors with no recorded use in the 12-week monitoring period were considered monitor failures (n = 17) and were excluded from the analysis because of lack of objective validation of nebulizer use. Electronic data were used to measure the length and frequency of nebulizer sessions.

## CHILD HEALTH OUTCOMES

Child health outcome and nebulizer practice measures were collected by face-to-face and telephone interviews conducted with the parent or caregiver at baseline and at the 12-month follow-up.

### Asthma Severity

Children were assigned an asthma severity level based on national guidelines[14,15,23] using frequency of child day and night symptoms based on caregiver responses to 2 specific questions, including "During the past 6 months on average, how many days per week did your child cough, wheeze or experience shortness of breath to limit exercise, ability to play sports or play with friends?" and "During the past 6 months on average, how many nights per month did your child wake up at night with cough, wheeze, shortness of breath, or tightness in chest?" Children who met the National Asthma Education and Prevention Program criteria for mild, moderate, or severe persistent asthma of daytime symptoms (>2 times per week) or nighttime symptoms (>2 times per month)[14,15] were included in the study. Children classified as having mild intermittent asthma based on symptom frequency, and reporting daily anti-inflammatory medication use, were reclassified as having mild persistent asthma based on premedication severity.[23]

### Asthma Morbidity and Health Care Use

Symptom frequency, number of ED visits, nonurgent or specialty care visits, and hospitalizations in the past 6 months were based on self-report. Specialty care visits were verified by medical record review, and nonurgent care visits were verified with the child's primary care provider.

## NEBULIZER USE PRACTICE

Nebulizer use practices, including sharing the nebulizer with family members, frequency of changing the nebulizer tubing and cleaning the nebulizer device, and home management of acute asthma exacerbations using a nebulizer, were ascertained by self-report.

## MEDICATION PRESCRIPTION PRACTICE OUTCOMES

Pharmacy records were obtained from all pharmacies used by each child, as reported by the parent or caregiver over the 12-month follow-up. Change in pharmacy use was ascertained every 6 months. Pharmacies were contacted for complete lists of all medications dispensed for each child. A database was created to capture the dispensing date, product name, strength, dosage form, quantity, and days supplied (if available). Before double entry in the database, all pharmacy records were reviewed by an asthma nurse specialist (K.E.M.) to ensure complete data retrieval. Discrepancies in data entries were adjudicated. Quick-relief medications were defined as short-acting β-agonist and oral corticosteroids, while controllers included inhaled corticosteroids, leukotriene modifiers, and mast cell stabilizers.

## STATISTICAL ANALYSIS

Standard $\chi^2$ tests for categorical variables and *t* tests for continuous variables were used to test for differences between groups (INT vs CON) at baseline and at the 12-month follow-up. To analyze differences between groups for variables with nonnormal distributions, we used nonparametric tests, including the Wilcoxon rank sum test. For comparison of asthma medication regimens by asthma severity and study group, children were categorized into 3 groups based on their prescribed asthma medication regimens over the 12-month follow-up: (1) no asthma medications dispensed, (2) quick-relief medications dispensed only, and (3) anti-inflammatory controller use and quick-relief medications dispensed. Statistical significance was accepted as $P \leq .05$. All analyses were performed using SAS statistical software (SAS V.8.0)[24] and Stata V.7.0[25] software.

# RESULTS

## SAMPLE CHARACTERISTICS

Children were primarily African American, male, Medicaid insured, and living in households with parents reporting at least a high school level of education and annual incomes of less than $20 000 (**Table 1**). Asthma severity and health care use were high at baseline (moderate or severe asthma severity, 34.8%; and mean [SD] ED visits in the past 6 months, 2.0 [2.7]). Most parents and caregivers (75.9%) correctly reported cleaning the nebulizer after every use at baseline, but fewer correctly reported the recommended frequency of changing the tubing at 1 time per month (27.9%) compared with when it looks dirty (28.8%). Almost all caregivers (93.6%) reported trying nebulizer treatments at home before taking their child to the ED, and most (63.4%) preferred a nebulizer to an MDI (20.3%) for home administration of asthma medications. Sharing the nebulizer with other family members by the child was reported by almost 1 in 5 (19.0%) parents and caregivers.

## NEBULIZER USE PRACTICE

Baseline and follow-up nebulized and MDI quick-relief medication was predominantly albuterol (baseline, 95%; and follow-up, 93%). Controller medications were nebulized less often (ie, budesonide, 20.8%; and cromolyn, 1.8%). The mean (SD) duration of all nebulizer sessions was 12.9 (8.5) minutes (range, 5-96 minutes), the number of sessions ranged from 0 to 8 times per day, and neither variable differed by group. The mean number of short-acting β-agonist and budesonide prescriptions did not differ by group for delivery device (ie, MDI, dry powder inhaler, or nebulizer). The accuracy for nebulizer cleaning frequency increased from 75.9% to 86.2%, and there was a 18.8% increase in the accuracy of changing nebulizer tubing once a month, yet these nebulizer use behavior items did not differ by group. Sharing of nebulizers decreased to 11.0% at follow-up from baseline, yet this change did not differ between groups.

**Table 1. Baseline Sociodemographic and Health Characteristics for 221 Children by Group Status***

| Characteristic | CON Group (n = 111) | INT Group (n = 110) | Total (N = 221) |
|---|---|---|---|
| Race/ethnicity | | | |
| African American | 103 (92.8) | 94 (85.5) | **197** (89.1) |
| White or other | 8 (7.2) | 16 (14.5) | **24** (10.9) |
| Male sex | 70 (63.1) | 75 (68.2) | **145** (65.6) |
| Child age (range, 2-9 y)† | 4.5 (2.0) | 4.6 (2.1) | 4.5 (2.1) |
| Medicaid health insurance | 87 (78.4) | 89 (80.9) | **176** (79.6) |
| Parent or guardian‡ | | | |
| Mother | 99 (89.2) | 101 (91.8) | **200** (90.5) |
| Legal guardian or other relative | 11 (9.9) | 9 (8.2) | **20** (9.0) |
| Parent or guardian educational level | | | |
| Some HS | 23 (20.7) | 30 (27.3) | **53** (24.0) |
| HS graduate or GED | 44 (39.6) | 41 (37.3) | **85** (38.5) |
| Some college or trade school or college graduate | 44 (39.6) | 39 (35.5) | **83** (37.6) |
| Mother employed outside the home | 72 (64.9) | 55 (50.0) | **127** (57.5) |
| Annual household income, $ | | | |
| <20 000 | 56 (50.5) | 50 (45.5) | **106** (48.0) |
| ≥20 000 | 47 (42.3) | 42 (38.2) | **89** (40.3) |
| Asthma severity | | | |
| Mild intermittent | 5 (4.5) | 5 (4.5) | **10** (4.5) |
| Mild persistent | 65 (58.6) | 69 (62.7) | **134** (60.6) |
| Moderate persistent | 27 (24.3) | 19 (17.3) | **46** (20.8) |
| Severe persistent | 14 (12.6) | 17 (15.5) | **31** (14.0) |
| Daytime symptom frequency | | | |
| <2 times per week | 43 (38.7) | 46 (41.8) | **89** (40.3) |
| ≥3 times per week | 43 (38.7) | 44 (40.0) | **87** (39.4) |
| Daily, not continual | 20 (18.0) | 13 (11.8) | **33** (14.9) |
| Continual | 5 (4.5) | 7 (6.4) | **12** (5.4) |
| Night symptom frequency | | | |
| <2 times per month | 41 (36.9) | 41 (37.3) | **82** (37.1) |
| ≥3 times per month | 38 (34.2) | 41 (37.3) | **79** (35.7) |
| >1 time per week | 21 (18.9) | 16 (14.5) | **37** (16.7) |
| Daily symptoms | 11 (9.9) | 12 (10.9) | **23** (10.4) |
| Health care use | | | |
| No. of hospitalizations for asthma† | 0.41 (0.8) | 0.34 (0.6) | 0.38 (0.7) |
| No. of ED visits for asthma† | 2.0 (2.9) | 1.9 (2.5) | 2.0 (2.7) |
| No. of regular or nonurgent visits for asthma† | 2.8 (2.5) | 3.3 (3.0) | 3.0 (2.8) |
| Specialty care for asthma in the past 2 y | 57 (51.4) | 50 (45.5) | **107** (48.4) |
| Asthma medication use in the past 6 mo (pharmacy data)† | | | |
| No. of short-acting β-agonist prescriptions | 1.7 (1.8) | 1.8 (2.0) | 1.8 (1.9) |
| No. of oral corticosteroid prescriptions | 0.6 (0.9) | 0.6 (0.8) | 0.6 (0.9) |
| No. of inhaled corticosteroid prescriptions | 1.0 (1.5) | 0.8 (1.3) | 0.9 (1.4) |

Abbreviations: CON, standard asthma education; ED, emergency department; GED, general equivalency diploma; HS, high school; INT, asthma educational intervention.

*Data are given as number (percentage) of each group unless otherwise indicated. Percentages may not total 100 because of rounding or because the number of children was fewer than the denominator given. At baseline, pharmacy data were available for 6 months before enrollment.

†Data are given as mean (SD).

‡N = 220.

## INTERVENTION EFFECTS AT 12 MONTHS IN 181 CHILDREN

Severity remained stable at follow-up (**Table 2**). Children in the CON group were more likely than those in the INT group to have had 1 or more hospitalizations and/or 1 or more ED visits for asthma during the past 6 months ($P<.05$ for both); however, the size of these effects remains uncertain. The mean number of nonurgent care visits over the past 6 months decreased from 3 to 2 from baseline to follow-up, with no differences by group.

Almost all children obtained inhaled quick-relief medications (93.4%), and most (59.1%) also received courses of oral corticosteroids. Most children (88.9%) had at least 1 albuterol prescription (range, 0-26 prescriptions) over the 12-month follow-up. More than one third of the children received 6 or more short-acting β-agonist prescriptions during the same period. The number of nebulizer and MDI quick-relief prescriptions did not differ by group over the follow-up. Although almost three quarters (71.8%) of the children obtained at least 1 prescription for an inhaled corticosteroid medication over the follow-up (**Table 3**), both groups had low exposure to inhaled corticosteroids, with a mean of 2.9 prescriptions over 12 months. The mean number of inhaled corticosteroid prescriptions was significantly higher for the CON vs the INT children at follow-up (3.30 vs 2.47 prescrip-

**Table 2. Health Characteristics by Group for 181 Children at Follow-up**

| Characteristic | CON Group (n = 86)* | INT Group (n = 95)* | Total (N = 181)* | Statistic† |
|---|---|---|---|---|
| Asthma morbidity and mortality over 12-mo follow-up | | | | |
| Severity at 12 mo‡ | | | | |
| Mild persistent | 57 (66.3) | 60 (63.2) | **117** (64.6) | 1.07 (0.93-1.22) |
| Moderate persistent | 7 (8.1) | 13 (13.7) | **20** (11.0) | 0.96 (0.50-1.83) |
| Severe persistent | 15 (17.4) | 10 (10.5) | **25** (13.8) | 1.50 (0.87-2.57) |
| Death | 1 (1.2) | 2 (2.1) | **3** (1.7) | 0.50 (0.05-5.39) |
| Health care use over 12-mo follow-up | | | | |
| Health insurance, medical assistance | 70 (81.4) | 78 (82.1) | **148** (81.8) | 0.98 (0.86-1.12) |
| Specialty care in the past 12 mo | 43 (50.0) | 37 (38.9) | **80** (44.2) | 1.28 (0.92-1.78) |
| Hospitalized in the past 6 mo (≥1 time) | 11 (12.8) | 4 (4.2) | **15** (8.3) | 3.03 (1.00-9.18) |
| ED visit in the past 6 mo (≥1 time) | 40 (46.5) | 27 (28.4) | **67** (37.0) | 1.60 (1.08-2.37) |
| No. of nonurgent clinic visits for asthma in the past 6 mo | 1.85 (1.20-2.49)§ | 2.36 (1.26-3.46)§ | 2.11 (4.40)‖ | *t* Test = 0.78, *P*=.44 |
| Asthma medication prescriptions over 12-mo follow-up | | | | |
| No. of short-acting β-agonist prescriptions (quick relief) (range, 0-26) | 3.88 (2.94-4.82)§ | 3.40 (2.74-4.06)§ | 3.65 (3.83)‖ | *z* = 0.50, *P*=.61¶ |
| No. of oral corticosteroid prescriptions (quick relief) (range, 0-8) | 1.20 (0.88-1.52)§ | 1.16 (0.84-1.48)§ | 1.20 (1.50)‖ | *z* = 0.48, *P*=.63¶ |
| No. of inhaled corticosteroid prescriptions (range, 0-14) | 3.30 (2.64-3.96)§ | 2.47 (1.84-3.11)§ | 2.90 (3.10)‖ | *z* = 2.38, *P*=.02¶ |

Abbreviations: See Table 1.
*Data are given as number (percentage) of each group unless otherwise indicated.
†Data are given as relative risk (95% confidence interval) unless otherwise indicated.
‡Reference includes mild intermittent severity.
§Data are given as mean (95% confidence interval).
‖Data are given as mean (SD).
¶Two-sided Wilcoxon rank sum test.

**Table 3. Specific Asthma Medication Regimens Over Follow-up by Study Group and Severity Level in 174 Children***

| Asthma Medication Regimen | CON Group Severity† | | INT Group Severity† | | |
|---|---|---|---|---|---|
| | Mild Persistent (n = 60) | Moderate or Severe Persistent (n = 32) | Mild Persistent (n = 54) | Moderate or Severe Persistent (n = 28) | Total (N = 174) |
| No medication | 2 (3.3) | 2 (6.3) | 4 (7.4) | 4 (14.3) | **12** (6.9) |
| Quick-relief medication only | | | | | |
| Short-acting β-agonist only | 7 (11.7) | 3 (9.4) | 11 (20.4) | 6 (21.4) | **27** (15.5) |
| Anti-inflammatory controller plus quick-relief use | | | | | |
| Inhaled corticosteroid plus quick-relief use‡ | 16 (26.7) | 9 (28.1) | 10 (18.5) | 8 (28.6) | **43** (24.7) |
| Leukotriene modifier plus quick-relief use | 2 (3.3) | 0 | 7 (13.0) | 1 (3.6) | **10** (5.7) |
| Inhaled corticosteroid plus leukotriene modifier or mast cell stabilizer plus quick relief‡ | 27 (45.0) | 14 (43.8) | 28 (51.9) | 13 (46.4) | **82** (47.1) |
| Oral corticosteroid use | | | | | |
| Oral corticosteroid bursts (≥1) | 34 (56.7) | 14 (43.8) | 38 (70.4) | 16 (57.1) | **102** (58.6) |

Abbreviations: See Table 1.
*Data are given as number (percentage) for those who received at least 1 prescription over 12 months. Data exclude 7 children with incomplete severity data at follow-up.
†All comparisons between groups and by severity were nonsignificant (*P* range, .13 to .94).
‡For any inhaled corticosteroid use alone or in combination, there were 125 (71.8%) of 174 children.

tions; $P=.02$). The frequency of inhaled corticosteroid refills was low for all children, with only 19.9% of children obtaining 6 or more inhaled corticosteroid prescriptions over the 12-month follow-up. Use of cromolyn was low (n=3).

## MORTALITY

Of the 3 deaths, 2 occurred in subjects assigned to the INT group, yet 1 INT child died before receiving any intervention education. The deaths occurred in children (mean [SD] age, 6.3 [2.5] years) with severe persistent asthma (66.6%), Medicaid insurance (100.0%), and low specialty care (33.3%). Health care use was also high in these children, with a mean (SD) of 2.0 (2.6) hospitalizations and a mean (SD) of 3.0 (1.7) ED visits over the past 6 months. Excessive quick-relief medication use (9 refills over 6 months) was noted in 1 child, yet only 1 child had adequate anti-inflammatory medication refills (4 refills) over 6 months. Neither asthma severity nor specialty care was associated with group assignment in the child deaths (severity: relative risk, 2.00 [95% confidence interval, 0.50-8.00]; and specialty care: relative risk, 4.50 [95% confidence interval, 0.32-63.94]).

## COMMENT

Our data indicate that most parents and caregivers preferred using a nebulizer device for home medication administration to their children even when they had a choice of medication delivery device. Preference for nebulizer use has been noted in more symptomatic high-risk adults with asthma,[26] suggesting that disease severity may be related to increased nebulizer use. We are unable to determine if preferential nebulizer use by parents was associated with the perception of more severe manifestations of disease in this sample; however, more than one third of the children had moderate or severe asthma.

Our results show that an INT targeting symptom recognition and appropriate nebulizer behavior had little effect on home nebulizer practice, asthma morbidity, or health care use outcomes over a 12-month follow-up. This lack of intervention effect may be due to not measuring other risks associated with nebulizer use, such as adequate storage of the device. Contamination of nebulizer equipment with cockroach allergen, resulting in antigen deposit directly into the small airways associated with severe asthma exacerbations, has been reported.[27] We did not ascertain nebulizer storage practice, yet it is plausible in these inner-city homes that some nebulizers were contaminated with mouse, cockroach, or mold antigen[27] and this may have indirectly contributed to the high asthma morbidity.

More important, this study indicates a high level of undertreatment and asthma mortality (1.4%) in this group of young inner-city children compared with the national asthma mortality rate of 0.7 per 100 000 in children younger than 18 years.[2] This study confirms the overreliance of young children with persistent asthma on quick-relief medication only (short-acting β-agonist and oral corticosteroid use) for asthma control, as previously reported in children with asthma-related ED visits.[28] Misuse of quick-relief medications has been associated with increased morbidity and mortality.[17,29] Although almost three quarters of the children in this study received some inhaled corticosteroids over the 12-month follow-up, a mean of 3 inhaled corticosteroid prescriptions over 12 months is inadequate for preventive asthma care. Patterns of inappropriate asthma medication use may result from parental misunderstanding of the role of inhaled anti-inflammatory medicines in asthma,[30] costly and overly complex medication regimens, worry about adverse effects,[30] lack of follow-up care,[31-33] underdiagnosis of asthma severity,[34] lack of specialty care,[35,36] psychosocial factors,[37] and the increased risk of violence, parental substance abuse, and poor housing associated with inner-city residence contributing to nonadherence to asthma management regimens.[38,39]

Most children in this sample had at least 2 opportunities (ie, nonurgent care visits) for assessment of symptoms, asthma control, and appropriate nebulizer and medication use by the child's health care providers (physicians, nurse practitioners, etc). The identification of young children requiring controller medication may decrease asthma morbidity[40,41] but relies on an accurate diagnosis of asthma severity. Spirometry measurement is impractical in young children, and parental symptom reports may be inaccurate. The public health implications of this study are to include standard assessment of the frequency of quick-relief medication use or review of pharmacy refill records to improve identification of children with "uncontrolled" asthma. In fact, pediatricians who received training in accurate diagnosis of asthma and patient communication not only had shorter patient-physician interactions compared with patients of physicians not receiving the training (22.8 vs 27.1 minutes) but also increased their rate of anti-inflammatory prescriptions.[42]

There are several limitations to be considered with this study. Although we were able to obtain pharmacy records regarding the number of prescriptions dispensed over a 12-month period, we are limited in determining actual medication use by the child or sharing of medication among household members. Prescription records do indicate drug availability and have been shown to be a reliable source of drug exposure.[43] Parent self-report indicates that quick-relief medication was the predominant nebulizer medication administered. Asthma severity may not be precise in that we based severity on parent recall of symptoms and report of anti-inflammatory medication use at 1 point. However, the severity classifications were consistent at baseline and 12 months. Last, some families assigned to the CON group may have been contaminated with content from the INT group in that nurses delivered the INT and CON to all families.

In summary, despite preference by most caregivers to use a nebulizer device for home asthma medication administration, an INT designed to teach symptom recognition and appropriate nebulizer use had little effect on asthma morbidity or health care use. Although nebulizer use remains prevalent in young children, the trend is toward increased use of MDIs. More important, this study reveals a high level of undertreatment and asthma mortality in a group of young children with persistent asthma despite most children being seen almost every 3 months for nonurgent care. We believe that a more multifaceted intervention may be necessary to improve health outcomes in this high-risk group of children.

**Accepted for Publication:** November 29, 2005.
**Correspondence:** Arlene M. Butz, RN, CRNP, ScD, The Johns Hopkins University Medical Institutions, 600 N Wolfe St, Park 358, Baltimore, MD 21287 (abutz@jhmi.edu).
**Author Contributions:** Dr Butz had full access to all the data in the study and takes responsibility for the integrity of the data and the accuracy of the data analysis.
**Funding/Support:** This study was supported by grant NR05060 from the National Institute of Nursing Research.
**Role of the Sponsor:** The funding body had no role in data extraction and analyses, in the writing of the manuscript, or in the decision to submit the manuscript for publication.
**Acknowledgment:** We thank the pharmacists for retrieving the pharmacy data and the families for their willingness to participate in this study.

## REFERENCES


1. American Lung Association Epidemiology and Statistics Unit. *Trends in Asthma Morbidity and Mortality*. New York, NY: American Lung Association; 2005:14-16.
2. National Center for Health Statistics, Centers for Disease Control and Prevention. Health data for all ages. Available at: http://www.cdc.gov/NCHS/Healthdataforall ages.htm. Accessed October 20, 2005.
3. Mannino DM, Homa DM, Akinbami LJ, Moorman JE, Gwynn C, Redd SC. Surveillance for asthma: United States, 1980-1999. *MMWR Surveill Summ.* 2002; 51:1-13.
4. Yoos HL, Kitzman H, McMullen A, Sidora K. Symptom perception in childhood asthma: how accurate are children and parents? *J Asthma.* 2003;40:27-39.
5. Zach MS, Karner U. Sudden death in asthma. *Arch Dis Child.* 1989;64:1446-1451.
6. Butz AM, Eggleston P, Huss K, Kolodner K, Rand C. Nebulizer use in inner-city children with asthma: morbidity, medication use, and asthma management practices. *Arch Pediatr Adolesc Med.* 2000;154:984-990.
7. Dawson KP, Jandera E, Penna AC. The prehospital management of children with acute asthma. *J Paediatr Child Health.* 1992;28:321-322.
8. Chou KJ, Cunningham SJ, Crain EF. Metered-dose inhalers with spacers vs nebulizers for pediatric asthma. *Arch Pediatr Adolesc Med.* 1995;149:201-205.
9. Schuh S, Johnson DW, Stephens D, Callahan S, Winders P, Canny GJ. Comparison of albuterol delivered by metered-dose inhaler with spacer versus a nebulizer in children with mild acute asthma. *J Pediatr.* 1999;135:22-25.
10. Lewis RA, Fleming SS. Fractional deposition from a jet nebulizer: how it differs from a metered dose inhaler. *Br J Dis Chest.* 1985;79:361-367.
11. Kerem E, Levison H, Schuh S. Efficacy of albuterol administered by nebulizer versus spacer device in children with acute asthma. *J Pediatr.* 1993;123:313-317.
12. Canny GJ, Levison H. Aersols: therapeutic use and delivery in childhood asthma. *Ann Allergy.* 1988;60:11-20.
13. Barry PW, O'Callaghan CO. Nebuliser therapy in childhood. *Thorax.* 1997;52(suppl 2):S78-S88.
14. National Heart, Lung, and Blood Institute. *National Asthma Education and Prevention Program: Expert Panel Report 2: Guidelines for the Diagnosis and Management of Asthma.* Bethesda, Md: National Institutes of Health, National Heart, Lung, and Blood Institute; 1997. National Institutes of Health publication 97-4051.
15. National Heart, Lung, and Blood Institute. Expert Panel Report: guidelines for the diagnosis and management of asthma: update on selected topics—2002. Bethesda, Md: US Dept of Health and Human Services; 2002.
16. Hannaway PJ. Demographic characteristics of patients experiencing near-fatal and fatal asthma: results of a regional survey of 400 asthma specialists. *Ann Allergy Asthma Immunol.* 2000;84:587-593.
17. Sears MR, Rea HH, Fenwick J, et al. 75 deaths in asthmatics prescribed home nebulisers. *BMJ.* 1987;294:477-480.
18. Wilson SR, Latini D, Starr NJ, et al. Education of parents of infants and very young children with asthma: a developmental evaluation of the Wee Wheezers Program. *J Asthma.* 1996;33:239-254.
19. Schneider SL, Richard M, Huss K, et al. Moving health care education into the community. *Nurs Manage.* 1997;28:40-43.
20. Yoos HL, McMullen A. Symptom perception and evaluation in childhood asthma. *Nurs Res.* 1999;48:2-8.
21. Butz AM, Syron L, Johnson B, Spaulding J, Walker M, Bollinger ME. Home-based asthma self-management education for inner city children. *Public Health Nurs.* 2005;22:189-199.
22. Butz AM, Donithan M, Bollinger ME, Rand C, Thompson RE. Monitoring nebulizer use in children: comparison of electronic and asthma diary data. *Ann Allergy Asthma Immunol.* 2005;94:360-365.
23. *Global Initiative for Asthma: Global Strategy for Asthma Management and Prevention: Revised 2002.* Bethesda, Md: National Institutes of Health, National Heart, Lung, and Blood Institute; 2002.
24. SAS Institute Inc. *SAS/STAT User's Guide: Version 8.01 Ed.* Cary, NC: SAS Institute Inc; 2000.
25. *Stata Statistical Software: Release 7.0.* College Station, Tex: Stata Corp; 2001.
26. Krishnan JA, Demott M, McCoy JV, Chanmugam A, Rand CS. Nebulized β2-agonist use in high-risk inner-city adults with asthma. *J Asthma.* 2003;40: 367-373.
27. Bollinger ME, Wolf B, Schwindt C, Hamilton RG. Contamination of nebulizer equipment with cockroach allergen: there's a bug in the system! *Ann Allergy Asthma Immunol.* 2004;92:475-477.
28. Stempel DA, McLaughlin TP, Stanford RH. Treatment patterns for pediatric asthma prior to and after emergency department events. *Pediatr Pulmonol.* 2005;40: 310-315.
29. Stempel DA, McLaughin TP, Stanford RH, Fuhlbrigge AL. Patterns of asthma control: a 3-year analysis of patient claims. *J Allergy Clin Immunol.* 2005;115: 935-939.
30. Bender BG, Bender SE. Patient-identified barriers to asthma treatment adherence: responses to interviews, focus groups, and questionnaires. *Immunol Allergy Clin North Am.* 2005;25:107-130.
31. Farber HJ, Capra AM, Finkelstein JA, et al. Misunderstanding of asthma controller medications: association with nonadherence. *J Asthma.* 2003;40:17-25.
32. Bender B, Milgrom H. Compliance with asthma therapy: a case for shared responsibility. *J Asthma.* 1996;33:199-202.
33. David C. Preventive therapy for asthmatic children under Florida Medicaid: changes during the 1990s. *J Asthma.* 2004;41:655-661.
34. Halterman JS, Aligne CA, Auinger P, McBride JT, Szilagyi PG. Inadequate therapy for asthma among children in the United States. *Pediatrics.* 2000;105:272-276.
35. Vollmer WM, O'Hollaren M, Ettinger KM, et al. Specialty differences in the management of asthma: a cross-sectional assessment of allergists' patients and generalists' patients in a large HMO. *Arch Intern Med.* 1997;157:1201-1208.
36. Mudd K, Bollinger ME, Donithan M, Butz AM. The impact of asthma action plans on quality of life and other asthma outcomes [abstract]. *J Allergy Clin Immunol.* 2004;113:S103.
37. Bartlett SJ, Kolodner K, Butz AM, Eggleston P, Malveaux FJ, Rand CS. Maternal depressive symptoms and emergency department use among inner-city children with asthma. *Arch Pediatr Adolesc Med.* 2001;155:347-353.
38. Wade S, Weil C, Holden G, et al. Psychosocial characteristics of inner-city children with asthma: a description of the NCICAS psychosocial protocol. *Pediatr Pulmonol.* 1997;24:263-276.
39. Morgan WJ, Crain EF, Gruchalla RS, et al. Results of a home-based environmental intervention among urban children with asthma. *N Engl J Med.* 2004;351: 1068-1080.
40. Childhood Asthma Management Program Research Group. Long-term effects of budesonide or nedocromil in children with asthma. *N Engl J Med.* 2000; 343:1054-1063.
41. Suissa S, Ernst P, Kezouh A. Regular use of inhaled corticosteroids and the long-term prevention of hospitalization for asthma. *Thorax.* 2002;57:880-884.
42. Clark NM, Gong M, Schork A, et al. Impact of education for physicians on patient outcomes. *Pediatrics.* 1998;101:831-836.
43. Lau HS, de Boer A, Beuning KS, Porsius A. Validation of pharmacy records in drug exposure assessment. *J Clin Epidemiol.* 1997;50:619-625.

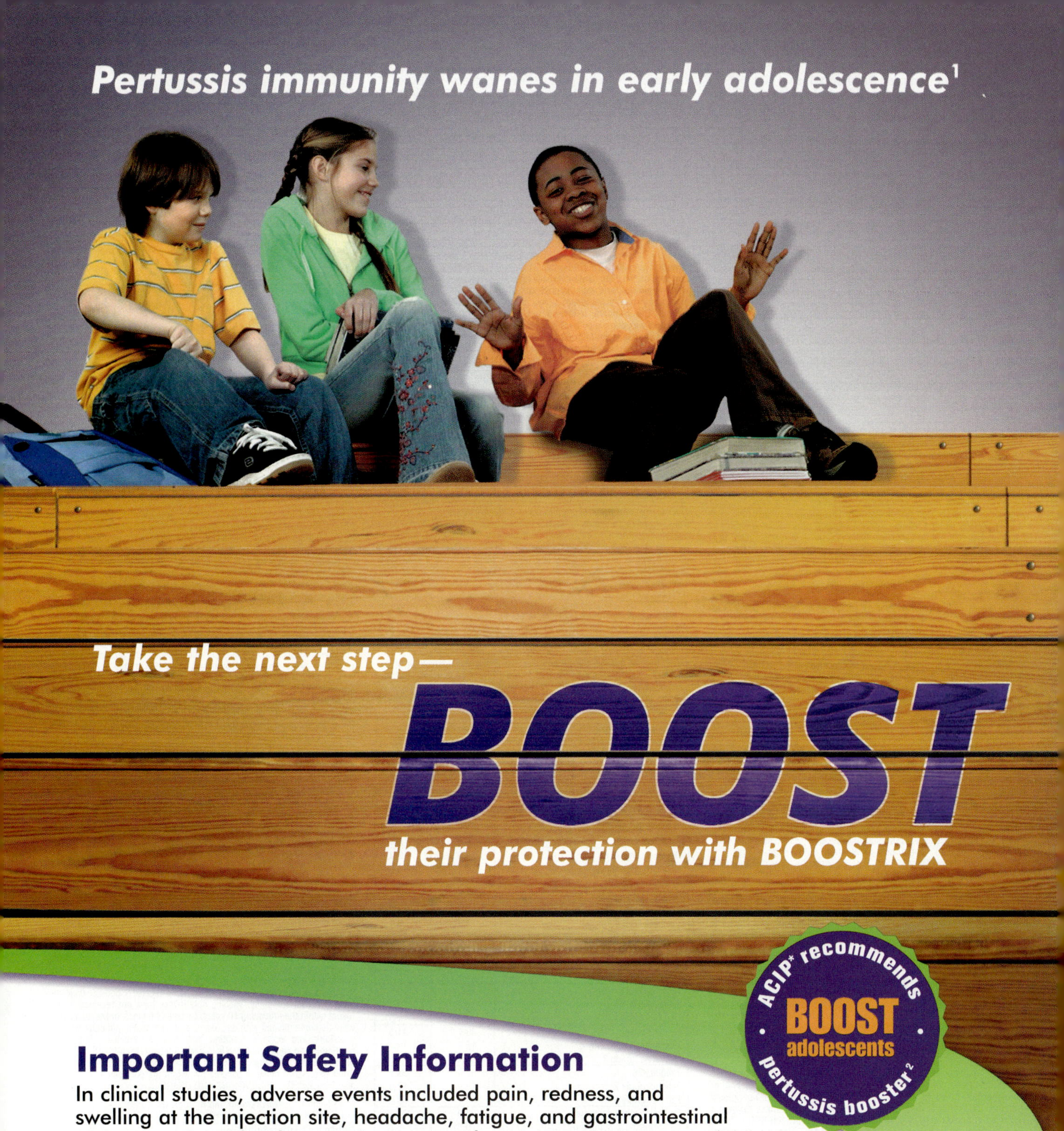


## Important Safety Information

In clinical studies, adverse events included pain, redness, and swelling at the injection site, headache, fatigue, and gastrointestinal symptoms. As with other vaccines, rare adverse events may occur. As with any vaccine, vaccination with BOOSTRIX may not protect 100% of susceptible individuals. Hypersensitivity to any component of BOOSTRIX is a contraindication.

*Advisory Committee on Immunization Practices.

gsk GlaxoSmithKline Vaccines

**BOOSTRIX®**

***Tetanus Toxoid, Reduced Diphtheria Toxoid and Acellular Pertussis Vaccine, Adsorbed***

**Please see references and brief summary of complete prescribing information on the adjacent page.**

# BOOSTRIX®

## (Tetanus Toxoid, Reduced Diphtheria Toxoid and Acellular Pertussis Vaccine, Adsorbed) (Tdap)

The following is a brief summary only; see full prescribing information for complete product information.

**INDICATIONS AND USAGE:** BOOSTRIX is indicated for active booster immunization against tetanus, diphtheria, and pertussis as a single dose in individuals 10 through 18 years of age. The use of BOOSTRIX as a primary series or to complete the primary series has not been studied. As with any vaccine, BOOSTRIX may not protect 100% of individuals receiving the vaccine.

**CONTRAINDICATIONS:** Hypersensitivity to any component of the vaccine is a contraindication (see DESCRIPTION in full prescribing information). Do not use BOOSTRIX after a serious allergic reaction (e.g., anaphylaxis) following any other tetanus toxoid, diphtheria toxoid or pertussis-containing vaccine, or any component of this vaccine (see DESCRIPTION in full prescribing information). Because of the uncertainty as to which component of the vaccine might be responsible, do not give further vaccination with any of these components; or, refer such individuals to an allergist for evaluation. The following events are contraindications to administration of BOOSTRIX: encephalopathy (e.g., coma, decreased level of consciousness, prolonged seizures) within 7 days of administration of a previous dose of a pertussis-containing vaccine that is not attributable to another identifiable cause; progressive neurologic disorder, uncontrolled epilepsy, or progressive encephalopathy. Do not vaccinate individuals with these conditions until a treatment regimen has been established and the condition has stabilized.

**WARNINGS:** The tip cap and the rubber plunger of the needleless prefilled syringes contain dry natural latex rubber that may cause allergic reactions in latex sensitive individuals. The vial stopper is latex-free. If any of the following events occurred in temporal relation to previous receipt of a Diphtheria and Tetanus Toxoids and Pertussis Vaccine Adsorbed (DTwP) vaccine or a vaccine containing an acellular pertussis component, consider carefully whether to give subsequent doses of BOOSTRIX: temperature of ≥40.5°C (105°F) within 48 hours not due to another identifiable cause; collapse or shock-like state (hypotonic-hyporesponsive episode) within 48 hours; persistent, inconsolable crying lasting ≥3 hours, occurring within 48 hours; seizures with or without fever occurring within 3 days. Persons who experienced serious Arthus-type hypersensitivity reactions following a prior dose of tetanus toxoid usually have high serum tetanus antitoxin levels and should not be given Tetanus and Diphtheria Toxoids Adsorbed For Adult Use (Td) or Tdap vaccines or even emergency doses of Td more frequently than every 10 years, even if the wound is neither clean nor minor. If Guillain-Barré syndrome has occurred within 6 weeks of receipt of prior vaccine containing tetanus toxoid, the decision to give BOOSTRIX or any vaccine containing tetanus toxoid should be based on careful consideration of the potential benefits and possible risks. The decision to administer a pertussis-containing vaccine to individuals with stable central nervous system (CNS) disorders must be made by the physician on an individual basis, with consideration of all relevant factors, and assessment of potential risks and benefits for that individual. Advise the patient, parent, or guardian of the potential increased risk involved (see PRECAUTIONS). A family history of seizures or other CNS disorders is not a contraindication to pertussis vaccine. The Advisory Committee on Immunization Practices (ACIP) has published guidelines for vaccination of persons with recent or acute illness (www.cdc.gov). Do not give BOOSTRIX to individuals with bleeding disorders such as hemophilia or thrombocytopenia, or to persons on anticoagulant therapy unless the potential benefit clearly outweighs the risk of administration. If the decision is made to administer BOOSTRIX to such persons, it should be given with caution with steps taken to avoid the risk of hematoma following the injection.

**PRECAUTIONS: General:** Before the injection of any biological, the physician should take all reasonable precautions to prevent allergic or other adverse reactions. Epinephrine injection (1:1,000) and other appropriate agents used for the control of immediate allergic reactions must be immediately available should an acute anaphylactic reaction occur. Immunosuppressed persons, including individuals receiving immunosuppressive therapy, may not develop the expected immune response. **Drug Interactions:** Do not mix BOOSTRIX with any other vaccine in the same syringe or vial. **Carcinogenesis, Mutagenesis, Impairment of Fertility:** BOOSTRIX has not been evaluated for carcinogenic or mutagenic potential, or for impairment of fertility. **Pregnancy:** Pregnancy Category C. Animal reproduction studies have not been conducted with BOOSTRIX. It is also not known whether BOOSTRIX can cause fetal harm when administered to a pregnant woman or can affect reproductive capacity. BOOSTRIX should be given to a pregnant woman only if clearly needed. Animal fertility studies have not been conducted with BOOSTRIX. In a developmental toxicity study, the effect of BOOSTRIX on embryo-fetal and pre-weaning development was evaluated in pregnant rats. Animals were administered INFANRIX® (Diphtheria and Tetanus Toxoids and Acellular Pertussis Vaccine Adsorbed) prior to gestation and BOOSTRIX during the period of organogenesis (gestation days 6, 8, 11) and later in pregnancy (gestation day 15), 0.1 mL/rat/occasion (a 45-fold increase compared to the human dose of BOOSTRIX on a body weight basis), by intramuscular injection. No adverse affect on pregnancy and lactation parameters, embryo-fetal or pre-weaning development was observed. There were no fetal malformations or other evidence of teratogenesis noted in this study. **Nursing Mothers:** It is not known whether BOOSTRIX is excreted in human milk. Because many drugs are excreted in human milk, caution should be exercised when BOOSTRIX is administered to a nursing woman. **Pregnancy Exposure Registry:** Healthcare providers are encouraged to register pregnant women who receive BOOSTRIX in the GlaxoSmithKline vaccination pregnancy registry by calling 1-888-825-5249. **Geriatric Use:** BOOSTRIX is not indicated for use in individuals older than 18 years. **Pediatric Use:** BOOSTRIX is not indicated for use in individuals younger than 10 years (see DOSAGE AND ADMINISTRATION in full prescribing information). For immunization of infants and children younger than 7 years against diphtheria, tetanus, and pertussis, refer to the manufacturers' package inserts for Diphtheria and Tetanus Toxoids and Acellular Pertussis Vaccine Adsorbed (DTaP) vaccines.

**ADVERSE REACTIONS:** A total of 3,608 adolescents were vaccinated with a single dose of BOOSTRIX during clinical trials. An additional 1,092 adolescents 10 to 18 years of age received a non-US formulation of BOOSTRIX (formulated to contain 0.5 mg aluminum per dose) in non-US clinical studies.

The primary safety study, conducted in the United States, was a randomized, observer-blinded, controlled study in which 3,080 adolescents 10 to 18 years of age received a single dose of BOOSTRIX and 1,034 received the control Td vaccine manufactured by Massachusetts Public Health Biologic Laboratories. There were no substantive differences in demographic characteristics between the vaccine groups. Among BOOSTRIX and control vaccine recipients approximately 75% were 10 to 14 years of age and approximately 25% were 15 to 18 years of age. Approximately 98% of participants in this study had received the recommended series of 4 or 5 doses of either DTwP or a combination of DTwP and DTaP in childhood. Data on adverse events were collected by the subjects, parents and/or guardians using standardized diaries for 15 consecutive days following the vaccine dose (i.e., day of vaccination and the next 14 days). Subjects were monitored for unsolicited adverse events that occurred within 31 days of vaccination (day 0-30) using diary cards (day 0-14) supplemented by spontaneous reports and a medical history as reported by subjects, parents, and/or guardians. Subjects were also monitored for 6 months post-vaccination for non-routine medical visits, visits to an emergency room, onset of new chronic illness, and serious adverse events. Information regarding late onset adverse events was obtained via a telephone call 6 months following vaccination. At least 97% of subjects completed the 6-month follow-up evaluation.

In a study conducted in Germany, BOOSTRIX was administered to 319 children 10 to 12 years of age previously vaccinated with 5 doses of acellular pertussis-containing vaccines, 193 of these subjects had previously received 5 doses of INFANRIX. Adverse events were recorded on diary cards during the 15 days following vaccination. Unsolicited adverse events that occurred within 31 days of vaccination (day 0-30) were recorded on the diary card or verbally reported to the investigator. Subjects were monitored for 6 months post-vaccination for physician office visits, emergency room visits, onset of new chronic illness, and serious adverse events. The 6-month follow-up evaluation, conducted via telephone interview, was completed by 90% of subjects.

The adverse event information from clinical trials provides a basis for identifying adverse events that appear to be related to vaccine use and for approximating rates. However, because clinical trials are conducted under widely varying conditions, adverse event rates observed in the clinical trials of a vaccine cannot be directly compared to rates in the clinical trials of another vaccine, and may not reflect the rates observed in practice.

**Serious Adverse Events in All Safety Studies:** In the US-safety study and German-safety study, no serious adverse events were reported to occur within 31 days of vaccination. During the 6-month extended safety evaluation period, no serious adverse events that were of potential autoimmune origin or new onset and chronic in nature were reported to occur. In non-US studies in which serious adverse events were monitored for up to 37 days, one subject was diagnosed with insulin dependent diabetes 20 days following administration of BOOSTRIX. No other serious adverse events of potential autoimmune origin or that were new onset and chronic in nature were reported to occur in these studies.

**Solicited Adverse Events in the US-Safety Study:** In a US study, the most common local adverse events following administration of BOOSTRIX were pain, redness, and swelling at the injection site. The most common general adverse events were headache and fatigue. Most of these events were reported at a similar frequency in recipients of both BOOSTRIX and Td. Any pain, grade 2 or 3 pain (but not grade 3 alone), and grade 2 or 3 headache (but not grade 3 alone) were reported at a higher rate in recipients of BOOSTRIX. The primary safety endpoint of the US study was the incidence of grade 3 pain (spontaneously painful and/or prevented normal activity) at the injection site within 15 days of vaccination. Grade 3 pain was reported in 4.6% of those who received BOOSTRIX compared with 4.0% of those who received the Td vaccine. The difference in rate of grade 3 pain was within the pre-defined clinical limit for non-inferiority (upper limit of the 95% CI for the difference ≤4%). These were the rates for solicited local and general adverse events within 15 days of vaccination with BOOSTRIX or Td vaccine for the total vaccinated cohort (all enrolled, vaccinated subjects with safety data available analyzed by vaccine received):

**Percentage of Individuals 10 to 18 Years of Age Reporting Solicited Local Adverse Events or Solicited General Adverse Events Within the 15-day* Post-Vaccination Period**

| | BOOSTRIX (N = 3,032) % | Td (N =1,013) % |
|---|---|---|
| **Local** | | |
| Pain,† any | 75.3 | 71.7 |
| Pain,† grade 2 or 3 | 51.2 | 42.5 |
| Pain,‡ grade 3 | 4.6 | 4.0 |
| Redness, any | 22.5 | 19.8 |
| Redness, >20 mm | 4.1 | 3.9 |
| Redness, ≥50 mm | 1.7 | 1.6 |
| Swelling, any | 21.1 | 20.1 |
| Swelling, >20 mm | 5.3 | 4.9 |
| Swelling, ≥50 mm | 2.5 | 3.2 |
| Arm circumference increase,§ >5 mm | 28.3 | 29.5 |
| Arm circumference increase,§ >20 mm | 2.0 | 2.2 |
| Arm circumference increase,§ >40 mm | 0.5 | 0.3 |
| **General** | | |
| Fever,‖ ≥99.5°F | 13.5 | 13.1 |
| Fever,‖ >100.4°F | 5.0 | 4.7 |
| Fever,‖ >102.2°F | 1.4 | 1.0 |
| Headache, any | 43.1 | 41.5 |
| Headache,† grade 2 or 3 | 15.7 | 12.7 |
| Headache, grade 3 | 3.7 | 2.7 |
| Fatigue, any | 37.0 | 36.7 |
| Fatigue, grade 2 or 3 | 14.4 | 12.9 |
| Fatigue, grade 3 | 3.7 | 3.2 |
| Gastrointestinal symptoms,¶ any | 26.0 | 25.8 |
| Gastrointestinal symptoms,¶ grade 2 or 3 | 9.8 | 9.7 |
| Gastrointestinal symptoms,¶ grade 3 | 3.0 | 3.2 |

Td = Tetanus and Diphtheria Toxoids Adsorbed For Adult Use manufactured by Massachusetts Public Health Biologic Laboratories.
N = number of subjects in the total vaccinated cohort with local/general symptoms sheets completed.
Grade 2 = Local: painful when the limb was moved; General: interfered with normal activity.
Grade 3 = Local: spontaneously painful and/or prevented normal activity; General: prevented normal activity.
*Day of vaccination and the next 14 days.
†Statistically significantly higher (P<0.05) following BOOSTRIX as compared to Td vaccine.
‡Grade 3 injection site pain following BOOSTRIX was not inferior to Td (upper limit of two-sided 95% CI for the difference in the percentage of subjects ≤4%).
§Mid-upper region of the vaccinated arm.
‖Oral temperatures or axillary temperatures.
¶Gastrointestinal symptoms included nausea, vomiting, diarrhea and/or abdominal pain.

Mid-upper arm circumference was measured by the adolescent or their parent/guardian prior to injection and daily for 15 days following vaccination. There was no significant difference between BOOSTRIX recipients and Td recipients in the proportion of subjects reporting an increase in mid-upper arm circumference in the vaccinated arm. The incidence of unsolicited adverse events reported in the 31 days after vaccination was comparable between the 2 groups.

**Solicited Adverse Events in the German Safety Study:** No cases of whole arm swelling were spontaneously reported. Two individuals (2/193) reported large injection site swelling (range 110 to 200 mm diameter), in one case associated with grade 3 pain. Neither individual sought medical attention. These episodes were reported to resolve without sequelae within 5 days. These were the rates of solicited local adverse events and fever within 15 days of vaccination for those subjects who had previously been vaccinated with 5 doses of INFANRIX:

**Rates of Solicited Adverse Events Reported Within the 15-day* Post-Vaccination Period Following Administration of BOOSTRIX in Individuals 10 to 12 Years of Age Who Had Previously Received 5 Doses of INFANRIX**

| Adverse Event | BOOSTRIX (N = 193) % (95% CI) |
|---|---|
| Pain, any | 62.2 (54.9-69.0) |
| Pain, grade 2 or 3 | 33.2 (26.6-40.3) |
| Pain, grade 3 | 5.7 (2.9-10.0) |
| Redness, any | 47.7 (40.4-55.0) |
| Redness, >20 mm | 15.0 (10.3-20.9) |
| Redness, ≥50 mm | 10.9 (6.9-16.2) |
| Swelling, any | 38.9 (31.9-46.1) |
| Swelling, >20 mm | 17.6 (12.5-23.7) |
| Swelling, ≥50 mm | 14.0 (9.4-19.7) |
| Fever, ≥99.5 | 8.8 (5.2-13.7) |
| Fever, >100.4 | 4.1 (1.8-8.0) |
| Fever, >102.2 | 1.0 (0.1-3.7) |

N = number of subjects with local/general symptoms sheets completed.
Grade 2 = Painful when the limb was moved.
Grade 3 = Spontaneously painful and/or prevented normal activity.
*Day of vaccination and the next 14 days.

As with any vaccine, there is the possibility that broad use of BOOSTRIX could reveal adverse events not observed in clinical trials.

**Postmarketing Reports:** Worldwide voluntary reports of adverse events received for BOOSTRIX in persons 10 to 18 years of age since market introduction of this vaccine are listed below. This list includes serious events or events which have causal connection to components of this or other vaccines or drugs. Because these events are reported voluntarily from a population of uncertain size, it is not possible to reliably estimate their frequency or establish a causal relationship to vaccine exposure. *Blood and lymphatic system disorders:* Lymphadenitis, lymphadenopathy. *Cardiac disorders:* Myocarditis. *Injection site reactions:* Induration, inflammation, mass, nodule, warmth, local reaction. *Metabolism and nutrition disorders:* Diabetes mellitus insulin-dependent. *Musculoskeletal and connective tissue disorders:* Arthralgia, back pain, myalgia. *Nervous system disorders:* Convulsion, encephalitis, facial palsy, paraesthesia. *Skin and subcutaneous tissue disorders:* Exanthem, Henoch-Schönlein purpura, rash. In addition, extensive swelling of the injected limb has been reported following administration of BOOSTRIX.

**Reporting Adverse Events:** Report the occurrence following immunization of any event set forth in the Vaccine Injury Table from the National Childhood Vaccine Injury Act including: Anaphylaxis or anaphylactic shock within 7 days, encephalopathy or encephalitis within 7 days, brachial neuritis within 28 days, or an acute complication or sequelae (including death) of an illness, disability, injury, or condition referred to above, or any events that would contraindicate further doses of vaccine, according to this prescribing information. These events should be reported to VAERS. The VAERS toll-free number is 1-800-822-7967. Reporting forms may also be obtained at the VAERS website at www.vaers.hhs.gov.

**DOSAGE AND ADMINISTRATION: Recommended Dose:** BOOSTRIX should be administered as a single 0.5 mL injection by the intramuscular route into the deltoid muscle of the upper arm in individuals 10 through 18 years of age. Do not administer this product subcutaneously or intravenously. There are no data to support repeat administration of BOOSTRIX. Five years should elapse between the subject's last dose of the recommended series of childhood DTwP and/or DTaP vaccine and the administration of BOOSTRIX. Limited data are available on the use of BOOSTRIX following Tetanus and Diphtheria Toxoids Adsorbed For Adult Use (Td) vaccine. **Additional Dosing Information:** ***Wound Management:*** Clinicians should refer to guidelines for tetanus prophylaxis in routine wound management. Adolescents 10 to 18 years of age who have completed a primary series against tetanus and who sustain wounds which are minor and uncomplicated, should receive a booster dose of a tetanus toxoid-containing vaccine only if they have not received tetanus toxoid within the preceding 10 years. In case of tetanus-prone injury (e.g., wounds contaminated with dirt, feces, soil, and saliva; puncture wounds; avulsions; and wounds resulting from missles, crushing, burns, and frostbite) in an adolescent who is in need of tetanus toxoid, BOOSTRIX can be used as an alternative to Tetanus and Diphtheria Toxoids Adsorbed For Adult Use (Td) vaccine in patients for whom the pertussis component is also indicated (see INDICATIONS AND USAGE).

Manufactured by **GlaxoSmithKline Biologicals**
Rixensart, Belgium, US License 1617

Distributed by **GlaxoSmithKline**
Research Triangle Park, NC 27709



Full prescribing information for BOOSTRIX is available at www.BOOSTRIX.com.
BRS-BO:L3

**References:** **1.** Centers for Disease Control and Prevention. Preventing tetanus, diphtheria, and pertussis among adolescents: use of tetanus toxoid, reduced diphtheria toxoid and acellular pertussis vaccines: recommendations of the Advisory Committee on Immunization Practices (ACIP). Early Release 2006;55(February 23, 2006):1–43. **2.** Centers for Disease Control and Prevention. Recommended childhood and adolescent immunization schedule—United States, 2006. *MMWR.* 2006;54(51&52):Q1–Q4.

ARTICLE

# Racial and Ethnic Disparities in Pediatric Tuberculosis in North Carolina

*Jason E. Stout, MD, MHS; Kapil K. Saharia, MD, MPH; Savithri Nageswaran, MD; Amina Ahmed, MD; Carol Dukes Hamilton, MD*

**Objectives:** To investigate an increase in active pediatric tuberculosis (TB) cases in North Carolina from 9 cases in 2001 to 32 cases in 2002, and to pilot test a screening tool for detection of latent TB infection in children.

**Design:** Retrospective cohort and cross-sectional study.

**Setting:** State of North Carolina and a county public health department pediatric clinic.

**Participants:** Children younger than 15 years with TB in North Carolina from January 1, 1994, to December 31, 2002, and children younger than 21 years initially seen in a primary care public health department pediatric clinic from July 16, 2004, to December 8, 2004.

**Interventions:** We reviewed medical records for 180 children (<15 years) with active TB reported in North Carolina. We subsequently initiated a screening project at a county public health department pediatric clinic.

**Main Outcome Measures:** Incidence of TB and prevalence of latent TB infection.

**Results:** One hundred eighty pediatric TB cases were reported from 1994 to 2002. Compared with 0.2 case per 100 000 non-Hispanic white children, the incidence rates were 3.0 cases per 100 000 non-Hispanic black children ($P = .003$) and 4.5 cases per 100 000 Hispanic children ($P = .01$); 88.3% of pediatric patients with TB were nonwhite. The screening project detected 2 cases of latent TB infection among 864 US-born children of foreign-born parents.

**Conclusions:** The burden of pediatric TB is almost entirely borne by black and Hispanic children in North Carolina. Tuberculin skin testing of US-born children of foreign-born parents is of low yield; more efficient screening strategies are necessary.

*Arch Pediatr Adolesc Med. 2006;160:631-637*

**Author Affiliations** are listed at the end of this article.

In 2002, for the first time since the inception of tuberculosis (TB) surveillance in 1951, foreign-born individuals accounted for most of the active TB cases in the United States.[1] Because most new immigrants come from countries where TB is endemic, many enter the country with latent TB infection (LTBI) that becomes active after settling in the United States. The effect of immigration on national TB case rates has been well described.[2,3] Epidemiological studies[4-6] of pediatric TB in many US jurisdictions conducted in the 1990s indicated that the increasing pediatric TB incidence was associated with the growing immigrant population.

Between 1990 and 2000, North Carolina experienced a 274% increase in its foreign-born population, the greatest percentage increase of any state in the United States.[7] The largest increase was observed in the Hispanic population, which rose almost 400% and by 2003 constituted more than 5% of the state's population.[8] Although the number of active TB cases in North Carolina children 0 to 14 years of age generally declined from 1994 to 2001, we observed a marked upsurge in reported pediatric TB cases, from 9 cases in 2001 to 32 cases in 2002. Given the recent demographic changes in North Carolina, we hypothesized that the state's 2002 increase in pediatric TB was attributable to the growing Hispanic population.

We conducted a retrospective cohort analysis of all pediatric TB cases reported in North Carolina from 1994 to 2002 to test this hypothesis and to characterize the epidemiology and clinical characteristics of the pediatric cases. Based on our findings, we implemented a screening project in a county public health department pediatric clinic to determine whether we could improve detection of LTBI among children at risk.

**Table 1. Demographic Characteristics of 180 Children Younger Than 15 Years With Tuberculosis in North Carolina From 1994 to 2002**

| Characteristic | No. (%) |
|---|---|
| Sex | |
| Male | 96 (53.3) |
| Female | 84 (46.7) |
| Age, y | |
| <5 | 97 (53.9) |
| 5-14 | 83 (46.1) |
| Race/ethnicity | |
| Non-Hispanic white | 21 (11.7) |
| Non-Hispanic black | 114 (63.3) |
| Asian/Pacific Islander | 12 (6.7) |
| Hispanic | 33 (18.3) |
| Country of birth | |
| United States | 155 (86.1) |
| Foreign | **25** (13.9) |
| Mexico | 10 (40.0) |
| Other Latin America/Carribean | 4 (16.0) |
| Asia | 6 (24.0) |
| Africa | 5 (20.0) |

## METHODS

### RETROSPECTIVE COHORT

#### Definitions

We used the Centers for Disease Control and Prevention TB surveillance case definition and age cutoff (<15 years) to define active pediatric TB cases.[9] We defined a source case as an individual 15 years or older with smear-positive or culture-positive pulmonary or laryngeal TB who was presumed to have transmitted TB to the youth. Interpretation of tuberculin skin test (TST) results was in accord with the Centers for Disease Control and Prevention recommendations.[10] We designated children as having a foreign association if they were foreign born, had at least 1 foreign-born parent, or had a foreign-born source case. Three modes of presentation among children were defined: (1) contact investigation (children brought in for evaluation because of suspected contact with a subject with TB), (2) symptomatic presentation (children with TB symptoms who were seen by health care providers), or (3) screening association (children directed for medical attention because of positive results on a TST performed for screening purposes [ie, school entry or immigration] or for an unrelated health problem). Race and ethnicity were classified by public health nurses.

#### Data Collection

All cases of pediatric TB reported from January 1, 1994, to December 31, 2002, were identified through the North Carolina Tuberculosis Information Management System database. North Carolina Tuberculosis Control Program staff reviewed medical records using a standardized record extraction form. We obtained information about sociodemographic factors, history of LTBI therapy, parents' country of birth, foreign travel within 2 years of TB diagnosis, and mode of presentation. For children diagnosed through a contact investigation, the degree of contact with and the relationship to the source case, as well as the interval between the time of identification as a contact to the time of TB evaluation, were abstracted. For children diagnosed through a screening association, the reason for screening was recorded.

### SCREENING PROJECT

The screening project was conducted in the pediatric clinic of Wake County Department of Health and Human Services. This clinic treats approximately 10 000 children (≤21 years) per year; 71% of these children are Hispanic, 25% are black, and 4% are white. Sixty percent of children treated in the clinic are aged 0 to 4 years, 29% are aged 5 to 10 years, and 11% are aged 11 to 21 years. The project was started in July 2004, and data collected between July 16, 2004, and December 8, 2004, were analyzed. Before this project, only foreign-born children the pediatric clinic had a TST performed on the initial visit. The screening project assessed the value of a TB screening questionnaire designed to identify the presence of any of the following TB risk factors: history of contact with a person with TB, foreign birth of the youth, foreign birth of the parent (if the child was <5 years), travel for longer than 1 month to a TB-endemic region, a compromised immune system, or exposure to high-risk individuals. The TB screening questionnaire was administered to all children aged 6 months to 5 years at each well-child examination and to all foreign-born children during their first visit, irrespective of age. If the answer to any question was affirmative, a TST was performed using the Mantoux method.

Institutional review boards at Duke University and The University of North Carolina at Chapel Hill approved the retrospective cohort analyses. The screening project was undertaken as a public health program activity and was exempted from institutional review board monitoring.

### STATISTICAL ANALYSIS

North Carolina population figures from 1994 to 1999 and from 2001 to 2002 were derived from intercensal estimates provided by the US Census Bureau.[8,11] The 2000 population data were derived from the 2000 US Census. Trends in the proportions of foreign-associated and Hispanic subjects with TB were analyzed in 3-year intervals using the $\chi^2$ test for trends. Differences in proportions were assessed using the $\chi^2$ test or the Fisher exact test, as appropriate. Risk ratios and 95% confidence intervals were calculated, where appropriate.

## RESULTS

### RETROSPECTIVE REVIEW OF PEDIATRIC TB CASES

One hundred eighty pediatric TB cases were reported in North Carolina from 1994 to 2002 (**Table 1**). In 1994, 28 cases were reported (an incidence of 1.93 cases per 100 000), but from 1995 to 2001, the number ranged from 9 to 21 cases per year, corresponding to incidence rates ranging from 0.53 to 1.32 cases per 100 000 (**Figure 1**). In 2002, 32 cases were reported, resulting in an incidence of 1.84 cases per 100 000 subjects.

Tuberculosis rates were 15- to 23-fold higher among minority children compared with non-Hispanic white children, and 88.3% of pediatric patients with TB were nonwhite. The median incidence of TB among non-Hispanic white children was 0.2 case per 100 000 person-years, compared with 3.0 cases per 100 000 person-years for non-Hispanic black children ($P = .003$) and 4.5 cases per 100 000 person-years for Hispanic children ($P = .01$). Although no trend was observed in the incidence of TB among Hispanic children, they represented an increasing proportion of North Carolina TB cases over time (8.2% in 1994-1996 vs 25.4% in 2000-2002, $P=.04$). The increase in Hispanic pediatric TB paralleled the rise in the Hispanic pediatric population in North Carolina, which increased from 2.5% of all children younger than 15 years in 1994, to 7.3% of all children younger than 15 years in 2002.

The primary site of TB disease varied by age group. Although older and younger children experienced similar proportions of extrapulmonary disease (21.7% for both groups), 7 (7.2%) of 97 subjects in the younger group experienced severe TB (disseminated or meningeal) compared with 1 (1.2%) of 83 subjects in the older group (risk ratio, 5.99; 95% confidence interval, 0.75-47.69). Two children died of meningeal TB 6 and 8 days after starting TB treatment. Of the total 180 pediatric cases, specimens were sent for culture in 44 cases (24.4%), and 14 (31.8%) of these specimens were culture positive. More children had specimens sent for culture from 2001 to 2002 (19/41 [46.3%]) than from 1994 to 2000 (25/139 [18.0%]).

Foreign-born children accounted for 13.9% of pediatric TB cases. Another 13.9% were US born but had a parent or a source case who was foreign born. Therefore, foreign-associated children accounted for 27.8% of all cases reported during the study period, rising over time from 18.0% of all pediatric TB cases from 1994 to 1996, to 35.6% of all pediatric TB cases from 2000 to 2002.

Source cases were identified much less frequently for foreign-associated children aged 5 to 14 years compared with children in this age group without a foreign association (19.1% vs 72.6%, $P<.001$). Most (81.0%) of these older foreign-associated children were foreign born and likely represented reactivation of LTBI acquired in their country of origin. In contrast, children younger than 5 years who had a foreign association were usually US born (72.4%), and a source case was identified as frequently as in pediatric cases without a foreign association (62.1% vs 67.7%, $P=.59$). **Figure 2** shows how the pediatric TB cases were identified. Children with a foreign association were less frequently identified through contact investigations than children without a foreign association (38.0% vs 56.9%, $P=.03$). No difference in the frequency of identification through contact tracing was noted when comparing non-Hispanic white children with minority children (42.9% vs 52.8%, $P=.39$).

## SOURCE CASE CHARACTERISTICS

Eighty-two unique source cases were believed to have infected 113 (62.8%) of 180 pediatric cases. The source case was a parent, guardian, or relative of the subject in 89 (78.8%) of 113 cases. Source cases were household contacts in 60 children (53.1%). An additional 42 children (37.2%) had close contact with the source case, while 5 children (4.4%) had casual contact with the source case. The extent of contact between 6 children (5.3%) and their source case was unknown. Source cases were more likely to be female and to have more infectious forms of TB (smear-positive and cavitary) than other patients with pulmonary or laryngeal TB (**Table 2**).

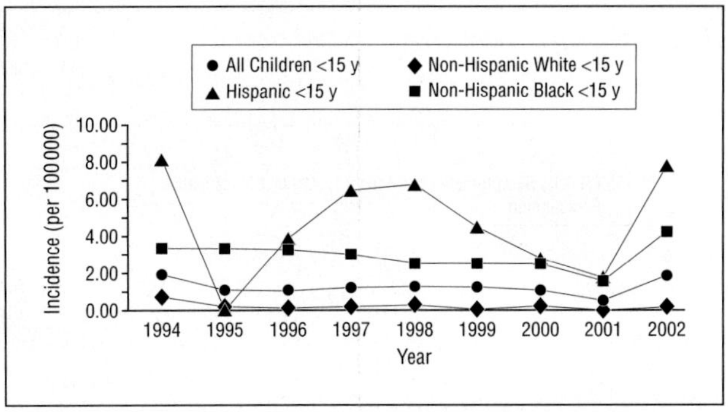


**Figure 1.** Incidence of pediatric (<15 years) tuberculosis (TB) in North Carolina, comparing the overall pediatric TB incidence with the incidence by race and ethnicity.

Thirty (16.7%) of 180 subjects were identified by contact investigations in which more than 1 subject with TB was presumably infected by the same source case. Two clusters with 4 children each involved adults who were symptomatic for more than 4 months before seeking health care.

## MISSED OPPORTUNITIES TO PREVENT TB TRANSMISSION OR DISEASE

We identified several missed opportunities to prevent progression to TB disease in children. Contact investigations were delayed for more than 2 weeks for 13 (7.2% of all cases) of 93 children eventually identified through contact investigations. An additional 8 children (4.4% of all cases) younger than 5 years exposed to TB had a negative TST on initial evaluation but failed to take or were not prescribed isoniazid during the 3-month window period before retesting at 3 months. Finally, 4 children (2.2% of all cases) who had a positive TST but no known TB exposure failed to complete a course of isoniazid and subsequently developed TB.

Opportunities to prevent disease transmission were also identified. Twelve children (6.7%) were not initially named as contacts to an adult TB case but were later found to be contacts during further investigation. Disease might have been prevented in 21 children (11.7%) had 16 of 24 source cases with a documented prior positive TST completed treatment for LTBI. In summary, 51 cases (28.3%) could have been prevented during the study period if all the tools available to treat and prevent TB had been used.

## SCREENING FOR LTBI

In the Wake County pediatric clinic, 1239 children (of 1917 initially seen for pediatric care) had a positive response to at least 1 of the 6 screening questions during the project period. Of these, 1213 (97.9%) had a TST placed, and 944 (77.8%) returned to have it read. Most subjects were younger than 5 years (73.2%) and Hispanic (87.5%); only 1.8% were non-Hispanic white, and 4.8% were non-Hispanic black. Seventeen (1.8%) of 944 subjects had new positive TSTs, and 1 child had a history of a positive TST. Foreign birth was the risk factor most highly associated with a reactive TST. Screening based on foreign birth alone would have identified 15 of

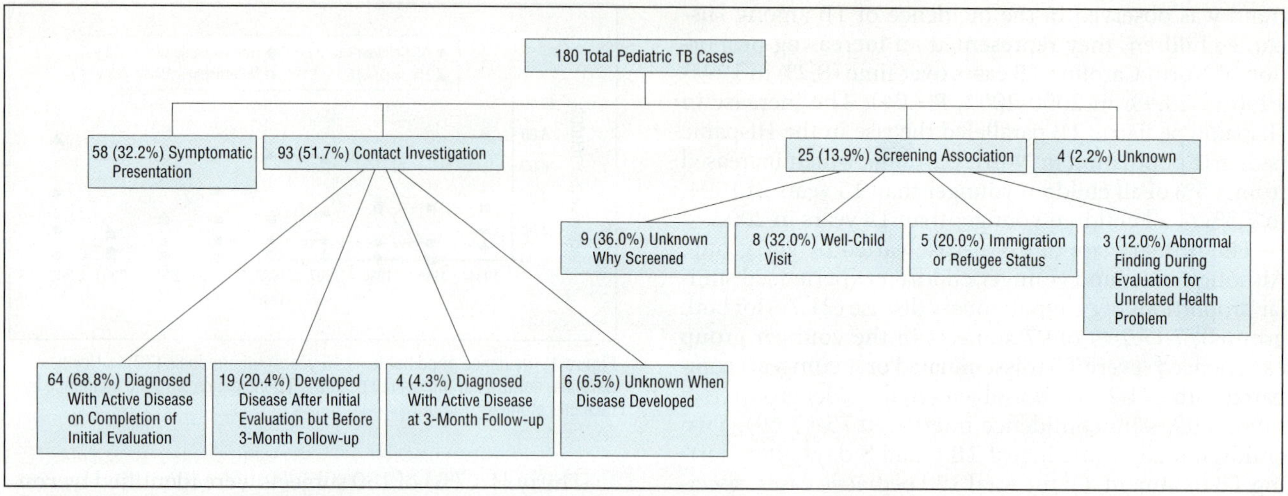


**Figure 2.** Manner in which children diagnosed with tuberculosis (TB) initially came to medical attention in North Carolina from 1994 to 2002.

**Table 2. Characteristics of Adult Patients With Tuberculosis (TB) Who Were Source Cases for at Least 1 Youth With TB, Compared With All Adults With Verified Pulmonary or Laryngeal TB in North Carolina From 1994 to 2002***

| Characteristic | Source Cases (n = 82) | All Adults With Pulmonary or Laryngeal TB (n = 3317) | Risk Ratio (95% Confidence Interval) |
|---|---|---|---|
| Sex | | | |
| Male | 44 (53.7) | 2333 (70.3) | 1.0 (Referent) |
| Female | 38 (46.3) | 984 (29.7) | 2.05 (1.34-3.14) |
| Race/ethnicity | | | |
| Non-Hispanic white | 15 (18.3) | 918 (27.7) | 1.0 (Referent) |
| Non-Hispanic black | 54 (65.9) | 1861 (56.1) | 1.78 (1.01-3.13) |
| Hispanic | 10 (12.2) | 350 (10.6) | 1.75 (0.79-3.86) |
| Asian/Pacific Islander | 3 (3.7) | 158 (4.8) | 1.16 (0.34-3.97) |
| Country of birth | | | |
| United States | 66 (80.5) | 2745 (82.8) | 1.0 (Referent) |
| Foreign | 16 (19.5) | 569 (17.2) | 1.17 (0.68-2.00) |
| Positive sputum smear | 72 (87.8) | 1708 (51.5) | 6.78 (3.51-13.10) |
| Cavitary lesion on x-ray film | 41 (50.0) | 972 (29.3) | 2.45 (1.60-3.76) |
| Human immunodeficiency virus positive | 4 (4.9) | 351 (10.6) | 0.44 (0.16-1.21) |
| Intravenous or other illicit drug use | 14 (17.1) | 345 (10.4) | 1.81 (1.03-3.19) |
| Alcohol use | 28 (34.1) | 967 (29.2) | 1.25 (0.80-1.97) |

*Data are given as number (percentage) unless otherwise indicated. Some characteristics do not sum to the heading totals because of missing data.

17 children with positive TSTs, yielding a "number needed to screen" of 17.5. There was considerable overlap among foreign birth, foreign parentage, and foreign travel (**Figure 3**). Screening US-born children whose parents were born in TB-endemic countries and who had not traveled outside the United States required 628 TSTs to identify 2 children with positive TSTs, for a marginal yield of 0.32%. No TST-positive children were immunosuppressed (0 of 8 positive subjects), had contact with high-risk individuals (0 of 16 positive subjects), or had a history of contact with a person with TB (0 of 13 positive subjects), but few children with these risk factors were identified. The rate of reactive TSTs increased significantly with age, and among foreign-born children, the rate correlated with the incidence of TB disease in the region of the subject's birth (**Table 3**).

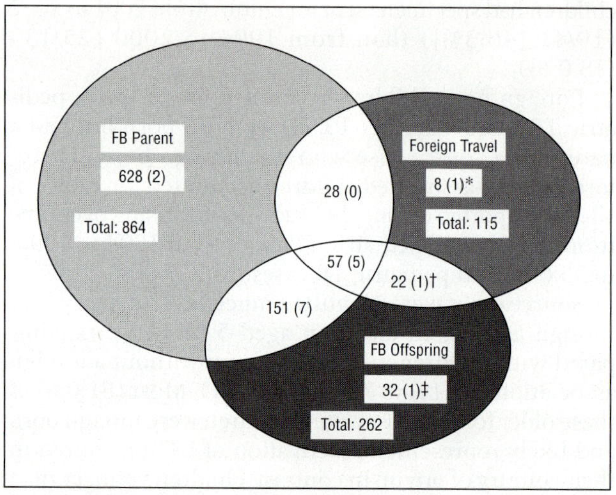


**Figure 3.** Overlap of foreign birth, foreign-born (FB) parentage, and foreign travel among 926 children who had at least 1 of these risk factors and who had a tuberculin skin test (TST) read at Wake County Human Services from July 16, 2004, to December 8, 2004. Numbers in parentheses indicate the number of children in that group with positive TST results (n=17). Asterisk indicates 8 children whose parents' place of birth was unknown; dagger, 20 children whose parents' place of birth was unknown; and double dagger, 29 children whose parents' place of birth was unknown.

## COMMENT

The burden of pediatric TB in North Carolina is almost entirely borne by its minority population. Furthermore, the greatest burden falls on the youngest cohort and causes the most severe disease.[12,13] In North Carolina, there are 2 separate but equally important phenomena driving ongoing disease in children. The first phenomenon is transmission among US-born non-Hispanic black adults, resulting in subsequent infection of non-Hispanic black children. The TB incidence among non-Hispanic black youth was 15-fold greater than that in non-Hispanic white children. Inequities in access to health care and declining familiarity with TB among health care providers may delay diagnosis, resulting in a higher likelihood of TB transmission by infectious adults.[14] The 2 clusters identified in 2002 illustrate this failure, as the adult source cases were symptomatic for longer than 4 months.

The second phenomenon, TB in foreign-associated children, is the result of a large wave of immigration from Latin America, where TB remains endemic.[15] The situation in North Carolina differs from the overall US situation because of the state's small population of non-Hispanic immigrants (who comprise a significant proportion of pediatric TB cases in states with high caseloads[16]) and because most Hispanics in North Carolina are recent immigrants or are children of recent immigrants.[11] Almost all Hispanic children with TB in North Carolina are foreign associated, whereas most pediatric patients with TB in the United States are US born and are likely to be a mix of foreign-associated and non–foreign-associated cases because of previously established Hispanic populations in many states.[16] Older US children who immigrated with their parents were likely infected in their native country and developed reactivation disease after immigration; most children (81.0%) aged 5 to 14 years with TB who had a foreign association were foreign born, and only 19.1% of these children had a source case identified. Conversely, TB among younger children more likely reflects recent transmission. In our study, 72.4% of children younger than 5 years with a foreign association were US born, and 62.1% had a source case identified. Understanding this difference should focus our contact investigation efforts on the youngest cohort, as they represent ongoing community transmission.

Reporting of pediatric TB cases as foreign born vs US born underestimates the effect of immigration on TB incidence. The proportion of foreign-born pediatric TB cases in North Carolina ranged between 13% and 15% from 1994 to 2002, with no temporal trend. By contrast, the proportion of foreign-associated pediatric TB cases in North Carolina doubled from 18.0% from 1994 to 1996, to 35.6% from 2000 to 2002. Children acquire TB infection from adults, and the country of birth of the parent or guardian is an important factor that is not collected by the national TB surveillance system.[16]

A source case was eventually identified in two thirds of our pediatric TB cases. Although most adults with TB in North Carolina (and in the United States in general) are male, source cases for children were more likely to be female adults and were more likely to be very infectious, as evidenced by a high rate of sputum smear–positive disease, a known risk factor for TB infection in youth contact.[17-19] However, 7 children acquired TB from 6 smear-negative source cases, demonstrating that smear-negative adults can still be infectious[20] and should be separated from contact with youth until the diagnosis of TB has been excluded or they demonstrate a response to treatment.

We identified several missed opportunities to prevent transmission or progression of disease in children. Twenty-eight percent of the pediatric TB cases could potentially have been prevented if the subjects or their adult sources had accepted and completed treatment of previously identified LTBI.[21,22] In the present study, the proportion of cases not treated with isoniazid (6.6%) was substantially less than others have reported[23] but represents a significant missed opportunity to prevent TB in children. Furthermore, infectious adults failed to name 12 children whom they had exposed, pointing to weaknesses in contact investigation methods that others have noted.[23-28] Better and continued training of TB field staff is needed to improve interviewing skills.

**Table 3. Results of Tuberculin Skin Tests (TST) Among 944 Children With at Least 1 Tuberculosis Risk Factor on Screening Who Returned for TST Reading at Wake County Department of Health and Human Services From July 16, 2004, to December 8, 2004***

| Characteristic | Positive TST Result (n = 17) | Negative TST Result (n = 927) | Risk Ratio (95% Confidence Interval) |
|---|---|---|---|
| Age, y | | | |
| 0-4 | 5 | 686 | 1.0 (Referent) |
| 5-14 | 7 | 224 | 4.19 (1.34-13.07) |
| 15-21 | 5 | 17 | 31.41 (9.80-100.66) |
| Sex | | | |
| Male | 9 | 492 | 1.0 (Referent) |
| Female | 8 | 429 | 1.02 (0.40-2.62) |
| Race/ethnicity | | | |
| Hispanic | 13 | 813 | 1.0 (Referent) |
| Non-Hispanic white | 0 | 17 | 0.00 (0.00-13.39) |
| Non-Hispanic black | 3 | 42 | 4.24 (1.25-14.33) |
| Asian/Pacific Islander | 1 | 47 | 1.32 (0.18-9.91) |
| Parent's country of birth | | | |
| United States | 1 | 16 | 1.0 (Referent) |
| Mexico | 8 | 638 | 0.21 (0.03-1.59) |
| Other Latin America/ Caribbean | 4 | 129 | 0.51 (0.06-4.31) |
| Sub-Saharan Africa | 2 | 36 | 0.89 (0.09-9.21) |
| Middle East | 1 | 11 | 1.42 (0.10-20.49) |
| Europe | 0 | 3 | 0 (0-108) |
| Asia | 1 | 3 | 4.25 (0.33-54.37) |
| Offspring's country of birth | | | |
| United States | 2 | 680 | 1.0 (Referent) |
| Mexico | 7 | 153 | 14.9 (3.13-71.1) |
| Other Latin America/ Caribbean | 4 | 48 | 26.23 (4.92-139.88) |
| Sub-Saharan Africa | 2 | 16 | 37.89 (5.65-254.16) |
| Middle East | 0 | 4 | 0 (0-660) |
| Europe | 0 | 2 | 0 (0-1520) |
| Asia | 1 | 15 | 21.31 (2.04-223.20) |

*Data are given as number of youth unless otherwise indicated. Some characteristics do not sum to the heading totals because of missing data.

Compared with a recently published risk assessment questionnaire,[29] our screening questionnaire detected a small number of additional children with LTBI. However, our approach was inefficient. Tuberculin skin test reactivity among these children (1.8%) was lower than that among low-risk adults in North Carolina who receive TSTs for "administrative" reasons (**Table 4**). Our highest yield came from screening children born in countries where TB is endemic, where we found 1 LTBI case per 17.5 children screened. Tuberculin skin test

**Table 4. Cumulative 2002 Data From North Carolina Public Health Department Clinics***

| Variable | Total No. of TSTs | Evaluated | TST Reactive | TB Found |
|---|---|---|---|---|
| Administrative† | 82 576 | 52 623 (63.7) | 1667 (3.2) | 1 (0.001) |
| Targeted testing‡ | 20 777 | 17 462 (84.0) | 2738 (15.7) | 19 (0.11) |
| Contacts§ | 3641 | 3366 (92.4) | 611 (18.2) | 42 (1.24) |

Abbreviations: TB, tuberculosis; TST, tuberculin skin test.
*Data are given as number (percentage) unless otherwise indicated.
†Tuberculin skin test in individuals who require testing because of employment or school regulations, without being referred by a clinician for a medical or epidemiological reason.
‡Tuberculin skin test among individuals who are at increased risk for exposure to TB (eg, foreign born) or are at risk to progress to active TB if exposed (eg, diagnosis of human immunodeficiency virus or AIDS).[10]
§Tuberculin skin test among individuals identified as having been exposed to a recent case of infectious TB, usually as part of an outbreak investigation.

screening among US-born children of foreign-born parents was inefficient and was discontinued. More effective strategies must be developed and tested, such as screening US-born children who have foreign-born visitors in the household.

The study had several limitations. The TB case analysis was retrospective, which constrained the nature of questions that could be asked of the existing data set. Medical records describing source cases and their contact with children were often incomplete. In addition, genotyping of TB isolates was not done, so the epidemiological links could not be confirmed with molecular data. However, an emphasis in obtaining culture confirmation in pediatric cases during the past several years decreases the chance that the increased number of cases in 2002 was secondary to clinical misdiagnoses.

The questionnaire used in the LTBI screening project could not be validated because TSTs were not performed in subjects with no identified risk characteristics. However, data from the North Carolina Tuberculosis Control Program provide a credible benchmark (Table 4). The fact that the youngest children, who would have most recently been vaccinated with bacille Calmette-Guérin, had low rates of TST reactivity further supports the current Centers for Disease Control and Prevention guidelines to disregard a subject's bacille Calmette-Guérin status when interpreting a TST.[29]

In conclusion, the pediatric TB caseload in North Carolina doubled in 2002 compared with the previous several years. Transmission among adults in poor communities, including US-born black citizens and a growing immigrant population, will likely contribute to new pediatric cases in the future. Additional public health resources are needed to identify and eliminate barriers to health care that delay evaluation and treatment of adults with TB. Effective TB education is needed among those likely to be exposed to TB, as well as among providers who may care for them. The public health community needs better tools for targeting socioeconomically disadvantaged communities in a culturally appropriate and supportive way to screen for LTBI and TB and to gain acceptance of proven treatment and prevention options.

**Accepted for Publication:** December 15, 2005.
**Author Affiliations:** Division of Infectious Diseases and International Health, Department of Medicine, Duke University Medical Center (Drs Stout and Dukes Hamilton), and Duke University School of Medicine (Dr Saharia), Durham; Tuberculosis Control Program, Wake County Department of Health and Human Services (Dr Stout), and North Carolina Tuberculosis Control Program, Communicable Disease Branch, Division of Public Health, Department of Health and Human Services (Dr Dukes Hamilton), Raleigh; School of Public Health (Dr Saharia) and Department of Preventive Medicine (Dr Nageswaran), The University of North Carolina at Chapel Hill; and Division of Infectious Diseases, Department of Pediatrics, Carolinas Medical Center, Charlotte (Dr Ahmed), NC. Dr Saharia is now in the Internal Medicine–Pediatrics Residency Program at Yale University, New Haven, Conn.
**Correspondence:** Jason E. Stout, MD, MHS, Division of Infectious Diseases and International Health, Department of Medicine, Duke University Medical Center, Box 3306, Durham, NC 27710 (stout002@mc.duke.edu).
**Funding/Support:** This study was supported by grant K23 AI51409 (Dr Stout) and by grant K24 AI001833-02 (Dr Dukes Hamilton) from the National Institute of Allergy and Infectious Diseases, National Institutes of Health.
**Acknowledgment:** We thank the North Carolina Tuberculosis Control Program nurse consultants (Dee Foster, Elizabeth Zeringue, Myra Allen, and Julie Luffman) and the TB nurses in the North Carolina county public health clinics (Ellen Fortenberry and Elizabeth Tilson, MD), without whose cooperation this study would not have been possible.

## REFERENCES

1. Centers for Disease Control and Prevention (CDC). Trends in tuberculosis morbidity—United States, 1992-2002 *MMWR Morb Mortal Wkly Rep.* 2003;52:217-222.
2. McKenna MT, McCray E, Onorato I. The epidemiology of tuberculosis among foreign-born persons in the United States, 1986 to 1993. *N Engl J Med.* 1995;332:1071-1076.
3. Talbot EA, Moore M, McCray E, Binkin NJ. Tuberculosis among foreign-born persons in the United States, 1993-1998. *JAMA.* 2000;284:2894-2900.
4. Kenyon TA, Driver C, Haas E, Valway SE, Moser KS, Onorato IM. Immigration and tuberculosis among children on the United States–Mexico border, County of San Diego, California. *Pediatrics.* 1999;104:e8.
5. Driver CR, Luallen JJ, Good WE, Valway SE, Frieden TR, Onorato IM. Tuberculosis in children younger than five years old: New York City. *Pediatr Infect Dis J.* 1995;14:112-117.
6. Ussery XT, Valway SE, McKenna M, Cauthen GM, McCray E, Onorato IM. Epidemiology of tuberculosis among children in the United States: 1985 to 1994. *Pediatr Infect Dis J.* 1996;15:697-704.
7. Migration Policy Institute. Fact sheet on the foreign born: North Carolina. http://www.migrationinformation.org/usfocus/statemap.cfm#. Accessed March 14, 2006.
8. US Population Bureau. Table 3: annual estimates of the population by sex, race and Hispanic or Latino origin for North Carolina: April 1, 2000 to July 1, 2003 (SC-EST2003-03-37). http://www.census.gov/popest/states/asrh/tables/SC-EST2003-03/SC-EST2003-03-37.pdf. Accessed June 21, 2005.
9. Centers for Disease Control and Prevention. Case definitions for infectious conditions under public health surveillance. *MMWR Recomm Rep.* 1997;46(RR-10):1-55.
10. Targeted tuberculin testing and treatment of latent tuberculosis infection. *Am J Respir Crit Care Med.* 2000;161(pt 2):S221-S247.
11. US Census Bureau. July 1, 2003 state and county characteristic population estimates. http://www.census.gov/popest/counties/files/CO-EST2003-alldata.csv. Accessed December 31, 2004.

12. Hussey G, Chisholm T, Kibel M. Miliary tuberculosis in children: a review of 94 cases. *Pediatr Infect Dis J.* 1991;10:832-836.
13. Steiner P, Portugaliza C. Tuberculosis meningitis in children. *Am Rev Respir Dis.* 1973;107:22-29.
14. Golub JE, Bur S, Cronin WA, et al. Patient and health care system delays in pulmonary tuberculosis diagnosis in a low-incidence state. *Int J Tuberc Lung Dis.* 2005;9:992-998.
15. Silberman P, Bazan-Manson A, Purves H. North Carolina Latino Health, 2003: a report from the Latino Health Task Force. *N C Med J.* 2003;64:113-121.
16. Nelson LJ, Schneider E, Wells CD, Moore M. Epidemiology of childhood tuberculosis in the United States, 1993-2001: the need for continued vigilance. *Pediatrics.* 2004;114:333-341.
17. Chapman JS, Dyerly MD. Social and other factors in intrafamilial transmission of tuberculosis. *Am Rev Respir Dis.* 1964;90:48-60.
18. Beyers N, Gie RP, Schaaf HS, et al. A prospective evaluation of children under the age of 5 years living in the same household as adults with recently diagnosed pulmonary tuberculosis. *Int J Tuberc Lung Dis.* 1997;1:38-43.
19. van Geuns HA, Meijer J, Styblo K. Results of contact examination in Rotterdam. *Bull Int Union Tuberc.* 1975;50:107-124.
20. Behr MA, Warren SA, Salamon H. Transmission of *Mycobacterium* tuberculosis from patients smear-negative for acid-fast bacilli [published correction appears in *Lancet.* 1999;353:1714]. *Lancet.* 1999;353:444-449.
21. Comstock GW, Livesay VT, Woolpert SF. The prognosis of a positive tuberculin reaction in childhood and adolescence. *Am J Epidemiol.* 1974;99:131-137.
22. Zeidberg LD, Dillon A, Gass RS. Risk of developing tuberculosis among children of tuberculous parents. *Am Rev Tuberc.* 1954;70:1009-1019.
23. Nolan RJ. Childhood tuberculosis in North Carolina: a study of the opportunities for intervention in the transmission of tuberculosis to children. *Am J Public Health.* 1986;76:26-30.
24. Mehta JB, Bentley S. Prevention of tuberculosis in children: missed opportunities. *Am J Prev Med.* 1992;8:283-286.
25. Starke JR, Taylor-Watts KT. Preventable childhood tuberculosis in Houston, Texas [abstract]. *Am Rev Respir Dis.* 1990;141:A336.
26. Kimerling ME, Barker JT, Bruce F, Brook NL, Dunlap NE. Preventable childhood tuberculosis in Alabama: implications and opportunity. *Pediatrics.* 2000;105:e53.
27. Lobato MN, Mohle-Boetani JC, Royce SE. Missed opportunities for preventing tuberculosis among children younger than five years of age. *Pediatrics.* 2000;106:e75.
28. Reichler MR, Reves R, Bur S, et al. Evaluation of investigations conducted to detect and prevent transmission of tuberculosis. *JAMA.* 2002;287:991-995.
29. Pediatric Tuberculosis Collaborative Group. Targeted tuberculin skin testing and treatment of latent tuberculosis infection in children and adolescents. *Pediatrics.* 2004;114(suppl 2):1175-1201.

# Effects of Antibullying School Program on Bullying and Health Complaints

*Minne Fekkes, MSc, PhD; Frans I. M. Pijpers, MD, PhD; S. Pauline Verloove-Vanhorick, MD, PhD*

**Objective:** To evaluate the effects of an antibullying school intervention in elementary schools.

**Design:** Two-year follow-up randomized intervention group–control group.

**Setting:** Forty-seven elementary schools in the Netherlands.

**Participants:** Three thousand eight hundred sixteen children aged 9 to 12 years.

**Intervention:** During the first study year, an antibullying school program was implemented in the schools in the intervention group.

**Main Outcome Measures:** A questionnaire measuring bullying behavior, depression, psychosomatic complaints, delinquent behavior, and satisfaction with school life and peer relationships was filled out by the students at 3 times to obtain the following data: a baseline measurement, a first-effect measurement at the end of the first year, and a second-effect measurement at the end of the second year.

**Results:** The number of bullied children decreased by 25% in the intervention group compared with the control group (relative risk, 0.75; 95% confidence interval, 0.57-0.98). The intervention group also showed a decline in the scale scores of victimization (−1.06 vs 0.28; *P*<.01) and active bullying behaviors (−0.47 vs 0.12, *P*<.05). Self-reported peer relationships also improved in the intervention schools (0.48 vs 0.11; *P*<.05), and there was a trend for a decrease in reported depression in the intervention schools (−0.33 vs −0.10; *P*<.10). At follow-up, there were no differences between the intervention and control groups for the outcome measures. Schools had also lowered their antibullying activities during the second study year.

**Conclusions:** An antibullying school policy can reduce bullying behavior. To keep bullying at a consistently low level, schools must continue antibullying measures every year. Continued counseling may help schools in their efforts to establish a lasting antibullying policy.

*Arch Pediatr Adolesc Med. 2006;160:638-644*

Author Affiliations: Youth Department, TNO (Netherlands Organization of Applied Scientific Research) Prevention and Health, Leiden (Drs Fekkes and Verloove-Vanhorick), Geneeskundige en GezondheidsDienst Amsterdam (Dr Pijpers), Department of Pediatrics and Child Health, Leiden University Medical Center (Dr Verloove-Vanhorick), the Netherlands.

BULLYING IS A FORM OF AGgressive behavior that is widespread among schoolchildren and is often characterized by repetition and an imbalance of power.[1] Bullying can take many forms, such as hitting, kicking, and name-calling, as well as more indirect forms such as exclusion and gossiping. One of the first large-scale studies on bullying behavior in Norway indicated that 1 of every 7 children was bullied regularly.[2,3] Subsequent studies in several countries have also shown that a substantial number of children are bullied.[4-7]

Several studies also show that children who are being bullied, and to a lesser degree the bullies, have higher incidences of health complaints and depression.[4,8-18] Other studies have found an association between bullying and suicidal thoughts.[10,19]

Since the 1980s, antibullying interventions have been implemented in schools in many countries.[20] A first large-scale intervention campaign was carried out in Norway and was evaluated by Olweus.[21] Results showed that schools implementing an antibullying policy had significant and lasting decreases in bullying behavior.[2,21] As a result, antibullying interventions were implemented in other countries.[20,22-25]

In the Netherlands, several antibullying measures have been developed to help schools prevent and diminish bullying. In 1995, school, teacher, and parent organizations joined in a collaborative effort to develop national standard antibullying guidelines for schools. This resulted in a protocol for schools to adopt antibullying measures that mirror many of the principles of the Olweus program.[26] Adoption of these antibullying measures was voluntary. Many schools adopted the guidelines and instituted an antibullying school policy, but a substantial number of schools did not develop a specific antibullying policy or implement antibullying activities.

The purpose of our study was to evaluate the effects of this antibullying school program in elementary schools. We studied effects on bullying behavior and on related outcome measures such as depression and health complaints. To evaluate the effects, we used a randomized intervention group–control group design. We hypothesized that bullying and related health complaints in schools that participated in the antibullying intervention would decrease compared with schools that did not participate in the intervention.

## METHODS

### PARTICIPATING SCHOOLS

To study the effect of an antibullying school program, the design included an intervention group and a control group (control group 1). For both groups, a baseline measurement (T0) and 2 follow-up measurements (T1 and T2) were obtained. In addition, another control group was added to the design (control group 2). This group was included in case the schools in control group 1 would start an antibullying school policy on their own during the first year as a result of the baseline measurement. However, this second control group did not contain any baseline measurement data and consequently was less than ideal for analysis. Therefore, control group 2 was included in the analyses only if schools in control group 1 started their own antibullying policy and had their staff trained.

Two hundred Dutch elementary schools were approached to participate in the study. Schools were eligible for participation if they did not have an antibullying school policy and their school staff was not recently trained in antibullying activities. Fifty schools agreed to participate. For logistic reasons, only 15 schools could participate in the intervention group. Schools were randomly assigned to either the intervention group or to 1 of the 2 control groups until each of the 3 groups contained 15 schools; the remaining schools were divided among the 2 control groups.

Children from the 3 highest grades (age, 9-12 years) participated by completing a questionnaire. The questionnaires were completed in classrooms under examinationlike conditions 3 times during the study: the first and second measurements were obtained during the school year, in November 1999 and May 2000, respectively, and the third measurement was obtained at the end of the follow-up school year in May 2001.

The design of the study was approved by the local medical ethics committee. All parental advisory boards of the participating schools were informed about the study and gave written informed consent for participation.

### BULLYING BEHAVIOR

Two questions were asked about general bullying behavior: How often did other children bully you in recent months? How often did you bully other children in recent months? Questions were based on the Dutch version of the Olweus Bully/Victim Questionnaire with somewhat modified answer categories.[27,28] Children could answer both questions on a 6-point scale: "not bullied at all," "1 or 2 times," "a few times a month," "once a week," "2 or 3 times a week," and "almost every day." Items were dichotomized into bullied ("a few times a month" or more often) and not bullied ("1 or 2 times" or less often). In addition, active and experienced bullying behavior was measured with items addressing 6 types of victimization: name-calling, exclusion, hitting or kicking, having things stolen or hidden, being rumored or gossiped about, and being teased.[29] Children were asked if they experienced or performed any of these behaviors during the last 4 weeks. Items were summed for both scales of active and experienced bullying behavior.

### PSYCHOSOMATIC COMPLAINTS

Students were asked about a series of health symptoms (eg, headache, sleeping problems, or abdominal pain) and for each symptom were asked to report whether in the last 4 weeks they had experienced the symptom never, sometimes, or often. Items were summed into a scale.

### DEPRESSION

Depression was evaluated with the Short Depression Inventory for Children.[30] This questionnaire contains 9 items, for example, "The last weeks I felt down." For each item, respondents answered whether this was true or not true. All items answered as true were summed.

### DELINQUENT BEHAVIOR

Delinquent behavior was measured with a 7-item scale.[29] Each item addressed a different form of delinquent behavior, such as "Have you stolen something at school?" All items that were answered positively were summed.

### SCHOOL SATISFACTION

Experience of school life was measured with 3 scales from the Dutch School Experience Questionnaire[31]: "satisfaction with contact with other students" (8 items, eg, "I would rather be in a classroom with other children"), general satisfaction with school life (10 items), and satisfaction with contact with teachers (15 items). For each item, answer options were always, often, sometimes, or never. Items were summed, with higher scores indicating more satisfaction.

### ANTIBULLYING ACTIVITIES

Compliance with the components of the intervention was measured by teacher reports. A questionnaire with questions regarding antibullying activities performed during the school year was distributed among teachers in the participating classes at the end of the second and third years (T1 and T2).

### STATISTICAL ANALYSES

Multilevel logistic and linear regression analyses (MLwiN; Multilevel Models Project, Institute of Education, London, England)[32] were used to calculate effects of the intervention at the end of the first and second years of the study. Three levels were included in the analyses: school, classroom, and individual. Outcomes were measured at the individual level, corrected for influences from a higher level, that is, classroom and school. Baseline levels of the outcome measure and grade, sex, and school size were included as covariates in the regression model. Odds ratios obtained from logistic regression were converted to relative risk by using the method described by Zhang and Yu.[33] $P$ values were 2-tailed. Significance levels for an effect were $P<.05$, and for a trend were $P<.10$.

### ANTIBULLYING PROGRAM

The antibullying program was developed in the Netherlands and mirrors many principles that also underlie antibullying programs in other countries, such as the Olweus program. The program aims to include teachers, bullied children, bullies, noninvolved children, and parents in the efforts to lower the bullying behavior.

An important part of the program is that teachers undergo training. Another important component is the development of a written antibullying school policy describing the activities that a school

**Table 1. Activities During First Year for Intervention and Control Schools**

| Activity | Intervention Group (n = 34) | Control Group 1 (n = 37) | Control Group 2 (n = 36) |
|---|---|---|---|
| Antibully training for teachers, %* | 97 | 0 | 3 |
| Bullying survey, %† | 71 | 26 | 14 |
| Antibullying rules, %‡ | 71 | 46 | 27 |
| Use of antibullying curriculum, % | 65 | 51 | 61 |
| Intensity of surveillance (mean No. of teachers per group of students during recess) | 0.42 | 0.36 | 0.42 |
| Organizing information meeting on bullying for parents, % | 9 | 5 | 3 |

*$\chi^2$ = 79.55; $P<.001$.
†$\chi^2$ = 14.60; $P<.001$.
‡$\chi^2$ = 14.27; $P<.001$.

**Table 2. Activities During Second Year for Intervention and Control Schools**

| Activity | Intervention Group (n = 29) | Control Group 1 (n = 41) | Control Group 2 (n = 35) |
|---|---|---|---|
| Bullying survey, % | 25 | 15 | 9 |
| Antibullying rules, % | 74 | 59 | 50 |
| Use of antibullying curriculum, % | 41 | 40 | 44 |
| Intensity of surveillance (mean No. of teachers per group of students during recess) | 0.41 | 0.41 | 0.64 |
| Organizing information meeting on bullying for parents, % | 4 | 10 | 3 |

plans to perform during the course of the school year and how to deal with bullying incidents. Training of teachers and assistance for the schools was given by the KPC group, an organization that specializes in training school staff and assisting schools with the implementation of new curricula and guidelines. Schools in the intervention group were assisted with the development of an antibullying school policy during the first year of the study.

At the beginning of the school year there was a meeting for school board supervisors to explain the program and create support. There was a 2-day training session for teachers to create awareness of bullying behavior, to assist them in applying antibullying measures, and to instruct them on how to deal with bullying incidents among children. During the intervention year, teachers could consult the training staff with questions about their antibullying activities.

Schools were supplied with the booklet *Bullying in School: How to Deal With It*,[26] which describes how a school can develop an antibullying policy and undertake various measures. They were also supplied with the Bullying Test,[26] a computerized questionnaire that children can complete anonymously in the classroom and that gives the teacher an insight into the bullying behavior of the students.

Schools were asked to develop a written antibullying school policy and to include in their activities the core program as described by Olweus[3]: set clear rules against bullying, have regular measurements of bullying behavior by means of a questionnaire, have a curriculum of lessons on bullying behavior and social skills, have good supervision during recess, and inform parents about and involve them in the antibullying policy of the school.

## RESULTS

The main criterion for including schools in the intervention group was that their teachers participate in the 2-day training. One school was originally part of the intervention group but indicated having no time for the training and, consequently, was excluded from the intervention group and the study.

### ANTIBULLYING ACTIVITIES DURING THE FIRST YEAR

The participating schools included 156 classes participating in the study during the first year. A questionnaire regarding the antibullying activities during the first year was returned for 107 classes (response rate, 69%). Results are given in **Table 1**. Most teachers in the intervention group participated in the training. None of the control schools had a substantial part of their staff trained in antibullying measures during the study. The results indicate further that intervention schools performed more antibullying activities, although not for all components of the intervention. Specifically, the use of an antibullying survey in the classrooms and the creation of antibullying rules were done significantly more often in the intervention group. At the end of the first year, 6 of the 14 schools in the intervention group had a written antibullying policy. One of the 18 schools in control group 1 had a written policy, and no school in control group 2 had a written antibullying policy.

### ANTIBULLYING ACTIVITIES DURING THE SECOND YEAR

The participating schools included 113 classes participating in the study during the second year. A questionnaire regarding the antibullying activities during this second year was returned for 105 classes (response rate, 93%). Results are given in **Table 2**. There was no significant difference in activities between the intervention group and the control groups. The main reasons why schools in the intervention group discontinued activities during the second year of the study were that they considered the antibullying activities to be a 1-year project, the school decided that an-

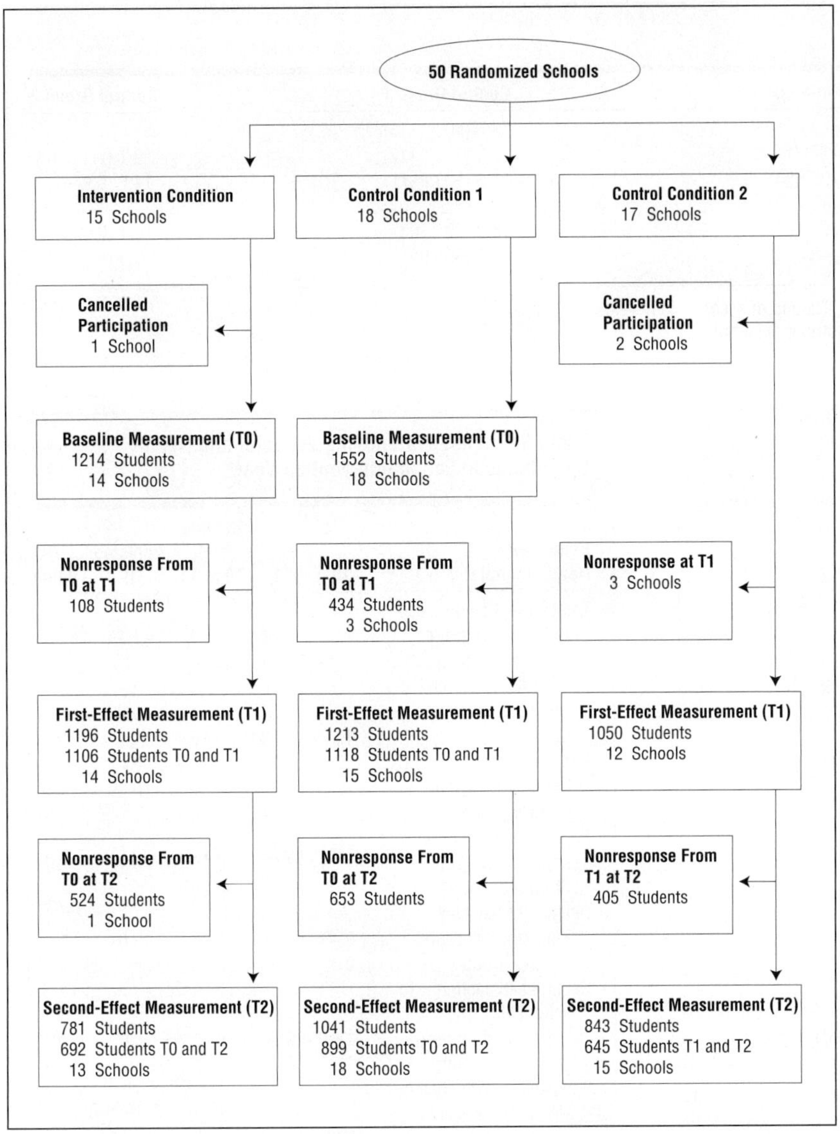


**Figure**. Flowchart shows school participation and follow-up data for students and schools. T1 & T2 are follow-up measurements obtained at the end of the second and third study years.

other issue should get priority during the following year, or simply that there was no time to perform the activities every year. Schools with a written antibullying policy performed more antibullying activities during the follow-up year than those without a written policy.

## EFFECTS OF ANTIBULLYING POLICY

A total of 3816 children participated in the study: 1214 students in the intervention group (at T0), 1552 students in control group 1 (at T0), and 1050 students in control group 2 (at T1) (**Figure**). Because most of the schools in both control groups did not have their staff trained and did not have a written antibullying school policy during the first year, control group 1 was used in the main effect analysis as the comparison group because this group also included a baseline measurement (T0).

## NONRESPONSE

The intervention group and control group 1 included 2848 students in the upper 3 grades; 2766 (97%) participated in the baseline measurement (T0), and 2224 (78%) participated in the first-effect measurement (T1). During the following school year children in the lower 2 grades of the initial sample, who were still in elementary school, participated in the second-effect measurement (T2), and 1591 children (58% of the initial total sample, 82% of the initial lower 2 grades) filled out the questionnaire (Figure).

For the nonresponders of the first-effect measurement (T1), there were no differences in outcome variables of the initial measurement between nonresponders from the intervention group and those from the control group. Nonresponders of the second-effect measurement (T2) differed only on the baseline scores of psychosomatic complaints (0.97 vs 1.21; $t$=2.71; $P$=.007).

## INITIAL SAMPLE

Mean (SD) age of students at the baseline measurement was 10.1 (1.1) years. Fifty percent of the sample were girls. **Table 3** gives data on general bullying behavior in intervention schools and control schools.

**Table 3. General Bullying Behavior***

| Behavior | Intervention Group | Control Group 1 | Control Group 2 |
|---|---|---|---|
| Being bullied, T0 | 17.7 (196/1106) | 14.6 (163/1115) | |
| Being bullied, T1 | 15.5 (171/1104) | 17.3 (192/1112) | 19.1 (122/640) |
| Being bullied, T2 | 14.0 (96/688) | 11.5 (103/897) | 14.5 (93/642) |
| Active bullying, T0 | 5.1 (56/1101) | 5.1 (57/1110) | |
| Active bullying, T1 | 7.9 (87/1098) | 8.9 (99/1108) | 10.2 (65/636) |
| Active bullying, T2 | 6.6 (45/686) | 7.3 (65/895) | 8.9 (57/643) |

Abbreviations: T0, baseline; T1, end of first study year; T2, end of second study year.
*Values indicate percentage (number in sample/total number in sample).

**Table 4. Relative Risk for General Bullying Behavior at End of Intervention Year***

| Behavior | RR (95% CI) |
|---|---|
| Being bullied | |
| Control group | 1.00 |
| Intervention group | 0.75 (0.57-0.98) |
| Active bullying | |
| Control group | 1.00 |
| Intervention group | 0.81 (0.55-1.15) |

Abbreviations: CI, confidence interval; RR, relative risk.
*Intervention group, n = 1106; control group 1, n = 1118.

## EFFECTS AFTER THE FIRST YEAR

At the end of the first year, the number of bullied children decreased significantly in the intervention schools compared with the control schools. In the intervention schools, the number of bullied children decreased from 17.7% to 15.5%, while the number of bullied children in the control group increased from 14.6% to 17.3%. Multilevel regression analyses indicated that children in the intervention group were at a relative risk of 0.75 (95% confidence interval, 0.57-0.98) of being bullied at the end of the first school year compared with the control group (**Table 4**). Thus, the number of bullied children decreased by 25% in the intervention group compared with the control group.

Scale scores on specific bullying behavior also indicated that children in the intervention schools experienced significantly less bullying behavior (**Table 5**). Children also indicated less active bullying behavior. Furthermore, there was a trend for fewer depressive symptoms in the intervention schools compared with the control schools at the end of the first year. Children in the intervention group also indicated higher satisfaction with contact with other students.

## EFFECTS AFTER THE SECOND YEAR

At the end of the follow-up year there were no significant differences in bullying behavior between schools in the intervention group and the control group (**Table 6**). There were also no differences between the groups in other outcome measures such as depression, psychosomatic complaints, and satisfaction with school life (**Table 7**).

**Table 5. Changes in Bullying Behavior and Health Complaints at End of Intervention Year***

| Behavior/ Health Complaint | T0 | T1 | Change from T0 to T1 | Adjusted β | P Value |
|---|---|---|---|---|---|
| Total scale, being bullied | | | | | |
| Intervention group | 2.85 | 1.79 | −1.06 | −1.18 | <.01 |
| Control group | 2.33 | 2.61 | 0.28 | | |
| Total scale, active bullying | | | | | |
| Intervention group | 1.78 | 1.31 | −0.47 | −0.62 | <.05 |
| Control group | 1.11 | 1.23 | 0.12 | | |
| Depression | | | | | |
| Intervention group | 2.10 | 1.77 | −0.33 | −0.16 | <.10 |
| Control group | 1.87 | 1.77 | −0.10 | | |
| Psychosomatic complaints | | | | | |
| Intervention group | 1.25 | 1.10 | −0.15 | −0.12 | NS |
| Control group | 1.08 | 1.06 | −0.02 | | |
| Delinquent behavior | | | | | |
| Intervention group | 0.43 | 0.49 | 0.06 | −0.01 | NS |
| Control group | 0.42 | 0.51 | 0.09 | | |
| General satisfaction with school life | | | | | |
| Intervention group | 21.47 | 20.64 | −0.83 | 0.43 | NS |
| Control group | 21.29 | 20.18 | −1.11 | | |
| Satisfaction with contact with other students | | | | | |
| Intervention group | 18.92 | 19.40 | 0.48 | 0.38 | <.05 |
| Control group | 19.30 | 19.41 | 0.11 | | |
| Satisfaction with contact with teachers | | | | | |
| Intervention group | 32.06 | 30.26 | −1.80 | 0.13 | NS |
| Control group | 32.23 | 30.48 | −1.75 | | |

Abbreviations: NS, not significant; T0, baseline; T1, end of first study year.
*Intervention group, n = 1106; control group 1, n = 1118.

## COMMENT

The results of this randomized control study indicate that schools can reduce the number of children being bullied. The number of bullied children decreased by 25% in the intervention group compared with the control group at the end of the first year. Self-reported peer relationships improved at the intervention schools, and there was a trend toward a decrease in reported depressive complaints in the intervention schools in comparison with the control schools.

Compliance in the intervention group was high for attending the 2-day training for teachers, using the bully-

**Table 6. Relative Risk for General Bullying Behavior at End of Second Study Year***

| Behavior | RR (95% CI) |
|---|---|
| Being bullied | |
| Control group A | 1.00 |
| Intervention group | 1.14 (0.81-1.59) |
| Active bullying | |
| Control group | 1.00 |
| Intervention group | 0.75 (0.43-1.29) |

Abbreviations: CI, confidence interval; RR, relative risk.
*Intervention group, n = 692; control group 1, n = 899.

ing questionnaire to establish levels of bullying behavior, and setting clear rules against bullying in the classroom. Compliance was low for some components of the intervention. For example, schools did not often involve the parents in their antibullying efforts. Awareness is considered important in combating bullying through a school-based intervention program.[3] It may well be that attending the training sessions and frequent use of the Bullying Test raised awareness of the bullying problem and made teachers more vigilant during the first year.

In the longer term, at the end of the second study year, there were no significant differences in outcome variables between the intervention and control schools. One explanation might be the decline of antibullying measures in the intervention schools during the second year. Although schools were asked to continue their activities, no training or counseling was given in the second year. This absence of ongoing support may have been an important reason for discontinuation of the activities in the second year. Another explanation is that not all schools in the intervention group developed a written antibullying school policy. Schools with a written policy did continue more of their antibullying measures. Furthermore, several schools indicated that they considered the antibullying activities part of a 1-year project and wanted to give their extra time and attention each year to a different health subject that needed special attention.

Other studies have found mixed results on antibullying school measures. Olweus[21] evaluated a nationally implemented antibullying intervention in Norway and found substantial (up to 50%) reductions in bullying victimization. However, other authors[34,35] evaluated the same program and found no overall effects. This difference in results is explained by the higher level of counseling given to schools in the Olweus study. Evaluation of similar programs in England and Belgium reported positive effects, although smaller than those reported in Norway.[23-25] A recent study in Finland found substantial reductions in bullying behavior, especially among schools with high levels of implementation of antibullying activities.[36]

Some strengths of our study are the randomized controlled design and the use of multilevel analysis, which controls for clustering effects at the group level. Effect analyses included baseline levels of bullying behavior to correct for initial differences between the groups. An adverse factor in the design was that schools in the control group performed several antibullying activities. All schools

**Table 7. Changes in Bullying Behavior and Health Complaints at End of Second Study Year***

| Behavior/ Health Complaint | T0 | T2 | Change from T0 to T2 | Adjusted β | *P* Value |
|---|---|---|---|---|---|
| Total scale, being bullied | | | | | |
| Intervention group | 2.96 | 2.09 | −0.87 | 0.42 | NS |
| Control group | 2.76 | 1.51 | −1.25 | | |
| Total scale, active bullying | | | | | |
| Intervention group | 1.86 | 1.23 | −0.63 | −0.16 | NS |
| Control group | 1.13 | 1.14 | 0.01 | | |
| Depression | | | | | |
| Intervention group | 2.19 | 1.64 | −0.55 | −0.03 | NS |
| Control group | 1.97 | 1.55 | −0.42 | | |
| Psychosomatic complaints | | | | | |
| Intervention group | 1.28 | 0.88 | −0.40 | −0.05 | NS |
| Control group | 1.16 | 0.88 | −0.28 | | |
| Delinquent behavior | | | | | |
| Intervention group | 0.44 | 0.65 | 0.21 | 0.05 | NS |
| Control group | 0.39 | 0.58 | 0.19 | | |
| General satisfaction with school life | | | | | |
| Intervention group | 21.65 | 21.26 | −0.39 | 0.51 | NS |
| Control group | 21.39 | 20.68 | −0.72 | | |
| Satisfaction with contact with other students | | | | | |
| Intervention group | 18.86 | 19.57 | 0.71 | 0.14 | NS |
| Control group | 19.08 | 19.59 | 0.51 | | |
| Satisfaction with contact with teachers | | | | | |
| Intervention group | 32.30 | 30.71 | −1.59 | 0.33 | NS |
| Control group | 32.37 | 30.73 | −1.64 | | |

Abbreviations: NS, not significant; T0, baseline; T2, end of second study year.
*Intervention group, n = 692; control group 1, n = 899.

were expected to be involved in some antibullying activities. However, these control schools can still be considered part of the control group because their staff did not undergo any antibullying training and most control schools did not develop a written antibullying policy.

Future implementation of the antibullying intervention in elementary schools should be more focused on developing a written antibullying policy and include regular follow-up counseling. A follow-up project is under way to investigate how schools can implement more antibullying activities and continue their activities each year with the help of ongoing consultation.

We conclude that an antibullying school intervention can reduce bullying victimization. However, to keep bullying behavior at a consistently low level, schools must continue antibullying measures every year. Regular follow-up counseling could help schools to continue their antibullying school policy.

**Accepted for Publication:** November 23, 2005.
**Correspondence:** Minne Fekkes, MSc, PhD, Youth Department, TNO (Netherlands Organization of Applied Scientific Research) Prevention and Health, PO Box 2215, 2301 CE Leiden, the Netherlands (m.fekkes@pg.tno.nl).
**Author Contributions:** Dr Fekkes had full access to all data in the study and takes responsibility for the integrity of the data and the accuracy of the data analysis.

**Funding/Support:** This study was supported by grant 22000061 from ZorgOnderzoek Nederland, The Hague, which had no role in the design or conduct of the study or in the preparation, review, or approval of the manuscript.

## REFERENCES


1. Olweus D. Sweden. In: Smith PK, Morita Y, Junger-Tas J, Olweus D, Catalano RF, Slee P, eds. *The Nature of School Bullying: A Cross-National Perspective.* New York, NY: Routledge; 1999:7-27.
2. Olweus D. Bully/victim problems among schoolchildren: basic facts and effects of a school based intervention program. In: Pepler DJ, Rubin KH, eds. *The Development and Treatment of Childhood Aggression.* Hillsdale, NY: Lawrence A Erlbaum Associates; 1991:411-448.
3. Olweus D. *Bullying at School: What We Know and What We Can Do.* Oxford, England: Blackwell Publishers Inc; 1993.
4. Kumpulainen K, Rasanen E, Henttonen I. Children involved in bullying: psychological disturbance and the persistence of the involvement. *Child Abuse Negl.* 1999;23:1253-1262.
5. Nansel TR, Overpeck M, Pilla RS, Ruan WJ, Simons-Morton B, Scheidt P. Bullying behaviors among US youth: prevalence and association with psychosocial adjustment. *JAMA.* 2001;285:2094-2100.
6. Rigby K, Slee PT. Bullying among Australian school children: reported behavior and attitudes toward victims. *J Soc Psychol.* 1991;131:615-627.
7. Wolke D, Woods S, Stanford K, Schulz H. Bullying and victimization of primary school children in England and Germany: prevalence and school factors. *Br J Psychol.* 2001;92:673-696.
8. Nishina A, Juvonen J, Witkow MR. Sticks and stones may break my bones, but names will make me feel sick: the psychosocial, somatic, and scholastic consequences of peer harassment. *J Clin Child Adolesc Psychol.* 2005;34:37-48.
9. Due P, Holstein BE, Lynch J, et al. Health behaviour in school-aged children bullying working group. Bullying and symptoms among school-aged children: international comparative cross sectional study in 28 countries. *Eur J Public Health.* 2005;15:128-132.
10. Kaltiala-Heino R, Rimpela M, Marttunen M, Rimpela A, Rantanen P. Bullying, depression, and suicidal ideation in Finnish adolescents: school survey. *BMJ.* 1999; 319:348-351.
11. Forero R, McLellan L, Rissel C, Bauman A. Bullying behavior and psychosocial health among school students in New South Wales, Australia: cross sectional survey. *BMJ.* 1999;319:344-348.
12. Kumpulainen K, Rasanen E, Henttonen I, et al. Bullying and psychiatric symptoms among elementary school-age children. *Child Abuse Negl.* 1998;22:705-717.
13. Rigby K. The relationship between reported health and involvement in bully/victim problems among male and female secondary school children. *J Health Psychol.* 1998;3:465-476.
14. Salmon G, James A, Smith DM. Bullying in schools: self reported anxiety, depression, and self esteem in secondary school children. *BMJ.* 1998;317:924-925.
15. Slee PT. Situational and interpersonal correlates of anxiety associated with peer victimisation. *Child Psychiatry Hum Dev.* 1994;25:97-107.
16. Williams K, Chambers M, Logan S, Robinson D. Association of common health symptoms with bullying in primary school children. *BMJ.* 1996;313:17-19.
17. Wolke D, Woods S, Bloomfield L, Karstadt L. Bullying involvement in primary school and common health problems. *Arch Dis Child.* 2001;85:197-201.
18. Bond L, Carlin JB, Thomas L, Rubin K, Patton G. Does bullying cause emotional problems? a prospective study of young teenagers. *BMJ.* 2001;323:480-484.
19. Cleary SD. Adolescent victimization and associated suicidal and violent behaviors. *Adolescence.* 2000;35:671-682.
20. Smith PK, Ananiadou K, Cowie H. Interventions to reduce school bullying. *Can J Psychiatry.* 2003;48:591-599.
21. Olweus D. Bullying at school: basic facts and effects of a school based intervention program. *J Child Psychol Psychiatry.* 1994;35:1171-1190.
22. Pepler DJ, Craig WM, Ziegler S, Charach A. An evaluation of an anti-bullying intervention in Toronto schools. *Can J Community Mental Health.* 1994;13:95-110.
23. Smith PK, Sharp S. *School Bullying: Insights and Perspectives.* London, England: Routledge; 1994.
24. Smith PK. Bullying in schools: the UK experience and the Sheffield anti-bullying project. *Ir J Psychol.* 1997;18:191-201.
25. Stevens V, De Bourdeaudhuij I, Van Oost P. Bullying in Flemish schools: an evaluation of anti-bullying intervention in primary and secondary schools. *Br J Educ Psychol.* 2000;70:195-210.
26. Limper R. Cooperation between parents, teachers, and school boards to prevent bullying in education: an overview of work done in the Netherlands. *Aggress Behav.* 2000;26:125-134.
27. Solberg M, Olweus D. Prevalence estimation of school bullying with the Olweus Bully/Victim Questionnaire. *Aggress Behav.* 2003;29:239-268.
28. Liebrand J, Van IJzerdoorn H, Van Lieshout C. *KRVL Klasgenoten Relatie Vragenlijst Junior.* Nijmegen, the Netherlands: Vakgroep Ontwikkelingspsychologie, Katholieke Universiteit Nijmegen; 1991.
29. Junger-Tas J, Van Kesteren JN. *Bullying and Delinquency in a Dutch School Population.* The Hague, the Netherlands: Kugler Publications; 1999.
30. Kroesbergen HT, De Wit CA, Stijnen TH. Detection of depressive complaints in children. *Eur J Public Health.* 1996;6:29-34.
31. Knuver JWM. *De Relatie tussen Klas: en Schoolkenmerken en het Affectief Functioneren van Leerlingen [The Relation Between Class and School Characteristics, and the Affective Functioning of Students].* Groningen, the Netherlands: RION; 1993.
32. Rasbash J, Browne W, Goldstein H, et al. *A User's Guide to MLwiN.* London, England: Multilevel Models Project, Institute of Education; 2000.
33. Zhang J, Yu KF. What's the relative risk? a method of correcting the odds ratio in cohort studies of common outcomes. *JAMA.* 1998;280:1690-1691.
34. Roland E, Munthe E. The 1996 Norwegian Program for preventing and managing bullying in schools. *Ir J Psychol.* 1997;18:233-247.
35. Roland E. Bullying in school: three national innovations in Norwegian schools in 15 years. *Aggress Behav.* 2000;26:135-143.
36. Salmivalli C, Kaukiainen A, Voeten M. Anti-bullying intervention: implementation and outcome. *Br J Educ Psychol.* 2005;75:465-487.


"The spirit of the Enlightenment of the eighteenth century and Rousseau's writings were among the incentives to concentrate on the [medical] problems of children. Nils von Rosenstein, George Armstrong, and William Cadogan were pioneers in this specialty."

—From *Medicine: An Illustrated History* by Albert S. Lyons, MD, and R. Joseph Petrucelli, MD, 1987

SECTION EDITOR: ALBERT C. YAN, MD; ASSISTANT SECTION EDITOR: SAMIR S. SHAH, MD

# Picture of the Month

*Sabrina J. Braham, BA; Amy E. Gilliam, MD*

A 4-YEAR-OLD BLACK GIRL PRESENTED TO THE pediatric dermatology clinic for evaluation of a growth on the right foot, first noted in "early childhood." Examination of the right heel revealed a well-circumscribed 3×5–mm white keratotic papule surrounded by a collarette of firm tissue with interruption of skin lines (**Figure 1**).

The lesion was assumed by the parents to be a wart and was treated with a topical salicylic acid preparation with complete resolution and subsequent recurrence within 1 month. The patient reported focal tenderness to pressure and discomfort while wearing shoes.

The child was born weighing 2090 g at 34 weeks' gestation by an otherwise uncomplicated vaginal delivery. Apgar scores were 8 and 9, and although the initial physical examination results were normal, the child was taken to the nursery for observation. The postnatal course was complicated by poor feeding, temperature instability, and hyperbilirubinemia, resulting in a prolonged hospital course of 11 days. At the time of discharge, the patient was healthy, and subsequent medical history is otherwise unremarkable.

At the time of the visit, a shave biopsy was performed on the lesion, which showed subepidermal calcification consistent with calcinosis cutis (**Figure 2**).

What is your diagnosis?

**Author Affiliations:** University of California, Davis, School of Medicine, Davis (Ms Braham); and Department of Dermatology and Pediatrics, University of California, San Francisco (Dr Gilliam).

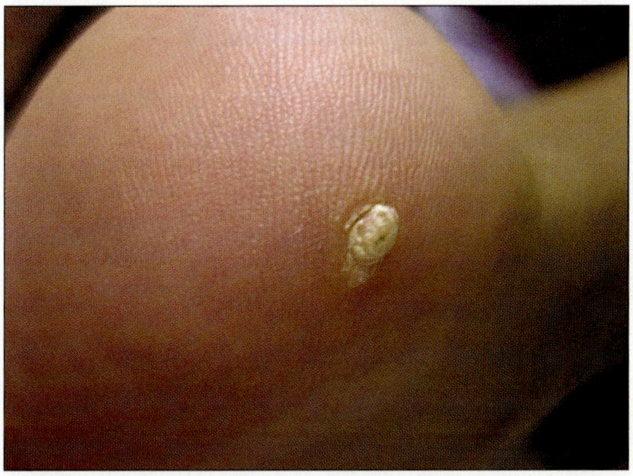

**Figure 1.** Well-circumscribed white keratotic papule on the right heel of a 4-year-old girl.

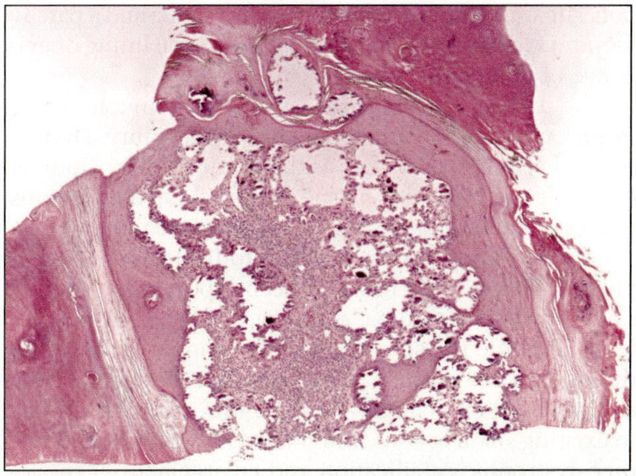

**Figure 2.** Histopathologic analysis of a shave biopsy specimen showing subepidermal calcification (hematoxylin-eosin, original magnification ×40).

# Denouement and Discussion

## *Calcified Nodule Secondary to Heel Sticks*

The first association between heel sticks to draw blood in the neonatal period and the development of calcified nodules of the heel was made by O'Doherty[1] and has since been fairly well-recognized in the neonatology community. Most reports of this entity have described it in association with high-risk neonates receiving multiple heel sticks in the nursery. However, more recently, Leung[2] and Rho et al[3] reported cases occurring following a single heel stick in healthy neonates.

Lesions may be multiple or solitary, white or yellowish verrucous papules or nodules, which are firm and often tender.[1-10] Typically, the lesions appear 4 to 12 months after birth[4-7] as multiple tiny specks that gradually enlarge and either persist or spontaneously extrude through the epidermis. Spontaneous resolution may occur within 18 to 30 months,[4,5,7,8] yet recurrence following removal with curettage has been reported.[6] Although previously thought to be largely asymptomatic, a protracted course with discomfort or tenderness may ensue.[3,6]

Plain films, if obtained, reveal opacity in the soft tissue.[5,6] Cases in which laboratory studies were obtained have reported normal serum calcium and phosphate levels.[3,4,7,8] As in our case, pathologic specimens characteristically show a cystic structure with irregular calcification, surrounded by fibrous connective tissue and a patchy mononuclear infiltrate without an epithelial lining or evidence of polarizable material.

The pathogenesis of these lesions likely involves dystrophic calcification following local tissue injury. Dystrophic calcification is defined as the abnormal deposition of insoluble calcium salts in dead or degenerated cutaneous tissues in the absence of abnormal serum calcium or phosphate concentrations. In addition to heel sticks, dystrophic calcinosis cutis has also been reported in scarring caused by burns, trauma, and surgery.[9] Injured tissue releases alkaline phosphatase, resulting in an elevation in the local pH and subsequent precipitation of calcium salts.[10] As suggested by Williamson and Holt,[6] repeated trauma to existing small lesions from footwear may promote further dystrophic calcification and enlargement of the lesions. However, it has also been suggested that these lesions may result from secondarily calcified epidermal inclusion cysts introduced by the heel sticks.[4,7] Although most authors describe the absence of an epithelial lining, which would argue against this etiology, one case did report the presence of an epithelial lining surrounding foci of calcification and fragments of keratin.[7]

For recurrent or symptomatic lesions, surgical excision or curettage may be warranted. As no abnormalities of calcium or phosphate have been reported to date in association with such lesions, further laboratory investigations do not appear to be warranted, although plain x-rays may help in making the diagnosis. This case describes a more chronic course, presenting as a symptomatic lesion later in childhood. In the case presented herein, the patient did receive 8 total heel sticks during her prolonged postnatal hospitalization.

**Accepted for Publication:** October 31, 2005.
**Correspondence:** Amy E. Gilliam, MD, Department of Dermatology, University of California, San Francisco, 1701 Divisadero St, 3rd Floor, San Francisco, CA 94143-0316 (gilliam@derm.ucsf.edu).
**Acknowledgment:** The clinical photograph was provided by Kelly M. Cordoro, MD, University of Virginia Health System, Charlottesville.

## REFERENCES

1. O'Doherty N. *Atlas of the Newborn.* Philadelphia, Pa: JB Lippincott Co; 1979: 166.
2. Leung A. Calcification following heel sticks. *J Pediatr.* 1985;106:168.
3. Rho NK, Youn SJ, Park HS, Kim WS, Lee ES. Calcified nodule on the heel of a child following a single heel stick in the neonatal period. *Clin Exp Dermatol.* 2003; 28:502-503.
4. Sell EJ, Hansen RC, Struck-Pierce S. Calcified nodules on the heel: a complication of neonatal intensive care. *J Pediatr.* 1980;96:473-475.
5. Cambiaghi S, Restano L, Imondi D. Calcified nodule of the heel. *Pediatr Dermatol.* 1997;14:494.
6. Williamson D, Holt PJ. Calcified cutaneous nodules on the heels of children: a complication of heel sticks as a neonate. *Pediatr Dermatol.* 2001;18:138-140.
7. Lemont H, Brady J. Infant heel nodules: calcification of epidermal cysts. *J Am Podiatr Med Assoc.* 2002;92:112-113.
8. Leung AK. Cutaneous nodule following heel pricks. *Can Med Assoc J.* 1985;132: 1163.
9. Walsh JS, Fairley JA. Calcifying disorders of the skin. *J Am Acad Dermatol.* 1995; 33:693-706.
10. Woods B, Kellaway TD. Cutaneous calculi: subepidermal calcified nodules. *Br J Dermatol.* 1963;75:1-11.

## Nearly 1 in 6 children did not receive all recommended DTaP doses*[1]

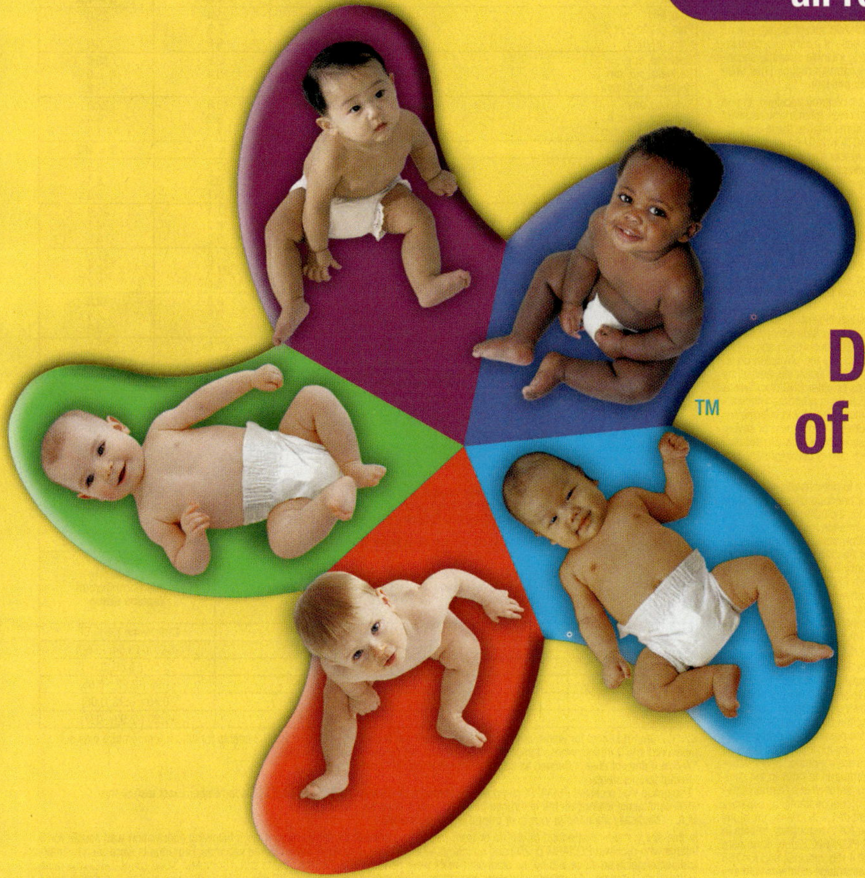


# Don't run the risk of letting one child get away

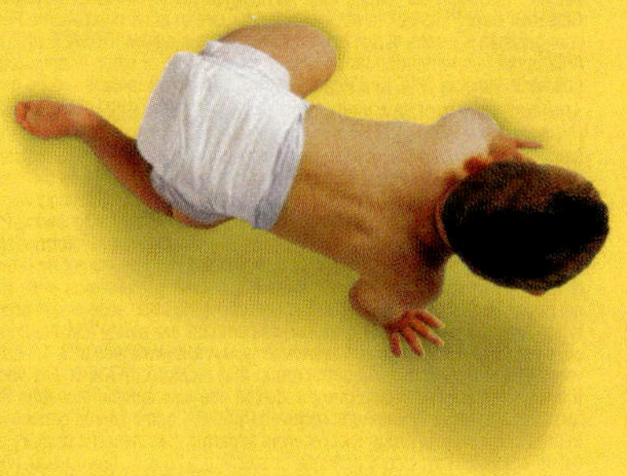

## PEDIARIX may help ensure timely vaccination with fewer injections

- With just 1 dose at 2, 4, and 6 months of age (in infants born of HBsAg-negative mothers)

*Based on analysis of the first four DTaP doses in the most recent National Immunization Survey (2003) of 21,210 children 19–35 months of age.

In clinical studies, adverse events in infants receiving PEDIARIX included injection-site reactions (pain, redness, or swelling), fever, and fussiness. Administration of PEDIARIX was associated with higher rates of fever relative to separately administered vaccines (see Adverse Reactions section of the brief summary). PEDIARIX is contraindicated in infants with known hypersensitivity to any component of the vaccine including yeast, neomycin, and polymyxin B. As with any vaccine, vaccination with PEDIARIX may not protect 100% of susceptible individuals.

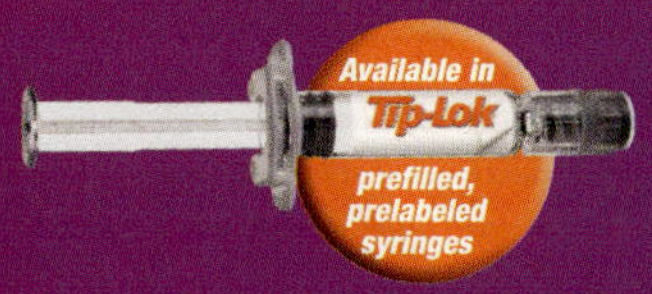


**Please see brief summary for PEDIARIX on the following page.**

**References: 1.** Centers for Disease Control and Prevention. National, state, and urban area vaccination coverage among children aged 19–35 months—United States, 2003. *MMWR.* 2004;53(29):658–661.



Manufactured by **GlaxoSmithKline Biologicals,** Rixensart, Belgium
Distributed by **GlaxoSmithKline,** Research Triangle Park, NC 27709

**Pediarix**

**Diphtheria and Tetanus Toxoids and Acellular Pertussis Adsorbed, Hepatitis B (Recombinant) and Inactivated Poliovirus Vaccine Combined**

gsk GlaxoSmithKline Vaccines

**PEDIARIX™ [Diphtheria and Tetanus Toxoids and Acellular Pertussis Adsorbed, Hepatitis B (Recombinant) and Inactivated Poliovirus Vaccine Combined]**

The following is a brief summary only; see full prescribing information for complete product information.

**CONTRAINDICATIONS:** Hypersensitivity to any component of the vaccine, including yeast, neomycin, and polymyxin B, is a contraindication (see DESCRIPTION in complete prescribing information). Do not use PEDIARIX after a serious allergic reaction (e.g., anaphylaxis) temporally associated with a previous dose of this vaccine or with any components of this vaccine. Because of the uncertainty as to which component of the vaccine might be responsible, do not give further vaccination with any of these components; or, refer such individuals to an allergist for evaluation. The following events are contraindications to administration of PEDIARIX: encephalopathy (e.g., coma, decreased level of consciousness, prolonged seizures) within 7 days of administration of a previous dose of a pertussis-containing vaccine that is not attributable to another identifiable cause; progressive neurologic disorder, including infantile spasms, uncontrolled epilepsy, or progressive encephalopathy. Do not vaccinate individuals with such conditions until a treatment regimen has been established and the condition has stabilized. PEDIARIX is not contraindicated for use in individuals with HIV infection.

**WARNINGS:** Administration of PEDIARIX is associated with higher rates of fever relative to separately administered vaccines. In one study that evaluated medically attended fever after the first dose of PEDIARIX or separately administered vaccines, infants who received PEDIARIX had a higher rate of medical encounters for fever within the first 4 days following vaccination. In some infants, these encounters included the performance of diagnostic studies to evaluate other causes of fever (see ADVERSE REACTIONS). The vial stopper is latex-free. The tip cap and the rubber plunger of the needleless prefilled syringes contain dry natural latex rubber that may cause allergic reactions in latex sensitive individuals. If any of the following events occur in temporal relation to receipt of whole-cell DTP or a vaccine containing an acellular pertussis component, consider carefully whether to give subsequent doses of PEDIARIX or any vaccine containing a pertussis component: temperature of ≥40.5°C (105°F) within 48 hours not due to another identifiable cause; collapse or shock-like state (hypotonic-hyporesponsive episode) within 48 hours; persistent, inconsolable crying lasting ≥3 hours, occurring within 48 hours; seizures with or without fever occurring within 3 days. If Guillain-Barré syndrome occurs within 6 weeks of receipt of prior vaccine containing tetanus toxoid, the decision to give subsequent doses of PEDIARIX or any vaccine containing tetanus toxoid should be based on careful consideration of the potential benefits and possible risks. A committee of the Institute of Medicine (IOM) has concluded that evidence is consistent with a causal relationship between whole-cell DTP vaccine and acute neurologic illness, and under special circumstances, between whole-cell DTP vaccine and chronic neurologic disease in the context of the National Childhood Encephalopathy Study (NCES) report; however, evidence was insufficient to indicate whether or not whole-cell DTP vaccine increased the overall risk of chronic neurologic disease. Acute encephalopathy and permanent neurologic damage have not been reported causally linked or in temporal association with administration of PEDIARIX, but the experience with PEDIARIX is insufficient to rule this out. Encephalopathy has been reported following INFANRIX® (Diphtheria and Tetanus Toxoids and Acellular Pertussis Vaccine Adsorbed) (see ADVERSE REACTIONS, Postmarketing Reports), but data are not sufficient to evaluate a causal relationship. The decision to administer a pertussis-containing vaccine to children with stable central nervous system (CNS) disorders must be made by the physician on an individual basis, with consideration of all relevant factors, and assessment of potential risks and benefits for that individual. Advise the parent or guardian of the potential increased risk involved (see PRECAUTIONS). A family history of seizures or other CNS disorders is not a contraindication to pertussis vaccine. For children at higher risk for seizures than the general population, an appropriate antipyretic may be administered at the time of vaccination and for the ensuing 24 hours according to the respective prescribing information recommended dosage to reduce the possibility of post-vaccination fever. Defer vaccination during the course of a moderate or severe illness with or without fever and vaccinate patients as soon as they have recovered from the acute phase of the illness. Do not give PEDIARIX to children on anticoagulant therapy or those with bleeding disorders unless the potential benefit clearly outweighs the risk of administration (see PRECAUTIONS in complete prescribing information).

**PRECAUTIONS:** Before the injection of any biological, the physician should take all reasonable precautions to prevent allergic or other adverse reactions. Epinephrine injection (1:1000) and other appropriate agents used for the control of immediate allergic reactions must be immediately available should an acute anaphylactic reaction occur. Immunosuppressed individuals, including those receiving immunosuppressive therapy, may not develop the expected immune response. **Drug Interactions:** For information regarding concomitant administration with other vaccines, refer to DOSAGE AND ADMINISTRATION in complete prescribing information. Do not mix PEDIARIX with any other vaccine in the same syringe or vial. **Carcinogenesis, Mutagenesis, Impairment of Fertility:** PEDIARIX has not been evaluated for carcinogenic or mutagenic potential, or for impairment of fertility. **Pregnancy:** Pregnancy Category C: PEDIARIX is not indicated for women of child-bearing age. Animal reproduction studies have not been conducted with PEDIARIX. It is not known whether PEDIARIX can cause fetal harm when administered to a pregnant woman or if PEDIARIX can affect reproductive capacity. **Geriatric Use:** PEDIARIX is not indicated for use in adult populations. **Pediatric Use:** Safety and effectiveness of PEDIARIX in infants younger than 6 weeks of age have not been evaluated (see DOSAGE AND ADMINISTRATION in complete prescribing information). PEDIARIX is not recommended for persons 7 years of age or older. Tetanus and Diphtheria Toxoids Adsorbed (Td) For Adult Use, inactivated poliovirus vaccine (IPV), and Hepatitis B Vaccine (Recombinant) should be used in individuals 7 years of age or older.

**ADVERSE REACTIONS:** A total of 20,739 doses of PEDIARIX have been administered to 7,028 infants as a 3-dose primary series. The most common adverse reactions observed in clinical trials were local injection site reactions (pain, redness, or swelling), fever, and fussiness. In comparative studies, administration of PEDIARIX was associated with higher rates of fever relative to separately administered vaccines (see WARNINGS). The prevalence of fever was highest on the day of vaccination and the day following vaccination. More than 98% of episodes of fever resolved within the 4-day period following vaccination (i.e., the period including the day of vaccination and the next 3 days). Rates of most other solicited adverse events following PEDIARIX were comparable to rates observed following separately administered US-licensed vaccines. The adverse event information from clinical trials provides a basis for identifying adverse events that appear to be related to vaccine use and for approximating rates. However, because clinical trials are conducted under widely varying conditions, adverse event rates observed in the clinical trials of a vaccine cannot be directly compared to rates in the clinical trials of another vaccine, and may not reflect the rates observed in practice. A total of 5,472 infants were enrolled in a German safety study that was originally designed to compare the safety and reactogenicity of PEDIARIX administered concomitantly at separate sites with 1 of 4 *Haemophilus influenzae* type b (Hib) vaccines at 3, 4, and 5 months of age. After enrollment of 1,569 infants, the study was amended to include a control group that received INFANRIX, Hib vaccine, and oral poliovirus vaccine (OPV) separately. Infants in the separate administration group received one less antigen (hepatitis B) than the infants who received PEDIARIX. Safety data were available for 4,666 infants who received PEDIARIX administered concomitantly at separate sites with 1 of 4 Hib vaccines and for 768 infants in the control group that received separate vaccines. The primary end-point of the study was the percentage of infants with any grade 3 solicited symptom (redness or swelling >20 mm, fever >103.1°F, or crying, pain, vomiting, diarrhea, loss of appetite, or restlessness that prevented normal daily activities) over the 3-dose primary series in infants who received PEDIARIX (4 groups that received PEDIARIX and Hib vaccines pooled) compared to the group that received INFANRIX and Hib vaccine separately with OPV. Analysis for the primary end-point was performed on the according-to-protocol (ATP) cohort that included only those infants who were enrolled after the protocol amendment to include a control group. Of 3,773 infants in the ATP cohort for whom safety data were available, 16.2% (95% CI: 14.9% to 17.5%) of 3,029 infants who received PEDIARIX and Hib vaccine compared to 20.3% (95% CI: 17.5% to 23.4%) of 744 infants who received separate vaccines were reported to have had at least one grade 3 solicited symptom within 4 days of vaccination (i.e., day of vaccination and the next 3 days). The difference between groups in the rate of grade 3 symptoms was 4.1% (90% CI: 1.4% to 7.1%). These were the rates for selected solicited symptoms within 4 days following each dose in a 3-dose primary series in infants who received PEDIARIX administered concomitantly with Hib vaccine and those who received separate concomitant administration of INFANRIX, Hib vaccine, and OPV for the intent-to-treat (ITT) cohort (includes all infants enrolled before and after the amendment who received the indicated vaccine and for whom at least one symptom sheet was completed):

**Percentage of German Infants With Solicited Local Reactions or Selected Systemic Adverse Events Within 4 Days of Vaccination* (ITT Cohort)**

| | PEDIARIX & Hib | | | INFANRIX, Hib, & OPV | | |
|---|---|---|---|---|---|---|
| | **Dose 1** | **Dose 2** | **Dose 3** | **Dose 1** | **Dose 2** | **Dose 3** |
| **N** | **4,666** | **4,619** | **4,574** | **768** | **757** | **750** |
| **Local†** | | | | | | |
| Pain, any | 14.0 | 10.2 | 9.9 | 14.2 | 9.8 | 8.1 |
| Pain, grade 2 or 3 | 2.9 | 1.2 | 1.5 | 3.6 | 1.7 | 1.1 |
| Pain, grade 3 | 0.7 | 0.3 | 0.3 | 1.3 | 0.4 | 0.1 |
| Redness, any | 18.6 | 26.6 | 25.6 | 16.1 | 21.4 | 20.8 |
| Redness, >5 mm | 6.7 | 9.9 | 9.0 | 5.9 | 8.2 | 7.7 |
| Redness, >20 mm | 1.2 | 1.0 | 1.1 | 1.8 | 0.7 | 1.1 |
| Swelling, any | 12.7 | 18.5 | 18.4 | 9.6 | 12.9 | 13.6 |
| Swelling, >5 mm | 5.6 | 7.7 | 7.8 | 3.6 | 5.2 | 4.8 |
| Swelling, >20 mm | 1.2 | 1.6 | 1.5 | 1.3 | 1.1 | 1.2 |
| **Systemic** | | | | | | |
| Restlessness, any | 41.4 | 32.0 | 26.7 | 46.4 | 35.0 | 27.6 |
| Restlessness, grade 2 or 3 | 14.4 | 10.0 | 8.9 | 20.2 | 11.5 | 8.4 |
| Restlessness, grade 3 | 3.0 | 1.5 | 1.6 | 5.7 | 3.0 | 1.7 |
| Fever‡, ≥100.4°F | 25.1 | 19.3 | 19.7 | 13.2 | 13.1 | 11.2 |
| Fever‡, >101.3°F | 5.8 | 4.1 | 4.6 | 2.2 | 2.8 | 2.1 |
| Fever‡, >103.1°F | 0.3 | 0.5 | 0.7 | 0.3 | 0.3 | 0.5 |
| Unusual cry§, any | 24.9 | 16.5 | 13.1 | 36.5 | 19.7 | 14.3 |
| Unusual cry§, grade 2 or 3 | 12.7 | 7.1 | 5.7 | 20.8 | 10.0 | 5.7 |
| Unusual cry§, grade 3 | 3.9 | 1.7 | 1.4 | 6.8 | 2.1 | 1.1 |
| Loss of appetite, any | 17.9 | 13.3 | 12.5 | 19.1 | 16.2 | 11.3 |
| Loss of appetite, grade 2 or 3 | 4.0 | 2.9 | 2.7 | 4.4 | 2.9 | 2.3 |
| Loss of appetite, grade 3 | 0.6 | 0.5 | 0.4 | 0.5 | 0.7 | 0.0 |

N = number of infants in the intent-to-treat (ITT) cohort.
Grade 2 defined as sufficiently discomforting to interfere with daily activities.
Grade 3 defined as preventing normal daily activities.
* Within 4 days of vaccination defined as day of vaccination and the next 3 days.
† Local reactions at the injection site for PEDIARIX or INFANRIX.
‡ Rectal temperatures.
§ Unusual cry lasting >1 hour.

In this study, infants were also monitored for unsolicited adverse events that occurred within 30 days following vaccination. Over the entire study period, 6 subjects in the group that received PEDIARIX reported seizures. Two of these subjects had a febrile seizure, 1 of whom also developed afebrile seizures. The remaining 4 subjects had afebrile seizures, including 2 with infantile spasms. Two subjects reported seizures within 7 days following vaccination (1 subject had both febrile and afebrile seizures, and 1 subject had afebrile seizures), corresponding to a rate of 0.22 seizures per 1,000 doses (febrile seizures 0.07 per 1,000 doses, afebrile seizures 0.14 per 1,000 doses). No subject who received concomitant INFANRIX, Hib vaccine, and OPV reported seizures. In a separate German study that evaluated the safety of INFANRIX in 22,505 infants who received 66,867 doses of INFANRIX administered as a 3-dose primary series, the rate of seizures within 7 days of vaccination with INFANRIX was 0.13 per 1,000 doses (febrile seizures 0.0 per 1,000 doses, afebrile seizures 0.13 per 1,000 doses). No cases of hypotonic-hyporesponsiveness, encephalopathy, or anaphylaxis were reported in the German study that evaluated the safety of PEDIARIX. Rates of serious adverse events that are less common than those reported in this safety study are not known at this time.

Additional safety data for PEDIARIX are available from a US study designed to evaluate lot-to-lot consistency and a bridge for a new manufacturing step. These were the rates for local reactions and selected adverse events within 4 days of vaccination with PEDIARIX administered concomitantly with a Hib vaccine at 2, 4, and 6 months of age:

**Percentage of US Infants With Solicited Local Reactions or Selected Systemic Adverse Events Within 4 Days of Vaccination* (ITT Cohort)**

| | PEDIARIX & Hib | | |
|---|---|---|---|
| | **Dose 1** | **Dose 2** | **Dose 3** |
| **Local†** | **N = 482** | **N = 469** | **N = 466** |
| Pain, any | 30.5 | 25.4 | 23.0 |
| Pain, grade 2 or 3 | 6.2 | 5.5 | 3.6 |
| Pain, grade 3 | 1.2 | 0.6 | 0.6 |
| Redness, any | 25.3 | 32.6 | 35.6 |
| Redness, >5 mm | 9.3 | 10.4 | 8.6 |
| Redness, >20 mm | 0.6 | 1.5 | 1.3 |
| Swelling, any | 15.1 | 16.6 | 22.3 |
| Swelling, >5 mm | 6.8 | 6.2 | 6.4 |
| Swelling, >20 mm | 1.0 | 1.3 | 1.3 |
| **Systemic** | **N = 482** | **N = 469** | **N = 467** |
| Restlessness, any | 28.8 | 30.3 | 28.5 |
| Restlessness, grade 2 or 3 | 7.1 | 9.0 | 9.4 |
| Restlessness, grade 3 | 1.0 | 1.1 | 0.6 |
| Fever‡, ≥100.4°F | 26.6 | 31.3 | 25.9 |
| Fever‡, >101.3°F | 2.9 | 6.2 | 4.7 |
| Fever‡, >103.1°F | 0.0 | 0.2 | 0.6 |
| Fussiness, any | 61.8 | 63.8 | 57.0 |
| Fussiness, grade 2 or 3 | 14.9 | 21.5 | 17.1 |
| Fussiness, grade 3 | 2.7 | 3.4 | 1.7 |
| Loss of appetite, any | 21.6 | 19.8 | 18.8 |
| Loss of appetite, grade 2 or 3 | 3.1 | 3.2 | 2.4 |
| Loss of appetite, grade 3 | 0.2 | 0.4 | 0.0 |
| Sleeping more than usual, any | 46.7 | 31.8 | 28.1 |
| Sleeping more than usual, grade 2 or 3 | 10.2 | 6.0 | 4.7 |
| Sleeping more than usual, grade 3 | 1.7 | 0.4 | 0.6 |

N = number of infants in the intent-to-treat (ITT) cohort (infants who received the indicated vaccine and for whom at least one symptom sheet was completed).
Grade 2 defined as sufficiently discomforting to interfere with daily activities.
Grade 3 defined as preventing normal daily activities.
* Within 4 days of vaccination defined as day of vaccination and the next 3 days.
† Local reactions at the injection site for PEDIARIX.
‡ Rectal temperatures.

In another US study, these were the rates for fever within 4 days following dose 1 (i.e., day of vaccination and the next 3 days) at 2 months of age in infants who received PEDIARIX when administered concomitantly at separate sites with Hib and pneumococcal conjugate vaccines and those who received INFANRIX, ENGERIX-B® [Hepatitis B Vaccine (Recombinant)], IPV, Hib vaccine, and pneumococcal conjugate vaccine:

**Percentage of US Infants With Fever Within 4 Days of Dose 1* (ITT Cohort)**

| | PEDIARIX, Hib, & Pneumococcal Conjugate (N = 667) | INFANRIX, ENGERIX-B, IPV, Hib, & Pneumococcal Conjugate (N = 333) | Separate Vaccine Group Minus Combination Vaccine Group |
|---|---|---|---|
| **Fever†** | **%** | **%** | **Difference (95% CI)** |
| ≥100.4°F‡ | 27.9 | 19.8 | -8.07 (-13.54, -2.60) |
| >101.3°F | 7.0 | 4.5 | -2.54 (-5.50, 0.41) |
| >102.2°F‡ | 2.2 | 0.3 | -1.95 (-3.22, -0.68) |
| >103.1°F | 0.4 | 0.0 | -0.45 (-0.96, 0.06) |
| M.A.‡ | 1.2 | 0.0 | -1.20 (-2.03, -037) |

N = number of infants for whom at least one symptom sheet was completed, excluding 3 infants for whom temperature was not measured and 3 infants whose temperature was measured by the tympanic method.
*Within 4 days of dose 1 defined as day of vaccination and the next 3 days.
† Rectal temperatures.
‡ The group that received PEDIARIX compared to separate vaccine group p value <0.05 (2-sided Fisher Exact test) or the 95% confidence interval on the difference between groups does not include 0.
M.A. = Medically attended (a visit to or from medical personnel).

In this study, medical attention (a visit to or from medical personnel) for fever within 4 days following vaccination was sought for 8 infants who received PEDIARIX (1.2%) and no infants who received separately administered vaccines. Four infants were seen by medical personnel in an office setting; no diagnostic tests were performed in 2 of the infants and a complete blood count (CBC) was done in the other 2 infants. Of 3 infants who were seen in an emergency room, all had a CBC and a blood and urine culture performed; chest X-rays were done in 2 of the infants and a nasopharyngeal specimen was tested for Respiratory Syncytial Virus in one of the infants. One infant was hospitalized for a work-up that included a CBC, blood and urine cultures, a lumbar puncture, and a chest X-ray. All episodes of medically attended fever resolved within 4 days post-vaccination.

Limited data are available from a study conducted in Moldova in which infants received a dose of hepatitis B vaccine within 48 hours of birth followed by 3 doses of PEDIARIX at 6, 10, and 14 weeks of age. No information was collected on the HBsAg status of mothers of enrolled infants. These were the rates for local reactions and selected adverse events within 4 days of vaccination with PEDIARIX administered comcomitantly with Hib vaccine following a birth dose of hepatitis B vaccine:

**Percentage of Moldovan Infants With Solicited Local Reactions or Selected Systemic Adverse Events Within 4 Days of Vaccination* (ITT Cohort)**

| | PEDIARIX & Hib | | |
|---|---|---|---|
| | **Dose 1** | **Dose 2** | **Dose 3** |
| **N** | **160** | **158** | **157** |
| **Local†** | | | |
| Pain, any | 25.6 | 18.4 | 14.0 |
| Pain, grade 3 | 3.1 | 0.6 | 1.9 |
| Redness, any | 41.9 | 41.8 | 47.1 |
| Redness, >20 mm | 1.9 | 2.5 | 4.5 |
| Swelling, any | 20.6 | 18.4 | 28.0 |
| Swelling, >20 mm | 4.4 | 2.5 | 7.0 |
| **Systemic** | | | |
| Restlessness, any | 13.1 | 10.8 | 8.9 |
| Restlessness, grade 3 | 1.3 | 0.6 | 0.6 |
| Fever‡, ≥100.4°F | 14.4 | 11.4 | 5.1 |
| Fever‡, >103.1°F | 0.0 | 0.6 | 0.0 |
| Fussiness, any | 25.0 | 21.5 | 17.8 |
| Fussiness, grade 3 | 2.5 | 0.6 | 0.6 |

N = number of infants in the intent-to-treat (ITT) cohort (infants who received the indicated vaccine and for whom at least one symptom sheet was completed).
Grade 3 defined as preventing normal daily activities.
*Within 4 days of vaccination defined as day of vaccination and the next 3 days.
† Local reactions at the injection site for PEDIARIX.
‡ Rectal temperatures.

Although there was no comparator group who received PEDIARIX without a birth dose of hepatitis B vaccine, available data suggest that some local adverse events may occur at a higher rate when PEDIARIX is administered after a birth dose of hepatitis B vaccine.

As with any vaccine, there is the possibility that broad use of PEDIARIX could reveal adverse events not observed in clinical trials.

**Postmarketing Reports:** Worldwide voluntary reports of adverse events received for INFANRIX and ENGERIX-B in children younger than 7 years of age since market introduction of these US-licensed vaccines are listed below. This list includes adverse events for which 20 or more reports were received with the exception of intussusception, idiopathic thrombocytopenic purpura, thrombocytopenia, anaphylactic reaction, angioedema, encephalopathy, hypotonic-hyporesponsive episode, and alopecia for which fewer than 20 reports were received. These latter events are included either because of the seriousness of the event or the strength of causal connection to components of this or other vaccines or drugs. *Body as a whole*: Asthenia[b], fever[a+b], lethargy[b], malaise[b], Sudden Infant Death Syndrome[a+b]. *Cardiovascular system*: Cyanosis[a+b], edema[b], pallor[b]. *Gastrointestinal system*: Abdominal pain[b], anorexia[b], diarrhea[a+b], intussusception[a+b], nausea[b], vomiting[a+b]. *Hematologic/lymphatic*: Idiopathic thrombocytopenic purpura[a+b], lymphadenopathy[a], thrombocytopenia[a+b]. *Hepatic*: Jaundice[b], liver function tests abnormal[b]. *Hypersensitivity*: Anaphylactic reaction[a+b], angioedema[b], hypersensitivity[a]. *Infections*: Cellulitis[a]. *Injection site reactions*: Injection site reactions[a+b]. *Musculoskeletal*: Arthralgia[b], limb swelling[a+b]. *Nervous system*: Convulsions[a+b], encephalopathy[a], headache[b], hypotonia[a+b], hypotonic-hyporesponsive episode[a], somnolence[a+b]. *Psychiatric*: Crying[a+b], irritability[a+b]. *Respiratory system*: Respiratory tract infection[a]. *Skin and appendages*: Alopecia[b], erythema[a+b], erythema multiforme[b], petechiae[b], pruritus[a+b], rash[a+b], urticaria[a+b]. *Special senses*: Ear pain[a]. [[a] Following INFANRIX; [b] Following ENGERIX-B; [a+b] Following either INFANRIX or ENGERIX-B.] These reactions were reported voluntarily from a population of uncertain size; therefore, it is not always possible to reliably estimate their frequency or establish a causal relationship to vaccination.

**Reporting Adverse Events:** Report the occurrence following immunization of any event set forth in the Vaccine Injury Table from the National Childhood Vaccine Injury Act including: Anaphylaxis or anaphylactic shock within 7 days, encephalopathy or encephalitis within 7 days, brachial neuritis within 28 days, or an acute complication or sequelae (including death) of an illness, disability, injury, or condition referred to above, or any events that would contraindicate further doses of PEDIARIX. The VAERS toll-free number is 1-800-822-7967.

Manufactured by **GlaxoSmithKline Biologicals**, Rixensart, Belgium, US License 1617

Distributed by **GlaxoSmithKline,** Research Triangle Park, NC 27709

PEDIARIX is a trademark and TIP-LOK, INFANRIX, and ENGERIX-B are registered trademarks of GlaxoSmithKline.

Full prescribing information for PEDIARIX is available at www.GSKVaccines.com/Pediarix. BRS-PE:L2

 PED583R0 June 2005

ARTICLE

# Evaluation of a Novel Web-Based Pediatric Advanced Life Support Course

*James M. Gerard, MD; Anthony J. Scalzo, MD; Steven P. Laffey, MD; Glen Sinks, RN, MSN, CS, FNP, EMT-P; Diana Fendya, RN, MSN; Patrice Seratti, BS*

**Objective:** To assess the educational efficacy of a Web-based pediatric advanced life support course (Web-PALS).

**Design:** Nonrandomized, prospective, cohort study.

**Setting:** University medical center.

**Participants:** Health care providers (includes physicians, nurses, paramedics, and respiratory therapists) taking either the Web-PALS or a traditional PALS course (Trad-PALS).

**Main Exposure:** Web-PALS.

**Main Outcome Measures:** Postcourse written examination scores and scored videotapes of students performing 5 PALS procedures were compared between study groups. Students completed precourse and postcourse questionnaires, rating on a 5-point Likert scale their self-confidence to perform PALS assessments and procedures. A structured, course satisfaction survey was given after students had taken the Web-PALS course.

**Results:** Eighty-six students completed the study (44 Web-PALS and 42 Trad-PALS). All students achieved a passing score on the written examination on their first attempt. Compared with students in the Trad-PALS group, students in the Web-PALS group scored slightly lower (97.1% vs 95.4%; difference, 1.7%; 95% confidence interval, 0.1-3.2). Mean overall videotape scores were similar among the Web-PALS and Trad-PALS groups (75.0% vs 73.0%; difference, 2.0%; 95% confidence interval, –2.0 to 6.0). After completing the Web-PALS course, the mean level of confidence improved from 3.77 to 4.28 (difference, 0.51; 95% confidence interval, 0.33-0.69). Ninety-six percent of respondents indicated that Web-PALS met all of the stated objectives of the PALS course. All respondents indicated that they would recommend Web-PALS to a colleague.

**Conclusions:** Students perceive Web-PALS as a positive educational experience. Though not identical to students taking the Trad-PALS course, they performed well on postcourse cognitive and psychomotor testing. These findings support Web-PALS as an acceptable format for administering the PALS course.

*Arch Pediatr Adolesc Med. 2006;160:649-655*

IN COOPERATION WITH THE AMERICAN Heart Association (AHA), in July 2002, we introduced a Web-based pediatric advanced life support course (Web-PALS)that teaches the cognitive portion of the PALS material via an Internet Web site. Through the Web site, students learn PALS concepts by completing 6 interactive, case-based modules. After completing online modules, students attend a 1-day course that provides the psychomotor training and testing components of the course. This format is similar to other self-directed, distance-taught life support courses such as the CD-ROM–based HeartCode advanced cardiac life support Anywhere course[1] and the online basic life support for health care providers[2] and electronic advanced cardiac life support[3] renewal courses. Web-PALS is offered to students taking an initial course and to those seeking recertification.

The Web-PALS course allows students to review the cognitive portion of the PALS material at a convenient time and at their own pace. The reduced onsite time lessens time away from home and office and has the potential to decrease travel-related expenses. The Web-PALS course offers advantages for PALS instructors and administrators by providing cognitive material online, thus decreasing the number of instructor-hours and related expenses to teach the PALS course. It ensures that the cognitive material is provided in a consistent manner, including the dissemination of PALS updates to all students. Finally, with the increasing availability of broadband Internet access, in the future,

***For editorial comment see page 658***

Author Affiliations: Departments of Pediatrics, Division of Pediatric Emergency Medicine, Saint Louis University School of Medicine (Drs Gerard, Scalzo, and Laffey), and Cardinal Glennon Children's Hospital (Mr Sinks and Mss Fendya and Seratti), St Louis, Mo.

Web-PALS will be ideally suited to present AHA-developed instructional videos to students taking the PALS course.

We describe the development of the Web-PALS course and a pilot study to assess its educational efficacy. The primary objective of the study was to compare the cognitive and psychomotor performance of students who completed the Web-PALS course with that of students who completed a traditional, classroom-based PALS course (Trad-PALS). Secondary goals were to assess the effect of the Web-PALS course on student self-confidence to perform PALS assessments and procedures and their overall satisfaction with the course.

## METHODS

### COURSE DEVELOPMENT

Core material from the PALS course was incorporated into 6 interactive, case-based modules: respiratory failure, shock, newly born, rhythm disturbances, trauma, and cardiac arrest. Each module contains a list of objectives, an interactive case, links to pertinent algorithms, and postmodule questions. Postmodule questions differ from those on the postcourse written examination. For each module, students select from a prehospital or hospital setting. Each module is designed to take approximately 1 to1½ hours to complete.

Students access the Web site at http://myamericanheart.org. The current charge for taking Web-PALS, including online and onsite components, is comparable to the charge for a traditional 2-day PALS course. A link for purchasing a hard-copy PALS textbook is provided on the Web site. Students must satisfactorily complete the AHA PALS pretest (minimum score, 85%) online before entering the modules. To complete each module, students must correctly answer 85% of the postmodule questions.

After completing the modules, students are eligible to take a 1-day skills/testing course, which is an 8-hour onsite class formatted to meet all of the AHA requirements for instruction of the psychomotor components of the PALS course.[4] During the 1-day skills/testing course, students rotate through skills instructional stations and case scenario practice stations. At the end of the course, students attend practical evaluation stations and complete the postcourse written examination. After satisfactory completion of the course, students receive an AHA course completion card.

### STUDY DESIGN AND SUBJECTS

Between July 16, 2002, and September 4, 2003, health care providers (includes physicians, nurses, paramedics, and respiratory therapists) taking either a Web-PALS or Trad-PALS course at the Saint Louis University Health Sciences Center were recruited into the study. The Trad-PALS course taught at our institution is a 3-day pediatric advanced cardiorespiratory and trauma support (PACTS)–PALS course that integrates all of the PALS elements with additional PACTS material. The PACTS curriculum, developed at our institution, consists of classroom lectures on topics such as surgical, neurosurgical, and toxicologic emergencies. In addition, students rotate through a practical trauma skills and scenario station.[5]

During the study, subjects were recruited from 14 PALS courses (8 Web-PALS and 6 Trad-PALS). All students, regardless of profession or previous PALS experience, were eligible to participate. Subjects were excluded from consideration if they were enrolled in a 1-day PALS recertification course. As an incentive, study subjects were reimbursed $50.00. The study was approved by the Institutional Review Board at Saint Louis University. All subjects provided written informed consent.

### DEMOGRAPHIC AND SELF-CONFIDENCE DATA

Before the start of each PALS course, study subjects completed questionnaires to provide demographic and self-confidence data. The self-confidence portion, adapted from a questionnaire developed by Craven and Froman,[6] consisted of 39 items on which students rated their confidence level to perform various PALS assessments and procedures on a 5-point Likert scale (1, very little; 5, quite a lot). Students taking the Web-PALS course completed the questionnaire online before being allowed into the educational modules. Students taking the Trad-PALS course completed the questionnaire at the beginning of the first day of each course. The self-confidence questionnaire was readministered to subjects immediately after completion of the course. Changes in self-confidence scores were assessed for students within each study group.

### COGNITIVE PERFORMANCE

To assess cognitive performance, scores from the AHA postcourse written examination were collected. The postcourse written examination consists of 33 multiple-choice questions developed and validated by the Pediatric Resuscitation Subcommittee of the AHA (Mary Fran Hazinski, MSN, written communication, January 2004). Successful completion of the written examination (minimum score, 84%) is required to receive PALS certification. Version A of the 2002 AHA PALS examination was used for both groups throughout the study. The frequency of correct responses for each examination question and overall mean examination scores were compared between groups.

### PSYCHOMOTOR PERFORMANCE

To assess psychomotor skills, videotapes were made of each subject performing a rapid cardiopulmonary assessment (RCPA) and 4 PALS procedures in a mock resuscitation setting. The videotaping protocol was modified from a protocol previously described by White et al[7] and Quan et al.[8] The procedures included bag-mask ventilation, tracheal intubation, intraosseous needle insertion, and rhythm assessment/defibrillation. Subjects participated in the videotaping sessions immediately after completion of each PALS course. The videotaping session was an additional station that study subjects participated in individually after completing the usual practical evaluation and written testing stations. Students were given a single opportunity to perform each task. Skill performance was not timed.

The videotaping sessions took place in a classroom setting with 4 Laerdal mannequins (Laerdal Medical Corp, Wappingers Falls, NY), a cardiac monitor/defibrillator with Laerdal 2000 HeartSim Rhythm Simulator, and standard PALS resuscitation equipment. Mannequin features included inflatable lungs, an intubatable airway, and an artificial tibia for intraosseous needle insertion. The room setup and equipment was identical for each videotaping session. One of 5 certified PALS instructors, trained in the study protocol, served as the moderator during each session. For practical considerations, moderators (including J.M.G., A.J. S. and S.P.L.) were not blinded to which course subjects had taken.

Each subject was given an identical scenario for the RCPA and each procedure. Reading from a prepared, written script, the moderator described the mock scenario, the age of the patient, and the specific task to be performed, for example, "You are asked to see a 6-month-old infant with a 2-day history of cough and trouble breathing. Please perform a rapid cardiopulmonary assessment." Moderators provided identical, scripted answers for all of the RCPA assessments and procedures. Moderators were instructed not to lead or prompt the students in any way during the videotaping sessions.

At the end of the study, videotapes were scored by a group of reviewers blinded to which course subjects had taken. The review group consisted of 3 certified PALS instructors or medical directors with extensive experience in this field. Reviewers were not involved in developing the Web-PALS program and were not instructors of any of the PALS courses.

A 41-item score sheet identifying key subcomponents of the RCPA and procedures was designed for this study. Each of these subcomponents is listed as a specific teaching point within the PALS instructor manual and is considered important for the optimal performance of the RCPA and each procedure.[4] Reviewers used this score sheet to grade each subject's performance. To score a subcomponent as being performed properly, the subcomponent had to be performed correctly and at an appropriate time in the given scenario. No partial credit was given.

To aid in scoring agreement, before scoring the videotapes, the reviewers met as a group with study investigators. Videotapes of 5 subjects were extensively reviewed and discussed for the scoring process. Disagreements on scoring of individual subcomponents were discussed and a consensus was reached on how subcomponents would be scored.

Over a 2-day period, each subject's videotape was independently scored by a single reviewer. These scores were used for comparisons between the study groups. After scoring the subjects' videotapes, each reviewer was given a copy of the videotapes of 10 randomly selected subjects. Each reviewer independently scored these same 10 subjects' videotapes, and the results were used to assess interrater agreement.

After completion of videotape scoring, study investigators (J.M.G. and P.S.) tabulated the score sheets. For each subject, an overall score (the number of all correctly performed subcomponents) as well as individual scores for the RCPA and each procedure were recorded. The frequency of correct performance for each subcomponent was compared between the study groups. In addition, group comparisons were made for mean overall score, RCPA score, and individual procedure score.

## WEB-PALS SURVEY

After completion of each Web-PALS course, to elicit feedback on the course, all students were given a 24-item, structured survey that addressed 3 main themes: technical aspects and usability of the Web-PALS site, content and flow of the online material, and content and flow of the 1-day skills/testing course. Many of the response formats used a continuous scale of 1 to 5 ("strongly disagree" or "really disliked" to "strongly agree or really liked," respectively) by which students rated the various aspects of the course. Partially completed surveys were included in the analyses. No attempt was made to elicit feedback from nonrespondents.

## STATISTICAL ANALYSIS

For written examination scores, based on data from previously taught Trad-PALS courses at our institution, we calculated that to detect a 2.5% difference in mean scores a sample size of 40 subjects in each study group would be needed to achieve a power of 80% at the .05 significance level. The study was not powered for other outcome measures.

Comparisons of proportions were made using the $\chi^2$ test or Fisher exact test. Because of a nonnormal distribution, the Mann-Whitney test was used to compare written examination scores. For the videotape component, mean overall scores and mean scores for the RCPA and each procedure were compared using independent-samples $t$ tests. Cohen's multirater $\kappa$ values were calculated to assess interrater agreement on videotape scoring. Paired-samples $t$ tests were used to compare precourse and postcourse self-confidence data. A 2-tailed $\alpha$ level of .05 was considered statistically significant for all analyses. Power analyses were performed using S-Plus Version 4.5 (Insightful Co, Seattle, Wash). All other analyses were performed using SPSS version 12 with the Exact Tests add-on module (SPSS Inc, Chicago, Ill). A macro titled mkappasc.sps was downloaded from the SPSS Web site that enables the base version of SPSS to calculate the Cohen multiple rater $\kappa$ values.

## RESULTS

During the study, excluding students enrolled in recertification classes, 349 students attended PALS courses (80 Web-PALS and 269 Trad-PALS) at our institution. Of this group, 88 subjects (46 Web-PALS and 42 Trad-PALS) were enrolled in the study. Two subjects from the Web-PALS group were excluded from the statistical analyses. One was excluded because of incomplete self-confidence data. The other was excluded because, after the course, it was discovered that the student had not completed all of the online modules; the student was inadvertently allowed to take the 1-day skills/testing session and mistakenly allowed in the study. Eighty-six subjects (44 Web-PALS and 42 Trad-PALS), therefore, make up the study groups for comparisons. There were no significant differences in demographic characteristics between the study groups (**Table 1**). Thirty-two students (73%) in the Web-PALS group were taking an online educational course for the first time.

All students in both groups successfully passed the postcourse written examination on the first attempt. Compared with students in the Trad-PALS group, students in the Web-PALS group scored slightly lower on the written examination (97.1% vs 95.4%; difference, 1.7%; 95% confidence interval [CI], 0.1-3.2). No significant differences were seen between groups for frequency of correct responses for any of the individual examination questions.

For interrater agreement of videotape scoring, using the classification scheme of Landis and Koch,[9] we rated agreement as poor or slight for 6 subcomponents, fair for 3, moderate for 7, substantial for 8, and nearly perfect for 17. Interrater agreement on overall videotape scores was substantial ($\kappa$=0.75). Agreement was nearly perfect for the RCPA ($\kappa$=0.86), substantial for the tracheal intubation, intraosseous needle insertion, and rhythm assessment/defibrillation procedures ($\kappa$=0.74, 0.69, and 0.75, respectively), and moderate for the bag-mask ventilation procedure ($\kappa$=0.58).

Students in the Web-PALS and Trad-PALS groups scored similarly on 38 of 41 skills subcomponents (**Table 2**). Differences between groups were seen for

**Table 1. Characteristics of Students in the Web-PALS and Trad-PALS Groups**

| Characteristic | Web-PALS (n = 44) No. (%) | Trad-PALS (n = 42) No. (%) | *P* Value |
|---|---|---|---|
| Occupation | | | |
| Physician | 12 (27) | 8 (19) | .61 |
| Nurse | 15 (34) | 16 (38) | |
| Paramedic | 16 (36) | 15 (36) | |
| Respiratory therapist | 1 (2) | 3 (7) | |
| Age, y | | | |
| ≤30 | 13 (29) | 16 (38) | .51 |
| 31-40 | 15 (34) | 14 (33) | |
| 41-50 | 10 (23) | 10 (24) | |
| >50 | 6 (14) | 2 (5) | |
| Male-female ratio | 24/20 (55) | 22/20 (52) | .84 |
| Primary work location | | | |
| Urban | 34 (77) | 31 (74) | .71 |
| Rural | 10 (23) | 11 (26) | |
| Experience, y | | | |
| ≤5 | 14 (32) | 14 (33) | .99 |
| 6-15 | 17 (39) | 16 (38) | |
| >15 | 13 (29) | 12 (29) | |
| Time caring for pediatric patients, % | | | |
| ≤10 | 18 (41) | 14 (33) | .82 |
| 11-50 | 12 (27) | 16 (38) | |
| >50 | 14 (32) | 12 (29) | |
| Had taken a previous PALS course | 32 (73) | 24 (57) | .13 |

Abbreviations: PALS, pediatric advanced life support course; Trad-PALS, traditional PALS, Web-PALS, Web-based PALS.

3 subcomponents. During the tracheal intubation procedure, students in the Web-PALS group more often inserted the tracheal tube to the proper depth (61% vs 38%; difference, 23%; $P = .03$) and more often properly secured the tracheal tube (77% vs 57%; $P = .046$). During bag-mask ventilation, students in the Web-PALS group used the proper-sized resuscitation bag less often than did students in the Trad-PALS group (34% vs 60%; $P = .02$).

Mean overall videotape scores were similar among the Web-PALS and Trad-PALS groups (75% vs 73%; difference, 2%; 95% CI, −2 to 6; **Table 3**). Students in the Web-PALS and Trad-PALS groups performed similarly on RCPA, bag-mask ventilation, and rhythm assessment/defibrillation procedures. Compared with students in the Trad-PALS group, those in the Web-PALS group scored higher on tracheal intubation (76% vs 68%; difference, 8%; 95% CI, 0.3-16) and intraosseous needle insertion (73% vs 64%; difference, 9%; 95% CI, 0.1-18).

Self-confidence to perform PALS assessments and procedures significantly improved in both groups after completion of the PALS course. In the Web-PALS group, mean self-confidence improved from 3.77 before the course to 4.28 after the course (difference, 0.51; 95% CI, 0.33-0.69). Among students in the Trad-PALS group, mean self-confidence improved from 3.57 before the course to 4.24 after the course (difference, 0.67; 95% CI, 0.52-0.81).

During the study, 60 students (75% of potential respondents) completed the Web-PALS postcourse survey (**Table 4** and **Table 5**). The results reveal that students seem to view the Web-PALS course as a posi-

**Table 2. Comparison of Correctly Performed Skills Subcomponents Among Web-PALS and Trad-PALS Groups**

| Subcomponent | Web-PALS (n = 44) No. (%) | Trad-PALS (n = 42) No. (%) | *P* Value |
|---|---|---|---|
| RCPA* | | | |
| Airway | 43 (98) | 40 (95) | .61 |
| Breathing | | | |
| Respiratory rate | 37 (84) | 35 (83) | .92 |
| Work of breathing | 27 (61) | 30 (71) | .32 |
| Air entry | 38 (86) | 39 (93) | .33 |
| Color | 35 (80) | 27 (64) | .12 |
| Attach pulse oximeter | 25 (57) | 24 (57) | .98 |
| Administer oxygen | 27 (61) | 30 (71) | .32 |
| Circulation | | | |
| Heart rate | 40 (91) | 32 (76) | .07 |
| Central pulse | 24 (55) | 30 (71) | .11 |
| Skin perfusion | 38 (86) | 39 (93) | .49 |
| Blood pressure | 22 (50) | 22 (52) | .83 |
| CNS perfusion | 34 (77) | 31 (74) | .71 |
| Bag-mask ventilation† | | | |
| Oxygen on | 14 (32) | 10 (24) | .41 |
| Proper bag size | 15 (34) | 25 (60) | .02 |
| Proper mask size | 41 (93) | 39 (93) | .99 |
| Position head (sniffing position) | 43 (98) | 39 (93) | .36 |
| Use E-C technique | 41 (93) | 40 (95) | .99 |
| No pressure on neck | 42 (96) | 42 (100) | .49 |
| Good mask seal | 39 (89) | 38 (91) | .99 |
| Assess chest rise | 41 (93) | 37 (88) | .48 |
| Tracheal intubation‡ | | | |
| Check laryngoscope light | 44 (100) | 38 (91) | >.05 |
| Correct tube size | 34 (77) | 27 (64) | .19 |
| Suction on | 23 (52) | 22 (52) | .99 |
| Preoxygenate | 32 (73) | 26 (62) | .28 |
| Correct tube depth | 27 (61) | 16 (38) | .03 |
| Assess chest rise | 36 (82) | 35 (83) | .85 |
| Auscultate | 35 (80) | 37 (88) | .28 |
| Place end-tidal $CO_2$ detector | 35 (80) | 30 (71) | .38 |
| Secure tube | 34 (77) | 24 (57) | .046 |
| Intraosseous needle insertion§ | | | |
| Prepare site | 21 (48) | 17 (41) | .499 |
| Twisting insertion motion | 38 (86) | 36 (86) | .93 |
| Needle stable in bone | 22 (50) | 14 (33) | .12 |
| Aspirate line | 38 (86) | 29 (69) | >.05 |
| Flush line | 41 (93) | 38 (91) | .71 |
| Defibrillation‖ | | | |
| Identify rhythm (VF) | 42 (96) | 36 (86) | .15 |
| Confirm pulselessness | 20 (46) | 19 (45) | .98 |
| Immediate defibrillation | 41 (93) | 37 (88) | .48 |
| Charge 2 J/kg (asynchronous mode) | 36 (82) | 37 (88) | .42 |
| Gel paddles | 29 (66) | 25 (60) | .54 |
| Proper paddle placement | 31 (71) | 30 (71) | .92 |
| Clear table | 27 (61) | 29 (69) | .46 |

Abbreviations: CNS, central nervous system; $CO_2$, carbon dioxide; RCPA, rapid cardiopulmonary assessment; Trad-PALS, traditional PALS; VF, ventricular fibrillation; Web-PALS, Web-based pediatric advanced life support course (PALS).

*Students were asked to perform RCPA on a 6-month-old infant with respiratory distress.

†Students were asked to perform bag-mask ventilation on a 6-month-old infant with apnea.

‡Students were asked to perform tracheal intubation on a 6-month-old infant with apnea.

§Students were asked to place an intraosseous needle in a 5-year-old child with sepsis.

‖Students were asked to identify and treat an arrhythmia (VF) in a 15-year-old patient.

**Table 3. Comparison of Mean Overall, RCPA, and Procedure Scores Among Web-PALS and Trad-PALS Groups**

| Variable | Web-PALS* (n = 44) | Trad-PALS* (n = 42) | Difference in No. % Between Groups (95% CI) | P Value |
|---|---|---|---|---|
| Overall | 75 (9) | 73 (10) | 2 (−2 to 6) | .27 |
| RCPA | 74 (14) | 75 (14) | −1 (−7 to 5) | .65 |
| Bag-mask ventilation | 78 (12) | 81 (17) | −3 (−9 to 4) | .42 |
| Tracheal intubation | 76 (18) | 68 (20) | 8 (0.3 to 16) | .04 |
| Intraosseous needle insertion | 73 (20) | 64 (21) | 9 (0.1 to 18) | .047 |
| Defibrillation | 73 (16) | 72 (17) | 1 (−6 to 8) | .80 |

Abbreviations: CI, confidence interval; RCPA, rapid cardiopulmonary assessment; Trad-PALS, traditional PALS; Web-PALS, Web-based pediatric advanced life support course (PALS).

*Data are given as percentage (SD).

**Table 4. Summary of Web-PALS Survey Questions***

| Question† | No. (%) Yes | No. (%) Somewhat |
|---|---|---|
| Were the following objectives of PALS course met?‡ (n = 50) | | |
| Learn to recognize infants and children at risk for pulmonary arrest | 50 (100) | 0 |
| Learn the information and strategies needed to prevent cardiopulmonary arrest in infants and children | 48 (96) | 2 (4) |
| Learn the cognitive and psychomotor skills needed to resuscitate and stabilize infants and children with respiratory failure, shock, or cardiopulmonary arrest | 48 (96) | 2 (4) |
| Would you recommend the Web-PALS course to a colleague? (n = 59)§ | 59 (100) | 0 |

Abbreviations: PALS, pediatric advanced life support course; Web-PALS, Web-based PALS.

*For clarity of presentation, the order and wording of some questions has been altered from the original survey.

†No students answered no to any questions.

‡This question was added to the survey during the study period.

§Students could select only yes or no for this question.

**Table 5. Summary of Web-PALS Survey Questions/Statements**

| Question/Statement (n = 60)* | Mean (SD)† |
|---|---|
| How did you like the registration process? | 4.3 (1.0) |
| How would you rate technical help? | 4.5 (0.8) |
| How did you like the flow of the online modules? | 4.3 (0.8) |
| The online modules maintained my interest. | 4.4 (0.8) |
| Time spent on skills stations was sufficient. | 4.7 (0.6) |
| How did you like the flow of the skills stations? | 4.5 (0.8) |
| Evaluation stations covered material taught in the modules. | 4.8 (0.5) |
| Overall, how did you like this educational experience? | 4.7 (0.5) |

Abbreviation: Web-PALS, Web-based pediatric advanced life support course.

*For these questions and statements, students rated responses on a continuous scale from 1 ("strongly disagree" or "really disliked") to 5 ("strongly agree" or "really liked").

†Owing to occasional omissions, mean ratings are based on valid responses.

tive educational experience. When asked to assess the overall educational experience, students gave a mean ±SD rating of 4.7±0.5. Ninety-six percent of respondents believed that the Web-PALS course met all of the stated objectives of the PALS course. All of the respondents indicated that they would recommend the Web-PALS course to a colleague. The lowest ratings were given for the registration process (4.3±1.0) and flow of the online modules (4.3±0.8) (Table 5).

## COMMENT

Despite their availability, the educational efficacy of distance-taught life support courses has largely not been studied. A limited number of studies have shown mixed results on self-instruction of basic life support and advanced cardiac life support material.[10-16] In the present study, students in the Web-PALS group compared favorably with students in the Trad-PALS group for cognitive (postcourse written examination scores) and psychomotor performance. The AHA-validated written examination is proportionally weighted to reflect the main teaching objectives of the PALS course and is an ideal tool to assess student knowledge of the most fundamental PALS concepts. Although their scores were slightly lower than those of students in the Trad-PALS group, students in the Web-PALS group performed well on the examination, achieving a mean±SD score of 95.4%±3.9%. All students in the Web-PALS group successfully passed the written examination on the first attempt and scored well above the minimum passing score of 84% mandated by the AHA.

Previous studies of Trad-PALS courses have reported somewhat lower written examination scores than those found in our study. In a study of 370 Israeli health care workers, Waisman et al[17] reported a postcourse mean score of 87%. In a smaller study of pediatric residents, Nadel et al[18] reported a mean score of 93% among pediatric residents who had taken a PALS course 6 months earlier. To our knowledge, however, this is the first report using the 2002 version of the examination. It is impossible, therefore, to accurately compare examination scores from the present study with any published data from courses administered outside of our institution.

Few studies have examined skills performance of students who have taken the PALS course.[7,8,17] To assess psychomotor skills, we modified a protocol previously described in studies by White et al[7] in 1998 and by Quan et al[8] in 2001. In addition to the 4 procedures examined in these studies, we assessed student performance on the RCPA. Our study is unique in its inclusion of the RCPA in the skills assessments.

Unlike these previous studies, we did not time students during psychomotor testing. The speed with which assessments and procedures are performed is critical during real resuscitations. In the present study, students typically performed tasks within a reasonable amount of time, consistent with what we would expect in a real setting. As an initial evaluation of the Web-PALS course, however, we were more interested in determining whether students had learned all of the concepts needed to properly perform psychomotor skills. By not timing students, we allowed them to focus their attention on being thorough and technically correct during the skills evaluations. This enabled us to better determine if the concepts needed to perform each task were sufficiently presented in the Web-PALS course.

In our study, psychomotor scores were somewhat lower than expected in both groups. We attribute this to the strict criteria that reviewers used when scoring videotaped performances. Students in the Web-PALS and Trad-PALS groups performed similarly in overall skills performance. Students in the Web-PALS group performed similarly or better than those in the Trad-PALS group on all but one of the skills subcomponents. When individual procedures were compared, students in the Web-PALS group performed better on tracheal intubation and intraosseous needle insertion. By enhancing the review of cognitive material before the day of skills training, students may have been able to better focus on skills acquisition during these sessions.

Several studies have examined student satisfaction with distance-taught life support courses.[12,16] Similar to these, we found that students who took the Web-PALS course generally seem to like this mode of studying the course material, especially because of its flexibility and self-directed learning format.

There are a number of limitations to our study. The study groups are a mixture of subjects from different professions and with different previous PALS experience. Though this demographic profile reflects what is typically seen in most PALS courses, the small number of subjects in our study prevents us from reaching any meaningful conclusions about the performance of individual subgroups. The study is underpowered to show how first-time students who have taken a Web-PALS course compare with first-time students who have taken a Trad-PALS course.

The potential for selection bias in our study cannot be overlooked. Students with previous PALS experience were more likely to participate in the study. This contributed, in part, to the disparity between the groups for the percentage of eligible students who participated in the study (44 [55%] in the Web-PALS group vs 42 [16%] in the Trad-PALS group). Such bias, coupled with nonrandomization of subjects, could potentially lead to overestimation of the true educational effect of the Web-PALS course.

Students in the Trad-PALS group received PACTS in addition to standard PALS training. We believe there is little overlap between the PACTS and PALS curriculae. It is possible, however, that, to some extent, PACTS reinforces some of the general PALS concepts. This may have led to somewhat higher scores than would otherwise be expected among traditional students. We believe, however, that the effect of this potential confounder does not change the main conclusions reached in our study.

Our study was limited by the artificial nature of mock resuscitation scenarios. Though previous studies have shown positive effects of life support courses on performance during actual resuscitations, it is unknown with certainty how subjects would perform in a real setting.[19,20] Inasmuch as moderators were not blinded to which course subjects had taken, we sought to overcome this potential for bias by adhering to a strict videotaping protocol and scoring process. Moderators read from a prepared, written script and were instructed not to lead or direct the students in any way during the videotaping sessions. Despite these safeguards, the potential for moderator bias in leading students during the skills evaluations cannot be excluded.

Because we did not directly observe students studying online, it is unknown how much time students spent reviewing cognitive material. Moreover, our study does not longitudinally address the retention of knowledge, skills ability, or perceived self-confidence among students who have taken the Web-PALS course. Long-term retention of learned concepts is a vital measure in the assessment of life support courses. Retention of knowledge and skills has been shown to diminish over time among students who have taken Trad-PALS courses.[21,22] We are unable to comment on this aspect of the Web-PALS course.

Despite its limitations, the present study contributes to the evolving knowledge of distance-taught life support courses. The findings in our study support the continued development and promotion of the Web-PALS course. Future studies, with larger numbers of subjects, are needed to address questions that are unanswered by our study. Of greatest importance is the need to determine whether the Web-PALS course is appropriate for first-time PALS students and the effect of the course on long-term retention of knowledge and skills performance.

**Accepted for Publication:** November 19, 2005.
**Correspondence:** James M. Gerard, MD, Department of Pediatrics, Division of Pediatric Emergency Medicine, Saint Louis University School of Medicine, 1465 S Grand Blvd, St Louis, MO 63104 (gerardjm@slu.edu).
**Author Contributions:** Dr Gerard had full access to all the data in the study and takes responsibility for the integrity of the data and the accuracy of the data analysis.
**Financial Disclosure:** Since the completion of this study, Ms Seratti has received financial compensation from the American Heart Association as a consultant to further develop the 1-day skills/testing course at PALS training sites.
**Funding/Support:** This study was funded by grant 1 H33 MC 00103 from the Health Resources and Services Administration and by a grant from the American Heart Association.
**Previous Presentation:** This study was presented at the Pediatric Academic Societies Meeting; May 15, 2005; Washington, DC.

**Acknowledgment:** We thank Steve Schexnayder, MD, for his insightful review of the manuscript.

## REFERENCES


1. HeartCode ACLS Anywhere: Inhospital [ACLS course on CD-ROM]. Dallas, Tex: American Heart Association; 2003.
2. American Heart Association. *National ECC Training Bulletin* [online basic life support for health care professionals renewal course]. Dallas, Tex: American Heart Association; 2004.
3. Electronic ACLS Web site. Available at: http://www.eacls.com. Accessed September 1, 2004.
4. Zaritsky AL, Nadkarni VM, Berg RA, Hickey RW, Schexnayder SM, eds. *Pediatric Advanced Life Support Instructor's Manual.* Dallas, Tex: American Heart Association; 2002.
5. Scalzo AJ, ed. *Pediatric Advanced Cardiorespiratory and Trauma Support for Life Textbook: Internal Publication.* St Louis, Mo: Saint Louis University; 2002.
6. Craven KO, Froman RD. Development of a pediatric skill self-efficacy scale. *J Nurs Meas.* 1993;1:125-133.
7. White JRM, Shugerman R, Brownlee C, et al. Performance of advanced resuscitation skills by pediatric housestaff. *Arch Pediatr Adolesc Med.* 1998;152:1232-1235.
8. Quan L, Shugerman RP, Kunkel NC, Quan L. Evaluation of resuscitation skills in new residents before and after pediatric advanced life support course. *Pediatrics.* 2001;108:e110. Available at: http://www.pediatrics.org. Accessed February 13, 2006.
9. Landis JR, Koch GG. The measurement of observer agreement for categorical data. *Biometrics.* 1977;33:159-174.
10. Todd KH, Braslow A, Brennan RT, et al. Randomized, controlled trial of video self-instruction versus traditional CPR training. *Ann Emerg Med.* 1998;31:364-369.
11. Todd KH, Heron SL, Thompson M, Dennis R, O'Connor J, Kellermann AL. Simple CPR: a randomized, controlled trial of video self-instructional cardiopulmonary resuscitation training in an African American church congregation. *Ann Emerg Med.* 1999;34:730-737.
12. Monsieurs KG, Vogels C, Bossaert LL, et al. Learning effect of a novel interactive basic life support CD: the JUST system. *Resuscitation.* 2004;62:159-165.
13. Clark LJ, Watson J, Cobbe SM, Reeve W, Swann IJ, Macfarlane PW. CPR '98: a practical multimedia computer-based guide to cardiopulmonary resuscitation for medical students. *Resuscitation.* 2000;44:109-117.
14. Polglase RF, Parish DC, Buckley RL, Smith RW, Joiner TA. Problem-based ACLS instruction: a model approach for undergraduate emergency medical education. *Ann Emerg Med.* 1989;18:997-1000.
15. Herrin TJ, Norman PF, Hill C, Crosby R. Modular approach to CPR training. *South Med J.* 1980;73:742-744.
16. Darr LR. Advanced cardiac life support education: a self-directed, scenario-based approach. *J Contin Educ Nurs.* 2000;31:116-120.
17. Waisman Y, Amir L, Mimouni M. Does the pediatric advanced life support course improve knowledge of pediatric resuscitation? *Pediatr Emerg Care.* 2002;18:168-170.
18. Nadel FM, Lavelle JM, Fein JA, Giardino AP, Decker JM, Durbin DR. Assessing pediatric senior residents' training in resuscitation: fund of knowledge, technical skills, and perception of confidence. *Pediatr Emerg Care.* 2000;16:73-76.
19. Camp BN, Parish DC, Andrews RH. Effect of advanced cardiac life support training on resuscitation efforts and survival in a rural hospital. *Ann Emerg Med.* 1997;29:529-533.
20. Lowenstein SR, Sabyan EM, Lassen CF, Kern DC. Benefits of training physicians in advanced cardiac life support. *Chest.* 1986;89:512-516.
21. Wolfram RW, Warren C, Doyle CR, Kerns R, Frye S. Retention of Pediatric Advanced Life Support (PALS) course concepts. *J Emerg Med.* 2003;25:475-479.
22. Su E, Schmidt TA, Mann NC, Zechnich AD. A randomized controlled trial to assess decay in acquired knowledge among paramedics completing a pediatric resuscitation course. *Acad Emerg Med.* 2000;7:779-786.


### *Announcement*

**Trial Registration Required.** In concert with the International Committee of Medical Journal Editors (ICMJE), *Archives of Pediatrics and Adolescent Medicine* will require, as a condition of consideration for publication, registration of all trials in a public trials registry (such as http://ClinicalTrials.gov). Trials must be registered at or before the onset of patient enrollment. This policy applies to any clinical trial starting enrollment after July 1, 2005. For trials that began enrollment before this date, registration will be required by September 13, 2005, before considering the trial for publication. The trial registration number should be supplied at the time of submission.

For details about this new policy, and for information on how the ICMJE defines a clinical trial, see the editorials by DeAngelis et al in the September 8, 2004 (2004;292:1363-1364) and June 15, 2005 (2005;293:2927-2929) issues of *JAMA*. Also see the Instructions to Authors on our Web site: www.archpediatrics.com.

# Obesity Among Latino Preschoolers

## *Do Children Outgrow the "Epidemiologic Paradox"?*

In recent decades, there has been an explosive increase in the number of overweight and obese adults and children in the United States and many other countries.[1] According to 1999-2002 data from the National Health and Nutrition Examination Survey, 15% of all children and adolescents in the United States were overweight, a 100% increase during a 20-year period.[2] Although we have become more sophisticated about recognizing obesity as a clinical and public health problem, we are surprisingly short on solutions or effective interventions.

*See also page 578*

Racial/ethnic differences in health outcomes have been consistently documented in the United States, and the article by Whitaker and Orzol[3] in this issue of the ARCHIVES highlights a critical but largely overlooked aspect of the domestic epidemic of childhood obesity.[4] Among urban families who participated in the 2001-2003 Fragile Families and Child Well-being Study, Latino preschoolers (aged 3 years) were twice as likely to be obese as white or African American preschoolers.[3] The elevated risk of obesity among young Latino children was not explained by 3 socioeconomic factors: maternal education, household income, and children's food security. The findings are consistent with national estimates of overweight in young children,[5,6] lending further support to the validity of the findings. Whereas perinatal studies have consistently documented more favorable outcomes among Latino children as compared with African American children,[7] the current study of overweight documented less favorable outcomes among Latino children.

However, the term *Latino preschoolers* is not specific enough to identify children who are overweight or obese because health outcomes in Latino individuals vary by national origin subgroup. For example, Puerto Rican–origin Latina women have substantially higher rates of low-birth-weight infants[7,8] and infant mortality[9] as compared with white women or Latina women of other national origin subgroups. Previous studies of overweight and obesity in children have analyzed Latino individuals as a single group[10] or included only Mexican-origin Latino individuals[6,11] so we lack a clear understanding of the risk of overweight and obesity among Latino children of Central/South American, Cuban, and Puerto Rican origins. Without detailed information about the national origin background of the Latino children who were included in the Fragile Families study population, it is not clear whether the elevated risk of obesity applies to all Latino children or only to specific subgroups. Thus, further study is needed before we can define all Latino children as high risk for overweight and obesity.

Maternal acculturation has been consistently identified as a significant risk factor for perinatal outcomes in Latino children[12] as well as early childhood outcomes such as immunization status,[13] but the Fragile Families study did not analyze maternal acculturation. Thus, it is not clear whether the risk of overweight among Latino children varies by maternal acculturation status. The importance of maternal acculturation is underscored by the fact that nearly two thirds of all childbearing Latina women in the United States are foreign born.[14] Further study is needed to determine whether acculturation status is an independent risk factor for overweight and obesity in children.

Maternal education was significantly associated with obesity only among the Latino subset in the Fragile Families study.[3] Latina women with less than a high school education had the highest rates of obese children, and Latina women with higher levels of educational attainment had similar rates of obese children. The relationship between maternal education and childhood obesity must be further studied in view of the fact that nearly half (47.5%) of childbearing Latina women in the United States have less than a high school education.[14] If the findings of the current study are replicated, pediatricians and child health professionals must urgently develop effective interventions to minimize the risk of obesity in the large subset of Latino children in the United States who are born to mothers with limited education.

The term *epidemiologic paradox* has been used for 20 years to describe the surprisingly low rates of adverse health outcomes among Latino relative to African American individuals.[15] The term is also used to describe the unexpected lack of a relationship between well-known sociodemographic risk factors, such as education and insurance status, and health outcomes in Latino individuals. The paradox has been documented for perinatal outcomes, where rates of low birth weight and infant mortality were similar between Latina and white women and the rates among Latina women were consistently lower than the rates among African American women.[7,9,16] In studies of adult mortality, the epidemiologic paradox has also been observed.[17] In the current study, on the other hand, Latino children were twice as likely to be obese as African American or white children, a direct contradiction to the epidemiologic paradox. The fact that Latino infants have surprisingly favorable outcomes at birth yet have higher obesity rates by early childhood, as documented in the Fragile Families study, suggests that the epidemiologic paradox no longer applies by the preschool years. The reversal of the relationship between ethnicity and health outcomes between infancy and early childhood requires further study.

The underlying explanation for the epidemiologic paradox remains elusive. Some have hypothesized that the paradox is related to religiosity or other cultural attributes,[18,19] while others have suggested that the paradox should be analyzed at a community level rather than as an individual-level phenomenon.[20] If there is no epidemiologic paradox among young Latino children, researchers need to develop new conceptual models to identify the factors that contribute to the paradox during pregnancy and infancy and/or the factors that override the paradox by early childhood.

There may be cultural differences in the "ideal" body image for children and adults[21] and these differences could contribute to the high rates of obesity among Latino children. For Latino immigrants, who may have experienced hunger as children or witnessed the adverse effects of malnutrition, the ideal image of a healthy baby or child may be an "overweight" image by current body mass standards.[22] Even among non-Latina mothers in the United States, it is commonly believed that heavy infants are healthier and indicate better parenting.[23] The interpretation of body mass is partially subjective, and unless parents believe their child is overweight, they may not be willing to make changes to their family lifestyle. The challenge of addressing childhood obesity was underscored by a recent study that documented that the majority of mothers of overweight children did not perceive their children as overweight.[24] It is difficult for health care professionals to directly assess parents' perceptions of body mass, but the anecdotal experiences of Latino parents complaining that their overweight child doesn't eat properly (*no come nada*)[22] offer indirect support for the hypothesis that ethnic differences in ideal body share are important.

The consequences of childhood overweight are social and health related. For example, overweight and obese children may be teased or subjected to other social pressures related to their weight.[25] However, the increasing proportion of overweight children may shift the body mass "norm" in the schoolyard and in other social settings. The main finding of the Fragile Families study, the elevated risk of obesity among young Latino children, is sobering and alarming. To mobilize health professionals and the population of Latino children and families affected by overweight and obesity, however, we need to understand the "modifiable root causes"[3] for this compelling problem. The research community must investigate the underlying risk factors and develop effective interventions to improve health and well-being for Latino children and their families.

*Elena Fuentes-Afflick, MD, MPH*

**Correspondence:** Dr Fuentes-Afflick, Departments of Pediatrics and Epidemiology and Biostatistics, San Francisco General Hospital, 1001 Potrero Ave, Mail Stop 6E, San Francisco, CA 94110 (efuentes@sfghpeds.ucsf.edu).

## REFERENCES

1. Olson E. UN warns that many children, rich and poor, are obese. *New York Times.* May 17, 2002; § A:9.
2. Dietz WH, Robinson TN. Overweight children and adolescents. *N Engl J Med.* 2005;352:2100-2109.
3. Whitaker RC, Orzol SM. Obesity among US urban preschool children: relationships to race, ethnicity, and socioeconomic status. *Arch Pediatr Adolesc Med.* 2006;160:578-584.
4. Flores G, Fuentes-Afflick E, Barbot O, et al. The health of Latino children. *JAMA.* 2002;288:82-90.
5. Sherry B, Mei Z, Scanlon K, Mokdad A, Grummer-Strawn L. Trends in state-specific prevalence of overweight and underweight in 2- through 4-year-old children from low-income families from 1989 through 2000. *Arch Pediatr Adolesc Med.* 2004;158:1116-1124.
6. Hedley AA, Ogden CL, Johnson CL, Carroll MD, Curtin LR, Flegal KM. Prevalence of overweight and obesity among US children, adolescents, and adults, 1999-2002. *JAMA.* 2004;291:2847-2850.
7. Fuentes-Afflick E, Hessol N, Perez-Stable E. Testing the epidemiologic paradox of low birth weight in Latinos. *Arch Pediatr Adolesc Med.* 1999;153:147-153.
8. Rosenberg TJ, Raggio TP, Chiasson MA. A further examination of the "epidemiologic paradox:" birth outcomes among Latinas. *J Natl Med Assoc.* 2005; 97:550-556.
9. Becerra JE, Hogue CJR, Atrash HK, Perez N. Infant mortality among Hispanics: a portrait of heterogeneity. *JAMA.* 1991;265:217-221.
10. Strauss RS, Pollack HA. Epidemic increase in childhood overweight, 1986-1998. *JAMA.* 2001;286:2845-2848.
11. Ogden CL, Flegal KM, Carroll MD, Johnson CL. Prevalence and trends in overweight among US children and adolescents, 1999-2000. *JAMA.* 2002;288: 1728-1732.
12. Fuentes-Afflick E, Hessol N, Perez-Stable E. Maternal birthplace, ethnicity, and low birth weight in California. *Arch Pediatr Adolesc Med.* 1998;152:1105-1112.
13. Anderson LM, Wood DL, Sherbourne CD. Maternal acculturation and childhood immunization levels among children in Latino families in Los Angeles. *Am J Public Health.* 1997;87:2018-2021.
14. Martin JA, Hamilton BE, Sutton PD, Ventura SJ, Menacker F, Munson ML. Births: final data for 2003. *Natl Vital Stat Rep.* 2005 Sep 8;54(2):1-116.
15. Markides KS, Coreil J. The health of Hispanics in the southwestern United States: an epidemiologic paradox. *Public Health Rep.* 1986;101:253-265.
16. Guendelman S, Gould JB, Hudes M, Eskenazi B. Generational differences in perinatal health among the Mexican American population: findings from HHANES 1982-84. *Am J Public Health.* 1990;80(suppl):61-65.
17. Abraido-Lanza AF, Dohrenwend BP, Ng-Mak DS, Turner JB. The Latino mortality paradox: a test of the "Salmon bias" and healthy migrant hypotheses. *Am J Public Health.* 1999;89:1543-1548.
18. Jones ME, Bond ML. Predictors of birth outcome among Hispanic immigrant women. *J Nurs Care Qual.* 1999;14:56-62.
19. Magana A, Clark N. Examining a paradox: does religiosity contribute to positive birth outcomes in Mexican American populations? *Health Educ Q.* 1995;22: 96-109.
20. Scribner R. Paradox as paradigm—the health outcomes of Mexican Americans. *Am J Public Health.* 1996;86:303-305.
21. Davis SP, Northington L, Kolar K. Cultural considerations for treatment of childhood obesity. *J Cult Divers.* 2000;7:128-132.
22. Garcia RS. No come nada. *Health Aff (Millwood).* 2004;23:215-219.
23. Baughcum AE, Burklow KA, Deeks CM, Powers SW, Whitaker RC. Maternal feeding practices and childhood obesity. *Arch Pediatr Adolesc Med.* 1998;152: 1010-1014.
24. Baughcum AE, Chamberlin LA, Deeks CM, Powers SW, Whitaker RC. Maternal perceptions of overweight preschool children. *Pediatrics.* 2000;106:1380-1386.
25. Navarro M. Playtime at the health club. *New York Times.* January 22, 2006; § 9:1.

# Pediatric Advanced Life Support Your Way

IN CASE YOU HAVEN'T NOTICED, THERE IS A REVOlution taking place in medical education that is unrivaled in significance since the release of the Flexner report in 1910. The Flexner report triggered reforms in the standards, organization, and curriculum of North American medical schools by proposing a system strong in biomedical sciences and hands-on clinical training. The current revolution directs us toward an approach that can be loosely defined by the buzz phrases of "student-centered learning," "competency-based evaluation," and "80-hour work rules." These winds of change in medical education are most associated with residency programs, but in reality, they affect us all.

*See also page 649*

In the subspecialty of pediatric emergency medicine, we are challenged with being responsive to the emergency medicine educational needs of physicians who practice outside of the emergency department. Perhaps foremost among those physicians are community pediatricians who must be able to competently respond to the office emergency. In our experience, pediatricians *want* to be prepared for the office emergency. They frequently seek our advice concerning equipment needs and stock medications. They care about training and express interest in ways to sharpen and maintain their resuscitation skills. They also provide the feedback that they want resuscitation courses that are relevant to their practice, are conveniently scheduled, and use their time efficiently. Time, after all, is a precious commodity, and courses such as the pediatric advanced life support course (PALS) can represent time away from the office and family. Most importantly, pediatricians want courses that improve self-efficacy so that at the end of training, they believe in their ability to care for a sick child. The educators, for their part, want courses that effectively impart the necessary knowledge, attitudes, behaviors, and skills required for resuscitation. To summarize, we believe community pediatricians want courses, like PALS for example, to be flexible, efficient, efficacious, and effective.

The study by Gerard et al[1] describes their experience with adapting traditional PALS to a Web-based format. As they point out, this distance learning format provides flexibility for the student. They provide data that the Web-based course is as effective in promoting cognitive and psychomotor learning as the traditional PALS course. All of the Web-PALS students passed the written examination, although at a slightly lower mean score than the traditional PALS students (mean score, 95.4% vs 97.1%, respectively). Overall procedure scores were the same in both groups for rapid cardiopulmonary assessment, bag-mask ventilation, and defibrillation and were significantly higher in the Web-PALS group for tracheal intubation and intraosseous needle insertion. Furthermore, satisfaction with the online concept was high, with 100% of responding participants acknowledging that they would recommend the Web-PALS course to colleagues. The students perceived the course as a highly positive educational experience.

We believe that this study represents only the first step in compelling resuscitation education to be more user friendly. There are other indications that resuscitation courses can be made more available to those with limited time without sacrificing learning. The American Heart Association, Dallas, Tex, recently developed a system for student-centered cardiopulmonary resuscitation education that can be completed in a fraction of the time of a traditional cardiopulmonary resuscitation course. This CPR Anytime kit includes a 30-minute instructional DVD, an easily inflatable mannequin, a program booklet, and supplies to clean and maintain the mannequin. The program is designed to be self-contained, practical, and eminently convenient. Its portability encourages use anywhere a DVD player is located at any time suitable to the user. Lynch et al[2] proved the utility and efficacy of a training kit with essentially the same contents for a group of lay responders. The researchers concluded that this kind of program could significantly increase the number of lay responders able to perform effective cardiopulmonary resuscitation.

Returning to the theme of Web-based learning, the advantages of such a system are clear. Not only does the Internet promote flexibility and convenience for the user, but it also allows the incorporation of multimedia presentations to enhance learning. Retention of information is promoted through seeing the concepts in words and pictures, hearing audio explanations, and evaluation by interactive testing throughout the educational module. Building Internet-based content can be difficult and very time consuming, but commercial products are available to facilitate the process. One such system, Blackboard (Blackboard Inc, Washington, DC), has been evaluated and found to be successful as an educational tool.[3,4]

Virtual reality is another technology that, in addition to the Internet, holds a vast, largely untapped potential for medical education. As the interface between human perception and computer-generated sensory input, virtual reality has been successfully used in fields outside of medicine, namely aviation, military, business, and nuclear energy.[5] Some medical applications of virtual reality simulation have been developed, particularly in the areas of anatomy education[6] and laparoscopic surgery.[7] Although it is expensive and labor intensive to create, virtual reality is recognized as an effective method of simulating high-stress scenarios[8] such as resuscitation in a nonthreatening manner.

Flexibility and choice are popular marketing strategies in modern American society. You can order a fast-food hamburger your way and buy services that give you the freedom to watch your favorite television shows anytime, anywhere. Why not tailor the options in resuscitation education to meet the needs of the student? Of course, this is easier said than done, and we are not suggesting that competence or interaction with an educator be sacrificed on the altar of flexibility and choice. However, dream of the possibilities for a moment.

Pediatric and infant human patient simulators are a reality. High-fidelity simulators are computer-controlled mannequins that can be programmed to elicit a wide variety of sensory responses to participant actions. Eyes blink or remain closed, palpable pulses increase and decrease their rate and quality, and laryngospasm causes intubation to be more difficult. Resuscitation scenarios are only limited by the programming capability of each simulation laboratory. Centers around the world are studying the application of high-fidelity simulation to medical education.[9,10] We believe that the data will be supportive, and we envision a world where physicians develop or refresh skills in pediatric resuscitation by scheduling a session convenient for them at a pediatric human patient simulation center or do it all using a virtual learning environment. We believe that PALS your way is possible, desirable, and just around the decade.

*Jane F. Knapp, MD*
*Robert D. Schremmer, MD*

**Correspondence:** Dr Knapp, Children's Mercy Hospital, 2401 Gillham Rd, Kansas City, MO 64108 (jknapp@cmh.edu).

## REFERENCES

1. Gerard JM, Scalzo AJ, Laffey SP, Sinks G, Fendya D, Seratti P. Evaluation of a novel Web-based pediatric advanced life support course. *Arch Pediatr Adolesc Med.* 2006;160:649-655.
2. Lynch B, Einspruch EL, Nichol G, Becker LB, Aufderheide TP, Idris A. Effectiveness of a 30-min CPR self-instruction program for lay responders: a controlled randomized study. *Resuscitation.* 2005;67:31-43.
3. Boberick KG. Creating a Web-enhanced interactive preclinic technique manual: case report and student response. *J Dent Educ.* 2004;68:1245-1257.
4. Stone VL, Bongiorno R, Hinegardner PG, Williams MA. Delivery of Web-based instruction using Blackboard: a collaborative project. *J Med Libr Assoc.* 2004;92:375-377.
5. Krummel TM. Surgical simulation and virtual reality: the coming revolution. *Ann Surg.* 1998;228:635-637.
6. Shaffer K. Teaching anatomy in the digital world. *N Engl J Med.* 2004;351:1279-1281.
7. Marescaux J, Clement JM, Tassetti V. Virtual reality applied to hepatic surgery simulation: the next revolution. *Ann Surg.* 1998;228:627-634.
8. Vozenilek J, Huff JS, Reznek M, Gordon JA. See one, do one, teach one: advanced technology in medical education. *Acad Emerg Med.* 2004;11:1149-1154.
9. Marsch SCU, Tschan F, Semmer N, Spychiger M, Breuer M, Hunziker PR. Performance of first responders in simulated cardiac arrests. *Crit Care Med.* 2005;33:963-967.
10. Mayo PH, Hackney JE, Mueck JT, Ribaudo V, Schneider RF. Achieving house staff competence in emergency airway management: results of a teaching program using a computerized patient simulator. *Crit Care Med.* 2004;32:2422-2427.

"The tobacco habit, while it does not compare with those just discussed in the seriousness of its results, is of no benefit, is of great and useless expense, and is often the direct cause of a derangement of the healthy actions of the body. Its use has been demonstrated to be very dangerous to the young. It is a habit easily avoided, and one that no one who has formed it would advise you to form."

—From *Advanced Lessons in Human Physiology*, Indiana State Series by Oliver P. Jenkins, PhD, 1891

## "I'm, Like, SO Fat!": Helping Your Teen Make Healthy Choices About Eating and Exercise in a Weight-Obsessed World

*by Dianne Newmark-Sztainer, PhD, 317 pages, $35, ISBN, 1593851677, New York, NY, The Guilford Press, 2005.*

Dr Newmark-Sztainer has written a wonderful book to guide parents through the triple threat of adolescent children in a food-toxic and weight-obsessed culture. Dr Newmark-Sztainer is a researcher and professor at the University of Minnesota School of Public Health and has been the principal investigator for Project EAT (Eating Among Teens). Her publications have included those on dietary practices and obesity of adolescents, weight control practices of adolescents, weight teasing and its potential implications, and family meals. She shares many of the findings from Project EAT in this very readable and enjoyable book.

The first half of the book presents an overview of the problem. She starts by setting up a context for discussing both eating disorders and obesity in the same book by putting these weight-related problems on opposite ends of a spectrum. She then discusses the different levels of influence on weight-related problems from a macrolevel (eg, national food policies, cultural norms for body image) to community (eg, availability of parks and grocery stores, built environment factors) to schools, peers, family, and individual characteristics. The next 5 chapters discuss the importance of parents, peer influences, the importance of physical activity, the dangers behind dieting, and 4 guiding principles for maintaining a child's healthy weight and body image.

The second half of the book gives more specific nutritional advice such as portion control, calorie counting, how to manage a teen who is vegetarian, family meals in the context of busy lives, fast food, and eating out. Her advice is refreshingly realistic and recognizes the time limitations of working parents, children in multiple activities, and lots of driving. The last 3 chapters tackle how to talk to kids about these difficult issues using pages of vignettes, how to help a teen who is already overweight, and how to identify signs of an eating disorder.

This book is written in a conversational style scattered with anecdotes of Dr Newmark-Sztainer's own experiences with her children. She integrates the best evidence with very practical approaches and positive, sound advice. Although the book is written for parents of adolescents and gives advice for youth at that developmental level, much of the content of the book (eating in moderation, integrating family activities, etc) is applicable to parents with children of all ages. Her messages are preventative and insightful.

Notably, she gently urges parents to look at their own eating and activity habits. In doing so, she acknowledges not only the challenges of changing habits but also the importance of parents modeling healthy behaviors. For example, she suggests, "Tell your family that you've given up dieting and instead are focusing on lifestyle changes." The other notable topic she discusses is "weightism"—in her words, "the last form of socially acceptable stigmatization tolerated in our society." And again, she urges parents to catch themselves when they make comments about their own appearance or others: "Don't make negative comments about your weight or appearance in front of your children. Resist the urge—it may be hard at first, but it is so important!" Which leads to my only criticism of this book—the title, "I'm, Like, SO Fat!" If I was concerned about my child, I wouldn't want this book lying around my house, and given her sensitivity on the weightism topic, I'm surprised this title was chosen.

Nonetheless, this excellent book should be read by all parents with children of all ages who are interested in integrating healthy nutrition and physical activity habits into their children's and their own lives. Her messages and advice on how to discuss this highly sensitive subject may also be helpful to health care professionals who regularly counsel families on the prevention and management of overweight and/or eating disorders.

*Lenna L. Liu, MD, MPH*

**Correspondence**: Dr Liu, Odessa Brown Children's Clinic, 2101 E Yesler Way, Seattle, WA 98122 (lennall@u.washington.edu).

"My sore throats, you know, are always worse than anybody's."
—Jane Austen

## HAVRIX®
## (Hepatitis A Vaccine, Inactivated)

The following is a brief summary only; see full prescribing information for complete product information.

**INDICATIONS AND USAGE:** HAVRIX is indicated for active immunization of persons ≥12 months of age against disease caused by hepatitis A virus (HAV). Primary immunization should be administered at least 2 weeks prior to expected exposure to HAV. When passive protection against hepatitis A is required either following exposure to hepatitis A virus or in persons requiring both immediate and long-term protection, HAVRIX may be administered concomitantly with immune globulin (IG) with different syringes and at different injection sites. Duration of immunity following a complete vaccination schedule has not been established.

**CONTRAINDICATIONS:** Hypersensitivity to any component of the vaccine, including neomycin, is a contraindication (see DESCRIPTION in full prescribing information). This vaccine is contraindicated in patients with previous hypersensitivity to any hepatitis A-containing vaccine.

**WARNINGS:** There have been rare reports of anaphylaxis/anaphylactoid reactions following commercial use of the vaccine. The tip cap and the rubber plunger of the needleless prefilled syringes contain dry natural latex rubber that may cause allergic reactions in latex sensitive individuals. The vial stopper is latex-free. Hepatitis A has a relatively long incubation period. Hepatitis A vaccine may not prevent hepatitis A infection in those who have an unrecognized hepatitis A infection at the time of vaccination. Additionally, it may not prevent infection in those who do not achieve protective antibody titers (although the lowest titer needed to confer protection has not been determined).

**PRECAUTIONS: General:** Prior to immunization with HAVRIX, the patient's current health status and medical history should be reviewed. The physician should review the patient's immunization history for possible vaccine sensitivity, previous vaccination-related adverse reactions and occurrence of any adverse–event-related symptoms and/or signs, in order to determine the existence of any contraindication to immunization with HAVRIX and to allow an assessment of benefits and risks. Appropriate medical treatment and supervision should be readily available for immediate use in case of a rare anaphylactic reaction following the administration of the vaccine. Epinephrine injection (1:1,000) and other appropriate agents used for the control of immediate allergic reactions must be immediately available. A separate, sterile syringe and needle or a sterile disposable unit should be used for each patient to prevent the transmission of other infectious agents from person to person. Needles should be disposed of properly and should not be recapped. As with any vaccine, if administered to immunosuppressed persons, including those receiving immunosuppressive therapy, the expected immune response may not be obtained. **Drug Interactions:** HAVRIX may be given concurrently with Hib conjugate vaccines in children 15 to 18 months of age (see CLINICAL PHARMACOLOGY in full prescribing information and ADVERSE REACTIONS). The safety of HAVRIX given concomitantly with INFANRIX has been evaluated (see ADVERSE REACTIONS). Insufficient data are available to assess the immune response of a fourth dose of DTaP vaccine when administered with HAVRIX. There are limited data to assess the concomitant use of HAVRIX with other vaccines. (See Immune Response to Concomitantly Administered Vaccines in full prescribing information.)

**Carcinogenesis, Mutagenesis, Impairment of Fertility:** HAVRIX has not been evaluated for its carcinogenic potential, mutagenic potential, or potential for impairment of fertility. **Pregnancy:** Pregnancy Category C. Animal reproduction studies have not been conducted with HAVRIX. It is also not known whether HAVRIX can cause fetal harm when administered to a pregnant woman or can affect reproduction capacity. Give HAVRIX to a pregnant woman only if clearly needed. **Nursing Mothers:** It is not known whether HAVRIX is excreted in human milk. Because many drugs are excreted in human milk, use caution when administering HAVRIX to a nursing woman. **Pediatric Use:** The safety and effectiveness of HAVRIX have been evaluated in 20,436 subjects 1 year to 18 years of age. (See CLINICAL PHARMACOLOGY and DOSAGE AND ADMINISTRATION in full prescribing information.) The safety and effectiveness of HAVRIX have not been established in subjects less than 12 months of age. **Geriatric Use:** Clinical studies of HAVRIX did not include sufficient numbers of subjects 65 years of age and older to determine whether they respond differently from younger subjects. Other reported clinical experience has not identified differences in overall safety between these subjects and younger adult subjects.

**ADVERSE REACTIONS:** As with all pharmaceuticals, however, it is possible that expanded commercial use of the vaccine could reveal rare adverse events. The adverse events most frequently reported by volunteers in clinical trials were injection-site soreness (56% of adults; 21% of children); headache (14% of adults; less than 9% of children). Other solicited and unsolicited events are listed below:

**Incidence 1% to 10% of Injections:** ***Local Reactions at Injection Site:*** Induration, redness, swelling; ***Body as a Whole:*** Fatigue, fever (>37.5°C), malaise; ***Gastrointestinal:*** Anorexia, nausea.

**Incidence <1% of Injections:** ***Local Reaction at Injection Site:*** Hematoma; ***Dermatologic:*** Pruritus, rash, urticaria; ***Respiratory:*** Pharyngitis, other upper respiratory tract infections; ***Gastrointestinal:*** Abdominal pain, diarrhea, dysgeusia, vomiting; ***Musculoskeletal:*** Arthralgia, elevation of creatine phosphokinase, myalgia; ***Hematologic:*** Lymphadenopathy; ***Central Nervous System:*** Hypertonic episode, insomnia, photophobia, vertigo.

**Additional safety data:** Safety data were obtained from 2 additional sources in which large populations were vaccinated. In an outbreak setting in which 4,930 individuals were immunized with a single dose of either 720 EL.U. or 1440 EL.U. of HAVRIX, the vaccine was well tolerated and no serious adverse events due to vaccination were reported. Overall, less than 10% of vaccinees reported solicited general adverse events following the vaccine. The most common solicited local adverse event was pain at the injection site, reported in 22.3% of subjects at 24 hours and decreasing to 2.4% by 72 hours.

In a field efficacy trial, 19,037 children received the 360 EL.U. dose of HAVRIX. The most commonly reported adverse events were injection-site pain (9.5%) and tenderness (8.1%), reported following first doses of HAVRIX. Other adverse events were infrequent and comparable to the control vaccine ENGERIX-B® [Hepatitis B Vaccine (Recombinant)].

In subjects with chronic liver disease, HAVRIX was safe and well tolerated. Local injection site reactions were similar among all 4 groups, and no serious adverse reactions attributed to the vaccine were reported in subjects with chronic liver disease.

***Safety Data for HAVRIX 720 EL.U./0.5 mL Beginning at 11 Months of Age:*** In the multicenter study described under CLINICAL PHARMACOLOGY in full prescribing information, parents/guardians recorded local and general symptoms on diary cards for 4 days (Days 0 to 3) after vaccination. In the 3 groups of children who received HAVRIX alone, safety data were available for 723 children who received 1,396 documented doses of HAVRIX. Additional safety data were available for 181 children who received HAVRIX coadministered with INFANRIX and Hib conjugate vaccine. Most adverse events were mild and transient. The frequencies of solicited local and systemic reactions following receipt of HAVRIX were monitored during the 4-day observation period.

The following rates of solicited adverse events in children who received their first dose of HAVRIX alone at between 11 and 25 months of age were observed. Among local reactions: pain was reported in 15-21% of subjects, redness in 16-21%, swelling in 8% of subjects. Among general reactions, irritability was reported in 24-36% of subjects, loss of appetite in 16-19% of subjects, drowsiness in 15-17% of subjects and fever >39.5°C in ≤2% of subjects. Following the booster dose of HAVRIX, among local reactions: pain was reported in 16-21% of subjects, redness in 17-22%, swelling in 8-10% of subjects. Following the booster dose of HAVRIX, among general reactions, irritability was reported in 19-29% of subjects, loss of appetite in 14-18% of subjects, drowsiness in 13-16% of subjects and fever >39.5°C in ≤1% of subjects.

Drowsiness and loss of appetite occurred at statistically significantly higher rates in subjects 15 to 18 months of age who received Hib conjugate vaccine (PRP-T) and INFANRIX concomitantly with HAVRIX as compared to subjects 15 to 18 months of age who received Hib conjugate vaccine (PRP-T) and INFANRIX (drowsiness 34% and 22% and loss of appetite 29% and 19%, respectively). With the exception of fever (>39.5°C), the solicited general symptoms occurred at statistically significantly higher rates in subjects 15 to 18 months of age who received Hib conjugate vaccine (PRP-T) and INFANRIX concomitantly with HAVRIX as compared to subjects 15 to 18 months of age who received HAVRIX alone (irritability 46% and 30%, drowsiness 34% and 17%, and loss of appetite 29% and 17%, respectively).

A febrile seizure was reported in an 18-month old subject two days after receiving the first dose of HAVRIX. Other serious adverse events reported during the course of this study included a single case each of hepatitis ~5 months post dose 1, insulin-dependent diabetes ~4 months post dose 1, and Kawasaki's disease ~3 1/2 months post dose 1. The association of these events with vaccination is unknown.

**Postmarketing Reports:** Rare voluntary reports of adverse events in people receiving HAVRIX since market introduction include the following: ***Local:*** Localized edema; ***Body as a Whole:*** Anaphylaxis/anaphylactoid reactions, somnolence; ***Cardiovascular:*** Syncope; ***Hepatobiliary:*** Jaundice, hepatitis; ***Dermatologic:*** Erythema multiforme, hyperhydrosis, angioedema; ***Respiratory:*** Dyspnea; ***Hematologic:*** Lymphadenopathy, thrombocytopenia; ***Central Nervous System:*** Convulsions, encephalopathy, dizziness, neuropathy, myelitis, paresthesia, Guillain-Barré syndrome, multiple sclerosis; ***Other:*** Congenital abnormality.

The US Department of Health and Human Services has established the Vaccine Adverse Events Reporting System (VAERS) to accept reports of suspected adverse events after the administration of any vaccine, including, but not limited to, the reporting of events required by the National Childhood Vaccine Injury Act of 1986. The toll-free number for VAERS forms and information is 1-800-822-7967. Reporting forms may also be obtained at the VAERS website at www.vaers.org.

Manufactured by **GlaxoSmithKline Biologicals**, Rixensart, Belgium

Distributed by **GlaxoSmithKline**, Research Triangle Park, NC 27709



BRS-HA:L20

**References: 1.** Centers for Disease Control and Prevention. Recommended childhood and adolescent immunization schedule—United States, 2006. *MMWR.* 2006;54(51&52):Q1–Q4. **2.** Bell BP, Shapiro CN. Hepatitis A virus. In: Long SS, Pickering LK, Prober CG, eds. *Principles and Practice of Pediatric Infectious Diseases.* 2nd ed. Philadelphia, Pa: Churchill Livingstone; 2003:1188–1192. **3.** Armstrong GL, Bell BP. Hepatitis A virus infection in the United States: model-based estimates and implication for childhood immunizations. *Pediatrics.* 2002;109:839–845.



Printed in USA. HAP283R0 February 2006

## FACULTY PHYSICIAN - General Pediatrics

St. Joseph's Hospital and Medical Center has been a symbol of quality healthcare in the Valley of the Sun for more than 111 years. This 536-bed teaching hospital, in downtown Phoenix, Arizona, is home to the internationally recognized Barrow Neurological Institute. The Children's Health Center includes a 79-bed general pediatrics unit, a 50-bed neonatal intensive care unit, a 24-bed pediatric intensive care unit, a dedicated children's emergency department, and the Pediatric Ambulatory Care Center. The program provides family-centered care to infants, children, and adolescents; our principal range of services includes general medical, surgery, cardiology, cardiac surgery, neurology, neurosurgery, orthopedics, craniofacial reconstruction, trauma, pulmonary, gastrointestinal, hematology and oncology, behavioral and developmental, and high risk delivery.

We are seeking a Faculty Pediatrician who is a hospital-based Physician to provide clinical services in general and acute care pediatrics. The successful candidate will supervise pediatric residents and medical students in general patient care and assume the role of mentor and teacher to these Physicians in training. This position requires unrestricted AZ MD or DO license, as well as Board certification/eligibility in pediatrics, and two years of general pediatric population experience. Background in academic setting preferred. For additional information please contact: **Bruce D. White, D.O., J.D., Interim Chief Pediatric Officer, 602-406-5199, bruce.white@chw.edu.** EOE

St. Joseph's Hospital
and Medical Center
CHW

## PEDIATRICS

**WE HAVE AN IMMEDIATE OPENING for a Pediatrician to join our highly respected Pediatric Group. Requires an IL License and Pediatric Board Certified or eligible. We have two offices located in the SW Suburbs of Chicago. We offer a highly competitive salary, benefit package and relocation assistance. Please E-mail your CV to drgsmd@aol.com or Fax: Attention George Skarpathiotis, MD, at 708-923-6949.**

PEDIATRIC OPPORTUNITIES AVAILABLE: NORTH SEATTLE Metro Area, Suburban Los Angeles, South Eastern Idaho. Single and multi specialty groups, very attractive compensation and benefits, partnership. Call Chris Warner 206-782-1277, E-mail: panther@seanet.com



## JOURNAL ADVERTISER INDEX


**CLASSIFIED ADVERTISING** ........ 663
http://www.amapublications.com

**GLAXOSMITHKLINE**
Boostrix ........ 629-630, COVER 3-4
Havrix ........ 589-590, 661-662
Pediarix ........ 565-566, 647-648

**MERCK & COMPANY**
Gardasil ........ 584A-C
Rotateq ........ 616A-D


*Demographic and "Mini" inserts and/or ROB ad pages

While every precaution is taken to ensure accuracy, we cannot guarantee against the possibility of an occasional change or omission in the preparation of this index.

ARCHIVES OF PEDIATRICS & ADOLESCENT MEDICINE

# CONTACT INFORMATION

## EDITORIAL OFFICE

**Editorial Office Information:** *Archives of Pediatrics & Adolescent Medicine*, Department of Pediatrics, Child Health Institute, University of Washington, 6200 NE 74th St, Suite 210, Seattle, WA 98115-8160, USA; phone: (206) 685-3573; fax: (206) 685-3572; e-mail: archpediatrics@jama-archives.org.

**Electronic Submission:** Manuscripts should be submitted via our online manuscript submission and review system (http://manuscripts.archpediatrics.com). Manuscripts submitted through our online system should not also be submitted by mail or fax. Signed authorship forms should be sent by regular mail or fax with the assigned manuscript number noted on each page in the upper right-hand corner. See the Instructions for Authors (www.archpediatrics.com) for more details.

## CONSORTIUM OF *JAMA* & *ARCHIVES* JOURNALS

The *Archives of Pediatrics & Adolescent Medicine* is a member of the consortium of AMA journals listed below.

The Journal of the American Medical Association (JAMA)
Archives of Dermatology
Archives of Facial Plastic Surgery
Archives of General Psychiatry
Archives of Internal Medicine
Archives of Neurology
Archives of Ophthalmology
Archives of Otolaryngology–Head & Neck Surgery
Archives of Pediatrics & Adolescent Medicine
Archives of Surgery

## *JAMA/ARCHIVES* MEDIA RELATIONS

Jann Ingmire; phone: (312) 464-5262; e-mail: mediarelations@jama-archives.org.

## *ARCHIVES OF PEDIATRICS* ONLINE

*Archives of Pediatrics & Adolescent Medicine* is available online at www.archpediatrics.com.

## *JAMA/ARCHIVES* REPRINTS

**Author/Educational Institution Reprints:** Anna Goins at (312) 464-2477; fax: (312) 464-5843; e-mail: anna.goins@ama-assn.org. Minimum order: 100 reprints.

**Commercial Reprints:** Phone: (312) 464-0776; fax: (312) 464-0708; e-mail: reprints@ama-assn.org. Minimum order: 100 reprints.

## PERMISSIONS

Information about obtaining permission to republish, reprint, or adapt material published in *Archives of Pediatrics & Adolescent Medicine* is available from Rhonda Bailey Brown; phone: (312) 464-2513; fax: (312) 464-5843; e-mail: permissions@ama-assn.org.

## DOCUMENT DELIVERY

Copies of individual articles are available online at www.archpediatrics.com and from the following: Infotrieve, phone: (800) 422-4633; fax: (310) 208-5971; URL: www.infotrieve.com; e-mail: orders@infotrieve.com; Institute for Scientific Information (ISI), phone: (800) 603-4367; fax: (856) 787-1679; URL: http://www.isidoc.com; e-mail: service@isidoc.com.

## ADVERTISING

Information about advertising is available from the following sales representatives and online at www.archpediatrics.com.

**Account Manager:** Tim Melroy (nationally); phone: (973) 263-9191 ext 213.

**Manager, Marketing Services:** Nancy Bell; phone: (973) 263-9191 ext 216.

**Advertising Office:** 119 Cherry Hill Rd, Suite 330, Parsippany, NJ 07054-1114; phone: (973) 263-9191.

**Classified Advertising:** Thalia Moss, Shana Brown, Kim Jenkins, Sophie Levandoski, 515 N State St, Chicago, IL 60610; phone: (800) 262-2260; e-mail: classifieds@jama-archives.org.

## ADVERTISING PRINCIPLES

Advertisements in this issue have been reviewed to comply with the principles governing advertising in AMA publications. A copy of these principles is available on request and online at www.archpediatrics.com. The appearance of advertising in AMA publications is not an AMA guarantee or endorsement of the product or the claims made for the product by the manufacturer.

## ADDRESS CHANGES

Send all address changes to *Archives of Pediatrics & Adolescent Medicine*, c/o the AMA Unified Service Center, American Medical Association, 515 N State St, Chicago, IL 60610. Notification of address changes must be made at least 6 weeks in advance; include both old and new addresses and a recent mailing label if sending via mail.

## SUBSCRIPTION RATES AND SERVICE

Subscription rates are shown in the table below. For service in the US and Americas, inquiries on pricing, address changes, missing issues, subscription billing, subscription renewal, and back issues, contact the AMA Unified Service Center, 24 hours a day, 7 days a week.

**AMA members:** phone: (800) 262-3211; e-mail: msc@ama-assn.org. **Other physicians and nonphysician customers, including subscription agents:** phone: (800) 262-2350 or (312) 670-7827; fax: (312) 464-5831; e-mail: ama-subs@ama-assn.org. **Inquiries:** Unified Service Center, American Medical Association, PO Box 10946, Chicago, IL 60610-0946. For subscribers with mailing addresses outside the United States & Americas: Contact *JAMA* & *Archives* Journals, c/o EMD GmbH, Birkenstr.67, 10559 Berlin, Germany. Phone: +49 (30) 33099828; fax: +49 (30) 33099829; e-mail: ama@emd-germany.de.

**Annual Subscription Rates**

| | United States | Americas | UK | Rest of World |
|---|---|---|---|---|
| INDIVIDUAL | | | | |
| Print and Online | $185 | $240 | £165 | €250 |
| INSTITUTION | | | | |
| Print and Online | $400 | $485 | £315 | €470 |

In Canada, US rate plus GST. Rates for residents and medical students available at pubs.ama-assn.org, or from the AMA Unified Service Center.

The ARCHIVES OF PEDIATRICS & ADOLESCENT MEDICINE (ISSN 01072–4710) is published monthly by the American Medical Association, 515 N State St, Chicago, IL 60610–0946, and is an official publication of the Association. The ARCHIVES OF PEDIATRICS & ADOLESCENT MEDICINE reaches more than 30 900 readers in over 83 countries each month. Periodicals postage paid at Chicago, Ill, and at additional mailing offices. GST registration number 12622 5556 RT. Canada Post International Publications Mail (Canadian Distribution) Sales Agreement No. 318728. POSTMASTER, send all address changes to *Archives of Pediatrics & Adolescent Medicine,* c/o the AMA Unified Service Center, American Medical Association, 515 N State St, Chicago, IL 60610. Printed in the USA.

# BOOSTRIX®

## (Tetanus Toxoid, Reduced Diphtheria Toxoid and Acellular Pertussis Vaccine, Adsorbed) (Tdap)

The following is a brief summary only; see full prescribing information for complete product information.

**INDICATIONS AND USAGE:** BOOSTRIX is indicated for active booster immunization against tetanus, diphtheria, and pertussis as a single dose in individuals 10 through 18 years of age. The use of BOOSTRIX as a primary series or to complete the primary series has not been studied. As with any vaccine, BOOSTRIX may not protect 100% of individuals receiving the vaccine.

**CONTRAINDICATIONS:** Hypersensitivity to any component of the vaccine is a contraindication (see DESCRIPTION in full prescribing information). Do not use BOOSTRIX after a serious allergic reaction (e.g., anaphylaxis) following any other tetanus toxoid, diphtheria toxoid or pertussis-containing vaccine, or any component of this vaccine (see DESCRIPTION in full prescribing information). Because of the uncertainty as to which component of the vaccine might be responsible, do not give further vaccination with any of these components; or, refer such individuals to an allergist for evaluation. The following events are contraindications to administration of BOOSTRIX: encephalopathy (e.g., coma, decreased level of consciousness, prolonged seizures) within 7 days of administration of a previous dose of a pertussis-containing vaccine that is not attributable to another identifiable cause; progressive neurologic disorder, uncontrolled epilepsy, or progressive encephalopathy. Do not vaccinate individuals with these conditions until a treatment regimen has been established and the condition has stabilized.

**WARNINGS:** The tip cap and the rubber plunger of the needleless prefilled syringes contain dry natural latex rubber that may cause allergic reactions in latex sensitive individuals. The vial stopper is latex-free. If any of the following events occurred in temporal relation to previous receipt of a Diphtheria and Tetanus Toxoids and Pertussis Vaccine Adsorbed (DTwP) vaccine or a vaccine containing an acellular pertussis component, consider carefully whether to give subsequent doses of BOOSTRIX: temperature of ≥40.5°C (105°F) within 48 hours not due to another identifiable cause; collapse or shock-like state (hypotonic-hyporesponsive episode) within 48 hours; persistent, inconsolable crying lasting ≥3 hours, occurring within 48 hours; seizures with or without fever occurring within 3 days. Persons who experienced serious Arthus-type hypersensitivity reactions following a prior dose of tetanus toxoid usually have high serum tetanus antitoxin levels and should not be given Tetanus and Diphtheria Toxoids Adsorbed For Adult Use (Td) or Tdap vaccines or even emergency doses of Td more frequently than every 10 years, even if the wound is neither clean nor minor. If Guillain-Barré syndrome has occurred within 6 weeks of receipt of prior vaccine containing tetanus toxoid, the decision to give BOOSTRIX or any vaccine containing tetanus toxoid should be based on careful consideration of the potential benefits and possible risks. The decision to administer a pertussis-containing vaccine to individuals with stable central nervous system (CNS) disorders must be made by the physician on an individual basis, with consideration of all relevant factors, and assessment of potential risks and benefits for that individual. Advise the patient, parent, or guardian of the potential increased risk involved (see PRECAUTIONS). A family history of seizures or other CNS disorders is not a contraindication to pertussis vaccine. The Advisory Committee on Immunization Practices (ACIP) has published guidelines for vaccination of persons with recent or acute illness (www.cdc.gov). Do not give BOOSTRIX to individuals with bleeding disorders such as hemophilia or thrombocytopenia, or to persons on anticoagulant therapy unless the potential benefit clearly outweighs the risk of administration. If the decision is made to administer BOOSTRIX to such persons, it should be given with caution with steps taken to avoid the risk of hematoma following the injection.

**PRECAUTIONS: General:** Before the injection of any biological, the physician should take all reasonable precautions to prevent allergic or other adverse reactions. Epinephrine injection (1:1,000) and other appropriate agents used for the control of immediate allergic reactions must be immediately available should an acute anaphylactic reaction occur. Immunosuppressed persons, including individuals receiving immunosuppressive therapy, may not develop the expected immune response. **Drug Interactions:** Do not mix BOOSTRIX with any other vaccine in the same syringe or vial. **Carcinogenesis, Mutagenesis, Impairment of Fertility:** BOOSTRIX has not been evaluated for carcinogenic or mutagenic potential, or for impairment of fertility. **Pregnancy:** Pregnancy Category C. Animal reproduction studies have not been conducted with BOOSTRIX. It is also not known whether BOOSTRIX can cause fetal harm when administered to a pregnant woman or can affect reproductive capacity. BOOSTRIX should be given to a pregnant woman only if clearly needed. Animal fertility studies have not been conducted with BOOSTRIX. In a developmental toxicity study, the effect of BOOSTRIX on embryo-fetal and pre-weaning development was evaluated in pregnant rats. Animals were administered INFANRIX® (Diphtheria and Tetanus Toxoids and Acellular Pertussis Vaccine Adsorbed) prior to gestation and BOOSTRIX during the period of organogenesis (gestation days 6, 8, 11) and later in pregnancy (gestation day 15), 0.1 mL/rat/occasion (a 45-fold increase compared to the human dose of BOOSTRIX on a body weight basis), by intramuscular injection. No adverse affect on pregnancy and lactation parameters, embryo-fetal or pre-weaning development was observed. There were no fetal malformations or other evidence of teratogenesis noted in this study. **Nursing Mothers:** It is not known whether BOOSTRIX is excreted in human milk. Because many drugs are excreted in human milk, caution should be exercised when BOOSTRIX is administered to a nursing woman. **Pregnancy Exposure Registry:** Healthcare providers are encouraged to register pregnant women who receive BOOSTRIX in the GlaxoSmithKline vaccination pregnancy registry by calling 1-888-825-5249. **Geriatric Use:** BOOSTRIX is not indicated for use in individuals older than 18 years. **Pediatric Use:** BOOSTRIX is not indicated for use in individuals younger than 10 years (see DOSAGE AND ADMINISTRATION in full prescribing information). For immunization of infants and children younger than 7 years against diphtheria, tetanus, and pertussis, refer to the manufacturers' package inserts for Diphtheria and Tetanus Toxoids and Acellular Pertussis Vaccine Adsorbed (DTaP) vaccines.

**ADVERSE REACTIONS:** A total of 3,608 adolescents were vaccinated with a single dose of BOOSTRIX during clinical trials. An additional 1,092 adolescents 10 to 18 years of age received a non-US formulation of BOOSTRIX (formulated to contain 0.5 mg aluminum per dose) in non-US clinical studies.

The primary safety study, conducted in the United States, was a randomized, observer-blinded, controlled study in which 3,080 adolescents 10 to 18 years of age received a single dose of BOOSTRIX and 1,034 received the control Td vaccine manufactured by Massachusetts Public Health Biologic Laboratories. There were no substantive differences in demographic characteristics between the vaccine groups. Among BOOSTRIX and control vaccine recipients approximately 75% were 10 to 14 years of age and approximately 25% were 15 to 18 years of age. Approximately 98% of participants in this study had received the recommended series of 4 or 5 doses of either DTwP or a combination of DTwP and DTaP in childhood. Data on adverse events were collected by the subjects, parents and/or guardians using standardized diaries for 15 consecutive days following the vaccine dose (i.e., day of vaccination and the next 14 days). Subjects were monitored for unsolicited adverse events that occurred within 31 days of vaccination (day 0-30) using diary cards (day 0-14) supplemented by spontaneous reports and a medical history as reported by subjects, parents, and/or guardians. Subjects were also monitored for 6 months post-vaccination for non-routine medical visits, visits to an emergency room, onset of new chronic illness, and serious adverse events. Information regarding late onset adverse events was obtained via a telephone call 6 months following vaccination. At least 97% of subjects completed the 6-month follow-up evaluation.

In a study conducted in Germany, BOOSTRIX was administered to 319 children 10 to 12 years of age previously vaccinated with 5 doses of acellular pertussis-containing vaccines, 193 of these subjects had previously received 5 doses of INFANRIX. Adverse events were recorded on diary cards during the 15 days following vaccination. Unsolicited adverse events that occurred within 31 days of vaccination (day 0-30) were recorded on the diary card or verbally reported to the investigator. Subjects were monitored for 6 months post-vaccination for physician office visits, emergency room visits, onset of new chronic illness, and serious adverse events. The 6-month follow-up evaluation, conducted via telephone interview, was completed by 90% of subjects.

The adverse event information from clinical trials provides a basis for identifying adverse events that appear to be related to vaccine use and for approximating rates. However, because clinical trials are conducted under widely varying conditions, adverse event rates observed in the clinical trials of a vaccine cannot be directly compared to rates in the clinical trials of another vaccine, and may not reflect the rates observed in practice.

**Serious Adverse Events in All Safety Studies:** In the US-safety study and German-safety study, no serious adverse events were reported to occur within 31 days of vaccination. During the 6-month extended safety evaluation period, no serious adverse events that were of potential autoimmune origin or new onset and chronic in nature were reported to occur. In non-US studies in which serious adverse events were monitored for up to 37 days, one subject was diagnosed with insulin dependent diabetes 20 days following administration of BOOSTRIX. No other serious adverse events of potential autoimmune origin or that were new onset and chronic in nature were reported to occur in these studies.

**Solicited Adverse Events in the US-Safety Study:** In a US study, the most common local adverse events following administration of BOOSTRIX were pain, redness, and swelling at the injection site. The most common general adverse events were headache and fatigue. Most of these events were reported at a similar frequency in recipients of both BOOSTRIX and Td. Any pain, grade 2 or 3 pain (but not grade 3 alone), and grade 2 or 3 headache (but not grade 3 alone) were reported at a higher rate in recipients of BOOSTRIX. The primary safety endpoint of the US study was the incidence of grade 3 pain (spontaneously painful and/or prevented normal activity) at the injection site within 15 days of vaccination. Grade 3 pain was reported in 4.6% of those who received BOOSTRIX compared with 4.0% of those who received the Td vaccine. The difference in rate of grade 3 pain was within the pre-defined clinical limit for non-inferiority (upper limit of the 95% CI for the difference ≤4%). These were the rates for solicited local and general adverse events within 15 days of vaccination with BOOSTRIX or Td vaccine for the total vaccinated cohort (all enrolled, vaccinated subjects with safety data available analyzed by vaccine received):

**Percentage of Individuals 10 to 18 Years of Age Reporting Solicited Local Adverse Events or Solicited General Adverse Events Within the 15-day* Post-Vaccination Period**

| | BOOSTRIX (N = 3,032) % | Td (N =1,013) % |
|---|---|---|
| **Local** | | |
| Pain,† any | 75.3 | 71.7 |
| Pain,† grade 2 or 3 | 51.2 | 42.5 |
| Pain,‡ grade 3 | 4.6 | 4.0 |
| Redness, any | 22.5 | 19.8 |
| Redness, >20 mm | 4.1 | 3.9 |
| Redness, ≥50 mm | 1.7 | 1.6 |
| Swelling, any | 21.1 | 20.1 |
| Swelling, >20 mm | 5.3 | 4.9 |
| Swelling, ≥50 mm | 2.5 | 3.2 |
| Arm circumference increase,§ >5 mm | 28.3 | 29.5 |
| Arm circumference increase,§ >20 mm | 2.0 | 2.2 |
| Arm circumference increase,§ >40 mm | 0.5 | 0.3 |
| **General** | | |
| Fever,‖ ≥99.5°F | 13.5 | 13.1 |
| Fever,‖ >100.4°F | 5.0 | 4.7 |
| Fever,‖ >102.2°F | 1.4 | 1.0 |
| Headache, any | 43.1 | 41.5 |
| Headache,† grade 2 or 3 | 15.7 | 12.7 |
| Headache, grade 3 | 3.7 | 2.7 |
| Fatigue, any | 37.0 | 36.7 |
| Fatigue, grade 2 or 3 | 14.4 | 12.9 |
| Fatigue, grade 3 | 3.7 | 3.2 |
| Gastrointestinal symptoms,¶ any | 26.0 | 25.8 |
| Gastrointestinal symptoms,¶ grade 2 or 3 | 9.8 | 9.7 |
| Gastrointestinal symptoms,¶ grade 3 | 3.0 | 3.2 |

Td = Tetanus and Diphtheria Toxoids Adsorbed For Adult Use manufactured by Massachusetts Public Health Biologic Laboratories.
N = number of subjects in the total vaccinated cohort with local/general symptoms sheets completed.
Grade 2 = Local: painful when the limb was moved; General: interfered with normal activity.
Grade 3 = Local: spontaneously painful and/or prevented normal activity; General: prevented normal activity.
*Day of vaccination and the next 14 days.
†Statistically significantly higher (P<0.05) following BOOSTRIX as compared to Td vaccine.
‡Grade 3 injection site pain following BOOSTRIX was not inferior to Td (upper limit of two-sided 95% CI for the difference in the percentage of subjects ≤4%).
§Mid-upper region of the vaccinated arm.
‖Oral temperatures or axillary temperatures.
¶Gastrointestinal symptoms included nausea, vomiting, diarrhea and/or abdominal pain.

Mid-upper arm circumference was measured by the adolescent or their parent/guardian prior to injection and daily for 15 days following vaccination. There was no significant difference between BOOSTRIX recipients and Td recipients in the proportion of subjects reporting an increase in mid-upper arm circumference in the vaccinated arm. The incidence of unsolicited adverse events reported in the 31 days after vaccination was comparable between the 2 groups.

**Solicited Adverse Events in the German Safety Study:** No cases of whole arm swelling were spontaneously reported. Two individuals (2/193) reported large injection site swelling (range 110 to 200 mm diameter), in one case associated with grade 3 pain. Neither individual sought medical attention. These episodes were reported to resolve without sequelae within 5 days. These were the rates of solicited local adverse events and fever within 15 days of vaccination for those subjects who had previously been vaccinated with 5 doses of INFANRIX:

**Rates of Solicited Adverse Events Reported Within the 15-day* Post-Vaccination Period Following Administration of BOOSTRIX in Individuals 10 to 12 Years of Age Who Had Previously Received 5 Doses of INFANRIX**

| Adverse Event | BOOSTRIX (N = 193) % (95% CI) |
|---|---|
| Pain, any | 62.2 (54.9-69.0) |
| Pain, grade 2 or 3 | 33.2 (26.6-40.3) |
| Pain, grade 3 | 5.7 (2.9-10.0) |
| Redness, any | 47.7 (40.4-55.0) |
| Redness, >20 mm | 15.0 (10.3-20.9) |
| Redness, ≥50 mm | 10.9 (6.9-16.2) |
| Swelling, any | 38.9 (31.9-46.1) |
| Swelling, >20 mm | 17.6 (12.5-23.7) |
| Swelling, ≥50 mm | 14.0 (9.4-19.7) |
| Fever, ≥99.5 | 8.8 (5.2-13.7) |
| Fever, >100.4 | 4.1 (1.8-8.0) |
| Fever, >102.2 | 1.0 (0.1-3.7) |

N = number of subjects with local/general symptoms sheets completed.
Grade 2 = Painful when the limb was moved.
Grade 3 = Spontaneously painful and/or prevented normal activity.
*Day of vaccination and the next 14 days.

As with any vaccine, there is the possibility that broad use of BOOSTRIX could reveal adverse events not observed in clinical trials.

**Postmarketing Reports:** Worldwide voluntary reports of adverse events received for BOOSTRIX in persons 10 to 18 years of age since market introduction of this vaccine are listed below. This list includes serious events or events which have causal connection to components of this or other vaccines or drugs. Because these events are reported voluntarily from a population of uncertain size, it is not possible to reliably estimate their frequency or establish a causal relationship to vaccine exposure. *Blood and lymphatic system disorders:* Lymphadenitis, lymphadenopathy. *Cardiac disorders:* Myocarditis. *Injection site reactions:* Induration, inflammation, mass, nodule, warmth, local reaction. *Metabolism and nutrition disorders:* Diabetes mellitus insulin-dependent. *Musculoskeletal and connective tissue disorders:* Arthralgia, back pain, myalgia. *Nervous system disorders:* Convulsion, encephalitis, facial palsy, paraesthesia. *Skin and subcutaneous tissue disorders:* Exanthem, Henoch-Schönlein purpura, rash. In addition, extensive swelling of the injected limb has been reported following administration of BOOSTRIX.

**Reporting Adverse Events:** Report the occurrence following immunization of any event set forth in the Vaccine Injury Table from the National Childhood Vaccine Injury Act including: Anaphylaxis or anaphylactic shock within 7 days, encephalopathy or encephalitis within 7 days, brachial neuritis within 28 days, or an acute complication or sequelae (including death) of an illness, disability, injury, or condition referred to above, or any events that would contraindicate further doses of vaccine, according to this prescribing information. These events should be reported to VAERS. The VAERS toll-free number is 1-800-822-7967. Reporting forms may also be obtained at the VAERS website at www.vaers.hhs.gov.

**DOSAGE AND ADMINISTRATION: Recommended Dose:** BOOSTRIX should be administered as a single 0.5 mL injection by the intramuscular route into the deltoid muscle of the upper arm in individuals 10 through 18 years of age. Do not administer this product subcutaneously or intravenously. There are no data to support repeat administration of BOOSTRIX. Five years should elapse between the subject's last dose of the recommended series of childhood DTwP and/or DTaP vaccine and the administration of BOOSTRIX. Limited data are available on the use of BOOSTRIX following Tetanus and Diphtheria Toxoids Adsorbed For Adult Use (Td) vaccine. **Additional Dosing Information:** ***Wound Management:*** Clinicians should refer to guidelines for tetanus prophylaxis in routine wound management. Adolescents 10 to 18 years of age who have completed a primary series against tetanus and who sustain wounds which are minor and uncomplicated, should receive a booster dose of a tetanus toxoid-containing vaccine only if they have not received tetanus toxoid within the preceding 10 years. In case of tetanus-prone injury (e.g., wounds contaminated with dirt, feces, soil, and saliva; puncture wounds; avulsions; and wounds resulting from missles, crushing, burns, and frostbite) in an adolescent who is in need of tetanus toxoid, BOOSTRIX can be used as an alternative to Tetanus and Diphtheria Toxoids Adsorbed For Adult Use (Td) vaccine in patients for whom the pertussis component is also indicated (see INDICATIONS AND USAGE).

Manufactured by **GlaxoSmithKline Biologicals**
Rixensart, Belgium, US License 1617

Distributed by **GlaxoSmithKline**
Research Triangle Park, NC 27709



Full prescribing information for BOOSTRIX is available at www.BOOSTRIX.com.
BRS-BO:L3

**References: 1.** Centers for Disease Control and Prevention. Preventing tetanus, diphtheria, and pertussis among adolescents: use of tetanus toxoid, reduced diphtheria toxoid and acellular pertussis vaccines: recommendations of the Advisory Committee on Immunization Practices (ACIP). Early Release 2006;55(February 23, 2006):1–43. **2.** Centers for Disease Control and Prevention. Recommended childhood and adolescent immunization schedule—United States, 2006. *MMWR.* 2006;54(51&52):Q1–Q4.

# ARCHIVES OF PEDIATRICS & ADOLESCENT MEDICINE

WWW.ARCHPEDIATRICS.COM

JULY 2006

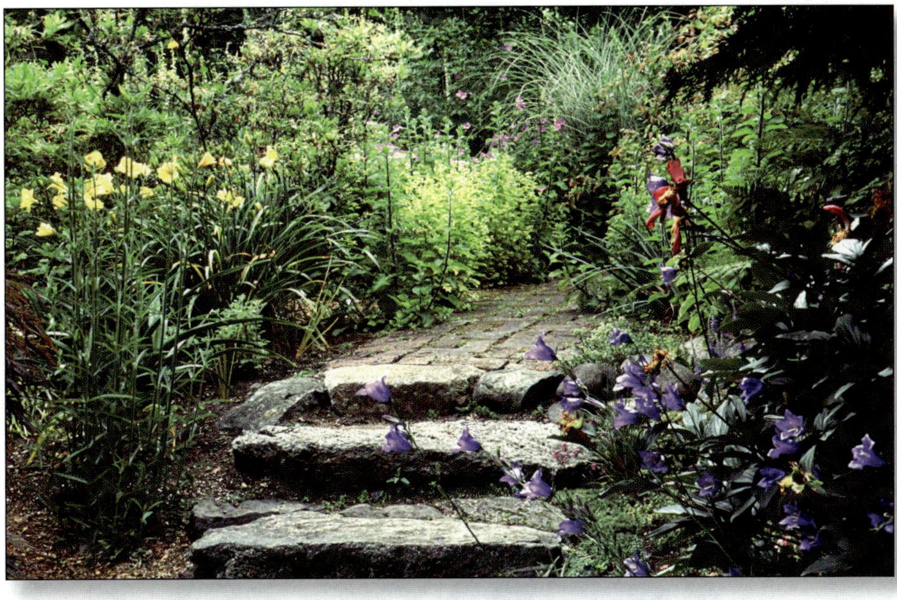

Summer in Lee Neff's Garden, Seattle, Wash, 2000. See page 669.

THE TRIAL OF INFANT RESPONSE TO DIPHENHYDRAMINE

RECOGNITION OF ADOLESCENT DEPRESSION IN PRIMARY CARE

HIV POSTEXPOSURE PROPHYLAXIS IN SEXUAL ASSAULT VICTIMS

AGE AT DRINKING ONSET AND ALCOHOL DEPENDENCE

COMPLETE TABLE OF CONTENTS ON PAGE 667



JAMA & ARCHIVES JOURNALS
American Medical Association

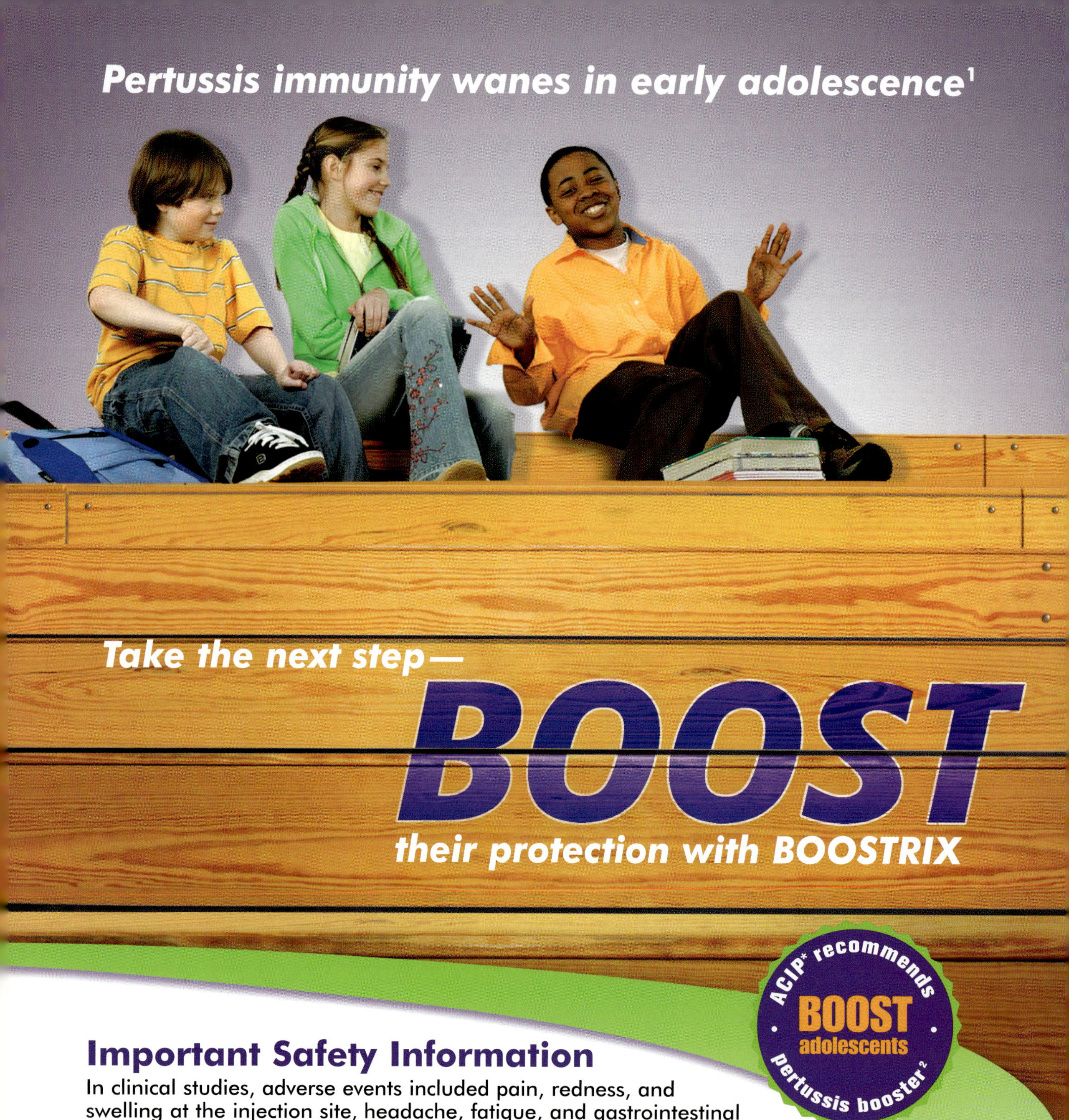


## Important Safety Information

In clinical studies, adverse events included pain, redness, and swelling at the injection site, headache, fatigue, and gastrointestinal symptoms. As with other vaccines, rare adverse events may occur. As with any vaccine, vaccination with BOOSTRIX may not protect 100% of susceptible individuals. Hypersensitivity to any component of BOOSTRIX is a contraindication.

*Advisory Committee on Immunization Practices.

**BOOSTRIX®**

***Tetanus Toxoid, Reduced Diphtheria Toxoid and Acellular Pertussis Vaccine, Adsorbed***

gsk GlaxoSmithKline Vaccines

**Please see references and brief summary of complete prescribing information on the adjacent page.**



Manufactured by **GlaxoSmithKline Biologicals,** Rixensart, Belgium

Distributed by **GlaxoSmithKline**, Research Triangle Park, NC 27709

# BOOSTRIX®

## (Tetanus Toxoid, Reduced Diphtheria Toxoid and Acellular Pertussis Vaccine, Adsorbed) (Tdap)

The following is a brief summary only; see full prescribing information for complete product information.

**INDICATIONS AND USAGE:** BOOSTRIX is indicated for active booster immunization against tetanus, diphtheria, and pertussis as a single dose in individuals 10 through 18 years of age. The use of BOOSTRIX as a primary series or to complete the primary series has not been studied. As with any vaccine, BOOSTRIX may not protect 100% of individuals receiving the vaccine.

**CONTRAINDICATIONS:** Hypersensitivity to any component of the vaccine is a contraindication (see DESCRIPTION in full prescribing information). Do not use BOOSTRIX after a serious allergic reaction (e.g., anaphylaxis) following any other tetanus toxoid, diphtheria toxoid or pertussis-containing vaccine, or any component of this vaccine (see DESCRIPTION in full prescribing information). Because of the uncertainty as to which component of the vaccine might be responsible, do not give further vaccination with any of these components; or, refer such individuals to an allergist for evaluation. The following events are contraindications to administration of BOOSTRIX: encephalopathy (e.g., coma, decreased level of consciousness, prolonged seizures) within 7 days of administration of a previous dose of a pertussis-containing vaccine that is not attributable to another identifiable cause; progressive neurologic disorder, uncontrolled epilepsy, or progressive encephalopathy. Do not vaccinate individuals with these conditions until a treatment regimen has been established and the condition has stabilized.

**WARNINGS:** The tip cap and the rubber plunger of the needleless prefilled syringes contain dry natural latex rubber that may cause allergic reactions in latex sensitive individuals. The vial stopper is latex-free. If any of the following events occurred in temporal relation to previous receipt of a Diphtheria and Tetanus Toxoids and Pertussis Vaccine Adsorbed (DTwP) vaccine or a vaccine containing an acellular pertussis component, consider carefully whether to give subsequent doses of BOOSTRIX: temperature of ≥40.5°C (105°F) within 48 hours not due to another identifiable cause; collapse or shock-like state (hypotonic-hyporesponsive episode) within 48 hours; persistent, inconsolable crying lasting ≥3 hours, occurring within 48 hours; seizures with or without fever occurring within 3 days. Persons who experienced serious Arthus-type hypersensitivity reactions following a prior dose of tetanus toxoid usually have high serum tetanus antitoxin levels and should not be given Tetanus and Diphtheria Toxoids Adsorbed For Adult Use (Td) or Tdap vaccines or even emergency doses of Td more frequently than every 10 years, even if the wound is neither clean nor minor. If Guillain-Barré syndrome has occurred within 6 weeks of receipt of prior vaccine containing tetanus toxoid, the decision to give BOOSTRIX or any vaccine containing tetanus toxoid should be based on careful consideration of the potential benefits and possible risks. The decision to administer a pertussis-containing vaccine to individuals with stable central nervous system (CNS) disorders must be made by the physician on an individual basis, with consideration of all relevant factors, and assessment of potential risks and benefits for that individual. Advise the patient, parent, or guardian of the potential increased risk involved (see PRECAUTIONS). A family history of seizures or other CNS disorders is not a contraindication to pertussis vaccine. The Advisory Committee on Immunization Practices (ACIP) has published guidelines for vaccination of persons with recent or acute illness (www.cdc.gov). Do not give BOOSTRIX to individuals with bleeding disorders such as hemophilia or thrombocytopenia, or to persons on anticoagulant therapy unless the potential benefit clearly outweighs the risk of administration. If the decision is made to administer BOOSTRIX to such persons, it should be given with caution with steps taken to avoid the risk of hematoma following the injection.

**PRECAUTIONS: General:** Before the injection of any biological, the physician should take all reasonable precautions to prevent allergic or other adverse reactions. Epinephrine injection (1:1,000) and other appropriate agents used for the control of immediate allergic reactions must be immediately available should an acute anaphylactic reaction occur. Immunosuppressed persons, including individuals receiving immunosuppressive therapy, may not develop the expected immune response. **Drug Interactions:** Do not mix BOOSTRIX with any other vaccine in the same syringe or vial. **Carcinogenesis, Mutagenesis, Impairment of Fertility:** BOOSTRIX has not been evaluated for carcinogenic or mutagenic potential, or for impairment of fertility. **Pregnancy:** Pregnancy Category C. Animal reproduction studies have not been conducted with BOOSTRIX. It is also not known whether BOOSTRIX can cause fetal harm when administered to a pregnant woman or can affect reproductive capacity. BOOSTRIX should be given to a pregnant woman only if clearly needed. Animal fertility studies have not been conducted with BOOSTRIX. In a developmental toxicity study, the effect of BOOSTRIX on embryo-fetal and pre-weaning development was evaluated in pregnant rats. Animals were administered INFANRIX® (Diphtheria and Tetanus Toxoids and Acellular Pertussis Vaccine Adsorbed) prior to gestation and BOOSTRIX during the period of organogenesis (gestation days 6, 8, 11) and later in pregnancy (gestation day 15), 0.1 mL/rat/occasion (a 45-fold increase compared to the human dose of BOOSTRIX on a body weight basis), by intramuscular injection. No adverse affect on pregnancy and lactation parameters, embryo-fetal or pre-weaning development was observed. There were no fetal malformations or other evidence of teratogenesis noted in this study. **Nursing Mothers:** It is not known whether BOOSTRIX is excreted in human milk. Because many drugs are excreted in human milk, caution should be exercised when BOOSTRIX is administered to a nursing woman. **Pregnancy Exposure Registry:** Healthcare providers are encouraged to register pregnant women who receive BOOSTRIX in the GlaxoSmithKline vaccination pregnancy registry by calling 1-888-825-5249. **Geriatric Use:** BOOSTRIX is not indicated for use in individuals older than 18 years. **Pediatric Use:** BOOSTRIX is not indicated for use in individuals younger than 10 years (see DOSAGE AND ADMINISTRATION in full prescribing information). For immunization of infants and children younger than 7 years against diphtheria, tetanus, and pertussis, refer to the manufacturers' package inserts for Diphtheria and Tetanus Toxoids and Acellular Pertussis Vaccine Adsorbed (DTaP) vaccines.

**ADVERSE REACTIONS:** A total of 3,608 adolescents were vaccinated with a single dose of BOOSTRIX during clinical trials. An additional 1,092 adolescents 10 to 18 years of age received a non-US formulation of BOOSTRIX (formulated to contain 0.5 mg aluminum per dose) in non-US clinical studies.

The primary safety study, conducted in the United States, was a randomized, observer-blinded, controlled study in which 3,080 adolescents 10 to 18 years of age received a single dose of BOOSTRIX and 1,034 received the control Td vaccine manufactured by Massachusetts Public Health Biologic Laboratories. There were no substantive differences in demographic characteristics between the vaccine groups. Among BOOSTRIX and control vaccine recipients approximately 75% were 10 to 14 years of age and approximately 25% were 15 to 18 years of age. Approximately 98% of participants in this study had received the recommended series of 4 or 5 doses of either DTwP or a combination of DTwP and DTaP in childhood. Data on adverse events were collected by the subjects, parents and/or guardians using standardized diaries for 15 consecutive days following the vaccine dose (i.e., day of vaccination and the next 14 days). Subjects were monitored for unsolicited adverse events that occurred within 31 days of vaccination (day 0-30) using diary cards (day 0-14) supplemented by spontaneous reports and a medical history as reported by subjects, parents, and/or guardians. Subjects were also monitored for 6 months post-vaccination for non-routine medical visits, visits to an emergency room, onset of new chronic illness, and serious adverse events. Information regarding late onset adverse events was obtained via a telephone call 6 months following vaccination. At least 97% of subjects completed the 6-month follow-up evaluation.

In a study conducted in Germany, BOOSTRIX was administered to 319 children 10 to 12 years of age previously vaccinated with 5 doses of acellular pertussis-containing vaccines, 193 of these subjects had previously received 5 doses of INFANRIX. Adverse events were recorded on diary cards during the 15 days following vaccination. Unsolicited adverse events that occurred within 31 days of vaccination (day 0-30) were recorded on the diary card or verbally reported to the investigator. Subjects were monitored for 6 months post-vaccination for physician office visits, emergency room visits, onset of new chronic illness, and serious adverse events. The 6-month follow-up evaluation, conducted via telephone interview, was completed by 90% of subjects.

The adverse event information from clinical trials provides a basis for identifying adverse events that appear to be related to vaccine use and for approximating rates. However, because clinical trials are conducted under widely varying conditions, adverse event rates observed in the clinical trials of a vaccine cannot be directly compared to rates in the clinical trials of another vaccine, and may not reflect the rates observed in practice.

**Serious Adverse Events in All Safety Studies:** In the US-safety study and German-safety study, no serious adverse events were reported to occur within 31 days of vaccination. During the 6-month extended safety evaluation period, no serious adverse events that were of potential autoimmune origin or new onset and chronic in nature were reported to occur. In non-US studies in which serious adverse events were monitored for up to 37 days, one subject was diagnosed with insulin dependent diabetes 20 days following administration of BOOSTRIX. No other serious adverse events of potential autoimmune origin or that were new onset and chronic in nature were reported to occur in these studies.

**Solicited Adverse Events in the US-Safety Study:** In a US study, the most common local adverse events following administration of BOOSTRIX were pain, redness, and swelling at the injection site. The most common general adverse events were headache and fatigue. Most of these events were reported at a similar frequency in recipients of both BOOSTRIX and Td. Any pain, grade 2 or 3 pain (but not grade 3 alone), and grade 2 or 3 headache (but not grade 3 alone) were reported at a higher rate in recipients of BOOSTRIX. The primary safety endpoint of the US study was the incidence of grade 3 pain (spontaneously painful and/or prevented normal activity) at the injection site within 15 days of vaccination. Grade 3 pain was reported in 4.6% of those who received BOOSTRIX compared with 4.0% of those who received the Td vaccine. The difference in rate of grade 3 pain was within the pre-defined clinical limit for non-inferiority (upper limit of the 95% CI for the difference ≤4%). These were the rates for solicited local and general adverse events within 15 days of vaccination with BOOSTRIX or Td vaccine for the total vaccinated cohort (all enrolled, vaccinated subjects with safety data available analyzed by vaccine received):

**Percentage of Individuals 10 to 18 Years of Age Reporting Solicited Local Adverse Events or Solicited General Adverse Events Within the 15-day* Post-Vaccination Period**

| | BOOSTRIX (N = 3,032) % | Td (N =1,013) % |
|---|---|---|
| **Local** | | |
| Pain,[†] any | 75.3 | 71.7 |
| Pain,[†] grade 2 or 3 | 51.2 | 42.5 |
| Pain,[‡] grade 3 | 4.6 | 4.0 |
| Redness, any | 22.5 | 19.8 |
| Redness, >20 mm | 4.1 | 3.9 |
| Redness, ≥50 mm | 1.7 | 1.6 |
| Swelling, any | 21.1 | 20.1 |
| Swelling, >20 mm | 5.3 | 4.9 |
| Swelling, ≥50 mm | 2.5 | 3.2 |
| Arm circumference increase,[§] >5 mm | 28.3 | 29.5 |
| Arm circumference increase,[§] >20 mm | 2.0 | 2.2 |
| Arm circumference increase,[§] >40 mm | 0.5 | 0.3 |
| **General** | | |
| Fever,[‖] ≥99.5°F | 13.5 | 13.1 |
| Fever,[‖] >100.4°F | 5.0 | 4.7 |
| Fever,[‖] >102.2°F | 1.4 | 1.0 |
| Headache, any | 43.1 | 41.5 |
| Headache,[†] grade 2 or 3 | 15.7 | 12.7 |
| Headache, grade 3 | 3.7 | 2.7 |
| Fatigue, any | 37.0 | 36.7 |
| Fatigue, grade 2 or 3 | 14.4 | 12.9 |
| Fatigue, grade 3 | 3.7 | 3.2 |
| Gastrointestinal symptoms,[¶] any | 26.0 | 25.8 |
| Gastrointestinal symptoms,[¶] grade 2 or 3 | 9.8 | 9.7 |
| Gastrointestinal symptoms,[¶] grade 3 | 3.0 | 3.2 |

Td = Tetanus and Diphtheria Toxoids Adsorbed For Adult Use manufactured by Massachusetts Public Health Biologic Laboratories.
N = number of subjects in the total vaccinated cohort with local/general symptoms sheets completed.
Grade 2 = Local: painful when the limb was moved; General: interfered with normal activity.
Grade 3 = Local: spontaneously painful and/or prevented normal activity; General: prevented normal activity.
*Day of vaccination and the next 14 days.
[†]Statistically significantly higher (P<0.05) following BOOSTRIX as compared to Td vaccine.
[‡]Grade 3 injection site pain following BOOSTRIX was not inferior to Td (upper limit of two-sided 95% CI for the difference in the percentage of subjects ≤4%).
[§]Mid-upper region of the vaccinated arm.
[‖]Oral temperatures or axillary temperatures.
[¶]Gastrointestinal symptoms included nausea, vomiting, diarrhea and/or abdominal pain.

Mid-upper arm circumference was measured by the adolescent or their parent/guardian prior to injection and daily for 15 days following vaccination. There was no significant difference between BOOSTRIX recipients and Td recipients in the proportion of subjects reporting an increase in mid-upper arm circumference in the vaccinated arm. The incidence of unsolicited adverse events reported in the 31 days after vaccination was comparable between the 2 groups.

**Solicited Adverse Events in the German Safety Study:** No cases of whole arm swelling were spontaneously reported. Two individuals (2/193) reported large injection site swelling (range 110 to 200 mm diameter), in one case associated with grade 3 pain. Neither individual sought medical attention. These episodes were reported to resolve without sequelae within 5 days. These were the rates of solicited local adverse events and fever within 15 days of vaccination for those subjects who had previously been vaccinated with 5 doses of INFANRIX:

**Rates of Solicited Adverse Events Reported Within the 15-day* Post-Vaccination Period Following Administration of BOOSTRIX in Individuals 10 to 12 Years of Age Who Had Previously Received 5 Doses of INFANRIX**

| Adverse Event | BOOSTRIX (N = 193) % (95% CI) |
|---|---|
| Pain, any | 62.2 (54.9-69.0) |
| Pain, grade 2 or 3 | 33.2 (26.6-40.3) |
| Pain, grade 3 | 5.7 (2.9-10.0) |
| Redness, any | 47.7 (40.4-55.0) |
| Redness, >20 mm | 15.0 (10.3-20.9) |
| Redness, ≥50 mm | 10.9 (6.9-16.2) |
| Swelling, any | 38.9 (31.9-46.1) |
| Swelling, >20 mm | 17.6 (12.5-23.7) |
| Swelling, ≥50 mm | 14.0 (9.4-19.7) |
| Fever, ≥99.5 | 8.8 (5.2-13.7) |
| Fever, >100.4 | 4.1 (1.8-8.0) |
| Fever, >102.2 | 1.0 (0.1-3.7) |

N = number of subjects with local/general symptoms sheets completed.
Grade 2 = Painful when the limb was moved.
Grade 3 = Spontaneously painful and/or prevented normal activity.
*Day of vaccination and the next 14 days.

As with any vaccine, there is the possibility that broad use of BOOSTRIX could reveal adverse events not observed in clinical trials.

**Postmarketing Reports:** Worldwide voluntary reports of adverse events received for BOOSTRIX in persons 10 to 18 years of age since market introduction of this vaccine are listed below. This list includes serious events or events which have causal connection to components of this or other vaccines or drugs. Because these events are reported voluntarily from a population of uncertain size, it is not possible to reliably estimate their frequency or establish a causal relationship to vaccine exposure. *Blood and lymphatic system disorders:* Lymphadenitis, lymphadenopathy. *Cardiac disorders:* Myocarditis. *Injection site reactions:* Induration, inflammation, mass, nodule, warmth, local reaction. *Metabolism and nutrition disorders:* Diabetes mellitus insulin-dependent. *Musculoskeletal and connective tissue disorders:* Arthralgia, back pain, myalgia. *Nervous system disorders:* Convulsion, encephalitis, facial palsy, paraesthesia. *Skin and subcutaneous tissue disorders:* Exanthem, Henoch-Schönlein purpura, rash. In addition, extensive swelling of the injected limb has been reported following administration of BOOSTRIX.

**Reporting Adverse Events:** Report the occurrence following immunization of any event set forth in the Vaccine Injury Table from the National Childhood Vaccine Injury Act including: Anaphylaxis or anaphylactic shock within 7 days, encephalopathy or encephalitis within 7 days, brachial neuritis within 28 days, or an acute complication or sequelae (including death) of an illness, disability, injury, or condition referred to above, or any events that would contraindicate further doses of vaccine, according to this prescribing information. These events should be reported to VAERS. The VAERS toll-free number is 1-800-822-7967. Reporting forms may also be obtained at the VAERS website at www.vaers.hhs.gov.

**DOSAGE AND ADMINISTRATION: Recommended Dose:** BOOSTRIX should be administered as a single 0.5 mL injection by the intramuscular route into the deltoid muscle of the upper arm in individuals 10 through 18 years of age. Do not administer this product subcutaneously or intravenously. There are no data to support repeat administration of BOOSTRIX. Five years should elapse between the subject's last dose of the recommended series of childhood DTwP and/or DTaP vaccine and the administration of BOOSTRIX. Limited data are available on the use of BOOSTRIX following Tetanus and Diphtheria Toxoids Adsorbed For Adult Use (Td) vaccine. **Additional Dosing Information:** ***Wound Management:*** Clinicians should refer to guidelines for tetanus prophylaxis in routine wound management. Adolescents 10 to 18 years of age who have completed a primary series against tetanus and who sustain wounds which are minor and uncomplicated, should receive a booster dose of a tetanus toxoid-containing vaccine only if they have not received tetanus toxoid within the preceding 10 years. In case of tetanus-prone injury (e.g., wounds contaminated with dirt, feces, soil, and saliva; puncture wounds; avulsions; and wounds resulting from missles, crushing, burns, and frostbite) in an adolescent who is in need of tetanus toxoid, BOOSTRIX can be used as an alternative to Tetanus and Diphtheria Toxoids Adsorbed For Adult Use (Td) vaccine in patients for whom the pertussis component is also indicated (see INDICATIONS AND USAGE).

Manufactured by **GlaxoSmithKline Biologicals**
Rixensart, Belgium, US License 1617

Distributed by **GlaxoSmithKline**
Research Triangle Park, NC 27709



Full prescribing information for BOOSTRIX is available at www.BOOSTRIX.com.
BRS-BO:L3

**References: 1.** Centers for Disease Control and Prevention. Preventing tetanus, diphtheria, and pertussis among adolescents: use of tetanus toxoid, reduced diphtheria toxoid and acellular pertussis vaccines: recommendations of the Advisory Committee on Immunization Practices (ACIP). Early Release 2006;55(February 23, 2006):1–43. **2.** Centers for Disease Control and Prevention. Recommended childhood and adolescent immunization schedule—United States, 2006. *MMWR.* 2006;54(51&52):Q1–Q4.

# ARCHIVES OF PEDIATRICS & ADOLESCENT MEDICINE

JULY 2006 VOLUME 160, NUMBER 7 PAGES 665-760


## ARTICLES


**Use of Human Immunodeficiency Virus Postexposure Prophylaxis in Adolescent Sexual Assault Victims** 674
*Elyse Olshen, MD, MPH; Katherine Hsu, MD, MPH; Elizabeth R. Woods, MD, MPH; Marvin Harper, MD; Brooke Harnisch, MA; Cathryn L. Samples, MD, MPH*

**The Effect of Peer Counselors on Breastfeeding Rates in the Neonatal Intensive Care Unit: Results of a Randomized Controlled Trial** 681
*Anne Merewood, MPH, IBCLC; Laura Beth Chamberlain, BA, IBCLC; John T. Cook, PhD; Barbara L. Philipp, MD; Kirsten Malone, BA, IBCLC; Howard Bauchner, MD, MPH*

**Prevalence of Coronary Artery Lesions on the Initial Echocardiogram in Kawasaki Syndrome** 686
*Aryeh Z. Baer, MD; Lorry G. Rubin, MD; Craig A. Shapiro, BA; Sunil K. Sood, MD; Sujatha Rajan, MD; Yehuda Shapir, MD; Angela Romano, MD; Fredrick Z. Bierman, MD*


## REVIEW ARTICLE


**Improving Recognition of Adolescent Depression in Primary Care** 694
*Rachel A. Zuckerbrot, MD; Peter S. Jensen, MD*


## SPECIAL FEATURE


**Picture of the Month** 705
*Kimberly A. Horii, MD; Amy Jo Nopper, MD; Vidya Sharma, MBBS, MPH*


## ARTICLES


**The Trial of Infant Response to Diphenhydramine: The TIRED Study—A Randomized, Controlled, Patient-Oriented Trial** 707
*Dan Merenstein, MD; Marie Diener-West, PhD; Ann C. Halbower, MD; Alex Krist, MD; Haya R. Rubin, MD, PhD*

**Accuracy and Impact of a Point-of-Care Rapid Influenza Test in Young Children With Respiratory Illnesses** 713
*Katherine A. Poehling, MD, MPH; Yuwei Zhu, MD, MS; Yi-Wei Tang, MD, PhD; Kathryn Edwards, MD*

**Work Hazards and Workplace Safety Violations Experienced by Adolescent Construction Workers** 721
*Carol W. Runyan, MPH, PhD; Janet Dal Santo, DrPH; Michael Schulman, PhD; Hester J. Lipscomb, PhD; Thomas A. Harris, JD*

**Postasphyxial Hypoxic-Ischemic Encephalopathy in Neonates: Outcome Prediction Rule Within 4 Hours of Birth** 729
*Prakesh S. Shah, FRCPC, MSc; Joseph Beyene, PhD; Teresa To, PhD; Arne Ohlsson, FRCPC, MSc; Max Perlman, FRCPC*

**Age at Drinking Onset and Alcohol Dependence: Age at Onset, Duration, and Severity** 739
*Ralph W. Hingson, ScD, MPH; Timothy Heeren, PhD; Michael R. Winter, MPH*

**Brain Death: Understanding of the Conceptual Basis by Pediatric Intensivists in Canada** 747
*Ari R. Joffe, MD, FRCPC; Natalie Anton, MD, FRCPC*


## EDITORIALS


**Human Immunodeficiency Virus Prophylaxis for Sexual Assault Survivors: What We Need to Know** 754
*Jonathan M. Ellen, MD*

**Screens and Doors: The Management of Adolescent Depression in Primary Care** 755
*David A. Brent, MD*

ARCHIVES OF PEDIATRICS & ADOLESCENT MEDICINE

## THE PEDIATRIC FORUM

**Concerns Over Alternating Acetaminophen and Ibuprofen for Fever** 757
*Barton D. Schmitt, MD*

**Alternating Acetaminophen and Ibuprofen in Children May Cause Parental Confusion and Is Dangerous** 757
*Phisit Saphyakhajon, MD; Gerald Greene, MD, MPH*

**In Reply** 757
*E. Michael Sarrell, MD; Eliahu Wielunsky, MD; Herman Avner Cohen, MD*

## CORRECTION

**Error in Byline: Dismissing Families: A Slippery Slope** 685
*Kathi J. Kemper, MD, MPH; Caryl J. Guth, MD*

## REGULAR DEPARTMENTS

**This Month in *Archives of Pediatrics & Adolescent Medicine*** 673

**Announcements** 680, 712, 736, 758

**Call for Papers** 752

**Classified Advertising** 759

**Journal Advertiser Index** 759

**Contact Information** 760

**Instructions for authors and the author and subject indexes are available on our Web site: http://www.archpediatrics.com. If you do not have access to the Web, contact Suzanne Shuey at (206) 685-3573.**

### About the Cover

*Summer in Lee Neff's Garden*, Seattle, Wash, 2000.

# ARCHIVES OF PEDIATRICS & ADOLESCENT MEDICINE


**Mission Statement:** *The Archives of Pediatrics & Adolescent Medicine* is a monthly, peer-reviewed journal for physicians and other health care professionals who contribute to the health of children and adolescents. The *Archives* provides an open forum for dialogue on a full range of clinical, scientific, advocacy, and humanistic issues relevant to the care of pediatric patients from infancy through young adulthood. The *Archives* is a vehicle for increased attention to adolescent health, the education of pediatric health care professionals, and disease prevention and health promotion. The *Archives* publishes original studies, editorials, reviews by experts, practice commentaries, case quizzes, and updates on clinical science and practice management. The Pediatric Forum provides our readers with opportunities to express their views. *Archives* incorporates *AJDC*, the oldest journal in US pediatric literature, which originated in 1911.



JAMA & ARCHIVES JOURNALS
American Medical Association

All articles published, including editorials, letters, and book reviews, represent the opinions of the authors and do not reflect the policy of the American Medical Association, the Editorial Board, or the institution with which the author is affiliated, unless this is clearly specified.

**ACIP *recommends vaccination of children against hepatitis A*[*1]**

# Hepatitis A spreads FAST... especially among children[2,3]

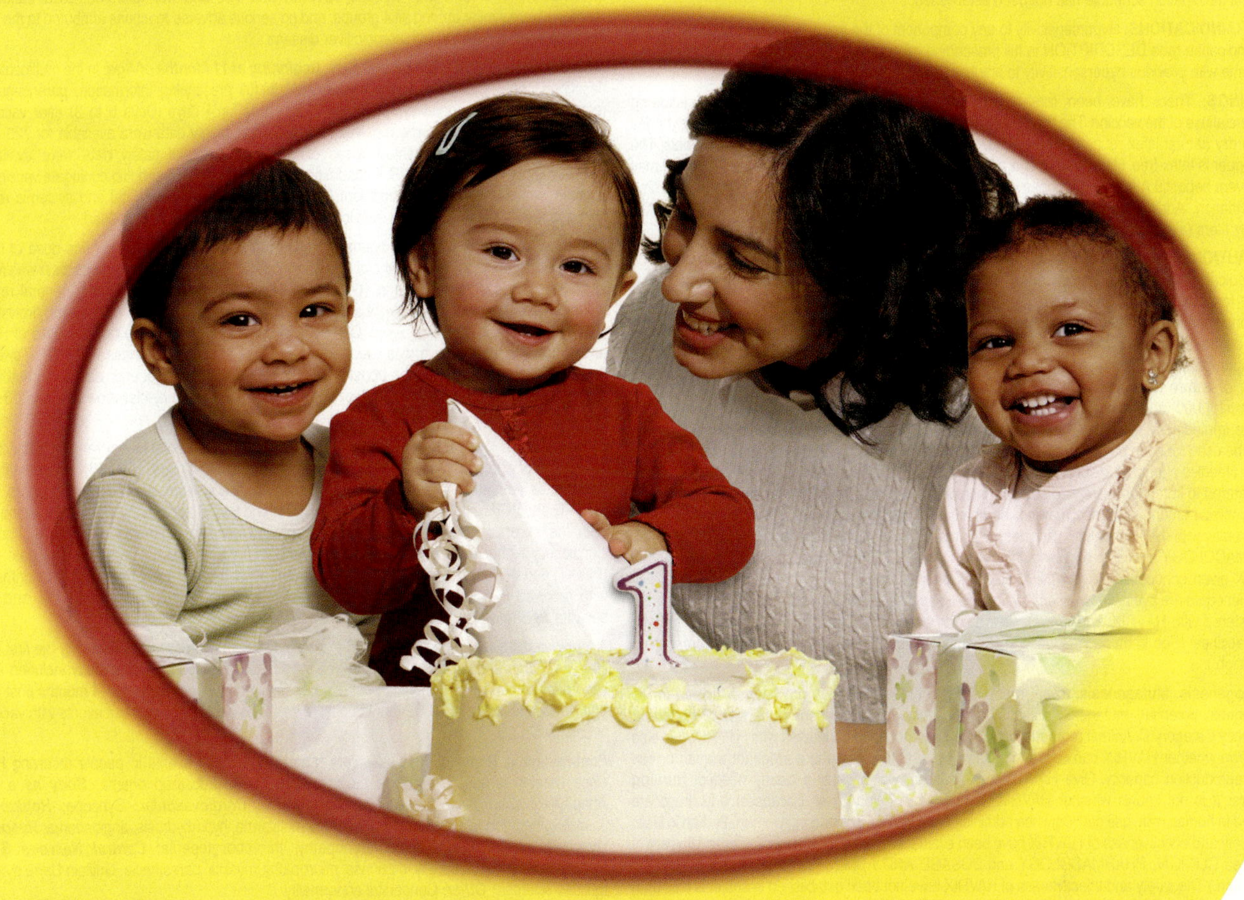

## HAVRIX provides excellent protection

HAVRIX is indicated for active immunization against hepatitis A virus in children 12 months of age and older.

## Important Safety Information

In clinical trials, the most common solicited adverse events were injection-site soreness and headache.

Greater incidences of general adverse events were observed in subjects who received HAVRIX at the same time as Hib conjugate and DTaP vaccines. As with any vaccine, rare adverse events may occur. (See Adverse Reactions section of the Prescribing Information for HAVRIX for potential side effects.) HAVRIX is contraindicated in people with hypersensitivity to any component of the vaccine, including neomycin.

* Advisory Committee on Immunization Practices recommends routine nationwide vaccination against hepatitis A in all children 1–2 years of age.

**Please see references and brief summary of complete prescribing information for HAVRIX on adjacent page.**

HAVRIX is a registered trademark of GlaxoSmithKline.

Manufactured by **GlaxoSmithKline Biologicals**, Rixensart, Belgium
Distributed by **GlaxoSmithKline**, Research Triangle Park, NC 27709

gsk GlaxoSmithKline Vaccines

**Havrix®**
**Hepatitis A Vaccine, Inactivated**

## HAVRIX®
## (Hepatitis A Vaccine, Inactivated)

The following is a brief summary only; see full prescribing information for complete product information.

**INDICATIONS AND USAGE:** HAVRIX is indicated for active immunization of persons ≥12 months of age against disease caused by hepatitis A virus (HAV). Primary immunization should be administered at least 2 weeks prior to expected exposure to HAV. When passive protection against hepatitis A is required either following exposure to hepatitis A virus or in persons requiring both immediate and long-term protection, HAVRIX may be administered concomitantly with immune globulin (IG) with different syringes and at different injection sites. Duration of immunity following a complete vaccination schedule has not been established.

**CONTRAINDICATIONS:** Hypersensitivity to any component of the vaccine, including neomycin, is a contraindication (see DESCRIPTION in full prescribing information). This vaccine is contraindicated in patients with previous hypersensitivity to any hepatitis A-containing vaccine.

**WARNINGS:** There have been rare reports of anaphylaxis/anaphylactoid reactions following commercial use of the vaccine. The tip cap and the rubber plunger of the needleless prefilled syringes contain dry natural latex rubber that may cause allergic reactions in latex sensitive individuals. The vial stopper is latex-free. Hepatitis A has a relatively long incubation period. Hepatitis A vaccine may not prevent hepatitis A infection in those who have an unrecognized hepatitis A infection at the time of vaccination. Additionally, it may not prevent infection in those who do not achieve protective antibody titers (although the lowest titer needed to confer protection has not been determined).

**PRECAUTIONS: General:** Prior to immunization with HAVRIX, the patient's current health status and medical history should be reviewed. The physician should review the patient's immunization history for possible vaccine sensitivity, previous vaccination-related adverse reactions and occurrence of any adverse–event-related symptoms and/or signs, in order to determine the existence of any contraindication to immunization with HAVRIX and to allow an assessment of benefits and risks. Appropriate medical treatment and supervision should be readily available for immediate use in case of a rare anaphylactic reaction following the administration of the vaccine. Epinephrine injection (1:1,000) and other appropriate agents used for the control of immediate allergic reactions must be immediately available. A separate, sterile syringe and needle or a sterile disposable unit should be used for each patient to prevent the transmission of other infectious agents from person to person. Needles should be disposed of properly and should not be recapped. As with any vaccine, if administered to immunosuppressed persons, including those receiving immunosuppressive therapy, the expected immune response may not be obtained. **Drug Interactions:** HAVRIX may be given concurrently with Hib conjugate vaccines in children 15 to 18 months of age (see CLINICAL PHARMACOLOGY in full prescribing information and ADVERSE REACTIONS). The safety of HAVRIX given concomitantly with INFANRIX has been evaluated (see ADVERSE REACTIONS). Insufficient data are available to assess the immune response of a fourth dose of DTaP vaccine when administered with HAVRIX. There are limited data to assess the concomitant use of HAVRIX with other vaccines. (See Immune Response to Concomitantly Administered Vaccines in full prescribing information.)

**Carcinogenesis, Mutagenesis, Impairment of Fertility:** HAVRIX has not been evaluated for its carcinogenic potential, mutagenic potential, or potential for impairment of fertility. **Pregnancy:** Pregnancy Category C. Animal reproduction studies have not been conducted with HAVRIX. It is also not known whether HAVRIX can cause fetal harm when administered to a pregnant woman or can affect reproduction capacity. Give HAVRIX to a pregnant woman only if clearly needed. **Nursing Mothers:** It is not known whether HAVRIX is excreted in human milk. Because many drugs are excreted in human milk, use caution when administering HAVRIX to a nursing woman. **Pediatric Use:** The safety and effectiveness of HAVRIX have been evaluated in 20,436 subjects 1 year to 18 years of age. (See CLINICAL PHARMACOLOGY and DOSAGE AND ADMINISTRATION in full prescribing information.) The safety and effectiveness of HAVRIX have not been established in subjects less than 12 months of age. **Geriatric Use:** Clinical studies of HAVRIX did not include sufficient numbers of subjects 65 years of age and older to determine whether they respond differently from younger subjects. Other reported clinical experience has not identified differences in overall safety between these subjects and younger adult subjects.

**ADVERSE REACTIONS:** As with all pharmaceuticals, however, it is possible that expanded commercial use of the vaccine could reveal rare adverse events. The adverse events most frequently reported by volunteers in clinical trials were injection-site soreness (56% of adults; 21% of children); headache (14% of adults; less than 9% of children). Other solicited and unsolicited events are listed below:

**Incidence 1% to 10% of Injections:** ***Local Reactions at Injection Site:*** Induration, redness, swelling; ***Body as a Whole:*** Fatigue, fever (>37.5°C), malaise; ***Gastrointestinal:*** Anorexia, nausea.

**Incidence <1% of Injections:** ***Local Reaction at Injection Site:*** Hematoma; ***Dermatologic:*** Pruritus, rash, urticaria; ***Respiratory:*** Pharyngitis, other upper respiratory tract infections; ***Gastrointestinal:*** Abdominal pain, diarrhea, dysgeusia, vomiting; ***Musculoskeletal:*** Arthralgia, elevation of creatine phosphokinase, myalgia; ***Hematologic:*** Lymphadenopathy; ***Central Nervous System:*** Hypertonic episode, insomnia, photophobia, vertigo.

**Additional safety data:** Safety data were obtained from 2 additional sources in which large populations were vaccinated. In an outbreak setting in which 4,930 individuals were immunized with a single dose of either 720 EL.U. or 1440 EL.U. of HAVRIX, the vaccine was well tolerated and no serious adverse events due to vaccination were reported. Overall, less than 10% of vaccinees reported solicited general adverse events following the vaccine. The most common solicited local adverse event was pain at the injection site, reported in 22.3% of subjects at 24 hours and decreasing to 2.4% by 72 hours.

In a field efficacy trial, 19,037 children received the 360 EL.U. dose of HAVRIX. The most commonly reported adverse events were injection-site pain (9.5%) and tenderness (8.1%), reported following first doses of HAVRIX. Other adverse events were infrequent and comparable to the control vaccine ENGERIX-B® [Hepatitis B Vaccine (Recombinant)].

In subjects with chronic liver disease, HAVRIX was safe and well tolerated. Local injection site reactions were similar among all 4 groups, and no serious adverse reactions attributed to the vaccine were reported in subjects with chronic liver disease.

***Safety Data for HAVRIX 720 EL.U./0.5 mL Beginning at 11 Months of Age:*** In the multicenter study described under CLINICAL PHARMACOLOGY in full prescribing information, parents/guardians recorded local and general symptoms on diary cards for 4 days (Days 0 to 3) after vaccination. In the 3 groups of children who received HAVRIX alone, safety data were available for 723 children who received 1,396 documented doses of HAVRIX. Additional safety data were available for 181 children who received HAVRIX coadministered with INFANRIX and Hib conjugate vaccine. Most adverse events were mild and transient. The frequencies of solicited local and systemic reactions following receipt of HAVRIX were monitored during the 4-day observation period.

The following rates of solicited adverse events in children who received their first dose of HAVRIX alone at between 11 and 25 months of age were observed. Among local reactions: pain was reported in 15-21% of subjects, redness in 16-21%, swelling in 8% of subjects. Among general reactions, irritability was reported in 24-36% of subjects, loss of appetite in 16-19% of subjects, drowsiness in 15-17% of subjects and fever >39.5°C in ≤2% of subjects. Following the booster dose of HAVRIX, among local reactions: pain was reported in 16-21% of subjects, redness in 17-22%, swelling in 8-10% of subjects. Following the booster dose of HAVRIX, among general reactions, irritability was reported in 19-29% of subjects, loss of appetite in 14-18% of subjects, drowsiness in 13-16% of subjects and fever >39.5°C in ≤1% of subjects.

Drowsiness and loss of appetite occurred at statistically significantly higher rates in subjects 15 to 18 months of age who received Hib conjugate vaccine (PRP-T) and INFANRIX concomitantly with HAVRIX as compared to subjects 15 to 18 months of age who received Hib conjugate vaccine (PRP-T) and INFANRIX (drowsiness 34% and 22% and loss of appetite 29% and 19%, respectively). With the exception of fever (>39.5°C), the solicited general symptoms occurred at statistically significantly higher rates in subjects 15 to 18 months of age who received Hib conjugate vaccine (PRP-T) and INFANRIX concomitantly with HAVRIX as compared to subjects 15 to 18 months of age who received HAVRIX alone (irritability 46% and 30%, drowsiness 34% and 17%, and loss of appetite 29% and 17%, respectively).

A febrile seizure was reported in an 18-month old subject two days after receiving the first dose of HAVRIX. Other serious adverse events reported during the course of this study included a single case each of hepatitis ~5 months post dose 1, insulin-dependent diabetes ~4 months post dose 1, and Kawasaki's disease ~3 1/2 months post dose 1. The association of these events with vaccination is unknown.

**Postmarketing Reports:** Rare voluntary reports of adverse events in people receiving HAVRIX since market introduction include the following: ***Local:*** Localized edema; ***Body as a Whole:*** Anaphylaxis/anaphylactoid reactions, somnolence; ***Cardiovascular:*** Syncope; ***Hepatobiliary:*** Jaundice, hepatitis; ***Dermatologic:*** Erythema multiforme, hyperhydrosis, angioedema; ***Respiratory:*** Dyspnea; ***Hematologic:*** Lymphadenopathy, thrombocytopenia; ***Central Nervous System:*** Convulsions, encephalopathy, dizziness, neuropathy, myelitis, paresthesia, Guillain-Barré syndrome, multiple sclerosis; ***Other:*** Congenital abnormality.

The US Department of Health and Human Services has established the Vaccine Adverse Events Reporting System (VAERS) to accept reports of suspected adverse events after the administration of any vaccine, including, but not limited to, the reporting of events required by the National Childhood Vaccine Injury Act of 1986. The toll-free number for VAERS forms and information is 1-800-822-7967. Reporting forms may also be obtained at the VAERS website at www.vaers.org.

Manufactured by **GlaxoSmithKline Biologicals**, Rixensart, Belgium

Distributed by **GlaxoSmithKline**, Research Triangle Park, NC 27709



BRS-HA:L20

**References:** **1.** Centers for Disease Control and Prevention. Recommended childhood and adolescent immunization schedule—United States, 2006. *MMWR.* 2006;54(51&52):Q1–Q4. **2.** Bell BP, Shapiro CN. Hepatitis A virus. In: Long SS, Pickering LK, Prober CG, eds. *Principles and Practice of Pediatric Infectious Diseases.* 2nd ed. Philadelphia, Pa: Churchill Livingstone; 2003:1188–1192. **3.** Armstrong GL, Bell BP. Hepatitis A virus infection in the United States: model-based estimates and implication for childhood immunizations. *Pediatrics.* 2002;109:839–845.



Printed in USA. HAP283R0 February 2006

### Use of Human Immunodeficiency Virus Postexposure Prophylaxis in Adolescent Sexual Assault Victims

Postexposure prophylaxis appears to be able to reduce the risk of human immunodeficiency virus transmission after sexual assault and national guidelines for its use have been published. Olshen and colleagues examined use of postexposure prophylaxis for 145 adolescents presenting to 2 urban emergency departments after sexual assault. Three fourths of patients were given prophylaxis for human immunodeficiency virus infection. The majority of these patients did not complete the prescribed 28-day course and 46% developed medication toxicity. A comprehensive follow-up system with case management will be necessary to encourage adherence to treatment and ensure follow-up.

See page 674 and page 754

### Improving Recognition of Adolescent Depression in Primary Care

As many as 20% of teenagers report that they have been depressed, but less than one third of these individuals receive treatment. To improve the identification and treatment of adolescent depression, primary care practitioners may need to adapt adult models of depression treatment. This systematic review examined methods used in primary care settings to identify adolescent depression. The review found that few practitioners use systematic depression identification methods despite growing evidence for the feasibility, validity, and effectiveness of this screening.

See page 694

### Age at Drinking Onset and Alcohol Dependence

More than one quarter of high school students begin drinking alcohol before the age of 13 years. Early onset of alcohol use is associated with many problems, both in adolescents and adults, including risk of injury, risk of unwanted and unprotected sex, other substance abuse, and school failure. This survey of 43 000 adults found that those who began drinking before the age of 14 years have nearly double the risk of alcohol dependence compared with those who started drinking after the age of 21 years. They were also 3 times more likely to have multiple episodes of alcohol dependence. For each additional year before the age of 21 years that individuals began drinking, the odds of developing alcohol dependence problems increased.

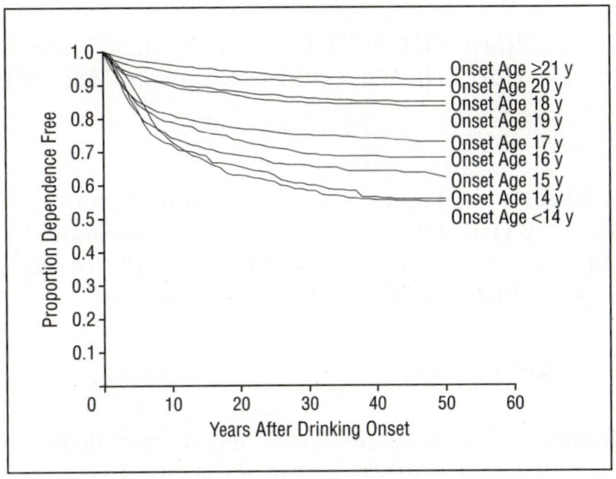

Kaplan-Meier survival curves describing the proportion of dependence-free individuals by age at drinking onset.

See page 739

### The Trial of Infant Response to Diphenhydramine

Many parents encounter frustration with poor infant sleep and often turn to their physician for advice and treatment. Half of the primary care pediatricians in this study reported prescribing antihistamines for sleep problems in infants in the past 6 months. This study was a randomized controlled trial of the use of diphenhydramine for infants 6 to 15 months of age who were reported to have sleep problems. The trial found no difference between diphenhydramine and placebo in decreased number of night awakenings. There was no difference in the time to fall asleep and no adverse effects were reported. Diphenhydramine appears to play no role in treating sleep problems in children.

See page 707

ARTICLE

# Use of Human Immunodeficiency Virus Postexposure Prophylaxis in Adolescent Sexual Assault Victims

*Elyse Olshen, MD, MPH; Katherine Hsu, MD, MPH; Elizabeth R. Woods, MD, MPH; Marvin Harper, MD; Brooke Harnisch, MA; Cathryn L. Samples, MD, MPH*

**Objectives:** To describe the use of human immunodeficiency virus (HIV) postexposure prophylaxis (PEP) in adolescent survivors of sexual assault and to explore barriers to PEP completion in this population.

**Design:** Chart review.

**Setting:** Two academic medical centers in Boston, Mass, between July 1, 2001, and June 30, 2003.

**Participants:** Adolescents presenting to 2 urban pediatric emergency departments within 72 hours of a penetrating sexual assault. Of 177 charts reviewed, adequate documentation of the sexual assault and medical management was available for 145 patients.

**Intervention:** Provision of HIV PEP.

**Main Outcome Measure:** Documented completion of a 28-day course of PEP.

**Results:** Among the 145 patients, 96% were female, 38% were black, and 14% were Hispanic. Many patients were uncertain regarding their exposures: 27% were unsure whether a condom had been used, 54% were unsure whether ejaculation had occurred, and 21% had blacked out during the assault. One hundred ten (76%) received HIV PEP. Of the 97 patients referred for follow-up at the academic centers, 37 returned for at least 1 visit and 13 completed a 28-day course of PEP. Sixteen (46%) of those taking PEP who returned for follow-up developed an adverse reaction to medication. Forty-seven percent of adolescent sexual assault survivors had carried a psychiatric diagnosis before the assault; adherence to PEP was lower among these adolescents.

**Conclusions:** We observed low rates of PEP completion among adolescent sexual assault survivors. Potential difficulties of using PEP in this population include uncertainties regarding exposure, high rates of psychiatric comorbidity, and low rates of return for follow-up care.

*Arch Pediatr Adolesc Med. 2006;160:674-680*

**Author Affiliations:** Divisions of Adolescent Medicine (Drs Olshen and Hsu) and Pediatric Infectious Disease (Dr Hsu and Ms Harnisch), Boston Medical Center, Boston University School of Medicine, Boston, Mass; and Divisions of Adolescent Medicine (Drs Olshen, Woods, and Samples), Pediatric Infectious Disease (Dr Harper), and Pediatric Emergency Medicine (Dr Harper), Children's Hospital Boston, Harvard Medical School. Dr Olshen is now with the Department of Pediatrics, Morgan Stanley Children's Hospital of New York-Presbyterian, Columbia University, New York, NY.

ADOLESCENTS SUFFER THE highest rates of sexual assault of any age group.[1] Up to 10% of adolescent females report a lifetime history of sexual assault.[2,3] Although the risk of contracting human immunodeficiency virus (HIV) is low after a single sexual exposure (0.1%-0.2% for receptive vaginal intercourse and 0.1%-3% for receptive anal intercourse),[4] HIV transmission has been reported after sexual assault.[5,6] Postexposure prophylaxis (PEP), the prescription of a 28-day course of antiretroviral medications, is an established intervention among health care workers to reduce the likelihood of HIV transmission after occupational exposures.[7] The use of PEP for nonoccupational exposures to HIV, including sexual assault, is an extension of this practice. Evidence on the efficacy of PEP for sexual exposures is limited. However, data from animal studies[8] and observational human studies[9,10] suggest that antiretroviral medications can reduce the risk of HIV transmission when administered within 72 hours after a sexual exposure to HIV.

During the past decade, physician attitudes and practices on providing PEP after sexual assault have varied,[11-14] likely because of the absence of uniform guidelines recommending that HIV prophylaxis be administered to sexual assault victims. In

*For editorial comment see page 754*

1998, an expert panel from the Centers for Disease Control and Prevention concluded that data at that time were lacking to recommend for or against the use of PEP for nonoccupational HIV exposures.[15] In the subsequent years, several states developed guidelines advising physicians to provide PEP after sexual assault.[16-19] National guidelines recommending that PEP be considered after sexual assault were only recently published, in January 2005.[20] At our 2 institutions, protocols for the use of

PEP in the pediatric emergency department (ED) were independently developed in 1997.[21] During the time covered by this retrospective study, both hospital protocols recommended that PEP be considered and offered on a case-by-case basis to adolescent survivors of sexual assault.

The use of PEP for survivors of sexual assault has been well described.[22-26] Postexposure prophylaxis is well tolerated among sexual assault survivors, with few reported serious adverse reactions.[23,24] Adherence to PEP among sexual assault survivors has varied from 16% to 85%.[22-24] Few studies to date have reported specifically on the use of PEP in adolescents.[27-29] It is likely that adolescent sexual assault survivors have unique issues complicating their adherence to PEP. The goals of the current retrospective study were to describe PEP use among adolescent sexual assault survivors, to determine rates of medication adherence and follow-up, and to explore potential obstacles to successful PEP completion in this population.

## METHODS

We reviewed charts for all adolescent visits after sexual assault to 2 pediatric EDs in Boston, Mass, during a 2-year period (July 1, 2001, through June 30, 2003). The 2 EDs are affiliated with urban academic medical centers and have a combined annual census of 75 000 visits per year. Both EDs have protocols for the management of sexual assault survivors that recommend HIV PEP be considered. Both EDs refer adolescents prescribed HIV PEP for follow-up with their primary care provider and/or with the sexual assault follow-up clinics affiliated with the medical centers. Location for follow-up care is based on patient and/or parental preference. The 2 adolescent sexual assault follow-up clinics are each staffed by a physician and a nurse or nurse practitioner with HIV medication expertise. The clinics have varying levels of social work involvement. Patients are advised to return for follow-up at 2 weeks, 6 weeks, 3 months, and 6 months after the assault. Testing for HIV antibody is recommended at baseline, 6 weeks, 3 months, and 6 months after the assault.

### IDENTIFYING PATIENTS FOR INCLUSION IN THE CHART REVIEW

Adolescents 12 to 22 years of age visiting 1 of the 2 participating EDs during the study period were included in the chart review if they were examined within 72 hours of a penetrating sexual assault. Patients were excluded from the chart review if they were examined for a nonpenetrating sexual assault, if they were examined more than 72 hours after a sexual assault, or if there was insufficient information in the medical record to determine the nature of the exposure and/or the ED management.

We identified patients for inclusion in the chart review by searching the electronic ED medical records using the keywords *trauma x*, *x*, *sexual assault*, *postexposure prophylaxis*, and *Combivir*. The most common *International Classification of Diseases, Ninth Revision*, codes found in charts identified by the text word search were then queried for all ED visits during the study period. Specific codes searched were: "V01.89—Exposure to infectious body fluid," "V07.9—Unspecified prophylactic measure," "V71.5—Observation following alleged rape or seduction," "V15.41—Psychological trauma," "995.53—Child maltreatment syndrome," "V15.85—Exposure to potentially hazardous body fluid," and "E960.1—Rape." We also reviewed social work log books, pharmacy databases, and records from the sexual assault follow-up clinics to further identify patients for inclusion.

### DATA COLLECTION

We abstracted data from medical records from the index ED visit and from previous and subsequent outpatient and ED visits within the 2 medical centers. Data were not available for visits outside of the 2 participating medical centers.

Data collected included demographic variables (age, race, and insurance), previous history of sexual assault, psychiatric comorbidity (defined as depression, bipolar disorder, substance abuse, suicidality, attention-deficit/hyperactivity disorder, conduct disorder, psychosis or schizophrenia, anxiety disorder, or posttraumatic stress disorder documented at the index ED visit or at previous outpatient visits), assault characteristics (penile-vaginal, penile-oral, and/or penile-rectal exposure; time from assault to ED visit; use of condom; ejaculation; number of assailants; whether victim knew assailant[s]; blacking out during assault; assailant HIV risk; and genital trauma), PEP information (whether PEP was recommended, medications offered, completion of 28-day course of PEP, and medication adverse reaction). Exposures were classified as being at risk for HIV transmission, in agreement with previous research,[24] if there was penile-rectal exposure, genital trauma, multiple assailants, or penile-vaginal or penile-oral exposure with ejaculation and no condom. We also collected data on whether patients returned for follow-up visits and repeat HIV testing within the 2 academic medical centers.

Assault characteristics were routinely recorded at both institutions on the Sexual Assault Evidence Collection Kit issued by the Massachusetts Executive Office of Public Safety. Demographic data, psychiatric illness, PEP provision, and medication adverse events were routinely recorded in the medical record as part of standard medical care. Charts were reviewed by 3 investigators (E.O., K.H., B.H.) and 1 research assistant, using a standardized data collection form. A subset of charts was reviewed by multiple investigators, resulting in no significant disagreements. All data entry was performed by a single investigator (E.O.).

### DATA ANALYSIS

We determined rates for demographic variables, assault characteristics, provision of PEP, and psychiatric comorbidity among the adolescent sexual assault survivors included in this chart review. We compared patients referred for care in the academic center vs those referred for follow-up care with their primary care provider. We also examined whether physician provision of PEP and patient agreement to initiate PEP were associated with specific demographic variables or assault characteristics.

We limited our evaluation of documented PEP completion and return for follow-up visits and HIV testing to patients referred to 2 academic medical centers. Patients who did not return for any follow-up visits were recorded as not completing a course of PEP. We further limited our evaluation of PEP toxic effects to patients agreeing to take PEP who returned for at least 1 follow-up visit. We explored the relationship between PEP completion and return for HIV testing independently with each of the demographic variables and assault characteristics. All bivariate analyses were conducted with Pearson $\chi^2$ test or Fisher exact test.

This chart review was approved by the institutional review boards of the 2 participating institutions.

**Table 1. Demographic Variables and Psychiatric Comorbidity**

| | No. (%)* | | | |
|---|---|---|---|---|
| | All Patients (N = 145) | Patients Referred for Follow-up at Academic Center (n = 97) | Patients Referred for Follow-up With PCP (n = 48) | *P* Value |
| Age <18 y | 101 (70) | 60 (62) | 41 (85) | .004 |
| Female sex | 139 (96) | 94 (97) | 45 (94) | .40 |
| Race/ethnicity | | | | |
| White | 54 (37) | 31 (32) | 23 (48) | .03 |
| Black | 55 (38) | 42 (43) | 13 (27) | |
| Hispanic | 21 (14) | 17 (18) | 4 (8) | |
| Other | 15 (10) | 7 (7) | 8 (17) | |
| Insurance | | | | |
| Medicaid | 67 (46) | 49 (51) | 18 (38) | .001 |
| Private | 39 (27) | 18 (19) | 21 (44) | |
| Uninsured | 39 (27) | 30 (31) | 9 (19) | |
| Site of ED visit | | | | |
| Site 1 | 80 (55) | 68 (70) | 12 (25) | <.001 |
| Site 2 | 65 (45) | 29 (30) | 36 (75) | |
| Past sexual assault | 18 (12) | 16 (16) | 2 (4) | .04 |
| ≥1 Previous psychiatric illness | 68 (47) | 48 (49) | 20 (42) | .38 |
| Depression | 37 (26) | 30 (31) | 7 (15) | .04 |
| Suicidality | 15 (10) | 12 (12) | 3 (6) | .39 |
| Bipolar disorder | 17 (12) | 13 (13) | 4 (8) | .43 |
| Conduct disorder | 9 (6) | 8 (8) | 1 (2) | .27 |
| ADHD | 12 (8) | 6 (6) | 6 (13) | .21 |
| Substance abuse | 17 (12) | 8 (6) | 9 (19) | .10 |
| Psychosis | 3 (2) | 2 (2) | 1 (2) | >.99 |
| Anxiety disorder | 4 (3) | 3 (3) | 1 (2) | >.99 |
| PTSD | 8 (6) | 6 (6) | 2 (4) | >.99 |

Abbreviations: ADHD, attention-deficit/hyperactivity disorder; ED, pediatric emergency department; PCP, primary care provider; PTSD, posttraumatic stress disorder.

*Because of rounding, percentages may not all total 100.

## RESULTS

Charts for 177 adolescents evaluated within 72 hours of a penetrating sexual assault were reviewed. Twenty-eight patients were excluded because of incomplete documentation of the sexual assault, 3 patients were excluded because they left the ED before medical evaluation, and 1 patient was excluded because the ED management was not documented. An additional 24 patients prescribed PEP were identified but not included in the chart review because their ED visit was outside the 72-hour window.

One hundred forty-five adolescent sexual assault survivors met study criteria and were included in the final study population. Patients were predominantly female, racially/ethnically diverse, and their insurance status varied (**Table 1**). Twenty-six percent had a history of depression and 47% had carried at least 1 psychiatric diagnosis before the assault. Ten patients (6%) were cognitively delayed. Ninety-seven patients were referred for follow-up at the 2 academic centers. Patients referred for follow-up at the academic centers differed significantly from those referred for follow-up with their primary care providers: they were older, were more likely to be nonwhite, were less likely to have private insurance, and had higher rates of previous sexual assault and depression (Table 1).

Assault characteristics for this cohort are detailed in **Table 2**. Most patients (74%) reported penile-vaginal exposure. More than one half of adolescent sexual assault survivors were unsure whether ejaculation had occurred and more than one quarter were unsure whether a condom had been used. For 38% of patients, risk of HIV transmission could not be determined from the available documentation. Twenty-one percent reported having blacked out during the assault; 14% reported assault by multiple perpetrators (Table 2). Nearly half reported knowing the perpetrator(s). None of the perpetrators were known to be HIV positive, and only 2% were thought to be at high risk for being HIV positive. There were no significant differences in the assault characteristics of patients referred for follow-up at the academic centers vs those referred for follow-up with their primary care providers.

Of the 145 adolescent sexual assault survivors included in this chart review, 129 (89%) were offered PEP and 110 (76%) agreed to take the PEP medications. Compared with patients not offered PEP, patients offered PEP were more likely to have an exposure classified as being at risk for HIV transmission. Other demographic and assault characteristics were not significantly associated with being offered PEP. Compared with patients who refused PEP, those agreeing to take PEP were more likely to have an exposure classified as being at risk for HIV transmission and less likely to report that a condom was used. Patients who were white were more likely to refuse the PEP medications (9 [17%] of 54 white patients, 4 [7%] of 55 black patients, and 1 [5%] of 21 Hispanic patients refused PEP; $P = .03$). Other demographic and assault characteristics were not associated with agreeing to take PEP. The 110 patients who agreed to take PEP were prescribed the following medications: lamivudine and zidovudine (94%); lamivudine, zidovudine, and nelfinavir (3%); and lamivudine, zidovudine, and indinavir (2%) (medications not documented for 1%).

Follow-up data are reported for the 97 patients who were referred for care at the 2 academic medical centers, of whom 86 (89%) agreed to take PEP. Only 37 (38%) returned for at least 1 follow-up visit, 35 of whom agreed to take PEP (34 were prescribed lamivudine and zidovudine). Medication toxicity data were available for the 35 patients taking PEP with at least 1 follow-up visit. Sixteen (46%) developed at least 1 adverse event related to PEP, including nausea in 13 (37%), diarrhea in 5 (14%), vomiting in 6 (17%), abdominal pain in 4 (11%), anemia in 3 (9%), and headaches in 2 (6%).

Of the 97 patients referred for follow-up at the academic medical centers, 23 (24%) had at least 1 follow-up HIV test and only 1 patient had all 3 recommended HIV tests. There were no seroconversions in this population. Of the 86 patients referred for follow-up at the academic medical centers who initiated PEP, 13 (15%) completed a full 28-day course of PEP.

On bivariate analysis, history of at least 1 previous psychiatric illness was associated with being less likely to complete a 28-day course of PEP (**Table 3**). No other demographic variables or assault characteristics were associated with PEP completion. No demographic or assault characteristics were associated with returning for follow-up HIV testing (**Table 4**).

**Table 2. Assault Characteristics**

| | No. (%)* (N = 145) |
|---|---|
| Time from assault to ED visit, h | |
| <24 | 84 (58) |
| 24-48 | 33 (23) |
| 48-72 | 28 (19) |
| Perpetrator known | 65 (45) |
| Blackout during episode | 30 (21) |
| Multiple assailants | 21 (14) |
| Use of condom | |
| Yes | 15 (10) |
| No | 70 (48) |
| Unsure | 39 (27) |
| Not documented | 21 (14) |
| Penile-vaginal exposure | |
| Yes | 108 (74) |
| No | 17 (12) |
| Unsure | 20 (14) |
| Not documented | 0 |
| Penile-rectal exposure | |
| Yes | 15 (10) |
| No | 96 (66) |
| Unsure | 23 (16) |
| Not documented | 11 (8) |
| Penile-oral exposure | |
| Yes | 34 (23) |
| No | 80 (55) |
| Unsure | 22 (15) |
| Not documented | 9 (6) |
| Ejaculation | |
| Yes | 44 (30) |
| No | 9 (6) |
| Unsure | 78 (54) |
| Not documented | 14 (10) |
| Genital trauma on examination | 52 (36) |
| Risk of HIV transmission† | |
| Yes | 48 (33) |
| No | 21 (14) |
| Could not be determined | 55 (38) |
| Not documented | 21 (14) |

Abbreviations: ED, pediatric emergency department; HIV, human immunodeficiency virus.

*Because of rounding, percentages may not all total 100.

†Risk of transmission was considered present if there was trauma, penile-rectal exposure, multiple assailants, or penile-vaginal or penile-oral exposure with ejaculation and no condom.

## COMMENT

In this chart review, we report on a large cohort of adolescent sexual assault survivors examined at 2 urban academic medical centers during a 2-year period. In accordance with hospital-based protocols, 89% of adolescent sexual assault survivors were offered HIV PEP, and 76% agreed to take the PEP medications. We observed a low rate of PEP completion among adolescent sexual assault survivors. Only 15% of patients who initiated PEP and were referred for follow-up at the academic medical centers were documented to complete a 28-day course of antiretroviral medications. This rate is comparable with that reported in 2 previous small series of adolescent patients who received PEP[27,28] and in 1 report of adult sexual assault survivors.[22] However, our rate of PEP completion is substantially lower than that reported among Brazilian (61%)[24] and South African (87%)[23] sexual assault survivors. The Brazilian and South African studies likely had improved adherence because patients were tracked prospectively and because the studies occurred in areas of high HIV prevalence, where the perceived risk of acquiring HIV after sexual assault was substantial. In contrast, in our population, none of the assailants were known to be HIV positive and only 2% were thought to be at high risk for being HIV positive. Furthermore, we assessed outcomes through retrospective chart review and thus may have underestimated our true adherence rate. Nevertheless, such low rates of medication adherence highlight the need for improved patient education and outreach.

Results of this study highlight some of the difficulties of administering PEP to adolescents after sexual assault. First, to assess the need for PEP, it is important to know specific details related to the assault. Recently released national guidelines on nonoccupational HIV PEP[20] recommend that when a source is of unknown HIV status, PEP should be provided on a case-by-case basis, after weighing the risks and benefits of treatment. However, in many cases of adolescent sexual assault, the risks of HIV transmission cannot be determined. Among patients in our study,

**Table 3. Factors Associated With Documented PEP Completion Among Patients Who Agreed to Initiate PEP and Were Referred for Follow-up at Academic Centers**

| | No. (%)* | | |
|---|---|---|---|
| | PEP Completed (n = 13) | PEP Not Completed (n = 73) | P Value |
| Age <18 y | 9 (69) | 42 (58) | .55 |
| Race | | | |
| White | 4 (31) | 24 (33) | .68 |
| Black | 7 (54) | 29 (40) | |
| Hispanic | 1 (8) | 15 (21) | |
| Other | 1 (8) | 5 (7) | |
| Insurance | | | |
| Medicaid | 5 (38) | 40 (55) | .28 |
| Private | 4 (31) | 10 (14) | |
| Uninsured | 4 (31) | 23 (32) | |
| Site of ED visit | | | |
| Site 1 | 11 (85) | 50 (68) | .33 |
| Site 2 | 2 (15) | 23 (32) | |
| History of ≥1 psychiatric illness | 3 (23) | 41 (56) | .04 |
| Perpetrator known | 7 (54) | 29 (40) | .48 |
| Blackout during episode | 2 (15) | 13 (18) | >.99 |
| Multiple assailants | 2 (15) | 12 (16) | >.99 |
| Genital trauma on examination | 4 (31) | 32 (44) | .54 |
| Ejaculation | | | |
| Yes | 2 (15) | 28 (38) | .28 |
| No | 2 (15) | 8 (11) | |
| Unsure | 9 (69) | 37 (51) | |
| Use of condom | | | |
| Yes | 1 (8) | 6 (8) | .94 |
| No | 9 (69) | 47 (64) | |
| Unsure | 3 (23) | 20 (27) | |
| Penile-vaginal exposure | | | |
| Yes | 10 (77) | 58 (80) | .89 |
| No | 1 (8) | 7 (10) | |
| Unsure | 2 (15) | 8 (11) | |
| Penile-rectal exposure | | | |
| Yes | 2 (15) | 11 (15) | .58 |
| No | 8 (62) | 53 (73) | |
| Unsure | 3 (23) | 9 (12) | |
| Risk of HIV transmission† | | | |
| Yes | 8 (62) | 49 (67) | .83 |
| No | 1 (8) | 3 (4) | |
| Could not be determined | 4 (31) | 21 (29) | |

Abbreviations: ED, pediatric emergency department; HIV, human immunodeficiency virus; PEP, postexposure prophylaxis.

*Because of rounding, percentages may not all total 100.

†Risk of transmission was considered present if there was trauma, penile-rectal exposure, multiple assailants, or penile-vaginal or penile-oral exposure with ejaculation and no condom.

**Table 4. Factors Associated With Return for HIV Testing Among Patients Referred for Follow-up at Academic Centers**

| | No. (%)* | | |
|---|---|---|---|
| | Returned for HIV Testing (n = 23) | Did Not Return for HIV Testing (n = 74) | P Value |
| Age <18 y | 14 (61) | 46 (62) | >.99 |
| Race | | | |
| White | 6 (26) | 25 (34) | .40 |
| Black | 13 (57) | 29 (39) | |
| Hispanic | 2 (9) | 15 (20) | |
| Other | 2 (9) | 5 (7) | |
| Insurance | | | |
| Medicaid | 9 (39) | 40 (54) | .07 |
| Private | 8 (35) | 10 (14) | |
| Uninsured | 6 (26) | 24 (32) | |
| Site of ED visit | | | |
| Site 1 | 18 (78) | 50 (68) | .44 |
| Site 2 | 5 (22) | 24 (32) | |
| History of ≥1 psychiatric illness | 8 (35) | 40 (54) | .15 |
| Perpetrator known | 13 (57) | 20 (27) | .34 |
| Blackout during episode | 1 (4) | 16 (22) | .07 |
| Multiple assailants | 4 (17) | 12 (16) | >.99 |
| Genital trauma on examination | 6 (26) | 33 (45) | .15 |
| Ejaculation | | | |
| Yes | 7 (30) | 25 (34) | .93 |
| No | 3 (13) | 8 (11) | |
| Unsure | 13 (57) | 41 (55) | |
| Use of condom | | | |
| Yes | 3 (13) | 7 (9) | .55 |
| No | 16 (70) | 46 (62) | |
| Unsure | 4 (17) | 21 (28) | |
| Penile-vaginal exposure | | | |
| Yes | 20 (87) | 55 (74) | .33 |
| No | 2 (9) | 7 (9) | |
| Unsure | 1 (4) | 12 (16) | |
| Penile-rectal exposure | | | |
| Yes | 4 (17) | 10 (14) | .86 |
| No | 16 (70) | 52 (70) | |
| Unsure | 3 (13) | 12 (16) | |
| Risk of HIV transmission† | | | |
| Yes | 15 (65) | 47 (64) | .54 |
| No | 3 (13) | 5 (7) | |
| Could not be determined | 5 (22) | 22 (30) | |

Abbreviations: ED, pediatric emergency department; HIV, human immunodeficiency virus.

*Because of rounding, percentages may not all total 100.

†Risk of transmission was considered present if there was trauma, penile-rectal exposure, multiple assailants, or penile-vaginal or penile-oral exposure with ejaculation and no condom.

21% reported having blacked out during the assault, 54% were unsure whether ejaculation had occurred, and 27% were unsure whether a condom had been used.

A second factor complicating the provision of PEP to adolescent sexual assault survivors is their high rate of psychiatric comorbidity. In our study, 47% of patients had a previous psychiatric diagnosis, including 26% with a history of depression and 10% with a history of suicidality. These rates are higher than previously reported rates of mental illness among sexual assault survivors.[30,31] Previous population-based studies[2,31] have shown an association in adolescents between sexual assault and depressive symptoms. Because of their cross-sectional design, these studies were unable to evaluate the temporal relationship between sexual assault and depression. Many have postulated that depression among sexual assault survivors is a response to the trauma of the assault. Indeed, 33% of sexual assault survivors develop posttraumatic stress disorder.[32] However, our high rates of psychiatric comorbidity before the assault suggest that mental illness may also be a risk factor for future victimization. Furthermore, in our study population, previous psychiatric illness was associated with decreased PEP adherence.

A third factor complicating the provision of PEP to adolescent sexual assault survivors is the low rate of return for follow-up care. Fewer than half of the patients who received PEP and were referred for follow-up at our institutions returned for at least 1 follow-up visit. Medical monitoring of patients taking PEP is important to promote medication adherence, to manage frequent medication side effects, and to monitor for acute seroconversion syndrome. Follow-up visits are also important for adolescents taking PEP to provide risk-reduction counseling and follow-up HIV testing. Our low follow-up rates also served as a study limitation because we were unable to fully evaluate medication adherence and medication toxic effects in this population.

Further limitations of this research should be noted. As a chart review, the study could report only on information documented in the medical records at the 2 participating academic centers. It is likely that certain variables were underreported in the medical records. Also, we were unable to assess outcomes for patients who sought care outside the 2 academic medical centers. The group of patients referred for follow-up with their primary care providers did differ demographically from those referred for follow-up at the academic medical centers, possibly affecting the generalizability of our findings.

A final limitation was that we reviewed charts only at 2 urban academic medical centers. Our cohort was diverse in racial/ethnic background and insurance coverage. Assault characteristics for our cohort (including whether the perpetrator was known, number of assailants, and presence of trauma on examination) were comparable with those in published reports of adolescent sexual assault.[33-36] However, our patients may have differed from adolescent sexual assault survivors seen in other clinical settings. Furthermore, provision of PEP was determined by hospital-based protocols and follow-up clinics. Factors associated with PEP initiation, PEP completion, and return for follow-up may be specific to our institutions.

Despite these limitations, our study provides further data on the use of PEP in adolescent sexual assault survivors. The use of PEP in this population can be difficult because of patient uncertainty regarding exposure, high rates of psychiatric comorbidity, and low rates of follow-up. We agree with published recommendations that PEP be offered to adolescent sexual assault survivors for exposures that pose a risk of HIV transmission. Patient education and a comprehensive follow-up system with extensive outreach and case management are necessary to encourage PEP adherence and return for follow-up care among adolescent sexual assault survivors.

**Accepted for Publication:** January 5, 2006.
**Correspondence:** Elyse Olshen, MD, MPH, Department of Pediatrics, Columbia University, 622 W 168th St, VC-402, New York, NY 10032 (Eo85@columbia.edu).
**Author Contributions:** *Study concept and design:* Olshen, Hsu, Woods, Harper, and Samples. *Acquisition of data:* Olshen, Hsu, Harper, and Harnisch. *Analysis and interpretation of data:* Olshen, Hsu, Harnisch, and Samples. *Drafting of the manuscript:* Olshen and Samples. *Critical revision of the manuscript for important intellectual content:* Olshen, Hsu, Woods, Harper, Harnisch, and Samples. *Statistical analysis:* Woods and Harper. *Obtained funding:* Olshen and Woods. *Administrative, technical, and material support:* Hsu, Harnisch, and Samples. *Study supervision:* Hsu, Woods, and Samples.
**Funding/Support:** This study was supported by the Aerosmith Endowment Fund for the Prevention and Treatment of HIV, Leadership Education in Adolescent Health Project, Maternal and Child Health Bureau, US Department of Health and Human Services (5T71-MC00009-13-00), and the Boston University School of Medicine Summer Research Scholarship Program.
**Previous Presentations:** This study was presented in part at the 2005 Annual Meeting of the Pediatric Academic Society; May 15, 2005; Washington, DC.
**Acknowledgment:** Hope Mitchell, MD, assisted with reviewing medical records.

## REFERENCES


1. Catalano SM. National crime victimization survey: criminal victimization, 2004. Office of Justice Program, US Department of Justice. http://www.ojp.usdoj.gov/bjs/pub/pdf/cv04.pdf. Accessed October 13, 2005.
2. Howard DE, Wang MQ. Psychosocial correlates of US adolescents who report a history of forced sexual intercourse. *J Adolesc Health.* 2005;36:372-379.
3. Champion HLO, Foley KL, Durant RH, Hensberry R, Wolfson M. Adolescent sexual victimization, use of other substances, and other health risk behaviors. *J Adolesc Health.* 2004;35:321-328.
4. Mastro TD, de Vincenzi I. Probabilities of sexual HIV-1 transmission. *AIDS.* 1996;10(suppl A):S75-S82.
5. Albert J, Wahlberg J, Leitner T, Escanilla D, Uhlen M. Analysis of a rape case by direct sequencing of the human immunodeficiency virus type I pol and gag genes. *J Virol.* 1994;68:5918-5924.
6. Murphy S, Kitchen V, Harris JR, Forster SM. Rape and subsequent seroconversion to HIV. *BMJ.* 1989;299:718.
7. Centers for Disease Control and Prevention. Updated U.S. Public Health Service guidelines for the management of occupational exposures to HBV, HCV and HIV and recommendations for post-exposure prophylaxis. *MMWR Morb Mortal Wkly Rep.* 2001;50(RR11):1-50.
8. Black RJ. Animal studies of prophylaxis. *Am J Med.* 1997;102:39-44.
9. Schechter M, do Lago RF, Mendelsohn AB, Moreira RI, Moulton LH, Harrison LH; Praca Onze Study Team. Behavioral impact, acceptability, and HIV incidence among homosexual men with access to postexposure chemoprophylaxis for HIV. *J Acquir Immune Defic Syndr.* 2004;35:519-525.
10. Wulfsohn A, Venter WDF, Schultze D, et al. Post-exposure prophylaxis after sexual assault in South Africa. Paper presented at: 10th Conference on Retroviruses and Opportunistic Infections; February 11, 2003; Boston, Mass.
11. Merchant RC, Keshavarz R. HIV postexposure prophylaxis practices by US ED practitioners. *Am J Emerg Med.* 2003;21:309-312.
12. McCausland JB, Linden JA, Degutis LC, Ramanujam P, Sullivan LM, D'onofrio G. Nonoccupational postexposure HIV prevention: emergency physicians' current practices, attitudes, and beliefs. *Ann Emerg Med.* 2003;42:651-656.
13. Babl FE, Cooper ER, Kastner B, Kharasch S. Prophylaxis against possible human immunodeficiency virus exposure after nonoccupational needlestick injuries or sexual assaults in children and adolescents. *Arch Pediatr Adolesc Med.* 2001;155:680-682.
14. Azikiwe N, Wright J, Cheng T, D'Angelo LJ. Management of rape victims (regarding STD treatment and pregnancy prevention): do academic emergency departments practice what they preach? *J Adolesc Health.* 2005;36:446-448.
15. Centers for Disease Control and Prevention. Management of possible sexual, injecting-drug-use, or other nonoccupational exposure to HIV, including considerations related to antiretroviral therapy public health service statement. *MMWR Morb Mortal Wkly Rep.* 1998;47(RR17):1-14.
16. New York State Coalition Against Sexual Assault. HIV prophylaxis following nonoccupational exposure including sexual assault. December 2004. http://www.hivguidelines.org/public_html/npep/npep.pdf. Accessed August 7, 2005.
17. Myles JE, Bamberger J; Housing and Urban Health of the San Francisco Department of Public Health; California HIV PEP After Sexual Assault Task Force; California State Office of AIDS. Offering HIV prophylaxis following sexual assault. 2001. http://www.dhs.ca.gov/ps/ooa/Reports/PDF/HIVProphylaxisFollowingSexualAssault.pdf. Accessed August 7, 2005.
18. Commonwealth of Massachusetts. Clinical advisory: HIV prophylaxis for nonoccupational exposures. October 20, 2000. http://www.mass.gov/dph/aids/guidelines/ca_exposure_nonwork.htm Accessed August 8, 2005.
19. Merchant RC, Mayer KH, Browning CA. Nonoccupational HIV post-exposure pro-

phylaxis: guidelines for Rhode Island from the Brown University AIDS Program and the RI Department of Health. *Med Health R I.* 2002;85:244-248.
20. Centers for Disease Control and Prevention. Antiretroviral postexposure prophylaxis after sexual, injection-drug use or other nonoccupational exposure to HIV in the United States. *MMWR Morb Mortal Wkly Rep.* 2005;54(RR02):1-20.
21. Olshen E, Samples CL. Postexposure prophylaxis: an intervention to prevent human immunodeficiency virus infection in adolescents. *Curr Opin Pediatr.* 2003; 15:379-384.
22. Wiebe ER, Comay SE, McGregor M, Ducceschi S. Offering HIV prophylaxis to people who have been sexually assaulted: 16 months' experience in a sexual assault service. *CMAJ.* 2000;162:641-645.
23. Roland M, Myers L, Chuunga R, et al. A prospective study of post-exposure prophylaxis following sexual assault in South Africa. Paper presented at: 12th Conference on Retroviruses and Opportunistic Infections; February 24, 2005; Boston, Mass. http://www.retroconference.org/2005/cd/PDFs/539.pdf. Accessed August 8, 2005.
24. Garcia MT, Figueiredo RM, Moretti ML, Resende MR, Bedoni AJ, Papaiordanou PM. Postexposure prophylaxis after sexual assaults: a prospective cohort study. *Sex Transm Dis.* 2005;32:214-219.
25. Myles JE, Hirozawa A, Katz MH, Kimmerling R, Bamberger JD. Postexposure prophylaxis for HIV after sexual assault. *JAMA.* 2000;284:1516-1518.
26. Herbert B. Sexual assault survivors: adherence to post-exposure prophylaxis. Paper presented at: XIII International AIDS Conference; July 2000; Durban, South Africa. http://www.iac2000.org/abdetail.asp?ID=WePeD4589. Accessed August 8, 2005.
27. Babl FE, Cooper ER, Damon B, Louie T, Kharasch S, Harris JA. HIV postexposure prophylaxis for children and adolescents. *Am J Emerg Med.* 2000;18:282-287.
28. Neu N, Heffernan S, Brown J, Stimell M. Pediatric and adolescent HIV prophylaxis after sexual assault. Presented at: Seventh Conference on Retroviruses and Opportunistic Infections; February 2, 2000; San Francisco, Calif. http://www.retroconference.org/2000/abstracts/491.htm. Accessed August 8, 2005.
29. Merchant RC, Keshavarz R, Low C. HIV post-exposure prophylaxis provided at an urban pediatric emergency department to female adolescents after sexual assault. *Emerg Med J.* 2004;21:449-451.
30. Kawsar M, Anfield A, Walters E, McCabe S, Forster GE. Prevalence of sexually transmitted infections and mental health needs of female child and adolescent survivors of rape and sexual assault attending a specialist clinic. *Sex Transm Infect.* 2004;80:138-141.
31. Wu ZH, Berenson AB, Wiemann CM. A profile of adolescent females with a history of sexual assault in Texas: familial environment, risk behaviors, and health status. *J Pediatr Adolesc Gynecol.* 2003;16:207-216.
32. Tjaden P, Thoennes N. *Full Report of the Prevalence, Incidence and Consequences of Violence Against Women: Findings From the National Violence Against Women Survey.* Washington, DC: National Institute of Justice, Office of Justice Program, US Dept of Justice and Centers for Disease Control and Prevention; 2000. NCJ183781.
33. Jones JS, Rossman L, Wynn BN, Dunnuck C, Schwartz N. Comparative analysis of adult versus adolescent sexual assault: epidemiology and patterns of anogenital injury. *Acad Emerg Med.* 2003;10:872-877.
34. Sugar NF, Fine DN, Eckert LO. Physical injury after sexual assault: findings of a large case series. *Am J Obstet Gynecol.* 2004;190:71-76.
35. Peipert JF, Domagalski LR. Epidemiology of adolescent sexual assault. *Obstet Gynecol.* 1994;84:867-871.
36. Muram D, Hostetler BR, Jones CE, Speck PM. Adolescent victims of sexual assault. *J Adolesc Health.* 1995;17:372-375.

## Announcement

**Trial Registration Required.** In concert with the International Committee of Medical Journal Editors (ICMJE), *Archives of Pediatrics and Adolescent Medicine* will require, as a condition of consideration for publication, registration of all trials in a public trials registry (such as http://ClinicalTrials.gov). Trials must be registered at or before the onset of patient enrollment. This policy applies to any clinical trial starting enrollment after July 1, 2005. For trials that began enrollment before this date, registration will be required by September 13, 2005, before considering the trial for publication. The trial registration number should be supplied at the time of submission.

For details about this new policy, and for information on how the ICMJE defines a clinical trial, see the editorials by DeAngelis et al in the September 8, 2004 (2004;292:1363-1364) and June 15, 2005 (2005;293: 2927-2929) issues of *JAMA*. Also see the Instructions to Authors on our Web site: www.archpediatrics.com.

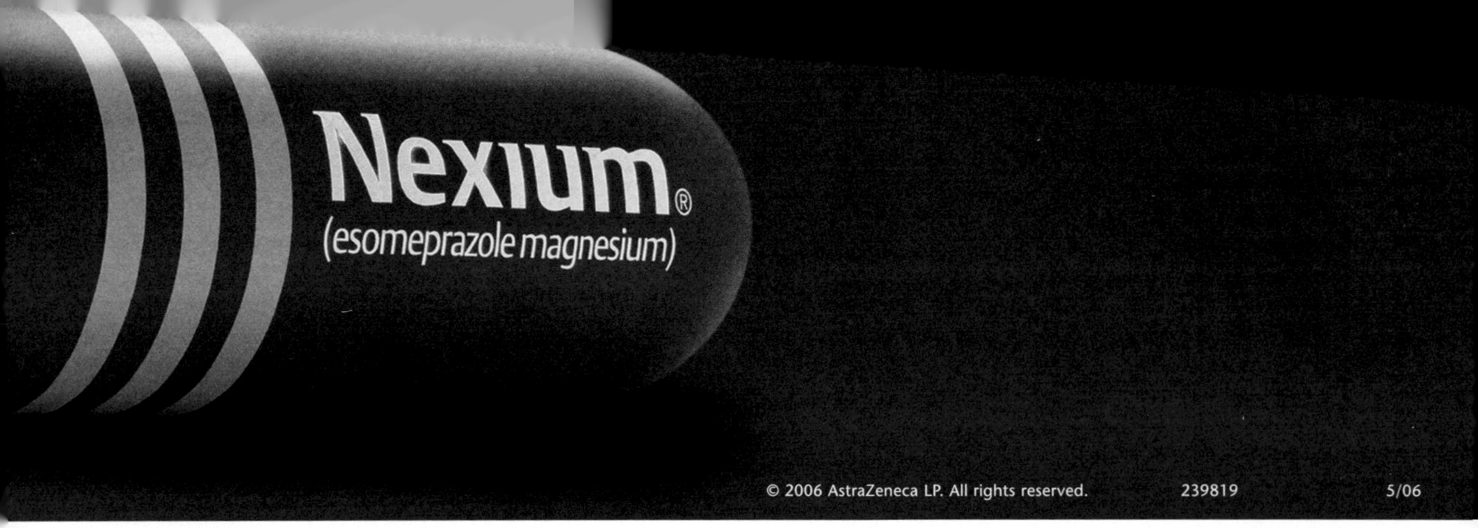


# NEXIUM® *(esomeprazole magnesium)*

## 20-mg, 40-mg Delayed-Release Capsules

**BRIEF SUMMARY** of Prescribing Information.

**INDICATIONS AND USAGE Treatment of GERD** NEXIUM is indicated for the short-term treatment (4 to 8 weeks) in the healing and symptomatic resolution of diagnostically confirmed erosive esophagitis; the maintenance of symptom resolution and healing of erosive esophagitis (controlled studies do not extend beyond 6 months); the treatment of heartburn and other symptoms associated with GERD; **Risk Reduction of NSAID-Associated Gastric Ulcer; *H.pylori* Eradication to Reduce the Risk of Duodenal Ulcer Recurrence.**

**CONTRAINDICATIONS** NEXIUM is contraindicated in patients with known hypersensitivity to any component of the formulation or to substituted benzimidazoles.

**PRECAUTIONS General** Symptomatic response to therapy with NEXIUM does not preclude the presence of gastric malignancy. Atrophic gastritis has been noted occasionally in gastric corpus biopsies from patients treated long-term with omeprazole, of which NEXIUM is an enantiomer. **Information for Patients** NEXIUM Delayed-Release Capsules should be swallowed whole and taken at least one hour before meals. For patients who have difficulty swallowing capsules, one tablespoon of applesauce can be added to an empty bowl and the NEXIUM Delayed-Release Capsule can be opened, and the pellets carefully emptied onto the applesauce. The pellets should be mixed with the applesauce and then swallowed immediately. The applesauce used should not be hot and should be soft enough to be swallowed without chewing. The pellets should not be chewed or crushed. The pellet/applesauce mixture should not be stored for future use. Antacids may be used while taking NEXIUM. **Drug Interactions** Esomeprazole is extensively metabolized in the liver by CYP2C19 and CYP3A4. *In vitro* and *in vivo* studies have shown that esomeprazole is not likely to inhibit CYPs 1A2, 2A6, 2C9, 2D6, 2E1 and 3A4. No clinically relevant interactions with drugs metabolized by these CYP enzymes would be expected. Drug interaction studies have shown that esomeprazole does not have any clinically significant interactions with phenytoin, warfarin, quinidine, clarithromycin or amoxicillin. Post-marketing reports of changes in prothrombin measures have been received among patients on concomitant warfarin and esomeprazole therapy. Increases in INR and prothrombin time may lead to abnormal bleeding and even death. Patients treated with proton pump inhibitors and warfarin concomitantly may need to be monitored for increases in INR and prothrombin time. Esomeprazole may potentially interfere with CYP2C19, the major esomeprazole metabolizing enzyme. Coadministration of esomeprazole 30 mg and diazepam, a CYP2C19 substrate, resulted in a 45% decrease in clearance of diazepam. Increased plasma levels of diazepam were observed 12 hours after dosing and onwards. However, at that time, the plasma levels of diazepam were below the therapeutic interval, and thus this interaction is unlikely to be of clinical relevance. Coadministration of oral contraceptives, diazepam, phenytoin, or quinidine did not seem to change the pharmacokinetic profile of esomeprazole. Concomitant administration of esomeprazole may reduce the plasma levels of atazanavir. Studies evaluating concomitant administration of esomeprazole and either naproxen (non-selective NSAID) or rofecoxib (COX-2 selective NSAID) did not identify any clinically relevant changes in the pharmacokinetic profiles of esomeprazole or these NSAIDs. Esomeprazole inhibits gastric acid secretion. Therefore, esomeprazole may interfere with the absorption of drugs where gastric pH is an important determinant of bioavailability (eg, ketoconazole, iron salts and digoxin). **Carcinogenesis, Mutagenesis, Impairment of Fertility** The carcinogenic potential of esomeprazole was assessed using omeprazole studies. In two 24-month oral carcinogenicity studies in rats, omeprazole at daily doses of 1.7, 3.4, 13.8, 44.0 and 140.8 mg/kg/day (about 0.7 to 57 times the human dose of 20 mg/day expressed on a body surface area basis) produced gastric ECL cell carcinoids in a dose-related manner in both male and female rats; the incidence of this effect was markedly higher in female rats, which had higher blood levels of omeprazole. Gastric carcinoids seldom occur in the untreated rat. In addition, ECL cell hyperplasia was present in all treated groups of both sexes. In one of these studies, female rats were treated with 13.8 mg omeprazole/kg/day (about 5.6 times the human dose on a body surface area basis) for 1 year, then followed for an additional year without the drug. No carcinoids were seen in these rats. An increased incidence of treatment-related ECL cell hyperplasia was observed at the end of 1 year (94% treated vs 10% controls). By the second year the difference between treated and control rats was much smaller (46% vs 26%) but still showed more hyperplasia in the treated group. Gastric adenocarcinoma was seen in one rat (2%). No similar tumor was seen in male or female rats treated for 2 years. For this strain of rat no similar tumor has been noted historically, but a finding involving only one tumor is difficult to interpret. A 78-week mouse carcinogenicity study of omeprazole did not show increased tumor occurrence, but the study was not conclusive. Esomeprazole was negative in the Ames mutation test, in the *in vivo* rat bone marrow cell chromosome aberration test, and the *in vivo* mouse micronucleus test. Esomeprazole, however, was positive in the *in vitro* human lymphocyte chromosome aberration test. Omeprazole was positive in the *in vitro* human lymphocyte chromosome aberration test, the *in vivo* mouse bone marrow cell chromosome aberration test, and the *in vivo* mouse micronucleus test. The potential effects of esomeprazole on fertility and reproductive performance were assessed using omeprazole studies. Omeprazole at oral doses up to 138 mg/kg/day in rats (about 56 times the human dose on a body surface area basis) was found to have no effect on reproductive performance of parental animals. **Pregnancy** *Teratogenic Effects. Pregnancy Category B* Teratology studies have been performed in rats at oral doses up to 280 mg/kg/day (about 57 times the human dose on a body surface area basis) and in rabbits at oral doses up to 86 mg/kg/day (about 35 times the human dose on a body surface area basis) and have revealed no evidence of impaired fertility or harm to the fetus due to esomeprazole. There are, however, no adequate and well-controlled studies in pregnant women. Because animal reproduction studies are not always predictive of human response, this drug should be used during pregnancy only if clearly needed. Teratology studies conducted with omeprazole in rats at oral doses up to 138 mg/kg/day (about 56 times the human dose on a body surface area basis) and in rabbits at doses up to 69 mg/kg/day (about 56 times the human dose on a body surface area basis) did not disclose any evidence for a teratogenic potential of omeprazole. In rabbits, omeprazole in a dose range of 6.9 to 69.1 mg/kg/day (about 5.5 to 56 times the human dose on a body surface area basis) produced dose-related increases in embryo-lethality, fetal resorptions, and pregnancy disruptions. In rats, dose-related embryo/ fetal toxicity and postnatal developmental toxicity were observed in offspring resulting from parents treated with omeprazole at 13.8 to 138.0 mg/kg/day (about 5.6 to 56 times the human doses on a body surface area basis). There are no adequate and well-controlled studies in pregnant women. Sporadic reports have been received of congenital abnormalities occurring in infants born to women who have received omeprazole during pregnancy. **Nursing Mothers** The excretion of esomeprazole in milk has not been studied. However, omeprazole concentrations have been measured in breast milk of a woman following oral administration of 20 mg. Because esomeprazole is likely to be excreted in human milk, because of the potential for serious adverse reactions in nursing infants from esomeprazole, and because of the potential for tumorigenicity shown for omeprazole in rat carcinogenicity studies, a decision should be made whether to discontinue nursing or to discontinue the drug, taking into account the importance of the drug to the mother. **Pediatric Use** Use of NEXIUM in adolescent patients 12 to 17 years of age for short-term treatment of GERD is supported by a) extrapolation of results, already included in the currently approved labeling, from adequate and well-controlled studies that supported the approval of NEXIUM for adults, and b) safety and pharmacokinetic studies performed in adolescent patients. (See **CLINICAL PHARMACOLOGY, Pharmacokinetics,** *Pediatric* for pharmacokinetic information.) The safety and effectiveness of NEXIUM for the treatment of symptomatic GERD in patients $<12$ years of age have not been established. The safety and effectiveness of NEXIUM for other pediatric uses have not been established. **12 to 17 Years of Age GERD** In a multi-center, randomized, double-blind, parallel-group study, 149 adolescent patients (12 to 17 years of age; 89 female; 124 Caucasian, 15 Black, 10 Other) with clinically diagnosed GERD were treated with either NEXIUM 20 mg or NEXIUM 40 mg once daily for up to 8 weeks to evaluate safety and tolerability. Patients were not endoscopically characterized as to the presence or absence of erosive esophagitis. The most frequently reported (at least 2%) treatment related adverse events in these patients were headache (8.1%), abdominal pain (2.7%), diarrhea (2%) and nausea (2%). No new safety concerns were identified. **Geriatric Use** Of the total number of patients who received NEXIUM in clinical trials, 1459 were 65 to 74 years of age and 354 patients were $\geq 75$ years of age. No overall differences in safety and efficacy were observed between the elderly and younger individuals, and other reported clinical experience has not identified differences in responses between the elderly and younger patients, but greater sensitivity of some older individuals cannot be ruled out.

**ADVERSE REACTIONS** The safety of NEXIUM was evaluated in over 15,000 patients (aged 18-84 years) in clinical trials worldwide including over 8,500 patients in the United States and over 6,500 patients in Europe and Canada. Over 2,900 patients were treated in long-term studies for up to 6-12 months. In general, NEXIUM was well tolerated in both short and long-term clinical trials. A study was performed evaluating the safety of NEXIUM in pediatric patients aged 12-17 for the treatment of symptomatic GERD (see **PRECAUTIONS – Pediatric Use**). The safety in the treatment of healing of erosive esophagitis was assessed in four randomized comparative clinical trials, which included 1,240 patients on NEXIUM 20 mg, 2,434 patients on NEXIUM 40 mg, and 3,008 patients on omeprazole 20 mg daily. The most frequently occurring adverse events ($\geq 1\%$) in all three groups was headache (5.5, 5.0, and 3.8, respectively) and diarrhea (no difference among the three groups). Nausea, flatulence, abdominal pain, constipation, and dry mouth occurred at similar rates among patients taking NEXIUM or omeprazole. Additional adverse events that were reported as possibly or probably related to NEXIUM with an incidence $<1\%$ are listed below by body system: ***Body as a Whole:*** abdomen enlarged, allergic reaction, asthenia, back pain, chest pain, chest pain substernal, facial edema, peripheral edema, hot flushes, fatigue, fever, flu-like disorder, generalized edema, leg edema, malaise, pain, rigors; ***Cardiovascular:*** flushing, hypertension, tachycardia; ***Endocrine:*** goiter; ***Gastrointestinal:*** bowel irregularity, constipation aggravated, dyspepsia, dysphagia, dysplasia GI, epigastric pain, eructation, esophageal disorder, frequent stools, gastroenteritis, GI hemorrhage, GI symptoms not otherwise specified, hiccup, melena, mouth disorder, pharynx disorder, rectal disorder, serum gastrin increased, tongue disorder, tongue edema, ulcerative stomatitis, vomiting; ***Hearing:*** earache, tinnitus; ***Hematologic:*** anemia, anemia hypochromic, cervical lymphoadenopathy, epistaxis, leukocytosis, leukopenia, thrombocytopenia; ***Hepatic:*** bilirubinemia, hepatic function abnormal, SGOT increased, SGPT increased; ***Metabolic/Nutritional:*** glycosuria, hyperuricemia, hyponatremia, increased alkaline phosphatase, thirst, vitamin B12 deficiency, weight increase, weight decrease; ***Musculoskeletal:*** arthralgia, arthritis aggravated, arthropathy, cramps, fibromyalgia syndrome, hernia, polymyalgia rheumatica; ***Nervous System/Psychiatric:*** anorexia, apathy, appetite increased, confusion, depression aggravated, dizziness, hypertonia, nervousness, hypoesthesia, impotence, insomnia, migraine, migraine aggravated, paresthesia, sleep disorder, somnolence, tremor, vertigo, visual field defect; ***Reproductive:*** dysmenorrhea, menstrual disorder, vaginitis; ***Respiratory:*** asthma aggravated, coughing, dyspnea, larynx edema, pharyngitis, rhinitis, sinusitis; ***Skin and Appendages:*** acne, angioedema, dermatitis, pruritus, pruritus ani, rash, rash erythematous, rash maculo-papular, skin inflammation, sweating increased, urticaria; ***Special Senses:*** otitis media, parosmia, taste loss, taste perversion; ***Urogenital:*** abnormal urine, albuminuria, cystitis, dysuria, fungal infection, hematuria, micturition frequency, moniliasis, genital moniliasis, polyuria; ***Visual:*** conjunctivitis, vision abnormal. Endoscopic findings that were reported as adverse events include: duodenitis, esophagitis, esophageal stricture, esophageal ulceration, esophageal varices, gastric ulcer, gastritis, hernia, benign polyps or nodules, Barrett's esophagus, and mucosal discoloration. Two placebo-controlled studies were conducted in 710 patients for the treatment of symptomatic gastroesophageal reflux disease. The most common adverse events that were reported as possibly or probably related to NEXIUM were diarrhea (4.3%), headache (3.8%), and abdominal pain (3.8%). Postmarketing Reports – There have been spontaneous reports of adverse events with postmarketing use of esomeprazole. These reports occurred rarely and are listed below by body system: ***Blood And Lymphatic System Disorders:*** agranulocytosis, pancytopenia; ***Eye Disorders:*** blurred vision; ***Gastrointestinal Disorders:*** pancreatitis; ***Hepatobiliary Disorders:*** hepatitis with or without jaundice; ***Immune System Disorders:*** anaphylactic reaction/shock; ***Musculoskeletal And Connective Tissue Disorders:*** myalgia; ***Psychiatric Disorders:*** depression; ***Skin and Subcutaneous Tissue Disorders:*** alopecia, erythema multiforme, Stevens-Johnson syndrome, toxic epidermal necrolysis (TEN, some fatal). Other adverse events not observed with NEXIUM, but occurring with omeprazole can be found in the omeprazole package insert, **ADVERSE REACTIONS** section.

**OVERDOSAGE** A single oral dose of esomeprazole at 510 mg/kg (about 103 times the human dose on a body surface area basis), was lethal to rats. The major signs of acute toxicity were reduced motor activity, changes in respiratory frequency, tremor, ataxia, and intermittent clonic convulsions. There have been some reports of overdosage with esomeprazole. Reports have been received of overdosage with omeprazole in humans. Doses ranged up to 2,400 mg (120 times the usual recommended clinical dose). Manifestations were variable, but included confusion, drowsiness, blurred vision, tachycardia, nausea, diaphoresis, flushing, headache, dry mouth, and other adverse reactions similar to those seen in normal clinical experience (see omeprazole package insert-**ADVERSE REACTIONS**). No specific antidote for esomeprazole is known. Since esomeprazole is extensively protein bound, it is not expected to be removed by dialysis. In the event of overdosage, treatment should be symptomatic and supportive. As with the management of any overdose, the possibility of multiple drug ingestion should be considered. For current information on treatment of any drug overdose, a certified Regional Poison Control Center should be contacted. Telephone numbers are listed in the Physicians' Desk Reference (PDR) or local telephone book. **DOSAGE AND ADMINISTRATION** Please see full Prescribing Information for recommended dosages and dosage adjustments for **Special Populations** for NEXIUM.


Distributed by: AstraZeneca LP, Wilmington, DE 19850
Product of France 31026-02 Rev. 04/06 240260

AstraZeneca

ARTICLE

# The Effect of Peer Counselors on Breastfeeding Rates in the Neonatal Intensive Care Unit

## *Results of a Randomized Controlled Trial*

*Anne Merewood, MPH, IBCLC; Laura Beth Chamberlain, BA, IBCLC; John T. Cook, PhD; Barbara L. Philipp, MD; Kirsten Malone, BA, IBCLC; Howard Bauchner, MD, MPH*

**Objective:** To determine whether peer counselors impacted breastfeeding duration among premature infants in an urban population.

**Design:** This was a randomized controlled clinical trial.

**Setting:** The trial was conducted in the Newborn Intensive Care Unit at Boston Medical Center, an inner-city teaching hospital with approximately 2000 births per year.

**Participants:** One hundred eight mother-infant pairs were enrolled between 2001 and 2004. Pairs were eligible if the mother intended and was eligible to breastfeed per the 1997 guidelines from the American Academy of Pediatrics and if the infant was 26 to 37 weeks' gestational age and otherwise healthy.

**Intervention:** Subjects were randomized to either a peer counselor who saw the mother weekly for 6 weeks or to standard of care.

**Main Outcome Measure:** The main outcome measure was any breast-milk feeding at 12 weeks postpartum.

**Results:** Intervention and control groups were similar on all measured sociodemographic factors. The average gestational age of infants was 32 weeks (range, 26.3-37 weeks) with a mean birth weight of 1875 g (range, 682-3005 g). At 12 weeks postpartum, women with a peer counselor had odds of providing any amount of breast milk 181% greater than women without a peer counselor (odds ratio, 2.81 [95% confidence interval, 1.11-7.14]; $P = .01$).

**Conclusions:** Peer counselors increased breastfeeding duration among premature infants born in an inner-city hospital and admitted to the neonatal intensive care unit. Peer counseling programs can help to increase breastfeeding in this vulnerable population.

*Arch Pediatr Adolesc Med. 2006;160:681-685*

NATIONAL DATA FOR BREASTfeeding rates among premature infants are not available, but regional data suggest these rates are low. In Massachusetts, the breastfeeding initiation rate among term infants in 2002 was 76%, while the initiation rate among premature infants was 68%.[1] Moreover, infants with the lowest gestational ages had the lowest breastfeeding rates (56% initiation among infants born between 24 and 27 weeks compared with 69% among infants born at 36 weeks' gestational age).[1] Nationally, breastfeeding rates are lowest,[2,3] and rates of prematurity highest,[4] among African American infants, suggesting that breastfeeding rates nationally in premature infants will be lower than average.[1]

The health risks associated with formula feeding for premature infants include increased incidence of necrotizing enterocolitis,[5] delayed brainstem maturation,[6] decreased scoring on cognitive and developmental tests,[7-10] and decreased visual development.[11,12] Thus, human-milk feeding of premature infants is desirable, and effective strategies to increase breastfeeding rates in this population are needed. Peer counseling programs have successfully raised breastfeeding rates among term infants in low-income families in a range of settings.[13-19] The objective of this study was to determine whether peer counselors improve breastfeeding duration rates among premature infants admitted to the neonatal intensive care unit (NICU). Secondary objectives were to determine whether peer counselors increased the number of women providing mostly breast milk and whether peer counselors increased rates of exclusive breastfeeding.

Author Affiliations: Boston University School of Medicine (Ms Merewood and Drs Cook, Philipp, and Bauchner) and The Breastfeeding Center, Boston Medical Center (Mss Chamberlain and Malone), Boston, Mass.

## METHODS

This randomized controlled trial was conducted between 2002 and 2004 in the level III, 15-bed NICU at Boston Medical Center, an in-

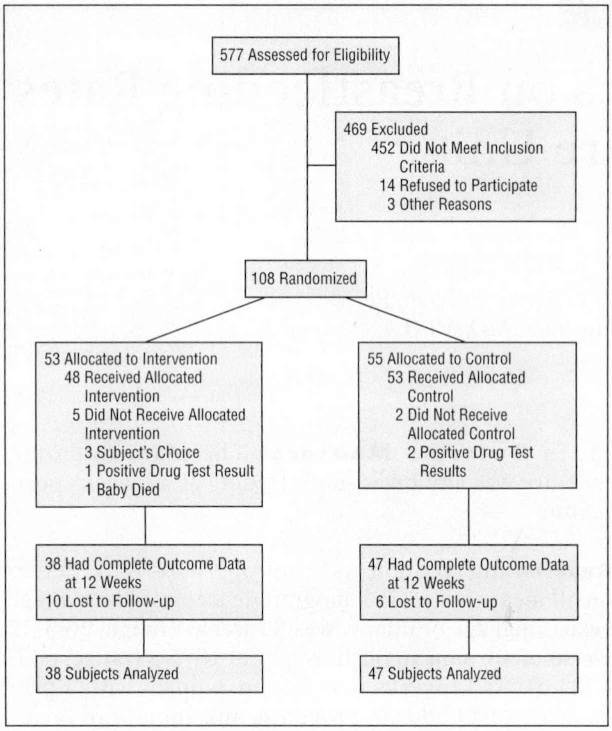


**Figure.** Design of randomized controlled trial.

ner-city teaching hospital and the only Baby-Friendly hospital in Massachusetts. Baby-Friendly status is awarded by the World Health Organization and the United Nations Children's Fund to hospitals that meet the Ten Steps to Successful Breastfeeding.[20] Women were enrolled between January 2001 and September 2004, and data analysis was completed in July 2005. Eligible women had an otherwise healthy premature infant (no congenital anomalies and no life-threatening condition in the immediate postpartum period) between 26 and 37 weeks' gestational age in the NICU; spoke English or Spanish; were eligible to breastfeed according to the 1997 guidelines from the American Academy of Pediatrics[21]; and chose to do so. Women were excluded when incapacitated by illness or birth complications preventing enrollment. Infants with gestational age younger than 26 weeks were excluded, because a relatively high percentage of infants in this age range die or experience severe medical complications. The study received approval from the Boston University Medical Center institutional review board.

Eligible women were approached about study participation within 72 hours postpartum and, if interested, provided consent. At the time of enrollment, consenting women were randomly assigned to receive peer support or standard of care (**Figure**). Randomization was performed using SAS (SAS Institute Inc, Cary, NC). The numbers 1 to 300 were randomized into 2 groups (intervention and control). Numbered envelopes were prepared by the primary investigator (A.M.) in groups of 50, containing either a red index card (intervention) or a green index card (control). After a research assistant enrolled the mother, she opened the sealed envelope to determine whether the subject would be in the intervention or control group. The research assistant then contacted the peer counselor for intervention group assignees; all initial peer counselor contacts with intervention mothers took place within the same 72-hour postpartum period. The reason for the 72-hour time frame was to ensure that the initial contact happened before the mother's hospital discharge. However, some flexibility within that 72 hours was necessary because these were generally high-risk deliveries and mothers were not always immediately available. Similarly, although a peer counselor was at the hospital every weekday morning, if the birth occurred on a weekend or at night, she was not immediately available.

Peer counselors were women with breastfeeding experience drawn from the local community. Over the course of the study, we used 2 US-born African American women; 1 non-US–born Mexican woman, 1 white US-born woman, and 1 white/Native American woman. Two of these women were also employed at the hospital as lay childbirth assistants, and 2 were former teenage mothers. Peer counselors were trained at a 5-day breastfeeding course (operated by The Center for Breastfeeding [http://www.healthychildren.cc/index4.htm]). They were also trained in the hospital about NICU procedures and breastfeeding techniques and at regular, mandatory breastfeeding training days for maternity staff throughout the course of their employment.[22]

After the initial face-to-face contact within 72 hours of the birth, the peer counselor was in contact with the mother thereafter on a weekly basis for 6 weeks. Control group women received standard of care treatment, which in our Baby-Friendly hospital includes referrals to the lactation consultant when needed, use of a pump in the hospital, access to 3 breastfeeding classes per week, staff who are highly trained in lactation management, and a free, high-grade electric breast pump for home use if the mother's insurance does not pay for a pump. The peer counseling model was based on published studies that demonstrate that, among peer counseling programs for low-income mothers of term infants, in-depth, in-person peer contacts are most effective.[13,15] Emphasis was thus placed on face-to-face contact, with meetings lasting at least 30 minutes. The program guidelines required peer counselors to meet in person with the mother, whenever possible, while the infant remained in the NICU. After the infant was discharged from the hospital, contact was by telephone unless the mother chose to come to the hospital to meet with the peer counselor. Peer counselors followed written guidelines (available on request) for each contact to establish consistency of care. The protocol required all peer counselors to maintain field records that could be reviewed to determine how completely the intervention was performed.

Infant feeding status was assessed by a research assistant unaware of the mother's group assignment at 2, 4, 8, and 12 weeks postpartum. Although data were gathered at 4 points, in part to ensure subject contact was maintained to the best of our ability, our analysis reports 12-week data because our focus was on duration. Data were obtained from the infant's medical records while the infant was hospitalized and by maternal recall by telephone after hospital discharge. The bedside feeding record was examined for the 48-hour period immediately preceding the date of the infant's 2-, 4-, 8-, and 12-week birthday. If an infant was not taking food at any observation point, the research assistant retraced the history in the infant's medical record and recorded data from the 48-hour period immediately prior to feeds being halted. In the case of telephone calls, mothers were called on the infant's 2-, 4-, 8-, and 12-week birthdays (or as soon as possible thereafter, if not reachable on the exact day) and asked to report the number of breast and/or formula feeds the infant had received in the previous 48 hours. On some occasions, mothers were not able to recall accurately the exact number of feeds in the previous 48 hours, in which case they were prompted to report categorically whether the baby received "only breast milk, mainly breast milk, mainly formula, or only formula."

## DEFINITION OF BREASTFEEDING AND PRIMARY OUTCOME MEASURES

Nationally, any amount of breastfeeding is used as a definition of breastfeeding to assess breastfeeding rates.[2,3] In keeping with this definition, we described breastfeeding as receiving any breast milk at 12 weeks as our primary outcome measure. However, this national definition is controversial. Thus, we collected more detailed data in the 4 categories listed earlier. Our final data are reported as any breast milk (combining the 3 categories of only breast milk, mostly breast milk, and mostly formula) and mostly and only breast milk, which adds useful and more detailed information. Mostly breast-milk feeders received equal to or greater than 50% of their feeds as breast milk; breast milk may have been received by gavage, bottle, or at the breast.

## DESCRIPTION OF ANALYSIS

Our sample-size calculation was based on a prestudy estimation that the proportion of infants breastfeeding would be 10% at 12 weeks with the intervention. We assumed that these proportions would rise to 40% at 12 weeks. Assuming an $\alpha$ of .05 and a power of 80%, the sample size necessary at 12 weeks would be 78. To have 2 groups stratified by gestational age, we would need a final sample size of 156 infants. In fact, we enrolled a total of 108 mother-infant pairs, after assessing 577 pairs for eligibility during 2 years. Fewer pairs than anticipated met the prematurity eligibility requirement, and when the project funding expired, we ended enrollment. As a result, stratification by gestational age was not pursued.

We examined differences in feeding behavior between mothers with and without peer counselors using logistic regression models with 3 separate dichotomous (yes or no) feeding outcome variables (any breast milk, mostly breast milk, and all breast milk). After determining that the 2 groups were similar on all measured sociodemographic variables using $\chi^2$ tests, data obtained at the 12-week follow-up observation point were analyzed. Because race is a factor in breastfeeding duration among term infants (39% of white US infants are breastfeeding at 6 months compared with 24% of African American infants[3]) and because of the high incidence of premature births among African American women, we performed a subgroup analysis on African American subjects.

We used Stata software version 8 (StataCorp, College Station, Tex) for all hypothesis tests, with a significance level of $\alpha = .05$.

## RESULTS

Overall, 577 mother-infant pairs were assessed for eligibility and 469 were excluded: 452 for not meeting inclusion criteria, 14 for refusing to participate, and 3 for other reasons (Figure). A total of 108 mother-infant pairs were enrolled and randomized; 53 were assigned to the intervention and 55 to the control groups. Of the 53 enrolled in the intervention group, 5 did not receive the allocated intervention; 3 subjects changed their mind after enrollment but before receiving the intervention, 1 mother had positive postpartum drug test results and was therefore not eligible to breastfeed, and 1 infant died, leaving a total of 48 women in the intervention group. Of the 55 women randomized to the control group, 2 were subsequently withdrawn from the study; both were found to have positive postpartum drug test results and were thus ineligible to breastfeed, leaving 53 in the control group. (Many women were not enrolled because of illicit drug use; those in whom drug use became apparent after enrollment had misled health care professionals regarding their drug use, which only became apparent through clinical symptoms afterward.) The 2 groups were similar on all measured characteristics, including maternal ethnicity, educational status, age, parity, breastfeeding history, and infant birth weight (intervention group, 1914.4 g; control group, 1840 g); gestational age; sex; and length of hospital stay (intervention group, mean 27.1 days [range, 2-81 days]; control group, mean 25.2 days [range, 1-104 days]) (**Table 1**). Most women (70 of 101; 69% of the total study population) were African American.

**Table 1. Baseline Characteristics of the Study Sample**

| | Intervention Group (n = 48) | Control Group (n = 53) | *P* Value |
|---|---|---|---|
| Infant characteristics | | | |
| Birth weight, g, mean (range) | 1914.4 (724-3320) | 1840 (682-3005) | .51 |
| Gestational age, wk | | | |
| Mean (range) | 32.6 (26.3-37) | 32.7 (26.4-36.3) | |
| ≥26 to <32, No. | 14 | 16 | .75 |
| ≥32 to ≤37, No. | 34 | 37 | |
| APGAR score | | | |
| 1 min, mean (range) | 6.6 (0-9) | 6.2 (0-9) | .36 |
| 5 min, mean (range) | 8.0 (3-9) | 7.8 (1-9) | .59 |
| Male, No. (%) | 25 (52) | 30 (57) | .65 |
| Mother characteristics | | | |
| Insurance status, No. (%) | | | |
| Medicaid | 27 (56.3) | 27 (50.9) | |
| Private/HMO | 8 (16.7) | 4 (7.5) | .33 |
| Other | 13 (27.1) | 22 (41.5) | |
| Race/ethnicity, No. (%) | | | |
| African American non-Hispanic | 35 (72.9) | 35 (66.0) | .14 |
| White non-Hispanic | 3 (6.2) | 2 (3.8) | |
| Hispanic | 5 (10.4) | 14 (26.4) | |
| Other | 5 (10.4) | 2 (3.8) | .43 |
| US born | 12 (25.0) | 17 (32.1) | |
| Non-US born | 36 (75.0) | 36 (67.9) | |

Abbreviations: APGAR, appearance (color), pulse (heart rate), grimace (reflex irritability), activity (muscle tone), and respiration (score reflecting condition of newborn); HMO, health maintenance organization.

Field records from the peer counselors were available for 43 of the 48 pairs in the intervention group. At the initial contact, peer counselors discussed pumping techniques in 100% of documented cases; helped the mother pump in 72.1% of cases; accompanied the mother to the NICU in 72.1% of cases; and helped the mother to breastfeed, kangaroo care, or both in 30.2% of cases (kangaroo care is skin-to-skin holding that has been practiced effectively with premature infants in many NICUs and shown to improve infants' outcomes[23-26]). After the initial contact, peer counselors' field records also included the infants' location and whether the intervention was performed by telephone or in person. For example, after 4 weeks, 37.2% of infants remained in the NICU, and 81.3% of their mothers were seen in person by the peer counselor in the NICU.

At 12 weeks, women with peer counselors had odds of providing any amount of breast milk 181% greater than those without peer counselors (odds ratio, 2.81 [95% confidence interval, 1.11-7.14]; $P = .03$) (**Table 2**). In our subgroup analysis of African American infants, at 12 weeks, African American mothers with peer counselors

**Table 2. Odds of Mothers Giving Different Amounts of Breast Milk at 12 Weeks' Follow-up**

| Breast Milk Category | Control Group (n = 47) | Intervention Group, OR (95% CI) (n = 38) | *P* Value |
|---|---|---|---|
| Any | 1.00 | 2.81 (1.11-7.14) | .03 |
| Mostly | 1.00 | 2.49 (0.97-6.40) | .006 |
| All | 1.00 | 1.30 (0.30-5.65) | .72 |

Abbreviations: CI, confidence interval; OR, odds ratio.

**Table 3. Odds of African American Mothers Giving Different Amounts of Breast Milk at Each Observation Point at 12 Weeks' Follow-up**

| Breast Milk Category | Control Group (n = 29) | Intervention Group, OR (95% CI) (n = 30) | *P* Value |
|---|---|---|---|
| Any | 1.00 | 3.59 (1.16-11.03) | .03 |
| Mostly | 1.00 | 1.94 (0.64-5.86) | .24 |
| All | 1.00 | 0.23 (0.02-2.26) | .21 |

Abbreviations: CI, confidence interval; OR, odds ratio.

had odds of providing any breast milk 249% greater than those for African American mothers without peer counselors (odds ratio, 3.59 [95% confidence interval, 1.16-11.03]; $P = .03$) (**Table 3**).

## COMMENT

In this randomized controlled trial, the use of peer counselors for breastfeeding mothers of premature infants increased breastfeeding duration, measured by the infants receiving any breast milk at 12 weeks. Because the benefits of breastfeeding are, in most studies, shown to be dose dependent, increasing the amount of breast milk consumed by premature infants, either through extending duration or increasing the number of breast vs formula feeds, is an important contribution to their short- and long-term health.

These results represent an important addition to the literature already describing the effectiveness of peer counseling programs at increasing breastfeeding rates.[13,15,16,27] Although operating a peer counseling program can be challenging,[22] it is manageable in a hospital setting. Not all peer counseling programs have equal success, and comparisons are difficult because peer counseling programs vary in their content and implementation. We believe that the effectiveness of this particular program was owing to a careful design incorporating elements shown to be most successful in previously published peer counseling studies. These elements included face-to-face contact, a checklist of goals for the peer counselors at their first meeting with mothers, carefully maintained field records, and close supervision of, and support for, the peer counselors. Peer counselors had immediate daily access to a lactation consultant working on the unit and to project managers. At the same time, the lactation consultant's and the project managers' presence helped to ensure peer counselor consistency, accuracy of knowledge, and reliability. In light of current investment at the national level by the US Department of Agriculture in breastfeeding peer counseling as part of the Women, Infants, and Children program, we strongly suggest that peer counseling programs be established with clear guidelines and an evaluation component.

This study has a number of limitations. Although we focused on premature infants, the majority of infants in this study were between 32 and 37 weeks' gestational age and were otherwise healthy. Infants with congenital anomalies or with life-threatening complications in the immediate postpartum period were excluded from the study. The study was conducted in a Baby-Friendly hospital. Baseline breastfeeding rates among both intervention and control groups were very high compared with state and national rates in this population. How much the environment of a Baby-Friendly hospital influenced findings cannot be determined; however, both intervention and control groups were exposed to the Baby-Friendly environment. Because breastfeeding is a desirable outcome, when feeding data were collected from the mother rather than the medical record of hospitalized infants, there may have been a tendency to overreport breastfeeding. It is also possible that nondifferential reporting inaccuracy might be expected to bias the effect of the intervention, and the direction of this bias would be unclear. The main limitation of the study is that 16 of 108 women were lost to follow-up at 12 weeks, and loss to follow-up was higher in the intervention arm than in the control group (10 and 6, respectively), although, in a cross-tabulation of number of mothers in each study arm by follow-up period, there was no statistically significant difference in loss to follow-up between the 2 groups ($P = .98$). Given the desirability of breastfeeding, it is possible that women in the intervention group felt more guilty about discontinuing breastfeeding than control women because of relationships developed with the peer counselor, and thus, they did not answer telephone calls when the research assistant called to ascertain feeding status. However, the peer counselor contact ended at week 6 and the majority of losses to follow-up occurred later than 6 weeks, and attempts to elaborate on reasons for loss to follow-up would be conjectural.

Many groups, including the American Academy of Pediatrics,[28] the American College of Obstetricians and Gynecologists,[29] the American Academy of Family Practice,[30] the US Department of Health and Human Services,[31] and the World Health Organization,[32] recognize the importance of prolonged breastfeeding. This is likely even more important in premature infants than in term infants because of the additional health risks they face. We found that NICU-based peer counselors increased breastfeeding duration among premature infants in an inner-city, Baby-Friendly hospital. Peer counseling programs can help to increase breastfeeding in this vulnerable population.

**Accepted for Publication:** January 6, 2006.
**Correspondence:** Anne Merewood, MPH, IBCLC, Division of General Pediatrics, Maternity Building, 4th Floor,

91 E Concord St, Boston Medical Center, Boston, MA 02118 (anne.merewood@bmc.org).
**Author Contributions:** *Study concept and design:* Merewood, Philipp, and Bauchner. *Acquisition of data:* Merewood, Chamberlain, and Malone. *Analysis and interpretation of data:* Cook. *Drafting of the manuscript:* Merewood, Chamberlain, and Bauchner. *Critical revision of the manuscript for important intellectual content*: Merewood, Cook, and Philipp. *Statistical analysis:* Cook. *Obtained funding:* Merewood and Philipp. *Study supervision:* Merewood and Bauchner.
**Funding/Support:** This study was supported by grant R40 MC 00252-03 from the Bureau of Maternal Child Health. Dr Bauchner was supported in part by grant K24HD 042489 from the National Institute of Child Health and Human Development.
**Acknowledgment:** We would like to thank our peer counselors, particularly Luz Lopez, Dawn Kennedy, and Karen Gunter, for their work on this project.

## REFERENCES

1. Merewood A, Brooks D, MacAuley L, Mehta SD. Breastfeeding rates among premature infants in Massachusetts: data from a model public health database. Paper presented at: American Public Health Association Annual Meeting; December 10-15, 2005; Philadelphia, Pa.
2. Ross Products Division. *Ross Mothers Survey.* Cleveland, Ohio: Abbott Laboratories; 2003.
3. Centers for Disease Control and Prevention. Breastfeeding: data and statistics: breastfeeding practices: results from the 2003 National Immunization Survey. http://www.cdc.gov/breastfeeding/data/NIS_data/data_2003.htm. Accessed January 2006.
4. Centers for Disease Control and Prevention. Infant mortality and low birth weight among black and white infants—United States, 1980-2000. *MMWR Morb Mortal Wkly Rep.* 2002;51:589-592.
5. Lucas A, Cole TJ. Breast milk and neonatal necrotising enterocolitis. *Lancet.* 1990; 336:1519-1523.
6. Amin SB, Merle KS, Orlando MS, Dalzell LE, Guillet R. Brainstem maturation in premature infants as a function of enteral feeding type. *Pediatrics.* 2000;106: 318-322.
7. Anderson JW, Johnstone BM, Remley DT. Breast-feeding and cognitive development: a meta-analysis. *Am J Clin Nutr.* 1999;70:525-535.
8. Lucas A, Morley R, Cole TJ, et al. Early diet in preterm babies and developmental status at 18 months. *Lancet.* 1990;335:1477-1481.
9. Lucas A, Morley R, Cole TJ, Lister G, Leeson-Payne C. Breast milk and subsequent intelligence quotient in children born preterm. *Lancet.* 1992;339:261-264.
10. Lucas A, Fewtrell MS, Morley R, et al. Randomized outcome trial of human milk fortification and developmental outcome in preterm infants. *Am J Clin Nutr.* 1996; 64:142-151.
11. Birch E, Birch D, Hoffman D, Hale L, Everett M, Uauy R. Breast-feeding and optimal visual development. *J Pediatr Ophthalmol Strabismus.* 1993;30:33-38.
12. Hylander MA, Strobino DM, Pezzullo JC, Dhanireddy R. Association of human milk feedings with a reduction in retinopathy of prematurity among very low birthweight infants. *J Perinatol.* 2001;21:356-362.
13. Grummer-Strawn LM, Rice SP, Dugas K, Clark LD, Benton-Davis S. An evaluation of breastfeeding promotion through peer counseling in Mississippi WIC clinics. *Matern Child Health J.* 1997;1:35-42.
14. Kistin N, Abramson R, Dublin P. Effect of peer counselors on breastfeeding initiation, exclusivity, and duration among low-income urban women. *J Hum Lact.* 1994;10:11-15.
15. Morrow AL, Guerrero ML, Shults J, et al. Efficacy of home-based peer counselling to promote exclusive breastfeeding: a randomised controlled trial. *Lancet.* 1999;353:1226-1231.
16. Martens PJ. Increasing breastfeeding initiation and duration at a community level: an evaluation of Sagkeeng First Nation's community health nurse and peer counselor programs. *J Hum Lact.* 2002;18:236-246.
17. Schafer E, Vogel MK, Viegas S, Hausafus C. Volunteer peer counselors increase breastfeeding duration among rural low-income women. *Birth.* 1998;25:101-106.
18. Chapman DJ, Damio G, Young S, Perez-Escamilla R. Effectiveness of breastfeeding peer counseling in a low-income, predominantly Latina population: a randomized controlled trial. *Arch Pediatr Adolesc Med.* 2004;158:897-902.
19. Guise JM, Palda V, Westhoff C, Chan BK, Helfand M, Lieu TA. The effectiveness of primary care-based interventions to promote breastfeeding: systematic evidence review and meta-analysis for the US Preventive Services Task Force. *Ann Fam Med.* 2003;1:70-78.
20. Protecting, promoting, and supporting breastfeeding: the special role of maternity services. a joint WHO/UNICEF statement. *Int J Gynaecol Obstet.* 1990; 31(suppl 1):171-183.
21. Work Group on Breastfeeding;American Academy of Pediatrics. Breastfeeding and the use of human milk. *Pediatrics.* 1997;100:1035-1039.
22. Merewood A, Philipp BL. Peer counselors for breastfeeding women in the hospital setting: trials, training, tributes, and tribulations. *J Hum Lact.* 2003;19: 72-76.
23. Charpak N, Ruiz-Pelaez JG, Figueroa de Calume Z. Current knowledge of Kangaroo Mother Intervention. *Curr Opin Pediatr.* 1996;8:108-112.
24. Hill PD, Aldag JC, Chatterton RT. Effects of pumping style on milk production in mothers of non-nursing preterm infants. *J Hum Lact.* 1999;15:209-216.
25. Hill PD, Aldag JC, Chatterton RT Jr. Breastfeeding experience and milk weight in lactating mothers pumping for preterm infants. *Birth.* 1999;26:233-238.
26. Kambarami RA, Chidede O, Pereira N. Long-term outcome of preterm infants discharged home on kangaroo care in a developing country. *Ann Trop Paediatr.* 2003;23:55-59.
27. Long DG, Funk-Archuleta MA, Geiger CJ, Mozar AJ, Heins JN. Peer counselor program increases breastfeeding rates in Utah Native American WIC population. *J Hum Lact.* 1995;11:279-284.
28. Gartner LM, Morton J, Lawrence RA, et al. Breastfeeding and the use of human milk. *Pediatrics.* 2005;115:496-506.
29. American College of Obstetricians and Gynecologists. *ACOG Educational Bulletin.* Washington, DC. American College of Obstetricians and Gynecologists; 2000.
30. American Academy of Family Physicians. Breastfeeding (position paper). http://www.aafp.org/x6633.xml. Accessed January 2006.
31. US Department of Health and Human Services Office on Women's Health. *Health and Human Services Blueprint for Action on Breastfeeding*; Washington, DC: US Dept of Health and Human Services; 2000.
32. World Health Organization UNCsFUS Agency of International Development; Swedish International Development Authority. *Innocenti Declaration on the Protection, Promotion, and Support of Breastfeeding.* New York, NY: UNICEF, Nutrition Section; 1990.

## *Correction*

**Error in Byline.** In the letter "Dismissing Families: A Slippery Slope" published in the April issue of the ARCHIVES (2006;160:452), a coauthor was mistakenly listed in the byline. The sole author of the letter was Kathi J. Kemper, MD, MPH.

ARTICLE

# Prevalence of Coronary Artery Lesions on the Initial Echocardiogram in Kawasaki Syndrome

*Aryeh Z. Baer, MD; Lorry G. Rubin, MD; Craig A. Shapiro, BA; Sunil K. Sood, MD; Sujatha Rajan, MD; Yehuda Shapir, MD; Angela Romano, MD; Fredrick Z. Bierman, MD*

**Objectives:** To determine whether coronary artery lesions (ectasia and aneurysm) are commonly observed on the initial echocardiogram of patients with acute Kawasaki syndrome, whether coronary artery ectasia and/or aneurysms occur more frequently in patients with incomplete Kawasaki syndrome than in those patients with complete findings, and whether earlier diagnosis and treatment of Kawasaki syndrome are associated with less frequent occurrence of coronary artery ectasia and/or aneurysm.

**Design:** A retrospective medical record review.

**Setting:** A tertiary care pediatric hospital.

**Participants:** One hundred patients treated for Kawasaki syndrome between July 1, 1998, and June 30, 2003, who were identified by a medical record search.

**Main Outcome Measure:** Prevalence of coronary artery lesions (ectasia and aneurysm) on the initial and subsequent echocardiograms.

**Results:** Forty-four percent of patients had a coronary artery lesion (31% with ectasia, 13% with aneurysm) on the initial echocardiogram. Patients with incomplete Kawasaki syndrome were treated significantly later (median, 10 days) and had a significantly higher occurrence of coronary artery aneurysms over the course of their illness (37%) than those with complete Kawasaki syndrome, who were treated at a median of 7 days ($P<.001$) and had a 12% aneurysm occurrence ($P=.009$). Patients treated by day 7 of illness had a less frequent occurrence of aneurysm (6%) compared with those patients treated between days 8 and 10 of illness (27%) ($P=.03$).

**Conclusions:** Coronary artery lesions are frequently detected on the initial echocardiogram of children with Kawasaki syndrome. If future studies show ectasia to have a relatively high degree of specificity for Kawasaki syndrome, the initial echocardiography may be a useful adjunctive diagnostic test.

*Arch Pediatr Adolesc Med. 2006;160:686-690*

KAWASAKI SYNDROME (KS) IS a systemic vasculitis with a predilection for the coronary arteries. It is currently the leading cause of acquired heart disease in children in the United States.[1] The etiology is unknown and there are no pathognomonic laboratory features. Diagnosis is therefore based on clinical criteria, the presence of fever for at least 5 days plus at least 4 of 5 typical physical findings, as well as supportive but nonspecific laboratory values. However, KS may be difficult to distinguish from common bacterial or viral infections. In addition, patients with KS may have fewer than 4 of the 5 criteria. These incomplete cases are more difficult to recognize and may have a higher incidence of coronary artery lesions (CALs).[2,3] Treatment with intravenous immunoglobulin (IVIG) and aspirin markedly reduces the development of coronary artery aneurysms.[4,5] Furthermore, there is evidence that earlier treatment leads to a lower incidence of aneurysm formation.[1,2,6,7] Timely diagnosis and treatment are therefore important.

Echocardiograms are often obtained at the time of diagnosis to serve as a baseline study of the coronary arteries and to screen for cardiac findings occasionally seen in acute KS, such as pericardial effusions, myocarditis, or valvular dysfunction. Echocardiography is repeated in the subacute phase of illness to detect development of CALs.[1] Until very recently, however, echocardiography has not been recommended as an adjunctive test to establish a diagnosis of KS.[1] Although earlier studies[4,5,8] reported low rates of CALs on the initial echocardiogram, more recent studies[9,10] suggest that previously applied definitions of aneurysm and ectasia may have significantly underestimated the true prevalence of CALs. If CALs are commonly detected on the initial echocardiogram, then echocardiography may be a useful adjunct in diagnosing KS. In this study, we evaluated the preva-

**Author Affiliations:** Divisions of Infectious Diseases (Drs Baer, Rubin, Sood, and Rajan and Mr Shapiro) and Cardiology (Drs Shapir, Romano, and Bierman), Department of Pediatrics, Schneider Children's Hospital of the North Shore–Long Island Jewish Health System, Albert Einstein College of Medicine, New Hyde Park, NY.

lence of CALs on the initial echocardiogram of patients with acute KS. In addition, we evaluated whether patients with incomplete KS were treated later in the course of their illness than patients with complete findings and whether CALs or the 2 subsets of CAL, ectasia and aneurysm, were observed more frequently in the patients with incomplete KS during the course of their illness than in patients with complete findings. To assess the potential impact of earlier diagnosis of KS, we also evaluated the relationship between the timing of the treatment for KS and the frequency of occurrences of CALs and the CAL subsets of ectasia and aneurysm.

## METHODS

We conducted a retrospective medical record review of all of the patients treated with IVIG and aspirin for KS at Schneider Children's Hospital, New Hyde Park, NY, between July 1, 1998, and June 30, 2003. Patients were identified by a search of medical records and a database of patients who underwent echocardiography in the Division of Cardiology. Inpatient and outpatient medical records and echocardiogram reports were reviewed for all of the patients. Patients were excluded if they had an alternative diagnosis that reasonably accounted for their illness. We recorded the following data for each patient: age, sex, duration of fever, presence or absence of each clinical criterion for KS, duration of illness to time of treatment, occurrence of periungual peeling in the subacute stage, and timing and findings of initial and subsequent echocardiograms. In addition, for each patient, we determined whether the initial echocardiogram influenced the diagnosis of KS. Patients in whom there was no documentation of a commitment to treat with IVIG prior to a report of abnormality on the echocardiogram were considered to have a diagnosis that was influenced by echocardiographic findings.

The fever criterion and the 5 other clinical criteria of KS were applied as previously described[1] with the following exceptions: (1) patients who defervesced following treatment with IVIG were considered to have fulfilled the fever criterion even if they were febrile for fewer than 5 days, and (2) periungual desquamation qualified as fulfilling the criterion for extremity changes only if present at the time of diagnosis.

An episode of KS was classified as complete if the patient fulfilled the fever criterion plus at least 4 of the 5 other clinical criteria. Episodes were classified as incomplete if either the fever criterion or presence of at least 4 of the other criteria were not fulfilled.

Echocardiograms were obtained with Sequoia echocardiographic imagers (Siemens Medical Solutions USA, Inc, Malvern, Pa). Performed projections included subxyphoid, parasternal long and short axis, and apical views. M-mode, 2-dimensional, Doppler flow, and color flow mapping studies were routinely performed. All of the studies were reviewed and reported by a pediatric cardiology attending (97% of the studies were interpreted by Y.S., A.R., or F.Z.B.). The echocardiographers distinguished between 2 subsets of CAL: ectasia and aneurysm. The echocardiographer found coronary artery ectasia if the vessel either was qualitatively dilated or tapered abnormally such that it did not taper as it progressed distally (distal ectasia) or such that it tapered precipitously from its origin (proximal ectasia). The echocardiographer found aneurysm if there was an isolated and distinct outpouching of a coronary artery segment. Based on the echocardiogram reports, results were classified as normal, ectasia, or aneurysm; a study with both ectasia and aneurysm was classified as aneurysm.

All of the echocardiogram reports were reviewed. The initial echocardiography was the first study performed at the time of diagnosis. For patients with more than 1 subsequent echocardiogram, the result of the study with the most marked abnormality was recorded. The final echocardiogram was the study most recently performed at the time of data collection and was included only if performed long enough into the course of the illness to be considered indicative of final coronary status, ie, at least 6 weeks from the onset of illness if the study results were normal and at least 90 days from the onset of illness if the study results were abnormal.

Proportions were compared using the Fisher exact test. Continuous variables (time to treatment and age at presentation) were analyzed using the nonparametric Mann-Whitney test. The institutional review board of Long Island Jewish Medical Center, New Hyde Park, approved the study protocol.

## RESULTS

One hundred three patients were treated for KS. Three were excluded because alternate diagnoses were established: 1 patient had systemic lupus erythematosus, 1 had Behçet syndrome, and 1 had enteroviral infection. All of the 3 patients had CALs. Of the remaining 100 patients, 7 had diagnoses of infectious diseases (4 patients with group A β-hemolytic streptococcal infection, 1 with parvovirus infection, 1 with adenovirus infection, and 1 with enterotoxin B–producing *Staphylococcus aureus* infection) but were still considered by the infectious diseases attending physician to have KS.

Sixty patients (60%) were male. The median age at diagnosis was 2.5 years. At the time of diagnosis, 73 patients (73%) fulfilled complete criteria (**Table 1**). A higher percentage of patients with incomplete KS (8 [30%] of 27 patients) were aged 12 months or younger compared with those with complete KS (10 [14%] of 73 patients), but this difference was not significant ($P = .08$). The median day of illness at the time of treatment was 8 days. Patients with complete KS were treated significantly earlier (median, 7 days; range, 3-19 days) than patients with incomplete KS (median, 10 days; range, 6-26 days; $P < .001$). In all but 5 patients, the initial echocardiogram was obtained within 24 hours of treatment; 4 of the 5 patients had an initial echocardiogram obtained within 48 hours of treatment and 1 within 72 hours of treatment. At some time during their course of illness, 75% of patients had documentation of aneurysm and/or periungual desquamation, findings highly characteristic of KS (Table 1).

Forty-four percent of patients had CALs on the initial echocardiogram; 31 (31%) had ectasia and 13 (13%) had aneurysms (**Table 2**). There was no significant difference in the prevalence of CALs ($P = .18$) or the CAL subset of ectasia ($P = .63$) on the initial echocardiogram between patients with complete and incomplete KS. However, the prevalence of the CAL subset of aneurysm on the initial echocardiogram in patients with incomplete KS (30%) was significantly higher than in patients with complete KS (7%) ($P = .006$). Findings on the initial echocardiogram influenced the diagnosis of KS or the timing of the diagnosis of KS in 14 patients. Of these patients, 6 had aneurysms, 7 had ectasia, and in 1 patient, the preliminary reading was ectasia but the official interpretation was normal coronary arteries.

To assess the prevalence of CALs on the initial echocardiogram in patients diagnosed early in the course of

**Table 1. Clinical Findings of Patients With Complete and Incomplete Kawasaki Syndrome**

| Clinical Finding | All Patients, No. (%) (N = 100) | Patients With Complete KS, No. (%) (n = 73) | Patients With Incomplete KS, No. (%) (n = 27) | Patients With Diagnosis by Echocardiogram, No. (%) (n = 14)* |
|---|---|---|---|---|
| Criteria fulfilled | | | | |
| Fever criterion | 98 (98) | 73 (100) | 25 (93) | 13 (93) |
| 0 of 5 clinical criteria | 1 (1) | NA | 1 (3) | 1 (7) |
| 1 of 5 clinical criteria | 3 (3) | NA | 3 (11) | 3 (21) |
| 2 of 5 clinical criteria | 4 (4) | NA | 4 (15) | 2 (14) |
| 3 of 5 clinical criteria | 19 (19) | NA | 19 (70) | 3 (21) |
| 4 of 5 clinical criteria | 52 (52) | 52 (71) | NA | 5 (36) |
| 5 of 5 clinical criteria | 21 (21) | 21 (29) | NA | 0 |
| Periungual peeling† | 67 (67) | 57 (78) | 10 (37) | 5 (36) |
| Presence of aneurysm† | 19 (19) | 9 (12) | 10 (37) | 8 (57) |
| Peeling or aneurysm† | 75 (75) | 57 (78) | 18 (67) | 11 (79) |

Abbreviations: KS, Kawasaki syndrome; NA, not applicable.
*Echocardiogram influenced either the diagnosis or the timing of the diagnosis of KS.
†Documented at any time during the patient's course of illness.

**Table 2. Comparison of Echocardiographic Findings in Patients With Complete and Incomplete Kawasaki Syndrome**

| Echocardiogram Finding | All Patients, No. (%) (N = 100) | Patients With Complete KS, No. (%) (n = 73) | Patients With Incomplete KS, No. (%) (n = 27) | *P* Value* |
|---|---|---|---|---|
| Initial echocardiogram | | | | |
| CAL† | 44 (44) | 29 (40) | 15 (56) | .18 |
| Ectasia | 31 (31) | 24 (33) | 7 (26) | .63 |
| Aneurysm‡ | 13 (13) | 5 (7) | 8 (30) | .006 |
| Presence of lesion on any echocardiogram | | | | |
| CAL† | 64 (64) | 45 (62) | 19 (70) | .49 |
| Ectasia§ | 45 (45) | 36 (49) | 9 (33) | .18 |
| Aneurysm‡‖ | 19 (19) | 9 (12) | 10 (37) | .009 |

Abbreviations: CAL, coronary artery lesion; KS, Kawasaki syndrome.
**P* values compare complete KS with incomplete KS.
†The number of patients with CAL is the sum of the patients with ectasia and aneurysm.
‡Some patients with aneurysm also had ectasia in another vessel.
§Ectasia was the most marked lesion at any point.
‖Finding includes 4 patients with initial ectasia who subsequently developed aneurysm (3 patients with complete KS, 1 with incomplete KS) and 1 patient with aneurysm that regressed to ectasia on a subsequent echocardiogram (incomplete KS).

their illness, we reanalyzed the data for patients presenting on or before the seventh day of illness and for those presenting between days 8 and 10 of illness. Considering only the 49 patients treated on or before day 7 of illness, 21 (43%) had a CAL (all of which were ectasia) on the initial echocardiogram. Similarly, of 26 patients treated on days 8 to 10 of illness, 11 (42%) had a CAL; 6 patients (23%) had ectasia and 5 (19%) had an aneurysm on the initial echocardiogram. Thus, CALs were commonly observed on the initial echocardiogram of patients diagnosed by the 7th and 10th days of illness.

The relationship between the findings on the initial and subsequent echocardiograms was examined (**Figure**). Coronary artery lesions were found on the subsequent echocardiogram in significantly higher percentages of patients who had an initial echocardiogram showing ectasia (77%) or aneurysm (85%) compared with those with normal initial echocardiographic results (36%). Sixty-four patients (64%) had a CAL at some point during their course of illness; however, only 11 patients (11%) had a CAL (6% of which were ectasia and 5% were aneurysm) on the final echocardiogram. Eighty-seven patients (87%) had normal coronary arteries on the final echocardiogram. In 2 patients, a CAL was detected on a final echocardiogram obtained before 90 days of illness; hence, their final coronary status could not be evaluated.

The frequency of occurrence of CALs over the course of illness was compared in patients with complete and incomplete KS (Table 2). Coronary artery lesions overall as well as the CAL subset of ectasia were observed in similar percentages of patients with complete and incomplete KS. In contrast, the CAL subset of aneurysm was observed in a significantly higher percentage of those with incomplete KS (10 [37%] of 27 patients) compared with those with complete KS (9 [12%] of 73 patients) ($P = .009$).

The relationship between the duration of illness before treatment and the frequency of occurrence of CALs was examined. Thirty-five (71%) of 49 patients treated on or before day 7 of illness had a CAL during their course compared with 14 (54%) of 26 patients treated on days 8 to 10 of illness and 15 (60%) of 25 patients treated after day 10 of illness. These differences were not statistically significant ($P = .29$ comparing patients treated on or before day 7 of illness, between days 8 and 10 of illness, and after day 10 of illness). In contrast, the CAL subset of aneurysm was observed significantly more often with a longer time to treatment. Three (6%) of 49 patients treated on or before day 7 of illness had an aneurysm during their course compared with 7 (27%) of 26 patients treated on days 8 to 10 of illness ($P=.03$). Similarly, a higher percentage of patients treated after 10 days of illness (9 [36%] of 25 patients) developed an aneurysm during their course compared with patients treated on or before day 10 of illness (10 [13%] of 75 patients) ($P=.02$).

Eighty-three percent of the initial echocardiograms were interpreted by 1 of 2 cardiologists (Y.S. and A.R.). The 2 cardiologists detected the presence of CALs at similar rates, with one finding CALs on 25 (51%) of 49 echocardiograms and the other finding CALs on 15 (44%) of 34 echocardiograms ($P=.66$).

Sixteen patients (10 with complete KS) were given more than 1 dose of IVIG for refractory KS. One patient received a third dose of IVIG, and 4 received steroids after 2 doses of IVIG. Twelve of the patients who received multiple doses of IVIG, including 4 patients with aneurysm, developed CALs during the course of their illness.

## COMMENT

Recently, the American Heart Association[1] (AHA) published guidelines on the diagnosis and treatment of KS that recommended the use of echocardiography as a diagnostic tool for patients with suspected incomplete KS. Of note, this recommendation is based on expert opinion, and the sensitivity and specificity of findings on the initial echocardiogram have not been clinically validated. In our study, we found a 44% prevalence of CALs on the initial echocardiogram. Other recent series[7,10,11] of patients with KS have found a similarly high prevalence of CALs on the initial echocardiogram. These findings suggest that echocardiography may be a useful adjunctive test for the diagnosis of KS. Diagnostic use of the echocardiogram may be particularly useful in those patients with incomplete KS in whom the diagnosis is more difficult and, as a consequence, often delayed.

Consistent with other reported series of patients with KS,[2,3,12] a substantial percentage of our patients had incomplete criteria for KS. In our study, these patients were treated significantly later and had a significantly higher rate of coronary artery aneurysms than those patients with complete KS. Benefit of treatment by day 10 of illness has been previously demonstrated.[1,2,4,5,13] Furthermore, some evidence suggests that treatment as early as day 6 to 7 confers a better coronary artery prognosis than later treatment.[6,7] The AHA guidelines recommend that treatment be initiated before the 10th day of illness and preferably before the 7th day of illness.[1] Considering treatment before and after these time points, we found that the percentage of patients with aneurysm increased significantly with a longer time to treatment. Based on the findings of our study, use of the echocardiogram as suggested by the AHA guidelines early in the course of illness in a patient with suspected incomplete KS may lead to earlier treatment and an improved coronary artery outcome.

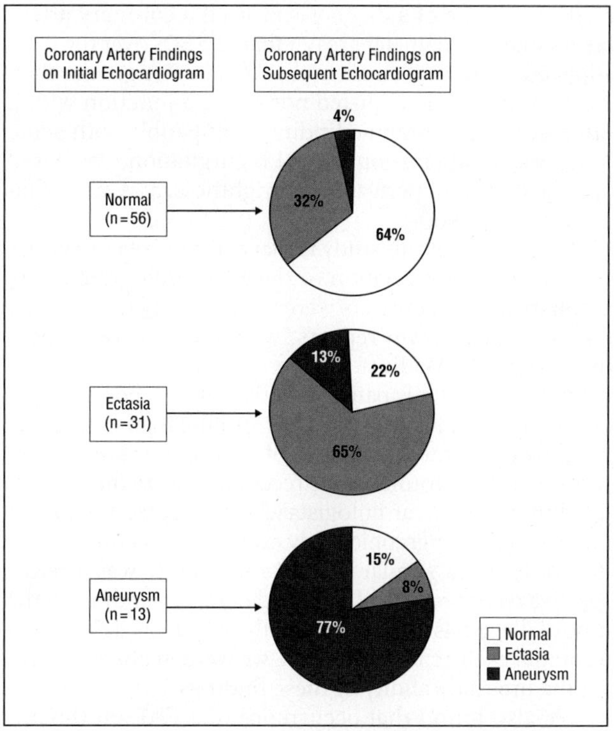


**Figure.** Coronary artery lesions (ectasia or aneurysm) were observed on subsequent echocardiograms in significantly more patients with ectasia ($P<.001$) or aneurysm ($P=.002$) on the initial echocardiograms than in patients with normal coronary arteries on the initial echocardiograms.

The prevalence of CALs on the initial echocardiogram of patients with acute KS that we report is much higher than that which had been reported in the literature during the 1980s and through much of the 1990s. In each of the 2 IVIG treatment studies by Newburger et al[4,5] in which only patients with complete KS treated in the first 10 days of illness were included, less than 4% of patients with KS had CALs on the initial echocardiogram. Similarly, Barron et al[8] found CALs on the initial echocardiogram in only 1 (2%) of 51 patients with complete KS treated by day 7 of illness. In comparison, of our patients with complete KS treated within 7 days of illness, CALs were present on the initial echocardiogram in 39%. Newer imaging technology that allows for a more accurate evaluation of the coronary arteries may partially explain the discrepancy. However, the evolution of the criteria used to define CALs is likely to be a more important factor. In earlier studies,[4-6,8] CAL was defined by a coronary artery diameter that exceeded an absolute measurement (ie, a 3- or 4-mm internal diameter). Two recent studies[9,10] suggest that these criteria may miss a significant proportion of abnormalities, and instead, they recommend the use of a CAL definition based on comparisons to body surface area (BSA)–adjusted norms of coronary artery internal diameters. Defining a CAL as a vessel with an internal diameter that is 2 or more SDs higher than the BSA-adjusted norm, 2 studies of patients with KS published in 2002 found prevalences of CALs on the initial echocardiogram of 34%[7] and 47%[10] of patients. The 2004 AHA guidelines also use BSA-adjusted criteria to define a CAL when the finding is used to diagnose a patient with incomplete KS. Using these guidelines, the results of echocardiography are considered supportive of a diagnosis of KS if a coronary artery has an internal diameter greater than 2.5 SDs over the BSA-adjusted norm or if an artery has a diameter greater than 2 SDs over the age-adjusted norm in conjunction with 2 other echocardiographic findings compatible with acute KS (pericardial effusion, mitral regurgitation, decreased systolic function, perivascular brightness, and lack of tapering of a vessel).

A limitation of this study is that a finding of ectasia was a subjective interpretation of the echocardiographer. As coronary artery diameters were not routinely recorded on the echocardiogram reports, we could not retrospectively apply BSA-adjusted criteria or the full AHA algorithm to most of our patients. Although it is possible that our definition of ectasia was less specific than ectasia defined by other methods, rates of CAL in our study were similar to those found in the recent literature on KS.[7,10,11] In addition, the 2 cardiologists who accounted for 83% of initial echocardiographic study evaluations recorded findings of CALs at similar rates. As this study was a retrospective record review of echocardiographic findings at the time of diagnosis and consequently only 1 cardiologist interpreted each echocardiogram, we were unable to evaluate the internal validity of these findings.

We also found that occurrence of a CAL on the initial echocardiogram was predictive of CAL occurrence on a subsequent echocardiogram in a given patient. Given that the echocardiographers for the subsequent echocardiograms were not blinded to the results of the initial echocardiogram, observer bias may have influenced this finding. However, our finding that the vast majority of patients with ectasia had normal coronary arteries on the final echocardiogram supports the validity of the diagnosis of ectasia rather than a misdiagnosed variant of a normal coronary artery.

As noted earlier, echocardiographic findings described in the AHA guidelines for diagnosis of KS are based on expert opinion, and the positive and negative predictive values of particular echocardiographic findings have not been validated in clinical trials. The specificity of a finding of ectasia must be ascertained before echocardiography can be validated as a diagnostic adjunct for KS. Although previously published studies have measured the dimensions of coronary arteries in healthy children, we are unaware of studies that compare artery dimensions of children with KS with those of similarly aged children with other acute febrile illnesses. Indeed, in our study, 3 children with CALs did not have KS, indicating that the specificity of a CAL was less than 100% for diagnosis of KS. In addition, a recent study[14] notes that patients with newly diagnosed juvenile rheumatoid arthritis may have coronary artery dilatation. If CALs may be found in other inflammatory diseases, the specificity of a finding of a CAL in KS may be limited.

A further limitation of this study is the retrospective design. As this study was a retrospective review of clinical data, the cardiologists were not blinded to the diagnosis of suspected KS. A reader-blinded case-control study comparing the coronary arteries of children with KS with the coronary arteries of age-matched febrile children would help to evaluate the positive and negative predictive values of the initial echocardiogram as an adjunctive test for diagnosing KS.

Our findings demonstrate that CALs are common on the initial echocardiogram of patients with acute KS. If these lesions are found to have a relatively high degree of specificity for KS, the initial echocardiogram may be a valuable tool in diagnosing the illness early in its course. Further studies are needed to help determine the utility of the initial echocardiogram in diagnosing KS and to determine echocardiographic findings that are most sensitive and specific for a diagnosis of KS.

**Accepted for Publication:** January 12, 2006.
**Correspondence:** Lorry G. Rubin, MD, Schneider Children's Hospital, 269-01 76th Ave, New Hyde Park, NY 11040 (lrubin@lij.edu).
**Author Contributions:** *Study concept and design:* Baer, Rubin, Sood, Rajan, Shapir, Romano, and Bierman. *Acquisition of data:* Baer, Shapiro, Sood, and Rajan. *Drafting of the manuscript:* Baer and Sood. *Critical revision of the manuscript for important intellectual content*: Baer, Rubin, Shapiro, Sood, Rajan, Shapir, Romano, and Bierman. *Administrative, technical, and material support:* Sood. *Study supervision:* Rubin, Sood, Rajan, Shapir, Romano, and Bierman. Dr Baer had full access to all of the data in the study and takes responsibility for the integrity of the data and the accuracy of the data analysis.

## REFERENCES


1. Newburger JW, Takahashi M, Gerber MA, et al; Committee on Rheumatic Fever, Endocarditis and Kawasaki Disease; Council on Cardiovascular Disease in the Young; American Heart Association; American Academy of Pediatrics. Diagnosis, treatment, and long-term management of Kawasaki disease. *Circulation.* 2004;110:2747-2771.
2. Witt MT, Minich LL, Bohnsack JF, Young PC. Kawasaki disease. *Pediatrics.* 1999; 104:e10.
3. Joffe A, Kabani A, Jadavji T. Atypical and complicated Kawasaki disease in infants. *West J Med.* 1995;162:322-327.
4. Newburger JW, Takahashi M, Burns JC, et al. The treatment of Kawasaki syndrome with intravenous gamma globulin. *N Engl J Med.* 1986;315:341-347.
5. Newburger JW, Takahashi M, Beiser AS, et al. A single intravenous infusion of gamma globulin as compared with four infusions in the treatment of acute Kawasaki syndrome. *N Engl J Med.* 1991;324:1633-1639.
6. Pallotto E, Shulman ST, Rowley AH, Goldberg C. Does the treatment of Kawasaki disease within the first 7 days of illness improve the long-term outcome compared to later (8-10th day) treatment? In: Kato H, ed. *Kawasaki Disease: Proceedings of the Fifth International Kawasaki Disease Symposium, Fukuoka, Japan.* Amsterdam, the Netherlands: Elsevier; 1995:305-309.
7. Tse SM, Silverman ED, McCrindle BW, Yeung RS. Early treatment with intravenous immunoglobulin in patients with Kawasaki disease. *J Pediatr.* 2002;140:450-455.
8. Barron KS, Murphy DJ, Silverman ED, Ruttenberg HD, Wright GB, Franklin W. Treatment of Kawasaki syndrome. *J Pediatr.* 1990;117:638-644.
9. De Zorzi A, Colan SD, Gauvreau K, Baker AL, Sundel RP, Newburger JW. Coronary artery dimensions may be misclassified as normal in Kawasaki disease. *J Pediatr.* 1998;133:254-258.
10. Kurotobi S, Nagai T, Kawakami N, Sano T. Coronary diameter in normal infants, children and patients with Kawasaki disease. *Pediatr Int.* 2002;44:1-4.
11. Han RK, Silverman ED, Newman A, McCrindle BW. Management and outcome of persistent or recurrent fever after initial intravenous gamma globulin therapy in acute Kawasaki disease. *Arch Pediatr Adolesc Med.* 2000;154:694-699.
12. Barone SR, Pontrelli LR, Krilov LR. The differentiation of classic Kawasaki disease, atypical Kawasaki disease, and acute adenoviral infection. *Arch Pediatr Adolesc Med.* 2000;154:453-456.
13. Miura M, Okhi H, Tsuchihashi T, Yamagishi H, Katada Y, Yamada K. Coronary risk factors in Kawasaki disease treated with additional gammaglobulin. *Arch Dis Child.* 2004;89:776-780.
14. Binstadt BA, Levine JC, Nigrovic PA, et al. Coronary artery dilation among patients presenting with systemic-onset juvenile idiopathic arthritis. *Pediatrics.* 2005; 116:e89-e93.

**PEDIARIX™ [Diphtheria and Tetanus Toxoids and Acellular Pertussis Adsorbed, Hepatitis B (Recombinant) and Inactivated Poliovirus Vaccine Combined]**

The following is a brief summary only; see full prescribing information for complete product information.

**CONTRAINDICATIONS:** Hypersensitivity to any component of the vaccine, including yeast, neomycin, and polymyxin B, is a contraindication (see DESCRIPTION in complete prescribing information). Do not use PEDIARIX after a serious allergic reaction (e.g., anaphylaxis) temporally associated with a previous dose of this vaccine or with any components of this vaccine. Because of the uncertainty as to which component of the vaccine might be responsible, do not give further vaccination with any of these components; or, refer such individuals to an allergist for evaluation. The following events are contraindications to administration of PEDIARIX: encephalopathy (e.g., coma, decreased level of consciousness, prolonged seizures) within 7 days of administration of a previous dose of a pertussis-containing vaccine that is not attributable to another identifiable cause; progressive neurologic disorder, including infantile spasms, uncontrolled epilepsy, or progressive encephalopathy. Do not vaccinate individuals with such conditions until a treatment regimen has been established and the condition has stabilized. PEDIARIX is not contraindicated for use in individuals with HIV infection.

**WARNINGS:** Administration of PEDIARIX is associated with higher rates of fever relative to separately administered vaccines. In one study that evaluated medically attended fever after the first dose of PEDIARIX or separately administered vaccines, infants who received PEDIARIX had a higher rate of medical encounters for fever within the first 4 days following vaccination. In some infants, these encounters included the performance of diagnostic studies to evaluate other causes of fever (see ADVERSE REACTIONS). The vial stopper is latex-free. The tip cap and the rubber plunger of the needleless prefilled syringes contain dry natural latex rubber that may cause allergic reactions in latex sensitive individuals. If any of the following events occur in temporal relation to receipt of whole-cell DTP or a vaccine containing an acellular pertussis component, consider carefully whether to give subsequent doses of PEDIARIX or any vaccine containing a pertussis component: temperature of ≥40.5°C (105°F) within 48 hours not due to another identifiable cause; collapse or shock-like state (hypotonic-hyporesponsive episode) within 48 hours; persistent, inconsolable crying lasting ≥3 hours, occurring within 48 hours; seizures with or without fever occurring within 3 days. If Guillain-Barré syndrome occurs within 6 weeks of receipt of prior vaccine containing tetanus toxoid, the decision to give subsequent doses of PEDIARIX or any vaccine containing tetanus toxoid should be based on careful consideration of the potential benefits and possible risks. A committee of the Institute of Medicine (IOM) has concluded that evidence is consistent with a causal relationship between whole-cell DTP vaccine and acute neurologic illness, and under special circumstances, between whole-cell DTP vaccine and chronic neurologic disease in the context of the National Childhood Encephalopathy Study (NCES) report; however, evidence was insufficient to indicate whether or not whole-cell DTP vaccine increased the overall risk of chronic neurologic disease. Acute encephalopathy and permanent neurologic damage have not been reported causally linked or in temporal association with administration of PEDIARIX, but the experience with PEDIARIX is insufficient to rule this out. Encephalopathy has been reported following INFANRIX® (Diphtheria and Tetanus Toxoids and Acellular Pertussis Vaccine Adsorbed) (see ADVERSE REACTIONS, Postmarketing Reports), but data are not sufficient to evaluate a causal relationship. The decision to administer a pertussis-containing vaccine to children with stable central nervous system (CNS) disorders must be made by the physician on an individual basis, with consideration of all relevant factors, and assessment of potential risks and benefits for that individual. Advise the parent or guardian of the potential increased risk involved (see PRECAUTIONS). A family history of seizures or other CNS disorders is not a contraindication to pertussis vaccine. For children at higher risk for seizures than the general population, an appropriate antipyretic may be administered at the time of vaccination and for the ensuing 24 hours according to the respective prescribing information recommended dosage to reduce the possibility of post-vaccination fever. Defer vaccination during the course of a moderate or severe illness with or without fever and vaccinate patients as soon as they have recovered from the acute phase of the illness. Do not give PEDIARIX to children on anticoagulant therapy or those with bleeding disorders unless the potential benefit clearly outweighs the risk of administration (see PRECAUTIONS in complete prescribing information).

**PRECAUTIONS:** Before the injection of any biological, the physician should take all reasonable precautions to prevent allergic or other adverse reactions. Epinephrine injection (1:1000) and other appropriate agents used for the control of immediate allergic reactions must be immediately available should an acute anaphylactic reaction occur. Immunosuppressed individuals, including those receiving immunosuppressive therapy, may not develop the expected immune response. **Drug Interactions:** For information regarding concomitant administration with other vaccines, refer to DOSAGE AND ADMINISTRATION in complete prescribing information. Do not mix PEDIARIX with any other vaccine in the same syringe or vial. **Carcinogenesis, Mutagenesis, Impairment of Fertility:** PEDIARIX has not been evaluated for carcinogenic or mutagenic potential, or for impairment of fertility. **Pregnancy:** Pregnancy Category C: PEDIARIX is not indicated for women of child-bearing age. Animal reproduction studies have not been conducted with PEDIARIX. It is not known whether PEDIARIX can cause fetal harm when administered to a pregnant woman or if PEDIARIX can affect reproductive capacity. **Geriatric Use:** PEDIARIX is not indicated for use in adult populations. **Pediatric Use:** Safety and effectiveness of PEDIARIX in infants younger than 6 weeks of age have not been evaluated (see DOSAGE AND ADMINISTRATION in complete prescribing information). PEDIARIX is not recommended for persons 7 years of age or older. Tetanus and Diphtheria Toxoids Adsorbed (Td) For Adult Use, inactivated poliovirus vaccine (IPV), and Hepatitis B Vaccine (Recombinant) should be used in individuals 7 years of age or older.

**ADVERSE REACTIONS:** A total of 20,739 doses of PEDIARIX have been administered to 7,028 infants as a 3-dose primary series. The most common adverse reactions observed in clinical trials were local injection site reactions (pain, redness, or swelling), fever, and fussiness. In comparative studies, administration of PEDIARIX was associated with higher rates of fever relative to separately administered vaccines (see WARNINGS). The prevalence of fever was highest on the day of vaccination and the day following vaccination. More than 98% of episodes of fever resolved within the 4-day period following vaccination (i.e., the period including the day of vaccination and the next 3 days). Rates of most other solicited adverse events following PEDIARIX were comparable to rates observed following separately administered US-licensed vaccines. The adverse event information from clinical trials provides a basis for identifying adverse events that appear to be related to vaccine use and for approximating rates. However, because clinical trials are conducted under widely varying conditions, adverse event rates observed in the clinical trials of a vaccine cannot be directly compared to rates in the clinical trials of another vaccine, and may not reflect the rates observed in practice. A total of 5,472 infants were enrolled in a German safety study that was originally designed to compare the safety and reactogenicity of PEDIARIX administered concomitantly at separate sites with 1 of 4 *Haemophilus influenzae* type b (Hib) vaccines at 3, 4, and 5 months of age. After enrollment of 1,569 infants, the study was amended to include a control group that received INFANRIX, Hib vaccine, and oral poliovirus vaccine (OPV) separately. Infants in the separate administration group received one less antigen (hepatitis B) than the infants who received PEDIARIX. Safety data were available for 4,666 infants who received PEDIARIX administered concomitantly at separate sites with 1 of 4 Hib vaccines and for 768 infants in the control group that received separate vaccines. The primary end-point of the study was the percentage of infants with any grade 3 solicited symptom (redness or swelling >20 mm, fever >103.1°F, or crying, pain, vomiting, diarrhea, loss of appetite, or restlessness that prevented normal daily activities) over the 3-dose primary series in infants who received PEDIARIX (4 groups that received PEDIARIX and Hib vaccines pooled) compared to the group that received INFANRIX and Hib vaccine separately with OPV. Analysis for the primary end-point was performed on the according-to-protocol (ATP) cohort that included only those infants who were enrolled after the protocol amendment to include a control group. Of 3,773 infants in the ATP cohort for whom safety data were available, 16.2% (95% CI: 14.9% to 17.5%) of 3,029 infants who received PEDIARIX and Hib vaccine compared to 20.3% (95% CI: 17.5% to 23.4%) of 744 infants who received separate vaccines were reported to have had at least one grade 3 solicited symptom within 4 days of vaccination (i.e., day of vaccination and the next 3 days). The difference between groups in the rate of grade 3 symptoms was 4.1% (90% CI: 1.4% to 7.1%). These were the rates for selected solicited symptoms within 4 days following each dose in a 3-dose primary series in infants who received PEDIARIX administered concomitantly with Hib vaccine and those who received separate concomitant administration of INFANRIX, Hib vaccine, and OPV for the intent-to-treat (ITT) cohort (includes all infants enrolled before and after the amendment who received the indicated vaccine and for whom at least one symptom sheet was completed):

**Percentage of German Infants With Solicited Local Reactions or Selected Systemic Adverse Events Within 4 Days of Vaccination* (ITT Cohort)**

| | PEDIARIX & Hib | | | INFANRIX, Hib, & OPV | | |
|---|---|---|---|---|---|---|
| | Dose 1 | Dose 2 | Dose 3 | Dose 1 | Dose 2 | Dose 3 |
| **N** | **4,666** | **4,619** | **4,574** | **768** | **757** | **750** |
| **Local†** | | | | | | |
| Pain, any | 14.0 | 10.2 | 9.9 | 14.2 | 9.8 | 8.1 |
| Pain, grade 2 or 3 | 2.9 | 1.2 | 1.5 | 3.6 | 1.7 | 1.1 |
| Pain, grade 3 | 0.7 | 0.3 | 0.3 | 1.3 | 0.4 | 0.1 |
| Redness, any | 18.6 | 26.6 | 25.6 | 16.1 | 21.4 | 20.8 |
| Redness, >5 mm | 6.7 | 9.9 | 9.0 | 5.9 | 8.2 | 7.7 |
| Redness, >20 mm | 1.2 | 1.0 | 1.1 | 1.8 | 0.7 | 1.1 |
| Swelling, any | 12.7 | 18.5 | 18.4 | 9.6 | 12.9 | 13.6 |
| Swelling, >5 mm | 5.6 | 7.7 | 7.8 | 3.6 | 5.2 | 4.8 |
| Swelling, >20 mm | 1.2 | 1.6 | 1.5 | 1.3 | 1.1 | 1.2 |
| **Systemic** | | | | | | |
| Restlessness, any | 41.4 | 32.0 | 26.7 | 46.4 | 35.0 | 27.6 |
| Restlessness, grade 2 or 3 | 14.4 | 10.0 | 8.9 | 20.2 | 11.5 | 8.4 |
| Restlessness, grade 3 | 3.0 | 1.5 | 1.6 | 5.7 | 3.0 | 1.7 |
| Fever‡, ≥100.4ºF | 25.1 | 19.3 | 19.7 | 13.2 | 13.1 | 11.2 |
| Fever‡, >101.3ºF | 5.8 | 4.1 | 4.6 | 2.2 | 2.8 | 2.1 |
| Fever‡, >103.1ºF | 0.3 | 0.5 | 0.7 | 0.3 | 0.3 | 0.5 |
| Unusual cry§, any | 24.9 | 16.5 | 13.1 | 36.5 | 19.7 | 14.3 |
| Unusual cry§, grade 2 or 3 | 12.7 | 7.1 | 5.7 | 20.8 | 10.0 | 5.7 |
| Unusual cry§, grade 3 | 3.9 | 1.7 | 1.4 | 6.8 | 2.1 | 1.1 |
| Loss of appetite, any | 17.9 | 13.3 | 12.5 | 19.1 | 16.2 | 11.3 |
| Loss of appetite, grade 2 or 3 | 4.0 | 2.9 | 2.7 | 4.4 | 2.9 | 2.3 |
| Loss of appetite, grade 3 | 0.6 | 0.5 | 0.4 | 0.5 | 0.7 | 0.0 |

N = number of infants in the intent-to-treat (ITT) cohort.
Grade 2 defined as sufficiently discomforting to interfere with daily activities.
Grade 3 defined as preventing normal daily activities.
* Within 4 days of vaccination defined as day of vaccination and the next 3 days.
† Local reactions at the injection site for PEDIARIX or INFANRIX.
‡ Rectal temperatures.
§ Unusual cry lasting >1 hour.

In this study, infants were also monitored for unsolicited adverse events that occurred within 30 days following vaccination. Over the entire study period, 6 subjects in the group that received PEDIARIX reported seizures. Two of these subjects had a febrile seizure, 1 of whom also developed afebrile seizures. The remaining 4 subjects had afebrile seizures, including 2 with infantile spasms. Two subjects reported seizures within 7 days following vaccination (1 subject had both febrile and afebrile seizures, and 1 subject had afebrile seizures), corresponding to a rate of 0.22 seizures per 1,000 doses (febrile seizures 0.07 per 1,000 doses, afebrile seizures 0.14 per 1,000 doses). No subject who received concomitant INFANRIX, Hib vaccine, and OPV reported seizures. In a separate German study that evaluated the safety of INFANRIX in 22,505 infants who received 66,867 doses of INFANRIX administered as a 3-dose primary series, the rate of seizures within 7 days of vaccination with INFANRIX was 0.13 per 1,000 doses (febrile seizures 0.0 per 1,000 doses, afebrile seizures 0.13 per 1,000 doses). No cases of hypotonic-hyporesponsiveness, encephalopathy, or anaphylaxis were reported in the German study that evaluated the safety of PEDIARIX. Rates of serious adverse events that are less common than those reported in this safety study are not known at this time.

Additional safety data for PEDIARIX are available from a US study designed to evaluate lot-to-lot consistency and a bridge for a new manufacturing step. These were the rates for local reactions and selected adverse events within 4 days of vaccination with PEDIARIX administered concomitantly with a Hib vaccine at 2, 4, and 6 months of age:

**Percentage of US Infants With Solicited Local Reactions or Selected Systemic Adverse Events Within 4 Days of Vaccination* (ITT Cohort)**

| | PEDIARIX & Hib | | |
|---|---|---|---|
| | Dose 1 | Dose 2 | Dose 3 |
| **Local†** | **N = 482** | **N = 469** | **N = 466** |
| Pain, any | 30.5 | 25.4 | 23.0 |
| Pain, grade 2 or 3 | 6.2 | 5.5 | 3.6 |
| Pain, grade 3 | 1.2 | 0.6 | 0.6 |
| Redness, any | 25.3 | 32.6 | 35.6 |
| Redness, >5 mm | 9.3 | 10.4 | 8.6 |
| Redness, >20 mm | 0.6 | 1.5 | 1.3 |
| Swelling, any | 15.1 | 16.6 | 22.3 |
| Swelling, >5 mm | 6.8 | 6.2 | 6.4 |
| Swelling, >20 mm | 1.0 | 1.3 | 1.3 |
| **Systemic** | **N = 482** | **N = 469** | **N = 467** |
| Restlessness, any | 28.8 | 30.3 | 28.5 |
| Restlessness, grade 2 or 3 | 7.1 | 9.0 | 9.4 |
| Restlessness, grade 3 | 1.0 | 1.1 | 0.6 |
| Fever‡, ≥100.4ºF | 26.6 | 31.3 | 25.9 |
| Fever‡, >101.3ºF | 2.9 | 6.2 | 4.7 |
| Fever‡, >103.1ºF | 0.0 | 0.2 | 0.6 |
| Fussiness, any | 61.8 | 63.8 | 57.0 |
| Fussiness, grade 2 or 3 | 14.9 | 21.5 | 17.1 |
| Fussiness, grade 3 | 2.7 | 3.4 | 1.7 |
| Loss of appetite, any | 21.6 | 19.8 | 18.8 |
| Loss of appetite, grade 2 or 3 | 3.1 | 3.2 | 2.4 |
| Loss of appetite, grade 3 | 0.2 | 0.4 | 0.0 |
| Sleeping more than usual, any | 46.7 | 31.8 | 28.1 |
| Sleeping more than usual, grade 2 or 3 | 10.2 | 6.0 | 4.7 |
| Sleeping more than usual, grade 3 | 1.7 | 0.4 | 0.6 |

N = number of infants in the intent-to-treat (ITT) cohort (infants who received the indicated vaccine and for whom at least one symptom sheet was completed).
Grade 2 defined as sufficiently discomforting to interfere with daily activities.
Grade 3 defined as preventing normal daily activities.
* Within 4 days of vaccination defined as day of vaccination and the next 3 days.
† Local reactions at the injection site for PEDIARIX.
‡ Rectal temperatures.

In another US study, these were the rates for fever within 4 days following dose 1 (i.e., day of vaccination and the next 3 days) at 2 months of age in infants who received PEDIARIX when administered concomitantly at separate sites with Hib and pneumococcal conjugate vaccines and those who received INFANRIX, ENGERIX-B® [Hepatitis B Vaccine (Recombinant)], IPV, Hib vaccine, and pneumococcal conjugate vaccine:

**Percentage of US Infants With Fever Within 4 Days of Dose 1* (ITT Cohort)**

| | PEDIARIX, Hib, & Pneumococcal Conjugate (N = 667) | INFANRIX, ENGERIX-B, IPV, Hib, & Pneumococcal Conjugate (N = 333) | Separate Vaccine Group Minus Combination Vaccine Group |
|---|---|---|---|
| **Fever†** | **%** | **%** | **Difference (95% CI)** |
| ≥100.4ºF‡ | 27.9 | 19.8 | -8.07 (-13.54, -2.60) |
| >101.3ºF | 7.0 | 4.5 | -2.54 (-5.50, 0.41) |
| >102.2ºF‡ | 2.2 | 0.3 | -1.95 (-3.22, -0.68) |
| >103.1ºF | 0.4 | 0.0 | -0.45 (-0.96, 0.06) |
| M.A.‡ | 1.2 | 0.0 | -1.20 (-2.03, -037) |

N = number of infants for whom at least one symptom sheet was completed, excluding 3 infants for whom temperature was not measured and 3 infants whose temperature was measured by the tympanic method.
*Within 4 days of dose 1 defined as day of vaccination and the next 3 days.
† Rectal temperatures.
‡ The group that received PEDIARIX compared to separate vaccine group p value <0.05 (2-sided Fisher Exact test) or the 95% confidence interval on the difference between groups does not include 0.
M.A. = Medically attended (a visit to or from medical personnel).

In this study, medical attention (a visit to or from medical personnel) for fever within 4 days following vaccination was sought for 8 infants who received PEDIARIX (1.2%) and no infants who received separately administered vaccines. Four infants were seen by medical personnel in an office setting; no diagnostic tests were performed in 2 of the infants and a complete blood count (CBC) was done in the other 2 infants. Of 3 infants who were seen in an emergency room, all had a CBC and a blood and urine culture performed; chest X-rays were done in 2 of the infants and a nasopharyngeal specimen was tested for Respiratory Syncytial Virus in one of the infants. One infant was hospitalized for a work-up that included a CBC, blood and urine cultures, a lumbar puncture, and a chest X-ray. All episodes of medically attended fever resolved within 4 days post-vaccination.

Limited data are available from a study conducted in Moldova in which infants received a dose of hepatitis B vaccine within 48 hours of birth followed by 3 doses of PEDIARIX at 6, 10, and 14 weeks of age. No information was collected on the HBsAg status of mothers of enrolled infants. These were the rates for local reactions and selected adverse events within 4 days of vaccination with PEDIARIX administered comcomitantly with Hib vaccine following a birth dose of hepatitis B vaccine:

**Percentage of Moldovan Infants With Solicited Local Reactions or Selected Systemic Adverse Events Within 4 Days of Vaccination* (ITT Cohort)**

| | PEDIARIX & Hib | | |
|---|---|---|---|
| | Dose 1 | Dose 2 | Dose 3 |
| **N** | **160** | **158** | **157** |
| **Local†** | | | |
| Pain, any | 25.6 | 18.4 | 14.0 |
| Pain, grade 3 | 3.1 | 0.6 | 1.9 |
| Redness, any | 41.9 | 41.8 | 47.1 |
| Redness, >20 mm | 1.9 | 2.5 | 4.5 |
| Swelling, any | 20.6 | 18.4 | 28.0 |
| Swelling, >20 mm | 4.4 | 2.5 | 7.0 |
| **Systemic** | | | |
| Restlessness, any | 13.1 | 10.8 | 8.9 |
| Restlessness, grade 3 | 1.3 | 0.6 | 0.6 |
| Fever‡, ≥100.4ºF | 14.4 | 11.4 | 5.1 |
| Fever‡, >103.1ºF | 0.0 | 0.6 | 0.0 |
| Fussiness, any | 25.0 | 21.5 | 17.8 |
| Fussiness, grade 3 | 2.5 | 0.6 | 0.6 |

N = number of infants in the intent-to-treat (ITT) cohort (infants who received the indicated vaccine and for whom at least one symptom sheet was completed).
Grade 3 defined as preventing normal daily activities.
*Within 4 days of vaccination defined as day of vaccination and the next 3 days.
† Local reactions at the injection site for PEDIARIX.
‡ Rectal temperatures.

Although there was no comparator group who received PEDIARIX without a birth dose of hepatitis B vaccine, available data suggest that some local adverse events may occur at a higher rate when PEDIARIX is administered after a birth dose of hepatitis B vaccine.

As with any vaccine, there is the possibility that broad use of PEDIARIX could reveal adverse events not observed in clinical trials.

**Postmarketing Reports:** Worldwide voluntary reports of adverse events received for INFANRIX and ENGERIX-B in children younger than 7 years of age since market introduction of these US-licensed vaccines are listed below. This list includes adverse events for which 20 or more reports were received with the exception of intussusception, idiopathic thrombocytopenic purpura, thrombocytopenia, anaphylactic reaction, angioedema, encephalopathy, hypotonic-hyporesponsive episode, and alopecia for which fewer than 20 reports were received. These latter events are included either because of the seriousness of the event or the strength of causal connection to components of this or other vaccines or drugs. *Body as a whole:* Asthenia[b], fever[a+b], lethargy[b], malaise[b], Sudden Infant Death Syndrome[a+b]. *Cardiovascular system:* Cyanosis[a+b], edema[b], pallor[b]. *Gastrointestinal system:* Abdominal pain[b], anorexia[b], diarrhea[a+b], intussusception[a+b], nausea[b], vomiting[a+b]. *Hematologic/lymphatic:* Idiopathic thrombocytopenic purpura[a+b], lymphadenopathy[a], thrombocytopenia[a+b]. *Hepatic:* Jaundice[b], liver function tests abnormal[b]. *Hypersensitivity:* Anaphylactic reaction[a+b], angioedema[b], hypersensitivity[a]. *Infections:* Cellulitis[a]. *Injection site reactions:* Injection site reactions[a+b]. *Musculoskeletal:* Arthralgia[b], limb swelling[a+b]. *Nervous system:* Convulsions[a+b], encephalopathy[a], headache[b], hypotonia[a+b], hypotonic-hyporesponsive episode[a], somnolence[a+b]. *Psychiatric:* Crying[a+b], irritability[a+b]. *Respiratory system:* Respiratory tract infection[a]. *Skin and appendages:* Alopecia[b], erythema[a+b], erythema multiforme[b], petechiae[b], pruritus[a+b], rash[a+b], urticaria[a+b]. *Special senses:* Ear pain[a]. [[a] Following INFANRIX; [b] Following ENGERIX-B; [a+b] Following either INFANRIX or ENGERIX-B.] These reactions were reported voluntarily from a population of uncertain size; therefore, it is not always possible to reliably estimate their frequency or establish a causal relationship to vaccination.

**Reporting Adverse Events:** Report the occurrence following immunization of any event set forth in the Vaccine Injury Table from the National Childhood Vaccine Injury Act including: Anaphylaxis or anaphylactic shock within 7 days, encephalopathy or encephalitis within 7 days, brachial neuritis within 28 days, or an acute complication or sequelae (including death) of an illness, disability, injury, or condition referred to above, or any events that would contraindicate further doses of PEDIARIX. The VAERS toll-free number is 1-800-822-7967.

Manufactured by **GlaxoSmithKline Biologicals**, Rixensart, Belgium, US License 1617

Distributed by **GlaxoSmithKline,** Research Triangle Park, NC 27709



Full prescribing information for PEDIARIX is available at www.GSKVaccines.com/Pediarix. BRS-PE:L2

 Printed in USA. PED583R0 June 2005

# Improving Recognition of Adolescent Depression in Primary Care

*Rachel A. Zuckerbrot, MD; Peter S. Jensen, MD*

**Objective:** To address the following questions: (1) What evidence (ie, psychometric data collected in pediatric primary care, patient outcome data) exists for the various methods used to identify adolescent depression in primary care? and (2) What identification practices are currently in use?

**Data Sources:** We systematically searched MEDLINE for English-language articles using specific search terms and examined relevant titles, abstracts, and articles.

**Study Selection:** We reviewed 1743 MEDLINE abstracts. Seventy-four articles were pulled for examination, with 30 articles meeting full criteria.

**Data Extraction:** Five studies had adequate psychometric data on various adolescent depression identification methods in primary care. Only 1 compared the diagnostic accuracy of physicians trained to ask depression questions vs physicians trained in the use of a diagnostic aid. Six studies reported on current practice. Evidence regarding sensitivity, specificity, positive predictive value, and negative predictive value was sought for question 1. Frequency of screening was sought for question 2.

**Data Synthesis:** Review of these articles found that few health care professionals use systematic depression identification methods, despite some growing evidence for their validity, feasibility, and possible efficacy.

**Conclusion:** Available evidence indicates that primary care professionals would improve their rates of depression diagnosis through training, but even more so by using adolescent symptom rating scales.

*Arch Pediatr Adolesc Med. 2006;160:694-704*

STUDIES HAVE FOUND THAT 3% to 9% of teenagers meet criteria for depression at any one time, and at the end of adolescence, as many as 20% of teenagers report a lifetime prevalence of depression.[1-4] Adolescent depression may affect the teen's socialization, family relations, and performance at school, often with potentially serious long-term consequences.[5] Adolescents with depression are at risk for increased hospitalizations, recurrent depressions, psychosocial impairment, alcohol abuse, and antisocial behaviors as they grow up.[6-8] Of course, the most devastating outcome of concern for adolescent depression is suicide, the third leading cause of death among older adolescents.[9]

Despite the severe morbidity and mortality associated with adolescent depression, most studies report that only 1 in 4 to 1 in 3 adolescents with depression are receiving treatment for this disorder.[10,11] Extant data suggest that depression is relatively common in pediatric settings[12,13] and is often unidentified by pediatric professionals.[14,15] Pediatricians, however, do feel responsible for identifying adolescent depression[16] and most of the major professional organizations have acknowledged the importance of identifying depression and suicidal behavior in youth.[17-19] To improve the identification and treatment of adolescent depression, primary care health professionals may need to adapt the service delivery models currently used in treating adults with depression. While depression screening and management are now considered to be an essential function of the primary care setting for adults,[20-22] no definitive recommendations have been made in support of adolescent depression screening in primary care.

*For editorial comment see page 755*

In light of the significant morbidity and mortality of adolescent depression; its high prevalence in pediatric primary care; the existence of promising treatments such as cognitive behavioral therapy,[23] interpersonal therapy for adolescents,[24] and medication[25] (despite the current "black box" warning[26]); and its underrecognition by pediatricians despite their good intentions, it is surprising that no literature, to our knowledge, has systematically reviewed the available evidence regarding the various methods available and in use for the identification of adolescent depression in pediatric primary care. We conducted a literature search to determine (1) What evidence exists for the various methods

**Author Affiliations:** Division of Child and Adolescent Psychiatry, Department of Psychiatry, Columbia University and Center for the Advancement of Children's Mental Health, Columbia University/New York State Psychiatric Institute, New York.

used to identify adolescent depression in primary care? and (2) What identification practices are currently in use? Question 1 includes the following: (1) the availability of psychometric data assessing adolescent depression screening and identification methods in pediatric primary care and (2) available evidence regarding the feasibility, acceptability, cost, and benefit to patients of available identification methods.

## METHODS

This search focused on psychometric data comparing the use of general psychosocial screening tools (eg, Child Behavior Checklist[27]), depression-specific tools (eg, self-reports, health care professional–rated checklists), reliance on chief complaints, and the use of parent and/or adolescent interview techniques to identify adolescent depression in primary care. Psychometric data sought included sensitivity (the proportion of those with the disease or condition, as measured by the gold standard, who have positive results by the test being studied), specificity (the proportion of those without the disease or condition, as measured by the gold standard, who have negative results by the method, criteria, or test being studied), positive predictive value (PPV), and negative predictive value (NPV) of different identification methods. While the gold standard depression diagnosis typically would involve experienced mental health professionals using high-quality assessment techniques and gathering information from multiple informants, the gold standard diagnosis may be a structured interview or other such approximation. We sought studies that clearly defined their gold standard in primary care. In addition, any available evidence regarding the feasibility, acceptability, cost, and outcome for the adolescent patient of any of the various identification methods was sought. Lastly, by identifying methods currently used in pediatric primary care settings, we hoped to find explanations for the current underrecognition.

We searched MEDLINE (English-language articles only) for all years up through December 28, 2004, using the following key words: primary care or pediatric$ ($ indicates a wild-card term) or family med$ or GP or health clinic or health center or teen clinic or teen center or adolescent clinic or adolescent center or family physician$ or family practi$ or adolescent medicine or ambulatory care and depress$ or mood$ and adolesc$ or teen$. Articles targeting populations with specific somatic symptoms, physical illnesses, or other risk factors; studies not focusing on adolescents; or those discussing children generally but not separating out older children (older than 10 years) were eliminated. Articles that dealt with general psychosocial issues, psychological distress, or suicidality, rather than depression, were included only if depression or mood disorders were also mentioned in the abstract and then specifically examined in the study as well. Population surveys and service use assessments were discarded because they did not take place in primary care, as were treatment articles that did not describe the mechanism of identification. Lastly, English-language articles that described screening conducted in non–English-speaking countries were discarded. In addition, a hand search of the references from the relevant articles found in the search was also conducted.

## RESULTS

We identified and hand reviewed 1743 titles (most with abstracts). Seventy-four full articles were selected for initial review based on relevance. Twenty-nine articles met criteria for final review: 24 addressed the first question regarding identification methods in primary care (**Table 1**) and 6 (including 1[49] from Table 1) focused on health care professional–reported current practices (**Table 2**). Final results from a previously published study[31] were published in January 2005 and that article is included as the 25th article[34] in Table 1.

## IDENTIFICATION DATA IN PRIMARY CARE (QUESTION 1 PART 1)

Of the 25 articles presented in Table 1, only 5 present data on the sensitivity, specificity, PPV, and NPV of a designated identification method in primary care. In the first of the 5 studies, Winter et al[82] trained pediatricians to administer the mood module of the Primary Care Evaluation of Mood Disorders[45] to 100 consecutive adolescents. Using the Primary Care Evaluation of Mood Disorders interview as the gold standard to validate a self-report (Beck Depression Inventory for Primary Care[83]), analyses demonstrated a sensitivity and specificity of 91% at a cutoff score of 4 or higher. With their sample prevalence of 11% for major depressive disorder, the PPV for the Beck Depression Inventory for Primary Care was 55.6% and the NPV, 98.7%.

In the second study, Johnson et al[43] attempted to validate the Patient Health Questionnaire for Adolescents, which assesses depression, eating disorders, and substance use. Using a mental health professional–administered telephone interview based mostly on the Primary Care Evaluation of Mood Disorders mood module as the gold standard diagnosis, the Patient Health Questionnaire for Adolescents yielded a sensitivity of 73%, specificity of 94%, and PPV of 56% for major depressive disorder, which rose to 62% for "any depressive disorder" (n=403).

In the third study, Schubiner and colleagues[72] examined the accuracy of physician diagnosis aided by a self-report questionnaire, as well as the accuracy of physician diagnosis based on a mnemonic verbal interview, comparing both with a gold standard, semistructured, psychologist-administered interview. Physicians at an urban adolescent clinic were randomized into 2 groups, 1 trained to use the Safe Times Questionnaire[73] (a 7-subscale screen with 1 subscale for depression/suicide comprising 5-7 items) vs 1 trained to conduct interviews based on the Safe Times Questionnaire mnemonic verbal interview. This latter group was not as accurate in depression identification as the Safe Times Questionnaire screening tool group, with area under the receiver operating characteristic curves of 88% for the screen vs 50% for the interview ($P<.05$), sensitivity of 80% vs 18% ($P<.05$), specificity of 91% vs 93%, PPV of 71% vs 43%, and NPV of 95% vs 80% ($P<.05$).[72] In this study, depression prevalence was 21%.

In the fourth study, Yates et al[84] administered the Mood and Feelings Questionnaire[40] to 267 adolescent primary care attendees in Great Britain, with the urban subgroup (n=130) also receiving the Schedule for Affective Disorders and Schizophrenia for School-Age Children[42] diagnostic interview. Full details of this study are described elsewhere.[15] Based on receiver operating characteristic curve analyses from an earlier study,[15] investigators chose a cutoff score of 17, rather than the accepted 26 in clinical samples, to

**Table 1. Identification Methods for Adolescent Depression Studied in Primary Care (in Alphabetical Order)**

| Source | Description of Sample | Study Identification Methods | Methods Integrated Clinically | Comparisons | Impact Assessed | Psychometric Data | Notes |
|---|---|---|---|---|---|---|---|
| Adams et al,[28] 2003 | Aged 11-19 y; N = 193; prevalence: high-risk mood, 4.2% and moderate-risk mood, 15.7% as per PARS[28]; variable setting: 69.9% of sample recruited from university-based adolescent medicine clinic, 14.5% from public middle school, and 15.5% from public high school | DSR (CDI[29]), GSR+ (PARS-SE,[28] GAPS[17]), HRCL (PARS), OSR (IC[30]) | No | Used CDI as GS to validate PARS; compared PARS with GAPS | No | Pearson correlations between mood and total CDI score, $r = 0.58$; $P<.01$ | Pearson correlations between PARS mood and GAPS mood, $r = 0.48$; $P<.01$ |
| Asarnow et al,[31] 2002 | Aged 13-22 y; sample size not reported; prevalence not reported; setting: 5 practices including managed care, academic, and public sector | DSR (CES-D[32]), HRCL (CIDI[33]) | No | GS (diagnostic interview) | Yes (usual care vs QI treatment; results published in Asarnow et al[34]) | Fewer than half with liberally defined positive screenings meet criteria for a depressive disorder as per preliminary reports | |
| Asarnow et al,[34] 2005 | Aged 13-21 y; N = 4002 screened; prevalence: NA; setting: 6 pediatric practice settings from 5 health care organizations | DSR (CES-D) (modified CIDI-12) | No | GS (diagnostic interview) | Yes; CES-D scores improved in QI group | NA | |
| Burns et al,[35] 2004 | Aged 12-18 y; N = 64; prevalence: 28.3%-31.25% (based on PARS screening variable); recruitment setting: university-affiliated pediatric and adolescent group practice clinic | DSR (CDI), HRCL (PARS) | OS (PARS only), PCP (PARS only) | No | Yes (longitudinal relationships between baseline depression variables, follow-up risk variables, and mental health intervention) | NA | |
| Cappelli et al,[36] 1995 | Aged 13-18 y; N = 104; prevalence: 41% (BDI[37] score > 16); setting: Canadian adolescent medicine clinic that often receives mental health referrals | DSR (BDI), OSR (SPS[38]) | No | CC | No | NA | |
| Gledhill et al,[39] 2003 | Aged 13-17 y; N = 10 GPs, 184 adolescents; prevalence: 11%; setting: central London GP practice | DSR (MFQ[40]), OSR (CSI[41]), AI+ HRCL (*DSM-IV* depression screen) | PCP (AI only + or − HRCL) | GS (K-SADS[42]) vs PCP-ID (AI + or − HRCL), PCP (AI) before and after training | Yes (3-mo follow-up for group with depression) | MFQ PPV (combined), 38% (n = 82); AI pretraining: sensitivity, 20%; specificity, 86%; PPV, 33%; AI posttraining: sensitivity, 43%; specificity, 87%; PPV, 75%; MFQ found 21 teens diagnosed with depression by the K-SADS vs GPs finding 9 teens diagnosed with depression by the K-SADS but falsely screened positive 20 teens not found to have depression on the K-SADS vs GPs falsely screening positive 3 teens not found to have depression on the K-SADS | While GPs trained in use of a *DSM-IV* depression screen, no mention of its use during the clinical interview is confirmed in the article |
| Johnson et al,[43] 2002 | Aged 13-18 y; N = 403; prevalence: 11.9% (any depressive disorder); setting: school clinics and primary care practices | DSR (Patient Health Questionnaire mood module), GSR (PHQ-A,[43] SF-20[44]) | No | GS (phone interview by MHP with PRIME-MD[45] mood module) | No | PHQ-A mood module major depressive disorder: sensitivity, 73%; specificity, 94%; PPV, 56%; NPV, 97% | Data also provided for depressive disorder and any mood disorder |

(continued)

**Table 1. Identification Methods for Adolescent Depression Studied in Primary Care (in Alphabetical Order) (cont)**

| Source | Description of Sample | Study Identification Methods | Methods Integrated Clinically | Comparisons | Impact Assessed | Psychometric Data | Notes |
|---|---|---|---|---|---|---|---|
| Joiner et al,[46] 2002 | Aged 15-24 y; N = 2851; prevalence: NA; setting: GP clinics | DSR (CES-D), GSR (GHQ-12[47]), OSR (DSI-SS[46]) | OS | CC | No | NA: distribution of scores, means, and comparisons between measures presented | |
| Joiner et al,[48] 2002 | Aged 15-24 y; N = 2851; prevalence: NA; setting: GP clinics | DSR (CES-D), GSR (GHQ-12), OSR (DSI-SS) | OS | CC | No | NA | |
| Klein et al,[49] 2001 | Aged 14-19 y; n = 318 teens preintervention, 331 teens postintervention; prevalence: NA; setting: 5 community and migrant health centers in 3 different states, 11 clinical sites in both urban and rural areas including 3 school-based health clinics and 1 teen clinic | GSR+ (GAPS), PR (GAPS) | OS, PCP | No | No | NA | |
| Kramer and Garralda,[15] 1998 | Aged 13-16 y; N = 131; prevalence: 21% (any depressive disorder); setting: GP clinics | PR (CBCL[27]), OSR (CSI and unspecified others), AI | PCP (AI) | GS (K-SADS) vs AI (for any psychiatric disorder) | No | AI pretraining vs any psychiatric disorder: sensitivity, 21%; specificity, 91%; PPV, 59% | Mean and total scores on the CSI were increased in adolescents with psychiatric disorder |
| Lipschitz et al,[50] 2000 | Aged 12-21 y; N=90; prevalence: NA; setting: urban adolescent primary care clinic | DSR (BDI), OSR (CEVC,[51] CTQ,[52] child PTSD checklist,[53] MASC,[54] PESQ,[55] FACESIII,[56] LEQ-A[57]) | No | BDI in those with PTSD and those without | No | NA | Mean BDI scores compared in adolescent females with full PTSD, partial PTSD, and no PTSD in an urban primary care clinic |
| Logan and King,[58] 2002 | Aged 12-18 y; N=477 screened; prevalence: 60 of 477 screened positive; setting: 2 general pediatric outpatient clinics | DSR (RADS[59]), PR (CAFAS,[60] CASA,[61] IPPA[62]) | No | GS (SCID[63] and parental DISC[64]) | No | 60 of 477 screened positive but only 50 consented to the SCID; 44 met *DSM-IV* criteria[65] for major depressive disorder, depressive disorder, or minor depression with an estimated PPV of at least 73.3% | |
| McKelvey et al,[66] 1998 | Aged 15-24 y; N=69; prevalence: 31.9% had score ≥16 on CES-D; setting: 5 GP clinics | DSR (CES-D), GSR (GHQ-12), OSR (DSI-SS) | OS | CC | No | NA | |
| McKelvey et al,[67] 2001 | Aged 15-24 y; N=2851; prevalence: 39.4% had score ≥16 on CES-D; setting: GP clinics | DSR (CES-D), GSR (GHQ-12), OSR (DSI-SS) | OS | CC | No | NA | |
| Pfaff et al,[68] 2001 | Aged 15-24 y; N=423; prevalence: 34.2% had score ≥16 on CES-D; setting: GP clinics | DSR (CES-D), GSR (GHQ-12), OSR (DSI-SS), AI | PCP (AI: GP underwent 1 day of training to recognize psychological distress and suicidal risk) | CC, PCP | Yes; patient treatment changes examined | NA | |
| Schichor et al,[69] 1994 | Mean age 15.5 y; N=966; prevalence: 22% reported feeling down frequently; setting: inner-city adolescent medicine service | GSR+ (unnamed) | OS, PCP | No | Yes; while no control or comparison, counseling and referral outcomes examined | NA | |
| Schubiner and Robin,[70] 1990 | Aged 13-23 y; N=226; prevalence: 14% moderate to severe BDI score; setting: center for high-risk inner-city adolescents and young adults | DSR (BDI, 7-item questionnaire with 3 depression-specific questions), OSR (CBQ[71]), AI | OS (unclear), PCP (AI only) | 3 screening questions vs BDI as GS, PCP vs BDI | No | 3 depression screening questions: PPV, 100%; NPV, 87%; sensitivity, 10%; specificity, 100%; physician: sensitivity, 23%; specificity, 93%; PPV, 33%, NPV, 89% | Receiver operating characteristic curve analysis presented and different data for varying cut points presented |

*(continued)*

**Table 1. Identification Methods for Adolescent Depression Studied in Primary Care (in Alphabetical Order) (cont)**

| Source | Description of Sample | Study Identification Methods | Methods Integrated Clinically | Comparisons | Impact Assessed | Psychometric Data | Notes |
|---|---|---|---|---|---|---|---|
| Schubiner et al,[72] 1994 | Aged 14-23 y; N=152; prevalence: 21%; setting: university-affiliated adolescent and young adult primary care center | DSR (STQ[73] with depression-specific questions), AI (STQ mnemonic-based interview) | OS (STQ and AI), PCP (STQ and AI) | GS (psychologist interview) | No | Area under the curve: AI, 50%; STQ, 88%; sensitivity: AI, 18%; STQ, 80%; specificity: AI, 93%; STQ, 91%; PPV: AI, 43%; STQ, 71% NPV: AI, 80%; STQ, 95% | |
| Slap et al,[74] 1992 | Aged 12-19 y; N=332; prevalence: 2% by YSR[75] in non–suicide attempters, 19% by YSR in suicide attempters; setting: teen health clinic in a large county hospital | GSR + (YSR), OSR (Offer family relationship subscale,[76] a brief pretested questionnaire about suicidal ideation and attempts, mental health care, and marijuana use), | None | CC (in suicide attempters vs nonattempters), PCP | No | NA | Depression as measured by the YSR subscale can help identify suicide attempters |
| Smith et al,[77] 2001 | Aged 16-30 y; N=51; prevalence: 10%-24% had sad/depressed feelings "a lot" to "all the time"; setting: teen health clinic in a large county hospital | GSR (problem area checklist with 8 areas and a problem symptom checklist) | OS | No | No | NA | |
| Smith et al,[78] 1990 | Aged 10-17 y; N=205; prevalence: 83 of 205 with any psychiatric disorder; setting: adolescent clinic | DSR (CDI), OSR (STAI[79]) | OS, PCP | CC, PCP | No | NA | |
| Walker et al,[80] 2002 | Aged 14-16 y; N=970; prevalence: 17.1% females and 11.9% males had score ≥16 on CES-D; setting: 8 GP practices | DSR (CES-DC[81]), GSR (packet of questionnaires) | No | No | Yes, 3- and 12-mo follow-up | NA | |
| Winter et al,[82] 1999 | Aged 12-17 y; N=100; prevalence: 11%; setting: suburban outpatient pediatric practice | DSR (BDI-PC[83]), AI (PRIME-MD mood module) | OS (BDI-PC), PCP (AI) | GS (PRIME-MD) | No | Score ≥4 : 91% sensitivity and specificity; area under the curve, 0.98; PPV, 55.6%; NPV, 98.7% | |
| Yates et al,[84] 2004 | Aged 13-16 y; N=267; prevalence: 15%-33% (MFQ cutoff score); setting: GP clinics, 1 urban and 2 suburban | DSR (MFQ), OSR (CSI), AI, PR (CBCL) | PCP (AI) | GS (K-SADS in urban group), CC, PCP | No | PPV, 38% (calculated from the article by Gledhill et al.[39]) and based on a cutoff score ≥17, chosen for optimal sensitivity and specificity using receiver operating characteristic curve MFQ data from the urban sample | |

Abbreviations: AI, adolescent interview; BDI, Beck Depression Inventory; BDI-PC, Beck Depression Inventory for Primary Care; CAFAS, Child and Adolescent Functional Assessment Scale; CASA, Child and Adolescent Services Assessment; CBCL, Child Behavior Checklist; CBQ, Conflict Behavior Questionnaire; CC, chief complaint; CES-D, Center for Epidemiologic Studies Depression Scale; CES-DC, Center for Epidemiologic Studies Depression Scale for Children; CDI, Children's Depression Inventory; CEVC, Child Exposure to Violence Checklist; Child PTSD Checklist, Child Post-Traumatic Stress Disorder Checklist; CIDI, Composite International Diagnostic Interview; CSI, Children's Somatization Inventory; CTQ, Childhood Trauma Questionnaire; DISC, Diagnostic Interview Schedule for Children Version 2.3; DSI-SS, Depression Symptom Inventory–suicidality subscale; *DSM-IV, Diagnostic and Statistical Manual of Mental Disorders, Fourth Edition*; DSR, depression self-report; FACES III, Family Adaptability and Cohesion Evaluation Scales; GAPS, Guidelines for Adolescent Preventive Services[17]; GHQ-12, General Health Questionnaire; GP, general practitioner; GS, gold standard; GSR, general self-report; HRCL, health care professional–rated checklist; IC, Issues Checklist; IPPA, Inventory of Parent and Peer Attachment; K-SADS, Schedule for Affective Disorders and Schizophrenia for School-Age Children; LEQ-A, Life Events Questionnaire for Adolescents; MASC, Multidimensional Anxiety Scale for Children; MFQ, Mood and Feelings Questionnaire; MHP, mental health professional; NA, not available; NPV, negative predictive value; OS, administered by office staff; OSR, other self-report; PARS, Perkins Adolescent Risk Screen; PARS-SE, Perkins Adolescent Risk Screen–Self-Evaluation; PCP, results used by primary care professionals; PCP-ID, primary care professional identification rates; PESQ, Personal Experience Screening Questionnaire; PHQ-A, Patient Health Questionnaire for Adolescents; PPV, positive predictive value; PR, parent report; PRIME-MD, Primary Care Evaluation of Mood Disorders; PTSD, posttraumatic stress disorder; QI, quality improvement; RADS, Reynolds Adolescent Depression Scale; SCID, Structured Clinical Interview for *DSM-IV* Axis I Disorders; SF-20, Medical Outcomes Study Short-Form General Health Survey; SPS, Suicide Probability Scale; STAI, State-Trait Anxiety Inventory; STQ, Safe Times Questionnaire; YSR, Youth Self-Report; +, with depression-specific questions; –, without depression-specific questions.

provide optimal sensitivity and specificity in their adolescent population with an estimated depression prevalence of 20%. Total and internalizing parent Child Behavior Checklist[27] scores were modestly correlated with adolescent-rated mood symptoms (Spearman $\rho$=0.203 and 0.239; $P$<.002 and <.001, respectively).[84] Recalculation of the data by Yates and colleagues, which is presented in Table 1 in a different article (by Gledhill et al[39], indicates that the Mood and Feelings Questionnaire yielded a PPV of 38% (n=82).

The fifth and final study[39] is a follow-up to the Yates et al study[80] and relied on Mood and Feelings Questionnaire cutoff scores of 17 for first-stage screening. Gledhill et al[39] trained 10 London general practitioners (GPs) in identification and management of adolescent depression and use of an unspecified, structured *Diagnostic and Statistical Manual of Mental Disorders, Fourth Edition*[65] *(DSM-IV)*–based depression questionnaire while interviewing the adolescent. Blinded-GP diagnosis was compared with gold standard diagnosis made by positive first-stage Mood and Feelings Questionnaire screens and follow-up Schedule for Affective Disorders and Schizophrenia for School-Age Children[42] interviews. Of 184 adolescents seen, physicians improved pretraining sensitivity and PPV (20% and 33%) to 43% and 75% posttraining, respectively. While improved, GPs still failed to identify more than half of adolescents with depression.

While, to our knowledge, these 5 articles represent the best psychometric data available, 2 other studies (3 articles) from Table 1 used a 2-stage screening method to provide some data on PPVs but not sensitivity or specificity. One of these studies is the Youth Partners in Care study,[31,34] in which Asarnow et al preliminarily report a PPV lower than 50% for any depressive disorder using the Center for Epidemiological Studies Depression Scale[32] (CES-D) and questions from the Composite International Diagnostic Interview.[33] In the second study, Logan and King[58] administered the Reynolds Adolescent Depression Scale[59] in a general pediatric clinic and obtained data suggesting PPVs of 73.3% to 88% for "any *DSM-IV* depressive disorder." Among youth identified as having depression based on the second-stage youth report, 79% of parents failed to endorse a single depression symptom.

In addition, another 6 studies provide some limited data about identification methods in primary care. Pfaff et al[68] trained primary care professionals to identify youths at risk for suicidality and found that physicians' ability to recognize high scorers on the CES-D (score ≥16) increased from 45.1% to 62.9% after training. No definitive diagnostic assessment was used, limiting firm conclusions about training. Another study, by Adams et al,[28] validated a health care professional–rated, general, psychosocial, adolescent risk screen that included 1 depression question, The Perkins Adolescent Risk Screen (PARS). Medical personnel were trained to use the PARS, while adolescents completed the Children's Depression Inventory[29] (CDI), a Periodic Adolescent Preventive Services Visit Form of the American Medical Association's Guidelines for Adolescent Preventive Services[17] (GAPS), and a PARS self-evaluation.[28] The single PARS mood item correlated significantly with total CDI score ($r$=0.58; $P$<.01) and with mood items from the GAPS ($r$=0.48; $P$<.01). The self-reported PARS mood item correlated significantly ($r$=0.47; $P$<.001; n=188) with the health care professional–rated mood item. In another adolescent medicine clinic study by Smith et al,[78] where positive State-Trait Anxiety Inventory[79] and CDI screens (n=205) were reassessed by physicians after their initial interview, screening identified 18 additional patients who were initially missed. Study health care professionals were so impressed by their inability to associate certain medical complaints with psychological issues that they decided to adopt the CDI into routine clinical care.[78] Similarly, 3 other studies[50,66,70] suggest that self-reports identify more youth at risk for depression than physician interviews alone. However, because these studies did not examine actual depression diagnoses, results are not definitive and may reflect some false-positive results.

Overall, of these 25 studies, only 1 study, the Schubiner et al[72] study, directly compared, through a randomized controlled study, physician diagnosis (based on self-report screening tools), physician identification (based on trained interview), and gold standard mental health interviews. Only 4 studies[49,50,58,84] collected information from parents about adolescents' mood symptoms, with only 2 of these studies[58,84] reporting a comparison of the results, limiting any information about this specific identification question.

Ten* of the 25 studies explored in different ways how patients' chief complaints could identify patients at risk for depression. All suggest that sole reliance on chief complaint misses many youth with depression. In 1 study of chief complaints in an adolescent clinic,[36] while depression and suicidality were more prominent in those initially seen with either psychological complaints or a combination of medical and psychological complaints, depression symptom prevalence in the patients only with medical chief complaints was still high: 21% of those with just medical complaints scored 16 or higher on the Beck Depression Inventory.[37] Similar results are described in other studies.[66-68,74,78,84]

## CHALLENGES IN INCORPORATION OF IDENTIFICATION METHODS INTO CLINICAL PRACTICE (QUESTION 1 PART 2)

Although researchers screen teenagers for study purposes, this does not necessarily suggest feasibility of screening in routine primary care. Ten studies[46,48,49,66-69,72,77,78] mention that the clinic or practice staff or receptionist administered the self-report identification tools to the adolescent patients, with an 11th study[35] having practice health care professionals administer and rate adolescent risk checklists. Of these 11, only 5[35,49,69,72,78] had health care professionals use results of the identification tools clinically, with a sixth[77] using clinic case managers to follow up on identified problems.

In 1 of these 11 studies, the Schubiner and colleagues[72] study of the Safe Times Questionnaire, less health care professional time was spent with patients given the questionnaire vs the interview, despite more sensitive and equally specific diagnosis with the questionnaire. The 23-second difference (75 seconds vs 98 seconds), however, was not found to be significant. In another of the 11 studies, the Burns et al study,[35] although the practice incorporated a health care professional–administered psychosocial risk screen (PARS) into routine care, a medical record review showed that only 49% of patients had a completed PARS.

**References 36, 46, 48, 50, 66-68, 74, 78, 84.*

**Table 2. Health Care Professional–Reported Current Adolescent Depression Identification Practice**

| Source, Year | Method | Response Rate, % | Sample Size | Screen for Depression | Screening Definition | Type of Visits |
|---|---|---|---|---|---|---|
| Halpern-Felsher et al,[85] 2000 | Mailed survey to health maintenance organization pediatricians asking about screening practices on 24 recommended services at routine visits | 66.2 | 366 | Seventeen percent of pediatricians report screening at least 80% of their adolescents for depression at preventive services visits; an estimated 46% of adolescents seen for preventive services visits were screened by all physicians together (SD, 36) | Screening was not defined but appears to mean asking about or assessing for depression in some form | Preventive services visit |
| Hodgman and Roberts,[86] 1982 | Mail/telephone survey to 55 practicing pediatricians in metropolitan Rochester, NY, and Syracuse, NY, asking abut experience with suicide, normal responses, and history-taking practices | 87 | 48 | In history taking, 20.8% report routinely including suicidal symptoms | "Did the pediatrician customarily interview patients to discover the suicide-prone or depressed individual in routine history taking?" | Not defined |
| Klein et al,[49] 2001 | Surveys distributed preimplementation at 5 community and migrant health centers participating in a preventive services implementation protocol | 97 | 79 | Sixty-four percent report screening for depression and 53% report screening for suicidal thoughts | Screening was not defined but appears to mean asking about or assessing for depression/suicidal thoughts in some form | Preventive visits = nonacute care visits including checkups, health maintenance, sports, work and camp physicals, and routine gynecological visits |
| Marks et al,[87] 1990 | Mail survey to 356 members of the pediatric societies of Nassau and Suffolk Counties, New York | 37 | 101 | Fourteen percent routinely discuss depression with their adolescent patients | "Routinely inquired about and provided anticipatory guidance" | "Routinely discuss" |
| Middleman et al,[88] 1995 | Pediatric residents at a university children's hospital were given 7 scenarios and asked to rate how likely they were to ask about and document high-risk behaviors | NA | 64 | Residents were most likely to ask about sexual activity (mean Likert = 2.6; median Likert = 2 [range, 1-5]; $P = .01$) and least likely to ask about depression (mean Likert = 3.8; median Likert = 4 [range, 1-5]; $P < .001$) | Defined as verbally asking about and documenting in the medical record | Seven scenarios ranged from an emergency visit for a finger laceration to a sports physical in a continuity clinic |
| Olson et al,[16] 2001 | National cross-sectional survey of randomly selected primary care pediatricians | 63 | 280 | Twenty-seven percent reported using a screening instrument for behavioral issues ever but did not report on how often; 90% felt it was their responsibility to recognize adolescent depression; 46% lacked confidence that they could recognize depression | When asked about their last remembered case of adolescent depression (n = 186), none reported detection using a screening questionnaire and 17% reported detection by routinely asking depression questions; 30% endorsed a family member raising concerns and 69% reported initial clinical problems associated with depression | Asked about their last remembered case of depression |

Abbreviations: NA, not available; SD, standard deviation.

Three[39,68,72] of the 11 studies trained physicians in identification methods, thus incorporating these techniques into routine practice as a research component, with 2 studies[39,68] showing improved identification after training. In addition, the Beck Depression Inventory for Primary Care validation study by Winter et al[82] had pediatricians administer the Primary Care Evaluation of Mood Disorders mood module in clinical practice, but unfortunately, no information was given about the feasibility of such endeavors in nonresearch settings.[82]

Two[49,69] of the 11 studies incorporated adolescent general self-reports that included depression questions into practice. In 1,[49] 5 community health centers implemented the American Medical Association's GAPS into clinical practice. While a medical record review found GAPS screening forms in 76% of the medical records, this study was limited by selection of health centers most likely to succeed, receipt of university-provided technical assistance, and financial support for health center staff. This study did not examine how many adolescents with depression were found, but it demonstrated that the routine protocol significantly increased (1) adolescents' reported receipt of depression and suicide preventive services (pre-GAPS, 16% and 7%; post-GAPS, 34% and 22%, respectively; $P<.001$), (2) medical record documentation of depression and suicide screening (pre-GAPS, 3% and 2%; post-GAPS, 79% and 78%, respectively; $P<.001$), and (3) medical record documentation of family history of mental illness (pre-GAPS, 40%; post-GAPS, 53%; $P<.001$). Sustained feasibility of this protocol was not examined.

In the second study that incorporated general self-reports,[69] 1012 adolescents attending an inner-city adolescent clinic for routine care completed questionnaires covering several health topics. Health care professionals reviewed questionnaires that were not part of the medical record. Adolescents responded (n=966) to questions regarding "being down or depressed," with 127 (22%) endorsing these items "weekly" or more often. Medical record review of 124 of 127 cases found physician documentation of youths' depressive symptoms in 81% (n=100) of medical records, demonstrating that most physicians examined the questionnaires.

## ASSESSMENT OF THE IMPACT OF IDENTIFICATION (QUESTION 1 PART 2)

### Patient Outcomes

Merely identifying adolescent depression may not lead to improved patient care or better mental health. Six[31,34,35,39,69,80] of the 25 articles in Table 1 did examine the impact of depression identification on patient outcomes. In the Burns et al study,[35] patients identified by medical record review as having been given a PARS previously were invited back to the clinic. At follow-up, a repeat PARS, CDI, and questionnaires studying mental health interventions were administered. While only 44% of follow-up youth reported "ever receiving a mental health intervention," 72% of those scoring "moderate" or higher on a baseline PARS and 50% of those scoring "moderate" or higher on a follow-up PARS reported receiving mental health interventions, although the study did not separate out the timing of the mental health intervention. Though this study did not make formal depression diagnoses, examine pathways to mental health intervention, and standardize the time between PARS scores, it does suggest that youth with previous positive PARS scores had higher rates of mental health intervention.

Only 1 (Asarnow et al Youth Partners in Care study[31,34]) of the 6 studies attempted to implement a clinical response in primary care to self-report screens and to measure patient impact. As part of their quality improvement research initiative, evidence-based management was initiated in 1 screened arm with usual care in the other; the quality improvement group fared better, with lower CES-D scores at follow-up. Likewise, another 1[39] of the 6 studies found improvement in Children's Global Assessment Scale[89] scores in adolescents receiving GP depression interventions among GPs completing training. Yet another study[80] used CES-D for Children[81] scores to measure the mental health impact of inviting teenagers to general practice consultations to discuss health behavior concerns and obtain appropriate follow-up care. While the CES-D for Children was not used as a screening tool per se, those with high scores (≥16) who came for the nurse consultation visits and were independently identified as having depression by the nurses had lower CES-D for Children scores on follow-up than those with high scores who never came for visits.

Finally, in another 1 of the 6 patient outcome studies, the Schichor et al[69] study, which incorporated general self-reports into clinical practice and did not have a comparison group, a medical record review demonstrated that of 100 adolescents with depression noted in the medical records, physicians counseled 33% (n=33) and referred 51% (n=51) for counseling. Follow-up showed that 55% (n=28) of those referred completed the referral process. In total, 61% of those identified as having depression by the physicians received some form of counseling in the end, suggesting that implementing routine depression identification can yield tangible increases in care actually delivered.

### Physician Management Outcomes

Two[68,69] of the 25 studies examined physician management outcomes on some level. While 61% of the patients in the Schichor et al[69] study received counseling, physicians actively intervened (either through counseling or referral) in 84% of the cases they identified as having depression and in 67.7% of the 124 patients with self-reported depressive symptoms. While there is no gold standard diagnosis and no comparison group in this study, these data suggest that systematic use of "trigger questions" or self-report scales can affect physician behavior.

In contrast, the Pfaff study et al[68] found no changes in management strategies despite improved GP identification of suicidal risk factors and high scorers on the CES-D after GP training. However, to truly understand whether there was no impact, studies would need to follow through on patient outcomes.

## CURRENT PRACTICE (QUESTION 2)

While the 25 articles from Table 1 provided some answers to our first question concerning the ways to identify adolescent depression in pediatric primary care, Table 2 represents the evidence for the second question concerning current practice. Six studies attempted to identify current depression identification practice by asking physicians directly either about their intentions or their reported activities (Table 2). In 1 study, Halpern-Felsher and colleagues[85] mail-surveyed pediatricians (n=366; response rate, 66.2%) within a health maintenance organization, with only 15% and 17% reporting screening all (defined as at least 80%) of their adolescent patients for suicide and depression, respectively, at preventive services visits. Likewise, in a second study, Olson and colleagues[16] surveyed a national sample of randomly selected pediatricians (response rate, 63%), finding that 46% lacked confidence that they could recognize depression, none recalling the use of any screening instrument during their last remembered case of adolescent depression and 17% using interview-based depression questions during their last remembered case of depression. Instead, identification was based mainly on chief complaints and family concerns. In a third study, Klein et al[49] reported that prior to GAPS implementation in several practices, health care professionals reported screening 64% and 53% of their patients for depression and suicidal thoughts, but medical record documentation of such practices was found in only 3% and 2%, respectively, rendering such high self-reported rates of questionable validity.

In a fourth study, Middleman et al[88] studied physicians' intentions to ask adolescents about high-risk behaviors. Using questionnaires, investigators presented 7 care scenarios to 64 pediatric residents, asking them to rate how likely they were to address 5 specific high-risk issues, including depression/suicide. Results indicated that residents were more likely to ask teens about sexual activity/birth control than any other high-risk behaviors. They were least likely to screen for suicide/depression and fighting/coping with anger.

Finally, 2 additional studies[86,87] of pediatric professionals from 1982 and 1990, which are older and may not reflect current practice, reflect lower rates of asking patients about depression (14%)[87] and suicide (20.8%),[86] suggesting that despite physicians' feelings of responsibility for[16] and good intentions to address depression and suicide, it usually does not happen.

## COMMENT

Complicating our understanding of comparisons between studies are the different criteria used for defining depression diagnoses. While no large studies randomized both physicians and youth and compared different identification methods against a gold standard, the studies examined suggest that adolescent self-report tools using recommended clinical cutoff scores identify more patients with depression than other methods and that some adolescent depression screening tools have adequate psychometric properties and feasibility characteristics for use in primary care. However, studies also suggest that using liberal screening criteria may result in overidentification and increase the burden of false-positive results.

While several of the reviewed articles used general psychosocial distress screening tools (vs instruments with depression-specific questions), and while others that screened for general adolescent distress were not included in our search specifically focused on depression, none of these articles addressed how well these questionnaires identified depression compared with a gold standard diagnosis. Thus, the use of general distress self-reports (eg, General Health Questionnaire) without depression-specific trigger questions in pediatric primary care to identify adolescent depression cannot be endorsed or repudiated herein.

Interestingly, training physicians improved their ability to identify depression through interview but not to levels as high as when self-report tools were available. While the HEADSS (home, education, activities, drug use and abuse, sexual behavior, suicidality and depression) interview[90] assessment is often discussed in adolescent medicine, no studies of its incorporation into routine primary care for depression identification were found. Thus, we do not have any evidence that even physicians who may have adequate training are successfully using their skills in a systematic fashion. The Schubiner et al study[72] is unique in that it studied physician diagnosis aided by a self-report tool, which approximates real-world clinical settings much more than just looking at the accuracy of cutoff scores for a screening instrument given in a vacuum with no additional clinical information. Lastly, the available evidence reviewed herein indicates that reliance on chief complaints alone is insufficient, because most patients with depression came in with medical complaints or for routine care.

## STUDIES INCORPORATING IDENTIFICATION METHODS INTO CLINICAL PRACTICE

Studies reviewed herein that incorporated identification methods into clinical practice were limited in number and implementation design. A look at the larger literature on psychosocial issues in pediatric primary care can give some practical suggestions for facilitating clinical incorporation[91-95] and information regarding cost.[96,97]

A final clinical issue not yet examined is how often adolescents need to be queried about their moods and at which type of visits. A study of psychosocial screening across ages showed that screening only at well-child visits misses a significant amount of psychosocial issues.[98] Our review also suggests that even at preventive services visits, physicians are often not screening for depression. Lastly, while self-reports may identify more teens with depression, the potential burden on practices of assessing false-positive results has not been adequately studied.

## IMPACT ON PHYSICIAN BEHAVIOR AND YOUTH OUTCOMES

More research is needed on the assessment of impact. While 1 study[72] did have physicians use depression self-report results to make diagnostic decisions, no single study combined all 3 necessary components: a screening component, an intervention, and an assessment of patient outcomes at follow-up. However, the Youth Partners in Care study[31,34] did show that screening and triaging done by specialized staff in primary care will lead to better outcomes when proper management is put into place.

## CURRENT PRACTICE

The studies cited herein suggest that not only is the use of adolescent depression self-reports rare but also that systematic physician inquiry into the moods of teenagers has been difficult to achieve. Failure to use systematic reliance screening tools or depression trigger questions may be a critical component of the problem, particularly if not coupled with increased pediatric training in this area.

## CONCLUSIONS

More research is needed to inform pediatric professionals about valid and feasible methods to identify adolescent depression and whether such identification will yield improved patient outcomes, but our review suggests that systematic use of adolescent self-reports with depression-specific questions may be a useful diagnostic aid to pediatric professionals. While improved pediatric diagnosis alone is unlikely to significantly change patient outcomes, recognizing teenagers with depression is the first step to improved depression management. The several studies available already suggest that adding primary care interventions for adolescent depression will be useful. With prolonged suffering and suicide as a potential consequence of undiagnosed depression, pediatric professionals may need to be more proactive and systematic in their depression identification methods.

**Accepted for Publication:** December 9, 2005.
**Correspondence:** Rachel A. Zuckerbrot, MD, 1051 Riverside Dr, Unit 78, New York, NY 10032 (raz1@columbia.edu).
**Author Contributions:** *Study concept and design:* Zuckerbrot and Jensen. *Acquisition of data:* Zuckerbrot and Jensen. *Drafting of the manuscript:* Zuckerbrot and Jensen. *Critical revision of the manuscript for important intellectual content:* Jensen. *Administrative, technical, and material support:* Zuckerbrot. *Study supervision:* Jensen.
**Funding/Support:** Dr Zuckerbrot was supported by research fellowship T-32 MH16434-22 from the National Institute of Mental Health.
**Acknowledgment:** We would like to acknowledge the support of David Shaffer, MD. We would also like to thank Lauren Zitner, BA, and Dana Pagar, BA, for their invaluable contribution to the current version of this article.

## REFERENCES

1. Garrison CZ, Addy CL, Jackson KL, McKeown RE, Waller JL. Major depressive disorder and dysthymia in young adolescents. *Am J Epidemiol.* 1992;135:792-802.
2. Lewinsohn PM, Hops H, Roberts RE, Seeley JR, Andrews JA. Adolescent psychopathology, I: prevalence and incidence of depression and other *DSM-III-R* disorders in high school students. *J Abnorm Psychol.* 1993;102:133-144.
3. Shaffer D, Fisher P, Dulcan MK, et al. The NIMH Diagnostic Interview Schedule for Children Version 2.3 (DISC-2.3): description, acceptability, prevalence rates, and performance in the MECA Study. Methods for the Epidemiology of Child and Adolescent Mental Disorders Study. *J Am Acad Child Adolesc Psychiatry.* 1996;35:865-877.
4. Whitaker A, Johnson J, Shaffer D, et al. Uncommon troubles in young people: prevalence estimates of selected psychiatric disorders in a nonreferred adolescent population. *Arch Gen Psychiatry.* 1990;47:487-496.
5. Fergusson DM, Woodward LJ. Mental health, educational, and social role outcomes of adolescents with depression. *Arch Gen Psychiatry.* 2002;59:225-231.
6. Aalto-Setala T, Marttunen M, Tuulio-Henriksson A, Poikolainen K, Lonnqvist J. Depressive symptoms in adolescence as predictors of early adulthood depressive disorders and maladjustment. *Am J Psychiatry.* 2002;159:1235-1237.
7. Rushton JL, Forcier M, Schectman RM. Epidemiology of depressive symptoms in the National Longitudinal Study of Adolescent Health. *J Am Acad Child Adolesc Psychiatry.* 2002;41:199-205.
8. Weissman MM, Wolk S, Goldstein RB, et al. Depressed adolescents grown up. *JAMA.* 1999;281:1707-1713.
9. Centers for Disease Control and Prevention National Center for Injury Prevention and Control. Web-based Injury Statistics Query and Reporting System (WISQARS). www.cdc.gov/ncipc/wisqars. Accessed June 27, 2003.
10. Burns BJ, Costello EJ, Angold A, et al. Children's mental health service use across service sectors. *Health Aff (Millwood).* 1995;14(3):147-159.
11. Leaf PJ, Alegria M, Cohen P, et al. Mental health service use in the community and schools: results from the four-community MECA study. *J Am Acad Child Adolesc Psychiatry.* 1996;35:889-897.
12. Bartlett JA, Schleifer SJ, Johnson RL, Keller SE. Depression in inner city adolescents attending an adolescent medicine clinic. *J Adolesc Health.* 1991;12:316-318.
13. Wortman RN, Donovan DS, Woodburn KE, et al. Depression and its relationship to somatic complaints in adolescent patients [abstract]. *J Adolesc Health Care.* 1986;7:295.
14. Chang G, Warner V, Weissman MM. Physicians' recognition of psychiatric disorders in children and adolescents. *AJDC.* 1988;142:736-739.
15. Kramer T, Garralda ME. Psychiatric disorders in adolescents in primary care. *Br J Psychiatry.* 1998;173:508-513.
16. Olson AL, Kelleher KJ, Kemper KJ, Zuckerman BS, Hammond CS, Dietrich AJ. Primary care pediatricians' roles and perceived responsibilities in the identification and management of depression in children and adolescents. *Ambul Pediatr.* 2001;1:91-98.
17. Elster AB, Kuznets NJ. *AMA Guidelines for Adolescent Preventive Services (GAPS): Recommendations and Rationale.* Baltimore, Md: Williams & Wilkins; 1994.
18. American Academy of Family Physicians. Recommended curriculum guidelines: adolescent health. http://www.aafp.org. Accessed June 27, 2003.
19. American Academy of Pediatrics; Committee on Psychosocial Aspects of Child and Family Health. *Guidelines for Health Supervision III.* 3rd ed. Elk Grove Village, Ill: American Academy of Pediatrics; 1997.
20. Agency for Healthcare Research and Quality. Screening for depression: recommendations and rationale. http://www.ahrq.gov. Accessed June 27, 2003.
21. Kroenke K, Taylor-Vaisey A, Dietrich AJ, Oxman TE. Interventions to improve provider diagnosis and treatment of mental disorders in primary care: a critical review of the literature. *Psychosomatics.* 2000;41:39-52.
22. Pignone MP, Gaynes BN, Rushton JL, et al. Screening for depression in adults: a summary of the evidence for the US Preventive Services Task Force. *Ann Intern Med.* 2002;136:765-776.
23. Brent DA, Holder D, Kolko D, et al. A clinical psychotherapy trial for adolescent depression comparing cognitive, family, and supportive therapy. *Arch Gen Psychiatry.* 1997;54:877-885.
24. Mufson L, Weissman MM, Moreau D, Garfinkel R. Efficacy of interpersonal psychotherapy for depressed adolescents. *Arch Gen Psychiatry.* 1999;56:573-579.
25. Emslie GJ, Heiligenstein JH, Wagner KD, et al. Fluoxetine for acute treatment of depression in children and adolescents: a placebo-controlled, randomized clinical trial. *J Am Acad Child Adolesc Psychiatry.* 2002;41:1205-1215.
26. US Food and Drug Administration. FDA launches a multi-pronged strategy to strengthen safeguards for children treated with antidepressant medications. http://www.fda.gov/bbs/topics/news/2004/NEW01124.html. Accessed November 2, 2005.
27. Achenbach TM. *Manual for the Child Behavior Checklist/4-18 and Profile.* Burlington: University of Vermont Dept of Psychiatry; 1991.
28. Adams CD, Perkins KC, Lumley V, Hughes C, Burns JJ, Omar HA. Validation of the Perkins Adolescent Risk Screen (PARS). *J Adolesc Health.* 2003;33:462-470.
29. Kovacs M. *Children's Depression Inventory.* North Tonawanda, NY: Multi-Health System; 1992.
30. Prinz RJ, Foster S, Kent RN, O'Leary KD. Multivariate assessment of conflict in distressed and non-distressed mother-adolescent dyads. *J Appl Behav Anal.* 1979;12:691-700.
31. Asarnow JR, Jaycox LH, Anderson M. Depression among youth in primary care models for delivering mental health services. *Child Adolesc Psychiatr Clin N Am.* 2002;11:477-497.
32. Radloff L. The CES-D scale: a self-report depression scale for research in the general population. *Appl Psychol Meas.* 1977;1:385-401.
33. *Composite International Diagnostic Interview Core Version 2.1 Interviewer's Manual.* Geneva, Switzerland: World Health Organization; 1997.
34. Asarnow JR, Jaycox LH, Duan N, et al. Effectiveness of a quality improvement intervention for adolescent depression in primary care clinics: a randomized controlled trial. *JAMA.* 2005;293:311-319.
35. Burns JJ, Cottrell L, Perkins K, et al. Depressive symptoms and health risk among rural adolescents. *Pediatrics.* 2004;113:1313-1320.
36. Cappelli M, Clulow MK, Goodman JT, et al. Identifying depressed and suicidal adolescents in a teen health clinic. *J Adolesc Health.* 1995;16:64-70.
37. Beck AT, Steer RA. *Manual for the Beck Depression Inventory.* San Antonio, Tex: The Psychological Corp; 1987.
38. Cull JG, Gill WS. *Suicide Probability Scale—Manual.* Los Angeles, Calif: Western Psychological Services; 1988.
39. Gledhill J, Kramer T, Iliffe S, Garralda ME. Training general practitioners in the identification and management of adolescent depression within the consultation: a feasibility study. *J Adolesc.* 2003;26:245-250.
40. Thapar A, McGuffin P. Validity of the shortened Mood and Feelings Question-

naire in a community sample of children and adolescents: a preliminary research note. *Psychiatry Res.* 1998;81:259-268.
41. Garber J, Walker L, Zeman J. Somatization symptoms in a community sample of children and adolescents: further validation of the Children's Somatization Inventory. *Psychol Assess.* 1991;3:588-595.
42. Ambrosini PJ. Historical development and present status of the Schedule for Affective Disorders and Schizophrenia for School-Age Children (K-SADS). *J Am Acad Child Adolesc Psychiatry.* 2000;39:49-58.
43. Johnson JG, Harris ES, Spitzer RL, Williams JB. The Patient Health Questionnaire for Adolescents: validation of an instrument for the assessment of mental disorders among adolescent primary care patients. *J Adolesc Health.* 2002;30:196-204.
44. Stewart AL, Hays RD, Ware JE Jr. The MOS Short-Form General Health Survey: reliability and validity in a patient population. *Med Care.* 1988;26:724-735.
45. Spitzer RL, Williams JB, Kroenke K, et al. Utility of a new procedure for diagnosing mental disorders in primary care: the PRIME-MD 1000 study. *JAMA.* 1994; 272:1749-1756.
46. Joiner TE Jr, Pfaff JJ, Acres JG. A brief screening tool for suicidal symptoms in adolescents and young adults in general health settings: reliability and validity data from the Australian National General Practice Youth Suicide Prevention Project. *Behav Res Ther.* 2002;40:471-481.
47. Goldberg DP, Gater R, Sartorius N, et al. The validity of two versions of the GHQ in the WHO study of mental illness in general health care. *Psychol Med.* 1997; 27:191-197.
48. Joiner TE Jr, Pfaff JJ, Acres JG. Characteristics of suicidal adolescents and young adults presenting to primary care with non-suicidal (indeed non-psychological) complaints. *Eur J Public Health.* 2002;12:177-179.
49. Klein JD, Allan MJ, Elster AB, et al. Improving adolescent preventive care in community health centers. *Pediatrics.* 2001;107:318-327.
50. Lipschitz DS, Rasmusson AM, Anyan W, Cromwell P, Southwick SM. Clinical and functional correlates of posttraumatic stress disorder in urban adolescent girls at a primary care clinic. *J Am Acad Child Adolesc Psychiatry.* 2000;39:1104-1111.
51. Amaya-Jackson L. *Child Exposure to Violence Checklist (adapted from Richters' Things I've Seen and Heard).* Durham, NC: Trauma Evaluation: Center for Child and Family Health; 1998.
52. Bernstein DP, Fink L. *Childhood Trauma Questionnaire Manual.* San Antonio, Tex: Psychological Corp; 1998.
53. Newman E, Amaya-Jackson L. Assessment of trauma instruments for children. Paper presented at: the Scientific Proceedings of the 12th International Conference for Traumatic Stress Studies; November 1996; San Francisco, Calif .
54. March JS, Parker JD, Sullivan K, Stallings P, Connors CK. The Multidimensional Anxiety Scale for Children (MASC): factor structure, reliability, and validity. *J Am Acad Child Adolesc Psychiatry.* 1997;36:554-565.
55. Winters KC. *Personal Experience Screening Questionnaire Manual.* Los Angeles, Calif: Western Psychological Services; 1991.
56. Olson DH, Portner J, Lavee Y. *FACES III (Family Adaptability and Cohesion Evaluation Scales).* St Paul: University of Minnesota Family Social Service; 1985.
57. Masten AS, Neemann J, Andenas S. Life events and adjustment in adolescents: the significance of event independence, desirability, and chronicity. *J Res Adolesc.* 1994;4:71-87.
58. Logan DE, King CA. Parental identification of depression and mental health service use among depressed adolescents. *J Am Acad Child Adolesc Psychiatry.* 2002;41:296-304.
59. Reynolds WM. *Reynolds Adolescent Depression Scale: Professional Manual.* Odessa, Fla: Psychological Assessment Resources; 1987.
60. Hodges K, Wong MM, Latessa M. Use of the Child and Adolescent Functional Assessment Scale (CAFAS) as an outcome measure in clinical settings. *J Behav Health Serv Res.* 1998;25:325-336.
61. Burns BJ, Angols A, Magruder-Habib K, Costello E, Patrick MKS. *The Child and Adolescent Services Assessment (CASA).* Durham, NC: Duke University Medical Center; 1992.
62. Armsden GC, Greenberg MT. The Inventory of Parent and Peer Attachment: individual differences and their relationship to psychological well-being in adolescence. *J Youth Adolesc.* 1987;16:427-454.
63. First MB, Spitzer R, Gibbon M, Williams J. *Structured Clinical Interview for* DSM-IV *Axis I Disorders.* New York: Biometrics Research Unit, New York State Psychiatric Institute; 1995.
64. Schwab-Stone ME, Shaffer D, Dulcan MK, et al. Criterion validity of the NIMH Diagnostic Interview Schedule for Children Version 2.3 (DISC-2.3). *J Am Acad Child Adolesc Psychiatry.* 1996;35:878-888.
65. American Psychiatric Association. *Diagnostic and Statistical Manual of Mental Disorders, Fourth Edition.* Washington, DC: American Psychiatric Association; 1994.
66. McKelvey RS, Davies LC, Pfaff JJ, Acres J, Edwards S. Psychological distress and suicidal ideation among 15-24-year-olds presenting to general practice: a pilot study. *Aust N Z J Psychiatry.* 1998;32:344-348.
67. McKelvey RS, Pfaff JJ, Acres JG. The relationship between chief complaints, psychological distress, and suicidal ideation in 15-24-year-old patients presenting to general practitioners. *Med J Aust.* 2001;175:550-552.
68. Pfaff JJ, Acres JG, McKelvey RS. Training general practitioners to recognise and respond to psychological distress and suicidal ideation in young people. *Med J Aust.* 2001;174:222-226.
69. Schichor A, Bernstein B, King S. Self-reported depressive symptoms in inner-city adolescents seeking routine health care. *Adolescence.* 1994;29:379-388.
70. Schubiner H, Robin A. Screening adolescents for depression and parent-teenager conflict in an ambulatory medical setting: a preliminary investigation. *Pediatrics.* 1990;85:813-818.
71. Foster SL, Robin AL. Family conflict and communication in adolescence. In: Mash EJ, Terdal LG, eds. *Behavioral Assessment of Childhood Disorders.* 2nd ed. New York, NY: Guilford Press; 1988.
72. Schubiner H, Tzelepis A, Wright K, Podany E. The clinical utility of the Safe Times Questionnaire. *J Adolesc Health.* 1994;15:374-382.
73. Schubiner H, Tzelpis A, Podany E. Development of the Safe Times Questionnaire [abstract]. *J Adolesc Health Care.* 1989;10:249.
74. Slap GB, Vorters DF, Khalid N, Margulies SR, Forke CM. Adolescent suicide attempters: do physicians recognize them? *J Adolesc Health.* 1992;13:286-292.
75. Achenbach TM, Edelbrock C. *Manual for the Youth Self-Report and Profile.* Burlington: University of Vermont Dept of Psychiatry; 1987.
76. Offer D, Ostrov E, Howard KI. *The Offer Self-Image Questionnaire for Adolescents: A Manual.* Chicago, Ill: Michael Reese Hospital and Medical Center Special Publication; 1977.
77. Smith PB, Buzi RS, Weinman ML. Mental health problems and symptoms among male adolescents attending a teen health clinic. *Adolescence.* 2001;36:323-332.
78. Smith MS, Mitchell J, McCauley EA, Calderon R. Screening for anxiety and depression in an adolescent clinic. *Pediatrics.* 1990;85:262-266.
79. Spielberger CD, Gorsuch RL, Lushene RE. *Manual for the State-Trait Anxiety Inventory.* Palo Alto, Calif: Consulting Psychologists Press; 1970.
80. Walker Z, Townsend J, Oakley L, et al. Health promotion for adolescents in primary care: randomised controlled trial. *BMJ.* 2002;325:524.
81. Fendrich M, Weissman MM, Warner V. Screening for depressive disorder in children and adolescents: validating the Center for Epidemiologic Studies Depression Scale for Children. *Am J Epidemiol.* 1990;131:538-551.
82. Winter LB, Steer RA, Jones-Hicks L, Beck AT. Screening for major depression disorders in adolescent medical outpatients with the Beck Depression Inventory for Primary Care. *J Adolesc Health.* 1999;24:389-394.
83. Beck AT, Guth D, Steer RA, Ball R. Screening for major depression disorders in medical inpatients with the Beck Depression Inventory for Primary Care. *Behav Res Ther.* 1997;35:785-791.
84. Yates P, Kramer T, Garralda E. Depressive symptoms amongst adolescent primary care attenders: levels and associations. *Soc Psychiatry Psychiatr Epidemiol.* 2004;39:588-594.
85. Halpern-Felsher BL, Ozer EM, Millstein SG, et al. Preventive services in a health maintenance organization: how well do pediatricians screen and educate adolescent patients? *Arch Pediatr Adolesc Med.* 2000;154:173-179.
86. Hodgman CH, Roberts FN. Adolescent suicide and the pediatrician. *J Pediatr.* 1982;101:118-123.
87. Marks A, Fisher M, Lasker S. Adolescent medicine in pediatric practice. *J Adolesc Health Care.* 1990;11:149-153.
88. Middleman AB, Binns HJ, DuRant RH. Factors affecting pediatric residents' intentions to screen for high risk behaviors. *J Adolesc Health.* 1995;17:106-112.
89. Shaffer D, Gould MS, Brasic J, et al. A children's global assessment scale (CGAS). *Arch Gen Psychiatry.* 1983;40:1228-1231.
90. Cohen E, Mackenzie RG, Yates GL. HEADSS, a psychosocial risk assessment instrument: implications for designing effective intervention programs for runaway youth. *J Adolesc Health.* 1991;12:539-544.
91. Metz JR, Allen CM, Barr G, Shinefield H. A pediatric screening examination for psychosocial problems. *Pediatrics.* 1976;58:595-606.
92. Jellinek MS, Murphy JM, Little M, Pagano ME, Comer DM, Kelleher KJ. Use of the Pediatric Symptom Checklist to screen for psychosocial problems in pediatric primary care: a national feasibility study. *Arch Pediatr Adolesc Med.* 1999; 153:254-260.
93. Murphy JM, Arnett HL, Bishop SJ, Jellinek MS, Reede JY. Screening for psychosocial dysfunction in pediatric practice: a naturalistic study of the Pediatric Symptom Checklist. *Clin Pediatr (Phila).* 1992;31:660-667.
94. Gardner W, Kelleher KJ, Pajer KA. Multidimensional adaptive testing for mental health problems in primary care. *Med Care.* 2002;40:812-823.
95. Jensen PS, Irwin RA, Josephson AM, et al. Data-gathering tools for "real world" clinical settings: a multisite feasibility study. *J Am Acad Child Adolesc Psychiatry.* 1996;35:55-66.
96. Valenstein M, Vijan S, Zeber JE, Boehm K, Buttar A. The cost-utility of screening for depression in primary care. *Ann Intern Med.* 2001;134:345-360.
97. Dobrez D, Sasso AL, Holl J, Shalowitz M, Leon S, Budetti P. Estimating the cost of developmental and behavioral screening of preschool children in general pediatric practice. *Pediatrics.* 2001;108:913-922.
98. Borowsky IW, Mozayeny S, Ireland M. Brief psychosocial screening at health supervision and acute care visits. *Pediatrics.* 2003;112:129-133.

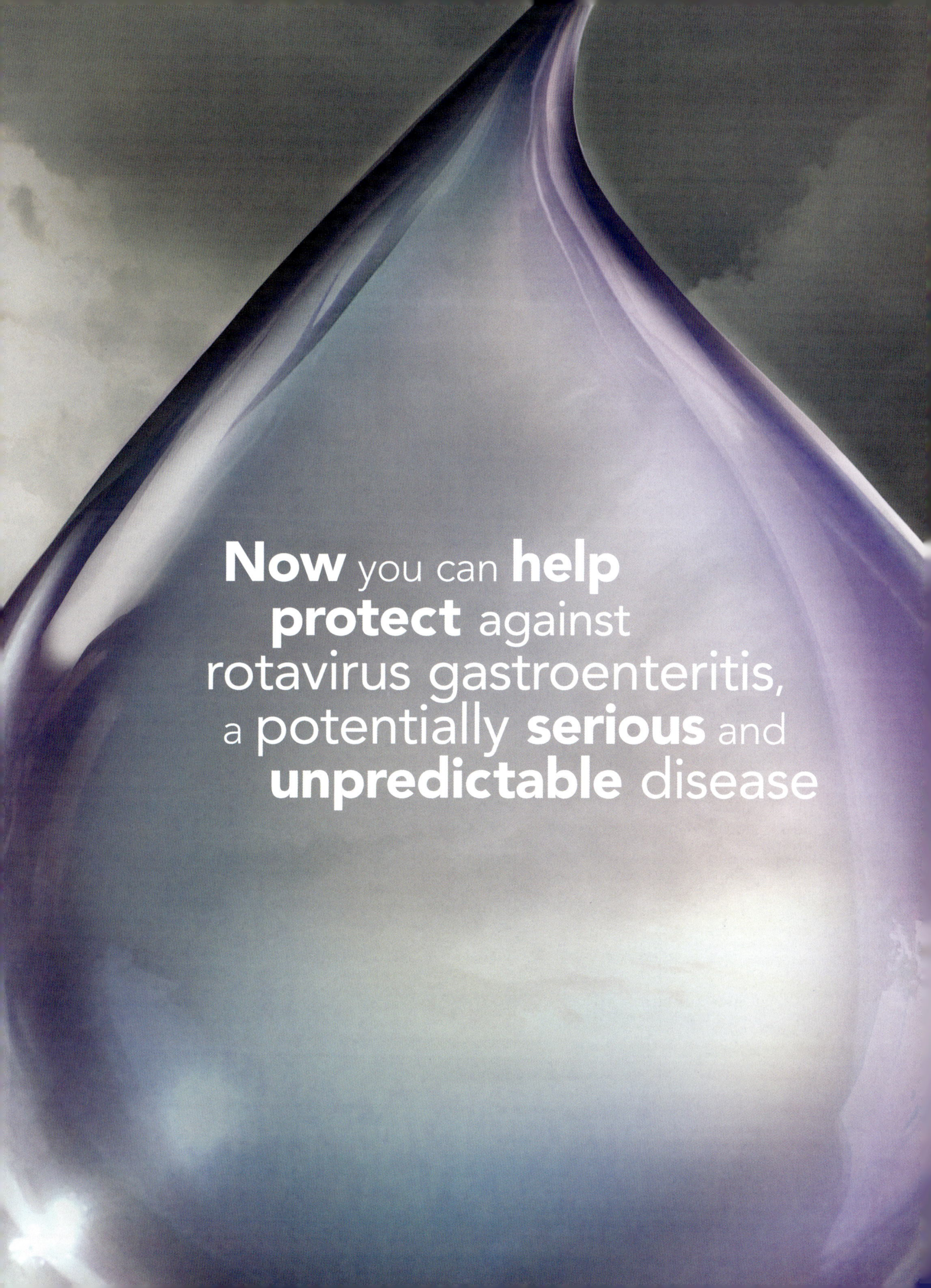
Now you can help
protect against
rotavirus gastroenteritis,
a potentially serious and
unpredictable disease

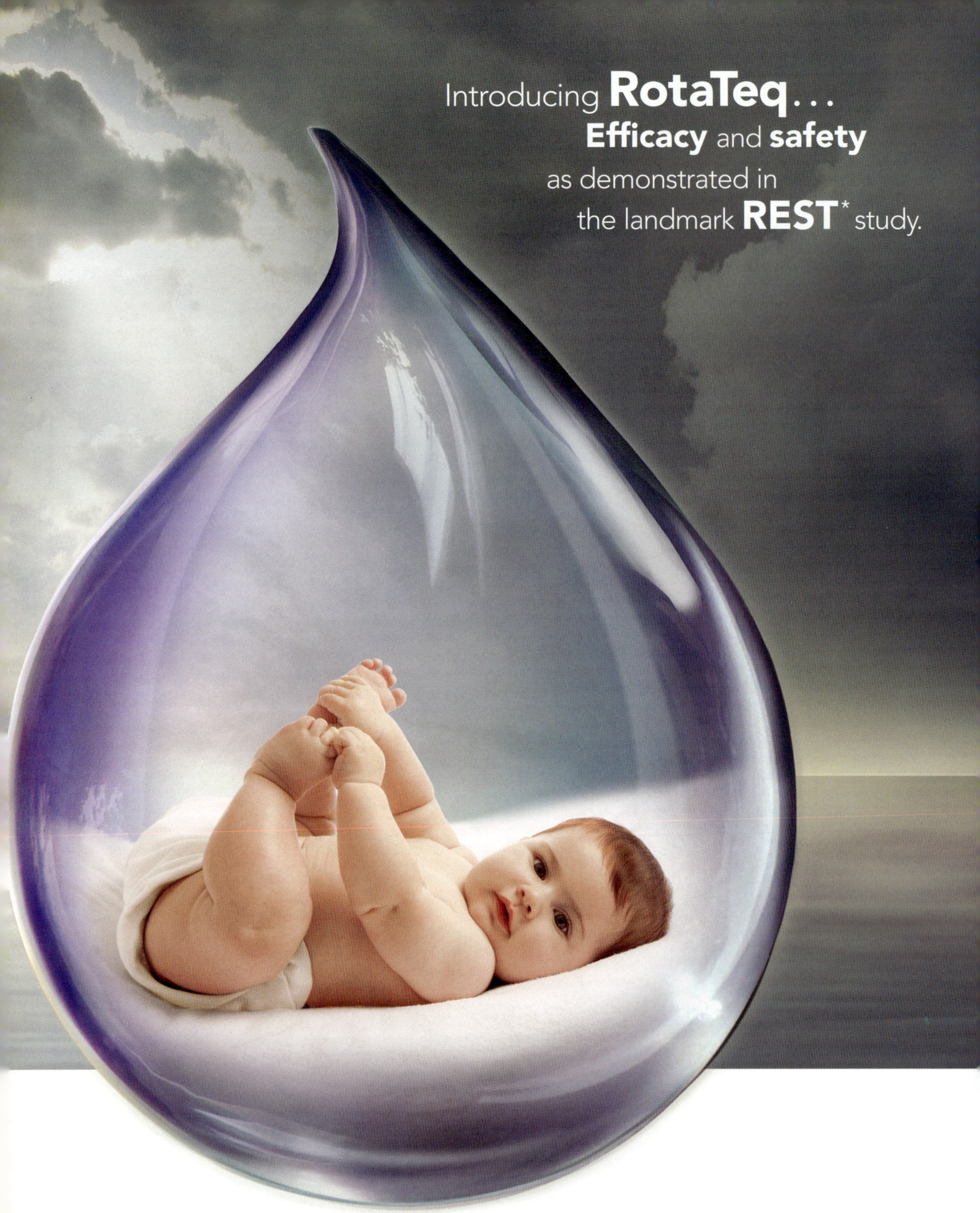
Introducing **RotaTeq**...
**Efficacy** and **safety**
as demonstrated in
the landmark **REST*** study.

SECTION EDITOR: ALBERT C. YAN, MD; ASSISTANT SECTION EDITOR: SAMIR S. SHAH, MD

# Picture of the Month

*Kimberly A. Horii, MD; Amy Jo Nopper, MD; Vidya Sharma, MBBS, MPH*

A 9-YEAR-OLD AFRICAN AMERICAN GIRL WAS seen in the dermatology clinic for evaluation of a lifelong history of easy bruising and scarring of the skin. She had an unremarkable medical history except for hypertension. On further discussion, she also had a history of increased flexibility of her joints but no history of joint dislocations, cardiac abnormalities, or ocular problems. There was no family history of any similar medical conditions. On examination, she was a healthy, developmentally appropriate girl. She had velvety, hyperextensible skin as well as atrophic scarring on the forehead, shins, and elbows (**Figure 1** and **Figure 2**). There was also joint hypermobility, particularly of her fingers, and she had a positive Gorlin sign (**Figure 3** and **Figure 4**). She was not noted to have hypotonia, scoliosis, atypical facial features, or body habitus. Ophthalmologic evaluation, echocardiography, and abdominal ultrasonography results were all normal.

**Author Affiliations:** Section of Dermatology, Children's Mercy Hospitals and Clinics, Kansas City, Mo.

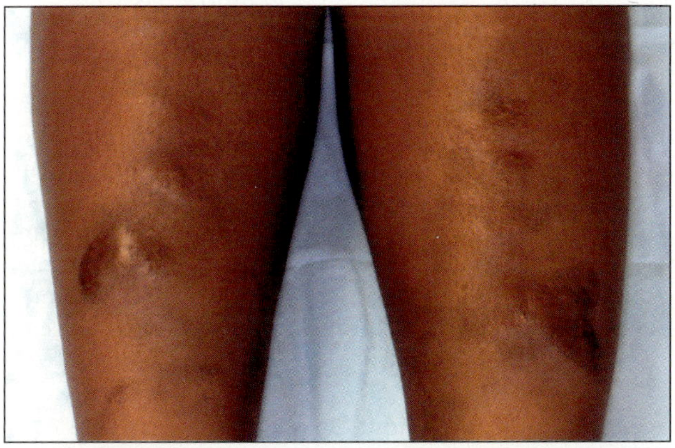

**Figure 1.** Large atrophic scars on bilateral shins.

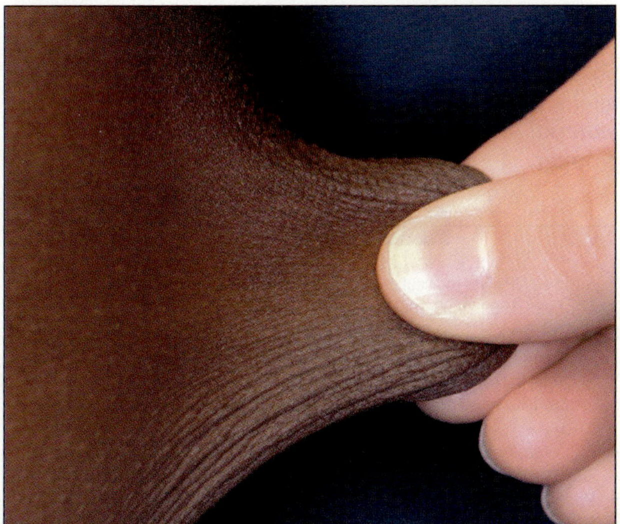

**Figure 2.** Hyperextensibility of skin on elbow.

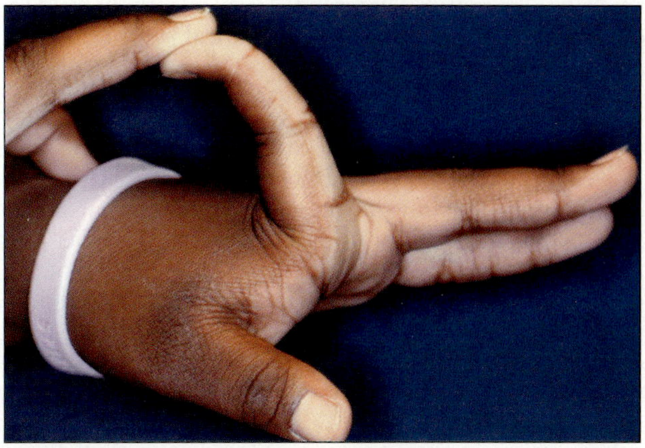

**Figure 3.** Joint hypermobility of index finger.

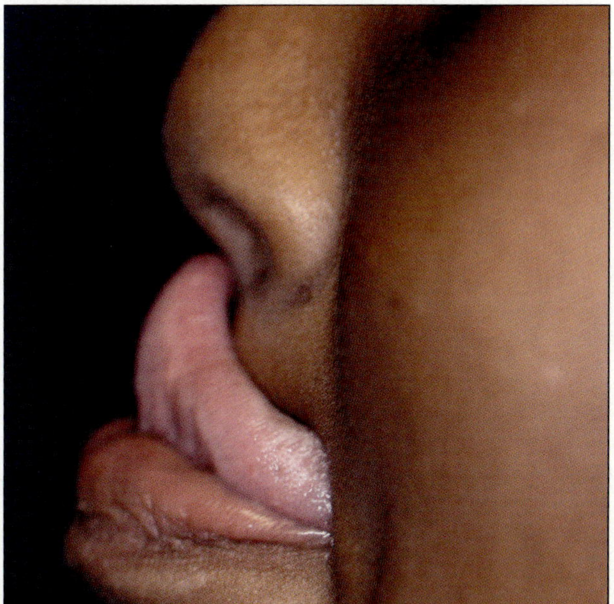

**Figure 4.** Positive Gorlin sign (tongue touching nose).

# Denouement and Discussion

## Ehlers-Danlos Syndrome, Classical Type

Ehlers-Danlos syndrome is a heterogenous group of inherited connective tissue disorders characterized by the variable expression of hyperextensible skin, joint hypermobility, and tissue fragility.[1] Ehlers-Danlos syndrome is thought to occur as frequently as 1 in 5000 and can affect any sex or race.[2] In 1997, a revised classification of Ehlers-Danlos syndrome resulted in a simplified classification of 6 types.[3] The new classification system proposed specific major and minor diagnostic criteria for each type and also included newly available molecular and biochemical data.[3] The 6 types include classical, hypermobility, vascular, kyphoscoliosis, arthrochalasia, dermatosparaxis, and other.[3] The inheritance pattern is either autosomal dominant or autosomal recessive depending on the specific subtype. Severity of symptoms can range from extremely mild to disabling. Because of the varied clinical symptoms, diagnosis can be difficult to make.

### CLINICAL FEATURES

The classical type of Ehlers-Danlos syndrome is the most common.[1] It is usually transmitted in an autosomal dominant pattern. The major clinical criteria for the classical type include skin hyperextensibility, widened atrophic scars (manifestation of tissue fragility), and joint hypermobility as assessed by the Beighton scale.[3] The presence of 1 or more major criteria is necessary to make a clinical diagnosis. Minor criteria are less specific but include smooth, velvety skin; molluscoid pseudotumors; subcutaneous spheroids; recurrent sprains, subluxations, or dislocations; muscle hypotonia; easy bruising; and history of surgical complications.[3] The skin manifestations can range in severity from barely perceivable to severe. Easy bruising and pronounced scar formation in areas of trauma are often the initial symptoms in early childhood. Because of increased bruising, affected children are frequently evaluated for a bleeding disorder before a diagnosis of Ehlers-Danlos syndrome is made.[4] The classical type usually does not have associated life-threatening systemic abnormalities; however, workup to rule out more severe types of Ehlers-Danlos syndrome is often warranted. The differential diagnosis for Ehlers-Danlos syndrome includes nonaccidental trauma (due to easy bruising and scarring), bleeding disorders, and cutis laxa.[4]

### ASSOCIATED SYSTEMIC FEATURES

Individuals with all types of Ehlers-Danlos syndrome are at risk for mitral valve prolapse and rarely, for aortic dilatation. In addition, individuals with the hypermobility type may have increased joint dislocations and chronic joint/limb pain. Individuals with the vascular type may be at risk for developing a life-threatening, medium-sized arterial rupture. Those with the kyphoscoliosis type may have associated hypotonia, scoliosis, and scleral fragility as well as an increased risk of ocular globe rupture.[1] Since some of these abnormalities may result in significant morbidity, appropriate diagnosis and anticipatory guidance are imperative.

### PATHOGENESIS

Ehlers-Danlos syndrome is a connective tissue disorder resulting from abnormal collagen synthesis. Type I, III, or V collagen can be affected, depending on the exact type of Ehlers-Danlos syndrome.[1] The classical type is due to an abnormality in the synthesis of collagen type V and has been linked to a mutation in the *COL5A1* or *COL5A2* gene.[5] Although identification of a gene mutation may confirm a diagnosis, absence of a mutation does not definitively rule out a diagnosis of classical Ehlers-Danlos syndrome, especially if suggestive clinical features are present.[3]

### MANAGEMENT

There is no effective treatment for Ehlers-Danlos syndrome. Palliative and preventive care are the mainstay of management.[6] Early diagnosis will allow the health care professional to monitor for possible future complications. Genetic counseling may be helpful for families of affected individuals.[4] Physical therapy and orthopedic care may be required for those with significant joint disease. Affected individuals are recommended to avoid high impact or contact sports and may need to modify their activities to limit stress on their joints.[6] The Ehlers-Danlos National Foundation can be a helpful source of information (www.ednf.org).

**Accepted for Publication:** October 31, 2005.
**Correspondence:** Kimberly A. Horii, MD, Section of Dermatology, Children's Mercy Hospital, 2401 Gillham Rd, Kansas City, MO 64108 (kahorii@cmh.edu).
**Author Contributions:** *Study concept and design:* Horii, Nopper, and Sharma. *Drafting of the manuscript:* Horii and Sharma. *Critical revision of the manuscript for important intellectual content*: Nopper. *Administrative, technical, and material support:* Horii and Sharma. *Study supervision:* Nopper.

### REFERENCES

1. Burrows NP. The molecular genetics of the Ehlers-Danlos syndrome. *Clin Exp Dermatol.* 1999;24:99-106.
2. Mao JR, Bristow J. The Ehlers-Danlos syndrome: on beyond collagens. *J Clin Invest.* 2001;107:1063-1069.
3. Beighton P, De Paepe A, Steinmann B, Tsipouras P, Wenstrup RJ. Ehlers-Danlos syndromes: revised nosology, Villefranche, 1997. *Am J Med Genet.* 1998;77:31-37.
4. Reichel JL, Weston WL, Bellus G, Morelli J. What syndrome is this? *Pediatr Dermatol.* 2001;18:156-158.
5. Burrows NP, Nicholls AC, Yates JR, et al. The gene encoding collagen $\alpha$1(V) (*COL5A1*) is linked to mixed Ehlers-Danlos syndrome type I/II. *J Invest Dermatol.* 1996;106:1273-1276.
6. Whitelaw SE. Ehlers-Danlos syndrome, classical type: case management. *Pediatr Nurs.* 2003;29:423-426.

# The Trial of Infant Response to Diphenhydramine

## *The TIRED Study—A Randomized, Controlled, Patient-Oriented Trial*

*Dan Merenstein, MD; Marie Diener-West, PhD; Ann C. Halbower, MD; Alex Krist, MD; Haya R. Rubin, MD, PhD*

**Objective:** To determine if infants aged 6 to 15 months with frequent parent-reported nighttime awakenings require reduced parental aid during a week of diphenhydramine hydrochloride treatment and 2 and 4 weeks after its discontinuation.

**Design:** Double-blind, randomized, controlled clinical trial.

**Setting:** The study was conducted from May 1, 2004, through May 1, 2005; patients were recruited nationally.

**Participants:** Forty-four participants aged 6 to 15 months.

**Interventions:** Placebo or diphenhydramine was administered in infants 30 minutes before anticipated bedtime.

**Main Outcome Measures:** The primary outcome was dichotomous: a parental report of improvement in the number of night awakenings requiring parental assistance during the intervention week, which ended on day 14. Secondary outcomes were improved sleep during the 2 weeks before days 29 and 43, parental overall happiness with sleep, and improved sleep latency.

**Results:** On June 6, 2005, the data safety monitoring board voted unanimously to stop the trial early because of lack of effectiveness of diphenhydramine over placebo. Only 1 of 22 children receiving diphenhydramine showed improvement compared with 3 of 22 receiving placebo. To reach the a priori determined sample size and have a positive outcome (ie, rejecting the null hypothesis), the trial would have needed to enroll 16 more participants in each arm, with 15 of the 16 in the diphenhydramine group and 0 of 16 in the placebo group improving.

**Conclusion:** During 1 week of therapy and at follow-up 2 and 4 weeks later, diphenhydramine was no more effective than placebo in reducing nighttime awakening or improving overall parental happiness with sleep for infants.

*Arch Pediatr Adolesc Med. 2006;160:707-712*

Author Affiliations: Robert Wood Johnson Clinical Scholars Program (Drs Merenstein and Diener-West) and Department of Pediatrics (Dr Halbower), The Johns Hopkins University School of Medicine, and Departments of Biostatistics and Epidemiology, The Johns Hopkins Bloomberg School of Public Health (Dr Diener-West), Baltimore, Md; Department of Family Medicine, Fairfax Family Practice Residency, Virginia Commonwealth University, Richmond (Dr Krist); and Department of Medicine and Healthcare Services and Quality Research Program, John A. Burns School of Medicine, University of Hawaii, Honolulu (Dr Rubin). Dr Merenstein is now with the Department of Family Medicine, Georgetown University, Washington, DC.

MANY PARENTS ENCOUNTER frustration coping with poor infant sleep, with 20% to 46% in various studies reporting that their infants have problems sleeping.[1-8] To confirm the importance that parents place on adequate infant sleep, one need only visit a local bookstore.[9-14] Most physicians have little formal training to help them advise new parents about sleep. In one study[15] of more than 600 pediatricians, the mean score on a test about sleep was 60%, whereas only 25% of primary care physicians report more than 6 hours of sleep education.[15-17]

Results of a few studies have shown controlled crying, prolonged crying, and parental education to be effective strategies for modifying infant sleep habits.[18-25] Although the extinction method (commonly referred to as *crying out*) is popular, professionals and lay authors have criticized it.[19,21,26] Another method, used with surprising frequency by parents and often recommended by physicians, is to use drugs to sedate infants before sleep. In one study in 62 children with recognized sleep difficulties, 71% of families reported using medicine for sleep.[27] The most widely studied sleep drugs in children are antihistamines, most of which are not readily available.[6,28-31] The antihistamine most often used, diphenhydramine hydrochloride (Benadryl; Pfizer Inc, Morris Plains, NJ), generally has been studied in adults, with only 1 study in children aged 2 to 12 years.[32-34] Although we could find no published studies in children younger than 2 years, a survey of 671 primary care pediatricians in the United States showed that 49% reported recommending antihistamines in children aged 0 to 2 years for sleep problems in the past 6 months.[35]

Because of the wide use of diphenhydramine and the lack of evidence in this setting, we investigated whether diphenhydramine improves infant sleep. Our goal was to undertake a practical clinical trial to examine short-term and long-term effects of diphenhydramine on infant sleep.[36] Because of the wide use and safety of diphenhydramine, we did not believe an efficacy study was indicated and thus undertook a patient-oriented effectiveness study.

We hypothesized that, on the basis of diphenhydramine's sedative properties, treated children would be more likely to fall asleep without their parents on nights they had been treated. In addition, we hypothesized that this treatment would lead children to associate the crib with sleep and comfort, and, therefore, they would need less assistance from their parents when they awakened during the night than would children receiving placebo. Finally, we hypothesized that because diphenhydramine would create a better association of the crib with sleep during the week of treatment, treated children would continue to have better sleeping habits at 2- and 4-week follow-up.

## METHODS

### STUDY DESIGN AND PARTICIPANTS

The Trial of Infant Response to Diphenhydramine (TIRED) study was a double-blind, randomized, controlled, clinical trial conducted at multiple centers with allocation concealment. This study was started and completed before registration in clinicaltrials.gov was required. Participants were recruited by using flyers in practice-based research networks, primary care offices, and day-care centers. In addition, national advertisements were placed in magazines and newspapers and on multiple Web sites targeted at parents throughout the United States. The Johns Hopkins University institutional review board approved the study. Written informed consent was obtained from all participating parents. Contact throughout the study was performed via telephone calls and mailings.

Children were eligible for enrollment if they (1) were aged 6 to 15 months, (2) had a parent or caregiver who spoke English or Spanish, (3) awoke 2 or more times per night, and (4) slept in a crib.

Children were ineligible if they (1) had chronic illness (defined as their taking medicine on a regular basis), (2) had seen a sleep or developmental specialist in the past, (3) were known to be allergic to diphenhydramine, (4) had a diagnosis of obstructive sleep apnea or snoring, (5) were actively ill, or (6) were born before 35 weeks of gestation.

### RANDOMIZATION, MASKING, AND ASSIGNMENT

A permuted block randomization scheme was used to balance the treatment assignments between diphenhydramine and placebo. In advance, a listing of random assignments was prepared, consisting of blocks of either 4 or 8 assignments. Each block consisted of an equal number of random assignments to each treatment. Two of us (D.M. and M.D.-W.) generated the sequence, and one (D.M.) was responsible for following this assignment and enrolling participants. Identical opaque bottles were labeled as either A or B and consisted of 100 mL of medicine or placebo, both cherry flavored. The pharmacist and a designated Johns Hopkins staff member not associated with the study were the only individuals privy to the label information. All other research personnel were blinded to treatment assignment, and at no time during the study did they obtain label information. Data were analyzed before revealing label information.

### INTERVENTIONS AND PROTOCOL

Diphenhydramine and placebo were randomly assigned after patient enrollment information and informed consent were obtained. The Community Drug Compounding Center (Pittsburgh, Pa) prepared and bottled the study medication and placebo. Parents were instructed, after a 7-day observation period, to give their children the study medication once daily, 30 minutes before anticipated bedtime, on study days 8 through 14 (the intervention week). Diphenhydramine concentration was 12.5 mg/5 mL and was prescribed at 1 mg per kilogram of body weight. Placebo was flavored purified water, colored to match diphenhydramine and was administered at 1 mg per kilogram of body weight. All researchers were blinded to interventions. Parents were informed of the proper dose by one of us (D.M.). Parents in both groups also were given a sleep brochure produced by the American Academy of Pediatrics (Elk Grove Village, Ill).

### MEASURES

The primary outcome was dichotomous: either improved or not improved number of night awakenings requiring parental intervention during the intervention week. Parents reported "yes," "no," or "unsure" when asked "Did your child require decreased parental intervention during the past week?" The responses of "no" and "unsure" were considered treatment failure in calculating differences between groups and the number needed to treat. Parents also tracked their child's sleep for the first 28 nights with a diary. If 2 parents lived with the child, they were encouraged to talk about outcomes, but only 1 parent relayed information to the study coordinator. In addition, on days 0, 15, 29, and 43, parents were asked, "On a scale of 1 to 10, where 1 is very unhappy and 10 is extremely happy, what would you rate your scale of happiness in regard to your child's overall sleep, in the past 2 weeks?"

All outcomes were assessed on days 15, 29, and 43. The primary outcome was improved sleep during intervention week, referred to as day 15. Secondary outcomes were improved sleep during the 2 weeks before days 29 and 43, parental overall happiness with sleep, and improved sleep latency.

### SAMPLE SIZE

Other successful interventions showed improvement in more than 50% of children per study.[29,31,37] Sample size was determined on the basis of the primary outcome of improvement of nighttime sleep after 1 week of intervention. We anticipated a 10% improvement in the placebo group and 40% in the intervention group. Setting statistical significance at .05 and 80% power, we calculated that the trial needed 38 participants per group to reject the null hypothesis.

### STATISTICAL ANALYSIS

Baseline characteristics were compared between the placebo and diphenhydramine groups by using either a $\chi^2$ test or Fisher exact test for categorical variables. For continuous variables, the *t* test was used; the Wilcoxon rank sum test was used for ordinal or skewed variables. All analysis was performed by using the intention-to-treat principle. The difference in the proportion improving between the placebo and diphenhydramine groups was estimated along with the associated 95% confidence interval (CI). The number needed to treat was calculated at the end of the study. All statistical analysis was conducted by using Stata 8.0 software.[38]

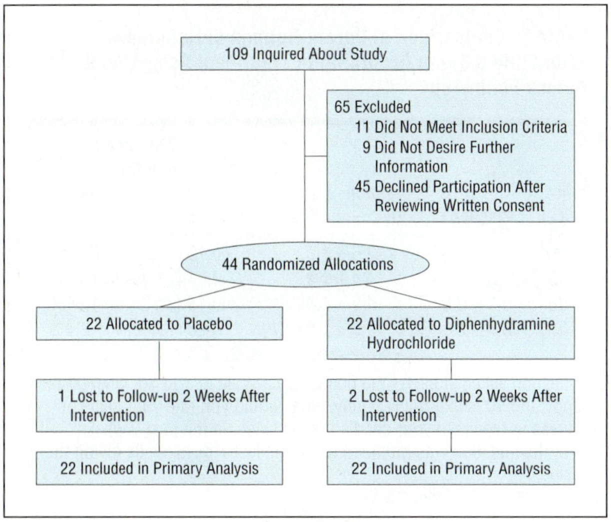


**Figure.** Participant flow diagram.

## RESULTS

### TRIAL MONITORING AND EARLY STOPPING

On June 6, 2005, approximately 1 year after the first participant was enrolled, a preplanned analysis was conducted by the data safety monitoring board, and they voted unanimously to stop the trial early. This decision was reached because of the lack of effectiveness diphenhydramine demonstrated in the multiple measured outcomes.

### RECRUITMENT, ENROLLMENT, AND PARTICIPANT FLOW

During the 12-month enrollment, from May 1, 2004, through May 1, 2005, 109 parents inquired about the study. Eleven infants did not meet inclusion criteria because of the child's age or because the child's sleep problem did not include nighttime awakenings. An additional 9 parents declined participation after receiving preliminary study information. Thus, 89 were mailed a written informed consent form, and 44 parents agreed to participate after reviewing it (**Figure**). One participant in the placebo group and 2 in the diphenhydramine group were lost to follow-up 2 weeks after the intervention. All 3 participants failed to improve immediately after the intervention and at days 29 and 43 treatment was considered to have failed ("not improved") in the intention-to-treat analysis.

### PRIMARY OUTCOME

There were no major differences with respect to any of the baseline characteristics between the treatment groups (**Table 1**). In the placebo group, 3 participants (14%) had improved nighttime awakening requiring parental aid compared with 1 (5%) in the diphenhydramine group after the intervention week (difference between treatment and placebo group, −9%; 95% CI, −26% to 8%, number needed to treat, 11; range, 12 to infinity) (**Table 2**).

**Table 1. Characteristics of Study Sample***

| Characteristic | Placebo (n = 22) | Diphenhydramine (n = 22) |
|---|---|---|
| Age of participants, mo | 10.6 ± 2.8 | 10.0 ± 2.6 |
| Age of parents, y | | |
| Mother | 31.9 ± 7.0 | 33.0 ± 6.1 |
| Father | 35.9 ± 5.6 | 32.7 ± 4.7 |
| Weight of participant, kg | 9.4 ± 1.0 | 9.4 ± 1.5 |
| No. of nighttime awakenings requiring parental aid | 3.6 ± 1.4 | 3.2 ± 1.0 |
| Sleep latency, min | 28.6 ± 39.4 | 23.4 ± 37.6 |
| Hours in crib at night | 10.7 ± 0.8 | 10.7 ± 1.0 |
| Girls | 12 (55) | 7 (32) |
| Boys | 10 (45) | 15 (68) |
| Mother, white† | 18 (82) | 20 (91) |
| Father, white† | 18 (82) | 19 (86) |
| Mother, non-Hispanic | 20 (91) | 19 (86) |
| Father, non-Hispanic | 21 (95) | 18 (82) |
| Participant sleeps alone in room | 17 (77) | 14 (64) |
| Positive smokers in household‡ | 3 (14) | 3 (14) |
| Parents married§ | 18 (82) | 17 (77) |
| Annual household income, $ | | |
| ≤25 000 | 2 (9) | 3 (14) |
| 25 001-74 999 | 9 (41) | 9 (41) |
| ≥75 000 | 11 (50) | 10 (45) |
| Hours per day napping | | |
| 1 to <2 | 4 (18) | 2 (9) |
| 2 to <3 | 8 (36) | 7 (32) |
| 3 to 4 | 10 (45) | 13 (59) |
| Participant is placed on back in crib‖ | 10 (45) | 13 (59) |
| Other children in household | | |
| 0 | 11 (50) | 8 (36) |
| 1 | 6 (27) | 13 (59) |
| >2 | 5 (23) | 1 (5) |

*Data are given as mean ± SD or number (percentage). Percentages do not always equal 100 because of missing data.
†Others were black, Asian, or other.
‡Positive smokers are anyone in the household who uses tobacco for smoking.
§Others were living with a partner, single, divorced, or widowed.
‖Others were placed on the stomach or side or no particular way.

### SECONDARY OUTCOMES

At intention-to-treat analysis at 29 and 43 days, a statistically significant difference emerged with 2 additional parents reporting improvement in the placebo group, an addition to the 3 who previously reported improvement. These 5 parents reported improvement at days 29 and 43 (Table 2). Parents also reported their overall happiness with their child's sleep on a scale of 1 (very unhappy) to 10 (extremely happy). The results on days 0, 15 (immediately after the intervention), 29, and 43 were nearly identical for the 2 groups (**Table 3**).

At day 0, parents in the placebo group reported a mean (SD) number of 3.6 (1.4) nighttime awakenings requiring intervention, whereas those in the diphenhydramine group reported 3.2 (1.0; estimated mean difference, 0.4 awakenings; 95% CI, −0.38 to 1.1). During the intervention week, parents in the placebo group reported a mean (SD) number of 2.1 (1.6) nighttime awakenings, compared with 2.0 (1.1) in the diphenhydramine group (estimated mean difference, 0.2 awakenings; 95% CI, −0.65 to 1.0).

**Table 2. Parental Report of Improved Nighttime Awakening According to Treatment Assignment Across Follow-up***

| Parental Report at Follow-up | Placebo Group | Diphenhydramine Hydrochloride Group | Difference Between Groups in Percentage of Improvement (95% Confidence Interval) |
|---|---|---|---|
| Day 15 | | | |
| Yes | 3 (14) | 1 (5) | −9 (−26% to 8%) |
| No | 16 (73) | 17 (77) | |
| Unsure | 3 (14) | 4 (18) | |
| Day 29 | | | |
| Yes | 5 (23) | 0 | −23 (−40% to −5%) |
| No | 16 (73) | 18 (82) | |
| Unsure | 1 (5)† | 4 (18)‡ | |
| Day 43 | | | |
| Yes | 5 (23) | 0 | −23 (−40% to −5%) |
| No | 14 (64) | 19 (86) | |
| Unsure | 3 (14)† | 3 (14)‡ | |

*Data are given as number (percentage).
†Includes 1 participant lost to follow-up.
‡Includes 2 participants lost to follow-up.

**Table 3. Comparison of Parent Ratings of Happiness With Child's Sleep According to Treatment Assignment Across Follow-up***

| Time, d | Placebo† | Diphenhydramine Hydrochloride† | Difference in Mean Ratings Between Groups (95% Confidence Interval) |
|---|---|---|---|
| 0 | 3.4 ± 1.6 | 3.6 ± 1.9 | −0.18 (−1.2% to 0.88%) |
| 15 | 4.3 ± 2.1 | 4.4 ± 1.9 | −0.08 (−1.3% to 1.2%) |
| 29 | 5.0 ± 2.6 | 4.9 ± 2.0 | 0.15 (−1.3% to 1.6%) |
| 43 | 5.8 ± 2.6 | 4.8 ± 1.8 | 0.96 (−0.46% to 2.4%) |

*Question asked at each time point, "On a scale of 1 to 10, where 1 is very unhappy and 10 is extremely happy, what would you rate your scale of happiness in regard to your child's overall sleep, in the past 2 weeks?" At day 15, the question was modified to "in the last 7 days, while giving the medicine."
†Data are given as mean ± SD.

Parental report of sleep latency, the time from when the child was placed in the crib until initial sleep, for the 7 days before intervention was a mean (SD) of 22.5 (17.9) minutes for the placebo group and 21.6 (38.5) minutes for the diphenhydramine group (estimated mean difference, 0.8 minutes; 95% CI, −17.8 to 19.5). During the week of intervention, the mean (SD) time in the placebo group decreased to 16.0 (13.5) minutes, whereas that in the diphenhydramine group decreased to 11.9 (15.2) minutes (estimated mean difference, 4.2 minutes; 95% CI, −4.7 to 13.0).

## SENSITIVITY ANALYSIS

The data safety monitoring board reviewed interim data, but the researchers remained blinded. To achieve power to detect the originally hypothesized effect of 40% improvement with diphenhydramine and 10% with placebo, we would need to enroll another 16 participants per group. The null hypothesis of no difference between groups then could be rejected only if no participants in the placebo group improved and 15 of the 16 in the diphenhydramine group improved. The data safety monitoring board considered this so unlikely that it advised us to stop the trial.

If the 3 people lost to follow-up were not considered treatment failure, thus not in accordance with conducting intention-to-treat analysis, our results at days 29 and 43 remain almost identical, with only a 1% difference. If we assumed that these children actually improved, then at days 29 and 43 there would no longer be a significant difference (−18%; 95% CI, −40% to 4%).

## ADVERSE EFFECTS AND MISSED DOSES

No parents reported adverse effects that caused them to stop study participation early. One patient in the diphenhydramine group acquired hand, foot, and mouth disease during the study and stopped after 5 days of intervention. Investigators and the data safety monitoring board judged that this was not related to study intervention. Two other children in the placebo group had mild adverse effects, one with hyperactivity and the other with diarrhea, and one in the diphenhydramine group also was reported as having hyperactivity. All conditions were reported by the parents to be mild.

According to parental report, 37 (84%) of the 44 infants complied with all 7 days of intervention. Four of the remaining 7 missed only 1 day of medicine, whereas the other 3 missed 2, 3, and 4 days.

## COMMENT

Many in the medical and lay community accept diphenhydramine as effective treatment for sleep problems.[39] Unfortunately, this attitude is based on anecdote and studies of adult physiological interactions. However, the TIRED study results demonstrated that at the most commonly used dose, diphenhydramine may play no role in treating infant sleep problems. Although parents did not report increased hyperactivity in the diphenhydramine group compared with the placebo group, it is also possible that diphenhydramine caused low-level hyperactivity in children, thereby negating the sleep benefits seen in some adults.

We believed that to evaluate diphenhydramine in the setting in which it is most commonly used and to assess effectiveness, a practical clinical trial would need to be conducted. Thus, we did not use methods such as actigraphy, video recording, or any measures foreign to the natural setting. In addition, we asked parents not to vary their routines, so the time the infant was placed in crib, bedtime routines, feeding schedules, and so on were not standardized, with the exception that parents were asked not to stay with the child once placed in the crib and to place the child in the crib awake. We asked parents not to stay with the infant because of the theory that changes in long-term sleep are achieved with the child learning to fall asleep alone. We believe that, rather than detracting from our study, this practical patient-oriented approach is an advantage of our study.

Our findings are consistent with those of a recent study by Paul et al,[40] who studied whether over-the-counter medications were superior to placebo for treating nocturnal cough and sleep difficulty. They enrolled patients aged 2 to 18 years who had respiratory tract infections, with 33 patients in the diphenhydramine group, 33 in the dextromethorphan group, and 34 in the placebo group. They found no differences in parental or child sleep in any of the groups. However, our results differed from those of the only other study with diphenhydramine solely meant to study sleep.[34] We can only speculate on the differences, but one of the major differences is that we enrolled only patients aged 6 to 15 months with difficulty staying asleep at night, whereas the other study's investigators enrolled children aged 2 to 12 years with various sleep disorders. The children in their study may have had more serious disease, and diphenhydramine may have positive results in these types of children and in older children. However, these investigators did not use intention-to-treat analysis, so they excluded 14% of patients from their final analyses.

Learning to fall asleep without parental intervention is the basis of most infant sleep theory.[10,41] Although the results of the TIRED study did not confirm this theory, we also examined other aspects of sleep such as parental happiness or satisfaction, parental belief that medicine worked, and sleep latency. Diphenhydramine was not superior to placebo for any of these outcomes. Although not statistically significant, the diphenhydramine group demonstrated a larger decrease in sleep latency (relative decrease of 45% vs 29% in placebo; data not reported). Such an observed decrease in the time it takes an infant to fall asleep may explain why some physicians and parents have believed diphenhydramine improves sleep.

Several important limitations of our study deserve mention. Most importantly, we used a dose of 1 mg per kilogram of body weight. Dose recommendations range from 1 to 1.5 mg per kilogram of body weight. We used a conservative dose for 2 reasons: (1) we consulted with many local physicians, and this dose was commonly used; (2) we could find no previous studies in this age group, so we wished to err on the side of safety. At a higher dose, diphenhydramine may be more sedating and would show some positive outcomes with infant sleep. Also, we used no biomarkers to assess compliance. However, parents had no incentives for participation in the study except to see their children's sleep improved, and they were highly motivated, as indicated by the fact that only 5 parents did not complete the entire 28-day diary. Our chosen effect size was purposely large, which may have resulted in our missing smaller effects of diphenhydramine on infant sleep and which was exacerbated by the data safety monitoring board's stopping the study early. Finally, as discussed, our study relied on parental reports of sleep behaviors, and no objective criterion to validate these reports was used. Proper infant sleep clearly is defined culturally, and many parents would never consider methods such as extinction or sedation; therefore, this selection bias needs to be considered when interpreting study results. However, regardless of the disease state being investigated, drug studies by definition are composed of a select population that not only has a disease but also is willing to take medicines.

Our study results reinforce the need for rigorous studies of common primary care interventions and illustrate that such studies are feasible.[36] Despite dozens of published books about infant sleep, we found only 10 level 1–evidence studies about sleep in healthy children. Because of a lack of evidence, parents and physicians often are forced to make important decisions on the basis of anecdotal experiences.

We have shown that it is possible to conduct quality patient-oriented primary care research in young children to provide parents and physicians with evidence to help them make their decisions. Important aspects of a young child's health care, such as proper food intake and sleep routine, often are based on assumptions. Our study results illustrate that such assumptions may be wrong and should be subjected to study in life laboratories not university laboratories. Increased emphasis on pediatric effectiveness research would allow treatment of children to become more evidence based.

**Accepted for Publication:** January 12, 2006.
**Correspondence:** Dan Merenstein, MD, Department of Family Medicine, Georgetown University, 3750 Reservoir Rd, 220 Kober Cogan, Washington, DC 20007 (djm23@georgetown.edu).
**Author Contributions:** *Study concept and design:* Merenstein, Diener-West, Halbower, and Rubin. *Acquisition of data:* Merenstein and Krist. *Analysis and interpretation of data:* Merenstein, Diener-West, Krist, Halbower, and Rubin. *Drafting of the manuscript:* Merenstein, Diener-West, and Krist. *Critical revision of the manuscript for important intellectual content:* Merenstein, Diener-West, Halbower, and Rubin. *Statistical analysis:* Merenstein and Diener-West. *Obtained funding:* Merenstein. *Administrative, technical, and material support:* Merenstein and Halbower. *Study supervision:* Merenstein, Diener-West, Halbower, and Rubin.
**Funding/Support:** The study was funded by the Robert Wood Johnson Clinical Scholars Program, Robert Wood Johnson Foundation (Drs Merenstein and Diener-West). All work was independent of funder.
**Acknowledgment:** We thank the data safety monitoring board members for their dedication and hard work: Alicia Bazzano, MD, MPH; Leigh Culver, PhD; Paul Lipkin, MD; and Thomas Newman, MD, MPH. We also thank Alicia I. Arbaje, MD, MPH, for invaluable help with translation and study input. We thank Community Drug Compounding Center of Pittsburgh, Pa, and pharmacist Susan Freedenberg, RPh, for drug development. We thank Fairfax Family Practice Centers, Southeast Denver Pediatrics, and Kathryn Casey, MD, for help with recruitment.

## REFERENCES

1. Zuckerman B, Stevenson J, Bailey V. Sleep problems in early childhood: continuities, predictive factors, and behavioral correlates. *Pediatrics.* 1987;80:664-671.
2. Armstrong KL, Quinn RA, Dadds MR. The sleep patterns of normal children. *Med J Aust.* 1994;161:202-206.
3. Lavigne JV, Arend R, Rosenbaum D, et al. Sleep and behavior problems among preschoolers. *J Dev Behav Pediatr.* 1999;20:164-169.

4. Hiscock H, Wake M. Infant sleep problems and postnatal depression: a community-based study. *Pediatrics*. 2001;107:1317-1322.
5. Ottaviano S, Giannotti F, Cortesi F, Bruni O, Ottaviano C. Sleep characteristics in healthy children from birth to 6 years of age in the urban area of Rome. *Sleep*. 1996;19:1-3.
6. France KG, Blampied NM, Wilkinson P. A multiple-baseline, double-blind evaluation of the effects of trimeprazine tartrate on infant sleep disturbance. *Exp Clin Psychopharmacol*. 1999;7:502-513.
7. Bax MC. Sleep disturbances in the young child. *BMJ*. 1980;280:1177-1179.
8. Johnson CM. Infant and toddler sleep: a telephone survey of parents in one community. *J Dev Behav Pediatr*. 1991;12:108-114.
9. Weissbluth M. *Healthy Sleep Habits, Happy Child*. New York, NY: Ballantine Publishing Group; 1999.
10. Ferber R. *Solve Your Child's Sleep Problems*. New York, NY: Simon & Schuster; 1986.
11. Ezzo G, Bucknam R. *On Becoming Baby Wise: Learn How Over 500,000 Babies Were Trained to Sleep Through the Night the Natural Way*. 2nd ed. Sisters, Ore: Multnomah Publishers; 1998.
12. Shelov SP, Hannemann RE. *Caring for Your Baby and Young Child: Birth to Age 5*. New York, NY; Bantam Books; 1991.
13. Hogg T, Blau M. *Secrets of the Baby Whisperer: How to Calm, Connect, and Communicate With Your Baby*. New York, NY: Ballantine Publishing Group; 2001.
14. Leach P. *Babyhood*. 2nd ed. New York, NY: Knopf Publishing; 1990.
15. Owens JA. The practice of pediatric sleep medicine: results of a community survey. *Pediatrics*. 2001;108:e51 http://pediatrics.aappublications.org/cgi/content/full/108/3/e51. Accessed July 2003.
16. Rosen RC, Rosekind M, Rosevear C, Cole WE, Dement WC. Physician education in sleep and sleep disorders: a national survey of U.S. medical schools. *Sleep*. 1993;16:249-254.
17. National Sleep Foundation. *Survey of Primary Care Physicians*. Prepared by WB&A Market Research; August 28, 2000; Crofton, Md.
18. Hiscock H, Wake M. Randomised controlled trial of behavioural infant sleep intervention to improve infant sleep and maternal mood. *BMJ*. 2002;324:1062-1065.
19. France KG, Henderson JMT, Hudson S. Fact, act and tact: a three-stage approach to treating the sleep problems of infants and young children. *Child Adolesc Psychiatr Clin N Am*. 1996;5:581-599.
20. Kerr SM, Jowett SA, Smith LN. Preventing sleep problems in infants: a randomized controlled trial. *J Adv Nurs*. 1996;24:938-942.
21. Rickert VI, Johnson CM. Reducing nocturnal awakening and crying episodes in infants and young children: a comparison between scheduled awakenings and systematic ignoring. *Pediatrics*. 1988;81:203-212.
22. Seymour FW, Brock P, During M, Poole G. Reducing sleep disruptions in young children: evaluation of therapist-guided and written information approaches—a brief report. *J Child Psychol Psychiatry*. 1989;30:913-918.
23. Scott G, Richards MP. Night waking in infants: effects of providing advice and support for parents. *J Child Psychol Psychiatry*. 1990;31:551-567.
24. Adams LA, Rickert VI. Reducing bedtime tantrums: comparison between positive routines and graduated extinction. *Pediatrics*. 1989;84:756-761.
25. Reid MJ, Walter AL, O'Leary SG. Treatment of young children's bedtime refusal and nighttime wakings: a comparison of "standard" and graduated ignoring procedures. *J Abnorm Child Psychol*. 1999;27:5-16.
26. Pantley E. *The No-Cry Sleep Solution: Gentle Ways to Help Your Baby Sleep Through the Night*. New York, NY: Contemporary Books; 2002.
27. Chavin W, Tinson S. The developing child: children with sleep difficulties. *Health Visit*. 1980;53:477-480.
28. Simonoff EA, Stores G. Controlled trial of trimeprazine tartrate for night waking. *Arch Dis Child*. 1987;62:253-257.
29. Ottaviano S, Giannotti F, Cortesi F. The effect of niaprazine on some common sleep disorders in children: a double-blind clinical trial by means of continuous home-videorecorded sleep. *Childs Nerv Syst*. 1991;7:332-335.
30. France KG, Blampied NM, Wilkinson P. Treatment of infant sleep disturbance by trimeprazine in combination with extinction. *J Dev Behav Pediatr*. 1991;12:308-314.
31. Montanari G, Schiaulini P, Covre A, Steffan A, Furlanut M. Niaprazine vs chlordesmethyldiazepam in sleep disturbances in pediatric outpatients. *Pharmacol Res*. 1992;25(suppl 1):83-84.
32. Teutsch G, Mahler DL, Brown CR, Forrest WH Jr, James KE, Brown BW. Hypnotic efficacy of diphenhydramine, methapyrilene, and pentobarbital. *Clin Pharmacol Ther*. 1975;17:195-201.
33. Kales J, Tan TL, Swearingen C, Kales A. Are over-the-counter sleep medications effective? all-night EEG studies. *Curr Ther Res Clin Exp*. 1971;13:143-151.
34. Russo RM, Gururaj VJ, Allen JE. The effectiveness of diphenhydramine HCL in pediatric sleep disorders. *J Clin Pharmacol*. 1976;16:284-288.
35. Owens JA, Rosen CL, Mindell JA. Medication use in the treatment of pediatric insomnia: results of a survey of community-based pediatricians. *Pediatrics*. 2003; 111(5, pt 1):e628-e635. http://pediatrics.aappublications.org/cgi/content/full/III/5/e628. Accessed May 18, 2006.
36. Tunis SR, Stryer DB, Clancy CM. Practical clinical trials: increasing the value of clinical research for decision making in clinical and health policy. *JAMA*. 2003; 290:1624-1632.
37. Wolfson A, Lacks P, Futterman A. Effects of parent training on infant sleeping patterns, parents' stress, and perceived parental competence. *J Consult Clin Psychol*. 1992;60:41-48.
38. Stata. *Stata Statistical Software, Release 8.0*. College Station, Tex: StataCorp; 2002.
39. American Academy of Pediatrics, Committee on Drugs. Use of codeine- and dextromethorphan-containing cough syrups in pediatrics. *Pediatrics*. 1978;62:118-122.
40. Paul IM, Yoder KE, Crowell KR, et al. Effect of dextromethorphan, diphenhydramine, and placebo on nocturnal cough and sleep quality for coughing children and their parents. *Pediatrics*. 2004;114:e85-e90. http://pediatrics.aappublications.org/cgi/content/full/114/1/e85. Accessed November 2005.
41. Minde K, Popiel K, Leos N, Falkner S, Parker K, Handley-Derry M. The evaluation and treatment of sleep disturbances in young children. *J Child Psychol Psychiatry*. 1993;34:521-533.

# GARDASIL®

## [Quadrivalent Human Papillomavirus (Types 6,11,16,18) Recombinant Vaccine]

# Available

To place an order, visit **www.MerckVaccines.com,** or call **1-800-MERCK-RX.**



20650396(1)-06/06-GRD
Printed in USA
Minimum 10% Recycled Paper

ARTICLE

# Accuracy and Impact of a Point-of-Care Rapid Influenza Test in Young Children With Respiratory Illnesses

*Katherine A. Poehling, MD, MPH; Yuwei Zhu, MD, MS; Yi-Wei Tang, MD, PhD; Kathryn Edwards, MD*

**Objective:** To determine whether a point-of-care rapid influenza test impacts the diagnostic evaluation and treatment of children with acute respiratory illnesses.

**Design:** Randomized controlled trial.

**Setting:** Pediatric emergency department and acute care clinic of a children's hospital.

**Participants:** Children aged younger than 5 years with fever or acute respiratory symptoms during 2 influenza seasons (2002 through 2004).

**Interventions:** Surveillance days were randomized to performance or no performance of a point-of-care rapid influenza test. All children had a nasal and throat swab obtained for laboratory tests. The rapid test group had another nasal swab obtained for the QuickVue Influenza Test (Quidel Corp, San Diego, Calif), which was performed by nurses; results were shared immediately with treating physicians.

**Main Outcome Measures:** Rapid test results were compared with results of the viral culture or 2 polymerase chain reaction assays for influenza. Diagnostic test ordering and antibiotic prescribing were compared for the groups.

**Results:** Of 468 enrolled children, 306 were from the emergency department and 162 from the clinic. Overall, 88 children (19%) had influenza infection. Of 205 children in the rapid test group, 51 (25%) had influenza infection. The rapid influenza test was 82% sensitive and 99% specific. In the emergency department, fewer children in the rapid test group had diagnostic tests ordered than in the no rapid test group (39% vs 51%, $P = .03$). There was no difference in test ordering in the clinic or in antibiotic prescribing in either setting. The use of antivirals was low.

**Conclusions:** Point-of-care rapid influenza tests were sensitive and specific and were associated with less diagnostic testing in the emergency department.

*Arch Pediatr Adolesc Med. 2006;160:713-718*

Author Affiliations: Departments of Pediatrics (Drs Poehling and Edwards), Biostatistics (Dr Zhu), and Medicine (Dr Tang), Vanderbilt University Medical Center, Nashville, Tenn.

INFLUENZA VIRUS CAUSES FEBRILE and respiratory illnesses in 10% to 30% of children each winter. Children aged younger than 2 years are hospitalized with influenza-related illnesses at rates that are comparable with rates for persons aged 65 years or older,[1,2] a group widely appreciated to have high morbidity from influenza. Although influenza infections are common among children, many remain undiagnosed because clinical manifestations of influenza disease can overlap significantly with those of other viral or bacterial infections. In addition, viral culture confirmation of influenza disease takes days to weeks and does not effectively support clinical decision making.

With the development and use of point-of-care rapid influenza tests, we hypothesized that such tests would impact patient care by reducing unnecessary diagnostic testing, decreasing antibiotic use, and increasing antiviral use. In this study, we evaluated the impact of using a rapid test for influenza among outpatient children with fever or acute respiratory symptoms and used viral culture and polymerase chain reactions assays to independently define influenza positive and negative. Because rapid tests for influenza have reported sensitivities of approximately 75%,[3] we evaluated the accuracy of the point-of-care rapid influenza test and accounted for the fact that a rapid influenza test will miss some children who have influenza infection. We also performed a randomized controlled trial of a point-of-care rapid influenza test to measure its impact on clinical care of young children who presented to the pediatric emergency department or an acute care clinic with fever or acute respiratory symptoms during 2 consecutive influenza seasons.

## METHODS

### STUDY POPULATION

Eligible children were younger than 5 years of age; resided in Davidson County, the county encompassing Nashville, Tenn; and presented to the university-based pediatric emergency department or acute care clinic with fever or acute respiratory symptoms during the 2002-2003 or 2003-2004 influenza season. The reason for the county restriction was that this study was part of a large surveillance effort of the New Vaccine Surveillance Network.[4] Eligible children presented with any of the following symptoms: cough, rhinorrhea, wheezing, difficulty breathing, fever, sore throat, apnea, or ear pain. Children were excluded if they were enrolled within the prior 4 days or had fever and neutropenia from chemotherapy. Enrollment times and days reflected the operational hours of each clinic setting. Children were enrolled 3 days per week in the pediatric emergency department and 1 day per week in the acute care clinic. During enrollment days, parents of consecutive eligible children were approached. Study days were prospectively randomized to the performance or no performance of a point-of-care rapid influenza test with equal numbers of study days for each group.

### STUDY DESIGN

Informed written consent was obtained from the parent/guardian of each enrolled child. A research nurse administered a standardized questionnaire containing demographic information, history of presenting illness, and medical history. Nasal and throat swabs were obtained from all enrolled children for viral culture and polymerase chain reactions (PCRs) for influenza virus and were performed by research laboratory personnel blinded to the results of the rapid influenza tests. An additional nasal swab, a recommended specimen according to the instructions for the QuickVue Influenza Test (Quidel Corp, San Diego, Calif), was obtained in those randomized to the performance of the point-of-care rapid test. After the patient visit, the medical record was reviewed to determine the diagnostic tests ordered and treatments prescribed.

The Vanderbilt Pediatric Emergency Department is the only pediatric emergency department in middle Tennessee and provides care for approximately 30 000 children per year. The majority of children reside in Davidson County and have Medicaid insurance. The university-based acute care clinic serves approximately 11 000 children, of which nearly 80% reside within Davidson County and have Medicaid insurance.

The study period included 2 consecutive influenza seasons. By definition, the influenza season began the first day of 2 weeks with 2 or more positive influenza cultures per week and ended the last day of the second week with fewer than 2 positive influenza cultures in hospital and research laboratories of Vanderbilt University Medical School.[5] For the 2 study years, this included the periods from January 28 to April 8, 2003, and December 1, 2003, to January 31, 2004.

Study days were randomized to rapid test or no rapid test days using blocks of 4 and 6. Block size and determination of which days the rapid test was performed were determined by a random number generator by Stata version 8.1 (Stata Corp, College Station, Tex). This study had 80% power to detect a 15% difference in diagnostic testing with 185 children in the rapid test group and the no rapid test group with an $\alpha$ of 0.05.

### INFLUENZA VIRUS DETERMINATION

#### Culture

Nasal and throat swabs were obtained from each enrolled child, combined into a test tube of veal-infusion broth transport medium, and inoculated onto primary rhesus monkey kidney cells. Cultures were incubated at 35°C and initially identified by cytopathic effect and hemadsorption. Cultures without cytopathic effect and hemadsorption were screened by immunofluorescent assay at 10 days.[6] A specimen was considered culture positive if either influenza A or B was identified.

#### Polymerase Chain Reaction

For reverse transcription–PCR (RT-PCR) testing, aliquots of the sample were placed in lysis buffer and the RNA was extracted and frozen at −70°C.[7] Duplicate aliquots of extracted RNA were tested by RT-PCR with previously described oligonucleotide primers and probes for influenza A and B viruses using colorimetric microtiter plate systems.[8] A specimen was considered PCR positive if both PCR determinations were positive for influenza A or B.

#### Criterion Standard

Influenza infection was defined as any sample with either a positive viral culture for influenza A or B or 2 consecutive positive PCRs for influenza A or B.[8] Approval to perform point-of-care rapid influenza testing was obtained from the Tennessee Medical Laboratory Board, and all study nurses completed formal training using the QuickVue Influenza Test. Laboratory proficiency tests from the American College of Pathologists were performed by the study nurses 3 times each year. Positive and negative controls were confirmed prior to use of each kit of 25 rapid influenza tests. A study nurse obtained a nasal swab with the QuickVue Influenza Test applicator, placed it in a test tube, and mixed it with kit reagent. The test was performed and interpreted at the point of care according to the manufacturer's instructions.

### STATISTICAL ANALYSIS

To measure the impact of the QuickVue Influenza Test, the primary study outcome was the proportion with any diagnostic tests, except a rapid influenza test, ordered by the treating physician in the performance and no performance of the rapid test groups using $\chi^2$ analysis. Secondary outcomes evaluated the performance of individual tests, including complete blood cell count and/or blood culture, urinanalysis and/or urine culture, and chest radiograph, which were compared using $\chi^2$ or Fisher exact tests. Antibiotic or antiviral prescriptions were also compared using $\chi^2$ or Fisher exact tests. Demographic variables (race and age) were analyzed using $\chi^2$ tests, and continuous variables were analyzed using a *t* test. Because excluding 10 children in the emergency department and 1 in the acute care clinic who were younger than 1 month of age did not change the statistically significant results, these 11 children were included in the study population. High-risk medical conditions were those conditions for which the influenza vaccine is specifically recommended according to the *2003 Red Book*.[9] Stata version 8.1 was used for all analyses.

**Table 1. Demographics of Study Population by Clinical Setting**

| Characteristic | Emergency Department: Rapid Test (n = 135), No. (%) | Emergency Department: No Rapid Test (n = 170), No. (%) | Acute Care Clinic: Rapid Test (n = 70), No. (%) | Acute Care Clinic: No Rapid Test (n = 93), No. (%) |
|---|---|---|---|---|
| Sex | | | | |
| Male | 66 (49) | 84 (49) | 33 (47) | 51 (55) |
| Female | 69 (51) | 86 (51) | 37 (53) | 42 (45) |
| Age, mo* | | | | |
| 0-5 | 33 (24) | 49 (29) | 10 (14) | 11 (12) |
| 6-23 | 57 (42) | 74 (44) | 27 (39) | 48 (52) |
| 24-59 | 45 (33) | 47 (28) | 33 (47) | 34 (37) |
| Race | | | | |
| Black | 73 (54) | 80 (47) | 45 (64) | 52 (56) |
| White | 46 (34) | 64 (38) | 14 (20) | 27 (29) |
| Other | 16 (12) | 26 (15) | 11 (16) | 14 (15) |
| High risk | 29 (21) | 34 (20) | 13 (19) | 13 (14) |

*Percentage sum might not equal 100% because of rounding.

The performance characteristics of the QuickVue Influenza Test were determined by comparing its results with that of the criterion standard. Intrarater and interrater reliability for 2 study nurses were ascertained by obtaining a second reading of 102 randomly selected test strips that were scanned and printed in color on the enrollment day.

## RESULTS

### PARTICIPANTS

Enrollment included 305 (92%) of 333 and 163 (84%) of 195 eligible children approached in the emergency department and acute care clinic, respectively. On days randomized to performance of the rapid test, 205 (89%) of 230 eligible children were enrolled. For each clinic setting, demographic characteristics of children enrolled on performance of rapid test days were similar to those on no rapid test days (**Table 1**). Demographic characteristics of children enrolled in the emergency department and the acute care clinic were similar with the exception that children in the emergency department were significantly younger than those in the clinic. Eighty-nine enrolled children (19%) had high-risk medical conditions and 71 (80%) had asthma.

Common presenting symptoms of enrolled included fever (77%) and cough (88%). Overall, the median symptom days prior to presentation was 3, and 38% of children had had symptoms for 2 or fewer days. Children with influenza infection by criterion standard had a mean of 3.9 symptom days prior to presentation to both the emergency department and the acute care clinic. None of the children enrolled in the clinic were subsequently hospitalized as compared with 41 children (13%) in the emergency department ($P<.001$). The mean number of diagnostic tests per child performed in the emergency department was significantly higher than in the clinic (1.1 vs 0.2, $P<.001$). Because of the significant difference in diagnostic test ordering between the 2 clinical settings, we analyzed the impact of the rapid test on clinical care for each clinical setting separately.

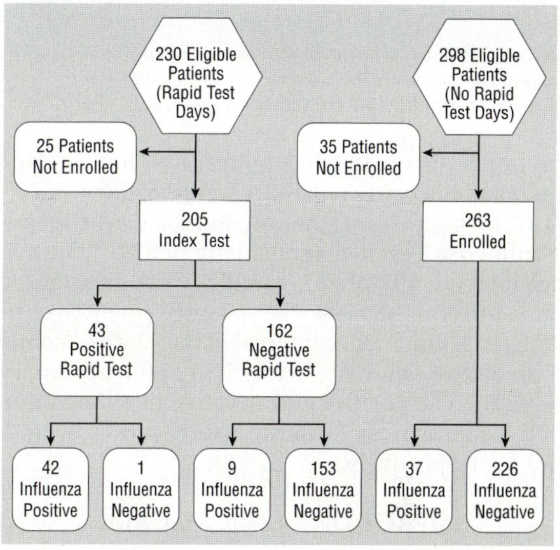


**Figure.** Flow diagram of children enrolled on days randomized to rapid influenza test and no rapid influenza test in emergency department or acute care clinic.

### RAPID INFLUENZA TEST CHARACTERISTICS

The nasal swab for the rapid influenza test and the nasal and throat swab for the criterion standard were obtained at enrollment and prior to any treatment. No adverse events were experienced with the performance of the rapid influenza test or criterion standard.

Because test characteristics were similar and the prevalence of influenza was 19% for both the emergency department and clinic settings, the data from both were combined to evaluate the diagnostic accuracy of the point-of-care rapid influenza test. Of 88 criterion-standard influenza infections, 87 (99%) had influenza A and 1 (1%) had influenza B. Of children enrolled on the performance of rapid test days, 51 (25%) were influenza positive by criterion standard and 43 (21%) were influenza positive by the point-of-care rapid test (**Figure**). Of 102

**Table 2. Impact of Rapid Test on Diagnostic Testing in the Emergency Department**

| | Overall | | | Influenza Positive* | | |
|---|---|---|---|---|---|---|
| | No. (%) | | | No. (%) | | |
| Diagnostic Test | Rapid Test (n = 135) | No Rapid Test (n = 170) | *P* Value† | Rapid Test (n = 28) | No Rapid Test (n = 29) | *P* Value† |
| Any diagnostic test | | | | | | |
| Yes | 53 (39) | 88 (52) | .03† | 9 (32) | 12 (41) | .47 |
| No | 82 (61) | 82 (48) | | 19 (68) | 17 (59) | |
| Chest radiograph | | | | | | |
| Yes | 31 (23) | 56 (33) | .06 | 3 (11) | 7 (24) | .18 |
| No | 104 (77) | 114 (67) | | 25 (89) | 22 (76) | |
| Blood count/culture | | | | | | |
| Yes | 14 (10) | 31 (18) | .05 | 1 (4) | 3 (10) | .61 |
| No | 121 (90) | 139 (82) | | 27 (96) | 26 (90) | |
| Urinanalysis/culture | | | | | | |
| Yes | 18 (13) | 27 (16) | .53 | 3 (11) | 3 (10) | 1.00 |
| No | 117 (87) | 143 (84) | | 25 (89) | 26 (90) | |
| Antibiotics | | | | | | |
| Yes | 43 (32) | 49 (29) | .57 | 4 (14) | 5 (17) | 1.00 |
| No | 92 (68) | 121 (71) | | 24 (86) | 24 (83) | |
| Antivirals | | | | | | |
| Yes | 1 (1) | 0 | .44 | 1 (4) | 0 | .49 |
| No | 134 (99) | 170 (100) | | 27 (96) | 29 (100) | |

*Influenza positive was determined by viral culture or reverse transcription–polymerase chain reaction.
†$\chi^2$ or Fisher exact tests are statistically significant at $P<.05$.

rapid test results read twice by research nurses, the intrarater and interrater reliability were excellent (κ=0.98, SE 0.02, for both). Using the criterion standard, the QuickVue Influenza Test had a sensitivity of 82% (95% confidence interval, 69%-92%), specificity of 99% (95% confidence interval, 96%-99.9%), positive predictive value of 98% (95% confidence interval, 88%-99.9%) and negative predictive value of 94% (95% confidence interval, 90%-97%). The positive and negative likelihood ratios, which are measures of discriminatory power, were 126 and 0.18, respectively.

### IMPACT ON CLINICAL CARE

In the emergency department, fewer children in the rapid test group, whether the rapid test had positive or negative results, had any diagnostic test ordered than those in the no rapid test group (39% vs 52%, *P*=.03, **Table 2**). Interestingly, fewer children without influenza infection had any diagnostic test ordered than those in the no rapid test group (41% vs 53%, *P*=.046). Although no one diagnostic test accounted for the differences in testing between the rapid and no rapid test groups, there was a trend for fewer chest radiographs and fewer blood cultures and/or complete blood counts in the rapid test group. Only 1 (5%) of 21 children who were positive for influenza met criteria for (symptoms for 1 or 2 days and at least 12 months of age) and was prescribed an antiviral medication; this child had a positive point-of-care rapid influenza test result. Overall, 13% of children in both the rapid and no rapid test groups were admitted to the hospital. In contrast to the emergency department, the performance and no performance of the rapid test groups did not differ in rates of diagnostic testing or antibiotic or antiviral prescribing in the acute care clinic setting (**Table 3**).

## COMMENT

To our knowledge, this is the first study to evaluate the impact of a rapid diagnostic test in an emergency department and an outpatient clinic using viral culture and PCR as the criterion standard. The QuickVue Influenza Test performed by trained nurses at the point-of-care in children younger than 5 years of age with fever or acute respiratory symptoms was sensitive, specific, and reliable. In addition, 12.5% fewer children in the emergency department had any diagnostic test performed in the rapid test group than in the no rapid test group; among children without influenza infections, those in the rapid test group had fewer diagnostic studies than those in the no rapid test group. There were no differences in diagnostic testing noted in the acute care clinic.

The point-of-care rapid influenza test characteristics in this report were very similar to those reported in earlier studies in children.[8,10-12] Although previous studies differed in age of population, sample collection methods, time between sample collection and test performance, influenza season, influenza strain, and the criterion standard, the QuickVue Influenza Test had comparable performance characteristics with sensitivity ranging from 37% to 96% (mean±SD, 75±18%) and specificity ranging from 81% to 98% (mean±SD, 88±10%).[3,8,10-17] Given the fact that younger children have higher viral titers, the sensitivity of the test is greater in the younger age groups.[8,17] Studies using frozen specimens or specimens delayed in testing have reported more false-positive results and thus a lower specificity.[13-17]

Two earlier studies in pediatric emergency departments found that children whose physicians were aware

**Table 3. Impact of Rapid Test on Diagnostic Testing in the Acute Care Clinic**

| Diagnostic Test | Overall No. (%) Rapid Test N = 70 | Overall No. (%) No Rapid Test N = 93 | Overall P Value† | Influenza Positive* No. (%) Rapid Test N = 23 | Influenza Positive* No. (%) No Rapid Test N = 8 | Influenza Positive* P Value† |
|---|---|---|---|---|---|---|
| Any diagnostic test | | | | | | |
| Yes | 12 (17) | 12 (13) | .45 | 2 (9) | 1 (13) | 1.00 |
| No | 58 (83) | 81 (87) | | 21 (91) | 7 (87) | |
| Chest radiograph | | | | | | |
| Yes | 6 (9) | 5 (5) | .42 | 2 (9) | 0 | 1.00 |
| No | 64 (91) | 88 (95) | | 21 (91) | 8 (100) | |
| Blood cell count/culture | | | | | | |
| Yes | 3 (4) | 3 (3) | 1.00 | 2 (9) | 1 (13) | 1.00 |
| No | 67 (96) | 90 (97) | | 21 (91) | 8 (100) | |
| Urinanalysis/culture | | | | | | |
| Yes | 5 (7) | 3 (3) | .29 | 2 (9) | 0 | 1.00 |
| No | 65 (93) | 90 (97) | | 21 (91) | 8 (100) | |
| Antibiotics | | | | | | |
| Yes | 18 (26) | 26 (29) | .75 | 6 (26) | 3 (38) | .54 |
| No | 52 (34) | 67 (71) | | 17 (74) | 5 (62) | |
| Antiviral | | | | | | |
| Yes | 0 | 0 | . . . | 0 | 0 | . . . |
| No | 70 (100) | 92 (100) | | 23 (100) | 8 (100) | |

*Influenza positive was determined by viral culture or reverse transcription–polymerase chain reaction.
†$\chi^2$ or Fisher exact test was used to determine *P* value.

of a positive rapid influenza test ordered fewer blood tests and urine tests as compared with physicians unaware of a positive rapid influenza test.[18,19] However, our study differed from these studies in 2 ways. First, we used an independent criterion standard instead of the results of the rapid influenza test to define influenza infection, which allowed us to account for the fact that rapid influenza tests are not 100% sensitive. Second, we evaluated the impact of the rapid influenza test in both the acute care clinic and the emergency department. In our study, fewer children in the emergency department had diagnostic tests ordered in the rapid test group compared with the no rapid test group. Although no differences between the groups in diagnostic testing were noted in the acute care clinic, this is likely due to the fact that fewer tests are ordered in the clinic than in the emergency department.

This study has some limitations. First, it was designed to evaluate the impact of the rapid influenza test on diagnostic testing and medication use. However, other factors such as alleviation of parental anxiety might have been impacted by the test and were not measured. Although the specific results of the diagnostic tests do dictate further evaluation and treatment, this study focused on whether 1 or more diagnostic studies were performed because ordering tests is associated with longer evaluation times. With increasing pediatric emergency department volumes and with long wait times due to overcrowding, especially during the respiratory season, factors influencing the performance of diagnostic testing are important. The sample size calculation was computed prior to the determination that the testing characteristics in the emergency department and acute care clinic were different. Although the acute care clinic study population had insufficient power to detect a difference in test ordering, this population would detect a significant difference only if 185 children were randomized to each group and the no rapid test group had a 22% higher rate of test ordering than the rapid test group. The impact of the rapid testing may vary by influenza season and between the beginning and end of each season. Finally, our results will likely be influenced by media coverage, pediatric influenza vaccination rate, and inherent prescribing practices of physicians.

Although 24% of all children with influenza infection met the criteria for antiviral treatment, the only child given antiviral medications was one who had a positive point-of-care rapid test. With effective antiviral agents, confirming influenza may be one major role for point-of-care tests. Persons who may benefit from antiviral therapy include individuals 12 months of age and older who arrive within 1 to 2 days of symptom onset of influenza infection or exposed family members and can be identified with rapid tests in a timely fashion. It is interesting to note that nearly 20% of children who tested positive for influenza from both study groups received antibiotics. Rapid influenza testing may provide timely data for influenza surveillance and impact public health decisions, including the decision to close schools during large outbreaks. Finally, with the expanding pediatric influenza vaccination recommendations, identifying children with influenza infections may impact the perceived value of influenza vaccinations for the child and family members.

In summary, point-of-care rapid influenza tests are readily available. A few studies have shown that positive rapid influenza test results impact clinical decision making in the pediatric emergency department. This study evaluated the impact of performing rapid influenza tests (both positive and negative results) on clinical decision making in a pediatric emergency department and an acute care clinic and used independent laboratory testing to define influenza infections.

We confirmed that the point-of-care QuickVue Influenza Test when performed by trained nurses was sensitive, specific, and reliable in young children who present to the outpatient setting with acute respiratory symptoms during the influenza season. The rapid influenza test results influenced the likelihood that a child had an influenza infection with positive and negative likelihood ratios of 126 and 0.18, respectively. The point-of-care rapid influenza test reduced unnecessary diagnostic testing in the emergency department by 12.5% among all children with respiratory symptoms during the influenza season when emergency department overcrowding is a common problem. Further assessment of the impact of rapid influenza testing is warranted.

**Accepted for Publication:** December 15, 2005.
**Correspondence:** Katherine A. Poehling, MD, MPH, Division of General Pediatrics, Vanderbilt University Medical Center, AA-0214 Medical Center North, Nashville, TN 37232-2504 (katherine.poehling@vanderbilt.edu).
**Author Contributions:** *Study concept and design:* Poehling and Edwards. *Acquisition of data:* Poehling, Zhu, and Tang. *Drafting of the manuscript:* Poehling. *Critical revision of the manuscript for important intellectual content:* Zhu, Tang, and Edwards. *Statistical analysis:* Poehling and Zhu. *Obtained funding:* Poehling. *Administrative, technical, and material support:* Poehling and Tang. *Study supervision:* Edwards.
**Funding/Support:** This study was supported in part by the New Vaccine Surveillance Network. Dr Poehling received support from the Robert Wood Johnson Generalist Physicians Faculty Scholars Program.
**Disclaimer:** The findings and conclusions in this manuscript are those of the authors and do not necessarily represent the views of the Centers for Disease Control and Prevention.
**Acknowledgment:** We thank the children and their parents who so willingly participated in this study; our nurses, Erin Keckley, RN; Ann Clay, RN; and Diane Kent, RN, who enrolled the patients, performed all the point-of-care rapid tests, and performed record reviews; Julia Francis Shaklee, who helped perform record reviews and entered data; Nayleen Whitehead, who entered all of the New Vaccine Surveillance Network questionnaire data; Robin McClenton, who entered the additional data about diagnostic testing; our clinical staff, under the leadership of Gregory Plemmons, MD, and Rebecca Swan, MD; and the pediatric emergency department staff, under the leadership of Andrea Bracikowski, MD. We also thank the anonymous reviewers for their helpful comments and suggestions.

## REFERENCES


1. Neuzil KM, Mellen BG, Wright PF, Mitchel EF Jr, Griffin MR. The effect of influenza on hospitalizations, outpatient visits, and courses of antibiotics in children. *N Engl J Med.* 2000;342:225-231.
2. Izurieta HS, Thompson WW, Kramarz P, et al. Influenza and the rates of hospitalization for respiratory disease among infants and young children. *N Engl J Med.* 2000;342:232-239.
3. Rodriguez WJ, Schwartz RH, Thorne MM. Evaluation of diagnostic tests for influenza in a pediatric practice. *Pediatr Infect Dis J.* 2002;21:193-196.
4. Iwane MK, Edwards KM, Szilagyi PG, et al. Population-based surveillance for hospitalizations associated with respiratory syncytial virus, influenza virus and parainfluenza viruses in young children. *Pediatrics.* 2004;113:1758-1764.
5. Griffin MR, Coffey CS, Neuzil KM, Mitchel EF Jr, Wright PF, Edwards KM. Winter viruses: influenza- and respiratory syncytial virus-related morbidity in chronic lung disease. *Arch Intern Med.* 2002;162:1229-1236.
6. Weinberg GA, Erdman DD, Edwards KM, et al. Superiority of reverse-transcription polymerase chain reaction to conventional viral culture in the diagnosis of acute respiratory tract infections in children. *J Infect Dis.* 2004;189:706-710.
7. Sefers SE, Rickmyre J, Blackman A, Li H, Edwards K, Tang YW. QIAamp MinElute Virus kit effectively extracts viral nucleic acids from cerebrospinal fluids and nasopharyngeal swabs. *J Clin Virol.* 2006;35:141-146.
8. Poehling KA, Griffin MR, Dittus RS, et al. Bedside diagnosis of influenzavirus infections in hospitalized children. *Pediatrics.* 2002;110:83-88.
9. American Academy of Pediatrics. Influenza. In: Pickering L, ed. *2003 Red Book: Report of the Committee on Infectious Diseases*, 26th ed. Elk Grove Village, Ill: American Academy of Pediatrics; 2003:382-391.
10. Cazacu AC, Greer J, Taherivand M, Demmler GJ. Comparison of lateral-flow immunoassay and enzyme immunoassay with viral culture for rapid detection of influenza virus in nasal wash specimens from children. *J Clin Microbiol.* 2003;41:2132-2134.
11. Yamazaki M, Mitamura K, Kimura K, et al. Clinical evaluation of an immunochromatography test for rapid diagnosis of influenza [in Japanese]. *Kansenshogaku Zasshi.* 2001;75:1047-1053.
12. Kawakami C, Shimizu H, Watanabe S, et al. Evaluation of immunochromatography method for rapid detection of influenza A and B viruses [in Japanese]. *Kansenshogaku Zasshi.* 2001;75:792-799.
13. Quach C, Newby D, Daoust G, Rubin E, McDonald J. QuickVue influenza test for rapid detection of influenza A and B viruses in a pediatric population. *Clin Diagn Lab Immunol.* 2002;9:925-926.
14. Bellei N, Benfica D, Perosa AH, Carlucci R, Barros M, Granato C. Evaluation of a rapid test (QuickVue) compared with the shell vial assay for detection of influenza virus clearance after antiviral treatment. *J Virol Methods.* 2003;109:85-88.
15. Pregliasco F, Puzelli S, Mensi C, et al. Influenza virological surveillance in children: the use of the QuickVue rapid diagnostic test. *J Med Virol.* 2004;73:269-273.
16. Ruest A, Michaud S, Deslandes S, Frost EH. Comparison of the Directigen flu A+B test, the QuickVue influenza test, and clinical case definition to viral culture and reverse transcription-PCR for rapid diagnosis of influenza virus infection. *J Clin Microbiol.* 2003;41:3487-3493.
17. Harnden A, Brueggemann A, Shepperd S, et al. Near patient testing for influenza in children in primary care: comparison with laboratory testing. *BMJ.* 2003;326:480.
18. Sharma V, Dowd MD, Slaughter AJ, Simon SD. Effect of rapid diagnosis of influenza virus type a on the emergency department management of febrile infants and toddlers. *Arch Pediatr Adolesc Med.* 2002;156:41-43.
19. Bonner AB, Monroe KW, Talley LI, Klasner AE, Kimberlin DW. Impact of the rapid diagnosis of influenza on physician decision-making and patient management in the pediatric emergency department: results of a randomized, prospective, controlled trial. *Pediatrics.* 2003;112:363-367.

## HAVRIX®
## (Hepatitis A Vaccine, Inactivated)

The following is a brief summary only; see full prescribing information for complete product information.

**INDICATIONS AND USAGE:** HAVRIX is indicated for active immunization of persons ≥12 months of age against disease caused by hepatitis A virus (HAV). Primary immunization should be administered at least 2 weeks prior to expected exposure to HAV. When passive protection against hepatitis A is required either following exposure to hepatitis A virus or in persons requiring both immediate and long-term protection, HAVRIX may be administered concomitantly with immune globulin (IG) with different syringes and at different injection sites. Duration of immunity following a complete vaccination schedule has not been established.

**CONTRAINDICATIONS:** Hypersensitivity to any component of the vaccine, including neomycin, is a contraindication (see DESCRIPTION in full prescribing information). This vaccine is contraindicated in patients with previous hypersensitivity to any hepatitis A-containing vaccine.

**WARNINGS:** There have been rare reports of anaphylaxis/anaphylactoid reactions following commercial use of the vaccine. The tip cap and the rubber plunger of the needleless prefilled syringes contain dry natural latex rubber that may cause allergic reactions in latex sensitive individuals. The vial stopper is latex-free. Hepatitis A has a relatively long incubation period. Hepatitis A vaccine may not prevent hepatitis A infection in those who have an unrecognized hepatitis A infection at the time of vaccination. Additionally, it may not prevent infection in those who do not achieve protective antibody titers (although the lowest titer needed to confer protection has not been determined).

**PRECAUTIONS: General:** Prior to immunization with HAVRIX, the patient's current health status and medical history should be reviewed. The physician should review the patient's immunization history for possible vaccine sensitivity, previous vaccination-related adverse reactions and occurrence of any adverse–event-related symptoms and/or signs, in order to determine the existence of any contraindication to immunization with HAVRIX and to allow an assessment of benefits and risks. Appropriate medical treatment and supervision should be readily available for immediate use in case of a rare anaphylactic reaction following the administration of the vaccine. Epinephrine injection (1:1,000) and other appropriate agents used for the control of immediate allergic reactions must be immediately available. A separate, sterile syringe and needle or a sterile disposable unit should be used for each patient to prevent the transmission of other infectious agents from person to person. Needles should be disposed of properly and should not be recapped. As with any vaccine, if administered to immunosuppressed persons, including those receiving immunosuppressive therapy, the expected immune response may not be obtained. **Drug Interactions:** HAVRIX may be given concurrently with Hib conjugate vaccines in children 15 to 18 months of age (see CLINICAL PHARMACOLOGY in full prescribing information and ADVERSE REACTIONS). The safety of HAVRIX given concomitantly with INFANRIX has been evaluated (see ADVERSE REACTIONS). Insufficient data are available to assess the immune response of a fourth dose of DTaP vaccine when administered with HAVRIX. There are limited data to assess the concomitant use of HAVRIX with other vaccines. (See Immune Response to Concomitantly Administered Vaccines in full prescribing information.)

**Carcinogenesis, Mutagenesis, Impairment of Fertility:** HAVRIX has not been evaluated for its carcinogenic potential, mutagenic potential, or potential for impairment of fertility. **Pregnancy:** Pregnancy Category C. Animal reproduction studies have not been conducted with HAVRIX. It is also not known whether HAVRIX can cause fetal harm when administered to a pregnant woman or can affect reproduction capacity. Give HAVRIX to a pregnant woman only if clearly needed. **Nursing Mothers:** It is not known whether HAVRIX is excreted in human milk. Because many drugs are excreted in human milk, use caution when administering HAVRIX to a nursing woman. **Pediatric Use:** The safety and effectiveness of HAVRIX have been evaluated in 20,436 subjects 1 year to 18 years of age. (See CLINICAL PHARMACOLOGY and DOSAGE AND ADMINISTRATION in full prescribing information.) The safety and effectiveness of HAVRIX have not been established in subjects less than 12 months of age. **Geriatric Use:** Clinical studies of HAVRIX did not include sufficient numbers of subjects 65 years of age and older to determine whether they respond differently from younger subjects. Other reported clinical experience has not identified differences in overall safety between these subjects and younger adult subjects.

**ADVERSE REACTIONS:** As with all pharmaceuticals, however, it is possible that expanded commercial use of the vaccine could reveal rare adverse events. The adverse events most frequently reported by volunteers in clinical trials were injection-site soreness (56% of adults; 21% of children); headache (14% of adults; less than 9% of children). Other solicited and unsolicited events are listed below:

**Incidence 1% to 10% of Injections:** ***Local Reactions at Injection Site:*** Induration, redness, swelling; ***Body as a Whole:*** Fatigue, fever (>37.5°C), malaise; ***Gastrointestinal:*** Anorexia, nausea.

**Incidence <1% of Injections:** ***Local Reaction at Injection Site:*** Hematoma; ***Dermatologic:*** Pruritus, rash, urticaria; ***Respiratory:*** Pharyngitis, other upper respiratory tract infections; ***Gastrointestinal:*** Abdominal pain, diarrhea, dysgeusia, vomiting; ***Musculoskeletal:*** Arthralgia, elevation of creatine phosphokinase, myalgia; ***Hematologic:*** Lymphadenopathy; ***Central Nervous System:*** Hypertonic episode, insomnia, photophobia, vertigo.

**Additional safety data:** Safety data were obtained from 2 additional sources in which large populations were vaccinated. In an outbreak setting in which 4,930 individuals were immunized with a single dose of either 720 EL.U. or 1440 EL.U. of HAVRIX, the vaccine was well tolerated and no serious adverse events due to vaccination were reported. Overall, less than 10% of vaccinees reported solicited general adverse events following the vaccine. The most common solicited local adverse event was pain at the injection site, reported in 22.3% of subjects at 24 hours and decreasing to 2.4% by 72 hours.

In a field efficacy trial, 19,037 children received the 360 EL.U. dose of HAVRIX. The most commonly reported adverse events were injection-site pain (9.5%) and tenderness (8.1%), reported following first doses of HAVRIX. Other adverse events were infrequent and comparable to the control vaccine ENGERIX-B® [Hepatitis B Vaccine (Recombinant)].

In subjects with chronic liver disease, HAVRIX was safe and well tolerated. Local injection site reactions were similar among all 4 groups, and no serious adverse reactions attributed to the vaccine were reported in subjects with chronic liver disease.

***Safety Data for HAVRIX 720 EL.U./0.5 mL Beginning at 11 Months of Age:*** In the multicenter study described under CLINICAL PHARMACOLOGY in full prescribing information, parents/guardians recorded local and general symptoms on diary cards for 4 days (Days 0 to 3) after vaccination. In the 3 groups of children who received HAVRIX alone, safety data were available for 723 children who received 1,396 documented doses of HAVRIX. Additional safety data were available for 181 children who received HAVRIX coadministered with INFANRIX and Hib conjugate vaccine. Most adverse events were mild and transient. The frequencies of solicited local and systemic reactions following receipt of HAVRIX were monitored during the 4-day observation period.

The following rates of solicited adverse events in children who received their first dose of HAVRIX alone at between 11 and 25 months of age were observed. Among local reactions: pain was reported in 15-21% of subjects, redness in 16-21%, swelling in 8% of subjects. Among general reactions, irritability was reported in 24-36% of subjects, loss of appetite in 16-19% of subjects, drowsiness in 15-17% of subjects and fever >39.5°C in ≤2% of subjects. Following the booster dose of HAVRIX, among local reactions: pain was reported in 16-21% of subjects, redness in 17-22%, swelling in 8-10% of subjects. Following the booster dose of HAVRIX, among general reactions, irritability was reported in 19-29% of subjects, loss of appetite in 14-18% of subjects, drowsiness in 13-16% of subjects and fever >39.5°C in ≤1% of subjects.

Drowsiness and loss of appetite occurred at statistically significantly higher rates in subjects 15 to 18 months of age who received Hib conjugate vaccine (PRP-T) and INFANRIX concomitantly with HAVRIX as compared to subjects 15 to 18 months of age who received Hib conjugate vaccine (PRP-T) and INFANRIX (drowsiness 34% and 22% and loss of appetite 29% and 19%, respectively). With the exception of fever (>39.5°C), the solicited general symptoms occurred at statistically significantly higher rates in subjects 15 to 18 months of age who received Hib conjugate vaccine (PRP-T) and INFANRIX concomitantly with HAVRIX as compared to subjects 15 to 18 months of age who received HAVRIX alone (irritability 46% and 30%, drowsiness 34% and 17%, and loss of appetite 29% and 17%, respectively).

A febrile seizure was reported in an 18-month old subject two days after receiving the first dose of HAVRIX. Other serious adverse events reported during the course of this study included a single case each of hepatitis ~5 months post dose 1, insulin-dependent diabetes ~4 months post dose 1, and Kawasaki's disease ~3 1/2 months post dose 1. The association of these events with vaccination is unknown.

**Postmarketing Reports:** Rare voluntary reports of adverse events in people receiving HAVRIX since market introduction include the following: ***Local:*** Localized edema; ***Body as a Whole:*** Anaphylaxis/anaphylactoid reactions, somnolence; ***Cardiovascular:*** Syncope; ***Hepatobiliary:*** Jaundice, hepatitis; ***Dermatologic:*** Erythema multiforme, hyperhydrosis, angioedema; ***Respiratory:*** Dyspnea; ***Hematologic:*** Lymphadenopathy, thrombocytopenia; ***Central Nervous System:*** Convulsions, encephalopathy, dizziness, neuropathy, myelitis, paresthesia, Guillain-Barré syndrome, multiple sclerosis; ***Other:*** Congenital abnormality.

The US Department of Health and Human Services has established the Vaccine Adverse Events Reporting System (VAERS) to accept reports of suspected adverse events after the administration of any vaccine, including, but not limited to, the reporting of events required by the National Childhood Vaccine Injury Act of 1986. The toll-free number for VAERS forms and information is 1-800-822-7967. Reporting forms may also be obtained at the VAERS website at www.vaers.org.

Manufactured by **GlaxoSmithKline Biologicals**, Rixensart, Belgium

Distributed by **GlaxoSmithKline**, Research Triangle Park, NC 27709



BRS-HA:L20

**References: 1.** Centers for Disease Control and Prevention. Recommended childhood and adolescent immunization schedule—United States, 2006. *MMWR.* 2006;54(51&52):Q1–Q4. **2.** Bell BP, Shapiro CN. Hepatitis A virus. In: Long SS, Pickering LK, Prober CG, eds. *Principles and Practice of Pediatric Infectious Diseases.* 2nd ed. Philadelphia, Pa: Churchill Livingstone; 2003:1188–1192. **3.** Armstrong GL, Bell BP. Hepatitis A virus infection in the United States: model-based estimates and implication for childhood immunizations. *Pediatrics.* 2002;109:839–845.

 Printed in USA. HAP283R0 February 2006

# Work Hazards and Workplace Safety Violations Experienced by Adolescent Construction Workers

*Carol W. Runyan, MPH, PhD; Janet Dal Santo, DrPH; Michael Schulman, PhD; Hester J. Lipscomb, PhD; Thomas A. Harris, JD*

**Objective:** To describe the working conditions of adolescents employed in construction in North Carolina, documenting hazards, safety practices, and prohibited activities.

**Design:** A cross-sectional telephone survey.

**Setting:** North Carolina.

**Participants:** Adolescents (aged <18 years) with work permits for the construction industry in North Carolina during summer 2001.

**Main Outcome Measures:** Types of jobs, work tasks, supervisory conditions, tools, equipment, and processes.

**Results:** A total of 187 survey respondents were in this study. Adolescents were employed in varied construction settings and business types. Nineteen of the 187 permitted workers were younger than 16 years, despite prohibitions against their employment in construction unless working for their parents. The remainder (n=168) were working legally based on age, but most performed prohibited tasks. In fact, 84% of all the 16- to 17-year-olds had performed at least 1 clearly prohibited task and 47% had performed 3 or more. Although most reported being supervised and working with others, approximately 19% of all respondents reported working where they were not in hearing distance of other workers. Data were collected from teenagers with work permits, suggesting that these adolescents may work for more responsible employers. If violations of child labor laws exist in this group, it is likely that adolescents without permits are exposed to even greater hazards and violations.

**Conclusion:** Involvement of teenagers in dangerous and/or prohibited tasks is cause for concern and suggests a pressing need to examine the enforcement of existing laws and the need for additional protection.

*Arch Pediatr Adolesc Med. 2006;160:721-727*

**Author Affiliations:** University of North Carolina Injury Prevention Research Center (Drs Runyan, Dal Santo, and Schulman) and Departments of Health Behavior and Health Education (Drs Runyan, Dal Santo, and Schulman) and Pediatrics (Dr Runyan), The University of North Carolina at Chapel Hill; Department of Sociology and Anthropology, North Carolina State University, Raleigh (Dr Schulman); Division of Occupational and Environmental Medicine, Department of Community and Family Medicine, Duke University Medical Center, Durham, NC (Dr Lipscomb); and State Employees Association of North Carolina Inc, Raleigh (Mr Harris).

DESPITE OCCUPATIONAL safety and health gains in recent decades, construction remains one of the most dangerous industries in the United States. Construction workers are exposed to a wide variety of dangerous circumstances or conditions, including work at heights, in trenches, and in confined spaces, exposure to motor vehicles and heavy equipment,[1,2] and a variety of other physical and chemical hazards.[3-5] Specific tasks and exposures vary based on trade (eg, painters vs electricians), the workers' level of experience or skill, and the work organization at any given work site.

Although only 3% of 15- to 17-year-old workers are employed in construction,[6] the industry ranks second only to agriculture in annual number of fatal injuries for workers younger than 18 years.[7] The part-time or seasonal nature of the work of most teenagers makes it difficult to estimate their actual time at risk. However, data suggest that teenagers employed in construction have fatality rates twice as high as construction workers 25 to 44 years of age.[8] The leading causes of death for construction workers, including those younger than 18 years, are falls, electrocutions, and being struck by objects.[9] Prior research has indicated that between 38% and 86% of work-related adolescent deaths are associated with performance of prohibited activities.[10,11]

Two sets of policies address safety for adolescent workers: child labor laws and Occupational Safety and Health Administration (OSHA) regulations. The Fair Labor Standards Act[12] and the US Department of Labor's regulations[13] adopted pursuant to the Fair Labor Standards Act provide the framework for all federal child labor provisions. Federal law, however, does not address all employers and employees. Therefore, like all other states, North Carolina has its own set of child labor laws[14] and regulations.[15] The North Carolina law extends the employment restrictions of the federal law to cover all employers and teenaged workers in the state not subject to the federal law. Additionally, North Carolina regulations define 9 detrimental occupations prohibited for all workers younger than 18 years at any business in the state.[16] The OSHA regulations[17] govern the safety of all workers regardless of age and provide a general backdrop for the more restrictive child labor laws.

Under both federal and North Carolina child labor law, teenagers younger than 16 years are prohibited from working in construction[18] unless for a business wholly owned by their parent(s).[19] Teenagers 16 and 17 years of age may work in construction and perform tasks not listed among either the 17 "hazardous occupations" identified in the federal regulations[20] or the 9 "detrimental" occupations identified in the North Carolina regulations.[16] For example, the federal rules prohibit teenagers of these ages from engaging in roofing work, trench and excavation work, operation of powered woodworking machines, and wrecking and demolition work, whereas the North Carolina rules add prohibitions for other work such as welding and work that requires the use of a respirator. Neither state nor federal child labor regulations apply to workers 18 years and older.

North Carolina is 1 of 41 states with a work permit system that regulates the employment of workers younger than 18 years. Typically, the employer initiates the process by completing a portion of the form that specifies the job for which the teenager is being hired. The adolescent then obtains the signature of a parent or legal guardian on the permit and takes it to the Department of Social Services, which, if the system works as prescribed, issues the certificate only after verifying the youth's age and the legality of the work proposed for a child of that age. Filed with the state's Department of Labor, a unique work permit is required each time an adolescent begins work for a new employer.

This descriptive study was performed to assess the work experiences and hazard exposures of adolescents working in construction jobs in North Carolina with an ultimate aim of identifying areas that need intervention to improve safety. Because prior research has noted that labor law violations are frequent among young construction worker fatalities,[21] we had a particular interest in examining lapses in adherence to child labor restrictions.

## METHODS

### SUBJECT IDENTIFICATION AND ELIGIBILITY

We collected data by telephone interview with working North Carolina teenagers younger than 18 years employed in construction during summer 2001. We identified study subjects by obtaining and sorting all work permits filed with North Carolina during a 4-month period and selecting the permits that indicated that a teenager was being hired to do construction work. These permits contain information on the worker's name, address, telephone number, age, and sex and a few words indicating the type of work the adolescent was being hired to do. Teenagers who filed for work permits between May and August 2001 were all eligible for inclusion. Workers were screened out at the time of interview if they had worked fewer than 10 days in construction, if they had been interviewed in the pilot study the prior summer, or if their work had been limited to office duties.

### PROTECTION OF HUMAN SUBJECTS

The interview protocol was reviewed and approved by the Public Health Institutional Review Board, The University of North Carolina at Chapel Hill. All subjects were minors, so interviewers first contacted a parent or guardian using the telephone number listed on the work permit and obtained oral permission to conduct the interview with their adolescent after reading a statement about the purpose of the study, risks and benefits, and confidentiality procedures. For those adolescents whose parents consented, interviewers obtained their assent in a similar manner. We provided both parents and teenagers with the local telephone number for the North Carolina Department of Labor for more information about child labor laws and worker safety issues.

### SURVEY INSTRUMENT

We consulted with staff from the North Carolina Department of Labor and used items from previous surveys and focus groups with teenagers in North Carolina to develop the survey instrument.[22-24] The instrument was pilot tested with a sample of 135 eligible North Carolina adolescents who had obtained work permits in 2000 for construction jobs. For the pilot test interviews, each respondent was debriefed at the conclusion of the interview to ascertain if there were questions that were confusing or offensive. The pilot interviews were carefully timed to allow adjustments in the length of the questionnaire to no more than 20 minutes. The final instrument consisted of 134 questions about work hours, training, exposure to chemicals, electrical hazards, supervision practices, and use of safety devices.

### DATA COLLECTION

We collected data by telephone survey using trained interviewers employed by The University of North Carolina Department of Biostatistics Survey Research Unit using a computer-assisted telephone interview program. Interviews were conducted between September and October 2001.

### DATA MANAGEMENT AND ANALYSIS

Once interviews were completed, we converted the CATI files to SAS files for data editing and analysis and generated basic descriptive statistics examining the teenagers' report of employer characteristics, their endorsement of work conditions and exposures, and safety practices. All analyses were conducted using SAS statistical software for Windows, version 8.2.[25] Data were analyzed depending on the age of the respondent as indicated on the work permit, with those aged 16 to 17 years combined and separated from those younger than 16 years.

## RESULTS

### THE RESPONDENTS

We identified 324 teenagers younger than 18 years with work permits that indicated construction jobs. Thirty-eight were determined to be ineligible because of language barriers (n=2), not taking the job in construction (n=8), not having worked 10 days for the employer (n=19), having participated in the pilot interview (n=3),

**Table 1. Demographics of 187 Adolescent Construction Worker Respondents, North Carolina, Summer 2001**

| Characteristics | No. (%) |
|---|---|
| Race | |
| White | 159 (85.0) |
| Black | 12 (6.4) |
| Other | 16 (8.6) |
| Age on work permit, y | |
| 14 | 5 (2.7) |
| 15 | 14 (7.5) |
| 16 | 101 (54.0) |
| 17 | 67 (35.8) |
| Last grade completed in school | |
| <9th | 7 (3.8) |
| 9th | 27 (14.6) |
| 10th | 64 (34.6) |
| 11th | 76 (41.1) |
| 12th | 11 (5.9) |
| Prior work in construction | 41 (21.9) |
| Has concurrent paid jobs outside of construction | 25 (13.4) |
| Ever participated in apprenticeship program related to construction | 50 (26.7) |

or lacking a telephone (n = 6). There also were 38 refusals, 24 because parents denied consent, 12 because teenagers refused to participate, and 2 because eligible teenagers with parental permission could not be reached. In addition, 19 households could not be reached, making it impossible to determine their eligibility. Interviews were conducted with 227 adolescents. Assuming those 19 we could not reach had the same proportion of eligibility as those we reached results in a response rate of 80%.

For this analysis, we restricted our study population to 187 respondents, eliminating those whose responses indicated predominantly office work (n = 1) or work that was not for construction firms (eg, working for colleges painting dorm rooms) as reported by 39 respondents. Demographics of the study population are given in **Table 1**.

## WORK ENVIRONMENTS

**Table 2** gives the type of construction work (not mutually exclusive) done by the businesses that employed the teenagers. Approximately half worked in businesses that were owned by members of their own families or in which family members also worked. Respondents indicated, on average, that they usually worked 8 hours a day, with a range of 3 to 12 hours.

## WORK TASKS

Teenagers performed a wide variety of tasks at work sites and under varying conditions. As indicated in **Table 3**, the most common legal tasks that 16- to 17-year-olds reported involved cleaning the work area and getting tools, equipment, and supplies (>90%). Although all the tasks presented in Table 3 are legal for teenagers 16 and 17 years old to perform, a number are dangerous activities, particularly in the hands of an unskilled worker, such as operating a jackhammer or working with equipment that could contact power lines.

**Table 2. Characteristics of the Work Environments of 187 Adolescent Construction Workers, North Carolina, Summer 2001**

| Primary Type of Construction | No. (%) |
|---|---|
| General carpentry, cabinetry, interior or exterior framing, sheetrock | 51 (27.3) |
| Concrete, masonry | 40 (21.4) |
| Electrical work | 37 (19.8) |
| Plumbing | 26 (13.9) |
| Trenching pipe laying | 18 (9.6) |
| Heating, air conditioning, venting | 15 (8.0) |
| Fence building, landscaping | 6 (3.2) |
| Excavation, grading | 13 (7.0) |
| Roofing | 11 (5.9) |
| Painting, wallpapering | 7 (3.7) |
| Demolition | 3 (1.6) |
| All other | 35 (18.7) |

**Table 3. Legal Work Tasks Engaged in by 16- and 17-Year-Old Construction Workers in North Carolina, Summer 2001***

| Tasks Reported | No. (%) |
|---|---|
| Clean work area | 161 (95.8) |
| Gone to get tools, equipment, supplies on the worksite | 156 (92.9) |
| Used shovel | 147 (87.5) |
| Used knife, box cutter, razor blades | 137 (81.6) |
| Worked as watcher or spotter | 125 (74.4) |
| Removed nails, rivets, screws | 116 (69.1) |
| Used sledgehammer | 113 (67.3) |
| Used handsaw | 107 (63.7) |
| Lifted more than 50 lb (22.5 kg) | 100 (59.5) |
| Used adhesives | 92 (54.8) |
| Mixed mortar, concrete, plaster | 67 (39.9) |
| Used jackhammer, hammer drill, or rotary hammer drill | 44 (26.2) |
| Worked with paint thinners or solvents | 27 (16.1) |
| Planted grass, shrubs, trees, other plants | 32 (19.1) |
| Sprayed paint | 27 (16.1) |
| Operated power lawnmower | 21 (12.5) |
| Mixed paint or polyurethane | 15 (8.9) |
| Worked with equipment where could come into contact with power line | 7 (4.2) |
| Used power-driven post hole digger | 6 (3.6) |

*Legal tasks for 168 adolescents working in construction in North Carolina are any tasks other than those listed in the federal hazardous Occupation Orders, 29 CFR §570E, and the North Carolina Detrimental Occupations rule, 13 NC Gen Stat §12.0406.

## PROHIBITED TASKS PERFORMED BY LEGALLY EMPLOYED ADOLESCENTS

Eighty-four percent of all the 16- to 17-year-old workers reported doing at least 1 task that is clearly prohibited (**Table 4**). Of those reporting doing prohibited activities, 19.1% reported just 1 activity, whereas 17.3% reported 2 activities and 47.0% reported 3 or more. More than a third reported operating power saws, whereas a quarter indicated working as an electrician's helper, being an outside helper on a motor vehicle, or working in trenches deeper than 4 ft (1.2 m).

**Table 4. Prohibited Tasks Reported by 16- to 17-Year-Old Construction Workers, North Carolina, Summer 2001***

| Activity | No. (%) |
|---|---|
| Used handheld circular saw, skill saw† | 60 (35.7) |
| Used any other reciprocating saw such as punch or jab saw or a Sawzall† | 61 (36.3) |
| Worked as electrician or electrician's helper† | 42 (25.0) |
| Worked in trenches, holes, or foundations deeper than 4 ft (1.2 m)† | 38 (22.6) |
| Used power nail guns or staple guns† | 34 (20.2) |
| Used power table saw† | 21 (12.5) |
| Used power drill† | 105 (62.5) |
| Operated forklift | 24 (14.3) |
| Put on shingles or other roofing materials† | 20 (11.9) |
| Used powder-activated tools (ie, using gun powder charge) | 10 (6.0) |
| Used chainsaws† | 1 (0.6) |
| Used explosives | 0 |
| Total No. of illegal activities reported | |
| 0 | 28 (16.7) |
| 1 | 32 (19.1) |
| 2 | 29 (17.3) |
| 3 | 23 (13.7) |
| ≥4 | 56 (33.3) |

*Illegal tasks for 168 adolescents listed in the federal Hazardous Occupation Orders, 29 CFR §570E, and the North Carolina Detrimental Occupations rule, 13 NC Gen Stat §12.0406. As illustrated by the tasks denoted by the dagger footnote, some of the federal Hazardous Occupation Orders and all North Carolina detrimental occupations contain exceptions for adolescents working under the supervision of bona fide apprenticeship and student learner programs.

†Legal for workers aged 16 and 17 years only if enrolled in a bona fide apprenticeship or student learner program.

**Table 5. Suspect Tasks for 16- to 17-Year-Old Construction Workers, North Carolina, Summer 2001***

| Activity | No. (%) |
|---|---|
| Drove motor vehicle† | 62 (36.9) |
| Worked on ladder, scaffold, or other structure higher than 6 ft (1.8 m) | 46 (27.4) |
| Outside helper on motor vehicle‡ | 35 (20.8) |
| Worked on open floor joists | 33 (19.6) |
| Worked on roofs doing other things (ie, besides shingles or roofing materials)§ | 28 (16.7) |
| Operated tractor or other heavy equipment† | 24 (14.3) |
| Used miscellaneous saws and drills | 10 (6.0) |
| Total No. of potentially illegal activities reported | |
| 0 | 34 (20.2) |
| 1 | 35 (20.8) |
| 2 | 32 (19.1) |
| 3 | 28 (16.7) |
| ≥4 | 39 (23.2) |

*Although the performance of these tasks by 168 adolescents could violate one of the Federal Hazardous Occupation Orders, 29 CFR §570E, or the North Carolina Detrimental Occupations rule, 13 NC Gen Stat §12.0406, insufficient information was gathered to make a firm determination of a violation.

†Adolescent workers 17 years and younger under federal law and adolescent workers aged 16 to 17 years under North Carolina law may legally drive a motor vehicle on public roads under certain restrictions and may also legally drive at a construction site, off public roads, except as noted here. Under federal law, adolescent workers aged 16 years may legally drive a motor vehicle if done at a construction site, off public roads. For both 16- and 17-year-old adolescents, motor vehicle driving is illegal in or around a mine, quarry, or logging or saw mill operation or in any excavation deeper than 4 ft (1.2 m), even if enrolled in a bona fide apprenticeship or student learner program, [29 CFR §570.52; NC Gen Stat §95-25.5(b) and (l)].

‡May be done at construction site, off public roads; illegal if on a public road, in or around a mine, quarry, or logging or saw mill operation, or in any excavation deeper than 4 ft (1.2 m), [29 CFR §570.52; NC Gen Stat §95-25.5(b)].

§Workers aged 16 to 17 years are permitted to work on roofs doing work on gutters and downspout work, construction of the sheathing or base of roofs, and the installation of television antennas and air conditioners, [29 CFR §570.67; NC Gen Stat §95-25.5(b)]. However, North Carolina law prohibits workers younger than 18 years from any work that involves the risk of falling a distance of 10 ft or more (≥3 m), so legality of these tasks depends on the height at which the work occurs, 13 NC Administrative Code §12.0406 (6).

Similarly, many of the respondents indicated performing a number of other tasks that, depending on the circumstances, may be illegal for workers younger than 18 years. We labeled these *suspect* tasks (**Table 5**) because we are unable to tell for sure if the activity was illegal without knowing more about the conditions under which it was performed. For example, 62 workers indicated they had driven a motor vehicle as part of the job. North Carolina law allows young workers to operate only certain motor vehicles on public roads but permits operation of most vehicles, except forklifts and other hoisting apparatus, on off-road sites (available at: http://www.nclabor.com/wh/fact%20sheets/joint_state_fed.htm). As another example, 46 teenagers indicated they had worked on a ladder, scaffold, or other structure at heights above 6 ft (1.8 m). It is noteworthy that this is the level at which OSHA mandates fall protection practices for all construction workers.

## WORKERS POTENTIALLY ILLEGALLY EMPLOYED

Although teenagers younger than 16 years are prohibited from working in construction, unless working for a business owned completely by their parents, our study population included 19 teenagers younger than 16 years. By definition, all had been issued work permits to do construction work. A higher proportion (13 [68%]) of these underaged workers were employed in businesses that also employed other family members compared with 49% (n=82) of the group in the 16- to 17-year age range. However, we cannot tell if the business was wholly owned by the teenager's parent (thus constituting legal employment) vs other family members (not legal employment) or if the business merely employed other family members in addition to the teenager.

These 19 adolescents were employed in varied types of construction businesses, including carpentry, interior and exterior framing, and hanging sheetrock (n=6), plumbing (n=3), trenching (n=1), heating and air conditioning (n=2), electrical work (n=2), roofing (n=2), concrete and masonry (n=2), excavation (n=2), and painting (n=1), with several of them reporting multiple types of construction work within the same business. Although 3 of the youngest workers reported spending some time working in the office of the firm, all spent at least part of their time doing construction labor.

As indicated in **Table 6**, these 14- to 15-year-olds performed a wide variety of tasks, with the group reporting a median of 13 of the tasks about which they were queried. Some of these youngest workers engaged in tasks illegal even for their 16- and 17-year-old counterparts and also not allowable for teenagers working for parents. These tasks include working in trenches, being an electrician's helper, or using powder-activated tools. Although not given in Table 6, 5 of the 14- and 15-year-olds reported having worked at elevations above 6 ft (1.8 m), and 1 indicated he had worked on scaffolding or ladders without fall protection. Thirteen of these workers younger than 16 years were given the responsibility of being a spotter for other workers.

### SUPERVISION PRACTICES

Consistent with much construction work, most of the teens worked in settings with few employees on site, with 54% indicating the business had fewer than 6 employees "usually present" at the worksite. Although most respondents indicated their work was checked more than once a day and that they were "told what to do and how to do it," nearly 20% of the respondents stated that they had worked completely alone, without being in hearing or sight distance of other workers.

## COMMENT

### MAJOR FINDINGS

Adolescent construction workers are exposed to numerous hazards, many working under illegal conditions and performing multiple types of illegal tasks. Most legally employed 16- and 17-year-old teenagers with permits to work in the construction industry in North Carolina in summer 2001 reported at least one activity that was illegal. A number of other activities these adolescents reported could have been illegal, depending on the circumstances. It was not uncommon for workers to report performance of multiple illegal or potentially illegal tasks. The illegal tasks reported by these adolescents include tasks that previous work has demonstrated to carry significant risk of morbidity, including high-cost injuries.[26] For example, the operation of nail guns was one of the prohibited tasks reported. The use of these easy-to-operate tools is often viewed as a relatively unskilled task assigned to new workers.[27] Suruda et al[21] found that fatal injuries among young construction workers were most commonly associated with electrocutions, being struck by falling objects or equipment, and falls and engagement in several specific prohibited activities, including being an outside helper, demolition work, or operating power saws or hoisting apparatus. According to our data, these types of hazards are common exposures that require more attention and enforcement.

Federal and state child labor laws and OSHA regulations are designed to enhance worker safety. However, the system does not appear to be working. Although laws clearly prohibit work on construction sites by teenagers younger than 16 years unless working for a business owned by the parent, 10% of our respondents were younger than 16 years. They came from 17 different counties, indicating failures of the permitting system in multiple locales. The data on illegal and suspect tasks, tools, and construction activities come from teenagers who report that they are told what to do and how to do it and that their work is supervised. Given that our sample of construction workers is based on work permits, the em-

**Table 6. Illegal Tasks Reported by 14- to 15-Year-Old Construction Workers, North Carolina, Summer 2001***

| Tasks Reported | No. (%) |
|---|---|
| Clean work area | 18 (95) |
| Used shovel | 17 (90) |
| Removed nails, rivets, or screws | 15 (79) |
| Gone to get tools, equipment, or supplies at the worksite | 15 (79) |
| Used knife, box cutter, or razor blades | 14 (74) |
| Worked as watcher or spotter | 13 (68) |
| Used power drill† | 12 (63) |
| Used sledgehammer | 12 (63) |
| Used adhesives | 11 (58) |
| Used handsaw | 9 (47) |
| Mixed mortar, concrete, or plaster | 8 (42) |
| Lifted more than 50 lb (22.5 kg) | 7 (37) |
| Worked with paint thinners or solvents | 5 (26) |
| Mixed paint or polyurethane | 4 (21) |
| Used power table saw† | 4 (21) |
| Worked in trenches, holes, or foundations deeper than 4 ft (1.2 m)† | 3 (16) |
| Used power nail guns or staple guns† | 3 (16) |
| Used handheld circular saw or skill saw† | 3 (16) |
| Used any other reciprocating saw such as a punch or jab saw or a Sawzall† | 3 (16) |
| Outside helper on motor vehicle | 3 (16) |
| Worked on roofs doing other things (ie, besides shingles or roofing materials) | 2 (10) |
| Sprayed paint | 2 (10) |
| Worked as electrician or electrician's helper† | 1 (5) |
| Used jackhammer, hammer drill, or rotary hammer drill | 1 (5) |
| Operated power lawnmower | 1 (5) |
| Used power-driven posthole digger | 1 (5) |
| Used powder-activated tools (ie, using gun powder charge)† | 1 (5) |
| Operated power lawnmower | 1 (5) |
| Worked on ladder, scaffold, or other structure higher than 6 ft (1.8 m) | 1 (5) |
| Worked on open floor joists | 1 (5) |
| Planted grass, shrubs, trees, or other plants | 0 |
| Worked with equipment where could come into contact with power line | 0 |
| Operated forklift† | 0 |
| Put on shingles or other roofing materials† | 0 |
| Used chainsaws† | 0 |
| Used explosives† | 0 |
| Drove motor vehicle | 0 |
| Operated tractor or other heavy equipment | 0 |
| Used miscellaneous saws and drills | 0 |
| Median No. of jobs (range) | 13 (2-19) |

*All work in construction (except for office and sales work) is illegal for 19 adolescents aged 14 to 15 years [29 CFR §570.33(f)(4); NC Gen Stat §95-25.5(c)] unless they are working for a business owned solely by one or both parents [29 CFR §203(l); NC Gen Stat §95-25.5]. There were 13 respondents who reported working at an establishment where other family members worked. For at least some of these, the parent may be the owner of the business, indicating the work was legal.

†Illegal tasks for adolescents aged 16 to 17 years (see Table 4 for details) and for all persons younger than 16 years, regardless of whether they are working for their parents or not.

ployers, by filling out the work permit, are demonstrating at least rudimentary understanding of the child labor laws. If the employers who are conforming with the work permit regulations are allowing illegal work and underaged workers, what illegal tasks or activities are being done by those teenagers employed by employers who do not comply with work permit regulations?

## STUDY LIMITATIONS

The study relied on self-reported information collected as part of a cross-sectional study. Consequently, data are limited by recall and clarity of the items to the adolescent respondents. However, the nature of the information obtained would have been nearly impossible to obtain in any other manner, and there is no reason to suspect that the respondents were misrepresenting their experiences. We were also only surveying teenaged workers with work permits. We had no access to those working in construction without permits. We are likely to have observed the best-case scenarios in that firms that employ adolescents without permits are likely to be more permissive than we observed. It is also unlikely that we have an accurate representation of the immigrant workforce in our population, and these workers may be at particularly high risk[28] for a variety of reasons, including limited health and safety training and language barriers associated with quality training and supervision.[29] If anything, the exposures reported herein are probably an underrepresentation of the true risk. Because of the nuances in the law with respect to specific circumstances, we were unable to detect with certainty all instances of illegal activity. For example, it is possible some of the teens reporting having worked at heights above 6 ft (1.8 m) actually may have been at heights of 10 ft or more (≥3 m). Likewise, some of our questions about powered equipment were not specific enough to ascertain if the respondents were reporting illegal practices. Consequently, we cannot say for sure which work is in violation of state or federal laws. Workers younger than 18 years who are in formal apprenticeship programs are legally able to engage in all but 10 types of tasks that are otherwise prohibited for all workers younger than 18 years.[19,20] Examples include being an outside helper on a motor vehicle, operating a forklift, using explosives, and using powder-activated tools (ie, using gunpowder charges).

Furthermore, although all respondents had worked at least 10 days, some had clearly worked longer than others, depending on when during the summer they began work. Although we cannot be sure, we suspect any biases associated with this factor are conservative, with more hazardous activities being undercounted given that some youth would not have had sufficient time to be assigned more difficult or dangerous tasks.

Finally, for the workers employed by family, our questions were not sensitive enough to differentiate those working for businesses owned wholly by the teenagers' parent vs businesses owned by other family members vs those not owned by family but employing other family members. Because of the allowance in the law for teenagers younger than 16 years to work for parent-owned businesses, we cannot tell which of the young workers were working legally. However, the mere presence of children this age working at construction sites is cause for concern, regardless of the legal nuances. Similarly, we were unable to determine if some of the adolescents were in apprenticeships at the time of the study vs prior apprenticeship involvement or if a teenager had a birthday, making them eligible for different work than that indicated by their age on the work permit.

## STUDY IMPLICATIONS

This research has uncovered areas in need of improvement in the regulation of a safer work environment for adolescents. First, underage teenagers (aged <16 years) are being given permits to work in an industry in which their employment is certainly dangerous and may be illegal. Second, adolescent workers aged 16 and 17 years are legally employed in construction but performing tasks that are unsafe, illegal, or both. These findings suggest the need for improved enforcement of existing regulations and efforts to increase safety awareness and advocacy for stronger safety regulations.

The existing restrictions are not adequate to protect teenagers in this dangerous industry. For example, although teenagers are prohibited in North Carolina from working as an electrician's helper, it is naïve to think this adequately protects them from electrical hazards. Suruda et al[21] identified electrocutions to be the largest single cause of deaths among teenagers in construction and not violating hazardous orders. Their findings are consistent with the findings of Lipscomb et al[30] that electrocutions among construction workers often involve workers other than electricians or linesmen.

Moreover, construction work is dynamic, because sites and work conditions change frequently, workers are exposed to a variety of hazards, including those associated with dangerous equipment, and work is frequently performed at heights and in inclement weather. Although more mature, career construction workers who have been involved in many construction projects may be accustomed to these changes, inexperienced workers may find the constantly changing site to be chaotic. This may help explain the finding of Breslin and Smith[31] that newer workers are more likely injured, regardless of age. However, even if the risks for younger workers may not be greater than for older workers, these young workers may require different interventions given the lack of overall maturity they bring to the job. The work permit system in North Carolina is intended to help screen youth from employment in prohibited work but also relies heavily on employers to correctly interpret and enforce the regulations. Without clearer employer education and sufficient enforcement, continuing violations are likely. It is critical that regulations be coupled with careful guidance from parents, teachers, and health care professionals.

## IMPLICATIONS FOR FUTURE RESEARCH

Additional investigation of the tasks and situations in which young people are engaged in construction would be valuable, particularly assessing the adequacy of laws for workers of this age group and the barriers associated with implementing and enforcing existing regulations or creating new ones. Understanding the challenges that employers face when hiring and supervising young workers and ensuring adherence to the laws could help point toward needed interventions. Studies of teenaged workers need to address both the formal and informal learning processes and also actual work practices on construction sites. Inexperienced workers learn from observation of other workers at the work sites, which means we must continue to try to understand safe and unsafe practices of more seasoned construction workers as well. Although it is more challenging to reach young workers without permits, we need to find ways to assess these workers to address their workplace safety as well. Dissemination research should explore how to improve the potential of teachers, parents, pediatricians, and other youth-oriented professionals and construction contractors to improve work safety for adolescents.

**Accepted for Publication:** December 9, 2005.
**Correspondence:** Carol W. Runyan, MPH, PhD, Injury Prevention Research Center, The University of North Carolina at Chapel Hill, Campus Box 7505, No. 500, 137 E Franklin St, Chapel Hill, NC 27599-7505 (carol_runyan@unc.edu).
**Author Contributions:** Drs Runyan (the principal investigator), Dal Santo, Schulman, and Lipscomb had full access to all the data in the study and take responsibility for the integrity of the data and the accuracy of the data analysis. *Study concept and design:* Runyan, Schulman, Lipscomb, and Harris. *Acquisition of data:* Runyan, Dal Santo, Schulman, and Harris. *Analysis and interpretation of data:* Runyan, Dal Santo, Schulman, Lipscomb, and Harris. *Drafting of the manuscript:* Runyan, Dal Santo, Schulman, and Lipscomb. *Critical revision of the manuscript for important intellectual content:* Runyan, Dal Santo, Schulman, Lipscomb, and Harris. *Statistical analysis:* Runyan, Schulman, and Lipscomb. *Obtained funding:* Runyan and Schulman. *Administrative, technical, and material support:* Runyan, Dal Santo, and Schulman. *Study supervision:* Runyan; *Epidemiology expertise:* Lipscomb. *Legal expertise:* Harris.
**Funding/Support:** This work was supported by Cooperative Agreement (U60-CCU417226) from the National Institute of Occupational Safety and Health to the University of North Carolina Injury Prevention Research Center.
**Acknowledgment:** We appreciate the assistance of Robin Argue, MPH, J. Michael Bowling, PhD, Stephanie Pratt, MM, MS, and Linda Treiber, MS, in helping with instrument development and sampling; Ashley Bowers, MS, for oversight of data collection; Robert Agans, PhD, Jose Sandoval, MS, Shankar Viswanathan, MS, and Xiaoyan Shi, MS, for help with data analyses; and Jennifer Cook, BA, for assistance in preparing the manuscript.

## REFERENCES

1. Center to Protect Workers' Rights. *The Construction Chart Book.* 3rd ed. Atlanta, Ga: Centers for Disease Control and Prevention; 2002.
2. Kisner S, Fosbroke D. Injury hazards in the construction industry. *J Occup Med.* 1994;36:137-143.
3. Schneider S, Susi P. Ergonomics and construction: a review of potential hazards in new construction. *Am Ind Hyg Assoc J.* 1994;55:635-649.
4. Burkhart G, Schulte PA, Robinson C, Sieber WK, Vossenas P, Ringen K. Job tasks, potential exposures, and health risks of laborers employed in the construction industry. *Am J Ind Med.* 1993;24:413-425.
5. Lipscomb HJ, Dement JM. Respiratory diseases among union carpenters: cohort and case-control analyses. *Am J Ind Med.* 1998;33:131-150.
6. National Institute of Occupational Safety and Health. Recommendations to the US Department of Labor for changes to hazardous orders. 2002. http://www.cdc.gov/niosh/docs/NIOSHRecsDOLHaz/default.html. Accessed August 26, 2005.
7. Castillo DN, Landen D, Layne L. Occupational injury deaths of 16- and 17-year-olds in the United States. *Am J Public Health.* 1994;84:646-649.
8. US Department of Labor. *Report on the Youth Labor Force.* Washington, DC: Bureau of Labor Statistics; 2000.
9. Windau J, Sygnatur E, Toscano G. Profile of work injuries incurred by young workers. *Mon Labor Rev.* 1999;122:3-10.
10. Dunn KA, Runyan CW. Deaths at work among children and adolescents. *AJDC.* 1993;147:1044-1047.
11. National Institute of Occupational Safety and Health. *Preventing Deaths and Injuries of Adolescent Workers.* Washington, DC: Dept of Health and Human Services; May 1995. Publication 95-125, NIOSH Alert.
12. 29 USC §201 *et seq.*
13. 29 CFR Part 570.
14. Youth employment. NC Gen Stat §95-25.5.
15. Youth employment. 13 NC Administrative Code §12.0400.
16. Detrimental Occupations. 13 NC Administrative Code §12.0406.
17. 29 CFR Parts 1910 (General Industry Standards) and 1926 (Construction Standards).
18. 29 CFR §570.33(f)(4); NCGS §95-25.5(c).
19. 29 USC §203(l); NCGS §95-25.5(i).
20. 29 CFR Part 570, Subpart E.
21. Suruda A, Philips P, Lillquist D, Sesek R. Fatal injuries to teenage construction workers in the US. *Am J Ind Med.* 2003;44:510-514.
22. Dunn KA, Runyan CW, Cohen LR, Schulman MD. Teens at work: a statewide study of jobs, hazards and injuries. *J Adolesc Health.* 1998;22:19-25.
23. Evensen CT, Schulman M, Runyan CW, Zakocs R, Dunn KA. The downside of adolescent employment: hazards and injuries among working teens in North Carolina. *J Adolesc.* 2000;23:545-560.
24. Zakocs RC, Runyan CW, Schulman M, Dunn KA, Evenson C. Improving safety for teens working in the retail trade sector: opportunities and obstacles. *Am J Ind Med.* 1998;34:342-350.
25. SAS Institute Inc. *SAS Version 8.2* [computer program]. Cary, NC: SAS Institute Inc; 1999.
26. Lipscomb HJ, Li L. Injuries among teens employed in the homebuilding industry in North Carolina. *Inj Prev.* 2001;7:205-209.
27. Lipscomb HJ, Dement JM, Nolan J, Patterson D, Li L. Nail gun injuries in residential carpentry: lessons from active injury surveillance. *Inj Prev.* 2003;9:20-24.
28. Dong X, Platner JW. Occupational fatalities of Hispanic construction workers from 1992 to 2000. *Am J Ind Med.* 2004;45:45-54.
29. O'Connor T, Loomis D, Runyan C, Dal Santo J, Schulman M. Adequacy of health and safety training among young Latino construction workers. *J Occup Environ Med.* 2005;47:272-277.
30. Lipscomb HJ, Dement J, Rodriguez-Acosta R. Deaths from external causes of injury among construction workers in North Carolina, 1988-1994. *Appl Occup Environ Hyg.* 2000;15:569-580.
31. Breslin C, Smith P. Age-related differences in work injuries: a multivariate, population-based study. *Am J Ind Med.* 2005;48:50-56.

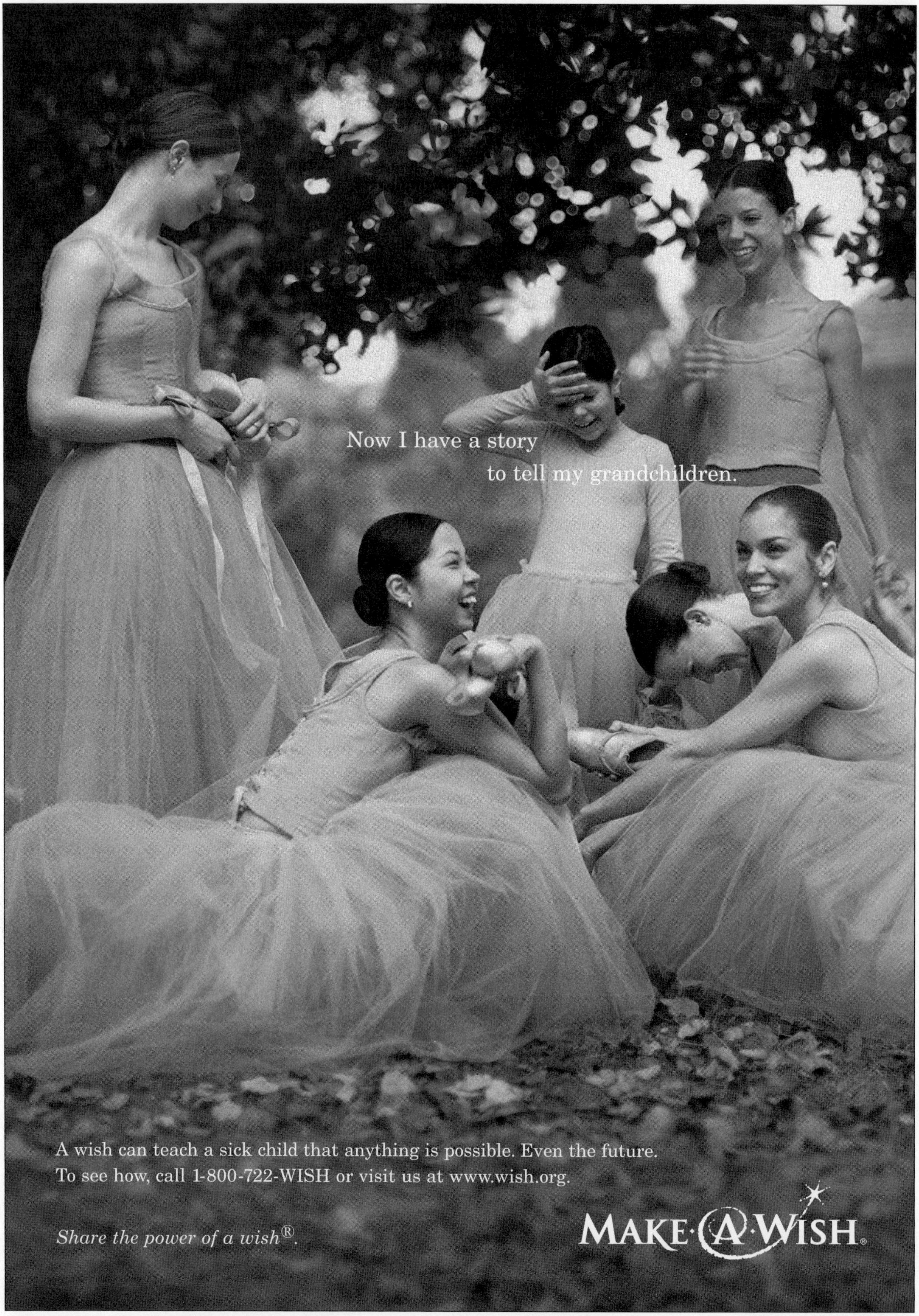
Now I have a story
to tell my grandchildren.
A wish can teach a sick child that anything is possible. Even the future.
To see how, call 1-800-722-WISH or visit us at www.wish.org.
Share the power of a wish®.
MAKE·A·WISH®

# Postasphyxial Hypoxic-Ischemic Encephalopathy in Neonates

## *Outcome Prediction Rule Within 4 Hours of Birth*

*Prakesh S. Shah, FRCPC, MSc; Joseph Beyene, PhD; Teresa To, PhD; Arne Ohlsson, FRCPC, MSc; Max Perlman, FRCPC*

**Objectives:** To construct and validate a model and derive a simple rule that is usable in any birth location for the prediction of outcome of term infants with severe asphyxia.

**Design:** Retrospective cohort study.

**Setting:** Regional outborn neonatal intensive care unit.

**Participants:** Infants with postintrapartum asphyxial hypoxic-ischemic encephalopathy (n=375).

**Main Exposures:** Clinical and laboratory predictors available at age 4 hours.

**Main Outcome Measures:** A logistic regression model was developed and internally validated (with random sampling and based on the year of birth) for severe adverse outcome, which was defined as death or severe disability (severe cerebral palsy, severe developmental delay, sensorineural deafness, or cortical blindness singly or in com bination). A simple prediction rule was derived from 3 variables.

**Results:** Complete data were available for 302 (92%) of the 345 infants with known outcomes (204 infants with severe adverse outcome). Six independent predictors of outcomes were identified. Using the 3 most significant predictors (chest compressions, age at onset of respiration, and base deficit), severe adverse outcome rates were 46% (95% confidence interval, 33%-58%) with none of the 3 predictors, 64% (95% confidence interval, 54%-73%) with any 1 predictor, 76% (95% confidence interval, 66%-85%) with any 2 predictors, and 93% (95% confidence interval, 81%-99%) with all of the 3 predictors present. The internal validations revealed a robust model.

**Conclusions:** This predictive model for neonatal hypoxic-ischemic encephalopathy provides a sliding scale of probabilities that could be used for prognostication and to design eligibility criteria for decision making including neuroprotective therapy.

*Arch Pediatr Adolesc Med. 2006;160:729-736*

APPROXIMATELY 23% OF THE 4 million annual global neonatal deaths are attributable to asphyxia.[1] Postasphyxial hypoxic-ischemic encephalopathy (HIE) occurs in approximately 1 to 2 infants per 1000 live term births.[2] Significant proportions of these infants die or survive with severe long-term morbidity. Among term infants, 6% to 23% of cases of cerebral palsy (CP) are attributable to intrapartum asphyxia.[3,4] Predictions of long-term outcome in the immediate neonatal period are based on clinical,[5-7] biochemical,[8,9] electrophysiological,[10,11] and imaging[12] findings. The predictive accuracy in the very early postnatal period is moderate.[5,13] Higher positive predictive values might be achieved with amplitude-integrated electroencephalography (EEG), but it is not available in many hospitals globally.

Certain strategies in experimental postasphyxial HIE prevent secondary neuronal injury when given within the therapeutic window of 5 to 6 hours from the insult.[14] Trials of hypothermia in humans have used clinical and/or amplitude-integrated EEG criteria for inclusion.[15-17] The choice of predictive inclusion criteria in research involves ethical and clinical considerations.[18] Early evaluation of risk is essential for appropriate selection of patients for neuroprotective therapies.[19] To decide on neuroprotective therapy within or outside of clinical trials, easily available, robust, and accurate prediction models are needed, preferably by age 4 hours to allow time for enrollment. Such a rule will also help to monitor the efficacy of interventions and for prognostication.

The objectives of this study were to develop and validate a prognostic model for term infants with postasphyxial HIE based on clinical and laboratory information available by age 4 hours and to develop a simple prediction rule based on the variables identified in the model.

Author Affiliations: Department of Paediatrics, Mount Sinai Hospital (Drs Shah and Ohlsson), Departments of Paediatrics (Drs Shah and Ohlsson) and Public Health Sciences (Drs Beyene and To), University of Toronto, and Division of Neonatology, Department of Paediatrics (Drs Shah and Perlman) and Research Institute (Drs Beyene and To), Hospital for Sick Children, Toronto, Ontario.

**Table 1. Definitions of Organ System Involvement and Time Courses of Asphyxia**

| Term | Definition |
|---|---|
| Organ system involvement | |
| Renal | 1 of the following: (1) anuria or oliguria (<1 mL/kg per hour) for 24 h or longer and a serum creatinine concentration >100 mmol/L; (2) anuria or oliguria for >36 h; (3) any serum creatinine concentration >125 mmol/L; or (4) serial serum creatinine levels that increased postnatally |
| Cardiovascular | Hypotension treated with inotrope for more than 24 h to maintain blood pressure within the normal range, or electrocardiographic evidence of transient myocardial ischemia |
| Pulmonary | Need for ventilator support with oxygen requirement >40% for at least the first 4 h after birth |
| Hepatic | Aspartate aminotransferase level >100 IU/L or alanine aminotransferase level >100 IU/L at any time during the first week after birth |
| Time course of asphyxia | |
| Prolonged partial | Frequent variable or late decelerations for >30 min prior to birth or placental abruption presenting to hospital with bleeding, abdominal pain, and bradycardia with >30 min between the onset of symptoms and birth |
| Acute near-total | Severe persistent fetal bradycardia for 10-30 min from the onset to birth associated with prolapsed cord, maternal shock during labor, ruptured uterus or tight nuchal cord, shoulder dystocia or other catastrophic events, or placental abruption documented in the hospital record and birth within 30 min |
| Combined or mixed | Prolonged partial asphyxia (as per criteria outlined earlier) followed by acute near-total asphyxia, or the reverse |

## METHODS

### INFANTS

We retrospectively reviewed the records of outborn infants with moderate to severe postasphyxial HIE who were admitted to the regional outborn neonatal intensive care unit at the Hospital for Sick Children, Toronto, Ontario (referral center for 55 000-60 000 births/y), between July 1, 1985, and December 31, 2000. The majority of infants were transported by our team and admitted between ages 3 and 8 hours.

### INCLUSION CRITERIA

The following inclusion criteria were adapted from the American College of Obstetricians and Gynecologists[20] and Society of Obstetricians and Gynecologists of Canada[21] statements. Infants who had an acute perinatal event were eligible if they met the following 3 criteria: (1) Apgar score of less than 5 at 5 minutes, metabolic acidosis (base deficit >16 mmol/L) in cord arterial blood or the first postnatal blood gas sample within 4 hours of birth, or delayed onset of breathing for more than 5 minutes; (2) need for mechanical ventilation immediately after birth; and (3) moderate to severe encephalopathy including altered state of consciousness and/or seizures.[22]

All of the infants had multisystem involvement[23] (encephalopathy and more than 1 other organ involved) identified as defined in **Table 1**. This was determined from the data beyond age 4 hours to ensure appropriate inclusion.

### EXCLUSION CRITERIA

Infants with encephalopathies associated with preterm birth, congenital abnormalities including subtle dysmorphism of unknown significance, a major single-organ anomaly, inborn errors of metabolism, congenital viral infection, septic shock, or cranial birth trauma, patients with evidence of antenatal events causing prenatal injury such as prolonged loss of fetal movements, arthrogryposis, or lack of fetal heart rate variability on admission of the mother to the hospital, and patients with severe meconium aspiration syndrome with persistent and prolonged postnatal hypoxemia were excluded to avoid the confounding effects on brain outcomes.

### NEONATAL DATA

Data were collected on custom-made forms from the patients' records by fully trained neonatal transport team members.[24,25] Data related to the maternal medical history, obstetric history, intrapartum details, and details of the resuscitation were collected. The time of onset of gasping, irregular breathing, regular breathing, or spontaneous breathing was recorded as available both in ventilated as well as unventilated infants. The age at onset of regular respiration was defined as the age at onset of spontaneous or regular breathing. The transport team members examined and recorded the neurological condition of the infant soon after arrival at the hospital of birth. The initial and subsequent neurological data included level of consciousness, presence of spontaneous movements and coma, altered muscle tone, the age at onset of seizures (subtle or tonic-clonic), and number and dosage of anticonvulsants received. This information along with a clinical description of the attending team was considered for determination of the degree of encephalopathy, which was classified according to the criteria by Sarnat and Sarnat.[22] None of the patients received prophylactic anticonvulsants. Use of muscle relaxants was not routine. Where data were available, the time course of the asphyxial insult was categorized for each subject as prolonged, acute near-total, or combined.[25] Two of us (P.S. and M.P.) assigned the time course of each subject independently, and discrepancies were resolved by consensus. When consensus was not reached or the time course could not be classified owing to insufficient data, the time course was categorized as indeterminate (Table 1). Blood gas analyses were performed at variable times during the first 4 hours after birth; therefore, each base deficit value was converted to the number of SDs from the mean normal values of full-term newborns for age at sampling[26] ($z$ score).

### OUTCOME DATA

Severe adverse outcome was defined in the research protocol as death or severe neurodevelopmental disability in survivors that was attributable to intrapartum asphyxial HIE. Cerebral palsy was defined as mild, moderate, or severe as suggested by Capute et al.[27] Developmental delay was defined as mild (developmental quotient, 81-90), moderate (developmental quotient, 71-80), or severe (developmental quotient, <70). Severe neurodevelopmental disability was defined as the following: (1) severe CP (probably nonambulatory) diagnosed by age 12 months by certified physical or occupational therapists and a pediatrician; (2) mild or moderate CP (likely ambulatory) but with severe cortical blindness or severe sensorineural deafness; or (3) moderate CP and suspected moderate or severe developmental delay at age 12 months confirmed by developmental testing between ages 18 and 36 months by certified occupational therapists or psychologists (Bayley scores >2 SD below the mean). The remaining children were classified as free of severe adverse outcome rather than good outcome, as some of these patients had minor disabilities.[28] All of the children with suspected motor or cognitive impairments were assessed by audiologists and ophthalmologists. Data regarding persistence of seizures and microcephaly were collected.

The outcome data were ascertained from health records of the neonatal follow-up clinic, neurology clinics, and readmissions when available. The neonatal follow-up clinic routinely assesses infants who had neonatal HIE at ages 4, 8, 12, and 18 to 24 months. If developmental delay or motor deficit was suspected on clinical grounds or on the basis of screening tests, developmental tests were performed at ages 18 to 30 months. Children unable to perform the developmental assessment tests owing to physical or cognitive deficits were classified in the severe adverse outcome group. The procedure for obtaining data for patients with incomplete follow-up was described previously.[24] The study was approved by the institutional research ethics board.

## STATISTICAL ANALYSES AND SAMPLE SIZE

Data were analyzed using SPSS version 12 statistical software (SPSS, Inc, Chicago, Ill). Patients with missing outcome data were excluded from analyses. Available data from patients with missing data were evaluated for randomness. Owing to the finding of nonrandomness of missing data, values were not imputed. Potential predictors selected on the basis of $P<.10$ in univariate logistic regression analyses were entered into multivariable models, and the odds ratios and 95% confidence intervals were computed. Goodness of fit of the model was assessed by the Hosmer-Lemeshow statistic and receiver operating characteristic curve. Internal validation was performed using 2 methods: (1) on a randomly selected derivation cohort comprising 70% of the cases and a validation cohort of the remaining 30%; and (2) temporally based by year of birth (1985-1995 as the derivation cohort and 1996-2000 as the validation cohort). Eight variables selected by univariate analyses were entered into the multivariate model. The sample size was adequate for the logistic model, as the number of events per variable exceeded 12 for both outcome categories.[29] An additional stepwise prediction rule was created using the 3 variables identified in multivariate logistic regression analysis to have the highest statistical significance based on the presence of none, any 1 or 2, or all of the 3 of these predictor variables, similar to the method used by Schmidt et al.[30] Predicted probabilities were then computed and compared with observed outcome rates. Likelihood ratios were calculated.

# RESULTS

## INFANTS

A total of 1195 patient records with relevant diagnoses (*birth asphyxia, asphyxia, HIE, birth hypoxia, perinatal depression, brain anoxia, hypoxic-ischemic encephalopathy*, or *hypoxic encephalopathy*) were reviewed; 375 patients met the eligibility criteria. Most of the exclusions (n=656) were owing to failure to meet the primary criteria of respiratory and/or neurological depression. These included most admissions with meconium aspiration syndrome. The remaining cases lacked evidence of moderate to severe encephalopathy (n=90) or had hemorrhagic shock (n=29), lack of fetal heart rate reactivity or absent fetal heart rate on admission (n=18), cranial trauma (n=17), congenital malformations (n=9), and congenital viral infection (n=1). The mean number of patients with moderate to severe postasphyxial HIE per year was 24 patients (range, 7-43 patients).

## OUTCOME

Outcome data were available for a total of 345 patients (327 from the hospital records, 4 from regional follow-up clinics, 13 from primary care physicians, and 1 from the mother). The mean age at follow-up assessment was 30 months (median age, 22 months; interquartile age range, 18-36 months). Of the 345 children with outcome data, 115 died; the median age at death was 48 hours (age range, 10 hours to 86 days), and the primary cause of death was HIE in all of the cases (due to withdrawal of life support in 105 infants based on high probability of adverse outcome; 10 infants died while receiving life-sustaining treatment). Of the survivors, 111 children had severe adverse outcome, and 119 children (34%) did not have this outcome. Thus, in total, 226 children (66%) had severe adverse outcome (**Figure 1**). A chronic seizure disorder or microcephaly was present at the time of assessment in 64 and 57 survivors, respectively.

## PREDICTOR VARIABLE ANALYSIS

Predictive data were not available for 43 children (21 children with severe adverse outcome and 22 free of severe adverse outcome). The missing data were type of asphyxia (n=30), blood gas analysis results (n=19), and time of onset of respiration (n=1) (some children had missing data for >1 variable). Comparisons of the predictive variables indicate that the 73 children lacking data (30 children who were missing outcome data and 43 who were missing predictor variable data) had less severe neonatal illness than the 302 children with complete data (**Table 2**).

For the remaining 302 children (204 children with severe adverse outcome and 98 free of severe adverse outcome), the results of univariate and multivariable logistic regression analyses with outcome as the dependent variable are respectively reported in **Table 3** and **Table 4**. Six independent predictors of outcome were identified. For severe adverse outcome, the accuracy, sensitivity, specificity, positive predictive value, and negative predictive value of the multivariable model were 73%, 89%, 41%, 76%, and 63%, respectively. The receiver operating characteristic curve (**Figure 2**) revealed an area under the curve of 0.74 (95% confidence interval, 0.69-0.80). The results of internal validation based on random case selection revealed accuracy, sensitivity, specificity, positive predictive value, and negative predictive value of 74%, 89%, 39%, 77%, and 62%, respectively, for the derivation cohort and 72%, 91%, 41%, 72%, and 72%, respectively, for the validation cohort. Validation based

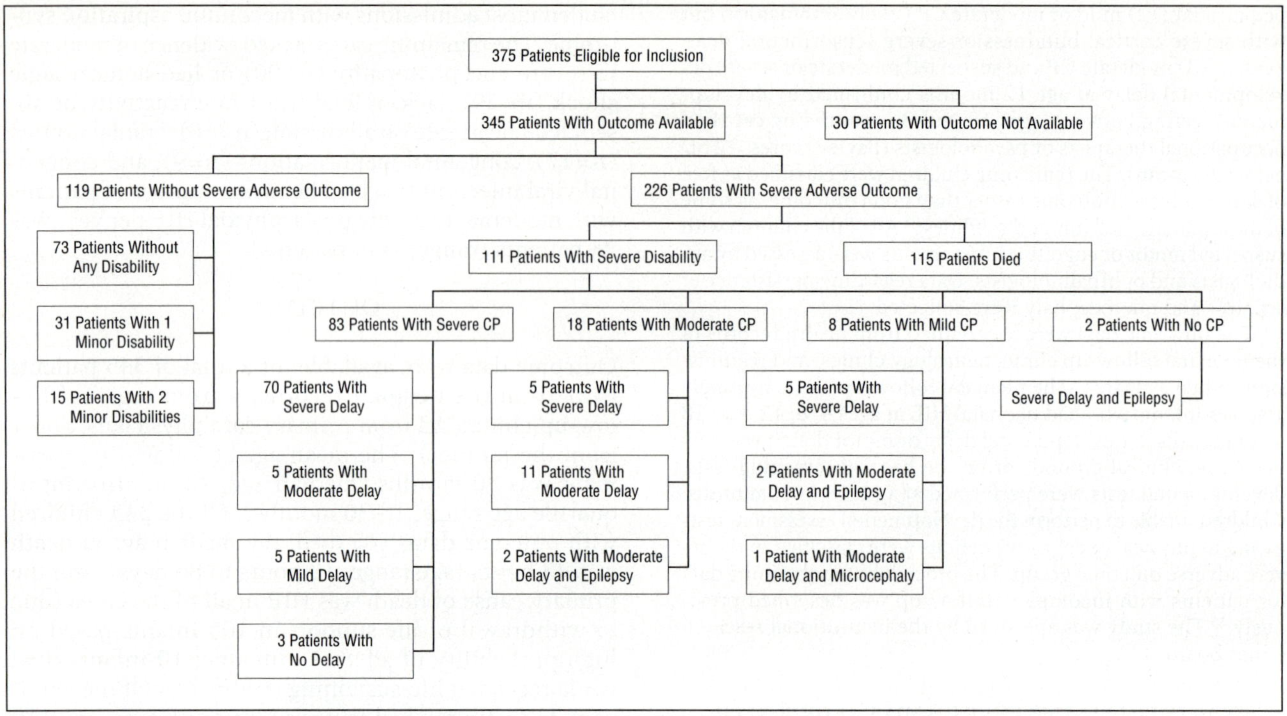


**Figure 1.** Outcome distribution of the entire cohort. CP indicates cerebral palsy.

**Table 2. Comparison of Patients With and Without Outcome Data**

| Variable | Complete Data (n = 302) | Missing Data (n = 73) | P Value* |
|---|---|---|---|
| Maternal age, mean ± SD, y | 29.1 ± 5.8 | 28.3 ± 5.3 | .43 |
| Gravida, median (range) | 2 (1-3) | 2 (1-3) | .38 |
| Para, median (range) | 0 (0-2) | 0 (0-1) | .47 |
| Gestational age, mean ± SD, wk | 40.0 ± 1.5 | 39.9 ± 1.4 | .37 |
| Birth weight, mean ± SD, g | 3480 ± 496 | 3404 ± 539 | .25 |
| Sex, male/female, No. | 179/123 | 35/38 | .09 |
| Apgar score at 5 min, median (interquartile range) | 3 (2-5) | 5 (4-6) | <.001† |
| Administration of chest compressions >1 min, % | 43 | 18 | <.001† |
| Administration of epinephrine, % | 29 | 12 | .002† |
| Age at onset of breathing ≥30 min, % | 33 | 7 | <.001† |
| Seizure or coma before age 4 h, % | 65 | 41 | <.001† |
| $PCO_2$ ≤30 mm Hg in the first blood gas analysis, % | 64 | 45 | .008† |
| $PO_2$ ≥200 mm Hg in the first blood gas analysis, % | 32 | 12 | .002† |
| Standardized base deficit for the age of sampling, mean ± SD, SD above mean | 5.7 ± 3.6 | 4.8 ± 2.5 | .10 |
| Renal involvement, % | 75 | 66 | .10 |
| Hepatic involvement, % | 84 | 78 | .32 |
| Cardiovascular involvement, % | 64 | 47 | .004† |
| Pulmonary involvement, % | 97 | 94 | .28 |

*Unpaired *t* test, $\chi^2$ test, and Wilcoxon rank sum test as appropriate.
†Significant at $P<.05$.

on temporal division of the cohort revealed accuracy, sensitivity, specificity, positive predictive value, and negative predictive value of 69%, 86%, 37%, 72%, and 58%, respectively, for the derivation cohort and 76%, 90%, 41%, 78%, and 60%, respectively, for the validation cohort.

## PREDICTION RULE

The results of the logistic regression model of only 3 predictors with high statistical significance (administration of chest compressions >1 minute, onset of breathing >30 minutes, and base deficit value >16 in any blood gas analysis within the first 4 hours from birth) and of the simple count of these variables are reported in **Table 5**. The observed and predicted rates of severe adverse outcome in subgroups with none, any 1, any 2, or all of the 3 of these predictors are reported in **Table 6**; a simple count of the variables individually and in various combinations correlated in a stepwise fashion with the observed (**Figure 3**) and predicted outcomes.

## COMMENT

Using a combination of 6 markers in this cohort, we developed a model with improved sensitivity (89%) and positive predictive value (76%) for severe adverse outcome compared with our previous prediction model that was based on a smaller sample.[5] Internal validation demonstrated the robustness of the model. The prediction rule derived by a simple count of 3 variables greatly improved predictive power. These 3 predictors are known to be associated with poor long-term outcome.[31] Individual estimates of odds of severe adverse outcome associated with each of these 3 variables were similar to that of the entire cohort; however, absence of all of the 3 variables reduced the probability of severe adverse out-

**Table 3. Univariate Logistic Analyses**

| Variable | Severe Adverse Outcome (n = 204) | Free of Severe Adverse Outcome (n = 98) | *P* Value | Severe Adverse Outcome Unadjusted OR (95% CI) |
|---|---|---|---|---|
| Birth weight, mean ± SD, g | 3459 ± 473 | 3523 ± 539 | .29 | 1.00 (0.99-1.00) |
| Sex, male/female, No. | 119/85 | 60/38 | .63 | 1.13 (0.69-1.85) |
| Delivery, vaginal/cesarean, No. | 73/131 | 49/49 | .02* | 1.80 (1.10-2.92) |
| Apgar score at 5 min, median (IQR) | 3 (2-4) | 4 (3-5) | .001* | NA |
| Administration of chest compression >1 min, % | 50 | 27 | <.001* | 2.82 (1.67-4.78) |
| Administration of epinephrine, % | 33 | 20 | .02* | 1.95 (1.10-3.46) |
| Age at onset of respiration ≥30 min, % | 40 | 18 | .001* | 2.99 (1.67-5.35) |
| Seizure or coma before age 4 h, % | 71 | 53 | .003* | 2.12 (1.29-3.49) |
| $PCO_2$ ≤30 mm Hg, % | 66 | 59 | .20 | 1.38 (0.84-2.27) |
| $PO_2$ ≥200 mm Hg, % | 33 | 29 | .41 | 1.25 (0.74-2.12) |
| Standardized base deficit, mean ± SD, SD above mean | 6.2 ± 3.4 | 4.5 ± 3.6 | <.001* | 1.16 (1.08-1.25) |
| Type of asphyxia | | | | |
| Acute near-total, % | 28 | 30 | .02* | 0.47 (0.27-0.99) |
| Prolonged partial, % | 44 | 56 | | 0.39 (0.20-0.77) |
| Combined, % | 28 | 14 | | Reference |

Abbreviations: CI, confidence interval; IQR, interquartile range; NA, not applicable; OR, odds ratio.
*Significant at $P<.05$.

come by 20% from baseline, and there was an approximately 15% risk for each variable added to the count.

Therapeutic decisions are based on the prognosis of the infant, which varies with the severity of illness. Gluckman et al[15] described their hesitations about enrolling babies with the most severe postasphyxial HIE (determined by amplitude-integrated EEG) to the head-cooling trial, and based on the results, they concluded that the therapy was probably not effective for patients with severe injury. Severe cases (eg, cases with 2 or all of the 3 predictor variables present) probably incur the risk of severe disability rather than death with neuroprotective therapy. In our opinion, prognostic models that offer a simple sliding scale of probability of severe adverse outcomes such as ours will be very useful in this regard for selection purposes. We agree with the speculation that clinical criteria are likely to complement amplitude-integrated EEG,[32] even when the latter is widely available.

To decide whether to institute neuroprotective therapy, predictive models are needed within the therapeutic window of 5 to 6 hours,[14] preferably by age 4 hours, to allow time for enrollment. Even a highly accurate predictive model or scoring system is not useful for experimental or clinical therapy beyond this therapeutic window.[7,33,34] Major issues with existing models include inadequate sample size, selection bias, timing of the model, outcome assessment, and lastly, attrition.[31,35] Perlman[36] reviewed the measures of diagnosis and severity of asphyxia that were used during labor and in the delivery room and suggested that these markers are useful in combination to identify infants who will progress to develop HIE or seizures. Apart from an earlier study from our institution,[5] few studies have built predictive models for the first 4 hours after birth. Perlman and Risser[35] studied 96 infants with asphyxia and identified a 5-minute Apgar score of less than 5, intubation in the delivery room, and fetal acidemia as predictors of risk of seizures within 4 hours of birth in 5 patients. Carter et al[37] developed a scoring system to predict

**Table 4. Logistic Regression Model***

| Variable | OR (95% CI) |
|---|---|
| Administration of chest compressions >1 min | 3.24 (1.44-7.32) |
| Administration of epinephrine | 2.64 (1.03-6.75) |
| Age at onset of respiration ≥30 min | 2.32 (1.22-4.39) |
| Seizure or coma before age 4 h | 2.03 (1.17-3.51) |
| Standardized base deficit, SD above mean | 1.17 (1.08-1.27) |
| Cesarean delivery | 1.97 (1.15-3.38) |

Abbreviations: CI, confidence interval; OR, odds ratio.
*Hosmer-Lemeshow statistics: $\chi^2_8 = 9.534$; $P = .30$.

**Table 5. Logistic Model Using 3 Variables and Their Counts**

| Model Type | OR (95% CI) | *P* Value |
|---|---|---|
| Individual variables | | |
| Administration of chest compression >1 min | 2.25 (1.30-3.89) | .004 |
| Base deficit >16 | 2.07 (1.24-3.45) | .005 |
| Age at onset of respiration ≥30 min | 2.33 (1.27-4.27) | .006 |
| Variable count | 2.20 (1.65-2.94) | <.001 |

multiorgan dysfunction based on fetal heart rate abnormalities, umbilical arterial acidosis, and 5-minute Apgar score. Other nonclinical markers such as serum or urine S100 levels,[9] urinary lactate-creatinine ratio,[8] and amplitude-integrated EEG results[10,38] have shown promise as early markers of severity of HIE, but their relationships to long-term outcome have not been tested. The need for a special assay and expertise to interpret the results may limit usefulness. Imaging modalities such as magnetic resonance imaging, magnetic resonance spectroscopy, and diffusion-weighted imaging are recommended between ages 2 to 8 days,[39] but their prognostic utility has not been established even on day 1.

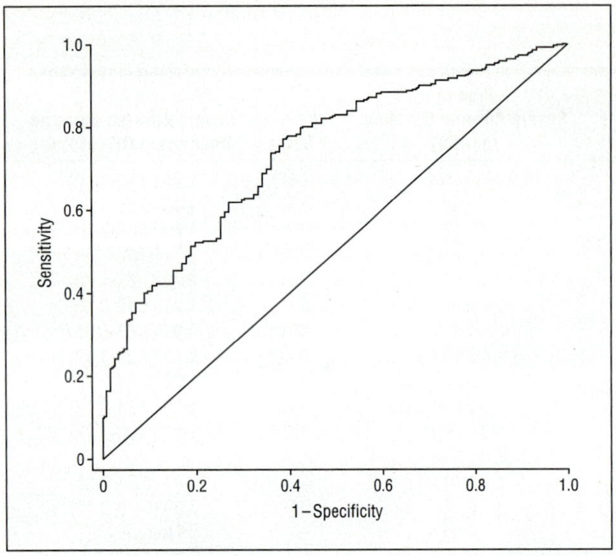


**Figure 2.** Receiver operating characteristic curve for predicted probabilities of severe adverse outcome.

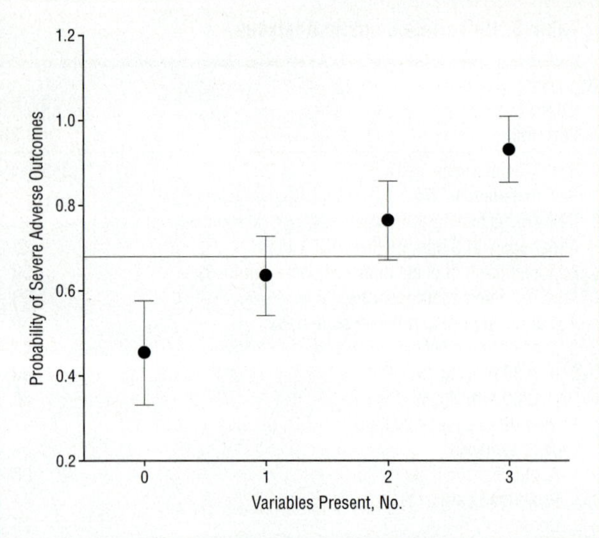


**Figure 3.** Stepwise prediction rule for severe adverse outcome. Error bars indicate 95% confidence intervals; horizontal line, observed adverse outcome rate of 68% for the entire cohort.

**Table 6. Simple Count of Presence of 3 Variables and Observed and Predicted Outcome Status**

| | Probability of Severe Adverse Outcome | | | | |
|---|---|---|---|---|---|
| | Observed Data | | Logistic Model Prediction | | |
| Variables | No./Total No. (%) | 95% CI | Individual Variables, % | Variable Count, % | LR, Positive, Negative |
| None | 30/66 (46) | 33-58 | 45 | 44 | Reference |
| 1 Variable | | | | | |
| CC | 18/26 (69) | NA | 64 | 64 | 1.3, 0.6 |
| Resp | 10/15 (67) | NA | 62 | | |
| BD | 40/66 (61) | NA | 65 | | |
| Overall | 68/107 (64) | 54-73 | NA | | |
| 2 Variables | | | | | |
| CC and Resp | 10/15 (67) | NA | 79 | 79 | 3.8, 0.7 |
| CC and BD | 34/44 (77) | NA | 81 | | |
| BD and Resp | 21/26 (81) | NA | 79 | | |
| Overall | 65/85 (77) | 66-85 | NA | | |
| 3 Variables | | | | | |
| CC and Resp and BD | 41/44 (93) | 81-99 | 90 | 89 | 6.6, 0.8 |
| All of the patients | 204/302 (68) | 62-73 | NA | NA | NA |

Abbreviations: BD, base deficit ≥16; CC, administration of chest compression for more than 1 minute; CI, confidence interval; LR, likelihood ratio; NA, not applicable; Resp, age at onset of respiration ≥30 min.

To interpret our results, methodological issues need consideration. Despite a rigorous selection method, we cannot exclude the presence of antenatal events in some infants. It could be argued that clinical practice and outcomes changed during the study period. However, we are not aware of any substantive change in therapy of postasphyxial HIE between 1985 and 2000 or of reports of secular changes in outcomes. No change in outcome, including the ratio of death to severe disability, was observed over time. Other factors that may cause instability of predictive models are changes in the diagnostic criteria of postasphyxial HIE[20,21,40-42] and the relatively low prevalence of intrapartum asphyxia as a cause of neonatal encephalopathy and CP.[18,43] Patients lost to follow-up exhibited less severe neonatal illness and were therefore more likely to have relatively good outcomes; however, their outcomes remain uncertain. The great majority of severe adverse outcomes are diagnosed by age 12 months. Shankaran et al[44] found that neurological examination at age 12 months can predict severe disability at age 5 years. We acknowledge that variability in developmental assessment may have introduced bias; however, the severe adverse outcomes defined in this study are far from subtle and have the ability to detect major differences between groups.

The referral patterns and the eligibility criteria for this study resulted in a cohort with characteristics including outcomes similar to those in infants enrolled in neuroprotective therapy trials[15-17] and infants admitted to children's hospitals providing similar regional services.[44,45] The inclusion of infants in our cohort with only moderate to severe encephalopathy is justified owing to the high likelihood of favorable outcomes in infants with mild encephalopathy.[46] Combining patients with moderate and severe encephalopathy allowed us to develop a pragmatic model; however, we are aware that the outcome spectrum is different for these 2 categories. The adverse outcome rate in patients with moderate and severe encephalopathy (66%) was somewhat higher than in the control groups in 2 recent clinical trials (60%[17] and 62%[15]), presumably owing to exclusion of infants in extremis.

The advantages of our model include selection of infants with moderate to severe HIE at high risk for adverse outcomes, a low attrition rate, simplicity of variables based on available clinical and biochemical criteria, and adequate power. Despite the selection bias against patients with most predictable outcomes (those with the most severe disease and the mildest disease), our results have high predictive values with narrow confidence limits and provide a sliding scale rather than categorical criteria.

Prognostic certainty is often unattainable. In patients referred to our center even with none of the 3 predictors present, there was a 46% possibility of poor outcome. Conversely, even with all of the 3 indicators present, there was a 7% possibility that the infant would remain free of severe adverse outcome. We caution that this prediction rule should be used only for the patients who meet the eligibility criteria outlined earlier. Improved models will depend on a better definition of asphyxia, precise data on predictors, and external validation.

**Accepted for Publication:** December 27, 2005.
**Correspondence:** Prakesh S. Shah, Department of Paediatrics, Mount Sinai Hospital, Room 775A, 600 University Ave, Toronto, Ontario, Canada M5G 1X5 (pshah@mtsinai.on.ca).
**Author Contributions:** *Study concept and design:* Shah, Beyene, To, and Ohlsson. *Acquisition of data:* Shah. *Drafting of the manuscript:* Shah. *Critical revision of the manuscript for important intellectual content:* Shah, Beyene, To, and Ohlsson. *Statistical analysis:* Beyene and To. *Administrative, technical, and material support:* Shah, Ohlsson, and Perlman. *Study supervision:* Beyene, Ohlsson, and Perlman.

## REFERENCES

1. Lawn JE, Cousens S, Zupan J. 4 million neonatal deaths: when? where? why? *Lancet.* 2005;365:891-900.
2. Low JA, Lindsay BG, Derrick EJ. Threshold of metabolic acidosis associated with newborn complications. *Am J Obstet Gynecol.* 1997;177:1391-1394.
3. Nelson KB. The epidemiology of cerebral palsy in term infants. *Ment Retard Dev Disabil Res Rev.* 2002;8:146-150.
4. Volpe JJ. Hypoxic-ischemic encephalopathy: intrauterine assessment. In: Volpe JJ, ed. *Neurology of the Newborn.* Philadelphia, Pa: WB Saunders Co; 2000:277-295.
5. Ekert P, Perlman M, Steinlin M, Hao Y. Predicting the outcome of postasphyxial hypoxic-ischemic encephalopathy within 4 hours of birth. *J Pediatr.* 1997;131:613-617.
6. van de Riet JE, Vandenbussche FP, Le Cessie S, Keirse MJ. Newborn assessment and long-term adverse outcome: a systematic review. *Am J Obstet Gynecol.* 1999;180:1024-1029.
7. Miller SP, Latal B, Clark H, et al. Clinical signs predict 30-month neurodevelopmental outcome after neonatal encephalopathy. *Am J Obstet Gynecol.* 2004;190:93-99.
8. Huang CC, Wang ST, Chang YC, Lin KP, Wu PL. Measurement of the urinary lactate: creatinine ratio for the early identification of newborn infants at risk for hypoxic-ischemic encephalopathy. *N Engl J Med.* 1999;341:328-335.
9. Nagdyman N, Komen W, Ko HK, Muller C, Obladen M. Early biochemical indicators of hypoxic-ischemic encephalopathy after birth asphyxia. *Pediatr Res.* 2001;49:502-506.
10. Hellstrom-Westas L, Rosen I, Svenningsen NW. Predictive value of early continuous amplitude integrated EEG recordings on outcome after severe birth asphyxia in full term infants. *Arch Dis Child Fetal Neonatal Ed.* 1995;72:F34-F38.
11. Taylor MJ, Murphy WJ, Whyte HE. Prognostic reliability of somatosensory and visual evoked potentials of asphyxiated term infants. *Dev Med Child Neurol.* 1992;34:507-515.
12. Rutherford MA, Pennock JM, Counsell SJ, et al. Abnormal magnetic resonance signal in the internal capsule predicts poor neurodevelopmental outcome in infants with hypoxic-ischemic encephalopathy. *Pediatrics.* 1998;102:323-328.
13. Shalak LF, Laptook AR, Velaphi SC, Perlman JM. Amplitude-integrated electroencephalography coupled with an early neurologic examination enhances prediction of term infants at risk for persistent encephalopathy. *Pediatrics.* 2003;111:351-357.
14. Gunn AJ. Cerebral hypothermia for prevention of brain injury following perinatal asphyxia. *Curr Opin Pediatr.* 2000;12:111-115.
15. Gluckman PD, Wyatt JS, Azzopardi D, et al. Selective head cooling with mild systemic hypothermia after neonatal encephalopathy: multicentre randomised trial. *Lancet.* 2005;365:663-670.
16. Inder TE, Hunt RW, Morley CJ, et al. Randomized trial of systemic hypothermia selectively protects the cortex on MRI in term hypoxic-ischemic encephalopathy. *J Pediatr.* 2004;145:835-837.
17. Shankaran S, Laptook AR, Ehrenkranz RA, et al; National Institute of Child Health and Human Development Neonatal Research Network. Whole-body hypothermia for neonates with hypoxic-ischemic encephalopathy. *N Engl J Med.* 2005;353:1574-1584.
18. Nelson KB, Grether JK. Selection of neonates for neuroprotective therapies: one set of criteria applied to a population. *Arch Pediatr Adolesc Med.* 1999;153:393-398.
19. Ferriero DM. Neonatal brain injury. *N Engl J Med.* 2004;351:1985-1995.
20. Committee on Obstetric Practice, American College of Obstetricians and Gynecologists. ACOG committee opinion: inappropriate uses of the terms fetal distress and birth asphyxia. *Int J Gynaecol Obstet.* 1998;61:309-310.
21. Policy statement: task force on cerebral palsy and neonatal asphyxia (part 1). *J SOGC.* 1996;18:1267-1279.
22. Sarnat HB, Sarnat MS. Neonatal encephalopathy following fetal distress: a clinical and electroencephalographic study. *Arch Neurol.* 1976;33:696-705.
23. Shah P, Riphagen S, Beyene J, Perlman M. Multiorgan dysfunction in infants with post-asphyxial hypoxic-ischaemic encephalopathy. *Arch Dis Child Fetal Neonatal Ed.* 2004;89:F152-F155.
24. Klinger G, Beyene J, Shah PS, Perlman M. Do hyperoxaemia or hypocapnia add to the risk of brain injury after intrapartum asphyxia? *Arch Dis Child Fetal Neonatal Ed.* 2005;90:F49-F53.
25. Shah PS, Raju NV, Beyene J, Perlman M. Recovery of metabolic acidosis in term infants with postasphyxial hypoxic-ischemic encephalopathy. *Acta Paediatr.* 2003;92:941-947.
26. Swanstrom S, Bratteby LE. Metabolic effects of obstetric regional analgesia and of asphyxia in the newborn infant during the first two hours after birth, III: adjustment of arterial blood gases and acid-base balance. *Acta Paediatr Scand.* 1981;70:811-818.
27. Capute AJ, Shapiro BK, Palmer FB. Spectrum of developmental disabilities: continuum of motor dysfunction. *Orthop Clin North Am.* 1981;12:3-22.
28. Robertson CM, Finer NN. Long-term follow-up of term neonates with perinatal asphyxia. *Clin Perinatol.* 1993;20:483-500.
29. Altman DG, Royston P. What do we mean by validating a prognostic model? *Stat Med.* 2000;19:453-473.
30. Schmidt B, Asztalos EV, Roberts RS, Robertson CM, Sauve RS, Whitfield MF. Impact of bronchopulmonary dysplasia, brain injury, and severe retinopathy on the outcome of extremely low-birth-weight infants at 18 months: results from the trial of indomethacin prophylaxis in preterms. *JAMA.* 2003;289:1124-1129.
31. Peliowski A, Finer NN. Birth asphyxia in the term infant. In: Sinclair JB, Bracken MB, eds. *Effective Care of the Newborn Infant.* Oxford, England: Oxford University Press; 1992:249-279.
32. Gunn AJ, Gluckman PD, Wyatt JS, Thoresen M, Edwards AD. Author's reply: se-

lective head cooling after neonatal encephalopathy. *Lancet.* 2005;365:1619-1620.
33. Caravale B, Allemand F, Libenson MH. Factors predictive of seizures and neurologic outcome in perinatal depression. *Pediatr Neurol.* 2003;29:18-25.
34. Kadri M, Shu S, Holshouser B, et al. Proton magnetic resonance spectroscopy improves outcome prediction in perinatal CNS insults. *J Perinatol.* 2003;23:181-185.
35. Perlman JM, Risser R. Can asphyxiated infants at risk for neonatal seizures be rapidly identified by current high-risk markers? *Pediatrics.* 1996;97:456-462.
36. Perlman JM. Intrapartum hypoxic-ischemic cerebral injury and subsequent cerebral palsy: medicolegal issues. *Pediatrics.* 1997;99:851-859.
37. Carter BS, McNabb F, Merenstein GB. Prospective validation of a scoring system for predicting neonatal morbidity after acute perinatal asphyxia. *J Pediatr.* 1998;132:619-623.
38. al Naqeeb N, Edwards AD, Cowan FM, Azzopardi D. Assessment of neonatal encephalopathy by amplitude-integrated electroencephalography. *Pediatrics.* 1999;103:1263-1271.
39. Ment LR, Bada HS, Barnes P, et al. Practice parameter: neuroimaging of the neonate: report of the Quality Standards Subcommittee of the American Academy of Neurology and the Practice Committee of the Child Neurology Society. *Neurology.* 2002;58:1726-1738.
40. Australian and New Zealand Perinatal Societies. The origin of cerebral palsy: a consensus statement. *Med J Aust.* 1995;162:85-90.
41. MacLennan A. A template for defining a causal relation between acute intrapartum events and cerebral palsy: international consensus statement. *BMJ.* 1999;319:1054-1059.
42. American College of Obstetricians and Gynecologists' Task Force on Neonatal Encephalopathy and Cerebral Palsy. *Neonatal Encephalopathy and Cerebral Palsy: Defining the Pathogenesis and Pathophysiology.* Washington, DC: American College of Obstetricians and Gynecologists; 2003:1-85.
43. Badawi N, Kurinczuk JJ, Keogh JM, et al. Intrapartum risk factors for newborn encephalopathy: the Western Australian case-control study. *BMJ.* 1998;317:1554-1558.
44. Shankaran S, Woldt E, Koepke T, Bedard MP, Nandyal R. Acute neonatal morbidity and long-term central nervous system sequelae of perinatal asphyxia in term infants. *Early Hum Dev.* 1991;25:135-148.
45. Cowan F, Rutherford M, Groenendaal F, et al. Origin and timing of brain lesions in term infants with neonatal encephalopathy. *Lancet.* 2003;361:736-742.
46. Robertson CM, Finer NN, Grace MG. School performance of survivors of neonatal encephalopathy associated with birth asphyxia at term. *J Pediatr.* 1989;114:753-760.

## Announcement

**Submissions.** The Editors welcome contributions to Picture of the Month. Submissions should describe common problems presenting uncommonly, rather than total zebras. Cases should be of interest to practicing pediatricians, highlighting problems that they are likely to at least occasionally encounter in the office or hospital setting. High-quality clinical images (in either 35-mm slide or electronic format) along with parent or patient permission to use these images must accompany the submission. The entire discussion should comprise no more than 750 words. Articles and photographs accepted for publication will bear the contributor's name. There is no charge for reproduction and printing of color illustrations. For details regarding electronic submission, please see: http://archpedi.ama-assn.org.

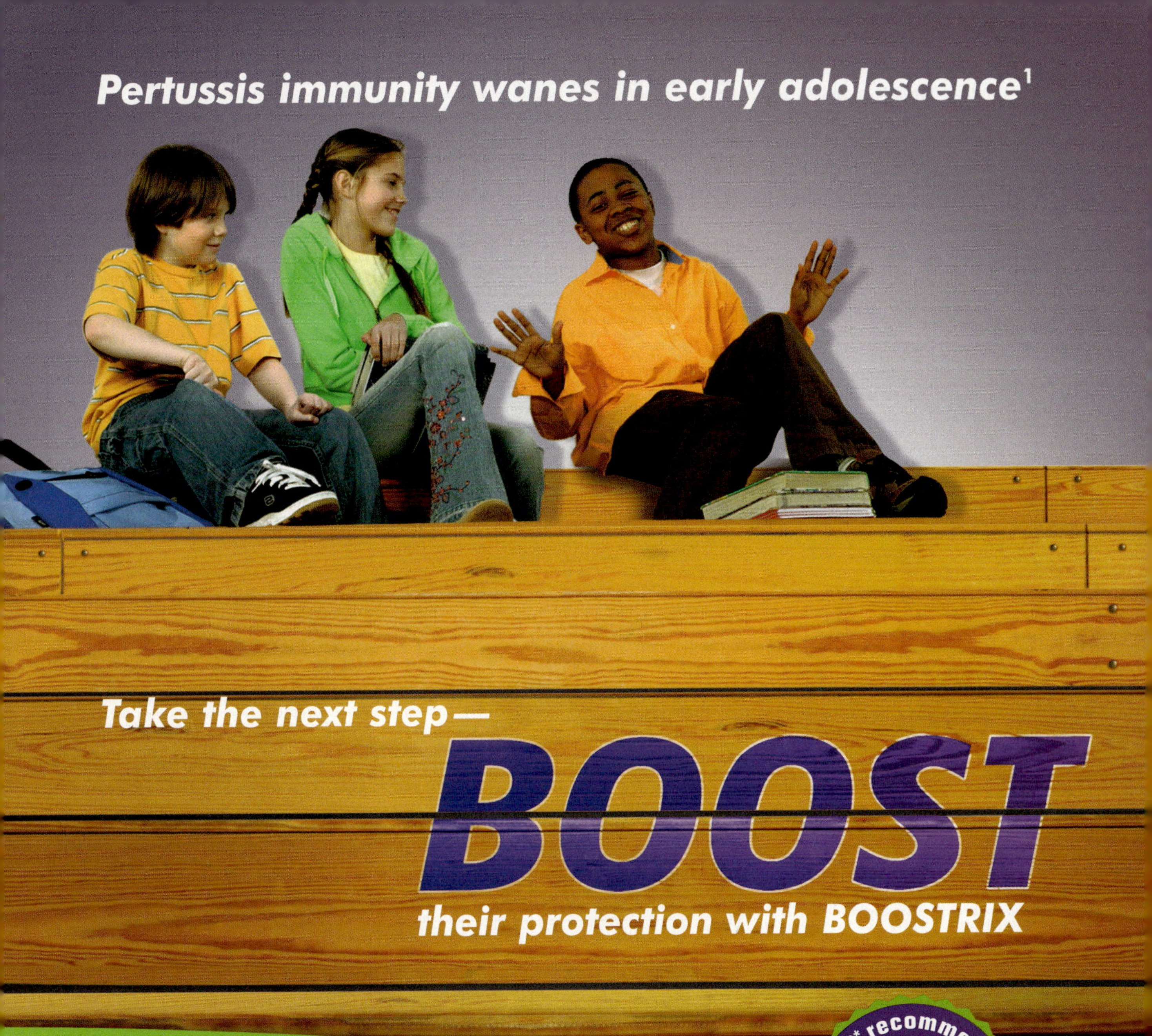


## Important Safety Information

In clinical studies, adverse events included pain, redness, and swelling at the injection site, headache, fatigue, and gastrointestinal symptoms. As with other vaccines, rare adverse events may occur. As with any vaccine, vaccination with BOOSTRIX may not protect 100% of susceptible individuals. Hypersensitivity to any component of BOOSTRIX is a contraindication.

*Advisory Committee on Immunization Practices.

**BOOSTRIX®**

***Tetanus Toxoid, Reduced Diphtheria Toxoid and Acellular Pertussis Vaccine, Adsorbed***

gsk GlaxoSmithKline Vaccines

**Please see references and brief summary of complete prescribing information on the adjacent page.**

BOOSTRIX is a registered trademark of GlaxoSmithKline.
Manufactured by **GlaxoSmithKline Biologicals,** Rixensart, Belgium

Distributed by **GlaxoSmithKline,** Research Triangle Park, NC 27709

# BOOSTRIX®

## (Tetanus Toxoid, Reduced Diphtheria Toxoid and Acellular Pertussis Vaccine, Adsorbed) (Tdap)

The following is a brief summary only; see full prescribing information for complete product information.

**INDICATIONS AND USAGE:** BOOSTRIX is indicated for active booster immunization against tetanus, diphtheria, and pertussis as a single dose in individuals 10 through 18 years of age. The use of BOOSTRIX as a primary series or to complete the primary series has not been studied. As with any vaccine, BOOSTRIX may not protect 100% of individuals receiving the vaccine.

**CONTRAINDICATIONS:** Hypersensitivity to any component of the vaccine is a contraindication (see DESCRIPTION in full prescribing information). Do not use BOOSTRIX after a serious allergic reaction (e.g., anaphylaxis) following any other tetanus toxoid, diphtheria toxoid or pertussis-containing vaccine, or any component of this vaccine (see DESCRIPTION in full prescribing information). Because of the uncertainty as to which component of the vaccine might be responsible, do not give further vaccination with any of these components; or, refer such individuals to an allergist for evaluation. The following events are contraindications to administration of BOOSTRIX: encephalopathy (e.g., coma, decreased level of consciousness, prolonged seizures) within 7 days of administration of a previous dose of a pertussis-containing vaccine that is not attributable to another identifiable cause; progressive neurologic disorder, uncontrolled epilepsy, or progressive encephalopathy. Do not vaccinate individuals with these conditions until a treatment regimen has been established and the condition has stabilized.

**WARNINGS:** The tip cap and the rubber plunger of the needleless prefilled syringes contain dry natural latex rubber that may cause allergic reactions in latex sensitive individuals. The vial stopper is latex-free. If any of the following events occurred in temporal relation to previous receipt of a Diphtheria and Tetanus Toxoids and Pertussis Vaccine Adsorbed (DTwP) vaccine or a vaccine containing an acellular pertussis component, consider carefully whether to give subsequent doses of BOOSTRIX: temperature of ≥40.5°C (105°F) within 48 hours not due to another identifiable cause; collapse or shock-like state (hypotonic-hyporesponsive episode) within 48 hours; persistent, inconsolable crying lasting ≥3 hours, occurring within 48 hours; seizures with or without fever occurring within 3 days. Persons who experienced serious Arthus-type hypersensitivity reactions following a prior dose of tetanus toxoid usually have high serum tetanus antitoxin levels and should not be given Tetanus and Diphtheria Toxoids Adsorbed For Adult Use (Td) or Tdap vaccines or even emergency doses of Td more frequently than every 10 years, even if the wound is neither clean nor minor. If Guillain-Barré syndrome has occurred within 6 weeks of receipt of prior vaccine containing tetanus toxoid, the decision to give BOOSTRIX or any vaccine containing tetanus toxoid should be based on careful consideration of the potential benefits and possible risks. The decision to administer a pertussis-containing vaccine to individuals with stable central nervous system (CNS) disorders must be made by the physician on an individual basis, with consideration of all relevant factors, and assessment of potential risks and benefits for that individual. Advise the patient, parent, or guardian of the potential increased risk involved (see PRECAUTIONS). A family history of seizures or other CNS disorders is not a contraindication to pertussis vaccine. The Advisory Committee on Immunization Practices (ACIP) has published guidelines for vaccination of persons with recent or acute illness (www.cdc.gov). Do not give BOOSTRIX to individuals with bleeding disorders such as hemophilia or thrombocytopenia, or to persons on anticoagulant therapy unless the potential benefit clearly outweighs the risk of administration. If the decision is made to administer BOOSTRIX to such persons, it should be given with caution with steps taken to avoid the risk of hematoma following the injection.

**PRECAUTIONS: General:** Before the injection of any biological, the physician should take all reasonable precautions to prevent allergic or other adverse reactions. Epinephrine injection (1:1,000) and other appropriate agents used for the control of immediate allergic reactions must be immediately available should an acute anaphylactic reaction occur. Immunosuppressed persons, including individuals receiving immunosuppressive therapy, may not develop the expected immune response. **Drug Interactions:** Do not mix BOOSTRIX with any other vaccine in the same syringe or vial. **Carcinogenesis, Mutagenesis, Impairment of Fertility:** BOOSTRIX has not been evaluated for carcinogenic or mutagenic potential, or for impairment of fertility. **Pregnancy:** Pregnancy Category C. Animal reproduction studies have not been conducted with BOOSTRIX. It is also not known whether BOOSTRIX can cause fetal harm when administered to a pregnant woman or can affect reproductive capacity. BOOSTRIX should be given to a pregnant woman only if clearly needed. Animal fertility studies have not been conducted with BOOSTRIX. In a developmental toxicity study, the effect of BOOSTRIX on embryo-fetal and pre-weaning development was evaluated in pregnant rats. Animals were administered INFANRIX® (Diphtheria and Tetanus Toxoids and Acellular Pertussis Vaccine Adsorbed) prior to gestation and BOOSTRIX during the period of organogenesis (gestation days 6, 8, 11) and later in pregnancy (gestation day 15), 0.1 mL/rat/occasion (a 45-fold increase compared to the human dose of BOOSTRIX on a body weight basis), by intramuscular injection. No adverse affect on pregnancy and lactation parameters, embryo-fetal or pre-weaning development was observed. There were no fetal malformations or other evidence of teratogenesis noted in this study. **Nursing Mothers:** It is not known whether BOOSTRIX is excreted in human milk. Because many drugs are excreted in human milk, caution should be exercised when BOOSTRIX is administered to a nursing woman. **Pregnancy Exposure Registry:** Healthcare providers are encouraged to register pregnant women who receive BOOSTRIX in the GlaxoSmithKline vaccination pregnancy registry by calling 1-888-825-5249. **Geriatric Use:** BOOSTRIX is not indicated for use in individuals older than 18 years. **Pediatric Use:** BOOSTRIX is not indicated for use in individuals younger than 10 years (see DOSAGE AND ADMINISTRATION in full prescribing information). For immunization of infants and children younger than 7 years against diphtheria, tetanus, and pertussis, refer to the manufacturers' package inserts for Diphtheria and Tetanus Toxoids and Acellular Pertussis Vaccine Adsorbed (DTaP) vaccines.

**ADVERSE REACTIONS:** A total of 3,608 adolescents were vaccinated with a single dose of BOOSTRIX during clinical trials. An additional 1,092 adolescents 10 to 18 years of age received a non-US formulation of BOOSTRIX (formulated to contain 0.5 mg aluminum per dose) in non-US clinical studies.

The primary safety study, conducted in the United States, was a randomized, observer-blinded, controlled study in which 3,080 adolescents 10 to 18 years of age received a single dose of BOOSTRIX and 1,034 received the control Td vaccine manufactured by Massachusetts Public Health Biologic Laboratories. There were no substantive differences in demographic characteristics between the vaccine groups. Among BOOSTRIX and control vaccine recipients approximately 75% were 10 to 14 years of age and approximately 25% were 15 to 18 years of age. Approximately 98% of participants in this study had received the recommended series of 4 or 5 doses of either DTwP or a combination of DTwP and DTaP in childhood. Data on adverse events were collected by the subjects, parents and/or guardians using standardized diaries for 15 consecutive days following the vaccine dose (i.e., day of vaccination and the next 14 days). Subjects were monitored for unsolicited adverse events that occurred within 31 days of vaccination (day 0-30) using diary cards (day 0-14) supplemented by spontaneous reports and a medical history as reported by subjects, parents, and/or guardians. Subjects were also monitored for 6 months post-vaccination for non-routine medical visits, visits to an emergency room, onset of new chronic illness, and serious adverse events. Information regarding late onset adverse events was obtained via a telephone call 6 months following vaccination. At least 97% of subjects completed the 6-month follow-up evaluation.

In a study conducted in Germany, BOOSTRIX was administered to 319 children 10 to 12 years of age previously vaccinated with 5 doses of acellular pertussis-containing vaccines, 193 of these subjects had previously received 5 doses of INFANRIX. Adverse events were recorded on diary cards during the 15 days following vaccination. Unsolicited adverse events that occurred within 31 days of vaccination (day 0-30) were recorded on the diary card or verbally reported to the investigator. Subjects were monitored for 6 months post-vaccination for physician office visits, emergency room visits, onset of new chronic illness, and serious adverse events. The 6-month follow-up evaluation, conducted via telephone interview, was completed by 90% of subjects.

The adverse event information from clinical trials provides a basis for identifying adverse events that appear to be related to vaccine use and for approximating rates. However, because clinical trials are conducted under widely varying conditions, adverse event rates observed in the clinical trials of a vaccine cannot be directly compared to rates in the clinical trials of another vaccine, and may not reflect the rates observed in practice.

**Serious Adverse Events in All Safety Studies:** In the US-safety study and German-safety study, no serious adverse events were reported to occur within 31 days of vaccination. During the 6-month extended safety evaluation period, no serious adverse events that were of potential autoimmune origin or new onset and chronic in nature were reported to occur. In non-US studies in which serious adverse events were monitored for up to 37 days, one subject was diagnosed with insulin dependent diabetes 20 days following administration of BOOSTRIX. No other serious adverse events of potential autoimmune origin or that were new onset and chronic in nature were reported to occur in these studies.

**Solicited Adverse Events in the US-Safety Study:** In a US study, the most common local adverse events following administration of BOOSTRIX were pain, redness, and swelling at the injection site. The most common general adverse events were headache and fatigue. Most of these events were reported at a similar frequency in recipients of both BOOSTRIX and Td. Any pain, grade 2 or 3 pain (but not grade 3 alone), and grade 2 or 3 headache (but not grade 3 alone) were reported at a higher rate in recipients of BOOSTRIX. The primary safety endpoint of the US study was the incidence of grade 3 pain (spontaneously painful and/or prevented normal activity) at the injection site within 15 days of vaccination. Grade 3 pain was reported in 4.6% of those who received BOOSTRIX compared with 4.0% of those who received the Td vaccine. The difference in rate of grade 3 pain was within the pre-defined clinical limit for non-inferiority (upper limit of the 95% CI for the difference ≤4%). These were the rates for solicited local and general adverse events within 15 days of vaccination with BOOSTRIX or Td vaccine for the total vaccinated cohort (all enrolled, vaccinated subjects with safety data available analyzed by vaccine received):

**Percentage of Individuals 10 to 18 Years of Age Reporting Solicited Local Adverse Events or Solicited General Adverse Events Within the 15-day* Post-Vaccination Period**

| | BOOSTRIX (N = 3,032) % | Td (N =1,013) % |
|---|---|---|
| **Local** | | |
| Pain,[†] any | 75.3 | 71.7 |
| Pain,[†] grade 2 or 3 | 51.2 | 42.5 |
| Pain,[‡] grade 3 | 4.6 | 4.0 |
| Redness, any | 22.5 | 19.8 |
| Redness, >20 mm | 4.1 | 3.9 |
| Redness, ≥50 mm | 1.7 | 1.6 |
| Swelling, any | 21.1 | 20.1 |
| Swelling, >20 mm | 5.3 | 4.9 |
| Swelling, ≥50 mm | 2.5 | 3.2 |
| Arm circumference increase,[§] >5 mm | 28.3 | 29.5 |
| Arm circumference increase,[§] >20 mm | 2.0 | 2.2 |
| Arm circumference increase,[§] >40 mm | 0.5 | 0.3 |
| **General** | | |
| Fever,[‖] ≥99.5°F | 13.5 | 13.1 |
| Fever,[‖] >100.4°F | 5.0 | 4.7 |
| Fever,[‖] >102.2°F | 1.4 | 1.0 |
| Headache, any | 43.1 | 41.5 |
| Headache,[†] grade 2 or 3 | 15.7 | 12.7 |
| Headache, grade 3 | 3.7 | 2.7 |
| Fatigue, any | 37.0 | 36.7 |
| Fatigue, grade 2 or 3 | 14.4 | 12.9 |
| Fatigue, grade 3 | 3.7 | 3.2 |
| Gastrointestinal symptoms,[¶] any | 26.0 | 25.8 |
| Gastrointestinal symptoms,[¶] grade 2 or 3 | 9.8 | 9.7 |
| Gastrointestinal symptoms,[¶] grade 3 | 3.0 | 3.2 |

Td = Tetanus and Diphtheria Toxoids Adsorbed For Adult Use manufactured by Massachusetts Public Health Biologic Laboratories.
N = number of subjects in the total vaccinated cohort with local/general symptoms sheets completed.
Grade 2 = Local: painful when the limb was moved; General: interfered with normal activity.
Grade 3 = Local: spontaneously painful and/or prevented normal activity; General: prevented normal activity.
*Day of vaccination and the next 14 days.
[†]Statistically significantly higher (P<0.05) following BOOSTRIX as compared to Td vaccine.
[‡]Grade 3 injection site pain following BOOSTRIX was not inferior to Td (upper limit of two-sided 95% CI for the difference in the percentage of subjects ≤4%).
[§]Mid-upper region of the vaccinated arm.
[‖]Oral temperatures or axillary temperatures.
[¶]Gastrointestinal symptoms included nausea, vomiting, diarrhea and/or abdominal pain.

Mid-upper arm circumference was measured by the adolescent or their parent/guardian prior to injection and daily for 15 days following vaccination. There was no significant difference between BOOSTRIX recipients and Td recipients in the proportion of subjects reporting an increase in mid-upper arm circumference in the vaccinated arm. The incidence of unsolicited adverse events reported in the 31 days after vaccination was comparable between the 2 groups.

**Solicited Adverse Events in the German Safety Study:** No cases of whole arm swelling were spontaneously reported. Two individuals (2/193) reported large injection site swelling (range 110 to 200 mm diameter), in one case associated with grade 3 pain. Neither individual sought medical attention. These episodes were reported to resolve without sequelae within 5 days. These were the rates of solicited local adverse events and fever within 15 days of vaccination for those subjects who had previously been vaccinated with 5 doses of INFANRIX:

**Rates of Solicited Adverse Events Reported Within the 15-day* Post-Vaccination Period Following Administration of BOOSTRIX in Individuals 10 to 12 Years of Age Who Had Previously Received 5 Doses of INFANRIX**

| Adverse Event | BOOSTRIX (N = 193) % (95% CI) |
|---|---|
| Pain, any | 62.2 (54.9-69.0) |
| Pain, grade 2 or 3 | 33.2 (26.6-40.3) |
| Pain, grade 3 | 5.7 (2.9-10.0) |
| Redness, any | 47.7 (40.4-55.0) |
| Redness, >20 mm | 15.0 (10.3-20.9) |
| Redness, ≥50 mm | 10.9 (6.9-16.2) |
| Swelling, any | 38.9 (31.9-46.1) |
| Swelling, >20 mm | 17.6 (12.5-23.7) |
| Swelling, ≥50 mm | 14.0 (9.4-19.7) |
| Fever, ≥99.5 | 8.8 (5.2-13.7) |
| Fever, >100.4 | 4.1 (1.8-8.0) |
| Fever, >102.2 | 1.0 (0.1-3.7) |

N = number of subjects with local/general symptoms sheets completed.
Grade 2 = Painful when the limb was moved.
Grade 3 = Spontaneously painful and/or prevented normal activity.
*Day of vaccination and the next 14 days.

As with any vaccine, there is the possibility that broad use of BOOSTRIX could reveal adverse events not observed in clinical trials.

**Postmarketing Reports:** Worldwide voluntary reports of adverse events received for BOOSTRIX in persons 10 to 18 years of age since market introduction of this vaccine are listed below. This list includes serious events or events which have causal connection to components of this or other vaccines or drugs. Because these events are reported voluntarily from a population of uncertain size, it is not possible to reliably estimate their frequency or establish a causal relationship to vaccine exposure. *Blood and lymphatic system disorders:* Lymphadenitis, lymphadenopathy. *Cardiac disorders:* Myocarditis. *Injection site reactions:* Induration, inflammation, mass, nodule, warmth, local reaction. *Metabolism and nutrition disorders:* Diabetes mellitus insulin-dependent. *Musculoskeletal and connective tissue disorders:* Arthralgia, back pain, myalgia. *Nervous system disorders:* Convulsion, encephalitis, facial palsy, paraesthesia. *Skin and subcutaneous tissue disorders:* Exanthem, Henoch-Schönlein purpura, rash. In addition, extensive swelling of the injected limb has been reported following administration of BOOSTRIX.

**Reporting Adverse Events:** Report the occurrence following immunization of any event set forth in the Vaccine Injury Table from the National Childhood Vaccine Injury Act including: Anaphylaxis or anaphylactic shock within 7 days, encephalopathy or encephalitis within 7 days, brachial neuritis within 28 days, or an acute complication or sequelae (including death) of an illness, disability, injury, or condition referred to above, or any events that would contraindicate further doses of vaccine, according to this prescribing information. These events should be reported to VAERS. The VAERS toll-free number is 1-800-822-7967. Reporting forms may also be obtained at the VAERS website at www.vaers.hhs.gov.

**DOSAGE AND ADMINISTRATION: Recommended Dose:** BOOSTRIX should be administered as a single 0.5 mL injection by the intramuscular route into the deltoid muscle of the upper arm in individuals 10 through 18 years of age. Do not administer this product subcutaneously or intravenously. There are no data to support repeat administration of BOOSTRIX. Five years should elapse between the subject's last dose of the recommended series of childhood DTwP and/or DTaP vaccine and the administration of BOOSTRIX. Limited data are available on the use of BOOSTRIX following Tetanus and Diphtheria Toxoids Adsorbed For Adult Use (Td) vaccine. **Additional Dosing Information:** ***Wound Management:*** Clinicians should refer to guidelines for tetanus prophylaxis in routine wound management. Adolescents 10 to 18 years of age who have completed a primary series against tetanus and who sustain wounds which are minor and uncomplicated, should receive a booster dose of a tetanus toxoid-containing vaccine only if they have not received tetanus toxoid within the preceding 10 years. In case of tetanus-prone injury (e.g., wounds contaminated with dirt, feces, soil, and saliva; puncture wounds; avulsions; and wounds resulting from missles, crushing, burns, and frostbite) in an adolescent who is in need of tetanus toxoid, BOOSTRIX can be used as an alternative to Tetanus and Diphtheria Toxoids Adsorbed For Adult Use (Td) vaccine in patients for whom the pertussis component is also indicated (see INDICATIONS AND USAGE).

Manufactured by **GlaxoSmithKline Biologicals**
Rixensart, Belgium, US License 1617
Distributed by **GlaxoSmithKline**
Research Triangle Park, NC 27709



Full prescribing information for BOOSTRIX is available at www.BOOSTRIX.com.
BRS-BO:L3

**References: 1.** Centers for Disease Control and Prevention. Preventing tetanus, diphtheria, and pertussis among adolescents: use of tetanus toxoid, reduced diphtheria toxoid and acellular pertussis vaccines: recommendations of the Advisory Committee on Immunization Practices (ACIP). Early Release 2006;55(February 23, 2006):1–43. **2.** Centers for Disease Control and Prevention. Recommended childhood and adolescent immunization schedule—United States, 2006. *MMWR.* 2006;54(51&52):Q1–Q4.

# Age at Drinking Onset and Alcohol Dependence

## *Age at Onset, Duration, and Severity*

*Ralph W. Hingson, ScD, MPH; Timothy Heeren, PhD; Michael R. Winter, MPH*

**Objective:** To examine whether starting to drink at an early age is associated with developing alcohol dependence at a younger age and chronic relapsing dependence, controlling for respondent demographics, smoking and illicit drug use, childhood antisocial behavior and depression, and family alcoholism history.

**Design:** Cross-sectional survey.

**Setting:** Nationwide face-to-face survey with a multistage probability sample.

**Participants:** A total of 43 093 adults were surveyed in 2001-2002.

**Main Outcome Measures:** Based on *Diagnostic and Statistical Manual of Mental Disorders, Fourth Edition,* criteria, lifetime alcohol dependence, dependence within 10 years of starting drinking, multiple episodes, an alcohol dependence episode in the past year, episodes exceeding 1 year, and meeting 6 or 7 dependence criteria.

**Results:** Relative to respondents who began drinking at 21 years or older, those who began drinking before age 14 years were more likely to experience alcohol dependence ever and within 10 years of first drinking (adjusted hazard ratios and 95% confidence intervals [CIs], 1.78 [1.51-2.11] and 1.69 [1.38-2.07], respectively). They also more often experienced past-year dependence and multiple dependence episodes (adjusted odds ratios, 1.93 [95% CI, 1.40-2.64] and 3.09 [95% CI, 2.19-4.35], respectively). Among alcohol-dependent persons, the odds were 2.62 (95% CI, 1.79-3.84) for having at least 1 episode exceeding 1 year and 2.89 (95% CI, 1.97-4.23) for meeting 6 or 7 dependence diagnostic criteria.

**Conclusion:** There is a need to screen and counsel adolescents about alcohol use and to implement policies and programs that delay alcohol consumption.

*Arch Pediatr Adolesc Med. 2006;160:739-746*

MORE THAN 75 000 DEATHS annually are attributable to excessive alcohol consumption, the third leading preventable cause of death in the United States.[1] Unhealthy alcohol use is found in 7% to 20% of outpatients, 30% to 40% of emergency department patients, and 50% of trauma patients.[2]

The Centers for Disease Control and Prevention's 2003 Youth Risk Behavior Survey of high school students nationwide revealed that 28% drank alcohol other than a few sips before age 13 years.[3] By age 17 years they were 7 times more likely to consume 5 or more drinks 6 or more times per month than those who waited until they were 17 years or older to begin drinking. The National Institute on Alcohol Abuse and Alcoholism has defined binge drinking as males consuming 5 or more and females 4 or more drinks in 2 hours.[4] Binge drinking for the average person on an empty stomach produces a blood alcohol level of 0.08% or higher, the legal level of intoxication in every state.[5] Thus, those who begin drinking before age 13 years are much more likely even in high school to frequently drink to intoxication. Compared with other students, the approximately 1 million frequent heavy drinkers more often exhibit behaviors that pose risk to themselves and others, such as riding with drinking drivers; driving after drinking; never wearing safety belts; carrying guns and other weapons; becoming injured in fights and suicide attempts; having unplanned and unprotected sex; becoming or making someone else pregnant; using tobacco, marijuana, and other illicit drugs; drinking and smoking marijuana at school; and earning mostly low grades (*D*'s and *F*'s) in school.[4]

Starting to drink at an early age is also associated with alcohol dependence and related problems during adult life. Accord-

**Author Affiliations:** Youth Alcohol Prevention Center, Boston University School of Public Health, Boston, Mass.

ing to analyses of the National Longitudinal Alcohol Epidemiologic Study (NLAES), a national survey of adults 18 years and older conducted in 1991-1992 (N=42 682; response rate, 90%), among persons who began drinking before age 14 years, 45% developed *Diagnostic and Statistical Manual of Mental Disorders, Fourth Edition (DSM-IV)*, diagnosable dependence compared with 10% of persons who waited until they were 21 years or older.[6] Those relations persisted after controlling analytically for family history of alcoholism, age, sex, race/ethnicity,[7] history of cigarette and other drug use, education, and marital status.[8]

Early drinking onset has also been linked, after episodes of drinking among both adolescents and adults, to unintentional injuries, motor vehicle crashes, physical fights, unplanned and unprotected sex,[8-12] nicotine dependence, illicit substance use, antisocial personality, conduct disorder, and academic underachievement.[13] Not all alcohol-dependent persons remain dependent throughout their lives. In the NLAES, whereas 12% experienced alcohol dependence at some point, 4% did so during the year preceding the survey.[6]

Unexplored has been whether starting to drink at a younger age is associated with developing dependence at a younger age and chronic relapsing dependence, characterized by multiple episodes, past-year dependence among adults of all ages, and among alcohol-dependent individuals, episodes of longer duration and a wider range of symptoms. This study examines these questions in a more recent national survey.

## METHODS

In 2001-2002, the National Institute on Alcohol Abuse and Alcoholism conducted the National Epidemiologic Survey on Alcohol and Related Conditions (NESARC).[14] Under contract, the US Census Bureau, supervised by the National Institute on Alcohol Abuse and Alcoholism, conducted face-to-face interviews with a multistage probability sample of 43 093 adults 18 years and older (response rate, 81%). The survey methods and other quality control procedures and test-retest reliability tests have been detailed by Grant et al.[14] The research protocol, including informed consent procedures, received full ethical review and approval from the US Census Bureau and the Office of Management and Budget.

### DIAGNOSTIC ASSESSMENT

The NESARC used the National Institute on Alcohol Abuse and Alcoholism's Alcohol Use Disorder and Associated Disabilities Interview Schedule *DSM-IV* version (AUDADIS-IV), a state-of-the-art structured diagnostic interview designed for use by nonclinician lay interviewers. Computer algorithms were designed to produce diagnoses of abuse and dependence consistent with the final *DSM-IV* criteria. Numerous national and international psychometric studies[14-25] have documented good to excellent reliability and validity of the AUDADIS-IV alcohol abuse and dependence criteria, including clinical reappraisals conducted by psychiatrists in clinical and general population samples.

On the basis of *DSM-IV* variables, lifetime and past-year alcohol dependence in the NESARC were defined by 7 diagnostic criteria: tolerance; the withdrawal syndrome or drinking to relieve or avoid withdrawal symptoms; drinking larger amounts or for a longer period than intended; persistent desire or unsuccessful attempts to cut down on drinking; spending a great deal of time obtaining alcohol, drinking, or recovering from effects of drinking; giving up important social, occupational, or recreational activities in favor of drinking; and continued drinking despite physical or psychological problems caused by drinking. Diagnosis of a 12-month alcohol dependence required that respondents satisfy 3 of the 7 *DSM-IV* criteria for dependence in the past year or during any year before the past year. Diagnosis of dependence before the past year also required clustering, as specified in the *DSM-IV*, of at least 3 dependence criteria in any 1 year of the respondent's life. Lifetime diagnosis includes all respondents who were dependent in the past year or before the past year. Alcohol dependence withdrawal criteria required at least 2 positive symptoms of withdrawal as defined by *DSM-IV* alcohol withdrawal diagnosis.

Duration criteria associated with dependence criteria in the NESARC define the repetitiveness with which these diagnostic criteria must occur to be positive. They were operationalized by means of qualifiers such as "recurrent," "often," and "persistent" and were embedded directly in the symptom questions. Several dependence-related outcomes were examined: lifetime dependence; dependence within 10 years of drinking onset, before age 25 years, and in the past year; experiencing 2 or more dependence episodes; episodes exceeding 1 year; and meeting 6 or 7 dependence symptom criteria.

Persons who met dependence criteria were asked how old they were the first time some of these experiences began to happen around the same time. We examined the incidence of dependence by years after drinking onset (for lifetime dependence and dependence within 10 years of drinking onset) and by chronological age (for dependence before age 25 years).

To determine the number of episodes, respondents who ever experienced dependence were asked, "In your entire life, how many separate periods like this did you have when some of these experiences were happening around the same time? By separate periods, I mean times that were separated by at least 1 year when you either stopped drinking entirely or you did not have any of the experiences you mentioned with alcohol at all." Duration of longest dependence was ascertained by asking diagnosed persons the longest period they had when some of these experiences were happening around the same time. Persons with lifetime and past-year dependence were stratified into those who met 6 or 7 vs 3 to 5 of the dependence diagnostic criteria.

Respondents were asked the age at which they first started drinking, not counting tastes or sips, which was categorized as younger than 14 years, separately for each year from 14 through 20 years old, and 21 years and older (the minimum legal drinking age in the United States). Family history of alcohol problems was positive if first-degree relatives (mother, father, sister, brother, son, or daughter) had an alcohol problem. Antisocial behavior was positive if respondents reported 3 or more antisocial behaviors before age 15 years, and depression was based on meeting *DSM-IV* criteria before age 14 years. The *DSM-IV* criteria for dysthymia and generalized anxiety were also examined. Test-retest reliability of AUDADIS-IV measures for depression, dysthmia, and antisocial behaviors were good ($\kappa$=0.65, 0.58, and 0.67, respectively; mean $\kappa$=0.64).[24]

Respondents were asked if they had ever and in the past year used 1 of 10 types of drugs: sedatives, tranquilizers, pain killers, stimulants, marijuana, cocaine, hallucinogens, inhalants, heroin, and other medicines. Persons who had ever smoked 100 cigarettes were considered cigarette users.

### DATA ANALYSIS

A software program (SUDAAN version 8.1; Research Triangle Institute, Research Triangle Park, NC) was used that applies Taylor series linearization to adjust for the complex survey

**Table. Dependence and, Among Dependents, Duration of Longest Dependence Episode and Number of Dependence Symptoms According to Age Started Drinking: National Epidemiologic Survey on Alcohol and Related Conditions***

| Age Started Drinking, y | Ever Drank, No. (%) (N = 26 829) | Dependence, % | | | | | | Among Persons Ever Alcohol Dependent, % | | | |
|---|---|---|---|---|---|---|---|---|---|---|---|
| | | Never | Lifetime† | Within 10 y† | Before Age 25 y† | Past Year | ≥2 Episodes | Duration of Longest Episode, mo <13 | 13-24 | ≥25 | 6-7 Dependence Symptoms |
| <14 | 1380 (5) | 53 | 47 | 27 | 33 | 13 | 15 | 42 | 17 | 41 | 54 |
| 14 | 956 (4) | 55 | 45 | 28 | 31 | 12 | 11 | 50 | 11 | 38 | 50 |
| 15 | 1516 (6) | 62 | 38 | 26 | 27 | 10 | 9 | 53 | 13 | 34 | 41 |
| 16 | 2925 (11) | 68 | 32 | 21 | 22 | 10 | 8 | 55 | 12 | 33 | 30 |
| 17 | 2761 (10) | 72 | 28 | 19 | 19 | 8 | 7 | 60 | 12 | 28 | 30 |
| 18 | 5834 (22) | 85 | 15 | 10 | 10 | 4 | 3 | 57 | 12 | 31 | 23 |
| 19 | 2063 (8) | 83 | 17 | 10 | 11 | 4 | 5 | 54 | 15 | 31 | 33 |
| 20 | 1978 (7) | 89 | 11 | 6 | 6 | 3 | 3 | 68 | 6 | 26 | 24 |
| ≥21 | 7416 (28) | 91 | 9 | 4 | 2 | 2 | 2 | 61 | 12 | 27 | 24 |

*$P<.001$ for all. *P* values refer to bivariate relationships between age started drinking and alcohol dependence outcomes tested using $\chi^2$ analysis.
†From Kaplan-Meier survival analysis.

sample design to estimate prevalence and standard errors for prevalence as well as odds ratios and 95% confidence intervals (CIs) using logistic regression. To be consistent with previous NLAES age at drinking onset analyses,[6-9] analyses focused only on respondents who drank 12 or more drinks in at least 1 year of their life. We used $\chi^2$ analyses to test the significance of relationships among age at drinking onset, background characteristics, and the various dependence outcomes.

Kaplan-Meier survival curves were calculated to describe the prevalence of alcohol dependence as a function of years since drinking onset, by age at drinking onset. Because of the cross-sectional nature of the NESARC sample, older respondents have longer follow-up after drinking onset and greater opportunity to develop dependence; survival data methods appropriately account for available follow-up, treating those without a history of dependence as censored at age of follow-up. Hazard ratios and 95% CIs from Cox proportional hazards multiple regression models assessed the increased risk of dependence for those with younger age at onset vs those with onset at 21 years or older (the reference group), controlling for demographic and other factors known to be related to age at drinking onset (expression of antisocial behaviors before age 15 years,[13] major depression before age 14 years,[26] and family history of alcohol dependence). Survival methods were also used to analyze dependence within 10 years of onset (censoring those who were dependence free 10 years after onset) and dependence before age 25 years (with chronological age at dependence as the outcome).

Controlling for demographic and background characteristics known to be related to age at drinking onset, logistic regression models examined relationships between age at drinking onset and the following outcomes: lifetime dependence, past-year dependence, experiencing 2 or more dependence episodes, and, among ever-dependent respondents, episodes exceeding 1 year and meeting 6 or 7 dependence symptom criteria. Odds ratios and 95% CIs were calculated describing the increased risk of dependence outcomes for those with drinking onset before age 14 years and at each age from 14 through 20 years relative to those who started drinking at or after age 21 years (the reference group).

## RESULTS

At some point in their lives, 12.5% of the NESARC sample met *DSM-IV* alcohol dependence criteria, 19% of ever drinkers, representing more than 26 million Americans. Eight

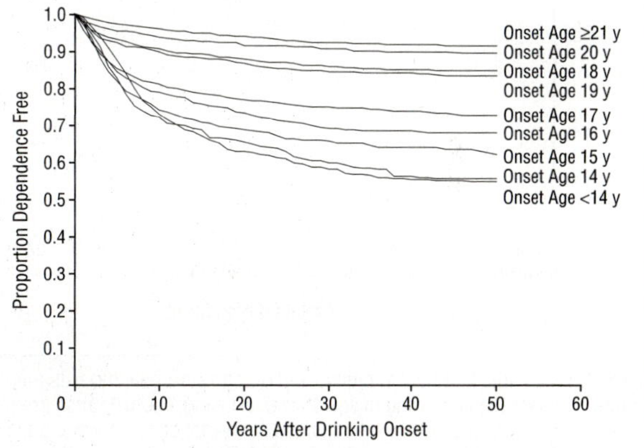


**Figure 1.** Kaplan-Meier survival curves describing the proportion of dependence-free individuals by age at drinking onset.

percent of the sample met the criteria before age 25 years, representing more than 16 million people. During the survey year, 3.8% of the sample, representing 7.9 million people, met the alcohol dependence criteria, one third of lifetime dependents. Three percent of the sample reported 2 or more episodes.

Among ever drinkers, 14% first became dependent within 10 years of drinking onset, 45% experienced an episode exceeding 1 year, and 33% had at least 6 of 7 potential dependence diagnostic criteria. Nine percent of ever drinkers met antisocial behavior criteria before age 15 years, 2% met depression criteria before age 14 years, and less than 1% met generalized anxiety or dysthmia criteria. The **Table** lists the percentages of ever drinkers who began before age 14 years and at each year from 14 through 21 years and older.

Early age at first drinking was strongly associated with the proportion of respondents who experienced alcohol dependence in their lifetime, within 10 years of drinking onset, before age 25 years, and during the survey year (when the average respondent age was 44 years) and who experienced multiple episodes of dependence (**Figure 1** and

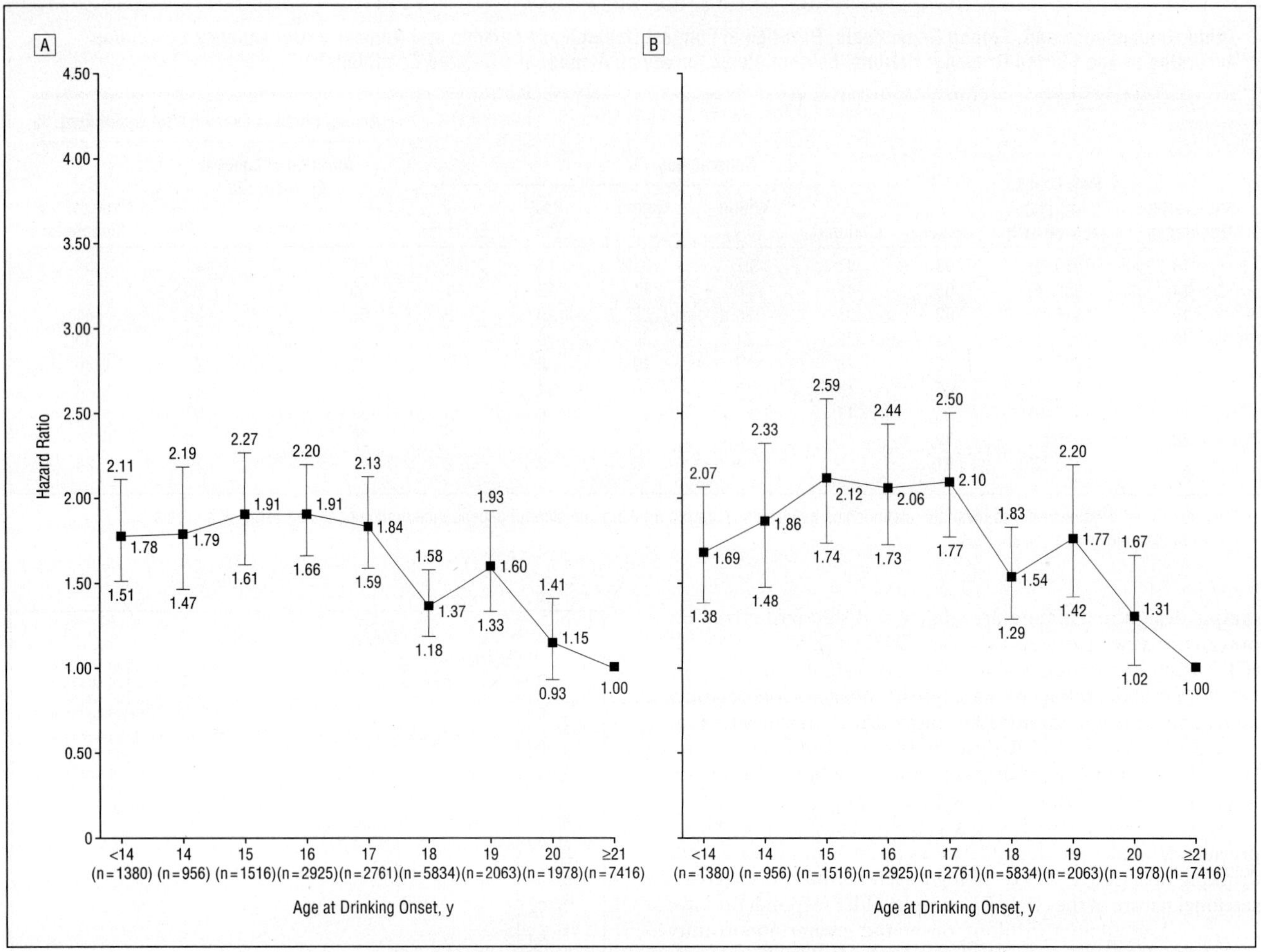


**Figure 2.** Mean adjusted hazard ratios from Cox proportional hazards multiple regressions for ever alcohol dependent (A) and alcohol dependent within 10 years of drinking onset (B) according to age started drinking. Hazard ratios are relative to those who started drinking at 21 years or older controlling for age, sex, race/ethnicity, highest grade in school, current marital status, former and current smoking, former and current drug use, family history of alcoholism, antisocial behavior before age 15 years, and depression before age 14 years. Error bars represent 95% confidence intervals.

Table). Comparing those who began drinking before age 14 years vs age 21 years or older, 47% vs 9% experienced lifetime dependence, 27% vs 4% within 10 years of onset, and 33% vs 2% before age 25 years (Kaplan-Meier survival estimates). Among persons who started to drink before age 14 years, 13% met the alcohol dependence criteria during the survey year, and 15% experienced 2 or more dependence episodes compared with only 2% of those who waited until they were 21 years or older (Table).

Individuals who began drinking at younger ages were more likely to experience multiple dependence episodes. However, among persons with lifetime dependence, early-onset drinkers were not more likely to experience multiple episodes, but they were more likely to experience episodes of longer duration (Table). Among those who began drinking before age 14 years, 58% experienced an episode lasting more than 1 year compared with 39% of those who waited until they were 21 years or older to begin drinking (Table).

Proportional hazards models and logistic regression analysis revealed that relative to those who waited until age 21 years or older, those who started drinking before age 14 years had elevated hazards of developing lifetime dependence (1.78; 95% CI, 1.51-2.11), dependence within 10 years of drinking onset (1.69; 95% CI, 1.38-2.07) (**Figure 2**), dependence before age 25 years (8.12; 95% CI, 6.33-10.43) (figure available on request), and past-year dependence (1.93; 95% CI, 1.40-2.64) (**Figure 3**) (proportional hazards regressions) and 3.09 (95% CI, 2.19-4.35) times the odds of experiencing 2 or more dependence episodes (logistic regressions) (Figure 3). These relationships held after controlling for age, sex, race/ethnicity, highest grade in school, marital status, former and current smoking, drug use, history of antisocial behavior before age 15 years, major depression before age 14 years, and family history of alcoholism.

Furthermore, among dependent persons relative to those who waited until they were 21 years or older, those who began drinking before age 14 years had 2.62 (95% CI, 1.79-3.84) times the odds of experiencing episodes exceeding 1 year and 2.89 (95% CI, 1.97-4.23) times the odds of experiencing 6 or 7 vs 3 to 5 dependence symptoms after controlling for the aforementioned covariates (**Figure 4**). Usually, each additional year earlier than age 21 years that a respondent began to drink, the greater the odds that he or she would develop the alcohol dependence outcomes examined.

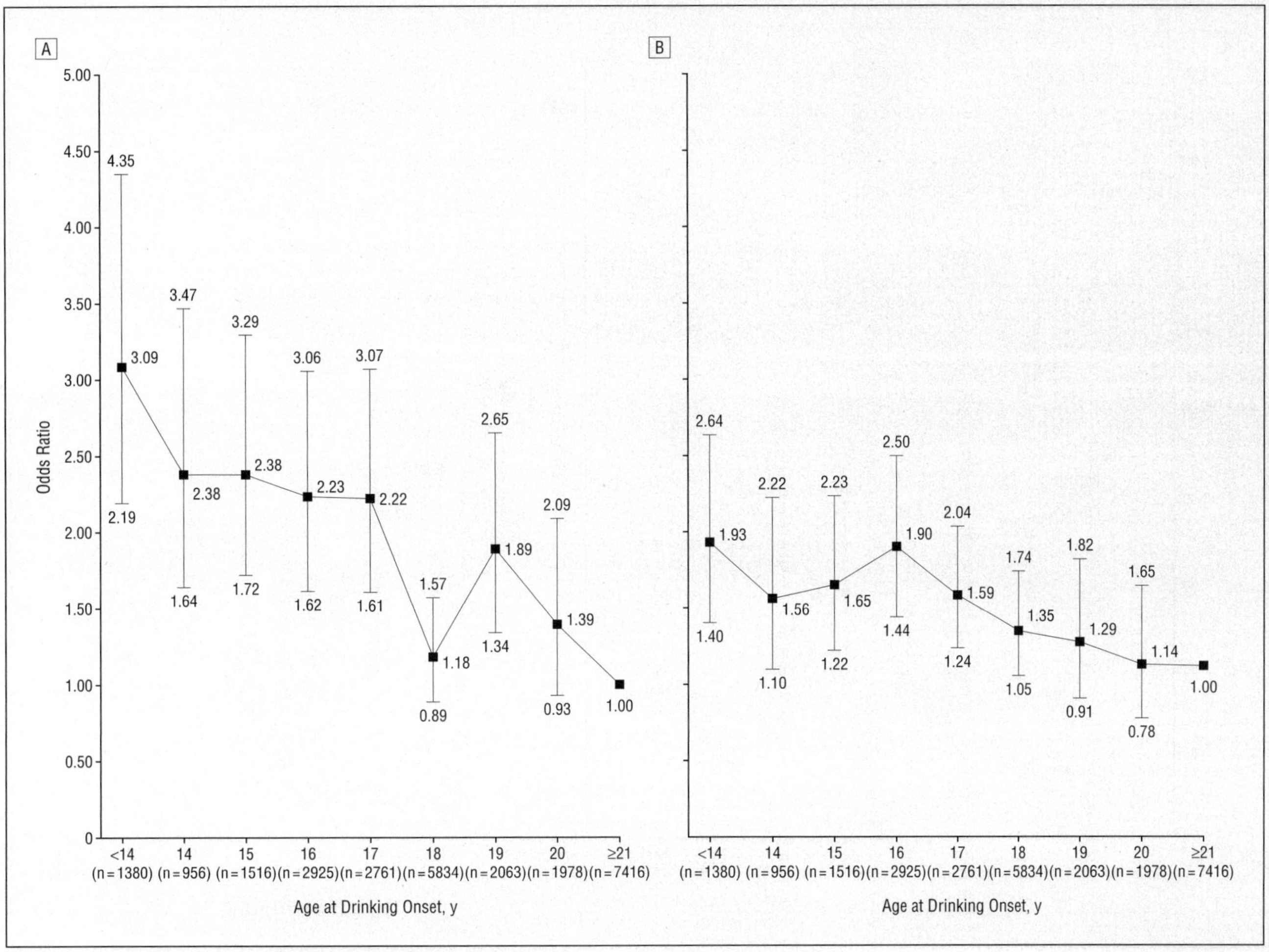


**Figure 3.** Mean adjusted odds ratios for 2 or more episodes of dependence vs 1 or fewer (A) and for past-year alcohol dependence (B) according to age started drinking. Odds ratios are relative to those who started drinking at 21 years or older controlling for age, sex, race/ethnicity, highest grade in school, current marital status, former and current smoking, former and current drug use, family history of alcoholism, antisocial behavior before age 15 years, and depression before age 14 years. Error bars represent 95% confidence intervals.

## COMMENT

This analysis underscores the importance of systematically exploring and counseling adolescent patients about their drinking practices. Because pediatric medical care providers considerably underdiagnose alcohol use, abuse, and dependence among patients aged 14 to 18 years, structured screening devices have been recommended to more accurately identify these conditions.[27] Among NESARC respondents, the percentage that experience onset of alcohol dependence peaks at age 18 years and rapidly declines after age 25 years.[28] Similar to results from the NLAES collected a decade earlier,[8] this study found that the younger respondents were when they began drinking, the greater their likelihood of experiencing lifetime alcohol dependence after analytically controlling for family history of alcoholism and numerous behavioral and personality characteristics related to the age at drinking onset. This persistence raises the possibility that this relationship may not be solely a by-product of greater risk-taking behavior among early drinkers reflected by tobacco or drug use or predisposing psychological characteristics or disorders that include childhood antisocial personality or major depression. Nearly half (46%) of drinkers who developed alcohol dependence began drinking at 16 years or younger, although only one quarter of drinkers started by that age. Other measures of adolescent risk taking not included in the survey could not be assessed as potential confounders.

This study identifies several new findings. First, the younger the age at which people started to drink, the greater their likelihood of developing alcohol dependence within 10 years of drinking onset and before age 25 years. Nearly half (47%) of the respondents who ever experienced alcohol dependence were first diagnosable by age 21 years, and two thirds by age 25 years. Furthermore, the younger the age at drinking onset, the stronger the subsequent association with chronic relapsing dependence, characterized by multiple episodes, past-year dependence, and, among dependent persons, episodes of longer duration and a wider range of symptoms.

Several issues should be considered in interpreting these results. First, this cross-sectional survey required recall many years earlier by some respondents of the age at which they began to drink and whether they experienced antisocial tendencies or major depression during childhood. The analyses indicate that age at drinking onset and dependence relationships were strongest among

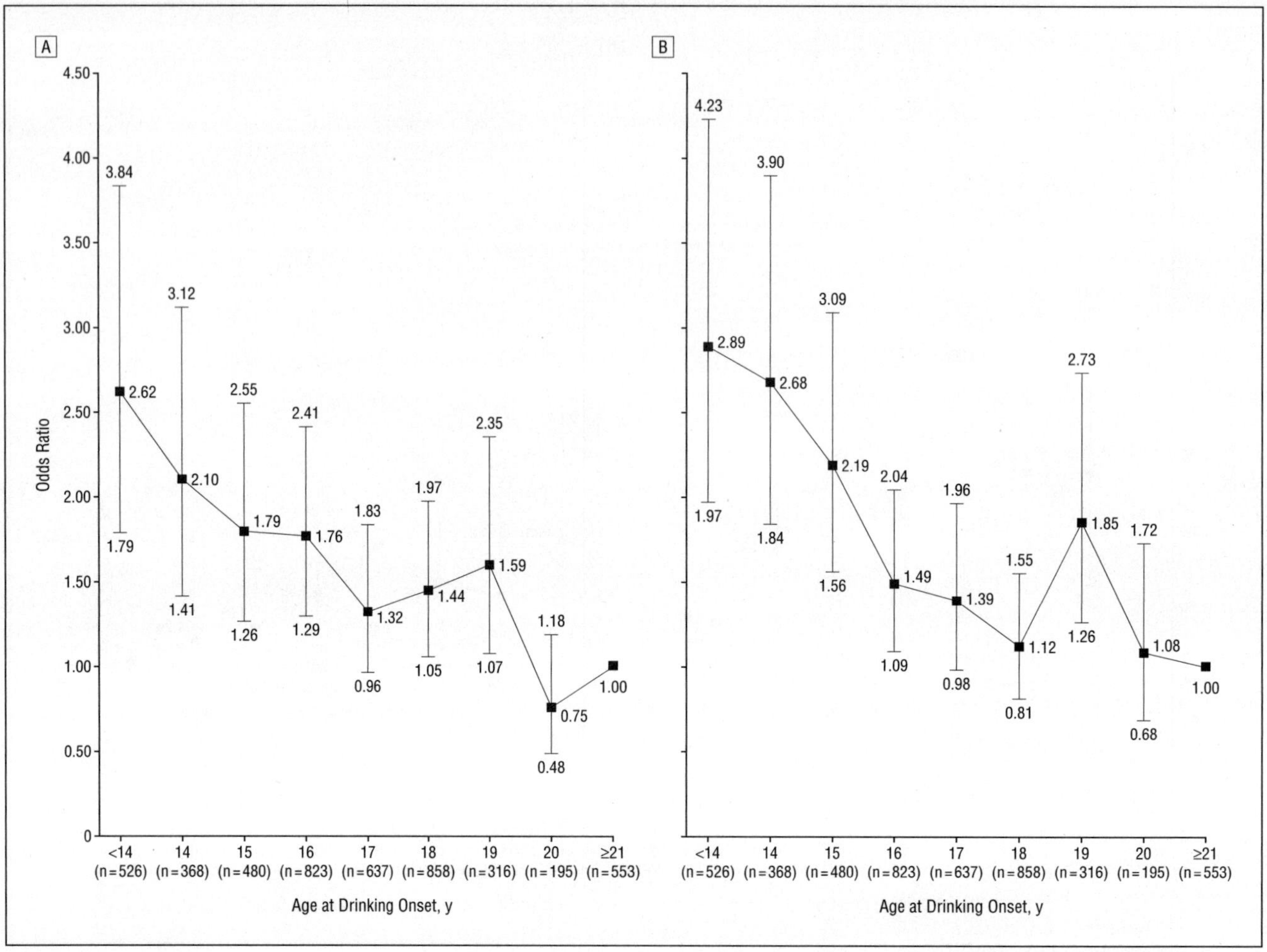


**Figure 4.** Mean adjusted odds ratios among persons ever alcohol dependent for duration of dependence of 1 year or more vs less than 1 year (A) and 6 or 7 dependence symptoms vs 3 to 5 (B) according to age started drinking. Odds ratios are relative to those who started drinking at 21 years or older controlling for age, sex, race/ethnicity, highest grade in school, current marital status, former and current smoking, former and current drug use, family history of alcoholism, antisocial behavior before age 15 years, and depression before age 14 years. Error bars represent 95% confidence intervals.

individuals younger than 34 years, for whom the recall period was shortest (data available on request).

Despite this survey's excellent response rates and analytic adjustments for respondent age and numerous personal and behavioral characteristics, longitudinal studies that begin during childhood, before drinking onset, and that follow adolescents into adult life would be preferable. They can prospectively test the potential age at drinking onset and alcohol dependence relation and may offer insights into mechanisms at work. A 12-year follow-up of the National Longitudinal Study of Youth found that earlier age at drinking onset is prospectively associated with alcohol dependence and abuse,[29] as did another analysis of a community sample followed longitudinally from age 12 to 30 years. That study found the strongest association among those who began drinking outside the home.[30]

Second, social desirability biases may foster underreporting of alcohol use and associated problems, prompting underdiagnosis of alcohol dependence. On the other hand, persons willing to report heavy drinking may be less hesitant than others to report adverse drinking consequences. Also, people with alcohol dependence may be more likely to remember when they started drinking because of consequences experienced later in life, thereby generating stronger relations between drinking onset age and alcohol dependence.

Third, consistent with age at earlier drinking onset research,[6-9] the present analyses focused on drinkers as defined in the NLAES: respondents who drank 12 or more drinks in at least 1 year of their life. In the NESARC, 27 324 respondents (63%) met those criteria. We repeated our analysis with the larger subset of NESARC respondents who reported ever having 1 or more drinks (n=38 827; 81%) and observed the same pattern of relationships between age at drinking onset and dependence outcomes (data available on request).

Fourth, although extensive research has established the reliability of lifetime and past-year alcohol dependence based on *DSM-IV* criteria using the AUDADIS-IV, the reliability of numbers of dependence episodes and duration of episodes has not received the same attention, and their association with drinking onset requires more cautious interpretation. Furthermore, some researchers question whether the meaning of *DSM-IV* criteria differs in adolescents and adults. During adolescence, increased tolerance to alcohol is probably a normal developmental phenomenon.[31] Also, the criteria "using more than intended" among adolescents may have more to do with social influences than the compulsion to drink.[32,33] In this study, almost all the persons diagnosed as being dependent reported these symptoms regardless of age at drinking onset.

Fifth, potential confounding variables not considered may have been responsible for the observed relations. Genetic factors, disinhibitory behavior patterns, and other psychiatric disorders may relate to early drinking onset and the development of alcohol dependence.[13] Also, children who experienced overt physical, sexual, or psychological abuse or whose parents exhibited psychiatric symptoms may start to drink at an earlier age and may drink larger amounts to cope with posttraumatic stress disorders. Of note, less than 1% of persons who ever drank met the *DSM-IV* criteria for dysthmia or generalized anxiety before age 14 years, and inclusion of these variables in regression analyses negligibly affected the study results.

A study[34] of sibling/twin/adopted adolescents aged 12 to 19 years reported that alcohol use in that age group is minimally affected by genetics but rather largely arises from environmental effects. Similar findings were reported in an analysis comparing persons with a family history of alcoholism and controls.[35] The strength of genetic effect on adolescent drinking has been found to increase from middle to late adolescence[36] and to overlap extensively with genetic effects on other disinhibited behaviors.[37,38] Thus, environmental factors may be most predictive of initial alcohol exposure, and environmental and genetic factors may interact in the development of lifetime, early-onset, and chronic relapsing dependence. Future research assessing these gene-environmental interactions should examine whether age at first drink or age at first alcohol dependence is more predictive of chronic relapsing dependence.

Sixth, although this analysis controlled for family history of alcoholism, many children born to nonalcoholic parents may nonetheless be raised in environments that allow youth easier access to alcohol. Also, some respondents may have had peers who engaged in heavy drinking and drug use that, in turn, contributed to earlier and heavier drinking, thereby fostering dependence.

Research is needed in different cultural settings. A Canadian study[39] found that early age at onset was related to subsequent alcohol dependence, despite a lower legal drinking age. Recent research[40] found that 29 of 30 European countries that have lower legal drinking ages than the United States had higher percentages of 15-year-olds who drink. Most of these countries also had a higher percentage of 15-year-olds who drink heavily (≥5 drinks per occasion) and to intoxication. However, Italy, France, Portugal, and Greece had similar or smaller percentages than the United States. Whether young people in those countries are more likely to drink with family and in meal settings and whether such practices moderate risks posed by early drinking warrant study.

These methodological considerations notwithstanding, this study reinforces important concerns about youth starting to drink at early ages. The human brain is still developing into the middle 20s. Some investigators have reported that compared with demographically matched nondependent adolescents from similar communities, adolescents who are dependent exhibit decrements in memory, spatial relations, and planning, and in magnetic resonance imaging studies exhibited less hippocampal development.[41,42] Whether these decrements preceded and contributed to the development of alcohol dependence and whether these problems will resolve if drinking is curtailed are not known. It is, however, known that alcohol dependence during the adult years is associated with visuospatial, executive, psychomotor, and memory decrements[43]; smaller brain volume[44-46]; and a host of social, work-related, and health problems.[47]

Recent clinical trials indicate that motivational counseling interventions can result in decreases in drinking and alcohol-related negative consequences among adolescents and college students.[48,49] Also, raising the legal drinking age to 21 years reduced drinking, alcohol-related traffic deaths, and deaths from other unintentional injuries among persons younger than 21 years.[50-52] A national analysis found that the law also reduced drinking among persons when they became 21 to 25 years of age,[52] but the effect of the law on the proportion of persons who develop alcohol dependence during adolescence or the adult years has not been studied. In addition studies have not examined whether other interventions that delay drinking onset also reduce the development of alcohol dependence during adolescence and adulthood. Although the results of this study suggest that such an impact is plausible, confirmatory longitudinal experimental research is needed. Whether interventions can delay the onset of alcohol use among adolescents and, in turn, reduce the development of alcohol dependence during adolescence and the adult years and its wide range of adverse consequences is a research question of vast medical, social, and public health importance.

**Accepted for Publication:** January 11, 2006.
**Correspondence:** Ralph W. Hingson, ScD, MPH, Youth Alcohol Prevention Center, Boston University School of Public Health, 715 Albany St, Boston, MA 02118 (rhingson@mail.nih.gov).
**Author Contributions:** *Study concept and design:* Hingson, Heeren, and Winter. *Acquisition of data:* Heeren. *Analysis and interpretation of data:* Hingson, Heeren, and Winter. *Drafting of the manuscript:* Hingson. *Critical revision of the manuscript for important intellectual content:* Heeren and Winter. *Statistical analysis:* Heeren and Winter. *Obtained funding:* Hingson. *Administrative, technical, and material support:* Hingson. *Study supervision:* Hingson.
**Financial Disclosure:** None reported.
**Funding/Support:** This study was supported by grant P60-AA013759 from the National Institute on Alcohol Abuse and Alcoholism.
**Additional Information:** This article is dedicated to Brian Paul McKelvey, who first sought treatment for alcohol problems at age 16 years. Two and a half years later, while in recovery, Brian was struck and fatally injured by an intoxicated driver.

## REFERENCES

1. Centers for Disease Control and Prevention. Alcohol-attributable deaths and years of potential life lost—United States, 2001. *MMWR Morb Mortal Wkly Rep.* 2004;53:866-870.
2. Saitz R. Unhealthy alcohol use. *N Engl J Med.* 2005;352:596-607.

3. Grunbaum J, Kaun L, Kinchen S, et al. Youth Risk Behavior Surveillance—United States, 2003. *MMWR Surveill Summ.* 2004;53:1-96.
4. Hingson R. Advances in measurement and intervention for excessive drinking. *Am J Prev Med.* 2004;27:261-263.
5. Hingson R, Winter M. Epidemiology and consequences of drinking and driving. *Alcohol Res Health.* 2003;27:63-78.
6. Grant BF, Dawson DA. Age at onset of alcohol use and its association with *DSM-IV* alcohol abuse and dependence: results from the National Longitudinal Alcohol Epidemiologic Survey. *J Subst Abuse.* 1997;9:103-110.
7. Grant BF. The impact of a family history of alcoholism on the relationship between age at onset of alcohol use and *DSM IV* dependence: results from the National Longitudinal Alcohol Epidemiologic Survey. *Alcohol Health Res World.* 1998;22:144-147.
8. Hingson RW, Heeren T, Jamanka A, Howland J. Age of drinking onset and unintentional injury involvement after drinking. *JAMA.* 2000;284:1527-1533.
9. Hingson R, Heeren T, Zakocs R. Age of drinking onset and involvement in physical fights after drinking. *Pediatrics.* 2001;108:872-877.
10. Hingson R, Heeren T, Levenson S, Jamanka A, Voas R. Age of drinking onset, driving after drinking, and involvement in alcohol related motor-vehicle crashes. *Accid Anal Prev.* 2002;34:85-92.
11. Hingson R, Heeren T, Winter M, Wechsler H. Early age of first drunkenness as a factor in college students' unplanned and unprotected sex due to drinking. *Pediatrics.* 2003;111:34-41.
12. Hingson R, Heeren T, Zakocs R, Winter M, Wechsler H. Age of first intoxication, heavy drinking, driving after drinking and risk of unintentional injury among U.S. college students. *J Stud Alcohol.* 2003;64:23-31.
13. McGue M, Iacono W, Legrand N, Elkins I. Origins and consequences of age at first drink, II: familial risk and heretability. *Alcohol Clin Exp Res.* 2001;25:1166-1173.
14. Grant BF, Dawson D, Stinson F, Chou S, Dufour M, Pickering R. The 12-month prevalence and trends in *DSM-IV* alcohol abuse and dependence: United States, 1991-1992 and 2001-2002. *Drug Alcohol Depend.* 2004;74:223-234.
15. Cottler LB, Grant BF, Blaine J, et al. Concordance of *DSM-IV* alcohol and drug use disorder criteria and diagnosis as measured by AUDADIS-ADR, CIDI, and SCAN. *Drug Alcohol Depend.* 1997;47:195-205.
16. Grant BF. *DSM-IV, DSM-III-R* and *ICD-10* alcohol and drug abuse/harmful use and dependence, United States, 1992: a nosological comparison. *Alcohol Clin Exp Res.* 1996;20:1481-1488.
17. Grant BF, Harford TC, Dawson DA, Chou PS, Pickering R. The Alcohol Use Disorder and Associated Disabilities Schedule (AUDADIS): reliability of alcohol and drug modules in a general population sample. *Drug Alcohol Depend.* 1995;39:37-44.
18. Hasin D, Li Q, McCloud S, Endicott J. Agreement between *DSM-III-R, DSM-IV* and *ICD-10* alcohol diagnosis in a US community-sample of heavy drinkers. *Addiction.* 1996;91:1517-1527.
19. Hasin D, Carpenter KM, McCloud S, Smith M, Grant BF. The Alcohol Use Disorder and Associated Disabilities Interview Schedule (AUDADIS): reliability of alcohol and drug modules in a clinical sample. *Drug Alcohol Depend.* 1997;44:133-141.
20. Hasin D, Grant BF, Cottler L, et al. Nosological comparisons of alcohol and drug diagnoses: a multisite, multi-instrument international study. *Drug Alcohol Depend.* 1997;47:217-226.
21. Hasin DS, Van Rossem R, McCloud S, Endicott J. Differentiating *DSM-IV* alcohol dependence and abuse by course: community heavy drinkers. *J Subst Abuse.* 1997;9:127-135.
22. Hasin D, Paykin A. Alcohol dependence and abuse diagnoses: concurrent validity in a nationally representative sample. *Alcohol Clin Exp Res.* 1999;23:144-150.
23. Ustun B, Compton W, Mager D, et al. WHO study on the reliability and validity of the alcohol and drug use disorder instruments: overview of methods and results. *Drug Alcohol Depend.* 1997;47:161-170.
24. Grant BF, Dawson DA, Stinson FS, Chou PS, Kay W, Pickering R. The Alcohol Use Disorder and Associated Disabilities Interview Schedule-IV (AUDADIS-IV): reliability of alcohol consumption, tobacco use, family history of depression and psychiatric diagnostic modules in a general population sample. *Drug Alcohol Depend.* 2003;71:7-16.
25. Grant BF, Stinson FS, Dawson DA, et al. Prevalence and co-occurrence of substance use disorders and independent mood and anxiety disorders: results from the National Epidemiologic Survey on Alcohol and Related Conditions. *Arch Gen Psychiatry.* 2004;61:807-816.
26. Kandel DB, Johnson JG, Bird HR, et al. Psychiatric disorders associated with substance use among children and adolescents: findings from the Methods for the Epidemiology of Child and Adolescent Mental Disorders (MECA) Study. *J Abnorm Child Psychol.* 1997;25:121-132.
27. Wilson CR, Sherritt L, Gates E, Knight JR. Are clinical impressions of adolescent substance abuse use accurate? *Pediatrics.* 2004;114:e536-e540.
28. Li TK, Hewett B, Grant B. Alcohol use disorders and mood disorders: a National Institute on Alcohol Abuse and Alcoholism perspective. *Biol Psychiatry.* 2004;56:718-720.
29. Grant BF, Stinson FS, Harford TC. Age at onset of alcohol use and *DSM-IV* alcohol abuse and dependence: a 12-year follow-up. *J Subst Abuse.* 2001;13:493-504.
30. Warner LA, White HR. Longitudinal effects of age at onset and first drinking solutions on problem drinking. *Subst Use Misuse.* 2003;38:1983-2003.
31. Martin CS, Winter KC. Diagnosis and assessment of alcohol use disorders among adolescents. *Alcohol Health Res World.* 1998;22:95-105.
32. Chung T, Martin C. Concurrent and discriminant validity of *DSM-IV* symptoms of impaired control over alcohol consumption in adolescents. *Alcohol Clin Exp Res.* 2002;26:485-492.
33. Cooper M. Motivations for alcohol use among adolescents: development and validation of a four factor model. *Psychol Assess.* 1994;6:117-128.
34. Rhee SH, Hewitt JK, Young SE, Corley RP, Crowley TJ, Stallings MC. Genetic and environmental influences on substance initiation, use, and problem use in adolescents. *Arch Gen Psychiatry.* 2003;60:1256-1264.
35. Kuperman S, Chan G, Kramer JR, et al. Relationship of age of first drink to child behavioral problems and family psychopathology. *Alcohol Clin Exp Res.* 2005;29:1869-1876.
36. Rose RJ, Dick DM, Viken RJ, Kaprio J. Gene-environment interaction in patterns of adolescent drinking: regional residency moderates longitudinal influences on alcohol use. *Alcohol Clin Exp Res.* 2001;25:637-643.
37. Krueger RF, Hickks BM, Patrick CJ, Carlson SR, Iacono WG, McGue M. Etiologic connections among substance dependence, antisocial behavior, and personality: modeling the externalizing spectrum. *J Abnorm Psychol.* 2002;111:411-424.
38. Young SE, Stallings MC, Corley RP, Krauter KS, Hewitt JK. Genetic and environmental influences on behavioral disinhibition. *Am J Med Genet.* 2000;96:684-695.
39. Dewit DJ, Adlaf DR, Offord DR, Ogcorne AC. Age of first alcohol use and a risk factor for development of alcohol disorders. *Am J Psychiatry.* 2000;157:745-750.
40. Hibell B, Anderson B, Bjarnason T, et al. *The ESPAD Report 2003: Alcohol and Other Drug Use Among Students in 35 European Countries.* Stockholm: Swedish Council for Information on Alcohol and Other Drugs; 2004.
41. Brown SA, Tapert SF, Grandholm E, Delis D. Neurocognitive functioning of adolescents: effects of protracted alcohol use. *Alcohol Clin Exp Res.* 2000;24:164-171.
42. De Bellis MD, Clark D, Beers S, et al. Hippocampal volume in adolescent-onset alcohol use disorders. *Am J Psychiatry.* 2000;157:737-744.
43. Grant I. Alcohol and the brain: neuropsychological correlates. *J Consult Clin Psychol.* 1987;55:310-324.
44. Jacobson R. The contributions of sex and drinking history to CT brain scan changes in alcoholics. *Psychol Med.* 1986;16:547-599.
45. Mann K, Batra A, Gunthner A, Schroth G. Do women develop alcohol brain damage more readily than men? *Alcohol Clin Exp Res.* 1992;16:1052-1056.
46. US Department of Health and Human Services. The neurotoxicity of alcohol. In: *10th Special Report to the US Congress on Alcohol and Health.* Rockville, Md: National Institute on Alcohol Abuse and Alcoholism; 2000:134-146. NIH publication 00-1580.
47. US Department of Health and Human Services; National Institute on Alcohol Abuse and Alcoholism. Alcohol's damaging effects on the brain. *Alcohol Alert.* 2004;63:1-7.
48. Tevyaw TO, Monti PM. Motivational enhancement and other brief interventions for adolescent substance abuse: foundations, applications and evaluations. *Addiction.* 2004;99(suppl 2):63-75.
49. Larimer ME, Cronce JM. Identification, prevention and treatment: a review of individual focused strategies to reduce problematic alcohol consumption by college students. *J Stud Alcohol Suppl.* 2002;14:148-163.
50. Shults RA, Elder RW, Sleet DA. Task Force on Community Preventive Services. Reviews of evidence regarding interventions to reduce alcohol-impaired driving. *Am J Prev Med.* 2001;21:66-88.
51. Wagenaar AC, Toomey TL. Effects of minimum drinking age laws: review and analysis of the literature from 1960 to 2000. *J Stud Alcohol Suppl.* 2002;14:206-225.
52. O'Malley PM, Wagenaar A. Effects of minimum drinking age laws on alcohol use, related behaviors and traffic crash involvement among American youth:1976-1987. *J Stud Alcohol.* 1991;52:478-491.

# Brain Death

## Understanding of the Conceptual Basis by Pediatric Intensivists in Canada

*Ari R. Joffe, MD, FRCPC; Natalie Anton, MD, FRCPC*

**Objective:** To determine whether pediatric intensivists in Canada are aware of the controversies regarding the concept of brain death (BD).

**Design:** Prospective survey.

**Setting:** From February to April 2004, a survey was mailed to each intensivist in the 15 pediatric intensive care units across the 8 provinces of Canada.

**Participants:** Sixty-four practicing pediatric intensivists.

**Main Outcome Measures:** Response rate, conceptual reasons to explain why BD is equivalent to death, and clinical findings that exclude a diagnosis of BD.

**Results:** Of the 64 surveys, 54 (84%) were returned. When asked to choose a conceptual reason to explain why BD is equivalent to death, 26 (48%) chose a higher brain concept, 17 (31%) chose a prognosis concept, and only 19 (35%) chose a loss of integration of the organism concept. More than half the respondents answered that BD is not compatible with electroencephalographic activity, brainstem evoked potential activity, or some cerebral blood flow. More than a third of respondents answered that a brainstem with minimal microscopic damage was not compatible with BD. Of the 36 respondents who answered they were comfortable diagnosing BD because "the conceptual basis of brain death makes it equivalent to death of the patient," in their own words, only 8 (22%) used a loss of integration of organism concept, 9 (25%) used a prognosis concept, 7 (19%) used a higher brain concept, and 13 (36%) did not articulate a concept.

**Conclusions:** There is significant confusion about the concept of BD among pediatric intensivists in Canada. The medical community should reconsider whether BD is equivalent to death.

*Arch Pediatr Adolesc Med. 2006;160:747-752*

BRAIN DEATH (BD) IS MEDICALLY and legally equivalent to death of the patient in most developed countries in the world.[1] Brain death is defined as the irreversible loss of critical functions in the entire brain, including the brainstem.[2] This, the many supporters of BD have argued, is considered to be conceptually equivalent to death because the brain is necessary for maintaining the integrative unity of the body.[3] Without the brain functions, it is claimed, the body functions will disintegrate. There are 2 justifications used to confirm that BD is irreversible and equivalent to death: the inevitability of cardiac arrest and somatic death within days and the pathologic verification of complete brain destruction in BD.[4,5] Higher BD, or neocortical death, with death of the "essence" or "soul" of humans or consciousness (but with preservation of brainstem function) is not BD, and is not accepted in any country medically or legally as equivalent to death of the patient.[3]

There are many problems with these statements about the concept of BD. Brain functions may continue in many brain-dead brains. For example, electroencephalographic (EEG) activity is documented in more than 20% of brain-dead patients,[6,7] evoked potentials are documented in more than 5% of brain-dead patients,[8,9] cerebral blood flow is documented in more than 5% of brain-dead patients,[10,11] diabetes insipidus does not occur in more than half of brain-dead patients,[12-14] and pituitary hormones (including hypothalamic hormones) are present in some studies in most of the brain-dead patients.[14] Moreover, somatic survival of patients with BD for months and years has been reported,[15] disproving the hypothesis that "loss of integrative function" of the brain leads to disintegration of the body.[16,17] Finally, pathologic destruction is not seen in at least 10% of brain-dead patients' brains, even when they have been maintained with circulation for more than 24 hours after BD occurred.[4,5,13,18-21]

These problems relate to the important components of a formulation about

**Author Affiliations:** Division of Pediatric Intensive Care, Department of Pediatrics, University of Alberta, Edmonton.

death.[22,23] A definition of death at the conceptual level is needed so that the question "criteria or tests of what?" can be answered.[22] A criterion for this definition of death is needed and, finally, bedside clinical tests that confirm this criterion is met are required.[22,23] In the case of BD as accepted, the definition of death is the irreversible absence of the body's capacity to organize and regulate itself.[3,22,23] The criterion for this definition is the cessation of whole-brain functioning.[3,22,23] The tests used are the medically accepted bedside tests to confirm BD.[24] The problems previously outlined involve these relationships. Questions arise about the loss of bodily integration in BD (the definition); about the pathologic destruction of the brain or persistent EEG, evoked potential, and hormonal activity of the brain (the criterion); and whether tests for BD ignore some persisting brain activity and integration (the tests). This study was designed to determine if staff pediatric intensivists in Canada, who pronounce BD frequently in the pediatric intensive care unit, are aware of these controversies.

## METHODS

### QUESTIONNAIRE ADMINISTRATION

This study was a prospective survey of pediatric intensivists' opinions regarding BD issues. Research staff created a mailing list of all practicing staff pediatric intensivists at the 15 pediatric intensive care units across Canada. Each staff intensivist was mailed the survey in February 2004, with a $2 gift certificate "so you can get a coffee while you fill out the questionnaire." A cover letter was sent asking to fill in the survey and mail it back in the self-addressed and stamped envelope. A second and third mailing was done at 3-week intervals to nonresponders. The cover letter stated "we are sending you a short questionnaire asking you your opinions around some of the concepts surrounding brain death determination. There are no right or wrong answers to the questions. We simply want to sample the opinions of pediatric intensivists across Canada regarding the concept of brain death. Your responses are voluntary and confidential." The study was approved by our university health research ethics board before mailing.

### QUESTIONNAIRE DEVELOPMENT

To generate the items for inclusion in the questionnaire, we searched MEDLINE from 1966 to 2004 for articles on BD, followed by review of the relevant article reference lists. Emphasis was placed on articles discussing the concept of BD, rather than the tests used to diagnose BD. Seven questions were generated, each with multiple possible answer boxes, with the instruction "in each question you may choose any/all of the responses that you consider correct." An additional question asked for a response in the practitioner's own words. The questionnaire started with the statement "All questions apply to a 14-year-old patient after severe head trauma in a motor vehicle collision. The patient fulfills all clinical brain death criteria unequivocally, including the suitable interval (in this case, 12 hours)." This statement was intended to convey that the tests for BD are not the focus of the study; rather, the concept is the issue. To ensure clarity, realism, validity, and ease of completion of the questionnaire, initial pilot testing of the instrument was done by having 5 local pediatric intensivists, 1 local pediatrician, and 1 local organ donation coordinator fill out the questionnaire. This was followed by a semistructured interview by us for feedback on the clarity of the questions and possible responses, and to confirm answers chosen reflected the intended response to the question. After minor modification, the questionnaire, 1 double-sided page, was mailed as previously described. The survey is available online (eFigure; available at http://www.archpediatrics.com).

### ANALYSIS

Certain definitions were agreed on a priori for 2 of the survey questions. The first question asked the respondent to choose from a list "stand-alone" reason(s) that "is/are an acceptable *conceptual* reason to explain why 'brain death' is equivalent to 'death.'" The seventh question asked, "This patient fulfills all brain death criteria unequivocally, including the suitable interval. *Conceptually*, why are they dead (ie, in your own words, what is it about loss of brain function including the brainstem that makes this patient dead)?" For analysis, we classified responses into categories that have been discussed in the literature: loss of integration concept of BD, higher brain concept of BD, prognosis concept of BD, and statement of the criterion only. Further detail is provided in the eFigure. We hypothesized that there would be variability in the stated conceptual reasons to explain why BD is equivalent to death and in the stated clinical findings that exclude a diagnosis of BD. In addition, it was hypothesized that most respondents would not state the medically accepted conceptual reason to explain why BD is equivalent to death or the clinical findings that exclude a diagnosis of BD.

Anonymous data were entered into a computer database (Microsoft Excel; Microsoft Corp, Redmond, Wash). We analyzed responses using standard tabulations. Qualitative variables expressed as percentages were used to report the proportion of respondents with the different answers.

## RESULTS

Surveys were mailed to all 64 practicing staff pediatric intensivists in 15 pediatric intensive care units across 8 provinces of Canada. Of the 64 surveys mailed, 54 (84%) were returned after the third mailing.

The first question asked which of several possibilities is an acceptable stand-alone conceptual reason to explain why BD is equivalent to death. Only 19 (35%) chose a loss of integration concept (**Table 1**).

The next 2 questions asked about which objective test results would not be compatible with BD. More than half answered that BD is not compatible with EEG activity that is not due to artifact (30 respondents [56%]); some visual, somatosensory, or auditory evoked potential activity (31 respondents [57%]); or some cerebral blood flow on technetium flow study (33 respondents [61%]). A significant minority also answered that normal regulatory pituitary hormones (3 respondents [6%]) and normal appearance of the brainstem grossly and microscopically (7 respondents [13%]) were not compatible with BD. In a patient who was brain dead for at least 48 hours, many answered that a brainstem (19 respondents [35%]) or cerebral cortex (13 respondents [24%]) that is structurally normal and microscopically with minimal damage was not compatible with BD; some (4 respondents [7%]) extended this to include a more moderately damaged brain (brainstem and cerebral cortex damaged; however, there are not widespread destructive changes typical of "respirator brain").

**Table 1. Responses to the Question on Conceptual Reasons to Explain Why Brain Death Is Equivalent to Death***

| Conceptual Reason | No. (%) of the 54 Respondents |
|---|---|
| Higher brain concept | 26 (48) |
| Irreversible loss of consciousness | 17 (31) |
| Irreversible loss of the soul or "the essence" of humans | 12 (22) |
| Irreversible loss of "personhood" | 14 (26) |
| Irreversible loss of the integration of body functions by the brain | 19 (35) |
| Prognosis concept | 17 (31) |
| The certainty of cardiac arrest within hours or days | 11 (20) |
| Further care is futile and/or degrading | 12 (22) |
| Statement of loss of brain function (the criterion) | 44 (81) |
| Irreversible loss of the function of the entire brain, including the brainstem | 30 (56) |
| Irreversible loss of the critical functions of the entire brain, including the brainstem | 34 (63) |
| Irreversible loss of the capacity for consciousness plus irreversible loss of the capacity to breathe | 22 (41) |
| Irreversible destruction of the brain, including the brainstem | 16 (30) |

*The exact question asked was as follows: "Which of the following is/are an acceptable *conceptual* reason to explain why 'brain death' is equivalent to 'death'"? Respondents could choose more than 1 answer; each answer had to be a stand-alone reason.

**Table 2. Response to the Question About What, in the Respondent's Own Words, Makes a Patient Dead***

| Concept Given to Justify Why Brain Death Is Death | No. (%) of the 54 Respondents |
|---|---|
| Higher brain concept | 9 (17) |
| Loss of integration of body concept | 12 (22) |
| Loss of integration alone | 6 (11) |
| Loss of integration combined with higher brain concept | 6 (11) |
| Prognosis concept | 12 (22) |
| Prognosis of death certain | 7 (13) |
| Quality-of-life statement | 5 (9) |
| Statement only: loss of brain function (the criterion) | 13 (24) |
| No response (blank) | 6 (11) |
| Other† | 3 (5) |

*The exact question was as follows: "This patient fulfills all brain death criteria unequivocally including the suitable interval. *Conceptually*, why are they dead (ie, in your own words, what is it about loss of brain function including the brainstem that makes this patient dead)?"
†Responses included "common sense," "it will not come back (no improvement)," and "life ≠ beating heart."

The next 3 questions asked about the timing of BD in different patient situations. When faced with a patient who has EEG activity yet fulfills all BD criteria, 15 (28%) would not consider the patient dead until the EEG became isoelectric 12 hours later. When faced with a pregnant brain-dead patient who is supported for 11 weeks until delivery, most agreed that the patient was brain dead by the second clinical BD examination (51 respondents [94%]); however, 3 respondents (6%) answered that the patient was not brain dead until after organs are harvested and the ventilator is stopped. When faced with a brain-dead patient who has no cerebral blood flow, yet a family that insists on continued "life support," only 25 respondents (46%) would tell the family that the patient is legally dead and that ventilation and inotropes will be withdrawn at a specified time; 20 respondents (37%) would continue support knowing that the patient will have a cardiac arrest soon (4 respondents [7%]) or to honor the family wishes (16 respondents [30%]). Most respondents answered that BD occurred after the second examination rather than after the first examination (22 respondents [41%] vs 16 respondents [30%] in the patient with EEG activity; and 27 respondents [50%] vs 24 respondents [44%] in the pregnant patient).

The next 2 questions asked again about the underlying conceptual basis of BD ("in your own words, what is it about loss of brain function including the brainstem that makes this patient dead?" and "prior to this survey, had you thought about why, at a conceptual level, brain death is equivalent to death of the patient?"). Of the respondents, 5 (9%) had not previously thought about why BD is equivalent to death. In their own words, only 12 (22%) used a loss of integration concept (**Table 2**). Finally, a question asked which choice "best describes why you are comfortable diagnosing death based on the criteria of brain death"; 36 (67%) responded "the conceptual basis of brain death makes it equivalent to death of the patient." Many responded that the reason is because it is a standard (22 respondents [41%]): an accepted medical standard (13 respondents [24%]), an accepted legal standard (14 respondents [26%]), and/or "the diagnosis of brain death was taught to me during my training" (3 respondents [6%]); only 1 respondent (2%) was not comfortable diagnosing death based on BD.

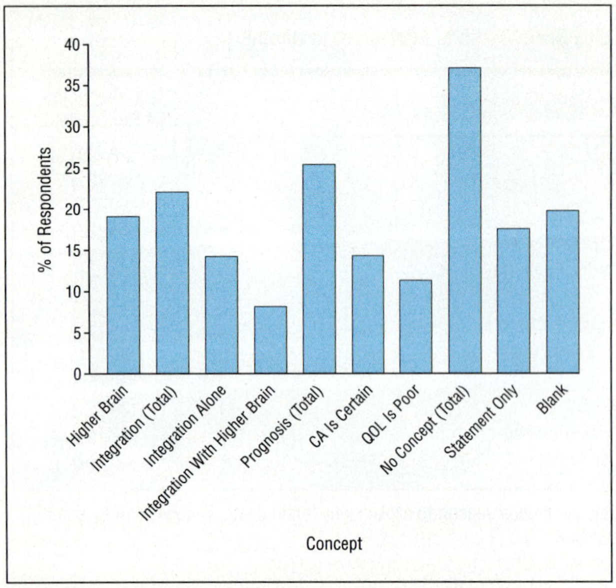


**Figure.** Concept used to justify brain death, used by the 36 respondents who agreed the conceptual basis makes brain death equivalent to death. The exact question asked was as follows: "This patient fulfills all brain death criteria unequivocally including the suitable interval. Conceptually, why are they dead?" CA indicates cardiac arrest; QOL, quality of life.

Further analysis was done for those 36 respondents (67%) who answered that they were comfortable diagnosing BD because "the conceptual basis of brain death makes it equivalent to death of the patient." Their response to the question asking to state the concept of BD in their own words is shown in the **Figure**. Only 8 (22%) used a loss of integration of body concept, and 13 (36%) did not articulate a concept (ie, used a statement of the criterion or left no response). On the first question, only 13 respondents (36%) considered "irreversible loss of the integration of body functions by the brain" as an acceptable conceptual reason to explain BD being equivalent to death and 11 (31%) considered a prognosis concept acceptable. Finally, when asked by family to continue "life support" on a brain-dead patient, 11 respondents (30%) would honor these wishes of the family.

## COMMENT

Brain death was defined originally to address 2 issues related to progress in intensive care: the need to withdraw ventilator support (ie, demand of scarce medical resources) in those patients with irreversible coma and advances in organ transplantation.[25,26] To define BD as death allowed withdrawal of intensive care and harvesting of organs for transplantation. Only after the clinical BD state was described was the underlying conceptual justification for it being equivalent to death of the patient described,[23] and endorsed by the President's Commission for the Study of Ethical Problems in Medicine and Biomedical and Behavioral Research[3]: the loss of integrative unity of the organism. This state was said to be present when there was irreversible loss of the functions of the entire brain, including the brainstem.[3]

In time, brain-dead patients who had persistent brain function were described, including EEG, evoked potential, and antidiuretic hormone activity.[6-13] Therefore, the BD criterion was adjusted to refer to the loss of the "critical functions" of the brain as a whole,[2] although who decides what is a critical function was debated.[22,27,28] Recently, it has been found that brain-dead bodies can "survive" for prolonged periods.[15] This and other arguments have shown that the BD state does not necessarily mean loss of integrative unity of the organism with resultant somatic death shortly thereafter.[16,17] In addition, the underlying reasons for "needing" a definition of BD are less needed: intensive care is withdrawn frequently from patients who are not brain dead and have a poor prognosis and organ donation occurs from non–heart-beating and living donors.

This survey documented significant confusion about the officially accepted concept of BD among pediatric intensivists in Canada. Only a minority (19 respondents [35%]) considered loss of integrative function of the organism a conceptual justification for BD. Many considered prognosis a conceptual justification for BD (17 respondents [31%]); however, imminent cardiac arrest or futile or degrading therapy is not justification for defining someone as already dead, even though the patient may be considered "as good as dead." Many used a higher brain concept of death (26 respondents [48%]), suggesting that permanent lack of consciousness or "personhood" is a concept of death. Although this has been suggested by a few ethicists,[29] it is not accepted by medical or legal bodies,[3,28] and would imply that patients in a permanent vegetative state or anencephalic infants could be cremated or buried while still awake, breathing, and moving.[14] The results were similar when asked to answer the following, "in your own words, what is it about loss of brain function including the brainstem that makes this patient dead?" Only 12 respondents (22%) used a loss of integration concept, 12 (22%) used a prognosis concept, and 13 (24%) used a statement that there is loss of brain function (the criterion of death, not the definition).

The conceptual confusion demonstrated in this survey included illogical statements, as in saying that a person is dead because the person will die soon, and philosophical differences of opinion, such as saying that loss of consciousness is death. Whether the philosophical differences of opinion reflect consideration of all the nuances of the various arguments cannot be answered by this survey. However, it would seem that the physicians are not well-informed of the philosophical debates about the concept of BD. In support of this is the finding that, when faced with a brain-dead patient who has no cerebral blood flow, yet a family that insists on continued "life support," 20 respondents (37%) would continue support. This is remarkably similar to a recent survey that asked 25 pediatric critical care attending physicians if "life supports should be withdrawn from a child who is legally brain dead even if the parents do not agree"; 34% responded that they disagree or are uncertain.[30] If similar support would not be continued on a patient after irreversible circulatory death, this suggests that BD is different from death.

There was also confusion regarding brain functions and pathologic features that are compatible with the accepted clinical criterion and tests for diagnosis of BD. More than half of respondents were not comfortable with the diagnosis of BD when there was any EEG activity, evoked potential activity, or cerebral blood flow, even though this is the case in 5% to 20% of patients diagnosed as being brain dead.[6-11] Many were not comfortable with the diagnosis of BD when there was only minimal brain pathologic damage, even though this is the case in at least 10% of patients diagnosed as being brain dead.[4,5,13,18-21] These concerns were reflected in the response to some specific patient scenarios that fulfilled all clinical tests for BD: 15 respondents (28%) would not diagnose BD until the EEG was isoelectric, 3 (6%) would not diagnose the pregnant patient as dead until after delivery of the neonate and the ventilator was turned off, and 16 (30%) would honor family requests to continue intensive care treatment of the brain-dead patient. Electroencephalography is not considered a confirmatory test in Canada, because it cannot test brainstem function; however, this ignores the common concern that cortical function on EEG may not be compatible with BD in the minds of those making the diagnosis. Because it is unlikely that the physicians were unaware of the legal requirements for BD, this empirical confusion demonstrates that many physicians were not aware of the problems with the BD tests themselves. The BD tests do not diagnose an irreversible loss of the function of the entire brain.

We found that 36 (67%) respondents were comfortable diagnosing death based on the tests of BD because "the conceptual basis of BD makes it equivalent to death of the patient." This subgroup of respondents demonstrated similar confusion about the concept of BD. Only 8 respondents (22%) used a loss of integration concept, 9 (25%) used a prognosis concept, 7 (19%) used a higher brain concept, and 13 (36%) did not articulate a concept (ie, used a statement of the BD criterion or left no response).

The strengths of this survey include the high response rate (54 [84%] of 64 subjects) and the rigorous survey development methods, including pretesting confirming the clarity of the questions and possible responses. The multicenter representation also enhances the generalizability of our findings. The limitations of the survey include the lack of demographic data on the respondents and the lack of open-ended questions allowing respondents to expand on their intended answers. In addition, there could be discrepancies between stated and actual practice regarding BD. However, we believe that these limitations would not affect the main conclusion of this study, that there is a limited awareness of the debates surrounding the BD concept among staff pediatric intensivists.

Others have found similar results in surveys of physicians and nurses[31-35] and, therefore, we believe the results herein can be generalized to the medical community beyond pediatric intensivists in Canada. For example, in 1989, Youngner et al[31] showed that one third of physicians and nurses involved in the management of brain-dead patients considered them dead because they had irreversible loss of cortical function, and another third because they had an unacceptable quality of life or were irreversibly dying. This lack of change in confusion over 35 years is concerning, and may reflect the irresistible utilitarian appeal of the BD diagnosis or ambivalence regarding the conceptual status of persons who are brain dead.

Many have elegantly discussed the inconsistencies in the concept of BD,[14,16,17,27,28,36-40] and to elaborate further herein is beyond the scope of this study. The discussion has been confined to academic ethics and philosophy communities,[41] and has not been seriously considered by the clinical medical community. This study confirms a limited knowledge among clinicians of the conceptual basis for BD and of the empirical problems with the tests used to confirm BD. The BD criterion does not fulfill the official theory for the definition/concept of death, and the tests used do not fulfill the criterion of BD. For these reasons, we and others[27,28,36,38,41,42] believe it is time for the medical community to reconsider whether BD is equivalent to death of the patient.

**Accepted for Publication:** January 6, 2006.
**Correspondence:** Ari R. Joffe, MD, FRCPC, 3A3.07 Walter Mackenzie Health Science Centre, Stollery Children's Hospital, 8440 112th St, Edmonton, Alberta, Canada T6G 2B7 (ajoffe@cha.ab.ca).
**Author Contributions:** *Study concept and design:* Joffe and Anton. *Acquisition of data:* Joffe and Anton. *Analysis and interpretation of data:* Joffe. *Drafting of the manuscript:* Joffe. *Critical revision of the manuscript for important intellectual content*: Joffe and Anton. *Statistical analysis:* Joffe. *Administrative, technical, and material support:* Joffe and Anton.
**Financial Disclosure:** None reported.
**Additional Resources:** The eFigure is available at http://www.archpediatrics.com.

## REFERENCES

1. Wijdicks EFM. Brain death worldwide: accepted fact but no global consensus in diagnostic criteria. *Neurology.* 2002;58:20-25.
2. Bernat JL. A defense of the whole brain concept of death. *Hastings Cent Rep.* 1998;28:14-23.
3. President's Commission for the Study of Ethical Problems in Medicine and Biomedical and Behavioral Research. *Defining Death: Medical, Legal and Ethical Issues in the Determination of Death.* Washington, DC: US Government Printing Office; 1981.
4. Black PM. Brain death (first of two parts). *N Engl J Med.* 1978;299:338-344.
5. Black PM. Brain death (second of two parts). *N Engl J Med.* 1978;299:393-401.
6. Grigg MM, Kelly MA, Celesia GG, Ghobrial MW, Ross ER. Electroencephalographic activity after brain death. *Arch Neurol.* 1987;44:948-954.
7. Paolin A, Manuali A, DiPaola F, et al. Reliability in diagnosis of brain death. *Intensive Care Med.* 1995;21:657-662.
8. Ruiz-Garcia M, Gonzalez-Astiazaran A, Collado-Corona MA, Rueda-Franco F, Sosa-de-Martinez C. Brain death in children: clinical, neurophysiological and radioisotopic angiography findings in 125 patients. *Childs Nerv Syst.* 2000;16:40-46.
9. Facco E, Munari M, Gallo F, et al. Role of short latency evoked potentials in the diagnosis of brain death. *Clin Neurophysiol.* 2002;113:1855-1866.
10. Kurtek RW, Lai KK, Tauxe WN, Eidelman BH, Fung JJ. Tc-99m hexamethylpropylene amine oxime scintigraphy in the diagnosis of brain death and its implications for the harvesting of organs used for transplantation. *Clin Nucl Med.* 2000;25:7-10.
11. Flowers WM, Patel BR. Persistence of cerebral blood flow after brain death. *South Med J.* 2000;93:364-370.
12. Staworn D, Lewison L, Marks J, Turner G, Levin D. Brain death in pediatric intensive care unit patients: incidence, primary diagnosis, and the clinical occurrence of Turner's triad. *Crit Care Med.* 1994;22:1301-1305.
13. Fackler JC, Troncoso JC, Gioia FR. Age-specific characteristics of brain death in children. *AJDC.* 1988;142:999-1003.
14. Truog RD. Is it time to abandon brain death? *Hastings Cent Rep.* 1997;27:29-37.

15. Shewmon DA. Chronic "brain death": meta-analysis and conceptual consequences. *Neurology.* 1998;51:1538-1545.
16. Shewmon DA. The brain and somatic integration: insights into the standard biological rationale for equating "brain death" with death. *J Med Philos.* 2001; 26:457-478.
17. Potts M. A requiem for whole brain death: a response to D. Alan Shewmon's "the brain and somatic integration." *J Med Philos.* 2001;26:479-491.
18. Walker AE, Diamond EL, Moseley J. The neuropathological findings in irreversible coma: a critique of the "respirator brain." *J Neuropathol Exp Neurol.* 1975; 34:295-323.
19. Schroder R. Later changes in brain death: signs of partial recirculation. *Acta Neuropathol (Berl).* 1983;62:15-23.
20. Mohandas A, Chou SN. Brain death: a clinical and pathological study. *J Neurosurg.* 1971;35:211-218.
21. Drake B, Ashwal S, Schneider S. Determination of cerebral death in the pediatric intensive care unit. *Pediatrics.* 1986;78:107-112.
22. Youngner SJ, Bartlett ET. Human death and high technology: the failure of the whole-brain formulations. *Ann Intern Med.* 1983;99:252-258.
23. Bernat JL, Culver CM, Gert B. On the definition and criterion of death. *Ann Intern Med.* 1981;94:389-394.
24. Guidelines for the determination of death: report of the medical consultants on the diagnosis of death to the President's Commission for the Study of Ethical Problems in Medicine and Biomedical and Behavioral Research. *JAMA.* 1981; 246:2184-2186.
25. A definition of irreversible coma: report of the Ad Hoc Committee of the Harvard Medical School to Examine the Definition of Brain Death. *JAMA.* 1968;205: 337-340.
26. Giacomini M. A change of heart and a change of mind? technology and the redefinition of death in 1968. *Soc Sci Med.* 1997;44:1465-1482.
27. Truog RD, Robinson WM. Role of brain death and the dead-donor rule in the ethics of organ transplantation. *Crit Care Med.* 2003;31:2391-2396.
28. Zamperetti N, Bellomo R, Defanti CA, Latronico N. Irreversible apnoeic coma 35 years later: towards a more rigorous definition of brain death? *Intensive Care Med.* 2004;30:1715-1722.
29. Veatch RM. Abandon the dead donor rule or change the definition of death? *Kennedy Inst Ethics J.* 2004;14:261-276.
30. Solomon MZ, Sellers DE, Heller KS, et al. New and lingering controversies in pediatric end-of-life care. *Pediatrics.* 2005;116:872-883.
31. Youngner SJ, Landefeld CS, Coulton CJ, Juknialis BW, Leary M. "Brain death" and organ retrieval: a cross-sectional survey of knowledge and concepts among health professionals. *JAMA.* 1989;261:2205-2210.
32. Youngner SJ, Allen M, Bartlett ET, et al. Psychosocial and ethical implications of organ retrieval. *N Engl J Med.* 1985;313:321-324.
33. Tomlinson T. Misunderstanding death on a respirator. *Bioethics.* 1990;4:253-264.
34. Kim JR, Elliott D, Hyde C. Korean health professionals' attitudes and knowledge toward organ donation and transplantation. *Int J Nurs Stud.* 2004;41:299-307.
35. White G. Intensive care nurses' perceptions of brain death. *Aust Crit Care.* 2003; 16:7-14.
36. Shewmon DA. Recovery from "brain death": a neurologist's apologia. *Linacre Q.* 1997;64:30-96.
37. Veatch RM. Impending collapse of the whole-brain definition of death. *Hastings Cent Rep.* 1993;23:18-24.
38. Kerridge IH, Saul P, Lowe M, McPhee J, Williams D. Death, dying and donation: organ transplantation and the diagnosis of death. *J Med Ethics.* 2002;28:89-94.
39. Halevy A, Brody B. Brain death: reconciling definitions, criteria, and tests. *Ann Intern Med.* 1993;119:519-525.
40. Byrne PA, O'Reilly S, Quay PM. Brain death: an opposing viewpoint. *JAMA.* 1979; 242:1985-1990.
41. Youngner SJ, Arnold RM. Philosophical debates about the definition of death: who cares? *J Med Philos.* 2001;26:527-537.
42. Potts M, Evans EW. Does it matter that organ donors are not dead? ethical and policy implications. *J Med Ethics.* 2005;31:406-409.

# Human Immunodeficiency Virus Prophylaxis for Sexual Assault Survivors

## *What We Need to Know*

Adolescent sexual assault is unfortunately all too common. An analysis of the 2001 Youth Risk Behavior Survey revealed that 10.2% of women and 5.1% of men reported forced sexual intercourse at least once in their lifetimes.[1] Recent National Criminal Victimization Survey results revealed that annually 1/10 of one percent of all individuals aged 12 or older had survived rape or sexual assault.[2] The ratio of male-female survivors is 1:10, and 29% of victims are 12 to 17 years old.

There is a general concern that survivors are at increased risk for acquiring human immunodeficiency virus (HIV) infection via the sexual assaults. Most reviews cite a case report by Murphy et al,[3] which describes HIV seroconversion related to rape. Epidemiological studies of consensual coitus have shown that the risk for heterosexual sexual transmission from 1 coital act ranges from 0.001 to 0.008.[4] Estimates vary by the stage of the infected person (eg, time since seroconversion: <5 months, 6-15 months, or >15 months) and type of exposure (eg, insertive anal intercourse, receptive vaginal intercourse).

*See also page 674*

There has been considerable debate around the costs and benefits of offering postexposure prophylaxis for HIV infection (PEP) to individuals who have been sexually assaulted. Animal models suggest that a 28-day course of antiretroviral therapy (ART) initiated within 72 hours of the transmission may be effective PEP.[5] The empirical basis for the PEP recommendations regarding timing of initiation, duration of treatment, and choice of antiretroviral therapy is weak, however. To date, no randomized controlled trials of PEP for nonoccupational exposures (such as rape) or for occupational exposures (such as those in the health care field) have been conducted. The most compelling study of PEP effectiveness is on occupational exposure and involves a case-controlled study of HIV seroconversion in health care workers.[6] The study included 33 case patients who received PEP and 679 controls who did not, people who were recruited from the United States and western European countries. The final logistic regression models revealed that, after controlling for the extent and nature of injury, there was no difference in rates at which patients were offered PEP (which was AZT [zidovudine] at the time of the study). But the investigators found that case patients were significantly less likely than controls to have taken PEP. The potential biases in this study—including reporting and ascertainment biases, the failure to control for differences in the infected patient's stage of infection, and an inability to test interaction because of small sample sizes—are sufficiently numerous to warrant caution regarding its findings.

In 2005, the Centers for Disease Control and Prevention (CDC) recommended a 2-pronged approach to management of nonoccupational exposures to HIV, including sexual assault exposure.[7] This approach is similar to the guidance provided by the American Academy of Pediatrics.[8] The CDC propose an algorithm for evaluation and treatment in which PEP should be recommended if the exposure has occurred within the past 72 hours and the source was known to be HIV positive. In cases where the exposure was greater than 72 hours, the CDC do not recommend PEP. Finally, in cases where the exposure is within the past 72 hours but the source is of unknown HIV status, they recommend a case-by-case determination. Factors to be considered in these situations include the nature of exposure and the source's risk profile. One additional consideration in the case of sexual assault survivors is the difficulty of obtaining a clinical history at the time of the postassault examination. The CDC recommend that if PEP is started, the clinician provide a 3- to 5-day ART starter pack and a follow-up evaluation at which time a better assessment of risk could be obtained.[1]

The other consideration is evidence of nonadherence to PEP among sexual assault survivors. Olshen et al[9] in this issue of the Archives found that only a small percentage of adolescents who were prescribed a 28-day course of ART completed the full course of treatment. The study used a retrospective medical-record review of all sexual assault survivors who had presented to either one of 2 urban academic pediatric emergency departments between July 2001 and July 2003. At the time, both emergency departments recommended that a 28-day prescription for PEP be considered for sexual assault survivors and that the survivors return to their primary care providers for follow-up evaluations at 2 weeks, 6 weeks, 3 months, and 6 months. The investigators found that 110 (76%) of 129 survivors offered PEP agreed to take medicine and 86 of these were referred to one of the 2 pediatric academic centers for follow-up. Only 35 of 86 returned for any care and a mere 13 completed the full 28-day course.

These results support earlier findings from a study conducted in Vancouver of sexual assault survivors (mean age, 26 years) presenting to the Vancouver General Hospital emergency department from 1996 through 1999.[10] Of the 71 individuals who accepted PEP, only 8 completed the 28-day course. In this study, instead of the full 28-day course, providers offered 5-day starter packs and recommended follow-up at 2 to 5 days for re-evaluation and possible additional prescription for 23 more days of PEP. Only 29 of 71 sexual assault survivors who accepted PEP returned at 2 to 5 days for reassessment.

These rates of nonadherence to prescribed ART and recommended follow-up are high enough to warrant concern. Nonadherence to ART may mitigate whatever effectiveness PEP possesses. Adolescents who are not consistently adherent to the regimen may fail to achieve the viral suppression necessary to prevent dissemination and established infection. In addition, nonadherence to ART may increase the likelihood that an HIV-infected sexual assault survivor develops viral resistance, complicating subsequent ART. The use of 3- to 5-day starter packs may mitigate some of the concerns about nonadherence and viral resistance by limiting exposure to ART.

Taken together, these 2 studies suggest that more than one half (approximately 60%) of sexual assault survivors who are prescribed PEP do not make any follow-up visits, and significantly fewer actually complete the 28-day treatment course. These findings coupled with CDC guidelines support a very judicious use of PEP in the case of sexual assault survivors. In accordance with the guidelines, centers and clinics that provide care to sexual assault survivors should offer a 5-day starter pack of PEP to survivors in cases when the source is known to be HIV positive and the exposure was within 72 hours. More importantly, additional consideration must be given to issues of nonadherence when making a case-by-case decision regarding PEP when the source's HIV infection status is unknown. Issues of nonadherence and the lack of resources to ensure follow-up and adherence weigh against starting PEP for adolescent sexual assault survivors. Although the saliency of HIV is great and the desire to offer treatment with any hope of benefit to someone traumatized by sexual assault is high, data support a restrained position.

*Jonathan M. Ellen, MD*

**Correspondence:** Dr Ellen, Division of General Pediatrics and Adolescent Medicine, Department of Pediatrics, Johns Hopkins School of Medicine, 600 N Wolfe St, Baltimore, MD 21287 (jellen@jhmi.edu).

1. Howard DE, Wang MQ. Psychosocial correlates of US adolescents who report a history of forced sexual intercourse. *J Adolesc Health*. 2005;36:372-379.
2. Catalano S. Criminal victimization. US Bureau of Justice Statistics. http://www.ojp.usdoj.gov/bjs. Accessed on May 12, 2006.
3. Murphy S, Kitchen V, Harris JRW, Forster SM. Rape and seroconversion to HIV. *BMJ*. 1989;299:718.
4. Wawer MJ, Gray RH, Sewankambo NK, et al. Rates of HIV-1 transmission per coital act, by stage of HIV-1 infection, in Rakai, Uganda. *J Infect Dis*. 2005;191:1403-1409.
5. Tsai CC, Emau P, Follis KE, et al. Effectiveness of postinoculation (R)-9-(2-phosphonylmethoxypropyl) adenine treatment for prevention of persistent simian immunodeficiency virus SIVmne infection depends critically on timing of initiation and duration of treatment. *J Virol*. 1998;72:4265-4273.
6. Cardo DM, Culver DH, Ciesielski CA, et al. A case-control study of HIV seroconversion in health care workers after percutaneous exposure. *N Engl J Med*. 1997;337:1485-1490.
7. Smith DK, Grohskopf LA, Black RJ, et al. Antiretroviral postexposure prophylaxis after sexual assault, injection-drug use, or other nonoccupational exposure to HIV in the United States: recommendations from the US Department of Health and Human Services. *MMWR Recomm Rep*. 2005;54(RR-2):1-20.
8. Havens PL. Postexposure prophylaxis in children and adolescents for nonoccupational exposure to human immunodeficiency virus. *Pediatrics*. 2003;111:1475-1489.
9. Olshen E, Hsu K, Woods ER, Harper M, Harnisch B, Samples CL. Use of human immunodeficiency virus postexposure prophylaxis in adolescent sexual assault victims. *Arch Pediatr Adolesc Med*. 2006;160:674-680.
10. Wiebe ER, Comay SE, McGregor M, Ducceschi S. Offering HIV prophylaxis to people who have been sexually assaulted: 16 months' experience in a sexual assault service. *CMAJ*. 2000;162:641-645.

# Screens and Doors

## *The Management of Adolescent Depression in Primary Care*

THE ARTICLE BY ZUCKERBROT AND JENSEN[1] IS both timely and thought-provoking. It is timely because all of us, both pediatricians and psychiatrists, are struggling to figure out how best to treat adolescent depression in light of the Food and Drug Administration "black box" warning and overall concerns about antidepressants. It is thought-provoking because this article explicitly conveys high expectations for the role of the pediatrician in the identification and management of depression and implicitly leads us to consider how primary care resources should best be allocated to ensure optimal psychosocial development for our pediatric patients.

*See also page 694*

The authors pose 3 questions. What do we know about screening for depression in pediatric primary care? Does screening make any difference in physician behavior or patient outcome? What is being done now as far as screening for depression in pediatric primary care?

The few studies examining screening for depression in primary care used either a brief interview, self-report, or a combination of the two. In one direct comparison between screening interviews and self-report, self-report showed performance equal or superior to physician interviews.[2] Although a number of the approaches made a respectable showing, the instrument that appeared to have the best psychometric properties was the self-reported Patient Health Questionnaire, which has a broader mental health focus on depression, substance abuse, and eating disorders. The screening sites that were reviewed by Zuckerbrot and Jensen[1] were most often adolescent clinics in teaching hospitals that tend to attract a patient population at higher risk for depression than might be typically seen in pediatric primary care.

With regard to the impact of screening, incorporating the screening procedure recommended by the American Medical Association[3] for an array of health risk behaviors into clinical practice resulted in increased rates of referrals for depression and suicide prevention and improved documentation of depression and suicide screening as well as family history of psychiatric disorder. However, patient outcome was not assessed.[4] In adult primary care, neither physician education nor screening for depression alone improves outcome.[5-7] A quality improvement study of the treatment of adolescent depression in primary care, in which screening plus on-site specialty mental health care was compared with screening alone for depressed adolescents, found results consistent to those found in adults. In this study, the rates of referral for psychotherapy and specialty mental health care after the intervention compared with the 6 months before the intervention were increased in the quality improvement but not in the screening-only group.[8] There are relatively little data on what practitioners are doing now, but the findings presented in this article suggest that pediatricians are not screening routinely for depression, in part because of their concerns about management and referral.

If the goal is to detect adolescent depression, is primary care the best venue? In primary care, many adolescents may be seen by their pediatricians once a year for a well-child visit, which may yield fewer positive screens than injury- or illness-related visits.[9] Although screening for mental health concerns is a reasonable part of a well-child visit, the low frequency of adolescent visits to primary care clinicians may result in incomplete detection of current depressive episodes. This may contrast with the yield in adolescent medicine clinics or in specialty programs for chronic diseases, where the rate of depression will be higher and the frequency of visits makes detection of a depressive episode more likely.

For pediatric primary care, a broader focus on emotional and behavioral problems and health risk behaviors, such as was used in the Guidelines for Adolescent Preventive Services program, may be a more efficient approach. Many health risk behaviors may co-occur with depression (eg, tobacco use, binge-drinking, abnormal eating habits, and having unprotected sex), each of which is potentially life-threatening or life-altering.[10,11] Perhaps a focus on functional impairment with peers, family, or school and a broader survey of health risk behaviors would give a greater yield for the same time devoted to screening. In addition, there may be other known risk factors for depression, such as parental depression, past depression or anxiety in the patient, and exposure to psychosocial stress, that can increase the pediatrician's index of suspicion for the presence of depression.

However, routine screening only makes sense if the pediatrician feels equipped to take the next step with those individuals who screen positive. As Zuckerbrot and Jensen[1] point out, many pediatricians do not feel comfortable managing adolescent depression because of a lack of training and experience, concern about the black box warning, or the time-consuming nature of chronic disease management. Many patients and their families may prefer psychotherapy over medication, the former of which pediatricians generally are not trained to provide. Moreover, even if pediatricians were to screen and diagnose depression optimally, a common and justified complaint of practitioners is the great difficulty gaining entrée for their patients to quality mental health care. Without the ability to care for the people who screen positive, screening will only be an exercise in frustration for everyone concerned.

One approach is midway between the pediatrician doing all the management and doing nothing at all: the collaborative care model, shown to be efficacious in trials with adults and most recently with depressed adolescents,[5,8,12] where on-site mental health care resulted in higher rates of receipt of specialty mental health care as well as better depressive outcome, presumably because the usual barriers to obtaining specialty treatment were removed by providing care on site. If such an approach can be shown to be economically sustainable, the colocation of a specialty mental health provider, such as a nurse clinician with available psychiatric consultation, may be able to meet the needs of patients, families, and pediatricians who require access to quality mental health care.[13] With access, there is then a built-in link between screening and outcome. We need screens, but we also need open doors to connect our patients with the care that they deserve.

*David A. Brent, MD*

**Correspondence:** Dr Brent, Department of Psychiatry, University of Pittsburgh School of Medicine, 3811 O'Hara St, Pittsburgh, PA 15213 (brentda@upmc.edu).

## REFERENCES

1. Zuckerbrot RA, Jensen PS. Improving recognition of adolescent depression in primary care. *Arch Pediatr Adolesc Med.* 2006;160:694-704.
2. Schubiner H, Tzelepis A, Wright K, Podany E. The clinical utility of the Safe Times Questionnaire. *J Adolesc Health.* 1994;15:374-382.
3. Elster AB, Kuznets NJ. *AMA Guidelines for Adolescent Preventive Services (GAPS): Recommendations and Rationale.* Baltimore, Md: Williams & Wilkins; 1994.
4. Klein JD, Allan MJ, Elster AB, et al. Improving adolescent preventive care in community health centers. *Pediatrics.* 2001;107:318-327.
5. Vergouwen AC, Bakker A, Katon WJ, Verheij TJ, Koerselman F. Improving adherence to antidepressants: a systematic review of interventions. *J Clin Psychiatry.* 2003;64:1415-1420.
6. Dowrick C, Buchan I. Twelve month outcome of depression in general practice: does detection or disclosure make a difference? *BMJ.* 1995;311:1274-1276.
7. Whooley MA, Simon GE. Managing depression in medical outpatients. *N Engl J Med.* 2000;343:1942-1950.
8. Asarnow JR, Jaycox LH, Duan N, et al. Effectiveness of a quality improvement intervention for adolescent depression in primary care clinics: a randomized controlled trial. *JAMA.* 2005;293:311-319.
9. Borowsky IW, Mozayeny S, Ireland M. Brief psychosocial screening at health supervision and acute care visits. *Pediatrics.* 2003;112:129-133.
10. Resnick MD, Bearman PS, Blum RW, et al. Protecting adolescents from harm: findings from the National Longitudinal Study on Adolescent Health. *JAMA.* 1997;278:823-832.
11. Borowsky IW, Ireland M, Resnick MD. Adolescent suicide attempts: risks and protectors. *Pediatrics.* 2001;107:485-493.
12. Pignone MP, Gaynes BN, Rushton JL, et al. Screening for depression in adults: a summary of the evidence for the U.S. Preventive Services Task Force. *Ann Intern Med.* 2002;136:765-776.
13. Hacker K, Weidner D, McBride J. Integrating pediatrics and mental health: the reality is in the relationships. *Arch Pediatr Adolesc Med.* 2004;158:833-834.

## Concerns Over Alternating Acetaminophen and Ibuprofen for Fever

The recent study by Sarrell et al[1] on alternating acetaminophen and ibuprofen for fever found significant benefits over monotherapy. Table 2 in their study reports a mean daily temperature approximately 1°C (1.8°F) lower with the alternating regimen. These findings beg to be implemented, but might there be repercussions?

I'm concerned that this approach might be applied to telephone care. The risk for dosage errors and poisoning due to caller confusion remains real on the telephone.[2] Telephone medicine is not practiced at research pace. This study had many safeguards: all patients were seen, written instructions on how to dose the 2 antipyretics (including the initial loading dose) were provided, and a pharmacist reinforced these instructions.

Emphasizing dual therapy also will probably increase parents' preoccupation with "controlling the fever" and their fear of elevated temperatures. More fever phobia in turn drives unnecessary phone calls and emergency department visits. Most children can be made comfortable with 1 antipyretic and increased fluids. Let's save dual therapy for unresponsive high fevers and continue our efforts to teach parents that fever is not a cosmic error but rather offers some benefits in fighting infections.

*Barton D. Schmitt, MD*

**Correspondence:** Dr Schmitt, The Children's Hospital, 1056 E 19th Ave, Denver, CO 80218 (schmitt.barton@tchden.org).

1. Sarrell EM, Wielunsky E, Cohen HA. Antipyretic treatment in young children with fever. *Arch Pediatr Adolesc Med.* 2006;160:197-202.
2. Mayoral CE, Marino RV, Rosenfeld W, Greensher J. Alternating antipyretics: is this an alternative? *Pediatrics.* 2000;105:1009-1012.

## Alternating Acetaminophen and Ibuprofen in Children May Cause Parental Confusion and Is Dangerous

We are concerned about "Antipyretic Treatment in Young Children With Fever: Acetaminophen, Ibuprofen, or Both Alternating in a Randomized, Double-Blind Study" reported by Sarrell et al[1] in the February issue of the ARCHIVES. The alternating of acetaminophen and ibuprofen for treating fever in children may cause parental confusion. The parent may give the child acetaminophen, acetaminophen, ibuprofen, ibuprofen rather than acetaminophen, ibuprofen, acetaminophen, ibuprofen.

The treatment may also be dangerous. One case report describes a 14-month-old, previously healthy girl who was admitted for febrile status epilepticus. Her seizure was controlled and her clinical course was improved, but she continued to have a fever. On hospital day 6, the patient spiked a temperature of 105.0°. An alternating regimen of acetaminophen and ibuprofen was initiated. On day 8 of hospitalization, she developed acute renal failure.

After a thorough renal investigation, the authors suggested that the combination of acetaminophen and ibuprofen could have synergistic and additive toxic effects on the kidneys in children who are mildly or moderately dehydrated.[2] The acetaminophen and ibuprofen act via a similar mechanism; both inhibit prostaglandin synthesis. In certain settings, such as hypovolemia, inhibition of prostaglandin synthesis may impair renal perfusion.[3] This may lead to acute renal failure.

Four children aged 16 to 36 months developed hematemesis after taking 1 or 2 age-appropriate doses of ibuprofen at home to treat fever. Two children had a cough, and 2 had rhinitis. A single dose was given to 3 children and 2 successive doses, to the fourth child. Hematemesis developed within 24 hours of the initial dose. Esophagogastroduodenoscopy showed an isolated ulcer in the gastric antrum of each child. The children had no underlying medical problems and were taking no other medications. Multiple gastric biopsy specimens from each child produced no histological or culture evidence of *Helicobacter pylori*.[4]

We recommend that alternating acetaminophen and ibuprofen should not be used for treating children for fever and ibuprofen alone should not be used in young children.

*Phisit Saphyakhajon, MD*
*Gerald Greene, MD, MPH*

**Correspondence:** Dr Saphyakhajon, Department of Pediatrics, Arrowhead Regional Medical Center, 400 N Pepper St, Colton, CA 92324 (phisitsaph@yahoo.com).

1. Sarrell EM, Wielunsky E, Cohen HA. Antipyretic treatment in young children with fever: acetaminophen, ibuprofen, or both alternating in a randomized, double-blind study. *Arch Pediatr Adolesc Med.* 2006;160:197-202.
2. Del Vecchio MT, Sundel ER. Alternating antipyretics: is this an alternate? *Pediatrics.* 2001;108:1236-1237.
3. Mayoral CE, Rosenfeld W, Marino RV, Greensher J. Alternating antipyretics: is this an alternative? *Pediatrics.* 2000;105:1009-1012.
4. Medow MS. Any ibuprofen may be too much in the young. *Pediatr News.* 2006;40:40.

### *In reply*

*We disagree with the comments made by Dr Saphyakhajon concerning the possible confusion of using both antipyretics in children with fever and their possible adverse effects in the doses studied. Furthermore, we disagree with Dr*

*Schmitt that dual therapy will increase parents' preoccupation with "controlling the fever" and increase fever phobia.*

*The recent study alternating acetaminophen and ibuprofen was prompted by parental concern with their child's fever, their confusion over the dosage and frequency of administration, and the fact that both medications are readily available and are widely used.[1] Studies have reported that 50% or more parents or caregivers administer both antipyretics to their children but their methods of alternation vary.[2] Furthermore, in about half the cases, the dose used is inaccurate.[3] We chose the dosages of 12.5 mg/kg of acetaminophen per dose (of 125 mg per 5 $cm^3$) alternating with 5 mg/kg of ibuprofen per dose (of 100 mg per 5 $cm^3$) every 4 hours. We chose this method because both antipyretic dosages are at the lower end of the recommended range (12-15 mg/kg every 6 hours for acetaminophen and 5-10 mg/kg every 8 hours for ibuprofen) and therefore minimize the adverse effects without sacrificing effectiveness. We chose an alternating regimen because it is easier for parents and medical personal to calculate and remember the amount of medication needed. In the standard formulation, it is 0.5 $cm^3$ of acetaminophen alternating with 0.25 $cm^3$ of ibuprofen per the child's own weight. Calculating the amount per the child weight in cubic centimeters and having the set regular interval decrease the confusion and inappropriate dosing or overdosing in comparison with medication that is used at different intervals. Furthermore, alternating dosage requires a lower total dose of acetaminophen (3 doses of acetaminophen in 24 hours rather than 6 as recommended), which further reduces adverse effects.*

*Crocetti et el,[4] in exploring the current parental attitudes toward fever and comparing these attitudes with those described by Schmitt in 1980, concluded that "fever phobia" persists in 91% of caregivers. Parents believed fever could cause harmful effects; 21% listed brain damage, and 14% listed death. Furthermore, 85% would awaken their child to give antipyretics. The investigators noted that 44% of the caregivers gave antipyretics at too frequent of dosing intervals.*

*We have used this mode of therapy for several years, as have other investigators,[5] and have not found any increase in gastrointestinal bleeding or renal abnormalities for the patients who use it for a short duration (3 days) and are well hydrated. We have recommended using the alternating antipyretics with extreme caution in children with any chronic illness malnutrition or dehydration until further studies are available.*

*We believe that parental education and reeducation on how and when to take a temperature, recommendation of sponging, increase of fluids, and other physical treatments of fever, along with instruction for when it is appropriate to use antipyretics, including clarification of the correct dosages, is the best way to alleviate anxiety and avoid fever phobia and excessive use of emergency department services.[6]*

*E. Michael Sarrell, MD*
*Eliahu Wielunsky, MD*
*Herman Avner Cohen, MD*

**Correspondence:** Dr Sarrell, General Health Care Services of Israel, 7 Hairis St, Moshav Gan-Haim 44910, Israel (michaelsar@clalit.org.il).

1. Vauzelle-Kervroedan F, d'Athis P, Pariente-Khayat A, Debregeas S, Olive G, Pons G. Equivalent antipyretic activity of ibuprofen and acetaminophen in febrile children. *J Pediatr.* 1997;131:683-687.
2. Li SF, Lacher B, Crain BF. Acetaminophen and ibuprofen dosing by parents. *Pediatr Emerg Care.* 2000;16:394-397.
3. Mayoral CE, Marino RV, Rosenfeld W, Greensher J. Alternating antipyretics: is this an alternative? *Pediatrics.* 2000;105:1009-1012.
4. Crocetti M, Moghbeli N, Serwint J. Fever phobia revisited: have parental misconceptions about fever changed in 20 years? *Pediatrics.* 2001;107:1241-1246.
5. Lesko SM, Mitchell A. The safety of acetaminophen and ibuprofen among children younger than two years old. *Pediatrics.* 1999;104:e39. http://pediatrics.aappublications.org/cgi/content/full/104/4/e39.
6. Sarrell EM, Kahan E. Impact of single-session parental education program on management of childhood fever. *Patient Educ Couns.* 2003;1532:12-18.

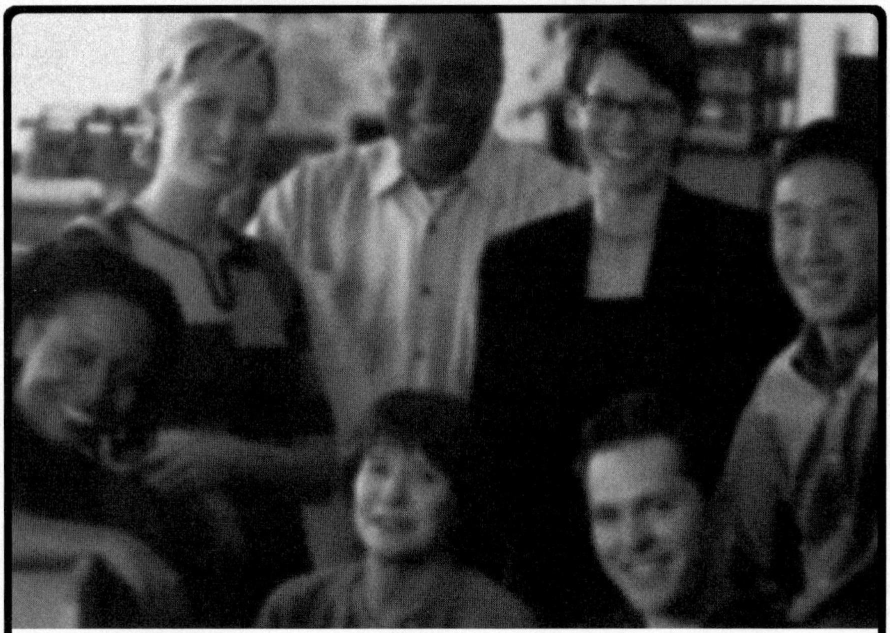

# *Move* Forward.
# *Move* Smart.
# *Move* Now.

**JAMACAREERNET**
*NetWorking for Physicians*

Are you a physician seeking a new position? Now, the leading family of clinical science journals is part of the most robust network of physician job listings in print and online. The single entry point for online recruitment listings of *JAMA & Archives* Journals is **jamacareernet.com**

JAMA CareerNet brings you a wide array of clinical and academic opportunities from every part of the nation. Whether you want a career move that takes you across the country or across the hall, make JAMA CareerNet your resource.

## PEDIATRICS

**FLORIDA: BC/BE Pediatrician Florida License required. Physician to join group practice in Central Florida. Competitive salary, malpractice insurance and benefits package. Fax CV to 352-567-3066 or E-mail to pmc1236@earthlink.net**

PEDIATRIC OPPORTUNITIES AVAILABLE: NORTH SEATTLE Metro Area, Suburban Los Angeles, South Eastern Idaho. Single and multi specialty groups, very attractive compensation and benefits, partnership. Call Chris Warner 206-782-1277, E-mail: panther@seanet.com

## PRACTICE FOR SALE

PRACTICE FOR SALE - WELL ESTABISHED PEDIATRICS AND ALLERGY practice for sale. Located 15 miles south of Boston close to major teaching hospitals. Owner will introduce. Call: 781-784-8403.

WESTERN CONNECTICUT PEDIATRIC PRACTICE FOR SALE. Established 50 years. Near excellent community Hospital. One hour to New York City, New Haven, Hartford. Reply to Box 2860, c/o PEDS, 515 N State St, 11th Fl, Chicago, IL 60610.

**BCHC** | **Brownsville Community Health Center**

Brownsville, TX: PEDIATRICIAN needed for a community health center starting August 1, 2006. Opportunity to "make a difference". Competitive compensation, benefits and incentives. Fax CV to Medical Director (956) 546-2056, or E-mail: **hlimperial@hotmail.com**

## ACKNOWLEDGMENT SERVICE

Acknowledgments in confirmation of advertising orders are sent each week. Upon receipt, please verify that your ad will be running under the appropriate heading and that your scheduling is correct. Changes to the schedule, cancellations or corrections must be communicated in writing by fax, e-mail, or regular mail prior to the published closing date of the scheduled issue.

## JOURNAL ADVERTISER INDEX


**ASTRAZENECA**
http://www.astrazeneca.com
Nexium .......... 680A-B

**CLASSIFIED ADVERTISING** .......... 759
http://www.amapublications.com

**GLAXOSMITHKLINE**
Boostrix .......... 737-738, COVER 2-665
Havrix .......... 671-672, 719-720
Pediarix .......... 691-692, COVER 3-4

**MERCK & COMPANY**
Gardasil .......... 712A-B
Rotateq .......... 704A-E


*Demographic and "Mini" inserts and/or ROB ad pages

While every precaution is taken to ensure accuracy, we cannot guarantee against the possibility of an occasional change or omission in the preparation of this index.

ARCHIVES OF PEDIATRICS & ADOLESCENT MEDICINE

# CONTACT INFORMATION

## EDITORIAL OFFICE

**Editorial Office Information:** *Archives of Pediatrics & Adolescent Medicine*, Department of Pediatrics, Child Health Institute, University of Washington, 6200 NE 74th St, Suite 210, Seattle, WA 98115-8160, USA; phone: (206) 685-3573; fax: (206) 685-3572; e-mail: archpediatrics@jama-archives.org.

**Electronic Submission:** Manuscripts should be submitted via our online manuscript submission and review system (http://manuscripts.archpediatrics.com). Manuscripts submitted through our online system should not also be submitted by mail or fax. Signed authorship forms should be sent by regular mail or fax with the assigned manuscript number noted on each page in the upper right-hand corner. See the Instructions for Authors (www.archpediatrics.com) for more details.

## CONSORTIUM OF *JAMA* & *ARCHIVES* JOURNALS

The *Archives of Pediatrics & Adolescent Medicine* is a member of the consortium of AMA journals listed below.

- The Journal of the American Medical Association (JAMA)
- Archives of Dermatology
- Archives of Facial Plastic Surgery
- Archives of General Psychiatry
- Archives of Internal Medicine
- Archives of Neurology
- Archives of Ophthalmology
- Archives of Otolaryngology–Head & Neck Surgery
- Archives of Pediatrics & Adolescent Medicine
- Archives of Surgery

## *JAMA/ARCHIVES* MEDIA RELATIONS

Jann Ingmire; phone: (312) 464-5262; e-mail: mediarelations@jama-archives.org.

## *ARCHIVES OF PEDIATRICS* ONLINE

*Archives of Pediatrics & Adolescent Medicine* is available online at www.archpediatrics.com.

## *JAMA/ARCHIVES* REPRINTS

**Author/Educational Institution Reprints:** Anna Goins at (312) 464-2477; fax: (312) 464-5843; e-mail: anna.goins@ama-assn.org. Minimum order: 100 reprints.

**Commercial Reprints:** Phone: (312) 464-0776; fax: (312) 464-0708; e-mail: reprints@ama-assn.org. Minimum order: 100 reprints.

## PERMISSIONS

Information about obtaining permission to republish, reprint, or adapt material published in *Archives of Pediatrics & Adolescent Medicine* is available from Rhonda Bailey Brown; phone: (312) 464-2513; fax: (312) 464-5843; e-mail: permissions@ama-assn.org.

## DOCUMENT DELIVERY

Copies of individual articles are available online at www.archpediatrics.com and from the following: Infotrieve, phone: (800) 422-4633; fax: (310) 208-5971; URL: www.infotrieve.com; e-mail: orders@infotrieve.com; Institute for Scientific Information (ISI), phone: (800) 603-4367; fax: (856) 787-1679; URL: http://www.isidoc.com; e-mail: service@isidoc.com.

The ARCHIVES OF PEDIATRICS & ADOLESCENT MEDICINE (ISSN 01072–4710) is published monthly by the American Medical Association, 515 N State St, Chicago, IL 60610–0946, and is an official publication of the Association. The ARCHIVES OF PEDIATRICS & ADOLESCENT MEDICINE reaches more than 30 900 readers in over 83 countries each month. Periodicals postage paid at Chicago, Ill, and at additional mailing offices. GST registration number 12622 5556 RT. Canada Post International Publications Mail (Canadian Distribution) Sales Agreement No. 318728. POSTMASTER, send all address changes to *Archives of Pediatrics & Adolescent Medicine,* c/o the AMA Unified Service Center, American Medical Association, 515 N State St, Chicago, IL 60610. Printed in the USA.

## ADVERTISING

Information about advertising is available from the following sales representatives and online at www.archpediatrics.com.

**Account Manager:** Tim Melroy (nationally); phone: (973) 263-9191 ext 213.

**Manager, Marketing Services:** Nancy Bell; phone: (973) 263-9191 ext 216.

**Advertising Office:** 119 Cherry Hill Rd, Suite 330, Parsippany, NJ 07054-1114; phone: (973) 263-9191.

**Classified Advertising:** Thalia Moss, Shana Brown, Kim Jenkins, Sophie Levandoski, 515 N State St, Chicago, IL 60610; phone: (800) 262-2260; e-mail: classifieds@jama-archives.org.

## ADVERTISING PRINCIPLES

Advertisements in this issue have been reviewed to comply with the principles governing advertising in AMA publications. A copy of these principles is available on request and online at www.archpediatrics.com. The appearance of advertising in AMA publications is not an AMA guarantee or endorsement of the product or the claims made for the product by the manufacturer.

## ADDRESS CHANGES

Send all address changes to *Archives of Pediatrics & Adolescent Medicine*, c/o the AMA Unified Service Center, American Medical Association, 515 N State St, Chicago, IL 60610. Notification of address changes must be made at least 6 weeks in advance; include both old and new addresses and a recent mailing label if sending via mail.

## SUBSCRIPTION RATES AND SERVICE

Subscription rates are shown in the table below. For service in the US and Americas, inquiries on pricing, address changes, missing issues, subscription billing, subscription renewal, and back issues, contact the AMA Unified Service Center, 24 hours a day, 7 days a week.

**AMA members:** phone: (800) 262-3211; e-mail: msc@ama-assn.org. **Other physicians and nonphysician customers, including subscription agents:** phone: (800) 262-2350 or (312) 670-7827; fax: (312) 464-5831; e-mail: ama-subs@ama-assn.org. **Inquiries:** Unified Service Center, American Medical Association, PO Box 10946, Chicago, IL 60610-0946. For subscribers with mailing addresses outside the United States & Americas: Contact *JAMA & Archives* Journals, c/o EMD GmbH, Birkenstr.67, 10559 Berlin, Germany. Phone: +49 (30) 33099828; fax: +49 (30) 33099829; e-mail: ama@emd-germany.de.

**Annual Subscription Rates**

| | United States | Americas | UK | Rest of World |
|---|---|---|---|---|
| INDIVIDUAL | | | | |
| Print and Online | $185 | $240 | £165 | €250 |
| INSTITUTION | | | | |
| Print and Online | $400 | $485 | £315 | €470 |

In Canada, US rate plus GST. Rates for residents and medical students available at pubs.ama-assn.org, or from the AMA Unified Service Center.

**PEDIARIX™ [Diphtheria and Tetanus Toxoids and Acellular Pertussis Adsorbed, Hepatitis B (Recombinant) and Inactivated Poliovirus Vaccine Combined]**

The following is a brief summary only; see full prescribing information for complete product information.

**CONTRAINDICATIONS:** Hypersensitivity to any component of the vaccine, including yeast, neomycin, and polymyxin B, is a contraindication (see DESCRIPTION in complete prescribing information). Do not use PEDIARIX after a serious allergic reaction (e.g., anaphylaxis) temporally associated with a previous dose of this vaccine or with any components of this vaccine. Because of the uncertainty as to which component of the vaccine might be responsible, do not give further vaccination with any of these components; or, refer such individuals to an allergist for evaluation. The following events are contraindications to administration of PEDIARIX: encephalopathy (e.g., coma, decreased level of consciousness, prolonged seizures) within 7 days of administration of a previous dose of a pertussis-containing vaccine that is not attributable to another identifiable cause; progressive neurologic disorder, including infantile spasms, uncontrolled epilepsy, or progressive encephalopathy. Do not vaccinate individuals with such conditions until a treatment regimen has been established and the condition has stabilized. PEDIARIX is not contraindicated for use in individuals with HIV infection.

**WARNINGS:** Administration of PEDIARIX is associated with higher rates of fever relative to separately administered vaccines. In one study that evaluated medically attended fever after the first dose of PEDIARIX or separately administered vaccines, infants who received PEDIARIX had a higher rate of medical encounters for fever within the first 4 days following vaccination. In some infants, these encounters included the performance of diagnostic studies to evaluate other causes of fever (see ADVERSE REACTIONS). The vial stopper is latex-free. The tip cap and the rubber plunger of the needleless prefilled syringes contain dry natural latex rubber that may cause allergic reactions in latex sensitive individuals. If any of the following events occur in temporal relation to receipt of whole-cell DTP or a vaccine containing an acellular pertussis component, consider carefully whether to give subsequent doses of PEDIARIX or any vaccine containing a pertussis component: temperature of ≥40.5°C (105°F) within 48 hours not due to another identifiable cause; collapse or shock-like state (hypotonic-hyporesponsive episode) within 48 hours; persistent, inconsolable crying lasting ≥3 hours, occurring within 48 hours; seizures with or without fever occurring within 3 days. If Guillain-Barré syndrome occurs within 6 weeks of receipt of prior vaccine containing tetanus toxoid, the decision to give subsequent doses of PEDIARIX or any vaccine containing tetanus toxoid should be based on careful consideration of the potential benefits and possible risks. A committee of the Institute of Medicine (IOM) has concluded that evidence is consistent with a causal relationship between whole-cell DTP vaccine and acute neurologic illness, and under special circumstances, between whole-cell DTP vaccine and chronic neurologic disease in the context of the National Childhood Encephalopathy Study (NCES) report; however, evidence was insufficient to indicate whether or not whole-cell DTP vaccine increased the overall risk of chronic neurologic disease. Acute encephalopathy and permanent neurologic damage have not been reported causally linked or in temporal association with administration of PEDIARIX, but the experience with PEDIARIX is insufficient to rule this out. Encephalopathy has been reported following INFANRIX® (Diphtheria and Tetanus Toxoids and Acellular Pertussis Vaccine Adsorbed) (see ADVERSE REACTIONS, Postmarketing Reports), but data are not sufficient to evaluate a causal relationship. The decision to administer a pertussis-containing vaccine to children with stable central nervous system (CNS) disorders must be made by the physician on an individual basis, with consideration of all relevant factors, and assessment of potential risks and benefits for that individual. Advise the parent or guardian of the potential increased risk involved (see PRECAUTIONS). A family history of seizures or other CNS disorders is not a contraindication to pertussis vaccine. For children at higher risk for seizures than the general population, an appropriate antipyretic may be administered at the time of vaccination and for the ensuing 24 hours according to the respective prescribing information recommended dosage to reduce the possibility of post-vaccination fever. Defer vaccination during the course of a moderate or severe illness with or without fever and vaccinate patients as soon as they have recovered from the acute phase of the illness. Do not give PEDIARIX to children on anticoagulant therapy or those with bleeding disorders unless the potential benefit clearly outweighs the risk of administration (see PRECAUTIONS in complete prescribing information).

**PRECAUTIONS:** Before the injection of any biological, the physician should take all reasonable precautions to prevent allergic or other adverse reactions. Epinephrine injection (1:1000) and other appropriate agents used for the control of immediate allergic reactions must be immediately available should an acute anaphylactic reaction occur. Immunosuppressed individuals, including those receiving immunosuppressive therapy, may not develop the expected immune response. **Drug Interactions:** For information regarding concomitant administration with other vaccines, refer to DOSAGE AND ADMINISTRATION in complete prescribing information. Do not mix PEDIARIX with any other vaccine in the same syringe or vial. **Carcinogenesis, Mutagenesis, Impairment of Fertility:** PEDIARIX has not been evaluated for carcinogenic or mutagenic potential, or for impairment of fertility. **Pregnancy:** Pregnancy Category C: PEDIARIX is not indicated for women of child-bearing age. Animal reproduction studies have not been conducted with PEDIARIX. It is not known whether PEDIARIX can cause fetal harm when administered to a pregnant woman or if PEDIARIX can affect reproductive capacity. **Geriatric Use:** PEDIARIX is not indicated for use in adult populations. **Pediatric Use:** Safety and effectiveness of PEDIARIX in infants younger than 6 weeks of age have not been evaluated (see DOSAGE AND ADMINISTRATION in complete prescribing information). PEDIARIX is not recommended for persons 7 years of age or older. Tetanus and Diphtheria Toxoids Adsorbed (Td) For Adult Use, inactivated poliovirus vaccine (IPV), and Hepatitis B Vaccine (Recombinant) should be used in individuals 7 years of age or older.

**ADVERSE REACTIONS:** A total of 20,739 doses of PEDIARIX have been administered to 7,028 infants as a 3-dose primary series. The most common adverse reactions observed in clinical trials were local injection site reactions (pain, redness, or swelling), fever, and fussiness. In comparative studies, administration of PEDIARIX was associated with higher rates of fever relative to separately administered vaccines (see WARNINGS). The prevalence of fever was highest on the day of vaccination and the day following vaccination. More than 98% of episodes of fever resolved within the 4-day period following vaccination (i.e., the period including the day of vaccination and the next 3 days). Rates of most other solicited adverse events following PEDIARIX were comparable to rates observed following separately administered US-licensed vaccines. The adverse event information from clinical trials provides a basis for identifying adverse events that appear to be related to vaccine use and for approximating rates. However, because clinical trials are conducted under widely varying conditions, adverse event rates observed in the clinical trials of a vaccine cannot be directly compared to rates in the clinical trials of another vaccine, and may not reflect the rates observed in practice. A total of 5,472 infants were enrolled in a German safety study that was originally designed to compare the safety and reactogenicity of PEDIARIX administered concomitantly at separate sites with 1 of 4 *Haemophilus influenzae* type b (Hib) vaccines at 3, 4, and 5 months of age. After enrollment of 1,569 infants, the study was amended to include a control group that received INFANRIX, Hib vaccine, and oral poliovirus vaccine (OPV) separately. Infants in the separate administration group received one less antigen (hepatitis B) than the infants who received PEDIARIX. Safety data were available for 4,666 infants who received PEDIARIX administered concomitantly at separate sites with 1 of 4 Hib vaccines and for 768 infants in the control group that received separate vaccines. The primary end-point of the study was the percentage of infants with any grade 3 solicited symptom (redness or swelling >20 mm, fever >103.1°F, or crying, pain, vomiting, diarrhea, loss of appetite, or restlessness that prevented normal daily activities) over the 3-dose primary series in infants who received PEDIARIX (4 groups that received PEDIARIX and Hib vaccines pooled) compared to the group that received INFANRIX and Hib vaccine separately with OPV. Analysis for the primary end-point was performed on the according-to-protocol (ATP) cohort that included only those infants who were enrolled after the protocol amendment to include a control group. Of 3,773 infants in the ATP cohort for whom safety data were available, 16.2% (95% CI: 14.9% to 17.5%) of 3,029 infants who received PEDIARIX and Hib vaccine compared to 20.3% (95% CI: 17.5% to 23.4%) of 744 infants who received separate vaccines were reported to have had at least one grade 3 solicited symptom within 4 days of vaccination (i.e., day of vaccination and the next 3 days). The difference between groups in the rate of grade 3 symptoms was 4.1% (90% CI: 1.4% to 7.1%). These were the rates for selected solicited symptoms within 4 days following each dose in a 3-dose primary series in infants who received PEDIARIX administered concomitantly with Hib vaccine and those who received separate concomitant administration of INFANRIX, Hib vaccine, and OPV for the intent-to-treat (ITT) cohort (includes all infants enrolled before and after the amendment who received the indicated vaccine and for whom at least one symptom sheet was completed):

**Percentage of German Infants With Solicited Local Reactions or Selected Systemic Adverse Events Within 4 Days of Vaccination* (ITT Cohort)**

| | PEDIARIX & Hib | | | INFANRIX, Hib, & OPV | | |
|---|---|---|---|---|---|---|
| | Dose 1 | Dose 2 | Dose 3 | Dose 1 | Dose 2 | Dose 3 |
| **N** | **4,666** | **4,619** | **4,574** | **768** | **757** | **750** |
| **Local†** | | | | | | |
| Pain, any | 14.0 | 10.2 | 9.9 | 14.2 | 9.8 | 8.1 |
| Pain, grade 2 or 3 | 2.9 | 1.2 | 1.5 | 3.6 | 1.7 | 1.1 |
| Pain, grade 3 | 0.7 | 0.3 | 0.3 | 1.3 | 0.4 | 0.1 |
| Redness, any | 18.6 | 26.6 | 25.6 | 16.1 | 21.4 | 20.8 |
| Redness, >5 mm | 6.7 | 9.9 | 9.0 | 5.9 | 8.2 | 7.7 |
| Redness, >20 mm | 1.2 | 1.0 | 1.1 | 1.8 | 0.7 | 1.1 |
| Swelling, any | 12.7 | 18.5 | 18.4 | 9.6 | 12.9 | 13.6 |
| Swelling, >5 mm | 5.6 | 7.7 | 7.8 | 3.6 | 5.2 | 4.8 |
| Swelling, >20 mm | 1.2 | 1.6 | 1.5 | 1.3 | 1.1 | 1.2 |
| **Systemic** | | | | | | |
| Restlessness, any | 41.4 | 32.0 | 26.7 | 46.4 | 35.0 | 27.6 |
| Restlessness, grade 2 or 3 | 14.4 | 10.0 | 8.9 | 20.2 | 11.5 | 8.4 |
| Restlessness, grade 3 | 3.0 | 1.5 | 1.6 | 5.7 | 3.0 | 1.7 |
| Fever‡, ≥100.4°F | 25.1 | 19.3 | 19.7 | 13.2 | 13.1 | 11.2 |
| Fever‡, >101.3°F | 5.8 | 4.1 | 4.6 | 2.2 | 2.8 | 2.1 |
| Fever‡, >103.1°F | 0.3 | 0.5 | 0.7 | 0.3 | 0.3 | 0.5 |
| Unusual cry§, any | 24.9 | 16.5 | 13.1 | 36.5 | 19.7 | 14.3 |
| Unusual cry§, grade 2 or 3 | 12.7 | 7.1 | 5.7 | 20.8 | 10.0 | 5.7 |
| Unusual cry§, grade 3 | 3.9 | 1.7 | 1.4 | 6.8 | 2.1 | 1.1 |
| Loss of appetite, any | 17.9 | 13.3 | 12.5 | 19.1 | 16.2 | 11.3 |
| Loss of appetite, grade 2 or 3 | 4.0 | 2.9 | 2.7 | 4.4 | 2.9 | 2.3 |
| Loss of appetite, grade 3 | 0.6 | 0.5 | 0.4 | 0.5 | 0.7 | 0.0 |

N = number of infants in the intent-to-treat (ITT) cohort.
Grade 2 defined as sufficiently discomforting to interfere with daily activities.
Grade 3 defined as preventing normal daily activities.
* Within 4 days of vaccination defined as day of vaccination and the next 3 days.
† Local reactions at the injection site for PEDIARIX or INFANRIX.
‡ Rectal temperatures.
§ Unusual cry lasting >1 hour.

In this study, infants were also monitored for unsolicited adverse events that occurred within 30 days following vaccination. Over the entire study period, 6 subjects in the group that received PEDIARIX reported seizures. Two of these subjects had a febrile seizure, 1 of whom also developed afebrile seizures. The remaining 4 subjects had afebrile seizures, including 2 with infantile spasms. Two subjects reported seizures within 7 days following vaccination (1 subject had both febrile and afebrile seizures, and 1 subject had afebrile seizures), corresponding to a rate of 0.22 seizures per 1,000 doses (febrile seizures 0.07 per 1,000 doses, afebrile seizures 0.14 per 1,000 doses). No subject who received concomitant INFANRIX, Hib vaccine, and OPV reported seizures. In a separate German study that evaluated the safety of INFANRIX in 22,505 infants who received 66,867 doses of INFANRIX administered as a 3-dose primary series, the rate of seizures within 7 days of vaccination with INFANRIX was 0.13 per 1,000 doses (febrile seizures 0.0 per 1,000 doses, afebrile seizures 0.13 per 1,000 doses). No cases of hypotonic-hyporesponsiveness, encephalopathy, or anaphylaxis were reported in the German study that evaluated the safety of PEDIARIX. Rates of serious adverse events that are less common than those reported in this safety study are not known at this time.

Additional safety data for PEDIARIX are available from a US study designed to evaluate lot-to-lot consistency and a bridge for a new manufacturing step. These were the rates for local reactions and selected adverse events within 4 days of vaccination with PEDIARIX administered concomitantly with a Hib vaccine at 2, 4, and 6 months of age:

**Percentage of US Infants With Solicited Local Reactions or Selected Systemic Adverse Events Within 4 Days of Vaccination* (ITT Cohort)**

| | PEDIARIX & Hib | | |
|---|---|---|---|
| | Dose 1 | Dose 2 | Dose 3 |
| **Local†** | **N = 482** | **N = 469** | **N = 466** |
| Pain, any | 30.5 | 25.4 | 23.0 |
| Pain, grade 2 or 3 | 6.2 | 5.5 | 3.6 |
| Pain, grade 3 | 1.2 | 0.6 | 0.6 |
| Redness, any | 25.3 | 32.6 | 35.6 |
| Redness, >5 mm | 9.3 | 10.4 | 8.6 |
| Redness, >20 mm | 0.6 | 1.5 | 1.3 |
| Swelling, any | 15.1 | 16.6 | 22.3 |
| Swelling, >5 mm | 6.8 | 6.2 | 6.4 |
| Swelling, >20 mm | 1.0 | 1.3 | 1.3 |
| **Systemic** | **N = 482** | **N = 469** | **N = 467** |
| Restlessness, any | 28.8 | 30.3 | 28.5 |
| Restlessness, grade 2 or 3 | 7.1 | 9.0 | 9.4 |
| Restlessness, grade 3 | 1.0 | 1.1 | 0.6 |
| Fever‡, ≥100.4°F | 26.6 | 31.3 | 25.9 |
| Fever‡, >101.3°F | 2.9 | 6.2 | 4.7 |
| Fever‡, >103.1°F | 0.0 | 0.2 | 0.6 |
| Fussiness, any | 61.8 | 63.8 | 57.0 |
| Fussiness, grade 2 or 3 | 14.9 | 21.5 | 17.1 |
| Fussiness, grade 3 | 2.7 | 3.4 | 1.7 |
| Loss of appetite, any | 21.6 | 19.8 | 18.8 |
| Loss of appetite, grade 2 or 3 | 3.1 | 3.2 | 2.4 |
| Loss of appetite, grade 3 | 0.2 | 0.4 | 0.0 |
| Sleeping more than usual, any | 46.7 | 31.8 | 28.1 |
| Sleeping more than usual, grade 2 or 3 | 10.2 | 6.0 | 4.7 |
| Sleeping more than usual, grade 3 | 1.7 | 0.4 | 0.6 |

N = number of infants in the intent-to-treat (ITT) cohort (infants who received the indicated vaccine and for whom at least one symptom sheet was completed).
Grade 2 defined as sufficiently discomforting to interfere with daily activities.
Grade 3 defined as preventing normal daily activities.
* Within 4 days of vaccination defined as day of vaccination and the next 3 days.
† Local reactions at the injection site for PEDIARIX.
‡ Rectal temperatures.

In another US study, these were the rates for fever within 4 days following dose 1 (i.e., day of vaccination and the next 3 days) at 2 months of age in infants who received PEDIARIX when administered concomitantly at separate sites with Hib and pneumococcal conjugate vaccines and those who received INFANRIX, ENGERIX-B® [Hepatitis B Vaccine (Recombinant)], IPV, Hib vaccine, and pneumococcal conjugate vaccine:

**Percentage of US Infants With Fever Within 4 Days of Dose 1* (ITT Cohort)**

| | PEDIARIX, Hib, & Pneumococcal Conjugate (N = 667) | INFANRIX, ENGERIX-B, IPV, Hib, & Pneumococcal Conjugate (N = 333) | Separate Vaccine Group Minus Combination Vaccine Group |
|---|---|---|---|
| **Fever†** | **%** | **%** | **Difference (95% CI)** |
| ≥100.4°F‡ | 27.9 | 19.8 | -8.07 (-13.54, -2.60) |
| >101.3°F | 7.0 | 4.5 | -2.54 (-5.50, 0.41) |
| >102.2°F‡ | 2.2 | 0.3 | -1.95 (-3.22, -0.68) |
| >103.1°F | 0.4 | 0.0 | -0.45 (-0.96, 0.06) |
| M.A.‡ | 1.2 | 0.0 | -1.20 (-2.03, -037) |

N = number of infants for whom at least one symptom sheet was completed, excluding 3 infants for whom temperature was not measured and 3 infants whose temperature was measured by the tympanic method.
*Within 4 days of dose 1 defined as day of vaccination and the next 3 days.
† Rectal temperatures.
‡ The group that received PEDIARIX compared to separate vaccine group p value <0.05 (2-sided Fisher Exact test) or the 95% confidence interval on the difference between groups does not include 0.
M.A. = Medically attended (a visit to or from medical personnel).

In this study, medical attention (a visit to or from medical personnel) for fever within 4 days following vaccination was sought for 8 infants who received PEDIARIX (1.2%) and no infants who received separately administered vaccines. Four infants were seen by medical personnel in an office setting; no diagnostic tests were performed in 2 of the infants and a complete blood count (CBC) was done in the other 2 infants. Of 3 infants who were seen in an emergency room, all had a CBC and a blood and urine culture performed; chest X-rays were done in 2 of the infants and a nasopharyngeal specimen was tested for Respiratory Syncytial Virus in one of the infants. One infant was hospitalized for a work-up that included a CBC, blood and urine cultures, a lumbar puncture, and a chest X-ray. All episodes of medically attended fever resolved within 4 days post-vaccination.

Limited data are available from a study conducted in Moldova in which infants received a dose of hepatitis B vaccine within 48 hours of birth followed by 3 doses of PEDIARIX at 6, 10, and 14 weeks of age. No information was collected on the HBsAg status of mothers of enrolled infants. These were the rates for local reactions and selected adverse events within 4 days of vaccination with PEDIARIX administered comcomitantly with Hib vaccine following a birth dose of hepatitis B vaccine:

**Percentage of Moldovan Infants With Solicited Local Reactions or Selected Systemic Adverse Events Within 4 Days of Vaccination* (ITT Cohort)**

| | PEDIARIX & Hib | | |
|---|---|---|---|
| | Dose 1 | Dose 2 | Dose 3 |
| **N** | **160** | **158** | **157** |
| **Local†** | | | |
| Pain, any | 25.6 | 18.4 | 14.0 |
| Pain, grade 3 | 3.1 | 0.6 | 1.9 |
| Redness, any | 41.9 | 41.8 | 47.1 |
| Redness, >20 mm | 1.9 | 2.5 | 4.5 |
| Swelling, any | 20.6 | 18.4 | 28.0 |
| Swelling, >20 mm | 4.4 | 2.5 | 7.0 |
| **Systemic** | | | |
| Restlessness, any | 13.1 | 10.8 | 8.9 |
| Restlessness, grade 3 | 1.3 | 0.6 | 0.6 |
| Fever‡, ≥100.4°F | 14.4 | 11.4 | 5.1 |
| Fever‡, >103.1°F | 0.0 | 0.6 | 0.0 |
| Fussiness, any | 25.0 | 21.5 | 17.8 |
| Fussiness, grade 3 | 2.5 | 0.6 | 0.6 |

N = number of infants in the intent-to-treat (ITT) cohort (infants who received the indicated vaccine and for whom at least one symptom sheet was completed).
Grade 3 defined as preventing normal daily activities.
*Within 4 days of vaccination defined as day of vaccination and the next 3 days.
† Local reactions at the injection site for PEDIARIX.
‡ Rectal temperatures.

Although there was no comparator group who received PEDIARIX without a birth dose of hepatitis B vaccine, available data suggest that some local adverse events may occur at a higher rate when PEDIARIX is administered after a birth dose of hepatitis B vaccine.

As with any vaccine, there is the possibility that broad use of PEDIARIX could reveal adverse events not observed in clinical trials.

**Postmarketing Reports:** Worldwide voluntary reports of adverse events received for INFANRIX and ENGERIX-B in children younger than 7 years of age since market introduction of these US-licensed vaccines are listed below. This list includes adverse events for which 20 or more reports were received with the exception of intussusception, idiopathic thrombocytopenic purpura, thrombocytopenia, anaphylactic reaction, angioedema, encephalopathy, hypotonic-hyporesponsive episode, and alopecia for which fewer than 20 reports were received. These latter events are included either because of the seriousness of the event or the strength of causal connection to components of this or other vaccines or drugs. *Body as a whole:* Asthenia[b], fever[a+b], lethargy[b], malaise[b], Sudden Infant Death Syndrome[a+b]. *Cardiovascular system:* Cyanosis[a+b], edema[b], pallor[b]. *Gastrointestinal system:* Abdominal pain[b], anorexia[b], diarrhea[a+b], intussusception[a+b], nausea[b], vomiting[a+b]. *Hematologic/lymphatic:* Idiopathic thrombocytopenic purpura[a+b], lymphadenopathy[a], thrombocytopenia[a+b]. *Hepatic:* Jaundice[b], liver function tests abnormal[b]. *Hypersensitivity:* Anaphylactic reaction[a+b], angioedema[b], hypersensitivity[a]. *Infections:* Cellulitis[a]. *Injection site reactions:* Injection site reactions[a+b]. *Musculoskeletal:* Arthralgia[b], limb swelling[a+b]. *Nervous system:* Convulsions[a+b], encephalopathy[a], headache[b], hypotonia[a+b], hypotonic-hyporesponsive episode[a], somnolence[a+b]. *Psychiatric:* Crying[a+b], irritability[a+b]. *Respiratory system:* Respiratory tract infection[a]. *Skin and appendages:* Alopecia[b], erythema[a+b], erythema multiforme[b], petechiae[b], pruritus[a+b], rash[a+b], urticaria[a+b]. *Special senses:* Ear pain[a]. [[a] Following INFANRIX; [b] Following ENGERIX-B; [a+b] Following either INFANRIX or ENGERIX-B.] These reactions were reported voluntarily from a population of uncertain size; therefore, it is not always possible to reliably estimate their frequency or establish a causal relationship to vaccination.

**Reporting Adverse Events:** Report the occurrence following immunization of any event set forth in the Vaccine Injury Table from the National Childhood Vaccine Injury Act including: Anaphylaxis or anaphylactic shock within 7 days, encephalopathy or encephalitis within 7 days, brachial neuritis within 28 days, or an acute complication or sequelae (including death) of an illness, disability, injury, or condition referred to above, or any events that would contraindicate further doses of PEDIARIX. The VAERS toll-free number is 1-800-822-7967.

Manufactured by **GlaxoSmithKline Biologicals**, Rixensart, Belgium, US License 1617

Distributed by **GlaxoSmithKline,** Research Triangle Park, NC 27709



Full prescribing information for PEDIARIX is available at www.GSKVaccines.com/Pediarix. BRS-PE:L2

 Printed in USA. PED583R0 June 2005

**Nearly 1 in 6 children did not receive all recommended DTaP doses*[1]**

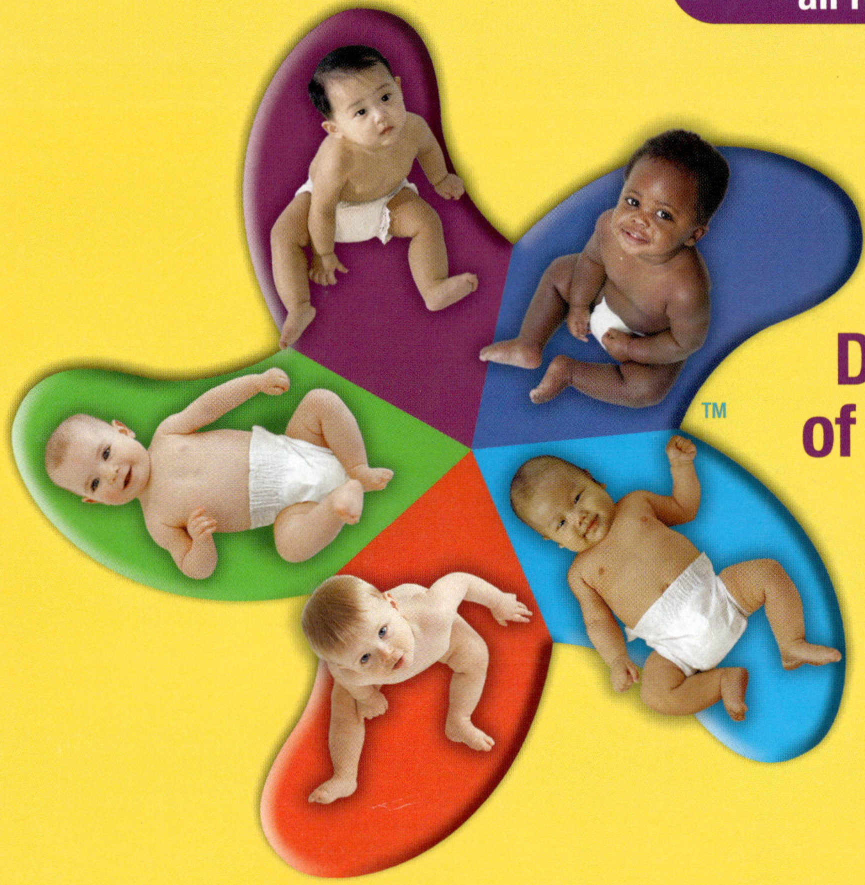


# Don't run the risk of letting one child get away

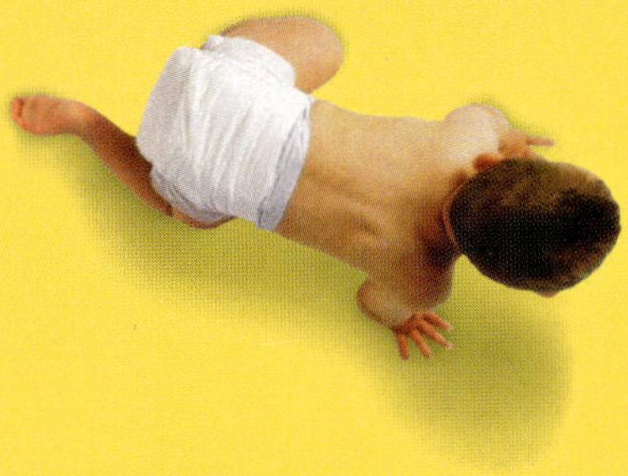

## PEDIARIX may help ensure timely vaccination with fewer injections

- With just 1 dose at 2, 4, and 6 months of age (in infants born of HBsAg-negative mothers)

*Based on analysis of the first four DTaP doses in the most recent National Immunization Survey (2003) of 21,210 children 19–35 months of age.

In clinical studies, adverse events in infants receiving PEDIARIX included injection-site reactions (pain, redness, or swelling), fever, and fussiness. Administration of PEDIARIX was associated with higher rates of fever relative to separately administered vaccines (see Adverse Reactions section of the brief summary). PEDIARIX is contraindicated in infants with known hypersensitivity to any component of the vaccine including yeast, neomycin, and polymyxin B. As with any vaccine, vaccination with PEDIARIX may not protect 100% of susceptible individuals.

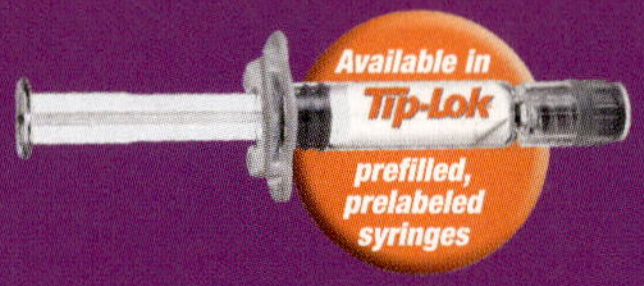


**Please see brief summary for PEDIARIX on the following page.**

**References: 1.** Centers for Disease Control and Prevention. National, state, and urban area vaccination coverage among children aged 19–35 months—United States, 2003. *MMWR.* 2004;53(29):658–661.



Manufactured by **GlaxoSmithKline Biologicals,** Rixensart, Belgium
Distributed by **GlaxoSmithKline,** Research Triangle Park, NC 27709

**Pediarix®**

**Diphtheria and Tetanus Toxoids and Acellular Pertussis Adsorbed, Hepatitis B (Recombinant) and Inactivated Poliovirus Vaccine Combined**

gsk GlaxoSmithKline Vaccines

ARCHIVES OF PEDIATRICS & ADOLESCENT MEDICINE

WWW.ARCHPEDIATRICS.COM

AUGUST 2006

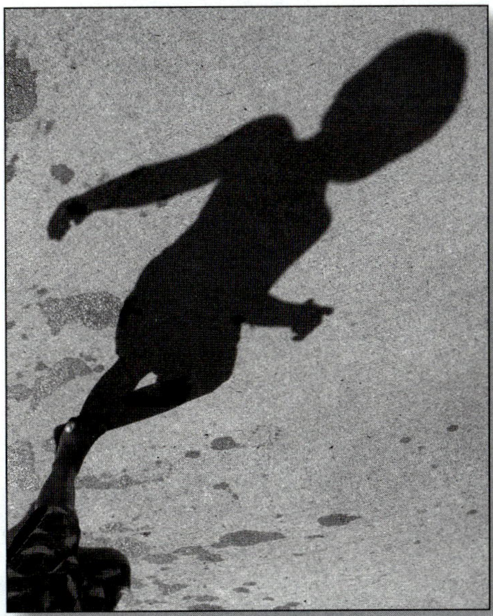

Shadow Play, Green Lake Wading Pool. Seattle, Wash, 2005. See page 765.

RANDOMIZED TRIAL OF HIV PREVENTION INTERVENTION FOR LATINOS

HEALTH CONDITIONS AND HEALTH CARE UTILIZATION AMONG CHILDREN WITH AUTISM

ARE HOUSEHOLD FIREARMS STORED LESS SAFELY IN HOMES WITH ADOLESCENTS?

THE IMPACT OF STAFFING ON BLOODSTREAM INFECTIONS IN THE NICU

COMPLETE TABLE OF CONTENTS ON PAGE 763

JAMA & ARCHIVES JOURNALS
American Medical Association

**PEDIARIX™ [Diphtheria and Tetanus Toxoids and Acellular Pertussis Adsorbed, Hepatitis B (Recombinant) and Inactivated Poliovirus Vaccine Combined]**

The following is a brief summary only; see full prescribing information for complete product information.

**CONTRAINDICATIONS:** Hypersensitivity to any component of the vaccine, including yeast, neomycin, and polymyxin B, is a contraindication (see DESCRIPTION in complete prescribing information). Do not use PEDIARIX after a serious allergic reaction (e.g., anaphylaxis) temporally associated with a previous dose of this vaccine or with any components of this vaccine. Because of the uncertainty as to which component of the vaccine might be responsible, do not give further vaccination with any of these components; or, refer such individuals to an allergist for evaluation. The following events are contraindications to administration of PEDIARIX: encephalopathy (e.g., coma, decreased level of consciousness, prolonged seizures) within 7 days of administration of a previous dose of a pertussis-containing vaccine that is not attributable to another identifiable cause; progressive neurologic disorder, including infantile spasms, uncontrolled epilepsy, or progressive encephalopathy. Do not vaccinate individuals with such conditions until a treatment regimen has been established and the condition has stabilized. PEDIARIX is not contraindicated for use in individuals with HIV infection.

**WARNINGS:** Administration of PEDIARIX is associated with higher rates of fever relative to separately administered vaccines. In one study that evaluated medically attended fever after the first dose of PEDIARIX or separately administered vaccines, infants who received PEDIARIX had a higher rate of medical encounters for fever within the first 4 days following vaccination. In some infants, these encounters included the performance of diagnostic studies to evaluate other causes of fever (see ADVERSE REACTIONS). The vial stopper is latex-free. The tip cap and the rubber plunger of the needleless prefilled syringes contain dry natural latex rubber that may cause allergic reactions in latex sensitive individuals. If any of the following events occur in temporal relation to receipt of whole-cell DTP or a vaccine containing an acellular pertussis component, consider carefully whether to give subsequent doses of PEDIARIX or any vaccine containing a pertussis component: temperature of ≥40.5°C (105°F) within 48 hours not due to another identifiable cause; collapse or shock-like state (hypotonic-hyporesponsive episode) within 48 hours; persistent, inconsolable crying lasting ≥3 hours, occurring within 48 hours; seizures with or without fever occurring within 3 days. If Guillain-Barré syndrome occurs within 6 weeks of receipt of prior vaccine containing tetanus toxoid, the decision to give subsequent doses of PEDIARIX or any vaccine containing tetanus toxoid should be based on careful consideration of the potential benefits and possible risks. A committee of the Institute of Medicine (IOM) has concluded that evidence is consistent with a causal relationship between whole-cell DTP vaccine and acute neurologic illness, and under special circumstances, between whole-cell DTP vaccine and chronic neurologic disease in the context of the National Childhood Encephalopathy Study (NCES) report; however, evidence was insufficient to indicate whether or not whole-cell DTP vaccine increased the overall risk of chronic neurologic disease. Acute encephalopathy and permanent neurologic damage have not been reported causally linked or in temporal association with administration of PEDIARIX, but the experience with PEDIARIX is insufficient to rule this out. Encephalopathy has been reported following INFANRIX® (Diphtheria and Tetanus Toxoids and Acellular Pertussis Vaccine Adsorbed) (see ADVERSE REACTIONS, Postmarketing Reports), but data are not sufficient to evaluate a causal relationship. The decision to administer a pertussis-containing vaccine to children with stable central nervous system (CNS) disorders must be made by the physician on an individual basis, with consideration of all relevant factors, and assessment of potential risks and benefits for that individual. Advise the parent or guardian of the potential increased risk involved (see PRECAUTIONS). A family history of seizures or other CNS disorders is not a contraindication to pertussis vaccine. For children at higher risk for seizures than the general population, an appropriate antipyretic may be administered at the time of vaccination and for the ensuing 24 hours according to the respective prescribing information recommended dosage to reduce the possibility of post-vaccination fever. Defer vaccination during the course of a moderate or severe illness with or without fever and vaccinate patients as soon as they have recovered from the acute phase of the illness. Do not give PEDIARIX to children on anticoagulant therapy or those with bleeding disorders unless the potential benefit clearly outweighs the risk of administration (see PRECAUTIONS in complete prescribing information).

**PRECAUTIONS:** Before the injection of any biological, the physician should take all reasonable precautions to prevent allergic or other adverse reactions. Epinephrine injection (1:1000) and other appropriate agents used for the control of immediate allergic reactions must be immediately available should an acute anaphylactic reaction occur. Immunosuppressed individuals, including those receiving immunosuppressive therapy, may not develop the expected immune response. **Drug Interactions:** For information regarding concomitant administration with other vaccines, refer to DOSAGE AND ADMINISTRATION in complete prescribing information. Do not mix PEDIARIX with any other vaccine in the same syringe or vial. **Carcinogenesis, Mutagenesis, Impairment of Fertility:** PEDIARIX has not been evaluated for carcinogenic or mutagenic potential, or for impairment of fertility. **Pregnancy:** Pregnancy Category C: PEDIARIX is not indicated for women of child-bearing age. Animal reproduction studies have not been conducted with PEDIARIX. It is not known whether PEDIARIX can cause fetal harm when administered to a pregnant woman or if PEDIARIX can affect reproductive capacity. **Geriatric Use:** PEDIARIX is not indicated for use in adult populations. **Pediatric Use:** Safety and effectiveness of PEDIARIX in infants younger than 6 weeks of age have not been evaluated (see DOSAGE AND ADMINISTRATION in complete prescribing information). PEDIARIX is not recommended for persons 7 years of age or older. Tetanus and Diphtheria Toxoids Adsorbed (Td) For Adult Use, inactivated poliovirus vaccine (IPV), and Hepatitis B Vaccine (Recombinant) should be used in individuals 7 years of age or older.

**ADVERSE REACTIONS:** A total of 20,739 doses of PEDIARIX have been administered to 7,028 infants as a 3-dose primary series. The most common adverse reactions observed in clinical trials were local injection site reactions (pain, redness, or swelling), fever, and fussiness. In comparative studies, administration of PEDIARIX was associated with higher rates of fever relative to separately administered vaccines (see WARNINGS). The prevalence of fever was highest on the day of vaccination and the day following vaccination. More than 98% of episodes of fever resolved within the 4-day period following vaccination (i.e., the period including the day of vaccination and the next 3 days). Rates of most other solicited adverse events following PEDIARIX were comparable to rates observed following separately administered US-licensed vaccines. The adverse event information from clinical trials provides a basis for identifying adverse events that appear to be related to vaccine use and for approximating rates. However, because clinical trials are conducted under widely varying conditions, adverse event rates observed in the clinical trials of a vaccine cannot be directly compared to rates in the clinical trials of another vaccine, and may not reflect the rates observed in practice. A total of 5,472 infants were enrolled in a German safety study that was originally designed to compare the safety and reactogenicity of PEDIARIX administered concomitantly at separate sites with 1 of 4 *Haemophilus influenzae* type b (Hib) vaccines at 3, 4, and 5 months of age. After enrollment of 1,569 infants, the study was amended to include a control group that received INFANRIX, Hib vaccine, and oral poliovirus vaccine (OPV) separately. Infants in the separate administration group received one less antigen (hepatitis B) than the infants who received PEDIARIX. Safety data were available for 4,666 infants who received PEDIARIX administered concomitantly at separate sites with 1 of 4 Hib vaccines and for 768 infants in the control group that received separate vaccines. The primary end-point of the study was the percentage of infants with any grade 3 solicited symptom (redness or swelling >20 mm, fever >103.1°F, or crying, pain, vomiting, diarrhea, loss of appetite, or restlessness that prevented normal daily activities) over the 3-dose primary series in infants who received PEDIARIX (4 groups that received PEDIARIX and Hib vaccines pooled) compared to the group that received INFANRIX and Hib vaccine separately with OPV. Analysis for the primary end-point was performed on the according-to-protocol (ATP) cohort that included only those infants who were enrolled after the protocol amendment to include a control group. Of 3,773 infants in the ATP cohort for whom safety data were available, 16.2% (95% CI: 14.9% to 17.5%) of 3,029 infants who received PEDIARIX and Hib vaccine compared to 20.3% (95% CI: 17.5% to 23.4%) of 744 infants who received separate vaccines were reported to have had at least one grade 3 solicited symptom within 4 days of vaccination (i.e., day of vaccination and the next 3 days). The difference between groups in the rate of grade 3 symptoms was 4.1% (90% CI: 1.4% to 7.1%). These were the rates for selected solicited symptoms within 4 days following each dose in a 3-dose primary series in infants who received PEDIARIX administered concomitantly with Hib vaccine and those who received separate concomitant administration of INFANRIX, Hib vaccine, and OPV for the intent-to-treat (ITT) cohort (includes all infants enrolled before and after the amendment who received the indicated vaccine and for whom at least one symptom sheet was completed):

**Percentage of German Infants With Solicited Local Reactions or Selected Systemic Adverse Events Within 4 Days of Vaccination* (ITT Cohort)**

| | PEDIARIX & Hib | | | INFANRIX, Hib, & OPV | | |
|---|---|---|---|---|---|---|
| | **Dose 1** | **Dose 2** | **Dose 3** | **Dose 1** | **Dose 2** | **Dose 3** |
| **N** | **4,666** | **4,619** | **4,574** | **768** | **757** | **750** |
| **Local[†]** | | | | | | |
| Pain, any | 14.0 | 10.2 | 9.9 | 14.2 | 9.8 | 8.1 |
| Pain, grade 2 or 3 | 2.9 | 1.2 | 1.5 | 3.6 | 1.7 | 1.1 |
| Pain, grade 3 | 0.7 | 0.3 | 0.3 | 1.3 | 0.4 | 0.1 |
| Redness, any | 18.6 | 26.6 | 25.6 | 16.1 | 21.4 | 20.8 |
| Redness, >5 mm | 6.7 | 9.9 | 9.0 | 5.9 | 8.2 | 7.7 |
| Redness, >20 mm | 1.2 | 1.0 | 1.1 | 1.8 | 0.7 | 1.1 |
| Swelling, any | 12.7 | 18.5 | 18.4 | 9.6 | 12.9 | 13.6 |
| Swelling, >5 mm | 5.6 | 7.7 | 7.8 | 3.6 | 5.2 | 4.8 |
| Swelling, >20 mm | 1.2 | 1.6 | 1.5 | 1.3 | 1.1 | 1.2 |
| **Systemic** | | | | | | |
| Restlessness, any | 41.4 | 32.0 | 26.7 | 46.4 | 35.0 | 27.6 |
| Restlessness, grade 2 or 3 | 14.4 | 10.0 | 8.9 | 20.2 | 11.5 | 8.4 |
| Restlessness, grade 3 | 3.0 | 1.5 | 1.6 | 5.7 | 3.0 | 1.7 |
| Fever[‡], ≥100.4°F | 25.1 | 19.3 | 19.7 | 13.2 | 13.1 | 11.2 |
| Fever[‡], >101.3°F | 5.8 | 4.1 | 4.6 | 2.2 | 2.8 | 2.1 |
| Fever[‡], >103.1°F | 0.3 | 0.5 | 0.7 | 0.3 | 0.3 | 0.5 |
| Unusual cry[§], any | 24.9 | 16.5 | 13.1 | 36.5 | 19.7 | 14.3 |
| Unusual cry[§], grade 2 or 3 | 12.7 | 7.1 | 5.7 | 20.8 | 10.0 | 5.7 |
| Unusual cry[§], grade 3 | 3.9 | 1.7 | 1.4 | 6.8 | 2.1 | 1.1 |
| Loss of appetite, any | 17.9 | 13.3 | 12.5 | 19.1 | 16.2 | 11.3 |
| Loss of appetite, grade 2 or 3 | 4.0 | 2.9 | 2.7 | 4.4 | 2.9 | 2.3 |
| Loss of appetite, grade 3 | 0.6 | 0.5 | 0.4 | 0.5 | 0.7 | 0.0 |

N = number of infants in the intent-to-treat (ITT) cohort.
Grade 2 defined as sufficiently discomforting to interfere with daily activities.
Grade 3 defined as preventing normal daily activities.
* Within 4 days of vaccination defined as day of vaccination and the next 3 days.
† Local reactions at the injection site for PEDIARIX or INFANRIX.
‡ Rectal temperatures.
§ Unusual cry lasting >1 hour.

In this study, infants were also monitored for unsolicited adverse events that occurred within 30 days following vaccination. Over the entire study period, 6 subjects in the group that received PEDIARIX reported seizures. Two of these subjects had a febrile seizure, 1 of whom also developed afebrile seizures. The remaining 4 subjects had afebrile seizures, including 2 with infantile spasms. Two subjects reported seizures within 7 days following vaccination (1 subject had both febrile and afebrile seizures, and 1 subject had afebrile seizures), corresponding to a rate of 0.22 seizures per 1,000 doses (febrile seizures 0.07 per 1,000 doses, afebrile seizures 0.14 per 1,000 doses). No subject who received concomitant INFANRIX, Hib vaccine, and OPV reported seizures. In a separate German study that evaluated the safety of INFANRIX in 22,505 infants who received 66,867 doses of INFANRIX administered as a 3-dose primary series, the rate of seizures within 7 days of vaccination with INFANRIX was 0.13 per 1,000 doses (febrile seizures 0.0 per 1,000 doses, afebrile seizures 0.13 per 1,000 doses). No cases of hypotonic-hyporesponsiveness, encephalopathy, or anaphylaxis were reported in the German study that evaluated the safety of PEDIARIX. Rates of serious adverse events that are less common than those reported in this safety study are not known at this time.

Additional safety data for PEDIARIX are available from a US study designed to evaluate lot-to-lot consistency and a bridge for a new manufacturing step. These were the rates for local reactions and selected adverse events within 4 days of vaccination with PEDIARIX administered concomitantly with a Hib vaccine at 2, 4, and 6 months of age:

**Percentage of US Infants With Solicited Local Reactions or Selected Systemic Adverse Events Within 4 Days of Vaccination* (ITT Cohort)**

| | PEDIARIX & Hib | | |
|---|---|---|---|
| | **Dose 1** | **Dose 2** | **Dose 3** |
| **Local[†]** | **N = 482** | **N = 469** | **N = 466** |
| Pain, any | 30.5 | 25.4 | 23.0 |
| Pain, grade 2 or 3 | 6.2 | 5.5 | 3.6 |
| Pain, grade 3 | 1.2 | 0.6 | 0.6 |
| Redness, any | 25.3 | 32.6 | 35.6 |
| Redness, >5 mm | 9.3 | 10.4 | 8.6 |
| Redness, >20 mm | 0.6 | 1.5 | 1.3 |
| Swelling, any | 15.1 | 16.6 | 22.3 |
| Swelling, >5 mm | 6.8 | 6.2 | 6.4 |
| Swelling, >20 mm | 1.0 | 1.3 | 1.3 |
| **Systemic** | **N = 482** | **N = 469** | **N = 467** |
| Restlessness, any | 28.8 | 30.3 | 28.5 |
| Restlessness, grade 2 or 3 | 7.1 | 9.0 | 9.4 |
| Restlessness, grade 3 | 1.0 | 1.1 | 0.6 |
| Fever[‡], ≥100.4°F | 26.6 | 31.3 | 25.9 |
| Fever[‡], >101.3°F | 2.9 | 6.2 | 4.7 |
| Fever[‡], >103.1°F | 0.0 | 0.2 | 0.6 |
| Fussiness, any | 61.8 | 63.8 | 57.0 |
| Fussiness, grade 2 or 3 | 14.9 | 21.5 | 17.1 |
| Fussiness, grade 3 | 2.7 | 3.4 | 1.7 |
| Loss of appetite, any | 21.6 | 19.8 | 18.8 |
| Loss of appetite, grade 2 or 3 | 3.1 | 3.2 | 2.4 |
| Loss of appetite, grade 3 | 0.2 | 0.4 | 0.0 |
| Sleeping more than usual, any | 46.7 | 31.8 | 28.1 |
| Sleeping more than usual, grade 2 or 3 | 10.2 | 6.0 | 4.7 |
| Sleeping more than usual, grade 3 | 1.7 | 0.4 | 0.6 |

N = number of infants in the intent-to-treat (ITT) cohort (infants who received the indicated vaccine and for whom at least one symptom sheet was completed).
Grade 2 defined as sufficiently discomforting to interfere with daily activities.
Grade 3 defined as preventing normal daily activities.
* Within 4 days of vaccination defined as day of vaccination and the next 3 days.
† Local reactions at the injection site for PEDIARIX.
‡ Rectal temperatures.

In another US study, these were the rates for fever within 4 days following dose 1 (i.e., day of vaccination and the next 3 days) at 2 months of age in infants who received PEDIARIX when administered concomitantly at separate sites with Hib and pneumococcal conjugate vaccines and those who received INFANRIX, ENGERIX-B® [Hepatitis B Vaccine (Recombinant)], IPV, Hib vaccine, and pneumococcal conjugate vaccine:

**Percentage of US Infants With Fever Within 4 Days of Dose 1* (ITT Cohort)**

| | PEDIARIX, Hib, & Pneumococcal Conjugate (N = 667) | INFANRIX, ENGERIX-B, IPV, Hib, & Pneumococcal Conjugate (N = 333) | Separate Vaccine Group Minus Combination Vaccine Group |
|---|---|---|---|
| **Fever[†]** | **%** | **%** | **Difference (95% CI)** |
| ≥100.4°F[‡] | 27.9 | 19.8 | -8.07 (-13.54, -2.60) |
| >101.3°F | 7.0 | 4.5 | -2.54 (-5.50, 0.41) |
| >102.2°F[‡] | 2.2 | 0.3 | -1.95 (-3.22, -0.68) |
| >103.1°F | 0.4 | 0.0 | -0.45 (-0.96, 0.06) |
| M.A.[‡] | 1.2 | 0.0 | -1.20 (-2.03, -037) |

N = number of infants for whom at least one symptom sheet was completed, excluding 3 infants for whom temperature was not measured and 3 infants whose temperature was measured by the tympanic method.
*Within 4 days of dose 1 defined as day of vaccination and the next 3 days.
† Rectal temperatures.
‡ The group that received PEDIARIX compared to separate vaccine group p value <0.05 (2-sided Fisher Exact test) or the 95% confidence interval on the difference between groups does not include 0.
M.A. = Medically attended (a visit to or from medical personnel).

In this study, medical attention (a visit to or from medical personnel) for fever within 4 days following vaccination was sought for 8 infants who received PEDIARIX (1.2%) and no infants who received separately administered vaccines. Four infants were seen by medical personnel in an office setting; no diagnostic tests were performed in 2 of the infants and a complete blood count (CBC) was done in the other 2 infants. Of 3 infants who were seen in an emergency room, all had a CBC and a blood and urine culture performed; chest X-rays were done in 2 of the infants and a nasopharyngeal specimen was tested for Respiratory Syncytial Virus in one of the infants. One infant was hospitalized for a work-up that included a CBC, blood and urine cultures, a lumbar puncture, and a chest X-ray. All episodes of medically attended fever resolved within 4 days post-vaccination.

Limited data are available from a study conducted in Moldova in which infants received a dose of hepatitis B vaccine within 48 hours of birth followed by 3 doses of PEDIARIX at 6, 10, and 14 weeks of age. No information was collected on the HBsAg status of mothers of enrolled infants. These were the rates for local reactions and selected adverse events within 4 days of vaccination with PEDIARIX administered comcomitantly with Hib vaccine following a birth dose of hepatitis B vaccine:

**Percentage of Moldovan Infants With Solicited Local Reactions or Selected Systemic Adverse Events Within 4 Days of Vaccination* (ITT Cohort)**

| | PEDIARIX & Hib | | |
|---|---|---|---|
| | **Dose 1** | **Dose 2** | **Dose 3** |
| **N** | **160** | **158** | **157** |
| **Local[†]** | | | |
| Pain, any | 25.6 | 18.4 | 14.0 |
| Pain, grade 3 | 3.1 | 0.6 | 1.9 |
| Redness, any | 41.9 | 41.8 | 47.1 |
| Redness, >20 mm | 1.9 | 2.5 | 4.5 |
| Swelling, any | 20.6 | 18.4 | 28.0 |
| Swelling, >20 mm | 4.4 | 2.5 | 7.0 |
| **Systemic** | | | |
| Restlessness, any | 13.1 | 10.8 | 8.9 |
| Restlessness, grade 3 | 1.3 | 0.6 | 0.6 |
| Fever[‡], ≥100.4°F | 14.4 | 11.4 | 5.1 |
| Fever[‡], >103.1°F | 0.0 | 0.6 | 0.0 |
| Fussiness, any | 25.0 | 21.5 | 17.8 |
| Fussiness, grade 3 | 2.5 | 0.6 | 0.6 |

N = number of infants in the intent-to-treat (ITT) cohort (infants who received the indicated vaccine and for whom at least one symptom sheet was completed).
Grade 3 defined as preventing normal daily activities.
*Within 4 days of vaccination defined as day of vaccination and the next 3 days.
† Local reactions at the injection site for PEDIARIX.
‡ Rectal temperatures.

Although there was no comparator group who received PEDIARIX without a birth dose of hepatitis B vaccine, available data suggest that some local adverse events may occur at a higher rate when PEDIARIX is administered after a birth dose of hepatitis B vaccine.

As with any vaccine, there is the possibility that broad use of PEDIARIX could reveal adverse events not observed in clinical trials.

**Postmarketing Reports:** Worldwide voluntary reports of adverse events received for INFANRIX and ENGERIX-B in children younger than 7 years of age since market introduction of these US-licensed vaccines are listed below. This list includes adverse events for which 20 or more reports were received with the exception of intussusception, idiopathic thrombocytopenic purpura, thrombocytopenia, anaphylactic reaction, angioedema, encephalopathy, hypotonic-hyporesponsive episode, and alopecia for which fewer than 20 reports were received. These latter events are included either because of the seriousness of the event or the strength of causal connection to components of this or other vaccines or drugs. *Body as a whole*: Asthenia[b], fever[a+b], lethargy[b], malaise[b], Sudden Infant Death Syndrome[a+b]. *Cardiovascular system*: Cyanosis[a+b], edema[b], pallor[b]. *Gastrointestinal system*: Abdominal pain[b], anorexia[b], diarrhea[a+b], intussusception[a+b], nausea[b], vomiting[a+b]. *Hematologic/lymphatic*: Idiopathic thrombocytopenic purpura[a+b], lymphadenopathy[a], thrombocytopenia[a+b]. *Hepatic*: Jaundice[b], liver function tests abnormal[b]. *Hypersensitivity*: Anaphylactic reaction[a+b], angioedema[b], hypersensitivity[a]. *Infections*: Cellulitis[a]. *Injection site reactions*: Injection site reactions[a+b]. *Musculoskeletal*: Arthralgia[b], limb swelling[a+b]. *Nervous system*: Convulsions[a+b], encephalopathy[a], headache[b], hypotonia[a+b], hypotonic-hyporesponsive episode[a], somnolence[a+b]. *Psychiatric*: Crying[a+b], irritability[a+b]. *Respiratory system*: Respiratory tract infection[a]. *Skin and appendages*: Alopecia[b], erythema[a+b], erythema multiforme[b], petechiae[b], pruritus[a+b], rash[a+b], urticaria[a+b]. *Special senses*: Ear pain[a]. [[a] Following INFANRIX;[b] Following ENGERIX-B;[a+b] Following either INFANRIX or ENGERIX-B.] These reactions were reported voluntarily from a population of uncertain size; therefore, it is not always possible to reliably estimate their frequency or establish a causal relationship to vaccination.

**Reporting Adverse Events:** Report the occurrence following immunization of any event set forth in the Vaccine Injury Table from the National Childhood Vaccine Injury Act including: Anaphylaxis or anaphylactic shock within 7 days, encephalopathy or encephalitis within 7 days, brachial neuritis within 28 days, or an acute complication or sequelae (including death) of an illness, disability, injury, or condition referred to above, or any events that would contraindicate further doses of PEDIARIX. The VAERS toll-free number is 1-800-822-7967.

Manufactured by **GlaxoSmithKline Biologicals**, Rixensart, Belgium, US License 1617

Distributed by **GlaxoSmithKline,** Research Triangle Park, NC 27709



Full prescribing information for PEDIARIX is available at www.GSKVaccines.com/Pediarix. BRS-PE:L2

 Printed in USA. PED583R0 June 2005

# ARCHIVES OF PEDIATRICS & ADOLESCENT MEDICINE

AUGUST 2006 VOLUME 160, NUMBER 8 PAGES 761-864



## ON MY MIND

**Beginnings and Endings** 770
*Maren Olson, MD*

## ARTICLES

**A Randomized Controlled Trial Testing an HIV Prevention Intervention for Latino Youth** 772
*Antonia M. Villarruel, PhD, RN; John B. Jemmott III, PhD; Loretta S. Jemmott, PhD, RN*

**Risk Factors for Opportunistic Illnesses in Children With Human Immunodeficiency Virus in the Era of Highly Active Antiretroviral Therapy** 778
*Nathalie Ylitalo, MD, PhD; Susan Brogly, PhD; Michael D. Hughes, PhD; Sharon Nachman, MD; Wayne Dankner, MD; Russell Van Dyke, MD; George R. Seage III, DSc, MPH; for the Pediatric AIDS Clinical Trials Group Protocol 219C Team*

**Are Household Firearms Stored Less Safely in Homes With Adolescents? Analysis of a National Random Sample of Parents** 788
*Renee M. Johnson, PhD; Matthew Miller, MD, ScD; Mary Vriniotis, MS; Deborah Azrael, PhD; David Hemenway, PhD*

**Healthy Steps in an Integrated Delivery System: Child and Parent Outcomes at 30 Months** 793
*Brian D. Johnston, MD, MPH; Colleen E. Huebner, PhD, MPH; Melissa L. Anderson, MS; Lynda T. Tyll, MS; Robert S. Thompson, MD*

## SPECIAL FEATURE

**Picture of the Month** 801
*Jason S. Reichenberg, MD; Mark D. P. Davis, MD*

## ARTICLES

**Socially Isolated Children 20 Years Later: Risk of Cardiovascular Disease** 805
*Avshalom Caspi, PhD; HonaLee Harrington, BS; Terrie E. Moffitt, PhD; Barry J. Milne, MSc; Richie Poulton, PhD*

**Association Between Severity of Musculoskeletal Injury and Risk of Subsequent Injury in Children and Adolescents on the Basis of Parental Recall** 812
*Glenn Keays, MS; Bonnie Swaine, PhD; Debbie Ehrmann-Feldman, PhD*

**Psychotropic Medication Use in Pediatric Patients With Cancer** 818
*Maryland Pao, MD; Elizabeth D. Ballard; Donald L. Rosenstein, MD; Lori Wiener, PhD; Alan S. Wayne, MD*

**Parental Report of Health Conditions and Health Care Use Among Children With and Without Autism: National Survey of Children's Health** 825
*James G. Gurney, PhD; Melissa L. McPheeters, PhD; Matthew M. Davis, MD, MAPP*

**Impact of Staffing on Bloodstream Infections in the Neonatal Intensive Care Unit** 832
*Jeannie P. Cimiotti, DNS, RN; Janet Haas, MS; Lisa Saiman, MD, MPH; Elaine L. Larson, PhD*

**Assessment of Immunization Registry Databases as Supplemental Sources of Data to Improve Ascertainment of Vaccination Coverage Estimates in the National Immunization Survey** 838
*Meena Khare, MS; Linda Piccinino, MPS (ID); Lawrence E. Barker, PhD; Robert W. Linkins, MPH, PhD*

**Classification of Asthma Severity in Children: The Contribution of Pulmonary Function Testing** 844
*James W. Stout, MD, MPH; Cynthia M. Visness, MA, MPH; Paul Enright, MD; Carin Lamm, MD; Gail Shapiro, MD; Vanthaya N. Gan, MD; G. Kenneth Adams III, PhD; Herman E. Mitchell, PhD*

ARCHIVES OF PEDIATRICS & ADOLESCENT MEDICINE

## THE PEDIATRIC FORUM

**Laboratory Testing for Drug Abuse** 854
*Elizabeth A. Warner, MD; Peter D. Friedmann, MD*

**In Reply** 854
*Sharon Levy, MD, MPH; Sion Kim Harris, PhD; Lon Sherritt, MPH; Michelle Angulo, BA; John R. Knight, MD*

**Use of a Partially Hydrolyzed Formula in the Dietary Prevention of Allergic Disease** 854
*Antonio Marini, MD; Massimo Agosti, MD; Carla Colombo, MD*

**In Reply** 855
*Tiffani Hays, MS, RD, LDN; Robert Wood, MD*

**Neonatal Adverse Reactions After In Utero Exposure to Selective Serotonin Reuptake Inhibitors: Still Controversial** 855
*Louise Beaulac-Baillargeon, BPharm, PhD; Nina Boucher, BPharm, MSc*

**In Reply** 856
*Gil Klinger, MD; Rachel Levinson-Castiel, MD; Paul Merlob, MD*

**Challenges to Study on Alcohol Advertising Effects on Youth Drinking** 857
*Don E. Schultz, PhD*

**Limitations of Study on Alcohol Advertising Effects on Youth Drinking** 857
*Reginald Smart, PhD*

**In Reply** 858
*Leslie B. Snyder, PhD; Michael Slater, PhD*

## BOOK REVIEWS AND OTHER MEDIA

**The Little Elephant With the Big Earache** 860
*Nkuchia M. M'ikanatha, DrPH, MPH*

## REGULAR DEPARTMENTS

**This Month in *Archives of Pediatrics & Adolescent Medicine*** 769

**In Other ARCHIVES Journals** 771

**Announcements** 777, 830, 858, 861

**Poetry in Pediatrics** 792

**Call for Papers** 822

**Classified Advertising** 863

**Journal Advertiser Index** 863

**Contact Information** 864

**Instructions for authors and the author and subject indexes are available on our Web site: http://www.archpediatrics.com. If you do not have access to the Web, contact Suzanne Shuey at (206) 685-3573.**

**About the Cover**

*Shadow Play, Green Lake Wading Pool.* Photographer: Greg Cooksey, PhD, Seattle, Wash, 2005.

# ARCHIVES OF PEDIATRICS & ADOLESCENT MEDICINE


**Mission Statement:** *The Archives of Pediatrics & Adolescent Medicine* is a monthly, peer-reviewed journal for physicians and other health care professionals who contribute to the health of children and adolescents. The *Archives* provides an open forum for dialogue on a full range of clinical, scientific, advocacy, and humanistic issues relevant to the care of pediatric patients from infancy through young adulthood. The *Archives* is a vehicle for increased attention to adolescent health, the education of pediatric health care professionals, and disease prevention and health promotion. The *Archives* publishes original studies, editorials, reviews by experts, practice commentaries, case quizzes, and updates on clinical science and practice management. The Pediatric Forum provides our readers with opportunities to express their views. *Archives* incorporates *AJDC*, the oldest journal in US pediatric literature, which originated in 1911.



JAMA & ARCHIVES JOURNALS
American Medical Association

All articles published, including editorials, letters, and book reviews, represent the opinions of the authors and do not reflect the policy of the American Medical Association, the Editorial Board, or the institution with which the author is affiliated, unless this is clearly specified.

# BOOSTRIX®

## (Tetanus Toxoid, Reduced Diphtheria Toxoid and Acellular Pertussis Vaccine, Adsorbed) (Tdap)

The following is a brief summary only; see full prescribing information for complete product information.

**INDICATIONS AND USAGE:** BOOSTRIX is indicated for active booster immunization against tetanus, diphtheria, and pertussis as a single dose in individuals 10 through 18 years of age. The use of BOOSTRIX as a primary series or to complete the primary series has not been studied. As with any vaccine, BOOSTRIX may not protect 100% of individuals receiving the vaccine.

**CONTRAINDICATIONS:** Hypersensitivity to any component of the vaccine is a contraindication (see DESCRIPTION in full prescribing information). Do not use BOOSTRIX after a serious allergic reaction (e.g., anaphylaxis) following any other tetanus toxoid, diphtheria toxoid or pertussis-containing vaccine, or any component of this vaccine (see DESCRIPTION in full prescribing information). Because of the uncertainty as to which component of the vaccine might be responsible, do not give further vaccination with any of these components; or, refer such individuals to an allergist for evaluation. The following events are contraindications to administration of BOOSTRIX: encephalopathy (e.g., coma, decreased level of consciousness, prolonged seizures) within 7 days of administration of a previous dose of a pertussis-containing vaccine that is not attributable to another identifiable cause; progressive neurologic disorder, uncontrolled epilepsy, or progressive encephalopathy. Do not vaccinate individuals with these conditions until a treatment regimen has been established and the condition has stabilized.

**WARNINGS:** The tip cap and the rubber plunger of the needleless prefilled syringes contain dry natural latex rubber that may cause allergic reactions in latex sensitive individuals. The vial stopper is latex-free. If any of the following events occurred in temporal relation to previous receipt of a Diphtheria and Tetanus Toxoids and Pertussis Vaccine Adsorbed (DTwP) vaccine or a vaccine containing an acellular pertussis component, consider carefully whether to give subsequent doses of BOOSTRIX: temperature of ≥40.5°C (105°F) within 48 hours not due to another identifiable cause; collapse or shock-like state (hypotonic-hyporesponsive episode) within 48 hours; persistent, inconsolable crying lasting ≥3 hours, occurring within 48 hours; seizures with or without fever occurring within 3 days. Persons who experienced serious Arthus-type hypersensitivity reactions following a prior dose of tetanus toxoid usually have high serum tetanus antitoxin levels and should not be given Tetanus and Diphtheria Toxoids Adsorbed For Adult Use (Td) or Tdap vaccines or even emergency doses of Td more frequently than every 10 years, even if the wound is neither clean nor minor. If Guillain-Barré syndrome has occurred within 6 weeks of receipt of prior vaccine containing tetanus toxoid, the decision to give BOOSTRIX or any vaccine containing tetanus toxoid should be based on careful consideration of the potential benefits and possible risks. The decision to administer a pertussis-containing vaccine to individuals with stable central nervous system (CNS) disorders must be made by the physician on an individual basis, with consideration of all relevant factors, and assessment of potential risks and benefits for that individual. Advise the patient, parent, or guardian of the potential increased risk involved (see PRECAUTIONS). A family history of seizures or other CNS disorders is not a contraindication to pertussis vaccine. The Advisory Committee on Immunization Practices (ACIP) has published guidelines for vaccination of persons with recent or acute illness (www.cdc.gov). Do not give BOOSTRIX to individuals with bleeding disorders such as hemophilia or thrombocytopenia, or to persons on anticoagulant therapy unless the potential benefit clearly outweighs the risk of administration. If the decision is made to administer BOOSTRIX to such persons, it should be given with caution with steps taken to avoid the risk of hematoma following the injection.

**PRECAUTIONS: General:** Before the injection of any biological, the physician should take all reasonable precautions to prevent allergic or other adverse reactions. Epinephrine injection (1:1,000) and other appropriate agents used for the control of immediate allergic reactions must be immediately available should an acute anaphylactic reaction occur. Immunosuppressed persons, including individuals receiving immunosuppressive therapy, may not develop the expected immune response. **Drug Interactions:** Do not mix BOOSTRIX with any other vaccine in the same syringe or vial. **Carcinogenesis, Mutagenesis, Impairment of Fertility:** BOOSTRIX has not been evaluated for carcinogenic or mutagenic potential, or for impairment of fertility. **Pregnancy:** Pregnancy Category C. Animal reproduction studies have not been conducted with BOOSTRIX. It is also not known whether BOOSTRIX can cause fetal harm when administered to a pregnant woman or can affect reproductive capacity. BOOSTRIX should be given to a pregnant woman only if clearly needed. Animal fertility studies have not been conducted with BOOSTRIX. In a developmental toxicity study, the effect of BOOSTRIX on embryo-fetal and pre-weaning development was evaluated in pregnant rats. Animals were administered INFANRIX® (Diphtheria and Tetanus Toxoids and Acellular Pertussis Vaccine Adsorbed) prior to gestation and BOOSTRIX during the period of organogenesis (gestation days 6, 8, 11) and later in pregnancy (gestation day 15), 0.1 mL/rat/occasion (a 45-fold increase compared to the human dose of BOOSTRIX on a body weight basis), by intramuscular injection. No adverse affect on pregnancy and lactation parameters, embryo-fetal or pre-weaning development was observed. There were no fetal malformations or other evidence of teratogenesis noted in this study. **Nursing Mothers:** It is not known whether BOOSTRIX is excreted in human milk. Because many drugs are excreted in human milk, caution should be exercised when BOOSTRIX is administered to a nursing woman. **Pregnancy Exposure Registry:** Healthcare providers are encouraged to register pregnant women who receive BOOSTRIX in the GlaxoSmithKline vaccination pregnancy registry by calling 1-888-825-5249. **Geriatric Use:** BOOSTRIX is not indicated for use in individuals older than 18 years. **Pediatric Use:** BOOSTRIX is not indicated for use in individuals younger than 10 years (see DOSAGE AND ADMINISTRATION in full prescribing information). For immunization of infants and children younger than 7 years against diphtheria, tetanus, and pertussis, refer to the manufacturers' package inserts for Diphtheria and Tetanus Toxoids and Acellular Pertussis Vaccine Adsorbed (DTaP) vaccines.

**ADVERSE REACTIONS:** A total of 3,608 adolescents were vaccinated with a single dose of BOOSTRIX during clinical trials. An additional 1,092 adolescents 10 to 18 years of age received a non-US formulation of BOOSTRIX (formulated to contain 0.5 mg aluminum per dose) in non-US clinical studies.

The primary safety study, conducted in the United States, was a randomized, observer-blinded, controlled study in which 3,080 adolescents 10 to 18 years of age received a single dose of BOOSTRIX and 1,034 received the control Td vaccine manufactured by Massachusetts Public Health Biologic Laboratories. There were no substantive differences in demographic characteristics between the vaccine groups. Among BOOSTRIX and control vaccine recipients approximately 75% were 10 to 14 years of age and approximately 25% were 15 to 18 years of age. Approximately 98% of participants in this study had received the recommended series of 4 or 5 doses of either DTwP or a combination of DTwP and DTaP in childhood. Data on adverse events were collected by the subjects, parents and/or guardians using standardized diaries for 15 consecutive days following the vaccine dose (i.e., day of vaccination and the next 14 days). Subjects were monitored for unsolicited adverse events that occurred within 31 days of vaccination (day 0-30) using diary cards (day 0-14) supplemented by spontaneous reports and a medical history as reported by subjects, parents, and/or guardians. Subjects were also monitored for 6 months post-vaccination for non-routine medical visits, visits to an emergency room, onset of new chronic illness, and serious adverse events. Information regarding late onset adverse events was obtained via a telephone call 6 months following vaccination. At least 97% of subjects completed the 6-month follow-up evaluation.

In a study conducted in Germany, BOOSTRIX was administered to 319 children 10 to 12 years of age previously vaccinated with 5 doses of acellular pertussis-containing vaccines, 193 of these subjects had previously received 5 doses of INFANRIX. Adverse events were recorded on diary cards during the 15 days following vaccination. Unsolicited adverse events that occurred within 31 days of vaccination (day 0-30) were recorded on the diary card or verbally reported to the investigator. Subjects were monitored for 6 months post-vaccination for physician office visits, emergency room visits, onset of new chronic illness, and serious adverse events. The 6-month follow-up evaluation, conducted via telephone interview, was completed by 90% of subjects.

The adverse event information from clinical trials provides a basis for identifying adverse events that appear to be related to vaccine use and for approximating rates. However, because clinical trials are conducted under widely varying conditions, adverse event rates observed in the clinical trials of a vaccine cannot be directly compared to rates in the clinical trials of another vaccine, and may not reflect the rates observed in practice.

**Serious Adverse Events in All Safety Studies:** In the US-safety study and German-safety study, no serious adverse events were reported to occur within 31 days of vaccination. During the 6-month extended safety evaluation period, no serious adverse events that were of potential autoimmune origin or new onset and chronic in nature were reported to occur. In non-US studies in which serious adverse events were monitored for up to 37 days, one subject was diagnosed with insulin dependent diabetes 20 days following administration of BOOSTRIX. No other serious adverse events of potential autoimmune origin or that were new onset and chronic in nature were reported to occur in these studies.

**Solicited Adverse Events in the US-Safety Study:** In a US study, the most common local adverse events following administration of BOOSTRIX were pain, redness, and swelling at the injection site. The most common general adverse events were headache and fatigue. Most of these events were reported at a similar frequency in recipients of both BOOSTRIX and Td. Any pain, grade 2 or 3 pain (but not grade 3 alone), and grade 2 or 3 headache (but not grade 3 alone) were reported at a higher rate in recipients of BOOSTRIX. The primary safety endpoint of the US study was the incidence of grade 3 pain (spontaneously painful and/or prevented normal activity) at the injection site within 15 days of vaccination. Grade 3 pain was reported in 4.6% of those who received BOOSTRIX compared with 4.0% of those who received the Td vaccine. The difference in rate of grade 3 pain was within the pre-defined clinical limit for non-inferiority (upper limit of the 95% CI for the difference ≤4%). These were the rates for solicited local and general adverse events within 15 days of vaccination with BOOSTRIX or Td vaccine for the total vaccinated cohort (all enrolled, vaccinated subjects with safety data available analyzed by vaccine received):

**Percentage of Individuals 10 to 18 Years of Age Reporting Solicited Local Adverse Events or Solicited General Adverse Events Within the 15-day* Post-Vaccination Period**

| | BOOSTRIX (N = 3,032) % | Td (N =1,013) % |
|---|---|---|
| **Local** | | |
| Pain,† any | 75.3 | 71.7 |
| Pain,† grade 2 or 3 | 51.2 | 42.5 |
| Pain,‡ grade 3 | 4.6 | 4.0 |
| Redness, any | 22.5 | 19.8 |
| Redness, >20 mm | 4.1 | 3.9 |
| Redness, ≥50 mm | 1.7 | 1.6 |
| Swelling, any | 21.1 | 20.1 |
| Swelling, >20 mm | 5.3 | 4.9 |
| Swelling, ≥50 mm | 2.5 | 3.2 |
| Arm circumference increase,§ >5 mm | 28.3 | 29.5 |
| Arm circumference increase,§ >20 mm | 2.0 | 2.2 |
| Arm circumference increase,§ >40 mm | 0.5 | 0.3 |
| **General** | | |
| Fever,‖ ≥99.5°F | 13.5 | 13.1 |
| Fever,‖ >100.4°F | 5.0 | 4.7 |
| Fever,‖ >102.2°F | 1.4 | 1.0 |
| Headache, any | 43.1 | 41.5 |
| Headache,† grade 2 or 3 | 15.7 | 12.7 |
| Headache, grade 3 | 3.7 | 2.7 |
| Fatigue, any | 37.0 | 36.7 |
| Fatigue, grade 2 or 3 | 14.4 | 12.9 |
| Fatigue, grade 3 | 3.7 | 3.2 |
| Gastrointestinal symptoms,¶ any | 26.0 | 25.8 |
| Gastrointestinal symptoms,¶ grade 2 or 3 | 9.8 | 9.7 |
| Gastrointestinal symptoms,¶ grade 3 | 3.0 | 3.2 |

Td = Tetanus and Diphtheria Toxoids Adsorbed For Adult Use manufactured by Massachusetts Public Health Biologic Laboratories.
N = number of subjects in the total vaccinated cohort with local/general symptoms sheets completed.
Grade 2 = Local: painful when the limb was moved; General: interfered with normal activity.
Grade 3 = Local: spontaneously painful and/or prevented normal activity; General: prevented normal activity.
*Day of vaccination and the next 14 days.
†Statistically significantly higher (P<0.05) following BOOSTRIX as compared to Td vaccine.
‡Grade 3 injection site pain following BOOSTRIX was not inferior to Td (upper limit of two-sided 95% CI for the difference in the percentage of subjects ≤4%).
§Mid-upper region of the vaccinated arm.
‖Oral temperatures or axillary temperatures.
¶Gastrointestinal symptoms included nausea, vomiting, diarrhea and/or abdominal pain.

Mid-upper arm circumference was measured by the adolescent or their parent/guardian prior to injection and daily for 15 days following vaccination. There was no significant difference between BOOSTRIX recipients and Td recipients in the proportion of subjects reporting an increase in mid-upper arm circumference in the vaccinated arm. The incidence of unsolicited adverse events reported in the 31 days after vaccination was comparable between the 2 groups.

**Solicited Adverse Events in the German Safety Study:** No cases of whole arm swelling were spontaneously reported. Two individuals (2/193) reported large injection site swelling (range 110 to 200 mm diameter), in one case associated with grade 3 pain. Neither individual sought medical attention. These episodes were reported to resolve without sequelae within 5 days. These were the rates of solicited local adverse events and fever within 15 days of vaccination for those subjects who had previously been vaccinated with 5 doses of INFANRIX:

**Rates of Solicited Adverse Events Reported Within the 15-day* Post-Vaccination Period Following Administration of BOOSTRIX in Individuals 10 to 12 Years of Age Who Had Previously Received 5 Doses of INFANRIX**

| Adverse Event | BOOSTRIX (N = 193) % (95% CI) |
|---|---|
| Pain, any | 62.2 (54.9-69.0) |
| Pain, grade 2 or 3 | 33.2 (26.6-40.3) |
| Pain, grade 3 | 5.7 (2.9-10.0) |
| Redness, any | 47.7 (40.4-55.0) |
| Redness, >20 mm | 15.0 (10.3-20.9) |
| Redness, ≥50 mm | 10.9 (6.9-16.2) |
| Swelling, any | 38.9 (31.9-46.1) |
| Swelling, >20 mm | 17.6 (12.5-23.7) |
| Swelling, ≥50 mm | 14.0 (9.4-19.7) |
| Fever, ≥99.5 | 8.8 (5.2-13.7) |
| Fever, >100.4 | 4.1 (1.8-8.0) |
| Fever, >102.2 | 1.0 (0.1-3.7) |

N = number of subjects with local/general symptoms sheets completed.
Grade 2 = Painful when the limb was moved.
Grade 3 = Spontaneously painful and/or prevented normal activity.
*Day of vaccination and the next 14 days.

As with any vaccine, there is the possibility that broad use of BOOSTRIX could reveal adverse events not observed in clinical trials.

**Postmarketing Reports:** Worldwide voluntary reports of adverse events received for BOOSTRIX in persons 10 to 18 years of age since market introduction of this vaccine are listed below. This list includes serious events or events which have causal connection to components of this or other vaccines or drugs. Because these events are reported voluntarily from a population of uncertain size, it is not possible to reliably estimate their frequency or establish a causal relationship to vaccine exposure. *Blood and lymphatic system disorders:* Lymphadenitis, lymphadenopathy. *Cardiac disorders:* Myocarditis. *Injection site reactions:* Induration, inflammation, mass, nodule, warmth, local reaction. *Metabolism and nutrition disorders:* Diabetes mellitus insulin-dependent. *Musculoskeletal and connective tissue disorders:* Arthralgia, back pain, myalgia. *Nervous system disorders:* Convulsion, encephalitis, facial palsy, paraesthesia. *Skin and subcutaneous tissue disorders:* Exanthem, Henoch-Schönlein purpura, rash. In addition, extensive swelling of the injected limb has been reported following administration of BOOSTRIX.

**Reporting Adverse Events:** Report the occurrence following immunization of any event set forth in the Vaccine Injury Table from the National Childhood Vaccine Injury Act including: Anaphylaxis or anaphylactic shock within 7 days, encephalopathy or encephalitis within 7 days, brachial neuritis within 28 days, or an acute complication or sequelae (including death) of an illness, disability, injury, or condition referred to above, or any events that would contraindicate further doses of vaccine, according to this prescribing information. These events should be reported to VAERS. The VAERS toll-free number is 1-800-822-7967. Reporting forms may also be obtained at the VAERS website at www.vaers.hhs.gov.

**DOSAGE AND ADMINISTRATION: Recommended Dose:** BOOSTRIX should be administered as a single 0.5 mL injection by the intramuscular route into the deltoid muscle of the upper arm in individuals 10 through 18 years of age. Do not administer this product subcutaneously or intravenously. There are no data to support repeat administration of BOOSTRIX. Five years should elapse between the subject's last dose of the recommended series of childhood DTwP and/or DTaP vaccine and the administration of BOOSTRIX. Limited data are available on the use of BOOSTRIX following Tetanus and Diphtheria Toxoids Adsorbed For Adult Use (Td) vaccine. **Additional Dosing Information:** ***Wound Management:*** Clinicians should refer to guidelines for tetanus prophylaxis in routine wound management. Adolescents 10 to 18 years of age who have completed a primary series against tetanus and who sustain wounds which are minor and uncomplicated, should receive a booster dose of a tetanus toxoid-containing vaccine only if they have not received tetanus toxoid within the preceding 10 years. In case of tetanus-prone injury (e.g., wounds contaminated with dirt, feces, soil, and saliva; puncture wounds; avulsions; and wounds resulting from missles, crushing, burns, and frostbite) in an adolescent who is in need of tetanus toxoid, BOOSTRIX can be used as an alternative to Tetanus and Diphtheria Toxoids Adsorbed For Adult Use (Td) vaccine in patients for whom the pertussis component is also indicated (see INDICATIONS AND USAGE).

Manufactured by **GlaxoSmithKline Biologicals**
Rixensart, Belgium, US License 1617

Distributed by **GlaxoSmithKline**
Research Triangle Park, NC 27709



Full prescribing information for BOOSTRIX is available at www.BOOSTRIX.com.
BRS-BO:L3

**References: 1.** Centers for Disease Control and Prevention. Preventing tetanus, diphtheria, and pertussis among adolescents: use of tetanus toxoid, reduced diphtheria toxoid and acellular pertussis vaccines: recommendations of the Advisory Committee on Immunization Practices (ACIP). Early Release 2006;55(February 23, 2006):1–43. **2.** Centers for Disease Control and Prevention. Recommended childhood and adolescent immunization schedule—United States, 2006. *MMWR.* 2006;54(51&52):Q1–Q4.

## Randomized Controlled Trial Testing an HIV Prevention Intervention for Latino Youth

Despite the high risk of sexually transmitted human immunodeficiency virus infection among Latino adolescents, few controlled intervention studies have been conducted with this population. This randomized controlled trial in 553 Latino adolescents aged 13 to18 years tested the efficacy of a cultural- and theory-based intervention delivered by adult facilitators to small groups of adolescents. It was designed to reduce sexual risk behavior. The intervention was successful in reducing the number of adolescents with multiple sexual partners and the number of days of unprotected intercourse and in increasing the consistent use of condoms. The effects of the intervention were greatest among those whose primary language was Spanish.

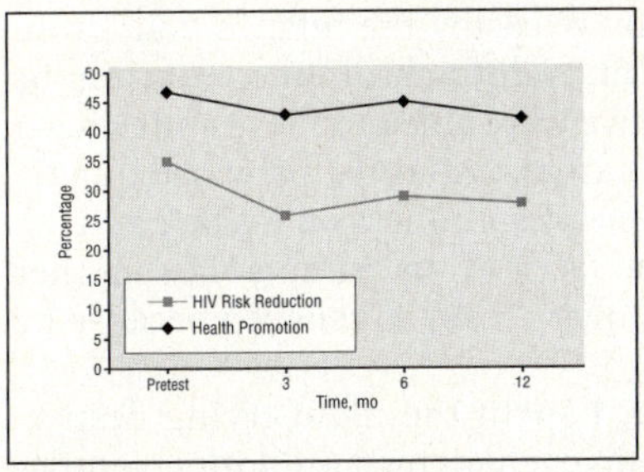


**Figure.** Consistent condom use in the past 3 months.

See page 772

## Are Household Firearms Stored Less Safely in Homes With Adolescents?

Firearms continue to be a major source of mortality for adolescents, accounting for the majority of adolescent suicides and homicides in this country. Firearms are kept in approximately one third of homes in which children and youth reside. In this random national survey, Johnson and colleagues found that guns kept in households with teenagers were 48% more likely to be stored unlocked, 25% more likely to be stored loaded, and 43% more likely to be stored both unlocked and loaded than are guns kept in households with younger children. This represents an important preventable risk for violent death in youth.

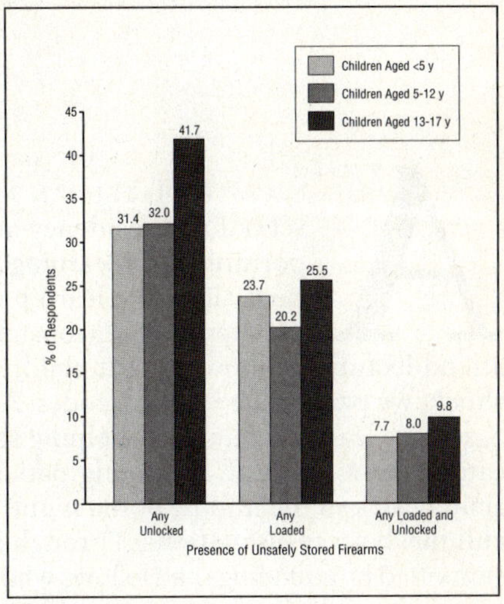


See page 788

## Parental Report of Health Conditions and Health Care Use Among Children With and Without Autism

Gurney and colleagues used data from the National Survey of Children's Health to examine the extent to which children with an autism spectrum disorder (ASD) have, according to parental report, a higher prevalence of common childhood conditions and health care use than children without an ASD. Children with an ASD had a significantly higher prevalence of depression or anxiety problems and behavioral or conduct problems and reported more respiratory, skin, and food allergies than children without an ASD. These children had higher health care use, especially for physical, occupational, and speech therapy. They were much more likely to need behavioral counseling and to be using long-term medications. The responsibilities that parents bear as they manage the diverse needs of their children with an ASD are enormous.

See page 825

## Impact of Staffing on Bloodstream Infections in the Neonatal Intensive Care Unit

Infants hospitalized in neonatal intensive care units have the highest rate of healthcare-associated infections in the pediatric population. Few studies have examined whether nurse staffing ratios are associated with bloodstream infections in this population. In this study of 2675 infants admitted to neonatal intensive care units for more than 48 hours, 224 had a bloodstream infection. The risk of infection was highest for the smallest infants and for those with peripherally inserted central venous catheters that were in place for longer periods of time. A greater number of registered nursing hours was associated with a markedly lower risk of infection.

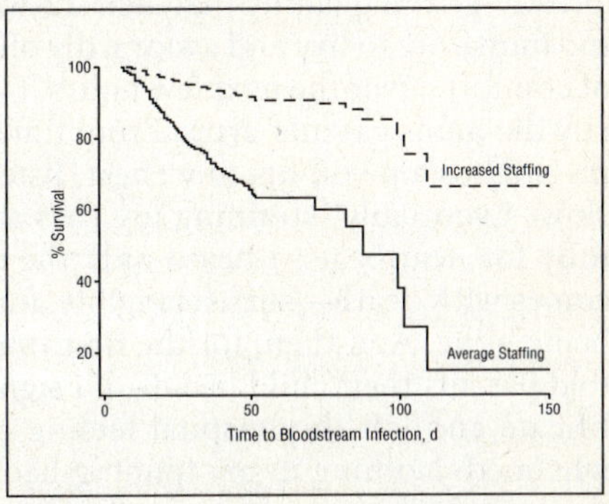


See page 832

# Beginnings and Endings

As any pediatrician knows, medical school and residency are filled with opportunities for learning how to keep a patient alive. We learn pediatric advanced life support and neonatal resuscitation, we attend lectures on how to treat children in cardiogenic shock, we participate in mock codes. And over and over again, we learn on our feet—helping stabilize a complicated trauma patient, managing patients who become acutely sick in the middle of the night, or running difficult newborn resuscitations. Through all of this, we are supported by attendings and fellows who answer our questions, give us feedback on our management decisions, and teach us new ways to care for critically ill children.

Sadly, not all children survive; as pediatricians we must also deal with death. But unlike the abundant teaching we receive on how to keep children alive, there is little formal instruction on what to do when a child is dying. This became painfully clear to me during my first month as a senior resident in the neonatal intensive care unit, when the very short life of a baby born far too early to live intersected with mine.

I was paged in the early hours of the morning to tend to an infant born at 22 weeks' gestation. Of course, it was not the infant who needed tending: I knew it was futile to try resuscitating a baby born so prematurely. My task was to help the parents understand why no resuscitative efforts were being undertaken while they watched the life of their tiny infant slowly ebb away. The situation was one I had never encountered before, one that no lecture had ever covered, and I struggled to figure out how to begin.

After a bit of fumbling, I began by reaffirming for the already-grieving family that their 22-week-old baby was too immature to live and awkwardly offered some words of comfort. Over the next few hours, I watched him quietly die in his parents' arms. From time to time, I placed my stethoscope on his tiny chest, listening to his heart slow. Eventually, straining my ears as I listened carefully for heartbeats, I heard only the eerie silence that comes with death—such a tangible, final sense of a soul being gone. And then, for the first time in my career, I told parents their child had died. I signed the death certificate and left the hospital feeling completely overwhelmed. Nothing in my training had prepared me for the night I had just experienced. I did not have a handy pocket card to pull out in case of impending death, and I had no memorized algorithm to follow. What I needed was to have been in such a situation before. I needed tangible examples of what to do and what to say.

Although we might conceivably benefit from more formal instruction on how to care for dying patients and their families, the best way to learn to navigate this critically important area of medicine is by following the examples of our teachers and mentors. We need to listen to the conversations they have with families about end-of-life issues, and we need to take time to talk with them about those conversations.

I am thankful that during the remainder of my month in the neonatal intensive care unit, a place where the beginning and ending of life sometimes overlap, I found myself surrounded by wonderful teachers. Several nights after that first baby's death, I watched a family realize that although their child was still alive (or, rather, was still being kept alive by machines and medications), their only hope was that their infant could die peacefully while they held him in their arms. After much conversation and gathering of family and friends, I watched the attending physician gently extubate the baby and wrap him in a blanket. She then wisely explained that death is not always a patient's worst fate. By releasing the infant's body from the imprisonment of an endotracheal tube, intravenous lines, and an isolette, we were able to relieve suffering—for both him and his parents. After the baby had quietly died, I was struck by the peacefulness on his face and the relief that colored the faces of his parents. His mother quietly said over and over, "I am so relieved because he is no longer suffering."

A few weeks later, I spent the night trying desperately to keep a child alive: changing antibiotics, ventilator settings, and intravenous fluids and increasing cardiac medications, anticonvulsants, dextrose, and respiratory support as vital signs and blood gas levels grew more concerning. I followed the recommendations of the specialists I had consulted as well as those of the neonatology fellow with whom I had multiple telephone conversations. Then, I did the only other thing left to do: I sat in a rocking chair by the baby's bedside and watched and hoped and prayed. Later in the night, I called the fellow again, not with any specific questions but for reassurance. He sensed that and immediately came in to help. Although he did not have much more medical insight to offer, I was amazingly thankful to have company in my bedside vigil. We pulled our chairs up and kept watch, following the waning blood pressures, the dropping oxygen saturation values, and the steadily worsening blood gas levels.

In the stillness of the long hours before dawn, it became clear that the infant was dying. So, at 4 o'clock in the morning, we summoned the parents to the hospital.

They arrived quickly, faces drawn, aware of the gravity of the situation even before we spoke. They stood at the bedside and clung to each other as the fellow told the family that although their child had been fighting hard for many days, his body simply could not fight anymore. I was struck with how few words he used and by the long silence that followed them—much needed space for the words to filter through and be heard. After a while, the baby's dad spoke up, barely able to get the words out because of his tears. "He's hurting more tonight, isn't he? He's suffering more?" His face made it clear that his questions were rhetorical; he knew the answers already. The fellow quietly talked through the options we had—that the child did not have to die attached to machines, lying alone in an incubator; that he could, instead, die in his parents' embrace. The parents agreed that it was time to allow the suffering to end and that to continue treatment would only prolong dying, not living. And so the infant died peacefully, cradled in the arms of his mother and father and surrounded by the love of many. But even the knowledge that death was the best thing for this child did not numb its sting. To lose a child is always a tragedy. Although the baby's mother later spoke to me of the relief she felt once her child's pain had ended, as we sat in that room she wept quiet, heart-wrenching sobs that spoke of a sorrow deep beyond imagining.

Walking out of the neonatal intensive care unit that morning utterly exhausted, I reflected on how death is often both a tragedy and a blessing. For many of the parents I've encountered, their child's death marks not only a life cut short, but also an end to suffering, thus bringing both sadness and relief. As I look ahead to years of working with critically ill children and their parents, I will carry these experiences with me. When I engage with families in discussions about difficult end-of-life decisions, I hope to follow the examples of my remarkable neonatology attending and fellow. Like them, I will strive to offer honesty and compassion for the journey of death and dying and thus help families find healing amidst mourning.

*Maren Olson, MD*

**Correspondence:** Dr Olson, University of Washington, Division of Neonatology, Box 356320, 1959 NE Pacific St, RR542, Seattle, WA 98195-6320 (marolson@u.washington.edu).

## IN OTHER ARCHIVES JOURNALS

### ARCHIVES OF DERMATOLOGY

**Development of Atopic Dermatitis During the First 3 Years of Life: The Copenhagen Prospective Study on Asthma in Childhood Cohort Study in High-Risk Children**

*Liselotte Brydensholt Halkjær, MD; Lotte Loland, MD, PhD; Frederik F. Buchvald, MD, PhD; Tove Agner, MD, DMSci; Lone Skov, MD, PhD; Matthew Strand, PhD; Hans Bisgaard, MD, DMSci*

**Objectives:** To describe the development of atopic dermatitis (AD) during the first 3 years of life and identify the localization of the early skin lesions that predicts the development of AD.
**Design:** Prospective, longitudinal, birth cohort study of children born to mothers with a history of asthma, followed up for 3 years with scheduled visits every 6 months as well as visits for onset or acute exacerbations of skin symptoms.
**Setting:** The cohort was recruited from greater Copenhagen, Denmark, and followed up at a clinical research unit, which controlled all diagnoses and treatment of skin diseases.
**Participants:** A total of 411 infants were enrolled in the cohort; 55 had incomplete follow-up and were excluded from certain analyses.
**Main Outcome Measures:** Atopic dermatitis was defined based on the criteria of Hanifin and Rajka, and severity was assessed by the SCORAD (Scoring Atopic Dermatitis) index. Predictive odds ratios of early skin lesions for those who developed AD vs those who did not were calculated.
**Results:** The cumulative incidence of AD by age 3 years was 44% (155/356). The prevalence rate peaked at age 2 years for boys and at age 2.5 years for girls, but there were no other sex differences in the proportion of children developing AD. Skin involvement in infants with AD was found to begin at the scalp, forehead, ear, and neck in a balaclava-like pattern and continue to the extensor sides and trunk, finally affecting the flexor sides of the extremities. Early skin lesions of arms and joints best predicted AD at age 3 years.
**Conclusions:** Atopic dermatitis begins at the scalp, forehead, ear, and neck in a balaclava-like pattern. Eczema at the arms and joints provides the highest predictive value for the development of AD at age 3 years. This may be used for early prediction and intervention of AD.

**Correspondence:** *Hans Bisgaard, MD, DMSci, Danish Pediatric Asthma Centre, Department of Pediatrics, Copenhagen University Hospital, Gentofte, Niels Andersens Vej 65, DK-2900 Hellerup, Denmark (Bisgaard@copsac.dk).*

# A Randomized Controlled Trial Testing an HIV Prevention Intervention for Latino Youth

*Antonia M. Villarruel, PhD, RN; John B. Jemmott III, PhD; Loretta S. Jemmott, PhD, RN*

**Objective:** To test the efficacy of a prevention intervention to reduce sexual risk behavior among Latino adolescents.

**Design:** Randomized controlled trial from April 2000 through March 2003, with data collection before and after intervention and at 3, 6, and 12 months.

**Setting:** Northeast Philadelphia schools.

**Participants:** Latinos aged 13 through 18 years (249 males and 304 females); 81.6% retained at 12-month follow-up.

**Interventions:** The HIV and health-promotion control interventions consisted of six 50-minute modules delivered by adult facilitators to small, mixed-gender groups in English or Spanish.

**Main Outcome Measure:** Self-reported sexual behavior.

**Results:** Analyses using generalized estimation equations over the follow-up period revealed that adolescents in the HIV intervention were less likely to report sexual intercourse (odds ratio, 0.66; 95% confidence interval [CI], 0.46-0.96), multiple partners (odds ratio, 0.53; 95% CI, 0.31-0.90), and days of unprotected intercourse (relative risk, 0.47; 95% CI, 0.26-0.84) and more likely to report using condoms consistently (odds ratio, 1.91; 95% CI, 1.24-2.93). Baseline sexual experience and language use moderated intervention efficacy. Adolescents assigned to the HIV intervention who were sexually inexperienced at baseline reported fewer days of unprotected sex (relative risk, 0.22; 95% CI, 0.08-0.63); Spanish speakers were more likely to have used a condom at last intercourse (odds ratio, 4.73; 95% CI, 1.72-12.97) and had a greater proportion of protected sex (mean difference, 0.35; $P<.01$) compared with similar adolescents in the health-promotion intervention.

**Conclusion:** Results provide evidence for the efficacy of HIV intervention in decreasing sexual activity and increasing condom use among Latino adolescents.

*Arch Pediatr Adolesc Med. 2006;160:772-777*

HUMAN IMMUNODEFICIENCY virus (HIV) and AIDS disproportionately affect Latino adolescents. The incidence of AIDS for adult and adolescent Latinos in 2001 was more than 3 times higher than that among their non-Hispanic white counterparts.[1,2] Heterosexual contact is the major mode of HIV transmission among Latino adolescents.[3] Data from the national Youth Risk Behavior Surveillance System show that the incidence of sexual intercourse before the age of 13 years, as well as multiple (>4) sexual partnerships, is higher among Latino youth than among non-Hispanic whites.[4] Furthermore, studies have consistently documented lower condom use by Latino adolescents than by African American or white adolescents.[4-6]

Despite the high risk of sexually transmitted HIV infection among Latino adolescents, few controlled intervention studies have been conducted in this population. In an electronic literature search, we identified only 5 intervention studies from 1994 through 2004 with sexual behavior outcomes that had sizable proportions (25% or more of the sample) of Latino adolescents.[7-11]

In 3 studies,[7-9] Latinos were included in tests of HIV risk-reduction curricula; however, the reported intervention effects on behavior were not consistent. Results from 1 study[9] indicated that an HIV risk-reduction intervention had no effect on sexual behavior among students in 6 Los Angeles middle schools. Conversely, a test of a 2-year comprehensive school-based HIV/sexually transmitted disease and pregnancy-prevention program indicated significant sexual behavior outcomes for Latino adolescents.[7] Latino adolescents in the intervention schools were significantly more likely to delay the initiation of sex, use condoms at last sex, and report fewer incidences of unprotected sex than those in the control schools. Because there was only 1 measure obtained 7 months after intervention, the long-term effects of the intervention are unknown.

**Author Affiliations:** School of Nursing, University of Michigan, Ann Arbor (Dr Villarruel); and Annenberg School for Communication (Dr J. B. Jemmott) and School of Nursing (Drs Villarruel and L. S. Jemmott), University of Pennsylvania, Philadelphia.

Latino adolescents were targeted in only 2 studies.[10,11] One study[11] included Spanish-speaking Latino adolescents but was not a randomized controlled trial, and only one[10] indicated that the intervention was culturally tailored for Latino adolescents. Sellers et al[11] reported mixed results from a community AIDS prevention program. The intervention did not significantly affect frequency of sex, the onset of sexual activity for girls, or number of partners among boys compared with those factors in a control group. However, in the intervention city, boys were less likely to initiate their first sexual intercourse, whereas girls were less likely to have multiple partners.

Mixed results also were reported in a test of a behavioral intervention conducted with a majority sample (78%) of pregnant adolescent Latina mothers (mean age, 16.7 years).[10] At 6 months post intervention, adolescents who participated in the HIV prevention program were significantly more likely than those in the control group to decrease the number of sex partners. However, there were no significant intervention effects on behavior at 12-month follow-up.

In summary, data about the efficacy of behavioral interventions to reduce sexual risk behavior among Latino adolescents are sparse. Moreover, no randomized controlled intervention trials have been conducted with Latino adolescents who are monolingual Spanish speakers. An important recommendation by Flores et al[12] and others[13] supports the need to address language and cultural barriers in interventions for Latino youth. Therefore, the purpose of this study was to test the efficacy of a culture- and theory-based intervention designed to reduce HIV sexual risk behavior among Latino adolescents.

## METHODS

### PARTICIPANTS

A total of 684 adolescents were eligible to participate; data analyzed for this study included 553 self-identified Latino adolescents (249 males and 304 females). Most participants were Puerto Rican (472 [85.4%]) with nearly half (249 [45.0%]) born outside the mainland United States. Participants had a mean (SD) age of 14.9 (1.49) years and a median of ninth grade in school, with 86.9% of the students in grades 8 through 11. About 235 (42.5%) reported ever having sexual intercourse, and the mean (SD) age of first intercourse was 13.5 (1.81) years.

### PROCEDURES

The study was a randomized controlled trial with data collection at preintervention; immediately after completion of the 2-day intervention; and at 3, 6, and 12 months after intervention. The human subjects committees of the University of Pennsylvania and the University of Michigan approved the study.

Latino students were recruited from 3 northeast Philadelphia high schools and community-based organizations within these neighborhoods. Students were invited to participate in "*¡Cuídate!* (Take Care of Yourself) The Latino Youth Health Promotion Program," an 8-hour program conducted over 2 consecutive Saturdays. The study was implemented with a pilot group, and 5 subsequent groups enrolled sequentially across 5 months. Youth were eligible to participate if they self-reported as being Latino, were aged 13 through 18 years, and provided assent and parental consent. Non-Latino students (n = 103) were not excluded from participation in the intervention but were excluded from the analysis. Students were asked their language preference and subsequently received the English or Spanish version of the questionnaires. The English versions were received by 412 adolescents and the Spanish versions by 141 adolescents.

Using a stratified permuted block randomization, we stratified adolescents according to gender, primary language, ethnicity (Latino and non-Latino), and age. On the basis of computer-generated random number sequences, adolescents were randomly assigned to the HIV risk-reduction intervention or the health-promotion intervention. Students received a T-shirt with the study logo for participating. In addition, they were compensated as much as $110 for participation: $40 after completion of the 2-session intervention, $20 for the 3- and 6-month follow-ups, and $30 for the12-month follow-up.

### INTERVENTION

The process of developing *¡Cuídate!* and details regarding the content of the curriculum have been previously described.[14] The HIV risk-reduction and health-promotion interventions were similar in organization, format, length, and delivery mode. Both interventions involved small-group discussions, videos, interactive exercises, and skill-building activities. Functionally equivalent versions of the HIV risk-reduction and health-promotion curriculum in English and Spanish were developed and pilot tested.

The HIV risk-reduction curriculum tested in this study was an adaptation of *Be Proud! Be Responsible!*[15] and similarly was based on social cognitive theory[16] and the theories of reasoned action and planned behavior.[17,18] *¡Cuídate!* also incorporated salient aspects of Latino culture, specifically familialism, or the importance of family, and gender-role expectations. Abstinence and condom use were presented as culturally accepted and effective ways to prevent sexually transmitted diseases, including HIV.

The health-promotion intervention focused on behaviors related to significant health issues affecting Latinos. These behaviors included diet; exercise and physical activity; and cigarette, alcohol, and drug use. Latino cultural values were presented as an important context that supported positive health behaviors.

### FACILITATORS AND FACILITATOR TRAINING

Facilitator recruitment, characteristics, and training have been described previously.[14] The bilingual facilitators (n = 41; 8 men and 33 women) had a mean (SD) age of 33.7 (10.23) years; and 34 (82.9%) self-identified as Puerto Rican. Facilitators were stratified according to age, gender, and ethnicity and were assigned according to computer-generated random number sequences to implement either the HIV risk-reduction intervention or the health-promotion intervention. This process ensured that there were no significant differences ($P > .05$) between facilitators in the interventions according to age, gender, or ethnicity. All facilitators received 2½ days of training designed to provide information and skills related to their specific intervention, to encourage and ensure implementation fidelity, and to generate high motivation and enthusiasm among all facilitators irrespective of their assigned intervention.

### QUALITY ASSURANCE

We took several measures to ensure the fidelity of intervention implementation. Project staff unobtrusively monitored facilitators and gave them cues to ensure fidelity to the time allotted for each activity. Facilitators completed a debriefing questionnaire to assess issues with implementation and their

**Table. Self-Reported Sexual Behavior According to Intervention Group at Baseline***

| Sexual Behavior | Intervention Group: HIV Risk Reduction, % (n = 263) | Health Promotion, % (n = 287) |
|---|---|---|
| Ever had sex | 40.9 | 44.7 |
| Sexual intercourse in the past 3 mo | 26.0 | 29.0 |
| Mean (SD) proportion of days of protected intercourse† | 0.67 (0.41) | 0.68 (0.39) |
| Multiple partners (≥2) | 21.0 | 15.6 |
| Consistent condom use† | 46.8 | 34.8 |
| Condom use at last intercourse† | 58.0 | 50.4 |

Abbreviation: HIV, human immunodeficiency virus.
*For all values, $P>.10$. The $P$ values for percentages are from $\chi^2$ tests; all others are from $t$ tests. Combined sample numbers vary because of missing data for baseline sexual experience.
†For the participants who were sexually active at baseline, 106 were in the HIV risk-reduction group and 127 were in the health-promotion group.

degree of fidelity to activities as written in the curriculum. Facilitators in both interventions reported a high degree of fidelity, implementing all activities in each module 87.8% (36/41) of the time. There were no significant differences among facilitators in relation to the number of modules completed.

## OUTCOME MEASURES

We used several self-report measures of sexual activity and condom use. Participants were asked if they ever had sexual intercourse ("your penis in a girl's vagina" or "boy's penis in your vagina") and whether they had done so in the past 3 months (yes or no). Given the past 3 months as a reference point, adolescents also were asked the number of days in which they had intercourse, the number of times they had sex, the number of days of sex without using a condom, and the number of sexual partners. For condom use, adolescents indicated on a 5-point Likert scale how often they used a condom (1 = never to 5 = always). Binary variables were created for consistent condom use (always used a condom; 0 = no; 1 = yes), and number of partners (0 = 1 or no partner; 1 = 2 or more partners). We also calculated the proportion of days of protected sex (1–number of days of sex without a condom/number of days of sex). We previously reported the procedures for the Spanish translation and pilot testing of these measures.[19]

We used several measures that had been used previously to increase the validity of self-reported sexual behavior.[20] First, we had trained project assistants, who were not involved in the delivery of the intervention, administer questionnaires. We stressed the confidentiality of participants' responses and used only code numbers on questionnaires. To facilitate the recall of sexual behaviors, we used a relatively brief follow-up (eg, 3 months) and provided calendars to mark the 3-month intervals. To minimize overreporting or underreporting of sexual behaviors, we stressed the importance of providing honest responses. Participants also signed a survey agreement form in which they pledged to answer questions honestly. Finally, we included a standard measure of social desirability bias,[21] which was used to examine statistically whether such bias could explain apparent intervention effects.

## STATISTICAL ANALYSES

We conducted a series of $\chi^2$ tests, Poisson and negative binomial regression analyses, and independent sample $t$ tests to identify significant differences between intervention groups in sociodemographic variables and preintervention measures of sexual behavior. In addition, we performed discrete time survival analysis[22] to model the likelihood of attrition and identify baseline factors influencing the likelihood of attrition.

Hypotheses regarding the effects of the HIV intervention on sexual behavior and condom use outcomes were tested in generalized linear model analyses. The models included the following covariates: intervention group (HIV risk reduction or health promotion), time (3-, 6-, and 12-month follow-up), sexual experience (ie, ever had intercourse) at baseline, baseline values for outcome variables, language (English or Spanish), and gender. Baseline values were not used as covariates for hypotheses regarding condom use because of the small number of participants who reported sexual intercourse at baseline.

In all analyses, generalized estimation equation methodology[23] was used to fit the generalized linear models to the type of longitudinal outcome data (continuous, count, or categorical measures). This method accounts for the likely correlations of repeated outcome measures for each participant. To determine potential moderators of intervention effects, we tested interactions between intervention and covariates hierarchically in the generalized linear models. Analyses were conducted by using an intention-to-treat approach in which participants were analyzed in their original randomized groups regardless of the number of intervention sessions they attended.

# RESULTS

## PREINTERVENTION COMPARABILITY OF CONDITIONS

There were no significant differences between adolescent intervention groups at baseline in gender, language use, or age. As seen in the **Table**, there were no significant differences in sexual behavior outcomes between the HIV risk-reduction group and the health-promotion group.

## ATTRITION

As shown in **Figure 1**, there was little attrition. Discrete time survival analyses[22] indicated there were no significant differences in attrition between the interventions. Among age, gender, primary language, and baseline sexual activity, the only significant predictor of attrition was primary language. English speakers were 90% more likely to attend a follow-up session than Spanish speakers (odds ratio [OR] = 1.91; 95% confidence interval [CI], 1.30-2.78).

## EFFECTS OF THE HIV RISK-REDUCTION INTERVENTION ON SEXUAL BEHAVIOR

The intervention had significant effects on sexual intercourse and multiple partners in the past 3 months. In **Figures 2**, **3**, and **4**, we provide a graphic representation of intervention results by showing the unadjusted means in each intervention group across time. Results of generalized estimation equation analyses indicate that adolescents in the HIV risk-reduction group were less likely to report having had sexual intercourse in the past 3 months during follow-up (OR, 0.66; 95% CI, 0.46-0.96) than were

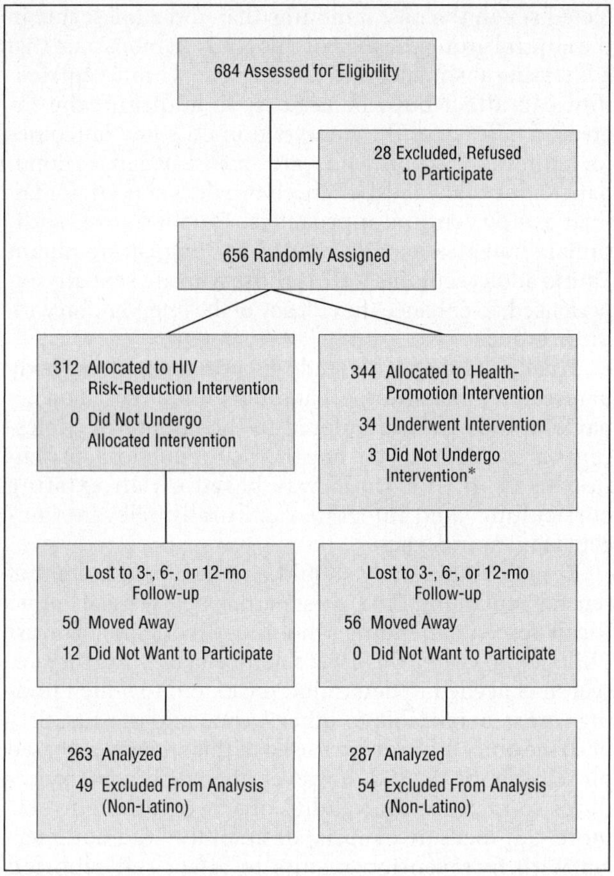


**Figure 1.** Progress of participants through the trial. Asterisk indicates reason unknown; HIV, human immunodeficiency virus.

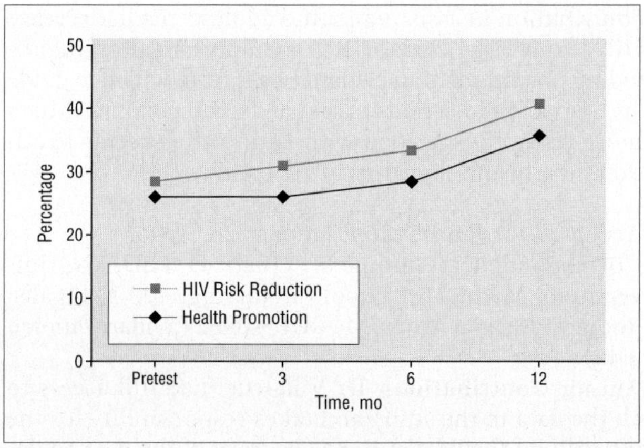


**Figure 2.** Self-report of sexual intercourse in the past 3 months. This graph does not represent results of generalized estimation equation analyses. The percentage (SE) was calculated for the outcome variable; unadjusted scores are presented for each time period. Values for the human immunodeficiency virus (HIV) risk-reduction group are as follows: pretest, 25.9% (0.44%); 3 mo, 26.0% (0.44%); 6 mo, 28.4% (0.45%); and 12 mo, 35.7% (0.48%). Values for the health-promotion group are as follows: pretest, 28.4% (0.45%); 3 mo, 31.0% (0.46%); 6 mo, 33.3% (0.47%); and 12 mo, 40.7% (0.49%).

those in the health-promotion intervention. Similarly, adolescents in the HIV risk-reduction intervention were less likely to report having multiple partners across follow-up compared with adolescents in the health-promotion intervention (OR, 0.53; 95% CI, 0.31-0.90).

The intervention also had significant effects related to consistent condom use and frequency of unprotected sex.

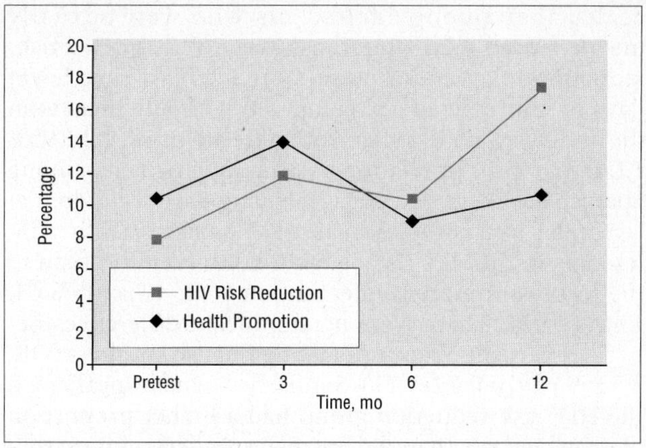


**Figure 3.** Self-report of multiple partners in the past 3 months. This graph does not represent results of generalized estimation equation analyses. The percentage (SE) was calculated for the outcome variable; unadjusted scores are presented for each time period. Values for the human immunodeficiency virus (HIV) risk-reduction group are as follows: pretest, 10.4% (0.31%); 3 mo, 14.0% (0.35%); 6 mo, 9.0% (0.29%); and 12 mo, 10.7% (0.31%). Values for the health-promotion group are as follows: pretest, 7.8% (0.27%); 3 mo, 11.7% (.0.32%); 6 mo, 10.3% (0.30%); and 12 mo, 17.3% (0.38%).

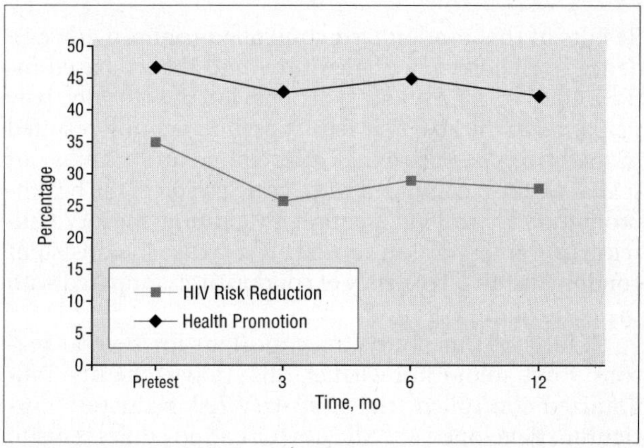


**Figure 4.** Consistent condom use in the past 3 months. This graph does not represent results of generalized estimation equation analyses. The percentage (SE) was calculated for the outcome variable; unadjusted scores are presented for each time period. Scores were calculated only for participants who were sexually active at baseline (human immunodeficiency virus [HIV] risk-reduction group [n = 106], health-promotion group [n = 127]). Values for the HIV risk-reduction group are as follows: pretest, 46.8% (0.50%); 3 mo, 42.6% (0.50%); 6 mo, 44.8% (0.50%); and 12 mo, 42.2% (0.50%). Values for the health-promotion group are as follows: pretest, 34.8% (0.48%); 3 mo, 25.7% (0.44%); 6 mo, 28.8% (0.46%); and 12 mo, 27.6% (0.45%).

Adolescents in the HIV risk-reduction group were more likely to report using condoms consistently (OR, 1.91; 95% CI, 1.24-2.93) and less likely to report days of unprotected sex (relative risk, 0.47; 95% CI, 0.26-0.84) than were adolescents in the health-promotion intervention. There were no significant effects for the outcomes of condom use at last sex (OR, 1.45; 95% CI, 0.97-2.15) and proportion of days of protected sex (B, 0.02; 95% CI, −0.07 to 0.12).

## MODERATORS OF THE INTERVENTION

Gender and social desirability did not moderate effects of the intervention. Sexual experience and primary language, however, had significant interactions with the intervention on selected outcomes. Additional analyses revealed that among adolescents who were sexually inexperienced at baseline, those assigned to the HIV risk-reduction intervention were more likely to have fewer days of unprotected sex compared with adolescents in the health-promotion intervention (relative risk, 0.22; 95% CI, 0.08-0.63). In relation to primary language, among Spanish speakers, the odds of having used a condom at last sexual intercourse were nearly 5 times higher for adolescents in the HIV risk-reduction intervention than in the health-promotion intervention (OR, 4.73; 95% CI, 1.72-12.97). There were no significant differences between intervention groups among English speakers (OR, 1.11; 95% CI, 0.72-1.71). Similarly, Spanish speakers in the HIV risk-reduction group had a higher proportion of protected sex than did Spanish speakers who participated in the health-promotion control intervention (mean difference, 0.35; $P<.01$). Conversely, there were no significant differences between intervention groups among English speakers (mean difference, −0.03; $P>.5$).

## COMMENT

Results of this randomized controlled trial provide evidence of the efficacy of a culture- and theory-based intervention on HIV sexual risk behavior. Specifically, participation in the HIV risk-reduction intervention resulted in fewer reports of sexual intercourse and number of sexual partners compared with participation in the health-promotion control intervention. In addition, the HIV risk-reduction intervention caused an increase in consistent condom use and frequency of condom use compared with the control intervention.

Results of this study are important for several reasons. First, to our knowledge, this study is the first randomized controlled trial of an HIV risk-reduction curriculum developed specifically for Latino adolescents to demonstrate long-term (12-month) effects on frequency of sexual intercourse and condom use. Other intervention studies that have included Latino adolescents either have been ineffective or have examined only short-term effects.[7-9,11]

Second, to our knowledge, this study is the first randomized controlled trial to demonstrate efficacy with Spanish-speaking Latino adolescents. The intervention used in this study was tailored to Latino culture, and we found that it had greater effects among Spanish-speaking adolescents on several outcomes. Specifically, Spanish speakers who participated in the HIV risk-reduction intervention had a higher proportion of days of protected sex and more frequent condom use at last sexual intercourse. To our knowledge, this is the first randomized controlled trial to demonstrate greater efficacy of a culturally tailored HIV risk-reduction intervention among people who speak the language of the culture for which it was tailored.

Third, results of this study demonstrate the efficacy of a safer sex intervention in decreasing sexual intercourse and increasing condom use. In addition, Latino adolescents who were sexually inexperienced before the intervention and who were assigned to the HIV risk-reduction intervention reported fewer days of unprotected sex in the past 3 months than did adolescents in the control group. Results of this study demonstrate that addressing abstinence and condom use within a curriculum can affect both behaviors. In addition, the increased efficacy of the intervention on some outcomes for Latino adolescents who were Spanish-language dominant and sexually inexperienced provides support for tailoring intervention approaches. Furthermore, additional strategies may be needed for English-dominant Latino adolescents, as well as those who are sexually experienced, to enhance the efficacy of the intervention with these groups.

Finally, results of this study support the growing body of research that indicates that interventions based on behavioral theories and tailored to the culture of adolescents are effective.[24-26] The HIV risk-reduction curriculum used in this study was based on an existing curriculum[15] and integrated culturally relevant concepts and approaches.[19]

Results of this study should be considered in light of several limitations. First, most participants were of Puerto Rican descent, attending school, and living in northeast Philadelphia, and they were self-selected. Further research is needed to determine the extent to which findings are generalizable to other Latino adolescents. Second, the outcome measures used in this study were based on self-report. We did, however, include several procedures to increase the validity of self-reports. Furthermore, our measure of social desirability[21] did not interact with intervention results to affect self-reported outcomes, suggesting that adolescents' responses were not motivated by the desire to please others.

Despite these limitations, this study is an important contribution in assisting Latino adolescents to decrease HIV sexual risk behavior. It is an important effort in providing practitioners an evidence base from which to guide and support adolescents in sexual decision making. Much more research is needed with Latino adolescents to address the health disparity in HIV and AIDS.

**Accepted for Publication:** January 28, 2006.
**Correspondence:** Antonia M. Villarruel, PhD, RN, University of Michigan, School of Nursing, 400 N Ingalls, Room 4320, Ann Arbor, MI 48109-0482 (avillarr@umich.edu).
**Author Contributions:** Dr Villarruel had full access to all the data in the study and takes responsibility for the integrity of the data and the accuracy of the data analysis. *Study concept and design:* Villarruel, J. B. Jemmott, and L. S. Jemmott. *Acquisition of data:* Villarruel and L. S. Jemmott. *Analysis and interpretation of data:* Villarruel and J. B. Jemmott. *Drafting of the manuscript:* Villarruel. *Critical revision of the manuscript for important intellectual content:* Villarruel, J. B. Jemmott, and L. S. Jemmott. *Statistical analysis:* Villarruel and J. B. Jemmott. *Obtained funding:* Villarruel, J. B. Jemmott, and L. S. Jemmott. *Administrative, technical, and material support:* Villarruel and L. S. Jemmott. *Study supervision:* Villarruel.
**Financial Disclosure:** None reported.
**Funding/Support:** The project described was supported by grant NR04855 from the National Institute of Nurs-

ing Research (Dr Villarruel). Its contents are solely the responsibility of the authors and do not necessarily represent the official views of the National Institute of Nursing Research or National Institutes of Health.

**Acknowledgment:** The authors gratefully acknowledge the support and contributions of staff, facilitators, project assistants, adolescents, and community members in the development and implementation of this project. In particular, we acknowledge the contributions of Margarita Bleier, MSW, Project Director, and Monique Howard, MS, PhD(c), HIV Curriculum Specialist. The authors also would like to acknowledge the contributions of Brady West, MA, BS, for his statistical consultation regarding the manuscript and Brenda L. Eakin, MS, in the preparation and editing of this article.

## REFERENCES


1. Centers for Disease Control and Prevention (CDC). Diagnosis of HIV/AIDS—32 states, 2000-2003. *MMWR Morb Mortal Wkly Rep.* 2004;53:1106-1110.
2. Centers for Disease Control and Prevention, National Center for HIV, STD and TB Prevention, Divisions of HIV/AIDS Prevention. HIV/AIDS among Hispanics. http://www.cdc.gov/hiv/pubs/facts/hispanic.htm. Accessed February 10, 2005.
3. Rosenberg PS, Biggar RJ. Trends in HIV incidence among young adults in the United States. *JAMA.* 1998;279:1894-1899.
4. Grunbaum JA, Kann L, Kinchen S, et al. Youth risk behavior surveillance—United States, 2003 [published corrections appear in *MMWR Morb Mortal Wkly Rep.* 2004;53:536; *MMWR Morb Mortal Wkly Rep.* 2005;54:608]. *MMWR Surveill Summ.* 2004;53:1-96.
5. Centers for Disease Control and Prevention (CDC). Trends in sexual risk behaviors among high school students—United States, 1991-2001. *MMWR Morb Mortal Wkly Rep.* 2002;51:856-859.
6. Kann L, Kinchen SA, Williams BI, et al. Youth risk behavior surveillance—United States, 1999. *MMWR CDC Surveill Summ.* 2000;49:1-32.
7. Kirby DB, Baumler E, Coyle KK, et al. The "Safer Choices" intervention: its impact on the sexual behaviors of different subgroups of high school students. *J Adolesc Health.* 2004;35:442-452.
8. Kennedy MG, Mizuno Y, Hoffman R, et al. The effect of tailoring a model HIV prevention program for local adolescent target audiences. *AIDS Educ Prev.* 2000; 12:225-238.
9. Kirby D, Korpi M, Adivi C, Weissman J. An impact evaluation of project SNAPP: an AIDS and pregnancy prevention middle school program. *AIDS Educ Prev.* 1997; 9(1 suppl):44-61.
10. Koniak-Griffin D, Lesser J, Nyamathi A, et al. Project CHARM: an HIV prevention program for adolescent mothers. *Fam Community Health.* 2003;26:94-107.
11. Sellers DE, McGraw SA, McKinlay J. Does the promotion and distribution of condoms increase teen sexual activity? evidence from an HIV prevention program for Latino youth. *Am J Public Health.* 1994;84:1952-1959.
12. Flores G, Fuentes-Afflick E, Barbot O, et al. The health of Latino children: urgent priorities, unanswered questions, and a research agenda. *JAMA.* 2002;288: 82-90.
13. National Institutes of Health (NIH). *NIH Consensus Development Statement-Interventions to Prevent HIV Risk Behaviors.* Bethesda, Md: NIH; 1997.
14. Villarruel AM, Jemmott LS, Jemmott JB III. Designing a culturally based intervention to reduce HIV sexual risk for Latino adolescents. *J Assoc Nurses AIDS Care.* 2005;16:23-31.
15. Jemmott LS, Jemmott JB III, McCaffree K. *Be Proud! Be Responsible! Strategies to Empower Youth to Reduce Their Risk for AIDS.* New York, NY: Select Media Publications; 1995.
16. Bandura A. *Social Foundations of Thought and Action: A Social Cognitive Theory.* Englewood Cliffs, NJ: Prentice-Hall; 1986.
17. Ajzen I, Madden T. Prediction of goal-directed behavior: attitudes, intentions, and perceived behavioral control. *J Exp Soc Psychol.* 1986;22:453-474.
18. Ajzen I. The theory of planned behavior. *Organ Behav Hum Decis Process.* 1991; 50:179-211.
19. Villarruel AM, Jemmott JB III, Jemmott LS, Ronis DL. Predictors of sexual intercourse and condom use intentions among Spanish-dominant Latino youth: a test of the planned behavior theory. *Nurs Res.* 2004;53:172-181.
20. Jemmott JB III, Jemmott LS, Fong GT. A randomized controlled trial of abstinence and safer sex HIV risk-reduction interventions for young African American adolescents. *JAMA.* 1998;279:1529-1536.
21. Crowne D, Marlowe D. *The Approval Motive.* New York, NY: John Wiley & Sons; 1964.
22. Allison P. *Survival Analysis Using the SAS System: A Practical Guide.* Cary, NC: SAS Institute Inc; 1995.
23. Diggle PJ, Heagerty P, Liang KY, Zeger SL. *The Analysis of Longitudinal Data.* 2nd ed. Oxford, England: Oxford University Press; 2002.
24. Jemmott JB III, Jones JM. Social psychology and AIDS among ethnic minority individuals: risk behaviors and strategies for changing them. In: Pryor J, Reeder G, eds. *Social Psychology of HIV Infection.* Hillsdale, NJ: Lawrence Erlbaum Associates; 1993:183-224.
25. Marín BV. *Analysis of AIDS Prevention Among African Americans and Latinos in the United States.* Washington, DC: Office of Technology Assessment; 1995.
26. Wingood GM, DiClemente RJ. HIV sexual risk reduction for women: a review. *Am J Prev Med.* 1996;12:209-217.


### *Announcement*

**Submissions.** The Editors welcome contributions to Picture of the Month. Submissions should describe common problems presenting uncommonly, rather than total zebras. Cases should be of interest to practicing pediatricians, highlighting problems that they are likely to at least occasionally encounter in the office or hospital setting. High-quality clinical images (in either 35-mm slide or electronic format) along with parent or patient permission to use these images must accompany the submission. The entire discussion should comprise no more than 750 words. Articles and photographs accepted for publication will bear the contributor's name. There is no charge for reproduction and printing of color illustrations. For details regarding electronic submission, please see: http://archpedi.ama-assn.org.

# Risk Factors for Opportunistic Illnesses in Children With Human Immunodeficiency Virus in the Era of Highly Active Antiretroviral Therapy

*Nathalie Ylitalo, MD, PhD; Susan Brogly, PhD; Michael D. Hughes, PhD; Sharon Nachman, MD; Wayne Dankner, MD; Russell Van Dyke, MD; George R. Seage III, DSc, MPH; for the Pediatric AIDS Clinical Trials Group Protocol 219C Team*

**Objective:** To examine the relationship between the use of highly active antiretroviral treatment (HAART) and the occurrence of opportunistic illnesses (OIs) among children perinatally infected with human immunodeficiency virus.

**Design:** Prospective cohort study.

**Setting:** Pediatric AIDS Clinical Trials Group 219C cohort.

**Participants:** From September 15, 2000, to August 31, 2003, 1927 children perinatally infected with human immunodeficiency virus and receiving HAART were followed up.

**Main Exposures:** Age at initiating HAART, duration of HAART use, $CD4^+$ T-lymphocyte percentage, and human immunodeficiency virus 1 viral load.

**Main Outcome Measures:** Incidence rates for Centers for Disease Control and Prevention OI category B and OI category C events were calculated. The association between main exposures and OI occurrence was estimated using proportional hazards regression.

**Results:** Of 1927 subjects, 226 (12.7%) developed OIs during follow-up. Incidence rates were 4.99 per 100 person-years (95% confidence interval, 4.30-5.76) for first OI category B events and 1.47 per 100 person-years (95% confidence interval, 1.12-1.91) for first OI category C events. Duration of HAART use was not related to OI risk. Older age (age >10 years) at HAART initiation was associated with increased risk of a first OI (hazard ratio, 2.48; 95% confidence interval, 1.23-5.00) compared with initiating HAART in children younger than 2 years. This increased risk diminished after adjusting for $CD4^+$ T-lymphocyte percentage and Centers for Disease Control and Prevention disease category at HAART initiation. More children with OIs than without OIs had a $CD4^+$ T-lymphocyte percentage of less than 15% at HAART initiation (49.6% of children with OIs vs 23.7% of children without OIs), at enrollment (41.2% of children with OIs vs 7.7% of children without OIs), and at the end of follow-up (41.2% of children with OIs vs 8.3% of children without OIs).

**Conclusions:** Opportunistic illnesses are occurring in the pediatric human immunodeficiency virus population in the HAART era, mainly in children with persistently low $CD4^+$ T-lymphocyte percentages. Lack of a sustained response to HAART rather than age at or duration of HAART use is predictive of OI risk.

*Arch Pediatr Adolesc Med. 2006;160:778-787*

THE INTRODUCTION OF HIGHLY active antiretroviral treatment (HAART) has resulted in a declining incidence of opportunistic illnesses (OIs) in individuals with human immunodeficiency virus (HIV).[1-8] However, OIs among some individuals treated with HAART continue to occur,[3,4] which may suggest a clinical failure of HAART. Generally, HAART causes a progressive improvement in immune function demonstrated by an increase in $CD4^+$ T-lymphocyte (CD4) counts and a decrease in HIV-1 viral load.[9,10] In children, HAART has been associated with a similar recovery in immunologic status,[11-14] although viral suppression is usually less evident in children compared with adults.[15] A combination of CD4 percentage or counts and HIV-1 viral load have proven to be the best predictors of future disease progression and mortality in both adults and children.[16-20]

Recently, the long-term effects of HAART on changes in the CD4 percentage were evaluated prospectively in the Pediatric AIDS Clinical Trials Group (PACTG) 219 cohort of children and adolescents with HIV in the United States.[2] The investigators reported a varied response to therapy according to the level of immunosuppression at the time of treatment initiation; children with the most severe im-

**Author Affiliations** are listed at the end of this article.
**Group Information:** The Pediatric AIDS Clinical Trials Group Protocol 219C personnel and Pediatric AIDS Clinical Trials Group centers are listed on page 785.

munosuppression experienced the greatest increase in CD4 percentage over time. However, only about one third of these children achieved a CD4 percentage within the normal range (CD4 percentage ≥25%) after 3 years. Furthermore, 16% of the children who initiated HAART while their CD4 percentages were in the normal range had decreases in their CD4 percentages to less than 25% during follow-up.[2]

Few studies have examined the occurrence of OIs in relation to HAART use in pediatric HIV infection. Thus, we used data from a large US cohort of children perinatally infected with HIV who initiated HAART at different ages and levels of immunosuppression to examine the relationship between HAART use and other clinical, demographic, and virologic factors and the occurrence of OIs in the pediatric HIV population.

## METHODS

The source population for this study was the PACTG 219C cohort, which began enrollment in September 2000 to assess the long-term effects of in utero, perinatal, and childhood exposure to antiretroviral therapy (ART) in children with HIV across the United States. The PACTG 219C protocol is a revised version of PACTG 219, a protocol initiated in 1993 and described in detail elsewhere.[21] Children eligible for the current study must have been perinatally infected with HIV and must have received HAART (as defined later) prior to or at enrollment in PACTG 219C. Institutional review board approval was obtained at all of the participating clinical centers, and the children's parents or guardians provided written informed consent. There were 2318 subjects perinatally infected with HIV enrolled in PACTG 219C between September 15, 2000, and August 31, 2003, and 1323 (57.1%) of them were previously enrolled in PACTG 219. Of the 2318 subjects, 12 (0.5%) were never treated with ART, 276 (11.9%) never received HAART, 101 (4.4%) initiated HAART after enrollment in PACTG 219C, and 2 (0.1%) had no follow-up after enrollment and thus were excluded. The remaining 1927 subjects (83.1%) met the eligibility criteria and were subsequently followed up for the occurrence of OIs until August 31, 2003.

At enrollment in PACTG 219C and every 3 months thereafter, participants underwent a physical examination and a medical history was obtained, including information on signs, symptoms, or diagnoses of any OIs (defined according to the Centers for Disease Control and Prevention [CDC] disease classification of pediatric HIV infection).[22,23] Information on treatment (including prophylactic treatment) or hospitalization for any OIs was also recorded. Measures of HIV-1 viral load and CD4 counts and percentages were also collected at each visit.

Detailed information on lifetime ART use, including start and stop dates of each drug, was obtained at enrollment in PACTG 219C. Use of HAART was defined as combination ART with at least 3 drugs, of which at least 1 was either a protease inhibitor (PI) or a nonnucleoside reverse transcriptase inhibitor.[8-10] Duration of HAART use was defined as time from HAART initiation to enrollment in PACTG 219C and was categorized into 3 groups: 0 to less than 1 year, 1 to less than 4 years, and 4 or more years. These categories were chosen to represent short-term, medium-term, and long-term HAART use. Subjects were further classified according to age at HAART initiation (ages 0 to <2 years, 2 to <10 years, and ≥10 years). In addition, treatment experience prior to initiating HAART, excluding zidovudine prophylaxis, was considered. Any change from one ART drug or combination of drugs to another was considered a change in regimen. Thus, subjects were categorized as treatment naïve, receiving 1 to 2 ART regimens, or receiving 3 or more different ART regimens prior to HAART. Subjects were also classified according to the number of different HAART regimens they received from HAART initiation to enrollment in PACTG 219C (1 HAART regimen and treatment naïve at HAART initiation, 1-2 different HAART regimens, and ≥3 different HAART regimens).

The main outcome was the first occurrence of an OI during follow-up in PACTG 219C (regardless of OI events before enrollment). All of the OI events were classified according to the CDC's criteria for pediatric HIV infection[22,23] as category B (OI-B) or category C (OI-C) events based on the type of OI and the subject's history of OIs. If a subject had a first OI-B event and a subsequent OI-C event, both the OI-B and OI-C events were considered in the respective incidence and regression analyses. However, if a subject had a first OI-C event and a subsequent OI-B event, only the OI-C event was considered. For pneumonias, only presumed events (with radiological and clinical evidence of pneumonia) or proven events (that were culture confirmed) were considered.

Incidence rates (per 100 person-years) and exact Poisson 95% confidence intervals (CIs) for the first OI (either OI-B or OI-C) event, the first OI-B event, and the first OI-C event were calculated for the period between September 15, 2000, and August 31, 2003. For these analyses, end of follow-up was defined as the date of the first OI event, date of loss to follow-up, or August 31, 2003, whichever came first. In addition, incidence rates (per 100 person-years) and exact Poisson 95% CIs for specific OIs (both OI-B and OI-C events) were calculated for the follow-up period.

The median CD4 percentage and HIV-1 viral load at enrollment and at the end of follow-up in PACTG 219C were determined for all of the study subjects. Subanalyses were performed among 741 study subjects previously enrolled in PACTG 219 for whom we had information on CD4 percentage at the time of HAART initiation. The HIV-1 RNA measurements were not recorded in the PACTG 219 protocol and thus could not be determined at HAART initiation. In addition, the proportion of subjects in different categories of CD4 percentage and HIV-1 viral load were determined by OI occurrence during follow-up.

The relationship between age at HAART initiation, duration of HAART use, and the risk of a first OI (either OI-B or OI-C) event during cohort follow-up was assessed using Cox proportional hazards regression while adjusting for the following potential confounders: age at enrollment, number of ART regimens prior to initiating HAART, number of HAART regimens before enrollment, adherence to HAART at enrollment, sex, and ethnicity. In a subanalysis including the 741 subjects with information on CD4 percentage at HAART initiation, CD4 percentage and CDC disease category at HAART initiation were added to the regression model to adjust for severity of illness at HAART initiation. The validity of the proportional hazards assumptions was assessed by examining residual plots to determine whether the hazards were approximately constant over time.[24] Hazard ratios (HRs), 95% CIs, and $P$ values were calculated using the likelihood ratio test.[24] All of the analyses were performed using SAS version 8.2 software (SAS Institute, Inc, Cary, NC).

## RESULTS

The characteristics of the 1927 subjects in the study population by OI occurrence during follow-up are summarized in **Table 1**. The risk of an OI during cohort follow-up was higher in children who were older, were

**Table 1. Characteristics of 1927 Children Perinatally Infected With Human Immunodeficiency Virus Enrolled in Pediatric AIDS Clinical Trials Group 219C Categorized by Opportunistic Illness Occurrence During Follow-up**

| Variable | Children Without OI, No. (%) (n = 1701) | Children With OI, No. (%) (n = 226) | *P* Value* |
|---|---|---|---|
| Age at enrollment, y | | | |
| 0 to <2 | 86 (5.1) | 12 (5.3) | .008 |
| 2 to <10 | 877 (51.6) | 92 (40.7) | |
| 10-21 | 738 (43.4) | 122 (54.0) | |
| Sex | | | |
| Female | 822 (48.3) | 118 (52.2) | .27 |
| Male | 879 (51.7) | 108 (47.8) | |
| Ethnicity | | | |
| Non-Hispanic white | 255 (15.0) | 19 (8.4) | .02 |
| Non-Hispanic black | 982 (57.7) | 138 (61.1) | |
| Hispanic | 438 (25.8) | 68 (30.1) | |
| Other | 26 (1.5) | 1 (0.4) | |
| CDC disease category at enrollment | | | |
| Asymptomatic or A | 688 (40.4) | 29 (12.8) | <.001 |
| B | 558 (32.8) | 79 (35.0) | |
| C | 429 (25.2) | 115 (50.9) | |
| Missing | 26 (1.5) | 3 (1.3) | |
| $CD4^+$ T lymphocytes at enrollment, % | | | |
| ≥25 | 1231 (72.4) | 89 (39.4) | <.001 |
| 15 to <25 | 330 (19.4) | 44 (19.5) | |
| <15 | 131 (7.7) | 93 (41.2) | |
| Missing | 9 (0.5) | 0 | |
| HIV-1 viral load at enrollment, copies/mL | | | |
| <400 | 471 (27.7) | 29 (12.8) | <.001 |
| 400 to <10 000 | 797 (46.9) | 64 (28.3) | |
| 10 000 to <100 000 | 321 (18.9) | 73 (32.3) | |
| ≥100 000 | 96 (5.6) | 60 (26.6) | |
| Missing | 16 (0.9) | 0 | |
| Age at HAART initiation, y | | | |
| 0 to <2 | 321 (18.9) | 26 (11.5) | .001 |
| 2 to <10 | 1091 (64.1) | 141 (62.4) | |
| 10-20 | 289 (17.0) | 59 (26.1) | |
| Duration of HAART use at enrollment, y | | | |
| 0 to <1 | 239 (14.1) | 29 (12.8) | .59 |
| 1 to <4 | 1178 (69.3) | 164 (72.6) | |
| 4-10 | 284 (16.7) | 33 (14.6) | |
| ART regimens prior to HAART initiation, No. | | | |
| 0 | 350 (20.6) | 37 (16.4) | <.001 |
| 1-2 | 833 (49.0) | 78 (34.5) | |
| ≥3 | 518 (30.4) | 111 (49.1) | |
| Different HAART regimens, No. | | | |
| 1† | 231 (13.6) | 19 (8.4) | <.001 |
| 1-2‡ | 1032 (60.7) | 102 (45.1) | |
| ≥3 | 438 (25.7) | 105 (46.5) | |
| Adherence to HAART regimen, %§ | | | |
| 100 | 1380 (81.1) | 168 (74.3) | .05 |
| 1-99 | 192 (11.3) | 39 (17.3) | |
| 0 | 64 (3.8) | 11 (4.9) | |
| Missing | 65 (3.8) | 8 (3.5) | |

Abbreviations: ART, antiretroviral therapy; CDC, Centers for Disease Control and Prevention; HAART, highly active antiretroviral treatment; HIV-1, human immunodeficiency virus 1.

**P* values are based on a statistical test of difference.

†Children who were treatment naïve at the time of initiating HAART.

‡Antiretroviral therapy–experienced children by the time of initiating HAART.

§Adherence was recorded during a 3-day period at the time of enrollment in Pediatric AIDS Clinical Trials Group 219C.

Hispanic or non-Hispanic black, were in CDC category C, had a CD4 percentage of less than 15%, had a higher HIV-1 viral load at enrollment, initiated HAART at an older age, and were treated with at least 3 different ART regimens before HAART initiation or at least 3 different HAART regimens before enrollment in PACTG 219C.

Median follow-up time was 28 months (range, 6 days to 35 months), and 316 subjects (16.4%) were censored prior to August 31, 2003. Reasons for censoring included site closure (n=227), subjects moving away from the site (n=41), death unrelated to OI (n=7), investigators being unable to contact the subjects (n=15), parents withdrawing consent (n=14), subjects being unable to adhere to the study protocol (n=8), subjects being too ill (n=3), and imprisonment (n=1).

Subjects were treated with a median of 2 (range, 0-12) different ART regimens prior to HAART initiation followed by a median of 1 (range, 1-17) different HAART regimen before PACTG 219C enrollment. Of the 387 subjects who were treatment naïve when initiating HAART, 250 (64.6%) continued to receive the same HAART regimen through enrollment in PACTG 219C. The first HAART regimen consisted of 2 nucleoside reverse transcriptase inhibitors and 1 PI for 1224 subjects (63.5%), 2 nucleoside reverse transcriptase inhibitors and 1 nonnucleoside reverse transcriptase inhibitor for 279 subjects (14.5%), 1 or 2 nucleoside reverse transcriptase inhibitors, 1 PI, and 1 nonnucleoside reverse transcriptase inhibitor for 395 subjects (20.5%), and other nucleoside reverse transcriptase inhibitor, PI, and nonnucleoside reverse transcriptase inhibitor combinations for 29 subjects (1.5%).

The OI incidence rates per 100 person-years of follow-up in PACTG 219C are shown in **Table 2**. In total, 185 first OI-B events and 57 first OI-C events occurred among 226 subjects during follow-up. The incidence rate was 6.21 (95% CI, 5.42-7.07) per 100 person-years for the first OI regardless of category, 4.99 (95% CI, 4.30-5.76) per 100 person-years for the first OI-B event, and 1.47 (95% CI, 1.12-1.91) per 100 person-years for the first OI-C event. The most frequently occurring OI-B event was bacterial pneumonia, and the most frequently occurring OI-C event was esophageal candidiasis. In 7 children, the OI-C event (2 *Pneumocystis jiroveci* pneumonia events, 3 culture-confirmed sepsis events, and 2 HIV encephalopathy events) led to death within a month after diagnosis. Ten additional children died from AIDS-related OIs after having had a prior OI-C event.

During follow-up, 721 (37.4%) of the participants received prophylaxis against *P jiroveci* pneumonia and 166 (8.6%) received prophylaxis against *Mycobacterium avium* complex infection. Children receiving *P jiroveci* pneumonia or *M avium* complex prophylaxis were significantly older at enrollment and HAART initiation and were more likely to be in CDC category C, have a lower CD4 percentage (<15%), and have a higher HIV-1 viral load (>10 000 copies/mL) at enrollment compared with subjects receiving no prophylaxis during follow-up (all $P<.001$).

The median CD4 percentage improved over time, from 22% (95% CI, 21%-23%) just prior to HAART initiation (among 741 subjects previously enrolled in PACTG 219) to 30% (95% CI, 29%-30%) at enrollment in PACTG 219C, and it persisted at 30% (95% CI, 29%-30%) until the end of follow-up. This increase in median CD4 percentage over time was observed across different subgroups, including sex, ethnic origin, age at HAART initiation, and age at enrollment. However, there were differences in median CD4 percentage levels within subgroups; girls had a significantly higher median CD4 percentage than boys when initiating HAART (25% vs 20%, respectively), at enrollment (31% vs 28%, respectively), and at the end of follow-up (31% vs 29%, respectively). Furthermore, subjects who initiated HAART when they were younger than 2 years had significantly higher median CD4 percentages compared with older children (aged >10 years) at HAART initiation (27% vs 17%, respectively), at enrollment (35% vs 23%, respectively), and at the end of follow-up (34% vs 23%, respectively). The HIV-1 viral load for the study population did not change substantially between enrollment (median viral load, 1081 copies/mL; 95% CI, 809-1397 copies/mL) and the end of follow-up (median viral load, 818 copies/mL; 95% CI, 574-1140 copies/mL).

The proportions of subjects in different categories of CD4 percentage at HAART initiation, at enrollment in PACTG 219C, and at the end of follow-up are shown by OI occurrence during follow-up in **Figure**, A. More subjects with OIs than without OIs were in the low CD4 percentage (<15%) category at HAART initiation (49.6% of subjects with OIs vs 23.7% of subjects without OIs), at enrollment (41.2% of subjects with OIs vs 7.7% of subjects without OIs), and at the end of follow-up (41.2% of subjects with OIs vs 8.3% of subjects without OIs). In addition, the proportion of subjects with normal CD4 percentages (≥25%) was more pronounced over time among subjects without an OI (from 48% to 71%) compared with those experiencing OIs (from 23% to 38%). The proportion of subjects in different categories of HIV-1 viral load at enrollment in PACTG 219C and at the end of fol-

**Table 2. Incidence Rates of Opportunistic Illnesses per 100 Person-Years During Follow-up for 1927 Children Perinatally Infected With Human Immunodeficiency Virus**

| Opportunistic Illness | Events, No. | Incidence Rate per 100 Person-Years (95% CI) |
|---|---|---|
| First opportunistic illness category B events | 185 | 4.99 (4.30-5.76) |
| Specific opportunistic illness category B events | | |
| Bacterial pneumonia | 139 | 3.67 (3.09-4.34) |
| Oral candidiasis | 44 | 1.13 (0.82-1.52) |
| Sepsis | 19 | 0.48 (0.29-0.76) |
| Herpes zoster virus | 8 | 0.20 (0.09-0.40) |
| Herpes simplex virus stomatitis | 7 | 0.18 (0.07-0.37) |
| Lymphoid interstitial pneumonia | 5 | 0.13 (0.04-0.30) |
| Bacterial meningitis | 2 | 0.05 (0.01-0.18) |
| First opportunistic illness category C events | 57 | 1.47 (1.12-1.91) |
| Specific opportunistic illness category C events | | |
| Esophageal candidiasis | 19 | 0.48 (0.29-0.76) |
| Bacterial infection (recurrent, culture confirmed) | 11 | 0.28 (0.14-0.50) |
| HIV encephalopathy | 11 | 0.28 (0.14-0.50) |
| HIV wasting syndrome | 11 | 0.28 (0.14-0.50) |
| *Pneumocystis jiroveci* pneumonia | 9 | 0.23 (0.10-0.43) |
| *Mycobacterium avium*, disseminated | 4 | 0.10 (0.03-0.26) |
| Non-Hodgkin lymphoma | 2 | 0.05 (0.01-0.18) |
| Hodgkin lymphoma | 2 | 0.05 (0.01-0.18) |
| Histoplasmosis, disseminated | 1 | 0.03 (0.001-0.14) |
| Herpes simplex virus, disseminated | 1 | 0.03 (0.001-0.14) |
| Cytomegalovirus retinitis | 1 | 0.03 (0.001-0.14) |
| Cryptosporidiosis, persistent | 1 | 0.03 (0.001-0.14) |

Abbreviations: CI, confidence interval; HIV, human immunodeficiency virus.

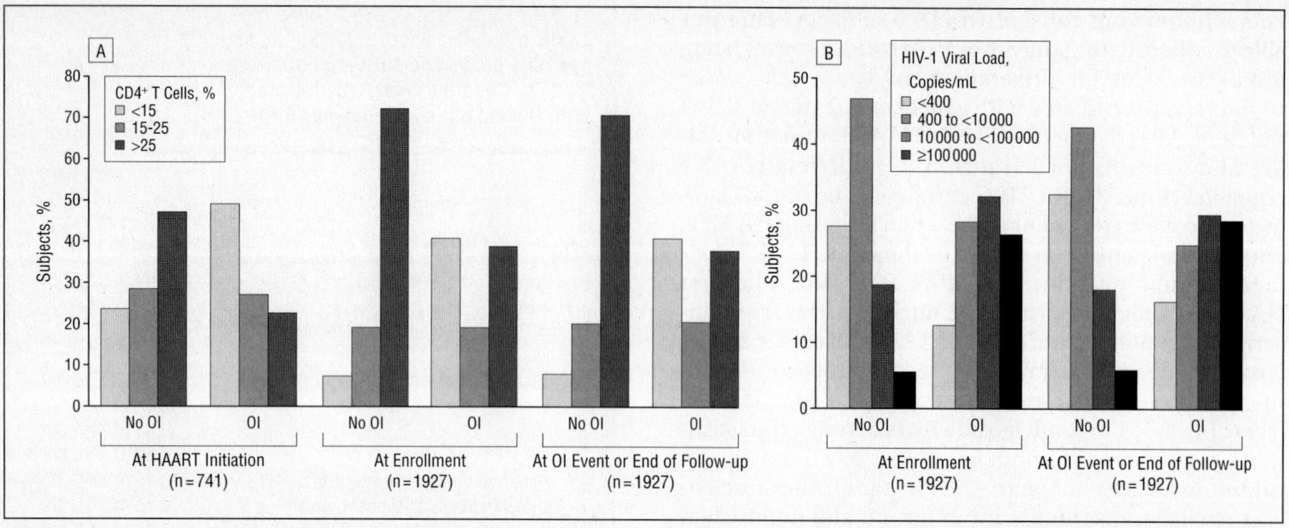


**Figure.** The proportion of subjects in different categories of CD4+ T-lymphocyte percentage at highly active antiretroviral treatment (HAART) initiation (calculated among the 741 subjects previously enrolled in Pediatric AIDS Clinical Trials Group 219), at enrollment in Pediatric AIDS Clinical Trials Group 219C, and at the end of follow-up in children with and without opportunistic illnesses (OIs) during follow-up (A) and in different categories of human immunodeficiency virus 1 (HIV-1) viral load at enrollment in Pediatric AIDS Clinical Trials Group 219C and at the end of follow-up in children with and without OIs during follow-up (B).

low-up did not change much over time (Figure, B). However, more subjects with OIs than without OIs were in the high viral load categories (≥100 000 copies/mL) both at enrollment (26.6% vs 5.7%, respectively) and at the end of follow-up (28.8% vs 6.1%, respectively). Also, the proportion of subjects with good viral suppression (<400 copies/mL) was lower among subjects with OIs compared with those without OIs at enrollment (12.8% vs 28.0%, respectively) and at the end of follow-up (16.4% vs 32.8%, respectively).

The risk of having a first OI (regardless of category) during follow-up in relation to HAART exposure was examined using Cox proportional hazards regression (**Table 3**). In the multivariate regression model, there was a significantly higher risk of a first OI during follow-up for non-Hispanic black subjects (HR, 2.09; 95% CI, 1.29-3.38) and Hispanic subjects (HR, 1.94; 95% CI, 1.16-3.23) compared with non-Hispanic white subjects. Subjects who enrolled in PACTG 219C when they were aged 10 years or older had a significantly lower risk of a first OI compared with subjects younger than 2 years at enrollment (HR, 0.37; 95% CI, 0.15-0.92). In contrast, subjects who initiated HAART when they were aged 10 years or older had a significantly higher risk of a first OI compared with those initiating HAART when they were younger than 2 years (HR, 2.48; 95% CI, 1.23-5.00). Subjects who switched between 3 or more HAART regimens had a significantly increased risk of a first OI compared with subjects who were treatment naïve at HAART initiation and continued to receive the same HAART regimen after HAART initiation (HR, 2.73; 95% CI, 1.40-5.32). There was no relationship between sex, duration of HAART use, number of ART regimens before initiating HAART, or short-term adherence to HAART and the risk of a first OI (Table 3). Regression analysis performed for OI-B and OI-C events separately gave similar results except for boys having a marginally significant lower risk of a first OI-B event during follow-up compared with girls (HR, 0.75; 95% CI, 0.56-1.00).

To control for severity of illness at HAART initiation, we performed separate Cox proportional hazards regression analyses for the 741 subjects previously enrolled in PACTG 219 for whom we had information on CD4 percentage at the time of initiating HAART. Initially, we ran the same multivariate model as shown in Table 3. The results were materially unchanged except for wider CIs, indicating no significant risk of OI according to race or ethnicity, age at HAART initiation, and age at enrollment. Subsequently, CD4 percentage and CDC disease category at HAART initiation were added to the multivariate model as indicators of severity of illness at the time of initiating combination therapy (**Table 4**). In this adjusted model, only CDC disease category and CD4 percentage at enrollment were related to OI risk during follow-up. Both CDC category B (HR, 3.21; 95% CI, 1.89-5.45) and category C (HR, 3.35; 95% CI, 1.77-6.35) at HAART initiation were associated with a higher risk of a first OI compared with being asymptomatic or in category A. A CD4 percentage of less than 15% at HAART initiation was associated with a 2-fold increased risk of a first OI compared with a normal CD4 percentage (≥25%) (HR, 2.04; 95% CI, 1.18-3.53).

## COMMENT

Given the fact that there are about 2.1 million children living with HIV or AIDS in the world and that combination therapies have become increasingly available and recommended, it is of greatest importance to define the optimal time to initiate HAART. Our findings that HAART initiation at an older age (age >10 years) was associated with an increased risk of OIs may have important clinical and policy implications. Despite the obvious risk of fast progression in young children, the question of when HAART should be initiated in children remains controversial. According to the US guidelines,[25] treatment intervention as early as possible regardless of the child's

**Table 3. Risk of First Opportunistic Illness Among 1927 Children Perinatally Infected With Human Immunodeficiency Virus Enrolled in Pediatric AIDS Clinical Trials Group 219C**

| Characteristic | Children, No. | Hazard Ratio (95% CI) Univariate Analysis | Hazard Ratio (95% CI) Multivariate Analysis* | P Value† |
|---|---|---|---|---|
| Sex | | | | |
| Female | 940 | Reference | Reference | .18 |
| Male | 987 | 0.85 (0.66-1.11) | 0.84 (0.64-1.09) | |
| Ethnicity | | | | |
| Non-Hispanic white | 274 | Reference | Reference | .005 |
| Non-Hispanic black | 1120 | 1.87 (1.16-3.02) | 2.09 (1.29-3.38) | |
| Hispanic | 506 | 1.88 (1.13-3.12) | 1.94 (1.16-3.23) | |
| Other | 27 | 0.52 (0.07-3.89) | 0.58 (0.08-4.34) | |
| Age at enrollment, y | | | | |
| 0 to <2 | 98 | Reference | Reference | .05 |
| 2 to <10 | 969 | 0.61 (0.34-1.12) | 0.35 (0.16-0.81) | |
| 10-21 | 860 | 0.98 (0.54-1.77) | 0.37 (0.15-0.92) | |
| Age at HAART initiation, y | | | | |
| 0 to <2 | 347 | Reference | Reference | .02 |
| 2 to <10 | 1232 | 1.40 (0.92-2.13) | 1.66 (0.92-3.01) | |
| 10-21 | 348 | 2.18 (1.37-3.45) | 2.48 (1.23-5.00) | |
| Duration of HAART use at enrollment, y | | | | |
| 0 to <1 | 268 | Reference | Reference | .96 |
| 1 to <4 | 1342 | 1.02 (0.69-1.51) | 0.97 (0.63-1.50) | |
| ≥4 | 317 | 1.19 (0.72-1.96) | 1.02 (0.58-1.80) | |
| ART regimens prior to HAART initiation, No. | | | | |
| 0 | 387 | Reference | Reference | <.001 |
| 1-2 | 911 | 0.80 (0.54-1.18) | 0.65 (0.38-1.11) | |
| ≥3 | 629 | 1.71 (1.18-2.48) | 1.21 (0.70-2.06) | |
| Different HAART regimens, No. | | | | |
| 1‡ | 250 | Reference | Reference | <.001 |
| 1-2§ | 1134 | 1.02 (0.63-1.67) | 1.20 (0.61-2.37) | |
| ≥3 | 543 | 2.45 (1.50-4.00) | 2.73 (1.40-5.32) | |
| Adherence to HAART regimen, %‖ | | | | |
| 100 | 1548 | Reference | Reference | .52 |
| 1-99 | 231 | 1.58 (1.11-2.23) | 1.31 (0.92-1.88) | |
| 0 | 75 | 1.31 (0.71-2.42) | 1.18 (0.64-2.18) | |
| Missing | 73 | 1.22 (0.60-2.47) | 1.05 (0.51-2.13) | |

Abbreviations: ART, antiretroviral therapy; CI, confidence interval; HAART, highly active antiretroviral treatment.
*Adjusted for all of the variables listed.
†The *P* values indicate whether there is any significant difference across the categories of each variable in the multivariate model.
‡Children who were treatment naïve at the time of initiating HAART.
§Antiretroviral therapy–experienced children by the time of initiating HAART.
‖Adherence was recorded during a 3-day period at the time of enrollment in Pediatric AIDS Clinical Trials Group 219C.

immune function is recommended. In contrast, European[26] and World Health Organization[27] guidelines recommend postponing treatment in children until the CD4 percentages fall below 15% or 20%.[25,26] Although some investigators have found that recovery to normal CD4 cell counts is independent of age,[28] the recovery of naïve CD4 cells is usually more rapid and effective in young children,[2,14,29] which may favor early intervention with HAART before severe immunosuppression has occurred.[14] Furthermore, from a long-term perspective, only a small fraction of children who start therapy when their CD4 percentages have fallen below 15% will reach normal CD4 percentages (≥25%). Again, this supports the view that HAART should be initiated as early as possible.[2]

The CD4 cell count at HAART initiation has previously been demonstrated as a strong predictor for subsequent OI risk.[4] In accordance, the significant association we found between older age (age >10 years) when initiating HAART and the risk of an OI during follow-up (Table 3) diminished when we controlled for the children's immunologic and clinical status (CD4 percentage and CDC disease category, respectively) at HAART initiation (Table 4). Subjects who already were in CDC category B or C at HAART initiation had a higher risk of additional OIs during follow-up compared with subjects who initiated HAART before development of clinical disease, even after adjustment for their CD4 percentages at HAART initiation (Table 4). In addition, more children with OIs than without OIs had a CD4 percentage of less than 15% at HAART initiation (49.6% of children with OIs vs 23.7% of children without OIs), at enrollment (41.2% of children with OIs vs 7.7% of children without OIs), and at the end of follow-up (41.2% of children with OIs vs 8.3% of children without OIs) (Figure, A). These results suggest that HAART initiation should not be delayed until the CD4 percentage has fallen below 15% or the child has already experienced an AIDS-defining illness.

**Table 4. Risk of First Opportunistic Illness Among 741 Children Perinatally Infected With Human Immunodeficiency Virus Enrolled in Pediatric AIDS Clinical Trials Group 219C Controlling for CD4⁺ T-Lymphocyte Percentage and Centers for Disease Control and Prevention Category***

| Characteristic | Children, No. | Hazard Ratio (95% CI): Univariate Analysis | Hazard Ratio (95% CI): Multivariate Analysis† | *P* Value‡ |
|---|---|---|---|---|
| Sex | | | | |
| Female | 353 | Reference | Reference | .06 |
| Male | 388 | 0.77 (0.53-1.11) | 0.70 (0.48-1.02) | |
| Ethnicity | | | | |
| Non-Hispanic white | 92 | Reference | Reference | .32 |
| Non-Hispanic black | 385 | 1.40 (0.71-2.75) | 1.50 (0.75-3.01) | |
| Hispanic | 258 | 1.83 (0.92-3.61) | 1.84 (0.92-3.67) | |
| Other | 6 | 1.58 (0.20-12.36) | 1.32 (0.16-10.63) | |
| Age at enrollment, y | | | | |
| 0 to <2 | 3 | 3.36 (0.46-24.49) | 4.95 (0.41-59.91) | .52 |
| 2 to <10 | 333 | Reference | Reference | |
| 10-21 | 405 | 1.72 (1.17-2.55) | 1.03 (0.63-1.70) | |
| CDC disease category at HAART initiation | | | | |
| Asymptomatic or A | 354 | Reference | Reference | <.001 |
| B | 251 | 4.59 (2.80-7.53) | 3.21 (1.89-5.45) | |
| C | 103 | 4.80 (2.69-8.58) | 3.35 (1.77-6.35) | |
| Missing | 33 | 2.13 (0.73-6.21) | 1.82 (0.60-5.53) | |
| CD4⁺ T lymphocytes at HAART initiation, % | | | | |
| ≥25 | 324 | Reference | Reference | .03 |
| 15 to <25 | 212 | 1.87 (1.11-3.15) | 1.35 (0.79-2.33) | |
| <15 | 205 | 3.96 (2.48-6.31) | 2.04 (1.18-3.53) | |
| Age at HAART initiation, y | | | | |
| 0 to <2 | 29 | Reference | Reference | .46 |
| 2 to <10 | 514 | 1.40 (0.44-4.45) | 1.12 (0.26-4.86) | |
| 10-21 | 198 | 2.20 (0.68-7.11) | 1.52 (0.32-7.24) | |
| Duration of HAART use at enrollment, y | | | | |
| 0 to <1 | 87 | Reference | Reference | .69 |
| 1 to <4 | 559 | 1.23 (0.65-2.30) | 0.86 (0.44-1.69) | |
| ≥4 | 95 | 1.77 (0.83-3.75) | 0.70 (0.30-1.65) | |
| ART regimens prior to HAART initiation, No. | | | | |
| 0 | 48 | Reference | Reference | .04 |
| 1-2 | 386 | 0.84 (0.36-1.98) | 0.56 (0.19-1.63) | |
| ≥3 | 307 | 1.82 (0.79-4.19) | 0.93 (0.32-2.66) | |
| Different HAART regimens, No. | | | | |
| 1§ | 30 | Reference | Reference | .001 |
| 1-2∥ | 504 | 1.71 (0.42-7.02) | 1.25 (0.21-7.32) | |
| ≥3 | 207 | 4.58 (1.12-18.79) | 2.71 (0.47-15.71) | |
| Adherence to HAART regimen, %¶ | | | | |
| 100 | 582 | Reference | Reference | .44 |
| 1-99 | 97 | 1.65 (1.03-2.65) | 1.50 (0.91-2.47) | |
| 0 | 29 | 1.24 (0.50-3.05) | 1.12 (0.44-2.87) | |
| Missing | 33 | 0.72 (0.23-2.29) | 0.76 (0.24-2.47) | |

Abbreviations: ART, antiretroviral therapy; CDC, Centers for Disease Control and Prevention; CI, confidence interval; HAART, highly active retroviral treatment.

*Subjects were those who were previously enrolled in Pediatric AIDS Clinical Trials Group 219 for whom information on CD4⁺ T-lymphocyte percentage at the time of HAART initiation was available.

†Adjusted for all of the variables listed.

‡The *P* values indicate whether there is any significant difference across the categories of each variable in the multivariate model.

§Children who were treatment naïve at the time of initiating HAART.

∥Antiretroviral therapy–experienced children by the time of initiating HAART.

¶Adherence was recorded during a 3-day period at the time of enrollment in Pediatric AIDS Clinical Trials Group 219C.

Our findings of an increased risk of OIs during follow-up among non-Hispanic black and Hispanic children (Table 3) compared with non-Hispanic white children have been previously observed yet not fully explained in the literature.[30] Genetic variation in immunologic status between ethnic groups has been suggested, especially since social disparities (such as access to treatment or adherence) have not been significantly associated with ethnic groups.[2,31] In accordance, we found lower median CD4 percentages among both non-Hispanic black and Hispanic subjects at HAART initiation, at enrollment, and at the OI event compared with non-Hispanic white subjects, and race or ethnicity was no longer predictive of risk in the model adjusted for the CD4 percentage at HAART initiation (Table 4). The relationship between sex, immunologic parameters, and clinical outcomes is less clear.[32,33] We found that girls had higher median CD4 percentages at all of the time points during

## Contributing Pediatric AIDS Clinical Trials Group 219C Site Personnel

*University of Medicine and Dentistry of New Jersey, Newark:* P. Palumbo, P. Andrew, A. Dieudonne, B. Dashefsky; *Robert Wood Johnson Medical School, Piscataway, NJ:* S. Gaur, P. Whitley-Williams, A. Malhotra, L. Cerracchio; *Harbor-UCLA Medical Center, Torrance, Calif:* M. Keller, J. Hayes, A. Gagajena, C. Mink; *Department of Pediatrics, Johns Hopkins University, Baltimore, Md:* N. Hutton, B. Griffith, M. Joyner, C. Kiefner; *Baylor Texas Children's Hospital, Houston, Tex:* F. Minglana, M. E. Paul, W. T. Shearer, C. D. Jackson; *Sinai Children's Hospital, Chicago, Ill:* D. C. Johnson, D. Kowalski, B. Wolfe, D. Ryan; *The Columbia Presbyterian Medical Center and Cornell University New York Presbyterian Hospital, New York:* A. Higgins, M. Foca, P. LaRussa, A. Gershon; *University of Miami, Coral Gables, Fla:* G. B. Scott, C. D. Mitchell, L. Taybo, C. Gamber; *Children's Hospital and Research Center, Oakland, Calif:* A. Petru, T. Courville, K. Gold, L. Johnson; *Phoenix Children's Hospital, Phoenix, Ariz:* J. P. Piatt, J. Foti, L. Clarke-Steffen; *University of North Carolina at Chapel Hill:* T. Belho, B. Pitkin, J. Eddleman; *Schneider Children's Hospital, New Hyde Park, NY:* V. R. Bonagura, S. J. Schuval, C. Colter; *Harlem Hospital, New York:* E. J. Abrams, M. Frere, D. Calo, S. Champion; *Children's Hospital at Downstate, Brooklyn, NY:* E. Handelsman, H. J. Moallem, D. M. Swindell, J. M. Kaye; *Jacobi Medical Center, New York:* M. Chin, K. Dorio, A. Wiznia, M. Donovan; *San Juan Hospital, San Juan, Puerto Rico:* M. Acevedo, M. Gonzalez, L. Fabregas, M. E. Texidor; *Yale University School of Medicine, New Haven, Conn:* W. A. Andiman, S. Romano, L. Hurst, J. de Jesus; *SUNY Upstate Medical University, Syracuse, NY:* L. B. Weiner, K. A. Contello, W. A. Holz, M. J. Famiglietti; *SUNY Stony Brook, Stony Brook, NY:* S. Nachman, D. Nikolic-Djokic, D. Ferraro, J. Perillo; *Howard University, Washington, DC:* S. Rana, H. Finke-Castro, P. H. Yu, J. C. Roa; *University of Florida Health Science Center, Jacksonville:* M. H. Rathore, A. Khayat, K. Champion, S. Cusic; *St Jude Children's Research Hospital, Memphis, Tenn:* P. M. Flynn, K. Knapp, N. Patel; *Vanderbilt University Medical Center, Nashville, Tenn:* G. Wilson; *Department of Pediatrics, Washington University School of Medicine, St Louis Children's Hospital, St Louis, Mo:* K. A. McGann, L. Pickering, G. A. Storch; *The Children's Hospital of Philadelphia, Philadelphia, Pa:* S. D. Douglas, G. Koutsoubis, R. M. Rutstein, C. A. Vincent; *Charity Hospital of New Orleans and Earl K. Long Early Intervention Clinic, New Orleans, La:* M. Silio, T. Alchediak, C. Boe, M. Cowie; *Baystate Medical Center Children's Hospital, Springfield, Mass:* B. W. Stechenberg, D. J. Fisher, A. M. Johnston, M. Toye; *Medical College of Georgia, Augusta:* C. S. Mani, S. Foshee, B. Kiean, S. Cobb; *University of Maryland Medical Center, Baltimore:* J. Farley, K. Klipner; *University of California, San Diego:* S. Spector, R. Viani, L. Stangl.

## Pediatric AIDS Clinical Trials Group Centers

Cooper Hospital–University Medical Center, Camden, NJ; Children's Hospital Boston, Boston, Mass; Boston Medical Center, Boston; University of California, Los Angeles, Medical Center, Los Angeles; Children's Hospital of Los Angeles, Los Angeles; Long Beach Memorial, Long Beach, Calif; Chicago Children's Memorial Hospital, Chicago; Cook County Hospital, Chicago; The University of Chicago Children's Hospital, Chicago; Women's and Children's HIV Program, Moffitt Hospital, University of California, San Francisco; Mother, Child, and Adolescent HIV Program, University of California, San Diego; Phoenix Children's Hospital; Duke University, Durham, NC; New York University School of Medicine Bellevue Hospital, New York; Children's National Medical Center, Washington; Children's Hospital and Regional Medical Center, Washington, DC; University of South Florida, Tampa; Oregon Health and Science University, Portland; Children's Hospital of the King's Daughters, Norfolk, Va; Lincoln Medical and Mental Health Center, New York; Mount Sinai Medical Center, Miami Beach, Fla; University of Illinois, Chicago; Children's Hospital of Michigan, Detroit; Children's Medical Center of Dallas, Dallas, Tex; Los Angeles County–University of Southern California Medical Center, Los Angeles; Children's Hospital, University of Colorado, Denver; North Broward Hospital District, Fort Lauderdale, Fla; University of Florida, Gainesville; University of Rochester Medical Center, Rochester, NY; University of Mississippi Medical Center, Jackson; Medical College of Virginia, Virginia Commonwealth University, Richmond, Va; University Children's Hospital AIDS Program, University of Puerto Rico, San Juan; St Christopher's Hospital for Children, Philadelphia; Bronx Lebanon Hospital Center, New York; St Luke's-Roosevelt Hospital Center, New York; Montefiore Medical, Albert Einstein College of Medicine, New York; Metropolitan Hospital Center, New York; University of Massachusetts Medical School, Worcester; Connecticut Children's Medical Center, Hartford; University of Alabama at Birmingham; University of South Alabama, Mobile; The Medical Center, Columbus, Ga; Incarnation Children's Center, New York; St Joseph's Hospital and Medical Center, Paterson, NJ; Wyler Hospital, Chicago; Children's Hospital of Oakland, Oakland; Emory University Hospital, Atlanta, Ga; Ruiz Arnau University Hospital, Bayamon, Puerto Rico; Medical University of South Carolina, Charleston; Children's Hospital at Albany Medical Center, Albany, NY; Columbus Children's Hospital, Columbus, Ohio; Public Health Unit, Palm Beach County, West Palm Beach, Fla.

follow-up whereas their viral loads were similar to those of boys. In contrast, the CD4 percentage–adjusted analyses showed that boys had a slightly lower risk of a first OI-B event compared with girls, a finding that has previously been reported for mortality in our pediatric cohort.[21]

This study has a number of potential limitations, including confounding by severity of illness. Previous analyses of this study population indicated that the most severely ill children were the first to start PI-based treatment.[21] To adjust for severity of illness, we included measures of immunologic (CD4 percentage) and clinical (CDC disease category) status at HAART initiation. These 2 measures, together with sex and age-adjusted weight, have recently been used in a Pediatric AIDS Severity System score and have proven to be highly predictive of mortality in children with HIV (W.M.D., G.R.S., Kate Buchacz, PhD, Geoffrey A. Weinberg, MD, Kenneth McIntosh, MD, unpublished data, December 31, 1996). Indeed, the increased risk of a first OI associated with an older age at initiating HAART disappeared when we adjusted for CD4 percentage and CDC disease category at the time of HAART initiation (Table 4). Unfortunately, HIV-1 RNA measurements at HAART initiation were unavailable for our subjects, which precluded adjustment for this variable in our analyses.

Other potential limitations include our measure of duration of HAART use, which was based on lifetime experience at enrollment and may not have represented HAART use at the actual time of OI occurrence. In addition, we did not take into account any interruptions or discontinuation of HAART after enrollment in PACTG 219C but rather used an intention-to-continue-treatment approach. However, previous data from the PACTG 219 cohort indicate that very few children (<5%) discontinue HAART once it has been initiated.[21] Furthermore, our risk estimates were based on the first OI to occur in PACTG 219C follow-up and may not have been the first OI while receiving HAART. Despite accrual of our study population from institutions across the United States, our results may not be generalizable to the underlying base population of children with HIV, especially since our study was conducted within a self-selective cohort of children who may have participated in previous ART clinical trials in the United States. Nevertheless, our study included 1927 children, thus representing a relatively large sample of children with HIV receiving care in the United States.

We conclude that OIs are still occurring in the pediatric HIV population after the introduction of HAART, but at lower incidence rates than in the pre-HAART era.[34] Low CD4 percentage (<15%) and CDC disease category B or C at the time of HAART initiation remained the strongest predictors of OIs in the pediatric HIV population in the era of HAART. A larger proportion of children with OIs than without OIs had a CD4 percentage of less than 15% at both HAART initiation and OI occurrence. Presumably, it is not the duration of HAART use or the age at HAART initiation but rather the sustained response to HAART that predicts the risk of OIs after HAART initiation. The optimal time to initiate HAART in children can only be, and needs to be, assessed in future randomized studies.

A related article was published in *JAMA* (Gona P, Van Dyke RB, Williams PL, et al. Incidence of opportunistic and other infections in HIV-infected children in the HAART era. *JAMA*. 2006;296;292-300).

**Accepted for Publication:** February 8, 2006.
**Author Affiliations:** Departments of Epidemiology (Drs Ylitalo and Seage) and Biostatistics (Dr Hughes) and Center for Biostatistics in AIDS Research (Dr Brogly), Harvard School of Public Health, Boston, Mass; Stony Brook Children's Service, Stony Brook University, New York, NY (Dr Nachman); Department of Pediatrics, Duke University Medical Center, Durham, NC (Dr Dankner); and Department of Pediatrics, Tulane School of Medicine, New Orleans, La (Dr Van Dyke).
**Corresponding Author:** Nathalie Ylitalo, MD, PhD, Department of Epidemiology, Harvard School of Public Health, 655 Huntington Ave, Boston, MA 02155 (nathalie.ylitalo@oncology.gu.se).
**Author Contributions:** *Study concept and design:* Ylitalo, Hughes, Dankner, Van Dyke, and Seage. *Acquisition of data:* Ylitalo, Hughes, Nachman, Dankner, Van Dyke, and Seage. *Analysis and interpretation of data:* Ylitalo, Brogly, Hughes, Nachman, Dankner, and Seage. *Drafting of the manuscript:* Ylitalo. *Critical revision of the manuscript for important intellectual content:* Brogly, Hughes, Nachman, Dankner, Van Dyke, and Seage. *Statistical analysis:* Ylitalo, Hughes, and Seage. *Obtained funding:* Hughes and Van Dyke. *Administrative, technical, and material support:* Ylitalo, Brogly, and Van Dyke. *Study supervision:* Hughes and Seage. Dr Ylitalo had full access to all of the data in the study and takes responsibility for the integrity of the data and the accuracy of the data analysis.
**Funding/Support:** This study was funded by the US National Institute of Allergy and Infectious Diseases, the National Institute of Child Health and Human Development, and the Center for Biostatistics in AIDS Research at the Harvard School of Public Health (the statistical and data analysis center of the Pediatric AIDS Clinical Trials Group) under cooperative agreement 5 U01 AI41110 with the US National Institute of Allergy and Infectious Diseases.
**Role of the Sponsors:** The US National Institute of Allergy and Infectious Diseases and the National Institute of Child Health and Human Development were involved in the design, data collection, and conduct of protocol 219C but were not involved in the present analysis, the interpretation of the data, the writing of the manuscript, or the decision to submit the manuscript for publication.
**Acknowledgment:** We acknowledge Shirley Traite and Matthew Manne at the Center for Biostatistics in AIDS Research at the Harvard School of Public Health for their invaluable programming support. We also thank all of the children, adolescents, and families for their participation in Pediatric AIDS Clinical Trials Group 219C.

## REFERENCES

1. Palella FJ Jr, Delaney KM, Moorman AC, et al; HIV Outpatient Study Investigators. Declining morbidity and mortality among patients with advanced human immunodeficiency virus infection. *N Engl J Med.* 1998;338:853-860.
2. Soh C-H, Oleske JM, Brady MT, et al. Long-term effects of protease-inhibitor-based combination therapy on CD4T-cell recovery in HIV-1 infected children and adolescents. *Lancet.* 2003;362:2045-2051.
3. Kaplan JE, Hanson D, Dworkin MS, et al. Epidemiology of human immunodeficiency virus-associated opportunistic infections in the United States in the era of highly active antiretroviral therapy. *Clin Infect Dis.* 2000;30(suppl 1):S5-S14.
4. Ledergerber B, Egger M, Erard V, et al. AIDS-related opportunistic illnesses occurring after initiation of potent antiretroviral therapy: the Swiss HIV Cohort Study. *JAMA.* 1999;282:2220-2226.
5. Detels R, Tarwater P, Phair JP, Margolick J, Riddler SA, Munoz A; Multicenter AIDS Cohort Study. Effectiveness of potent antiretroviral therapies on the incidence of opportunistic infections before and after AIDS diagnosis. *AIDS.* 2001;15:347-355.
6. Cameron DW, Heath-Chiozzi M, Danner S, et al; Advanced HIV Disease Ritonavir Study Group. Randomised placebo-controlled trial of ritonavir in advanced HIV-1 disease. *Lancet.* 1998;351:543-549.
7. Ives NJ, Gazzard BG, Easterbrook PJ. The changing pattern of AIDS-defining illnesses with the introduction of highly active antiretroviral therapy (HAART) in a London clinic. *J Infect.* 2001;42:134-139.
8. Moore RD, Chaisson RE. Natural history of HIV infection in the era of combination antiretroviral therapy. *AIDS.* 1999;13:1933-1942.
9. Collier AC, Coombs RW, Schoenfeld DA, et al. Treatment of human immunodeficiency virus infection with saquinavir, zidovudine and zalcitrabine. *N Engl J Med.* 1996;334:1011-1017.
10. Li TS, Tubiana R, Katlama C, Calvez V, Ait Mohand H, Autran B. Long-lasting recovery in CD4 T-cell function and viral-load reduction after highly active antiretroviral therapy in advanced HIV-1 disease. *Lancet.* 1998;351:1682-1686.

11. Rutstein RM, Feingold A, Meislich D, Word B, Rudy B. Protease inhibitor therapy in children with perinatally acquired HIV infection. *AIDS.* 1997;11:F107-F111.
12. Cohen Stuart JW, Slieker WA, Rijkers GT, et al; Dutch Study Group for Children With HIV Infections. Early recovery of CD4+ T lymphocytes in children on highly active antiretroviral therapy. *AIDS.* 1998;12:2155-2159.
13. Gibb DM, Newberry A, Klein N, de Rossi A, Grosch-Woerner I, Bab A; Paediatric European Network for Treatment of AIDS (PENTA) Steering Committee. Immune repopulation after HAART in previously untreated HIV-1-infected children. *Lancet.* 2000;355:1331-1332.
14. Hainaut M, Ducarme M, Schandene L, et al. Age-related immune reconstitution during highly active antiretroviral therapy in human immunodeficiency virus type 1 infected children. *Pediatr Infect Dis J.* 2003;22:62-69.
15. van Rossum AM, Fraaij PL, de Groot R. Efficacy of highly active antiretroviral therapy in HIV-1 infected children. *Lancet Infect Dis.* 2002;2:93-102.
16. O'Brien WA, Hartigan PM, Martin D, et al; Veterans Affairs Cooperative Study Group on AIDS. Changes in plasma HIV-1 RNA and CD4+ lymphocyte counts and the risk of progression to AIDS. *N Engl J Med.* 1996;334:426-431.
17. Mellors JW, Munoz A, Giorgi JV, et al. Plasma viral load and CD4+ lymphocytes as prognostic markers of HIV-1 infection. *Ann Intern Med.* 1997;126:946-954.
18. Mofenson LM, Korelitz J, Meyer WA III, et al; National Institute of Child Health and Human Development Intravenous Immunoglobulin Clinical Trial Study Group. The relationship between serum human immunodeficiency virus type 1 (HIV-1) RNA level, CD4 lymphocyte percent, and long-term mortality risk in HIV-1-infected children. *J Infect Dis.* 1997;175:1029-1038.
19. Palumbo PE, Raskino C, Fiscus S, et al. Predictive value of quantitative plasma HIV RNA and CD4+ lymphocyte count in HIV-infected infants and children. *JAMA.* 1998;279:756-761.
20. Dunn D; HIV Paediatric Prognostic Markers Collaborative Study Group. Short-term risk of disease progression in HIV-1 infected children receiving no antiretroviral therapy or zidovudine monotherapy: a meta-analysis. *Lancet.* 2003; 362:1605-1611.
21. Gortmaker SL, Hughes M, Cervia J, et al; Pediatric AIDS Clinical Trials Group Protocol 219 Team. Effect of combination therapy including protease inhibitors on mortality among children and adolescents infected with HIV-1. *N Engl J Med.* 2001;345:1522-1528.
22. Centers for Disease Control and Prevention. 1993 revised classification system for HIV infection and expanded surveillance case definition for AIDS among adolescents and adults. *MMWR Recomm Rep.* 1992;41(RR-17):1-19.
23. Centers for Disease Control and Prevention. 1994 revised classification system for human immunodeficiency virus infection in children less than 13 years of age. *MMWR Recomm Rep.* 1994;43(RR-12):1-10.
24. Kalbfleisch JD, Prentice RL. The Statistical Analysis of Failure Time Data. New York, NY: John Wiley & Sons; 1980:22-23, 79-81.
25. Working Group on Antiretroviral Therapy and Medical Management of HIV-Infected Children. Guidelines for the use of antiretroviral agents in pediatric HIV infection. http://www.aidsinfo.nih.gov. Accessed November 30, 2004.
26. Sharland M, di Zub GC, Ramos JT, Blanche S, Gibb DM; Pediatric European Network for Treatment of AIDS. PENTA guidelines for the use of antiretroviral therapy in paediatric HIV infection. *HIV Med.* 2002;3:215-226.
27. World Health Organization. Scaling up antiretroviral therapy in resource-limited settings: guidelines for a public health approach: executive summary. http://www.who.int/hiv/pub/guidelines/en. Accessed November 30, 2003.
28. van Rossum A-M, Scherpbier H, van Lochem E, et al. Therapeutic immune reconstitution in HIV-1-infected children is independent of their age and pretreatment immune status. *AIDS.* 2001;15:2267-2275.
29. Walker AS, Doerholt K, Sharland M, Gibb DM; Collaborative HIV Paediatric Study (CHIPS) Steering Committee. Response to highly active antiretroviral therapy varies with age: the UK and Ireland Collaborative HIV Paediatric Study. *AIDS.* 2004; 18:1915-1924.
30. European Collaborative Study. Are there gender and race differences in cellular immunity patterns over age in infected and uninfected children born to HIV-infected women? *J Acquir Immune Defic Syndr.* 2003;33:635-641.
31. Van Dyke RB, Lee S, Johnson GM, et al; Pediatric AIDS Clinical Trials Group Adherence Subcommittee Pediatric AIDS Clinical Trials Group 377 Study Team. Reported adherence as a determinant of response to highly active antiretroviral therapy in children who have human immunodeficiency virus infection. *Pediatrics.* 2002;109:e61.
32. European Collaborative Study. Level and pattern of RNA viral load over age: differences between girls and boys? *AIDS.* 2002;16:97-104.
33. Anastos K, Gange SJ, Lau B, et al. Association of race and gender with quantitative HIV-1 RNA levels and immunological progression. *J Acquir Immune Defic Syndr.* 2000;24:218-226.
34. Dankner WM, Lindsey JC, Levin MJ; Pediatric AIDS Clinical Trials Group Protocol Teams 051, 128, 138, 144, 152, 179, 190, 220, 240, 245, 254, 300, and 327. Correlates of opportunistic infections in children infected with the human immunodeficiency virus managed before highly active antiretroviral therapy. *Pediatr Infect Dis J.* 2001;20:40-48.

### *Atkins Diet in 1906?*

Diet is alone sufficient to improve the condition; its chief feature is the exclusion of the two elements, starch and sugar, from the food. In one year, on this diet, Mr Banting reduced his weight 46 pounds. Meat Diet, very successful in 42 cases, the diet being confined to rump-steak, hot water and codfish, for 14 days, excluding absolutely everything else.

—From *Materia Medica Pharmacy and Therapeutics*, 1906

# Are Household Firearms Stored Less Safely in Homes With Adolescents?

## *Analysis of a National Random Sample of Parents*

*Renee M. Johnson, PhD; Matthew Miller, MD, ScD; Mary Vriniotis, MS; Deborah Azrael, PhD; David Hemenway, PhD*

**Objective:** To examine whether firearms are more frequently stored loaded, unlocked, or both in households with adolescents only (aged 13-17 years) compared with households with younger children only (aged 0-12 years).

**Design:** Random-digit-dial survey on firearms (n=2770). We computed bivariate associations between the presence of adolescents and firearm storage practices. Statistical significance was assessed using prevalence ratios with 95% confidence intervals.

**Setting:** United States.

**Participants:** Survey respondents with children (aged <18 years) who reported the presence of a household firearm.

**Main Outcome Measures:** Prevalence of firearms in the home stored loaded and/or unlocked.

**Results:** Of the 392 respondents, 22% had a loaded firearm, 32% had an unlocked firearm, and 8% had a firearm stored loaded and unlocked. Compared with households with younger children, households with adolescents only were somewhat more likely to store a firearm unlocked (42% vs 29%; prevalence ratio, 1.48; 95% confidence interval, 1.04-2.02), loaded (26% vs 20%; prevalence ratio, 1.25; 95% confidence interval, 0.82-1.91), or both (10% vs 8%; prevalence ratio, 1.43; 95% confidence interval, 0.64-3.19).

**Conclusions:** Parents of adolescents appear to be more likely to keep household firearms stored unsafely, especially with regard to keeping firearms unlocked. This is of concern because most youth firearm injuries happen to adolescents. Firearm injury prevention programs should directly target parents of adolescents to promote safe firearm storage.

*Arch Pediatr Adolesc Med. 2006;160:788-792*

FIREARMS ARE PRESENT IN about one third of US households with children and youth.[1-4] Therefore, safe firearm storage practices—including keeping firearms stored unloaded and locked up—represent important safety behaviors. Research suggests that safe storage may confer a degree of protection in the risks for suicide and unintentional injury.[5-8] In keeping with these findings, professional organizations, including the American Academy of Pediatrics[9] and the Society for Adolescent Medicine,[10] recommend that parents keep firearms stored unloaded and locked up.

In the United States, 14% to 30% of households with guns and young or adolescent children (aged <18 years) have at least 1 loaded firearm, and about 43% contain an unlocked firearm.[1,3,4,11,12] A recent study[13] estimated that nearly 2 million US children live in homes with loaded, unlocked firearms. The home is the primary place from which young people obtain firearms that are used in unintentional and violent injuries, as well as a primary setting in which pediatric firearm injuries, especially suicides, take place.[7,8,14-16]

Keeping children and youth safe represents a strong motivation for parents to not have firearms in the home or to store them locked up and unloaded.[2-4,17,18] However, parents' perceptions of how likely their children are to get hurt with a firearm may vary based on characteristics of the child. Qualitative research shows that parents' expectations that their children will not play with or touch guns are based on beliefs about their children having the wherewithal to act responsibly.[18] When asked whether their children would handle firearms, parents who disagreed said things such as "My child knows better" or "has common sense."[18] In the same vein, parents are more apt to believe that older children are old enough to act responsibly and use good judgment when there are fire-

**Author Affiliations:** Harvard Injury Control Research Center, Harvard School of Public Health, Boston, Mass.

arms in the home[18-20]; parents may therefore be less likely to use safe firearm storage practices when the only young people in the home are adolescents.[3,4,18-20]

A few studies have explored how firearm storage practices vary by the age of the children in the home; their results suggest that parents of adolescents have less safe firearm storage practices than parents of younger children.[3,4,18] In 1 national random-digit-dial study, authors found that, among gun owners with children (n=252), those with children younger than 13 years were less likely than those with adolescent children to store at least 1 gun loaded and unlocked (6% vs 17%; $P<.01$).[3] Similarly, a separate national study showed that parents whose youngest children were aged 13 to 17 years were significantly more likely to report the presence of a firearm that was stored loaded and unlocked than parents who had children younger than 13 years.[4] Unfortunately, neither study examined these 2 firearm storage practices individually. A third study, which was based on a sample of parents of children aged 5 to 15 years in northeastern Ohio, showed that parents with at least 1 child aged 5 to 9 years were significantly less likely than those whose children were all aged 10 to 15 years to have a firearm stored loaded and unlocked (12% vs 30%; $P=.046$).[18]

Additional research is needed to confirm how parents' firearm storage practices vary on the basis of the ages of children in the home. The purpose of this study was to examine the prevalence of having a firearm in the home that is loaded, unlocked, or both among a national sample of parents with children 17 years or younger. On the basis of findings from previous studies, we expected that parents of adolescents (aged 13-17 years) would be more likely to have a loaded and/or unlocked firearm in the home than those with younger children (aged 0-12 years).

## METHODS

Data for this investigation come from the National Firearms Study 2004, a telephone survey in which adults (aged ≥18 years) in the United States were randomly selected for participation from a list-assisted sampling frame.[21] Those who were unable to complete an interview in English were excluded. Data collection was performed by Fact Finders Inc, a social science research firm in Albany, NY. The number of interviews designated for each state was determined by that state's population relative to the total population of the United States. In multiadult households, 1 adult was randomly selected to take part in the study.

Of the 31 302 telephone numbers called for the study, 91.1% did not result in an interview. Of these, 41.4% were ineligible numbers (eg, nonresidential, line out of service, quota reached for the particular state). For an additional 39.2%, an interview did not take place after the maximum number of calls (ie, 10) had been made for 1 of the following reasons: only an answering machine picked up, the line was always busy, the line was never answered, or the potential respondent was never available. Only 19.0%[5,21] of the numbers called that did not result in an interview were refusals. The total National Firearms Study 2004 sample included 2770 adults.

The instrument included some 100 items and was designed to be completed in approximately 15 minutes. A verbal informed consent procedure was conducted before beginning the interview. Items inquired about included attitudes and beliefs regarding firearms, firearm ownership and storage practices, and demographic characteristics of the respondent and members of the household. To inquire about firearm ownership, we asked the following question: "Do you have any guns in your home or motor vehicle?" We then asked about how those firearms were stored (eg, "How many of those guns are currently loaded?"). Data were collected in the spring of 2004 using computer-assisted telephone interviewing technology.[22-24] The study was approved by the Institutional Review Board at the Harvard School of Public Health, Boston, Mass.

For this investigation, the National Firearms Study 2004 sample was restricted to the 405 respondents who had at least 1 child younger than 18 years living with them and who also indicated that there was a firearm in the home. Thirteen of the 405 eligible respondents were excluded because they had not provided information on the ages of children in their households, leaving a total number of respondents in the analysis sample of 392. Descriptive statistics were generated for demographic characteristics, firearm storage practices (presence of any firearm in the home that was loaded, unlocked, or both), and ages of the children (<5, 5-12, and 13-17 years). We calculated cross-tabulated frequency distributions to examine the relationship between the ages of the children in the home and firearm storage practices. Next, we compared the prevalence of an unsafe firearm storage practice (storing a firearm loaded, unlocked, or both) in homes in which all of the children were aged 13 to 17 years with that in homes in which all of the children were younger than 13 years. We excluded households that contained children in both age groups from this analysis. We tested the statistical significance of the associations by estimating prevalence ratios (PRs) with 95% confidence intervals.[25,26] Analyses were conducted using SAS statistical software, version 9.1.2.[27]

## RESULTS

Of the 392 respondents in the analysis sample, 58.7% were male, 78.5% were married, 66.5% were aged 30 to 49 years, and 87.1% were white. By design, all respondents in the study sample had firearms in the home and children younger than 18 years. Ages of children ranged from a few weeks to 17 years. Nearly half (47.7%) had at least 1 teenager in the home. For 110 (28.1%) of the 392 respondents, all of the children in the home were aged 13 to 17 years (**Table 1**).

The number of guns respondents had in their homes ranged from 1 to 70; more than three quarters (78.1%) reported having more than 1 gun. Of the respondents, 70.8% indicated that they personally owned at least 1 of the household firearms, and 64.9% reported the presence of a handgun. In terms of storage practices, 21.7% had a loaded gun, 31.5% had an unlocked gun, and 8.3% had a gun that was loaded and unlocked (**Table 2**).

Respondents whose children were all aged 13 to 17 years had the highest prevalence of unsafe firearm storage practices (**Figure**). Whereas 28.8% of parents whose children were all 12 years or younger had an unlocked firearm in the home, 41.7% of parents whose children were all aged 13 to 17 years did (PR, 1.48; 95% confidence interval, 1.04-2.02). Although not statistically significant at the .05 level, the PRs suggest that having a teenager as opposed to a younger child is associated with an increased likelihood of having a household firearm stored loaded (PR, 1.25) or loaded and unlocked (PR, 1.43) (Table 2).

## COMMENT

Previous research suggests that parents with children older than 12 years may be more likely to store firearms unsafely than those with younger children.[3,4,18] We tested those findings by investigating whether parents of adolescents were more likely to have firearms stored unsafely. Our results were consistent with those of previous research. We found that parents of adolescents were significantly more likely than parents of children 12 years or younger to have an unlocked firearm in the home (41.7% vs 28.8%; $P<.05$). Findings were similar, but not statistically significant, for keeping firearms stored loaded and both loaded and unlocked.

An alternative explanation for the associations between children's ages and firearm storage practices is that parents of older children are less likely to have safe storage practices. Because parents whose children were all aged 13 to 17 years were about 10 years older on average than parents whose children were all younger than 13 years, we sought to test this alternative explanation. When we examined storage practices by mean age of respondents, we did not find evidence that older parents had less safe firearm storage practices. When we analyzed all 392 respondents, the mean age of the respondents with unsafe storage practices was not substantially different than the mean age of the respondents without unsafe storage practices (data not shown).

A secondary finding is that children of all ages have access to unsafely stored firearms in their homes. More than one third of the parents in this sample said there was a gun in their home that was stored loaded, unlocked, or both. This represents a threat to the safety of young people.

As with most survey research, these data may be subject to bias because of inaccurate recall, lack of knowledge, or social desirability. An additional limitation is that some respondents chose not to disclose information about how firearms were stored, or about how old their children were. This resulted in missing data, including 14.3% of the respondents with missing data on the presence of a firearm stored unlocked; 10.5% with missing data on the presence of a firearm stored loaded and unlocked; and 4.8% with missing data on the presence of a firearm stored loaded. It is unclear how the results would differ with complete information. Because of this limitation, it is important for future studies examining firearm storage practices to report information on the ages of children to confirm the validity of our findings. Nevertheless, the proportion of respondents with a loaded firearm (21.7%) or an unlocked firearm (31.5%) obtained from this investigation were comparable to estimates from other studies (14%-30% and 43% respectively).[1]

As young people become adolescents, parents may become less vigilant about keeping firearms stored securely. This assertion is supported by the present research, as well as by studies on parents' attitudes about firearm safety,[18-20,28] in which authors concluded that parents were more likely to believe that adolescents, com-

**Table 1. Demographic Characteristics of the Study Sample**

| Characteristic | No. (%) of Sample* |
|---|---|
| Age of respondent, y (n = 388) | |
| <20 | 5 (1.3) |
| 20-29 | 61 (15.7) |
| 30-39 | 122 (31.4) |
| 40-49 | 136 (35.1) |
| 50-59 | 54 (13.9) |
| >60 | 10 (2.6) |
| Age of children in the home, not mutually exclusive, y (n = 392) | |
| Any <5 | 117 (29.8) |
| Any 5-12 | 216 (55.1) |
| Any 13-17 | 187 (47.7) |
| Mutually exclusive child age groups, y (n = 333)† | |
| All <13 (n = 333) | 223 (67.0) |
| All <5 (n = 223) † | 60 (26.9) |
| All 5-12 (n = 223) † | 106 (47.5) |
| All 13-17 (n = 333) | 110 (33.0) |
| Marital status (n = 391) | |
| Not married or living with a partner | 54 (13.8) |
| Not married, living with a partner | 30 (7.7) |
| Married | 307 (78.5) |
| Race (n = 389) | |
| White | 339 (87.1) |
| Black | 18 (4.6) |
| Hispanic | 14 (3.6) |
| Other | 18 (4.6) |
| Sex (n = 392) | |
| Male | 230 (58.7) |
| Female | 162 (41.3) |
| Level of educational attainment (n = 391) | |
| Attended or completed high school | 130 (33.2) |
| Attended college or another type of higher education | 154 (39.4) |
| Completed a 4-y college degree | 107 (27.4) |

*Totals may not sum to 392 because of missing data.
†Excludes 59 respondents with children in multiple age groups.

**Table 2. Comparison of Firearm Storage Practices in Homes With Younger Children vs Adolescents***

| | Total (N = 392) | Children Age Groups, y† All 0-12 (n = 223) | All 13-17 (n = 110) | PR (95% CI)† |
|---|---|---|---|---|
| Any unlocked firearm (n = 336) | 106/336 (31.5) | 57/198 (28.8) | 35/84 (41.7) | 1.48 (1.04-2.02) |
| Any loaded firearm (n = 373) | 81/373 (21.7) | 44/216 (20.4) | 26/102 (25.5) | 1.25 (0.82-1.91) |
| Any unlocked and loaded firearm (n = 351) | 29/351 (8.3) | 14/205 (6.8) | 9/92 (9.8) | 1.43 (0.64-3.19) |

Abbreviations: CI, confidence interval; PR, prevalence ratio.
*Data are expressed as number (percentage) of respondents unless otherwise indicated. The listed numbers of subjects represent only nonmissing observations.
†Excludes the 59 respondents with children in both age groups.

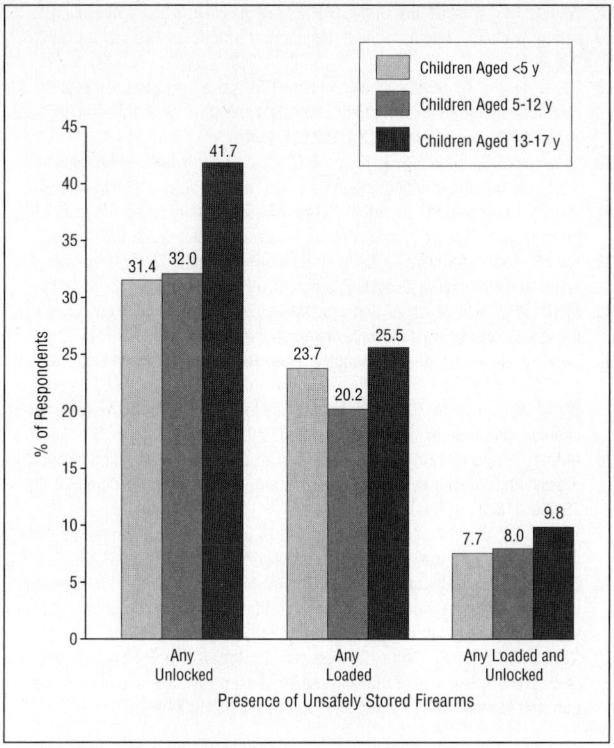


**Figure.** Reported firearm storage practices stratified by the age of the young people living in the home. Age categories are mutually exclusive. Respondents with children in more than 1 age group were excluded from the analyses.

pared with younger children, are old enough to exhibit good judgment around firearms. This belief creates a situation in which adolescents have easy access to a lethal means with which to kill themselves or to hurt others. Unfortunately, our study did not inquire about parents' perceptions of their children being injured with a firearm in the home, limiting our ability to assess whether the perception of susceptibility is, in fact, the intervening variable between the age of the children in the home and storage practices.

Safe storage practices have the potential to reduce the risk of death by limiting access to the most lethal means of injury.[5-8] In recent years, public health and medical professionals have worked to educate gun owners, and gun-owning parents in particular, about the importance of safe storage practices through face-to-face counseling, mass media campaigns, and legislation.[29-37] Anticipatory guidance by pediatricians has been a leading strategy for promoting safe firearm storage.[30,33,34,38,39] Although important, most of these promotional efforts focus on preventing unintentional injury (rather than suicide) and may have the greatest influence on parents of children younger than 13 years. As an example, a billboard for 1 media campaign included a child-sized coffin and the slogan: "Buy a box for your gun, not for your kid."[37] In our attempts to keep young children safe, we may be leaving behind adolescents, who are significantly more at risk for gun injuries than younger children. In the future, it may be important for educational efforts to purposefully include messages that are directly targeted to parents of adolescents. A specific recommendation for reaching parents of adolescents is more firearm safety education outside of pediatric clinics because many adolescents do not visit pediatricians or their parents do not accompany them to the physicians' offices.

**Accepted for Publication:** February 15, 2006.
**Correspondence:** Renee M. Johnson, PhD, Harvard Injury Control Research Center, Harvard School of Public Health, 677 Huntington Ave, Kresge Building, Room 318, Boston, MA 02115 (rejohnso@hsph.harvard.edu).
**Author Contributions:** *Study concept and design:* Johnson, Miller, and Hemenway. *Acquisition of data:* Miller, Azrael, and Hemenway. *Analysis and interpretation of data:* Johnson, Miller, Vriniotis, Azrael, and Hemenway. *Drafting of the manuscript:* Johnson and Miller. *Critical revision of the manuscript for important intellectual content:* Miller, Vriniotis, Azrael, and Hemenway. *Statistical analysis:* Johnson, Vriniotis, and Azrael. *Obtained funding:* Miller, Azrael, and Hemenway. *Administrative, technical, and material support:* Hemenway. *Study supervision:* Miller and Hemenway.
**Funding/Support:** The National Firearms Study 2004 was supported by a grant from the Joyce Foundation to the Harvard Injury Control Research Center (principal investigator, Dr Miller).
**Previous Presentations:** This study was presented as a poster at the CDC National Injury Prevention and Control Conference; May 9, 2005; Denver, Colo.
**Acknowledgment:** We thank Jenny Hochstadt, MS, MSW, of the Harvard Injury Control Research Center for assistance with data analysis.

## REFERENCES


1. Johnson RM, Coyne-Beasley T, Runyan CW. Firearm ownership and storage practices, US households, 1992-2002: a systematic review. *Am J Prev Med.* 2004; 27:173-182.
2. Stennies G, Ikeda R, Ledbetter S, Houston B, Sacks J. Firearm storage practices and children in the home, United States, 1994. *Arch Pediatr Adolesc Med.* 1999; 153:586-590.
3. Azrael D, Miller M, Hemenway D. Are household firearms stored safely? it depends on whom you ask. *Pediatrics.* 2000;106:e31.
4. Schuster MA, Franke T, Bastian A, Sor S, Halfon N. Firearm storage patterns in US homes with children. *Am J Public Health.* 2000;90:588-594.
5. Miller M, Azrael D, Hemenway D, Vriniotis M. Firearm storage practices and rates of unintentional firearm deaths in the United States. *Accid Anal Prev.* 2005; 37:661-667.
6. Grossman DC, Mueller BA, Riedy C, et al. Gun storage practices and risk of youth suicide and unintentional firearm injuries. *JAMA.* 2005;293:707-714.
7. Brent DA, Perper JA, Allman CJ, Moritz GM, Wartella ME, Zelenak JP. The presence and accessibility of firearms in the homes of adolescent suicides: a case-control study. *JAMA.* 1991;266:2989-2995.
8. Shah S, Hoffman RE, Wake L, Marine WM. Adolescent suicide and household access to firearms in Colorado: results of a case-control study. *J Adolesc Health.* 2000;26:157-163.
9. American Academy of Pediatrics Committee on Injury and Poison Prevention. Firearm-related injuries affecting the pediatric population. *Pediatrics.* 2000; 105:888-895.
10. Duke N, Resnick MD, Borowsky IW. Adolescent firearm violence: position paper of the Society for Adolescent Medicine. *J Adolesc Health.* 2005;37:171-174.
11. Hemenway D, Solnick SJ, Azrael DR. Firearm training and storage. *JAMA.* 1995; 273:46-50.
12. Weil DS, Hemenway D. Loaded guns in the home: analysis of a national random survey of gun owners. *JAMA.* 1992;267:3033-3037.
13. Okoro CA, Nelson DE, Mercy JA, Balluz LS, Crosby AE, Mokdad AH. Prevalence of household firearms and firearm-storage practice in the 50 states and the District of Columbia: findings from the Behavioral Risk Factor Surveillance System, 2002. *Pediatrics.* 2005;116:e370-e376.
14. Centers for Disease Control and Prevention. Source of firearms used by stu-

dents in school-associated violent deaths: United States, 1992-1999. *MMWR Morb Mortal Wkly Rep.* 2003;52:169-172.
15. Grossman DC, Reay DT, Baker SA. Self-inflicted and unintentional firearm injuries among children and adolescents: the source of the firearm. *Arch Pediatr Adolesc Med.* 1999;153:875-878.
16. Wintemute GJ, Teret SP, Kraus JF, Wright MA, Bradfield G. When children shoot children: 88 unintended deaths in California. *JAMA.* 1987;257:3107-3109.
17. Smith TW. *1997-98 National Gun Policy Survey of the National Opinion Research Center: Research Findings.* Chicago, Ill: National Opinion Research Center, University of Chicago; 1998.
18. Connor SM, Wesolowski KL. "They're too smart for that": predicting what children would do in the presence of guns. *Pediatrics.* 2003;111:e109-e114.
19. Farah MM, Simon HK, Kellermann AL. Firearms in the home: parental perceptions. *Pediatrics.* 1999;104:1059-1063.
20. Webster DW, Wilson MEH, Duggan AK, Pakula LC. Parents' beliefs about preventing gun injuries to children. *Pediatrics.* 1992;89:908-914.
21. Waksberg J. Sampling methods for random digit dialing. *J Am Stat Assoc.* 1978; 73:40-46.
22. Groves RM, Biemer PP, Lyberg LE, Massey JT, Nicholls WL, Waksberg J, eds. *Telephone Survey Methodology.* New York, NY: John Wiley & Sons; 2001.
23. Marcus AC, Crane LA. Telephone surveys in public health research. *Med Care.* 1986;24:97-112.
24. Sainsbury R, Ditch J, Hutton S. Computer-assisted personal interviewing. *Soc Res Update.* 1993;3:1-11.
25. Spiegelman D, Hertzmark E. Easy SAS calculations for risk or prevalence ratios and differences. *Am J Epidemiol.* 2005;162:199-200.
26. Cummings P, Rivara FP. Reporting statistical information in medical journal articles. *Arch Pediatr Adolesc Med.* 2003;157:321-324.
27. SAS Institute Inc. *Statistical Applications Software, Version 9.1.2.* Cary, NC: SAS Institute Inc; 2004.
28. Webster DW, Wilson MEH, Duggan AK, Pakula LC. Firearm injury prevention counseling: a study of pediatricians' beliefs and practices. *Pediatrics.* 1992;89: 902-907.
29. Coyne-Beasley T, Schoenbach VJ, Johnson RM. "Love Our Kids, Lock Your Guns": a community-based firearm safety counseling and gun lock distribution program. *Arch Pediatr Adolesc Med.* 2001;155:659-664.
30. Grossman DC, Cummings P, Koepsell TD, et al. Firearm safety counseling in primary care pediatrics: a randomized controlled trial. *Pediatrics.* 2000;106:22-26.
31. Horn A, Grossman DC, Jones W, Berger LR. Community based program to improve firearm storage practices in rural Alaska. *Inj Prev.* 2003;9:231-234.
32. Kunz Howard P. An overview of a few well-known national children's gun safety programs and ENA's newly developed program. *J Emerg Nurs.* 2001;27:485-488.
33. McGee KS, Coyne-Beasley T, Johnson RM. Review of evaluations of educational approaches to promote safe storage of firearms. *Inj Prev.* 2003;9:108-111.
34. Oatis PJ, Buderer NMF, Cummings P, Fleitz R. Pediatric practice based evaluation of the Steps to Prevent Firearm Injury program. *Inj Prev.* 1999;5:48-52.
35. Wafer MS, Carruth A. "Locks for Life": a gun lock distribution community health intervention program. *J Emerg Nurs.* 2003;29:349-351.
36. Meyer G, Roberto AJ, Atkin C. A radio-based approach to promoting gun safety: process and outcome evaluation implications and insights. *Health Commun.* 2003; 15:299-318.
37. Sidman EA, Grossman DC, Koepsell T, et al. Evaluation of a community-based handgun safe-storage campaign. *Pediatrics.* 2005;115:e654-e661.
38. Coyne-Beasley T, Baccaglini L, Johnson RM, Webster B, Wiebe DJ. Do partners with children know about firearms in their home? evidence of a gender gap and implications for practitioners. *Pediatrics.* 2005;115:e662-e667.
39. Stevens MM, Olson AL, Gaffney CA, Tosteson TD, Mott LA, Starr P. A pediatric, practice-based, randomized trial of drinking and smoking prevention, and bicycle helmet, gun, and seatbelt safety promotion. *Pediatrics.* 2002;109:490-497.

## *Poetry in Pediatrics*

### Evidence-Based Relief for Grandparents

They're all asleep now so that each of my elderly
alpha synuclein particles snuggles gently against its chosen
dendritic spray, waiting for the first of five grandchildren
to wake up frightened, look for school clothes, look for
their mom, and ask for water, while ignoring a grandparent's
slowly capitulating struggle with his overwhelming sense of
entropy, which can be delightfully stalled for a few
nanoseconds while watching a middle-school dance
recital, or a seven-boy tag-team football
game, or even by listening to precise
'structions for making
cherry tapioca.

*Ed Spudis, MD*

*Alpha synuclein tauopathy references are available from recognized journals.

# GARDASIL®

**[Quadrivalent Human Papillomavirus (Types 6,11,16,18) Recombinant Vaccine]**

# Available

# GARDASIL®

**[Quadrivalent Human Papillomavirus (Types 6,11,16,18) Recombinant Vaccine]**

# Available

To place an order, visit **www.MerckVaccines.com,** or call **1-800-MERCK-RX.**

MERCK
Vaccine Division



20650396(1)-06/06-GRD
Printed in USA
Minimum 10% Recycled Paper

ARTICLE

# Healthy Steps in an Integrated Delivery System

## *Child and Parent Outcomes at 30 Months*

*Brian D. Johnston, MD, MPH; Colleen E. Huebner, PhD, MPH; Melissa L. Anderson, MS; Lynda T. Tyll, MS; Robert S. Thompson, MD*

**Objective:** To test the effects of the Healthy Steps for Young Children program (HS) (which supports parents managing children's developmental and behavioral issues)—with and without a prenatal component—on child health and development, parenting practices, and parental well-being.

**Design:** A concurrent comparison with clinic-level assignment to intervention or usual care status. Nested in the intervention arm, a randomized trial compared HS with and without a prenatal component.

**Setting:** Five primary care clinics in an integrated delivery system in the Pacific Northwest.

**Participants:** A consecutive sample of 439 pregnant women (80% of eligible) were enrolled. Follow-up data were obtained for 78% when the child was 30 months old.

**Intervention:** Families in intervention clinics received HS services, including developmental and behavioral advice and risk factor screening. In addition, those randomized to prenatal services received 3 home visits during pregnancy.

**Main Outcome Measures:** Assessed by telephone interview in the 3 domains of child health and development, parenting practices, and parental well-being.

**Results:** Intervention was associated with positive outcomes in timely well-child care, immunization rates, breastfeeding, television viewing, injury prevention, and discipline strategies. Prenatal initiation of services was associated with larger expressive vocabularies at age 24 months. Mothers who received the intervention reported more depressive symptoms, but there was no increase in the proportion with clinically significant depression.

**Conclusions:** For members of an integrated delivery system, the HS intervention was associated with positive effects on children's health and parenting practices. There was little evidence of any additional benefit of HS services initiated during the prenatal period.

*Arch Pediatr Adolesc Med. 2006;160:793-800*

THE HEALTHY STEPS FOR Young Children program (HS) was designed to support families of young children using a new type of health care provider, the HS specialist (HSS), in a practice-based intervention.[1] The HS consists of risk reduction activities and universal components, including developmental screening, anticipatory guidance, and follow-up services, offered to all families receiving care.[2-5] Expected benefits of HS include improved parental promotion of child development,[6] parenting practices, child development, and health care utilization. Evaluation of the program to date has demonstrated improved timeliness and quality of pediatric services, parenting practices, and parent satisfaction with services.[5,7,8]

In this trial, we investigated pediatric usual care (UC) vs HS implemented with and without PrePare (PP), a prenatal component designed to begin the therapeutic HSS-parent relationship during pregnancy. PrePare was delivered as 3 home visits. The objective was to introduce the HSS to the parents as a knowledgeable and caring resource, helping them prepare for the arrival of their newborn. The content of the prenatal visits included information about fetal and infant development, home safety, and the material needs of newborns and infants.[9] Families who received PP services continued to receive the standard HS intervention from the same HSS during the postnatal period.

Our tests of this intervention package found no incremental benefits of PP (compared with HS only) on parental well-being, knowledge, or parenting practices when the infants were 3 months of age.[8] However, families who received PP were more satisfied with their pediatric care and were less likely to disenroll from the health plan in the 12 months following the child's birth. We hypothesized that organiza-

Author Affiliations:
Department of Pediatrics (Dr Johnston) and Maternal and Child Health Program and Department of Health Services (Dr Huebner), University of Washington, and Center for Health Studies (Mss Anderson and Tyll and Dr Thompson) and Department of Preventive Care (Dr Thompson), Group Health Cooperative, Seattle.

tional bonding might explain these positive effects of the prenatal intervention and theorized, in turn, that benefits for children and parents would become apparent during infancy and toddlerhood.

Herein, we report results of tests for intervention effects on child health and development, parenting practices, and parental well-being when enrolled children were 30 months old. A quasi-experimental design was used to compare intervention families with families who received the health plan's usual complement of pregnancy and pediatric services. Within intervention clinics, a nested randomized trial compared PP+HS with HS only.

## METHODS

### SETTING AND DESIGN

This clinical trial was conducted from July 20, 1998, through November 7, 2003, in a large integrated delivery system that provides services to approximately 550 000 people located in the Pacific Northwest. Three clinics received the intervention while 2 other geographically distant clinics served as comparison sites. Within intervention clinics, enrolled families were individually randomized to receive services beginning prenatally (PP+HS) or postnatally (HS only). Data analysis was performed in 2004.

### RECRUITMENT AND ENROLLMENT

Recruitment was by review of obstetrical records in the second trimester, followed by a letter of invitation, telephone screening, and an enrollment visit with study staff. To be eligible, pregnant women had to be at less than 22 weeks' gestation at study enrollment, younger than 45 years, English speaking, and planning to use a study clinic for pediatric care. Enrollment occurred from July 20, 1998, through September 29, 2000. Individual randomization was performed centrally, stratified by clinic, and blocked in groups of 4.

### INTERVENTIONS

Four master's-level trained HSSs provided most of the intervention program's services. Two HSSs had backgrounds in nursing, one in clinical social work and one in mental health practice. All received additional training and ongoing education in early child development and in specific aspects of HS.[9] Key clinicians and other personnel from intervention clinic sites also received intervention-related training. Enrollees randomized to HS were eligible to receive postnatal home visits from an HSS; developmental advice and parent-initiated telephone support; developmental assessments conducted in tandem with scheduled well-child care, the Reach Out and Read literacy program, and other risk-based screening services[9]; and parenting classes delivered by HSSs.

The PP participants began the intervention by receiving 3 home visits with their HSS when they were at approximately 20, 27, and 34 weeks' gestation.[10] The conceptual framework for PP drew on findings of the psychological transition to parenthood,[11] in which adjustment to the maternal role requires renegotiation of the current family structure to incorporate the unavoidable changes that accompany the birth of a baby. In keeping with this framework, the 3 home visits were structured to help parents create a safe, knowing, and welcoming environment for their newborn.[9] In addition, the PP participants received screening and intervention for targeted risk factors, such as smoking, depression, and domestic violence. The HSS who provided prenatal services continued to provide the standard package of HS services following the birth of the infant. Comparison clinic enrollees received the health plan's standard package of well-child pediatric care, outreach, and support services.

The Group Health Cooperative Human Subjects Review Committee reviewed the study. Informed consent was obtained from all participating families.

### DATA COLLECTION

Most outcome data were collected by telephone interview of mothers at enrollment to the study (at 16-20 weeks' gestation), at 7 to 10 days post partum, when enrolled children were 3 months of age, and again when these children were at 30 months of age. Data on language acquisition were obtained by mailed questionnaire at age 24 months. Health plan utilization data were extracted from administrative databases.

The overall intervention goal was to improve child health and developmental attainment by supporting appropriate parenting practices. Herein, we present findings grouped into the following 3 domains: child health and development, parenting practices, and parental well-being.

### OUTCOME MEASURES

#### Child Health and Development

We used immunization delivery and attainment of timely age-appropriate well-child care as intermediate health outcomes. Well-child visits occurring within 60-day windows centered around the health plan's recommended visits at 2, 4, 6, 10, 15, and 24 months were counted as "timely" preventive care. Among those continuously enrolled for the first 2 years of life, the health plan's standard Health Plan Employer Data and Information Set measure was used to identify children whose immunizations were up-to-date at age 24 months (4 diphtheria and tetanus toxoids and pertussis vaccines [or diphtheria and tetanus toxoids with acellular pertussis vaccines], 3 oral polio vaccines or inactivated poliovirus vaccines, 1 measles-mumps-rubella vaccine, 2 *Haemophilus influenzae* type b vaccines, and 3 hepatitis B vaccines).[12]

When enrolled children were 24 months old, parents completed a questionnaire that included elements of the short and long forms of the MacArthur Communicative Development Inventories[13] assessing single-word expressive vocabulary, word combining (≥2 words), use of 3 or more word endings, and mean length (in morphemes) of the child's 3 longest phrases.

Parental perception of child behavior problems was assessed at 30 months by telephone using 3 subscales from the Child Behavior Checklist.[14] These included aggressive behavior, sleep problems, and symptoms related to an anxious or depressed mood.

#### Parenting Practices

The PP and HS interventions promoted parental knowledge of child development, self-efficacy, and developmentally supportive parenting practices. **Table 1** gives an overview of the continuous measures used to assess these constructs. For parenting practices, we used established scales of nurturing behavior[15] and parenting sense of competence.[16] We developed and used a brief measure of self-efficacy for pediatric health care (Table 1). Other measures of parenting practices reported herein include frequency of activities to promote child development (including reading or playing with the child), maintaining routines around bedtime and meal times, and limiting television viewing. The proportion of mothers initiating breastfeeding and engaging in any breastfeeding beyond 6 months is reported.

**Table 1. Selected Continuous Measures Used in Assessment of Child Health and Development, Parenting Practices, and Parental Well-being***

| Outcome Assessed | Instrument Used | Items | Potential Range | Cronbach α† | Source |
|---|---|---|---|---|---|
| | | | **Child Health and Development** | | |
| Parental perceptions of problem child behaviors | Subscales of the Child Behavior Checklist | | | | Achenbach,[14] 1992 |
| | Aggressive behavior | 15 | 0-30 | .85 | |
| | Anxious or depressed mood | 11 | 0-22 | .68 | |
| | Sleep problems | 7 | 0-14 | .68 | |
| | | | **Parenting Practices** | | |
| Nurturing parental style | Nurturing subscale of parenting behavior checklist | 18 | 18-72 | .79 | Fox et al,[15] 1995 |
| Parenting self-efficacy | Parenting sense of competence | 16 | 16-64 | .79 | Johnston and Marsh,[16] 1989 |
| Health care self-efficacy | Self-care scale | 5 | 5-20 | .82 | Instrument developed for this study |
| Child safety | Injury prevention index | 5 | 0-5 | ... | Instrument developed for this study |
| | | | **Parental Well-being** | | |
| Maternal depressive symptoms | Modified CESD | 14 | 0-42 | .83 | Radloff,[17] 1977 |

Abbreviation: CESD, Center for Epidemiological Studies Depression Scale.
*Binary outcome measures are described in the text. All instruments were Likert-response type except for the injury prevention index, which sums binary items.
†In the present study sample.

Mothers' reports of child injury prevention practices were summed to create a 5-point index that reflected the presence of a functioning smoke detector (1 point), regular use of a car seat (1 point) in the correct position (1 point), and absence of firearms in the home (2 points) or safe storage of any firearms reported (1 point). We also asked about the use of 4 common household safety items (safety latches, electrical outlet covers, stair gates, and poison control center telephone number).

Mothers were asked about specific discipline strategies. The proportion reporting any unusually harsh discipline (ie, slapping on the face or spanking with an object) is reported.

### Parental Well-being

The PP and HS interventions offered screening and referral for maternal depression along with general social support from the HSS. Maternal depressive symptoms were assessed using a modification of the Center for Epidemiological Studies Depression Scale[17] (Table 1); the scores are reported herein along with the proportion of respondents who reported "feelings of sadness" that were discussed with someone in the pediatric practice.

Other measures of maternal well-being included self-reported use of any illicit drug and the presence or absence of significant physical domestic violence in the preceding 12 months ("Did your partner hit you, shove you, or kick you?"). "Problem drinkers" were identified according to accepted definitions based on reported alcohol consumption.[18] Exposure to environmental tobacco smoke was assessed as the proportion of households with current smokers.

## SAMPLE SIZE

Sample size estimates indicated that 100 enrollees per study group were needed for analysis of our primary outcomes at 30 months. For example, with a total sample of 300, we could detect (with 80% power at $\alpha = .05$) a difference of 0.28 SD when the outcome measured was continuous.

## STATISTICAL ANALYSIS

We based all analyses on initial group assignment and made adjustments to minimize differences due to the quasi-experimental design. We used generalized linear models with robust variance estimates to account for within-clinic clustering effects. To identify a parsimonious and consistent set of covariates for use in adjusted analyses, we examined all demographic data collected. No enrolled family had missing data at baseline for these variables. One variable was selected from any highly correlated pairs. Covariates were included if they differed statistically between the intervention and comparison groups at baseline or if inclusion in an analytic model caused point estimates of effect size to vary by more than 10%. Based on these criteria, maternal education, family income, and status as a first-time parent were used as covariates in our adjusted analyses. To account for norms used in scoring language outcomes, these were also adjusted for the child's sex and age at the time of the assessment. For all outcomes measured at baseline, we used statistical adjustment for these baseline scores, providing a test of the intervention's effect on change after enrollment.

For dichotomous outcomes, rate ratios (RRs) from Poisson models are presented. For continuous outcome variables, we report adjusted linear regression coefficients. All estimates are reported with 95% confidence intervals (CIs). All analyses were performed using Stata 8.0 (StataCorp LP, College Station, Tex).

# RESULTS

## STUDY RESPONSE AND DEMOGRAPHICS

Women who agreed to participate in the study (N=439) represented about 80% of those who were eligible.[10] Participants in the intervention groups (PP+HS vs HS only)

**Table 2. Baseline Demographic Characteristics of Respondents by Treatment Group***

| Characteristic | Usual Care (n = 104) | Intervention (n = 239) | *P* Value† | HS Only (n = 117) | PP+HS (n = 122) | *P* Value† |
|---|---|---|---|---|---|---|
| | 30-mo Respondents | | | | | |
| Maternal education | | | | | | |
| High school or vocational school | 15.4 | 7.1 | | 4.3 | 9.8 | |
| Some college or college graduate | 64.4 | 57.3 | <.01 | 62.4 | 52.5 | .14 |
| Graduate school | 20.2 | 35.6 | | 33.3 | 37.7 | |
| Paternal education | | | | | | |
| High school or vocational school | 15.5 | 14.2 | | 12.8 | 15.6 | |
| Some college or college graduate | 60.2 | 53.1 | .30 | 51.3 | 54.9 | .55 |
| Graduate school | 24.3 | 32.6 | | 35.9 | 29.5 | |
| Family income, $ | | | | | | |
| <40 000 | 13.6 | 17.1 | | 13.9 | 20.2 | |
| 40 000-75 000 | 38.8 | 45.7 | .20 | 46.1 | 45.4 | .40 |
| >75 000 | 47.6 | 37.2 | | 40.0 | 34.5 | |
| White maternal race | 80.6 | 78.6 | .68 | 75.9 | 81.2 | .32 |
| First-time parent | 52.9 | 51.9 | .86 | 53.0 | 50.8 | .74 |
| No spouse or partner | 5.8 | 4.6 | .65 | 1.7 | 7.4 | .04 |
| Receiving public assistance | 9.6 | 9.2 | .90 | 5.1 | 13.1 | .03 |
| Male child | 55.5 | 51.7 | .53 | 50.0 | 53.3 | .61 |
| Maternal age, mean ± SD, y | 30.9 ± 5.1 | 32.5 ± 4.8 | <.01 | 32.5 ± 4.8 | 32.5 ± 5.0 | .90 |
| Child age at "24-mo" interview, mean ± SD, mo | 23.5 ± 0.5 | 23.4 ± 0.5 | .38 | 23.4 ± 0.5 | 23.4 ± 0.6 | .81 |

Abbreviations: HS, Healthy Steps for Young Children program; PP, PrePare.
*Data are given as percentages unless otherwise indicated.
†Between-group differences.

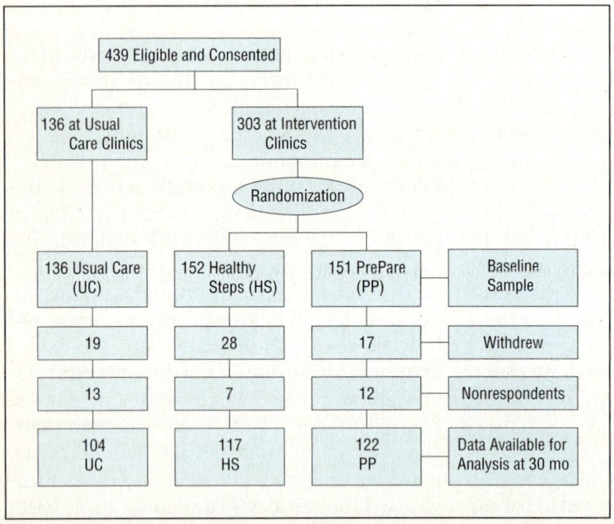


**Figure.** Treatment group assignment, randomization, and follow-up of eligible enrolled subjects.

differed from those in the UC group on 2 potential confounds, maternal education and maternal age (**Table 2**). Therefore, we report unadjusted and adjusted comparisons for intervention vs comparison group outcomes.

The telephone interview at 30 months was completed by 77% of enrollees assigned to HS only, 81% of those assigned to PP+HS, and 77% of those assigned to UC (**Figure**). Nonrespondents at 30 months had less maternal education and lower family incomes compared with respondents. Nonrespondents in the intervention group were more likely than comparison group nonrespondents to be first-time parents (67% vs 53%) and be without a spouse or partner (13% vs 3%). The mailed paper survey was completed at 24 months by 71% of the HS-only group, 74% of the PP+HS group, and 68% of the UC group.

## OUTCOMES BY DOMAIN

Throughout this article, intervention vs UC comparisons are presented first. These are followed by results of the randomized contrast between the PP+HS and HS-only groups.

### Child Health and Development

Receipt of well-child care within specified time intervals was more likely among intervention recipients than comparison enrollees at 4, 6, and 15 months (**Table 3**). Among the intervention recipients, the PP+HS group was more likely than the HS-only group to make a timely 24-month visit (adjusted RR, 1.17 [95% CI, 1.08-1.27]). At 24 months, more intervention recipients than comparison enrollees were up to date for immunizations (90% vs 85%; adjusted RR, 1.06 [95% CI, 1.02-1.09]); among intervention recipients, full immunization was significantly more common in the PP+HS group (92%) than in the HS-only group (88%).

Attainment of developmentally appropriate language skills at 24 months did not differ between the intervention and UC groups for vocabulary size, sentence length, the proportion of children using 3 or more word endings, or the proportion combining 2 or more words (Table 3). Within the intervention group, the vocabulary score of PP+HS children, on average, exceeded that

**Table 3. Child Health and Development Outcomes**

| Variable | Unadjusted Estimates: Usual Care (n = 104) | Intervention (n = 239) | HS Only (n = 117) | PP+HS (n = 122) | Adjusted Analyses*: Intervention vs Usual Care | PP+HS vs HS Only |
|---|---|---|---|---|---|---|
| **Continuous Outcomes, Mean ± SD or β (95% Confidence Interval)** | | | | | | |
| MCDI, 24 mo | (n = 92) | (n = 219) | (n = 108) | (n = 111) | ... | ... |
| Vocabulary checklist, 0-100 | 50.4 ± 26.2 | 53.4 ± 24.6 | 52.3 ± 24.2 | 54.4 ± 25.1 | −1.64 (−5.55 to 227) | 4.08 (0.69 to 7.47)† |
| Length of child's 3 longest phrases, morphemes | 3.86 ± 2.12 | 4.42 ± 2.28 | 4.57 ± 2.46 | 4.29 ± 2.10 | 0.14 (−0.07 to 0.35) | −0.22 (−0.47 to 0.04) |
| Child Behavior Checklist subscales | | | | | | |
| Aggressive behavior | 6.80 ± 4.35 | 7.74 ± 4.45 | 7.46 ± 4.49 | 8.01 ± 4.40 | 0.83 (0.37 to 1.30)† | 0.54 (0.00 to 1.08) |
| Sleep problems | 2.89 ± 2.55 | 3.12 ± 2.70 | 2.88 ± 2.61 | 3.35 ± 2.77 | 0.09 (−0.29 to 0.48) | 0.39 (−0.12 to 0.90) |
| Anxious or depressed mood | 3.83 ± 2.59 | 3.92 ± 2.36 | 3.71 ± 2.08 | 4.12 ± 2.60 | 0.03 (−0.44 to 0.50) | 0.40 (0.07 to 0.73)† |
| **Dichotomous Outcomes, % or Rate Ratio (95% Confidence Interval)** | | | | | | |
| Age-appropriate well-child care, visit month | | | | | | |
| 2 (n = 375) | 93.6 | 94.3 | 95.5 | 93.1 | 1.00 (0.97 to 1.03) | 0.97 (0.92 to 1.03) |
| 4 (n = 377) | 93.6 | 96.6 | 97.8 | 95.5 | 1.03 (1.02 to 1.04)† | 0.97 (0.89 to 1.07) |
| 6 (n = 372) | 87.2 | 93.9 | 93.9 | 94.0 | 1.08 (1.00 to 1.17)† | 1.01 (0.86 to 1.18) |
| 10 (n = 351) | 92.0 | 93.6 | 93.4 | 93.8 | 1.02 (0.98 to 1.06) | 1.01 (0.93 to 1.09) |
| 15 (n = 330) | 77.8 | 88.3 | 89.0 | 87.7 | 1.13 (1.04 to 1.22)† | 0.99 (0.95 to 1.03) |
| 24 (n = 306) | 72.6 | 81.5 | 75.7 | 87.4 | 1.09 (0.97 to 1.22) | 1.17 (1.08 to 1.27)† |
| Immunization status up-to-date at 24 mo | 84.6 | 89.9 | 88.0 | 92.0 | 1.06 (1.02 to 1.09)† | 1.03 (1.01 to 1.06)† |
| MCDI, 24 mo | (n = 92) | (n = 219) | (n = 108) | (n = 111) | ... | ... |
| 2 Word endings, ≥3 vs <3 | 43.3 | 55.2 | 55.2 | 55.1 | 1.10 (0.82 to 1.50) | 1.09 (0.92 to 1.30) |
| Combining ≥2 words, sometimes/often vs not yet | 88.5 | 91.0 | 89.4 | 92.5 | 1.02 (0.94 to 1.12) | 1.05 (1.02 to 1.08)† |

Abbreviations: HS, Healthy Steps for Young Children program; MCDI, MacArthur Communicative Development Inventories (language outcomes include additional adjustments for age and sex); PP, PrePare.

*Include adjustment for maternal education, family income, status as first-time parent, baseline measures of the outcome when available, and clustering at the level of the clinic.

†Statistically significant comparisons (*P*<.05).

of HS-only children by 4.08 (95% CI, 0.69-7.74) words, and the proportion combining words in the PP+HS group exceeded the proportion in the HS-only group (93% vs 89%; adjusted RR, 1.05 [95% CI, 1.02-1.08]).

Group differences in the Child Behavior Checklist scores showed that parents in the intervention group reported higher scores than those in the UC group on the aggressive behavior subscale (7.74 vs 6.80; adjusted β, 0.83 [95% CI, 0.37-1.30]), although neither group reached a subscale score of clinical significance (the cutoff for this age is 22 years) (Table 3).[14] There were no group differences in reported sleep problems or problems with depression or anxiety. Although children in the PP+HS group were reported to have more anxious or depressed behaviors than those in HS-only group (β level, 0.40 [95% CI, 0.07-0.73]), the mean scores were well below the range of clinical significance.

### Parenting Practices

Within the intervention group, 97% of mothers initiated breastfeeding compared with 91% in the UC group (adjusted RR, 1.06 [95% CI, 1.00-1.11]) (**Table 4**). Intervention recipients who initiated breastfeeding also breastfed their infants longer on average than the UC recipients (13.4 vs 11.2 months; adjusted β, 1.30 [95% CI, 0.18-2.43]). The proportion of intervention mothers who breastfed for 6 months or longer[19] was higher (82%) than that of UC mothers (64%). No difference was found between the PP+HS and the HS-only groups.

There were no group differences in parents' nurturing behavior or self-efficacy for pediatric health care. Parenting sense of competence was slightly lower among intervention recipients (β level, −0.92 [95% CI, −1.40 to −0.44]), an effect driven by lower scores on the satisfaction subscale rather than by differences in self-efficacy (Table 4).

Parents in the intervention group were more likely to report the use of routines in the home (adjusted RR, 1.12 [95% CI, 1.03-1.22]) and were 25% less likely than those in the UC group to allow more than 1 hour of daily television viewing (34% vs 50%; adjusted RR, 0.75 [95% CI, 0.62-0.90]). Within the intervention group, recipients of PP+HS reported that they were less likely to read to their child daily (88% vs 95%) and were more likely to allow more than 1 hour of television viewing (39% vs 28%) compared with recipients of HS only.

Respondents in the intervention group were almost 20% more likely than those in the UC group to score the full 5 points on the index of injury control behaviors (smoke detector function, car seat use, and gun safety items). Intervention families were also more likely to use stair gates (adjusted RR, 1.19 [95% CI, 1.15-1.23]) and to have access to the local poison control center's telephone number (adjusted RR, 1.08 [95% CI, 1.03-1.12]), but they were less likely to report having safety

**Table 4. Parenting Practices Outcomes**

| Variable | Unadjusted Estimates: Usual Care (n = 104) | Intervention (n = 239) | HS Only (n = 117) | PP+HS (n = 122) | Adjusted Analyses: Intervention vs Usual Care | PP+HS vs HS Only |
|---|---|---|---|---|---|---|
| **Continuous Outcomes, Mean ± SD or β (95% Confidence Interval)** | | | | | | |
| Breastfeeding duration, mo | 11.2 ± 9.5 (n = 91) | 13.4 ± 8.8 (n = 232) | 13.9 ± 8.7 (n = 116) | 13.0 ± 8.9 (n = 116) | 1.30 (0.18 to 2.43)* | −0.64 (−1.13 to −0.16)* |
| Parenting behavior checklist nurturing subscale | 59.6 ± 6.3 | 59.4 ± 6.6 | 60.2 ± 5.6 | 58.7 ± 7.3 | −0.06 (−0.42 to 0.31) | −1.35 (−3.11 to 0.41) |
| Parenting sense of competence | | | | | | |
| Efficacy subscale | 21.4 ± 2.2 | 21.1 ± 2.2 | 21.2 ± 2.2 | 21.1 ± 2.2 | −0.06 (−0.47 to 0.34) | −0.17 (−0.56 to 0.22) |
| Satisfaction subscale | 26.8 ± 3.0 | 26.2 ± 3.3 | 26.4 ± 3.5 | 26.0 ± 3.1 | −0.55 (−0.96 to −0.14)* | −0.61 (−1.32 to 0.09) |
| **Total** | **48.2** ± 4.5 | **47.3** ± 4.8 | **47.6** ± 4.9 | **47.1** ± 4.6 | −0.92 (−1.40 to −0.44)* | −0.69 (−1.46 to 0.09) |
| Health care self-efficacy | 16.9 ± 2.0 | 17.0 ± 2.0 | 17.0 ± 1.9 | 17.0 ± 2.0 | 0.04 (−0.28 to 0.36) | −0.14 (−0.52 to 0.25) |
| Injury prevention index | 4.68 ± 0.56 | 4.84 ± 0.43 | 4.81 ± 0.45 | 4.86 ± 0.41 | 0.15 (0.05 to 0.25)* | −0.02 (−0.04 to 0.08) |
| **Dichotomous Outcomes, % or Rate Ratio (95% Confidence Interval)** | | | | | | |
| Breastfeeding | (n = 91) | (n = 232) | (n = 116) | (n = 116) | ... | ... |
| Ever breastfed | 91.4 | 97.1 | 99.2 | 95.1 | 1.06 (1.00 to 1.11)* | 0.96 (0.93 to 0.99)* |
| Duration >6 mo | 64.4 | 81.6 | 83.8 | 79.5 | 1.18 (1.11 to 1.26)* | 0.96 (0.83 to 1.11) |
| Child activities | | | | | | |
| Read to child at least daily | 88.5 | 91.2 | 94.9 | 87.7 | 1.03 (0.96 to 1.10) | 0.92 (0.91 to 0.94)* |
| Play with child at least daily | 97.1 | 97.9 | 99.2 | 96.7 | 1.01 (0.99 to 1.02) | 0.98 (0.93 to 1.03) |
| Watch television >1 h/d | 50.0 | 33.6 | 28.3 | 38.7 | 0.75 (0.62 to 0.90)* | 1.35 (1.08 to 1.70)* |
| Followed 3 routines, 2 if no nap | 86.5 | 85.2 | 90.6 | 80.0 | 1.12 (1.03 to 1.22)* | 1.02 (0.96 to 1.08) |
| Injury prevention index (5 vs <5) | 72.1 | 86.2 | 83.8 | 88.5 | 1.19 (1.09 to 1.28)* | 1.04 (0.99 to 1.08) |
| Household safety items | | | | | | |
| Use stair gate | 30.2 | 33.2 | 34.4 | 32.1 | 1.19 (1.15 to 1.23)* | 0.99 (0.59 to 1.66) |
| Covers on electrical outlets | 92.3 | 92.9 | 90.6 | 95.0 | 1.00 (0.98 to 1.03) | 1.06 (1.02 to 1.10)* |
| Safety latches on cabinets | 77.9 | 66.8 | 70.9 | 62.8 | 0.88 (0.83 to 0.93)* | 0.87 (0.82 to 0.91)* |
| Poison control center telephone number | 90.4 | 95.8 | 95.7 | 95.9 | 1.08 (1.03 to 1.12)* | 1.01 (1.00 to 1.01) |
| Discipline by ever slapping face or spanking with object | 2.9 | 2.1 | 3.4 | 0.8 | 0.46 (0.29 to 0.73)* | 0.20 (0.02 to 1.90) |

Abbreviations: HS, Healthy Steps for Young Children program; PP, PrePare.
*Statistically significant comparisons ($P<.05$).

latches on cabinets (Table 4). Intervention families were 54% less likely to report the use of extreme disciplinary measures (ie, slapping the child's face or spanking with an object) than UC families (adjusted RR, 0.46 [95% CI, 0.29-0.73]).

## Parental Well-being

When the study children were 30 months old, maternal depressive symptoms scores on the Center for Epidemiological Studies Depression Scale were generally low (**Table 5**). The intervention respondents reported slightly more distress than the UC respondents on these measures (adjusted β, 0.75 [95% CI, 0.20-1.31]) but were no more likely to score above the clinical cutoff for an affective disorder. The elevated 30-month Center for Epidemiological Studies Depression Scale scores in the intervention group were driven by a higher prevalence of depressive symptoms among the PP+HS group (a difference not present at baseline). Among those who were self-identified as having problems with depression or sadness, 53% in the HS-only group and 49% in the PP+HP group said that they had discussed these concerns with someone in the pediatric practice, compared with only 35% of those in the UC group (adjusted RR, 1.45 [95% CI, 0.95-2.21]).

Only a small proportion of respondents reported any use of illicit drugs or exposure to significant physical domestic violence in the preceding year. No group differences in these outcomes were detected. Although screening and referral for smoking cessation services were included in both arms, the low proportion of house-

**Table 5. Parental Well-being Outcomes**

| Variable | Unadjusted Estimates: Usual Care (n = 104) | Intervention (n = 239) | HS Only (n = 117) | PP+HS (n = 122) | Adjusted Analyses: Intervention vs Usual Care | PP+HS vs HS Only |
|---|---|---|---|---|---|---|
| | **Continuous Outcome, Mean ± SD or β (95% Confidence Interval)** | | | | | |
| CESD maternal depressive symptoms | 3.50 ± 3.93 | 4.28 ± ±4.47 | 3.80 ± 4.42 | 4.74 ± 4.49 | 0.75 (0.20-1.31)* | 0.55 (0.31-0.78)* |
| | **Dichotomous Outcomes, % or Rate Ratio (95% Confidence Interval)** | | | | | |
| Maternal depressive symptoms | | | | | | |
| Clinically significant depressive symptoms, CESD >11 | 6.7 | 8.4 | 6.8 | 9.9 | 1.21 (0.80-1.82) | 0.93 (0.67-1.30) |
| Discussed sadness with someone in pediatric practice† | 35.3 (n = 34) | 50.6 (n = 83) | 52.6 (n = 38) | 48.9 (n = 45) | 1.45 (0.95-2.21) | 1.04 (0.53-2.04) |
| Risky parental health behaviors | | | | | | |
| Any drug use | 4.8 | 6.3 | 5.1 | 7.4 | 1.61 (0.71-3.64) | 1.02 (0.50-2.09) |
| Domestic violence in past year | 4.8 | 1.7 | 0.9 | 2.5 | 0.40 (0.16-1.05) | 2.09 (0.73-6.01) |
| Environment with tobacco smoke | 9.6 | 8.4 | 6.8 | 9.8 | 0.76 (0.48-1.22) | 1.05 (0.70-1.58) |

Abbreviations: CESD, Center for Epidemiological Studies Depression Scale; HS, Healthy Steps for Young Children program; PP, PrePare.
*Statistically significant comparisons ($P<.05$).
†Among those self-identified as "needing help with sadness or depression."

holds with adult smokers in the intervention group (8%) did not differ from the proportion in the UC group (10%).

## COMMENT

The HS has been shown to improve the quality of child health services and parental satisfaction in diverse practice settings.[7] When children in this study were 3 months old, an evaluation demonstrated that HS with or without PP was associated with improved parental knowledge, practice, well-being, and satisfaction.[8] When the children were 30 months old, there were additional positive effects on the receipt of timely well-child care, immunization rates, duration of breastfeeding, and parenting practices to prevent childhood injury, to increase the use of household daily living routines, to minimize television viewing, and to reduce the use of inappropriate discipline techniques.

An important feature of HS is the universal nature of the intervention. Parenting support programs have been shown to have positive effects among families with young infants at high psychosocial risk.[20-25] Our results suggest a benefit from the universal provision of parenting and child development support services to an unselected sample of families with health coverage, who ranged from the affluent and employed to those at greater socioeconomic and psychosocial risk. This is a meaningful result.

There was no difference in response to the intervention according to the HSS assigned (data not shown). All were experienced master's-level clinicians. Whether paraprofessionals with other backgrounds could produce similar outcomes is unknown and should not be assumed.[26] Dose-response analyses are an appealing strategy to identify the intensity of intervention required to elicit desired effects; however, they are not applicable in this trial. The intervention was clinic based, involving office staff, providers, and systems of care. The effect of these changes in the milieu of care cannot easily be delineated from the effect of countable visits or encounters with the HSS.

Despite the noted improvements in child health and parenting practices, the intervention was associated with some undesirable effects. Intervention recipients reported more depressive symptoms and a diminished parenting sense of competence that stemmed from less satisfaction in the parenting role. Whether this reflects an increase in symptoms or an increased accuracy and willingness to identify and report symptoms is unknown. Differences in neither baseline rates of depression nor maternal education explain these findings. Fortunately, the number of depressive symptoms in any group was low when enrolled children reached 2½ years old. Nevertheless, more investigation of the interaction among the intervention, parenting experience, and maternal mental health outcomes seems warranted.

A major objective of this study was to test a new model for delivering HS services capitalizing on the strengths of an integrated delivery system. To do so, we added a prenatal component. Despite increased member satisfaction and decreased health plan disenrollment in the early postnatal period, the only long-term health benefits from PP seemed to be (1) greater compliance with the 24-month well-child visit, with a concurrent improvement in immunization status, and (2) modestly increased vocabulary production and word combination at 24 months. Paradoxically, these developmental attainments were seen in a group that reported more depressive symptoms, more television viewing, and less daily reading to the children. These findings in the PP+HS arm cannot be explained using the data available to us.

There are several potential limitations in this trial. Although we were gratified to achieve a 78% retention rate in the study during 3 years, there remain significant differences in the demographic composition of nonrespondents in the intervention group compared with the UC group, and within the randomized treatment groups as well. The comparisons between the combined intervention and UC groups were limited by the quasi-experimental design. Although we adjusted for several important baseline covariates and for clustering within clinics, unmeasured residual confounding likely exists.

Overall, we believe that our implementation of HS in an integrated delivery system resulted in positive effects for parents and their children. These must be weighed against costs of the intervention, its effects on utilization, provider satisfaction, and satisfaction of health plan enrollees. These outcomes will be assessed in future studies, and policy implications of the findings will be discussed in subsequent publications.

**Accepted for Publication:** February 8, 2006.
**Correspondence:** Brian D. Johnston, MD, MPH, Department of Pediatrics, University of Washington, Harborview Medical Center, 325 Ninth Ave, Box 359774, Seattle, WA 98104 (bdj@u.washington.edu).
**Author Contributions:** Dr Johnston had full access to all the data in the study and takes responsibility for the integrity of the data and the accuracy of the data analysis. *Study concept and design*: Huebner and Thompson. *Acquisition of data*: Johnston and Tyll. *Analysis and interpretation of data*: Anderson. *Drafting of the manuscript*: Johnston and Huebner. *Critical revision of the manuscript for important intellectual content*: Johnston, Huebner, Anderson, Tyll, and Thompson. *Statistical analysis*: Anderson. *Obtained funding*: Tyll and Thompson. *Administrative, technical, and material support*: Huebner and Tyll. *Study supervision*: Tyll and Thompson.
**Funding/Support:** This work was supported by a generous grant during 6 years from the Kaiser Foundation Health Plan. Additional financial support was provided by the Group Health Community Foundation, the Nesholm Family Foundation, and the Group Health Administration Employees Community Fund of Boeing, Puget Sound.
**Financial Disclosure:** None reported.
**Acknowledgements**: We acknowledge William Barlow for statistical consultation, Malia Oliver for programming work, and Eve Adams for assistance in manuscript preparation. We thank the participating Group Health Cooperative clinics and their staff along with the following HSSs who delivered their services with dedication and compassion: Susan Anderson, MA, CMHC; Jolyn Bien, MA, CMHC; Lori Roehl, RN, MSN; Sara Schott, MSW; and Nancy Kaplan, MSSW.

## REFERENCES

1. Zuckerman B, Parker S, Kaplan-Sanoff M, Augustyn M, Barth MC. Healthy Steps: a case study of innovation in pediatric practice. *Pediatrics.* 2004;114:820-826.
2. Kaplan-Sanoff M, Zuckerman B, Parker S. *Healthy Steps: Strategies for Change: Child Development in Primary Care for Young Children.* Boston, Mass: Boston University School of Medicine; 1999.
3. Lawrence PR, Magee T, Bernard A. Reshaping primary care: the Healthy Steps Initiative. *J Pediatr Health Care.* 2001;15:58-62.
4. Zuckerman B, Kaplan-Sanoff M, Parker S, Young K. *The Healthy Steps for Young Children Program: Zero to Three.* Washington, DC: Zero to Three National Center for Infants, Toddlers, and Families; June/July 1997:20-25.
5. Minkovitz C, Strobino D, Hughart N, Scharfstein D, Guyer B. Early effects of the Healthy Steps for Young Children Program. *Arch Pediatr Adolesc Med.* 2001; 155:470-479.
6. McLearn KT, Zuckerman BS, Parker S, Yellowitz M, Kaplan-Sanoff M. Child development and pediatrics for the 21st century: the Healthy Steps approach. *J Urban Health.* 1998;75:704-723.
7. Minkovitz CS, Hughart N, Strobino D, et al. A practice-based intervention to enhance quality of care in the first 3 years of life: the Healthy Steps for Young Children Program. *JAMA.* 2003;290:3081-3091.
8. Johnston BD, Huebner CE, Tyll L, Barlow WE, Thompson RS. Expanding developmental and behavioral services for newborns in primary care: effects on parental well-being, practice, and satisfaction. *Am J Prev Med.* 2004;26:356-366.
9. Huebner CE, Tyll L, Luallen J, Johnston BD, Thompson RS. PrePare: a program of enhanced prenatal services within health-maintenance organization settings. *Health Educ Res.* 2001;16:71-80.
10. Huebner CE, Barlow WE, Tyll LT, Johnston BD, Thompson RS. Expanding developmental and behavioral services for newborns in primary care: program design, delivery, and evaluation framework. *Am J Prev Med.* 2004;26:344-355.
11. Rubin R. *Maternal Identity and the Maternal Experience.* New York, NY: Springer Publishing Co Inc; 1984.
12. Health Plan Employer Data and Information Set (HEDIS). http://www.ncqa.org/somc2001/child_imm_2001_cis.html. Accessed February 2003.
13. Fenson L, Dale P, Resnick JS, et al. *MacArthur Communicative Development Inventories: User's Guide and Technical Manual.* San Diego, Calif: Singular Publishing Co; 1993.
14. Achenbach T. *Manual for the Child Behavior Checklist/2-3 and 1992 Profile.* Burlington: University of Vermont; 1992.
15. Fox RA, Platz DL, Bentley KS. Maternal factors related to parenting practices, developmental expectations, and perceptions of child behavior problems. *J Genet Psychol.* 1995;156:431-441.
16. Johnston C, Mash E. A measure of parenting satisfaction and efficacy. *J Clin Child Psychol.* 1989;18:167-175.
17. Radloff L. The CES-D Scale: a self-report depression scale for research in the general population. *Appl Psychol Meas.* 1977;1:385-401.
18. Institute of Medicine. *Broadening the Base for Treatment for Alcohol Problems.* Washington, DC: National Academy Press; 1990.
19. American Academy of Pediatrics, Work Group on Breastfeeding. Breastfeeding and the use of human milk. *Pediatrics.* 1997;100:1035-1039.
20. Armstrong KL, Fraser JA, Dadds MR, Morris J. Promoting secure attachment, maternal mood and child health in a vulnerable population: a randomized controlled trial. *J Paediatr Child Health.* 2000;36:555-562.
21. Infant Health and Development Program. Enhancing the outcomes of low-birth-weight, premature infants: a multisite, randomized trial. *JAMA.* 1990;263:3035-3042.
22. Hardy JB, Streett R. Family support and parenting education in the home: an effective extension of clinic-based preventive health care services for poor children. *J Pediatr.* 1989;115:927-931.
23. Kitzman H, Olds DL, Henderson CR Jr, et al. Effect of prenatal and infancy home visitation by nurses on pregnancy outcomes, childhood injuries, and repeated childbearing: a randomized controlled trial. *JAMA.* 1997;278:644-652.
24. Morrell CJ, Spiby H, Stewart P, Walters S, Morgan A. Costs and effectiveness of community postnatal support workers: randomised controlled trial. *BMJ.* 2000; 321:593-598.
25. Lyons-Ruth K, Connell DB, Grunebaum HU, Botein S. Infants at social risk: maternal depression and family support services as mediators of infant development and security of attachment. *Child Dev.* 1990;61:85-98.
26. Olds DL, Robinson J, Pettitt L, et al. Effects of home visits by paraprofessionals and by nurses: age 4 follow-up results of a randomized trial. *Pediatrics.* 2004; 114:1560-1568.

Now:
The Purple Pill™ is FDA-approved for use in kids 12 to 17 years old with GERD

# NEXIUM for the NEXT GENERATION

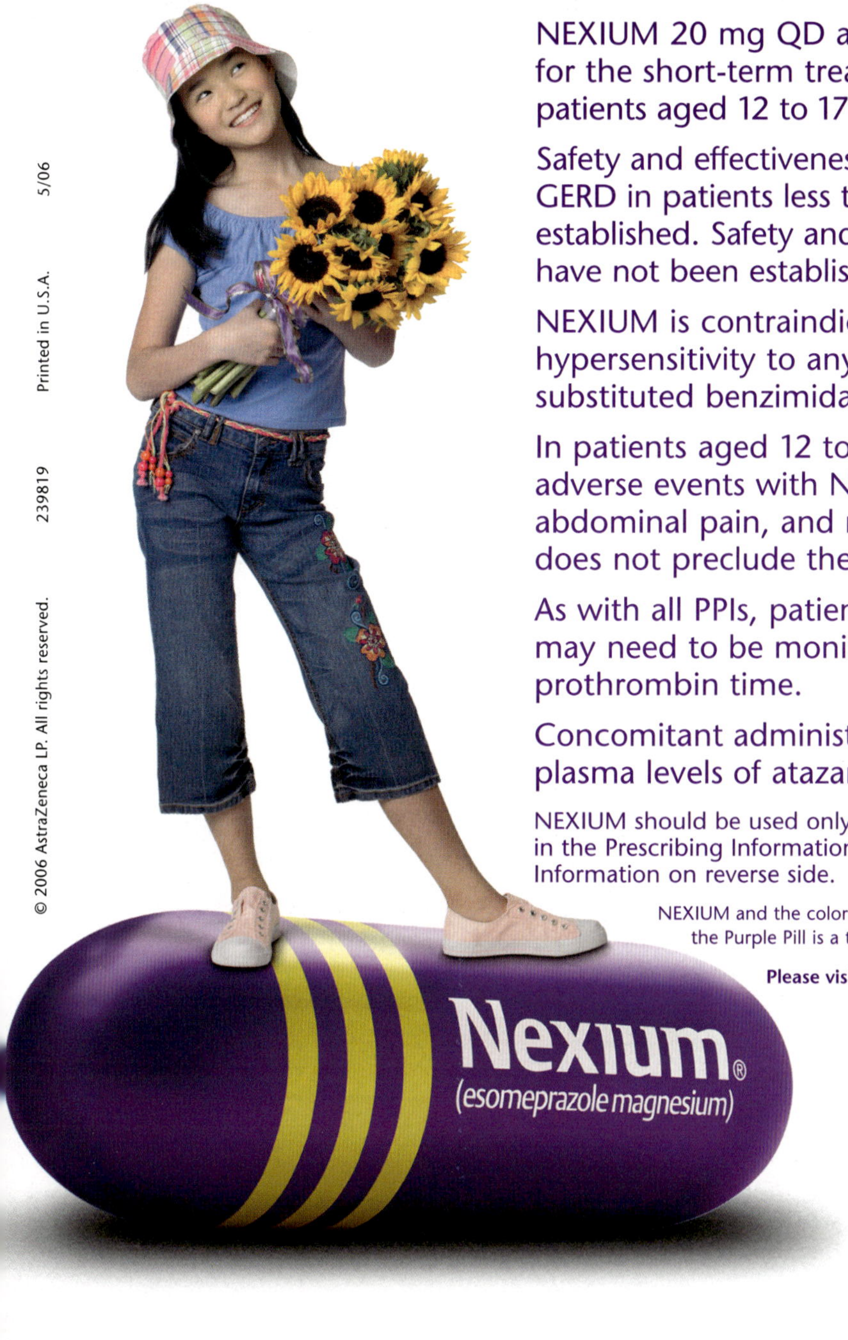


NEXIUM 20 mg QD and NEXIUM 40 mg QD are approved for the short-term treatment (up to 8 weeks) of GERD in patients aged 12 to 17 years.

Safety and effectiveness for the treatment of symptomatic GERD in patients less than 12 years of age have not been established. Safety and effectiveness for other pediatric uses have not been established.

NEXIUM is contraindicated in patients with known hypersensitivity to any component of the formulation or to substituted benzimidazoles.

In patients aged 12 to 17 years, the most frequently reported adverse events with NEXIUM include headache, diarrhea, abdominal pain, and nausea. Symptomatic response to therapy does not preclude the presence of gastric malignancy.

As with all PPIs, patients treated concomitantly with warfarin may need to be monitored for increases in INR and prothrombin time.

Concomitant administration of esomeprazole may reduce the plasma levels of atazanavir.

NEXIUM should be used only for the conditions, dosages, and durations specified in the Prescribing Information. Please see the brief summary of full Prescribing Information on reverse side.

NEXIUM and the color purple as applied to the capsule are registered trademarks and the Purple Pill is a trademark of the AstraZeneca group of companies.

**Please visit our Web site at www.Nexium-us.com**

Nexium®
(esomeprazole magnesium)

AstraZeneca

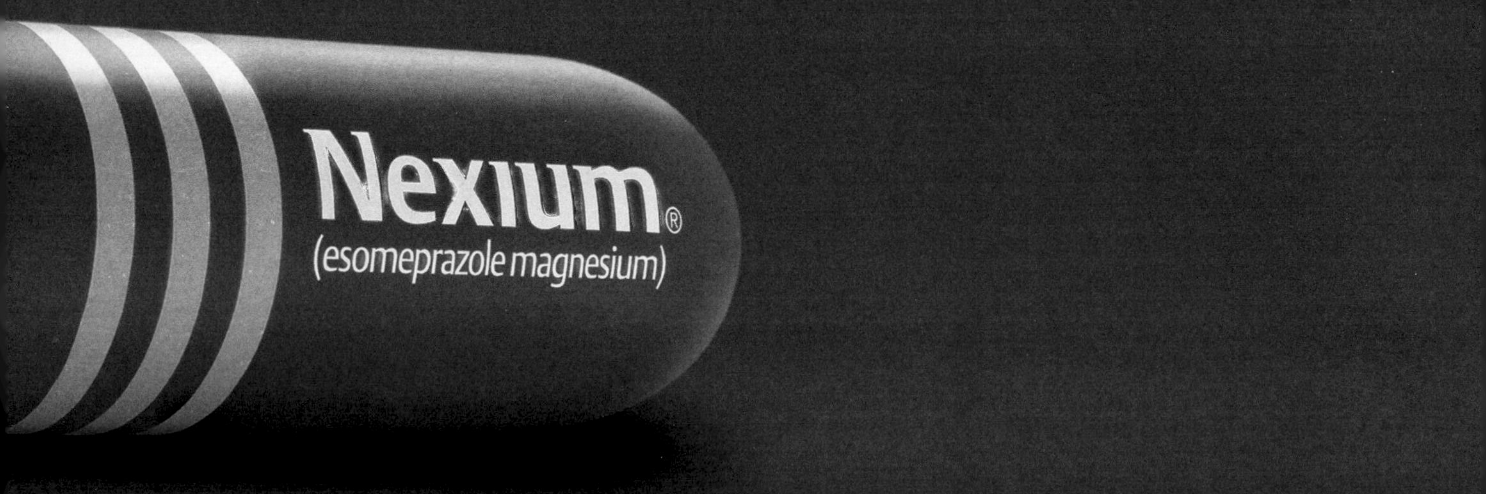




# NEXIUM® *(esomeprazole magnesium)*

## 20-mg, 40-mg Delayed-Release Capsules

**BRIEF SUMMARY** of Prescribing Information.

**INDICATIONS AND USAGE Treatment of GERD** NEXIUM is indicated for the short-term treatment (4 to 8 weeks) in the healing and symptomatic resolution of diagnostically confirmed erosive esophagitis; the maintenance of symptom resolution and healing of erosive esophagitis (controlled studies do not extend beyond 6 months); the treatment of heartburn and other symptoms associated with GERD; **Risk Reduction of NSAID-Associated Gastric Ulcer; *H.pylori* Eradication to Reduce the Risk of Duodenal Ulcer Recurrence.**

**CONTRAINDICATIONS** NEXIUM is contraindicated in patients with known hypersensitivity to any component of the formulation or to substituted benzimidazoles.

**PRECAUTIONS General** Symptomatic response to therapy with NEXIUM does not preclude the presence of gastric malignancy. Atrophic gastritis has been noted occasionally in gastric corpus biopsies from patients treated long-term with omeprazole, of which NEXIUM is an enantiomer. **Information for Patients** NEXIUM Delayed-Release Capsules should be swallowed whole and taken at least one hour before meals. For patients who have difficulty swallowing capsules, one tablespoon of applesauce can be added to an empty bowl and the NEXIUM Delayed-Release Capsule can be opened, and the pellets carefully emptied onto the applesauce. The pellets should be mixed with the applesauce and then swallowed immediately. The applesauce used should not be hot and should be soft enough to be swallowed without chewing. The pellets should not be chewed or crushed. The pellet/applesauce mixture should not be stored for future use. Antacids may be used while taking NEXIUM. **Drug Interactions** Esomeprazole is extensively metabolized in the liver by CYP2C19 and CYP3A4. *In vitro* and *in vivo* studies have shown that esomeprazole is not likely to inhibit CYPs 1A2, 2A6, 2C9, 2D6, 2E1 and 3A4. No clinically relevant interactions with drugs metabolized by these CYP enzymes would be expected. Drug interaction studies have shown that esomeprazole does not have any clinically significant interactions with phenytoin, warfarin, quinidine, clarithromycin or amoxicillin. Post-marketing reports of changes in prothrombin measures have been received among patients on concomitant warfarin and esomeprazole therapy. Increases in INR and prothrombin time may lead to abnormal bleeding and even death. Patients treated with proton pump inhibitors and warfarin concomitantly may need to be monitored for increases in INR and prothrombin time. Esomeprazole may potentially interfere with CYP2C19, the major esomeprazole metabolizing enzyme. Coadministration of esomeprazole 30 mg and diazepam, a CYP2C19 substrate, resulted in a 45% decrease in clearance of diazepam. Increased plasma levels of diazepam were observed 12 hours after dosing and onwards. However, at that time, the plasma levels of diazepam were below the therapeutic interval, and thus this interaction is unlikely to be of clinical relevance. Coadministration of oral contraceptives, diazepam, phenytoin, or quinidine did not seem to change the pharmacokinetic profile of esomeprazole. Concomitant administration of esomeprazole may reduce the plasma levels of atazanavir. Studies evaluating concomitant administration of esomeprazole and either naproxen (non-selective NSAID) or rofecoxib (COX-2 selective NSAID) did not identify any clinically relevant changes in the pharmacokinetic profiles of esomeprazole or these NSAIDs. Esomeprazole inhibits gastric acid secretion. Therefore, esomeprazole may interfere with the absorption of drugs where gastric pH is an important determinant of bioavailability (eg, ketoconazole, iron salts and digoxin). **Carcinogenesis, Mutagenesis, Impairment of Fertility** The carcinogenic potential of esomeprazole was assessed using omeprazole studies. In two 24-month oral carcinogenicity studies in rats, omeprazole at daily doses of 1.7, 3.4, 13.8, 44.0 and 140.8 mg/kg/day (about 0.7 to 57 times the human dose of 20 mg/day expressed on a body surface area basis) produced gastric ECL cell carcinoids in a dose-related manner in both male and female rats; the incidence of this effect was markedly higher in female rats, which had higher blood levels of omeprazole. Gastric carcinoids seldom occur in the untreated rat. In addition, ECL cell hyperplasia was present in all treated groups of both sexes. In one of these studies, female rats were treated with 13.8 mg omeprazole/kg/day (about 5.6 times the human dose on a body surface area basis) for 1 year, then followed for an additional year without the drug. No carcinoids were seen in these rats. An increased incidence of treatment-related ECL cell hyperplasia was observed at the end of 1 year (94% treated vs 10% controls). By the second year the difference between treated and control rats was much smaller (46% vs 26%) but still showed more hyperplasia in the treated group. Gastric adenocarcinoma was seen in one rat (2%). No similar tumor was seen in male or female rats treated for 2 years. For this strain of rat no similar tumor has been noted historically, but a finding involving only one tumor is difficult to interpret. A 78-week mouse carcinogenicity study of omeprazole did not show increased tumor occurrence, but the study was not conclusive. Esomeprazole was negative in the Ames mutation test, in the *in vivo* rat bone marrow cell chromosome aberration test, and the *in vivo* mouse micronucleus test. Esomeprazole, however, was positive in the *in vitro* human lymphocyte chromosome aberration test. Omeprazole was positive in the *in vitro* human lymphocyte chromosome aberration test, the *in vivo* mouse bone marrow cell chromosome aberration test, and the *in vivo* mouse micronucleus test. The potential effects of esomeprazole on fertility and reproductive performance were assessed using omeprazole studies. Omeprazole at oral doses up to 138 mg/kg/day in rats (about 56 times the human dose on a body surface area basis) was found to have no effect on reproductive performance of parental animals. **Pregnancy** *Teratogenic Effects. Pregnancy Category B* Teratology studies have been performed in rats at oral doses up to 280 mg/kg/day (about 57 times the human dose on a body surface area basis) and in rabbits at oral doses up to 86 mg/kg/day (about 35 times the human dose on a body surface area basis) and have revealed no evidence of impaired fertility or harm to the fetus due to esomeprazole. There are, however, no adequate and well-controlled studies in pregnant women. Because animal reproduction studies are not always predictive of human response, this drug should be used during pregnancy only if clearly needed. Teratology studies conducted with omeprazole in rats at oral doses up to 138 mg/kg/day (about 56 times the human dose on a body surface area basis) and in rabbits at doses up to 69 mg/kg/day (about 56 times the human dose on a body surface area basis) did not disclose any evidence for a teratogenic potential of omeprazole. In rabbits, omeprazole in a dose range of 6.9 to 69.1 mg/kg/day (about 5.5 to 56 times the human dose on a body surface area basis) produced dose-related increases in embryo-lethality, fetal resorptions, and pregnancy disruptions. In rats, dose-related embryo/ fetal toxicity and postnatal developmental toxicity were observed in offspring resulting from parents treated with omeprazole at 13.8 to 138.0 mg/kg/day (about 5.6 to 56 times the human doses on a body surface area basis). There are no adequate and well-controlled studies in pregnant women. Sporadic reports have been received of congenital abnormalities occurring in infants born to women who have received omeprazole during pregnancy. **Nursing Mothers** The excretion of esomeprazole in milk has not been studied. However, omeprazole concentrations have been measured in breast milk of a woman following oral administration of 20 mg. Because esomeprazole is likely to be excreted in human milk, because of the potential for serious adverse reactions in nursing infants from esomeprazole, and because of the potential for tumorigenicity shown for omeprazole in rat carcinogenicity studies, a decision should be made whether to discontinue nursing or to discontinue the drug, taking into account the importance of the drug to the mother. **Pediatric Use** Use of NEXIUM in adolescent patients 12 to 17 years of age for short-term treatment of GERD is supported by a) extrapolation of results, already included in the currently approved labeling, from adequate and well-controlled studies that supported the approval of NEXIUM for adults, and b) safety and pharmacokinetic studies performed in adolescent patients. (See **CLINICAL PHARMACOLOGY, Pharmacokinetics,** *Pediatric* for pharmacokinetic information.) The safety and effectiveness of NEXIUM for the treatment of symptomatic GERD in patients <12 years of age have not been established. The safety and effectiveness of NEXIUM for other pediatric uses have not been established. **12 to 17 Years of Age GERD** In a multi-center, randomized, double-blind, parallel-group study, 149 adolescent patients (12 to 17 years of age; 89 female; 124 Caucasian, 15 Black, 10 Other) with clinically diagnosed GERD were treated with either NEXIUM 20 mg or NEXIUM 40 mg once daily for up to 8 weeks to evaluate safety and tolerability. Patients were not endoscopically characterized as to the presence or absence of erosive esophagitis. The most frequently reported (at least 2%) treatment related adverse events in these patients were headache (8.1%), abdominal pain (2.7%), diarrhea (2%) and nausea (2%). No new safety concerns were identified. **Geriatric Use** Of the total number of patients who received NEXIUM in clinical trials, 1459 were 65 to 74 years of age and 354 patients were ≥75 years of age. No overall differences in safety and efficacy were observed between the elderly and younger individuals, and other reported clinical experience has not identified differences in responses between the elderly and younger patients, but greater sensitivity of some older individuals cannot be ruled out.

**ADVERSE REACTIONS** The safety of NEXIUM was evaluated in over 15,000 patients (aged 18-84 years) in clinical trials worldwide including over 8,500 patients in the United States and over 6,500 patients in Europe and Canada. Over 2,900 patients were treated in long-term studies for up to 6-12 months. In general, NEXIUM was well tolerated in both short and long-term clinical trials. A study was performed evaluating the safety of NEXIUM in pediatric patients aged 12-17 for the treatment of symptomatic GERD (see **PRECAUTIONS – Pediatric Use**). The safety in the treatment of healing of erosive esophagitis was assessed in four randomized comparative clinical trials, which included 1,240 patients on NEXIUM 20 mg, 2,434 patients on NEXIUM 40 mg, and 3,008 patients on omeprazole 20 mg daily. The most frequently occurring adverse events (≥1%) in all three groups was headache (5.5, 5.0, and 3.8, respectively) and diarrhea (no difference among the three groups). Nausea, flatulence, abdominal pain, constipation, and dry mouth occurred at similar rates among patients taking NEXIUM or omeprazole. Additional adverse events that were reported as possibly or probably related to NEXIUM with an incidence <1% are listed below by body system: ***Body as a Whole:*** abdomen enlarged, allergic reaction, asthenia, back pain, chest pain, chest pain substernal, facial edema, peripheral edema, hot flushes, fatigue, fever, flu-like disorder, generalized edema, leg edema, malaise, pain, rigors; ***Cardiovascular:*** flushing, hypertension, tachycardia; ***Endocrine:*** goiter; ***Gastrointestinal:*** bowel irregularity, constipation aggravated, dyspepsia, dysphagia, dysplasia GI, epigastric pain, eructation, esophageal disorder, frequent stools, gastroenteritis, GI hemorrhage, GI symptoms not otherwise specified, hiccup, melena, mouth disorder, pharynx disorder, rectal disorder, serum gastrin increased, tongue disorder, tongue edema, ulcerative stomatitis, vomiting; ***Hearing:*** earache, tinnitus; ***Hematologic:*** anemia, anemia hypochromic, cervical lymphoadenopathy, epistaxis, leukocytosis, leukopenia, thrombocytopenia; ***Hepatic:*** bilirubinemia, hepatic function abnormal, SGOT increased, SGPT increased; ***Metabolic/Nutritional:*** glycosuria, hyperuricemia, hyponatremia, increased alkaline phosphatase, thirst, vitamin B12 deficiency, weight increase, weight decrease; ***Musculoskeletal:*** arthralgia, arthritis aggravated, arthropathy, cramps, fibromyalgia syndrome, hernia, polymyalgia rheumatica; ***Nervous System/Psychiatric:*** anorexia, apathy, appetite increased, confusion, depression aggravated, dizziness, hypertonia, nervousness, hypoesthesia, impotence, insomnia, migraine, migraine aggravated, paresthesia, sleep disorder, somnolence, tremor, vertigo, visual field defect; ***Reproductive:*** dysmenorrhea, menstrual disorder, vaginitis; ***Respiratory:*** asthma aggravated, coughing, dyspnea, larynx edema, pharyngitis, rhinitis, sinusitis; ***Skin and Appendages:*** acne, angioedema, dermatitis, pruritus, pruritus ani, rash, rash erythematous, rash maculo-papular, skin inflammation, sweating increased, urticaria; ***Special Senses:*** otitis media, parosmia, taste loss, taste perversion; ***Urogenital:*** abnormal urine, albuminuria, cystitis, dysuria, fungal infection, hematuria, micturition frequency, moniliasis, genital moniliasis, polyuria; ***Visual:*** conjunctivitis, vision abnormal. Endoscopic findings that were reported as adverse events include: duodenitis, esophagitis, esophageal stricture, esophageal ulceration, esophageal varices, gastric ulcer, gastritis, hernia, benign polyps or nodules, Barrett's esophagus, and mucosal discoloration. Two placebo-controlled studies were conducted in 710 patients for the treatment of symptomatic gastroesophageal reflux disease. The most common adverse events that were reported as possibly or probably related to NEXIUM were diarrhea (4.3%), headache (3.8%), and abdominal pain (3.8%). Postmarketing Reports – There have been spontaneous reports of adverse events with postmarketing use of esomeprazole. These reports occurred rarely and are listed below by body system: ***Blood And Lymphatic System Disorders:*** agranulocytosis, pancytopenia; ***Eye Disorders:*** blurred vision; ***Gastrointestinal Disorders:*** pancreatitis; ***Hepatobiliary Disorders:*** hepatitis with or without jaundice; ***Immune System Disorders:*** anaphylactic reaction/shock; ***Musculoskeletal And Connective Tissue Disorders:*** myalgia; ***Psychiatric Disorders:*** depression; ***Skin and Subcutaneous Tissue Disorders:*** alopecia, erythema multiforme, Stevens-Johnson syndrome, toxic epidermal necrolysis (TEN, some fatal). Other adverse events not observed with NEXIUM, but occurring with omeprazole can be found in the omeprazole package insert, **ADVERSE REACTIONS** section.

**OVERDOSAGE** A single oral dose of esomeprazole at 510 mg/kg (about 103 times the human dose on a body surface area basis), was lethal to rats. The major signs of acute toxicity were reduced motor activity, changes in respiratory frequency, tremor, ataxia, and intermittent clonic convulsions. There have been some reports of overdosage with esomeprazole. Reports have been received of overdosage with omeprazole in humans. Doses ranged up to 2,400 mg (120 times the usual recommended clinical dose). Manifestations were variable, but included confusion, drowsiness, blurred vision, tachycardia, nausea, diaphoresis, flushing, headache, dry mouth, and other adverse reactions similar to those seen in normal clinical experience (see omeprazole package insert-**ADVERSE REACTIONS**). No specific antidote for esomeprazole is known. Since esomeprazole is extensively protein bound, it is not expected to be removed by dialysis. In the event of overdosage, treatment should be symptomatic and supportive. As with the management of any overdose, the possibility of multiple drug ingestion should be considered. For current information on treatment of any drug overdose, a certified Regional Poison Control Center should be contacted. Telephone numbers are listed in the Physicians' Desk Reference (PDR) or local telephone book. **DOSAGE AND ADMINISTRATION** Please see full Prescribing Information for recommended dosages and dosage adjustments for **Special Populations** for NEXIUM.



Distributed by: AstraZeneca LP, Wilmington, DE 19850
Product of France 31026-02 Rev. 04/06 240260

AstraZeneca

SECTION EDITOR: ALBERT C. YAN, MD; ASSISTANT SECTION EDITOR: SAMIR S. SHAH, MD

# Picture of the Month

*Jason S. Reichenberg, MD; Mark D. P. Davis, MD*

A PREVIOUSLY HEALTHY 15-YEAR-OLD BOY came to the emergency department with severe prostration associated with a worsening rash. The eruption had begun as red macules on his palms 4 days previously and rapidly progressed to involve all areas of his skin. He also had painful ulcerations in his mouth and uncomfortable redness of his eyes.

**Author Affiliations:** Department of Dermatology, Mayo Clinic, Rochester, Minn.

On physical examination, he was lethargic and hypotensive, with a blood pressure of 80/30 mm Hg. Discrete and confluent erythematous patches and plaques, many of which were targetoid (**Figure 1**), involved 95% of his skin. There was distinct palmar involvement (**Figure 2**) and central facial swelling with bilateral conjunctivitis (**Figure 3**). He had ulcerations in his mouth and on his glans penis.

What is your diagnosis?

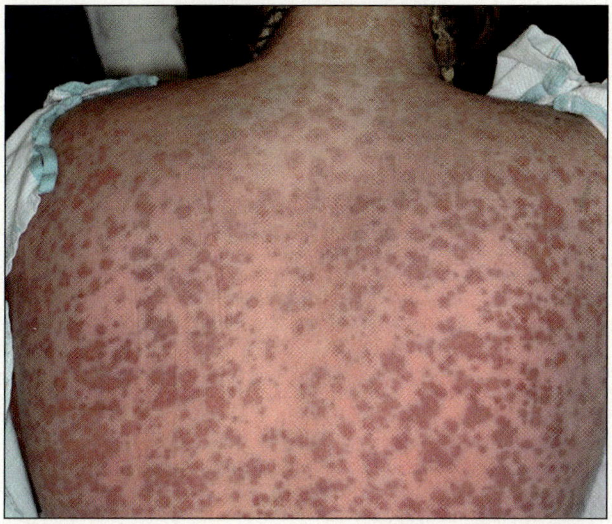

**Figure 1.** Patient's back showing discrete and confluent erythematous patches, many with a targetoid appearance, that involved approximately 95% of the trunk and extremities.

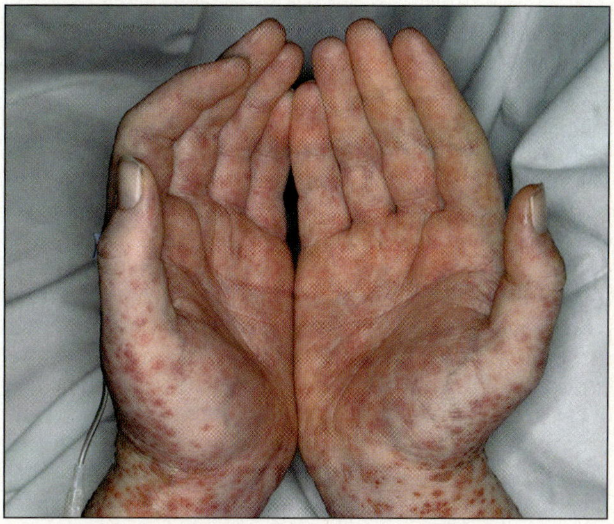

**Figure 2.** Targetoid macules and patches involving the palms.

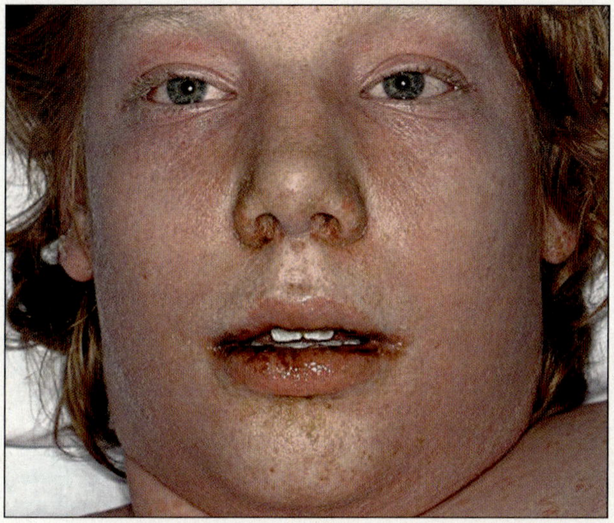

**Figure 3.** Facial edema, conjunctival injection, erosions, and crusting of lips.

# Denouement and Discussion

## *Stevens-Johnson Syndrome*

On the basis of the clinical findings, a diagnosis of Stevens-Johnson syndrome was made. The cause was identified to be a nonsteroidal anti-inflammatory drug, nabumetone, that the patient had begun taking 4 days before the skin eruption occurred for muscle soreness after a motor vehicle crash. Nabumetone administration was discontinued.

The patient was transferred to the intensive care unit for fluid resuscitation and pain control. Intravenous immunoglobulin was initiated at a dosage of 0.7 g/kg per day for 3 days. The patient's general condition stabilized. After 24 hours, new skin lesions stopped appearing. The lesions that were already present resolved over the following 3 to 4 weeks. The patient was discharged on hospital day 8 in good health with no sequelae.

Stevens-Johnson syndrome is a severe reactive condition affecting skin and mucosal surfaces. By definition, Stevens-Johnson syndrome has extensive skin involvement accompanied by erosions of at least 2 mucosal surfaces. It is often triggered by the administration of a medication, such as sulfamethoxazole, carbamazepine, phenytoin, nonsteroidal anti-inflammatory drugs, or allopurinol,[1,2] or by infection, such as with mycoplasma. Targetoid skin lesions, as in this patient, are characteristic. Individual lesions classically demonstrate central violaceous color bounded by pallor and a rim of erythema. Stevens-Johnson syndrome is associated with a high mortality rate. Intensive multidisciplinary supportive management and discontinuation of the causative drug or treatment of the underlying infection leading to the condition are the cornerstones of management. The use of corticosteroids in the treatment of Stevens-Johnson syndrome has been controversial because some case series[3-5] have shown increased mortality in these patients. This may be owing to the immunosuppressive effect of prolonged treatment and an increased susceptibility to infection. Although the use of intravenous immunoglobulin is not yet the standard of care, several small studies[6,7] have suggested that it may halt the progression of and decrease morbidity and mortality from toxic epidermal necrolysis; isolated case reports and a recent case series have documented similar benefits of intravenous immunoglobulin in Stevens-Johnson syndrome.[8]

**Accepted for Publication:** November 8, 2005.
**Correspondence:** Mark D. P. Davis, MD, Department of Dermatology, Mayo Clinic, 200 First Street SW, Rochester, MN 55905 (davis.mark2@mayo.edu).
**Author Contributions:** *Study concept and design:* Reichenberg and Davis. *Acquisition of data:* Reichenberg and Davis. *Drafting of the manuscript:* Reichenberg and Davis. *Critical revision of the manuscript for important intellectual content:* Reichenberg and Davis.

## REFERENCES

1. Roujeau JC, Kelly JP, Naldi L, et al. Medication use and the risk of Stevens-Johnson syndrome or toxic epidermal necrolysis. *N Engl J Med.* 1995;333:1600-1607.
2. Lin MS, Dai YS, Pwu RF, Chen YH, Chang NC. Risk estimates for drugs suspected of being associated with Stevens-Johnson syndrome and toxic epidermal necrolysis: a case-control study. *Intern Med J.* 2005;35:188-190.
3. Rasmussen JE. Erythema multiforme in children: response to treatment with systemic corticosteroids. *Br J Dermatol.* 1976;95:181-186.
4. Corticosteroids for erythema multiforme? *Pediatr Dermatol.* 1989;6:229-250.
5. Halebian PH, Corder VJ, Madden MR, Finklestein JL, Shires GT. Improved burn center survival of patients with toxic epidermal necrolysis managed without corticosteroids. *Ann Surg.* 1986;204:503-512.
6. Viard I, Wehrli P, Bullani R, et al. Inhibition of toxic epidermal necrolysis by blockade of CD95 with human intravenous immunoglobulin. *Science.* 1998;282:490-493.
7. Trent JT, Kirsner RS, Romanelli P, Kerdel FA. Analysis of intravenous immunoglobulin for the treatment of toxic epidermal necrolysis using SCORTEN: the University of Miami experience. *Arch Dermatol.* 2003;139:39-43.
8. Metry DW, Jung P, Levy ML. Use of intravenous immunoglobulin in children with Stevens-Johnson syndrome and toxic epidermal necrolysis: seven cases and review of the literature. *Pediatrics.* 2003;112:1430-1436.

### *Early Treatment for Hernia*

"Coffee, large doses, has certainly a remarkable influence in aiding or causing reduction of strangulated hernia."
—From *Materia Medica Pharmacy and Therapeutics*, 1906

**ACIP recommends vaccination of children against hepatitis A*[1]**

## Hepatitis A spreads FAST... especially among children[2,3]

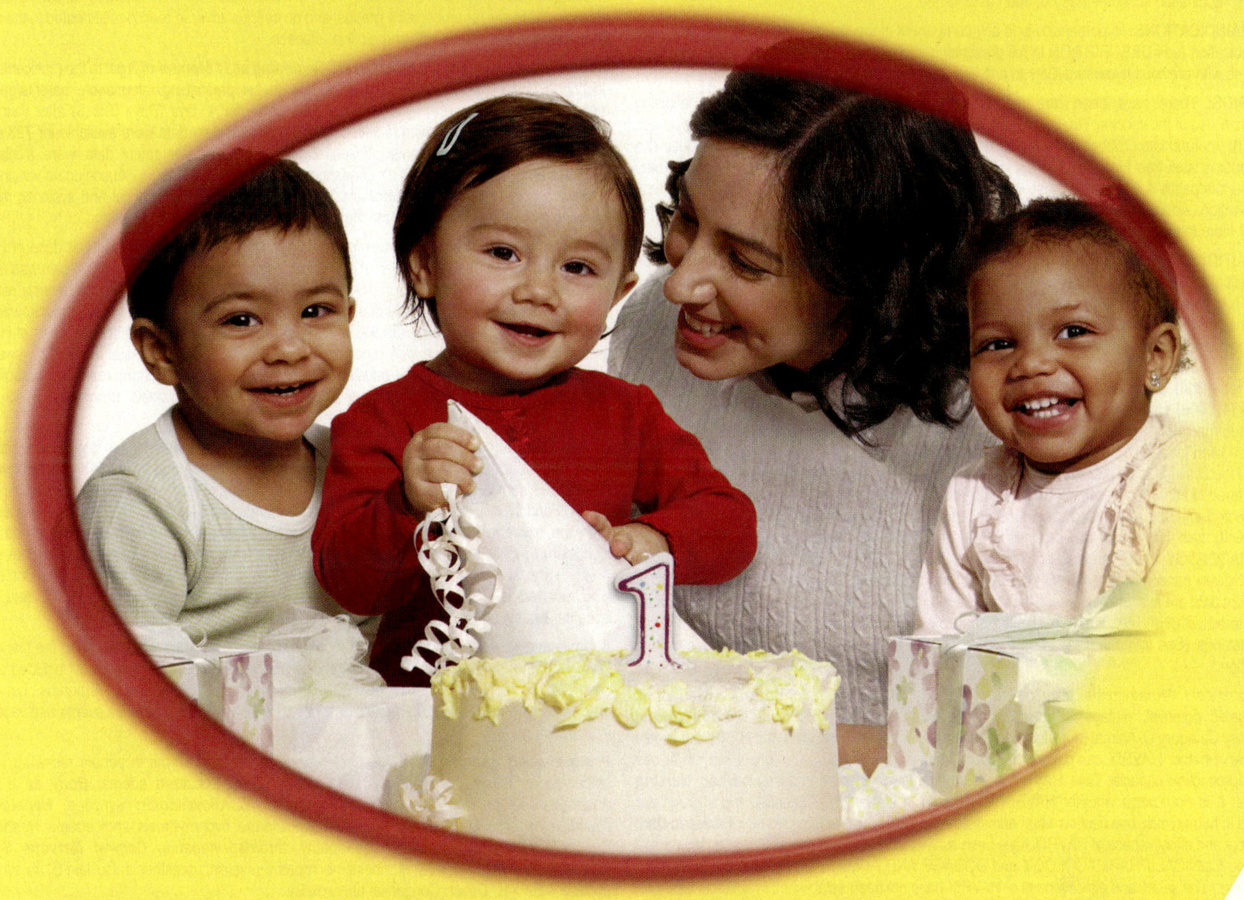

## HAVRIX provides excellent protection

HAVRIX is indicated for active immunization against hepatitis A virus in children 12 months of age and older.

## Important Safety Information

In clinical trials, the most common solicited adverse events were injection-site soreness and headache.

Greater incidences of general adverse events were observed in subjects who received HAVRIX at the same time as Hib conjugate and DTaP vaccines. As with any vaccine, rare adverse events may occur. (See Adverse Reactions section of the Prescribing Information for HAVRIX for potential side effects.) HAVRIX is contraindicated in people with hypersensitivity to any component of the vaccine, including neomycin.

* Advisory Committee on Immunization Practices recommends routine nationwide vaccination against hepatitis A in all children 1–2 years of age.

**Please see references and brief summary of complete prescribing information for HAVRIX on adjacent page.**



Manufactured by **GlaxoSmithKline Biologicals**, Rixensart, Belgium
Distributed by **GlaxoSmithKline**, Research Triangle Park, NC 27709

gsk GlaxoSmithKline Vaccines

**Havrix®**
**Hepatitis A Vaccine, Inactivated**

## HAVRIX®
## (Hepatitis A Vaccine, Inactivated)

The following is a brief summary only; see full prescribing information for complete product information.

**INDICATIONS AND USAGE:** HAVRIX is indicated for active immunization of persons ≥12 months of age against disease caused by hepatitis A virus (HAV). Primary immunization should be administered at least 2 weeks prior to expected exposure to HAV. When passive protection against hepatitis A is required either following exposure to hepatitis A virus or in persons requiring both immediate and long-term protection, HAVRIX may be administered concomitantly with immune globulin (IG) with different syringes and at different injection sites. Duration of immunity following a complete vaccination schedule has not been established.

**CONTRAINDICATIONS:** Hypersensitivity to any component of the vaccine, including neomycin, is a contraindication (see DESCRIPTION in full prescribing information). This vaccine is contraindicated in patients with previous hypersensitivity to any hepatitis A-containing vaccine.

**WARNINGS:** There have been rare reports of anaphylaxis/anaphylactoid reactions following commercial use of the vaccine. The tip cap and the rubber plunger of the needleless prefilled syringes contain dry natural latex rubber that may cause allergic reactions in latex sensitive individuals. The vial stopper is latex-free. Hepatitis A has a relatively long incubation period. Hepatitis A vaccine may not prevent hepatitis A infection in those who have an unrecognized hepatitis A infection at the time of vaccination. Additionally, it may not prevent infection in those who do not achieve protective antibody titers (although the lowest titer needed to confer protection has not been determined).

**PRECAUTIONS: General:** Prior to immunization with HAVRIX, the patient's current health status and medical history should be reviewed. The physician should review the patient's immunization history for possible vaccine sensitivity, previous vaccination-related adverse reactions and occurrence of any adverse–event-related symptoms and/or signs, in order to determine the existence of any contraindication to immunization with HAVRIX and to allow an assessment of benefits and risks. Appropriate medical treatment and supervision should be readily available for immediate use in case of a rare anaphylactic reaction following the administration of the vaccine. Epinephrine injection (1:1,000) and other appropriate agents used for the control of immediate allergic reactions must be immediately available. A separate, sterile syringe and needle or a sterile disposable unit should be used for each patient to prevent the transmission of other infectious agents from person to person. Needles should be disposed of properly and should not be recapped. As with any vaccine, if administered to immunosuppressed persons, including those receiving immunosuppressive therapy, the expected immune response may not be obtained. **Drug Interactions:** HAVRIX may be given concurrently with Hib conjugate vaccines in children 15 to 18 months of age (see CLINICAL PHARMACOLOGY in full prescribing information and ADVERSE REACTIONS). The safety of HAVRIX given concomitantly with INFANRIX has been evaluated (see ADVERSE REACTIONS). Insufficient data are available to assess the immune response of a fourth dose of DTaP vaccine when administered with HAVRIX. There are limited data to assess the concomitant use of HAVRIX with other vaccines. (See Immune Response to Concomitantly Administered Vaccines in full prescribing information.)

**Carcinogenesis, Mutagenesis, Impairment of Fertility:** HAVRIX has not been evaluated for its carcinogenic potential, mutagenic potential, or potential for impairment of fertility. **Pregnancy:** Pregnancy Category C. Animal reproduction studies have not been conducted with HAVRIX. It is also not known whether HAVRIX can cause fetal harm when administered to a pregnant woman or can affect reproduction capacity. Give HAVRIX to a pregnant woman only if clearly needed. **Nursing Mothers:** It is not known whether HAVRIX is excreted in human milk. Because many drugs are excreted in human milk, use caution when administering HAVRIX to a nursing woman. **Pediatric Use:** The safety and effectiveness of HAVRIX have been evaluated in 20,436 subjects 1 year to 18 years of age. (See CLINICAL PHARMACOLOGY and DOSAGE AND ADMINISTRATION in full prescribing information.) The safety and effectiveness of HAVRIX have not been established in subjects less than 12 months of age. **Geriatric Use:** Clinical studies of HAVRIX did not include sufficient numbers of subjects 65 years of age and older to determine whether they respond differently from younger subjects. Other reported clinical experience has not identified differences in overall safety between these subjects and younger adult subjects.

**ADVERSE REACTIONS:** As with all pharmaceuticals, however, it is possible that expanded commercial use of the vaccine could reveal rare adverse events. The adverse events most frequently reported by volunteers in clinical trials were injection-site soreness (56% of adults; 21% of children); headache (14% of adults; less than 9% of children). Other solicited and unsolicited events are listed below:

**Incidence 1% to 10% of Injections:** ***Local Reactions at Injection Site:*** Induration, redness, swelling; ***Body as a Whole:*** Fatigue, fever (>37.5°C), malaise; ***Gastrointestinal:*** Anorexia, nausea.

**Incidence <1% of Injections:** ***Local Reaction at Injection Site:*** Hematoma; ***Dermatologic:*** Pruritus, rash, urticaria; ***Respiratory:*** Pharyngitis, other upper respiratory tract infections; ***Gastrointestinal:*** Abdominal pain, diarrhea, dysgeusia, vomiting; ***Musculoskeletal:*** Arthralgia, elevation of creatine phosphokinase, myalgia; ***Hematologic:*** Lymphadenopathy; ***Central Nervous System:*** Hypertonic episode, insomnia, photophobia, vertigo.

**Additional safety data:** Safety data were obtained from 2 additional sources in which large populations were vaccinated. In an outbreak setting in which 4,930 individuals were immunized with a single dose of either 720 EL.U. or 1440 EL.U. of HAVRIX, the vaccine was well tolerated and no serious adverse events due to vaccination were reported. Overall, less than 10% of vaccinees reported solicited general adverse events following the vaccine. The most common solicited local adverse event was pain at the injection site, reported in 22.3% of subjects at 24 hours and decreasing to 2.4% by 72 hours.

In a field efficacy trial, 19,037 children received the 360 EL.U. dose of HAVRIX. The most commonly reported adverse events were injection-site pain (9.5%) and tenderness (8.1%), reported following first doses of HAVRIX. Other adverse events were infrequent and comparable to the control vaccine ENGERIX-B® [Hepatitis B Vaccine (Recombinant)].

In subjects with chronic liver disease, HAVRIX was safe and well tolerated. Local injection site reactions were similar among all 4 groups, and no serious adverse reactions attributed to the vaccine were reported in subjects with chronic liver disease.

***Safety Data for HAVRIX 720 EL.U./0.5 mL Beginning at 11 Months of Age:*** In the multicenter study described under CLINICAL PHARMACOLOGY in full prescribing information, parents/guardians recorded local and general symptoms on diary cards for 4 days (Days 0 to 3) after vaccination. In the 3 groups of children who received HAVRIX alone, safety data were available for 723 children who received 1,396 documented doses of HAVRIX. Additional safety data were available for 181 children who received HAVRIX coadministered with INFANRIX and Hib conjugate vaccine. Most adverse events were mild and transient. The frequencies of solicited local and systemic reactions following receipt of HAVRIX were monitored during the 4-day observation period.

The following rates of solicited adverse events in children who received their first dose of HAVRIX alone at between 11 and 25 months of age were observed. Among local reactions: pain was reported in 15-21% of subjects, redness in 16-21%, swelling in 8% of subjects. Among general reactions, irritability was reported in 24-36% of subjects, loss of appetite in 16-19% of subjects, drowsiness in 15-17% of subjects and fever >39.5°C in ≤2% of subjects. Following the booster dose of HAVRIX, among local reactions: pain was reported in 16-21% of subjects, redness in 17-22%, swelling in 8-10% of subjects. Following the booster dose of HAVRIX, among general reactions, irritability was reported in 19-29% of subjects, loss of appetite in 14-18% of subjects, drowsiness in 13-16% of subjects and fever >39.5°C in ≤1% of subjects.

Drowsiness and loss of appetite occurred at statistically significantly higher rates in subjects 15 to 18 months of age who received Hib conjugate vaccine (PRP-T) and INFANRIX concomitantly with HAVRIX as compared to subjects 15 to 18 months of age who received Hib conjugate vaccine (PRP-T) and INFANRIX (drowsiness 34% and 22% and loss of appetite 29% and 19%, respectively). With the exception of fever (>39.5°C), the solicited general symptoms occurred at statistically significantly higher rates in subjects 15 to 18 months of age who received Hib conjugate vaccine (PRP-T) and INFANRIX concomitantly with HAVRIX as compared to subjects 15 to 18 months of age who received HAVRIX alone (irritability 46% and 30%, drowsiness 34% and 17%, and loss of appetite 29% and 17%, respectively).

A febrile seizure was reported in an 18-month old subject two days after receiving the first dose of HAVRIX. Other serious adverse events reported during the course of this study included a single case each of hepatitis ~5 months post dose 1, insulin-dependent diabetes ~4 months post dose 1, and Kawasaki's disease ~3 1/2 months post dose 1. The association of these events with vaccination is unknown.

**Postmarketing Reports:** Rare voluntary reports of adverse events in people receiving HAVRIX since market introduction include the following: ***Local:*** Localized edema; ***Body as a Whole:*** Anaphylaxis/anaphylactoid reactions, somnolence; ***Cardiovascular:*** Syncope; ***Hepatobiliary:*** Jaundice, hepatitis; ***Dermatologic:*** Erythema multiforme, hyperhydrosis, angioedema; ***Respiratory:*** Dyspnea; ***Hematologic:*** Lymphadenopathy, thrombocytopenia; ***Central Nervous System:*** Convulsions, encephalopathy, dizziness, neuropathy, myelitis, paresthesia, Guillain-Barré syndrome, multiple sclerosis; ***Other:*** Congenital abnormality.

The US Department of Health and Human Services has established the Vaccine Adverse Events Reporting System (VAERS) to accept reports of suspected adverse events after the administration of any vaccine, including, but not limited to, the reporting of events required by the National Childhood Vaccine Injury Act of 1986. The toll-free number for VAERS forms and information is 1-800-822-7967. Reporting forms may also be obtained at the VAERS website at www.vaers.org.

Manufactured by **GlaxoSmithKline Biologicals**, Rixensart, Belgium

Distributed by **GlaxoSmithKline**, Research Triangle Park, NC 27709



BRS-HA:L20

**References: 1.** Centers for Disease Control and Prevention. Recommended childhood and adolescent immunization schedule—United States, 2006. *MMWR.* 2006;54(51&52):Q1–Q4. **2.** Bell BP, Shapiro CN. Hepatitis A virus. In: Long SS, Pickering LK, Prober CG, eds. *Principles and Practice of Pediatric Infectious Diseases.* 2nd ed. Philadelphia, Pa: Churchill Livingstone; 2003:1188–1192. **3.** Armstrong GL, Bell BP. Hepatitis A virus infection in the United States: model-based estimates and implication for childhood immunizations. *Pediatrics.* 2002;109:839–845.



Printed in USA. HAP283R0 February 2006

ARTICLE

# Socially Isolated Children 20 Years Later

## *Risk of Cardiovascular Disease*

*Avshalom Caspi, PhD; HonaLee Harrington, BS; Terrie E. Moffitt, PhD; Barry J. Milne, MSc; Richie Poulton, PhD*

**Objective:** To test the hypothesis that children who occupy peripheral or isolated roles in their peer groups (isolated children) are at risk of poor adult health.

**Design:** Longitudinal study of an entire birth cohort.

**Setting:** Dunedin, New Zealand.

**Participants:** A total of 1037 children who were followed up from birth to age 26 years.

**Interventions:** Measurement of social isolation in childhood, adolescence, and adulthood.

**Main Outcome Measures:** When study members were 26 years old, we measured adult cardiovascular multifactorial risk status (overweight, elevated blood pressure, elevated total cholesterol level, low high-density lipoprotein level, elevated glycated hemoglobin concentration, and low maximum oxygen consumption).

**Results:** Socially isolated children were at significant risk of poor adult health compared with nonisolated children (risk ratio, 1.37; 95% confidence interval, 1.17-1.61). This association was independent of other well-established childhood risk factors for poor adult health (low childhood socioeconomic status, low childhood IQ, childhood overweight), was not accounted for by health-damaging behaviors (lack of exercise, smoking, alcohol misuse), and was not attributable to greater exposure to stressful life events. In addition, longitudinal findings showed that chronic social isolation across multiple developmental periods had a cumulative, dose-response relationship to poor adult health (risk ratio, 2.58; 95% confidence interval, 1.46-4.56).

**Conclusions:** Longitudinal findings about children followed up to adulthood suggest that social isolation has persistent and cumulative detrimental effects on adult health. The findings underscore the usefulness of a life-course approach to health research, by focusing attention on the effect of the timing of psychosocial risk factors in relation to adult health.

*Arch Pediatr Adolesc Med. 2006;160:805-811*

THE NEED TO BELONG IS A fundamental human motivation that, when thwarted, compromises psychological health.[1,2] Loneliness and social isolation can also compromise physical health. Prospective studies have documented that lack of social support and social isolation in adulthood predict the future onset of coronary artery disease[3-5] and are related to the prognosis for adult patients with preexisting coronary artery disease.[6,7] However, emerging evidence from life-course epidemiology points to the importance of early life experiences in shaping adult disease.[8-10] In the present study, we observed a 1972-1973 cohort of children from birth to young adulthood and tested the hypothesis that children who occupy peripheral or isolated roles in their peer group are at significant risk of poor adult health. Because the cohort was still too young to present adverse clinical end points of cardiovascular disease (eg, myocardial infarction), we focused on multiple risk-factor clustering as a measure of adverse cardiovascular risk.[11-13]

Our first aim was to test whether childhood social isolation was an independent risk factor for poor adult health. We thus tested 3 alternative explanations for the link between social isolation and poor adult health.

A first alternative explanation, the *co-occurring risk hypothesis*, is that links between childhood isolation and poor adult health are spurious because both are associated with other well-established childhood risk factors for adult disease. We tested 4 such risk factors. First, some children may be socially isolated from their peers because they come from socioeconomically disadvantaged families, and children who grow up in families with low socioeconomic status (SES) have poor health in adulthood.[14] Second, some children may be

Author Affiliations: Department of Psychology, University of Wisconsin, Madison (Drs Caspi and Moffitt and Ms Harrington); Social, Genetic, and Developmental Psychiatry Centre, Institute of Psychiatry, King's College, London, England (Drs Caspi and Moffitt and Mr Milne); and Dunedin Multidisciplinary Health and Development Research Unit, Dunedin School of Medicine, University of Otago, Dunedin, New Zealand (Dr Poulton).

isolated because they are overweight,[15] and childhood overweight is a risk factor for poor adult health.[16,17] Third, some children may be isolated because they are mentally retarded or simply not very bright, and recent longitudinal research suggests that intelligence (as measured by IQ tests) predicts adult morbidity and mortality, including cardiovascular diseases.[18] Fourth, some children are isolated because they are aggressive and are thus rejected by their peers,[19] and longitudinal research suggests that aggression may be a risk factor for all-cause morbidity.[20] If childhood social isolation is an independent risk factor for adult poor health, it should survive controlling for all of these co-occurring childhood risk factors.

A second alternative explanation, the *health-behavior hypothesis,* is that socially isolated children develop poor health because they engage in health-compromising behaviors as adolescents or adults.[21] For example, they may become so socially disengaged that they lead increasingly sedentary lives and refrain from exercise. In addition, lonely children may smoke and drink more, possibly as a form of self-medication or as a way to gain approval from peers. In the present study, we measured these behaviors and tested whether childhood social isolation is related to poor adult health because isolated young people engage in more health-compromising behaviors.

According to the *differential-exposure hypothesis*, lonely children grow up to be exposed to more stress.[21] In the present study, we measured 3 potential stressors (low status attainment, stressful life events, and depression) and tested whether childhood social isolation is related to poor adult health because lonely children experience more stressful lives when they grow up.

Our second aim was to test the cumulative effects of social isolation on adult health, testing 2 interrelated hypotheses. First, we examined the *early-timing hypothesis,* testing whether childhood social isolation has an influence on adult health because it contributes to adult social isolation or because it may establish psychological and biological tendencies that independently affect adult health.[22] If childhood social isolation is linked to poor adult health simply because it is a developmental precursor of later social isolation, the association between childhood social isolation and poor adult health should be attenuated once adult social isolation is factored into the longitudinal analysis. If the longitudinal association remains significant, it would suggest that the distress created by social isolation early in life may erode health over time. Second, we examined the *cumulative stress hypothesis*, testing whether the duration of social isolation across multiple developmental periods bears a dose-response relationship to poor adult health.

## METHODS

### SAMPLE

Participants were members of the Dunedin Multidisciplinary Health and Development Study, a longitudinal investigation of health and behavior in a complete birth cohort.[23] Study members were born in Dunedin, New Zealand, between April 1, 1972, and March 31, 1973. Of these, 1037 children (91% of eligible births; 52% male) participated in the first follow-up assessment at age 3 years, constituting the base sample for the remainder of the study. Cohort families represented the full range of SES in the general population of New Zealand's South Island and were primarily white. Follow-up examinations were carried out at ages 5, 7, 9, 11, 13, 15, 18, 21, and, most recently, 26 years, when we assessed 980 (96.2%) of the 1019 study members still alive. Participants attended the research unit within 60 days of their birthday for a full day of individual data collection. The unit assumed study members' costs to remove all barriers to their participation, eg, travel, lost wages, and child care. The Otago Ethics Committee granted ethical approval for each phase of this longitudinal study. Study members gave informed consent before participating.

### SOCIAL ISOLATION MEASURES

#### Childhood Social Isolation

When study members were 5, 7, 9, and 11 years old, their parents and teachers completed the Rutter Child Scales.[24] Two items measure peer problems ("tends to do things on his/her own; is rather solitary" and "not much liked by other children"). Scores on these 2 items were averaged across the 4 time periods and by 2 reporters (Cronbach $\alpha$=0.77). Evidence shows that children who chronically experience negative peer relations have the worst prognosis, and repeated assessments of children's peer experiences are recommended for research purposes.[25]

#### Adolescent Social Isolation

When study members were 15 years old, they completed the inventory of peer attachment,[26,27] which assesses the extent to which adolescents feel integrated with their peers (eg, "I feel alone or apart when I am with friends" and "friends are concerned about my well-being" [reverse coded]). Scores were summed to derive a scale of adolescent social isolation (Cronbach $\alpha$=0.80).

#### Adult Social Isolation

When study members were 26 years old, we used 2 sources of information to identify socially isolated study members. First, we identified those who were not involved with any partner and/or had not dated at all in the past year (5%). Second, study members were interviewed about their social support networks and asked how many people (1) "make you feel liked or loved," (2) "can comfort you or calm you down," (3) "you can trust to keep the things you talk about private," and (4) "you can talk to when you are feeling down or blue." We identified those who said they had no one to provide any one of these emotional support roles (4%). We classified as "isolated" those who said they were not involved with any partner and had not dated at all in the past year or those who had no one to provide emotional support; 8% of the sample was so classified.

### CO-OCCURRING RISK FACTORS AND POTENTIAL MEDIATING VARIABLES

The SES of study members' families was measured with a 6-point scale assessing parents' occupational status. The scale places each occupation into 1 of 6 categories (from 1, professional to 6, unskilled laborer) on the basis of educational levels and income associated with that occupation in data from the New Zealand census.[9]

Height and weight measurements were taken at ages 5, 7, 9, and 11 years. Body mass index was calculated and standardized within each age and averaged across the 4 time periods to yield an index of childhood overweight.

The Wechsler Intelligence Scale for Children[28] was administered by trained psychometrists at ages 7, 9, and 11 years.[29] We averaged scores from the 3 age periods to form an overall score (mean, 106.4; SD, 14.46).

When study members were 5, 7, 9, and 11 years old, their parents and teachers rated whether each child "frequently fights with other children."[24] We created a childhood aggression scale by averaging these ratings (Cronbach $\alpha = 0.70$).[23]

We measured 3 health-damaging behaviors. First, the lack of vigorous exercise was assessed at age 26 years by asking study members to report how much time, in a typical week, they spent engaged in physical activity that "caused you to breathe hard or puff a lot, eg, working out at the gym, playing [a] sport, digging in the garden, or activity at work."[30] Because of the skewed nature of reported activity levels, quartiles were formed. Second, heavy smoking at age 26 years was defined as smoking 20 or more cigarettes per day (10% of the sample). Third, alcohol dependence was assessed at age 26 years using a reporting period of the past 12 months; 17% of the study members met *Diagnostic and Statistical Manual of Mental Disorders, Fourth Edition*[31] criteria for alcohol dependence.

We measured 3 adult stressors. First, low adult SES was measured with a 6-point scale assessing occupational status, as described in the first paragraph of this section. Second, stressful life events during the past 5 years (including problems with employment, finances, housing, disabling injuries, and partner relationships) were assessed at age 26 years.[32] Third, depression was assessed at age 26 years using a reporting period of the past 12 months; 17% of the study members met *Diagnostic and Statistical Manual of Mental Disorders, Fourth Edition*[31] criteria for a major depressive disorder.

## ADULT PHYSICAL HEALTH MEASURES

Physical examinations were conducted at age 26 years. We assessed health risk-factor clustering by measuring 6 biomarkers: weight, blood pressure, total cholesterol level, high-density lipoprotein cholesterol level, glycated hemoglobin concentration, and maximum oxygen consumption. (Pregnant women were excluded from the reported analyses.)

To determine overweight, we assessed body mass index (calculated as weight in kilograms divided by the square of height in meters) and waist girth (in centimeters). Study members were considered overweight if their body mass index was 30 or more or if their waist measurement was 88 cm or more for women or 102 cm or more for men[33,34]; 16% of the women and 10% of the men in the sample met this criterion.

Blood pressure (in millimeters of mercury) was assessed according to standard protocols.[35] Study members were considered to have high blood pressure if their systolic reading was 130 mm Hg or higher or if their diastolic reading was 85 mm Hg or higher[34]; 6% of the women and 26% of the men met this criterion.

Venipuncture was conducted at the same time each day (4:15-4:45 PM). Ninety percent of the sample consented. Nonfasting total cholesterol, high-density lipoprotein cholesterol, and glycated hemoglobin levels were measured in the serum.

Study members were considered to have an elevated total cholesterol level if their total cholesterol reading was 240 mg/dL (6.22 mmol/L) or greater[34]; 12% of the women and 12% of the men met this criterion.

Study members were considered to have a low high-density lipoprotein cholesterol level if the value was 40 mg/dL (1.04 mmol/L) or lower for men and 50 mg/dL (1.3 mmol/L) or less for women[34]; 32% of the women and 27% of the men met this criterion.

Glycated hemoglobin concentrations (expressed as a percentage of total hemoglobin) were measured by ion exchange high-performance liquid chromatography (Variant II; Bio-Rad, Hercules, Calif) (coefficient of variation, 2.4%), a method certified by the US National Glycohemoglobin Standardization Program (http://www.missouri.edu/~diabetes/ngsp.html). Following Blake et al,[36] study members were designated as having this health risk if their scores were in the top quartile (≥5.2%) of the cohort's distribution.

Maximum oxygen consumption adjusted for body weight (in milliliters per minute per kilogram) was assessed by measuring heart rate in response to a submaximal exercise test on a friction-braked cycle ergometer, and calculated by standard protocols.[37] Sex-specific quartiles were formed. Following Carnethon et al,[38] study members in the lowest quartile were considered to have this health risk.

We assessed multiple risk-factor clustering by summing the number of biomarkers on which the study member was at risk (range, 0-6; 35% of the study members had 0 risks; 35%, 1 risk; 16%, 2 risks; 10%, 3 risks; 3%, 4 risks; and 1%, ≥5 risks). Study members were "clustered" if they had at least 3 risk factors: 14% of the study members were clustered (13% of the women and 15% of the men).

## DATA ANALYSIS

We estimated the effect of social isolation on adult health, controlling for sex. We then expanded the regression equation to control for co-occurring childhood risk factors, health-damaging behaviors, and adult stress exposure. For these analyses linking childhood social to adult health outcomes, the total number in the cohort was 841. For sensitivity analyses, we conducted all analyses twice. First, we estimated regression models where the outcome was binary (1, clustered; 0, nonclustered), and in this article we report risk ratios (RRs) and 95% confidence intervals (CIs). Second, we estimated negative binomial regressions where the outcome was the summed number of biomarkers (0-6). The same pattern of associations was observed across both methods examined; tables showing the results from negative binomial regressions are available from the authors.

We tested the cumulative effects of social isolation on multiple risk-factor clustering in adulthood by using 2 steps. First, we conducted a regression analysis to estimate the unique effects of childhood social isolation, adolescent social isolation, and adult social isolation on adult clustering. Second, we estimated the effect of the linear combination of these 3 variables on adult risk-factor clustering. For these analyses, we had complete data for 810 study members.

# RESULTS

## CHILDHOOD ISOLATION AND ADULT HEALTH

**Table 1** shows the biomarker and risk-factor characteristics of nonclustered vs clustered participants. The regression analysis in **Table 2** (model 1) shows that a 1-SD change in childhood social isolation increased the risk of adult risk-factor clustering (defined as having adverse levels of ≥3 of the 6 adult biomarkers) by 1.37 (95% CI, 1.17-1.61). We tested whether the longitudinal association between childhood social isolation and adult clustering was confounded by 4 well-established risk factors for poor adult health (the co-occurring risk hypothesis). The regression analysis in Table 2 (model 2) shows that, even after controlling for these 4 childhood risk factors for poor adult health, the association between child-

**Table 1. Biomarker Characteristics and Risk-Factor Characteristics of Study Participants, According to Adult Cardiovascular Multifactorial Risk Status (Nonclustered vs Clustered)***

| | Full Sample (n = 841) | Nonclustered (n = 722) | Clustered (n = 119) |
|---|---|---|---|
| Biomarkers | | | |
| Overweight | | | |
| BMI | 25.1 (4.4) | 24.2 (3.5) | 30.2 (5.5) |
| Waist girth, cm | 80.3 (10.0) | 78.4 (8.2) | 92.1 (11.7) |
| Blood pressure, mm Hg | | | |
| Systolic | 116.9 (11.0) | 115.8 (10.1) | 123.8 (13.7) |
| Diastolic | 71.8 (9.4) | 71.1 (8.9) | 76.0 (11.5) |
| Total cholesterol, mg/dL | 193.0 (38.7) | 189.5 (34.8) | 224.3 (46.4) |
| HDL cholesterol, mg/dL | 54.1 (15.5) | 54.1 (15.5) | 42.5 (11.6) |
| Glycated hemoglobin, % of total hemoglobin | 5.0 (0.3) | 4.9 (0.3) | 5.1 (0.3) |
| $\dot{V}O_{2max}$, mL/min per kilogram | 44.4 (11.1) | 46.1 (10.6) | 34.1 (8.5) |
| Risk factors | | | |
| Sex, % F | 46.8 | 47.5 | 42.5 |
| Childhood social isolation† | 0 (1) | −0.11 (0.9) | 0.30 (1.1) |
| Low childhood social class† | 0 (1) | −0.05 (1.0) | 0.11 (1.1) |
| Childhood overweight† | 0 (1) | −0.07 (0.9) | 0.57 (1.3) |
| Low childhood IQ† | 0 (1) | −0.12 (0.9) | 0.14 (1.0) |
| Childhood aggression† | 0 (1) | −0.05 (1.0) | 0.26 (1.1) |
| Alcohol dependence, %‡ | 17.7 | 18.0 | 15.8 |
| Lack of exercise† | 0 (1) | −0.06 (1.0) | 0.22 (1.0) |
| Heavy smoking, %‡ | 10.2 | 9.5 | 14.3 |
| Low adult SES† | 0 (1) | −0.07 (1.0) | 0.20 (1.0) |
| Adult stressors† | 0 (1) | −0.01 (1.0) | 0.04 (1.0) |
| Diagnosis of depression, %‡ | 16.6 | 16.6 | 16.7 |
| Adolescent social isolation†§ | 0 (1) | −0.04 (1.0) | 0.25 (1.1) |
| Adult social isolation, %‡§ | 7.6 | 6.5 | 14.3 |

Abbreviations: BMI, body mass index (calculated as weight in kilograms divided by the square of height in meters); HDL, high-density lipoprotein; SES, socioeconomic status; $\dot{V}O_{2max}$, maximum oxygen consumption.

SI conversion factor: To convert cholesterol values to millimoles per liter, multiply by 0.0259.

*Multiple risk-factor clustering was defined in terms of a study member having at least 3 of the following 6 risk factors: overweight, elevated systolic and/or diastolic blood pressure, elevated serum total cholesterol level, low serum HDL cholesterol level, elevated glycated hemoglobin level, and low $\dot{V}O_{2max}$. Values are mean (SD) unless otherwise specified.

†These predictor variables were measured as continuous variables and entered into the analyses as *z* scores.

‡These predictor variables were measured as binary variables and entered into the analyses as dummy variables.

§For analyses using these social isolation variables, n = 810.

hood social isolation and adult clustering remained statistically significant: RR, 1.34; 95% CI, 1.10-1.64. Thus, the link between childhood social isolation and adult risk-factor clustering appeared to be independent of other well-established childhood risk factors for poor health.

We also tested whether the longitudinal association between childhood social isolation and adult risk-factor clustering was accounted for by the fact that isolated children later engaged in more health-damaging behaviors (the health-behavior hypothesis). After controlling for these potential health-damaging behaviors, the association between childhood social isolation and adult risk-factor clustering remained statistically significant: RR, 1.33; 95% CI, 1.13-1.56 (Table 2; model 3).

Finally, we tested whether the longitudinal association between childhood social isolation and adult clustering was mediated by isolated children's greater exposure to stress in adulthood (the differential-exposure hypothesis). After controlling for these potential mediators, the association between childhood isolation and adult risk-factor clustering remained statistically significant: RR, 1.37; 95% CI, 1.16-1.62 (Table 2; model 4).

## CUMULATIVE INFLUENCE OF SOCIAL ISOLATION ON ADULT HEALTH

Social isolation showed some continuity across the life course. Children who were rated by adults as socially isolated were likely to self-report that they were socially isolated in adolescence ($r=0.16$, $P<.001$), and social isolation in both childhood and adolescence increased the risk of social isolation in adulthood (RR, 1.37; 95% CI, 1.13-1.66; and RR, 1.61; 95% CI, 1.30-1.99, respectively).

**Table 3** shows the links between these 3 developmentally distinct assessments of social isolation and adult risk-factor clustering. The table highlights 4 findings. First, column A shows that social isolation was robustly linked to adult risk-factor clustering, whether isolation was assessed in childhood (RR, 1.37; 95% CI, 1.17-1.60), in adolescence (RR, 1.26; 95% CI, 1.04-1.52), or in adulthood (RR, 2.01; 95% CI, 1.20-3.36). Second, column A also shows that social isolation was linked to adult risk-factor clustering, whether isolation was measured via adults' reports about children's social isolation or via adolescents' and adults' own self-reports. Third, column B shows that, even after taking into account adult social isolation, child-

**Table 2. Association Between Childhood Social Isolation and Adult Cardiovascular Multifactorial Risk Status***

| | RR (95% CI) | | | |
|---|---|---|---|---|
| **Predictor Variables** | **Model 1: Baseline Bivariate Associations** | **Model 2: Co-occurring Childhood Risk Factors Hypothesis†** | **Model 3: Health-Damaging Behavior Hypothesis‡** | **Model 4: Differential Stress-Exposure Hypothesis§** |
| Sex | 1.19 (0.83-1.71) | 1.19 (0.80-1.86) | 1.27 (0.87-1.86) | 1.17 (0.79-1.74) |
| Childhood isolation‖ | 1.37 (1.17-1.61) | 1.34 (1.10-1.64) | 1.33 (1.13-1.56) | 1.37 (1.16-1.62) |
| Low childhood social class‖ | 1.15 (0.96-1.38) | 0.93 (0.76-1.15) | ... | ... |
| Childhood overweight‖ | 1.56 (1.35-1.81) | 1.54 (1.32-1.79) | ... | ... |
| Low childhood IQ‖ | 1.30 (1.07-1.58) | 1.27 (1.02-1.58) | ... | ... |
| Childhood aggression‖ | 1.27 (1.08-1.49) | 0.98 (0.79-1.21) | ... | ... |
| Alcohol dependence¶ | 0.88 (0.54-1.43) | ... | 0.81 (0.48-1.36) | ... |
| Lack of exercise‖ | 1.29 (1.07-1.55) | ... | 1.24 (1.02-1.49) | ... |
| Heavy smoking¶ | 1.47 (0.88-2.46) | ... | 1.36 (0.80-2.32) | ... |
| Low adult SES‖ | 1.27 (1.05-1.53) | ... | ... | 1.20 (0.98-1.47) |
| Adult stressors‖ | 1.05 (0.88-1.25) | ... | ... | 0.99 (0.81-1.20) |
| Diagnosis of depression¶ | 1.00 (0.62-1.62) | ... | ... | 1.03 (0.62-1.72) |

Abbreviations: CI, confidence interval; RR, risk radio; SES, socioeconomic status; ellipses, variable not included in model.

*Multiple risk-factor clustering was defined in terms of a study member having at least 3 of the following 6 risk factors: overweight, elevated systolic and/or diastolic blood pressure, elevated serum total cholesterol level, low serum high-density lipoprotein cholesterol level, elevated glycated hemoglobin level, and low maximum oxygen consumption.

†For model 2, −2 (log likelihood) = 594.1.

‡For model 3, −2 (log likelihood) = 675.2.

§For model 4, −2 (log likelihood) = 637.6.

‖These predictor variables were measured as continuous variables and entered into the regression equations as *z* scores.

¶These predictor variables were measured as binary variables and entered into the regression equations as dummy variables.

**Table 3. Cumulative Influence of Social Isolation on Adult Cardiovascular Multifactorial Risk Status***

| | RR (95% CI) | |
|---|---|---|
| | **A. Individual Contributions at Each Age†** | **B. Independent Contributions From All Ages‡** |
| Measured in childhood, via adults' reports§ | 1.37 (1.17-1.60) | 1.31 (1.11-1.56) |
| Measured in adolescence, via self-reports§ | 1.26 (1.04-1.52) | 1.16 (0.95-1.40) |
| Measured in adulthood, via self-reports‖ | 2.01 (1.20-3.36) | 1.70 (0.98-2.95) |
| Cumulative isolation across all ages¶ | ... | 2.58 (1.46-4.56) |

Abbreviations: CI, confidence interval; RR, risk ratio; ellipses, variable not included in model.

*Multiple risk-factor clustering was defined in terms of a study member having at least 3 of the following 6 risk factors: overweight, elevated systolic and/or diastolic blood pressure, elevated serum total cholesterol level, low serum high-density lipoprotein cholesterol level, elevated glycated hemoglobin level, and low maximum oxygen consumption.

†The individual contributions were estimated in 3 separate regression models, with sex as a covariate.

‡The independent contributions were estimated in a multivariate regression, with all measures of social isolation entered simultaneously along with sex as a covariate.

§These predictor variables were measured as continuous variables and entered into the regression equations as *z* scores.

‖This predictor variable was measured as a binary variable and entered into the regression equation as a dummy variable.

¶The effect of cumulative isolation was estimated as the combined effect of childhood social isolation plus adolescent social isolation plus adult social isolation, with sex as a covariate.

hood social isolation continued to be linked significantly to adult risk-factor clustering (RR, 1.31; 95% CI, 1.11-1.56). Fourth, the bottom row of Table 3 shows that social isolation was cumulatively linked to adult clustering; study members who occupied peripheral or isolated roles in their networks at multiple developmental periods were in worse health in adulthood (RR, 2.58; 95% CI, 1.46-4.56). The **Figure** documents the association between cumulative social isolation and adult clustering.

## COMMENT

The findings from this prospective longitudinal study are novel in 2 ways. First, whereas clinical and research interest in the association between social isolation and poor health has been generated by studies of adults,[7] the findings from this study provide, to our knowledge, the first evidence linking childhood social isolation to poor adult health. Our findings are consistent with a handful of retrospective studies reporting associations between chronic health conditions in adulthood and adults' retrospective reports of a perceived lack of social support in childhood.[39,40] There has been concern about the accuracy of long-term recall of childhood experiences,[41] but that is not an issue in this study because we collected data about childhood social isolation contemporaneously during childhood in the context of the longitudinal prospective investigation. In addition, the association between childhood social isolation and poor adult health was independent of other well-established childhood risk fac-

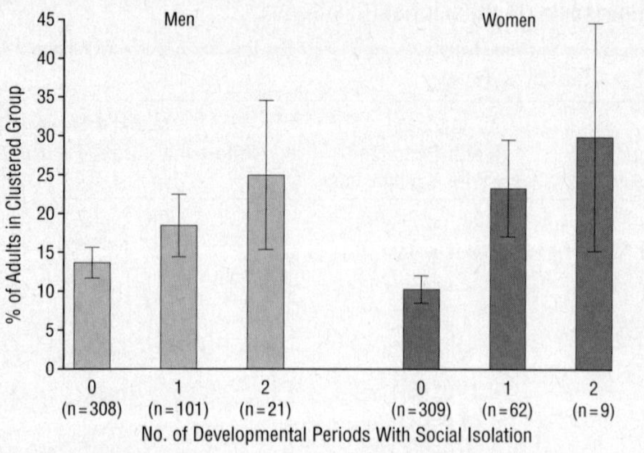


**Figure.** Association between cumulative social isolation and risk-factor clustering in adulthood. For illustrative purposes, study participants were considered isolated if they were in the top decile in each developmental period. Limit lines indicate standard error.

tors for poor adult health, including low childhood SES, low childhood IQ, and childhood overweight. Moreover, health-damaging behaviors did not account for the association between childhood social isolation and poor adult health. This is consistent with studies of adults[21,42] in which health-damaging behaviors did not account for the poor health of socially isolated individuals. Finally, the association between childhood social isolation and poor adult health was not accounted for by a greater exposure to stressful life circumstances among isolated children in adulthood.

Second, whereas studies of adults have pointed to an inverse gradient between social support and clinical outcomes,[7] the present study additionally documents that social isolation during multiple developmental periods (in childhood, adolescence, and adulthood) had a cumulative, dose-response relationship to poor adult health. A useful concept for understanding how repeated social isolation can lead to poor health is allostatic load,[43] which refers to the cumulative wear and tear caused by repeated adaptations to psychosocial stressors (such as social isolation) in childhood, adolescence, and adulthood. The experience of social isolation may be a form of chronic stress that activates the sympathetic nervous and hypothalamic-pituitary-adrenocortical systems and induces a variety of pathophysiologic responses that contribute to the clustering of risk factors for coronary artery disease (hypertension, insulin resistance, and central adiposity).[44,45] It is also possible that social isolation disrupts constructive and restorative processes that enhance physiological capacities, as suggested by evidence that lonely individuals experience disrupted sleep[46] and engage in passive rather than active coping strategies in their everyday lives.[47]

The new findings should be evaluated alongside several limitations. First, because we studied a cohort of children born only in the early 1970s, we are not yet able to assess disease outcomes; the study members are still too young. Instead, we focused on intermediate health risks that are known to predict future disease in midlife and old age.[11,12] Second, findings from this New Zealand cohort require replication in other parts of the world. However, there is reason to believe that these findings about the effect of childhood social isolation may be generalizable to other settings, given that our findings about the significance of other well-established childhood risk factors for poor adult health (eg, low childhood SES and childhood overweight) are consistent with findings reported from North American and European population-based studies.[48] Third, we do not know whether these findings can be generalized to all ethnic groups.

The findings from the present study underscore the usefulness of a life-course approach to health research.[8] The influence of psychosocial risk factors on the course of coronary artery disease is now well documented.[49] However, adult risk factors are the target of most research into the effect of psychosocial risk factors on poor adult health and on the pathogenesis of cardiovascular disease in particular. In contrast, a life-course perspective focuses attention on the effect of the developmental timing of psychosocial factors on adult health.[50,51] The findings from this longitudinal, observational study of children followed up from childhood to adulthood suggest that social isolation has persistent and cumulative effects on poor adult health. The findings appear to meet several criteria suggestive of a causal association between social isolation and adult health[52]: social isolation preceded the outcome, the association between isolation and health appeared to be independent of a wide range of correlated risk factors, the findings were consistent with reports from studies of adults about the link between their social isolation and poor health, and there was evidence of a dose-response relationship between duration of exposure to social isolation and poor adult health. The epidemiologic evidence cannot identify the mechanisms involved but is consistent with emerging evidence that social isolation and social exclusion may have tangible neurobiological effects on lifelong development.[2,53,54]

**Accepted for Publication:** January 28, 2006.
**Correspondence:** Avshalom Caspi, PhD, Institute of Psychiatry, SGDP Centre Mailbox P080, De Crespigny Park, London SE5 8AF, England (a.caspi@iop.kcl.ac.uk).
**Author Contributions:** *Study concept and design:* Caspi, Harrington, Moffitt, and Poulton. *Acquisition of data:* Caspi, Moffitt, and Poulton. *Analysis and interpretation of data:* Harrington and Milne. *Drafting of the manuscript:* Caspi, Harrington, and Milne. *Critical revision of the manuscript for important intellectual content:* Moffitt and Poulton. *Statistical analysis:* Caspi, Harrington, and Milne. *Obtained funding:* Caspi, Moffitt, and Poulton. *Administrative, technical, and material support:* Poulton. *Study supervision:* Moffitt.
**Funding/Support:** This study was supported by grants from the UK Medical Research Council, the National Institute of Mental Health, the William T. Grant Foundation, the National Heart Foundation of New Zealand, and the Health Research Council of New Zealand. Dr Moffitt is a Royal-Society Wolfson Research Merit Award holder.

## REFERENCES

1. Baumeister RF, Leary MR. The need to belong: desire for interpersonal attachments as a fundamental human motivation. *Psychol Bull.* 1995;117:497-529.
2. MacDonald G, Leary MR. Why does social exclusion hurt? the relationship between social and physical pain. *Psychol Bull.* 2005;131:202-223.
3. Berkman LF, Syme SL. Social networks, host resistance, and mortality: a nine-year follow-up study of Alameda County residents. *Am J Epidemiol.* 1979;109:186-204.
4. House JS, Robbins C, Metzner HL. The association of social relationships and activities with mortality: prospective evidence from the Tecumseh Community Health Study. *Am J Epidemiol.* 1982;116:123-140.
5. Kaplan GA, Wilson TW, Cohen RD, Kauhanen J, Wu M, Salonen JT. Social functioning and overall mortality: prospective evidence from the Kuopio Ischemic Heart Disease Risk Factor Study. *Epidemiology.* 1994;5:495-500.
6. Williams RB, Barefoot JC, Califf RM, et al. Prognostic importance of social and economic resources among medically treated patients with angiographically documented coronary artery disease. *JAMA.* 1992;267:520-524.
7. Rozanski A, Blumenthal JA, Kaplan J. Impact of psychological factors on the pathogenesis of cardiovascular disease and implications for therapy. *Circulation.* 1999;99:2192-2217.
8. Kuh D, Ben-Shlomo Y. *A Life Course Approach to Chronic Disease Epidemiology.* Oxford, England: Oxford University Press; 2004.
9. Poulton R, Caspi A, Milne BJ, et al. Association between children's experience of socioeconomic disadvantage and adult health: a life-course study. *Lancet.* 2002;360:1640-1645.
10. Wadsworth MEJ. Health inequalities in the life course perspective. *Soc Sci Med.* 1997;44:859-870.
11. Grundy SM, Pasternak R, Greenland P, Smith S Jr, Fuster V. Assessment of cardiovascular risk by use of multiple-risk-factor assessment equations: a statement for healthcare professionals from the American Heart Association and the American College of Cardiology. *J Am Coll Cardiol.* 1999;34:1348-1359.
12. Munoz A, Gange SJ. Methodological issues for biomarkers and intermediate outcomes in cohort studies. *Epidemiol Rev.* 1998;20:29-42.
13. Myers L, Coughlin SS, Webber LS, Srinivasan SR, Berenson GS. Prediction of adult cardiovascular multifactorial risk status from childhood risk factor levels: the Bogalusa heart study. *Am J Epidemiol.* 1995;142:918-924.
14. Galobardes B, Lynch JW, Davey SG. Childhood socioeconomic circumstances and cause-specific mortality in adulthood: systematic review and interpretation. *Epidemiol Rev.* 2004;26:7-21.
15. Strauss RS, Pollack HA. Social marginalization of overweight children. *Arch Pediatr Adolesc Med.* 2003;157:746-752.
16. Gunnell DJ, Frankel SJ, Nanchahal K, Peters TJ, Davey SG. Childhood obesity and adult cardiovascular mortality: a 57-y follow-up study based on the Boyd Orr cohort. *Am J Clin Nutr.* 1998;67:1111-1118.
17. Freedman DS, Dietz WH, Srinivasan SR, Berenson GS. The relation of overweight to cardiovascular risk factors among children and adolescents: the Bogalusa Heart Study. *Pediatrics.* 1999;103:1175-1182.
18. Gottfredson LS, Deary IJ. Intelligence predicts health and longevity, but why? *Curr Dir Psychol Sci.* 2004;13:1-4.
19. Rubin KH, Bukowski W, Parker JG. Peer interactions, relationships and groups. In: Eisenberger N, ed. *Social, Emotional and Personality Development.* New York, NY: John Wiley & Sons Inc; 1998:619-700. Damon W, ed. *Handbook of Child Psychology;* vol 3.
20. Laub JH, Vaillant GE. Delinquency and mortality: a 50-year follow-up study of 1,000 delinquent and nondelinquent boys. *Am J Psychiatry.* 2000;157:96-102.
21. Cacioppo JT, Hawkley LC, Bernston GG. The anatomy of loneliness. *Curr Dir Psychol Sci.* 2003;12:71-74.
22. Adler NE, Snibbe AC. The role of psychosocial processes in explaining the gradient between socioeconomic status and health. *Curr Dir Psychol Sci.* 2003;12:119-123.
23. Moffitt TE, Caspi A, Rutter M, Silva PA. *Sex Differences in Antisocial Behaviour: Conduct Disorder, Delinquency, and Violence in the Dunedin Longitudinal Study.* Cambridge, England: Cambridge University Press; 2001.
24. Elander J, Rutter M. Use and development of the Rutter parents' and teachers' scale. *Int J Methods Psychiatr Res.* 1996;6:63-78.
25. Asher SR, Paquette JA. Loneliness and peer relations in childhood. *Curr Dir Psychol Sci.* 2003;12:75-78.
26. Armsden GC, Greenberg MT. The inventory of parent and peer attachment: individual differences and their relationship to psychological well-being in adolescence. *J Youth Adolesc.* 1987;16:427-454.
27. Nada-Raja S, McGee R, Stanton WR. Perceived attachments to parents and peers and psychological well-being in adolescence. *J Youth Adolesc.* 1992;21:471-485.
28. Wechsler D. *Manual for the Wechsler Intelligence Scale for Children–Revised.* New York, NY: Psychological Corp; 1974.
29. Moffitt TE, Caspi A, Harkness AR, Silva PA. The natural history of change in intellectual performance: who changes? how much? is it meaningful? *J Child Psychol Psychiatry.* 1993;34:455-506.
30. Hopkins WG, Wilson NC, Russell DG. Validation of the physical activity instrument for the Life in New Zealand national survey. *Am J Epidemiol.* 1991;133:73-82.
31. American Psychiatric Association. *Diagnostic and Statistical Manual of Mental Disorders.* 4th ed. Washington, DC: American Psychiatric Association; 1994.
32. Caspi A, Sugden K, Moffitt TE, et al. Influence of life stress on depression: moderation by a polymorphism in the 5-HTT gene. *Science.* 2003;301:386-389.
33. National Institutes of Health. *Clinical Guidelines on the Identification, Evaluation, and Treatment of Overweight and Obesity in Adults.* Bethesda, Md: Dept of Health and Human Services, National Heart, Lung and Blood Institute, National Institutes of Health; 1998.
34. National Institutes of Health. *Third Report of the National Cholesterol Education Program (NCEP) Expert Panel on Detection, Evaluation and Treatment of Cholesterol in Adults (Adult Treatment Panel III).* Bethesda, Md: National Cholesterol Education Program, National Heart, Lung and Blood Institute, National Institutes of Health; 2001.
35. Perloff D, Grim C, Flack J, et al. Human blood pressure determination by sphygmomanometry. *Circulation.* 1993;88:2460-2470.
36. Blake GJ, Pradhan AD, Manson JE, et al. Hemoglobin $A_{1c}$ level and future cardiovascular events among women. *Arch Intern Med.* 2004;164:757-761.
37. Cullinane EM, Siconolfi S, Carleton RA, Thompson PD. Modification of the Astrand-Rhyming sub-maximal bicycle test for estimating VO2max of inactive men and women. *Med Sci Sports Exerc.* 1988;20:317-318.
38. Carnethon MR, Gidding SS, Nehgme R, Sidney S, Jacobs DR Jr, Liu K. Cardiorespiratory fitness in young adulthood and the development of cardiovascular disease risk factors. *JAMA.* 2003;290:3092-3100.
39. Russek LG, Schwartz GE. Perceptions of parental caring predict health status in midlife: a 35-year follow-up of the Harvard Mastery of Stress Study. *Psychosom Med.* 1997;59:144-149.
40. Shaw BA, Krause N, Chatters LM, Connell CM, Ingersoll-Dayton B. Emotional support from parents early in life, aging, and health. *Psychol Aging.* 2004;19:4-12.
41. Hardt J, Rutter M. Validity of adult retrospective reports of adverse childhood experiences: review of the evidence. *J Child Psychol Psychiatry.* 2004;45:260-273.
42. Seeman TE. Health promoting effects of friends and family on health outcomes in older adults. *Am J Health Promot.* 2000;14:362-370.
43. McEwen B. *The End of Stress as We Know It.* Washington, DC: Joseph Henry Press; 2002.
44. Rozanski A, Blumenthal JA, Davidson KW, Saab PG, Kubzansky L. The epidemiology, pathophysiology, and management of psychosocial risk factors in cardiac practice: the emerging field of behavioral cardiology. *J Am Coll Cardiol.* 2005;45:637-651.
45. Steptoe A, Owen N, Kunz-Ebrecht SR, Brydon L. Loneliness and neuroendocrine, cardiovascular, and inflammatory stress responses in middle-aged men and women. *Psychoneuroendocrinology.* 2004;29:593-611.
46. Cacioppo JT, Hawkley LC, Berntson GG, et al. Do lonely days invade the nights? potential social modulation of sleep efficiency. *Psychol Sci.* 2002;13:384-387.
47. Cacioppo JT, Hawkley LC, Crawford LE, et al. Loneliness and health: potential mechanisms. *Psychosom Med.* 2002;64:407-417.
48. Power C, Graham H, Due P, et al. The contribution of childhood and adult socioeconomic position to adult obesity and smoking behaviour: an international comparison. *Int J Epidemiol.* 2005;34:335-344.
49. Rosengren A, Hawken S, Ounpuu S, et al. Association of psychosocial risk factors with risk of acute myocardial infarction in 11 119 cases and 13 648 controls from 52 countries (the INTERHEART study). *Lancet.* 2004;364:953-962.
50. Elder GH, Johnson MK, Crosnoe R. The emergence and development of life course theory. In: Mortimer JT, Shanahan MJ, eds. *Handbook of the Life Course.* New York, NY: Plenum Publishing Corp; 2003:3-22.
51. Elder GH Jr, Shanahan MJ. The life course and human development. In: Lerner RM, ed. *Theoretical Models of Human Development.* New York, NY: John Wiley & Sons Inc; 2006:chap 12. Damon W, ed. *Handbook of Child Psychology;* vol 1.
52. Grimes DA, Schulz KF. Bias and causal associations in observational research. *Lancet.* 2002;359:248-252.
53. Eisenberger NI, Lieberman MD, Williams KD. Does rejection hurt? an fMRI study of social exclusion. *Science.* 2003;302:290-292.
54. McCabe PM, Gonzales JA, Zaias J, et al. Social environment influences the progression of atherosclerosis in the Watanabe heritable hyperlipidemic rabbit. *Circulation.* 2002;105:354-359.

ARTICLE

# Association Between Severity of Musculoskeletal Injury and Risk of Subsequent Injury in Children and Adolescents on the Basis of Parental Recall

*Glenn Keays, MS; Bonnie Swaine, PhD; Debbie Ehrmann-Feldman, PhD*

**Objectives:** To describe the frequency of subsequent injuries in children who were seen at an emergency department (ED) for a musculoskeletal injury and to explore factors associated with sustaining a subsequent injury within a year.

**Design:** This was a prospective cohort study of children aged 1 through 17 years who sought care at an ED for an injury. Subsequent injuries were assessed through telephone interviews.

**Setting:** Subjects were recruited from a national database of childhood injury after they presented to a hospital ED at 1 of the 2 pediatric trauma centers in Montreal, Quebec.

**Patients/Participants:** A consecutive sample of 7640 children aged 1 through 17 years who sought care for a fracture or a soft-tissue injury to an arm or a leg; 6182 completed both telephone interviews (80.9% response rate).

**Main Exposure:** Having a more severe injury was defined in 2 ways: (1) fracture of a limb or (2) injury that required follow-up or admission.

**Main Outcome Measure:** Having a subsequent injury during 12-month follow-up.

**Results:** : Subjects with an index fracture were at lower risk of subsequent injury than were those with a soft-tissue injury (13.5% compared with 17.7%; adjusted odds ratio, 0.74; 95% confidence interval, 0.63-0.87). Subjects whose injury needed a follow-up were also at lower risk of subsequent injury than those whose injury was treated only in the ED (17.7% compared with 14.3%; adjusted odds ratio, 0.79; 95% confidence interval, 0.67-0.93) as were those who were admitted (17.7% compared with 8.7%; adjusted odds ratio, 0.51; 95% confidence interval, 0.26-0.99).

**Conclusions:** Having had a severe musculoskeletal injury may be associated with a decreased risk of subsequent injury in children and adolescents. A possible explanation could be reduced exposure to risk.

*Arch Pediatr Adolesc Med. 2006;160:812-816*

AMONG CHILDREN WHO SEEK medical care for an injury, an estimated 73% have done so for more than 1 injury by age 9 years.[1] Between 15% and 32% of children younger than 18 years visited an emergency department (ED) within a year for at least 2 separate injury events.[2,3] Among children who had a fracture, 40% had another fracture before adulthood.[4]

In children, determinants of injury risk such as sex and age,[2,5] socioeconomic status,[6,7] and type of activity at the time of injury[8] are well known. Factors associated with risk of reinjury are somewhat similar to those associated with risk of injury and include sex,[1,2,9,10] age,[11,12] and socioeconomic status.[9,12,13]

Although information about the influence of severity of an initial injury on subsequent injury in children is scant, results of studies among adults suggest that severity of the first injury may be associated with risk of subsequent injuries. Results of one study[14] indicated that patients (mean age, 28.5 years) with severe injuries such as intracranial injury, fractures, and wounds to the head and neck, tend to have fewer subsequent injuries than do patients with more minor injuries such as muscle sprains. Authors of a study on injured soldiers observed that subjects who saw only a medic, as opposed to a physician, for their injury were at a 72% increased risk of sustaining a subsequent injury.[15]

It is important to identify additional characteristics of the children who are most at risk of subsequent injuries so appropriate prevention strategies can be developed. It is plausible that compared with children who have a mild injury, children who have a severe injury may learn ways to avoid future injury or may receive better medical and rehabilitation services that reduce potential residual motor problems and thus their risk of subsequent injury. The objectives of this

**Author Affiliations:** School of Public Health (Mr Keays) and Faculty of Medicine, School of Rehabilitation, Physiotherapy Program (Drs Swaine and Ehrmann-Feldman), University of Montreal, Quebec.

study were, therefore, to describe the frequency of subsequent injuries in children who were seen at an ED according to severity (defined by injury type and level of treatment) and to explore factors associated with sustaining a subsequent injury within a year.

## METHODS

Subjects were recruited through an injury surveillance system, the Canadian Hospitals Injury Reporting and Prevention Program,[16] in place at 2 tertiary care pediatric hospitals (Montreal Children's Hospital and Sainte-Justine Hospital) in Montreal, Quebec. These hospitals are designated trauma centers and have both participated in the program for more than a decade. Parents of children presenting for an injury to one of the participating hospital's EDs are asked to fill out a questionnaire detailing the circumstances of the injury event. For each patient, the diagnosis and site of the injury, as noted by the attending physician, are coded on the back of the form. Disposition is also coded according to level of treatment provided by the ED physician: treated only in ED, return appointment scheduled, or admitted to hospital.

Subjects were patients and their parents who filled out a Canadian Hospitals Injury Reporting and Prevention Program form between December 14, 2000, and March 31, 2003, at the participating hospitals and gave their consent to be telephoned with regard to the child's injury. They represent a subsample of children recruited as part of a larger study examining the risk of second head injury in children. In the context of this larger study, controls were recruited among those presenting to the ED with a musculoskeletal injury (fracture, laceration, sprain, and soft-tissue injury) to the extremities. Children who presented with any other injury were excluded. The present study examines risk of subsequent injuries among the total sample of controls (ie, children aged 1-17 years who did not have a head injury but who presented to the ED with a musculoskeletal injury to an arm or a leg). Of the consecutive sample of 7640 children (mean age, 10 years), 6182 completed both telephone interviews (80.9% response rate at 12 months) and thus were retained for analysis. Responders and nonresponders were highly comparable with respect to sex, age, type of index injury, treatment received for index injury, and body part involved.

Severity scores, such as the Abbreviated Injury Score and the Injury Severity Score, offer little help when trying to differentiate severity from a fracture from that of a sprain or a bruise of the forearm because both would be coded as minor (ie, less than 2 on a scale from 1 to 6).[17] We therefore chose to define severity according to type of injury (ie, we contend that upper or lower limb fractures usually require more medical services than do lacerations, bruises, and sprains) or level of treatment.

In addition to the injury data, telephone interviews with the parents were conducted by trained individuals at 6 and 12 months after the index ED visit to provide information about subsequent injuries. Parents were asked questions about whether their child sought medical care for any injury during the last 6 months. They also provided details about discharge recommendations for the index injury regarding activity restrictions, as well as the usual level of activity of their child compared with that of children of the same age, sex, and sociodemographic data (mother's educational level and parental structure). There were no specific questions pertaining to subsequent exposure (ie, whether the child stopped participating in some activities) among children with musculoskeletal index injuries.

The institutional review boards at both hospitals approved this study, and parents gave verbal consent to be interviewed.

The rate of subsequent injuries is reported according to the severity of the index injury by using 2 proxy measures: type of musculoskeletal injury (fracture vs soft tissue) and level of treatment provided in the ED. Univariate analyses were performed to determine the factors associated with subsequent injuries. These factors were patient related (age, sex, family structure, maternal educational level, and child's level of activity compared with children of the same age and sex) and index injury related (injury type, extremity injured, whether the child was involved in a recreational activity at time of injury, and if the child received discharge information about activity restrictions).

Multivariate analysis included the calculation of 2 logistic regression models to evaluate factors associated with risk of subsequent injuries: one with index injury type (fracture vs soft tissue) as the independent variable and the other with level of treatment received (treated only in ED, return appointment scheduled, or admitted to hospital) for the index injury. Covariates included patient-related and index injury–related variables. Statistical analyses were conducted with commercially available software (SPSS version 11.0; SPSS Inc, Chicago, Ill).

## RESULTS

There were 6182 children in our cohort: 58.5% were boys and 41.5% were girls; their mean ± SD age was 10 ± 4.5 years. The type of injuries were distributed as follows: 3262 had an index fracture (52.8%), and 2920 (47.2%) had an index soft-tissue injury (eg, laceration, sprain, or bruise). The overall rate of having a subsequent injury within a year of the index injury was 15.5% (n = 958); 513 patients (8.3%) reported a subsequent injury during the first 6 months and 445 patients (7.2%) reported another injury between 6 and 12 months following the index injury. Of those whose index injury was a fracture (n = 3262), 440 children (13.5%) reported seeking medical care for another injury within the following year compared with 518 children (17.7%) who had an initial soft-tissue injury. Across 12 months, children who sustained an index fracture were less likely to seek care for another injury compared with children who had an initial soft-tissue injury (odds ratio [OR], 0.72; 95% confidence interval [CI], 0.63-0.83).

Although there were more boys among the children who had index fractures than who had soft-tissue injuries (62.0% compared with 54.6%), for boys and girls, fractures were associated with a lower risk of subsequent injury. **Table 1** summarizes the results of the univariate analyses for 12 months.

Multiple logistic regression analysis confirmed that having had a fracture was associated with a lower risk of subsequent injury after adjusting for sex, age, lower extremity vs upper extremity, receipt of discharge information about return to activities, involvement in recreational activity at the time of index injury, activity level in comparison with that of other children of the same age and sex, maternal educational level, and parental structure (adjusted OR, 0.74; $P < .001$). Other factors associated with lower risk of subsequent injury were being less active than or equally as active as other children of the same age and sex, lower maternal education, and being aged 1 through 4 years (**Table 2**).

Compared with the OR for children who were treated only in the ED for their index injury, the OR for those who had a return appointment scheduled was 0.77 (95% CI, 0.67-0.89), and the OR for those admitted to the hospital was 0.45 (95% CI, 0.24-0.83) (Table 1). Control-

**Table 1. Univariate Analyses to Determine Association Between Index Injury and Patient-Related Variables and Subsequent Injuries**

| Characteristic | No. of Patients (N=6182) | Subsequent Injury, % Yes | Subsequent Injury, % No | Odds Ratio (95% Confidence Interval) |
|---|---|---|---|---|
| Type of injury | | | | |
| Soft-tissue injury | 2920 | 17.7 | 82.3 | 1.00 |
| Fracture | 3262 | 13.5 | 86.5 | 0.72* (0.63-0.83) |
| Level of treatment | | | | |
| Treated only in the emergency department | 2424 | 17.7 | 82.3 | 1.00 |
| Return appointment scheduled | 3632 | 14.3 | 85.7 | 0.77* (0.67-0.89) |
| Admitted to hospital | 126 | 8.7 | 91.3 | 0.45* (0.24-0.83) |
| Circumstances of the first injury | | | | |
| Received discharge information about when to return to physical activities | | | | |
| No | 2205 | 13.8 | 86.2 | 1.00 |
| Yes | 3977 | 16.4 | 83.6 | 1.22* (1.06-1.42) |
| Involved in recreational activity at time of index injury | | | | |
| No | 2886 | 12.9 | 87.1 | 1.00 |
| Yes | 3296 | 17.8 | 82.2 | 1.47* (1.28-1.69) |
| Extremity injured | | | | |
| Upper | 3838 | 14.6 | 85.4 | 1.00 |
| Lower | 2344 | 17.0 | 83.0 | 1.20* (1.05-1.38) |
| Patient characteristics | | | | |
| Age, y | | | | |
| 1 | 277 | 14.8 | 85.2 | 1.00 |
| 2-4 | 804 | 8.5 | 91.5 | 0.53* (0.35-0.81) |
| 5-9 | 1644 | 11.7 | 88.3 | 0.76 (0.53-1.10) |
| 10-14 | 2599 | 18.8 | 81.2 | 1.33 (0.94-1.89) |
| 15-18 | 858 | 19.6 | 80.4 | 1.40 (0.97-2.03) |
| Female | 2565 | 14.5 | 85.5 | 1.00 |
| Male | 3617 | 16.2 | 83.8 | 1.15 (0.99-1.32) |
| Child is considered more active than children of same age† | | | | |
| No | 3370 | 12.6 | 87.4 | 1.00 |
| Yes | 2796 | 19.0 | 81.0 | 1.63* (1.41-1.87) |
| Child lives with both parents† | | | | |
| No | 1167 | 16.6 | 83.4 | 1.00 |
| Yes | 4989 | 15.2 | 84.8 | 1.11 (0.94-1.32) |
| Mother has postsecondary education† | | | | |
| No | 1812 | 13.7 | 86.3 | 1.00 |
| Yes | 4189 | 16.0 | 84.0 | 1.20* (1.02-1.40) |

*Data are statistically significant at $P<.05$.
†Data do not add up to 6182 cases because some patients or parents did not answer.

ling for confounding factors in the multiple logistic regression model, this classification of severity yielded adjusted ORs that still were associated with lower risk of subsequent injury as the severity of index injury increased (**Table 3**). Other similarly associated factors were being aged 1 through 4 years, lower maternal education, and being less active than or equally as active as children of the same sex and age.

Finally, because a fractured limb, compared with a soft-tissue injury, is often immobilized for a longer time, thus limiting a child's exposure to participating fully in regular activities, we also examined the association between risk of subsequent injury and severity of index injury during the 6 to 12 months after the index injury. Of all the children who had a fracture, only 6.3% (205/3262) sought medical care for a subsequent injury during this period compared with 8.3% (242/2920) for those with a soft-tissue injury (OR, 0.75; 95% CI, 0.62-0.91). Although not a statistically significant finding, of the children whose index injury required follow-up or hospital admission, 6.6% sought medical care for a subsequent injury compared with 8.2% for those whose index injury was treated only in the ED (OR, 0.70; 95% CI, 0.42-1.17).

## COMMENT

The present study's results suggest that having had a severe index injury, defined by either injury type or level of treatment, compared with having had a minor injury to an extremity reduces the risk of subsequent injury. The observed overall rate of 15.5% for subsequent injury lies within the range found in other studies in which children with all types of injuries to all body regions (eg, 15%[2] and 32%[3]) were examined. Our results also concur with those of Williams et al[14] who found that patients (mean age, 28.5 years) with more severe injuries (defined as intracranial injury, fractures, and wounds to the head and neck) tended to have less subsequent injury than those with more minor injuries such as muscle sprains; their explanation involves a reduction of exposure because of limited activity levels in the more severely injured group. The level of treat-

**Table 2. Multiple Logistic Regression: Association Between Index Injury and Subsequent Injury**

| Type of Injury | Adjusted Odds Ratio (95% Confidence Interval) |
|---|---|
| Index injury (fracture) | 0.74* (0.63-0.87) |
| Circumstances of the first injury | |
| Received discharge information about when to return to physical activities | 1.01 (0.85-1.20) |
| Involved in recreational activity at time of index injury | 1.17 (0.99-1.37) |
| Lower extremity injured (vs upper) | 0.99 (0.84-1.17) |
| Patient characteristics | |
| Age, y | |
| 1 | 1.00 |
| 2-4 | 0.55* (0.36-0.83) |
| 5-9 | 0.76 (0.52-1.13) |
| 10-14 | 1.24 (0.85-1.81) |
| 15-18 | 1.16 (0.77-1.74) |
| Female | 1.00 |
| Male | 1.10 (0.95-1.27) |
| Child is considered more active than children of same age | 1.51* (1.31-1.75) |
| Child lives with both parents | 1.10 (0.92-1.32) |
| Mother has postsecondary education | 1.19* (1.01-1.40) |

*Data are statistically significant.

**Table 3. Multiple Logistic Regression: Association Between Level of Treatment and Subsequent Injury**

| Association Between Level of Treatment and Subsequent Injury | Adjusted Odds Ratio (95% Confidence Interval) |
|---|---|
| Level of treatment | |
| Treated only in the emergency department | 1.00 |
| Return appointment scheduled | 0.79* (0.67-0.93) |
| Admitted to hospital | 0.51 (0.26-0.99) |
| Circumstances of the first injury | |
| Received discharge information about when to return to physical activities | 1.00 (0.84-1.20) |
| Involved in recreational activity at time of index injury | 1.17 (0.99-1.37) |
| Lower extremity injured (vs upper) | 1.03 (0.88-1.21) |
| Patient characteristics | |
| Age, y | |
| 1 | 1.00 |
| 2-4 | 0.55* (0.36-0.83) |
| 5-9 | 0.76 (0.52-1.13) |
| 10-14 | 1.24 (0.85-1.81) |
| 15-18 | 1.17 (0.78-1.77) |
| Female | 1.00 |
| Male | 1.09 (0.94-1.27) |
| Child is considered more active than children of same age | 1.51* (1.31-1.75) |
| Child lives with both parents | 1.10 (0.92-1.32) |
| Mother has postsecondary education | 1.19* (1.01-1.40) |

*Data are statistically significant.

ment also was reported as a factor by Schneider et al[15] who observed a lower risk of subsequent injury for soldiers who sought more care for their injuries. As an explanation for these results, the authors remarked that these patients might not have sought sufficient care because medics are limited in the level of care they can provide, especially regarding activity restrictions.

Our results showed that the reduced risk of a severe injury was present as long as 12 months after the index injury. Although a severe injury could limit a child physically and diminish the child's exposure to further injuries, the follow-up of a year allowed for a potentially complete recovery from the index injury. In other words, the child's injury probably did not prevent the child from participating in sports for a whole year. Investigators in one study[18] found that children with fractures of long bones in their arms and legs reported being restricted in their activities for a maximum of 71 days.

The reduced exposure to risk can be explained from many angles. Physically, children with fractures in this study may have had a persistent reduced exposure. Psychologically, children with more severe injuries may have adopted safer behaviors when they returned to their activities to avoid a similar traumatic event. Also possible is a shift in parental attitude toward more risky activities; children with more severe injury may find themselves forbidden to continue practicing activities parents deem too dangerous.

Changes in behavior have been observed after milder as well as more serious injuries.[19] Gagnon et al[20] found that children who had a mild head injury appear to lack confidence in their ability to perform physical activities compared with their attitude before their injury. Subtle problems of balance and response time can persist for 12 weeks in children having sustained only a mild head injury.[20] It is unclear whether this difficulty is a result of a physiological effect (immature bone structure) or the result of behavioral or environmental differences in this age group.

When controlling for either injury type or level of treatment for the index injury, we found that being less active than or equally as active as other children of the same age and sex was associated with a lower risk of subsequent injury. Such children may participate less in high-risk activities such as sports or recreational activities (eg, skateboarding or cycling), thus reducing their risk of subsequent injury. Our findings of an association between mother's educational level and risk of subsequent injury do not concur with those of Brook and Heim.[12] Mothers with postsecondary education may be more likely to work outside the home, so their children receive less supervision. However, we believe that the relationship is better explained by mothers with postsecondary education being more easily able to afford the fees associated with organized sports activities, so these children have a greater exposure to injury-related events.

Our study has several limitations. We may not have collected all pertinent data to assess the influence of injury severity on possible subsequent injury. For example, data about preexisting medical conditions could not be collected (eg, osteogenesis imperfecta renders bones more susceptible to fractures[21]). The children classified with minor injuries may have had fractures that were undiagnosed at the time of presentation to the ED (ie, the calcium deposition was not yet visible on a radiograph). However, it is unlikely they were classified with minor injuries rather than more severe injuries because of lack of appropriate medical care. There also may be a bias toward parents of children classified with severe index injury being more inclined to seek medical care for a subsequent injury, even a minor one, than children whose index injury was not severe. In other words, the results may be explained partly by the possibility of confounding by health care use (ie, higher use by those with minor injury). Both of these scenarios, however, would lead to underestimation of the true association between a severe injury and the risk of subsequent injury. Finally, because this study was conducted in children who visited an urban trauma pediatric hospital within a universal health care system, generalizing these findings may be limited to these specific types of settings.

We were not able to identify specific reasons why a severe injury is associated with a lower risk of subsequent injuries. Psychological factors related to a child's return to activities might have played a role. Possibly, having had a severe injury may generate fear in children or parents so that they subsequently adopt safer behaviors.

Finally, these data are based on parental recall, so there is a potential for recall bias. Parents' recall of their child's injury diminishes with time and differs with the severity of the injury.[22] We cannot exclude the possibility that parents of children with soft-tissue injury were less able to recall consulting for a subsequent injury. If this is the case, it would not diminish the relationship but rather lead to underestimation of its true value.

This study's results suggest that children who had minor injuries are more likely to injure themselves again compared with children who had severe injuries. Possible explanations could include the minimization of some injuries, such as lacerations, bruises, and sprains, by society and clinicians. These results highlight the need for appropriate interventions in targeting children with injuries to prevent them from repeatedly injuring themselves. The time spent in the ED, although often short, could be an ideal setting for injury prevention. In conclusion, the results provide evidence that the severity of an injury to an arm or a leg is associated with the risk of sustaining another injury within the next 12 months.

**Accepted for Publication:** February 1, 2006.
**Correspondence:** Bonnie Swaine, PhD, School of Rehabilitation, Physiotherapy Program, University of Montreal, C.P. 6128, Succursale Centre-Ville, Montreal, Quebec, Canada H3C 3J7 (bonnie.swaine@umontreal.ca).
**Author Contributions:** *Study concept and design:* Keays, Swaine, and Ehrmann-Feldman. *Acquisition of data:* Keays and Swaine. *Analysis and interpretation of data:* Keays, Swaine, and Ehrmann-Feldman. *Drafting of the manuscript:* Keays, Swaine, and Ehrmann-Feldman. *Critical revision of the manuscript for important intellectual content:* Keays, Swaine, and Ehrmann-Feldman. *Statistical analysis:* Keays, Swaine, and Ehrmann-Feldman. *Obtained funding:* Swaine. *Administrative, technical, and material support:* Swaine. *Study supervision:* Keays, Swaine, and Ehrmann-Feldman.
**Funding/Support:** We acknowledge the financial support of the Canadian Institutes of Health Research. This research was conducted at the Research Center of the Centre de recherche interdisciplinaire en réadaption.

## REFERENCES


1. Spady DW, Saunders DL, Schopflocher DP, et al. Patterns of injury in children: a population-based approach. *Pediatrics.* 2004;113:522-529.
2. Scheidt PC, Harel Y, Trumble AC, et al. The epidemiology of nonfatal injuries among US children and youth. *Am J Public Health.* 1995;85:932-938.
3. Taylor BW, MacIntyre J, Forgeron P. Trauma recurrence in the pediatric emergency population. *J Trauma.* 1999;46:479-482.
4. Jones IE, Williams SM, Dow N, Goulding A. How many children remain fracture-free during growth? a longitudinal study of children and adolescents participating in the Dunedin Multidisciplinary Health and Development Study. *Osteoporos Int.* 2002;13:990-995.
5. Rivara FP, Bergman AB, LoGerfo JP, Weiss NS. Epidemiology of childhood injuries, II: sex differences in injury rates. *Am J Dis Child.* 1982;136:502-506.
6. Danseco ER, Miller TR, Spicer RS. Incidence and costs of 1987-1994 childhood injuries: demographic breakdowns. *Pediatrics.* 2000;105:e27. http://pediatrics.aappublications.org/cgi/content/full/105/2/e27. Accessed May 5, 2006.
7. Durkin MS, Davidson LL, Kuhn L, O'Connor P, Barlow B. Low-income neighborhoods and the risk of severe pediatric injury: a small-area analysis in northern Manhattan. *Am J Public Health.* 1994;84:587-592.
8. Rivara FP, Calonge N, Thompson RS. Population-based study of unintentional injury incidence and impact during childhood. *Am J Public Health.* 1989;79:990-994.
9. Sayfan J, Berlin Y. Previous trauma as a risk factor for recurrent trauma in rural northern Israel. *J Trauma.* 1997;43:123-125.
10. Kaufmann CR, Branas CC, Brawley ML. A population-based study of trauma recidivism. *J Trauma.* 1998;45:325-332.
11. Pless IB, Millar W. Unintentional injuries in childhood: results from Canadian health surveys. 2000. http://www.phac-aspc.gc.ca/dca-dea/publications/pdf/unintentional_e.pdf. Accessed May 5, 2006.
12. Brook U, Heim M. Accidents among high school pupils in Israel: a recurrent disease? *Patient Educ Couns.* 1997;31:237-242.
13. Wilkins R, Houle C, Berthelot J, et al. *The Changing Health Status of Canada's Children.* Montreal, Quebec: Presses de l'Université de Montréal; 2000.
14. Williams JM, Furbee PM, Hungerford DW, et al. Injury recidivism in a rural ED. *Ann Emerg Med.* 1997;30:176-180.
15. Schneider GA, Bigelow C, Amoroso PJ. Evaluating risk of re-injury among 1214 army airborne soldiers using a stratified survival model. *Am J Prev Med.* 2000;18:156-163.
16. Mackenzie SG, Pless IB. CHIRPP: Canada's principal injury surveillance program—Canadian Hospitals Injury Reporting and Prevention Program. *Inj Prev.* 1999;5:208-213.
17. Durbin DR, Winston FK, Applegate SM, et al. Development and validation of the injury severity assessment survey/parent report: a new injury severity assessment survey. *Arch Pediatr Adolesc Med.* 1999;153:404-408.
18. Kopjar B, Wickizer TM. Fractures among children: incidence and impact on daily activities. *Inj Prev.* 1998;4:194-197.
19. Shalev AY, Freedman S, Peri T, et al. Prospective study of posttraumatic stress disorder and depression following trauma. *Am J Psychiatry.* 1998;155:630-637.
20. Gagnon I, Swaine B, Friedman D, Forget R. Exploring children's self-efficacy related to physical activity performance after a mild traumatic brain injury. *J Head Trauma Rehabil.* 2005;20:436-449.
21. Kocher MS, Shapiro F. Osteogenesis imperfecta. *J Am Acad Orthop Surg.* 1998;6:225-236.
22. Cummings P, Rivara FP, Thompson RS, Reid RJ. Ability of parents to recall the injuries of their young children. *Inj Prev.* 2005;11:43-47.


"It's kind of fun to do the impossible."
–Walt Disney

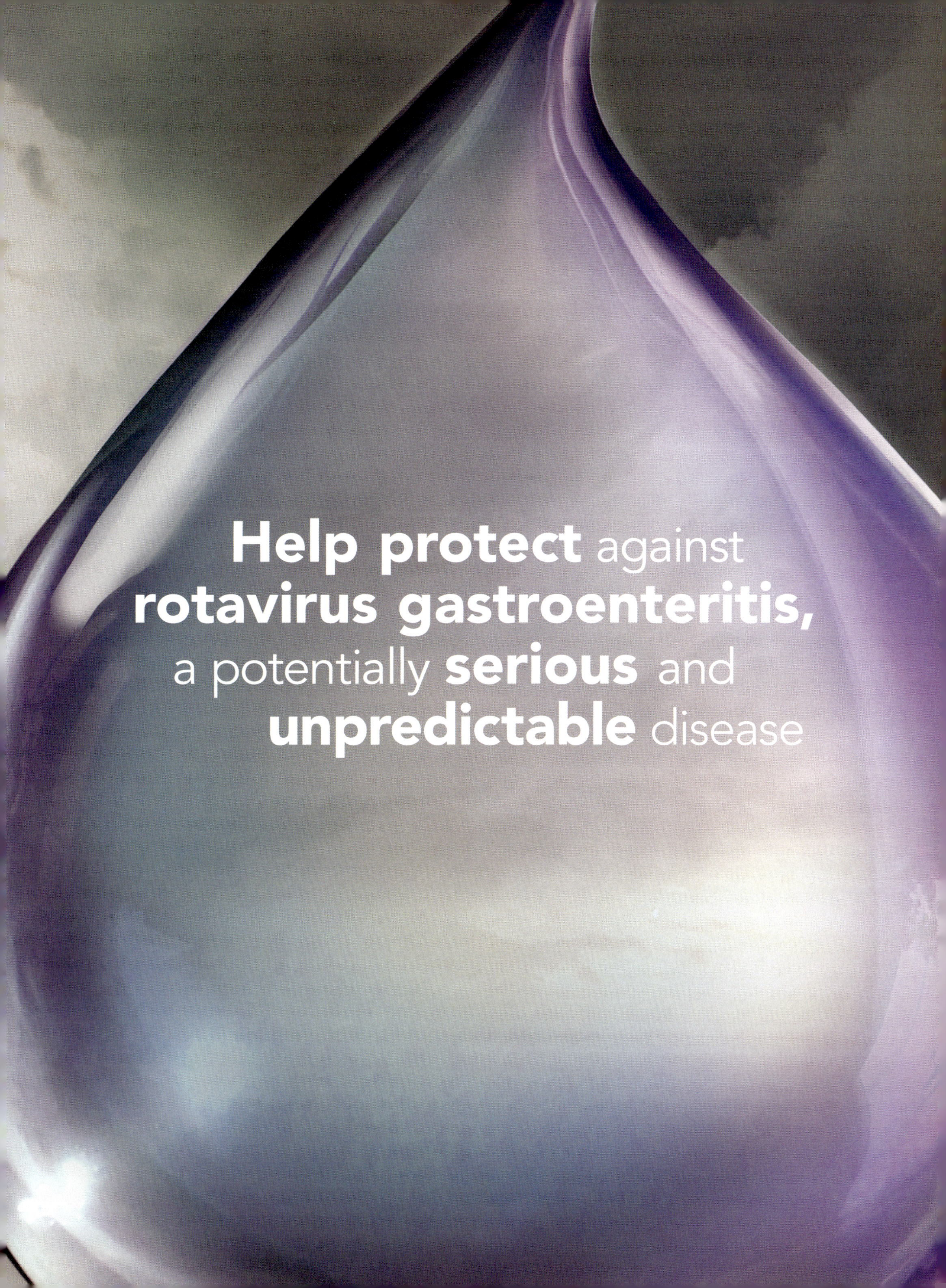

Help protect against
rotavirus gastroenteritis,
a potentially serious and
unpredictable disease

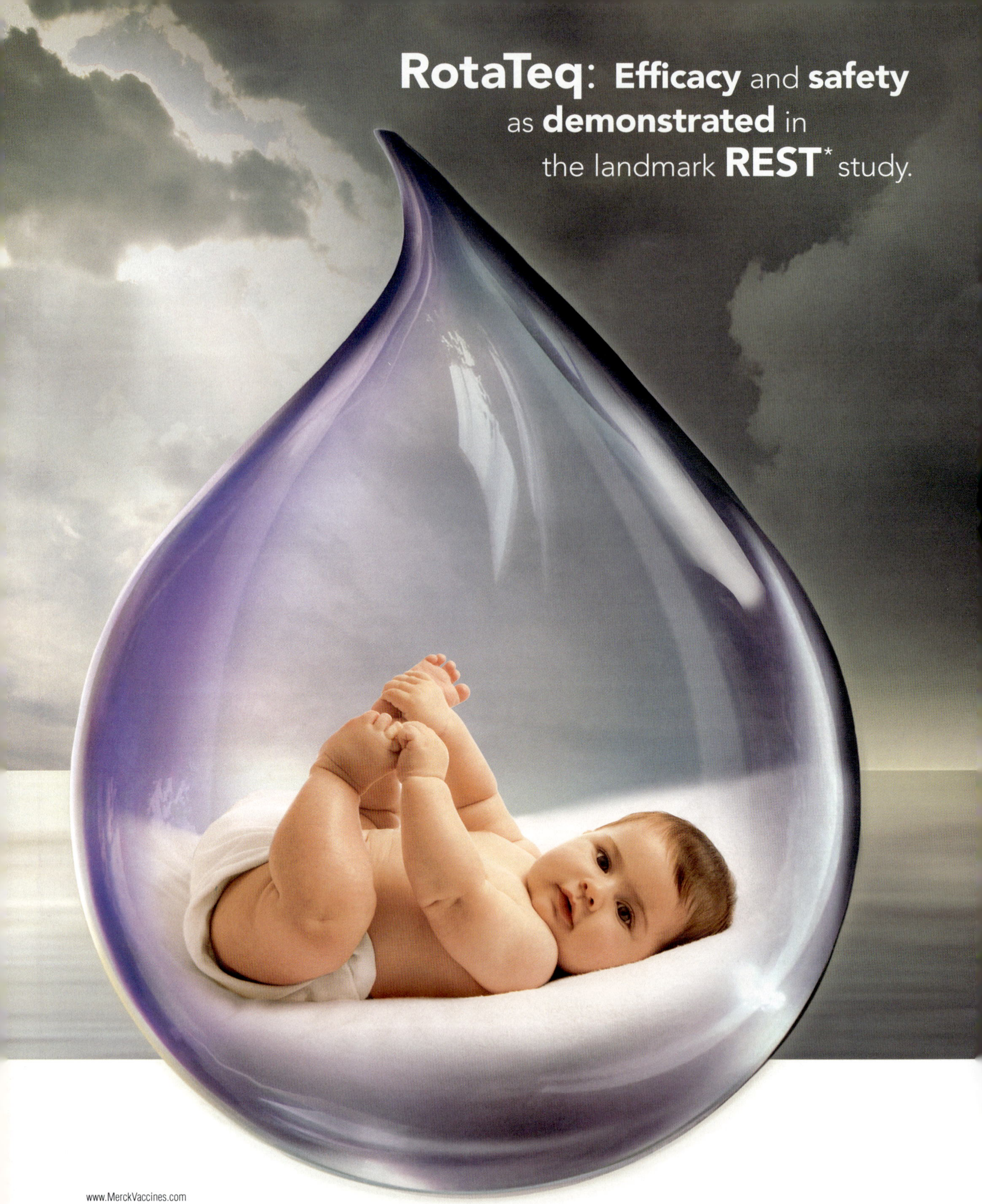
RotaTeq: Efficacy and safety
as demonstrated in
the landmark REST* study.

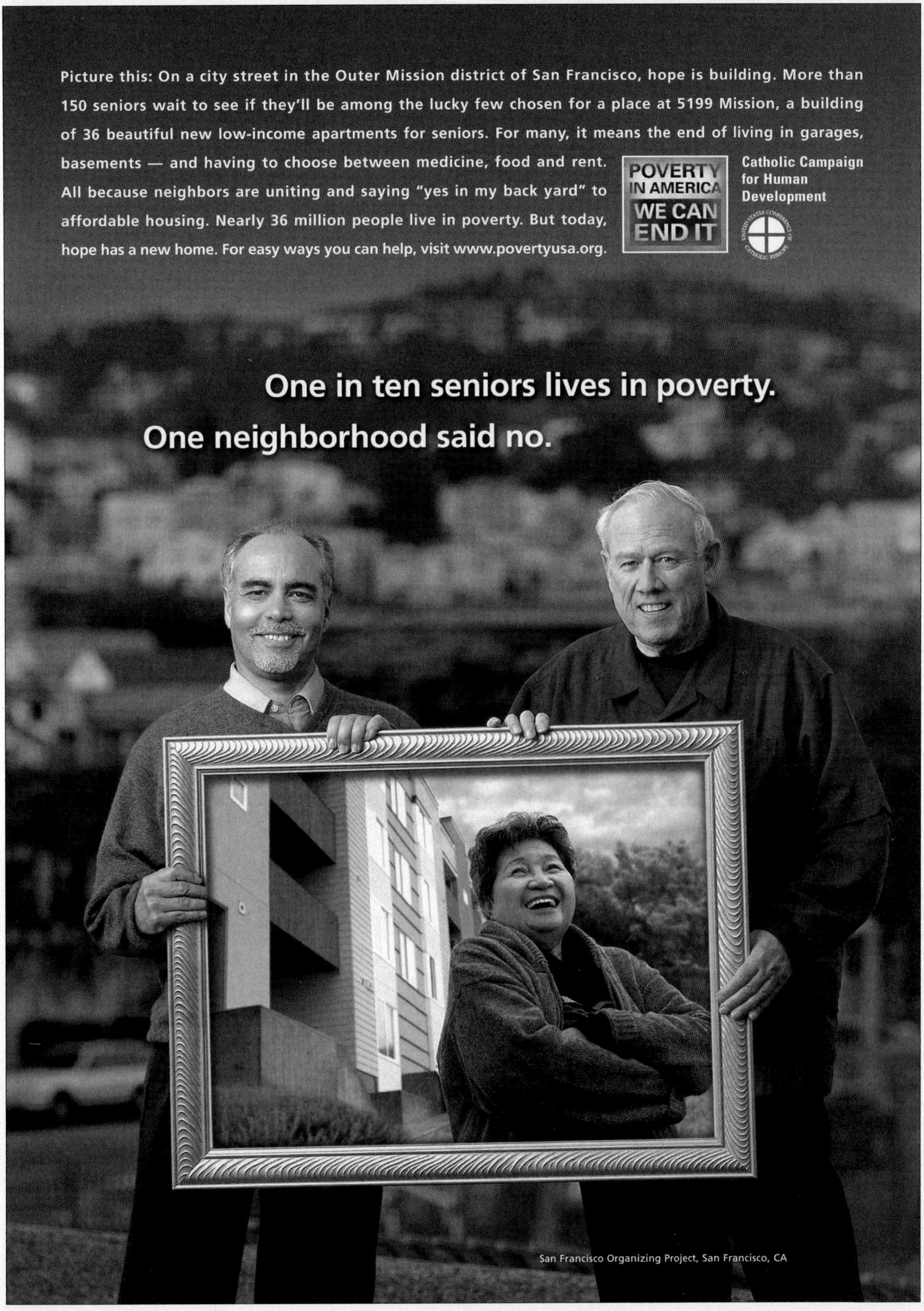
Picture this: On a city street in the Outer Mission district of San Francisco, hope is building. More than 150 seniors wait to see if they'll be among the lucky few chosen for a place at 5199 Mission, a building of 36 beautiful new low-income apartments for seniors. For many, it means the end of living in garages, basements — and having to choose between medicine, food and rent. All because neighbors are uniting and saying "yes in my back yard" to affordable housing. Nearly 36 million people live in poverty. But today, hope has a new home. For easy ways you can help, visit www.povertyusa.org.
POVERTY IN AMERICA
WE CAN END IT
Catholic Campaign for Human Development
UNITED STATES CONFERENCE OF CATHOLIC BISHOPS
One in ten seniors lives in poverty.
One neighborhood said no.
San Francisco Organizing Project, San Francisco, CA

ARTICLE

# Psychotropic Medication Use in Pediatric Patients With Cancer

*Maryland Pao, MD; Elizabeth D. Ballard; Donald L. Rosenstein, MD; Lori Wiener, PhD; Alan S. Wayne, MD*

**Background:** Use of psychotropic medication in medically ill adults, in particular, patients with cancer, is common. While increased use of psychotropic medications in children and adolescents in the general population has been reported, little is known about the prescribing practices for these medications in medically ill children.

**Objective:** To examine the frequency and types of psychotropic medications used in a population of children and adolescents with cancer.

**Design:** Retrospective review of the National Institutes of Health Medical Information System.

**Setting:** Pediatric Oncology Branch of the National Cancer Institute, National Institutes of Health.

**Participants:** Three hundred forty-seven patients aged 1 to 21 years who were enrolled in clinical research trials at the Pediatric Oncology Branch between January 2000 and December 2003.

**Main Outcome Measures:** Psychotropic medication use was analyzed according to cancer diagnosis and patient age.

**Results:** Fourteen percent of identified patients had been prescribed at least 1 psychotropic medication at the time of National Cancer Institute clinical trial enrollment. The most commonly used medications were anticonvulsant agents (8%) and antidepressant medications (7%), in particular, selective serotonin reuptake inhibitors. Anxiolytic medications could not be accurately assessed because of their frequent use as antiemetic agents in many chemotherapy regimens. Psychostimulant use was rare.

**Conclusions:** This study suggests that psychotropic medications are commonly prescribed to children and adolescents with cancer. Clinical safety and efficacy trials are needed in medically ill children at high risk for mood and anxiety symptoms.

*Arch Pediatr Adolesc Med. 2006;160:818-822*

CANCER IS THE SECOND leading cause of death in children aged 5 to 14 years and is the leading cause of nonacute death in children.[1] Nevertheless, more children are surviving into adulthood, with 5-year survival rates significantly improving from 59% in 1974-1976 to 79% in 1995-2000.[2] The diagnosis of a life-threatening illness in a child or adolescent is frequently associated with anxiety and depression. The judicious use of psychotropic medications may improve the quality of life for some youth with cancer who have persistent distress or posttreatment psychological and physical symptoms.

Use of psychotropic medications in children and adolescents has been a controversial topic over the last few decades.[3-6] The prescription rate for psychotropic drugs in the pediatric population has reached an estimated 5.9% to 6.3%, with stimulant and antidepressant agents most commonly prescribed.[7] Even as the frequency of use of psychotropic medications in children approaches that in adults, little research data exist on the efficacy, safety, and pharmacokinetics of these medications in children.[8]

Data on the administration of psychotropic medications in medically ill children are even more elusive. To our knowledge, no cross-sectional study has examined use of psychotropic medications in children with medical illness, specifically, cancer. A 2005 report by Kersun and Kazak[9] found that half of pediatric oncologists at a major children's hospital reported prescribing selective serotonin reuptake inhibitors for pediatric patients. Most oncologists who prescribed these antidepressants had prescribed more than 1 selective serotonin reuptake inhibitor, often without input from a psychologist or a psychiatrist. Beyond this study and clinical case reports on behav-

**Author Affiliations:** Office of the Clinical Director, National Institute of Mental Health (Drs Pao and Rosenstein and Ms Ballard), Pediatric Oncology Branch, Center for Cancer Research, National Cancer Institute (Drs Wiener and Wayne), National Institutes of Health, Bethesda, Md.

ioral effects of psychotropic medications,[10-15] little psychopharmacologic research has been reported in children with cancer or other medical illnesses.

Recognition of the need to treat distress, particularly depression, in adults with cancer began in the 1970s.[16] A study from 1979 reported that more than half of adult patients with cancer from 5 medical centers were given at least 1 psychotropic agent.[17] By 1998, an investigation by Cullivan et al[18] of adult patients with cancer referred to a psycho-oncology service showed that in more than half, a psychotropic medication had been started before referral; the most common agents were tranquilizers, followed by antidepressants. Despite numerous trials, treatment of depression with antidepressants in adult patients with cancer has shown encouraging trends toward effectiveness, but with no definitive conclusions.[19]

Despite the absence of definitive clinical data, antidepressants may be useful in treating symptoms of depressed mood in patients with cancer, such as pain, gastrointestinal tract distress, wasting, fatigue, anxiety, and cognitive impairment.[20] Symptom researchers, including Cleeland et al,[20] have posited that these symptoms might be biologically associated with a type of sickness behavior similar to behavior produced in animals with lipopolysaccharide-induced bacterial infections. Sickness behavior and concomitant depressed mood may be considered an expected outcome of cancer.[21] Recent data suggest that prophylaxis with selective serotonin reuptake inhibitors might be beneficial in preventing symptoms of depression in patients with cancer receiving chemotherapy.[22] In a recent open-label trial (n=15), fluvoxamine was shown to improve symptoms of depression and anxiety in children and adolescents with cancer.[23] Antidepressants and other psychotropic medications can be used as tools to improve the quality of life in patients with cancer.

Published studies of depression and anxiety in children with chronic medical problems, including cancer, are highly limited. While depression has not been shown to be more common in medically ill children compared with healthy children, symptoms of depression are commonly reported in this population.[24,25] The difficulty in assessing and treating depression in medically ill children underscores the need for further investigation.[24-27] This retrospective study examines the use of psychotropic medication in pediatric patients with cancer enrolled in clinical trials and suggests new directions for further research.

## METHODS

The Medical Information System of the National Institutes of Health (NIH) was reviewed retrospectively for all patients aged 1 to 21 years entering Pediatric Oncology Branch, National Cancer Institute (POB-NCI) clinical research trials between January 1, 2000, and December 31, 2003. The study was approved by the NIH Office of Human Subjects Research. Three hundred forty-seven patients were identified, and their electronic medical records were reviewed further for cancer diagnoses and psychotropic medication information. Oncologic diagnoses were grouped as sarcomas, leukemias and lymphomas, brain tumors, and other cancers. No distinction was made between recurrent and nonrecurrent cancers. While many patients (>50) participated in multiple clinical trials at the NIH, only the psychotropic medication regimen active at the time of a patient's first trial enrollment during the study period was recorded. The duration and dosage of treatment, and indications and efficacies of the prescriptions were unavailable through the Medical Information System and could not be reported. Ten additional patients who received psychotropic medication only during subsequent years were excluded from the study analysis. The psychotropic medications reviewed are listed in **Table 1**; the category of antidepressants includes selective serotonin reuptake inhibitors, tricyclic antidepressants, and novel antidepressants. Lorazepam, diphenhydramine, opiate agents, and zolpidem were excluded from the review because these medications are commonly used in protocols for cancer treatment. Univariate analyses were used to describe demographic characteristics and the prevalence of psychotropic medication use.

**Table 1. Medications Reviewed***

| Type of Medication | |
|---|---|
| Antidepressants | |
| Fluoxetine† | Mirtazapine† |
| Sertraline† | Bupropion |
| Paroxetine† | Trazodone† |
| Citalopram† | Amitriptyline† |
| Escitalopram† | Desipramine† |
| Fluvoxamine | Nortriptyline† |
| Venlafaxine† | |
| Antianxiolytics | |
| Clonazepam† | Alprazolam† |
| Mood stabilizers | |
| Lithium | Oxcarbazepine |
| Valproate | Gabapentin† |
| Carbamazepine† | Lamotrigine |
| Antipsychotics | |
| Haloperidol† | Quetiapine |
| Risperidone | Ziprasidone |
| Olanzapine | Aripiprazole |
| Stimulants | |
| Methylphenidate† | Dextroamphetamine |
| Other | |
| Atomoxetine | Guanfacine |
| Clonidine† | Propranolol |

*Nefazodone, thorazine, and clozapine were excluded from the search because of black box warnings or possible neutropenia. Diphenhydramine, lorazepam, opiates, and zolpidem are commonly prescribed and were excluded.

†Prescribed in study population.

## RESULTS

Patient demographics are given in **Table 2**. Cancer diagnoses are shown in the **Figure**. Diagnoses are representative of the research focus of the POB-NCI and do not represent the prevalence of cancer in the general pediatric oncology population. The older age of the patients with sarcoma (mean age, 14.6 years) compared with patients with brain tumors (mean age, 9 years), leukemia or lymphomas (mean age, 10.3 years), and other cancers (mean age, 11.8 years) reflects the expected age distribution of pediatric cancers.

The rate of psychotropic medication use in children entering NCI pediatric oncology protocols was 14% over-

**Table 2. Demographic Characteristics of Study Subjects***

| Characteristic | Total Patients | Patients Receiving Medications |
|---|---|---|
| Patients | 347 | 49 (14) |
| Age, y | | |
| Range | 1-21 | 3-21 |
| Mean | 12.3 | 15.9 |
| Sex | | |
| Female | 142 (41) | 20 (41) |
| Male | 205 (59) | 29 (59) |
| Diagnoses | | |
| Sarcoma | 153 (44) | 37 (76) |
| Leukemia/lymphoma | 109 (32) | 3 (6) |
| Brain tumor | 42 (12) | 3 (6) |
| Other cancer | 43 (12) | 6 (12) |

*Data are expressed as number (percentage) unless otherwise indicated.

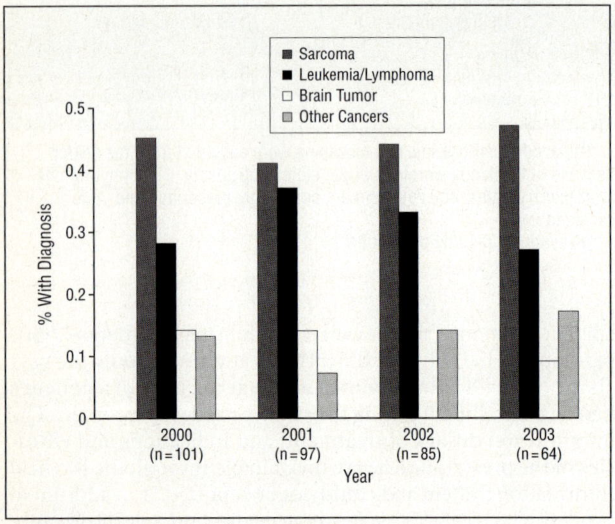


**Figure.** Diagnoses of the patient population.

all, ranging from 12% to 16% by study year. Patients receiving psychotropic medications tended to be older ($t=-5.76$; $P<.001$), with only 6 patients younger than 12 years. The most commonly prescribed medications in these patients were anticonvulsants (37%), with gabapentin (n=36) the most prescribed agent in this class. Antidepressants (35%) followed, with sertraline (n=13) being the most commonly prescribed agent. Use of stimulant, antipsychotic, or other psychotropic medications was rare. Forty-five percent (n=22) of the patients prescribed psychotropic medications were prescribed more than 1 class of psychotropic medication.

## COMMENT

The NIH Clinical Center provides a unique setting for evaluation of the use of psychotropic medications in children during participation in cancer treatment trials. Our data show that this population of pediatric patients with cancer are prescribed psychotropic medications at more than twice the rate in children in the general population (5.9%-6.3%).[7] Sarcoma was the most common cancer in our patients prescribed psychotropic medications (n=37), which may reflect disease-specific factors. For example, patients with sarcoma often require multimodal treatment including surgery, chemotherapy, and radiation therapy. In addition, pain and altered body image are common consequences of these therapies (Patrick Mansky, MD and colleagues; unpublished data, 2006). While not included in the univariate analysis, 10 additional patients received psychotropic medications after enrolling in protocols at the NCI. Together, these findings suggest a possible relationship between psychotropic medication use and illness severity, duration, and treatment intensity. Furthermore, these statistics may underestimate rates of psychotropic medication use in the pediatric oncology population because anxiolytic drugs such as lorazepam and opiate medications were excluded.

Certain results from this retrospective review are striking. The rare use of psychostimulants was unexpected, especially in comparison with prevalence rates in the non–medically ill pediatric population. These patients, in particular, might have had low rates of behavioral, attentional, or internalizing problems, which may account for the low frequency of antipsychotic and psychostimulant use. Also, the physicians might have had an unknown preference for antidepressant and anticonvulsant agents. An analysis by Jensen et al[28] has shown stimulants to be one of the best researched classes of psychotropic medications in children for both efficacy and safety. While these agents have been suggested to have limited clinical applications in children without a psychiatric disorder,[29] psychostimulants may still be useful in pediatric patients with cancer by treating fatigue, poor concentration, and opiate-induced sedation.

The frequent use of mood stabilizers and antidepressants in this population of children with cancer was not unexpected. Mood stabilizers, such as gabapentin, are used in the treatment of peripheral neuropathy, which is commonly associated with both cancer and adverse effects of therapy (eg, tumor compression, surgery, and treatment with vinca alkaloids). Gabapentin has been shown to be well tolerated in childhood epilepsy and has applications in pediatric pain relief.[30] Although gabapentin is a less potent mood stabilizer, it has been associated with treatment of mood in children.[31] Other mood stabilizers, such as carbamazepine and valproic acid, are thought to be less clinically useful in medically ill pediatric patients because of delayed onset of action, drug interactions, and multiple toxicities (eg, hepatic, hematologic, and metabolic abnormalities).[29] Tricyclic antidepressants are also often used to treat insomnia and pain in pediatric populations.

Despite controversy about the use of antidepressants in children and adolescents, a published report suggests that these agents are prescribed by approximately half of pediatric oncologists.[9] This practice suggests that physicians are responding to clinically significant symptoms. Most children with terminal cancer have been described by their parents as having fatigue, pain, dyspnea, gastrointestinal tract symptoms, and "no fun" toward the end of life.[32] While end-of-life issues were not addressed in this study, all children with cancer have these symptoms at some point, and some may find relief from the use of psychotropic medications during the course of their cancer treatment. Treatment of symptom clusters such as depressed mood and fatigue in cancer has been gaining acceptance[33] because psychopharmacologic treatment for subthreshold psychiatric disorders may improve the quality of life in pediatric patients with cancer.

Multiple contributions to symptoms of mood and anxiety disorders, such as illness severity, duration of illness, school absences, parental separation, activity limitations, and adverse effects of cancer treatments, are not ameliorated by psychotropic medication. Psychopharmacologic management is not intended to replace other comprehensive and multimodal interdisciplinary support or treatment of psychological symptoms and pain but to serve as an adjunct treatment when symptoms become debilitating. Further research to determine the efficacy of each medication class is needed to close the clinical practice gap[28] in this medically ill population.

This retrospective investigation has a number of limitations. The method used to identify patients could not account for repeat patients who were enrolled before 2000. Anxiolytic agents could not be adequately assessed because of the frequent use of lorazepam in cancer treatment. Multiple medication use, cancer onset, and treatment, and neither the onset nor duration of cancer were assessed. Medication treatment and duration and the indications for and efficacy of the medication use could not be assessed beyond the point of entry into a protocol. While patients with brain tumors are at risk for seizures, no patients with brain tumors in this study (n=42) received an anticonvulsant drug from the NIH. Since the black box warning on antidepressants in October 2004, a substantial decline in antidepressant prescription frequency has been reported, with a possible increase in atypical antipsychotic prescription in children and adolescents.[34] It is unclear whether these changes will be found in medically ill populations as well. Medications prescribed by non-NIH providers may not have been recorded in the computer records, leading to underestimation of usage.

Children and adolescents participating in NCI trials comprise a select population of families within a single institution with the motivation to participate in clinical trials. Consequently, these patients may not be representative of or directly generalizable to the general population. Many of these patients have more severe illness than seen in the general population with cancer, but yearly, on average, 13 patients with newly diagnosed sarcoma were enrolled in pediatric oncology trials at the NCI, showing that the study population is comparable with pediatric oncology clinic samples.

This study was undertaken as an initial step in investigating the psychopharmacologic treatment of mood and anxiety symptoms in children with cancer. While symptom relief is a concern in this population, we recommend a comprehensive assessment for psychiatric syndromes when treating pediatric patients with cancer. Medications are not a substitute for respectful and open communication with patients. Psychological support, with or without psychotropic medications, is always indicated in a depressed or anxious child with cancer. Brain development[35] and medical complications such as absorption difficulties and drug-drug interactions[36] are additional considerations when giving a child psychotropic medication. We believe that the judicious prescription of psychotropic medications is an essential component of the comprehensive care of children and adolescents with cancer. Prospective treatment and prophylaxis investigations using psychotropic medications in pediatric patients with cancer should be considered, and such data should be collected in future pediatric cancer trials.

**Accepted for Publication:** February 1, 2006.
**Correspondence:** Maryland Pao, MD, National Institute of Mental Health, Clinical Research Center, 6-5340, Bethesda, MD 20892 (paom@mail.nih.gov).
**Author Contributions:** Dr Pao had full access to all the data in the study and takes responsibility for the integrity of the data and the accuracy of the data analysis.
**Financial Disclosure:** None reported.
**Funding/Support:** This study was supported by the Intramural Research Programs of the National Institute of Mental Health and the National Cancer Institute.
**Acknowledgment:** We thank Chantal Champaloux, Inna D'Empaire, MD, Haven Battles, PhD, and Michelle Hendry for their help, and the patients who shared their experiences.

## REFERENCES

1. National Center for Health Statistics. Leading causes of death for 2001. http://www.cdc.gov/nchs/data/dvs/LCWK1_2001.pdf. Accessed October 14, 2005.
2. Surveillance Epidemiology and End Results, National Cancer Institute. SEER Cancer Statistics Review, 1975-2002. http://seer.cancer.gov/csr/1975_2002/. Accessed November 14, 2005.
3. Conrad P. Prescribing more psychotropic medications for children: what does the increase mean? *Arch Pediatr Adolesc Med.* 2004;158:829-830.
4. Jellinek MS. Mirror, mirror on the wall: are we prescribing the right psychotropic medications to the right children using the right treatment plan? *Arch Pediatr Adolesc Med.* 2003;157:14-16.
5. Walkup JT. Increasing use of psychotropic medications in children and adolescents: what does it mean? *J Child Adolesc Psychopharmacol.* 2003;13:1-3.
6. Vitiello B. Psychopharmacology for young children: clinical needs and research opportunities. *Pediatrics.* 2001;108:983-989.
7. Zito JM, Safer DJ, Dosreis S, et al. Psychotropic practice patterns for youth: a 10 year perspective. *Arch Pediatr Adolesc Med.* 2003;157:17-25.
8. Mental Health: A report of the Surgeon General. http://www.surgeongeneral.gov/library/mentalhealth/chapter3/sec3.html. Accessed November 18, 2005.
9. Kersun LS, Kazak AE. Prescribing practices of selective serotonin reuptake inhibitors (SSRIs) among pediatric oncologists: a single institution experience [published online ahead of print]. Pediatr Blood Cancer. http://www3.interscience.wiley.com/cgi-bin/fulltext/110560614/PDFSTART. Accessed November 30, 2005.
10. Bealke JM, Meighen KG. Risperidone treatment of three seriously medically ill children with secondary mood disorders. *Psychosomatics.* 2005;46:254-258.
11. Pelletier G. Lacroix Y, Moghrabi A, Robaey P. Double-blind crossover study of chlorpromazine and lorazepam in the treatment of behavioral problems during treatment of children with acute lymphoblastic leukemia receiving glucocorticoids. *Med Pediatr Oncol.* 2000;34:276-277.
12. Brown RL, Henke A, Greenhalgh DG, Warden GD. The use of haloperidol in the agitated, critically ill pediatric patient with burns. *J Burn Care Rehabil.* 1996;17:34-38.
13. Pfefferbaum B, Overall JE, Boren HA, Frankel LS, Sullivan MP, Johnson K. Alprazolam in the treatment of anticipatory and acute situational anxiety in children with cancer. *J Am Acad Child Adolesc Psychiatry.* 1987;26:532-535.
14. Maisami M, Sohmer BH, Coyle JT. Combined use of tricyclic antidepressants and neuroleptics in the management of terminally ill children: a report on three cases. *J Am Acad Child Psychiatry.* 1985;24:487-489.
15. Pfefferbaum-Levine B, Kumor K, Cangir A, Choroszy M, Roseberry EA. Tricyclic antidepressants for children with cancer. *Am J Psychiatry.* 1983;140:1074-1076.

16. Holland JC. IPOS Sutherland Memorial Lecture. An international perspective on the development of psychosocial oncology: overcoming cultural and attitudinal barriers to improve psychosocial care. *Psychooncology.* 2004;13:445-459.
17. Derogatis LR, Feldstein M, Morrow G, et al. A survey of psychotropic drug prescriptions in an oncology population. *Cancer.* 1979;44:1919-1920.
18. Cullivan R, Crown J, Walsh N. The use of psychotropic medication in patients referred to a psycho-oncology service. *Psychooncology.* 1998;7:301-306.
19. Fisch M. Treatment of depression in cancer. *J Natl Cancer Inst Monogr.* 2004;(32): 105-111.
20. Cleeland CS, Bennett GJ, Dantzer R, et al. Are the symptoms of cancer and cancer treatment due to a shared biologic mechanism? a cytokine-immunologic model of cancer symptoms. *Cancer.* 2003;97:2919-2925.
21. Lee BN, Dantzer R, Langley KE, et al. A cytokine-based neuroimmunologic mechanism of cancer-related symptoms. *Neuroimmunomodulation.* 2004;11: 279-292.
22. Musselman DL, Lawson DH, Gumnick JF, et al. Paroxetine for the prevention of depression induced by high-dose interferon alpha. *N Engl J Med.* 2001;344: 961-966.
23. Gothelf D, Rubinstein M, Shemesh E, et al. Pilot study: fluvoxamine treatment for depression and anxiety disorders in children and adolescents with cancer. *J Am Acad Child Adolesc Psychiatry.* 2005;44:1258-1262.
24. Shemesh E, Bartell A, Newcorn JH. Assessment and treatment of depression in medically ill children. *Curr Psychiatry Rep.* 2002;4:88-92.
25. Bennett DS. Depression among children with chronic medical problems: a meta-analysis. *J Pediatr Psychol.* 1994;19:149-169.
26. Shemesh E, Yehuda R, Rockmore L, et al. Assessment of depression in medically ill children presenting to pediatric specialty clinics. *J Am Acad Child Adolesc Psychiatry.* 2005;44:1249-1257.
27. Harris ES, Canning RD, Kelleher KJ. A comparison of measures of adjustment, symptoms, and impairment among children with chronic medical conditions. *J Am Acad Child Adolesc Psychiatry.* 1996;35:1025-1032.
28. Jensen PS, Bhatara VS, Vitiello B, Hoagwood K, Feil M, Burke LB. Psychoactive medication prescribing practices for U.S. children: gaps between research and clinical practice. *J Am Acad Child Adolesc Psychiatry.* 1999;38:557-565.
29. Cummings MR, Miller BD. Pharmacologic management of behavioral instability in medically ill pediatric patients. *Curr Opin Pediatr.* 2004;16:516-522.
30. Keskinbora K, Pekel AF, Aydinli I. The use of gabapentin in a 12-year old boy with cancer pain. *Acta Anaesthesiol Scand.* 2004;48:663-664.
31. Bhangoo RK, Lowe CH, Myers FS, et al. Medication use in children and adolescents treated in the community for bipolar disorder. *J Child Adolesc Psychopharmacol.* 2003;13:515-522.
32. Wolfe J, Grier HE, Klar N et al. Symptoms and suffering at the end of life in children with cancer. *N Engl J Med.* 2000;342:326-333.
33. Fleishman SB. Treatment of symptom clusters: pain, depression and fatigue. *J Natl Cancer Inst Monogr.* 2004;(32):119-123.
34. Rosack J. New data show declines in antidepressant prescribing. *Psychiatr News.* 2005;40:1-39.
35. Vitiello B. Pediatric psychopharmacology and the interaction between drugs and the developing brain. *Can J Psychiatry.* 1998;43:582-584.
36. Buclin T, Mazzocato C, Berney A, Stiefel F. Psychopharmacology in supportive care of cancer: a review for the clinician, IV: other psychotropic agents. *Support Care Cancer.* 2001;9:213-222.

**PEDIARIX™ [Diphtheria and Tetanus Toxoids and Acellular Pertussis Adsorbed, Hepatitis B (Recombinant) and Inactivated Poliovirus Vaccine Combined]**

The following is a brief summary only; see full prescribing information for complete product information.

**CONTRAINDICATIONS:** Hypersensitivity to any component of the vaccine, including yeast, neomycin, and polymyxin B, is a contraindication (see DESCRIPTION in complete prescribing information). Do not use PEDIARIX after a serious allergic reaction (e.g., anaphylaxis) temporally associated with a previous dose of this vaccine or with any components of this vaccine. Because of the uncertainty as to which component of the vaccine might be responsible, do not give further vaccination with any of these components; or, refer such individuals to an allergist for evaluation. The following events are contraindications to administration of PEDIARIX: encephalopathy (e.g., coma, decreased level of consciousness, prolonged seizures) within 7 days of administration of a previous dose of a pertussis-containing vaccine that is not attributable to another identifiable cause; progressive neurologic disorder, including infantile spasms, uncontrolled epilepsy, or progressive encephalopathy. Do not vaccinate individuals with such conditions until a treatment regimen has been established and the condition has stabilized. PEDIARIX is not contraindicated for use in individuals with HIV infection.

**WARNINGS:** Administration of PEDIARIX is associated with higher rates of fever relative to separately administered vaccines. In one study that evaluated medically attended fever after the first dose of PEDIARIX or separately administered vaccines, infants who received PEDIARIX had a higher rate of medical encounters for fever within the first 4 days following vaccination. In some infants, these encounters included the performance of diagnostic studies to evaluate other causes of fever (see ADVERSE REACTIONS). The vial stopper is latex-free. The tip cap and the rubber plunger of the needleless prefilled syringes contain dry natural latex rubber that may cause allergic reactions in latex sensitive individuals. If any of the following events occur in temporal relation to receipt of whole-cell DTP or a vaccine containing an acellular pertussis component, consider carefully whether to give subsequent doses of PEDIARIX or any vaccine containing a pertussis component: temperature of ≥40.5°C (105°F) within 48 hours not due to another identifiable cause; collapse or shock-like state (hypotonic-hyporesponsive episode) within 48 hours; persistent, inconsolable crying lasting ≥3 hours, occurring within 48 hours; seizures with or without fever occurring within 3 days. If Guillain-Barré syndrome occurs within 6 weeks of receipt of prior vaccine containing tetanus toxoid, the decision to give subsequent doses of PEDIARIX or any vaccine containing tetanus toxoid should be based on careful consideration of the potential benefits and possible risks. A committee of the Institute of Medicine (IOM) has concluded that evidence is consistent with a causal relationship between whole-cell DTP vaccine and acute neurologic illness, and under special circumstances, between whole-cell DTP vaccine and chronic neurologic disease in the context of the National Childhood Encephalopathy Study (NCES) report; however, evidence was insufficient to indicate whether or not whole-cell DTP vaccine increased the overall risk of chronic neurologic disease. Acute encephalopathy and permanent neurologic damage have not been reported causally linked or in temporal association with administration of PEDIARIX, but the experience with PEDIARIX is insufficient to rule this out. Encephalopathy has been reported following INFANRIX® (Diphtheria and Tetanus Toxoids and Acellular Pertussis Vaccine Adsorbed) (see ADVERSE REACTIONS, Postmarketing Reports), but data are not sufficient to evaluate a causal relationship. The decision to administer a pertussis-containing vaccine to children with stable central nervous system (CNS) disorders must be made by the physician on an individual basis, with consideration of all relevant factors, and assessment of potential risks and benefits for that individual. Advise the parent or guardian of the potential increased risk involved (see PRECAUTIONS). A family history of seizures or other CNS disorders is not a contraindication to pertussis vaccine. For children at higher risk for seizures than the general population, an appropriate antipyretic may be administered at the time of vaccination and for the ensuing 24 hours according to the respective prescribing information recommended dosage to reduce the possibility of post-vaccination fever. Defer vaccination during the course of a moderate or severe illness with or without fever and vaccinate patients as soon as they have recovered from the acute phase of the illness. Do not give PEDIARIX to children on anticoagulant therapy or those with bleeding disorders unless the potential benefit clearly outweighs the risk of administration (see PRECAUTIONS in complete prescribing information).

**PRECAUTIONS:** Before the injection of any biological, the physician should take all reasonable precautions to prevent allergic or other adverse reactions. Epinephrine injection (1:1000) and other appropriate agents used for the control of immediate allergic reactions must be immediately available should an acute anaphylactic reaction occur. Immunosuppressed individuals, including those receiving immunosuppressive therapy, may not develop the expected immune response. **Drug Interactions:** For information regarding concomitant administration with other vaccines, refer to DOSAGE AND ADMINISTRATION in complete prescribing information. Do not mix PEDIARIX with any other vaccine in the same syringe or vial. **Carcinogenesis, Mutagenesis, Impairment of Fertility:** PEDIARIX has not been evaluated for carcinogenic or mutagenic potential, or for impairment of fertility. **Pregnancy:** Pregnancy Category C: PEDIARIX is not indicated for women of child-bearing age. Animal reproduction studies have not been conducted with PEDIARIX. It is not known whether PEDIARIX can cause fetal harm when administered to a pregnant woman or if PEDIARIX can affect reproductive capacity. **Geriatric Use:** PEDIARIX is not indicated for use in adult populations. **Pediatric Use:** Safety and effectiveness of PEDIARIX in infants younger than 6 weeks of age have not been evaluated (see DOSAGE AND ADMINISTRATION in complete prescribing information). PEDIARIX is not recommended for persons 7 years of age or older. Tetanus and Diphtheria Toxoids Adsorbed (Td) For Adult Use, inactivated poliovirus vaccine (IPV), and Hepatitis B Vaccine (Recombinant) should be used in individuals 7 years of age or older.

**ADVERSE REACTIONS:** A total of 20,739 doses of PEDIARIX have been administered to 7,028 infants as a 3-dose primary series. The most common adverse reactions observed in clinical trials were local injection site reactions (pain, redness, or swelling), fever, and fussiness. In comparative studies, administration of PEDIARIX was associated with higher rates of fever relative to separately administered vaccines (see WARNINGS). The prevalence of fever was highest on the day of vaccination and the day following vaccination. More than 98% of episodes of fever resolved within the 4-day period following vaccination (i.e., the period including the day of vaccination and the next 3 days). Rates of most other solicited adverse events following PEDIARIX were comparable to rates observed following separately administered US-licensed vaccines. The adverse event information from clinical trials provides a basis for identifying adverse events that appear to be related to vaccine use and for approximating rates. However, because clinical trials are conducted under widely varying conditions, adverse event rates observed in the clinical trials of a vaccine cannot be directly compared to rates in the clinical trials of another vaccine, and may not reflect the rates observed in practice. A total of 5,472 infants were enrolled in a German safety study that was originally designed to compare the safety and reactogenicity of PEDIARIX administered concomitantly at separate sites with 1 of 4 *Haemophilus influenzae* type b (Hib) vaccines at 3, 4, and 5 months of age. After enrollment of 1,569 infants, the study was amended to include a control group that received INFANRIX, Hib vaccine, and oral poliovirus vaccine (OPV) separately. Infants in the separate administration group received one less antigen (hepatitis B) than the infants who received PEDIARIX. Safety data were available for 4,666 infants who received PEDIARIX administered concomitantly at separate sites with 1 of 4 Hib vaccines and for 768 infants in the control group that received separate vaccines. The primary end-point of the study was the percentage of infants with any grade 3 solicited symptom (redness or swelling >20 mm, fever >103.1°F, or crying, pain, vomiting, diarrhea, loss of appetite, or restlessness that prevented normal daily activities) over the 3-dose primary series in infants who received PEDIARIX (4 groups that received PEDIARIX and Hib vaccines pooled) compared to the group that received INFANRIX and Hib vaccine separately with OPV. Analysis for the primary end-point was performed on the according-to-protocol (ATP) cohort that included only those infants who were enrolled after the protocol amendment to include a control group. Of 3,773 infants in the ATP cohort for whom safety data were available, 16.2% (95% CI: 14.9% to 17.5%) of 3,029 infants who received PEDIARIX and Hib vaccine compared to 20.3% (95% CI: 17.5% to 23.4%) of 744 infants who received separate vaccines were reported to have had at least one grade 3 solicited symptom within 4 days of vaccination (i.e., day of vaccination and the next 3 days). The difference between groups in the rate of grade 3 symptoms was 4.1% (90% CI: 1.4% to 7.1%). These were the rates for selected solicited symptoms within 4 days following each dose in a 3-dose primary series in infants who received PEDIARIX administered concomitantly with Hib vaccine and those who received separate concomitant administration of INFANRIX, Hib vaccine, and OPV for the intent-to-treat (ITT) cohort (includes all infants enrolled before and after the amendment who received the indicated vaccine and for whom at least one symptom sheet was completed):

**Percentage of German Infants With Solicited Local Reactions or Selected Systemic Adverse Events Within 4 Days of Vaccination* (ITT Cohort)**

| | PEDIARIX & Hib | | | INFANRIX, Hib, & OPV | | |
|---|---|---|---|---|---|---|
| | Dose 1 | Dose 2 | Dose 3 | Dose 1 | Dose 2 | Dose 3 |
| **N** | **4,666** | **4,619** | **4,574** | **768** | **757** | **750** |
| **Local†** | | | | | | |
| Pain, any | 14.0 | 10.2 | 9.9 | 14.2 | 9.8 | 8.1 |
| Pain, grade 2 or 3 | 2.9 | 1.2 | 1.5 | 3.6 | 1.7 | 1.1 |
| Pain, grade 3 | 0.7 | 0.3 | 0.3 | 1.3 | 0.4 | 0.1 |
| Redness, any | 18.6 | 26.6 | 25.6 | 16.1 | 21.4 | 20.8 |
| Redness, >5 mm | 6.7 | 9.9 | 9.0 | 5.9 | 8.2 | 7.7 |
| Redness, >20 mm | 1.2 | 1.0 | 1.1 | 1.8 | 0.7 | 1.1 |
| Swelling, any | 12.7 | 18.5 | 18.4 | 9.6 | 12.9 | 13.6 |
| Swelling, >5 mm | 5.6 | 7.7 | 7.8 | 3.6 | 5.2 | 4.8 |
| Swelling, >20 mm | 1.2 | 1.6 | 1.5 | 1.3 | 1.1 | 1.2 |
| **Systemic** | | | | | | |
| Restlessness, any | 41.4 | 32.0 | 26.7 | 46.4 | 35.0 | 27.6 |
| Restlessness, grade 2 or 3 | 14.4 | 10.0 | 8.9 | 20.2 | 11.5 | 8.4 |
| Restlessness, grade 3 | 3.0 | 1.5 | 1.6 | 5.7 | 3.0 | 1.7 |
| Fever‡, ≥100.4ºF | 25.1 | 19.3 | 19.7 | 13.2 | 13.1 | 11.2 |
| Fever‡, >101.3ºF | 5.8 | 4.1 | 4.6 | 2.2 | 2.8 | 2.1 |
| Fever‡, >103.1ºF | 0.3 | 0.5 | 0.7 | 0.3 | 0.3 | 0.5 |
| Unusual cry§, any | 24.9 | 16.5 | 13.1 | 36.5 | 19.7 | 14.3 |
| Unusual cry§, grade 2 or 3 | 12.7 | 7.1 | 5.7 | 20.8 | 10.0 | 5.7 |
| Unusual cry§, grade 3 | 3.9 | 1.7 | 1.4 | 6.8 | 2.1 | 1.1 |
| Loss of appetite, any | 17.9 | 13.3 | 12.5 | 19.1 | 16.2 | 11.3 |
| Loss of appetite, grade 2 or 3 | 4.0 | 2.9 | 2.7 | 4.4 | 2.9 | 2.3 |
| Loss of appetite, grade 3 | 0.6 | 0.5 | 0.4 | 0.5 | 0.7 | 0.0 |

N = number of infants in the intent-to-treat (ITT) cohort.
Grade 2 defined as sufficiently discomforting to interfere with daily activities.
Grade 3 defined as preventing normal daily activities.
* Within 4 days of vaccination defined as day of vaccination and the next 3 days.
† Local reactions at the injection site for PEDIARIX or INFANRIX.
‡ Rectal temperatures.
§ Unusual cry lasting >1 hour.

In this study, infants were also monitored for unsolicited adverse events that occurred within 30 days following vaccination. Over the entire study period, 6 subjects in the group that received PEDIARIX reported seizures. Two of these subjects had a febrile seizure, 1 of whom also developed afebrile seizures. The remaining 4 subjects had afebrile seizures, including 2 with infantile spasms. Two subjects reported seizures within 7 days following vaccination (1 subject had both febrile and afebrile seizures, and 1 subject had afebrile seizures), corresponding to a rate of 0.22 seizures per 1,000 doses (febrile seizures 0.07 per 1,000 doses, afebrile seizures 0.14 per 1,000 doses). No subject who received concomitant INFANRIX, Hib vaccine, and OPV reported seizures. In a separate German study that evaluated the safety of INFANRIX in 22,505 infants who received 66,867 doses of INFANRIX administered as a 3-dose primary series, the rate of seizures within 7 days of vaccination with INFANRIX was 0.13 per 1,000 doses (febrile seizures 0.0 per 1,000 doses, afebrile seizures 0.13 per 1,000 doses). No cases of hypotonic-hyporesponsiveness, encephalopathy, or anaphylaxis were reported in the German study that evaluated the safety of PEDIARIX. Rates of serious adverse events that are less common than those reported in this safety study are not known at this time.

Additional safety data for PEDIARIX are available from a US study designed to evaluate lot-to-lot consistency and a bridge for a new manufacturing step. These were the rates for local reactions and selected adverse events within 4 days of vaccination with PEDIARIX administered concomitantly with a Hib vaccine at 2, 4, and 6 months of age:

**Percentage of US Infants With Solicited Local Reactions or Selected Systemic Adverse Events Within 4 Days of Vaccination* (ITT Cohort)**

| | PEDIARIX & Hib | | |
|---|---|---|---|
| | Dose 1 | Dose 2 | Dose 3 |
| **Local†** | **N = 482** | **N = 469** | **N = 466** |
| Pain, any | 30.5 | 25.4 | 23.0 |
| Pain, grade 2 or 3 | 6.2 | 5.5 | 3.6 |
| Pain, grade 3 | 1.2 | 0.6 | 0.6 |
| Redness, any | 25.3 | 32.6 | 35.6 |
| Redness, >5 mm | 9.3 | 10.4 | 8.6 |
| Redness, >20 mm | 0.6 | 1.5 | 1.3 |
| Swelling, any | 15.1 | 16.6 | 22.3 |
| Swelling, >5 mm | 6.8 | 6.2 | 6.4 |
| Swelling, >20 mm | 1.0 | 1.3 | 1.3 |
| **Systemic** | **N = 482** | **N = 469** | **N = 467** |
| Restlessness, any | 28.8 | 30.3 | 28.5 |
| Restlessness, grade 2 or 3 | 7.1 | 9.0 | 9.4 |
| Restlessness, grade 3 | 1.0 | 1.1 | 0.6 |
| Fever‡, ≥100.4ºF | 26.6 | 31.3 | 25.9 |
| Fever‡, >101.3ºF | 2.9 | 6.2 | 4.7 |
| Fever‡, >103.1ºF | 0.0 | 0.2 | 0.6 |
| Fussiness, any | 61.8 | 63.8 | 57.0 |
| Fussiness, grade 2 or 3 | 14.9 | 21.5 | 17.1 |
| Fussiness, grade 3 | 2.7 | 3.4 | 1.7 |
| Loss of appetite, any | 21.6 | 19.8 | 18.8 |
| Loss of appetite, grade 2 or 3 | 3.1 | 3.2 | 2.4 |
| Loss of appetite, grade 3 | 0.2 | 0.4 | 0.0 |
| Sleeping more than usual, any | 46.7 | 31.8 | 28.1 |
| Sleeping more than usual, grade 2 or 3 | 10.2 | 6.0 | 4.7 |
| Sleeping more than usual, grade 3 | 1.7 | 0.4 | 0.6 |

N = number of infants in the intent-to-treat (ITT) cohort (infants who received the indicated vaccine and for whom at least one symptom sheet was completed).
Grade 2 defined as sufficiently discomforting to interfere with daily activities.
Grade 3 defined as preventing normal daily activities.
* Within 4 days of vaccination defined as day of vaccination and the next 3 days.
† Local reactions at the injection site for PEDIARIX.
‡ Rectal temperatures.

In another US study, these were the rates for fever within 4 days following dose 1 (i.e., day of vaccination and the next 3 days) at 2 months of age in infants who received PEDIARIX when administered concomitantly at separate sites with Hib and pneumococcal conjugate vaccines and those who received INFANRIX, ENGERIX-B® [Hepatitis B Vaccine (Recombinant)], IPV, Hib vaccine, and pneumococcal conjugate vaccine:

**Percentage of US Infants With Fever Within 4 Days of Dose 1* (ITT Cohort)**

| | PEDIARIX, Hib, & Pneumococcal Conjugate (N = 667) | INFANRIX, ENGERIX-B, IPV, Hib, & Pneumococcal Conjugate (N = 333) | Separate Vaccine Group Minus Combination Vaccine Group |
|---|---|---|---|
| **Fever†** | **%** | **%** | **Difference (95% CI)** |
| ≥100.4ºF‡ | 27.9 | 19.8 | -8.07 (-13.54, -2.60) |
| >101.3ºF | 7.0 | 4.5 | -2.54 (-5.50, 0.41) |
| >102.2ºF‡ | 2.2 | 0.3 | -1.95 (-3.22, -0.68) |
| >103.1ºF | 0.4 | 0.0 | -0.45 (-0.96, 0.06) |
| M.A.‡ | 1.2 | 0.0 | -1.20 (-2.03, -037) |

N = number of infants for whom at least one symptom sheet was completed, excluding 3 infants for whom temperature was not measured and 3 infants whose temperature was measured by the tympanic method.
*Within 4 days of dose 1 defined as day of vaccination and the next 3 days.
† Rectal temperatures.
‡ The group that received PEDIARIX compared to separate vaccine group p value <0.05 (2-sided Fisher Exact test) or the 95% confidence interval on the difference between groups does not include 0.
M.A. = Medically attended (a visit to or from medical personnel).

In this study, medical attention (a visit to or from medical personnel) for fever within 4 days following vaccination was sought for 8 infants who received PEDIARIX (1.2%) and no infants who received separately administered vaccines. Four infants were seen by medical personnel in an office setting; no diagnostic tests were performed in 2 of the infants and a complete blood count (CBC) was done in the other 2 infants. Of 3 infants who were seen in an emergency room, all had a CBC and a blood and urine culture performed; chest X-rays were done in 2 of the infants and a nasopharyngeal specimen was tested for Respiratory Syncytial Virus in one of the infants. One infant was hospitalized for a work-up that included a CBC, blood and urine cultures, a lumbar puncture, and a chest X-ray. All episodes of medically attended fever resolved within 4 days post-vaccination.

Limited data are available from a study conducted in Moldova in which infants received a dose of hepatitis B vaccine within 48 hours of birth followed by 3 doses of PEDIARIX at 6, 10, and 14 weeks of age. No information was collected on the HBsAg status of mothers of enrolled infants. These were the rates for local reactions and selected adverse events within 4 days of vaccination with PEDIARIX administered comcomitantly with Hib vaccine following a birth dose of hepatitis B vaccine:

**Percentage of Moldovan Infants With Solicited Local Reactions or Selected Systemic Adverse Events Within 4 Days of Vaccination* (ITT Cohort)**

| | PEDIARIX & Hib | | |
|---|---|---|---|
| | Dose 1 | Dose 2 | Dose 3 |
| **N** | **160** | **158** | **157** |
| **Local†** | | | |
| Pain, any | 25.6 | 18.4 | 14.0 |
| Pain, grade 3 | 3.1 | 0.6 | 1.9 |
| Redness, any | 41.9 | 41.8 | 47.1 |
| Redness, >20 mm | 1.9 | 2.5 | 4.5 |
| Swelling, any | 20.6 | 18.4 | 28.0 |
| Swelling, >20 mm | 4.4 | 2.5 | 7.0 |
| **Systemic** | | | |
| Restlessness, any | 13.1 | 10.8 | 8.9 |
| Restlessness, grade 3 | 1.3 | 0.6 | 0.6 |
| Fever‡, ≥100.4ºF | 14.4 | 11.4 | 5.1 |
| Fever‡, >103.1ºF | 0.0 | 0.6 | 0.0 |
| Fussiness, any | 25.0 | 21.5 | 17.8 |
| Fussiness, grade 3 | 2.5 | 0.6 | 0.6 |

N = number of infants in the intent-to-treat (ITT) cohort (infants who received the indicated vaccine and for whom at least one symptom sheet was completed).
Grade 3 defined as preventing normal daily activities.
*Within 4 days of vaccination defined as day of vaccination and the next 3 days.
† Local reactions at the injection site for PEDIARIX.
‡ Rectal temperatures.

Although there was no comparator group who received PEDIARIX without a birth dose of hepatitis B vaccine, available data suggest that some local adverse events may occur at a higher rate when PEDIARIX is administered after a birth dose of hepatitis B vaccine.

As with any vaccine, there is the possibility that broad use of PEDIARIX could reveal adverse events not observed in clinical trials.

**Postmarketing Reports:** Worldwide voluntary reports of adverse events received for INFANRIX and ENGERIX-B in children younger than 7 years of age since market introduction of these US-licensed vaccines are listed below. This list includes adverse events for which 20 or more reports were received with the exception of intussusception, idiopathic thrombocytopenic purpura, thrombocytopenia, anaphylactic reaction, angioedema, encephalopathy, hypotonic-hyporesponsive episode, and alopecia for which fewer than 20 reports were received. These latter events are included either because of the seriousness of the event or the strength of causal connection to components of this or other vaccines or drugs. *Body as a whole*: Asthenia[b], fever[a+b], lethargy[b], malaise[b], Sudden Infant Death Syndrome[a+b]. *Cardiovascular system*: Cyanosis[a+b], edema[b], pallor[b]. *Gastrointestinal system*: Abdominal pain[b], anorexia[b], diarrhea[a+b], intussusception[a+b], nausea[b], vomiting[a+b]. *Hematologic/lymphatic*: Idiopathic thrombocytopenic purpura[a+b], lymphadenopathy[a], thrombocytopenia[a+b]. *Hepatic*: Jaundice[b], liver function tests abnormal[b]. *Hypersensitivity*: Anaphylactic reaction[a+b], angioedema[b], hypersensitivity[a]. *Infections*: Cellulitis[a]. *Injection site reactions*: Injection site reactions[a+b]. *Musculoskeletal*: Arthralgia[b], limb swelling[a+b]. *Nervous system*: Convulsions[a+b], encephalopathy[a], headache[b], hypotonia[a+b], hypotonic-hyporesponsive episode[a], somnolence[a+b]. *Psychiatric*: Crying[a+b], irritability[a+b]. *Respiratory system*: Respiratory tract infection[a]. *Skin and appendages*: Alopecia[b], erythema[a+b], erythema multiforme[b], petechiae[b], pruritus[a+b], rash[a+b], urticaria[a+b]. *Special senses*: Ear pain[a]. [[a] Following INFANRIX; [b] Following ENGERIX-B; [a+b] Following either INFANRIX or ENGERIX-B.] These reactions were reported voluntarily from a population of uncertain size; therefore, it is not always possible to reliably estimate their frequency or establish a causal relationship to vaccination.

**Reporting Adverse Events:** Report the occurrence following immunization of any event set forth in the Vaccine Injury Table from the National Childhood Vaccine Injury Act including: Anaphylaxis or anaphylactic shock within 7 days, encephalopathy or encephalitis within 7 days, brachial neuritis within 28 days, or an acute complication or sequelae (including death) of an illness, disability, injury, or condition referred to above, or any events that would contraindicate further doses of PEDIARIX. The VAERS toll-free number is 1-800-822-7967.

Manufactured by **GlaxoSmithKline Biologicals**, Rixensart, Belgium, US License 1617

Distributed by **GlaxoSmithKline,** Research Triangle Park, NC 27709



Full prescribing information for PEDIARIX is available at www.GSKVaccines.com/Pediarix. BRS-PE:L2

 Printed in USA. PED583R0 June 2005

# Parental Report of Health Conditions and Health Care Use Among Children With and Without Autism

## *National Survey of Children's Health*

*James G. Gurney, PhD; Melissa L. McPheeters, PhD; Matthew M. Davis, MD, MAPP*

**Objective:** To compare parent-reported prevalence of health conditions and health care use between children with and without autism.

**Design:** Cross-sectional analysis of the 2003 to 2004 National Survey of Children's Health.

**Setting:** Population-based sample across the United States.

**Participants:** More than 100 000 parents. The main exposure was "autism" (not further defined), from response to the question: "Has a doctor or health professional every told you that your child has autism?"

**Main Outcome Measures:** Medical and mental health conditions and measures of health care use.

**Results:** Autism prevalence among children aged 3 to 17 years was 53 per 10 000 (95% confidence interval, 45-61 per 10 000), equating to a national estimate of 324 000 children (95% confidence interval, 274 000-375 000 children). Children with autism had a significantly ($P$<.001) higher prevalence of depression or anxiety problems (38.9% vs 4.2%) and behavioral or conduct problems (58.9% vs 5.2%) than children without autism. Respiratory, food, and skin allergies were reported by parents more often for children with autism, with food allergies having the strongest relative difference between the groups (odds ratio, 4.5; 95% confidence interval, 3.0-7.0). Children with autism had significantly ($P$<.001) higher mean physician visits over 12 months for preventive care, nonemergency care, and hospital emergency care, and were far more likely than children without autism to receive physical, occupational, or speech therapy (76.0% vs 6.3%), to need treatment or counseling for an emotional, developmental, or behavioral problem (75.4% vs 7.0%), and, among those taking a prescribed medication, to be using a medication long-term (51.4% vs 14.5%).

**Conclusion:** We found markedly higher reports of concurrent conditions and health care use associated with childhood autism in this study.

*Arch Pediatr Adolesc Med. 2006;160:825-830*

**Author Affiliations:** Child Health Evaluation and Research Unit, Department of Pediatrics, University of Michigan (Drs Gurney, McPheeters, and Davis), and Division of General Internal Medicine and Gerald R. Ford School of Public Policy, University of Michigan (Dr Davis), Ann Arbor.

AUTISM SPECTRUM DISORDERS (ASDs) represent a wide range of neurobehavioral conditions that, depending on phenotype, are characterized by limitations in reciprocal social interactions and social functioning, stereotypical repetitive behaviors, and language and speech impairments.[1(pp65-78)2] Autism spectrum disorders, with subtypes classified under the rubric of "pervasive developmental disorders" in the *Diagnostic and Statistical Manual of Mental Disorders, Fourth Edition*,[1(pp65-78)] are generally identifiable by the age of 3 years and are lifelong chronic conditions. In the clinical and psychological literature, children with ASD are often described as having 1 or more of a variety of medical and psychological comorbidities,[3] including higher than expected rates of mental retardation,[4] epilepsy,[5,6] gastrointestinal problems,[7,8] attention-deficit/hyperactivity disorder (ADHD),[9] depression,[10] anxiety, and sleep disorders.[11]

The term *comorbidities*, however, implies a condition that is distinct from the disease itself. Many conditions associated with ASD may not be discrete from the phenotypic expression of the disorder, so henceforth we use the term *concurrent conditions* to include the spectrum of physical and mental health disorders evaluated in this study. If, in fact, this propensity for concurrent conditions is true, children with ASD likely require a high degree of health care and mental health services, with associated costs and burdens to their families and to health care systems. To our knowledge, however, no prior study has attempted to broadly characterize concurrent condi-

**Table 1. Descriptive Characteristics of US Children Aged 3 to 17 Years, From the National Survey of Children's Health***

| Characteristic | Children With Autism (n = 324 000) | Children Without Autism (n = 61 100 000) | *P* Value |
|---|---|---|---|
| Age, y | | | |
| 3-5 | 15.0 | 20.5 | <.001 |
| 6-10 | 52.8 | 38.8 | |
| 11-17 | 32.3 | 40.6 | |
| Sex | | | |
| Male | 79.0 | 51.0 | <.001 |
| Female | 21.0 | 49.0 | |
| Missing | 0 | 0.07 | |
| Race | | | |
| White | 73.9 | 67.3 | .25 |
| Black | 15.3 | 15.0 | |
| Multiracial | 1.6 | 3.2 | |
| Other | 2.6 | 4.6 | |
| Missing | 6.7 | 9.9 | |
| Primary language | | | |
| English | 98.0 | 87.9 | <.001 |
| Other | 2.1 | 12.1 | |
| Missing | 0 | 0 | |
| Respondent | | | |
| Mother | 83.2 | 79.3 | .18 |
| Father | 13.8 | 16.1 | |
| Other relative | 3.0 | 4.6 | |
| Poverty level of household, % | | | |
| <100 | 27.7 | 22.3 | .24 |
| 100-199 | 9.2 | 13.5 | |
| 200-299 | 14.2 | 16.0 | |
| 300-399 | 16.1 | 14.0 | |
| ≥400 | 24.9 | 24.1 | |
| Missing | 7.9 | 10.1 | |
| Highest level of educational attainment in household | | | |
| <High school | 2.2 | 7.6 | .02 |
| High school graduate (12 y) | 23.2 | 26.3 | |
| >High school | 72.3 | 65.6 | |
| Missing | 2.3 | 0.5 | |
| Medical insurance during the past 12 mo | | | |
| Fully insured | | | |
| Private | 57.3 | 64.7 | <.001 |
| Medicaid or S-CHIP | 32.8 | 23.7 | |
| Insured part of the year | 9.5 | 6.3 | |
| No insurance throughout the year | 0.4 | 5.3 | |

Abbreviation: S-CHIP, State Children's Health Insurance Program.
*Data are given as percentage of each group unless otherwise indicated. Percentages may not total 100 because of rounding. Prevalences are based on sampling fractions and weighted extrapolation from parent report of 483 children with autism and 84 789 children without autism.

tions of children with autism or, in particular, to compare their health care use with that of children without autism.

This study describes and evaluates the extent to which children with an ASD have, according to parental report, a higher prevalence of common childhood conditions and higher health care use than children without an ASD. To accomplish this aim, we analyzed data from the National Survey of Children's Health (NSCH), a population-based survey of more than 100 000 randomly selected parents or guardians in the United States. This study includes information on 483 children described by the parent to have been diagnosed as having autism by a doctor or other health professional. The data set includes weighting measures to allow extrapolation of prevalence estimates to the general pediatric population of the United States.

## METHODS

The NSCH was a population-based, cross-sectional, telephone survey using a complex, multicluster, probability sampling design.[12] The NSCH was sponsored by the Maternal and Child Health Bureau in partnership with the National Center for Health Statistics, which is part of the Centers for Disease Control and Prevention. The purpose of the NSCH was to produce national and state-specific prevalence estimates of health indicators and children's experiences with the health care system.[12] The telephone survey includes questions about sociodemographics, physical and mental health status, health insurance coverage, and access to and use of health care services. The NSCH public use data set contains no information on the personal identity of participants, and this analysis was approved as exempt by the University of Michigan Human Subjects Review Board.

The NSCH used random-digit dialing to recruit and survey households with children younger than 18 years. One child in each household was randomly selected to be the subject of the survey, and the respondent for the interview was the parent or guardian (hereafter termed parent) who was most familiar with the child's health and health care. Interviews were conducted in English or Spanish. Estimates reported herein are based on 85 272 interviews completed from January 2003 through July 2004; the NSCH had with a weighted response of 55.3%.

Autism was ascertained through a question to the parent, "Has a doctor or health professional ever told you that your child has autism?" Inquiries about other medical and mental health conditions used the same question format. No questions were asked to help distinguish subtype or phenotype of ASD, so we use the terminology of the questionnaire and refer to autism henceforth throughout the article. The 483 affirmative answers produced the autism group for this analysis, and all other children in the survey sample composed the comparison group (N = 84 789).

Prevalence proportions of selected variables were calculated and adjusted using the stratified weighted sampling fractions provided in the NSCH public use data set.[12] Multivariable logistic regression techniques were used to estimate the relative odds of selected outcomes after adjusting for the potentially confounding effects of child's age and sex, the primary language spoken in the home (English or other), the highest level of educational attainment in the household, and insurance status (categorized as shown in **Table 1**). Missing data were assessed for their differential distribution in the autism and nonautism groups and for their potential influence on the measures of effect. Of the covariates examined, only race and poverty level had missing responses of more than 3%. Neither race nor household poverty level met the criteria as a confounder in this data set, so these variables were not included in our regression models and no information was lost because of missing data from them. Those with missing data for other variables of interest (Table 1) were excluded from the regression models under the untested assumption that they were missing at random.

As measures of health care use, parents were first asked whether during the past 12 months their child saw a doctor, nurse, or other health professional. If they answered yes, parents were queried about the number of preventive care visits,

**Table 2. Parental Description of Health Status and Therapy and Services Use, From the National Survey of Children's Health**

| Variable | Children With Autism (n = 324 000)* | Children Without Autism (n = 61 100 000)* | OR (95% CI)† |
|---|---|---|---|
| Would you say your child's health is | | | |
| Excellent | 33.7 | 60.2 | 1.0 |
| Very good | 22.8 | 23.5 | 1.8 (1.2-2.7) |
| Good | 32.7 | 13.0 | 5.9 (3.9-9.1) |
| Fair | 7.4 | 2.9 | 7.7 (4.3-13.8) |
| Poor | 3.5 | 0.4 | 21.1 (9.3-47.9) |
| Does the child use more medical care, mental health or educational services than is usual for most children of the same age? | 89.6 | 11.8 | 52.8 (34.7-80.4) |
| Is the child limited or prevented in the ability to do the things most children the same age can do? | 68.5 | 5.7 | 36.2 (24.9-52.6) |
| Does the child get special therapy, such as physical, occupational, or speech therapy? | 76.0 | 6.3 | 44.4 (31.9-61.8) |
| Does the child have any emotional, developmental, or behavioral problem for which she needs treatment or counseling? | 75.4 | 7.0 | 36.9 (25.7-53.1) |
| Does the child currently need or use medicine prescribed by a doctor, other than vitamins? | 54.7 | 21.1 | 3.5 (2.6-4.7) |
| If yes, is this for a condition expected to last 12 mo or longer? | 51.4 | 14.5 | 11.0 (1.6-76.9) |

Abbreviations: CI, confidence interval; OR, odds ratio.
*Data are given as the percentage of each group and are based on sampling fractions and weighted extrapolation from parent report of 483 children with autism and 84 789 children without autism.
†Data are adjusted for sex, primary language, age, insurance, and household educational attainment.

hospital emergency department visits, and nonemergency visits in that 12-month period. Where the answer to the initial question was no, we ascribed 0 visits in each category. We then used a 2-equation modeling technique[13] to provide an adjusted mean number of visits for each type of physician visit. This model accounts for the strong right skewing of the data because of the high frequency of those with no visits and relatively few high users of health care services. Because variances are not directly produced in the 2-equation modeling method, we calculated 95% confidence intervals for the means after bootstrapping standard errors, drawing 1000 samples from the data.

## RESULTS

The weighted prevalence of reported autism among children aged 3 to 17 years was 53 per 10 000 (95% confidence interval, 45-61 per 10 000), equating to a US national estimate of 324 000 children with autism (95% confidence interval, 274 000-375 000 children with autism). Table 1 compares the distribution of sociodemographic characteristics among those with and without autism in the study population. The male-female ratio was 3.8:1 among children with autism, compared with 1:1 in children without autism. The annual household income distribution, relative to the federal poverty level, showed little evidence of differences between the comparison groups. Similarly, any difference in race distribution was not statistically significant, and black children composed about 15% of those with and without autism in the study population. Non–English-speaking parents, however, were underrepresented in the autism group relative to the nonautism group, and the educational level of parents with children with autism was, on average, higher than that of the comparison parents.

Parental perceptions of their child's health status and need for therapies and services are shown in **Table 2**. Parents with a child with autism were much more likely to report their child's health as fair or poor, rather than excellent, compared with other parents in the study. Strong differences in measures of reported use of or need for mental and physical health therapies were also observed between the study groups. During the preceding 12 months, children with autism were far more likely than children without autism to receive physical, occupational, or speech therapy; to need treatment or counseling for an emotional, developmental, or behavioral problem; and to be using medication. Among children using prescribed medication, many more parents of children with autism reported that the use was for a condition expected to last at least 12 months.

A variety of conditions were more frequently reported by parents of children with autism than parents of children without autism (**Table 3**), including depression or anxiety problems, behavioral or conduct problems, and ADHD or attention-deficit disorder. No differences between the study groups were observed for diabetes mellitus or asthma. Allergies, however, whether respiratory, food, or skin, were reported more often for children with autism, with food allergies having the strongest relative difference between the study groups.

The relative frequencies and adjusted means of physician visits for preventive care, nonemergency care, and hospital emergency care are shown in **Table 4**. On average, parents reported significantly more visits for their children with autism in the previous 12 months for each type of physician visit than did parents of children without autism. The largest differences were observed for visits involving preventive care and nonemergency care; for the latter, the adjusted mean number of visits was 2.80 for children with autism, compared with 1.56 for children without autism (*P*<.001).

**Table 3. Parental Report of Clinical Conditions Among Children With and Without Autism, From the National Survey of Children's Health**

| Variable | Children With Autism (n = 324 000)* | Children Without Autism (n = 61 100 000)* | OR (95% CI)† |
|---|---|---|---|
| Has a doctor or health professional ever told you that he/she has | | | |
| Behavioral or conduct problems | 58.9 | 5.2 | 23.4 (16.9-32.4) |
| Attention-deficit disorder or attention-deficit/hyperactive disorder, that is, ADD or ADHD | 45.1 | 7.0 | 8.0 (5.6-11.4) |
| Stuttering, stammering, or other speech problems | 40.1 | 3.3 | 16.7 (12.0-23.1) |
| Depression or anxiety problems | 38.9 | 4.2 | 15.0 (10.1-22.3) |
| Bone, joint, or muscle problems | 23.0 | 3.4 | 7.5 (4.7-12.1) |
| Three or more ear infections | 13.2 | 4.8 | 3.1 (2.1-4.7) |
| Hearing problems or vision problems that cannot be corrected with glasses or contact lenses | 10.7 | 2.8 | 3.7 (2.4-5.7) |
| Asthma | 17.6 | 13.5 | 0.9 (0.6-1.4) |
| Diabetes | 0.4 | 0.3 | 1.1 (0.4-3.1) |
| During the last 12 mo, have you been told by a doctor or other health professional that he/she has | | | |
| Hay fever or any kind of respiratory allergy | 27.0 | 16.2 | 1.6 (1.1-2.4) |
| Any kind of food or digestive allergy | 14.1 | 3.2 | 4.5 (3.0-7.0) |
| Frequent or severe headaches, including migraines | 12.0 | 5.5 | 2.4 (1.2-5.0) |
| Eczema or any kind of skin allergy | 14.9 | 9.2 | 1.4 (1.0-2.1) |

Abbreviations: See Table 2.

*Data are given as the percentage of each group and are based on sampling fractions and weighted extrapolation from parent report of 483 children with autism and 84 789 children without autism.

†Data are adjusted for sex, primary language, age, insurance, and household educational attainment.

**Table 4. Data for Physician Visits in the Past 12 Months as a Measure of Health Care Use Among Children With and Without Autism, From the National Survey of Children's Health***

| Variable | Children With Autism (n = 324 000)† | Children Without Autism (n = 61 100 000)† |
|---|---|---|
| No. of visits for preventive care | | |
| 0 | 16.4 | 25.0 |
| 1-2 | 56.3 | 60.9 |
| 3-5 | 19.4 | 12.2 |
| ≥6 | 7.9 | 1.9 |
| Mean (95% CI) | 3.89 (3.57-4.21) | 2.51 (2.49-2.53) |
| No. of hospital emergency department visits | | |
| 0 | 70.3 | 83.4 |
| 1 | 19.7 | 11.7 |
| ≥2 | 10.0 | 4.9 |
| Mean (95% CI) | 0.18 (0.12-0.23) | 0.10 (0.09-0.10) |
| No. of nonemergency visits | | |
| 0 | 29.5 | 42.0 |
| 1 | 16.3 | 19.8 |
| ≥2 | 54.2 | 38.2 |
| Mean (95% CI) | 2.80 (2.44-3.16) | 1.56 (1.54-1.58) |

Abbreviation: See Table 2.

*Data are adjusted for sex, primary language, age, insurance, and household educational attainment. $P<.001$ for the difference between the 2 groups for all variables.

†Data are given as the percentage of each group and are based on sampling fractions and weighted extrapolation from parent report of 483 children with autism and 84 789 children without autism.

## COMMENT

Results from this large national survey of children's health suggest a consistent pattern of substantially higher health care needs and use among children with autism, relative to other children. Parents of children with autism reported needing markedly more services for emotional or behavioral problems; for physical, occupational, or speech therapy; and for prescribed medications meant for long-term use. Internally consistent with these results for children with autism were the concordant parental reports of higher average numbers of hospital emergency department, preventive care, and nonemergency physician visits and higher prevalences of behavioral and conduct problems, ADHD, anxiety or depression, allergies, and several other conditions. Indeed, parents reported their children with autism to be in fair or poor health far more frequently on average than did other parents (10.9% vs 3.3%), despite the fact that autism is not considered a medical disorder per se.

This study serves to highlight the breadth of health care challenges that are faced by children with autism and their families. In addition to the conditions asked about in this survey, it is well documented that epilepsy is common in children with autism, perhaps occurring in up to 29%.[14] Although more controversial,[15,16] a high frequency of chronic gastrointestinal problems also has been reported in several autism studies.[7] Molloy and Manning-Courtney[8] estimated the prevalence of gastrointestinal symptoms in a clinic population of children with autism at 24%, with chronic diarrhea being the most common at 12%. In addition, several rare clinical conditions are associated with autism, including Rett disorder, fragile X syndrome, and tuberous sclerosis.[17,18] Rutter et al[19] suggest that 10% to 12% of individuals with autism have congenital conditions affecting the central nervous system. The prevalence of these conditions in children with autism seems to vary with IQ, with increased frequency among those with lower intellectual capacities.[20] Other researchers[20,21] also describe the association of concurrent conditions with IQ and, with broader definitions, note that between 24% and 37% of children with autism were associated with another medical condition. They included in their definition of a medical condition metabolic, immune-related, and other diseases beyond those that directly affect the central nervous system.[3]

Comparing the range of concurrent conditions across studies is difficult because studies differ in their inclusion criteria for autism subtypes and differ in methods for identifying and defining what constitutes a comorbid condition. The latter issue is important when considering the high prevalence of parent-reported concurrent ADHD with autism in our study. The *Diagnostic and Statistical Manual of Mental Disorders, Fourth Edition*,[1(p78)] states in reference to ADHD, "The disturbance does not occur exclusively during the course of a Pervasive Developmental Disorder," suggesting that ADHD should not be diagnosed concurrently with autism. However, as discussed in detail by Ghaziuddin,[22] this *Diagnostic and Statistical Manual of Mental Disorders, Fourth Edition*, instruction is based on untenable clinical assumptions about autism, and ADHD certainly is diagnosed in children with autism in current practice, particularly for Asperger disorder.[23-27] Nevertheless, the frequency of parent-reported dual diagnoses of ADHD and autism in our study is high and should be interpreted cautiously. Also, given the rigorous testing required for a clinical diagnosis of food allergies and the scant evidence in the medical literature to support our finding that food allergies are more common among children with ASD, caution should be exercised when interpreting this finding as well.

Although the omission of survey questions related to medical and mental health conditions more specific to autism, such as epilepsy and mental retardation, is an important limitation of this analysis, these data illustrate the need for a comprehensive evaluation of the full spectrum of concurrent conditions among children with autism. The Council on Children With Disabilities of the American Academy of Pediatrics[28(p1223)] stated that "although children with ASD have the same health care needs as children without disabilities, they are at greater risk of concurring psychiatric problems." Our data are consistent with the observation of higher rates of several psychiatric challenges, including depression, anxiety, and ADHD, but, in contrast to the American Academy of Pediatrics council statement, we also found a substantially higher proportion of a range of medical ailments than would be expected based on the comparison group. Presumably, the effects from epilepsy, gastrointestinal problems, mental retardation, and other medical and psychological conditions not asked about in this survey are reflected in our results through reported medication use, physician visits, need for therapies, and other measures of health care use. A formal investigation of economic and resource use related to autism would provide important information for future planning within health care systems.

The complex presentation of many children with autism, as suggested by the findings in our study, poses a potential dilemma in the pediatric primary care setting, particularly when considering the characteristic sensory sensitivities that may be present in the child.[29,30] Children with autism, along with their need for sameness and predictability, may be unusually reactive to the lighting, sounds, or odors of the clinic. They also may be very uncomfortable with being touched by instruments or by persons, including nurses and physicians, whom they do not know well. Given the relative infrequency of seeing autistic patients in most primary care practices, it may be unrealistic to design a clinical setting to specifically accommodate the special needs of these children. It might be possible, however, for large practices or health care systems to implement a coordinated care or case management plan (ie, a medical home model[31,32]) for children with autism that would provide a knowledgeable central contact person who is familiar with the child's specific medical and psychological needs. Also, having office management procedures in place to alert staff, nurses, and physicians in anticipation of a visit and to minimize the social and sensory difficulties of the child with autism might improve the efficiency and effectiveness of the visit and of the patient/parent satisfaction level. Clinical research to evaluate these ideas could be informative.

The nature of the cross-sectional data in the survey (ie, unvalidated parental report with lack of specificity on type of ASD or method of diagnosis) is another limitation that needs to be considered when interpreting our findings. Although the possibility of false positives and false negatives for ASD is likely, the study's prevalence estimate of autism at 53 per 10 000 children aged 3 through 17 years is reasonably consistent with the range reported in recent studies.[33,34] In addition, the weighted mean number of visits reported by parents for nonurgent care (preventive and nonemergency combined) of 3.46 among the children aged 3 through 17 years without autism in our study (data not shown) is also reasonably close to the 2.88 reported for children younger than 18 years in the National Ambulatory Medical Care Study.[35]

In conclusion, the findings we report herein document an important pattern of high parent-reported rates of concurrent conditions and high health care use associated with childhood autism on a national scale that warrants systematic assessment in more specific detail, from the standpoint of health systems and effect on the family. The responsibilities that parents bear as they manage the diverse needs of their child with autism are likely to be enormous from economic, psychosocial, and caregiving perspectives. Likewise, an economic evaluation of health services related to ASD across health care systems would be valuable to understand and plan for present and future resource needs, perhaps including special training of primary care providers in the diverse management requirements of these pediatric patients. Given the striking trends of increasing prevalence of childhood ASD[34,36] during the past decade, a more comprehensive understanding is needed on the impact of ASD on public and private health care systems.

**Accepted for Publication:** January 24, 2006.
**Correspondence:** James G. Gurney, PhD, Department of Pediatrics, University of Michigan, 300 N Ingalls St, Room

6E02, Ann Arbor, MI 48109-0456 (jamegurn@umich.edu).

**Author Contributions:** *Study concept and design:* Gurney, McPheeters, and Davis. *Acquisition of data:* McPheeters. *Analysis and interpretation of data:* McPheeters. *Drafting of the manuscript:* Gurney and McPheeters. *Critical revision of the manuscript for important intellectual content:* Gurney, McPheeters, and Davis. *Statistical analysis:* Gurney and McPheeters. *Administrative, technical, and material support:* Gurney and Davis. *Study supervision:* Gurney.

**Financial Disclosure:** None reported.

## REFERENCES


1. American Psychiatric Association. *Diagnostic and Statistical Manual of Mental Disorders, Fourth Edition.* Washington, DC: American Psychiatric Association; 1994.
2. Lord C, Rutter M, Le Couteur A. Autism Diagnostic Interview–Revised: a revised version of a diagnostic interview for caregivers of individuals with possible pervasive developmental disorders. *J Autism Dev Disord.* 1994;24:659-685.
3. Gillberg C, Billstedt E. Autism and Asperger syndrome: coexistence with other clinical disorders. *Acta Psychiatr Scand.* 2000;102:321-330.
4. Rutter M. Cognitive deficits in the pathogenesis of autism. *J Child Psychol Psychiatry.* 1983;24:513-531.
5. Danielsson S, Gillberg IC, Billstedt E, Gillberg C, Olsson I. Epilepsy in young adults with autism: a prospective population-based follow-up study of 120 individuals diagnosed in childhood. *Epilepsia.* 2005;46:918-923.
6. Canitano R, Luchetti A, Zappella M. Epilepsy, electroencephalographic abnormalities, and regression in children with autism. *J Child Neurol.* 2005;20:27-31.
7. Horvath K, Perman JA. Autistic disorder and gastrointestinal disease. *Curr Opin Pediatr.* 2002;14:583-587.
8. Molloy CA, Manning-Courtney P. Prevalence of chronic gastrointestinal symptoms in children with autism and autistic spectrum disorders. *Autism.* 2003;7:165-171.
9. Castillo M. Autism and ADHD: common disorders, elusive explanations. *Acad Radiol.* 2005;12:533-534.
10. Ghaziuddin M, Ghaziuddin N, Greden J. Depression in persons with autism: implications for research and clinical care. *J Autism Dev Disord.* 2002;32:299-306.
11. Malow BA. Sleep disorders, epilepsy, and autism. *Ment Retard Dev Disabil Res Rev.* 2004;10:122-125.
12. NCHS. National Survey of Children's Health. http://www.cdc.gov/nchs/about/major/slaits/nsch.htm. Accessed January 23, 2006.
13. Duan N, Manning W, Morris C, Newhouse J. A comparison of alternative models for the demand for medical care. *J Bus Econ Stat.* 1983;1:115-126.
14. Kielinen M, Rantala H, Timonen E, Linna SL, Moilanen I. Associated medical disorders and disabilities in children with autistic disorder: a population-based study. *Autism.* 2004;8:49-60.
15. Kuddo T, Nelson KB. How common are gastrointestinal disorders in children with autism? *Curr Opin Pediatr.* 2003;15:339-343.
16. Black C, Kaye JA, Jick H. Relation of childhood gastrointestinal disorders to autism: nested case-control study using data from the UK General Practice Research Database. *BMJ.* 2002;325:419-421.
17. Fombonne E. The epidemiology of autism: a review. *Psychol Med.* 1999;29:769-786.
18. Baker P, Piven J, Sato Y. Autism and tuberous sclerosis complex: prevalence and clinical features. *J Autism Dev Disord.* 1998;28:279-285.
19. Rutter M, Bailey A, Bolton P, Le Couteur A. Autism and known medical conditions: myth and substance. *J Child Psychol Psychiatry.* 1994;35:311-322.
20. Barton M, Volkmar F. How commonly are known medical conditions associated with autism? *J Autism Dev Disord.* 1998;28:273-278.
21. Gillberg C, Coleman M. Autism and medical disorders: a review of the literature. *Dev Med Child Neurol.* 1996;38:191-202.
22. Ghaziuddin M. *Mental Health Aspects of Autism and Asperger Syndrome.* London, England: Jessica Kingsley Publishers; 2005:109-126.
23. Gillberg IC, Gillberg C, Ahlsen G. Autistic behaviour and attention deficits in tuberous sclerosis: a population-based study. *Dev Med Child Neurol.* 1994;36:50-56.
24. Goldstein S, Schwebach AJ. The comorbidity of pervasive developmental disorder and attention deficit hyperactivity disorder: results of a retrospective chart review. *J Autism Dev Disord.* 2004;34:329-339.
25. Ghaziuddin M, Weidmer-Mikhail E, Ghaziuddin N. Comorbidity of Asperger syndrome: a preliminary report. *J Intellect Disabil Res.* 1998;42:279-283.
26. Hastings RP, Beck A, Daley D, Hill C. Symptoms of ADHD and their correlates in children with intellectual disabilities. *Res Dev Disabil.* 2005;26:456-468.
27. Sturm H, Fernell E, Gillberg C. Autism spectrum disorders in children with normal intellectual levels: associated impairments and subgroups. *Dev Med Child Neurol.* 2004;46:444-447.
28. American Academy of Pediatrics. The pediatrician's role in the diagnosis and management of autistic spectrum disorder in children. *Pediatrics.* 2001;107:1221-1226.
29. Harrison J, Hare DJ. Brief report: assessment of sensory abnormalities in people with autistic spectrum disorders. *J Autism Dev Disord.* 2004;34:727-730.
30. O'Neill M, Jones RS. Sensory-perceptual abnormalities in autism: a case for more research? *J Autism Dev Disord.* 1997;27:283-293.
31. American Academy of Pediatrics Council on Children With Disabilities. Care coordination in the medical home: integrating health and related systems of care for children with special health care needs. *Pediatrics.* 2005;116:1238-1244.
32. Cooley WC. Redefining primary pediatric care for children with special health care needs: the primary care medical home. *Curr Opin Pediatr.* 2004;16:689-692.
33. Yeargin-Allsopp M, Rice C, Karapurkar T, Doernberg N, Boyle C, Murphy C. Prevalence of autism in a US metropolitan area. *JAMA.* 2003;289:49-55.
34. Gurney JG, Fritz MS, Ness KK, Sievers P, Newschaffer CJ, Shapiro EG. Analysis of prevalence trends of autism spectrum disorder in Minnesota. *Arch Pediatr Adolesc Med.* 2003;157:622-627.
35. NCHS. Health, United States, 2004: chartbook on trends in the health of Americans. Available at: http://www.cdc.gov/nchs/data/hus/hus04.pdf#083. Accessed January 23, 2006.
36. Newschaffer CJ, Falb MD, Gurney JG. National autism prevalence trends from United States special education data. *Pediatrics.* 2005;115:e277-e282. doi:10.1542/peds.2004-1958. Accessed May 10, 2006.

# Impact of Staffing on Bloodstream Infections in the Neonatal Intensive Care Unit

*Jeannie P. Cimiotti, DNS, RN; Janet Haas, MS; Lisa Saiman, MD, MPH; Elaine L. Larson, PhD*

**Objective:** To examine the association between registered nurse staffing and healthcare-associated bloodstream infections in infants in the neonatal intensive care unit (NICU).

**Design:** Prospective cohort study.

**Setting:** Two level III-IV NICUs in New York, NY, from March 1, 2001, through January 31, 2003.

**Participants:** A total of 2675 infants admitted to the NICUs for more than 48 hours and all registered nurses who worked in the same NICUs during the study period.

**Intervention:** Hours of care provided by registered nurses.

**Main Outcome Measure:** Time to first episode of healthcare-associated bloodstream infection.

**Results:** A total of 224 infants had an infection that met the study definition of healthcare-associated bloodstream infection. In a multivariate analysis, after controlling for infants' intrinsic and extrinsic risk factors, a greater number of hours of care provided by registered nurses in NICU 2 was associated with a decreased risk of bloodstream infection in these infants (hazard ratio, 0.21; 95% confidence interval, 0.06-0.79).

**Conclusion:** Our findings suggest that registered nurse staffing is associated with the risk of bloodstream infection in infants in the NICU.

*Arch Pediatr Adolesc Med. 2006;160:832-836*

HEALTHCARE-ASSOCIATED infections are a significant cause of morbidity and mortality among infants in the neonatal intensive care unit (NICU).[1,2] Infants hospitalized in the NICU have the highest rates of healthcare-associated infection among the pediatric population, with infection rates ranging from 6 to more than 30 infections per 100 patient discharges.[3] Among infants in the NICU, the bloodstream is the most common site of healthcare-associated infection in all birth weight groups.[4]

Evidence of a significant association between nurse staffing and adverse patient outcomes has been reported.[5-7] However, to date only a few studies have examined the association between nurse staffing and healthcare-associated infections in infants.[8-11] Furthermore, no prospective studies, to our knowledge, have specifically examined the association between nurse staffing and bloodstream infections in the NICU. This study examined the association between registered nurse staffing and bloodstream infections among infants in the NICU.

**Author Affiliations:** Center for Health Outcomes and Policy Research, School of Nursing, University of Pennsylvania, Philadelphia (Dr Cimiotti); School of Nursing (Ms Haas and Dr Larson) and Department of Pediatrics, College of Physicians and Surgeons (Dr Saiman), Columbia University, and Department of Epidemiology, New York–Presbyterian Hospital (Dr Saiman), New York, NY.

## METHODS

### DESIGN

This cohort study used data collected as part of a larger clinical trial to assess the effects of 2 hand hygiene regimens on healthcare-associated infections in infants in the NICU.[12] The study used a randomly assigned crossover design in which either a traditional antiseptic soap containing 2% chlorhexidine gluconate or a waterless hand rinse containing 61% ethyl alcohol was used by all staff and visitors sequentially for half of the study period (11 months for each product).

### SAMPLE AND SETTING

The study was conducted in 2 level III-IV NICUs located in New York, NY. Both NICU 1 (43 beds) and NICU 2 (50 beds) are affiliated with the New York–Presbyterian Hospital and provide specialized medical treatment to severely compromised infants. Data on nurse staffing were provided by the nurse staffing office of each NICU, and data were classified as follows: hours per day for full-time registered nurses, full-time other (ie, nurse managers), per-diem registered nurses, float registered nurses, and agency registered nurses. Staffing data were collected on all infants who were hospitalized in the NICU for more than 48 hours from March 1, 2001, through January 31, 2003. Institutional review board approval was obtained from the participating institutions.

## DATA COLLECTION

In this study, we examined only the first episode of healthcare-associated bloodstream infection. Data on bloodstream infections were collected by the study nurse epidemiologist, and the National Nosocomial Infection Surveillance System definitions were used.[13] Clinical data were obtained from infants' medical records, and laboratory, radiology, and pharmacy data were collected from the hospitals' computer information systems (ECLIPSYS; Eclipsys Corp, Boca Raton, Fla; WEBCIS; Columbia University Department of Informatics, New York; HealthQuest; McKesson Information Solutions, Alpharetta, Ga; and Eagle; Siemens AG, Munich, Germany). A computerized list of all blood cultures positive for organisms from infants was generated by the clinical microbiology laboratories and reviewed twice weekly by the nurse epidemiologist, who also made unit rounds at least once weekly.

Interrater agreement ($\kappa$=0.97) regarding presence or absence of bloodstream infection was established by comparing data collected simultaneously by the study nurse epidemiologist and the hospital infection control staff for 3 months. Discrepancies regarding infection status were resolved by the consensus of 2 physician coinvestigators (including L.S.).

## RISK FACTORS

Four risk factors reported to be associated with bloodstream infection in infants were examined: birth weight,[14-17] intravascular catheterization,[16-19] major surgery,[20,21] and total parenteral nutrition.[17,19] Birth weight was stratified into 4 groups: less than 1000 g, 1000 to 1500 g, 1501 to 2500 g, and more than 2500 g. Catheters were classified as umbilical, tunneled (Hickman and Broviac), and peripherally inserted central. The performance of major surgery, defined as an operating room procedure other than circumcision or minor abdominal surgery,[22] was determined from the infant's diagnosis related group. Total parenteral nutrition was recorded as the number of days of total parenteral nutrition received before bloodstream infection, or on discharge in infants without a bloodstream infection.

Two additional variables were examined: (1) the hand hygiene product used by staff when each bloodstream infection was diagnosed and (2) registered nurse hours, defined as registered nurse care hours per infant per day. Registered nurse hours were adjusted for patient case mix based on diagnosis related group and nursing intensity weight as described elsewhere.[5-7,23] The 2001 nursing intensity weights, which reflect the amount of nursing care required for typical patients in each diagnosis related group, ranged from 1.96 to 32.40.

## DATA ANALYSIS

Continuous variables were presented as the mean and standard deviation and categorical variables were expressed as percentages. Infant characteristics were compared by $\chi^2$, Fisher exact, and unpaired $t$ tests. Data from each day of each infant's admission were linked with the corresponding registered nurse staffing data (adjusted for case mix) for the same days before bloodstream infection or censoring (eg, death or discharged with no infection). The window of exposure was calculated as the mean of registered nurse hours from 48 to 144 hours before bloodstream infection.

A Cox proportional hazards regression model was used to identify risk factors associated with bloodstream infection. The proportional hazards assumption was validated both graphically and through fitting a discrete-time model as described by Allison.[24] Confounder selection was based on the criteria described by Mickey and Greenland[25]; variables significant ($P<.25$) in the preliminary analysis were included in the multivariate model. Intravascular catheterization, total parenteral nutrition, and registered nurse hours were modeled as time-dependent covariates.

In this analysis, the risk of bloodstream infection was modeled for each infant, and then parameter estimates of the covariates birth weight, intravascular catheterization, total parenteral nutrition, hand hygiene product, NICU site, and adjusted registered nurse hours were calculated for that same infant. If a neonate had more than one bloodstream infection, only the first was included in these analyses.

Because intravascular catheters in infants have been reported as a risk factor for bloodstream infection,[16-18] the incidence density was also defined as number of bloodstream infections per 1000 catheter days, as per National Nosocomial Infections Surveillance System protocol.[3] All calculations were performed with Stata release 9 statistical software (StataCorp LP, College Station, Tex).

# RESULTS

A total of 3155 admissions to the study NICU were recorded during the study period. After excluding infants who were admitted for 48 hours or less, the final sample included 2675 admissions. Of these, 224 infants (8.4%) had a total of 298 bloodstream infections. Coagulase-negative staphylococci (45.0%) were the most common pathogens, followed by gram-negative bacteria (23.2%), yeast (13.5%), *Staphylococcus aureus* (9.5%), and enterococci (7.7%). The incidence rate of bloodstream infection was 6.11 per 1000 patient days and 16.56 per 1000 catheter days. Of the 48 infant deaths that occurred during this study, 16 involved infants with a bloodstream infection.

## CHARACTERISTICS OF INFANTS

The characteristics of infants enrolled in this study are summarized in **Table 1**. Overall, 55.9% of the infants in this sample were male, their mean gestational age was 34.8 weeks (range, 23-42 weeks), and their mean birth weight was 2401 g (range, 428-5513 g). Overall, 309 infants (11.6%) had a birthweight of less than 1000 g; 330 (12.3%), 1000 to 1500 g; 812 (30.3%), 1501 to 2500 g; and 1224 (45.8%), greater than 2500 g. The length of stay before bloodstream infection ranged from 2 to 312 days (mean, 14.7 days). Central venous catheters were inserted in 1543 infants (57.6%): 783 (50.7%) were umbilical, 45 (2.9%) tunneled, and 715 (46.3%) peripherally inserted central catheters. In addition, 468 infants (17.5%) had major surgery and 1284 (48.0%) received total parenteral nutrition during their hospitalization.

## CHARACTERISTICS OF REGISTERED NURSE STAFFING

Nursing acuity and registered nurse hours are summarized in **Table 2**. Overall, the mean nursing acuity in the 2 NICUs was 5.3 (range, 2.04-32.4). The mean number of infants occupying beds in the NICUs was 37 (range, 21-49), and the mean number of registered nurse hours per infant per day was 10.8 (range, 7.3-15.0).

**Table 1. Characteristics of Study Population by Neonatal Intensive Care Unit (NICU)***

| Characteristic | NICU 1 (n = 1550) No Infection | NICU 1 (n = 1550) Infection | NICU 2 (n = 1125) No Infection | NICU 2 (n = 1125) Infection |
|---|---|---|---|---|
| No. (%) of infants | 1388 (89.5) | 162 (10.5) | 1063 (94.5) | 62 (5.5) |
| Birth weight, No. (%), g | | | | |
| <1000 | 134 (9.7) | 75 (46.3) | 66 (6.2) | 34 (54.8) |
| 1000-1500 | 153 (11.0) | 32 (19.8) | 131 (12.3) | 14 (22.6) |
| 1501-2500 | 433 (31.2) | 22 (13.6) | 349 (32.8) | 8 (12.9) |
| >2500 | 668 (48.1) | 33 (20.4) | 517 (48.6) | 6 (9.7) |
| Catheter, No. (%) | | | | |
| Umbilical | 394 (28.4) | 98 (60.5) | 253 (23.8) | 38 (61.3) |
| Tunneled | 18 (1.3) | 4 (2.5) | 15 (1.4) | 8 (12.9) |
| Peripherally inserted central | 372 (26.8) | 116 (71.6) | 178 (16.7) | 49 (79.0) |
| Catheter days, mean (SD) | 5.3 (11.4) | 16.4 (16.7)† | 3.8 (10.8) | 19.0 (13.5)† |
| Total parenteral nutrition, No. (%) | 823 (59.3) | 154 (95.1) | 200 (23.5) | 57 (91.9) |
| Total parenteral nutrition days, mean (SD) | 6.9 (20.0) | 15.0 (13.4)† | 3.0 (20.0) | 15.9 (13.4)† |
| Surgery, No. (%) | 305 (22.0) | 39 (24.1) | 111 (10.4) | 13 (21.0) |
| Length of stay, mean (SD), d | 12.8 (17.6) | 16.7 (13.3)† | 16.5 (17.6) | 23 (13.3)† |

*Because of rounding, percentages may not all total 100.
†Days to bloodstream infection.

**Table 2. Nursing Acuity and Registered Nurse Staffing by Neonatal Intensive Care Unit (NICU)**

| Characteristic | Mean (SD) NICU 1 No Infection | Mean (SD) NICU 1 Infection | Mean (SD) NICU 2 No Infection | Mean (SD) NICU 2 Infection |
|---|---|---|---|---|
| Nursing intensity weight | 5.3 (2.6) | 7.8 (3.0) | 4.7 (2.1) | 8.5 (3.7) |
| Registered nurse h/d* | 10.7 (1.0) | 10.7 (1.0) | 11.0 (1.0) | 10.7 (1.2) |
| Infant census | 39 (4) | 39 (4) | 34 (5) | 34 (6) |

*Indicates registered nurse hours per infant per day.

**Table 3. Hazard Ratios Estimating the Risk of Bloodstream Infection**

| Variable | Hazard Ratio (95% CI) |
|---|---|
| Birth weight, g | |
| <1000 | 2.64 (1.77-3.94) |
| 1000-1500 | 1.82 (1.15-2.89) |
| 1501-2500 | 1.42 (0.85-2.38) |
| >2500 | 1.00 |
| Peripherally inserted central catheter | 1.83 (1.31-2.56) |
| Umbilical catheter | 1.33 (0.88-2.02) |
| Total parenteral nutrition | 12.62 (6.93-22.98) |
| Alcohol hand rub | 1.15 (0.84-1.58) |
| Chlorhexidine gluconate | 1.00 |
| NICU 1 | 0.07 (0.005-1.02) |
| NICU 2 | 1.00 |
| Registered nurse hours, NICU 1 | 1.53 (0.39-6.07) |
| Registered nurse hours, NICU 2 | 0.21 (0.06-0.79) |

Abbreviations: CI, confidence interval; NICU, neonatal intensive care unit.

## MULTIVARIATE ANALYSIS

In the preliminary analysis, surgery, tunneled catheters, and the hand hygiene product used by staff were not significantly associated with bloodstream infection (all *P*>.25). Risk factors significant in the preliminary analyses included birth weight, 2 catheter types (umbilical and peripherally inserted central catheters), total parenteral nutrition, NICU site, and registered nurse hours. We found a significant NICU site × registered nurse hours interaction effect (hazard ratio [HR], 7.12; 95% confidence interval [CI], 1.23-41.42). On the basis of this finding, we adjusted our model in an attempt to obtain an accurate representation of registered nurse staffing in each NICU as described by Greenland and Rothman.[26]

These significant variables and the hand hygiene product were further analyzed in the multivariate Cox regression model. The hand hygiene product, although not significant in the preliminary analysis (*P*=.26), was included in the multivariate model because it was the intervention in the parent clinical trial. A summary of results from the multivariate Cox regression model is provided in **Table 3**. In this model, 3 risk factors were independently associated with bloodstream infection. Birth weight of less than 1000 g (HR, 2.64; 95% CI, 1.77-3.94), birth weight of 1000 to 1500 g (HR, 1.82; 95% CI, 1.15-2.89), number of days of peripherally inserted central catheter use (HR, 1.83; 95% CI, 1.31-2.56), and number of days of total parenteral nutrition use (HR, 12.62; 95% CI, 6.93-22.98) were significantly associated with an increased risk of bloodstream infection. Among the 4 birth weight groups, infants weighing less than 1000 g were 2.64 times more likely to develop bloodstream infection than the highest birth weight group (>2500 g). Further analysis of the catheter data showed that infants with bloodstream infection had peripherally inserted central catheters in place for significantly more days than uninfected infants (mean, 12 and 3 days, respectively; $P<.001$).

In addition, the number of registered nurse hours in NICU 2 was significantly associated with a decreased risk (HR, 0.21; 95% CI, 0.06-0.79) of bloodstream infection. We found that more registered nurse hours per nursing intensity weight was associated with a 79% reduction in the risk of bloodstream infection in NICU 2. Umbilical catheter use, hand hygiene product, NICU site, and registered nurse hours in NICU 1 were not associated with risk of bloodstream infection. A survival curve comparing registered nurse hours at NICU 2 and number of days to first bloodstream infection is shown in the **Figure**.

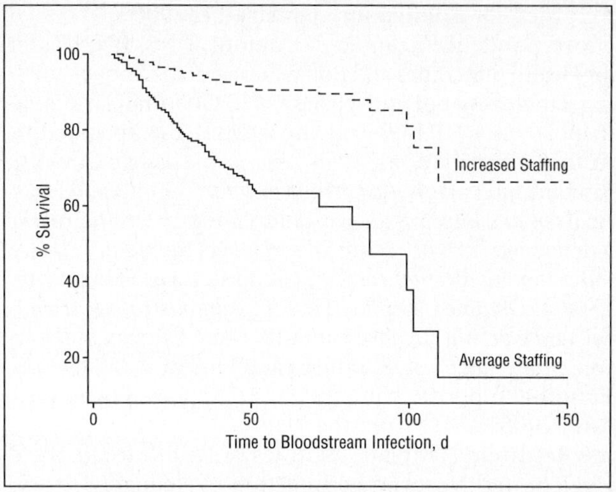


**Figure.** Survival estimates of 1125 infants in neonatal intensive care unit 2, showing the typical changes in survival after increasing registered nurse hours.

## COMMENT

To our knowledge, this is the first prospective study to examine registered nurse staffing and the risk of endemic bloodstream infection in infants in the NICU. We found low birth weight, peripherally inserted central catheters, and total parenteral nutrition to be significantly associated with bloodstream infection. These findings are consistent with previous research on infants in the NICU.[17,19,27-33]

After controlling for infants' intrinsic and extrinsic risk factors, we found that the number of hours of care provided by registered nurses was significantly associated with the risk of bloodstream infection in one of our study NICUs. This finding is consistent with other studies on nurse staffing. Nursing workload has been associated with higher rates of infection[34-36] and increased mortality.[37,38] The use of pooled or temporary nurses has been significantly associated with infection,[8,34,39,40] possibly because of lapses in aseptic technique by those unfamiliar with the routine care policies of the nursing unit. In the NICU, it has been reported that bloodstream infection is associated with understaffing, overcrowding, and the moving of infants between rooms.[8,9,11] Furthermore, understaffing has been linked to several infectious outbreaks[8,11] and the transmission of antibiotic-resistant organisms among premature infants.[8,10] Our findings suggest that increasing registered nurse staffing by 1 full-time equivalent could possibly reduce the risk of bloodstream infection by 11% in NICU 2.

The fact that the number of registered nurse hours was not associated with bloodstream infection in NICU 1 (HR, 1.53; 95% CI, 0.39-6.07) may have several explanations. When compared with the infants in NICU 2, those in NICU 1 were significantly smaller and more acutely ill, with more invasive devices, which could outweigh the effect of registered nurse staffing. In addition, the infants in NICU 1 had consistently fewer registered nurse hours of care per day than those in NICU 2. This lack of variation in registered nurse hours in NICU 1 may have made it more difficult to detect an association between registered nurse hours and bloodstream infection in these infants. Surprisingly, we found that when nursing acuity increased, registered nurse hours remained the same in NICU 1 and decreased in NICU 2. This unrecognized increase in nursing acuity could have increased the risk of bloodstream infection in both NICUs. It has been reported that scores on acuity measures are associated with the risk of healthcare-associated infection in infants. Gray and colleagues[41] report in a study of low-birth-weight infants that assessing illness severity with the Score for Neonatal Acute Physiology provides information on the risk of bloodstream infection beyond that provided by birth weight alone. Griffin and Moorman[42] reported that Score for Neonatal Acute Physiology values rise 24 hours before bloodstream infection. It has also been reported that the Clinical Risk Index for Babies is predictive of bloodstream infection in low-birth-weight infants.[43] Hospital staffing decisions are typically determined by the number of patients in a unit; however, the foregoing findings suggest that hospitals should consider implementing a patient classification system that is acuity driven to determine nurse staffing need.

This study had several limitations. First, it was conducted in 2 NICUs with high-risk infants, which limits generalizability to other hospital units and patient populations. Second, although the level of nurse education has been associated with adverse patient outcomes,[44] the educational level of nurses was unmeasured in this study. Third, the 2 study NICUs were environmentally different in a number of ways (NICU 2 was newly renovated and more spacious than NICU 1).

In conclusion, our findings suggest that registered nurse staffing is associated with the risk of bloodstream infection among infants in the NICU. We hypothesize that inadequate nurse staffing and increased nurse workload in a critical care environment results in poor hand hygiene compliance, breaks in aseptic technique, or compromises in practice that might increase the risk of transmitting infection. Further research is warranted that examines the association between registered nurse staffing and healthcare-associated infection to improve the quality of care and the outcomes of infants in the NICU.

**Accepted for Publication:** January 17, 2006.
**Correspondence:** Jeannie P. Cimiotti, DNS, RN, Center for Health Outcomes and Policy Research, School of Nursing, University of Pennsylvania, 420 Guardian Dr, Philadelphia, PA 19104-6096 (jcimiott@nursing.upenn.edu).
**Author Contributions:** *Study concept and design:* Cimiotti, Saiman, and Larson. *Acquisition of data:* Cimiotti and Haas. *Analysis and interpretation of data:* Cimiotti. *Drafting of the manuscript:* Cimiotti. *Critical revision of the manuscript for important intellectual content*: Cimiotti, Haas, Saiman, and Larson. *Obtained funding:* Larson. *Administrative, technical, and material support:* Cimiotti, Haas, Saiman, and Larson. *Study supervision:* Saiman and Larson.
**Funding/Support:** This study was supported by grant 1 R01 NR05197-03 from the National Institute of Nursing Research, National Institutes of Health (Staff Hand Hygiene and Nosocomial Infection in Neonates).
**Acknowledgment:** Leo Lichtig, PhD (vice president, Aon Consulting), and Jack Needleman, PhD (associate professor, University of California at Los Angeles), acted as expert consultants on this study. John E. Marcotte, PhD (director, Statistical Computing Group, University of Pennsylvania), and Tim Cheney (data analyst, Center for Health Outcomes and Policy Research, School of Nursing, University of Pennsylvania) provided statistical support, and 3M Health Information Systems provided the DRG Finder software that was used in analysis. We are extremely grateful to the neonatal nurses and the management staff of New York–Presbyterian Hospital.

## REFERENCES


1. Pessoa-Silva CL, Miyasaki CH, de Almeida MF, Kopelman BI, Raggio RL, Wey SB. Neonatal late-onset bloodstream infection: attributable mortality, excess of length of stay and risk factors. *Eur J Epidemiol.* 2001;17:715-720.
2. Stoll BJ, Hansen N. Infections in VLBW infants: studies from the NICHD Neonatal Research Network. *Semin Perinatol.* 2003;27:293-301.
3. NNIS System. National Nosocomial Infections Surveillance (NNIS) System Report, data summary from January 1992 through June 2003, issued August 2003. *Am J Infect Control.* 2003;31:481-498.
4. Gaynes RP, Edwards JR, Jarvis WR, Culver DH, Tolson JS, Martone WJ. Nosocomial infections among neonates in high-risk nurseries in the United States: National Nosocomial Infections Surveillance System. *Pediatrics.* 1996;98:357-361.
5. Knauf RA, Lichtig LK, Risen-McCoy R, Singer AD, Wozniak L. *Implementing Nursing's Report Card: A Study of RN Staffing, Length of Stay and Patient Outcomes.* Washington, DC: American Nurses Association; 1997.
6. Lichtig LK, Knauf RA, Milholland DK. Some impacts of nursing on acute care hospital outcomes. *J Nurs Adm.* 1999;29:25-33.
7. Needleman J, Buerhaus P, Mattke S, Stewart M, Zelevinsky K. Nurse-staffing levels and the quality of care in hospitals. *N Engl J Med.* 2002;346:1715-1722.
8. Andersen BM, Lindemann R, Bergh K, et al. Spread of methicillin-resistant *Staphylococcus aureus* in a neonatal intensive unit associated with understaffing, overcrowding and mixing of patients. *J Hosp Infect.* 2002;50:18-24.
9. Haley RW, Bregman DA. The role of understaffing and overcrowding in recurrent outbreaks of staphylococcal infection in a neonatal special-care unit. *J Infect Dis.* 1982;145:875-885.
10. Haley RW, Cushion NB, Tenover FC, et al. Eradication of endemic methicillin-resistant *Staphylococcus aureus* infections from a neonatal intensive care unit. *J Infect Dis.* 1995;171:614-624.
11. Harbarth S, Sudre P, Dharan S, Cadenas M, Pittet D. Outbreak of *Enterobacter cloacae* related to understaffing, overcrowding, and poor hygiene practices. *Infect Control Hosp Epidemiol.* 1999;20:598-603.
12. Larson EL, Cimiotti J, Haas J, et al. Effect of antiseptic handwashing vs alcohol sanitizer on health care–associated infections in neonatal intensive care units. *Arch Pediatr Adolesc Med.* 2005;159:377-383.
13. Horan TC, Emori TG. Definitions of key terms used in the NNIS System. *Am J Infect Control.* 1997;25:112-116.
14. Lehner R, Leitich H, Jirecek S, Weninger M, Kaider A. Retrospective analysis of early-onset neonatal sepsis in very low birth-weight infants. *Eur J Clin Microbiol Infect Dis.* 2001;20:830-832.
15. Watson RS, Carcillo JA, Linde-Zwirble WT, Clermont G, Lidicker J, Angus DC. The epidemiology of severe sepsis in children in the United States. *Am J Respir Crit Care Med.* 2003;167:695-701.
16. Urrea M, Iriondo M, Thio M, et al. A prospective incidence study of nosocomial infections in a neonatal care unit. *Am J Infect Control.* 2003;31:505-507.
17. Nagata E, Brito AS, Matsuo T. Nosocomial infections in a neonatal intensive care unit: incidence and risk factors. *Am J Infect Control.* 2002;30:26-31.
18. Wisplinghoff H, Seifert H, Tallent SM, Bischoff T, Wenzel RP, Edmond MB. Nosocomial bloodstream infections in pediatric patients in United States hospitals: epidemiology, clinical features and susceptibilities. *Pediatr Infect Dis J.* 2003;22:686-691.
19. Brodie SB, Sands KE, Gray JE, et al. Occurrence of nosocomial bloodstream infections in six neonatal intensive care units. *Pediatr Infect Dis J.* 2000;19:56-65.
20. Oppido G, Napoleone CP, Formigari R, et al. Outcome of cardiac surgery in low birth weight and premature infants. *Eur J Cardiothorac Surg.* 2004;26:44-53.
21. Christie C, Hammond J, Reising S, Evans-Patterson J. Clinical and molecular epidemiology of enterococcal bacteremia in a pediatric teaching hospital. *J Pediatr.* 1994;125:392-399.
22. *AP-DRGs: All Patient Diagnosis Related Groups Definitions Manual.* Version 18.0. Wallingford, Conn: 3M Health Information Systems; 2000.
23. Lichtig LK, Knauf RA, Risen-McCoy R, Wozniak L. *Nurse Staffing and Patient Outcomes in the Inpatient Hospital Setting.* Washington, DC: American Nurses Association; 2000.
24. Allison PA. *Event History Analysis Regression for Longitudinal Event Data.* Newbury Park, Calif: Sage Publications; 1984.
25. Mickey RM, Greenland S. The impact of confounder selection criteria on effect estimation. *Am J Epidemiol.* 1989;129:125-137.
26. Greenland S, Rothman KJ. Concepts in interaction. In: Rothman KJ, Greenland S, eds. *Modern Epidemiology.* Philadelphia, Pa: Lippincott Williams & Wilkins; 1998:329-342.
27. Carrieri MP, Stolfi I, Moro ML; Italian Study Group on Hospital Acquired Infections in Neonatal Intensive Care Units. Intercenter variability and time of onset: two crucial issues in the analysis of risk factors for nosocomial sepsis. *Pediatr Infect Dis J.* 2003;22:599-609.
28. Pawa AK, Ramji S, Prakash K, Thirupuram S. Neonatal nosocomial infection: profile and risk factors. *Indian Pediatr.* 1997;34:297-302.
29. Moro ML, De Toni A, Stolfi I, Carrieri MP, Braga M, Zunin C. Risk factors for nosocomial sepsis in newborn intensive and intermediate care units. *Eur J Pediatr.* 1996;155:315-322.
30. Stoll BJ, Hansen N, Fanaroff AA, et al. Late-onset sepsis in very low birth weight neonates: the experience of the NICHD Neonatal Research Network. *Pediatrics.* 2002;110:285-291.
31. Stoll BJ, Gordon T, Korones SB, et al. Late-onset sepsis in very low birth weight neonates: a report from the National Institute of Child Health and Human Development Neonatal Research Network. *J Pediatr.* 1996;129:63-71.
32. Avila-Figueroa C, Goldmann DA, Richardson DK, Gray JE, Ferrari A, Freeman J. Intravenous lipid emulsions are the major determinant of coagulase-negative staphylococcal bacteremia in very low birth weight newborns. *Pediatr Infect Dis J.* 1998;17:10-17.
33. Beck-Sague CM, Azimi P, Fonseca SN, et al. Bloodstream infections in neonatal intensive care unit patients: results of a multicenter study. *Pediatr Infect Dis J.* 1994;13:1110-1116.
34. Fridkin SK, Pear SM, Williamson TH, Galgiani JN, Jarvis WR. The role of understaffing in central venous catheter-associated bloodstream infections. *Infect Control Hosp Epidemiol.* 1996;17:150-158.
35. Vicca AF. Nursing staff workload as a determinant of methicillin-resistant *Staphylococcus aureus* spread in an adult intensive therapy unit. *J Hosp Infect.* 1999;43:109-113.
36. Arnow P, Allyn PA, Nichols EM, Hill DL, Pezzlo M, Bartlett RH. Control of methicillin-resistant *Staphylococcus aureus* in a burn unit: role of nurse staffing. *J Trauma.* 1982;22:954-959.
37. Aiken LH, Clarke SP, Sloane DM, Sochalski J, Silber JH. Hospital nurse staffing and patient mortality, nurse burnout, and job dissatisfaction. *JAMA.* 2002;288:1987-1993.
38. Tarnow-Mordi WO, Hau C, Warden A, Shearer AJ. Hospital mortality in relation to staff workload: a 4-year study in an adult intensive-care unit. *Lancet.* 2000;356:185-189.
39. Li J, Birkhead GS, Strogatz DS, Coles FB. Impact of institution size, staffing patterns, and infection control practices on communicable disease outbreaks in New York State nursing homes. *Am J Epidemiol.* 1996;143:1042-1049.
40. Robert J, Fridkin SK, Blumberg HM, et al. The influence of the composition of the nursing staff on primary bloodstream infection rates in a surgical intensive care unit. *Infect Control Hosp Epidemiol.* 2000;21:12-17.
41. Gray JE, Richardson DK, McCormick MC, Goldman DA. Coagulase-negative staphylococcal bacteremia among very low birth weight infants: relation to admission illness severity, resource use, and outcome. *Pediatrics.* 1995;95:225-230.
42. Griffin MP, Moorman JR. Toward the early diagnosis of neonatal sepsis and sepsis-like illness using a novel heart rate analysis. *Pediatrics.* 2001;107:97-103.
43. Auriti C, Maccallini A, DiLiso G, DiCiommo V, Ronchetti MP, Orazalesi M. Risk factors for nosocomial infections in the neonatal intensive-care unit. *J Hosp Infect.* 2003;53:25-30.
44. Aiken LH, Clarke SP, Cheung RB, Sloane DM, Silber JH. Educational levels of hospital nurses and surgical patient mortality. *JAMA.* 2003;290:1617-1623.

ARTICLE

# Assessment of Immunization Registry Databases as Supplemental Sources of Data to Improve Ascertainment of Vaccination Coverage Estimates in the National Immunization Survey

Meena Khare, MS; Linda Piccinino, MPS (ID); Lawrence E. Barker, PhD; Robert W. Linkins, MPH, PhD

**Objective:** To evaluate the use of immunization registry data to supplement missing or incomplete vaccination data reported by immunization providers (referred to as "providers" hereafter) in the National Immunization Survey.

**Design:** Cross-sectional, random-digit–dialing, telephone survey to measure vaccination coverage among children aged 19 to 35 months in the United States.

**Setting:** Four sites with mature (with >67% of provider participation in the area) immunization registries.

**Participants:** Of the 639 children with complete household interviews, interviewers had consent from the respondents for 569 (89.0%) children to contact their providers and for 556 (87.0%) children to contact both providers and registries.

**Main Outcome Measures:** Percentages of children up-to-date for vaccines based on data from providers, registries, and both sources combined.

**Results:** According to provider-reported data, weighted estimates of coverage for the recommended childhood vaccine series 4:3:1:3 at the 4 sites were 65.6%, 78.8%, 81.6%, and 77.0%. According to registry data, these coverage rates were consistently lower: 31.7% ($P<.05$), 65.4%, 71.9%, and 61.8%, respectively. When all unique vaccine doses were combined from both sources, the pooled 4:3:1:3 coverage rates increased to 72.0%, 92.0%, 88.7%, and 80.2%, respectively. The quality and completeness of vaccination histories from the registries were inconsistent and varied by sites.

**Conclusions:** Vaccination coverage estimates were the lowest when only registry-reported data were used and were the highest when provider- and registry-reported histories were combined. Although registries enrolled and matched more children, vaccination histories were missing, incomplete, and inconsistent. The quality and completeness of the registry data must be improved and must be comparable across all states before further consideration may be given to supplement or replace the provider-reported National Immunization Survey data.

*Arch Pediatr Adolesc Med. 2006;160:838-842*

**Author Affiliations:** National Center for Health Statistics, Centers for Disease Control and Prevention, Hyattsville, Md (Ms Khare); Abt Associates Inc, Bethesda, Md (Ms Piccinino); and National Immunization Program (Drs Barker and Linkins), Centers for Disease Control and Prevention, Atlanta, Ga. Dr Barker is now with the National Center for Injury Prevention and Control, and Dr Linkins is now with the National Center for HIV, STD, and TB Prevention, both at the Centers for Disease Control and Prevention.

THE NATIONAL IMMUNIZATION Survey (NIS), a large, ongoing, nationwide telephone survey conducted by the Centers for Disease Control and Prevention since 1994, monitors the results of efforts to achieve and maintain Healthy People 2010 objectives for childhood vaccination coverage.[1] The goal is to achieve 90% or more vaccination coverage among children aged 19 to 35 months for 4 or more doses of diphtheria and tetanus toxoids and pertussis vaccine (DTaP), 3 or more doses of poliovirus vaccine, 1 or more doses of measles-mumps-rubella vaccine, 3 or more doses of *Haemophilus influenzae* type B vaccine, 3 or more doses of hepatitis B vaccine, and 1 dose of varicella vaccine.

The NIS collects data in 2 phases. In phase 1, a household telephone interview collects immunization histories and sociodemographic information from the respondent and obtains consent to contact the child's immunization provider (referred to as "provider" hereafter). In phase 2, an immunization history questionnaire is mailed to the immunization provider identified in the interview to collect the child's vaccination history. The NIS uses the same method to collect and process vaccination data in 50 states and 28 large urban areas; this enables researchers to compare vaccination coverage rates across 78 immunization action plan areas. Details of the NIS design and estimation methods are published elsewhere.[2]

In the NIS, approximately 21% of the children with a complete household interview had a missing provider-reported immunization history because the household respondent did not give consent to contact providers; an additional 12% had a missing vaccination history because their immunization provider(s) either did not respond to the mailed questionnaire or did not report an adequate vaccination history to determine the child's up-to-date (UTD) status. Thus, while about 67% of the children had adequate vaccination histories from the providers, this percentage varied across 78 immunization action plan areas (range, 51%-80%).

Another Healthy People 2010 goal is to increase to 95% the proportion of children younger than 6 years in a fully operational population-based immunization registry.[1] Immunization registries are confidential, population-based, computerized information systems that collect vaccination data on children younger than 6 years within a state or local area; the age group varies by the registry. Since the measles outbreak in the early 1990s, a concerted effort has been made by federal, state, and local governments and nonprofit foundations to develop immunization registries that track vaccinations received by age-eligible children.[3,4] As of 2002, 36 states and the District of Columbia had registries targeting the entire state, 7 states had regional or countywide registries, and the remaining 7 states were planning statewide systems.[5] Nationwide, approximately 43% of children younger than 6 years had 2 or more vaccinations recorded in a registry. Methods to collect and process immunization histories by those 43 state and regional registries varied considerably from site to site. Consequently, there are interstate and intrastate differences in the quality and completeness of immunization histories collected from the registries. Several previously published studies[6-8] also reported inconsistencies in data quality and underestimation in coverage rates because of missing dose information (range,10%-40%) in computerized immunization tracking systems.

The objective of the Centers for Disease Control and Prevention–sponsored registry data query project was to explore whether vaccination data could be collected from mature (with >67% of provider participation in the area) registries in the United States and whether these data would be of sufficient quality so that missing or incomplete vaccination histories in the NIS could be supplemented with the registry data in a state.[9,10] Before this study, it was not known how complete or of what quality the data were from the mature registries. It was hoped, however, that these mature registries could consistently demonstrate that they could provide high-quality vaccination data to replace or supplement survey data in order to produce reliable and comparable estimates of vaccination coverage across states in the United States.

The goals of the 2002 NIS registry data query project were to (1) assess whether consent to contact registries can be obtained from the NIS respondents, (2) measure match rates for the NIS children in the registries, (3) evaluate the quality and completeness of the vaccination histories from mature registries, and (4) assess the potential for registry data to replace missing or supplement incomplete vaccination data from the providers.

To achieve these goals, 3 states and 1 urban immunization action plan area with mature registries were selected for this study. Registry sites were selected for geographic diversity and to represent a mix of mandated vs voluntary provider participation. To maintain confidentiality, these 4 sites are referred to as A, B, C, and D in this article.

## METHODS

Quarterly data from the 2002 NIS were used in this study. For 1 of the sites, interview data were used from the first quarter of 2002; and for the other 3 sites, from the third quarter of 2002. After completing the household interview part of the questionnaire, interviewers request consent to contact immunization providers and, if granted, obtain their contact information from the respondents. For this study, household respondents in the 4 areas who consented to contact providers were also requested to grant permission to contact the immunization registry to obtain the child's vaccination history. Following the NIS protocol, immunization history questionnaires with the child's name, sex, and date of birth were mailed to the providers and the same information was also mailed to the registries. Providers were asked to report vaccinations and administration dates for all vaccines given before the date of the household interview. Registries in the 4 areas (A-D) were also searched to locate vaccination records for the NIS-sampled children. This study was approved by the Research Ethics Review Board of the National Center for Health Statistics, Centers for Disease Control and Prevention.

Any registry record or provider response with at least 1 vaccine dose for the matched child was included in this assessment. For comparison, we created 3 subgroups of children who had vaccination data available: (1) only from the providers, (2) only from the registries, and (3) from either providers or registries. For comparability of estimates across the 3 subgroups, simple poststratification was used to adjust the quarterly weights within each subgroup to represent all age-eligible children in the sampling area. (None of the estimates from these 3 subgroups resemble the published NIS estimates because of differences in the weighting procedures.) We compared the weighted proportions of children UTD for the series 4:3:1:3 (with ≥4 DTaP doses, ≥3 poliovirus vaccine doses, ≥1 measles-mumps-rubella vaccine or measles-containing vaccine dose, and ≥3 *Haemophilus influenzae* type B vaccine doses) according to provider data, registry data, and combined provider and registry data. Counting each unique shot date as a single dose for a vaccine from either source created the total number of combined doses for the vaccine. We also substituted missing dose information from the providers with a valid registry-reported dose (shot dates within vaccine schedule or with at least 14 days' lag between 2 unique shot dates), if available. Thus, for example, using the "combined" pooled-dose approach, the total number of DTaP UTD children with 4 or more doses of DTaP included all children classified as DTaP UTD from the provider(s), all children described as DTaP UTD from the registry, and a subset of not UTD children from either source who had incomplete data from both sources and became UTD with the pooled DTaP doses.

A 2-way distribution of the reported number of doses from both sources was examined to assess agreement in and completeness of the dose information for each vaccine type and vaccine series.[10] Generally, multidose vaccines are more likely to have missing doses than a single-dose vaccine when vaccination data are collected from multiple sources; also, medical records or registries are more likely to have missing vaccination data for multidose vaccines when they are administered by multiple providers. In this article, we present the pattern of missing doses for a multidose vaccine, DTaP, and examine the distribution of the number of doses reported by the registries among children who were UTD (ie, having ≥4 doses of DTaP) according to the provider-reported data. We also examine the distribution of the number of doses reported by the providers among those children who were UTD from the registries.

**Table 1. Consent Status and Source of Vaccination Data Among Children With Complete Household Interviews by Registry Site: National Immunization Survey, 2002**

| | Registry Site | | | | |
|---|---|---|---|---|---|
| Variable | A (n = 217) | B (n = 107) | C (n = 217) | D (n = 98) | Total (N = 639) |
| Have consent to contact providers | 189 (87.1) | 94 (87.9) | 197 (90.8) | 89 (90.8) | **569** (89.0) |
| Have consent to contact registry* | 189 (87.1) | 92 (86.0) | 189 (87.1) | 86 (87.8) | **556** (87.0) |
| Children matched in registry† | 171 (78.8) | 79 (73.8) | 172 (79.3) | 71 (72.4) | **493** (77.2) |
| Have registry data‡ | 159 (73.3) | 62 (57.9) | 156 (71.9) | 50 (51.0) | **427** (66.8) |
| Have provider data§ | 129 (59.4) | 67 (62.6) | 141 (65.0) | 65 (66.3) | **402** (62.9) |
| Have provider and/or registry data | 171 (78.8) | 80 (74.8) | 181 (83.4) | 73 (74.5) | **505** (79.0) |
| Have provider and registry data | 116 (53.5) | 49 (45.8) | 116 (53.5) | 42 (42.9) | **323** (50.5) |

*Consent to contact the registry was obtained after receiving the consent to contact the provider (eg, physicians, nurses, hospitals, clinics, others).
†Match based on child's date of birth, sex, and name.
‡One or more doses of vaccine in the registry.
§One or more doses of vaccine reported by the immunization provider(s).

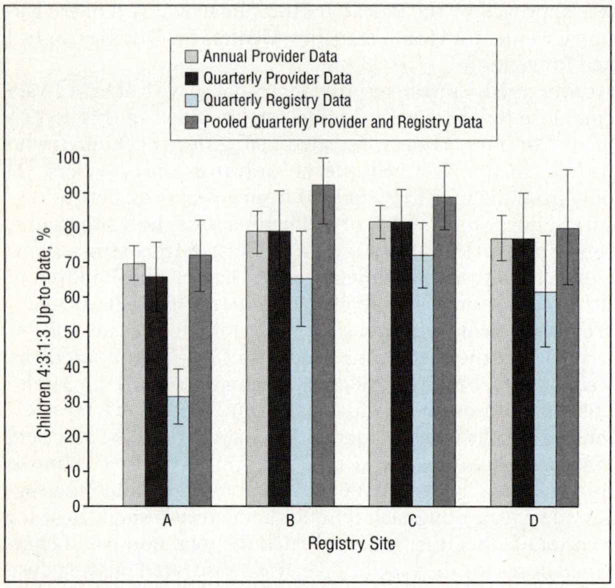


**Figure.** Comparison of the annual coverage estimate for the 4:3:1:3 series and the estimates based on quarterly data from the immunization providers (eg, physicians, nurses, hospitals, clinics, others), the registries, and the pooled provider and registry data reported: National Immunization Survey, 2002. The 4:3:1:3 series includes 4 or more diphtheria and tetanus toxoids and pertussis vaccine doses, 3 or more poliovirus vaccine doses, 1 or more measles-mumps-rubella vaccine or measles-containing vaccine doses, and 3 or more *Haemophilus influenzae* type B vaccine doses.

## RESULTS

In the 2002 NIS, a total of 639 children from the 4 selected areas had complete household interview data. Of these children, interviewers had consent from the respondents for 569 (89.0%) children to contact their providers and for 556 (87.0%) children to contact both providers and registries (**Table 1**). In 2002, the overall NIS consent rate was 87.6% across all 78 immunization action plan areas.

For each selected site, Table 1 shows the number and percentage of children with complete household interviews, consent, and registry- or provider-reported vaccination data. Among the 639 children with interview data, 505 (79.0%; range, 74.5%-83.4%) had vaccination data from at least 1 source: 402 (62.9%; range, 59.4%-66.3%) had information from providers, 427 (66.8%; range, 51.0%-73.3%) had information from the registries, and 323 (50.5%; range, 42.9%-53.5%) had information from both sources. Thus, for 79 (402−323) children (12.4%; range, 6.0%-23.5%), provider-reported data were the only source of vaccination information; and for 104 (427−323) children (16.3%; range, 8.2%-19.8%), registries were the only source of vaccination histories.

From the provider-reported data, the weighted estimates of coverage (and 95% confidence limits) for the vaccine series 4:3:1:3 were as follows: 65.6% (±10.0%), 78.8% (±11.5%), 81.6% (±9.5%), and 77.0% (±13.2%), in sites A through D, respectively. The same weighted estimates based on only registry data were consistently lower, with coverage rates as follows: 31.7% (±8.2%), 65.4% (±13.7%), 71.9% (±9.5%), and 61.8% (±16.2%), respectively (**Figure**). These estimates were not statistically different from the provider-based estimates, except for the estimate for site A ($P<.05$). Vaccination coverage rates were the highest, with the pooled estimates at 72.0% (±10.2%), 92.0% (±11.1%), 88.7% (±9.1%), and 80.2% (±16.4%), respectively, and were not statistically different from the provider-based estimates. The pooled estimates included all 4:3:1:3 UTD children according to providers or registries and a subset of the not UTD children who became UTD after combining vaccine doses from both sources.

**Table 2** compares the registry- and provider-reported number of DTaP doses to assess agreement and completeness of the registry data. It shows that 47.2% to 62.2% of children (across the 4 sites) who were described as DTaP UTD (with ≥4 DTaP doses) by the providers were also DTaP UTD according to the registries. However, 7.7% to 39.6% of children who were described as DTaP UTD from the providers had missing dose information from the registries for 1 to 3 DTaP doses, and 9.9% to 38.5% of children could not be matched in the registry database and, therefore, had all DTaP doses missing from the registries. Similar results were also observed on completeness of other individual vaccines[8] (data not shown). These results show that missing records (when children could not be matched) and incomplete dose information (among matched cases) are the major causes of the lower coverage rates from the registries.

**Table 2. Distribution of the Number of DTaP Doses Reported From the Registry Among Children Who Are UTD for DTaP According to Immunization Providers by Registry Site: National Immunization Survey, 2002**

| Registry Data: Reported No. of Doses of DTaP | Provider Data: UTD for DTaP, With ≥4 Doses, by Site* A (n = 91) | B (n = 58) | C (n = 119) | D (n = 52) |
|---|---|---|---|---|
| Missing record | 9.9 | 31.0 | 18.5 | 38.5 |
| 0 (no dose information) | 3.3 | 0 | 2.5 | 3.8 |
| 1-3 | 39.6 | 12.1 | 16.8 | 7.7 |
| ≥4 (UTD) | 47.2 | 56.9 | 62.2 | 50.0 |

Abbreviations: DTaP, diphtheria and tetanus toxoids and pertussis vaccine; UTD, up-to-date.
*Data are given as percentage of all children at each site. Providers include physicians, nurses, hospitals, clinics, and others.

**Table 3. Distribution of the Number of DTaP Doses Reported by the Immunization Providers Among Children Who Are UTD for DTaP According to Registries by Site: National Immunization Survey, 2002***

| Provider Data: Reported No. of Doses of DTaP | Registry Data: UTD for DTaP, With ≥4 Doses, by Site† A (n = 66) | B (n = 45) | C (n = 102) | D (n = 31) |
|---|---|---|---|---|
| Missing record | 27.7 | 17.8 | 21.6 | 12.9 |
| 1-3 | 7.7 | 8.9 | 5.9 | 3.2 |
| ≥4 (UTD) | 64.6 | 73.3 | 72.5 | 83.9 |

Abbreviations: See Table 2.
*Provider includes physicians, nurses, hospitals, clinics, and others.
†Data are given as percentage of all children at each site.

Conversely, to assess completeness of the provider data, we examined the distribution of provider-reported DTaP doses among children who were DTaP UTD according to the registries. **Table 3** shows that many children (range, 64.6%-83.9%) who were described as DTaP UTD from registries were also DTaP UTD from the provider reports. This implies that if a registry contains complete vaccination history for a child, it is highly likely that the child's provider has the complete vaccination history. However, this agreement varies considerably across the 4 sites. Furthermore, only a few of the DTaP UTD children (range, 3.2%-8.9%) had incomplete histories, with missing information on 1 to 3 doses of DTaP from the providers. One of the key benefits of collecting vaccination data from the registries was that 12.9% to 27.7% of the children who were described as DTaP UTD from the registries had all dose information missing from the providers.

## COMMENT

A stable source of comparable vaccination data is the cornerstone of ensuring continuous monitoring of nationwide and statewide coverage. The NIS uses the same sample design and standardized data collection and processing methods that are comparable across all 78 areas to monitor national, state, and urban area vaccination coverage. Although the NIS faces many challenges in collecting immunization histories, it provides the only national source for monitoring many important issues with childhood immunization, including gaps in coverage by socioeconomic status and geography.[2] The NIS uses the provider-reported data to publish national and state-specific estimates of vaccination coverage.

The NIS registry data query project was conducted to evaluate the quality and completeness of the vaccination histories collected from mature registries and to assess the potential for registry data to supplement missing and incomplete vaccination data from providers. Most household respondents who gave consent to contact providers also gave consent to contact registries. Match rates for the NIS-sampled children were high (>70%) in all 4 registries.

Missing vaccination records (when children could not be matched) and incomplete or inconsistent dose information (among matched cases) were 2 major causes of lower coverage rates from the registries when compared with the coverage rates from the providers. The analysis also shows that despite incomplete histories reported by registries (or providers), the combined-dose method increased the overall pooled vaccination coverage rates in all 4 sites. Because of large standard errors, none of the pooled estimates were statistically different from the provider-based estimates. However, the increase in coverage estimates shows that supplementing missing or incomplete provider-reported vaccination histories with the data from mature registries has the potential to improve the completeness of vaccination histories.

For regional studies (eg, to identify population subgroups with low vaccination coverage in an area), it may be desirable to use pooled estimates by combining the registry- and provider-reported histories. However, supplementing incomplete or inconsistent registry data to the provider data could jeopardize the comparability of results from state to state (because availability and completeness of registry data vary among states) and over time (because enrollment and completeness of vaccination data in registries may change over time). With many immunization registries operating throughout the United States, several of them have progressed to high levels of enrollment of children in their catchment areas. A recent survey of the Centers for Disease Control and Prevention's 56 grantees in 50 states and 6 cities that receive funding under section 317b of the Public Health Service Act indicated that by 2004 approximately 48% of US children younger than 6 years were enrolled in an immunization registry. Of the 56 grantees, only 10 (18%) had greater than 95% and 7 (13%) had 81% to 94% of children enrolled in the registries.[11] Thus, to ensure comparability of vaccination coverage estimates, state and regional registries must be able to sustain high levels of enrollment, data completeness, and accuracy over time.

Finally, there are limitations to both sources of the vaccination data. Because some households with young children move in and out of the state where children were born, it is difficult for registries and for providers to keep track of the vaccination information for these children, leading to incomplete or missing records. Sometimes registries have missing or incomplete records because not all providers have complete data to submit for those children who have previously lived in another state or recently moved out to another state. Conversely, some children who had missing vaccination data from the providers had complete histories from the registry. In addition, sometimes there is a lag between the time when a vaccination is administered to the child and the time the provider submits the vaccination information to the registry and the registry enters the information in the database. Immunization records maintained by providers and by registries are not always of sufficient or consistent quality. Therefore, an adequate vaccination history may not be available for some children from either source because of missing doses, inconsistent quality, transcription errors, or misclassification errors.[6,12-14]

In conclusion, vaccination coverage estimates were the lowest when only registry-reported data were used, and increased when all unique vaccine doses from provider- and registry-reported data were combined. Although registries enrolled and matched more children, missing, incomplete, and inconsistent vaccination histories were the major causes for the lower coverage rates. The completeness of dose information varied considerably by registry, and the quality of the information was unknown and inconsistent. The quality and completeness of the registry data must be improved and must be comparable across all states before further consideration may be given to supplement or replace the provider-reported data in the NIS. Immunization information systems that record standardized vaccination data at the time and point of service may greatly enhance the completeness and quality of the registry data.[7,8]

**Accepted for Publication:** January 19, 2006.
**Correspondence:** Meena Khare, MS, National Center for Health Statistics, Centers for Disease Control and Prevention, 3311 Toledo Rd, Room 3218, Hyattsville, MD 20782 (mkhare@cdc.gov).
**Author Contributions:** Ms Khare has full access to all the data used in the study, and all coauthors take responsibility for the integrity and the accuracy of the data. *Study concept and design:* Khare, Piccinino, Barker, and Linkins. *Acquisition of data:* Khare, Piccinino, Barker, and Linkins. *Analysis and interpretation of data:* Khare, Piccinino, Barker, and Linkins. *Drafting of the manuscript:* Khare, Piccinino, Barker, and Linkins. *Critical revision of the manuscript for important intellectual content*: Khare, Piccinino, Barker, and Linkins. *Statistical analysis:* Khare, Piccinino, and Barker. *Administrative, technical, and material support:* Khare, Piccinino, and Linkins. *Study supervision:* Khare, Barker, and Linkins.
**Financial Disclosure:** None reported.
**Disclaimer:** The findings and conclusions in this article are those of the authors and do not necessarily represent the views of the Centers for Disease Control and Prevention.
**Acknowledgments:** We acknowledge Michael P. Battaglia, MS, Abt Associates Inc, for his assistance in designing and implementing the study; Diana Bartlett, MPH, National Immunization Program, Centers for Disease Control and Prevention, for providing consultation and coordinating data collection from registries; and Mary McCauley, MTSC, National Immunization Program, Centers for Disease Control and Prevention, for helping to edit the early drafts of the manuscript.

## REFERENCES

1. US Department of Health and Human Services. *Healthy People 2010: Understanding and Improving Health.* 2nd ed. Washington, DC: US Government Printing Office; 2000.
2. Smith PJ, Hoaglin DC, Battaglia MP, Khare M, Barker LE; Centers for Disease Control and Prevention. Statistical methodology of the National Immunization Survey, 1994-2002. *Vital Health Stat 2.* 2005;(No. 138):1-55.
3. Linkins RW. Immunization registries: progress and challenges in reaching the 2010 national objective. *J Public Health Manag Pract.* 2001;7:67-74.
4. Centers for Disease Control and Prevision (CDC). *Implementing a National Strategy to Improve the Quality of Immunization Practices Among VFC Providers, 2001 Annual Report: National Immunization Program.* Atlanta, Ga: CDC; 2002.
5. Centers for Disease Control and Prevention (CDC). Immunization registry progress: United States, January-December 2002. *MMWR Morb Mortal Wkly Rep.* 2004; 53:431-433.
6. Wilton R, Pennisi AJ. Evaluating the accuracy of transcribed computer-stored immunization data. *Pediatrics.* 1994;94:902-906.
7. Adams WG, Conners WP, Mann AM, Palfrey S. Immunization entry at the point of service improves quality, saves time, and is well-accepted. *Pediatrics.* 2000; 106:489-492.
8. Samuels RC, Appel L, Reddy SI, Tilson RS. Improving accuracy in a computerized immunization registry. *Ambul Pediatr.* 2002;2:187-192.
9. Centers for Disease Control and Prevention (CDC). *The National Immunization Survey: 2003 Annual Methodology Report.* Cambridge, Mass: Abt Associates Inc; 2003.
10. Centers for Disease Control and Prevention (CDC). *The National Immunization Survey Registry Query Pretest: Final Analysis Reports (Sites A-D).* Chicago, Ill: Abt Associates Inc; 2003.
11. Centers for Disease Control and Prevention (CDC). Immunization information system progress: United States, 2004. *MMWR Morb Mortal Wkly Rep.* 2005;54: 1156-1157.
12. Khare M, Piccinino L, Battaglia MP. An assessment of the quality of health data collected from multiple sources: registries, provider records, and household reports. Paper presented at: American Association for Public Opinion Research Meeting; May 14, 2005; Miami, Fla.
13. Khare M, Battaglia MP, Huggins VJ, et al. Accuracy of vaccination dates reported by immunization providers in the National Immunization Survey. In: *2000 Proceedings of the Section on Survey Research Methods.* Alexandria, Va: American Statistical Association; 2000. http://www.amstat.org/sections/SRMS/Proceedings/. Accessed May 11, 2006.
14. Khare M, Ezzati-Rice TM, Battaglia MP, Zell ER. An assessment of misclassification error in provider-reported vaccination histories. In: *2001 Proceedings of the Section on Survey Research Methods.* Alexandria, Va: American Statistical Association; 2001. http://www.amstat.org/sections/SRMS/Proceedings/. Accessed May 11, 2006.

ARTICLE

# Classification of Asthma Severity in Children

## *The Contribution of Pulmonary Function Testing*

*James W. Stout, MD, MPH; Cynthia M. Visness, MA, MPH; Paul Enright, MD; Carin Lamm, MD; Gail Shapiro, MD; Vanthaya N. Gan, MD; G. Kenneth Adams III, PhD; Herman E. Mitchell, PhD*

**Background:** Despite increasing awareness of the National Asthma Education and Prevention Program guidelines, the relative contribution of symptom frequency or pulmonary function to the recommended asthma severity levels remains poorly understood.

**Objective:** To determine whether adding lung function measurements to clinical history substantially changes the asthma severity classification, thereby influencing treatment decisions.

**Design:** Baseline data were studied from children enrolled in 2 multicenter studies: phase 1 of the National Cooperative Inner-City Asthma Study (1992-1994) (cohort 1) and the Inner-City Asthma Study (1998-2001) (cohort 2).

**Setting:** Fifteen (8 for cohort 1 and 7 for cohort 2) major metropolitan inner-city areas in the United States.

**Participants:** Inner-city children aged 8 through 11 years with asthma.

**Main Outcome Measures:** Proportion of children reclassified from less severe asthma categories based on symptom frequency into more severe categories because of lung function.

**Results:** Of children with symptoms of mild intermittent asthma, 22.8% in cohort 1 and 27.7% in cohort 2 would be reclassified as having either moderate or severe persistent asthma. Of children with symptoms of mild persistent asthma, 31.2% in cohort 1 and 33.3% in cohort 2 would be similarly reclassified.

**Conclusions:** In 2 different studies of inner-city children with asthma, approximately one third of the participants were reclassified into higher National Asthma Education and Prevention Program asthma severity categories when pulmonary function was considered in addition to symptom frequency. This may have direct implications for the undertreatment of asthma.

*Arch Pediatr Adolesc Med. 2006;160:844-850*

THE NATIONAL ASTHMA EDUcation and Prevention Program (NAEPP) guidelines recommend that medical professionals use a combination of clinical findings and objective measurement of lung function for the diagnosis of asthma.[1] According to these guidelines, asthma is classified into 4 levels at initial diagnosis: mild intermittent, mild persistent, moderate persistent, and severe persistent based on symptom frequency and either spirometric (forced expiratory volume in 1 second [$FEV_1$]) or peak expiratory flow (PEF) measurements (**Table 1**). Despite increasing awareness of these guidelines, the relative contribution of symptom frequency and pulmonary function to the recommended asthma severity levels remains poorly understood.

Choice of therapy depends on an accurate determination of asthma severity because underestimation will result in suboptimal treatment and increased morbidity.[2,3] In a study of more than 4000 asthmatic patients in managed care, Wolfenden et al[4] found that physicians systematically underestimate asthma severity. In addition, Baker et al[5] provided 24 board-certified allergists and pulmonologists with 8 asthma case summaries and found low levels of agreement for NAEPP guideline asthma severity classification.

In a sample of more than 200 hospitalized asthmatic patients, Warman et al[6] showed that 83% should be classified as having persistent asthma but that only 35% were receiving daily anti-inflammatory agents. They reported ascertainment of severity using symptom frequency. The potential contribution of pulmonary function was not addressed.[6]

Peak expiratory flow and $FEV_1$ are commonly used measures of lung function, and they are used particularly for assessment of the airway obstruction typically seen with asthma. Both are recommended in the NAEPP guidelines as measures of severity assessment. The PEF meter is a simple and inexpensive device that is widely available

**Author Affiliations:** Department of Pediatrics, University of Washington School of Medicine, Seattle (Drs Stout and Shapiro); Rho Federal Systems Division Inc, Chapel Hill, NC (Dr Mitchell and Ms Visness); Respiratory Sciences Center, University of Arizona, Tucson (Dr Enright); Departments of Pediatrics, Mount Sinai School of Medicine, New York, NY (Dr Lamm), and University of Texas Southwestern Medical Center at Dallas (Dr Gan); and National Institute of Allergy and Infectious Diseases, Bethesda, Md (Dr Adams).

but has several limitations compared with the spirometer. Peak expiratory flow is effort dependent, and several studies[7-10] have shown that it underestimates the degree of airway obstruction. Eid et al[11] found that PEF had poor negative predictive value for patients with air trapping as determined by elevated residual volume/total lung capacity. Patients with air trapping can generate a peak burst of airflow, yielding a normal PEF measurement, but as exhalation continues, abnormalities in measurements such as $FEV_1$ and forced expiratory flow between 25% and 75% are detected. The spirometric measurement, $FEV_1$, is reliable and has good correlation with degree of airway obstruction.[12]

Despite the NAEPP recommendations to assess lung function by means of $FEV_1$ or peak flow, these measurements, particularly $FEV_1$, which requires a spirometer, are not routinely determined.[13] Picken et al[14] reported that when primary care physicians were given the opportunity to adapt the NAEPP guidelines for their own local use, they included clinical criteria and PEF measurement. Spirometry was recommended only for patients with an incomplete response to inhaled corticosteroids as determined by clinical examination, for "unusual" patients, or for patients in whom an alternate diagnosis was suspected. In a survey[13] of primary care physicians, only 21% reported using $FEV_1$ to establish the diagnosis of asthma, and only 8% used $FEV_1$ measurements in routine follow-up. In contrast, 75% reported using PEF in the initial diagnosis or follow-up.[13] In a study by Diette et al,[15] only half of the patients reported ever undergoing pulmonary function testing.

The NAEPP guidelines organize asthma severity into 4 categories, using "or" criteria for daytime and nighttime symptom frequency, office-based pulmonary functions ($FEV_1$ or PEF rate [PEFR]), and home-based diurnal variability in PEFR (Table 1). The purpose of this study is to determine whether asthma severity classification based on clinical history alone is changed by the addition of spirometric measures of lung function. If more patients needing treatment are identified in this manner, it could reduce the problem of undertreatment of asthma.

## METHODS

To increase the generalizability of the findings, we included children enrolled in 2 separate but related multicenter studies: phase 1 of the National Cooperative Inner-City Asthma Study (NCICAS), conducted between January 2, 1993, and November 12, 1994, and the Inner-City Asthma Study (ICAS), conducted between July 24, 1998, and August 9, 2001. For both studies, each participating site received approval from the human subjects review committee at their institution. Informed consent was obtained from all the parents or legal guardians, and the children provided age-appropriate assent.

Pulmonary function findings are based on predicted values for height, race, and for certain measures, the sex of the child, and the findings are expressed as a percentage of the predicted value. We chose the third National Health and Nutrition Examination Survey normative data set for the study population's pulmonary function values.[16] These spirometric reference values include data from 7429 asymptomatic nonsmoking participants and compare white, African American, and Mexican American individuals aged 8 to 80 years. Of the available normative data sets, these comparisons are the most relevant to our study populations. Because of the age range of the reference values, our analyses are restricted to children aged 8 to 11 years.

**Table 1. Asthma Severity Classifications According to the Expert Panel Report 2 National Asthma Guidelines**

| Asthma Classification | Days With Symptoms | Nights With Symptoms | Children >5 y Who Can Use a Spirometer or Peak Flowmeter, %: $FEV_1$ or PEF (Predicted Normal) | PEF Variability |
|---|---|---|---|---|
| Severe persistent | Continual | Frequent | ≤60 | >30 |
| Moderate persistent | Daily | ≥5/mo | >60 to <80 | >30 |
| Mild persistent | >2/wk | 3-4/mo | ≥80 | 20-30 |
| Mild intermittent | ≤2/wk | ≤2/mo | ≥80 | <20 |

Abbreviations: $FEV_1$, forced expiratory volume in 1 second; PEF, peak expiratory flow.

## NATIONAL COOPERATIVE INNER-CITY ASTHMA STUDY

Phase 1 of the NCICAS (cohort 1) enrolled 1528 children aged 4 to 9 years who resided in 8 major metropolitan inner-city areas in the United States.[17] The NCICAS asthma inclusion criteria were a combination of physician diagnosis and symptom history (**Table 2**). Participants in the NCICAS sample resided in census tracts in which approximately 20% to 40% of the households had incomes below the 1990 federal poverty level. Of the 1376 previously diagnosed asthmatic children, 327 children aged 8 to 9 years attempted spirometry. Acceptable measurements for $FEV_1$ and PEFR were available for 257 participants.

## INNER-CITY ASTHMA STUDY

The ICAS (cohort 2) enrolled 937 children aged 5 to 11 years with moderate to severe asthma using inclusion criteria intended to result in participants with more severe asthma than those in the NCICAS sample. Children and their families were eligible for the ICAS if the child had at least 1 hospitalization or 2 urgent care visits for asthma during the 6 months before screening and had a positive skin test reaction to at least 1 of 11 common indoor allergens (Table 2).[18] Except for 1 site, where alternate criteria for poverty were used, children enrolled in the ICAS had to live in a census tract in which at least 20% of households reported a household income below the federal poverty level, and they had to sleep in the intervention home at least 5 nights of every week. Of the 455 participants aged 8 to 11 years, complete data were available for 383.

For both study cohorts, a comprehensive baseline evaluation was conducted at enrollment. A variety of questions were asked of the caregiver, including the child's medication use and adherence, home environment and smoking history, perceived stress and stressful life events, mental health measures for the caregiver and the child participant, and recent morbidity. Morbidity measures included asthma symptoms in the past 2 weeks, school days missed in the past 2 weeks, and use of health care services in the past 2 months. In addition, each child answered questions regarding stress and quality of life and underwent allergy skin testing. In the NCICAS, pulmonary function testing was performed using a Pulmonary Screen IIE/VRS system (S&H Instrument, Doylestown, Pa), and in the ICAS, a Renaissance II spirometer (Nellcor Puritan Bennett, Pleasanton, Calif) was used. The pulmonary function measures reported in this article, including PEFRs, were obtained from these respective instruments. All test-

**Table 2. Eligibility Criteria for Cohorts 1 and 2**

| Criterion | Cohort 1 (National Cooperative Inner-City Asthma Study) | Cohort 2 (Inner-City Asthma Study) |
|---|---|---|
| Age, y | 4-9 | 5-11 |
| Residence | Selected census tracts with >40% of household incomes below the 1990 poverty level | Selected census tracts with at least 20%-40% of household incomes below the 1990 poverty level *and* sleeps overnight at 1 address ≥5 times per week |
| Recruitment sites | Emergency departments and community primary care sites | Hospitals, emergency departments, and clinics |
| Definition of asthma | 1. Physician diagnosis of asthma *and* asthma symptoms (cough, wheeze, shortness of breath, or whistling or tightness in the chest) for >3 d in the past 12 mo *or*<br>2. Asthma symptoms (cough, wheeze, or shortness of breath) for >6 wk in the past 12 mo *and* that met 3 of the 5 following conditions:<br>a. Cough, wheeze, or shortness of breath was present more than half the days and nights during the 6-wk period<br>b. Cough, wheeze, or shortness of breath was aggravated by exercise or cold air<br>c. There is a parent or sibling with asthma<br>d. Child does not have a history of antibiotic therapy for sinusitis accompanying the cough<br>e. Cough, wheeze, or shortness of breath that resulted in disturbance of the child's sleep | Physician diagnosis of asthma *and*<br>1. At least 1 hospitalization related to asthma in the past 6 mo *or*<br>2. At least 2 unscheduled visits to an emergency department or clinic related to asthma in the past 6 mo |
| Other | None | Positive allergen skin test reaction to at least 1 indoor allergen (eg, dust mites, cockroaches, mold, rodents, or pets) |

ing was performed by trained technicians and followed American Thoracic Society guidelines.[19]

We classified the asthma severity of study participants according to the Expert Panel Report 2 national asthma guidelines.[1] Using the symptom frequency categories given in Table 1, we placed participants into 3 severity levels: mild intermittent, mild persistent, and moderate and severe persistent asthma. Using 14-day reports, children who had 0 to 4 days with symptoms and 0 to 1 night with symptoms were classified as mild intermittent. Children who had 5 to 13 days with symptoms or 2 nights with symptoms were classified as mild persistent. Children who had 14 days with symptoms or 3 to 14 nights with symptoms were classified as moderate or severe persistent. The 2 most severe categories (moderate and severe persistent asthma) were collapsed into 1 because with this data set we could not reliably differentiate moderate from severe persistent asthma based on patient symptom frequency self-report alone (ie, differentiating between "daily" and "continual" daytime symptoms or defining "frequent" nights with symptoms).[1,20]

We examined the pulmonary function test results at the baseline evaluation for each study to determine the proportion of children in each asthma severity category who would be reclassified from symptom-only severity categories based on the addition of these lung function results. Consistent with the NAEPP guidelines, we examined $FEV_1$ and PEFR separately and together as "or" criteria along with symptom frequency so that the addition of lung function could result either in no change in asthma severity categories if pulmonary function was normal or in an increase in asthma severity categories if pulmonary function findings were abnormal.

## RESULTS

### CHARACTERISTICS OF THE STUDY SAMPLES

The NCICAS population is designated cohort 1, and the ICAS population is cohort 2. For this analysis, cohort 1 included 257 children, and cohort 2 included 383 children. The study samples for both cohorts were demographically similar (**Table 3**). The mean age for cohort 1 was 8.5 years and for cohort 2 was 9.5 years, reflecting their different age inclusion criteria. Approximately 60% of the participants in both cohorts were boys. In cohort 1, most study participants (74.4%) were African American. In cohort 2, Hispanic and African American children were enrolled in similar proportions (almost 40% for each). In both cohorts, approximately 70% of the caregivers reported graduating from high school, and almost 60% of respondents in each study reported household incomes of less than $15 000. Caregivers in cohort 2 were more likely to report being married (35.2% vs 23.4%) and, consistent with recent reforms in welfare legislation, were also more likely to report at least 1 currently employed household member (76.1% vs 50.2%).

### ASTHMA SEVERITY ACCORDING TO SYMPTOM FREQUENCY

We first examined the distribution of participants into asthma severity categories based on symptom frequency categories alone and on daytime symptoms and nighttime symptoms separately and together as "or" criteria, consistent with the NAEPP guidelines (**Table 4**). As expected, given the eligibility criteria, a greater proportion of cohort 1 children fell into the mild intermittent category compared with cohort 2 children (47.9% vs 38.6%; $P = .02$) (Table 4). The proportion of children in the mild persistent category was similar in cohorts 1 and 2 (18.7% vs 18.8%; $P = .97$). Finally, a smaller proportion of cohort 1 vs cohort 2 children were in the moderate or severe persistent category (33.5% vs 42.6%; $P = .02$).

For both cohorts, consideration of nighttime symptoms alone places more participants in the moderate or severe persistent categories than use of daytime symptoms alone (cohort 1: 29.6% vs 10.1%; cohort 2: 36.3% vs 19.8%; $P < .001$ for both).

## ASTHMA SEVERITY ACCORDING TO PULMONARY FUNCTION

We then examined the distribution of children into normal (≥80% of predicted) or abnormal (<80% of predicted) categories of $FEV_1$ and PEFR according to the NAEPP guidelines. For $FEV_1$, a smaller proportion of children in cohort 1 vs cohort 2 had abnormal lung function (16.7% vs 28.2%; $P<.001$) (**Table 5**). The PEFR was less sensitive to differences in cohort severity, with the difference between cohorts only approaching significance (19.5% vs 25.3%; $P=.08$). When either $FEV_1$ or PEFR was considered (the recommended NAEPP guidelines approach), 24.5% of children in cohort 1 had abnormal lung function compared with 35.8% in cohort 2 ($P=.003$).

## INFLUENCE OF PULMONARY FUNCTION IN CHANGING THE SEVERITY CLASSIFICATION

To address the main study question, we examined how the severity distribution would change when abnormal pulmonary function—either $FEV_1$ or PEFR—is also considered (Table 5). Among children with symptoms consistent with mild intermittent asthma, 22.8% in cohort 1 and 27.7% in cohort 2 would be reclassified as having moderate or severe persistent asthma. Among children with symptoms consistent with mild persistent asthma, 31.2% in cohort 1 and 33.3% in cohort 2 would be reclassified as having moderate or severe persistent asthma. Among children who were already classified as having moderate or severe persistent asthma by symptoms alone, 23.3% in cohort 1 and 44.2% in cohort 2 had abnormal pulmonary function. **Figure 1** shows the overall distribution of severity classifications when using the differing criteria.

## COMMENT

These 2 cohorts of inner-city children with asthma differed somewhat in severity, reflecting the differences in eligibility criteria. Regardless, approximately one third of the children in each cohort were reclassified to higher NAEPP asthma severity categories when pulmonary function was considered in addition to symptom frequency. These results demonstrate that the NAEPP severity assessment algorithm is highly dependent on the availability of symptom frequency and pulmonary function data.

The findings are from 2 populations of relatively severe asthmatic children living in an inner-city environment and may not be generalizable to all asthmatic children. The participants from the ICAS, for example, were included only if they had 1 hospitalization or 2 acute care visits for asthma in the past 6 months (Table 2). Most of the children in this analysis were in the moderate and severe asthma categories, which is consistent with our strategy to enroll children with significant and active asthma morbidity for this study.

It may be that, at least for some patients, PEF and $FEV_1$ are not the most sensitive indicators of small-airway obstruction. Klein et al[21] found that some children with symptoms suggestive of moderately severe asthma had normal PEF and $FEV_1$ measurements but decreased forced expiratory flow between 25% and 75%. Moy and colleagues[22] found that intensity of shortness of breath was

**Table 3. Description of Study Samples: National Cooperative Inner-City Study (Cohort 1) and Inner-City Asthma Study (Cohort 2)***

| Characteristic | Cohort 1 (n = 257) | Cohort 2 (n = 383) |
|---|---|---|
| Demographic characteristics | | |
| Child's age, mean (SD) [range], y | 8.5 (0.5) [8-9] | 9.5 (1.1) [8-11] |
| Child's sex, No. (%) | | |
| M | 156 (60.7) | 241 (62.9) |
| F | 101 (39.3) | 142 (37.1) |
| Race/ethnicity, No. (%) | | |
| Hispanic | 45 (17.7) | 148 (38.6) |
| African American | 189 (74.4) | 151 (39.4) |
| White | 0 | 28 (7.3) |
| Asian/Pacific Islander | 0 | 2 (0.5) |
| American Indian | 0 | 13 (3.4) |
| Mixed/other | 20 (7.9) | 41 (10.7) |
| Caregiver is high school graduate, No. (%) | 171 (67.3) | 274 (72.1) |
| Caregiver is married, No. (%) | 60 (23.4) | 134 (35.2) |
| Household income <$15 000, No. (%) | 139 (57.9) | 215 (59.4) |
| Household employment, No. (%) | 128 (50.2) | 290 (76.1) |
| Medication use at baseline, No. (%) | | |
| Using inhaled corticosteroids | 37 (14.8) | 115 (30.0) |
| Using β-agonists | 207 (82.8) | 328 (85.6) |
| Baseline morbidity, mean (SD) | | |
| Days with wheeze in past 14 d | 3.4 (3.9) | 4.4 (4.4) |
| Days with slowed activity in past 14 d | 2.7 (3.8) | 4.1 (4.8) |
| Nights child woke in past 14 d | 2.1 (3.5) | 2.7 (3.8) |
| School days missed† | 0.10 (0.13) | 0.93 (1.83) |
| Hospitalizations in past 3 or 2 mo‡ | 0.11 (0.40) | 0.17 (0.45) |
| Unscheduled visits in past 3 or 2 mo‡ | 0.79 (1.0) | 0.96 (1.19) |

*Numbers do not always add up to the total because of sporadic missing data.

†In cohort 1, school days missed is the proportion of days missed of the number of days school was in session in the previous 3 months. In cohort 2, school days missed is the actual number of days missed in the previous 2 weeks, typically 10 school days. Thus, the average of 1 of 10 days missed is comparable with the 10% in cohort 1.

‡In cohort 1, hospitalizations and unscheduled visits were measured for 3 months, and in cohort 2 they were measured for 2 months.

**Table 4. Asthma Severity Distribution According to Symptom Frequency: National Cooperative Inner-City Study (Cohort 1) and Inner-City Asthma Study (Cohort 2)**

| Symptoms Classified by | Mild Intermittent | Mild Persistent | Moderate or Severe Persistent |
|---|---|---|---|
| Cohort 1, % (n = 257) | | | |
| Daytime | 70.0 | 19.8 | 10.1 |
| Nighttime | 57.6 | 12.8 | 29.6 |
| Daytime or nighttime | 47.9 | 18.7 | 33.5 |
| Cohort 2, % (n = 383) | | | |
| Daytime | 52.0 | 28.2 | 19.8 |
| Nighttime | 51.2 | 12.5 | 36.3 |
| Daytime or nighttime | 38.6 | 18.8 | 42.6 |

**Table 5. Children With Abnormal Lung Function by Symptom Category: National Cooperative Inner-City Study (Cohort 1) and Inner-City Asthma Study (Cohort 2)***

| Severity Classification by Symptoms | Participants, No. | <80% of Predicted | | |
|---|---|---|---|---|
| | | $FEV_1$ | PEF | Either $FEV_1$ or PEF |
| **Cohort 1 Symptoms (n = 257)** | | | | |
| Severity by daytime symptoms | | | | |
| Mild intermittent | 180 | 12.8 | 15.6 | 20.6 |
| Mild persistent | 51 | 27.4 | 31.4 | 35.3 |
| Moderate or severe persistent | 26 | 23.1 | 23.1 | 30.8 |
| Severity by nighttime symptoms | | | | |
| Mild intermittent | 148 | 15.5 | 21.0 | 25.7 |
| Mild persistent | 33 | 15.2 | 18.2 | 24.2 |
| Moderate or severe persistent | 76 | 19.7 | 17.1 | 22.4 |
| Severity by daytime + nighttime symptoms | | | | |
| Mild intermittent | 123 | 14.6 | 17.9 | 22.8 |
| Mild persistent | 48 | 18.8 | 27.1 | 31.2 |
| Moderate or severe persistent | 86 | 18.6 | 17.4 | 23.3 |
| Overall | 257 | 16.7 | 19.5 | 24.5 |
| **Cohort 2 Symptoms (n = 383)** | | | | |
| Severity by daytime symptoms | | | | |
| Mild intermittent | 199 | 23.6 | 21.1 | 30.6 |
| Mild persistent | 108 | 26.8 | 22.2 | 33.3 |
| Moderate or severe persistent | 76 | 42.1 | 40.8 | 52.6 |
| Severity by nighttime symptoms | | | | |
| Mild intermittent | 196 | 22.4 | 20.4 | 28.1 |
| Mild persistent | 48 | 35.4 | 27.1 | 41.7 |
| Moderate or severe persistent | 139 | 33.8 | 31.6 | 44.6 |
| Severity by daytime + nighttime symptoms | | | | |
| Mild intermittent | 148 | 22.3 | 19.6 | 27.7 |
| Mild persistent | 72 | 27.8 | 22.2 | 33.3 |
| Moderate or severe persistent | 163 | 33.7 | 31.9 | 44.2 |
| Overall | 383 | 28.2 | 25.3 | 35.8 |

Abbreviations: $FEV_1$, forced expiratory volume in 1 second; PEF, peak expiratory flow.
*Data are given as percentages.

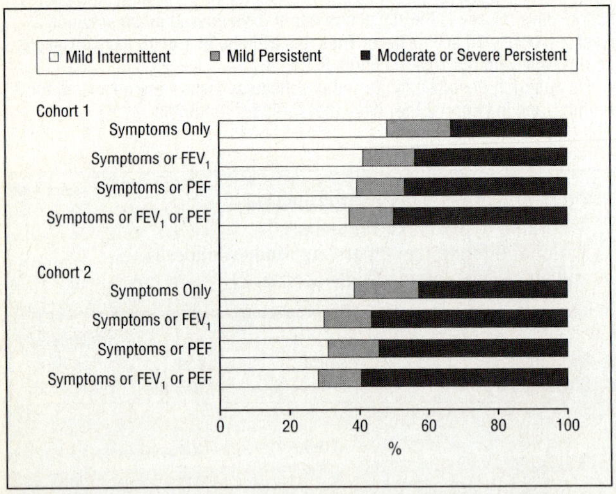


**Figure 1.** Asthma severity distribution in each cohort according to symptom frequency and lung function. $FEV_1$ indicates forced expiratory volume in 1 second; PEF, peak expiratory flow.

a predictor of quality of life at all severity levels in contrast to lung function, which did not independently predict quality of life at any asthma severity level. A recent environmental intervention was demonstrated to reduce symptoms but had no effect on lung function.[23]

Other studies have shown the weakness of symptoms alone as a predictor of asthma severity. For example, Osborne et al[24] found that a 2-year review of medical records, including exacerbations, urgent care visits, hospitalizations, and medications, correlated well with pulmonary function and glucocorticoid use but not with asthma symptoms.

There are inherent limitations with the assessment of asthma, a dynamic chronic illness, at any given point. Calhoun et al[25] found that in repeated assessments of asthma severity based on symptoms and PEF, a single point-in-time classification of asthma was highly unreliable. Unfortunately, initial therapeutic decisions must be based on such limited information.

Within the symptom frequency categories, many more participants in this study were classified as severe according to nighttime vs daytime symptoms, a finding corroborated by Colice et al.[26] This raises the importance of a careful nocturnal symptom history, realizing that this history may be an underestimate of what is really occurring. For example, variables such as the location of the historian's (ie, parent's) bed to the patient's bed and whether the historian is a deep sleeper can affect the accuracy of recall and thus the accuracy of asthma severity classification and the resulting treatment.

Bacharier et al[27] described a weak relationship among symptom frequency, medication use, and $FEV_1$. However, they also demonstrated a decrease in the $FEV_1$/forced vital capacity ratio as asthma severity increased. Their findings underscore the imperfect overlap between symptom frequency and pulmonary function at a moment in time, and the value of using multiple domains when diagnosing and assessing asthma.

Nair et al[28] recently corroborated our finding, demonstrating that the use of spirometry identified a large proportion of asthmatic children with abnormal lung function who otherwise had mild asthma based on history or physical examination findings alone. Fuhlbrigge et al[29] demonstrated a strong association between decreased $FEV_1$ and risk of an asthma attack in the subsequent year. Juniper et al[30] demonstrated via factor analysis that airway caliber (ie, pulmonary function) was 1 of 4 distinct domains of asthma health status, along with quality of life, daytime symptoms and β-agonist use, and nighttime symptoms.

These findings support the use of spirometry when assessing patients with asthma. Administering the forced expiratory maneuver requires good patient coaching, which in turn requires careful and adequate support staff and provider training. If well-trained personnel are in place and quality criteria are diligently used, the increased availability of reliable and user-friendly spirometers may make possible the incorporation of pulmonary function testing in primary care settings. Spirometry is often problematic for children, and 16% to 21% of our curves were unacceptable, underscoring the importance of ensuring that a good-quality flow volume curve is being interpreted.

Approximately the same number of children with "abnormal" lung function were identified using PEFR as using $FEV_1$. However, these 2 subsets of children do not overlap completely. The $FEV_1$ and $FEV_1$/forced vital capacity, when performed and interpreted properly, provide an objective view of the expiratory phase that may help identify patients with airway obstruction otherwise missed by history and physical examination. A single measure of PEF, however, is considered to be of limited value when using predicted equations.[31] In addition, PEFR determined using a mechanical peak flowmeter is likely to differ from peak flow determined using an automated spirometer, as reported in our study.[32] Hankinson et al[33,34] found that differences in the frequency response and accuracy of mechanical peak flowmeters and spirometers often produce values that may be 15% higher or lower than the comparison instrument. In cohort 1, we had same-day measurements of PEFR using both instruments and found that the correlation between them was only 0.60. Because of the inexact nature of asthma severity assessment and the lack of a universal gold standard, we may also need additional discriminators. Miller et al[35] recently highlighted the potential contribution of asthma-related health care and medication use as additional discriminators of asthma severity. Exhaled nitric oxide concentration, as another example, is a biomarker of inflammation that may eventually prove to be a better predictor of current or future asthma severity.[36]

This study has several limitations. The PEF values were obtained using an automated spirometer and may differ from values obtained using a handheld mechanical peak flowmeter. In the lowest ranges (<200 L/min), our data show a significant discrepancy between values obtained using these 2 methods. The findings from an inner-city population may or may not be generalizable to other populations. It is also possible that findings from children in a limited age range (8-11 years) may not be generalizable to other age groups. The inclusion criterion of a recent hospitalization or 2 acute care visits was meant to identify asthmatic children with significant morbidity. This recruitment strategy partially explains the high proportion of these participants who were in the more severe asthma categories.

We show that using symptom frequency alone to classify asthma severity underestimates the number of children with moderate to severe persistent asthma. This finding suggests that the often described phenomenon of undertreatment of more severe asthma with controller medications, most notably inhaled corticosteroids, may be due, in part, to an underestimate of asthma severity. Increased use of spirometry may lead to better identification of asthma severity and thereby improve treatment with daily anti-inflammatory medication.

**Accepted for Publication:** March 3, 2006.
**Correspondence:** James W. Stout, MD, Department of Pediatrics, University of Washington School of Medicine, Box 354920, Seattle, WA 98195-4920 (jstout@u.washington.edu).
**Author Contributions:** Dr Mitchell, principal investigator, Data Coordinating Center, had full access to all the data in the study and takes responsibility for the integrity of the data and the accuracy of the data analysis. *Study concept and design:* Stout, Enright, Shapiro, and Mitchell. *Acquisition of data:* Stout, Enright, Gan, and Lamm. *Analysis and interpretation of data:* Stout, Visness, Enright, Gan, Adams, and Mitchell. *Drafting of the manuscript:* Stout, Visness, Lamm, Shapiro, Gan, and Mitchell. *Critical revision of the manuscript for important intellectual content:* Stout, Visness, Enright, Gan, Adams, and Mitchell. *Statistical analysis:* Visness and Mitchell. *Obtained funding:* Stout and Mitchell. *Administrative, technical, and material support:* Stout, Visness, Enright, Adams, and Mitchell. *Study supervision:* Stout, Lamm, and Mitchell.
**Group Members:** The Inner-City Asthma Study was a collaboration of the following institutions and investigators. *Boston University School of Medicine, Boston, Mass*: George O'Connor, MD (principal investigator [PI], Suzanne Steinbach, MD, Amy Lang Zapata, MPH, Jodie Cline Casagrande, MSW, MPH, and Linda Schneider, MD (Children's Hospital, Boston); *Albert Einstein College of Medicine/Jacobi Medical Center, Bronx, NY*: Ellen Crain, MD, PhD (PI), Laurie Bauman, PhD, Yvonne Senturia, MD, and David Rosenstreich, MD; *Children's Memorial Hospital, Chicago, Ill*: Richard Evans III, MD (PI), Jacqueline Pongracic, MD, Anne Sawyer, and Kristin Koridek; *University of Texas Southwestern Medical Center at Dallas*: Rebecca S. Gruchalla, MD, PhD (PI), Vanthaya Gan, MD Yvonne Coyle, MD, and Nina F. Gorham; *Mount Sinai School of Medicine, New York, NY*: Meyer Kattan, MD, CM (PI), Carin Lamm, MD, Morton Lippmann, PhD, Elisabeth Luder, PhD, Mark Chassin,

MD, and Gloria Xanthos; *University of Washington School of Medicine and Public Health, Seattle*: James Stout, MD (PI), Gail Shapiro, MD, Lenna Liu, MD, Jane Koenig, PhD, Mary Lasley, MD, Sandra Randels, and Helen Powell, MS; *The University of Arizona College of Medicine, Tucson*: Wayne Morgan, MD, CM (PI), Paul Enright, MD, Jamie Goodwin, PhD, and Terri Garcia (El Rio Health Clinic, Tucson); *Data Coordinating Center, Rho Inc, Chapel Hill*: Herman Mitchell, PhD (PI), Michelle Walter, MS, Henry Lynn, MS, Sheri Hart, William Tolbert, and Elizabeth Nuebler; *Allergen Assay Laboratories, Harvard School of Public Health, Boston*: Harriet Burge, PhD, Michael Muilenberg, MS, and Diane Gold, MD; *The Johns Hopkins Dermatology, Allergy and Clinical Immunology Reference Laboratory, Johns Hopkins University School of Medicine, Baltimore, Md*: Robert Hamilton, PhD; *National Institute of Allergy and Infectious Diseases, Bethesda, Md*: Marshall Plaut, MD, Ernestine Smartt, RN, and G. Kenneth Adams, PhD; and *National Institute of Environmental Health Sciences, Research Triangle Park, NC*: George Malindzak, PhD, and Patrick Mastin, PhD.

**Financial Disclosure:** Dr Stout received funding from the Centers for Disease Control for production of a CD-ROM entitled "Spirometry Fundamentals: A Basic Guide to Lung Function Testing." He plans to license this tool through the University of Washington's Office of Tech Transfer.

**Funding/Support:** This research was supported by grants AI-39769, AI-39900, AI-39902, AI-39789, AI-39901, AI-39761, AI-39785, and AI-39776 from the National Institute of Allergy and Infectious Diseases and by the National Institute of Environmental Health Sciences, National Institutes of Health, Department of Health and Human Services; and by grant M01 RR00533 from the National Center for Research Resources.

## REFERENCES


1. National Asthma Education and Prevention Program. *Expert Panel Report: Guidelines for the Diagnosis and Management of Asthma.* Bethesda, Md: US Dept of Health and Human Services, Public Health Service; April 1997. NIH publication 97-4051.
2. Piecoro LT, Potoski M, Talbert JC, Doherty DE. Asthma prevalence, cost, and adherence with expert guidelines on the utilization of health care services and costs in a state Medicaid population. *Health Serv Res.* 2001;36:357-371.
3. Nestor A, Calhoun AC, Dickson M, Kalik CA. Cross-sectional analysis of the relationship between national guideline recommended asthma drug therapy and emergency/hospital use within a managed care population. *Ann Allergy Asthma Immunol.* 1998;81:327-330.
4. Wolfenden LL, Diette GB, Krishnan JA, Skinner EA, Steinwachs DM, Wu AW. Lower physician estimate of underlying asthma severity leads to undertreatment. *Arch Intern Med.* 2003;163:231-236.
5. Baker KM, Brand DA, Hen J Jr. Classifying asthma: disagreement among specialists. *Chest.* 2003;124:2156-2163.
6. Warman KL, Silver EJ, Stein RE. Asthma symptoms, morbidity, and antiinflammatory use in inner-city children. *Pediatrics.* 2001;108:277-282.
7. Vaughan TR, Weber RW, Tipton WR, Nelson HS. Comparison of PEFR and $FEV_1$ in patients with varying degrees of airway obstruction: effect of modest altitude. *Chest.* 1989;95:558-562.
8. Ferguson AC. Persisting airway obstruction in asymptomatic children with asthma with normal peak expiratory flow rates. *J Allergy Clin Immunol.* 1988;82:19-22.
9. Cross D, Nelson HS. The role of the peak flow meter in the diagnosis and management of asthma. *J Allergy Clin Immunol.* 1991;87:120-128.
10. Meltzer AA, Smolensky MH, D'Alonzo GE, Harrist RB, Scott PH. An assessment of peak expiratory flow as a surrogate measurement of $FEV_1$ in stable asthmatic children. *Chest.* 1989;96:329-333.
11. Eid N, Yandell B, Howell L, Eddy M, Sheikh S. Can peak expiratory flow predict airflow obstruction in children with asthma? *Pediatrics.* 2000;105:354-358.
12. Enright PL, Lebowitz MD, Cockroft DW. Physiologic measures: pulmonary function tests: asthma outcome. *Am J Respir Crit Care Med.* 1994;149:S9-S18.
13. Finkelstein JA, Lozano P, Shulruff R, et al. Self-reported physician practices for children with asthma: are national guidelines followed? *Pediatrics.* 2000;106(4)(suppl):886-896.
14. Picken HA, Greenfield S, Teres D, Hirway PS, Landis JN. Effect of local standards on the implementation of national guidelines for asthma: primary care agreement with national asthma guidelines. *J Gen Intern Med.* 1998;13:659-663.
15. Diette GB, Skinner EA, Markson LE, et al. Consistency of care with national guidelines for children with asthma in managed care. *J Pediatr.* 2001;138:59-64.
16. Hankinson JL, Odencrantz JR, Fedan KB. Spirometric reference values from a sample of the general U.S. population. *Am J Respir Crit Care Med.* 1999;159:179-187.
17. Mitchell H, Senturia Y, Gergen P, et al. Design and methods of the National Cooperative Inner-City Asthma Study. *Pediatr Pulmonol.* 1997;24:237-252.
18. Crain EF, Walter M, O'Connor GT, et al. Home and allergic characteristics of children with asthma in seven U.S. urban communities and design of an environmental intervention: the Inner-City Asthma Study. *Environ Health Perspect.* 2002;110:939-945.
19. American Thoracic Society. Standardization of spirometry, 1994 update. *Am J Respir Crit Care Med.* 1995;152:1107-1136.
20. American Academy of Asthma, Allergy, and Immunology. *Pediatric Asthma: Promoting Best Practice.* Milwaukee, Wis: American Academy of Asthma, Allergy, and Immunology; 1999.
21. Klein RB, Fritz GK, Yeung A, McQuaid EL, Mansell A. Spirometric patterns in childhood asthma: peak flow compared with other indices. *Pediatr Pulmonol.* 1995;20:372-379.
22. Moy ML, Fuhlbrigge AL, Blumenschein K, et al. Association between preference-based health-related quality of life and asthma severity. *Ann Allergy Asthma Immunol.* 2004;92:329-334.
23. Morgan WJ, Crain EF, Gruchalla RS, et al. Results of a home-based environmental intervention among urban children with asthma. *N Engl J Med.* 2004;351:1068-1080.
24. Osborne ML, Vollmer WM, Pedula KL, Wilkins J, Buist AS, O'Hollaren M. Lack of correlation of symptoms with specialist-assessed long-term asthma severity. *Chest.* 1999;115:85-91.
25. Calhoun WJ, Sutton LB, Emmett A, Dorinsky PM. Asthma variability in patients previously treated with $\beta_2$-agonists alone. *J Allergy Clin Immunol.* 2003;112:1088-1094.
26. Colice GL, Burgt JV, Song J, Stampone P, Thompson PJ. Categorizing asthma severity. *Am J Respir Crit Care Med.* 1999;160:1962-1967.
27. Bacharier LB, Strunk RC, Mauger D, White D, Lemanske RF Jr, Sorkness CA. Classifying asthma severity in children: mismatch between symptoms, medication use, and lung function. *Am J Respir Crit Care Med.* 2004;170:426-432.
28. Nair SJ, Daigle KL, DeCuir P, Lapin CD, Schramm CM. The influence of pulmonary function testing on the management of asthma in children. *J Pediatr.* 2005;147:797-801.
29. Fuhlbrigge AL, Kitch BT, Paltiel AD, et al. $FEV_1$ is associated with risk of asthma attacks in a pediatric population. *J Allergy Clin Immunol.* 2001;107:61-67.
30. Juniper EF, Wisniewski ME, Cox FM, Emmett AH, Nielsen KE, O'Byrne PM. Relationship between quality of life and clinical status in asthma: a factor analysis. *Eur Respir J.* 2004;23:287-291.
31. Quanjer PH, Lebowitz MD, Gregg I, Miller MR, Pedersen OF. Peak expiratory flow: conclusions and recommendations of a Working Party of the European Respiratory Society. *Eur Respir J Suppl.* 1997;24:2S-8S.
32. Gardner RM, Crapo RO, Jackson BR, Jensen RL. Evaluation of accuracy and reproducibility of peak flowmeters at 1,400 m. *Chest.* 1992;101:948-952.
33. Hankinson JL, Das MK. Frequency response of portable PEF meters. *Am J Respir Crit Care Med.* 1995;152:702-706.
34. Hankinson JL, Filios MS, Kinsley KB, Petsonk EL. Comparing MiniWright and spirometer measurements of peak expiratory flow. *Chest.* 1995;108:407-410.
35. Miller MK, Johnson C, Miller DP, Deniz Y, Bleecker ER, Wenzel SE. Severity assessment in asthma: an evolving concept. *J Allergy Clin Immunol.* 2005;116:990-995.
36. Delgado-Corcoran C, Kissoon N, Murphy SP, Duckworth LJ. Exhaled nitric oxide reflects asthma severity and asthma control. *Pediatr Crit Care Med.* 2004;5:48-52.

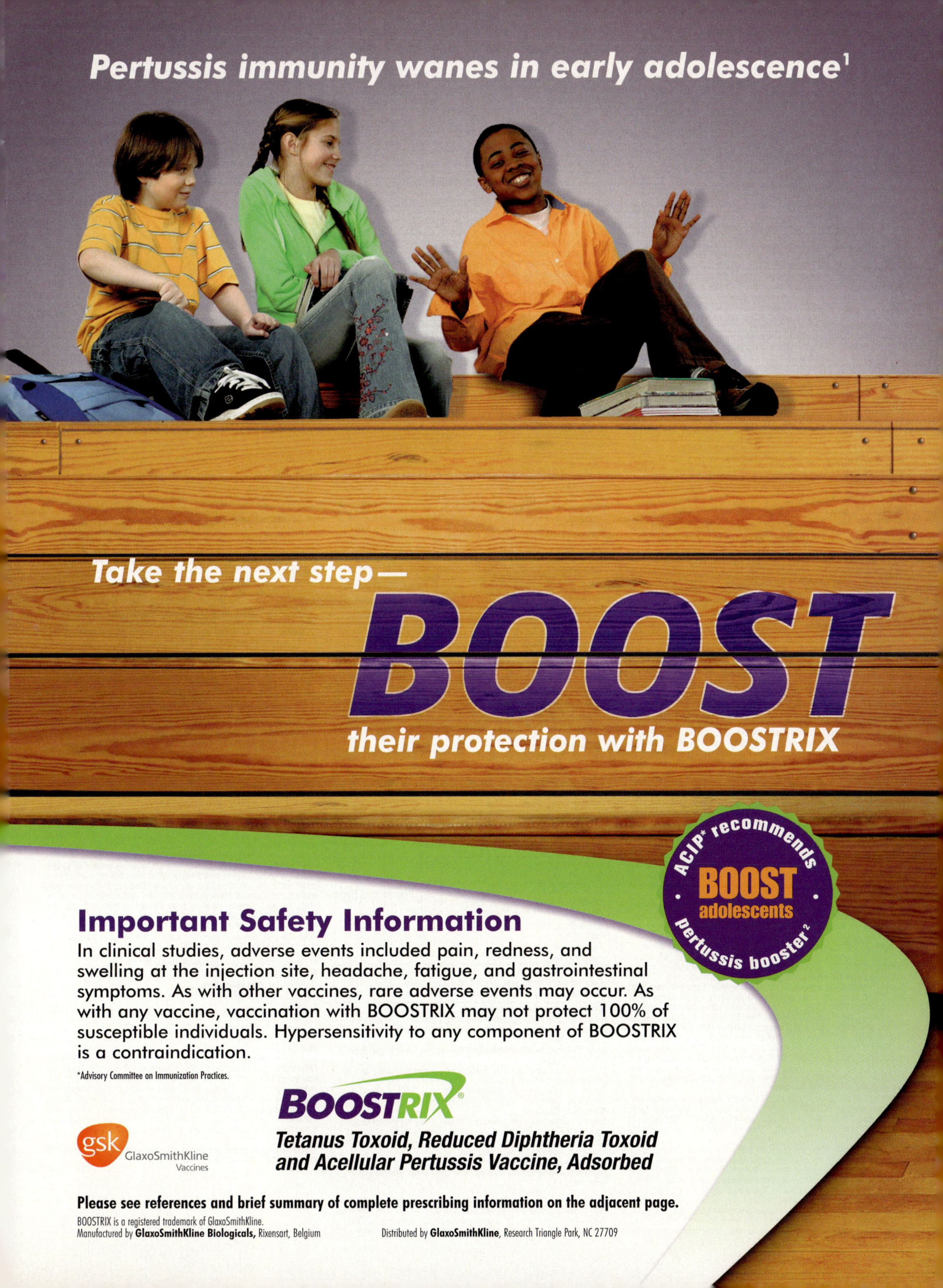

# BOOSTRIX®

## (Tetanus Toxoid, Reduced Diphtheria Toxoid and Acellular Pertussis Vaccine, Adsorbed) (Tdap)

The following is a brief summary only; see full prescribing information for complete product information.

**INDICATIONS AND USAGE:** BOOSTRIX is indicated for active booster immunization against tetanus, diphtheria, and pertussis as a single dose in individuals 10 through 18 years of age. The use of BOOSTRIX as a primary series or to complete the primary series has not been studied. As with any vaccine, BOOSTRIX may not protect 100% of individuals receiving the vaccine.

**CONTRAINDICATIONS:** Hypersensitivity to any component of the vaccine is a contraindication (see DESCRIPTION in full prescribing information). Do not use BOOSTRIX after a serious allergic reaction (e.g., anaphylaxis) following any other tetanus toxoid, diphtheria toxoid or pertussis-containing vaccine, or any component of this vaccine (see DESCRIPTION in full prescribing information). Because of the uncertainty as to which component of the vaccine might be responsible, do not give further vaccination with any of these components; or, refer such individuals to an allergist for evaluation. The following events are contraindications to administration of BOOSTRIX: encephalopathy (e.g., coma, decreased level of consciousness, prolonged seizures) within 7 days of administration of a previous dose of a pertussis-containing vaccine that is not attributable to another identifiable cause; progressive neurologic disorder, uncontrolled epilepsy, or progressive encephalopathy. Do not vaccinate individuals with these conditions until a treatment regimen has been established and the condition has stabilized.

**WARNINGS:** The tip cap and the rubber plunger of the needleless prefilled syringes contain dry natural latex rubber that may cause allergic reactions in latex sensitive individuals. The vial stopper is latex-free. If any of the following events occurred in temporal relation to previous receipt of a Diphtheria and Tetanus Toxoids and Pertussis Vaccine Adsorbed (DTwP) vaccine or a vaccine containing an acellular pertussis component, consider carefully whether to give subsequent doses of BOOSTRIX: temperature of ≥40.5°C (105°F) within 48 hours not due to another identifiable cause; collapse or shock-like state (hypotonic-hyporesponsive episode) within 48 hours; persistent, inconsolable crying lasting ≥3 hours, occurring within 48 hours; seizures with or without fever occurring within 3 days. Persons who experienced serious Arthus-type hypersensitivity reactions following a prior dose of tetanus toxoid usually have high serum tetanus antitoxin levels and should not be given Tetanus and Diphtheria Toxoids Adsorbed For Adult Use (Td) or Tdap vaccines or even emergency doses of Td more frequently than every 10 years, even if the wound is neither clean nor minor. If Guillain-Barré syndrome has occurred within 6 weeks of receipt of prior vaccine containing tetanus toxoid, the decision to give BOOSTRIX or any vaccine containing tetanus toxoid should be based on careful consideration of the potential benefits and possible risks. The decision to administer a pertussis-containing vaccine to individuals with stable central nervous system (CNS) disorders must be made by the physician on an individual basis, with consideration of all relevant factors, and assessment of potential risks and benefits for that individual. Advise the patient, parent, or guardian of the potential increased risk involved (see PRECAUTIONS). A family history of seizures or other CNS disorders is not a contraindication to pertussis vaccine. The Advisory Committee on Immunization Practices (ACIP) has published guidelines for vaccination of persons with recent or acute illness (www.cdc.gov). Do not give BOOSTRIX to individuals with bleeding disorders such as hemophilia or thrombocytopenia, or to persons on anticoagulant therapy unless the potential benefit clearly outweighs the risk of administration. If the decision is made to administer BOOSTRIX to such persons, it should be given with caution with steps taken to avoid the risk of hematoma following the injection.

**PRECAUTIONS: General:** Before the injection of any biological, the physician should take all reasonable precautions to prevent allergic or other adverse reactions. Epinephrine injection (1:1,000) and other appropriate agents used for the control of immediate allergic reactions must be immediately available should an acute anaphylactic reaction occur. Immunosuppressed persons, including individuals receiving immunosuppressive therapy, may not develop the expected immune response. **Drug Interactions:** Do not mix BOOSTRIX with any other vaccine in the same syringe or vial. **Carcinogenesis, Mutagenesis, Impairment of Fertility:** BOOSTRIX has not been evaluated for carcinogenic or mutagenic potential, or for impairment of fertility. **Pregnancy:** Pregnancy Category C. Animal reproduction studies have not been conducted with BOOSTRIX. It is also not known whether BOOSTRIX can cause fetal harm when administered to a pregnant woman or can affect reproductive capacity. BOOSTRIX should be given to a pregnant woman only if clearly needed. Animal fertility studies have not been conducted with BOOSTRIX. In a developmental toxicity study, the effect of BOOSTRIX on embryo-fetal and pre-weaning development was evaluated in pregnant rats. Animals were administered INFANRIX® (Diphtheria and Tetanus Toxoids and Acellular Pertussis Vaccine Adsorbed) prior to gestation and BOOSTRIX during the period of organogenesis (gestation days 6, 8, 11) and later in pregnancy (gestation day 15), 0.1 mL/rat/occasion (a 45-fold increase compared to the human dose of BOOSTRIX on a body weight basis), by intramuscular injection. No adverse affect on pregnancy and lactation parameters, embryo-fetal or pre-weaning development was observed. There were no fetal malformations or other evidence of teratogenesis noted in this study. **Nursing Mothers:** It is not known whether BOOSTRIX is excreted in human milk. Because many drugs are excreted in human milk, caution should be exercised when BOOSTRIX is administered to a nursing woman. **Pregnancy Exposure Registry:** Healthcare providers are encouraged to register pregnant women who receive BOOSTRIX in the GlaxoSmithKline vaccination pregnancy registry by calling 1-888-825-5249. **Geriatric Use:** BOOSTRIX is not indicated for use in individuals older than 18 years. **Pediatric Use:** BOOSTRIX is not indicated for use in individuals younger than 10 years (see DOSAGE AND ADMINISTRATION in full prescribing information). For immunization of infants and children younger than 7 years against diphtheria, tetanus, and pertussis, refer to the manufacturers' package inserts for Diphtheria and Tetanus Toxoids and Acellular Pertussis Vaccine Adsorbed (DTaP) vaccines.

**ADVERSE REACTIONS:** A total of 3,608 adolescents were vaccinated with a single dose of BOOSTRIX during clinical trials. An additional 1,092 adolescents 10 to 18 years of age received a non-US formulation of BOOSTRIX (formulated to contain 0.5 mg aluminum per dose) in non-US clinical studies.

The primary safety study, conducted in the United States, was a randomized, observer-blinded, controlled study in which 3,080 adolescents 10 to 18 years of age received a single dose of BOOSTRIX and 1,034 received the control Td vaccine manufactured by Massachusetts Public Health Biologic Laboratories. There were no substantive differences in demographic characteristics between the vaccine groups. Among BOOSTRIX and control vaccine recipients approximately 75% were 10 to 14 years of age and approximately 25% were 15 to 18 years of age. Approximately 98% of participants in this study had received the recommended series of 4 or 5 doses of either DTwP or a combination of DTwP and DTaP in childhood. Data on adverse events were collected by the subjects, parents and/or guardians using standardized diaries for 15 consecutive days following the vaccine dose (i.e., day of vaccination and the next 14 days). Subjects were monitored for unsolicited adverse events that occurred within 31 days of vaccination (day 0-30) using diary cards (day 0-14) supplemented by spontaneous reports and a medical history as reported by subjects, parents, and/or guardians. Subjects were also monitored for 6 months post-vaccination for non-routine medical visits, visits to an emergency room, onset of new chronic illness, and serious adverse events. Information regarding late onset adverse events was obtained via a telephone call 6 months following vaccination. At least 97% of subjects completed the 6-month follow-up evaluation.

In a study conducted in Germany, BOOSTRIX was administered to 319 children 10 to 12 years of age previously vaccinated with 5 doses of acellular pertussis-containing vaccines, 193 of these subjects had previously received 5 doses of INFANRIX. Adverse events were recorded on diary cards during the 15 days following vaccination. Unsolicited adverse events that occurred within 31 days of vaccination (day 0-30) were recorded on the diary card or verbally reported to the investigator. Subjects were monitored for 6 months post-vaccination for physician office visits, emergency room visits, onset of new chronic illness, and serious adverse events. The 6-month follow-up evaluation, conducted via telephone interview, was completed by 90% of subjects.

The adverse event information from clinical trials provides a basis for identifying adverse events that appear to be related to vaccine use and for approximating rates. However, because clinical trials are conducted under widely varying conditions, adverse event rates observed in the clinical trials of a vaccine cannot be directly compared to rates in the clinical trials of another vaccine, and may not reflect the rates observed in practice.

**Serious Adverse Events in All Safety Studies:** In the US-safety study and German-safety study, no serious adverse events were reported to occur within 31 days of vaccination. During the 6-month extended safety evaluation period, no serious adverse events that were of potential autoimmune origin or new onset and chronic in nature were reported to occur. In non-US studies in which serious adverse events were monitored for up to 37 days, one subject was diagnosed with insulin dependent diabetes 20 days following administration of BOOSTRIX. No other serious adverse events of potential autoimmune origin or that were new onset and chronic in nature were reported to occur in these studies.

**Solicited Adverse Events in the US-Safety Study:** In a US study, the most common local adverse events following administration of BOOSTRIX were pain, redness, and swelling at the injection site. The most common general adverse events were headache and fatigue. Most of these events were reported at a similar frequency in recipients of both BOOSTRIX and Td. Any pain, grade 2 or 3 pain (but not grade 3 alone), and grade 2 or 3 headache (but not grade 3 alone) were reported at a higher rate in recipients of BOOSTRIX. The primary safety endpoint of the US study was the incidence of grade 3 pain (spontaneously painful and/or prevented normal activity) at the injection site within 15 days of vaccination. Grade 3 pain was reported in 4.6% of those who received BOOSTRIX compared with 4.0% of those who received the Td vaccine. The difference in rate of grade 3 pain was within the pre-defined clinical limit for non-inferiority (upper limit of the 95% CI for the difference ≤4%). These were the rates for solicited local and general adverse events within 15 days of vaccination with BOOSTRIX or Td vaccine for the total vaccinated cohort (all enrolled, vaccinated subjects with safety data available analyzed by vaccine received):

**Percentage of Individuals 10 to 18 Years of Age Reporting Solicited Local Adverse Events or Solicited General Adverse Events Within the 15-day* Post-Vaccination Period**

| | BOOSTRIX (N = 3,032) % | Td (N =1,013) % |
|---|---|---|
| **Local** | | |
| Pain,† any | 75.3 | 71.7 |
| Pain,† grade 2 or 3 | 51.2 | 42.5 |
| Pain,‡ grade 3 | 4.6 | 4.0 |
| Redness, any | 22.5 | 19.8 |
| Redness, >20 mm | 4.1 | 3.9 |
| Redness, ≥50 mm | 1.7 | 1.6 |
| Swelling, any | 21.1 | 20.1 |
| Swelling, >20 mm | 5.3 | 4.9 |
| Swelling, ≥50 mm | 2.5 | 3.2 |
| Arm circumference increase,§ >5 mm | 28.3 | 29.5 |
| Arm circumference increase,§ >20 mm | 2.0 | 2.2 |
| Arm circumference increase,§ >40 mm | 0.5 | 0.3 |
| **General** | | |
| Fever,‖ ≥99.5°F | 13.5 | 13.1 |
| Fever,‖ >100.4°F | 5.0 | 4.7 |
| Fever,‖ >102.2°F | 1.4 | 1.0 |
| Headache, any | 43.1 | 41.5 |
| Headache,† grade 2 or 3 | 15.7 | 12.7 |
| Headache, grade 3 | 3.7 | 2.7 |
| Fatigue, any | 37.0 | 36.7 |
| Fatigue, grade 2 or 3 | 14.4 | 12.9 |
| Fatigue, grade 3 | 3.7 | 3.2 |
| Gastrointestinal symptoms,¶ any | 26.0 | 25.8 |
| Gastrointestinal symptoms,¶ grade 2 or 3 | 9.8 | 9.7 |
| Gastrointestinal symptoms,¶ grade 3 | 3.0 | 3.2 |

Td = Tetanus and Diphtheria Toxoids Adsorbed For Adult Use manufactured by Massachusetts Public Health Biologic Laboratories.
N = number of subjects in the total vaccinated cohort with local/general symptoms sheets completed.
Grade 2 = Local: painful when the limb was moved; General: interfered with normal activity.
Grade 3 = Local: spontaneously painful and/or prevented normal activity; General: prevented normal activity.
*Day of vaccination and the next 14 days.
†Statistically significantly higher (P<0.05) following BOOSTRIX as compared to Td vaccine.
‡Grade 3 injection site pain following BOOSTRIX was not inferior to Td (upper limit of two-sided 95% CI for the difference in the percentage of subjects ≤4%).
§Mid-upper region of the vaccinated arm.
‖Oral temperatures or axillary temperatures.
¶Gastrointestinal symptoms included nausea, vomiting, diarrhea and/or abdominal pain.

Mid-upper arm circumference was measured by the adolescent or their parent/guardian prior to injection and daily for 15 days following vaccination. There was no significant difference between BOOSTRIX recipients and Td recipients in the proportion of subjects reporting an increase in mid-upper arm circumference in the vaccinated arm. The incidence of unsolicited adverse events reported in the 31 days after vaccination was comparable between the 2 groups.

**Solicited Adverse Events in the German Safety Study:** No cases of whole arm swelling were spontaneously reported. Two individuals (2/193) reported large injection site swelling (range 110 to 200 mm diameter), in one case associated with grade 3 pain. Neither individual sought medical attention. These episodes were reported to resolve without sequelae within 5 days. These were the rates of solicited local adverse events and fever within 15 days of vaccination for those subjects who had previously been vaccinated with 5 doses of INFANRIX:

**Rates of Solicited Adverse Events Reported Within the 15-day* Post-Vaccination Period Following Administration of BOOSTRIX in Individuals 10 to 12 Years of Age Who Had Previously Received 5 Doses of INFANRIX**

| Adverse Event | BOOSTRIX (N = 193) % (95% CI) |
|---|---|
| Pain, any | 62.2 (54.9-69.0) |
| Pain, grade 2 or 3 | 33.2 (26.6-40.3) |
| Pain, grade 3 | 5.7 (2.9-10.0) |
| Redness, any | 47.7 (40.4-55.0) |
| Redness, >20 mm | 15.0 (10.3-20.9) |
| Redness, ≥50 mm | 10.9 (6.9-16.2) |
| Swelling, any | 38.9 (31.9-46.1) |
| Swelling, >20 mm | 17.6 (12.5-23.7) |
| Swelling, ≥50 mm | 14.0 (9.4-19.7) |
| Fever, ≥99.5 | 8.8 (5.2-13.7) |
| Fever, >100.4 | 4.1 (1.8-8.0) |
| Fever, >102.2 | 1.0 (0.1-3.7) |

N = number of subjects with local/general symptoms sheets completed.
Grade 2 = Painful when the limb was moved.
Grade 3 = Spontaneously painful and/or prevented normal activity.
*Day of vaccination and the next 14 days.

As with any vaccine, there is the possibility that broad use of BOOSTRIX could reveal adverse events not observed in clinical trials.

**Postmarketing Reports:** Worldwide voluntary reports of adverse events received for BOOSTRIX in persons 10 to 18 years of age since market introduction of this vaccine are listed below. This list includes serious events or events which have causal connection to components of this or other vaccines or drugs. Because these events are reported voluntarily from a population of uncertain size, it is not possible to reliably estimate their frequency or establish a causal relationship to vaccine exposure. *Blood and lymphatic system disorders:* Lymphadenitis, lymphadenopathy. *Cardiac disorders:* Myocarditis. *Injection site reactions:* Induration, inflammation, mass, nodule, warmth, local reaction. *Metabolism and nutrition disorders:* Diabetes mellitus insulin-dependent. *Musculoskeletal and connective tissue disorders:* Arthralgia, back pain, myalgia. *Nervous system disorders:* Convulsion, encephalitis, facial palsy, paraesthesia. *Skin and subcutaneous tissue disorders:* Exanthem, Henoch-Schönlein purpura, rash. In addition, extensive swelling of the injected limb has been reported following administration of BOOSTRIX.

**Reporting Adverse Events:** Report the occurrence following immunization of any event set forth in the Vaccine Injury Table from the National Childhood Vaccine Injury Act including: Anaphylaxis or anaphylactic shock within 7 days, encephalopathy or encephalitis within 7 days, brachial neuritis within 28 days, or an acute complication or sequelae (including death) of an illness, disability, injury, or condition referred to above, or any events that would contraindicate further doses of vaccine, according to this prescribing information. These events should be reported to VAERS. The VAERS toll-free number is 1-800-822-7967. Reporting forms may also be obtained at the VAERS website at www.vaers.hhs.gov.

**DOSAGE AND ADMINISTRATION: Recommended Dose:** BOOSTRIX should be administered as a single 0.5 mL injection by the intramuscular route into the deltoid muscle of the upper arm in individuals 10 through 18 years of age. Do not administer this product subcutaneously or intravenously. There are no data to support repeat administration of BOOSTRIX. Five years should elapse between the subject's last dose of the recommended series of childhood DTwP and/or DTaP vaccine and the administration of BOOSTRIX. Limited data are available on the use of BOOSTRIX following Tetanus and Diphtheria Toxoids Adsorbed For Adult Use (Td) vaccine. **Additional Dosing Information:** ***Wound Management:*** Clinicians should refer to guidelines for tetanus prophylaxis in routine wound management. Adolescents 10 to 18 years of age who have completed a primary series against tetanus and who sustain wounds which are minor and uncomplicated, should receive a booster dose of a tetanus toxoid-containing vaccine only if they have not received tetanus toxoid within the preceding 10 years. In case of tetanus-prone injury (e.g., wounds contaminated with dirt, feces, soil, and saliva; puncture wounds; avulsions; and wounds resulting from missles, crushing, burns, and frostbite) in an adolescent who is in need of tetanus toxoid, BOOSTRIX can be used as an alternative to Tetanus and Diphtheria Toxoids Adsorbed For Adult Use (Td) vaccine in patients for whom the pertussis component is also indicated (see INDICATIONS AND USAGE).

Manufactured by **GlaxoSmithKline Biologicals**
Rixensart, Belgium, US License 1617

Distributed by **GlaxoSmithKline**
Research Triangle Park, NC 27709

BOOSTRIX and INFANRIX are registered trademarks of GlaxoSmithKline.

Full prescribing information for BOOSTRIX is available at www.BOOSTRIX.com.
BRS-BO:L3

**References: 1.** Centers for Disease Control and Prevention. Preventing tetanus, diphtheria, and pertussis among adolescents: use of tetanus toxoid, reduced diphtheria toxoid and acellular pertussis vaccines: recommendations of the Advisory Committee on Immunization Practices (ACIP). Early Release 2006;55(February 23, 2006):1–43. **2.** Centers for Disease Control and Prevention. Recommended childhood and adolescent immunization schedule—United States, 2006. *MMWR.* 2006;54(51&52):Q1–Q4.

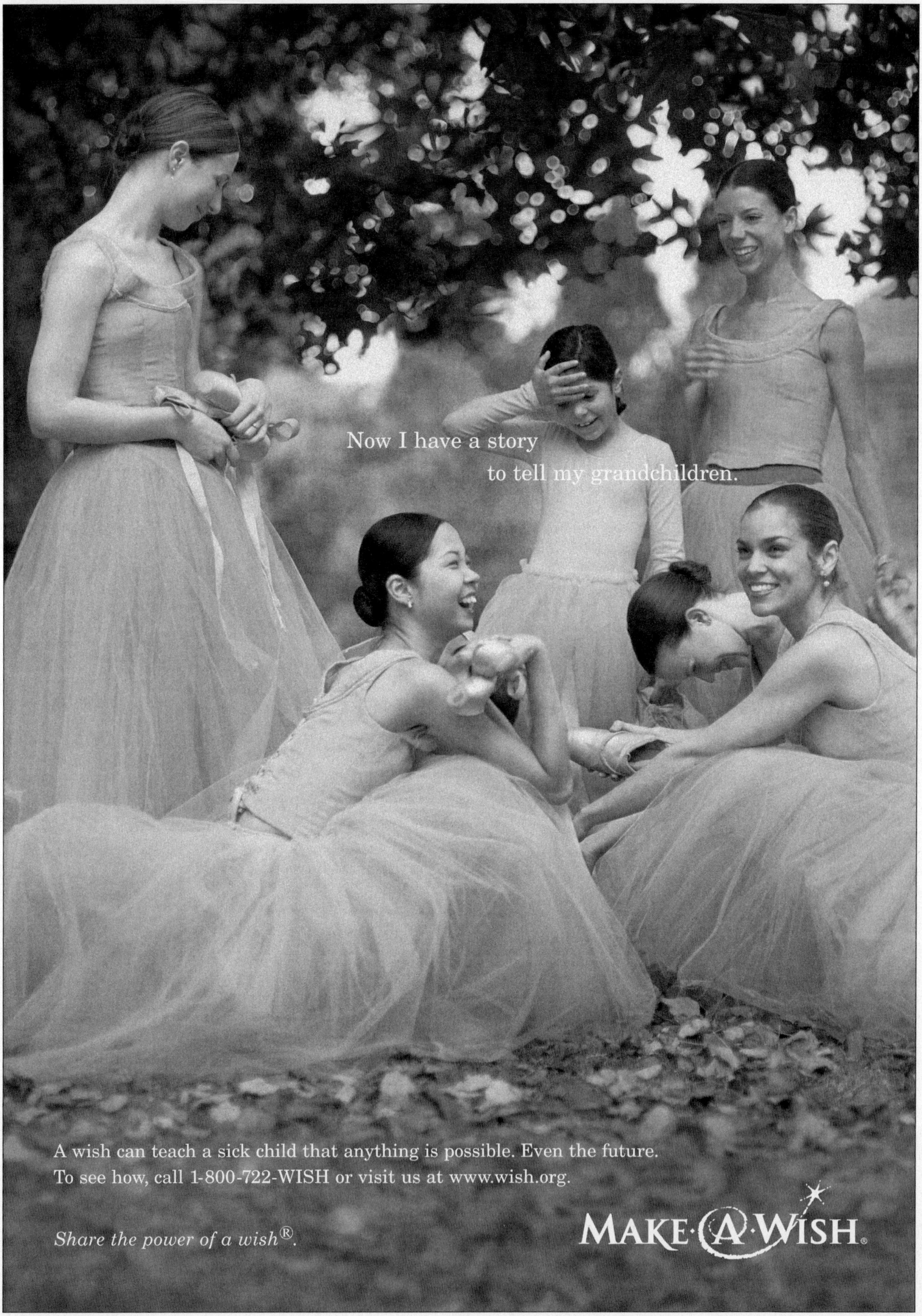
Now I have a story
to tell my grandchildren.
A wish can teach a sick child that anything is possible. Even the future.
To see how, call 1-800-722-WISH or visit us at www.wish.org.
Share the power of a wish®.
MAKE·A·WISH®

## Laboratory Testing for Drug Abuse

The Levy et al article[1] on adolescent physicians' knowledge of the practices of screening for drug abuse is timely. We have long felt that practicing physicians' knowledge of drug testing has not recognized the technical and ethical issues involved.[2] In our experience, clinical testing for drug abuse does not follow the policies and procedures outlined for federal workplace testing. In fact, most hospital laboratories do not have established policies for validation of specimens and many do not have the ability to perform confirmatory testing, which in federal testing requires gas chromatography/mass spectroscopy. We disagree with the blanket statement of Levy et al that urine drug screenings do not detect oxycodone and ecstasy (3,4-methylenedioxymethamphetamine). The ability to detect these substances depends on the cross-reactivity of the particular immunoassay used. The technology for immunoassays is continually evolving and many of the currently used assays do, in fact, detect these substances. Physicians who order drug screens can review the package inserts provided to the laboratory by the manufacturer of the immunoassay to determine the sensitivity of the assay for detecting oxycodone, ecstasy, and other specific substances.[3] Another important question, which the authors did not address, is whether the physicians obtain informed consent before performing laboratory screening for drug abuse.

*Elizabeth A. Warner, MD*
*Peter D. Friedmann, MD*

**Correspondence:** Dr Warner, Department of Internal Medicine, University of South Florida, 12901 Bruce B. Downs Blvd, MDC 80, Tampa, FL 33612 (ewarner@hsc.usf.edu).

1. Levy S, Harris SK, Sherritt L, Angulo M, Knight JR. Drug testing of adolescents in ambulatory medicine physician practices and knowledge. *Arch Pediatr Adolesc Med.* 2006;160:146-150.
2. Warner EA, Walker RM, Friedmann PD. Should informed consent be required for testing for drug of abuse in medical settings? *Am J Med.* 2003;115:54-58.
3. Warner EA. Laboratory diagnosis. In: Graham AW, Schultz TK, Mayo-Smith M, Ries RK, Wilford BB, eds. *Principles of Addiction Medicine.* 3rd ed. Chevy Chase, Md: American Society of Addiction Medicine; 2003:337-348.

### In reply

*We agree with Drs Warner and Friedmann that the detection of illicit substances such as oxycodone and ecstasy (3,4 methylenedioxymethamphetamine) by immunoassay screens depends on the particular screen used, and indeed, some commercial products are able to detect these compounds in urine. Our study was conducted in 2004 when the preferred assays used in standard drug-testing laboratories did not reliably detect ecstasy, as noted in the footnote to Table 2, and to date, the majority of opioid screens do not include oxycodone. However, even if we discount these items from our questionnaire analysis, our conclusion that the primary care workforce is not currently prepared to support widespread implementation of urine drug testing would not change. Moreover, the variability in what is included in a "standard panel" among available urine screening products underscores the complexity of this procedure. Furthermore, prior research by our team examined Internet-based information regarding home drug-testing kits as well as product inserts. We found that the information companies provided regarding which drugs are detected by their testing products was often conflicting or incomplete.[1] Therefore, physicians who use point-of-service test kits may have difficulty in determining which substances are detected even after examining the information provided. The question of whether physicians obtain consent prior to performing laboratory screening was beyond the scope of our article, which focused on the technical challenges of drug testing. Analysis of physician attitudes and practices is reported in a subsequent article.[2]*

*Sharon Levy, MD, MPH*
*Sion Kim Harris, PhD*
*Lon Sherritt, MPH*
*Michelle Angulo, BA*
*John R. Knight, MD*

**Correspondence:** Dr Levy, Center for Adolescent Substance Abuse Research, Children's Hospital Boston, 300 Longwood Ave, Boston, MA 02115 (sharon.levy@childrens.harvard.edu).

1. Levy S, van Hook S, Knight J. A review of internet-based home drug-testing products for parents. *Pediatrics.* 2004;113:720-726.
2. Levy S, Harris SK, Sherritt L, Angulo M, Knight JR. Drug testing of adolescents in general medical clinics, in school and at home: physician attitudes and practices. *J Adolesc Health.* 2006;38:336-342.

## Use of a Partially Hydrolyzed Formula in the Dietary Prevention of Allergic Disease

We read with particular interest the article by Hays and Wood "A Systematic Review of the Role of Hydrolyzed Infant Formulas in Allergy Prevention"[1] and appreciate being quoted twice. We confirm our preference for the use of partially hydrolyzed formula (PHF) for the nutritional prevention of allergy, but only in highly atopic subjects. Extensively hydrolyzed formulas are more expensive, have a bad taste, and do not satisfy the nutritional needs of the growing baby.[2]

Changes in intestinal microflora[3] should be taken into account because of their influence on the future development of allergies, which is similar to that observed in breastfed babies; peptides have a bifidogenic effect. Adding prebiotics to infant formula has a permanent bifidogenic effect as it increases lactobacilli and markedly decreases previously present pathogen germs.[4] However, to obtain a clear advantage, any intervention must be part of a more general nutritional program and environmental advice.

We do not agree with widespread use of hydrolyzed formulas for the general population because of some long-term possible concerns regarding an unusual nutritional exposure. In guinea pigs fed from birth to adolescence with mother's milk, intact protein formula, and PHF, we found, in PHF-fed animals at the last evaluation, signs of exocrine pancreatic hypoplasia, partially corrected by the cellular content of zymogen granules.[5]

Examining the development of atherosclerosis in growing rabbits, we found that the worst results, with similar lipid blood values, were observed with PHF (whey), with no difference between vegetal- and intact casein–fed animals. Analysis of the products showed that the concentration of asymmetric dimethylarginine is 10 times higher in PHF than in intact casein. Asymmetric dimethylarginine is toxic for the endothelium and can damage arteries. However, our animals received high quantities of proteins because of the nitrogen nutritional needs for the growth of guinea pigs and rabbits, and we might have seen the phenomenon through a magnifying glass.

Therefore, we feel that a word of caution should be considered for generalized use of hydrolyzed formulas. The use of PHF must to be limited to the prevention of allergic disease in high-risk atopic subjects only when breast milk is lacking.

*Antonio Marini, MD*
*Massimo Agosti, MD*
*Carla Colombo, MD*

**Correspondence:** Prof Marini, Institute of Pediatrics and Neonatology, University of Milan, Via della Commenda 9, Milan, Italy (antonio.marini@unimi.it).

1. Hays T, Wood RA. A systematic review of the role of hydrolyzed infant formulas in allergy prevention. *Arch Pediatr Adolesc Med*. 2005;159:810-816.
2. Zeiger RS. Food allergen avoidance in the prevention of food allergy in infants and children. *Pediatrics*. 2003;111:1662-1671.
3. Björkstén B. The intrauterine and postnatal environment. *J Allergy Clin Immunol*. 1999;104:1119-1127.
4. Marini A, Boehm G, Negretti F, Agosti M. Probiotics, prebiotics, or both in a very low birth weight infant. *Pediatrics*. 2005;116:522-523.
5. Colombo C, Biffi A, Agosti M, Crosignani A, Bennato V, Marini A. Pancreatic development in newborn guinea pigs fed intact or low-hydrolyzed protein formulas. *J Pediatr Gastroenterol Nutr*. 2005;41:644-649.

*In reply*

*We thank you for the thoughtful comments. We agree that the long-term consequences of partially hydrolyzed cow's milk formula are not fully known and that the use of PHF for the general population remains controversial. However, the whey-based hydrolysate, which was shown to reduce allergy in high-risk infants, has been approved and used as a routine infant formula in North America for 20 years.*

*We do not know every potential characteristic or component in formulas (intact protein formulas included) that could be detrimental. It is also clear that not all hydrolysates are compositionally or functionally the same. The formula leading to adverse effects in animals discussed by Professor Marini[1] is a hydrolyzed formula with a median molecular weight of 5000 and made with a combination of casein and whey. This formula is significantly different than either the casein-based extensive hydrolysate or whey-based hydrolysate, which have been studied for primary prevention.[2] Casein/whey hydrolysates have not been shown to be effective in allergy risk reduction.[3] Recommendations for allergy prevention should only be made for formulas that have demonstrated efficacy in clinical trials and have a good safety record.*

*Who should we target for allergy prevention? It is commonly suggested that we target infants at risk for atopic disease and most studies on allergy prevention have focused on these high-risk populations. However, the majority of infants who develop allergy do not have a positive family history,[4] and the thorough family history needed to identify atopic risk is not routinely used to screen infants in the general population. Therefore, in standard clinical practice, most infants at risk for atopy remain unidentified. Until more comprehensive methods of risk assessment are available, it makes more sense to offer prevention strategies to the general population.*

*No nutritional intervention is 100% efficacious or risk free; but for infants who get formula, our goal should be to minimize the risks that come from not exclusively breastfeeding, and we should aim to do this in the greatest number of infants possible. Decisions on infant feeding should always be made carefully, and thoughtfully, between a health care professional and an informed parent, taking all aspects of health care into consideration.*

*Tiffani Hays, MS, RD, LDN*
*Robert Wood, MD*

**Correspondence:** Ms Hays, Johns Hopkins Children's Center, Brady 302, 600 N Wolfe St, Baltimore, MD 21287 (thays@jhmi.edu).

1. Colombo C, Biffi A, Agosti M, Crosignani A, Bennato V, Marini A. Pancreatic development in newborn guinea pigs fed intact or low-hydrolyzed protein formulas. *J Pediatr Gastroenterol Nutr*. 2005;41:644-649.
2. Hays T, Wood RA. A systematic review of the role of hydrolyzed infant formulas in allergy prevention. *Arch Pediatr Adolesc Med*. 2005;159:810-816.
3. von Berg A, Koletzko A, Grubl A, et al. The effect of hydrolyzed cow's milk formula for allergy prevention in the first year of life. *J Allergy Clin Immunol*. 2003;111:533-540.
4. Bergmann RL, Edenharter G, Bergmann KE, et al. Predictability of early atopy by cord blood-IgE and parental history. *Clin Exp Allergy*. 1997;27:752-760.

## Neonatal Adverse Reactions After In Utero Exposure to Selective Serotonin Reuptake Inhibitors: Still Controversial

Levinson-Castiel et al[1] reported neonatal abstinence syndrome (NAS) in 30% of selective serotonin reuptake inhibitor (SSRI)–exposed neonates in late pregnancy using the Finnegan NAS score. Although other reports exist of antidepressant-exposed neonates having a positive Finnegan score,[2] the score was designed to assess opiates and not SSRI withdrawal. Moreover, the fact that newborns exposed to SSRIs in late pregnancy share some clinical features compatible with NAS does not indicate that the Finnegan score is representative of the same prevalence of symptoms or that all important symptoms are taken into account. We are currently analyzing data from a retrospective cohort of 66 SSRI- or serotonin-norepinephrine reuptake inhibitor–exposed newborns in late pregnancy; more than 20% showed decreased reactivity and/or decreased tonus during the first 72 hours of life, symptoms that are not assessed by the Finnegan score. Newborns also showed symptoms compatible with NAS in that time frame. Decreased reactivity or tonus have been reported in other cases and studies.[3] This discrepancy shows that the etiology of these symptoms is still unclear.

An important point is that symptoms could be related either to serotonergic toxic effects,[4] withdrawal syndrome, or adverse effects. Using the terms *withdrawal* or *abstinence* is assuming that the drug has disappeared, or nearly so, from the newborn's serum. The correlation between higher SSRI doses in the mother and higher Finnegan score does not demonstrate that symptoms are related to withdrawal. In fact, neonates' serum levels are essential to establish differential diagnosis between a toxic reaction and withdrawal[5] and to decide treatment if necessary.

Time elapsed between birth and the emergence of symptoms should be interpreted with caution. It is unlikely that symptoms in the first days of life will be linked to withdrawal from fluoxetine because this drug and its active metabolite have a long half-life (4-6 days and 4-16 days, respectively) and, most likely, are still present in the newborn's serum. On the other hand, the fact that symptoms have not appeared during the first 24 hours of life does not demonstrate that it was a withdrawal reaction. Here again, drug levels may be helpful. However, drug action, which is slow to appear, may be slow to disappear, and relation to drug concentration might be hard to interpret.

Controversy remains on whether neonatal adverse reaction is due to a toxic reaction or to a form of withdrawal. Because both entities could be present,[5] each case is unique and generalization is not yet possible.

*Louise Beaulac-Baillargeon, BPharm, PhD*
*Nina Boucher, BPharm, MSc*

**Correspondence:** Dr Beaulac-Baillargeon, Faculty of Pharmacy, Laval University, Pavillon Vandry, 2230, Quebec G1K 7P4, Canada (louise.beaulac-baillargeon@pha.ulaval.ca).
**Funding/Support:** Dr Boucher received a doctorate scholarship from St-Francois d'Assise Hospital Research Center.

1. Levinson-Castiel R, Merlob P, Linder N, Sirota L, Klinger G. Neonatal abstinence syndrome after in utero exposure to selective serotonin reuptake inhibitors in term infants. *Arch Pediatr Adolesc Med*. 2006;160:173-176.
2. Rampono J, Proud S, Hackett LP, Kristensen JH, Ilett KF. A pilot study of newer antidepressant concentrations in cord and maternal serum and possible effects in the neonate. *Int J Neuropsychopharmacol*. 2004;7:329-334.
3. Nordeng H, Spigset O. Treatment with selective serotonin reuptake inhibitors in the third trimester of pregnancy: effects on the infant. *Drug Saf*. 2005; 28:565-581.
4. Hegerl U, Bottlender R, Jurgen G, et al. The serotonin syndrome scale: first results on validity. *Eur Arch Psychiatry Clin Neurosci*. 1998;248:96-103.
5. Koren G. A new indication for therapeutic drug monitoring in the neonate. *Ther Drug Monit*. 2006;28:1.

## *In reply*

*We read with interest the letter by Beaulac-Baillargeon and Boucher regarding our article[1] on NAS following in utero exposure to SSRIs in term infants.*

*Our study clearly showed that 30% of infants exposed to SSRIs had symptoms of NAS as measured by the Finnegan score and that the symptoms were related to SSRI exposure because they were absent in nonexposed infants. The Finnegan score is an objective method used to monitor onset, progression, and improvement of NAS symptoms in passively exposed infants. Although the Finnegan score was designed for assessment of opiate withdrawal, NAS scores have been similarly used for SSRI-exposed infants.[2,3] This score captures most NAS symptoms; however, we observed in some infants, and especially in preterm infants, additional symptoms such as hypotonia, decreased activity, and weak cry as Beaulac-Baillargeon and Boucher also report. Inclusion of these additional symptoms would probably increase the accuracy of NAS assessment.*

*Beaulac-Baillargeon and Boucher are correct to repeat the same point that we discussed at large in our article regarding the possibility that neonatal symptoms may be due to abstinence or in some cases to serotoninergic hyperstimulation. This point is important for deciding how to treat symptomatic infants. Pharmacologic reasoning would suggest treatment of abstinence symptoms with the same medication that infants were previously exposed to; however, this is presently unacceptable because the safety of giving SSRIs to infants is unknown. In the few infants who had extreme NAS, we elected to treat symptomatically with sedation (phenobarbital).*

*It is correctly stated that for the minority of our exposed infants, theoretically, a long half-life should decrease the likelihood of early symptoms, yet Beaulac-Baillargeon and Boucher themselves have observed symptoms in 20% of their cohort within 72 hours of birth.*

*Although some aspects of NAS in SSRI-exposed infants may seem controversial, today it is a well-recognized postnatal clinical syndrome that needs close monitoring using a standardized protocol.*

*Gil Klinger, MD*
*Rachel Levinson-Castiel, MD*
*Paul Merlob, MD*

**Correspondence:** Dr Klinger, Neonatal Intensive Care Unit, Schneider Children's Medical Center of Israel, 14 Kaplan St, Petah Tiqwa, 49202 Israel (gilkl@post.tau.ac.il).

1. Levinson-Castiel R, Merlob P, Linder N, Sirota L, Klinger G. Neonatal abstinence syndrome after in utero exposure to selective serotonin reuptake inhibitors in term infants. *Arch Pediatr Adolesc Med*. 2006;160: 173-176.
2. Nordeng H, Lindemann R, Perminov KV, Reikvam A. Neonatal withdrawal syndrome after in utero exposure to selective serotonin reuptake inhibitors. *Acta Paediatr*. 2001;90:288-291.
3. Nijhuis IJ, Kok-Van Rooij GW, Bosschaart AN. Withdrawal reactions of a premature neonate after maternal use of paroxetine [letter]. *Arch Dis Child Fetal Neonatal Ed*. 2001;84:F77.

## Challenges to Study on Alcohol Advertising Effects on Youth Drinking

I challenge the Snyder et al study[1] examining alcohol advertising effects on drinking behaviors. The study refutes decades of very sophisticated advertising, marketing communication, and consumer behavior research. For example, during the past 50 years, researchers, globally, have not been able to demonstrate a direct and measurable effect of mass media advertising on consumer behavior except in certain instances of direct response–type appeals.

Primary issues I have with the Snyder et al research include:

- A Hierarchy of Effects model (circa 1961) apparently underlies the study (ie, the assumption of a linear, 1-way, outbound model in which marketer investments result in advertising exposure that results in consumer behavioral changes). While intuitively appealing, this conditioned-response, behaviorist model has been challenged for years, most recently by new studies in cognitive science.
- Correlations do not mean causality. The authors carefully skirt this issue, relying on correlations in some instances and causality in others but drawing a final conclusion of causality.
- Starting with 1872 respondents and ending with 588 respondents results in a massive attrition rate (68%). One can only wonder at the representativeness of the final group compared with the original sample.
- Assuming that certain levels of marketplace advertising expenditures result in certain levels of in-market advertising media weight that then result in certain levels of message distribution that then result in certain levels of consumer exposure that then result in actual consumer behavioral changes is tenuous at best. These linkages simply cannot be made and no amount of statistical magic can make them appear.
- Averaging media investments to a per capita base ignores the fact that media exposure is unique among audiences and individuals. Self-reporting does not mediate the problem.
- Four-week respondent recall is fraught with problems. Asking people to recall what advertising they saw and what alcohol beverages they consumed during the past month commonly invites respondent speculation and guessing.

*Don E. Schultz, PhD*

**Correspondence:** Dr Schultz, Integrated Marketing Communications Department, Northwestern University, 1870 Campus Dr, Evanston, IL 60208 (dschultz@northwestern.edu).

**Funding/Support:** Dr Schultz received funding from the Distilled Spirits Council.

1. Snyder LB, Milici FF, Slater M, Sun H, Strizhakova . Effects of alcohol advertising exposure on drinking among youth. *Arch Pediatr Adolesc Med.* 2006; 160:18-24.

## Limitations of Study on Alcohol Advertising Effects on Youth Drinking

The Snyder et al study[1] examines drinking by youth and young adults, segments of special interest in alcohol advertising research. However, the study has serious limitations in planning and execution.

- The study often refers to a "youth sample" but 50% were 21 years and older. Although the study is called "longitudinal," two thirds of the sample were not followed up through the 4 interview periods.
- Although the study is correlational and cannot show causality, alcohol advertising is assumed to be the cause of drinking. The analyses are limited to demographic and advertising variables, but variables that best explain youth alcohol consumption (eg, peer drinking, parents drinking, and religion) are left out.
- The study claims that more advertising leads to more drinking. However, Table 2 in the Snyder et al study[1] shows that those who saw the most advertising actually decreased their drinking.
- There is no reference to experimental, economic, and advertising-ban studies, predominantly showing negative effects on alcohol consumption. This suggests a biased, 1-sided view of alcohol advertising effects.
- The measurement of alcohol use combines average and maximum number of drinks, giving the same weight to maximum, although most drinkers rarely drink their maximum and also take maximums into account when reporting averages. The reliability and validity of the measure have not been assessed and must be suspect.
- In areas where there was more drinking, there was more alcohol advertising, but religious and alcohol-availability factors were omitted.
- The study had major problems with attrition because the sample went from 1872 to 588 in 21 months or 31% at time 4. The nonattriters were different than the attriters in drinking levels. With 24 media areas and less than 50% of respondents younger than 21 years, smaller areas would have few youth by time 4. There is no power analysis and the power to detect real results for youth would then be low.
- Anomalies appear in the alcohol consumption data (eg, at baseline, black and Hispanic individuals drank substantially more than white individuals). Also, those younger than 23 years drank far more than those aged 23 to 26 years. These results suggest sampling biases, because their findings are different from large, well-established data sets.

The study has limitations that make it impossible to understand or interpret the results. It will not change thinking in the alcohol-advertising debate.

*Reginald Smart, PhD*

**Correspondence:** Dr Smart, Social Science Consulting, 90 Wimbleton Rd, Toronto M9A3S6, Canada (smartreg@idirect.com).

**Funding/Support:** Dr Smart received funding from the Distilled Spirits Council.

1. Snyder LB, Milici FF, Slater M, Sun H, Strizhakova Y. Effects of alcohol advertising exposure on drinking among youth. *Arch Pediatr Adolesc Med.* 2006; 160:18-24.

### In reply

*Our study,[1] which among other results found that drinking rates were higher among youth aged 15 to 20 years in the United States living in markets with more alcohol advertising than among those living in markets with less advertising, was one of several large studies funded since 1997 to examine alcohol advertising effects over time. Despite differences in design, the 4 studies are fairly consistent in their findings. Seventh-grade alcohol advertising exposure was related to greater beer drinking in eighth grade in Los Angeles, Calif,[2] and initiating drinking by ninth grade in South Dakota.[3] The large sample from 24 markets, longitudinal design, and objective measure of advertising spending per market in addition to self-reports of advertising exposure and analysis of markets, individuals, and over time per person simultaneously are strengths of our study.*

*Drs Smart and Schultz, both of whom have received funding from the alcohol industry, have a number of concerns about the study. First, Dr Schultz's unsubstantiated claim that advertising does not directly affect consumer behavior seems to negate the value of advertising, yet it remains a vibrant industry and clients expect advertising to help sales.[4] The research literature shows that advertising is effective at least some of the time.[5]*

*Dr Smart was concerned about the lack of reference to some prior research. As cited in the article, recent studies show that alcohol advertising bans lead to a reduction in drinking over time. Econometric studies examine total sales, which are predominantly to adults, so they are less relevant to the debate about youth drinking; moreover, they do not allow for cumulative effects. The experimental literature, to which Dr Smart contributed in the 1980s, found inconsistent effects of ads on drinking in a laboratory, but experiments are weak on generalizability to the real world. Furthermore, our study found that drinking was related to ongoing patterns in alcohol advertising exposure rather than immediate or contemporaneous exposure as is tested in experiments and econometric studies. The current generation of studies has advanced from the limitations of the prior literature.*

*In answer to other concerns, sample ages are well specified in the article; trends are better examined in the simultaneous analyses than without controls; the interaction between market expenditures, time, and age is still significant when alcohol use is measured by frequency×quantity; and the impact of gradual attrition was minimized by using all the available data on each person.*

*Our study provides associational, prospective evidence regarding alcohol advertising effects on youth drinking. It is, of course, subject to the common concerns regarding nonexperimental designs; limitations are noted in the article. Our research, however, does address some key limitations of prior research—notably, the use of market-level data to validate findings from individual self-reports of alcohol exposure in a multilevel model, test of cumulative exposure, and a national sample—and in so doing provides substantial additional support to the body of research suggesting that alcohol advertising does influence adolescent alcohol use behavior.*

*Leslie B. Snyder, PhD*
*Michael Slater, PhD*

**Correspondence:** Dr Snyder, Department of Communication Sciences, University of Connecticut, Storrs, CT 06269-1085 (leslie.snyder@uconn.edu).

1. Snyder LB, Milici FF, Slater M, Sun H, Strizhakova Y. Effects of alcohol advertising exposure on drinking among youth. *Arch Pediatr Adolesc Med.* 2006; 160:18-24.
2. Stacy AW, Zogg JB, Unger JB, Dent CW. Exposure to televised alcohol ads and subsequent adolescent alcohol use. *Am J Health Behav.* 2004;28:498-509.
3. Ellickson PL, Collins RL, Hambarsoomians K, McCaffrey DF. Does alcohol advertising promote adolescent drinking? Results from a longitudinal assessment. *Addiction.* 2005;100:235-246.
4. Shimp T. *Advertising, Promotion, and Supplemental Aspects of Integrated Marketing Communications.* 6th ed. Orlando, Fla: Harcourt; 2000.
5. Kim P. Does advertising work: a review of the evidence. *J Consum Mark.* 1992; 9:5-21.

### Announcement

**Topic Collections**. The *Archives* offers collections of articles in specific topic areas to make it easier for physicians to find the most recent publications in a field. These are available by subspecialty, study type, disease, or problem. In addition, you can sign up to receive a Collection E-Mail Alert when new articles on specific topics are published. Go to http://archpedi.ama-assn.org/collections to see these collections of articles.

SECTION EDITOR: ABRAHAM BERGMAN, MD

## The Little Elephant With the Big Earache

*by Charlotte Cowan, MD, 30 pp, $17.95, ISBN 0-9753516-0-5, Concord, Mass, The Hippocratic Press, 2004.*

Overuse of antibiotics for acute otitis media, one of the most common illnesses of preschool-aged children, contributes to antimicrobial resistance.[1] Physicians cite parental expectations as one of the factors that influences overprescription of antibiotics to children. Multifaceted campaigns that include printed materials such as pamphlets and posters have been helpful in directing messages on appropriate use of antibiotics to parents. For example, public health officials in Tennessee documented an 11% reduction in antibiotic prescriptions to children that was attributed to a community-wide intervention in which "Antibiotics and Your Child," a Centers for Disease Control and Prevention pamphlet, was mailed to parents.[2]

While direct messages are useful for public health campaigns, less direct but engaging stories could also be used to promote positive values and reduce parental expectations for antibiotics. Children's books have been an attractive means for conveying values through generations, and the shared experience of reading books aloud has the potential to communicate to both children and their parents.[3] *The Little Elephant With the Big Earache*, a book by Charlotte Cowan for children aged 2 to 7 years, is an example of a new tool that could be used in combination with other appropriate antibiotics use interventions directed to parents. In the book, when the little elephant Eddie develops an earache the night before his birthday, his mother gives him an over-the-counter medication and comforts him until he falls asleep (**Figure**). The next morning, the mother arranges for Eddie to be seen by the pediatrician, Dr Hippo, who diagnoses the child's illness as an early ear infection. But instead of prescribing antibiotics, Dr Hippo asks the mother to watch Eddie and return if his condition either fails to improve or worsens.

Many parents and their preschool-aged children, especially those who have experienced the pain of an ear infection, would identify with the story of Eddie and his mother. The colorful scenes and playful imagery of an earache in an animal known for its big ears are appealing. However, the book's depiction of a parent who readily accepts the pediatrician's decision to monitor a child without reflexively initiating antibiotics suggests a shift in a cultural norm where antibiotics are often expected. Eddie's mother is believable because she comes across as an experienced parent who does not panic but instead gives pain medication and comforts her child overnight until the child is evaluated by a pediatrician the next morning. Thus, the author advocates adherence to official guidelines using a story that can engage the audience, perhaps more than didactics.

The subtle message is both the book's strength and weakness. Without being aware of the subject, it is unlikely that after reading this book a parent would understand its implication regarding appropriate antibiotics use. This limitation is partially addressed in the accompanying parent's guide *Ear Infections Made Easy: Answers to Common Questions.* This laminated insert covers official guidelines concerning diagnosis and management of acute otitis media,[4] as well as appropriate use of

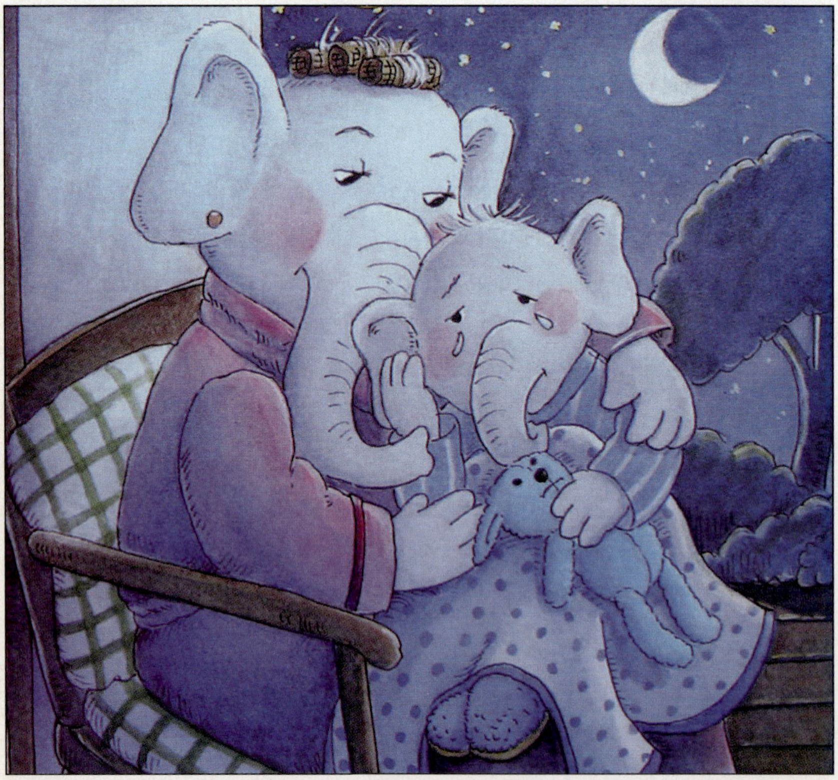

**Figure.** Eddie, the little elephant with the big earache, is comforted by his mother at night. Illustration by Elaine Garvin, 2004.

the telephone, the emergency department, and the pediatrician's office. After engaging the audience in a sympathetic story, the supplemental didactics clarify what might otherwise be too subtle a message. In this guide, parents will find answers to common questions such as "What do I do if I think my child has an ear infection?" and "When should I take my child to the doctor?" As a pediatrician at Massachusetts General Hospital (Boston) and Harvard Medical School (Boston), Dr Cowan has concisely responded to the most common questions for parents.

For this reviewer, *The Little Elephant With the Big Earache* is not a quick solution to parental expectations for antibiotics. Instead, making copies of the book available in pediatricians' offices, libraries, and parents' groups can complement existing appropriate antibiotics-use interventions. A separate facilitator's guide, *A Trunkful of Tips,* is also available for use by group leaders or health educators. Public health officials working on appropriate antibiotics use in several states are considering this book as a tool to educate parents, and at least one state, Wyoming, has provided a copy for every pediatrician's office. In summary, *The Little Elephant With the Big Earache* is a well-written story that could serve as one way to promote appropriate antibiotics use among parents who read to their children. This secondary objective can be achieved without compromising the book's primary purpose: to educate and entertain children.

*Nkuchia M. M'ikanatha, DrPH, MPH*

**Correspondence:** Dr M'ikanatha, Division of Infectious Disease Epidemiology, Pennsylvania Department of Health, Health and Welfare Building, PO Box 90, Harrisburg, PA 17108 (nmikanatha@state.pa.us).
**Acknowledgment:** I wish to acknowledge David and Dawning Welliver for sharing a parent and child perspective of *The Little Elephant With the Big Earache.*

1. Dowell SF, March SM, Phillips WR, Gerber MA, Schwartz B. Otitis media—principles of judicious use of antimicrobial agents. *Pediatrics.* 1998; 101(suppl):165-171.
2. Perz JF, Craig AS, Coffey CS, et al. Changes in antibiotic prescribing for children after a community-wide campaign. *JAMA.* 2002;287:3103-3109.
3. Spitz EH. *Inside Picture Books.* New Haven, Conn: Yale University Press; 1999.
4. Diagnosis and management of acute otitis media [American Academy of Family Physicians Web site]. Available at: http://www.aafp.org/x26481.xml.

**Announcement**

**Trial Registration Required.** In concert with the International Committee of Medical Journal Editors (ICMJE), *Archives of Pediatrics and Adolescent Medicine* will require, as a condition of consideration for publication, registration of all trials in a public trials registry (such as http://ClinicalTrials.gov). Trials must be registered at or before the onset of patient enrollment. This policy applies to any clinical trial starting enrollment after July 1, 2005. For trials that began enrollment before this date, registration will be required by September 13, 2005, before considering the trial for publication. The trial registration number should be supplied at the time of submission.

For details about this new policy, and for information on how the ICMJE defines a clinical trial, see the editorials by DeAngelis et al in the September 8, 2004 (2004;292:1363-1364) and June 15, 2005 (2005;293: 2927-2929) issues of *JAMA*. Also see the Instructions to Authors on our Web site: www.archpediatrics.com.

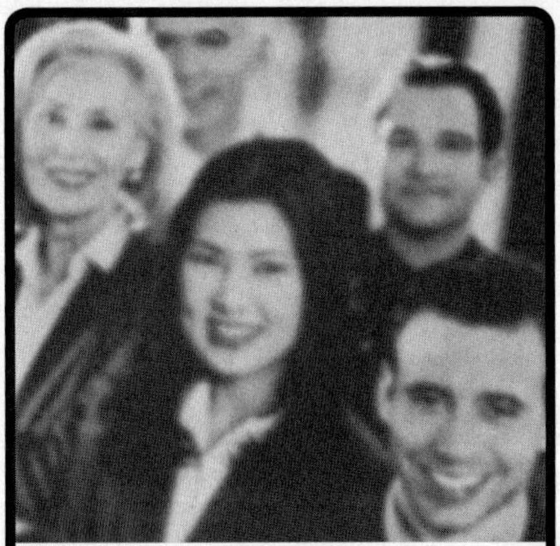

*Move* Forward.
*Move* Smart.
*Move* Now.

**JAMACAREERNET**
*NetWorking for Physicians*

*It's Your Move.*

**Fondation Jérôme LEJEUNE**
pour la recherche sur les maladies génétiques de l'intelligence

The main target of the Fondation Jerome Lejeune, a state-recommended foundation, is research into Intelligence Disability.

"Searching, Healing, Defending"

**GRANTS**

The Fondation Jerome Lejeune invites interested teams and researchers to submit projects to its Scientific Committee, on fundamental or applied research programs (genetics, molecular biology, neurosciences, adult or cord blood stem cells, clinics, therapeutics, behaviour, etc.) aimed at leading to the discovery of treatments for genetic intelligence diseases, of which includes the trisomy 21 (Down syndrome), in order to improve the intelligence disease symptoms. A part of these call for tender grants will be dedicated to research on the Smith-Magenis syndrome. The Fondation also considers support for congresses organization.

**PRACTICAL INFORMATION**

Please fill in the "on-line" application form on www.fondationlejeune.org
or e-mail: conseilscientifique@fondationlejeune.org
(validation deadline: 22/09/2006):

Conseil Scientifique - Fondation Jerome Lejeune
48, rue Galande - 75005 PARIS - France
Tel: +33 1 5310 0830 Fax: +33 1 5310 8598

## PRACTICE FOR SALE

PRACTICE FOR SALE - WELL ESTABISHED PEDIATRICS AND ALLERGY practice for sale. Located 15 miles south of Boston close to major teaching hospitals. Owner will introduce. Call: 781-784-8403.

**BCHC** Brownsville Community Health Center

Brownsville, TX: PEDIATRICIAN needed for a community health center starting August 1, 2006. Opportunity to "make a difference". Competitive compensation, benefits and incentives. Fax CV to Medical Director (956) 546-2056, or E-mail: **hlimperial@hotmail.com**

## ACKNOWLEDGMENT SERVICE

Acknowledgments in confirmation of advertising orders are sent each week. Upon receipt, please verify that your ad will be running under the appropriate heading and that your scheduling is correct. Changes to the schedule, cancellations or corrections must be communicated in writing by fax, e-mail, or regular mail prior to the published closing date of the scheduled issue.

***Osler Institute 69th to 72nd***

# Ped Board Reviews

***approved for AMA/PRA category 1 credit***

- 6-day seminar with outstanding faculty
- Comprehensive lecture-note syllabus

August 14-19 – San Francisco
September 25-30 – Philadelphia
October 16-21, 2006 – Dallas
Spring 2007 – To be announced

***New – Best of Pediatrics Audio***

**Call Today: (800) 356-7537**
**www.osler.org/b68c**

## JOURNAL ADVERTISER INDEX


**ASTRAZENECA**
http://www.astrazeneca.com
Nexium ........ 800A-B
**CLASSIFIED ADVERTISING** ........ 863
http://www.amapublications.com
**GLAXOSMITHKLINE**
Boostrix ........ 767-768, 851-852
Havrix ........ 803-804, COVER 3-4
Pediarix ........ 823-824, COVER 2-761
**MERCK & COMPANY**
Gardasil ........ 792A-B
Rotateq ........ 816A-E


*Demographic and "Mini" inserts and/or ROB ad pages

While every precaution is taken to ensure accuracy, we cannot guarantee against the possibility of an occasional change or omission in the preparation of this index.

ARCHIVES OF PEDIATRICS & ADOLESCENT MEDICINE

# CONTACT INFORMATION

## EDITORIAL OFFICE

**Editorial Office Information:** *Archives of Pediatrics & Adolescent Medicine*, Department of Pediatrics, Child Health Institute, University of Washington, 6200 NE 74th St, Suite 210, Seattle, WA 98115-8160, USA; phone: (206) 685-3573; fax: (206) 685-3572; e-mail: archpediatrics@jama-archives.org.

**Electronic Submission:** Manuscripts should be submitted via our online manuscript submission and review system (http://manuscripts.archpediatrics.com). Manuscripts submitted through our online system should not also be submitted by mail or fax. Signed authorship forms should be sent by regular mail or fax with the assigned manuscript number noted on each page in the upper right-hand corner. See the Instructions for Authors (www.archpediatrics.com) for more details.

## CONSORTIUM OF *JAMA* & *ARCHIVES* JOURNALS

The *Archives of Pediatrics & Adolescent Medicine* is a member of the consortium of AMA journals listed below.

- The Journal of the American Medical Association (JAMA)
- Archives of Dermatology
- Archives of Facial Plastic Surgery
- Archives of General Psychiatry
- Archives of Internal Medicine
- Archives of Neurology
- Archives of Ophthalmology
- Archives of Otolaryngology–Head & Neck Surgery
- Archives of Pediatrics & Adolescent Medicine
- Archives of Surgery

## *JAMA/ARCHIVES* MEDIA RELATIONS

Jann Ingmire; phone: (312) 464-5262; e-mail: mediarelations@jama-archives.org.

## *ARCHIVES OF PEDIATRICS* ONLINE

*Archives of Pediatrics & Adolescent Medicine* is available online at www.archpediatrics.com.

## *JAMA/ARCHIVES* REPRINTS

**Author/Educational Institution Reprints:** Anna Goins at (312) 464-2477; fax: (312) 464-5843; e-mail: anna.goins@ama-assn.org. Minimum order: 100 reprints.

**Commercial Reprints:** Phone: (312) 464-0776; fax: (312) 464-0708; e-mail: reprints@ama-assn.org. Minimum order: 100 reprints.

## PERMISSIONS

Information about obtaining permission to republish, reprint, or adapt material published in *Archives of Pediatrics & Adolescent Medicine* is available from Rhonda Bailey Brown; phone: (312) 464-2513; fax: (312) 464-5843; e-mail: permissions@ama-assn.org.

## DOCUMENT DELIVERY

Copies of individual articles are available online at www.archpediatrics.com and from the following: Infotrieve, phone: (800) 422-4633; fax: (310) 208-5971; URL: www.infotrieve.com; e-mail: orders@infotrieve.com; Institute for Scientific Information (ISI), phone: (800) 603-4367; fax: (856) 787-1679; URL: http://www.isidoc.com; e-mail: service@isidoc.com.

## ADVERTISING

Information about advertising is available from the following sales representatives and online at www.archpediatrics.com.

**Account Manager:** Tim Melroy (nationally); phone: (973) 263-9191 ext 213.

**Manager, Marketing Services:** Nancy Bell; phone: (973) 263-9191 ext 216.

**Advertising Office:** 119 Cherry Hill Rd, Suite 330, Parsippany, NJ 07054-1114; phone: (973) 263-9191.

**Classified Advertising:** Thalia Moss, Shana Brown, Kim Jenkins, Sophie Levandoski, 515 N State St, Chicago, IL 60610; phone: (800) 262-2260; e-mail: classifieds@jama-archives.org.

## ADVERTISING PRINCIPLES

Advertisements in this issue have been reviewed to comply with the principles governing advertising in AMA publications. A copy of these principles is available on request and online at www.archpediatrics.com. The appearance of advertising in AMA publications is not an AMA guarantee or endorsement of the product or the claims made for the product by the manufacturer.

## ADDRESS CHANGES

Send all address changes to *Archives of Pediatrics & Adolescent Medicine*, c/o the AMA Unified Service Center, American Medical Association, 515 N State St, Chicago, IL 60610. Notification of address changes must be made at least 6 weeks in advance; include both old and new addresses and a recent mailing label if sending via mail.

## SUBSCRIPTION RATES AND SERVICE

Subscription rates are shown in the table below. For service in the US and Americas, inquiries on pricing, address changes, missing issues, subscription billing, subscription renewal, and back issues, contact the AMA Unified Service Center, 24 hours a day, 7 days a week.

**AMA members:** phone: (800) 262-3211; e-mail: msc@ama-assn.org. **Other physicians and nonphysician customers, including subscription agents:** phone: (800) 262-2350 or (312) 670-7827; fax: (312) 464-5831; e-mail: ama-subs@ama-assn.org. **Inquiries:** Unified Service Center, American Medical Association, PO Box 10946, Chicago, IL 60610-0946. For subscribers with mailing addresses outside the United States & Americas: Contact *JAMA* & *Archives* Journals, c/o EMD GmbH, Birkenstr.67, 10559 Berlin, Germany. Phone: +49 (30) 33099828; fax: +49 (30) 33099829; e-mail: ama@emd-germany.de.

**Annual Subscription Rates**

| | United States | Americas | UK | Rest of World |
|---|---|---|---|---|
| INDIVIDUAL | | | | |
| Print and Online | $185 | $240 | £165 | €250 |
| INSTITUTION | | | | |
| Print and Online | $400 | $485 | £315 | €470 |

In Canada, US rate plus GST. Rates for residents and medical students available at pubs.ama-assn.org, or from the AMA Unified Service Center.

The ARCHIVES OF PEDIATRICS & ADOLESCENT MEDICINE (ISSN 01072–4710) is published monthly by the American Medical Association, 515 N State St, Chicago, IL 60610–0946, and is an official publication of the Association. The ARCHIVES OF PEDIATRICS & ADOLESCENT MEDICINE reaches more than 30 900 readers in over 83 countries each month. Periodicals postage paid at Chicago, Ill, and at additional mailing offices. GST registration number 12622 5556 RT. Canada Post International Publications Mail (Canadian Distribution) Sales Agreement No. 318728. POSTMASTER, send all address changes to *Archives of Pediatrics & Adolescent Medicine,* c/o the AMA Unified Service Center, American Medical Association, 515 N State St, Chicago, IL 60610. Printed in the USA.

# HAVRIX®
# (Hepatitis A Vaccine, Inactivated)

The following is a brief summary only; see full prescribing information for complete product information.

**INDICATIONS AND USAGE:** HAVRIX is indicated for active immunization of persons ≥12 months of age against disease caused by hepatitis A virus (HAV). Primary immunization should be administered at least 2 weeks prior to expected exposure to HAV. When passive protection against hepatitis A is required either following exposure to hepatitis A virus or in persons requiring both immediate and long-term protection, HAVRIX may be administered concomitantly with immune globulin (IG) with different syringes and at different injection sites. Duration of immunity following a complete vaccination schedule has not been established.

**CONTRAINDICATIONS:** Hypersensitivity to any component of the vaccine, including neomycin, is a contraindication (see DESCRIPTION in full prescribing information). This vaccine is contraindicated in patients with previous hypersensitivity to any hepatitis A-containing vaccine.

**WARNINGS:** There have been rare reports of anaphylaxis/anaphylactoid reactions following commercial use of the vaccine. The tip cap and the rubber plunger of the needleless prefilled syringes contain dry natural latex rubber that may cause allergic reactions in latex sensitive individuals. The vial stopper is latex-free. Hepatitis A has a relatively long incubation period. Hepatitis A vaccine may not prevent hepatitis A infection in those who have an unrecognized hepatitis A infection at the time of vaccination. Additionally, it may not prevent infection in those who do not achieve protective antibody titers (although the lowest titer needed to confer protection has not been determined).

**PRECAUTIONS: General:** Prior to immunization with HAVRIX, the patient's current health status and medical history should be reviewed. The physician should review the patient's immunization history for possible vaccine sensitivity, previous vaccination-related adverse reactions and occurrence of any adverse–event-related symptoms and/or signs, in order to determine the existence of any contraindication to immunization with HAVRIX and to allow an assessment of benefits and risks. Appropriate medical treatment and supervision should be readily available for immediate use in case of a rare anaphylactic reaction following the administration of the vaccine. Epinephrine injection (1:1,000) and other appropriate agents used for the control of immediate allergic reactions must be immediately available. A separate, sterile syringe and needle or a sterile disposable unit should be used for each patient to prevent the transmission of other infectious agents from person to person. Needles should be disposed of properly and should not be recapped. As with any vaccine, if administered to immunosuppressed persons, including those receiving immunosuppressive therapy, the expected immune response may not be obtained. **Drug Interactions:** HAVRIX may be given concurrently with Hib conjugate vaccines in children 15 to 18 months of age (see CLINICAL PHARMACOLOGY in full prescribing information and ADVERSE REACTIONS). The safety of HAVRIX given concomitantly with INFANRIX has been evaluated (see ADVERSE REACTIONS). Insufficient data are available to assess the immune response of a fourth dose of DTaP vaccine when administered with HAVRIX. There are limited data to assess the concomitant use of HAVRIX with other vaccines. (See Immune Response to Concomitantly Administered Vaccines in full prescribing information.)

**Carcinogenesis, Mutagenesis, Impairment of Fertility:** HAVRIX has not been evaluated for its carcinogenic potential, mutagenic potential, or potential for impairment of fertility. **Pregnancy:** Pregnancy Category C. Animal reproduction studies have not been conducted with HAVRIX. It is also not known whether HAVRIX can cause fetal harm when administered to a pregnant woman or can affect reproduction capacity. Give HAVRIX to a pregnant woman only if clearly needed. **Nursing Mothers:** It is not known whether HAVRIX is excreted in human milk. Because many drugs are excreted in human milk, use caution when administering HAVRIX to a nursing woman. **Pediatric Use:** The safety and effectiveness of HAVRIX have been evaluated in 20,436 subjects 1 year to 18 years of age. (See CLINICAL PHARMACOLOGY and DOSAGE AND ADMINISTRATION in full prescribing information.) The safety and effectiveness of HAVRIX have not been established in subjects less than 12 months of age. **Geriatric Use:** Clinical studies of HAVRIX did not include sufficient numbers of subjects 65 years of age and older to determine whether they respond differently from younger subjects. Other reported clinical experience has not identified differences in overall safety between these subjects and younger adult subjects.

**ADVERSE REACTIONS:** As with all pharmaceuticals, however, it is possible that expanded commercial use of the vaccine could reveal rare adverse events. The adverse events most frequently reported by volunteers in clinical trials were injection-site soreness (56% of adults; 21% of children); headache (14% of adults; less than 9% of children). Other solicited and unsolicited events are listed below:

**Incidence 1% to 10% of Injections:** ***Local Reactions at Injection Site:*** Induration, redness, swelling; ***Body as a Whole:*** Fatigue, fever (>37.5°C), malaise; ***Gastrointestinal:*** Anorexia, nausea.

**Incidence <1% of Injections:** ***Local Reaction at Injection Site:*** Hematoma; ***Dermatologic:*** Pruritus, rash, urticaria; ***Respiratory:*** Pharyngitis, other upper respiratory tract infections; ***Gastrointestinal:*** Abdominal pain, diarrhea, dysgeusia, vomiting; ***Musculoskeletal:*** Arthralgia, elevation of creatine phosphokinase, myalgia; ***Hematologic:*** Lymphadenopathy; ***Central Nervous System:*** Hypertonic episode, insomnia, photophobia, vertigo.

**Additional safety data:** Safety data were obtained from 2 additional sources in which large populations were vaccinated. In an outbreak setting in which 4,930 individuals were immunized with a single dose of either 720 EL.U. or 1440 EL.U. of HAVRIX, the vaccine was well tolerated and no serious adverse events due to vaccination were reported. Overall, less than 10% of vaccinees reported solicited general adverse events following the vaccine. The most common solicited local adverse event was pain at the injection site, reported in 22.3% of subjects at 24 hours and decreasing to 2.4% by 72 hours.

In a field efficacy trial, 19,037 children received the 360 EL.U. dose of HAVRIX. The most commonly reported adverse events were injection-site pain (9.5%) and tenderness (8.1%), reported following first doses of HAVRIX. Other adverse events were infrequent and comparable to the control vaccine ENGERIX-B® [Hepatitis B Vaccine (Recombinant)].

In subjects with chronic liver disease, HAVRIX was safe and well tolerated. Local injection site reactions were similar among all 4 groups, and no serious adverse reactions attributed to the vaccine were reported in subjects with chronic liver disease.

***Safety Data for HAVRIX 720 EL.U./0.5 mL Beginning at 11 Months of Age:*** In the multicenter study described under CLINICAL PHARMACOLOGY in full prescribing information, parents/guardians recorded local and general symptoms on diary cards for 4 days (Days 0 to 3) after vaccination. In the 3 groups of children who received HAVRIX alone, safety data were available for 723 children who received 1,396 documented doses of HAVRIX. Additional safety data were available for 181 children who received HAVRIX coadministered with INFANRIX and Hib conjugate vaccine. Most adverse events were mild and transient. The frequencies of solicited local and systemic reactions following receipt of HAVRIX were monitored during the 4-day observation period.

The following rates of solicited adverse events in children who received their first dose of HAVRIX alone at between 11 and 25 months of age were observed. Among local reactions: pain was reported in 15-21% of subjects, redness in 16-21%, swelling in 8% of subjects. Among general reactions, irritability was reported in 24-36% of subjects, loss of appetite in 16-19% of subjects, drowsiness in 15-17% of subjects and fever >39.5°C in ≤2% of subjects. Following the booster dose of HAVRIX, among local reactions: pain was reported in 16-21% of subjects, redness in 17-22%, swelling in 8-10% of subjects. Following the booster dose of HAVRIX, among general reactions, irritability was reported in 19-29% of subjects, loss of appetite in 14-18% of subjects, drowsiness in 13-16% of subjects and fever >39.5°C in ≤1% of subjects.

Drowsiness and loss of appetite occurred at statistically significantly higher rates in subjects 15 to 18 months of age who received Hib conjugate vaccine (PRP-T) and INFANRIX concomitantly with HAVRIX as compared to subjects 15 to 18 months of age who received Hib conjugate vaccine (PRP-T) and INFANRIX (drowsiness 34% and 22% and loss of appetite 29% and 19%, respectively). With the exception of fever (>39.5°C), the solicited general symptoms occurred at statistically significantly higher rates in subjects 15 to 18 months of age who received Hib conjugate vaccine (PRP-T) and INFANRIX concomitantly with HAVRIX as compared to subjects 15 to 18 months of age who received HAVRIX alone (irritability 46% and 30%, drowsiness 34% and 17%, and loss of appetite 29% and 17%, respectively).

A febrile seizure was reported in an 18-month old subject two days after receiving the first dose of HAVRIX. Other serious adverse events reported during the course of this study included a single case each of hepatitis ~5 months post dose 1, insulin-dependent diabetes ~4 months post dose 1, and Kawasaki's disease ~3 1/2 months post dose 1. The association of these events with vaccination is unknown.

**Postmarketing Reports:** Rare voluntary reports of adverse events in people receiving HAVRIX since market introduction include the following: ***Local:*** Localized edema; ***Body as a Whole:*** Anaphylaxis/anaphylactoid reactions, somnolence; ***Cardiovascular:*** Syncope; ***Hepatobiliary:*** Jaundice, hepatitis; ***Dermatologic:*** Erythema multiforme, hyperhydrosis, angioedema; ***Respiratory:*** Dyspnea; ***Hematologic:*** Lymphadenopathy, thrombocytopenia; ***Central Nervous System:*** Convulsions, encephalopathy, dizziness, neuropathy, myelitis, paresthesia, Guillain-Barré syndrome, multiple sclerosis; ***Other:*** Congenital abnormality.

The US Department of Health and Human Services has established the Vaccine Adverse Events Reporting System (VAERS) to accept reports of suspected adverse events after the administration of any vaccine, including, but not limited to, the reporting of events required by the National Childhood Vaccine Injury Act of 1986. The toll-free number for VAERS forms and information is 1-800-822-7967. Reporting forms may also be obtained at the VAERS website at www.vaers.org.

Manufactured by **GlaxoSmithKline Biologicals**, Rixensart, Belgium

Distributed by **GlaxoSmithKline**, Research Triangle Park, NC 27709



BRS-HA:L20

**References: 1.** Centers for Disease Control and Prevention. Recommended childhood and adolescent immunization schedule—United States, 2006. *MMWR.* 2006;54(51&52):Q1–Q4. **2.** Bell BP, Shapiro CN. Hepatitis A virus. In: Long SS, Pickering LK, Prober CG, eds. *Principles and Practice of Pediatric Infectious Diseases.* 2nd ed. Philadelphia, Pa: Churchill Livingstone; 2003:1188–1192. **3.** Armstrong GL, Bell BP. Hepatitis A virus infection in the United States: model-based estimates and implication for childhood immunizations. *Pediatrics.* 2002;109:839–845.

 Printed in USA. HAP283R0 February 2006

# ARCHIVES OF PEDIATRICS & ADOLESCENT MEDICINE

WWW.ARCHPEDIATRICS.COM

SEPTEMBER 2006


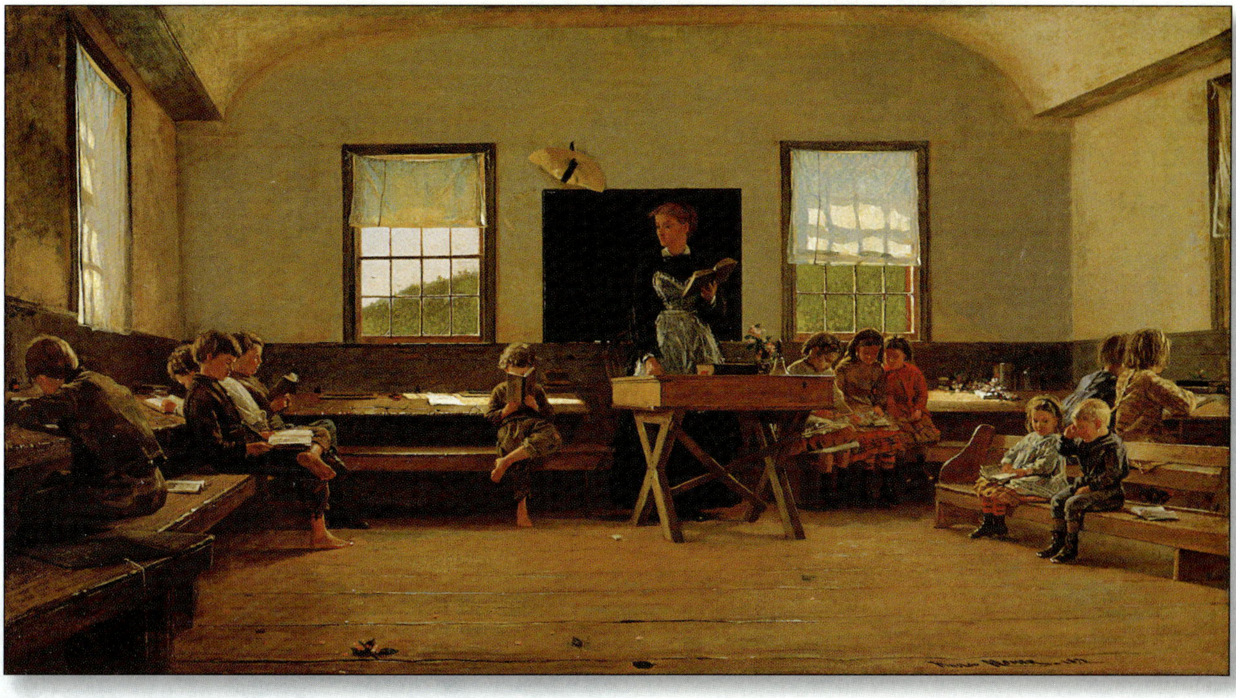

Winslow Homer (1836-1910), American, *The Country School*, 1871. See page 875.

ARCHIVES EXPRESS LONG-TERM EFFECTS OF INTERVENTIONS FOR METHAMPHETAMINE USE

EFFECT OF OPEN ACCESS SCHEDULING FOR INFANT WELL-CHILD CARE VISITS

A SYSTEMATIC REVIEW OF DIETETIC INTERVENTIONS IN CHILD OBESITY

CHILDREN TREATED AT AN EXPEDITIONARY MILITARY HOSPITAL IN IRAQ


COMPLETE TABLE OF CONTENTS ON PAGE 867





JAMA & ARCHIVES JOURNALS

American Medical Association

**References: 1.** Centers for Disease Control and Prevention. Pertussis Surveillance Report—2004 (final data). Issued 8/12/05. **2.** Centers for Disease Control and Prevention. *Epidemiology and Prevention of Vaccine-Preventable Diseases*. Reported Cases and Deaths from Vaccine Preventable Diseases, United States, 1950-2003. Available at http://www.cdc.gov/nip/publications/pink/appendices/G/cases&deaths.pdf. Accessed May 10, 2006. **3.** Centers for Disease Control and Prevention. *Epidemiology and Prevention of Vaccine-Preventable Diseases*. Atkinson W, Hamborsky J, McIntyre L, Wolfe S, eds. 9th ed. Washington, DC: Public Health Foundation;2006: 84. **4.** PEDIARIX Prescribing Information.

**PEDIARIX® [Diphtheria and Tetanus Toxoids and Acellular Pertussis Adsorbed, Hepatitis B (Recombinant) and Inactivated Poliovirus Vaccine Combined]**

The following is a brief summary only; see full prescribing information for complete product information.

**CONTRAINDICATIONS:** Hypersensitivity to any component of the vaccine, including yeast, neomycin, and polymyxin B, is a contraindication (see DESCRIPTION in complete prescribing information). Do not use PEDIARIX after a serious allergic reaction (e.g., anaphylaxis) temporally associated with a previous dose of this vaccine or with any components of this vaccine. Because of the uncertainty as to which component of the vaccine might be responsible, do not give further vaccination with any of these components; or, refer such individuals to an allergist for evaluation. The following events are contraindications to administration of PEDIARIX: encephalopathy (e.g., coma, decreased level of consciousness, prolonged seizures) within 7 days of administration of a previous dose of a pertussis-containing vaccine that is not attributable to another identifiable cause; progressive neurologic disorder, including infantile spasms, uncontrolled epilepsy, or progressive encephalopathy. Do not vaccinate individuals with these conditions until a treatment regimen has been established and the condition has stabilized.

**WARNINGS:** Administration of PEDIARIX is associated with higher rates of fever relative to separately administered vaccines. In a safety study that evaluated medically attended fever after PEDIARIX or separately administered vaccines when coadministered with 7-valent pneumococcal and Hib conjugate vaccines, infants who received PEDIARIX had a higher rate of medical encounters for fever within the first 4 days following the first vaccination. In some infants, these encounters included the performance of diagnostic studies to evaluate other causes of fever (see ADVERSE REACTIONS). The tip cap and the rubber plunger of the needleless prefilled syringes contain dry natural latex rubber that may cause allergic reactions in latex sensitive individuals. The vial stopper is latex-free. If any of the following events occur in temporal relation to receipt of DTwP or a vaccine containing an acellular pertussis component, consider carefully whether to give any pertussis vaccine, including PEDIARIX: temperature of ≥40.5°C (105°F) within 48 hours not due to another identifiable cause; collapse or shock-like state (hypotonic-hyporesponsive episode) within 48 hours; persistent, inconsolable crying lasting ≥3 hours, occurring within 48 hours; seizures with or without fever occurring within 3 days. If Guillain-Barré syndrome occurs within 6 weeks of receipt of prior vaccine containing tetanus toxoid, the decision to give any tetanus toxoid-containing vaccine, including PEDIARIX, should be based on careful consideration of the potential benefits and possible risks. If tetanus toxoid is withheld, other available vaccines should be given, as indicated. The decision to administer a pertussis-containing vaccine to individuals with stable central nervous system (CNS) disorders must be made by the physician on an individual basis, with consideration of all relevant factors, and assessment of potential risks and benefits for that individual. Advise the parent or guardian of the potential increased risk involved (see PRECAUTIONS). For children at higher risk for seizures than the general population, an appropriate antipyretic may be administered at the time of vaccination and for the ensuing 24 hours according to the respective prescribing information recommended dosage to reduce the possibility of post-vaccination fever. The ACIP has published guidelines for vaccination of persons with recent or acute illness (www.cdc.gov/nip).

**PRECAUTIONS:** PEDIARIX should be given with caution in children with bleeding disorders such as hemophilia or thrombocytopenia and in children on anticoagulant therapy, with steps taken to avoid the risk of hematoma following the injection. Before the injection of any biological, the physician should take all reasonable precautions to prevent allergic or other adverse reactions. Epinephrine injection (1:1,000) and other appropriate agents used for the control of immediate allergic reactions must be immediately available should an acute anaphylactic reaction occur. Immunosuppressed individuals, including those receiving immunosuppressive therapy, may not develop the expected immune response. The ACIP has published guidelines for vaccination of persons on such therapies (www.cdc.gov/nip). **Drug Interactions:** For information regarding concomitant administration with other vaccines, refer to DOSAGE AND ADMINISTRATION in complete prescribing information. Do not mix PEDIARIX with any other vaccine in the same syringe or vial. **Carcinogenesis, Mutagenesis, Impairment of Fertility:** PEDIARIX has not been evaluated for carcinogenic or mutagenic potential, or for impairment of fertility. **Pregnancy:** Pregnancy Category C: PEDIARIX is not indicated for women of child-bearing age. Animal reproduction studies have not been conducted with PEDIARIX. It is not known whether PEDIARIX can cause fetal harm when administered to a pregnant woman or if PEDIARIX can affect reproductive capacity. **Geriatric Use:** PEDIARIX is not indicated for use in adult populations. **Pediatric Use:** Safety and effectiveness of PEDIARIX in infants younger than 6 weeks of age have not been evaluated. PEDIARIX is not recommended for persons 7 years of age or older.

**ADVERSE REACTIONS:** A total of 23,849 doses of PEDIARIX have been administered to 8,088 infants who received one or more doses as part of a 3-dose primary series during 14 clinical studies. The most common adverse reactions observed in clinical trials were local injection site reactions (pain, redness, or swelling), fever, and fussiness. In comparative studies, administration of PEDIARIX was associated with higher rates of fever relative to separately administered vaccines (see WARNINGS and ADVERSE REACTIONS Table 1). The prevalence of fever was highest on the day of vaccination and the day following vaccination. More than 96% of episodes of fever resolved within the 4-day period following vaccination (i.e., the period including the day of vaccination and the next 3 days). In the largest of the 14 studies, conducted in Germany, safety data were available for 4,666 infants who received PEDIARIX administered concomitantly at separate sites with 1 of 4 *Haemophilus influenzae* type b (Hib) vaccines at 3, 4, and 5 months of age and for 768 infants in the control group that received INFANRIX® (Diphtheria and Tetanus Toxoids and Acellular Pertussis Vaccine Adsorbed), Hib conjugate vaccine, and oral poliovirus vaccine (OPV) separately. Data on adverse events were collected by parents using standardized diary cards for 4 consecutive days following each vaccine dose (i.e., day of vaccination and the next 3 days). Infants were also monitored for unsolicited adverse events that occurred within 30 days following vaccination using diaries which were returned at subsequent visits and were supplemented by spontaneous reports and a medical history as reported by parents. More than 95% of study participants were white.

In a US study, the safety of PEDIARIX administered to 673 infants was compared to the safety of separately administered INFANRIX, ENGERIX-B® [Hepatitis B Vaccine (Recombinant)], inactivated poliovirus vaccine (IPV) in 335 infants. In both groups, infants received Hib and 7-valent pneumococcal conjugate vaccines concomitantly at separate sites. All vaccines were administered at 2, 4, and 6 months of age. The study was powered to evaluate fever >101.3° F following dose 1. Data on solicited adverse events were collected by parents using standardized diary cards for 4 consecutive days following each vaccine dose (i.e., day of vaccination and the next 3 days) and are presented in Table 1. Telephone follow-up was conducted 1 month and 6 months after the third vaccination to inquire about serious adverse events. At the 6-month follow-up, information also was collected on new onset of chronic illnesses. 638 subjects who received PEDIARIX and 313 subjects who received INFANRIX, ENGERIX-B, and IPV completed the 6-month follow-up. Among subjects in both study groups combined, 69% were white, 18% were Hispanic, 7% were black, 3% were Oriental, and 3% were of other racial/ethnic groups.

The adverse event information from clinical trials provides a basis for identifying adverse events that appear to be related to vaccine use and for approximating rates. However, because clinical trials are conducted under widely varying conditions, adverse event rates observed in the clinical trials of a vaccine cannot be directly compared to rates in the clinical trials of another vaccine, and may not reflect the rates observed in practice. As with any vaccine, there is the possibility that broad use of PEDIARIX could reveal adverse events not observed in clinical trials.

**Deaths:** In 14 clinical trials, 5 deaths were reported among 8,088 (0.06%) recipients of PEDIARIX and 1 death was reported among 2,287 (0.04%) recipients of comparator vaccines. Causes of death in the group that received PEDIARIX included 2 cases of Sudden Infant Death Syndrome (SIDS) and one case of each of the following: Convulsive disorder, congenital immunodeficiency with sepsis, and neuroblastoma. One case of SIDS was reported in the comparator group. The rate of SIDS among all recipients of PEDIARIX across the 14 trials was 0.25/1,000. The rate of SIDS observed for recipients of PEDIARIX in the German safety study was 0.2/1,000 infants (reported rate of SIDS in Germany in the latter part of the 1990s was 0.7/1,000 newborns). The reported rate of SIDS in the United States from 1990 to 1994 was 1.2/1,000 live births. By chance alone, some cases of SIDS can be expected to follow receipt of pertussis-containing vaccines.

**Serious Adverse Events:** Within 30 days following any dose of vaccine in the US safety study in which all subjects received concomitant pneumococcal and Hib conjugate vaccines, 7 serious adverse events were reported in 7 subjects (1% [7/673]) who received PEDIARIX (1 case each of pyrexia, gastroenteritis, and culture negative clinical sepsis and 4 cases of bronchiolitis) and 5 serious adverse events were reported in 4 subjects (1% [4/335]) who received INFANRIX, ENGERIX-B, and IPV (uteropelvic junction obstruction and testicular atrophy in one subject and 3 cases of bronchiolitis).

**Onset of Chronic Illnesses:** In the US safety study in which all subjects received concomitant pneumococcal and Hib conjugate vaccines, 21 subjects (3%) who received PEDIARIX and 14 subjects (4%) who received INFANRIX, ENGERIX-B, and IPV reported new onset of a chronic illness during the period from 1 to 6 months following the last dose of study vaccines. Among the chronic illnesses reported in the subjects who received PEDIARIX, there were 4 cases of asthma and 1 case each of diabetes mellitus and chronic neutropenia. There were 4 cases of asthma in subjects who received INFANRIX, ENGERIX-B, and IPV.

**Seizures:** In the German safety study over the entire study period, 6 subjects in the group that received PEDIARIX reported seizures. Two of these subjects had a febrile seizure, 1 of whom also developed afebrile seizures. The remaining 4 subjects had afebrile seizures, including 2 with infantile spasms. Two subjects reported seizures within 7 days following vaccination (1 subject had both febrile and afebrile seizures, and 1 subject had afebrile seizures), corresponding to a rate of 0.22 seizures per 1,000 doses (febrile seizures 0.07 per 1,000 doses, afebrile seizures 0.14 per 1,000 doses). No subject who received concomitant INFANRIX, Hib vaccine, and OPV reported seizures. In a separate German study that evaluated the safety of INFANRIX in 22,505 infants who received 66,867 doses of INFANRIX administered as a 3-dose primary series, the rate of seizures within 7 days of vaccination with INFANRIX was 0.13 per 1,000 doses (febrile seizures 0.0 per 1,000 doses, afebrile seizures 0.13 per 1,000 doses). Over the entire study period in the US safety study in which all subjects received concomitant pneumococcal and Hib conjugate vaccines, 4 subjects in the group that received PEDIARIX reported seizures. Three of these subjects had a febrile seizure and 1 had an afebrile seizure. Over the entire study period, 2 subjects in the group that received INFANRIX, ENGERIX-B, and IPV reported febrile seizures. There were no afebrile seizures in this group. No subject in either study group had seizures within 7 days following vaccination.

**Other Neurological Events of Interest:** No cases of hypotonic-hyporesponsiveness or encephalopathy were reported in either the German safety study or the US safety study.

**Solicited Adverse Events:** Table 1 presents data from the US safety study on solicited local and systemic adverse events within 4 days of vaccination with PEDIARIX or INFANRIX, ENGERIX-B, and IPV, administered concomitantly with Hib and 7-valent pneumococcal conjugate vaccines. In this study, medical attention (a visit to or from medical personnel) for fever within 4 days following vaccination was sought in the group who received PEDIARIX for 8 infants after the first dose (1.2%), 1 infant following the second dose (0.2%), and 5 infants following the third dose (0.8%) (Table 1). Following dose 2, medical attention for fever was sought for 2 infants (0.6%) who received separately administered vaccines (Table 1). Among infants who had a medical visit for fever within 4 days following vaccination, 9 of 14 who received PEDIARIX and 1 of 2 who received separately administered vaccines, had one or more diagnostic studies performed to evaluate the cause of fever.

**Safety of PEDIARIX after a previous dose of hepatitis B vaccine:** Limited data are available on the safety of administering PEDIARIX after a previous dose of hepatitis B vaccine. In 2 separate studies, 160 Moldovan infants and 96 US infants, respectively, received 3 doses of PEDIARIX following 1 previous dose of hepatitis B vaccine. Neither study was designed to detect significant differences in rates of adverse events associated with PEDIARIX administered after a previous dose of hepatitis B vaccine compared to PEDIARIX administered without a previous dose of hepatitis B vaccine.

**Table 1. Percentage of US Infants With Solicited Local Reactions or Systemic Adverse Events Within 4 Days of Vaccination* at 2, 4, and 6 Months of Age With PEDIARIX Administered Concomitantly With Hib Conjugate Vaccine and 7-valent Pneumococcal Conjugate Vaccine (PCV7) or With Separate Concomitant Administration of INFANRIX, ENGERIX-B, IPV, Hib Conjugate Vaccine, and PCV7 (Modified ITT cohort)**

| | PEDIARIX, Hib Vaccine, & PCV7 | | | INFANRIX, ENGERIX-B, IPV, Hib Vaccine, & PCV7 | | |
|---|---|---|---|---|---|---|
| | **Dose 1** | **Dose 2** | **Dose 3** | **Dose 1** | **Dose 2** | **Dose 3** |
| **Local[†]** | | | | | | |
| **N** | **671** | **653** | **648** | **335** | **323** | **315** |
| Pain, any | 36.1 | 36.1 | 31.2 | 31.9 | 30.0 | 29.8 |
| Pain, grade 2 or 3 | 11.5 | 10.9 | 10.6 | 9.0 | 8.7 | 8.9 |
| Pain, grade 3 | 2.4 | 2.5 | 1.7 | 2.7 | 1.5 | 1.3 |
| Redness, any | 29.9[§] | 37.2 | 40.1 | 18.2 | 32.8 | 39.0 |
| Redness, >5 mm | 6.0[§] | 9.6[§] | 12.7[§] | 1.8 | 5.9 | 7.3 |
| Redness, >20 mm | 0.9 | 1.2[§] | 2.8 | 0.3 | 0.0 | 1.9 |
| Swelling, any | 17.3[§] | 26.5[§] | 28.7 | 9.6 | 20.4 | 24.8 |
| Swelling, >5 mm | 5.8[§] | 9.6[§] | 9.3[§] | 1.8 | 5.0 | 4.1 |
| Swelling, >20 mm | 1.9 | 2.5[§] | 3.1 | 0.6 | 0.0 | 1.3 |
| **Systemic** | | | | | | |
| **N** | **667** | **644** | **645** | **333** | **321** | **311** |
| Fever[‡], ≥100.4°F | 27.9[§] | 38.8[§] | 33.5[§] | 19.8 | 30.2 | 23.8 |
| Fever[‡], >101.3°F | 7.0 | 14.1[§] | 8.8 | 4.5 | 9.7 | 5.8 |
| Fever[‡], >102.2°F | 2.2[§] | 3.6 | 3.4 | 0.3 | 3.1 | 2.3 |
| Fever[‡], >103.1°F | 0.4 | 1.4 | 1.1 | 0.0 | 0.3 | 0.3 |
| Fever[‡], M.A. | 1.2[§] | 0.2 | 0.8 | 0.0 | 0.6 | 0.0 |
| **N** | **671** | **653** | **648** | **335** | **323** | **315** |
| Drowsiness, any | 57.2 | 51.6 | 40.9 | 54.0 | 48.3 | 38.4 |
| Drowsiness, grade 2 or 3 | 15.8 | 13.8 | 11.4 | 17.6 | 12.4 | 11.1 |
| Drowsiness, grade 3 | 2.5 | 1.2 | 0.9 | 3.6 | 0.6 | 1.9 |
| Irritability/Fussiness, any | 60.5 | 64.9 | 61.1 | 61.5 | 61.6 | 56.5 |
| Irritability/Fussiness, grade 2 or 3 | 19.8 | 27.9[§] | 25.2[§] | 19.4 | 21.1 | 19.4 |
| Irritability/Fussiness, grade 3 | 3.4 | 4.4 | 3.5 | 3.9 | 3.4 | 3.2 |
| Loss of appetite, any | 30.4 | 30.6 | 26.2 | 27.8 | 26.6 | 23.8 |
| Loss of appetite, grade 2 or 3 | 6.6 | 7.8[§] | 5.9 | 5.1 | 3.4 | 5.4 |
| Loss of appetite, grade 3 | 0.7 | 0.3 | 0.2 | 0.6 | 0.3 | 0.0 |

Modified ITT cohort = all vaccinated subjects for whom safety data were available
N = number of infants for whom at least one symptom sheet was completed; for fever, numbers exclude missing temperature recordings or tympanic measurements.
M.A. = Medically attended (a visit to or from medical personnel).
Grade 2 defined as sufficiently discomforting to interfere with daily activities.
Grade 3 defined as preventing normal daily activities.
* Within 4 days of vaccination defined as day of vaccination and the next 3 days.
† Local reactions at the injection site for PEDIARIX or INFANRIX.
‡ Rectal temperatures or axillary temperatures increased by 1°C to derive equivalent rectal temperature.
§ Rate significantly higher in the group that received PEDIARIX compared to separately administered vaccines [p value < 0.05 (2-sided Fisher Exact test) or the 95% CI on the difference between groups (Separate minus PEDIARIX) does not include 0].

**Postmarketing Reports With PEDIARIX:** Worldwide voluntary reports of adverse events received for PEDIARIX since market introduction of this vaccine are listed below. This list includes serious adverse events or events which have a suspected causal connection to components of PEDIARIX or other vaccines or drugs. Because these events are reported voluntarily from a population of uncertain size, it is not always possible to reliably estimate their frequency or establish a causal relationship to vaccine exposure. *Cardiac Disorders:* Cyanosis. *Gastrointestinal Disorders:* Diarrhea, vomiting. *General Disorders and Administrative Site Conditions:* Fatigue, injection site cellulitis, injection site induration, injection site itching, injection site nodule/lump, injection site pain, injection site reactions, injection site redness, injection site swelling, injection site warmth, irritability, limb pain, limb swelling, pyrexia, Sudden Infant Death Syndrome. *Immune System Disorders:* Anaphylactic reaction, anaphylactoid reaction, hypersensitivity. *Infections and Infestations:* Upper respiratory tract infection. *Investigations:* Abnormal liver function tests. *Metabolism and Nutrition Disorders:* Anorexia. *Nervous System Disorders:* Bulging fontanelle, convulsions, depressed level of consciousness, febrile convulsion, hypotonia, hypotonic-hyporesponsive episode, lethargy, somnolence. *Psychiatric Disorders:* Crying, insomnia, irritability, nervousness, restlessness, screaming, unusual crying. *Respiratory, Thoracic and Mediastinal Disorders:* Apnea, dyspnea. *Skin and Subcutaneous Tissue Disorders:* Angioedema, erythema, rash, urticaria. *Vascular Disorders:* Pallor, petechiae.

**Postmarketing Reports With INFANRIX and/or ENGERIX-B:** Worldwide voluntary reports of adverse events received for INFANRIX and/or ENGERIX-B in children younger than 7 years of age but not already reported for PEDIARIX are listed below. This list includes serious adverse events or events which have a suspected causal connection to components of INFANRIX and/or ENGERIX-B or other vaccines or drugs. Because these events are reported voluntarily from a population of uncertain size, it is not always possible to reliably estimate their frequency or establish a causal relationship to vaccine exposure. *Blood and Lymphatic System Disorders:* Idiopathic thrombocytopenic purpura[a,b], lymphadenopathy[a], thrombocytopeni[a,b]. *Gastrointestinal Disorders:* Abdominal pain[b], intussusception[a,b], nausea[b]. *General Disorders and Administrative Site Conditions:* Asthenia[b], malaise[b]. *Hepatobiliary Disorders:* Jaundice[b]. *Immune System Disorders:* Anaphylactic shock[a], serum sickness–like disease[b]. *Musculoskeletal and Connective Tissue Disorders:* Arthralgia[b], myalgia[b]. *Nervous System Disorders:* Encephalopathy[a], headache[b]. *Skin and Subcutaneous Tissue Disorders:* Alopecia[b], erythema multiforme[b], pruritus[a,b], Stevens-Johnson syndrome[a]. [[a] Following INFANRIX; [b] Following ENGERIX-B]

**Reporting Adverse Events:** Report the occurrence following immunization of any event set forth in the Vaccine Injury Table from the National Childhood Vaccine Injury Act including: Anaphylaxis or anaphylactic shock within 7 days, encephalopathy or encephalitis within 7 days, brachial neuritis within 28 days, or an acute complication or sequelae (including death) of an illness, disability, injury, or condition referred to above, or any events that would contraindicate further doses of PEDIARIX. These events should be reported to VAERS. The VAERS toll-free number is 1-800-822-7967. Reporting forms may also be obtained at the VAERS website at www.vaers.hhs.gov.

Manufactured by **GlaxoSmithKline Biologicals**, Rixensart, Belgium, US License 1617
Distributed by **GlaxoSmithKline,** Research Triangle Park, NC 27709

Full prescribing information for PEDIARIX is available at www.GSKVaccines.com/Pediarix.

BRS-PE:L3

 Printed in USA. PED644R0 May 2006

# ARCHIVES
OF
# PEDIATRICS & ADOLESCENT MEDICINE

SEPTEMBER 2006 VOLUME 160, NUMBER 9 PAGES 865-992

## COVER ART

**Winslow Homer (1836-1910): *The Country School*, 1871** 875
*Thomas D. Koepsell, MD, MPH*

## ARTICLES

**Long-term Effects of Universal Preventive Interventions on Methamphetamine Use Among Adolescents** 876
ARCHIVES EXPRESS
*Richard L. Spoth, PhD; Scott Clair, PhD; Chungyeol Shin, PhD; Cleve Redmond, PhD*

**Televised Movie Trailers: Undermining Restrictions on Advertising Tobacco to Youth** 885
*Cheryl G. Healton, DrPH; Ella S. Watson-Stryker, BA; Jane Appleyard Allen, MA; Donna M. Vallone, PhD; Peter A. Messeri, PhD; Philip R. Graham, MBS; Anna M. Stewart, BS; M. David Dobbins, JD; Stanton A. Glantz, PhD*

**Effect of Open Access Scheduling on Missed Appointments, Immunizations, and Continuity of Care for Infant Well-Child Care Visits** 889
*Mary E. O'Connor, MD, MPH; Bethany S. Matthews, MSPH; Dexiang Gao, PhD*

**Total Body Weight and Waist Circumference Associated With Chronic Periodontitis Among Adolescents in the United States** 894
*Anne F. Reeves, MPH; Jane M. Rees, PhD, MS, RD; Melissa Schiff, MD, MPH; Philippe Hujoel, DDS, PhD*

**Nutrition and Exercise Environment Available to Outpatients, Visitors, and Staff in Children's Hospitals in Canada and the United States** 900
*Christine M. McDonald, RD; Tara Karamlou, MD; James G. Wengle, MSc; Jennifer Gibson, RD; Brian W. McCrindle, MD, MPH*

## REVIEW ARTICLE

**Measuring Effectiveness of Dietetic Interventions in Child Obesity: A Systematic Review of Randomized Trials** 906
*Clare E. Collins, PhD, BSc, Dip(Nutr&Diet), Dip(ClinEpi), AdvAPD; Janet Warren, PhD, BSc, RD; Melinda Neve, BND, APD; Penelope McCoy, BHSc(Nutr&Diet), APD; Barrie J. Stokes, BSc, MMath*

## ARTICLES

**Hispanic Concentration and the Conditional Influence of Collective Efficacy on Adolescent Childbearing** 925
*Sandra Way, PhD; Brian K. Finch, PhD; Deborah Cohen, MD, MPH*

**Obese Children and Adolescents: A Risk Group for Low Vitamin $B_{12}$ Concentration** 933
*Orit Pinhas-Hamiel, MD; Noa Doron-Panush, RD; Brian Reichman, MD; Dorit Nitzan-Kaluski, MD, MPH, RD; Shlomit Shalitin, MD; Liat Geva-Lerner, MD*

**Human Herpesvirus 8 Infection Among Adolescents in the REACH Cohort** 937
*Corey Casper, MD, MPH; Amalia S. Meier, PhD; Anna Wald, MD, MPH; Rhoda Ashley Morrow, PhD; Lawrence Corey, MD; Anna-Barbara Moscicki, MD*

**Ruling Out the Need for Antibiotics: Are We Sending the Right Message?** 945
*Rita Mangione-Smith, MD, MPH; Marc N. Elliott, PhD; Tanya Stivers, PhD; Laurie L. McDonald, MS; John Heritage, PhD*

**Randomized Controlled Trial of a Prenatal and Postnatal Lactation Consultant Intervention on Infant Health Care Use** 953
*Karen A. Bonuck, PhD; Katherine Freeman, DrPH; Michelle Trombley, MPH*

**Relationship Between the Decision to Take a Child to the Clinic for Abdominal Pain and Maternal Psychological Distress** 961
*Rona L. Levy, MSW, PhD, MPH; Shelby L. Langer, PhD; Lynn S. Walker, PhD; Lauren D. Feld; William E. Whitehead, PhD*

**Effect of Missed Opportunities on Influenza Vaccination Rates Among Children With Asthma** 966
*Kevin J. Dombkowski, DrPH, MS; Matthew M. Davis, MD, MAPP; Lisa M. Cohn, MS; Sarah J. Clark, MPH*

**Children Treated at an Expeditionary Military Hospital in Iraq** 972
*Lt Col Christopher P. Coppola, USAF, MC; Maj Brian E. Leininger, USAF, MC; Lt Col Todd E. Rasmussen, USAF, MC; Col David L. Smith, USAF, MC*

**Fetal Origin of Childhood Disease: Intrauterine Growth Restriction in Term Infants and Risk for Hypertension at 6 Years of Age** 977
*Seetha Shankaran, MD; Abhik Das, PhD; Charles R. Bauer, MD; Henrietta Bada, MD, MPH; Barry Lester, PhD; Linda Wright, MD; Rosemary Higgins, MD; Kenneth Poole, PhD*

## SPECIAL FEATURE

**Picture of the Month** 983
*Jennifer A. Jewell, MD, MS; Lorraine L. McElwain, MD; Amy S. Blake, BS*

## BOOK REVIEWS AND OTHER MEDIA

**Immunizations & Infectious Diseases: An Informed Parent's Guide** 986
*Tina Kelley, BA*

## THE PEDIATRIC FORUM

**Denial of Insurance Authorization at a Subspecialty Office as a Cause of Missed Opportunities for Influenza Vaccination in Children With Asthma** 987
*Ronald M. Ferdman, MD, MEd; Joseph A. Church, MD*

**Internet Cigarette Vendors' Lack of Compliance With a California State Law Designed to Prevent Tobacco Sales to Minors** 988
*Rebecca S. Williams, PhD; Kurt M. Ribisl, PhD; Ellen C. Feighery, MS*

## CORRECTIONS

**Omission in: *About the Cover*** 905

**Incorrect Terminology in: Effectiveness of Child Safety Seats vs Seat Belts in Reducing Risk for Death in Children in Passenger Vehicle Crashes** 952
*Michael R. Elliott, PhD; Michael J. Kallan, MS; Dennis R. Durbin, MD, MSCE; Flaura K. Winston, MD, PhD*

## REGULAR DEPARTMENTS

**This Month in *Archives of Pediatrics & Adolescent Medicine*** 874

**Announcements** 882, 888, 942, 985

**Poetry in Pediatrics** 976

**Classified Advertising** 990

**Journal Advertiser Index** 991

**Contact Information** 992

**Instructions for authors and the author and subject indexes are available on our Web site: http://www.archpediatrics.com. If you do not have access to the Web, contact Suzanne Shuey at (206) 685-3573.**

### About the Cover

Winslow Homer (1836-1910), American. *The Country School*, 1871. Oil on canvas. Photo credit: Saint Louis Art Museum, St Louis, Mo.

# ARCHIVES OF PEDIATRICS & ADOLESCENT MEDICINE


**Mission Statement:** *The Archives of Pediatrics & Adolescent Medicine* is a monthly, peer-reviewed journal for physicians and other health care professionals who contribute to the health of children and adolescents. The *Archives* provides an open forum for dialogue on a full range of clinical, scientific, advocacy, and humanistic issues relevant to the care of pediatric patients from infancy through young adulthood. The *Archives* is a vehicle for increased attention to adolescent health, the education of pediatric health care professionals, and disease prevention and health promotion. The *Archives* publishes original studies, editorials, reviews by experts, practice commentaries, case quizzes, and updates on clinical science and practice management. The Pediatric Forum provides our readers with opportunities to express their views. *Archives* incorporates *AJDC*, the oldest journal in US pediatric literature, which originated in 1911.




JAMA & ARCHIVES JOURNALS
American Medical Association

**PROFESSIONAL BRIEF SUMMARY-CONSULT PACKAGE INSERT FOR FULL PRESCRIBING INFORMATION.**
03-5435-Rev. July, 2005
(Nos. 3769, 3771, 6151)

# Omnicef® (cefdinir) capsules
# Omnicef® (cefdinir) for oral suspension

## Rx only

## INDICATIONS AND USAGE

To reduce the development of drug-resistant bacteria and maintain the effectiveness of OMNICEF and other antibacterial drugs, OMNICEF should be used only to treat or prevent infections that are proven or strongly suspected to be caused by susceptible bacteria. When culture and susceptibility information are available, they should be considered in selecting or modifying antibacterial therapy. In the absence of such data, local epidemiology and susceptibility patterns may contribute to the empiric selection of therapy.

OMNICEF (cefdinir) capsules and OMNICEF (cefdinir) for oral suspension are indicated for the treatment of patients with mild to moderate infections caused by susceptible strains of the designated microorganisms in the conditions listed below.

### Adults and Adolescents

**Community-Acquired Pneumonia** caused by *Haemophilus influenzae* (including β-lactamase producing strains), *Haemophilus parainfluenzae* (including β-lactamase producing strains), *Streptococcus pneumoniae* (penicillin-susceptible strains only), and *Moraxella catarrhalis* (including β-lactamase producing strains).

**Acute Exacerbations of Chronic Bronchitis** caused by *Haemophilus influenzae* (including β-lactamase producing strains), *Haemophilus parainfluenzae* (including β-lactamase producing strains), *Streptococcus pneumoniae* (penicillin-susceptible strains only), and *Moraxella catarrhalis* (including β-lactamase producing strains).

**Acute Maxillary Sinusitis** caused by *Haemophilus influenzae* (including β-lactamase producing strains), *Streptococcus pneumoniae* (penicillin-susceptible strains only), and *Moraxella catarrhalis* (including β-lactamase producing strains).

**NOTE:** For information on use in pediatric patients, see **Pediatric Use** and **DOSAGE AND ADMINISTRATION**.

**Pharyngitis/Tonsillitis** caused by *Streptococcus pyogenes*.

**NOTE:** Cefdinir is effective in the eradication of *S. pyogenes* from the oropharynx. Cefdinir has not, however, been studied for the prevention of rheumatic fever following *S. pyogenes* pharyngitis/tonsillitis. Only intramuscular penicillin has been demonstrated to be effective for the prevention of rheumatic fever.

**Uncomplicated Skin and Skin Structure Infections** caused by *Staphylococcus aureus* (including β-lactamase producing strains) and *Streptococcus pyogenes*.

### Pediatric Patients

**Acute Bacterial Otitis Media** caused by *Haemophilus influenzae* (including β-lactamase producing strains), *Streptococcus pneumoniae* (penicillin-susceptible strains only), and *Moraxella catarrhalis* (including β-lactamase producing strains).

**Pharyngitis/Tonsillitis** caused by *Streptococcus pyogenes*.

**NOTE:** Cefdinir is effective in the eradication of *S. pyogenes* from the oropharynx. Cefdinir has not, however, been studied for the prevention of rheumatic fever following *S. pyogenes* pharyngitis/tonsillitis. Only intramuscular penicillin has been demonstrated to be effective for the prevention of rheumatic fever.

**Uncomplicated Skin and Skin Structure Infections** caused by *Staphylococcus aureus* (including β-lactamase producing strains) and *Streptococcus pyogenes*.

## CONTRAINDICATIONS

OMNICEF (cefdinir) is contraindicated in patients with known allergy to the cephalosporin class of antibiotics.

## WARNINGS

**BEFORE THERAPY WITH OMNICEF (CEFDINIR) IS INSTITUTED, CAREFUL INQUIRY SHOULD BE MADE TO DETERMINE WHETHER THE PATIENT HAS HAD PREVIOUS HYPERSENSITIVITY REACTIONS TO CEFDINIR, OTHER CEPHALOSPORINS, PENICILLINS, OR OTHER DRUGS. IF CEFDINIR IS TO BE GIVEN TO PENICILLIN-SENSITIVE PATIENTS, CAUTION SHOULD BE EXERCISED BECAUSE CROSS-HYPERSENSITIVITY AMONG β-LACTAM ANTIBIOTICS HAS BEEN CLEARLY DOCUMENTED AND MAY OCCUR IN UP TO 10% OF PATIENTS WITH A HISTORY OF PENICILLIN ALLERGY. IF AN ALLERGIC REACTION TO CEFDINIR OCCURS, THE DRUG SHOULD BE DISCONTINUED. SERIOUS ACUTE HYPERSENSITIVITY REACTIONS MAY REQUIRE TREATMENT WITH EPINEPHRINE AND OTHER EMERGENCY MEASURES, INCLUDING OXYGEN, INTRAVENOUS FLUIDS, INTRAVENOUS ANTIHISTAMINES, CORTICOSTEROIDS, PRESSOR AMINES, AND AIRWAY MANAGEMENT, AS CLINICALLY INDICATED.**

**Pseudomembranous colitis has been reported with nearly all antibacterial agents, including cefdinir, and may range in severity from mild- to life-threatening. Therefore, it is important to consider this diagnosis in patients who present with diarrhea subsequent to the administration of antibacterial agents.**

Treatment with antibacterial agents alters the normal flora of the colon and may permit overgrowth of clostridia. Studies indicate that a toxin produced by *Clostridium difficile* is a primary cause of "antibiotic-associated colitis."

After the diagnosis of pseudomembranous colitis has been established, appropriate therapeutic measures should be initiated. Mild cases of pseudomembranous colitis usually respond to drug discontinuation alone. In moderate to severe cases, consideration should be given to management with fluids and electrolytes, protein supplementation, and treatment with an antibacterial drug clinically effective against *Clostridium difficile*.

## PRECAUTIONS

### General

Prescribing OMNICEF in the absence of a proven or strongly suspected bacterial infection or a prophylactic indication is unlikely to provide benefit to the patient and increases the risk of the development of drug-resistant bacteria.

As with other broad-spectrum antibiotics, prolonged treatment may result in the possible emergence and overgrowth of resistant organisms. Careful observation of the patient is essential. If superinfection occurs during therapy, appropriate alternative therapy should be administered.

Cefdinir, as with other broad-spectrum antimicrobials (antibiotics), should be prescribed with caution in individuals with a history of colitis.

In patients with transient or persistent renal insufficiency (creatinine clearance <30 mL/min), the total daily dose of OMNICEF should be reduced because high and prolonged plasma concentrations of cefdinir can result following recommended doses.

### Information for Patients

Patients should be counseled that antibacterial drugs including OMNICEF should only be used to treat bacterial infections. They do not treat viral infections (e.g., the common cold). When OMNICEF is prescribed to treat a bacterial infection, patients should be told that although it is common to feel better early in the course of therapy, the medication should be taken exactly as directed. Skipping doses or not completing the full course of therapy may (1) decrease the effectiveness of the immediate treatment and (2) increase the likelihood that bacteria will develop resistance and will not be treatable by OMNICEF or other antibacterial drugs in the future.

Antacids containing magnesium or aluminum interfere with the absorption of cefdinir. If this type of antacid is required during OMNICEF therapy, OMNICEF should be taken at least 2 hours before or after the antacid.

Iron supplements, including multivitamins that contain iron, interfere with the absorption of cefdinir. If iron supplements are required during OMNICEF therapy, OMNICEF should be taken at least 2 hours before or after the supplement.

Iron-fortified infant formula does not significantly interfere with the absorption of cefdinir. Therefore, OMNICEF for Oral Suspension can be administered with iron-fortified infant formula.

Diabetic patients and caregivers should be aware that the oral suspension contains 2.86 g of sucrose per teaspoon.

### Drug Interactions

**Antacids:** (aluminum- or magnesium-containing): Concomitant administration of 300-mg cefdinir capsules with 30 mL Maalox® TC suspension reduces the rate ($C_{max}$) and extent (AUC) of absorption by approximately 40%. Time to reach $C_{max}$ is also prolonged by 1 hour. There are no significant effects on cefdinir pharmacokinetics if the antacid is administered 2 hours before or 2 hours after cefdinir. If antacids are required during OMNICEF therapy, OMNICEF should be taken at least 2 hours before or after the antacid.

**Probenecid:** As with other β-lactam antibiotics, probenecid inhibits the renal excretion of cefdinir, resulting in an approximate doubling in AUC, a 54% increase in peak cefdinir plasma levels, and a 50% prolongation in the apparent elimination $t_{1/2}$.

**Iron Supplements and Foods Fortified With Iron:** Concomitant administration of cefdinir with a therapeutic iron supplement containing 60 mg of elemental iron (as $FeSO_4$) or vitamins supplemented with 10 mg of elemental iron reduced extent of absorption by 80% and 31%, respectively. If iron supplements are required during OMNICEF therapy, OMNICEF should be taken at least 2 hours before or after the supplement.

The effect of foods highly fortified with elemental iron (primarily iron-fortified breakfast cereals) on cefdinir absorption has not been studied.

Concomitantly administered iron-fortified infant formula (2.2 mg elemental iron/6 oz) has no significant effect on cefdinir pharmacokinetics. Therefore, OMNICEF for Oral Suspension can be administered with iron-fortified infant formula.

There have been reports of reddish stools in patients receiving cefdinir. In many cases, patients were also receiving iron-containing products. The reddish color is due to the formation of a nonabsorbable complex between cefdinir or its breakdown products and iron in the gastrointestinal tract.

### Drug/Laboratory Test Interactions

A false-positive reaction for ketones in the urine may occur with tests using nitroprusside, but not with those using nitroferricyanide. The administration of cefdinir may result in a false-positive reaction for glucose in urine using Clinitest®, Benedict's solution, or Fehling's solution. It is recommended that glucose tests based on enzymatic glucose oxidase reactions (such as Clinistix® or Tes-Tape®) be used. Cephalosporins are known to occasionally induce a positive direct Coombs' test.

### Carcinogenesis, Mutagenesis, Impairment of Fertility

The carcinogenic potential of cefdinir has not been evaluated. No mutagenic effects were seen in the bacterial reverse mutation assay (Ames) or point mutation assay at the hypoxanthine-guanine phosphoribosyltransferase locus (HGPRT) in V79 Chinese hamster lung cells. No clastogenic effects were observed *in vitro* in the structural chromosome aberration assay in V79 Chinese hamster lung cells or *in vivo* in the micronucleus assay in mouse bone marrow. In rats, fertility and reproductive performance were not affected by cefdinir at oral doses up to 1000 mg/kg/day (70 times the human dose based on mg/kg/day, 11 times based on mg/m$^2$/day).

### Pregnancy - Teratogenic Effects

**Pregnancy Category B:** Cefdinir was not teratogenic in rats at oral doses up to 1000 mg/kg/day (70 times the human dose based on mg/kg/day, 11 times based on mg/m$^2$/day) or in rabbits at oral doses up to 10 mg/kg/day (0.7 times the human dose based on mg/kg/day, 0.23 times based on mg/m$^2$/day). Maternal toxicity (decreased body weight gain) was observed in rabbits at the maximum tolerated dose of 10 mg/kg/day without adverse effects on offspring. Decreased body weight occurred in rat fetuses at ≥ 100 mg/kg/day, and in rat offspring at ≥ 32 mg/kg/day. No effects were observed on maternal reproductive parameters or offspring survival, development, behavior, or reproductive function.

There are, however, no adequate and well-controlled studies in pregnant women. Because animal reproduction studies are not always predictive of human response, this drug should be used during pregnancy only if clearly needed.

### Labor and Delivery

Cefdinir has not been studied for use during labor and delivery.

### Nursing Mothers

Following administration of single 600-mg doses, cefdinir was not detected in human breast milk.

### Pediatric Use

Safety and efficacy in neonates and infants less than 6 months of age have not been established. Use of cefdinir for the treatment of acute maxillary sinusitis in pediatric patients (age 6 months through 12 years) is supported by evidence from adequate and well-controlled studies in adults and adolescents, the similar pathophysiology of acute sinusitis in adult and pediatric patients, and comparative pharmacokinetic data in the pediatric population.

### Geriatric Use

Efficacy is comparable in geriatric patients and younger adults. While cefdinir has been well-tolerated in all age groups, in clinical trials geriatric patients experienced a lower rate of adverse events, including diarrhea, than younger adults. Dose adjustment in elderly patients is not necessary unless renal function is markedly compromised.

## ADVERSE EVENTS

**Clinical Trials - OMNICEF Capsules (Adult and Adolescent Patients):**

In clinical trials, 5093 adult and adolescent patients (3841 US and 1252 non-US) were treated with the recommended dose of cefdinir capsules (600 mg/day). Most adverse events were mild and self-limiting. No deaths or permanent disabilities were attributed to cefdinir. One hundred forty-seven of 5093 (3%) patients discontinued medication due to adverse events thought by the investigators to be possibly, probably, or definitely associated with cefdinir therapy. The discontinuations were primarily for gastrointestinal disturbances, usually diarrhea or nausea. Nineteen of 5093 (0.4%) patients were discontinued due to rash thought related to cefdinir administration.

In the US, the following adverse events were thought by investigators to be possibly, probably, or definitely related to cefdinir capsules in multiple-dose clinical trials (N = 3841 cefdinir-treated patients):

**ADVERSE EVENTS ASSOCIATED WITH CEFDINIR CAPSULES US TRIALS IN ADULT AND ADOLESCENT PATIENTS (N=3841)[a]**

| | | |
|---|---|---|
| Incidence ≥ 1% | Diarrhea | 15% |
| | Vaginal moniliasis | 4% of women |
| | Nausea | 3% |
| | Headache | 2% |
| | Abdominal pain | 1% |
| | Vaginitis | 1% of women |
| Incidence <1% but >0.1% | Rash | 0.9% |
| | Dyspepsia | 0.7% |
| | Flatulence | 0.7% |
| | Vomiting | 0.7% |
| | Abnormal stools | 0.3% |
| | Anorexia | 0.3% |
| | Constipation | 0.3% |
| | Dizziness | 0.3% |
| | Dry mouth | 0.3% |
| | Asthenia | 0.2% |
| | Insomnia | 0.2% |
| | Leukorrhea | 0.2% of women |
| | Moniliasis | 0.2% |
| | Pruritus | 0.2% |
| | Somnolence | 0.2% |

[a] 1733 males, 2108 females

The following laboratory value changes of possible clinical significance, irrespective of relationship to therapy with cefdinir, were seen during clinical trials conducted in the US:

**LABORATORY VALUE CHANGES OBSERVED WITH CEFDINIR CAPSULES US TRIALS IN ADULT AND ADOLESCENT PATIENTS (N=3841)**

| | | |
|---|---|---|
| Incidence ≥ 1% | ↑ Urine leukocytes | 2% |
| | ↑ Urine protein | 2% |
| | ↑ Gamma-glutamyltransferase[a] | 1% |
| | ↓ Lymphocytes, ↑ Lymphocytes | 1%, 0.2% |
| | ↑ Microhematuria | 1% |
| Incidence <1% but >0.1% | ↑ Glucose[a] | 0.9% |
| | ↑ Urine glucose | 0.9% |
| | ↑ White blood cells, ↓ White blood cells | 0.9%, 0.7% |
| | ↑ Alanine aminotransferase (ALT) | 0.7% |
| | ↑ Eosinophils | 0.7% |
| | ↑ Urine specific gravity, ↓ Urine specific gravity[a] | 0.6%, 0.2% |
| | ↓ Bicarbonate[a] | 0.6% |
| | ↑ Phosphorus, ↓ Phosphorus[a] | 0.6%, 0.3% |
| | ↑ Aspartate aminotransferase (AST) | 0.4% |
| | ↑ Alkaline phosphatase | 0.3% |
| | ↑ Blood urea nitrogen (BUN) | 0.3% |
| | ↓ Hemoglobin | 0.3% |
| | ↑ Polymorphonuclear neutrophils (PMNs), ↓ PMNs | 0.3%, 0.2% |
| | ↑ Bilirubin | 0.2% |
| | ↑ Lactate dehydrogenase[a] | 0.2% |
| | ↑ Platelets | 0.2% |
| | ↑ Potassium[a] | 0.2% |
| | ↑ Urine pH[a] | 0.2% |

[a] N<3841 for these parameters

**Clinical Trials - OMNICEF for Oral Suspension (Pediatric Patients):**

In clinical trials, 2289 pediatric patients (1783 US and 506 non-US) were treated with the recommended dose of cefdinir suspension (14 mg/kg/day). Most adverse events were mild and self-limiting. No deaths or permanent disabilities were attributed to cefdinir. Forty of 2289 (2%) patients discontinued medication due to adverse events considered by the investigators to be possibly, probably, or definitely associated with cefdinir therapy. Discontinuations were primarily for gastrointestinal disturbances, usually diarrhea. Five of 2289 (0.2%) patients were discontinued due to rash thought related to cefdinir administration.

In the US, the following adverse events were thought by investigators to be possibly, probably, or definitely related to cefdinir suspension in multiple-dose clinical trials (N=1783 cefdinir-treated patients):

**ADVERSE EVENTS ASSOCIATED WITH CEFDINIR SUSPENSION US TRIALS IN PEDIATRIC PATIENTS (N=1783)[a]**

| | | |
|---|---|---|
| Incidence ≥ 1% | Diarrhea | 8% |
| | Rash | 3% |
| | Vomiting | 1% |
| Incidence <1% but >0.1% | Cutaneous moniliasis | 0.9% |
| | Abdominal pain | 0.8% |
| | Leukopenia[b] | 0.3% |
| | Vaginal moniliasis | 0.3% of girls |
| | Vaginitis | 0.3% of girls |
| | Abnormal stools | 0.2% |
| | Dyspepsia | 0.2% |
| | Hyperkinesia | 0.2% |
| | Increased AST[b] | 0.2% |
| | Maculopapular rash | 0.2% |
| | Nausea | 0.2% |

[a] 977 males, 806 females

[b] Laboratory changes were occasionally reported as adverse events.

NOTE: In both cefdinir- and control-treated patients, rates of diarrhea and rash were higher in the youngest pediatric patients. The incidence of diarrhea in cefdinir-treated patients ≤2 years of age was 17% (95/557) compared with 4% (51/1226) in those >2 years old. The incidence of rash (primarily diaper rash in the younger patients) was 8% (43/557) in patients ≤2 years of age compared with 1% (8/1226) in those >2 years old.

The following laboratory value changes of possible clinical significance, irrespective of relationship to therapy with cefdinir, were seen during clinical trials conducted in the US:

**LABORATORY VALUE CHANGES OF POSSIBLE CLINICAL SIGNIFICANCE OBSERVED WITH CEFDINIR SUSPENSION US TRIALS IN PEDIATRIC PATIENTS (N=1783)**

| | | |
|---|---|---|
| Incidence ≥ 1% | ↑ Lymphocytes, ↓ Lymphocytes | 2%, 0.8% |
| | ↑ Alkaline phosphatase | 1% |
| | ↓ Bicarbonate[a] | 1% |
| | ↑ Eosinophils | 1% |
| | ↑ Lactate dehydrogenase | 1% |
| | ↑ Platelets | 1% |
| | ↑ PMNs, ↓ PMNs | 1%, 1% |
| | ↑ Urine protein | 1% |
| Incidence <1% but >0.1% | ↑ Phosphorus, ↓ Phosphorus | 0.9%, 0.4% |
| | ↑ Urine pH | 0.8% |
| | ↓ White blood cells, ↑ White blood cells | 0.7%, 0.3% |
| | ↓ Calcium[a] | 0.5% |
| | ↓ Hemoglobin | 0.5% |
| | ↑ Urine leukocytes | 0.5% |
| | ↑ Monocytes | 0.4% |
| | ↑ AST | 0.3% |
| | ↑ Potassium[a] | 0.3% |
| | ↑ Urine specific gravity, ↓ Urine specific gravity | 0.3%, 0.1% |
| | ↓ Hematocrit[a] | 0.2% |

[a] N=1387 for these parameters

**Postmarketing Experience**

The following adverse experiences and altered laboratory tests, regardless of their relationship to cefdinir, have been reported during extensive postmarketing experience, beginning with approval in Japan in 1991: Stevens-Johnson syndrome, toxic epidermal necrolysis, exfoliative dermatitis, erythema multiforme, erythema nodosum, serum sickness-like reactions, conjunctivitis, stomatitis, acute hepatitis, cholestasis, fulminant hepatitis, hepatic failure, jaundice, increased amylase, shock, anaphylaxis, facial and laryngeal edema, feeling of suffocation, acute enterocolitis, bloody diarrhea, hemorrhagic colitis, melena, pseudomembranous colitis, pancytopenia, granulocytopenia, leukopenia, thrombocytopenia, idiopathic thrombocytopenic purpura, hemolytic anemia, acute respiratory failure, asthmatic attack, drug-induced pneumonia, eosinophilic pneumonia, idiopathic interstitial pneumonia, fever, acute renal failure, nephropathy, bleeding tendency, coagulation disorder, disseminated intravascular coagulation, upper GI bleed, peptic ulcer, ileus, loss of consciousness, allergic vasculitis, possible cefdinir-diclofenac interaction, cardiac failure, chest pain, myocardial infarction, hypertension, involuntary movements, and rhabdomyolysis.

**Cephalosporin Class Adverse Events**

The following adverse events and altered laboratory tests have been reported for cephalosporin-class antibiotics in general:

> Allergic reactions, anaphylaxis, Stevens-Johnson syndrome, erythema multiforme, toxic epidermal necrolysis, renal dysfunction, toxic nephropathy, hepatic dysfunction including cholestasis, aplastic anemia, hemolytic anemia, hemorrhage, false-positive test for urinary glucose, neutropenia, pancytopenia, and agranulocytosis. Pseudomembranous colitis symptoms may begin during or after antibiotic treatment (see **WARNINGS**).

Several cephalosporins have been implicated in triggering seizures, particularly in patients with renal impairment when the dosage was not reduced (see **OVERDOSAGE**). If seizures associated with drug therapy occur, the drug should be discontinued. Anticonvulsant therapy can be given if clinically indicated.

## OVERDOSAGE

Information on cefdinir overdosage in humans is not available. In acute rodent toxicity studies, a single oral 5600-mg/kg dose produced no adverse effects. Toxic signs and symptoms following overdosage with other β-lactam antibiotics have included nausea, vomiting, epigastric distress, diarrhea, and convulsions. Hemodialysis removes cefdinir from the body. This may be useful in the event of a serious toxic reaction from overdosage, particularly if renal function is compromised.

**Rx only**

Ref: 03-5435-Rev. July, 2005
(Nos. 3769, 3771, 6151)



05J-034-L150-2 **MASTER**

Manufactured by:
**CEPH** International Corporation
Carolina, Puerto Rico 00986

For:
**Abbott Laboratories**
North Chicago, IL 60064, U.S.A.

Under License of:
astellas
Astellas Pharma Inc.
Tokyo, Japan

06F-034-Q068-1
Printed in U.S.A.

## Long-term Effects of Universal Preventive Interventions on Methamphetamine Use Among Adolescents

Methamphetamine use among adolescents increased dramatically during the 1990s with those in rural areas and small towns particularly vulnerable. Spoth and colleagues conducted 2 randomized controlled trials of the longitudinal effects on methamphetamine use of partnership-based universal preventive interventions. The studies involved sixth and seventh grade students and their families in a Midwestern state. The interventions focused on both the adolescents and their families; more than 1200 families participated in the study. At grades 11 and 12, the intervention students had almost no methamphetamine use compared with 3% to 5% among control students. These results indicate that large-scale trials of such universal preventive interventions should be conducted to protect future adolescents against drug abuse and its attendant consequences.

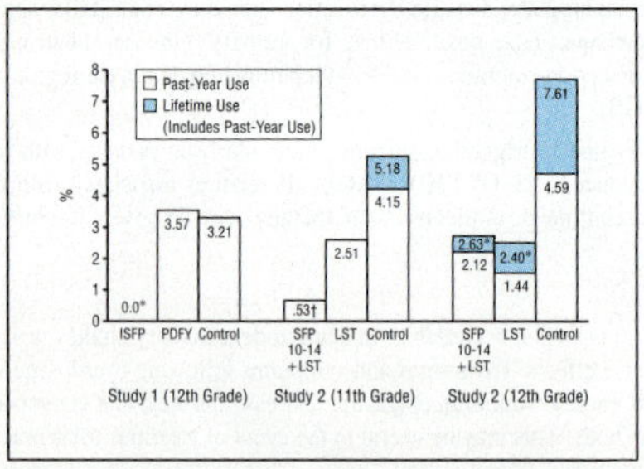


**Figure.** Lifetime and past-year methamphetamine use 4½ to 6½ years past baseline. No lifetime use data were available from study 1; in study 2 at 11th grade, lifetime use is equal to past-year use for both intervention conditions. For study 2, the 12th-grade sample size differs from 11th grade because of sample attrition. ISFP indicates Iowa Strengthening Families Program; LST, Life Skills Training; PDFY, Preparing for the Drug Free Years; and SFP 10-14 + LST, Strengthening Families Program: For Parents and Youth 10-14 plus Life Skills Training. *, $P \leq .05$. †, $P \leq .01$.

See page 876

## Measuring Effectiveness of Dietetic Interventions in Child Obesity: A Systematic Review of Randomized Trials

The response to the obesity epidemic will require primary prevention as well as weight reduction programs. This systematic review was conducted to evaluate the best available evidence on the effectiveness of dietetic treatment and management for overweight children or adolescents. Of the 1310 original articles identified, 37 studies met inclusion criteria, involving a total of 2262 participants. Among the 8 studies suitable for meta-analysis, dietetic intervention by itself or in conjunction with increased physical activity was successful in reducing weight by as much as 8%. However, the effect of the interventions appeared to wane over time.

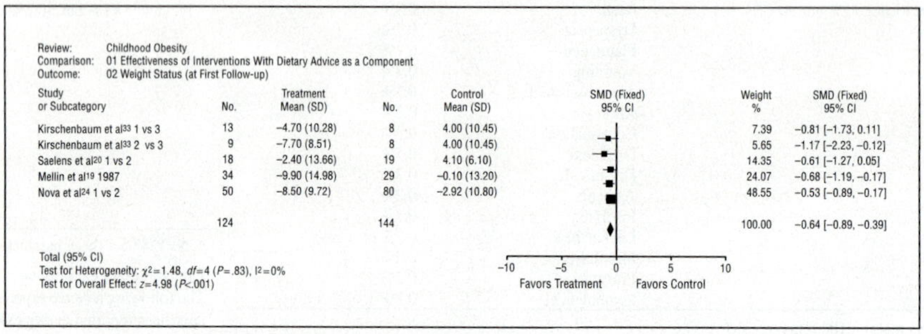


**Figure.** Meta-analysis of 3 randomized controlled trials of interventions for child obesity where a "true" control arm was used and results were reported after a period of follow-up.

See page 906

## Effect of Open Access Scheduling on Missed Appointments, Immunizations, and Continuity of Care for Infant Well-Child Visits

Open access scheduling attempts to provide access to care at the point it is needed. Under open access, when a parent calls to schedule a well-child visit, the patient would be seen within 1 or 2 days in contrast to usual systems of 4- to 6-week delays. In this randomized controlled trial involving 10 providers and 878 infants, providers were randomized to either open access for future visits or open access for current visits. In both groups, missed appointment rates dropped dramatically, although more so among the same-day open access group. Immunization rates increased in both groups; provider continuity was higher in the group with open access for future visits.

See page 889

## Children Treated at an Expeditionary Military Hospital in Iraq

Coppola and colleagues report on their experiences caring for children at a level III expeditionary hospital in Iraq. Over a 17-month period, 85 children were treated, representing 5% of all patients treated at the hospital. Approximately half were treated for trauma, most commonly due to injuries from explosions. Overall, 6% of the children died.

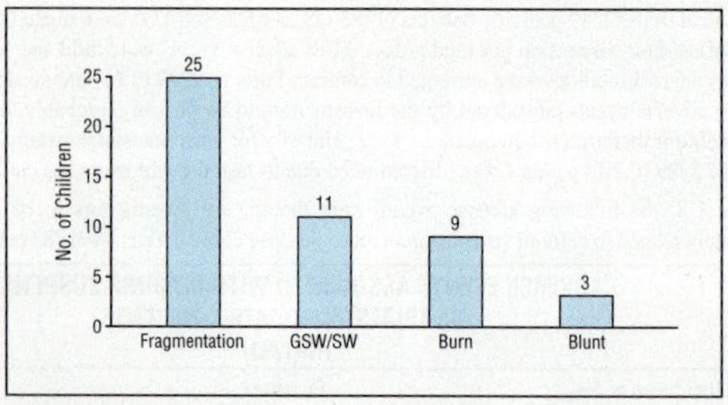


**Figure.** Mechanism of injury in 48 children treated at an expeditionary military hospital. GSW/SW indicates gunshot wound and stab wound.

See page 972

# Winslow Homer (1836-1910)

## The Country School, *1871*

THROUGHOUT THE 1800S, AS SETTLERS SPREAD across the American prairies and turned them into farmland, the first public building to be erected in a new community was often a 1-room schoolhouse. By the century's end, more than 200 000 1-room schools dotted the nation's landscape, and half of all American schoolchildren attended them.[1]

In Winslow Homer's *The Country School*, class is in session. According to custom, boys sit on one side and girls on the other. An exception is the boy and girl on the low bench at the right, who may be brother and sister. Siblings were allowed to sit together so that they could share the same books (or maybe not, in this case). Some of the older children read by themselves or in small groups. Others practice writing or work on arithmetic problems, using a long sloped shelf on the back and side walls for writing in lieu of a desk.

At the center of this orderly scene is the prim young woman framed against the blackboard. In the 1870s, most schoolteachers were women. Men were in short supply after the Civil War, and many were lured away from teaching by higher pay in business or other professions. Teaching was a respectable first job for a young woman while waiting for a marriage prospect to come along. Teachers of either sex were usually hired for just a single school term. They often "boarded around," staying for a week or two with the family of 1 of their students before moving on to stay with another family. At the end of the school term, the teacher organized a public presentation in which children could show off what they had learned. They recited famous orations or poetry, competed in "spell downs," or displayed their knowledge of geography by drawing maps or naming the state capitals. Soon afterward, the teacher and students said goodbye.

Here, the teacher and the 3 boys on her right may be engaged in a recitation session in which pupils take turns reading aloud while the others follow along. What might they be reading? Chances are good that it is a *McGuffey Reader*. Volume 1 of this venerable 6-volume series was a thin book with big print, starting with the alphabet. Once a student mastered a volume and could read it fluently, regardless of age, he or she was moved up to the next book in the series. Volume 6 was a thick, eclectic collection including biographical essays about famous men and women, stories about chivalry, descriptions of faraway natural wonders, and excerpts from great works of world literature by Longfellow, Poe, Dickens, and Shakespeare, among others.[2] For children growing up in the cloistered world of a small settlement on the prairie, the *McGuffey Readers* opened the children's minds to the world beyond, including the world of ideas.

A sprig of cherry blossoms on the teacher's desk suggests that it is springtime. On such a sunny day, even the most interesting book or math problem might have a hard time keeping a young person's attention indoors. In another well-known picture from his series about children and schools, Homer turned the youngsters loose for recess and showed them playing a lively game of "snap the whip." This same 1-room schoolhouse appears in the background with its door open, waiting for legs to tire, the teacher to ring the school bell, and young minds to be drawn back again to the business of learning.

*Thomas D. Koepsell, MD, MPH*

**Correspondence:** Dr Koepsell, Department of Epidemiology, University of Washington, F-261F Health Sciences, Box 357236, Seattle, WA 98195-7236 (koepsell@u.washington.edu).

## REFERENCES

1. Bial R. *One-Room School.* Boston, Mass: Houghton Mifflin; 1999:36.
2. McGuffey WH. *McGuffey's Sixth Eclectic Reader.* New York, NY: Van Antwerp, Bragg & Co; 1879.

ARTICLE

ARCHIVES EXPRESS

# Long-term Effects of Universal Preventive Interventions on Methamphetamine Use Among Adolescents

*Richard L. Spoth, PhD; Scott Clair, PhD; Chungyeol Shin, PhD; Cleve Redmond, PhD*

**Objective:** To examine the long-term effects of universal preventive interventions on methamphetamine use by adolescents in the general population during their late high school years.

**Design:** Two randomized, controlled prevention trials.

**Setting:** Public schools in the Midwest from 1993 to 2004.

**Participants:** Study 1 began with 667 sixth grade students from 33 rural public schools; the follow-up included 457 students. Study 2 began with 679 seventh grade students from 36 rural public schools; the follow-up assessment included 597 students.

**Interventions:** In study 1, schools were assigned to the Iowa Strengthening Families Program (ISFP), Preparing for the Drug Free Years, or a control condition. In study 2, schools were assigned to a revised ISFP (SFP 10-14) plus Life Skills Training (SPF 10-14 + LST), LST alone, or a control condition.

**Results:** Self-reports of lifetime and past-year methamphetamine use were collected at 6½ years past baseline (study 1) and at 4½ and 5½ years past baseline (study 2). In study 1, the ISFP past-year rate was 0.0% compared with 3.2% in the control condition ($P = .04$). In study 2, SFP 10-14 + LST showed significant effects on lifetime and past-year use at the 4½ year follow-up (eg, 0.5% lifetime use in the intervention condition vs 5.2% in the control condition, $P = .006$); both SFP 10-14 + LST and LST alone had significant lifetime use effects at the 5½ year follow-up.

**Conclusion:** Brief universal interventions have potential for public health impact by reducing methamphetamine use among adolescents.

*Arch Pediatr Adolesc Med. 2006;160:876-882*

METHAMPHETAMINE USE has been characterized as having reached epidemic proportions in the United States by the mid 1990s,[1,2] posing a substantial threat to public health. The unique characteristics of the methamphetamine problem—including its widespread use, its ready production, and its low cost—suggest a pernicious, long-term public health problem.[3]

Methamphetamine use among adolescents increased dramatically during the 1990s; although the rates have decreased since that time, the 2004 lifetime prevalence of use for seniors was more than 6%.[4-6] The unique and substantial social and health consequences of methamphetamine addiction, including social dysfunction and a wide range of medical problems, underscore the importance of preventing early use.[2] Adolescents in smaller towns and rural areas are particularly vulnerable, given potentially powerful peer influences in rural environments and the historical appeal of stimulants to rural youth.[2] The threat to adolescents in the rural Midwest has been particularly acute since methamphetamines spread to this region in the 1980s with surges in methamphetamine-related problems by the 1990s.[3,7,8] The 2 randomized studies reported in this article both involve adolescent high school students residing in a rural midwestern state.

Researchers summarizing the case for the likely persistence of the methamphetamine problem have argued strongly in favor of a preventive approach.[3] Guided by etiological research, a number of preventive interventions have been designed to modify the 2 primary socializing environments of youth, family and school, or to build youth competencies in the school setting.[9-13] Although these preventive interventions have shown effects on reduced adolescent alcohol, tobacco, and marijuana use, no studies could be found that examined effects of any kind of preven-

Author Affiliations:
Partnerships in Prevention Science Institute, Iowa State University, Ames.

tive interventions on methamphetamine use; only randomized, controlled studies of treatment outcomes were found in the published literature.[14]

A key feature of the tested preventive interventions is that they were implemented via community-university partnerships. Positive outcomes of universal interventions are strongly associated with high-quality implementation; earlier reports have described the importance of these partnerships in achieving such high-quality implementation and have demonstrated their value in this connection.[12,15-20]

To summarize, the persistent public health problem of methamphetamine use warrants more emphasis on evidence-based prevention among adolescents in the general population, particularly in rural areas. In consideration of reports of increasing prevalence of adolescent methamphetamine use and the need to examine the role of preventive interventions, items specific to methamphetamine use were added to annual assessments in our ongoing prevention trials (see http://www.ppsi.iastate.edu). Results for alcohol-related outcomes, including drunkenness, and cigarette, marijuana, and other illicit drug use were reported earlier,[12,13] but not the results of the methamphetamine items that were added following the pretest. The objective of the present article is to report findings of 2 randomized, controlled studies of the longitudinal effects on methamphetamine use of partnership-based preventive interventions for adolescents in the general population and their families residing in a rural midwestern state.

## METHODS

Both studies reported were randomized, controlled studies of the outcomes of universal preventive interventions designed to reduce substance use and other problem behaviors with a focus on delaying substance use onset. Both were implemented in rural communities. A key difference in the studies is that study 1 tested 2 different family-focused interventions whereas study 2 examined a multicomponent family-focused and school-based intervention along with a school-based intervention alone. Institutional review board approval for human subject procedures in both studies was obtained from Iowa State University, Ames.

## STUDY 1

### Sample

Families of all sixth-graders enrolled in 33 rural schools in 19 contiguous counties in a midwestern state were recruited for participation in a family-focused preventive intervention evaluation project. School selection was based on school lunch program eligibility (greater than 15%) and community size (population less than 8500) prior to randomization. After blocking on school size and the proportion of lower-income families, the schools were randomly assigned to either a minimal contact control group or 1 of 2 experimental groups, the latter of which entailed either implementation of the 7-session Iowa Strengthening Families Program (ISFP) or the 5-session Preparing for the Drug Free Years (PDFY). Of 1309 families recruited from the 33 schools, 667 (51%) completed pretesting. This level of participation is relatively high for multisession interventions requiring both parent and youth involvement.[12] Among the 667 families completing pretesting were 238 ISFP, 221 PDFY, and 208 control group families. The 12th-grade follow-up (6½ years past baseline) was completed by 457 families (151 ISFP, 149 PDFY, 157 control) (**Figure 1**).

Among the families who completed the pretest, there was an average of 3.1 children per family. Representative of the study region, 86% of the families were dual-parent. Nearly all participants (98%) were white. Data from a prospective telephone survey conducted in the region supported the representativeness of the study sample.[21]

### Procedures

Families willing to participate were interviewed in their homes by a project staff member. During the in-home visit, a household composition interview was conducted, followed by the administration of confidentially and independently completed written questionnaires for the parent(s) and participating young adolescent (60-80 minutes to complete).

### Intervention Implementation

Preparing for the Drug Free Years is a family competency training program based on the social development model.[22,23] Its primary objectives are to enhance protective parent-child interactions and to reduce children's risk for early substance use initiation. Preparing for the Drug Free Years is a 5-session program with an average session length of 2 hours. One session requires the child's attendance; the other 4 sessions are solely for parents. A detailed description of PDFY is provided in earlier reports.[12,13]

The ISFP is based on empirically supported family risk and protective factor models.[24] With these conceptual underpinnings, ISFP targets the enhancement of family protective factors and the reduction of family risk processes.[24] The ISFP includes seven 2-hour sessions. Each of the first 6 sessions includes separate, concurrent youth and parent skills-building curricula (1 hour) followed by a conjoint family curriculum (1 hour). The seventh session includes only the 1-hour family interaction session. See earlier reports for a detailed ISFP program description.[13,24]

## STUDY 2

### Sample

Study 2 participants included seventh-graders enrolled in 36 rural schools in a different region of the same midwestern state in which study 1 was conducted. Criteria for selection of the schools were eligibility for the free and reduced-cost school lunch program (approximately 20% or more); community size/school district enrollment (fewer than 1200 students); and middle school structure (grades 6-8 taught at only 1 location).

Schools were matched on several factors to form 12 blocks of 3 schools each.[25] The 3 schools in each block were then randomly assigned to the 3 experimental groups: the Strengthening Families Program: For Parents and Youth 10-14 combined with the Life Skills Training (LST) program (SFP 10-14 + LST), the LST only, or a minimal-contact control group.

Randomly selected families with seventh-grade students in participating schools were recruited for participation. Of the 1017 eligible families contacted for recruitment for the in-home assessment, 679 (67%) completed pretesting (226 SFP 10-14 + LST group families, 231 LST-only group families, and 222 control group families) (**Figure 2**). Although a total of 691 families completed the pretest assessments, 12 families moved from a school in one condition to a school in another condition and were dropped from the sample. At the 11th grade follow-up (4½ years past baseline), a total of 588 families participated. Those included 190 SFP 10-14 + LST group families, 202 LST-only fami-

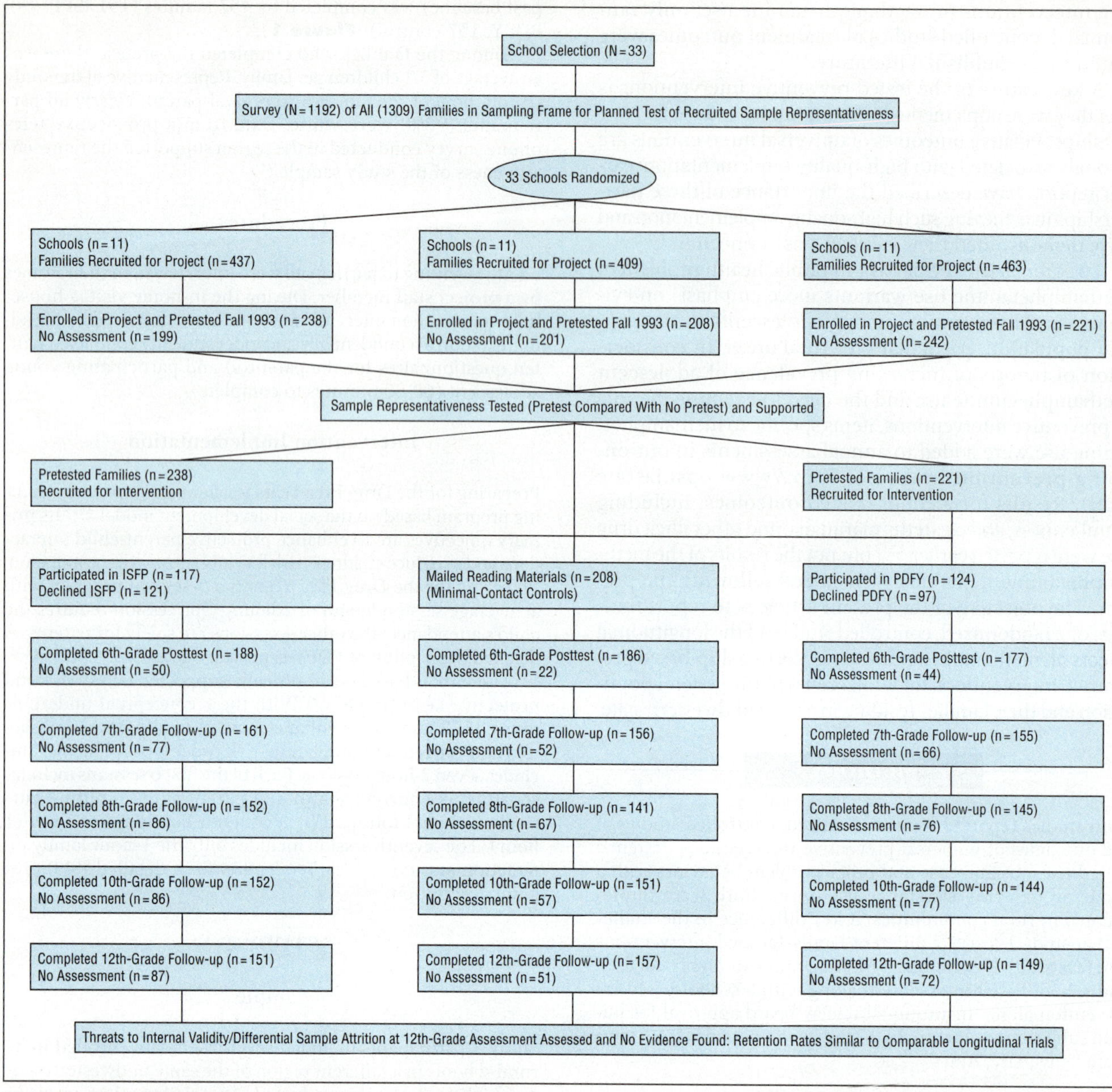


**Figure 1.** Study 1 participation summary. ISFP indicates Iowa Strengthening Families Program; PDFY, Preparing for the Drug Free Years.

lies, and 196 control group families. At the 12th-grade follow-up (5½ years past baseline), a total of 597 families participated. Those included 191 SFP 10-14 + LST group families, 209 LST-only families, and 197 control group families.

Among families who completed the pretest, there was an average of 3.2 children. The majority of families (87%) were dual-parent families. Of these dual-parent families, 83% included both of the target child's biological parents. Virtually all participants were white (99%).

## Procedures

Eligible families were contacted to schedule an in-home recruitment visit from a staff member. Those who accepted the visit and indicated a willingness to participate in the project pretest were scheduled for the in-home assessment visit. Approximately 60 to 80 minutes were required to complete the questionnaires. The same data collection procedures were employed across all data collection points.

## Intervention Implementation

The multicomponent intervention in this study entailed the LST program and a revision of the ISFP (previously described for study 1, now called the Strengthening Families Program: For Parents and Youth 10-14) that includes the same essential content as in the original program.[24] Theoretical underpinnings of the LST program are described elsewhere.[26,27] The LST program consists of 15 sessions taught during regular classroom periods and 5 booster sessions taught 1 year later. Each session includes a major goal along with corresponding, measurable student objectives.

## STUDY 1 AND STUDY 2 MEASURES AND ANALYSES

Adolescent past-year methamphetamine use was assessed with a single item. In study 1, the question read, "For each sub-

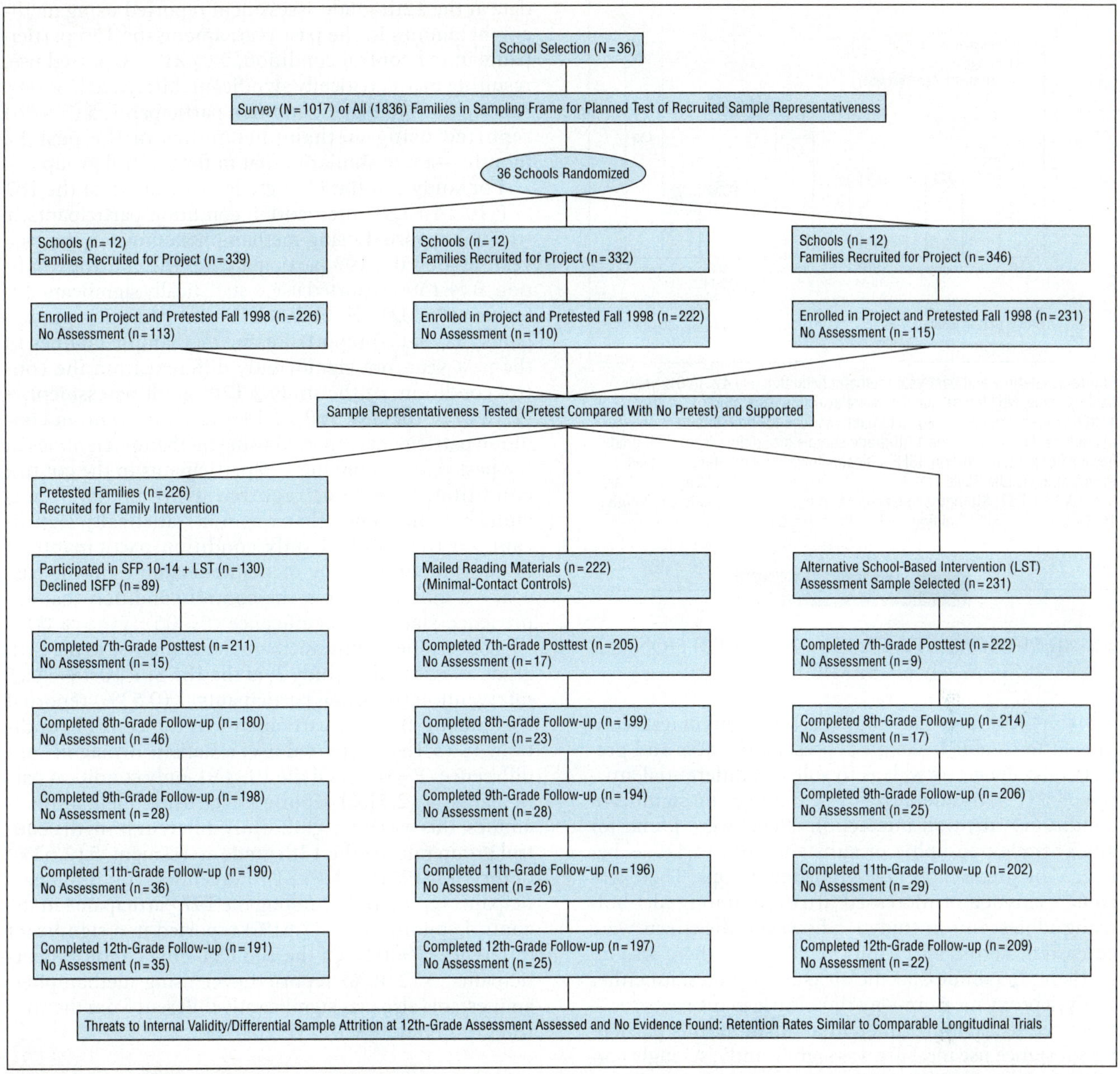


**Figure 2.** Study 2 participation summary. ISFP indicates Iowa Strengthening Families Program; LST, Life Skills Training; SFP 10-14 + LST, Strengthening Families Program: For Parents and Youth 10-14 plus Life Skills Training.

stance listed below, please write down the number of times you used it during the past 12 months . . . took methamphetamines (meth)." For study 2, the question read: "In the past 12 months, how many times have you used methamphetamines (meth)?" In addition, study 2 included a separate item on lifetime use of methamphetamines ("Have you ever used methamphetamine [meth]?"). These items were then dichotomized and recoded into 0 for respondents who did not use methamphetamines and 1 for those who did. These items were not included in the pretest surveys of either of the 2 studies but were added at later waves in consideration of epidemiological reports of increasing methamphetamine use. Specifically, among the waves of data collected during the middle and high school years for study 1, only data on use in the past year was collected at the 12th-grade assessment. In study 2, both past-year and lifetime use items were included at the seventh-grade spring semester data collection point (posttest) and all subsequent waves of middle and high school data collection. Because methamphetamine use rates at the seventh-, eighth-, and ninth-grade assessment points in study 2 were all less than 0.5% across conditions, analyses of intervention effects at those waves were precluded. Statistical significance testing was conducted only for those waves in which at least 5 participants reported methamphetamine use in at least 1 of the 3 conditions.

Analyses for the current article used intent-to-treat analyses. Because of the small cell sizes, the Fisher exact test[28] was used to assess differences in methamphetamine use between the intervention and control conditions in each study. In addition, given the small numbers of methamphetamine users, a multilevel analysis to address the nested structure of the data was not feasible. An examination of methamphetamine user frequencies by school, however, showed minimal evidence of within-school dependence of user rates and thus little need for multilevel analyses. For example, the 25 respondents reporting lifetime use at the 12th-grade assessment in study 2 were distributed across 18 schools; at the 11th-grade assessment, the 16 lifetime users were distributed across 13 schools.

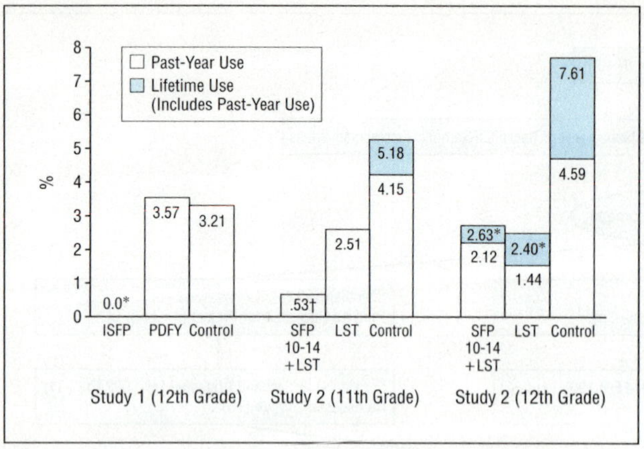


**Figure 3.** Lifetime and past-year methamphetamine use 4½ to 6½ years past baseline. No lifetime use data were available from study 1; in study 2 at 11th grade, lifetime use is equal to past-year use for both intervention conditions. For study 2, the 12th-grade sample size differs from 11th grade because of sample attrition. ISFP indicates Iowa Strengthening Families Program; LST, Life Skills Training; PDFY, Preparing for the Drug Free Years; SFP 10-14 + LST, Strengthening Families Program: For Parents and Youth 10-14 plus Life Skills Training. *, $P \leq .05$. †, $P \leq .01$.

## RESULTS

### REPRESENTATIVENESS AND ATTRITION OF SAMPLE

Earlier reports provide detailed descriptions of tests conducted to establish sample representativeness and pretest equivalence, as well as to rule out differential attrition.[13,21,25,29] To summarize these findings, no significant condition × attrition interaction effects were found for any sociodemographic or substance use variables between the pretest and 12th-grade follow-ups. There was some evidence of increased attrition among alcohol-using adolescents in study 1[13]; however, the effects were consistent across all conditions. Because there was no methamphetamine-specific measure at pretest for either study, a proxy measure—marijuana use in the past year—was used to examine differential attrition; this particular substance use measure was significantly, strongly correlated with methamphetamine use in the past year. Pretest equivalence was found for this proxy measure and there was no evidence of differential attrition.

### CONTROL COMPARISON WITH NATIONAL RATES

The control groups in the current sample reported methamphetamine use rates roughly comparable with those found in national surveys. For example, the Monitoring the Future study reported annual use rates of methamphetamines by 12th-graders of 4.3% in 2000 and 3.4% in 2004 and lifetime use of methamphetamines by 6.2% of 12th-graders in 2004.[5]

### EXPERIMENTAL DIFFERENCES IN METHAMPHETAMINE USE

Concerning past-year use in study 1, none of the 148 participants in the ISFP intervention condition with valid data at the 12th-grade assessment reported using methamphetamines in the past year; among the 156 participants in the control condition, 5 (3.21%) reported use, resulting in a statistically significant difference ($P = .04$). Among the 140 PDFY condition participants, 5 (3.57%) reported using methamphetamines in the past 12 months—a rate similar to that in the control group.

For study 2 at the 11th-grade assessment, of the 187 SFP 10-14 + LST intervention condition participants, 1 (0.53%) reported using methamphetamines in the past year; among the 193 participants in the control condition, 8 (4.15%) reported use, a statistically significant difference ($P = .02$). Of the 199 LST-only condition participants, 5 (2.51%) reported using methamphetamines in the past year, not significantly different from the control condition. At the study 2 12th-grade assessment, 4 (2.12%) of the 189 SFP 10-14 + LST intervention condition participants reported using methamphetamines in the past year; among the 196 participants in the control condition, 9 (4.59%) reported using methamphetamines, a difference that was not statistically significant. Of the 208 LST-only condition participants, 3 (1.44%) reported using methamphetamines in the past year—a difference from the control condition that approached statistical significance ($P = .06$) (**Figure 3**).

Concerning lifetime methamphetamine use in the 11th grade as assessed in study 2, of the 187 SFP 10-14 + LST intervention condition participants, 1 (0.53%) reported use; among the 193 participants in the control condition, 10 (5.18%) reported use, a statistically significant difference ($P = .006$). Of the 199 LST-only condition participants, 5 (2.51%) reported ever using methamphetamines; this was not significantly different from the control group rate. At the 12th grade assessment, 5 (2.63%) of the 190 SFP 10-14 + LST intervention condition participants reported use; among the 197 participants in the control condition, 15 (7.61%) reported it, a significant difference ($P = .02$). Of the 208 LST-only condition participants, 5 (2.40%) reported ever using methamphetamines; this also was significantly different from the control group rate ($P = .01$) (Figure 3).

## COMMENT

As the problem of methamphetamine use has persisted, the need to identify effective universal prevention efforts to counter this problem has become clearer. In preparing the current article we were not able to identify any previously documented long-term effects for general population preventive interventions. The current studies extend earlier reports on these universal preventive intervention studies that showed positive longitudinal effects on other drug and alcohol outcomes.[12,13,25] Given the lack of previous preventive intervention outcome research on methamphetamine use, the results of the current study are welcome, indicating the effectiveness of 3 of 4 universal interventions on lifetime or annual methamphetamine use across 2 randomized studies. It is noteworthy in this context that none of the interventions had content specific to the prevention of methamphetamine use; the observed intervention effects were obtained by addressing general risk and protective factors for drug use associated with family and school environments.

Differential outcomes from the ISFP and PDFY interventions in study 1 are noteworthy. Earlier findings do indicate positive PDFY results for other types of substance use.[13] In cases where ISFP has shown stronger effects, the relative differences in effects have been attributed to the higher number of ISFP intervention sessions and the involvement of young adolescents in all of the ISFP sessions, among other factors.[13] Other differential effects were seen in the SFP 10-14 + LST vs control comparisons in contrast with the LST-alone vs control comparison. It was expected that the combination of the family-focused and school-based universal intervention would produce stronger effects than the school-based intervention alone, as was the case for the study 2 11th-grade assessment. Although the relatively stronger effects for the SFP 10-14 + LST were no longer in evidence at the 12th-grade assessment on either measure, the single point at which the differences are observed and the lack of a statistically significant difference between the 2 intervention conditions render it problematic to draw any conclusions about this pattern of results.

Results from studies 1 and 2 underscore the argument for greater emphasis on preventive interventions, particularly universal ones.[3] Epidemiological literature indicates that methamphetamine use has been sustained at the higher levels it attained in the 1990s and that it has been particularly problematic in rural areas, like the settings for the studies reported here. The epidemiology of use in rural midwestern populations suggests it as an important population to target; because no methamphetamine-specific preventive intervention outcome study with rural adolescents was uncovered, the selected samples constitute a strength of the studies reported.

To further address the practical significance of the current findings, it is useful to express those findings in terms of relative reduction of methamphetamine use. Considering lifetime use at the 12th-grade assessment in study 2 for the SFP 10-14 + LST condition as a conservative example, the relative reduction in use was 65%. In practical terms, if such rates held in general population implementation of the intervention in study 2, this relative reduction rate means that for every 100 adolescents in the general population who reported methamphetamine use, there would be only 35 in the intervention population reporting use during that same period. Furthermore, earlier economic analyses of results for study 1, which considered only estimated reductions in costs of alcohol disorders associated with delayed onset of alcohol use among adolescents, estimated a return of $9.60 for every dollar invested in the intervention in the reference case.[30] There is, however, evidence that a substantial percentage of methamphetamine users do not have alcohol disorders.[31] With additional positive effects on the reduction of other drug use, including methamphetamines, it would be reasonable to expect a comparable or higher rate of return, depending on the degree to which the estimated costs of alcohol disorder-related problems also capture costs of methamphetamine abuse for those who abuse both types of substances. Even with the diminution of effect that occurs when preventive interventions are scaled up to the general population, effects are sufficiently strong and sufficiently generalizable that the public health potential of such universal interventions warrants further investigation.

The production of positive results from universal family and school preventive intervention requires high-quality implementation of those interventions, the type of implementation that benefits from effective partnerships among families, schools, and communities.[15,16] As noted earlier, prior reports have demonstrated the key role of partnerships in quality implementation. Moreover, community-based preventive interventions have the advantage of using multifaceted approaches implemented in a manner that are sensitive to local culture and conditions. The community-university partnership-based prevention trials reported here entailed implementation through existing delivery systems, under relatively more "real world" community conditions, in a way that helps overcome barriers to large-scale implementation of evidence-based interventions.[16-18,32] Thus, they allow for greater confidence in the generalizability of the findings to those conditions; also, partnership process evaluations have provided useful information for scaling up the interventions for greater public health impact.[12,14,33,34]

Although the study of prevention of methamphetamine use among rural populations is clearly warranted, there may be a limitation in the degree to which findings generalize to nonrural populations, rural populations in other regions of the country, or populations with different ethnic compositions. Another cautionary note concerns the frequency of methamphetamine use in adolescent populations. First, given the relatively small numbers of adolescents per condition who reported methamphetamine use, specific estimates of use rates are sensitive to small changes in numbers of users, although the observed pattern across time and conditions was generally stable. A related caution concerns the nested structure of the data; that is, students were nested within schools. As noted in the data analysis section, a multilevel analysis was not possible because of the limited numbers of methamphetamine users in the sample. However, there also was an indication it was unnecessary, given minimal evidence of within-school dependence of methamphetamine use rates.

Considering additional necessary steps to be taken in the scaling up of universal preventive interventions, a critically important research question concerns whether positive results would occur when sustained implementation of the universal interventions is solely the province of local implementation teams supported by university-based technical assistance. This question will be addressed in a future study.

**Accepted for Publication:** April 12, 2006.
**Correspondence:** Richard L. Spoth, PhD, Partnerships in Prevention Science Institute, ISU Research Park, Bldg 2, Suite 500, 2625 North Loop Dr, Iowa State University, Ames, IA 50010 (rlspoth@iastate.edu).
**Author Contributions:** *Study concept and design:* Spoth and Redmond. *Acquisition of data:* Spoth. *Analysis and interpretation of data:* Spoth, Clair, Shin, and Redmond. *Drafting of the manuscript:* Spoth and Clair. *Critical revision of the manuscript for important intellectual content:*

Spoth, Clair, Shin, and Redmond. *Statistical analysis:* Clair and Shin. *Obtained funding:* Spoth and Redmond. *Study supervision:* Spoth and Redmond.

**Funding/Support:** This study was supported by research grant DA010815 from the National Institute on Drug Abuse, by grant MH 49217 from the National Institute of Mental Health, and by grant AA 014702 from the National Institute on Alcohol Abuse and Alcoholism.

## REFERENCES

1. Cunningham JK, Thielemeir MA. Trends and regional variations in amphetamine-related emergency admissions: California, 1984-1993. Los Angeles, Calif: Public Statistics Institute; 1995.
2. Wermuth L. Methamphetamine use: hazards and social influences. *J Drug Educ.* 2000;30:423-433.
3. Rawson RA, Anglin MD, Ling W. Will the methamphetamine problem go away? *J Addict Dis.* 2002;21:5-19.
4. Johnston LD, O'Malley PM, Bachman JG. *The Monitoring the Future National Survey Results on Adolescent Drug Use: Overview of Key Findings, 2001* [publication NIH02-5105]. Bethesda, Md: National Institute on Drug Abuse; 2002.
5. Johnston LD, O'Malley PM, Bachman JG, Schulenberg JE. *Monitoring the Future National Results on Adolescent Drug Use: Overview of Key Findings, 2004.* Bethesda, Md: National Institute on Drug Abuse; 2005. http://monitoringthefuture.org/pubs/monographs/overview2004.pdf. Accessed on May 17, 2006.
6. Oetting ER, Deffenbacher JL, Taylor MJ, Luther N, Beauvais F, Edwards RW. Methamphetamine use by high school students: recent trends, gender and ethnicity differences, and use of other drugs. *J Child Adolesc Subst Abuse.* 2000; 10:33-50.
7. Hall JN, Broderick PM. Community networks for response to abuse outbreaks of methamphetamine and its analogs. In: Miller MA, Kozel NJ, eds. *Methamphetamine Abuse: Epidemiologic Issues and Implications* [research monograph No. 115]. Rockville, Md: National Institute on Drug Abuse; 1991.
8. The Methamphetamine Challenge: Threatening Communities Coast-to-Coast [telecast downlink]. US Department of Health and Human Services. SAMSHA National Clearinghouse for Alcohol and Drug Information. June 19, 1997.
9. Spoth RL, Kavanagh K, Dishion T. Family-centered preventive intervention science: toward benefits to larger populations of children, youth, and families. *Prev Sci.* 2002;3:145-152.
10. Romer D, ed. *Reducing Adolescent Risk: Toward an Integrated Approach.* Thousand Oaks, Calif: Sage; 2002.
11. Vakalahi HF. Adolescent substance use and family-based risk and protective factors: a literature review. *J Drug Educ.* 2001;31:29-46.
12. Spoth RL, Redmond C. Project Family prevention trials based in community-university partnerships: toward scaled-up preventive interventions. *Prev Sci.* 2002; 3:203-221.
13. Spoth RL, Redmond C, Shin C. Randomized trial of brief family interventions for general populations: adolescent substance use outcomes 4 years following baseline. *J Consult Clin Psychol.* 2001;69:627-642.
14. Rawson RA, Gonzales R, Brethen P. Treatment of methamphetamine use disorders: an update. *J Subst Abuse Treat.* 2002;23:145-150.
15. Spoth R, Molgaard V. Project Family: a partnership integrating research with the practice of promoting family and youth competencies. In: Chibucos T, Lerner R, eds. *Serving Children and Families Through Community-University Partnerships: Success Stories.* Boston, Mass: Kluwer Academic Publishers; 1999:127-137.
16. Spoth R, Guyll M, Trudeau L, Goldberg-Lillehoj C. Two studies of proximal outcomes and implementation quality of universal preventive interventions in a community-university collaboration context. *J Community Psychol.* 2002;30:499-518.
17. Spoth R, Guyll M, Lillehoj CJ, Redmond C, Greenberg M. PROSPER community-university partnership implementation quality study: toward better translation of science into practice. *J Community Psychol.* In press.
18. Spoth RL, Greenberg MT. Toward a comprehensive strategy for effective practitioner-scientist partnerships and larger-scale community health and well-being. *Am J Community Psychol.* 2005;35:107-126.
19. Altshuler SJ. Drug-endangered children need a collaborative community response. *Child Welfare.* 2005;84:171-190.
20. Spoth R, Greenberg M, Bierman K, Redmond C. PROSPER community-university partnership model for public education systems: capacity-building for evidence-based, competence-building prevention. *Prev Sci.* 2004;5:31-39.
21. Spoth RL, Redmond C, Kahn J, Shin C. A prospective validation study of inclination, belief, and context predictors of family-focused prevention involvement. *Fam Process.* 1997;36:403-429.
22. Catalano RF, Hawkins JD. The Social Development Model: a theory of antisocial behavior. In: Hawkins JD, ed. *Delinquency and Crime: Current Theories.* New York, NY: Cambridge University Press; 1996:149-197.
23. Catalano RF, Kosterman R, Hawkins JD, Newcomb MD, Abbot RD. Modeling the etiology of adolescent substance use: a test of the social development model. *J Drug Issues.* 1996;26:429-455.
24. Molgaard VM, Spoth R, Redmond C. Competency Training: The Strengthening Families Program for Parents and Youth 10-14 [OJJDP Juvenile Justice Bulletin NCJ 182208]. Washington, DC: US Department of Justice, Office of Juvenile Justice and Delinquency Prevention; 2000.
25. Spoth RL, Redmond C, Trudeau L, Shin C. Longitudinal substance initiation outcomes for a universal preventive intervention combining family and school programs. *Psychol Addict Behav.* 2002;16:129-134.
26. Botvin GJ. *Life Skills Training.* Princeton, NJ: Princeton Health Press, Inc; 2000.
27. Botvin GJ, Baker E, Renick NL, Filazzola AD, Botvin EM. A cognitive-behavioral approach to substance abuse prevention. *Addict Behav.* 1984;9:137-147.
28. Snedecor GW, Cochran WG. *Statistical Methods,* 8th ed. Ames, Iowa: Iowa State University Press; 1989.
29. Spoth R, Redmond C, Shin C. Direct and indirect latent-variable parenting outcomes of two universal family-focused preventive interventions: extending a public health-oriented research base. *J Consult Clin Psychol.* 1998;66:385-399.
30. Spoth RL, Guyll M, Day SX. Universal family-focused interventions in alcohol-use disorder prevention: cost-effectiveness and cost-benefit analyses of two interventions. *J Stud Alcohol.* 2002;63:219-228.
31. Simons JS, Oliver MNI, Gaher RM, Ebel G, Brummels P. Methamphetamine and alcohol abuse and dependence symptoms: associations with affect lability and impulsivity in a rural treatment population. *Addict Behav.* 2005;30:1370-1381.
32. Chibucos T, Lerner R, eds. *Serving Children and Families Through Community-University Partnerships: Success Stories.* Boston, Mass: Kluwer Academic Publishers; 1999.
33. Sandler I, Ostrom A, Bitner MJ, Ayers TS, Wolchik S, Daniels VS. Developing effective prevention services for the real world: a prevention service development model. *Am J Community Psychol.* 2005;35:127-142.
34. Klesges LM, Estabrooks PA, Dzewaltowski DA, Bull SS, Glasgow RE. Beginning with the application in mind: designing and planning health behavior change interventions to enhance dissemination. *Ann Behav Med.* 2005;29(suppl):66-75.

**ACIP recommends vaccination of children against hepatitis A*[1]**

# Hepatitis A spreads FAST... especially among children[2,3]

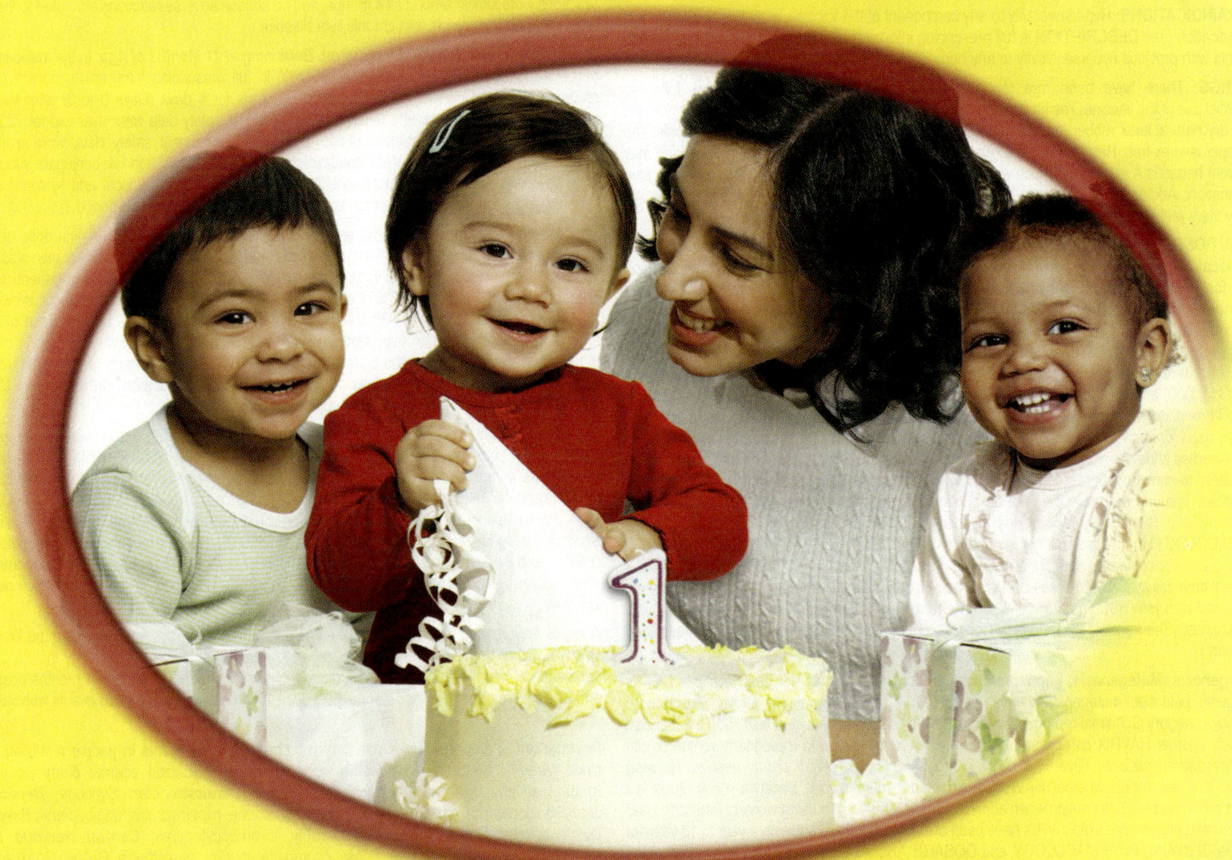

# HAVRIX provides excellent protection

HAVRIX is indicated for active immunization against hepatitis A virus in children 12 months of age and older.

## Important Safety Information

In clinical trials, the most common solicited adverse events were injection-site soreness and headache.

Greater incidences of general adverse events were observed in subjects who received HAVRIX at the same time as Hib conjugate and DTaP vaccines. As with any vaccine, rare adverse events may occur. (See Adverse Reactions section of the Prescribing Information for HAVRIX for potential side effects.) HAVRIX is contraindicated in people with hypersensitivity to any component of the vaccine, including neomycin.

* Advisory Committee on Immunization Practices recommends routine nationwide vaccination against hepatitis A in all children 1–2 years of age.

**Please see references and brief summary of complete prescribing information for HAVRIX on adjacent page.**

HAVRIX is a registered trademark of GlaxoSmithKline.

Manufactured by **GlaxoSmithKline Biologicals**, Rixensart, Belgium
Distributed by **GlaxoSmithKline**, Research Triangle Park, NC 27709

gsk GlaxoSmithKline Vaccines

**Havrix®**
**Hepatitis A Vaccine, Inactivated**

## HAVRIX®
## (Hepatitis A Vaccine, Inactivated)

The following is a brief summary only; see full prescribing information for complete product information.

**INDICATIONS AND USAGE:** HAVRIX is indicated for active immunization of persons ≥12 months of age against disease caused by hepatitis A virus (HAV). Primary immunization should be administered at least 2 weeks prior to expected exposure to HAV. When passive protection against hepatitis A is required either following exposure to hepatitis A virus or in persons requiring both immediate and long-term protection, HAVRIX may be administered concomitantly with immune globulin (IG) with different syringes and at different injection sites. Duration of immunity following a complete vaccination schedule has not been established.

**CONTRAINDICATIONS:** Hypersensitivity to any component of the vaccine, including neomycin, is a contraindication (see DESCRIPTION in full prescribing information). This vaccine is contraindicated in patients with previous hypersensitivity to any hepatitis A-containing vaccine.

**WARNINGS:** There have been rare reports of anaphylaxis/anaphylactoid reactions following commercial use of the vaccine. The tip cap and the rubber plunger of the needleless prefilled syringes contain dry natural latex rubber that may cause allergic reactions in latex sensitive individuals. The vial stopper is latex-free. Hepatitis A has a relatively long incubation period. Hepatitis A vaccine may not prevent hepatitis A infection in those who have an unrecognized hepatitis A infection at the time of vaccination. Additionally, it may not prevent infection in those who do not achieve protective antibody titers (although the lowest titer needed to confer protection has not been determined).

**PRECAUTIONS: General:** Prior to immunization with HAVRIX, the patient's current health status and medical history should be reviewed. The physician should review the patient's immunization history for possible vaccine sensitivity, previous vaccination-related adverse reactions and occurrence of any adverse–event-related symptoms and/or signs, in order to determine the existence of any contraindication to immunization with HAVRIX and to allow an assessment of benefits and risks. Appropriate medical treatment and supervision should be readily available for immediate use in case of a rare anaphylactic reaction following the administration of the vaccine. Epinephrine injection (1:1,000) and other appropriate agents used for the control of immediate allergic reactions must be immediately available. A separate, sterile syringe and needle or a sterile disposable unit should be used for each patient to prevent the transmission of other infectious agents from person to person. Needles should be disposed of properly and should not be recapped. As with any vaccine, if administered to immunosuppressed persons, including those receiving immunosuppressive therapy, the expected immune response may not be obtained. **Drug Interactions:** HAVRIX may be given concurrently with Hib conjugate vaccines in children 15 to 18 months of age (see CLINICAL PHARMACOLOGY in full prescribing information and ADVERSE REACTIONS). The safety of HAVRIX given concomitantly with INFANRIX has been evaluated (see ADVERSE REACTIONS). Insufficient data are available to assess the immune response of a fourth dose of DTaP vaccine when administered with HAVRIX. There are limited data to assess the concomitant use of HAVRIX with other vaccines. (See Immune Response to Concomitantly Administered Vaccines in full prescribing information.)

**Carcinogenesis, Mutagenesis, Impairment of Fertility:** HAVRIX has not been evaluated for its carcinogenic potential, mutagenic potential, or potential for impairment of fertility. **Pregnancy:** Pregnancy Category C. Animal reproduction studies have not been conducted with HAVRIX. It is also not known whether HAVRIX can cause fetal harm when administered to a pregnant woman or can affect reproduction capacity. Give HAVRIX to a pregnant woman only if clearly needed. **Nursing Mothers:** It is not known whether HAVRIX is excreted in human milk. Because many drugs are excreted in human milk, use caution when administering HAVRIX to a nursing woman. **Pediatric Use:** The safety and effectiveness of HAVRIX have been evaluated in 20,436 subjects 1 year to 18 years of age. (See CLINICAL PHARMACOLOGY and DOSAGE AND ADMINISTRATION in full prescribing information.) The safety and effectiveness of HAVRIX have not been established in subjects less than 12 months of age. **Geriatric Use:** Clinical studies of HAVRIX did not include sufficient numbers of subjects 65 years of age and older to determine whether they respond differently from younger subjects. Other reported clinical experience has not identified differences in overall safety between these subjects and younger adult subjects.

**ADVERSE REACTIONS:** As with all pharmaceuticals, however, it is possible that expanded commercial use of the vaccine could reveal rare adverse events. The adverse events most frequently reported by volunteers in clinical trials were injection-site soreness (56% of adults; 21% of children); headache (14% of adults; less than 9% of children). Other solicited and unsolicited events are listed below:

**Incidence 1% to 10% of Injections:** ***Local Reactions at Injection Site:*** Induration, redness, swelling; ***Body as a Whole:*** Fatigue, fever (>37.5°C), malaise; ***Gastrointestinal:*** Anorexia, nausea.

**Incidence <1% of Injections:** ***Local Reaction at Injection Site:*** Hematoma; ***Dermatologic:*** Pruritus, rash, urticaria; ***Respiratory:*** Pharyngitis, other upper respiratory tract infections; ***Gastrointestinal:*** Abdominal pain, diarrhea, dysgeusia, vomiting; ***Musculoskeletal:*** Arthralgia, elevation of creatine phosphokinase, myalgia; ***Hematologic:*** Lymphadenopathy; ***Central Nervous System:*** Hypertonic episode, insomnia, photophobia, vertigo.

**Additional safety data:** Safety data were obtained from 2 additional sources in which large populations were vaccinated. In an outbreak setting in which 4,930 individuals were immunized with a single dose of either 720 EL.U. or 1440 EL.U. of HAVRIX, the vaccine was well tolerated and no serious adverse events due to vaccination were reported. Overall, less than 10% of vaccinees reported solicited general adverse events following the vaccine. The most common solicited local adverse event was pain at the injection site, reported in 22.3% of subjects at 24 hours and decreasing to 2.4% by 72 hours.

In a field efficacy trial, 19,037 children received the 360 EL.U. dose of HAVRIX. The most commonly reported adverse events were injection-site pain (9.5%) and tenderness (8.1%), reported following first doses of HAVRIX. Other adverse events were infrequent and comparable to the control vaccine ENGERIX-B® [Hepatitis B Vaccine (Recombinant)].

In subjects with chronic liver disease, HAVRIX was safe and well tolerated. Local injection site reactions were similar among all 4 groups, and no serious adverse reactions attributed to the vaccine were reported in subjects with chronic liver disease.

***Safety Data for HAVRIX 720 EL.U./0.5 mL Beginning at 11 Months of Age:*** In the multicenter study described under CLINICAL PHARMACOLOGY in full prescribing information, parents/guardians recorded local and general symptoms on diary cards for 4 days (Days 0 to 3) after vaccination. In the 3 groups of children who received HAVRIX alone, safety data were available for 723 children who received 1,396 documented doses of HAVRIX. Additional safety data were available for 181 children who received HAVRIX coadministered with INFANRIX and Hib conjugate vaccine. Most adverse events were mild and transient. The frequencies of solicited local and systemic reactions following receipt of HAVRIX were monitored during the 4-day observation period.

The following rates of solicited adverse events in children who received their first dose of HAVRIX alone at between 11 and 25 months of age were observed. Among local reactions: pain was reported in 15-21% of subjects, redness in 16-21%, swelling in 8% of subjects. Among general reactions, irritability was reported in 24-36% of subjects, loss of appetite in 16-19% of subjects, drowsiness in 15-17% of subjects and fever >39.5°C in ≤2% of subjects. Following the booster dose of HAVRIX, among local reactions: pain was reported in 16-21% of subjects, redness in 17-22%, swelling in 8-10% of subjects. Following the booster dose of HAVRIX, among general reactions, irritability was reported in 19-29% of subjects, loss of appetite in 14-18% of subjects, drowsiness in 13-16% of subjects and fever >39.5°C in ≤1% of subjects.

Drowsiness and loss of appetite occurred at statistically significantly higher rates in subjects 15 to 18 months of age who received Hib conjugate vaccine (PRP-T) and INFANRIX concomitantly with HAVRIX as compared to subjects 15 to 18 months of age who received Hib conjugate vaccine (PRP-T) and INFANRIX (drowsiness 34% and 22% and loss of appetite 29% and 19%, respectively). With the exception of fever (>39.5°C), the solicited general symptoms occurred at statistically significantly higher rates in subjects 15 to 18 months of age who received Hib conjugate vaccine (PRP-T) and INFANRIX concomitantly with HAVRIX as compared to subjects 15 to 18 months of age who received HAVRIX alone (irritability 46% and 30%, drowsiness 34% and 17%, and loss of appetite 29% and 17%, respectively).

A febrile seizure was reported in an 18-month old subject two days after receiving the first dose of HAVRIX. Other serious adverse events reported during the course of this study included a single case each of hepatitis ~5 months post dose 1, insulin-dependent diabetes ~4 months post dose 1, and Kawasaki's disease ~3 1/2 months post dose 1. The association of these events with vaccination is unknown.

**Postmarketing Reports:** Rare voluntary reports of adverse events in people receiving HAVRIX since market introduction include the following: ***Local:*** Localized edema; ***Body as a Whole:*** Anaphylaxis/anaphylactoid reactions, somnolence; ***Cardiovascular:*** Syncope; ***Hepatobiliary:*** Jaundice, hepatitis; ***Dermatologic:*** Erythema multiforme, hyperhydrosis, angioedema; ***Respiratory:*** Dyspnea; ***Hematologic:*** Lymphadenopathy, thrombocytopenia; ***Central Nervous System:*** Convulsions, encephalopathy, dizziness, neuropathy, myelitis, paresthesia, Guillain-Barré syndrome, multiple sclerosis; ***Other:*** Congenital abnormality.

The US Department of Health and Human Services has established the Vaccine Adverse Events Reporting System (VAERS) to accept reports of suspected adverse events after the administration of any vaccine, including, but not limited to, the reporting of events required by the National Childhood Vaccine Injury Act of 1986. The toll-free number for VAERS forms and information is 1-800-822-7967. Reporting forms may also be obtained at the VAERS website at www.vaers.org.

Manufactured by **GlaxoSmithKline Biologicals**, Rixensart, Belgium

Distributed by **GlaxoSmithKline**, Research Triangle Park, NC 27709



BRS-HA:L20

**References: 1.** Centers for Disease Control and Prevention. Recommended childhood and adolescent immunization schedule—United States, 2006. *MMWR.* 2006;54(51&52):Q1–Q4. **2.** Bell BP, Shapiro CN. Hepatitis A virus. In: Long SS, Pickering LK, Prober CG, eds. *Principles and Practice of Pediatric Infectious Diseases.* 2nd ed. Philadelphia, Pa: Churchill Livingstone; 2003:1188–1192. **3.** Armstrong GL, Bell BP. Hepatitis A virus infection in the United States: model-based estimates and implication for childhood immunizations. *Pediatrics.* 2002;109:839–845.



Printed in USA. HAP283R0 February 2006

# Televised Movie Trailers

## *Undermining Restrictions on Advertising Tobacco to Youth*

*Cheryl G. Healton, DrPH; Ella S. Watson-Stryker, BA; Jane Appleyard Allen, MA; Donna M. Vallone, PhD; Peter A. Messeri, PhD; Philip R. Graham, MBS; Anna M. Stewart, BS; M. David Dobbins, JD; Stanton A. Glantz, PhD*

**Objective:** To determine the proportion of televised movie trailers that included images of tobacco use during 1 year and the extent of youth exposure to those trailers.

**Design:** Content analysis combined with Nielsen data measuring media exposure. All movie trailers (N = 216) shown on television from August 1, 2001, through July 31, 2002.

**Main Outcome Measures:** Exposure among youth aged 12 to 17 years to televised movie trailers that included smoking imagery.

**Results:** Of the movie trailers televised during the study period, 14.4% (31 trailers) included images of tobacco use. Tobacco use was shown in 24.0% of the 23 trailers for R-rated (restricted) movies and 7.5% of the 8 trailers for PG-13– and PG-rated (parental guidance) movies. Ninety-five percent of all youth aged 12 to 17 years in the United States saw at least 1 movie trailer depicting tobacco use on television during this 1 year, and 88.8% saw at least 1 of these trailers 3 or more times.

**Conclusions:** Nearly all US youth aged 12 to 17 years were exposed to images of tobacco use on television in the context of a movie trailer during the study period. Given the relationship between youth exposure to tobacco use in movies and smoking initiation, the public health community should work to enact policy to reduce or eliminate the influence of tobacco use in televised movie trailers.

*Arch Pediatr Adolesc Med. 2006;160:885-888*

**Author Affiliations:** American Legacy Foundation, Washington, DC (Drs Healton and Vallone, Mss Watson-Stryker, Allen, and Stewart, and Mr Dobbins); Department of Sociomedical Sciences, Columbia University, Mailman School of Public Health, New York, NY (Drs Healton and Messeri); Center for Tobacco Control Research and Education and Department of Medicine, University of California, San Francisco (Dr Glantz); and Mother, New York (Mr Graham).

ALTHOUGH TOBACCO ADVERTISING was banned from television in 1971,[1] tobacco use can still be seen across a spectrum of programming, including televised movie trailers (movie advertisements aired on television). Trailers pair tobacco use with popular movie stars and edgy action shots. These images translate into positive images of tobacco that are conveyed to a broad audience, including a large population younger than 18 years. To our knowledge, this is the first study to examine the extent of youth exposure to tobacco use in televised movie trailers.

This research is conducted in the context of a growing body of literature on the prevalence of tobacco use in movies and the association between exposure to tobacco use in movies and youth smoking.[2] Recent research indicates that images of tobacco use in movies are common,[3] even in youth-oriented movies,[4-7] and that youth are exposed to and recall these tobacco images.[8] The most recent data regarding prevalence of smoking in movies are from a 2004 study by Polansky and Glantz.[9] This study, which includes all US-produced, live-action movies released from 1999 through 2003, indicates that 90% of R-rated (restricted) movies, 80% of PG-13–rated movies, and 50% of PG- and G-rated movies include images of smoking (PG-13 indicates parents strongly cautioned; PG, parental guidance suggested; and G, general audiences).[9]

A number of studies have documented the relationship between exposure to movie stars' use of tobacco in films and youth smoking initiation or susceptibility to tobacco use.[10-14] Pechmann and Shih[10] demonstrated that ninth grade nonsmokers who watched a movie in which the lead characters smoke were more likely to report intentions to smoke compared with their peers who watched the same movie from which the smoking images had been removed. This study showed that seeing an antitobacco advertisement before viewing the movie eradicated this association.[10] A 1999 survey of more than 6000 youth by Distefan et al[11] found tobacco use of favorite movie stars to be associated with youth smoking status.[11] A longitudinal study expanding on this research demonstrated that, among girls who did not smoke at baseline, those with a favorite movie star who smoked had double the risk of smoking 3 years later.[12] Girls may be more likely than boys to see role models smoking; a study by Escamilla et al[14] shows that female stars smoke as often in PG- and PG-13–rated movies as they do in R-rated movies.

Frequency of exposure to tobacco use in movies also has a role in susceptibility to smoking. Sargent et al[15] demonstrated a positive, dose-response association between exposure to tobacco use in movies and susceptibility to smoking. Longitudinal follow-up of these students more than a year later indicated that 17% of those in the highest quartile of exposure had begun smoking compared with 3% of those in the lowest quartile. Multivariate analysis indicated that 52% of these initiations were a result of having seen tobacco use in movies.[16] A recent national cross-sectional study[17] confirmed these results.

The goals of this study were to determine the proportion of movie trailers televised during a 1-year period from August 1, 2001, to July 31, 2002, that included images of tobacco use and to assess the extent of youth exposure to those trailers. The public health community is urged to work for the enactment of policy that will reduce or eliminate youth exposure to televised images of tobacco use in movie trailers.

## METHODS

### SAMPLE

The sample for this study consisted of all movie trailers (movie advertisements aired on television) televised in the United States from August 1, 2001, through July 31, 2002. Only trailers advertising movies released to theaters were included in the sample. Video Monitoring Service, a media content monitoring company used by corporations to assess their marketing and public relations efforts, was hired to identify all of the movie trailers televised during this period. The trailers were also purchased from Video Monitoring Service so they could be analyzed for this study. The analysis included the full-length, uncut versions of each of the trailers. The final sample included 216 trailers.

### CONTENT AND STATISTICAL ANALYSIS

A content analysis of the trailers was conducted to determine whether they included images of tobacco use. Tobacco use was defined as use of any tobacco product by any character. The tobacco product (eg, cigarette or pipe) had to be clearly displayed to be registered as an instance of tobacco use; visible smoke from an unseen source was not considered tobacco use. Each trailer was viewed and coded twice, each time by a different trained analyst (E.S.W.-S. and A.M.S.) working independently. Differences in tobacco use coding occurred in 5 instances. In these 5 cases, the trailers were reexamined by the analysts and differences were resolved. Simple frequencies were calculated to determine the proportion of trailers that included images of tobacco use, overall and by movie rating, and tabulated with Stata 7 software (StataCorp, College Station, Tex).

### MEASUREMENT OF EXPOSURE

Youth exposure to the trailers that included images of smoking was measured using gross rating points (GRPs) and gross impressions among youth aged 12 to 17 years. Gross rating points are the standard unit of measurement for television exposure and are a function of the reach of an advertisement multiplied by the frequency with which the target audience was exposed to it. Advertisement reach is a measure of the scope of the target audience; that is, it describes the population that is exposed to the advertisement. Frequency is a measure of the number of times individuals in the target audience are exposed to an advertisement. One GRP equals 1% of exposure among the intended audience, on average. For example, if a movie trailer aired at 250 GRPs, everyone in the target audience saw it, on average, 2.5 times. Gross impressions represent the number of times an advertisement was seen by the collective target audience. Data were purchased from Nielsen Media Research, the primary source of television ratings in the United States, used by all major television broadcasters to assess program performance and to set prices for advertising. Nielsen data are reported as they were received, with no additional analysis conducted.

## RESULTS

Overall, of the 216 movie trailers televised from August 1, 2001, through July 31, 2002, 14.4% (31 trailers) included images of tobacco use. Tobacco use was most common in trailers advertising R-rated movies: 24.0% of R-rated movie trailers (23 trailers) included images of tobacco use. Among trailers for PG-13– and PG-rated movies, 7.5% (8 trailers) included tobacco use. There were no images of tobacco use in trailers for G-rated movies.

Nielsen data indicate that 95.0% of all youth aged 12 to 17 years in the United States saw at least 1 movie trailer depicting tobacco use on television during this 1 year (**Table**). Nearly 89.0% (88.8%) of these youth saw at least 1 of these trailers 3 or more times. In total, these 31 trailers generated more than 270 million impressions among US youth aged 12 to 17 years. This means that, over the course of a single year, movie trailers showing tobacco use were seen 270 million times among youth aged 12 to 17 years. At 11 090 GRPs, this translates into 111 advertisement exposures per youth, on average. The trailer for the PG-13–rated movie *The Sum of All Fears,* which contained numerous images of smoking, alone achieved more than 48 million impressions among 91.1% of all US youth aged 12 to 17 years. In terms of GRPs, this means that the advertisement was seen 20 times per youth, on average.

## COMMENT

This study demonstrates that nearly all youth in the United States see tobacco use on television in the context of movie trailers. All available research suggests that these images increase the likelihood of tobacco use among youth. For most youth, tobacco use will be cigarette smoking, and among those who smoke, one third will eventually die of tobacco-related disease.[18,19] To reduce the number of today's youth who will ultimately die as a result of tobacco use, the influence of televised movie trailers on youth smoking must be addressed.

There are 2 steps the public health community should take to reduce or eliminate the influence of tobacco use in televised movie trailers. First, the public health community should call on the motion picture industry to eliminate tobacco imagery from movie trailers. There is precedent for such a recommendation: in 2000, the Federal Trade

**Table. Exposure of Youth Aged 12 to 17 Years to Tobacco Use in Movie Trailers Televised From August 1, 2001, Through July 31, 2002***

| Movie (Rating)† | Gross Rating Points | Gross Impressions | Saw Trailer ≥1 Times, % | Saw Trailer ≥3 Times, % |
|---|---|---|---|---|
| *The Sum of All Fears* (PG-13) | 1967 | 48 391 398 | 91 | 83 |
| *Zoolander* (PG-13) | 1149 | 28 265 400 | 89 | 76 |
| *Big Fat Liar* (PG) | 1144 | 28 142 400 | 90 | 80 |
| *Reign of Fire* (PG-13) | 1000 | 24 597 294 | 87 | 73 |
| *Black Hawk Down* (R) | 860 | 21 163 380 | 88 | 75 |
| *How High* (R) | 830 | 20 418 000 | 87 | 73 |
| *A Beautiful Mind* (PG-13) | 721 | 17 736 600 | 86 | 70 |
| *Baby Boy* (R) | 583 | 14 339 340 | 85 | 66 |
| *Slackers* (R) | 550 | 13 530 000 | 85 | 64 |
| *Hart's War* (R) | 528 | 12 979 944 | 84 | 63 |
| *The Majestic* (PG) | 476 | 11 709 600 | 83 | 61 |
| *The Royal Tenenbaums* (R) | 370 | 9 104 460 | 78 | 50 |
| *The Wash* (R) | 268 | 6 596 244 | 73 | 40 |
| *Deuces Wild* (R) | 265 | 6 510 636 | 74 | 41 |
| *The Curse of the Jade Scorpion* (PG-13) | 214 | 5 264 400 | 68 | 33 |
| *Birthday Girl* (R) | 139 | 3 429 732 | 60 | 20 |
| *Y Tu Mama Tambien* (R) | 17 | 410 328 | 14 | 0 |
| *The Man Who Wasn't There* (R) | 5 | 123 000 | 5 | 0 |
| *Happy Accidents* (R) | 3 | 73 800 | 3 | 0 |
| *Big Bad Love* (R) | 1 | 22 878 | 1 | 0 |
| **Total** | **11 090** | **272 808 834** | 95 | 89 |

Abbreviations: PG, parental guidance suggested; PG-13, parents strongly cautioned; R, restricted.
*Data from Nielsen ADVIEWS, Nielsen Media Research, 2005.
†The following movie trailers generated no gross rating points (and minimal gross impressions) among youth aged 12 to 17 years: *High Heels and Low Lifes* (R); *The Devil's Backbone* (R); *Devious Beings* (R); *Greenfingers* (R); *Crush* (R); *How To Kill Your Neighbor's Dog* (R); *The Importance of Being Earnest* (PG); *Lantana* (R); *Proof of Life* (R); *The Salton Sea* (R); *Sexy Beast* (R).

Commission found that the motion picture industry was intentionally marketing violent, R-rated movies to children and teenagers.[20] The recommendation of the investigating committee was to "establish or expand codes that prohibit target marketing to children and impose sanctions for violations."[20(p54)] The Federal Trade Commission recommended that the industry trade associations "monitor and encourage their members' compliance with these policies and impose meaningful sanctions for noncompliance."[20(p54)] A 2004 update on progress in this area showed little change on the part of the motion picture industry.[21] The public health community should join with those who would like to see the 2000 Federal Trade Commission recommendation enforced and should insist that the recommendation be expanded to prevent youth exposure to tobacco imagery in all motion picture marketing, including televised movie trailers.

Second, the public health community should call on networks to refuse to air movie trailers that include smoking imagery. Network standards and practices groups routinely disallow content that is considered inappropriate. Because recent research suggests that televised movie trailers function as de facto tobacco advertisements in terms of their effect on public health, networks should be urged to treat them as they would traditional tobacco advertising.

Because of the consolidation of the media industry, parent companies in many cases own both motion picture companies and a major television network. Working toward the aforementioned policies should, therefore, exert pressure on these companies from 2 fronts, which may provide the incentive needed to change practices regarding airing images of smoking. Taking these important first steps to reduce youth exposure to televised images of tobacco use could prevent many youth from smoking.

The extent of youth exposure to tobacco use via televised trailers described here is likely an underestimate. This study incorporates data only for youth aged 12 to 17 years, although children younger than 12 years are also exposed to these images. Exposure of youth younger than 12 years to these images may have an even greater influence on their future tobacco use behavior than it does on older youth.

This study focuses on a single media channel: televised movie trailers. However, images of tobacco use appear to be common throughout other television programming. Future research should document the extent to which youth are exposed to images of tobacco use through other television programming, and policies to prevent youth from being exposed to televised tobacco images should ultimately include all relevant television programming.

**Accepted for Publication:** March 24, 2006.
**Correspondence:** Jane Appleyard Allen, MA, American Legacy Foundation, 2030 M St NW, Sixth Floor, Washington, DC 20036 (jallen@americanlegacy.org).
**Author Contributions:** Dr Healton had full access to all the data in the study and takes responsibility for the integrity of the data and the accuracy of the data analysis. *Study concept and design:* Healton, Watson-Stryker,

Vallone, Messeri, and Glantz. *Acquisition of data:* Watson-Stryker, Graham, and Stewart. *Analysis and interpretation of data:* Allen and Dobbins. *Drafting of the manuscript:* Healton, Watson-Stryker, and Allen. *Critical revision of the manuscript for important intellectual content:* Healton, Watson-Stryker, Allen, Messeri, Graham, Stewart, Dobbins, and Glantz. *Statistical analysis:* Messeri, Graham, and Glantz. *Administrative, technical, and material support:* Watson-Stryker, Allen, Stewart, and Dobbins. *Study supervision:* Allen and Vallone.

**Funding/Support:** This study was supported by the American Legacy Foundation and by grant CA-61021 from the National Cancer Institute.

**Acknowledgment:** We thank Kelly Healton at Columbia University, New York, NY, and Margaret Brown at the University of Wisconsin, Madison, for assistance with this study.

## REFERENCES

1. US Department of Health and Human Services. *Reducing the Health Consequences of Smoking: 25 Years of Progress: A Report of the Surgeon General.* Rockville, Md: US Dept of Health and Human Services, Public Health Service, Centers for Disease Control and Prevention, Center for Chronic Disease Prevention and Health Promotion, Office on Smoking and Health; 1989. DHHS Publication No. (CDC)89-8411.
2. Sargent JD. Smoking in movies: impact on adolescent smoking. *Adolesc Med Clin.* 2005;16:345-370.
3. Dalton MA, Tickle JJ, Sargent JD, Beach ML, Ahrens MB, Heatherton TF. The incidence and context of tobacco use in popular movies from 1988 to 1997. *Prev Med.* 2002;34:516-523.
4. Charlesworth A, Glantz SA. Smoking in the movies increases adolescent smoking: a review. *Pediatrics.* 2005;116:1516-1528.
5. Goldstein AO, Sobel RA, Newman GR. Tobacco and alcohol use in G-rated children's animated films. *JAMA.* 1999;28:1131-1136.
6. Thompson KM, Yokota F. Depiction of alcohol, tobacco, and other substances in G-rated animated feature movies. *Pediatrics.* 2001;107:1369-1374.
7. Mekemson C, Glik D, Titus K, et al. Tobacco use in popular movies during the past decade. *Tob Control.* 2004;13:400-402.
8. Centers for Disease Control and Prevention. Tobacco use, access and exposure to tobacco in the media among middle and high school students: United States, 2004. *MMWR Morb Mortal Wkly Rep.* 2005;54:297-301.
9. Polansky JR, Glantz SA. First-run smoking presentations in U.S. movies 1999-2003. University of California, San Francisco: Center for Tobacco Control Research and Education;2004. http://repositories.cdlib.org/ctcre/tcpmus/Movies2004/. Accessed November 14, 2005.
10. Pechmann C, Shih CF. Smoking scenes in movies and antismoking advertisements before movies: effects on youth. *J Mark.* 1999;63:1-13.
11. Distefan JM, Gilpin EA, Sargent JD, Pierce JP. Do movie stars encourage adolescents to start smoking? evidence from California. *Prev Med.* 1999;28:1-11.
12. Distefan JM, Pierce JP, Gilpin EA. Do favorite movie stars influence adolescent smoking initiation? [published correction appears in *Am J Public Health.* 2004;94:1296]. *Am J Public Health.* 2004;94:1239-1244.
13. Tickle JJ, Sargent JD, Dalton MA, Beach ML, Heatherton TF. Favourite movie stars, their tobacco use in contemporary movies, and its association with adolescent smoking. *Tob Control.* 2001;10:16-22.
14. Escamilla G, Cradock AL, Kawachi I. Women and smoking in Hollywood movies: a content analysis. *Am J Public Health.* 2000;90:412-414.
15. Sargent JD, Dalton MA, Beach ML, et al. Viewing tobacco use in movies: does it shape attitudes that mediate adolescent smoking? *Am J Prev Med.* 2002;22:137-145.
16. Dalton MA, Sargent JD, Beach ML, et al. Effect of viewing smoking in movies on adolescent smoking initiation: a cohort study. *Lancet.* 2003;362:281-285.
17. Sargent JD, Beach ML, Adachi-Mejia AM, et al. Exposure to movie smoking: its relation to smoking initiation among US adolescents. *Pediatrics.* 2005;116:1183-1191.
18. Centers for Disease Control and Prevention. Tobacco use among middle and high school students: United States, 2002. *MMWR Morb Mortal Wkly Rep.* 2003;512:1096-1098.
19. Centers for Disease Control and Prevention. Projected smoking-related deaths among youth. *MMWR Morb Mortal Wkly Rep.* 1996;45:971-974.
20. Federal Trade Commission. *Marketing Violent Entertainment to Children: A Review of Self-regulation and Industry Practices in the Motion Picture, Music Recording and Electronic Game Industries: Report of the Federal Trade Commission*; September 2000.
21. Federal Trade Commission. *Marketing Violent Entertainment to Children: A Fourth Follow-up Review of Industry Practices in the Motion Picture, Music Recording and Electronic Game Industries: A report to Congress*; July 2004.

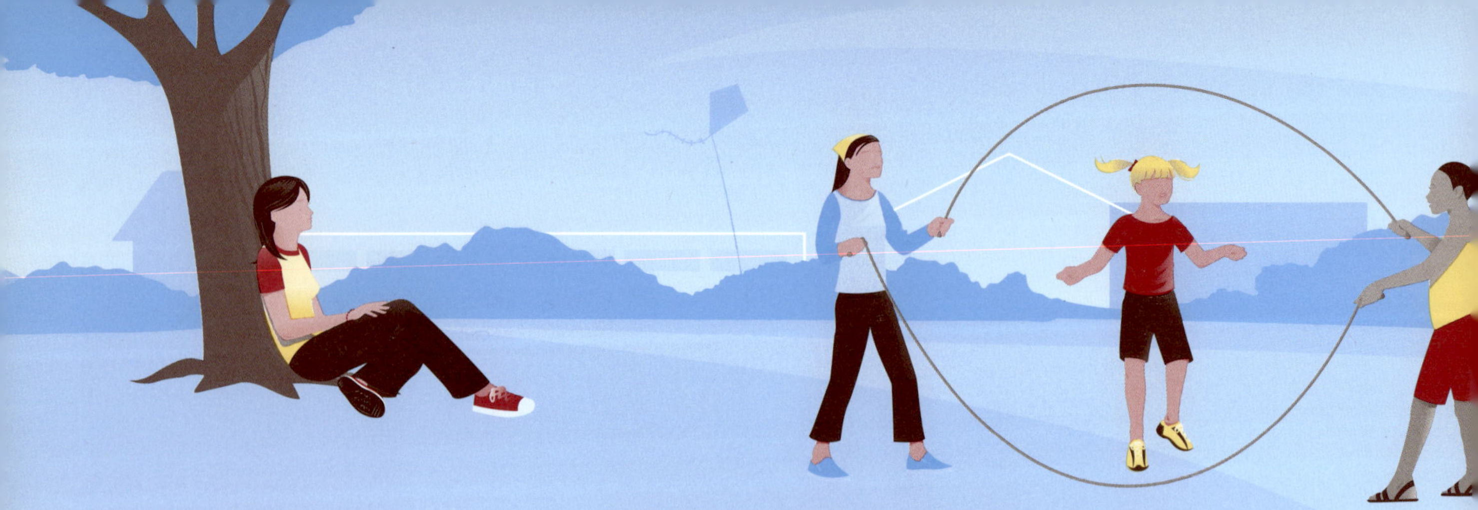

# Introducing GARDASIL—helping you

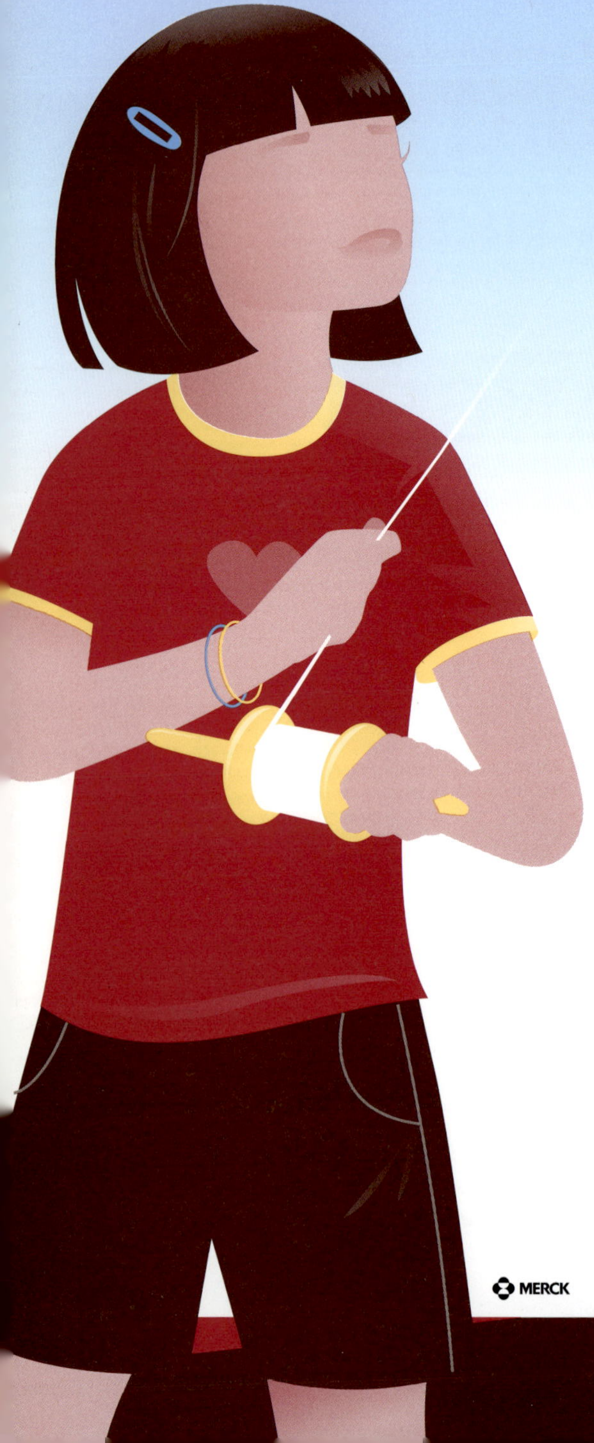

- GARDASIL is a vaccine indicated in girls and women 9 to 26 years of age for the prevention of cervical cancer, precancerous or dysplastic lesions, and genital warts caused by human papillomavirus (HPV) Types 6, 11, 16, and 18.
- A complete vaccination regimen of GARDASIL consists of a 3-dose schedule.

## Select safety information

GARDASIL is contraindicated in individuals who are hypersensitive to the active substances or to any of the excipients of the vaccine.

GARDASIL does not substitute for routine cervical cancer screening, and women who receive GARDASIL should continue to undergo screening per standard of care.

Vaccination with GARDASIL may not result in protection in all vaccine recipients.

GARDASIL is not intended to be used for treatment of active genital warts; cervical cancer; cervical intraepithelial neoplasia, vulvar intraepithelial neoplasia, or vaginal intraepithelial neoplasia.

To place an order, call **1-800-MERCK-RX,** or visit **www.MerckVaccines.com.**

MERCK

# Effect of Open Access Scheduling on Missed Appointments, Immunizations, and Continuity of Care for Infant Well-Child Care Visits

*Mary E. O'Connor, MD, MPH; Bethany S. Matthews, MSPH; Dexiang Gao, PhD*

**Objective:** To examine the effect of open access scheduling (OA) on infant well-child care (WCC).

**Design:** Cluster randomization of 2 methods of OA compared with a baseline group (prior to OA).

**Setting:** Community health center pediatric clinic, August 1, 2003, to January 31, 2004.

**Participants:** Ten providers (pediatricians and physician assistants) and 878 infants; 2-, 4-, and 6-month WCC visits were scheduled.

**Interventions:** Two scheduling methods were compared under the OA model: the OA future visit group scheduled their infant's next WCC visit when leaving the visit, and the OA same day group called for a same-day appointment.

**Main Outcome Measures:** Missed appointment rates, on-time immunization rates, and continuity of care.

**Results:** Missed appointment rates decreased from 21% in the baseline group to 14% and 9% in the OA future visit and OA same day groups, respectively ($P<.02$). For 630 infants older than 5 months at study end, on-time immunization rates were 59% in the baseline group and 74% in both OA groups ($P<.006$). Of 412 infants with 2 or more WCC visits, 75% in the OA future visit group and 60% in the OA same day group saw the same provider for all visits ($P=.001$). This difference was due to differences among providers, not to the different scheduling methods.

**Conclusion:** Open access scheduling decreases missed appointments for infant WCC visits and appears to increase on-time immunizations.

*Arch Pediatr Adolesc Med. 2006;160:889-893*

**Author Affiliations:** Denver Health (Dr O'Connor and Ms Matthews), Departments of Pediatrics (Dr O'Connor) and Family Medicine (Ms Matthews), University of Colorado School of Medicine, and The Research Institute, The Children's Hospital (Dr Gao), Denver.

OPEN ACCESS SCHEDULING (OA) is an appointment scheduling system that attempts to provide access to care at the time it is needed.[1,2] In OA, when a parent calls to schedule a well-child care (WCC) visit, the patient receives an appointment within 1 to 2 days. When OA is not used, the next available WCC visit appointment is often in 4 to 6 weeks. In OA, since more than 50% of appointments are available for the same day, ill children can receive a same-day appointment without overbooking. Overbooking usually results in long wait times. Without overbooking, doctors' time may not be filled because of cancellations or missed appointments. Open access scheduling was developed in the early 1990s to address these issues.[1-3] Open access scheduling systems have decreased missed appointment rates, improved continuity of care, and improved patient satisfaction.[2,4-6] We found no published data on the effect of OA on infant WCC visits.

Immunization rates, a marker of effective pediatric care, remain lower than the Healthy People 2010 goal of 90% of all children aged 19 to 35 months having received 4 diphtheria and tetanus toxoids and acellular pertussis vaccines; 3 inactivated poliovirus vaccines; 1 measles, mumps, and rubella vaccine; 3 *Haemophilus influenzae* type b vaccines; 3 hepatitis B vaccines; and 1 varicella vaccine (4:3:1:3:3:1). Despite use of immunization registries,[7] improved insurance coverage,[8] and reminder recall systems for parents and health care professionals,[9-13] only 76% of 19- to 35-month-old children had completed the 4:3:1:3:3:1 series in 2004.[14] Parents report that inability to get timely appointments impedes their ability to get care.[15,16] The National Vaccine Advisory Committee recommends minimizing delays in scheduling appointments to improve immunization rates.[17] If OA improves access to care and decreases missed appointment rates, immunization rates should improve. If parents forget to call

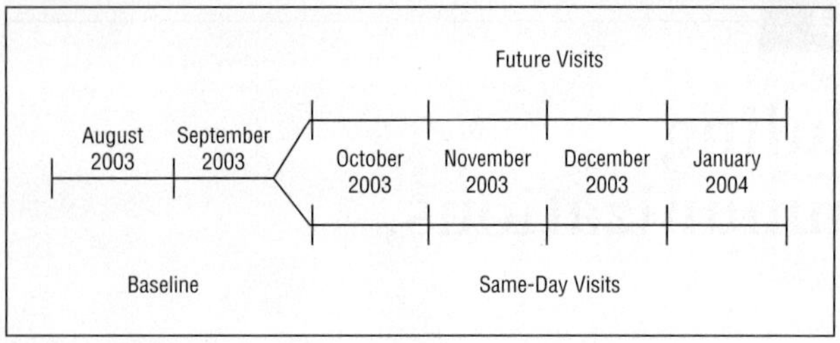


**Figure.** Timeline for open access study.

for an appointment in OA, immunization rates might decrease. We found no published data on the effect of OA on immunization rates or whether it is better to schedule infant WCC visits in advance compared with same-day scheduling.

The hypotheses for this project include: (1) The missed appointment rate for WCC visits will be reduced from the estimated baseline (non-OA) rate of 25% to 16% in OA. (2) There will be no difference in on-time immunizations in the baseline group compared with the OA group.

## METHODS

### STUDY SETTING AND POPULATION

This study was conducted in a pediatric clinic of a community health center, Westside Family Health Center (WFHC), that is part of Denver Health, an integrated health system. The system includes a safety-net hospital, 9 community health centers, and other entities. The WFHC clinic is staffed by pediatricians, physician assistants, residents, and support staff. More than 25 000 immunizations are administered annually at approximately 25 000 visits. About two thirds of the patients have Medicaid, one third are uninsured, and less than 5% have commercial insurance. The patients are largely of Mexican origin. Prior to the start of OA in October 2003, all infants were scheduled for the next 2-, 4-, or 6-month WCC visit at the end of the prior visit.

### BASELINE PERIOD

For the 2 months preceding the change to OA, missed appointments and immunizations were tracked for all infants scheduled for 2-, 4-, and 6-month WCC visits.

### OPEN ACCESS PERIOD

Ten pediatricians and physician assistants caring for infants were divided into 4 groups of 2 or 4 providers each by sessions worked per week, Spanish-language fluency, and education (physician assistant or physician degree). Residents and pediatricians not working throughout the study period were excluded. Half of each group was randomized (by cluster) to the OA future visit group. Families needing a 2-, 4-, or 6-month WCC visit prescheduled their next appointment (same scheduling system as during baseline). The other half was randomized to the OA same day group, whose families called for an appointment the week it was needed. Informed consent was obtained from all providers.

The clinic began OA for all patients on October 1, 2003. Beginning at the 2-week WCC visit, providers in the OA future visit group gave parents an appointment slip for the clerk to schedule their next appointment prior to leaving the clinic. Providers in the OA same day group gave parents a reminder slip with their pediatrician's or physician assistant's name and the proper week to call for their infant's next appointment. Under OA, 50% to 75% of appointments were available at the beginning of each day.

Standard procedures for infant WCC visits included the following:

- Standardized forms were used to document WCC visits.
- At all clinic visits, the Denver Health immunization registry was queried. Immunization history and recommended immunizations were printed for the provider to review.
- The immunization registry printed recall postcards that were mailed monthly when infants were more than 30 days overdue for immunizations. Mailings were repeated every 3 months until the appropriate immunizations were recorded or the infant was inactivated from the registry.
- When infants did not attend a WCC visit, the medical assistant made a telephone call or sent a postcard to remind parents to reschedule.
- Standard immunizations for infants during the study included the administration of combined diphtheria and tetanus toxoids and acellular pertussis–inactivated poliovirus–hepatitis B vaccine, *H influenzae* type b vaccine, and 7-valent pneumococcal conjugate vaccine at 2-, 4-, and 6-month WCC visits.

### DATA COLLECTION

Data were collected for all infants attending 2-, 4-, and 6-month WCC visits from August through September 2003 (baseline) and during the first 4 months of OA from October 1, 2003, through January 31, 2004 (**Figure**). All data were collected from computerized information systems. The clerks scheduling appointments noted which infants were scheduled for 2-, 4-, or 6-month WCC visits. On a biweekly basis during the study, 1 research assistant searched the daily schedule for each study provider. For any patient having a 2-, 4-, or 6-month WCC appointment, the medical record number, patient name, provider name, visit date, date the appointment was scheduled, and appointment attendance were recorded in a spreadsheet. The date of birth, sex, insurance, and race/ethnicity (by parental report) were collected from registration data. The immunization registry was checked for immunizations administered. Data were generally collected within 2 weeks of the visit date.

Any infant who had a 2-, 4-, or 6-month WCC visit scheduled with 1 of the study providers during the study period was included. Infants completed the study when they received their 6-month immunizations or on January 31, 2004, whichever came first. After January 31, 2004, the immunization registry was queried on all children whose immunizations were not up-to-date. Immunizations given at nonstudy visits or given elsewhere were included in the data collection and analysis. At the end of data collection, the patient name and hospital number were removed to deidentify the data.

### DATA ANALYSIS

Statistical analysis was performed using SPSS for Windows version 12.0 (SPSS Inc, Chicago, Ill) and SAS version 8.2 (SAS Institute Inc, Cary, NC).[18] Categorical variables were compared by $\chi^2$ test, and nonnormally distributed continuous variables were compared by Kruskal-Wallis test.

Ethnic group was reported by families as Hispanic; however, it was transformed into Mexican American based on prior research at WFHC. Providers were identified as being fluent in Spanish or not. Insurance was dichotomized into having any insurance (Medicaid, State Children's Health Insurance Program, or private insurance) vs self-pay or being a Medicaid applicant. When insurance was used as a variable in the regression models for analysis of immunization rates and continuity of care, the insurance status at the last appointment was used.

Three outcomes were analyzed. The missed appointment status was tabulated for each scheduled visit. Repeated logistic regression was used to examine the effect of the risk variables, group (baseline, OA future visit, and OA same day), insurance status, and Spanish-speaking provider on the missed appointment status. Correlation due to the repeated measurements on the same subjects (possible 2-, 4-, and 6-month visits) was taken into account during modeling.[19]

On-time immunization rates based on all immunizations in the registry assessed the proportion of infants older than 153 days (5 months) at study completion who had received their most recent immunizations within 30 days of the recommended age for that immunization. The Luman definition of being younger than 153 days for the receipt of 4-month immunizations or younger than 214 days for the receipt of 6-month immunizations was used.[20] Infants were coded as being in the baseline, OA future visit, or OA same day group by the group they were in for the last study visit. Logistic regression was used to examine the effect of the risk variables, group (baseline, OA future visit, and OA same day), insurance status, and Spanish-speaking provider on the on-time immunization rate.

Continuity of care was assessed for all infants having 2 or more visits during the study. Infants were coded as having perfect continuity (being seen by the same provider for all visits) or not (being seen by > 1 provider). For the comparison of rates of perfect continuity between the 2 OA groups, the match effect for provider and cluster effect for patients nested within providers were taken into consideration during modeling. Logit link function and binomial distribution[21] were applied to the outcome variable in the nonlinear effect model.

The project was approved by the Colorado Multiple Institutional Review Board and a Health Insurance Portability and Accountability Act of 1996 waiver was obtained.

## RESULTS

Between August 1, 2003, and January 31, 2004, 1563 appointments for 2-, 4-, or 6-month WCC visits were scheduled for or attended by 878 infants. **Table 1** compares the demographic information of the infants and the Spanish fluency of the providers among the 3 groups.

The 2 different methods of OA used in this study resulted in significant differences among the baseline and the 2 OA groups for the median number of days ahead that the appointments were scheduled and the number of appointments scheduled the same day and within 36 hours of the appointment. There were 228 missed appointments (15%). The missed appointment rate decreased by 30% in the OA future visit group and by more than 50% in the OA same day group (**Table 2**). Variables associated with the decreased missed appointment rate for 1539 visits included being in the OA future visit group vs the baseline group (adjusted odds ratio [OR], 0.58 [95% confidence interval (CI), 0.42-0.80]), being in the OA same day group vs the baseline group (adjusted OR, 0.38 [95% CI, 0.26-0.55]), being seen by a Spanish-speaking provider (adjusted OR, 0.58 [95% CI, 0.43-0.79]), and having insurance (adjusted OR, 0.57 [95% CI, 0.40-0.82]).

Of the 630 infants who were older than 5 months at study end, 59% of the baseline group and 74% of both OA groups had on-time immunizations (Table 2). Variables associated with on-time immunizations for 628 infants included being in the OA future visit group vs the baseline group (adjusted OR, 2.12 [95% CI, 1.34-3.36]), being in the OA same day group vs the baseline

**Table 1. Comparison of Demographic Factors and Visit Characteristics During Baseline and OA Periods for 1563 Appointments**

| | No./Total No. (%) | | |
|---|---|---|---|
| Demographic Factor | Baseline (n = 483) | OA Future Visit (n = 522) | OA Same Day (n = 558) |
| Male | 235/483 (49) | 275/522 (53) | 280/558 (50) |
| Has Medicaid/insurance | 399/483 (83) | 443/519 (85) | 460/553 (83) |
| Mexican American | 452/479 (94) | 466/511 (91) | 532/553 (96)* |
| WCC visit | | | |
| 2 mo | 183/483 (38) | 198/522 (38) | 202/558 (36) |
| 4 mo | 178/483 (37) | 179/522 (34) | 192/558 (35) |
| 6 mo | 122/483 (25) | 145/522 (28) | 164/558 (29) |
| Seen by Spanish-fluent pediatrician/physician assistant | 311/483 (64)† | 279/522 (53) | 418/558 (75)† |

Abbreviations: OA, open access scheduling; WCC, well-child care.

*$P<.003$ by $\chi^2$ test, with the significant difference being between OA future visit and OA same-day groups.

†$P<.001$ by $\chi^2$ test, with each group being significantly different from the other 2 groups. There was no significant difference among the 3 groups for the other variables.

**Table 2. Comparison of Outcome Variables and Characteristics of Appointment Scheduling During Baseline and OA**

| | No./Total No. (%)* | | |
|---|---|---|---|
| | Baseline | OA Future Visit | OA Same Day |
| No. of days ahead appointment was scheduled, median (n = 1563) | 48 | 15 | 0† |
| No. of appointments scheduled same day or day before (n = 1563) | 10/483 (2) | 176/522 (34) | 398/558 (71)‡ |
| No. of appointments scheduled same day (n = 1563) | 6/483 (1) | 126/522 (24) | 279/558 (50)‡ |
| Missed appointment rate (n = 1563) | 101/483 (21) | 74/522 (14) | 53/558 (9)§ |
| On-time immunization rate (n = 630) | 94/158 (59) | 161/218 (74) | 187/254 (74)‖ |
| Perfect continuity of care (n = 412) | NA | 135/180 (75) | 138/232 (60)¶ |

Abbreviations: NA, not applicable; OA, open access scheduling.

*Data so given unless otherwise indicated.

†$P<.001$ by Kruskal-Wallis test, with each group being significantly different from the other 2 groups.

‡$P<.001$ by $\chi^2$ test, with each group being significantly different from the other 2 groups.

§$P<.02$ by $\chi^2$ test, with each group being significantly different from the other 2 groups.

‖$P<.006$ by $\chi^2$ test, with the baseline group being significantly different from the 2 OA groups.

¶$P<.001$ by $\chi^2$ test.

group (adjusted OR, 1.89 [95% CI, 1.22-2.93]), having insurance (adjusted OR, 2.95 [95% CI, 1.68-5.19]), and being seen by a Spanish-speaking provider (adjusted OR, 1.55 [95% CI, 1.06-2.26]).

Of the 412 infants having 2 or more WCC visits, 274 (67%) had perfect continuity. In the OA future visit group, 136 (75%) of 180 infants had perfect continuity compared with 138 (60%) of 232 infants in the OA same day group ($P = .001$). This difference in perfect continuity was not due to the difference between the OA methods ($P = .90$) but was due to variation among the providers.

## COMMENT

Use of OA decreased missed appointment rates for WCC visits from 21% in the baseline period to 14% in the OA future visit group and to 9% in the OA same day group. The decrease in the missed appointment rate in the OA future visit group was unexpected. The OA future visit group had a significant increase in appointments scheduled within 36 hours of the visit compared with the baseline period (Table 2). Only 50 (8%) of the 584 appointments scheduled within 36 hours of the visit were missed, compared with 177 (18%) of 978 missed appointments scheduled more than 1 day in advance. Scheduling appointments within 36 hours of the visit was associated with decreased missed appointments.

High missed appointment rates affect patient flow, the availability of appointments, and productivity. Missed appointment rates of 8% to more than 50% have been found in patients insured by Medicaid.[9,22-25] Belardi et al[4] did not find a decrease in missed appointment rates after implementation of OA in a family practice clinic; however, their baseline missed appointment rate of 9% was much less than the baseline missed appointment rate of 21% for infants at WFHC. Bundy et al[6] found that missed appointment rates decreased from 16% to 11% in 4 pediatric and family practice clinics after the introduction of OA. With the decreased missed appointment rate at WFHC, we have decreased the number of appointments scheduled and increased the number of patients seen in a session. This increases access to care.

Three factors were associated with decreased missed appointment rates: being in either of the OA groups, being seen by a Spanish-speaking provider (a proxy for our patients who are monolingual Spanish speakers), and having insurance. Monolingual Spanish-speaking families at WFHC are recent immigrants from Mexico and their infants, born in the United States, are eligible for Medicaid. Having health insurance is a marker of their ability to complete the Medicaid paperwork. Inability to complete the Medicaid paperwork may be associated with other problems in accessing care. Families without Medicaid may not have attended a visit for fear of getting a bill.

On-time immunizations improved by 25% between the baseline group and the 2 OA groups. The decreased missed appointment rates in the OA groups should increase immunization rates. Irigoyen et al[9] found that children who attended their appointment after a reminder call were 2.3 times more likely to be up-to-date on immunizations than children who missed the visit. LeBaron et al[10] improved immunization rates by 3% to 6% by using an automated appointment reminder/recall system; however, the major reason for delayed immunizations remained missed appointments. In OA, if an appointment is canceled or missed, it can be promptly rescheduled. Of 176 appointments in the OA future visit group that were scheduled within 36 hours of the visit, 42 (24%) were scheduled after a prior missed appointment. Before OA at WFHC, the next available WCC visit appointment would have been in 3 to 6 weeks.

Randolph et al[2] hypothesized that OA should improve immunization rates by decreasing the time between scheduling the appointment and the appointment date. Lannon et al[15] found that the long wait between scheduling an appointment and the appointment date impeded the ability of low-income mothers to get medical care for their children. Our results support the hypothesis of Randolph et al.

In addition to OA, having insurance and being seen by a Spanish-speaking provider were also associated with improved on-time immunization rates. Our results support the importance of insurance in improving immunization rates found by others.[8,26] The variable "Spanish-speaking provider" is a marker for the importance of immunizations for families who have recently immigrated from Mexico. Anderson et al[27] found that Latino children whose mothers were the least acculturated were 3 to 5 times more likely to be up-to-date on immunizations as Latino children whose mothers were more acculturated.

The Denver Health system, with its access to an organization-wide immunization registry, assessment of immunizations at each visit, printed provider reminders of immunizations needed, follow-up after missed appointments, and mailed parent recalls for delayed immunizations, has attempted to optimize immunization rates. Open access scheduling appears to improve immunization rates further.

Practices using OA for at least 6 to 12 months report increased continuity of care.[4,5] We found less continuity of care in the infants seen in the OA same day group than in the OA future visit group. The reason for this was differences in continuity among providers, not differences between the OA groups. One provider on maternity leave during part of the study may have accounted for some of the difference among providers. Our study duration was only 4 months.

This study had several limitations. Because of time and financial constraints, we were unable to randomize the infants, so we used a cluster design with provider randomization. Since the baseline group had no cluster randomization and we compared the 3 groups for missed appointment rates and on-time immunizations, we could not include the cluster randomization in this data analysis. However, comparison of the missed appointment and on-time immunization rates between the 2 OA groups including the effect of the cluster randomization yielded similar results as the comparison of the 3 groups without the cluster randomization. With randomization of the providers, some patients crossed between the 2 OA groups. In the analysis of continuity and immunization rates, infants were grouped based on the group they were in at their last visit. We have no data that the crossing between the 2 OA groups occurred more 1 way than the other. The time frame of the study was short and results could have been affected by seasonal variations. However, quarterly monitoring of missed appointment and immunization rates of 1-year-old children has shown no seasonal variations.

The increased on-time immunization rates in the OA groups could be because of infants who never had an appointment scheduled, never got immunizations, and were not included in the study. Since the infants in the baseline and OA future visit groups had their appointments for WCC visits scheduled in the same manner, this was not a factor in the OA future visit group results. There was only a small number of infants who attended a 2-week visit, and who were not included in the study. There was no difference between the number of these infants who were not seen during the baseline period or during the OA period.

Our study population was low income and largely Mexican American. An evaluation of OA needs to be replicated in other ethnic and socioeconomic groups. Using a study design with complete cohorts seen in a non-OA and an OA system would give more robust data results for comparison of immunization rates.

## CONCLUSIONS

Open access scheduling decreased the missed appointment rates for infant WCC visits. Scheduling 2-, 4-, and 6-month WCC visits 2 months ahead within an OA system allows the same improvement in on-time immunizations as scheduling same-day infant WCC. In a community health center that is part of a health care system that has attempted to optimize immunization rates, OA appears to have increased on-time immunization rates.

At WFHC, we have continued to offer future-visit appointments for 2-, 4-, and 6-month WCC visits in OA. This allows parents to schedule ahead or the same day, whichever they prefer. Open access scheduling has improved access to care.

**Accepted for Publication:** April 20, 2006.
**Correspondence:** Mary E. O'Connor, MD, MPH, Westside Family Health Center, 1100 Federal Blvd, Denver, CO 80204 (mary.o'connor@dhha.org).
**Author Contributions:** Dr O'Connor had full access to all the data in the study and takes responsibility for the integrity of the data and the accuracy of the data analysis. *Study concept and design:* O'Connor and Matthews. *Acquisition of data:* O'Connor and Matthews. *Analysis and interpretation of data:* O'Connor and Gao. *Drafting of the manuscript:* O'Connor, Matthews, and Gao. *Critical revision of the manuscript for important intellectual content:* O'Connor, Matthews, and Gao. *Statistical analysis:* O'Connor and Gao.
**Funding/Support:** This study was funded in part by Health Resources and Services Administration grant 2D54HP0054-04-00 to the Primary Care Research Unit, University of Colorado Health Sciences Center.
**Acknowledgment:** Thanks go to Stephen Vogler, MD, for persistently asking the question "How will we know that our infants are coming for care?"; Pete Gutierrez, BA, and Jeff Brown, MD, MPH, for their support of this project; the providers, nursing staff, and especially to Celina Magallanes and Joann Rios for their ability to accurately schedule patients in the 2 different open access systems; and Simon Hambidge, MD, PhD, and the other reviewers for their suggestions.

## REFERENCES

1. Murray M, Tantau C. Same-day appointments: exploding the access paradigm. *Fam Pract Manag.* 2000;7:45-53. www.aafp.org/fpm. Accessed February 28, 2006.
2. Randolph GD, Murray M, Swanson JA, Margolis PA. Behind schedule, improving access to care for children one practice at a time. *Pediatrics.* 2004;113:e230-e236. http://pediatrics.aappublications.org/cgi/content/full/113/3/e230. Accessed June 26, 2006.
3. Murray M, Bodenheimer T, Rittenhouse D, Grumbach K. Improving timely access to primary care: case studies of the advanced access model. *JAMA.* 2003;289:1042-1046.
4. Belardi FG, Weir S, Craig FW. A controlled trial of an Advanced Access appointment system in a residency family medicine center. *Fam Med.* 2004;36:341-345.
5. O'Hare CD, Corlett J. The outcomes of Open-Access scheduling. *Fam Pract Manag.* 2004;11:35-40. www.aafp.org/fpm. Accessed December 28, 2005.
6. Bundy DG, Randolph GD, Murray M, Anderson J, Margolis PA. Open Access in primary care: results of a North Carolina pilot project. *Pediatrics.* 2005;116:82-87.
7. Kempe A, Beaty BL, Steiner JF, et al. The regional immunization registry as a public health tool for improving clinical practice and guiding immunization delivery policy. *Am J Public Health.* 2004;94:967-972.
8. Holl JL, Szilagyi PG, Rodewald LE, et al. Evaluation of New York State's Child Health Care Plus: access, utilization, quality of health care, and health status. *Pediatrics.* 2000;105:711-718.
9. Irigoyen MM, Findley S, Earle B, Stambaugh K, Vaughan R. Impact of appointment reminders on vaccination coverage at an urban clinic. *Pediatrics.* 2000;106:919-923.
10. LeBaron CW, Starnes DM, Rask KJ. The impact of reminder-recall interventions on low vaccination coverage in an inner-city population. *Arch Pediatr Adolesc Med.* 2004;158:255-261.
11. Rodewald LE, Szilagyi PG, Humiston SG, Barth R, Kraus R, Raubertas RF. A randomized study of tracking with outreach and provider prompting to improve immunization coverage and primary care. *Pediatrics.* 1999;103:31-38.
12. Minkovitz CS, Belote AD, Higman SM, Servint JR, Weiner JP. Effectiveness of a practice-based intervention to increase vaccination rates and reduce missed opportunities. *Arch Pediatr Adolesc Med.* 2001;155:382-386.
13. Szilagyi PG, Schaffer S, Shone L, et al. Reducing geographic, racial, and ethnic disparities in childhood immunization rates by using reminder/recall interventions in urban primary care practices. *Pediatrics.* 2002;110:e58. www.pediatrics.org/cgi/content/full/110/5/e58. Accessed June 26, 2006.
14. Centers for Disease Control and Prevention. National, state, and urban area vaccination coverage among children aged 19-35 months, United States, 2004. *MMWR Morb Mortal Wkly Rep.* 2005;54:717-721.
15. Lannon C, Brack V, Stuart J, et al. What mothers say about why poor children fall behind on immunizations. *Arch Pediatr Adolesc Med.* 1995;149:1070-1075.
16. Morrow AL, Rosenthal J, Lakkis HD, et al. A population-based study of access to immunization among urban Virginia children served by public, private, and military health care systems. *Pediatrics.* 1998;101:e5. www.pediatrics.org/cgi/content/full/101/2/e5. Accessed June 26, 2006.
17. National Vaccine Advisory Committee. Standards for child and adolescent immunization practices. *Pediatrics.* 2003;112:958-963.
18. SAS Institute. *SAS/STAT User's Guide.* Cary, NC: SAS Institute; 1999.
19. Wolfinger R, O'Connell M. Generalized linear mixed models: a pseudo-likelihood approach. *J Stat Computation Simulation.* 1993;48:233-243.
20. Luman ET, Barker LE, Shaw KM, McCauley MM, Buehler JW, Pickering LK. Timeliness of childhood vaccinations in the United States. *JAMA.* 2005;293:1204-1211.
21. McCullagh P, Nelder JA. *Generalized Linear Models.* Baca Raton, Fla: Chapman Hall/CRC; 1989.
22. Lamberth EF, Rothstein EP, Hipp TJ, et al. Rates of missed appointments among pediatric patients in a private practice: Medicaid compared with private insurance. *Arch Pediatr Adolesc Med.* 2002;156:86-87.
23. Moore CG, Wilson-Witherspoon P, Probst JC. Time and money: effects of no-shows at a family practice residency clinic. *Fam Med.* 2001;33:522-527.
24. Hixon AL, Chapman RW, Nuovo J. Failure to keep clinic appointments: implications for residency education and productivity. *Fam Med.* 1999;31:627-630.
25. Specht EM, Powell KR, Dormo CA. Factors affecting missed appointment rates for pediatric patients insured by Medicaid in a traditional hospital-based resident clinic and hospital-owned practice settings. *Clin Pediatr (Phila).* 2004;43:749-752.
26. Santoli JM, Huet NJ, Smith PJ, et al. Insurance status and vaccination coverage among US preschool children. *Pediatrics.* 2004;113:1959-1964.
27. Anderson LM, Wood DF, Sherbourne CD. Maternal acculturation and childhood immunization levels among children in Latino families on Los Angeles. *Am J Public Health.* 1997;87:2018-2021.

ARTICLE

# Total Body Weight and Waist Circumference Associated With Chronic Periodontitis Among Adolescents in the United States

*Anne F. Reeves, MPH; Jane M. Rees, PhD, MS, RD; Melissa Schiff, MD, MPH; Philippe Hujoel, DDS, PhD*

**Objective:** To investigate whether measures of obesity are associated with periodontitis.

**Design:** A case-control study.

**Setting:** A nationally representative sample using data from the Third National Health and Nutrition Examination Survey.

**Participants:** The sample included 2452 nonsmokers, aged 13 to 21 years, who received a periodontal examination and had complete information for age, sex, and smoking habits.

**Main Exposures:** Skinfold thickness, weight, and waist circumference were examined as independent variables in logistic regression models. Final models were adjusted for sex, race/ethnicity, poverty index ratio, last dental visit, and self-reported calcium intake.

**Main Outcome Measures:** Cases were subjects with the presence of 1 or more periodontal sites with both a loss of tissue attachment of 3 mm and a probing depth of 3 mm (n=111). Subjects who did not meet these criteria were classified as controls (n=2341).

**Results:** Total body weight and waist circumference were associated with periodontitis, but the association varied by age. Adolescents aged 13 to 16 years were not at increased risk of chronic periodontitis, while adolescents aged 17 to 21 years had an increased risk per 1-kg increase in body weight (adjusted odds ratio, 1.06 [95% confidence interval, 1.01-1.09]). Similarly, adolescents aged 13 to 16 years were not at increased risk for periodontal disease, while adolescents aged 17 to 21 years were at an increased risk of periodontal disease per 1-cm increase in waist circumference (adjusted odds ratio, 1.05 [95% confidence interval, 1.01-1.08]).

**Conclusion:** Periodontitis may follow patterns similar to other chronic conditions that originate early in life and are related to central adiposity.

*Arch Pediatr Adolesc Med. 2006;160:894-899*

An increasing prevalence of overweight is well documented among US adolescents of all ages and ethnicities.[1] As a result, serious medical and psychosocial comorbidities are emerging early in life. The onset of type 2 diabetes mellitus in overweight adolescents demonstrates that traditionally age-dependent, chronic diseases can begin earlier in life than once thought. While previous studies have examined numerous physical and psychological consequences of adiposity during adolescence, little is known about the effects on oral health.

Periodontitis is commonly defined as a condition where the tissue supporting the teeth is destroyed. The disease is slow to progress and has been defined in adolescents as the presence of loss of tissue attachment of 3 mm or more on 1 or more teeth.[2] Risk factors include diabetes, older age, genetics, smoking, African American and Mexican American ethnicity, oral factors, lack of dental care, and socioeconomic status.[3,4] Oral diseases disproportionately affect low-income and minority populations who are often lacking access to preventive oral health education and services.[5] Unfortunately, primary care professionals treating underserved adolescents generally lack time and training to perform oral health education and screening.[6]

Periodontitis is estimated to affect only 2% to 5% of US adolescents compared with more than 50% of adults.[4] However, untreated oral disease leads to tooth loss, pain, suffering, and problems eating, speaking, and learning as well as absence from school.[7] More than 51 million US school hours are lost each year to dental-related disease.

Recent US and Japanese studies report associations between obesity and periodontal disease in adults.[8-11] Central skin-

Author Affiliations: Primary, Maternal, and Child Health Program, Departments of Health Services (Ms Reeves and Dr Rees), Pediatric Dentistry (Ms Reeves), Pediatrics, Adolescent Medicine Section (Dr Rees), Epidemiology (Dr Schiff), and Dental Public Health Sciences, School of Dentistry (Dr Hujoel), University of Washington, Seattle. Ms Reeves is now a dental student at the School of Dentistry, Center for Health Sciences, University of California, Los Angeles.

fold thickness and body mass index (BMI) (calculated as weight in kilograms divided by height in meters squared) were significant predictors of periodontal disease. However, to our knowledge, no study has investigated how early the relationship between adiposity and periodontitis arises among adolescents. We examined whether periodontitis, following traditionally age-dependent, chronic diseases patterns, was associated with overweight in adolescents.

## METHODS

### STUDY DESIGN AND SAMPLE

We used a case-control design to test whether adiposity was associated with periodontitis among US adolescents aged 13 to 21 years. All subjects received a periodontal examination and had complete information on sex, age, and smoking habits. Since smoking is strongly related to both systemic health and periodontal disease, control for confounding can best be achieved by restricting subjects to nonsmokers.[12] Accordingly, this study was restricted to self-reported nonsmokers. Data were collected on 3466 subjects aged 13 to 21 years; 2452 (71%) met the criteria.

### DATA SOURCE

Adolescent body measurements and oral health status were taken from data collected in the Third National Health and Nutrition Examination Survey (NHANES III), a cross-sectional examination conducted by the National Center for Health Statistics and Centers for Disease Control and Prevention from 1988 to 1994. The NHANES III was designed to obtain nationally representative data on health and nutritional status in the United States through surveys, as well as medical and dental examinations in a mobile clinic. Nutritional data were collected by a trained interviewer administering a 24-hour recall. The US civilian, noninstitutionalized population 2 months or older is represented in NHANES III. Data were collected from 33 994 individuals. As part of the stratified, multistage probability design, African American and Mexican American subjects were oversampled. Details about the survey and its methods have been previously published.[13]

### INDEPENDENT VARIABLES: ANTHROPOMETRIC INDEXES

Adiposity was assessed by triceps, subscapular, suprailiac, thigh, and sum of skinfold thickness (triceps + subscapular) measures. Skinfold thickness measures were log transformed in the event of a skewed distribution. Weight, height, and waist circumference were examined as continuous independent variables. We did not use BMI as an independent variable. Although BMI is a useful screening tool, it may be a poor proxy for fat distribution and central adiposity in children and adolescents.[14,15] Moreover, use of BMI in statistical models can lead to incorrect inferences, inadequately adjusting for each variable in the ratio.[16,17] In this study, BMI was initially examined as an interaction term, with weight and height ($1/m^2$) included as main effects.[16] No significant relationship was found between BMI and periodontitis.

### OUTCOME VARIABLE: PERIODONTITIS

Oral health data from 1 randomly assigned upper and lower quadrant per mouth were collected on each subject in NHANES III. Measures of periodontal loss of tissue attachment and probing depth from mesiofacial and midfacial sites (28 sites per individual) were recorded to determine periodontal status. Third molars, partially erupted teeth, and retained roots were excluded. Cases of periodontitis were defined as the presence of 1 or more periodontal sites with both a loss of tissue attachment of 3 mm or more and a probing depth of 3 mm or more. Subjects not meeting these criteria were classified as controls.

### STATISTICAL METHODS

Statistical software Stata 8.0 (StataCorp, College Station, Tex) was used for all analyses, allowing inclusion of population weights, calculation of the standard errors, and adjustment for the complex sampling design. Following the National Center for Health Statistics and Centers for Disease Control and Prevention guidelines, statistical sample weights were used to account for both oversampling and nonresponse. The final sample weight variable from the mobile clinic was used to obtain nationally representative estimates.

Demographic, dental, and nutritional variables of cases and controls were compared. Possible associations of skinfold thickness, weight, and waist circumference with periodontitis were examined in a series of logistic regression models. Crude odds ratios (ORs) and 95% confidence intervals (CIs) were estimated using logistic regression, with sociodemographic variables and periodontitis risk factors as potential confounding factors. Covariates included in the final models a priori were age, sex, race/ethnicity, poverty index ratio, last dental visit, and self-reported calcium intake. Ethnicity (non-Hispanic white, non-Hispanic black, Mexican American, and others) was obtained from the NHANES III race/ethnicity variable. The poverty index in NHANES III (family income divided by the poverty threshold) was categorized as high (≥3.5), medium (1.851-3.499), and low (0-1.850) based on federal eligibility for free and reduced-price lunch services. History of dental care was categorized as less than 1 year, 2 to 3 years, more than 3 years, and never visited. Self-reported calcium intakes were divided into quartiles.

Selection of additional potential confounding variables was based on forward selection with the decision to include or delete based on changes in ORs of the exposure effects. Potential confounders examined using this method were insulin use (yes/no), nonfasting serum glucose level, and self-reported vitamin C intake. A glucose level of 200 mg/dL (11.1 mmol/L) or higher was considered elevated regardless of length of fast.[18] Vitamin C intakes were divided into quartiles. Exposure coefficients did not change when insulin use, serum glucose level, and vitamin C intake were added to the respective models. Final models included sex, race/ethnicity, poverty index ratio, last dental visit, and calcium intake as confounding factors.

## RESULTS

National estimates based on weighted data and the unweighted sample size on which these estimates were based are presented in **Table 1**. Of 2452 adolescents examined, 111 were classified as having periodontitis, yielding an overall weighted prevalence of 3.3%. Adolescents with periodontitis were more likely to be 17 to 21 years of age, male, African American or other race, in the lowest socioeconomic group, and without a dental visit for 3 years or more. Those with periodontitis were more likely to have self-reported calcium and vitamin C intakes in the lowest quartiles and less likely to have upper-quartile calcium intake. Subjects aged 17 to 21 years with

**Table 1. Characteristics of Adolescents Aged 13 to 21 Years Sampled in the National Health and Nutrition Examination Survey III* (1988-1994) by Chronic Periodontitis Status**

| Characteristic | Sample Size (N = 2452)† | No. (%) Cases (n = 111) | No. (%) Controls (n = 2341) |
|---|---|---|---|
| Age, y | | | |
| 13-16 | 1022 | 28 (24.5) | 994 (41.1) |
| 17-21 | 1430 | 83 (75.6) | 1347 (58.0) |
| Sex | | | |
| Male | 1093 | 51 (64.7) | 1042 (47.1) |
| Female | 1359 | 60 (35.2) | 1299 (52.8) |
| Race/ethnicity | | | |
| Non-Hispanic white | 532 | 9 (37.1) | 523 (62.0) |
| Non-Hispanic black | 922 | 55 (28.2) | 867 (17.4) |
| Mexican American | 857 | 41 (11.8) | 816 (9.2) |
| Other | 141 | 6 (23.0) | 135 (11.4) |
| Poverty index ratio | | | |
| 0-1.850 | 1369 | 69 (66.2) | 1300 (41.8) |
| 1.851-3.499 | 581 | 23 (26.9) | 558 (34.6) |
| ≥3.5 | 256 | 2 (6.9) | 254 (23.6) |
| Last dental visit, y | | | |
| <1 | 1494 | 52 (54.1) | 1442 (72.6) |
| 1-3 | 449 | 23 (23.6) | 426 (15.0) |
| >3 | 252 | 14 (13.1) | 238 (7.6) |
| Never | 234 | 20 (9.3) | 214 (5.0) |
| Quartile calcium intake‡ | | | |
| 0-24 | 565 | 29 (28.1) | 565 (20.3) |
| 25-49 | 597 | 30 (25.0) | 567 (23.5) |
| 50-74 | 603 | 32 (32.7) | 571 (25.6) |
| 75-100 | 593 | 19 (14.1) | 574 (30.6) |
| Quartile vitamin C intake‡ | | | |
| 0-24 | 577 | 29 (31.1) | 548 (24.9) |
| 25-49 | 589 | 28 (29.0) | 561 (26.2) |
| 50-74 | 606 | 20 (11.8) | 586 (25.8) |
| 75-100 | 615 | 33 (28.1) | 582 (23.1) |
| Insulin use | | | |
| Yes | 6 | 1 (0.02) | 5 (0.034) |
| No | 2359 | 106 (99.8) | 2253 (99.6) |
| Nonfasting glucose level, mg/dL | | | |
| <200 | 2218 | 103 (100) | 2115 (99.8) |
| ≥200 | 3 | 0 | 3 (0.02) |

SI conversion factor: To convert nonfasting glucose level to micromoles per liter, multiply by 0.0555.
*Weighted to produce nationally representative estimates.
†Total differs in some cells because of missing data.
‡Nutrient intakes were self-reported by the 24-hour recall method.

periodontitis were, on average, 7 kg heavier, with a waist circumference 8 cm larger than controls of the same age (data not shown). Few of the 2452 adolescents reported taking insulin or had elevated serum glucose levels.

Interaction between age and weight, as well as age and waist circumference, was tested for significance using the Wald test with $P<.05$. Interaction between age and weight ($P<.009$) and age and waist circumference ($P<.02$) was significant. Therefore, final models evaluating weight and waist circumference were stratified by age. There were no significant interactions between race/ethnicity and weight, race/ethnicity and waist circumference, poverty index and weight, or poverty index ratio and waist circumference.

**Table 2. Crude and Adjusted ORs for Weight and Chronic Periodontitis in 2109 Adolescents**

| Age, y | Crude OR (95% CI) | Adjusted OR* (95% CI) |
|---|---|---|
| 13-16 | 1.0 (0.98-1.0) | 0.99 (0.97-1.0) |
| 17-21 | 1.03 (1.0-1.05) | 1.06 (1.01-1.09) |

Abbreviations: CI, confidence interval; OR, odds ratio.
*Adjusted for height, age, sex, race/ethnicity, poverty index ratio, last dental visit, and calcium intake.

**Table 3. Crude and Adjusted ORs for Waist Circumference and Chronic Periodontitis in 2079 Adolescents**

| Age, y | Crude OR (95% CI) | Adjusted OR* (95% CI) |
|---|---|---|
| 13-16 | 1.0 (0.98-1.02) | 1.0 (0.98-1.01) |
| 17-21 | 1.04 (1.0-1.07) | 1.05 (1.01-1.08) |

Abbreviations: See Table 2.
*Adjusted for sex, race/ethnicity, poverty index ratio, last dental visit, and calcium intake.

Triceps, subscapular, suprailiac, and thigh skinfolds; sum of skinfold thickness; and log sum of skinfold thickness were not associated with periodontitis (data not shown). Adolescents aged 13 to 16 years were not at increased risk of periodontitis with each unit increase in weight (OR, 0.99 [95% CI, 0.97-1.0]), while adolescents aged 17 to 21 years were at a 6% increased risk of periodontitis for each 1-kg weight increase (adjusted OR, 1.06 [95% CI, 1.01-1.09]) (**Table 2**). Similarly, adolescents aged 13 to 16 years were not at increased risk of periodontitis (OR, 1.0 [95% CI, 0.98-1.04]) with each unit waist circumference increase, while adolescents aged 17 to 21 years were at a 5% increased risk of disease for each 1-cm increase in waist circumference (adjusted OR, 1.05 [95% CI, 1.01-1.08]) (**Table 3**). Of 432 smokers excluded, 25 had periodontitis. Results were unchanged with smokers included in the analysis and smoking controlled in the model (data not shown).

## COMMENT

### RESULTS AND COMPARISONS WITH PREVIOUS REPORTS

In a representative sample of US adolescents, weight and waist circumference were associated with increased risk of periodontitis among those aged 17 to 21 years. Skinfold thickness measures were not associated with periodontal disease among US adolescents.

Among adolescents aged 17 to 21 years, each 1-kg increase was associated with a 6% increase in risk of disease. Similarly, each 1-cm increase in waist circumference was associated with a 5% increase in risk of periodontitis. The risk of disease varied with age. No relationship was found between waist circumference or weight and risk of periodontitis for adolescents aged 13 to 16 years. These results extend previous findings of a relationship between central adiposity and periodontal disease to include adolescents aged 17 to 21 years.[8,10] This suggests that periodontitis could be an age-dependent, chronic condition clinically recognizable after the age of 16 years and associated with excess fat accumulated by adolescence.

In a previous analysis, young adults aged 18 to 34 years with a BMI greater than 30 had a 76% increased risk for periodontal disease, and those with a large waist circumference had a 127% increased risk of disease.[8] Others found obesity and central adiposity predictive of periodontal disease in Japanese adults.[9] Reportedly, the relationship between obesity and periodontal disease was even greater for adults who had insulin resistance.[11]

In the United Kingdom, trends of waist-circumference increases have surpassed trends of BMI increases among adolescents aged 11 to 16 years.[14] In the United States, increasing central adiposity rates from adolescence to adulthood are greatest among children of low socioeconomic status.[19] Adiposity and related disease risk also differ between ethnicities.[20-22] Low-income and minority communities generally lack access to oral health education and services and may be disproportionately affected by the possible relationship between excess central adiposity and periodontal disease.

Unlike adults,[10] skinfold thickness and periodontitis were not associated among adolescents in this study. Skinfold measures may not appropriately assess body composition among a heterogeneous population undergoing growth and development. The thickness of subcutaneous adipose tissue may not reflect a constant proportion of total body fat, since the relationship between subcutaneous fat and fat stores around organs is nonlinear and varies by body weight and age. Subcutaneous fat distribution also varies by sex, race, and age.[23]

## MECHANISMS

A variety of potential mechanisms could account for an association between obesity and periodontitis, including noncausal mechanisms related to health risk behaviors. Overweight adolescents may have unhealthy dietary patterns with insufficient micronutrient and excess sugar and fat content increasing the risk for periodontal disease.[8] Other possible mechanisms include changes in host immunity and/or increased stress levels,[8] often related to gaining excess fat early in life.

Poor dietary patterns may affect oral tissues and the immune response. Calcium and vitamin C are important cofactors for maintaining these systems in animals and humans.[24] Obesity and periodontal disease were strongly related in young but not in middle-age or older adults.[8] We propose that a cohort effect whereby less healthy dietary patterns among young adults (compared with patterns among older generations) may explain the increased periodontal disease risk. If this is true, the total population oral disease burden could be significantly affected as adolescents continue to consume unhealthy diets into adulthood, deposit fat earlier in life, and maintain excess weight as they age.

It has been proposed that obesity triggers the immune response, generating a state of chronic subclinical systemic inflamation.[25] Adipocytes have been identified as active producers of cytokines, including tumor necrosis factor α, a powerful producer of IL-6, and to some degree IL-1.[26] Increases in cytokines stimulate a variety of acute immune responses by the liver such as C-reactive protein and fibrinogen production. In overweight children, elevated C-reactive protein levels have been documented, suggesting systemic inflammation may occur early in life.[27] In children as young as 11 years, obesity has been related to impaired microvascular functioning.[28,29] Periodontal blood vessels and tissues may be affected by alterations in the inflammatory response as well as decreased blood flow; both can affect cell signaling and host immunity.

Insulin resistance may mediate the relationship between obesity and periodontal disease.[11] Dietary free fatty acids may cause insulin resistance by increasing apoptosis of pancreatic β cells. In turn, the immune response may interfere with glucose transporters, inhibiting insulin signaling and causing the body to develop an inflammatory state. An increased inflammatory state "sets the stage for increased levels of periodontal disease triggered by oral pathogens."[11(p2082)]

Psychosocial stress associated with adolescent overweight may affect periodontal health through physiological and behavioral pathways. Physiological responses to stress may alter blood and salivary flow, decreasing the immune response to oral pathogens.[30] Psychosocial stress related to teasing about body weight[31,32] may affect oral health behaviors such as regular brushing, flossing, fluoride use, and and/or seeking preventive dental services. Overweight adolescents report engaging in significantly more unhealthy behaviors compared with their nonoverweight peers.[33] However, little is known about these relationships among teens. Among adults, oral health behaviors and general health characteristics are correlated; a lack of daily flossing is a strong marker of obesity.[34,35] Thus, the observed association between obesity and periodontitis may be due to factors associated with health awareness rather than a biological mechanism.

## LIMITATIONS

This study had several limitations. First, the cross-sectional design precluded determining the temporal sequence. Whether adolescents with periodontitis had accumulated excess fat during childhood is unknown. Second, the role of genetics, oral health behaviors (eg, brushing or flossing), or "local factors" (eg, gingival inflammation, active caries, dental plaque, and calculus) were not considered in periodontitis etiology. Therefore, results may have been confounded by uncontrolled factors. Nonresponse and missing values for variables may have led to bias, though several authors have indicated little bias due to nonresponse to HANES and NHANES III surveys.[36-39]

Despite its limitations, the current study raises questions about the role of early excess central adiposity in oral disease etiology. Sample representativeness and weighting provide generalizability of the results to the

US adolescent population. Many covariates that could have confounded the relationship between weight, central adiposity, and periodontal disease were controlled. Since smokers were excluded, we can be confident that our results were not due to residual confounding by smoking, a strong causal factor for periodontitis.

## CONCLUSIONS

The results of this study have implications for the care of overweight adolescents, an increasing proportion of youth. Periodontitis appears to be yet another disease associated with overweight and obesity. Our research suggests periodontal disease follows risk patterns similar to other age-dependent, chronic conditions originating early in life and is related to lifestyles associated with central adiposity. Increasing adiposity during childhood may potentially affect adolescent periodontal health through a variety of mechanisms including unhealthy dietary habits, alterations in host immunity, and increased psychosocial stress. Alternatively, adiposity may be a marker for unhealthy lifestyles that cause periodontitis.

The results described earlier and related research indicate that obesity is a potential marker for periodontal disease among youth. Medical and dental professionals should develop interdisciplinary approaches for identifying and treating early signs of oral disease among children and adolescents. Since oral and general health behaviors are related, it is important to query parents, children, and teens about their oral hygiene practices when assessing health/risk behaviors and offer oral health education and care when necessary.

Like other health conditions, periodontal disease and overweight disproportionately affect low-socioeconomic and minority youth and/or those lacking access to health care. Primary care and other medical and dental professionals can potentially promote adolescent oral health by screening overweight teens, especially those with central adiposity, for early signs of gum disease and referring them for appropriate care. Since waist circumference is a simple, accurate measure for identifying youth at risk for chronic disease, health care professionals can use it to screen adolescents with or without a high BMI, especially in high-risk populations. To appropriately screen, professionals serving adolescents should be well informed about the connections between oral and systemic health, which historically have been believed to have little overlap.[6]

From a public health perspective, longitudinal studies can further explore associations between overweight and periodontitis in youth, such as whether hormonal changes related to physical maturation influence periodontal disease. Ethnic differences in periodontal disease risk can also be investigated. If associations between obesity, periodontal disease, and maturation are confirmed, the fat distribution patterns among low-income and minority adolescents could be recognized as increasing the oral disease burden in African American, Hispanic, and Native American communities. Since it is known that dietary, oral hygiene, and other behavioral practices during this period are likely to influence long-term health, public health planners should consider including oral health education and care in childhood and adolescent health programs.

**Accepted for Publication:** April 20, 2006.

**Correspondence:** Anne F. Reeves, MPH, School of Dentistry, Center for Health Sciences, University of California Los Angeles, 10833 Le Conte Ave, Box 160, Los Angeles, CA (afreeves@ucla.edu).

**Author Contributions:** *Study concept and design:* Reeves, Rees, Schiff, and Hujoel. *Acquisition of data:* Reeves, Rees, and Schiff. *Drafting of the manuscript:* Reeves, Rees, Schiff, and Hujoel. *Critical revision of the manuscript for important intellectual content:* Reeves, Rees, Schiff, and Hujoel. *Statistical analysis:* Reeves, Rees, Schiff, and Hujoel. *Obtained funding:* Rees. *Administrative, technical, and material support:* Rees. *Study supervision:* Rees, Schiff, and Hujoel.

**Funding/Support:** This study was supported in part by project T76 MC 00011 from the Maternal and Child Health Bureau (Title V, Social Security Act), Health Resources and Services Administration, US Department of Health and Human Services.

**Acknowledgment:** We thank Mary L. Hediger, PhD, investigator, Epidemiology Branch/Division of Epidemiology, Statistics, and Prevention Research, National Institute of Child, Health, and Human Development, National Institutes of Health, for assistance with this article and Bill O'Brien, data records coordinator, Department of Epidemiology, University of Washington, for help with acquisition of the data set.

## REFERENCES

1. Ogden CL, Flegal KM, Carroll MD, Johnson CL. Prevalence and trends in overweight among US children and adolescents, 1999-2000. *JAMA.* 2002;288:1728-1732.
2. Lopez R, Baelum V. Classifying periodontitis among adolescents: implications for epidemiological research. *Community Dent Oral Epidemiol.* 2003;31:136-143.
3. Albandar JM. Global risk factors and risk indicators for periodontal diseases. *Periodontol 2000.* 2002;29:177-206.
4. Albandar JM, Tinoco EM. Global epidemiology of periodontal diseases in children and young persons. *Periodontol 2000.* 2002;29:153-176.
5. Mouradian WE, Wehr E, Crall JJ. Disparities in children's oral health and access to dental care. *JAMA.* 2000;284:2625-2631.
6. Mouradian WE, Reeves A, Kim S, et al. An oral health curriculum for medical students at the University of Washington. *Acad Med.* 2005;80:434-442.
7. Oral Health in America. *A Report of the Surgeon General: Executive Summary.* Rockville, Md: US Dept of Health and Human Services, National Institute of Dental and Craniofacial Research, National Institutes of Health; 2000:2-13.
8. Al-Zahrani MS, Bissada NF, Borawskit EA. Obesity and periodontal disease in young, middle-aged, and older adults. *J Periodontol.* 2003;74:610-615.
9. Saito T, Shimazaki Y, Koga T, Tsuzuki M, Ohshima A. Relationship between upper body obesity and periodontitis. *J Dent Res.* 2001;80:1631-1636.
10. Wood N, Johnson RB, Streckfus CF. Comparison of body composition and periodontal disease using nutritional assessment techniques: Third National Health and Nutrition Examination Survey (NHANES III). *J Clin Periodontol.* 2003;30:321-327.
11. Genco RJ, Grossi SG, Ho A, Nishimura F, Murayama Y. A proposed model linking inflammation to obesity, diabetes, and periodontal infections. *J Periodontol.* 2005;76(11)(suppl):2075-2084.
12. Hujoel PP, Drangsholt M, Spiekerman C, DeRouen TA. Periodontitis-systemic disease associations in the presence of smoking—causal or coincidental? *Periodontol 2000.* 2002;30:51-60.
13. National Center for Health Statistics; Centers for Disease Control and Prevention. Analytic and reporting guidelines: the Third Nutritional Health and Nutrition

Examination Survey, NHANES III (1988-94). October 1996. http://www.cdc.gov/nchs/data/nhanes/nhanes3/cdrom/nchs/manuals/nh3guide.pdf. Accessed June 20, 2006.
14. McCarthy HD, Ellis SM, Cole TJ. Central overweight and obesity in British youth aged 11-16 years: cross sectional surveys of waist circumference. *BMJ.* 2003; 326:624.
15. Daniels SR, Khoury PR, Morrison JA. The utility of body mass index as a measure of body fatness in children and adolescents: differences by race and gender. *Pediatrics.* 1997;99:804-807.
16. Kronmal RA. Spurious correlation and the fallacy of the ratio standard revisited. *J R Stat Soc Ser A.* 1993;156:379-392.
17. Tanner JM. Fallacy of per-weight and per-surface area standards, and their relation to spurious correlation. *J Appl Physiol.* 1949;2:1-15.
18. Fagot-Campagna A, Saaddine JB, Flegal KM, Beckles GL. Diabetes, impaired fasting glucose, and elevated HbA1c in US adolescents: the Third National Health and Nutrition Examination Survey. *Diabetes Care.* 2001;24:834-837.
19. Dekkers JC, Podolsky RH, Treiber FA, et al. Development of general and central obesity from childhood into early adulthood in African American and European American males and females with a family history of cardiovascular disease. *Am J Clin Nutr.* 2004;79:661-668.
20. Cruz ML, Bergman RN, Goran MI. Unique effect of visceral fat on insulin sensitivity in obese Hispanic children with a family history of type 2 diabetes. *Diabetes Care.* 2002;25:1631-1636.
21. Goran MI, Ball GD, Cruz ML. Obesity and risk of type 2 diabetes and cardiovascular disease in children and adolescents. *J Clin Endocrinol Metab.* 2003;88: 1417-1427.
22. Gower BA. Syndrome X in children: influence of ethnicity and visceral fat. *Am J Hum Biol.* 1999;11:249-257.
23. Gibson RS. *Principles of Nutritional Assessment.* Oxford, England: Oxford University Press; 1990:187-262.
24. Neiva RF, Steigenga J, Al-Shammari KF, Wang HL. Effects of specific nutrients on periodontal disease onset, progression and treatment. *J Clin Periodontol.* 2003; 30:579-589.
25. Das UN. Is obesity an inflammatory condition? *Nutrition.* 2001;17:953-966.
26. Zoccali C, Mallamaci F, Tripepi G. Adipose tissue as a source of inflammatory cytokines in health and disease: focus on end stage renal disease. *Kidney Int Suppl.* 2003;(84):S65-S68.
27. Ford ES, Galuska DA, Gillespie C, et al. C-reactive protein and body mass index in children: findings from the Third National Health and Nutrition Examination Survey, 1988-1994. *J Pediatr.* 2001;138:486-492.
28. Tounian P, Aggoun Y, Dubern B, et al. Presence of increased stiffness of the common carotid artery and endothelial dysfunction in severely obese children: a prospective study. *Lancet.* 2001;358:1400-1404.
29. Khan F, Green FC, Forsyth JS, et al. Impaired microvascular function in normal children: effects of adiposity and poor glucose handling. *J Physiol.* 2003;551: 705-711.
30. da Silva AM, Newman HN, Oakley DA. Psychosocial factors in inflammatory periodontal diseases: a review. *J Clin Periodontol.* 1995;22:516-526.
31. Eisenberg ME, Neumark-Sztainer D, Story M. Associations of weight-based teasing and emotional well-being among adolescents. *Arch Pediatr Adolesc Med.* 2003; 157:733-738.
32. Ackard DM, Neumark-Sztainer D, Story M, Perry C. Overeating among adolescents: prevalence and associations with weight-related characteristics and psychological health. *Pediatrics.* 2003;111:67-74.
33. Mellin AE, Neumark-Sztainer D, Story M, Ireland M, Resnick MD. Unhealthy behaviors and psychosocial difficulties among overweight adolescents: the potential impact of familial factors. *J Adolesc Health.* 2002;31:145-153.
34. Hujoel PP, Cunha-Cruz J, Kressin NR. Spurious associations in oral epidemiological research: the case of dental flossing and obesity. *J Clin Periodontol.* In press.
35. Toneatto A, Binik YM. Internal structure of prevention and dental health behaviors. *J Behav Med.* 1990;13:481-487.
36. Troiano RP, Flegal KM. Overweight children and adolescents: description, epidemiology, and demographics. *Pediatrics.* 1998;101:497-504.
37. Winkleby MA, Robinson TN, Sundquist J, Kraemer HC. Ethnic variation in cardiovascular disease risk factors among children and young adults: findings from the Third National Health and Nutrition Examination Survey, 1988-1994. *JAMA.* 1999;281:1006-1013.
38. Landis JR, Lepkowski JM, Eklund SA, Stehouwer SA. A statistical methodology for analyzing data from a complex survey: the first National Health and Nutrition Examination Survey. *Vital Health Stat 2.* 1982;92:1-52.
39. LaVange LM, Stearns SC, Lafata JE, Koch GG, Shah BV. Innovative strategies using SUDAAN for analysis of health surveys with complex samples. *Stat Methods Med Res.* 1996;5:311-329.

**Who's Got Cooties?**

"Cooties are 'imaginary germs' or 'contaminated bugs.' All a child does to start a game is touch someone and say, 'You've got cooties!' Or he may specify the source of the infection: 'You've got Larry's cooties!' He may add, 'No tag backs.' Children mimic immunization shots with ballpoint pens or mark a magic 'X' on their hands with an appropriately named Magic Marker. They write 'C. P.' on their tennis shoes—for 'Cootie Protection.'"
—From *One Potato, Two Potato: The Secret Education of American Children* by Mary and Herbert Knapp, 1976

# Nutrition and Exercise Environment Available to Outpatients, Visitors, and Staff in Children's Hospitals in Canada and the United States

*Christine M. McDonald, RD; Tara Karamlou, MD; James G. Wengle, MSc; Jennifer Gibson, RD; Brian W. McCrindle, MD, MPH*

**Background:** Children's hospitals should advocate for children's health by modeling optimum health environments.

**Objectives:** To determine whether children's hospitals provide optimum health environments and to identify associated factors.

**Design:** Telephone survey.

**Setting:** Canadian and US hospitals with accredited pediatric residency programs.

**Participants:** Food services directors or administrative dietitians.

**Main Outcome Measures:** Health environment grades as determined for 4 domains quantifying (1) the amount of less nutritious food sold at cafeterias (cafeteria grade), (2) the presence of fast food outlets (outlet grade), (3) the amount of nutritious food alternatives available (healthful alternative grade), and (4) the presence of patient obesity or employee exercise programs (program grade).

**Results:** The overall response rate was 87%. Compared with Canadian hospitals, US hospitals had more food outlets (89% vs 50%) and more snack/beverage vending machines (median, 16 vs 12) ($P=.001$ for both), despite equivalent consumer numbers. External companies managed more outlets at US vs Canadian hospitals (65% vs 14%; $P=.01$), and, generally, US hospitals recuperated more revenue from their outlets. Worst cafeteria grade was associated with US hospital location (odds ratio [OR], 8.9; 95% confidence interval [CI], 1.6-50; $P=.01$) and lower healthful alternative grade (OR, 0.016; 95% CI, 0.002-0.15; $P<.001$). Lower grade in any domain was related to whether hospitals received more revenue from noncafeteria food outlets (OR, 1.7; 95% CI, 1.06-2.72; $P=.03$) and the presence of more internally operated cafeterias (OR, 2.3 per cafeteria; 95% CI, 1.53-3.36; $P<.001$).

**Conclusions:** Children's hospitals provide suboptimal health environments. Reliance on revenue may be an important motivating factor encouraging the adoption of outlets that serve less nutritious food.

*Arch Pediatr Adolesc Med. 2006;160:900-905*

THE INCREASING PREVALENCE of overweight and obesity in North American children is a serious public health concern. Children's hospitals are uniquely positioned to advocate for the improved general health of children and should, therefore, provide an environment that encourages the consumption of nutritious food and emphasizes physical activity. The objective of this study was to survey the food services and health programs available to visitors, outpatients, and staff in Canadian and US children's hospitals to determine whether an optimum nutrition and exercise environment is present and, if not, what factors are associated with the adoption and tolerance of less optimum environments.

**Author Affiliations:** Division of Cardiology, Department of Pediatrics, University of Toronto, The Hospital for Sick Children, Toronto, Ontario.

## METHODS

### HOSPITALS AND THE SURVEY INSTRUMENT

All hospitals with pediatric residency programs accredited by either the Royal College of Physicians and Surgeons of Canada or the American Medical Association and with membership in the Canadian Association of Pediatric Health Centers or the National Association of Children's Hospitals and Related Institutions were eligible for the study (N=116). After obtaining ethics approval from The Hospital for Sick Children's Research Ethics Board, data were collected between June 1, 2004, and August 31, 2005. We obtained basic hospital demographic information, including the location of the hospital, the number of inpatient beds, the estimated number of outpatient clinic and day-surgery visits, the number of emergency department visits, and the number of staff members, by conducting telephone interviews with each hospital's appropriate public relations representative or from the public affairs report if it was accessible from institutional Internet-based resources.

Three of us (C.M.M., J.G.W., and J.G.) used a standardized closed-ended questionnaire and conducted telephone interviews with each hospital's food service director or administrative dietitian to obtain information regarding the food services available to outpatients, visitors, and staff members at each facility. In some cases, when it was not possible to conduct the interview by telephone, the appropriate contact person completed the questionnaire by hand and returned it to the investigators by fax. Data were obtained about the main cafeteria, other commercial and noncommercial food outlets, and vending machines in each hospital. For each main cafeteria and food service outlet, we requested information regarding the hours of operation, whether it was operated by an external company, whether all revenue was recuperated by the hospital, whether nutritional information was displayed or available on request, and the specific food choices available. We also collected data regarding the number of dietitians employed at each hospital, whether the hospital operated an obesity clinic or program for children, and whether an exercise program was available for hospital employees. Interviewees were also invited to make comments about what, if any, measures their hospital was taking to improve their current environment.

We made every attempt to avoid value judgments regarding food quality. The terms *good, suboptimal*, and *bad* pertaining to food were specifically avoided because of their inherent subjectivity and the lack of uniform agreement of their constituents. Instead, we used the terms *less nutritious, healthful*, and *not healthful* to describe food items that met the accepted criteria (defined in the following subsection). The criteria used in this study for the classification of food items as healthful or not healthful were formulated based on a synthesis of currently available nutritional guidelines.[1-3] For specific vendor items (eg, McDonald's, Burger King, or Starbucks coffee options), we determined, when available, the caloric content, number of calories from fat, *trans*-fat content, and saturated fat content of food items using nutritional information provided by the specific food outlets and restaurants.[4-7]

## GRADING SYSTEM

The overall nutritional "health" of each hospital was measured by the responses in 4 separate domains: cafeteria grade, outlet grade, healthful alternative grade, and program grade. Cafeteria grade quantifies the number of food items of less nutritional value marketed in the cafeteria(s). To calculate cafeteria grade, a total grade was derived from the sum of less nutritional food items available in the cafeteria. Less nutritious food items included (1) nutrient-poor foods, such as candy bars, potato chips, and soda pop; (2) items containing 1 g or more of *trans*-fat; (3) foods in which more than 30% of the calories are derived from fat; (4) items that provided more than 33% of the recommended saturated fat per day, defined as 65 g for a 2000-cal/d diet; (5) processed foods made with hydrogenated oils or shortening, such as commercial baked goods, donuts, and cakes; and (6) fast food items, such as burgers and french fries. This total grade was then subdivided into an ordinal 4-level grade based on rank quartiles (1 = worst and 4 = best).

Outlet grade quantifies the proportion of fast food franchises and other noncafeteria food service outlets serving food items of less nutritional value in the hospital. To calculate outlet grade, a total grade was derived on the basis of the proportion of fast food franchises and other noncafeteria food service outlets serving food items of less nutritional value divided by the total number of outlets. This total grade was then subdivided into an ordinal 4-level grade (1 = worst and 4 = best). Quartile ranks could not be used because 68% of the hospitals had no outlets serving food items of suboptimal nutritional value and were assigned a grade of 4. To validate the grouping of different food outlets, such as Starbucks and fast food restaurants, together as serving food that is not healthful, we performed a comparative analysis of the nutritional content of 22 popular menu items (using nonfat milk for the drink options) to ensure that no significant differences existed among the outlets. For example, there was no significant difference between Starbucks and McDonald's with respect to either caloric content (median, 330 vs 345; $P = .72$) or saturated fat (median, 6 vs 3.8 g; $P = .47$). Both outlets provided high levels of saturated fat, with Starbucks drink options providing a slightly higher level of saturated fat despite the use of nonfat milk drink options in these comparisons. We included a domain score, the healthful alternative grade discussed in the following paragraph, into the analysis to improve the discrimination among outlets based on the number of healthful food options. This grade quantified the number of healthful alternative choices available at the outlets and provided each food outlet with a mechanism to achieve a higher nutritional score if they had comparatively more healthful options.

Healthful alternative grade quantifies the number of more optimal nutritious food items available in the hospital. To calculate this grade, a total grade was derived from the sum of the amount of nutritious food available in all food sources in the hospital. Healthful food items included the following: (1) nutrient-rich foods, such as fresh fruits, vegetables, and salad; (2) items containing 1 g or less of *trans*-fat; (3) fat-free (0.5 g of fat per serving) or low-fat (≤3 g of total fat per 100-g serving) items; (4) tuna, turkey, or vegetarian sandwiches; and (5) nonfried fish or poultry items. This total grade was then subdivided into an ordinal 4-level grade based on rank quartiles (1 = worst and 4 = best).

Program grade quantifies the availability of overweight and obesity programs for children and exercise programs for staff. Score assignment was as follows: obesity and exercise programs present = 4, obesity program only = 3, exercise program only = 2, and neither = 1.

## DATA ANALYSIS

Data are presented as frequency, median (range), or mean ± SD as appropriate. Because some interviewees could not answer some questions, where there are missing data, the number of nonmissing values is given. Percentages, odds ratios (ORs), and estimates are presented with 95% confidence intervals (CIs). All the data analyses were performed using statistical software (SAS version 9; SAS Institute Inc, Cary, NC). Multivariable logistic regression models and multivariable linear regression models were constructed initially to explore the relationship between factors and the derived domain grades. However, because we expected important intrainstitutional correlation among the 4 domain grades (cafeteria, outlet, healthful alternative, and program grades), these grades were then treated as repeated measurements. Therefore, to accurately account for this correlation and the repeated nature of measurement, generalized estimating equations were used to identify factors associated with having a lower (worse) grade value. Independent correlation structures were used for the generalized estimating equation models, and the assumption of proportional odds was verified by cumulative logit plots.

# RESULTS

## HOSPITAL CHARACTERISTICS

There were 116 children's hospitals that met the inclusion criteria. Demographic data for all of the hospitals

**Table 1. Demographic Characteristics of 116 Children's Hospitals**

| Variable | Value | No. Missing |
|---|---|---|
| Location, No. | | 0 |
| Canada | 12 | |
| United States | 104 | |
| Completed survey, No. (%) | 101 (87) | 15 |
| Inpatient beds, median (range), No. | 175 (26-666) | 4 |
| Outpatient visits per day, median (range), No. | 220 (3-1500) | 55 |
| ED visits per day, median (range), No. | 130 (25-11 476) | 58 |
| Employees, median (range), No. | 2200 (220-8500) | 41 |
| Dietitians, median (range), No. | 9 (1-32) | 32 |
| Food resources | | |
| Cafeterias in hospital, median (range), No. | 1 (0-8) | 1 |
| Food outlets in hospital, median (range), No. | 1 (0-6) | 16 |
| Hospitals with a noncafeteria food outlet, No. (%) | 82 (81) | 19 |
| Snack/beverage vending machines, median, (range), No. | 15 (0-235) | 29 |
| Types of food available in cafeteria, No. (%) | | |
| Not healthful food choices (n = 114) | | 2 |
| Chocolate/candy | 105 (92) | |
| Pies/cake | 90 (79) | |
| Potato chips | 104 (91) | |
| Beef burgers/french fries | 99 (87) | |
| Meat pizza | 93 (82) | |
| Healthful food choices (n = 100) | | 16 |
| Low-fat yogurt | 96 (96) | |
| Fruits/vegetables | 97 (97) | |
| Low-fat desserts | 34 (34) | |
| Low-fat baked goods | 46 (46) | |
| Salad | 92 (92) | |
| Chicken/fish dishes | 90 (90) | |
| Hospital programs for staff, No. (%) (n = 94) | | 24 |
| Both obesity and exercise programs | 16 (17) | |
| Obesity program only | 25 (27) | |
| Exercise program only | 29 (31) | |
| No obesity or exercise program | 23 (25) | |
| Cafeteria revenue, No. (%) (n = 113) | | 3 |
| All revenue recuperated | 88 (78) | |
| Some revenue recuperated | 12 (11) | |
| No revenue recuperated | 12 (11) | |
| Food outlet revenue, No. (%) (n = 72) | | 45 |
| All revenue recuperated | 28 (39) | |
| Some revenue recuperated | 21 (29) | |
| No revenue recuperated | 23 (32) | |

Abbreviation: ED, emergency department.

are given in **Table 1**. The response rate for conducting the interviews was 87% overall (n=101) and was slightly better for Canadian vs US hospitals (100% vs 86%). Reasons for noncompletion of the interview were refusal to participate for 2 hospitals and inability to contact the person identified at the respective hospital for the remaining 13 hospitals.

## FOOD RESOURCES

Of 99 hospitals with cafeterias, 82 (83%) had noncafeteria food service outlets as well. Although many hospitals had cafeterias that operated until 2 or 3 AM, food was also available for purchase on the hospital inpatient wards for 35 hospitals. Snack and beverage vending machines were present in all but 4 hospitals, with a median of 15 machines (ranging up to 235) per hospital. Less nutritious food choices predominated in hospital cafeterias, including 92% selling chocolates and candy; 79% selling pies, cakes, or other dessert items; 91% selling potato chips; 87% selling beef burgers and french fries; and 82% selling meat pizza (Table 1). In contrast, healthful alternatives, such as low-fat desserts or baked goods, were present in only 34% and 46% of hospitals, respectively. A total of 29 fast food franchise outlets were found in 24 hospitals, with 2 hospitals having more than 1 such outlet. Hospital cafeterias were externally operated in 54% of the hospitals, with 79% of the hospitals having their noncafeteria food service outlets operated by external management companies.

## BEVERAGE CHOICES

Regular soft drinks were sold at all times in 99% of the hospital cafeterias and in 75% of the noncafeteria food service outlets. Regular fruit juice was sold in 99% of the cafeterias and in 81% of the noncafeteria outlets. In contrast, only 47% of the noncafeteria outlets sold skim milk, and 75% sold diet soft drinks. Coffee vendors, including Starbucks, were found in 69% of hospitals.

## HOSPITAL PROGRAMS

Obesity programs for children and exercise programs for staff were both present in only 13 hospitals. An obesity or exercise program alone existed in 45 hospitals, and 19 hospitals had neither type of program. Information regarding programs was unavailable for 24 hospitals. Although several respondents mentioned health promotion initiatives that their hospitals were undertaking, these tended to be in hospitals that were combined adult and child facilities. Many respondents cited their hospital's increasing demands for revenue as a major factor limiting the availability and affordability of more nutritious alternatives.

## REVENUE

All the revenue from the cafeterias was recuperated by 76 (78%) of 98 responding hospitals, and an additional 11 hospitals (11%) recuperated a percentage of the revenue from the sale of cafeteria items. Of 56 responding hospitals, 22 (39%) recuperated all of the revenue generated from the noncafeteria food service outlets, and an additional 16 (29%) recuperated a percentage of the revenue from outlet sales (Table 1).

## DOMAIN GRADES

Distribution of the 4 domain grades is shown in the **Figure**. The cafeteria and healthful alternative grades were calculated for 98% of the hospitals (n=99). The median total cafeteria score before conversion to a quartile grade was 10 (range, 1-14). Similarly, the median healthful alternative score was 19 (range, 4-40.5) before conver-

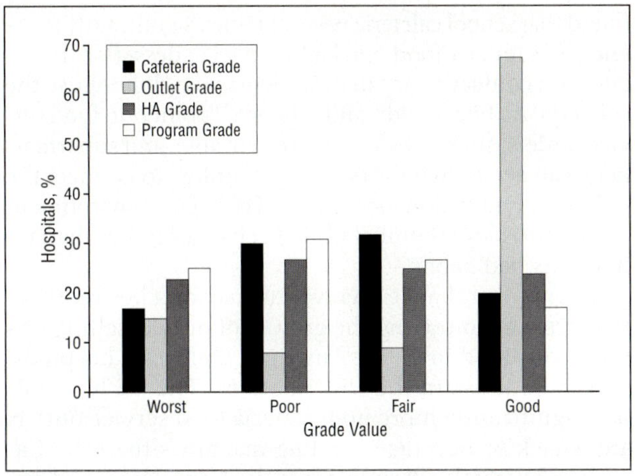


**Figure.** Distribution of the domain grades for hospitals. Ordinal grade assignment was based on rank quartile groups for the cafeteria and healthful alternative (HA) grades. For the outlet grade, however, there were 52 hospitals with no noncafeteria outlets serving predominantly less nutritious food, and, therefore, these hospitals all received a grade of good. Similarly, the program grade was assigned on the basis of other criteria, and so distributions could not be grouped according to rank quantiles.

sion to a quartile grade. Data to generate program and outlet grades were available for 76% of the hospitals (n=77). Of hospitals with available scores, only 8 had a final program grade of good, indicating the presence of both an obesity program for patients and an exercise program for staff. Although fast food franchise outlets were present in several of the large hospitals, 52 (68%) of the 77 hospitals received a final outlet grade of good, indicating that none of the noncafeteria food service outlets at that hospital sold predominantly food with suboptimal nutritional value.

Important differences existed between US and Canadian hospitals (**Table 2**). The US hospitals had significantly more noncafeteria food service outlets serving food of suboptimal nutritional value compared with the Canadian hospitals (89% vs 50%) and more snack and beverage vending machines than the Canadian hospitals (median, 16 vs 12; $P=.001$ for both), despite equivalent employee and patient numbers. Noncafeteria food service outlets in US hospitals were more likely to be managed by external companies (65%) than such outlets in Canadian hospitals (14%; $P=.01$), and, in general, US hospitals recuperated a greater proportion of the revenues generated from these outlets. Similarly, multivariable logistic regression analysis determined that US hospital location was independently associated with worst cafeteria grade (grade 1) (OR, 8.9; 95% CI, 1.6-50; $P=.01$; area under the curve, 0.85). Worst cafeteria grade was also inversely related to the healthful alternative grade (OR, 0.016; 95% CI, 0.002-0.15; $P<.001$; area under the curve, 0.85), indicating a marked imbalance for cafeterias selling the greatest proportion of items with suboptimal nutritional value. Lower program score tended to be positively correlated with increased number of noncafeteria food service outlets serving items of suboptimal nutritional value ($r=0.48$; $P=.07$), suggesting that hospitals with no exercise or obesity programs were most likely to have more outlets with suboptimal choices.

**Table 2. Characteristics of US Hospitals vs Canadian Hospitals***

| Variable | US Hospitals (n = 104) | Canadian Hospitals (n = 12) | P Value |
|---|---|---|---|
| Full-time employees, median (range), No. | 2114 (300-8500) | 2400 (220-6300) | .58 |
| Inpatient beds, median (range), No. | 186 (26-666) | 144 (60-450) | .38 |
| ED visits, median (range), No. | 135 (25-11 476) | 118 (39-185) | .55 |
| Outpatient visits, median (range), No. | 203 (3-1500) | 289 (40-875) | .79 |
| Dietitians, median (range), No. | 8 (1-32) | 11 (3-25) | .27 |
| Cafeterias, median (range), No. | 1 (0-8) | 1 (1-3) | .33 |
| Food outlets, % | 89 | 50 | .001 |
| Beverage vending machines, median (range), No. | 8 (0-215) | 5 (0-10) | .004 |
| Total vending machines, median (range), No. | 16 (0-235) | 12 (0-15) | <.001 |
| Obesity program, % | 50 | 27 | .20 |
| Exercise program, % | 45 | 64 | .26 |
| All or some revenue recuperated from food outlets, % | 70 | 50 | .24 |
| All or some revenue recuperated from cafeteria, % | 87 | 100 | .38 |
| Externally operated cafeterias, % | 37 | 17 | .21 |
| Externally operated food outlets, % | 65 | 14 | .01 |

Abbreviation: ED, emergency department.
*Values are based on the number of responders.

## FACTORS ASSOCIATED WITH INCREASING DOMAIN GRADES

Independent factors associated with lower (worse) grades were sought. Hospitals receiving more revenue from noncafeteria food service outlets were more likely to have lower grade values compared with hospitals receiving no revenue from outlets (OR, 1.7; 95% CI, 1.06-2.72; $P=.03$). Domain grade was also significantly lower in hospitals with more internally operated cafeterias (OR, 2.3 per cafeteria; 95% CI, 1.53-3.36; $P<.001$).

## COMMENT

We used a telephone interview with an 87% response rate to show that most university-affiliated pediatric hospitals in Canada and the United States provide a suboptimal nutrition and exercise environment for their patients, patients' families, and employees. Although several studies have investigated the quality and availability of food services provided to inpatients, we extended this analysis to outpatients, staff, and visitors. We also included the presence of obesity programs and staff exercise programs as a measure of the hospital's commitment to overall nutritional health. We found that no children's hospitals received a "perfect" grade in all 4 domains. Although children's hospitals are in a unique position to advocate for the general health of children from a position of authority and example, especially in the face of a growing epidemic of childhood obesity, they seem to be failing.

The increasing prevalence of overweight and obesity in North American society continues to be a serious public health concern. Results of the 2004 Canadian Community Health Survey[8,9] show that 59% of Canadian adults 18 years or older and 26% of children and adolescents aged 2 to 17 years were overweight or obese. In the United States, results of the 1999-2002 National Health and Nutrition Examination Survey[10] revealed that 65% of American adults 20 years or older were overweight or obese, whereas 32% of children 6 to 19 years of age were at risk for overweight or were overweight.

Environmental factors that affect lifestyle and consequently dietary choices are among the many variables contributing to this epidemic. St. Onge et al[11] note that time limitations have become an important factor in determining the types of food consumed. The food industry has responded by increasing the number of convenience foods and prepared meals available to customers.[12] Several hospitals have recently integrated commercial food outlets into their food service systems in hopes of generating more sales, of which a variable proportion of revenue is often contributed back to the hospital. We have shown, in agreement with this trend, that most (85%) of the university-affiliated children's hospitals have either fast food franchise outlets or other outlets selling items of less nutritional value. These hospitals also prominently featured less nutritious food choices in their cafeterias while providing few healthier alternatives. The adverse effect of this unwholesome environment may be magnified because hospital staff, patients, and their families represent a relatively captive consumer market. This increased reliance on foods consumed away from home and the decreased expense associated with less nutritious convenience food, food advertising, marketing, and promotion have changed the way North Americans eat.[13] Between 1977 and 1995, the percentage of meals and snacks eaten at fast food restaurants increased by 200%, and in 1998, 46% of all US adults ate at a restaurant on any given day.[13] Lin et al[14] found that away-from-home foods are higher in fat and energy compared with foods prepared and eaten at home. Furthermore, increased fast food restaurant use has been associated with higher energy and fat intake among adolescents[15] and an increased prevalence of obesity.[16,17] Based on our nutritional analysis, an average meal at McDonald's, consisting of a Big Mac, medium french fries, and a medium shake, contains 1520 total calories and 22 g of saturated fat.

Although we cannot provide direct evidence that the amount of food of suboptimal nutritional value consumed is increased by the predominance of commercial food service outlets and unwholesome food choices, it is certainly a plausible conclusion that people eat what is readily available and least expensive. This notion is supported by previous studies[18-20] that explicitly demonstrate the influential role that the nutrition environment plays in the health and nutritional status of the public. Bell and Swinburn[18] found that school cafeteria users obtained significantly more energy from fast food, packaged snacks, desserts, chocolate, and confectionary than students who did not use the cafeteria. As Fitzgerald[20] and others[21-23] point out, food service outlets, such as cafeterias, restaurants, and supermarkets, can act as "windows of opportunity" to connect the public with nutrition messages and can act as environmental supports for continual lifestyle changes rather than reinforcing bad habits.

Economic reliance on revenue may be a key motivating factor encouraging the growth of outlets selling less nutritious food in North American children's hospitals, especially those in the United States. The US hospitals had significantly more noncafeteria food service outlets and snack or beverage vending machines than the Canadian hospitals, despite equivalent employee and patient numbers. Furthermore, our data determined that 78% of the hospitals recuperated at least a percentage of the revenues generated from these food outlets, with a greater proportion of US hospitals recuperating all of the revenue from food outlet sales compared with their Canadian counterparts. Hospitals in the United States also relied more on external companies to manage their food outlets. Increased dependence on external companies may directly encourage the sale of less nutritious items because these items are the least expensive to purchase, distribute, and store, therefore generating the best profit-loss ratio for external companies.

Consumption of sweetened beverages such as soft drinks also has been linked to childhood diabetes mellitus and obesity in North American children.[18,24-26] Of further concern is the finding that soft drinks may be displacing milk and fruit juice in the diets of children and adolescents, particularly because only 5% of 7- to 14-year-old children meet the national recommendations for servings of fruit and only 9% of children meet the recommendations for dairy.[21] Despite the clear evidence that sweetened beverages promote childhood disease, we found an alarmingly high number of soft drink vending machines at many children's hospitals, with only 2 hospitals having none. Gazibarich[27] notes that hospitals have the potential to be models for healthful environments, a mission that should be reflected in the food that is made available to patrons. In Australia, this mission was articulated by setting a target to increase the proportion of health service users, visitors, and employees who have access to catering services that supply a range of food consistent with good dietary guidelines.[27] However, North American literature has failed to reveal any similar objectives.

A limitation of this study concerns the use of self-report to measure the outcome variable: the overall nutrition environment of each children's hospital. Financial considerations obviously precluded the possibility of visiting every children's hospital and directly validating respondents' self-report. Although our overall response rate was excellent at 87%, we cannot assume that nonparticipants were similar to participants. However, the repeated nature of grade assessment and the intragrade correlation apparent from the exploratory analysis allowed the use of generalized estimating equations to amplify the sample size. In addition, we considered only variables with robust response rates to minimize the introduction of bias. The lack of direct evidence that unwholesome hospital environments foster the choice of items of suboptimal nutritional value is another potential limitation.

In conclusion, children's hospitals frequently have available a plethora of unwholesome food and beverage choices, and these choices contribute to revenue in most of these hospitals. Economic reliance on this revenue may be a key motivating factor encouraging the growth of unwholesome food outlets in North American children's hospitals. Coupled with revenue dependence, increased corporate control over the food services at many children's hospitals also makes it difficult to ensure that more healthful foods are available and being marketed to outpatients and visitors. Political and legislative initiatives should be actively pursued by children's hospitals to eliminate environmental factors that foster excess caloric consumption and threaten the general health of children.

**Accepted for Publication:** March 23, 2006.
**Correspondence:** Brian W. McCrindle, MD, MPH, The Hospital for Sick Children, 555 University Ave, Toronto, Ontario, Canada M5G 1X8 (brian.mccrindle@sickkids.ca).
**Author Contributions:** *Study concept and design:* McDonald, Karamlou, and McCrindle. *Acquisition of data:* McDonald, Karamlou, Wengle, and Gibson. *Analysis and interpretation of data:* McDonald, Karamlou, and McCrindle. *Drafting of the manuscript:* McDonald, Karamlou, and McCrindle. *Critical revision of the manuscript for important intellectual content:* Karamlou, Wengle, Gibson, and McCrindle. *Statistical analysis:* Karamlou, Wengle, and McCrindle. *Administrative, technical, and material support:* Wengle, Gibson, and McCrindle. *Study supervision:* McCrindle.

## REFERENCES


1. Dietary guidelines for Americans 2005. http://www.cnpp.usda.gov/dietary_guidelines.html. Accessed August 21, 2005.
2. Canada's food guide to healthy eating. http://www.hc-sc.gc.ca/fn-an/food-guide-aliment/fg_rainbow-arc_en_ciel_ga_e.html. Accessed August 21, 2005.
3. McCrindle BW, Wengle JG. *Get a Healthy Weight for Your Child: A Parent's Guide to Better Eating and Exercise.* Toronto, Ontario: Robert Rose Inc; 2005.
4. Starbucks beverage nutrition guide. http://starbucks.co.uk/en-GB/_Favorite+Beverages/Beverage+Nutrition.htm. Accessed August 21, 2005.
5. McDonald's USA nutrition facts for popular menu items. http://www.mcdonalds.com/app_controller.nutrition.index1.html. Accessed August 21, 2005.
6. Have it your way: Burger King nutritional information. http://www.burgerking.ca/imagelibrary/PDF/nutritional.pdf. Accessed August 21, 2005.
7. Tim Horton's nutritional information. http://www.timhortons.com/en/menu/menu_info.html. Accessed August 21, 2005.
8. Tjepkema M. Nutrition: findings from the Canadian Community Health Survey—adult obesity in Canada: measured height and weight. http://www.statcan.ca/english/research/82-620-MIE/2005001/pdf/aobesity.pdf. Accessed October 2005.
9. Shields M. Nutrition: findings from the Canadian Community Health Survey—overweight Canadian children and adolescents. http://www.statcan.ca/english/research/82-620-MIE/2005001/pdf/cobesity.pdf. Accessed October 2005.
10. Hedley AA, Ogden CL, Johnson CL, Carroll MD, Curtin CR, Flegal KM. Prevalence of overweight and obesity among US children, adolescents, and adults, 1999-2002. *JAMA.* 2004;291:2847-2850.
11. St. Onge MP, Keller KL, Heymsfield SB. Changes in childhood food consumption patterns: a cause for concern in light of increasing body weights. *Am J Clin Nutr.* 2003;78:1068-1073.
12. Schluter G, Lee C. Changing food consumption patterns: their effects on the US food system, 1972-92. *Food Rev.* 1999;22:35-37.
13. French SA, Story M, Jeffery RW. Environmental influences on eating and physical activity. *Annu Rev Public Health.* 2001;22:309-335.
14. Lin BH, Guthrie J, Frazao E. Quality of children's diets at and away from home: 1994-1996. *Food Rev.* 1999;22:2-10.
15. French SA, Story M, Neumark-Sztainer D, Fulkerson JA, Hannan P. Fast food restaurant use among adolescents: associations with nutrient intake, food choices and behavioral and psychosocial variables. *Int J Obes Relat Metab Disord.* 2001;25:1823-1833.
16. Maddock J. The relationship between obesity and the prevalence of fast food restaurants: state-level analysis. *Am J Health Promot.* 2004;19:137-143.
17. French SA, Harnack L, Jeffery RW. Fast food restaurant use among women in the Pound of Prevention study: dietary, behavioral and demographic correlates. *Int J Obes Relat Metab Disord.* 2000;24:1353-1359.
18. Bell AC, Swinburn BA. What are the key food groups to target for preventing obesity and improving nutrition in schools? *Eur J Clin Nutr.* 2004;58:258-263.
19. Snyder P, Anliker J, Cunningham-Sabo L, et al. The Pathways study: a model for lowering the fat in school meals. *Am J Clin Nutr.* 1999;69(4)(suppl):810S-815S.
20. Fitzgerald CM, Kannan S, Sheldon S, Allen Eagle K. Effect of a promotional campaign on heart-healthy menu choices in community restaurants. *J Am Diet Assoc.* 2004;104:429-432.
21. American Academy of Pediatrics. National Cholesterol Education Program: report of the Expert Panel on Blood Cholesterol Levels in Children and Adolescents. *Pediatrics.* 1992;89:525-584.
22. Gidding SS, Dennison BA, Birch LL, et al. Dietary recommendations for children and adolescents: a guide for practitioners: consensus statement from the American Heart Association. *Circulation.* 2005;112:2061-2075.
23. Fried EJ, Nestle M. The growing political movement against soft drinks in schools. *JAMA.* 2002;288:2181.
24. Sturm R. Childhood obesity: what we can learn from existing data on societal trends, part 2. *Prev Chronic Dis.* 2005;2:A20. http://www.cdc.gov/pcd/issues/2005/apr/04_0039.htm. Accessed November 2005.
25. Nicklas TA, Yang SJ, Baranowski T, Zakeri I, Berenson G. Eating patterns and obesity in children: the Bogalusa Heart Study. *Am J Prev Med.* 2003;25:9-16.
26. Harnack L, Stang J, Story M. Soft drink consumption among US children and adolescents: nutritional consequences. *J Am Diet Assoc.* 1999;99:436-441.
27. Gazibarich B. A framework for the measurement of healthy hospital menus. *Australian J Nutr Dietetics.* 1997;54:70-77.


## *Correction*

**Omission in *About the Cover*.** In *About the Cover* for the photograph *Summer in Lee Neff's Garden* in the July issue of the ARCHIVES (2006;160:669), the photographer was mistakenly omitted. The photographer was John Neff, MD.

REVIEW ARTICLE

# Measuring Effectiveness of Dietetic Interventions in Child Obesity

## *A Systematic Review of Randomized Trials*

*Clare E. Collins, PhD, BSc, Dip(Nutr&Diet), Dip(ClinEpi), AdvAPD; Janet Warren, PhD, BSc, RD; Melinda Neve, BND, APD; Penelope McCoy, BHSc(Nutr&Diet), APD; Barrie J. Stokes, BSc, MMath*

**Objectives:** To assess the effectiveness of dietetic treatment for obese children and to report details of dietary interventions.

**Data Sources:** English-language articles from 1975 to 2003 available from health and medical databases.

**Study Selection:** Randomized controlled trials with subjects younger than 18 years of age that included a dietary intervention in isolation or in combination with lifestyle modifications and/or psychological therapies. One person searched the databases; 2 people independently critically appraised the articles for methodological quality and then extracted data using standardized tools.

**Data Extraction:** Thirty-seven randomized controlled trials met the inclusion criteria; 17 contained sufficient information for a Forest plot of the standardized effects. Eight studies had a true control and were included in a meta-analysis. The random effects model was reported if the Q noncombinability $\chi^2$ statistic was significant at the 10% level because it has low power as a strict test of homogeneity.

**Data Synthesis:** The 2 strongly qualified meta-analyses suggest that interventions that include a dietary treatment do achieve relative weight loss. Details of the dietary intervention or participant food intake are rarely described.

**Conclusions:** It is not possible to evaluate the effectiveness of dietary treatment for childhood obesity because of the lack of high-quality studies and the heterogeneity of designs, treatment combinations, outcome measures, and follow-up. There is an urgent need to improve the quality of studies in this area because childhood obesity poses major health risks for populations, yet there is limited evidence on which to base treatment strategies.

*Arch Pediatr Adolesc Med. 2006;160:906-922*

**Author Affiliations:** School of Health Sciences (Drs Collins and Warren and Mss Neve and McCoy) and Discipline of Clinical Pharmacology (Mr Stokes), University of Newcastle, Callaghan, Australia; and Food and Nutrition Australia, Sydney (Ms McCoy).

OBESITY IN CHILDREN IS INcreasing rapidly around the world. The associated major adverse health consequences have been systematically reviewed[1] and the psychological consequences and social marginalization reported.[2]

Prevention is clearly the ideal solution to the problem. However, for those already overweight or obese, or at an increased risk of becoming so, effective interventions will offer the only chance of reducing the probability of progression to adult obesity, its associated comorbidities, and the increased risk of premature mortality.[3] Essential elements of interventions are likely to include diet and food intake modification,[4] and these have been identified for adult interventions. The efficacy of such interventions in the pediatric population is not known. An examination of successful interventions along with the key dietary changes achieved by participants would inform the optimal dietary treatment for broad dissemination. Therefore, the objective of this review was to identify and present the best available evidence on the effectiveness of dietetic treatment and management for overweight or obese children and adolescents. A secondary goal was to specifically describe the elements of successful dietary treatments.

## METHODS

### SEARCH STRATEGY

We performed a systematic review of the published English-language literature from 1975 to 2003. These limits were set to contain costs and maintain timelines. Because the prevalence of child obesity has increased predominantly since the late 1970s,[5] it was considered likely that few relevant studies would have been published before then. An additional author search was carried out in 2004 for the most up-to-date results of specific studies identified in the original search.

Electronic databases were searched (CINAHL [Cumulative Index to Nursing and Allied Health Literature], MEDLINE, PREMEDLINE, DARE [Database of Abstracts of Review of Effectiveness], Cochrane, EMBASE [Excerpta Medica Database], Austrom, Current Concepts, and Dissertation Abstracts). In addition, we searched nutrition and dietetics journals by hand (the *Journal of the Dietitians Association of Australia*, the *International Journal of Obesity*, and the *Journal of Human Nutrition and Dietetics*) and government reports from the United States, United Kingdom, and Australia along with the reference lists and bibliographies of retrieved articles. The MeSH (Medical Subject Headings of the National Library of Medicine) keyword search terms were dietetic, paediatric (pediatric), child, adolescent, family, parent, school, overweight, obesity, intervention, weight control or weight management or weight loss, and healthy weight.

## SELECTION OF STUDIES

The current report is limited to the randomized controlled trials (RCTs) identified for a more extensive review undertaken for the Joanna Briggs Institute (JBI), Adelaide, Australia. Any trial that evaluated the effectiveness of nutrition or dietary interventions for treating overweight or obesity in children and adolescents was included for the JBI review.

Participants aged younger than 18 years who were defined as overweight or obese were included. We also included programs that were directed exclusively at parents of overweight or obese children and adolescents. Participants were free-living outpatients; inpatients in clinical obesity units; or students attending community programs, one-off programs, camps, or schools. Studies that reported at least one of the following primary outcomes were included: percentile of body mass index (BMI), calculated as weight in kilograms divided by height in meters squared; BMI $z$ score; percentage of children overweight for age; waist measurement; skin folds; percentage of body fat; or percentage of lean body mass.

We considered interventions aimed at the treatment of elevated body weight delivered by any health professional or nutrition scientist. Initially, the aim was to review only studies that compared dietary modification with a standard control (ie, no treatment). Because of the limited number of such studies, we also reviewed interventions that included dietary modification both as part of an intervention and/or control with various combinations of lifestyle modifications (physical activity and/or sedentary behavior modification) and psychological components (cognitive and/or behavioral therapy).

Studies that did not report a weight-related variable as a primary outcome were excluded from the review. Those studies that were assessed as being of poor methodological quality using the JBI tools[6] or that did not meet the inclusion criteria were excluded from the review.

Articles were retrieved if the information contained in the title, abstract, and descriptor/MeSH headings appeared to meet the inclusion criteria. Working independently, 2 reviewers critically appraised the articles for methodological quality using the JBI critical appraisal tools.[6] Particular attention was paid to sources of bias in the studies.[7] If disagreement between reviewers occurred in any of these steps, a third person repeated the procedure to achieve consensus.

We used Review Manager (RevMan 4.2, The Cochrane Collaboration, Oxford, England) to manage the systematic review. Interventions and study design defined comparability of the studies. Heterogeneity was assessed using the standard Q statistic for heterogeneity and visual interpretation of graphs. Significant heterogeneity was assumed when $P < .10$. All outcome data reported were continuous, but because studies variously reported changes in percentage overweight, BMI $z$ score, percentage body fat, or body weight, standardized mean differences were used in the analyses. The standardized mean difference has the important property that its value does not depend on the measurement scale. This enabled comparisons of differences in mean weight loss when expressed in percentage body fat, weight for height, or another outcome measure. Studies were excluded from the analyses if they did not report numbers of participants or standard deviations.

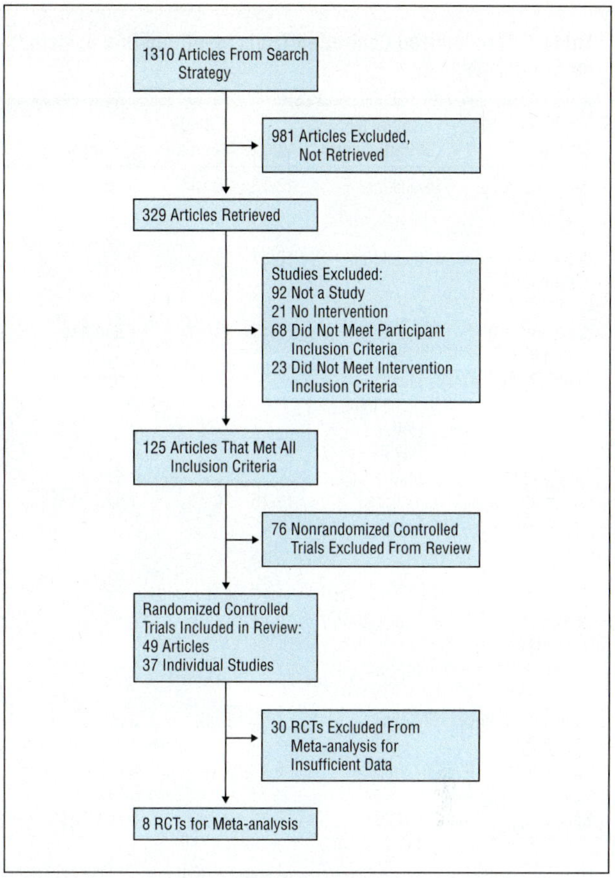


**Figure 1.** Randomized controlled trials (RCTs) for inclusion in a meta-analysis of effectiveness of dietetic interventions in child and adolescent obesity.

## RESULTS

There were 1310 articles identified by the search strategy (**Figure 1**). After excluding studies due to duplication and assessing titles and abstracts to meet inclusion criteria, we retrieved 329 full text articles for reviewing. One hundred twenty-five articles met the inclusion criteria for the main review and details will be reported through JBI publications. After we excluded the nonrandomized trials, there were 49 articles arising from 37 individual studies because some reported the results of the same study more than once. These 37 RCTs are reported here.

The total number of participants across all studies was 2262. The focus of the interventions was diet with various combinations of modifications to physical activity and/or sedentary behavior or behavioral and/or cognitive therapy. Of the 37 studies, 18 had two intervention arms,[8-25] 11 had three,[26-35] 6 had four,[36-41] and 1 had five arms (**Table 1**).[43]

**Table 1. Randomized Controlled Trials Identified in a Systematic Review of the Effectiveness of Dietetic Interventions for Child Obesity**

| Source | Initial No. of Participants | Age, y | Study Length | Follow-up | Study Arms* | Retention, %† | Intention-to-Treat Analysis |
|---|---|---|---|---|---|---|---|
| Becque et al (1988)[26] | 36 children | 12-13 | 20 wk | None | (1) Control<br>(2) DA + BT<br>(3) DA + BT + PA | 100 | Yes |
| Botvin and Cantlon (1979)[42] | 119 children | 12-17 | 10 wk | None | (1) Control<br>(2) DA + PA + BT | 89 | No |
| Braet and Van Winckel (1997)[43]‡ | 259 children (1-y follow-up study); 136 children (4.6-y follow-up study) | 7-17 | Varied | 1 and 4.6 y (not group 5) | (1) CBT + DA + PA (individual treatment)<br>(2) CBT + DA + PA (outpatient group treatment)<br>(3) CBT + DA + PA (summer camp training)<br>(4) CBT + DA + PA (typical care)<br>(5) Control group (nonclinically obese) | 81 at 1 y<br>80 at 4.6 y | Yes at 1 y<br>No at 4.6 y |
| Brownell et al (1983)[27] | 42 children | 12-16 | 16 wk | 1 y | (1) BT + DA + PA (mother and child in separate groups)<br>(2) BT + DA + PA (mother and child in same group)<br>(3) BT + DA + PA (child alone) | 86 at 1 y | Unclear |
| Coates et al (1983)[41] | 42 children | 13-17 | 15 wk | 6 mo | (1) DA (daily contact, weight loss focus)<br>(2) DA (weekly contact, weight loss focus)<br>(3) DA (daily contact, kcal change focus)<br>(4) DA (weekly contact, kcal change focus) | 79 at 6 mo | Yes |
| Duffy and Spence (1992)[8] | 27 children | 7-13 | 8 wk | 3 and 6 mo | (1) DA + PA + CBT<br>(2) DA + PA + BT | 63 at 6 mo | No |
| Epstein et al (1980)[9] | 16 families | 6-12 | 7 wk | 3 mo | (1) BT + DA + PA<br>(2) DA + PA | 69 at 3 mo | Yes |
| Epstein et al[35,44-46]* | 76 families; 86 children | 6-12 | 8 mo | 5 and 10 y | (1) BT + PA + DA (parent and child were targets)<br>(2) BT + PA + DA (child was target)<br>(3) BT + PA + DA (nonspecific target) | 88 at 5 y<br>80 at 10 y | No at 5 y<br>No at 10 y |
| Epstein et al (1982)[40] | 51 families | 8-12 | 2 mo | 6 and 17 mo | (1) DA + PA (lifestyle)<br>(2) DA + PA (programmed)<br>(3) PA (lifestyle)<br>(4) PA (programmed) | 75 at 17 mo | No |
| Epstein et al[35,44]* | 53 families | 8-12 | 6 mo | 1 y (not controls) | (1) DA<br>(2) DA + PA<br>(3) Control (waiting list) | 94 at 1 y | No |
| Epstein et al (1985)[10] | 23 girls | 8-12 | 2 mo | 6 and 12 mo | (1) DA + BT<br>(2) DA + BT + PA | 83 at 12 mo | No |
| Epstein et al (1985)[11] | 24 children | 5-8 | 6 wk | 8 and 12 mo | (1) DA + PA<br>(2) BT + DA + PA | 75 at 12 mo | No |
| Epstein et al[12,35,44,46] | 41 families | 8-12 | 1 y | 3 and 5 y | (1) DA + PA (parent)<br>(2) DA + PA (child) | 93 at 3 y<br>80 at 5 y | No |
| Epstein et al (1994)[13] | 44 families | 8-12 | 1 y | 12 and 24 mo | (1) DA + PA + BT (parents mastered skills before progressing)<br>(2) DA + PA + BT (control parents not required to master skills) | 89 at 24 mo | No |
| Epstein et al (1995)[28] | 61 families | 8-12 | 6 mo | 1 y | (1) DA + SB<br>(2) DA + PA<br>(3) DA + PA + SB | 90 at 1 y | No |
| Epstein et al (2000)[39] | 90 families | 8-12 | 6 mo | 1 and 2 y | (1) PA (high dose) + DA<br>(2) PA (low dose) + DA<br>(3) SB (high dose) + DA<br>(4) SB (low dose) + DA | 84 at 2 y | Yes |
| Epstein et al (2000)[29] | 67 families | 8-12 | 6 mo | 1 and 2 y | (1) BT + DA + PA (parent and child taught problem solving)<br>(2) BT + DA + PA (child only taught problem solving)<br>(3) BT + DA + PA (no problem solving) | 78 at 2 y | No |
| Epstein et al (2001)[14] | 67 families | 8-12 | 6 mo | 12 mo | (1) PA + DA<br>(2) PA + DA + SB | 84 at 12 mo | No |
| Epstein et al (2004)[15] | 63 families | 8-12 | 6 mo | 12 mo | (1) SB (stimulus control) + DA<br>(2) SB (reinforce) + DA | 95 at 12 mo | No |
| Flodmark et al (1993)[30] | 94 children | 10-11 | 14-18 mo | 1 y (intervention only) | (1) Untreated control (nonrandomized)<br>(2) DA (conventional treatment)<br>(3) DA (family therapy) | 84 at 1 y | Yes |

(*continued*)

**Table 1. Randomized Controlled Trials Identified in a Systematic Review of the Effectiveness of Dietetic Interventions for Child Obesity (cont)**

| Source | Initial No. of Participants | Age, y | Study Length | Follow-up | Study Arms* | Retention, %† | Intention-to-Treat Analysis |
|---|---|---|---|---|---|---|---|
| Golan et al[25,47]‡ | 60 children | 6-11 | 12 mo | 2 and 7 y | (1) DA + SB + BT (parents only)<br>(2) DA + SB + BT (child only) | 83 at 7 y | Yes |
| Goldfield et al (2001)[16] | 31 families | 8-12 | 5 mo | 6 and 12 mo | (1) DA + PA + BT (individual and group sessions)<br>(2) DA + PA + BT (group) | 77 at 12 mo | No |
| Graves et al (1988)[31] | 40 children | 6-12 | 8 wk | 1, 2, 3, and 6 mo | (1) DA + PA + BT<br>(2) DA + PA + BT + CBT<br>(3) DA + PA (instruction only) | 78 at 6 mo | Unclear |
| Gutin et al (2002)[32] | 80 children | 13-16 | 8 mo | None | (1) LSE<br>(2) LSE + moderate-intense PA<br>(3) LSE + high-intense PA<br>(LSE involved BT + DA + PA) | 71 | Yes |
| Hills and Parker (1988)[17] | 35 children | Prepubertal | 16 wk | None | (1) DA<br>(2) DA + PA<br>(3) Control (nonobese) | 100 | Yes |
| Kirschenbaum et al (1984)[33] | 40 families | 9-13 | 9 wk | 3 and 12 mo | (1) DA + PA + CBT (parent and child)<br>(2) DA + PA + CBT (child only)<br>(3) Waiting list control | 83 at 12 mo | No |
| Lansky and Brownell (1982)[18] | 71 children | 12-15 | 3.5 mo | None | (1) DA + PA + BT<br>(2) DA + PA (instruction only) | 75 | Yes |
| Mellin et al (1987)[19] | 66 children | 12-18 | 3 mo | 6 and 15 mo | (1) CBT + DA + PA<br>(2) Control group | 84 at 1 y | Yes |
| Nova et al (2001)[24] | 186 children | 3-12 | 1 appointment | Varied | (1) Control (general advice DA + PA)<br>(2) DA + PA (enhanced approach) | 70 at 12 mo | Unclear |
| Rocchini et al (1987)[38] | 60 children | 10-16 | 20 wk | None | (1) Control group (nonobese)<br>(2) DA + BT<br>(3) DA + PA + BT<br>(4) Obese control group | 100 | Yes |
| Rocchini et al (1988)[37] | 82 children | 10-16 | 20 wk | None | (1) Control group (nonobese)<br>(2) DA + BT<br>(3) Diet + PA + BT<br>(4) Obese control group | 88 | No |
| Saelens et al (2002)[20] | 44 children | 12-16 | 4 mo | 3 mo | (1) DA + BT + PA (intensive follow-up)<br>(2) Typical care (single physician session) | 84 at 3 mo | Yes |
| Schwingshandl et al (1999)[21] | 30 children | 6-18 | 12 wk | 6 and 12 mo | (1) DA + PA<br>(2) DA | 66 at 12 mo | Yes |
| Senediak and Spence (1985)[36] | 45 children | 6-12.5 | 4 and 15 wk | 15 and 26 wk | (1) DA + PA + BT (rapid behavioral group)<br>(2) DA + PA + BT (nonspecific behavioral control)<br>(3) DA + PA (control)<br>(4) Control group (waiting list) | 77 at 15 wk<br>71 at 26 wk | No |
| Sondike et al (2003)[22] | 39 children | 12-18 | 12 wk | None | (1) DA (low fat)<br>(2) DA (low carbohydrate) | 77 | No |
| Sung et al (2002)[23] | 82 children | 8-11 | 6 wk | None | (1) DA + PA<br>(2) DA | 100 | Yes |
| Wadden et al (1990)[34] | 47 girls | 12-16 | 16 wk | 6 mo | (1) DA + PA + BT (child alone)<br>(2) DA + PA + BT (mother and child together)<br>(3) DA + PA + BT (child and mother separately) | 77 at 6 mo | No |

Abbreviations: BT, behavioral therapy; CBT, cognitive behavioral therapy; DA, dietary advice; LSE, lifestyle education; PA, physical activity; SB, sedentary behavior.
*Numbers in study arms may be different from number of participants because of dropouts, and numbers were not given for specific interventions.
†Retention rates reported postintervention if no follow-up or at latest point of follow-up.
‡Selected references cited; a complete reference list is available from the authors.

Thirty-two studies* included physical activity as a component of at least 1 of the study arms while 14 studies† included behavioral therapy as a component of at least 1 of the study arms. Six studies[8,19,29,31,33,43] included cognitive behavioral therapy specifically as a component of at least 1 of the study arms. Six studies[12,14,15,25,28,39] included decreasing sedentary behavior as a component of at least 1 of the study arms. The length of intervention in each RCT ranged from 6 weeks to 18 months with the majority (n=17) between 3 months and 6 months.‡ Nine

*References 8-14, 16-21, 23, 24, 26-29, 31-40, 42, 43.
†References 8, 9, 11, 13, 16, 18, 20, 26, 27, 31, 32, 34, 35, 42.
‡References 14-20, 26-29, 34, 35, 37-39, 41.

studies[8-10,21-23,31,33,40] described interventions that were run for up to 3 months, and 7 studies[12,13,25,30,32,35,43] had interventions that ran for longer than 6 months. The length of intervention was unclear or varied in 3 studies.[11,24,36] The length of follow-up was very diverse among the studies. The shortest was 1 month[38] while the longest was 10 years.[44] Nine studies§ included no follow-up of participants postintervention. Table 1 also reports the retention rates at the longest point of follow-up except for the 5 studies with a follow-up exceeding 2 years where interim rates are given.[24,25,35,43,45] Studies undertaking intention-to-treat analyses are also highlighted in Table 1. The majority of studies were conducted in the United States (n=29), 5 were in different European countries,[21,24,25,30,43] 2 were in Australia,[8,17] and 1 was in Hong Kong.[23]

Because of the various combinations of treatments that included a dietary intervention and the variable composition of the control groups, a meta-analysis to show the effectiveness of dietetic interventions per se was not possible. Results of the main weight outcomes for each of the 37 RCTs are presented in **Table 2** with the significance indicated. A Forest plot of the standardized effects for the studies that contained sufficient information (n=17) highlights the heterogeneity of the interventions (**Figure 2**). It was not appropriate to report a meta-analysis result because only a minority of studies had an adequate control group and the treatments reported were highly diverse. However, a meta-analysis was undertaken on the subset of studies (n=8) that included both a dietary intervention component and an adequate control group (**Figure 3**). In these studies, diet was a component of the interventions and the control group either received no intervention, was placed on a waiting list, or received usual care. Caution must be exercised in the interpretation of the analysis because diet was only a component of the interventions, making its contribution difficult to evaluate. In addition, the number of studies is limited. The meta-analysis suggests that interventions that contain a dietary component are effective in achieving relative weight loss in overweight/obese children and adolescents (pooled standardized mean difference, −1.82; 95% confidence interval, −2.40 to −1.23) (Figure 3). The 2 studies with the greatest standardized effect were those of Rochini et al[38] and Becque et al[26] (Figure 2). Becque et al reported that in adolescents, a reduction in the percentage body fat of approximately 3% was achieved after 20 weeks of treatment with diet and behavior change with or without exercise.[26] Postintervention, participants in the study by Rochini et al of obese adolescents significantly decreased their percentage body fat by 3% to 6%[38] (Table 2). Only 4 studies had follow-up data, and a meta-analysis of the outcomes of these results suggests a diminishing effect of the intervention over time (pooled standardized mean difference, −0.64; 95% confidence interval, −0.89 to −0.39) (**Figure 4**).

A summary of the dietary interventions and the studies that measured and reported dietary compliance and outcomes is given in **Table 3**. Sixteen studies|| used the Stoplight/Traffic Light diet (or a variation of it) as their dietary intervention. Five studies[18,26,36-38] included food or calorie exchange programs while only 1 study[22] compared 2 different dietary interventions (low fat vs low carbohydrate). Compliance with the dietary intervention was reported in only 3 studies[13,22,28] although reported as having been measured by food diaries or records in 23 studies. An attempt to describe the dietary intake of those participating in or completing an intervention was made in most studies, but the level of detail was of variable quality. A dietitian was reported to be involved in the formulation and/or delivery of the dietary intervention in 13 primary studies¶ (Table 3).

All 37 RCTs had at least 1 methodological weakness using the JBI critical appraisal tools.[6] Although all studies reported randomization of participants to study groups, the method of randomization was described in a minority of studies. Allocation concealment was unclear in 24 studies, adequate in 11 studies,# and not used in 2 studies. The number of participants in the studies varied but was generally low; 16 had fewer than 50 participants and only 2 studies had sample sizes greater than 150.[24,43] The nature of dietary and lifestyle interventions prevents the blinding of participants. Only 1 study mentions assessor blinding and this was only for some of the assessments.[23] Outcomes were measured using varying scales among the studies but within each study were reported as being measured in the same manner for all participants. The retention rates were greater than 80% for 17 of 37 RCTs; the lowest rate was 63% at 1-year follow-up after a long intervention period of 14 to 18 months.[27] The retention rate was unclear in 1 study and difficult to ascertain at various stages of the intervention and/or follow-up in several studies.

## COMMENT

The initial aim of this review was to assess the effectiveness of dietary interventions in the management of overweight and obesity in children and adolescents. Only a very limited number of studies (n=7)[17,21-23,30,35,41] tested a dietary intervention as the sole component of treatment and compared this with a nonintervention control group or a treatment group with a different approach or intensity. Therefore, we evaluated studies that comprised dietary treatments in combination with other treatments. This resulted in a diverse set of studies that made it impossible to report the effectiveness of dietary interventions in childhood/adolescent overweight and obesity. Although the Forest plot and the results in Table 2 indicate significant reductions in weight in many studies, the study quality, range of outcome measures, and short time span of most studies limit the conclusions that can be drawn. This review further highlights the paucity of quality research in this area that has recently been acknowledged in a Cochrane Review.[49] The analyses undertaken suggest that interventions that include a dietary treatment can be effective in this group, but many caveats apply, including most importantly the limited number of quality studies undertaken to date and inadequate long-term follow-up data.

§*References 17, 18, 22, 23, 26, 32, 37, 38, 42.*

||*References 8-16, 22, 28, 29, 35, 36, 39, 40.*

¶*References 9, 16-19, 21-23, 25, 26, 30, 34, 35.*

#*References 9, 10, 13, 18, 23, 25, 27, 31, 34, 39-41.*

**Table 2. Results of the Main Weight Outcomes in Studies Included in a Systematic Review of the Effectiveness of Dietetic Interventions for Child Obesity**

| Source | Measurement of Weight Status | Weight Status Results | Significance of Results |
|---|---|---|---|
| Becque et al (1988)[26] | Mean (SD) percentage body fat at baseline and postintervention | Group 1, n = 14; B, 39.8 (1.8), Post, 40.5 (2.0)<br>Group 2, n = 11; B, 38.3 (1.2), Post, 35.3 (1.6)<br>Group 3, n = 11; B, 44.0, Post, 40.5 (1.9) | No significant differences between baseline and post measurements in any group or between groups |
| Botvin and Cantlon (1979)[42] | % of participants ≥130% and <130% of ideal weight at baseline and postintervention | Group 1, n = 69; B, >130% 39, <130% 61; Post, n = 69; >130% 35, <130% 65<br>Group 2, B, n = 37; >130% 38, <130% 62; Post, n = 37; >130% 17, <130% 83 | Significant decrease in percentage overweight of the intervention (group 2), $P<.05$<br>No significant change in percentage overweight of group 1 (control) |
| Braet and Van Winckel (1997)[43]* | 1-y follow-up paper; mean percentage weight loss at 3-mo, 6-mo, and 1-y follow-ups | Group 1, n = 48; 3 mo, 0.57, 6 mo, 8.34, 1 y, 9.84<br>Group 2, n = 45; 3 mo, 3.31, 6 mo, 8.44, 1 y, 13.08<br>Group 3, n = 57; 1 y, 6.84<br>Group 4, n = 55; 3 mo, 8.22, 6 mo, 15.59, 1 y, 14.67<br>Group 5, n = 54; 1 y, −2.52 | Significant weight loss at 3 mo, 6 mo, and 1 y, $P<.001$, in groups 1, 2, and 4<br>Significant weight loss at 1 y in group 3<br>Significant weight gain at 1 y in group 5 |
| | 4.6-y follow-up; percentage overweight at baseline, 1-y follow-up, and 4.6-y follow-up | Group 1, n = 13; B, 50 (19), 1 y, 42 (13), 4.6 y, 39 (24)<br>Group 2, n = 19; B, 52 (13), 1 y, 40 (14), 4.6 y, 34 (19)<br>Group 3, n = 30; B, 60 (23), 1 y, 42 (21), 4.6 y, 45 (21)<br>Group 4, n = 47; B, 52 (22), 1 y, 46 (22), 4.6 y, 45 (30) | Significant decrease in percentage overweight in all groups: 1 $P<.001$, 2 $P<.05$, 3 $P<.001$, and 4 $P<.05$ |
| Brownell et al (1983)[27] | Mean (SD) percentage overweight at baseline, 16 wk, and 1 y | Group 1: B, n = 14, 59.9 (6.1); 16 wk, n = 13, −17.1 (2.4); 1 y, n = 12; −20.5 (6.5)<br>Group 2: B, n = 15, 50.4 (9.9); 16 wk, n = 13, −7.0 (9.4); 1 y, n = 12; −5.5 (3.5)<br>Group 3: B, n = 13, 57.4 (8.3); 16 wk, n = 12, −6.8 (2.0); 1 y, n = 12, −6.0 (3.8) | Significantly greater weight change in mother-child separately (group 1) than child-alone (group 3) at 16 wk<br>No significant difference between mother-child together (group 2) and group 1 or 3 at 16 wk<br>Mother-child separately (group 1) significantly greater reduction in percentage overweight at 1 y compared with groups 2 and 3 |
| Coates et al (1983)[41] | Mean (SD) percentage overweight at baseline, postintervention (15 wk), and 6 mo postintervention | Group 1, n = 8; B, 37.3 (22.3), 15 wk, 25.3 (17.5), 6 mo, 29.3 (27.2)<br>Group 2, n = 8; B, 39.4 (25.6), 15 wk, 34.2 (23.7), 6 mo, 49.8 (30.5)<br>Group 3, n = 11; B, 37.3 (23.9), 15 wk, 31.1 (25.2), 6 mo, 34.9 (30.9)<br>Group 4, n = 11; B, 46.1 (23.9), 15 wk, 41.1 (29.6), 6 mo, 51.9 (49.9) | Daily contact weight reward (group 1) only group with significant decreases in percentage overweight from baseline to postintervention, $P<.02$, and follow-up, $P<.04$ |
| Duffy and Spence (1992)[8] | Percentage overweight at baseline and postintervention, 3-mo follow-up, and 6-mo follow-up (divided into those with all data and those with data up to 3-mo follow-up only) | Group 1, n = 11; B, 45.48 (17.52), Post, 42.43 (25.45), 3 mo, 42.84 (24.90)<br>Group 2, n = 10; B, 51.33 (26.92), Post, 42.43 (25.45), 3 mo, 42.84 (24.90)<br>Group 1, n = 9; B, 45.96 (18.55), Post, 37.62 (19.64), 3 mo, 39.13 (19.31), 6 mo, 37.02 (24.58)<br>Group 2, n = 8; B, 46.28 (19.32), Post, 36.99 (18.32), 3 mo, 38.15 (20.72), 6 mo, 37.09 (21.71) | Significant reduction from baseline for percentage overweight at postintervention ($P<.01$), 3 mo ($P<.01$), and 6 mo ($P<.01$) follow-up in all participants but not for either group separately |
| Epstein et al (1980)[9] | Percentage overweight at baseline, postintervention, and 3-mo follow-up | Group 1, B, 68.4, Post, 58.7, 3 mo, 50.9<br>Group 2, B, 60.9, Post, 55.2, 3 mo, 54.5 (group No. not reported) | Significant effect for all participants only ($P<.05$)<br>No significant effect in either group |
| Epstein et al[35,44,45,48]* | Change in percentage overweight at baseline, 2 mo, 8 mo, and 21 mo | Reported in figure (group No. not reported) | Significant decrease in percentage overweight from baseline to 2 mo, $P<.01$, 2 mo to 8 mo, $P<.01$, and baseline to 2 y, $P<.01$, in all groups |
| | Mean (SD) percentage overweight at baseline and 5 y postintervention | Group 1, n = 24; B, 41.0 (28.3), 5 y, 28.3 (19.6)<br>Group 2, n = 21; B, 39.7 (15.2), 5 y, 44.0 (26.0)<br>Group 3, n = 22; B, 45.5 (16.1), 5 y, 53.7 (24.0) | Analysis of n = 34 who had data available at 2, 8, 21, and 60 mo showed children in the parent + child (group 1) maintained the intervention effects at 5 y; groups 2 and 3 did not |
| | Percentage overweight at baseline, 8 mo, 21 mo, 5 y, and 10 y | Reported in figure (group No. not reported) | Parent and child (group 1) showed significant decreases in percentage overweight at 5 and 10 y, $P<.05$<br>Groups 2 and 3 did not |

(*continued*)

**Table 2. Results of the Main Weight Outcomes in Studies Included in a Systematic Review of the Effectiveness of Dietetic Interventions for Child Obesity (cont)**

| Source | Measurement of Weight Status | Weight Status Results | Significance of Results |
|---|---|---|---|
| Epstein et al (1982)[40] | Mean (SEM) percentage overweight at baseline, postintervention, 6 mo, and 17 mo | Group 1, n = 10; B, 40.5 (4.3), Post, 32.4 (4.0), 6 mo, 21.5 (4.0), 17 mo, 26.7 (4.3)<br>Group 2, n = 8; B, 37.2 (4.0), Post, 28.6 (4.5), 6 mo, 26.9 (4.2), 17 mo, 37.3 (6.1)<br>Group 3, n = 8; B, 34.0 (5.3), Post, 29.2 (5.7), 6 mo, 20.8 (6.1), 17 mo, 22.8 (4.9)<br>Group 4, n = 11; B, 38.7 (5.4), Post, 32.7 (5.0), 6 mo, 24.8 (5.5), 17 mo, 29.0 (6.4) | All groups together showed significant changes in percentage overweight over time, $P<.001$<br>Significant decreases in percentage overweight in all groups combined from postintervention to 6 mo and from baseline to 17 mo, $P<.01$<br>Greater changes in percentage overweight in program exercise (group 4) at 17 mo compared with group 2<br>No significant difference between changes of groups 1 and 2 at any point |
| Epstein et al[35,44]* | Change in percentage overweight at 2, 6, and 12 mo | Reported in figure (group No. not reported) | Diet and diet + exercise (groups 1 and 2) significantly lower percentage overweight at 6 mo than group 3 control<br>No differences in changes in percentage overweight of diet and diet + exercise groups |
| | Percentage overweight at baseline and change at 5 y | Group 1, B, 43.6, 5 y, −6.8<br>Group 2, B, 45.1, 5 y, −1.8 (group No. not reported) | No significant difference between diet and diet + exercise group at 5 y |
| | Change in percentage overweight at 10 y | Group 1, 10 y, −8.4%<br>Group 2, 10 y, −10% (group No. not reported) | No significant difference between diet and diet + exercise group at 10 y |
| Epstein et al (1985)[10] | Mean (SD) percentage overweight at baseline, postintervention, and 6- and 12-mo follow-up | Group 1, B, 48.1 (17.6), Post, 36.2 (19.0), 6 mo, 29.3 (22.3), 12 mo, 29.4 (22.5)<br>Group 2, B, 48.0 (23.2), Post, 30.7 (21.5), 6 mo, 20.5 (22.6), 12 mo, 29.4 (22.5) (group No. not reported) | At 2 mo, both diet (group 1) and diet + exercise (group 2) showed significant decreases in percentage overweight, $P<.05$, $P<.01$<br>At 6 mo, both groups showed significant differences from baseline, $P<.01$<br>Significant between-group differences: diet + exercise (group 2) significantly lower percentage overweight than diet alone (group 1), $P<.05$<br>At 6 mo, only the diet + exercise (group 2) had significant decreases in percentage overweight from 2 mo, $P<.01$<br>At 12 mo, both groups showed significant decreases in percentage overweight from baseline, $P<.01$ |
| Epstein et al (1985)[11] | Mean (SD) percentage overweight at baseline and 4, 8, and 12 mo | Group 1, B, 39.2 (17.1), 4 mo, 25.8 (16.2), 8 mo, 27.6 (17.1), 12 mo, 28.0 (16.7)<br>Group 2, B, 41.9 (13.6), 4 mo, 22.1 (12.7), 8 mo, 18.2 (16.2), 12 mo, 15.6 (15.2) (group No. not reported) | Significant differences between groups in percentage overweight at 8 and 12 mo lower in group 2 |
| Epstein et al[12,35,44,48] | Change in percentage overweight from baseline to 6 mo, 1 y, 3 y, or 5 y | Group 1, 6 mo, −17.4, 1 y, −12.4, 3 y, −5.7, 5 y, −3.6<br>Group 2, 6 mo, −14.7, 1 y, −11.7, 3 y, +0.1, 5 y, +3.3 (group No. not reported) | No significance between groups at any point |
| | Change in percentage overweight from baseline at 10 y | Group 1, − 11.1<br>Group 2, + 3.1 (group No. not reported) | No significant difference between group changes at 10 y, $P = .12$ |
| Epstein et al (1994)[13] | Change in percentage overweight at 6, 12, and 24 mo | Group 1, 6 mo, −30.1, 12 mo, −26.5, 24 mo, −15.4<br>Group 2, 6 mo, −20.0, 12 mo, −16.7, 24 mo, −10.6 (group No. not reported) | Significant differences between groups at 6 and 12 mo, $P<.05$<br>No significant difference between groups at 24 mo, $P = .29$ |
| Epstein et al (1995)[28] | Percentage overweight at baseline and 4, 8, and 12 mth | Reported in graph (group No. not reported) | Significant differences in percentage overweight between the exercise (group 1) and sedentary (group 2) at 4 mo, with lower percentage in group 2<br>Significant differences in percentage overweight between the sedentary (group 2) and the 2 other groups at 1 y, with lower percentage in group 2 |
| Epstein et al (2000)[39] | Mean (SD) change in percentage overweight from baseline to 6 mo and from baseline to 2 y | Group 1, 6 mo, −26.4 (10.5), 2 y, −13.2 (16.4)<br>Group 2, 6 mo, −25.6 (8.1), 2 y, −12.4 (13.3)<br>Group 3, 6 mo, −27.4 (10.7), 2 y, −14.3 (16.9)<br>Group 4, 6 mo, −22.4 (12.6), 2 y, −11.6 (21.9) (No. not reported) | Overall significant decreases across groups in percentage overweight at 6 mo and 2 y, $P<.001$ |
| Epstein et al (2000)[29] | Mean (SD) BMI *z* score at baseline, postintervention, 12 mo, and 24 mo | Group 1, n = 17; B, 2.8 (0.9), Post, 1.5 (0.9), 12 mo, 1.7 (1.0), 24 mo, 2.3 (1.1)<br>Group 2, n = 18; B, 2.6 (0.9), Post, 1.2 (0.8), 12 mo, 1.3 (0.9), 24 mo, 1.7 (0.9)<br>Group 3, n = 17; B, 2.7 (0.8), Post, 1.2 (0.8), 12 mo, 1.4 (0.9), 24 mo, 1.6 (1.0) | Linear changes between the parent and child (group 1) vs no problem solving (group 3), $P<.03$ |

(*continued*)

**Table 2. Results of the Main Weight Outcomes in Studies Included in a Systematic Review of the Effectiveness of Dietetic Interventions for Child Obesity (cont)**

| Source | Measurement of Weight Status | Weight Status Results | Significance of Results |
|---|---|---|---|
| Epstein et al (2001)[14] | Mean (SEM) change in percentage overweight at 6 and 12 mo (divided into boys/girls for each group) | Reported in figure (group No. not reported) | Boys in combined (group 2) had greater reduction in percentage overweight compared with girls in the same group, P<.001, and either sex in the increased activity (group 1) |
| Epstein et al (2004)[15] | Mean (SD) BMI *z* score baseline to 6 and 12 mo | Group 1, n = 30; B, 3.3 (1.0), 6 mo, 2.3 (1.0), 12 mo, 2.4 (1.0)<br>Group 2, n = 32; B, 3.2 (1.0), 6 mo, 2.2 (1.1), 12 mo, 2.6 (1.0) | Significant intervention effects at 6 and 12 mo, P<.001<br>No differences between groups |
| Flodmark et al (1993)[30] | Mean (SEM) BMI at baseline, postintervention, and 1-y follow-up | Group 1, B, n = 50, 25.1 (0.35); 1 y, n = 48; 27.9 (0.61)<br>Group 2, B, n = 19, 25.5 (0.53); Post, n = 19, 26.1 (0.72); 1 y, n = 19, 27.1 (0.88)<br>Group 3, B, n = 24, 24.7 (0.36); Post, n = 22, 25.0 (0.53); 1 y, n = 20, 25.8 (0.73) | Significantly lower increase in BMI in family therapy (group 3), then conventional intervention (group 2) at postintervention, P = .04<br>At 1-y follow-up, significantly smaller increase in BMI in the family therapy (group 3) compared with the control (group 1), P = .02<br>No significant differences between control (group 1) or family therapy (group 3) and conventional intervention (group 2) at 1 y |
| Golan et al[25] and Golan and Crow (1998)[47]* | Mean (SEM) change in percentage overweight at 3, 5, 8, 10, 12, and 18 mo | Recorded in figure for groups combined (group No. not reported) | Significant decrease in percentage overweight in both groups at postprogram (P<.001, group 1, and P<.01, group 2)<br>Weight reduction significantly greater in family intervention (group 2), P<.05, at 5, 8, 10, 12, and 18 mo |
| | Mean percentage overweight at baseline; postintervention; and 1-y, 2-y, and 7-y follow-up | Group 1, n = 30; B, 39.1, Post, 25.1, 1 y, 26.0, 2 y, 24.6, 7 y, 10.4<br>Group 2, n = 30; B, 39.6, Post, 31.5, 1 y, 39.8, 2 y, 42.0, 7 y, 18.87 | Significantly greater weight loss in parent-only intervention (group 2) at postintervention (P<.01) and 1 y (P<.01), 2 y (P<.01), and 7 y (P<.05) follow-up |
| Goldfield et al (2001)[16] | Mean (SD) changes BMI *z* score at 6 and 12 mo (from baseline) | Group 1, n = 12, 6 mo, −0.59 (0.51), 12 mo, −0.62 (0.62)<br>Group 2, n = 12, 6 mo, −0.60 (0.49), 12 mo, −0.66 (0.69) | Significance of results not reported |
| Graves et al (1988)[31] | Mean (SD) percentage overweight at baseline, postintervention, and 3- and 6-mo follow-up | Group 1, B, 56.30 (36.30), Post, 47.70 (35.71), 3 mo, 43.20 (35.60), 6 mo, 46.10 (39.13)<br>Group 2, B, 53.00 (21.00), Post, 39.55 (19.85), 3 mo, 28.73 (19.19), 6 mo, 46.10 (39.13)<br>Group 3, B, 51.80 (22.03), Post, 47.10 (23.49), 3 mo, 41.50 (17.85), 6 mo, 42.30 (18.57) (group No. not reported) | Significantly greater reductions in percentage overweight in behavioral (group 1) and problem solving (group 2) interventions compared with instruction only (group 3) at postintervention maintained at 3 and 6 mo |
| Gutin et al (2002)[32] | Mean (SEM) change in percentage of body fat from baseline to 8 mo | Group 1, n = 17 to 19; 0.19 (0.62)<br>Groups 2 and 3, n = 20 to 22; −3.57 (0.80) | Significant difference between group differences in percentage body fat at 8 mo<br>(No significant difference between 3 groups in intention-to-treat analysis) |
| Hills and Parker (1988)[17] | Mean (SE) body mass at baseline and postintervention | Group 1, n = 10; B, 51.6 (2.68), Post, 46.1 (2.46)<br>Group 2, n = 10; B, 50.2 (2.81), Post, 52.8 (3.02)<br>Group 3, n = 15; B, 30.7 (1.81), Post, 30.6 (1.75) | No significant difference between intervention groups' weight changes |
| Kirschenbaum et al (1984)[33] | Mean (SD) percentage overweight at baseline, postintervention, and 3-mo and 1-y follow-up | Group 1, n = 13, B, 58.1 (26.2), Post, 51.8 (24.3), 3 mo, 53.4 (26.2), 1 y, 50.5 (27.9)<br>Group 2, n = 9, B, 39.0 (18.4), Post, 31.9 (18.1), 3 mo, 31.3 (17.7), 1 y, 32.8 (18.1)<br>Group 3, n = 8, B, 42.4 (20.4), Post, 43.0 (24.1), 3 mo, 46.4 (21.4) | Significant differences between control (group 3) and child and child and parent (groups 1 and 2) at postintervention, 3 mo, and 1 y, P>.01 |
| Lansky and Brownell (1982)[18] | Mean change in percentage overweight at postintervention | Group 1, n = 36; −3.0<br>Group 2, n = 35; −2.1 | No significant difference between groups |
| Mellin et al (1987)[19] | Mean (SD) change in relative weight at 3, 6, and 15 mo | Group 1, n = 34; 3 mo, −5.9 (6.75), 6 mo, −6.2, 15 mo, −9.9 (14.98)<br>Group 2, n = 29; 3 mo, −0.3 (6.61), 6 mo, −5.2, 15 mo, −0.1 (13.20) | At 3 mo, P<.001, and 15 mo, P<.01, the behavioral, diet, and physical activity intervention (group 1) showed significant improvements in relative weight<br>No significant differences in control (group 2) |
| Nova et al (2001)[24] | Mean (SD) change in percentage overweight from baseline to 12 mo, baseline to 6 mo, and 6 mo to 12 mo | Group 1, 12 mo, n = 80, −2.92 (10.8), 6 mo, n = 92, −2.95 (8.47), 12 mo, n = 73, 0.30 (6.19)<br>Group 2, 12 mo, n = 50, −8.50 (9.72), 6 mo, n = 51, −8.80 (6.62), 12 mo, n = 45, 0.64 (8.05) | Statistically greater reduction in percentage overweight in enhanced approach (group 2) from baseline to 6 mo, P<.001, and baseline to 12 mo, P<.001<br>No significant difference in between-group changes in percentage overweight between 6 and 12 mo |

(*continued*)

**Table 2. Results of the Main Weight Outcomes in Studies Included in a Systematic Review of the Effectiveness of Dietetic Interventions for Child Obesity (cont)**

| Source | Measurement of Weight Status | Weight Status Results | Significance of Results |
|---|---|---|---|
| Rocchini et al (1987)[38] | Mean (SD) percentage body fat at baseline and postintervention | Group 2, n = 15; B, 42 (6), Post, 39 (6)<br>Group 3, n = 18; B, 40 (5), Post, 34 (4)<br>Group 4, n = 17; B, 40 (6), Post, 41 (7) | Significant reductions in percentage body fat from baseline in diet + exercise and diet + exercise + behavioral therapy intervention groups (groups 2 and 3), $P<.05$<br>Significantly greater improvements in percentage body fat in both intervention groups (groups 2 and 3) compared with control (group 1), $P<.05$<br>Significantly greater improvements in percentage body fat in diet + exercise + behavioral therapy (group 3) than in diet and behavioral therapy alone (group 2), $P<.05$ |
| Rocchini et al (1988)[37] | Mean (SD) percentage body fat at baseline and postintervention | Group 2, n = 22; B, 43 (8), Post, 39 (8)<br>Group 3, n = 23; B, 41 (6), Post, 35 (4)<br>Group 4, n = 18; B, 41 (6), Post, 42 (8) | Significantly decreases in percentage body fat from baseline in diet + exercise and diet + exercise + behavioral therapy intervention groups (groups 2 and 3), $P<.05$<br>Significantly greater improvements in percentage body fat in both intervention groups (groups 2 and 3) compared with control (group 1), $P<.05$ |
| Saelens et al (2002)[20] | Mean (SD) percentage overweight at baseline, postintervention, and 3-mo follow-up | Group 1, B, n = 20, 62.0 (20.5); Post, n = 20, 59.8 (21.8); 3 mo, n = 19, 59.6 (24.6)<br>Group 2, B, n = 19, 62.3 (17.4); Post, n = 19, 66.2 (18.6); 3 mo, n = 19, 66.4 (20.1) | Results for BMI *z* score reported in graph showed significant group × time interaction for BMI *z* score with decreases in scores of intensive follow-up (group 1)<br>No significant differences between group changes in percentage overweight at any point |
| Schwingshandl et al (1999)[21] | Mean (SEM) change in BMI standard deviation score from baseline to 12 mo | Group 1, n = 14, −0.53 (0.11)<br>Group 2, n = 16, −0.51 (0.18) | Both groups showed significant improvements in BMI standard deviation score at 12 mo: group 1, $P<.001$; group 2, $P=.01$ |
| Senediak and Spence (1985)[36] | Mean (SD) percentage overweight at 1, 4, 15, and 26 wk | Group 1, 1 wk, n = 12, 34.63 (13.42); 4 wk, n = 12, 29.37 (14.74); 15 wk, n = 9, 20.99 (12.04); 26 wk, n = 8, 19.94 (14.22)<br>Group 2, 1 wk, n = 12, 34.63 (13.67); 4 wk, n = 12, 30.70 (13.97); 15 wk, n = 9, 17.84 (12.62); 26 wk, n = 10, 16.64 (11.46)<br>Group 3, 1 wk, n = 11, 41.68 (10.62); 4 wk, n = 12, 40.32 (8.50); 15 wk, n = 9, 86.72 (10.47); 26 wk, n = 7, 30.80 (10.4)<br>Group 4, 1 wk, n = 10, 37.64 (12.77); 4 wk, n = 10, 39.95 (14.52); no further contact | No analysis of the significance of these results conducted |
| Sondike et al (2003)[22] | Mean change in BMI *z* score postintervention | Group 1, n = 14; −0.20 (0.14)<br>Group 2, n = 16; −0.14 (0.27) | Significantly greater change in low carbohydrate diet (group 2) compared with low fat diet (group 1) |
| Sung et al (2002)[23] | Mean change in BMI at postintervention | Group 1, n = 41; −0.2 (1.5)<br>Group 2, n = 41; −0.5 (0.9) | No significant differences in BMI changes within or between groups |
| Wadden et al (1990)[34] | Mean change in weight at postintervention | Group 1, 1.6<br>Group 2, 3.7<br>Group 3, 3.1 (group No. not reported) | No significant differences between-group changes in weight at postintervention |

Abbreviations: B, baseline; BMI, body mass index (calculated as weight in kilograms divided by height in meters squared); Post, postintervention.
*Selected references cited; a complete reference list is available on request.

Many studies inadequately described the details of the dietary intervention itself, making replication almost impossible without assistance from study authors. The Stoplight/Traffic Light diet[50] was the most commonly reported dietary intervention strategy. It is calorie controlled and categorizes food into different colored groups, red (very limited), green (eat freely), and yellow (limited). It then prescribes a recommended number of daily/weekly servings of each of these food groups. Although the Stoplight diet as described originally by Epstein and Squires[51] is frequently used as the dietary prescription in studies conducted in the United States, these studies do predominantly arise from a single research group and the applicability to other settings has not been established. From Table 3, the evolution within the Stoplight/Traffic Light diet is apparent, both in terms of the gradual increase in the number of red foods allowed per week, the reduced focus on tight calorie restriction, a redefinition of the food groups to align more closely to the food pyramid, and the integration of behavioral therapy.

Given that the rationale and objectives of the dietary interventions were rarely described, it was not surprising that the quality of most of the studies was poor in terms of assessing changes in dietary intake in response to the intervention at either the individual or group level. Many studies did not report dietary outcomes, and it is unclear whether food intake data was not collected or was collected but not used because it was of poor quality or because the focus in reporting was only on changes in the primary outcome of weight status.

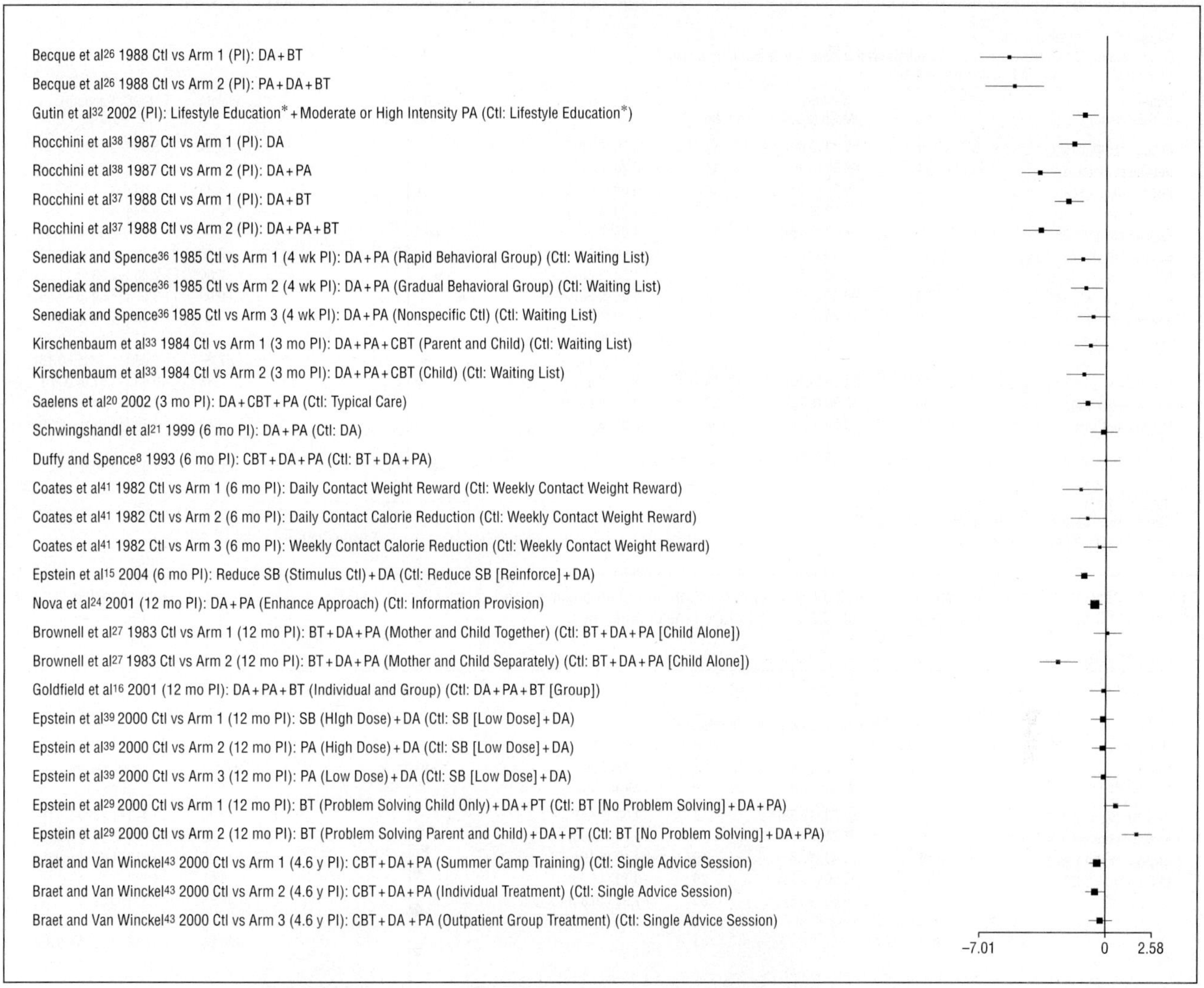


**Figure 2.** Heterogeneity among 17 randomized controlled trials of interventions for child obesity highlighting the variability of study components and follow-up periods. BT indicates behavioral therapy; CBT, cognitive behavioral therapy; Ctl, control; DA, dietary advice; PA, physical activity; PI, postintervention; SB, sedentary behavior. * indicates lifestyle education included behavioral therapy plus dietary advice plus physical activity.

A challenge for researchers will be in estimating and validating changes in food intake, for example, through the use of dietary biomarkers. The inherent difficulties of dietary assessment in children are well recognized[52] and researchers have recently made attempts to validate dietary changes within their studies.[22,38]

In adult obesity, long-term studies indicate that following a low-fat diet in conjunction with modest daily energy intake restriction (500-1000 kcal/d) results in approximately 5% weight loss after 2 years of follow-up.[53] For children, no such evidence is available. Only 3 studies in the meta-analysis had a follow-up of longer than a year. To date, the changes achieved in the dietary intakes of children and adolescents who have successfully lost weight, even in the short-term, have not been described qualitatively or quantitatively. This presents additional challenges when designing dietary interventions for child obesity trials. An attempt to address this gap has been made recently through the use of dietary modeling of food intakes from a reference population to achieve a reduction in energy density.[54]

In the absence of consensus of expert opinion, a rational approach is to base interventions on observational and epidemiological data. Targeting an increase in fruit and vegetable consumption may be more effective than focusing on a reduction in high-energy, low-nutrient-dense foods.[55] Beverage intake may also be a particular problem in children, and consumption of soft drinks has been linked to obesity.[48] Behaviors that could be targeted in children to achieve energy reduction and an increase in nutrient density have recently been described.[4]

## METHODOLOGICAL CONSIDERATIONS FOR FUTURE STUDIES

There are practical and ethical considerations about conducting a trial with a no-intervention control. However, the following methodological considerations are important when addressing the significant gaps in the evidence and weaknesses in study design on this serious public health issue. A number of trials in this review have no clear reference arm with the treatment (ie, dietary modification) under test often present in both the treatment and the control arms. This makes it difficult for cli-

Review: Childhood Obesity
Comparison: 01 Effectiveness of Interventions With Dietary Advice as a Component
Outcome: 01 Weight Status (Postintervention)

| Study or Subcategory | No. | Treatment Mean (SD) | No. | Control Mean (SD) | Weight % | SMD (Random) 95% CI |
|---|---|---|---|---|---|---|
| Becque et al[26] 2 vs 1 | 11 | −3.00 (0.60) | 14 | 0.70 (0.72) | 4.84 | −5.34 [−7.13 to −3.54] |
| Becque et al[26] 3 vs 1 | 11 | −3.50 (0.90) | 14 | 0.70 (0.72) | 5.03 | −5.06 [−6.78 to −3.34] |
| Kirschenbaum et al[33] 1 vs 3 | 13 | −6.30 (9.91) | 8 | 0.60 (11.16) | 7.32 | −0.64 [−1.54 to 0.27] |
| Kirschenbaum et al[33] 2 vs 3 | 9 | −7.10 (8.60) | 8 | 0.60 (11.16) | 7.07 | −0.74 [−1.73 to 0.25] |
| Rocchini et al[38] 1987 2 vs 1 | 15 | −3.00 (2.19) | 17 | 1.00 (2.24) | 7.52 | −1.76 [−2.59 to −0.93] |
| Rocchini et al[38] 1987 3 vs 1 | 18 | −6.00 (1.61) | 17 | 1.00 (2.24) | 6.76 | −3.52 [−4.62 to −2.42] |
| Rocchini et al[37] 1988 2 vs 1 | 22 | −4.00 (2.41) | 18 | 1.00 (2.36) | 7.66 | −2.05 [−2.83 to −1.27] |
| Rocchini et al[37] 1988 3 vs 1 | 23 | −6.00 (1.50) | 18 | 1.00 (2.36) | 6.99 | −3.57 [−4.59 to −2.55] |
| Saelens et al[20] 1 vs 2 | 20 | −2.20 (6.69) | 19 | 3.90 (5.84) | 7.96 | −0.95 [−1.62 to −0.28] |
| Senediak and Spence[36] 1 vs 4 | 12 | −5.26 (5.75) | 10 | 2.31 (6.12) | 7.25 | −1.23 [−2.16 to −0.30] |
| Senediak and Spence[36] 2 vs 4 | 12 | −4.23 (5.64) | 10 | 2.31 (6.12) | 7.31 | −1.07 [−1.98 to −0.16] |
| Senediak and Spence[36] 3 vs 4 | 11 | −1.36 (4.10) | 10 | 2.31 (6.12) | 7.38 | −0.68 [−1.57 to 0.20] |
| Mellin et al[19] 1987 | 34 | −5.90 (6.75) | 29 | −0.30 (6.61) | 8.30 | −0.83 [−1.34 to −0.31] |
| Nova et al[24] 1 vs 2 | 51 | −8.80 (6.62) | 92 | −2.95 (8.47) | 8.60 | −0.74 [−1.09 to −0.39] |
| Total (95% CI) | 262 | | 284 | | 100.00 | −1.82 [−2.40 to −1.23] |

Test for Heterogeneity: $\chi^2=96.38$, $df=13$ ($P<.001$), $I^2=86.5\%$
Test for Overall Effect: $z=6.07$ ($P<.001$)

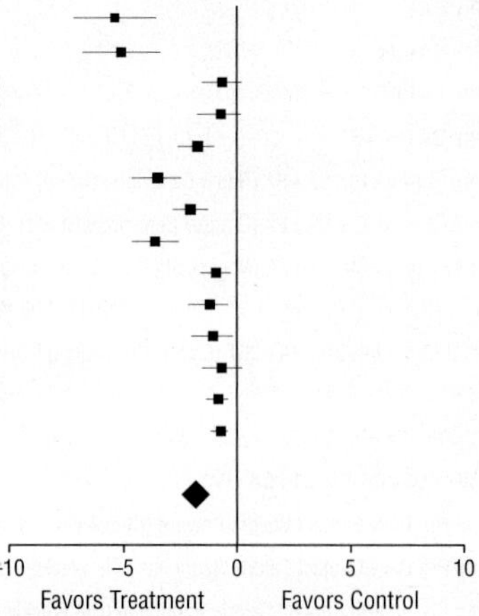


**Figure 3.** Meta-analysis of 7 randomized controlled trials of interventions for child obesity where a "true" control arm was used and results were reported postintervention. CI indicates confidence interval; SMD, standardized mean difference.

Review: Childhood Obesity
Comparison: 01 Effectiveness of Interventions With Dietary Advice as a Component
Outcome: 02 Weight Status (at First Follow-up)

| Study or Subcategory | No. | Treatment Mean (SD) | No. | Control Mean (SD) | Weight % | SMD (Fixed) 95% CI |
|---|---|---|---|---|---|---|
| Kirschenbaum et al[33] 1 vs 3 | 13 | −4.70 (10.28) | 8 | 4.00 (10.45) | 7.39 | −0.81 [−1.73 to 0.11] |
| Kirschenbaum et al[33] 2 vs 3 | 9 | −7.70 (8.51) | 8 | 4.00 (10.45) | 5.65 | −1.17 [−2.23 to −0.12] |
| Saelens et al[20] 1 vs 2 | 18 | −2.40 (13.66) | 19 | 4.10 (6.10) | 14.35 | −0.61 [−1.27 to 0.05] |
| Mellin et al[19] 1987 | 34 | −9.90 (14.98) | 29 | −0.10 (13.20) | 24.07 | −0.68 [−1.19 to −0.17] |
| Nova et al[24] 1 vs 2 | 50 | −8.50 (9.72) | 80 | −2.92 (10.80) | 48.55 | −0.53 [−0.89 to −0.17] |
| Total (95% CI) | 124 | | 144 | | 100.00 | −0.64 [−0.89 to −0.39] |

Test for Heterogeneity: $\chi^2=1.48$, $df=4$ ($P=.83$), $I^2=0\%$
Test for Overall Effect: $z=4.98$ ($P<.001$)

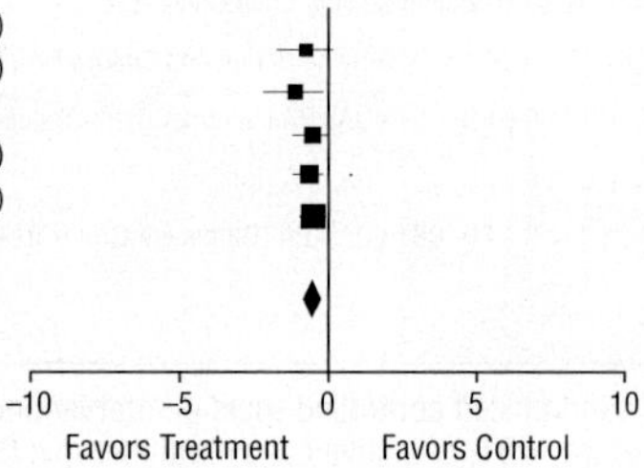


**Figure 4.** Meta-analysis of 3 randomized controlled trials of interventions for child obesity where a "true" control arm was used and results were reported after a period of follow-up. CI indicates confidence interval; SMD, standardized mean difference.

nicians to extract meaningful results and strategies applicable in general patient settings.

The variety of outcome measures in the trials included body weight, percentage overweight, BMI, and BMI *z* score with some investigators using a number of different measures. To make direct comparisons of effectiveness, we recommend that BMI *z* score be reported in all intervention studies in child obesity as a clinically meaningful outcome measure along with the proportion of subjects whose final (follow-up) BMI *z* score is in the healthy weight range for the appropriate population demographic.

## TRIAL SIZES

The small arm sizes in many of the trials in this study raise statistical concerns. It would seem that a standard power calculation (using readily available freeware such as PS[56] available from http://biostat.mc.vanderbilt.edu/twiki/bin/view/Main/PowerSampleSize) is rarely performed. This is important because the large standard deviations commonly reported indicate that sample sizes well in excess of those commonly used would be required to achieve 80% power. We therefore recommend that studies be powered (ie, employ sample sizes) to have an 80% chance of rejecting a null hypothesis or no-intervention effect if the true intervention effect is more than a specified clinically important value.

## AGE RANGES

Within the 37 trials reported, the age ranges in the subgroups varied from 3 to 12 years to 12 to 18 years with numerous prepubescent and postpubescent subgroup age ranges. One of the authors (B.J.S.) has previously noticed broadly in medical research this use of incompatible age ranges across studies, often by the same researchers. Such inconsistency makes valid meta-analysis difficult to achieve because the assumption then has to be made that age has no effect on weight outcomes when we know

**Table 3. Description of Dietary Interventions, Measurement and Report of Compliance, and Dietary Outcomes in Studies Included in a Systematic Review of the Effectiveness of Dietetic Interventions for Child Obesity**

| | | Compliance to Diet Intervention | | Dietary Outcomes | | |
|---|---|---|---|---|---|---|
| **Source** | **Dietary Intervention** | **How Measured** | **Reported** | **How Measured** | **Reported** | **Dietetic Involvement Reported** |
| Becque et al (1988)[26] | American Dietetic Association Exchange Program with kcal prescription to give weight loss of 1-2 lb/wk<br>Weekly adjustment of eating pattern and kcal intake<br>Weekly nutrition education materials (food, energy, general eating behavior, and cooking) | Weekly food records with rewards for compliance | No | Not measured | No | Yes, weekly nutrition instruction |
| Botvin and Cantlon (1979)[42] | Healthy food selection, prudent diet, preplanning, and changing eating patterns | Daily food and exercise log | No | Not measured | No | Not specifically |
| Braet and Van Winckel (1997)[43]* | Healthy eating and 3 midmeal snacks<br>Unhealthy/favorite meals limited to 1/mo or small amount weekly<br>Food preparation, shopping habits, increasing vegetable intake, and reducing sugar and fat<br>No kcal counting<br>Summer camp: balanced healthy food 1500 kcal/d<br>Advice in 1 session: how to lose weight in a reasonable way | Not measured | No | Actual food intake not measured<br>Eating habits form for child | No<br>Mentions results of a pilot study only | No |
| Brownell et al (1983)[27] | Basic food groups with emphasis on reducing sugar, salt, and fat intake and information on shopping, preparing, storing, and serving food and misconceptions about diet and nutrition | Not measured | No | Not measured | No | No |
| Coates et al (1983)[41] | Caloric goals based on estimates of amount needed to lose 1 lb/wk<br>Instructed to weigh food portions and learn kcal values, choose low-kcal foods, and calculate daily kcal needed to achieve a 1-2 lb/wk weight loss<br>Discussed advantages of diets higher in complex CHO and PS fat and lower in cholesterol, sugar, and saturated fat | Estimated by self-reported kcal | No | Not measured | No | No |
| Duffy and Spence (1992)[8] | Traffic Light with no strict energy restrictions<br>Emphasized aim of gradual weight reduction through healthy eating and exercise habits | Not measured | No | 7-d food record at preintervention and postintervention only, not follow-up<br>Red foods (No./day) | Report a significant reduction over time, $P<.001$, but table reports an increase of 0.15/d | No |
| Epstein et al (1980)[9] | Traffic Light<br>Red food = in each food category (fruit, vegetable, dairy and protein) any food with an energy value >20 kcal than the average for the food group<br>Yellow food = basic reference foods for balanced nutrition<br>Green = free foods, very low kcal and eat freely<br>Restrict total kcal to 1200-1500/d<br>Eliminate high caloric density food using 3 diet rules<br>(1) Eat core 900 kcal/d<br>(2) Do not exceed 1200-1500 kcal/d<br>(3) No more than 4 red foods/wk | Daily self-monitoring of kcal and weight in food diaries<br>(BT arm only) | No | Food diaries | No | Yes, adults only were seen by dietitian |
| Epstein et al[35,44,45,48]* | Traffic Light<br>Foods divided into 11 groups and then in each group; red (any food >20 kcal above the standard for this group + all sweets and sugared beverages), yellow (no more than 20 kcal per average serving above the group average), green (<20 kcal than the average serving)<br>2 diet rules:<br>(1) 1200- to 1500-kcal limit<br>(2) Limit to 4 red foods/wk<br>Daily minimum of 2 servings high-protein food plus 2 dairy servings, 2 servings of starches, 4 servings of fruit and vegetables | Self-monitoring diary + chart to record daily weight, kcal, and red foods<br>Basic diet picture chart | No | 7-d self-recorded food intake at preintervention and postintervention | Yes<br>Total food servings from 42 to 31 foods/wk<br>Preintervention and postintervention servings of red foods (53.3-12.6) | Yes, food records scored by dietitian |
| Epstein et al (1982)[40] | Diet intervention for children, Traffic Light diet; 11 food groups divided into 3 colors. Aim to cut down red foods, keep yellow foods constant, and increase green foods, with 1200-1500 kcal/d<br>2 diet rules:<br>(1) Keep below kcal limit<br>(2) Limit to 4 red foods/wk<br>Control children given general advice on dieting and no advice on behavior change | Daily nutrition recording sheets | No | Not measured | No | No |

(*continued*)

**Table 3. Description of Dietary Interventions, Measurement and Report of Compliance, and Dietary Outcomes in Studies Included in a Systematic Review of the Effectiveness of Dietetic Interventions for Child Obesity (cont)**

| Source | Dietary Intervention | Compliance to Diet Intervention | | Dietary Outcomes | | Dietetic Involvement Reported |
|---|---|---|---|---|---|---|
| | | How Measured | Reported | How Measured | Reported | |
| Epstein et al[35,44]* | Traffic Light<br>Foods divided into 11 groups and then in each group; red (any food >20 kcal above the standard for this group + all sweets and sugared beverages), yellow (no more than 20 kcal per average serving above the group average), green (<20 kcal than the average serving)<br>2 diet rules:<br>(1) 1200- to 1500-kcal limit<br>(2) Limit to 4 red foods/wk<br>Daily minimum of 2 servings high protein food plus 2 dairy servings, 2 servings of starches, 4 servings of fruit and vegetables | Red foods per wk, d/wk under the kcal limit; d/wk with complete recordings | Yes | Habits book for children | Yes<br>3.0 red foods/wk; 6.5 wk, <4 red food limit; 5.4 wk, < kcal limit; 6.7 wk with complete recordings | No |
| Epstein et al (1985)[10] | Traffic Light<br>Foods divided into 5 groups; red (any food >20 kcal above the standard for this group + all sweets and sugared beverages), yellow (no more than 20 kcal per average serving above the group average), green (<20 kcal than the average serving)<br>2 diet rules:<br>(1) Stay within prescribed kcal range<br>(2) Limit to 4 red foods/wk<br>Goal to reduce kcal intake and to provide most nutrition for lowest kcal<br>Minimum of 900 kcal and max of 1200 kcal | Food diary recording food preparation serving size, kcal, time, and color code | No | Not measured | No | No |
| Epstein et al (1985)[11] | Traffic Light diet<br>Foods divided into 5 groups; red (any food >20 kcal above the standard for this group + all sweets and sugared beverages), yellow (no more than 20 kcal per average serving above the group average), green (<20 kcal than the average serving)<br>2 diet rules:<br>(1) Stay within prescribed kcal range<br>(2) Limit to 4 red foods/wk<br>Minimum, 900 kcal/d, children <7 y, max, 1000 kcal, and >7 y, 1200 kcal | Food diary (BT arm only) recording food eaten, serving size, kcal, and color code | No | Not measured | No | No |
| Epstein et al[12,35,44,48] | Traffic Light<br>Foods divided into 5 groups; red (any food >20 kcal above the standard for this group + all sweets and sugared beverages), yellow (no more than 20 kcal per average serving above the group average), green (<20 kcal than the average serving)<br>2 diet rules:<br>(1) Stay within prescribed kcal range (1200 kcal/d)<br>(2) Limit to 4 red foods/wk | Daily habit record for first 2 mo | Obese children with nonobese parents had better kcal compliance | Not measured | No | No |
| Epstein et al (1994)[13] | Traffic Light<br>Foods divided into 5 groups; red (any food >20 kcal above the standard for this group + all sweets and sugared beverages), yellow (no more than 20 kcal per average serving above the group average), green (<20 kcal than the average serving)<br>2 diet rules:<br>(1) Stay within prescribed kcal range<br>(2) Limit to 4 red foods/wk<br>Gradual reduction in kcal intake range from 900-1800 on level 1 to 900-1200 by level 4 | Daily food records: red foods/wk, days in kcal range, complete recordings | Yes | Not measured | No | No |
| Epstein et al (1995)[28] | Traffic Light (modified)<br>Maintain nutrient balance by eating recommended servings using the 1992 US food pyramid or the basic 4 food groups<br>5-level system used to shape changes in the targeted behaviors<br>1000-1200 kcal/d<br>Limit red foods to ≤7/wk | Habits book: food kcal and number red foods intake | Yes<br>No difference in compliance, $P > .05$ | Yes<br>Estimated energy intake from habit book | Greater energy for PA (1124.1 ± 28.0 kcal) vs combined (973.2 ± 26.2 kcal) vs sedentary (983.9 ± 27.1), $P < .001$ | No |
| Epstein et al (2000)[39] | Traffic Light with recommended food servings from the food pyramid with foods color-coded based on nutrient density. Green (very low calorie), yellow (higher in calories and include dietary staples needed for a balanced diet), red (higher in calories and low nutrient density)<br>4184-5012 kJ/d<br>Red foods limited to <11/wk | Not measured | No | No | No | No |
| Epstein et al (2000)[29] | Traffic Light with 1200 kcal/d based on food pyramid with foods color-coded based on nutrient density. Red (any food >20 kcal above the standard for this group + all sweets and sugared beverages), yellow (no more than 20 kcal per average serving above the group average), green (<20 kcal than the average serving) | Not measured | No | Not measured | No | No |

(*continued*)

**Table 3. Description of Dietary Interventions, Measurement and Report of Compliance, and Dietary Outcomes in Studies Included in a Systematic Review of the Effectiveness of Dietetic Interventions for Child Obesity (cont)**

| Source | Dietary Intervention | Compliance to Diet Intervention | | Dietary Outcomes | | Dietetic Involvement Reported |
|---|---|---|---|---|---|---|
| | | How Measured | Reported | How Measured | Reported | |
| Epstein et al (2001)[14] | Traffic Light with recommended food servings from the food pyramid with foods color-coded based on nutrient density. Green (very low calorie), yellow (higher in calories and include dietary staples needed for a balanced diet), red (higher in calories and low nutrient density) 1200-1500 kcal/d Red foods limited to <11/wk | 25-item questionnaire for diet and PA | No | Not measured | No | No |
| Epstein et al (2004)[15] | Traffic Light (modified) Green food <2 g fat per serving Yellow 2-5 g fat/serving Red >5 g fat/serving + all foods at top of 1992 US food pyramid Starting diet, 800-1200 kcal/d Weight loss goal for children, 0.5 lb/wk Goal to gradually reduce red foods to 15/wk or less Praise and reinforcement for meeting goals and contract reinforcement system to motivate behavior change | Habit book: food diary, food description, amount, kcal, No. red foods | No | Yes Validated food intake questionnaire (baseline and 6 mo) Red foods per day and fruit and vegetables per day | Decreased red foods at 6 mo (−2.6 ± 2.2), $P<.001$, and increased fruit and vegetables (0.6 ± 2.3), $P<.05$ | No |
| Flodmark et al (1993)[30] | Energy reduction, 1500-1700 kcal, low fat (<30% of energy) Dietary counseling by a dietitian and/or pediatrician in both groups | Not measured | No | Not measured | No | Yes |
| Golan et al[25] and Golan and Crow (1998)[47]* | Prudent diet (reduce total fat, saturated fat and increase monounsaturated fat) Child only group: energy prescription (1500 kcal/d) Parent only group: no energy restriction | Not measured | No | Yes 7-d food records, validated by 24-h recall (preintervention and postintervention) | Greater reduction in energy intake per day in parent group, 26% vs 17%, $P<.001$ | Yes, led the groups and did the 24-h recalls |
| Goldfield et al (2001)[16] | Traffic Light: red food (>5 g fat/serving and/or low nutrient density); yellow (2-5 g fat/serving); green (0-1 g fat/serving and nutrient dense) 1000-1200 kcal/d, maximum of 15 red foods/wk, recommended servings from the US food pyramid. Once nonobese, subject could add 100 kcal per day per wk until weight maintenance | Habit book; food and kcal intake and number of red foods/d | No | Yes 3 × telephone 24-h diet recalls (preintervention, 6 mo, and 1 y) using measuring cups and ruler prompt | At 1 y, fewer red foods (34.7 ± 16.2 vs 18.6 ± 9.2), $P<.001$; fewer total servings, $P<.005$; less total energy, $P<.001$ (1881 ± 462 kcal vs 1338 ± 444) | Yes, collected 24-h recalls |
| Graves et al (1988)[31] | Dietary information provided is not clear | Color-coded record charts at 1 and 8 wk | No | Yes | Parent and child reported greater increase in green foods and reduction in red foods in intervention groups vs instruction only | No |
| Gutin et al (2002)[32] | Lifestyle education, including nutrition; no details given | Not measured | No | 2-d standardized recalls at preintervention, 4 mo, and 8 mo (self-recorded) | Yes Increase in kcal/d in both moderate- and high-intensity PA groups | No |
| Hills and Parker (1988)[17] | Nutrition education after baseline diet data collection to identify individual diet and food behavior goals Ongoing nutrition education and parent support | Energy balance record sheet | No | Not measured | No | Yes, an individual consult prior to exercise program and halfway through program |
| Kirschenbaum et al (1984)[33] | Nutrition education; no details given | Self-monitoring | No | Not measured | No | No |
| Lansky and Brownell (1982)[18] | Food exchange (1200 kcal/d-food exchange) plus appropriate nutrition habits | Self-recorded food intake | No | Not measured | No | Yes, advised on the diet program to be implemented |
| Mellin et al (1987)[19] | "Shapedown": self-directed, successive, sustainable, small modifications in diet | Not measured | No | Habit inventory; questions on caloric density, frequency, and quantity of food consumed at preintervention, 3 mo, and 15 mo | No | Yes, 3 of 4 group leaders were registered dietitians |
| Nova et al (2001)[24] | Routine group: general advice on healthy eating Intervention: energy prescription approximately 1400 kcal/d | Food diary with accuracy rated by family pediatrician as good, sufficient, or poor | Yes (group 2 only) | Not measured | No | No |
| Rocchini et al (1987)[38] | Modified kcal exchange program to produce weight loss of 1 lb/wk | Record keeping | No | 24-h urinary sodium excretion preintervention and postintervention (20 wk) | No significant difference | No |

(*continued*)

**Table 3. Description of Dietary Interventions, Measurement and Report of Compliance, and Dietary Outcomes in Studies Included in a Systematic Review of the Effectiveness of Dietetic Interventions for Child Obesity (cont)**

| | | Compliance to Diet Intervention | | Dietary Outcomes | | |
|---|---|---|---|---|---|---|
| **Source** | **Dietary Intervention** | **How Measured** | **Reported** | **How Measured** | **Reported** | **Dietetic Involvement Reported** |
| Rocchini et al (1988)[37] | Modified kcal exchange program to produce weight loss | Record keeping | No | Not measured | No | No |
| Saelens et al (2002)[20] | Computer-based program: assessment of eating with individual plan to decrease fat or increase fruit and vegetables or decrease overeating/snacking<br>Printed action plans with foods divided into red (≥5 g fat or diet versions of high-fat foods) or green (≤1 g fat, <150 kcal and nutrient dense)<br>1200-1500 kcal/d and weekly goal of 40 green and <15 red foods | Food diary, type and amount of food, kcal and number of red/green foods | No | 2-d dietary recall interview at preintervention, postintervention, and follow-up | Yes<br>No significant difference in total energy or percentage energy from fat | No |
| Schwingshandl et al (1999)[21] | General dietary advice (20% protein, 30% fat, 50% CHO)<br>Energy restricted to 1000-1400 kcal/d with daily allowances for each food component | Not measured | No | Not measured | No | Yes, all received diet advice at baseline and 4, 8, and 12 wk |
| Senediak and Spence (1985)[36] | Modified Traffic Light plus modified food exchange system | Self-reported, 7-d kcal intake per d pretreatment and posttreatment in the intervention groups only | No | 7-d food records at pretreatment and posttreatment | Yes<br>Total energy intake/d reported as significantly different from baseline in the intervention groups, a deficit of 456 and 362 kcal in groups 1 and 2 ($P<.01$) | No |
| Sondike et al (2003)[22] | Stoplight approach<br>Low CHO group: max 20 g CHO/d + ad libitum protein, fat, and energy for 2 wk, then 10 wk, 40 g CHO/d + multivitamin + water + potassium + fiber supplements<br>Low-fat group, <40 g/d + 5 servings/d of starches + ad libitum fat-free dairy food, fruit, and vegetable + multivitamin | 3-d food records at baseline and biweekly<br>Daily urinary ketones | Yes<br>Significantly more fat, $P=.001$, in low CHO group<br>Low CHO (ketotic most days) vs none in low-fat group | 3-d food records | Yes<br>Greater mean energy, fat, and protein and lower mean CHO in low CHO group, $P<.001$ | Yes, monitoring of diet adherence at baseline and biweekly |
| Sung et al (2002)[23] | Low energy, 900-1200 kcal/d, low fat (20%-25%), high complex CHO (50%-60%), and sufficient protein (25%-30%) | 3-d record at baseline and biweekly using volume, size, and atlas of low kcal food portions | No | 3-d record pretreatment and posttreatment | Yes<br>Percentage fat lower ($P<.05$) and percentage CHO higher ($P<.05$) at 6 wk | Yes, gave all children the same diet advice |
| Wadden et al (1990)[34] | WRAP (Weight Reduction and Pride) program: measuring foods and beverages; recording food and kcal intake; low-fat, well-balanced meals of 1000-1500 kcal/d; limiting high-kcal snacks and fast foods | Not measured | No | Not measured | No | Registered dietitian investigator but not therapist |

Abbreviations: BT, behavior therapy; CHO, carbohydrate; PA, physical activity; PS, polyunsaturated.
*Selected references cited; a complete reference list is available from the authors.

that body composition does indeed vary with age and pubertal status. We recommend that pediatric weight loss researchers seek consensus on age group targets for children and adolescents younger than 20 years so that later meta-analyses can be facilitated.

## FOLLOW-UP DURATION

Most of the trials reported results immediately postintervention and at 1 or more follow-up times. There is wide variation in both intervention lengths and the follow-up intervals and duration. Some trials employ follow-up durations as short as 3, 6, or 8 months. We suggest that the success of a weight loss intervention designed ultimately to produce lasting improvements in the health states of obese patients cannot be established clinically, as opposed to statistically, in as short a time frame as 8 months. More consistent intervention and follow-up durations across the field would facilitate informal as well as more formal comparisons of trial results via meta-analysis. We therefore recommend that professional bodies lobby major funding agencies to raise awareness of these issues and advocate for priority funding of large intervention trials with adequate follow-up periods.

## GENERAL HETEROGENEITY OF TRIAL DESIGN

The fact that only 2 strongly qualified meta-analyses could be presented in this article is in itself an indication of the significant heterogeneity of interventions for weight management in children and adolescents. Consistency of patient attributes, treatment types, and trial protocols is essential if the meta-analytic calculations are to yield results that can be relied on and incorporated into the knowledge base of the field.

Many trials in weight loss research are small in comparison with other areas, such as cancer treatment research. This may be because funding is generally limited, because it is difficult to recruit into lifestyle interventions particularly for child obesity due to its multifactorial etiology, or because the research is opportunistic.

## CONCLUSIONS

Although there is insufficient evidence to determine the effectiveness of dietary interventions in treating excessive weight gain in children and adolescents, this systematic review does indicate that interventions that include dietary modification, both as part of an intervention or control and in various treatment combinations, are effective in gaining improvements in weight-related outcomes. This effect appeared to diminish with time. It is difficult to make evidence-based dietary recommendations for child weight management because details of the dietary interventions or the changes made by those who are successful are lacking. The evidence base for pediatric weight management research would increase if researchers considered carefully the methodological quality of their trials, including sample size, at the earliest planning stage. This article has highlighted current gaps in knowledge and limitations in current study designs. Researchers in clinical, public health, and research settings are encouraged to fully describe the rationale and aims of their dietary interventions, evaluate whether subjects adhere to the dietary recommendations, and report dietary outcomes to address the urgent need to develop effective dietary interventions for both childhood obesity treatment and prevention.

**Accepted for Publication:** February 16, 2006.
**Correspondence:** Clare E. Collins, PhD, BSc, Dip (Nutr&Diet), Dip(ClinEpi), APD, School of Health Sciences, Mail Box 38, Hunter Building, University of Newcastle, Callaghan, NSW 2308, Australia (clare.collins@newcastle.edu.au).
**Author Contributions:** *Study concept and design:* Collins, Warren, Neve, McCoy, and Stokes. *Acquisition of data:* Collins, Warren, Neve, and McCoy. *Analysis and interpretation of data:* Collins, Warren, Neve, McCoy, and Stokes. *Drafting of the manuscript:* Collins, Warren, McCoy, and Stokes. *Critical revision of the manuscript for important intellectual content:* Collins, Warren, Neve, McCoy, and Stokes. *Statistical analysis:* Neve and Stokes. *Administrative, technical, and material support:* Collins, Warren, Neve, McCoy, and Stokes.
**Funding/Support:** This study was supported by a grant from the Joanna Briggs Institute, Adelaide, Australia.
**Acknowledgment:** We thank Susan Day, AUDIS, for assistance with search and retrieval strategy; Paul Carless, MMedSc(ClinEpi), for methodological and statistical advice; and Tracy Burrows, BHSc(N&D), and Rachel Sutherland, MPH, for identification and retrieval of references and for creating Figure 1 (T.B.).

## REFERENCES

1. Reilly JJ, Methven E, McDowell Z, et al. Health consequences of obesity. *Arch Dis Child.* 2003;88:748-752.
2. Strauss RS, Pollack HA. Social marginalization of overweight children. *Arch Pediatr Adolesc Med.* 2003;157:746-752.
3. Dietz WH. Childhood weight affects adult morbidity and mortality. *J Nutr.* 1998;128:411S-414S.
4. Kirk S, Scott BJ, Daniels SR. Pediatric obesity epidemic: treatment options. *J Am Diet Assoc.* 2005;105(suppl 1):44-51.
5. Kumanyika SK. Minisymposium on obesity: overview and some strategic considerations. *Annu Rev Public Health.* 2001;22:293-308.
6. Experimental critical appraisal form 4.1. Joanna Briggs Institute, Adelaide, Australia. 2003.
7. Data extraction form 5. Joanna Briggs Institute, Adelaide, Australia. 2003.
8. Duffy G, Spence SH. The effectiveness of cognitive self-management as an adjunct to a behavioural intervention for childhood obesity: a research note. *J Child Psychol Psychiatry.* 1993;34:1043-1050.
9. Epstein LH, Wing RR, Steranchak L, Dickson B, Michelson J. Comparison of family-based behavior modification and nutrition education for childhood obesity. *J Pediatr Psychol.* 1980;5:25-36.
10. Epstein LH, Wing RR, Penner B, Kress MJ. Effect of diet and controlled exercise on weight loss in obese children. *J Pediatr.* 1985;107:358-361.
11. Epstein LH, Wing RR, Woodall K, Penner BC, Kress MJ, Koeske R. Effects of family-based behavioural treatment on obese 5-to-8-year-old children. *Behav Ther.* 1985;16:205-212.
12. Epstein LH, Wing RR, Koeske R, Valoski A. Effect of parent weight on weight loss in obese children. *J Consult Clin Psychol.* 1986;54:400-401.
13. Epstein LH, McKenzie SJ, Valoski A, Klein KR, Wing RR. Effects of mastery criteria and contingent reinforcement for family-based child weight control. *Addictive Behav.* 1994;19:135-145.
14. Epstein LH, Paluch R, Raynor H. Sex differences in obese children and siblings in family-based obesity treatment. *Obes Res.* 2001;9:746-753.
15. Epstein LH, Paluch RA, Kilanowski CK, Raynor HA. The effect of reinforcement or stimulus control to reduce sedentary behaviour in the treatment of pediatric obesity. *Health Psychol.* 2004;23:371-380.
16. Goldfield GS, Epstein LH, Kilanowski CK, Paluch RA, Kogut-Bossler B. Cost-effectiveness of group and mixed family-based treatment for childhood obesity. *Int J Obes Relat Meta Disord.* 2001;25:1843-1849.
17. Hills AP, Parker AW. Obesity management via diet and exercise intervention. *Child Care Health Dev.* 1988;14:409-416.
18. Lansky D, Brownell KD. Comparison of school-based treatments for adolescent obesity. *J Sch Health.* 1982;52:384-387.
19. Mellin LM, Slinkard LA, Irwin CE Jr. Adolescent obesity intervention: validation of the SHAPEDOWN program. *J Am Diet Assoc.* 1987;87:333-338.
20. Saelens BE, Sallis JF, Wilfley DE, Patrick K, Cella JA, Buchta R. Behavioral weight control for overweight adolescents initiated in primary care. *Obes Res.* 2002;10:22-32.
21. Schwingshandl J, Sudi K, Eibl B, Wallner S, Borkenstein M. Effect of an individualised training programme during weight reduction on body composition: a randomised trial. *Arch Dis Child.* 1999;81:426-428.
22. Sondike SB, Copperman N, Jacobson MS. Effects of a low-carbohydrate diet on weight loss and cardiovascular risk factor in overweight adolescents. *J Pediatr.* 2003;142:253-258.
23. Sung RYT, Yu CW, Chang SKY, Mo SW, Woo KS, Lam CWK. Effects of dietary intervention and strength training on blood lipid level in obese children. *Arch Dis Child.* 2002;86:407-410.
24. Nova A, Russo A, Sala E. Long-term management of obesity in paediatric office practice: experimental evaluation of two different types of intervention. *Ambul Child Health.* 2001;7:239-247.
25. Golan M, Weizman A, Apter A, Fainaru M. Parents as the exclusive agents of change in the treatment of childhood obesity. *Am J Clin Nutr.* 1998;67:1130-1135.
26. Becque MD, Katch VL, Rocchini AP, Marks CR, Moorehead C. Coronary risk incidence of obese adolescents: reduction by exercise plus diet intervention. *Pediatrics.* 1988;81:605-612.
27. Brownell KD, Kelman JH, Stunkard AJ. Treatment of obese children with and without their mothers: changes in weight and blood pressure. *Pediatrics.* 1983;71:515-523.
28. Epstein LH, Valoski AM, Vara LS, et al. Effects of decreasing sedentary behavior and increasing activity on weight change in obese children. *Health Psychol.* 1995;14:109-115.
29. Epstein LH, Paluch RA, Gordy CC, Saelens BE, Ernst MM. Problem solving in the treatment of childhood obesity. *J Consult Clin Psychol.* 2000;68:717-721.

30. Flodmark CE, Ohlsson T, Ryden O, Sveger T. Prevention of progression to severe obesity in a group of obese schoolchildren treated with family therapy. *Pediatrics.* 1993;91:880-884.
31. Graves T, Meyers AW, Clark L. An evaluation of parental problem-solving training in the behavioral treatment of childhood obesity. *J Consult Clin Psychol.* 1988; 56:246-250.
32. Gutin B, Barbeau P, Owens S, et al. Effects of exercise intensity on cardiovascular fitness, total body composition, visceral adiposity of obese adolescents. *Am J Clin Nutr.* 2002;75:818-826.
33. Kirschenbaum D, Harris E, Tomarken A. Effects of parental involvement in behavioural weight loss therapy for preadolescents. *Behav Ther.* 1984;15:485-500.
34. Wadden TA, Stunkard AJ, Rich L, Rubin CJ, Sweidel G, McKinney S. Obesity in black adolescent girls: a controlled clinical trial of treatment by diet, behavior modification, and parental support. *Pediatrics.* 1990;85:345-352.
35. Epstein LH, McCurley J, Wing RR, Valoski A. Five-year follow-up of family-based behavioral treatments for childhood obesity. *J Consult Clin Psychol.* 1990; 58:661-664.
36. Senediak C, Spence SH. Rapid versus gradual scheduling of therapeutic contact in a family based behavioural weight control programme for children. *Behav Psychother.* 1985;13:285-287.
37. Rocchini AP, Katch V, Anderson J, et al. Blood pressure in obese adolescents: effect of weight loss. *Pediatrics.* 1988;82:16-23.
38. Rocchini AP, Katch V, Schork A, Kelch RP. Insulin and blood pressure during weight loss in obese adolescents. *Hypertension.* 1987;10:267-273.
39. Epstein LH, Paluch RA, Gordy CC, Dorn J. Decreasing sedentary behaviors in treating pediatric obesity. *Arch Pediatr Adolesc Med.* 2000;154:220-226.
40. Epstein LH, Wing RR, Koeske R, Ossip D, Beck S. A comparison of lifestyle change and programmed aerobic exercise on weight and fitness changes in obese children. *Behav Ther.* 1982;13:651-665.
41. Coates T, Jeffrey R, Slinkard LA, Killen JD, Danaher BG. Frequency of monetary contact and monetary reward in weight loss; lipid change and blood pressure reduction. *Behav Ther.* 1982;13:175-185.
42. Botvin GJ, Cantlon A. Reducing adolescent obesity through a school health program. *J Pediatr.* 1979;95:1060-1062.
43. Braet C, Van Winckel M. Long-term follow-up of a cognitive behavioral treatment program for obese children. *Behav Ther.* 2000;31:55-74.
44. Epstein LH, Valoski A, Wing RR, McCurley J. Ten-year outcomes of behavioral family-based treatment for childhood obesity. *Health Psychol.* 1994;13:373-383.
45. Epstein LH, Valoski A, Wing RR, McCurley J. Ten-year follow-up of behavioral, family-based treatment for obese children. *JAMA.* 1990;264:2519-2523.
46. Epstein LH, Wing RR, Koeske R, Valoski A. Long-term effects of family-based treatment of childhood obesity. *J Consult Clin Psychol.* 1987;55:91-95.
47. Golan M, Crow S. Targeting parents exclusively in the treatment of childhood obesity: long-term results. *Obes Res.* 2004;12:357-361.
48. Ludwig DS, Peterson KE, Gortmaker SL. Relation between consumption of sugar-sweetened drinks and childhood obesity: a prospective, observational analysis. *Lancet.* 2001;357:505-509.
49. Summerbell C, Ashton V, Campbell K, Edmunds L, Kelly S, Waters E. Interventions for treating obesity in children. *Cochrane Database Syst Rev.* 2003;(3): CD001872.
50. Epstein LH, Myers MD, Raynor HA, Saelens BE. Treatment of pediatric obesity. *Pediatrics.* 1998;101(3 II suppl):554-570.
51. Epstein LH, Squires S. *The Stoplight Diet for Children.* Boston, Mass: Little, Brown and Co; 1977.
52. Livingstone MB, Robson PJ. Measurement of dietary intake in children. *Proc Nutr Soc.* 2000;59:279-293.
53. National Institute of Health National Heart Lung and Blood Institute. Clinical guidelines on the identification, evaluation, and treatment of overweight and obesity in adults: the evidence report [published correction appears in *Obes Res.* 1998;6:464]. *Obesity Res.* 1998;6(suppl 2):51S-209S.
54. Gehling RK, Magarey AM, Daniels LA. Food-based recommendations to reduce fat intake: an evidence-based approach to the development of a family-focused child weight management programme. *J Paediatr Child Health.* 2005;41:112-118.
55. Epstein LH, Gordy CC, Raynor HA, Beddome M, Kilanowski CK, Paluch R. Increasing fruit and vegetable intake and decreasing fat and sugar intake in families at risk for childhood obesity. *Obes Res.* 2001;9:171-178.
56. Dupont W, Plummer W. PS Power and sample size program available for free on the internet. *Control Clin Trials.* 1997;18:274.


## What Was Done for Colds in the Early 1900s?

Catarrh, Acute Nasal

"Menthol, 1 or 2 parts dissolved in 20 of chloroform, of which a few drops in the follow of the hand, the hands then rubbed together and placed before the face, the remedy being inhaled alternately through the nose and the mouth, will arrest the progress of a cold in its initial stages."

—From *Materia Medica Pharmacy and Therapeutics*, 1906

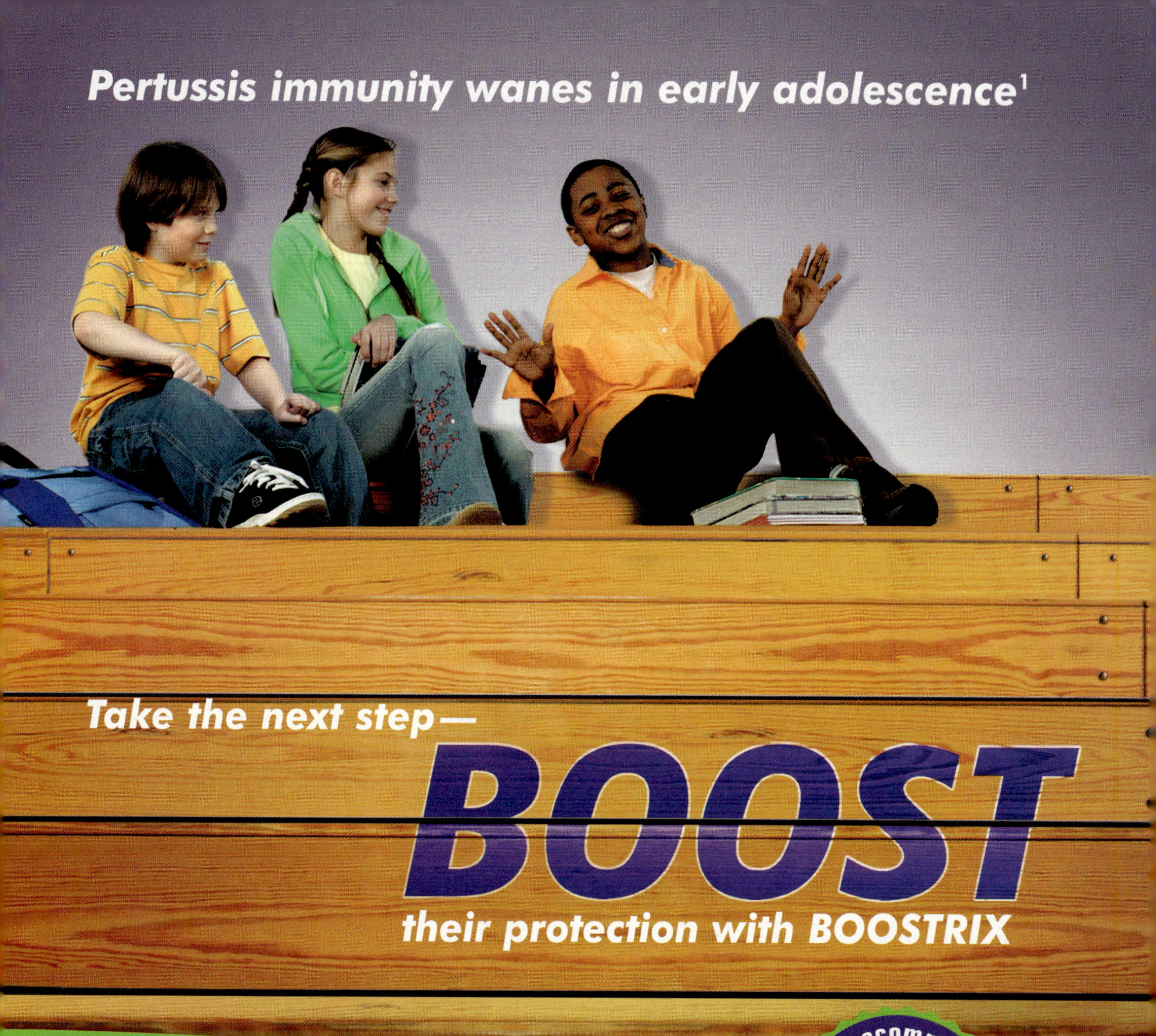


## Important Safety Information

In clinical studies, adverse events included pain, redness, and swelling at the injection site, headache, fatigue, and gastrointestinal symptoms. As with other vaccines, rare adverse events may occur. As with any vaccine, vaccination with BOOSTRIX may not protect 100% of susceptible individuals. Hypersensitivity to any component of BOOSTRIX is a contraindication.

*Advisory Committee on Immunization Practices.

**BOOSTRIX®**

***Tetanus Toxoid, Reduced Diphtheria Toxoid and Acellular Pertussis Vaccine, Adsorbed***

gsk GlaxoSmithKline Vaccines

**Please see references and brief summary of complete prescribing information on the adjacent page.**



Manufactured by **GlaxoSmithKline Biologicals,** Rixensart, Belgium

Distributed by **GlaxoSmithKline**, Research Triangle Park, NC 27709

# BOOSTRIX®

## (Tetanus Toxoid, Reduced Diphtheria Toxoid and Acellular Pertussis Vaccine, Adsorbed) (Tdap)

The following is a brief summary only; see full prescribing information for complete product information.

**INDICATIONS AND USAGE:** BOOSTRIX is indicated for active booster immunization against tetanus, diphtheria, and pertussis as a single dose in individuals 10 through 18 years of age. The use of BOOSTRIX as a primary series or to complete the primary series has not been studied. As with any vaccine, BOOSTRIX may not protect 100% of individuals receiving the vaccine.

**CONTRAINDICATIONS:** Hypersensitivity to any component of the vaccine is a contraindication (see DESCRIPTION in full prescribing information). Do not use BOOSTRIX after a serious allergic reaction (e.g., anaphylaxis) following any other tetanus toxoid, diphtheria toxoid or pertussis-containing vaccine, or any component of this vaccine (see DESCRIPTION in full prescribing information). Because of the uncertainty as to which component of the vaccine might be responsible, do not give further vaccination with any of these components; or, refer such individuals to an allergist for evaluation. The following events are contraindications to administration of BOOSTRIX: encephalopathy (e.g., coma, decreased level of consciousness, prolonged seizures) within 7 days of administration of a previous dose of a pertussis-containing vaccine that is not attributable to another identifiable cause; progressive neurologic disorder, uncontrolled epilepsy, or progressive encephalopathy. Do not vaccinate individuals with these conditions until a treatment regimen has been established and the condition has stabilized.

**WARNINGS:** The tip cap and the rubber plunger of the needleless prefilled syringes contain dry natural latex rubber that may cause allergic reactions in latex sensitive individuals. The vial stopper is latex-free. If any of the following events occurred in temporal relation to previous receipt of a Diphtheria and Tetanus Toxoids and Pertussis Vaccine Adsorbed (DTwP) vaccine or a vaccine containing an acellular pertussis component, consider carefully whether to give subsequent doses of BOOSTRIX: temperature of ≥40.5°C (105°F) within 48 hours not due to another identifiable cause; collapse or shock-like state (hypotonic-hyporesponsive episode) within 48 hours; persistent, inconsolable crying lasting ≥3 hours, occurring within 48 hours; seizures with or without fever occurring within 3 days. Persons who experienced serious Arthus-type hypersensitivity reactions following a prior dose of tetanus toxoid usually have high serum tetanus antitoxin levels and should not be given Tetanus and Diphtheria Toxoids Adsorbed For Adult Use (Td) or Tdap vaccines or even emergency doses of Td more frequently than every 10 years, even if the wound is neither clean nor minor. If Guillain-Barré syndrome has occurred within 6 weeks of receipt of prior vaccine containing tetanus toxoid, the decision to give BOOSTRIX or any vaccine containing tetanus toxoid should be based on careful consideration of the potential benefits and possible risks. The decision to administer a pertussis-containing vaccine to individuals with stable central nervous system (CNS) disorders must be made by the physician on an individual basis, with consideration of all relevant factors, and assessment of potential risks and benefits for that individual. Advise the patient, parent, or guardian of the potential increased risk involved (see PRECAUTIONS). A family history of seizures or other CNS disorders is not a contraindication to pertussis vaccine. The Advisory Committee on Immunization Practices (ACIP) has published guidelines for vaccination of persons with recent or acute illness (www.cdc.gov). Do not give BOOSTRIX to individuals with bleeding disorders such as hemophilia or thrombocytopenia, or to persons on anticoagulant therapy unless the potential benefit clearly outweighs the risk of administration. If the decision is made to administer BOOSTRIX to such persons, it should be given with caution with steps taken to avoid the risk of hematoma following the injection.

**PRECAUTIONS: General:** Before the injection of any biological, the physician should take all reasonable precautions to prevent allergic or other adverse reactions. Epinephrine injection (1:1,000) and other appropriate agents used for the control of immediate allergic reactions must be immediately available should an acute anaphylactic reaction occur. Immunosuppressed persons, including individuals receiving immunosuppressive therapy, may not develop the expected immune response. **Drug Interactions:** Do not mix BOOSTRIX with any other vaccine in the same syringe or vial. **Carcinogenesis, Mutagenesis, Impairment of Fertility:** BOOSTRIX has not been evaluated for carcinogenic or mutagenic potential, or for impairment of fertility. **Pregnancy:** Pregnancy Category C. Animal reproduction studies have not been conducted with BOOSTRIX. It is also not known whether BOOSTRIX can cause fetal harm when administered to a pregnant woman or can affect reproductive capacity. BOOSTRIX should be given to a pregnant woman only if clearly needed. Animal fertility studies have not been conducted with BOOSTRIX. In a developmental toxicity study, the effect of BOOSTRIX on embryo-fetal and pre-weaning development was evaluated in pregnant rats. Animals were administered INFANRIX® (Diphtheria and Tetanus Toxoids and Acellular Pertussis Vaccine Adsorbed) prior to gestation and BOOSTRIX during the period of organogenesis (gestation days 6, 8, 11) and later in pregnancy (gestation day 15), 0.1 mL/rat/occasion (a 45-fold increase compared to the human dose of BOOSTRIX on a body weight basis), by intramuscular injection. No adverse affect on pregnancy and lactation parameters, embryo-fetal or pre-weaning development was observed. There were no fetal malformations or other evidence of teratogenesis noted in this study. **Nursing Mothers:** It is not known whether BOOSTRIX is excreted in human milk. Because many drugs are excreted in human milk, caution should be exercised when BOOSTRIX is administered to a nursing woman. **Pregnancy Exposure Registry:** Healthcare providers are encouraged to register pregnant women who receive BOOSTRIX in the GlaxoSmithKline vaccination pregnancy registry by calling 1-888-825-5249. **Geriatric Use:** BOOSTRIX is not indicated for use in individuals older than 18 years. **Pediatric Use:** BOOSTRIX is not indicated for use in individuals younger than 10 years (see DOSAGE AND ADMINISTRATION in full prescribing information). For immunization of infants and children younger than 7 years against diphtheria, tetanus, and pertussis, refer to the manufacturers' package inserts for Diphtheria and Tetanus Toxoids and Acellular Pertussis Vaccine Adsorbed (DTaP) vaccines.

**ADVERSE REACTIONS:** A total of 3,608 adolescents were vaccinated with a single dose of BOOSTRIX during clinical trials. An additional 1,092 adolescents 10 to 18 years of age received a non-US formulation of BOOSTRIX (formulated to contain 0.5 mg aluminum per dose) in non-US clinical studies.

The primary safety study, conducted in the United States, was a randomized, observer-blinded, controlled study in which 3,080 adolescents 10 to 18 years of age received a single dose of BOOSTRIX and 1,034 received the control Td vaccine manufactured by Massachusetts Public Health Biologic Laboratories. There were no substantive differences in demographic characteristics between the vaccine groups. Among BOOSTRIX and control vaccine recipients approximately 75% were 10 to 14 years of age and approximately 25% were 15 to 18 years of age. Approximately 98% of participants in this study had received the recommended series of 4 or 5 doses of either DTwP or a combination of DTwP and DTaP in childhood. Data on adverse events were collected by the subjects, parents and/or guardians using standardized diaries for 15 consecutive days following the vaccine dose (i.e., day of vaccination and the next 14 days). Subjects were monitored for unsolicited adverse events that occurred within 31 days of vaccination (day 0-30) using diary cards (day 0-14) supplemented by spontaneous reports and a medical history as reported by subjects, parents, and/or guardians. Subjects were also monitored for 6 months post-vaccination for non-routine medical visits, visits to an emergency room, onset of new chronic illness, and serious adverse events. Information regarding late onset adverse events was obtained via a telephone call 6 months following vaccination. At least 97% of subjects completed the 6-month follow-up evaluation.

In a study conducted in Germany, BOOSTRIX was administered to 319 children 10 to 12 years of age previously vaccinated with 5 doses of acellular pertussis-containing vaccines, 193 of these subjects had previously received 5 doses of INFANRIX. Adverse events were recorded on diary cards during the 15 days following vaccination. Unsolicited adverse events that occurred within 31 days of vaccination (day 0-30) were recorded on the diary card or verbally reported to the investigator. Subjects were monitored for 6 months post-vaccination for physician office visits, emergency room visits, onset of new chronic illness, and serious adverse events. The 6-month follow-up evaluation, conducted via telephone interview, was completed by 90% of subjects.

The adverse event information from clinical trials provides a basis for identifying adverse events that appear to be related to vaccine use and for approximating rates. However, because clinical trials are conducted under widely varying conditions, adverse event rates observed in the clinical trials of a vaccine cannot be directly compared to rates in the clinical trials of another vaccine, and may not reflect the rates observed in practice.

**Serious Adverse Events in All Safety Studies:** In the US-safety study and German-safety study, no serious adverse events were reported to occur within 31 days of vaccination. During the 6-month extended safety evaluation period, no serious adverse events that were of potential autoimmune origin or new onset and chronic in nature were reported to occur. In non-US studies in which serious adverse events were monitored for up to 37 days, one subject was diagnosed with insulin dependent diabetes 20 days following administration of BOOSTRIX. No other serious adverse events of potential autoimmune origin or that were new onset and chronic in nature were reported to occur in these studies.

**Solicited Adverse Events in the US-Safety Study:** In a US study, the most common local adverse events following administration of BOOSTRIX were pain, redness, and swelling at the injection site. The most common general adverse events were headache and fatigue. Most of these events were reported at a similar frequency in recipients of both BOOSTRIX and Td. Any pain, grade 2 or 3 pain (but not grade 3 alone), and grade 2 or 3 headache (but not grade 3 alone) were reported at a higher rate in recipients of BOOSTRIX. The primary safety endpoint of the US study was the incidence of grade 3 pain (spontaneously painful and/or prevented normal activity) at the injection site within 15 days of vaccination. Grade 3 pain was reported in 4.6% of those who received BOOSTRIX compared with 4.0% of those who received the Td vaccine. The difference in rate of grade 3 pain was within the pre-defined clinical limit for non-inferiority (upper limit of the 95% CI for the difference ≤4%). These were the rates for solicited local and general adverse events within 15 days of vaccination with BOOSTRIX or Td vaccine for the total vaccinated cohort (all enrolled, vaccinated subjects with safety data available analyzed by vaccine received):

**Percentage of Individuals 10 to 18 Years of Age Reporting Solicited Local Adverse Events or Solicited General Adverse Events Within the 15-day* Post-Vaccination Period**

| | BOOSTRIX (N = 3,032) % | Td (N =1,013) % |
|---|---|---|
| **Local** | | |
| Pain,[†] any | 75.3 | 71.7 |
| Pain,[†] grade 2 or 3 | 51.2 | 42.5 |
| Pain,[‡] grade 3 | 4.6 | 4.0 |
| Redness, any | 22.5 | 19.8 |
| Redness, >20 mm | 4.1 | 3.9 |
| Redness, ≥50 mm | 1.7 | 1.6 |
| Swelling, any | 21.1 | 20.1 |
| Swelling, >20 mm | 5.3 | 4.9 |
| Swelling, ≥50 mm | 2.5 | 3.2 |
| Arm circumference increase,[§] >5 mm | 28.3 | 29.5 |
| Arm circumference increase,[§] >20 mm | 2.0 | 2.2 |
| Arm circumference increase,[§] >40 mm | 0.5 | 0.3 |
| **General** | | |
| Fever,[‖] ≥99.5°F | 13.5 | 13.1 |
| Fever,[‖] >100.4°F | 5.0 | 4.7 |
| Fever,[‖] >102.2°F | 1.4 | 1.0 |
| Headache, any | 43.1 | 41.5 |
| Headache,[†] grade 2 or 3 | 15.7 | 12.7 |
| Headache, grade 3 | 3.7 | 2.7 |
| Fatigue, any | 37.0 | 36.7 |
| Fatigue, grade 2 or 3 | 14.4 | 12.9 |
| Fatigue, grade 3 | 3.7 | 3.2 |
| Gastrointestinal symptoms,[¶] any | 26.0 | 25.8 |
| Gastrointestinal symptoms,[¶] grade 2 or 3 | 9.8 | 9.7 |
| Gastrointestinal symptoms,[¶] grade 3 | 3.0 | 3.2 |

Td = Tetanus and Diphtheria Toxoids Adsorbed For Adult Use manufactured by Massachusetts Public Health Biologic Laboratories.
N = number of subjects in the total vaccinated cohort with local/general symptoms sheets completed.
Grade 2 = Local: painful when the limb was moved; General: interfered with normal activity.
Grade 3 = Local: spontaneously painful and/or prevented normal activity; General: prevented normal activity.
*Day of vaccination and the next 14 days.
†Statistically significantly higher (P<0.05) following BOOSTRIX as compared to Td vaccine.
‡Grade 3 injection site pain following BOOSTRIX was not inferior to Td (upper limit of two-sided 95% CI for the difference in the percentage of subjects ≤4%).
§Mid-upper region of the vaccinated arm.
‖Oral temperatures or axillary temperatures.
¶Gastrointestinal symptoms included nausea, vomiting, diarrhea and/or abdominal pain.

Mid-upper arm circumference was measured by the adolescent or their parent/guardian prior to injection and daily for 15 days following vaccination. There was no significant difference between BOOSTRIX recipients and Td recipients in the proportion of subjects reporting an increase in mid-upper arm circumference in the vaccinated arm. The incidence of unsolicited adverse events reported in the 31 days after vaccination was comparable between the 2 groups.

**Solicited Adverse Events in the German Safety Study:** No cases of whole arm swelling were spontaneously reported. Two individuals (2/193) reported large injection site swelling (range 110 to 200 mm diameter), in one case associated with grade 3 pain. Neither individual sought medical attention. These episodes were reported to resolve without sequelae within 5 days. These were the rates of solicited local adverse events and fever within 15 days of vaccination for those subjects who had previously been vaccinated with 5 doses of INFANRIX:

**Rates of Solicited Adverse Events Reported Within the 15-day* Post-Vaccination Period Following Administration of BOOSTRIX in Individuals 10 to 12 Years of Age Who Had Previously Received 5 Doses of INFANRIX**

| Adverse Event | BOOSTRIX (N = 193) % (95% CI) |
|---|---|
| Pain, any | 62.2 (54.9-69.0) |
| Pain, grade 2 or 3 | 33.2 (26.6-40.3) |
| Pain, grade 3 | 5.7 (2.9-10.0) |
| Redness, any | 47.7 (40.4-55.0) |
| Redness, >20 mm | 15.0 (10.3-20.9) |
| Redness, ≥50 mm | 10.9 (6.9-16.2) |
| Swelling, any | 38.9 (31.9-46.1) |
| Swelling, >20 mm | 17.6 (12.5-23.7) |
| Swelling, ≥50 mm | 14.0 (9.4-19.7) |
| Fever, ≥99.5 | 8.8 (5.2-13.7) |
| Fever, >100.4 | 4.1 (1.8-8.0) |
| Fever, >102.2 | 1.0 (0.1-3.7) |

N = number of subjects with local/general symptoms sheets completed.
Grade 2 = Painful when the limb was moved.
Grade 3 = Spontaneously painful and/or prevented normal activity.
*Day of vaccination and the next 14 days.

As with any vaccine, there is the possibility that broad use of BOOSTRIX could reveal adverse events not observed in clinical trials.

**Postmarketing Reports:** Worldwide voluntary reports of adverse events received for BOOSTRIX in persons 10 to 18 years of age since market introduction of this vaccine are listed below. This list includes serious events or events which have causal connection to components of this or other vaccines or drugs. Because these events are reported voluntarily from a population of uncertain size, it is not possible to reliably estimate their frequency or establish a causal relationship to vaccine exposure. *Blood and lymphatic system disorders:* Lymphadenitis, lymphadenopathy. *Cardiac disorders:* Myocarditis. *Injection site reactions:* Induration, inflammation, mass, nodule, warmth, local reaction. *Metabolism and nutrition disorders:* Diabetes mellitus insulin-dependent. *Musculoskeletal and connective tissue disorders:* Arthralgia, back pain, myalgia. *Nervous system disorders:* Convulsion, encephalitis, facial palsy, paraesthesia. *Skin and subcutaneous tissue disorders:* Exanthem, Henoch-Schönlein purpura, rash. In addition, extensive swelling of the injected limb has been reported following administration of BOOSTRIX.

**Reporting Adverse Events:** Report the occurrence following immunization of any event set forth in the Vaccine Injury Table from the National Childhood Vaccine Injury Act including: Anaphylaxis or anaphylactic shock within 7 days, encephalopathy or encephalitis within 7 days, brachial neuritis within 28 days, or an acute complication or sequelae (including death) of an illness, disability, injury, or condition referred to above, or any events that would contraindicate further doses of vaccine, according to this prescribing information. These events should be reported to VAERS. The VAERS toll-free number is 1-800-822-7967. Reporting forms may also be obtained at the VAERS website at www.vaers.hhs.gov.

**DOSAGE AND ADMINISTRATION: Recommended Dose:** BOOSTRIX should be administered as a single 0.5 mL injection by the intramuscular route into the deltoid muscle of the upper arm in individuals 10 through 18 years of age. Do not administer this product subcutaneously or intravenously. There are no data to support repeat administration of BOOSTRIX. Five years should elapse between the subject's last dose of the recommended series of childhood DTwP and/or DTaP vaccine and the administration of BOOSTRIX. Limited data are available on the use of BOOSTRIX following Tetanus and Diphtheria Toxoids Adsorbed For Adult Use (Td) vaccine. **Additional Dosing Information:** ***Wound Management:*** Clinicians should refer to guidelines for tetanus prophylaxis in routine wound management. Adolescents 10 to 18 years of age who have completed a primary series against tetanus and who sustain wounds which are minor and uncomplicated, should receive a booster dose of a tetanus toxoid-containing vaccine only if they have not received tetanus toxoid within the preceding 10 years. In case of tetanus-prone injury (e.g., wounds contaminated with dirt, feces, soil, and saliva; puncture wounds; avulsions; and wounds resulting from missles, crushing, burns, and frostbite) in an adolescent who is in need of tetanus toxoid, BOOSTRIX can be used as an alternative to Tetanus and Diphtheria Toxoids Adsorbed For Adult Use (Td) vaccine in patients for whom the pertussis component is also indicated (see INDICATIONS AND USAGE).

Manufactured by **GlaxoSmithKline Biologicals**
Rixensart, Belgium, US License 1617

Distributed by **GlaxoSmithKline**
Research Triangle Park, NC 27709



Full prescribing information for BOOSTRIX is available at www.BOOSTRIX.com.

BRS-BO:L3

**References: 1.** Centers for Disease Control and Prevention. Preventing tetanus, diphtheria, and pertussis among adolescents: use of tetanus toxoid, reduced diphtheria toxoid and acellular pertussis vaccines: recommendations of the Advisory Committee on Immunization Practices (ACIP). Early Release 2006;55(February 23, 2006):1–43. **2.** Centers for Disease Control and Prevention. Recommended childhood and adolescent immunization schedule—United States, 2006. *MMWR.* 2006;54(51&52):Q1–Q4.

# Hispanic Concentration and the Conditional Influence of Collective Efficacy on Adolescent Childbearing

*Sandra Way, PhD; Brian K. Finch, PhD; Deborah Cohen, MD, MPH*

**Objective:** To determine how Hispanic residential concentration moderates the relationship between neighborhood collective efficacy and teenage birth rates.

**Design:** Cross-sectional analysis of census tract level survey data and birth records.

**Setting:** Sixty-five Los Angeles (California) County census tracts in 2000 and 2001.

**Participants:** Measures of neighborhood collective efficacy from 2600 adults from the Los Angeles Family and Neighborhood Study (LAFANS) survey were linked with demographic information from the US 2000 Census and Los Angeles County birth records for 10- through 19-year-old mothers.

**Main Exposures:** Collective efficacy and Hispanic residential concentration.

**Main Outcome Measures:** Married and unmarried teenage birth rates.

**Results:** In census tracts with less than a 50% Hispanic population, a 1-SD increase in collective efficacy was associated with a 5.07 births per 1000 decrease in the unmarried teenage birth rate ($P<.05$). In census tracts with a 50% or greater Hispanic population, a 1-SD increase in collective efficacy was not statistically related to unmarried rates, but it was associated with a 3.43 increase in the married teenage birth rate ($P<.05$).

**Conclusions:** Collective efficacy may help reduce adolescent childbearing in some, but not all, neighborhoods. An interaction between collective efficacy and Hispanic population concentration suggests cultural variation may play a role in how collective efficacy influences adolescent fertility. Possible explanations for the positive relationship between collective efficacy and married birth rates found in segregated Hispanic neighborhoods include profertility orientations and availability of childrearing networks for young parents. To help harness social capital to improve public health outcome, we suggest future studies examine the role of community cultural variation.

*Arch Pediatr Adolesc Med. 2006;160:925-930*

RECENT RESEARCH EXAMINES how the social characteristics or contexts of neighborhoods can influence residents' health outcomes.[1,2] Emphasis has been focused on how neighborhood poverty or disadvantage may influence the health of residents.[2] A less studied neighborhood attribute that could potentially ameliorate negative health outcomes, however, is that of collective efficacy, or the degree to which communities exhibit social cohesion and informal social control. Seminal research on collective efficacy theory by Sampson et al[3] suggests that neighborhoods characterized by solidarity and mutual trust, in which neighbors watch out for one another and are willing to intervene, have less criminal activity. Extending collective efficacy theory to more general social behavior, researchers have found associations with respiratory disease,[4] premature mortality,[5] self-rated health,[6] and adolescent sexual activity.[7] We explore how neighborhood collective efficacy may be related to teenage birth rates.

Adolescent childbearing is generally regarded as a social problem. Early motherhood has been linked to lower educational achievement and worse employment outcomes.[8,9] In addition, children born to teenage mothers tend to experience less positive educational and health outcomes than their counterparts in more traditional families.[10,11] Although some scholars have questioned the negative effects of teenage parenting, there is still substantial support for defining teenage pregnancy and childbirth as a public health issue.[12-14]

Teenage fertility rates are strongly related to race/ethnicity; Hispanic and black women are significantly more likely than white or Asian women to have children during adolescence.[15] These higher rates remain even after traditional measures of

Author Affiliations:
Department of Sociology/Anthropology, New Mexico State University, Las Cruces (Dr Way); Department of Sociology, San Diego State University, San Diego, Calif (Dr Finch); and RAND Corporation, Santa Monica, Calif (Dr Cohen).

**Table 1. Numbers of Respondents, Means, and Standard Deviations for Collective Efficacy Measure by Race/Ethnicity**

| Race/Ethnicity | No. of Respondents | Mean (SD) Collective Efficacy |
|---|---|---|
| Hispanic | 1435 | 3.34 (0.66) |
| White | 677 | 3.70 (0.65) |
| Black | 247 | 3.38 (0.73) |
| Asian | 173 | 3.53 (0.64) |
| Other | 33 | 3.35 (0.76) |

socioeconomic status are statistically controlled.[16,17] Persistent differences have led some researchers to suggest that cultural norms may be partially accountable.[18] If Hispanic or black communities implicitly condone adolescent childbearing, then collective efficacy is unlikely to suppress teenage birth rates. Consequently, as an ethnic population becomes increasingly influential within a community, cultural orientations may moderate the influence of neighborhood collective efficacy on adolescent childbearing. We explored this possibility by examining the relationship between collective efficacy and married and unmarried teenage birth rates in Hispanic and non-Hispanic neighborhoods. Hispanics have the highest teenage birth rates and are the largest and fastest-growing minority group in the United States, making the study of this population particularly important.[15,19]

Hispanic women across age groups have comparatively high fertility, both in the United States and Latin America, particularly Mexico to which approximately 72% of the Los Angeles (California) County Hispanic population identify their ancestry.[20] One popular explanation links high fertility with adherence to pronatalist norms that value motherhood and discourage contraception and abortion.[21] In one study, lower prevalence of contraception and abortion accounted for higher rates of Mexican American adolescent childbearing.[22] Ethnographic studies in Southern California have found that for disadvantaged Hispanic teenagers a normative environment that is less critical of premarital sex and childbearing coexists with traditional ideals stressing marriage, motherhood, and sexual discretion.[23,24] This is consistent with general accounts of acculturation where Hispanic teenagers simultaneously grapple with traditional cultural norms and mainstream American culture.[25] The fact that Mexican American adolescents have higher fertility rates than Mexican adolescents and evidence that teenage pregnancy risk increases with US acculturation suggests that adolescent childbearing is more than an extension of immigrant pronatalist norms.[26]

Other profamily norms such as familism, an orientation that stresses the importance of emotional and social relations with extended family and children, may also play a role.[27] Familism is consistent with a willingness on the part of older community members to provide material and care-giving support to young mothers. Familism coupled with the social cohesion found in efficacious neighborhoods may provide a supportive environment for early childbearing.

As suggested by collective efficacy theory, we expect collective efficacy will be associated with lower teenage birth rates for integrated and non-Hispanic white neighborhoods. Because childbirth among married adolescents is more socially acceptable, the negative relationship should be weaker than for unmarried births. We suspect collective efficacy operates differently in Hispanic neighborhoods. Based on a review of the literature, we hypothesize that collective efficacy will have less of an effect on adolescent birth rates in neighborhoods with high concentrations of Hispanic residents. Birth rates may even increase if conservative norms and familism are activated by collective efficacy, encouraging pregnant teenagers to marry and give birth.

## METHODS

This study links data from 3 different sources across 65 US census tracts in Los Angeles County: the 2001 Los Angeles Family and Neighborhood Study (LAFANS), the 2000 US Census, and Los Angeles County birth records. The LAFANS is a study of families in Los Angeles County designed in part to address questions about how neighborhoods affect a broad set of family outcomes for adults and children. Based on a presurvey assessment, neighborhoods were defined by US census tract boundaries. Between April 2000 and December 2002, researchers interviewed adults and children in 3085 households in a stratified probability sample of 65 census tracts throughout Los Angeles County. To develop a measure of collective efficacy, the current analysis uses responses from 2565 adult residents, with a response rate of approximately 85%. On average, there were 40 respondents per census tract, with none of the tracts having fewer than 27 respondents. Among other questions, respondents were asked to provide perceptions of current neighborhood characteristics. A detailed methodology of the LAFANS survey is available elsewhere.[28]

### INDEPENDENT MEASURES

The collective efficacy variable combines measures of social cohesion and informal social control constructed from LAFANS survey responses. Social cohesion includes respondents' agreement with the following statements about their neighborhoods: (1) this is a close-knit neighborhood; (2) there are adults children can look up to; (3) people are willing to help their neighbors; (4) neighbors generally do not get along with each other; (5) you can count on adults to watch out that children are safe and do not get in trouble; and (6) neighbors do not share the same values. Informal social control is captured by asking residents to estimate the likelihood that neighbors would do something if: (1) neighborhood children were skipping school and hanging out on a street corner; (2) children were spray-painting graffiti on a local building; and (3) a child was showing disrespect to an adult. All items were represented by a 5-item Likert scale. Possible responses to the social cohesion items were strongly agree, agree, unsure, disagree, or strongly disagree and possible responses to the informal social control items were very likely, likely, unsure, unlikely, or very unlikely. To obtain a neighborhood measure of collective efficacy, we combined the 9 items to form a single scale (Cronbach $\alpha = 0.79$) and aggregated individual scores up to the census tract level. **Table 1** provides descriptive statistics for the collective efficacy measure by the ethnic category of the respondents. This measure of collective efficacy is based on standard items and aggregation techniques used by Sampson et al[3] and Browning et al.[29]

We assigned demographic and socioeconomic characteristics to each of the 65 census tracts based on 2000 US census

**Table 2. Numbers of Respondents, Means, and Standard Deviations for Multiple Regression Variables by Hispanic Concentration**

| Variables | Total Mean (SD) | High (≥50%) Hispanic Concentration, Mean (SD) | Low (<50%) Hispanic Concentration, Mean (SD) |
|---|---|---|---|
| Sample size: census tracts | **65** | 39 | 26 |
| Dependent variables: teenage (10-19 y) birth rates | | | |
| Married | 8.76 (6.29) | 11.85 (4.89) | 4.13 (5.28) |
| Unmarried | 14.49 (8.69) | 18.85 (6.99) | 7.95 (6.66) |
| Independent variable | | | |
| Collective efficacy | 3.46 (0.313) | 3.27 (0.198) | 3.73 (0.245) |
| Control variables: neighborhood composition | | | |
| % of Hispanics who are foreign born | 0.47 (0.15) | 0.54 (0.10) | 0.37 (0.14) |
| % of non-Hispanics who are black | 0.26 (0.31) | 0.36 (0.36) | 0.10 (0.09) |
| Socioeconomic disadvantage, % | 0.13 (0.07) | 0.17 (0.06) | 0.08 (0.05) |
| Household receiving public assistance | 0.09 (0.07) | 0.13 (0.07) | 0.04 (0.04) |
| Female-headed household | 0.14 (0.07) | 0.17 (0.07) | 0.09 (0.05) |
| Household living in poverty | 0.23 (0.14) | 0.31 (0.11) | 0.11 (0.09) |
| Male unemployment | 0.07 (0.04) | 0.07 (0.03) | 0.06 (0.06) |

data. Neighborhood composition was captured by measuring the percentage of households in a census tract that possess specific demographic characteristics, including the percentage of residents who are Hispanic, the percentage of non-Hispanic residents who are black, and the percentage of Hispanic residents who are foreign born. Because black and Hispanic fertility rates follow similar patterns, we included the measure of black concentration as a covariate. While we believe a similar relationship may exist between black concentration and collective efficacy, there were insufficient numbers of black residents across census tracts to conduct a similar analysis. We also included a variable to capture socioeconomic disadvantage within each census tract. The socioeconomic disadvantage measure is constructed from the following 4 items: percentage of male unemployment, female-headed households, families in poverty, and families receiving public assistance.[30]

## DEPENDENT VARIABLES: BIRTH RATES

The California Department of Health Services, Center for Health Statistics, Sacramento, provided the age, marital status, and census tract of residence for all women in Los Angeles County who gave birth in 2000 and 2001. With these data we computed married and unmarried teenage birth rates for each of the 65 census tracts. Rates were standardized as the number of births per year to 10- through 19-year-old females for every 1000 10- through 19-year-old females in the population, averaged for the years 2000 and 2001.

## STATISTICAL ANALYSIS

We used ordinary least-squared regression to test for significant relationships between census tract characteristics and corresponding birth rates, including interactions between Hispanic concentration and collective efficacy. Estimates were calculated using the SAS PROC REG (SAS Institute Inc, Cary, NC) procedure. A multiple regression model was run for each of the 2 birth rate measures—marital and nonmarital. In addition to our explanatory collective efficacy variable, the analyses include the following census level covariates: socioeconomic disadvantage, percentage of the non-Hispanic population that is black, percentage of the Hispanic population that is foreign born, and a dummy variable indicating whether the population of the census tract is greater or less than 50% Hispanic. For the analysis, we converted collective efficacy into standardized *z* scores with a mean (SD) of 0 (1).

To determine whether the effect of collective efficacy varied by Hispanic concentration, an interaction term composed of the dummy 50% Hispanic and collective efficacy variable was also included in the model. The nondummy independent variables were mean centered to facilitate the interpretation of the coefficients. Consequently, the coefficients can be understood as the slope of the corresponding measure when all other covariates are at their mean. Statistically significant interactions ($P<.05$) were followed up to evaluate whether the simple collective efficacy slopes for high and low Hispanic tracts were significantly different from 0 (*t* test, $P<.05$). Since less than 50% Hispanic concentration is the comparison group (<50%=0 and ≥50%=1), the regression coefficient for collective efficacy is the simple slope for census tracts with less than 50% Hispanic concentration. By substituting a recoded dummy variable (≥50%=0 and <50%=1) and rerunning the regression model, we obtained the simple slope for census tracts with a greater than 50% Hispanic concentration.[31]

## RESULTS

**Table 2** gives descriptive statistics for each of the census tract variables for all tracts and by Hispanic concentration. Consistent with the Los Angeles population, the concentration of Hispanic residents in the sampled census tracts was high, with a mean concentration of 55.2%. In the mean census tract, 47.2% of the Hispanic residents were foreign born and 25.7% of the non-Hispanic residents were black. On average, the 39 census tracts in which 50% or more of the population was Hispanic had higher married and unmarried birthrates, lower collective efficacy, higher concentrations of foreign-born Hispanics and black non-Hispanics, and were more socioeconomically disadvantaged than the 26 census tracts with lower Hispanic resident concentrations. Hispanic neighborhoods in our sample had a mix of immigrant and native Hispanic residents. Within the 39 high Hispanic census tracts, foreign-born residents were less than 40% of the total Hispanic population in only 2 tracts and more than 70% in only 1 tract.

Los Angeles County Hispanic teenagers account for a disproportionate amount of teenage childbearing. While in 2000 approximately 53% of Los Angeles County females aged 10- through 19-years-old were Hispanic, 77%

of unmarried teenage births and 81% of married teenage births were to Hispanic mothers. Within the sampled census tracts, highly populated Hispanic tracts had significantly higher married and unmarried birthrates than low Hispanic tracts ($P<.001$). High Hispanic tracts averaged 11.85 married births and 18.50 unmarried births per 1000 adolescent females while the low Hispanic tracts, averaged 4.13 married and 7.95 unmarried births per 1000 adolescent females. In addition, in high Hispanic tracts a greater percentage of total teenage births were to married adolescents; 38% vs 29% in low Hispanic tracts ($P<.001$).

To provide a description of mean birth rates by Hispanic concentration and collective efficacy, we created 4 types of census tracts: low collective efficacy/low Hispanic concentration, low collective efficacy/high Hispanic concentration, high collective efficacy/low Hispanic concentration, and high collective efficacy/high Hispanic concentration. **Table 3** lists the unadjusted means and margins of error for the 4 groups. Consistent with our hypothesis, census tracts with lower concentrations of Hispanic residents and higher levels of collective efficacy had the lowest mean birthrates. High Hispanic tracts had higher rates with less difference between the collective efficacy categories.

**Table 4** gives the results of the multiple regression analyses. The interaction terms are significant ($\beta=5.49$, $P<.05$; and $\beta=4.36$, $P<.05$), indicating the relationship between collective efficacy and adolescent childbearing depends on the Hispanic composition of the neighborhood. The simple slopes indicate that in census tracts with less than a 50% Hispanic population a 1-SD increase in collective efficacy was associated with a 5.07 births per 1000 decrease in the unmarried birth rate ($P<.05$). In census tracts with more than a 50% Hispanic population, a 1-SD increase in collective efficacy was not statistically related to unmarried rates but was instead associated with a 3.43 births per 1000 increase in the married birth rate ($P<.05$).

The **Figure** shows the interaction by graphing the calculated regression equations for unmarried and married birth rates, respectively. The lines represent the corresponding simple collective efficacy slopes after statistically controlling for the covariates. Figure A shows that as collective efficacy increased, unmarried teenage birth rates decreased in the census tracts with less than a 50% Hispanic population. Figure B shows that as collective efficacy increased, married teenage birth rates increased in census tracts with 50% or greater Hispanic populations. The fact that the lines for the 50% or greater Hispanic unmarried birth rates and the less than 50% Hispanic married birth rates run parallel to the y-axis reflects the finding in Table 1 that the simple collective efficacy slopes for these 2 groups were not significantly different from 0. Note that the pattern for married rates is similar to that of unmarried, only shifted upward.

**Table 3. ANOVA for Unadjusted Mean Birth Rates by Collective Efficacy and Percentage of Hispanics**

| | | | Mean ± SD Teenage Birth Rate per 1000 Females Aged 10 to 19 Years | |
|---|---|---|---|---|
| Collective Efficacy* | % Hispanics† | Sample Size | Unmarried‡ | Married‡ |
| Low | Low | 5 | 13.95 ± 5.98 | 8.79 ± 4.38 |
| Low | High | 32 | 19.13 ± 2.36 | 12.03 ± 1.73 |
| High | Low | 21 | 6.52 ± 2.92 | 3.02 ± 2.14 |
| High | High | 7 | 17.56 ± 5.06 | 11.01 ± 3.71 |

Abbreviation: ANOVA, analysis of variation.

*For collective efficacy, low is defined as below the mean; high, above the mean.

†For percentage of Hispanics, low is defined as less than 50% in the census tract; high, 50% or higher in the census tract.

‡Least squares means test with Tukey-Kramer adjustment for multiple comparisons indicate married and unmarried teenage birth rates for the high-low group are significantly lower than those for both the high-high and the low-high group. Married (mean difference = high-high group: −7.99 [95% confidence interval, −13.64 to −2.34], low-high group: 1.02 [95% confidence interval, −4.38 to 6.42]). Unmarried (mean difference = high-high group: 11.03 [95% confidence interval, −18.74 to −3.32], low-high group: 12.61 ([95% confidence interval, 7.65 to 17.57]).

## COMMENT

In this study, we used collective efficacy theory to explore how neighborhoods influence married and unmar-

**Table 4. Multivariate Analysis for the Effects of Collective Efficacy and Hispanic Concentration on Married and Unmarried Teenage (10- Through 19-Year-Old) Birth Rates**

| | β (95% Confidence Interval) Teenage Birth Rate per 1000 Females Aged 10 to 19 Years | |
|---|---|---|
| Variable | Unmarried | Married |
| Intercept | 12.48† (8.67 to 16.3) | 7.79† (5.11 to 10.46) |
| Collective efficacy | −5.07* (−8.83 to −1.31) | −0.93 (−3.57 to 1.72) |
| Socioeconomic disadvantage | −27.77 (−71.97 to 16.42) | 34.54* (3.50 to 65.58) |
| % Hispanic foreign born | −2.74 (−16.77 to 11.28) | −1.60 (−11.44 to 8.25) |
| % Non-Hispanic black | 12.09† (5.71 to 18.48) | 6.63† (2.14 to 11.12) |
| ≥50% Hispanic | 6.57* (1.84 to 11.29) | 4.18* (0.87 to 7.5) |
| ≥50% Hispanic* collective efficacy | 5.49* (0.94 to 10.03) | 4.36* (1.16 to 7.55) |
| Adjusted $R^2$ | 0.51 | 0.54 |
| Simple slopes: collective efficacy | | |
| ≥50% Hispanic | 0.42 (−3.85 to 4.68) | 3.43* (0.43 to 6.43) |
| <50% Hispanic | −5.07* (−8.83 to −1.31) | −0.93 (−3.57 to 1.72) |

*$P<.05$.
†$P<.01$.

ried teenage birth rates in a sample of 65 Los Angeles County US census tracts. As predicted, we found differential effects of collective efficacy on adolescent childbearing based on Hispanic residential homogeneity. Collective efficacy was associated with lower unmarried birth rates in census tracts where the population was less than 50% Hispanic. In census tracts in which the population was 50% or greater Hispanic, however, collective efficacy was not associated with lower unmarried teenage birth rates but instead was linked to higher married teenage birth rates.

Collective efficacy theory has increasingly been applied to public health issues and, in general, the findings have supported the conclusion that cohesive communities in which neighbors reproach inappropriate behaviors may be potential allies in promoting positive public health outcomes. Our findings are consistent with this conclusion. This study indicates that neighborhood collective efficacy may be capable of influencing adolescent behaviors. The results also suggest, however, that collective efficacy may not improve public health outcomes in all settings. Collective efficacy seems to have a complex relationship with teenage childbearing; one that is likely conditioned by neighborhood cultural norms.

Our analysis does not allow us to speak directly to why the relationship between collective efficacy and adolescent childbearing differed by ethnic homogeneity. Consequently, we can only speculate about the underlying explanations for our findings. One possibility is that Hispanic normative orientations help define how collective efficacy in a neighborhood is manifested. If communities view behaviors as less problematic, social control motivators are absent. This explanation is probably most applicable to marital adolescent childbearing where cross-cultural variation in acceptability has been noted.[32] Consistent with this reasoning, teenage mothers in high percentage Hispanic census tracts were more likely to be married than other teenage mothers. Norms do not have to directly encourage adolescent childbearing to have an effect. Pronatalist views might be extended to adolescent nonmarital childbearing under certain circumstances, such as when adolescents observe peer behavior or when there are few economic incentives to delay childbearing. Assimilation into the more liberal sexual and gender norms of the wider US society, acceptance of profamily norms, negative or ambivalent views on birth control and abortion, and disadvantaged socioeconomic conditions may combine to create an environment conducive to adolescent childbearing. Such an environment may override concurrent norms that value marriage and condemn premarital sex.

Another, more structural, explanation is that social cohesion found in high collective efficacy neighborhoods provides material and emotional support for adolescent parenting. Communities with high collective efficacy and familism may provide young mothers with needed resources. Some scholars have argued that early childbearing can function as a healthy adaptive strategy in populations where delaying childbearing has fewer economic returns, especially when family members are available to assist with childrearing.[33,34] Higher teenage

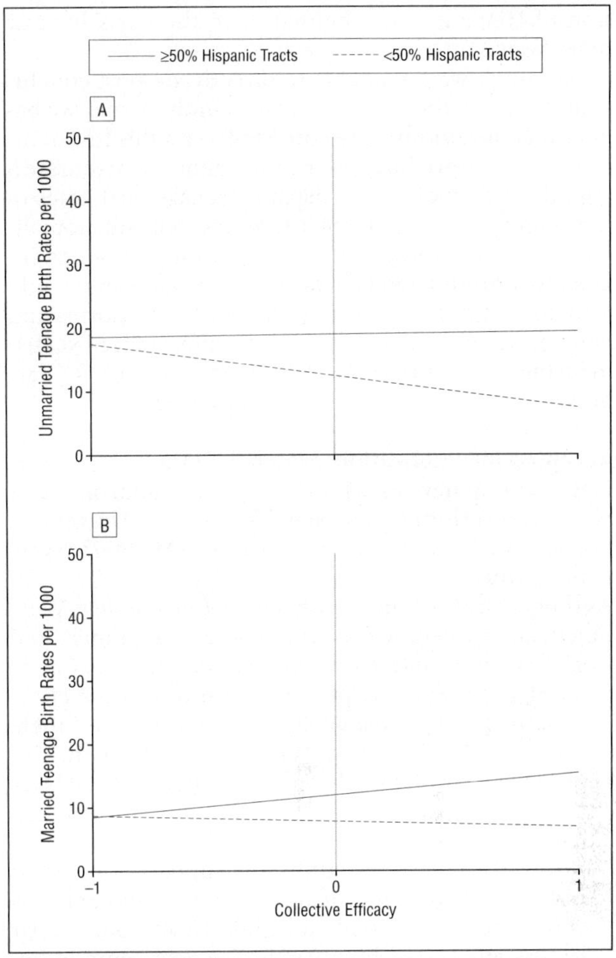


**Figure.** Effects of collective efficacy on unmarried (A) and married (B) teenage birth rates by Hispanic concentration in 65 US census tracts in Los Angeles (California) County from 2000 through 2001.

birth rates may be less problematic in such neighborhoods.

There are several limitations in our analysis. First, as an ecological study, the analysis is limited to interpretation at the neighborhood, in this case, census tract level. Therefore, one must be careful not to directly infer a relationship between individual experiences of collective efficacy and the likelihood of giving birth as an adolescent. Second, the analysis is cross-sectional in nature and consequently limited in its ability to differentiate between correlation and causation. By including characteristics that may be related to both Hispanic concentration and teenage birth rates such as socioeconomic disadvantage and immigrant and black population concentrations, we try to account for some of these factors. In general, however, almost all neighborhoods in Los Angeles County that have a high concentration of Hispanics are comparatively disadvantaged, making it difficult to untangle issues of ethnicity and economic conditions. In addition, while our analysis suggests neighborhood cultural differences based on Hispanic concentration, cultural differences are never directly measured or modeled. Based on a reading of the previous literature, profamily and fertility norms are believed to be present in neighborhoods with a high concentration of Hispanics and helped form the basis for our hypothesis.

Although we are unable to directly support conclusions based on the role of Hispanic family norms, we believe that our findings are consistent with this line of inquiry and contribute to a more general discussion regarding the increasing Hispanic teenage birth rates in the United States. We hope future research will more directly examine these issues by including questions related to attitudes and beliefs about sexuality and family formation. Examining variations in cultural norms and neighborhood dynamics may be an important next step in further elucidating how collective efficacy may be harnessed to improve public health outcomes.

**Accepted for Publication:** March 8, 2006.
**Correspondence:** Sandra Way, PhD, Department of Sociology/Anthropology, New Mexico State University, PO Box 30001, MSC 3BV, Las Cruces, NM 88003 (sway@nmsu.edu).
**Author Contributions:** *Study concept and design:* Way, Finch, and Cohen. *Acquisition of data:* Way, Finch, and Cohen. *Analysis and interpretation of data:* Way and Finch. *Drafting of the manuscript:* Way. *Critical revision of the manuscript for important intellectual content:* Way, Finch, and Cohen. *Statistical analysis:* Way and Finch. *Obtained funding:* Cohen. *Administrative, technical, and material support:* Way and Finch. *Study supervision:* Finch and Cohen.
**Funding/Support:** This study was supported by grant R40MC00303 from the Health Resources and Services Administration, Maternal and Child Health Bureau. Dr Way was supported by a RAND/Spencer Foundation Postdoctoral Fellowship during the time of the analysis.
**Acknowledgment:** We thank Aimee Bower, BS, for her assistance in preparing these data for analyses.

## REFERENCES

1. Diez Roux AV. Investigating neighborhood and area effects on health. *Am J Public Health.* 2001;91:1783-1789.
2. Robert S. Socioeconomic position and health: the independent contribution of community socioeconomic context. *Annu Rev Sociol.* 1999;25:489-516.
3. Sampson RJ, Raudenbush SW, Earls F. Neighborhoods and violent crime: a multilevel study of collective efficacy. *Science.* 1997;277:918-924.
4. Cagney KA, Browning CR. Exploring neighborhood-level variation in asthma and other respiratory diseases. *J Gen Intern Med.* 2004;19:229-236.
5. Cohen DA, Farley TA, Mason K. Why is poverty unhealthy? social and physical mediators. *Soc Sci Med.* 2003;57:1631-1641.
6. Browning CR, Cagney KA. Moving beyond poverty: neighborhood structure, social processes, and health. *J Health Soc Behav.* 2003;44:552-571.
7. Browning CR, Leventhal T, Brooks-Gunn J. Neighborhood context and racial differences in early adolescent sexual activity. *Demography.* 2004;41:697-720.
8. Klepinger DH, Lundberg S, Plotnick RD. Adolescent fertility and the education attainment of young women. *Fam Plann Perspect.* 1995;27:23-28.
9. Hayes CD. *Risking the Future.* Vol 1. Washington, DC: National Academy Press; 1987.
10. Haveman R, Wolfe B, Wilson K. Childhood poverty and adolescent schooling and fertility outcomes: reduced-form and structural estimates. In: Duncan GJ, Brooks-Gunn J, eds. *Consequences of Growing Up Poor.* New York, NY: Russell Sage Foundation; 1997:419-460.
11. Maynard RA, ed. *Kids Having Kids: Economic Costs and Social Consequences of Teen Pregnancy.* Washington, DC: Urban Institute Press; 1997.
12. Luker K. *Dubious Conceptions: The Politics of Teenage Pregnancy.* Cambridge, Mass: Harvard University Press; 1996.
13. Lawlor DA, Shaw M. Too much too young? teenage pregnancy is not a public health problem. *Int J Epidemiol.* 2002;31:552-554.
14. Scally G. Too much too young? teenage pregnancy is a public health, not a clinical, problem. *Int J Epidemiol.* 2002;31:554-555.
15. Martin JA, Hamilton BE, Sutton PD, Ventura SJ, Menacker F, Munson ML. *Births: Final Data for 2003.* Hyattsville, Md: National Center for Health Statistics; 2005. National Vital Statistics Reports, No. 2. http://www.cdc.gov/nchs/data/nvsr54/nvsr54_02.pdf. Accessed December 6, 2005.
16. South SJ, Crowder KD. Neighborhood effects on family formation: concentrated poverty and beyond. *Am Soc Rev.* 1999;64:113-132.
17. Moore KA, Simms MC, Betsey CL. *Choice and Circumstance: Racial Differences in Adolescent Sexuality and Fertility.* New Brunswick, Conn: Transaction Books; 1986.
18. St. John C, Rowe D. Adolescent background and fertility norms: implications for racial differences in early childbearing. *Soc Sci Q.* 1990;71:152-162.
19. Driscoll AK, Biggs MA, Brindis CD, Yankah E. Adolescent Latino reproductive health: a review of the literature. *Hisp J Behav Sci.* 2001;23:255-326.
20. United Nations Population Division. *World Population Prospects: The 2004 Revision.* New York, NY: United Nations Division of Economics and Social Affairs, Population Division; 2005.
21. Marcum JP. Comment on "Untangling structural and normative aspects of the minority status-fertility hypothesis" by Lopez and Sabagh. *Am J Sociol.* 1980;86:377-382.
22. Aneshensel CS, Fielder EP, Becerra RM. Fertility and fertility-related behavior among Mexican-American and non-Hispanic white female adolescents. *J Health Soc Behav.* 1989;30:56-76.
23. Deitrich LC. *Chicana Adolescents; Bitches, 'Hos's' and Schoolgirls.* Westport, Conn: Praeger Publishers; 1998.
24. Erickson P. *Latina Adolescent Childbearing in East Los Angeles.* Austin: University of Texas Press; 1998.
25. Marin G, Sabogal F, Marin BV, Otero-Sabogal R, Perez-Stable EJ. Development of a short acculturation scale for Hispanics. *Hisp J Behav Sci.* 1987;9:182-205.
26. Frank R, Heuveline P. A crossover in Mexican and Mexican-American fertility rates: evidence and explanations for an emerging paradox. *Demogr Res.* 2005;12:78-101.
27. Vega W. Hispanic families in the 1980's: a decade of research. *J Marriage Fam.* 1990;52:1015-1024.
28. Sastry N, Ghosh-Dastider B, Adams J, Pebley A. *The Design of a Multilevel Longitudinal Survey of Children, Families, and Communities: The Los Angeles Family and Neighborhood Survey.* Santa Monica, Calif: RAND Corp; 2000. Labor and Population Program, Working Paper 00-18.
29. Browning CR, Feinberg SL, Dietz RD. The paradox of social organization: networks, collective efficacy, and violent crime in urban neighborhoods. *Soc Forces.* 2004;83:503-534.
30. Ricketts R, Sawhill IV. Defining and measuring the underclass. *J Policy Anal Manage.* 1988;7:316-325.
31. Aiken LS, West SG. *Multiple Regression: Testing and Interpreting Interactions.* Thousand Oaks, Calif: Sage Publications; 1991.
32. Geronimus AT. Damned if you do: culture, identity, privilege, and teenage childbearing in the United States. *Soc Sci Med.* 2003;57:881-893.
33. Geronimus AT. The weathering hypothesis and the health of African American women and infants. *Ethn Dis.* 1992;2:207-221.
34. Stack CB. *All Our Kin.* New York, NY: Harper & Row; 1974.

There is no short cut nor "royal road" to the attainment of medical knowledge.
—Huntarian Oration, 1819

**PEDIARIX® [Diphtheria and Tetanus Toxoids and Acellular Pertussis Adsorbed, Hepatitis B (Recombinant) and Inactivated Poliovirus Vaccine Combined]**

The following is a brief summary only; see full prescribing information for complete product information.

**CONTRAINDICATIONS:** Hypersensitivity to any component of the vaccine, including yeast, neomycin, and polymyxin B, is a contraindication (see DESCRIPTION in complete prescribing information). Do not use PEDIARIX after a serious allergic reaction (e.g., anaphylaxis) temporally associated with a previous dose of this vaccine or with any components of this vaccine. Because of the uncertainty as to which component of the vaccine might be responsible, do not give further vaccination with any of these components; or, refer such individuals to an allergist for evaluation. The following events are contraindications to administration of PEDIARIX: encephalopathy (e.g., coma, decreased level of consciousness, prolonged seizures) within 7 days of administration of a previous dose of a pertussis-containing vaccine that is not attributable to another identifiable cause; progressive neurologic disorder, including infantile spasms, uncontrolled epilepsy, or progressive encephalopathy. Do not vaccinate individuals with these conditions until a treatment regimen has been established and the condition has stabilized.

**WARNINGS:** Administration of PEDIARIX is associated with higher rates of fever relative to separately administered vaccines. In a safety study that evaluated medically attended fever after PEDIARIX or separately administered vaccines when coadministered with 7-valent pneumococcal and Hib conjugate vaccines, infants who received PEDIARIX had a higher rate of medical encounters for fever within the first 4 days following the first vaccination. In some infants, these encounters included the performance of diagnostic studies to evaluate other causes of fever (see ADVERSE REACTIONS). The tip cap and the rubber plunger of the needleless prefilled syringes contain dry natural latex rubber that may cause allergic reactions in latex sensitive individuals. The vial stopper is latex-free. If any of the following events occur in temporal relation to receipt of DTwP or a vaccine containing an acellular pertussis component, consider carefully whether to give any pertussis vaccine, including PEDIARIX: temperature of ≥40.5°C (105°F) within 48 hours not due to another identifiable cause; collapse or shock-like state (hypotonic-hyporesponsive episode) within 48 hours; persistent, inconsolable crying lasting ≥3 hours, occurring within 48 hours; seizures with or without fever occurring within 3 days. If Guillain-Barré syndrome occurs within 6 weeks of receipt of prior vaccine containing tetanus toxoid, the decision to give any tetanus toxoid-containing vaccine, including PEDIARIX, should be based on careful consideration of the potential benefits and possible risks. If tetanus toxoid is withheld, other available vaccines should be given, as indicated. The decision to administer a pertussis-containing vaccine to individuals with stable central nervous system (CNS) disorders must be made by the physician on an individual basis, with consideration of all relevant factors, and assessment of potential risks and benefits for that individual. Advise the parent or guardian of the potential increased risk involved (see PRECAUTIONS). For children at higher risk for seizures than the general population, an appropriate antipyretic may be administered at the time of vaccination and for the ensuing 24 hours according to the respective prescribing information recommended dosage to reduce the possibility of post-vaccination fever. The ACIP has published guidelines for vaccination of persons with recent or acute illness (www.cdc.gov/nip).

**PRECAUTIONS:** PEDIARIX should be given with caution in children with bleeding disorders such as hemophilia or thrombocytopenia and in children on anticoagulant therapy, with steps taken to avoid the risk of hematoma following the injection. Before the injection of any biological, the physician should take all reasonable precautions to prevent allergic or other adverse reactions. Epinephrine injection (1:1,000) and other appropriate agents used for the control of immediate allergic reactions must be immediately available should an acute anaphylactic reaction occur. Immunosuppressed individuals, including those receiving immunosuppressive therapy, may not develop the expected immune response. The ACIP has published guidelines for vaccination of persons on such therapies (www.cdc.gov/nip). **Drug Interactions:** For information regarding concomitant administration with other vaccines, refer to DOSAGE AND ADMINISTRATION in complete prescribing information. Do not mix PEDIARIX with any other vaccine in the same syringe or vial. **Carcinogenesis, Mutagenesis, Impairment of Fertility:** PEDIARIX has not been evaluated for carcinogenic or mutagenic potential, or for impairment of fertility. **Pregnancy:** Pregnancy Category C: PEDIARIX is not indicated for women of child-bearing age. Animal reproduction studies have not been conducted with PEDIARIX. It is not known whether PEDIARIX can cause fetal harm when administered to a pregnant woman or if PEDIARIX can affect reproductive capacity. **Geriatric Use:** PEDIARIX is not indicated for use in adult populations. **Pediatric Use:** Safety and effectiveness of PEDIARIX in infants younger than 6 weeks of age have not been evaluated. PEDIARIX is not recommended for persons 7 years of age or older.

**ADVERSE REACTIONS:** A total of 23,849 doses of PEDIARIX have been administered to 8,088 infants who received one or more doses as part of a 3-dose primary series during 14 clinical studies. The most common adverse reactions observed in clinical trials were local injection site reactions (pain, redness, or swelling), fever, and fussiness. In comparative studies, administration of PEDIARIX was associated with higher rates of fever relative to separately administered vaccines (see WARNINGS and ADVERSE REACTIONS Table 1). The prevalence of fever was highest on the day of vaccination and the day following vaccination. More than 96% of episodes of fever resolved within the 4-day period following vaccination (i.e., the period including the day of vaccination and the next 3 days). In the largest of the 14 studies, conducted in Germany, safety data were available for 4,666 infants who received PEDIARIX administered concomitantly at separate sites with 1 of 4 *Haemophilus influenzae* type b (Hib) vaccines at 3, 4, and 5 months of age and for 768 infants in the control group that received INFANRIX® (Diphtheria and Tetanus Toxoids and Acellular Pertussis Vaccine Adsorbed), Hib conjugate vaccine, and oral poliovirus vaccine (OPV) separately. Data on adverse events were collected by parents using standardized diary cards for 4 consecutive days following each vaccine dose (i.e., day of vaccination and the next 3 days). Infants were also monitored for unsolicited adverse events that occurred within 30 days following vaccination using diaries which were returned at subsequent visits and were supplemented by spontaneous reports and a medical history as reported by parents. More than 95% of study participants were white.

In a US study, the safety of PEDIARIX administered to 673 infants was compared to the safety of separately administered INFANRIX, ENGERIX-B® [Hepatitis B Vaccine (Recombinant)], inactivated poliovirus vaccine (IPV) in 335 infants. In both groups, infants received Hib and 7-valent pneumococcal conjugate vaccines concomitantly at separate sites. All vaccines were administered at 2, 4, and 6 months of age. The study was powered to evaluate fever >101.3° F following dose 1. Data on solicited adverse events were collected by parents using standardized diary cards for 4 consecutive days following each vaccine dose (i.e., day of vaccination and the next 3 days) and are presented in Table 1. Telephone follow-up was conducted 1 month and 6 months after the third vaccination to inquire about serious adverse events. At the 6-month follow-up, information also was collected on new onset of chronic illnesses. 638 subjects who received PEDIARIX and 313 subjects who received INFANRIX, ENGERIX-B, and IPV completed the 6-month follow-up. Among subjects in both study groups combined, 69% were white, 18% were Hispanic, 7% were black, 3% were Oriental, and 3% were of other racial/ethnic groups.

The adverse event information from clinical trials provides a basis for identifying adverse events that appear to be related to vaccine use and for approximating rates. However, because clinical trials are conducted under widely varying conditions, adverse event rates observed in the clinical trials of a vaccine cannot be directly compared to rates in the clinical trials of another vaccine, and may not reflect the rates observed in practice. As with any vaccine, there is the possibility that broad use of PEDIARIX could reveal adverse events not observed in clinical trials.

**Deaths:** In 14 clinical trials, 5 deaths were reported among 8,088 (0.06%) recipients of PEDIARIX and 1 death was reported among 2,287 (0.04%) recipients of comparator vaccines. Causes of death in the group that received PEDIARIX included 2 cases of Sudden Infant Death Syndrome (SIDS) and one case of each of the following: Convulsive disorder, congenital immunodeficiency with sepsis, and neuroblastoma. One case of SIDS was reported in the comparator group. The rate of SIDS among all recipients of PEDIARIX across the 14 trials was 0.25/1,000. The rate of SIDS observed for recipients of PEDIARIX in the German safety study was 0.2/1,000 infants (reported rate of SIDS in Germany in the latter part of the 1990s was 0.7/1,000 newborns). The reported rate of SIDS in the United States from 1990 to 1994 was 1.2/1,000 live births. By chance alone, some cases of SIDS can be expected to follow receipt of pertussis-containing vaccines.

**Serious Adverse Events:** Within 30 days following any dose of vaccine in the US safety study in which all subjects received concomitant pneumococcal and Hib conjugate vaccines, 7 serious adverse events were reported in 7 subjects (1% [7/673]) who received PEDIARIX (1 case each of pyrexia, gastroenteritis, and culture negative clinical sepsis and 4 cases of bronchiolitis) and 5 serious adverse events were reported in 4 subjects (1% [4/335]) who received INFANRIX, ENGERIX-B, and IPV (uteropelvic junction obstruction and testicular atrophy in one subject and 3 cases of bronchiolitis).

**Onset of Chronic Illnesses:** In the US safety study in which all subjects received concomitant pneumococcal and Hib conjugate vaccines, 21 subjects (3%) who received PEDIARIX and 14 subjects (4%) who received INFANRIX, ENGERIX-B, and IPV reported new onset of a chronic illness during the period from 1 to 6 months following the last dose of study vaccines. Among the chronic illnesses reported in the subjects who received PEDIARIX, there were 4 cases of asthma and 1 case each of diabetes mellitus and chronic neutropenia. There were 4 cases of asthma in subjects who received INFANRIX, ENGERIX-B, and IPV.

**Seizures:** In the German safety study over the entire study period, 6 subjects in the group that received PEDIARIX reported seizures. Two of these subjects had a febrile seizure, 1 of whom also developed afebrile seizures. The remaining 4 subjects had afebrile seizures, including 2 with infantile spasms. Two subjects reported seizures within 7 days following vaccination (1 subject had both febrile and afebrile seizures, and 1 subject had afebrile seizures), corresponding to a rate of 0.22 seizures per 1,000 doses (febrile seizures 0.07 per 1,000 doses, afebrile seizures 0.14 per 1,000 doses). No subject who received concomitant INFANRIX, Hib vaccine, and OPV reported seizures. In a separate German study that evaluated the safety of INFANRIX in 22,505 infants who received 66,867 doses of INFANRIX administered as a 3-dose primary series, the rate of seizures within 7 days of vaccination with INFANRIX was 0.13 per 1,000 doses (febrile seizures 0.0 per 1,000 doses, afebrile seizures 0.13 per 1,000 doses). Over the entire study period in the US safety study in which all subjects received concomitant pneumococcal and Hib conjugate vaccines, 4 subjects in the group that received PEDIARIX reported seizures. Three of these subjects had a febrile seizure and 1 had an afebrile seizure. Over the entire study period, 2 subjects in the group that received INFANRIX, ENGERIX-B, and IPV reported febrile seizures. There were no afebrile seizures in this group. No subject in either study group had seizures within 7 days following vaccination.

**Other Neurological Events of Interest:** No cases of hypotonic-hyporesponsiveness or encephalopathy were reported in either the German safety study or the US safety study.

**Solicited Adverse Events:** Table 1 presents data from the US safety study on solicited local and systemic adverse events within 4 days of vaccination with PEDIARIX or INFANRIX, ENGERIX-B, and IPV, administered concomitantly with Hib and 7-valent pneumococcal conjugate vaccines. In this study, medical attention (a visit to or from medical personnel) for fever within 4 days following vaccination was sought in the group who received PEDIARIX for 8 infants after the first dose (1.2%), 1 infant following the second dose (0.2%), and 5 infants following the third dose (0.8%) (Table 1). Following dose 2, medical attention for fever was sought for 2 infants (0.6%) who received separately administered vaccines (Table 1). Among infants who had a medical visit for fever within 4 days following vaccination, 9 of 14 who received PEDIARIX and 1 of 2 who received separately administered vaccines, had one or more diagnostic studies performed to evaluate the cause of fever.

**Safety of PEDIARIX after a previous dose of hepatitis B vaccine:** Limited data are available on the safety of administering PEDIARIX after a previous dose of hepatitis B vaccine. In 2 separate studies, 160 Moldovan infants and 96 US infants, respectively, received 3 doses of PEDIARIX following 1 previous dose of hepatitis B vaccine. Neither study was designed to detect significant differences in rates of adverse events associated with PEDIARIX administered after a previous dose of hepatitis B vaccine compared to PEDIARIX administered without a previous dose of hepatitis B vaccine.

**Table 1. Percentage of US Infants With Solicited Local Reactions or Systemic Adverse Events Within 4 Days of Vaccination* at 2, 4, and 6 Months of Age With PEDIARIX Administered Concomitantly With Hib Conjugate Vaccine and 7-valent Pneumococcal Conjugate Vaccine (PCV7) or With Separate Concomitant Administration of INFANRIX, ENGERIX-B, IPV, Hib Conjugate Vaccine, and PCV7 (Modified ITT cohort)**

| | PEDIARIX, Hib Vaccine, & PCV7 | | | INFANRIX, ENGERIX-B, IPV, Hib Vaccine, & PCV7 | | |
|---|---|---|---|---|---|---|
| | **Dose 1** | **Dose 2** | **Dose 3** | **Dose 1** | **Dose 2** | **Dose 3** |
| **Local[†]** | | | | | | |
| **N** | **671** | **653** | **648** | **335** | **323** | **315** |
| Pain, any | 36.1 | 36.1 | 31.2 | 31.9 | 30.0 | 29.8 |
| Pain, grade 2 or 3 | 11.5 | 10.9 | 10.6 | 9.0 | 8.7 | 8.9 |
| Pain, grade 3 | 2.4 | 2.5 | 1.7 | 2.7 | 1.5 | 1.3 |
| Redness, any | 29.9[§] | 37.2 | 40.1 | 18.2 | 32.8 | 39.0 |
| Redness, >5 mm | 6.0[§] | 9.6[§] | 12.7[§] | 1.8 | 5.9 | 7.3 |
| Redness, >20 mm | 0.9 | 1.2[§] | 2.8 | 0.3 | 0.0 | 1.9 |
| Swelling, any | 17.3[§] | 26.5[§] | 28.7 | 9.6 | 20.4 | 24.8 |
| Swelling, >5 mm | 5.8[§] | 9.6[§] | 9.3[§] | 1.8 | 5.0 | 4.1 |
| Swelling, >20 mm | 1.9 | 2.5[§] | 3.1 | 0.6 | 0.0 | 1.3 |
| **Systemic** | | | | | | |
| **N** | **667** | **644** | **645** | **333** | **321** | **311** |
| Fever[‡], ≥100.4°F | 27.9[§] | 38.8[§] | 33.5[§] | 19.8 | 30.2 | 23.8 |
| Fever[‡], >101.3°F | 7.0 | 14.1[§] | 8.8 | 4.5 | 9.7 | 5.8 |
| Fever[‡], >102.2°F | 2.2[§] | 3.6 | 3.4 | 0.3 | 3.1 | 2.3 |
| Fever[‡], >103.1°F | 0.4 | 1.4 | 1.1 | 0.0 | 0.3 | 0.3 |
| Fever[‡], M.A. | 1.2[§] | 0.2 | 0.8 | 0.0 | 0.6 | 0.0 |
| **N** | **671** | **653** | **648** | **335** | **323** | **315** |
| Drowsiness, any | 57.2 | 51.6 | 40.9 | 54.0 | 48.3 | 38.4 |
| Drowsiness, grade 2 or 3 | 15.8 | 13.8 | 11.4 | 17.6 | 12.4 | 11.1 |
| Drowsiness, grade 3 | 2.5 | 1.2 | 0.9 | 3.6 | 0.6 | 1.9 |
| Irritability/Fussiness, any | 60.5 | 64.9 | 61.1 | 61.5 | 61.6 | 56.5 |
| Irritability/Fussiness, grade 2 or 3 | 19.8 | 27.9[§] | 25.2[§] | 19.4 | 21.1 | 19.4 |
| Irritability/Fussiness, grade 3 | 3.4 | 4.4 | 3.5 | 3.9 | 3.4 | 3.2 |
| Loss of appetite, any | 30.4 | 30.6 | 26.2 | 27.8 | 26.6 | 23.8 |
| Loss of appetite, grade 2 or 3 | 6.6 | 7.8[§] | 5.9 | 5.1 | 3.4 | 5.4 |
| Loss of appetite, grade 3 | 0.7 | 0.3 | 0.2 | 0.6 | 0.3 | 0.0 |

Modified ITT cohort = all vaccinated subjects for whom safety data were available
N = number of infants for whom at least one symptom sheet was completed; for fever, numbers exclude missing temperature recordings or tympanic measurements.
M.A. = Medically attended (a visit to or from medical personnel).
Grade 2 defined as sufficiently discomforting to interfere with daily activities.
Grade 3 defined as preventing normal daily activities.
* Within 4 days of vaccination defined as day of vaccination and the next 3 days.
† Local reactions at the injection site for PEDIARIX or INFANRIX.
‡ Rectal temperatures or axillary temperatures increased by 1°C to derive equivalent rectal temperature.
§ Rate significantly higher in the group that received PEDIARIX compared to separately administered vaccines [p value < 0.05 (2-sided Fisher Exact test) or the 95% CI on the difference between groups (Separate minus PEDIARIX) does not include 0].

**Postmarketing Reports With PEDIARIX:** Worldwide voluntary reports of adverse events received for PEDIARIX since market introduction of this vaccine are listed below. This list includes serious adverse events or events which have a suspected causal connection to components of PEDIARIX or other vaccines or drugs. Because these events are reported voluntarily from a population of uncertain size, it is not always possible to reliably estimate their frequency or establish a causal relationship to vaccine exposure. *Cardiac Disorders:* Cyanosis. *Gastrointestinal Disorders:* Diarrhea, vomiting. *General Disorders and Administrative Site Conditions:* Fatigue, injection site cellulitis, injection site induration, injection site itching, injection site nodule/lump, injection site pain, injection site reactions, injection site redness, injection site swelling, injection site warmth, irritability, limb pain, limb swelling, pyrexia, Sudden Infant Death Syndrome. *Immune System Disorders:* Anaphylactic reaction, anaphylactoid reaction, hypersensitivity. *Infections and Infestations:* Upper respiratory tract infection. *Investigations:* Abnormal liver function tests. *Metabolism and Nutrition Disorders:* Anorexia. *Nervous System Disorders:* Bulging fontanelle, convulsions, depressed level of consciousness, febrile convulsion, hypotonia, hypotonic-hyporesponsive episode, lethargy, somnolence. *Psychiatric Disorders:* Crying, insomnia, irritability, nervousness, restlessness, screaming, unusual crying. *Respiratory, Thoracic and Mediastinal Disorders:* Apnea, dyspnea. *Skin and Subcutaneous Tissue Disorders:* Angioedema, erythema, rash, urticaria. *Vascular Disorders:* Pallor, petechiae.

**Postmarketing Reports With INFANRIX and/or ENGERIX-B:** Worldwide voluntary reports of adverse events received for INFANRIX and/or ENGERIX-B in children younger than 7 years of age but not already reported for PEDIARIX are listed below. This list includes serious adverse events or events which have a suspected causal connection to components of INFANRIX and/or ENGERIX-B or other vaccines or drugs. Because these events are reported voluntarily from a population of uncertain size, it is not always possible to reliably estimate their frequency or establish a causal relationship to vaccine exposure. *Blood and Lymphatic System Disorders:* Idiopathic thrombocytopenic purpura[a,b], lymphadenopathy[a], thrombocytopenia[a,b]. *Gastrointestinal Disorders:* Abdominal pain[b], intussusception[a,b], nausea[b]. *General Disorders and Administrative Site Conditions:* Asthenia[b], malaise[b]. *Hepatobiliary Disorders:* Jaundice[b]. *Immune System Disorders:* Anaphylactic shock[a], serum sickness–like disease[b]. *Musculoskeletal and Connective Tissue Disorders:* Arthralgia[b], myalgia[b]. *Nervous System Disorders:* Encephalopathy[a], headache[b]. *Skin and Subcutaneous Tissue Disorders:* Alopecia[b], erythema multiforme[b], pruritus[a,b], Stevens-Johnson syndrome[a]. [[a] Following INFANRIX; [b] Following ENGERIX-B]

**Reporting Adverse Events:** Report the occurrence following immunization of any event set forth in the Vaccine Injury Table from the National Childhood Vaccine Injury Act including: Anaphylaxis or anaphylactic shock within 7 days, encephalopathy or encephalitis within 7 days, brachial neuritis within 28 days, or an acute complication or sequelae (including death) of an illness, disability, injury, or condition referred to above, or any events that would contraindicate further doses of PEDIARIX. These events should be reported to VAERS. The VAERS toll-free number is 1-800-822-7967. Reporting forms may also be obtained at the VAERS website at www.vaers.hhs.gov.

Manufactured by **GlaxoSmithKline Biologicals**, Rixensart, Belgium, US License 1617
Distributed by **GlaxoSmithKline,** Research Triangle Park, NC 27709



Full prescribing information for PEDIARIX is available at www.GSKVaccines.com/Pediarix.

BRS-PE:L3

ARTICLE

# Obese Children and Adolescents

## *A Risk Group for Low Vitamin $B_{12}$ Concentration*


*Orit Pinhas-Hamiel, MD; Noa Doron-Panush, RD; Brian Reichman, MD; Dorit Nitzan-Kaluski, MD, MPH, RD; Shlomit Shalitin, MD; Liat Geva-Lerner, MD*



**Objective:** To assess whether overweight children and adolescents are at an increased risk for vitamin $B_{12}$ deficiency.

**Design:** Prospective descriptive study.

**Setting:** Two pediatric endocrine centers in Israel.

**Participants:** Three hundred ninety-two children and adolescents were divided into 2 groups as follows: the normal-weight group had body mass indexes, calculated as weight in kilograms divided by height in meters squared, under the 95th percentile (<1.645 standard deviation scores; n=228); the obese group had body mass indexes equal to or above the 95th percentile (≥1.645 standard deviation scores; n=164).

**Intervention:** We measured vitamin $B_{12}$ concentrations. Low serum $B_{12}$ was defined as a $B_{12}$ concentration less than 246 pg/mL, and vitamin $B_{12}$ deficiency was defined as a concentration below 211 pg/mL.

**Main Outcome Measure:** Vitamin $B_{12}$ concentrations corrected for body mass index standard deviation scores, age, and sex.

**Results:** Median concentration of serum $B_{12}$ in normal-weight children was 530 pg/mL and in obese children, 400 pg/mL ($P<.001$). Low $B_{12}$ concentrations were noted in 10.4% of the obese children compared with only 2.2% of the normal weight group ($P<.001$). Vitamin $B_{12}$ deficiency was noted in 12 children, 8 (4.9%) of the obese subjects and 4 (1.8%) of the normal weight group ($P=.08$). After we adjusted for age and sex, obesity was associated with a 4.3-fold risk for low serum $B_{12}$, and each unit increase in body mass index standard deviation score resulted in an increased risk of 1.24 (95% confidence interval, 0.99-1.56).

**Conclusions:** Obesity in children and adolescents was associated with an increased risk of low vitamin $B_{12}$ concentration. We recommend that dietary assessment of obese children should include an estimation of vitamin $B_{12}$ intake. The possibility of vitamin $B_{12}$ deficiency in addition to other micronutrient deficiencies should be considered in obese children.



*Arch Pediatr Adolesc Med. 2006;160:933-936*



**Author Affiliations** are listed at the end of this article.


IN GENERAL, FOOD HABITS OF ADOLESCENTS are characterized by an irregular meal pattern with skipped meals.[1] In a national survey among youth in the United States, the percentage of youth meeting national dietary recommendations was approximately 30% for the fruit, grain, meat, and dairy pyramid groups. Sixteen percent of youth did not meet any recommendations, and only 1% met all dietary recommendations.[2] Dietary intakes of several micronutrients were found to be inadequate among adolescents in several studies.[2,3]

Although it is hard to conceive of a nutritional deficiency occurring in subjects with excessive dietary and caloric intake, obese children tend to consume foods rich in carbohydrates and fat and thus may be at increased risk of micronutrient deficiency. For example, obesity has been associated with poor dietary calcium intake both in adults and in children.[4] We have reported that 38.8% of obese children had low iron levels compared with only 4.4% of normal-weight children.[5] Iron levels showed a significant negative correlation with greater standard deviation scores (SDSs) of body mass index (BMI), calculated as weight in kilograms divided by height in meters squared. Similarly, the National Health and Nutrition Examination Survey III (1988 through 1994), providing cross-sectional data on iron deficiency among children aged 2 to 16 years, showed that the prevalence of iron deficiency increased with increasing BMI and iron deficiency was particularly common among obese adolescents (9.1% compared with 3.5% in nonobese adolescents).[6]

Vitamin $B_{12}$, also known as cobalamin, is a required nutrient; its main source

**Table 1. Age, Sex, and Vitamin $B_{12}$ Levels According to Weight Status**

| Characteristic | Normal Weight (n = 228) | Obese (n = 164) | P Value |
|---|---|---|---|
| Age, mean ± SD, y | 11.4 ± 2.7 | 12.4 ± 3.3 | .002 |
| Age, No. (%) | | | |
| <12 y | 137 (60.1) | 69 (42.1) | <.001 |
| ≥12 y | 91 (39.9) | 95 (57.9) | <.001 |
| Body mass index, median (interquartile range)* | 16.8 (15.2-18.7) | 31.5 (27.0-36.3) | <.001 |
| Sex, No. (%) | | | |
| Male | 86 (37.7) | 70 (42.7) | |
| Female | 142 (62.3) | 94 (57.3) | .32 |
| Vitamin $B_{12}$ concentration, median, pg/mL (interquartile range) | | | |
| All | 530 (410-663) | 400 (304-518) | <.001 |
| Boys | 526 (384-695) | 410 (304-520) | <.001 |
| Girls | 530 (420-635) | 396 (304-504) | <.001 |
| Age <12 y | 541 (425-709) | 490 (401-598) | .02 |
| Age ≥12 y | 504 (385-614) | 337 (279-439) | <.001 |

*Body mass index is calculated as weight in kilograms divided by height in meters squared.

is from foods of animal origin. Vitamin $B_{12}$ deficiency is associated with hematologic, neurologic, and psychiatric manifestations.[7] Furthermore, vitamin $B_{12}$ deficiency results in hyperhomocystinemia, which is an independent risk factor for atherosclerotic disease.[8] This study aimed to assess whether obese children are at increased risk for vitamin $B_{12}$ deficiency.

## METHODS

The study population comprised 392 children and adolescents aged 6 to 19 years of Sephardic and Ashkenazi Jewish origin. One hundred sixty-four were obese subjects referred to the obesity clinics of 2 endocrine centers in Israel. Two hundred twenty-eight were normal weight children referred to the endocrine clinics because of familial short stature, precocious or delayed puberty, or hirsutism and in whom no endocrine disorder was subsequently detected. Celiac disease was excluded in 103 of 128 children with short stature. We excluded children who had chronic diseases, those using vitamin supplements, those who were declared vegetarians, and those treated with metformin.

Subjects were divided into 2 groups on the basis of BMI for age and sex according to the National Institutes of Health data[9] as follows: the normal weight group had BMIs under the 95th percentile (<1.645 SDSs) for age and sex, and the obese group had BMIs at or above the 95th percentile (≥1.645 SDSs) for age and sex.

The study protocol was approved by the human experimentation committees of Sheba and Schneider medical centers (Tel Hashomer and Petah Tikva, Israel, respectively). Written parental informed consent and child assent were obtained from obese participants. Serum $B_{12}$ concentrations were routinely taken from patients as part of initial blood test screening following an overnight fast. Serum $B_{12}$ concentration was measured using the ADVIA Centaur System, a competitive immunoassay using direct chemiluminescent technology (Bayer Diagnostics, Tarrytown, NY). Serum $B_{12}$ concentrations above 246 pg/mL were deemed normal, results between 211 and 246 pg/mL borderline were considered low, and concentrations less than 211 pg/mL indicated a $B_{12}$ deficiency as recommended by the manufacturer.

Data were analyzed with SAS software version 8.0 (SAS Institute, Cary, NC). Variables were compared using a $\chi^2$ test for discrete variables and *t* test or Wilcoxon rank sum test for continuous variables. All tests were 2-tailed and *P* values below .05 were considered statistically significant. Adjusted odds ratios and 95% confidence intervals were obtained from logistic regression models with low serum $B_{12}$ concentration (<246 pg/mL) as a dependent variable and age, sex, and obesity as predictors. Goodness-of-fit of the models was estimated by a Hosmer-Lemeshow test and c statistics.

**Table 2. Multivariate Analysis for Low Serum Vitamin $B_{12}$ Levels***

| Characteristic | No. | Low $B_{12}$, No. (%) | Adjusted OR (95% CI) | P Value |
|---|---|---|---|---|
| BMI SDSs | | | | |
| Normal | 228 | 5 (2.9) | 1 | |
| Obese | 164 | 17 (10.4) | 4.33 (1.54-12.2) | <.01 |
| Age | | | | |
| <12 y | 206 | 4 (1.9) | 1 | |
| ≥12 y | 186 | 18 (9.7) | 4.46 (1.46-13.6) | <.01 |
| Sex | | | | |
| Male | 156 | 7 (4.5) | 1 | |
| Female | 236 | 15 (6.4) | 1.67 (0.45-4.31) | .29 |

Abbreviations: BMI, body mass index (calculated as weight in kilograms divided by height in meters squared); CI, confidence interval; OR, odds ratio; SDSs, standard deviation scores.

*Serum $B_{12}$ concentration was less than 246 pg/mL.

## RESULTS

Of 392 study participants, 228 were of normal weight, and 164 were obese. Age and sex distribution, BMI, and vitamin $B_{12}$ concentrations of each group are shown in **Table 1**. The median serum $B_{12}$ concentration of obese children was significantly lower than that of normal weight children; 400 vs 530 pg/mL, respectively ($P<.001$). This difference was especially marked in children aged 12 years and older.

Low vitamin $B_{12}$ concentrations (<246 pg/mL) were present in 22 subjects (5.6%), 17 (10.4%) of whom were obese and 5 (2.2%) of whom were normal-weight children ($P<.001$). Vitamin $B_{12}$ concentrations below 246 pg/mL were noted in 18 (9.7%) of 186 children older than 12 years of age compared with 4 (1.9%) of 206 children aged 6 to 11 years ($P=.001$). The percentages of boys (4.5%) and girls (6.4%) with $B_{12}$ concentrations below 246 pg/mL were not statistically different.

Vitamin $B_{12}$ deficiency (<211 pg/mL) occurred in 12 children, 8 of whom were aged 12 to 19 years. Vitamin $B_{12}$ deficiency was present in 8 (4.9%) of the obese subjects and in 4 (1.8%) of the normal weight group ($P=.08$).

On multivariant analysis (**Table 2**), obesity was associated with an excess risk for low vitamin $B_{12}$ levels (odds ratio, 4.33) after adjustment for age and sex. The Hosmer-Lemeshow goodness-of-fit test and c statistics showed that the model fitted well ($P=.90$, $c=0.77$). A similar model was conducted with BMI SDSs and age as continuous variables. An increase of 1 BMI SDS resulted in increased risk for low $B_{12}$ levels of 1.24 (95% confidence interval, 0.99-1.56), and an increase in 1 year of age resulted in increased risk of 1.35 (95% confidence interval, 1.13-1.61). Linear regression that included BMI SDSs, age, and sex ($r=-0.42$) revealed that an increase of each unit of BMI SDSs decreased vitamin $B_{12}$ concentration by 28 pg/mL ($P<.001$). Each increase in 1 year of age decreased vitamin $B_{12}$ concentration by 22 pg/mL ($P<.001$). There was no sex effect on vitamin $B_{12}$ level ($P=.33$).

## COMMENT

Our results show that obese children and adolescents had significantly lower $B_{12}$ concentrations than normal-weight children and that 10% of obese children had low serum $B_{12}$ concentrations. Obesity was associated with a greater than 4-fold risk for low vitamin $B_{12}$ concentrations, and for each unit increase in BMI SDS, there was a 24% increase risk of low serum $B_{12}$ concentrations. To the best of our knowledge, this is the first report of low $B_{12}$ concentrations in obese children. Lower serum $B_{12}$ concentrations were detected in overweight Brazilian adolescents compared with those of normal-weight adolescents; however, this difference did not reach statistical significance.[10] Among Thai adults, no statistically significant difference in vitamin $B_{12}$ concentrations was found in overweight and obese subjects compared with normal control subjects.[11] Among adult Turkish patients with metabolic syndrome, serum $B_{12}$ concentrations were significantly lower than those of healthy subjects.[12]

Vitamin $B_{12}$ deficiency results from decreased intake, abnormal nutrient absorption, and rare inborn errors of vitamin $B_{12}$ metabolism.[13-15] Abnormal absorption may be due to medications that decrease gastric acid secretion, pernicious anemia, infection with giardia lamblia, and any disruption of the ileal mucosa such as Crohn and celiac disease. Because obese children gain weight easily, there is no reason to suspect they have a problem with absorption. Although declared vegetarians were excluded from our study, dietary habits of obese children may be high in carbohydrate and fat and low in proteins from animal sources that contain vitamin $B_{12}$. Indeed in a recent study, low-nutrient-density foods contributed more than 30% of daily energy intake,[16] and intake of micronutrients related inversely to intake of low-nutrient-density foods. In the present study, although obese children were new to our clinic and had not yet been started on a weight-loss diet, it is possible that some of them had tried unbalanced diets prior to their referral to the clinic. Furthermore, it is possible that obese children have increased vitamin $B_{12}$ needs compared with nonobese children because of their increased growth and body surface area.[17] Finally, $B_{12}$ concentrations noted reflect the status in Israeli children and may not be comparable with data from other countries. For example, in our cohort, the mean $B_{12}$ concentration of normal-weight children aged 6 to 11 years was 541 pg/mL and in the 12- to 18-year-old group, 504 pg/mL, compared with 708 and 528 pg/mL in same age groups in the United States.[18]

Vitamin $B_{12}$ is a cofactor in the synthesis of methionine from homocysteine; therefore, deficiency in vitamin $B_{12}$ leads to hyperhomocystinemia. Longitudinal cohort studies have established that even mild hyperhomocystinemia both predicts and precedes the development of cardiovascular morbidity and mortality.[19,20] Hyperhomocystinemia correlated with insulin resistance in obese prepubertal children.[21] Among adults with the metabolic syndrome, levels of homocysteine were significantly higher and levels of vitamin $B_{12}$ were significantly lower compared with those of healthy subjects.[12] Homocysteine-lowering treatments have resulted in improvement of cardiovascular reactivity and coagulation factors.[22] It is thus possible that vitamin $B_{12}$ deficiency may further contribute to the high risk of developing cardiovascular disease among obese children. Folate and vitamin $B_{12}$ treatment improved insulin resistance and endothelial dysfunction, along with decreasing homocysteine levels, in patients with metabolic syndrome.[23]

In assessing the results of this study, a number of limitations should be considered. First, although measurement of serum vitamin $B_{12}$ concentration has been widely used as the standard screening test for deficiency, the test has poor positive and negative predictive values.[24] A "normal" concentration does not reliably exclude deficiency and low serum of vitamin $B_{12}$ concentration does not necessarily indicate deficiency. Other assays are expensive, such as those for methylmalonic acid and homocysteine, which seem to provide greater sensitivity and specificity, and concerns about the use of these assays and the interpretation of their results are emerging.[25] Second, in the absence of an Israeli population-based reference, we used the manufacturer reference for definitions of low and deficient. Vitamin $B_{12}$ concentrations in serum vary with the analytical method used and the laboratory conducting the analysis. Data from the National Health Examination Survey in the United States (1988-1994) defined $B_{12}$ deficiency as levels lower than the fifth percentile for age, which in the US population aged 4 years and older corresponded to 233 pg/mL.[18] The fifth percentile for children aged 6 to 11 years was 380 pg/mL and for those aged 12 to 19 years was 289 pg/mL. These values are higher than our cutoff levels. A detailed dietary questionnaire was not obtained from the children, so we could not correlate $B_{12}$ levels with intake.

Third, vitamin $B_{12}$ levels reflect results in Israeli children and may not be comparable with data from other countries. Lower $B_{12}$ levels have been reported in a population of young adult men in Israel compared with those of the United States.[26] Unfortunately, $B_{12}$ levels of healthy children in Israel have not been reported. Finally, although low vitamin $B_{12}$ levels were significantly more prevalent among obese children, $B_{12}$ deficiency was more prevalent only with borderline significance, maybe because of the relatively small sample size. These results are therefore preliminary observations and need further investigation.

In summary, our findings show that obese children are at high risk for low serum vitamin $B_{12}$ levels. We speculate that causes may include poor dietary content, repeated short-term restrictive diets, and increased requirements. We recommend that dietary assessment of obese children should include an estimation of vitamin $B_{12}$ and other micronutrient intakes.

**Accepted for Publication:** March 24, 2006.
**Author Affiliations:** Pediatric Endocrinology and Diabetes Unit, Edmond and Lily Safra Children's Hospital, Sheba Medical Center, Tel Hashomer, Israel (Dr Pinhas-Hamiel, Ms Doron-Panush, and Dr Reichman); Pediatric Endocrinology and Metabolism Unit, Schneider Children's Medical Center, Petah Tikva, Israel (Ms Doron-Panush and Dr Shatilin); Women and Children's Health Research Unit, Gertner Institute, Tel Hashomer (Drs Reichman and Geva-Lerner); Food and Nutrition Administration and Department of Epidemiology and Preventive Medicine, Ministry of Health, Jerusalem, Israel (Dr Nitzan-Kaluski); and Sackler School of Medicine, Tel-Aviv University, Tel-Aviv, Israel (Dr Pinhas-Hamiel, Ms Doron-Panush, and Drs Reichman, Nitzan-Kaluski, Shalitin, and Geva-Lerner).
**Correspondence**: Orit Pinhas-Hamiel, MD, Pediatric Endocrine and Diabetes Unit, Sheba Medical Center, Ramat-Gan, 52621, Israel (orithami@sheba.health.gov.il).
**Author Contributions:** *Study concept and design:* Pinhas-Hamiel, Doron-Panush, and Nitzan-Kaluski. *Acquisition of data:* Pinhas-Hamiel, Doron-Panush, and Shalitin. *Analysis and interpretation of data:* Pinhas-Hamiel, Reichman, and Geva-Lerner. *Drafting of the manuscript:* Pinhas-Hamiel, Reichman, and Geva-Lerner. *Critical revision of the manuscript for important intellectual content:* Pinhas-Hamiel, Reichman, Nitzan-Kaluski, and Geva-Lerner. *Statistical analysis:* Geva-Lerner. *Study supervision:* Pinhas-Hamiel.

## REFERENCES

1. Samuelson G. Dietary habits and nutritional status in adolescents over Europe: an overview of current studies in the Nordic countries. *Eur J Clin Nutr.* 2000; 54(suppl 1):S21-S28.
2. Munoz KA, Krebs-Smith SM, Ballard-Barbash R, Cleveland LE. Food intakes of US children and adolescents compared with recommendations. *Pediatrics.* 1997; 100:323-329.
3. Ganji V, Hampl JS, Betts NM. Race-, gender- and age-specific differences in dietary micronutrient intakes of US children. *Int J Food Sci Nutr.* 2003;54:485-490.
4. Zemel MB. Mechanisms of dairy modulation of adiposity. *J Nutr.* 2003;133:252S-256S.
5. Pinhas-Hamiel O, Newfield RS, Koren I, Agmon A, Lilos P, Phillip M. Greater prevalence of iron deficiency in overweight and obese children and adolescents. *Int J Obes Relat Metab Disord.* 2003;27:416-418.
6. Nead KG, Halterman JS, Kaczorowski JM, Auinger P, Weitzman M. Overweight children and adolescents: a risk group for iron deficiency. *Pediatrics.* 2004; 114:104-108.
7. Oh R, Brown DL. Vitamin B12 deficiency. *Am Fam Physician.* 2003;67:979-986.
8. Strain JJ, Dowey L, Ward M, Pentieva K, McNulty H. B-vitamins, homocysteine metabolism and CVD. *Proc Nutr Soc.* 2004;63:597-603.
9. CDC growth charts. US National Center for Health Statistics. http://www.cdc.gov/nchs/about/major/nhanes/growthcharts/charts.htm. Accessed January 9, 2006.
10. Brasileiro RS, Escrivao MA, Taddei JA, D'Almeida V, Ancona-Lopez F, Carvalhaes JT. Plasma total homocysteine in Brazilian overweight and non-overweight adolescents: a case-control study. *Nutr Hosp.* 2005;20:313-319.
11. Tungtrongchitr R, Pongpaew P, Tongboonchoo C, et al. Serum homocysteine, B12 and folic acid concentration in Thai overweight and obese subjects. *Int J Vitam Nutr Res.* 2003;73:8-14.
12. Guven A, Inanc F, Kilinc M, Ekerbicer H. Plasma homocysteine and lipoprotein (a) levels in Turkish patients with metabolic syndrome. *Heart Vessels.* 2005; 20:290-295.
13. Allen LH. Folate and vitamin B12 status in the Americas. *Nutr Rev.* 2004;62:S29-S33.
14. Rasmussen SA, Fernhoff PM, Scanlon KS. Vitamin B12 deficiency in children and adolescents. *J Pediatr.* 2001;138:10-17.
15. Goraya JS. Vitamin B12 deficiency in childhood and adolescence. *J Pediatr.* 2002; 140:636.
16. Kant AK. Reported consumption of low-nutrient-density foods by American children and adolescents: nutritional and health correlates, NHANES III, 1988 to 1994. *Arch Pediatr Adolesc Med.* 2003;157:789-796.
17. Food and nutrition guidelines for healthy adolescents. New Zealand Ministry of Health. http://www.moh.govt.nz. Accessed on July 7, 2006.
18. Wright JD, Bialostosky K, Gunter EW, et al. Blood folate and vitamin B12: United States, 1988-94. *Vital Health Stat 11.* 1998;243:1-78.
19. Herrmann W. The importance of hyperhomocysteinemia as a risk factor for diseases: an overview. *Clin Chem Lab Med.* 2001;39:666-674.
20. Homocysteine Studies Collaboration. Homocysteine and risk of ischemic heart disease and stroke: a meta-analysis. *JAMA.* 2002;288:2015-2022.
21. Martos R, Valle M, Morales R, Canete R, Gavilan MI, Sanchez-Margalet V. Hyperhomocysteinemia correlates with insulin resistance and low-grade systemic inflammation in obese prepubertal children. *Metabolism.* 2006;55:72-77.
22. Setola E, Monti LD, Galluccio E, et al. Insulin resistance and endothelial function are improved after folate and vitamin B12 therapy in patients with metabolic syndrome: relationship between homocysteine levels and hyperinsulinemia. *Eur J Endocrinol.* 2004;151:483-489.
23. Schnyder G, Roffi M, Flammer Y, Pin R, Hess OM. Effect of homocysteine-lowering therapy with folic acid, vitamin B12, and vitamin B6 on clinical outcome after percutaneous coronary intervention: the Swiss Heart Study: a randomized controlled trial. *JAMA.* 2002;228:973-979.
24. Green R. Unreliability of current assays to detect cobalamin deficiency: "nothing gold can stay." *Blood.* 2005;105:910-911.
25. Solomon LR. Cobalamin-responsive disorders in the ambulatory care setting: unreliability of cobalamin, methylmalonic acid, and homocysteine testing. *Blood.* 2005;105:978-985.
26. Nitzan Kaluski D. Impact of government in nutrition epidemiology for nutrition and health policy. Presented at: 25th ESPEN Congress; September 20, 2003; Cannes, France.

Now:
The Purple Pill™ is FDA-approved for use in kids 12 to 17 years old with GERD

# NEXIUM for the NEXT GENERATION

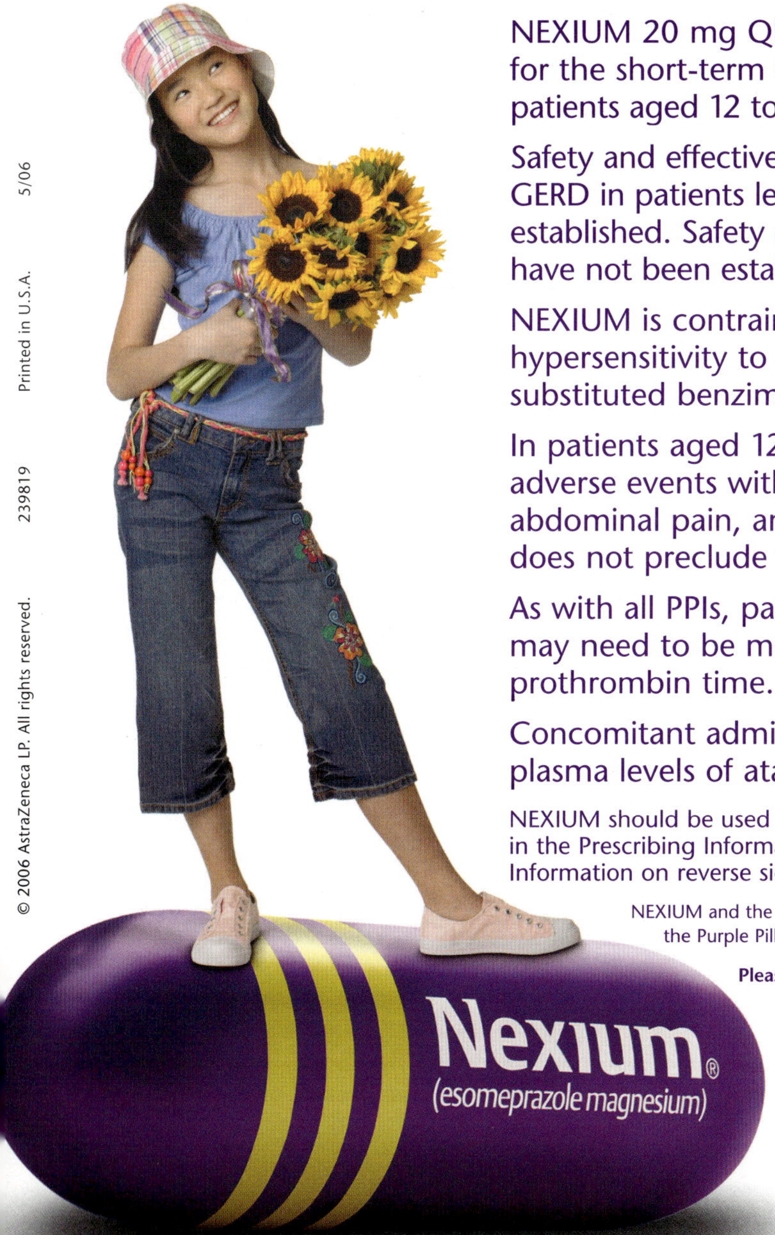


NEXIUM 20 mg QD and NEXIUM 40 mg QD are approved for the short-term treatment (up to 8 weeks) of GERD in patients aged 12 to 17 years.

Safety and effectiveness for the treatment of symptomatic GERD in patients less than 12 years of age have not been established. Safety and effectiveness for other pediatric uses have not been established.

NEXIUM is contraindicated in patients with known hypersensitivity to any component of the formulation or to substituted benzimidazoles.

In patients aged 12 to 17 years, the most frequently reported adverse events with NEXIUM include headache, diarrhea, abdominal pain, and nausea. Symptomatic response to therapy does not preclude the presence of gastric malignancy.

As with all PPIs, patients treated concomitantly with warfarin may need to be monitored for increases in INR and prothrombin time.

Concomitant administration of esomeprazole may reduce the plasma levels of atazanavir.

NEXIUM should be used only for the conditions, dosages, and durations specified in the Prescribing Information. Please see the brief summary of full Prescribing Information on reverse side.

NEXIUM and the color purple as applied to the capsule are registered trademarks and the Purple Pill is a trademark of the AstraZeneca group of companies.

**Please visit our Web site at www.Nexium-us.com**

Nexium®
(esomeprazole magnesium)

AstraZeneca

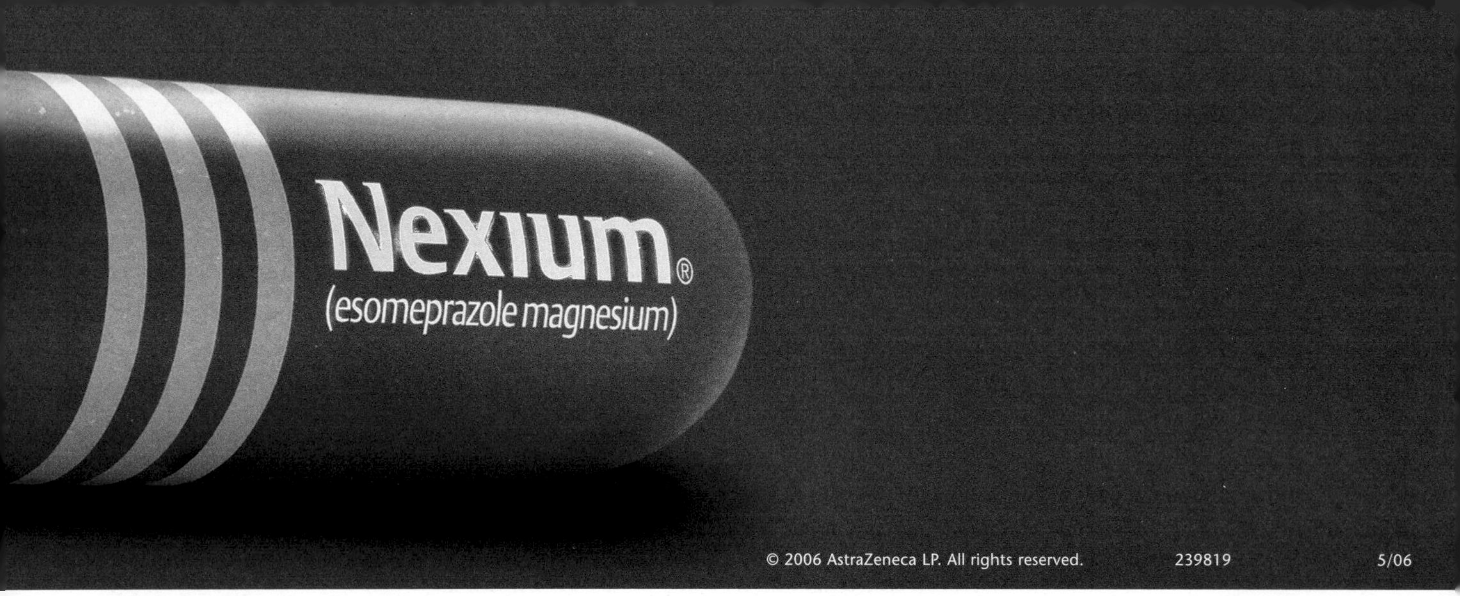


# NEXIUM® *(esomeprazole magnesium)*

## 20-mg, 40-mg Delayed-Release Capsules

**BRIEF SUMMARY** of Prescribing Information.

**INDICATIONS AND USAGE Treatment of GERD** NEXIUM is indicated for the short-term treatment (4 to 8 weeks) in the healing and symptomatic resolution of diagnostically confirmed erosive esophagitis; the maintenance of symptom resolution and healing of erosive esophagitis (controlled studies do not extend beyond 6 months); the treatment of heartburn and other symptoms associated with GERD; **Risk Reduction of NSAID-Associated Gastric Ulcer; *H.pylori* Eradication to Reduce the Risk of Duodenal Ulcer Recurrence.**

**CONTRAINDICATIONS** NEXIUM is contraindicated in patients with known hypersensitivity to any component of the formulation or to substituted benzimidazoles.

**PRECAUTIONS General** Symptomatic response to therapy with NEXIUM does not preclude the presence of gastric malignancy. Atrophic gastritis has been noted occasionally in gastric corpus biopsies from patients treated long-term with omeprazole, of which NEXIUM is an enantiomer. **Information for Patients** NEXIUM Delayed-Release Capsules should be swallowed whole and taken at least one hour before meals. For patients who have difficulty swallowing capsules, one tablespoon of applesauce can be added to an empty bowl and the NEXIUM Delayed-Release Capsule can be opened, and the pellets carefully emptied onto the applesauce. The pellets should be mixed with the applesauce and then swallowed immediately. The applesauce used should not be hot and should be soft enough to be swallowed without chewing. The pellets should not be chewed or crushed. The pellet/applesauce mixture should not be stored for future use. Antacids may be used while taking NEXIUM. **Drug Interactions** Esomeprazole is extensively metabolized in the liver by CYP2C19 and CYP3A4. *In vitro* and *in vivo* studies have shown that esomeprazole is not likely to inhibit CYPs 1A2, 2A6, 2C9, 2D6, 2E1 and 3A4. No clinically relevant interactions with drugs metabolized by these CYP enzymes would be expected. Drug interaction studies have shown that esomeprazole does not have any clinically significant interactions with phenytoin, warfarin, quinidine, clarithromycin or amoxicillin. Post-marketing reports of changes in prothrombin measures have been received among patients on concomitant warfarin and esomeprazole therapy. Increases in INR and prothrombin time may lead to abnormal bleeding and even death. Patients treated with proton pump inhibitors and warfarin concomitantly may need to be monitored for increases in INR and prothrombin time. Esomeprazole may potentially interfere with CYP2C19, the major esomeprazole metabolizing enzyme. Coadministration of esomeprazole 30 mg and diazepam, a CYP2C19 substrate, resulted in a 45% decrease in clearance of diazepam. Increased plasma levels of diazepam were observed 12 hours after dosing and onwards. However, at that time, the plasma levels of diazepam were below the therapeutic interval, and thus this interaction is unlikely to be of clinical relevance. Coadministration of oral contraceptives, diazepam, phenytoin, or quinidine did not seem to change the pharmacokinetic profile of esomeprazole. Concomitant administration of esomeprazole may reduce the plasma levels of atazanavir. Studies evaluating concomitant administration of esomeprazole and either naproxen (non-selective NSAID) or rofecoxib (COX-2 selective NSAID) did not identify any clinically relevant changes in the pharmacokinetic profiles of esomeprazole or these NSAIDs. Esomeprazole inhibits gastric acid secretion. Therefore, esomeprazole may interfere with the absorption of drugs where gastric pH is an important determinant of bioavailability (eg, ketoconazole, iron salts and digoxin). **Carcinogenesis, Mutagenesis, Impairment of Fertility** The carcinogenic potential of esomeprazole was assessed using omeprazole studies. In two 24-month oral carcinogenicity studies in rats, omeprazole at daily doses of 1.7, 3.4, 13.8, 44.0 and 140.8 mg/kg/day (about 0.7 to 57 times the human dose of 20 mg/day expressed on a body surface area basis) produced gastric ECL cell carcinoids in a dose-related manner in both male and female rats; the incidence of this effect was markedly higher in female rats, which had higher blood levels of omeprazole. Gastric carcinoids seldom occur in the untreated rat. In addition, ECL cell hyperplasia was present in all treated groups of both sexes. In one of these studies, female rats were treated with 13.8 mg omeprazole/kg/day (about 5.6 times the human dose on a body surface area basis) for 1 year, then followed for an additional year without the drug. No carcinoids were seen in these rats. An increased incidence of treatment-related ECL cell hyperplasia was observed at the end of 1 year (94% treated vs 10% controls). By the second year the difference between treated and control rats was much smaller (46% vs 26%) but still showed more hyperplasia in the treated group. Gastric adenocarcinoma was seen in one rat (2%). No similar tumor was seen in male or female rats treated for 2 years. For this strain of rat no similar tumor has been noted historically, but a finding involving only one tumor is difficult to interpret. A 78-week mouse carcinogenicity study of omeprazole did not show increased tumor occurrence, but the study was not conclusive. Esomeprazole was negative in the Ames mutation test, in the *in vivo* rat bone marrow cell chromosome aberration test, and the *in vivo* mouse micronucleus test. Esomeprazole, however, was positive in the *in vitro* human lymphocyte chromosome aberration test. Omeprazole was positive in the *in vitro* human lymphocyte chromosome aberration test, the *in vivo* mouse bone marrow cell chromosome aberration test, and the *in vivo* mouse micronucleus test. The potential effects of esomeprazole on fertility and reproductive performance were assessed using omeprazole studies. Omeprazole at oral doses up to 138 mg/kg/day in rats (about 56 times the human dose on a body surface area basis) was found to have no effect on reproductive performance of parental animals. **Pregnancy** *Teratogenic Effects. Pregnancy Category B* Teratology studies have been performed in rats at oral doses up to 280 mg/kg/day (about 57 times the human dose on a body surface area basis) and in rabbits at oral doses up to 86 mg/kg/day (about 35 times the human dose on a body surface area basis) and have revealed no evidence of impaired fertility or harm to the fetus due to esomeprazole. There are, however, no adequate and well-controlled studies in pregnant women. Because animal reproduction studies are not always predictive of human response, this drug should be used during pregnancy only if clearly needed. Teratology studies conducted with omeprazole in rats at oral doses up to 138 mg/kg/day (about 56 times the human dose on a body surface area basis) and in rabbits at doses up to 69 mg/kg/day (about 56 times the human dose on a body surface area basis) did not disclose any evidence for a teratogenic potential of omeprazole. In rabbits, omeprazole in a dose range of 6.9 to 69.1 mg/kg/day (about 5.5 to 56 times the human dose on a body surface area basis) produced dose-related increases in embryo-lethality, fetal resorptions, and pregnancy disruptions. In rats, dose-related embryo/ fetal toxicity and postnatal developmental toxicity were observed in offspring resulting from parents treated with omeprazole at 13.8 to 138.0 mg/kg/day (about 5.6 to 56 times the human doses on a body surface area basis). There are no adequate and well-controlled studies in pregnant women. Sporadic reports have been received of congenital abnormalities occurring in infants born to women who have received omeprazole during pregnancy. **Nursing Mothers** The excretion of esomeprazole in milk has not been studied. However, omeprazole concentrations have been measured in breast milk of a woman following oral administration of 20 mg. Because esomeprazole is likely to be excreted in human milk, because of the potential for serious adverse reactions in nursing infants from esomeprazole, and because of the potential for tumorigenicity shown for omeprazole in rat carcinogenicity studies, a decision should be made whether to discontinue nursing or to discontinue the drug, taking into account the importance of the drug to the mother. **Pediatric Use** Use of NEXIUM in adolescent patients 12 to 17 years of age for short-term treatment of GERD is supported by a) extrapolation of results, already included in the currently approved labeling, from adequate and well-controlled studies that supported the approval of NEXIUM for adults, and b) safety and pharmacokinetic studies performed in adolescent patients. (See **CLINICAL PHARMACOLOGY, Pharmacokinetics,** *Pediatric* for pharmacokinetic information.) The safety and effectiveness of NEXIUM for the treatment of symptomatic GERD in patients $<$12 years of age have not been established. The safety and effectiveness of NEXIUM for other pediatric uses have not been established. **12 to 17 Years of Age GERD** In a multi-center, randomized, double-blind, parallel-group study, 149 adolescent patients (12 to 17 years of age; 89 female; 124 Caucasian, 15 Black, 10 Other) with clinically diagnosed GERD were treated with either NEXIUM 20 mg or NEXIUM 40 mg once daily for up to 8 weeks to evaluate safety and tolerability. Patients were not endoscopically characterized as to the presence or absence of erosive esophagitis. The most frequently reported (at least 2%) treatment related adverse events in these patients were headache (8.1%), abdominal pain (2.7%), diarrhea (2%) and nausea (2%). No new safety concerns were identified. **Geriatric Use** Of the total number of patients who received NEXIUM in clinical trials, 1459 were 65 to 74 years of age and 354 patients were $\geq$75 years of age. No overall differences in safety and efficacy were observed between the elderly and younger individuals, and other reported clinical experience has not identified differences in responses between the elderly and younger patients, but greater sensitivity of some older individuals cannot be ruled out.

**ADVERSE REACTIONS** The safety of NEXIUM was evaluated in over 15,000 patients (aged 18-84 years) in clinical trials worldwide including over 8,500 patients in the United States and over 6,500 patients in Europe and Canada. Over 2,900 patients were treated in long-term studies for up to 6-12 months. In general, NEXIUM was well tolerated in both short and long-term clinical trials. A study was performed evaluating the safety of NEXIUM in pediatric patients aged 12-17 for the treatment of symptomatic GERD (see **PRECAUTIONS – Pediatric Use**). The safety in the treatment of healing of erosive esophagitis was assessed in four randomized comparative clinical trials, which included 1,240 patients on NEXIUM 20 mg, 2,434 patients on NEXIUM 40 mg, and 3,008 patients on omeprazole 20 mg daily. The most frequently occurring adverse events ($\geq$1%) in all three groups was headache (5.5, 5.0, and 3.8, respectively) and diarrhea (no difference among the three groups). Nausea, flatulence, abdominal pain, constipation, and dry mouth occurred at similar rates among patients taking NEXIUM or omeprazole. Additional adverse events that were reported as possibly or probably related to NEXIUM with an incidence $<$1% are listed below by body system: ***Body as a Whole:*** abdomen enlarged, allergic reaction, asthenia, back pain, chest pain, chest pain substernal, facial edema, peripheral edema, hot flushes, fatigue, fever, flu-like disorder, generalized edema, leg edema, malaise, pain, rigors; ***Cardiovascular:*** flushing, hypertension, tachycardia; ***Endocrine:*** goiter; ***Gastrointestinal:*** bowel irregularity, constipation aggravated, dyspepsia, dysphagia, dysplasia GI, epigastric pain, eructation, esophageal disorder, frequent stools, gastroenteritis, GI hemorrhage, GI symptoms not otherwise specified, hiccup, melena, mouth disorder, pharynx disorder, rectal disorder, serum gastrin increased, tongue disorder, tongue edema, ulcerative stomatitis, vomiting; ***Hearing:*** earache, tinnitus; ***Hematologic:*** anemia, anemia hypochromic, cervical lymphoadenopathy, epistaxis, leukocytosis, leukopenia, thrombocytopenia; ***Hepatic:*** bilirubinemia, hepatic function abnormal, SGOT increased, SGPT increased; ***Metabolic/Nutritional:*** glycosuria, hyperuricemia, hyponatremia, increased alkaline phosphatase, thirst, vitamin B12 deficiency, weight increase, weight decrease; ***Musculoskeletal:*** arthralgia, arthritis aggravated, arthropathy, cramps, fibromyalgia syndrome, hernia, polymyalgia rheumatica; ***Nervous System/Psychiatric:*** anorexia, apathy, appetite increased, confusion, depression aggravated, dizziness, hypertonia, nervousness, hypoesthesia, impotence, insomnia, migraine, migraine aggravated, paresthesia, sleep disorder, somnolence, tremor, vertigo, visual field defect; ***Reproductive:*** dysmenorrhea, menstrual disorder, vaginitis; ***Respiratory:*** asthma aggravated, coughing, dyspnea, larynx edema, pharyngitis, rhinitis, sinusitis; ***Skin and Appendages:*** acne, angioedema, dermatitis, pruritus, pruritus ani, rash, rash erythematous, rash maculo-papular, skin inflammation, sweating increased, urticaria; ***Special Senses:*** otitis media, parosmia, taste loss, taste perversion; ***Urogenital:*** abnormal urine, albuminuria, cystitis, dysuria, fungal infection, hematuria, micturition frequency, moniliasis, genital moniliasis, polyuria; ***Visual:*** conjunctivitis, vision abnormal. Endoscopic findings that were reported as adverse events include: duodenitis, esophagitis, esophageal stricture, esophageal ulceration, esophageal varices, gastric ulcer, gastritis, hernia, benign polyps or nodules, Barrett's esophagus, and mucosal discoloration. Two placebo-controlled studies were conducted in 710 patients for the treatment of symptomatic gastroesophageal reflux disease. The most common adverse events that were reported as possibly or probably related to NEXIUM were diarrhea (4.3%), headache (3.8%), and abdominal pain (3.8%). Postmarketing Reports – There have been spontaneous reports of adverse events with postmarketing use of esomeprazole. These reports occurred rarely and are listed below by body system: ***Blood And Lymphatic System Disorders:*** agranulocytosis, pancytopenia; ***Eye Disorders:*** blurred vision; ***Gastrointestinal Disorders:*** pancreatitis; ***Hepatobiliary Disorders:*** hepatitis with or without jaundice; ***Immune System Disorders:*** anaphylactic reaction/shock; ***Musculoskeletal And Connective Tissue Disorders:*** myalgia; ***Psychiatric Disorders:*** depression; ***Skin and Subcutaneous Tissue Disorders:*** alopecia, erythema multiforme, Stevens-Johnson syndrome, toxic epidermal necrolysis (TEN, some fatal). Other adverse events not observed with NEXIUM, but occurring with omeprazole can be found in the omeprazole package insert, **ADVERSE REACTIONS** section.

**OVERDOSAGE** A single oral dose of esomeprazole at 510 mg/kg (about 103 times the human dose on a body surface area basis), was lethal to rats. The major signs of acute toxicity were reduced motor activity, changes in respiratory frequency, tremor, ataxia, and intermittent clonic convulsions. There have been some reports of overdosage with esomeprazole. Reports have been received of overdosage with omeprazole in humans. Doses ranged up to 2,400 mg (120 times the usual recommended clinical dose). Manifestations were variable, but included confusion, drowsiness, blurred vision, tachycardia, nausea, diaphoresis, flushing, headache, dry mouth, and other adverse reactions similar to those seen in normal clinical experience (see omeprazole package insert-**ADVERSE REACTIONS**). No specific antidote for esomeprazole is known. Since esomeprazole is extensively protein bound, it is not expected to be removed by dialysis. In the event of overdosage, treatment should be symptomatic and supportive. As with the management of any overdose, the possibility of multiple drug ingestion should be considered. For current information on treatment of any drug overdose, a certified Regional Poison Control Center should be contacted. Telephone numbers are listed in the Physicians' Desk Reference (PDR) or local telephone book. **DOSAGE AND ADMINISTRATION** Please see full Prescribing Information for recommended dosages and dosage adjustments for **Special Populations** for NEXIUM.


Distributed by: AstraZeneca LP, Wilmington, DE 19850
Product of France 31026-02 Rev. 04/06 240260

AstraZeneca

# Human Herpesvirus 8 Infection Among Adolescents in the REACH Cohort

*Corey Casper, MD, MPH; Amalia S. Meier, PhD; Anna Wald, MD, MPH; Rhoda Ashley Morrow, PhD; Lawrence Corey, MD; Anna-Barbara Moscicki, MD*

**Objective:** Human herpesvirus 8 (HHV-8) infection is common among children in areas where Kaposi sarcoma is endemic. Human herpesvirus 8 is uncommon in children but prevalent in adults at risk for human immunodeficiency virus (HIV) infection in the United States, including men who have sex with men (MSM) and women who engage in high-risk sexual behavior. We examined the prevalence and predictors of HHV-8 infection among adolescents with or at high risk for acquiring HIV infection.

**Design:** Cross-sectional analysis.

**Setting:** National study of HIV infection among adolescents in primary care.

**Participants:** A total of 537 young adults practicing high-risk sexual behavior, of which 403 were women and 134 were men; among the 134 men, 75% were MSM.

**Interventions:** Detailed questionnaires and testing for serum antibodies to HHV-8.

**Outcome Measure:** Detection of serum antibodies to HHV-8.

**Results:** Sixty (11.2%) of 537 young adults were HHV-8 seropositive, including 20 MSM (19.6%), 2 male heterosexuals (6.5%), and 27 female heterosexuals (8.2%). The prevalence of HHV-8 in HIV-positive MSM (17/74 [23.0%]) was twice as high as that in HIV-negative MSM (3/28 [10.7%]) ($P=.18$), but no characteristic predicted HHV-8 infection among MSM. In multivariate analysis, history of gonorrhea (odds ratio [OR], 2.8; 95% confidence interval [CI], 1.4-5.7; $P<.01$), history of having sex with women (OR, 2.4; 95% CI, 1.1-5.3; $P=.03$), and African American race (OR, 3.4; 95% CI, 1.1-10.0; $P=.03$) were associated with HHV-8 infection among women.

**Conclusions:** Human herpesvirus 8 is common among US adolescents practicing high-risk sexual behaviors. Sexual identity, race, and sexual behavior may influence the risk of infection with HHV-8 in women.

*Arch Pediatr Adolesc Med. 2006;160:937-942*

Author Affiliations: Departments of Medicine (Drs Casper, Wald, and Corey), Laboratory Medicine (Drs Meier, Morrow, and Corey), and Epidemiology (Dr Wald), University of Washington, Seattle; the Programs in Infectious Diseases (Drs Casper, Wald, and Corey) and Biostatistics (Dr Meier), Fred Hutchinson Cancer Research Center, Seattle; and Department of Pediatrics, University of California, San Francisco (Dr Moscicki).

HUMAN HERPESVIRUS 8 (HHV-8) (also known as Kaposi sarcoma [KS]–associated herpesvirus) was first identified in 1994.[1] In the United States and western Europe, the virus is likely acquired through sexual contact and is largely restricted to men who have sex with men (MSM)[2] and women at high risk for sexually transmitted or parenteral infections.[3] Infection is rare among US children[4] but ranges from 30% to 100% in African children, who typically acquire HHV-8 before the onset of puberty but after the perinatal period.[5-7] In many parts of Africa, KS is a tumor endemic among children with and without human immunodeficiency virus (HIV) infection,[8-10] but most HHV-8 infections worldwide are asymptomatic.

Human herpesvirus 8 is shed frequently in the oropharynx.[11] Contact with saliva during sex is associated with incident HHV-8 infection in adult MSM,[11-14] whereas household contact with saliva may be a mode of HHV-8 transmission in African children.[15] Children contract other HHV infections through contact with saliva, including herpes simplex virus type 1 (HSV-1),[16] cytomegalovirus,[17] and Epstein-Barr virus,[18] which are all ubiquitous worldwide. If some or all HHV-8 transmission is explained by contact with saliva, it remains unclear why HHV-8 infection is not more prevalent in most parts of the developed world.

We hypothesized that HIV-positive adolescents and young adults and those practicing high-risk sexual behavior may be at substantial risk of HHV-8 infection because of homosexual contact and multiple sex partners. We therefore examined the seroprevalence and predictors of HHV-8 infection among such individuals.

## METHODS

### STUDY POPULATION

The REACH (Reaching for Excellence in Adolescent Care and Health) project recruited adolescents aged 13 to 18 years from 15 clinical sites in 13 US cities to evaluate the biomedical and behavioral characteristics of HIV infection.[19] Eligible adolescents either had acquired HIV sexually or parenterally or were HIV negative but with similar age and risk behaviors. Participants or their guardians provided informed consent, as approved by each site's institutional review board and human experimentation guidelines of the US Department of Health and Human Services. Subjects underwent physical examination, questionnaire collection, and phlebotomy at 3-month intervals for HIV-positive and at 6-month intervals for HIV-negative persons.

### LABORATORY ANALYSIS

A combined whole-virus enzyme immunoassay with immunofluorescence assay detected serum HHV-8 antibodies from the last study visit available.[20] Antigens derived from purified viral lysate (Advanced Biotechnologies Inc, Columbia, Md) are plated on 96-well plates. After application of human serum, bound antibodies are detected by horseradish peroxidase–conjugated goat anti–human IgG Fc (Chemicon, Temecula, Calif) and TMB (3,3′,5,5′-tetramethylbenzidine) substrate (KPL Inc, Gaithersburg, Md). Optical densities are determined in a standard enzyme-linked immunosorbent assay plate reader. Samples with intermediate enzyme immunoassay values are rerun with a standard immunofluorescence assay for antibodies to latent and lytic antigens in body cavity–based B-cell lymphoma 1 cells. This testing strategy was found to be 88% sensitive and 97% specific for the identification of HHV-8 infection.

Laboratory tests for gonorrhea, chlamydia, and syphilis were performed biannually. For HIV-positive participants, the AIDS Clinical Trials Group laboratories determined T-cell lymphocyte counts by flow cytometry, and HIV plasma RNA levels were quantified by nucleic acid sequence-based amplification (Organon Technika, Westchester, Pa).

### STATISTICAL METHODS

For each potential predictor of HHV-8 infection, we selected data from the period closest to the date of HHV-8 antibody assessment, with the exception of some characteristics collected only at baseline.

The analysis was restricted to participants previously identified as having a high HHV-8 prevalence among adults, that is, MSM (defined by self-identification as being homosexual or bisexual or reporting any history of anal receptive sex) and all women (who by inclusion in the cohort were at risk for or had HIV infection). Men reporting exclusively heterosexual partners and behaviors were excluded.

Statistical analysis was performed using SAS for Windows Version 8.2 software (SAS Institute Inc, Cary, NC). Associations with HHV-8 status were evaluated using univariate and multivariate logistic regression. Multivariate model selection proceeded by including all factors univariately associated with HHV-8 at $P<.1$ and eliminating factors until all remaining predictors were significant at $P\leq.05$.

## RESULTS

### DEMOGRAPHIC CHARACTERISTICS OF STUDY PARTICIPANTS

Of the 550 adolescents enrolled in the REACH project, 537 (97.6%) had serum samples available for HHV-8 testing. Participants had a median follow-up time of 33 months (range, 0-57 months) prior to the HHV-8 serologic assessment. Of the 537 participants, 134 (25.0%) were men and 403 (75.0%) were women. Among the 134 men, 102 (76.1%) were classified as MSM.

The median age of participants at the time of HHV-8 serologic assessment was 19 years (range, 18-21 years), with most (71.1%) identifying themselves as African American (**Table 1**). A greater proportion of women study participants were African American when compared with MSM (75.4% of women vs 53.9% of MSM; $P<.001$).

### RISK BEHAVIOR OF STUDY COHORT

Most (82.1%) of the women identified themselves as heterosexual (Table 1), whereas 47.8% of the men identified themselves as homosexual. Men who have sex with men were more likely to report a history of sex with a commercial sex worker (20.6% of MSM vs 7.9% of women [$P<.01$]) but had similar exposure to HIV-positive sex partners (24.5% of MSM vs 19.6% of women [$P=.34$]). Anal sex was common among both MSM and women. At the time of HHV-8 serologic testing, 12.7% of women and 8.8% of MSM had a concurrent diagnosis of chlamydia; 5.2% of women and 3.9% of MSM, of gonorrhea; and 2.2% of women and 3.9% of MSM, of syphilis. Intravenous drug use was uncommon among the study youth, reported by 0.5% of women and 6.9% of MSM.

At the time of enrollment, 64.3% of women and 70.6% of MSM were HIV-positive, and an additional 2 MSM acquired HIV during the study. The median CD4 count was 601 cells/μL (interquartile range, 398-839 cells/μL), and the median HIV plasma RNA level was 3.9 log copies/mL. Only 7 participants reported having an AIDS-defining illness[21] and no participant had KS.

### FREQUENCY AND PREDICTORS OF HHV-8 INFECTION

Overall, 60 (11.2%) of 537 participants were HHV-8 seropositive, including 20 (19.6%) of 102 MSM, 2 (6.5%) of 31 heterosexual men (data not shown), and 38 (9.4%) of 403 women ($\chi^2$ test, $P<.01$). The **Figure** depicts the prevalence of HHV-8 infection by demographic group and HIV status (26 [10.0%] of 259 HIV-positive women vs 12 [8.3%] of 144 HIV-negative women; odds ratio [OR], 1.2; 95% confidence interval [CI], 0.6-2.5; $P=.58$; 1 [7.1%] of 14 vs 1 [5.9%] of 17 heterosexual males; OR, 1.2; 95% CI, 0.1-23.8; $P=.89$; 17 [23.0%] of 74 vs 3 [10.7%] of 28 MSM; OR, 2.5; 95% CI, 0.7-9.4; $P=.18$). There was no significant difference in the prevalence of HHV-8 infection among HIV-negative women and HIV-negative MSM (8.3% vs 10.7%, $P=.68$). In a univariate analysis, only 3 factors were significantly associated with an increased risk of HHV-8 infection among women, including a history of gonorrhea (OR, 2.8; 95% CI, 1.4-5.7; $P=.002$) and sex with other women (WSW) (OR, 2.4; 95% CI, 1.1-5.3; $P=.03$) (**Table 2**). In a multivariate model restricted to female participants, these factors remained significantly associated with an elevated risk of HHV-8 infection. No factors were significantly associated with HHV-8 infection among MSM.

In subset analyses of 331 HIV-positive subjects separated by sex, neither HIV RNA level (modeled continuously, OR, 1.4; 95% CI, 0.9-2.1; $P=.12$ among women,

**Table 1. Demographic and Risk Behaviors Among the Study Cohort***

| | Women | | MSM | | |
|---|---|---|---|---|---|
| | HHV-8 Negative (n = 365) | HHV-8 Positive (n = 38) | HHV-8 Negative (n = 82) | HHV-8 Positive (n = 20) | Total (N = 505) |
| Median age at visit (IQR), y | 19 (18-21) | 19 (18-20) | 20 (19-21) | 20 (19-21) | 19 (18-21) |
| Race | | | | | |
| African American | 270 (73.9)† | 34 (89.5)† | 43 (52.4) | 12 (60.0) | **359** (71.1) |
| Native American/Alaskan native | 1 (0.3) | 0 | 1 (1.2) | 1 (5.0) | **3** (0.6) |
| White | 27 (7.4) | 0 | 10 (12.2) | 4 (20.0) | **41** (8.1) |
| Other or mixed race | 67 (18.4) | 4 (10.5) | 28 (34.1) | 3 (15.0) | **102** (20.2) |
| Completed high school | 220 (60.3) | 22 (57.9) | 59 (72.0) | 14 (70.0) | **315** (62.4) |
| Place of residence | | | | | |
| Independent living | 137 (37.5) | 16 (42.1) | 42 (51.2) | 10 (50.0) | **205** (40.6) |
| Family | 198 (54.2) | 20 (52.6) | 36 (43.9) | 8 (40.0) | **262** (51.9) |
| Institution | 22 (6.0) | 1 (2.6) | 3 (3.7) | 2 (10.0) | **28** (5.5) |
| Homeless | 1 (0.3) | 0 | 0 | 0 | **1** (0.2) |
| Other place | 7 (1.9) | 1 (2.6) | 1 (1.2) | 0 | **9** (1.8) |
| Sexual preference | | | | | |
| Heterosexual | 304 (83.3)‡ | 27 (71.1)‡ | 13 (15.9) | 3 (15.0) | **347** (68.7) |
| Bisexual | 37 (10.1)‡ | 6 (15.8)‡ | 17 (20.7) | 3 (15.0) | **63** (12.5) |
| Homosexual | 10 (2.7)‡ | 2 (5.3)‡ | 51 (62.2) | 13 (65.0) | **76** (15.0) |
| Not sure | 13 (3.6) | 3 (7.9) | 1 (1.2) | 1 (5.0) | **18** (3.6) |
| Median age at first sex (IQR), y | 14 (13-15) | 14 (13-15) | 13 (12-15) | 14 (12-16) | 14 (13-15) |
| Ever received anal sex | 86 (23.6) | 9 (23.7) | 62 (75.6) | 17 (85.0) | **174** (34.5) |
| Ever performed anal sex | NA | NA | 57 (69.5) | 17 (85.0) | **74** (14.7) |
| Median total No. of lifetime partners (IQR) | 9 (4-18) | 11 (4-17) | 20 (12-42) | 28 (9-35) | 11 (5-21) |
| Sex with CSW | 31 (8.5) | 1 (2.6) | 16 (19.5) | 5 (25.0) | **53** (10.5) |
| History of HIV-positive partners | 75 (20.5) | 4 (10.5) | 20 (24.4) | 5 (25.0) | **104** (20.6) |
| History of IVDU partner | 19 (5.2) | 0 | 8 (9.8) | 3 (15.0) | **30** (5.9) |
| Positive syphilis test results§ | 7 (1.9) | 2 (5.3) | 4 (4.9) | 0 | **13** (2.6) |
| Chlamydia infection§ | 151 (41.4) | 16 (42.1) | 28 (34.1) | 7 (35.0) | **202** (40.0) |
| Gonorrhea infection§ | 67 (18.4)‖ | 16 (42.1)‖ | 20 (24.4) | 7 (35.0) | **110** (21.8) |
| Established HIV infection | 233 (63.8) | 26 (68.4) | 57 (69.5) | 15 (75.0) | **331** (65.5) |
| Incident HIV infection | 0/132 | 0/12 | 0/25 | 2/5 (40.0) | **2/174** (1.1) |
| History of IV drug use | 2 (0.5) | 0 | 7 (8.5) | 0 | **9** (1.8) |

Abbreviations: CSW, commercial sex worker; HHV-8, human herpesvirus 8; HIV, human immunodeficiency virus; IQR, interquartile range; IV, intravenous; IVDU, IV drug user; MSM, men who have sex with men; NA, not applicable.

*Data are presented as number (percentage) unless otherwise indicated. All $P > .1$ for HHV-8–positive vs HHV-8–negative participants except as noted.

†$P = .04$.

‡$P = .06$ for homosexual or bisexual vs heterosexual women.

§Since study enrollment.

‖$P = .001$.

and OR, 0.8; 95% CI, 0.4-1.4; $P = .40$ among MSM) nor highly active antiretroviral treatment (HAART) use (OR, 0.5; 95% CI, 0.1-1.2; $P = .15$ among women, and OR, 1.5; 95% CI, 0.5-4.8; $P = .46$ among MSM) was associated with HHV-8 infection.

## COMMENT

A decade after the initial identification of HHV-8, many questions still remain about its epidemiology.[22] The restriction of HHV-8 infection to specific geographic and demographic "pockets" is perplexing given the evidence for the transmission of HHV-8 through saliva and the comparative ubiquity of other HHVs.[12] We found antibodies to HHV-8 in 11.2% of adolescents with HIV infection and/or high-risk sexual and substance use behavior. Our results provide several important insights into the epidemiology of HHV-8 in adolescents.

In the United States and western Europe, 2% to 10% of the general population have serum antibodies to HHV-8,[23] but little is known about the timing of HHV-8 acquisition. One previous study[24] found a low rate of infection among MSM aged 16 to 22 years in the United States, which was comparable to the rate in a matched population of young heterosexual males and females.

We found the highest rates of HHV-8 infection in HIV-positive adolescent MSM, but this rate is lower than the 30% to 75% prevalence previously observed in populations of adult HIV-positive MSM.[14,25] In a cross-sectional study, the relationship between the timing of HHV-8 and HIV infection could not be assessed. The lower prevalence of HHV-8 in HIV-positive adolescent MSM compared with adult MSM suggests that they acquire HIV prior to HHV-8. This may be clinically relevant because the incidence of KS appears to be higher among MSM who acquire HHV-8 after HIV infection compared with those first infected with HHV-8.[26]

The rarity of KS among women in the pre-HAART era led many to speculate that HHV-8 infection was uncommon among women.[27] Recent data, however, suggest rates that are 2 to 4 times higher than the rate among the general population of the United States and similar to that among HIV-negative MSM.[3,28,29] We identified 2 novel risk factors for HHV-8 infection among young women.

We found a high HHV-8 prevalence among WSW but did not specifically ask about their behaviors. Previous studies offer potential explanations for the higher prevalence in this group. First, WSW in this study infrequently reported exclusively female sex partners, and WSW are more likely to have sex with bisexual males.[30-32] Second, some WSW practice riskier sexual behavior, including concurrent substance abuse with sex.[32] Third, exposure of the oral cavity to genital or oral secretions during sex is nearly universal among WSW[33] and the use of protective barriers is uncommon.[34] Human herpesvirus 8 infects epithelial cells, which may be the site of primary infection.[11,35] Limited studies in women find HHV-8 in oral and genital secretions.[36-39] Whether HHV-8 shed in saliva is transmissible through other mucosal sites, such as the genital epithelium, has yet to be determined. Taken together, it is possible that sexual mixing between WSW and other demographic groups with high HHV-8 prevalence may allow transmission to female partners during oro-oral or orogenital sex.

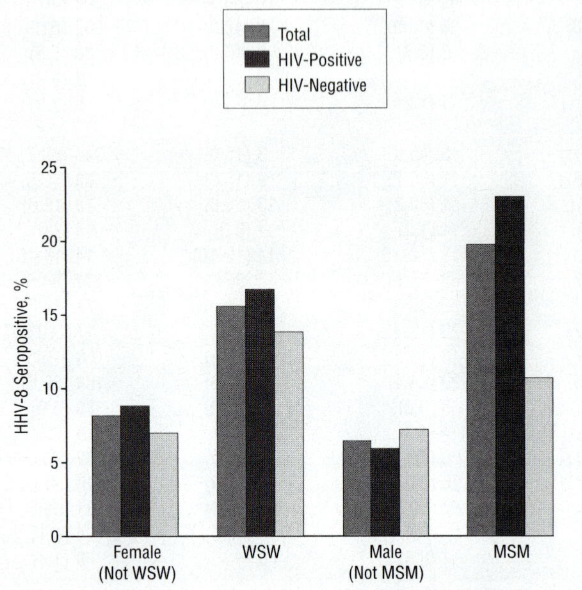


**Figure.** Seroprevalence of human herpesvirus 8 (HHV-8) among high-risk adolescents, stratified by risk group and human immunodeficiency virus (HIV) status. MSM indicates men who have sex with men; WSW, women who have sex with women.

The association between HHV-8 and gonorrhea has been reported in both men[40,41] and women,[42] but the small number of participants in our study infected with both HHV-8 and gonorrhea precluded a comprehensive analysis. Sexual networks could also help explain the relationship between HHV-8 prevalence and gonorrhea in women because previous studies[43] have found that persons infected with *Neisseria gonorrhoeae* have larger, more demographically discordant sexual networks.

Our observed association between African American race and HHV-8 infection has been corroborated by 2 other cohorts of adult women[3,28] and, to our knowledge, has not been described in men.[44] Studies of sexual networks among African American adolescents show that most report their typical sex partner to be older and sex with these partners to be often unprotected.[45] This "disassortive mixing" by age increases the risk of sexually transmitted infections in adolescents[46] and of HSV-2 infection in adults.[47]

The findings of this study must be taken in the context of the included study population. Specifically, the relatively small number of MSM limits the ability to detect predictors of HHV-8 infection among this group. Conversely, the overrepresentation of female or African American youths may have allowed us to identify previously uncharacterized risks for HHV-8 in these groups. Fi-

**Table 2. Risk Factors for HHV-8 Seropositivity Among High-Risk Adolescents**

| | OR (95% CI) | | |
|---|---|---|---|
| | Women | | MSM |
| Covariate | Univariate | Multivariate* | Univariate |
| Demographic characteristics | | | |
| African American vs all others | 3.0 (1.0-8.7)† | 3.4 (1.1-10.0)† | 1.4 (0.5-3.7) |
| Homosexual or bisexual vs heterosexual | 2.1 (1.0-4.4)† | 2.4 (1.1-5.3)† | NA |
| Risk behavior | | | |
| Age at first sexual experience | 1.1 (0.9-1.4) | . . . | 1.1 (0.8-1.4) |
| No. of lifetime partners ≥10 | 1.2 (0.6-2.3) | . . . | 0.5 (0.1-1.6) |
| Ever performed anal sex | NA | NA | 2.5 (0.7-9.4) |
| Ever received anal sex | 1 (0.5-2.3) | . . . | 1.8 (0.5-7.0) |
| Sexually transmitted infection | | | |
| Gonorrhea | 3.2 (1.6-6.4)† | 2.8 (1.4-5.7)† | 1.4 (0.1-14.0) |
| Chlamydia | 1 (0.5-2.0) | . . . | 1 (0.4-2.8) |
| HIV | 1.2 (0.6-2.5) | . . . | 2.5 (0.7-9.4) |
| HSV-2 IgG positive | 1.3 (0.7-2.6) | . . . | 1.8 (0.6-5.2) |
| CMV IgG positive | 3.1 (0.7-13.3) | . . . | 3.6 (0.4-29.7) |

Abbreviations: CI, confidence interval; CMV, cytomegalovirus; HHV-8, human herpesvirus 8; HIV, human immunodeficiency virus; HSV-2, herpes simplex virus 2; MSM, men who have sex with men; NA, not applicable; OR, odds ratio; ellipses, not included in the model.
*Adjusted for race, positive test results for gonorrhea, and sexual identity.
†$P<.05$.

nally, the lack of information on behaviors specifically associated with the exchange of saliva is a limitation of previous studies and our current investigation.

In sum, we found HHV-8 infection to be common among US adolescents practicing high-risk sexual behavior and identified novel risk factors for HHV-8 infection in females. The incidence of KS in the United States and western Europe has declined dramatically in the HAART era,[48] with little change in the prevalence of HHV-8 infection.[49] The long-term sequelae of infection with HHV-8, a known oncogenic virus, are still undetermined, and specific therapy for HHV-8 infection is lacking. Consequently, prevention of HHV-8 infection remains important, and future studies should examine the mode of HHV-8 transmission and acquisition.

**Accepted for Publication:** April 27, 2006.
**Correspondence:** Corey Casper, MD, MPH, Program in Infectious Diseases, Fred Hutchinson Cancer Research Center, 1100 Fairview Ave N, Mail Stop D3-100, Seattle, WA 98109 (ccasper@u.washington.edu).
**Author Contributions:** *Study concept and design:* Casper, Wald, Corey, and Moscicki. *Acquisition of data:* Morrow and Moscicki. *Analysis and interpretation of data:* Casper, Meier, Wald, Corey, and Moscicki. *Drafting of the manuscript:* Casper, Meier, and Moscicki. *Critical revision of the manuscript for important intellectual content*: Meier, Wald, Morrow, Corey, and Moscicki. *Statistical analysis:* Casper and Meier. *Obtained funding:* Corey and Moscicki. *Administrative, technical, and material support:* Casper, Morrow, Corey, and Moscicki. *Study supervision:* Wald, Morrow, and Corey.
**Funding/Support:** This study was supported in part by National Institutes of Health (NIH) grant U01-HD32830 from the National Institute of Child Health and Human Development with cofunding from the National Institutes on Drug Abuse, of Allergy and Infectious Diseases, and of Mental Health; NIH grants K23 AI54162 and U19 AI31448 from the National Institute of Allergy and Infectious Diseases; and a Clinical Scientist Development Award from the Doris Duke Charitable Foundation.
**Acknowledgment:** We thank the investigators and staff of the Adolescent Medicine HIV/AIDS Research Network (1994-2001) (listed in the *Journal of Adolescent Health* [2001;29(suppl):5-60]), and the adolescents and young adults who participated in the REACH project, for their valuable contributions.

## REFERENCES


1. Chang Y, Cesarman E, Pessin MS, et al. Identification of herpesvirus-like DNA sequences in AIDS-associated Kaposi's sarcoma. *Science.* 1994;266:1865-1869.
2. Martin JN, Ganem DE, Osmond DH, Page-Shafer KA, Macrae D, Kedes DH. Sexual transmission and the natural history of human herpesvirus 8 infection. *N Engl J Med.* 1998;338:948-954.
3. Cannon MJ, Dollard SC, Smith DK, et al; HIV Epidemiology Research Study Group. Blood-borne and sexual transmission of human herpesvirus 8 in women with or at risk for human immunodeficiency virus infection. *N Engl J Med.* 2001;344:637-643.
4. Martro E, Bulterys M, Stewart JA, et al. Comparison of human herpesvirus 8 and Epstein-Barr virus seropositivity among children in areas endemic and non-endemic for Kaposi's sarcoma. *J Med Virol.* 2004;72:126-131.
5. Mayama S, Cuevas LE, Sheldon J, et al. Prevalence and transmission of Kaposi's sarcoma–associated herpesvirus (human herpesvirus 8) in Ugandan children and adolescents. *Int J Cancer.* 1998;77:817-820.
6. Gessain A, Mauclere P, van Beveren M, et al. Human herpesvirus 8 primary infection occurs during childhood in Cameroon, Central Africa. *Int J Cancer.* 1999;81:189-192.
7. Brayfield BP, Phiri S, Kankasa C, et al. Postnatal human herpesvirus 8 and human immunodeficiency virus type 1 infection in mothers and infants from Zambia. *J Infect Dis.* 2003;187:559-568.
8. Taylor JF, Templeton AC, Vogel CL, Ziegler JL, Kyalwazi SK. Kaposi's sarcoma in Uganda: a clinico-pathological study. *Int J Cancer.* 1971;8:122-135.
9. Burkitt D, O'Conor GT. Malignant lymphoma in African children, I: a clinical syndrome. *Cancer.* 1961;14:258-269.
10. Wabinga HR, Parkin DM, Wabwire-Mangen F, Nambooze S. Trends in cancer incidence in Kyadondo County, Uganda, 1960-1997. *Br J Cancer.* 2000;82:1585-1592.
11. Pauk J, Huang ML, Brodie SJ, et al. Mucosal shedding of human herpesvirus 8 in men. *N Engl J Med.* 2000;343:1369-1377.
12. Corey L, Brodie S, Huang ML, Koelle DM, Wald A. HHV-8 infection: a model for reactivation and transmission. *Rev Med Virol.* 2002;12:47-63.
13. Casper C, Wald A, Pauk J, Tabet SR, Corey L, Celum CL. Correlates of prevalent and incident Kaposi's sarcoma–associated herpesvirus infection in men who have sex with men. *J Infect Dis.* 2002;185:990-993.
14. Casper C, Redman M, Huang ML, et al. HIV infection and human herpesvirus-8 oral shedding among men who have sex with men. *J Acquir Immune Defic Syndr.* 2004;35:233-238.
15. Plancoulaine S, Abel L, van Beveren M, et al. Human herpesvirus 8 transmission from mother to child and between siblings in an endemic population. *Lancet.* 2000;356:1062-1065.
16. Stanberry L, Rosenthal S. The epidemiology of herpes simplex virus infections in adolescents. *Herpes.* 1999;6:12-15.
17. Adler SP. Molecular epidemiology of cytomegalovirus: viral transmission among children attending a day care center, their parents, and caretakers. *J Pediatr.* 1988;112:366-372.
18. Fleisher GR, Pasquariello PS, Warren WS, et al. Intrafamilial transmission of Epstein-Barr virus infections. *J Pediatr.* 1981;98:16-19.
19. Wilson CM, Houser J, Partlow C, Rudy BJ, Futterman DC, Friedman LB. The REACH (Reaching for Excellence in Adolescent Care and Health) project: study design, methods, and population profile. *J Adolesc Health.* 2001;29(3)(suppl):8-18.
20. Casper C, Krantz E, Taylor H, et al. Assessment of a combined testing strategy for detection of antibodies to human herpesvirus 8 (HHV-8) in persons with Kaposi's sarcoma, persons with asymptomatic HHV-8 Infection, and persons at low risk for HHV-8 infection. *J Clin Microbiol.* 2002;40:3822-3825.
21. 1993 Revised classification system for HIV infection and expanded surveillance case definition for AIDS among adolescents and adults. *MMWR Recomm Rep.* 1992;41(RR-17):1-19.
22. Dukers NH, Rezza G. Human herpesvirus 8 epidemiology: what we do and do not know. *AIDS.* 2003;17:1717-1730.
23. Chatlynne LG, Ablashi DV. Seroepidemiology of Kaposi's sarcoma–associated herpesvirus (KSHV). *Semin Cancer Biol.* 1999;9:175-185.
24. Diamond C, Thiede H, Perdue T, MacKellar D, Valleroy LA, Corey L. Seroepidemiology of human herpesvirus 8 among young men who have sex with men. *Sex Transm Dis.* 2001;28:176-183.
25. Schulz TF. Epidemiology of Kaposi's sarcoma–associated herpesvirus/human herpesvirus 8. *Adv Cancer Res.* 1999;76:121-160.
26. Renwick N, Halaby T, Weverling GJ, et al. Seroconversion for human herpesvirus 8 during HIV infection is highly predictive of Kaposi's sarcoma. *AIDS.* 1998;12:2481-2488.
27. Kedes DH, Ganem D, Ameli N, Bacchetti P, Greenblatt R. The prevalence of serum antibody to human herpesvirus 8 (Kaposi sarcoma–associated herpesvirus) among HIV-seropositive and high-risk HIV-seronegative women. *JAMA.* 1997;277:478-481.
28. Greenblatt RM, Jacobson LP, Levine AM, et al. Human herpesvirus 8 infection and Kaposi's sarcoma among human immunodeficiency virus-infected and -uninfected women. *J Infect Dis.* 2001;183:1130-1134.
29. de Sanjose S, Marshall V, Sola J, et al. Prevalence of Kaposi's sarcoma–associated herpesvirus infection in sex workers and women from the general population in Spain. *Int J Cancer.* 2002;98:155-158.
30. Scheer S, Peterson I, Page-Shafer K, et al. Sexual and drug use behavior among women who have sex with both women and men: results of a population-based survey. *Am J Public Health.* 2002;92:1110-1112.
31. Bauer GR, Welles SL. Beyond assumptions of negligible risk: sexually transmitted diseases and women who have sex with women. *Am J Public Health.* 2001;91:1282-1286.
32. Koh AS, Gomez CA, Shade S, Rowley E. Sexual risk factors among self-

identified lesbians, bisexual women, and heterosexual women accessing primary care settings. *Sex Transm Dis.* 2005;32:563-569.
33. Marrazzo JM, Koutsky LA, Stine KL, et al. Genital human papillomavirus infection in women who have sex with women. *J Infect Dis.* 1998;178:1604-1609.
34. Kennedy M, Moore J, Schuman P, et al. Sexual behavior of HIV-infected women reporting recent sexual contact with women. *JAMA.* 1998;280:29-30.
35. Duus KM, Lentchitsky V, Wagenaar T, Grose C, Webster-Cyriaque J. Wild-type Kaposi's sarcoma–associated herpesvirus isolated from the oropharynx of immune-competent individuals has tropism for cultured oral epithelial cells. *J Virol.* 2004; 78:4074-4084.
36. Lampinen TM, Kulasingam S, Min J, et al. Detection of Kaposi's sarcoma–associated herpesvirus in oral and genital secretions of Zimbabwean women. *J Infect Dis.* 2000;181:1785-1790.
37. Calabro ML, Fiore JR, Favero A, et al. Detection of human herpesvirus 8 in cervicovaginal secretions and seroprevalence in human immunodeficiency virus type 1–seropositive and –seronegative women. *J Infect Dis.* 1999;179:1534-1537.
38. Monini P, Howard MR, Rimessi P, de Lellis L, Schulz TF, Cassai E. Human herpesvirus DNA in prostate and semen from HIV-negative individuals in Italy [letter]. *AIDS.* 1997;11:1530-1532.
39. Taylor MM, Chohan B, Lavreys L, et al. Shedding of human herpesvirus 8 in oral and genital secretions from HIV-1-seropositive and -seronegative Kenyan women. *J Infect Dis.* 2004;190:484-488.
40. Armenian HK, Hoover DR, Rubb S, et al. Composite risk score for Kaposi's sarcoma based on a case-control and longitudinal study in the Multicenter AIDS Cohort Study (MACS) population. *Am J Epidemiol.* 1993;138:256-265.
41. Jacobson LP, Munoz A, Fox R, et al; Multicenter AIDS Cohort Study Group. Incidence of Kaposi's sarcoma in a cohort of homosexual men infected with the human immunodeficiency virus type 1. *J Acquir Immune Defic Syndr.* 1990; 3(suppl 1):S24-S31.
42. Lavreys L, Chohan B, Ashley R, et al. Human herpesvirus 8: seroprevalence and correlates in prostitutes in Mombasa, Kenya. *J Infect Dis.* 2003;187:359-363.
43. Stoner BP, Whittington WL, Hughes JP, Aral SO, Holmes KK. Comparative epidemiology of heterosexual gonococcal and chlamydial networks: implications for transmission patterns. *Sex Transm Dis.* 2000;27:215-223.
44. Crum NF, Wallace MR, Stephan K, et al. Correlates of human herpesvirus-8 seropositivity among U.S. military members recently infected with human immunodeficiency virus. *Sex Transm Dis.* 2003;30:713-718.
45. Doherty IA, Padian NS, Marlow C, Aral SO. Determinants and consequences of sexual networks as they affect the spread of sexually transmitted infections. *J Infect Dis.* 2005;191(suppl 1):S42-S54.
46. Lee JK, Jennings JM, Ellen JM. Discordant sexual partnering: a study of high-risk adolescents in San Francisco. *Sex Transm Dis.* 2003;30:234-240.
47. Catania JA, Binson D, Stone V. Relationship of sexual mixing across age and ethnic groups to herpes simplex virus-2 among unmarried heterosexual adults with multiple sexual partners. *Health Psychol.* 1996;15:362-370.
48. Eltom MA, Jemal A, Mbulaiteye SM, Devesa SS, Biggar RJ. Trends in Kaposi's sarcoma and non-Hodgkin's lymphoma incidence in the United States from 1973 through 1998. *J Natl Cancer Inst.* 2002;94:1204-1210.
49. Osmond DH, Buchbinder S, Cheng A, et al. Prevalence of Kaposi sarcoma–associated herpesvirus infection in homosexual men at beginning of and during the HIV epidemic. *JAMA.* 2002;287:221-225.

*Announcement*

**Trial Registration Required.** In concert with the International Committee of Medical Journal Editors (ICMJE), *Archives of Pediatrics and Adolescent Medicine* will require, as a condition of consideration for publication, registration of all trials in a public trials registry (such as http://ClinicalTrials.gov). Trials must be registered at or before the onset of patient enrollment. This policy applies to any clinical trial starting enrollment after July 1, 2005. For trials that began enrollment before this date, registration will be required by September 13, 2005, before considering the trial for publication. The trial registration number should be supplied at the time of submission.

For details about this new policy, and for information on how the ICMJE defines a clinical trial, see the editorials by DeAngelis et al in the September 8, 2004 (2004;292:1363-1364) and June 15, 2005 (2005;293: 2927-2929) issues of *JAMA*. Also see the Instructions to Authors on our Web site: www.archpediatrics.com.

**ACIP recommends vaccination of children against hepatitis A*[1]**

# Hepatitis A spreads FAST... especially among children[2,3]

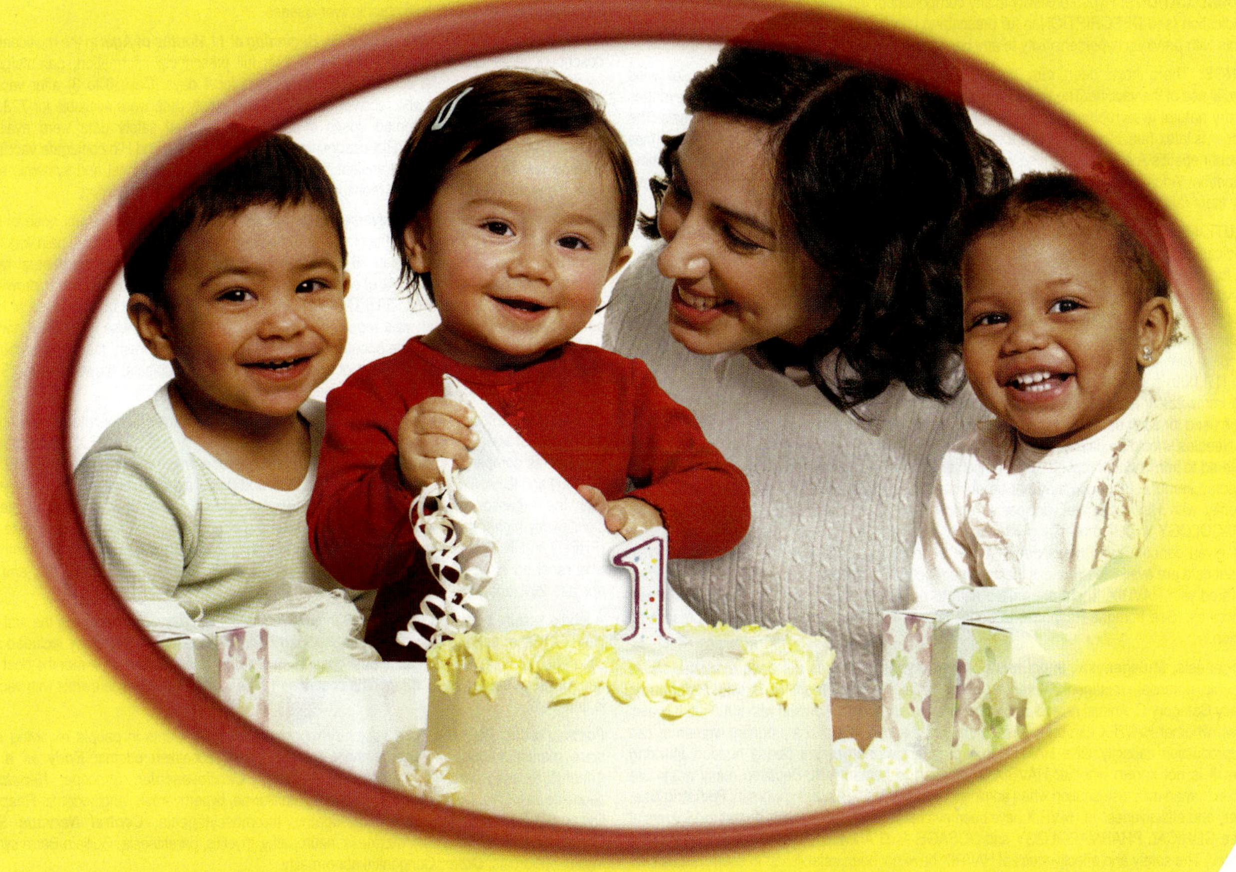

## HAVRIX provides excellent protection

HAVRIX is indicated for active immunization against hepatitis A virus in children 12 months of age and older.

## Important Safety Information

In clinical trials, the most common solicited adverse events were injection-site soreness and headache.

Greater incidences of general adverse events were observed in subjects who received HAVRIX at the same time as Hib conjugate and DTaP vaccines. As with any vaccine, rare adverse events may occur. (See Adverse Reactions section of the Prescribing Information for HAVRIX for potential side effects.) HAVRIX is contraindicated in people with hypersensitivity to any component of the vaccine, including neomycin.

* Advisory Committee on Immunization Practices recommends routine nationwide vaccination against hepatitis A in all children 1–2 years of age.

**Please see references and brief summary of complete prescribing information for HAVRIX on adjacent page.**

HAVRIX is a registered trademark of GlaxoSmithKline.

Manufactured by **GlaxoSmithKline Biologicals**, Rixensart, Belgium
Distributed by **GlaxoSmithKline**, Research Triangle Park, NC 27709

gsk GlaxoSmithKline Vaccines

**Havrix®**
**Hepatitis A Vaccine, Inactivated**

## HAVRIX®
## (Hepatitis A Vaccine, Inactivated)

The following is a brief summary only; see full prescribing information for complete product information.

**INDICATIONS AND USAGE:** HAVRIX is indicated for active immunization of persons ≥12 months of age against disease caused by hepatitis A virus (HAV). Primary immunization should be administered at least 2 weeks prior to expected exposure to HAV. When passive protection against hepatitis A is required either following exposure to hepatitis A virus or in persons requiring both immediate and long-term protection, HAVRIX may be administered concomitantly with immune globulin (IG) with different syringes and at different injection sites. Duration of immunity following a complete vaccination schedule has not been established.

**CONTRAINDICATIONS:** Hypersensitivity to any component of the vaccine, including neomycin, is a contraindication (see DESCRIPTION in full prescribing information). This vaccine is contraindicated in patients with previous hypersensitivity to any hepatitis A-containing vaccine.

**WARNINGS:** There have been rare reports of anaphylaxis/anaphylactoid reactions following commercial use of the vaccine. The tip cap and the rubber plunger of the needleless prefilled syringes contain dry natural latex rubber that may cause allergic reactions in latex sensitive individuals. The vial stopper is latex-free. Hepatitis A has a relatively long incubation period. Hepatitis A vaccine may not prevent hepatitis A infection in those who have an unrecognized hepatitis A infection at the time of vaccination. Additionally, it may not prevent infection in those who do not achieve protective antibody titers (although the lowest titer needed to confer protection has not been determined).

**PRECAUTIONS: General:** Prior to immunization with HAVRIX, the patient's current health status and medical history should be reviewed. The physician should review the patient's immunization history for possible vaccine sensitivity, previous vaccination-related adverse reactions and occurrence of any adverse–event-related symptoms and/or signs, in order to determine the existence of any contraindication to immunization with HAVRIX and to allow an assessment of benefits and risks. Appropriate medical treatment and supervision should be readily available for immediate use in case of a rare anaphylactic reaction following the administration of the vaccine. Epinephrine injection (1:1,000) and other appropriate agents used for the control of immediate allergic reactions must be immediately available. A separate, sterile syringe and needle or a sterile disposable unit should be used for each patient to prevent the transmission of other infectious agents from person to person. Needles should be disposed of properly and should not be recapped. As with any vaccine, if administered to immunosuppressed persons, including those receiving immunosuppressive therapy, the expected immune response may not be obtained. **Drug Interactions:** HAVRIX may be given concurrently with Hib conjugate vaccines in children 15 to 18 months of age (see CLINICAL PHARMACOLOGY in full prescribing information and ADVERSE REACTIONS). The safety of HAVRIX given concomitantly with INFANRIX has been evaluated (see ADVERSE REACTIONS). Insufficient data are available to assess the immune response of a fourth dose of DTaP vaccine when administered with HAVRIX. There are limited data to assess the concomitant use of HAVRIX with other vaccines. (See Immune Response to Concomitantly Administered Vaccines in full prescribing information.)

**Carcinogenesis, Mutagenesis, Impairment of Fertility:** HAVRIX has not been evaluated for its carcinogenic potential, mutagenic potential, or potential for impairment of fertility. **Pregnancy:** Pregnancy Category C. Animal reproduction studies have not been conducted with HAVRIX. It is also not known whether HAVRIX can cause fetal harm when administered to a pregnant woman or can affect reproduction capacity. Give HAVRIX to a pregnant woman only if clearly needed. **Nursing Mothers:** It is not known whether HAVRIX is excreted in human milk. Because many drugs are excreted in human milk, use caution when administering HAVRIX to a nursing woman. **Pediatric Use:** The safety and effectiveness of HAVRIX have been evaluated in 20,436 subjects 1 year to 18 years of age. (See CLINICAL PHARMACOLOGY and DOSAGE AND ADMINISTRATION in full prescribing information.) The safety and effectiveness of HAVRIX have not been established in subjects less than 12 months of age. **Geriatric Use:** Clinical studies of HAVRIX did not include sufficient numbers of subjects 65 years of age and older to determine whether they respond differently from younger subjects. Other reported clinical experience has not identified differences in overall safety between these subjects and younger adult subjects.

**ADVERSE REACTIONS:** As with all pharmaceuticals, however, it is possible that expanded commercial use of the vaccine could reveal rare adverse events. The adverse events most frequently reported by volunteers in clinical trials were injection-site soreness (56% of adults; 21% of children); headache (14% of adults; less than 9% of children). Other solicited and unsolicited events are listed below:

**Incidence 1% to 10% of Injections:** ***Local Reactions at Injection Site:*** Induration, redness, swelling; ***Body as a Whole:*** Fatigue, fever (>37.5°C), malaise; ***Gastrointestinal:*** Anorexia, nausea.

**Incidence <1% of Injections:** ***Local Reaction at Injection Site:*** Hematoma; ***Dermatologic:*** Pruritus, rash, urticaria; ***Respiratory:*** Pharyngitis, other upper respiratory tract infections; ***Gastrointestinal:*** Abdominal pain, diarrhea, dysgeusia, vomiting; ***Musculoskeletal:*** Arthralgia, elevation of creatine phosphokinase, myalgia; ***Hematologic:*** Lymphadenopathy; ***Central Nervous System:*** Hypertonic episode, insomnia, photophobia, vertigo.

**Additional safety data:** Safety data were obtained from 2 additional sources in which large populations were vaccinated. In an outbreak setting in which 4,930 individuals were immunized with a single dose of either 720 EL.U. or 1440 EL.U. of HAVRIX, the vaccine was well tolerated and no serious adverse events due to vaccination were reported. Overall, less than 10% of vaccinees reported solicited general adverse events following the vaccine. The most common solicited local adverse event was pain at the injection site, reported in 22.3% of subjects at 24 hours and decreasing to 2.4% by 72 hours.

In a field efficacy trial, 19,037 children received the 360 EL.U. dose of HAVRIX. The most commonly reported adverse events were injection-site pain (9.5%) and tenderness (8.1%), reported following first doses of HAVRIX. Other adverse events were infrequent and comparable to the control vaccine ENGERIX-B® [Hepatitis B Vaccine (Recombinant)].

In subjects with chronic liver disease, HAVRIX was safe and well tolerated. Local injection site reactions were similar among all 4 groups, and no serious adverse reactions attributed to the vaccine were reported in subjects with chronic liver disease.

***Safety Data for HAVRIX 720 EL.U./0.5 mL Beginning at 11 Months of Age:*** In the multicenter study described under CLINICAL PHARMACOLOGY in full prescribing information, parents/guardians recorded local and general symptoms on diary cards for 4 days (Days 0 to 3) after vaccination. In the 3 groups of children who received HAVRIX alone, safety data were available for 723 children who received 1,396 documented doses of HAVRIX. Additional safety data were available for 181 children who received HAVRIX coadministered with INFANRIX and Hib conjugate vaccine. Most adverse events were mild and transient. The frequencies of solicited local and systemic reactions following receipt of HAVRIX were monitored during the 4-day observation period.

The following rates of solicited adverse events in children who received their first dose of HAVRIX alone at between 11 and 25 months of age were observed. Among local reactions: pain was reported in 15-21% of subjects, redness in 16-21%, swelling in 8% of subjects. Among general reactions, irritability was reported in 24-36% of subjects, loss of appetite in 16-19% of subjects, drowsiness in 15-17% of subjects and fever >39.5°C in ≤2% of subjects. Following the booster dose of HAVRIX, among local reactions: pain was reported in 16-21% of subjects, redness in 17-22%, swelling in 8-10% of subjects. Following the booster dose of HAVRIX, among general reactions, irritability was reported in 19-29% of subjects, loss of appetite in 14-18% of subjects, drowsiness in 13-16% of subjects and fever >39.5°C in ≤1% of subjects.

Drowsiness and loss of appetite occurred at statistically significantly higher rates in subjects 15 to 18 months of age who received Hib conjugate vaccine (PRP-T) and INFANRIX concomitantly with HAVRIX as compared to subjects 15 to 18 months of age who received Hib conjugate vaccine (PRP-T) and INFANRIX (drowsiness 34% and 22% and loss of appetite 29% and 19%, respectively). With the exception of fever (>39.5°C), the solicited general symptoms occurred at statistically significantly higher rates in subjects 15 to 18 months of age who received Hib conjugate vaccine (PRP-T) and INFANRIX concomitantly with HAVRIX as compared to subjects 15 to 18 months of age who received HAVRIX alone (irritability 46% and 30%, drowsiness 34% and 17%, and loss of appetite 29% and 17%, respectively).

A febrile seizure was reported in an 18-month old subject two days after receiving the first dose of HAVRIX. Other serious adverse events reported during the course of this study included a single case each of hepatitis ~5 months post dose 1, insulin-dependent diabetes ~4 months post dose 1, and Kawasaki's disease ~3 1/2 months post dose 1. The association of these events with vaccination is unknown.

**Postmarketing Reports:** Rare voluntary reports of adverse events in people receiving HAVRIX since market introduction include the following: ***Local:*** Localized edema; ***Body as a Whole:*** Anaphylaxis/anaphylactoid reactions, somnolence; ***Cardiovascular:*** Syncope; ***Hepatobiliary:*** Jaundice, hepatitis; ***Dermatologic:*** Erythema multiforme, hyperhydrosis, angioedema; ***Respiratory:*** Dyspnea; ***Hematologic:*** Lymphadenopathy, thrombocytopenia; ***Central Nervous System:*** Convulsions, encephalopathy, dizziness, neuropathy, myelitis, paresthesia, Guillain-Barré syndrome, multiple sclerosis; ***Other:*** Congenital abnormality.

The US Department of Health and Human Services has established the Vaccine Adverse Events Reporting System (VAERS) to accept reports of suspected adverse events after the administration of any vaccine, including, but not limited to, the reporting of events required by the National Childhood Vaccine Injury Act of 1986. The toll-free number for VAERS forms and information is 1-800-822-7967. Reporting forms may also be obtained at the VAERS website at www.vaers.org.

Manufactured by **GlaxoSmithKline Biologicals**, Rixensart, Belgium

Distributed by **GlaxoSmithKline**, Research Triangle Park, NC 27709



BRS-HA:L20

**References: 1.** Centers for Disease Control and Prevention. Recommended childhood and adolescent immunization schedule—United States, 2006. *MMWR.* 2006;54(51&52):Q1–Q4. **2.** Bell BP, Shapiro CN. Hepatitis A virus. In: Long SS, Pickering LK, Prober CG, eds. *Principles and Practice of Pediatric Infectious Diseases.* 2nd ed. Philadelphia, Pa: Churchill Livingstone; 2003:1188–1192. **3.** Armstrong GL, Bell BP. Hepatitis A virus infection in the United States: model-based estimates and implication for childhood immunizations. *Pediatrics.* 2002;109:839–845.

 Printed in USA. HAP283R0 February 2006

# Ruling Out the Need for Antibiotics

## *Are We Sending the Right Message?*

*Rita Mangione-Smith, MD, MPH; Marc N. Elliott, PhD; Tanya Stivers, PhD; Laurie L. McDonald, MS; John Heritage, PhD*

**Objectives:** To examine the relationships among physician-parent communication practices, physicians' perceptions of parental expectations for antibiotic treatment, and inappropriate antibiotic prescribing for viral upper respiratory tract infections.

**Design:** Cross-sectional study of pediatric encounters motivated by cold symptoms between October 1, 2000, and June 30, 2001. Each encounter was videotaped. Physicians completed a postvisit survey that measured whether they perceived the parent as expecting antibiotics. Coded communication variables were merged with survey variables. Multivariate analyses identified key predictors of parent-physician communication practices, physician perceptions of parents' expectations for antibiotics, and inappropriate antibiotic prescribing for viral conditions.

**Setting:** Twenty-seven pediatric practices in Los Angeles, Calif.

**Participants:** Thirty-eight pediatricians and 522 consecutively approached parents of children with cold symptoms.

**Main Outcome Measures:** Physicians' perceptions of parental expectations for antibiotics, inappropriate antibiotic prescribing, and parental questioning of nonantibiotic treatments.

**Results:** Physicians were 20.2% more likely to perceive parents as expecting antibiotics when they questioned the physician's treatment plan ($P = .004$; 95% confidence interval, 6.3%-34.0%). When physicians perceived parents as expecting antibiotics, they were 31.7% more likely to inappropriately prescribe them ($P < .001$; 95% confidence interval, 16.0%-47.3%). Parents were 24.0% more likely to question the treatment plan when the physician ruled out the need for antibiotics ($P = .004$; 95% confidence interval, 7.7%-40.3%).

**Conclusions:** Parental questioning of the treatment plan increases physicians' perceptions that antibiotics are expected and thus increases inappropriate antibiotic prescribing. Treatment plans that focus on what can be done to make a child feel better, rather than on what is not needed, ie, antibiotics, may decrease inappropriate antibiotic prescribing.

*Arch Pediatr Adolesc Med. 2006;160:945-952*

Author Affiliations: Departments of Pediatrics (Dr Mangione-Smith) and Sociology (Dr Heritage), University of California–Los Angeles; RAND Corporation, Santa Monica, Calif (Dr Elliott and Ms McDonald); and Max Planck Institute for Psycholinguistics, Nijmegen, the Netherlands (Dr Stivers). Dr Mangione-Smith is now with the Department of Pediatrics, University of Washington, Seattle.

INAPPROPRIATE ANTIBIOTIC PREscribing for viral upper respiratory tract infections (URIs) is common.[1-7] Nearly one third of patients diagnosed as having the common cold receive an antibiotic prescription, and prescribing for bronchitis and other viral illnesses is estimated to be as high as 60%.[2] Based on the prevalence of bacterial infections, 55% of antibiotic prescriptions for acute respiratory illnesses in 1998 were in excess of expected prescribing rates.[2] Although a number of recent studies indicate that antibiotic prescribing may have peaked in the early 1990s,[6,8-10] evidence suggests that declining prescribing rates are primarily driven by decreased rates of office visits for respiratory tract infections.[6] For patients presenting with URIs, physicians' rates of prescribing show a relatively modest and uneven decrease,[6] together with increased reliance on broad-spectrum agents.[10,11] The inappropriate use of antibiotics has led to increased resistance among many strains of bacteria that commonly infect children and adults,[12-19] posing risks to the individual and the community.[18,20-24]

Upper respiratory tract infections are the most common reason that parents seek medical care for their children.[25] Results from the National Ambulatory Medical Care Survey show that acute respiratory conditions account for approximately 75% of children's antibiotic prescriptions.[6] Although 50% to 70% of parents report a previsit expectation that their child will be given antibiotics,[5,26] 65% to 70% of these infections are viral and thus cannot effectively be so treated.[27-32]

Previous research has shown associations between patient-parent reports of an expectation for antibiotics and physician prescribing,[33-39] but physician perceptions of parental expectations have been demonstrated to be a stronger predictor of actual prescribing behavior.[5,26,33-35] Similarly, although physicians commonly cite parent pressure as a reason for prescribing,[40-44] recordings of actual encounters between parents and physicians show that explicit demands or requests for antibiotics are relatively infrequent.[45,46] Nevertheless, previous research[47] has identified a number of indirect parental communication behaviors that are associated with physician perceptions of parental expectations, although that research was limited by a small physician sample and a homogeneous parent sample.

This study has the following 2 main objectives: (1) to test the relationships between previously identified parental communication practices[47] and physician perceptions of parental expectations for antibiotics using a larger and more heterogeneous sample of physicians and parents and (2) to investigate the relationship between new qualitatively identified physician communication practices[48-50] and parental questioning of nonantibiotic treatments for URI.

## METHODS

### STUDY DESIGN

We conducted a nested cross-sectional study of 522 pediatric encounters clustered among 38 pediatricians (approximately 15 encounters per physician) in 27 community pediatric practices in Los Angeles County, California. Details regarding recruitment of the physician and parent samples have been reported elsewhere.[5] For parents to be eligible, children had to present with respiratory tract infection symptoms (cough, nasal congestion, ear pain, or throat pain). The child had to be between the ages of 6 months and 10 years and to not have taken antibiotics during the preceding 2 weeks. The parent had to be able to speak and read English, and the visit had to occur between October 1, 2000, and June 30, 2001.

As previously reported, 38 of the 59 invited eligible pediatricians agreed to participate (64.4% participation rate), 1 to 4 from each of the 27 practices.[5] Of the 678 parents invited to participate, 570 agreed (84.1%). Twenty-seven participating parents were later determined to be ineligible because their children did not have an eligible diagnosis (eg, earwax impaction or gastroenteritis), yielding a sample of 543 participating parents of 651 invited eligible parents (eligible participation rate, 83.4%). Twenty-one encounters were not conducted in English, thus yielding a sample of 522 complete encounters for the present communication analysis.

All physician and parent participants gave written informed consent. All study procedures were reviewed and approved by the general campus institutional review board of the University of California–Los Angeles.

### DATA COLLECTION PROCEDURES

Before the visit, parents completed a self-administered questionnaire. Each pediatric visit was then videotaped. After the visit, physicians completed a self-administered questionnaire. A detailed list of survey variables collected can be found in our previous report.[5] For the purposes of the present study, the following diagnoses were coded as viral: bronchitis, bronchiolitis, croup, viral pharyngitis, viral pneumonia, viral stomatitis, and viral URI. Oral and injectable antibacterial drugs were considered antibiotics for analysis purposes. Inappropriate antibiotic prescribing was defined as the prescription of antibiotics for a viral respiratory diagnosis.

Parental expectations for antibiotic treatment were assessed by responses to the following question, "How necessary do you think it is for the physician to prescribe an antibiotic for your child?" This item was scored on a 5-point scale (response options: definitely necessary, probably necessary, uncertain, probably unnecessary, and definitely unnecessary). Responses were dichotomized such that the first 2 ratings were labeled "antibiotics expected," whereas the other ratings were labeled "antibiotics not expected."

Physician perceptions of parental expectations for antibiotics were measured by physicians' responses to the statement, "At the beginning of this visit, this parent expected me to prescribe an antibiotic." This item was scored on a 5-point Likert scale (response options: strongly agree, somewhat agree, uncertain, somewhat disagree, and strongly disagree). Responses were dichotomized such that the first 2 ratings were labeled "physician perceives a parental expectation for antibiotics," whereas the other ratings were labeled "physician perceives no parental expectation for antibiotics."

### COMMUNICATION CONDUCT

The qualitative method of conversation analysis was used to analyze the videotaped data.[51-53] Both of the conversation analysts (T.S. and J.H.) were initially blinded as to whether antibiotics were prescribed for a given encounter. Through conversation analysis, we identified 3 relevant communication practices that constituted our interaction analysis coding scheme. Two trained research assistants each coded approximately half of the 522 videotaped encounters, and one of us (R.M.-S.) coded a 15% random sample of the encounters to test interrater reliability of the coding scheme, as measured by the κ statistic. The communication behaviors we focused on emerge in the problem presentation and counseling phases of the visit. We examined whether (1) the parent offered a candidate bacterial diagnosis during the presentation of the child's illness to the physician, (2) the physician's treatment recommendation explicitly ruled out the need for antibiotics, and (3) the parent questioned the physician's treatment recommendation. These communication behaviors are summarized and exemplified in **Table 1** and the eFigure (available at: http://www.archpediatrics.com). Weighted κ statistics calculated to examine interrater reliability for coding the 3 communication behaviors revealed moderate to near-perfect agreement beyond that of chance: 0.84, 0.77, and, 0.55 respectively.[54]

### ANALYTIC METHODS

For all analyses, the physician-parent encounter, clustered within physicians in practices, was the unit of analysis. All multivariate analyses corrected for this hierarchical structure. We tested the bivariate relationships between our hypothesized categorical predictor and outcome variables using the $\chi^2$ test of independence.

Bivariate relationships were examined between each of a common set of candidate predictor variables and (1) parental expectations for antibiotics and (2) physician perceptions of parental expectations. The predictor variables included parental communication practices as summarized in Table 1, symptoms, whether antibiotics had previously been prescribed for a cold or sore throat, and child, parent, and physician demographics. Predictor variables having significant bivariate relationships ($P<.05$) with these outcome variables were retained for multivariate models. The final models included (1) parents who were not initially offered antibiotics for their child and who did not question the treatment plan and (2) parents

**Table 1. Communication Conduct**

| Speaker | Communication Behavior | Definition | Example | Frequency |
|---|---|---|---|---|
| Parent | Candidate diagnosis at problem presentation | Parent presents child's problem by suggesting a bacterial diagnosis | "He's had a terrible sore throat, so I thought maybe it was strep." | 31/522 (5.9%) |
| Parent | Questioning the treatment plan | Parent questions the treatment plan or states a preference for a treatment other than the one the physician recommended | After a suggestion to use over-the-counter cough medicine, a parent questions the treatment being recommended (eg, "The Robitussin just isn't working."), or after a recommendation of over-the-counter medication the parent asks, "So, you don't think he needs any antibiotics?" | 52/325 (16.0%)* |
| Physician | Recommendation against antibiotic treatment | Physician's treatment plan includes a recommendation against the use of an antibiotic | "I think we're in good shape here." "I don't think he needs antibiotics because it wouldn't work." or "We can make him more comfortable, but there's no antibiotic that will touch it." | 48/297 (16.2%)† |

*Excludes cases in which the parent did not question the treatment plan but did receive antibiotics because, for the purposes of this analysis, this parental communication practice was only relevant in cases where antibiotics were not initially suggested as part of the treatment plan.
†Includes only those cases in which the initial diagnosis was nonbacterial, ie, viral or other (eg, asthma).

who were not initially offered antibiotics for their child but did question the treatment plan. This latter group of parents was included regardless of whether they successfully negotiated with the physician to ultimately obtain antibiotics for their children. We excluded from these analyses 204 cases (39.1%) in which both of the following exclusion criteria were met: (1) physicians recommended antibiotics as part of their initial treatment plan and (2) parents did not question the treatment plan. In other words, we excluded cases in which parents did not need to negotiate with the physician to obtain a prescription for antibiotics because the physician's initial treatment recommendation already included antibiotics. This yielded a subsample of 318 encounters for analysis in which physician-parent communication had reasonable potential to influence physician perceptions and ultimately to lead to inappropriate antibiotic prescribing.

Bivariate relationships were also examined between a set of candidate predictor variables and prescribing antibiotics for a viral condition. This set of predictor variables included parental expectations for antibiotic treatment, physician perceptions of parental expectations, symptoms, duration of illness, parent anxiety level (extremely or very worried vs somewhat or not very worried about the child's illness), history of chronic illness, past experience with the physician regarding antibiotic treatment for colds and sore throat, physical examination findings, the physician's level of diagnostic uncertainty, presence of a local influenza epidemic, patient load for the day (slow, average, very busy, or extremely busy), day of the week, whether the child could attend day care when sick, length of the relationship with the child's physician, and child, parent, and physician demographics. Predictor variables having significant bivariate relationships ($P<.05$) with prescribing antibiotics for a viral condition were retained for the multivariate model.

Parental questioning of nonantibiotic treatment recommendations was modeled using a subset of variables, including physician and parent demographics and 2 physician communication variables that were significant in bivariate analyses ($P<.05$).

Because of the strong confounding of the parent's race/ethnicity and socioeconomic status (SES) in the sample, independent estimates of race/ethnicity and SES in multivariate models were not well identified, and large standard errors resulted when both were included simultaneously. Thus, we constructed a combined variable with 8 mutually exclusive categories having sufficient sample size for precise estimates. These categories included very low SES with any race/ethnicity (65 of 74 parents in this category were Hispanic), low SES with Hispanic ethnicity, low SES with other race/ethnicity, medium SES with white race (reference group), medium SES with Hispanic ethnicity, medium SES with African American race, medium SES with Asian race, and high SES with any race/ethnicity (60 of 105 parents in this category were non-Hispanic white).

All multivariate models were logistic regressions that allowed independent practice-site intercepts. These intercept effects were not reported for individual sites, but their magnitudes were summarized to assess the importance of unmeasured site characteristics. For each model, odds ratios and 95% confidence intervals (CIs) were estimated for all predictor variables. Multivariate adjusted proportions with 95% CIs were then calculated to estimate the marginal effects of each significant predictor variable, holding all other independent variables constant. These proportions estimate the change in the probability of the outcome associated with a change in a single predictor.

## RESULTS

Parents in the sample were on average 34 years of age, with a median annual income of approximately $40 000. Of the 522 parents, 86.0% were female, 52.9% were Hispanic, and 68.4% had attended at least some college (**Table 2**). As previously reported,[5] 27 (71.1%) of the participating physicians were male, 27 (71.1%) were non-Hispanic white or Asian (Table 2), and 16 (42.1%) were aged 40 to 65 years.

### PARENTAL EXPECTATIONS FOR ANTIBIOTICS

Of the 318 parents involved in encounters in which the physians did not recommend antibiotics as part of their initial treatment plan and who either did or did not question the treatment plan, 203 (63.8%) reported an expectation for antibiotic treatment, whereas physicians perceived such an expectation in 70 (22.0%) of the 318 encounters. Parents who expected antibiotics were more likely to use a candidate diagnosis during the initial presentation of their child's problem (Table 1), with the rate of parental expectations for antibiotics 27.0% higher (93.1% vs 66.1%) in those who used candidate diagnoses than those who did not (**Table 3**; $P=.02$; 95% CI,

**Table 2. Parent and Physician Demographics***

| Demographic Characteristics | No. (%) of Subjects: Parents (n = 522) | Physicians (n = 38) |
|---|---|---|
| Female | 449 (86.0) | 11 (28.9) |
| Race/ethnicity | | |
| White (non-Hispanic) | 144 (27.6) | 16 (42.1) |
| Hispanic | 276 (52.9) | 5 (13.2) |
| African American | 63 (12.1) | 3 (7.9) |
| Asian | 39 (7.5) | 11 (28.9) |
| Other | 0 | 3 (7.9) |
| Education | | NA |
| Less than high school | 81 (15.5) | |
| High school graduate | 84 (16.1) | |
| Some college | 231 (44.3) | |
| Bachelor's degree or more | 126 (24.1) | |
| Income | | NA |
| <\$20 000 | 96 (18.4) | |
| \$20 000-\$40 000 | 169 (32.4) | |
| \$41 000-\$80 000 | 155 (29.7) | |
| >\$80 000 | 102 (19.5) | |

Abbreviation: NA, not applicable.
*The physician demographic data have been presented previously in Mangione-Smith et al.[5]

4.6%-49.4%). However, no significant association was found between parents questioning the treatment plan and their expectations for antibiotics. Parents who reported that they were very anxious about their child's illness before the visit were 29.3% more likely to expect antibiotics for their child (Table 3; $P=.001$; 95% CI, 12.3%-46.3%). Hispanic parents with low SES were 20.7% more likely to expect antibiotics for their child's illness than were non-Hispanic white parents with medium SES (Table 3; $P=.02$; 95% CI, 3.0%-38.5%). Parents of chronically ill children and parents attending visits with male physicians were significantly less likely to expect antibiotics (Table 3).

## PHYSICIAN PERCEPTIONS OF EXPECTATIONS

Adjusted results indicated that physicians were 9.3% more likely (25.6% vs 16.3%) to perceive a parent as expecting antibiotics if the parent offered a candidate bacterial diagnosis during the presentation of their child's problem (Table 3; $P=.02$; 95% CI, 1.8%-16.9%). Physicians were also 20.2% more likely to perceive an expectation for antibiotics if the parent questioned the physician's treatment plan (Table 3; $P=.004$; 95% CI, 6.3%-34.0%). Hispanic parents with medium SES were 14.3% less likely to be perceived as expecting antibiotics when compared with non-Hispanic white parents with medium SES (Table 3; $P=.02$; 95% CI, −26.6% to −2.0%), after controlling for other predictors, including these 2 parental communication behaviors.

## INAPPROPRIATE ANTIBIOTIC PRESCRIBING

Antibiotics were prescribed in 41 (15.8%) of 260 cases with viral diagnoses. Multivariate models showed that when physicians perceived a parent as expecting antibiotics, they were 31.7% more likely (33.7% vs 2.0%) to inappropriately prescribe them (**Table 4**; $P<.001$; 95% CI, 16.0%-47.3%). In addition, when physicians reported the presence of rhonchi or wheezing on examination, the probability that they would inappropriately prescribe an-

**Table 3. Multivariate-Adjusted Probabilities of Parental Expectations for Antibiotics and Physician Perceptions of Parental Expectations for Antibiotics***

| Characteristics of the Clinical Encounter | Change in Probability, % (95% CI): Parent Expecting Antibiotics† | Physician Perceives an Expectation for Antibiotics‡ |
|---|---|---|
| Parent offers a candidate diagnosis during problem presentation | 27.0 (4.6 to 49.4) | 9.3 (1.8 to 16.9) |
| Parent questions the physician's treatment recommendation | −6.2 (−16.7 to 4.3) | 20.2 (6.3 to 34.0) |
| Child or parent reports fever | −0.2 (−1.2 to 0.8) | −3.8 (−13.0 to 5.5) |
| Child or parent reports that child has ear pain | 11.1 (−4.2 to 26.4) | −5.5 (−25.9 to 14.9) |
| Child presents with ≥2 symptoms | 11.8 (−11.6 to 35.2) | 9.6 (−2.7 to 21.9) |
| Child has been sick for <2 d | 1.5 (−7.9 to 10.9) | −0.8 (−4.3 to 2.7) |
| Child has any chronic condition | −15.3 (−25.1 to −5.5) | −4.9 (−12.4 to 2.6) |
| Antibiotics previously prescribed for cold | 20.7 (−3.9 to 45.2) | 8.3 (−2.6 to 19.2) |
| Antibiotics previously prescribed for sore throat | 14.6 (−35.5 to 64.1) | −1.1 (−3.0 to 0.8) |
| Parents with high SES§ | −29.3 (−79.3 to 20.7) | 4.1 (−17.4 to 25.5) |
| Parents with medium SES§ | | |
| Hispanic | 13.6 (−2.0 to 29.2) | −14.3 (−26.6 to −2.0) |
| African American | 5.3 (−3.9 to 14.5) | 26.3 (−12.5 to 65.1) |
| Asian | 11.7 (−12.7 to 36.1) | 11.8 (−6.7 to 30.3) |
| Parents with low SES§ | | |
| Hispanic | 20.7 (3.0 to 38.5) | 1.9 (−4.7 to 8.4) |
| Non-Hispanic | 14.2 (−12.5 to 40.8) | NA‖ |
| Parents with very low SES§ | 10.8 (−7.0 to 28.6) | 0.4 (−0.3 to 1.1) |
| Parent has known physician for ≥1 y | 10.5 (−58.0 to 78.9) | 4.1 (−11.5 to 19.7) |
| Parent is anxious about the child's current illness | 29.3 (12.3 to 46.3) | 3.9 (−8.7 to 16.6) |
| Physician age <45 y¶ | −1.0 (−11.5 to 9.6) | −6.3 (−39.7 to 27.1) |
| Physician age >65 y¶ | −23.1 (−73.1 to 26.9) | −2.1 (−13.4 to 9.1) |
| Physician is male | −14.9 (−28.8 to −1.1) | 6.3 (−6.3 to 19.0) |

Abbreviations: CI, confidence interval; NA, not applicable; SES, socioeconomic status.
*Analysis excludes cases in which antibiotics were recommended as part of the initial treatment plan
†Base rate is 64%.
‡Base rate is 22%.
§Analysis is relative to non-Hispanic white parents with medium SES. The SES group definitions are as follows: high, education greater than a bachelor's degree and annual income of \$40 000 to \$80 000 or more than \$80 000; low, high school education and annual income less than \$40 000; very low, less than a high school education and annual income less than \$40 000; and medium, all others.
‖None of the 16 parents in this group were perceived as expecting antibiotics. This perfect prediction precluded their inclusion in this multivariate model.
¶Analysis is relative to physicians aged 45 to 65 years.

**Table 4. Multivariate-Adjusted Predictors of Prescribing Antibiotics for Viral Conditions**

| Predictor Variable | Change in Probability of Physician Inappropriately Prescribing Antibiotics, % (95% CI)* |
|---|---|
| Parent expects to receive antibiotics | 3.7 (−25.5 to 33.0) |
| Physician perceives parent as expecting antibiotics | 31.7 (16.0 to 47.3) |
| Child presents with ≥2 symptoms | 1.8 (−0.7 to 4.3) |
| Child has been sick for <2 d | 2.5 (67.1 to −72.0) |
| Abnormal appearance of the tympanic membranes | 4.3 (−29.7 to 38.4) |
| Rhonchi or wheezing on lung examination | 20.7 (7.4 to 34.1) |
| Presence of purulent rhinorrhea | 25.8 (−10.1 to 61.85) |
| Erythematous pharynx in a patient with sore throat | 11.7 (−11.0 to 34.3) |
| Patient febrile at home and in physician's office | 12.7 (−4.6 to 30.0) |
| Parents with high SES† | −0.2 (−0.5 to 0.1) |
| Parents with medium SES† | |
| Hispanic | 4.4 (−1.3 to 10.1) |
| African American | −3.4 (−8.1 to 1.3) |
| Asian | −2.2 (−7.7 to 3.3) |
| Parents with low SES† | |
| Hispanic | −4.9 (−22.8 to 12.9) |
| Non-Hispanic | 25.4 (5.6 to 45.1) |
| Parents with very low SES† | 24.2 (3.5 to 44.9) |
| Parent is anxious about the child's current illness | 11.8 (1.5 to 22.1) |

Abbreviations: CI, confidence interval; SES, socioeconomic status.
*Base rate is 16%.
†Analysis is relative to non-Hispanic white parents with medium SES. The SES group definitions appear in a footnote to Table 3.

tibiotics increased by 20.7% (Table 4; $P=.002$; 95% CI, 7.4%-34.1%). Parents who reported that they were very anxious about their child's illness before the visit were also significantly more likely to receive an inappropriate antibiotic prescription for their child's viral illness (Table 4). Children of non-Hispanic parents with low SES and all children of parents with very low SES were significantly more likely to receive an inappropriate antibiotic prescription than were children of white parents with medium SES (Table 4). Inappropriate prescribing was not associated with actual parental expectations for antibiotics after controlling for these other factors.

## PARENTAL QUESTIONING OF PHYSICIAN NONANTIBIOTIC TREATMENT RECOMMENDATIONS

Among parents who received nonantibiotic treatment recommendations for their children, none of the 40 African American parents but 53 of the 285 non–African American parents questioned the physician's treatment plan ($P=.02$). This perfect prediction did not allow the inclusion of race/ethnicity in subsequent logistic regressions, so subsequent multivariate modeling was restricted to non–African American parents.

Adjusted results showed that the only additional significant predictor of parents questioning a nonantibiotic treatment plan was the physician's ruling out the need for antibiotics when discussing his or her treatment recommendations (Table 1). Parents were 24.0% more likely to question the physician's treatment plan when physicians exclusively ruled out the need for antibiotics or when their treatment plan consisted of ruling out antibiotics in combination with positive treatment recommendations for symptomatic medications or home remedies (**Figure**; 41.4% vs 17.4%; $P=.004$; 95% CI, 7.7%-40.3%). This increase in the probability of parents questioning the treatment plan occurred whether the statement ruling out the need for antibiotics was positioned before or after any positive treatment recommendations provided by the physician.

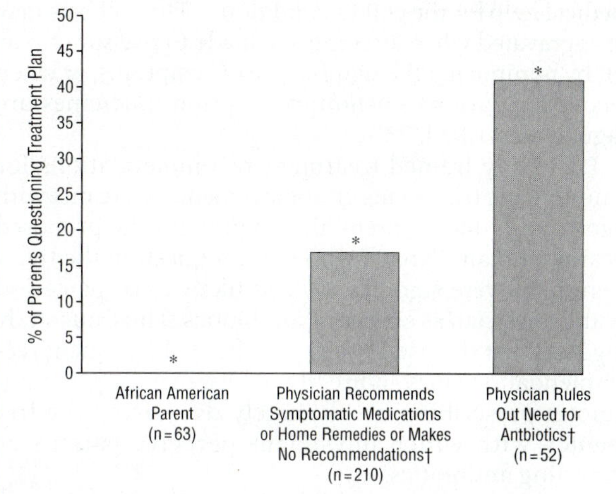


**Figure.** Covariate-adjusted frequencies for parents questioning the physician's treatment plan. Adjustments include child age, parental socioeconomic status, and physician age. The analysis excludes parents who received antibiotics without questioning the treatment recommendation.
*$P<.01$ for all subgroup comparisons.
†Includes only non–African American parents.

## COMMENT

Inappropriate antibiotic prescribing is primarily driven by physicians' perceptions that parents expect an antibiotic for their child.[5,26] In the present study, we hypothesized that these perceptions would be positively associated with a variety of parental communication practices, including the use of candidate diagnoses and parental questioning of physicians' diagnoses and treatment recommendations.[47-50] Our results indicate that physician perceptions of parental expectations for antibiotic treatment are strongly related to both candidate diagnoses being offered and parental questioning of non–antibiotic treatment recommendations. Although the offering of candidate diagnoses was also associated with a preexisting parental expectation for antibiotic treatment, questioning the physician's treatment plan was not. Instead, parental questioning of the treatment plan was strongly associated with the physician communication practice of ruling out the need for antibiotics. Qualitative analyses of these exchanges suggested that these rule-out statements may motivate such questioning because they seem to delegitimize the parent's decision to seek medical help for the child's condition.[48] These effects may be aggravated when attempts are made to reassure a parent by minimizing the significance of symptoms, or when recommendations for nonprescription medicines are vaguely described.[48-50]

Positively framed treatment recommendations for symptomatic treatments or home remedies were met with significantly more parent alignment with the proposed treatment plan. Parents who did not question the treatment plan were significantly less likely to be perceived by the physician as expecting antibiotics. Thus, our study suggests that the use of positively framed treatment recommendations may indirectly reduce inappropriate antibiotic prescribing by ultimately decreasing the frequency with which physicians perceive parents as expecting antibiotics.

Parents who used candidate diagnoses when presenting their child's problem were more likely to expect and be perceived as expecting antibiotics. Because these presentations are the first event to occur in the visit, education about what would support the diagnosis proposed by the parent might best be addressed during this first phase of the visit, shortly after the parent has raised the issue. The physician might tell the parent what findings from the physical examination he or she will be focusing on to evaluate the suggested diagnosis, as well as address which of these findings would require antibiotic treatment. For example, if the parent offers "strep throat" as a candidate diagnosis, the physician could briefly explain that if the child has white spots on the tonsils this would raise his suspicion of streptococcus infection, and a throat culture or rapid test would be used to confirm the diagnosis. If the actual examination reveals only a red throat and the physician states that the tonsils do not have white spots on them, the parent has already been prepared for the possibility of a different diagnosis that may not require a test or antibiotics.[55]

Low-SES Hispanic parents were significantly more likely to expect antibiotics than were medium-SES white parents who were otherwise similar (20.7% more likely; $P = .02$), but physicians did not perceive these higher expectations (1.9% more likely; $P = .58$) (Table 3). The higher expectations of low-SES Hispanic parents did not translate into higher-level use of the 2 key parental communication practices we identified in this study as having the potential to influence physician perceptions and behavior; their use of these behaviors was similar to their use by parents in other SES and racial/ethnic groups (data not shown). This finding suggests that any additional unmeasured communication practices used by this group of parents to convey expectations for antibiotics are unlikely to have substantial effects on physician perceptions and behavior.

Physicians were significantly more likely to inappropriately prescribe antibiotics to children of all parents in the very-low-SES group (n=74; 87.8% Hispanic and 12.2% African American parents) and to children of parents in the low-SES group who were African American (n=7) or white (n=6). However, physicians did not perceive these parents as being more likely to expect antibiotics and, in fact, they were no more likely to expect antibiotics than were medium-SES white parents. The families in the very-low- and low-SES groups were primarily seen in high-volume safety-net clinics in East or South Central Los Angeles. Physicians providing care in these clinics may view the practice of prescribing inappropriate antibiotics as more efficient than explaining how to provide symptomatic over-the-counter treatments or home remedies to these families. However, 1 recent study does not support the presumed efficiency of such prescribing practices.[56] Using data from the National Ambulatory Medical Care Survey, Coco and Mainous[56] found that pediatric visits in which antibiotics were prescribed for colds and bronchitis were 3.6 seconds longer on average (14.24 vs 14.18 minutes; $P > .05$) than were visits in which no antibiotics were provided.

This study has several limitations. First, it was conducted in Los Angeles, so the results may not be generalizable to different populations of parents and physicians in different geographic locations. We had a small physician sample (n=38), which underrepresented non-Hispanic white physicians (42.1%) and female physicians (28.9%). Second, it is possible that under normal circumstances, when these particular physicians are not being observed, pressure to prescribe antibiotics may be acted on more frequently. In a previous study[57] with a similar study design, a significant Hawthorne effect was observed on antibiotic prescribing patterns. It is our expectation that Hawthorne effects are more likely to cause us to underestimate the strength of associations between parental communication practices and physician perceptions and behavior than they are to cause the reverse. Finally, our results indicate that other unmeasured factors contribute to physician-perceived expectations for antibiotics and inappropriate antibiotic prescribing.

## CONCLUSIONS

Although many physicians may understandably wish to educate parents about the circumstances in which antibiotics are an appropriate treatment option, our results suggest that the final phase of the visit, when treatment recommendations are being made, may be an ineffective context in which to begin physician-initiated education for which the parent is unprepared. Although changing the way treatment recommendations are made (ie, avoiding statements that rule out the need for antibiotics) will not eliminate inappropriate prescribing in response to perceived parental expectations, changing physician communication in this regard will likely help to diminish the problem. Future interventions should consider alternative communication practices by which physicians can educate parents about the appropriateness of antibiotic medications early in the visit and prepare parents for the subsequent diagnosis and treatment recommendation. Because inappropriate antibiotic prescribing to children from families with low and very low SES does not appear to be primarily driven by physician-perceived pressure to prescribe, future work should examine the determinants of prescribing antibiotics to these children to better inform the development of interventions aimed at physicians caring for them.

**Accepted for Publication:** April 27, 2006.
**Correspondence:** Rita Mangione-Smith, MD, MPH, Department of Pediatrics, University of Washington, Child Health Institute, 6200 NE 74th St, Suite 210, Seattle, WA 98115-8160 (ritams@u.washington.edu).
**Author Contributions:** Dr Mangione-Smith had full access to all of the data in the study and takes responsibility for the integrity of the data and the accuracy of the data analysis. *Study concept and design:* Mangione-Smith, Elliott, Stivers, and Heritage. *Acquisition of data:* Mangione-Smith and Stivers. *Analysis and interpretation of data:* Mangione-Smith, Elliott, Stivers, McDonald, and Heritage. *Drafting of the manuscript:* Mangione-Smith, Elliott, Stivers, and Heritage. *Critical revision of the manuscript for important intellectual content:* Mangione-Smith, Elliott, Stivers, and Heritage. *Obtained funding:* Mangione-Smith. *Administrative, technical, and material support:* Mangione-Smith, Elliott, Stivers, McDonald, and Heritage. *Study supervision:* Mangione-Smith and Heritage.
**Funding/Support:** This study was supported by grant 039189 from the Robert Wood Johnson Foundation and grant KO2-HS13299-01 from the Agency for Healthcare Research and Quality.
**Role of the Sponsor:** The funding agencies did not participate in the design or conduct of the study; in the collection, analysis, or interpretation of the data; or in the preparation, review, or approval of the manuscript.
**Additional Information:** The eFigure is available at: http://www.archpediatrics.com.
**Acknowledgment:** We thank Andrea Richardson, MPH, for her assistance with programming for analyses on this project.

## REFERENCES


1. Finkelstein JA, Metlay J, Davis RI, Dowell SF, Platt R. Antimicrobial use in defined populations of infants and young children. *Arch Pediatr Adolesc Med.* 2000;154:395-400.
2. Gonzales R, Malone DC, Maselli JH, Sande MA. Excessive antibiotic use for acute respiratory infections in the United States. *Clin Infect Dis.* 2001;33:757-762.
3. Gonzales R, Steiner JF, Sande MA. Antibiotic prescribing for adults with colds, upper respiratory tract infections, and bronchitis by ambulatory care physicians. *JAMA.* 1997;278:901-904.
4. Mainous AG, Hueston WJ, Clark JR. Antibiotics and upper respiratory infection: do some folks think there is a cure for the common cold? *J Fam Pract.* 1996;42:357-361.
5. Mangione-Smith R, Elliott MN, Stivers T, McDonald L, Heritage J, McGlynn EA. Racial/ethnic variation in parent expectations for antibiotics: implications for public health campaigns. *Pediatrics.* 2004;113:e385-e394. http://pediatrics.aapublications.org/cgi/content/full/113/e385-e394. Accessed November 18, 2005.
6. McCaig LF, Besser RE, Hughes JM. Trends in antimicrobial prescribing rates for children and adolescents. *JAMA.* 2002;287:3096-3102.
7. Pennie RA. Prospective study of antibiotic prescribing for children. *Can Fam Physician.* 1998;44:1850-1856.
8. Finkelstein JA, Stille C, Nordin J, et al. Reduction in antibiotic use among US children, 1996-2000. *Pediatrics.* 2003;112:620-627.
9. Nash DR, Harman J, Wald ER, Kelleher KJ. Antibiotic prescribing by primary care physicians for children with upper respiratory tract infections. *Arch Pediatr Adolesc Med.* 2002;156:1114-1119.
10. Steinman MA, Gonzales R, Linder JA, Landefeld CS. Changing use of antibiotics in community-based outpatient practice. *Ann Intern Med.* 2003;138:525-533.
11. McCaig LF, Besser RE, Hughes JM. Antimicrobial drug prescriptions in ambulatory care settings, United States, 1992-2000. *Emerg Infect Dis.* 2003;9:432-437.
12. Cristino JM. Correlation between consumption of antimicrobials in humans and development of resistance in bacteria. *Int J Antimicrob Agents.* 1999;12:199-202.
13. Deeks SL, Palacio R, Ruvinsky R, et al; *Streptococcus pneumoniae* Working Group. Risk factors and course of illness among children with invasive penicillin-resistant *Streptococcus pneumoniae. Pediatrics.* 1999;103:409-413.
14. Gomez J, Banos V, Gomez JR, et al. Clinical significance of pneumococcal bacteraemias in a general hospital: a prospective study 1989-1993. *J Antimicrob Chemother.* 1995;36:1021-1030.
15. Nava JM, Bella F, Garau J, et al. Predictive factors for invasive disease due to penicillin-resistant *Streptococcus pneumoniae*: a population-based study. *Clin Infect Dis.* 1994;19:884-890.
16. Pihlajamaki M, Kotilainen P, Kaurila T, Klaukka T, Palva E, Huovinen P. Macrolide-resistant *Streptococcus pneumoniae* and use of antimicrobial agents. *Clin Infect Dis.* 2001;33:483-488.
17. Seppala H, Klaukka T, Vuopiio-Varikila J. The effect of changes in the consumption of macrolide antibiotics on erythromycin resistance in group A streptococci in Finland. *N Engl J Med.* 1997;337:441-446.
18. Watanabe H, Sato S, Kawakami K, et al. A comparative clinical study of pneumonia by penicillin-resistant and sensitive *Streptococcus pneumoniae* in a community hospital. *Respirology.* 2000;5:59-64.
19. Whitney CG, Farley MM, Hadler J, et al. Increasing prevalence of multidrug-resistant *Streptococcus pneumoniae* in the United States. *N Engl J Med.* 2000;343:1917-1924.
20. Dagan R. Clinical significance of resistant organisms in otitis media. *Pediatr Infect Dis J.* 2000;19:378-382.
21. Feikin DR, Schuchat A, Kolczak M, et al. Mortality from invasive pneumococcal pneumonia in the era of antibiotic resistance, 1995-1997. *Am J Public Health.* 2000;90:223-229.
22. Friedland IR. Comparison of the response to antimicrobial therapy of penicillin-resistant and penicillin-susceptible pneumococcal disease. *Pediatr Infect Dis J.* 1995;14:885-890.
23. Gums JG. Assessing the impact of antimicrobial resistance. *Am J Health Syst Pharm.* 2002;59(suppl 3):S4-S6.
24. Holmberg SD, Solomon SL, Blake PA. Health and economic impacts of antimicrobial resistance. *Rev Infect Dis.* 1987;9:1065-1078.
25. Benson V, Marano MA. *Current Estimates from the National Health Interview Survey: Vital Health Statistics Series 10, No. 189.* Hyattsville, Md: National Center for Health Statistics; 1994.
26. Mangione-Smith R, McGlynn EA, Elliott MN, Krogstad P, Brook RH. The relationship between perceived parental expectations and pediatrician antimicrobial prescribing behavior. *Pediatrics.* 1999;103:711-718.
27. Gadomski AM. Potential interventions for preventing pneumonia among young children: lack of effect of antibiotic treatment for upper respiratory infections. *Pediatr Infect Dis J.* 1993;12:115-120.
28. Howie JGR, Clark GA. Double-blind trial of early demethylchlortetracycline in minor respiratory illness in general practice. *Lancet.* 1970;2:1099-1102.
29. Orr PH, Scherer K, MacDonald A, Moffatt MEK. Randomized placebo-controlled trials of antibiotics for acute bronchitis: a critical review of the literature. *J Fam Pract.* 1993;36:507-512.
30. Stott NCH, West RR. Randomised controlled trial of antibiotics in patients with cough and purulent sputum. *BMJ.* 1976;2:556-559.
31. Taylor B, Abbot GD, Kerr MM, Ferguson D. Amoxycillin and co-trimoxazole in presumed viral upper respiratory infections of childhood: placebo-controlled trial. *BMJ.* 1977;2:552-554.
32. Todd JK, Todd N, Damato J, Todd W. Bacteriology and treatment of purulent nasopharyngitis: a double blind, placebo-controlled evaluation. *Pediatr Infect Dis.* 1984;3:226-232.
33. Britten N, Ukoumunne O. The influence of patients' hopes of receiving a prescription on doctors' perceptions and the decision to prescribe: a questionnaire study. *BMJ.* 1997;315:1506-1510.
34. Cockburn J, Pit S. Prescribing behaviour in clinical practice: patients' expectations and doctors' perceptions of patients' expectations—a questionnaire study. *BMJ.* 1997;315:520-523.
35. Hamm RM, Hicks RJ, Bemben DA. Antibiotics and respiratory infections: are patients more satisfied when expectations are met? *J Fam Pract.* 1996;43:56-62.
36. Himmel W, Lippert-Urbanke E, Kochen MM. Are patients more satisfied when they receive a prescription? the effect of patient expectations in general practice. *Scand J Prim Health Care.* 1997;15:118-122.
37. Macfarlane J, Holmes W, Macfarlane R, Britten N. Influence of patients' expectations on antibiotic management of acute lower respiratory tract illness in general practice: questionnaire study. *BMJ.* 1997;315:1211-1214.
38. Virji A, Britten N. A study of the relationship between patients' attitudes and doctors' prescribing. *Fam Pract.* 1991;8:314-319.
39. Webb S, Lloyd M. Prescribing and referral in general practice: a study of patients' expectations and doctors' actions. *Br J Gen Pract.* 1994;44:165-169.
40. Barden LS, Dowell SF, Schwartz B, Lackey C. Current attitudes regarding use of antimicrobial agents: results from physicians' and parents' focus group discussions. *Clin Pediatr (Phila).* 1998;37:665-672.

41. Butler CC, Rollnick S, Pill R, Maggs-Rapport F, Stott N. Understanding the culture of prescribing: qualitative study of general practitioners' and patients' perceptions of antibiotics for sore throats. *BMJ.* 1998;317:637-642.
42. Palmer DA, Bauchner H. Patients' and physicians' views on antibiotics. *Pediatrics.* 1997;99:E6.
43. Schwartz B. Preventing the spread of antimicrobial resistance among bacterial respiratory pathogens in industrialized countries: the case for judicious antimicrobial use. *Clin Infect Dis.* 1999;28:211-213.
44. Schwartz RH, Freij BJ, Ziai M, Sheridan MJ. Antimicrobial prescribing for acute purulent rhinitis in children: a survey of pediatricians and family practitioners. *Pediatr Infect Dis J.* 1997;16:185-190.
45. Mangione-Smith R, McGlynn EA, Elliott MN, McDonald L, Franz CE, Kravitz RL. Parent expectations for antibiotics, doctor-parent communication, and satisfaction. *Arch Pediatr Adolesc Med.* 2001;155:800-806.
46. Stivers T. Participating in decisions about treatment: overt parent pressure for antibiotic medication in pediatric encounters. *Soc Sci Med.* 2002;54:1111-1130.
47. Stivers T, Mangione-Smith R, Elliott MN, McDonald L, Heritage J. Why do physicians think parents expect antibiotics? what parents report versus what physicians believe. *J Fam Pract.* 2003;52:140-147.
48. Stivers T. Non–antibiotic treatment recommendations: delivery formats and implications for parent resistance. *Soc Sci Med.* 2005;60:949-964.
49. Stivers T. Treatment decisions: negotiations between doctors and patients in acute care encounters. In: Heritage J, Maynard D, eds. *Communication in Medical Care: Interaction Between Primary Care Physicians and Patients.* Cambridge, England: Cambridge University Press; 2006:279-312.
50. Stivers T. Parent resistance to physicians' treatment recommendations: one resource for initiating a negotiation of the treatment decision. *Health Commun.* 2005; 18:41-74.
51. Atkinson JM, Heritage J. *Structures of Social Action: Studies in Conversation Analysis.* New York, NY: Cambridge University Press; 1984.
52. Heritage J, Maynard D. Analyzing interaction between doctors and patients in primary care encounters. In: Heritage J, Maynard D, eds. *Communication in Medical Care: Interaction Between Primary Care Physicians and Patients.* Cambridge, England: Cambridge University Press; 2006:1-21.
53. Schegloff EA. *A Primer of Conversation Analysis: Sequence Organization.* New York, NY: Cambridge University Press; 2005.
54. Maclure M, Willett WC. Misinterpretation and misuse of the kappa statistic. *Am J Epidemiol.* 1987;126:161-169.
55. Heritage J, Stivers T. Online commentary in acute medical visits: a method of shaping patient expectations. *Soc Sci Med.* 1999;49:1501-1517.
56. Coco A, Mainous AG. Relation of time spent in an encounter with the use of antibiotics in pediatric office visits for viral respiratory infections. *Arch Pediatr Adolesc Med.* 2005;159:1145-1149.
57. Mangione-Smith R, Elliott MN, McDonald L, McGlynn EA. An observational study of antibiotic prescribing behavior and the Hawthorne effect. *Health Serv Res.* 2002; 37:1603-1623.

## *Correction*

**Incorrect Terminology.** In the article titled "Effectiveness of Child Safety Seats vs Seat Belts in Reducing Risk for Death in Children in Passenger Vehicle Crashes," by Elliott et al published in the June issue of the ARCHIVES (2006;160:617-621) the term *tow-away* was incorrectly changed to the term *two-way*. Thus, on page 617, in the "Participants" subsection of the "Abstract," the sentence should have read as follows: "Children in tow-away crashes occurring between 1998 and 2003." The same error occurred on page 621, left-hand column, lines 1 and 2. These should have read ". . . of the NASS CDS to obtain a representative sample of the full tow-away crash population may suffer from confounding. . . ." Further down on the same page and in the same column, the last sentence of that paragraph should have read as follows: "The restriction of NASS CDS to tow-away crashes and use of adjustment factors such as vehicle type, model year, age of driver, and, especially, survival status of the driver should reduce this confounding."

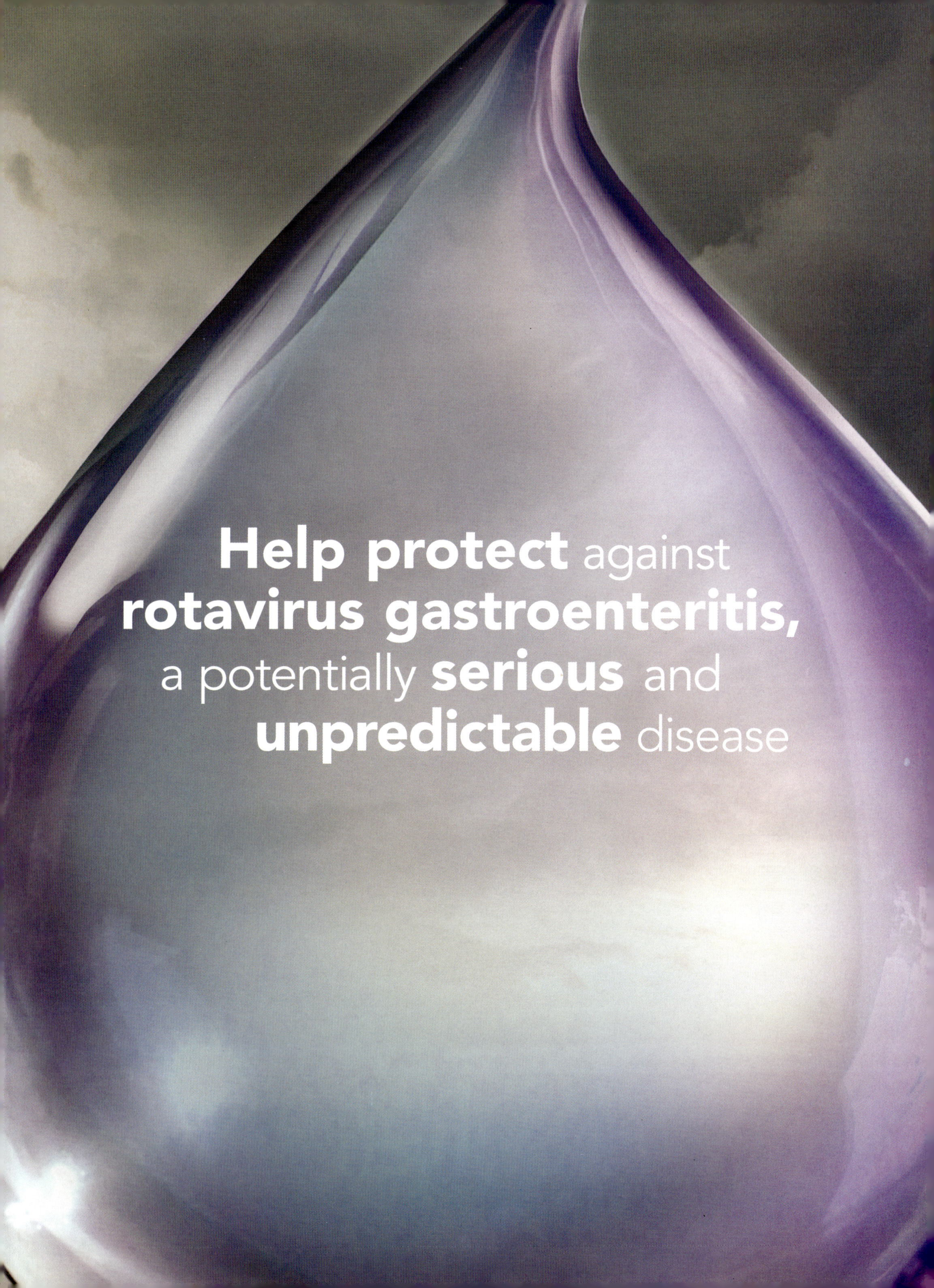
**Help protect** against
**rotavirus gastroenteritis,**
a potentially **serious** and
**unpredictable** disease

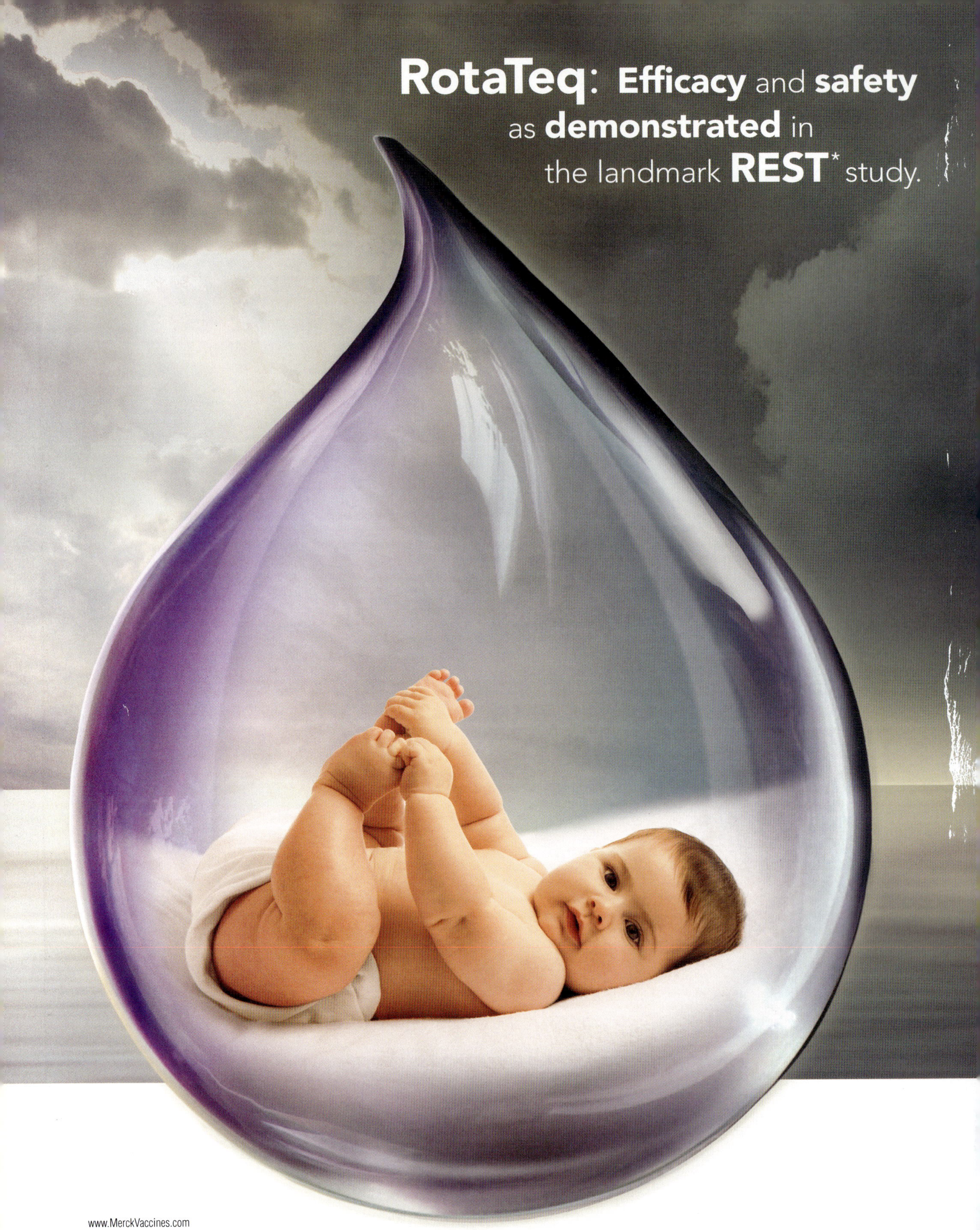
RotaTeq: Efficacy and safety
as demonstrated in
the landmark REST* study.

# Randomized Controlled Trial of a Prenatal and Postnatal Lactation Consultant Intervention on Infant Health Care Use

Karen A. Bonuck, PhD; Katherine Freeman, DrPH; Michelle Trombley, MPH

**Objective:** To determine whether infants of women randomized to a prenatal and postpartum lactation support intervention incur fewer otitis media–, respiratory tract–, or gastrointestinal-related visits than controls.

**Design:** Randomized, unmasked controlled trial recruiting women from prenatal care settings. Breastfeeding sensitive (BFS) illness visits for otitis media or respiratory tract or gastrointestinal complaints were obtained up to 12 months.

**Setting:** Two urban community health centers.

**Participants:** Analytic sample of 338 low-income, primarily Hispanic and/or black mother-infant dyads (n=163 for the intervention group and n=175 for the control group).

**Intervention:** Study lactation consultants attempted 2 prenatal meetings, 1 postpartum hospital and/or home visit, and telephone calls as needed. Controls received the standard of care.

**Main Outcome Measures:** Combined outpatient and emergency department visits with illness and BFS illness diagnoses.

**Results:** There was a significant interaction between treatment and Medicaid; among those not receiving Medicaid, the number of otitis media visits was higher among controls ($P \leq .03$). Visits for any illness and BFS, gastrointestinal, or respiratory tract illnesses did not differ by treatment group. Intervention group infants received more breast milk than controls, but exclusive breastfeeding rates remained low and did not differ between groups at any point.

**Conclusions:** Only the number of otitis media visits was reduced, in a subset of the intervention group. The intervention did not reduce visits for respiratory tract or gastrointestinal illness. Limited intervention contact and low exclusive breastfeeding rates may have attenuated intervention effects. Future interventions designed to yield markedly increased breastfeeding rates may show greater effects in low-income multiethnic samples. Health coverage for visits may moderate intervention effects.

*Arch Pediatr Adolesc Med. 2006;160:953-960*

OVERWHELMING EPIDEMIOLOGICAL evidence exists that "even in developed countries, breastfeeding protects against gastrointestinal and (to a lesser extent) respiratory tract infection, and that the protective effect is enhanced with greater duration and exclusivity of breastfeeding."[1(p8)] In the first year of life, protective effects are reported for otitis media,[2-8] respiratory tract infections,[9-15] and gastrointestinal illnesses.[13-17] Still, US breastfeeding rates at 6 months (35%) and 12 months (16%)[18] do not meet the *Healthy People 2010* goals of 50% and 25%, respectively.[19] Exclusive breastfeeding rates remain low and stagnant.[20]

It is infeasible and unethical to perform random assignment of breastfeeding. There are only 4 randomized controlled trials (RCTs) of breastfeeding intervention effects on child morbidity. In a multisite RCT in Belarus, the intervention group had less gastrointestinal infection and atopic eczema but no differences in respiratory tract infection up to 12 months.[21] An intensive peer counselor intervention (up to 13 contacts) yielded a reduced incidence of diarrhea, 38% vs 12% in controls.[22] A small US-based RCT[23] reported that the $301 cost of a postpartum community nurse or peer counselor intervention was partially offset by formula and health care cost savings. In Mexico, infants of mothers who received home peer support for breastfeeding had a lower incidence of diarrhea than controls, 26% vs 12%.[14]

We conducted an unmasked RCT of a best-practices[24] prenatal and postnatal lac-

Author Affiliations:
Department of Epidemiology and Population Health, Montefiore Medical Center/Albert Einstein College of Medicine, Bronx, NY.

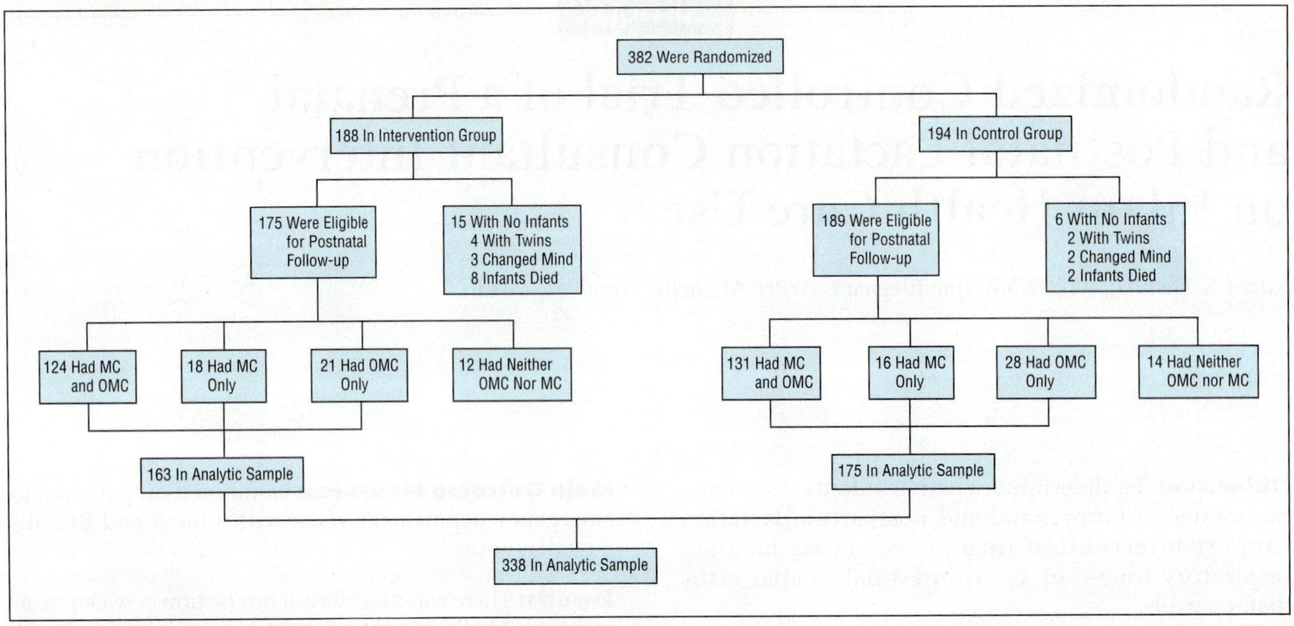


**Figure.** Trial enrollment and infant health care use outcomes. MC indicates infants with 1 or more encounter identified in the computerized medical center data for any reason, exclusive of predischarge newborn data, up to 12 months of age; OMC, outside medical center data for infant, self-reported by mother during follow-up interviews, up to 12 months of age.

tation consultant (LC) intervention on infant emergency department (ED) and outpatient site care for up to 12 months. Maternal self-report of health care use for symptoms of otitis media, respiratory tract illness, and gastrointestinal illness and computerized medical center (MC) data for these breastfeeding sensitive (BFS) illnesses were obtained. Weekly breastfeeding outcomes up to 12 months were assessed via a standardized tool that measured 7 levels of breastfeeding.

## METHODS

### RECRUITMENT

The Moms into Learning About Kids (MILK) study assessed breastfeeding and infant health care use outcomes up to 12 months. This article reports on infant health care use outcomes. Breastfeeding outcomes and detailed methods are reported elsewhere.[25] Briefly, prenatal care patients at 2 Bronx, NY, sites were recruited from August 1, 2000, through November 30, 2002. Eligibility criteria included English or Spanish speaking, twin or singleton pregnancy, and gestation before 24 weeks. Exclusion criteria included medical or obstetric complications for which breastfeeding is contraindicated and long-term use of medications incompatible with breastfeeding.

Eligible, consenting women were randomized by a research assistant. Randomization used an undisclosed blocking factor, stratified by center, with sealed, coded envelopes. All study materials were professionally translated into Spanish. The MC's institutional review board approved the study.

### TRIAL ENROLLMENT

As shown in the **Figure**, 382 women were randomized into the study (188 into the intervention group and 194 into the control group). Of these, 21 were excluded at postnatal follow-up (15 in the intervention group and 6 in the control group). Of the remaining 364 mother-infant dyads, 26 were lost to all follow-up (both self-reported and computerized MC infant health visit data) and are excluded from analysis.

Of the remaining 338 infants who comprise the analytic sample, 304 mothers had 1 or more follow-up interviews (145 in the intervention group and 159 in the control group) at which time they reported infant ED or outpatient visits to sites outside the MC (OMC) for up to 12 months. We obtained computerized data of ED and outpatient visits to MC-affiliated sites for 289 of the 338 infants (142 in the intervention group and 147 in the control group). Well-child care visits for MC and OMC visits were excluded. Thus, outcome data are available for 93% of eligible mother-infant dyads ([364−26]100/364=93%).[26] Data were not collected for women who were approached but did not enroll.

### DATA COLLECTION

A prenatal baseline interview obtained data on demographics and breastfeeding experience and intentions. Postpartum telephone interviews at 1, 2, 3, 4, 6, 8, 10, and 12 months assessed infant feeding and health care use. The 1-month interview collected details about the immediate postpartum experience, whereas subsequent interviews focused on weekly feeding and infant health care use. Participants were compensated.

### MASKING

The research assistants were not masked to treatment group. To minimize bias, research assistants were trained in standard procedures for classifying outcomes and completed follow-up with women in both groups. The MC data were extracted from the MC database by an analyst masked to treatment group. The LCs who provided the intervention were not masked to treatment group.

### POWER ANALYSIS

The power analysis assumed that infants who are primarily breastfed up to 6 months would incur \$901 in health care costs in the first year of life vs \$1105 for exclusively bottle-fed children. These data come from 2 samples in which 34% and 14% of infants were primarily breastfed at 3 months.[27] Under these assumptions, 138 women per group are needed to detect a difference ($\alpha = .05$; $\beta = .20$; 2-tailed test).

## ASSESSMENT OF INFANT HEALTH CARE OUTCOMES

### OMC Data

Postnatal follow-up interviews asked women to recall any OMC ED or outpatient visits for symptoms of illness in general and for symptoms of gastrointestinal, respiratory tract, or otitis media conditions in particular. Maternal report of gastrointestinal, respiratory tract, and otitis media symptoms (classified separately from respiratory tract illness by design) was based on definitions used by others.[10] The recall period was the time since the last interview or postdischarge from birth if at the first follow-up interview.

### MC Data

The MC computerized data identified the date, site, and diagnoses (*International Classification of Diseases, Ninth Revision* [*ICD-9*]) of all infant visits to the 2 EDs or 21 health clinics affiliated with the MC, including the 2 recruitment sites.

## DESCRIPTION OF THE INTERVENTION

After the baseline interview, the MILK research assistant referred intervention participants to a study LC, who arranged to meet at an upcoming clinic visit or the participant's home. Per protocol, the LC was to meet individually with each intervention participant twice prenatally and attempt 1 postpartum hospital and/or 1 home visit. Prenatal and home visits averaged 60 minutes; hospital visits averaged 90 minutes. The LCs also provided postpartum telephone support as needed for up to 12 months.

One LC, of Dominican descent, was en route to obtaining International Board of Certified Lactation Consultants certification. The other LC, born in Trinidad, was certified at the study's inception. Those LCs who are certified by the International Board of Lactation Consultant Examiners[28] are trained in lactation physiology and support and management of breastfeeding. Neither LC had other allied health training.

The initial prenatal meeting provided basic breastfeeding education. The second meeting addressed what to expect in the postpartum period and specifics about initiating breastfeeding in the hospital. During initial hospital and home visits, women were instructed how to avoid common breastfeeding complications. After breastfeeding was established, topics included frequency of feeding, confidence, stooling patterns, determining adequate intake, and maternal nutrition.

Control group women received the health center standard of care and had no contact with the study LCs. One site conducted mandatory prenatal classes, which did not address breastfeeding in detail. The other site had no routine prenatal education. Most (85%) of the sample gave birth at the MC hospital, which was not a designated infant-friendly hospital. The hospital's mother-infant unit nursing staff had received various levels of breastfeeding education.

## ASSESSMENT OF BREASTFEEDING

Women reported the intensity of breast vs artificial milk or solid feedings for each week since the prior interview using a standardized schema.[29,30] The 7 levels in the schema are mutually exclusive. Exclusive breastfeeding was defined as no artificial milk (ie, formula) or solids. Intake of water, liquids other than artificial milk, and vitamin drops was not assessed. Thus, our definition of exclusive breastfeeding does not conform to the stricter World Health Organization definition.[31] The 7 levels in the schema are as follows:

1. 100% Breast milk
2. More than 80% breast milk combined with less than 20% artificial milk or solids
3. More than 50% to 80% breast milk and the rest artificial milk or solids
4. 50% Breast milk and 50% artificial milk or solids
5. More than 20% to 50% breast milk and the rest artificial milk or solids
6. Less than 20% breast milk combined with more than 80% artificial milk or solids
7. 100% Artificial milk or solids (includes weaned).

## SELECTION OF BFS DIAGNOSES

A physician panel reviewed the list of *ICD-9* codes found in the MC data (masked to treatment group) and classified those for which breastfeeding might reduce the incidence or severity as otitis media (all BFS illnesses), respiratory tract and BFS illnesses, and gastrointestinal and BFS illnesses. Respiratory BFS diagnoses included viral enteritis not otherwise specified (008.80), unspecified viral infection (079.99), acute pharyngitis (462.00), croup (464.40), acute upper respiratory infections (465.90), acute bronchitis (466.00), nasal and sinus disease not elsewhere classified (478.10), pneumonia organism, unspecified (486.00), bronchitis (490.00), asthma (493.90), cough (786.20), and respiratory syncytial virus (466.11).[32] Gastrointestinal BFS diagnoses included esophageal reflux (530.81), gastritis/gastroduodenitis (535.50), noninfectious gastroenteritis not elsewhere classified (558.90), unspecified constipation (564.00), vomiting alone (787.03.91), and reflux esophagitis (530.11).[32] Otitis media BFS diagnoses included suppurative otitis media not otherwise specified (382.40) and unspecified otitis media (382.90).[32]

We did not assess breastfeeding-associated hypernatremia of the infant because proper diagnosis and treatment require hospitalization, which was not an outcome measure.[33] Although jaundice rates are higher in breastfed children,[34] there was no jaundice reported in the OMC data and just 2 cases (*ICD-9* code 774.60), 1 per group, in the MC data.

## STATISTICAL ANALYSES

Differences between women randomized into the intervention and control groups, as well as within-treatment group differences between those excluded and the analytic sample, were tested for statistical significance. Descriptive statistics are shown as mean (SD) or number (percentage). Only foreign birth differed between the sites (K. A. B., unpublished data, November 2004) and was thus controlled for in multivariate analyses, which pooled data for the 2 sites. No significant differences were found between the analytic (ie, outcomes) sample and the randomized sample.

Treatment group differences in the proportion of women reporting any breastfeeding (combined levels 1-6), 50% or more breastfeeding (combined levels 1-4), and exclusive breastfeeding (level 1) for postpartum weeks 1 to 52 were tested by the Mantel-Haenszel $\chi^2$ or $\chi^2$ test.

We computed the rate of all sick care visits and those with BFS illness diagnoses for 52 person-weeks of observation. For the MC data, we assumed a 52-week observation period (ie, no participant missing any computerized MC data). For OMC data, the date of the last interview denoted the end of each infant's observation period. For women missing all OMC data, we imputed OMC data by treatment group. The MC and OMC

**Table 1. Demographics of Sample***

| Demographic | Intervention Randomized (n = 188) | Intervention Outcome (n = 163) | Control Randomized (n = 194) | Control Outcome (n = 175) | Total Randomized (N = 382) | Total Outcome (N = 338) |
|---|---|---|---|---|---|---|
| Age, mean (SD), y | 25.7 (6.4) | 26 (6.4) | 24.8 (5.9) | 25.0 (5.0) | 25.2 (6.1) | 25.2 (6.2) |
| High school graduate | 110 (58.5) | 95 (58.3) | 123 (63.4) | 109 (62.3) | 233 (61.0) | 204 (60.4) |
| Married or has partner | 94 (50.3) | 79 (48.8) | 106 (54.6) | 81 (46.3) | 200 (52.5) | 160 (47.5) |
| Foreign born | 83 (44.1) | 73 (44.8) | 67 (34.5) | 63 (36.0) | 150 (39.3) | 136 (40.2) |
| Race/ethnicity | | | | | | |
| African American | 67 (35.6) | 58 (35.6) | 75 (38.7) | 62 (35.4) | 142 (37.2) | 120 (35.5) |
| Hispanic | 103 (54.8) | 90 (55.2) | 107 (55.2) | 101 (57.7) | 210 (55.0) | 191 (56.5) |
| Other | 18 (9.6) | 15 (9.2) | 12 (6.2) | 12 (6.9) | 30 (7.9) | 27 (8.0) |
| Medicaid recipient | 101 (53.7) | 87 (53.4) | 113 (58.2) | 107 (61.1) | 214 (56.0) | 194 (57.4) |
| Other children | 109 (59.9) | 94 (59.9) | 116 (62.0) | 106 (63.1) | 225 (61.0) | 200 (61.5) |
| Previously breastfed | 74 (67.9) | 68 (72.3) | 80 (67.8) | 73 (67.6) | 154 (67.8) | 141 (69.8) |
| Intentions | | | | | | |
| Only breast milk | 62 (33.0) | 55 (33.7) | 47 (32.4) | 49 (28.0) | 118 (30.9) | 104 (30.8) |
| Both | 89 (47.3) | 78 (47.9) | 73 (50.3) | 84 (48.0) | 818 (47.4) | 162 (47.9) |
| Only formula | 16 (8.5) | 15 (9.2) | 112 (7.6) | 17 (9.7) | 36 (9.4) | 32 (11.8) |
| Do not know | 21 (11.2) | 15 (9.2) | 14 (9.7) | 25 (14.3) | 47 (12.3) | 40 (9.5) |

*Data are presented as number (percentage) unless otherwise indicated. Outcomes include mother-infant dyads with medical center and/or outside medical center self-reported data. Outcome samples exclude the 21 mother-infant dyads who were ineligible for follow-up and the 26 infants for whom neither any medical center nor outside medical center infant health care use data were obtained.

**Table 2. Retention and Use of Infant Health Care by Data Source and Treatment Group***

| Data Source | Intervention | Control | Total |
|---|---|---|---|
| OMC data at follow-up | | | |
| ≤3 mo | 131 (80.4) | 147 (84.0) | **278** (82.2) |
| ≤6 mo | 114 (69.9) | 138 (78.9) | **252** (74.6) |
| ≤9 mo | 102 (62.6) | 125 (71.4) | **227** (67.2) |
| ≤12 mo | 92 (56.4) | 107 (61.1) | **199** (58.9) |
| MC data with any visits | | | |
| 0-3 mo | 139 (85.3) | 144 (82.3) | **283** (83.7) |
| 3-6 mo | 120 (73.6) | 117 (66.9) | **237** (70.1) |
| 6-9 mo | 106 (65.0) | 108 (61.7) | **214** (63.3) |
| 9-12 mo | 100 (61.3) | 98 (56.0) | **198** (58.6) |

Abbreviations: MC, medical care; OMC, outside medical care.

*Data are presented as number (percentage). The OMC data consist of infant emergency department and outpatient visits to non–medical center–affiliated sites obtained during that period. The MC data connote participants' infants with 1 or more encounter identified in the computerized MC data for any reason, not including predischarge newborn data, up to 12 months of age.

data were combined. Data for ED and outpatient visits were combined after reviewing *ICD-9* diagnosis codes for ED visits, many of which were for nonemergent sick care.

We examined the bivariate associations between visits with any illness, any BFS illness, and specific BFS illness diagnoses (dependent variables) and variables potentially related to these outcomes (independent variables). Maternal variables included age, educational level, marital status, race/ethnicity, country of origin (mainland United States vs other), Medicaid status, other children (ie, siblings), and recruitment site. Infant variables included sex, low birth weight, neonatal intensive care unit admission, newborn health problems (maternal report), day care for infants 1 month or younger, and age at last interview. We did not include maternal smoking as a covariate, given that less than 5% of the sample reported any cigarette use at baseline. Assessment of day care use was restricted to 1 month or less, given varying observation periods after the 1-month follow-up visit.

Variables with bivariate associations yielding $P \leq .20$ were used in initial multiple linear regression models, which also tested for interactions with treatment group. Given the nonnormal distributions of the health care outcomes data, each variable was transformed logarithmically (log[total number of visits + 1]). Independent variables were assessed for significance using a monitored backward stepwise procedure. Using data from all participants regardless of treatment group, covariates and treatment group interactions with associations of $P < .05$ were retained in the final multivariate models to assess the significance of the intervention. All tests of significance were 2-tailed, with $\alpha = .05$. Analyses were based on an intent-to-treat model.

## RESULTS

### BASELINE CHARACTERISTICS

Baseline characteristics for the analytic sample of 338 women are given in **Table 1**. No significant treatment group differences were found. The sample was primarily Hispanic (56%) and African American (36%) according to participant-reported, investigator-defined options, and 40% were foreign born. Nearly two thirds were multiparous (62%). Combined breast milk and formula was the most common prenatal breastfeeding intention (48%). Detailed data about the birth and immediate postpartum experience, reported elsewhere, did not differ by treatment group, including low birth weight (<2500 g, 8% for sample) and neonatal intensive care unit admissions (13% for sample).[25]

### RETENTION IN AND USE OF INFANT HEALTH CARE BY DATA SOURCE

**Table 2** indicates the retention in and use of OMC and MC data by treatment group. The OMC data in Table 2 indicate the proportion of the outcomes sample re-

**Table 3. Any, 50%, and Exclusive Breastfeeding by Selected Weekly Intervals up to 52 Weeks by Treatment Group***

| | Breast Milk Feedings | | | | | | | | |
|---|---|---|---|---|---|---|---|---|---|
| | Any | | | 50% or More | | | Exclusive | | |
| Interval | Intervention | Control | *P* Value | Intervention | Control | *P* Value | Intervention | Control | *P* Value |
| 2 wk (n = 300) | 124 (86.7) | 102 (65.0) | ≤.001 | 94 (65.7) | 72 (45.9) | ≤.001 | 29 (20.3) | 30 (19.1) | .80 |
| 6 wk (n = 292) | 99 (72.3) | 85 (54.8) | .002 | 71 (51.8) | 58 (37.4) | .01 | 21 (15.3) | 25 (16.1) | .85 |
| 13 wk (n = 273) | 79 (60.8) | 66 (46.2) | .02 | 55 (42.3) | 48 (33.6) | .14 | 11 (8.5) | 16 (11.2) | .45 |
| 20 wk (n = 257) | 62 (53.0) | 55 (39.3) | .03 | 37 (31.6) | 33 (23.6) | .15 | 9 (6.2) | 14 (8.8) | .38 |
| 26 wk (n = 251) | 51 (44.3) | 45 (33.1) | .07 | 34 (29.6) | 30 (22.1) | .17 | 6 (5.2) | 11 (8.1) | .37 |
| 52 wk (n = 181) | 15 (18.3) | 15 (15.2) | .57 | 12 (14.6) | 13 (13.1) | .77 | 5 (6.1) | 5 (5.1) | .76 |

*Data are presented as number (percentage).

tained in follow-up through those periods. At follow-up, respondents were asked only about OMC sick care visits, not well-child care. The MC data in Table 2 indicate the proportion of the outcomes samples using the MC for infant care for any reason, exclusive of the birth hospitalization. However, our MC outcomes exclude visits solely for well-child care. We assume that the computerized MC data results in 100% retention for the study period for the outcomes sample.

Both OMC (retention) and MC (use) data were available for more than 80% of the sample through 3 months, declining to just more than 70% at 6 months, approximately 65% at 9 months, and 59% by 12 months. With regard to treatment group, rates for both OMC and MC data appear roughly comparable through the 12 months.

## DETECTION OF BIAS IN INFANT HEALTH OUTCOMES DATA

To detect potential surveillance and/or selection biases in the MC and OMC data, we performed a series of treatment group comparisons (data not shown).

### Follow-up for OMC Data

We compared baseline characteristics of participants with OMC data at 13, 26, 39, 48, and 52 weeks (ie, retained in follow-up interview) with those without OMC data (ie, lost to follow-up interview) at those weeks, both within and across treatment groups. These baseline characteristics included age, educational level, foreign birth, race/ethnicity, marriage or partner status, Medicaid use, parity, prior breastfeeding experience, and infant feeding intention at baseline. Both attrition rates and characteristics of those retained at quarterly periods were similar for the 2 groups.

### Any OMC Data vs Any MC Data

We compared baseline characteristics of participants with any OMC data (n=304) with those with any MC data (n=289) by treatment group. No significant differences were detected.

### Use of MC as Primary Source of Care

To examine treatment group differences in reliance on the MC as a routine source of infant care, we examined rates of well-child visits (*ICD-9* code V-20) up to 12 months. Similar proportions had any MC well-child visits (81% in the intervention group vs 76% of controls), 1 to 2 visits (7% in the intervention group vs 6% of controls), and 3 or more visits (67% in the intervention group vs 70% of controls).

## WEEKLY BREASTFEEDING OUTCOMES

**Table 3** presents data for any breastfeeding, breastfeeding 50% or more of the time, and exclusive breastfeeding by treatment group for selected weeks for the 304 women with self-reported data (MC data). At 2 weeks, significantly more intervention group women were breastfeeding (87% in the intervention group vs 65% of controls; $P \leq .001$) and giving their infants 50% or more breast milk (66% in the intervention group vs 46% of controls; $P \leq .001$). The intervention group was significantly more likely to breastfeed at each week, up to and including week 20 (53.0% vs 39.3% for controls; $P \leq .03$), except for week 18 (data not shown). Group differences for 50% or more breast milk remained statistically significant for each week, up to and including week 9 (45.8% vs 33.1% for controls; $P \leq .03$; data not shown). There were no differences in exclusive breastfeeding rates at any time, which peaked for both groups at 2 weeks.

## INTERVENTION COMPONENT RECEIVED BY SOURCE OF INFANT HEALTH OUTCOMES DATA

We compared intervention participants with MC data, OMC data, or either data with regard to their receipt of the intervention's various prenatal and postnatal components. As indicated in **Table 4**, 124 (76%) of the intervention group outcomes sample received any intervention. Ninety-nine (61%) had prenatal intervention, 97 (60%) had postnatal intervention, and 72 (44%) had both prenatal and postnatal intervention. Participants with MC and those with OMC data had similar patterns of receiving the prenatal and postnatal interventions.

## VISITS WITH BFS ILLNESS DIAGNOSES BY DATA SOURCE: DESCRIPTIVE DATA

**Table 5** presents descriptive data by treatment site (ED or outpatient), data source (OMC vs MC), and type of

**Table 4. Intervention by Source of Infant Health Care Use Data***

| Intervention | OMC (n = 145) | MC (n = 142) | Either MC or OMC (n = 163) |
|---|---|---|---|
| Prenatal | | | |
| Any prenatal contact | 93 (64.1) | 91 (64.1) | 99 (60.7) |
| 2 Prenatal contacts | 77 (53.1) | 75 (52.8) | 81 (49.7) |
| Postnatal | | | |
| Any postnatal contact | 92 (63.4) | 87 (61.3) | 97 (59.5) |
| Hospital visits | 36 (24.8) | 34 (23.9) | 38 (23.3) |
| Home visits | 71 (49.0) | 66 (46.5) | 73 (44.8) |
| Telephone calls | 80 (55.2) | 73 (51.4) | 81 (49.7) |
| Prenatal and postnatal | | | |
| Any contact | 117 (80.7) | 111 (78.2) | 124 (76.1) |
| Both | 68 (46.9) | 67 (47.2) | 72 (44.2) |

Abbreviations: MC, medical care; OMC, outside medical care.
*Data are presented as number (percentage). The MC data connote participants' infants with 1 or more encounters identified in the computerized medical center data for any reason, not including predischarge newborn data, up to 12 months of age. The OMC data connote participants who ever provided self-reported data about their infant's use of health care up to 12 months of age.

BFS illness (gastrointestinal [>1], respiratory tract including asthma [>2], respiratory tract excluding asthma [>2], and otitis media [>1]). Both treatment groups had similar patterns of OMC and MC visits, suggesting limited surveillance bias.

### VISITS WITH ILLNESS AND BFS ILLNESS DIAGNOSES: MULTIVARIATE LINEAR REGRESSION

**Table 6** presents the multivariate linear regression analysis of factors associated with any illness and BFS illness diagnosis–related visits. Results are shown for analyses after adjustment for any covariates that were associated with the outcomes at $P \leq .20$ in bivariate analysis. Apart from treatment group, adjusted and unadjusted β coefficients and 95% confidence intervals are given only for variables with adjusted β coefficients ($P < .05$).

Only otitis media visits were reduced, in a subset of the intervention group. Infants of controls without Medicaid had significantly more ($P \leq .03$) otitis media–related visits (mean [SD]=0.88 [1.73]; data not shown) than infants of intervention group participants without Medicaid (mean [SD]=0.36 [0.98]; data not shown) (ie, a Medicaid-by–treatment group interaction). Treatment group was not associated with reduced visits for respiratory tract or gastrointestinal illness. Gastrointestinal illness visits were reduced in infants of multiparous women (multiparous mean [SD]=0.85 [1.57]; primiparous mean [SD]=0.71 [3.06]; data not shown). The number of respiratory tract illness visits was greater for boys.

Boys had more visits with illness diagnoses (boys: mean [SD]=7.77 [8.84]; girls: mean [SD]=5.27 [5.93]; data not shown) and more visits with any BFS illness diagnoses (boys: mean [SD]=6.14 [9.68]; girls: mean [SD]=3.77 [4.83]; data not shown). Medicaid was associated with more BFS illness diagnosis–related visits in the intervention group (mean [SD]=5.56 [9.13] vs mean [SD]=3.91 [6.91] for those without Medicaid; data not shown), but there was no such difference among controls (ie, a Medicaid-by–treatment group interaction).

## COMMENT

This RCT assessed the effect of a prenatal and postnatal LC intervention on infant respiratory tract–, gastrointestinal-, and otitis media–related outpatient and ED visits up to 12 months. In multivariate analysis, treatment effects for respiratory tract, gastrointestinal, any BFS, and any illness visits were not statistically significant. For otitis media, there was a significant treatment group–by-Medicaid interaction, with reduced visits for the intervention group's non-Medicaid participants relative to its Medicaid participants. Possibly, lack of coverage for health visits in this low-income sample combined with the intervention to reduce the number of otitis media–related visits. Infant visits for otitis media (39% in the intervention group vs 47% of controls) are comparable to national data; 44% of infants 12 months or younger have an episode of otitis media.[35] As reported elsewhere, the intervention group had significantly greater breastfeeding intensity in multivariate analysis.[25]

Boys, who have greater susceptibility to infections,[36] had more sick care, combined BFS illness, and respiratory tract illness visits than the sample's girls. Infants of multiparous vs primiparous mothers in our sample had more gastrointestinal illness visits, consistent with other data.[12,17] The BFS illness visits were reduced in the intervention group's non-Medicaid participants relative to its Medicaid participants. It is not clear why no such difference was found among controls.

Our finding of only modest effects is undoubtedly related to relatively low LC contact in the intervention group. Analyses were based on intent to treat. The MILK LCs were part-time consultants. Just 44% of the intervention group had both prenatal and postnatal LC contact; 24% had no LC contact at all. Some declined LC assistance when contacted; others were difficult to locate in a timely manner. Immediate postpartum assistance is critical for establishing breastfeeding. This lack of a routine physical presence, and integration with clinic staff in particular, impeded the LCs' ability to contact women. Greater intervention contact would likely have led to greater breastfeeding intensity and reduced infant illness.

In addition, the low rate and lack of group difference in exclusive breastfeeding rates may have blunted the intervention's effect. Power analyses were based on data comparing infants exclusively breastfed for 3 months (34% and 14% in 2 middle-class, primarily non-Hispanic white samples) to never-breastfed infants.[27] In sharp contrast, exclusive breastfeeding in the MILK study declined from a high at 2 weeks (20% in the intervention group and 19% in the control group; $P \leq .80$) to half that at 3 months (9% in the intervention group and 11% in the control group; $P \leq .45$).

Findings from our sample (low-income, multiethnic women; 60% multiparous) may have limited generaliz-

**Table 5. Visits for Breastfeeding Sensitive Diagnoses by Data Source: Descriptive Data***

| Visit | Intervention (n = 163) OMC | MC | Total | Control (n = 175) OMC | MC | Total |
|---|---|---|---|---|---|---|
| ED visits | | | | | | |
| >1 GI illness | 0 | 4 (2.3) | 4 (2.3) | 0 | 4 (2.1) | 4 (2.1) |
| >2 Respiratory tract illnesses | 0 | 10 (5.7) | 10 (5.7) | 0 | 9 (4.8) | 9 (4.8) |
| >1 Case of otitis media | 0 | 2 (1.1) | 2 (1.1) | 0 | 7 (3.7) | 7 (3.7) |
| Outpatient visits | | | | | | |
| >1 GI illness | 0 | 33 (8.9) | 33 (18.9) | 0 | 41 (21.7) | 41 (21.7) |
| >2 Respiratory tract illnesses | 38 (21.7) | 77 (44.0) | 115 (65.7) | 56 (29.6) | 81 (42.9) | 137 (72.5) |
| >1 Case of otitis media | 32 (18.3) | 37 (21.1) | 69 (39.4) | 48 (25.4) | 41 (21.7) | 89 (47.1) |

Abbreviations: ED, emergency department; GI, gastrointestinal; MC, medical care; OMC, outside medical care.
*Data are presented as number (percentage).

**Table 6. Visits With Illness and BFS Illness Diagnoses: Multiple Linear Regression Analysis***

| Characteristic | β (95% CI) Illness | BFS Illness | GI Illness | Respiratory Tract Illness | Otitis Media |
|---|---|---|---|---|---|
| Treatment group | | | | | |
| Adjusted | −0.06 (−0.29 to 0.17) | 0.25 (−0.10 to 0.59) | 0.03 (−0.09 to 0.16) | 0.22 (−0.09 to 0.53) | 0.20 (0.00 to 0.39)†‡ |
| Unadjusted | −0.07 (−0.28 to 0.14) | 0.01 (−0.20 to 0.23) | 0.03 (−0.10 to 0.16) | −0.02 (−0.21 to 0.18) | 0.02 (−0.11 to 0.15) |
| Maternal Medicaid use by treatment group | | | | | |
| Adjusted | | −0.49 (−0.95 to 0.03)† | | −0.48 (−0.89 to −0.06)† | −0.32 (−0.58 to −0.05)† |
| Unadjusted | | −0.41 (−0.84 to 0.03) | | −0.39 (−0.78 to 0.00) | −0.32 (−0.58 to −0.05) |
| Maternal parity | | | | | |
| Adjusted | | | −0.13 (−0.26 to 0.00)† | | |
| Unadjusted | | | −0.13 (−0.26 to 0.00) | | |
| Infant sex | | | | | |
| Adjusted | 0.30 (0.07 to 0.53)† | 0.24 (0.02 to 0.47)† | | 0.22 (0.01 to 0.43)† | |
| Unadjusted | 0.30 (0.07 to 0.53) | 0.26 (0.03 to 0.49) | | 0.23 (0.03 to 0.44) | |

Abbreviations: BFS, breastfeeding sensitive; CI, confidence interval; GI, gastrointestinal.
*The β coefficients refer to regression models for which the outcome is the log of the number of visits +1. None of the following were associated with the outcomes and are therefore excluded from the Table: maternal variables: age, educational level, marital status, US born, race/ethnicity, previously breastfed, and baseline breastfeeding intention; infant variables: low birth weight, neonatal intensive care unit admission, maternal perception of newborn health problem, day care use, and age at last interview.
†$P<.05$.
‡There was a significant interaction between treatment and Medicaid. In this model, treatment group was significant for non-Medicaid participants ($P\leq.03$) but not for Medicaid participants ($P\leq.20$).

ability to other groups. Certainly, Medicaid's interaction with treatment group suggests that findings might differ in samples with equal coverage for health visits. Our intervention had a stronger effect on breastfeeding among multiparous women.[25] Simultaneously, infants of multiparous women had more gastrointestinal illness visits. Thus, there are likely to be differences by parity in terms of both infant illness and patterns of health care use.

A study strength is the combination of both MC computerized data and self-reported OMC visits. Nationally, the average number of office visits for children at less than 200% of the federal poverty level is 5.08 for children younger than 1 year. Rates for children above the federal poverty level are similar (Suk-fong Tang, PhD, American Academy of Pediatrics, written communication, December 19, 2003). Our sample's mean (SD) number of sick care visits alone (MC and OMC) was 7.04 (7.38), suggesting relatively high ascertainment of infant health outcomes.

In comparison with previous data on breastfeeding interventions and child health, our findings differ with regard to exclusive breastfeeding and health care outcomes. In the large Belarus trial of a hospital-based intervention, intervention site infants vs controls were more likely to be exclusively breastfed at 3 months (43.3% vs 6.4%; $P\leq.001$) and 6 months (7.9% vs 0.6%; $P\leq.001$). The incidence of gastrointestinal illness was reduced, but that of respiratory tract infections and otitis media were not.[21] In a Mexican home-based peer counselor trial, rates of exclusive breastfeeding were increased and diarrhea incidence decreased by more than half.[14]

Our intervention group's increased breastfeeding intensity was apparently sufficient to yield a reduction in otitis media–related visits, at least among participants without Medicaid. We found no treatment group differences in exclusive breastfeeding, which remained low throughout the study. On the basis of these trials, we posit that had there been differences in exclusive breastfeeding rates, gastrointestinal illness–related visits might also have been reduced.

In conclusion, future interventions with low-income, multiethnic women must increase breastfeeding intensity significantly if they are to demonstrably affect infant health. At the same time, intervention levels need to be feasible in practice.[37] Clearly, achieving the proposed *Healthy People 2010* goal of 60% of women exclusively breastfeeding at 3 months will be challenging.[38]

**Accepted for Publication:** April 22, 2006.
**Correspondence:** Karen A. Bonuck, PhD, Department of Epidemiology and Population Health, Montefiore Medical Center/Albert Einstein College of Medicine, 111 E 210th St, Bronx, NY 10467 (kbonuck@montefiore.org).
**Author Contributions:** *Study concept and design:* Bonuck, Freeman, and Trombley. *Acquisition of data:* Bonuck and Trombley. *Analysis and interpretation of data:* Freeman. *Drafting of the manuscript:* Bonuck and Freeman. *Critical revision of the manuscript for important intellectual content*: Bonuck, Freeman, and Trombley. *Statistical analysis:* Freeman and Trombley. *Obtained funding:* Bonuck. *Administrative, technical, and material support:* Bonuck and Trombley. *Study supervision:* Bonuck.
**Funding/Support:** This study was supported by grants from the US Department of Agriculture, the Maternal and Child Health Bureau, and the Agency for Healthcare Quality and Research.

## REFERENCES


1. Kramer MS, Kakuma R. *The Optimal Duration of Exclusive Breastfeeding: A Systematic Review.* Geneva, Switzerland: Dept of Nutrition for Health and Development, Dept of Child and Adolescent Health and Development; 2002.
2. Aniansson G, Alm B, Andersson B, et al. A prospective cohort study on breastfeeding and otitis media in Swedish infants. *Pediatr Infect Dis J.* 1994;13:183-188.
3. Pisacane A, Impagliazzo N, De Caprio C, Criscuolo L, Inglese A, Pereira de Silva MC. Breastfeeding and tonsillectomy. *BMJ.* 1996;312:746-747.
4. Duncan B, Ey J, Holberg CJ, Wright AL, Martinez FD, Taussig LM. Exclusive breastfeeding for at least 4 months protects against otitis media. *Pediatrics.* 1993;91:867-872.
5. Knishkowy B, Palti H, Adler B, Tepper D. Effect of otitis media on development: a community-based study. *Early Hum Dev.* 1991;26:101-111.
6. Scariati PD, Grummer-Strawn LM, Fein SB. A longitudinal analysis of infant morbidity and the extent of breast-feeding in the United States. *Pediatrics.* 1997;99:e5.
7. Alho OP, Koivu M, Sorri M, Rantakallio P. Risk factors for recurrent acute otitis media and respiratory infection in infancy. *Int J Pediatr Otorhinolaryngol.* 1990;19:151-161.
8. Duffy LC, Faden H, Wasielewski R, Wolf J, Krystofik D. Exclusive breastfeeding protects against bacterial colonization and day care exposure to otitis media. *Pediatrics.* 1997;100:e7.
9. Chantry CJ, Howard CR, Auinger P. Full breastfeeding duration and associated decrease in respiratory tract infection in US children. *Pediatrics.* 2006;117:425-432.
10. Beaudry M, Dufour R, Marcoux S. Relation between infant feeding and infections during the first six months of life. *J Pediatr.* 1995;126:191-197.
11. Pisacane A, Graziano L, Zona G, et al. Breastfeeding and acute lower respiratory infection. *Acta Paediatr.* 1994;83:714-718.
12. Sinha A, Madden J, Ross-Degnan D, et al. Reduced risk of respiratory infections among breastfed girls but not boys. *Pediatrics.* 2003;112:e303-e307.
13. Dewey KG, Heinig MJ, Nommsen-Rivers LA. Differences in morbidity between breast-fed and formula-fed infants. *J Pediatr.* 1995;126:696-702.
14. López-Alarcón M, Villalpandro S, Fajardo A. Breast-feeding lowers the frequency and duration of acute respiratory infection and diarrhea in infants under six months of age. *J Nutr.* 1997;127:436-443.
15. Cushing AH, Samet JM, Lambert WE, et al. Breastfeeding reduces risk of respiratory illness in infants. *Am J Epidemiol.* 1998;147:863-870.
16. Baker D, Taylor H, Henderson H. Inequality in infant mortality: causes and consequences in England in the 1990s. *J Epidemiol Community Health.* 1998;52:451-458.
17. Raisler J, Alexander C, O'Campo C. Breast-feeding and infant illness: a dose-response relationship. *Am J Public Health.* 1999;90:1478-1479.
18. Li R, Darling N, Maurice E, Barker L, Grummer-Strawn LM. Breastfeeding rates in the United States by characteristics of the child, mother, or family: the 2002 National Immunization Survey. *Pediatrics.* 2005;115:e31-e37.
19. US Department of Health and Human Services. *Healthy People 2010, Volumes I and II.* Washington, DC: US Dept of Health and Human Services, Public Health Service, Office of the Assistant Secretary for Health; 2000.
20. Ryan AS, Wenjun Z, Acosta A. Breastfeeding continues to increase into the new millennium. *Pediatrics.* 2002;110:1103-1109.
21. Kramer MS, Chalmers B, Hodnett E, et al. Promotion of Breastfeeding Intervention Trial (PROBIT): a randomized trial in the Republic of Belarus. *JAMA.* 2001;285:413-420.
22. Anderson AK, Damio G, Young S, Chapman DJ, Perez-Escamilla R. A randomized trial assessing the efficacy of peer counseling on exclusive breastfeeding in a predominantly Latina low-income community. *Arch Pediatr Adolesc Med.* 2005;159:836-841.
23. Pugh LC, Milligan RA, Frick KD, Spatz D, Bronner Y. Breastfeeding duration, costs, and benefits of a support program for low-income breast-feeding women. *Birth.* 2002;29:95-100.
24. US Preventive Services Task Force. Behavioral Intentions to Promote Breastfeeding: Recommendations and Rationale. July 2003. http://www.ahrq.gov/clinic/3rduspstf/brstfeed/brfeedrr.htm. Accessed June 5, 2006.
25. Bonuck KA, Trombley M, Freeman K, McKee D. Randomized controlled trial of a pre- and post-natal lactation consultant intervention upon duration and intensity of breastfeeding up to 12 months. *Pediatrics.* 2005;116:1413-1426.
26. American Association for Public Opinion Research. *Standard Definitions: Final Dispositions of Case Codes and Outcome Rate for Surveys.* Ann Arbor, Mich: American Association for Public Opinion Research; 2000.
27. Perrin JM, Ball TM, Wright AL. Health care costs of formula feeding in the first year of life. *J Ambul Pediatr Assoc.* 1999;103(suppl):870-876.
28. International Board of Lactation Consultant Examiners. http://www.iblce.org. Accessed April 7, 2006.
29. Labbok M, Krasovek K. Toward consistency in breastfeeding definition. *Stud Fam Plann.* 1991;12:226-230.
30. Labbok MH, Coffin CJ. A call for consistency in definition of breastfeeding behaviors. *Soc Sci Med.* 1997;44:1931-1932.
31. World Health Organization. *Indicators for Assessing Breast-feeding Practices.* Geneva, Switzerland: World Health Organization; 1991.
32. Wikipedia. List of ICD-9 codes. http://en.wikipedia.org/wiki/List_of_ICD-9_codes. Accessed June 9, 2006.
33. Moritz ML, Manole MD, Bogen DL, Ayus JC. Breastfeeding-associated hypernatremia: are we missing the diagnosis? *Pediatrics.* 2005;116:e343-e347.
34. Gourley GR, Li Z, Kreamer BL, Kosorok MR. A controlled, randomized double-blind trial of prophylaxis against jaundice among breastfed newborns. *Pediatrics.* 2005;116:385-391.
35. Auinger P, Lamphear BP, Kalwarf HJ, Mansour ME. Trends in otitis media among children in the United States. *Pediatrics.* 2003;112:514-520.
36. Green MS. The male predominance in the incidence of infectious diseases in children: a postulated explanation for disparities in the literature [published correction appears in *Int J Epidemiol.* 1992;21:1199]. *Int J Epidemiol.* 1992;21:381-386.
37. Bonuck KA. Increased exclusive breastfeeding rates fall short of proposed Healthy People 2010 goals. *Arch Pediatr Adolesc Med.* 2006;160:324.
38. Department of Health and Human Services. Healthy People 2010 Midcourse Review: Revised Objectives for 16-19: Breastfeeding. http://www.healthypeople.gov/data/midcourse/comments/faobjective.asp?id=16&subid=19. Accessed October 7, 2005.

ARTICLE

# Relationship Between the Decision to Take a Child to the Clinic for Abdominal Pain and Maternal Psychological Distress

*Rona L. Levy, MSW, PhD, MPH; Shelby L. Langer, PhD; Lynn S. Walker, PhD; Lauren D. Feld; William E. Whitehead, PhD*

**Background:** Among adults with functional gastrointestinal disorders, psychological distress influences who consults a physician, but little is known about predictors of consultation when the patient is a child.

**Objective:** To determine the relative contributions of psychological symptoms of the mother, psychological symptoms of the child, severity of child abdominal pain, and family stress to consultation.

**Design:** Observational study.

**Setting:** Health maintenance organization.

**Participants:** Two hundred seventy-five mothers of 334 children who had abdominal pain in the past 2 weeks, as per child self-report.

**Main Outcome Measures:** Mothers completed questionnaires about themselves (Symptom Checklist 90–Revised) and their children (school absences, medication use, and the Child Behavior Checklist). Children completed the Pain Beliefs Questionnaire to assess perceived pain severity.

**Results:** Thirty-nine children had been taken to the clinic for abdominal pain symptoms at least once in the past 3 months (consulters), whereas 295 were nonconsulters. Logistic regression analyses revealed that both the child's self-report of perceived pain severity ($P<.001$) and maternal psychological symptoms ($P=.006$) predicted consultation. Although children who visited physicians had significantly more psychological symptoms, this was not a significant predictor of consultation after adjusting for maternal psychological symptoms. Family stress did not predict consultation.

**Conclusion:** The decision to take a child to the clinic for abdominal pain is best predicted by maternal psychological distress and the child's perceived pain severity.

*Arch Pediatr Adolesc Med. 2006;160:961-965*

**Author Affiliations:** School of Social Work (Drs Levy and Langer) and School of Medicine and Department of Psychology (Dr Levy), University of Washington, and Lakeside School (Ms Feld), Seattle; Department of Adolescent Medicine and Behavioral Science, Vanderbilt University Medical Center, Nashville, Tenn (Dr Walker); and Center for Functional GI and Motility Disorders, University of North Carolina at Chapel Hill (Dr Whitehead).

AMONG ADULTS WITH UNEXplained (functional) abdominal pain, it has been reported that consulting behavior is influenced by the severity of abdominal pain,[1] the presence of distressing psychological symptoms,[2-4] and exposure to stressful life events.[5] A variety of studies have investigated the determinants of physician consultation when the patient is a child. In some of these studies, predictors of physician consultation included child demographic characteristics (younger age or lower educational level), pain intensity, pain frequency, and school absenteeism.[6,7] Because the actual decision to consult is made by parents, a related body of research has focused on the psychological traits of the parents instead of, or in addition to, the sociodemographic characteristics, traits, and symptoms of the child. This research has suggested that child health care utilization is related to parental anxiety, somatization, or maternal health care utilization.[8-15] However, limitations exist in all of these studies, including (1) relatively small sample sizes; (2) reliance on volunteers from the community rather than randomly selected participants, which could lead to biased sampling; (3) parent rather than child report of children's symptoms, potentially confounding parental perceptions and psychological distress; and (4) failure to assess the relative contribution of parental, family, and child distress. Furthermore, most of this research has focused on general consulting rather than abdominal pain in children, a common reason for seeking health care for children and the most frequent reason for visits to pediatric gastroenterologists.[16] Therefore, the aim of this study was to assess the relative contribution of the following variables to physician consultation for a child's abdominal pain:

severity of the child's self-reported abdominal pain, the child's psychological symptoms, the mother's psychological symptoms, and family stress.

## METHODS

### SUBJECTS

This study was part of a larger study[17] looking at children of parents who either did or did not have irritable bowel syndrome (IBS). Families with IBS were identified by reviewing the automated database of a large health maintenance organization to identify all women who had received a diagnosis of IBS or abdominal pain at a clinic visit during the preceding 2 years. Non-IBS families were selected from the same database by identifying women who did not have a clinic visit during the preceding 2 years for IBS, abdominal pain, constipation, or diarrhea. Additionally, only families who had 1 or more children between the ages of 8 and 15 years were selected from the database. All potential study subjects were further screened by trained telephone interviewers to determine whether the mother met Rome II criteria for IBS diagnosis.[18] Other inclusion criteria ascertained in the telephone interview were that (1) the mother was the child's legal guardian and the child had lived with her for at least half of the time during the preceding 2 years, (2) no interviewed child had a developmental disability requiring full-time special education, and (3) no family member had a diagnosis of ulcerative colitis or Crohn disease.

This process resulted in 1447 families being initially selected from the database. Of these, 789 (54.5%) agreed to be further screened by telephone, and 857 (59.2%) of the initial 1447 families were then determined to be eligible. The participation rate was 97% among those determined to be eligible during the telephone interview. This resulted in a final sample of 334 children and 275 mothers.

The study was reviewed and approved by the human subjects review boards for the Group Health Cooperative, the University of Washington, and the University of North Carolina at Chapel Hill (the data management site).

### PROCEDURE AND MEASURES

All assessments were conducted by means of a single interview in the home. Child assessments were administered orally, face to face. These assessments were conducted by graduate-level mental health professionals who received extensive training in standardized questionnaire administration. Mothers independently completed a battery of pencil-and-paper questionnaires (in the home while the child was being interviewed). Measures are described as follows.

### CHILD REPORT MEASURES

#### Abdominal Pain in the Past 2 Weeks

This symptom was assessed with an item from the Children's Somatization Inventory,[19,20] a measure of children's nonspecific somatic symptoms. Ratings were made on a 0-4 scale: not at all (0), a little (1), some (2), a lot (3) and a whole lot (4) for the single item of "pain in your stomach or abdomen." As described previously, the sample was limited to those children who provided a rating of 1 or higher; that is, those who experienced at least "a little" pain in the past 2 weeks. Stated conversely, children with no pain were excluded. The Children's Somatization Inventory has excellent reliability and validity.

#### Perceived Pain Severity

The Pain Beliefs Questionnaire[21] contains 32 statements about stomachaches. Sample items are "My stomachaches mean I have a serious illness," and "When I have a bad stomachache, it usually lasts a long time." Children were asked to respond to each statement by rating how true it was for their stomachaches (in general). There were 5 possible answers ranging from "not at all true" to "very true." The 32 questions are scored for 5 different subscales that describe different dimensions of symptom severity (eg, condition seriousness, condition duration, condition frequency, episode intensity, and episode duration) and 2 subscales that describe how the child copes (eg, problem-focused coping potential and emotion-focused coping potential). The 5 symptom severity dimensions can be summed together to form a total score; this summary index was used as the measure of severity of the child's abdominal pain. The Pain Beliefs Questionnaire was found to have adequate validity and reliability.[21]

### PARENT REPORT MEASURES

#### Maternal Psychological Distress

Mothers were asked to complete the anxiety, depression, and somatization subscales of the Symptom Checklist 90–Revised (a total of 35 items).[22] These 3 subscales were summed together to create a single index of overall psychological distress, as is recommended in the Brief Symptom Inventory-18, which is the short form of the Symptom Checklist 90–Revised. The Global Symptom Index of the Brief Symptom Inventory-18, computed in this way, was shown to be valid and reliable.[22]

#### Child Psychological Distress

Mothers completed the Child Behavior Checklist for children aged 4 to 18 years.[23,24] This is a valid, reliable, and frequently used scale to assess behavioral problems in children. The Child Behavior Checklist is conventionally scored for 2 broad dimensions of behavioral problems: internalizing and externalizing. The Internalizing scale is the sum of 3 subscales (withdrawn, somatic complaints, and anxious/depressed) that correspond to the dimensions measured in the mothers. For the purposes of this study, the Internalizing scale was used as an index of psychological distress in the child, and this score was converted to a sex-appropriate T score to facilitate pooling of boys and girls.

#### Family Stress

The Family Inventory of Life Events is a parental report form that assesses potentially stressful negative life events experienced by family members in the previous year. McCubbin et al[25] report that internal consistency reliability is 0.81 and 4-week test-retest reliability is 0.80. Agreement between family members on the occurrence of events supports the validity of the Family Inventory of Life Events.

#### Consultation for Abdominal Pain

Mothers were asked, "In the past 3 months, how many times did your child go to the doctor for abdominal pain?" Choices were "none," "1-3 days," "4-6 days," "7-9 days," and "10 or more days." Children were classified as consulting a physician for abdominal pain if the response was anything other than "none."

**Table 1. Demographic Characteristics of the Sample***

| Characteristic | Value |
|---|---|
| Maternal characteristics | |
| No. of subjects | 275 |
| Age, mean ± SD, y | 42.9 ± 5.8 |
| Ethnicity, No. (%) | |
| White | 225 (82) |
| African American | 16 (6) |
| Asian | 17 (6) |
| Hispanic | 6 (2) |
| Other | 7 (3) |
| Unknown | 4 (2) |
| Educational status, No. (%) | |
| <High school | 5 (2) |
| High school degree | 27 (10) |
| Some college or technical school | 115 (42) |
| 4-year college degree | 51 (18) |
| Graduate school | 75 (27) |
| Unknown | 2 (1) |
| Employment status, No. (%) | |
| Not employed | 52 (19) |
| Employed part-time | 69 (25) |
| Employed full-time | 150 (54) |
| Unknown | 4 (2) |
| Living situation, No. (%) | |
| Married or cohabiting | 220 (80) |
| Adult roommates or adult family members | 10 (4) |
| No other adults in the home | 36 (13) |
| Separated | 5 (2) |
| Unknown | 4 (2) |
| Child characteristics | |
| No. of subjects | 334 |
| Age, mean ± SD, y | 12.1 ± 2.5 |
| Age, range, y | 8-17 |
| Sex, No. (%) | |
| Male | 149 (45) |
| Female | 185 (55) |
| Ethnicity, No. (%) | |
| White | 271 (81) |
| African American | 20 (6) |
| Asian | 19 (6) |
| Hispanic | 9 (3) |
| Other | 11 (3) |
| Unknown | 4 (1) |
| Severity of abdominal pain in past 2 wk, No. (%) | |
| A little | 207 (62) |
| Some | 80 (24) |
| A lot | 41 (12) |
| A whole lot | 6 (2) |

*Percentages may not total 100 because of rounding.

## DATA ANALYSIS

Unpaired *t* tests and $\chi^2$ tests were used to compare consulters (those taken to the medical clinic for gastrointestinal symptoms at least once in the past 3 months) and nonconsulters (those not taken to the medical clinic for gastrointestinal symptoms in the past 3 months) with respect to demographic, clinical, and psychosocial variables. Bivariate correlations were used to examine relationships among the predictor variables. Logistic regression was used to determine which of 4 variables (abdominal pain symptom severity, maternal psychological distress, child psychological distress, and family stress) contributed significantly to consulting behavior. This was a 2-step process. Each variable was first analyzed via univariate regression, with just that predictor entered into the model. Those variables that significantly predicted consultation in univariate regressions were then analyzed via stepwise regression. For all analyses, $\alpha = .05$.

**Table 2. Clinical and Psychosocial Characteristics as a Function of Gastrointestinal Consulting Behavior***

| | Consulters | Nonconsulters | *P* Value |
|---|---|---|---|
| No. of subjects | 39 | 295 | NA |
| Maternal psychological distress (parent)† | 2.82 (2.03) | 1.95 (1.59) | .002 |
| Perceived pain severity (child)‡ | 32.59 (13.46) | 25.47 (9.5) | .003 |
| Child psychological distress (parent)§ | 56.67 (7.34) | 52.47 (10.57) | .002 |
| Family stress (parent)‖ | 13.21 (6.67) | 11.62 (6.25) | .14 |
| No. of school absences, past 3 mo | 1.03 (0.84) | 0.31 (0.60) | <.001 |
| No. of times took medicine for abdominal pain, past 3 mo | 1.41 (1.21) | 0.30 (0.64) | <.001 |

Abbreviation: NA, not applicable.
*Results are expressed as mean (SD) unless otherwise indicated.
†Sum of anxiety, depression, and somatization subscales of the Symptom Checklist 90–Revised.
‡Pain Beliefs Questionnaire total severity score.
§Child Behavior Checklist Internalizing scale.
‖Family Inventory of Life Events.

## RESULTS

### CHARACTERISTICS OF THE SAMPLE

Demographic and clinical characteristics of the sample are listed in **Table 1**. Mothers were, on average, 42 years old. Most mothers were white (82%), as were their children (81%). Just under one half of the mothers had received at least a 4-year college degree (45%, with 27% having attended graduate school). Employment status was mixed, with 19% unemployed, 25% employed part-time, and 55% employed full-time. Finally, 80% of mothers were married or cohabiting with a partner.

The mean child age was 12.1 years; sex distribution was fairly even (55% female). Children varied in their reports of abdominal pain during the past 2 weeks: 207 (62%) reported "a little pain"; 80 (24%), "some pain"; 41 (12%), "a lot of pain"; and just 6 (2%), "a whole lot of pain."

**Table 2** compares clinical and psychosocial characteristics of consulters and nonconsulters. Children who were brought to the clinic for stomachaches perceived greater pain severity than children with stomachaches who were not brought to the clinic, as per the Pain Beliefs Questionnaire ($P = .003$). They were also more likely to miss school and to take medicine for abdominal pain ($P < .001$ for both). Mothers of consulters reported greater psychological distress than did mothers of nonconsulters ($P = .002$). Similarly, consulting children were rated higher on the Child Behavior Checklist (our measure of child psychological distress) by their parents as compared with nonconsulting children ($P = .002$). Consulters and nonconsulters did not differ with respect to family stress ($P = .14$).

**Table 3. Pearson Correlations Among the Predictor Variables***

| | Maternal Psychological Distress | Perceived Pain Severity | Child Psychological Distress | Family Stress |
|---|---|---|---|---|
| Maternal psychological distress (parent) | NA | .078 | .390† | .408† |
| Perceived pain severity (child) | NA | NA | .171† | .027 |
| Child psychological distress (parent) | NA | NA | NA | .381† |
| Family stress (parent) | NA | NA | NA | NA |

Abbreviation: NA, not applicable.
*Sample sizes range from 328 to 334.
†$P<.01$.

**Table 4. Logistic Regressions for Gastrointestinal Consulting Behavior**

| | Univariate | | | Multivariate | | |
|---|---|---|---|---|---|---|
| | β (SE) | OR | P Value* | β (SE) | OR | P Value |
| Maternal psychological distress (parent)† | .27 (.09) | 1.31 | .003 | .26 (.10) | 1.30 | .006 |
| Perceived pain severity (child)‡ | .06 (.02) | 1.06 | <.001 | .06 (.02) | 1.06 | <.001 |
| Child psychological distress (parent)§ | .04 (.02) | 1.04 | .02 | NA | NA | NA |
| Family stress (parent)‖ | .04 (.03) | 1.04 | .15 | NA | NA | NA |

Abbreviations: NA, not applicable; OR, odds ratio.
*Predictors associated with the outcome at $P<.05$ in univariate models were entered into a multivariate model.
†Sum of anxiety, depression, and somatization subscales of the Symptom Checklist 90–Revised.
‡Pain Beliefs Questionnaire total severity score.
§Child Behavior Checklist Internalizing scale.
‖Family Inventory of Life Events.

## RELATIONSHIPS AMONG PREDICTOR VARIABLES

**Table 3** displays Pearson correlations among the predictor variables. Significant positive correlations were found among maternal psychological distress, child psychological distress, and family stress (all rated by the mother). In addition, perceived pain severity (as rated by the child) was significantly related to child psychological distress (as rated by the mother). Perceived pain severity was unrelated to both maternal psychological distress and family stress.

## PREDICTORS OF CONSULTATION

Results of the logistic regressions are displayed in **Table 4**. In univariate regressions, maternal psychological symptoms, child psychological symptoms, and perceived pain severity all predicted consultation. However, in stepwise regression analysis, only maternal psychological symptoms and perceived pain severity were found to be significant predictors ($P=.006$ and $P<.001$, respectively).

To further support our findings, we conducted the same regressions using a slightly different sample based on maternal vs child ratings of pain severity in the past 2 weeks (again, excluding children with no pain). This sample included 323 children: 58 consulters and 265 nonconsulters. Results were the same. Only maternal psychological symptoms and perceived pain severity were entered into the final model ($\beta=.28$; odds ratio = 1.33; $P=.001$ for the former and $\beta=.04$; odds ratio = 1.04; $P=.02$ for the latter).

## COMMENT

A principal finding of this study is that a child's visit to the clinic for abdominal pain is best predicted by symptoms of psychological distress in the mother and severity of abdominal pain as reported by the child, rather than psychological distress in the child or family stress. The fact that most of the children in our sample were only in "a little" pain adds interest to this finding. It suggests that these parents are seeking health care even when their children's complaints are minor.

The correlations among the predictor variables are also of interest. Mothers' psychological distress did not correlate with child-reported pain severity, yet both were related to utilization. This lends support to the regression findings; both factors independently predict utilization.

As stated earlier, previous studies have found that some parental psychological factors as well as parental health care utilization are related to children's health care utilization. This study has demonstrated that these findings were replicated in the area of abdominal pain, a chronic and common childhood complaint. Furthermore, more recently, Janicke and Finney[26] refined the investigations of general children's health care utilization by determining that parental self-efficacy, in interaction with parental stress, contributed to children's utilization. They, along with others, have recommended that interventions targeted to reducing family stress were therefore a reasonable direction to reduce health care utilization. Our study suggests that these efforts might be more efficient when directed at parents, rather than efforts to reduce child distress or overall family stress factors, since neither child distress nor family stress appeared to be significant determinants of health care utilization, at least within this population.

One limitation of our study is that whereas other research has demonstrated that the father may have a significant influence on the illness behavior of the child,[8,27] the current study was limited by our ability to obtain data only from mothers. It is possible that had we measured the psychological traits of fathers in the group of parents, our findings may have been more robust.

Another area where a question might be raised concerns the subsample used and whether these findings would generalize to children with more severe pain. As mentioned previously, most children (62%) reported "a little pain," followed by "some pain" (24%), "a lot of pain" (12%), and "a whole lot of pain" (2%). To address this potential issue, we repeated the regression analyses and included all children with at least some pain (n=127). The findings did not change; maternal psychological distress and perceived pain severity both significantly predicted consultation.

In conclusion, this study adds support to the mounting evidence that children's health care utilization cannot be seen in isolation from environmental influences. Consulting for health care is based on a myriad of factors, from the child's response to physical symptoms to the way those in his or her environment react to this response. Ultimately, a parent's decision to consult is subjective, and psychological state can have a major effect on this decision. When the parent is distressed, this factor can have paramount influence on this decision. Our study has presented further evidence of which factors are the most important to focus on in assessing children's health care utilization. Future research should assess how addressing parental psychological distress could affect children's health care use patterns.

**Submitted for Publication:** December 22, 2005; final revision received March 28, 2006; accepted May 7, 2006.
**Correspondence:** Rona L. Levy, MSW, PhD, MPH, School of Social Work, University of Washington, 4101 15th Avenue NE, Box 354900, Seattle, WA, 98105 (rlevy@u.washington.edu).
**Author Contributions:** *Study concept and design:* Levy, Walker, and Whitehead. *Acquisition of data:* Levy, Walker, and Feld. *Analysis and interpretation of data:* Levy, Langer, Walker, and Whitehead. *Drafting of the manuscript:* Levy, Langer, and Walker. *Critical revision of the manuscript for important intellectual content*: Levy, Langer, Walker, Feld, and Whitehead. *Statistical analysis:* Levy, Langer, and Whitehead. *Obtained funding:* Levy. *Administrative, technical, and material support:* Levy, Feld, and Whitehead. *Study supervision:* Levy.
**Funding/Support:** This study was supported by grants RO1 HD36069, RO1 DK31369, and R24DK67674 from the National Institutes of Health.

## REFERENCES

1. Koloski NA, Talley NJ, Boyce PM. Predictors of health care seeking for irritable bowel syndrome and nonulcer dyspepsia: a critical review of the literature on symptom and psychosocial factors. *Am J Gastroenterol.* 2001;96:1340-1349.
2. Drossman DA, Mckee DC, Sandler RS, et al. Psychosocial factors in the irritable bowel syndrome: a multivariate study of patients and nonpatients with irritable bowel syndrome. *Gastroenterology.* 1988;95:701-708.
3. Whitehead WE, Bosmajian L, Zonderman AB, Costa PT, Schuster MM. Symptoms of psychologic distress associated with irritable bowel syndrome: comparison of community and medical clinic samples. *Gastroenterology.* 1988; 95:709-714.
4. Smith RC, Greenbaum DS, Vancouver JB, et al. Psychosocial factors associated with health care seeking rather than diagnosis in irritable bowel syndrome. *Gastroenterology.* 1990;98:293-301.
5. Whitehead WE, Crowell MD, Robinson JC, Heller BR, Schuster MM. Effects of stressful life events on bowel symptoms: subjects with irritable-bowel-syndrome compared with subjects without bowel dysfunction. *Gut.* 1992;33:825-830.
6. Perquin CW, Hazebroek-Kampschreur AA, Hunfeld JA, van Suijlekom-Smit LW, Passchier J, van der Wouden JC. Chronic pain among children and adolescents: physician consultation and medication use. *Clin J Pain.* 2000;16:229-235.
7. Perquin CW, Hunfeld JA, Hazebroek-Kampschreur AA, et al. Insights in the use of health care services in chronic benign pain in childhood and adolescence. *Pain.* 2001;94:205-213.
8. Levy RL, Whitehead WW, Von Korff M, Feld AD. Intergenerational transmission of gastrointestinal illness behavior. *Am J Gastroenterol.* 2000;95:451-456.
9. Berkanovic E, Telesky C. Social networks, beliefs and the decision to seek medical care: an analysis of congruent and incongruent patterns. *Med Care.* 1982; 20:1018-1026.
10. Garralda ME, Bailey D. Psychosomatic aspects of children's consultation in primary care. *Eur Arch Psychiatry Neurol Sci.* 1987;236:319-322.
11. Johnsen N, Engelstad F, Bruusgard D. The general practitioner and the family: a case study of the use of general practitioners' services by families with children. *Scand J Prim Health Care.* 1988;6:155-160.
12. Cafferata GL, Kasper JD. Family structure and children's use of ambulatory physician services. *Med Care.* 1985;23:350-360.
13. Lewis CE, Lewis MA, Lorimer A, Palmer BB. Child initiated care: the use of school nursing services by children in an "adult free" system. *Pediatrics.* 1977;60: 499-507.
14. Janicke DM, Finney JW, Riley AW. Children's health care use: a prospective investigation of factors related to care-seeking. *Med Care.* 2001;39:990-1001.
15. Riley AW, Finney JW, Mellits ED, et al. Determinants of children's health care use: an investigation of psychosocial factors. *Med Care.* 1993;31:767-783.
16. Fleisher DR, Feldman EJ. The biopsychosocial model of clinical practice in functional gastrointestinal disorder. In: Hyman PE, ed. *Pediatric Functional Gastrointestinal Disorders.* New York, NY: Academy Professional Information Services; 1999:1-20.
17. Levy RL, Whitehead WE, Walker LS, et al. Increased somatic complaints and health-care utilization in children: effects of parent IBS status and parent response to gastrointestinal symptoms. *Am J Gastroenterol.* 2004;99:2442-2451.
18. Thompson WG, Longstreth G, Drossman DA, Heaton K, Irvine EJ, Muller-Lissner S. Functional bowel disorders and functional abdominal pain. In: Drossman DA, Corazziari E, Talley NJ, Thompson WG, Whitehead WE, eds. *Rome II: The Functional Gastrointestinal Disorders.* 2nd ed. McLean, Va: Degnon Associates; 2000:351-432.
19. Garber J, Walker LS, Zeman JL. Somatization symptoms in a community sample of children and adolescents: further validation of the Children's Somatization Inventory. *Psychol Assess.* 1991;3:588-595.
20. Walker L, Garber J. *Manual for the Children's Somatization Inventory.* Nashville, Tenn: Vanderbilt University Medical Center, Department of Pediatrics; 2003.
21. Walker LS, Smith CA, Garber J, Claar RL. Testing a model of pain appraisal and coping in children with recurrent abdominal pain. *Health Psychol.* 2005;24:364-374.
22. Derogatis LR, Fitzpatrick M. The SCL-90-R, the Brief Symptom Inventory (BSI), and the BSI-18. In: Maruish ME, ed. *The Use of Psychological Testing for Treatment Planning and Outcomes Assessment: Volume 3: Instruments for Adults.* 3rd ed. Mahwah, NJ: Lawrence Erlbaum Associates; 2004:1-41.
23. Achenbach TM, Brown JS. *Bibliography of Published Studies Using the Child Behavior Checklist and Related Material.* Burlington, Vt: University Associates in Psychiatry; 1988.
24. Achenbach TM, Edelbrock C. *Manual for the Child Behavior Checklist and revised child behavior profile.* Burlington: University of Vermont; 1983.
25. McCubbin H, Patterson J, Wilson L. Family Inventory of Life Events and Changes (FILE). In: McCubbin HI, Thompson AI, McCubbin MA, eds. *Family Assessment: Resiliency, Coping and Adaptation-Inventories for Research and Practice.* Madison: University of Wisconsin System; 1996:103-178.
26. Janicke DM, Finney JW. Children's primary health care services: social-cognitive factors related to utilization. *J Pediatr Psychol.* 2003;28:547-557.
27. Lackner JM, Gudleski GB, Blanchard EB. Beyond abuse: the association among parenting style, abdominal pain and somatization in IBS patients. *Behav Res Ther.* 2004;42:41-56.

ARTICLE

# Effect of Missed Opportunities on Influenza Vaccination Rates Among Children With Asthma

*Kevin J. Dombkowski, DrPH, MS; Matthew M. Davis, MD, MAPP; Lisa M. Cohn, MS; Sarah J. Clark, MPH*

**Objectives:** To assess rates of influenza vaccination among children with asthma; document the frequency, timing, and patterns of missed opportunities to vaccinate during successive influenza seasons; and project potential influenza vaccination rates that could be achieved by reducing or eliminating missed opportunities.

**Setting:** Michigan Medicaid program during the 2001-2002 and 2002-2003 influenza seasons.

**Design:** Retrospective cohort analysis of administrative claims.

**Participants:** We evaluated the claims of 4358 children aged 5 to 18 years with persistent asthma who were continuously enrolled in Medicaid.

**Main Outcome Measures:** Influenza vaccinations and missed opportunities assessed using procedure and diagnosis codes.

**Results:** During the 2001-2002 season, 16.7% of children with asthma received an influenza vaccination; during 2002-2003, 21.8% received the vaccine (9.5% vaccinated in both seasons). However, 76.5% of children had at least 1 office visit during the 2001-2002 influenza season (75.3% during 2002-2003). Among children without influenza vaccination, 72.9% had at least 1 missed opportunity for vaccination during the 2001-2002 season and 69.3% during 2002-2003. The most common outcome was having at least 1 missed opportunity (39.6%) in each of 2 successive influenza seasons. Eliminating missed opportunities prior to the historical peak of influenza season would have increased the influenza vaccination rate among this population of children to 76%.

**Conclusions:** Missed opportunities for influenza vaccination among children with asthma are common and are often repeated from one influenza season to the next. Future studies should assess how interventions could be aimed at patients and health care professionals to improve awareness of the need for annual influenza vaccination.

*Arch Pediatr Adolesc Med. 2006;160:966-971*

ASTHMA IS A COMMON chronic disease that affects 9 million children in the United States.[1] The health services burden of asthma is substantial—especially among minority populations—often requiring physician office visits, emergency department (ED) visits, and hospitalizations.[2] Children with asthma are at increased risk for influenza-related morbidity and mortality[3-6] and consequently are recommended to receive an annual influenza vaccination.[7,8]

Despite these long-standing recommendations, many high-risk children remain unvaccinated each influenza season. Prior studies have reported vaccination rates ranging from 7% to 26%.[9-12] Somewhat higher rates have been observed among children with asthma in practice settings using reminder-recall notices for influenza vaccination, although even the most favorable of rates reported by primary care clinics are well below 50%.[13-15] One important factor that may influence influenza vaccination rates is missed opportunities to vaccinate. Missed opportunities are visits when a vaccine-eligible child is seen by a health care professional, yet no vaccine is administered. Missed opportunities are a well-documented barrier to primary vaccinations among children.[16-20] Prior studies of influenza vaccinations among children with asthma suggest that missed opportunities occur frequently and, if eliminated, could improve vaccination rates markedly.[10-12] However, this work has primarily focused on privately insured children in a single influenza season. We are unaware of any previous studies that have assessed missed opportunities for influenza vaccination among economically disadvantaged children or have considered the degree to which individuals experience missed opportunities during successive influenza seasons.

Our objective in this study was to characterize missed opportunities for influenza vaccination among a population of children with asthma enrolled in Medicaid. We were interested in identifying chil-

**Author Affiliations:** Child Health Evaluation and Research Unit, Division of General Pediatrics (Drs Dombkowski and Davis and Mss Cohn and Clark), and the Division of General Internal Medicine and the Gerald R. Ford School of Public Policy (Dr Davis), University of Michigan, Ann Arbor.

dren who missed opportunities for influenza vaccination in successive seasons to better understand the potential for improving and sustaining vaccination rates through interventions targeted at high-risk groups. Specifically, we sought to (1) assess influenza vaccination rates among children with asthma, (2) describe patterns of influenza vaccination and missed opportunities to vaccinate during successive influenza seasons, and (3) project potential improvements in influenza vaccination rates among this population by reducing missed opportunities to vaccinate during influenza season.

## METHODS

This study is based on a retrospective analysis of administrative claims data for the Michigan Medicaid program and was approved by the University of Michigan institutional review board.

### STUDY POPULATION

We identified a total of 4358 children between 5 and 18 years of age who were continuously enrolled in the Michigan Medicaid program, had no other source of health insurance, and had persistent asthma based on Health Plan Employer Data and Information Set (HEDIS) criteria for calendar years 2001 and 2002. The HEDIS persistent asthma criteria require administrative claims evidence of a child having any of the following within 2 consecutive calendar years: at least 4 asthma medication–dispensing events, at least 1 inpatient or 1 ED claim with a primary diagnosis of asthma, or at least 4 outpatient visits with an asthma diagnosis and at least 2 asthma medication–dispensing events.[21] The HEDIS criteria, detailed in a comprehensive list from the National Committee for Quality Assurance, classify an asthma medication–dispensing event as 1 prescription of a supply lasting 30 days or less.[22] Evidence suggests that the identification of asthma cases using claims from 2 consecutive years improves asthma classification specificity.[23,24]

Children younger than 5 years were excluded because the diagnosis of asthma is difficult among young children and administrative claims records may not reliably reflect persistent asthma cases for these age groups.[24] We excluded children with other health insurance in addition to Medicaid to ensure that claims for all health services during the study period were available in the Medicaid administrative data files. Medicaid program eligibility and demographic characteristics were obtained for each subject from the Medicaid administrative files, including all children enrolled in either a fee-for-service or managed care health plan during the study period.

### OUTCOME MEASURES

Four outcomes were measured for the 2001-2002 and 2002-2003 influenza seasons: (1) outpatient office visits, (2) influenza vaccinations, (3) missed opportunities for influenza vaccination, and (4) asthma ED visits. The date at which each outcome occurred was determined for the period from October 1 through January 31, which was considered the influenza vaccination season for this study. The Advisory Committee on Immunization Practices indicates that the optimal time to vaccinate is during October and November,[25] and evidence from a prior national study suggests that only a small proportion of physicians continue to administer influenza vaccine beyond the end of January, which is historically when the peak number of influenza cases occur.[26] No substantial vaccine shortages were experienced in Michigan during either of the observed influenza seasons, although a temporary delay was experienced early in the 2001-2002 season.[27]

Outpatient visits were identified based on *Current Procedural Terminology* (*CPT*) procedure codes or *International Classification of Diseases, Ninth Revision, Clinical Modification* (*ICD-9-CM*)[28] diagnosis codes, and the visit was classified as being for short-term or long-term care (ie, evaluation and management) or preventive medicine (including general medical examinations); home visits were not considered in this study. Office visits with *ICD-9-CM* diagnosis codes 493.0-493.9 were classified as asthma visits, and the date of each outpatient visit was recorded; information on physician specialty was not available. Similarly, asthma ED visits during each influenza season were also classified using *ICD-9-CM* diagnosis codes and CPT procedure codes (99281-99285). Influenza vaccinations were identified using CPT procedure codes (90657-90660 and 90724) and *ICD-9-CM* diagnosis codes (V048 and V066). In addition, vaccination records were obtained for calendar years 2001-2002 from the Michigan Childhood Immunization Registry (MCIR); MCIR data were not available for January 2003. The MCIR is a population-based registry that automatically initiates a record for each child born in Michigan based on input from electronic birth certificates. Health care professionals who provide vaccinations are required by Michigan law to report these to the MCIR. Vaccination records from the MCIR were merged with Medicaid claims by beneficiary identifier. If more than 1 influenza dose was administered during an influenza season, the first date of influenza vaccination (from either Medicaid claims or MCIR data) was recorded as the vaccination date. Missed opportunities were classified as the initial office visit occurring during the influenza vaccination season among children with no influenza vaccination; subsequent missed opportunities for each influenza season were not counted. The date of missed opportunity was recorded as the date of the index office visit during the influenza season at which an influenza vaccination was not administered.

### STATISTICAL ANALYSIS

We performed $\chi^2$ tests to assess differences in each outcome measured by demographic characteristics. Simulated influenza vaccination rates were estimated based on observed vaccination rates and the date of missed opportunities during the influenza seasons. The potential achievable influenza vaccination rate was estimated for 3 scenarios of potential reductions in missed opportunities (25%, 50%, and 100%) using the observed dates for first missed opportunities. For each scenario, a corresponding proportion of initial missed opportunities at any point in time (eg, every fourth, every other, or every missed opportunity) were classified as being immunized. Claims data reduction and summarization were conducted using SAS version 9 statistical software (SAS Institute Inc, Cary, NC).

## RESULTS

**Table 1** summarizes the demographic characteristics of our study population of 4358 children with persistent asthma; most (74.6%) of our study population was enrolled in the same Medicaid health plan throughout the 2-year study period. During the 2001-2002 influenza season, the 4358 children had a total of 14 609 office visits: 3335 children (76.5%) had at least 1 office visit, and 2828 (64.9%) had 2 or more visits. During the 2002-2003 influenza season, there were a total of 13 219 office visits: 3280 children (75.3%) had at least 1 office visit and 2682 (61.5%) had 2 or more visits. Most children (64.5%) had an office visit during both influenza seasons, whereas 12.7% had no visit during either season. Overall, the vast majority of children had at least 1 short-term or long-term care visit (74.5% for 2001-2002 and 72.8% for 2002-2003), followed by those with preventive medicine or general medical examinations (18.7% and 18.9%). During the 2001-2002 influenza season, 2025 children (46.5%) had at least 1 office visit with an asthma diagnosis reported (2039 [46.8%] in 2002-2003).

During the 2001-2002 season, 16.7% of children with asthma had an influenza vaccination; among the 3630 children not vaccinated, 2647 (72.9%) had at least 1 missed opportunity during that influenza season. During the 2002-2003 season, 21.8% of children with asthma had an influenza vaccination; among the 3408 children not vaccinated, 2363 (69.3%) had at least 1 missed opportunity. Two thirds of children with missed opportunities during the 2001-2002 season had at least 1 office visit with an asthma diagnosis (58.2% during 2002-2003).

**Figure 1** summarizes the proportion of children with influenza vaccination or missed opportunities during both influenza seasons. Less than 10% of children received influenza vaccinations in both seasons; the vast majority (71.0%) were not vaccinated in either season. The most common outcome during the 2 influenza seasons was having at least 1 missed opportunity in each season (39.6%). The timing of the first missed opportunity for unvaccinated children among those with at least 1 office visit is illustrated in **Table 2**. In both seasons, approximately half of the children experienced their initial missed opportunity in October, and nearly three quarters had their first missed opportunity by the end of November.

**Figure 2** contrasts outcomes for 3 groups of children during the 2002-2003 season: those having an influenza vaccination, a missed opportunity, or no office visit during the prior influenza season. For children with no office visits during the second influenza season, the figure also summarizes the frequency of asthma ED use. The figure illustrates that for each outcome observed during the first season, the same outcome was most common during the second season. For example, among the 728 children having an influenza vaccination during the first season, 414 (56.9%) also had an influenza vaccination during the following season. Children with a missed opportunity during the 2001-2002 season were most likely (65.1%) to also have a missed opportunity during the second season; similarly, children with no office visit during the first season were most likely (53.4%) to also have no office visit during the second season. Figure 2 illustrates that asthma ED use varied among children who had no office visits during the 2002-2003 influenza season, with the highest rates for the 525 children with no office visits in either influenza season. Compared with all other outcome groups, this group of children had the highest proportion of asthma ED users during the 2002-2003 season (23%; *P*=.004).

**Table 1. Characteristics of the Study Population**

| Characteristic | No. (%) |
|---|---|
| No. of subjects | 4358 |
| Age, y | |
| 5-9 | 1614 (37.1) |
| 10-14 | 1976 (45.3) |
| 15-18 | 768 (17.6) |
| Sex | |
| Male | 2571 (59.0) |
| Female | 1787 (41.0) |
| Race | |
| White | 1804 (41.4) |
| Black | 2299 (52.8) |
| All others | 255 (5.9) |
| Residence | |
| Urban | 3693 (84.7) |
| Nonurban | 665 (15.3) |
| Continuous enrollment in same Medicaid plan, mo | |
| <22 | 1108 (25.4) |
| ≥22 | 3250 (74.6) |

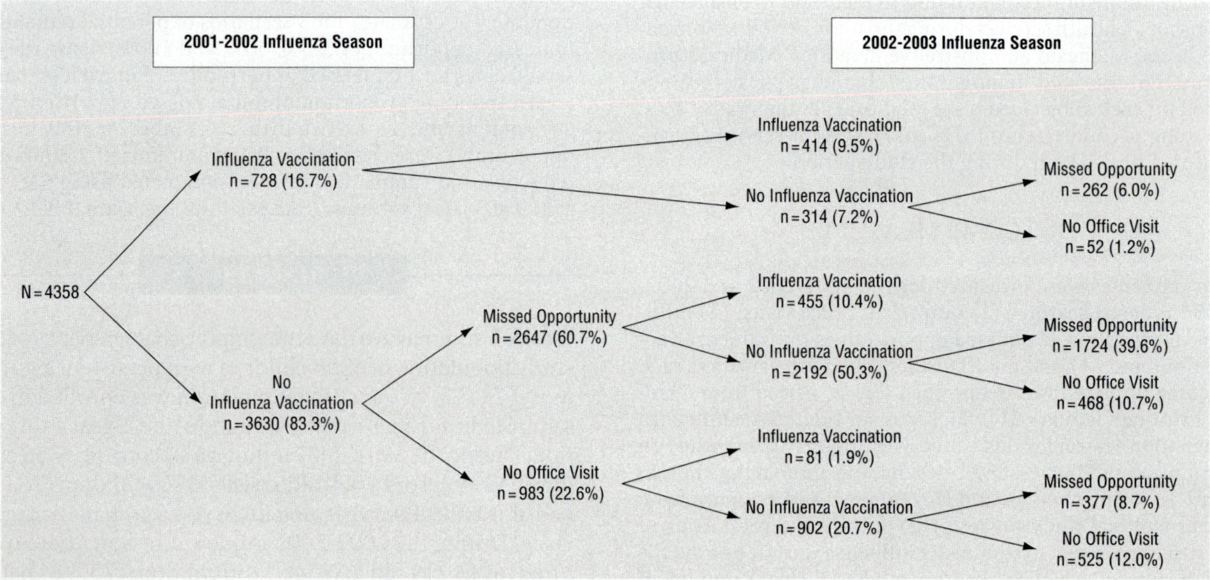


**Figure 1.** Influenza vaccination and missed opportunities for children in successive influenza seasons.

**Figure 3** illustrates the influenza vaccination rates potentially achievable through the reduction or elimination of missed opportunities based on rates observed during the 2002-2003 influenza season. The figure illustrates that a 25% reduction in missed opportunities could result in an overall 35% influenza vaccination rate among children with asthma. Similarly, a 50% reduction in missed opportunities would translate into an influenza vaccination rate of 49% by the end of January. Complete elimination of missed opportunities would yield a 77% influenza vaccination rate.

## COMMENT

Our findings confirm previous studies demonstrating low influenza vaccination rates among children with asthma in both Medicaid and commercial health plans[9-12]; however, missed opportunities occurred more frequently among children in our study population. We found that most missed opportunities occurred early in the influenza season, well before the historical peak,[7] and that even modest reductions in missed opportunities could sharply increase influenza vaccination rates among children with asthma.

**Table 2. Missed Opportunities by Month of Influenza Season***

| Month of First Missed Opportunity | Influenza Season 2001-2002 | Influenza Season 2002-2003 |
|---|---|---|
| No. of subjects | 2647 | 2363 |
| October | 1326 (50.1) | 1154 (48.8) |
| November | 661 (25.0) | 520 (22.0) |
| December | 325 (12.3) | 340 (14.4) |
| January | 335 (12.7) | 349 (14.8) |

*The initial office visit occurring during influenza vaccination season among unvaccinated children; this excludes emergency department visits. Data are presented as number (percentage).

An important and unique component of our study was to document patterns of office visits and influenza vaccination across 2 successive influenza seasons, thereby demonstrating the pathways of care that characterize Medicaid-enrolled children with asthma. We found that children often experienced the same outcome during successive influenza seasons. The majority of children in this study had at least 1 office visit in each influenza season; therefore, these patterns may reflect consistent underrecognition (by either parents or physicians) of the need for annual influenza vaccination for children with asthma. Previous reports have suggested that the most common reasons for children with asthma not receiving an influenza vaccination include the vaccine not being recommended by a physician and parents not perceiving the risk of influenza for their children with asthma.[11] Future studies should assess the extent to which certain patient and physician triggers are effective in reducing missed opportunities for influenza vaccination.

We also found that the lack of an office visit was a pattern that repeated itself from one influenza season to the next. For children without office visits during influenza season, these consistent patterns from season to season likely reflect health care–seeking behaviors on the part of these patients and families. Among these children, rates of missed opportunities in the office setting are nil since (by definition) a missed opportunity requires an office visit. On the other hand, we found that many unvaccinated children with no office visits had an asthma ED visit during influenza season. These ED visits may reflect differences in care seeking or severity of illness or may be an indicator of limited access to primary care for this group of children. These visits may represent a different form of missed opportunity, one with unique challenges. Using ED visits to improve childhood vaccination rates has historically proved difficult although it may represent the most commonly used source of care for some children.[29,30] Vaccines may not be readily available in EDs,

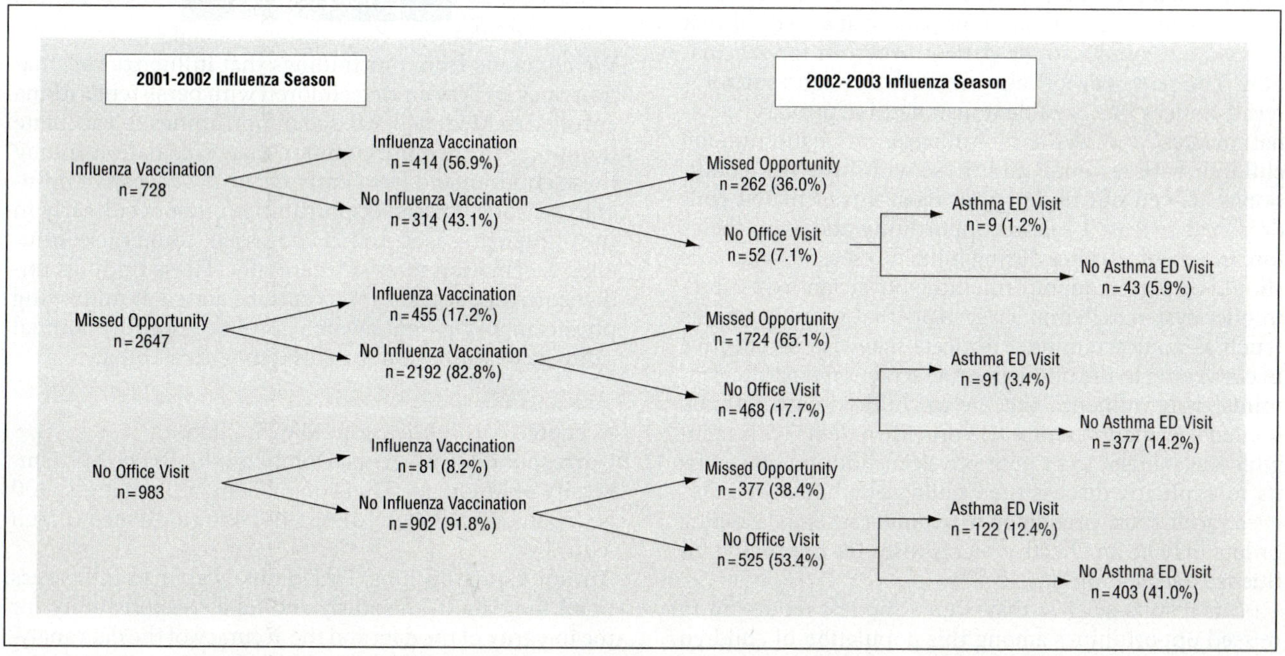


**Figure 2.** Asthma emergency department (ED) use based on history of influenza vaccination, missed opportunities, and office visits.

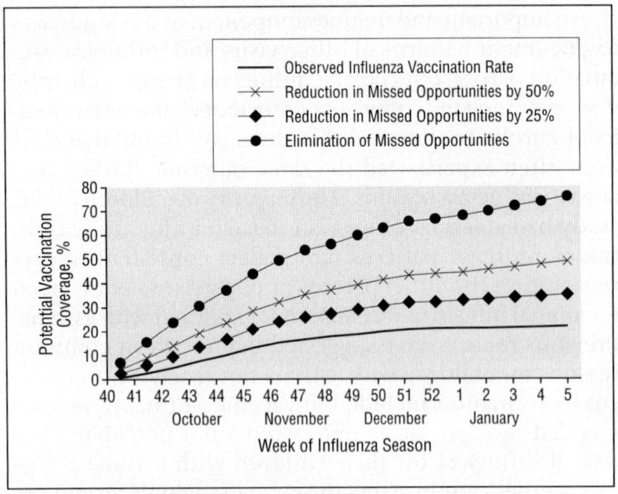


**Figure 3.** Potential influenza vaccination rates with reduction in missed opportunities based on observed timing of initial office visits occurring during influenza vaccination season among unvaccinated children. Emergency department visits are excluded.

and therefore these visits may reflect opportunities for referrals to patients' primary care physicians for appropriate follow-up, including influenza vaccination.[8]

Strategies to reduce missed opportunities, such as standing orders and reminder-recall systems, have been explored in previous studies[13,31-40]; these approaches may be applicable to reducing missed opportunities for influenza vaccination among children with asthma. These strategies may be beneficial for families and health care professionals by establishing expectations and routines for influenza vaccination year after year among children with asthma. The Task Force on Community Preventive Services has supported the use of reminder-recall systems that can be integrated within immunization registries or clinical information systems and can be directed to cue physicians and patients (or their parents) into action.[31] Using this information, the health care professional can either recommend a vaccination to the patient at a medical visit or send a reminder to the patient to return for vaccination. The potential for improvement through reminder-recall notices has been demonstrated for primary vaccination rates[41-45] as well as for influenza vaccination among children with asthma[15] and those with high-risk conditions.[13] Given our finding that most unvaccinated children had at least 1 missed opportunity and were therefore in a medical office during influenza season, emphasis should be placed on implementing physician-focused reminder systems. Reminder systems that prompt parents (such as mailed reminder notices) may also be effective in conveying to the physician cues to action regarding administering influenza vaccine to children with asthma. Mailed vaccination reminders provide parents with a tangible mechanism to prompt physicians during office visits to explicitly discuss their child's eligibility for influenza vaccination. In addition to reminder systems, standing orders may be an effective mechanism for improving influenza vaccination rates.[31,38,39]

Our results suggest that even a modest reduction in missed opportunities among this population of children could substantially increase influenza vaccination rates prior to the historical peak of influenza activity,[7] consistent with findings for a primarily privately insured group of children with asthma.[11] We also found that many children do not receive influenza vaccination and have missed opportunities in successive years, suggesting that these occurrences do not reflect isolated events and may be more deeply rooted in physician attitudes and behaviors. Interventions aimed at eliminating the underlying cause of these missed opportunities could result in an influenza vaccination rate higher than 60% and potentially help to establish for families and physicians an expectation for, and a long-term pattern of, annual influenza vaccination.

This study has several limitations. We used a HEDIS-based approach with administrative claims data, since this method is used widely in the United States and is familiar to physicians and health plans. Prior studies have shown that the HEDIS classification for persistent asthma that we used in this study generally has high sensitivity but lower specificity for distinguishing asthma severity.[46] Because the HEDIS case definition for persistent asthma is not based on objective clinical criteria, our findings may have limited generalizability to settings that use alternative asthma classification criteria (eg, symptoms or pulmonary function testing) to distinguish intermittent cases from severe asthma cases. These data did not allow us to determine cases in which an influenza vaccination was recommended but refused by the parent, a valid contraindication existed, or children may have obtained influenza vaccinations through health fairs or free clinics. In addition, we were unable to distinguish whether office visits made were with specialists or primary care physicians. Although the completeness of the data reported by Michigan Medicaid managed care plans is generally good, there are variations in the timeliness, accuracy, and thoroughness of plans' claims data. In an effort to maximize the completeness of vaccination records, we augmented Medicaid administrative claims data with immunization registry information.

## CONCLUSIONS

We conclude from our findings that influenza vaccination rates are low among children with persistent asthma enrolled in Medicaid. Missed opportunities to vaccinate for influenza are more common than vaccination among these children and frequently occur in successive influenza seasons. Missed opportunities often occur early in the influenza season and, if addressed, could raise influenza vaccination rates substantially. These findings underscore the need for interventions aimed at improving physician and parent awareness of the need for annual influenza vaccination for children with asthma.

**Accepted for Publication:** May 8, 2006.
**Correspondence:** Kevin J. Dombkowski, DrPH, MS, University of Michigan, Division of General Pediatrics, 300 N. Ingalls, Ann Arbor, MI 48109-0456 (kjd@med.umich.edu).
**Author Contributions:** Dr Dombkowski had full access to all the data in the study and takes responsibility for the integrity of the data and the accuracy of the data analysis. *Study concept and design:* Dombkowski and Clark. *Ac-*

*quisition of data:* Dombkowski and Cohn. *Analysis and interpretation of data:* Dombkowski, Clark, and Davis. *Drafting of the manuscript:* Dombkowski, Clark, and Cohn. *Critical revision of the manuscript for important intellectual content:* Dombkowski, Clark, and Davis. *Statistical analysis:* Dombkowski. *Obtained funding:* Dombkowski and Clark. *Administrative, technical, and material support:* Clark. *Study supervision:* Dombkowski.

**Funding/Support:** This study was supported by the Michigan Department of Community Health and the Blue Cross Blue Shield of Michigan Foundation.

**Previous Presentation:** Portions of this study were presented at the 39th National Immunization Conference, March 22, 2005, Washington, DC; and the Pediatric Academic Societies' Annual Meeting, May 14, 2005, Washington, DC.

**Acknowledgment:** We thank Susan Moran, BSN, MPH, of the Michigan Department of Community Health for her insights and comments regarding this study.

## REFERENCES

1. Dey A. Summary health statistics for US children: National Health Interview Survey, 2004. *Vital Health Stat 10.* 2006(227):18 Bloom B.
2. National Center for Health Statistics. Asthma prevalence, health care use and mortality, 2002. http://www.cdc.gov/nchs/products/pubs/pubd/hestats/asthma/asthma.htm. Accessed October 4, 2005.
3. Glezen WP, Greenberg SB, Atmar RL, Piedra PA, Couch RB. Impact of respiratory virus infections on persons with chronic underlying conditions. *JAMA.* 2000;283:499-505.
4. Barker WH. Excess pneumonia and influenza associated hospitalization during influenza epidemics in the United States, 1970-78. *Am J Public Health.* 1986;76:761-765.
5. Neuzil KM, Wright PF, Mitchel EF Jr, Griffin MR. The burden of influenza illness in children with asthma and other chronic medical conditions. *J Pediatr.* 2000;137:856-864.
6. Menec VH, Black C, MacWilliam L, Aoki FY. The impact of influenza-associated respiratory illnesses on hospitalizations, physician visits, emergency room visits, and mortality. *Can J Public Health.* 2003;94:59-63.
7. Centers for Disease Control and Prevention. Prevention and control of influenza: recommendations of the Advisory Committee on Immunization Practices (ACIP). *MMWR Morb Mortal Wkly Rep.* 2005;54(RR-8):9-10.
8. National Asthma Education and Prevention Program. *Guidelines for the Diagnosis and Management of Asthma.* Bethesda, Md: National Institutes of Health, National Heart, Lung, and Blood Institute; 1997. Publication 97-4051.
9. Chung EK, Casey R, Pinto-Martin JA, Pawlowski NA, Bell LM. Routine and influenza vaccination rates in children with asthma. *Ann Allergy Asthma Immunol.* 1998;80:318-322.
10. Kramarz P, DeStefano F, Gargiullo PM, et al. Influenza vaccination in children with asthma in health maintenance organizations: Vaccine Safety Datalink Team. *Vaccine.* 2000;18:2288-2294.
11. Daley MF, Beaty BL, Barrow J, et al. Missed opportunities for influenza vaccination in children with chronic medical conditions. *Arch Pediatr Adolesc Med.* 2005;159:986-991.
12. Szilagyi PG, Rodewald LE. Missed opportunities for influenza vaccination among children with asthma. *Pediatr Infect Dis J.* 1992;11:705-708.
13. Daley MF, Barrow J, Pearson K, et al. Identification and recall of children with chronic medical conditions for influenza vaccination. *Pediatrics.* 2004;113:e26-e33.
14. Gaglani M, Riggs M, Kamenicky C, Glezen WP. A computerized reminder strategy is effective for annual influenza immunization of children with asthma or reactive airway disease. *Pediatr Infect Dis J.* 2001;20:1155-1160.
15. Szilagyi PG, Rodewald LE, Savageau J, Yoos L, Doane C. Improving influenza vaccination rates in children with asthma: a test of a computerized reminder system and an analysis of factors predicting vaccination compliance. *Pediatrics.* 1992;90:871-875.
16. American Academy of Pediatrics. Implementation of the immunization policy. *Pediatrics.* 1995;96:360-361.
17. Holt E, Guyer B, Hughart N, et al. The contribution of missed opportunities to childhood underimmunization in Baltimore. *Pediatrics.* 1996;97:474-480.
18. Kimmel SR, Madlon-Kay D, Burns IT, Admire B. Breaking the barriers to childhood immunization. *Am Fam Physician.* 1996;53:1648-1656.
19. National Vaccine Advisory Committee. The measles epidemic: the problems, barriers, and recommendations. *JAMA.* 1991;266:1547-1552.
20. Szilagyi PG, Rodewald LE. Missed opportunities for immunizations: a review of the evidence. *J Public Health Manag Pract.* 1996;2:18-25.
21. National Committee for Quality Assurance. *Use of Appropriate Medications for People With Asthma: HEDIS 2003.* Vol 2. Washington, DC: National Committee for Quality Assurance; 2003.
22. National Committee for Quality Assurance. Use of appropriate medications for people with asthma denominator. http://www.ncqa.org/programs/hedis/asthmadenominator.xls. Accessed December 5, 2003.
23. Berger WE, Legorreta AP, Blaiss MS, et al. The utility of the Health Plan Employer Data and Information Set (HEDIS) asthma measure to predict asthma-related outcomes. *Ann Allergy Asthma Immunol.* 2004;93:538-545.
24. Dombkowski KJ, Wasilevich E, Lyon-Callo S. Pediatric asthma surveillance using Medicaid claims. *Public Health Rep.* 2005;120:515-524.
25. Centers for Disease Control and Prevention. Prevention and control of asthma: recommendations of the Advisory Committee on Immunization Practices (ACIP). *MMWR Morb Mortal Wkly Rep.* 2005;54(RR-8):19-21.
26. Davis MM, McMahon SR, Santoli JM, Schwartz B, Clark SJ. A national survey of physician practices regarding influenza vaccine. *J Gen Intern Med.* 2002;17:670-676.
27. Centers for Disease Control and Prevention. Notice to readers: delayed influenza vaccine availability for 2001-02 season and supplemental recommendations of the Advisory Committee on Immunization Practices. *MMWR Morb Mortal Wkly Rep.* 2001;50:582-585.
28. *International Classification of Diseases, Ninth Revision, Clinical Modification.* Washington, DC: Public Health Service, US Dept of Health and Human Services; 1988.
29. Callahan JM, Reed D, Meguid V, Wojcik S, Reed K. Utility of an immunization registry in a pediatric emergency department. *Pediatr Emerg Care.* 2004;20:297-301.
30. Cetta F, Ros SP, Beck AM. Are routine immunizations in the emergency department a realistic goal? *Clin Pediatr (Phila).* 1993;32:161-162.
31. Briss PA, Rodewald LE, Hinman AR, et al. Reviews of evidence regarding interventions to improve vaccination coverage in children, adolescents, and adults. *Am J Prev Med.* 2000;18(1S):97-140.
32. Szilagyi PG, Schaffer S, Shone L, et al. Reducing geographic, racial, and ethnic disparities in childhood immunization rates by using reminder/recall interventions in urban primary care practices. *Pediatrics.* 2002;110:e58.
33. LeBaron CW, Starnes DM, Rask KJ. The impact of reminder-recall interventions on low vaccination coverage in an inner-city population. *Arch Pediatr Adolesc Med.* 2004;158:255-261.
34. Lieu TA, Capra AM, Makol J, Black SB, Shinefield HR. Effectiveness and cost-effectiveness of letters, automated telephone messages, or both for underimmunized children in a health maintenance organization. *Pediatrics.* 1998;101:E3.
35. Szilagyi PG, Schaffer S, Barth R, et al. Effect of telephone reminder/recall on adolescent immunization and preventive visits: results from a randomized clinical trial. *Arch Pediatr Adolesc Med.* 2006;160:157-163.
36. Franzini L, Rosenthal J, Spears W, et al. Cost-effectiveness of childhood immunization reminder/recall systems in urban private practices. *Pediatrics.* 2000;106:177-183.
37. Rodewald LE, Szilagyi PG, Humiston SG, Barth R, Kraus R, Raubertas RF. A randomized study of tracking with outreach and provider prompting to improve immunization coverage and primary care. *Pediatrics.* 1999;103:31-38.
38. Brimberry R. Vaccination of high-risk patients for influenza: a comparison of telephone and mail reminder methods. *J Fam Pract.* 1988;26:397-400.
39. Kimmel SR, Burns IT, Zimmerman RK. Addressing immunization barriers, benefits, and risks. *J Fam Pract.* 2003;52(1 suppl):S47-S55.
40. Wood DL; American Academy of Pediatrics Committee on Community Health Services; American Academy of Pediatrics Committee on Practice and Ambulatory Medicine. Increasing immunization coverage. *Pediatrics.* 2003;112:993-996.
41. Centers for Disease Control and Prevention. Recommendations of the Advisory Committee on Immunization Practices, the American Academy of Pediatrics, and the American Academy of Family Physicians: use of reminder and recall by vaccination providers to increase vaccination rates. *MMWR Morb Mortal Wkly Rep.* 1998;47:715-717.
42. Gostin LO, Lazzarini Z. Childhood immunization registries: a national review of public health information systems and the protection of privacy. *JAMA.* 1995;274:1793-1799.
43. Linkins RW, Dini EF, Watson G, Patriarca PA. A randomized trial of the effectiveness of computer-generated telephone messages in increasing immunization visits among preschool children. *Arch Pediatr Adolesc Med.* 1994;148:908-914.
44. Szilagyi PG, Bordley C, Vann JC, et al. Effect of patient reminder/recall interventions on immunization rates: a review. *JAMA.* 2000;284:1820-1827.
45. Young SA, Halpin TJ, Johnson DA, Irvin JJ, Marks JS. Effectiveness of a mailed reminder on the immunization levels of infants at high risk of failure to complete immunizations. *Am J Public Health.* 1980;70:422-424.
46. Cabana MD, Slish KK, Nan B, Clark NM. Limits of the HEDIS criteria in determining asthma severity for children. *Pediatrics.* 2004;114:1049-1055.

# Children Treated at an Expeditionary Military Hospital in Iraq

*Lt Col Christopher P. Coppola, USAF, MC; Maj Brian E. Leininger, USAF, MC; Lt Col Todd E. Rasmussen, USAF, MC; Col David L. Smith, USAF, MC*

**Objective:** To describe the treatment of children at an expeditionary military hospital in wartime Iraq.

**Design:** Descriptive, retrospective study.

**Setting:** The 332nd Air Force Theater Hospital in Balad, Iraq, January 1, 2004, to May 31, 2005.

**Patients:** All 85 children (of 1626 total patients) evaluated and treated at the hospital during the study period.

**Interventions:** Indicated surgical procedures performed on children.

**Main Outcome Measures:** Age, sex, diagnosis, injury, operations, and complications for children during the study period.

**Results:** The 85 children (age range, 1 day to 17 years; mean, 8 years) represented 5.2% of all patients. Thirty-four (61%) of the 56 children for whom sex was recorded were male. Injury was the diagnosis for 48 children (56%). Of these, the cause was fragmentation wound in 25 children (52%), penetrating trauma in 11 (23%), burn in 9 (19%), and blunt trauma in 3 (6%). The site of injury was the lower extremity in 18 children (38%), head in 11 (23%), upper extremity in 8 (17%), abdomen in 8 (17%), and chest in 3 (6%). Nontraumatic conditions had congenital, infectious, gastrointestinal, and neoplastic causes. During the study, 134 operations were performed on 63 children. There were 5 deaths.

**Conclusions:** Expeditionary military hospitals will encounter both injured and noninjured children seeking medical care. To optimize the care of these children, it will be necessary to provide the proper personnel, training, and equipment.

*Arch Pediatr Adolesc Med. 2006;160:972-976*

Modern warfare occurs in territories with a civilian population, resulting in injuries to noncombatants, including children.[1-6] Sometimes, children are employed as combatants or used as human shields.[7] Therefore, it is inevitable that military medical units will encounter injured children. Because local health care is often disrupted near sites of conflict, children with other problems also may seek care at military hospitals. Just as it is important for military medical services to recognize and prepare for traumatic injuries incurred by combatants and noncombatants, it is also important to prepare for medical illnesses that may be encountered.

United States and coalition forces entered Iraq in 2003 and were accompanied by medical personnel and facilities. Combat medical echelons of care are as follows: level I, battalion aid stations; level II, forward surgical teams; level III, hospital facilities in the theater of combat; level IV, Landstuhl Regional Medical Center in Germany; and level V, Walter Reed Army Medical Center, Washington, DC.[8]

The level III hospitals in the theater of combat are the highest-acuity facilities available to civilian casualties, including children. The absence of adequate national medical facilities creates difficulty in discharging children from expeditionary military hospitals if they have ongoing medical needs.[9] The lack of infrastructure, supplies, and personnel compromise the effectiveness of Iraqi hospitals. Early in the conflict, the decision was made to offer US military hospital care to injured civilians in instances of life-, limb-, and vision-threatening injury. In addition, on a case-by-case basis, the hospital commander could approve admission for children with medical needs beyond the scope of the Iraqi civilian medical system. This report details a 17-month experience with

**Author Affiliations:** Department of Surgery, Wilford Hall Medical Center, Lackland Air Force Base, Tex.

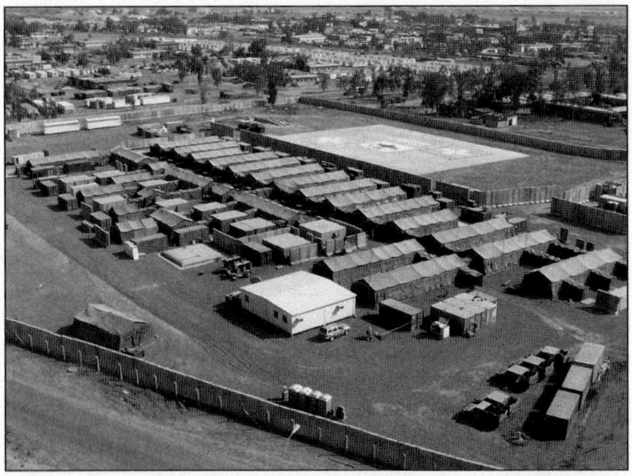

Figure 1. The 332nd Expeditionary Medical Support Air Force Theater Hospital in Balad, Iraq. The network of tents includes 3 operating rooms, which can each accommodate 2 simultaneous operations. The adjoining helipad is visible in the background.

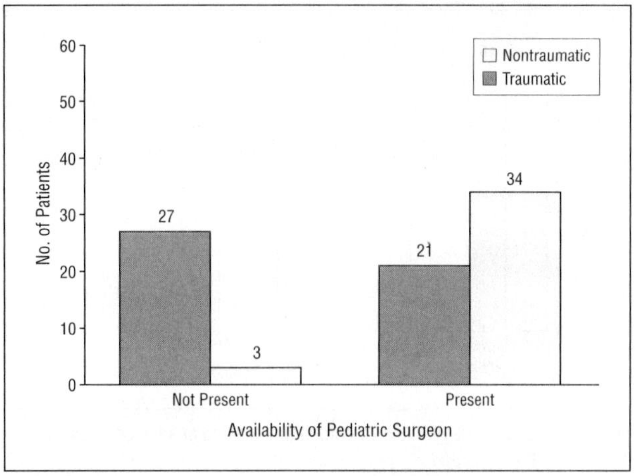


Figure 2. Children presenting to an expeditionary military hospital for traumatic and nontraumatic conditions during the 12 months before and the 5 months after a pediatric surgeon arrived at the facility.

children treated at a level III expeditionary military hospital in Balad, Iraq.

## METHODS

This study is a descriptive, retrospective study, for which institutional review board approval was obtained from the hospital command section. All patients presented to the 332nd Air Force Theater Hospital in Balad, approximately 40 miles north of Baghdad. The facility consists of a series of tents, linked by corridors, and a concrete floor (**Figure 1**).

The structure includes metal containers used as operating rooms. In each of these 3 operating rooms, 2 operations can occur simultaneously, so that 6 procedures can be performed at a time. The hospital is capable of up to 24 intensive care unit beds and 80 ward beds, depending on how it is configured. A multinational staff of approximately 420 personnel enables surgical and medical care across numerous specialties.

The period studied was 17 months from January 1, 2004, through May 31, 2005. This period was chosen because an electronic record of all patients was initiated in January 2004 and the authors left the hospital in May 2005. Data were collected from the surgical logs of the hospital and reviewed retrospectively. The record included all patients presenting to the hospital for care. The diagnosis was determined by the admitting surgeon. Demographic data were obtained from patients and relatives, with assistance from translators, and recorded by the admitting nurse. Pediatric age was defined as being younger than 18 years. Data collected were age, sex, diagnosis, treatment, and complications. An *International Classification of Diseases, Ninth Edition (ICD-9)* code and Injury Severity Score (ISS) were assigned for all children. The ISS was calculated using ICDMAP-90 software (Tri-Analytics, Inc, Bel Air, Md). Statistical analysis was by $\chi^2$ for distributions and unpaired, 2-tailed *t* test for numerical data.

## RESULTS

The conditions of a total of 85 children were evaluated and the children were treated during the study period, representing 5.2% of all 1626 patients in the surgical logs and approximately 18% of the Iraqi civilians treated. Their age range was 1 day to 17 years (mean age, 8 years). Sex was recorded for 56 of the 85 children. Of these, 34 (61%) were male, 21 (38%) were female, and 1 child with intersexuality had indeterminate sex.

Overall, 48 (56%) of the 85 children were treated for a traumatic condition (ISS range, 1-29; mean, 8.5). The remaining 37 children (44%) were treated for nontraumatic diagnoses. From January 1, 2004, through December 31, 2004, when no pediatric surgeon was present, 3 (10%) of 30 children were treated for nontraumatic diagnoses. From January 1, 2005, through May 31, 2005, when a pediatric surgeon was present, 34 (62%) of 55 children were treated for nontraumatic diagnoses ($P<.001$) (**Figure 2**).

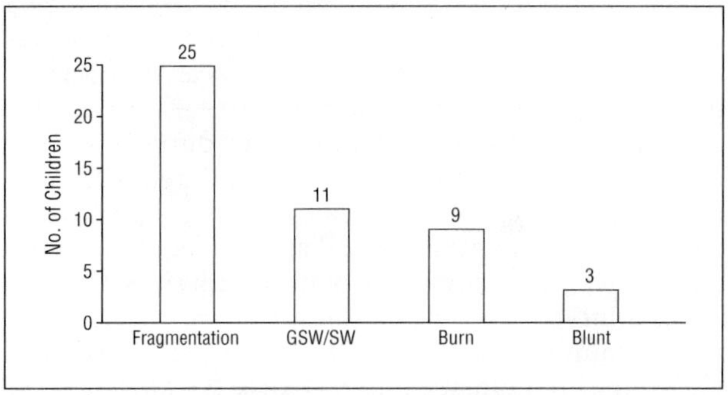


Figure 3. Mechanism of injury in 48 children treated at an expeditionary military hospital. GSW/SW indicates gunshot wound and stab wound.

### INJURIES AND OTHER CONDITIONS

The most common cause of trauma was fragmentation injury (25 [52%] of the 48 injured children) (**Figure 3**). This category includes improvised explosive devices, unexploded ordnance, indirect fire (mortars, rockets, and rocket-propelled grenades), mines, and blast injuries. Most of the children with fragmentation injury were injured in improvised explosive device attacks. Most of the 48 injured children had multiple sites of injury, with the most common site of primary injury being the lower extremity (18 children [38%]) (**Figure 4**).

Nontraumatic conditions were grouped into the broad categories of those having congenital, infectious, gastrointestinal and feeding, and neoplastic causes (**Table 1**).

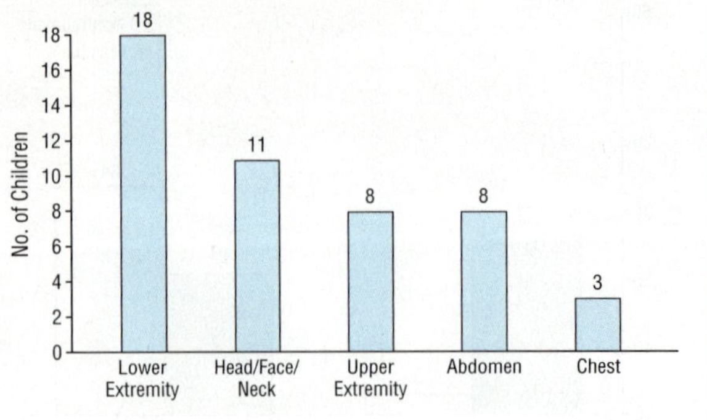


**Figure 4.** Primary site of injury in 48 children treated at an expeditionary military hospital.

## OPERATIONS AND OUTCOMES

At least 1 operation was required by 63 (74%) of the 85 children examined at our hospital. A total of 134 operations were performed on 63 children (mean number, 2.1 operations per child). These represented 4.4% of the 3036 total operations recorded at the hospital during the study period. Forty-seven (98%) of the 48 children with traumatic injury required an operation. Only 16 (43%) of 37 children with a nontraumatic diagnosis required an operation ($P<.001$ compared with children with traumatic injury).

One hundred eleven operations were performed in 47 children with traumatic injury (**Table 2**). Most of these children required procedures at multiple sites of injury. The most common operation performed was skin or soft tissue wound care (which included irrigation, debridement, fasciotomy, escharotomy, skin graft, dressing change, and splint application). Twenty-three operations or procedures were performed on 16 children with nontraumatic diagnoses.

Three complications occurred during the study period. A 14-year-old child with a comminuted left femur fracture developed osteomyelitis. An 18-month-old child developed pneumonia after hepatoportojejunostomy for biliary atresia. A 3-year-old child presenting with pneumonia and malnutrition went into cardiorespiratory arrest when her endotracheal tube was dislodged, but she was revived with cardiopulmonary resuscitation.

There were 5 deaths during the study period. Two were the result of burns: a 10-year-old child with burns covering 65% of the total body surface area and a 2-year-old child with burns covering 40% of the total body surface area. Two deaths resulted from infectious causes: an 8-day-old newborn with neonatal sepsis and a 3-year-old boy with visceral leishmaniasis. The remaining death occurred in a 12-year-old girl with traumatic head injury who required tracheostomy and placement of a gastrostomy tube. She was transferred to a civilian facility where she asphyxiated when her tracheostomy became plugged with secretions. For the 3 children who died after injury, the mean ISS was 26.7, whereas the 45 children who survived their injuries had a mean ISS of 7.3 ($P<.05$). Thirty-day operative mortality was 6% (5 children) for the entire group of 85 children. There was 1 late death when the child who underwent portoenterostomy died of liver failure 15 months after operation.

**Table 1. Nontraumatic Diagnoses in Children***

| Diagnosis by Category (*ICD-9* Code) | No. of Children |
|---|---|
| Congenital (n = 22) | |
| Genitourinary (ambiguous genitalia [752.7], hypospadias [753.8], cryptorchidism [752.89]) | 3 |
| Hernia (inguinal [550.9], ventral [553.2]) | 3 |
| Vascular (228.01)/lymphatic (457.9) malformation | 3 |
| Craniofacial malformation (756) | 3 |
| CNS (encephalocele [742], meningomyelocele [741.93]) | 2 |
| Thalassemia (282.49) | 2 |
| Cardiac (hypoplastic left heart) (745.3) | 1 |
| Biliary atresia (751.61) | 1 |
| Cystic fibrosis (277) | 1 |
| Spondylolisthesis (756.14) | 1 |
| Calcific keratopathy (366.8) | 1 |
| Spastic contractures (718.4) | 1 |
| Infectious (n = 7) | |
| Visceral leishmaniasis (085.9) | 2 |
| Pneumonia (486) | 2 |
| Neonatal sepsis (771.81) | 1 |
| Infectious diarrhea (009.2) | 1 |
| Otitis media (382.9) | 1 |
| Gastrointestinal/feeding (n = 5) | |
| Gastroesophageal reflux (530.81) | 1 |
| Rectal prolapse (569.1) | 1 |
| Aspirated foreign object (934) | 1 |
| Dehydration (276.5) | 1 |
| Failure to thrive (783.41) | 1 |
| Neoplastic (n = 3) | |
| Central nervous system (239.6) | 1 |
| Mastoid (239.2) | 1 |
| Maxillary sinus (239.1) | 1 |
| **Total** | **37** |

Abbreviations: CNS, central nervous system; *ICD-9*, *International Classification of Diseases, Ninth Revision.*

## COMMENT

This report describes the care of children by an expeditionary hospital in Iraq. Our primary mission as a level III hospital was to provide evaluation, resuscitation, and surgical care to combat-injured troops. When stabilized, American troops were evacuated to the regional medical center in Germany. However, our facility experienced "mission creep" because of the presence of injured civilians, including children. Children additionally had dehydration and malnutrition, which contribute to increased mortality.[10] After January 1, 2005, a pediatric surgeon was available and a broader range of nontraumatic conditions were treated in children.

Our experience mirrors that of other military medical providers in Afghanistan and Iraq in that fragmentation and blast injuries were the most common mechanisms of injury.[11] This is the typical pattern of injury in victims of improvised explosive devices and suicide bombers. Children are particularly vulnerable to unexploded ordnance and land mines.[12,13] Blast and fragmentation devices produce multiple injuries over different regions of the body. This is especially true in civilians, who lack the body armor worn by combatants.[14] The injuries are a combination of penetration and crush of the soft tissues, often accompanied by fractures. The wounds are contaminated by fragments of the explosive device, vehicle shrapnel, clothing, and dirt. This requires extensive debridement and high-pressure irrigation to clear the wounds of debris and devitalized tissue. The fragments from improvised explosive devices and land mines produce a cone of injury larger than the entry wound.[15] Injured children at our facility required multiple procedures for debridement of necrotic tissue, which delayed primary closure of the wounds.

The lower extremity was the most common site of injury, followed by the head. This differs from reports of injured adults, who sustain upper and lower extremity injuries more often than head injuries.[8,11,14,16] This pattern may differ in children owing to their shorter stature and the proportionately larger size of the head. These factors make the head a more likely target of fragmentation devices. The third most common operation performed, after soft tissue wound operations and fracture fixation, was craniotomy for head injury.

Nontraumatic conditions were treated at our facility. Some children were referred by Iraqi institutions unable to provide the acuity of care required. Others chose to seek care at the American military base because of financial hardship, another family member being treated at our hospital, or referral after an encounter with American soldiers. Through the initiative and innovation of the hospital personnel, we were able to make the most of the austere conditions and limited resources, and we optimized the care provided for these children.

Some deficiencies in resources became manifest. There was a short supply of the smallest endotracheal tubes, sizes 3.5 to 5.0. Twenty-two– and 24-gauge catheters were quickly depleted following intravenous access in the hands of providers not accustomed to pediatric care. Finally, personnel experienced in pediatric anesthesiology, critical care, and critical care nursing were rare in our facility. The few individuals with this experience were often hard-pressed to cover prolonged periods when extremely ill children were present in the hospital.

Military pediatric specialists were dispersed throughout the theater of combat, assigned responsibility for adult combat troops. Once we discovered their presence, these providers represented a valuable resource for the care of children. This pool of pediatric expertise was also present during the first Gulf War.[17] On one occasion, a pediatric anesthesiologist, who was assigned north of our location, traveled to our base to anesthetize a child for portoenterostomy. One pediatrician, officially assigned as the battalion surgeon for helicopter personnel on our base, participated in our weekly clinic. Another example of pooled resources was the case of the 2-year-old girl who underwent resection of a cervical cystic hygroma at our hospital and later received radiofrequency ablation treatment of her enlarged tongue at a different combat support hospital.[18,19]

Our experiences have demonstrated several important lessons in the care of children in a war zone. Any hospital near conflict should expect to receive civilian casualties, including children. The most common mechanism of injury in children is fragmentation injury, and the most common sites are the lower extremity and head. Fragmentation injuries are contaminated, resulting in necrotic tissue and requiring careful and repeated debridement. The neurosurgeons assigned to the facility were surprised by the excellent outcomes after penetrating head trauma in this setting. Local health resources may be so disrupted that children cannot be safely discharged until they are well enough to survive under the care of their families. To provide adequate care for children during war, expeditionary medical hospitals must prepare for them by providing the proper personnel, training, and equipment.

**Table 2. Operations and Procedures Performed on Children**

| Operation | No. of Operations |
|---|---|
| **For Traumatic Injuries** | |
| Skin and soft tissue wound care | 83 |
| Fracture fixation | 10 |
| Craniotomy/cranioplasty | 6 |
| Exploratory laparotomy | 4 |
| Vascular exploration/repair | 3 |
| Thoracotomy | 2 |
| Bronchoscopy/esophagoscopy | 1 |
| Enucleation | 1 |
| Sural nerve graft | 1 |
| **Total** | **111** |
| **For Nontraumatic Conditions** | |
| Vascular access | 4 |
| CNS (resection of tumor, meningomyelocele repair, decompression) | 3 |
| Bronchoscopy | 2 |
| Excision of head and neck mass | 2 |
| Orthopedic fixation | 2 |
| Hernia repair | 2 |
| Computed tomography while under general anesthesia | 2 |
| Orchidopexy | 1 |
| Repair of rectal prolapse | 1 |
| Roux-en-Y hepatoportojejunostomy | 1 |
| Bone marrow biopsy | 1 |
| Thoracoscopic decortication | 1 |
| Ophthalmologic evaluation while under general anesthesia | 1 |
| **Total** | **23** |

Abbreviation: CNS, central nervous system.

**Accepted for Publication:** May 8, 2006.
**Correspondence:** Lt Col Christopher P. Coppola, USAF, MC, Department of Surgery, Wilford Hall Medical Center, 2200 Bergquist Dr, Suite 1/MCSG, Lackland Air Force Base, TX 78236 (ccoppola@pol.net).
**Author Contributions:** *Study concept and design:* Coppola. *Acquisition of data:* Coppola, Leininger, Rasmussen, and Smith. *Analysis and interpretation of data:* Coppola. *Drafting of the manuscript:* Coppola. *Critical revision of the manuscript for important intellectual content:* Coppola, Leininger, Rasmussen, and Smith. *Statistical analysis:* Coppola. *Administrative, technical, and material support:* Coppola. *Study supervision:* Coppola.

**Acknowledgment:** We thank Martin Eichelberger, MD, of George Washington University (Professor of Surgery and Pediatrics), Children's National Medical Center, and Safe Kids Worldwide (President and CEO), Washington, DC, for his advice and counsel during the preparation of this manuscript. We also acknowledge Mitchell Strait, of the Section of Trauma Services, Wilford Hall Medical Center (Trauma Statistician), for his assistance in calculating Injury Severity Scores.

## REFERENCES


1. Pearn J. Pediatric diseases and operational deployments. *Mil Med.* 2000;165:283-286.
2. Chmatal P, Bohonek M, Dobiasova M, Hasek R, Cernohous M. A humanitarian mission in southern Iraq: utilization of the 7th Field Hospital of the Army of the Czech Republic—a report on its medical activities and working conditions. *Mil Med.* 2005;170:473-475.
3. Hinsley DE, Rosell PA, Rowlands TK, Clasper JC. Penetrating missile injuries during asymmetric warfare in the 2003 Gulf conflict. *Br J Surg.* 2005;92:637-642.
4. Gurney I. Paediatric casualties during OP TELIC. *J R Army Med Corps.* 2004;150:270-272.
5. Lockey DJ, Nordmann GR, Field JM, Clough D, Henning JD. The deployment of an intensive care facility with a military field hospital to the 2003 conflict in Iraq. *Resuscitation.* 2004;62:261-265.
6. Rew DA, Clasper J, Kerr G. Surgical workload from an integrated UK field hospital during the 2003 Gulf conflict. *J R Army Med Corps.* 2004;150:99-106.
7. Uppard S. Child soldiers and children associated with the fighting forces. *Med Confl Surviv.* 2003;19:121-127.
8. Montgomery SP, Swiecki CW, Shriver CD. The evaluation of casualties from Operation Iraqi Freedom on return to the continental United States from March to June 2003. *J Am Coll Surg.* 2005;201:7-13.
9. Paine GF, Bonnema CL, Stambaugh TA, Capacchione JF, Sipe PS. Anesthesia services aboard USNS Comfort (T-AH-20) during Operation Iraqi Freedom. *Mil Med.* 2005;170:476-482.
10. Reyna TM. Observations of a pediatric surgeon in the Persian Gulf War. *J Pediatr Surg.* 1993;28:209-213.
11. Bilski TR, Baker BC, Grove JR, et al. Battlefield casualties treated at Camp Rhino, Afghanistan: lessons learned. *J Trauma.* 2003;54:814-822.
12. Pearn J. War zone paediatrics in Rwanda. *J Paediatr Child Health.* 1996;32:290-295.
13. Bilukha OO, Brennan M, Woodruff BA. Death and injury from landmines and unexploded ordnance in Afghanistan. *JAMA.* 2003;290:650-653.
14. Patel TH, Wenner KA, Price SA, Weber MA, Leveridge A, McAtee SJ. A U.S. Army Forward Surgical Team's experience in Operation Iraqi Freedom. *J Trauma.* 2004;57:201-207.
15. Radonic V, Giunio L, Boric T, Mimica Z, Furlan D, Definis-Gojanovic M. Antipersonnel mine injuries in southern Croatia. *Mil Med.* 2004;169:313-319.
16. Place RJ, Rush RM Jr, Arrington ED. Forward surgical team (FST) workload in a special operations environment: the 250th FST in Operation ENDURING FREEDOM. *Curr Surg.* 2003;60:418-422.
17. Pierce JR. The role of the United States Army active component pediatricians in Operations Desert Shield, Desert Storm, and Provide Comfort. *Mil Med.* 1993;158:105-108.
18. Coppola M. Someday this war will be over and we'll have to go home. In: *Made a Difference for That One: A Surgeon's Letters Home from Iraq.* Lincoln, Neb: iUniverse Inc; 2005:111-118.
19. Hodierne R. Mission of mercy. *Air Force Times.* June 20, 2005:26.


## *Poetry in Pediatrics*

### Emeritus Eavesdropping

Listening to 4 sophomores at lunch behind a lacy
screen, arguing. "So, define schizoid and why we
have 35 meds for 1 disease. That teacher
is a Freudian relic with feeble antisense
oligonucleotides."
I must be in that old minority who can no longer
activate those chubby polyribosomes or totipotents,
quite wistful over lost oligos, but still hopefully
anticipating a durable concept of international
peace, and perhaps the universal acceptance of
our modern concepts of prose poetry. I am trying.
And, I suspect that they knew I was listening.

*Ed Spudis, MD*

# Fetal Origin of Childhood Disease

## Intrauterine Growth Restriction in Term Infants and Risk for Hypertension at 6 Years of Age

*Seetha Shankaran, MD; Abhik Das, PhD; Charles R. Bauer, MD; Henrietta Bada, MD, MPH; Barry Lester, PhD; Linda Wright, MD; Rosemary Higgins, MD; Kenneth Poole, PhD*

**Objective:** To examine the association between intrauterine growth restriction (IUGR) status at birth among full-term infants, exposure to substance use during pregnancy, and risk of hypertension at 6 years of age.

**Design:** Prospective evaluation of high-risk children.

**Setting:** Four centers of the National Institute of Child Health and Human Development Neonatal Research Network.

**Participants:** One thousand three hundred eighty-eight infants (600 cocaine exposed, 781 nonexposed, and 7 indeterminate, matched by gestational age, race, and sex), were enrolled at these sites. Nine hundred fifty children (415 exposed, 535 nonexposed) were followed up for 6 years.

**Intervention:** Right arm blood pressure was measured using the Dinamap portable adult/pediatric monitor with appropriate cuff size.

**Main Outcome Measure:** Blood pressure levels. Hypertension was defined as either systolic or diastolic blood pressure higher than the 95th percentile for sex, age, and height.

**Results:** Eight hundred ninety-one children had blood pressure data at 6 years of age: 516 were born at full term; 144 (28%) of the 516 children had a diagnosis of IUGR at birth. At 6 years of age, 93 (19%) of 516 children had hypertension. Of 144 children with IUGR, 35 (24%) had hypertension as compared with 58 (16%) of 372 children without IUGR ($P<.05$). Twenty percent of cocaine-exposed children had hypertension as compared with 16% of nonexposed children ($P=.20$). Intrauterine growth restriction status at birth was significantly associated with hypertension (relative risk, 1.8 [95% confidence interval, 1.2-2.7]) when multivariable Poisson regression analysis was performed adjusting for site; maternal race, education, and tobacco, marijuana, alcohol, and cocaine use during pregnancy; and child's current body mass index (calculated as weight in kilograms divided by height in meters squared).

**Conclusion:** In term infants, IUGR is linked to risk of hypertension in early childhood, which may be a marker for adult cardiovascular disease.

*Arch Pediatr Adolesc Med. 2006;160:977-981*

ADULTS WHO WERE NOTED at birth to have low birth weight have been found to have hypertension in retrospective analysis of the relationship between current blood pressure (BP) and birth weight.[1] A prospective study (Perinatal Collaborative Project) studied 137 black Americans and found BP and birth weight are not correlated at age 28 years.[2] Hinchliffe et al[3] proposed a potential pathogenesis for the linkage between low birth weight and hypertension in adulthood: the undernourished, growth-retarded fetus becomes a low-birth-weight newborn whose kidneys have a reduced number of nephrons. To our knowledge, the risk of hypertension in early childhood among infants who were of normal gestation but growth restricted at birth has not been examined in a prospective manner.

Prenatal cocaine exposure is associated with growth restriction at birth in both full-term and preterm pregnancies.[4-6] The deleterious effect of prenatal cocaine exposure may be greater in full-term compared with preterm pregnancies,[7] with growth deceleration in cocaine-exposed infants evident after 32 weeks' gestation.[4]

The association between prenatal cocaine exposure and BP in early childhood appears to be unclear. In the study by Horn,[8] high BP was noted among cocaine-exposed infants (n=12), while the study by Needlman et al[9] evaluating BP in 32 cocaine-exposed and 23 nonexposed infants found no differences in BP between groups.

**Author Affiliations:** National Institute of Child Health and Human Development Neonatal Research Network, Bethesda, Md.

**Table 1. Baseline Characteristics of 6-Year-Old, Full-Term Children**

| Characteristic | Children Born at Term and Evaluated at Age 6 Years (n = 516) | Children Born at Term and Not Evaluated at Age 6 Years (n = 295) |
|---|---|---|
| Maternal characteristic, No. (%) | | |
| Prenatal care | 483 (93.60) | 270 (91.53) |
| Race* | | |
| White | 83 (16.09) | 63 (21.36) |
| Black | 399 (77.33) | 210 (71.19) |
| Other | 34 (6.59) | 22 (7.46) |
| Smoking during pregnancy | 271 (52.52) | 163 (55.25) |
| Alcohol during pregnancy | 320 (62.02) | 180 (61.02) |
| Marijuana during pregnancy | 112 (21.71) | 72 (24.49) |
| Cocaine during pregnancy | 220 (42.64) | 121 (41.02) |
| Opiates during pregnancy | 39 (7.56) | 33 (11.19) |
| Maternal education, y | | |
| <12 | 204 (39.53) | 106 (36.18) |
| 12 | 205 (39.73) | 117 (39.93) |
| >12 | 107 (20.74) | 70 (23.89) |
| Socioeconomic status: Hollingshead Index of Social Status[18] score, mean (SD)† | 27.98 (10.46) | 29.78 (10.47) |
| Neonatal characteristic, No.(%) | | |
| Neonatal birth weight, g, mean (SD) | 3100.94 (535.99) | 3141.9 (490.97) |
| IUGR status | 144 (27.91) | 66 (22.37) |
| Sex of infant | | |
| M | 275 (53.29) | 174 (58.98) |
| F | 241 (46.71) | 121 (41.02) |
| Length of hospital stay, d, mean (SD) | 4.24 (4.82) | 4.62 (5.99) |

Abbreviation: IUGR, intrauterine growth restriction.
*Race was identified by mother.
†Statistically significant difference ($P<.05$) between term children whose cases were evaluated and not evaluated at age 6 years.

The objective of this study was to examine the association between intrauterine growth restriction (IUGR) status at birth among full-term infants, substance use during pregnancy, and risk for hypertension at 6 years of age in a multisite, prospective, longitudinal study.

## METHODS

This analysis is part of the ongoing Maternal Life Style study, evaluating the impact of maternal lifestyle during pregnancy on childhood outcome. The study is performed at Brown University, University of Miami, University of Tennessee (Memphis), and Wayne State University. The 4 clinical sites are participating centers of the National Institute of Child Health and Human Development Neonatal Research Network. The study was approved by the institutional review board at each site and informed consent was obtained from the parents prior to participation.

Infants were prospectively recruited into the study between May 1993 and May 1995. Infants born to women who used cocaine during pregnancy (exposed group) were matched to non–cocaine exposed (comparison group) infants by gestational age, race, and sex within the same institution during the same recruitment year. Inclusion criteria were maternal age 18 years or older, inborn birth, singleton birth, and gestational age of 43 weeks or less. Exclusion criteria were maternal psychiatric disorders or developmental delay and language barriers to informed consent. Cocaine and opiate exposure were determined by maternal admission of use during pregnancy and/or a positive screen for meconium metabolites confirmed with gas chromatography/mass spectroscopy. Prenatal exposure to alcohol, tobacco, and marijuana existed in both cocaine-exposed and non–cocaine exposed groups.[10] Gestational age was assessed by the Ballard examination.[11] The children were categorized at birth to have a normal birth weight for gestational age or IUGR if birth weight was lower than the 10th percentile.[12] Only full-term infants were participants in the present study, since prematurity is a risk factor for elevated BP in adolescents and adulthood.[13,14] Infants were prospectively followed up at each site with annual visits. At the 6-year visit to each clinical center, BP was measured as the average of 3 measurements of the right arm BP using the Dinamap portable adult/pediatric monitor (Critikon, Tampa, Fla) with the appropriate cuff size for the upper arm, with the width of the cuff bladder that was 40% of mid upper arm circumference. The child was seated during the measurements. The child's height was obtained using a stadiometer and weight, with the pediatric digital scale. The child's body mass index (BMI) (calculated as weight in kilograms divided by height in meters squared) was noted on the growth charts established by the National Center for Health Statistics in collaboration with the Centers for Disease Control and Prevention.[15] Hypertension was defined as systolic BP or diastolic BP in the 95th percentile or higher for sex, age, and height based on the National High Blood Pressure Education Working Group on High Blood Pressure in Children and Adolescents.[16] The growth measurements and BP measurements were obtained by the study research nurse at each clinical center. Prior to each annual clinic visit, the study center primary investigator and research nurse reviewed the manual of operations developed, and each center's research nurse was certified to obtain BP measurements.

Poisson regression with robust standard errors[17] was used to examine the effect of IUGR status at birth and BP at 6 years of age, adjusting for (1) clinical center, maternal race and education, and preeclampsia, and (2) use of tobacco, marijuana, alcohol, and cocaine during pregnancy and child's BMI at 6 years of age. Maternal BP levels were not obtained at the child's 6-year visit to the clinic.

## RESULTS

Of the 19 079 women screened, 11 811 consented to participate in the acute phase of the study evaluating neonatal effects of cocaine exposure during pregnancy.[6] For the longitudinal phase of the study, 1388 infants were enrolled at 1 month; there were 600 infants in the cocaine-exposed group, 781 in the comparison group, and 7 infants with indeterminate cocaine exposure who were subsequently excluded from this analysis. There were 811 full-term infants with a gestational age of more than 36 weeks enrolled at 1 month. Infants were examined at 4 and 8 months and annually thereafter until 6 years of age. The children were evaluated for the 6-year visit between November 1999 and November 2001. Of the children enrolled at the onset of the longitudinal study, 891 had BP and growth parameters at 6 years of age. Among these 891 children, 516 were born at full-term gestation. These 516 children are the subject of this report. Intrauterine growth restriction status at birth was noted in 144 (27.91%) of the 516 children. The clinical and demographic characteristics of the full-term children evaluated at 6 years of age and those not examined (lost to follow-up) are noted in **Table 1**. Only socioeconomic status was different between the children whose cases were evaluated at 6 years of age and those not evaluated.

**Table 2. Clinical Characteristics of Children With and Without IUGR**

| Characteristic | With IUGR (n = 144) | Without IUGR (n = 372) |
|---|---|---|
| Maternal characteristic, No. (%) | | |
| Race | | |
| White | 15 (10.42) | 68 (18.28) |
| Black | 121 (84.03) | 278 (74.73) |
| Other | 8 (5.56) | 26 (6.99) |
| Maternal age, y, mean (SD)* | 29.10 (6.08) | 27.96 (5.76) |
| Marital status | | |
| Married | 20 (13.89) | 77 (20.75) |
| Single | 117 (81.25) | 282 (76.01) |
| Divorced | 7 (4.86) | 8 (2.16) |
| Widowed | 0 | 4 (1.08) |
| Insurance | | |
| Private health insurance | 6 (4.17) | 28 (7.53) |
| Medical assistance or Medicaid | 121 (84.03) | 296 (79.57) |
| Prepaid HMO | 8 (5.56) | 28 (7.53) |
| Self-pay | 8 (5.56) | 16 (4.30) |
| Unknown | 1 (0.69) | 4 (1.08) |
| Maternal education, y | | |
| <12 | 58 (40.28) | 146 (39.25) |
| 12 | 62 (43.06) | 143 (38.44) |
| >12 | 24 (16.67) | 83 (22.31) |
| Prenatal care | 130 (90.28) | 353 (94.89) |
| Substance use | | |
| Alcohol | 96 (66.67) | 224 (60.22) |
| Tobacco* | 97 (67.36) | 174 (46.77) |
| Cocaine* | 79 (54.86) | 141 (37.90) |
| Marijuana | 36 (25.00) | 76 (20.43) |
| Other | 3 (2.08) | 4 (1.08) |
| Chronic hypertension | 5 (3.47) | 7 (1.88) |
| Preeclampsia | 7 (4.86) | 14 (3.76) |
| Oligohydramnios | 10 (6.94) | 13 (3.49) |
| Polyhydramnios | 0 | 2 (0.54) |
| Prolonged rupture of membranes | 3 (2.08) | 5 (1.34) |
| Treated for chorioamnionitis | 4 (2.78) | 11 (2.96) |
| Cesarean section delivery | 32 (22.22) | 56 (15.05) |
| Neonatal characteristic | | |
| Birth weight, g, mean (SD)* | 2472.94 (241.65) | 3344.03 (404.91) |
| Gestational age, wk, mean (SD) | 38.75 (1.34) | 38.99 (1.33) |
| Major congenital anomaly, No. (%) | 0 | 0 |
| Proven in utero infections, No. (%) | 8 (5.56) | 15 (4.03) |

Abbreviations: HMO, health maintenance organization; IUGR, intrauterine growth restriction.
*Statistically significant difference ($P<.05$) between children with and without IUGR.

**Table 3. Risk for Hypertension at Age 6 Years**

| | No. (%) | | Unadjusted Relative Risk (95% Confidence Interval)* |
|---|---|---|---|
| | Hypertension (n = 93) | No Hypertension (n = 423) | |
| Site | | | |
| A (n = 187) | 26 (14) | 161 (86) | 2.5 (1.4-3.3) |
| B (n = 13) | 34 (26) | 99 (74) | 1.2 (0.8-2.0) |
| C (n = 97) | 30 (31) | 67 (69) | 5.0 (2.0-10.0) |
| D (n = 99) | 7 (7) | 92 (93) | 1.0 |
| Sex | | | |
| M (n = 275) | 45 (16) | 229 (84) | 0.8 (0.6-1.2) |
| F (n = 241) | 48 (20) | 193 (80) | 1.0 |
| Race | | | |
| Black (n = 399) | 76 (19) | 323 (81) | 1.4 (0.8-2.6) |
| Other (n = 34) | 6 (18) | 28 (82) | 1.3 (0.5-3.3) |
| White (n = 83) | 11 (13) | 71 (87) | 1.0 |
| Maternal education, y | | | |
| <12 (n = 204) | 31 (15) | 173 (85) | 0.9 (0.5-1.4) |
| 12 (n = 205) | 43 (21) | 161 (79) | 1.2 (0.7-1.9) |
| >12 (n = 107) | 19 (18) | 88 (82) | 1.0 |
| Substance use during pregnancy | | | |
| Smoking | | | |
| Yes (n = 271) | 54 (20) | 216 (80) | 1.3 (0.9-1.8) |
| No (n = 245) | 39 (16) | 206 (84) | 1.0 |
| Alcohol | | | |
| Yes (n = 320) | 51 (16) | 269 (84) | 0.7 (0.5-1.1) |
| No (n = 196) | 42 (22) | 153 (78) | 1.0 |
| Marijuana | | | |
| Yes (n = 112) | 21 (19) | 91 (81) | 1.0 (0.7-1.6) |
| No (n = 404) | 72 (18) | 331 (82) | 1.0 |
| Cocaine | | | |
| Yes (n = 220) | 45 (20) | 175 (80) | 1.3 (0.9-1.8) |
| No (n = 295) | 48 (16) | 247 (84) | 1.0 |
| Opiates | | | |
| Yes (n = 38) | 7 (18) | 31 (82) | 1.1 (0.5-2.2) |
| No (n = 421) | 70 (17) | 351 (83) | 1.0 |
| Preeclampsia | | | |
| Yes (n = 21) | 4 (19) | 17 (81) | 1.1 (0.4-2.6) |
| No (n = 494) | 89 (18) | 405 (82) | 1.0 |
| IUGR status at birth | | | |
| Yes (n = 144) | 35 (24) | 109 (76) | 1.6 (1.1-2.3) |
| No (n = 372) | 58 (16) | 313 (84) | 1.0 |
| BMI at age 6 y, mean (SD) | 17.8 (3.9) | 16.2 (2.2) | 1.6 (1.0-2.1)* |

Abbreviations: BMI, body mass index (calculated as weight in kilograms divided by height in meters squared); IUGR, intrauterine growth restriction.
*Value is expressed as mean difference (95% confidence interval).

The clinical and demographic characteristics of the children born with IUGR and those without IUGR status are presented in **Table 2**. Maternal age was higher and tobacco and cocaine use during pregnancy were higher among the women with infants who had IUGR at birth as compared with those infants who did not have growth restriction at birth. The average weight of the infants who had IUGR at birth was 871 g less than those who did not have IUGR at birth.

## MEASUREMENTS AT 6 YEARS OF AGE

A systolic BP in the 95th percentile or higher was noted among 90 (17.4%) of 516 children born full term. A diastolic BP in the 95th percentile or higher was recorded among 14 (2.7%) of 516 children born full term. A systolic or diastolic BP in the 95th percentile or higher was seen among 93 (18.0%) of 516 children. These measurements were the mean of 3 readings. The first reading was the highest of 3 systolic BP readings in 44% of the children, while the first reading was the highest of 3 diastolic BP readings in 36% of the children.

The characteristics of the children with and without hypertension are presented in **Table 3**. The rate of hypertension at 6 years of age was greater among children who had IUGR at birth as compared with those who were of normal weight. Center differences in the rate of hypertension were also noted. The rate of hypertension did not differ among children exposed to maternal use of to-

**Table 4. Adjusted Relative Risk of Hypertension at Age 6 Years**

| Risk Factor | Adjusted Relative Risk* (95% Confidence Interval) |
|---|---|
| Site | |
| A vs D | 0.2 (0.1-0.5) |
| B vs D | 0.5 (0.3-0.8) |
| C vs D | 0.8 (0.5-1.2) |
| Race | |
| Black vs white | 1.0 (0.5-2.0) |
| Other vs white | 1.2 (0.5-3.1) |
| Sex | |
| F vs M | 1.0 (0.7-1.5) |
| Maternal education, y | |
| <12 vs >12 | 0.8 (0.5-1.3) |
| 12 vs >12 | 1.0 (0.6-1.5) |
| Maternal preeclampsia | 0.7 (0.3-1.7) |
| BMI at age 6 y, per unit increase | 1.1 (1.1-1.2) |
| IUGR | 1.8 (1.2-2.7) |
| Tobacco exposure | 1.4 (0.8-2.4) |
| Alcohol exposure | 0.8 (0.5-1.1) |
| Marijuana exposure | 0.9 (0.5-1.4) |
| Cocaine exposure | 1.2 (0.7-1.8) |

Abbreviations: See Table 3.
*Adjusted relative risks are obtained from Poisson regression modeling risk of hypertension at 6 years of age, adjusting for all the factors presented in Table 4.

bacco, alcohol, marijuana, cocaine, and opiates during pregnancy as compared with those not exposed to these substances. Maternal educational status did not influence rate of hypertension.

The mean (SD) BMI at 6 years of age among children who had IUGR at birth was 15.3 (2.0) as compared with those who did not have growth restriction at birth (16.9 [2.8]) ($P<.001$).

The multivariable logistic regression analyses evaluating model of risk for hypertension show that IUGR status at birth (relative risk, 1.8 [95% confidence interval, 1.2-2.7]) and BMI (per unit increase, relative risk, 1.1 [95% CI, 1.1-1.2]) increase risk for hypertension (**Table 4**). Again, center differences were noted in the risk for hypertension at 6 years of age.

## COMMENT

In this report, we have demonstrated that in full-term infants, IUGR status at birth appears to be linked to risk for hypertension in childhood after adjusting for potential confounders. These results suggest that IUGR status at birth may result in lifelong consequences because hypertension is a marker for adult cardiovascular disease.

We excluded preterm infants in this study because preterm birth has effects on the vascular system that persist to adult life. Kistner et al[13] have demonstrated that preterm birth affects the retinal vascular system, both functionally and structurally, resulting in a lower threshold for the development of vascular disease. Another reason for excluding children who were born preterm was that BP has been found to be significantly higher in very low-birth-weight subjects in late adolescence as compared with normal-birth-weight subjects.[14]

Blood pressure was measured in our study by the portable Dinamap monitor, an oscillometric device, and compared with normative data obtained by the sphygmomanometer auscultatory method.[16] Relationships between BP measurements using the Dinamap monitor and the sphygmomanometer method have been debated. Earlier reports by investigators have noted the accuracy of BP measurements by the Dinamap monitor in infants and children.[19,20] Most recent data, however, have shown that higher readings are obtained by the Dinamap monitor as compared with the sphygmomanometer.[21] However, the Dinamap monitor is the most common instrument used in current clinical practice. The BP cuffs used in this study were based on the recommendations established by the National High Blood Pressure Education Program Working Group on High Blood Pressure in Children and Adolescents.[16] By doing so, we believe we have avoided the pitfalls of inappropriate cuff selection.[22]

In this study, an association between increases in BMI and elevation in BP was noted. The systolic BP of children, adolescents, and adults is affected by BMI measured at corresponding ages.[23-26] Although overweight and obesity status were not seen in the 6-year-old children in this report, we anticipate the frequency of these conditions to increase as the children continue to be evaluated at older ages,[27,28] when it is anticipated a greater association of BMI with hypertension can be demonstrated.

Race and socioeconomic factors have been shown to influence hypertension. Black Americans are at higher risk for hypertension than white Americans, and an increase in overweight and obesity in Hispanic individuals has been reported.[25,26,29] Among minorities, the relative risk for hypertension is significant for both sex and overweight status. The majority of the children in our study were black; however, no risk for hypertension was attributed to race. Unfortunately, we did not measure maternal BP at the child's 6-year clinic visit because this is an important confounder. We are currently obtaining BP measurements at the 9-year visit of the children. We did find clinical site differences, which need to be explored. In our study, at 6 years of age, we did not find a relationship between sex and hypertension. Socioeconomic status was measured as maternal education in our study and was not associated with hypertension.

The association between maternal lifestyle during pregnancy and risk for hypertension in the offspring is unclear when examining prenatal cocaine exposure and elevated BP in childhood. Horn[8] examined 12 infants following intrauterine cocaine exposure and noted that half of the infants had hypertension or normal BP. Needlman et al[9] found no differences in BP between 32 cocaine-exposed and 23 nonexposed infants at 8 to 26 months of age. Echocardiography of infants born to women following cocaine exposure and comparison infants (total of 87 infants evaluated) has not demonstrated any difference in the shortening fraction of the left ventricle or abnormalities in cardiac rhythm.[30] Prenatal exposure to cigarettes has been associated with elevated BP at birth and at 12 months of age.[31] We did not find any association with either cocaine, opiate, marijuana, tobacco, or alcohol use during pregnancy and hypertension at 6 years of age.

Additional risk factors for hypertension are diet[32,33] and genetic determinant of cardiovascular risk.[34] New arteriosclerosis risk factors in obese children and adolescents and children and adolescents with hypertension and diabetes are now available.[35] As we follow up our cohort longitudinally we will obtain data on these risk factors.

Sixteen percent of children who did not have growth restriction at birth were found to have hypertension at 6 years of age. We suggest that this high rate reflects an atypical study group that is predominantly inner city and African American and has a low socioeconomic status.

In summary, in this study we have demonstrated an association between IUGR status at birth and elevated BP at 6 years of age among full-term infants. Six years of age may be too young to label a child at risk for hypertension; however, an awareness of the prehypertensive status in childhood may serve as a signal to institute healthful lifestyle changes that might avert future cardiovascular disease.[36]

**Accepted for Publication:** June 24, 2006.
**Correspondence:** Seetha Shankaran, MD, Neonatal-Perinatal Medicine, Children's Hospital of Michigan, 3901 Beaubien Blvd, Detroit, MI 48201 (sshankar@med.wayne.edu).
**Author Contributions:** *Study concept and design:* Shankaran, Das, Bauer, Bada, Lester, Wright, Higgins, and Poole. *Acquisition of data:* Shankaran, Das, Bauer, Bada, Lester, Wright, Higgins, and Poole. *Analysis and interpretation of data:* Shankaran, Das, Bauer, Bada, Lester, Wright, Higgins, and Poole. *Drafting of the manuscript:* Shankaran. *Critical revision of the manuscript for important intellectual content:* Shankaran, Das, Bauer, Bada, Lester, Wright, Higgins, and Poole. *Statistical analysis:* Shankaran and Das. *Obtained funding:* Shankaran, Das, Bauer, Bada, Lester, and Poole. *Administrative, technical, and material support:* Shankaran, Das, Bauer, Bada, Lester, Wright, Higgins, and Poole. *Study supervision:* Shankaran, Das, Bauer, Bada, Lester, Wright, Higgins, and Poole.
**Funding/Support:** This study was supported by National Institute of Child Health and Human Development (NICHD) grants U10 HD 27904 (Dr Lester), U10 HD 21397 (Dr Bauer), U10 HD 21415 (Dr Bada), U10 HD 21385 (Dr Shankaran), and U01 HD 36790 (Dr Poole) and National Institute on Drug Abuse (NIDA) grant N01-HD-2-3159 (Dr Lester).
**Acknowledgment:** We thank the research coordinators and research nurses involved with the Maternal Lifestyle Study: Brown University: Susan Schibler, RN, Melissa Ambrosia, RN, and Linda LaGasse, PhD; University of Miami: Wendy Griffin, RN, and Elizabeth Jacque, RN; University of Tennessee: Charlotte Bursi, MSSW, Claudia Duncan, RN, PNP, and Andrea Simmons, RN, PNP; Wayne State University: Eunice Woldt, MSN, and Jay Ann Nelson, BSN; Research Triangle Institute International: Jane Hammond, PhD; NICHD: Linda L. Wright, MD; NIDA: Vincent L Smeriglio, PhD.

## REFERENCES

1. Barker DJP, Osmond C, Winter PD, Margetts B, Simmonds SJ. Weight in infancy and death from ischaemic heart disease. *Lancet.* 1989;2:577-580.
2. Falkner B, Hulman S, Kushner H. Birth weight versus childhood growth as determinants of adult blood pressure. *Hypertension.* 1998;31:145-150.
3. Hinchliffe SA, Lynch MRJ, Sargent PH, Howard CV, Velzen DV. The effect of intrauterine growth retardation on the development of renal nephrons. *Br J Obstet Gynaecol.* 1992;99:296-301.
4. Bada HS, Das A, Bauer CR, et al. Gestational cocaine exposure and intrauterine growth: Maternal Lifestyle Study. *Obstet Gynecol.* 2002;100:916-924.
5. Bandstra ES, Morrow CE, Anthony JC, et al. Intrauterine growth of full-term infants: impact of prenatal cocaine exposure. *Pediatrics.* 2001;108:1309-1319.
6. Bauer CR, Langer JC, Shankaran S, et al. Acute neonatal effects of cocaine exposure during pregnancy. *Arch Pediatr Adolesc Med.* 2005;159:824-834.
7. Brown JV, Bakeman R, Coles CD, Sexson WR, Demi AS. Maternal drug use during pregnancy: are preterm and full-term infants affected differently? *Dev Psychol.* 1998;34:540-554.
8. Horn PT. Persistent hypertension after prenatal cocaine exposure. *J Pediatr.* 1992;121:288-291.
9. Needlman R, Frank DA, Cabral H, Mirochnick M, Kwon C, Zuckerman B. Blood pressure in children exposed prenatally to cocaine. *Clin Pediatr (Phila).* 1998;37:659-664.
10. Messinger DS, Bauer CR, Das A, et al. The Maternal Lifestyle Study: cognitive, motor, and behavioral outcomes of cocaine-exposed and opiate-exposed infants through three years of age. *Pediatrics.* 2004;113:1677-1685.
11. Ballard JL, Khoury JC, Wedig K, Wang L, Eilers-Walsmans BL, Lipp R. New Ballard Score, expanded to include extremely premature infants. *J Pediatr.* 1991;119:417-423.
12. Alexander GR, Himes JH, Kaufman RB, Mor J, Kogan M. A United States national reference for fetal growth. *Obstet Gynecol.* 1996;87:163-168.
13. Kistner A, Jacobson L, Jacobson SH, Svensson E, Hellström A. Low gestational age associated with abnormal retinal vascularization and increased blood pressure in adult women. *Pediatr Res.* 2002;51:675-680.
14. Doyle LW, Faber B, Callanan C, Morley R. Blood pressure in late adolescence and very low birth weight. *Pediatrics.* 2003;111:252-257.
15. Kuczmarski RJ, Ogden CL, Grummer-Strawn LM, et al. CDC growth charts: United States. *Adv Data.* 2000;314:1-27.
16. National High Blood Pressure Education Program Working Group on High Blood Pressure in Children and Adolescents. The fourth report on the diagnosis, evaluation, and treatment of high blood pressure in children and adolescents. *Pediatrics.* 2004;114:555-576.
17. Zou G. A modified Poisson regression approach to prospective studies with binary data. *Am J Epidemiol.* 2004;159:702-706.
18. Hollingshead AB. *Four Factor Index of Social Status.* New Haven, Conn: Yale University; 1975.
19. Park MK, Menard SM. Accuracy of blood pressure measurement by the Dinamap monitor in infants and children. *Pediatrics.* 1987;79:907-914.
20. Weaver MG, Park MK, Lee D. Differences in blood pressure levels obtained by auscultatory and oscillometric methods. *AJDC.* 1990;144:911-914.
21. Park MK, Menard SW, Yuan C. Comparison of auscultatory and oscillometric blood pressures. *Arch Pediatr Adolesc Med.* 2001;155:50-53.
22. Arafat M, Mattoo JK. Measurement of blood pressure in children: recommendations and perceptions on cuff selection. *Pediatrics.* 1999;104:e30. http://pediatrics.aappublications.org/cgi/content/full/104/3/e30. Accessed November 2, 2005.
23. Muntner P, He J, Cutler JA, Wildman RP, Whelton PK. Trends in blood pressure among children and adolescents. *JAMA.* 2004;291:2107-2113.
24. Update on the 1987 Task Force Report on high blood pressure in children and adolescents: a working group report from the National High Blood Pressure Education Program. *Pediatrics.* 1996;98:649-658.
25. Hardy R, Kuh D, Langenberg C, Wadsworth MEJ. Birthweight, childhood social class, and change in adult blood pressure in the 1946 British birth cohort. *Lancet.* 2003;362:1178-1183.
26. Sorof JM, Lai D, Turner JT, Poffenbarger T, Portman RJ. Overweight, ethnicity, and the prevalence of hypertension in school-aged children. *Pediatrics.* 2004;113:475-482.
27. Ebbeling CB, Pawlak DB, Ludwig DS. Childhood obesity: public-health crisis, common sense cure. *Lancet.* 2002;360:473-482.
28. Committee on Nutrition. Prevention of pediatric overweight and obesity. *Pediatrics.* 2003;112:424-430.
29. Wilson DK, Kliewer W, Plybon L, Sica DA. Socioeconomic status and blood pressure reactivity in healthy black adolescents. *Hypertension.* 2000;35:496-500.
30. Tuboku-Metzger AJ, O'Shea JA, Campbell RM, et al. Cardiovascular effects of cocaine in neonates exposed prenatally. *Am J Perinatol.* 1996;13:1-4.
31. Beratis NG, Panagoulias D, Varvarigou A. Increased blood pressure in neonates and infants whose mothers smoked during pregnancy. *J Pediatr.* 1996;128:806-812.
32. Falkner B, Sheriff K, Michel S, Kushner H. Dietary nutrients and blood pressure in urban minority adolescents at risk for hypertension. *Arch Pediatr Adolesc Med.* 2000;154:918-922.
33. Simons-Morton DG, Hunsberger SA, Van Horn L, et al. Nutrient intake and blood pressure in the dietary intervention study in children. *Hypertension.* 1997;29:930-936.
34. Lloyd-Jones DM, Nam BH, D'Agostino RB, et al. Parental cardiovascular disease as a risk factor for cardiovascular disease in middle-aged adults. *JAMA.* 2004;291:2204-2211.
35. Glowinska B, Urban M, Koput A, Galar M. New atherosclerosis risk factors in obese, hypertensive and diabetic children and adolescents. *Atherosclerosis.* 2003;167:275-286.
36. Ingelfinger JR. Pediatric antecedents of adult cardiovascular disease-awareness and intervention. *N Engl J Med.* 2004;350:2123-2126.

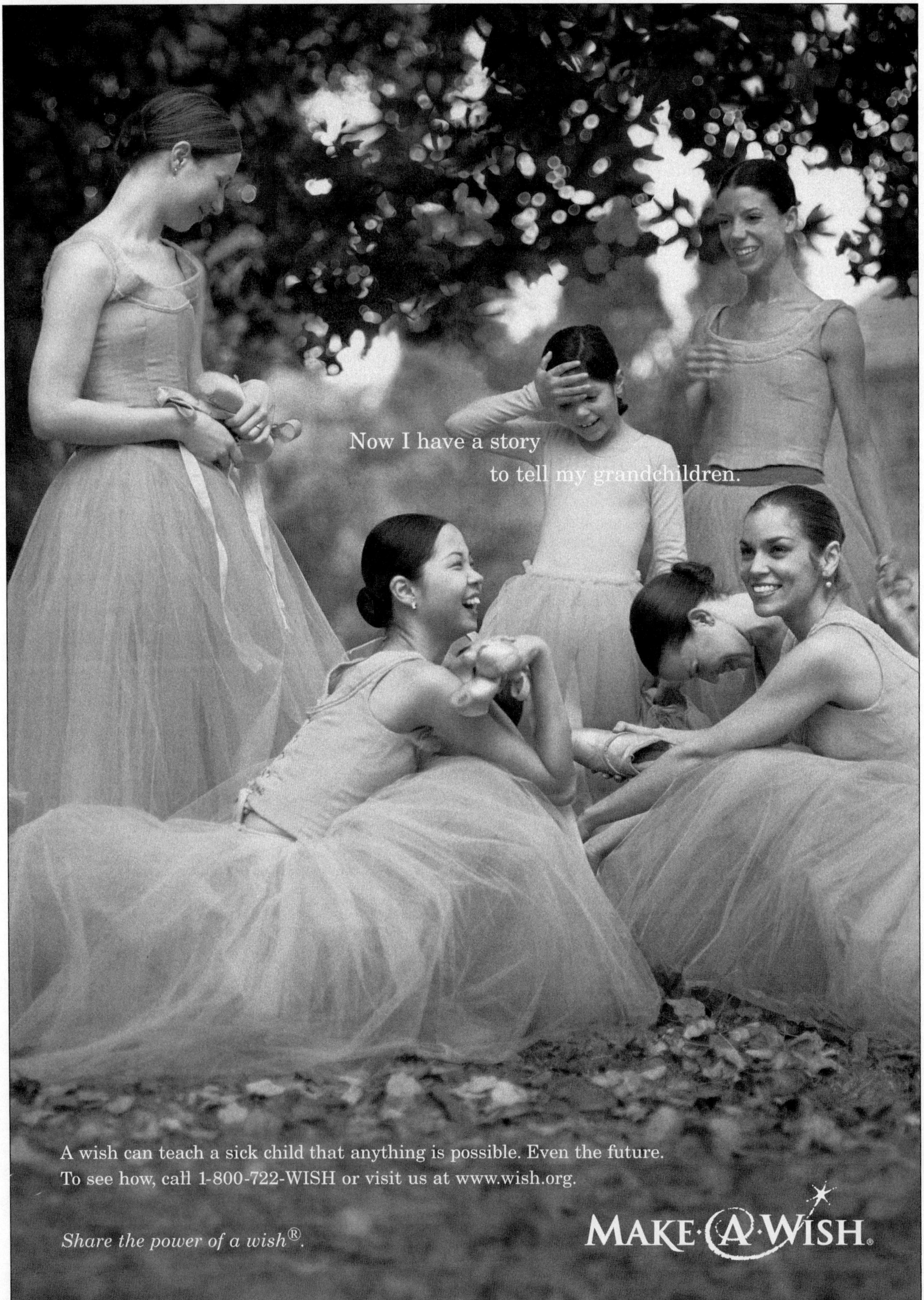
Now I have a story
to tell my grandchildren.
A wish can teach a sick child that anything is possible. Even the future.
To see how, call 1-800-722-WISH or visit us at www.wish.org.
*Share the power of a wish®.*
MAKE·A·WISH

SECTION EDITOR: ALBERT C. YAN, MD; ASSISTANT SECTION EDITOR: SAMIR S. SHAH, MD

# Picture of the Month

*Jennifer A. Jewell, MD, MS; Lorraine L. McElwain, MD; Amy S. Blake, BS*

A 23-MONTH-OLD SUDANESE GIRL HAD FAILure to thrive and an unusual gait. She was noted to be a happy, developmentally appropriate child (**Figure**, A) with bowed legs (Figure, B), thick wrists (Figure, C), and dental caries. Her weight (8.7 kg) and height (72.5 cm) were below the third percentiles for her age. Her diet consisted predominantly of breastfeeding 5 times daily; however, she did consume 500 mL of juice, 4 teaspoons of rice, and a few bites of a sandwich most days. Her medical history included iron-deficiency anemia that was corrected with oral iron supplementation. She was receiving no other medications. The patient was born in the United States after an unremarkable prenatal, delivery, and postnatal course. She resided in the northeastern United States with her parents. Laboratory studies revealed an elevated total alkaline phosphatase level (1151 U/L) and an elevated intact parathyroid hormone level (16.2 pmol/L [reference range, 1.6-6.8 pmol/L]). The 25-hydroxyvitamin D level was decreased (19 nmol/L [reference range, 25-137 nmol/L). The complete blood cell count, remainder of the comprehensive metabolic profile, ionized calcium level, and phosphorous level were unremarkable. Plain radiographs of the patient's knees (Figure, D) and wrists (Figure, E) demonstrated osseous changes including metaphyseal cupping and flaring, epiphyseal irregularities, and widening of the physeal plates. A chest radiograph was unremarkable.

What is your diagnosis?

**Author Affiliations:** The Barbara Bush Children's Hospital, Portland, Me (Drs Jewell and McElwain); Dartmouth Medical School, Hanover, NH (Drs Jewell and McElwain); and University of Vermont College of Medicine, Burlington (Drs Jewell and McElwain and Ms Blake).

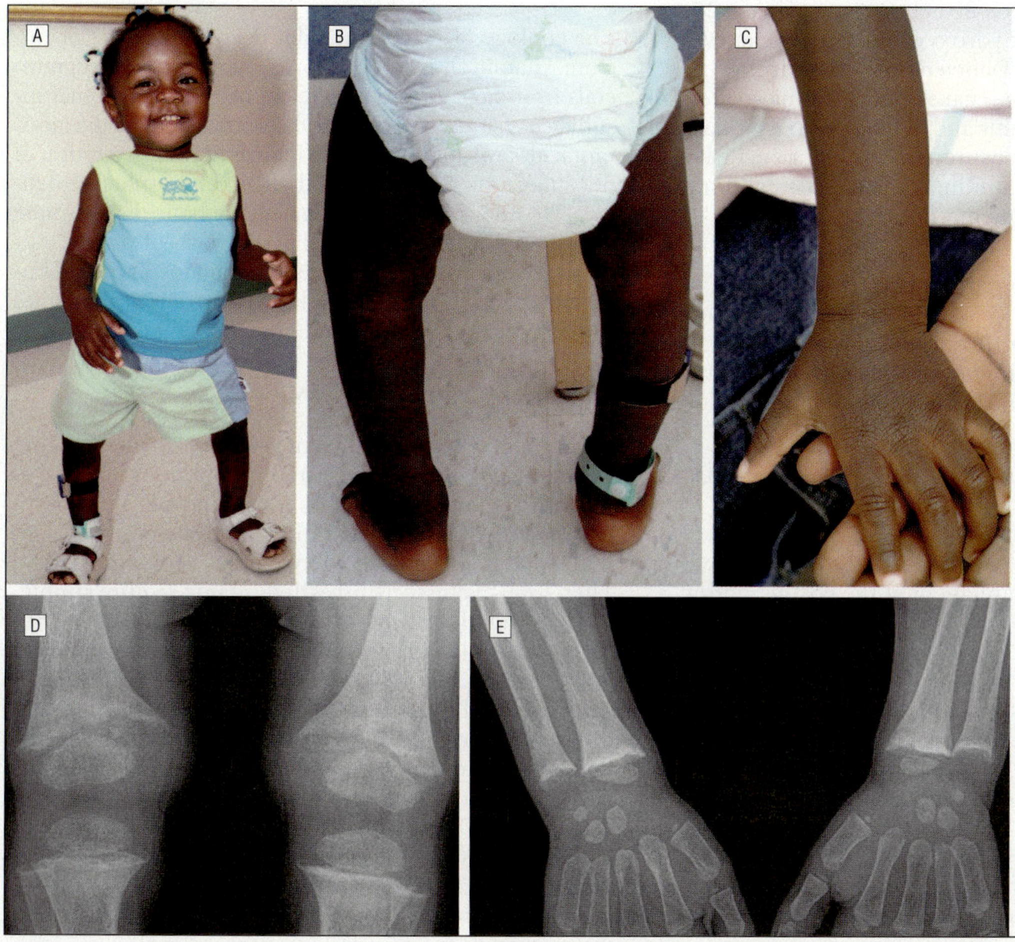


**Figure.** A well-appearing 23-month-old patient has failure to thrive (A), bowing of bilateral extremities (B), and a thickened left wrist (C). D, A bilateral knee radiograph shows femoral cupping and flaring, epiphyseal irregularities, and widened physes. E, A bilateral wrist radiograph shows radial and ulnar cupping and flaring, epiphyseal irregularities, and widened physes.

# Denouement and Discussion

## *Nutritional Rickets*

Nutritional rickets has a prevalence rate between 5% and 10% in developing countries.[1,2] By the mid 1900s, nutritional rickets was virtually eliminated in the United States. However, a recent reemergence has been witnessed by health care providers in the United States and other developed countries.[3-6] Because rickets is not a reportable disease, the exact incidence in US children is unknown.

Rickets occurs when calcium and/or phosphorus deficiency results in inadequate bone mineralization. Both 1,25-dihydroxyvitamin D and parathyroid hormone are essential to calcium and phosphorus homeostasis. The 1,25-dihydroxyvitamin D increases calcium and phosphorus absorption from the gastrointestinal tract. Parathyroid hormone increases the serum calcium level by bone resorption and decreases the serum phosphorus level by increased urinary excretion. Together, these mechanisms maintain serum calcium and phosphorus concentrations at the expense of bone mineralization.[7] Rickets occurs in patients with disorders in calcium, phosphorus, and vitamin D metabolism.

Nutritional rickets occurs when 1,25-dihydroxyvitamin D, calcium, or both are deficient. Because 25-hydroxyvitamin D is the direct precursor to 1,25-dihydroxyvitamin D, 25-hydroxyvitamin D deficiency is a direct cause of rickets. Deficiency of 25-hydroxyvitamin D is the most common cause of nutritional rickets and is associated with infants and toddlers who have dark skin, limited sunlight exposure, prolonged or exclusive breastfeeding, diets with minimal dairy intake, and improper vitamin D supplementation.[3-5]

### CLINICAL FEATURES

Most of the clinical manifestations of rickets occur secondary to either impaired mineralization of the bony matrix or hypocalcemia. Skeletal findings include the following:

- Craniotabes (softening of the skull and occipital flattening)
- Delayed fontanelle closure
- Frontal bossing
- Rachitic rosary (enlargement at the costochondral junction)
- Harrison sulcus (groove in the lower ribs where the diaphragm attaches)
- Scoliosis and/or kyphosis
- Genu varum or genu valgum (in ambulatory patients)
- Bowing of the radius and ulna (in nonambulatory patients)
- Saber shin deformity (anterior bowing of the tibia)
- Thickened wrists and ankles
- Bone pain and tenderness
- Hypotonia

Extraskeletal features include the following:

- Late teeth eruption and poor enamelization of teeth
- Seizures and/or tetany (related to hypocalcemia)
- Failure to thrive or short stature
- Developmental delay
- Secondary immunodeficiency

Laboratory evaluation reveals a significantly elevated alkaline phosphatase level in all types of rickets. The calcium (total and ionized) and phosphorus levels are frequently decreased whereas the parathyroid hormone level is frequently increased in hypocalcemic rickets. The 25-hydroxyvitamin D level is decreased in vitamin D deficiency and hypocalcemic rickets.

Radiographic findings are noted in the growth plates of long bones, especially the distal ulnar, radius, and femur and the proximal tibia. In these locations, metaphyseal widening, cupping, fraying, and flaring are common. Bowing of the upper and lower extremities, depending on the weight-bearing status of the patient, is another frequent radiographic finding. Cortical thinning and osteopenia of the long bone diaphyses can be seen.

### DIFFERENTIAL DIAGNOSIS

The etiology of rickets includes decreased intake of calcium, vitamin D, and phosphorus, poor absorption of minerals from hepatic and pancreatic insufficiency, renal insufficiency, interference with absorption from medications (antacids and antiepileptics), increased renal excretion of phosphorus and calcium, and alkaline phosphatase deficiency. Other rare causes of metabolic bone disease must be considered in the differential diagnosis of rickets. Additionally, Blount disease, neurofibromatosis type I, fibular hemimelia, and congenital lower extremity anomalies can result in genu varum and other bowing deformities.

### TREATMENT

To prevent vitamin D deficiency, it is recommended that all infants who do not ingest a minimum of 500 mL of vitamin D–containing formula or milk receive vitamin D supplementation. Breast milk contains minimal vitamin D and is not considered a vitamin D–containing milk. Therefore, exclusively breastfed infants require supplementation before 2 months of age. Additionally, children and adolescents who do not drink a minimum of 500 mL of vitamin D–containing milk, do not have adequate sunlight exposure, or do not receive a multivitamin with at least 200 IU of vitamin D require supplementation. The prophylactic dose of vitamin D is 200 IU daily.[8] To treat nutritional rickets, high doses of oral vitamin D (2000-10 000 IU of ergocalciferol daily) and calcium (300-1000 mg of elemental calcium daily) are suggested for 3 months. Consultation with an endocrinologist or other health care provider with an interest in bone disorders may be warranted.

Because a positive correlation between maternal and child vitamin D status has been demonstrated,[9] especially with breastfed infants,[10] a diagnosis of rickets strongly suggests maternal vitamin D deficiency. If a child at high risk for vitamin D deficiency is diagnosed with rickets, routine management should include analysis of maternal vitamin D status and appropriate therapy for the mother.[11] A daily maternal intake of approximately 2000 to 4000 IU of vitamin D is recommended since this supplementation appears to safely provide sufficient vitamin D to enter the breast milk and increase the infant's circulating 25-hydroxyvitamin D level.[12] In our case, the mother was receiving no vitamin D supplementation despite limited sun exposure, darkly pigmented skin, and inadequate diet and had a decreased 25-hydroxyvitamin D level (27 nmol/L [optimal range, 62-200 nmol/L]).

**Accepted for Publication:** November 22, 2005.
**Correspondence:** Jennifer A. Jewell, MD, MS, The Barbara Bush Children's Hospital, 22 Bramhall St, Portland, ME 04102 (jewelj@mmc.org).
**Author Contributions:** *Study concept and design:* Jewell, McElwain, and Blake. *Acquisition of data:* Jewell, McElwain, and Blake. *Drafting of the manuscript:* Jewell, McElwain, and Blake. *Critical revision of the manuscript for important intellectual content:* Jewell, McElwain, and Blake. *Administrative, technical, and material support:* Jewell, McElwain, and Blake. *Study supervision:* Jewell and McElwain.

## REFERENCES


1. Meisner C, Welch R, Duxbury JM, Lauren JG. Making a greener revolution: a nutrient delivery system for food production to address malnutrition through crop science. http://www.cropscience.org.au/icsc2004/poster/5/1/3/1944_meisner.htm. Accessed July 26, 2005.
2. Pfitzner MA, Thackher TD, Pettifor JM, et al. Absence of vitamin D deficiency in young Nigerian children. *J Pediatr.* 1998;133:740-744.
3. Weisberg P, Scanlon KS, Li R, Cogswell ME. Nutritional rickets among children in the United States: review of cases reported between 1996 and 2003. *Am J Clin Nutr.* 2004;80:1697S-1705S.
4. Tomashek KM, Nesby S, Scanlon KS, et al. Nutritional rickets in Georgia. *Pediatrics.* 2001;107:e45 http://www.pediatrics.org/cgi/content/full/107/4/e45. Accessed July 26, 2005.
5. DeLucia MC, Mitnick ME, Carpenter TO. Nutritional rickets with normal circulating 25-hydroxyvitamin D: a call for reexamining the role of dietary calcium intake in North American infants. *J Clin Endocrinol Metab.* 2003;88:3539-3545.
6. Cowell CT. Comment: seizures as the presenting feature of rickets in an infant. *Med J Aust.* 2003;178:467-468.
7. Behrman RE, Kliegman RM, Jenson HB. *Nelson Textbook of Pediatrics.* 17th ed. Philadelphia, Pa: Saunders; 2004.
8. Gartner LM, Greer FR. Prevention of rickets and vitamin D deficiency: new guidelines for vitamin D intake. *Pediatrics.* 2003;111:908-910.
9. Nozza JM, Rodda CP. Vitamin D deficiency in mothers of infants with rickets. *Med J Aust.* 2001;175:253-255.
10. Daaboul J, Sanderson S, Kristensen K, Kitson H. Vitamin D deficiency in pregnant and breast-feeding women and their infants. *J Perinatol.* 1997;17:10-14.
11. Dawodu A, Agarwal M, Sankarankutty M, Hardy D, Kochiyil J, Badrinath P. Higher prevalence of vitamin D deficiency in mothers of rachitic than nonrachitic children. *J Pediatr.* 2005;147:109-111.
12. Hollis BW, Wagner CL. Vitamin D requirements during lactation: high-dose maternal supplementation as therapy to prevent hypovitaminosis D for both mother and the nursing infant. *Am J Clin Nutr.* 2004;80:1752S-1758S.


### *Announcement*

**Submissions.** The Editors welcome contributions to Picture of the Month. Submissions should describe common problems presenting uncommonly, rather than total zebras. Cases should be of interest to practicing pediatricians, highlighting problems that they are likely to at least occasionally encounter in the office or hospital setting. High-quality clinical images (in either 35-mm slide or electronic format) along with parent or patient permission to use these images must accompany the submission. The entire discussion should comprise no more than 750 words. Articles and photographs accepted for publication will bear the contributor's name. There is no charge for reproduction and printing of color illustrations. For details regarding electronic submission, please see: http://archpedi.ama-assn.org.

SECTION EDITOR: ABRAHAM BERGMAN, MD

## Immunizations & Infectious Diseases: An Informed Parent's Guide

*by Margaret C. Fisher, MD, editor, 328 pages, $14.95, ISBN 1581101392, Elk Grove Village, Ill, American Academy of Pediatrics, 2005.*

This book contains information about things that I as a parent might wish were true but aren't, like antibacterial soaps (herein debunked) and the BRAT diet, in which bananas, rice, applesauce, and toast are supposed to help a nauseous child.

Then there are the facts I wish were not true but are: children are supposed to wash their hands after every time they touch a pet. They are never ever to be left alone with animals. And you don't want rodents, or their traces, anywhere near you. Baby turtles or (gasp!) cookie dough or sprouts, either. The last bit of bad news: if it involves making a mess, as do most verbs of childhood, you must wash your hands afterward. So, unfortunately, since the cover price does not include a full-time governess, I must resign myself to the nagging knowledge that my children are at constant risk. They will have to develop any obsessive-compulsive handwashing disorder on their own. I will scrub them whenever I can, short of making myself crazy. But the good news is many of the infectious diseases described in detail in this new volume can be prevented by frequent applications of soap and water.

Of course, many parents will be turning to this book for the first part of its title, looking for a factual assessment of the passionate debate over the safety of immunizations. You'll get answers to questions like how safe are vaccines, which ones are needed, and how do I keep my newborn protected? Based on the American Academy of Pediatrics *Red Book*,[1] this evidence-based guide promises to "save hours of practice time answering questions that parents are asking."

When it comes to vaccines, I admit I have a bias, having spent a few sleepless nights with my 4-month-old son while visiting a community where unimmunized children were experiencing a pertussis outbreak. How dare those parents, with their fears of "unnatural" medicine, put my child at risk? As the authors note, "The greatest risks come when children are not immunized." While it could have likely been more convincing if they had taken on, one by one, more of the concerns of the Internet's antivaccine contingent, they present unbiased studies that form a decisive argument for immunizing your children.

The authors alternate fairly between male and female pronouns but suddenly stop in the section on sexually transmitted diseases (STDs). As parents, we are to "make sure she knows" that AIDS is the leading cause of death in people aged 15 to 24 years, that "saying 'no' today is better than doing something she will regret tomorrow," "that using alcohol or drugs can affect her ability to make a good decision," and that "if a teenager starts having sex, it is important for her to practice safe sex." We should talk to our teenager "about how she can reduce her risk of STDs by limiting the number of lifetime sexual partners." Please. If we are not also teaching our sons how to protect themselves, we are putting their health, and the health of their girlfriends or boyfriends, at serious risk. The American Academy of Pediatrics should know that. And it should spread the word instead of falling back on quaint wording and obsolete assumptions.

But aside from that, the authors lead the lay reader to have more respect for the pediatrician. What baroque sort of decision-making flowchart must there be for physicians making decisions about when a barfy night is just something to wait out and when it is an early sign of something life threatening?

The warnings (in the section on *Haemophilus influenzae* type b infections, for example) to call your physician if any of the symptoms appear are a bit frightening, as one of them (fever) is something that a reasonably careful mother (me) would wait a bit on, at least for someone older than 1 year. One of my pediatricians does not really believe in putting too much stock in the numbers on a thermometer, because, he says, they do not really tell you much (and, I suspect, because people like me tend to call people like him when people like him would rather be asleep).

The authors' careful descriptions of everything from chicken pox through mad cow disease leave me wondering how many times I should have called about an upset stomach and what diagnoses those lingering toddler viral illnesses might have warranted. The careful discussion of the dangerous overuse of antibiotics was also enlightening—who knew that physicians prescribe antibacterials 65% of the time when they think parents want them but only 12% of the time if they think parents do not? "Just say no" can apply to amoxicillin as well as marijuana.

Overall, this is a comprehensive volume, useful for parents who want to keep their little ones safe and healthy.

*Tina Kelley, BA*

**Correspondence:** Ms Kelley (tinapetekate@yahoo.com).

1. Pickering LK, ed. *Red Book: 2003 Report of the Committee on Infectious Diseases*. 26th ed. Elk Grove Village, Ill: American Academy of Pediatrics; 2003. http://aapredbook.aappublications.org/current.shtml.

## Denial of Insurance Authorization at a Subspecialty Office as a Cause of Missed Opportunities for Influenza Vaccination in Children With Asthma

Despite American Academy of Pediatrics (AAP) recommendations that children with asthma receive yearly influenza vaccines,[1] vaccination rates remain low.[2] Visits to allergists are opportunities to vaccinate children with asthma, yet insurance authorization for vaccination is not uniformly granted to subspecialists. We prospectively followed up children with asthma for whom we could not obtain insurance authorization for influenza vaccinations in our allergy clinic to determine how many eventually received the vaccine.

**Methods.** During the 2003-2004 influenza vaccination season, all patients with asthma initially seen in a hospital-based allergy clinic who met AAP-defined criteria for vaccination were identified. Vaccination season was defined as starting on receipt of the vaccine, approximately September 22, 2003, through January 31, 2004. Patients for whom insurance authorization was obtained were vaccinated, while those for whom authorization could not be obtained were advised to get vaccinated by their primary care physician as soon as possible. In March 2004, patients not vaccinated in the allergy clinic were contacted to determine their vaccination status. This study was approved by the hospital institutional review board.

Differences in vaccination rates between groups with different insurance plans were analyzed using the 2-sided Fisher exact test. The mean delay until vaccination between the Medicaid and private insurance groups was compared using the *t* test. A *P* value of $<.05$ was considered significant.

**Results.** Two hundred twenty-nine eligible patients (61.4% female; mean age, 9.9 years [range, 1.5-18.9 years]) were identified. Vaccination was contraindicated in 7 with egg allergy, 5 refused vaccination, and 17 were lost to follow-up, leaving 200 evaluable subjects (**Figure**). Most patients (160) had Medicaid (29 of 160) or a Medicaid health maintenance organization (HMO) (131 of 160) insurance, and the remainder had various commercial insurances. Fourteen were vaccinated prior to their first in-season allergy clinic visit. Eighty-five (42.5%) were not authorized to receive their vaccine in our allergy clinic, the majority (64 [75.3%]) of whom had Medicaid HMO plans.

Forty-one (48.2%) of the 85 denied patients ultimately received the vaccine. Of these, 31 were vaccinated by their primary physician, while 10 paid out-of-pocket for the vaccine even though their insurance would have covered the vaccine at their primary care physician's office. Forty-four (51.8%) (22% of all 200 evaluable patients) never received the vaccine. Denied patients with commercial HMOs were more likely to eventually get the vaccine (66.7% vs 42.4%) and to pay out-of-pocket for the vaccine (23.8% vs 7.8%) compared with patients with Medicaid HMOs, but this trend

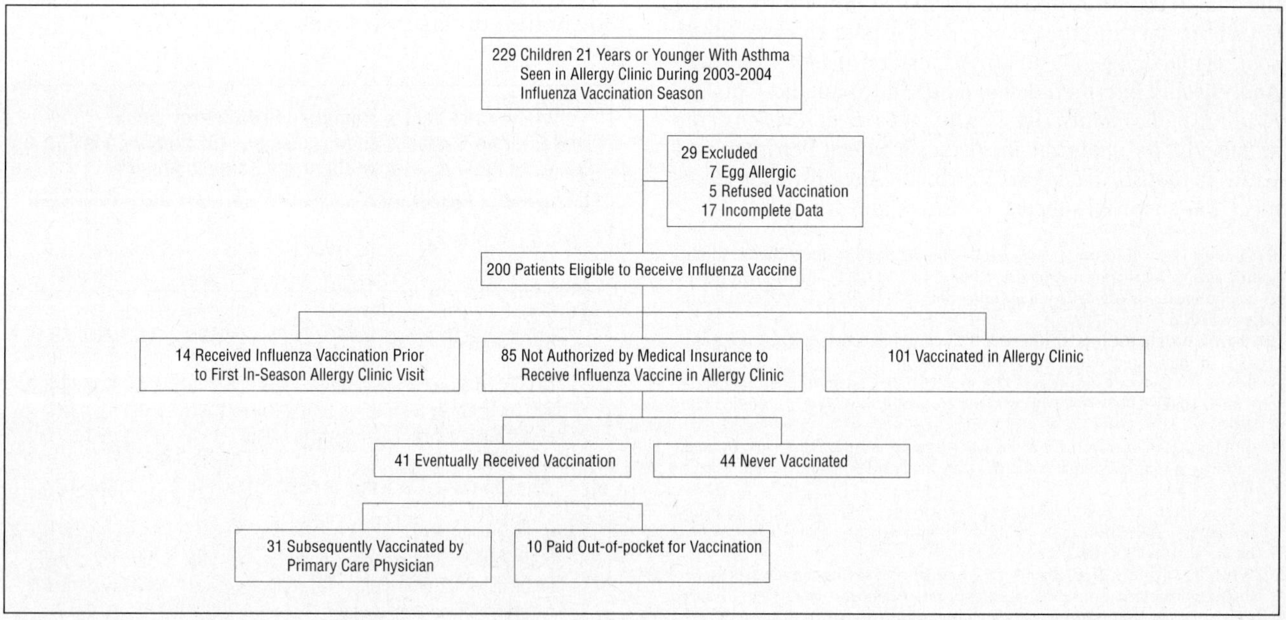


**Figure.** Flow diagram of study.

did not reach statistical significance. The mean delay to vaccine administration was 30.1 days (range, 0-114 days). The reasons for nonvaccination were no return to their primary physician's office (24 [77.4%]), their primary physician running out of vaccine (5 [16.1%]), or refusal to vaccinate (2 [6.5%]).

**Comment.** A substantial percentage of children in this study (22%) never received their influenza vaccine because of lack of insurance authorization. This may actually be an underestimation of the problem because there may have been increased demand for vaccination compared with previous seasons because of increased media reports of pediatric deaths from influenza that season.[3] There was a trend toward less vaccination in children with Medicaid HMOs, which could be a factor in the poorer asthma outcome seen in children with asthma with Medicaid.[4]

Children with chronic medical disorders are at high risk for influenza-associated morbidity[2] yet paradoxically have lower vaccination rates.[5] Subspecialty clinic visits represent opportunities for vaccination of these patients, and an AAP policy statement[1] recommends that influenza immunization be started as early in the season as possible and at all visits—not just well-child visits. In addition, requiring extra physician visits solely for immunization increases costs to families and the health care system and makes influenza vaccination less cost-effective.[6]

Changes in authorization procedures and policies should be implemented to allow vaccinations by subspecialty physician offices in the same manner as primary care physician offices.

*Ronald M. Ferdman, MD, MEd*
*Joseph A. Church, MD*

**Correspondence:** Dr Ferdman, Division of Clinical Immunology and Allergy, Childrens Hospital Los Angeles, 4650 Sunset Blvd, MS 75, Los Angeles, CA 90027 (rferdman@chla.usc.edu).

**Author Contributions:** Dr Ferdman had full access to all the data in the study and takes responsibility for the integrity of the data and the accuracy of the data analysis. *Study concept and design:* Ferdman. *Acquisition of data:* Ferdman. *Analysis and interpretation of data:* Ferdman and Church. *Drafting of the manuscript:* Ferdman. *Critical revision of the manuscript for important intellectual content:* Ferdman and Church. *Statistical analysis:* Ferdman. *Administrative, technical, and material support:* Ferdman and Church.

1. Committee on Infectious Diseases. Recommendations for influenza immunization in children. *Pediatrics*. 2004;113:1441-1447. http://aappolicy.aappublications.org/cgi/content/full/pediatrics;113/5/1441. Accessed February 2, 2006.
2. Bhat N, Wright JG, Broder KR, et al. Influenza-associated deaths among children in the United States, 2003-2004. *N Engl J Med*. 2005;353:2559-2567.
3. Centers for Disease Control and Prevention (CDC). Update: influenza activity—United States, 2003-04 season. *MMWR Morb Mortal Wkly Rep*. 2004;53:284-287.
4. Shields AE, Comstock C, Weiss KB. Variations in asthma care by race/ethnicity among children enrolled in a state Medicaid program. *Pediatrics*. 2004;113:496-504.
5. Chung EK, Casey R, Pinto-Martin JA, Pawlowski NA, Bell LM. Routine and influenza vaccination rates in children with asthma. *Ann Allergy Asthma Immunol*. 1998;80:318-322.
6. White T, Lavoie S, Nettleman MD. Potential cost savings attributable to influenza vaccination of school-aged children. *Pediatrics*. 1999;103:e73. http://pediatrics.aappublications.org/cgi/content/full/103/6/e73. Accessed February 2, 2006.

## Internet Cigarette Vendors' Lack of Compliance With a California State Law Designed to Prevent Tobacco Sales to Minors

Efforts by public health and law enforcement officials in recent years have had a substantial impact on reducing youth access to cigarettes through retail stores, leading to growing concern over youth access to cigarettes from Internet cigarette vendors (ICVs). This has led some states to pass legislation governing Internet tobacco sales to minors. California Business and Professions Code § 22963[1] (BP § 22963) is currently one of the most stringent ICV youth access laws because it requires vendors to comply with 6 provisions designed to reduce youth purchases of cigarettes via the Internet. This study, unlike others that have assessed compliance with existing state laws regulating retail store cigarette sales, assessed vendor compliance with a new state law specifically regulating Internet cigarette sales.

**Methods.** An adult research assistant purchased cigarettes from 101 ICVs randomly selected from a January 2003 sample identified as part of an ongoing longitudinal study examining the sales practices of ICVs.[2] Data were collected at each step of the ordering/package receipt process to determine the level of vendor compliance with the 6 provisions of BP § 22963: (1) verifying the buyer's age either by using a government database to verify name, address, and date of birth or by collecting a copy of a government-issued photo identification and a signed age attestation statement; (2) delivering packages only to the address used for age verification, which must match the buyer's credit card billing address; (3) requiring a 2-carton or more minimum order; (4) refusing to accept money orders; (5) including the words "tobacco product" on credit card statements; and (6) calling buyers after 5 PM to confirm orders prior to shipping.

**Table. Internet Vendor Compliance With Provisions of California Business and Professions (BP) Code § 22963,[1] a Law to Prevent Internet Cigarette Sales to Minors**

| | No. | % (95% Confidence Interval) |
|---|---|---|
| Provision | | |
| Did not accept money orders | 50 | 49.5 (40.0-59.1) |
| Required ≥2-carton minimum purchase | 25 | 24.8 (17.4-34.0) |
| Age verified as specified in BP § 22963 | 0 | 0.0 (0.0-3.7) |
| Called buyer after 5 PM to confirm order | 0 | 0.0 (0.0-3.7) |
| Delivered packages only to verified billing address | 0 | 0.0 (0.0-3.7) |
| "Tobacco product" included on credit card statement | 0 | 0.0 (0.0-3.7) |
| Level of compliance | | |
| Complied with at least 1 provision | 63 | 62.4 (52.6-71.2) |
| Complied with 2 provisions | 11 | 10.9 (6.2-18.5) |
| Complied with all provisions | 0 | 0.0 (0.0-3.7) |

**Results.** All of the 101 purchases made in this study were successfully received. None of the vendors fully complied with all 6 provisions of the law. Some vendors complied with 2 of the provisions: nearly half (49.5%) of the vendors did not accept money orders, and about one quarter (24.8%) required a 2-carton or more minimum purchase (**Table**). No vendors complied with the other 4 provisions.

**Comment.** Our results indicating zero compliance with BP § 22963 are discouraging. Comparatively, recent Food and Drug Administration compliance checks in retail stores yielded an overall 26.6% rate of cigarette sales to minors.[3] The low rate of compliance in our study indicates that either ICVs were unaware of the law or they did not believe compliance was important. The California Attorney General's office sent letters to more than 200 ICVs seeking compliance with BP § 22963 in September 2002 and February 2003, making the former possibility unlikely (Laura Kaplan, California Deputy Attorney General, written communication, November 2005).

The high rate of noncompliance may be due to the fact that the state of California had not yet actively enforced this law prior to our purchase study. As a result, vendors had little motivation to comply. In the retail environment, merchant education efforts combined with enforcement have had substantial success in increasing vendor compliance with youth access laws.[4]

After this study was conducted, the state of California filed lawsuits against several vendors for not complying with BP § 22963.[5] Whether these enforcement efforts will lead to increased compliance with BP § 22963 should be examined. A follow-up compliance survey needs to be done to assess whether California's enforcement efforts have improved vendor compliance and to determine whether more aggressive enforcement and the imposition of high fines on offenders achieves the goal of effectively reducing youth access to cigarettes via the Internet.

*Rebecca S. Williams, PhD*
*Kurt M. Ribisl, PhD*
*Ellen C. Feighery, MS*

**Correspondence:** Dr Williams, UNC Center for Health Promotion and Disease Prevention, 1700 Martin Luther King Jr Blvd, CB 7426, Chapel Hill, NC 27599-7426 (rebeccawilliams@unc.edu).
**Author Contributions:** Dr Williams had full access to all the data in the study and takes responsibility for the integrity of the data and the accuracy of the data analysis. *Study concept and design:* Williams, Ribisl, and Feighery. *Acquisition of data:* Williams, Ribisl, and Feighery. *Analysis and interpretation of data:* Williams. *Drafting of the manuscript:* Williams. *Critical revision of the manuscript for important intellectual content:* Williams, Ribisl, and Feighery. *Statistical analysis:* Williams. *Obtained funding:* Williams and Ribisl. *Administrative, technical, and material support:* Williams, Ribisl, and Feighery. *Study supervision:* Ribisl.
**Funding/Support:** This study was supported by grants from The Robert Wood Johnson Foundation and the Association of Schools of Public Health's American Legacy Foundation–funded Scholarship, Training, and Education Program for Tobacco Use Prevention (STEP UP).
**Acknowledgment:** We thank Sonya Sutton, MA, for assistance in copyediting this article.

1. Stop Tobacco Access to Kids Enforcement Act. California Business and Professions Code. § 22950-22963 (2002).
2. Ribisl KM, Kim AE, Williams RS. Sales and marketing of cigarettes on the Internet: emerging threats to tobacco control and promising policy solutions. In: *Reducing Tobacco Use: Strategies, Barriers, and Consequences*. Washington, DC: National Academy Press. In press.
3. Clark PI, Natanblut SL, Schmitt CL, Wolters C, Iachan R. Factors associated with tobacco sales to minors: lessons learned from the FDA compliance checks. *JAMA*. 2000;284:729-734.
4. Stead LF, Lancaster T. Interventions for preventing tobacco sales to minors. *Cochrane Database Syst Rev*. 2005;(1):CD001497.
5. Attorney General Lockyer files lawsuits against five retailers for Internet sales to minors [press release]. Sacramento, Calif: Office of the Attorney General; April 1, 2003.

## PEDIATRICS

**WE HAVE AN IMMEDIATE OPENING for a Pediatrician to join our Pediatric Group. Requires an IL License and Pediatric Board Certified or eligible. We have two offices located in the SW Suburbs of Chicago. We offer a highly competitive salary, benefit package and relocation assistance. Please E-mail your CV to drgsmd@aol.com or Fax: Attn Kathy McCollam at 708-923-6949.**

## PRACTICE FOR SALE

PRACTICE FOR SALE - WELL ESTABISHED PEDIATRICS AND ALLERGY practice for sale. Located 15 miles south of Boston close to major teaching hospitals. Owner will introduce. Call: 781-784-8403.

## ACKNOWLEDGMENT SERVICE

Acknowledgments in confirmation of advertising orders are sent each week. Upon receipt, please verify that your ad will be running under the appropriate heading and that your scheduling is correct. Changes to the schedule, cancellations or corrections must be communicated in writing by fax, e-mail, or regular mail prior to the published closing date of the scheduled issue.

## Childhood Obesity Prevention Researcher

The Department of Epidemiology and Prevention in the Division of Public Health Sciences and the Department of Pediatrics, Wake Forest University School of Medicine, invite applications for a tenure-track faculty position (open rank). The successful candidate will be expected to conduct an active program of independent and collaborative research in the prevention of childhood obesity. We especially invite candidates with an interest in community-based behavioral research who may also have interests in nutrition, physical activity, diabetes, cardiovascular disease, and minority health/health disparities. The position also includes some support for the role of Executive Director of an ongoing academic-community partnership to strengthen families and neighborhoods. In this role, the selected candidate will have the opportunity to shape the development of this unique academic-community initiative.

The Division of Public Health Sciences has an active group of 45 faculty collaborating in these, and other research areas. Funded research includes etiologic epidemiology, pharmacologic and behavioral intervention studies, community research, and health services research. The Division is ranked first nationally in NIH research funding among similar medical school departments. The Department of Pediatrics has 63 faculty with multiple specialties who collaborate on various research studies, including office-based interventions, obesity prevention and intervention, and complementary and alternative medicine.

Applicants should have a PhD, MD, or other doctoral degree with expertise in behavioral medicine or other relevant fields such as epidemiology, psychology, health education, medicine, exercise physiology/exercise science, physical education, nutrition, or public health. MDs with strong research interest are particularly encouraged to apply. Experience in collaborative research in a multidisciplinary setting is desirable. Excellent written and oral communication skills are required.

Applicants should send a letter, curriculum vitae, and a summary of research interests to:

**Dr Lynne Wagenknecht, Chair**
Department of Epidemiology and Prevention
Division of Public Health Sciences
Medical Center Blvd
Wake Forest University School of Medicine
Winston-Salem, NC 27157
336-716-5770 lwgnkcht@wfubmc.edu

WAKE FOREST
UNIVERSITY
HEALTH SCIENCES

*Applications will be accepted until the position is filled. The Wake Forest University School of Medicine is an equal opportunity/affirmative action employer. Applications from women and minority candidates are encouraged.*

**JOURNAL ADVERTISER INDEX**


**ABBOTT LABS**
Omnicef OS ........ 871-873

**ASTRAZENECA**
http://www.astrazeneca.com
Nexium ........ 936A-B

**CLASSIFIED ADVERTISING**
http://www.amapublications.com ........ 990-991

**GLAXOSMITHKLINE**
Boostrix ........ 923-924, COVER 3-4
Havrix ........ 883-884, 943-944
Pediarix ........ 931-932, COVER 2-865

**MERCK & COMPANY**
Gardasil ........ 888A-E
Rotateq ........ 952A-E


*Demographic and "Mini" inserts and/or ROB ad pages

While every precaution is taken to ensure accuracy, we cannot guarantee against the possibility of an occasional change or omission in the preparation of this index.

# ARCHIVES OF PEDIATRICS & ADOLESCENT MEDICINE

## CONTACT INFORMATION

### EDITORIAL OFFICE

**Editorial Office Information:** *Archives of Pediatrics & Adolescent Medicine*, Department of Pediatrics, Child Health Institute, University of Washington, 6200 NE 74th St, Suite 210, Seattle, WA 98115-8160, USA; phone: (206) 685-3573; fax: (206) 685-3572; e-mail: archpediatrics@jama-archives.org.

**Electronic Submission:** Manuscripts should be submitted via our online manuscript submission and review system (http://manuscripts.archpediatrics.com). Manuscripts submitted through our online system should not also be submitted by mail or fax. Signed authorship forms should be sent by regular mail or fax with the assigned manuscript number noted on each page in the upper right-hand corner. See the Instructions for Authors (www.archpediatrics.com) for more details.

### CONSORTIUM OF *JAMA* & *ARCHIVES* JOURNALS

The *Archives of Pediatrics & Adolescent Medicine* is a member of the consortium of AMA journals listed below.

The Journal of the American Medical Association (JAMA)
Archives of Dermatology
Archives of Facial Plastic Surgery
Archives of General Psychiatry
Archives of Internal Medicine
Archives of Neurology
Archives of Ophthalmology
Archives of Otolaryngology–Head & Neck Surgery
Archives of Pediatrics & Adolescent Medicine
Archives of Surgery

### *JAMA/ARCHIVES* MEDIA RELATIONS

Jann Ingmire; phone: (312) 464-5262; e-mail: mediarelations@jama-archives.org.

### *ARCHIVES OF PEDIATRICS* ONLINE

*Archives of Pediatrics & Adolescent Medicine* is available online at www.archpediatrics.com.

### *JAMA/ARCHIVES* REPRINTS

**Author/Educational Institution Reprints:** Anna Goins at (312) 464-2477; fax: (312) 464-5843; e-mail: anna.goins@ama-assn.org. Minimum order: 100 reprints.

**Commercial Reprints:** Phone: (312) 464-0776; fax: (312) 464-0708; e-mail: reprints@ama-assn.org. Minimum order: 100 reprints.

### PERMISSIONS

Information about obtaining permission to republish, reprint, or adapt material published in *Archives of Pediatrics & Adolescent Medicine* is available from Rhonda Bailey Brown; phone: (312) 464-2513; fax: (312) 464-5843; e-mail: permissions@ama-assn.org.

### DOCUMENT DELIVERY

Copies of individual articles are available online at www.archpediatrics.com and from the following: Infotrieve, phone: (800) 422-4633; fax: (310) 208-5971; URL: www.infotrieve.com; e-mail: orders@infotrieve.com; Institute for Scientific Information (ISI), phone: (800) 603-4367; fax: (856) 787-1679; URL: http://www.isidoc.com; e-mail: service@isidoc.com.

The ARCHIVES OF PEDIATRICS & ADOLESCENT MEDICINE (ISSN 01072–4710) is published monthly by the American Medical Association, 515 N State St, Chicago, IL 60610–0946, and is an official publication of the Association. The ARCHIVES OF PEDIATRICS & ADOLESCENT MEDICINE reaches more than 30 900 readers in over 83 countries each month. Periodicals postage paid at Chicago, Ill, and at additional mailing offices. GST registration number 12622 5556 RT. Canada Post International Publications Mail (Canadian Distribution) Sales Agreement No. 318728. POSTMASTER, send all address changes to *Archives of Pediatrics & Adolescent Medicine,* c/o the AMA Unified Service Center, American Medical Association, 515 N State St, Chicago, IL 60610. Printed in the USA.

### ADVERTISING

Information about advertising is available from the following sales representatives and online at www.archpediatrics.com.

**Account Manager:** Tim Melroy (nationally); phone: (973) 263-9191 ext 213.

**Manager, Marketing Services:** Nancy Bell; phone: (973) 263-9191 ext 216.

**Advertising Office:** 119 Cherry Hill Rd, Suite 330, Parsippany, NJ 07054-1114; phone: (973) 263-9191.

**Classified Advertising:** Thalia Moss, Shana Brown, Kim Jenkins, Sophie Levandoski, 515 N State St, Chicago, IL 60610; phone: (800) 262-2260; e-mail: classifieds@jama-archives.org.

### ADVERTISING PRINCIPLES

Advertisements in this issue have been reviewed to comply with the principles governing advertising in AMA publications. A copy of these principles is available on request and online at www.archpediatrics.com. The appearance of advertising in AMA publications is not an AMA guarantee or endorsement of the product or the claims made for the product by the manufacturer.

### ADDRESS CHANGES

Send all address changes to *Archives of Pediatrics & Adolescent Medicine*, c/o the AMA Unified Service Center, American Medical Association, 515 N State St, Chicago, IL 60610. Notification of address changes must be made at least 6 weeks in advance; include both old and new addresses and a recent mailing label if sending via mail.

### SUBSCRIPTION RATES AND SERVICE

Subscription rates are shown in the table below. For service in the US and Americas, inquiries on pricing, address changes, missing issues, subscription billing, subscription renewal, and back issues, contact the AMA Unified Service Center, 24 hours a day, 7 days a week.

**AMA members:** phone: (800) 262-3211; e-mail: msc@ama-assn.org. **Other physicians and nonphysician customers, including subscription agents:** phone: (800) 262-2350 or (312) 670-7827; fax: (312) 464-5831; e-mail: ama-subs@ama-assn.org. **Inquiries:** Unified Service Center, American Medical Association, PO Box 10946, Chicago, IL 60610-0946. For subscribers with mailing addresses outside the United States & Americas: Contact *JAMA & Archives* Journals, c/o EMD GmbH, Birkenstr.67, 10559 Berlin, Germany. Phone: +49 (30) 33099828; fax: +49 (30) 33099829; e-mail: ama@emd-germany.de.

**Annual Subscription Rates**

| | United States | Americas | UK | Rest of World |
|---|---|---|---|---|
| INDIVIDUAL | | | | |
| Print and Online | $185 | $240 | £165 | €250 |
| INSTITUTION | | | | |
| Print and Online | $400 | $485 | £315 | €470 |

In Canada, US rate plus GST. Rates for residents and medical students available at pubs.ama-assn.org, or from the AMA Unified Service Center.

# BOOSTRIX®

## (Tetanus Toxoid, Reduced Diphtheria Toxoid and Acellular Pertussis Vaccine, Adsorbed) (Tdap)

The following is a brief summary only; see full prescribing information for complete product information.

**INDICATIONS AND USAGE:** BOOSTRIX is indicated for active booster immunization against tetanus, diphtheria, and pertussis as a single dose in individuals 10 through 18 years of age. The use of BOOSTRIX as a primary series or to complete the primary series has not been studied. As with any vaccine, BOOSTRIX may not protect 100% of individuals receiving the vaccine.

**CONTRAINDICATIONS:** Hypersensitivity to any component of the vaccine is a contraindication (see DESCRIPTION in full prescribing information). Do not use BOOSTRIX after a serious allergic reaction (e.g., anaphylaxis) following any other tetanus toxoid, diphtheria toxoid or pertussis-containing vaccine, or any component of this vaccine (see DESCRIPTION in full prescribing information). Because of the uncertainty as to which component of the vaccine might be responsible, do not give further vaccination with any of these components; or, refer such individuals to an allergist for evaluation. The following events are contraindications to administration of BOOSTRIX: encephalopathy (e.g., coma, decreased level of consciousness, prolonged seizures) within 7 days of administration of a previous dose of a pertussis-containing vaccine that is not attributable to another identifiable cause; progressive neurologic disorder, uncontrolled epilepsy, or progressive encephalopathy. Do not vaccinate individuals with these conditions until a treatment regimen has been established and the condition has stabilized.

**WARNINGS:** The tip cap and the rubber plunger of the needleless prefilled syringes contain dry natural latex rubber that may cause allergic reactions in latex sensitive individuals. The vial stopper is latex-free. If any of the following events occurred in temporal relation to previous receipt of a Diphtheria and Tetanus Toxoids and Pertussis Vaccine Adsorbed (DTwP) vaccine or a vaccine containing an acellular pertussis component, consider carefully whether to give subsequent doses of BOOSTRIX: temperature of ≥40.5°C (105°F) within 48 hours not due to another identifiable cause; collapse or shock-like state (hypotonic-hyporesponsive episode) within 48 hours; persistent, inconsolable crying lasting ≥3 hours, occurring within 48 hours; seizures with or without fever occurring within 3 days. Persons who experienced serious Arthus-type hypersensitivity reactions following a prior dose of tetanus toxoid usually have high serum tetanus antitoxin levels and should not be given Tetanus and Diphtheria Toxoids Adsorbed For Adult Use (Td) or Tdap vaccines or even emergency doses of Td more frequently than every 10 years, even if the wound is neither clean nor minor. If Guillain-Barré syndrome has occurred within 6 weeks of receipt of prior vaccine containing tetanus toxoid, the decision to give BOOSTRIX or any vaccine containing tetanus toxoid should be based on careful consideration of the potential benefits and possible risks. The decision to administer a pertussis-containing vaccine to individuals with stable central nervous system (CNS) disorders must be made by the physician on an individual basis, with consideration of all relevant factors, and assessment of potential risks and benefits for that individual. Advise the patient, parent, or guardian of the potential increased risk involved (see PRECAUTIONS). A family history of seizures or other CNS disorders is not a contraindication to pertussis vaccine. The Advisory Committee on Immunization Practices (ACIP) has published guidelines for vaccination of persons with recent or acute illness (www.cdc.gov). Do not give BOOSTRIX to individuals with bleeding disorders such as hemophilia or thrombocytopenia, or to persons on anticoagulant therapy unless the potential benefit clearly outweighs the risk of administration. If the decision is made to administer BOOSTRIX to such persons, it should be given with caution with steps taken to avoid the risk of hematoma following the injection.

**PRECAUTIONS: General:** Before the injection of any biological, the physician should take all reasonable precautions to prevent allergic or other adverse reactions. Epinephrine injection (1:1,000) and other appropriate agents used for the control of immediate allergic reactions must be immediately available should an acute anaphylactic reaction occur. Immunosuppressed persons, including individuals receiving immunosuppressive therapy, may not develop the expected immune response. **Drug Interactions:** Do not mix BOOSTRIX with any other vaccine in the same syringe or vial. **Carcinogenesis, Mutagenesis, Impairment of Fertility:** BOOSTRIX has not been evaluated for carcinogenic or mutagenic potential, or for impairment of fertility. **Pregnancy:** Pregnancy Category C. Animal reproduction studies have not been conducted with BOOSTRIX. It is also not known whether BOOSTRIX can cause fetal harm when administered to a pregnant woman or can affect reproductive capacity. BOOSTRIX should be given to a pregnant woman only if clearly needed. Animal fertility studies have not been conducted with BOOSTRIX. In a developmental toxicity study, the effect of BOOSTRIX on embryo-fetal and pre-weaning development was evaluated in pregnant rats. Animals were administered INFANRIX® (Diphtheria and Tetanus Toxoids and Acellular Pertussis Vaccine Adsorbed) prior to gestation and BOOSTRIX during the period of organogenesis (gestation days 6, 8, 11) and later in pregnancy (gestation day 15), 0.1 mL/rat/occasion (a 45-fold increase compared to the human dose of BOOSTRIX on a body weight basis), by intramuscular injection. No adverse affect on pregnancy and lactation parameters, embryo-fetal or pre-weaning development was observed. There were no fetal malformations or other evidence of teratogenesis noted in this study. **Nursing Mothers:** It is not known whether BOOSTRIX is excreted in human milk. Because many drugs are excreted in human milk, caution should be exercised when BOOSTRIX is administered to a nursing woman. **Pregnancy Exposure Registry:** Healthcare providers are encouraged to register pregnant women who receive BOOSTRIX in the GlaxoSmithKline vaccination pregnancy registry by calling 1-888-825-5249. **Geriatric Use:** BOOSTRIX is not indicated for use in individuals older than 18 years. **Pediatric Use:** BOOSTRIX is not indicated for use in individuals younger than 10 years (see DOSAGE AND ADMINISTRATION in full prescribing information). For immunization of infants and children younger than 7 years against diphtheria, tetanus, and pertussis, refer to the manufacturers' package inserts for Diphtheria and Tetanus Toxoids and Acellular Pertussis Vaccine Adsorbed (DTaP) vaccines.

**ADVERSE REACTIONS:** A total of 3,608 adolescents were vaccinated with a single dose of BOOSTRIX during clinical trials. An additional 1,092 adolescents 10 to 18 years of age received a non-US formulation of BOOSTRIX (formulated to contain 0.5 mg aluminum per dose) in non-US clinical studies.

The primary safety study, conducted in the United States, was a randomized, observer-blinded, controlled study in which 3,080 adolescents 10 to 18 years of age received a single dose of BOOSTRIX and 1,034 received the control Td vaccine manufactured by Massachusetts Public Health Biologic Laboratories. There were no substantive differences in demographic characteristics between the vaccine groups. Among BOOSTRIX and control vaccine recipients approximately 75% were 10 to 14 years of age and approximately 25% were 15 to 18 years of age. Approximately 98% of participants in this study had received the recommended series of 4 or 5 doses of either DTwP or a combination of DTwP and DTaP in childhood. Data on adverse events were collected by the subjects, parents and/or guardians using standardized diaries for 15 consecutive days following the vaccine dose (i.e., day of vaccination and the next 14 days). Subjects were monitored for unsolicited adverse events that occurred within 31 days of vaccination (day 0-30) using diary cards (day 0-14) supplemented by spontaneous reports and a medical history as reported by subjects, parents, and/or guardians. Subjects were also monitored for 6 months post-vaccination for non-routine medical visits, visits to an emergency room, onset of new chronic illness, and serious adverse events. Information regarding late onset adverse events was obtained via a telephone call 6 months following vaccination. At least 97% of subjects completed the 6-month follow-up evaluation.

In a study conducted in Germany, BOOSTRIX was administered to 319 children 10 to 12 years of age previously vaccinated with 5 doses of acellular pertussis-containing vaccines, 193 of these subjects had previously received 5 doses of INFANRIX. Adverse events were recorded on diary cards during the 15 days following vaccination. Unsolicited adverse events that occurred within 31 days of vaccination (day 0-30) were recorded on the diary card or verbally reported to the investigator. Subjects were monitored for 6 months post-vaccination for physician office visits, emergency room visits, onset of new chronic illness, and serious adverse events. The 6-month follow-up evaluation, conducted via telephone interview, was completed by 90% of subjects.

The adverse event information from clinical trials provides a basis for identifying adverse events that appear to be related to vaccine use and for approximating rates. However, because clinical trials are conducted under widely varying conditions, adverse event rates observed in the clinical trials of a vaccine cannot be directly compared to rates in the clinical trials of another vaccine, and may not reflect the rates observed in practice.

**Serious Adverse Events in All Safety Studies:** In the US-safety study and German-safety study, no serious adverse events were reported to occur within 31 days of vaccination. During the 6-month extended safety evaluation period, no serious adverse events that were of potential autoimmune origin or new onset and chronic in nature were reported to occur. In non-US studies in which serious adverse events were monitored for up to 37 days, one subject was diagnosed with insulin dependent diabetes 20 days following administration of BOOSTRIX. No other serious adverse events of potential autoimmune origin or that were new onset and chronic in nature were reported to occur in these studies.

**Solicited Adverse Events in the US-Safety Study:** In a US study, the most common local adverse events following administration of BOOSTRIX were pain, redness, and swelling at the injection site. The most common general adverse events were headache and fatigue. Most of these events were reported at a similar frequency in recipients of both BOOSTRIX and Td. Any pain, grade 2 or 3 pain (but not grade 3 alone), and grade 2 or 3 headache (but not grade 3 alone) were reported at a higher rate in recipients of BOOSTRIX. The primary safety endpoint of the US study was the incidence of grade 3 pain (spontaneously painful and/or prevented normal activity) at the injection site within 15 days of vaccination. Grade 3 pain was reported in 4.6% of those who received BOOSTRIX compared with 4.0% of those who received the Td vaccine. The difference in rate of grade 3 pain was within the pre-defined clinical limit for non-inferiority (upper limit of the 95% CI for the difference ≤4%). These were the rates for solicited local and general adverse events within 15 days of vaccination with BOOSTRIX or Td vaccine for the total vaccinated cohort (all enrolled, vaccinated subjects with safety data available analyzed by vaccine received):

**Percentage of Individuals 10 to 18 Years of Age Reporting Solicited Local Adverse Events or Solicited General Adverse Events Within the 15-day* Post-Vaccination Period**

| | BOOSTRIX (N = 3,032) % | Td (N = 1,013) % |
|---|---|---|
| **Local** | | |
| Pain,[†] any | 75.3 | 71.7 |
| Pain,[†] grade 2 or 3 | 51.2 | 42.5 |
| Pain,[‡] grade 3 | 4.6 | 4.0 |
| Redness, any | 22.5 | 19.8 |
| Redness, >20 mm | 4.1 | 3.9 |
| Redness, ≥50 mm | 1.7 | 1.6 |
| Swelling, any | 21.1 | 20.1 |
| Swelling, >20 mm | 5.3 | 4.9 |
| Swelling, ≥50 mm | 2.5 | 3.2 |
| Arm circumference increase,[§] >5 mm | 28.3 | 29.5 |
| Arm circumference increase,[§] >20 mm | 2.0 | 2.2 |
| Arm circumference increase,[§] >40 mm | 0.5 | 0.3 |
| **General** | | |
| Fever,[‖] ≥99.5°F | 13.5 | 13.1 |
| Fever,[‖] >100.4°F | 5.0 | 4.7 |
| Fever,[‖] >102.2°F | 1.4 | 1.0 |
| Headache, any | 43.1 | 41.5 |
| Headache,[†] grade 2 or 3 | 15.7 | 12.7 |
| Headache, grade 3 | 3.7 | 2.7 |
| Fatigue, any | 37.0 | 36.7 |
| Fatigue, grade 2 or 3 | 14.4 | 12.9 |
| Fatigue, grade 3 | 3.7 | 3.2 |
| Gastrointestinal symptoms,[¶] any | 26.0 | 25.8 |
| Gastrointestinal symptoms,[¶] grade 2 or 3 | 9.8 | 9.7 |
| Gastrointestinal symptoms,[¶] grade 3 | 3.0 | 3.2 |

Td = Tetanus and Diphtheria Toxoids Adsorbed For Adult Use manufactured by Massachusetts Public Health Biologic Laboratories.
N = number of subjects in the total vaccinated cohort with local/general symptoms sheets completed.
Grade 2 = Local: painful when the limb was moved; General: interfered with normal activity.
Grade 3 = Local: spontaneously painful and/or prevented normal activity; General: prevented normal activity.
*Day of vaccination and the next 14 days.
[†]Statistically significantly higher (P<0.05) following BOOSTRIX as compared to Td vaccine.
[‡]Grade 3 injection site pain following BOOSTRIX was not inferior to Td (upper limit of two-sided 95% CI for the difference in the percentage of subjects ≤4%).
[§]Mid-upper region of the vaccinated arm.
[‖]Oral temperatures or axillary temperatures.
[¶]Gastrointestinal symptoms included nausea, vomiting, diarrhea and/or abdominal pain.

Mid-upper arm circumference was measured by the adolescent or their parent/guardian prior to injection and daily for 15 days following vaccination. There was no significant difference between BOOSTRIX recipients and Td recipients in the proportion of subjects reporting an increase in mid-upper arm circumference in the vaccinated arm. The incidence of unsolicited adverse events reported in the 31 days after vaccination was comparable between the 2 groups.

**Solicited Adverse Events in the German Safety Study:** No cases of whole arm swelling were spontaneously reported. Two individuals (2/193) reported large injection site swelling (range 110 to 200 mm diameter), in one case associated with grade 3 pain. Neither individual sought medical attention. These episodes were reported to resolve without sequelae within 5 days. These were the rates of solicited local adverse events and fever within 15 days of vaccination for those subjects who had previously been vaccinated with 5 doses of INFANRIX:

**Rates of Solicited Adverse Events Reported Within the 15-day* Post-Vaccination Period Following Administration of BOOSTRIX in Individuals 10 to 12 Years of Age Who Had Previously Received 5 Doses of INFANRIX**

| Adverse Event | BOOSTRIX (N = 193) % (95% CI) |
|---|---|
| Pain, any | 62.2 (54.9-69.0) |
| Pain, grade 2 or 3 | 33.2 (26.6-40.3) |
| Pain, grade 3 | 5.7 (2.9-10.0) |
| Redness, any | 47.7 (40.4-55.0) |
| Redness, >20 mm | 15.0 (10.3-20.9) |
| Redness, ≥50 mm | 10.9 (6.9-16.2) |
| Swelling, any | 38.9 (31.9-46.1) |
| Swelling, >20 mm | 17.6 (12.5-23.7) |
| Swelling, ≥50 mm | 14.0 (9.4-19.7) |
| Fever, ≥99.5 | 8.8 (5.2-13.7) |
| Fever, >100.4 | 4.1 (1.8-8.0) |
| Fever, >102.2 | 1.0 (0.1-3.7) |

N = number of subjects with local/general symptoms sheets completed.
Grade 2 = Painful when the limb was moved.
Grade 3 = Spontaneously painful and/or prevented normal activity.
*Day of vaccination and the next 14 days.

As with any vaccine, there is the possibility that broad use of BOOSTRIX could reveal adverse events not observed in clinical trials.

**Postmarketing Reports:** Worldwide voluntary reports of adverse events received for BOOSTRIX in persons 10 to 18 years of age since market introduction of this vaccine are listed below. This list includes serious events or events which have causal connection to components of this or other vaccines or drugs. Because these events are reported voluntarily from a population of uncertain size, it is not possible to reliably estimate their frequency or establish a causal relationship to vaccine exposure. *Blood and lymphatic system disorders:* Lymphadenitis, lymphadenopathy. *Cardiac disorders:* Myocarditis. *Injection site reactions:* Induration, inflammation, mass, nodule, warmth, local reaction. *Metabolism and nutrition disorders:* Diabetes mellitus insulin-dependent. *Musculoskeletal and connective tissue disorders:* Arthralgia, back pain, myalgia. *Nervous system disorders:* Convulsion, encephalitis, facial palsy, paraesthesia. *Skin and subcutaneous tissue disorders:* Exanthem, Henoch-Schönlein purpura, rash. In addition, extensive swelling of the injected limb has been reported following administration of BOOSTRIX.

**Reporting Adverse Events:** Report the occurrence following immunization of any event set forth in the Vaccine Injury Table from the National Childhood Vaccine Injury Act including: Anaphylaxis or anaphylactic shock within 7 days, encephalopathy or encephalitis within 7 days, brachial neuritis within 28 days, or an acute complication or sequelae (including death) of an illness, disability, injury, or condition referred to above, or any events that would contraindicate further doses of vaccine, according to this prescribing information. These events should be reported to VAERS. The VAERS toll-free number is 1-800-822-7967. Reporting forms may also be obtained at the VAERS website at www.vaers.hhs.gov.

**DOSAGE AND ADMINISTRATION: Recommended Dose:** BOOSTRIX should be administered as a single 0.5 mL injection by the intramuscular route into the deltoid muscle of the upper arm in individuals 10 through 18 years of age. Do not administer this product subcutaneously or intravenously. There are no data to support repeat administration of BOOSTRIX. Five years should elapse between the subject's last dose of the recommended series of childhood DTwP and/or DTaP vaccine and the administration of BOOSTRIX. Limited data are available on the use of BOOSTRIX following Tetanus and Diphtheria Toxoids Adsorbed For Adult Use (Td) vaccine. **Additional Dosing Information:** ***Wound Management:*** Clinicians should refer to guidelines for tetanus prophylaxis in routine wound management. Adolescents 10 to 18 years of age who have completed a primary series against tetanus and who sustain wounds which are minor and uncomplicated, should receive a booster dose of a tetanus toxoid-containing vaccine only if they have not received tetanus toxoid within the preceding 10 years. In case of tetanus-prone injury (e.g., wounds contaminated with dirt, feces, soil, and saliva; puncture wounds; avulsions; and wounds resulting from missles, crushing, burns, and frostbite) in an adolescent who is in need of tetanus toxoid, BOOSTRIX can be used as an alternative to Tetanus and Diphtheria Toxoids Adsorbed For Adult Use (Td) vaccine in patients for whom the pertussis component is also indicated (see INDICATIONS AND USAGE).

Manufactured by **GlaxoSmithKline Biologicals**
Rixensart, Belgium, US License 1617

Distributed by **GlaxoSmithKline**
Research Triangle Park, NC 27709

BOOSTRIX and INFANRIX are registered trademarks of GlaxoSmithKline.

Full prescribing information for BOOSTRIX is available at www.BOOSTRIX.com.
BRS-BO:L3

**References: 1.** Centers for Disease Control and Prevention. Preventing tetanus, diphtheria, and pertussis among adolescents: use of tetanus toxoid, reduced diphtheria toxoid and acellular pertussis vaccines: recommendations of the Advisory Committee on Immunization Practices (ACIP). Early Release 2006;55(February 23, 2006):1–43. **2.** Centers for Disease Control and Prevention. Recommended childhood and adolescent immunization schedule—United States, 2006. *MMWR.* 2006;54(51&52):Q1–Q4.

# ARCHIVES OF PEDIATRICS & ADOLESCENT MEDICINE

WWW.ARCHPEDIATRICS.COM

OCTOBER 2006

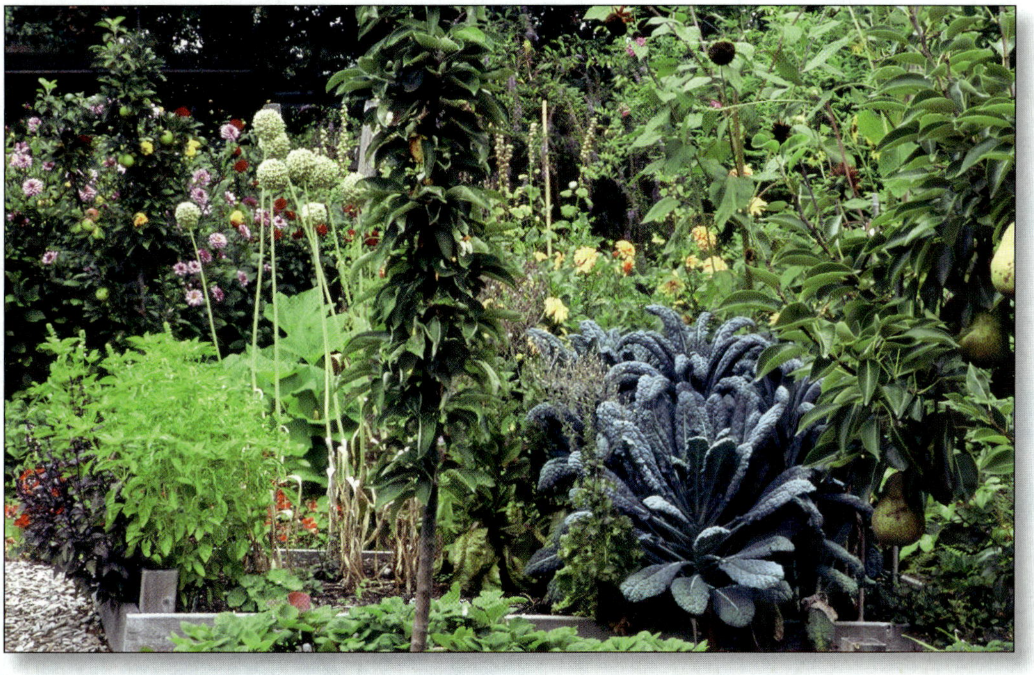

Fall in Lee Neff's Garden, Seattle, Washington, 2004. See page 997.

CARDIORESPIRATORY FITNESS LEVELS AMONG US YOUTH

A RANDOMIZED TRIAL OF CLINICIAN PROMPTING IN PEDIATRIC OFFICES FOR ASTHMA

ATTENTION-DEFICIT/HYPERACTIVITY DISORDER IN CHILDREN: EXCESS COSTS

ADOLESCENT BONE HEALTH

COMPLETE TABLE OF CONTENTS ON PAGE 995



JAMA & ARCHIVES JOURNALS
American Medical Association

# Xopenex HFA™

(levalbuterol tartrate) Inhalation Aerosol

FOR ORAL INHALATION ONLY

## BRIEF SUMMARY

**INDICATIONS AND USAGE**

XOPENEX HFA (levalbuterol tartrate) Inhalation Aerosol is indicated for the treatment or prevention of bronchospasm in adults, adolescents, and children 4 years of age and older with reversible obstructive airway disease.

**CONTRAINDICATIONS**

XOPENEX HFA (levalbuterol tartrate) Inhalation Aerosol is contraindicated in patients with a history of hypersensitivity to levalbuterol, racemic albuterol, or any other component of XOPENEX HFA Inhalation Aerosol.

**WARNINGS**

1. Paradoxical Bronchospasm: Like other inhaled beta-adrenergic agonists, XOPENEX HFA Inhalation Aerosol can produce paradoxical bronchospasm, which may be life-threatening. If paradoxical bronchospasm occurs, XOPENEX HFA (levalbuterol tartrate) Inhalation Aerosol should be discontinued immediately and alternative therapy instituted. It should be recognized that paradoxical bronchospasm, when associated with inhaled formulations, frequently occurs with the first use of a new canister. 2. Deterioration of Asthma: Asthma may deteriorate acutely over a period of hours or chronically over several days or longer. If the patient needs more doses of XOPENEX HFA Inhalation Aerosol than usual, this may be a marker of destabilization of asthma and requires reevaluation of the patient and treatment regimen, giving special consideration to the possible need for anti-inflammatory treatment, e.g., corticosteroids.
3. Use of Anti-Inflammatory Agents: The use of a beta-adrenergic agonist alone may not be adequate to control asthma in many patients. Early consideration should be given to adding anti-inflammatory agents, e.g., corticosteroids, to the therapeutic regimen. 4. Cardiovascular Effects: XOPENEX HFA Inhalation Aerosol, like other beta-adrenergic agonists, can produce clinically significant cardiovascular effects in some patients, as measured by heart rate, blood pressure, and/or symptoms. Although such effects are uncommon after administration of XOPENEX HFA Inhalation Aerosol at recommended doses, if they occur, the drug may need to be discontinued. In addition, beta-agonists have been reported to produce electrocardiogram (ECG) changes, such as flattening of the T wave, prolongation of the QTc interval, and ST segment depression. The clinical significance of these findings is unknown. Therefore, XOPENEX HFA Inhalation Aerosol, like all sympathomimetic amines, should be used with caution in patients with cardiovascular disorders, especially coronary insufficiency, cardiac arrhythmias, and hypertension. 5. Do Not Exceed Recommended Dose: Fatalities have been reported in association with excessive use of inhaled sympathomimetic drugs in patients with asthma. The exact cause of death is unknown, but cardiac arrest following an unexpected development of a severe acute asthmatic crisis and subsequent hypoxia is suspected.
6. Immediate Hypersensitivity Reactions: Immediate hypersensitivity reactions may occur after administration of racemic albuterol, as demonstrated by rare cases of urticaria, angioedema, rash, bronchospasm, anaphylaxis, and oropharyngeal edema. The potential for hypersensitivity must be considered in the clinical evaluation of patients who experience immediate hypersensitivity reactions while receiving XOPENEX HFA Inhalation Aerosol.

**PRECAUTIONS**

**General**

XOPENEX HFA (levalbuterol tartrate) Inhalation Aerosol, like all sympathomimetic amines, should be used with caution in patients with cardiovascular disorders, especially coronary insufficiency, hypertension, and cardiac arrhythmias; in patients with convulsive disorders, hyperthyroidism, or diabetes mellitus; and in patients who are unusually responsive to sympathomimetic amines. Clinically significant changes in systolic and diastolic blood pressure have been seen in individual patients and could be expected to occur in some patients after the use of any beta-adrenergic bronchodilator.

Large doses of intravenous racemic albuterol have been reported to aggravate preexisting diabetes mellitus and ketoacidosis. As with other beta-adrenergic agonist medications, XOPENEX HFA Inhalation Aerosol may produce significant hypokalemia in some patients, possibly through intracellular shunting, which has the potential to produce adverse cardiovascular effects. The decrease is usually transient, not requiring supplementation.

**Information for Patients**

The action of XOPENEX HFA Inhalation Aerosol should last for 4 to 6 hours. XOPENEX HFA Inhalation Aerosol should not be used more frequently than recommended. Do not increase the dose or frequency of doses of XOPENEX HFA Inhalation Aerosol without consulting your physician. If you find that treatment with XOPENEX HFA Inhalation Aerosol becomes less effective for symptomatic relief, your symptoms become worse, and/or you need to use the product more frequently than usual, you should seek medical attention immediately. While you are using XOPENEX HFA Inhalation Aerosol, other inhaled drugs and asthma medications should be taken only as directed by your physician.

Common adverse effects of treatment with inhaled beta-agonists include palpitations, chest pain, rapid heart rate, tremor, and nervousness. If you are pregnant or nursing, contact your physician about use of XOPENEX HFA Inhalation Aerosol. Effective and safe use of XOPENEX HFA Inhalation Aerosol includes an understanding of the way that it should be administered.

Use XOPENEX HFA Inhalation Aerosol only with the actuator supplied with the product. Discard the canister after 200 sprays have been used. Never immerse the canister in water to determine how full the canister is ("float test").

In general, the technique for administering XOPENEX HFA Inhalation Aerosol to children is similar to that for adults. Children should use XOPENEX HFA Inhalation Aerosol under adult supervision, as instructed by the patient's physician.

**Drug Interactions**

Other short-acting sympathomimetic aerosol bronchodilators or epinephrine should be used with caution with XOPENEX HFA Inhalation Aerosol. If additional adrenergic drugs are to be administered by any route, they should be used with caution to avoid deleterious cardiovascular effects.

1. Beta-blockers: Beta-adrenergic receptor-blocking agents not only block the pulmonary effect of beta-adrenergic agonists, such as XOPENEX HFA Inhalation Aerosol, but may produce severe bronchospasm in asthmatic patients. Therefore, patients with asthma should not normally be treated with beta-blockers. However, under certain circumstances, e.g., as prophylaxis after myocardial infarction, there may be no acceptable alternatives to the use of beta-adrenergic blocking agents in patients with asthma. In this setting, cardioselective beta-blockers should be considered, although they should be administered with caution. 2. Diuretics: The ECG changes and/or hypokalemia that may result from the administration of non–potassium-sparing diuretics (such as loop and thiazide diuretics) can be acutely worsened by beta-agonists, especially when the recommended dose of the beta-agonist is exceeded. Although the clinical significance of these effects is not known, caution is advised in the coadministration of beta-agonists with non–potassium-sparing diuretics. 3. Digoxin: Mean decreases of 16% to 22% in serum digoxin levels were demonstrated after single-dose intravenous and oral administration of racemic albuterol, respectively, to normal volunteers who had received digoxin for 10 days. The clinical significance of these findings for patients with obstructive airway disease who are receiving XOPENEX HFA Inhalation Aerosol and digoxin on a chronic basis is unclear. Nevertheless, it would be prudent to carefully evaluate the serum digoxin levels in patients who are currently receiving digoxin and XOPENEX HFA Inhalation Aerosol. 4. Monoamine Oxidase Inhibitors or Tricyclic Antidepressants: XOPENEX HFA Inhalation Aerosol should be administered with extreme caution to patients being treated with monoamine oxidase inhibitors or tricyclic antidepressants, or within 2 weeks of discontinuation of such agents, because the action of albuterol on the vascular system may be potentiated.

**Carcinogenesis, Mutagenesis, and Impairment of Fertility** No carcinogenesis or impairment of fertility studies have been carried out with levalbuterol tartrate. However, racemic albuterol sulfate has been evaluated for its carcinogenic potential and ability to impair fertility.

In a 2-year study in Sprague-Dawley rats, racemic albuterol sulfate caused a significant dose-related increase in the incidence of benign leiomyomas of the mesovarium at, and above, dietary doses of 2 mg/kg/day (approximately 30 times the maximum recommended daily inhalation dose of levalbuterol tartrate for adults on a mg/m$^2$ basis and approximately 15 times the maximum recommended daily inhalation dose of levalbuterol tartrate for children on a mg/m$^2$ basis). In another study, this effect was blocked by the coadministration of propranolol, a nonselective beta-adrenergic antagonist. In an 18-month study in CD-1 mice, racemic albuterol sulfate showed no evidence of tumorigenicity at dietary doses up to 500 mg/kg/day (approximately 3800 times the maximum recommended daily inhalation dose of levalbuterol tartrate for adults on a mg/m$^2$ basis and approximately 1800 times the maximum recommended daily inhalation dose of levalbuterol tartrate for children on a mg/m$^2$ basis). In a 22-month study in the Golden hamster, racemic albuterol sulfate showed no evidence of tumorigenicity at dietary doses up to 50 mg/kg/day (approximately 500 times the maximum recommended daily inhalation dose of levalbuterol tartrate for adults on a mg/m$^2$ basis and approximately 240 times the maximum recommended daily inhalation dose of levalbuterol tartrate for children on a mg/m$^2$ basis).

Levalbuterol HCl was not mutagenic in the Ames test or the CHO/HPRT Mammalian Forward Gene Mutation Assay.

Levalbuterol HCl was not clastogenic in the in vivo micronucleus test in mouse bone marrow. Racemic albuterol sulfate was negative in an in vitro chromosomal aberration assay in CHO cell cultures.

Reproduction studies in rats using racemic albuterol sulfate demonstrated no evidence of impaired fertility at oral doses up to 50 mg/kg/day (approximately 750 times the maximum recommended daily inhalation dose of levalbuterol tartrate for adults on a mg/m$^2$ basis).

**Teratogenic Effects - Pregnancy Category C** A reproduction study in New Zealand White rabbits demonstrated that levalbuterol HCl was not teratogenic when administered orally at doses up to 25 mg/kg/day (approximately 750 times the maximum recommended daily inhalation dose of levalbuterol tartrate for adults on a mg/m$^2$ basis).

However, racemic albuterol sulfate has been shown to be teratogenic in mice and rabbits. A study in CD-1 mice given racemic albuterol sulfate subcutaneously showed cleft palate formation in 5 of 111 (4.5%) fetuses at 0.25 mg/kg/day (approximately 2 times the maximum recommended daily inhalation dose of levalbuterol tartrate for adults on a mg/m$^2$ basis) and in 10 of 108 (9.3%) fetuses at 2.5 mg/kg/day (approximately 20 times the maximum recommended daily inhalation dose of levalbuterol tartrate for adults on a mg/m$^2$ basis). The drug did not induce cleft palate formation when administered subcutaneously at a dose of 0.025 mg/kg/day (less than the maximum recommended daily inhalation dose of levalbuterol tartrate for adults on a mg/m$^2$ basis). Cleft palate also occurred in 22 of 72 (30.5%) fetuses from females treated subcutaneously with 2.5 mg/kg/day of isoproterenol (positive control).

A reproduction study in Stride Dutch rabbits revealed cranioschisis in 7 of 19 (37%) fetuses when racemic albuterol sulfate was administered orally at a dose of 50 mg/kg/day (approximately 1500 times the maximum recommended daily inhalation dose of levalbuterol tartrate for adults on a mg/m$^2$ basis).

A study in which pregnant rats were dosed with radiolabeled racemic albuterol sulfate demonstrated that drug-related material is transferred from the maternal circulation to the fetus.

There are no adequate and well-controlled studies of XOPENEX HFA Inhalation Aerosol in pregnant women. Because animal reproduction studies are not always predictive of human response, XOPENEX HFA Inhalation Aerosol should be used during pregnancy only if the potential benefit justifies the potential risk to the fetus.

During marketing experience of racemic albuterol, various congenital anomalies, including cleft palate and limb defects, have been rarely reported in the offspring of patients being treated with racemic albuterol. Some of the mothers were taking multiple medications during their pregnancies. No consistent pattern of defects can be discerned, and a relationship between racemic albuterol use and congenital anomalies has not been established.

**Use in Labor and Delivery** Because of the potential for beta-adrenergic agonists to interfere with uterine contractility, the use of XOPENEX HFA Inhalation Aerosol for the treatment of bronchospasm during labor should be restricted to those patients in whom the benefits clearly outweigh the risk.

**Tocolysis** XOPENEX HFA Inhalation Aerosol has not been approved for the management of preterm labor. The benefit:risk ratio when levalbuterol tartrate is administered for tocolysis has not been established. Serious adverse reactions, including maternal pulmonary edema, have been reported during or following treatment of premature labor with beta2-agonists, including racemic albuterol.

**Nursing Mothers** Plasma concentrations of levalbuterol after inhalation of therapeutic doses are very low in humans. It is not known whether levalbuterol is excreted in human milk.

Because of the potential for tumorigenicity shown for racemic albuterol in animal studies and the lack of experience with the use of XOPENEX HFA Inhalation Aerosol by nursing mothers, a decision should be made whether to discontinue nursing or to discontinue the drug, taking into account the importance of the drug to the mother. Caution should be exercised when XOPENEX HFA Inhalation Aerosol is administered to a nursing woman.

**Pediatrics** The safety and efficacy of XOPENEX HFA Inhalation Aerosol have been established in pediatric patients 4 years of age and older in an adequate and well-controlled clinical trial. Use of XOPENEX HFA Inhalation Aerosol in children is also supported by evidence from adequate and well-controlled studies of XOPENEX HFA Inhalation Aerosol in adults, considering that the pathophysiology, systemic exposure of the drug, and clinical profile in pediatric and adult patients are substantially similar. Safety and effectiveness of XOPENEX HFA Inhalation Aerosol in pediatric patients below the age of 4 years have not been established.

**Geriatrics** Clinical studies of XOPENEX HFA Inhalation Aerosol did not include sufficient numbers of subjects aged 65 and older to determine whether they respond differently from younger subjects. Other reported clinical experience has not identified differences in responses between the elderly and younger patients. In general, dose selection for an elderly patient should be cautious, usually starting at the low end of the dosing range, reflecting the greater frequency of decreased hepatic, renal, or cardiac function, and of concomitant diseases or other drug therapy.

Albuterol is known to be substantially excreted by the kidney, and the risk of toxic reactions may be greater in patients with impaired renal function. Because elderly patients are more likely to have decreased renal function, care should be taken in dose selection, and it may be useful to monitor renal function.

**ADVERSE REACTIONS** Adverse event information concerning XOPENEX HFA (levalbuterol tartrate) Inhalation Aerosol in adults and adolescents is derived from two 8-week, multicenter, randomized, double-blind, active- and placebo-controlled trials in 748 adult and adolescent patients with asthma that compared XOPENEX HFA Inhalation Aerosol, a marketed albuterol HFA inhaler, and an HFA-134a placebo inhaler. The following lists the incidence (% XOPENEX HFA 90 mcg, marketed albuterol HFA inhaler 180 mcg, placebo, respectively) of all adverse events (whether considered by the investigator to be related or unrelated to drug) from these trials that occurred at a rate of 2% or greater in the group treated with XOPENEX HFA Inhalation Aerosol and more frequently than in the HFA-134a placebo inhaler group. Body as a whole: pain (4.0%, 3.4%, 3.6%). Central nervous system: dizziness (2.7%, 0.6%, 1.8%). Respiratory system: asthma (9.4%, 7.3%, 6.0%), pharyngitis (7.9%, 2.2%, 2.4%), rhinitis (7.4%, 2.2%, 3.0%).

Adverse events reported by less than 2% and at least 2 or more of the adolescent and adult patients receiving XOPENEX HFA Inhalation Aerosol and by a greater proportion than receiving HFA-134a placebo inhaler include cyst, flu syndrome, viral infection, constipation, gastroenteritis, myalgia, hypertension, epistaxis, lung disorder, acne, herpes simplex, conjunctivitis, ear pain, dysmenorrhea, hematuria, and vaginal moniliasis. There were no significant laboratory abnormalities observed in these studies.

Adverse event information concerning XOPENEX HFA Inhalation Aerosol in children is derived from a 4-week, randomized, double-blind trial of XOPENEX HFA Inhalation Aerosol, a marketed albuterol HFA inhaler, and an HFA-134a placebo inhaler in 150 children aged 4 to 11 years with asthma. The following lists the adverse events (% XOPENEX HFA 90 mcg, marketed albuterol HFA inhaler 180 mcg, placebo, respectively) reported for XOPENEX HFA Inhalation Aerosol in children at a rate of 2% or greater and more frequently than for placebo. Body as a whole: accidental injury (9.2%, 10.3%, 5.7%). Digestive system: vomiting (10.5%, 7.7%, 5.7%). Respiratory system: bronchitis (2.6%, 0%, 0%), pharyngitis (6.6%, 12.8%, 5.7%).

The incidence of systemic beta-adrenergic adverse effects (e.g., tremor, nervousness) was low and comparable across all treatment groups, including placebo.

**Postmarketing** In addition to the adverse events reported in clinical trials, the following adverse events have been observed in postapproval use of levalbuterol inhalation solution. These events have been chosen for inclusion due to their seriousness, their frequency of reporting, or their likely beta-mediated mechanism: angioedema, anaphylaxis, arrhythmias (including atrial fibrillation, supraventricular tachycardia, extrasystoles), asthma, chest pain, cough increased, dyspnea, nausea, nervousness, rash, tachycardia, tremor, urticaria. Because these events have been reported spontaneously from a population of unknown size, estimates of frequency cannot be made.

In addition, XOPENEX HFA Inhalation Aerosol, like other sympathomimetic agents, can cause adverse reactions such as hypertension, angina, vertigo, central nervous system stimulation, sleeplessness, headache, and drying or irritation of the oropharynx.

Rx only.

# ARCHIVES OF PEDIATRICS & ADOLESCENT MEDICINE

OCTOBER 2006 VOLUME 160, NUMBER 10 PAGES 993-1088

## ARTICLES

**Cardiorespiratory Fitness Levels Among US Youth 12 to 19 Years of Age: Findings From the 1999-2002 National Health and Nutrition Examination Survey** 1005
*Russell R. Pate, PhD; Chia-Yih Wang, PhD; Marsha Dowda, DrPH; Stephen W. Farrell, PhD; Jennifer R. O'Neill, MPH*

**Attenuating Growth in Children With Profound Developmental Disability: A New Approach to an Old Dilemma** 1013
*Daniel F. Gunther, MD, MA; Douglas S. Diekema, MD, MPH*

**Improved Preventive Care for Asthma: A Randomized Trial of Clinician Prompting in Pediatric Offices** 1018
*Jill S. Halterman, MD, MPH; Susan Fisher, PhD; Kelly M. Conn, MPH; Maria Fagnano, BA; Kathleen Lynch, BA; Andrew Marky, BA; Peter G. Szilagyi, MD, MPH*

## REVIEW ARTICLES

**Adolescent Bone Health** 1026
*Keith J. Loud, MDCM, MSc; Catherine M. Gordon, MD, MSc*

**Tall Girls: The Social Shaping of a Medical Therapy** 1035
*Joyce M. Lee, MD, MPH; Joel D. Howell, MD, PhD*

## ARTICLES

**Motor and Cognitive Outcomes in Nondisabled Low-Birth-Weight Adolescents: Early Determinants** 1040
*Agnes H. Whitaker, MD; Judith F. Feldman, PhD; John M. Lorenz, MD; Sa Shen, PhD; Fiona McNicholas, MD; Marlon Nieto, BA; Dawn McCulloch, MSEd; Jennifer A. Pinto-Martin, PhD; Nigel Paneth, MD, MPH*

**Ethanol-Lock Technique for Persistent Bacteremia of Long-term Intravascular Devices in Pediatric Patients** 1049
*Wes Onland, MD; Cathy E. Shin, MD; Stana Fustar, RN, CRNI; Teresa Rushing, PharmD, BCPS; Wing-Yen Wong, MD*

**Inpatient Health Care Use Among Adult Survivors of Chronic Childhood Illnesses in the United States** 1054
*Megumi J. Okumura, MD; Andrew D. Campbell, MD; Samya Z. Nasr, MD; Matthew M. Davis, MD, MAPP*

**Attention-Deficit/Hyperactivity Disorder in Children: Excess Costs Before and After Initial Diagnosis and Treatment Cost Differences by Ethnicity** 1063
*G. Thomas Ray, MBA; Peter Levine, MD; Lisa A. Croen, PhD; Farasat A. S. Bokhari, PhD; Teh-wei Hu, PhD; Laurel A. Habel, PhD*

**Cost-effectiveness Analysis of Palivizumab in Premature Infants Without Chronic Lung Disease** 1070
*Nahed O. ElHassan, MD, MPH; Melony E. S. Sorbero, PhD, MS, MPH; Caroline B. Hall, MD; Timothy P. Stevens, MD, MPH; Andrew W. Dick, PhD*

ARCHIVES
OF
PEDIATRICS &
ADOLESCENT MEDICINE

## EDITORIALS

**Growth Attenuation: A Diminutive Solution to a Daunting Problem** 1077
*Jeffrey P. Brosco, MD, PhD; Chris Feudtner, MD, PhD, MPH*

**At What Cost?** 1079
*John Reiss, PhD; Robert W. Gibson, PhD, MSOTR/L*

## SPECIAL FEATURE

**Picture of the Month** 1081
*Jeffrey S. Gerber, MD, PhD; Samir S. Shah, MD*

## BOOK REVIEWS AND OTHER MEDIA

**A Generation at Risk: The Global Impact of HIV/AIDS on Orphans and Vulnerable Children** 1084
*Gabriel Berson, MD*

## REGULAR DEPARTMENTS

**This Month in *Archives of Pediatrics & Adolescent Medicine*** 1002

**Announcements** 1012, 1025, 1053, 1083

**Classified Advertising** 1085

**Journal Advertiser Index** 1087

**Contact Information** 1088

**Instructions for authors and the author and subject indexes are available on our Web site: http://www.archpediatrics.com. If you do not have access to the Web, contact Suzanne Shuey at (206) 685-3573.**

***About the Cover***

Photographer: John Neff, MD, Seattle, Wash, 2004.

ARCHIVES
OF
PEDIATRICS &
ADOLESCENT MEDICINE

**Mission Statement:** *The Archives of Pediatrics & Adolescent Medicine* is a monthly, peer-reviewed journal for physicians and other health care professionals who contribute to the health of children and adolescents. The *Archives* provides an open forum for dialogue on a full range of clinical, scientific, advocacy, and humanistic issues relevant to the care of pediatric patients from infancy through young adulthood. The *Archives* is a vehicle for increased attention to adolescent health, the education of pediatric health care professionals, and disease prevention and health promotion. The *Archives* publishes original studies, editorials, reviews by experts, practice commentaries, case quizzes, and updates on clinical science and practice management. The Pediatric Forum provides our readers with opportunities to express their views. *Archives* incorporates *AJDC*, the oldest journal in US pediatric literature, which originated in 1911.



JAMA & ARCHIVES JOURNALS
American Medical Association

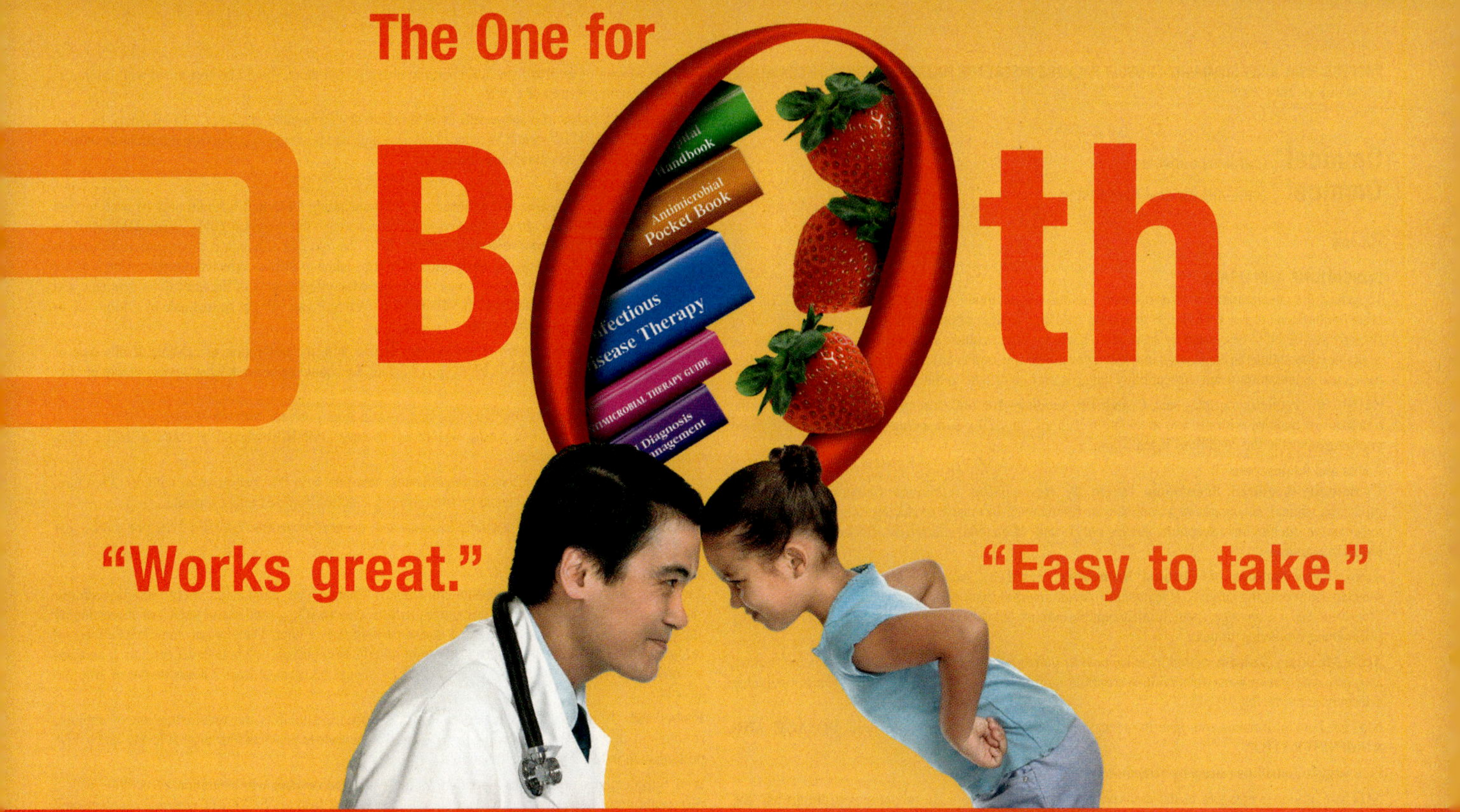


# 250 mg/5 mL* — Half the Volume†

**According to published peer-reviewed literature,[1-3] compliance factors that make an antibiotic easy to take include:**

- **Taste (palatability)**
- **Tolerability**
- **Short duration of treatment**
- **Number of daily doses**

**Indications** OMNICEF (cefdinir) for Oral Suspension is indicated in patients 6 months through 12 years for mild to moderate **Acute Bacterial Otitis Media** caused by susceptible strains of *H influenzae* (including ß-lactamase producing strains), *S pneumoniae* (penicillin-susceptible strains only), and *M catarrhalis* (including ß-lactamase producing strains).[4]

**Important Safety Information**[4]

- To reduce the development of drug-resistant bacteria and maintain the effectiveness of OMNICEF and other antibacterial drugs, OMNICEF should be used only to treat or prevent infections that are proven or strongly suspected to be caused by bacteria
- OMNICEF is contraindicated in patients with known allergy to the cephalosporin class of antibiotics
- For patients with previous hypersensitivity reaction to penicillins, caution should be exercised because cross-hypersensitivity among ß-lactam antibiotics has been clearly documented. If an allergic reaction to cefdinir occurs, the drug should be discontinued
- Safety and efficacy in neonates and infants less than 6 months of age have not been established
- 2% of 2,289 pediatric patients discontinued medication due to adverse events in US and non-US clinical trials. Discontinuations were primarily for gastrointestinal disturbance, usually diarrhea
- The most common reported adverse events occurring in ≥1% of pediatric patients in US clinical trials (N=1,783) were diarrhea (8%), rash (3%), and vomiting (1%)
- Maximum dose of OMNICEF for pediatric patients weighing ≥43 kg is 600 mg/day. For pediatric patients with a creatinine clearance of <30 mL/min/1.73 m$^2$ and not requiring hemodialysis, the dose of cefdinir should be 7 mg/kg (up to 300 mg) given once daily
- Antacids that contain magnesium or aluminum and iron supplements, including multivitamins that contain iron, should be taken at least 2 hours before or 2 hours after taking OMNICEF

***For pediatric patients weighing 20 lbs, use the 125 mg/5 mL product.[4]**
**†Of the 125 mg/5 mL formulation.**

**References: 1.** Brixner DI. Improving acute otitis media outcomes through proper antibiotic use and adherence. *Am J Manag Care.* 2005;11:S202-S210. **2.** Kardas P. Patient compliance with antibiotic treatment for respiratory tract infections. *J Antimicrob Chemother.* 2002;49:897-903. **3.** Ramgoolam A, Steele R. Formulations of antibiotics for children in primary care. *Pediatr Drugs.* 2002;4:323-333. **4.** OMNICEF (cefdinir) Capsules and for Oral Suspension Prescribing Information, Abbott Laboratories.

**Please see adjacent brief summary of full prescribing information.**

OMNICEF®
(cefdinir) for oral suspension
*125 mg/5 mL and 250 mg/5 mL*
"Works great." "Easy to take."

astellas
Under License of
**Astellas Pharma Inc.**
Japan

**Abbott**
A Promise for Life

**PROFESSIONAL BRIEF SUMMARY-CONSULT PACKAGE INSERT FOR FULL PRESCRIBING INFORMATION.**
03-5435-Rev. July, 2005
(Nos. 3769, 3771, 6151)

# Omnicef® (cefdinir) capsules
# Omnicef® (cefdinir) for oral suspension

**Rx only**

## INDICATIONS AND USAGE

To reduce the development of drug-resistant bacteria and maintain the effectiveness of OMNICEF and other antibacterial drugs, OMNICEF should be used only to treat or prevent infections that are proven or strongly suspected to be caused by susceptible bacteria. When culture and susceptibility information are available, they should be considered in selecting or modifying antibacterial therapy. In the absence of such data, local epidemiology and susceptibility patterns may contribute to the empiric selection of therapy.

OMNICEF (cefdinir) capsules and OMNICEF (cefdinir) for oral suspension are indicated for the treatment of patients with mild to moderate infections caused by susceptible strains of the designated microorganisms in the conditions listed below.

### Adults and Adolescents

**Community-Acquired Pneumonia** caused by *Haemophilus influenzae* (including β-lactamase producing strains), *Haemophilus parainfluenzae* (including β-lactamase producing strains), *Streptococcus pneumoniae* (penicillin-susceptible strains only), and *Moraxella catarrhalis* (including β-lactamase producing strains).

**Acute Exacerbations of Chronic Bronchitis** caused by *Haemophilus influenzae* (including β-lactamase producing strains), *Haemophilus parainfluenzae* (including β-lactamase producing strains), *Streptococcus pneumoniae* (penicillin-susceptible strains only), and *Moraxella catarrhalis* (including β-lactamase producing strains).

**Acute Maxillary Sinusitis** caused by *Haemophilus influenzae* (including β-lactamase producing strains), *Streptococcus pneumoniae* (penicillin-susceptible strains only), and *Moraxella catarrhalis* (including β-lactamase producing strains).

**NOTE:** For information on use in pediatric patients, see **Pediatric Use** and **DOSAGE AND ADMINISTRATION**.

**Pharyngitis/Tonsillitis** caused by *Streptococcus pyogenes*.

**NOTE:** Cefdinir is effective in the eradication of *S. pyogenes* from the oropharynx. Cefdinir has not, however, been studied for the prevention of rheumatic fever following *S. pyogenes* pharyngitis/tonsillitis. Only intramuscular penicillin has been demonstrated to be effective for the prevention of rheumatic fever.

**Uncomplicated Skin and Skin Structure Infections** caused by *Staphylococcus aureus* (including β-lactamase producing strains) and *Streptococcus pyogenes*.

### Pediatric Patients

**Acute Bacterial Otitis Media** caused by *Haemophilus influenzae* (including β-lactamase producing strains), *Streptococcus pneumoniae* (penicillin-susceptible strains only), and *Moraxella catarrhalis* (including β-lactamase producing strains).

**Pharyngitis/Tonsillitis** caused by *Streptococcus pyogenes*.

**NOTE:** Cefdinir is effective in the eradication of *S. pyogenes* from the oropharynx. Cefdinir has not, however, been studied for the prevention of rheumatic fever following *S. pyogenes* pharyngitis/tonsillitis. Only intramuscular penicillin has been demonstrated to be effective for the prevention of rheumatic fever.

**Uncomplicated Skin and Skin Structure Infections** caused by *Staphylococcus aureus* (including β-lactamase producing strains) and *Streptococcus pyogenes*.

## CONTRAINDICATIONS

OMNICEF (cefdinir) is contraindicated in patients with known allergy to the cephalosporin class of antibiotics.

## WARNINGS

**BEFORE THERAPY WITH OMNICEF (CEFDINIR) IS INSTITUTED, CAREFUL INQUIRY SHOULD BE MADE TO DETERMINE WHETHER THE PATIENT HAS HAD PREVIOUS HYPERSENSITIVITY REACTIONS TO CEFDINIR, OTHER CEPHALOSPORINS, PENICILLINS, OR OTHER DRUGS. IF CEFDINIR IS TO BE GIVEN TO PENICILLIN-SENSITIVE PATIENTS, CAUTION SHOULD BE EXERCISED BECAUSE CROSS-HYPERSENSITIVITY AMONG β-LACTAM ANTIBIOTICS HAS BEEN CLEARLY DOCUMENTED AND MAY OCCUR IN UP TO 10% OF PATIENTS WITH A HISTORY OF PENICILLIN ALLERGY. IF AN ALLERGIC REACTION TO CEFDINIR OCCURS, THE DRUG SHOULD BE DISCONTINUED. SERIOUS ACUTE HYPERSENSITIVITY REACTIONS MAY REQUIRE TREATMENT WITH EPINEPHRINE AND OTHER EMERGENCY MEASURES, INCLUDING OXYGEN, INTRAVENOUS FLUIDS, INTRAVENOUS ANTIHISTAMINES, CORTICOSTEROIDS, PRESSOR AMINES, AND AIRWAY MANAGEMENT, AS CLINICALLY INDICATED.**

**Pseudomembranous colitis has been reported with nearly all antibacterial agents, including cefdinir, and may range in severity from mild- to life-threatening. Therefore, it is important to consider this diagnosis in patients who present with diarrhea subsequent to the administration of antibacterial agents.**

Treatment with antibacterial agents alters the normal flora of the colon and may permit overgrowth of clostridia. Studies indicate that a toxin produced by *Clostridium difficile* is a primary cause of "antibiotic-associated colitis."

After the diagnosis of pseudomembranous colitis has been established, appropriate therapeutic measures should be initiated. Mild cases of pseudomembranous colitis usually respond to drug discontinuation alone. In moderate to severe cases, consideration should be given to management with fluids and electrolytes, protein supplementation, and treatment with an antibacterial drug clinically effective against *Clostridium difficile*.

## PRECAUTIONS

### General

Prescribing OMNICEF in the absence of a proven or strongly suspected bacterial infection or a prophylactic indication is unlikely to provide benefit to the patient and increases the risk of the development of drug-resistant bacteria.

As with other broad-spectrum antibiotics, prolonged treatment may result in the possible emergence and overgrowth of resistant organisms. Careful observation of the patient is essential. If superinfection occurs during therapy, appropriate alternative therapy should be administered.

Cefdinir, as with other broad-spectrum antimicrobials (antibiotics), should be prescribed with caution in individuals with a history of colitis.

In patients with transient or persistent renal insufficiency (creatinine clearance <30 mL/min), the total daily dose of OMNICEF should be reduced because high and prolonged plasma concentrations of cefdinir can result following recommended doses.

### Information for Patients

Patients should be counseled that antibacterial drugs including OMNICEF should only be used to treat bacterial infections. They do not treat viral infections (e.g., the common cold). When OMNICEF is prescribed to treat a bacterial infection, patients should be told that although it is common to feel better early in the course of therapy, the medication should be taken exactly as directed. Skipping doses or not completing the full course of therapy may (1) decrease the effectiveness of the immediate treatment and (2) increase the likelihood that bacteria will develop resistance and will not be treatable by OMNICEF or other antibacterial drugs in the future.

Antacids containing magnesium or aluminum interfere with the absorption of cefdinir. If this type of antacid is required during OMNICEF therapy, OMNICEF should be taken at least 2 hours before or after the antacid.

Iron supplements, including multivitamins that contain iron, interfere with the absorption of cefdinir. If iron supplements are required during OMNICEF therapy, OMNICEF should be taken at least 2 hours before or after the supplement.

Iron-fortified infant formula does not significantly interfere with the absorption of cefdinir. Therefore, OMNICEF for Oral Suspension can be administered with iron-fortified infant formula.

Diabetic patients and caregivers should be aware that the oral suspension contains 2.86 g of sucrose per teaspoon.

### Drug Interactions

**Antacids:** (aluminum- or magnesium-containing): Concomitant administration of 300-mg cefdinir capsules with 30 mL Maalox® TC suspension reduces the rate ($C_{max}$) and extent (AUC) of absorption by approximately 40%. Time to reach $C_{max}$ is also prolonged by 1 hour. There are no significant effects on cefdinir pharmacokinetics if the antacid is administered 2 hours before or 2 hours after cefdinir. If antacids are required during OMNICEF therapy, OMNICEF should be taken at least 2 hours before or after the antacid.

**Probenecid:** As with other β-lactam antibiotics, probenecid inhibits the renal excretion of cefdinir, resulting in an approximate doubling in AUC, a 54% increase in peak cefdinir plasma levels, and a 50% prolongation in the apparent elimination $t_{1/2}$.

**Iron Supplements and Foods Fortified With Iron:** Concomitant administration of cefdinir with a therapeutic iron supplement containing 60 mg of elemental iron (as $FeSO_4$) or vitamins supplemented with 10 mg of elemental iron reduced extent of absorption by 80% and 31%, respectively. If iron supplements are required during OMNICEF therapy, OMNICEF should be taken at least 2 hours before or after the supplement.

The effect of foods highly fortified with elemental iron (primarily iron-fortified breakfast cereals) on cefdinir absorption has not been studied.

Concomitantly administered iron-fortified infant formula (2.2 mg elemental iron/6 oz) has no significant effect on cefdinir pharmacokinetics. Therefore, OMNICEF for Oral Suspension can be administered with iron-fortified infant formula.

There have been reports of reddish stools in patients receiving cefdinir. In many cases, patients were also receiving iron-containing products. The reddish color is due to the formation of a nonabsorbable complex between cefdinir or its breakdown products and iron in the gastrointestinal tract.

### Drug/Laboratory Test Interactions

A false-positive reaction for ketones in the urine may occur with tests using nitroprusside, but not with those using nitroferricyanide. The administration of cefdinir may result in a false-positive reaction for glucose in urine using Clinitest®, Benedict's solution, or Fehling's solution. It is recommended that glucose tests based on enzymatic glucose oxidase reactions (such as Clinistix® or Tes-Tape®) be used. Cephalosporins are known to occasionally induce a positive direct Coombs' test.

### Carcinogenesis, Mutagenesis, Impairment of Fertility

The carcinogenic potential of cefdinir has not been evaluated. No mutagenic effects were seen in the bacterial reverse mutation assay (Ames) or point mutation assay at the hypoxanthine-guanine phosphoribosyltransferase locus (HGPRT) in V79 Chinese hamster lung cells. No clastogenic effects were observed *in vitro* in the structural chromosome aberration assay in V79 Chinese hamster lung cells or *in vivo* in the micronucleus assay in mouse bone marrow. In rats, fertility and reproductive performance were not affected by cefdinir at oral doses up to 1000 mg/kg/day (70 times the human dose based on mg/kg/day, 11 times based on mg/m$^2$/day).

### Pregnancy - Teratogenic Effects

**Pregnancy Category B:** Cefdinir was not teratogenic in rats at oral doses up to 1000 mg/kg/day (70 times the human dose based on mg/kg/day, 11 times based on mg/m$^2$/day) or in rabbits at oral doses up to 10 mg/kg/day (0.7 times the human dose based on mg/kg/day, 0.23 times based on mg/m$^2$/day). Maternal toxicity (decreased body weight gain) was observed in rabbits at the maximum tolerated dose of 10 mg/kg/day without adverse effects on offspring. Decreased body weight occurred in rat fetuses at ≥ 100 mg/kg/day, and in rat offspring at ≥ 32 mg/kg/day. No effects were observed on maternal reproductive parameters or offspring survival, development, behavior, or reproductive function.

There are, however, no adequate and well-controlled studies in pregnant women. Because animal reproduction studies are not always predictive of human response, this drug should be used during pregnancy only if clearly needed.

### Labor and Delivery

Cefdinir has not been studied for use during labor and delivery.

### Nursing Mothers

Following administration of single 600-mg doses, cefdinir was not detected in human breast milk.

### Pediatric Use

Safety and efficacy in neonates and infants less than 6 months of age have not been established. Use of cefdinir for the treatment of acute maxillary sinusitis in pediatric patients (age 6 months through 12 years) is supported by evidence from adequate and well-controlled studies in adults and adolescents, the similar pathophysiology of acute sinusitis in adult and pediatric patients, and comparative pharmacokinetic data in the pediatric population.

### Geriatric Use

Efficacy is comparable in geriatric patients and younger adults. While cefdinir has been well-tolerated in all age groups, in clinical trials geriatric patients experienced a lower rate of adverse events, including diarrhea, than younger adults. Dose adjustment in elderly patients is not necessary unless renal function is markedly compromised.

## ADVERSE EVENTS

**Clinical Trials - OMNICEF Capsules (Adult and Adolescent Patients):**

In clinical trials, 5093 adult and adolescent patients (3841 US and 1252 non-US) were treated with the recommended dose of cefdinir capsules (600 mg/day). Most adverse events were mild and self-limiting. No deaths or permanent disabilities were attributed to cefdinir. One hundred forty-seven of 5093 (3%) patients discontinued medication due to adverse events thought by the investigators to be possibly, probably, or definitely associated with cefdinir therapy. The discontinuations were primarily for gastrointestinal disturbances, usually diarrhea or nausea. Nineteen of 5093 (0.4%) patients were discontinued due to rash thought related to cefdinir administration.

In the US, the following adverse events were thought by investigators to be possibly, probably, or definitely related to cefdinir capsules in multiple-dose clinical trials (N = 3841 cefdinir-treated patients):

**ADVERSE EVENTS ASSOCIATED WITH CEFDINIR CAPSULES US TRIALS IN ADULT AND ADOLESCENT PATIENTS (N=3841)[a]**

| | | |
|---|---|---|
| Incidence ≥ 1% | Diarrhea | 15% |
| | Vaginal moniliasis | 4% of women |
| | Nausea | 3% |
| | Headache | 2% |
| | Abdominal pain | 1% |
| | Vaginitis | 1% of women |
| Incidence <1% but >0.1% | Rash | 0.9% |
| | Dyspepsia | 0.7% |
| | Flatulence | 0.7% |
| | Vomiting | 0.7% |
| | Abnormal stools | 0.3% |
| | Anorexia | 0.3% |
| | Constipation | 0.3% |
| | Dizziness | 0.3% |
| | Dry mouth | 0.3% |
| | Asthenia | 0.2% |
| | Insomnia | 0.2% |
| | Leukorrhea | 0.2% of women |
| | Moniliasis | 0.2% |
| | Pruritus | 0.2% |
| | Somnolence | 0.2% |

[a] 1733 males, 2108 females

The following laboratory value changes of possible clinical significance, irrespective of relationship to therapy with cefdinir, were seen during clinical trials conducted in the US:

**LABORATORY VALUE CHANGES OBSERVED WITH CEFDINIR CAPSULES US TRIALS IN ADULT AND ADOLESCENT PATIENTS (N=3841)**

| | | |
|---|---|---|
| Incidence ≥ 1% | ↑ Urine leukocytes | 2% |
| | ↑ Urine protein | 2% |
| | ↑ Gamma-glutamyltransferase[a] | 1% |
| | ↓ Lymphocytes, ↑ Lymphocytes | 1%, 0.2% |
| | ↑ Microhematuria | 1% |
| Incidence <1% but >0.1% | ↑ Glucose[a] | 0.9% |
| | ↑ Urine glucose | 0.9% |
| | ↑ White blood cells, ↓ White blood cells | 0.9%, 0.7% |
| | ↑ Alanine aminotransferase (ALT) | 0.7% |
| | ↑ Eosinophils | 0.7% |
| | ↑ Urine specific gravity, ↓ Urine specific gravity[a] | 0.6%, 0.2% |
| | ↓ Bicarbonate[a] | 0.6% |
| | ↑ Phosphorus, ↓ Phosphorus[a] | 0.6%, 0.3% |
| | ↑ Aspartate aminotransferase (AST) | 0.4% |
| | ↑ Alkaline phosphatase | 0.3% |
| | ↑ Blood urea nitrogen (BUN) | 0.3% |
| | ↓ Hemoglobin | 0.3% |
| | ↑ Polymorphonuclear neutrophils (PMNs), ↓ PMNs | 0.3%, 0.2% |
| | ↑ Bilirubin | 0.2% |
| | ↑ Lactate dehydrogenase[a] | 0.2% |
| | ↑ Platelets | 0.2% |
| | ↑ Potassium[a] | 0.2% |
| | ↑ Urine pH[a] | 0.2% |

[a] N<3841 for these parameters

**Clinical Trials - OMNICEF for Oral Suspension (Pediatric Patients):**

In clinical trials, 2289 pediatric patients (1783 US and 506 non-US) were treated with the recommended dose of cefdinir suspension (14 mg/kg/day). Most adverse events were mild and self-limiting. No deaths or permanent disabilities were attributed to cefdinir. Forty of 2289 (2%) patients discontinued medication due to adverse events considered by the investigators to be possibly, probably, or definitely associated with cefdinir therapy. Discontinuations were primarily for gastrointestinal disturbances, usually diarrhea. Five of 2289 (0.2%) patients were discontinued due to rash thought related to cefdinir administration.

In the US, the following adverse events were thought by investigators to be possibly, probably, or definitely related to cefdinir suspension in multiple-dose clinical trials (N=1783 cefdinir-treated patients):

**ADVERSE EVENTS ASSOCIATED WITH CEFDINIR SUSPENSION US TRIALS IN PEDIATRIC PATIENTS (N=1783)[a]**

| | | |
|---|---|---|
| Incidence ≥ 1% | Diarrhea | 8% |
| | Rash | 3% |
| | Vomiting | 1% |
| Incidence <1% but >0.1% | Cutaneous moniliasis | 0.9% |
| | Abdominal pain | 0.8% |
| | Leukopenia[b] | 0.3% |
| | Vaginal moniliasis | 0.3% of girls |
| | Vaginitis | 0.3% of girls |
| | Abnormal stools | 0.2% |
| | Dyspepsia | 0.2% |
| | Hyperkinesia | 0.2% |
| | Increased AST[b] | 0.2% |
| | Maculopapular rash | 0.2% |
| | Nausea | 0.2% |

[a] 977 males, 806 females

[b] Laboratory changes were occasionally reported as adverse events.

NOTE: In both cefdinir- and control-treated patients, rates of diarrhea and rash were higher in the youngest pediatric patients. The incidence of diarrhea in cefdinir-treated patients ≤2 years of age was 17% (95/557) compared with 4% (51/1226) in those >2 years old. The incidence of rash (primarily diaper rash in the younger patients) was 8% (43/557) in patients ≤2 years of age compared with 1% (8/1226) in those >2 years old.

The following laboratory value changes of possible clinical significance, irrespective of relationship to therapy with cefdinir, were seen during clinical trials conducted in the US:

**LABORATORY VALUE CHANGES OF POSSIBLE CLINICAL SIGNIFICANCE OBSERVED WITH CEFDINIR SUSPENSION US TRIALS IN PEDIATRIC PATIENTS (N=1783)**

| | | |
|---|---|---|
| Incidence ≥ 1% | ↑ Lymphocytes, ↓ Lymphocytes | 2%, 0.8% |
| | ↑ Alkaline phosphatase | 1% |
| | ↓ Bicarbonate[a] | 1% |
| | ↑ Eosinophils | 1% |
| | ↑ Lactate dehydrogenase | 1% |
| | ↑ Platelets | 1% |
| | ↑ PMNs, ↓ PMNs | 1%, 1% |
| | ↑ Urine protein | 1% |
| Incidence <1% but >0.1% | ↑ Phosphorus, ↓ Phosphorus | 0.9%, 0.4% |
| | ↑ Urine pH | 0.8% |
| | ↓ White blood cells, ↑ White blood cells | 0.7%, 0.3% |
| | ↓ Calcium[a] | 0.5% |
| | ↓ Hemoglobin | 0.5% |
| | ↑ Urine leukocytes | 0.5% |
| | ↑ Monocytes | 0.4% |
| | ↑ AST | 0.3% |
| | ↑ Potassium[a] | 0.3% |
| | ↑ Urine specific gravity, ↓ Urine specific gravity | 0.3%, 0.1% |
| | ↓ Hematocrit[a] | 0.2% |

[a] N=1387 for these parameters

**Postmarketing Experience**

The following adverse experiences and altered laboratory tests, regardless of their relationship to cefdinir, have been reported during extensive postmarketing experience, beginning with approval in Japan in 1991: Stevens-Johnson syndrome, toxic epidermal necrolysis, exfoliative dermatitis, erythema multiforme, erythema nodosum, serum sickness-like reactions, conjunctivitis, stomatitis, acute hepatitis, cholestasis, fulminant hepatitis, hepatic failure, jaundice, increased amylase, shock, anaphylaxis, facial and laryngeal edema, feeling of suffocation, acute enterocolitis, bloody diarrhea, hemorrhagic colitis, melena, pseudomembranous colitis, pancytopenia, granulocytopenia, leukopenia, thrombocytopenia, idiopathic thrombocytopenic purpura, hemolytic anemia, acute respiratory failure, asthmatic attack, drug-induced pneumonia, eosinophilic pneumonia, idiopathic interstitial pneumonia, fever, acute renal failure, nephropathy, bleeding tendency, coagulation disorder, disseminated intravascular coagulation, upper GI bleed, peptic ulcer, ileus, loss of consciousness, allergic vasculitis, possible cefdinir-diclofenac interaction, cardiac failure, chest pain, myocardial infarction, hypertension, involuntary movements, and rhabdomyolysis.

**Cephalosporin Class Adverse Events**

The following adverse events and altered laboratory tests have been reported for cephalosporin-class antibiotics in general:

Allergic reactions, anaphylaxis, Stevens-Johnson syndrome, erythema multiforme, toxic epidermal necrolysis, renal dysfunction, toxic nephropathy, hepatic dysfunction including cholestasis, aplastic anemia, hemolytic anemia, hemorrhage, false-positive test for urinary glucose, neutropenia, pancytopenia, and agranulocytosis. Pseudomembranous colitis symptoms may begin during or after antibiotic treatment (see **WARNINGS**).

Several cephalosporins have been implicated in triggering seizures, particularly in patients with renal impairment when the dosage was not reduced (see **OVERDOSAGE**). If seizures associated with drug therapy occur, the drug should be discontinued. Anticonvulsant therapy can be given if clinically indicated.

## OVERDOSAGE

Information on cefdinir overdosage in humans is not available. In acute rodent toxicity studies, a single oral 5600-mg/kg dose produced no adverse effects. Toxic signs and symptoms following overdosage with other β-lactam antibiotics have included nausea, vomiting, epigastric distress, diarrhea, and convulsions. Hemodialysis removes cefdinir from the body. This may be useful in the event of a serious toxic reaction from overdosage, particularly if renal function is compromised.

**Rx only**

Ref: 03-5435-Rev. July, 2005
(Nos. 3769, 3771, 6151)



05J-034-L150-2 **MASTER**

Manufactured by:
**CEPH** International Corporation
Carolina, Puerto Rico 00986

Under License of:
astellas Astellas Pharma Inc.
Tokyo, Japan

For:
**Abbott Laboratories**
North Chicago, IL 60064, U.S.A.

06F-034-Q068-1
Printed in U.S.A.

## Cardiorespiratory Fitness Levels Among US Youth 12 to 19 Years of Age

Increasing scrutiny on the problem of obesity in children and youth involves analysis of the levels of physical activity and concomitant cardiorespiratory fitness of youth. This study presents data on 3287 youth aged 12 to 19 years who had fitness measured as part of the National Health and Nutrition Examination Survey. Youth who reported higher levels of physical activity had higher levels of cardiorespiratory fitness. On the treadmill test, males and females in the overweight and at risk for overweight groups had lower cardiorespiratory fitness than their peers in the normal weight group. Approximately one third of youth aged 12 to 19 years in the United States fail to meet the levels of cardiorespiratory fitness deemed appropriate by experts. This is an important public health problem because low physical fitness during adolescence tracks into adulthood, increasing the risk for later chronic morbidity and early mortality.

**See page 1005**

## Attention-Deficit/Hyperactivity Disorder in Children: Excess Costs Before and After Initial Diagnosis and Treatment Cost Differences by Ethnicity

Ray and his colleagues at Kaiser Permanente of Northern California compared the health care costs among 3122 children with attention-deficit/hyperactivity disorder (ADHD) with those among 15 899 children without ADHD. Children with ADHD had health care costs that were nearly twice that of children without ADHD in the year prior to their initial diagnosis of ADHD and nearly 3 times as costly in the year after their initial diagnosis. Health care for children with ADHD and coexisting mental health disorders was much costlier than that for children without such comorbidities. The higher costs were due primarily to increased psychiatric and pediatric care as well as increased costs for medication. Nonwhite children were less likely to use ADHD medication in the year after their diagnosis than were white children, and among users, less medication was used.

**See page 1063**

## Improved Preventive Care for Asthma: A Randomized Trial of Clinician Prompting in Pediatric Offices

Despite the availability of effective medications to treat asthma, many providers do not follow established guidelines for their use. Halterman and colleagues conducted a randomized controlled trial in 2 inner-city pediatric practices among children aged 2 to 12 years with persistent asthma. Clinicians who received a written prompt including the child's symptoms and guideline recommendations at the time of the child's visit were more likely to deliver an asthma action plan, perform smoking-reduction counseling, discuss asthma with the family, and recommend a follow-up visit than clinicians who did not receive the prompt. Children in the clinician-prompting group had a 3-fold greater odds of receiving any preventive action than children in the control group. Because guidelines-based asthma care can improve outcomes, the implications of this study are great.

**See page 1018**

## Adolescent Bone Health

Pediatric and adolescent health care providers have increasingly recognized the importance of understanding the skeletal health of their patients. At least one fourth of adult total bone mineral is acquired during the 4-year period surrounding peak height velocity with up to 60% during the remaining peripubertal years. This review outlines the known conditions that are associated with impaired bone mineral accrual and clinical settings in which the evaluation of the "at-risk" adolescents should be considered. The article provides current recommendations regarding physical activity and nutrition for all adolescents as well as therapeutic options for patients identified as having low bone mineral density.

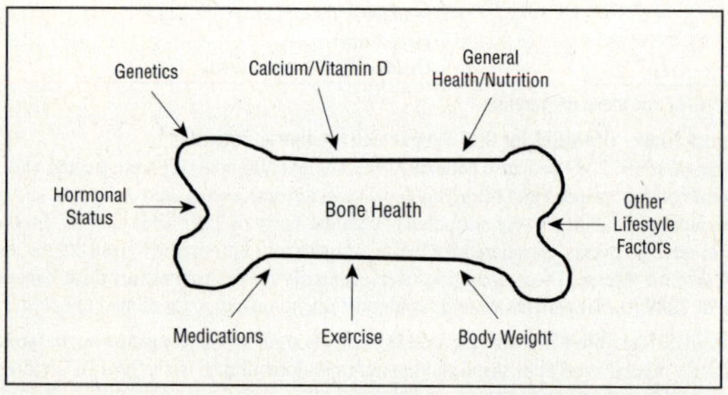


**Figure.** Factors affecting bone health. Reprinted with permission.

**See page 1026**

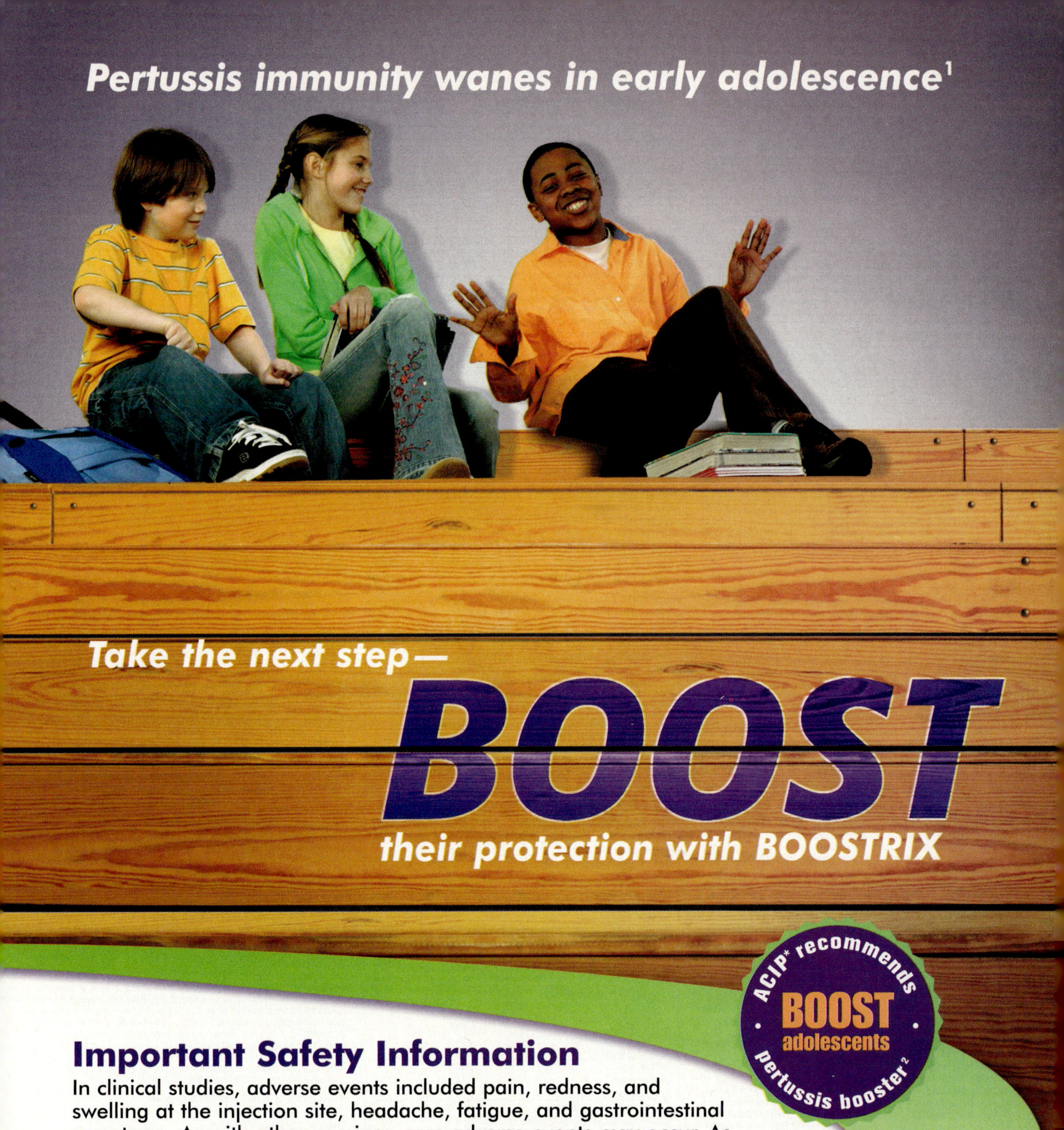


## Important Safety Information

In clinical studies, adverse events included pain, redness, and swelling at the injection site, headache, fatigue, and gastrointestinal symptoms. As with other vaccines, rare adverse events may occur. As with any vaccine, vaccination with BOOSTRIX may not protect 100% of susceptible individuals. Hypersensitivity to any component of BOOSTRIX is a contraindication.

*Advisory Committee on Immunization Practices.

gsk GlaxoSmithKline Vaccines

**BOOSTRIX®**

***Tetanus Toxoid, Reduced Diphtheria Toxoid and Acellular Pertussis Vaccine, Adsorbed***

**Please see references and brief summary of complete prescribing information on the adjacent page.**


Manufactured by **GlaxoSmithKline Biologicals,** Rixensart, Belgium    Distributed by **GlaxoSmithKline**, Research Triangle Park, NC 27709

# BOOSTRIX®

## (Tetanus Toxoid, Reduced Diphtheria Toxoid and Acellular Pertussis Vaccine, Adsorbed) (Tdap)

The following is a brief summary only; see full prescribing information for complete product information.

**INDICATIONS AND USAGE:** BOOSTRIX is indicated for active booster immunization against tetanus, diphtheria, and pertussis as a single dose in individuals 10 through 18 years of age. The use of BOOSTRIX as a primary series or to complete the primary series has not been studied. As with any vaccine, BOOSTRIX may not protect 100% of individuals receiving the vaccine.

**CONTRAINDICATIONS:** Hypersensitivity to any component of the vaccine is a contraindication (see DESCRIPTION in full prescribing information). Do not use BOOSTRIX after a serious allergic reaction (e.g., anaphylaxis) following any other tetanus toxoid, diphtheria toxoid or pertussis-containing vaccine, or any component of this vaccine (see DESCRIPTION in full prescribing information). Because of the uncertainty as to which component of the vaccine might be responsible, do not give further vaccination with any of these components; or, refer such individuals to an allergist for evaluation. The following events are contraindications to administration of BOOSTRIX: encephalopathy (e.g., coma, decreased level of consciousness, prolonged seizures) within 7 days of administration of a previous dose of a pertussis-containing vaccine that is not attributable to another identifiable cause; progressive neurologic disorder, uncontrolled epilepsy, or progressive encephalopathy. Do not vaccinate individuals with these conditions until a treatment regimen has been established and the condition has stabilized.

**WARNINGS:** The tip cap and the rubber plunger of the needleless prefilled syringes contain dry natural latex rubber that may cause allergic reactions in latex sensitive individuals. The vial stopper is latex-free. If any of the following events occurred in temporal relation to previous receipt of a Diphtheria and Tetanus Toxoids and Pertussis Vaccine Adsorbed (DTwP) vaccine or a vaccine containing an acellular pertussis component, consider carefully whether to give subsequent doses of BOOSTRIX: temperature of ≥40.5°C (105°F) within 48 hours not due to another identifiable cause; collapse or shock-like state (hypotonic-hyporesponsive episode) within 48 hours; persistent, inconsolable crying lasting ≥3 hours, occurring within 48 hours; seizures with or without fever occurring within 3 days. Persons who experienced serious Arthus-type hypersensitivity reactions following a prior dose of tetanus toxoid usually have high serum tetanus antitoxin levels and should not be given Tetanus and Diphtheria Toxoids Adsorbed For Adult Use (Td) or Tdap vaccines or even emergency doses of Td more frequently than every 10 years, even if the wound is neither clean nor minor. If Guillain-Barré syndrome has occurred within 6 weeks of receipt of prior vaccine containing tetanus toxoid, the decision to give BOOSTRIX or any vaccine containing tetanus toxoid should be based on careful consideration of the potential benefits and possible risks. The decision to administer a pertussis-containing vaccine to individuals with stable central nervous system (CNS) disorders must be made by the physician on an individual basis, with consideration of all relevant factors, and assessment of potential risks and benefits for that individual. Advise the patient, parent, or guardian of the potential increased risk involved (see PRECAUTIONS). A family history of seizures or other CNS disorders is not a contraindication to pertussis vaccine. The Advisory Committee on Immunization Practices (ACIP) has published guidelines for vaccination of persons with recent or acute illness (www.cdc.gov). Do not give BOOSTRIX to individuals with bleeding disorders such as hemophilia or thrombocytopenia, or to persons on anticoagulant therapy unless the potential benefit clearly outweighs the risk of administration. If the decision is made to administer BOOSTRIX to such persons, it should be given with caution with steps taken to avoid the risk of hematoma following the injection.

**PRECAUTIONS: General:** Before the injection of any biological, the physician should take all reasonable precautions to prevent allergic or other adverse reactions. Epinephrine injection (1:1,000) and other appropriate agents used for the control of immediate allergic reactions must be immediately available should an acute anaphylactic reaction occur. Immunosuppressed persons, including individuals receiving immunosuppressive therapy, may not develop the expected immune response. **Drug Interactions:** Do not mix BOOSTRIX with any other vaccine in the same syringe or vial. **Carcinogenesis, Mutagenesis, Impairment of Fertility:** BOOSTRIX has not been evaluated for carcinogenic or mutagenic potential, or for impairment of fertility. **Pregnancy:** Pregnancy Category C. Animal reproduction studies have not been conducted with BOOSTRIX. It is also not known whether BOOSTRIX can cause fetal harm when administered to a pregnant woman or can affect reproductive capacity. BOOSTRIX should be given to a pregnant woman only if clearly needed. Animal fertility studies have not been conducted with BOOSTRIX. In a developmental toxicity study, the effect of BOOSTRIX on embryo-fetal and pre-weaning development was evaluated in pregnant rats. Animals were administered INFANRIX® (Diphtheria and Tetanus Toxoids and Acellular Pertussis Vaccine Adsorbed) prior to gestation and BOOSTRIX during the period of organogenesis (gestation days 6, 8, 11) and later in pregnancy (gestation day 15), 0.1 mL/rat/occasion (a 45-fold increase compared to the human dose of BOOSTRIX on a body weight basis), by intramuscular injection. No adverse affect on pregnancy and lactation parameters, embryo-fetal or pre-weaning development was observed. There were no fetal malformations or other evidence of teratogenesis noted in this study. **Nursing Mothers:** It is not known whether BOOSTRIX is excreted in human milk. Because many drugs are excreted in human milk, caution should be exercised when BOOSTRIX is administered to a nursing woman. **Pregnancy Exposure Registry:** Healthcare providers are encouraged to register pregnant women who receive BOOSTRIX in the GlaxoSmithKline vaccination pregnancy registry by calling 1-888-825-5249. **Geriatric Use:** BOOSTRIX is not indicated for use in individuals older than 18 years. **Pediatric Use:** BOOSTRIX is not indicated for use in individuals younger than 10 years (see DOSAGE AND ADMINISTRATION in full prescribing information). For immunization of infants and children younger than 7 years against diphtheria, tetanus, and pertussis, refer to the manufacturers' package inserts for Diphtheria and Tetanus Toxoids and Acellular Pertussis Vaccine Adsorbed (DTaP) vaccines.

**ADVERSE REACTIONS:** A total of 3,608 adolescents were vaccinated with a single dose of BOOSTRIX during clinical trials. An additional 1,092 adolescents 10 to 18 years of age received a non-US formulation of BOOSTRIX (formulated to contain 0.5 mg aluminum per dose) in non-US clinical studies.

The primary safety study, conducted in the United States, was a randomized, observer-blinded, controlled study in which 3,080 adolescents 10 to 18 years of age received a single dose of BOOSTRIX and 1,034 received the control Td vaccine manufactured by Massachusetts Public Health Biologic Laboratories. There were no substantive differences in demographic characteristics between the vaccine groups. Among BOOSTRIX and control vaccine recipients approximately 75% were 10 to 14 years of age and approximately 25% were 15 to 18 years of age. Approximately 98% of participants in this study had received the recommended series of 4 or 5 doses of either DTwP or a combination of DTwP and DTaP in childhood. Data on adverse events were collected by the subjects, parents and/or guardians using standardized diaries for 15 consecutive days following the vaccine dose (i.e., day of vaccination and the next 14 days). Subjects were monitored for unsolicited adverse events that occurred within 31 days of vaccination (day 0-30) using diary cards (day 0-14) supplemented by spontaneous reports and a medical history as reported by subjects, parents, and/or guardians. Subjects were also monitored for 6 months post-vaccination for non-routine medical visits, visits to an emergency room, onset of new chronic illness, and serious adverse events. Information regarding late onset adverse events was obtained via a telephone call 6 months following vaccination. At least 97% of subjects completed the 6-month follow-up evaluation.

In a study conducted in Germany, BOOSTRIX was administered to 319 children 10 to 12 years of age previously vaccinated with 5 doses of acellular pertussis-containing vaccines, 193 of these subjects had previously received 5 doses of INFANRIX. Adverse events were recorded on diary cards during the 15 days following vaccination. Unsolicited adverse events that occurred within 31 days of vaccination (day 0-30) were recorded on the diary card or verbally reported to the investigator. Subjects were monitored for 6 months post-vaccination for physician office visits, emergency room visits, onset of new chronic illness, and serious adverse events. The 6-month follow-up evaluation, conducted via telephone interview, was completed by 90% of subjects.

The adverse event information from clinical trials provides a basis for identifying adverse events that appear to be related to vaccine use and for approximating rates. However, because clinical trials are conducted under widely varying conditions, adverse event rates observed in the clinical trials of a vaccine cannot be directly compared to rates in the clinical trials of another vaccine, and may not reflect the rates observed in practice.

**Serious Adverse Events in All Safety Studies:** In the US-safety study and German-safety study, no serious adverse events were reported to occur within 31 days of vaccination. During the 6-month extended safety evaluation period, no serious adverse events that were of potential autoimmune origin or new onset and chronic in nature were reported to occur. In non-US studies in which serious adverse events were monitored for up to 37 days, one subject was diagnosed with insulin dependent diabetes 20 days following administration of BOOSTRIX. No other serious adverse events of potential autoimmune origin or that were new onset and chronic in nature were reported to occur in these studies.

**Solicited Adverse Events in the US-Safety Study:** In a US study, the most common local adverse events following administration of BOOSTRIX were pain, redness, and swelling at the injection site. The most common general adverse events were headache and fatigue. Most of these events were reported at a similar frequency in recipients of both BOOSTRIX and Td. Any pain, grade 2 or 3 pain (but not grade 3 alone), and grade 2 or 3 headache (but not grade 3 alone) were reported at a higher rate in recipients of BOOSTRIX. The primary safety endpoint of the US study was the incidence of grade 3 pain (spontaneously painful and/or prevented normal activity) at the injection site within 15 days of vaccination. Grade 3 pain was reported in 4.6% of those who received BOOSTRIX compared with 4.0% of those who received the Td vaccine. The difference in rate of grade 3 pain was within the pre-defined clinical limit for non-inferiority (upper limit of the 95% CI for the difference ≤4%). These were the rates for solicited local and general adverse events within 15 days of vaccination with BOOSTRIX or Td vaccine for the total vaccinated cohort (all enrolled, vaccinated subjects with safety data available analyzed by vaccine received):

**Percentage of Individuals 10 to 18 Years of Age Reporting Solicited Local Adverse Events or Solicited General Adverse Events Within the 15-day* Post-Vaccination Period**

| | BOOSTRIX (N = 3,032) % | Td (N = 1,013) % |
|---|---|---|
| **Local** | | |
| Pain,† any | 75.3 | 71.7 |
| Pain,† grade 2 or 3 | 51.2 | 42.5 |
| Pain,‡ grade 3 | 4.6 | 4.0 |
| Redness, any | 22.5 | 19.8 |
| Redness, >20 mm | 4.1 | 3.9 |
| Redness, ≥50 mm | 1.7 | 1.6 |
| Swelling, any | 21.1 | 20.1 |
| Swelling, >20 mm | 5.3 | 4.9 |
| Swelling, ≥50 mm | 2.5 | 3.2 |
| Arm circumference increase,§ >5 mm | 28.3 | 29.5 |
| Arm circumference increase,§ >20 mm | 2.0 | 2.2 |
| Arm circumference increase,§ >40 mm | 0.5 | 0.3 |
| **General** | | |
| Fever,‖ ≥99.5°F | 13.5 | 13.1 |
| Fever,‖ >100.4°F | 5.0 | 4.7 |
| Fever,‖ >102.2°F | 1.4 | 1.0 |
| Headache, any | 43.1 | 41.5 |
| Headache,† grade 2 or 3 | 15.7 | 12.7 |
| Headache, grade 3 | 3.7 | 2.7 |
| Fatigue, any | 37.0 | 36.7 |
| Fatigue, grade 2 or 3 | 14.4 | 12.9 |
| Fatigue, grade 3 | 3.7 | 3.2 |
| Gastrointestinal symptoms,¶ any | 26.0 | 25.8 |
| Gastrointestinal symptoms,¶ grade 2 or 3 | 9.8 | 9.7 |
| Gastrointestinal symptoms,¶ grade 3 | 3.0 | 3.2 |

Td = Tetanus and Diphtheria Toxoids Adsorbed For Adult Use manufactured by Massachusetts Public Health Biologic Laboratories.
N = number of subjects in the total vaccinated cohort with local/general symptoms sheets completed.
Grade 2 = Local: painful when the limb was moved; General: interfered with normal activity.
Grade 3 = Local: spontaneously painful and/or prevented normal activity; General: prevented normal activity.
*Day of vaccination and the next 14 days.
†Statistically significantly higher (P<0.05) following BOOSTRIX as compared to Td vaccine.
‡Grade 3 injection site pain following BOOSTRIX was not inferior to Td (upper limit of two-sided 95% CI for the difference in the percentage of subjects ≤4%).
§Mid-upper region of the vaccinated arm.
‖Oral temperatures or axillary temperatures.
¶Gastrointestinal symptoms included nausea, vomiting, diarrhea and/or abdominal pain.

Mid-upper arm circumference was measured by the adolescent or their parent/guardian prior to injection and daily for 15 days following vaccination. There was no significant difference between BOOSTRIX recipients and Td recipients in the proportion of subjects reporting an increase in mid-upper arm circumference in the vaccinated arm. The incidence of unsolicited adverse events reported in the 31 days after vaccination was comparable between the 2 groups.

**Solicited Adverse Events in the German Safety Study:** No cases of whole arm swelling were spontaneously reported. Two individuals (2/193) reported large injection site swelling (range 110 to 200 mm diameter), in one case associated with grade 3 pain. Neither individual sought medical attention. These episodes were reported to resolve without sequelae within 5 days. These were the rates of solicited local adverse events and fever within 15 days of vaccination for those subjects who had previously been vaccinated with 5 doses of INFANRIX:

**Rates of Solicited Adverse Events Reported Within the 15-day* Post-Vaccination Period Following Administration of BOOSTRIX in Individuals 10 to 12 Years of Age Who Had Previously Received 5 Doses of INFANRIX**

| Adverse Event | BOOSTRIX (N = 193) % (95% CI) |
|---|---|
| Pain, any | 62.2 (54.9-69.0) |
| Pain, grade 2 or 3 | 33.2 (26.6-40.3) |
| Pain, grade 3 | 5.7 (2.9-10.0) |
| Redness, any | 47.7 (40.4-55.0) |
| Redness, >20 mm | 15.0 (10.3-20.9) |
| Redness, ≥50 mm | 10.9 (6.9-16.2) |
| Swelling, any | 38.9 (31.9-46.1) |
| Swelling, >20 mm | 17.6 (12.5-23.7) |
| Swelling, ≥50 mm | 14.0 (9.4-19.7) |
| Fever, ≥99.5 | 8.8 (5.2-13.7) |
| Fever, >100.4 | 4.1 (1.8-8.0) |
| Fever, >102.2 | 1.0 (0.1-3.7) |

N = number of subjects with local/general symptoms sheets completed.
Grade 2 = Painful when the limb was moved.
Grade 3 = Spontaneously painful and/or prevented normal activity.
*Day of vaccination and the next 14 days.

As with any vaccine, there is the possibility that broad use of BOOSTRIX could reveal adverse events not observed in clinical trials.

**Postmarketing Reports:** Worldwide voluntary reports of adverse events received for BOOSTRIX in persons 10 to 18 years of age since market introduction of this vaccine are listed below. This list includes serious events or events which have causal connection to components of this or other vaccines or drugs. Because these events are reported voluntarily from a population of uncertain size, it is not possible to reliably estimate their frequency or establish a causal relationship to vaccine exposure. *Blood and lymphatic system disorders:* Lymphadenitis, lymphadenopathy. *Cardiac disorders:* Myocarditis. *Injection site reactions:* Induration, inflammation, mass, nodule, warmth, local reaction. *Metabolism and nutrition disorders:* Diabetes mellitus insulin-dependent. *Musculoskeletal and connective tissue disorders:* Arthralgia, back pain, myalgia. *Nervous system disorders:* Convulsion, encephalitis, facial palsy, paraesthesia. *Skin and subcutaneous tissue disorders:* Exanthem, Henoch-Schönlein purpura, rash. In addition, extensive swelling of the injected limb has been reported following administration of BOOSTRIX.

**Reporting Adverse Events:** Report the occurrence following immunization of any event set forth in the Vaccine Injury Table from the National Childhood Vaccine Injury Act including: Anaphylaxis or anaphylactic shock within 7 days, encephalopathy or encephalitis within 7 days, brachial neuritis within 28 days, or an acute complication or sequelae (including death) of an illness, disability, injury, or condition referred to above, or any events that would contraindicate further doses of vaccine, according to this prescribing information. These events should be reported to VAERS. The VAERS toll-free number is 1-800-822-7967. Reporting forms may also be obtained at the VAERS website at www.vaers.hhs.gov.

**DOSAGE AND ADMINISTRATION: Recommended Dose:** BOOSTRIX should be administered as a single 0.5 mL injection by the intramuscular route into the deltoid muscle of the upper arm in individuals 10 through 18 years of age. Do not administer this product subcutaneously or intravenously. There are no data to support repeat administration of BOOSTRIX. Five years should elapse between the subject's last dose of the recommended series of childhood DTwP and/or DTaP vaccine and the administration of BOOSTRIX. Limited data are available on the use of BOOSTRIX following Tetanus and Diphtheria Toxoids Adsorbed For Adult Use (Td) vaccine. **Additional Dosing Information:** ***Wound Management:*** Clinicians should refer to guidelines for tetanus prophylaxis in routine wound management. Adolescents 10 to 18 years of age who have completed a primary series against tetanus and who sustain wounds which are minor and uncomplicated, should receive a booster dose of a tetanus toxoid-containing vaccine only if they have not received tetanus toxoid within the preceding 10 years. In case of tetanus-prone injury (e.g., wounds contaminated with dirt, feces, soil, and saliva; puncture wounds; avulsions; and wounds resulting from missles, crushing, burns, and frostbite) in an adolescent who is in need of tetanus toxoid, BOOSTRIX can be used as an alternative to Tetanus and Diphtheria Toxoids Adsorbed For Adult Use (Td) vaccine in patients for whom the pertussis component is also indicated (see INDICATIONS AND USAGE).

Manufactured by **GlaxoSmithKline Biologicals**
Rixensart, Belgium, US License 1617
Distributed by **GlaxoSmithKline**
Research Triangle Park, NC 27709



Full prescribing information for BOOSTRIX is available at www.BOOSTRIX.com.
BRS-BO:L3

**References: 1.** Centers for Disease Control and Prevention. Preventing tetanus, diphtheria, and pertussis among adolescents: use of tetanus toxoid, reduced diphtheria toxoid and acellular pertussis vaccines: recommendations of the Advisory Committee on Immunization Practices (ACIP). Early Release 2006;55(February 23, 2006):1–43. **2.** Centers for Disease Control and Prevention. Recommended childhood and adolescent immunization schedule—United States, 2006. *MMWR.* 2006;54(51&52):Q1–Q4.

# Cardiorespiratory Fitness Levels Among US Youth 12 to 19 Years of Age

## *Findings From the 1999-2002 National Health and Nutrition Examination Survey*

*Russell R. Pate, PhD; Chia-Yih Wang, PhD; Marsha Dowda, DrPH; Stephen W. Farrell, PhD; Jennifer R. O'Neill, MPH*

**Objectives:** To assess cardiorespiratory fitness levels in youth aged 12 to 19 years and to examine associations between fitness and age, sex, race/ethnicity, and self-reported physical activity in this age group.

**Design:** Cross-sectional study.

**Setting:** The National Health and Nutrition Examination Survey's mobile examination center, throughout the United States from 1999-2002.

**Participants:** A representative sample of 4732 youth aged 12 to 19 years was examined; 3287 completed the treadmill test and were included in the analysis. The National Center for Health Statistics conducted the survey.

**Main Exposures:** Age, sex, race/ethnicity, weight status, self-reported physical activity, and television viewing.

**Main Outcome Measure:** Estimated maximal oxygen uptake ($\dot{V}O_{2max}$) determined by a submaximal treadmill exercise test.

**Results:** Estimated $\dot{V}O_{2max}$ ($mL \cdot kg^{-1} \cdot min^{-1}$) was higher in males (mean ± SE, 46.4 ± 0.4) than in females (mean ± SE, 38.7 ± 0.3) but did not differ across race/ethnicity groups. Among males, older participants had higher $\dot{V}O_{2max}$ values, while in females, younger participants had higher values. For both males and females, those in the normal weight group had higher fitness levels than those in the at risk for overweight and overweight groups. Approximately one third of both males and females failed to meet recommended standards for cardiorespiratory fitness.

**Conclusions:** In US youth, cardiorespiratory fitness is lower in males and females who are overweight than in those of normal weight, but fitness is not related to race/ethnicity. Youth who have low levels of physical activity and high levels of sedentary behavior are also more likely to have lower cardiorespiratory fitness.

*Arch Pediatr Adolesc Med. 2006;160:1005-1012*

In children and adolescents, cardiorespiratory fitness is inversely associated with physiologic risk factors for chronic disease including high blood pressure,[1] hyperinsulinemia,[2] fat mass,[3] atherogenic lipid profile,[4] insulin resistance,[5] hemostatic and inflammatory markers,[6] and clustering of metabolic risk factors.[7] Also, higher levels of fitness support participation in sports and other physically demanding leisure activities. Attainment of fitness standards is a common prerequisite for entry into occupations such as law enforcement, firefighting, the military, and many other jobs that involve physically demanding labor.[8,9]

Between the 1950s and the 1980s, surveys of physical fitness were conducted regularly in the US population of children and adolescents.[10] During each of those 4 decades, the President's Council on Physical Fitness and Sports sponsored national surveys of youth physical fitness.[10,11] Also, in the 1980s, the National Children and Youth Fitness Study was conducted under the auspices of the US Department of Health and Human Services.[12,13] Both the National Children and Youth Fitness Study and the various President's Council on Physical Fitness and Sports surveys used field measures of physical fitness.[10,12,13] The 1966-1970 Health Examination Survey Cycle III included a treadmill exercise test for 12- to 17-year-olds to measure cardiorespiratory fitness.[14,15]

Obesity rates in US children and adolescents have increased dramatically since the 1980s,[16,17] and it seems likely that decreased physical activity is a major factor explaining that trend.[18,19] If contemporary American youth are fatter and less ac-

**Author Affiliations:**
Department of Exercise Science, Arnold School of Public Health, University of South Carolina, Columbia (Drs Pate and Dowda and Ms O'Neill); National Center for Health Statistics, Centers for Disease Control and Prevention, Hyattsville, Md (Dr Wang); and The Cooper Institute, Dallas, Tex (Dr Farrell).

**Table 1. Characteristics of Participants Aged 12 to 19 Years Examined at the NHANES MEC in 1999-2002**

| Characteristic | Examined in the MEC (n = 4732) Sample Size | % (SE)* | Study Sample (n = 3287) Sample Size | % (SE)* |
|---|---|---|---|---|
| Male | 2361 | 51.1 (0.9) | 1686 | 52.6 (1.5) |
| Race/ethnicity† | | | | |
| Non-Hispanic white | 1208 | 60.4 (2.1) | 826 | 59.5 (2.0) |
| Non-Hispanic black | 1398 | 14.4 (1.6) | 951 | 14.0 (1.6) |
| Mexican American | 1767 | 10.9 (1.4) | 1246 | 11.2 (1.4) |
| Age, y, mean | 4732 | 15.5 (0.1) | 3287 | 15.4 (0.1) |
| BMI, mean | 4642 | 23.2 (0.1) | 3287 | 23.0 (0.1) |
| Moderate physical activity, past 30 d (yes) | 4591 | 61.6 (1.1) | 3248 | 63.7 (1.3) |
| Vigorous physical activity, past 30 d (yes) | 4596 | 69.5 (1.1) | 3249 | 72.9 (1.2) |

Abbreviations: BMI, body mass index (calculated as weight in kilograms divided by height in meters squared); MEC, mobile examination center; NHANES, National Health and Nutrition Examination Surveys.

*Unless otherwise indicated.

†No separate estimates were presented for persons classified as "other," but they are included in the total population estimates.

tive than previous generations, it is possible that physical fitness has also declined in this population. A key component of overall physical fitness is cardiorespiratory endurance.[19] Between 1999 and 2002, the National Health and Nutrition Examination Surveys (NHANES) included a measure of cardiorespiratory fitness, which was administered to participants between ages 12 and 49 years. The purpose of this article is to present findings of NHANES for youth between ages 12 and 19 years. Associations between cardiorespiratory fitness and demographic characteristics will be reported as well as associations with select self-reported physical activity behaviors.

## METHODS

### SURVEY DESIGN AND STUDY POPULATION

The NHANES is designed to monitor the health and nutritional status of the US civilian, noninstitutionalized population. The surveys are conducted by the National Center for Health Statistics of the Centers for Disease Control and Prevention.[20] Since 1999, a nationally representative sample has been selected annually using a stratified multistage probability cluster sample design. Data are released in 2-year periods (eg, 1999-2000, 2001-2002). Mexican American and black individuals, adolescents aged 12 to 19 years, persons 60 years and older, low-income white individuals, and pregnant women were oversampled in 1999-2002 to allow for more precise estimates for these groups. This report is based on data from the 1999-2002 NHANES.[21,22] The 1999-2002 NHANES protocol was approved by the National Center for Health Statistics institutional review board, and written informed consent was obtained from all participants 18 years and older. In addition to the consent provided by parents or guardians, written informed assent was also obtained for adolescents younger than 18 years.

### SUBJECTS

The NHANES protocol consists of a household interview followed by an examination at a mobile examination center. In 1999-2002, 4902 individuals aged 12 to 19 years were interviewed at home, and of these, 4732 individuals (97%) were examined at the mobile examination center. Of those, 522 (11%) were excluded from the fitness test for a variety of reasons, including pregnancy, physical limitations, and cardiovascular and asthma conditions or symptoms.[23] Of those eligible to participate in the fitness test, 923 (20%) did not have their fitness level estimated for a variety of reasons, including insufficient time to conduct the test, refusal, equipment problems, prematurely terminated tests because of safety concerns, and insufficient heart rate response to classify fitness level (ie, the change in heart rate between the 2 exercise stages was less than 8 beats/min). Complete fitness data on 3287 individuals (69%) are included in the present analyses. Sex, race/ethnicity, age, body mass index (BMI) (calculated as weight in kilograms divided by height in meters squared), and activity levels of this analytic sample were comparable with the overall sample that was examined in the mobile examination center (**Table 1**).

### CARDIORESPIRATORY FITNESS TEST

Cardiorespiratory fitness was assessed by a submaximal treadmill exercise test. The treadmill test consisted of a 2-minute warm-up, followed by two 3-minute work stages, and a 2-minute cooldown period. Blood pressure, rating of perceived exertion,[24] and heart rate were obtained during each of the stages. The Jackson nonexercise test formula was used to predict each participant's fitness level prior to the treadmill test, based on his or her age, sex, BMI, and self-reported physical activity level.[25] From this prediction, 1 of the 8 protocols was selected for each participant.[23] The goal of the test was to elicit a heart rate that is approximately 80% of age-predicted maximum (220 − age) by the end of the second exercise stage.[23]

The main outcome of the cardiorespiratory fitness test is estimated maximal oxygen uptake ($\dot{V}O_{2max}$). It was estimated by extrapolation to an expected age-specific maximal heart rate using measured heart rate responses to the two 3-minute exercise stages.[26] It was assumed that the relationship between heart rate and oxygen consumption is linear during treadmill exercise. Because true $\dot{V}O_{2max}$ values greater than 75 $mL \cdot kg^{-1} \cdot min^{-1}$ are quite rare, we assumed such values to be overestimates and they were coded as 75 $mL \cdot kg^{-1} \cdot min^{-1}$ in the analysis (n=29). Equipment included a Quinton MedTrack ST65 Treadmill (Quinton, Deerfield, Wis) and a Colin STBP-780 Automatic Blood Pressure Monitor (Colin Medical Instruments Corp, San Antonio, Tex) to measure heart rate and blood pressure. All technicians were trained by exercise physiologists from the Cooper Institute, were monitored twice a year, and participated in an annual retraining session to assure quality control.

## COVARIATES

### Demographic Variables

Participants were placed in 4 age groups: 12 to 13, 14 to 15, 16 to 17, and 18 to 19 years of age. Self-reported information on race and ethnicity was categorized as non-Hispanic white, non-Hispanic black, Mexican American, and other. Because of the small sample size of the "other" group, no separate estimates were presented for persons classified as "other," but they are included in the total population estimates. Measured weight and height were used to calculate BMI. The 2000 Centers for Disease Control and Prevention Growth Charts for the United States were used to define normal weight, at risk for overweight, and overweight.[27] Normal weight is defined as less than the 85th percentile of BMI for age, at risk for overweight is defined as at or higher than the 85th percentile but less than the 95th percentile of BMI for age, and overweight is defined as at or higher than the 95th percentile of BMI for age.

### Physical Activity Variables

Self-reported physical activity variables were dichotomized into yes or no for activities performed during the last 30 days. The activities included walking or biking as part of getting to and from work, school, or errands; moderate-intensity physical activities performed for at least 10 minutes that cause light sweating or slight to moderate increase in breathing or heart rate; vigorous-intensity physical activities performed for at least 10 minutes that cause heavy sweating or large increases in breathing or heart rate; and physical activities specifically designed to strengthen muscles, such as lifting weights, push-ups, or sit-ups. Additionally, participants were asked if their amount of activity during the past 30 days was more, less, or about the same as others of the same age and sex.

Sedentary activity questions differed by age group. Participants aged 16 to 19 years reported the amount of time on a typical day during the past 30 days that they spent sitting and watching television or videos or using a computer outside of work. Children aged 12 to 15 years were asked about television viewing and computer use/computer games separately, in reference to the previous day. The 2 questions were summed. Responses were dichotomized into fewer than 3 hours and 3 or more hours per day.

Participants were also asked to identify the type, frequency, and duration of moderate and vigorous physical activities they participated in during the past 30 days. All reported activities were assigned a MET (metabolic equivalent unit) (1 MET = 3.5 mL $O_2 \cdot kg^{-1} \cdot min^{-1}$) value based on reported intensity.[28] The number of times an activity was performed was multiplied by the number of minutes and the MET value. The total MET score was then divided by 30 to obtain MET minutes per day for each reported activity. To correct for gross errors, reported frequency and duration higher than the 99th percentile (90 times per 30 days and 240 minutes each time, respectively) were coded to 90 and 240, respectively, for the analysis. MET minutes of moderate to vigorous physical activity (MVPA) were calculated by totaling activities with a MET value of 3 or more. MET minutes of vigorous physical activity (VPA) were calculated by totaling the activities with a MET value of 6 or more. Participants received a score of zero if they did not report any individual activity and responded no to participation in moderate physical activity or VPA during the past 30 days (n=503 [15.3%] for MVPA; n=824 [25.1%] for VPA). Participants were categorized into tertiles (low, intermediate, high) of MVPA and VPA for analyses.

Participants were classified into 2 fitness levels based on the FITNESSGRAM Standards for Healthy Fitness Zone.[29,30] Males aged 12 to 19 years with a $\dot{V}O_{2max}$ of 42 $mL \cdot kg^{-1} \cdot min^{-1}$ or higher were classified as meeting the FITNESSGRAM standards. Girls aged 12 and 13 years with a $\dot{V}O_{2max}$ of 37 and 36 $mL \cdot kg^{-1} \cdot min^{-1}$, respectively, were classified as meeting the FITNESSGRAM standards. Females aged 14 to 19 with a $\dot{V}O_{2max}$ of 35 $mL \cdot kg^{-1} \cdot min^{-1}$ or higher were classified as meeting the FITNESSGRAM standards.

## STATISTICAL ANALYSES

All analyses were conducted separately for males and females. Means and deciles of estimated $\dot{V}O_{2max}$ were calculated for 4 age groups. One-way analyses of variance using estimated $\dot{V}O_{2max}$ as the dependent variable were conducted for demographic, weight status, and physical activity variables and by tertiles of MET minutes of physical activity. The trends of $\dot{V}O_{2max}$ by tertiles of MET minutes of MVPA and VPA were also tested. Sample weights were used to account for differential probabilities of selection, noncoverage, and nonresponse to the examination.[31] Standard errors were calculated using the Taylor series linearization method. Statistical significance was defined as $\alpha = .05$. Paired comparisons were done within each category when the testing for analysis of variance was significant. The Bonferroni method was used to adjust for multiple comparisons. Thus, for age group comparisons, $\alpha = .008$ was used and for weight status, MVPA, and VPA, $\alpha = .017$ was used for significance level. All statistical analyses were conducted using SAS for Windows[32] and SUDAAN.[33]

## RESULTS

Percentiles for estimated $\dot{V}O_{2max}$ are presented in **Table 2** by sex and age group. Generally, among males, older participants had higher $\dot{V}O_{2max}$ values, while in females, younger participants had higher values.

Estimated $\dot{V}O_{2max}$ is presented by demographic groups, weight status, and FITNESSGRAM categories in **Table 3**. Estimated $\dot{V}O_{2max}$ was higher in males than females. In males, estimated $\dot{V}O_{2max}$ was significantly lower in 12- and 13-year-olds than in the other age groups. Males in the normal weight group had significantly higher estimated $\dot{V}O_{2max}$ than those in the at risk for overweight and overweight groups, and a higher percentage of older males (aged 14-19 years) than younger males (aged 12-13 years) met the FITNESSGRAM standards. In females, estimated $\dot{V}O_{2max}$ was significantly lower in older females (aged 18-19 years) than in younger females (aged 12-13 years). Females in the normal weight group had higher estimated $\dot{V}O_{2max}$ than the females in the at risk for overweight and overweight groups. There were no differences among the age groups for females meeting the FITNESSGRAM standards.

**Table 4** shows the comparison of the estimated $\dot{V}O_{2max}$ among physical activity variable categories. Males who commuted through walking or biking, participated in VPA, or did strengthening exercise during the past 30 days were fitter than males who did not report these activities. Females who reported walking or biking during the past 30 days were more fit than females who did not report walking or biking. Males and females who reported fewer than 3 hours of television, video, or computer use per day had higher fitness levels compared with those who participated in 3 or more hours. Those who considered themselves to be more active than their peers

**Table 2. Deciles of Estimated $\dot{V}O_{2max}$ by Sex and Age Groups**

| | Sample Size | Decile, Mean $\dot{V}O_{2max}$ (95% Confidence Interval), mL · kg⁻¹ · min⁻¹ | | | | | | | | |
|---|---|---|---|---|---|---|---|---|---|---|
| | | 10th | 20th | 30th | 40th | 50th | 60th | 70th | 80th | 90th |
| Males | | | | | | | | | | |
| Ages 12-13 y | 393 | 34.7 (33.6-36.1) | 37.3 (36.2-38.9) | 39.0 (38.3-40.3) | 41.0 (39.5-42.2) | 43.0 (42.1-44.5) | 45.0 (44.1-46.9) | 47.3 (46.2-50.2) | 51.5 (49.5-55.3) | 56.2 (53.5-60.2) |
| Ages 14-15 y | 424 | 38.1 (36.8-39.4) | 40.0 (39.5-41.0) | 41.9 (40.3-43.6) | 43.8 (42.6-45.0) | 45.8 (44.2-48.1) | 48.2 (46.6-49.3) | 50.2 (48.5-51.5) | 52.5 (51.3-54.4) | 58.8 (54.9-61.7) |
| Ages 16-17 y | 486 | 36.4 (35.0-37.8) | 38.9 (38.2-41.0) | 42.0 (41.0-43.5) | 44.4 (42.8-45.9) | 46.2 (45.1-47.3) | 47.9 (46.5-49.4) | 50.2 (48.8-51.9) | 53.8 (51.5-55.4) | 58.3 (56.8-60.5) |
| Ages 18-19 y | 383 | 37.6 (36.7-39.0) | 40.3 (39.2-41.3) | 43.0 (40.9-43.9) | 44.4 (43.9-45.4) | 46.3 (45.2-47.6) | 48.7 (47.1-50.5) | 50.8 (49.4-52.7) | 53.7 (51.9-55.6) | 58.4 (55.3-63.3) |
| Females | | | | | | | | | | |
| Ages 12-13 y | 465 | 31.0 (30.5-32.4) | 33.2 (32.5-34.9) | 35.8 (34.8-36.7) | 37.2 (36.4-38.5) | 39.3 (37.8-39.9) | 40.4 (39.6-42.6) | 43.2 (41.3-44.6) | 45.1 (43.6-46.7) | 48.4 (45.8-51.6) |
| Ages 14-15 y | 434 | 30.6 (29.8-31.4) | 32.1 (31.7-33.1) | 34.5 (33.0-35.6) | 36.2 (35.2-37.1) | 38.0 (37.2-38.4) | 38.9 (38.3-39.9) | 40.5 (39.3-41.7) | 43.2 (41.3-43.9) | 47.2 (44.2-49.1) |
| Ages 16-17 y | 379 | 30.5 (29.6-32.0) | 32.8 (32.0-34.2) | 34.5 (33.5-36.0) | 36.1 (35.1-37.3) | 37.6 (36.5-38.8) | 39.4 (38.1-40.5) | 41.4 (40.2-42.8) | 44.2 (42.4-45.6) | 48.8 (45.3-53.4) |
| Ages 18-19 y | 323 | 28.9 (28.2-30.1) | 31.0 (29.6-32.8) | 33.5 (31.5-35.4) | 35.4 (33.8-36.4) | 36.7 (35.7-37.8) | 38.3 (37.0-39.4) | 39.6 (38.9-40.6) | 41.9 (40.0-44.4) | 47.2 (44.0-52.5) |

Abbreviation: $\dot{V}O_{2max}$, maximal oxygen uptake.

**Table 3. Estimated $\dot{V}O_{2max}$ by Age, Race/Ethnicity, Weight Status, and Percentage Meeting Fitness Standards for Males and Females Aged 12 to 19 Years**

| Variables | Males: Sample Size | Males: $\dot{V}O_{2max}$, Mean (SE), mL · kg⁻¹ · min⁻¹ | Males: *P* Value* | Females: Sample Size | Females: $\dot{V}O_{2max}$, Mean (SE), mL · kg⁻¹ · min⁻¹ | Females: *P* Value* |
|---|---|---|---|---|---|---|
| Total† | 1686 | 46.6 (0.4) | | 1601 | 38.7 (0.3) | |
| Age, y | | | | | | |
| 12-13 | 393 | 44.6 (0.7) | .001 | 465 | 39.7 (0.5) | .02 |
| 14-15 | 424 | 47.1 (0.6) | | 434 | 38.3 (0.4) | |
| 16-17 | 486 | 46.9 (0.6) | | 379 | 38.9 (0.6) | |
| 18-19 | 383 | 47.6 (0.6) | | 323 | 37.5 (0.6) | |
| Race/ethnicity‡ | | | | | | |
| Non-Hispanic white | 436 | 46.7 (0.6) | .27 | 390 | 39.0 (0.4) | .15 |
| Non-Hispanic black | 486 | 46.9 (0.5) | | 465 | 37.9 (0.4) | |
| Mexican American | 635 | 46.1 (0.5) | | 611 | 39.3 (0.6) | |
| Weight status§ | | | | | | |
| Normal weight | 1141 | 48.2 (0.5) | <.001 | 1010 | 39.6 (0.3) | <.001 |
| At risk for overweight | 249 | 43.5 (0.6) | | 278 | 37.6 (0.7) | |
| Overweight | 296 | 41.6 (1.0) | | 313 | 35.9 (0.6) | |
| Percentage meeting fitness standards‖ | Yes/Total No. | % (SE) | | Yes/Total No. | % (SE) | |
| Ages 12-13 y | 232/393 | 55.3 (2.5) | <.001 | 284/465 | 64.1 (3.1) | .82 |
| Ages 14-15 y | 287/424 | 70.0 (3.6) | | 297/434 | 66.6 (2.9) | |
| Ages 16-17 y | 330/486 | 70.1 (2.7) | | 256/379 | 67.9 (3.8) | |
| Ages 18-19 y | 256/383 | 71.7 (2.9) | | 189/323 | 62.3 (4.6) | |

Abbreviations: BMI, body mass index (calculated as weight in kilograms divided by height in meters squared); $\dot{V}O_{2max}$, maximal oxygen uptake.
**P* values refer to sex-specific comparisons within each age, race/ethnicity, weight status, or fitness standard groups using 1-way analysis of variance.
†Males>females; *P*<.001.
‡No separate estimates were presented for persons classified as "other," but they are included in the total population estimates.
§The 2000 Centers for Disease Control and Prevention Growth Charts were used to define normal weight, at risk for overweight, and overweight as follows: less than 85th percentile of BMI for age = normal weight; 85th to less than 95th percentile of BMI for age = at risk for overweight; 95th percentile or higher of BMI for age = overweight.
‖FITNESSGRAM Standards for Healthy Fitness Zone.[29,30]

were more fit than those who considered themselves to be less active or about the same as others. For both males and females, there was a statistically significant positive trend for higher levels of fitness with increasing tertiles of both MVPA and VPA.

## COMMENT

The NHANES is conducted in nationally representative samples of American youth, and in the 1999-2002 survey cycle, the protocol included a submaximal tread-

**Table 4. Estimated $\dot{V}O_{2max}$ by Physical Activity Categories for Males and Females Aged 12 to 19 Years**

| | Males | | | Females | | |
|---|---|---|---|---|---|---|
| Variables | Sample Size | $\dot{V}O_{2max}$, Mean (SE), $mL \cdot kg^{-1} \cdot min^{-1}$ | *P* Value | Sample Size | $\dot{V}O_{2max}$, Mean (SE), $mL \cdot kg^{-1} \cdot min^{-1}$ | *P* Value |
| Commuted by walking/biking, past 30 d | | | | | | |
| Yes | 816 | 47.6 (0.5) | .005* | 742 | 39.3 (0.4) | .05* |
| No | 848 | 45.7 (0.5) | | 842 | 38.2 (0.3) | |
| Moderate physical activity, past 30 d | | | | | | |
| Yes | 938 | 46.7 (0.6) | .61* | 953 | 38.8 (0.4) | .42* |
| No | 726 | 46.4 (0.5) | | 631 | 38.3 (0.4) | |
| VPA, past 30 d | | | | | | |
| Yes | 1282 | 47.1 (0.5) | .001* | 959 | 39.0 (0.4) | .06* |
| No | 383 | 44.7 (0.6) | | 625 | 37.9 (0.3) | |
| Strength exercise, past 30 d | | | | | | |
| Yes | 1146 | 47.1 (0.5) | .04* | 825 | 39.2 (0.4) | .08* |
| No | 518 | 45.4 (0.7) | | 758 | 38.1 (0.4) | |
| Television/video/computer use, h/d | | | | | | |
| <3 | 751 | 47.4 (0.7) | .04* | 775 | 39.5 (0.3) | .005* |
| ≥3 | 914 | 45.8 (0.4) | | 808 | 37.8 (0.5) | |
| Compared with others | | | | | | |
| More active | 567 | 49.2 (0.5) | <.001* | 429 | 40.1 (0.4) | <.001* |
| About the same | 938 | 45.7 (0.5) | | 866 | 38.6 (0.4) | |
| Less active | 158 | 41.9 (1.3) | | 289 | 36.5 (0.6) | |
| Tertiles of MET-min/d MVPA activities† | | | | | | |
| Low | 555 | 44.3 (0.5) | <.001‡ | 529 | 37.6 (0.4) | .002‡ |
| Intermediate | 557 | 46.6 (0.7) | | 527 | 38.4 (0.6) | |
| High | 553 | 48.6 (0.4) | | 528 | 39.7 (0.4) | |
| Tertiles of MET-min/d VPA activities§ | | | | | | |
| Low | 555 | 44.4 (0.7) | <.001‡ | 527 | 38.1 (0.4) | .008‡ |
| Intermediate | 555 | 46.9 (0.5) | | 530 | 37.9 (0.5) | |
| High | 555 | 48.3 (0.6) | | 527 | 39.8 (0.4) | |

Abbreviations: MET, metabolic equivalent unit; MVPA, moderate to vigorous activity; $\dot{V}O_{2max}$, maximal oxygen uptake; VPA, vigorous physical activity.
**P* values refer to sex-specific comparisons within each activity category using 1-way analysis of variance.
†For females, low = 0 to 48, intermediate = 49 to 247.5, and high = 248 to 10573 MET-min/d. For males, low = 0 to 139, intermediate = 139.2 to 510, and high = 510.5 to 8904 MET-min/d.
‡*P* values refer to sex-specific trend testing within each activity category.
§For females, low = 0 to 3.7, intermediate = 4 to 168, and high = 170 to 10373.5 MET-min/d. For males, low = 0 to 86.7, intermediate = 89 to 417, and high = 420 to 8904 MET-min/d.

mill exercise test. An accepted criterion measure of cardiorespiratory fitness is maximal oxygen consumption, $\dot{V}O_{2max}$, measured by gas exchange during performance of exhaustive exercise. The submaximal treadmill test used in NHANES involves applying the slope of the heart rate response to submaximal exercise in estimating $\dot{V}O_{2max}$, a procedure that has been well validated.[34] As such, the data presented in this report provide a valid characterization of the cardiorespiratory fitness levels of contemporary American youth. This information is important because it provides a basis for monitoring future trends in physical fitness in the population of 12- to 19-year-old youth in the United States. In addition, these data provide population norms against which individuals and groups of youth can be compared.

National population-based surveys in the United States have monitored body weight status in youth since 1963.[35] Recent surveys have demonstrated a marked increase in the prevalence of obesity in young people.[17,36,37] In addition, many have suggested that physical fitness has declined in American youth during this same period.[38] Physical fitness was surveyed in representative samples of American youth on several occasions between the late 1950s and mid 1980s.[10,12,13] Unfortunately, the procedures used to measure physical fitness varied from survey to survey, and none of the previous national surveys used controlled testing procedures such as those used in the present survey. Consequently, it is not possible to determine whether there have been population-level changes in fitness in American youth during the past several decades. However, the present study includes some information that may bear on this issue. As shown by the data in Table 3, weight status was associated with fitness, with overweight and at-risk-for-overweight males and females showing lower cardiorespiratory fitness than their normal-weight peers. This suggests that population-level increases in the prevalence of obesity are likely to be associated with decreased cardiorespiratory fitness. This would be expected when fitness is measured with a weight-bearing task such as treadmill walking or running, because greater weight requires more energy to be expended at any specified speed of movement. Nonetheless, a clear demonstration of a secular decline in physical fitness in American youth must await the result of future surveys using methods comparable with those used in this and/or earlier surveys.

One method for interpreting physical fitness levels of youth is to apply criterion-referenced standards that are linked to functional and/or health outcomes. Such an approach is used by FITNESSGRAM, a fitness testing program that has been used by more than 18 000 schools and school districts nationally. The criterion-referenced standards used by FITNESSGRAM were developed by an expert panel, and for cardiorespiratory fitness, the standards for maximal oxygen uptakes are 42 $mL \cdot kg^{-1} \cdot min^{-1}$ for males and 35 to 37 $mL \cdot kg^{-1} \cdot min^{-1}$ (depending on age) for females.[29] When these standards are applied to the group measured in this study, approximately 65% of both males and females meet the standards. This indicates that roughly one third of US youth aged 12 to 19 years fail to meet the levels of cardiorespiratory fitness deemed appropriate by experts.

The findings presented in this report confirm the frequently observed sex difference in cardiorespiratory endurance. Mean estimated $\dot{V}O_{2max}$ was approximately 17% lower in girls than boys in the overall sample, and the sex difference increased with increasing age from about 11% in 12- and 13-year-olds to more than 21% in 18- and 19-year-olds. These differences are comparable with those reported in previous surveys.[14,39] The widening sex difference with increasing age was due to countervailing age-related differences in the 2 sexes. Fitness increased with age in males but decreased with age in females, and these changes were statistically significant in both sexes. This may be explained by physical developmental factors, such as sex-related changes in lean weight and fat weight during puberty.[40] However, some studies have shown that the sex difference in physical activity levels widens during adolescence, so it may be that rapidly declining physical activity in females may partially explain the age-related trends in physical fitness.[41,42]

In this study, fitness did not differ across the 3 race/ethnicity groups observed. Most previous national surveys of fitness in children and youth did not report data for race/ethnicity subgroups.[10,12,13] However, 1 national survey in the 1960s did find higher cardiorespiratory fitness in black youth than white youth.[14] That observation is inconsistent with the findings of most studies using smaller samples that were not nationally representative. Several of these studies have observed higher fitness in white than black adolescents.[2,43] The present study is unique because the sampling protocol ensured that nationally representative samples of non-Hispanic white, non-Hispanic black, and Mexican American males and females were included. The findings provide no indication that cardiorespiratory fitness varied across those 3 population subgroups in 1999-2002.

In general, youth who reported higher levels of physical activity had higher levels of cardiorespiratory fitness. Those who reported participating in VPA during the past 30 days and those who were in the upper tertile of MET minutes per day of MVPA and VPA were more fit than other participants. Although these findings suggest that higher levels of physical activity result in higher levels of fitness, the data are cross-sectional and the direction of causality cannot be determined. It may be that young people who have higher cardiorespiratory fitness find it easier or more enjoyable to participate in physical activity. The only exception to the activity-fitness pattern was for moderate physical activity in the past 30 days; those who reported participating in moderate physical activity during the past 30 days did not have higher fitness levels than those who did not report such activity. This may be due to inaccuracies in the classification and reporting of moderate activity by children and youth or to the fact that VPA explains more of the variance in fitness than moderate activity.[44] In addition to a positive relationship between physical activity and fitness, we also observed a negative relationship between sedentary activity and fitness. Participants who reported 3 or more hours per day of television, video, and computer use had lower levels of fitness than those who reported less than 3 hours of these activities. This finding differs from previous studies that found no significant relationship between television watching and fitness.[45,46] The inclusion of other electronic media, in addition to television, in the present study may provide a more accurate estimate of the amount of time that children and youth spend in sedentary activity.

The findings of this study suggest that one third of youth aged 12 to 19 years in the United States has low levels of cardiorespiratory fitness. Low cardiorespiratory fitness, a strong and independent risk factor for cardiovascular disease,[47,48] is known to track from adolescence to adulthood.[49,50] Further, it has been shown that low cardiorespiratory fitness in adolescence predicts adult body fatness,[51] large-artery stiffness,[52] poor lipid profiles,[53,54] and low physical activity levels.[55] Accordingly, because highly active youth tend to manifest higher levels of cardiorespiratory fitness, several expert panels have recommended that physicians counsel pediatric and adolescent patients and their parents about the importance of meeting current physical activity guidelines.[19,56,57] Identifying youth who are at elevated risk for low cardiovascular fitness is important because fitness testing is impractical in most clinical settings. The findings of this study suggest that youth who have high BMI, low levels of physical activity, and high levels of sedentary behavior are likely to have low cardiorespiratory fitness.

Strengths of this study include the large sample size, the racial and ethnic diversity of the participants, and the use of a standardized testing protocol. The use of a submaximal exercise test for estimating $\dot{V}O_{2max}$ is a potential weakness of this study, because submaximal tests are less accurate than maximal exercise tests. However, maximal exercise tests are considered impractical for use in population-based studies. Another potential limitation is the response rate of 69%; however, as demonstrated in Table 1, youth included in our study sample were demographically comparable with the total sample examined in the mobile examination center.

## CONCLUSIONS

In conclusion, estimated $\dot{V}O_{2max}$ ($mL \cdot kg^{-1} \cdot min^{-1}$) was higher in males than females and lower in overweight than normal weight youth but not different across the 3 race/ethnic groups observed (non-Hispanic black, Mexican American, non-Hispanic white). More physically active youth tended to manifest higher fitness levels than those reporting less activity. Approximately one third of males and females aged 12 to 19 years failed to meet current standards for acceptable cardiorespiratory endurance. This represents a significant public health problem because low physical fitness during adolescence tends to track into adulthood, and low-fit adults are at substantially increased risk for chronic disease morbidity and mortality.

**Accepted for Publication:** May 26, 2006.
**Correspondence:** Russell R. Pate, PhD, Department of Exercise Science, University of South Carolina, 921 Assembly St, Columbia, SC 29208 (rpate@gwm.sc.edu).
**Author Contributions:** Dr Pate had full access to all the data in the study and takes responsibility for the integrity of the data and the accuracy of the data analysis. *Study concept and design:* Pate, Wang, Dowda, and O'Neill. *Acquisition of data:* Wang, Dowda, and Farrell. *Analysis and interpretation of data:* Pate, Wang, Dowda, Farrell, and O'Neill. *Drafting of the manuscript:* Pate, Wang, Dowda, Farrell, and O'Neill. *Critical revision of the manuscript for important intellectual content:* Wang, Dowda, and O'Neill. *Statistical analysis:* Wang and Dowda. *Administrative, technical, and material support:* Farrell and O'Neill. *Study supervision:* Pate and Farrell.
**Funding/Support:** This study was funded by grant 5R01HL057775 from the National Heart, Lung, and Blood Institute (Dr Pate) and grant 5R01HD043125 from the National Institute of Child Health and Human Development (Dr Pate).
**Acknowledgment:** We thank Gaye Groover Christmus, MPH, and Felipe Lobelo, MD, for assistance in the development of this article.

## REFERENCES


1. Sallis JF, Patterson TL, Buono MJ, Nader PR. Relation of cardiovascular fitness and physical activity to cardiovascular disease risk factors in children and adults. *Am J Epidemiol.* 1988;127:933-941.
2. Gutin B, Yin Z, Humphries MC, Hoffman WH, Gower B, Barbeau P. Relations of fatness and fitness to fasting insulin in black and white adolescents. *J Pediatr.* 2004;145:737-743.
3. Ball GD, Shaibi GQ, Cruz ML, Watkins MP, Weigensberg MJ, Goran MI. Insulin sensitivity, cardiorespiratory fitness, and physical activity in overweight Hispanic youth. *Obes Res.* 2004;12:77-85.
4. Gutin B, Islam S, Manos T, Cucuzzo N, Smith C, Stachura ME. Relation of percentage of body fat and maximal aerobic capacity to risk factors for atherosclerosis and diabetes in black and white seven- to eleven-year-old children. *J Pediatr.* 1994;125:847-852.
5. Kasa-Vubu JZ, Lee CC, Rosenthal A, Singer K, Halter JB. Cardiovascular fitness and exercise as determinants of insulin resistance in postpubertal adolescent females. *J Clin Endocrinol Metab.* 2005;90:849-854.
6. Barbeau P, Litaker MS, Woods KF, et al. Hemostatic and inflammatory markers in obese youths: effects of exercise and adiposity. *J Pediatr.* 2002;141:415-420.
7. Brage S, Wedderkopp N, Ekelund U, et al. Features of the metabolic syndrome are associated with objectively measured physical activity and fitness in Danish children: the European Youth Heart Study (EYHS). *Diabetes Care.* 2004;27:2141-2148.
8. Knapik J. The Army Physical Fitness Test (APFT): a review of the literature. *Mil Med.* 1989;154:326-329.
9. National Fire Protection Association. *Standard on Health-Related Fitness Programs for Fire Fighters.* Quincy, Mass: NFPA; 2000.
10. Reiff GG, Dixon W, Jacoby D, Ye G, Spain CG, Hunsicker P. *The President's Council on Physical Fitness and Sports National School Population Fitness Survey.* Ann Arbor: University of Michigan; 1986.
11. President's Council on Physical Fitness and Sports. President's Council history. http://www.fitness.gov/about_history.htm. Accessed June 28, 2005.
12. US Department of Health and Human Services. National Children and Youth Fitness Study. *J Physical Educ Recreation Dance.* 1985;56:44-90.
13. US Department of Health and Human Services. National Children and Youth Fitness Study. *J Physical Educ Recreation Dance.* 1987;58:50-96.
14. Gillum RF. The relationship of treadmill test performance to blood pressure and other cardiovascular risk factors in adolescents. *Am Heart J.* 1989;118:161-171.
15. McDowell A. Cardiovascular endurance, strength, and lung function tests in the NCHS National Health and Nutrition Surveys. In: Drury T, ed. *Assessing Physical Fitness and Activity Patterns in General Populations Surveys.* Hyattsville, Md: National Center for Health Statistics; 1989:21-35.
16. Jolliffe D. Extent of overweight among US children and adolescents from 1971 to 2000. *Int J Obes Relat Metab Disord.* 2004;28:4-9.
17. Strauss RS, Pollack HA. Epidemic increase in childhood overweight, 1986-1998. *JAMA.* 2001;286:2845-2848.
18. US Department of Health and Human Services. *Healthy People 2010.* 2nd ed. Washington, DC: US Government Printing Office; 2000.
19. US Department of Health and Human Services. *Physical Activity and Health: A Report of the Surgeon General.* Atlanta, Ga: US Dept of Health and Human Services, Centers for Disease Control and Prevention; 1996.
20. Centers for Disease Control and Prevention; National Center for Health Statistics. *National Health and Nutrition Examination Surveys.* Hyattsville, Md: US Dept of Health and Human Services, Centers for Disease Control and Prevention. www.cdc.gov/nchs/nhanes.htm. Accessed June 1, 2005.
21. Centers for Disease Control and Prevention; National Center for Health Statistics. *National Health and Nutrition Examination Survey 1999-2000 Data.* Hyattsville, Md: US Dept of Health and Human Services, Centers for Disease Control and Prevention; 2004. http://www.cdc.gov/nchs/about/major/nhanes/nhanes99_00.htm. Accessed May 13, 2005.
22. Centers for Disease Control and Prevention; National Center for Health Statistics. *National Health and Nutrition Examination Survey 2001-2002 Data.* Hyattsville, Md: US Dept of Health and Human Services, Centers for Disease Control and Prevention; 2004. http://www.cdc.gov/nchs/about/major/nhanes/nhanes01-02.htm. Accessed June 23, 2005.
23. Centers for Disease Control and Prevention; National Center for Health Statistics. *National Health and Nutrition Examination Cardiovascular Fitness Procedures Manual.* Hyattsville, Md: US Dept of Health and Human Services, Centers for Disease Control and Prevention; 2004.
24. Borg GA. Psychophysical bases of perceived exertion. *Med Sci Sports Exerc.* 1982;14:377-381.
25. Jackson AS, Blair SN, Mahar MT, Wier LT, Ross RM, Stuteville JE. Prediction of functional aerobic capacity without exercise testing. *Med Sci Sports Exerc.* 1990;22:863-870.
26. American College of Sports Medicine. *ACSM's Guidelines for Exercise Testing and Prescription.* 7th ed. Philadelphia, Pa: Lippincott Williams & Wilkins; 2005.
27. Kuczmarski RJ, Ogden CL, Grummer-Strawn LM, et al. CDC Growth Charts: United States. *Adv Data.* 2000;314:1-27.
28. Centers for Disease Control and Prevention; National Center for Health Statistics. *NHANES 2001-2002 Data Documentation: Physical Activity Individual Activities File.* Hyattsville, Md: US Dept of Health and Human Services, Centers for Disease Control and Prevention; 2004. http://www.cdc.gov. Accessed June 1, 2005.
29. Cureton KJ, Warren GL. Criterion-referenced standards for youth health-related fitness tests: a tutorial. *Res Q Exerc Sport.* 1990;61:7-19.
30. The Cooper Institute. *FITNESSGRAM Test Administration Manual.* 3rd ed. Champaign, Ill: Human Kinetics; 2004.
31. Centers for Disease Control and Prevention; National Center for Health Statistics. *NHANES Analytic Guidelines.* Hyattsville, Md: US Dept of Health and Human Services, Centers for Disease Control and Prevention; 2004. http://www.cdc.gov. Accessed June 1, 2005.
32. SAS Online DOC. *Version 8 With PDF Files.* Cary, NC: SAS Institute; 2000.
33. Research Triangle Institute. *SUDAAN Language Manual, Release 9.0.* Research Triangle Park, NC: Research Triangle Institute; 2004.
34. Astrand PO, Rhyming I. A nomogram for calculation of aerobic capacity (physical fitness) from pulse rate during submaximal work. *J Appl Physiol.* 1954;7:218-221.
35. Plan, operation, and response results of a program of children's examinations. *Vital Health Stat 1.* 1967;(5):1-56.
36. Troiano RP, Flegal KM, Kuczmarski RJ, Campbell SM, Johnson CL. Overweight prevalence and trends for children and adolescents: the National Health and Nutrition Examination Surveys, 1963 to 1991. *Arch Pediatr Adolesc Med.* 1995;149:1085-1091.
37. Ogden CL, Carroll MD, Curtin LR, McDowell MA, Tabak CJ, Flegal KM. Prevalence of overweight and obesity in the United States, 1999-2004. *JAMA.* 2006;295:1549-1555.
38. Rowland T. Declining cardiorespiratory fitness in youth: fact or supposition? *Pediatr Exerc Sci.* 2002;14:1-8.

39. Armstrong N, Welsman JR. Assessment and interpretation of aerobic fitness in children and adolescents. *Exerc Sport Sci Rev.* 1994;22:435-476.
40. Krahenbuhl GS, Skinner JS, Kohrt WM. Developmental aspects of maximal aerobic power in children. *Exerc Sport Sci Rev.* 1985;13:503-538.
41. Pate RR, Long BJ, Heath G. Descriptive epidemiology of physical activity in adolescents. *Pediatr Exerc Sci.* 1994;6:434-447.
42. Sallis JF. Epidemiology of physical activity and fitness in children and adolescents. *Crit Rev Food Sci Nutr.* 1993;33:403-408.
43. Pivarnik JM, Fulton JE, Taylor WC, Snider SA. Aerobic capacity in black adolescent girls. *Res Q Exerc Sport.* 1993;64:202-207.
44. Gutin B, Yin Z, Humphries MC, Barbeau P. Relations of moderate and vigorous physical activity to fitness and fatness in adolescents. *Am J Clin Nutr.* 2005; 81:746-750.
45. Katzmarzyk PT, Malina RM, Song TM, Bouchard C. Television viewing, physical activity, and health-related fitness of youth in the Quebec Family Study. *J Adolesc Health.* 1998;23:318-325.
46. Grund A, Krause H, Siewers M, Rieckert H, Muller MJ. Is TV viewing an index of physical activity and fitness in overweight and normal weight children? *Public Health Nutr.* 2001;4:1245-1251.
47. Blair SN, Kohl HWI, Paffenbarger RS Jr, Clark DG, Cooper KH, Gibbons LW. Physical fitness and all-cause mortality: a prospective study of healthy men and women. *JAMA.* 1989;262:2395-2401.
48. Williams PT. Physical fitness and activity as separate heart disease risk factors: a meta-analysis. *Med Sci Sports Exerc.* 2001;33:754-761.
49. Malina RM. Tracking of physical activity and physical fitness across the lifespan. *Res Q Exerc Sport.* 1996;67:S48-S57.
50. Twisk JWR, Kemper HCG, Snel J. Tracking of cardiovascular risk factors in relation to lifestyle. In: Kemper HCG, ed. *The Amsterdam Growth Study: A Longitudinal Analysis of Health, Fitness, and Lifestyle.* Champaign, Ill: Human Kinetics; 1995:203-204.
51. Eisenmann JC, Wickel EE, Welk GJ, Blair SN. Relationship between adolescent fitness and fatness and cardiovascular disease risk factors in adulthood: the Aerobics Center Longitudinal Study (ACLS). *Am Heart J.* 2005;149:46-53.
52. Ferreira I, Twisk JW, Stehouwer CD, van Mechelen W, Kemper HC. Longitudinal changes in VO2max: associations with carotid IMT and arterial stiffness. *Med Sci Sports Exerc.* 2003;35:1670-1678.
53. Hasselstrom H, Hansen SE, Froberg K, Andersen LB. Physical fitness and physical activity during adolescence as predictors of cardiovascular disease risk in young adulthood—Danish Youth and Sports Study: an eight-year follow-up study. *Int J Sports Med.* 2002;23:S27-S31.
54. Twisk JW, Kemper HC, van Mechelen W. The relationship between physical fitness and physical activity during adolescence and cardiovascular disease risk factors at adult age: the Amsterdam Growth and Health Longitudinal Study. *Int J Sports Med.* 2002;23:S8-14.
55. Glenmark B, Hedberg G, Jansson E. Prediction of physical activity level in adulthood by physical characteristics, physical performance and physical activity in adolescence: an 11-year follow-up study. *Eur J Appl Physiol Occup Physiol.* 1994; 69:530-538.
56. Strong WB, Malina RM, Blimkie CJ, et al. Evidence based physical activity for school-age youth. *J Pediatr.* 2005;146:732-737.
57. US Department of Agriculture. Nutrition and Your Health: Dietary Guidelines for Americans, 2005 Dietary Guidelines Advisory Committee Report. 2004. http://www.health.gov/dietaryguidelines/dga2005/report/default.htm. Accessed November 29, 2004.


## Announcement

**Trial Registration Required.** In concert with the International Committee of Medical Journal Editors (ICMJE), *Archives of Pediatrics and Adolescent Medicine* will require, as a condition of consideration for publication, registration of all trials in a public trials registry (such as http://ClinicalTrials.gov). Trials must be registered at or before the onset of patient enrollment. This policy applies to any clinical trial starting enrollment after July 1, 2005. For trials that began enrollment before this date, registration will be required by September 13, 2005, before considering the trial for publication. The trial registration number should be supplied at the time of submission.

For details about this new policy, and for information on how the ICMJE defines a clinical trial, see the editorials by DeAngelis et al in the September 8, 2004 (2004;292:1363-1364) and June 15, 2005 (2005;293: 2927-2929) issues of *JAMA*. Also see the Instructions to Authors on our Web site: www.archpediatrics.com.

# Attenuating Growth in Children With Profound Developmental Disability

## *A New Approach to an Old Dilemma*

*Daniel F. Gunther, MD, MA; Douglas S. Diekema, MD, MPH*

Caring for children with profound developmental disabilities can be difficult and demanding. For nonambulatory children with severe, combined neurologic and cognitive impairment, all the necessities of life must be provided by caregivers, usually parents, and these tasks become more difficult as the child grows to adolescence and adulthood. Many parents would like to continue caring for their child with special needs at home but find it difficult to do so as the child increases in size. If growth could be permanently arrested while the child was still small, both child and parent would likely benefit because this would facilitate the option of continued care in the home. Treatment of the child with high-dose estrogen, initiated at an early age, could provide this option. High-dose estrogen both inhibits growth and rapidly advances maturation of the epiphyseal growth plates, bringing about permanent attenuation in size after a relatively short period of treatment. We present a case report and discuss the medical and ethical considerations of such an intervention strategy. We suggest that after proper screening and informed consent, growth-attenuation therapy should be a therapeutic option available to these children should their parents request it.
*Arch Pediatr Adolesc Med. 2006;160:1013-1017*

The American Academy of Pediatrics recently endorsed the goal of *Healthy People 2010* to reduce the number of children and youth with disabilities in congregate care facilities to zero by the year 2010.[1] The American Academy of Pediatrics Committee/Section on Children With Disabilities notes that "most parents desire to raise their children with special health care needs at home"[1(p507)] and supports a shifting emphasis away from placement strategies to permanency planning in the "belief that all children, regardless of the presence of a disability, belong in families."[1(p508)]

However, caring for a nonambulatory child with severe, combined developmental and cognitive disabilities can be a daunting task for parents, especially as the child increases in size.[2] The difficulties of caring for these children—dressing, bathing, diapering, transferring from bed to wheelchair, transporting—increase exponentially as the children grow to adolescence and adulthood. Despite medical and technological advances, many parents who would like to continue caring for their child with special needs at home find it difficult to do so given the physical limitations imposed by continued growth. Achieving permanent growth attenuation while the child is still young and of manageable size would remove one of the major obstacles to family care and might extend the time that parents with the ability, resources, and inclination to care for their child at home might be able to do so.

***For editorial comment see page 1077***

Treatment with high-dose estrogen could accomplish this goal. In high doses, estrogen both arrests growth and rapidly advances maturation of the epiphyseal growth plates. This combined effect should bring about permanent attenuation in size after a relatively short period of treatment.

**Author Affiliations:** Division of Pediatric Endocrinology (Dr Gunther) and Center for Pediatric Bioethics (Dr Diekema), Department of Pediatrics, Children's Hospital and Regional Medical Center, University of Washington School of Medicine, Seattle.

At our institution, we have begun such a treatment protocol in a child who meets the criteria for severe, irreversible neurologic and cognitive impairment. The treatment was requested by the parents and initiated after careful consultation and review by our institutional ethics committee. Other children are being considered for treatment as part of a comprehensive program that includes review by pediatric specialists in endocrinology, neurology, development, surgery, and ethics.

In this article, we present the child's case, discuss the history of growth-attenuation therapy, and make an argument for the careful application of such a treatment strategy in nonambulatory, profoundly impaired children. We believe that foreshortening growth in these children could result in a positive benefit in the quality of life for both child and caregiver, and we propose that in situations in which parents request such an intervention, it is both medically feasible and ethically defensible.

## CASE REPORT

The patient is a 6-year-7-month-old white female initially referred to the pediatric endocrine service for early pubertal development. She had been the full-term product of an unremarkable pregnancy followed by an uncomplicated birth. After the first month of life, she began to display symptoms of hypotonia, feeding difficulties, choreoathetoid movements, and developmental delay. Extensive subsequent evaluation by specialists in neurology, medical genetics, and developmental pediatrics failed to uncover a specific cause. Static encephalopathy with marked global developmental deficits eventually was diagnosed. In the ensuing years, her development never progressed beyond that of an infant. At the age of 6 years, she cannot sit up, ambulate, or use language. She is gastrostomy-tube dependent for nutrition. However, she clearly responds to others—vocalizing and smiling in response to care and affection. The combined opinion of the specialists involved in her care is that there will be no significant future improvement in her cognitive or neurologic baseline.

Since birth, the patient has been cared for in the home by her parents, both of whom are college-educated professionals. She has 2 healthy siblings. Despite her severe disability, she clearly is an integral, and much loved, member of the family.

The patient presented for endocrine evaluation with a 1-year history of pubic hair development and 3-month history of breast budding. The parents were particularly concerned about accelerated growth, the patient having advanced from the 50th to the 75th percentile for length during the previous 6 months. After some probing, it was clear that the onset of puberty had awakened parental fears for their daughter's long-term future. The parents particularly feared that continued growth eventually would make it untenable for them to care for their daughter at home, despite their strong desire to do so. They were concerned that care might eventually have to be "put in the hands of strangers." There were also concerns about the complications of puberty, particularly the onset of menses.

After extensive consultation between parents and physician, a plan was devised to attenuate growth by using high-dose estrogen and to reduce the long-term complications of puberty in general, and treatment adverse effects in particular, by performing pretreatment hysterectomy. Because a growth-attenuating treatment regimen is unconventional, and bound to be controversial, the case was referred to our institutional ethics committee. The committee met with the family, the patient, and the patient's physicians and carefully explored the family's reasons for their request. After a lengthy discussion, the committee reached consensus that both the requests for growth attenuation and hysterectomy were ethically appropriate in this case. The committee also recognized that, although justified in this patient, growth attenuation should be considered in future patients only after careful evaluation of the risks and benefits on a case-by-case basis. Toward that end, plans were instituted to convene an interdisciplinary review panel that includes pediatric specialists in endocrinology, neurology, development, surgery, and ethics.

After uneventful surgery, the patient began a course of 400 μg of transdermal estradiol daily. She is followed up every 3 months and carefully monitored for growth, bone age, insulin-like growth factor I, estrogen and prolactin levels, and thrombotic factors. She is now a little more than a year into therapy and approaching the end of her growth. As of yet, there have been no treatment complications.

## THE HISTORY OF GROWTH-ATTENUATION THERAPY

Physicians long have appreciated that one consequence of early puberty is its deleterious effect on growth. In children who are exposed to sex steroids prematurely, final adult height is seriously attenuated because of acceleration in epiphyseal (growth plate) maturation.[3] The earlier the onset of puberty, the greater the reduction in final height.[4] Although both estrogens and androgens accelerate growth, it is now appreciated that estrogen is the dominant hormone in the advancement of skeletal maturation in both boys and girls and seems exclusively responsible for bringing about epiphyseal fusion and an end to growth.[5]

The effect of estrogen on growth appears to be biphasic. Although physiologic levels of estrogen accelerate growth (the pubertal growth spurt), supraphysiologic doses paradoxically tend to inhibit growth.[4,6,7] The mechanism by which high levels of estrogen interfere with growth is not completely understood but may be caused, at least in part, by estrogen's suppression of insulin-like growth factor I (or somatomedin C), the peptide that mediates the growth-promoting effects of growth hormone.[8-10]

It is not surprising that this biphasic effect of estrogen eventually would be exploited therapeutically in situations in which attenuating growth was thought to be desirable. Tall adolescent girls wishing to minimize any further gain in height represented one such population. The first use of high-dose estrogen in girls with constitutional tall stature was reported by Goldzieher in 1956.[11] In the ensuing years, this practice became an established, if somewhat controversial, strategy for attenuating growth in these girls, and many reports have appeared in the literature.[12-15] The practice continues to this day, although less commonly, no doubt because of a decreasing sense of stigma associated with tall stature in women.[16] Most of what is known about the effectiveness and potential adverse effects of high-dose estrogen treatment comes from these reports in this population.

The estrogen compounds used for growth attenuation, and the dosages used, have evolved across time and varied by region. In western and northern Europe, injectable estrogen compounds initially were used before being replaced by oral stilbestrol and eventually oral ethinyl estradiol (the estrogen most commonly used in oral contraceptives today). In the United States, the conjugated estrogen Premarin (Wyeth Pharmaceuticals Inc, Philadelphia, Pa; a combination of different estrogenic compounds derived from the urine of pregnant horses) was used predominantly.[12,13] Initially, doses greater than 10 to 15 times physiologic (or what was thought to be so at the time) were used, but eventually more modest doses were found to be as effective.[15] In most cases, severe uterine breakthrough bleeding occurred in girls taking estrogen alone, and a progestin was added at the end of the monthly cycle to induce normal menstrual periods.[12]

Although all reports claimed varying degrees of success in reducing adult stature, the amount of success varied. Most reported decreases in adult height were between 2 and 10 cm.[12-14] In most cases, treatment was not initiated until the girls were in early adolescence, and many had already had their first menses (a point at which girls will, on average, have already achieved 93% of their final adult height). Not surprisingly, the greatest reductions in height were seen when treatment was started earliest.[12]

How much reduction in height could we expect to achieve in young children using high-dose estrogen? Without prior experience, we can only reasonably speculate, and it would obviously depend on the child's age at the start of treatment. The younger the child at the beginning of treatment, the greater the reduction in height. We believe it a reasonable prediction, for example, that treatment beginning in a 5-year-old boy of average height and weight might result in a reduction in final length of as much as 24 inches (60 cm) and in weight of more than 100 pounds (45 kg). Older, larger children will see less of an effect.

## THE RISKS OF TREATMENT

Because we have no direct experience with high-dose estrogen treatment in young children, the possible adverse effects and risks are difficult to assess with certainty. In adolescent girls treated for constitutional tall stature, reported adverse effects included nausea, headache, and weight gain, but these were generally mild and virtually never a reason for discontinuing treatment. Hyperprolactinemia has been reported but is generally of no clinical significance and resolves after treatment.[17] There is one report of a girl with a prolactinoma after high-dose estrogen treatment, but it is unclear whether this was a preexisting condition.[18] Recently, concerns about long-term effects on fertility in treated girls have been raised,[19] but clearly this is not relevant to our population.

The consequence of introducing high-dose estrogen in young prepubertal children will be significant. In boys, the only likely outward manifestation of estrogen exposure would be the development of gynecomastia. In girls, there will be rapid advancement of isosexual secondary sexual characteristics—most notably breast development and uterine bleeding. Uterine bleeding might be controlled by a combination of concurrent estrogen/progesterone treatment, but breakthrough bleeding is likely.[20] Although monthly or quarterly injections of depot medroxyprogesterone acetate are often used to control menses in some patients with severe developmental disabilities,[21,22] an alternative for these children is pretreatment hysterectomy, as was performed in our patient.

A word here about hysterectomy is probably appropriate. Hysterectomy in children, particularly in the disabled, is controversial and invariably associated with the negative connotations and history of forced "sterilization." But in these profoundly impaired children, with no realistic reproductive aspirations, prophylactic hysterectomy has several advantages as an adjunct to high-dose estrogen treatment. This onetime procedure eliminates the complications of menses, and in many cases, will spare the individual and her caregivers the expense, pain, and inconvenience of a lifetime of hormone injections. Hysterectomy also eliminates the need to give concurrent progesterone during the treatment phase, potentially reducing the risks of thrombosis.[23,24] It also eliminates the possibility of future uterine and cervical cancer. With the ovaries left in situ, hormones continue to be produced, providing some protection from osteoporosis. The risks of this surgical procedure in prepubertal girls, and the risks of long-term complications, are minimal—certainly they do not exceed the risk of similar procedures many of these children will experience as part of their medical care. The decision to perform hysterectomy should be made carefully, and the ethical (and legal) considerations important in making this decision have been discussed elsewhere.[25]

The most significant safety concern regarding high-dose estrogen treatment is the risk of thrombosis, most commonly deep vein thrombosis. The increased risk for developing deep vein thrombosis among women taking oral contraceptives is somewhere between 2- and 5-fold, increasing with age, although it is still relatively uncommon.[26,27] The risk of thrombosis also is increased among postmenopausal women receiving hormone therapy.[28] The mechanism through which estrogen increases thrombogenesis is not completely clear but probably is related to its direct effects on thrombotic factors.[29-32] Although concerns about the risk of thrombosis have been raised in the treatment of adolescent girls of tall stature,[33] few actual events have been reported. In combined reports of more than 700 girls with tall stature treated at 2 different centers, there was only 1 report of a mild deep vein thrombosis in a girl with a strong family history.[14,15] Weimann and Brack[34] also reported a case of deep vein thrombosis in a girl who had undergone arthroscopy during her treatment.

The actual risk of thrombosis in developmentally delayed children is difficult to assess. On the one hand, the risk of thrombosis seems decreased in the young; on the other, the risk is greater in those who are nonambulatory. Some evidence suggests that spasticity, a not uncommon finding in this population, might provide a measure of protection against thrombosis.[35] The risk might also be reduced by using transdermal estrogen, which we elected to do in our patient, and by performing pretreatment hysterectomy, thus eliminating the need for progesterone. The risk in boys taking estrogen is probably similar to the risk in girls.[36]

## THE ETHICAL DEBATE

There is not much doubt that growth can be attenuated significantly by using high-dose estrogen, particularly if undertaken in patients at an early age. But should it be? Is such an intervention in the best interest of these children?

There are good historical reasons to proceed cautiously when considering any intervention directed at persons with developmental disabilities. Past abuses against this population are well documented. During the late 19th and early 20th centuries, for example, many persons who had mental retardation (or who were thought to have mental retardation) were subject to involuntary sterilization because of the belief that they were genetically "unfit" and would pass their "defects" on to future generations.[37,38] In many cases, these individuals were capable of living independently, marrying, and raising children. These decisions were based not on the best interest of the patient but rather on the perceived interest of society and, in some cases, the interests of parents or caretakers.

The lessons of these and other abuses must be remembered, but past abuses should not dissuade us from exploring novel therapies that offer the potential for benefit. The population we propose to treat—children like our patient with profound cognitive and neurologic impairment, who are nonambulatory and wholly dependent on others for every need—is different from the mildly to moderately impaired. Nevertheless, we recognize the concern about inappropriate application of these procedures in children who are less severely disabled. To guard against the arbitrary application of growth-limiting therapy, it seems appropriate, even perhaps necessary, that a formal mechanism exists to ensure proper application of treatment. At our institution, we are convening an interdisciplinary group consisting of pediatric specialists in endocrinology, neurology, development, surgery, and ethics to consider each case on its merits. This same group will also carefully consider whether any additional procedures, such as hysterectomy, are appropriate and serve the interests of the child. Ideally, this approach might be combined with a research protocol approved by an institutional review board. Growth attenuation should be considered only after careful consideration of the risks and benefits to each patient on an individual basis.

When deciding whether it is ethically appropriate to attenuate growth in these children, there are 2 primary considerations. First, does growth attenuation offer the patient benefit? And second, does growth attenuation do any harm to the patient? The question here, then, is whether there is a reasonable expectation of improved quality of life for a nonambulatory child with profound developmental disability, and at what risk?

The primary benefit offered by growth attenuation is the potential to make caring for the child less burdensome and therefore more accessible. A smaller person is not as difficult to move and transfer from place to place. Although this may seem to be an advantage that accrues to the caretakers rather than the child, it offers several distinct benefits to the child as well. A child who is easier to move will in all likelihood be moved more frequently. Being easier to move means more stimulation, fewer medical complications, and more social interaction. Physical contact between parent and child is likely to be more direct and personal without the need for hoisting apparatus or other devices. Being easier to move and transfer also makes it more likely that the child will be included in family activities and family outings.

Finally, as we have already argued, parents often wish to continue caring for an older child but find themselves unable to manage the physical demands as their child grows to adult size. Although size may not be the only consideration, and not all parents will choose this option, growth attenuation may offer some parents at least the opportunity to extend the time they can care for their child at home, whereas otherwise institutionalization, or foster care, might be the only alternative.

For all of these reasons, growth attenuation in the nonambulatory child with severe developmental disability seems mutually beneficial to caretakers and patient. There does not appear to be a conflict between the interests of the parents and the interests of the child.

Having established a probable benefit to small stature, the second consideration derives from the ethical principle of nonmaleficence, *primum non nocere*, to "do no harm." Could growth attenuation cause harm to these children?

Several potential harms should be considered. Already mentioned are the possible medical adverse effects of high-dose estrogen, the most significant of which is the risk of thrombosis. Although these are real risks, they do not appear to be excessive and probably do not significantly exceed the risks of similar therapies used in this population to control menstruation or prevent pregnancy.

Can one imagine harm to this population from simply being small? Height and normal stature clearly have social value for most individuals. Being taller has been associated with enhanced social stature, greater pay, greater success in attracting a mate, and other social benefits.[39] However, a nonambulatory, severely impaired child is not someone who will experience these benefits of tall stature and therefore will not suffer their loss if kept short. For an individual who will never be capable of holding a job, establishing a romantic relationship, or interacting as an adult, it is hard to imagine how being smaller would be socially disadvantageous.

One might argue that being smaller might alter the way others interact with an older disabled person, perhaps tending to treat that person as a child instead of an adult. Whereas this might be an important issue for a short-statured adult who is capable of normal adult interactions, it is unlikely that such "infantilization" harms a person whose mental capacity will always remain that of a young child. In fact, for a person with a developmental age of an infant, smaller stature may actually constitute an advantage because others probably would be more likely to interact in ways that are more appropriate to that person's developmental age.

In summary, the harms associated with growth attenuation for persons with severe developmental disability are primarily those associated with the medical risks of treatment. These risks do not appear to be unreasonable and are not out of line with the risks of other medical interventions these children undergo.

## CONCLUSIONS

A parent's desire to seek growth attenuation for a permanently nonambulatory child with profound developmental, neurologic, and cognitive impairment would seem reasonable and understandable. We have argued that a compelling case can be made that the child will benefit from such treatment, that the risks of harm are limited to the adverse effects of the therapy, and that such risks do not significantly exceed those of other standard medical interventions.

To prevent the possibility of abuse and to ensure the safe administration and follow-up of therapy, we suggest that treatment should proceed only after evaluation by a pediatric neurodevelopmental specialist and with the supervision of a pediatric endocrinologist, preferably after review by the institution's ethics committee or in the context of a study reviewed by an institutional review board. Parents should be made aware of the risks and uncertainties of a novel, untested medical intervention. In the presence of those safeguards, we suggest that such treatment is both ethical and feasible and should be an option available to parents.

**Accepted for Publication:** March 2, 2006.
**Correspondence:** Daniel F. Gunther, MD, MA, Division of Pediatric Endocrinology, Department of Pediatrics, Children's Hospital and Regional Medical Center, 4800 Sand Point Way NE M1-3, Seattle, WA 98105 (Dan.Gunther@seattlechildrens.org).
**Author Contributions:** *Study concept and design:* Gunther and Diekema. *Acquisition of data:* Gunther and Diekema. *Drafting of the manuscript:* Gunther and Diekema. *Critical revision of the manuscript for important intellectual content*: Gunther and Diekema. *Administrative, technical, and material support:* Gunther and Diekema. *Study supervision:* Gunther and Diekema.

## REFERENCES


1. Johnson CP, Kastner TA. Helping families raise children with special health care needs at home. *Pediatrics.* 2005;115:507-511.
2. Taanila A, Syrjala L, Kokkonen J, Jarvelin MR. Coping of parents with physically and/or intellectually disabled children. *Child Care Health Dev.* 2002; 28:73-86.
3. Thamdrup E. *Precocious Sexual Development: A Clinical Study of 100 Children.* Springfield, Ill: Charles C Thomas; 1961.
4. Bourguignon JP. Linear growth as a function of age at onset of puberty and sex steroid dosage: therapeutic implications. *Endocr Rev.* 1988;9:467-488.
5. Grumbach MM. Estrogen, bone, growth and sex: a sea change in conventional wisdom. *J Pediatr Endocrinol Metab.* 2000;13(suppl 6):1439-1455.
6. Ross JL, Cassorla FG, Skerda MC, Valk IM, Loriaux DL, Cutler GB Jr. A preliminary study of the effect of estrogen dose on growth in Turner's syndrome. *N Engl J Med.* 1983;309:1104-1106.
7. Ohlsson C, Isgaard J, Tornell J, Nilsson A, Isaksson OG, Lindahl A. Endocrine regulation of longitudinal bone growth. *Acta Paediatr Suppl.* 1993; 82(suppl 391):33-40.
8. Meyer WJ, Furlanetto RW, Walker PA. The effect of sex steroids on radioimmunoassayable plasma somatomedin C concentrations. *J Clin Endocrinol Metab.* 1982;55:1184-1187.
9. Schwartz E, Echemendia E, Schiffer M, Panariello VA. Mechanisms of estrogenic action in acromegaly. *J Clin Invest.* 1969;48:260-270.
10. Wiedemann E, Schwartz E. Suppression of growth hormone-dependent human serum sulfation factor by estrogen. *J Clin Endocrinol.* 1972;34:51-58.
11. Goldzieher MA. Treatment of excessive growth in the adolescent female. *J Clin Endocrinol Metab.* 1956;16:249-252.
12. Bailey JD, Park E, Cowell C. Estrogen treatment of girls with constitutional tall stature. *Pediatr Clin North Am.* 1981;28:501-512.
13. Drop SL, De Waal WJ, De Muinck Keizer-Schrama SM. Sex steroid treatment of constitutionally tall stature. *Endocr Rev.* 1998;19:540-558.
14. Normann EK, Trygstad O, Larsen S, Dahl-Jorgensen K. Height reduction in 539 tall girls treated with three different dosages of ethinyloestradiol. *Arch Dis Child.* 1991;66:1275-1278.
15. Wettenhall HN, Cahill C, Roche AF. Tall girls: a survey of 15 years of management and treatment. *J Pediatr.* 1975;86:602-610.
16. Barnard ND, Scialli AR, Bobela SB. The current use of estrogens for growth-suppressant therapy in adolescent girls. *J Pediatr Adolesc Gynecol.* 2002; 15:23-26.
17. Houdijk EC, Delemarre-van de Waal HA. Increase of serum prolactin during combined high-dose estrogen and progestin treatment in girls with constitutional tall stature [letter]. *Acta Paediatr.* 2000;89:1504-1505.
18. Panteon E, Loumaye E, Maes M, Malvaux P. Occurrence of prolactinoma after estrogen treatment in a girl with constitutional tall stature. *J Pediatr.* 1988; 113:337-339.
19. Venn A, Bruinsma F, Werther G, et al. Oestrogen treatment to reduce the adult height of tall girls: long-term effects on fertility. *Lancet.* 2004;364:1513-1518.
20. Nand SL, Webster MA, Baber R, O'Connor V. Bleeding pattern and endometrial changes during continuous combined hormone replacement therapy: the Ogen/Provera Study Group. *Obstet Gynecol.* 1998;91(5, pt 1):678-684.
21. Bigrigg A, Evans M, Gbolade B, et al. Depo Provera: position paper on clinical use, effectiveness and side effects. *Br J Fam Plann.* 1999;25:69-76.
22. Backeljauw PF, Rose SR, Lawson M. Clinical management of menstruation in adolescent females with developmental delay. *Endocrinologist.* 2004; 14:87-92.
23. Bladbjerg EM, Skouby SO, Andersen LF, Jespersen J. Effects of different progestin regimens in hormone replacement therapy on blood coagulation factor VII and tissue pathway inhibitor. *Hum Reprod.* 2002;17:3235-3241.
24. Girolami A, Spiezia L, Rossi F, Zanon E. Oral contraceptives and venous thromboembolism: which are the safest preparations available? *Clin Appl Thromb Hemost.* 2002;8:157-162.
25. Diekema DS. Involuntary sterilization of persons with mental retardation: an ethical analysis. *Ment Retard Dev Disabil Res Rev.* 2003;9:21-26.
26. Lidegaard O, Edstrom B, Kreiner S. Oral contraceptives and venous thromboembolism: a five-year national case-control study. *Contraception.* 2002;65: 187-196.
27. Weiss G. Risk of venous thromboembolism with third-generation oral contraceptives: a review. *Am J Obstet Gynecol.* 1999;180(2, pt 2):295-301.
28. Daly E, Vessey MP, Hawkins MM, Carson JL, Gough P, Marsh R. Risk of venous thromboembolism in users of hormone replacement therapy. *Lancet.* 1996; 348:977-980.
29. Post MS, Christella M, Thomassen LG, et al. Effect of oral and transdermal estrogen replacement therapy on hemostatic variables associated with venous thrombosis: a randomized, placebo-controlled study in postmenopausal women. *Arterioscler Thromb Vasc Biol.* 2003;23:1116-1121.
30. van Ommen CH, Fijnvandraat K, Vulsma T, Delemarre-Van De Waal HA, Peters M. Acquired protein S deficiency caused by estrogen treatment of tall stature. *J Pediatr.* 1999;135:477-481.
31. Oger E, Alhenc-Gelas M, Lacut K, et al. Differential effects of oral and transdermal estrogen/progesterone regimens on sensitivity to activated protein C among postmenopausal women: a randomized trial. *Arterioscler Thromb Vasc Biol.* 2003; 23:1671-1676.
32. Mishell DR Jr. Oral contraception: past, present, and future perspectives. *Int J Fertil.* 1991;36(suppl 1):7-18.
33. Blomback M, Hall K, Ritzen EM. Estrogen treatment of tall girls: risk of thrombosis? *Pediatrics.* 1983;72:416-419.
34. Weimann E, Brack C. Severe thrombosis during treatment with ethinylestradiol for tall stature. *Horm Res.* 1996;45:261-263.
35. Rousseau MC, Guillotel B. Risk factors for deep venous thrombosis in tetraparesic mentally retarded patients. *Brain Inj.* 2001;15:1041-1044.
36. Toorians AW, Thomassen MC, Zweegman S, et al. Venous thrombosis and changes of hemostatic variables during cross-sex hormone treatment in transsexual people. *J Clin Endocrinol Metab.* 2003;88:5723-5729.
37. Park DC, Radford JP. From the case files: reconstructing a history of involuntary sterilization. *Disabil Soc.* 1998;13:317-342.
38. Reilly PR. *The Surgical Solution: A History of Involuntary Sterilization in the United States.* Baltimore, Md: Johns Hopkins University Press; 1991.
39. Diekema DS. Is taller really better? growth hormone therapy in short children. *Perspect Biol Med.* 1990;34:109-123.

ARTICLE

# Improved Preventive Care for Asthma

## *A Randomized Trial of Clinician Prompting in Pediatric Offices*

*Jill S. Halterman, MD, MPH; Susan Fisher, PhD; Kelly M. Conn, MPH; Maria Fagnano, BA; Kathleen Lynch, BA; Andrew Marky, BA; Peter G. Szilagyi, MD, MPH*

**Objective:** To determine whether clinician prompting regarding a child's symptom severity and guideline recommendations at the time of an office visit improves the delivery of preventive asthma care.

**Design:** Randomized controlled trial.

**Setting:** Two inner-city pediatric practices in Rochester, NY.

**Participants:** Two hundred twenty-six children with persistent asthma (aged 2-12 years) presenting to the clinics for well-child care, asthma care, or non–asthma-related illness care.

**Intervention:** We assigned children randomly to a clinician-prompting group (single-page prompt including the child's symptoms and guideline recommendations given to the clinician at the time of the visit) or a standard-care group (no prompt given). Interviewers called parents after the visit to inquire about preventive measures taken, and medical charts were reviewed.

**Main Outcome Measures:** Any preventive action related to asthma taken at the visit.

**Results:** Children in the clinician-prompting group were more likely to have had any preventive measures taken at the visit compared with children in the standard-care group (87% vs 69%). Specifically, visits for children in the clinician-prompting group were more likely to include delivery of an action plan (50% vs 24%), discussions regarding asthma (87% vs 76%), and recommendations for an asthma follow-up visit (54% vs 37%). In a regression model, children in the clinician-prompting group had 3-fold greater odds of receiving any preventive action compared with the standard-care group.

**Conclusion:** Clinician prompting regarding asthma severity and care guidelines at the time of an office visit significantly improved the delivery of preventive asthma care.

*Arch Pediatr Adolesc Med. 2006;160:1018-1025*

ASTHMA IS THE MOST COMmon chronic illness of childhood,[1] and morbidity has increased despite improvements in therapy.[2] National guidelines for the management of asthma are available,[3-5] and use of these guidelines can reduce morbidity and mortality due to asthma.[5-10] However, several studies have documented poor physician adherence to the guidelines,[11-15] likely contributing to otherwise preventable illness. Children from poor or minority backgrounds suffer the greatest morbidity from asthma[16-18] and are the least likely to receive appropriate preventive treatment.[19-21]

An office visit provides an opportunity for the clinician to apply asthma guidelines to clinical care.[4] Unfortunately, during many patient encounters, opportunities to provide guideline-based preventive care are missed. We know, for example, that many providers fail to document symptom severity in the medical record[22] and underestimate the severity of their patient's symptoms.[13,23] Similarly, written action plans[22,24] and asthma education are not provided consistently.[24] Several barriers associated with poor implementation of the guidelines have been documented.[11,25]

Provider prompts can be effective in stimulating action regarding clinical issues and improving preventive care.[26-28] The objective of this study was to determine whether clinician prompting regarding asthma symptom severity and guideline recommendations at the time of an office visit improves preventive care delivery for inner-city children with persistent asthma.

**Author Affiliations:** Departments of Pediatrics (Drs Halterman and Szilagyi; Mss Conn, Fagnano, and Lynch; and Mr Marky) and Community and Preventive Medicine (Dr Fisher), University of Rochester School of Medicine and Dentistry, and the Strong Children's Research Center (Drs Halterman and Szilagyi; Mss Conn, Fagnano, and Lynch; and Mr Marky), Rochester, NY.

## METHODS

### SETTING

We conducted this study in 2 inner-city pediatric practices in Rochester, NY, from November 20, 2003, through September 14, 2005. The practices are training sites for the residency program at the University of Rochester, are staffed by attending physicians and nurse practitioners, and provide care primarily for low-income, minority patients. Children aged 2 to 12 years with at least 2 asthma exacerbations in the preceding 2 years were identified as potential study subjects. We reviewed medical charts daily for children with scheduled visits for well-child care, asthma care, or non–asthma-related illness care. A study team member approached parents of identified children in the waiting room before their visit with the clinician and completed a detailed survey to assess eligibility. The institutional review board of the University of Rochester approved the study protocol.

## PARTICIPANTS

Eligibility required children to have symptoms consistent with mild persistent or more severe asthma[5] and thus to need enhanced preventive care. Parents were asked the following specific questions about their child's current asthma symptoms: (1) During the past 2 weeks, how often has your child had coughing, wheezing, or shortness of breath during the day (less than twice a week, twice a week, more than twice a week but not every day, everyday but not all the time, or everyday/all the time)? and (2) During the past 2 weeks, how often has your child had coughing, wheezing, or shortness of breath during the night (never, once every 2 weeks or less, once a week, more than 1 night a week, or frequently/every night)? Children of parents who indicated daytime symptoms of at least more than twice a week but not everyday or nighttime symptoms at least once a week were considered to have persistent asthma and were eligible to participate. Because of a lack of available resources, Spanish-speaking families were enrolled into the study only on days when a Spanish-speaking interviewer was available. Eligible children had to be accompanied by a parent or legal guardian. We excluded children with other medical illnesses that would complicate the assessment of asthma symptoms (eg, cystic fibrosis or heart disease).

## ENROLLMENT AND RANDOMIZATION

After written informed consent was obtained, a baseline survey was conducted with the parent to obtain information regarding household demographic characteristics, asthma symptom severity, medication use, and environmental tobacco smoke (ETS) exposure.

After completion of the baseline assessment, each child was assigned randomly to the clinician-prompting group or the standard-care group. Randomization was stratified by office site and preventive asthma medication use at baseline and was blocked in groups of 6 to ensure an equal number of subjects in each group for each seasonal time period. Only 1 child was randomly selected for enrollment from eligible sibling pairs who arrived together for an office visit. Randomization cards were made from a table of random numbers and were kept in sealed, opaque, sequentially numbered envelopes until after the baseline assessment.

### Clinician-Prompting Group

The study team member enrolling the child in the waiting room prepared an asthma report and action recommendation form to serve as the prompt for each child in the clinician-prompting group (**Figure 1**). This prompt included information regarding the child's current asthma symptoms, as obtained from the baseline survey conducted in the waiting room, the classification of the child's asthma severity, and recommendations for treatment based on the national guidelines.[5] The prompt also included information regarding the child's exposure to ETS, with recommendations for discussion of ETS reduction.

The prompt was given to the parent in the waiting room, and the parent was instructed to hand it to the clinician when the child was called back for the office visit. We also included a blank asthma action plan form along with the prompt for the health care provider to complete and return to the family at the end of the visit. Parents were specifically instructed to hand these forms to the clinician in the examination room, rather than to the nurse or the aide who might be initiating the visit with the child.

### Standard-Care Group

Parents of children in the standard-care group completed the baseline assessment in the waiting room, but no asthma prompt was created, and no information regarding the interview was shared with the provider. After the baseline assessment, the office visit proceeded according to usual care.

Before the initiation of the study, the principal investigator (J.S.H.) met with health care providers in both offices to describe the intervention and orient them to the prompt. Each practice was given a donation of $500 to thank them for their participation.

## ASSESSMENT OF OUTCOME MEASURES

Interviewers blinded to the child's group assignment called the parent or guardian who accompanied the child to the office visit to assess the outcome measures for the study. To optimize recall, we excluded interview follow-up data for children who did not complete a follow-up within 60 days of the intervention or who had another office visit between the time of enrollment and follow-up (n = 10 in the clinician-prompting group and n = 10 in the standard-care group). The follow-up data included in the analyses were collected, on average, 11 days after the visit (range, 0-57 days). We asked parents to think about the office visit and answer specific questions about what occurred during the visit. The interview included inquiries regarding whether the clinician discussed asthma symptoms, emergency visits and absenteeism due to asthma, medication compliance, environmental triggers, and how to properly use medications. We also asked whether the clinician recommended a specific asthma follow-up visit or a visit with an asthma or allergy specialist, and whether parents were given a written asthma action plan. We inquired about whether the child received a new preventive medication different from the one he or she was already taking or if a dosage of a preventive medication he or she was already taking was changed. Finally, we asked parents whether anything else was done at the office visit to help their child's asthma.

We also performed blinded reviews of the children's medical records from that office visit to assess these same preventive measures on the basis of the health care provider's report. A study team member used a standardized chart abstraction form to collect data from the medical record, and any documentation of asthma care was recorded. The principal investigator (J.S.H.) performed a second blinded review of all medical records and completed medical chart abstraction forms to ensure accuracy of the medical-related data.

Preventive actions included provision of an asthma action plan, treatment of a comorbid condition (eg, allergies, sinusitis, or gastroesophageal reflux), recommendation of a follow-up visit for asthma, referral to a specialist, discussions related to asthma (inquiries regarding emergency visits and absenteeism due to asthma, environmental changes, and adherence to preventive medications), and changes in the pre-

**Asthma Report and Action Recommendations for Today's Visit**

Child's Name:________ ________

***Below are parent-reported asthma symptoms for your patient. These symptoms were reported today through a brief survey while the patient was waiting to be seen.***

**During the past 2 weeks**, the child has had coughing, wheezing, or shortness of breath *during the day:*

- ☐ **Twice a week or less**
- ☐ **More than 2 times a week, but not every day**
- ☐ **Everyday, but not all the time**
- ☐ **Everyday, all the time**

**During the past 2 weeks**, the child has had coughing, wheezing, or shortness of breath *during the night:*

- ☐ **Once every 2 weeks or less**
- ☐ **Once a week**
- ☐ **More than 1 night a week**
- ☐ **Frequently/every night**

According to National Guidelines, this child ☐**DOES** / ☐**DOES NOT** have symptoms consistent with mild persistent to severe persistent asthma and preventive medications ☐ **SHOULD** / ☐**SHOULD NOT** be considered.

**Recommended Actions:**

***Mild Intermittent***

**Review use of medications, provide refills as needed**

**Discuss environmental triggers**

***Mild Persistent to Severe Persistent***

**Consider starting preventive medication (inhaled steroid) if child is not currently using one**

**If child is already using a preventive medication you may want to:**

**Review technique/discuss compliance**

**Step up therapy**

**Discuss environmental triggers**

**Provide action plan**

**Additionally, the parent ☐ DID / ☐ DID NOT report that the child is exposed to smoke in the home and/or car.**

**Recommended actions for all children with asthma:**

Ask the caregiver specifically about the child's secondhand smoke exposure in various settings (home, car, or day care)
Educate the caregiver about the negative effect of smoke on asthma symptoms
Suggest ways to decrease the child's exposure to secondhand smoke, such as implementing smoking bans (no smoking in the home or car with no exceptions)
For caregivers who smoke, encourage cessation and provide resources as appropriate

**Figure 1.** Sample clinician prompt used in the intervention.

ventive medication (prescription of a new preventive medication or increase of the dose of a current preventive medication). We defined smoke reduction counseling as any discussion regarding smoke avoidance or smoking cessation or education regarding the harm of ETS exposure for those households where 1 or more members smoked.

The primary outcome for this study was any preventive action occurring during the study visit (defined as any of the actions listed in the preceding paragraph). If the parent or the medical record indicated the occurrence of a preventive action, we assumed for the purposes of this study that an action had been taken. The parent interview and medical chart review data yielded the same result for this primary outcome measure in 75% of cases.

## ASSESSMENT OF COVARIATES

Independent variables included sex, age, race (white, African American, or other), ethnicity (Hispanic or not Hispanic), Medicaid insurance (yes or no), caretaker education (less than high school or high school or more), asthma severity (mild persistent, moderate persistent, or severe persistent), type of provider conducting the visit (attending physician, nurse practitioner, or resident), whether the visit was conducted by the child's usual health care provider (yes or no), and the number of smokers living in the home (0 or ≥1).

## STATISTICAL ANALYSIS

All randomized subjects were kept in their originally assigned treatment groups for analysis. Analysis was performed using commercially available statistical software (SPSS, version 14.0; SPSS Inc, Chicago, Ill). We used $\chi^2$ analyses to compare the dependent variables between the 2 groups. A single post hoc analysis was performed with data stratified by the type of office visit (asthma visit, well-child visit, or non–asthma-related illness visit). We also performed multiple logistic regression analyses to predict the key outcome variables after controlling for the child's age, sex, race, ethnicity, and asthma severity; a smoker living in the home; and the provider's characteristics.

In planning this study, the sample size calculations were based on the ability to detect a change of 20% in the primary outcome variable (any preventive action) (improvement from a baseline of action being taken in 56% of visits[29] to occurrence in 76% of visits). A total sample of 200 patients was required ($\alpha = .05$; $\beta = 0.20$; 2-sided test).

# RESULTS

We reviewed the medical charts of 722 children who visited the clinics and approached 510 (70.6%) of these subjects, who were potentially eligible. Of the 510 ap-

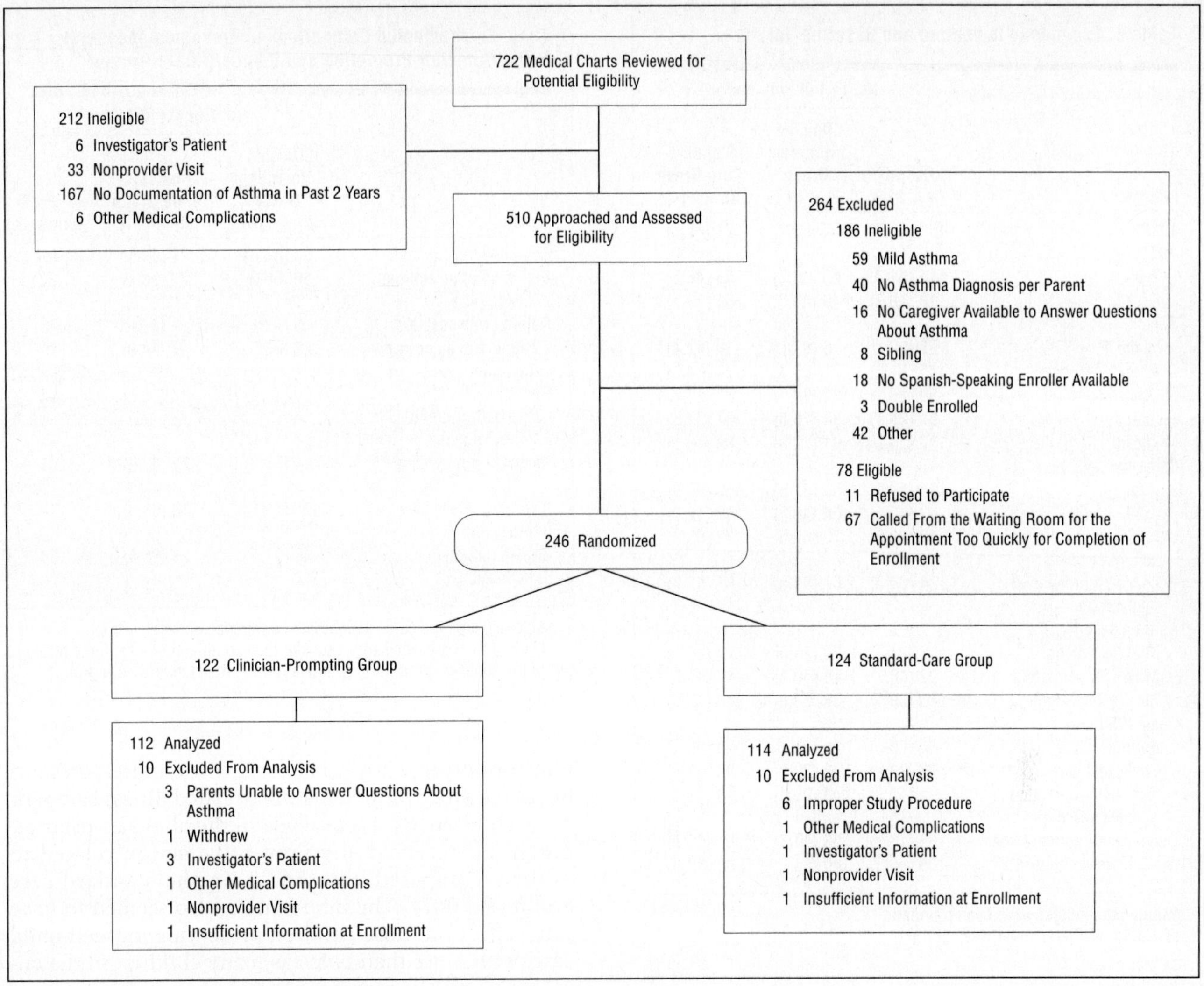


**Figure 2.** Flow diagram of enrollment into the trial.

proached, 186 were ineligible for reasons such as lack of an asthma diagnosis according to the parent, mild asthma symptoms, or lack of Spanish-speaking enrollers (**Figure 2**). Among the 324 eligible children, 78 were not enrolled because of parent refusal (n = 11) or lack of time in the waiting room to complete enrollment before the office visit began (n = 67). The remaining 246 children were enrolled in the program for a response rate of 75.9%. One hundred twenty-two children were randomized into the clinician-prompting group and 124 were randomized into the standard-care group. After randomization, 20 subjects were determined to be ineligible (n = 10 in the clinician-prompting group and n = 10 in the standard-care group) and were removed from further analysis (Figure 2). Seventy-nine different health care providers participated in the trial and 37 had patients in each treatment arm.

Two hundred twenty-six children had data available for analysis for the primary outcome (n = 112 in the clinician-prompting group and n = 114 in the standard-care group). We were able to include data for a subject if an eligible follow-up was completed with the parent or if a medical record abstraction was available. The overall response rate for parent follow-up interviews was 78.3% (78.5% in the clinician-prompting group and 78.1% in the standard-care group). We reviewed the medical charts for all 226 subjects.

**Table 1** describes the demographic characteristics for the children and caregivers. Most of the children were male (58.0%), African American (64.2%), and insured by Medicaid (75.2%). Overall, 51.3% of the children were aged 2 to 5 years and 29.6% were Hispanic. Most of the caretakers had at least a high school education (62.8%). Among the children, 59.3% were using a preventive medication at baseline and 38.1% had severe persistent symptoms. On the day of the studied visit, 26.5% of the children were presenting to the office for asthma-related care, 33.2% for well-child care, and 40.3% for care for an illness other than asthma. Approximately half of the children (48.2%) saw their usual health care provider at the visit.

After randomization, there were fewer boys in the clinician-prompting group compared with the standard-care group (49.1% vs 66.7%). In addition, a smaller proportion of children in the clinician-prompting group lived with 1 or more smokers compared with children in the standard-care group (35.7% vs 57.0%). There were no significant differences in other baseline measures between the 2 groups.

**Table 1. Prognostic Indicators and Baseline Values**

| Indicator | No. (%) of Patients* Overall (N = 226) | Clinician-Prompting Group (n = 112) | Standard-Care Group (n = 114) |
|---|---|---|---|
| Male† | 131 (58.0) | 55 (49.1) | 76 (66.7) |
| Age, y | | | |
| 2-5 | 116 (51.3) | 63 (56.2) | 53 (46.5) |
| 6-12 | 110 (48.7) | 49 (43.8) | 61 (53.5) |
| Race | | | |
| White | 22 (9.7) | 9 (8.0) | 13 (11.4) |
| African American | 145 (64.2) | 71 (63.4) | 74 (64.9) |
| Other | 59 (26.1) | 32 (28.6) | 27 (23.7) |
| Hispanic | 67 (29.6) | 30 (26.8) | 37 (32.5) |
| Medicaid | 170 (75.2) | 81 (72.3) | 89 (78.1) |
| Caretaker age, y | | | |
| <30 | 124 (54.9) | 58 (51.8) | 66 (57.9) |
| ≥30 | 102 (45.1) | 54 (48.2) | 48 (42.1) |
| Caretaker education of high school or more | 142 (62.8) | 70 (62.5) | 72 (63.2) |
| Receiving a preventive medication | 134 (59.3) | 67 (59.8) | 67 (58.8) |
| Asthma severity | | | |
| Mild persistent | 48 (21.2) | 29 (25.9) | 19 (16.7) |
| Moderate persistent | 92 (40.7) | 45 (40.2) | 47 (41.2) |
| Severe persistent | 86 (38.1) | 38 (33.9) | 48 (42.1) |
| Reason for visit | | | |
| Asthma | 60 (26.5) | 31 (27.7) | 29 (25.4) |
| Well-child care | 75 (33.2) | 38 (33.9) | 37 (32.5) |
| Non–asthma-related illness care | 91 (40.3) | 43 (38.4) | 48 (42.1) |
| Usual health care provider | 109 (48.2) | 53 (47.3) | 56 (49.1) |
| ≥1 Smoker in home† | 105 (46.5) | 40 (35.7) | 65 (57.0) |

*Some percentages have been rounded.
†*P*<.05 for difference between groups.

**Table 2. Unadjusted Comparison of Preventive Measures in the Clinician-Prompting and Standard-Care Groups**

| Action | No. (%) of Patients Clinician-Prompting Group (n = 112) | Standard-Care Group (n = 114) | *P* Value* |
|---|---|---|---|
| Any preventive action | 97 (86.6) | 79 (69.3) | **.002** |
| Provision of an asthma action plan | 56 (50.0) | 27 (23.7) | **<.001** |
| Referral to a specialist | 5 (4.5) | 4 (3.5) | .75 |
| Treatment of a comorbid condition | 23 (20.5) | 17 (14.9) | .30 |
| Recommendation of a specific asthma follow-up visit | 60 (53.6) | 42 (36.8) | **.02** |
| Discussion regarding asthma | 84 (75.0) | 72 (63.2) | **.05** |
| Change in preventive medication | 46 (41.1) | 38 (33.3) | .27 |
| Smoke reduction counseling† | 23 (57.5) | 23 (35.4) | **.04** |

*Boldface type indicates a significant difference between groups.
†Limited to 105 participants exposed to secondhand smoke in the home (40 in the clinician-prompting group and 65 in the standard-care group).

**Table 2** shows the overall results of the intervention for the 226 children included in the analysis. The children in the clinician-prompting group were more likely to have any preventive action related to asthma taken at the visit compared with children in the standard-care group (86.6% vs 69.3%; *P*=.002). Specifically, visits for children in the clinician-prompting group were more likely to include the delivery of an action plan (50.0% vs 23.7%; *P*<.001), recommendation for a specific asthma follow-up visit (53.6% vs 36.8%; *P*=.02), and discussions regarding asthma (75.0% vs 63.2%; *P*=.05) compared with visits for children in the standard-care group. Among children with 1 or more smokers in the home (n=105), those in the clinician-prompting group received smoke reduction counseling more frequently than those in the standard-care group (57.5% vs 35.4%; *P*=.04). There were no statistical differences in referrals for specialist care, treatment of comorbid conditions, or changes in preventive medication between the 2 groups.

**Table 3** shows the results of the intervention stratified by type of office visit. Among the 60 children presenting for an asthma-related visit, there were no differences between the clinician-prompting and the standard-care groups, and preventive actions were taken for most of the children. The greatest effect of the intervention appeared to be for the 91 children presenting to the office for non–asthma-related illness care. For these children, 81.4% of those in the clinician-prompting group received any preventive action related to asthma, compared with 54.2% in the standard-care group (*P*=.007). The intervention also seemed to have some effect on those children presenting for well-child care, with more than twice as many children in the clinician-prompting group receiving an asthma action plan compared with children in the standard-care group (57.9% vs 27%; *P*<.01).

Almost all of the significant findings from the overall analysis remained statistically significant in multivariate regression analyses after we controlled for baseline asthma severity, provider characteristics, child demographic factors (age, sex, race, and ethnicity), and exposure to ETS (**Table 4**). In these analyses, children in the clinician-prompting group had 3-fold greater odds of having any preventive action taken at the visit compared with children in the standard-care group (odds ratio, 3.1; 95% confidence interval, 1.4-6.6).

## COMMENT

This study demonstrates that prompting clinicians about asthma severity and care guidelines at the time of an office visit results in improved preventive care delivery for inner-city children. Visits for the children in the clinician-prompting group were more likely to include discussions of asthma prevention, recommendations for specific asthma follow-up, and the delivery of an action plan at the time of the visit compared with visits for children receiving standard care. Prompting also improved smoke reduction counseling for patients whose households in-

**Table 3. Preventive Measures Stratified by Visit Type**

| | Type of Visit, No. (%) of Patients | | | | | |
|---|---|---|---|---|---|---|
| | Asthma Care (n = 60) | | Well-Child Care (n = 75) | | Non–Asthma-Related Illness Care (n = 91) | |
| Action | Clinician-Prompting Group (n = 31) | Standard-Care Group (n = 29) | Clinician-Prompting Group (n = 38) | Standard-Care Group (n = 37) | Clinician-Prompting Group (n = 43) | Standard-Care Group (n = 48) |
| Any preventive action | 30 (97) | 25 (86) | 32 (84) | 28 (76) | 35 (81) | 26 (54)† |
| Provision of an asthma action plan | 16 (52) | 10 (34) | 22 (58) | 10 (27)† | 18 (42) | 7 (15)† |
| Treatment of a comorbid condition | 8 (26) | 4 (14) | 7 (18) | 4 (11) | 8 (19) | 9 (19) |
| Recommendation of a specific asthma follow-up visit | 20 (65) | 12 (41) | 20 (53) | 18 (49) | 20 (47) | 12 (25)‡ |
| Discussion regarding asthma | 28 (90) | 24 (83) | 28 (74) | 27 (73) | 28 (65) | 21 (44) |
| Change in preventive medication | 12 (39) | 11 (38) | 19 (50) | 16 (43) | 15 (35) | 11 (23) |

*Some percentages have been rounded.
†$P<.01$ for the difference between groups.
‡$P<.05$ for the difference between groups.

cluded a smoker. The benefits of the intervention were seen primarily among children presenting for non–asthma-related illness care or for well-child care because most children presenting for asthma care received preventive actions regardless of their group allocation.

Although the intervention improved the delivery of preventive care, one could argue that a large percentage of the children in the clinician-prompting group still had no follow-up visit recommended (46.4%), received no action plan (50.0%), and had no discussions related to asthma (25.0%). In addition, we found no difference between groups with regard to a change in the prescription of preventive medications. In part, this may be because our symptom inquiry was restricted to the 2 weeks preceding the visit; thus, some providers may have interpreted the child's symptoms as a manifestation of viral respiratory infection rather than of persistent asthma. This would not necessarily warrant guideline-based preventive care.[30] The prompt was designed to serve as a screen for current persistent symptoms, not as a definitive diagnostic measure. In addition, because we considered actions taken during only 1 visit, it is possible that patients received a preventive intervention at a different visit.

Several studies[31-34] have evaluated other methods to improve preventive care delivery to inner-city children with asthma in the office setting. A few studies[23,32,35] have suggested that physician education regarding asthma management and quality improvement can improve adherence to care guidelines. However, Homer et al[36] recently evaluated a quality improvement educational intervention for asthma in primary care offices and found no significant effect on care for children with asthma. Lozano et al[34] evaluated a multilevel intervention involving clinician education regarding care guidelines combined with nurse-led case management. That combined intervention was effective in improving asthma care for subjects in the intervention group, including greater adherence to controller medications. However the clinician-education component of the intervention was not sufficient to yield significant benefit for the intervention group; the additional resources provided by a trained nurse clinician for individual case management were required. Novel methods to improve asthma care within the time demands and financial constraints of a primary care office are needed.

**Table 4. Impact of Intervention on Preventive Measures in Logistic Regression**

| Action | OR (95% CI)* | P Value† |
|---|---|---|
| Any preventive action | 3.1 (1.4-6.6) | **.004** |
| Provision of an asthma action plan | 4.0 (2.1-7.8) | **<.001** |
| Treatment of a comorbid condition | 1.4 (0.6-3.1) | .38 |
| Recommendation of a specific asthma follow-up visit | 2.3 (1.2-4.3) | **.009** |
| Discussion regarding asthma | 1.8 (0.9-3.3) | .08 |
| Change in preventive medication | 1.6 (0.9-3.0) | .12 |
| Smoke reduction counseling‡ | 3.0 (1.1-8.1) | **.03** |

Abbreviations: CI, confidence interval; OR, odds ratio.
*Indicates odds of action for children in the clinician-prompting group compared with children in the standard-care group, controlling for baseline asthma severity, type of health care provider, whether visit is with the child's usual health care provider, the child's demographic factors (age, sex, race, and ethnicity), and exposure to secondhand smoke in the home.
†Boldface type indicates a significant difference between groups.
‡Limited to 105 participants exposed to secondhand smoke in the home.

The concept of missed opportunities at an office visit implies that individuals eligible for a particular health-related intervention are seen for care but do not receive that particular intervention. Studies have focused on identifying and reducing missed opportunities during office visits for routine immunizations,[37,38] influenza immunization,[39-41] and screening and counseling for health risks.[42-44] Missed opportunities to improve asthma care are common[22,24] and, if exploited properly, can enhance preventive care within the context of the child's usual place for medical care.

The institution of symptom screening and prompting used in the present study is relatively simple and inexpensive and yielded a significant increase in the delivery of preventive care for children with persistent asthma. This type of intervention could be implemented into routine practice with the use of electronic medical records, which are increasingly available in many pediatric offices. On their arrival for an office visit, patients with asthma could be identified by codes from the *International Classification of Diseases, Ninth Revision*, and parents could enter the current symptom information into computerized templates. This information could be translated electronically into a prompt for the clinician as a computerized printout or a prompt on the screen of an examination room computer. Alternatively, in the absence of electronic medical records, one could design a manual system by using written forms and medical charts to establish symptoms, severity classification, and guideline recommendations. Forms could be given to the parent at the time he or she checks in for an appointment, completed in the waiting room by the parent, and delivered to the health care provider at the time of the visit. The translation of symptom information into the guideline recommendations would be facilitated by appropriately designed screening forms with simple algorithms for the provider. Such changes to the system of care would allow the clinician to avoid missed opportunities and to provide guideline-based asthma care within the context of a busy practice.

## LIMITATIONS

There are some potential limitations to this study. Blinding of parents and clinicians to the allocated treatment groups was not possible, and self-reported responses could have been biased. Furthermore, although the study team specifically asked the parents in the clinician-prompting group to give the prompt to their health care provider during the visit, this did not occur in all cases and thus may have led to an underestimation of the intervention effect.

Although physician education was not a key feature of the intervention, clinicians were oriented to the prompt and reminded of care guidelines before the start of the study. Because randomization was on the patient level rather than the clinician level, clinicians of patients in both treatment arms received this orientation. This may have served as a reminder to the clinicians to use guideline-based care and thus may have created a conservative bias, making differences between the 2 treatment groups more difficult to detect.

Medical chart review data often lack details of the clinical encounter[22,45]; thus, we may have missed some preventive care actions that occurred. However, we also used parent-reported data, which is more accurate in determining what happens at a visit.[45] The clinicians for children in the intervention group received a prompt during only 1 visit, and the prompt included only general recommendations based on the guidelines. Prompting at multiple visits with detailed recommendations tailored to individual patients (eg, suggesting specialist referrals for children with severe persistent asthma) may have yielded even more significant findings with improvements across additional areas of preventive care. Finally, only 2 urban clinics in Rochester were included in the study; thus, the findings can be generalized only to similar practice sites.

## IMPLICATIONS

This study demonstrates improved delivery of preventive care for urban children with asthma with the use of symptom-based clinician prompting in primary care offices. Because guideline-based care can improve asthma outcomes,[5-10] the potential implications of these findings are great. In addition, because urban children are at highest risk for receiving suboptimal care, incorporating such a method of systematic screening and prompting into routine visits for these children may substantially reduce asthma morbidity.

**Accepted for Publication:** May 27, 2006.
**Correspondence:** Jill S. Halterman, MD, MPH, Department of Pediatrics, University of Rochester School of Medicine and Dentistry, PO Box 777, 601 Elmwood Ave, Rochester, NY 14642 (jill_halterman@urmc.rochester.edu).
**Author Contributions:** Dr Halterman had full access to all of the data in the study and takes responsibility for the integrity of the data and the accuracy of the data analysis. *Study concept and design:* Halterman, Fisher, and Szilagyi. *Acquisition of data:* Halterman, Conn, Fagnano, Lynch, and Marky. *Analysis and interpretation of data:* Halterman, Fisher, Conn, and Szilagyi. *Drafting of the manuscript:* Halterman, Fagnano, and Lynch. *Critical revision of the manuscript for important intellectual content:* Halterman, Fisher, Conn, Marky, and Szilagyi. *Statistical analysis:* Fisher and Conn. *Obtained funding:* Halterman. *Administrative, technical, and material support:* Conn, Fagnano, and Lynch. *Study supervision:* Szilagyi.
**Funding/Support:** The study was supported by grants from the Halcyon Hill Foundation and the Robert Wood Johnson Foundation's Generalist Physician Faculty Scholars Program.
**Acknowledgment:** We thank George B. Segel, MD, for his insightful review of the manuscript.

## REFERENCES

1. Newacheck PW, Halfon N. Prevalence, impact and trends in childhood disability due to asthma. *Arch Pediatr Adolesc Med.* 2000;154:287-293.
2. Mannino DM, Homa DM, Akinbami LJ, Moorman JE, Gwynn C, Redd SC. Surveillance for asthma: United States, 1980-1999. *MMWR Surveill Summ.* 2002; 51(1):1-13.
3. National Asthma Education and Prevention Program. *Expert Panel Report: Guidelines for the Diagnosis and Management of Asthma*. Bethesda, Md: National Institutes of Health; 1991. Publication 91-3642.
4. National Asthma Education and Prevention Program. *Expert Panel Report 2: Guidelines for the Diagnosis and Management of Asthma*. Bethesda, Md: National Institutes of Health; 1997. Publication 97-4051.
5. National Asthma Education Program. *Expert Panel Report II: Guidelines for the Diagnosis and Management of Asthma—Update on Selected Topics 2002.* Bethesda, Md: US Dept of Health and Human Services, National Institutes of Health; 2002. Publication 02-5075.
6. Suissa S, Ernst P, Benayoun S, Baltzan M, Cai B. Low-dose inhaled corticosteroids and the prevention of death from asthma. *N Engl J Med.* 2000;343:332-336.
7. Donahue JG, Weiss S, Livingston J, Goetsch M, Greineder D, Platt R. Inhaled steroids and the risk of hospitalization for asthma. *JAMA.* 1997;277:887-891.
8. Kelly CS, Morrow AL, Shults J, Nakas N, Strope GL, Adelman RD. Outcomes evaluation of a comprehensive intervention program for asthmatic children enrolled in Medicaid. *Pediatrics.* 2000;105:1029-1035.
9. Guevara JP, Wolf FM, Crum CM, Clark NM. Effects of educational interventions for self management of asthma in children and adolescents: systematic review and meta-analysis. *BMJ.* 2003;326:1308-1309.

10. Schatz M, Zeiger RS, Mosen M, et al. Improved asthma outcomes from allergy specialist care: a population-based cross-sectional analysis. *J Allergy Clin Immunol.* 2005;116:1307-1313.
11. Cabana MD, Ebel B, Cooper-Patrick L, Powe N, Rubin H, Rand C. Barriers pediatricians face when using asthma practice guidelines. *Arch Pediatr Adolesc Med.* 2000;154:685-693.
12. Diette GB, Skinner E, Markson L, et al. Consistency of care with national guidelines for children with asthma in managed care. *J Pediatr.* 2001;138:59-64.
13. Halterman JS, Yoos HL, Kaczorowski JM, et al. Providers underestimate symptom severity among urban children with asthma. *Arch Pediatr Adolesc Med.* 2002;156:141-146.
14. Roghmann MC, Sexton M. Adherence to asthma guidelines in general practice. *J Asthma.* 1999;36:381-387.
15. Finkelstein JA, Lozano P, Shulruff R, et al. Self-reported physician practices for children with asthma: are national guidelines being followed? *Pediatrics.* 2000;106:886-896.
16. Carr W, Zeitel L, Weiss K. Variations in asthma hospitalizations and deaths in New York City. *Am J Public Health.* 1992;82:59-65.
17. Weiss KB, Wagener DK. Changing patterns of asthma mortality: identifying target populations at high risk. *JAMA.* 1990;264:1683-1687.
18. Akinbami LJ, Schoendorf KC. Trends in childhood asthma: prevalence, health care utilization, and mortality. *Pediatrics.* 2002;110:315-322.
19. Kattan M, Mitchell H, Eggleston P, et al. Characteristics of inner-city children with asthma: the National Cooperative Inner-City Asthma Study. *Pediatr Pulmonol.* 1997;24:253-262.
20. Eggleston PA, Malveaux FJ, Butz AM, et al. Medications used by children with asthma living in the inner city. *Pediatrics.* 1998;101:349-354.
21. Warman KL, Silver EJ, McCourt MP, Stein REK. How does home management of asthma exacerbation by parents of inner-city children differ from NHLBI guideline recommendations? *Pediatrics.* 1999;103:422-427.
22. Cabana MD, Bruckman D, Meister K, Bradley FJ, Clark N. Documentation of asthma severity in pediatric outpatient clinics. *Clin Pediatr (Phila).* 2003;42:121-125.
23. Moonie SA, Strunk FC, Crocker S, Curtis V, Schechtman K, Castro M. Community asthma program improves appropriate prescribing in moderate to severe asthma. *J Asthma.* 2005;42:281-289.
24. Tsuyuki RT, Sin DD, Sharpe HM, et al. Management of asthma among community-based primary care physicians. *J Asthma.* 2005;42:163-167.
25. Cabana MD, Rand C, Powe N, Wu A, Abboud P, Rubin H. Why don't physicians follow clinical practice guidelines? a framework for improvement. *JAMA.* 1999;282:1458-1465.
26. Harris RP, O'Malley MS, Fletcher SW, Knight BP. Prompting physicians for preventive procedures: a five-year study of manual and computer reminders. *Am J Prev Med.* 1990;6:145-152.
27. Minkovitz CS, Belote AD, Higman SM, Serwint JR, Weiner JP. Effectiveness of practice-based intervention to increase vaccination rates and reduce missed opportunities. *Arch Pediatr Adolesc Med.* 2001;155:382-386.
28. Chang HC, Zimmerman LH, Beck JM. Impact of chart reminders on smoking cessation practices of pulmonary physicians. *Am J Respir Crit Care Med.* 1995;152:984-987.
29. Halterman JS, McConnochie KM, Conn KM, et al. A randomized trial of provider prompting to enhance preventive asthma therapy. *Arch Pediatr Adolesc Med.* 2005;159:422-427.
30. Weinberger M. Consensus statement from a conference on treatment of viral respiratory infection–induced asthma in young children. *J Pediatr.* 2003;142:S45-S46.
31. Premaratne UN, Sterne JA, Marks C, Webb GB, Burney RJ. Clustered randomized trial of an intervention to improve management of asthma: Greenwich asthma study. *BMJ.* 1999;318:1251-1255.
32. Clark NM, Gong M, Schork A, et al. Impact of education for physicians on patient outcomes. *Pediatrics.* 1998;101:831-836.
33. Evans D, Mellins R, Lobach K, et al. Improving care for minority children with asthma: professional education in public health clinics. *Pediatrics.* 1997;99:157-164.
34. Lozano P, Finkelstein JA, Carey VJ, et al. A multi-site randomized trial of the effects of physician education and organizational change in chronic asthma care: health outcomes of the Pediatric Asthma Care PORT study. *Arch Pediatr Adolesc Med.* 2004;158:875-883.
35. Brown R, Bratton SL, Cabana MD, Kaciroti N, Clark NM. Physician asthma education program improves outcomes for children of low-income families. *Chest.* 2004;126:369-374.
36. Homer CJ, Forbes P, Horvitz SM, Peterson LE, Wypij D, Heinrich P. Impact of a quality improvement program on care and outcomes for children with asthma. *Arch Pediatr Adolesc Med.* 2005;159:464-469.
37. Szilagyi PG, Rodewald LE. Missed opportunities for immunizations: a review of the evidence. *J Public Health Manag Pract.* 1996;2:18-25.
38. Santoli JM, Szilagyi PG, Rodewald LE. Barriers to immunization and missed opportunities. *Pediatr Ann.* 1998;27:366-374.
39. Daley MF, Beaty BL, Barrow J, et al. Missed opportunities for influenza vaccination in children with chronic medical conditions. *Arch Pediatr Adolesc Med.* 2005;159:986-991.
40. Szilagyi PG, Rodewald LE, Savageau J, Yoos L, Doane C. Improving influenza vaccination rates in children with asthma: a test of a computerized reminder system and an analysis of factors predicting vaccination compliance. *Pediatrics.* 1992;90:871-875.
41. Kramarz P, DeStefano F, Gargiullo PM, et al; Vaccine Safety Datalink Team. Influenza vaccination in children with asthma in health maintenance organizations. *Vaccine.* 2000;18:2288-2294.
42. Petersen R, Clark KA, Hartmann KE, Melvin CL. Getting focused: missed opportunities for smoking interventions for pregnant women receiving Medicaid. *Prev Med.* 2005;40:209-215.
43. Coups EJ, Gaba A, Orleans CT. Physician screening for multiple behavioral health risk factors. *Am J Prev Med.* 2004;27:34-41.
44. Liddicoat RV, Horton NJ, Urban R, Maier E, Christiansen D, Samet JH. Assessing missed opportunities for HIV testing in medical settings. *J Gen Intern Med.* 2004;19:349-356.
45. Senturia YD, Bauman LJ, Coyle YM, et al. The use of parent report to assess the quality of care in primary care visits among children with asthma. *Ambul Pediatr.* 2001;1:194-200.

# Adolescent Bone Health

*Keith J. Loud, MDCM, MSc; Catherine M. Gordon, MD, MSc*

Pediatric and adolescent care professionals have increasingly recognized the importance of understanding the skeletal health of their patients. Peak bone mass, the "bone bank" on which an individual will draw for their entire adult life, is likely achieved by late adolescence, with the critical window for accumulation occurring much earlier. This review outlines the known conditions that are associated with impaired bone mineral accrual and clinical settings in which the evaluation of "at-risk" adolescents should be considered. We describe the methods available to the health care professional for evaluating bone density, along with the limitations of each technology. Potential therapeutic options for patients identified to have a low bone mineral density are discussed. Finally, current recommendations regarding physical activity and nutrition, beneficial interventions for all adolescents, are presented.

*Arch Pediatr Adolesc Med. 2006;160:1026-1032*

## BONE ACQUISITION IN ADOLESCENCE

Peak bone mass (PBM) is one of the most significant predictors of postmenopausal osteoporosis[1,2] and is likely achieved early in the third decade of life.[3,4] At least 26% of adult total bone mineral is acquired during the 4-year period surrounding peak height velocity,[5,6] with up to 60% acquired during the remaining peripubertal years.[7,8] Addressing modifiable risk factors (**Figure 1**) that may predispose to a low bone mass during this critical window for bone accrual could therefore prevent future osteoporosis,[10] a major national public health goal.

### Physical Activity

It has long been observed that immobilized and other non–weight-bearing individuals (eg, astronauts) rapidly lose bone mass, suggesting the importance of skeletal loading for bone health.[11] Classic studies in animal models have demonstrated that bone mineral acquisition requires forces that vary in intensity and are dynamic.[12] Two recent comprehensive literature reviews by expert panels in which both retrospective and prospective studies were evaluated concluded that adult bone mass is positively correlated with childhood activity and that most clinical trials of exercise interventions confirm a positive association between activity and the bone health of children, adolescents, and adults.[13,14] The benefits are noted to be "site specific," meaning that the response of the skeleton varies depending on the type of exercise studied (eg, weight bearing),[15] and may also be modified by nutritional factors.[16]

### Nutrition

Interest and controversy surround the effects of nutritional factors on bone density and bone accretion during adolescence.[16,17] Within a healthy weight range, there is a direct, positive relationship between body mass index (calculated as weight in kilograms divided by height in meters squared) and bone mineral den-

**Author Affiliations:** Divisions of Adolescent Medicine and Sports Medicine, Children's Hospital Medical Center of Akron, Akron, Ohio (Dr Loud); and Divisions of Adolescent Medicine and Endocrinology, Children's Hospital Boston, Boston, Mass (Dr Gordon).

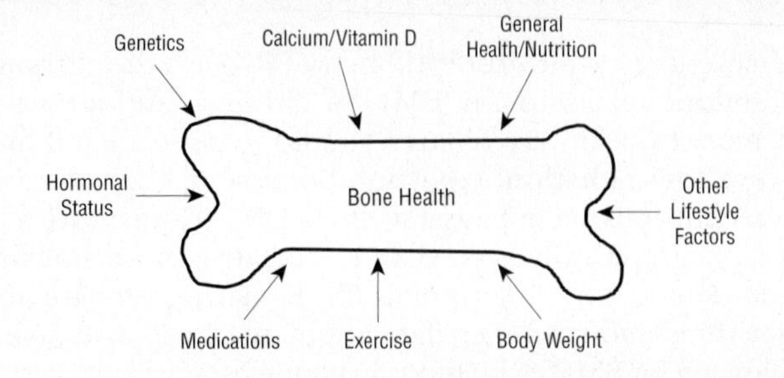


**Figure 1.** Factors affecting bone health. Reprinted with permission.[9]

sity (BMD).[18] Recent studies have demonstrated that overweight children have an increased incidence of fractures, suggesting a deleterious effect of excess adiposity on skeletal development and resilience.[16,19] At the other end of the spectrum, illnesses that are characterized by weight loss, such as anorexia nervosa, illustrate the detrimental effect of malnutrition on bone density in teenagers.[20-23] Questions have arisen regarding the applicability of findings from such studies of malnourished youth with chronic disease to the bone health of well adolescents. In particular, the skeletal effects of calcium and vitamin D in all children and adolescents is an issue that has received attention in many recent reports, including a position statement by the American Academy of Pediatrics.[16,24-30]

The effect of calcium intake during adolescence is one of the most intensely studied areas of pediatric bone health. Calcium is needed for normal mineralization of the bone and cartilage matrix. Once calcium intake is adequate to prevent rickets (disordered organization of the cartilage matrix) or osteomalacia (defective bone mineralization), provision of additional calcium may increase bone density by affecting bone turnover and the size of the remodeling space.[30,31] Controversy arises because some, but not all, studies of calcium intake and measures of bone health show a positive relationship.[24] However, because adolescence is the most critical period for bone mineral accrual, experts currently advocate for the provision of optimal calcium intake to maximize peak bone mass.[16,17] These recommendations are driven by the fact that calcium absorption is known to be enhanced during puberty,[6,32,33] with an optimal calcium balance achieved at an intake of approximately 1300 mg/d.[34] Few data are available regarding the appropriate intake level for racial groups other than white adolescents.[16] One study showed that compared with white adolescent girls, black teenagers exhibit more efficient calcium absorption and may achieve the same PBM with less calcium intake.[35] Because of the potential skeletal benefits of calcium, it is concerning that the majority of adolescents fail to achieve the recommended daily intake.[16,36]

Several research papers and policy statements have also examined the role of vitamin D, which is needed for efficient bodily absorption of calcium, on the bone health of children and adolescents. Vitamin D deficiency has been linked to fracture and a low bone mass in elderly men and women.[37-41] Recent research has documented vitamin D deficiency to be a common problem among otherwise

Chronic medical conditions (multifactorial etiologies)
- Prolonged immobilization
- Anorexia nervosa
- Asthma
- Celiac disease
- Cerebral palsy and other neuromuscular conditions
- Chronic renal failure
- Cranial irradiation (particularly pituitary)
- Cystic fibrosis*
- Diabetes mellitus
- Epilepsy
- Human immunodeficiency virus infection
- Inflammatory bowel disease
- Malignancies
- Organ transplantation (solid and bone marrow)
- Rheumatologic diseases
- Sickle cell disease
- Thalassemia
- Turner syndrome

Specific endocrinopathies
- Cushing syndrome (hypercortisolemia)
- Growth hormone deficiency
- Hyperthyroidism
- Hyperparathyroidism
- Hyperprolactinemia
- Hypopituitarism
- Hypothyroidism
- Sex hormone deficiency/hypogonadism (acquired or genetic)

Medications (medium- to long-term use)
- Anticonvulsants
- Glucocorticoids
- Cyclosporine A
- Gonadotropin-releasing hormone agonists
- Heparin
- Lithium
- Depot medroxyprogesterone acetate
- Methotrexate
- Other chemotherapeutic agents

Deleterious behaviors
- Female athlete triad,* defined as the interrelationship among disordered eating, amenorrhea, and osteoporosis in female athletes competing in activities that emphasize a lean physique
- Excessive alcohol consumption
- Tobacco use

**Figure 2.** Clinical settings that potentially confer skeletal "risk" to adolescents. * Indicates that an official position statement has been published (cystic fibrosis[44]; female athlete triad[45]).

healthy young patients, including adolescents,[27-29] but have not definitively correlated this deficiency with decreased bone density in youth, often because of the lack of BMD measurements in some studies.

## Hormonal Status

A number of hormones affect bone formation and remodeling. Endogenous circulating estrogens and androgens exert independently positive effects on bone growth, development, and mineral acquisition among both male and female adolescents.[42,43] Patients with hormonal deficiencies or receptor abnormalities demonstrate lower than expected BMD.[18] Similarly, growth hormone deficiency negatively impacts bone size and mass.[18] Other endocrinopathies (**Figure 2**) affect the bone remodeling cycle by influencing osteoclasts and osteoblasts directly (eg, thyroid or parathyroid hormone, cortisol) or indirectly via their effects on the sex steroids (eg, hyperprolactinemia, hypopituitarism). Finally, ongoing studies are investigating the role of leptin as a primary or secondary messenger that modulates bone remodeling.[46]

## General Health and Genetics

In addition to exercise, proper nutrition, and maintaining a normal hormonal milieu, avoidance of excessive alcohol and any tobacco use is beneficial to bone health.[18] The vast majority, between 60% and 80%, of the variance in PBM can be attributed to inherited and, likely, polygenetic factors,[47] including putative, but unproven, receptor polymorphisms for vitamin D, estrogen, type I collagen, insulin-like growth factor I, transforming growth factor-β, and IL-6.[18]

## WHICH PATIENTS ARE AT RISK FOR POOR SKELETAL HEALTH?

Important conditions that are currently believed to place adolescents at risk for poor skeletal health—other than intrinsic bone diseases such as osteogenesis imperfecta—are listed in Figure 2. Some diseases (such as cystic fibrosis and inflammatory bowel disease) are associated with increased secretion of proinflammatory cytokines such as IL-1β, tumor necrosis factor α, and IL-6 that may directly inflict harm to the skeleton by increasing bone resorption.[48,49] Many of these illnesses also require use of medications with deleterious skeletal effects (Figure 2). Finally, any condition that negatively affects the factors described previously (Figure 1) could impair bone mineral accrual.

Although the concept of "athletic amenorrhea" and its detrimental skeletal effects had been described earlier,[50,51] it was not until 1992 that the term *female athlete triad* was coined (definition in Figure 2).[45] Estimates of the prevalence of the triad have varied dramatically depending on the population studied[18]; it may remain elusive until, as some experts have recommended, the skeletal component "osteoporosis" is redefined to allow for a more meaningful assessment in young athletes.[52] While the earlier term implicated the stress of exercise to be the cause of menstrual irregularity and a consequent hypoestrogenic state, more recent work has demonstrated that even subtle imbalances between caloric intake and energy expenditure alter luteinizing hormone pulsatility and amplitude, triggering the cascade that results in luteal phase defects or frank hypothalamic amenorrhea.[53] Those who exhibit the female athlete triad may be at increased risk for stress fracture,[54] but it is yet to be determined if this injury is a sentinel event for low BMD, warranting further evaluation.

## HOW TO EVALUATE SKELETAL STATUS

### Measures of BMD

Bone mineral density has been the most commonly used outcome measure to address skeletal status because bone mass predicts 80% to 90% of its strength in vitro,[11] which translates into a high predictive value for osteoporotic fractures in postmenopausal women.[55,56] Among children and adolescents, the association is not as strong, although the majority of case-control studies of healthy children suggest that the BMD *z* score (number of standard deviations higher or lower than the mean of peers matched for age, sex, and ethnicity) is predictive of fractures of the distal forearm (the most common fracture site during the pubertal growth spurt), with each standard deviation decrease from the mean significantly associated with an increased risk.[56] The relationship is less clear among children and adolescents with chronic illness.[56]

### Dual-Energy X-ray Absorptiometry (DXA)

Dual-energy x-ray absorptiometry (DXA) is the current standard for assessing BMD in children and adolescents. The scans are relatively rapid to perform and involve low radiation exposure. Because of their use in screening postmenopausal women, DXA scanners are often geographically accessible to pediatric professionals and demonstrate high precision. Pediatric software algorithms and reference data are increasingly available, allowing for BMD evaluations in young patients from early childhood up through adolescence.[57,58] Using x-ray beams at 2 photon energies to differentiate soft tissue from bone, DXA can measure bone mineral content (in grams) and areal BMD—a 2-dimensional measurement of bone mineral per unit of area (grams divided by centimeters squared)—and estimate total body lean vs fat mass.

There are several caveats that arise as DXA is used in adolescents. A pediatric normative database must be used to interpret properly the measurement for either bone mineral content or BMD. The normative data must have been generated on a similar instrument[58,59] and should account for sex[58] and ethnicity,[60,61] as each can influence bone mass. Since the *z* score is based on chronologic age, "correcting" the BMD for an adolescent with a delayed bone age (interpreting for that age) can be a helpful maneuver to avoid the overestimation of skeletal deficits.[17,62] Even with appropriately matched databases and age adjustment, DXA does not adequately account for the influence of bone shape and size on its measurements.[17,63-65] In essence, DXA estimates bone mineral content by measuring the "shadow" cast by bone within a fan-shaped x-ray beam. This shadow is influenced not only by the composition of the bone, but its depth, which is not measured, and the distance of the bone from the beam.[63,66] Attempts to correct for these limitations include obtaining 2 orthogonal scans (ie, anteroposterior and lateral), mathematical formulas to estimate volumetric BMD (eg, bone mineral apparent density),[67,68] and more advanced regression models,[69,70] none of which have been adopted uniformly. The bones of an adolescent are also changing continuously because of growth, which only further complicates the BMD interpretation.

In recognition of these challenges, a 2004 position statement of the International Society for Clinical Densitometry issued guidance for the use of DXA in the diagnosis of osteoporosis in children[56] (**Table 1**). Perhaps the most pertinent recommendation was that T scores, which compare bone density to PBM (assumed to occur between ages 20-29 years) and which are the basis of the World Health Organization definition of postmenopausal osteoporosis, should not appear in DXA reports for children and adolescents. Therefore, the diagnosis of osteoporosis in children requires evidence of skeletal fragility; it should not be made based on DXA measurements alone.[56]

### Quantitative Computed Tomography

The current "gold standard" for noninvasive bone evaluation is quantitative computed tomography (QCT), which can evaluate bone in 3 dimensions, thereby providing a direct measure of "true" volumetric BMD (in grams per centimeters cubed).[71] Differentiating cortical from trabecular bone, QCT can also precisely track the pubertal changes in bone size and shape that occur during adolescence.[72] Performed on standard computed tomography scanners, QCT requires specific software algorithms that are not widely available, in part because of cost. The greatest drawback to QCT is its moderately high radiation dose. As a consequence, normative pediatric data are sparse, with their use reserved predominantly for research. Peripheral QCT, which only evaluates BMD of the extremities, uses much lower radiation doses than those associated with axial QCT but is hindered by the same factors.[73]

### Ultrasound

Quantitative ultrasound is attractive in that it involves no radiation exposure, is portable, and potentially allows for inexpensive, office-based bone health screening.[74] Unfortunately, not all quantitative ultrasound devices are appropriately sized for use in children and younger adolescents, and most devices do not have adequate normative pediatric databases.[75] Furthermore, correlation with BMD as measured by DXA or QCT has been inconsistent. Further research is needed to determine if this technique captures intrinsic qualities of bone (eg, elasticity, trabecular separation) that are not detected by other modalities but still may affect fracture risk.[76,77]

### Assessment of Bone Strength

One of the most clinically relevant properties of bone is its strength, which is dependent not only on bone mass, but size, geometry, and microarchitecture. Quantitative computed tomography is able to measure all of these parameters and is capable of generating numeric estimates of bone strength.[78] Magnetic resonance imaging is also being investigated as a radiation-free modality to evaluate both bone geometry and quality,[79] and there are mathematical models that use DXA data to estimate bone strength at the hip (ie, hip structural analysis).[80]

### Measurement of Bone Turnover

Serum and urinary markers of bone turnover are sensitive to changes in bone formation and resorption. They are increasingly available for clinical use in reference laboratories, but normal growth and development during adolescence increase the variability in these measures such that their use should be restricted to monitoring treatment effects, not diagnosis.[17] Common measures of calcium homeostasis such as serum calcium, magnesium, phosphorus, 25-hydroxyvitamin D, parathyroid hormone, and urinary spot calcium-creatinine ratio do not directly reflect bone turnover. They may be useful, however, when evaluating low BMD, but only to complement thorough medical, menstrual, and family histories; a complete review of systems; and a directed objective examination, including body mass index calculation and Tanner staging. Finally, bone biopsy to obtain computer-assisted histomorphometric information may rarely be requested by skeletal health specialists for particularly challenging cases.[17]

**Table 1. Guidance on Dual-Energy X-ray Absorptiometry Interpretation in Children and Adolescents Younger Than 20 Years***

| |
|---|
| Only *z* scores, which compare BMD with age- and sex-matched peers, should be used. |
| T scores, which compare BMD with the PBM of healthy young adults aged 20-29 years, should not be used and should not appear in reports or on dual-energy x-ray absorptiometry printouts. |
| The diagnosis of osteoporosis should not be made on the basis of densitometric criteria alone. |
| Terms such as *low bone density for chronologic age* or *below the expected range for age* may be used if the *z* score is lower than −2.0; use of the term *osteopenia* is discouraged. |
| Spine and total body are the preferred skeletal sites for measurements. |
| The value of BMD to predict fractures in children and adolescents is not clearly determined. |
| Adjustments made to BMD or BMC for bone size, pubertal stage, skeletal maturity, or body composition should be clearly stated in the report; there is no agreement on standards for such adjustments. |
| Serial BMD studies should be done on the same machine using the same scanning mode, software, and analysis. |

Abbreviations: BMC, bone mineral content; BMD, bone mineral density; PBM, peak bone mass.

*Modified from the International Society for Clinical Densitometry Position Development Conference[3] (http://www.iscd.org/Visitors/positions/OfficialPositionsText.cfm).

## WHEN SHOULD ONE CONSIDER A BONE DENSITY MEASUREMENT?

At the present time, no evidence-based clinical guidelines exist to help health care professionals determine when BMD screening is warranted, although a number of groups have published recommendations. The Cystic Fibrosis Foundation recently published an official position regarding bone health[44] including an assessment and treatment protocol with baseline DXA scans obtained as young as 8 years. The British Paediatric and Adolescent Bone Group has also published guidelines for bone density screening and treatment in adolescents who they consider to be at risk, including those who have sustained recurrent fractures or a low-impact fracture, back pain, spinal deformity, loss of height, or a change in mobility or nutrition.[73] The varied recommendations of these and other groups reflect the fundamental uncertainty over what constitutes a "fracture threshold" for children and adolescents at this time. Our clinical practice is to consider DXA scanning for an adolescent who has an underlying chronic condition that predisposes to a low BMD (Figure 2), with the presence of multiple risk factors or a strong family history of osteoporosis lowering our threshold for evaluation.

An example of the complexity of the decisions facing health care professionals regarding appropriate BMD screening practices is the debate stimulated by the recent Food and Drug Administration decision to issue a "black box" warning label on depot medroxyprogesterone acetate because of bone loss attributable to this agent.[81,82] There is some evidence to suggest that adoles-

**Table 2. Recommended Dietary Intake of Calcium for Adolescents in the United States***

| Age, y | Calcium AI, mg/d |
|---|---|
| 9-18 | 1300 |
| 19-50 | 1000 |

Abbreviation: AI, adequate intake (used if sufficient scientific evidence is not available to derive a recommended daily allowance).
*Adapted from the Institute of Medicine and Food and Nutrition Board.[34]

cents regain bone density after discontinuing depot medroxyprogesterone acetate use,[81,83] so the advantages of short-term use generally outweigh theoretical safety concerns regarding fracture risk in this population. However, the World Health Organization has stated that data are currently insufficient to determine if this also applies to long-term use of this agent, especially in adolescent girls.[82] As with other at-risk adolescents, the decision to obtain a bone density measurement should be individualized, taking into account other potential risk factors for a low bone mass. More information will become available from continued research, both in depot medroxyprogesterone acetate users and other patient groups, to afford information regarding appropriate and evidence-based practice algorithms for this agent and other areas of pediatric bone health.

## USE OF SKELETAL AGENTS IN ADOLESCENTS

There are few skeletal agents (medications designed to augment BMD by either inhibiting bone resorption and/or increasing bone formation) available for potential use in adolescents. The unknown effects of some of these medications on a growing skeleton and the disappointing efficacy of others has hindered their use by pediatric professionals. Bisphosphonates are prescribed commonly to adults for postmenopausal and glucocorticoid-induced osteoporosis and offer a life-changing therapy for children with osteogenesis imperfecta[84-87] and low bone mass and fractures secondary to cerebral palsy.[88] With the exception of recent information on oral alendronate sodium,[89] there is little experience with agents other than intravenous pamidronate for these diagnoses.[84-88] Nonetheless, given the apparent positive tolerability of bisphosphonates in these populations, there is interest in expanding their use to indications for which efficacy is currently unknown. For example, alendronate sodium and risedronate sodium have been investigated in small studies of adolescents and young women with anorexia nervosa.[90,91] Information is lacking on the long-term (>10 years) adverse effects of these agents, optimal duration of treatment, or appropriate maximal dose. Because it is known that bisphosphonates remain in the skeleton for several years, perhaps indefinitely, and that they cross the placenta, health care professionals should proceed with caution until more definitive safety and efficacy data are available.

The role of estrogen and/or progestin therapy in adolescent girls with anorexia nervosa or hypothalamic amenorrhea is yet another area of both controversy and active investigation.[20,92] Several reports have documented no significant change in BMD in this group after estrogen therapy, often provided in the form of an oral contraceptive.[21,93,94] Some subgroups of patients may be protected from bone loss with this therapy, especially young women with an extremely low body mass index (<70% of ideal body weight).[93] The balance of data from several research studies suggests that the lack of efficacy of estrogen therapy in this population is because the observed bone loss may be attributable to other abnormalities beyond that of estrogen deficiency. Recent studies have explored the roles of insulin-like growth factor I,[95] alone or in concert with an oral contraceptive,[96] and androgen therapy (dehydroepiandrosterone[21] and transdermal testosterone[97]).

## POTENTIALLY BENEFICIAL INTERVENTIONS FOR ALL ADOLESCENTS

### Physical Activity

If physical activity is to be prescribed for bone mineral accrual, the questions to be answered include "how" and "when"? MacKelvie et al[98] suggest that the benefits of exercise may be most pronounced in premenarchal girls experiencing their peak height velocity and boys in comparably early puberty, or ages 10 to 12 years in girls and 12 to 14 years in boys, on average. MacKelvie et al[98] call for further research to clarify this "critical window" for bone accretion, as well as to determine whether benefits persist into adulthood. Another important area of inquiry in this field includes the interaction between physical activity and hormonal status, particularly the effect of estrogen status on bone mass in young women. Finally, the optimal types and duration of exercise have yet to be defined, leaving the American College of Sports Medicine, in its recent position stand on "Physical Activity and Bone Health," unable to outline a prescription more detailed than high-intensity impact activities (such as running, jumping, gymnastics, or basketball) for 10 to 20 minutes, at least 3 days per week.[13]

### Nutrition

The minimal amount of calcium that results in bone accretion is unclear, and the effect of calcium intake also varies by skeletal site, with cortical bone appearing to respond more significantly than trabecular bone.[30] Recommendations for teenagers are further complicated by the fact that the skeletal effects of calcium may be dependent on the level of physical activity.[99] However, the best available evidence was summarized by the National Academy of Sciences in 1997 to produce the dietary reference intake ranges (**Table 2**).[34]

In 2003, the American Academy of Pediatrics adopted the National Academy of Sciences recommendation that all children from infancy to adolescence receive 200 IU of vitamin D supplementation daily, a policy that has been met with some controversy.[29] This recommendation was reiterated in the recent position statement by the American Academy of Pediatrics on bone health.[16] In addition, the appropriate supplementation requirement for certain adolescents who may be at higher risk for this deficiency (eg, African American adolescents, those residing in northern latitudes) is currently unknown but is likely significantly greater than the American Academy of Pediatrics recommendation. Provision of larger doses (eg, 800-1000 IU) may be needed for these groups, especially during winter. There is a critical need to reconvene an expert panel to evaluate the dietary reference intake for vitamin D for young patients.

## CONCLUSIONS

Adolescence is the most critical period across the life span for bone health because more than half of PBM is accumulated during the teenage years. Recent and ongoing studies have highlighted the increasing number of clinical settings in which an adolescent may potentially lose bone density and are beginning to fill gaps in knowledge regarding the roles of physical activity and calcium and vitamin D intake in healthy adolescents, as well as the appropriate use of pharmacologic skeletal agents in those with chronic illness. Unfortunately, research has not yet generated evidence to identify appropriate candidates for both baseline bone density screening and continued monitoring. Nonetheless, although there still seem to be more questions than answers in this new field, adolescent health care professionals are on the cusp of an exciting era in which they can have a major role in improving the skeletal health of our nation.

**Accepted for Publication:** April 20, 2006.
**Correspondence:** Catherine M. Gordon, MD, MSc, Children's Hospital Bone Health Program, Children's Hospital Boston, 300 Longwood Ave, Boston, MA 02115 (catherine.gordon@childrens.harvard.edu).
**Author Contributions:** *Study concept and design:* Loud and Gordon. *Drafting of the manuscript:* Loud and Gordon. *Critical revision of the manuscript for important intellectual content*: Loud and Gordon. *Administrative, technical, and material support:* Loud. *Study supervision:* Gordon.
**Funding/Support:** This work was supported in part by National Institutes of Health grant RO1 HD 043869 and project 5 T71-MC-00009-14 00 from the Maternal and Child Health Bureau (Title V, Social Security Act), Health Resources and Services Administration, Department of Health and Human Services.

## REFERENCES

1. Hui SL, Slemenda CW, Johnston CC. The contribution of bone loss of postmenopausal osteoporosis. *Osteoporos Int.* 1990;1:30-34.
2. Seeman E. Reduced bone density in women with fractures: contribution of low peak bone density and rapid bone loss. *Osteoporos Int.* 1994;4(suppl 1):15-25.
3. Ferretti JL. On new opportunities for absorptiometry. *J Clin Densitom.* 1998;1:41-53.
4. Henry YM, Fatayerji D, Eastell R. Attainment of peak bone mass at the lumbar spine, femoral neck, and radius in men and women: relative contributions of bone size and volumetric bone mineral density. *Osteoporos Int.* 2004;15:263-273.
5. Bailey DA. The Saskatchewan Pediatric Bone Mineral Accrual Study: bone mineral acquisition during the growing years. *Int J Sports Med.* 1997;18(suppl 3):S191-S194.
6. Bailey DA, Martin AD, McKay HA, et al. Calcium accretion in girls and boys during puberty: a longitudinal analysis. *J Bone Miner Res.* 2000;15:2245-2250.
7. Bonjour JP, Thientz G, Buchs B, et al. Critical years and stages of puberty for spinal and femoral bone mass accumulation during adolescence. *J Clin Endocrinol Metab.* 1991;73:555-563.
8. Theintz G, Buchs G, Rizzoli R, et al. Longitudinal monitoring of bone mass accumulation in healthy adolescents: evidence for a marked reduction after 16 years of age at the levels of lumbar spine and femoral neck in female subjects. *J Clin Endocrinol Metab.* 1992;75:1060-1065.
9. Loud KJ, Gordon CM. Bone and nutrition in health and disease. *International Seminars in Pediatric Gastroenterology and Nutrition.* 2002;11:1-7.
10. Etherington J, Harris PA, Nandra D, et al. The effect of weightbearing exercise on bone mineral density: a study of female ex-athletes and the general population. *J Bone Miner Res.* 1996;11:1333-1338.
11. Mazess RB, Whedon GD. Immobilization and bone. *Calcif Tissue Int.* 1983;35:265-267.
12. Burr DB, Robling AG, Turner CH. Effects of biomechanical stress on bones in animals. *Bone.* 2002;30:781-786.
13. Kohrt WM, Bloomfield SA, Little KD, et al. American College of Sports Medicine Position Stand: physical activity and bone health. *Med Sci Sports Exerc.* 2004;36:1985-1996.
14. Strong WB, Malina RM, Blimkie CJR, et al. Evidence based physical activity for school-age youth. *J Pediatr.* 2005;146:732-737.
15. Turner CH, Robling AG. Exercises for improving bone strength. *Br J Sports Med.* 2005;39:188-189.
16. Greer FR, Krebs NF; Committee on Nutrition, American Academy of Pediatrics. Optimizing bone health and calcium intakes of infants, children and adolescents. *Pediatrics.* 2006;117:578-585.
17. Gordon CM, Bachrach LK, Carpenter TO, et al. Bone health in children and adolescents: a symposium at the annual meeting of the Pediatric Academic Societies/Lawson Wilkins Pediatric Endocrine Society, May 2003. *Curr Probl Pediatr Adolesc Health Care.* 2004;34:226-242.
18. Loud KJ, Gordon CM. Adolescence: bone disease. In: Walker WA, Watkins JB, Duggan C, eds. *Nutrition in Pediatrics.* 3rd ed. Hamilton, Ontario: BC Decker; 2003:883-896.
19. Goulding A, Taylor RW, Jones IE, et al. Overweight and obese children have low bone mass and area for their weight. *Int J Obes Relat Metab Disord.* 2000;24:627-632.
20. Gordon CM, Nelson LM. Amenorrhea and bone heath in adolescents and young women. *Curr Opin Obstet Gynecol.* 2003;15:377-384.
21. Gordon CM, Grace E, Emans SJ, et al. Effects of oral dehydroepiandrosterone on bone density in young women with anorexia nervosa: a randomized trial. *J Clin Endocrinol Metab.* 2002;87:4935-4941.
22. Soyka LA, Grinspoon S, Levitsky L, Herzog DB, Klibanski A. The effects of anorexia nervosa on bone metabolism in female adolescents. *J Clin Endocrinol Metab.* 1999;84:4489-4496.
23. Golden NH. Osteopenia and osteoporosis in anorexia nervosa. *Adolesc Med.* 2003;14:97-108.
24. Lanou AJ, Berkow SE, Barnard ND. Calcium, dairy products and bone health in children and young adults: a reevaluation of the evidence. *Pediatrics.* 2005;115:736-743.
25. Guillemant J, Taupin P, Le HT, et al. Vitamin D status during puberty in French health male adolescents. *Osteoporos Int.* 1999;10:222-225.
26. Lehtonen-Veromaa M, Mottonen T, Irjala K, et al. Vitamin D intake is low and hypovitaminosis D common in healthy 9- to 15-year-old Finnish girls. *Eur J Clin Nutr.* 1999;53:746-751.
27. Looker AC, Dawson-Hughes B, Calvo MS, Gunter EW, Sahyoun NR. Serum 25-hydroxyvitamin D status of adolescents and adults in two seasonal subpopulations from NHANES III. *Bone.* 2002;30:771-777.
28. El-Hajj Fuleihan G, Nabulsi M, Choucair M, et al. Hypovitaminosis D in healthy schoolchildren. *Pediatrics.* 2001;107:E53. http://pediatrics.aappublications.org/cgi/content/full/107/4/e53. Accessed March 10, 2006.
29. Gordon CM, DePeter KC, Feldman HA, Grace E, Emans SJ. Prevalence of vitamin D deficiency among healthy adolescents. *Arch Pediatr Adolesc Med.* 2004;158:531-537.
30. Wosje KS, Specker BL. Role of calcium in bone health during childhood. *Nutr Rev.* 2000;58:253-268.
31. Slemenda CW, Peacock M, Hui S, Zhou L, Johnston CC. Reduced rates of skeletal remodeling are associated with increased bone mineral density during the development of peak skeletal mass. *J Bone Miner Res.* 1997;12:676-682.
32. Ellis KJ, Abrams SA, Wong WW. Body composition in a young multiethnic female population. *Am J Clin Nutr.* 1997;65:724-731.
33. Abrams SA, Grusak MA, Stuff J, O'Brien KO. Calcium and magnesium balance in 9-14 year-old children. *Am J Clin Nutr.* 1997;66:1172-1177.
34. Institute of Medicine; Food and Nutrition Board. *Dietary Reference Intakes for Calcium, Phosphorus, Magnesium, Vitamin D, and Fluoride.* Washington, DC: National Academy Press; 1997.
35. Bryant RJ, Wastney ME, Martin BR, et al. Racial differences in bone turnover and calcium metabolism in adolescent females. *J Clin Endocrinol Metab.* 2003;88:1043-1047.
36. US Department of Agriculture; Agricultural Research Service. The Continuing Survey of Food Intakes by Individuals (CSFII) and the Diet and Health Knowledge Survey (DHKS), 1994-96. www.ars.usda.gov/services/docs.htm?docid=7760. Accessed February 16, 2006.
37. Dawson-Hughes B, Harris SS, Krall EA, Dallal GE. Effect of withdrawal of calcium and vitamin D supplements on bone mass in elderly men and women. *Am J Clin Nutr.* 2000;72:745-750.
38. Dawson-Hughes B, Harris SS, Krall EA, Dallal GE. Effect of calcium and vitamin D

supplementation on bone density in men and women 65 years of age or older. *N Engl J Med.* 1997;337:670-676.
39. LeBoff MS, Kohlmeier L, Hurwitz S, et al. Occult vitamin D deficiency in post-menopausal US women with acute hip fracture. *JAMA.* 1999;281:1505-1511.
40. Parfitt AM, Gallagher JC, Heaney RP, et al. Vitamin D and bone health in the elderly. *Am J Clin Nutr.* 1982;36(5)(suppl):1014-1031.
41. Tsai K-S, Ebeling PR, Riggs BL. Impaired vitamin D metabolism with aging in women. *J Clin Invest.* 1984;73:1668-1672.
42. Slemenda CW, Reister TK, Hui SL, et al. Influences on skeletal mineralization in children and adolescents: evidence for varying effects of sexual maturation and physical activity. *J Pediatr.* 1994;125:201-207.
43. Kasperk CH, Wakley GK, Hierl T, Ziegler R. Gonadal and adrenal androgens are potent regulators of human bone cell metabolism in vitro. *J Bone Miner Res.* 1997;12:464-471.
44. Aris RM, Merkel PA, Bachrach LK, et al. Consensus statement: guide to bone health and disease in cystic fibrosis. *J Clin Endocrinol Metab.* 2005;90:1888-1896.
45. Otis CL, Drinkwater BL, Johnson M, et al. American College of Sports Medicine Position Stand: the female athlete triad. *Med Sci Sports Exerc.* 1997;29:i-ix.
46. Chan JL, Mantzoros CS. Role of leptin in energy-deprivation states: normal human physiology and clinical implications for hypothalamic amenorrhea and anorexia nervosa. *Lancet.* 2005;366:74-85.
47. Steelman J, Zeitler P. Osteoporosis in pediatrics. *Pediatr Rev.* 2001;22:56-64.
48. Teramoto S, Matsuse T, Ouchi Y. Increased production of TNF-$\alpha$ may play a role in osteoporosis in cystic fibrosis patients. *Chest.* 1997;112:574.
49. Schulte C, Dignass AU, Mann K, Goeball H. Reduced bone mineral density and unbalanced bone metabolism in patients with inflammatory bowel disease. *Inflamm Bowel Dis.* 1998;4:268-275.
50. Mansfield MJ, Emans SJ. Anorexia nervosa, athletics, and amenorrhea. *Pediatr Clin North Am.* 1989;36:533-549.
51. Drinkwater BL, Breumner B, Chestnut CH. Menstrual history as a determinant of current bone density in young athletes. *JAMA.* 1990;263:545-548.
52. Khan KM, Liu-Ambrose T, Sran MM, et al. New criteria for female athlete triad syndrome? *Br J Sports Med.* 2002;36:10-13.
53. Loucks AB. Energy availability, not body fatness, regulates reproductive function in women. *Exerc Sport Sci Rev.* 2003;31:144-148.
54. Myburgh KH, Hutchins J, Fataar AB, Hough SF, Noakes TD. Low bone density is an etiologic factor for stress fractures in athletes. *Ann Intern Med.* 1990;113:754-759.
55. Wasnich R. Bone mass measurement: prediction of risk. *Am J Med.* 1993;95:6S-10S.
56. Writing Group for the ISCD Position Development Conference. Diagnosis of osteoporosis in men, premenopausal women, and children. *J Clin Densitom.* 2004;7:17-26.
57. Bachrach LK. Dual energy x-ray absorptiometry (DXA) measurements of bone density and body composition: promise and pitfalls. *J Pediatr Endocrinol Metab.* 2000;13:983-988.
58. Leonard MB, Propert KJ, Zemel BS, Stallings VA, Feldman HI. Discrepancies in pediatric bone mineral density reference data: potential for misdiagnosis of osteopenia. *J Pediatr.* 1999;135:182-188.
59. Wang J, Thornton JC, Horlick M, Formica C, Wang W, Pierson RN Jr. Dual x-ray absorptiometry in pediatric studies: changing scan modes alters bone and body composition measurements. *J Clin Densitom.* 1999;2:135-141.
60. Bachrach LK, Hastie T, Wang MC, Narasimhan B, Marcus R. Bone mineral acquisition in healthy Asian, Hispanic, Black and Caucasian youth: a longitudinal study. *J Clin Endocrinol Metab.* 1999;84:4702-4712.
61. Gilsanz V. Bone density in children: a review of the available techniques and indications. *Eur J Radiol.* 1998;26:177-182.
62. Bachrach LK. Osteoporosis and measurement of bone mass in children and adolescents. *Endocrinol Metab Clin North Am.* 2005;34:521-535.
63. Cole JH, Scerpella TA, van der Meulen MCH. Fan-beam densitometry of the growing skeleton. *J Clin Densitom.* 2005;8:57-64.
64. Koo WWK, Hammami M, Shypailo RJ, Ellis KJ. Bone and body composition measurements of small subjects: discrepancies from software for fan beam dual energy x-ray absorptiometry. *J Am Coll Nutr.* 2004;23:647-650.
65. Hammami M, Koo WWK, Hockman EM. Technical considerations for fan-beam dual-energy x-ray absorptiometry body composition measurements in pediatric studies. *JPEN J Parenter Enteral Nutr.* 2004;28:328-333.
66. Pocock NA, Noakes KA, Majerovic Y, Griffiths MR. Magnification error of femoral geometry using fan beam densitometers. *Calcif Tissue Int.* 1997;60:8-10.
67. Carter DR, Bouxsein ML, Marcus R. New approaches for interpreting projected bone densitometry data. *J Bone Miner Res.* 1992;7:137-145.
68. Kroger H, Kotaniemi A, Vainio P, Alhava E. Bone densitometry of the spine and femur in children by dual-energy x-ray absorptiometry. *Bone Miner.* 1992;17:75-85.
69. Molgaard C, Thomsen BL, Prentie A, Cole TJ, Michaelsen KF. Whole body bone mineral content in healthy children and adolescents. *Arch Dis Child.* 1997;76:9-15.
70. Horlick M, Wang J, Pierson RN Jr, Thornton JC. Prediction models for evaluation of total-body bone mass with dual-energy x-ray absorptiometry among children and adolescents. *Pediatrics.* 2004;114:e337-e345. http://pediatrics.aappublications.org/cgi/content/full/114/3/e337. Accessed March 12, 2006.
71. Genant HK, Engelke K, Fuerst T, et al. Noninvasive assessment of bone mineral and structure: state of the art. *J Bone Miner Res.* 1996;11:707-2730.
72. Mora S, Gilsanz V. Establishment of peak bone mass. *Endocrinol Metab Clin North Am.* 2003;32:39-63.
73. Specker BL, Schoenau E. Quantitative bone analysis in children: current methods and recommendations. *J Pediatr.* 2005;146:726-731.
74. Malavolta N, Mule R, Frigato M. Quantitative ultrasound assessment of bone. *Aging Clin Exp Res.* 2004;16:23-28.
75. Fricke O, Tutlewski B, Schwahn B, Schoenau E. Speed of sound: relation to geometric characteristics of bone in children, adolescents, and adults. *J Pediatr.* 2005;146:764-768.
76. Hartman C, Shamir R, Eshach-Adiv O, Iosilevsky G, Brik R. Assessment of osteoporosis by quantitative ultrasound versus dual energy x-ray absorptiometry in children with chronic rheumatic diseases *J Rheumatol.* 2004;31:981-985.
77. Hartman C, Hino B, Lerner A, et al. Bone quantitative ultrasound and bone mineral density in children with celiac disease. *J Pediatr Gastroenterol Nutr.* 2004;39:504-510.
78. Schiessl H, Ferretti JL, Tysarczyk-Niemeyer G, et al. Non-invasive bone strength index as analyzed by peripheral quantitative computed tomography (pQCT). In: Schonau E, ed. *Paediatric Osteology: New Developments in Diagnostics and Therapy.* Amsterdam, the Netherlands: Elsevier; 1996:141-146.
79. McKay HA, Sievanen H, Petit MA, et al. Application of magnetic resonance imaging to evaluation of femoral neck structure in growing girls. *J Clin Densitom.* 2004;7:161-168.
80. Beck TJ, Ruff CB, Warden KE, et al. Predicting femoral neck strength from bone mineral data: a structural approach. *Invest Radiol.* 1990;25:6-18.
81. Kaunitz AM. Depo-Provera's black box: time to reconsider? *Contraception.* 2005;72:165-167.
82. WHO. WHO statement on hormonal contraception and bone health. *Wkly Epidemiol Rec.* 2005;80:302-304.
83. Scholes D, LaCroix AZ, Ichikawa LE, Barlow WE, Ott SM. Change in bone mineral density among adolescent women using and discontinuing depot medroxyprogesterone acetate contraception. *Arch Pediatr Adolesc Med.* 2005;159:139-144.
84. Glorieux FH, Bishop NJ, Plotkin H, Chabot G, Lanoue G, Travers R. Cyclic administration of pamidronate in children with severe osteogenesis imperfecta. *N Engl J Med.* 1998;339:947-952.
85. Rauch F, Travers R, Plotkin H, Glorieux FH. The effects of intravenous pamidronate on the bone tissue of children and adolescents with osteogenesis imperfecta. *J Clin Invest.* 2002;110:1293-1299.
86. Rauch F, Plotkin H, Travers R, Zeitlin L, Glorieux FH. Osteogenesis imperfecta types I, III, and IV: effect of pamidronate therapy on bone and mineral metabolism. *J Clin Endocrinol Metab.* 2003;88:986-992.
87. Rauch F, Plotkin H, Zeitlin L, Glorieux FH. Bone mass, size, and density in children and adolescents with osteogenesis imperfecta: effect of intravenous pamidronate therapy. *J Bone Miner Res.* 2003;18:610-614.
88. Henderson RC, Lark RK, Keskemethy HH, Miller F, Harcke HT, Bachrach J. Bisphosphonates to treat osteopenia in children with quadriplegic cerebral palsy: a randomized placebo-controlled clinical trial *J Pediatr.* 2002;141:644-651.
89. Ward LM, Denker AE, Porras A, et al. Single-dose pharmacokinetics and tolerability of alendronate 35- and 70-milligram tablets in children and adolescents with osteogenesis imperfecta type I. *J Clin Endocrinol Metab.* 2005;90:4051-4056.
90. Miller KK, Grieco KA, Mulder J, et al. Effects of risedronate on bone density in anorexia nervosa. *J Clin Endocrinol Metab.* 2004;89:3903-3906.
91. Golden NH, Iglesias EA, Jacobson MS, et al. Alendronate for the treatment of osteopenia in anorexia nervosa: a randomized, double-blind, placebo-controlled trial. *J Clin Endocrinol Metab.* 2005;90:3179-3185.
92. Liu SL, Lebrun CM. Effect of oral contraceptives and hormone replacement therapy on bone mineral density in premenopausal and perimenopausal women: a systematic review. *Br J Sports Med.* 2006;40:11-24.
93. Klibanski A, Biller BMK, Schoenfeld DA, Herzog DB, Saxe VC. The effects of estrogen administration on trabecular bone in young women with anorexia nervosa. *J Clin Endocrinol Metab.* 1995;80:898-904.
94. Golden NH, Lanzkowsky L, Schebendach J, Palestro CJ, Jacobson MS, Shekner IR. The effect of estrogen-progestin treatment on bone mineral density in anorexia nervosa. *J Pediatr Adolesc Gynecol.* 2002;15:135-143.
95. Grinspoon S, Baum H, Lee K, Anderson E, Herzog D, Klibanski A. Effects of short-term recombinant human insulin-like growth factor I administration on bone turnover in osteopenic women with anorexia nervosa. *J Clin Endocrinol Metab.* 1996;81:3864-3870.
96. Grinspoon S, Thomas L, Miller K, Herzog D, Klibanski A. Effects of recombinant human IGF-I and oral contraceptive administration on bone density in anorexia nervosa. *J Clin Endocrinol Metab.* 2002;87:2883-2891.
97. Miller KK, Grieco KA, Klibanski A. Testosterone administration in women with anorexia nervosa. *J Clin Endocrinol Metab.* 2005;90:1428-1433.
98. MacKelvie KJ, Khan KM, McKay HA. Is there a critical period for bone response to weight-bearing exercise in children and adolescents? a systematic review. *Br J Sports Med.* 2002;36:250-257.
99. Specker B, Binkley T. Randomized trial of physical activity and calcium supplementation on bone mineral content in 3- to 5-year-old children. *J Bone Miner Res.* 2003;18:885-892.

Now:

The Purple Pill™ is FDA-approved for use in kids 12 to 17 years old with GERD

# NEXIUM for the NEXT GENERATION

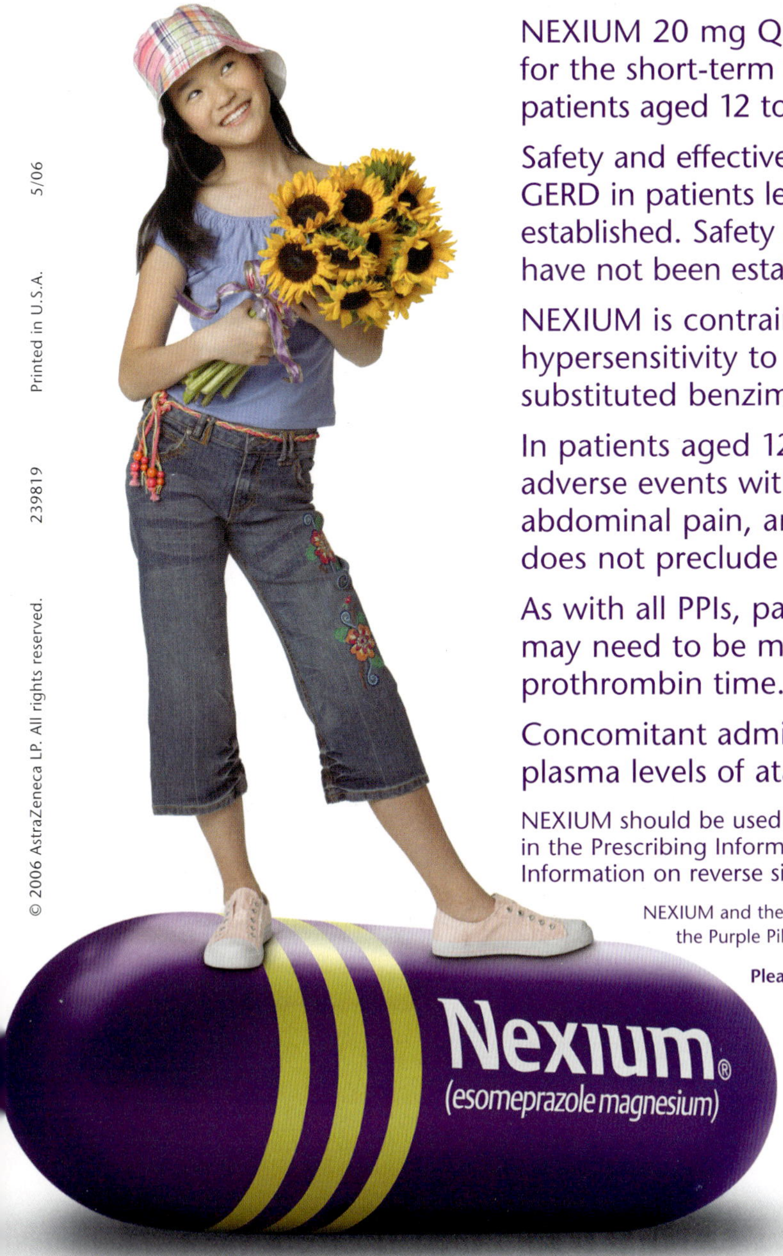


NEXIUM 20 mg QD and NEXIUM 40 mg QD are approved for the short-term treatment (up to 8 weeks) of GERD in patients aged 12 to 17 years.

Safety and effectiveness for the treatment of symptomatic GERD in patients less than 12 years of age have not been established. Safety and effectiveness for other pediatric uses have not been established.

NEXIUM is contraindicated in patients with known hypersensitivity to any component of the formulation or to substituted benzimidazoles.

In patients aged 12 to 17 years, the most frequently reported adverse events with NEXIUM include headache, diarrhea, abdominal pain, and nausea. Symptomatic response to therapy does not preclude the presence of gastric malignancy.

As with all PPIs, patients treated concomitantly with warfarin may need to be monitored for increases in INR and prothrombin time.

Concomitant administration of esomeprazole may reduce the plasma levels of atazanavir.

NEXIUM should be used only for the conditions, dosages, and durations specified in the Prescribing Information. Please see the brief summary of full Prescribing Information on reverse side.



**Please visit our Web site at www.Nexium-us.com**

**Nexium®**
(esomeprazole magnesium)

AstraZeneca

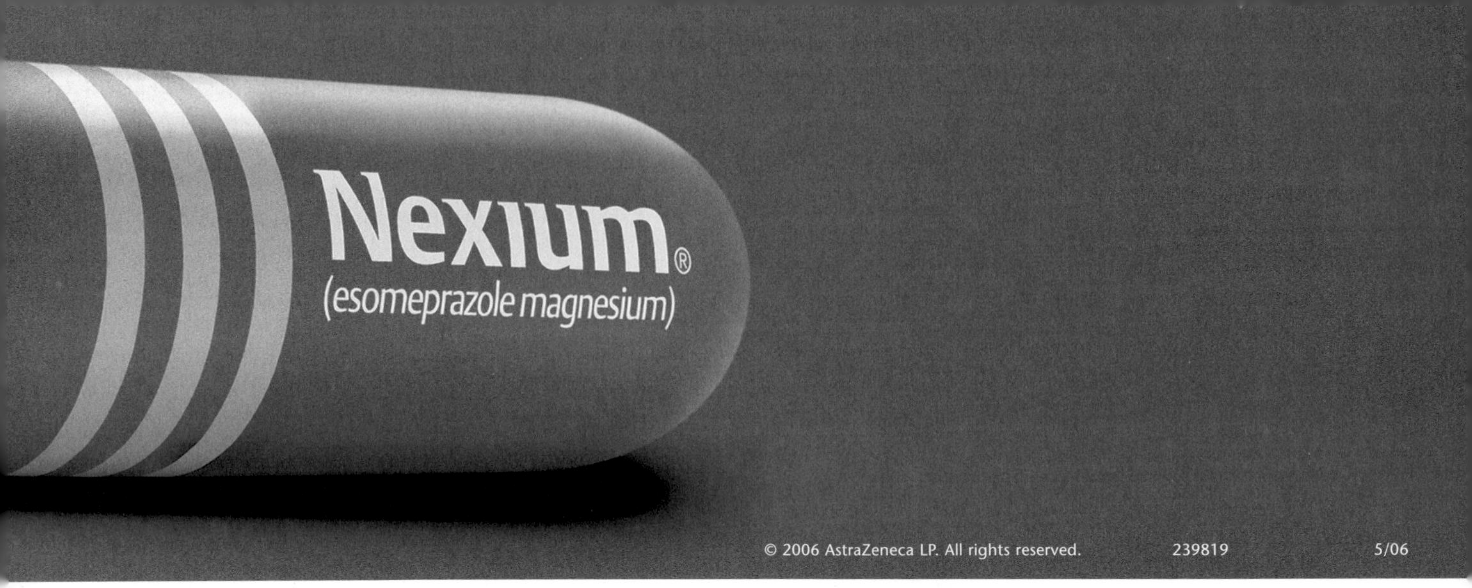


# NEXIUM® *(esomeprazole magnesium)*

## 20-mg, 40-mg Delayed-Release Capsules

**BRIEF SUMMARY** of Prescribing Information.

**INDICATIONS AND USAGE** **Treatment of GERD** NEXIUM is indicated for the short-term treatment (4 to 8 weeks) in the healing and symptomatic resolution of diagnostically confirmed erosive esophagitis; the maintenance of symptom resolution and healing of erosive esophagitis (controlled studies do not extend beyond 6 months); the treatment of heartburn and other symptoms associated with GERD; **Risk Reduction of NSAID-Associated Gastric Ulcer; *H.pylori* Eradication to Reduce the Risk of Duodenal Ulcer Recurrence.**

**CONTRAINDICATIONS** NEXIUM is contraindicated in patients with known hypersensitivity to any component of the formulation or to substituted benzimidazoles.

**PRECAUTIONS General** Symptomatic response to therapy with NEXIUM does not preclude the presence of gastric malignancy. Atrophic gastritis has been noted occasionally in gastric corpus biopsies from patients treated long-term with omeprazole, of which NEXIUM is an enantiomer. **Information for Patients** NEXIUM Delayed-Release Capsules should be swallowed whole and taken at least one hour before meals. For patients who have difficulty swallowing capsules, one tablespoon of applesauce can be added to an empty bowl and the NEXIUM Delayed-Release Capsule can be opened, and the pellets carefully emptied onto the applesauce. The pellets should be mixed with the applesauce and then swallowed immediately. The applesauce used should not be hot and should be soft enough to be swallowed without chewing. The pellets should not be chewed or crushed. The pellet/applesauce mixture should not be stored for future use. Antacids may be used while taking NEXIUM. **Drug Interactions** Esomeprazole is extensively metabolized in the liver by CYP2C19 and CYP3A4. *In vitro* and *in vivo* studies have shown that esomeprazole is not likely to inhibit CYPs 1A2, 2A6, 2C9, 2D6, 2E1 and 3A4. No clinically relevant interactions with drugs metabolized by these CYP enzymes would be expected. Drug interaction studies have shown that esomeprazole does not have any clinically significant interactions with phenytoin, warfarin, quinidine, clarithromycin or amoxicillin. Post-marketing reports of changes in prothrombin measures have been received among patients on concomitant warfarin and esomeprazole therapy. Increases in INR and prothrombin time may lead to abnormal bleeding and even death. Patients treated with proton pump inhibitors and warfarin concomitantly may need to be monitored for increases in INR and prothrombin time. Esomeprazole may potentially interfere with CYP2C19, the major esomeprazole metabolizing enzyme. Coadministration of esomeprazole 30 mg and diazepam, a CYP2C19 substrate, resulted in a 45% decrease in clearance of diazepam. Increased plasma levels of diazepam were observed 12 hours after dosing and onwards. However, at that time, the plasma levels of diazepam were below the therapeutic interval, and thus this interaction is unlikely to be of clinical relevance. Coadministration of oral contraceptives, diazepam, phenytoin, or quinidine did not seem to change the pharmacokinetic profile of esomeprazole. Concomitant administration of esomeprazole may reduce the plasma levels of atazanavir. Studies evaluating concomitant administration of esomeprazole and either naproxen (non-selective NSAID) or rofecoxib (COX-2 selective NSAID) did not identify any clinically relevant changes in the pharmacokinetic profiles of esomeprazole or these NSAIDs. Esomeprazole inhibits gastric acid secretion. Therefore, esomeprazole may interfere with the absorption of drugs where gastric pH is an important determinant of bioavailability (eg, ketoconazole, iron salts and digoxin). **Carcinogenesis, Mutagenesis, Impairment of Fertility** The carcinogenic potential of esomeprazole was assessed using omeprazole studies. In two 24-month oral carcinogenicity studies in rats, omeprazole at daily doses of 1.7, 3.4, 13.8, 44.0 and 140.8 mg/kg/day (about 0.7 to 57 times the human dose of 20 mg/day expressed on a body surface area basis) produced gastric ECL cell carcinoids in a dose-related manner in both male and female rats; the incidence of this effect was markedly higher in female rats, which had higher blood levels of omeprazole. Gastric carcinoids seldom occur in the untreated rat. In addition, ECL cell hyperplasia was present in all treated groups of both sexes. In one of these studies, female rats were treated with 13.8 mg omeprazole/kg/day (about 5.6 times the human dose on a body surface area basis) for 1 year, then followed for an additional year without the drug. No carcinoids were seen in these rats. An increased incidence of treatment-related ECL cell hyperplasia was observed at the end of 1 year (94% treated vs 10% controls). By the second year the difference between treated and control rats was much smaller (46% vs 26%) but still showed more hyperplasia in the treated group. Gastric adenocarcinoma was seen in one rat (2%). No similar tumor was seen in male or female rats treated for 2 years. For this strain of rat no similar tumor has been noted historically, but a finding involving only one tumor is difficult to interpret. A 78-week mouse carcinogenicity study of omeprazole did not show increased tumor occurrence, but the study was not conclusive. Esomeprazole was negative in the Ames mutation test, in the *in vivo* rat bone marrow cell chromosome aberration test, and the *in vivo* mouse micronucleus test. Esomeprazole, however, was positive in the *in vitro* human lymphocyte chromosome aberration test. Omeprazole was positive in the *in vitro* human lymphocyte chromosome aberration test, the *in vivo* mouse bone marrow cell chromosome aberration test, and the *in vivo* mouse micronucleus test. The potential effects of esomeprazole on fertility and reproductive performance were assessed using omeprazole studies. Omeprazole at oral doses up to 138 mg/kg/day in rats (about 56 times the human dose on a body surface area basis) was found to have no effect on reproductive performance of parental animals. **Pregnancy** *Teratogenic Effects. Pregnancy Category B* Teratology studies have been performed in rats at oral doses up to 280 mg/kg/day (about 57 times the human dose on a body surface area basis) and in rabbits at oral doses up to 86 mg/kg/day (about 35 times the human dose on a body surface area basis) and have revealed no evidence of impaired fertility or harm to the fetus due to esomeprazole. There are, however, no adequate and well-controlled studies in pregnant women. Because animal reproduction studies are not always predictive of human response, this drug should be used during pregnancy only if clearly needed. Teratology studies conducted with omeprazole in rats at oral doses up to 138 mg/kg/day (about 56 times the human dose on a body surface area basis) and in rabbits at doses up to 69 mg/kg/day (about 56 times the human dose on a body surface area basis) did not disclose any evidence for a teratogenic potential of omeprazole. In rabbits, omeprazole in a dose range of 6.9 to 69.1 mg/kg/day (about 5.5 to 56 times the human dose on a body surface area basis) produced dose-related increases in embryo-lethality, fetal resorptions, and pregnancy disruptions. In rats, dose-related embryo/ fetal toxicity and postnatal developmental toxicity were observed in offspring resulting from parents treated with omeprazole at 13.8 to 138.0 mg/kg/day (about 5.6 to 56 times the human doses on a body surface area basis). There are no adequate and well-controlled studies in pregnant women. Sporadic reports have been received of congenital abnormalities occurring in infants born to women who have received omeprazole during pregnancy. **Nursing Mothers** The excretion of esomeprazole in milk has not been studied. However, omeprazole concentrations have been measured in breast milk of a woman following oral administration of 20 mg. Because esomeprazole is likely to be excreted in human milk, because of the potential for serious adverse reactions in nursing infants from esomeprazole, and because of the potential for tumorigenicity shown for omeprazole in rat carcinogenicity studies, a decision should be made whether to discontinue nursing or to discontinue the drug, taking into account the importance of the drug to the mother. **Pediatric Use** Use of NEXIUM in adolescent patients 12 to 17 years of age for short-term treatment of GERD is supported by a) extrapolation of results, already included in the currently approved labeling, from adequate and well-controlled studies that supported the approval of NEXIUM for adults, and b) safety and pharmacokinetic studies performed in adolescent patients. (See **CLINICAL PHARMACOLOGY, Pharmacokinetics,** *Pediatric* for pharmacokinetic information.) The safety and effectiveness of NEXIUM for the treatment of symptomatic GERD in patients <12 years of age have not been established. The safety and effectiveness of NEXIUM for other pediatric uses have not been established. **12 to 17 Years of Age GERD** In a multicenter, randomized, double-blind, parallel-group study, 149 adolescent patients (12 to 17 years of age; 89 female; 124 Caucasian, 15 Black, 10 Other) with clinically diagnosed GERD were treated with either NEXIUM 20 mg or NEXIUM 40 mg once daily for up to 8 weeks to evaluate safety and tolerability. Patients were not endoscopically characterized as to the presence or absence of erosive esophagitis. The most frequently reported (at least 2%) treatment related adverse events in these patients were headache (8.1%), abdominal pain (2.7%), diarrhea (2%) and nausea (2%). No new safety concerns were identified. **Geriatric Use** Of the total number of patients who received NEXIUM in clinical trials, 1459 were 65 to 74 years of age and 354 patients were ≥75 years of age. No overall differences in safety and efficacy were observed between the elderly and younger individuals, and other reported clinical experience has not identified differences in responses between the elderly and younger patients, but greater sensitivity of some older individuals cannot be ruled out.

**ADVERSE REACTIONS** The safety of NEXIUM was evaluated in over 15,000 patients (aged 18-84 years) in clinical trials worldwide including over 8,500 patients in the United States and over 6,500 patients in Europe and Canada. Over 2,900 patients were treated in long-term studies for up to 6-12 months. In general, NEXIUM was well tolerated in both short and long-term clinical trials. A study was performed evaluating the safety of NEXIUM in pediatric patients aged 12-17 for the treatment of symptomatic GERD (see **PRECAUTIONS – Pediatric Use**). The safety in the treatment of healing of erosive esophagitis was assessed in four randomized comparative clinical trials, which included 1,240 patients on NEXIUM 20 mg, 2,434 patients on NEXIUM 40 mg, and 3,008 patients on omeprazole 20 mg daily. The most frequently occurring adverse events (≥1%) in all three groups was headache (5.5, 5.0, and 3.8, respectively) and diarrhea (no difference among the three groups). Nausea, flatulence, abdominal pain, constipation, and dry mouth occurred at similar rates among patients taking NEXIUM or omeprazole. Additional adverse events that were reported as possibly or probably related to NEXIUM with an incidence <1% are listed below by body system: ***Body as a Whole:*** abdomen enlarged, allergic reaction, asthenia, back pain, chest pain, chest pain substernal, facial edema, peripheral edema, hot flushes, fatigue, fever, flu-like disorder, generalized edema, leg edema, malaise, pain, rigors; ***Cardiovascular:*** flushing, hypertension, tachycardia; ***Endocrine:*** goiter; ***Gastrointestinal:*** bowel irregularity, constipation aggravated, dyspepsia, dysphagia, dysplasia GI, epigastric pain, eructation, esophageal disorder, frequent stools, gastroenteritis, GI hemorrhage, GI symptoms not otherwise specified, hiccup, melena, mouth disorder, pharynx disorder, rectal disorder, serum gastrin increased, tongue disorder, tongue edema, ulcerative stomatitis, vomiting; ***Hearing:*** earache, tinnitus; ***Hematologic:*** anemia, anemia hypochromic, cervical lymphoadenopathy, epistaxis, leukocytosis, leukopenia, thrombocytopenia; ***Hepatic:*** bilirubinemia, hepatic function abnormal, SGOT increased, SGPT increased; ***Metabolic/Nutritional:*** glycosuria, hyperuricemia, hyponatremia, increased alkaline phosphatase, thirst, vitamin B12 deficiency, weight increase, weight decrease; ***Musculoskeletal:*** arthralgia, arthritis aggravated, arthropathy, cramps, fibromyalgia syndrome, hernia, polymyalgia rheumatica; ***Nervous System/Psychiatric:*** anorexia, apathy, appetite increased, confusion, depression aggravated, dizziness, hypertonia, nervousness, hypoesthesia, impotence, insomnia, migraine, migraine aggravated, paresthesia, sleep disorder, somnolence, tremor, vertigo, visual field defect; ***Reproductive:*** dysmenorrhea, menstrual disorder, vaginitis; ***Respiratory:*** asthma aggravated, coughing, dyspnea, larynx edema, pharyngitis, rhinitis, sinusitis; ***Skin and Appendages:*** acne, angioedema, dermatitis, pruritus, pruritus ani, rash, rash erythematous, rash maculo-papular, skin inflammation, sweating increased, urticaria; ***Special Senses:*** otitis media, parosmia, taste loss, taste perversion; ***Urogenital:*** abnormal urine, albuminuria, cystitis, dysuria, fungal infection, hematuria, micturition frequency, moniliasis, genital moniliasis, polyuria; ***Visual:*** conjunctivitis, vision abnormal. Endoscopic findings that were reported as adverse events include: duodenitis, esophagitis, esophageal stricture, esophageal ulceration, esophageal varices, gastric ulcer, gastritis, hernia, benign polyps or nodules, Barrett's esophagus, and mucosal discoloration. Two placebo-controlled studies were conducted in 710 patients for the treatment of symptomatic gastroesophageal reflux disease. The most common adverse events that were reported as possibly or probably related to NEXIUM were diarrhea (4.3%), headache (3.8%), and abdominal pain (3.8%). Postmarketing Reports – There have been spontaneous reports of adverse events with postmarketing use of esomeprazole. These reports occurred rarely and are listed below by body system: ***Blood And Lymphatic System Disorders:*** agranulocytosis, pancytopenia; ***Eye Disorders:*** blurred vision; ***Gastrointestinal Disorders:*** pancreatitis; ***Hepatobiliary Disorders:*** hepatitis with or without jaundice; ***Immune System Disorders:*** anaphylactic reaction/shock; ***Musculoskeletal And Connective Tissue Disorders:*** myalgia; ***Psychiatric Disorders:*** depression; ***Skin and Subcutaneous Tissue Disorders:*** alopecia, erythema multiforme, Stevens-Johnson syndrome, toxic epidermal necrolysis (TEN, some fatal). Other adverse events not observed with NEXIUM, but occurring with omeprazole can be found in the omeprazole package insert, **ADVERSE REACTIONS** section.

**OVERDOSAGE** A single oral dose of esomeprazole at 510 mg/kg (about 103 times the human dose on a body surface area basis), was lethal to rats. The major signs of acute toxicity were reduced motor activity, changes in respiratory frequency, tremor, ataxia, and intermittent clonic convulsions. There have been some reports of overdosage with esomeprazole. Reports have been received of overdosage with omeprazole in humans. Doses ranged up to 2,400 mg (120 times the usual recommended clinical dose). Manifestations were variable, but included confusion, drowsiness, blurred vision, tachycardia, nausea, diaphoresis, flushing, headache, dry mouth, and other adverse reactions similar to those seen in normal clinical experience (see omeprazole package insert-**ADVERSE REACTIONS**). No specific antidote for esomeprazole is known. Since esomeprazole is extensively protein bound, it is not expected to be removed by dialysis. In the event of overdosage, treatment should be symptomatic and supportive. As with the management of any overdose, the possibility of multiple drug ingestion should be considered. For current information on treatment of any drug overdose, a certified Regional Poison Control Center should be contacted. Telephone numbers are listed in the Physicians' Desk Reference (PDR) or local telephone book. **DOSAGE AND ADMINISTRATION** Please see full Prescribing Information for recommended dosages and dosage adjustments for **Special Populations** for NEXIUM.


Distributed by: AstraZeneca LP, Wilmington, DE 19850
Product of France 31026-02 Rev. 04/06 240260

AstraZeneca

**Pertussis is on the rise[1,2]...**

***Infants may be at risk when they are not vaccinated on time[3]***

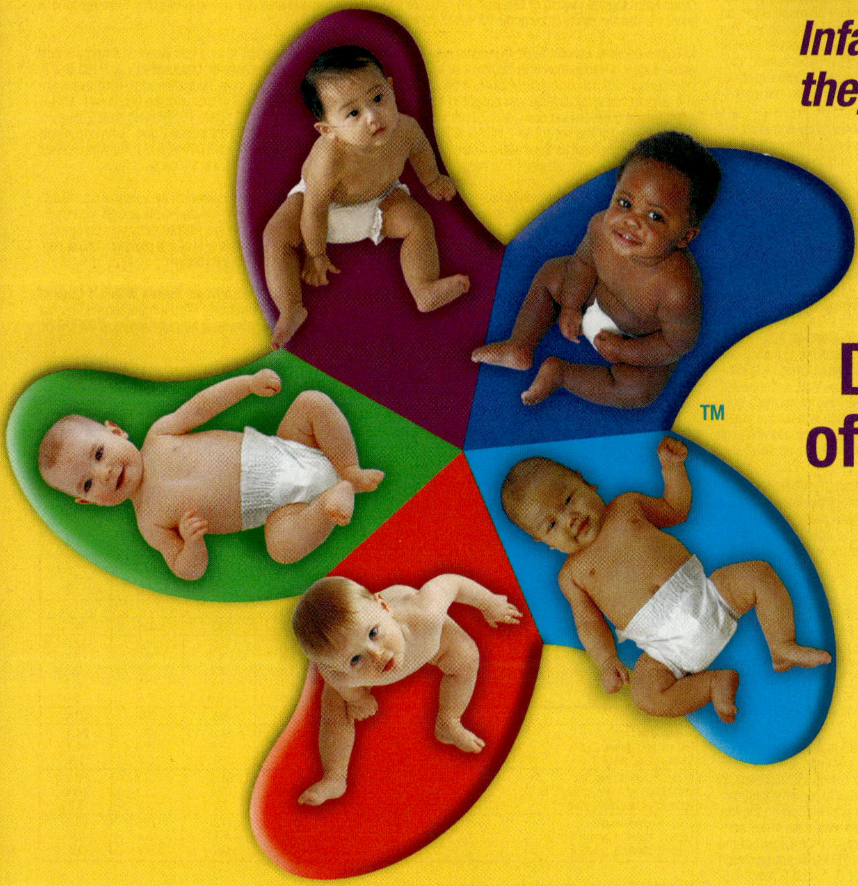


# Don't run the risk of letting one child get away

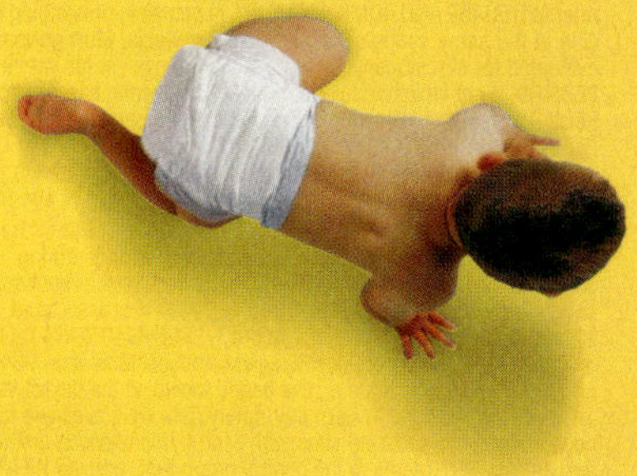

## PEDIARIX may help ensure timely vaccination with fewer injections

- 5 serious childhood diseases—1 combination vaccine*[4]
- With just 1 dose at 2, 4, and 6 months of age (in infants born of HBsAg-negative mothers)

## Important Safety information

In clinical studies, adverse events in infants receiving PEDIARIX included injection-site reactions (pain, redness, or swelling), fever, and fussiness. Administration of PEDIARIX was associated with higher rates of fever relative to separately administered vaccines (see Adverse Reactions section of the Brief Summary). PEDIARIX is contraindicated in infants with known hypersensitivity to any component of the vaccine including yeast, neomycin, and polymyxin B. As with any vaccine, vaccination with PEDIARIX may not protect 100% of susceptible individuals.

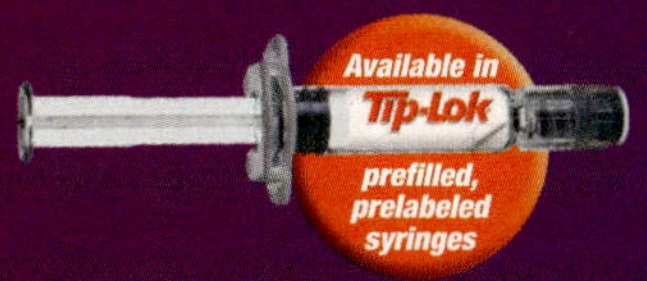


**Please see brief summary for PEDIARIX on adjacent page.**

Pediarix

**Diphtheria and Tetanus Toxoids and Acellular Pertussis Adsorbed, Hepatitis B (Recombinant) and Inactivated Poliovirus Vaccine Combined**

**References: 1.** Centers for Disease Control and Prevention. Pertussis Surveillance Report—2004 (final data). Issued 8/12/05. **2.** Centers for Disease Control and Prevention. *Epidemiology and Prevention of Vaccine-Preventable Diseases.* Reported Cases and Deaths from Vaccine Preventable Diseases, United States, 1950-2003. Available at http://www.cdc.gov/nip/publications/pink/appendices/G/cases&deaths.pdf. Accessed May 10, 2006. **3.** Centers for Disease Control and Prevention. *Epidemiology and Prevention of Vaccine-Preventable Diseases.* Atkinson W, Hamborsky J, McIntyre L, Wolfe S, eds. 9th ed. Washington, DC: Public Health Foundation;2006: 84. **4.** PEDIARIX Prescribing Information.

*Does not require reconstitution.



Manufactured by **GlaxoSmithKline Biologicals,** Rixensart, Belgium
Distributed by **GlaxoSmithKline,** Research Triangle Park, NC 27709

gsk GlaxoSmithKline Vaccines

**PEDIARIX® [Diphtheria and Tetanus Toxoids and Acellular Pertussis Adsorbed, Hepatitis B (Recombinant) and Inactivated Poliovirus Vaccine Combined]**

The following is a brief summary only; see full prescribing information for complete product information.

**CONTRAINDICATIONS:** Hypersensitivity to any component of the vaccine, including yeast, neomycin, and polymyxin B, is a contraindication (see DESCRIPTION in complete prescribing information). Do not use PEDIARIX after a serious allergic reaction (e.g., anaphylaxis) temporally associated with a previous dose of this vaccine or with any components of this vaccine. Because of the uncertainty as to which component of the vaccine might be responsible, do not give further vaccination with any of these components; or, refer such individuals to an allergist for evaluation. The following events are contraindications to administration of PEDIARIX: encephalopathy (e.g., coma, decreased level of consciousness, prolonged seizures) within 7 days of administration of a previous dose of a pertussis-containing vaccine that is not attributable to another identifiable cause; progressive neurologic disorder, including infantile spasms, uncontrolled epilepsy, or progressive encephalopathy. Do not vaccinate individuals with these conditions until a treatment regimen has been established and the condition has stabilized.

**WARNINGS:** Administration of PEDIARIX is associated with higher rates of fever relative to separately administered vaccines. In a safety study that evaluated medically attended fever after PEDIARIX or separately administered vaccines when coadministered with 7-valent pneumococcal and Hib conjugate vaccines, infants who received PEDIARIX had a higher rate of medical encounters for fever within the first 4 days following the first vaccination. In some infants, these encounters included the performance of diagnostic studies to evaluate other causes of fever (see ADVERSE REACTIONS). The tip cap and the rubber plunger of the needleless prefilled syringes contain dry natural latex rubber that may cause allergic reactions in latex sensitive individuals. The vial stopper is latex-free. If any of the following events occur in temporal relation to receipt of DTwP or a vaccine containing an acellular pertussis component, consider carefully whether to give any pertussis vaccine, including PEDIARIX: temperature of ≥40.5°C (105°F) within 48 hours not due to another identifiable cause; collapse or shock-like state (hypotonic-hyporesponsive episode) within 48 hours; persistent, inconsolable crying lasting ≥3 hours, occurring within 48 hours; seizures with or without fever occurring within 3 days. If Guillain-Barré syndrome occurs within 6 weeks of receipt of prior vaccine containing tetanus toxoid, the decision to give any tetanus toxoid-containing vaccine, including PEDIARIX, should be based on careful consideration of the potential benefits and possible risks. If tetanus toxoid is withheld, other available vaccines should be given, as indicated. The decision to administer a pertussis-containing vaccine to individuals with stable central nervous system (CNS) disorders must be made by the physician on an individual basis, with consideration of all relevant factors, and assessment of potential risks and benefits for that individual. Advise the parent or guardian of the potential increased risk involved (see PRECAUTIONS). For children at higher risk for seizures than the general population, an appropriate antipyretic may be administered at the time of vaccination and for the ensuing 24 hours according to the respective prescribing information recommended dosage to reduce the possibility of post-vaccination fever. The ACIP has published guidelines for vaccination of persons with recent or acute illness (www.cdc.gov/nip).

**PRECAUTIONS:** PEDIARIX should be given with caution in children with bleeding disorders such as hemophilia or thrombocytopenia and in children on anticoagulant therapy, with steps taken to avoid the risk of hematoma following the injection. Before the injection of any biological, the physician should take all reasonable precautions to prevent allergic or other adverse reactions. Epinephrine injection (1:1,000) and other appropriate agents used for the control of immediate allergic reactions must be immediately available should an acute anaphylactic reaction occur. Immunosuppressed individuals, including those receiving immunosuppressive therapy, may not develop the expected immune response. The ACIP has published guidelines for vaccination of persons on such therapies (www.cdc.gov/nip). **Drug Interactions:** For information regarding concomitant administration with other vaccines, refer to DOSAGE AND ADMINISTRATION in complete prescribing information. Do not mix PEDIARIX with any other vaccine in the same syringe or vial. **Carcinogenesis, Mutagenesis, Impairment of Fertility:** PEDIARIX has not been evaluated for carcinogenic or mutagenic potential, or for impairment of fertility. **Pregnancy:** Pregnancy Category C: PEDIARIX is not indicated for women of child-bearing age. Animal reproduction studies have not been conducted with PEDIARIX. It is not known whether PEDIARIX can cause fetal harm when administered to a pregnant woman or if PEDIARIX can affect reproductive capacity. **Geriatric Use:** PEDIARIX is not indicated for use in adult populations. **Pediatric Use:** Safety and effectiveness of PEDIARIX in infants younger than 6 weeks of age have not been evaluated. PEDIARIX is not recommended for persons 7 years of age or older.

**ADVERSE REACTIONS:** A total of 23,849 doses of PEDIARIX have been administered to 8,088 infants who received one or more doses as part of a 3-dose primary series during 14 clinical studies. The most common adverse reactions observed in clinical trials were local injection site reactions (pain, redness, or swelling), fever, and fussiness. In comparative studies, administration of PEDIARIX was associated with higher rates of fever relative to separately administered vaccines (see WARNINGS and ADVERSE REACTIONS Table 1). The prevalence of fever was highest on the day of vaccination and the day following vaccination. More than 96% of episodes of fever resolved within the 4-day period following vaccination (i.e., the period including the day of vaccination and the next 3 days). In the largest of the 14 studies, conducted in Germany, safety data were available for 4,666 infants who received PEDIARIX administered concomitantly at separate sites with 1 of 4 *Haemophilus influenzae* type b (Hib) vaccines at 3, 4, and 5 months of age and for 768 infants in the control group that received INFANRIX® (Diphtheria and Tetanus Toxoids and Acellular Pertussis Vaccine Adsorbed), Hib conjugate vaccine, and oral poliovirus vaccine (OPV) separately. Data on adverse events were collected by parents using standardized diary cards for 4 consecutive days following each vaccine dose (i.e., day of vaccination and the next 3 days). Infants were also monitored for unsolicited adverse events that occurred within 30 days following vaccination using diaries which were returned at subsequent visits and were supplemented by spontaneous reports and a medical history as reported by parents. More than 95% of study participants were white.

In a US study, the safety of PEDIARIX administered to 673 infants was compared to the safety of separately administered INFANRIX, ENGERIX-B® [Hepatitis B Vaccine (Recombinant)], inactivated poliovirus vaccine (IPV) in 335 infants. In both groups, infants received Hib and 7-valent pneumococcal conjugate vaccines concomitantly at separate sites. All vaccines were administered at 2, 4, and 6 months of age. The study was powered to evaluate fever >101.3° F following dose 1. Data on solicited adverse events were collected by parents using standardized diary cards for 4 consecutive days following each vaccine dose (i.e., day of vaccination and the next 3 days) and are presented in Table 1. Telephone follow-up was conducted 1 month and 6 months after the third vaccination to inquire about serious adverse events. At the 6-month follow-up, information also was collected on new onset of chronic illnesses. 638 subjects who received PEDIARIX and 313 subjects who received INFANRIX, ENGERIX-B, and IPV completed the 6-month follow-up. Among subjects in both study groups combined, 69% were white, 18% were Hispanic, 7% were black, 3% were Oriental, and 3% were of other racial/ethnic groups.

The adverse event information from clinical trials provides a basis for identifying adverse events that appear to be related to vaccine use and for approximating rates. However, because clinical trials are conducted under widely varying conditions, adverse event rates observed in the clinical trials of a vaccine cannot be directly compared to rates in the clinical trials of another vaccine, and may not reflect the rates observed in practice. As with any vaccine, there is the possibility that broad use of PEDIARIX could reveal adverse events not observed in clinical trials.

**Deaths:** In 14 clinical trials, 5 deaths were reported among 8,088 (0.06%) recipients of PEDIARIX and 1 death was reported among 2,287 (0.04%) recipients of comparator vaccines. Causes of death in the group that received PEDIARIX included 2 cases of Sudden Infant Death Syndrome (SIDS) and one case of each of the following: Convulsive disorder, congenital immunodeficiency with sepsis, and neuroblastoma. One case of SIDS was reported in the comparator group. The rate of SIDS among all recipients of PEDIARIX across the 14 trials was 0.25/1,000. The rate of SIDS observed for recipients of PEDIARIX in the German safety study was 0.2/1,000 infants (reported rate of SIDS in Germany in the latter part of the 1990s was 0.7/1,000 newborns). The reported rate of SIDS in the United States from 1990 to 1994 was 1.2/1,000 live births. By chance alone, some cases of SIDS can be expected to follow receipt of pertussis-containing vaccines.

**Serious Adverse Events:** Within 30 days following any dose of vaccine in the US safety study in which all subjects received concomitant pneumococcal and Hib conjugate vaccines, 7 serious adverse events were reported in 7 subjects (1% [7/673]) who received PEDIARIX (1 case each of pyrexia, gastroenteritis, and culture negative clinical sepsis and 4 cases of bronchiolitis) and 5 serious adverse events were reported in 4 subjects (1% [4/335]) who received INFANRIX, ENGERIX-B, and IPV (uteropelvic junction obstruction and testicular atrophy in one subject and 3 cases of bronchiolitis).

**Onset of Chronic Illnesses:** In the US safety study in which all subjects received concomitant pneumococcal and Hib conjugate vaccines, 21 subjects (3%) who received PEDIARIX and 14 subjects (4%) who received INFANRIX, ENGERIX-B, and IPV reported new onset of a chronic illness during the period from 1 to 6 months following the last dose of study vaccines. Among the chronic illnesses reported in the subjects who received PEDIARIX, there were 4 cases of asthma and 1 case each of diabetes mellitus and chronic neutropenia. There were 4 cases of asthma in subjects who received INFANRIX, ENGERIX-B, and IPV.

**Seizures:** In the German safety study over the entire study period, 6 subjects in the group that received PEDIARIX reported seizures. Two of these subjects had a febrile seizure, 1 of whom also developed afebrile seizures. The remaining 4 subjects had afebrile seizures, including 2 with infantile spasms. Two subjects reported seizures within 7 days following vaccination (1 subject had both febrile and afebrile seizures, and 1 subject had afebrile seizures), corresponding to a rate of 0.22 seizures per 1,000 doses (febrile seizures 0.07 per 1,000 doses, afebrile seizures 0.14 per 1,000 doses). No subject who received concomitant INFANRIX, Hib vaccine, and OPV reported seizures. In a separate German study that evaluated the safety of INFANRIX in 22,505 infants who received 66,867 doses of INFANRIX administered as a 3-dose primary series, the rate of seizures within 7 days of vaccination with INFANRIX was 0.13 per 1,000 doses (febrile seizures 0.0 per 1,000 doses, afebrile seizures 0.13 per 1,000 doses). Over the entire study period in the US safety study in which all subjects received concomitant pneumococcal and Hib conjugate vaccines, 4 subjects in the group that received PEDIARIX reported seizures. Three of these subjects had a febrile seizure and 1 had an afebrile seizure. Over the entire study period, 2 subjects in the group that received INFANRIX, ENGERIX-B, and IPV reported febrile seizures. There were no afebrile seizures in this group. No subject in either study group had seizures within 7 days following vaccination.

**Other Neurological Events of Interest:** No cases of hypotonic-hyporesponsiveness or encephalopathy were reported in either the German safety study or the US safety study.

**Solicited Adverse Events:** Table 1 presents data from the US safety study on solicited local and systemic adverse events within 4 days of vaccination with PEDIARIX or INFANRIX, ENGERIX-B, and IPV, administered concomitantly with Hib and 7-valent pneumococcal conjugate vaccines. In this study, medical attention (a visit to or from medical personnel) for fever within 4 days following vaccination was sought in the group who received PEDIARIX for 8 infants after the first dose (1.2%), 1 infant following the second dose (0.2%), and 5 infants following the third dose (0.8%) (Table 1). Following dose 2, medical attention for fever was sought for 2 infants (0.6%) who received separately administered vaccines (Table 1). Among infants who had a medical visit for fever within 4 days following vaccination, 9 of 14 who received PEDIARIX and 1 of 2 who received separately administered vaccines, had one or more diagnostic studies performed to evaluate the cause of fever.

**Safety of PEDIARIX after a previous dose of hepatitis B vaccine:** Limited data are available on the safety of administering PEDIARIX after a previous dose of hepatitis B vaccine. In 2 separate studies, 160 Moldovan infants and 96 US infants, respectively, received 3 doses of PEDIARIX following 1 previous dose of hepatitis B vaccine. Neither study was designed to detect significant differences in rates of adverse events associated with PEDIARIX administered after a previous dose of hepatitis B vaccine compared to PEDIARIX administered without a previous dose of hepatitis B vaccine.

**Table 1. Percentage of US Infants With Solicited Local Reactions or Systemic Adverse Events Within 4 Days of Vaccination* at 2, 4, and 6 Months of Age With PEDIARIX Administered Concomitantly With Hib Conjugate Vaccine and 7-valent Pneumococcal Conjugate Vaccine (PCV7) or With Separate Concomitant Administration of INFANRIX, ENGERIX-B, IPV, Hib Conjugate Vaccine, and PCV7 (Modified ITT cohort)**

| | PEDIARIX, Hib Vaccine, & PCV7 | | | INFANRIX, ENGERIX-B, IPV, Hib Vaccine, & PCV7 | | |
|---|---|---|---|---|---|---|
| | **Dose 1** | **Dose 2** | **Dose 3** | **Dose 1** | **Dose 2** | **Dose 3** |
| **Local[†]** | | | | | | |
| **N** | **671** | **653** | **648** | **335** | **323** | **315** |
| Pain, any | 36.1 | 36.1 | 31.2 | 31.9 | 30.0 | 29.8 |
| Pain, grade 2 or 3 | 11.5 | 10.9 | 10.6 | 9.0 | 8.7 | 8.9 |
| Pain, grade 3 | 2.4 | 2.5 | 1.7 | 2.7 | 1.5 | 1.3 |
| Redness, any | 29.9[§] | 37.2 | 40.1 | 18.2 | 32.8 | 39.0 |
| Redness, >5 mm | 6.0[§] | 9.6[§] | 12.7[§] | 1.8 | 5.9 | 7.3 |
| Redness, >20 mm | 0.9 | 1.2[§] | 2.8 | 0.3 | 0.0 | 1.9 |
| Swelling, any | 17.3[§] | 26.5[§] | 28.7 | 9.6 | 20.4 | 24.8 |
| Swelling, >5 mm | 5.8[§] | 9.6[§] | 9.3[§] | 1.8 | 5.0 | 4.1 |
| Swelling, >20 mm | 1.9 | 2.5[§] | 3.1 | 0.6 | 0.0 | 1.3 |
| **Systemic** | | | | | | |
| **N** | **667** | **644** | **645** | **333** | **321** | **311** |
| Fever[‡], ≥100.4°F | 27.9[§] | 38.8[§] | 33.5[§] | 19.8 | 30.2 | 23.8 |
| Fever[‡], >101.3°F | 7.0 | 14.1[§] | 8.8 | 4.5 | 9.7 | 5.8 |
| Fever[‡], >102.2°F | 2.2[§] | 3.6 | 3.4 | 0.3 | 3.1 | 2.3 |
| Fever[‡], >103.1°F | 0.4 | 1.4 | 1.1 | 0.0 | 0.3 | 0.3 |
| Fever[‡], M.A. | 1.2[§] | 0.2 | 0.8 | 0.0 | 0.6 | 0.0 |
| **N** | **671** | **653** | **648** | **335** | **323** | **315** |
| Drowsiness, any | 57.2 | 51.6 | 40.9 | 54.0 | 48.3 | 38.4 |
| Drowsiness, grade 2 or 3 | 15.8 | 13.8 | 11.4 | 17.6 | 12.4 | 11.1 |
| Drowsiness, grade 3 | 2.5 | 1.2 | 0.9 | 3.6 | 0.6 | 1.9 |
| Irritability/Fussiness, any | 60.5 | 64.9 | 61.1 | 61.5 | 61.6 | 56.5 |
| Irritability/Fussiness, grade 2 or 3 | 19.8 | 27.9[§] | 25.2[§] | 19.4 | 21.1 | 19.4 |
| Irritability/Fussiness, grade 3 | 3.4 | 4.4 | 3.5 | 3.9 | 3.4 | 3.2 |
| Loss of appetite, any | 30.4 | 30.6 | 26.2 | 27.8 | 26.6 | 23.8 |
| Loss of appetite, grade 2 or 3 | 6.6 | 7.8[§] | 5.9 | 5.1 | 3.4 | 5.4 |
| Loss of appetite, grade 3 | 0.7 | 0.3 | 0.2 | 0.6 | 0.3 | 0.0 |

Modified ITT cohort = all vaccinated subjects for whom safety data were available

N = number of infants for whom at least one symptom sheet was completed; for fever, numbers exclude missing temperature recordings or tympanic measurements.

M.A. = Medically attended (a visit to or from medical personnel).

Grade 2 defined as sufficiently discomforting to interfere with daily activities.

Grade 3 defined as preventing normal daily activities.

*Within 4 days of vaccination defined as day of vaccination and the next 3 days.

[†] Local reactions at the injection site for PEDIARIX or INFANRIX.

[‡] Rectal temperatures or axillary temperatures increased by 1°C to derive equivalent rectal temperature.

[§] Rate significantly higher in the group that received PEDIARIX compared to separately administered vaccines [p value < 0.05 (2-sided Fisher Exact test) or the 95% CI on the difference between groups (Separate minus PEDIARIX) does not include 0].

**Postmarketing Reports With PEDIARIX:** Worldwide voluntary reports of adverse events received for PEDIARIX since market introduction of this vaccine are listed below. This list includes serious adverse events or events which have a suspected causal connection to components of PEDIARIX or other vaccines or drugs. Because these events are reported voluntarily from a population of uncertain size, it is not always possible to reliably estimate their frequency or establish a causal relationship to vaccine exposure. *Cardiac Disorders:* Cyanosis. *Gastrointestinal Disorders:* Diarrhea, vomiting. *General Disorders and Administrative Site Conditions:* Fatigue, injection site cellulitis, injection site induration, injection site itching, injection site nodule/lump, injection site pain, injection site reactions, injection site redness, injection site swelling, injection site warmth, irritability, limb pain, limb swelling, pyrexia, Sudden Infant Death Syndrome. *Immune System Disorders:* Anaphylactic reaction, anaphylactoid reaction, hypersensitivity. *Infections and Infestations:* Upper respiratory tract infection. *Investigations:* Abnormal liver function tests. *Metabolism and Nutrition Disorders:* Anorexia. *Nervous System Disorders:* Bulging fontanelle, convulsions, depressed level of consciousness, febrile convulsion, hypotonia, hypotonic-hyporesponsive episode, lethargy, somnolence. *Psychiatric Disorders:* Crying, insomnia, irritability, nervousness, restlessness, screaming, unusual crying. *Respiratory, Thoracic and Mediastinal Disorders:* Apnea, dyspnea. *Skin and Subcutaneous Tissue Disorders:* Angioedema, erythema, rash, urticaria. *Vascular Disorders:* Pallor, petechiae.

**Postmarketing Reports With INFANRIX and/or ENGERIX-B:** Worldwide voluntary reports of adverse events received for INFANRIX and/or ENGERIX-B in children younger than 7 years of age but not already reported for PEDIARIX are listed below. This list includes serious adverse events or events which have a suspected causal connection to components of INFANRIX and/or ENGERIX-B or other vaccines or drugs. Because these events are reported voluntarily from a population of uncertain size, it is not always possible to reliably estimate their frequency or establish a causal relationship to vaccine exposure. *Blood and Lymphatic System Disorders:* Idiopathic thrombocytopenic purpura[a,b], lymphadenopathy[a], thrombocytopeni[a,b]. *Gastrointestinal Disorders:* Abdominal pain[b], intussusception[a,b], nausea[b]. *General Disorders and Administrative Site Conditions:* Asthenia[b], malaise[b]. *Hepatobiliary Disorders:* Jaundice[b]. *Immune System Disorders:* Anaphylactic shock[a], serum sickness–like disease[b]. *Musculoskeletal and Connective Tissue Disorders:* Arthralgia[b], myalgia[b]. *Nervous System Disorders:* Encephalopathy[a], headache[b]. *Skin and Subcutaneous Tissue Disorders:* Alopecia[b], erythema multiforme[b], pruritus[a,b], Stevens-Johnson syndrome[a]. [[a] Following INFANRIX; [b] Following ENGERIX-B]

**Reporting Adverse Events:** Report the occurrence following immunization of any event set forth in the Vaccine Injury Table from the National Childhood Vaccine Injury Act including: Anaphylaxis or anaphylactic shock within 7 days, encephalopathy or encephalitis within 7 days, brachial neuritis within 28 days, or an acute complication or sequelae (including death) of an illness, disability, injury, or condition referred to above, or any events that would contraindicate further doses of PEDIARIX. These events should be reported to VAERS. The VAERS toll-free number is 1-800-822-7967. Reporting forms may also be obtained at the VAERS website at www.vaers.hhs.gov.

Manufactured by **GlaxoSmithKline Biologicals**, Rixensart, Belgium, US License 1617

Distributed by **GlaxoSmithKline,** Research Triangle Park, NC 27709



Full prescribing information for PEDIARIX is available at www.GSKVaccines.com/Pediarix.

BRS-PE:L3

# Tall Girls

## *The Social Shaping of a Medical Therapy*

*Joyce M. Lee, MD, MPH; Joel D. Howell, MD, PhD*

During the latter half of the 20th century, estrogen therapy was administered to prevent otherwise healthy girls with tall stature from becoming tall adults by inhibiting further linear growth. We explore how decisions to treat tall girls with estrogen were influenced by both scientific knowledge and sociologic norms. Estrogen therapy represented the logical application of scientific knowledge regarding the role of estrogen for closure of the growth plates, but it also reflected prevailing societal and political beliefs about what it meant to be a tall girl. We discuss the rise and fall in popularity of this therapy and suggest that insight into the present-day treatment of short stature can be gained by comparing the use of estrogen therapy for tall girls with the use of growth hormone therapy for short boys. We suggest that this case study illustrates how scientific knowledge is always created and applied within a particular social context.

*Arch Pediatr Adolesc Med. 2006;160:1035-1039*

The therapeutic use of sex steroids dates back to the late 19th century, when medical practitioners such as midwives used ovarian extracts to treat a variety of female disorders. For example, the filtered juice of guinea pigs' ovaries was used for women with hysteria, debility, and abnormal menstruation. Thus, even prior to the discovery of specific substances derived from the ovaries, practitioners attempted to harness their therapeutic potential.[1,2]

**For editorial comment see page 1077**

Changes in scientific understanding led to the concept of hormones, substances that were produced in a particular organ but acted throughout the body in a complex web of interactions. By the 1930s, scientists had identified specific hormones produced by the ovaries and testes.[3] The pharmaceutical industry soon began manufacturing ovarian and testicular preparations, and physicians began exploring a wide range of therapeutic applications.[2]

One such application in the pediatric arena was the use of sex steroids for influencing growth. By the 1940s, physicians began to understand hormonal influences on the growth plate through 2 important clinical observations. First, they observed that children with early exposure to sex hormones due to precocious puberty had premature epiphyseal closure and developed short stature as adults. Physicians also found that children with pituitary disease who lacked sex hormones had open epiphyses with a prolonged period of growth.[4] Based on these clinical observations, it was postulated that gonadal steroids were responsible for closing the epiphyses.[5]

Children at risk for tall stature due to acromegaly thus became the first recipients of estrogen and testosterone therapy for prevention of excess growth during the 1940s.[6] Clinical trials revealed that estrogen preparations, in contrast to testosterone preparations, were particularly successful for preventing tall stature in children with acromegaly. As a consequence, physicians naturally considered

**Author Affiliations:** Division of Pediatric Endocrinology (Dr Lee), Child Health Evaluation and Research Unit (Dr Lee), and Departments of Internal Medicine, History, and Health Management and Policy (Dr Howell), University of Michigan, Ann Arbor.

whether the same treatment could be applied in other settings. Girls with constitutional tall stature represented a potential group of patients for whom hormone therapy might prevent further growth, an outcome that some considered desirable.

In 1946, a brief abstract was published about the clinical experience of estrogen treatment in tall girls who were "becoming alarmed and unhappy about the extremes to which their exuberant, albeit normal growth was carrying them."[5] A decade later, Goldzieher[7] published the first formal clinical study of the use of estrogen therapy for the treatment of constitutional tall stature in girls. Goldzieher cast his research in terms of the application of new scientific advances; he claimed that estrogen treatment of girls destined to be tall as adults was a logical next step following the estrogen treatment of children with acromegaly and hence represented "no novelty." In his initial case series, 14 girls aged 9 to 16 years were treated with oral forms (2 mg daily of stilbestrol or 2.5-5.0 mg daily of premarin) or injected forms (1.6 mg of estradiol monobenzoate every 5 days) of estrogen for anywhere from 3 months to 5 years. Criteria for treatment included a current height of 168 cm (66 in) with open epiphyses or a current height less than 168 cm (66 in) but with a predicted height 10 cm (4 in) above the average. In his article, Goldzieher concluded that growth was successfully arrested based on his observation that the majority of girls had growth of no more than 5 cm (2 in) from the start of therapy.

## SCIENTIFIC AND SOCIAL RATIONALE FOR STANDARD THERAPY FOR TALL GIRLS

These observations appear to have attracted considerable interest within the scientific community. Two years after Goldzieher's initial article, an article by Freed entitled "Suppression of Growth in Excessively Tall Girls" was published in *JAMA* in 1958.[8] Freed noted that "some tall young girls are self-conscious about their height because of the great difference between them and their classmates and friends. By bringing this procedure to the attention of physicians, it is hoped that girls whose height is embarrassing to them may receive medical aid in preventing continued rapid growth."[8] The topic appears to have continued to interest *JAMA* readers (and editors), for in 1959[9] and again in 1961,[10] queries about the treatment of girls with excessive height were published in the "Questions and Answers" section of the journal, a section that offered expert medical opinion to the practicing clinician. By 1962, a scientific review[11] referencing these 3 *JAMA* articles emphasized that the "problem of excessive height in otherwise normal girls is evident,"[11] highlighting the legitimacy of this medical condition while at the same time documenting the efficacy of the treatment. This review was followed by the publication of a number of scientific articles about the treatment in the mid to late 1960s[12-16] that supported a consensus within the medical community that estrogen therapy was a standard treatment for tall girls. These articles scarcely mentioned the treatment of tall boys.

Why was this therapy seen to be useful and interesting enough to attract multiple articles and scientific reviews? It represented newfound knowledge regarding the effects of sex hormones on human growth and development and—perhaps most important—the power to use that knowledge to alter the appearance of potentially tall girls. Many articles detailed how estrogen treatment could bring tall girls' height into or closer to the normal range. But, why should tall girls be made shorter? And, why was the treatment almost exclusively focused on girls but not boys?

The scientific literature details that parents were concerned about the social implications of their daughters being too tall, including difficulty and expense in finding clothes that fit, lack of interest in schoolwork and play, and future difficulty in finding employment in some careers, such as air hostess, classical ballet dancer, or military or airline pilot.[17] There was also discussion of the negative psychosocial effects of excessively tall stature, which included depression, social withdrawal, and even "kyphosis [from] an effort to appear smaller and more like the others."[18]

However, the single most commonly cited social reason for reducing the height of tall girls was social attractiveness. Part of those concerns were contemporaneous with childhood; parents worried about how tall stature was contributing to their daughter's self-consciousness and shyness[9] or that her size might "jeopardize her social contacts."[10] But, tall girls usually became tall women, and the biggest concern seemed to be that tall women would have a hard time fitting in, being comfortable in social situations, and perhaps most important, finding permanent male partners. As one article stated:

> Some girls feel so embarrassed with boys shorter than themselves that they believe that their choice of male companions, both in the immediate future and as adults, will be seriously jeopardized.[17]

If we want to understand why this rationale for treatment had the sort of widespread resonance it did in the 1950s and early 1960s and why the treatment was for girls but not boys, we need to look at the importance of heterosexual marriage for American society in that period.

## SOCIAL CONTEXT

In the 1950s, the most important "career" for women to pursue was that of homemaker and mother. Individuals who did not marry were considered "immoral, selfish, or neurotic,"[19] and even Federal Bureau of Investigation director J. Edgar Hoover suggested that women should marry early and have children to fight "the twin enemies of freedom—crime and Communism."[20] Popular magazines such as *Life* emphasized homemaking for women as a full-time profession, home economics textbooks offered women practical advice about how to be a good wife,[21] and Hollywood movies reinforced the sentiment that "marriage is the most important thing in the world"[22] to women. If a woman's ideal goal was to be successful at marriage, girls who became excessively tall and who did not embody the feminine ideal would have difficulty in finding marriage partners.

A 1954 psychology study by Beigel[23] gives insight into cultural assumptions regarding height and female attractiveness. When 410 persons were surveyed about what characteristics made up a good mate, 59% of the individuals made references to body height as an important and desirable characteristic. Beigel explained the observation that men are almost always taller than women among lovers and married couples by the fact that "most men do not feel attracted to taller women."[23] In this study, desirable women were almost never described as tall and attractive men were almost never described as short.[23]

This was a relational view of height in which women's height was seen in relation to men's height. These sorts of norms were reflected in the medical rationale for estrogen treatment of girls but not boys. Tall girls were said to be dissatisfied with the "prospect of towering over the average male."[24] They were "less attractive than their shorter, more graceful sisters."[25] Thus, physicians were charged with preventing excess growth to increase a girl's physical desirability and her chances of a successful marriage.

## INCREASING SCIENTIFIC KNOWLEDGE ABOUT ESTROGEN THERAPY

Published scientific literature[5,11-18,24,26-35] written mostly by prominent pediatric endocrinologists about "tall girl therapy" proliferated in the 1960s and peaked in the 1970s. Case reports and physician surveys from the United States, Australia, and Europe discussed the administration of estrogen therapy to girls aged 9 to 16 years (mean age, 12 or 13 years) until fusion of the epiphyses was documented, which occurred for most girls at age 15 or 16 years.[5,11-18,24,26-35] Diethylstilbestrol was 1 of the estrogens initially used, at a dose of 1 to 10 mg/d.[5,28] However, the discovery of the association of maternal diethylstilbestrol treatment during pregnancy with vaginal carcinoma in teenaged daughters in 1969 gave way to the use of other estrogen preparations, including conjugated estrogens (0.3-20 mg/d), ethinyl estradiol (0.02-0.5 mg/d), and intramuscular estradiol, which were prescribed as interrupted courses, continuous estrogen therapy, or estrogens in combination with progesterone.[5,28]

Most articles suggested that if administered until fusion of the epiphyses was achieved, estrogen treatment was efficacious, with a diminution of height that ranged anywhere from 3.6 to 7.1 cm (1.4-2.8 in).[14,17,18,24,26,34] Patients who initiated treatment earlier had a greater reduction in height compared with patients who initiated treatment later with regard to chronologic age[11] and pubertal stage.[26] However, the lack of controlled clinical trials led some to doubt its effectiveness. Some studies noted particular difficulty in accurately predicting the adult heights of girls.[35] One study[12] did not find statistically significant differences between predicted and observed adult height, suggesting that individual variations could be misinterpreted as therapeutic results, although the small numbers in this study caused some[17] to question its findings.

Reported positive effects of the therapy included rapid slowing of linear growth, improved self-confidence and self-image, improved performance in school and sports, and disappearance of acne.[5,18,32] However, only slowing of linear growth was formally documented.

Physicians carefully commented on the adverse physiologic events associated with the treatment, including mild adverse effects such as nausea, headaches, weight gain, and breakthrough bleeding as well as more potentially serious adverse effects such as mild hypertension, benign breast disease, ovarian cysts, posttherapeutic amenorrhea, and rare events of thromboembolism. Although there were no reports of malignancy in treated girls, the potential role of estrogen in carcinogenesis was mentioned by a number of studies[5,18,25] and may have subdued some of the initial enthusiasm for estrogen treatment.

## CHANGING DEFINITION OF TALL STATURE

Near the end of 1977, a Conference on Estrogen Treatment of the Young was held in California.[27] The existence of this conference may be taken as a marker of both the maturity of the field and the presence of a critical mass of people doing work in the area. The 1980s and 1990s saw fewer articles extolling the values of estrogen therapy,[36-44] and the literature about estrogen therapy changed, marked by a much more critical commentary.[45-47] Prior to the 1980s, discussions were fairly typical of the literature for most new therapies. Articles discussed whether the therapy worked as indicated, detailed the adverse effects, and explained different medications or dosages that might help improve results while minimizing adverse effects. Later, the debate changed from whether the therapy was effective and how practitioners could minimize its adverse effects to whether tall girls ought to be treated at all. Rather than debating the scientific merit of the practice, critics were increasingly skeptical about the ethics.

One physician wrote in response to a report of estrogen treatment:

> One has to question seriously the right of physicians or parents to determine the ultimate height of a girl. One wonders whether women do not have the right to be tall, just as boys have the right to be short.[47]

Another article concluded that although estrogen therapy would probably work, it should be attempted in a "small number of very tall girls" for whom losing an inch or two in their final height would be a "great comfort."[33] Still others called the procedure "the height of medical hybris" and suggested that the procedure be discontinued.[47] Articles became much more cautious and called for more work in what was now termed an unsettled area.[25] New scientific literature suggesting a link between estrogens and breast and uterine cancer in postmenopausal women[48,49] raised theoretical concerns of an increased risk of cancer due to estrogen treatment, which was highlighted both in the medical literature[5] and in popular newspapers such as the *New York Times*.[50,51]

This skepticism may have led to a diminishing interest in the estrogen treatment of tall girls, which was reflected in physician surveys. A 1977 survey of the Lawson Wilkins Pediatric Endocrine Society found that 50% of respondents reported having treated tall girls with estrogen therapy, with 34% treating only rarely.[28] This contrasts with a 1999 survey of respondents from the same pediatric endocrine society that found that only 23% of respondents had treated tall girls in the previous 5 years and only 1% had treated more than 5 cases.[52] Another marked change was a continuous rise in the predicted height of girls thought to need therapy. For the initial clinical report from 1956, a height prediction of approximately 175 cm (5 ft 9 in) was an indication for treatment,[7] whereas in 1977, therapy was indicated for a predicted adult height of 180 cm (5 ft 11 in) according to the majority of clinicians.[28] In comparison, by 1999, some clinicians required a predicted adult height of 188 cm (6 ft 2 in) before starting therapy.[52]

The increasing reluctance of physicians to prescribe the therapy may have also been mirrored by decreasing requests for therapy from parents and girls, likely influenced by changing societal definitions of tall stature. For example, when girls being seen in a clinic for possible estrogen therapy were asked by their physicians, "How tall is too tall?" the response most frequently given was 173 cm (5 ft 8 in) during the mid 1960s, which rose to 178 cm (5 ft 10 in) during the late 1960s and to 183 cm (6 ft) in the 1970s.[5]

Therefore, just as the rise in estrogen treatment of tall girls was influenced by the social context in which the science was discovered, the decline in prescribing patterns was also influenced by changing societal norms regarding girls, women, and height. Those changing norms had much to do with the cultural upheavals and changing ideas about gender in the 1960s and 1970s.

The feminist movement in particular had a transformative effect on American society. Leaders of the feminist movement exhorted women to assert their own identity, questioning the centrality of the traditional nuclear family and encouraging women to not define their success in terms of male partners. Organizations such as the National Organization for Women actively supported women's participation in the workforce.[53] Work outside the home gave many women a potential for independence that they had not experienced before and enabled them to define their success in terms other than marriage.

The number of women working outside the home in the United States doubled from 15% to 30% between 1940 and 1960.[54] In 1950, 12% of women with preschool-aged children were employed outside the home; by 1995, that percentage was 65%.[55] With this changing demographic, new magazines such as *New York Woman*, *Self*, and *Working Woman* appeared in popular culture, aimed at the young working woman and exhorting the professional woman to adopt a "tailored male look" signaling authority and power,[56] a look that was not inconsistent with being tall.

Increasing opportunities for tall girls also expanded into the athletic arena. Enacted in 1972, Title IX required that federally funded educational organizations such as universities allocate resources equally by sex, which led to increased women's participation in sports and increased media coverage of female athletes. Being tall, once seen as a problem, is now a key part of increasingly successful collegiate athletic enterprises such as volleyball and basketball.[57] Tall women may pursue professional sports careers such as playing for the Women's National Basketball Association, whose players have an average height of 180 cm (5 ft 11 in), with the tallest player measuring 218 cm (7 ft 2 in).[58]

Sociologic studies are also now confirming that tall women are finally reaping the benefits of their stature, at both personal and economic levels. Recent studies show that height positively influences character perception of women; compared with their shorter counterparts, taller women were rated to be more intelligent, affluent, assertive, and ambitious.[59] Just as is the case for men, tall women now enjoy higher incomes than shorter women.[60]

## IMPLICATIONS FOR FUTURE ALTERATION OF HEIGHT IN CHILDREN

Although estrogen therapy for tall girls appears from our early 21st-century vantage point to be largely a therapeutic experiment of the past, it was once considered an appropriate application of scientific progress. Newfound knowledge about the role of estrogen in growth plate physiology led to its therapeutic application to modify height. Estrogen was first used in children with abnormal forms of tall stature, such as acromegaly, and then primarily in otherwise healthy tall girls to prevent them from becoming tall adults.

The use of growth hormone (GH) therapy for short stature has followed a similar pattern thus far. The discovery of the instrumental role of GH for normal statural growth led to the use of cadaveric human GH extracts or recombinant GH for children with abnormal forms of short stature due to GH deficiency,[61] with exclusive treatment of children with the most severe forms of GH deficiency.[62,63] However, with the wide availability of recombinant GH and the recent Food and Drug Administration approval of GH therapy for idiopathic short stature in 2003,[64] GH is now being used for otherwise healthy short children to prevent them from becoming short adults.[63]

The most striking difference between the use of estrogen for tall stature and the use of GH for short stature is sex. Whereas mostly girls were evaluated for tall stature and were treated with estrogen in the past, twice as many boys than girls are evaluated for short stature and are treated with GH today.[65,66] In his book *Better Than Well: American Medicine Meets the American Dream*, philosopher Carl Elliott argues that one of the sociologic reasons for the use of estrogen in tall girls and the use of GH in short boys relates to the topic of sexual partners.[67] He states that "neither tall girls nor short boys . . . can compete successfully for mates,"[67] asking the critical question that gets to the heart of the debate about stature, "In the great homecoming dance of life, how does a short boy get a date with the head cheerleader?"[67]

Although the increasing social value of height for girls as well as the increasing concern about the adverse effects of estrogen therapy likely influenced the decline in the use of estrogen therapy, the use of GH therapy for short males has replaced estrogen therapy as a means for preventing what was and might still be considered the union most offensive to taste: the union of a tall woman with a short man.[23] In essence, GH treatment of short stature in boys could be considered the 21st-century counterpart to estrogen treatment of tall stature in girls.

As we continue to explore the powers of science for modifying height for both boys and girls, we should keep in mind historical examples such as estrogen treatment for tall girls. These examples should help us realize that scientific advances are always applied within a specific social context, and within that context, idealized gender relations may be as important as scientific studies in determining what we will do as practicing clinicians.

**Accepted for Publication:** June 22, 2006.
**Correspondence:** Joyce M. Lee, MD, MPH, 300 NIB, Room 6E05, Campus Box 0456, Ann Arbor, MI 48109-0456 (joyclee@umich.edu).
**Author Contributions:** *Study concept and design:* Lee and Howell. *Acquisition of data:* Lee and Howell. *Analysis and interpretation of data:* Lee and Howell. *Drafting of the manuscript:* Lee and Howell. *Critical revision of the manuscript for important intellectual content*: Lee and Howell. *Administrative, technical, and material support:* Lee and Howell. *Study supervision:* Lee and Howell.
**Funding/Support:** Dr Lee was supported by Pediatric Health Services Research Training Grant T32HD 07534-05 from the National Institute of Child Health and Human Development, National Institutes of Health.
**Acknowledgment:** We thank Regina Morantz-Sanchez, PhD, for her thoughtful contributions to the manuscript.

## REFERENCES

1. Corner GW. The early history of the oestrogenic hormones. *J Endocrinol.* 1965; 31:III-XVII.
2. Oudshoorn N. On measuring sex hormones: the role of biological assays in sexualizing chemical substances. *Bull Hist Med.* 1990;64:243-261.
3. Borell M. Organotherapy, British physiology, and discovery of the internal secretions. *J Hist Biol.* 1985;18:1-30.
4. Fancher TK. Some observations on anterior lobe hyperpituitarism. *Endocrinology.* 1932;16:611.
5. Crawford JD. Treatment of tall girls with estrogen. *Pediatrics.* 1978;62:1189-1195.
6. Kirklin OL, Wilder RM. Follicular hormone administration in acromegaly. *Proc Staff Meet Mayo Clin.* 1936;11:121-125.
7. Goldzieher MA. Treatment of excessive growth in the adolescent female. *J Clin Endocrinol Metab.* 1956;16:249-252.
8. Freed SC. Suppression of growth in excessively tall girls. *JAMA.* 1958;166:1322-1323.
9. Questions and answers. *JAMA.* 1959;169:305.
10. Questions and answers. *JAMA.* 1961;175:1036.
11. Whitelaw MJ, Foster TN. Treatment of excessive height in girls: a long-term study. *J Pediatr.* 1962;61:566-570.
12. Bayley N, Gordon GS, Bayer LM. Attempt to suppress excessive growth in girls by estrogen treatment: statistical evaluation. *J Clin Endocrinol Metab.* 1962; 22:1127-1129.
13. Whitelaw MJ, Foster TN, Graham WH. Estradiol valerate: its effects on anabolism and skeletal age in the prepubertal girl. *J Clin Endocrinol.* 1963;23:1125-1129.
14. Greenblatt RB, McDonough PG, Mahesh VB. Estrogen therapy in inhibition of growth. *J Clin Endocrinol.* 1966;26:1185-1191.
15. Whitelaw MJ. Experiences in treating excessive height in girls with cyclic oestradiol valerate: a ten year survey. *Acta Endocrinol (Copenh).* 1967;54:473-484.
16. Frasier SD, Smith FG. Effect of estrogens on mature height in tall girls: a controlled study. *J Clin Endocrinol.* 1968;28:416-419.
17. Wettenhall HNB, Roche AF. Tall girls assessment and management. *Aust Paediatr J.* 1965;1:210-216.
18. Prader A, Zachmann M. Treatment of excessively tall girls and boys with sex hormones. *Pediatrics.* 1978;62(suppl):1202-1210.
19. Rosen R. *The World Split Open.* New York, NY: Penguin Group; 2000.
20. Hoover JE. The twin enemies of freedom: crime and communism: address before the 28th Annual Convocation of the National Council of Catholic Women. *Vital Speeches Day.* 1956;23:104-107.
21. Mikkelson B, Mikkelson DP. Urban legends reference pages: how to be a good wife. http://www.snopes.com/language/document/goodwife.htm. Accessed June 13, 2006.
22. Rosen R. *The World Split Open.* New York, NY: Penguin Group; 2000:13.
23. Beigel HG. Body height in mate selection. *J Soc Psychol.* 1954;39:257-268.
24. Tall girl therapy. *CMAJ.* 1976;114:9.
25. Bailey JD, Park E, Cowell C. Estrogen treatment of girls with constitutional tall stature. *Pediatr Clin North Am.* 1981;28:501-512.
26. Bierich JR. Estrogen treatment of girls with constitutional tall stature. *Pediatrics.* 1978;62:1196-1201.
27. Report of the Conference on Estrogen Treatment of the Young. *Pediatrics.* 1978; 62:1087-1217.
28. Conte FA, Grumbach MM. Estrogen use in children and adolescents: a survey. *Pediatrics.* 1978;62:1091-1097.
29. Colle ML. The tall girl: prediction of mature height and management. *Arch Dis Child.* 1977;52:118-120.
30. Kuhn N, Blunck W, Stahnke N, Wiebel J, Willig RP. Estrogen treatment in tall girls. *Acta Paediatr Scand.* 1977;66:161-167.
31. Zachmann M, Ferrandez A, Murset G, Prader A. Estrogen treatment of excessively tall girls. *Helv Paediatr Acta.* 1975;30:11-30.
32. Excessive height [editorial]. *BMJ.* 1975;2:648-649.
33. Marshall WA. What can we do about tall girls? *Arch Dis Child.* 1975;50:671-673.
34. Schoen EJ, Solomon IL, Warner O, Wingerd J. Estrogen treatment of tall girls. *AJDC.* 1973;125:71-74.
35. Roche AF, Wettenhall HNB. The prediction of adult stature in tall girls. *Aust Paediatr J.* 1969;5:13-22.
36. Weimann E, Bergmann S, Bohles HJ. Oestrogen treatment of constitutional tall stature: a risk-benefit ratio. *Arch Dis Child.* 1998;78:148-151.
37. Binder G, Grauer ML, Wehner AV, Wehner F, Ranke MB. Outcome in tall stature: final height and psychological aspects in 220 patients with and without treatment. *Eur J Pediatr.* 1997;156:905-910.
38. de Waal WJ, Greyn-Fokker MH, Stijnen T, et al. Accuracy of final height prediction and effect of growth-reductive therapy in 362 constitutionally tall children. *J Clin Endocrinol Metab.* 1996;81:1206-1216.
39. de Waal WJ, Torn M, de Muinck Keizer-Schrama SMPF, Aarsen RSR, Drop SLS. Long term sequelae of sex steroid treatment in the management of constitutionally tall stature. *Arch Dis Child.* 1995;73:311-315.
40. Joss EE, Zeuner J, Zurbrugg RP, Mullis PE. Impact of different doses of ethinyl oestradiol on reduction of final height in constitutionally tall girls. *Eur J Pediatr.* 1994;153:797-801.
41. Normann EK, Trygstad O, Larsen S, Dahl-Jorgensen K. Height reduction in 539 tall girls treated with three different dosages of ethinyloestradiol. *Arch Dis Child.* 1991;66:1275-1278.
42. Gruters A, Heidemann P, Schluter H, Stubbe P, Weber B, Helge H. Effect of different oestrogen doses on final height reduction in girls with constitutional tall stature. *Eur J Pediatr.* 1989;149:11-13.
43. Bartsch O, Weschke B, Weber B. Oestrogen treatment of constitutionally tall girls with 0.1 mg/day ethinyl oestradiol. *Eur J Pediatr.* 1988;147:59-63.
44. Sorgo W, Scholler K, Heinze F, Heinze E, Teller WM. Critical analysis of height reduction in oestrogen-treated tall girls. *Eur J Pediatr.* 1984;142:260-265.
45. Brook CG, Stanhope R, Preece MA, Green AA, Hindmarsh PC. Oestrogen treatment of tall stature [letter]. *Arch Dis Child.* 1998;79:199.
46. Lecointre C, Toublanc JE. Psychological indications for treatment of tall stature in adolescent girls. *J Pediatr Endocrinol Metab.* 1997;10:529-531.
47. Stickler GB. Reduction of adult height in tall girls [letter]. *Eur J Pediatr.* 1980;134:91.
48. Lipsett MB. Estrogen use and cancer risk. *JAMA.* 1977;237:1112-1115.
49. Hoover R, Gray LA Sr, Cole P, MacMahon B. Menopausal estrogens and breast cancer. *N Engl J Med.* 1976;295:401-405.
50. Brozan N. The use of estrogen as a growth inhibitor in over-tall girls is being questioned. *New York Times.* February 11, 1976:55.
51. Haines A. Controlling height. *New York Times.* April 4, 1976:19.
52. Barnard ND, Scialli AR, Bobela S. The current use of estrogens for growth-suppressant therapy in adolescent girls. *J Pediatr Adolesc Gynecol.* 2002;15: 23-26.
53. Rosen R. *The World Split Open.* New York, NY: Penguin Group; 2000:74-81.
54. Rosen R. *The World Split Open.* New York, NY: Penguin Group; 2000:19.
55. Metzl JM. *Prozac on the Couch: Prescribing Gender in the Era of Wonder Drugs.* Durham, NC: Duke University Press; 2003.
56. Rosen R. *The World Split Open.* New York, NY: Penguin Group; 2000:312-314.
57. Shakib S, Dunbar MD. The social construction of female and male high school basketball participation: reproducing the gender order through a two-tiered sporting institution. *Sociol Perspect.* 2002;45:353-378.
58. WNBA Enterprises LLC. 2003 WNBA player survey results: height. http://www.wnba.com/statistics/survey_height_2003.html. Accessed June 4, 2006.
59. Chu S, Geary K. Physical stature influences character perception in women. *Pers Individ Dif.* 2005;38:1927-1934.
60. Judge TA, Cable DM. The effect of physical height on workplace success and income: preliminary test of a theoretical model. *J Appl Psychol.* 2004;89:428-441.
61. Raben MS. Treatment of a pituitary dwarf with human growth hormone. *J Clin Endocrinol Metab.* 1958;18:901-903.
62. Allen DB, Fost N. hGH for short stature: ethical issues raised by expanded access. *J Pediatr.* 2004;144:648-652.
63. Cuttler L, Silvers JB. Growth hormone treatment for idiopathic short stature: implications for practice and policy. *Arch Pediatr Adolesc Med.* 2004;158:108-110.
64. US Food and Drug Administration. FDA talk paper: FDA approves Humatrope for short stature. http://www.fda.gov/bbs/topics/ANSWERS/2003/ANS01242.html. Accessed July 7, 2004.
65. Grimberg A, Kutikov JK, Cucchiara AJ. Sex differences in patients referred for evaluation of poor growth. *J Pediatr.* 2005;146:212-216.
66. Wyatt D. Lessons from the national cooperative growth study. *Eur J Endocrinol.* 2004;151(suppl 1):S55-S59.
67. Elliott C. *Better Than Well: American Medicine Meets the American Dream.* New York, NY: WW Norton Co & Inc; 2003.

# Motor and Cognitive Outcomes in Nondisabled Low-Birth-Weight Adolescents

## *Early Determinants*

*Agnes H. Whitaker, MD; Judith F. Feldman, PhD; John M. Lorenz, MD; Sa Shen, PhD; Fiona McNicholas, MD; Marlon Nieto, BA; Dawn McCulloch, MSEd; Jennifer A. Pinto-Martin, PhD; Nigel Paneth, MD, MPH*

**Objectives:** To describe motor and cognitive outcomes in nondisabled low-birth-weight (LBW) adolescents and to determine the relation of specific prenatal, perinatal, and neonatal risk factors to these outcomes.

**Design:** A prospective epidemiological study.

**Setting:** An adolescent follow-up of a regional LBW (<2000 g) cohort born in or admitted to 3 hospitals between September 1, 1984, and June 30, 1987 (n=1105). Of 862 eligible survivors, 628 (72.9%) underwent assessment at a mean age of 16 years; of these, 33 had severe disability that precluded psychometric evaluation. The 474 nondisabled adolescents undergoing assessment at home had slightly less social risk at birth than did all other nondisabled eligible adolescents.

**Participants:** The 474 nondisabled LBW adolescents assessed at home.

**Main Exposures:** Basic birth characteristics (social risk, sex, fetal growth ratio, and gestational age), neonatal cranial ultrasound abnormalities, and other early medical complications.

**Main Outcome Measures:** Riley Motor Problems Inventory and Wechsler Abbreviated Scales of Intelligence.

**Results:** Nondisabled LBW adolescents had an excess of motor problems compared with the normative sample. The IQ scores, although within the normal range, were significantly lower than population norms. Independent predictors of total motor problems included male sex, white matter injury on neonatal ultrasound, and days of ventilation. Independent predictors of lower Full Scale IQ scores included social disadvantage, fetal growth ratio, and white matter injury on neonatal ultrasound.

**Conclusions:** Specific prenatal, perinatal, and neonatal risk factors influence motor and cognitive performance in nondisabled LBW survivors well into adolescence, even when controlling for social risk. Advances in maternal-fetal and neonatal care can substantially improve these long-term outcomes.

*Arch Pediatr Adolesc Med. 2006;160:1040-1046*

**Author Affiliations:** Division of Child and Adolescent Psychiatry, Columbia University and New York State Psychiatric Institute (Drs Whitaker and Feldman, Mr Nieto, and Ms McCulloch), and Departments of Psychiatry (Dr Whitaker), Pediatrics (Dr Lorenz), and Neuroscience in Psychiatry (Dr Shen), Columbia University, New York, NY; Department of Child Psychiatry, University College, Dublin, Ireland (Dr McNicholas); Schools of Nursing and Medicine, University of Pennsylvania, Philadelphia (Dr Pinto-Martin); and Departments of Epidemiology and Pediatrics and Human Development, College of Human Medicine, Michigan State University, East Lansing (Dr Paneth).

MOUNTING EVIDENCE suggests that low birth weight (LBW) increases risk for not only major disabilities such as cerebral palsy and mental retardation[1,2] but also subtler motor and cognitive problems in nondisabled survivors by school age[3-6] and, with some exceptions,[7] even as late as adolescence.[8-13] The most commonly studied prenatal, perinatal, and neonatal risk factors for motor and cognitive outcomes in nondisabled LBW adolescents are the basic birth characteristics that are readily available at or before birth: social disadvantage, sex, birth weight for gestational age, and gestational age.[8,9,13] With rare exception,[12] the relation of early medical complications to these subtler outcomes has not been examined, to our knowledge. Such information could help identify potential targets for preventive intervention with respect to long-term outcomes.

The regional LBW cohort assembled for the Neonatal Brain Hemorrhage Study[14] provides an unprecedented opportunity to examine the relation between specific early risk factors and adolescent motor and cognitive outcomes. This cohort is unique in the following respects: (1) it was geographically defined, representing nearly all infants with birth weights of less than 2000 g in a 3-county region during a 3-year period; (2) all members underwent neonatal cranial ultrasound (US) screening for evidence of neonatal brain injury; and (3) a large database of other prenatal, perinatal, and neonatal risk factors was collected systematically at birth on the entire cohort. The objectives of the present study were to describe motor and cognitive outcomes in nondisabled LBW adolescents and to determine the relation of specific prenatal, perinatal, and neonatal risk factors to these outcomes.

**Table 1. Risk Factors**

**Basic Risk Variables**

**Maternal social disadvantage:** Based on the Social Risk Index of Hack et al,[15] this composite score is a count of the number of maternal risk conditions out of 5 (age <19 y, <high school education, unmarried status, minority status, and receipt of public assistance) that were present at the time of the infant's birth.

**Sex:** Ascertained from physical examination at birth as recorded in the infant's medical chart.

**Gestational age:** Estimated using a hierarchical algorithm[16] with data from multiple sources—prenatal ultrasound images (preferably before 20 weeks of gestation), prenatal and postnatal medical records, and postnatal maternal interview—with attention to consistency across records.

**Fetal growth ratio:** Calculated as birth weight divided by median weight for gestational age according to Yudkin et al.[17]

**Early Medical Complications**

**Neonatal ultrasound abnormalities:**

Serial cranial ultrasound performed at 4 and 24 h and 7 d of life, according to a research protocol.[18] Scans read independently by ≥2 radiologists blinded to all clinical information except birth weight; disagreements (only 6% of cases) resolved with a third reading. Two types of ultrasound abnormalities were identified:

**GMH/IVH:** Isolated germinal matrix hemorrhage and/or intraventricular hemorrhage (GMH/IVH).

**PL/VE:** Parenchymal lesions and/or ventricular enlargement with or without GMH/IVH.

**Other early medical complications:**

**Maternal smoking:** Maternal report of number of cigarettes smoked per day during pregnancy (log-transformed for analysis).

**Placental abruption:** Determined from medical record; recorded as clinically evident.

**Chorioamnionitis:** Determined from medical record; recorded as clinically evident.

**Active labor:** According to Qiu et al.[19]

**5-min Apgar score:** Sum of 5 ratings (0-2, with 2 being best) at 5 min post partum.

**Base excess:** Metabolic acid-base status, calculated from pH and bicarbonate ion concentrations in the first blood gas measurement after birth.[20] Positive values indicate metabolic alkalosis; negative values indicate metabolic acidosis. In the immediate perinatal period, having more negative values (greater acidosis) indicates less adequate oxygen delivery to the tissues.

**Seizures:** Any notation of seizure during the first 24 h of life in the infant's medical chart.

**Thyroid status:** Standardized *z* score derived from newborn blood thyroxine and thyrotrophic screening results according to the criteria of Reuss et al.[21] (There were no known cases of congenital hypothyroidism in our cohort.)

**Hypocapnia exposure:** Time- and severity-weighted variable defined by Collins et al[20] as the number of hours of exposure to $Pco_2$ <35 mm Hg ($\kappa$ = 4.7) multiplied by the number of millimeters of mercury of $Pco_2$ <35; higher values indicate more prolonged and/or severe exposure.

**Hyperoxia exposure:** Time- and severity-weighted variable defined by Collins et al[20] as the number of hours of exposure to $Po_2$ >60 ($\kappa$ = 8.0) multiplied by the number of $Po_2$ units >60; higher values indicate more prolonged and/or severe exposure.

**Low systolic blood pressure:** Number of days with a systolic blood pressure >2 SDs below the mean for that day as defined for this cohort by Hegyi et al.[22,23]

**Peak bilirubin:** Highest bilirubin level recorded during the first 8 neonatal days.

**Neonatal infection:** Any positive blood, cerebrospinal fluid, or urine culture during the neonatal intensive care unit stay.

**Ventilator days:** Number of days with any mechanical ventilation.[20]

## METHODS

### BIRTH COHORT

Participants belonged to the Neonatal Brain Hemorrhage Study birth cohort.[14] The original study prospectively enrolled 1105 consecutive infants with birth weights of less than 2000 g born in or admitted to 3 New Jersey hospitals between September 1, 1984, and June 30, 1987. During that period, the neonatal intensive care units at these hospitals provided neonatal care for 83% of all infants with birth weights of less than 2000 g and 90% of those with birth weights of less than 1500 g in 3 New Jersey counties. Compared with the nation as a whole, this 3-county region had a slightly higher per capita income and slightly lower proportion of minorities.[14]

### SAMPLE AT 16 YEARS OF AGE

The adolescent follow-up was approved by the institutional review board of the New York State Psychiatric Institute. Informed consent was obtained from legal guardians for all of the adolescents before participation. The mean±SD age at assessment was 16.0±0.5 years (range, 14.8-19.4 years). By age 16 years, 212 (19.2%) of the original birth cohort were known to have died and 31 (2.8%) had been adopted or were in foster care, leaving 862 enrollees who were potentially eligible for follow-up. Of the eligible enrollees, 628 (72.9%) participated in the 16-year follow-up, whereas 83 (9.6%) refused and 151 (17.5%) could not be located. Of the latter group, 68 (45.0%) had been lost to follow-up since hospital discharge.

Of the 628 adolescent participants, 33 (5.3%) had a severe major disability, defined as the inability to walk without assistance (n=24), an IQ score of less than 55 (>3 SDs below the population mean; n=28), or neurosensory impairment severe enough to preclude outcome testing (deaf or blind; n=4). Of the 595 nondisabled participants, 474 (79.7%) were assessed during home visits and 121 by telephone. Adolescents assessed by telephone were slightly older, on average, than those assessed in the home. The focus of this report is the 474 nondisabled adolescents assessed in the home.

### EARLY RISK FACTORS

**Table 1** gives the definitions of the risk factors used in this study.

#### Basic Risk

These variables, readily available at or before birth, are commonly used to predict later outcomes. It is not yet established, however, that they are related to outcome in nondisabled adolescents independently of neonatal brain injury and other early medical complications.

#### Neonatal Brain Injury

In view of the unique nature of the neonatal brain injury information in this cohort, US status was considered as a separate set of early medical complications. Ninety-eight percent of the cohort was scanned with US at least once in the first week

**Table 2. Risk Exposure in Nondisabled LBW Adolescents Undergoing Assessment at Home vs Other Eligible LBW Adolescents***

| Risk Factor | Assessed at Home (n = 474) | Other Eligible Adolescents (n = 347)† |
|---|---|---|
| Basic risk | | |
| Maternal social risk (number of risk conditions at child's birth) | 0.89 ± 1.26 | 1.40 ± 1.49‡ |
| Male, % | 51.27 | 48.99 |
| Fetal growth ratio | 0.88 ± 0.21 | 0.90 ± 0.23 |
| Gestational age, wk | 31.27 ± 3.10 | 31.19 ± 3.14 |
| US abnormalities, % | | |
| GM/IVH | 14.56 | 14.70 |
| PL/VE | 4.85 | 4.61 |
| Other early medical complications | | |
| Maternal smoking during pregnancy (number of cigarettes a day) | 3.72 ± 7.15 | 3.85 ± 6.74 |
| Placental abruption, % | 7.73 | 8.48 |
| Chorioamnionitis, % | 4.42 | 5.15 |
| Active labor, % | 58.85 | 62.09 |
| 5-min Apgar Score | 7.84 ± 1.44 | 7.88 ± 1.41 |
| Base excess (first determination), mEq/L | −4.69 ± 4.22 | −4.54 ± 3.60 |
| Seizure in first 24 h, % | 0.42 | 1.44 |
| Thyroxine level, *z* score | −1.43 ± 1.03 | −1.48 ± 1.10 |
| Cumulative hypocapnia in first 8 d, mm Hg × hours | 138.48 ± 233.83 | 132.75 ± 197.96 |
| Cumulative hyperoxia in first 8 d, mm Hg × hours | 1487.72 ± 1557.99 | 1615.44 ± 1795.80 |
| Systolic BP, number of days >2 SDs below mean in first week | 0.83 ± 1.50 | 0.86 ± 1.52 |
| Peak bilirubin level in first 8 d | 9.20 ± 2.67 | 9.12 ± 2.52 |
| Neonatal infection, % | 30.80 | 26.51 |
| Days on ventilator | 5.39 ± 12.14 | 4.86 ± 12.61 |

Abbreviations: BP, blood pressure; GM/IVH, germinal matrix and/or intraventricular hemorrhage; LBW, low-birth-weight; PL/VE, parenchymal lesion and/or ventricular enlargement with or without GM/IVH; US, ultrasound.

*Unless otherwise indicated, data are expressed as mean ± SD. Risk factors are described in Table 1.

†Includes those undergoing assessment only by telephone, those lost to follow-up, and those who refused participation. For telephone interview assessments (n = 129), severe major disability was defined as a Vineland Adaptive Behavior Composite score lower than 55 and/or a parental report of an inability to walk without assistance at 16 years of age; 8 were excluded on these grounds. For those lost to follow-up (n = 151) and those who refused participation (n = 80), major motor disability was defined as parental report at 6 years of age of an inability to walk without assistance; 3 were excluded on these grounds. No information regarding major disability was available for those not assessed at 6 years of age (n = 165). An additional 5 were excluded on grounds of major mental disability, which was defined as a score in the moderate to profound mental retardation range on a test of general cognitive ability from the most proximal earlier follow-up age (2, 6, or 9 years) and/or a Vineland Adaptive Behavior Composite score lower than 55 at the most proximal earlier age. For those lost to follow-up since birth-hospital discharge (n = 45), no information was available.

‡Assessed vs not assessed, $P<.01$.

after birth, and 47% was also scanned between the third and fifth weeks of hospitalization and at or before discharge. The US abnormalities were classified from the scan showing the most severe abnormality, using the criteria of Paneth et al[14] (Table 1).

### Other Early Medical Complications

Early medical complications other than US abnormalities were selected from an extensive database that included information abstracted from prenatal, perinatal, and neonatal medical records and from a maternal interview conducted soon after birth.[18] Some of these complications (hypothyroxinemia,[21] hypocapnia,[20] hypotension,[24] hyperbilirubinemia,[25] seizures,[24] and ventilation days or indices of chronic lung disease[26]) have previously been shown to predict major disability and might reasonably be expected to cause subtler problems as well. Others, such as metabolic acidosis,[20] appear not to increase risk for major disability[27] but might increase subtler problems.

### Motor and Cognitive Assessment

All assessors were blinded to birth history and trained to reliability. Motor function was assessed with the Riley Motor Problems Inventory,[28] which tests for oral, fine, and gross motor problems. Area scores are weighted counts of errors in performing an area's tasks (3 tasks each for the oral and fine motor areas and 4 for the gross motor area), with errors weighted as 0 (no errors serious enough to be counted), 1, and 2. The maximum scores for the oral, fine, and gross motor areas are 6, 6, and 8, respectively. The total score is the sum of the 3 area scores (maximum, 20 points). The total score for persons 9 years or older has a median, upper tenth centile, and upper second centile, in the standardization sample, of 1, 5, and 7 points, respectively. For oral, fine, and gross motor area scores, these centiles are 3, 0, and 2 points, respectively. Full Scale, Verbal, and Performance IQ scores were assessed with the Wechsler Abbreviated Scales of Intelligence.[29] For all 3 scales, mean ± SD is 100 ± 15.

## STATISTICAL ANALYSIS

Bivariate relations were examined with Pearson product moment correlations (and with regressions, using $k-1$ dummy variables for categorical variables with more than 2 categories). However, multiple regression was the principal method used to evaluate the relation of predictors to outcomes.

To keep the number of predictors small relative to the number of cases in the sample, the prenatal, perinatal, and neonatal predictors used for this study were selected from a larger set that had been chosen on the basis of a priori theoretical interest or some indication in the literature that they were related to the studied outcomes. Selection for inclusion in these analyses was based on bivariate relations among predictors and between predictors and outcomes in this data set. Variables unrelated to any outcomes and those highly correlated or redundant with more meaningful ones were excluded. To maintain the sample size and power, missing values of predictors were replaced and dichotomous missing value indicators were included in regressions for predictors that were missing more than 3% of their values.[30] The probability level (α criterion) for statistical significance was set at .01 for all analyses. We used SPSS[31] and SAS[32] statistical software.

## RESULTS

### STUDY SAMPLE

Except for having slightly less social risk at birth, the nondisabled adolescents assessed at home were similar to those nondisabled adolescents who were eligible for the study but were not assessed at home (**Table 2**).

### MOTOR PROBLEMS AND IQ SCORES IN THE NONDISABLED SAMPLE

The means for the total, oral, fine, and gross motor problem scores (**Table 3**) place the sample of nondisabled adolescents as a whole between the median and upper tenth centile of the standardization sample. Total motor problem scores were 5 or greater for 22.4% of these adolescents, placing them in the top 10% of the standardization sample, and 7 or greater for 11.3%, placing them in the top 2%.

Although the mean IQ scores in Table 3 were all within the average range, the distributions were shifted downward. The means for the Full Scale and Performance IQ scores were significantly lower than those for the population norm ($t=-3.96$ and $t=-6.91$, respectively; both $P<.001$).

### MULTIPLE REGRESSIONS

The standardized partial regression coefficients in **Table 4** show the relation of each risk factor to outcome after controlling for all other risk factors. These coefficients indicate how much of a change in outcome (in standard deviation units) is uniquely associated with 1 SD of change in the risk factor.

#### Basic Risk

Greater maternal social risk at birth was significantly associated with lower Full Scale, Verbal, and Performance IQ scores, but not with any type of motor problem. For each additional condition of maternal social risk, the IQ scores were depressed by 3.6 points on the Full Scale IQ, 3.6 points on the Verbal IQ, and 2.6 points on the Performance IQ. Male sex was significantly associated with more total, oral, and fine motor problems, but not with lower IQ. Gestational age was not associated with any aspect of motor problems or IQ score, whereas a lower fetal growth ratio was significantly associated with lower Full Scale and Performance IQ scores.

#### Neonatal Cranial US Abnormalities

Compared with those who had no US abnormalities, nondisabled adolescents with germinal matrix and/or intraventricular hemorrhage (GM/IVH) had higher scores on the oral motor problems scale by half a point, whereas those with parenchymal lesions and/or ventricular enlargement (PL/VE) had higher scores on the total, oral, fine, and gross motor problem scales by 3.7, 0.8, 0.9, and 2.0 points, respectively, and lower Full Scale and Performance IQ scores by 1.6 and 2.2 points, respectively.

**Table 3. Motor Problems and Cognitive Ability in Nondisabled LBW Adolescents**

| Domain (Outcome Measure) | No. of Adolescents | Mean ± SD Score |
|---|---|---|
| Motor problems* | | |
| Total | 464 | 3.58 ± 3.27 |
| Oral | 464 | 0.75 ± 1.22 |
| Fine | 464 | 1.80 ± 1.48 |
| Gross | 464 | 1.03 ± 1.65 |
| Cognitive performance† | | |
| Full Scale | 474 | 97.27 ± 14.57 |
| Verbal | 468 | 99.56 ± 14.57 |
| Performance | 468 | 95.21 ± 14.57 |

Abbreviation: LBW, low-birth-weight.
*Scores from the Rily Motor Problems Inventory.
†IQ scores from the Wechsler Abbreviated Scales of Intelligence.

#### Other Early Medical Complications

Except for placental abruption and ventilator days, the independent relations of these risk factors to motor problems were nonsignificant. The average fine motor problems score was 0.7 points higher among those with placental abruption. For every additional week of mechanical ventilation, total and oral motor problem scores were higher by 0.33 and 0.14 points, respectively. Other medical complications had no independent relation to IQ scores.

#### Relations of Risk to IQ Score Among Nondisabled LBW Adolescents of Normal Intelligence

To determine whether the relations described in Table 4 were primarily due to the inclusion of adolescents with Full Scale IQ scores in the mildly retarded or borderline range (55-84), analyses were repeated excluding those adolescents. In this sample (n=385), the following 5 relations between risk factors and intelligence scores dropped below the significance threshold, although they differed only minimally in magnitude from those in the less restricted sample: age at test with Full Scale IQ ($\beta=-0.12$) and Verbal IQ ($\beta=-0.16$), fetal growth ratio with Full Scale IQ ($\beta=0.11$), and PL/VE with Full Scale IQ ($\beta=-0.08$) and Performance IQ ($\beta=-0.11$). Other significant relations with IQ scores in Table 4 remained, and a new relation emerged between low thyroxine levels and lower Full Scale IQ scores ($\beta=0.16$; $P<.01$).

## COMMENT

The finding that nondisabled LBW adolescents had an excess of motor problems relative to the normative sample is consistent with results of 2 case-control studies of motor skills

**Table 4. Independent Relations of Prenatal, Perinatal, and Neonatal Risk Factors to Motor Problems and General Cognitive Ability in Nondisabled LBW Adolescents***

| | | RMPI‡ | | | | WASI‡ | | |
|---|---|---|---|---|---|---|---|---|
| **Risk Factor†** | **Missing Values, %** | **Total** | **Oral** | **Fine** | **Gross** | **Full Scale** | **Verbal** | **Performance** |
| Age at test (control) | 0 | −0.04 | −0.01 | −0.02 | −0.05 | **−0.12§** | **−0.17‖** | −0.05 |
| Basic | | | | | | | | |
| Maternal social risk | 0 | 0.01 | 0.01 | 0.02 | −0.01 | **−0.31‖** | **−0.32‖** | **−0.23‖** |
| Male | 0 | **0.14‖** | **0.13§** | **0.15‖** | 0.05 | 0.03 | 0.03 | 0.01 |
| Fetal growth ratio | 0 | −0.14 | −0.10 | −0.14 | −0.08 | **0.18§** | 0.05 | **0.29‖** |
| Gestational age | 0 | −0.16 | −0.13 | −0.18 | −0.05 | 0.03 | −0.08 | 0.14 |
| US abnormalities | | | | | | | | |
| GM/IVH | 0 | 0.03 | **0.15§** | −0.01 | −0.03 | −0.07 | −0.05 | −0.09 |
| PL/VE | 0 | **0.25‖** | **0.15‖** | **0.13§** | **0.26‖** | **−0.11§** | −0.06 | **−0.15‖** |
| Other early medical complications | | | | | | | | |
| Maternal smoking during pregnancy | 13 | 0.03 | 0.03 | 0.03 | 0.01 | −0.07 | −0.09 | −0.02 |
| Placental abruption | 5 | 0.08 | 0.07 | **0.13§** | −0.02 | −0.06 | −0.08 | −0.05 |
| Chorioamnionitis | 5 | −0.03 | 0.03 | −0.05 | −0.04 | −0.01 | 0.02 | −0.03 |
| Active labor | 1 | 0.05 | 0.03 | 0.04 | 0.05 | 0.03 | 0.03 | 0.01 |
| 5-min Apgar score | 2 | 0.00 | 0.11 | −0.01 | −0.06 | 0.05 | 0.03 | 0.06 |
| Base excess (first determination) | 23 | −0.09 | −0.11 | −0.05 | −0.06 | 0.09 | 0.09 | 0.08 |
| Seizure in first 24 h | 0 | 0.06 | 0.07 | 0.00 | 0.06 | −0.08 | −0.04 | −0.11 |
| Thyroxine level (*z* score) | 5 | 0.05 | 0.05 | −0.02 | 0.07 | 0.03 | 0.05 | 0.00 |
| Cumulative hypocapnia in first 8 d | 16 | 0.03 | 0.00 | 0.02 | 0.04 | −0.08 | −0.11 | −0.04 |
| Cumulative hyperoxia in first 8 d | 16 | 0.06 | 0.04 | −0.01 | 0.09 | −0.02 | 0.03 | −0.06 |
| Systolic BP (lowest in first week) | 4 | 0.08 | 0.02 | 0.07 | 0.09 | −0.04 | −0.05 | −0.03 |
| Peak bilirubin level in first 8 days | 7 | −0.05 | −0.02 | 0.03 | −0.11 | 0.05 | 0.06 | 0.04 |
| Neonatal infection | 0 | 0.01 | −0.01 | −0.03 | 0.06 | 0.00 | 0.01 | −0.01 |
| Days on Ventilator | 0 | **0.18§** | **0.20‖** | 0.10 | 0.11 | −0.09 | −0.10 | −0.06 |

Abbreviations: GM/IVH, germinal matrix and/or intraventricular hemorrhage; LBW, low-birth-weight; PL/VE, parenchymal lesion; and/or ventricular enlargement with or without GM/IVH; RMPI, Riley Motor Problems Inventory; US, ultrasound; WASI, Wechsler Abbreviated Scales of Intelligence.

*Risk factors are described in Table 1. Data are expressed as standardized partial regression coefficients (βs) controlling for age at test, all other risk factors, and missing value indicators. Missing value indicators, coded 1 (missing) or 0 (otherwise), were included in the regression equations for all variables with 3% or more of their values missing. For all variables, the mean (or mode, for categorical variables) was substituted for missing values (as described in the "Statistical Analysis" subsection of the "Methods" section). To simplify Table 4, the coefficients associated with the missing value indicators are not presented; none were significant, indicating that missing values were not due to any systematic factors related to outcome. Significant relations are expressed in boldface.

†Risk factors excluded from these regressions because they were unrelated to outcome in preliminary bivariate analyses included born in vs transferred to study hospitals, maternal alcohol intake in pregnancy, maternal hypertension, duration of ruptured membranes, and fetal presentation. Those risk factors excluded because they were highly correlated with listed ones were birth weight (redundant with gestational age when fetal growth ratio is also included as a risk factor), head circumference ratio (correlated with fetal growth ratio), multiple birth (also correlated with fetal growth ratio), diastolic blood pressure (correlated with systolic blood pressure), and chronic lung disease (correlated with days on ventilator).

‡For the RMPI, higher scores indicate more problems (worse performance); for the WASI, higher scores indicate better performance.

§$P \leq .01$.

‖$P \leq .001$.

in nondisabled very-LBW adolescents.[8,13] Motor problems in nondisabled adolescents have clinically important correlates because such problems are significantly associated with poor self-esteem[33] and, in this LBW cohort, with lower overall adaptive functioning (A.H.W., unpublished data, November 2005). The finding that the IQ scores of these nondisabled LBW adolescents were in the average range is consistent with studies of extremely LBW[11,34] and very LBW[12,35] adolescents. Here, this finding is extended to a broader range of birth weight. In this sample, as in the studies just cited, however, the slight downward shift of the means indicates an extra public health burden when these findings are extrapolated to the general population.[36]

When other risk factors were controlled for, gestational age alone was not an independent predictor of adolescent motor or cognitive outcomes. This finding runs counter to the view that, in the absence of medical complications, premature exposure to the extrauterine environment per se alters brain development in LBW infants.[37]

Major independent determinants of motor outcomes in these LBW adolescents without severe disabilities were male sex, evidence of white matter injury on neonatal brain US, and number of ventilation days. The finding of an adverse effect of male sex, despite control for so many other risk factors, suggests a need to look beyond the association of maleness with greater prevalence and severity of neonatal complications[38] to explain this male vulnerability effect. One possibility is that hormonal differences between the sexes affect acute response to and long-term recovery from brain injury.[39] Although gestational age appeared to have a protective effect on motor problems, this effect is an artifact of the inverse relation between gestational age and fetal growth ratio in this birth-weight–truncated sample.[40]

In this study, neonatal US evidence of focal white matter injury (PL/VE) was found to be associated with all types of motor problems. These pervasive effects on motor outcomes are difficult to understand, given an apparently localized lesion on US. Evidence from magnetic resonance imaging studies, however, suggests that focal white matter injury may also be a marker for diffuse white matter injury and may be related to minor motor impairments. Abernethy et al[41] found that preterm school-age children without major neurodisability had, in addition to visible lesions on magnetic resonance images, a diffuse abnormality of cerebral white matter (manifested as an increase in T2 relaxation time) that was highly related to minor motor impairment but not to Full Scale IQ scores. The finding that GM/IVH was related selectively to oral motor problems is consistent with the location of this injury near the head of the caudate nucleus, which is now being implicated in oromotor control.[42]

Of the other early medical complications, only placental abruption and ventilator days were independently related to motor outcomes. Placental abruption has been widely reported to be associated with cerebral palsy; thus, an association with fine motor problems is not surprising. The relation of ventilator days could be explained by the duration of mechanical ventilation being considered a marker for severity of illness; this could explain its disappearance as a factor when the adolescents with below-normal IQ scores were deleted from the sample. Duration of mechanical ventilation could also be associated with an increased risk of exposure to some ventilation-related practice that itself is detrimental. (Hypocapnia and hyperoxia might be reasonable candidates for such exposure.[20]) This hypothesis is attractive because it suggests that, if we could identify the practice and modify it, outcome could be improved.

Major independent predictors of intelligence were social disadvantage at birth, fetal growth ratio, and white matter injury as seen on neonatal US images of the brain. Although this latter factor was no longer significant in the smaller sample (those with an IQ score at or above 85), the magnitude of its association with cognitive outcome was only minimally reduced. An adverse effect of early social disadvantage on intelligence that occurs as late as adolescence in LBW survivors is a well-replicated finding.[43,44] On the other hand, the finding that biological risk factors also predicted adolescent cognitive outcome suggests that effects of early biological insult are not completely overwhelmed by the environment over time.

The finding that slow growth in utero (as indexed by fetal growth ratio) was highly associated with intelligence in adolescence—in particular with the Performance IQ score—is consistent with findings from a population cohort study of Swedish men showing that all studied indices of slow fetal growth were independently associated with increased risk of poor cognitive performance at 18 to 19 years of age.[45] The present finding is inconsistent with that of an earlier literature review,[46] which concluded that, by adolescence and adulthood, the deleterious effect of intrauterine growth retardation sometimes found at earlier ages was inconsequential compared with environmental influences. In the present study, low fetal growth ratio was highly correlated with fetal head circumference ratio; 77.7% of the infants in the sample who were small for gestational age also had a head circumference ratio that was in the lowest tenth percentile for age. Thus, it is not possible to discern from these data whether the effect on cognition was related to fetal growth ratio in general or rather, more specifically, to fetal head growth retardation. This issue requires further exploration.

Several caveats apply to these findings. First, although only a few of the early medical complications examined were independently related to motor or cognitive outcomes, their possible importance to these outcomes in adolescence cannot be dismissed. It may well be that several of these early complications share the same determinative path, and thus account for similar aspects of motor problems and/or cognitive performance. In consequence, any independent relation of these risk factors to outcome would be precluded. Second, inasmuch as the present regression findings apply to entire distributions of exposures, they do not rule out an effect of being at the extreme of the distribution for some risk factor (eg, <26 weeks of gestation). In addition, interactions between medical complications (eg, between Apgar scores and mechanical ventilation) cannot be ruled out. Third, although subject loss was within the expected range for such a long-term follow-up in a population-based sample, some bias might be expected. In particular, the caretakers of infants with identified problems are more likely to participate in follow-up visits, thereby possibly inflating the estimates of dysfunction.[47]

The strengths of this study remain (1) the use of a regional birth cohort, (2) the prospective and systematic ascertainment of a rich set of early medical complications, (3) the rigor of the US protocol, and (4) the inclusion of a wider spectrum of LBW survivors than is usually examined in modern follow-up studies.

The finding that, independent of social risk, specific prenatal, perinatal, and neonatal biological risk factors are associated with cognitive and motor outcomes as late as adolescence runs counter to the view that, absent severe disability, early biological risk factors are of little importance in later life.[43,48] The prevention of white matter injury and the need for mechanical ventilation may be key to improving motor outcomes, whereas the prevention of intrauterine growth retardation (or perhaps impaired head growth) and white matter injury may be key to improving cognitive outcomes. Taken together, these findings suggest that enhanced maternal-fetal and neonatal care have the potential to substantially improve cognitive and motor outcomes for nondisabled LBW adolescents.

**Accepted for Publication:** June 5, 2006.
**Correspondence:** Agnes H. Whitaker, MD, Division of Child and Adolescent Psychiatry, Unit 74, New York State Psychiatric Institute, 1051 Riverside Dr, New York, NY 10032 (whitakea@childpsych.columbia.edu).
**Author Contributions:** Drs Whitaker and Feldman had full access to all of the data in the study and take full responsibility for the integrity of the data and the accuracy of the data analysis. *Study concept and design:* Whitaker, Feldman, Lorenz, Shen, McNicholas, Pinto-Martin, and Paneth. *Acquisition of data:* Whitaker, McNicholas, Nieto, McCulloch, and Paneth. *Analysis and interpretation of data:* Whitaker, Feldman, Lorenz, Shen, and Paneth. *Drafting of the manuscript:* Whitaker, Feldman, Lorenz, Nieto, and Paneth. *Critical revision of the*

*manuscript for important intellectual content:* Whitaker, Feldman, Shen, Pinto-Martin, and Paneth. *Statistical analysis:* Feldman and Shen. *Obtained funding:* Whitaker, Feldman and Pinto-Martin, and Paneth. *Administrative, technical, and material support:* Whitaker, Feldman, McNicholas, Nieto, McCulloch, and Pinto-Martin. *Study supervision:* Whitaker.

**Funding/Support:** This study was supported by grant 5 R01 MH57514-05 from the National Institute of Mental Health and grant 12-FY03-46 from the March of Dimes.

**Acknowledgment:** We thank the participating adolescents and their families, who made this study possible, and Janet Baxendale, for study coordination.

## REFERENCES

1. Pinto-Martin JA, Riolo SA, Cnaan A, Holzman C, Susser MW, Paneth N. Cranial ultrasound prediction of disabling and non-disabling cerebral palsy in a low birth weight population. *Pediatrics.* 1995;95:249-254.
2. Whitaker AH, Feldman JF, Van Rossem R, et al. Neonatal cranial ultrasound abnormalities in LBW infants: relation to cognitive outcomes at age six. *Pediatrics.* 1996;98:719-729.
3. Pinto-Martin JA, Whitaker AH, Feldman JF, Van Rossem R, Paneth N. Relation of cranial ultrasound abnormalities in low-birthweight infants to motor or cognitive performance at ages 2, 6, and 9 years. *Dev Med Child Neurol.* 1999;41:826-833.
4. Marlow N, Roberts BL, Cooke RWI. Motor skills in extremely low birthweight children at the age of 6 years. *Arch Dis Child.* 1989;64:839-847.
5. Crowe TK, Deitz JC, Bennett FC, TeKolste K. Preschool motor skills of children born prematurely and not diagnosed as having cerebral palsy. *J Dev Behav Pediatr.* 1988;9:189-193.
6. Bhutta AT, Cleves MA, Casey PH, Cradock MM, Anand KJS. Cognitive and behavioral outcomes of school-aged children who were born preterm: a meta-analysis. *JAMA.* 2002;288:728-737.
7. Tideman E. Longitudinal follow-up of children born preterm: cognitive development at age 19. *Early Hum Dev.* 2000;58:81-90.
8. Powls A, Botting N, Cooke RW, Marlow N. Motor impairment in children 12 to 13 years old with a birthweight of less than 1250 g. *Arch Dis Child Fetal Neonatal Ed.* 1995;73:F62-F66.
9. Saigal S. Follow-up of very low birthweight babies to adolescence. *Semin Neonatol.* 2000;5:107-118.
10. Rickards AL, Kelly EA, Doyle LW, Callanan C. Cognition, academic progress, behavior, and self-concept at 14 years of very low birth weight children. *J Dev Behav Pediatr.* 2001;22:11-18.
11. Grunau RE, Whitfield MF, Fay TB. Psychosocial and academic characteristics of extremely low birth weight (≤800 g) adolescents who are free of major impairment compared with term-born control subjects. *Pediatrics.* 2004;114:e725-e732.
12. Taylor HG, Minich N, Bangert B, Filipek P, Hack M. Long-term neuropsychological outcomes of very low birth weight: associations with early risks for periventricular brain insults. *J Int Neuropsychol Soc.* 2004;10:987-1004.
13. Evensen KAI, Vik T, Helbostad J, Indredavik MS, Kulseng S, Brubakk AM. Motor skills in adolescents with low birth weight. *Arch Dis Child Fetal Neonatal Ed.* 2004; 89:F451-F455.
14. Paneth N, Rudelli R, Kazam E, Monte WA. *Brain Damage in the Preterm Infant.* London, England: MacKeith Press; 1994.
15. Hack M, Taylor G, Klein N, Eiben R, Schatschneider C, Mercuri-Minich N. School-age outcomes in children with birth weights under 750 g. *N Engl J Med.* 1994; 331:753-759.
16. Holzman C, Paneth N, Little R, Pinto-Martin J. Perinatal brain injury in premature infants born to mothers using alcohol in pregnancy. *Pediatrics.* 1995;95:66-73.
17. Yudkin PL, Aboualfa M, Eyre JA, Redman CWG, Wilkinson AR. New birthweight and head circumference centiles for gestational ages 24 and 42 weeks. *Early Hum Dev.* 1987;15:45-52.
18. Pinto-Martin J, Paneth N, Witomski T, et al. The central New Jersey neonatal brain hemorrhage study: design of the study and reliability of ultrasound diagnosis. *Paediatr Perinat Epidemiol.* 1992;6:273-284.
19. Qiu H, Paneth N, Lorenz JM, Collins M. Labor and delivery factors in brain damage, disabling cerebral palsy, and neonatal death in low-birth-weight infants. *Am J Obstet Gynecol.* 2003;189:1143-1149.
20. Collins MP, Lorenz JM, Jetton JR, Paneth N. Hypocapnia and other ventilation-related risk factors for cerebral palsy in low birth weight infants. *Pediatr Res.* 2001;50:712-719.
21. Reuss ML, Paneth N, Pinto-Martin JA, Lorenz JM, Susser M. The relation of transient hypothyroxemia in preterm infants to neuorologic development at two years of age. *N Engl J Med.* 1996;334:821-827.
22. Hegyi T, Carbone MT, Anwar M, et al. Blood pressure ranges in premature infants, I: the first hours of life. *J Pediatr.* 1994;124:627-633.
23. Hegyi T, Carbone MT, Anwar M, et al. Blood pressure ranges in premature infants, II: the first week of life. *Pediatrics.* 1996;97:336-342.
24. Murphy DJ, Hope PL, Johnson A. Neonatal risk factors for cerebral palsy in very preterm babies: case-control study. *BMJ.* 1997;314:404-408.
25. Byers RK, Paine RS, Crothers B. Extrapyradimal cerebral palsy with hearing loss following erythroblastosis. *Pediatrics.* 1955;15:248-254.
26. Pinto-Martin JA, Riolo S, Cnaan A, Holzman C, Susser MW, Paneth N. Cranial ultrasound prediction of disabling and non-disabling cerebral palsy in a low birth weight population [published correction appears in *Pediatrics.* 2001;108:238]. *Pediatrics.* 1995;95:249-254.
27. Holcroft CJ, Lakemore KJ, Allen M, Graham E. Association of prematurity and neonatal infection with neurologic morbidity in very low birth weight infants. *Obstet Gynecol.* 2003;101:1249-1253.
28. Riley GD. *Riley Motor Problems Inventory Manual.* Los Angeles, Calif: Western Psychological Services; 1976.
29. Wechsler D. *WASI: Wechsler Abbreviated Scales of Intelligence.* San Antonio, Tex: Psychological Corp; 1999.
30. Cohen J, Cohen P. *Applied Multiple Regression/Correlation Analysis for the Behavioral Sciences.* 2nd ed. Hillsdale, NJ: Lawrence A Erlbaum Associates; 1983.
31. *SPSS for Windows.* Chicago, Ill: SPSS Inc; 2004.
32. *SAS/STAT.* Cary, NC: SAS Institute Inc; 2003.
33. Skinner RA, Piek JP. Psychosocial implications of poor motor coordination in children and adolescents. *Hum Mov Sci.* 2001;20:73-94.
34. Saigal S, Hoult LA, Streiner DL, Stoskopf BL, Rosenbaum PL. School difficulties at adolescence in a regional cohort of children who were extremely low birth weight. *Pediatrics.* 2000;105:325-331.
35. Rickards AL, Kelly EA, Doyle LW, Callanan C. Cognition, academic progress, behavior and self-concept at 14 years of very low birth weight children. *J Dev Behav Pediatr.* 2001;22:11-18.
36. Breslau N, DelDotto JE, Brown GG, et al. A gradient relationship between low birth weight and IQ at age 6 years. *Arch Pediatr Adolesc Med.* 1994;148:377-383.
37. de Haan M, Bauer PJ, Georgieff MK, Nelson CA. Explicit memory in low-risk infants aged 19 months born between 27 and 42 weeks of gestation. *Dev Med Child Neurol.* 2000;42:304-312.
38. Hack M, Wilson-Costello D, Friedman H, Taylor GH, Schluchter M, Fanaroff AA. Neurodevelopment and predictors of outcomes of children with birth weights of less than 1000 g: 1992-1995. *Arch Pediatr Adolesc Med.* 2000;154:725-731.
39. Nuñez JL, McCarthy MM. Sex differences and hormonal effects in a model of preterm infant brain injury. *Ann N Y Acad Sci.* 2003;1008:281-284.
40. Arnold CC, Kramer MS, Hobbs CA, McLean FH, Usher RH. Very low birth weight: a problematic cohort for epidemiologic studies of very small or immature neonates. *Am J Epidemiol.* 1991;134:604-613.
41. Abernethy LJ, Klafkowski G, Foulder-Hughes L, Cooke RW. Magnetic resonance imaging and T2 relaxometry of cerebral white matter and hippocampus in children born preterm. *Pediatr Res.* 2003;54:868-874.
42. Watkins KE, Vargha-Khadem F, Ashburner J, et al. MRI analysis of an inherited speech and language disorder: structural brain abnormalities. *Brain.* 2002; 125 (pt 3):465-478.
43. Sameroff AJ. Longitudinal studies of preterm infants: a review of chapters 17-20. In: Friedman S, Sigman M, eds. *Preterm Birth and Psychological Development.* Orlando, Fla: Academic Press Inc; 1981:387-393.
44. Shenkin SD, Starr J, Deary I. Birth weight and cognitive ability in childhood: a systematic review. *Psychol Bull.* 2004;130:989-1013.
45. Bergvall N, Iliadou A, Tuvemo T, Cnattingius S. Birth characteristics and risk of low intellectual performance in early adulthood: are the associations confounded by socioeconomic factors in adolescence or familial effects? *Pediatrics.* 2006;117:714-721.
46. Hack M. Effects of intrauterine growth retardation on mental performance and behavior, outcomes during adolescence and adulthood. *Eur J Clin Nutr.* 1998; 52(suppl 1):S65-S70.
47. Aylward GP. Methodological issues in outcome studies of at-risk infants. *J Pediatr Psychol.* 2002;27:37-45.
48. Sameroff AJ, Chandler MJ. Reproductive risk and the continuum of caretaking casualty. In: Horowitz FD, ed. *Review of Child Development Research.* Chicago, Ill: University of Chicago Press; 1975:187-244.

**Orapred ODT™**
(prednisolone sodium phosphate orally disintegrating tablets)

**BRIEF SUMMARY:** Please see full prescribing information.

**DESCRIPTION:**
Orapred ODT orally disintegrating tablets are available in strengths containing 13.4 mg, 20.2 mg, and 40.3 mg prednisolone sodium phosphate (equivalent to 10 mg, 15 mg, or 30 mg prednisolone base, respectively).
**PRECAUTIONS: General: Do not break or use partial Orapred ODT tablets.** The lowest possible dose of corticosteroid should be used to control the condition under treatment, and when reduction in dosage is possible, the reduction should be gradual.
Since complications of treatment with glucocorticoids are dependent on the size of the dose and the duration of treatment, a risk/benefit decision must be made in each individual case as to dose and duration of treatment and as to whether daily or intermittent therapy should be used.
There is an enhanced effect of corticosteroids in patients with hypothyroidism and in those with cirrhosis
Kaposi's sarcoma has been reported to occur in patients receiving corticosteroid therapy, most often for chronic conditions. Discontinuation of corticosteroids may result in clinical improvement.
**Cardio-renal:** As sodium retention with resultant edema and potassium loss may occur in patients receiving corticosteroids, these agents should be used with caution in patients with hypertension, congestive heart failure, or renal insufficiency.
**Endocrine:** Drug-induced secondary adrenocortical insufficiency may be minimized by gradual reduction of dosage. This type of relative insufficiency may persist for months after discontinuation of therapy; therefore, in any situation of stress occurring during that period, hormone therapy should be reinstituted. Since mineralocorticoid secretion may be impaired, salt and/or a mineralocorticoid should be administered concurrently.
**Gastrointestinal:** Steroids should be used with caution in nonspecific ulcerative colitis, if there is a probability of impending perforation, abscess or other pyogenic infection;
diverticulitis; fresh intestinal anastomoses; active or latent peptic ulcer. Signs of peritoneal irritation following gastrointestinal perforation in patients receiving corticosteroids may be minimal or absent.
**Musculoskeletal:** Corticosteroids decrease bone formation and increase bone resorption both through their effect on calcium regulation (i.e., decreasing absorption and increasing excretion) and inhibition of osteoblast function. This, together with a decrease in the protein matrix of the bone secondary to an increase in protein catabolism, and reduced sex hormone production, may lead to inhibition of bone growth in children and adolescents and the development of osteoporosis at any age. Special consideration should be given to patients at increased risk of osteoporosis (i.e., postmenopausal women) before initiating corticosteroid therapy.
**Neuro-psychiatric:** Although controlled clinical trials have shown corticosteroids to be effective in speeding the resolution of acute exacerbations of multiple sclerosis, they do not show that they affect the ultimate outcome or natural history of the disease. The studies do show that relatively high doses of corticosteroids are necessary to demonstrate a significant effect. (See DOSAGE AND ADMINISTRATION.)
An acute myopathy has been observed with the use of high doses of corticosteroids, most often occurring in patients with disorders of neuromuscular transmission (e.g., myasthenia gravis), or in patients receiving concomitant therapy with neuromuscular blocking drugs (e.g., pancuronium). This acute myopathy is generalized, may involve ocular and respiratory muscles, and may result in quadriparesis. Elevation of creatinine kinase may occur. Clinical improvement or recovery after stopping corticosteroids may require weeks to years.
Psychic derangements may appear when corticosteroids are used, ranging from euphoria, insomnia, mood swings, personality changes, and severe depression, to frank psychotic manifestations. Also, existing emotional instability or psychotic tendencies may be aggravated by corticosteroids.
**Ophthalmic:** Intraocular pressure may become elevated in some individuals. If steroid therapy is continued for more than 6 weeks, intraocular pressure should be monitored.
**Information For Patients:** Patients should be warned not to discontinue the use of Orapred abruptly or without medical supervision, to advise any medical attendants that they are taking it, and to seek medical advice at once should they develop fever or other signs of infection.
Persons who are on immunosuppressant doses of corticosteroids should be warned to avoid exposure to chickenpox or measles. Patients should also be advised that if they are exposed, medical advice should be sought without delay.
**Drug Interactions:** Drugs such as barbiturates, phenytoin, ephedrine, and rifampin, which induce hepatic microsomal drug metabolizing enzyme activity may enhance metabolism of prednisolone and require that the dosage of Orapred be increased.
Increased activity of both cyclosporin and corticosteroids may occur when the two are used concurrently. Convulsions have been reported with this concurrent use.
Estrogens may decrease the hepatic metabolism of certain corticosteroids thereby increasing their effect.
Ketoconazole has been reported to decrease the metabolism of certain corticosteroids by up to 60% leading to an increased risk of corticosteroid side effects.
Coadministration of corticosteroids and warfarin usually results in inhibition of response to warfarin, although there have been some conflicting reports. Therefore, coagulation indices should be monitored frequently to maintain the desired anticoagulant effect.
Concomitant use of aspirin (or other non-steroidal anti-inflammatory agents) and corticosteroids increases the risk of gastrointestinal side effects. Aspirin should be used cautiously in conjunction with corticosteroids in hypoprothrombinemia. The clearance of salicylates may be increased with concurrent use of corticosteroids.
When corticosteroids are administered concomitantly with potassium-depleting agents (i.e., diuretics, amphotericin-B), patients should be observed closely for development of
hypokalemia. Patients on digitalis glycosides may be at increased risk of arrhythmias due to hypokalemia.
Concomitant use of anticholinesterase agents and corticosteroids may produce severe weakness in patients with myasthenia gravis. If possible, anticholinesterase agents should be withdrawn at least 24 hours before initiating corticosteroid therapy.
Due to inhibition of antibody response, patients on prolonged corticosteroid therapy may exhibit a diminished response to toxoids and live or inactivated vaccines. Corticosteroids may also potentiate the replication of some organisms contained in live attenuated vaccines. If possible, routine administration of vaccines or toxoids should be deferred until corticosteroid therapy is discontinued.
Because corticosteroids may increase blood glucose concentrations, dosage adjustments of antidiabetic agents may be required.
Corticosteroids may suppress reactions to skin tests.
**Pregnancy: Teratogenic Effects:** *Pregnancy Category C.*
Prednisolone has been shown to be teratogenic in many species when given in doses equivalent to the human dose. Animal studies in which prednisolone has been given to pregnant mice, rats, and rabbits have yielded an increased incidence of cleft palate in the offspring. There are no adequate and well-controlled studies in pregnant women. Orapred should be used during pregnancy only if the potential benefit justifies the potential risk to the fetus. Infants born to mothers who have received corticosteroids during pregnancy should be carefully observed for signs of hypoadrenalism.
**Nursing Mothers:** Systemically administered corticosteroids appear in human milk and could suppress growth, interfere with endogenous corticosteroid production, or cause other untoward effects. Caution should be exercised when Orapred is administered to a nursing woman.
**Pediatric Use:** The efficacy and safety of prednisolone in the pediatric population are based on the well-established course of effect of corticosteroids, which is similar in pediatric and adult populations. Published studies provide evidence of efficacy and safety in pediatric patients for the treatment of nephrotic syndrome (>2 years of age), and aggressive lymphomas and leukemias (>1 month of age). However, some of these conclusions and other indications for pediatric use of corticosteroid, e.g., severe asthma and wheezing, are based on adequate and well-controlled trials conducted in adults, on the premises that the course of the diseases and their pathophysiology are considered to be substantially similar in both populations.
The adverse effects of prednisolone in pediatric patients are similar to those in adults (see ADVERSE REACTIONS). Like adults, pediatric patients should be carefully observed with frequent measurements of blood pressure, weight, height, intraocular pressure, and clinical evaluation for the presence of infection, psychosocial disturbances, thromboembolism, peptic ulcers, cataracts, and osteoporosis. Children, who are treated with corticosteroids by any route, including systemically administered corticosteroids, may experience a decrease in their growth velocity. This negative impact of corticosteroids on growth has been observed at low systemic doses and in the absence of laboratory evidence of HPA axis suppression (i.e., cosyntropin stimulation and basal cortisol plasma levels). Growth velocity may therefore be a more sensitive indicator of systemic corticosteroid exposure in children than some commonly used tests of HPA axis function. The linear growth of children treated with corticosteroids by any route should be monitored, and the potential growth effects of prolonged treatment should be weighed against clinical benefits obtained and the availability of other treatment alternatives. In order to minimize the potential growth effects of corticosteroids, children should be *titrated* to the lowest effective dose.
**Geriatric Use:** Clinical studies of prednisolone sodium phosphate oral solution did not include sufficient numbers of subjects aged 65 and over to determine whether they respond differently from younger subjects. Other reported clinical experience with prednisolone sodium phosphate has not identified differences in responses between the elderly and younger patients. However, the incidence of corticosteroid-induced side effects may be increased in geriatric patients and appear to be dose-related. Osteoporosis is the most frequently encountered complication, which occurs at a higher incidence rate in corticosteroid-treated geriatric patients as compared to younger populations and in agematched controls. Losses of bone mineral density appear to be greatest early on in the course of treatment and may recover over time after steroid withdrawal or use of lower doses (i.e., 5 mg/day).
Prednisolone doses of 7.5 mg/day or higher, have been associated with an increased relative risk of both vertebral and nonvertebral fractures, even in the presence of higher bone density compared to patients with involutional osteoporosis.
Routine screening of geriatric patients, including regular assessments of bone mineral density and institution of fracture prevention strategies, along with regular review of Orapred indication should be undertaken to minimize complications and keep the Orapred dose at the lowest acceptable level. Co-administration of bisphosphonates has been shown to retard the rate of bone loss in corticosteroid-treated males and postmenopausal females, and these agents are recommended in the prevention and treatment of corticosteroid-induced osteoporosis.
It has been reported that equivalent weight-based doses yield higher total and unbound prednisolone plasma concentrations and reduced renal and non-renal clearance in elderly patients compared to younger populations. However, it is not clear whether dosing reductions would be necessary in elderly patients, since these pharmacokinetic alterations may be offset by age-related differences in responsiveness of target organs and/or less pronounced suppression of adrenal release of cortisol. Dose selection for an elderly patient should be cautious, usually starting at the low end of the dosing range, reflecting the greater frequency of decreased hepatic, renal, or cardiac function, and of concomitant disease or other drug therapy.
This drug is known to be substantially excreted by the kidney, and the risk of toxic reactions to this drug may be greater in patients with impaired renal function. Because elderly patients are more likely to have decreased renal function, care should be taken in dose selection, and it may be useful to monitor renal function (see CLINICAL PHARMACOLOGY).
**ADVERSE REACTIONS: (listed alphabetically under each subsection):**
**Cardiovascular:** Hypertrophic cardiomyopathy in premature infants.
**Dermatologic:** Facial erythema; increased sweating; impaired wound healing; may suppress reactions to skin tests; petechiae and ecchymoses; thin fragile skin; urticaria; edema.
**Endocrine:** Decreased carbohydrate tolerance; development of cushingoid state; hirsutism; increased requirements for insulin or oral hypoglycemic agents in diabetic patients; manifestations of latent diabetes mellitus; menstrual irregularities; secondary adrenocortical and pituitary unresponsiveness, particularly in times of stress, as in trauma, surgery or illness; suppression of growth in children.
**Fluid and Electrolyte Disturbances:** Congestive heart failure in susceptible patients; fluid retention; hypertension; hypokalemic alkalosis; potassium loss; sodium retention.
**Gastrointestinal:** Abdominal distention; elevation in serum liver enzyme levels (usually reversible upon discontinuation); pancreatitis; peptic ulcer with possible perforation and hemorrhage; ulcerative esophagitis.
**Metabolic:** Negative nitrogen balance due to protein catabolism.
**Musculoskeletal:** Aseptic necrosis of femoral and humeral heads; loss of muscle mass; muscle weakness; osteoporosis; pathologic fracture of long bones; steroid myopathy; tendon rupture; vertebral compression fractures.
**Neurological:** Convulsions; headache; increased intracranial pressure with papilledema
(pseudotumor cerebri) usually following discontinuation of treatment; psychic disorders; vertigo.
**Ophthalmic:** Exophthalmos; glaucoma; increased intraocular pressure; posterior subcapsular cataracts.
**Other:** Increased appetite; malaise; nausea; weight gain.
In clinical trials with ORAPRED ODT, the following adverse reactions were seen.
Facial edema, pharyngolaryngeal pain, blood in stool, eye irritation, eyelid edema.
**OVERDOSAGE:** The effects of accidental ingestion of large quantities of prednisolone over a very short period of time have not been reported, but prolonged use of the drug can produce mental symptoms, moon face, abnormal fat deposits, fluid retention, excessive appetite, weight gain, hypertrichosis, acne, striae, ecchymosis, increased sweating, pigmentation, dry scaly skin, thinning scalp hair, increased blood pressure, tachycardia, thrombophlebitis, decreased resistance to infection, negative nitrogen balance with delayed bone and wound healing, headache, weakness, menstrual disorders, accentuated menopausal symptoms, neuropathy, fractures, osteoporosis, peptic ulcer, decreased glucose tolerance, hypokalemia, and adrenal insufficiency. Hepatomegaly and abdominal distention have been observed in children.

Treatment of acute overdosage is by immediate gastric lavage or emesis followed by supportive and symptomatic therapy. For chronic overdosage in the face of severe disease requiring continuous steroid therapy, the dosage of prednisolone may be reduced only temporarily, or alternate day treatment may be introduced.

**Do not break or use partial Orapred ODT tablets.** Keep out of the reach of children.

**Rx only**
Revised May 2006.

Manufactured for Alliant Pharmaceuticals, Inc.
Alpharetta, GA 30022

by CIMA LABS INC., Eden Prairie, MN 55344 (Orapred ODT)

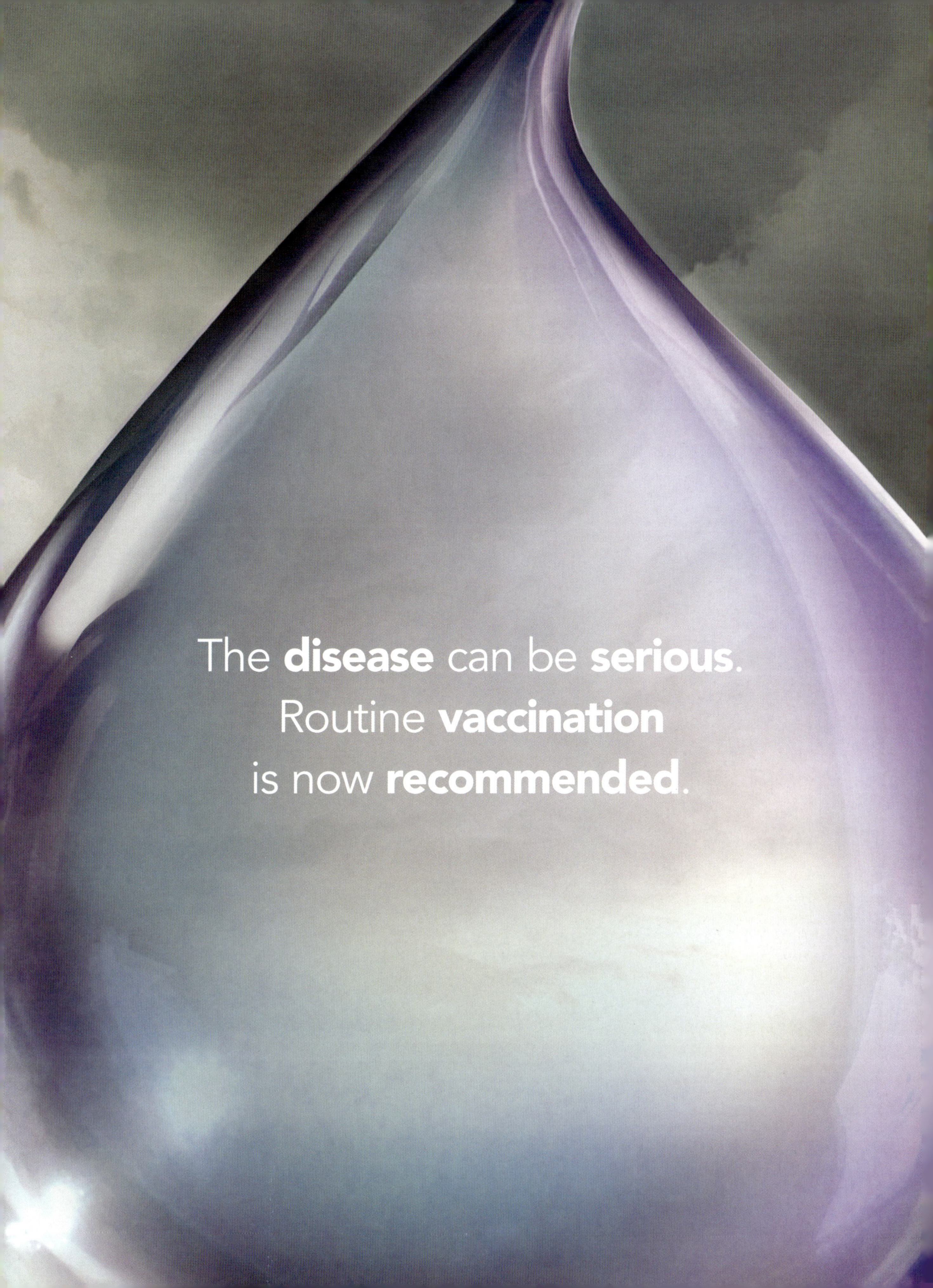
The disease can be serious.
Routine vaccination
is now recommended.

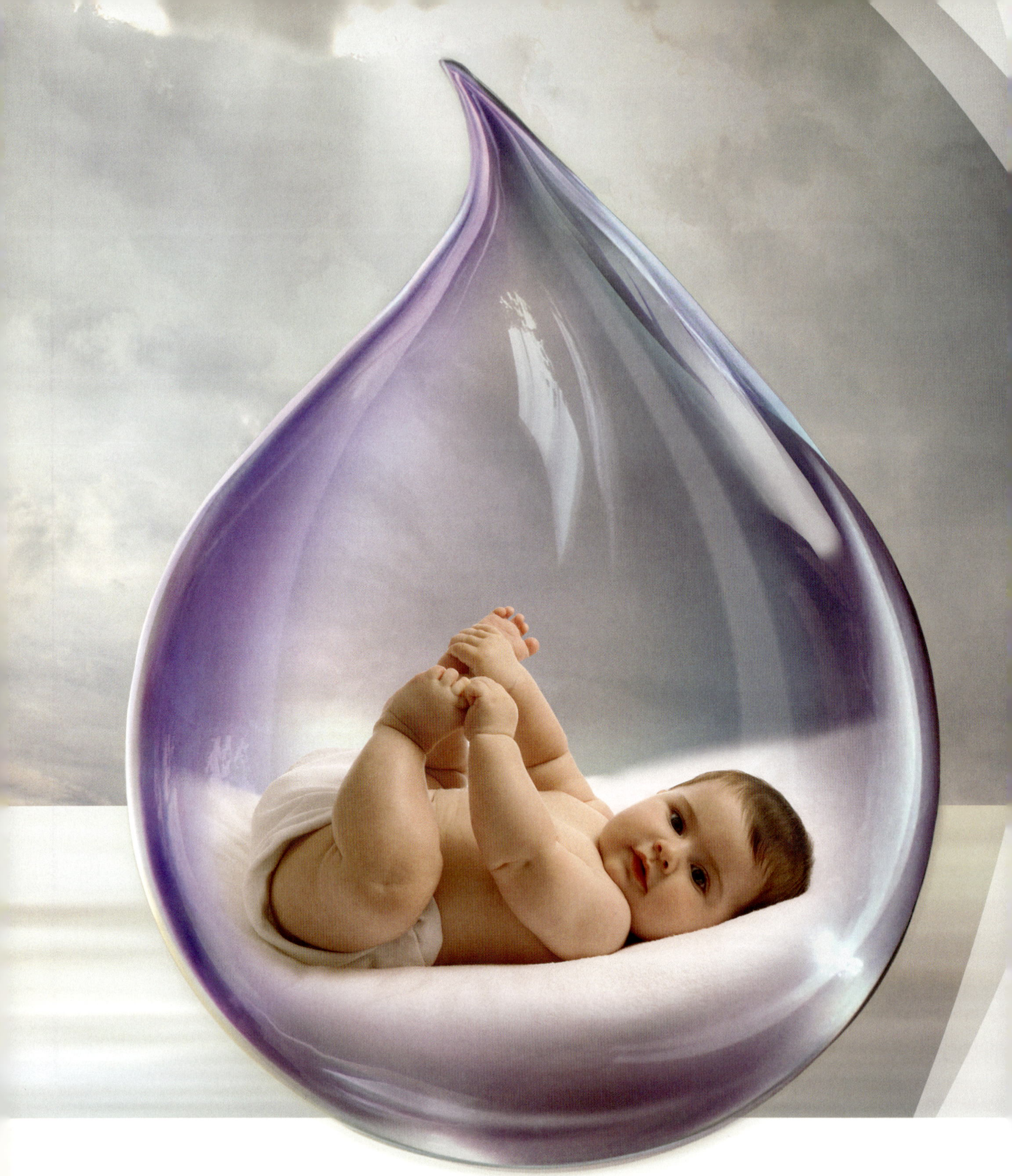

ARTICLE

# Ethanol-Lock Technique for Persistent Bacteremia of Long-term Intravascular Devices in Pediatric Patients

*Wes Onland, MD; Cathy E. Shin, MD; Stana Fustar, RN, CRNI; Teresa Rushing, PharmD, BCPS; Wing-Yen Wong, MD*

**Objectives:** To use the ethanol-lock technique (in conjunction with systemic antibiotics) to salvage central lines from removal and to prevent persistence of catheter-related infections among pediatric patients with long-term intravascular devices.

**Design:** Medical records of patients treated with ethanol locks were retrospectively reviewed from June 1, 2004, through June 22, 2005.

**Setting:** Childrens Hospital Los Angeles, Los Angeles, Calif, a tertiary care pediatric hospital.

**Patients:** Forty children with diverse underlying disorders were treated for 51 catheter-related infections using the Childrens Hospital Los Angeles ethanol-lock technique.

**Interventions:** Eligible infected central lines were instilled with a dose volume of 0.8 to 1.4 mL of 70% ethanol into the catheter lumen during 12 to 24 hours and then withdrawn. The volume of ethanol used was based on the type of intravascular device.

**Main Outcome Measures:** Clearance of infection and incidence of recurrence.

**Results:** Of the 51 ethanol-lock treatments in 40 children, no catheters were removed because of persistent infection. Eighty-eight percent (45/51) of the treated episodes cleared without recurrence (defined as a relapse within 30 days with the same pathogen). Twelve (75%) of 16 polymicrobial isolates and 33 (94%) of 35 monomicrobial isolates were successfully treated. There were no adverse reactions or adverse effects reported.

**Conclusion:** This retrospective study supports the use of the ethanol-lock technique in conjunction with systemic antibiotics as an effective and safe method to retain the use of a previously infected central venous catheter, decrease the need for line removal, and eradicate persistent pathogens in catheter-related infections.

*Arch Pediatr Adolesc Med. 2006;160:1049-1053*

LONG-TERM INTRAVASCULAR devices (IVDs) are crucial for the care of children requiring chemotherapy, apheresis, parenteral nutrition, frequent transfusion of blood products, or prolonged intravenous medications. However, catheter-related infections (CRIs) are a major complication of IVDs, necessitating removal and replacement when venous access sites are severely limited. Most nosocomial bloodstream infections in pediatric patients are related to the use of an IVD.[1] Bacterial colonization of the catheter hub and lumen is a significant problem in patients with long-term IVDs,[2,3] leading to increased patient morbidity, costs and length of hospitalization,[4-6] and mortality in critically ill patients.[7] The incidence of IVD-related infection ranges from 3% to 60%, with a rate of 0.2 to 2.4 infections per 1000 catheter-days.[8-12]

Repeated replacement of IVDs should be prevented because of the added cost of care, the delay in therapy, and (most important) the problem of limited access sites, especially in young children. To salvage infected IVDs, several methods of prophylaxis or treatment have been developed, such as antibiotic locks with or without anticoagulation agents or antiseptic chamber–containing hubs, with variable success.[13-15] Dannenberg et al[16] used ethanol locks in oncology patients with CRIs, in conjunction with systemic antibiotics. To our knowledge, there have been no other reports on the use of ethanol-lock techniques for the treatment of CRIs. The ethanol-lock technique was introduced at Childrens Hospital Los Angeles, Los Angeles, Calif, in early 2004. In this study, we report our experience with the ethanol-lock technique, as an adjunctive therapy to systemic antibiotics, to intraluminally

Author Affiliations: Department of Pediatrics, Emma Children's Hospital, Academic Medical Center, Amsterdam, the Netherlands (Dr Onland); and Divisions of Pediatric Surgery (Dr Shin), Hematology-Oncology (Ms Fustar and Drs Rushing and Wong), and Pharmacy (Dr Rushing), Childrens Hospital Los Angeles, Los Angeles, Calif.

**Table 1. Protocol of the Childrens Hospital Los Angeles Ethanol-Lock Technique**

Withdraw 1 mL of 98% dehydrated ethanol with filter needle into a 10-mL syringe
Add 0.4 mL of sterile saline (0.9% sodium chloride) to withdrawn syringe containing 98% ethanol (final concentration, 1.4 mL of 70% ethanol)
Assemble 3-way stopcock
Administration of ethanol lock
1. Attach a 3-way stopcock to injection cap
2. Unclamp the catheter and gently flush with isotonic sodium chloride solution to ensure patency of the catheter
3. Instill ethanol into the catheter to fill volume
4. Remove 3-way stopcock and clamp the catheter; ethanol should remain within the lumen a minimum of 12 h (24 h for best results)

Doses are based on the intravascular device intraluminal volume
Type of catheter
1. Single-lumen tunneled
   - Broviac
     - 4.2F (ID, 0.7 mm) (dose volume, 0.8 mL)
     - 6.6F (ID, 1 mm) (dose volume, 0.8 mL)
   - Medcomp (dose volume, 1.2 mL)
2. Double-lumen tunneled
   - Hickman
     - 7F distal (red) (ID, 1 mm) (dose volume, 1.2 mL)
     - 9F proximal (white) (ID, 0.7 mm) (dose volume, 1.2 mL)
   - Medcomp 8F or 10F (dose volume, 1.2 mL)
3. Port-A-Cath
   - Any port (dose volume, 1.4 mL)

Repeat procedure for 5 d

Abbreviation: ID, inner diameter.

disinfect and salvage long-term IVDs among children with CRIs.

## METHODS

A retrospective review of patients' medical records and pharmacy dispensing records of ethanol locks from June 1, 2004, through June 22, 2005, was undertaken after appropriate approval from the Childrens Hospital Los Angeles Institutional Review Board. Catheter-related infections were as defined by the Centers for Disease Control and Prevention.[12] No concomitant peripheral blood cultures were obtained.

Eligibility criteria for ethanol-lock treatment included age older than 6 months, a patent lumen before initiation of ethanol locks, a negative history of allergy to ethanol, and persistence of positive blood cultures (persistent positive blood cultures after 48 hours' administration of appropriate intravenous antimicrobial therapy) or incidence of multiple CRIs. Only silicone catheters qualified for ethanol-lock procedures.

The instilled ethanol lock had to dwell for 12 to 24 hours in a single-lumen IVD. After this period, the ethanol lock was withdrawn and discarded, followed by an isotonic sodium chloride solution flush. This procedure was repeated for 5 consecutive days. A separate peripheral line was placed for intravenous antibiotics. With double-lumen IVDs, ethanol was instilled in one lumen for 24 hours, while the other lumen was used for infusion. During the next 24 hours, the other lumen was locked with ethanol, while the first lumen was used for infusions. Both lumens were alternately treated for 10 days. Any adverse effects of the treatment were documented. Details of the ethanol-lock procedure are summarized in **Table 1**.

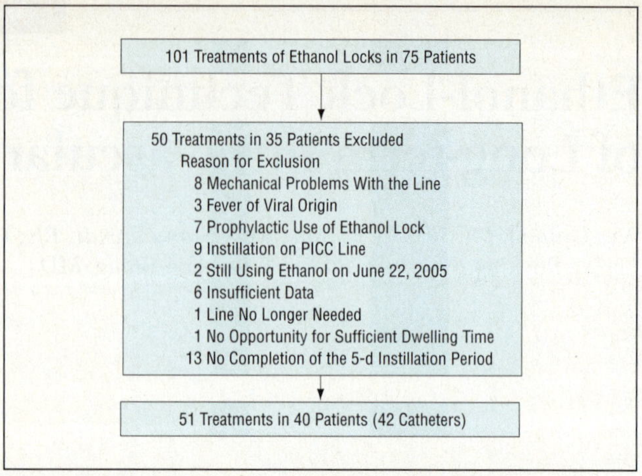


**Figure.** Study sample inclusions and exclusions. PICC indicates peripherally inserted central catheter.

Data of CRIs treated with ethanol locks were reviewed from the first day of insertion (or the beginning of the study period) until the end of the study period. When the subsequent CRI in the same catheter was not treated with ethanol locks, the consecutive data were excluded.

A total of 101 ethanol-lock treatments were dispensed to 75 patients. Fifty treatments in 35 patients were excluded (**Figure**). Eleven treatments had no documented CRI but were associated with mechanical problems with the line (n=8) or with fever of viral origin (n=3). Nine treatments were carried out on peripherally inserted central catheters, 6 had inadequate data documentation, and 7 had prophylactic ethanol locks instilled before any proven infection. In 2 treatments, the patients were still receiving ethanol locks on the last day of the study period. In 1 treatment, the line was deemed clinically expendable after ethanol had been instilled, and it was removed halfway through the treatment protocol. One treatment was excluded because the patient's medical management required the use of both lumens for continuous infusion of parenteral nutrition and systemic antibiotics, leaving no opportunity for the minimum dwelling period of 12 to 24 hours. Of the 50 excluded ethanol-lock treatments, 13 were judged to be unevaluable because the patients' medical records showed that the IVDs were ordered to be removed before completion of the 5-day instillation period.

*Treatment success* was defined as resolution of fever within 24 hours, no recurrence of positive blood cultures with the same organism, and retention of the IVD. *Treatment failure* was defined as recurrence within 30 days with the same pathogen or removal of the IVD because of a persistent infection. When the catheter was removed because of a mechanical event or completion of therapy, it was not classified as a treatment failure. Data were analyzed using Intercooled STATA version 8.0 (StataCorp LP, College Station, Tex).

## RESULTS

Data from 51 ethanol-lock treatments on 40 patients and 42 catheters were analyzed. Two patients received a second IVD of the same type that they previously had, and in both cases the catheter was removed after a CRI that was not treated with ethanol locks. The patients' characteristics are summarized in **Table 2**. There were more boys than girls. The median age was 3.9 years (age range, 1.9-13.5 years). Solid tumors accounted for 38% (15/40) of the underlying diagnoses. Other diagnoses included severe immunocompromise after bone marrow or

**Table 2. Characteristics Among 40 Patients**

| Characteristic | Total No. |
|---|---|
| Male/female ratio | 24:16 |
| Age, median (interquartile range), y | 3.9 (1.9-13.5) |
| Diagnosis (n = 40) | |
| Oncology, solid tumors | 15 |
| Oncology, malignant hematology | 3 |
| Hematology, benign | 3 |
| Bone marrow or small-bowel transplantation | 9 |
| Metabolic disorder | 1 |
| Gastroenterological disorder | 9 |
| Type of catheter (n = 42) | |
| Broviac single lumen | 11 |
| Hickman double lumen | 17 |
| Port-A-Cath | 9 |
| Medcomp double lumen | 5 |
| Catheter-days | |
| Mean ± SD | 201.4 ± 201.5 |
| Total | 8045 |
| Infection rate per 1000 catheter-days | 6.3 |
| Median (25%-75% interquartile range) | 126.5 (70-258) |
| No. of treatments (n = 51) | |
| 1 | 34 |
| 2 | 5 |
| 7 | 1 |

small-bowel transplantation (23% [9/40]) and gastroenterological disorders requiring long-term dependence on parenteral nutrition associated with short-bowel syndrome, pseudo-obstruction syndrome, or microvillous inclusion syndrome (23% [9/40]). Most of the 42 catheters were Hickman catheters (40% [17/42]), followed by Broviac catheters (26% [11/42]) and Port-A-Cath catheters (21% [9/42]).

Among the 40 patients, 34 were treated once with ethanol locks, 5 were treated twice, and 1 received the therapy 7 times during the study period. We registered 3863 catheter-days in 40 patients from the day of insertion (or the previous CRI not treated with ethanol locks) until the date of the first positive CRI, an infection rate of 10 per 1000 catheter-days. The total number of catheter-days among 42 catheters was 8054 days, with an infection rate of 6.3 per 1000 catheter-days (Table 2). The distribution of catheter-days from insertion to the first CRI (median, 34.5 catheter-days [interquartile range, 16-85 catheter-days] and the total catheter-days (median, 126.5 catheter-days [interquartile range, 70-258 catheter-days]) were not normally divided.

**Table 3** lists the organisms isolated. Monomicrobial culture was isolated in 69% of the CRIs. Gram-positive organisms accounted for 57% of 51 infections; 35% of them were coagulase-negative staphylococci. Polymicrobial isolates grew in 16 CRIs (31%); 1 CRI (2%) was a mixed culture of yeast and bacteria. In 38% of the polymicrobial isolates, there were more than 2 different bacteria. More gram-negative isolates grew out of the polymicrobial cultures (49%) than out of the monomicrobial cultures.

All of the IVDs treated with ethanol locks were successfully retained and used. Five of the catheters were later removed when patients ended their chemotherapy or before allogenic bone marrow transplantation, as standard practice. All of these removals occurred after 30 days (**Table 4**). One of the patients died of disease progression unrelated to a CRI.

**Table 3. Monomicrobial or Polymicrobial Pathogens Isolated in 51 Catheter-Related Infections**

| Pathogen | No. of Cases |
|---|---|
| Monomicrobial cultures | |
| Gram-positive isolates (n = 29) | |
| Coagulase-negative staphylococci | 18 |
| *Enterococcus faecalis* (group D) | 4 |
| *Enterococcus faecium* | 1 |
| Methicillin-resistant *Staphylococcus aureus* | 2 |
| *S aureus* | 3 |
| *Bacillus* species (not *Bacillus anthracis*) | 1 |
| Gram-negative isolates (n = 5) | |
| *Enterobacter cloacae* | 1 |
| *Klebsiella oxytoca* | 1 |
| *Klebsiella pneumoniae* | 1 |
| *Serratia marcescens* | 1 |
| *Actinobacter* species | 1 |
| Yeast (n = 1) | |
| *Candida glabrata* | 1 |
| Polymicrobial cultures (n = 16) | |
| Gram-positive isolates | 19 |
| Gram-negative isolates | 19 |
| Yeast | 1 |

**Table 4. Removal of Intravascular Device for Reason Other Than Catheter-Related Infection (CRI) in 5 Patients**

| Patient No. | No. of CRIs | Reason for Removal | Interval Between Last CRI and Removal, d |
|---|---|---|---|
| 1 | 1 | No longer in use | 136 |
| 2 | 1 | No longer in use | 74 |
| 3 | 1 | No longer in use | 65 |
| 4 | 2 | Upcoming ABMT | 53 |
| 5 | 1 | Died of disease progression | 85 |

Abbreviation: ABMT, allogenic bone marrow transplantation.

In 6 cases, bacteremia recurred within 30 days with the same pathogen (**Table 5**). These recurrences occurred in 3 patients and comprised 4 different polymicrobial isolates in the first CRIs that recurred in the subsequent CRIs. In patient 8 in Table 5, the pathogen (*Klebsiella pneumoniae*) recurred twice with different pathogens in a polymicrobial isolate.

Ethanol-lock treatments were well tolerated in all children. No adverse effects were reported.

## COMMENT

Infection of long-term IVDs results from invasion of organisms present at insertion sites, contaminated infusates, hematogenous seeding of the catheter tips, and contamination of the hubs, the hubs being the most common site of CRIs. Microorganisms causing CRIs are en-

**Table 5. Recurrence Within 30 Days With the Same Pathogen in 3 Patients**

| Patient No. | Interval Between CRIs, d | Pathogen of First CRI | Pathogen of Subsequent CRI |
|---|---|---|---|
| 6 | 19 | MRSA | MRSA* |
| 7 | 27 | CNS | CNS |
| | 29 | CNS† | CNS |
| 8 | 30 | *Serratia marcescens*† | *S marcescens* |
| | 17 | *Klebsiella pneumoniae*† | *K pneumoniae*† |
| | 28 | *K pneumoniae*† | *K pneumoniae*† |

Abbreviations: CNS, coagulase-negative staphylococci; CRI, catheter-related infection; MRSA, methicillin-resistant *Staphylococcus aureus*.

*At the subsequent CRI, no ethanol locks were used, and the intravascular device was removed.

†In polymicrobial isolate.

countered in 2 forms, the planktonic free-floating form and the sessile form, with bacteria embedded in a biofilm.[17] In most cases, the planktonic free-floating form can effectively be eradicated by appropriate systemic antibiotics. The sessile form poses a significant and often persistent problem. Bacteria adherent to implanted medical devices or damaged tissue can cause persistent infections by forming a biofilm. These bacteria encase themselves in a hydrated matrix of polysaccharide and protein, causing their inherent resistance to antibiotic therapy, neutrophil function, phagocytes, and antibodies.[18,19] Another part of this biofilm that is composed of host-derived glycoproteins, such as fibrinogen, fibronectin, collagen, and laminin, enhances bacterial adherence to foreign material.[6,17] Susceptibility tests using in vitro biofilm models have shown survival of bacterial biofilms after treatment with antibiotics at concentrations hundreds of times (or even 1000 times) the minimum inhibitory concentration of the bacteria measured in a suspension culture.[20,21]

We performed a retrospective review of the efficacy and safety of ethanol locks as an adjunctive therapy to systemic antibiotics in persistent CRIs among children with long-term IVDs. Ethanol is an effective disinfectant against a broad range of microorganisms, including bacteria and fungi. Two hours of exposure to 70% ethanol is required to kill established biofilms of gram-positive bacteria, gram-negative bacteria, and *Candida* species in vitro.[22]

The number of infections in our study period per 1000 catheter-days (6.3 infections) is higher than that reported in the study by Dannenberg et al.[16] This is probably because 5 of the 42 catheters were inserted before the beginning of the study period, and these catheter-days without CRIs were excluded in the analyses. Other reasons may include our inclusion of younger and sicker children, different groups of underlying illnesses, and various types of catheters at high risk for CRIs. To minimize venipunctures in these children with significant venous access difficulties, no peripheral blood cultures were obtained. Cultures of blood samples, drawn from an indwelling IVD, were assessed in a study by Martinez et al.[23] The positive predictive value of IVD and peripheral blood cultures was low (63% and 73%, respectively) and required clinical interpretation and conformation; however, the negative predictive values were 99% and 98%, respectively, obviating the need for a concomitant separate peripheral blood culture.

None of the catheters treated with ethanol were removed, and 45 (88%) of the 51 CRIs showed no recurrence within 30 days with the same pathogen. Of the recurrences in 3 patients (Table 5), patient 6 had methicillin-resistant *Staphylococcus aureus* at the time of the catheter insertion. After the recurrence of methicillin-resistant *S aureus* in patient 6, ethanol locks were not instilled and the IVD was removed. Patient 7, with stage IV neuroblastoma requiring intensive chemotherapy, had a recurrence of coagulase-negative staphylococci 27 days after the first CRI, which was treated with ethanol locks, and a second recurrence 29 days after the first recurrence. Patient 8, with 3 recurrences in 7 CRIs, had short-bowel syndrome and was dependent on parenteral nutrition. Five of the 7 CRIs were treated with ethanol locks for a second or third time, with good effect. The IVDs in patients 2 and 3 were not removed. Because this was a retrospective review, we could not evaluate the DNA type of each pathogen and whether the CRI was localized intraluminally.

Coagulase-negative staphylococci, *S aureus*, aerobic gram-negative bacilli, and *Candida albicans* are most commonly associated with CRIs.[24,25] We found equal numbers of the different bacteria but also found a considerable amount of polymicrobial isolates, constituting 49% of the gram-negative bacteria grown, and a mixed bacterial and fungal isolate. Of the polymicrobial isolates, 75% (12/16) did not show a recurrence, and of the 35 monomicrobial isolates, 94% (33/35) were successfully treated. The treatments of 2 yeast isolates were also successful.

## CONCLUSIONS

Despite the limitations of this retrospective study, our results suggest that using the ethanol-lock technique for persistent CRIs in children with long-term IVDs is effective in salvaging the line, with a low rate of recurrences. It is a safe, well-tolerated, and low-cost method, without risks of inducing multiresistant bacteria. A prospective, randomized, double-blind trial comparing the ethanol-lock technique with placebo and the alternatives would be needed to determine the best method to treat persistent CRIs.

**Accepted for Publication:** June 13, 2006.

**Correspondence:** Wing-Yen Wong, MD, Division of Hematology-Oncology, Childrens Hospital Los Angeles, 4650 Sunset Blvd, Mail Stop 54, Los Angeles, CA 90027 (wwong@chla.usc.edu).

**Author Contributions:** *Study concept and design:* Onland, Shin, Rushing, and Wong. *Acquisition of data:* Onland, Shin, Rushing, and Wong. *Analysis and interpretation of data:* Onland, Fustar, and Wong. *Drafting of the manuscript:* Onland, Fustar, and Wong. *Critical revision of the manuscript for important intellectual content:* Onland,

Shin, Rushing, and Wong. *Administrative, technical, and material support:* Onland and Rushing. *Study supervision:* Shin and Wong.

## REFERENCES


1. Jarvis WR, Edwards JR, Culver DH, et al. Nosocomial infection rates in adult and pediatric intensive care units in the United States: National Nosocomial Infections Surveillance System. *Am J Med.* 1991;91:185S-191S.
2. Maki DG, Mermel LA. Infections due to infusion therapy. In: Bennet JV, Brachman PS, eds. *Hospital Infections.* Philadelphia, Pa: Lippincott-Raven Publishers; 1998:689-724.
3. Mayhall CG. Diagnosis and management of infections of implantable devices used for prolonged venous access. *Curr Clin Top Infect Dis.* 1992;12:83-110.
4. Digiovine B, Chenoweth C, Watts C, Higgins M. The attributable mortality and costs of primary nosocomial bloodstream infections in the intensive care unit. *Am J Respir Crit Care Med.* 1999;160:976-981.
5. Rello J, Ochagavia A, Sabanes E, et al. Evaluation of outcome of intravenous catheter-related infections in critically ill patients. *Am J Respir Crit Care Med.* 2000; 162:1027-1030.
6. Eggimann P, Sax H, Pittet D. Catheter-related infections. *Microbes Infect.* 2004; 6:1033-1042.
7. Pittet D, Tarara D, Wenzel RP. Nosocomial bloodstream infection in critically ill patients: excess length of stay, extra costs, and attributable mortality. *JAMA.* 1994; 271:1598-1601.
8. Develter W, De Cubber A, Van Biesen W, Vanholder R, Lameire N. Survival and complications of indwelling venous catheters for permanent use in hemodialysis patients. *Artif Organs.* 2005;29:399-405.
9. Wiener ES. Catheter sepsis: the central venous line Achilles' heel. *Semin Pediatr Surg.* 1995;4:207-214.
10. Stovroff M, Teague WG. Intravenous access in infants and children. *Pediatr Clin North Am.* 1998;45:1373-1393, viii.
11. Crnich CJ, Maki DG. The promise of novel technology for the prevention of intravascular device–related bloodstream infection, II: long-term devices. *Clin Infect Dis.* 2002;34:1362-1368.
12. de Jonge RC, Polderman KH, Gemke RJ. Central venous catheter use in the pediatric patient: mechanical and infectious complications. *Pediatr Crit Care Med.* 2005;6:329-339.
13. Berrington A, Gould FK. Use of antibiotic locks to treat colonized central venous catheters. *J Antimicrob Chemother.* 2001;48:597-603.
14. Leon C, Alvarez-Lerma F, Ruiz-Santana S, et al. Antiseptic chamber–containing hub reduces central venous catheter-related infection: a prospective, randomized study. *Crit Care Med.* 2003;31:1318-1324.
15. Bestul MB, Vandenbussche HL. Antibiotic lock technique: review of the literature. *Pharmacotherapy.* 2005;25:211-227.
16. Dannenberg C, Bierbach U, Rothe A, Beer J, Korholz D. Ethanol-lock technique in the treatment of bloodstream infections in pediatric oncology patients with Broviac catheter. *J Pediatr Hematol Oncol.* 2003;25:616-621.
17. Raad I. Intravascular-catheter–related infections. *Lancet.* 1998;351:893-898.
18. Stewart PS, Costerton JW. Antibiotic resistance of bacteria in biofilms. *Lancet.* 2001;358:135-138.
19. Donlan RM. Biofilm formation: a clinically relevant microbiological process. *Clin Infect Dis.* 2001;33:1387-1392.
20. Ceri H, Olson ME, Stremick C, Read RR, Morck D, Buret A. The Calgary Biofilm Device: new technology for rapid determination of antibiotic susceptibilities of bacterial biofilms. *J Clin Microbiol.* 1999;37:1771-1776.
21. Williams I, Venables WA, Lloyd D, Paul F, Critchley I. The effects of adherence to silicone surfaces on antibiotic susceptibility in *Staphylococcus aureus*. *Microbiology.* 1997;143:2407-2413.
22. Metcalf SC, Chambers ST, Pithie AD. Use of ethanol locks to prevent recurrent central line sepsis. *J Infect.* 2004;49:20-22.
23. Martinez JA, DesJardin JA, Aronoff M, Supran S, Nasraway SA, Snydman DR. Clinical utility of blood cultures drawn from central venous or arterial catheters in critically ill surgical patients. *Crit Care Med.* 2002;30:7-13.
24. Raad II, Hanna HA. Intravascular catheter–related infections: new horizons and recent advances. *Arch Intern Med.* 2002;162:871-878.
25. Mermel LA, Farr BM, Sherertz RJ, et al. Guidelines for the management of intravascular catheter–related infections. *Clin Infect Dis.* 2001;32:1249-1272.

ARTICLE

# Inpatient Health Care Use Among Adult Survivors of Chronic Childhood Illnesses in the United States

*Megumi J. Okumura, MD; Andrew D. Campbell, MD; Samya Z. Nasr, MD; Matthew M. Davis, MD, MAPP*

**Objectives:** To describe the inpatient length of stay and related charges for adults in the United States with childhood-onset chronic disease and to examine patterns with respect to different hospital settings.

**Design:** We analyzed data from the 2002 Nationwide Inpatient Sample, a nationally representative data set of hospital discharges. We performed a case-mix–adjusted, sample-weighted regression analysis as well as descriptive statistics of hospital use among adults with childhood-onset chronic disease.

**Setting:** United States.

**Participants:** We identified hospitalizations for persons aged 18 years or older with a diagnosis of complex congenital heart disease, cystic fibrosis, sickle cell disease, or spina bifida.

**Main Exposure:** Childhood chronic illness.

**Main Outcome Measures:** Length of stay and total charges among pediatric, adult, and mixed hospitals.

**Results:** In multivariate adjusted analyses, patients with complex congenital heart disease and cystic fibrosis had a significantly longer length of stay in pediatric hospitals than in adult or mixed hospitals ($P<.001$); no similar difference was found for sickle cell disease and spina bifida. For all of the 4 conditions, hospital charges were significantly greater in pediatric hospitals than in adult or mixed hospitals ($P<.001$ for cystic fibrosis, complex congenital heart disease, and sickle cell disease, and $P<.01$ for spina bifida).

**Conclusions:** The vast majority of persons who have survived to adulthood with complex congenital heart disease, cystic fibrosis, spina bifida, or sickle cell disease are hospitalized in hospitals that predominantly care for adults, where charges for care appear to be lower than in pediatric hospitals.

*Arch Pediatr Adolesc Med. 2006;160:1054-1060*

THROUGHOUT THE LAST 30 years, life expectancy has climbed for many children with chronic illnesses. For example, in 1973, children with cystic fibrosis (CF) had an average lifespan of 7 years; by 2000, the median age of survival was 31 years.[1] Similarly, the survival for sickle cell disease (SCD) has improved during the past 20 years primarily owing to the success of penicillin prophylaxis in children.[2,3] As a result, there has been an increase in the number of patients with SCD entering their third decade of life.

With improved survival to adulthood today, the American Academy of Pediatrics, Elk Grove Village, Ill, American College of Physicians–American Society of Internal Medicine, Philadelphia, Pa, and American Academy of Family Physicians, Leawood, Kan, advocate the transitioning of adolescents with chronic conditions into an adult-centered heath care system.[4] This recommendation has also been supported by many subspecialty societies.[5,6] Despite these recommendations, many adults continue to use the pediatric health care system.[7] In fact, a recent study[8] estimated that approximately 6.3% of total inpatient charges in pediatric hospital settings were attributable to care for adults.

*For editorial comment see page 1079*

To our knowledge, no prior study has examined the health care use of adults with chronic childhood illnesses in the adult health care setting or has compared use in pediatric vs predominantly adult health care systems. In this study, we examine measures of hospital use (length of stay [LOS] and associated total charges) among adults (aged ≥18 years) with complex congenital heart disease (CCHD), CF, SCD, and spina bifida (SB) between predomi-

**Author Affiliations:** Division of General Internal Medicine (Drs Okumura and Davis), Child Health Evaluation and Research Unit, Division of General Pediatrics (Drs Okumura and Davis), Sections of Pediatric Hematology (Dr Campbell) and Pediatric Pulmonology (Dr Nasr), Department of Pediatrics, and Gerald R. Ford School of Public Policy (Dr Davis), University of Michigan, Ann Arbor. Dr Okumura is now with the Division of General Pediatrics, University of California, San Francisco.

nantly pediatric and nonpediatric facilities. These are 4 chronic conditions of childhood onset with genetic or in utero origins whose adult survivors frequently require hospital care for progressively severe symptoms with increasing age. Our rationale for this study was that pediatric hospitals may have greater familiarity with these childhood disease processes, but institutions predominantly seeing adults would be more familiar with problems specific to older patients regardless of the condition. Therefore, we investigated whether such differences across pediatric and adult health care settings manifest as differences in LOS or charges, 2 readily available measures that have been used previously to describe differences in hospital care for similar diseases between pediatric and adult institutions.[9,10]

## METHODS

### SAMPLE

We used the 2002 Nationwide Inpatient Sample (NIS), a component of the Healthcare Cost and Utilization Project (HCUP), a set of health care databases developed through partnership among federal and state governments and health care institutions and sponsored by the Agency for Healthcare Research and Quality, Rockville, Md.[11] The NIS is the largest publicly available all-payer inpatient database in the United States.

The NIS contains deidentified, patient-level clinical and resource use data included in a standard discharge abstract. The 2002 NIS includes 7 853 982 sampled discharges representative of 37 804 021 discharges. These data reflect discharge data from 995 hospitals located in 35 states, approximating a 20%-stratified sample of nonfederal community hospitals including public hospitals, pediatric hospitals, and academic medical centers but excluding long-term hospitals, psychiatric hospitals, and chemical dependency treatment facilities. Stratification also includes the profit status for each hospital. The sampling frame for the NIS composes approximately 90% of all hospital discharges in the United States. Sampling from the universe of US hospitals is stratified based on 5 hospital characteristics: US region, urban or rural location, ownership or control, bed size, and teaching status. Discharge weights are provided by the HCUP to permit national estimates of hospitalization frequencies. Documentation of the generation of discharge weights is available online through the HCUP.[12] Total charges are expressed in 2002 US dollars. Analyses did not include Pennsylvania discharges because they did not have comorbidities specified.

### IDENTIFICATION OF CASES

We searched for CCHD, CF, SCD, and SB discharges in any of the 15 diagnostic positions included for each discharge in the NIS among patients aged 18 years or older. Complex congenital heart disease was identified with the *International Classification of Diseases, Ninth Revision, Clinical Modification*[13] (*ICD-9-CM*) codes 745-745.39, 745.6-745.60, 745.69-745.9, 746-746.5, 746.7-746.9, and 747.1-747.49. As isolated atrial septal defect and ventricular septal defects are often followed up clinically and do not have as complex a course as tetralogy of Fallot or other significant malformations, we excluded individuals who were coded only for atrial septal defect or ventricular septal defect. The CF discharges were identified with the *ICD-9-CM* codes 277.00-277.09. The SCD discharges were identified with the *ICD-9-CM* codes 282.60-282.69. Spina bifida was identified with the *ICD-9-CM* codes 741-741.99 and 756.17.

### IDENTIFICATION OF PEDIATRIC, ADULT, AND MIXED HOSPITALS

Pediatric hospitals were identified using NIS-provided hospital identifiers and were cross-referenced with listings from the National Association of Children's Hospitals and Related Institutions, Alexandria, Va. For those hospitals not labeled in the NIS, if more than 75% of the discharges for any diagnosis (not just CCHD, CF, SCD, and SB) were for individuals younger than 18 years, the hospital was designated as a pediatric hospital. For those hospitals with more than 75% of the discharges for individuals older than 18 years, the hospital was categorized as an adult hospital. All of the others were designated as mixed hospitals. Hospitals classified via cross-referencing with the National Association of Children's Hospitals and Related Institutions list were also checked with the age-at-discharge method. Of the 18 hospitals identified by the methods described earlier as possible pediatric hospitals, 5 National Association of Children's Hospitals and Related Institutions–identified hospitals were pediatric hospitals within adult hospitals. Since the discharges from the pediatric hospital could not be separated from the adult hospital discharges, we coded these hospitals as mixed hospitals for purposes of this analysis.

### CASE-MIX ADJUSTMENT

We used the comorbidity measure provided by the HCUP; it is a comprehensive set of 30 comorbidity measures developed for use with large administrative inpatient data sets that are associated with LOS, hospital charges, and in-hospital death in adults.[14] Because of the small number of patients with CF identified with each specific comorbidity, initial regressions were run using individual dummy variables for comorbidities, then the dummy variables were consolidated to form a singular comorbidity composite (count) variable for the analyses. There were no differences in regression fit or in interpretation of the models with the individual comorbidity vs the composite form, so for consistency across diseases, we used the composite measure for all of the analyses.

Analyses were also adjusted for procedures reported during the hospitalizations that were identified via the *ICD-9-CM* procedure codes. We categorized procedures by those that were most frequently identified for patients with CCHD, CF, SCD, and SB because those were the diagnoses of chief analytic interest across conditions. Blood transfusions, venous catheterization, use of antibiotics, and cardiac catheterization or cardiac procedures were the most common, so these were included as separate procedures in analyses. Intubation was also coded separately because it would identify patients with severe illness requiring intensive care. All of the other procedures were collapsed into an "other" category. Procedures were categorized in mutually exclusive categories.

### DATA ANALYSIS

We examined differences in LOS and total charges for each category of hospital (pediatric, adult, and mixed) and chronic condition, controlling for patient age and sex, procedures, mortality, payer type, comorbidity measures, hospital volume, and patient annual income by ZIP code. Race is not reported reliably in the NIS and was missing in approximately 36% of the sample, so we were unable to use race or ethnicity as a covariate. Hospital teaching status (as specified in the NIS) and hospital volume (for all of the diagnoses) were found to be colinear in the analysis, so hospital volume was used in the final analysis to control for both teaching status and differences in care accounted for by larger patient volumes. In our charge analy-

**Table 1. Description of Patients 18 Years or Older Included in the 2002 Nationwide Inpatient Sample***

| Characteristic | Complex Congenital Heart Disease | Cystic Fibrosis | Sickle Cell Disease | Spina Bifida |
|---|---|---|---|---|
| Discharges, No. | 28 072 | 10 863 | 72 800 | 16 453 |
| Female, No. (%) | 13 963 (49.7) | 5780 (53.2) | 42 005 (57.7) | 9749 (59.3) |
| Age, mean, y | 50.8 | 29.0 | 33.0 | 37.7 |
| Age by hospital type, mean, y | | | | |
| Pediatric | 26.4 | 20.4 | 20.0 | 21.1 |
| Mixed | 49.4 | 27.9 | 31.4 | 35.9 |
| Adult | 52.0 | 30.1 | 33.9 | 39.4 |
| Use by hospital type, No. (%) | | | | |
| Pediatric | 761 (2.7) | 658 (6.0) | 1260 (1.7) | 692 (4.2) |
| Mixed | 6303 (22.5) | 2907 (26.8) | 18 336 (25.2) | 4 050 (24.6) |
| Adult | 21 009 (74.8) | 7299 (67.2) | 53 203 (73.1) | 11 709 (71.2) |
| Procedures, No. (%)† | | | | |
| No procedure | 8400 (29.9) | 4614 (42.5) | 39 594 (54.4) | 5589 (34.0) |
| Antibiotic | 130 (0.5) | 290 (2.7) | 330 (0.5) | 130 (0.8) |
| Transfusion | 540 (1.9) | 138 (1.3) | 13 588 (18.7) | 513 (3.1) |
| Cardiac or venous procedure | 12 154 (43.3) | 3221 (29.7) | 9697 (13.3) | 2319 (14.1) |
| Intubated | 307 (1.1) | 215 (2.0) | 383 (0.5) | 248 (1.5) |
| Procedure NOS | 6541 (23.3) | 2383 (21.9) | 9208 (12.6) | 7651 (46.5) |
| LOS, mean, d | 5.3 | 8.5 | 6.5 | 7.2 |
| Inpatient death, No. (%) | 638 (2.3) | 314 (2.9) | 658 (0.9) | 240 (1.5) |
| Income by ZIP code, No. (%) | | | | |
| <$25 000 | 1315 (4.8) | 391 (3.7) | 8431 (11.8) | 973 (6.0) |
| $25 000-$34 999 | 5110 (18.8) | 1929 (18.2) | 20 416 (28.7) | 3415 (21.2) |
| $35 000-$44 999 | 7033 (25.8) | 2413 (22.7) | 18 755 (26.4) | 4036 (25.1) |
| ≥$45 000 | 13 796 (50.6) | 5888 (55.4) | 23 522 (33.1) | 7665 (47.6) |
| Primary payer, No. (%) | | | | |
| Medicare | 9610 (34.3) | 2055 (18.9) | 19 776 (27.2) | 5713 (34.8) |
| Medicaid | 3544 (12.7) | 2296 (21.1) | 32 877 (45.2) | 4616 (28.1) |
| Private | 12 677 (45.2) | 5694 (52.4) | 14 861 (20.4) | 5273 (32.1) |
| Self-pay | 2177 (7.8) | 808 (7.4) | 5219 (7.2) | 813 (5.0) |
| Charge per discharge, mean, US $ | 31 740 | 34 865 | 18 163 | 24 145 |

Abbreviations: LOS, length of stay; NOS, not otherwise specified.
*All of the data are presented as national estimates. The proportions are based on those who reported values.
†The categories are exclusive.

sis, we also included a model with LOS to determine the percentage of charge difference between hospital types that could be accounted for by LOS (see the "Comment" section).

Using Stata version 8.2 software (Stata Corp, College Station, Tex), we performed weighted linear regression on log-transformed total charges and LOS, controlling for the earlier-mentioned covariates. Taylor series linearization was used for variance estimation. Postregression adjustment of the log-transformed case-mix–adjusted charges and LOS was done to estimate real charges and LOS between hospital types.[15] We considered alternative models for analyzing the significantly right-skewed dependent variable, such as Poisson and negative binomial regression, but the best-fit model was achieved in the log-transformed linear model.

Because pediatric hospitals care for few older adults compared with mixed and adult hospitals, we also ran the regression analysis limiting the age range from 18 to 35 years across all of the hospital types. Also, to address potential bias introduced by outliers, additional sensitivity analyses were done on subsets without procedures, eliminating charges greater than $100 000 and patients having LOS greater than 30 days. None of these separate analyses affected our model significantly. These are reported as additional analyses, the details of which can be requested directly from Dr Okumura.

We also attempted to conduct additional analysis of economic significance using the cost-to-charge information that has been released by the HCUP for the 2002 NIS. However, hospital-specific cost-to-charge information for our patients of interest was missing in approximately 30% of the cases and was disproportionately missing for pediatric hospitals; therefore, we state all of the economic findings in this article as charges.

## RESULTS

### SAMPLE CHARACTERISTICS

The analytic sample for the regression model included 5597 discharges (unweighted) with CCHD, 2182 with CF, 14 897 with SCD, and 3278 with SB. The numbers of unweighted discharges in the pediatric hospitals were 158 for CCHD, 137 for CF, 236 for SCD, and 152 for SB.

The weighted sample sizes and sociodemographic characteristics used for the multivariate analysis for patients hospitalized with these 4 conditions appear in **Table 1** along with the mean ages per hospital type. Age ranges in the pediatric hospitals in this data set were as follows: 18 to 64 years for CCHD, 18 to 40 years for CF, 18 to 50 years for SCD, and 18 to 33 years for SB.

### HOSPITAL CHARACTERISTICS

The hospital characteristics for each condition across hospital types are presented in **Table 2**. We report the survey-weighted proportions or averages of the differences be-

**Table 2. Description of Patients by Hospital Type***

| Characteristic | Cystic Fibrosis | | | Complex Congenital Heart Disease | | | Sickle Cell Disease | | | Spina Bifida | | |
|---|---|---|---|---|---|---|---|---|---|---|---|---|
| | Pediatric Hospital | Mixed Hospital | Adult Hospital | Pediatric Hospital | Mixed Hospital | Adult Hospital | Pediatric Hospital | Mixed Hospital | Adult Hospital | Pediatric Hospital | Mixed Hospital | Adult Hospital |
| Patients aged 18-35 y, % (SE) | 99.4 (0.6) | 82.1 (3.1) | 76.6 (1.8) | 84.5 (3.5) | 28.1 (2.0) | 24.1 (1.1) | 99.7 (0.3) | 68.9 (2.0) | 60.1 (1.2) | 100 | 55.9 (3.1) | 45.9 (1.5) |
| Comorbidities | | | | | | | | | | | | |
| Comorbidities, mean No. (SE) | 0.93 (0.18) | 1.07 (0.10) | 1.14 (0.06) | 0.47 (0.06) | 1.49 (0.04) | 1.49 (0.04) | 0.38 (0.14) | 0.71 (0.04) | 0.83 (0.02) | 0.63 (0.07) | 1.16 (0.05) | 1.41 (0.04) |
| Patients with any comorbidities, % (SE) | 55.3 (10.4) | 61.9 (3.8) | 63.9 (3.0) | 29.1 (3.3) | 73.6 (1.5) | 68.2 (1.5) | 20.7 (8.2) | 45.2 (1.8) | 48.6 (1.1) | 32.3 (4.2) | 65.9 (2.1) | 66.8 (1.5) |
| Comorbidities among patients with any comorbidities, mean No. (SE) | 1.54 (0.07) | 1.73 (0.05) | 1.73 (0.05) | 1.47 (0.12) | 2.02 (0.04) | 2.04 (0.04) | 1.44 (0.13) | 1.58 (0.03) | 1.67 (0.02) | 1.78 (0.09) | 1.76 (0.04) | 1.96 (0.04) |
| Procedures, % (SE) | | | | | | | | | | | | |
| None | 34.3 (10.6) | 43.4 (6.6) | 42.8 (2.8) | 15.0 (4.0) | 31.3 (2.3) | 30.0 (1.3) | 55.2 (9.3) | 53.0 (3.5) | 54.9 (1.6) | 17.0 (3.0) | 30.6 (2.1) | 36.1 (1.5) |
| Antibiotic | 2.0 (1.2) | 0.8 (0.6) | 3.4 (2.4) | 0 | 0.5 (0.3) | 0.5 (0.2) | 0.4 (0.3) | 0.6 (0.4) | 0.4 (0.2) | 0.7 (0.8) | 1.7 (1.3) | 0.4 (0.2) |
| Transfusion | 0.7 (0.4) | 1.1 (0.8) | 1.4 (0.3) | 1.3 (0.6) | 2.3 (0.5) | 1.8 (0.3) | 26.7 (4.1) | 20.6 (2.6) | 17.8 (1.5) | 1.3 (0.9) | 2.5 (0.6) | 3.4 (0.5) |
| Cardiac or venous | 31.4 (7.7) | 32.5 (3.4) | 28.4 (2.1) | 55.5 (3.4) | 41.1 (2.6) | 43.5 (1.6) | 3.5 (1.1) | 13.6 (2.3) | 13.6 (0.9) | 10.4 (3.6) | 14.0 (1.3) | 14.3 (0.9) |
| Intubation | 0.6 (0.6) | 2.2 (0.7) | 2.0 (0.4) | 0.5 (0.5) | 1.5 (0.3) | 1.0 (0.1) | 0 | 0.7 (0.1) | 0.5 (0.1) | 0.6 (0.3) | 2.1 (0.5) | 1.4 (0.2) |
| NOS | 30.9 (6.4) | 20.0 (2.8) | 21.9 (1.4) | 27.7 (5.1) | 23.3 (1.4) | 23.1 (0.8) | 14.2 (4.7) | 11.5 (1.4) | 13.0 (1.7) | 69.9 (2.3) | 49.1 (1.8) | 44.2 (1.4) |
| Teaching status, % (SE) | | | | | | | | | | | | |
| Rural | 0 | 2.8 (2.3) | 12.5 (4.4) | 0 | 14.3 (2.7) | 12.1 (1.4) | 0.6 (0.7) | 13.2 (4.3) | 8.0 (1.6) | 0 | 18.7 (4.8) | 14.5 (1.5) |
| Urban nonteaching | 17.0 (15.4) | 7.9 (5.5) | 20.4 (5.9) | 1.2 (1.1) | 20.3 (4.3) | 39.6 (3.0) | 1.8 (1.5) | 21.2 (6.1) | 38.7 (3.5) | 18.0 (13.6) | 17.6 (3.8) | 36 (2.5) |
| Urban teaching | 83.0 (15.4) | 89.3 (6.1) | 67.2 (7.5) | 98.8 (1.1) | 65.4 (5.2) | 48.2 (3.3) | 97.6 (1.8) | 65.6 (7.7) | 53.4 (3.7) | 82.0 (13.6) | 63.6 (6.0) | 49.5 (3.0) |
| Payer, % (SE) | | | | | | | | | | | | |
| Medicare | 1.9 (1.3) | 20.1 (2.6) | 20.0 (1.7) | 6.1 (4.5) | 36.1 (2.0) | 34.8 (1.1) | 1.6 (0.5) | 22.6 (2.3) | 28.0 (1.1) | 4.2 (1.1) | 33.0 (2.5) | 37.3 (1.5) |
| Medicaid | 24.9 (7.3) | 26.5 (3.6) | 18.7 (2.2) | 24.7 (3.9) | 14.4 (1.5) | 11.7 (0.8) | 79.8 (5.2) | 47.5 (2.8) | 43.6 (1.5) | 44.6 (6.6) | 33.6 (2.5) | 25.2 (1.5) |
| Private | 61.3 (6.3) | 47.0 (3.0) | 53.8 (2.9) | 59.8 (3.5) | 38.1 (2.5) | 46.9 (1.3) | 13.9 (4.2) | 19.2 (2.0) | 21.0 (1.3) | 48.1 (5.3) | 28.1 (2.9) | 32.6 (1.5) |
| Self | 11.9 (4.1) | 6.3 (1.9) | 7.5 (1.7) | 9.4 (4.3) | 11.4 (1.6) | 6.6 (0.6) | 4.6 (2.2) | 6.7 (1.2) | 7.4 (0.8) | 3.0 (1.3) | 5.3 (0.6) | 4.9 (0.6) |

Abbreviation: NOS, not otherwise specified.
*All of the proportions are survey weighted and based on those who reported values. Standard errors are given in the same units as the point estimates. This table also includes discharges from Pennsylvania who were not included in the regression model.

**Table 3. Length of Stay for Adults With Chronic Conditions by Hospital Type***

| Hospital Type | LOS for CCHD, d | | LOS for CF, d | | LOS for SCD, d | | LOS for SB, d | |
|---|---|---|---|---|---|---|---|---|
| | Unadjusted | Adjusted† | Unadjusted | Adjusted† | Unadjusted | Adjusted† | Unadjusted | Adjusted† |
| Pediatric | 7.7‡ | 7.7‡ | 10.9‡ | 12.0‡ | 6.8 | 6.8 | 6.1 | 6.7 |
| Mixed | 5.8 | 5.3 | 10.9 | 9.5‡ | 7.3 | 7.0 | 7.3 | 7.2 |
| Adult | 4.9 | 5.1 | 7.6 | 7.7 | 6.2 | 6.2 | 7.3 | 7.0 |

Abbreviations: CCHD, complex congenital heart disease; CF, cystic fibrosis; LOS, length of stay; SB, spina bifida; SCD, sickle cell disease.
*All of the data are weighted.
†Adjusted data reflect estimates adjusted for sex, age, whether inpatient death occurred, procedures, income, health insurance, and comorbidities.
‡$P \leq .001$.

tween pediatric, mixed, and adult hospitals for the proportion of patients aged 18 to 35 years, the mean number of comorbidities reported, the proportion of patients with comorbidities reported, the proportion with different procedures, teaching status, and payer mix. Patients in pediatric hospitals had lower rates of comorbidity than those in adult hospitals and slightly higher rates of procedures for some diseases. Because of these differences, we controlled for these variables in the regression model described later. Pediatric hospitals generally had higher proportions of discharges with Medicaid as the primary payer, although this varied widely between disease states. Higher proportions of discharges from pediatric hospitals than from adult and mixed hospitals were at teaching institutions.

## DIFFERENCES IN LOS

After case-mix adjustment, LOS was significantly longer for patients with CCHD and CF in pediatric hospitals as compared with those in adult hospitals (both $P < .001$). There was no significant difference in LOS between adult and pediatric hospitals in patients treated for SCD or SB (**Table 3**).

## DIFFERENCES IN TOTAL CHARGES

Significant differences in total charges were found for all of the 4 study conditions across the hospital types ($P < .001$ for CF, CCH, and SCD, and $P < .01$ for SB), with pediatric hospital charges consistently higher than those of

**Table 4. Mean Hospital Charges for Adults With Chronic Conditions by Hospital Type***

| Hospital Type | Hospital Charges for CCHD, Mean, $ | | Hospital Charges for CF, Mean, $ | | Hospital Charges for SCD, Mean, $ | | Hospital Charges for SB, Mean, $ | |
|---|---|---|---|---|---|---|---|---|
| | Unadjusted | Adjusted† | Unadjusted | Adjusted† | Unadjusted | Adjusted† | Unadjusted | Adjusted† |
| Pediatric | 68 345‡ | 63 498‡ | 56 742‡ | 69 213‡ | 33 925‡ | 28 891‡ | 30 214‡ | 30 900§ |
| Mixed | 34 160 | 34 312 | 35 108 | 31 831 | 18 473 | 17 963 | 23 561 | 24 876 |
| Adult | 29 687 | 28 904 | 32 766 | 30 668 | 17 677 | 16 697 | 23 994 | 22 467 |

Abbreviations: CCHD, complex congenital heart disease; CF, cystic fibrosis; SB, spina bifida; SCD, sickle cell disease.
*All of the data are weighted.
†Adjusted data reflect estimates adjusted for sex, age, whether inpatient death occurred, procedures, income, health insurance, and comorbidities.
‡$P \leq .001$
§$P < .01$.

mixed and adult hospitals (**Table 4**). To examine how much of the charge difference could be accounted for by LOS, LOS was included in the charge regression model as a covariate in separate analyses. Approximately 60% of the charge difference found between pediatric and adult hospitals could be accounted for by prolonged LOS in the pediatric hospitals for CF, and 44% was accounted for by LOS for CCHD. In comparison, less than 10% of the difference in charges across hospital categories could be attributed to LOS differences for SCD and SB discharges. In general, patterns in the mixed hospitals appeared to mirror patterns in the adult hospitals.

## AGE-STRATIFIED ANALYSES

A subanalysis was performed by restricting the data set to discharges for patients aged 18 to 35 years to help control for other immeasurable factors that may be related to increased comorbidity rates in an aging population and to allow the subsamples to be more comparable across hospital types with respect to age. Length of stay remained significantly longer in pediatric hospitals for CCHD and CF. In addition, LOS was significantly longer in pediatric hospitals vs adult hospitals for SCD (7.0 vs 6.0 days, respectively; $P = .004$) in this subgroup. Total charges remained significantly higher in pediatric hospitals as compared with adult hospitals for all of the 4 diagnoses (all $P \leq .001$).

## COMMENT

In this nationally representative sample, we found that case-mix–adjusted hospital charges were significantly higher for adult survivors of CCHD, CF, SCD, and SB in pediatric hospitals as compared with those admitted to other hospitals. Lengths of stay were significantly longer for individuals with CCHD and CF discharged from pediatric hospitals. In addition, the differences in total charges and LOS remained consistent or even more pronounced when limiting the analysis age group to ages 18 to 35 years. Overall, these findings have several implications for understanding patterns of hospital care for adult survivors of chronic conditions originating in childhood, and they raise additional questions about how care delivery differs by hospital type for individuals with the same diagnoses.

## DIFFERENCES IN LOS AND TOTAL CHARGES AMONG HOSPITAL TYPES

We hypothesized that pediatric hospitals would have more experience with disease-specific care for patients with chronic illnesses of childhood whereas adult hospitals would have more experience in addressing more common comorbidities and care of adult patients. However, it was unclear how differences in familiarity with specific childhood diseases vs familiarity with general adult care would be related to hospital charges and LOS. Our findings suggest that there are processes of care differences that influence LOS and charge outcomes. Whether this is because of familiarity, practice variation between providers, hospital variation in provision of specific services, or other reasons could not be examined with these data and remains unknown.

This pattern contrasts with a prior article[16] regarding SCD hospitalizations that indicated shorter LOS on pediatric services as compared with adult services. However, this earlier study did not separate children from adults in the analyses. Children, who stay almost exclusively in pediatric settings and pediatric ward services, would be expected to have shorter LOS than adults,[17] who would tend to have more comorbidities that are often progressive in nature. For example, patients with SCD who survive to adulthood are more likely to have end organ damage than pediatric patients, typically resulting in longer admissions for adult patients.

Our findings are more similar to those in other studies[9,10] that examined children treated in pediatric hospitals vs community hospitals or nonpediatric hospitals and found that charges were higher overall in pediatric hospitals as compared with nonpediatric hospitals, although LOS was similar. However, those studies considered acute diseases among children whereas we measured hospital use for chronic illnesses in the adult population.

Our study also has implications for the health economic impact of adult survivors of chronic conditions originating in childhood. Goodman et al[8] estimated that adult survivors in pediatric hospitals with all diagnoses have at least $1 billion in annual charges. However, in our study, adults with SCD alone incurred inpatient charges exceeding $1 billion in 2002 nationally. Overall, higher total charges in pediatric hospitals are consistent with other recent studies[18,19] that also found higher mean charges in pediatric hospitals as compared with nonpediatric hospitals across a fixed set of discharge diagnoses.

Such variation in charges may correspond to differences in quality of care or outcomes. Processes of care for the same diagnosis may vary substantively between adult and pediatric hospitals for reasons that are independent of LOS and subsequent charges. Moreover, there are several possible explanations for higher mean charges at pediatric vs other hospitals. It is possible that higher staffing ratios in pediatric hospitals or lower thresholds for intensive care service account for the difference in charges. Another hypothesis is that pediatric hospitals may provide more ancillary services for patients, such as child-life services and social work support, and hence the charges are higher for each patient. It is also plausible that higher charges in pediatric hospitals may be attributable to higher operational costs per discharge compared with adult-predominant institutions such that pediatric hospitals would need to charge greater amounts per discharge to cover overhead costs.

Although it is also possible that there are unmeasured comorbidities and disease severity that explain the differences we found, this seems unlikely because case-mix adjustment resulted in greater rather than smaller differences between the hospitals. However, if adult hospitals are systematically better at coding and reporting comorbid conditions, this could have resulted in biasing our results against pediatric hospitals. Unfortunately, we are not able to explore these hypotheses with this data set.

## LIMITATIONS

This is an observational study in which we attempted to control for multiple factors that would potentially confound analyses of LOS and hospital charges. Optimally, we would be able to prospectively study differences of care for similar patients randomly assigned to admission to a pediatric hospital vs other hospital types, but such a study would not be feasible or ethical. As with any observational study, we cannot exclude the possibility that associations we described are confounded by unmeasured illness severity, even though our study controlled for a host of comorbidities and other patient attributes. It is also possible that some differences we observed between hospitals are attributable to patient selection bias, but our model remained robust despite additions of illness severity measures and case-mix adjustment. There are other pressures that may keep an adult in a pediatric hospital, such as treatment resource availability, personal provider, or special needs of the patient, but those cannot be measured in this data set.

We were also unable to determine in mixed and adult hospitals whether a patient was admitted to adult or pediatric ward services or whether subspecialty services were consulted and influenced practice variation. In addition, we could not ascertain within the pediatric hospitals group whether institutions had different policies regarding admission of adult patients; this limits the ability of our study to inform pediatric hospitals about their specific policies. Despite these limitations of our observational design, we feel that our study provides key insights to possible differences in care for adults with complex illness of childhood origin admitted to different care settings.

Data in the NIS are based on discharges, not on individual patients; therefore, we are unable to assess readmission rates or functional status after discharge. It is possible, for instance, that discharges for adults with CF from pediatric hospitals had longer LOS but lower rates of readmission than discharges from adult hospitals, resulting in comparable or even lower total annual charges at the person level. This may be true for patients with SCD because readmissions are common, especially among adults. A recent large prospective study[20] reported that 50% of adult patients with SCD were readmitted within 1 month of discharge, but the hospital types were not compared in that study.

Finally, as with any study that relies on diagnostic codes for case findings, it is possible that there were attribution errors that led to misclassification of discharges in one analytic group or another. We believe, however, that this probability is mitigated by the clinical prominence of the conditions on which we focused. It should be noted that we only examined 4 disease states and therefore cannot generalize specific findings to all chronic illnesses of childhood.

## CONCLUSIONS

Despite concerns that adult survivors of chronic childhood illnesses have difficulty accessing and continuing care in the adult health care setting,[1,21-23] the vast majority of adults with chronic conditions originating in childhood receive inpatient care in the adult health care setting. Some practitioners may admit adults to a pediatric hospital with the assumption that their patients have specific disease care needs that require a pediatric hospital whereas other patients are still cared for in outpatient settings by pediatricians who admit to the ward services where they have privileges. Patient preference can also be a factor in the hospital to which a patient is admitted.

Our findings also indicate that adults cared for at pediatric hospitals have higher total charges and longer LOS than in adult hospitals despite case-mix adjustment. Currently, whether and how these hospital resource use differences translate into differences in quality of care, decreased morbidity, or future savings in health care expenditures is unknown. Of note, shorter LOS cannot be automatically equated with improved care.[24]

Based on the increasing numbers of adult survivors with chronic conditions of childhood,[25,26] further research is warranted to evaluate reasons for differences or similarities that are associated with better inpatient care. Although interest in the research and care of adults with illnesses originating in childhood has largely occurred in pediatrics,[22,27] our findings are a reminder that pediatricians compose the minority of providers for this growing population. Further elucidation of the reasons for interinstitutional differences we have described offers the opportunity to improve care across hospitals with patients of all ages with chronic conditions.

**Accepted for Publication:** May 27, 2006.
**Correspondence:** Megumi Okumura, MD, Division of General Pediatrics, University of California, San Francisco, 3333 California St, Suite 245, Box 0503, San Francisco, CA 94143-0503 (okumuram@peds.ucsf.edu).
**Author Contributions:** *Study concept and design:* Okumura, Nasr, and Davis. *Acquisition of data:* Okumura. *Analysis and interpretation of data:* Okumura, Campbell, and Davis. *Drafting of the manuscript:* Okumura. *Critical revision of the manuscript for important intellectual content:* Okumura, Campbell, Nasr, and Davis. *Statistical analysis:* Okumura. *Obtained funding:* Okumura. *Administrative, technical, and material support:* Okumura, Nasr, and Davis. *Study supervision:* Okumura, Nasr, and Davis.
**Funding/Support:** This work was supported by the Robert Wood Johnson Clinical Scholars Program at the University of Michigan, Ann Arbor.
**Acknowledgment:** We thank Sonya Demonner, MPH, Myra Kim, PhD, and Achamyeleh Gebremariam, MS, for their assistance with the data set. We especially thank Rodney Hayward, MD, for his wisdom and guidance with the analysis and the manuscript.

## REFERENCES

1. Reiss J, Gibson R. Health care transition: destinations unknown. *Pediatrics.* 2002;110:1307-1314.
2. Gaston MH, Verter JI, Woods G, et al. Prophylaxis with oral penicillin in children with sickle cell anemia: a randomized trial. *N Engl J Med.* 1986;314:1593-1599.
3. Platt OS, Brambilla DJ, Rosse WF, et al. Mortality in sickle cell disease: life expectancy and risk factors for early death. *N Engl J Med.* 1994;330:1639-1644.
4. American Academy of Pediatrics; American Academy of Family Physicians; American College of Physicians–American Society of Internal Medicine. A consensus statement on health care transitions for young adults with special health care needs. *Pediatrics.* 2002;110:1304-1306.
5. Foster E, Graham TP Jr, Driscoll DJ, et al. Task force 2: special health care needs of adults with congenital heart disease. *J Am Coll Cardiol.* 2001;37:1176-1183.
6. Cystic Fibrosis Foundation Center Committee and Guidelines Subcommittee. Cystic Fibrosis Foundation guidelines for patient services, evaluation, and monitoring in cystic fibrosis centers. *AJDC.* 1990;144:1311-1312.
7. Lam PY, Fitzgerald BB, Sawyer SM. Young adults in children's hospitals: why are they there? *Med J Aust.* 2005;182:381-384.
8. Goodman DM, Mendez E, Throop C, Ogata ES. Adult survivors of pediatric illness: the impact on pediatric hospitals. *Pediatrics.* 2002;110:583-589.
9. Merenstein D, Egleston B, Diener-West M. Lengths of stay and costs associated with children's hospitals. *Pediatrics.* 2005;115:839-844.
10. Samuels BN, Novack AH, Martin DP, Connell FA. Comparison of length of stay for asthma by hospital type. *Pediatrics.* 1998;101:E13.
11. Agency for Healthcare Research and Quality. Healthcare Cost and Utilization Project. http://www.hcup-us.ahrq.gov/home.jsp. Accessed January 24, 2006.
12. Houchens R, Elixhauser A, Sommers J. *Changes in the NIS Sampling and Weighting Strategy for 1998.* Rockville, Md: Agency for Healthcare Research and Quality; 2002. Healthcare Cost and Utilization Project Methods Series Report No. 2002-1. http://www.hcup-us.ahrq.gov/reports/1998ChangesintheNISRedesignFinal.pdf. Accessed July 18, 2006.
13. *International Classification of Diseases, Ninth Revision, Clinical Modification.* Washington, DC: Public Health Service, US Dept of Health and Human Services; 1988.
14. Elixhauser A, Steiner C, Harris DR, Coffey RM. Comorbidity measures for use with administrative data. *Med Care.* 1998;36:8-27.
15. Duan N. Smearing estimate: a nonparametric retransformation method. *J Am Stat Assoc.* 1983;78:605-610.
16. Mayer ML, Konrad TR, Dvorak CC. Hospital resource utilization among patients with sickle cell disease. *J Health Care Poor Underserved.* 2003;14:122-135.
17. Agency for Healthcare Research and Quality. HCUPnet . http://hcup.ahrq.gov/HCUPnet.asp. Accessed January 24, 2006.
18. Silber JH, Rosenbaum PR, Even-Shoshan O, et al. Length of stay, conditional length of stay, and prolonged stay in pediatric asthma. *Health Serv Res.* 2003;38:867-886.
19. Srivastava R, Homer CJ. Length of stay for common pediatric conditions: teaching vs nonteaching hospitals. *Pediatrics.* 2003;112:278-281.
20. Ballas SK, Lusardi M. Hospital readmission for adult acute sickle cell painful episodes: frequency, etiology, and prognostic significance. *Am J Hematol.* 2005;79:17-25.
21. Fox A. Physicians as barriers to successful transitional care. *Int J Adolesc Med Health.* 2002;14:3-7.
22. Reid GJ, Irvine MJ, McCrindle BW, et al. Prevalence and correlates of successful transfer from pediatric to adult health care among a cohort of young adults with complex congenital heart defects. *Pediatrics.* 2004;113:e197-e205.
23. Reiss JG, Gibson RW, Walker LR. Health care transition: youth, family, and provider perspectives. *Pediatrics.* 2005;115:112-120.
24. Hayward RA, Bernard AM, Rosevear JS, Anderson JE, McMahon LF Jr. An evaluation of generic screens for poor quality of hospital care on a general medicine service. *Med Care.* 1993;31:394-402.
25. Davis H, Moore RM Jr, Gergen PJ. Cost of hospitalizations associated with sickle cell disease in the United States. *Public Health Rep.* 1997;112:40-43.
26. Lakdawalla DN, Bhattacharya J, Goldman DP. Are the young becoming more disabled? *Health Aff (Millwood).* 2004;23:168-176.
27. McManus MA, Newacheck PW, Greaney AM. Young adults with special health care needs: prevalence, severity, and access to health services. *Pediatrics.* 1990;86:674-682.

Why call the vehicle for moving people an *ambulance* when walking cases are *ambulant*? An ambulance once brought the hospital to the patient. The French devised the term and applied it to their early field hospitals, which they called "hospitals ambulants." From this the name ambulance was applied to the vehicle and maintained when it reversed the process and brought patients to the hospital.

—From *Why Do We Say It?*, Castle Books, 1985

## Pertussis immunity wanes in early adolescence[1]

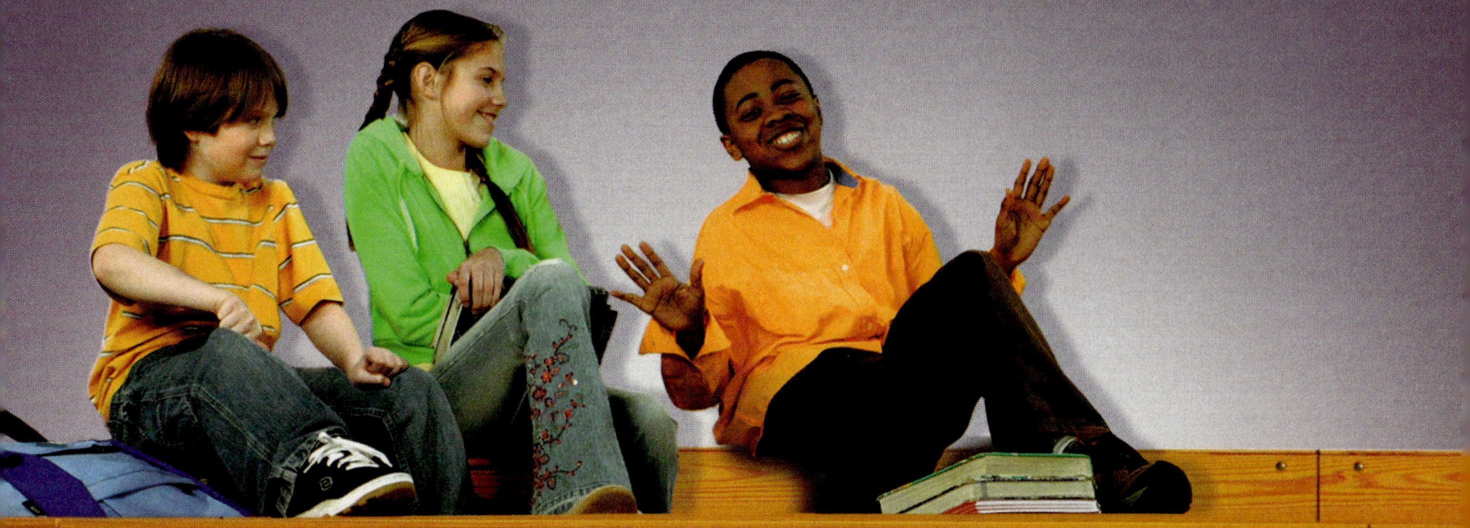

**Take the next step—**

# BOOST

**their protection with BOOSTRIX**

ACIP* recommends
**BOOST**
adolescents
pertussis booster[2]

## Important Safety Information

In clinical studies, adverse events included pain, redness, and swelling at the injection site, headache, fatigue, and gastrointestinal symptoms. As with other vaccines, rare adverse events may occur. As with any vaccine, vaccination with BOOSTRIX may not protect 100% of susceptible individuals. Hypersensitivity to any component of BOOSTRIX is a contraindication.

*Advisory Committee on Immunization Practices.

gsk GlaxoSmithKline Vaccines

**BOOSTRIX®**

***Tetanus Toxoid, Reduced Diphtheria Toxoid and Acellular Pertussis Vaccine, Adsorbed***

**Please see references and brief summary of complete prescribing information on the adjacent page.**


Manufactured by **GlaxoSmithKline Biologicals,** Rixensart, Belgium
Distributed by **GlaxoSmithKline**, Research Triangle Park, NC 27709

# BOOSTRIX®

## (Tetanus Toxoid, Reduced Diphtheria Toxoid and Acellular Pertussis Vaccine, Adsorbed) (Tdap)

The following is a brief summary only; see full prescribing information for complete product information.

**INDICATIONS AND USAGE:** BOOSTRIX is indicated for active booster immunization against tetanus, diphtheria, and pertussis as a single dose in individuals 10 through 18 years of age. The use of BOOSTRIX as a primary series or to complete the primary series has not been studied. As with any vaccine, BOOSTRIX may not protect 100% of individuals receiving the vaccine.

**CONTRAINDICATIONS:** Hypersensitivity to any component of the vaccine is a contraindication (see DESCRIPTION in full prescribing information). Do not use BOOSTRIX after a serious allergic reaction (e.g., anaphylaxis) following any other tetanus toxoid, diphtheria toxoid or pertussis-containing vaccine, or any component of this vaccine (see DESCRIPTION in full prescribing information). Because of the uncertainty as to which component of the vaccine might be responsible, do not give further vaccination with any of these components; or, refer such individuals to an allergist for evaluation. The following events are contraindications to administration of BOOSTRIX: encephalopathy (e.g., coma, decreased level of consciousness, prolonged seizures) within 7 days of administration of a previous dose of a pertussis-containing vaccine that is not attributable to another identifiable cause; progressive neurologic disorder, uncontrolled epilepsy, or progressive encephalopathy. Do not vaccinate individuals with these conditions until a treatment regimen has been established and the condition has stabilized.

**WARNINGS:** The tip cap and the rubber plunger of the needleless prefilled syringes contain dry natural latex rubber that may cause allergic reactions in latex sensitive individuals. The vial stopper is latex-free. If any of the following events occurred in temporal relation to previous receipt of a Diphtheria and Tetanus Toxoids and Pertussis Vaccine Adsorbed (DTwP) vaccine or a vaccine containing an acellular pertussis component, consider carefully whether to give subsequent doses of BOOSTRIX: temperature of ≥40.5°C (105°F) within 48 hours not due to another identifiable cause; collapse or shock-like state (hypotonic-hyporesponsive episode) within 48 hours; persistent, inconsolable crying lasting ≥3 hours, occurring within 48 hours; seizures with or without fever occurring within 3 days. Persons who experienced serious Arthus-type hypersensitivity reactions following a prior dose of tetanus toxoid usually have high serum tetanus antitoxin levels and should not be given Tetanus and Diphtheria Toxoids Adsorbed For Adult Use (Td) or Tdap vaccines or even emergency doses of Td more frequently than every 10 years, even if the wound is neither clean nor minor. If Guillain-Barré syndrome has occurred within 6 weeks of receipt of prior vaccine containing tetanus toxoid, the decision to give BOOSTRIX or any vaccine containing tetanus toxoid should be based on careful consideration of the potential benefits and possible risks. The decision to administer a pertussis-containing vaccine to individuals with stable central nervous system (CNS) disorders must be made by the physician on an individual basis, with consideration of all relevant factors, and assessment of potential risks and benefits for that individual. Advise the patient, parent, or guardian of the potential increased risk involved (see PRECAUTIONS). A family history of seizures or other CNS disorders is not a contraindication to pertussis vaccine. The Advisory Committee on Immunization Practices (ACIP) has published guidelines for vaccination of persons with recent or acute illness (www.cdc.gov). Do not give BOOSTRIX to individuals with bleeding disorders such as hemophilia or thrombocytopenia, or to persons on anticoagulant therapy unless the potential benefit clearly outweighs the risk of administration. If the decision is made to administer BOOSTRIX to such persons, it should be given with caution with steps taken to avoid the risk of hematoma following the injection.

**PRECAUTIONS: General:** Before the injection of any biological, the physician should take all reasonable precautions to prevent allergic or other adverse reactions. Epinephrine injection (1:1,000) and other appropriate agents used for the control of immediate allergic reactions must be immediately available should an acute anaphylactic reaction occur. Immunosuppressed persons, including individuals receiving immunosuppressive therapy, may not develop the expected immune response. **Drug Interactions:** Do not mix BOOSTRIX with any other vaccine in the same syringe or vial. **Carcinogenesis, Mutagenesis, Impairment of Fertility:** BOOSTRIX has not been evaluated for carcinogenic or mutagenic potential, or for impairment of fertility. **Pregnancy:** Pregnancy Category C. Animal reproduction studies have not been conducted with BOOSTRIX. It is also not known whether BOOSTRIX can cause fetal harm when administered to a pregnant woman or can affect reproductive capacity. BOOSTRIX should be given to a pregnant woman only if clearly needed. Animal fertility studies have not been conducted with BOOSTRIX. In a developmental toxicity study, the effect of BOOSTRIX on embryo-fetal and pre-weaning development was evaluated in pregnant rats. Animals were administered INFANRIX® (Diphtheria and Tetanus Toxoids and Acellular Pertussis Vaccine Adsorbed) prior to gestation and BOOSTRIX during the period of organogenesis (gestation days 6, 8, 11) and later in pregnancy (gestation day 15), 0.1 mL/rat/occasion (a 45-fold increase compared to the human dose of BOOSTRIX on a body weight basis), by intramuscular injection. No adverse affect on pregnancy and lactation parameters, embryo-fetal or pre-weaning development was observed. There were no fetal malformations or other evidence of teratogenesis noted in this study. **Nursing Mothers:** It is not known whether BOOSTRIX is excreted in human milk. Because many drugs are excreted in human milk, caution should be exercised when BOOSTRIX is administered to a nursing woman. **Pregnancy Exposure Registry:** Healthcare providers are encouraged to register pregnant women who receive BOOSTRIX in the GlaxoSmithKline vaccination pregnancy registry by calling 1-888-825-5249. **Geriatric Use:** BOOSTRIX is not indicated for use in individuals older than 18 years. **Pediatric Use:** BOOSTRIX is not indicated for use in individuals younger than 10 years (see DOSAGE AND ADMINISTRATION in full prescribing information). For immunization of infants and children younger than 7 years against diphtheria, tetanus, and pertussis, refer to the manufacturers' package inserts for Diphtheria and Tetanus Toxoids and Acellular Pertussis Vaccine Adsorbed (DTaP) vaccines.

**ADVERSE REACTIONS:** A total of 3,608 adolescents were vaccinated with a single dose of BOOSTRIX during clinical trials. An additional 1,092 adolescents 10 to 18 years of age received a non-US formulation of BOOSTRIX (formulated to contain 0.5 mg aluminum per dose) in non-US clinical studies.

The primary safety study, conducted in the United States, was a randomized, observer-blinded, controlled study in which 3,080 adolescents 10 to 18 years of age received a single dose of BOOSTRIX and 1,034 received the control Td vaccine manufactured by Massachusetts Public Health Biologic Laboratories. There were no substantive differences in demographic characteristics between the vaccine groups. Among BOOSTRIX and control vaccine recipients approximately 75% were 10 to 14 years of age and approximately 25% were 15 to 18 years of age. Approximately 98% of participants in this study had received the recommended series of 4 or 5 doses of either DTwP or a combination of DTwP and DTaP in childhood. Data on adverse events were collected by the subjects, parents and/or guardians using standardized diaries for 15 consecutive days following the vaccine dose (i.e., day of vaccination and the next 14 days). Subjects were monitored for unsolicited adverse events that occurred within 31 days of vaccination (day 0-30) using diary cards (day 0-14) supplemented by spontaneous reports and a medical history as reported by subjects, parents, and/or guardians. Subjects were also monitored for 6 months post-vaccination for non-routine medical visits, visits to an emergency room, onset of new chronic illness, and serious adverse events. Information regarding late onset adverse events was obtained via a telephone call 6 months following vaccination. At least 97% of subjects completed the 6-month follow-up evaluation.

In a study conducted in Germany, BOOSTRIX was administered to 319 children 10 to 12 years of age previously vaccinated with 5 doses of acellular pertussis-containing vaccines, 193 of these subjects had previously received 5 doses of INFANRIX. Adverse events were recorded on diary cards during the 15 days following vaccination. Unsolicited adverse events that occurred within 31 days of vaccination (day 0-30) were recorded on the diary card or verbally reported to the investigator. Subjects were monitored for 6 months post-vaccination for physician office visits, emergency room visits, onset of new chronic illness, and serious adverse events. The 6-month follow-up evaluation, conducted via telephone interview, was completed by 90% of subjects.

The adverse event information from clinical trials provides a basis for identifying adverse events that appear to be related to vaccine use and for approximating rates. However, because clinical trials are conducted under widely varying conditions, adverse event rates observed in the clinical trials of a vaccine cannot be directly compared to rates in the clinical trials of another vaccine, and may not reflect the rates observed in practice.

**Serious Adverse Events in All Safety Studies:** In the US-safety study and German-safety study, no serious adverse events were reported to occur within 31 days of vaccination. During the 6-month extended safety evaluation period, no serious adverse events that were of potential autoimmune origin or new onset and chronic in nature were reported to occur. In non-US studies in which serious adverse events were monitored for up to 37 days, one subject was diagnosed with insulin dependent diabetes 20 days following administration of BOOSTRIX. No other serious adverse events of potential autoimmune origin or that were new onset and chronic in nature were reported to occur in these studies.

**Solicited Adverse Events in the US-Safety Study:** In a US study, the most common local adverse events following administration of BOOSTRIX were pain, redness, and swelling at the injection site. The most common general adverse events were headache and fatigue. Most of these events were reported at a similar frequency in recipients of both BOOSTRIX and Td. Any pain, grade 2 or 3 pain (but not grade 3 alone), and grade 2 or 3 headache (but not grade 3 alone) were reported at a higher rate in recipients of BOOSTRIX. The primary safety endpoint of the US study was the incidence of grade 3 pain (spontaneously painful and/or prevented normal activity) at the injection site within 15 days of vaccination. Grade 3 pain was reported in 4.6% of those who received BOOSTRIX compared with 4.0% of those who received the Td vaccine. The difference in rate of grade 3 pain was within the pre-defined clinical limit for non-inferiority (upper limit of the 95% CI for the difference ≤4%). These were the rates for solicited local and general adverse events within 15 days of vaccination with BOOSTRIX or Td vaccine for the total vaccinated cohort (all enrolled, vaccinated subjects with safety data available analyzed by vaccine received):

**Percentage of Individuals 10 to 18 Years of Age Reporting Solicited Local Adverse Events or Solicited General Adverse Events Within the 15-day* Post-Vaccination Period**

| | BOOSTRIX (N = 3,032) % | Td (N =1,013) % |
|---|---|---|
| **Local** | | |
| Pain,† any | 75.3 | 71.7 |
| Pain,† grade 2 or 3 | 51.2 | 42.5 |
| Pain,‡ grade 3 | 4.6 | 4.0 |
| Redness, any | 22.5 | 19.8 |
| Redness, >20 mm | 4.1 | 3.9 |
| Redness, ≥50 mm | 1.7 | 1.6 |
| Swelling, any | 21.1 | 20.1 |
| Swelling, >20 mm | 5.3 | 4.9 |
| Swelling, ≥50 mm | 2.5 | 3.2 |
| Arm circumference increase,§ >5 mm | 28.3 | 29.5 |
| Arm circumference increase,§ >20 mm | 2.0 | 2.2 |
| Arm circumference increase,§ >40 mm | 0.5 | 0.3 |
| **General** | | |
| Fever,‖ ≥99.5°F | 13.5 | 13.1 |
| Fever,‖ >100.4°F | 5.0 | 4.7 |
| Fever,‖ >102.2°F | 1.4 | 1.0 |
| Headache, any | 43.1 | 41.5 |
| Headache,† grade 2 or 3 | 15.7 | 12.7 |
| Headache, grade 3 | 3.7 | 2.7 |
| Fatigue, any | 37.0 | 36.7 |
| Fatigue, grade 2 or 3 | 14.4 | 12.9 |
| Fatigue, grade 3 | 3.7 | 3.2 |
| Gastrointestinal symptoms,¶ any | 26.0 | 25.8 |
| Gastrointestinal symptoms,¶ grade 2 or 3 | 9.8 | 9.7 |
| Gastrointestinal symptoms,¶ grade 3 | 3.0 | 3.2 |

Td = Tetanus and Diphtheria Toxoids Adsorbed For Adult Use manufactured by Massachusetts Public Health Biologic Laboratories.
N = number of subjects in the total vaccinated cohort with local/general symptoms sheets completed.
Grade 2 = Local: painful when the limb was moved; General: interfered with normal activity.
Grade 3 = Local: spontaneously painful and/or prevented normal activity; General: prevented normal activity.
*Day of vaccination and the next 14 days.
†Statistically significantly higher (P<0.05) following BOOSTRIX as compared to Td vaccine.
‡Grade 3 injection site pain following BOOSTRIX was not inferior to Td (upper limit of two-sided 95% CI for the difference in the percentage of subjects ≤4%).
§Mid-upper region of the vaccinated arm.
‖Oral temperatures or axillary temperatures.
¶Gastrointestinal symptoms included nausea, vomiting, diarrhea and/or abdominal pain.

Mid-upper arm circumference was measured by the adolescent or their parent/guardian prior to injection and daily for 15 days following vaccination. There was no significant difference between BOOSTRIX recipients and Td recipients in the proportion of subjects reporting an increase in mid-upper arm circumference in the vaccinated arm. The incidence of unsolicited adverse events reported in the 31 days after vaccination was comparable between the 2 groups.

**Solicited Adverse Events in the German Safety Study:** No cases of whole arm swelling were spontaneously reported. Two individuals (2/193) reported large injection site swelling (range 110 to 200 mm diameter), in one case associated with grade 3 pain. Neither individual sought medical attention. These episodes were reported to resolve without sequelae within 5 days. These were the rates of solicited local adverse events and fever within 15 days of vaccination for those subjects who had previously been vaccinated with 5 doses of INFANRIX:

**Rates of Solicited Adverse Events Reported Within the 15-day* Post-Vaccination Period Following Administration of BOOSTRIX in Individuals 10 to 12 Years of Age Who Had Previously Received 5 Doses of INFANRIX**

| Adverse Event | BOOSTRIX (N = 193) % (95% CI) |
|---|---|
| Pain, any | 62.2 (54.9-69.0) |
| Pain, grade 2 or 3 | 33.2 (26.6-40.3) |
| Pain, grade 3 | 5.7 (2.9-10.0) |
| Redness, any | 47.7 (40.4-55.0) |
| Redness, >20 mm | 15.0 (10.3-20.9) |
| Redness, ≥50 mm | 10.9 (6.9-16.2) |
| Swelling, any | 38.9 (31.9-46.1) |
| Swelling, >20 mm | 17.6 (12.5-23.7) |
| Swelling, ≥50 mm | 14.0 (9.4-19.7) |
| Fever, ≥99.5 | 8.8 (5.2-13.7) |
| Fever, >100.4 | 4.1 (1.8-8.0) |
| Fever, >102.2 | 1.0 (0.1-3.7) |

N = number of subjects with local/general symptoms sheets completed.
Grade 2 = Painful when the limb was moved.
Grade 3 = Spontaneously painful and/or prevented normal activity.
*Day of vaccination and the next 14 days.

As with any vaccine, there is the possibility that broad use of BOOSTRIX could reveal adverse events not observed in clinical trials.

**Postmarketing Reports:** Worldwide voluntary reports of adverse events received for BOOSTRIX in persons 10 to 18 years of age since market introduction of this vaccine are listed below. This list includes serious events or events which have causal connection to components of this or other vaccines or drugs. Because these events are reported voluntarily from a population of uncertain size, it is not possible to reliably estimate their frequency or establish a causal relationship to vaccine exposure. *Blood and lymphatic system disorders:* Lymphadenitis, lymphadenopathy. *Cardiac disorders:* Myocarditis. *Injection site reactions:* Induration, inflammation, mass, nodule, warmth, local reaction. *Metabolism and nutrition disorders:* Diabetes mellitus insulin-dependent. *Musculoskeletal and connective tissue disorders:* Arthralgia, back pain, myalgia. *Nervous system disorders:* Convulsion, encephalitis, facial palsy, paraesthesia. *Skin and subcutaneous tissue disorders:* Exanthem, Henoch-Schönlein purpura, rash. In addition, extensive swelling of the injected limb has been reported following administration of BOOSTRIX.

**Reporting Adverse Events:** Report the occurrence following immunization of any event set forth in the Vaccine Injury Table from the National Childhood Vaccine Injury Act including: Anaphylaxis or anaphylactic shock within 7 days, encephalopathy or encephalitis within 7 days, brachial neuritis within 28 days, or an acute complication or sequelae (including death) of an illness, disability, injury, or condition referred to above, or any events that would contraindicate further doses of vaccine, according to this prescribing information. These events should be reported to VAERS. The VAERS toll-free number is 1-800-822-7967. Reporting forms may also be obtained at the VAERS website at www.vaers.hhs.gov.

**DOSAGE AND ADMINISTRATION: Recommended Dose:** BOOSTRIX should be administered as a single 0.5 mL injection by the intramuscular route into the deltoid muscle of the upper arm in individuals 10 through 18 years of age. Do not administer this product subcutaneously or intravenously. There are no data to support repeat administration of BOOSTRIX. Five years should elapse between the subject's last dose of the recommended series of childhood DTwP and/or DTaP vaccine and the administration of BOOSTRIX. Limited data are available on the use of BOOSTRIX following Tetanus and Diphtheria Toxoids Adsorbed For Adult Use (Td) vaccine. **Additional Dosing Information:** ***Wound Management:*** Clinicians should refer to guidelines for tetanus prophylaxis in routine wound management. Adolescents 10 to 18 years of age who have completed a primary series against tetanus and who sustain wounds which are minor and uncomplicated, should receive a booster dose of a tetanus toxoid-containing vaccine only if they have not received tetanus toxoid within the preceding 10 years. In case of tetanus-prone injury (e.g., wounds contaminated with dirt, feces, soil, and saliva; puncture wounds; avulsions; and wounds resulting from missles, crushing, burns, and frostbite) in an adolescent who is in need of tetanus toxoid, BOOSTRIX can be used as an alternative to Tetanus and Diphtheria Toxoids Adsorbed For Adult Use (Td) vaccine in patients for whom the pertussis component is also indicated (see INDICATIONS AND USAGE).

Manufactured by **GlaxoSmithKline Biologicals**
Rixensart, Belgium, US License 1617

Distributed by **GlaxoSmithKline**
Research Triangle Park, NC 27709



Full prescribing information for BOOSTRIX is available at www.BOOSTRIX.com.
BRS-BO:L3

**References: 1.** Centers for Disease Control and Prevention. Preventing tetanus, diphtheria, and pertussis among adolescents: use of tetanus toxoid, reduced diphtheria toxoid and acellular pertussis vaccines: recommendations of the Advisory Committee on Immunization Practices (ACIP). Early Release 2006;55(February 23, 2006):1–43. **2.** Centers for Disease Control and Prevention. Recommended childhood and adolescent immunization schedule—United States, 2006. *MMWR.* 2006;54(51&52):Q1–Q4.

ARTICLE

# Attention-Deficit/Hyperactivity Disorder in Children

## Excess Costs Before and After Initial Diagnosis and Treatment Cost Differences by Ethnicity

*G. Thomas Ray, MBA; Peter Levine, MD; Lisa A. Croen, PhD; Farasat A. S. Bokhari, PhD; Teh-wei Hu, PhD; Laurel A. Habel, PhD*

**Objectives:** To estimate the excess costs for children in the years surrounding initial diagnosis of attention-deficit/hyperactivity disorder (ADHD) and to estimate differences in treatment costs by ethnicity.

**Design:** We identified children diagnosed with ADHD and estimated their health service costs in the 2 years before and 2 years after initial diagnosis of ADHD. Costs were compared with those for children without ADHD. We adjusted for age, sex, ethnicity, pharmacy co-pay, estimated family income, coexisting mental health disorders, and chronic medical conditions.

**Setting:** Nonprofit, integrated health care delivery system in northern California from January 1, 1996, to December 31, 2004.

**Participants:** Children aged 2 to 10 years with (n=3122) and without (n=15 899) ADHD.

**Main Exposure:** Attention-deficit/hyperactivity disorder.

**Main Outcome Measures:** Health care costs and use in the years before and after initial ADHD diagnosis as well as costs of ADHD-related services.

**Results:** Compared with children without ADHD, children with ADHD had mean costs that were $488 more in the second year before their ADHD diagnosis, $678 more in the year before their diagnosis, $1328 more in the year after their diagnosis, and $1040 more in the second year after their diagnosis. Asian Americans diagnosed with ADHD had lower total ADHD-related mean costs per year than white Americans diagnosed with ADHD ($221 lower), and Asian Americans, African Americans, and Hispanic Americans all had lower ADHD-related pharmacy mean costs than white Americans ($95, $63, and $77 lower, respectively).

**Conclusions:** Children with ADHD use significantly more health services before and after their diagnosis than children without ADHD. Among children diagnosed with ADHD, nonwhite Americans (especially Asian Americans) use fewer ADHD-related services than white Americans.

*Arch Pediatr Adolesc Med. 2006;160:1063-1069*

**Author Affiliations:** Division of Research, Kaiser Permanente Medical Care Program, Northern California Region, Oakland, Calif (Mr Ray and Drs Croen and Habel); Department of Pediatrics, The Permanente Medical Group, Inc, Walnut Creek, Calif (Dr Levine); Department of Economics, Florida State University, Tallahassee (Dr Bokhari); and School of Public Health, University of California, Berkeley (Dr Hu).

ATTENTION-DEFICIT/HYPERACTIVITY DISORDER (ADHD) is one of the most common psychiatric disorders of childhood, with an estimated prevalence of nearly 8% in US children aged 4 to 17 years.[1] It is known to have significant morbidity affecting academic achievement, social behaviors, and work success.[2,3] Treatment to help ameliorate those problems includes medication and behavioral approaches,[4,5] both of which can be costly.[6,7]

Although there have been a number of cost studies related to ADHD,[6-12] we are aware of no studies that indicate the pattern of excess health service cost and use both before and after initial diagnosis of ADHD, and few have analyzed cost or use differences by ethnicity—none of which included significant numbers of Asian Americans. Excess use of services prior to an ADHD diagnosis may signal an existing problem for which the family may be seeking a diagnosis and may indicate that assessment protocols are not identifying these children early enough. Ethnic differences in the use of ADHD services among children who are diagnosed may lead to determining whether there is undertreatment or overtreatment of certain groups.

## METHODS

### SETTING

Kaiser Permanente (KP) of Northern California (KPNC), Oakland, is a nonprofit, integrated health care delivery system providing care to more than 3 million members, about 700 000 of whom are younger than 18 years.

Kaiser Permanente of Northern California provides comprehensive health services in more than 15 counties throughout northern California. The guideline for all providers at KP is to use the *Diagnostic and Statistical Manual of Mental Disorders, Fourth Edition*[13] criteria for diagnosing ADHD. An assessment should take place, but there is some diversity with respect to the tools used. Generally, an ADHD-specific questionnaire is filled out by parents and the child's teacher(s), a developmental history questionnaire (usually with a KP-developed tool) is filled out by the parents, and the parents and children are interviewed. Patients generally receive medication treatment from either their primary care pediatrician or a child psychiatrist.

## SELECTION OF STUDY POPULATION

Using KPNC electronic databases, we selected all of the children from January 1, 1996, to December 31, 2004, who either were dispensed an ADHD-related medication (psychostimulants or atomoxetine) in a KPNC outpatient pharmacy or had an outpatient visit at a KPNC facility that included the diagnosis or management of ADHD (*International Classification of Diseases, Ninth Revision, Clinical Modification*[14] code 314.0). The first date that the child was seen for ADHD or had a prescription filled for an ADHD medication within this 9-year period was considered the diagnosis or index date for that child. Our goal was to identify the first time that children in the health plan were diagnosed with or treated for ADHD. Therefore, our study population was restricted to children who were no older than 2 years on January 1, 1996 (when KPNC began capturing outpatient visit diagnoses electronically) and were born in a KP hospital (so as to capture race, which is recorded in the KP hospitalization database). We further required that all of the study children were continuous members of the health plan from age 2 years until their index date. As a result of these selection criteria, children in this study were between ages 2 and 10 years on their index date. Although our primary study population included children with ADHD who were seen or treated for ADHD at least once, we also identified the subset of these children who met the more stringent requirement of having 2 or more ADHD-related visits or 2 or more ADHD-related medication prescriptions within a 1-year period.

For each ADHD case, we selected approximately 6 children who met all of the criteria stated earlier but were not diagnosed or treated for ADHD between January 1, 1996, and December 31, 2004. These children were matched to the cases by age and sex. Each child in the comparison group was assigned a pseudoindex date that was the same as that of the matched case.

For each year period in relation to the index date, we determined the child's pharmacy co-pay and the family's estimated median income based on census block group according to 2000 US Census data.

## COST AND USE DATA

Costs for services provided by KPNC were obtained from the Cost Management Information System, an automated system that integrates use and financial databases. Costs (including program and facility overhead) are generated for services using standard accounting methods and program-specific relative value units. From these data, we estimated the average cost of the following: (1) hospitalizations by diagnosis-related group and by length of stay within the diagnosis-related group; (2) emergency department visits; and (3) outpatient office visits by department and provider type (eg, physician, registered nurse). Hospitalizations, emergency department visits, and office visits were extracted from the health plan's automated databases and were assigned the costs described earlier. Visits were considered to be ADHD-related if at least 1 of the diagnoses assigned by the provider as relating to the cause of the visit was *International Classification of Diseases, Ninth Revision, Clinical Modification* code 314.0.

Pharmacy costs were obtained from KPNC's Pharmacy Information Management System, which records information on all of the prescription drugs dispensed at KPNC outpatient pharmacies, including dose, days' supply, and acquisition cost of the medications dispensed. Medication costs were separated into 3 categories: (1) ADHD-related medications (psychostimulants and atomoxetine); (2) non–ADHD-related psychotropic medications (some of which may occasionally be used to treat ADHD, but most of which—eg, antidepressants, anxiolytics, antipsychotics, and mood stabilizers—are primarily used for other psychiatric conditions); and (3) all other medications. Medication quantity was measured by the days' supply dispensed.

For services covered by KPNC but provided by non-KPNC vendors, we used the payments made to those vendors as the cost of those services. This study does not include any patient out-of-pocket costs. The Consumer Price Index was used to adjust all costs to 2004 dollars.

## COEXISTING MENTAL HEALTH DISORDERS AND OTHER CHRONIC CONDITIONS

Using outpatient visit diagnosis codes, we identified (in each year) whether the child was seen for any of the following mental health disorders (MHDs): substance abuse disorder, psychoses, unipolar mood disorders, bipolar mood disorders, pervasive developmental disorders, anxiety disorders, obsessive-compulsive disorders, tic or Tourette syndrome, posttraumatic stress disorder, conduct disorder, oppositional or defiant disorder, or learning disorders (excluding speech and language problems). Because the health plan's system for capturing diagnoses made it somewhat more difficult for pediatricians (as opposed to psychiatrists) to record this information and because KPNC providers do not generally assess for learning disabilities, MHDs may have been underestimated.

We used the Johns Hopkins Ambulatory Care Group casemix system software[15] to identify children with other chronic medical conditions. This software assigns diagnosis codes into 32 mutually exclusive diagnostic morbidity clusters known as ambulatory diagnostic groups (ADGs). We considered children whose diagnoses fell into 1 or more of the following ADGs to have a chronic condition: ADG06 ("asthma"), ADG10 ("chronic medical: stable"), ADG11 ("chronic medical: unstable"), ADG12 ("chronic specialty: stable orthopedic"), ADG13 ("chronic specialty: stable ear, nose, throat"), ADG14 ("chronic specialty: stable eye"), ADG16 ("chronic specialty: unstable orthopedic"), ADG17 ("chronic specialty: unstable ear, nose, throat), and ADG18 ("chronic specialty: unstable eye"). This classification scheme includes relatively common conditions such as myopia and obesity. In addition, we included ADG32 ("malignancy") because of the potential severity and costliness of that condition. These ADGs were assigned to each child in each year of the study based on diagnoses received in that year.

## ANALYSES

Our analytic data set consisted of 1 observation per child per year for each of the 2 years before and after the index date as long as the entire year fell between January 1, 1996, and December 31, 2004. *Year −1* was defined as the year prior to the index date. *Year 1* was defined as the year starting with the index date. Yearly records were only included in analyses if the child was a continuous member throughout that year and had pharmacy benefits in that year (more than 95% of KPNC members have pharmacy benefits). Thus, a child whose index date was June 15, 1997, could contribute to year −1 but not year −2 because cost data only went back to 1996. Likewise, a child whose index date was June 15, 2004, could contribute to the analysis of year −1 but not year 1 because we did not include cost data after 2004. This algorithm allowed us to retain the maximum number of complete annual records.

To estimate the annual excess costs to the health plan of children with ADHD as compared with children without ADHD in relation to when they were first diagnosed with ADHD, we ran a general linear model in which cost was the dependent variable and all of the years for all of the eligible children were included. We included an interaction term for the ADHD–non-ADHD indicator by year in relation to index date. Because we had yearly repeated cost measures on the children, we used a generalized estimating equation approach with an autoregressive covariance structure to account for correlation among records for the same child. We also adjusted for sex, race or ethnicity (white, black, Hispanic, Asian, and other), age (continuous), income (categories), pharmacy copay (yes or no), the presence or absence of a non-ADHD MHD, and the presence or absence of any chronic medical conditions. All but sex and ethnicity were time-changing covariables. The subgroups of costs assessed were hospital-related costs, emergency department costs, psychiatry department costs where the visit included a diagnosis code for ADHD, pediatric department costs where the visit included a diagnosis code for ADHD, other psychiatric department costs, other pediatric department costs, other clinic-related costs (specialty department visits such as neurology as well as outpatient services provided by non-KP vendors), costs of medications used to treat ADHD, costs of other psychotropic medications, and other medication costs. In an auxiliary analysis, we ran the model described earlier but did not adjust for coexisting MHDs or chronic medical conditions. To test the model's sensitivity to very high-cost children, we ran a sensitivity analysis in which the 15 most costly children (those with costs greater than $100 000) were excluded.

A separate model was run to examine whether the cost of ADHD-related services varied depending on the race or sex of the child. To increase power in this analysis, we combined the 2 years following the index date and estimated the mean annual costs during those 2 years. All of the statistical analyses were performed using SAS version 9 software (SAS Institute, Inc, Cary, NC).

## RESULTS

### SUBJECT CHARACTERISTICS

There were 3122 children with ADHD and 15 899 children without ADHD who met the study criteria. By design, each child had at least 1 year of continuous KP membership during the 4 years being analyzed, although only a subset had continuous membership in any given year. **Table 1** describes the characteristics of the children with ADHD (n = 2014) and the children without ADHD (n = 9342) who had continuous KP membership during the year after the index date. Because we matched by age and sex, children with ADHD had age and sex distributions similar to those without ADHD. The average age at the index date was 6.7 years, and the majority of study children were male. Children with ADHD were more likely than children without ADHD to be white American (69% vs 53%, respectively) and to have lower pharmacy copays. They were also more likely than children without ADHD to be seen for a coexisting MHD (30% vs 2%, respectively) and to be diagnosed with a chronic medical condition (35% vs 27%, respectively).

**Table 1. Demographic Characteristics of Children With and Without Attention-Deficit/Hyperactivity Disorder in the Year After the Index Date***

| Characteristic | Children With ADHD (n = 2014)† | Children Without ADHD (n = 9342)† |
|---|---|---|
| Age at index date, mean, y | 6.7 | 6.7 |
| Sex | | |
| Male | 1569 (78) | 7141 (77) |
| Female | 445 (22) | 2102 (23) |
| Race‡ | | |
| Asian American | 123 (6) | 1590 (17) |
| African American | 186 (9) | 817 (9) |
| Hispanic American | 277 (14) | 1713 (18) |
| White American | 1381 (69) | 4941 (53) |
| Other or unknown | 47 (2) | 281 (3) |
| Pharmacy co-pays, $‡ | | |
| 0 | 277 (14) | 880 (9) |
| 1-7 | 834 (41) | 3794 (41) |
| 10-25 | 282 (14) | 1293 (14) |
| 5 Generic + 10-20 brand | 244 (12) | 1198 (13) |
| 10 Generic + 10-20 brand | 190 (9) | 1006 (11) |
| 10 Generic + 25 brand | 118 (6) | 720 (8) |
| Other | 69 (3) | 451 (5) |
| Income based on census block group, quintile | | |
| First (bottom) | 285 (14) | 1208 (13) |
| Second | 362 (18) | 1678 (18) |
| Third | 385 (19) | 1721 (18) |
| Fourth | 444 (22) | 2125 (23) |
| Fifth (top) | 461 (23) | 2268 (24) |
| Unknown | 77 (4) | 342 (4) |
| Diagnosed with a non-ADHD mental health condition‡ | 614 (30) | 164 (2) |
| Diagnosed with a non–mental health, chronic condition‡ | 696 (35) | 2553 (27) |

Abbreviation: ADHD, attention-deficit/hyperactivity disorder.

*For ADHD cases, the index date was the date that the child was first seen or treated for ADHD. Each comparison non-ADHD case was assigned an index date equivalent to that of the matched ADHD case. Because of selection criteria, all of the children in this study were between ages 2 and 10 years.

†Values are expressed as number (percentage) unless otherwise indicated.

‡The ADHD group was significantly different from the non-ADHD group at $P \leq .05$.

**Table 2** indicates the numbers of children contributing to the analysis in each year as well as the baseline unadjusted mean annual total costs. Children with ADHD were nearly twice as costly as children without ADHD in the year prior to their initial diagnosis of ADHD (mean cost, $1456 vs $751, respectively) and nearly 3 times as costly in the year after their initial ADHD diagnosis (mean cost, $2091 vs $701, respectively). Only 387 (13%) of 3067 children with ADHD were diagnosed with a coexisting MHD in the year before they were diagnosed with ADHD compared with 614 (30%) of 2014 children and 275 (23%) of 1215 children in the first and second years, respectively, after being diagnosed with ADHD.

Children with ADHD who had coexisting MHDs were much more costly than children with ADHD who did not

**Table 2. Sample Size and Mean Unadjusted Cost by Year in Relation to Index Date**

| Variable* | All Children: Children With ADHD | All Children: Children Without ADHD | Children With ADHD: Children With Coexisting Mental Health Conditions | Children With ADHD: Children Without Coexisting Mental Health Conditions |
|---|---|---|---|---|
| Children meeting study criteria in each year, No. | | | | |
| Year −2 | 2950 | 15 036 | 125 | 2825 |
| Year −1 | 3067 | 15 572 | 387 | 2680 |
| Year +1 | 2014 | 9342 | 614 | 1400 |
| Year +2 | 1215 | 4679 | 275 | 940 |
| Annual total cost per child by year, mean, $† | | | | |
| Year −2‡ | 1340 | 839 | 2335 | 1296 |
| Year −1‡ | 1456 | 751 | 2432 | 1315 |
| Year +1‡ | 2091 | 701 | 3018 | 1685 |
| Year +2‡ | 1859 | 742 | 3366 | 1418 |

Abbreviation: ADHD, attention-deficit/hyperactivity disorder.

*For ADHD cases, the index date was the date that the child was first seen or treated for ADHD. Each comparison non-ADHD case was assigned an index date equivalent to that of the matched ADHD case. Year −2 indicates the second year before the index date; year −1, the year before the index date; year +1, the year after the index date; and year +2, the second year after the index date.

†Costs are unadjusted mean values. However, because the non-ADHD comparison group was matched by age and sex to the ADHD group, cost differences between the 2 groups reflect similar age and sex distributions.

‡Costs for the ADHD group were significantly different from the non-ADHD group at $P \leq .05$, and costs for children with ADHD with coexisting mental health conditions were significantly different from children with ADHD without coexisting mental health conditions at $P \leq .05$.

have coexisting MHDs. Mean costs in the year after initial ADHD diagnosis, for example, were $3018 for children with ADHD who had coexisting MHDs and $1685 for children with ADHD who did not have coexisting MHDs.

## EXCESS COST AND USE

Children with ADHD were substantially more costly than children without ADHD—both before and after their initial diagnosis of ADHD—after adjusting for all of the covariables (**Table 3**). In the second year prior to the index date, children with ADHD cost an average of $302 more than children without ADHD, and in the year prior, they cost an average of $383 more. During these years, emergency, pediatric, and psychiatric department costs were all higher for children with ADHD, as were other kinds of outpatient visit costs and pharmacy costs. In the year prior to their initial ADHD diagnosis, children with ADHD averaged 1.7 more outpatient visits per year and 29 more days' use of outpatient medications than children without ADHD.

After the index date, children with ADHD incurred substantial costs for ADHD-specific visits and medications as well as somewhat higher costs for psychiatric-related visits and psychotropic medications (Table 3). In the first year after the index date, children with ADHD had excess mean costs of $860, which fell to $672 in the second year. The decrease in the second year was due to a tapering off of ADHD-related visits that were somewhat offset by increased cost of medications.

Excess costs associated with ADHD were approximately 50% higher when coexisting MHDs and chronic medical conditions were not included in the model. For example, in the year after initial diagnosis, the excess mean cost of children with ADHD was $860 when adjusting for these other conditions and $1328 when not adjusting for them. When the 15 children with the highest costs were excluded (those with costs >$100 000), the excess mean costs in year −2, year −1, year +1, and year +2 were $274, $284, $959, and $783, respectively, compared with $302, $383, $860, and $672, respectively, in the primary analysis. When we included only those children with ADHD who met the more stringent requirement of having at least 2 ADHD-related visits or 2 ADHD-related medication prescriptions within 1 year (74% of the children with ADHD), the excess mean costs in year −2, year −1, year +1, and year +2 were $315, $447, $1052, and $862, respectively.

Sixty-seven percent of the children with ADHD were dispensed ADHD-related medications during the year after the initial diagnosis whereas a significantly smaller number (57%) were dispensed such medications during the second year after diagnosis ($P < .001$). Among children who were dispensed ADHD-related medications, the average total days' supply dispensed increased from 275 days' supply in year 1 to 294 days' supply in year 2 ($P = .01$).

Girls with ADHD had lower annual ADHD-related psychiatry department visit mean costs than boys with ADHD ($72 lower), but their other ADHD costs were similar (**Table 4**). Asian Americans, African Americans, and Hispanic Americans all had lower yearly mean costs for ADHD medications compared with white Americans ($95, $63, and $77 lower, respectively). Nonwhite Americans were less likely than white Americans to receive any ADHD-related medications in year 1 (61% vs 70%, respectively; $P < .001$), and among those who did receive them, they tended to receive fewer days' supplies (250 days' supply vs 285 days' supply, respectively; $P < .001$). Only 57% of Asian Americans with ADHD received ADHD-related medications in the year after their index date compared with 70% of white Americans ($P = .004$). Asian Americans also had lower ADHD-related psychiatry department mean costs compared with white Americans ($105 lower) as well as lower overall ADHD-related mean costs ($221 lower). The annual ADHD-related mean

**Table 3. Adjusted Excess Costs and Use for Children With vs Without Attention-Deficit/Hyperactivity Disorder by Year in Relation to Index Date**

| Variable | Year −2* | Year −1* | Year +1* | Year +2* |
|---|---|---|---|---|
| Children contributing to analysis, No. | | | | |
| Children with ADHD | 2950 | 3067 | 2014 | 1215 |
| Children without ADHD | 15 036 | 15 572 | 9342 | 4679 |
| Adjusted excess costs for children with ADHD compared with costs for children without ADHD, mean (95% CI), $ | | | | |
| All hospital-related costs | 65 (−45 to 175) | 84 (−80 to 248) | −72 (−200 to 56) | −72 (−361 to 218) |
| ED-related costs | 20 (9 to 31) | 19 (9 to 28) | 9 (−2 to 20) | 13 (−1 to 27) |
| Psychiatry department ADHD visit costs | † | † | 384 (355 to 413) | 219 (194 to 245) |
| Pediatric department ADHD visit costs | † | † | 201 (190 to 211) | 97 (88 to 106) |
| Psychiatry department other costs | 34 (26 to 43) | 133 (121 to 146) | 58 (42 to 75) | 18 (1 to 35) |
| Pediatric department other costs | 111 (95 to 128) | 115 (100 to 130) | 31 (15 to 48) | 36 (14 to 57) |
| Other clinic-related costs | 75 (52 to 99) | 51 (30 to 71) | 25 (−7 to 57) | 48 (13 to 83) |
| ADHD-related pharmacy costs | † | † | 186 (173 to 198) | 222 (205 to 239) |
| Other psychotropic pharmacy costs | −1 (−2 to 0) | 1 (−1 to 4) | 24 (17 to 32) | 46 (33 to 60) |
| Other pharmacy costs | 25 (5 to 46) | 31 (10 to 51) | 43 (22 to 64) | 76 (40 to 111) |
| Total‡ | 302 (166 to 437) | 383 (206 to 560) | 860 (708 to 1013) | 672 (354 to 991) |
| Total excess cost without adjusting for coexisting conditions, mean (95% CI), $§ | 488 (336 to 641) | 678 (470 to 887) | 1328 (1183 to 1473) | 1040 (687 to 1394) |
| Excess use by children with ADHD compared with that of children without ADHD, mean (95% CI) | | | | |
| Outpatient visits, No. | 1.2 (1.1 to 1.3) | 1.7 (1.6 to 1.8) | 3.8 (3.6 to 4.0) | 2.1 (1.9 to 2.4) |
| Days' supply of all outpatient drugs | 29 (20 to 37) | 29 (21 to 37) | 237 (224 to 251) | 240 (224 to 257) |

Abbreviations: ADHD, attention-deficit/hyperactivity disorder; CI, confidence interval; ED, emergency department.
*Year −2 indicates the second year before the index date; year −1, the year before the index date; year +1, the year after the index date; and year +2, the second year after the index date. For ADHD cases, the index date was the date that the child was first seen or treated for ADHD. Each comparison non-ADHD case was assigned an index date equivalent to that of the matched ADHD case
†Because children with ADHD were identified by virtue of ADHD-related use, neither children with ADHD nor those without ADHD had ADHD-related costs prior to the index year, and children without ADHD had no ADHD-related costs in any year of the study.
‡Owing to the use of the generalized estimating equation modeling approach, total excess costs are not precisely the sum of the component costs.
§Excess costs after adjusting for all of the covariables except those indicating the presence or absence of mental health disorders and chronic medical conditions.

**Table 4. Adjusted Differences in Mean Annual Attention-Deficit/Hyperactivity Disorder–Related Costs by Race or Ethnicity and Sex In 2 Years After Index Date Among Children Diagnosed With Attention-Deficit/Hyperactivity Disorder***

| | Race or Ethnicity† | | | |
|---|---|---|---|---|
| Cost Type | Asian American, Mean (95% CI) | African American, Mean (95% CI) | Hispanic American, Mean (95% CI) | Girls vs Boys, Mean (95% CI) |
| Psychiatry department ADHD visit cost difference, $ | −105 (−191 to −18) | −8 (−92 to 75) | 99 (18 to 180) | −72 (−128 to −16) |
| Pediatric department ADHD visit cost difference, $ | −23 (−54 to 9) | −11 (−40 to 17) | −36 (−62 to −11) | 1 (−19 to 21) |
| ADHD-related pharmacy cost difference, $ | −95 (−140 to −51) | −63 (−103 to −23) | −77 (−109 to −44) | 8 (−23 to 38) |
| All outpatient ADHD-related cost difference, $ | −221 (−335 to −109) | −82 (−194 to 30) | −112 (−113 to 89) | −63 (−138 to 12) |

Abbreviations: ADHD, attention-deficit/hyperactivity disorder; CI, confidence interval.
*The index date was the date that the child was first seen or treated for ADHD. Confidence intervals that do not cross 0 indicate that cost differences are significant at $P<.05$. Costs are reported in 2004 US dollars.
†The reference group was white American.

cost for white Americans was about $750. Thus, among children diagnosed with ADHD, per-person ADHD-related costs for Asian Americans were about 70% of those for white Americans. When this analysis was restricted to children who were prescribed an ADHD-related medication at least once, the differences remained, although they were somewhat attenuated. Excess mean costs for Asian Americans as compared with those for white Americans went from $221 less to $184 less ($P=.04$). The mean age at first diagnosis was the same for children in each ethnicity. To account for the possibility that the racial differences might be confounded by the site where the different groups most commonly received care, we also ran the model adjusting for clinic and found no substantial change to the results.

## COMMENT

Parents commonly state that behavioral problems predate their child's ADHD diagnosis, often by several years,[16,17] and these problems may affect their use of health services. In our study sample, costs were significantly higher in the 2 years before the index date among children subsequently diagnosed with ADHD, and costs remained higher for at least 2 years following the initial ADHD diagnosis. Much of the excess cost was due to increased pediatric and psychiatric services, which were higher in the first year after diagnosis than in the second year. Medication treatment visits for ADHD tend to be more frequent in the first year after diagnosis, as that is the time when determining the correct medication and making the most dosage adjustments tend to occur.[4] Behavioral treatments for ADHD also tend to be short term. The majority of treatments are less than 2 months in duration[18,19] and may result in increases in costs for ADHD care in the first year of treatment with a decline during the second year.

Our finding of higher costs and use for children with ADHD who have coexisting MHDs has been reported by others.[10,12] Children with ADHD and coexisting MHDs have more complex problems, have a poorer long-term prognosis, commonly require more care, and may need more medications.[20-22]

Our study also found that after being diagnosed with ADHD, Asian Americans, African Americans, and Hispanic Americans use fewer ADHD-related medications than white Americans and that Asian-American children have lower overall ADHD-related costs. Although some of these per-person differences are modest, the total differences summed across the population may be substantial. Our results indicate that alongside the case-mix factor, ethnicity is another important factor contributing to cost differences. A number of studies[23-27] have shown that rates of ADHD diagnosis or treatment are lower for African Americans and Hispanic Americans, although not all agree on the disparity of medication use. Stevens et al[25] found no ethnic differences in the likelihood of receiving a stimulant during a visit in which the child had been diagnosed with ADHD. However, Rowland et al[26] and Stevens et al[24] found that among children diagnosed with ADHD, African Americans[24,26] and Hispanic Americans[26] were less likely than white Americans to receive stimulants. To our knowledge, though, our study is the first to look at ethnic differences in all types of medical use and costs among children diagnosed with ADHD and the first to look at any use and costs among Asian Americans with ADHD. These findings of lower use and cost are not confounded by differences in health insurance coverage or by the age at which the children were diagnosed, and differences in income have also been accounted for to some extent. Given the evidence that response to treatment does not vary by ethnicity[28] and that our population had similar medical coverage and access to care, our data suggest that lower use of medications among ethnic minorities may be explained in part by cultural differences in the acceptance of ADHD diagnoses and treatment.[28-30] Future studies, particularly those involving interviews of the parents of children with ADHD and their health care providers, could shed light on the reasons for these differences.

Although no study to our knowledge has analyzed costs over time in relation to the initial ADHD diagnosis, our study is comparable in design to the study by Guevara et al,[10] who also studied members of an integrated health plan. Our findings of excess mean costs of $860 in the year following the initial ADHD diagnosis are higher than the $495 (when children with and without coexisting conditions are combined) reported by Guevara and colleagues. This difference is likely owing in part to differences in methods—that study adjusted for non–mental health–related comorbidities using a different method, restricted the category of children without ADHD to those who used some medical services in the study year, and included children up to age 17 years. It is possible that the excess costs for older children are lower than those for younger children, although some evidence suggests that this may not be so.[7] Differences in study findings may also be owing in part to recent increases in the cost of ADHD drug formulations. Studies by Swensen et al[8] and Birnbaum et al[11] (using fee-for-service claims) found excess costs of $1033 and $1265, respectively, although again, these studies included older children and had somewhat different sample selection criteria.

Our estimate of excess cost for children with ADHD may underestimate true excess costs seen today and in the future. New, more expensive ADHD medications and formulations have been introduced in recent years, but our cost estimates represent a blending of the older, less expensive medications and newer medications. Because this was a study of children who were diagnosed with or treated for ADHD, we cannot make conclusions about those children who have ADHD but are not diagnosed with it. However, by analyzing years prior to diagnosis, we do provide some data, to our knowledge unavailable in the current literature, on health care costs among undiagnosed children. We did not independently assess the validity of the ADHD diagnoses made by providers; thus, there may be some misclassification. Nevertheless, the children with ADHD in our sample were considered by the health system (and probably by the family) to have ADHD. Diagnosis of ADHD is likely to drive physician prescribing patterns and behavioral treatments and thus be important from the health system perspective. Our cohort reflects the actual way that ADHD diagnoses are given, and the percentage of all of the children receiving medication treatment in KPNC is similar to that recently reported for California by the Centers for Disease Control and Prevention, Atlanta, Ga (about 2%).[1] Rates of ADHD diagnosis and treatment with medication are lower in California than in other states.[1] If the children who are diagnosed in California tend to be the more severe cases, excess costs associated with these children may be higher than in other states.

It is possible that once a child is diagnosed with ADHD, he or she may be more likely to be assessed for and diagnosed with other medical disorders and MHDs. In our main analysis, we chose to adjust for coexisting mental health conditions and chronic medical conditions; thus, excess cost estimates derived from those analyses might be considered conservative.

Our estimates of excess cost may be high if families who are more likely to seek a diagnosis for and treatment of their child's ADHD are also prone to seeking treatment in general. This propensity to use services may partly explain the excess costs for these children. Because of data constraints, this study was limited to children younger than 11 years. Older children may have different excess costs.

## CONCLUSIONS

Children with ADHD have excess medical costs compared with similar children without ADHD. Our study shows that these excess costs precede the initial diagnosis of ADHD by at least 2 years, indicating the presence of problems well in advance of the initial diagnosis. Once these children are diagnosed, the excess costs for them are even higher owing primarily to increased psychiatric and pediatric care as well as increased costs for medication. Consistent with prior studies, we found that African-American and Hispanic children with ADHD have lower ADHD-related medication costs than white children with ADHD. Our study extends this finding to Asian Americans and also shows that compared with white Americans, not only are they less likely to use ADHD-related medications after their diagnosis but their total use of ADHD services (medications and visits) during this period is less than that of white Americans. Future evaluation should be considered to determine the reasons for these differences.

**Accepted for Publication:** June 22, 2006.
**Correspondence:** G. Thomas Ray, MBA, Division of Research, Kaiser Permanente, 2000 Broadway, Oakland, CA 94612 (tom.ray@kp.org).
**Author Contributions:** *Study concept and design:* Ray, Levine, Croen, Bokhari, Hu, and Habel. *Acquisition of data:* Ray and Levine. *Analysis and interpretation of data:* Ray, Levine, Croen, Bokhari, Hu, and Habel. *Drafting of the manuscript:* Ray, Levine, Bokhari, and Hu. *Critical revision of the manuscript for important intellectual content:* Ray, Levine, Croen, Hu, and Habel. *Statistical analysis:* Ray, Bokhari, and Hu. *Obtained funding:* Bokhari and Habel. *Administrative, technical, and material support:* Ray, Levine, and Habel. *Study supervision:* Ray and Habel. Mr Ray had full access to all of the data in the study and takes responsibility for the integrity of the data and the accuracy of the data analysis.
**Funding/Support:** This work was funded by grant R01 MH067084 from the National Institute of Mental Health.
**Acknowledgment:** We thank Richard Scheffler, PhD, Steve Hinshaw, PhD, Susan Stone, PhD, and Timothy Brown, PhD, for their roles in developing the research questions addressed in this study, their helpful comments on preliminary results, and their reviews of the manuscript.

## REFERENCES

1. Centers for Disease Control and Prevention. Mental health in the United States: prevalence of diagnosis and medication treatment for attention-deficit/hyperactivity disorder: United States, 2003. *MMWR Morb Mortal Wkly Rep.* 2005;54:842-847.
2. Mannuzza S, Klein RG, Bessler A, Malloy P, Hynes ME. Educational and occupational outcome of hyperactive boys grown up. *J Am Acad Child Adolesc Psychiatry.* 1997;36:1222-1227.
3. Barkley RA, Fischer M, Edelbrock CS, Smallish L. The adolescent outcome of hyperactive children diagnosed by research criteria, I: an 8-year prospective follow-up study. *J Am Acad Child Adolesc Psychiatry.* 1990;29:546-557.
4. Jensen PS, Hinshaw SP, Swanson JM, et al. Findings from the NIMH Multimodal Treatment Study of ADHD (MTA): implications and applications for primary care providers. *J Dev Behav Pediatr.* 2001;22:60-73.
5. Dulcan M; American Academy of Child and Adolescent Psychiatry. Practice parameters for the assessment and treatment of children, adolescents, and adults with attention-deficit/hyperactivity disorder. *J Am Acad Child Adolesc Psychiatry.* 1997;36:85S-121S.
6. Leibson CL, Katusic SK, Barbaresi WJ, Ransom J, O'Brien PC. Use and costs of medical care for children and adolescents with and without attention-deficit/hyperactivity disorder. *JAMA.* 2001;285:60-66.
7. Burd L, Klug MG, Coumbe MJ, Kerbeshian J. Children and adolescents with attention deficit-hyperactivity disorder, 1: prevalence and cost of care. *J Child Neurol.* 2003;18:555-561.
8. Swensen AR, Birnbaum HG, Secnik K, Marynchenko M, Greenberg P, Claxton A. Attention-deficit/hyperactivity disorder: increased costs for patients and their families. *J Am Acad Child Adolesc Psychiatry.* 2003;42:1415-1423.
9. Chan E, Zhan C, Homer CJ. Health care use and costs for children with attention-deficit/hyperactivity disorder: national estimates from the medical expenditure panel survey. *Arch Pediatr Adolesc Med.* 2002;156:504-511.
10. Guevara J, Lozano P, Wickizer T, Mell L, Gephart H. Utilization and cost of health care services for children with attention-deficit/hyperactivity disorder. *Pediatrics.* 2001;108:71-78.
11. Birnbaum HG, Kessler RC, Lowe SW, et al. Costs of attention deficit-hyperactivity disorder (ADHD) in the US: excess costs of persons with ADHD and their family members in 2000. *Curr Med Res Opin.* 2005;21:195-206.
12. DeBar LL, Lynch FL, Boles M. Healthcare use by children with attention deficit/hyperactivity disorder with and without psychiatric comorbidities. *J Behav Health Serv Res.* 2004;31:312-323.
13. American Psychiatric Association. *Diagnostic and Statistical Manual of Mental Disorders, Fourth Edition.* Washington, DC: American Psychiatric Association; 1994.
14. *International Classification of Diseases, Ninth Revision, Clinical Modification.* Washington, DC: Public Health Service, US Dept of Health and Human Services; 1988.
15. Health Services Research and Development Center, Johns Hopkins University. *Johns Hopkins ACG Case-Mix System Documentation and Application Manual, Version 5.0.* Baltimore, Md: Johns Hopkins University; 2001.
16. Campbell SB. *Behavior Problems in Preschool Children.* 2nd ed. New York, NY: Guilford Press; 2002.
17. Barkley RA. Attention-deficit hyperactivity disorder. In: Mash EJ, Barkley RA, eds. *Child Psychopathology.* 2nd ed. New York, NY: Guilford Press; 1996.
18. Barkley RA, Guevremont DC, Anastopoulos AD, Fletcher KE. A comparison of three family therapy programs for treating family conflicts in adolescents with attention-deficit hyperactivity disorder. *J Consult Clin Psychol.* 1992;60:450-462.
19. Tutty S, Gephart H, Wurzbacher K. Enhancing behavioral and social skill functioning in children newly diagnosed with attention-deficit hyperactivity disorder in a pediatric setting. *J Dev Behav Pediatr.* 2003;24:51-57.
20. Thiruchelvam D, Charach A, Schachar RJ. Moderators and mediators of long-term adherence to stimulant treatment in children with ADHD. *J Am Acad Child Adolesc Psychiatry.* 2001;40:922-928.
21. Satterfield JH, Schell A. A prospective study of hyperactive boys with conduct problems and normal boys: adolescent and adult criminality. *J Am Acad Child Adolesc Psychiatry.* 1997;36:1726-1735.
22. Hinshaw SP. Academic underachievement, attention deficits, and aggression: comorbidity and implications for intervention. *J Consult Clin Psychol.* 1992;60:893-903.
23. Olfson M, Gameroff MJ, Marcus SC, Jensen PS. National trends in the treatment of attention deficit hyperactivity disorder. *Am J Psychiatry.* 2003;160:1071-1077.
24. Stevens J, Harman JS, Kelleher KJ. Race/ethnicity and insurance status as factors associated with ADHD treatment patterns. *J Child Adolesc Psychopharmacol.* 2005;15:88-96.
25. Stevens J, Harman JS, Kelleher KJ. Ethnic and regional differences in primary care visits for attention-deficit hyperactivity disorder. *J Dev Behav Pediatr.* 2004;25:318-325.
26. Rowland AS, Umbach DM, Stallone L, Naftel AJ, Bohlig EM, Sandler DP. Prevalence of medication treatment for attention deficit-hyperactivity disorder among elementary school children in Johnston County, North Carolina. *Am J Public Health.* 2002;92:231-234.
27. Hoagwood K, Jensen PS, Feil M, Vitiello B, Bhatara VS. Medication management of stimulants in pediatric practice settings: a national perspective. *J Dev Behav Pediatr.* 2000;21:322-331.
28. Arnold LE, Elliot M, Sachs L, et al. Effects of ethnicity on treatment attendance, stimulant response/dose, and 14-month outcome in ADHD. *J Consult Clin Psychol.* 2003;71:713-727.
29. Leslie LK, Weckerly J, Landsverk J, Hough RL, Hurlburt MS, Wood PA. Racial/ethnic differences in the use of psychotropic medication in high-risk children and adolescents. *J Am Acad Child Adolesc Psychiatry.* 2003;42:1433-1442.
30. Bussing R, Gary FA, Mills TL, Garvan CW. Parental explanatory models of ADHD: gender and cultural variations. *Soc Psychiatry Psychiatr Epidemiol.* 2003;38:563-575.

ARTICLE

# Cost-effectiveness Analysis of Palivizumab in Premature Infants Without Chronic Lung Disease

*Nahed O. ElHassan, MD, MPH; Melony E. S. Sorbero, PhD, MS, MPH; Caroline B. Hall, MD; Timothy P. Stevens, MD, MPH; Andrew W. Dick, PhD*

**Objectives:** To evaluate the cost-effectiveness of palivizumab as respiratory syncytial virus prophylaxis in premature infants without chronic lung disease and to evaluate the impact on cost-effectiveness of a potential reduction in risk of asthma following respiratory syncytial virus infection among infants receiving palivizumab.

**Design:** Two decision analytic models were designed, one with and the other without accounting for increased risk of asthma following respiratory syncytial virus infection.

**Setting:** A hypothetical community or university hospital.

**Participants:** Hypothetical cohorts of infants without chronic lung disease born at 26 to 32 weeks' gestation.

**Interventions:** Palivizumab prophylaxis vs no prophylaxis.

**Main Outcome Measures:** Expected costs and incremental cost-effectiveness ratio expressed as cost per quality-adjusted life-year.

**Results:** The expected costs were higher for palivizumab prophylaxis as compared with no prophylaxis. The incremental cost-effectiveness ratios were high for all gestations and are not considered cost-effective by today's standards (<$200 000 per quality-adjusted life-year). Both models were sensitive to variation in the cost of palivizumab. The model that included asthma was sensitive to variation in quality of life for children with asthma. In instances where asthma was considered severe with profound worsening in quality of life compared with life without asthma, some infants had an incremental cost per quality-adjusted life-year that was less than $200 000.

**Conclusions:** Our model supports implementing more restrictive guidelines for palivizumab prophylaxis. Palivizumab was cost-effective for some infants in an analysis that accounted for increased risk of severe asthma following respiratory syncytial virus infection.

*Arch Pediatr Adolesc Med. 2006;160:1070-1076*

Respiratory syncytial virus (RSV) is the most important pathogen in lower respiratory tract infection in infants and young children.[1] By age 2 years, approximately 80% to 90% of children experience at least 1 episode of RSV infection. Although the majority of RSV infections resolve uneventfully in otherwise healthy children, high-risk populations such as premature infants may develop severe and sometimes fatal lower respiratory tract infections.[1] Long-term complications of RSV infections are unclear. Although there is an established association between RSV infection and recurrent wheezing, a cause-effect relationship has not been demonstrated.[2-4] Palivizumab (Synagis; MedImmune, Inc, Gaithersburg, Md), a humanized monoclonal antibody, is effective in reducing the risk of hospitalization secondary to RSV infection.[5] The American Academy of Pediatrics (AAP), Elk Grove Village, Ill, developed guidelines[6] for the use of palivizumab for RSV prophylaxis in 1998 and revised these guidelines in 2003.[7] In part owing to cost concerns, the AAP policy recommended the use of palivizumab only in infants at highest risk for severe RSV infection. A number of economic analyses of RSV intravenous immunoglobulin and palivizumab have been performed in the United States and in other countries.[8-20] Multiple economic analyses of palivizumab performed outside of the United States concluded that the use of the prophylaxis is not cost-effective,[17-19] but analyses performed in the United States have generated mixed results.[8-14,16,20] A systematic review[15] of economic analyses of RSV intravenous immunoglobulin and palivizumab found a significant difference in results by funding source ($P = .002$); all of the 4 studies with pharmaceutical funding reported that

**Author Affiliations:** Division of Neonatology, Department of Pediatrics, College of Medicine, University of Arkansas for Medical Sciences, Little Rock (Dr ElHassan); RAND Corp, Pittsburgh, Pa (Drs Sorbero and Dick); and Divisions of Infectious Disease (Dr Hall) and Neonatology (Dr Stevens), Department of Pediatrics, Strong Children's Research Center, Rochester, NY.

the prophylaxis was either cost-effective or cost-saving for a high-risk infant population whereas none of the 8 studies without pharmaceutical funding reported similar findings.[15] None of these analyses considered potential long-term sequelae, ie, the possible increased risk of asthma following RSV infection in infancy and its impact on quality of life.[21]

The objectives of this study were to evaluate the cost-effectiveness of palivizumab as RSV prophylaxis in premature infants without chronic lung disease and to evaluate the impact on cost-effectiveness of a potential reduction in risk of asthma following RSV infection among infants receiving palivizumab. To our knowledge, our model is the first to study the cost-effectiveness of RSV prophylaxis by specific gestational age, to evaluate the implication of the possible increased risk of asthma with RSV infection, and to integrate measures of morbidity (quality-adjusted life-years).

## METHODS

### MODEL SETTING AND ASSUMPTIONS

This study was an economic evaluation using decision analytic modeling. The DATA 3.5 for Healthcare software package (TreeAge Software, Williamstown, Mass) was used to combine data from secondary data sources, including publications and government documents, and to simulate costs and outcomes for the intervention.

A hypothetical cohort of premature infants born at 26 to 32 weeks' gestation was assumed to be discharged from the neonatal intensive care unit at 36 weeks' postconceptional age based on unpublished data from the University of Rochester Medical Center, Rochester, NY (T.P.S., 2003). We assumed that an infant had an equal probability of being discharged from the neonatal intensive care unit at different months of the year. Each infant's weight at the time of discharge was assumed to be 2000 g (10% of the growth curve for an infant at 36 weeks' postconceptional age).[22] Because the association between RSV infection and asthma remains unclear, we completed 2 sets of analyses, one with and the other without asthma included in the models. The models including asthma used time-dependent Markov processes to allow the risk of asthma to vary with the age of the cohort.[23] Analyses were conducted from the societal perspective[24] and therefore included all of the relevant costs and outcomes regardless of to whom they accrued. A separate decision analytic model was constructed for each gestational age. Sensitivity analyses were performed to test the robustness of the results.

The model combined published data on the risk of RSV hospitalization by gestational age, the seasonal pattern of RSV hospitalization, the efficacy of palivizumab in reducing the risk of RSV hospitalization, national costs of RSV hospitalizations, costs of palivizumab injection visits, costs of emergency department visits, drug costs, and costs of work hours missed by parents for visits and hospitalization. In the base-case analysis with asthma, the model also included the risk of asthma, reduction in quality of life due to asthma, and national estimates of the cost of asthma for a child with the disease. There is no current evidence that palivizumab reduces the probability of death in infants; therefore, we did not include risk of death secondary to RSV hospitalization in the models.[6,7]

Analyses without asthma had a time horizon of 1 year's postconception age because palivizumab has not been shown to affect other long-term health outcomes; these were cost-benefit analyses. Cost-effectiveness analyses were performed on the models that included asthma. The model with asthma had a time horizon of 8 years in the base-case analysis and was varied up to 10 years in sensitivity analyses to reflect the length of increased risk of asthma following RSV bronchiolitis.[25-27] Future benefits and costs were discounted at 3% annually. The use of RSV prophylaxis was evaluated using the incremental cost-effectiveness ratio (ICER), defined as the additional costs associated with the use of palivizumab divided by the additional quality-adjusted life-years associated with its use. Based on recent recommendations,[28] we considered an ICER of less than \$200 000 per quality-adjusted life-year to be cost-effective.

**Table 1. Point Estimates for Noncost Variables**

| Variable | Estimate | Values for Sensitivity Analysis, Range |
|---|---|---|
| Average probability of RSV hospitalization in the no-prophylaxis group[5,29-35] | | |
| 26-wk gestation | 0.206 | 0.073-0.206 |
| 27- to 28-wk gestation | 0.146 | 0.073-0.146 |
| 29- to 30-wk gestation | 0.113 | 0.113-0.120 |
| 31- to 32-wk gestation | 0.064 | 0.064-0.120 |
| Efficacy of palivizumab in infants without chronic lung disease[5] | | |
| <32-wk gestation | 0.747 | 0.747-0.950 |
| 32-wk gestation | 0.820 | 0.820-0.950 |
| Average probability of RSV hospitalization in the prophylaxis group[5,30]* | | |
| 26-wk gestation | 0.052 | NA |
| 27- to 28-wk gestation | 0.037 | NA |
| 29- to 30-wk gestation | 0.028 | NA |
| 31-wk gestation | 0.016 | NA |
| 32-wk gestation | 0.011 | NA |
| Length of RSV hospitalization, d[30,34,36,37] | 6.8 | 4.9-8.7 |
| Probability of asthma in control group, %[26,27] | | |
| Age 1 y | 0.0 | 0.0-6.2 |
| Age 3 y | 1.0 | 1.0-6.2 |
| Age 7.5 y | 3.0 | 1.0-6.2 |
| Probability of asthma in RSV group, %[26,27,38] | | |
| Age 1 y | 11 | 11-45 |
| Age 3 y | 23 | 23-45 |
| Age 7.5 y | 30 | 30-45 |
| Duration of increased risk of asthma following RSV infection during infancy, y[25-27,38] | 7.5 | 7.5-10.0 |

Abbreviations: NA, not applicable; RSV, respiratory syncytial virus.

*Average probability of RSV hospitalization in the prophylaxis group = average probability of RSV hospitalization in the no-prophylaxis group × (1 − efficacy).

### NONCOST PARAMETERS

The values of noncost parameters included in the model are shown in **Table 1**. The table shows base-case values and ranges of values used for sensitivity analyses.

#### Probability of RSV Hospitalization by Gestational Age

We calculated the probability of RSV hospitalization by specific gestational age and month of neonatal intensive care unit discharge[29,30] by using gestational age–specific RSV hospitalization rates and the seasonal pattern of respiratory hospitalization. We used gestational age–specific risks (ie, at ≤26, 27-28, 29-30, and 31-32 weeks' gestation) of RSV hospitalization

**Table 2. Point Estimates of Cost Variables**

| Variable | Estimate, US $ |
|---|---|
| Cost of palivizumab[49] | |
| 50-mg vial | 725.00 |
| 100-mg vial | 1370.00 |
| Cost of visit for palivizumab injection[50] | 70.00 |
| Cost of RSV hospitalization[16,51,52] | 9260.00 |
| Cost of emergency department visit by local estimates | 405.00 |
| Cost of 1 h of work lost by parents[53] | 16.63 |
| Cost of work time lost by 1 parent during RSV hospitalization[53]* | 907.00 |
| Cost of work time lost by parents during emergency department visit[53]† | 49.90 |
| Costs of asthma[52,54,55] | 859.00 |

Abbreviation: RSV, respiratory syncytial virus.
*Cost of work time lost by 1 parent during RSV hospitalization = length of hospitalization × 8 × cost of 1 hour of work lost by parents.
†Cost of work time lost by parents during emergency department visit = cost of 1 hour of work lost by parents × 3.

as reported by Stevens et al[30] in the only study to provide detailed gestational age–specific risks. We applied a monthly adjustment factor based on the seasonal relationship between hospitalization owing to respiratory illness and month of neonatal intensive care unit discharge reported by Cunningham et al.[29] The probability of RSV hospitalization was varied across the range of risk reported in the literature[5,29-35] for premature infants in sensitivity analyses.

We calculated the gestational age–specific estimates of the efficacy of palivizumab in reducing risk of RSV hospitalization among infants without chronic lung disease using data from the IMpact-RSV study,[5] the only randomized trial of palivizumab. The probability of RSV hospitalization for the noprophylaxis group was calculated as the probability of hospitalization without prophylaxis multiplied by (1 − efficacy). In the sensitivity analysis, we allowed the efficacy of palivizumab to improve to 95% to determine whether prophylaxis would be cost-effective with very high efficacy rates.

### Length of RSV Hospitalization

From reported values, an average length of stay of 6.8 days[30,34,36,37] for RSV hospitalization was included in our base-case analysis. The entire range of values reported in the literature was considered in sensitivity analyses.

### Probability of Asthma and Length of Increased Risk of Asthma following RSV Bronchiolitis

We based our estimates of the increased risk of asthma on data by Sigurs et al[26,27] in the only study to prospectively evaluate the risk of asthma among children who had been hospitalized with RSV bronchiolitis as infants relative to controls (data shown in Table 1). A linear extrapolation was performed to calculate the risk of asthma at ages not included in these articles by Sigurs and colleagues. In the sensitivity analysis, we considered the range of values of increased risk of asthma following RSV bronchiolitis reported in retrospective studies.[38-46]

### Quality of Life With and Without Asthma

Quality of life data have been increasingly used to evaluate the benefits of health care options. In this approach, patients' preferences for a condition are multiplied by the duration spent with the condition to generate a quality-adjusted life-year. Quality-of-life estimates for children with symptomatic asthma (0.89)[47] and the absolute difference in quality of life with and without asthma (0.03)[48] were obtained from articles and measured using the Health Utility Index. In sensitivity analyses, the quality of life with asthma was varied by 1 SD.[47]

## MODEL COSTS

The costs included in the model are shown in **Table 2**. Costs are reported in 2002 US dollars and estimates were updated with relevant portions of the Consumer Price Index[51,52,54] as necessary.

### Drug Costs

The current recommended palivizumab dosage is 15-mg/kg intramuscular injections once per month for a total of 5 doses during the RSV season, which is November through March. The costs of 50-mg and 100-mg vials of palivizumab were derived from published wholesale prices.[49] Once reconstituted, the shelf life of palivizumab is estimated at 6 hours[21]; hence, drug wastage was accounted for in the base-case analysis.

We predicted the weight that a 2000-g infant would attain at each recommended palivizumab injection visit using standard growth curves[22] to calculate the total amount and the cost of the drug. Assumptions about drug wastage and costs were varied in sensitivity analyses.

### Costs of Drug Injection

Palivizumab injections were assumed to take place during office visits coded as "established patient, intermediate," and the cost of these visits was assigned the lowest reimbursement rate by local private insurers.[50] The total administration costs were obtained by multiplying the cost of each visit by the number of recommended palivizumab injections, calculated as described in our previous article.[56]

### Hospitalization Costs

Stang et al[16] estimated the cost of an infant hospitalized with RSV infection using a National Inpatient Sample. The 95% confidence interval ($8000-$10 520) of the estimate was used in our sensitivity analyses.

### Emergency Department Visit Costs

We assumed that infants hospitalized with RSV infection were admitted through the emergency department with a visit coded as being of moderate severity. The cost of an emergency department visit of moderate severity was obtained from local estimates in Rochester, NY. Medicare reimbursement rates were not used owing to this being a pediatric population.

### Nonmedical Costs

We assumed that 1 parent lost an average of 8 hours of work per day during RSV hospitalization as well an average of 3 hours of work per day for palivizumab injection visits and emergency department visits. The national costs of time lost from work were based on US Bureau of Labor Statistics data.[53]

**Table 3. Expected and Incremental Costs per Quality-Adjusted Life-Year for Gestational Ages**

| Variable | Gestational Age at Birth, wk 26 | 27 | 28 | 29-30 | 31 | 32 |
|---|---|---|---|---|---|---|
| **Cost-benefit Analysis for No Increased Risk of Asthma** | | | | | | |
| Expected costs, US $ | | | | | | |
| No prophylaxis | 2184 | 1548 | 1548 | 1198 | 678 | 678 |
| Palivizumab prophylaxis | 7298 | 7137 | 8000 | 3725 | 3530 | 4092 |
| Incremental* | 5114 | 5589 | 6452 | 2527 | 2852 | 3414 |
| **Cost-effectiveness Analysis for Increased Risk of Asthma** | | | | | | |
| Expected costs, US $ | | | | | | |
| No prophylaxis | 2493 | 1790 | 1790 | 1403 | 925 | 829 |
| Palivizumab prophylaxis | 7435 | 7257 | 8120 | 3852 | 3711 | 4185 |
| Change in QALY | 0.0060 | 0.0042 | 0.0042 | 0.0036 | 0.0023 | 0.0018 |
| ICER† | 830 152 | 1 295 781 | 1 500 351 | 675 780 | 1 212 497 | 1 855 000 |

Abbreviations: ICER, incremental cost-effectiveness ratio; QALY, quality-adjusted life-year.
*Incremental expected costs = expected costs for prophylaxis group − expected costs for no-prophylaxis group.
†Incremental cost-effectiveness ratio = (cost of palivizumab prophylaxis − cost of no prophylaxis)/(QALY for palivizumab prophylaxis − QALY for no prophylaxis).

### Costs of Asthma

Estimates of per capita costs of asthma for persons younger than 18 years were taken from the study by Weiss et al.[55] These estimates included the costs of inpatient and outpatient hospital services, emergency department visits, office-based physician services, and pharmaceuticals as well as time lost from work.

### TARGETED USE POLICY

In addition to the 2 scenarios and 1-way sensitivity analyses described earlier, we generated estimates for a targeted best-case scenario for the use of palivizumab prophylaxis. The current AAP recommendations for the use of palivizumab result in treating many infants who are at low risk for RSV hospitalization, leading us to conduct additional simulations modifying the current recommendations to seek more cost-effective alternatives using the following parameters: no drug wastage; application of prophylaxis restricted to only the infant's first RSV season; younger chronological age cutoffs, ie, those infants assumed to be discharged from September through March; and infants born at 27 weeks' gestation or earlier if discharged before the RSV season and infants born at 30 weeks' gestation or earlier if discharged during the RSV season.

## RESULTS

### COST-BENEFIT ANALYSIS ASSUMING NO CAUSAL RELATIONSHIP WITH ASTHMA

The results for the different gestational ages are summarized in **Table 3**. The results for infants born at 29 and 30 weeks' gestation are reported together since the estimates of the cost and probabilities are identical for infants born at these gestational ages.

Irrespective of the gestational age at birth, we found that the added costs of prophylaxis are greater than the savings from reduced hospitalizations. The expected costs for the prophylaxis group are greatest for infants born at 28 weeks' gestation ($8000 in the model with no increased risk of asthma). Thereafter, the expected costs decrease markedly.

### COST-EFFECTIVENESS ANALYSIS ASSUMING A CAUSAL RELATIONSHIP WITH ASTHMA

The ICERs for the different gestational ages are summarized in Table 3. The ICERs are higher than $200 000 per quality-adjusted life-year for all gestations and reach a maximum of $1 855 000 per quality-adjusted life-year for infants born at 32 weeks' gestation when palivizumab is used in accordance with AAP recommendations.

### SENSITIVITY ANALYSES

The results of the most significant sensitivity analyses are summarized in **Table 4** for the models without increased risk of asthma and in **Table 5** for the models with increased risk of asthma. These analyses were shown for 5 different gestational ages to display the trend of varying a specific quantity in the model on ICERs and incremental expected costs. In the model without asthma, the use of RSV prophylaxis did not result in cost savings for any of the sensitivity analyses performed. The model that included asthma was sensitive to varying the quality of life for children with asthma and costs of palivizumab vials. When the quality of life with asthma was reduced to 0.8, the ICER was approximately $200 000 per quality-adjusted life-year for infants born at 26 and 29 to 30 weeks' gestation (Table 5). Reductions in palivizumab costs to 25% of their current values result in an ICER less than $100 000 per quality-adjusted life-year for infants born at 26 and 29 weeks' gestation.

### TARGETED USE POLICY

The alterations included in the targeted policy dramatically improved the ICER for the use of palivizumab, with the ICER ranging from $103 053 per quality-adjusted life-year for infants born at 26 weeks' gestation to $280 083 per quality-adjusted life-year for infants born at 29 and 30 weeks' gestation. With the targeted policy, the ICER

**Table 4. One-way Sensitivity Analysis in the Model Without Increased Risk of Asthma**

| Variable (Range) | Incremental Expected Costs, Range, US $* | | | |
|---|---|---|---|---|
| | 26-wk Gestation | 28-wk Gestation | 29- to 30-wk Gestation | 32-wk Gestation |
| Efficacy of palivizumab (0.75-0.95) | 5114-4671 | 6452-6138 | 2381-2137 | 3396-3258 |
| Costs of RSV hospitalization ($8000-$10 520) | 5308-7119 | 6590-6315 | 2945-1883 | 341-3280 |
| Cost of palivizumab assuming no drug wastage | 4254 | 5475 | 1758 | 2671 |
| Costs of palivizumab vials (25%-200% of current price) | 511-11 251 | 1240-13 402 | 337-5448 | 795-6905 |

Abbreviation: RSV, respiratory syncytial virus.
*Incremental expected costs = expected costs for prophylaxis group − expected costs for no-prophylaxis group.

**Table 5. Sensitivity Analysis in the Model With Increased Risk of Asthma**

| Variable (Range) | Incremental Expected Costs, Range, US $* | | | |
|---|---|---|---|---|
| | 26-wk Gestation | 28-wk Gestation | 29- to 30-wk Gestation | 32-wk Gestation |
| Efficacy of palivizumab (0.75-0.95)† | 830 152-678 015 | 1 500 351-1 068 307 | 675 780-442 594 | 1 855 000-1 516 839 |
| Increased risk of asthma† | 830 152-560 297 | 1 500 351-1 019 971 | 675 780-454 458 | 1 587 525-1 079 368 |
| Length of increased risk of asthma (7.5-10.0 y)† | 830 152-545 404 | 1 500 351-993 385 | 675 780-458 472 | 1 587 525-1 058 103 |
| Quality of life in infants with asthma (0.80-0.89)† | 199 529-830 152 | 360 611-1 500 351 | 216 092-906 309 | 450 593-1 855 000 |
| Cost of palivizumab assuming no drug wastage‡ | 685 720 | 1 268 679 | 657 780 | 1 481 965 |
| Cost of RSV hospitalization ($8000-$10 520)‡ | 862 721-797 583 | 1 532 920-1 467 782 | 708 683-642 876 | 1 887 132-1 822 868 |
| Costs of palivizumab vials (25%-200% of current price)‡ | 56 938-1 861 103 | 264 952-3 147 549 | 37 858-1 526 3421 | 407 583-3 784 891 |
| Targeted use policy | 103 053 | 216 830 | 280 083 | NA§ |

Abbreviations: NA, not applicable; RSV, respiratory syncytial virus.
*Incremental cost-effectiveness ratio = (cost of palivizumab prophylaxis − cost of no prophylaxis)/(quality-adjusted life-years for palivizumab prophylaxis − quality-adjusted life-years for no prophylaxis).
†The base-case values of the variables are reported in Table 1.
‡The base-case values of the variables are reported in Table 2.
§Under the targeted policy, these infants would not receive palivizumab.

is less than $200 000 per quality-adjusted life-year for infants born at 26 or 27 weeks' gestation.

## COMMENT

This decision analytic model compared the costs and effects of palivizumab prophylaxis for RSV and no prophylaxis for a hypothetical cohort of premature infants without chronic lung disease. Our results show that palivizumab prophylaxis is not cost-effective for these infants. Under the first scenario in which we assumed that RSV had no effect on asthma rates, we found that for all gestational ages, the increased costs associated with the use of prophylaxis were greater than the cost savings from reduced hospitalizations and other costs. The decrease in expected costs for infants born at more than 28 weeks' gestation reflects the AAP policy for RSV prophylaxis: infants born at 29 to 32 weeks' gestation receive palivizumab if they are younger than 6 months at the start of the RSV season, and infants born at 26 to 28 weeks' gestation receive prophylaxis if they are younger than 12 months at the start of the RSV season, ie, infants born at 26 to 28 weeks' gestation generally received a higher total number of palivizumab injections and, thereafter, a higher cost of RSV prophylaxis than infants born at 29 to 32 weeks' gestation.[6,7] With the second scenario in which we included the health effects associated with the potential increase in asthma rates among children with RSV infections, we found that the ICERs are greater than $200 000 per quality-adjusted life-year for all gestational ages. Our model was most sensitive to variation in the quality of life with asthma, with ICERs less than $200 000 per quality-adjusted life-year for some gestational ages (infants born at 26 and 29 to 30 weeks' gestation) when the quality of life with asthma was reduced to 0.80, and to variation in the cost of palivizumab, with ICERs less than $100 000 per quality-adjusted life-year for some gestational ages (infants born at 26 and 29 weeks' gestation) when palivizumab costs were only 25% of their current values. The cost-effectiveness of the current guideline for RSV prophylaxis does not compare favorably with many accepted interventions,[57] numerous vaccinations for children,[58,59] or other health care for premature infants.[60]

Our analyses reveal 2 main explanations for these findings. First, the use of palivizumab results in substantially increased expected costs. Second, the use of palivizumab results in very small increases in expected quality-adjusted life-years for 3 reasons: (1) there is no evidence of, nor did we model, a mortality benefit to the use of the prophylaxis; (2) there is no evidence of long-term improvement in the quality of life associated with its use; and (3) if there is an improvement in quality-adjusted life-years owing to a reduced prevalence of asthma, the value of the improvement is likely to be small. These explanations for the relatively small potential long-term quality of life effects suggest that the overall welfare effects of the prophylaxis strategy will be driven by the cost consequences. Given the current costs of palivizumab, the reduction in other medical and nonmedical costs is simply not great enough to offset the drug costs. Our formulation of a targeted use policy, however, would be considered cost-effective for more restricted use among infants born at 26 or 27 weeks' gestation, but it is based on the assumption that drug wastage could be eliminated.

Our study has several limitations. First, the cost and length of hospitalization was assumed to be equal for all gestational ages. This assumption will bias our base-case model findings toward improved cost-effectiveness in the more premature infants and worse cost-effectiveness in the less premature infants. Second, the costs of asthma were based on data collected during 1985 to 1994. Finally, 1 assumption was made in our base-case analysis that deliberately biased our results toward improved cost-effectiveness of RSV prophylaxis. We assumed that the weights of the infant at the time of discharge and the time of injections are at 10% of the growth curve. This assumption will markedly reduce the cost of prophylaxis for different gestational ages.

## CONCLUSIONS

In conclusion, our model is the first to our knowledge to study the cost-effectiveness of RSV prophylaxis by specific gestational age, to evaluate the implication of the possible increased risk of asthma on the economic analysis of RSV prophylaxis, and to integrate measures of morbidity (quality of life). We found that the current AAP recommendations for the use of palivizumab as RSV prophylaxis in premature infants without chronic lung disease are not cost-effective by today's standards. Our analyses support the implementation of more restrictive guidelines for RSV prophylaxis for these infants. Additional studies are needed to identify the best way to target RSV prophylaxis guidelines to enhance the cost-effectiveness of palivizumab. We found evidence that long-term health consequences of RSV are central to the determination of the cost-effectiveness of the intervention. In analyses where asthma following RSV infection was considered severe with profound worsening in quality of life (0.8) compared with quality of life without asthma (0.92), palivizumab was marginally cost-effective only for infants born at 26, 29, or 30 weeks' gestation.

**Accepted for Publication:** June 22, 2006.
**Correspondence:** Melony E. S. Sorbero, PhD, MS, MPH, RAND Corp, 4570 Fifth Ave, Suite 600, Pittsburgh, PA 15213 (msorbero@rand.org).
**Author Contributions:** *Study concept and design:* ElHassan, Sorbero, Hall, Stevens, and Dick. *Acquisition of data:* ElHassan, Sorbero, and Stevens. *Analysis and interpretation of data:* ElHassan, Sorbero, Hall, Stevens, and Dick. *Drafting of the manuscript:* ElHassan, Sorbero, Hall, and Stevens. *Critical revision of the manuscript for important intellectual content:* ElHassan, Hall, and Dick. *Statistical analysis:* ElHassan and Dick. *Administrative, technical, and material support:* ElHassan and Sorbero. *Study supervision:* Hall and Dick.
**Acknowledgment:** We acknowledge Kenneth McConnochie, MD, MPH, and Kristine Palmer, MD, for their help in reviewing the manuscript.

## REFERENCES

1. Hall CB. Respiratory syncytial virus. In: Feign RD, Cherry JD, Demmler GJ, Kaplan S, eds. *Textbook of Pediatric Infectious Diseases.* 5th ed. Philadelphia, Pa: WB Saunders Co; 2003.
2. Sly PD, Hibbert ME. Childhood asthma following hospitalization with acute viral bronchiolitis in infancy. *Pediatr Pulmonol.* 1989;7:153-158.
3. Twiggs JT, Larson LA, O'Connell EJ, Ilstrup DM. Respiratory syncytial virus infection: ten-year follow-up. *Clin Pediatr (Phila).* 1981;20:187-190.
4. Long CE, McBride JT, Hall CB. Sequelae of respiratory syncytial virus infections: a role for intervention studies. *Am J Respir Crit Care Med.* 1995;151:1678-1681.
5. IMpact-RSV Study Group. Palivizumab, a humanized respiratory syncytial virus monoclonal antibody, reduces hospitalization from respiratory syncytial virus infection in high-risk infants. *Pediatrics.* 1998;102:531-537.
6. American Academy of Pediatrics Committee on Infectious Diseases and Committee on Fetus and Newborn. Prevention of respiratory syncytial virus infections: indications for the use of palivizumab and update on the use of RSV-IGIV. *Pediatrics.* 1998;102:1211-1216.
7. American Academy of Pediatrics. Respiratory syncytial virus. In: Pickering LK, ed. *Red Book: 2003 Report of the Committee on Infectious Diseases.* 26th ed. Elk Grove Village, Ill: American Academy of Pediatrics; 2003.
8. Storch GA. Humanized monoclonal antibody for prevention of respiratory syncytial virus infection. *Pediatrics.* 1998;102:648-651.
9. Joffe S, Ray GT, Escobar GJ, Black SB, Lieu TA. Cost-effectiveness of respiratory syncytial virus prophylaxis among preterm infants. *Pediatrics.* 1999;104:419-427.
10. Marchetti A, Lau H, Magar R, Wang L, Devercelli G. Impact of palivizumab on expected costs of respiratory syncytial virus infection in preterm infants: potential for savings. *Clin Ther.* 1999;21:752-766.
11. Lofland JH, Touch SM, O'Connor JP, et al. Palivizumab for respiratory syncytial virus prophylaxis in high-risk infants: a cost-effectiveness analysis. *Clin Ther.* 2000;22:1357-1369.
12. Barton LL, Grant KL, Lemen RJ. Respiratory syncytial virus immune globulin: decisions and costs. *Pediatr Pulmonol.* 2001;32:20-28.
13. Schrand LM, Elliott JM, Ross MB, Bell EF, Mutnick AH. A cost-benefit analysis of RSV prophylaxis in high-risk infants. *Ann Pharmacother.* 2001;35:1186-1193.
14. Shireman TI, Braman KS. Impact and cost-effectiveness of respiratory syncytial virus prophylaxis for Kansas Medicaid's high-risk children. *Arch Pediatr Adolesc Med.* 2002;156:1251-1255.
15. Kamal-Bahl S, Doshi J, Campbell J. Economic analyses of respiratory syncytial virus immunoprophylaxis in high-risk infants: a systematic review. *Arch Pediatr Adolesc Med.* 2002;156:1034-1041.
16. Stang P, Brandenburg N, Carter B. The economic burden of respiratory syncytial virus-associated bronchiolitis hospitalizations. *Arch Pediatr Adolesc Med.* 2001;155:95-96.
17. Vogel AM, McKinlay MJ, Ashton T, et al. Cost-effectiveness of palivizumab in New Zealand. *J Paediatr Child Health.* 2002;38:352-357.
18. Numa A. Outcome of respiratory syncytial virus infection and a cost-benefit analysis of prophylaxis. *J Paediatr Child Health.* 2000;36:422-427.
19. Farina D, Rodriguez SP, Bauer G, et al. Respiratory syncytial virus prophylaxis: cost-effective analysis in Argentina. *Pediatr Infect Dis J.* 2002;21:287-291.
20. Moler FW, Brown RW, Faix RG, Gilsdorf JR. Comments on palivizumab (Synagis). *Pediatrics.* 1999;103:495-497.
21. Sanchez PJ. Immunoprophylaxis for respiratory syncytial virus. *Pediatr Infect Dis J.* 2002;21:473-478.
22. Battaglia FC, Lubchenco LO. A practical classification of newborn infants by weight and gestational age. *J Pediatr.* 1967;71:159-163.
23. Keeler E. Decision trees and Markov models in cost-effectiveness research. In: Sloan FA, ed. *Valuing Health Care: Costs, Benefits, and Effectiveness of Pharmaceuticals and Other Medical Technologies.* New York, NY: Cambridge University Press; 1998.
24. Luce BR, Manning WG, Siegel JE, Lipscomb J. Estimating costs in cost-

effectiveness analysis. In: Gold MR, Siegel JE, Russell LB, Weinstein MC, eds. *Cost-Effectiveness in Health and Medicine.* New York, NY: Oxford University Press; 1996.
25. Pullan CR, Hey EN. Wheezing, asthma, and pulmonary dysfunction 10 years after infection with respiratory syncytial virus in infancy. *BMJ.* 1982;284:1665-1669.
26. Sigurs N, Bjarnarson R, Sigurbergsson F, Kjellman B, Bjorksten B. Asthma and immunoglobulin E antibodies after respiratory syncytial virus bronchiolitis: a prospective cohort study with matched controls. *Pediatrics.* 1995;95:500-505.
27. Sigurs N, Bjarnason R, Sigurbergsson F, Kjellman B. Respiratory syncytial virus bronchiolitis in infancy is an important risk factor for asthma and allergy at age 7. *Am J Respir Crit Care Med.* 2000;161:1501-1507.
28. Ubel PA, Hirth RA, Chernew ME, Fendrick AM. What is the price of life and why doesn't it increase at the rate of inflation? *Arch Intern Med.* 2003;163:1637-1641.
29. Cunningham CK, McMillan JA, Gross SJ. Rehospitalization for respiratory illness in infants of less than 32 weeks' gestation. *Pediatrics.* 1991;88:527-532.
30. Stevens TP, Sinkin RA, Hall CB, Maniscalco WM, McConnochie KM. Respiratory syncytial virus and premature infants at 32 weeks' gestation or earlier: hospitalization and economic implications of prophylaxis. *Arch Pediatr Adolesc Med.* 2000;154:55-61.
31. PREVENT Study Group. Reduction of respiratory syncytial virus hospitalization among premature infants and infants with bronchopulmonary dysplasia using respiratory syncytial virus immune globulin prophylaxis. *Pediatrics.* 1997;99:93-99.
32. O'Shea TM, Sevick MA, Givner LB. Costs and benefits of respiratory syncytial virus immunoglobulin to prevent hospitalization for lower respiratory tract illness in very low birth weight infants. *Pediatr Infect Dis J.* 1998;17:587-593.
33. Shay DK, Holman RC, Newman RD, Liu LL, Stout JW, Anderson LJ. Bronchiolitis-associated hospitalizations among US children, 1980-1996. *JAMA.* 1999;282:1440-1446.
34. Joffe S, Escobar GJ, Black SB, Armstrong MA, Lieu TA. Rehospitalization for respiratory syncytial virus among premature infants. *Pediatrics.* 1999;104:894-899.
35. Boyce TG, Mellen BG, Mitchel EF, Wright PF, Griffin MR. Rates of hospitalization for respiratory syncytial virus infection among children in Medicaid. *J Pediatr.* 2000;137:865-870.
36. Howard TS, Hoffman LH, Stang PE, Simoes EAF. Respiratory syncytial virus pneumonia in the hospital setting: length of stay, charges, and mortality. *J Pediatr.* 2000;137:227-232.
37. Romero JR. Palivizumab prophylaxis of respiratory syncytial virus disease from 1998 to 2002: results from four years of palivizumab usage. *Pediatr Infect Dis J.* 2003;22:S46-S54.
38. Kneyber MCJ, Steyerberg EW, de Groot R, Moll HA. Long-term effects of respiratory syncytial virus (RSV) bronchiolitis in infants and young children: a quantitative review. *Acta Paediatr.* 2000;89:654-660.
39. Sims DG, Downham MA, Gardner PS, Webb JK, Weightman D. Study of 8-year old children with a history of respiratory syncytial virus bronchiolitis in infancy. *BMJ.* 1978;1:11-14.
40. McConnochie KM, Roghmann KJ. Bronchiolitis as a possible cause of wheezing in childhood: new evidence. *Pediatrics.* 1984;74:1-10.
41. Mok JYQ, Simpson H. Outcome for acute bronchitis, bronchiolitis, and pneumonia in infancy. *Arch Dis Child.* 1984;59:306-309.
42. Carlsen KH, Larsen S, Bjerve O, Leegaard J. Acute bronchiolitis: predisposing factors and characterization of infants at risk. *Pediatr Pulmonol.* 1987;3:153-160.
43. Murray M, Webb MSC, O'Callaghan C, Swarbrick AS, Milner AD. Respiratory status and allergy after bronchiolitis. *Arch Dis Child.* 1992;67:482-487.
44. Osundwa VM, Dawod ST, Ehlayel M. Recurrent wheezing in children with respiratory syncytial virus (RSV) bronchiolitis in Qatar. *Eur J Pediatr.* 1993;152:1001-1003.
45. Noble V, Murray M, Webb MSC, Alexander J, Swarbrick AS, Milner AD. Respiratory status and allergy nine to 10 years after acute bronchiolitis. *Arch Dis Child.* 1997;76:315-319.
46. Stein RT, Sherrill D, Morgan WJ, et al. Respiratory syncytial virus in early life and risk of wheeze and allergy by age 13 years. *Lancet.* 1999;354:541-545.
47. Juniper EF, Guyatt GH, Feeney DH, Griffith LE, Ferrie PJ. Minimum skills required by children to complete health-related quality of life instruments for asthma: comparison of measurement properties. *Eur Respir J.* 1997;10:2285-2294.
48. Gold M, Franks P, Erickson P. Assessing the health of the nation: the predictive validity of a preference-based measure and self-rated health. *Med Care.* 1996;34:163-177.
49. Medical Economics Co; Thomson Healthcare. *Drug Topics Red Book.* Montvale, NJ: Medical Economics Co Inc; 2002.
50. American Hospital Directory. Current data sources. http://www.ahd.com/data_sources.html. Accessed November 3, 2003.
51. Bureau of Labor Statistics, US Department of Labor. Consumer Price Index: December 1998. ftp://ftp.bls.gov/pub/news.release/History/cpi.011499.news. Accessed November 4, 2003.
52. Bureau of Labor Statistics, US Department of Labor. Consumer Price Index: December 2002. http://www.bls.gov. Accessed November 4, 2003.
53. Bureau of Labor Statistics, US Department of Labor. National compensation survey: occupational wages in the United States, July 2002. http://www.bls.gov/ncs/ocs/compub.htm#National. Accessed November 3, 2003.
54. Bureau of Labor Statistics, US Department of Labor. Consumer Price Index: December 1994. ftp://ftp.bls.gov/pub/news.release/History/cpi.011195.news. Accessed March 27, 2002.
55. Weiss KB, Sullivan SD, Lyttle CS. Trends in the cost of illness for asthma in the United States, 1985-1994. *J Allergy Clin Immunol.* 2000;106:493-499.
56. Elhassan NO, Stevens TP, Sorbero MES, Dick AW, Guillet R, Hall CB. Guidelines for palivizumab prophylaxis: are they based on infant's risk of hospitalization for respiratory syncytial viral disease? *Pediatr Infect Dis J.* 2003;22:939-942.
57. Tengs TO, Adams ME, Pliskin JS, et al. Five-hundred life-saving interventions and their cost-effectiveness. *Risk Anal.* 1995;15:369-390.
58. Bloom BS, Hillman AL, Fendrick AM, Schwartz JS. A reappraisal of Hepatitis B virus vaccination strategies using cost-effectiveness analysis. *Ann Intern Med.* 1993;118:298-306.
59. Lieu TA, Ray GT, Black SB, et al. Projected cost-effectiveness of pneumococcal conjugate vaccination of healthy infants and young children. *JAMA.* 2000;283:1460-1468.
60. Zupancic JAF, Richardson DK, O'Brien BJ, Eichenwald EC, Weinstein MC. Cost-effectiveness analysis of predischarge monitoring for apnea of prematurity. *Pediatrics.* 2003;111:146-152.

"In the midst of your illness, you will promise a goat, but when you have recovered, a chicken will seem sufficient."
—African proverb

# Growth Attenuation

## *A Diminutive Solution to a Daunting Problem*

SHOULD HORMONE THERAPY BE USED TO MAKE children with profound impairment smaller? This question—having within it the key elements of a modern tragedy—needs to be handled with supreme care regarding both the predicament it addresses and the treatment it proposes.

Consider the predicament: among the many extraordinary problems confronted by parents of children with profound cognitive and physical disabilities, figuring out how to provide care as the child grows into an adult is among the most difficult to solve and distressing to contemplate. When parents age and face disability themselves, many find increasingly difficult the tasks of bathing, diapering, and transferring their adolescent and adult children, who have grown larger, heavier, and perhaps stronger. Additionally, as the child transitions from the pediatric into the adult system of medical and social services care, parents often have less access to personal care aids or to useful but expensive devices such as mechanical lifts. Having devoted much of their lives to meeting the basic daily needs of their child, many parents find themselves forced to find out-of-home placements for their son or daughter.

*See also pages 1013 and 1035*

Now examine the proposed treatment: in this issue of the ARCHIVES, Gunther and Diekema[1] offer a medical solution to families who will likely face the harrowing choice of what to do when their child becomes too big to care for at home. Specifically, the authors suggest that high-dose estrogen could be used to attenuate the growth of children with profound developmental disabilities (which they characterize as a combination of severe neurologic and cognitive impairment). They present a case study and some historical context and describe the risks and benefits of treatment with high-dose estrogen. Gunther and Diekema conclude that growth attenuation may be appropriate "when parents request it." They urge caution in the wider implementation of growth attenuation, suggesting that a developmental specialist and an ethics committee be involved in each case.

Combined together, the predicament and the proposed intervention raise 4 central questions.

First, quite practically, will the treatment work? More precisely, will the administration of high-dose estrogen to children with profound disabilities enable them to remain at home under the care of their parents for a longer period? And will this improve the quality of their lives? The answers to these pivotal questions are unknown, which underscores the highly speculative aspect to the medical strategy proposed by Gunther and Diekema. While there are data that high-dose estrogen treatment will make extremely tall-for-age (but otherwise normal) girls shorter as adults, this effect may be different in the population of children with severe disabilities. More needs to be known. What is the typical velocity of linear growth over time and final adult height in this population? When in a child's growth trajectory would estrogen have to be given to achieve a clinically significant reduction in height but without making them excessively short? What is the correlation between final adult height (which might be reduced by high-dose estrogen treatment) and weight (which may not be limited by this treatment), since weight is likely as important a factor as height with regard to the physical burdens of care? Furthermore, given the association between low-dose estrogen therapy and seizures, consideration of potential adverse effects of high-dose therapy should be studied in this population that is predisposed to or has epilepsy. And ultimately, the motivating hypothesis—namely, that young adults with profound impairment who are shorter and lighter stay at home longer and are (on their own terms) happier than their taller and heavier peers—should be tested through a randomized controlled trial or other rigorous methods with adequate follow-up.

Second, more generally, is manipulating nature in this heavy-handed manner acceptable? Some readers might recoil from the idea of "shortening" people, feeling that it seems just plain wrong to so dramatically change a person's physical stature. In truth, though, American society is fairly accepting—even encouraging—of other forms of medical therapy that seek to enhance one's existence. If in the pursuit of a more perfect appearance, adults and even teenagers can readily enlist plastic surgeons to fix noses or augment breasts—and there is no moral outrage over this unnatural modification—then perhaps we should be more circumspect about decrying the treatment proposed by Gunther and Diekema as unnatural or abnormal. Indeed, as Lee and Howell[2] point out in this issue of the ARCHIVES, estrogen has long been used to attenuate growth in girls destined to be taller than average. Furthermore, if what offends us is simply the idea of a small adult, we are wise to recall the lessons of the late 20th-century disability rights movement in the United States: there is value in every human life regardless of how closely any of us approximates average size, function, or appearance.[3] Persons with a medical or genetic condition that results in severe short stature typically reject the idea that they are any less "normal" than average-sized persons, and exceedingly few opt for surgical fixes to lengthen limbs and appear taller. Is it right to reject the Gunther and Diekema plan simply because the potential results—a smaller adult—strike some of us as odd? Not if we truly believe that the worth of a person goes deeper than his or her physical appearance.

Third, somewhat speculatively, might the treatment be misused? Given the history of persons with disabilities over the past 100 years—as mentioned by Gunther and Diekema—concern on this front is warranted. The eugenic movement of the first half of the 20th century, although now routinely castigated, was at the time championed by mainstream scholars and societal leaders across the political spectrum.[4] Well-meaning eugenic advocates hoped to eliminate pain from disease and inequity in US society by allowing "defective" infants to die, encouraging certain couples to marry, and discouraging others from parenthood. Because they believed that persons with mental retardation could not be trusted to understand the wisdom of eugenics, many states passed laws that led to the involuntary sterilization of adults with mental retardation. Upheld by the US Supreme Court in their 1927 *Buck v Bell* decision, such laws resulted in more than 60 000 individuals being sterilized. Although eugenics was viewed with mounting disdain after World War II, sterilizations of persons with mental retardation continued in the United States through the 1960s, and it was still routine practice in the 1970s to allow a child with Down syndrome to die of lack of surgical correction of duodenal atresia. In this historical context, the proposal to radically alter the growth patterns of a child with severe disabilities demands the utmost scrutiny and, if implemented, the most thorough safeguards and protections.

Finally, and most broadly, does the proposed treatment do justice to the scope of the problem? American society in general, and the medical community in particular, has traditionally sought simple technical fixes for seemingly intractable problems, which often combine biological and social aspects of human existence.[5] In the end, what might be most distressing about attempts to shorten children with profound disabilities and thus lighten the load on their parents is not only that it might not work or cause undesired adverse effects or be misused; no, more distressing is how this solution fails to situate the plight of these parents, struggling to care for their children, in the larger context of a society failure to provide adequate social support in this most admirable of undertakings. Without this broader reframing of the core predicament, high-dose estrogen therapy to prevent out-of-home placement simply creates a new Sophie's Choice for parents to confront, where neither letting the child grow unchecked nor imposing shortness is without peril. If we as a society want to fundamentally revise the nature of the harrowing predicament that these parents face, then, in the end, more funds for home-based services, not more medication, is what is called for.

As Lee and Howell argue in their recounting of the history of hormone therapy for attenuating growth in tall girls, judgments regarding the appropriateness of medical therapy reflect broad appraisals of social and political values as well as specific individualized assessments of health risks and benefits. Treating girls who had idiopathic tall stature with high-dose estrogen arose as a practice in the mid-20th century in the United States, conforming to then prevailing expectations that adult women would fulfill certain gender roles, and declined starting in the 1970s with the rise of the feminist movement. Similarly, the appropriateness of attenuating growth in children with profound developmental disabilities will be judged not only in the privacy of clinical offices or within the confines of institutional review boards but also in the social-political context of both the disability rights movement and the woefully impoverished options for high-quality long-term residential care of children or adults with profound developmental disabilities.

Although we believe that attempts to attenuate growth are ill advised, we applaud Gunther and Diekema for publishing this case report. By focusing on a critical issue and beginning the debate, they help to advance our ethical dialogue as we struggle to define our core values in words, laws, and deeds. If high-dose estrogen treatment is on the right track, the collective community response will bestow general approval on growth attenuation; if not, the criticism may suffice to proscribe this mode of treatment. Only with further research and public discussion will we learn whether attempts to attenuate growth run with or against our fundamental values in caring for children with profound developmental disabilities.

*Jeffrey P. Brosco, MD, PhD*
*Chris Feudtner, MD, PhD, MPH*

**Correspondence**: Dr Brosco, Department of Pediatrics, University of Miami, PO Box 016820 (D-820), Miami, FL 33101 (jbrosco@miami.edu).

## REFERENCES

1. Gunther DF, Diekema DS. Attenuating growth in children with profound developmental disability: a new approach to an old dilemma. *Arch Pediatr Adolesc Med.* 2006;160:1013-1017.
2. Lee JM, Howell JD. Tall girls: the social shaping of a medical therapy. *Arch Pediatr Adolesc Med.* 2006;160:1035-1039.
3. Shapiro JP. *No Pity: People With Disabilities Forging a New Civil Rights Movement.* New York, NY: Times Books; 1994.
4. Pernick MS. *The Black Stork: Eugenics and the Death of "Defective" Babies in American Medicine and Motion Pictures Since 1915.* New York, NY: Oxford University Press; 1996.
5. Rosenberg CE. *The Care of Strangers: The Rise of America's Hospital System.* New York, NY: Basic Books; 1987.

# At What Cost?

It is encouraging to see the financing aspects of health care for young adults with chronic health conditions and disabilities becoming a focus of health services research, and study findings are providing new perspectives on the cost and benefits of moving children with special health care needs from pediatric to adult-oriented medical systems. Nonetheless, transitioning young adults to adult-oriented medicine, or for that matter any transition in medicine,[1,2] is a complex phenomenon and financial measures alone cannot adequately reflect short- and long-term consequences at the patient, health care professional, and health system levels.

*See also page 1054*

In this issue of the ARCHIVES, Okumura et al[3] present an analysis of differences in charges and length of stay for adult patients (18-64 years of age) with 1 of 4 pediatric-onset disabling conditions who received inpatient care from either pediatric, mixed, or adult-oriented hospitals. The authors found that after controlling for a variety of confounding variables, charges and length of stay for adults with these 4 conditions were lower following treatment in adult-oriented hospitals. This study was not able to explain why charges were higher in pediatric facilities.

These findings appear to provide a fiscal justification for the rapid transfer of young adults with chronic conditions to adult-oriented hospitals for inpatient treatment. However, the literature on health care transition clearly shows that it is important to look beyond the finances. The remainder of this editorial briefly highlights 3 important aspects of health care transition, access to health insurance and health care, patient satisfaction, and the preparation for transition, which are not included in the financial perspective offered by Okumura et al.[3]

## ACCESS TO HEALTH INSURANCE AND HEALTH CARE

In their study, Okumura et al[3] reported that only a small percentage of the patients in their sample were self-pay (5%-7.8%). The remaining patients had health care coverage provided by Medicare, Medicaid, or private insurance. Study design also excluded all individuals who did not have access to inpatient care. A recent analysis of health insurance status and access to care[4] presents a very different picture of access to health care for the general population of young adults. Using data from the 1999-2002 National Health Survey, it was determined that 35% of all young adults aged 19 to 29 years with disabling chronic conditions reported an unmet health care need because of cost. Uninsurance rates for young adults with and without disabling conditions were very high, 26% vs 28%, respectively. More than two thirds of uninsured respondents with a disabling condition reported an unmet health need and 45% reported no usual source of care. After adjusting for sociodemographic factors, uninsured young adults with disabling chronic conditions had 8 times greater odds of reporting unmet health care needs and 6 times greater odds of having no usual source of care relative to insured young adults with disabling chronic conditions.[4(p178)]

This study, as well as the findings from others,[5-8] suggests there are many young adults with special health care needs who are not receiving the health care they need from the adult-oriented medical system because of a lack of insurance. Thus, the sample used by Okumura et al[3] may not be representative of the general population of young adults with disabilities.

## PATIENT SATISFACTION AND EXCELLENCE IN HEALTH CARE

Our research has focused on the process of transitioning youth and families out of pediatric care and the associated health care transition experiences of patients, families, and health care professionals. This research, and that of others,[9,10] has identified a variety of forces and factors that negatively impact continuity and quality of care during the move to adult-oriented health care professionals and facilities. In addition to the lack of health care insurance, a significant problem is the lack of adult-oriented health care professionals who have up-to-date training and experience in treating conditions that have historically been the purview of pediatrics. This dilemma is highlighted in the recounting of a conversation with an adult-oriented physician by a young adult with cystic fibrosis (CF).

Young adult: "I was asked, while an inpatient, how I got CF—yes, believe it! This is how the conversation went:

Doctor: 'So which one of your parents has CF?'

Young adult: 'Neither one of my parents have CF.'

Doctor: 'Well then, how did you get CF?'

Young adult: 'Um, my parents each have a CF gene.'

Doctor: 'They each have a CF gene?'

Young adult: 'Yes.'

Doctor: 'Wow, that's really interesting that both your parents have a CF gene.'

Young adult: (thinking to myself, 'um, you are going to take care of me?')

Doctor: 'Is your sister healthy?'

Young adult: 'She has CF too.'

Doctor: 'That's unbelievable that 2 siblings have CF. What are the chances of that happening?'

Young adult: 'I know a lot of siblings that have CF.'

Doctor: 'Very interesting.'"

The young adult with CF went on to state that they could not get over the doctor's lack of knowledge of the illness he was there to treat.

"I feel like the adults with CF are being punished. Because we are adults with CF we cannot get good care. The children with CF are getting excellent care. . . . Why is it so difficult to find a good doctor who will listen to their patients?" the young adult said.

Although this is the reflection of only 1 young adult, stories like this abound in discussions of transition to adult-oriented care. When the transfer to adult-oriented care means not only a break in continuity but also a loss of clinical expertise, young adults pay the price, not only in a reduced level of satisfaction with their medical care but also in an increased risk of receiving care that is clinically inferior to the care they received from their pediatric care professionals. This can only have a deleterious effect on their health and independence.

## PREPARATION FOR TRANSITION

There are significant differences in the treatment practices of pediatrics and adult-oriented medicine and they can be considered distinct medical subcultures.[11,12] These differences are not necessarily good or bad and are the results of differences in medical training and professional enculturation. Transitioning out of pediatrics requires young adults with chronic disabling conditions to leave medical systems that are familiar, comfortable, and supportive. By virtue of their long-term relationships, patients and families are often viewed by health care professionals as experts and are treated as partners in care and decision making. In the new world of adult-oriented medicine, these young people are strangers. Adult-oriented medicine often involves new or different treatment practices and protocols. These changes in treatment are often questioned and not viewed in a positive light by patients. In addition, transfer to adult-oriented health care professionals often occurs around the time a patient turns 18 years of age and legal responsibility for medical decision making transfers to the young adult. Because of these and many other changes not highlighted herein, young people need to be knowledgeable about their condition and how to advocate for themselves if they are to successfully navigate the adult-oriented health care system. This requires a significant amount of preparation and training

Preparing a young person and his or her family for their new roles and responsibilities is the hard work of transition. We believe that an assessment of a young person's capacity to negotiate the adult system, and the adult system's capacity to provide high-quality care as well as potential cost savings, should be included in the equation for assessing the costs and benefits of transferring a patient out of the pediatric system.

## CONCLUSIONS

In providing heath care as well as educational and other related services, society has made a significant investment in children and youth with special needs. As a result of these investments, children with chronic health conditions and disabilities are not only surviving into adulthood, many are thriving. Currently, more than 90% of young people with childhood-onset chronic health conditions and disabilities live long enough to age out of pediatric care and transition to adult-oriented medicine.

In thinking about the move from pediatric to adult-oriented medicine, it is important to distinguish transfer from transition. Transfer attends only to the outcome of moving young adults to adult-oriented care. Transition encompasses the process of preparing young adults to take responsibility for their own care and learn how to interact successfully with the adult-oriented medical system. Transition also encompasses the process of preparing adult-oriented health care professionals and facilities to provide high-quality care.

We also need to address the differences in the way health care is funded for children and adults and develop mechanisms that guarantee continued access to health insurance and quality care. We must be careful not to let the prospect of a short-term reduction in inpatient costs precipitate a rushed transfer of young adults out of the pediatric system. It is the long-term return on investment, as measured by the level of participation in society and quality of life, that is the true measure of transition success.

The question we now have to answer is, do we as health care professionals and a society want to see these young people continue to be as healthy as possible so that they can work, have families of their own, and live independently in the community and make a contribution to society? If so, health services research must not only look at the bottom line (cost and length of stay) but must also look carefully at what it takes to assure that the investments we have made in the health of children and youth come to full fruition as these young people grow into adulthood.

*John Reiss, PhD*
*Robert W. Gibson, PhD, MSOTR/L*

**Correspondence**: Dr Reiss, Institute for Child Health Policy, University of Florida, PO Box 100147, Gainesville, FL 32610-0147 (jgr@ichp.ufl.edu).

## REFERENCES

1. Coleman EA, Berenson R. Lost in transition: challenges and opportunities for improving the quality of transitional care. *Ann Intern Med.* 2004;141:533-536.
2. Coleman EA, Min S, Chomiak A, Kramer A. Posthospital care transitions: pattern, complications and risk identification. *Health Serv Res.* 2004;39:1449-1465.
3. Okumura MJ, Campbell AD, Nasr SZ, Davis MM. Inpatient health care utilization among adult survivors of chronic childhood illnesses in the United States. *Arch Pediatr Adolesc Med.* 2006;160:1054-1060.
4. Callahan ST, Cooper W. Access to health care for young adults with disabling chronic conditions. *Arch Pediatr Adolesc Med.* 2006;160:178-182.
5. Center for Disease Control and Prevention; National Center for Health Statistics. Early release of selected estimates based on data from the 2003 National Health Interview Survey 19. June 2004. www.cdc.gov/nchs/data/nhis/earlyrelease/earlyrelease200406.pdf. Accessed July 21, 2006.
6. Collins SR, Schoen C, Kriss J, Doty M, Mahato B. Rite of passage? why young adults become uninsured and how new policies can help. *Issue Brief (Commonw Fund).* 2006 May;20:1-14. http://www.cmwf.org. Accessed July 21, 2006.
7. Fishman E. Aging out of coverage: young adults with special health care needs. *Health Aff (Millwood).* 2001;20:254-266.
8. White PH. Access to health care: health insurance considerations for young adults with special health care needs/disabilities. *Pediatrics.* 2002;110:1328-1335.
9. Betz CL. Transition of adolescents with special health care needs: review and analysis of the literature. *Issues Compr Pediatr Nurs.* 2004;27:179-241.
10. Forbes A, While A, Ullman R, Lewis S, Mathes L, Griffiths P. *A Multi-Method Review to Identify Components of Practice Which May Promote Continuity in the Transition From Child to Adult Care for Young People With Chronic Illness or Disability: Report for the National Co-ordination Centre for National Health Service Delivery and Organisation R & D.* London, England: NCCSDO; 2001.
11. Reiss JG, Gibson R, Walker L. Health care transition: youth family and providers perspectives. *Pediatrics.* 2005;115:112-120.
12. Rosen D. Between two worlds: bridging the cultures of child health and adult medicine. *J Adolesc Health.* 1995;17:10-16.

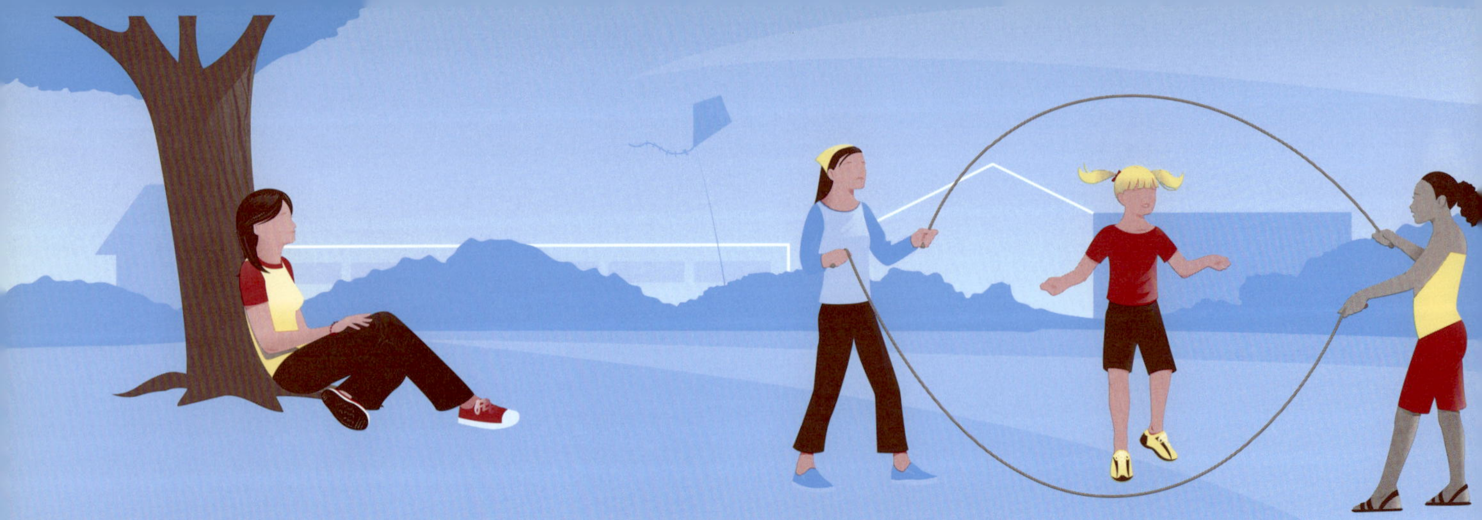

# Introducing GARDASIL—helping you

- **GARDASIL is a vaccine indicated in girls and women 9 to 26 years of age for the prevention of cervical cancer, precancerous or dysplastic lesions, and genital warts caused by human papillomavirus (HPV) Types 6, 11, 16, and 18.**
- **A complete vaccination regimen of GARDASIL consists of a 3-dose schedule.**

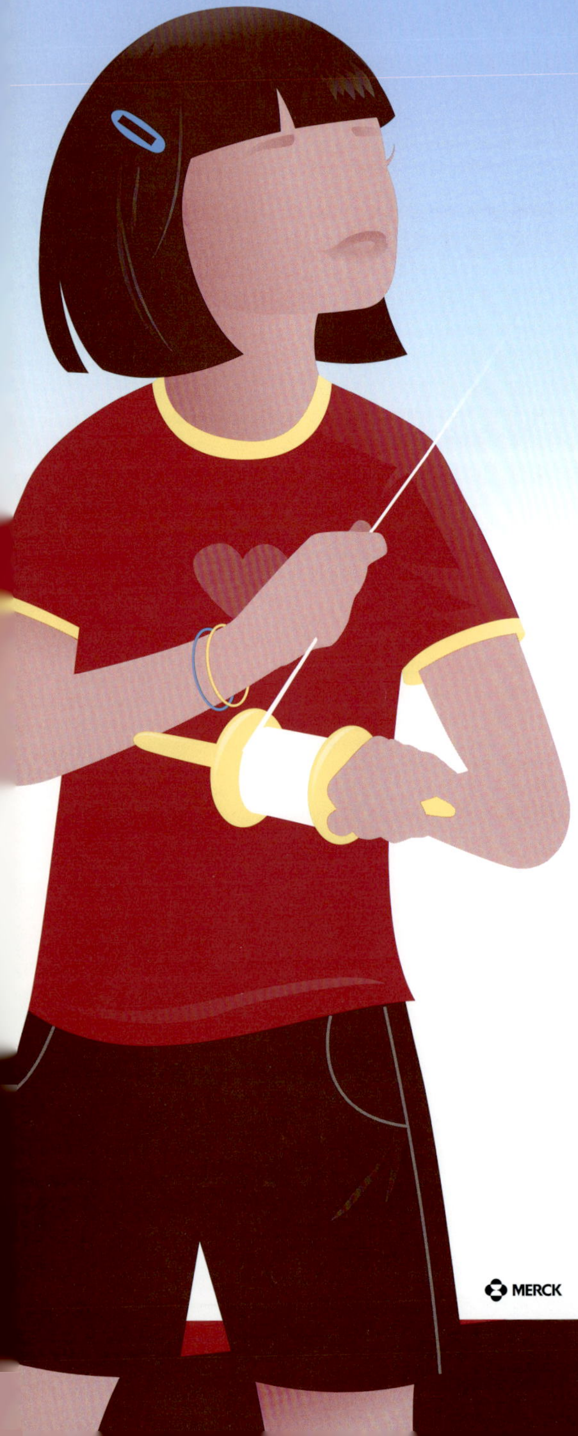

## Select safety information

GARDASIL is contraindicated in individuals who are hypersensitive to the active substances or to any of the excipients of the vaccine.

GARDASIL does not substitute for routine cervical cancer screening, and women who receive GARDASIL should continue to undergo screening per standard of care.

Vaccination with GARDASIL may not result in protection in all vaccine recipients.

GARDASIL is not intended to be used for treatment of active genital warts; cervical cancer; cervical intraepithelial neoplasia, vulvar intraepithelial neoplasia, or vaginal intraepithelial neoplasia.

To place an order, call **1-800-MERCK-RX,** or visit **www.MerckVaccines.com.**

MERCK

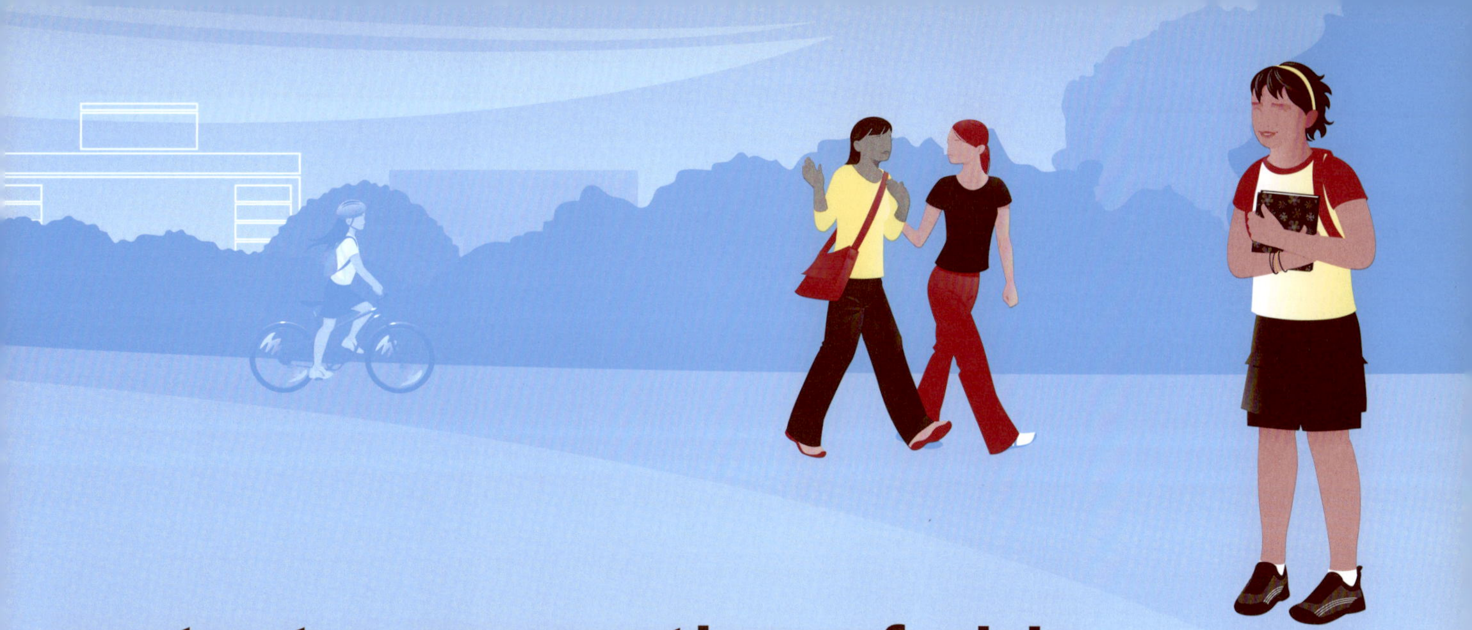

# protect a generation of girls

**The only quadrivalent vaccine that prevents disease caused by significant human papillomavirus (HPV) types: 6, 11, 16, and 18**

- **CERVICAL CANCER**
- **CERVICAL DYSPLASIA**
- **GENITAL WARTS**

- **Now is the time to vaccinate girls and young women 9 to 26 years of age.**

The vaccine-related adverse experiences that were observed among recipients of GARDASIL at a frequency of at least 1.0% and greater than placebo were pain, swelling, erythema, fever, nausea, pruritus, and dizziness.

Please see Brief Summary of Prescribing Information on adjacent page.

GARDASIL®

**[Quadrivalent Human Papillomavirus (Types 6,11,16,18) Recombinant Vaccine]**

# GARDASIL®

## [Quadrivalent Human Papillomavirus (Types 6, 11, 16, 18) Recombinant Vaccine]



**BRIEF SUMMARY OF PRESCRIBING INFORMATION**

**CONTRAINDICATIONS:** Hypersensitivity to the active substances or to any of the excipients of the vaccine.

Individuals who develop symptoms indicative of hypersensitivity after receiving a dose of GARDASIL should not receive further doses of GARDASIL.

**PRECAUTIONS:** ***General:*** As for any vaccine, vaccination with GARDASIL may not result in protection in all vaccine recipients.

This vaccine is not intended to be used for treatment of active genital warts; cervical cancer; cervical intraepithelial neoplasia (CIN), vulvar intraepithelial neoplasia (VIN), or vaginal intraepithelial neoplasia (VaIN).

This vaccine will not protect against diseases that are not caused by human papillomavirus (HPV).

GARDASIL has not been shown to protect against diseases due to non-vaccine HPV types.

As with all injectable vaccines, appropriate medical treatment should always be readily available in case of rare anaphylactic reactions following the administration of the vaccine.

The decision to administer or delay vaccination because of a current or recent febrile illness depends largely on the severity of the symptoms and their etiology. Low-grade fever itself and mild upper respiratory infection are not generally contraindications to vaccination.

Individuals with impaired immune responsiveness, whether due to the use of immunosuppressive therapy, a genetic defect, Human Immunodeficiency Virus (HIV) infection, or other causes, may have reduced antibody response to active immunization (see PRECAUTIONS, ***Drug Interactions***).

As with other intramuscular injections, GARDASIL should not be given to individuals with bleeding disorders such as hemophilia or thrombocytopenia, or to persons on anticoagulant therapy unless the potential benefits clearly outweigh the risk of administration. If the decision is made to administer GARDASIL to such persons, it should be given with steps to avoid the risk of hematoma following the injection.

*Information for the Patient, Parent, or Guardian:* The health care provider should inform the patient, parent, or guardian that vaccination does not substitute for routine cervical cancer screening. Women who receive GARDASIL should continue to undergo cervical cancer screening per standard of care.

The health care provider should provide the vaccine information required to be given with each vaccination to the patient, parent, or guardian.

The health care provider should inform the patient, parent, or guardian of the benefits and risks associated with vaccination. For risks associated with vaccination, see PRECAUTIONS and ADVERSE REACTIONS.

GARDASIL is not recommended for use in pregnant women.

The health care provider should inform the patient, parent, or guardian of the importance of completing the immunization series unless contraindicated.

Patients, parents, or guardians should be instructed to report any adverse reactions to their health care provider.

***Drug Interactions:*** *Use with Other Vaccines:* Results from clinical studies indicate that GARDASIL may be administered concomitantly (at a separate injection site) with hepatitis B vaccine (recombinant) (see CLINICAL PHARMACOLOGY, *Studies with Other Vaccines*). Co-administration of GARDASIL with other vaccines has not been studied.

*Use with Hormonal Contraceptives:* In clinical studies, 13,293 subjects (vaccine = 6644; placebo = 6649) who had post-Month 7 follow-up used hormonal contraceptives for a total of 17,597 person-years (65.1% of the total follow-up time in the study for these subjects). Use of hormonal contraceptives or lack of use of hormonal contraceptives among study participants did not alter vaccine efficacy in the per-protocol efficacy (PPE) population.

*Use with Systemic Immunosuppressive Medications:* Immunosuppressive therapies, including irradiation, antimetabolites, alkylating agents, cytotoxic drugs, and corticosteroids (used in greater than physiologic doses), may reduce the immune responses to vaccines (see PRECAUTIONS, ***General***).

*Carcinogenesis, Mutagenesis, Impairment of Fertility:* GARDASIL has not been evaluated for the potential to cause carcinogenicity or genotoxicity.

GARDASIL administered to female rats at a dose of 120 mcg total protein, which corresponds to approximately 300-fold excess relative to the projected human dose, had no effects on mating performance, fertility, or embryonic/fetal survival.

***Pregnancy:*** *Pregnancy Category B:* Reproduction studies have been performed in female rats at doses up to 300 times the human dose (on a mg/kg basis) and have revealed no evidence of impaired female fertility or harm to the fetus due to GARDASIL. However, it is not known whether GARDASIL can cause fetal harm when administered to a pregnant woman or if it can affect reproductive capacity. GARDASIL should be given to a pregnant woman only if clearly needed. An evaluation of the effect of GARDASIL on embryo-fetal, pre- and postweaning development was conducted using rats. One group of rats was administered GARDASIL twice prior to gestation, during the period of organogenesis (gestation day 6) and on lactation day 7. A second group of pregnant rats was administered GARDASIL during the period of organogenesis (gestation day 6) and on lactation day 7 only. GARDASIL was administered at 0.5 mL/rat/occasion (approximately 300-fold excess relative to the projected human dose on a mg/kg basis) by intramuscular injection. No adverse effects on mating, fertility, pregnancy, parturition, lactation, embryo-fetal or pre- and postweaning development were observed. There were no vaccine-related fetal malformations or other evidence of teratogenesis noted in this study. In addition, there were no treatment-related effects on developmental signs, behavior, reproductive performance, or fertility of the offspring. The effect of GARDASIL on male fertility has not been studied.

In clinical studies, women underwent urine pregnancy testing prior to administration of each dose of GARDASIL. Women who were found to be pregnant before completion of a 3-dose regimen of GARDASIL were instructed to defer completion of their vaccination regimen until resolution of the pregnancy.

During clinical trials, 2266 women (vaccine = 1115 vs. placebo = 1151) reported at least 1 pregnancy each. Overall, the proportions of pregnancies with an adverse outcome were comparable in subjects who received GARDASIL and subjects who received placebo. Overall, 40 and 41 subjects in the group that received GARDASIL or placebo, respectively (3.6% and 3.6% of all subjects who reported a pregnancy in the respective vaccination groups), experienced a serious adverse experience during pregnancy. The most common events reported were conditions that can result in Caesarean section (e.g., failure of labor, malpresentation, cephalopelvic disproportion), premature onset of labor (e.g., threatened abortions, premature rupture of membranes), and pregnancy-related medical problems (e.g., pre-eclampsia, hyperemesis). The proportions of pregnant subjects who experienced such events were comparable between the vaccination groups.

There were 15 cases of congenital anomaly in pregnancies that occurred in subjects who received GARDASIL and 16 cases of congenital anomaly in pregnancies that occurred in subjects who received placebo.

Further sub-analyses were conducted to evaluate pregnancies with estimated onset within 30 days or more than 30 days from administration of a dose of GARDASIL or placebo. For pregnancies with estimated onset within 30 days of vaccination, 5 cases of congenital anomaly were observed in the group that received GARDASIL compared to 0 cases of congenital anomaly in the group that received placebo. The congenital anomalies seen in pregnancies with estimated onset within 30 days of vaccination included pyloric stenosis, congenital megacolon, congenital hydronephrosis, hip dysplasia and club foot. Conversely, in pregnancies with onset more than 30 days following vaccination, 10 cases of congenital anomaly were observed in the group that received GARDASIL compared with 16 cases of congenital anomaly in the group that received placebo. The types of anomalies observed were consistent (regardless of when pregnancy occurred in relation to vaccination) with those generally observed in pregnancies in women aged 16 to 26 years.

*Pregnancy Registry for GARDASIL:* Merck & Co., Inc. maintains a Pregnancy Registry to monitor fetal outcomes of pregnant women exposed to GARDASIL. Patients and health care providers are encouraged to report any exposure to GARDASIL during pregnancy by calling (800) 986-8999.

*Lactation:* It is not known whether vaccine antigens or antibodies induced by the vaccine are excreted in human milk.

Because many drugs are excreted in human milk, caution should be exercised when GARDASIL is administered to a nursing woman.

A total of 995 nursing mothers (vaccine = 500, placebo = 495) were given GARDASIL or placebo during the vaccination period of the clinical trials. Geometric mean titers (GMTs) in nursing and non-nursing mothers were as follows:

The GMTs in nursing mothers were 595.9 (95% CI: 522.5, 679.5) for anti-HPV 6, 864.3 (95% CI: 754.0, 990.8) for anti-HPV 11, 3056.9 (95% CI: 2594.4, 3601.8) for anti-HPV 16, and 527.2 (95% CI: 450.9, 616.5) for anti-HPV 18. The GMTs for women who did not nurse during vaccine administration were 540.1 (95% CI: 523.5, 557.2) for anti-HPV 6, 746.3 (95% CI: 720.4, 773.3) for anti-HPV 11, 2290.8 (95% CI: 2180.7, 2406.3) for anti-HPV 16, and 456.0 (95% CI: 438.4, 474.3) for anti-HPV 18.

Overall, 17 and 9 infants of subjects who received GARDASIL or placebo, respectively (representing 3.4% and 1.8% of the total number of subjects who were breast-feeding during the period in which they received GARDASIL or placebo, respectively), experienced a serious adverse experience. None was judged by the investigator to be vaccine related.

In clinical studies, a higher number of breast-feeding infants (n = 6) whose mothers received GARDASIL had acute respiratory illnesses within 30 days post-vaccination of the mother as compared to infants (n = 2) whose mothers received placebo. In these studies, the rates of other adverse experiences in the mother and the nursing infant were comparable between vaccination groups.

*Pediatric Use:* The safety and efficacy of GARDASIL have not been evaluated in children younger than 9 years.

*Geriatric Use:* The safety and efficacy of GARDASIL have not been evaluated in adults above the age of 26 years.

**ADVERSE REACTIONS:** In 5 clinical trials (4 placebo-controlled), subjects were administered GARDASIL or placebo on the day of enrollment, and approximately 2 and 6 months thereafter. Few subjects (0.1%) discontinued due to adverse experiences. In all except 1 of the clinical trials, safety was evaluated using vaccination report card (VRC)-aided surveillance for 14 days after each injection of GARDASIL or placebo. The subjects who were monitored using VRC-aided surveillance included 5088 girls and women 9 through 26 years of age at enrollment who received GARDASIL and 3790 girls and women who received placebo.

***Common Adverse Experiences:*** *Vaccine-related Common Adverse Experiences:* The vaccine-related adverse experiences that were observed among female recipients of GARDASIL at a frequency of at least 1.0% and also at a greater frequency than that observed among placebo recipients are shown in Table 1.

**Table 1. Vaccine-related Injection-site and Systemic Adverse Experiences***

| Adverse Experience (1 to 5 Days Postvaccination) | GARDASIL (N = 5088) % | Aluminum-Containing Placebo (N = 3470) % | Saline Placebo (N = 320) % |
|---|---|---|---|
| *Injection Site* | | | |
| Pain | 83.9 | 75.4 | 48.6 |
| Swelling | 25.4 | 15.8 | 7.3 |
| Erythema | 24.6 | 18.4 | 12.1 |
| Pruritus | 3.1 | 2.8 | 0.6 |
| **Adverse Experience (1 to 15 Days Postvaccination)** | **GARDASIL (N = 5088) %** | **Placebo (N = 3790) %** | |
| *Systemic* | | | |
| Fever | 10.3 | 8.6 | |

*The vaccine-related adverse experiences that were observed among recipients of GARDASIL were at a frequency of at least 1.0% and also at a greater frequency than that observed among placebo recipients.

*All-cause Common Systemic Adverse Experiences:* All-cause systemic adverse experiences for female subjects reported 1 to 15 days postvaccination and observed at a frequency of ≥1% with incidence in the GARDASIL group (N = 5088) ≥ that of the placebo group (N = 3790), respectively, were: pyrexia (13.0% vs. 11.2%), nausea (6.7% vs. 6.6%), nasopharyngitis (6.4% vs. 6.4%), dizziness (4.0% vs. 3.7%), diarrhea (3.6% vs. 3.5%), vomiting (2.4% vs. 1.9%), myalgia (2.0% vs. 2.0%), cough (2.0% vs. 1.5%), toothache (1.5% vs. 1.4%), upper respiratory tract infection (1.5% vs. 1.5%), malaise (1.4% vs. 1.2%), arthralgia (1.2% vs. 0.9%), insomnia (1.2% vs. 0.9%), and nasal congestion (1.1% vs. 0.9%).

*Evaluation of Injection-site Adverse Experiences by Dose:* An analysis of injection-site adverse experiences in female subjects by dose is shown in Table 2. Overall, 94.3% of subjects who received GARDASIL judged their injection-site adverse experience to be mild or moderate in intensity.

**Table 2. Postdose Evaluation of Injection-site Adverse Experiences**

| Adverse Experience | Vaccine (% occurrence) Post-dose 1 | Post-dose 2 | Post-dose 3 | Post Any Dose |
|---|---|---|---|---|
| **Pain** | 63.4 | 60.7 | 62.7 | 83.9 |
| Mild/Moderate | 62.5 | 59.7 | 61.2 | 81.1 |
| Severe | 0.9 | 1.0 | 1.5 | 2.8 |
| **Swelling*** | 10.2 | 12.8 | 15.1 | 25.4 |
| Mild/Moderate | 9.6 | 11.9 | 14.3 | 23.3 |
| Severe | 0.6 | 0.8 | 0.8 | 2.0 |
| **Erythema*** | 9.2 | 12.1 | 14.7 | 24.7 |
| Mild/Moderate | 9.0 | 11.7 | 14.3 | 23.7 |
| Severe | 0.2 | 0.3 | 0.4 | 0.9 |

*Intensity of swelling and erythema was measured by size (inches): Mild = 0 to ≤1; Moderate = >1 to ≤2; Severe = >2.

| | Aluminum-Containing Placebo (% occurrence) | | | | Saline Placebo (% occurrence) | | | |
|---|---|---|---|---|---|---|---|---|
| **Adverse Experience** | Post-dose 1 | Post-dose 2 | Post-dose 3 | Post Any Dose | Post-dose 1 | Post-dose 2 | Post-dose 3 | Post Any Dose |
| **Pain** | 57.0 | 47.8 | 49.5 | 75.4 | 33.7 | 20.3 | 27.3 | 48.6 |
| Mild/Moderate | 56.6 | 47.3 | 48.9 | 74.1 | 33.3 | 20.3 | 27.0 | 48.0 |
| Severe | 0.4 | 0.5 | 0.6 | 1.3 | 0.3 | 0.0 | 0.3 | 0.6 |
| **Swelling*** | 8.2 | 7.5 | 7.6 | 15.8 | 4.4 | 3.0 | 3.3 | 7.3 |
| Mild/Moderate | 8.0 | 7.2 | 7.3 | 15.2 | 4.4 | 3.0 | 3.3 | 7.3 |
| Severe | 0.2 | 0.3 | 0.2 | 0.6 | 0.0 | 0.0 | 0.0 | 0.0 |
| **Erythema*** | 9.8 | 8.4 | 8.9 | 18.4 | 7.3 | 5.3 | 5.7 | 12.1 |
| Mild/Moderate | 9.5 | 8.3 | 8.8 | 18.0 | 7.3 | 5.3 | 5.7 | 12.1 |
| Severe | 0.3 | 0.1 | 0.1 | 0.4 | 0.0 | 0.0 | 0.0 | 0.0 |

*Evaluation of Fever by Dose:* An analysis of fever in girls and women by dose is shown in Table 3.

**Table 3. Postdose Evaluation of Fever**

| | Vaccine (% occurrence) | | | Placebo (% occurrence) | | |
|---|---|---|---|---|---|---|
| **Temperature (°F)** | Post-dose 1 | Post-dose 2 | Post-dose 3 | Post-dose 1 | Post-dose 2 | Post-dose 3 |
| ≥100 to <102 | 3.7 | 4.1 | 4.4 | 3.1 | 3.8 | 3.6 |
| ≥102 | 0.3 | 0.5 | 0.5 | 0.3 | 0.4 | 0.6 |

*Serious Adverse Experiences:* A total of 102 subjects out of 21,464 total subjects (9- to 26-year-old girls and women and 9- to 15-year-old boys) who received both GARDASIL and placebo reported a serious adverse experience on Day 1-15 following any vaccination visit during the clinical trials for GARDASIL. The most frequently reported serious adverse experiences regardless of causality for GARDASIL compared to placebo, respectively, were: headache (0.03% vs. 0.02%), gastroenteritis (0.03% vs. 0.01%), appendicitis (0.02% vs. 0.01%), and pelvic inflammatory disease (0.02% vs. 0.01%).

One case of bronchospasm and 2 cases of asthma were reported as serious adverse experiences that occurred during Day 1-15 of any vaccination visit.

*Deaths:* Across the clinical studies, 17 deaths were reported in 21,464 male and female subjects. The events reported were consistent with events expected in healthy adolescent and adult populations. The most common cause of death was motor vehicle accident (4 subjects who received GARDASIL and 3 placebo subjects), followed by overdose/suicide (1 subject who received GARDASIL and 2 subjects who received placebo), and pulmonary embolus/deep vein thrombosis (1 subject who received GARDASIL and 1 placebo subject). In addition, there were 2 cases of sepsis, 1 case of pancreatic cancer, and 1 case of arrhythmia in the group that received GARDASIL, and 1 case of asphyxia in the placebo group.

*Systemic Autoimmune Disorders:* In the clinical studies, subjects were evaluated for new medical conditions that occurred over the course of up to 4 years of follow up. The number of subjects who received both GARDASIL and placebo and developed a new medical condition potentially indicative of a systemic immune disorder is shown in Table 4.

**Table 4. Summary of Subjects Who Reported an Incident Condition Potentially Indicative of a Systemic Autoimmune Disorder After Enrollment in Clinical Trials of GARDASIL**

| Potential Autoimmune Disorder | GARDASIL (N = 11,813) | Placebo (N = 9701) |
|---|---|---|
| Specific Terms | 3 (0.025%) | 1 (0.010%) |
| Juvenile arthritis | 1 | 0 |
| Rheumatoid arthritis | 2 | 0 |
| Systemic lupus erythematosus | 0 | 1 |
| Other Terms | 6 (0.051%) | 2 (0.021%) |
| Arthritis | 5 | 2 |
| Reactive Arthritis | 1 | 0 |

N = Number of subjects enrolled

*Safety in Concomitant Use with Other Vaccines:* The safety of GARDASIL when administered concomitantly with hepatitis B vaccine (recombinant) was evaluated in a placebo-controlled study. There were no statistically significant higher rates in systemic or injection-site adverse experiences among subjects who received concomitant vaccination compared with those who received GARDASIL or hepatitis B vaccine alone.

*Reporting of Adverse Events:* The US Department of Health and Human Services has established a Vaccine Adverse Event Reporting System (VAERS) to accept all reports of suspected adverse events after the administration of any vaccine, including but not limited to the reporting of events required by the National Childhood Vaccine Injury Act of 1986. For information or a copy of the vaccine reporting form, call the VAERS toll-free number at 1-800-822-7967 or report on line to www.vaers.hhs.gov.

For more detailed information, please read the Prescribing Information.
GARDASIL is a registered trademark of Merck & Co., Inc.

MERCK



20650343(2)(300)-GRD

SECTION EDITOR: ALBERT C. YAN, MD; ASSISTANT SECTION EDITOR: SAMIR S. SHAH, MD

# Picture of the Month

*Jeffrey S. Gerber, MD, PhD; Samir S. Shah, MD*

A 15-YEAR-OLD BOY WAS INITIALLY SEEN IN the emergency department with complaints of right facial twitching accompanied by drooling and inability to speak. The spells lasted for approximately 2 minutes, having occurred 3 times per day for the past 2 weeks, and were associated with mild headaches. There was no fever, nausea, vomiting, weight loss, or trauma. There was no medical history of seizures or family history of epilepsy. The patient had immigrated to the northeastern United States from Mexico 1½ months previously, where he had lived on a farm housing chickens and pigs. Vital signs were within normal limits for age. Mental status, strength, tone, and deep tendon reflexes were all normal. Cranial nerve examination demonstrated rightward deviation of the tongue but results were otherwise normal, as were results of cerebellar and Babinski tests. Complete blood cell count and serum electrolyte levels, including calcium, were normal. Cerebrospinal fluid contained 3 white blood cells and 143 red blood cells per microliter, a protein level of 37 mg/dL, and a glucose level of 56 mg/dL (3.11 mmol/L). Computed tomography (CT) (**Figure 1**) and magnetic resonance imaging (MRI) (**Figure 2**) of the brain were performed.

**Author Affiliations:** Division of Infectious Diseases, The Children's Hospital of Philadelphia, and the Department of Pediatrics, University of Pennsylvania School of Medicine, Philadelphia.

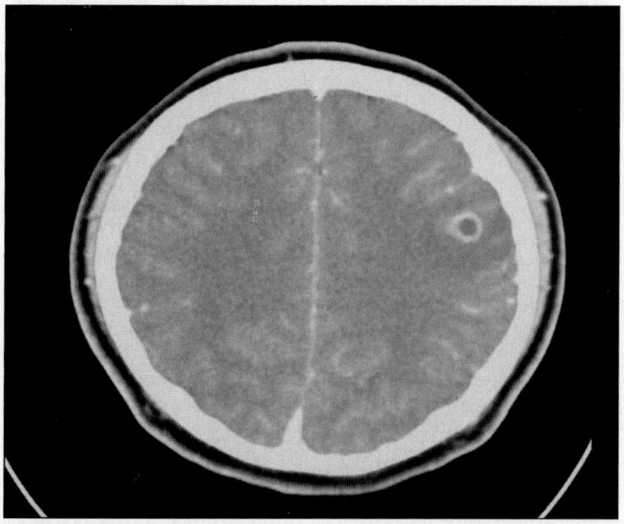

**Figure 1.** Contrast-enhanced computed tomographic scan of the brain, demonstrating a 1-cm focal hypodensity in the left frontal lobe with rim enhancement and an associated zone of vasogenic edema.

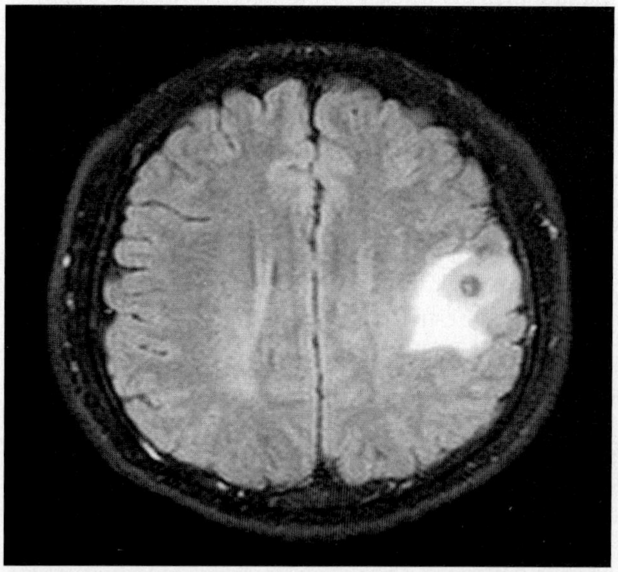

**Figure 2.** Sagittal midline view of postcontrast T1-weighted magnetic resonance imaging of the brain, demonstrating a left frontal cystic lesion with a thick rim of surrounding enhancement and surrounding vasogenic edema.

# Denouement and Comment

## *Neurocysticercosis*

The 1-cm focal hypodensity in the left frontal lobe with rim enhancement and associated zone of vasogenic edema shown in Figure 1 and the left frontal cystic lesion with a thick rim of surrounding enhancement and surrounding vasogenic edema shown in Figure 2 are characteristic of a degenerating parenchymal cysticercus; Figure 2 also shows a punctate area of central high signal, likely representing the scolex of a parasite. Neurocysticercosis is the most common parasitic disease of the central nervous system and the leading cause of acquired epilepsy worldwide.[1] The causative pathogen, *Taenia solium*, is harbored by an estimated 20 million people, most of whom live in Mexico, Latin America, sub-Saharan Africa, India, and Southeast Asia. Though most prevalent in these areas, increased rates of travel and immigration have made neurocysticercosis more common in developed nations. It is an emerging infectious disease in the United States, where approximately 1000 new cases are diagnosed each year.[2] Infection can occur at any age, but the clinical manifestations peak in the third and fourth decade of life. Ten percent of patients are children.[3]

### PATHOGENESIS

The life cycle of *T solium* revolves around its 2 developmental forms: the adult segmented worm causes taeniasis, an intestinal tapeworm infection, while the larval stage causes cysticercosis, an invasive form of infection. Pigs ingest *T solium* eggs. However, humans are the only host of both forms of the parasite, and pigs serve only as intermediates by harboring the cysticerci. In the intestine, the eggs release embryos, which penetrate the intestinal mucosa, enter the bloodstream, and burrow into tissues where they mature into cysticerci (infective larvae). Humans, as the definitive host, ingest the cysticerci in undercooked pork. The cysticerci mature into adult worms in the small intestine, where they attach and produce eggs (taeniasis) to continue the parasite life cycle. Cysticercosis occurs when humans act as the intermediate host. In such instances, humans ingest *T solium* eggs through fecal-oral contact with humans with taeniasis. The eggs hatch in the human intestine, liberating embryos that then penetrate the intestinal mucosa and disseminate to various organs (eg, brain, eye, muscle) via the bloodstream. The clinical manifestations of cysticercosis reflect the location of these cysticerci.

Central nervous system disease (neurocysticercosis) is influenced by the parasite load, location, and the patient's immune status. In most cases, neurocysticercosis in children manifests as a single cystic parenchymal brain lesion (multiple cysts are more common in adults) that is either clinically silent and self-resolving or characterized by partial seizures with or without secondary generalization. Though rare in children, extraparenchymal disease can cause hydrocephalus or encephalitis with headaches, mental status changes, and even life-threatening intracranial pressures. Spinal cord involvement is extremely rare at any age.[2,4]

### DIAGNOSIS

Accurate diagnosis of neurocysticercosis requires clinical and epidemiologic data to direct radiological imaging and serologic testing. Proposed diagnostic criteria are complex[5] and yet to be validated and, therefore, are not universally accepted. The only absolute criteria—biopsy specimen of a brain lesion, direct visualization of parasites by funduscopic examination, or scolex identification on CT or MRI—are rarely met. However, within the right context, CT and MRI are quite helpful. Initially, the cysticercus appears as a hypodense, fluid-filled cystic structure without surrounding inflammation or edema; the patient is usually clinically asymptomatic at this stage. Invocation of the host immune response results in parasite degeneration creating annular enhancement around the cyst (Figure 1), increasing fluid density within, and surrounding edema (Figure 2). Seizures are a common manifestation during this stage. This intermediate stage is followed by granulomatous change and, ultimately, calcification and occasionally disappearance. Computed tomography best visualizes granulomas and calcifications, while MRI (T2-weighted or gadolinium-enhanced) better defines surrounding edema (immune response) and fluid content (viability) and is superior for extraparenchymal disease. Many serologic assays are fraught with error related to poor specificity and to the high rate of seropositivity in endemic areas among those exposed but without active central nervous system disease. Enzyme-linked immunotransfer blot has a specificity approaching 100%, but the sensitivity is less than 50% in patients with solitary cystic lesions. Inflammatory changes in cerebrospinal fluid are nonspecific and only present in extraparenchymal disease. An ophthalmologic examination should always be performed to exclude eye disease, which alters treatment.

### TREATMENT

Although safe and effective drugs are readily available, antiparasitic treatment of neurocysticercosis is controversial. Both praziquantel and albendazole are appropriate, though albendazole (15 mg/kg per day for 28 days) is favored as the first-line agent secondary to its lower price, increased cysticidal activity, increased plasma levels during concomitant corticosteroid therapy (by contrast, corticosteroid therapy leads to lower praziquantel levels), and minimal toxic effects. Steroids are recommended as coagents to reduce the inflammation triggered by parasite destruction. Appropriate antiepileptic therapy should also be used in conjunction with these drugs. The theoretical argument against treatment lies in the belief that the inflammatory immune response to the parasite—not the mass effect of the parasite—triggers seizure activity. Thus, if a viable cyst resides in

**Table. Comparison of Randomized Controlled Trials of Albendazole Compared With Placebo for Small, Enhancing Parenchymal Brain Lesions by Computed Tomography in Children With New-Onset Focal Seizures**

| Source | Sample Size | No. of Lesions | Lesion Resolution Compared With Placebo | Seizure Frequency Compared With Placebo |
|---|---|---|---|---|
| Baranwal et al,[8] 1998 | 63 | 1 | Increased | No significant difference |
| Kalra et al,[9] 2003 | 123 | 1-2 | Increased | Decreased |
| Gogia et al,[10] 2003 | 72 | 1-2* | No significant difference | No significant difference |
| Singhi et al,[7] 2004 | 133 | 1 | No significant difference | Decreased |

*Sixteen percent of patients in this study had more than 2 lesions. Seventy percent of the patients had solitary lesions.

the brain evading a significant immune response, it might be detrimental to induce parasite destruction and subsequent inflammation. Also, the cysts and seizures often spontaneously resolve without specific therapy.[6] Some data support this stance, but most studies were not randomized and include patients of varying ages, different numbers and locations of cysts, and a multitude of outcomes. Four randomized controlled trials[7-10] have been conducted in children with 1 or 2 parenchymal cysts and new-onset partial seizures (**Table**). The results are mixed; 2 of the 4 albendazole treatment groups displayed better lesion resolution and improved seizure control, while the other 2 were not statistically different. The high rate of spontaneous resolution of both radiographic and clinical manifestations of this common manifestation of neurocysticercosis may require larger patient groups and meta-analyses to definitively show statistical significance higher than the apparent trend gleaned from these few pediatric studies.

**Accepted for Publication:** November 8, 2005.
**Correspondence:** Samir S. Shah, MD, Division of Infectious Diseases, The Children's Hospital of Philadelphia, 34th Street and Civic Center Boulevard, North Campus Room 1526, Philadelphia, PA 19104 (shahs@email.chop.edu).
**Author Contributions:** *Study concept and design:* Gerber and Shah. *Acquisition of data:* Shah. *Drafting of the manuscript:* Gerber. *Critical revision of the manuscript for important intellectual content:* Gerber and Shah. *Administrative, technical, and material support:* Shah. *Study supervision:* Shah.

## REFERENCES

1. White AC Jr. Neurocysticercosis: a major cause of neurological disease worldwide. *Clin Infect Dis.* 1997;24:101-113.
2. Carpio A. Neurocysticercosis: an update. *Lancet Infect Dis.* 2002;2:751-762.
3. Sotelo J. Taenia solium and Taenia saginata (taeniasis and cysticercosis). In: Long SL, ed. *Principles and Practice of Pediatric Infectious Diseases.* 2nd ed. London, England: Churchill Livingstone; 2002.
4. Singhi P, Singhi S. Neurocysticercosis in children. *J Child Neurol.* 2004;19:482-492.
5. Del Brutto OH, Rajshekhar V, White AC Jr, et al. Proposed diagnostic criteria for neurocysticercosis. *Neurology.* 2001;57:177-183.
6. Singh MK, Garg RK, Nath G, Verma DN, Misra S. Single small enhancing computed tomographic (CT) lesions in Indian patients with new-onset seizures: a prospective follow-up in 75 patients. *Seizure.* 2001;10:573-578.
7. Singhi P, Jain V, Khandelwal N. Corticosteroids versus albendazole for treatment of single small enhancing computed tomographic lesions in children with neurocysticercosis. *J Child Neurol.* 2004;19:323-327.
8. Baranwal AK, Singhi PD, Khandelwal N, Singhi SC. Albendazole therapy in children with focal seizures and single small enhancing computerized tomographic lesions: a randomized, placebo-controlled, double blind trial. *Pediatr Infect Dis J.* 1998;17:696-700.
9. Kalra V, Dua T, Kumar V. Efficacy of albendazole and short-course dexamethasone treatment in children with 1 or 2 ring-enhancing lesions of neurocysticercosis: a randomized controlled trial. *J Pediatr.* 2003;143:111-114.
10. Gogia S, Talukdar B, Choudhury V, Arora BS. Neurocysticercosis in children: clinical findings and response to albendazole therapy in a randomized, double-blind, placebo-controlled trial in newly diagnosed cases. *Trans R Soc Trop Med Hyg.* 2003;97:416-421.

### Announcement

**Topic Collections.** The *Archives* offers collections of articles in specific topic areas to make it easier for physicians to find the most recent publications in a field. These are available by subspecialty, study type, disease, or problem. In addition, you can sign up to receive a Collection E-Mail Alert when new articles on specific topics are published. Go to http://archpedi.ama-assn.org/collections to see these collections of articles.

## A Generation at Risk: The Global Impact of HIV/AIDS on Orphans and Vulnerable Children

*edited by Geoff Foster, Carol Levine, and John Williamson, 332 pp, $75. ISBN 0521652642, Cambridge, Mass, Cambridge University Press, 2005.*

As pediatricians, we are trained to approach disease from a medical perspective—diagnosing illness, treating symptoms and guiding patients back to health. But what can be done when a disease ravages whole nations, affecting the lives of millions of children? We are forced to widen our focus, look beyond the traditional medical model, and examine the socioeconomic components of health. The millions of children affected by HIV/AIDS include not only those who are infected, but those whose countries, communities, families, and homes are devastated by illness. *A Generation at Risk: The Global Impact of HIV/AIDS on Orphans and Vulnerable Children* provides information and perspective on their plight, and what is being done to change it.

The editors have done an admirable job of assembling an internationally known and respected team of authors. After a preface by Archbishop Emeritus Desmond Tutu, the subject matter is well introduced in a chapter entitled "HIV/AIDS and Its Long-Term Impact on Children." The numbers of infected people, now estimated at 40 million globally, are staggering, as are the "cascading impacts" of the disease on the lives of children. An estimated 5 million people a year become newly infected with HIV, including 700 000 under the age of fifteen. By 2010, an estimated 20 million children will have lost one or both parents to AIDS. With these numbers in mind, the next chapter, a cogent exploration of family and community-based care, demonstrates the importance of maintaining cohesive family structure in the face of the pandemic. Most orphans are cared for by immediate or extended family in improvised arrangements. Supporting them will require reframing the idea of family in the legal and cultural sense, while developing new institutions dedicated to their development.

Assisting these new families will also require substantial economic and educational reform. The actions taken today, for better or worse, will have tremendous impact on the course of national and world events in the years to come. A chapter on strengthening households and communities explores the economic effects of HIV in regions where many families were already struggling to survive. There is a desperate need to educate children affected by HIV/AIDS, and a chapter on education discusses efforts to alleviate the burden of school fees, improve school attendance, and maintain a cadre of healthy teachers. Chapters on the psychosocial and human-rights impacts of the disease stress the importance of defending not only children, but the very concept of childhood against a pandemic that traumatizes whole societies.

While the threat of the HIV/AIDS is universal, effective interventions require a deep understanding of local conditions and culture. In many nations, faith-based organizations have traditionally tended to the needy and the ill, and form a vital part of the safety net for vulnerable children. A chapter explores religious traditions relating to the care of orphans and discusses strategies for expanding the role of local faith-based groups. Chapters on the Asia-Pacific region and the United States reinforce our understanding of the disease's global impact on children and the work that remains to be done, even in the most developed of nations.

If there is one theme that permeates *A Generation at Risk*, it is the fragile and precarious nature of childhood affected by disease. HIV/AIDS disproportionately disables and kills those of parenting age, leaving behind the young and the elderly to survive as best they can. In much of the world, it affects communities that already have a profound lack of resources, where what some would consider societal basics—clean water, public education, a legal system that protects children—cannot be taken for granted. The loss of parental support through death or disability quickly depletes whatever economic, social, or psychological reserve a child may have.

Caring for orphans and vulnerable children requires not just medicine and clinical expertise, but an understanding of social structures, economic incentives, education and human rights. The closing chapters of the book highlight the need for basic research in these areas, as well as the difficulty of identifying vulnerable children, meeting their needs, and creating structures that will be sustainable in the long term. While it does not address the specifics of antiretroviral medication regimens, clinic construction, or community health networks, *A Generation at Risk* is most definitely a book about children's health. It provides valuable information on the social and economic context in which health care is delivered to vulnerable children. It is a worthy read for anyone interested in the global response to HIV/AIDS and the children it affects.

*Gabriel Berson, MD*

**Correspondence**: Dr Berson, University of Washington, 1806 NE 73rd St, Seattle, WA 98115 (gberson@u.washington.edu).

## THE UNIVERSITY OF SOUTH DAKOTA

### CHAIR OF PEDIATRICS/CHIEF PEDIATRIC MEDICAL OFFICER

The Sanford School of Medicine of The University of South Dakota (http://www.usd.edu/med) in conjunction with Sioux Valley Hospitals and Health System (http://www.siouxvalley.org) seeks a dynamic, experienced academic and clinical leader to serve as Chair of the Sanford School of Medicine Department of Pediatrics and the Chief Pediatric Medical Officer for Sioux Valley and the Sanford Children's Hospital. The Sanford School of Medicine was founded in 1907 and is responsible for medical education for the State. Sanford Children's Specialty Clinic, a comprehensive pediatric specialty group, fulfills the academic goals of the School and serves as its Department of Pediatrics for Sioux Valley Hospital University of South Dakota Medical Center. Sioux Valley is nationally recognized for excellence in care with a significant commitment to research. A new facility, the Sanford Children's Hospital will be built on the medical campus. As Chief Pediatric Medical Officer, this physician will play a critical role in the development and medical direction for this new state of the art pediatric hospital.

**QUALIFICATIONS:** M.D./D.O. Pediatrician with appropriate Board Certification, academic qualification for appointment at Full Professor, and demonstrated skills in education, scholarship, clinical service, research, and administration are mandatory. Priority will be given to candidates with a proven track record in medical education, especially of medical students, and medical staff administration. Excellent leadership and interpersonal skills are necessary to administer a program which depends on the resources of community practitioners, and affiliated institutions and is spread across a wide geographic area. Support for faculty and departmental involvement in research is necessary. Applicants must have experience in the clinical practice of pediatrics or one of its specialties and be licensable in South Dakota.

**SALARY/COMPENSATION:** Commensurate with education and experience.

Apply on-line at www.yourfuture.sdbor.edu or by submitting a letter of application, vita, and names, addresses and phone numbers of three professional references to: **Sanford School of Medicine, The University of South Dakota, Pediatrics Chair Search, ATTN: Lisa Sorensen, Human Resources, 1400 W. 22nd St., Sioux Falls, SD 57105, Email: lisa.sorensen@usd.edu, Phone: 605-357-1388, Fax: 605-357-1311**

Screening of applications will begin on October 30, 2006 and continue until a suitable candidate is hired.

The University of South Dakota is an Equal Opportunity / Affirmative Action educator and employer committed to increasing the diversity of its faculty, staff and students.

Sioux Valley

SANFORD SCHOOL OF MEDICINE
The University of South Dakota

## Associate Professor/Professor

*(Clinical or Tenure Track)*

## Chief of the Division General Pediatrics

*at the University at Buffalo and the Women and Children's Hospital of Buffalo*

The Department of Pediatrics is searching for a new Chief for our General Pediatrics Division. Potential candidates must be board certified in Pediatrics and have clinical and administrative skills, experience in an academic teaching environment, and evidence of scholarly activity. This Division of 11 faculty and 6 nurse practitioners currently has 3 clinic sites that together have over 30,000 visits per year. The division oversees the hospitalist group which covers inpatients and 1100 normal newborns per year from its own clinics as well as children referred from primary care physicians in the Western New York region. Additional responsibilities include 11 school based health clinics, the largest school based health clinic system in New York. The Division has an extensive teaching program for residents and medical students which takes place in all of its inpatient and outpatient sites as well as several community-based private practices. Applicants will have great opportunity to conduct clinical research and clinical trials. State University of New York at Buffalo is an Equal Opportunity, Affirmative Action Employer/Recruiter. Women and minorities are encouraged to apply.

*Interested candidates should send a letter of intent and curriculum vitae to:*

Drucy Borowitz, MD
Chief, Pediatric Pulmonology
Professor of Clinical Pediatrics
State University of New York at Buffalo
University Pediatric Associates, Inc.
Women and Children's Hospital of Buffalo
219 Bryant Street
Buffalo, NY 14222

Tel: 716-878-7524
Fax: 716-888-3945
Email: dborowitz@upa.chob.edu

University at Buffalo
The State University of New York

WOMEN & CHILDREN'S HOSPITAL of BUFFALO

JAMACareerNet *NetWorking for Physicians*

BrownMed
BROWN MEDICAL SCHOOL

MEMORIAL HOSPITAL OF RHODE ISLAND

# General Pediatrician

The Department of Pediatrics is seeking a General Pediatrician to join its growing academic faculty. The successful candidate will have opportunities for family-centered care, teaching and clinical research. Memorial Hospital is a major teaching hospital for Brown Medical School. The Division of General Pediatrics provides clinical care and medical homes for community children as well as medical support to community schools. The Division pursues excellence in clinical care and in the teaching and mentoring of medical students, resident and fellows. The successful candidate will have a unique opportunity for professional growth and will be encouraged to develop innovative forward-looking healthcare programs or resident educational programs that will be needed by Pediatric training programs in the future.

Candidates must be BC/BE in Pediatrics and eligible for a faculty appointment at the assistant or associate professor level at Brown Medical school. Research experience is valued but not required.

Interested candidates should forward correspondence and curriculum vitae to: **Joseph J Hallett, M.D., c/o Rose Tremblay, Department of Pediatrics, Memorial Hospital, 111 Brewster Street, Pawtucket, RI 02860 or email Rose_Tremblay@mhri.org.**

We are an equal opportunity employer M/F/D/V.

MAYO CLINIC

## Academic Primary Care Pediatrician

Rochester, Minnesota

The Department of Pediatric and Adolescent Medicine, Mayo Clinic, Rochester, Minnesota, is seeking three (3) board-certified/board-eligible pediatricians with interests in academic, community-based primary care to join its Division of Community Pediatric and Adolescent Medicine. The Division consists of seventeen (17) pediatricians and five (5) pediatric nurse practitioners and is fully integrated within a department that includes all pediatric subspecialties.

This is a unique opportunity to join a large, multispecialty, integrated practice with a strong commitment to primary care and academic medicine. Mayo Clinic has a medical school, a pediatric residency program, pediatric fellowship programs and the Mayo Eugenio Litta Children's Hospital.

This position includes primary care in an active group practice, adolescent medicine interests, and primary care research and/or health care services research, as well as education and mentoring of medical students, residents, and nurse practitioners. Academic rank and salary will depend on certification, academic accomplishments, and experience.

To learn more about Mayo Clinic and Rochester, MN, please visit **www.mayoclinic.org**.

For information, please include a curriculum vita and write to:

**Dr. Daniel Broughton**, Search Committee Chair
Division of Community Pediatric and Adolescent Medicine
**Mayo Clinic and Foundation**
200 First Street, SW
Rochester, MN 55905-0001
Telephone: 507-284-4466
Fax: 507-284-9744
e-mail: dbroughton@mayo.edu

**Mayo Foundation is an affirmative action and equal opportunity educator and employer. Post-offer/pre-employment drug screening is required.**

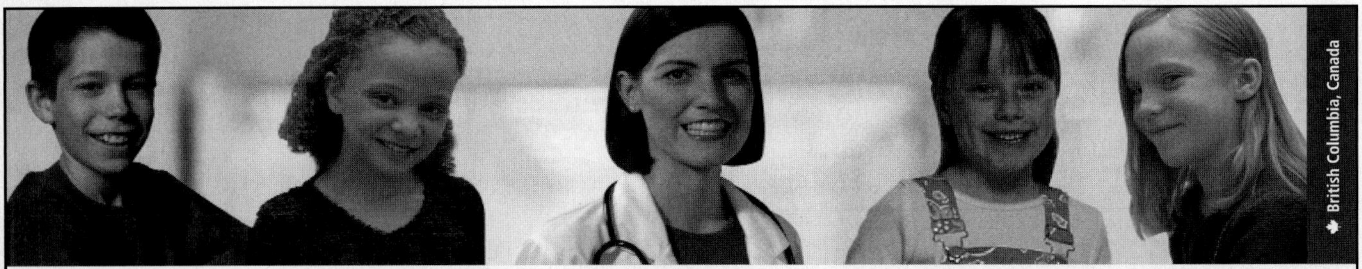


**Sunny Hill Health Centre for Children (SHHCC)** is a leading provincial facility offering specialized services to children and youth with developmental disabilities from birth to the age of 19. Sunny Hill focuses on the child, their family and supports health care professionals in their community, providing specific knowledge in the consultation, diagnosis and treatment within pediatric rehabilitation.

**SHHCC** is an organization within the **Provincial Health Services Authority (PHSA)**, which plans, manages and evaluates selected specialty and province-wide health care services across BC.

## Developmental Pediatrician

**Sunny Hill Health Centre for Children**

An outstanding opportunity is available to join the Division of Developmental Pediatrics at BC Children's Hospital/Sunny Hill Health Centre for Children and the University of British Columbia and take a central role as a clinician investigator in the area of neuromotor disabilities.

The Child Development and Rehabilitation Program at Sunny Hill is a provincial resource providing consultation and community support for the management of children with disabilities. As the academic medical leader, you will be expected to work with the inter-disciplinary team and take a leadership role in developing provincially focused evidence-based services to children with neuromotor disabilities, as well as initiate and support a range of clinical and health services research, and quality improvement activities.

The Division has 12 faculty members and works within a program management model with excellent inter-professional collaborative opportunities. The Division has strong research and education programs and expects to have a Royal College approved training program in Developmental Pediatrics within the next year. The Division has an excellent compensation and professional support program within a department practice plan.

The successful candidate will also be eligible for an appointment at UBC in Pediatrics (rank commensurate with experience) and will participate in clinical care, teaching, clinical research and quality improvement. The anticipated start date is February 1, 2007. Salary will be commensurate with qualifications and experience.

SHHCC and the University of British Columbia hire on the basis of merit and are committed to employment equality. We encourage all qualified persons to apply; however, Canadian and permanent residents of Canada will be given priority.

Applications, accompanied by a detailed curriculum vitae and names and or contact details of three references, should be directed by **October 31, 2006** to: **Dr. Robert Armstrong, MD PhD FRCPC, Head, Department of Paediatrics, University of British Columbia Room 2D15, 4480 Oak Street, Vancouver, B.C., V6H 3V4, Canada; E-mail: barmstrong@cw.bc.ca**

UBC

Sunny Hill HEALTH CENTRE FOR CHILDREN
A program of BC Children's Hospital

PROVINCIAL Health Services AUTHORITY
*Province-wide solutions. Better health.*

**www.bcchildrens.ca** **careers.phsa.ca**

www.jamacareernet.com

## PRACTICE FOR SALE

PRACTICE FOR SALE - WELL ESTABISHED PEDIATRICS AND ALLERGY practice for sale. Located 15 miles south of Boston close to major teaching hospitals. Owner will introduce. Call: 781-784-8403.



## JOURNAL ADVERTISER INDEX

**ABBOTT LABS**
Omnicef OS ..... 999-1001

**ALLIANT PHARMACEUTICALS**
Orapred Odt ..... 1047-1048

**ASTRAZENECA**
http://www.astrazeneca.com
Nexium ..... 1032A-B

**CLASSIFIED ADVERTISING** ..... 1085-1087
http://www.amapublications.com

**GLAXOSMITHKLINE**
Boostrix ..... 1003-1004, 1061-1062
Pediarix ..... 1033-1034, COVER 3-4

**MERCK & COMPANY**
Gardasil ..... 1080A-D
Rotateq ..... 1048A-E

**SEPRACOR**
Xopenex ..... COVER 2-993

*Demographic and "Mini" inserts and/or ROB ad pages
While every precaution is taken to ensure accuracy, we cannot guarantee against the possibility of an occasional change or omission in the preparation of this index.

ARCHIVES OF PEDIATRICS & ADOLESCENT MEDICINE

# CONTACT INFORMATION

## EDITORIAL OFFICE

**Editorial Office Information:** *Archives of Pediatrics & Adolescent Medicine*, Department of Pediatrics, Child Health Institute, University of Washington, 6200 NE 74th St, Suite 210, Seattle, WA 98115-8160, USA; phone: (206) 685-3573; fax: (206) 685-3572; e-mail: archpediatrics@jama-archives.org.

**Electronic Submission:** Manuscripts should be submitted via our online manuscript submission and review system (http://manuscripts.archpediatrics.com). Manuscripts submitted through our online system should not also be submitted by mail or fax. Signed authorship forms should be sent by regular mail or fax with the assigned manuscript number noted on each page in the upper right-hand corner. See the Instructions for Authors (www.archpediatrics.com) for more details.

## CONSORTIUM OF *JAMA* & *ARCHIVES* JOURNALS

The *Archives of Pediatrics & Adolescent Medicine* is a member of the consortium of AMA journals listed below.

- The Journal of the American Medical Association (JAMA)
- Archives of Dermatology
- Archives of Facial Plastic Surgery
- Archives of General Psychiatry
- Archives of Internal Medicine
- Archives of Neurology
- Archives of Ophthalmology
- Archives of Otolaryngology–Head & Neck Surgery
- Archives of Pediatrics & Adolescent Medicine
- Archives of Surgery

## *JAMA/ARCHIVES* MEDIA RELATIONS

Jann Ingmire; phone: (312) 464-5262; e-mail: mediarelations@jama-archives.org.

## *ARCHIVES OF PEDIATRICS* ONLINE

*Archives of Pediatrics & Adolescent Medicine* is available online at www.archpediatrics.com.

## *JAMA/ARCHIVES* REPRINTS

**Author/Educational Institution Reprints:** Anna Goins at (312) 464-2477; fax: (312) 464-5843; e-mail: anna.goins@ama-assn.org. Minimum order: 100 reprints.

**Commercial Reprints:** Phone: (312) 464-0776; fax: (312) 464-0708; e-mail: reprints@ama-assn.org. Minimum order: 100 reprints.

## PERMISSIONS

Information about obtaining permission to republish, reprint, or adapt material published in *Archives of Pediatrics & Adolescent Medicine* is available from Rhonda Bailey Brown; phone: (312) 464-2513; fax: (312) 464-5843; e-mail: permissions@ama-assn.org.

## DOCUMENT DELIVERY

Copies of individual articles are available online at www.archpediatrics.com and from the following: Infotrieve, phone: (800) 422-4633; fax: (310) 208-5971; URL: www.infotrieve.com; e-mail: orders@infotrieve.com; Institute for Scientific Information (ISI), phone: (800) 603-4367; fax: (856) 787-1679; URL: http://www.isidoc.com; e-mail: service@isidoc.com.

## ADVERTISING

Information about advertising is available from the following sales representatives and online at www.archpediatrics.com.

**Account Manager:** Tim Melroy (nationally); phone: (973) 263-9191 ext 213.

**Manager, Marketing Services:** Nancy Bell; phone: (973) 263-9191 ext 216.

**Advertising Office:** 119 Cherry Hill Rd, Suite 330, Parsippany, NJ 07054-1114; phone: (973) 263-9191.

**Classified Advertising:** Thalia Moss, Shana Brown, Kim Jenkins, Sophie Levandoski, 515 N State St, Chicago, IL 60610; phone: (800) 262-2260; e-mail: classifieds@jama-archives.org.

## ADVERTISING PRINCIPLES

Advertisements in this issue have been reviewed to comply with the principles governing advertising in AMA publications. A copy of these principles is available on request and online at www.archpediatrics.com. The appearance of advertising in AMA publications is not an AMA guarantee or endorsement of the product or the claims made for the product by the manufacturer.

## ADDRESS CHANGES

Send all address changes to *Archives of Pediatrics & Adolescent Medicine*, c/o the AMA Unified Service Center, American Medical Association, 515 N State St, Chicago, IL 60610. Notification of address changes must be made at least 6 weeks in advance; include both old and new addresses and a recent mailing label if sending via mail.

## SUBSCRIPTION RATES AND SERVICE

Subscription rates are shown in the table below. For service in the US and Americas, inquiries on pricing, address changes, missing issues, subscription billing, subscription renewal, and back issues, contact the AMA Unified Service Center, 24 hours a day, 7 days a week.

**AMA members:** phone: (800) 262-3211; e-mail: msc@ama-assn.org. **Other physicians and nonphysician customers, including subscription agents:** phone: (800) 262-2350 or (312) 670-7827; fax: (312) 464-5831; e-mail: ama-subs@ama-assn.org. **Inquiries:** Unified Service Center, American Medical Association, PO Box 10946, Chicago, IL 60610-0946. For subscribers with mailing addresses outside the United States & Americas: Contact *JAMA & Archives* Journals, c/o EMD GmbH, Birkenstr.67, 10559 Berlin, Germany. Phone: +49 (30) 33099828; fax: +49 (30) 33099829; e-mail: ama@emd-germany.de.

**Annual Subscription Rates**

| | United States | Americas | UK | Rest of World |
|---|---|---|---|---|
| INDIVIDUAL | | | | |
| Print and Online | $185 | $240 | £165 | €250 |
| INSTITUTION | | | | |
| Print and Online | $400 | $485 | £315 | €470 |

In Canada, US rate plus GST. Rates for residents and medical students available at pubs.ama-assn.org, or from the AMA Unified Service Center.

The ARCHIVES OF PEDIATRICS & ADOLESCENT MEDICINE (ISSN 01072–4710) is published monthly by the American Medical Association, 515 N State St, Chicago, IL 60610–0946, and is an official publication of the Association. The ARCHIVES OF PEDIATRICS & ADOLESCENT MEDICINE reaches more than 30 900 readers in over 83 countries each month. Periodicals postage paid at Chicago, Ill, and at additional mailing offices. GST registration number 12622 5556 RT. Canada Post International Publications Mail (Canadian Distribution) Sales Agreement No. 318728. POSTMASTER, send all address changes to *Archives of Pediatrics & Adolescent Medicine*, c/o the AMA Unified Service Center, American Medical Association, 515 N State St, Chicago, IL 60610. Printed in the USA.

**PEDIARIX® [Diphtheria and Tetanus Toxoids and Acellular Pertussis Adsorbed, Hepatitis B (Recombinant) and Inactivated Poliovirus Vaccine Combined]**

The following is a brief summary only; see full prescribing information for complete product information.

**CONTRAINDICATIONS:** Hypersensitivity to any component of the vaccine, including yeast, neomycin, and polymyxin B, is a contraindication (see DESCRIPTION in complete prescribing information). Do not use PEDIARIX after a serious allergic reaction (e.g., anaphylaxis) temporally associated with a previous dose of this vaccine or with any components of this vaccine. Because of the uncertainty as to which component of the vaccine might be responsible, do not give further vaccination with any of these components; or, refer such individuals to an allergist for evaluation. The following events are contraindications to administration of PEDIARIX: encephalopathy (e.g., coma, decreased level of consciousness, prolonged seizures) within 7 days of administration of a previous dose of a pertussis-containing vaccine that is not attributable to another identifiable cause; progressive neurologic disorder, including infantile spasms, uncontrolled epilepsy, or progressive encephalopathy. Do not vaccinate individuals with these conditions until a treatment regimen has been established and the condition has stabilized.

**WARNINGS:** Administration of PEDIARIX is associated with higher rates of fever relative to separately administered vaccines. In a safety study that evaluated medically attended fever after PEDIARIX or separately administered vaccines when coadministered with 7-valent pneumococcal and Hib conjugate vaccines, infants who received PEDIARIX had a higher rate of medical encounters for fever within the first 4 days following the first vaccination. In some infants, these encounters included the performance of diagnostic studies to evaluate other causes of fever (see ADVERSE REACTIONS). The tip cap and the rubber plunger of the needleless prefilled syringes contain dry natural latex rubber that may cause allergic reactions in latex sensitive individuals. The vial stopper is latex-free. If any of the following events occur in temporal relation to receipt of DTwP or a vaccine containing an acellular pertussis component, consider carefully whether to give any pertussis vaccine, including PEDIARIX: temperature of ≥40.5°C (105°F) within 48 hours not due to another identifiable cause; collapse or shock-like state (hypotonic-hyporesponsive episode) within 48 hours; persistent, inconsolable crying lasting ≥3 hours, occurring within 48 hours; seizures with or without fever occurring within 3 days. If Guillain-Barré syndrome occurs within 6 weeks of receipt of prior vaccine containing tetanus toxoid, the decision to give any tetanus toxoid-containing vaccine, including PEDIARIX, should be based on careful consideration of the potential benefits and possible risks. If tetanus toxoid is withheld, other available vaccines should be given, as indicated. The decision to administer a pertussis-containing vaccine to individuals with stable central nervous system (CNS) disorders must be made by the physician on an individual basis, with consideration of all relevant factors, and assessment of potential risks and benefits for that individual. Advise the parent or guardian of the potential increased risk involved (see PRECAUTIONS). For children at higher risk for seizures than the general population, an appropriate antipyretic may be administered at the time of vaccination and for the ensuing 24 hours according to the respective prescribing information recommended dosage to reduce the possibility of post-vaccination fever. The ACIP has published guidelines for vaccination of persons with recent or acute illness (www.cdc.gov/nip).

**PRECAUTIONS:** PEDIARIX should be given with caution in children with bleeding disorders such as hemophilia or thrombocytopenia and in children on anticoagulant therapy, with steps taken to avoid the risk of hematoma following the injection. Before the injection of any biological, the physician should take all reasonable precautions to prevent allergic or other adverse reactions. Epinephrine injection (1:1,000) and other appropriate agents used for the control of immediate allergic reactions must be immediately available should an acute anaphylactic reaction occur. Immunosuppressed individuals, including those receiving immunosuppressive therapy, may not develop the expected immune response. The ACIP has published guidelines for vaccination of persons on such therapies (www.cdc.gov/nip). **Drug Interactions:** For information regarding concomitant administration with other vaccines, refer to DOSAGE AND ADMINISTRATION in complete prescribing information. Do not mix PEDIARIX with any other vaccine in the same syringe or vial. **Carcinogenesis, Mutagenesis, Impairment of Fertility:** PEDIARIX has not been evaluated for carcinogenic or mutagenic potential, or for impairment of fertility. **Pregnancy:** Pregnancy Category C: PEDIARIX is not indicated for women of child-bearing age. Animal reproduction studies have not been conducted with PEDIARIX. It is not known whether PEDIARIX can cause fetal harm when administered to a pregnant woman or if PEDIARIX can affect reproductive capacity. **Geriatric Use:** PEDIARIX is not indicated for use in adult populations. **Pediatric Use:** Safety and effectiveness of PEDIARIX in infants younger than 6 weeks of age have not been evaluated. PEDIARIX is not recommended for persons 7 years of age or older.

**ADVERSE REACTIONS:** A total of 23,849 doses of PEDIARIX have been administered to 8,088 infants who received one or more doses as part of a 3-dose primary series during 14 clinical studies. The most common adverse reactions observed in clinical trials were local injection site reactions (pain, redness, or swelling), fever, and fussiness. In comparative studies, administration of PEDIARIX was associated with higher rates of fever relative to separately administered vaccines (see WARNINGS and ADVERSE REACTIONS Table 1). The prevalence of fever was highest on the day of vaccination and the day following vaccination. More than 96% of episodes of fever resolved within the 4-day period following vaccination (i.e., the period including the day of vaccination and the next 3 days). In the largest of the 14 studies, conducted in Germany, safety data were available for 4,666 infants who received PEDIARIX administered concomitantly at separate sites with 1 of 4 *Haemophilus influenzae* type b (Hib) vaccines at 3, 4, and 5 months of age and for 768 infants in the control group that received INFANRIX® (Diphtheria and Tetanus Toxoids and Acellular Pertussis Vaccine Adsorbed), Hib conjugate vaccine, and oral poliovirus vaccine (OPV) separately. Data on adverse events were collected by parents using standardized diary cards for 4 consecutive days following each vaccine dose (i.e., day of vaccination and the next 3 days). Infants were also monitored for unsolicited adverse events that occurred within 30 days following vaccination using diaries which were returned at subsequent visits and were supplemented by spontaneous reports and a medical history as reported by parents. More than 95% of study participants were white.

In a US study, the safety of PEDIARIX administered to 673 infants was compared to the safety of separately administered INFANRIX, ENGERIX-B® [Hepatitis B Vaccine (Recombinant)], inactivated poliovirus vaccine (IPV) in 335 infants. In both groups, infants received Hib and 7-valent pneumococcal conjugate vaccines concomitantly at separate sites. All vaccines were administered at 2, 4, and 6 months of age. The study was powered to evaluate fever >101.3° F following dose 1. Data on solicited adverse events were collected by parents using standardized diary cards for 4 consecutive days following each vaccine dose (i.e., day of vaccination and the next 3 days) and are presented in Table 1. Telephone follow-up was conducted 1 month and 6 months after the third vaccination to inquire about serious adverse events. At the 6-month follow-up, information also was collected on new onset of chronic illnesses. 638 subjects who received PEDIARIX and 313 subjects who received INFANRIX, ENGERIX-B, and IPV completed the 6-month follow-up. Among subjects in both study groups combined, 69% were white, 18% were Hispanic, 7% were black, 3% were Oriental, and 3% were of other racial/ethnic groups.

The adverse event information from clinical trials provides a basis for identifying adverse events that appear to be related to vaccine use and for approximating rates. However, because clinical trials are conducted under widely varying conditions, adverse event rates observed in the clinical trials of a vaccine cannot be directly compared to rates in the clinical trials of another vaccine, and may not reflect the rates observed in practice. As with any vaccine, there is the possibility that broad use of PEDIARIX could reveal adverse events not observed in clinical trials.

**Deaths:** In 14 clinical trials, 5 deaths were reported among 8,088 (0.06%) recipients of PEDIARIX and 1 death was reported among 2,287 (0.04%) recipients of comparator vaccines. Causes of death in the group that received PEDIARIX included 2 cases of Sudden Infant Death Syndrome (SIDS) and one case of each of the following: Convulsive disorder, congenital immunodeficiency with sepsis, and neuroblastoma. One case of SIDS was reported in the comparator group. The rate of SIDS among all recipients of PEDIARIX across the 14 trials was 0.25/1,000. The rate of SIDS observed for recipients of PEDIARIX in the German safety study was 0.2/1,000 infants (reported rate of SIDS in Germany in the latter part of the 1990s was 0.7/1,000 newborns). The reported rate of SIDS in the United States from 1990 to 1994 was 1.2/1,000 live births. By chance alone, some cases of SIDS can be expected to follow receipt of pertussis-containing vaccines.

**Serious Adverse Events:** Within 30 days following any dose of vaccine in the US safety study in which all subjects received concomitant pneumococcal and Hib conjugate vaccines, 7 serious adverse events were reported in 7 subjects (1% [7/673]) who received PEDIARIX (1 case each of pyrexia, gastroenteritis, and culture negative clinical sepsis and 4 cases of bronchiolitis) and 5 serious adverse events were reported in 4 subjects (1% [4/335]) who received INFANRIX, ENGERIX-B, and IPV (uteropelvic junction obstruction and testicular atrophy in one subject and 3 cases of bronchiolitis).

**Onset of Chronic Illnesses:** In the US safety study in which all subjects received concomitant pneumococcal and Hib conjugate vaccines, 21 subjects (3%) who received PEDIARIX and 14 subjects (4%) who received INFANRIX, ENGERIX-B, and IPV reported new onset of a chronic illness during the period from 1 to 6 months following the last dose of study vaccines. Among the chronic illnesses reported in the subjects who received PEDIARIX, there were 4 cases of asthma and 1 case each of diabetes mellitus and chronic neutropenia. There were 4 cases of asthma in subjects who received INFANRIX, ENGERIX-B, and IPV.

**Seizures:** In the German safety study over the entire study period, 6 subjects in the group that received PEDIARIX reported seizures. Two of these subjects had a febrile seizure, 1 of whom also developed afebrile seizures. The remaining 4 subjects had afebrile seizures, including 2 with infantile spasms. Two subjects reported seizures within 7 days following vaccination (1 subject had both febrile and afebrile seizures, and 1 subject had afebrile seizures), corresponding to a rate of 0.22 seizures per 1,000 doses (febrile seizures 0.07 per 1,000 doses, afebrile seizures 0.14 per 1,000 doses). No subject who received concomitant INFANRIX, Hib vaccine, and OPV reported seizures. In a separate German study that evaluated the safety of INFANRIX in 22,505 infants who received 66,867 doses of INFANRIX administered as a 3-dose primary series, the rate of seizures within 7 days of vaccination with INFANRIX was 0.13 per 1,000 doses (febrile seizures 0.0 per 1,000 doses, afebrile seizures 0.13 per 1,000 doses). Over the entire study period in the US safety study in which all subjects received concomitant pneumococcal and Hib conjugate vaccines, 4 subjects in the group that received PEDIARIX reported seizures. Three of these subjects had a febrile seizure and 1 had an afebrile seizure. Over the entire study period, 2 subjects in the group that received INFANRIX, ENGERIX-B, and IPV reported febrile seizures. There were no afebrile seizures in this group. No subject in either study group had seizures within 7 days following vaccination.

**Other Neurological Events of Interest:** No cases of hypotonic-hyporesponsiveness or encephalopathy were reported in either the German safety study or the US safety study.

**Solicited Adverse Events:** Table 1 presents data from the US safety study on solicited local and systemic adverse events within 4 days of vaccination with PEDIARIX or INFANRIX, ENGERIX-B, and IPV, administered concomitantly with Hib and 7-valent pneumococcal conjugate vaccines. In this study, medical attention (a visit to or from medical personnel) for fever within 4 days following vaccination was sought in the group who received PEDIARIX for 8 infants after the first dose (1.2%), 1 infant following the second dose (0.2%), and 5 infants following the third dose (0.8%) (Table 1). Following dose 2, medical attention for fever was sought for 2 infants (0.6%) who received separately administered vaccines (Table 1). Among infants who had a medical visit for fever within 4 days following vaccination, 9 of 14 who received PEDIARIX and 1 of 2 who received separately administered vaccines, had one or more diagnostic studies performed to evaluate the cause of fever.

**Safety of PEDIARIX after a previous dose of hepatitis B vaccine:** Limited data are available on the safety of administering PEDIARIX after a previous dose of hepatitis B vaccine. In 2 separate studies, 160 Moldovan infants and 96 US infants, respectively, received 3 doses of PEDIARIX following 1 previous dose of hepatitis B vaccine. Neither study was designed to detect significant differences in rates of adverse events associated with PEDIARIX administered after a previous dose of hepatitis B vaccine compared to PEDIARIX administered without a previous dose of hepatitis B vaccine.

**Table 1. Percentage of US Infants With Solicited Local Reactions or Systemic Adverse Events Within 4 Days of Vaccination* at 2, 4, and 6 Months of Age With PEDIARIX Administered Concomitantly With Hib Conjugate Vaccine and 7-valent Pneumococcal Conjugate Vaccine (PCV7) or With Separate Concomitant Administration of INFANRIX, ENGERIX-B, IPV, Hib Conjugate Vaccine, and PCV7 (Modified ITT cohort)**

| | PEDIARIX, Hib Vaccine, & PCV7 | | | INFANRIX, ENGERIX-B, IPV, Hib Vaccine, & PCV7 | | |
|---|---|---|---|---|---|---|
| | **Dose 1** | **Dose 2** | **Dose 3** | **Dose 1** | **Dose 2** | **Dose 3** |
| **Local**† | | | | | | |
| **N** | **671** | **653** | **648** | **335** | **323** | **315** |
| Pain, any | 36.1 | 36.1 | 31.2 | 31.9 | 30.0 | 29.8 |
| Pain, grade 2 or 3 | 11.5 | 10.9 | 10.6 | 9.0 | 8.7 | 8.9 |
| Pain, grade 3 | 2.4 | 2.5 | 1.7 | 2.7 | 1.5 | 1.3 |
| Redness, any | 29.9§ | 37.2 | 40.1 | 18.2 | 32.8 | 39.0 |
| Redness, >5 mm | 6.0§ | 9.6§ | 12.7§ | 1.8 | 5.9 | 7.3 |
| Redness, >20 mm | 0.9 | 1.2§ | 2.8 | 0.3 | 0.0 | 1.9 |
| Swelling, any | 17.3§ | 26.5§ | 28.7 | 9.6 | 20.4 | 24.8 |
| Swelling, >5 mm | 5.8§ | 9.6§ | 9.3§ | 1.8 | 5.0 | 4.1 |
| Swelling, >20 mm | 1.9 | 2.5§ | 3.1 | 0.6 | 0.0 | 1.3 |
| **Systemic** | | | | | | |
| **N** | **667** | **644** | **645** | **333** | **321** | **311** |
| Fever‡, ≥100.4°F | 27.9§ | 38.8§ | 33.5§ | 19.8 | 30.2 | 23.8 |
| Fever‡, >101.3°F | 7.0 | 14.1§ | 8.8 | 4.5 | 9.7 | 5.8 |
| Fever‡, >102.2°F | 2.2§ | 3.6 | 3.4 | 0.3 | 3.1 | 2.3 |
| Fever‡, >103.1°F | 0.4 | 1.4 | 1.1 | 0.0 | 0.3 | 0.3 |
| Fever‡, M.A. | 1.2§ | 0.2 | 0.8 | 0.0 | 0.6 | 0.0 |
| **N** | **671** | **653** | **648** | **335** | **323** | **315** |
| Drowsiness, any | 57.2 | 51.6 | 40.9 | 54.0 | 48.3 | 38.4 |
| Drowsiness, grade 2 or 3 | 15.8 | 13.8 | 11.4 | 17.6 | 12.4 | 11.1 |
| Drowsiness, grade 3 | 2.5 | 1.2 | 0.9 | 3.6 | 0.6 | 1.9 |
| Irritability/Fussiness, any | 60.5 | 64.9 | 61.1 | 61.5 | 61.6 | 56.5 |
| Irritability/Fussiness, grade 2 or 3 | 19.8 | 27.9§ | 25.2§ | 19.4 | 21.1 | 19.4 |
| Irritability/Fussiness, grade 3 | 3.4 | 4.4 | 3.5 | 3.9 | 3.4 | 3.2 |
| Loss of appetite, any | 30.4 | 30.6 | 26.2 | 27.8 | 26.6 | 23.8 |
| Loss of appetite, grade 2 or 3 | 6.6 | 7.8§ | 5.9 | 5.1 | 3.4 | 5.4 |
| Loss of appetite, grade 3 | 0.7 | 0.3 | 0.2 | 0.6 | 0.3 | 0.0 |

Modified ITT cohort = all vaccinated subjects for whom safety data were available

N = number of infants for whom at least one symptom sheet was completed; for fever, numbers exclude missing temperature recordings or tympanic measurements.

M.A. = Medically attended (a visit to or from medical personnel).

Grade 2 defined as sufficiently discomforting to interfere with daily activities.

Grade 3 defined as preventing normal daily activities.

* Within 4 days of vaccination defined as day of vaccination and the next 3 days.

† Local reactions at the injection site for PEDIARIX or INFANRIX.

‡ Rectal temperatures or axillary temperatures increased by 1°C to derive equivalent rectal temperature.

§ Rate significantly higher in the group that received PEDIARIX compared to separately administered vaccines [p value < 0.05 (2-sided Fisher Exact test) or the 95% CI on the difference between groups (Separate minus PEDIARIX) does not include 0].

**Postmarketing Reports With PEDIARIX:** Worldwide voluntary reports of adverse events received for PEDIARIX since market introduction of this vaccine are listed below. This list includes serious adverse events or events which have a suspected causal connection to components of PEDIARIX or other vaccines or drugs. Because these events are reported voluntarily from a population of uncertain size, it is not always possible to reliably estimate their frequency or establish a causal relationship to vaccine exposure. *Cardiac Disorders:* Cyanosis. *Gastrointestinal Disorders:* Diarrhea, vomiting. *General Disorders and Administrative Site Conditions:* Fatigue, injection site cellulitis, injection site induration, injection site itching, injection site nodule/lump, injection site pain, injection site reactions, injection site redness, injection site swelling, injection site warmth, irritability, limb pain, limb swelling, pyrexia, Sudden Infant Death Syndrome. *Immune System Disorders:* Anaphylactic reaction, anaphylactoid reaction, hypersensitivity. *Infections and Infestations:* Upper respiratory tract infection. *Investigations:* Abnormal liver function tests. *Metabolism and Nutrition Disorders:* Anorexia. *Nervous System Disorders:* Bulging fontanelle, convulsions, depressed level of consciousness, febrile convulsion, hypotonia, hypotonic-hyporesponsive episode, lethargy, somnolence. *Psychiatric Disorders:* Crying, insomnia, irritability, nervousness, restlessness, screaming, unusual crying. *Respiratory, Thoracic and Mediastinal Disorders:* Apnea, dyspnea. *Skin and Subcutaneous Tissue Disorders:* Angioedema, erythema, rash, urticaria. *Vascular Disorders:* Pallor, petechiae.

**Postmarketing Reports With INFANRIX and/or ENGERIX-B:** Worldwide voluntary reports of adverse events received for INFANRIX and/or ENGERIX-B in children younger than 7 years of age but not already reported for PEDIARIX are listed below. This list includes serious adverse events or events which have a suspected causal connection to components of INFANRIX and/or ENGERIX-B or other vaccines or drugs. Because these events are reported voluntarily from a population of uncertain size, it is not always possible to reliably estimate their frequency or establish a causal relationship to vaccine exposure. *Blood and Lymphatic System Disorders:* Idiopathic thrombocytopenic purpura[a,b], lymphadenopathy[a], thrombocytopeni[a,b]. *Gastrointestinal Disorders:* Abdominal pain[b], intussusception[a,b], nausea[b]. *General Disorders and Administrative Site Conditions:* Asthenia[b], malaise[b]. *Hepatobiliary Disorders:* Jaundice[b]. *Immune System Disorders:* Anaphylactic shock[a], serum sickness–like disease[b]. *Musculoskeletal and Connective Tissue Disorders:* Arthralgia[b], myalgia[b]. *Nervous System Disorders:* Encephalopathy[a], headache[b]. *Skin and Subcutaneous Tissue Disorders:* Alopecia[b], erythema multiforme[b], pruritus[a,b], Stevens-Johnson syndrome[a]. [[a] Following INFANRIX; [b] Following ENGERIX-B]

**Reporting Adverse Events:** Report the occurrence following immunization of any event set forth in the Vaccine Injury Table from the National Childhood Vaccine Injury Act including: Anaphylaxis or anaphylactic shock within 7 days, encephalopathy or encephalitis within 7 days, brachial neuritis within 28 days, or an acute complication or sequelae (including death) of an illness, disability, injury, or condition referred to above, or any events that would contraindicate further doses of PEDIARIX. These events should be reported to VAERS. The VAERS toll-free number is 1-800-822-7967. Reporting forms may also be obtained at the VAERS website at www.vaers.hhs.gov.

Manufactured by **GlaxoSmithKline Biologicals**, Rixensart, Belgium, US License 1617

Distributed by **GlaxoSmithKline**, Research Triangle Park, NC 27709



Full prescribing information for PEDIARIX is available at www.GSKVaccines.com/Pediarix.

BRS-PE:L3

**References: 1.** Centers for Disease Control and Prevention. Pertussis Surveillance Report—2004 (final data). Issued 8/12/05. **2.** Centers for Disease Control and Prevention. *Epidemiology and Prevention of Vaccine-Preventable Diseases*. Reported Cases and Deaths from Vaccine Preventable Diseases, United States, 1950-2003. Available at http://www.cdc.gov/nip/publications/pink/appendices/G/cases&deaths.pdf. Accessed May 10, 2006. **3.** Centers for Disease Control and Prevention. *Epidemiology and Prevention of Vaccine-Preventable Diseases*. Atkinson W, Hamborsky J, McIntyre L, Wolfe S, eds. 9th ed. Washington, DC: Public Health Foundation;2006: 84. **4.** PEDIARIX Prescribing Information.


*Does not require reconstitution.

# ARCHIVES OF PEDIATRICS & ADOLESCENT MEDICINE

WWW.ARCHPEDIATRICS.COM

NOVEMBER 2006

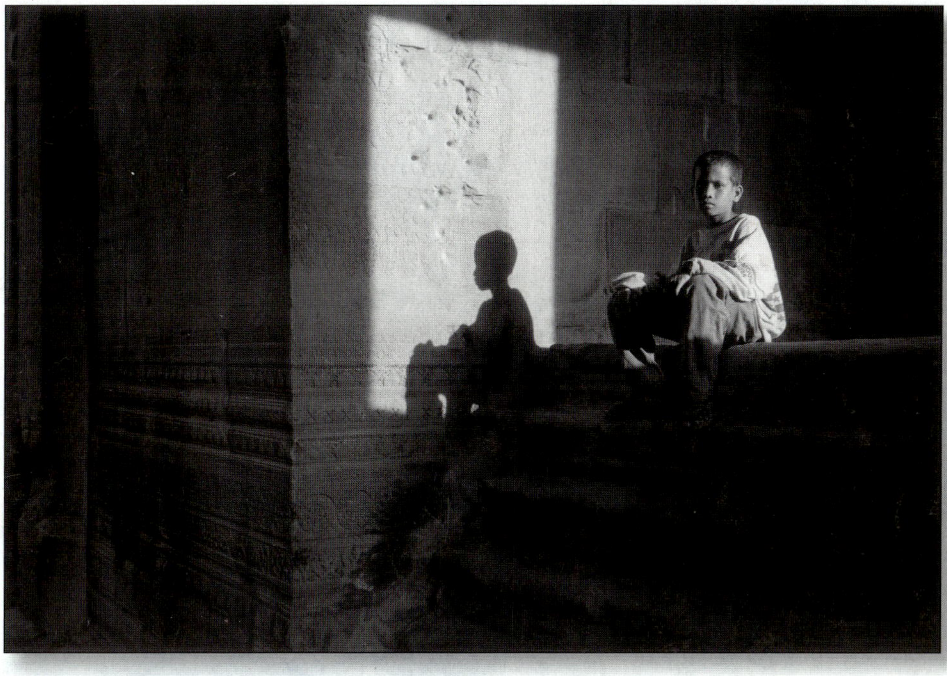

Boy sitting in temple in Angkor Wat, Cambodia, 2000. See page 1095.

PUBLIC OPINION ON SEX EDUCATION IN SCHOOLS

PARENTAL REACTIONS TO INFORMATION ABOUT GENETIC RISK FOR DIABETES IN THE NEWBORN

DOUBLE BURDEN OF IRON DEFICIENCY IN INFANCY AND LOW SOCIOECONOMIC STATUS

AUTISM: A REVIEW OF THE STATE OF THE SCIENCE

COMPLETE TABLE OF CONTENTS ON PAGE 1093



JAMA & ARCHIVES JOURNALS
American Medical Association

**References: 1.** Centers for Disease Control and Prevention. Pertussis Surveillance Report—2004 (final data). Issued 8/12/05. **2.** Centers for Disease Control and Prevention. *Epidemiology and Prevention of Vaccine-Preventable Diseases.* Reported Cases and Deaths from Vaccine Preventable Diseases, United States, 1950-2003. Available at http://www.cdc.gov/nip/publications/pink/appendices/G/cases&deaths.pdf. Accessed May 10, 2006. **3.** Centers for Disease Control and Prevention. *Epidemiology and Prevention of Vaccine-Preventable Diseases.* Atkinson W, Hamborsky J, McIntyre L, Wolfe S, eds. 9th ed. Washington, DC: Public Health Foundation;2006: 84. **4.** PEDIARIX Prescribing Information.

**PEDIARIX® [Diphtheria and Tetanus Toxoids and Acellular Pertussis Adsorbed, Hepatitis B (Recombinant) and Inactivated Poliovirus Vaccine Combined]**

The following is a brief summary only; see full prescribing information for complete product information.

**CONTRAINDICATIONS:** Hypersensitivity to any component of the vaccine, including yeast, neomycin, and polymyxin B, is a contraindication (see DESCRIPTION in complete prescribing information). Do not use PEDIARIX after a serious allergic reaction (e.g., anaphylaxis) temporally associated with a previous dose of this vaccine or with any components of this vaccine. Because of the uncertainty as to which component of the vaccine might be responsible, do not give further vaccination with any of these components; or, refer such individuals to an allergist for evaluation. The following events are contraindications to administration of PEDIARIX: encephalopathy (e.g., coma, decreased level of consciousness, prolonged seizures) within 7 days of administration of a previous dose of a pertussis-containing vaccine that is not attributable to another identifiable cause; progressive neurologic disorder, including infantile spasms, uncontrolled epilepsy, or progressive encephalopathy. Do not vaccinate individuals with these conditions until a treatment regimen has been established and the condition has stabilized.

**WARNINGS:** Administration of PEDIARIX is associated with higher rates of fever relative to separately administered vaccines. In a safety study that evaluated medically attended fever after PEDIARIX or separately administered vaccines when coadministered with 7-valent pneumococcal and Hib conjugate vaccines, infants who received PEDIARIX had a higher rate of medical encounters for fever within the first 4 days following the first vaccination. In some infants, these encounters included the performance of diagnostic studies to evaluate other causes of fever (see ADVERSE REACTIONS). The tip cap and the rubber plunger of the needleless prefilled syringes contain dry natural latex rubber that may cause allergic reactions in latex sensitive individuals. The vial stopper is latex-free. If any of the following events occur in temporal relation to receipt of DTwP or a vaccine containing an acellular pertussis component, consider carefully whether to give any pertussis vaccine, including PEDIARIX: temperature of ≥40.5°C (105°F) within 48 hours not due to another identifiable cause; collapse or shock-like state (hypotonic-hyporesponsive episode) within 48 hours; persistent, inconsolable crying lasting ≥3 hours, occurring within 48 hours; seizures with or without fever occurring within 3 days. If Guillain-Barré syndrome occurs within 6 weeks of receipt of prior vaccine containing tetanus toxoid, the decision to give any tetanus toxoid-containing vaccine, including PEDIARIX, should be based on careful consideration of the potential benefits and possible risks. If tetanus toxoid is withheld, other available vaccines should be given, as indicated. The decision to administer a pertussis-containing vaccine to individuals with stable central nervous system (CNS) disorders must be made by the physician on an individual basis, with consideration of all relevant factors, and assessment of potential risks and benefits for that individual. Advise the parent or guardian of the potential increased risk involved (see PRECAUTIONS). For children at higher risk for seizures than the general population, an appropriate antipyretic may be administered at the time of vaccination and for the ensuing 24 hours according to the respective prescribing information recommended dosage to reduce the possibility of post-vaccination fever. The ACIP has published guidelines for vaccination of persons with recent or acute illness (www.cdc.gov/nip).

**PRECAUTIONS:** PEDIARIX should be given with caution in children with bleeding disorders such as hemophilia or thrombocytopenia and in children on anticoagulant therapy, with steps taken to avoid the risk of hematoma following the injection. Before the injection of any biological, the physician should take all reasonable precautions to prevent allergic or other adverse reactions. Epinephrine injection (1:1,000) and other appropriate agents used for the control of immediate allergic reactions must be immediately available should an acute anaphylactic reaction occur. Immunosuppressed individuals, including those receiving immunosuppressive therapy, may not develop the expected immune response. The ACIP has published guidelines for vaccination of persons on such therapies (www.cdc.gov/nip). **Drug Interactions:** For information regarding concomitant administration with other vaccines, refer to DOSAGE AND ADMINISTRATION in complete prescribing information. Do not mix PEDIARIX with any other vaccine in the same syringe or vial. **Carcinogenesis, Mutagenesis, Impairment of Fertility:** PEDIARIX has not been evaluated for carcinogenic or mutagenic potential, or for impairment of fertility. **Pregnancy:** Pregnancy Category C: PEDIARIX is not indicated for women of child-bearing age. Animal reproduction studies have not been conducted with PEDIARIX. It is not known whether PEDIARIX can cause fetal harm when administered to a pregnant woman or if PEDIARIX can affect reproductive capacity. **Geriatric Use:** PEDIARIX is not indicated for use in adult populations. **Pediatric Use:** Safety and effectiveness of PEDIARIX in infants younger than 6 weeks of age have not been evaluated. PEDIARIX is not recommended for persons 7 years of age or older.

**ADVERSE REACTIONS:** A total of 23,849 doses of PEDIARIX have been administered to 8,088 infants who received one or more doses as part of a 3-dose primary series during 14 clinical studies. The most common adverse reactions observed in clinical trials were local injection site reactions (pain, redness, or swelling), fever, and fussiness. In comparative studies, administration of PEDIARIX was associated with higher rates of fever relative to separately administered vaccines (see WARNINGS and ADVERSE REACTIONS Table 1). The prevalence of fever was highest on the day of vaccination and the day following vaccination. More than 96% of episodes of fever resolved within the 4-day period following vaccination (i.e., the period including the day of vaccination and the next 3 days). In the largest of the 14 studies, conducted in Germany, safety data were provided for 4,666 infants who received PEDIARIX administered concomitantly at separate sites with 1 of 4 *Haemophilus influenzae* type b (Hib) vaccines at 3, 4, and 5 months of age and for 768 infants in the control group that received INFANRIX® (Diphtheria and Tetanus Toxoids and Acellular Pertussis Vaccine Adsorbed), Hib conjugate vaccine, and oral poliovirus vaccine (OPV) separately. Data on adverse events were collected by parents using standardized diary cards for 4 consecutive days following each vaccine dose (i.e., day of vaccination and the next 3 days). Infants were also monitored for unsolicited adverse events that occurred within 30 days following vaccination using diaries which were returned at subsequent visits and were supplemented by spontaneous reports and a medical history as reported by parents. More than 95% of study participants were white.

In a US study, the safety of PEDIARIX administered to 673 infants was compared to the safety of separately administered INFANRIX, ENGERIX-B® [Hepatitis B Vaccine (Recombinant)], inactivated poliovirus vaccine (IPV) in 335 infants. In both groups, infants received Hib and 7-valent pneumococcal conjugate vaccines concomitantly at separate sites. All vaccines were administered at 2, 4, and 6 months of age. The study was powered to evaluate fever >101.3° F following dose 1. Data on solicited adverse events were collected by parents using standardized diary cards for 4 consecutive days following each vaccine dose (i.e., day of vaccination and the next 3 days) and are presented in Table 1. Telephone follow-up was conducted 1 month and 6 months after the third vaccination to inquire about serious adverse events. At the 6-month follow-up, information also was collected on new onset of chronic illnesses. 638 subjects who received PEDIARIX and 313 subjects who received INFANRIX, ENGERIX-B, and IPV completed the 6-month follow-up. Among subjects in both study groups combined, 69% were white, 18% were Hispanic, 7% were black, 3% were Oriental, and 3% were of other racial/ethnic groups.

The adverse event information from clinical trials provides a basis for identifying adverse events that appear to be related to vaccine use and for approximating rates. However, because clinical trials are conducted under widely varying conditions, adverse event rates observed in the clinical trials of a vaccine cannot be directly compared to rates in the clinical trials of another vaccine, and may not reflect the rates observed in practice. As with any vaccine, there is the possibility that broad use of PEDIARIX could reveal adverse events not observed in clinical trials.

**Deaths:** In 14 clinical trials, 5 deaths were reported among 8,088 (0.06%) recipients of PEDIARIX and 1 death was reported among 2,287 (0.04%) recipients of comparator vaccines. Causes of death in the group that received PEDIARIX included 2 cases of Sudden Infant Death Syndrome (SIDS) and one case of each of the following: Convulsive disorder, congenital immunodeficiency with sepsis, and neuroblastoma. One case of SIDS was reported in the comparator group. The rate of SIDS among all recipients of PEDIARIX across the 14 trials was 0.25/1,000. The rate of SIDS observed for recipients of PEDIARIX in the German safety study was 0.2/1,000 infants (reported rate of SIDS in Germany in the latter part of the 1990s was 0.7/1,000 newborns). The reported rate of SIDS in the United States from 1990 to 1994 was 1.2/1,000 live births. By chance alone, some cases of SIDS can be expected to follow receipt of pertussis-containing vaccines.

**Serious Adverse Events:** Within 30 days following any dose of vaccine in the US safety study in which all subjects received concomitant pneumococcal and Hib conjugate vaccines, 7 serious adverse events were reported in 7 subjects (1% [7/673]) who received PEDIARIX (1 case each of pyrexia, gastroenteritis, and culture negative clinical sepsis and 4 cases of bronchiolitis) and 5 serious adverse events were reported in 4 subjects (1% [4/335]) who received INFANRIX, ENGERIX-B, and IPV (uteropelvic junction obstruction and testicular atrophy in one subject and 3 cases of bronchiolitis).

**Onset of Chronic Illnesses:** In the US safety study in which all subjects received concomitant pneumococcal and Hib conjugate vaccines, 21 subjects (3%) who received PEDIARIX and 14 subjects (4%) who received INFANRIX, ENGERIX-B, and IPV reported new onset of a chronic illness during the period from 1 to 6 months following the last dose of study vaccines. Among the chronic illnesses reported in the subjects who received PEDIARIX, there were 4 cases of asthma and 1 case each of diabetes mellitus and chronic neutropenia. There were 4 cases of asthma in subjects who received INFANRIX, ENGERIX-B, and IPV.

**Seizures:** In the German safety study over the entire study period, 6 subjects in the group that received PEDIARIX reported seizures. Two of these subjects had a febrile seizure, 1 of whom also developed afebrile seizures. The remaining 4 subjects had afebrile seizures, including 2 with infantile spasms. Two subjects reported seizures within 7 days following vaccination (1 subject had both febrile and afebrile seizures, and 1 subject had afebrile seizures), corresponding to a rate of 0.22 seizures per 1,000 doses (febrile seizures 0.07 per 1,000 doses, afebrile seizures 0.14 per 1,000 doses). No subject who received concomitant INFANRIX, Hib vaccine, and OPV reported seizures. In a separate German study that evaluated the safety of INFANRIX in 22,505 infants who received 66,867 doses of INFANRIX administered as a 3-dose primary series, the rate of seizures within 7 days of vaccination with INFANRIX was 0.13 per 1,000 doses (febrile seizures 0.0 per 1,000 doses, afebrile seizures 0.13 per 1,000 doses). Over the entire study period in the US safety study in which all subjects received concomitant pneumococcal and Hib conjugate vaccines, 4 subjects in the group that received PEDIARIX reported seizures. Three of these subjects had a febrile seizure and 1 had an afebrile seizure. Over the entire study period, 2 subjects in the group that received INFANRIX, ENGERIX-B, and IPV reported febrile seizures. There were no afebrile seizures in this group. No subject in either study group had seizures within 7 days following vaccination.

**Other Neurological Events of Interest:** No cases of hypotonic-hyporesponsiveness or encephalopathy were reported in either the German safety study or the US safety study.

**Solicited Adverse Events:** Table 1 presents data from the US safety study on solicited local and systemic adverse events within 4 days of vaccination with PEDIARIX or INFANRIX, ENGERIX-B, and IPV, administered concomitantly with Hib and 7-valent pneumococcal conjugate vaccines. In this study, medical attention (a visit to or from medical personnel) for fever within 4 days following vaccination was sought in the group who received PEDIARIX for 8 infants after the first dose (1.2%), 1 infant following the second dose (0.2%), and 5 infants following the third dose (0.8%) (Table 1). Following dose 2, medical attention for fever was sought for 2 infants (0.6%) who received separately administered vaccines (Table 1). Among infants who had a medical visit for fever within 4 days following vaccination, 9 of 14 who received PEDIARIX and 1 of 2 who received separately administered vaccines, had one or more diagnostic studies performed to evaluate the cause of fever.

**Safety of PEDIARIX after a previous dose of hepatitis B vaccine:** Limited data are available on the safety of administering PEDIARIX after a previous dose of hepatitis B vaccine. In 2 separate studies, 160 Moldovan infants and 96 US infants, respectively, received 3 doses of PEDIARIX following 1 previous dose of hepatitis B vaccine. Neither study was designed to detect significant differences in rates of adverse events associated with PEDIARIX administered after a previous dose of hepatitis B vaccine compared to PEDIARIX administered without a previous dose of hepatitis B vaccine.

**Table 1. Percentage of US Infants With Solicited Local Reactions or Systemic Adverse Events Within 4 Days of Vaccination* at 2, 4, and 6 Months of Age With PEDIARIX Administered Concomitantly With Hib Conjugate Vaccine and 7-valent Pneumococcal Conjugate Vaccine (PCV7) or With Separate Concomitant Administration of INFANRIX, ENGERIX-B, IPV, Hib Conjugate Vaccine, and PCV7 (Modified ITT cohort)**

| | PEDIARIX, Hib Vaccine, & PCV7 | | | INFANRIX, ENGERIX-B, IPV, Hib Vaccine, & PCV7 | | |
|---|---|---|---|---|---|---|
| | **Dose 1** | **Dose 2** | **Dose 3** | **Dose 1** | **Dose 2** | **Dose 3** |
| **Local†** | | | | | | |
| **N** | **671** | **653** | **648** | **335** | **323** | **315** |
| Pain, any | 36.1 | 36.1 | 31.2 | 31.9 | 30.0 | 29.8 |
| Pain, grade 2 or 3 | 11.5 | 10.9 | 10.6 | 9.0 | 8.7 | 8.9 |
| Pain, grade 3 | 2.4 | 2.5 | 1.7 | 2.7 | 1.5 | 1.3 |
| Redness, any | 29.9§ | 37.2 | 40.1 | 18.2 | 32.8 | 39.0 |
| Redness, >5 mm | 6.0§ | 9.6§ | 12.7§ | 1.8 | 5.9 | 7.3 |
| Redness, >20 mm | 0.9 | 1.2§ | 2.8 | 0.3 | 0.0 | 1.9 |
| Swelling, any | 17.3§ | 26.5§ | 28.7 | 9.6 | 20.4 | 24.8 |
| Swelling, >5 mm | 5.8§ | 9.6§ | 9.3§ | 1.8 | 5.0 | 4.1 |
| Swelling, >20 mm | 1.9 | 2.5§ | 3.1 | 0.6 | 0.0 | 1.3 |
| **Systemic** | | | | | | |
| **N** | **667** | **644** | **645** | **333** | **321** | **311** |
| Fever‡, ≥100.4°F | 27.9§ | 38.8§ | 33.5§ | 19.8 | 30.2 | 23.8 |
| Fever‡, >101.3°F | 7.0 | 14.1§ | 8.8 | 4.5 | 9.7 | 5.8 |
| Fever‡, >102.2°F | 2.2§ | 3.6 | 3.4 | 0.3 | 3.1 | 2.3 |
| Fever‡, >103.1°F | 0.4 | 1.4 | 1.1 | 0.0 | 0.3 | 0.3 |
| Fever‡, M.A. | 1.2§ | 0.2 | 0.8 | 0.0 | 0.6 | 0.0 |
| **N** | **671** | **653** | **648** | **335** | **323** | **315** |
| Drowsiness, any | 57.2 | 51.6 | 40.9 | 54.0 | 48.3 | 38.4 |
| Drowsiness, grade 2 or 3 | 15.8 | 13.8 | 11.4 | 17.6 | 12.4 | 11.1 |
| Drowsiness, grade 3 | 2.5 | 1.2 | 0.9 | 3.6 | 0.6 | 1.9 |
| Irritability/Fussiness, any | 60.5 | 64.9 | 61.1 | 61.5 | 61.6 | 56.5 |
| Irritability/Fussiness, grade 2 or 3 | 19.8 | 27.9§ | 25.2§ | 19.4 | 21.1 | 19.4 |
| Irritability/Fussiness, grade 3 | 3.4 | 4.4 | 3.5 | 3.9 | 3.4 | 3.2 |
| Loss of appetite, any | 30.4 | 30.6 | 26.2 | 27.8 | 26.6 | 23.8 |
| Loss of appetite, grade 2 or 3 | 6.6 | 7.8§ | 5.9 | 5.1 | 3.4 | 5.4 |
| Loss of appetite, grade 3 | 0.7 | 0.3 | 0.2 | 0.6 | 0.3 | 0.0 |

Modified ITT cohort = all vaccinated subjects for whom safety data were available
N = number of infants for whom at least one symptom sheet was completed; for fever, numbers exclude missing temperature recordings or tympanic measurements.
M.A. = Medically attended (a visit to or from medical personnel).
Grade 2 defined as sufficiently discomforting to interfere with daily activities.
Grade 3 defined as preventing normal daily activities.
* Within 4 days of vaccination defined as day of vaccination and the next 3 days.
† Local reactions at the injection site for PEDIARIX or INFANRIX.
‡ Rectal temperatures or axillary temperatures increased by 1°C to derive equivalent rectal temperature.
§ Rate significantly higher in the group that received PEDIARIX compared to separately administered vaccines [p value < 0.05 (2-sided Fisher Exact test) or the 95% CI on the difference between groups (Separate minus PEDIARIX) does not include 0].

**Postmarketing Reports With PEDIARIX:** Worldwide voluntary reports of adverse events received for PEDIARIX since market introduction of this vaccine are listed below. This list includes serious adverse events or events which have a suspected causal connection to components of PEDIARIX or other vaccines or drugs. Because these events are reported voluntarily from a population of uncertain size, it is not always possible to reliably estimate their frequency or establish a causal relationship to vaccine exposure. *Cardiac Disorders:* Cyanosis. *Gastrointestinal Disorders:* Diarrhea, vomiting. *General Disorders and Administrative Site Conditions:* Fatigue, injection site cellulitis, injection site induration, injection site itching, injection site nodule/lump, injection site pain, injection site reactions, injection site redness, injection site swelling, injection site warmth, irritability, limb pain, limb swelling, pyrexia, Sudden Infant Death Syndrome. *Immune System Disorders:* Anaphylactic reaction, anaphylactoid reaction, hypersensitivity. *Infections and Infestations:* Upper respiratory tract infection. *Investigations:* Abnormal liver function tests. *Metabolism and Nutrition Disorders:* Anorexia. *Nervous System Disorders:* Bulging fontanelle, convulsions, depressed level of consciousness, febrile convulsion, hypotonia, hypotonic-hyporesponsive episode, lethargy, somnolence. *Psychiatric Disorders:* Crying, insomnia, irritability, nervousness, restlessness, screaming, unusual crying. *Respiratory, Thoracic and Mediastinal Disorders:* Apnea, dyspnea. *Skin and Subcutaneous Tissue Disorders:* Angioedema, erythema, rash, urticaria. *Vascular Disorders:* Pallor, petechiae.

**Postmarketing Reports With INFANRIX and/or ENGERIX-B:** Worldwide voluntary reports of adverse events received for INFANRIX and/or ENGERIX-B in children younger than 7 years of age but not already reported for PEDIARIX are listed below. This list includes serious adverse events or events which have a suspected causal connection to components of INFANRIX and/or ENGERIX-B or other vaccines or drugs. Because these events are reported voluntarily from a population of uncertain size, it is not always possible to reliably estimate their frequency or establish a causal relationship to vaccine exposure. *Blood and Lymphatic System Disorders:* Idiopathic thrombocytopenic purpura[a,b], lymphadenopathy[a], thrombocytopeni[a,b]. *Gastrointestinal Disorders:* Abdominal pain[b], intussusception[a,b], nausea[b]. *General Disorders and Administrative Site Conditions:* Asthenia[b], malaise[b]. *Hepatobiliary Disorders:* Jaundice[b]. *Immune System Disorders:* Anaphylactic shock[a], serum sickness–like disease[b]. *Musculoskeletal and Connective Tissue Disorders:* Arthralgia[b], myalgia[b]. *Nervous System Disorders:* Encephalopathy[a], headache[b]. *Skin and Subcutaneous Tissue Disorders:* Alopecia[b], erythema multiforme[b], pruritus[a,b], Stevens-Johnson syndrome[a]. [[a] Following INFANRIX; [b] Following ENGERIX-B]

**Reporting Adverse Events:** Report the occurrence following immunization of any event set forth in the Vaccine Injury Table from the National Childhood Vaccine Injury Act including: Anaphylaxis or anaphylactic shock within 7 days, encephalopathy or encephalitis within 7 days, brachial neuritis within 28 days, or an acute complication or sequelae (including death) of an illness, disability, injury, or condition referred to above, or any events that would contraindicate further doses of PEDIARIX. These events should be reported to VAERS. The VAERS toll-free number is 1-800-822-7967. Reporting forms may also be obtained at the VAERS website at www.vaers.hhs.gov.

Manufactured by **GlaxoSmithKline Biologicals**, Rixensart, Belgium, US License 1617

Distributed by **GlaxoSmithKline,** Research Triangle Park, NC 27709



Full prescribing information for PEDIARIX is available at www.GSKVaccines.com/Pediarix.

BRS-PE:L3

**Orapred ODT™**
(prednisolone sodium phosphate orally disintegrating tablets)

**BRIEF SUMMARY:** Please see full prescribing information.

**DESCRIPTION:**
Orapred ODT orally disintegrating tablets are available in strengths containing 13.4 mg, 20.2 mg, and 40.3 mg prednisolone sodium phosphate (equivalent to 10 mg, 15 mg, or 30 mg prednisolone base, respectively).
**PRECAUTIONS: General: Do not break or use partial Orapred ODT tablets.** The lowest possible dose of corticosteroid should be used to control the condition under treatment, and when reduction in dosage is possible, the reduction should be gradual.
Since complications of treatment with glucocorticoids are dependent on the size of the dose and the duration of treatment, a risk/benefit decision must be made in each individual case as to dose and duration of treatment and as to whether daily or intermittent therapy should be used.
There is an enhanced effect of corticosteroids in patients with hypothyroidism and in those with cirrhosis
Kaposi's sarcoma has been reported to occur in patients receiving corticosteroid therapy, most often for chronic conditions. Discontinuation of corticosteroids may result in clinical improvement.
**Cardio-renal:** As sodium retention with resultant edema and potassium loss may occur in patients receiving corticosteroids, these agents should be used with caution in patients with hypertension, congestive heart failure, or renal insufficiency.
**Endocrine:** Drug-induced secondary adrenocortical insufficiency may be minimized by gradual reduction of dosage. This type of relative insufficiency may persist for months after discontinuation of therapy; therefore, in any situation of stress occurring during that period, hormone therapy should be reinstituted. Since mineralocorticoid secretion may be impaired, salt and/or a mineralocorticoid should be administered concurrently.
**Gastrointestinal:** Steroids should be used with caution in nonspecific ulcerative colitis, if there is a probability of impending perforation, abscess or other pyogenic infection;
diverticulitis; fresh intestinal anastomoses; active or latent peptic ulcer. Signs of peritoneal irritation following gastrointestinal perforation in patients receiving corticosteroids may be minimal or absent.
**Musculoskeletal:** Corticosteroids decrease bone formation and increase bone resorption both through their effect on calcium regulation (i.e., decreasing absorption and increasing excretion) and inhibition of osteoblast function. This, together with a decrease in the protein matrix of the bone secondary to an increase in protein catabolism, and reduced sex hormone production, may lead to inhibition of bone growth in children and adolescents and the development of osteoporosis at any age. Special consideration should be given to patients at increased risk of osteoporosis (i.e., postmenopausal women) before initiating corticosteroid therapy.
**Neuro-psychiatric:** Although controlled clinical trials have shown corticosteroids to be effective in speeding the resolution of acute exacerbations of multiple sclerosis, they do not show that they affect the ultimate outcome or natural history of the disease. The studies do show that relatively high doses of corticosteroids are necessary to demonstrate a significant effect. (See DOSAGE AND ADMINISTRATION.)
An acute myopathy has been observed with the use of high doses of corticosteroids, most often occurring in patients with disorders of neuromuscular transmission (e.g., myasthenia gravis), or in patients receiving concomitant therapy with neuromuscular blocking drugs (e.g., pancuronium). This acute myopathy is generalized, may involve ocular and respiratory muscles, and may result in quadriparesis. Elevation of creatinine kinase may occur. Clinical improvement or recovery after stopping corticosteroids may require weeks to years.
Psychic derangements may appear when corticosteroids are used, ranging from euphoria, insomnia, mood swings, personality changes, and severe depression, to frank psychotic manifestations. Also, existing emotional instability or psychotic tendencies may be aggravated by corticosteroids.
**Ophthalmic:** Intraocular pressure may become elevated in some individuals. If steroid therapy is continued for more than 6 weeks, intraocular pressure should be monitored.
**Information For Patients:** Patients should be warned not to discontinue the use of Orapred abruptly or without medical supervision, to advise any medical attendants that they are taking it, and to seek medical advice at once should they develop fever or other signs of infection. Persons who are on immunosuppressant doses of corticosteroids should be warned to avoid exposure to chickenpox or measles. Patients should also be advised that if they are exposed, medical advice should be sought without delay.
**Drug Interactions:** Drugs such as barbiturates, phenytoin, ephedrine, and rifampin, which induce hepatic microsomal drug metabolizing enzyme activity may enhance metabolism of prednisolone and require that the dosage of Orapred be increased.
Increased activity of both cyclosporin and corticosteroids may occur when the two are used concurrently. Convulsions have been reported with this concurrent use.
Estrogens may decrease the hepatic metabolism of certain corticosteroids thereby increasing their effect.
Ketoconazole has been reported to decrease the metabolism of certain corticosteroids by up to 60% leading to an increased risk of corticosteroid side effects.
Coadministration of corticosteroids and warfarin usually results in inhibition of response to warfarin, although there have been some conflicting reports. Therefore, coagulation indices should be monitored frequently to maintain the desired anticoagulant effect.
Concomitant use of aspirin (or other non-steroidal anti-inflammatory agents) and corticosteroids increases the risk of gastrointestinal side effects. Aspirin should be used cautiously in conjunction with corticosteroids in hypoprothrombinemia. The clearance of salicylates may be increased with concurrent use of corticosteroids. When corticosteroids are administered concomitantly with potassium-depleting agents (i.e., diuretics, amphotericin-B), patients should be observed closely for development of
hypokalemia. Patients on digitalis glycosides may be at increased risk of arrhythmias due to hypokalemia.
Concomitant use of anticholinesterase agents and corticosteroids may produce severe weakness in patients with myasthenia gravis. If possible, anticholinesterase agents should be withdrawn at least 24 hours before initiating corticosteroid therapy.
Due to inhibition of antibody response, patients on prolonged corticosteroid therapy may exhibit a diminished response to toxoids and live or inactivated vaccines. Corticosteroids may also potentiate the replication of some organisms contained in live attenuated vaccines. If possible, routine administration of vaccines or toxoids should be deferred until corticosteroid therapy is discontinued.
Because corticosteroids may increase blood glucose concentrations, dosage adjustments of antidiabetic agents may be required.
Corticosteroids may suppress reactions to skin tests.
**Pregnancy: Teratogenic Effects:** *Pregnancy Category C.*
Prednisolone has been shown to be teratogenic in many species when given in doses equivalent to the human dose. Animal studies in which prednisolone has been given to pregnant mice, rats, and rabbits have yielded an increased incidence of cleft palate in the offspring. There are no adequate and well-controlled studies in pregnant women. Orapred should be used during pregnancy only if the potential benefit justifies the potential risk to the fetus. Infants born to mothers who have received corticosteroids during pregnancy should be carefully observed for signs of hypoadrenalism.
**Nursing Mothers:** Systemically administered corticosteroids appear in human milk and could suppress growth, interfere with endogenous corticosteroid production, or cause other untoward effects. Caution should be exercised when Orapred is administered to a nursing woman.
**Pediatric Use:** The efficacy and safety of prednisolone in the pediatric population are based on the well-established course of effect of corticosteroids, which is similar in pediatric and adult populations. Published studies provide evidence of efficacy and safety in pediatric patients for the treatment of nephrotic syndrome (>2 years of age), and aggressive lymphomas and leukemias (>1 month of age). However, some of these conclusions and other indications for pediatric use of corticosteroid, e.g., severe asthma and wheezing, are based on adequate and well-controlled trials conducted in adults, on the premises that the course of the diseases and their pathophysiology are considered to be substantially similar in both populations.
The adverse effects of prednisolone in pediatric patients are similar to those in adults (see ADVERSE REACTIONS). Like adults, pediatric patients should be carefully observed with frequent measurements of blood pressure, weight, height, intraocular pressure, and clinical evaluation for the presence of infection, psychosocial disturbances, thromboembolism, peptic ulcers, cataracts, and osteoporosis. Children, who are treated with corticosteroids by any route, including systemically administered corticosteroids, may experience a decrease in their growth velocity. This negative impact of corticosteroids on growth has been observed at low systemic doses and in the absence of laboratory evidence of HPA axis suppression (i.e., cosyntropin stimulation and basal cortisol plasma levels). Growth velocity may therefore be a more sensitive indicator of systemic corticosteroid exposure in children than some commonly used tests of HPA axis function. The linear growth of children treated with corticosteroids by any route should be monitored, and the potential growth effects of prolonged treatment should be weighed against clinical benefits obtained and the availability of other treatment alternatives. In order to minimize the potential growth effects of corticosteroids, children should be *titrated* to the lowest effective dose.
**Geriatric Use:** Clinical studies of prednisolone sodium phosphate oral solution did not include sufficient numbers of subjects aged 65 and over to determine whether they respond differently from younger subjects. Other reported clinical experience with prednisolone sodium phosphate has not identified differences in responses between the elderly and younger patients. However, the incidence of corticosteroid-induced side effects may be increased in geriatric patients and appear to be dose-related. Osteoporosis is the most frequently encountered complication, which occurs at a higher incidence rate in corticosteroid-treated geriatric patients as compared to younger populations and in agematched controls. Losses of bone mineral density appear to be greatest early on in the course of treatment and may recover over time after steroid withdrawal or use of lower doses (i.e., 5 mg/day). Prednisolone doses of 7.5 mg/day or higher, have been associated with an increased relative risk of both vertebral and nonvertebral fractures, even in the presence of higher bone density compared to patients with involutional osteoporosis.
Routine screening of geriatric patients, including regular assessments of bone mineral density and institution of fracture prevention strategies, along with regular review of Orapred indication should be undertaken to minimize complications and keep the Orapred dose at the lowest acceptable level. Co-administration of bisphosphonates has been shown to retard the rate of bone loss in corticosteroid-treated males and postmenopausal females, and these agents are recommended in the prevention and treatment of corticosteroid-induced osteoporosis.
It has been reported that equivalent weight-based doses yield higher total and unbound prednisolone plasma concentrations and reduced renal and non-renal clearance in elderly patients compared to younger populations. However, it is not clear whether dosing reductions would be necessary in elderly patients, since these pharmacokinetic alterations may be offset by age-related differences in responsiveness of target organs and/or less pronounced suppression of adrenal release of cortisol. Dose selection for an elderly patient should be cautious, usually starting at the low end of the dosing range, reflecting the greater frequency of decreased hepatic, renal, or cardiac function, and of concomitant disease or other drug therapy.
This drug is known to be substantially excreted by the kidney, and the risk of toxic reactions to this drug may be greater in patients with impaired renal function. Because elderly patients are more likely to have decreased renal function, care should be taken in dose selection, and it may be useful to monitor renal function (see CLINICAL PHARMACOLOGY).
**ADVERSE REACTIONS: (listed alphabetically under each subsection):**
**Cardiovascular:** Hypertrophic cardiomyopathy in premature infants.
**Dermatologic:** Facial erythema; increased sweating; impaired wound healing; may suppress reactions to skin tests; petechiae and ecchymoses; thin fragile skin; urticaria; edema.
**Endocrine:** Decreased carbohydrate tolerance; development of cushingoid state; hirsutism; increased requirements for insulin or oral hypoglycemic agents in diabetic patients; manifestations of latent diabetes mellitus; menstrual irregularities; secondary adrenocortical and pituitary unresponsiveness, particularly in times of stress, as in trauma, surgery or illness; suppression of growth in children.
**Fluid and Electrolyte Disturbances:** Congestive heart failure in susceptible patients; fluid retention; hypertension; hypokalemic alkalosis; potassium loss; sodium retention.
**Gastrointestinal:** Abdominal distention; elevation in serum liver enzyme levels (usually reversible upon discontinuation); pancreatitis; peptic ulcer with possible perforation and hemorrhage; ulcerative esophagitis.
**Metabolic:** Negative nitrogen balance due to protein catabolism.
**Musculoskeletal:** Aseptic necrosis of femoral and humeral heads; loss of muscle mass; muscle weakness; osteoporosis; pathologic fracture of long bones; steroid myopathy; tendon rupture; vertebral compression fractures.
**Neurological:** Convulsions; headache; increased intracranial pressure with papilledema
(pseudotumor cerebri) usually following discontinuation of treatment; psychic disorders; vertigo.
**Ophthalmic:** Exophthalmos; glaucoma; increased intraocular pressure; posterior subcapsular cataracts.
**Other:** Increased appetite; malaise; nausea; weight gain.
In clinical trials with ORAPRED ODT, the following adverse reactions were seen.
Facial edema, pharyngolaryngeal pain, blood in stool, eye irritation, eyelid edema.
**OVERDOSAGE:** The effects of accidental ingestion of large quantities of prednisolone over a very short period of time have not been reported, but prolonged use of the drug can produce mental symptoms, moon face, abnormal fat deposits, fluid retention, excessive appetite, weight gain, hypertrichosis, acne, striae, ecchymosis, increased sweating, pigmentation, dry scaly skin, thinning scalp hair, increased blood pressure, tachycardia, thrombophlebitis, decreased resistance to infection, negative nitrogen balance with delayed bone and wound healing, headache, weakness, menstrual disorders, accentuated menopausal symptoms, neuropathy, fractures, osteoporosis, peptic ulcer, decreased glucose tolerance, hypokalemia, and adrenal insufficiency. Hepatomegaly and abdominal distention have been observed in children.

Treatment of acute overdosage is by immediate gastric lavage or emesis followed by supportive and symptomatic therapy. For chronic overdosage in the face of severe disease requiring continuous steroid therapy, the dosage of prednisolone may be reduced only temporarily, or alternate day treatment may be introduced.

**Do not break or use partial Orapred ODT tablets.** Keep out of the reach of children.

**Rx only**
Revised May 2006.

Manufactured for Alliant Pharmaceuticals, Inc.
Alpharetta, GA 30022

by CIMA LABS INC., Eden Prairie, MN 55344 (Orapred ODT)

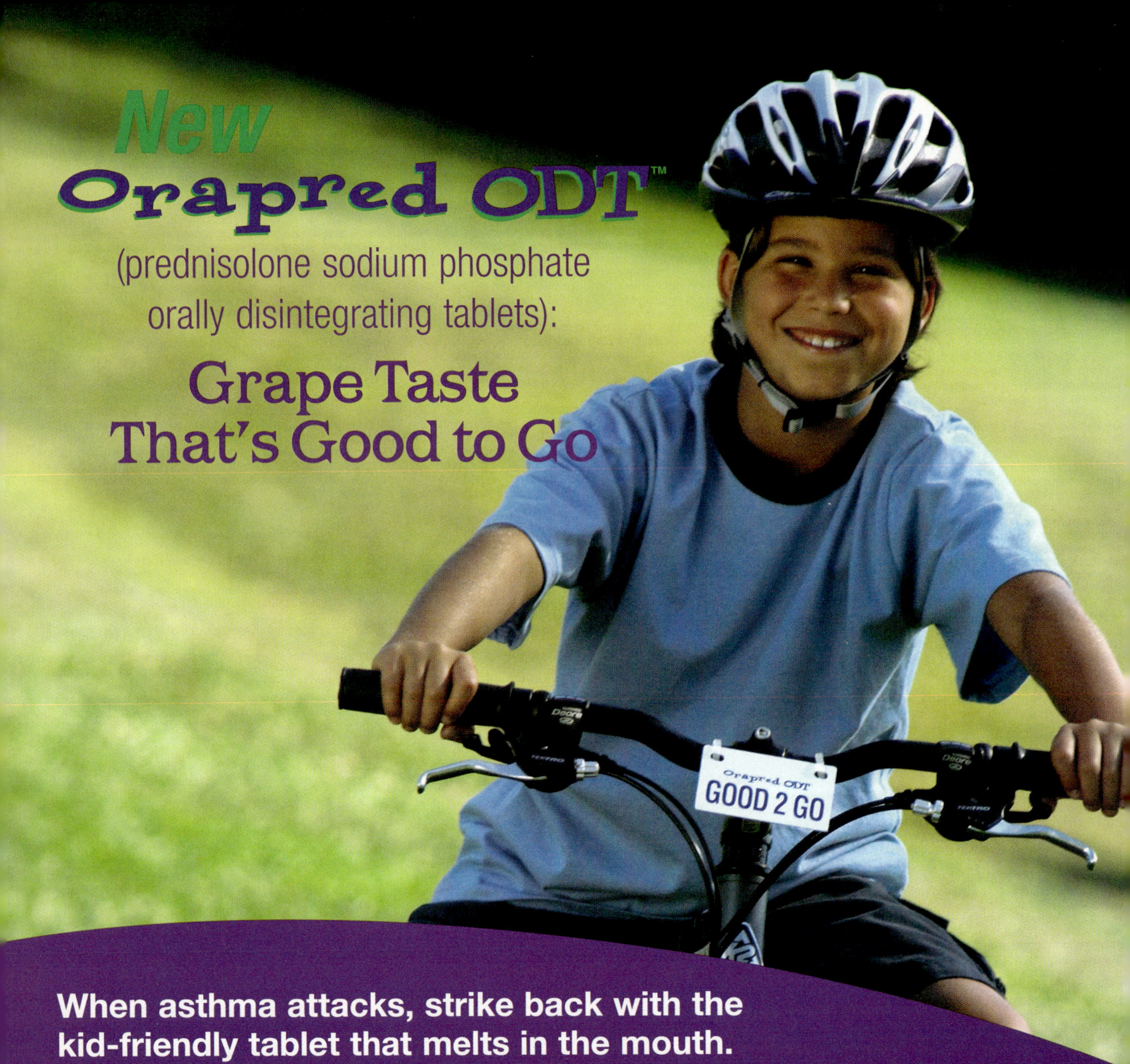


New

# Orapred ODT™

(prednisolone sodium phosphate orally disintegrating tablets):

## Grape Taste That's Good to Go

**When asthma attacks, strike back with the kid-friendly tablet that melts in the mouth.**

**The first and only orally disintegrating prednisolone tablet**

**Disintegrates on the tongue without water or messy spoon**

**Kid-preferred grape taste**

**Natural flavors and sweeteners neutralize prednisolone's unpleasant taste**

As with all glucocorticoids, Orapred ODT is contraindicated in persons with systemic fungal infections. In clinical trials of Orapred ODT, the following adverse events were seen: facial edema, pharyngolaryngeal pain, blood in stool, eye irritation, and eyelid edema. Please see accompanying full prescribing information for a complete list of all adverse events, such as dermatological and gastrointestinal disturbances. Do not break or use partial Orapred ODT tablets.

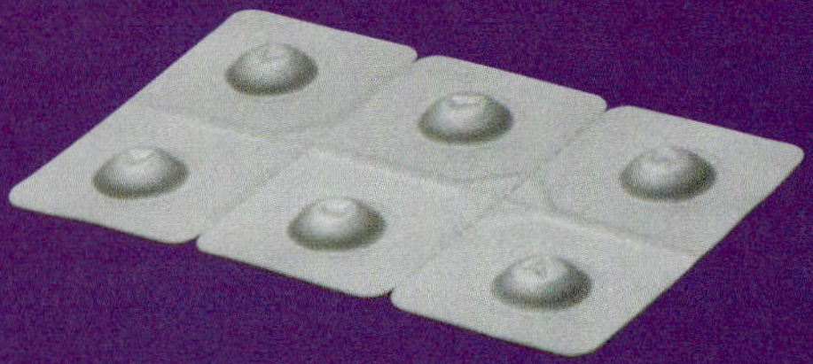

Orapred ODT™

(prednisolone sodium phosphate orally disintegrating tablets)

Equivalent to prednisolone 15mg

# ARCHIVES OF PEDIATRICS & ADOLESCENT MEDICINE

NOVEMBER 2006 VOLUME 160, NUMBER 11 PAGES 1089-1192


## ARTICLES


**Home-Visiting Intervention to Improve Child Care Among American Indian Adolescent Mothers: A Randomized Trial** 1101
*Allison Barlow, MA, MPH; Elena Varipatis-Baker, MPH, MSW; Kristen Speakman, MA, MPH; Golda Ginsburg, PhD; Ingrid Friberg, MHS; Novalene Goklish; Brandii Cowboy; Pauline Fields; Ranelda Hastings; William Pan, DrPH; Raymond Reid, MD, MPH; Mathuram Santosham, MD, MPH; John Walkup, MD*

**Double Burden of Iron Deficiency in Infancy and Low Socioeconomic Status: A Longitudinal Analysis of Cognitive Test Scores to Age 19 Years** 1108
*Betsy Lozoff, MD; Elias Jimenez, MD; Julia B. Smith, EdD*

**Iron Depletion Is Associated With Daytime Bottle-feeding in the Second and Third Years of Life** 1114
*Trenna L. Sutcliffe, MSc, MD, FRCPC; Amina Khambalia, MSc; Shelley Westergard, RN; Sheila Jacobson, MBBCh, FRCPC; Michael Peer, MD, FRCPC; Patricia C. Parkin, MD, FRCPC*

**Efficacy of Duct Tape vs Placebo in the Treatment of Verruca Vulgaris (Warts) in Primary School Children** 1121
*Marloes de Haen, MD; Marcus G. Spigt, PhD; Caro J. T. van Uden, PhD; Pierre van Neer, MD; Frans J. M. Feron, MD; André Knottnerus, PhD*


## EVIDENCE-BASED JOURNAL CLUB


**Interpreting Negative Results From an Underpowered Clinical Trial: Warts and All** 1126
*Jeanne Van Cleave, MD; Alex R. Kemper, MD, MPH, MS; Matthew M. Davis, MD, MAPP*


## ARTICLES


**Parental Reactions to Information About Increased Genetic Risk of Type 1 Diabetes Mellitus in Infants** 1131
*Paula Simonen, PhLic; Tapio Korhonen, PhD; Tuula Simell, MPH, PhD; Päivi Keskinen, MD, PhD; Maarit Kärkkäinen, MHSci; Mikael Knip, MD, PhD; Jorma Ilonen, MD, PhD; Olli Simell, MD, PhD*

**The Association Between Parents' Past Agricultural Injuries and Their Children's Risk of Injury: Analyses From the Regional Rural Injury Study–II** 1137
*Kathleen Ferguson Carlson, PhD; Deborah Langner, MS; Bruce H. Alexander, PhD; James G. Gurney, PhD; Susan G. Gerberich, PhD; Andrew D. Ryan, MS; Colleen M. Renier, BS; Steven J. Mongin, MS*

**The Interpreter as Cultural Educator of Residents: Improving Communication for Latino Parents** 1145
*Ann Chen Wu, MD; John M. Leventhal, MD; Jacqueline Ortiz, MPhil; Ernesto E. Gonzalez, BS; Brian Forsyth, MBChB*

**Public Opinion on Sex Education in US Schools** 1151
*Amy Bleakley, PhD, MPH; Michael Hennessy, PhD, MPH; Martin Fishbein, PhD*

**Adolescent and Parent Perceptions on Youth Participation in Risk Behavior Research** 1159
*Ryan H. Pasternak, MD, MPH; Gail Geller, ScD; Catherine Parrish, MD; Tina L. Cheng, MD*

## REVIEW ARTICLE

**Autism: A Review of the State of the Science for Pediatric Primary Health Care Clinicians** **1167**
*William J. Barbaresi, MD; Slavica K. Katusic, MD; Robert G. Voigt, MD*

## SPECIAL FEATURE

**Picture of the Month** **1177**
*Jon M. Burnham, MD; Portia A. Kreiger, MD; Michele Paessler, DO; Leslie S. Kersun, MD; Randy Q. Cron, MD, PhD*

## EDITORIALS

**Understanding Shared Injury Risk on the Family Farm** **1180**
*Brian D. Johnston, MD, MPH*

**Comprehensive Sex Education: Strong Public Support and Persuasive Evidence of Impact, but Little Funding** **1182**
*Douglas Kirby, PhD*

## THE PEDIATRIC FORUM

**Primum Non Nocere** **1185**
*David Dickens, MD; Dianne Sinsabaugh, RPh; Brenda Winger, PharmD*

**In Reply** **1185**
*George R. Kim, MD; Allen R. Chen, MD, PhD; Robert J. Arceci, MD, PhD; Christoph U. Lehmann, MD*

## CORRECTION

**Errors in Figures in: A Randomized Controlled Trial Testing an HIV Prevention Intervention for Latino Youth** **1187**
*Antonia M. Villarruel, PhD, RN; John B. Jemmott III, PhD; Loretta S. Jemmott, PhD, RN*

## REGULAR DEPARTMENTS

**This Month in *Archives of Pediatrics & Adolescent Medicine*** **1100**

**Announcements** **1129, 1142, 1156, 1184**

**Classified Advertising** **1190**

**Journal Advertiser Index** **1191**

**Contact Information** **1192**


**Instructions for authors and the author and subject indexes are available on our Web site: http://www.archpediatrics.com. If you do not have access to the Web, contact Suzanne Shuey at (206) 685-3573.**

**About the Cover**

Photographer: Gary M. Reisfield, MD, Jacksonville, Fla, 2000.

# ARCHIVES OF PEDIATRICS & ADOLESCENT MEDICINE

**Mission Statement:** *The Archives of Pediatrics & Adolescent Medicine* is a monthly, peer-reviewed journal for physicians and other health care professionals who contribute to the health of children and adolescents. The *Archives* provides an open forum for dialogue on a full range of clinical, scientific, advocacy, and humanistic issues relevant to the care of pediatric patients from infancy through young adulthood. The *Archives* is a vehicle for increased attention to adolescent health, the education of pediatric health care professionals, and disease prevention and health promotion. The *Archives* publishes original studies, editorials, reviews by experts, practice commentaries, case quizzes, and updates on clinical science and practice management. The Pediatric Forum provides our readers with opportunities to express their views. *Archives* incorporates *AJDC*, the oldest journal in US pediatric literature, which originated in 1911.



JAMA & ARCHIVES JOURNALS
American Medical Association

# The One for Both

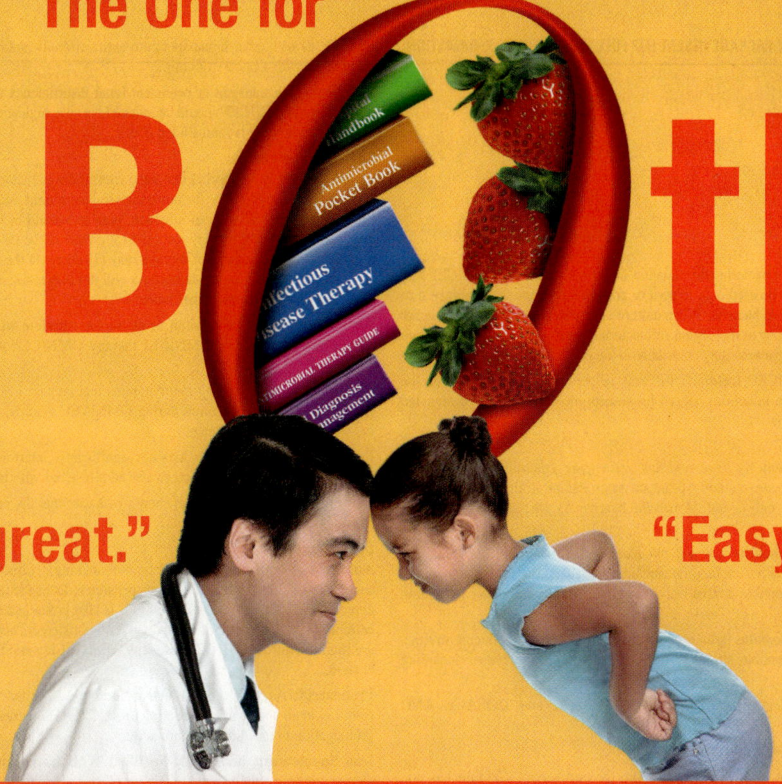


"Works great." "Easy to take."

## 250 mg/5 mL* — Half the Volume†

**According to published peer-reviewed literature,[1-3] compliance factors that make an antibiotic easy to take include:**

- **Taste (palatability)**
- **Tolerability**
- **Short duration of treatment**
- **Number of daily doses**

**Indications** OMNICEF (cefdinir) for Oral Suspension is indicated in patients 6 months through 12 years for mild to moderate **Acute Bacterial Otitis Media** caused by susceptible strains of *H influenzae* (including ß-lactamase producing strains), *S pneumoniae* (penicillin-susceptible strains only), and *M catarrhalis* (including ß-lactamase producing strains).[4]

**Important Safety Information**[4]

- To reduce the development of drug-resistant bacteria and maintain the effectiveness of OMNICEF and other antibacterial drugs, OMNICEF should be used only to treat or prevent infections that are proven or strongly suspected to be caused by bacteria
- OMNICEF is contraindicated in patients with known allergy to the cephalosporin class of antibiotics
- For patients with previous hypersensitivity reaction to penicillins, caution should be exercised because cross-hypersensitivity among ß-lactam antibiotics has been clearly documented. If an allergic reaction to cefdinir occurs, the drug should be discontinued
- Safety and efficacy in neonates and infants less than 6 months of age have not been established
- 2% of 2,289 pediatric patients discontinued medication due to adverse events in US and non-US clinical trials. Discontinuations were primarily for gastrointestinal disturbance, usually diarrhea
- The most common reported adverse events occurring in ≥1% of pediatric patients in US clinical trials (N=1,783) were diarrhea (8%), rash (3%), and vomiting (1%)
- Maximum dose of OMNICEF for pediatric patients weighing ≥43 kg is 600 mg/day. For pediatric patients with a creatinine clearance of <30 mL/min/1.73 $m^2$ and not requiring hemodialysis, the dose of cefdinir should be 7 mg/kg (up to 300 mg) given once daily
- Antacids that contain magnesium or aluminum and iron supplements, including multivitamins that contain iron, should be taken at least 2 hours before or 2 hours after taking OMNICEF

***For pediatric patients weighing 20 lbs, use the 125 mg/5 mL product.[4]**
**†Of the 125 mg/5 mL formulation.**


**References: 1.** Brixner DI. Improving acute otitis media outcomes through proper antibiotic use and adherence. *Am J Manag Care.* 2005;11:S202-S210. **2.** Kardas P. Patient compliance with antibiotic treatment for respiratory tract infections. *J Antimicrob Chemother.* 2002;49:897-903. **3.** Ramgoolam A, Steele R. Formulations of antibiotics for children in primary care. *Pediatr Drugs.* 2002;4:323-333. **4.** OMNICEF (cefdinir) Capsules and for Oral Suspension Prescribing Information, Abbott Laboratories.


**Please see adjacent brief summary of full prescribing information.**

OMNICEF®
(cefdinir) for oral suspension
*125 mg/5 mL and 250 mg/5 mL*
"Works great." "Easy to take."

astellas
Under License of **Astellas Pharma Inc.** Japan

**Abbott**
A Promise for Life

**PROFESSIONAL BRIEF SUMMARY-CONSULT PACKAGE INSERT FOR FULL PRESCRIBING INFORMATION.**
03-5435-Rev. July, 2005
(Nos. 3769, 3771, 6151)

# Omnicef® (cefdinir) capsules
# Omnicef® (cefdinir) for oral suspension

**Rx only**

## INDICATIONS AND USAGE

To reduce the development of drug-resistant bacteria and maintain the effectiveness of OMNICEF and other antibacterial drugs, OMNICEF should be used only to treat or prevent infections that are proven or strongly suspected to be caused by susceptible bacteria. When culture and susceptibility information are available, they should be considered in selecting or modifying antibacterial therapy. In the absence of such data, local epidemiology and susceptibility patterns may contribute to the empiric selection of therapy.

OMNICEF (cefdinir) capsules and OMNICEF (cefdinir) for oral suspension are indicated for the treatment of patients with mild to moderate infections caused by susceptible strains of the designated microorganisms in the conditions listed below.

### Adults and Adolescents

**Community-Acquired Pneumonia** caused by *Haemophilus influenzae* (including β-lactamase producing strains), *Haemophilus parainfluenzae* (including β-lactamase producing strains), *Streptococcus pneumoniae* (penicillin-susceptible strains only), and *Moraxella catarrhalis* (including β-lactamase producing strains).

**Acute Exacerbations of Chronic Bronchitis** caused by *Haemophilus influenzae* (including β-lactamase producing strains), *Haemophilus parainfluenzae* (including β-lactamase producing strains), *Streptococcus pneumoniae* (penicillin-susceptible strains only), and *Moraxella catarrhalis* (including β-lactamase producing strains).

**Acute Maxillary Sinusitis** caused by *Haemophilus influenzae* (including β-lactamase producing strains), *Streptococcus pneumoniae* (penicillin-susceptible strains only), and *Moraxella catarrhalis* (including β-lactamase producing strains).

**NOTE:** For information on use in pediatric patients, see **Pediatric Use** and **DOSAGE AND ADMINISTRATION**.

**Pharyngitis/Tonsillitis** caused by *Streptococcus pyogenes*.

**NOTE:** Cefdinir is effective in the eradication of *S. pyogenes* from the oropharynx. Cefdinir has not, however, been studied for the prevention of rheumatic fever following *S. pyogenes* pharyngitis/tonsillitis. Only intramuscular penicillin has been demonstrated to be effective for the prevention of rheumatic fever.

**Uncomplicated Skin and Skin Structure Infections** caused by *Staphylococcus aureus* (including β-lactamase producing strains) and *Streptococcus pyogenes*.

### Pediatric Patients

**Acute Bacterial Otitis Media** caused by *Haemophilus influenzae* (including β-lactamase producing strains), *Streptococcus pneumoniae* (penicillin-susceptible strains only), and *Moraxella catarrhalis* (including β-lactamase producing strains).

**Pharyngitis/Tonsillitis** caused by *Streptococcus pyogenes*.

**NOTE:** Cefdinir is effective in the eradication of *S. pyogenes* from the oropharynx. Cefdinir has not, however, been studied for the prevention of rheumatic fever following *S. pyogenes* pharyngitis/tonsillitis. Only intramuscular penicillin has been demonstrated to be effective for the prevention of rheumatic fever.

**Uncomplicated Skin and Skin Structure Infections** caused by *Staphylococcus aureus* (including β-lactamase producing strains) and *Streptococcus pyogenes*.

## CONTRAINDICATIONS

OMNICEF (cefdinir) is contraindicated in patients with known allergy to the cephalosporin class of antibiotics.

## WARNINGS

**BEFORE THERAPY WITH OMNICEF (CEFDINIR) IS INSTITUTED, CAREFUL INQUIRY SHOULD BE MADE TO DETERMINE WHETHER THE PATIENT HAS HAD PREVIOUS HYPERSENSITIVITY REACTIONS TO CEFDINIR, OTHER CEPHALOSPORINS, PENICILLINS, OR OTHER DRUGS. IF CEFDINIR IS TO BE GIVEN TO PENICILLIN-SENSITIVE PATIENTS, CAUTION SHOULD BE EXERCISED BECAUSE CROSS-HYPERSENSITIVITY AMONG β-LACTAM ANTIBIOTICS HAS BEEN CLEARLY DOCUMENTED AND MAY OCCUR IN UP TO 10% OF PATIENTS WITH A HISTORY OF PENICILLIN ALLERGY. IF AN ALLERGIC REACTION TO CEFDINIR OCCURS, THE DRUG SHOULD BE DISCONTINUED. SERIOUS ACUTE HYPERSENSITIVITY REACTIONS MAY REQUIRE TREATMENT WITH EPINEPHRINE AND OTHER EMERGENCY MEASURES, INCLUDING OXYGEN, INTRAVENOUS FLUIDS, INTRAVENOUS ANTIHISTAMINES, CORTICOSTEROIDS, PRESSOR AMINES, AND AIRWAY MANAGEMENT, AS CLINICALLY INDICATED.**

**Pseudomembranous colitis has been reported with nearly all antibacterial agents, including cefdinir, and may range in severity from mild- to life-threatening. Therefore, it is important to consider this diagnosis in patients who present with diarrhea subsequent to the administration of antibacterial agents.**

Treatment with antibacterial agents alters the normal flora of the colon and may permit overgrowth of clostridia. Studies indicate that a toxin produced by *Clostridium difficile* is a primary cause of "antibiotic-associated colitis."

After the diagnosis of pseudomembranous colitis has been established, appropriate therapeutic measures should be initiated. Mild cases of pseudomembranous colitis usually respond to drug discontinuation alone. In moderate to severe cases, consideration should be given to management with fluids and electrolytes, protein supplementation, and treatment with an antibacterial drug clinically effective against *Clostridium difficile*.

## PRECAUTIONS

### General

Prescribing OMNICEF in the absence of a proven or strongly suspected bacterial infection or a prophylactic indication is unlikely to provide benefit to the patient and increases the risk of the development of drug-resistant bacteria.

As with other broad-spectrum antibiotics, prolonged treatment may result in the possible emergence and overgrowth of resistant organisms. Careful observation of the patient is essential. If superinfection occurs during therapy, appropriate alternative therapy should be administered.

Cefdinir, as with other broad-spectrum antimicrobials (antibiotics), should be prescribed with caution in individuals with a history of colitis.

In patients with transient or persistent renal insufficiency (creatinine clearance <30 mL/min), the total daily dose of OMNICEF should be reduced because high and prolonged plasma concentrations of cefdinir can result following recommended doses.

### Information for Patients

Patients should be counseled that antibacterial drugs including OMNICEF should only be used to treat bacterial infections. They do not treat viral infections (e.g., the common cold). When OMNICEF is prescribed to treat a bacterial infection, patients should be told that although it is common to feel better early in the course of therapy, the medication should be taken exactly as directed. Skipping doses or not completing the full course of therapy may (1) decrease the effectiveness of the immediate treatment and (2) increase the likelihood that bacteria will develop resistance and will not be treatable by OMNICEF or other antibacterial drugs in the future.

Antacids containing magnesium or aluminum interfere with the absorption of cefdinir. If this type of antacid is required during OMNICEF therapy, OMNICEF should be taken at least 2 hours before or after the antacid.

Iron supplements, including multivitamins that contain iron, interfere with the absorption of cefdinir. If iron supplements are required during OMNICEF therapy, OMNICEF should be taken at least 2 hours before or after the supplement.

Iron-fortified infant formula does not significantly interfere with the absorption of cefdinir. Therefore, OMNICEF for Oral Suspension can be administered with iron-fortified infant formula.

Diabetic patients and caregivers should be aware that the oral suspension contains 2.86 g of sucrose per teaspoon.

### Drug Interactions

**Antacids:** (aluminum- or magnesium-containing): Concomitant administration of 300-mg cefdinir capsules with 30 mL Maalox® TC suspension reduces the rate ($C_{max}$) and extent (AUC) of absorption by approximately 40%. Time to reach $C_{max}$ is also prolonged by 1 hour. There are no significant effects on cefdinir pharmacokinetics if the antacid is administered 2 hours before or 2 hours after cefdinir. If antacids are required during OMNICEF therapy, OMNICEF should be taken at least 2 hours before or after the antacid.

**Probenecid:** As with other β-lactam antibiotics, probenecid inhibits the renal excretion of cefdinir, resulting in an approximate doubling in AUC, a 54% increase in peak cefdinir plasma levels, and a 50% prolongation in the apparent elimination $t_{1/2}$.

**Iron Supplements and Foods Fortified With Iron:** Concomitant administration of cefdinir with a therapeutic iron supplement containing 60 mg of elemental iron (as $FeSO_4$) or vitamins supplemented with 10 mg of elemental iron reduced extent of absorption by 80% and 31%, respectively. If iron supplements are required during OMNICEF therapy, OMNICEF should be taken at least 2 hours before or after the supplement.

The effect of foods highly fortified with elemental iron (primarily iron-fortified breakfast cereals) on cefdinir absorption has not been studied.

Concomitantly administered iron-fortified infant formula (2.2 mg elemental iron/6 oz) has no significant effect on cefdinir pharmacokinetics. Therefore, OMNICEF for Oral Suspension can be administered with iron-fortified infant formula.

There have been reports of reddish stools in patients receiving cefdinir. In many cases, patients were also receiving iron-containing products. The reddish color is due to the formation of a nonabsorbable complex between cefdinir or its breakdown products and iron in the gastrointestinal tract.

### Drug/Laboratory Test Interactions

A false-positive reaction for ketones in the urine may occur with tests using nitroprusside, but not with those using nitroferricyanide. The administration of cefdinir may result in a false-positive reaction for glucose in urine using Clinitest®, Benedict's solution, or Fehling's solution. It is recommended that glucose tests based on enzymatic glucose oxidase reactions (such as Clinistix® or Tes-Tape®) be used. Cephalosporins are known to occasionally induce a positive direct Coombs' test.

### Carcinogenesis, Mutagenesis, Impairment of Fertility

The carcinogenic potential of cefdinir has not been evaluated. No mutagenic effects were seen in the bacterial reverse mutation assay (Ames) or point mutation assay at the hypoxanthine-guanine phosphoribosyltransferase locus (HGPRT) in V79 Chinese hamster lung cells. No clastogenic effects were observed *in vitro* in the structural chromosome aberration assay in V79 Chinese hamster lung cells or *in vivo* in the micronucleus assay in mouse bone marrow. In rats, fertility and reproductive performance were not affected by cefdinir at oral doses up to 1000 mg/kg/day (70 times the human dose based on mg/kg/day, 11 times based on $mg/m^2$/day).

### Pregnancy - Teratogenic Effects

**Pregnancy Category B:** Cefdinir was not teratogenic in rats at oral doses up to 1000 mg/kg/day (70 times the human dose based on mg/kg/day, 11 times based on $mg/m^2$/day) or in rabbits at oral doses up to 10 mg/kg/day (0.7 times the human dose based on mg/kg/day, 0.23 times based on $mg/m^2$/day). Maternal toxicity (decreased body weight gain) was observed in rabbits at the maximum tolerated dose of 10 mg/kg/day without adverse effects on offspring. Decreased body weight occurred in rat fetuses at ≥ 100 mg/kg/day, and in rat offspring at ≥ 32 mg/kg/day. No effects were observed on maternal reproductive parameters or offspring survival, development, behavior, or reproductive function.

There are, however, no adequate and well-controlled studies in pregnant women. Because animal reproduction studies are not always predictive of human response, this drug should be used during pregnancy only if clearly needed.

### Labor and Delivery

Cefdinir has not been studied for use during labor and delivery.

### Nursing Mothers

Following administration of single 600-mg doses, cefdinir was not detected in human breast milk.

### Pediatric Use

Safety and efficacy in neonates and infants less than 6 months of age have not been established. Use of cefdinir for the treatment of acute maxillary sinusitis in pediatric patients (age 6 months through 12 years) is supported by evidence from adequate and well-controlled studies in adults and adolescents, the similar pathophysiology of acute sinusitis in adult and pediatric patients, and comparative pharmacokinetic data in the pediatric population.

### Geriatric Use

Efficacy is comparable in geriatric patients and younger adults. While cefdinir has been well-tolerated in all age groups, in clinical trials geriatric patients experienced a lower rate of adverse events, including diarrhea, than younger adults. Dose adjustment in elderly patients is not necessary unless renal function is markedly compromised.

## ADVERSE EVENTS

**Clinical Trials - OMNICEF Capsules (Adult and Adolescent Patients):**

In clinical trials, 5093 adult and adolescent patients (3841 US and 1252 non-US) were treated with the recommended dose of cefdinir capsules (600 mg/day). Most adverse events were mild and self-limiting. No deaths or permanent disabilities were attributed to cefdinir. One hundred forty-seven of 5093 (3%) patients discontinued medication due to adverse events thought by the investigators to be possibly, probably, or definitely associated with cefdinir therapy. The discontinuations were primarily for gastrointestinal disturbances, usually diarrhea or nausea. Nineteen of 5093 (0.4%) patients were discontinued due to rash thought related to cefdinir administration.

In the US, the following adverse events were thought by investigators to be possibly, probably, or definitely related to cefdinir capsules in multiple-dose clinical trials (N = 3841 cefdinir-treated patients):

**ADVERSE EVENTS ASSOCIATED WITH CEFDINIR CAPSULES US TRIALS IN ADULT AND ADOLESCENT PATIENTS (N=3841)[a]**

| | | |
|---|---|---|
| Incidence ≥ 1% | Diarrhea | 15% |
| | Vaginal moniliasis | 4% of women |
| | Nausea | 3% |
| | Headache | 2% |
| | Abdominal pain | 1% |
| | Vaginitis | 1% of women |
| Incidence <1% but >0.1% | Rash | 0.9% |
| | Dyspepsia | 0.7% |
| | Flatulence | 0.7% |
| | Vomiting | 0.7% |
| | Abnormal stools | 0.3% |
| | Anorexia | 0.3% |
| | Constipation | 0.3% |
| | Dizziness | 0.3% |
| | Dry mouth | 0.3% |
| | Asthenia | 0.2% |
| | Insomnia | 0.2% |
| | Leukorrhea | 0.2% of women |
| | Moniliasis | 0.2% |
| | Pruritus | 0.2% |
| | Somnolence | 0.2% |

[a] 1733 males, 2108 females

The following laboratory value changes of possible clinical significance, irrespective of relationship to therapy with cefdinir, were seen during clinical trials conducted in the US:

**LABORATORY VALUE CHANGES OBSERVED WITH CEFDINIR CAPSULES US TRIALS IN ADULT AND ADOLESCENT PATIENTS (N=3841)**

| | | |
|---|---|---|
| Incidence ≥ 1% | ↑ Urine leukocytes | 2% |
| | ↑ Urine protein | 2% |
| | ↑ Gamma-glutamyltransferase[a] | 1% |
| | ↓ Lymphocytes, ↑ Lymphocytes | 1%, 0.2% |
| | ↑ Microhematuria | 1% |
| Incidence <1% but >0.1% | ↑ Glucose[a] | 0.9% |
| | ↑ Urine glucose | 0.9% |
| | ↑ White blood cells, ↓ White blood cells | 0.9%, 0.7% |
| | ↑ Alanine aminotransferase (ALT) | 0.7% |
| | ↑ Eosinophils | 0.7% |
| | ↑ Urine specific gravity, ↓ Urine specific gravity[a] | 0.6%, 0.2% |
| | ↓ Bicarbonate[a] | 0.6% |
| | ↑ Phosphorus, ↓ Phosphorus[a] | 0.6%, 0.3% |
| | ↑ Aspartate aminotransferase (AST) | 0.4% |
| | ↑ Alkaline phosphatase | 0.3% |
| | ↑ Blood urea nitrogen (BUN) | 0.3% |
| | ↓ Hemoglobin | 0.3% |
| | ↑ Polymorphonuclear neutrophils (PMNs), ↓ PMNs | 0.3%, 0.2% |
| | ↑ Bilirubin | 0.2% |
| | ↑ Lactate dehydrogenase[a] | 0.2% |
| | ↑ Platelets | 0.2% |
| | ↑ Potassium[a] | 0.2% |
| | ↑ Urine pH[a] | 0.2% |

[a] N<3841 for these parameters

**Clinical Trials - OMNICEF for Oral Suspension (Pediatric Patients):**

In clinical trials, 2289 pediatric patients (1783 US and 506 non-US) were treated with the recommended dose of cefdinir suspension (14 mg/kg/day). Most adverse events were mild and self-limiting. No deaths or permanent disabilities were attributed to cefdinir. Forty of 2289 (2%) patients discontinued medication due to adverse events considered by the investigators to be possibly, probably, or definitely associated with cefdinir therapy. Discontinuations were primarily for gastrointestinal disturbances, usually diarrhea. Five of 2289 (0.2%) patients were discontinued due to rash thought related to cefdinir administration.

In the US, the following adverse events were thought by investigators to be possibly, probably, or definitely related to cefdinir suspension in multiple-dose clinical trials (N=1783 cefdinir-treated patients):

**ADVERSE EVENTS ASSOCIATED WITH CEFDINIR SUSPENSION US TRIALS IN PEDIATRIC PATIENTS (N=1783)[a]**

| | | |
|---|---|---|
| Incidence ≥ 1% | Diarrhea | 8% |
| | Rash | 3% |
| | Vomiting | 1% |
| Incidence <1% but >0.1% | Cutaneous moniliasis | 0.9% |
| | Abdominal pain | 0.8% |
| | Leukopenia[b] | 0.3% |
| | Vaginal moniliasis | 0.3% of girls |
| | Vaginitis | 0.3% of girls |
| | Abnormal stools | 0.2% |
| | Dyspepsia | 0.2% |
| | Hyperkinesia | 0.2% |
| | Increased AST[b] | 0.2% |
| | Maculopapular rash | 0.2% |
| | Nausea | 0.2% |

[a] 977 males, 806 females

[b] Laboratory changes were occasionally reported as adverse events.

NOTE: In both cefdinir- and control-treated patients, rates of diarrhea and rash were higher in the youngest pediatric patients. The incidence of diarrhea in cefdinir-treated patients ≤2 years of age was 17% (95/557) compared with 4% (51/1226) in those >2 years old. The incidence of rash (primarily diaper rash in the younger patients) was 8% (43/557) in patients ≤2 years of age compared with 1% (8/1226) in those >2 years old.

The following laboratory value changes of possible clinical significance, irrespective of relationship to therapy with cefdinir, were seen during clinical trials conducted in the US:

**LABORATORY VALUE CHANGES OF POSSIBLE CLINICAL SIGNIFICANCE OBSERVED WITH CEFDINIR SUSPENSION US TRIALS IN PEDIATRIC PATIENTS (N=1783)**

| | | |
|---|---|---|
| Incidence ≥ 1% | ↑ Lymphocytes, ↓ Lymphocytes | 2%, 0.8% |
| | ↑ Alkaline phosphatase | 1% |
| | ↓ Bicarbonate[a] | 1% |
| | ↑ Eosinophils | 1% |
| | ↑ Lactate dehydrogenase | 1% |
| | ↑ Platelets | 1% |
| | ↑ PMNs, ↓ PMNs | 1%, 1% |
| | ↑ Urine protein | 1% |
| Incidence <1% but >0.1% | ↑ Phosphorus, ↓ Phosphorus | 0.9%, 0.4% |
| | ↑ Urine pH | 0.8% |
| | ↓ White blood cells, ↑ White blood cells | 0.7%, 0.3% |
| | ↓ Calcium[a] | 0.5% |
| | ↓ Hemoglobin | 0.5% |
| | ↑ Urine leukocytes | 0.5% |
| | ↑ Monocytes | 0.4% |
| | ↑ AST | 0.3% |
| | ↑ Potassium[a] | 0.3% |
| | ↑ Urine specific gravity, ↓ Urine specific gravity | 0.3%, 0.1% |
| | ↓ Hematocrit[a] | 0.2% |

[a] N=1387 for these parameters

**Postmarketing Experience**

The following adverse experiences and altered laboratory tests, regardless of their relationship to cefdinir, have been reported during extensive postmarketing experience, beginning with approval in Japan in 1991: Stevens-Johnson syndrome, toxic epidermal necrolysis, exfoliative dermatitis, erythema multiforme, erythema nodosum, serum sickness-like reactions, conjunctivitis, stomatitis, acute hepatitis, cholestasis, fulminant hepatitis, hepatic failure, jaundice, increased amylase, shock, anaphylaxis, facial and laryngeal edema, feeling of suffocation, acute enterocolitis, bloody diarrhea, hemorrhagic colitis, melena, pseudomembranous colitis, pancytopenia, granulocytopenia, leukopenia, thrombocytopenia, idiopathic thrombocytopenic purpura, hemolytic anemia, acute respiratory failure, asthmatic attack, drug-induced pneumonia, eosinophilic pneumonia, idiopathic interstitial pneumonia, fever, acute renal failure, nephropathy, bleeding tendency, coagulation disorder, disseminated intravascular coagulation, upper GI bleed, peptic ulcer, ileus, loss of consciousness, allergic vasculitis, possible cefdinir-diclofenac interaction, cardiac failure, chest pain, myocardial infarction, hypertension, involuntary movements, and rhabdomyolysis.

**Cephalosporin Class Adverse Events**

The following adverse events and altered laboratory tests have been reported for cephalosporin-class antibiotics in general:

Allergic reactions, anaphylaxis, Stevens-Johnson syndrome, erythema multiforme, toxic epidermal necrolysis, renal dysfunction, toxic nephropathy, hepatic dysfunction including cholestasis, aplastic anemia, hemolytic anemia, hemorrhage, false-positive test for urinary glucose, neutropenia, pancytopenia, and agranulocytosis. Pseudomembranous colitis symptoms may begin during or after antibiotic treatment (see **WARNINGS**).

Several cephalosporins have been implicated in triggering seizures, particularly in patients with renal impairment when the dosage was not reduced (see **OVERDOSAGE**). If seizures associated with drug therapy occur, the drug should be discontinued. Anticonvulsant therapy can be given if clinically indicated.

## OVERDOSAGE

Information on cefdinir overdosage in humans is not available. In acute rodent toxicity studies, a single oral 5600-mg/kg dose produced no adverse effects. Toxic signs and symptoms following overdosage with other β-lactam antibiotics have included nausea, vomiting, epigastric distress, diarrhea, and convulsions. Hemodialysis removes cefdinir from the body. This may be useful in the event of a serious toxic reaction from overdosage, particularly if renal function is compromised.

**Rx only**

Ref: 03-5435-Rev. July, 2005
(Nos. 3769, 3771, 6151)



05J-034-L150-2 **MASTER**

Manufactured by:
**CEPH** International Corporation
Carolina, Puerto Rico 00986
Under License of:
astellas Astellas Pharma Inc.
Tokyo, Japan

For:
**Abbott Laboratories**
North Chicago, IL 60064, U.S.A.

06F-034-Q068-1
Printed in U.S.A.

## Parental Reactions to Information About Increased Genetic Risk for Type 1 Diabetes Mellitus in Infants

Although genetic screening for type 1 diabetes mellitus cannot be done, testing whether infants have an increased risk for type 1 diabetes is feasible. Such screening has a sensitivity of approximately 70% for identifying those at risk of developing type 1 diabetes before age 15 years but a positive predictive value of only 3% to 7%. In this study from Finland in which parents were told of their newborns' risk for diabetes, families of 523 high-risk babies were compared with 506 families of low-risk babies 1 to 2 weeks after learning the risk status. The amount of anxiety in the 2 sets of families was similar, and more than 90% were grateful to know the risk status. Increased anxiety was related to other life stress.

See page 1131

## Autism: A Review of the State of the Science for Pediatric Primary Health Care Clinicians

Autism and related conditions in the "autism spectrum" have become the focus of intense interest, fueled by concerns about the apparent increase in the number of children affected by these developmental disorders. Pediatricians have an important role in the identification and ongoing management of children with autism. Barbaresi and colleagues in this comprehensive review article examine the epidemiology of autism, examine the approaches to identifying and diagnosing children suspected of having the disorder, and discuss treatment strategies for the child and family.

See page 1167

## Public Opinion on Sex Education in US Schools

Sex education for adolescents is necessary to prevent the spread of sexually transmitted infections. Although the federal government's current policy is to promote abstinence-only education, there are limited data to support its effectiveness. This study used a random-digit dialing household survey to examine the type of school-based sex education preferred by the public. Approximately 82% of respondents indicated support for programs that teach students about both abstinence and other methods of preventing pregnancy and sexually transmitted infections. Abstinence-only education programs received the lowest level of support and the highest level of opposition. Regardless of political ideology, adults in the United States preferred a balanced approach to sex education.

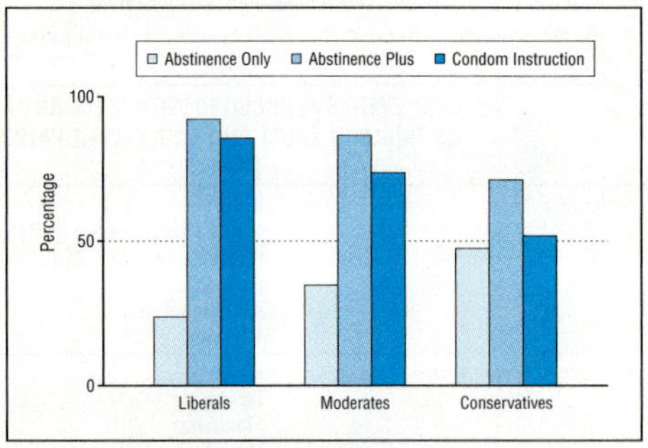


**Figure.** Percentage of support for sex education programs by political ideology.

See page 1151

## Double Burden of Iron Deficiency in Infancy and Low Socioeconomic Status: A Longitudinal Analysis of Cognitive Test Scores to Age 19 Years

Prior studies from around the world have consistently shown that infants with iron deficiency have lower cognitive test scores than infants with good iron stores. The present study assessed change in cognitive test performance from the second year of life to age 19 years among 185 individuals from Costa Rica. In individuals with chronic iron deficiency in infancy from families of middle socioeconomic status, their cognitive test scores at age 19 years averaged 9 points lower than those of comparable individuals without a history of iron deficiency. Among individuals from low socioeconomic status backgrounds, this cognitive difference at age 19 years was 25 points. The chronic iron deficiency group did not exhibit a catch-up in their cognitive scores over time. The gap for individuals from low socioeconomic status backgrounds widened. These results underscore the need for prevention and treatment of iron deficiency.

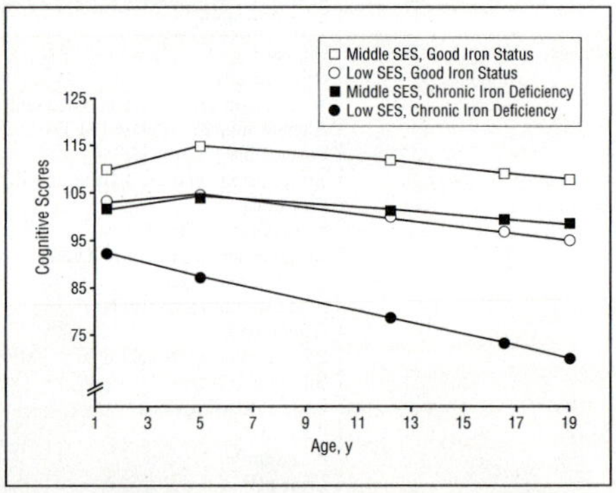


**Figure.** Cognitive composite scores over time comparing infant iron status groups within middle- and low-socioeconomic status (SES) families. Iron status group and SES level each affected initial scores ($P$=.01 for chronic iron deficiency difference within middle-SES families and $P$=.003 for chronic iron deficiency difference within low-SES families). Change over time differed only for the chronic iron deficiency group in low-SES families ($P$=.02 for change from infancy to age 5 years and $P$=.04 for change from ages 5 to 19 years). Each participant is represented once: good iron status (n=67) compared with chronic iron deficiency (n=20) in middle-SES families and good iron status (n=65) compared with chronic iron deficiency (n=33) in low-SES families. Symbols are placed at the average age for each assessment.

See page 1108

# Home-Visiting Intervention to Improve Child Care Among American Indian Adolescent Mothers

## *A Randomized Trial*

*Allison Barlow, MA, MPH; Elena Varipatis-Baker, MPH, MSW; Kristen Speakman, MA, MPH; Golda Ginsburg, PhD; Ingrid Friberg, MHS; Novalene Goklish; Brandii Cowboy; Pauline Fields; Ranelda Hastings; William Pan, DrPH; Raymond Reid, MD, MPH; Mathuram Santosham, MD, MPH; John Walkup, MD*

**Objective:** To assess the impact of a paraprofessional-delivered home-visiting intervention to promote child care knowledge, skills, and involvement among pregnant American Indian adolescents.

**Design:** Randomized controlled trial comparing a family-strengthening intervention with a breastfeeding education program.

**Setting:** One Apache and 3 Navajo communities.

**Participants:** Fifty-three pregnant American Indian adolescents were randomly assigned to intervention (n=28) or control (n=25) groups. Follow-up data were available for 19 intervention and 22 control participants.

**Intervention:** Paraprofessionals delivered 41 prenatal and infant care lessons in participants' homes from 28 weeks' gestation to 6 months post partum.

**Main Outcome Measures:** Child care knowledge, skills, and involvement.

**Results:** Mothers in the intervention compared with the control group had significantly higher parent knowledge scores at 2 months (adjusted mean difference [AMD], +14.9 [95% confidence interval (CI), +7.5 to +22.4]) and 6 months post partum (AMD, +15.3 [95% CI, +5.9 to +24.7]). Intervention group mothers scored significantly higher on maternal involvement scales at 2 months post partum (AMD, +1.5 [95% CI, −0.02 to +3.02]), and scores approached significance at 6 months post partum (AMD, +1.1 [95% CI, −0.06 to +2.2]). No between-group differences were found for child care skills.

**Conclusions:** A paraprofessional-delivered, family-strengthening home-visiting program significantly increased mothers' child care knowledge and involvement. A longer and larger trial is needed to understand the intervention's potential to improve adolescent parenting and related child outcomes in American Indian communities.

*Arch Pediatr Adolesc Med. 2006;160:1101-1107*

ADOLESCENT CHILDBEARING has been linked to negative parenting patterns and poor health and behavior outcomes for teen mothers and their children.[1,2] Approximately 46% of American Indian women vs 25% of all women in the United States have their first child during adolescence[3] and twice as many have 2 or more births during adolescence.[3] Expectant American Indian mothers, regardless of age, receive inadequate prenatal care.[4] Almost twice as many American Indian women compared with other US women receive no prenatal care (31.2% vs 17.3%).[5] Of those who receive prenatal care, reservation-based teens do not seek prenatal care until late in their second and sometimes not until their third trimester.[6] Compounding the problems associated with teen parenthood, American Indian adolescents have greater health and behavior risks than other US ethnic and racial groups: at least 31% of reservation-based adolescents live in poverty; 37% do not complete high school, and only 2% will obtain a bachelor's degree.[7] American Indian adolescents compared with other US racial groups also have elevated rates of drug abuse, suicide, domestic violence, and injuries.[3] Although the health and behavior risks for American Indian youth are well documented, protective factors related to child rearing within reservation communities are often not acknowledged. In general, native traditions promote strong extended family networks and cultural practices that reinforce the value of family-centered healing and prevention.[8-10]

Numerous studies support the short- and long-term efficacy of home-visiting programs delivered during pregnancy and early childhood for low-income, at-risk families with poor access to services.[11-19]

Author Affiliations: Johns Hopkins Center for American Indian Health and Johns Hopkins Bloomberg School of Public Health, Baltimore, Md.

Home-visiting interventions have documented improvements in parenting and the home environment[20]; maternal life outcomes[15,16,21-23]; children's health and behavior outcomes[12,24-28]; and reduced lifetime drug use and legal problems for mothers and children.[18,22,29] However, to our knowledge, no home-visiting studies have included American Indian individuals as the target population. Nurse- vs paraprofessional-delivered home-visiting programs have been more rigorously evaluated and have demonstrated more positive outcomes.[17] Because of a severe shortage of nurses on reservations and the greater cost of nurse vs paraprofessional home visitors, nurse home-visiting programs are not feasible for reservation communities at this time.[30-32]

We conducted a randomized controlled trial to evaluate the short-term impact of a paraprofessional-delivered home-visiting intervention among rural Navajo and Apache pregnant teens. Primary outcomes included mothers' child care (1) knowledge, (2) skills, and (3) involvement. Secondary outcomes included psychological and behavior risks that could interfere with child care: (1) family conflict and cohesion, (2) social support, (3) self-esteem, (4) locus of control, and (5) drug use.

## METHODS

### PARTICIPANTS

All pregnant American Indian adolescents aged 12 to 19 years at conception and at 28 weeks' or earlier gestation were potentially eligible for participation. The expectant teens were recruited from 4 American Indian health service catchment areas on the Navajo and White Mountain Apache reservations in New Mexico and Arizona. Expectant teens were not eligible if they had serious medical, legal, or social problems that would preclude their ability to fully participate in the intervention and assessments. Recruitment occurred between July 2001 and February 2002.

The study protocol was approved by the Johns Hopkins institutional review boards, the Navajo Nation Human Research Review Board and appropriate Navajo community health boards, the White Mountain Apache Health Board and Tribal Council, the Whiteriver Service Unit, and the Phoenix Area Indian Health Service. If the participant was younger than 18 years, informed consent was obtained from the parent or guardian and assent, from the participant. If the participant was 18 years or older, consent was obtained from the participant alone.

### SAMPLE SIZE

The sample size was based on the number of eligible teens who enrolled during an 8-month recruitment period (n=50). Formal sample-size calculations were not done.

### RANDOMIZATION

Study participants were randomly assigned to the intervention or control conditions within each site. Randomization stratified by site was determined by the Randomization.com Web site[33] prior to enrolling any study participants. Although we did not balance by site, the number of intervention and control participants per site was similar. The randomization sequence for each site was stored in Baltimore, Md, by our data manager and was concealed from the key investigators and on-site educators at all times. After each participant signed consent/assent forms and completed the baseline assessment, the educators faxed these materials to the data manager in Baltimore. The data manager checked that all assessments were properly completed, confirmed that the teen met inclusion criteria and no exclusion criteria, and then informed the educator of the participant's group assignment. The participants and evaluators were not blind to intervention assignment.

### INTERVENTION AND CONTROL

#### Intervention Arm

The home-visiting intervention was modeled on "Healthy Families America." Healthy Families America is a national program founded on 12 research-based principles to ensure quality of home-visiting interventions for at-risk families. The content of the home-visiting intervention was derived from extensive community input on what teen parents needed to learn and was based on the *American Academy of Pediatrics Guide to Baby Care: Caring for Your Baby and Young Child: Birth to Age 5*.[34] Lessons covered prenatal care, labor, delivery, breastfeeding, nutrition, parenting, home safety, immunizations, well-baby care, family planning, sexually transmitted disease prevention, and maternal goal setting for personal and family development. The curricular content was scheduled chronologically to provide key instruction at developmentally appropriate times for participants' children. The protocol included 25 home visits and 41 discrete lessons taught from 28 weeks' gestation until 6 months post partum (about 9 months total) by the educators using tabletop flip charts. Home visits were scheduled to last approximately 1.5 hours. Cultural adaptations—including style, graphics, delivery, and content—were achieved through a community-based participatory process.

#### Control Arm

Control participants received a breastfeeding education program that was developed in 1996-1997 by Johns Hopkins Center for American Indian Health and the participating communities. Participants assigned to the control arm were scheduled to receive 23 home visits covering 20 breastfeeding lessons. The expected visit duration was 1 to 1.5 hours.

#### Educators

After randomization, participants (both intervention and control) were served by a single educator in their respective community. The educators (n=4) were bilingual American Indian women who had a job history in tribal health and human services, passed a background screening, and had been teen mothers themselves or had special interest in this population. The educators participated in more than 500 hours of training and were tested to ensure they had mastered lesson content and delivery strategies prior to study implementation. Educators received daily supervision at the site and weekly supervision through cross-site conference calls. Ongoing training occurred bimonthly throughout the study. Every 3 months, supervisors observed educators with participants and rated educators' professionalism, rapport, interpersonal skills, and adherence to the home-visitation protocol.

### DATA COLLECTION

Data collected included child care knowledge and skills test scores and maternal self-reports at 3 intervals: baseline (≤28 weeks' gestation) and 2 months and 6 months post partum.

## Description of Key Measures

For all measures, higher scores are better, unless noted.

**Primary Outcome Measures.** The primary outcome measures were as follows:

- Knowledge. A 51-item multiple-choice test developed by the study team with a possible score of 0% to 100%.
- Skills. Educators asked participants to complete 9 exercises to demonstrate infant care skills, using dolls at baseline and their own infants at 2 and 6 months post partum. Educators scored the results. Possible scores ranged from 0% to 100%.
- Involvement. Five selected self-report items scored on a 4-point scale with a possible score of 5 to 20.

**Secondary Outcome Measures.** The secondary outcome measures were as follows:

- Family conflict.[35] Five self-report items scored on a 4-point scale with a possible score of 5 to 20; higher scores are worse.
- Family cohesion.[35] Three self-report items scored on a 4-point scale with a possible score of 3 to 12.
- Social support. A 10-item self-report scored on a 5-point scale with a possible score of 10 to 50.
- Self-esteem.[36] A 10-item self-report scored on a 4-point scale with a possible score of 10 to 40.
- Depression.[37] A 20-item self-report scored on a 4-point scale with a possible score of 0 to 60; higher scores are worse.[38-45]
- Locus of control.[46] A 7-item self-report scored on a 4-point scale with a possible score of 7 to 28.
- Drug use.[47] Eight self-report items scored on a 4-point scale with a possible score of 8 to 32.

## ANALYSIS

The study sample was defined as those mothers who were randomized and provided at least 1 follow-up evaluation, regardless of the degree of intervention received. For baseline comparisons, we used *t* tests for continuous variables and $\chi^2$ tests for categorical variables. We adjusted for baseline scores and compared outcomes for the intervention and control groups at 2 months and 6 months post partum. We adjusted for baseline scores using PROC REG in SAS 8.0 (SAS Institute Inc, Cary, NC).

For attrition analyses, differences between participants who dropped out (n=12) and those who continued (n=41) were assessed with *t* tests and $\chi^2$ tests (data not shown). It was not necessary to control for educator bias since 1 educator per site (n=4) implemented the intervention and control conditions. Similarly, clustering by site was not necessary because baseline characteristics between sites were comparable (data not shown). Few observations had missing values (<11%), and differences between those participants with known and missing data did not yield any significant differences.

# RESULTS

## PARTICIPANT FLOW

Of the 77 participants who were initially contacted, 61 (79%) met eligibility criteria and agreed to enroll (**Figure**). Of the 61 enrolled, 8 (13%) dropped out before randomization. Twenty-eight were randomly assigned to the intervention arm and 25, to the control. Of those randomized, 19 (68%) of the intervention mothers and 22 (88%) of the control mothers completed at least 1 of 2 follow-up assessments, and 17 intervention (61%) and 22 control (88%) participants completed both follow-up assessments.

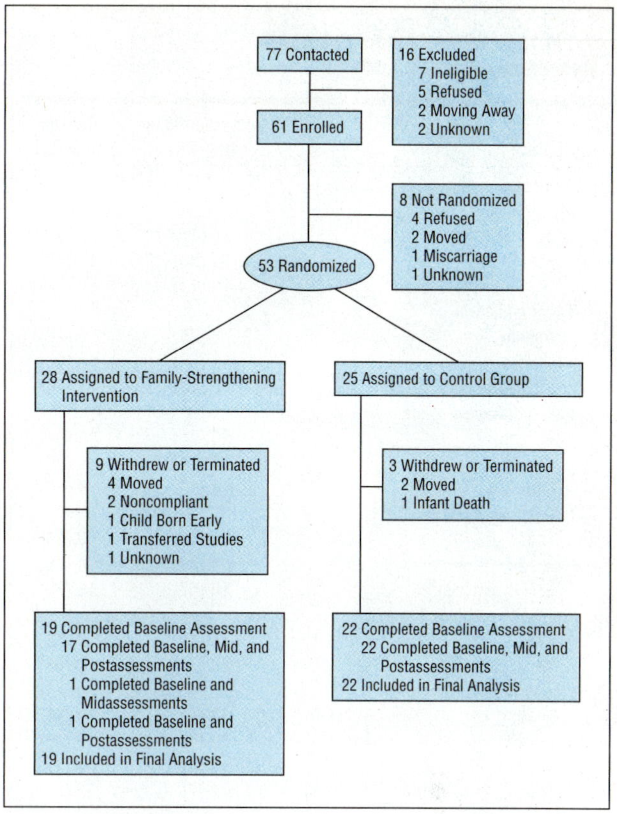


**Figure.** Study flowchart.

## PARTICIPANT CHARACTERISTICS

Randomized participants (N=53) ranged in age from 14 to 20 years (median age, 17.1 years) and all were 19 years or younger at conception. Fifty-one (96%) had never married; twelve (23%) (8 intervention participants, 4 controls) had completed high school and 36 (68%) (20 intervention participants, 16 controls) lived with their parents. Forty mothers (75%) (21 intervention participants, 19 controls) were pregnant with their first child, and 7 (13%) (4 intervention participants, 3 controls) had 1 previous child; data on parity was missing for 6 participants (11%). Among all baseline characteristics, only median gestational age at recruitment differed between the 2 groups (intervention, 20 weeks; control, 25 weeks) (**Table 1**). There were no important differences between arms in baseline outcome variables, with the exception of self-esteem score (mean, intervention, 28.6 vs control, 26.3 [95% confidence interval (CI), –4.4 to –0.3]). Those with known data were not substantially different from those with missing data in terms of baseline characteristics and outcome variables. Twelve participants dropped out prior to follow-up (9 intervention participants and 3 controls); the dropouts by study arm appeared similar in age, tribal affiliation, employment, and father involvement, as well as baseline outcome variables. However, dropouts in the intervention group tended to live with their parents (8 intervention participants vs

**Table 1. Baseline Comparison of All Randomized Participants***

| Variable | Intervention (n = 28) | Control (n = 25) |
|---|---|---|
| Demographics | | |
| Age, y | | |
| ≤14 | 2 (7) | 2 (8) |
| 15-17 | 14 (50) | 15 (60) |
| ≥18 | 12 (43) | 8 (32) |
| Tribal affiliation | | |
| Apache | 7 (25) | 5 (20) |
| Navajo | 19 (68) | 15 (60) |
| Mixed affiliations | 2 (17) | 5 (20) |
| Living situation | | |
| Parents | 20 (71) | 16 (64) |
| Significant other | 4 (14) | 5 (20) |
| Others | 4 (15) | 4 (16) |
| Education, y | | |
| <12 | 3 (11) | 6 (24) |
| ≥12 | 8 (29) | 4 (16) |
| Still in school | 16 (57) | 15 (60) |
| Currently employed | | |
| Yes | 4 (14) | 3 (12) |
| No | 20 (71) | 22 (88) |
| Age at first alcohol use, y | | |
| ≤14 | 12 (43) | 9 (36) |
| 15-17 | 13 (46) | 9 (36) |
| ≥18 | 1 (4) | 1 (4) |
| Never used alcohol | 2 (7) | 5 (20) |
| Parity | | |
| 0 | 21 (75) | 19 (76) |
| 1 | 4 (14) | 3 (12) |
| Gestational age, wk | | |
| ≤20 | 14 (50) | 4 (16) |
| 21-28 | 10 (36) | 12 (48) |
| ≥29† | 2 (7) | 7 (28) |
| Median gestational age, wk | 20 | 25 |
| Father involved | | |
| Yes | 16 (57) | 11 (44) |
| No | 12 (43) | 14 (56) |
| Parenting, mean score | | |
| Knowledge | 46.4 | 46.5 |
| Skills | 73.9 | 77.8 |
| Involvement | 16.8 | 16.1 |
| Family relationships, mean score | | |
| Conflict | 7.5 | 7.3 |
| Cohesion | 8.4 | 7.9 |
| Mental/behavioral health, mean score | | |
| Social support | 24.2 | 24.2 |
| Self-esteem† | 28.6 | 26.3 |
| Depression | 17.7 | 18.4 |
| Locus of control | 21.0 | 19.4 |
| Drug use | 24.4 | 22.3 |

*Values are expressed as number (percentage) of participants unless otherwise indicated. Some data were missing for some variables.
†$P<.05$.

0 controls), still be enrolled in school (8 intervention participants vs 0 controls), and were recruited at a younger gestational age (7 intervention participants ≤20 gestational weeks vs 0 controls).

## FIDELITY TO DOSE OF INTERVENTION

The intervention group completed 82% of 41 lessons and 85% of 25 expected home visits. The control group completed 86% of 20 lessons and 63% of 23 expected home visits.

## PRIMARY OUTCOMES

The adjusted mean difference (AMD) for knowledge scores among mothers in the intervention compared with the control arm at 2 months post partum was +14.9 (95% CI, +7.5 to +22.4) and at 6 months post partum, +15.3 (95% CI, +5.9 to +24.7) (**Table 2**). The AMD for maternal skill scores at 2 months post partum was +5.8 (95% CI, −2.4 to +14.0) and at 6 months post partum, +4.1 (95% CI, −4.0 to +12.3). The AMD for maternal involvement scores at 2 months post partum was +1.5 (95% CI, −0.02 to +3.02) and at 6 months post partum, +1.1 (95% CI, −0.06 to +2.2).

## SECONDARY OUTCOMES

There were no within- or between-group changes in family conflict or cohesion scores from baseline to postintervention (Table 2). Regarding psychological and behavioral risk scores, social support, self-esteem, and locus of control, there were no within- or between-group differences from baseline to postintervention. Depression scores were elevated in both groups at baseline (intervention, 16.8 vs control, 18.8, with a cutoff score of <16 as symptomatic). Mothers in the intervention experienced a larger drop in depressive symptoms at both 2 months and 6 months post partum (AMD, at 2 months post partum, −3.1 [95% CI, −8.8 to +2.5] and at 6 months post partum, −6.1 [95% CI, −13.0 to +0.85]); however, the CIs do include zero. Mothers in both groups reported low drug use (data not shown) and high levels of perceived risk at baseline and follow-up.

## LIMITATIONS

The study had 4 major limitations. (1) We were not able to measure the full extent of teen mothers' child care capacity. Parenting knowledge and involvement could be indicators for capacity but the links are not yet proven. The primary outcome measure that would be the closest proxy—the observed child care skill exercises—had implementation difficulties. (2) There was a notable number of dropouts, particularly in the intervention arm (9 of 28 intervention mothers vs 3 of 25 controls). The imbalance in dropouts between arms is potentially a significant source of bias, even if underlying reasons do not appear to favor the intervention arm (see "Comment" section). (3) Most measures were a type of self-report. Thus, respondents may have given socially desirable answers. (4) The study lacked evaluators blind to the intervention group. Although most of the outcomes were self-reports, the educators supervised the self-reports and conducted the 1 observation skill assessment, which may have biased reported outcomes.

## COMMENT

To our knowledge, this is the first published randomized trial assessing the impact of a family-strengthening

**Table 2. Mean Outcome Scores for Each Study Arm at 2 and 6 Months Post Partum, With Mean Differences Adjusted for Baseline**

| | Unadjusted Mean (SD) | | Adjusted Outcomes | |
|---|---|---|---|---|
| Outcome Score | Intervention (n = 19) | Control (n = 22) | Difference (95% CI) | *P* Value |
| Parenting | | | | |
| Knowledge (range, 0-100) | | | | |
| 2 mo | 71.9 (10) | 58.1 (13) | 14.9 (+7.5 to +22.4) | <.001 |
| 6 mo | 71.1 (14) | 57.2 (15) | 15.3 (+5.9 to +24.7) | .002 |
| Skills (range, 0-100) | | | | |
| 2 mo | 92.4 (10) | 86.9 (15) | 5.8 (−2.4 to +14.0) | .16 |
| 6 mo | 91.1 (24) | 86.4 (15) | 4.1 (−4.0 to +12.3) | .31 |
| Involvement (range, 5-20) | | | | |
| 2 mo | 16.9 (1) | 15.4 (3) | 1.5 (−0.02 to +3.02) | .05 |
| 6 mo | 16.8 (1) | 15.7 (2) | 1.1 (−0.06 to +2.2) | .06 |
| Family relationships | | | | |
| Conflict (range, 5-20; higher score is worse) | | | | |
| 2 mo | 6.9 (2) | 6.6 (2) | 0.2 (−0.9 to +1.3) | .68 |
| 6 mo | 6.8 (2) | 6.5 (3) | 0.4 (−1.4 to +2.2) | .68 |
| Cohesion (range, 3-12) | | | | |
| 2 mo | 8.2 (2) | 7.3 (2) | 0.6 (−0.3 to +1.5) | .18 |
| 6 mo | 8.0 (2) | 8.3 (2) | −0.4 (−1.4 to +0.7) | .45 |
| Mental/behavioral health | | | | |
| Social support (range, 10-50) | | | | |
| 2 mo | 22.2 (6) | 24.0 (5) | −2.3 (−5.4 to +0.97) | .16 |
| 6 mo | 23.1 (7) | 22.5 (5) | 0.41 (−3.4 to +4.2) | .83 |
| Self-esteem (range, 10-40) | | | | |
| 2 mo | 27.7 (4) | 27.2 (3) | −0.84 (−2.9 to +1.2) | .41 |
| 6 mo | 29.4 (4) | 26.4 (3) | 1.6 (−0.77 to +4.1) | .17 |
| Depression (range, 0-60; higher score is worse) | | | | |
| 2 mo | 11.6 (10) | 15.2 (8) | −3.1 (−8.8 to +2.5) | .27 |
| 6 mo | 8.4 (10) | 14.2 (11) | −6.1 (−13.0 to +0.85) | .08 |
| Locus of control (range, 7-28) | | | | |
| 2 mo | 20.8 (3) | 20.1 (4) | −0.23 (−2.5 to +2.0) | .84 |
| 6 mo | 21.3 (4) | 20.9 (4) | 0.17 (−2.3 to +2.6) | .89 |
| Drug abuse (range, 4-32) | | | | |
| 2 mo | 23.9 (8) | 22.5 (7) | 1.1 (−3.9 to +6.0) | .67 |
| 6 mo | 25.1 (6) | 22.4 (8) | 2.6 (−2.2 to +7.4) | .27 |

Abbreviation: CI, confidence interval.

home-visiting intervention on American Indian pregnant teens as a target population.

Intervention mothers had significantly higher knowledge scores at 2 and 6 months post partum. Consistent with numerous behavior change theories, mothers' increased knowledge could lead to increased parental competence, more positive parenting, and better outcomes for mothers and children.[48-50]

Although we originally expected the intervention to affect child care skill scores, the small positive differences we observed at 2 months post partum were even less at 6 months post partum. If the intervention was responsible for skill improvement for some individuals, it was transitory. The modest change in skills may be related to high scores at baseline (ie, a ceiling effect). The skills test was difficult to implement and rate and requires further development and evaluation.

Intervention mothers had significantly higher involvement scores at 2 months post partum, and scores approached significance at 6 months post partum. These differences were associated with positive maternal self-image and characteristics relating to maternal role attainment. Maternal role attainment is a process whereby a woman integrates her new child care responsibilities into her existing behavioral repertoire.[51-53] Studies have linked maternal role attainment to parent competence, sensitive caregiving, and positive involvement over the long-term.[54-56] Adolescent mothers often have complications with maternal role attainment because of their own developmental needs.[53]

Larger decreases in depression scores at 2 and 6 months post partum for intervention mothers were not significant. However, the magnitude of both unadjusted and adjusted mean score differences between groups suggests the intervention may help reduce mothers' depressive symptoms, although our small sample size resulted in imprecise estimates and wide confidence intervals. Depression during pregnancy and post partum has been associated with significant impairments in functioning for both the mother and, ultimately, her child.[57-59] High baseline scores for expectant teens in both groups (>16.0) provide evidence that the study population may be at high risk for depression and invites further investigation of the intervention's impact on depressive symptoms.

With respect to family relationships, there were no differences between groups at end point. One explanation is that baseline scores identified few problems, with little room for either group to improve. Educators observed levels of family conflict that were higher than participants reported. Family relationship measures may be influenced by cultural beliefs that discourage individuals from speaking negatively about one's family. More appropriate family assessment measures will be required for future studies in this population.

There were no observed intervention effects on psychological or behavioral risks. Locus of control, a measure of psychological self-sufficiency, was not affected in this or other home-visitation studies.[16] Lack of impact on social support was not surprising since each group received a large dose of home visitation. The fact that mothers reported low substance use at baseline and follow-up was not expected. National and local studies have described high endemic substance abuse rates in both participating tribes.[60,61] Further, onset of alcohol use before age 15 years predicts higher risk for substance use in adulthood,[62] and our baseline rates of "first drink" averaged 14.5 years of age for all participants. Because the participants were pregnant and legally underage, they may not have been actively using; may have stopped using when they found out they were pregnant; or may have given socially desirable answers. Or the measure for drug use may not have been adequate to assess substance use in this population.

Previous evaluations of home-visiting programs have noted problems with high attrition and adherence to number of expected visits.[63,64] Effective programs generally planned an average of 60 visits over a 1- to 5-year period but averaged between 22 to 33 visits.[63] Our intervention had 25 planned visits covering 41 lessons over a 9-month period. More than 80% of home visits and lessons were completed. However, as illustrated in the Figure, there was a significant number of dropouts from the intervention arm (32%) vs the control arm (12%). Our analyses of the dropouts revealed that the intervention dropouts compared with the control dropouts were more likely to live with their parents, to be currently enrolled in school, and to be recruited earlier in their pregnancies (<20 weeks' gestation). These varying characteristics may suggest that the intervention dropouts had adequate resources (help from their family) to cope with their pregnancy or that the duration and intensity of the intervention was untenable for those still in school or those recruited early in their pregnancy.

Overall, this study indicated that trained American Indian paraprofessionals were able to identify, recruit, obtain consent from, and effectively implement a family-strengthening home-visiting intervention with expectant and postpartum teen mothers. The intervention improved mothers' child care knowledge and involvement and may reduce maternal risk for depression. Firm conclusions cannot yet be drawn because of study limitations. A larger, longer randomized controlled trial incorporating lessons learned from this study is under way to estimate short- and long-term impacts of this paraprofessional-delivered intervention on parenting and health and behavior outcomes for American Indian teen mothers and their children.

**Accepted for Publication:** April 4, 2006.
**Correspondence:** Allison Barlow, MA, MPH, Johns Hopkins Center for American Indian Health, 621 N Washington St, Baltimore, MD 21205 (abarlow@jhsph.edu).
**Author Contributions:** Dr Walkup, the primary investigator for this work, had full access to the study data and takes responsibility for the data integrity and accuracy of the analyses. *Study concept and design:* Barlow, Varipatis-Baker, Speakman, Ginsburg, Pan, Reid, Santosham, and Walkup. *Acquisition of data:* Goklish, Cowboy, Fields, and Hastings. *Analysis and interpretation of data:* Friberg and Pan. *Drafting of the manuscript:* Barlow, Varipatis-Baker, Ginsburg, Friberg, Santosham, and Walkup. *Critical revision of the manuscript for important intellectual content:* Varipatis-Baker, Speakman, Ginsburg, Goklish, Cowboy, Fields, Hastings, Pan, Reid, and Walkup. *Statistical analysis:* Ginsburg, Friberg, and Pan. *Obtained funding:* Barlow, Varipatis-Baker, Speakman, Ginsburg, and Walkup. *Administrative, technical, and material support:* Barlow, Varipatis-Baker, Speakman, Ginsburg, Reid, and Walkup. *Study supervision:* Barlow, Goklish, Cowboy, Fields, Hastings, Reid, Santosham, and Walkup.
**Financial Disclosure:** None reported.
**Funding/Support:** Generous financial support for this work was provided by the Substance Abuse Mental Health Services Administration, the Ford Foundation, the Annie E. Casey Foundation, and the C. S. Mott Foundation. These organizations funded all aspects of this work, from training to formative research, development, implementation, and evaluation.
**Disclaimer:** The opinions expressed are those of the authors and do not necessarily reflect the views of the Indian Health Service.
**Acknowledgment:** We owe the success of this project to our partner organizations, the Navajo Nation and White Mountain Apache Tribe, and the 53 Navajo and Apache families who agreed to take part.

## REFERENCES

1. Elfenbein DS, Felice ME. Adolescent pregnancy. *Pediatr Clin North Am.* 2003;50:781-800.
2. Furstenberg FF, Brooks-Gunn J, Morgan SP. Adolescent mothers and their children in later life. *Fam Plann Perspect.* 1987;19:142-151.
3. US DHHS. *Trends in Indian Health 2000-2001.* Rockville, Md: Public Health Service, Indian Health Service; 2004.
4. Baldwin LM, Grossman DC, Casey S, et al. Perinatal and infant health among rural and urban American Indians/Alaska Natives. *Am J Public Health.* 2002;92:1491-1497.
5. Keppel KG, Pearcy JN, Wagener DK. Trends in racial and ethnic-specific rates for the health status indicators: United States, 1990-1998. *Healthy People 2000 Stat Notes.* 2002;23:1-16.
6. Barlow A, Walkup JT. Developing mental health services for Native American children. *Child Adolesc Psychiatr Clin N Am.* 1998;7:555-577.
7. Census US. *2000 Census American Indian and Alaska Native Area Data.* Washington, DC: Census Bureau; 2000.
8. Bayne SL. Culture materials in schools' programs for Indian students. *J Am Ind Education.* 1969;9:1-6.
9. Sanchez-Way R, Johnson S. Cultural practices in American Indian prevention programs. *Juvenile Justice J.* 2000;7:20-30. http://www.ncjrs.gov/html/ojjdp/jjnl_2000_12/cult.html.
10. Oetting ER, Beauvais F. Orthogonal cultural identification theory: the cultural identification of minority adolescents. *Int J Addict.* 1990-91;25:655-685.
11. Duggan AK, McFarlane EC, Windham AM. Evaluation of Hawaii's Healthy Start Program. *Future Child.* 1999;9:66-90, discussion 177-178.
12. Eckenrode J, Ganzel B, Henderson CR Jr, et al. Preventing child abuse and ne-

glect with a program of nurse home visitation: the limiting effects of domestic violence. *JAMA*. 2000;284:1385-1391.
13. Olds DL, Henderson CR Jr, Kitzman HJ, Eckenrode JJ, Cole RE, Tatelbaum RC. Prenatal and infancy home visitation by nurses: recent findings. *Future Child.* 1999;9:44-65, 190-191.
14. Koniak-Griffin D, Anderson N, Verzemnieks I, Brecht M. A public health nursing early intervention program for adolescent mothers: outcomes from pregnancy through 6 weeks postpartum. *Nurs Res.* 2000;49:130-138.
15. Kitzman H, Olds DL, Sidora K, et al. Enduring effects of nurse home visitation on maternal life course: a 3-year follow-up of a randomized trial. *JAMA*. 2000; 283:1983-1989.
16. Olds DL. Prenatal and infancy home visiting by nurses: from randomized trials to community replication. *Prev Sci.* 2002;3:153-172.
17. Olds DL, Robinson J, O'Brien R, et al. Home visiting by paraprofessionals and by nurses: a randomized, controlled trial. *Pediatrics.* 2002;110:486-496.
18. Kumpfer KL, Alvarado R, Whiteside HO. Family-based interventions for substance use and misuse prevention. *Subst Use Misuse.* 2003;38:1759-1787.
19. Gomby DS. Understanding evaluations of home visitation programs. *Future Child.* 1999;9:27-43.
20. Kendrick D, Elkan R, Hewitt M, et al. Does home visiting improve parenting and the quality of the home environment? a systematic review and meta analysis. *Arch Dis Child.* 2000;82:443-451.
21. Olds DL, Henderson CR Jr, Tatelbaum R, Chamberlin R. Improving the life-course development of socially disadvantaged mothers: a randomized trial of nurse home visitation. *Am J Public Health.* 1988;78:1436-1445.
22. Kumpfer KL, Alexander J, McDonald L, Olds DL. Family-focused substance prevention: what has been learned from other fields. In: Ashery RS, Robertson EB, Kumpfer KL, eds. *Drug Abuse Prevention Through Family Intervention.* Rockville, Md: US Dept of Health and Human Services; 1998:78-102. NIDA Research Monograph 177.
23. McCurdy K. Can home visitation enhance maternal social support? *Am J Community Psychol.* 2001;29:97-112.
24. Eckenrode J, Zielinski D, Smith E, et al. Child maltreatment and the early onset of problem behaviors: can a program of nurse home visitation break the link? *Dev Psychopathol.* 2001;13:873-890.
25. Hahn RA, Bilukha OO, Crosby A, et al. First reports evaluating the effectiveness of strategies for preventing violence: early childhood home visitation: findings from the Task Force on Community Preventive Services. *MMWR Recomm Rep.* 2003;52(RR-14):1-9.
26. Koniak-Griffin D, Anderson N, Brecht M, Verzemnieks I, Lesser J, Kim S. Public health nursing care for adolescent mothers: impact on infant health and selected maternal outcomes at 1 year postbirth. *J Adolesc Health.* 2002;30:44-54.
27. Olds DL, Kitzman H. Can home visitation improve the health of women and children at environmental risk? *Pediatrics.* 1990;86:108-116.
28. Olds D, Henderson CR Jr, Kitzman HJ, Cole RE. Effects of prenatal and infancy nurse home visitation on surveillance of child maltreatment. *Pediatrics.* 1995; 95:365-372.
29. Olds D, Henderson CR Jr, Cole RE, et al. Long-term effects of nurse home visitation on children's criminal and antisocial behavior: 15-year follow-up of a randomized controlled trial. *JAMA.* 1998;280:1238-1244.
30. Armstrong F. Australia needs more indigenous nurses. *Aust Nurs J.* 2001;8(9): 28-30.
31. Hagengruber J. Native nurse. *Billings Gazette.* October 22, 2001. http://www.billingsgazette.com/newdex.php?display=rednews/2001/10/22/build/community/cOMMUN.inc.
32. Yurkovich EE. Working with American Indians toward educational success. *J Nurs Educ.* 2001;40:259-269.
33. Randomization.com Web site. http://randomization.com/. Accessed May 2001.
34. American Academy of Pediatrics. *American Academy of Pediatrics Guide to Baby Care: Caring for Your Baby and Young Child: Birth to Age 5.* New York, NY: Bantam Books; 1998.
35. Bloom BL. A factor analysis of self-report measures of family functioning. *Fam Process.* 1985;24:225-239.
36. Rosenberg M. *Society and the Adolescent Self-Image.* Rev ed. Middletown, Conn: Wesleyan University Press; 1989.
37. Weissman MM, Pottenger M, Kleber I, Ruber HL, Williams D. Symptom patterns in primary and secondary depression: a comparison of primary depressives with depressed opiate addicts, alcoholics, and schizophrenics. *Arch Gen Psychiatry.* 1977;34:854-862.
38. Dick RW, Beals J, Keane EM, Manson SM. Factorial structure of the CES-D among American Indian adolescents. *J Adolesc.* 1994;17:73-79.
39. Garrison CZ, Jackson KL, Marsteller F, McKeown R, Addy C. A longitudinal study of depressive symptomatology in young adolescents. *J Am Acad Child Adolesc Psychiatry.* 1990;29:581-585.
40. Garrison CZ, Addy CL, Jackson KL, McKeown R, Waller JL. The CES-D as a screen for depression and other psychiatric disorders in adolescence. *J Am Acad Child Adolesc Psychiatry.* 1991;30:636-641.
41. Prescott CA, McArdle JJ, Hishinuma ES, et al. Prediction of major depression and dysthymia from CES-D scores among ethnic minority adolescents. *J Am Acad Child Adolesc Psychiatry.* 1998;37:495-503.
42. Somervell PD, Beals J, Kinzie JD, Boehnlein J, Leung P, Manson SM. Use of the CES-D in an American Indian village. *Cult Med Psychiatry.* 1992;16:503-517.
43. Somervell PD, Beals J, Kinzie JD, Boehnlein J, Leung P, Manson SM. Criterion validity of the Center for Epidemiologic Studies Depression scale in a population sample from an American Indian village. *Psychiatry Res.* 1993;47:255-266.
44. Wilcox H, Field T, Prodromidis M, Scafidi F. Correlations between the BDI and CES-D in a sample of adolescent mothers. *Adolescence.* 1998;33:565-573.
45. Beals J, Manson SM, Keane E, et al. Factorial structure of the Center for Epidemiologic Studies Depression Scale among American Indian college students. *Psychol Assess.* 1991;3:623-627.
46. Pearlin LI, Lieberman MA, Menaghan EG, Mullan JT. The stress process. *J Health Soc Behav.* 1981;22:337-356.
47. SAMHSA Measures and Instruments Resource Web site. Measure: CSAP GPRA attitudes and beliefs—youth (2005). June 22, 2005. http://preventionplatform.samhsa.gov/macro/csap/mir_search_create/redesign/measures/detail.cfm?MeasureID=27b198f0-7304-41e0-814a-572733ccf6f8. Accessed June 22, 2005.
48. Ajzen I. The theory of planned behavior. *Organ Behav Hum Decis Process.* 1991; 50:179-211.
49. Bandura A. Self-efficacy: toward a unifying theory of behavioral change. *Psychol Rev.* 1977;84:191-215.
50. Prochaska JO. *Systems of Psychotherapy: a Transtheoretical Analysis.* 2nd ed. Pacific Grove, Calif: Brooks-Cole; 1984.
51. Mercer RT, Ferketich SL. Experienced and inexperienced mothers' maternal competence during infancy. *Res Nurs Health.* 1995;18:333-343.
52. Rubin R. Attainment of the maternal role, part I: processes. *Nurs Res.* 1967;14: 237-245.
53. Sartore AT. Maternal role attainment in adolescent mothers: foundations and implications. *Online J Knowl Synth Nurs.* 1996;E3:86-96.
54. Ishii K, Mori E, Maehara S. The relationship between maternal role attainment during pregnancy and empathy. *Nihon Kango Kagakkaishi.* 1997;17:37-45.
55. Jirapaet V. Factors affecting maternal role attainment among low-income, Thai, HIV-positive mothers. *J Transcult Nurs.* 2001;12:25-33.
56. Dukewich TL, Borkowski JG, Whitman TL. Adolescent mothers and child abuse potential: an evaluation of risk factors. *Child Abuse Negl.* 1996;20:1031-1047.
57. Lundy B, Jones N, Field T, et al. Prenatal depression effects on neonates. *Infant Behav Dev.* 1999;22:121-131.
58. Martins C, Gaffan EA. Effects of early maternal depression on patterns of infant-mother attachment: a meta-analytic investigation. *J Child Psychol Psychiatry.* 2000;41:737-746.
59. Steer RA, Scholl TO, Hediger ML, Fischer RL. Self-reported depression and negative pregnancy outcomes. *J Clin Epidemiol.* 1992;45:1093-1099.
60. *Navajo Nation Youth Risk Behavior Survey.* Window Rock, Ariz: Navajo Health Promotion Office and Indian Health Service; 2005.
61. May PA. Substance abuse and American Indians: prevalence and susceptibility. *Int J Addict.* 1982;17:1185-1209.
62. Dishion TJ, Kavanagh K, Kiesner J. Prevention of early adolescent substance abuse among high-risk youth: a multiple gating approach to parent intervention. In: Ashery RS, Robertson EB, Kumpfer KL, eds. *Drug Abuse Prevention Through Family Interventions.* Rockville, Md: US Dept of Health and Human Services; 1998: 208-228. NIDA Research Monograph 177.
63. Gomby DS, Culross PL, Behrman RE. Home visiting: recent program evaluation—analysis and recommendations. *Future Child.* 1999;9:4-26.
64. St Pierre RG, Layzer JI. Using home visits for multiple purposes: the Comprehensive Child Development Program. *Future Child.* 1999;9:134-151.

# Double Burden of Iron Deficiency in Infancy and Low Socioeconomic Status

## *A Longitudinal Analysis of Cognitive Test Scores to Age 19 Years*

*Betsy Lozoff, MD; Elias Jimenez, MD; Julia B. Smith, EdD*

**Objective:** To assess change in cognitive functioning after iron deficiency in infancy, depending on socioeconomic status (SES; middle vs low).

**Design:** Longitudinal study.

**Setting:** Urban community in Costa Rica (infancy phase [July 26, 1983, through February 28, 1985] through 19-year follow-up [March 19, 2000, through November 4, 2002]).

**Participants:** A total of 185 individuals enrolled at 12 to 23 months of age (no preterm or low-birth-weight infants or infants with acute or chronic health problems). The participants were assessed in infancy and at 5, 11 to 14, 15 to 18, and 19 years of age. A total of 97% were evaluated at 5 or 11 to 14 years and 78% at 15 to 18 or 19 years. Individuals who had chronic iron deficiency in infancy (iron deficiency with hemoglobin concentrations ≤10.0 g/dL or, with higher hemoglobin concentrations, not fully corrected within 3 months of iron therapy) were compared with those who had good iron status as infants (hemoglobin concentrations ≥12.0 g/dL and normal iron measures before and/or after therapy).

**Main Outcome Measures:** Cognitive change over time (composite of standardized scores at each age).

**Results:** For middle-SES participants, scores averaged 101.2 in the group with chronic iron deficiency vs 109.3 in the group with good iron status in infancy and remained 8 to 9 points lower through 19 years (95% confidence interval [CI], −10.1 to −6.2). For low-SES participants, the gap widened from 10 points (93.1 vs 102.8; 95% CI for difference, −12.8 to −6.6) to 25 points (70.4 vs 95.3; 95% CI for difference, 20.6 to 29.4).

**Conclusions:** The group with chronic iron deficiency in infancy did not catch up to the group with good iron status in cognitive scores over time. There was a widening gap for those in low-SES families. The results suggest the value of preventing iron deficiency in infancy.

*Arch Pediatr Adolesc Med. 2006;160:1108-1113*

INFANTS WITH IRON DEFICIENCY anemia or other indications of chronic, severe iron deficiency have shown lower cognitive test scores than infants with good iron status in all but 1 of 14 studies that assessed overall cognitive functioning, from countries around the world.[1,2] The few available follow-up studies at school age or early adolescence report persisting lower scores despite iron therapy in infancy.[3-7] A recent meta-analysis estimated the long-term effects on IQ to be 1.73 points lower for each 1.0-g/dL decrease in hemoglobin.[8] Differences in group means raise questions about stability and change over time. Is there evidence of catch-up or further decline? Does the impact of iron deficiency in infancy vary over time depending on socioeconomic circumstances? These issues pertain to millions of children.[8] An estimated 20% to 25% of infants worldwide have iron deficiency anemia, and more have iron deficiency without anemia.[9-11] Poor, minority, and/or immigrant infants in industrialized countries are also at increased risk for iron deficiency.[12]

To address questions about change over time depending on iron status in infancy and socioeconomic status (SES), we applied techniques of longitudinal analysis[13] to data from an ongoing study in Costa Rica. Previous cross-sectional analyses showed that cognitive test scores for the group with chronic, severe iron deficiency in infancy (see the "Methods" section) were lower than the group with good iron status in infancy[14] and at ages 5 and 11 to 14 years.[6,15] By 11 to 14 years, a higher proportion of children in the group with chronic iron deficiency had repeated a grade in school and/or been referred for special services.[6] The present study assessed change in cognitive test performance from the second year of life to the transition to adulthood (19 years) according to SES.

**Author Affiliations:** Center for Human Growth and Development and Department of Pediatrics and Communicable Diseases, University of Michigan, Ann Arbor (Dr Lozoff); Department of Hematology, Hospital Nacional de Niños, San Jose, Costa Rica (Dr Jimenez); and Department of Educational Leadership, Oakland University, Rochester, Mich (Dr Smith). Dr Jimenez is currently with the Department of Pediatrics, Hospital CIMA San Jose, San Jose, Costa Rica.

## METHODS

### SAMPLE

The analysis used data from a longitudinal study in Costa Rica that included evaluations in infancy and 4 subsequent follow-ups (5, 11-14, 15-18, and 19 years of age). Enrollment in the original infant study was conducted from July 26, 1983, through February 28, 1985, in an urban community near San Jose, the capital of Costa Rica.[14] The 19-year evaluation was conducted from March 19, 2000, through November 4, 2002. The community was mixed middle and lower class, and parents of study infants averaged 8 to 10 years of education. Enrollment entailed door-to-door screening, inviting study participation for all 12- to 23-month-old infants who had a birth weight of 2.5 kg or higher and a singleton, full-term, uncomplicated birth who were free of acute or chronic medical problems and had normal physical examination results. The refusal rate was 11.6%. Infants enrolled in the study had no evidence of growth failure or other nutrient deficiencies.[14] The mean age at study entry was 17 months. Iron deficiency was thus likely to have lasted for months, especially since the local feeding practice at the time was to introduce unmodified cow's milk in the first months of life (along with breastfeeding). Of the 191 infants in the initial study, 185 provided data for this longitudinal analysis (6 were excluded because of lack of information about their iron status after iron therapy).

**Figure 1** shows a flowchart of the number and percentage of participants at each subsequent assessment. From the 5-year follow-up study,[15] 161 children provided data for the longitudinal analysis. All but 15 received the comprehensive psychoeducational assessment within 2 weeks of their fifth birthday (age range, 59-63 months). From the reevaluation at age 11 to 14 years,[6] 162 children provided data (mean age, 12.3 years; range, 10.9-13.7 years). Overall, 97% of the original sample participated in assessments either at age 5 years or early adolescence. A brief follow-up in late adolescence provided data for 133 participants (mean age, 16.4 years; range, 15.0-17.9 years). A comprehensive assessment at 19 years provided data for 121 participants (mean age, 19.0 years; range, 18.0-20.0 years). A total of 145 (78%) of the original 185 participants were evaluated at 15 to 18 years and/or 19 years. Participants who were not tested at a given age often participated subsequently (Figure 1). Lack of participation was primarily due to difficulty in locating a family.

Parental signed informed consent for each phase of the study was obtained by the project pediatrician. Assent or consent of the adolescent was obtained beginning with the early-adolescent follow-up. The infancy and 5-year protocols were approved by the institutional review board of Case Western Reserve University, Cleveland, Ohio, and subsequent protocols were approved by the institutional review board of the University of Michigan. All protocols were approved by ethics committees of the Hospital Nacional de Niños or Instituto Costarricense de Investigationes Clinicas (for the 19-year evaluation) and the Ministry of Health, San Jose, Costa Rica.

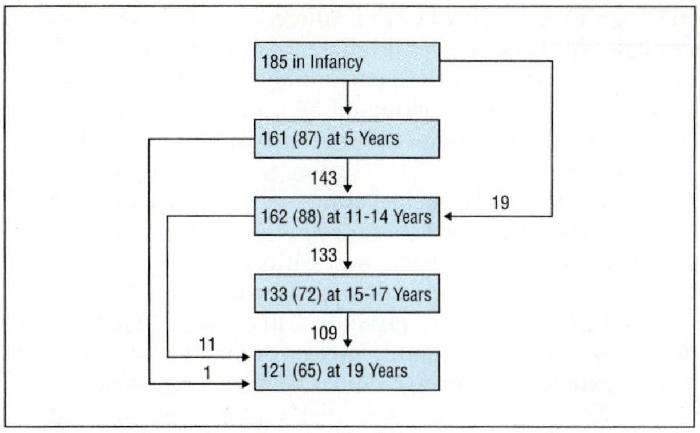


**Figure 1.** Flowchart of study participation. The number (percentage) of participants at each time point is shown, indicating that participants who missed an assessment were often available subsequently. Numbers between boxes indicate number of children studied at both ages in connected boxes. Numbers by outer arrows are children who missed 1 or more assessments but were evaluated at the ages shown.

### MEASURES

#### Iron Status

Iron status in infancy was determined by venous concentrations of hemoglobin, transferrin saturation, free erythrocyte protoporphyrin, and serum ferritin. Iron deficiency was defined as 2 or more abnormal iron measures (a serum ferritin concentration of <12 ng/mL [<27.0 pmol/L] and either a free erythrocyte protoporphyrin level of ≥100 μg/dL [≥1.77 μmol/L] of red blood cells or a transferrin saturation of <10%)."[16-18] Iron sufficiency was defined as a hemoglobin concentration of 12.0 g/dL or more and normal values on all iron status measures. Hematologic response to iron therapy in infancy was excellent, with a mean hemoglobin increase of 3.7 g/dL among iron-deficient infants with a hemoglobin concentration of 10.5 g/dL or less. Anemia in all infants resolved following 3 months of iron therapy, but as might be expected, those with indications of more severe or chronic iron deficiency still had biochemical alterations, such as elevated erythrocyte protoporphyrin values.[14] At the subsequent follow-ups that included blood collection (5, 11-14, and 19 years),[6,15] iron deficiency was present in less than 5%, and no one had iron deficiency anemia except for 4 women at 19 years, 2 of whom were pregnant. These data indicate that the Costa Rican diet at the time provided adequate iron to correct any iron parameters that were still altered after treatment in infancy and to maintain good iron status thereafter.

Following the approach in the 5-year follow-up and subsequent reports,[6,15,19] we compared participants who had chronic, severe iron deficiency in infancy (with or without anemia) with the rest of the sample who were iron sufficient before and/or after iron therapy in infancy. For simplicity, the chronic, severe iron-deficient group will be referred to as "chronic iron deficiency" and the rest of the sample as "good iron status." The chronic–iron deficiency group consisted of participants who had marked iron deficiency anemia in infancy (hemoglobin ≤10.0 g/dL) and those with higher hemoglobin concentrations and iron deficiency that did not fully correct after 3 months of iron therapy.[15] Analyses compared the chronic–iron deficiency (n=53) and good–iron status (n=132) groups. There was no differential attrition; the chronic–iron deficiency group constituted 28% to 29% of the sample in both infancy and the late-adolescent follow-up.

#### Cognitive Assessments

In infancy, the Mental Development Index of the Bayley Scales of Infant Development[20] was administered before and after iron treatment. At the 5-year follow-up, the overall tests of cognitive function were the Wechsler Preschool and Primary Scale of Intelligence[21] and the Woodcock-Johnson Psychoeducational Battery.[22] At 11 to 14 years, the general cognitive measures were the Wechsler Intelligence Scale for Children–Revised,[23] the Wide Range Achievement Test–Revised (arithmetic and reading),[24] and the Directed Writing Task.[25] At 15 to 18 years, the measures were arithmetic and reading achievement[24] and the Directed Writing Task.[25] At 19 years, the general cognitive measures were arithmetic achievement[24] and 5 subscales of the Wechsler Intelligence Scale for Adults,[26] prorated to estimate verbal and performance intelligence scores.[27] All assessments were conducted by trained Costa Rican psychologists who were unaware of participants' hematologic status at any age.

Factor analyses (principal components with Varimax rotation[28]) showed that the general cognitive measures at each assessment were closely associated with each other. Each set of measures yielded a single factor that explained 62% (5 years) to 78% (19 years) of the variance. This data reduction information warranted combining measures into a composite cognitive score for a given age. Since all tests were standardized or could be rescaled to a mean of 100 and an SD of 15 to 16, analyses could be conducted across ages and differing tests. In the longitudinal model structure described herein, all analyses were adjusted for each individual's exact age at each follow-up. Results report change relative to age-normed scores based on US standardization samples at each time point. Thus, a "decline" is relative to norms for age, rather than in actual knowledge or absolute cognitive performance.

### Environmental Factors

Iron deficiency often goes along with other individual, family, and/or environmental disadvantages, some of which could affect cognitive development.[1,29-31] The critical comparison of our study considers the impact of infant iron status depending on family SES. Measures of family SES generally assess such factors as family structure, economic circumstances, education, and occupation. We used the Hollingshead Four Factor Index,[32] which considers parental education and occupation and father presence and is widely used. We compared individuals whose family SES in infancy was low (levels 4 and 5: unskilled and semiskilled workers) or middle to high (levels 1-3: professional, managerial, clerical, and skilled workers).[32]

## STATISTICAL ANALYSIS

Longitudinal analysis using hierarchical linear modeling (HLM) was the primary statistical approach.[13,33] This class of analytic techniques has not previously been applied to change in cognitive scores over time with iron deficiency in infancy. By considering the within-individual correlations between measures, longitudinal analysis provides relatively unbiased estimates for each individual of the starting level (intercept), change over time (slope), and acceleration or deceleration (curvature). The study's analyses were conducted with HLM software.[33] Hierarchical linear modeling estimates the covariance structure appropriately in data sets that, like ours, have incomplete and unbalanced time parameters, with a varying number of assessments and intervals between assessments for different individuals, resulting in a varying variance structure.[13] The analysis used measures nested within individuals (level 1), comparing differences between individuals in the good–iron status and chronic–iron deficiency groups (level 2). The level 1 model used individual age at testing as the time parameter, with the change estimated specific to the amount of time between assessments for each individual. We tested for the possibility of curvilinear components or multiple growth trajectories, as well as single linear change, and selected the most parsimonious and best-fitting model based on the lowest deviance relative to the *df*.[13] The best model estimated 2 distinct slopes: one for change from infancy to age 5 years and another for change from 5 to 19 years of age. Models were anchored to actual test scores at the beginning and end of these intervals (infancy, age 5 years, and age 19 years).

We tested for an interaction between iron status in infancy and SES (middle vs low) in an overall model. The interactions were statistically significant for intercept ($P$=.02) and both slopes ($P$=.003 for change from infancy to age 5 years and $P$=.01 for change from age 5 to 19 years). To facilitate interpretation, we present results comparing change over time in the chronic–iron deficiency and good–iron status groups separately for middle- and low-SES families (for middle-SES families, 67 had good iron status and 20 had chronic iron deficiency; for low-SES families, 65 had good iron status and 33 had chronic iron deficiency). The estimated intercepts and change over time for these analyses match the estimates from the overall model. Where appropriate, we conducted post hoc tests of common parameters for significant differences by examining the difference in parameter estimate relative to the pooled SE of the estimate (a form of $t$ test comparison).[13]

## RESULTS

A higher proportion of the chronic–iron deficiency group was male (75% vs 48% in the good–iron status group; $P$=.005), as noted in previous reports.[6,14] These individuals also weighed 200 g less at birth (mean [SD] birth weight: 3.1 [0.3] kg vs 3.3 [0.4] kg in the good–iron status group; $P$=.02). Sex and birth weight were therefore covaried in all analyses. The sample was reasonably balanced between middle- and low-SES families (87 middle-SES families and 98 low-SES families). Socioeconomic status was lower in the chronic–iron deficiency group when analyzed as a continuous variable (mean [SD] Hollingshead score: 27.2 [10.8] vs 31.0 [12.6] in the good–iron status group; $P$=.02). However, the difference in the proportion in low-SES families did not reach statistical significance. Sixty-two percent of the chronic–iron deficiency group came from low-SES families compared with 49% of the good–iron status group ($P$=.11).

**Figure 2** shows the relationship between iron deficiency and cognitive test scores over time depending on SES. In middle-SES families, initial cognitive scores for participants who had chronic iron deficiency in infancy averaged 8 points lower than those with good iron status (101.2 vs 109.3; difference in infancy, −8.15; 95% CI, −10.1 to −6.2; effect size, 0.54 SD). No statistically significant differences were found between groups in change from infancy to age 5 years or from 5 to 19 years of age. Thus, the magnitude of difference was maintained; at 19 years, their scores averaged 9 points lower (98.2 vs 107.6; 95% CI for the difference, −11.0 to −7.0).

In low-SES families, initial cognitive scores for participants with chronic iron deficiency in infancy averaged 10 points lower than those with good iron status (93.1 vs 102.8; difference in infancy, −9.7; 95% CI, −12.8 to −6.6; effect size, 0.67 SD). Scores for the chronic–iron deficiency group declined from infancy to age 5 years (difference in rate of change, −1.8; 95% CI, −2.6 to −1.1), whereas those for the good–iron status group did not. Although a pattern of decline in cognitive test scores from 5 to 19 years was generally observed, in low-SES families, the decline among individuals with chronic iron deficiency in infancy was steeper than for those in the good–iron status group (difference in rate of change, −0.6; 95% CI, −0.8 to −0.3). This resulted in mean scores of 70.4 vs 95.3 by 19 years—a 25-point gap (95% CI, 20.6 to 29.4;

effect size, 1.67 SD)—between chronic–iron deficiency and good–iron status groups with low-SES backgrounds.

In light of our interest in environmental disadvantage, we also compared iron status groups across SES levels in a post hoc comparison of models. For the good–iron status group, those in low-SES families had scores in infancy 7 points (95% CI, 4.0 to 10.0; effect size, 0.47 SD) lower than those in middle-SES families, increasing to 12 points (95% CI, 8.4 to 15.6) by age 19 years. For the chronic–iron deficiency group, individuals from middle-SES families started with scores in infancy like those of the good–iron status group in low-SES families: in between those with good iron status from middle-SES families and those with chronic iron deficiency from low-SES families. The chronic–iron deficiency group from middle-SES families showed a pattern over time like that of the good–iron status group in middle-SES families except 8 to 9 points lower (95% CI, 5.2 to 11.8; effect sizes, 0.53 to 0.60 SD). In contrast, the cognitive test score gap for individuals in the chronic–iron deficiency group from low-SES families (compared with those in middle-SES families) widened from 8 points (95% CI, 5.4 to 10.8) in infancy to 28 points at age 19 years (95% CI, 23.6 to 32.4; effect size, 1.87 SD).

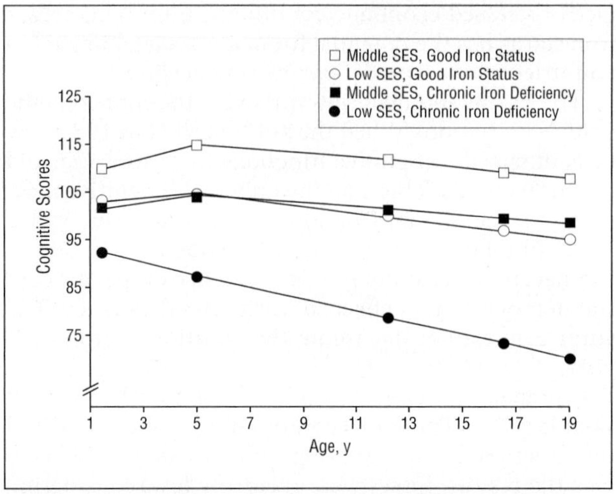


**Figure 2.** Cognitive composite scores over time, comparing infant iron status groups within middle- and low-socioeconomic status (SES) families. Iron status group and SES level each affected initial scores ($P=.01$ for chronic–iron deficiency difference within middle-SES families and $P=.003$ for chronic–iron deficiency difference within low-SES families). Change over time differed only for the chronic–iron deficiency group in low-SES families ($P=.02$ for change from infancy to age 5 years and $P=.04$ for change from age 5 to 19 years). Each participant is represented once: good iron status (n=67) compared with chronic iron deficiency (n=20) in middle-SES families and good iron status (n=65) compared with chronic iron deficiency (n=33) in low-SES families. Symbols are placed at the average age for each assessment.

## COMMENT

Using longitudinal analytic techniques, this study showed no evidence of catch-up in cognitive test performance for individuals with chronic iron deficiency in infancy and a widening gap for those in low-SES families. This finding was observed despite iron therapy in infancy sufficient to correct anemia for those who had been anemic and good iron status thereafter. A gap of the observed magnitude (25-28 points) is likely to correspond to major differences in life course.

The observed pattern appears to make sense in terms of the cumulative and transactional nature of cognitive development.[34-36] Acquisition of new skills is intimately linked to mastery of skills at an earlier developmental level. If direct and indirect effects of early iron deficiency on the brain[37] disrupted or delayed basic developmental processes, there could be a snowball effect. In an economically stressed family environment, there might not be the resources or capacity to help children compensate. Together, these factors could contribute to earlier school failure[6] and less advanced cognitive processes in individuals with chronic iron deficiency in infancy in low-SES families. Thus, our results fit with the concept of "double jeopardy" or "double hazard"[38,39] (ie, worse outcome among individuals who experience both an early biological insult or stressor and more disadvantaged background[40]).

As expected, individuals from disadvantaged backgrounds showed lower cognitive test scores. This was confirmed for both the good–iron status and chronic–iron deficiency groups. Even with good iron status in infancy, low-SES individuals showed a decline in test scores like that observed in the United States.[41] Our observation that SES differences in cognitive test performance appeared to be set by preschool age and not improved by schooling has also been reported in the United States and elsewhere.[42,43] This has sometimes been called the Matthew effect[44,45] in reference to the biblical quotation "To all those who have, more will be given, and they will have an abundance, but from those who have nothing, even what they have will be taken away." However, there was a differential effect of iron status on change over time in low-SES families. Individuals in the chronic–iron deficiency group not only tested lower in infancy but also showed a more marked decline, and hence an increasing gap, in subsequent cognitive test performance. Thus, good iron status before and/or after iron therapy in infancy appeared to attenuate the decline.

A major food supplementation trial in Guatemala found that early nutritional supplementation eliminated the decline in test scores associated with low SES.[46] Although the interventions differed (single micronutrient in our study and energy plus multimicronutrients in the Guatemala study), both studies provide support for long-term cognitive benefits of improved nutrition in infancy. Several investigators have assessed the likelihood that improved nutrition contributes to the rising IQs observed in many countries.[47] IQ tests and other such measures have had to be restandardized to adjust for rising scores. Because infant iron status has improved markedly in the United States and elsewhere in the past several decades,[48,49] a reduction in iron deficiency might play a role in the continued phenomenon of rising IQs. If the pattern we observed among individuals with good iron status before or after iron therapy in infancy applies elsewhere (ie, higher cognitive test scores later on), there might be corresponding population-level increases in cognitive test scores with improved iron status in infancy. If replicated, the results would suggest that even in the face of stressed economic conditions, improving infant iron status has the potential for major societal impact in countries where iron deficiency is widespread.

The results should be interpreted in the context of the study's limitations. When the study started in 1981, few tests of specific cognitive functions in 1- to 2-year-old infants were available, and the only early cognitive measure was the Mental Development Index of the Bayley Scales of Infant Development. Consequently, this longitudinal analysis cannot provide evidence of specific central nervous system effects of early iron deficiency. The study also cannot determine the duration of iron deficiency; it could have started in the first year or even earlier (prenatally). The study is further limited by its small sample size and potential confounding by measured and unmeasured factors. Although missing data could also bias the results, losses were relatively low, considering follow-up from infancy to the transition to adulthood.

Socioeconomic status may exert its effects in different ways in various societies and cultures. Thus, the relationships observed in this Costa Rican sample may not generalize to other parts of the world. Furthermore, study participants were full-term infants, free of chronic or acute illnesses, and growing normally by US standards. Children who are not in such good overall health might not show the same effects. Conversely, children who experience briefer or milder iron deficiency in infancy might not show the pattern of declining cognitive test scores we observed. However, most infants in the world are not tested for anemia or iron deficiency and thus may experience even more prolonged or severe and/or untreated iron deficiency. Their outcome might be poorer than what we observed.

## CONCLUSIONS

In this study in Costa Rica, participants who had chronic, severe iron deficiency in infancy (moderate iron deficiency anemia or hemoglobin concentrations >100 g/L with abnormal iron measures after treatment) did not catch up in cognitive test scores over time to those who were iron sufficient before and/or after treatment in infancy. For individuals from middle-SES families who had chronic iron deficiency in infancy, the magnitude of the gap remained the same from infancy to age 19 years (8-9 points lower). However, those in lower-SES families seemed doubly burdened; the gap widened substantially from 10 points in infancy to 25 points at age 19 years. Such a difference is likely to be functionally significant regarding educational attainment and career choices in adulthood. The analysis also suggested a protective effect of good iron status in infancy in low-SES families. In light of potential adverse effects at the level of the individual and the society in settings where iron deficiency is widespread, it seems reasonable to prevent iron deficiency in infancy and treat it before it becomes chronic or severe.

**Accepted for Publication:** July 8, 2006.
**Correspondence:** Betsy Lozoff, MD, Center for Human Growth and Development, 300 N Ingalls, University of Michigan, Ann Arbor, MI 48109-0406 (blozoff@umich.edu).
**Author Contributions:** Dr Lozoff had full access to all study data and takes responsibility for data integrity and accuracy of data analysis. *Study concept and design:* Lozoff and Jimenez. *Acquisition of data:* Lozoff and Jimenez. *Analysis and interpretation of data:* Lozoff and Smith. *Drafting of the manuscript:* Lozoff. *Critical revision of the manuscript for important intellectual content:* Lozoff, Jimenez, and Smith. *Statistical analysis:* Smith. *Obtained funding:* Lozoff. *Administrative, technical, and material support:* Lozoff and Jimenez. *Study supervision:* Lozoff and Jimenez.
**Financial Disclosure:** None reported.
**Funding/Support:** All phases of the study were supported by grants from the US National Institute of Child Health and Human Development. The longitudinal analysis was supported by a MERIT (Method to Extend Research in Time) Award to Dr Lozoff (R37 HD31606).
**Previous Presentation:** Preliminary results were presented at the Pediatric Academic Societies annual meeting; May 2, 2004; San Francisco, Calif.
**Acknowledgment:** We are grateful to study families for commitment and continued participation, to the skilled psychologists who meticulously performed the cognitive tests over 2 decades, and to Agustin Calatroni, MS, Niko Kaciroti, PhD, and Stephen Raudenbush, PhD, for heated discussion and good advice on longitudinal analysis.

## REFERENCES

1. Grantham-McGregor S, Ani C. A review of studies on the effect of iron deficiency on cognitive development in children. *J Nutr.* 2001;131:649S-668S.
2. Lozoff B, Georgieff MK. Iron deficiency and brain development. *Semin Pediatr Neurol.* In press.
3. Cantwell RJ. The long term neurological sequelae of anemia in infancy [abstract]. *Pediatr Res.* 1974;342:68.
4. Palti H, Meijer A, Adler B. Learning achievement and behavior at school of anemic and non-anemic infants. *Early Hum Dev.* 1985;10:217-223.
5. Hurtado EK, Claussen AH, Scott KG. Early childhood anemia and mild or moderate mental retardation. *Am J Clin Nutr.* 1999;69:115-119.
6. Lozoff B, Jimenez E, Hagen J, Mollen E, Wolf AW. Poorer behavioral and developmental outcome more than 10 years after treatment for iron deficiency in infancy. *Pediatrics.* 2000;105:E51.
7. Antunes H. *Iron Deficiency Anaemia in Infants: A Prospective Neurodevelopment Evaluation.* Porto: Faculty of Medicine, University of Portugal; 2004.
8. Stoltzfus RJ, Mullany L, Black RE. Iron deficiency anaemia. In: Ezzati M, Lopez AD, Rodgers A, Murray CJL, eds. *Comparative Quantification of Health Risks: Global and Regional Burden of Disease Attributable to Selected Major Risk Factors.* Vol 1. Geneva, Switzerland: World Health Organization; 2004:163-209.
9. deMaeyer E, Adiels-Tegman M. The prevalence of anaemia in the world. *World Health Stat Q.* 1985;38:302-316.
10. Florentino RF, Guirriec RM. Prevalence of nutritional anemia in infancy and childhood with emphasis on developing countries. In: Steckel A, ed. *Iron Nutrition in Infancy and Childhood.* New York, NY: Raven Press; 1984:61-74.
11. Mannar V, Bellamy C. *Vitamin and Mineral Deficiency: A Global Progress Report.* New York, NY: UNICEF; 2004.
12. Brotanek JM, Halterman J, Auinger P, Flores G, Weitzman M. Iron deficiency, prolonged bottle-feeding, and racial/ethnic disparities in young children. *Arch Pediatr Adolesc Med.* 2005;159:1038-1042.
13. Raudenbush SW, Bryk A. *Hierarchical Linear Models Applications and Data Analysis Methods.* 2nd ed. Thousand Oaks, Calif: Sage Publications; 2002.
14. Lozoff B, Brittenham GM, Wolf AW, et al. Iron deficiency anemia and iron therapy: effects on infant developmental test performance. *Pediatrics.* 1987;79:981-995.
15. Lozoff B, Jimenez E, Wolf AW. Long-term developmental outcome of infants with iron deficiency. *N Engl J Med.* 1991;325:687-694.
16. Cook JD, Finch CA. Assessing iron status of a population. *Am J Clin Nutr.* 1979;32:2115-2119.
17. Deinard AS, Schwartz S, Yip R. Developmental changes in serum ferritin and eryth-

rocyte protoporphyrin in normal (nonanemic) children. *Am J Clin Nutr.* 1983; 38:71-75.
18. Saarinen UM, Siimes MA. Developmental changes in serum iron, total iron-binding capacity, and transferrin saturation in infancy. *J Pediatr.* 1977;91:875-877.
19. Felt B, Jimenez E, Smith J, et al. Iron deficiency in infancy predicts altered serum prolactin response 10 years later. *Pediatr Res.* In press.
20. Bayley N. *Bayley Scales of Infant Development.* New York, NY: Psychological Corp; 1969.
21. Wechsler D. *Manual for the Wechsler Preschool and Primary Scale of Intelligence.* San Antonio, Tex: Psychological Corp; 1967.
22. Woodcock RW. *Woodcock Spanish Psycho-educational Battery.* Allen, Tex: DLM Teaching Resources; 1982.
23. Wechsler D. *Wechsler Intelligence Scale for Children.* 3rd ed. San Antonio, Tex: Psychological Corp; 1991.
24. Jastak S, Wilkinson GS. *Wide Range Achievement Test-Revised.* Wilmington, Del: Jastak Associates Inc; 1984.
25. Wechsler D. *Wechsler Individual Achievement Test.* San Antonio, Tex: Psychological Corp; 1992.
26. Wechsler D. *Manual for the Wechsler Adult Intelligence Scale–Revised.* San Antonio, Tex: Psychological Corp; 1981.
27. Tellegen A, Briggs PF. Old wine in new skins: grouping Wechsler subtests into new scales. *J Consult Psychol.* 1967:31:499-506.
28. Brown TA. *Confirmatory Factor Analysis for Applied Research: Methodology in the Social Sciences.* New York, NY: Guilford Press; 2006.
29. Lozoff B. Has iron deficiency been shown to cause altered behavior in infants? In: Dobbing J, ed. *Brain, Behaviour, and Iron in Infant Diet.* New York, NY: Springer-Verlag; 1990:107-131.
30. Martins S, Logan S, Gilbert R. Iron therapy for improving psychomotor development and cognitive function in children under the age of three with iron deficiency anaemia. *Cochrane Database Syst Rev.* 2001;(2):CD001444.
31. Pollitt E. Developmental sequel from early nutritional deficiencies: conclusive and probability judgments. *J Nutr.* 2000;130:350S-353S.
32. Hollingshead AB. *Four Factor Index of Social Status.* New Haven, Conn: Yale University; 1975.
33. Raudenbush SW, Bryk AS, Cheong YF, Congdon R. *Hierarchical Linear and Nonlinear Modeling.* Lincolnwood, Ill: SSI Scientific Software International; 2004.
34. Sameroff AJ, MacKenzie MJ. Research strategies for capturing transactional models of development: the limits of the possible. *Dev Psychopathol.* 2003;15: 613-640.
35. Williams WM, Ceci SJ. A person-process-context-time approach to understanding intellectual development. *Rev Gen Psychol.* 1997;1:288-310.
36. Rutter M. Statistical and personal interactions: facets and perspectives. In: Magnusson D, Allen VL, eds. *Human Development: An Interactional Perspective.* New York, NY: Academic Press; 1983:295-319.
37. Lozoff B, Beard J, Connor J, Felt B, Georgieff M, Schallert T. Long-lasting neural and behavioral effects of iron deficiency in infancy. *Nutr Rev.* 2006;64:S34-S43.
38. Parker S, Greer S, Zuckerman B. Double jeopardy: the impact of poverty on early child development. *Pediatr Clin North Am.* 1988;35:1227-1240.
39. Escalona SK. Babies at double hazard: early development of infants at biological and social risk. *Pediatrics.* 1982;70:670-676.
40. Sameroff AJ, Seifer R, Baldwin A, Baldwin C. Stability of intelligence from preschool to adolescence: the influence of social and family risk factors. *Child Dev.* 1993;64:80-97.
41. Breslau N, Chilcoat H, Susser ES, Matte T, Liang K, Peterson EL. Stability and change in children's Intelligence Quotient scores: a comparison of two socioeconomically disparate communities. *Am J Epidemiol.* 2001;154:711-717.
42. Bond GC. Social economic status and educational achievement: a review article. *Anthropol Educ Q.* 1981;12:227-257.
43. Harris A. The contradictions of education policy: disadvantage and achievement. *Br Educ Res J.* 2005;31:571-587.
44. Merton RK. The Matthew effect in science. *Science.* 1968;159:56-63.
45. Shaywitz BA, Holford TR, Holahan JM, et al. A Matthew effect for IQ but not for reading: results from a longitudinal study. *Reading Res Q.* 1995;30:894-906.
46. Pollitt E, Gorman KS, Engle PL, Rivera JA, Martorell R. Nutrition in early life and the fulfillment of intellectual potential. *J Nutr.* 1995;125:1111S-1118S.
47. Neisser U, ed. *The Rising Curve: Long-Term Gains in IQ and Related Measures.* Washington, DC: American Psychological Association; 1998.
48. Sherry B, Bister D, Yip R. Continuation of decline in prevalence of anemia in low-income children: the Vermont experience. *Arch Pediatr Adolesc Med.* 1997; 151:928-930.
49. Male C, Persson LA, Freeman V, Guerra A, van't Hof MA, Haschke F; Euro-Growth Iron Study Group. Prevalence of iron deficiency in 12-mo-old infants from 11 European areas and influence of dietary factors on iron status (Euro-Growth study). *Acta Paediatr.* 2001;90:492-498.

There are few experiences more deeply disturbing for the inexperienced mother than the sight of her child in the grip of some unexplained illness.

—From *A Parent's Guide to Children's Illnesses*, by Dr John Henderson, 1957

ARTICLE

# Iron Depletion Is Associated With Daytime Bottle-feeding in the Second and Third Years of Life

*Trenna L. Sutcliffe, MSc, MD, FRCPC; Amina Khambalia, MSc; Shelley Westergard, RN; Sheila Jacobson, MBBCh, FRCPC; Michael Peer, MD, FRCPC; Patricia C. Parkin, MD, FRCPC*

**Objective:** To measure the association between daytime bottle-feeding and iron depletion in young children.

**Design:** Cross-sectional design with concurrent measurement of exposure and outcome. The exposure was the current container (bottle or cup) used for daytime milk consumption. Child, maternal, and dietary variables were collected.

**Setting:** Community-based pediatric practice serving a diverse population in an urban Canadian city.

**Participants:** One hundred fifty healthy children, aged 12 to 38 months, attending a well-child care visit.

**Main Outcome Measure:** Iron depletion (serum ferritin level, <10 µg/L]).

**Results:** Of the 150 children, 82 (55%) were bottle-fed and 68 (45%) were cup fed. Iron depletion occurred in 29 (37%) of 78 bottle-fed and in 12 (18%) of 67 cup-fed children. The crude relative risk for iron depletion was 1.81 (95% confidence interval, 1.09-3.01). In the final logistic regression model, a significant association between bottle use and iron depletion was identified, beginning after the age of 16 months. At 18 months, the relative risk, adjusted for several child, maternal, and dietary variables, for the association between bottle use and iron depletion was 1.31 (95% confidence interval,1.24-1.47); at 24 months, the adjusted relative risk was 2.50 (95% confidence interval, 2.46-2.53). Milk consumption of more than 16 oz/d occurred in 55 (67%) of the 82 bottle-fed and in 22 (32%) of the 68 cup-fed children ($P<.001$).

**Conclusions:** In the second and third years of life, there is an almost 2-fold association between iron depletion and daytime bottle-feeding compared with cup feeding. The child's age may be a modifier, and milk volume consumed may be a mediator, of this association. Duration of bottle use is a potentially modifiable practice.

*Arch Pediatr Adolesc Med. 2006;160:1114-1120*

**Author Affiliations:** Departments of Pediatrics, University of Toronto Faculty of Medicine, Toronto, Ontario (Drs Sutcliffe and Parkin), and Stanford University, Stanford, Calif (Dr Sutcliffe); Pediatric Outcomes Research Team (Ms Khambalia and Dr Parkin), Division of Pediatric Medicine (Drs Jacobson, Peer, and Parkin), and Child Health Evaluative Sciences (Dr Parkin), Hospital for Sick Children Research Institute, Toronto; and Clairhurst Medical Centre (Ms Westergard and Drs Jacobson and Peer), Toronto.

CHILDREN IN THE SECOND and third years of life are vulnerable to iron depletion, which may progress to iron deficiency anemia (IDA).[1] Infants with iron deficiency are at risk for developmental delay and poor academic performance, which may not improve with iron therapy.[2-5] Iron depletion occurs in up to 30% of young children in developed countries.[6-8]

Data from the 1991 US National Health Interview Survey indicate that about 95% of children aged 6 months to 5 years have ever used a baby bottle.[9] Bottle weaning is recommended between the ages of 12 and 18 months.[10,11] However, families and physicians demonstrate considerable variation regarding the age of bottle weaning, and single-site studies[12-15] suggest that 40% of children aged 24 months and 18% of children aged 42 months continue bottle-feeding. Previous studies[16-19] suggest that prolonged bottle-feeding may contribute to iron depletion; however, the contribution of volume of milk consumed and other dietary variables were not considered.

Our study objective was to examine the association between daytime bottle-feeding and iron depletion in healthy young children in the second and third years of life, assessing the role of the child's age and volume of milk consumed, while controlling for maternal and other dietary variables.

## METHODS

### STUDY POPULATION, SETTING, AND STUDY PROCEDURE

Children were recruited from a 2-physician (S.J. and M.P.) community-based pediatric practice in Toronto, from November 1, 2002, to

March 31, 2004. The practice is hospital and university affiliated, and provides primary care for approximately 10 000 children, with approximately 500 office visits per week.

Healthy children, aged 12 to 38 months, drinking nonfortified milk, were included. Exclusion criteria were as follows: acute febrile illness at enrollment, which may increase serum ferritin level; history of illness or medication associated with iron deficiency or anemia; previous diagnosis of iron depletion or anemia; current use of iron supplements; and breast milk or formula as the primary source of milk at or within 8 weeks of enrollment, which provides more available iron.

The office computerized appointment book was used to identify age-eligible children with a scheduled well-child care visit. An information letter was sent to parents 2 weeks before their scheduled appointment, informing them that the study objective was to assess the association between toddler feeding habits and iron depletion, without specific reference to bottle use to minimize reporting bias. At the appointment, the attending pediatrician and study nurse (S.W.) identified those children meeting all eligibility criteria, and asked parents to participate. Informed consent was obtained from the child's parent.

At enrollment, using a standardized data collection form, the study nurse collected data on child and maternal characteristics, child's dietary history during the first year of life, child's current use of a bottle or cup, and current diet (see details later). The study was approved by the Research Ethics Board of the Hospital for Sick Children.

## CHILD AND MATERNAL CHARACTERISTICS

Child characteristics collected included the following: age, sex, birth weight, prematurity (<37 weeks' gestation), and current weight. Maternal characteristics collected included the following: age and achievement of high school–level education or greater. The child's dietary history during the first year of life was collected as dichotomous variables (yes or no) and included the following: ever breastfed, introduction of solids at or before the age of 6 months, and introduction of cow's milk at or after the age of 12 months.

## CHILD'S CURRENT DIET

To collect data on current diet, the study team developed 8 diet questions based on the Canadian nutrition guidelines for healthy infants.[20] These questions quantified consumption of the following variables: milk; pure fruit juice; fruit drinks; cereals or breads; meat, fish, poultry, or legumes; red meat; vegetables and fruit; and chips, fried snacks, or sweets.

## BOTTLE USE: EXPOSURE

The definition of exposure incorporated time of day and type of liquid. Parents were asked the following: Has your child been completely weaned yet from daytime bottle drinking of milk? Children whose parents responded "no" were categorized as bottle-fed, and children whose parents responded "yes" were categorized as cup fed. No attempt was made to further categorize children according to nighttime bottle use or according to type of cup used.

## SERUM FERRITIN LEVEL: PRIMARY OUTCOME

Phlebotomy was completed in a single laboratory concurrently with determination of exposure. A venous blood sample was drawn for measurements of serum ferritin level, mean corpuscular volume, and hemoglobin level. The primary outcome, iron depletion, was defined as a serum ferritin level of less than 10 μg/L. It was anticipated that IDA would be much less prevalent than iron depletion alone, but an important outcome to explore. Iron deficiency anemia was defined as a serum ferritin level of less than 10 μg/L, a mean corpuscular volume of less than 73 $\mu m^3$, and a hemoglobin level of less than 11 g/dL. These cutoff values were derived by an expert panel for the Second and Third National Health and Nutrition Examination Surveys.[21,22]

## DATA ANALYSIS

The sample size calculation was based on the following estimates: $\alpha$ error=.05; $\beta$ error=.20 (80% power); prevalence of iron depletion in the bottle-fed group, 35%; and prevalence of iron depletion in the cup-fed group, 15%. Based on these assumptions, at least 70 subjects were required per group.

The characteristics of the bottle- and cup-fed groups were compared using the Fisher exact test and the Mann-Whitney test for categorical and continuous variables, respectively. A relative risk (RR) and 95% confidence interval (CI) were calculated for iron depletion (serum ferritin level, <10 vs ≥10 μg/L).

Two distinct logistic regression models were developed. The first step was the development of a logistic regression model, predicting bottle or cup use, to calculate a propensity score for each subject. The propensity score for an individual is defined as the conditional probability of receiving the treatment given the individual's covariates.[23] The score can balance the covariates in the 2 groups and, thus, reduce bias, which can occur in observational studies. The score can then be included as a predicted probability in a subsequent logistic regression model predicting outcome. In this analysis, the propensity score logistic regression model contained variables found significant at the univariate level, to model the propensity of a child to use the bottle. Four variables were included in the score: maternal educational level, ever breastfed, daily volume of pure fruit juice consumed, and weekly servings of chips, fried snacks, or sweets. The propensity score was subsequently used as a covariate in the final model predicting iron depletion.

The second step was the development of a logistic regression model predicting iron depletion (ferritin level, <10 μg/L). The model contained 4 variables potentially related to iron depletion: bottle or cup use, the propensity score, child's age, and daily volume of milk consumed. Given the sample size, no further variables were entered into the final model. This model was examined for interaction and collinearity.

Child's age was entered into the final model rather than the propensity score to explore age as a moderator of the effect of bottle or cup use on iron depletion. A moderator variable is an effect modifier, which specifies on whom or under what conditions another variable will operate to produce the outcome.[24] Daily volume of milk consumed was entered into the final model to explore milk volume as a mediator of the effect of bottle use on iron depletion. A mediator variable is one that occurs in a causal pathway, causes variation in the outcome variable, and itself is caused to vary by the exposure variable.

A 2-sided $P$=.05 indicated statistical significance. All statistical analyses were performed using SAS statistical software, version 9.1 (SAS Institute Inc, Cary, NC).

# RESULTS

## STUDY POPULATION

A total of 458 children met the age criteria, of whom 332 (72%) met the full eligibility criteria. Of these children, 150 had questionnaire and blood work completed and

**Table 1. Characteristics of 150 Bottle- or Cup-Fed Children**

| Characteristic | Bottle-fed Children (n = 82)* | Cup-Fed Children (n = 68)* | RR (95% CI) |
|---|---|---|---|
| Child | | | |
| Age, mo† | 18 (12-36) | 24 (12-38) | 0.94 (0.92-0.96) |
| Male sex | 53 (65) | 42 (62) | 1.06 (0.78-1.44) |
| Birth weight, g† | 3235 (780-4675) | 3402 (2087-4905) | 1.00 (0.99-1.00) |
| Prematurity | 8 (10) | 4 (6) | 0.80 (0.52-1.24) |
| Current weight, kg† | 11.63 (8.05-18.54) | 12.20 (8.73-18.50) | 1.01 (0.93-1.08) |
| Maternal | | | |
| Secondary education is the highest level attained | 24 (29) | 9 (13) | 1.12 (1.02-1.17) |
| Age, y† | 33 (20-44) | 33 (23-48) | 0.99 (0.96-1.02) |
| First-year diet | | | |
| Ever breastfed | 69 (84) | 64 (96)‡ | 1.57 (1.18-2.09) |
| Solids introduced at the age of ≤6 mo | 68 (83) | 51 (75) | 0.79 (0.52-1.20) |
| Cow's milk introduced at the age of ≥12 mo | 45 (58)§ | 39 (59)‖ | 1.03 (0.76-1.39) |

Abbreviations: CI, confidence interval; RR, relative risk.
*Data are given as number (percentage) of each group unless otherwise indicated.
†Data are given as median (range).
‡The denominator used was 67.
§The denominator used was 78.
‖The denominator used was 66.

were enrolled in the study. Maternal age ranged from 20 to 48 years, secondary education was the highest level of educational attainment for 22% of mothers, and 45% of child participants had at least 1 older sibling. Approximately 50% of mothers reported their ethnicity as other than Canadian or European, including Asian (13%), Latin American (8%), African (3%), Middle Eastern (3%), Mediterranean (2%), East Indian (1%), West Indian (1%), and First Nations (1%).

## CHARACTERISTICS

Of the 150 subjects, 82 (55%) were drinking milk from a bottle and 68 (45%) were drinking milk from a cup. The characteristics of bottle- and cup-fed children are found in **Table 1** and **Table 2**. There were no significant differences between the bottle- and cup-fed children for sex, birth weight, prematurity, current weight, maternal age, introduction of solids by the age of 6 months, introduction of cow's milk at or after the age of 12 months, and current consumption of fruit drinks, red meat, vegetables and fruit, cereals or breads, and milk, fish, poultry, or legumes. The characteristics that were significantly different between bottle- and cup-fed children included age, secondary school as the highest level of maternal education, ever breastfed in the first year of life, and current consumption of milk, pure juice, and chips, fried snacks, or sweets.

## ASSOCIATION BETWEEN CONTAINER USE AND IRON DEPLETION

Because of insufficient blood quantities, iron status could not be determined in 5 children (4 bottle-fed and 1 cup fed) and IDA could not be determined in 10 children (4 bottle-fed and 6 cup fed). Iron depletion (n=145) occurred in 29 (37%) of 78 bottle-fed children and in 12 (18%) of 67 cup-fed children (RR, 1.81; 95% CI, 1.09-3.01). Iron deficiency anemia (n=140) occurred in 3 (4%) of 78 bottle-fed children and in 1 (2%) of 62 cup-fed children (*P*=.40).

The propensity score logistic regression model contained variables found significant at the univariate level: maternal educational level, ever breastfed, daily volume of pure fruit juice consumed, and weekly servings of chips, fried snacks, or sweets.

The final logistic regression model contained the propensity score, current bottle use, child's age, and daily volume of milk consumed. No significant association was found between iron depletion and the propensity score (RR, 0.68; 95% CI, 0.10-2.83). Significant statistical interaction between bottle use and child's age was identified, with significant association between bottle use and iron depletion beginning after the age of 16 months (Hosmer-Lemeshow goodness-of-fit test, *P*=.59). The relationship between bottle use, child's age, and iron depletion is demonstrated in **Figure 1**. The bottle × age interaction variable was included in the model (RR, 1.13; 95% CI, 1.02-1.28), indicating that, on average, for every 1-month increase in age, bottle-fed children were 13% more likely to be iron depleted compared with cup-fed children. For example, at the age of 18 months, the RR was 1.31 (95% CI, 1.24-1.47) for the association between bottle use and iron depletion; at the age of 24 months, the RR was 2.50 (95% CI, 2.46-2.53).

In the final logistic regression model, there was no significant association between iron depletion and daily volume of milk consumed (RR, 1.03; 95% CI, 0.87-1.22). There was no evidence of interaction or collinearity when the variable measuring daily milk volume consumed was entered into the final logistic regression model. Further exploratory analysis identified that bottle or cup use was significantly associated with daily volume of milk consumed (Table 2 and **Figure 2**); 55 (67%) of 82 bottle-fed children and 22 (32%) of 68 cup-fed children consumed more than 16 oz/d (*P*<.001). At all volumes of

**Table 2. Current Diet Characteristics of 150 Bottle- or Cup-Fed Children**

| Characteristic | Bottle-fed Children (n = 82)* | Cup-Fed Children (n = 68)* | RR (95% CI) |
|---|---|---|---|
| Milk consumption, oz/d | | | |
| <8 | 3 | 14 | 1.00 |
| 9-12 | 8 | 16 | 0.53 (0.16-1.71) |
| 13-16 | 16 | 16 | 0.35 (0.12-1.03) |
| 17-20 | 18 | 7 | 0.25 (0.09-0.70) |
| 21-24 | 10 | 9 | 0.36 (0.01-1.02) |
| 25-28 | 8 | 3 | 0.24 (0.08-0.72) |
| 29-32 | 13 | 3 | 0.22 (0.08-0.62) |
| ≥33 | 6 | 0 | NA |
| Pure juice consumption, oz/d | | | |
| <8 | 54 | 27 | 1.00 |
| 9-12 | 18 | 25 | 1.59 (1.08-2.34) |
| 13-16 | 6 | 11 | 1.89 (0.98-3.66) |
| ≥17 | 4 | 5 | 1.50 (0.71-3.16) |
| Fruit drinks, glasses per day | | | |
| ≤1 | 64 | 53 | 1.00 |
| 2 | 11 | 11 | 1.09 (0.70-1.71) |
| 3 | 6 | 3 | 0.82 (0.50-1.34) |
| ≥4 | 1 | 1 | 1.09 (0.27-4.42) |
| Red meat, servings per week | | | |
| 0 | 13 | 7 | 1.00 |
| 1-2 | 44 | 32 | 1.12 (0.77-1.63) |
| 3-4 | 21 | 22 | 1.33 (0.85-2.07) |
| 5-6 | 3 | 5 | 1.73 (0.67-4.48) |
| ≥7 | 1 | 2 | 1.95 (0.38-9.98) |
| Vegetables and fruits, servings per day | | | |
| 0-3 | 42 | 28 | 1.00 |
| 4-6 | 38 | 35 | 1.15 (0.86-1.54) |
| ≥7 | 2 | 5 | 2.10 (0.64-6.88) |
| Cereals or breads, servings per day | | | |
| 0-3 | 61 | 43 | 1.00 |
| 4-6 | 18 | 20 | 1.24 (0.85-1.80) |
| ≥7 | 3 | 5 | 1.56 (0.63-3.88) |
| Meat, fish, poultry, or legumes, servings per week | | | |
| 0 | 1 | 2 | 1.00 |
| 1-3 | 17 | 10 | 0.53 (0.10-2.69) |
| 4-7 | 37 | 38 | 0.68 (0.13-3.40) |
| 8-13 | 26 | 16 | 0.54 (0.11-2.71) |
| ≥14 | 1 | 2 | 1.00 (0.10-9.61) |
| Chips, fried snacks, or sweets, servings per week | | | |
| 0-2 | 67 | 40 | 1.00 |
| 3-5 | 15 | 21 | 1.50 (0.99-2.27) |
| ≥6 | 0 | 7 | NA |

Abbreviations: CI, confidence interval; NA, data not applicable; RR, relative risk.
*Data are given as number of children.

milk consumed, bottle-fed children had an increased probability of iron depletion compared with cup-fed children (**Figure 3**).

## COMMENT

In this sample of healthy children, aged 12 to 38 months, 55% were bottle-fed in the daytime, 51% consumed greater than 16 oz/d of milk, 28% had iron depletion, and 3% had IDA. Children drinking milk from a bottle during the daytime were almost twice as likely to be iron depleted compared with cup-fed children. The association remained after analyses accounted for several child characteristics, diet variables, and maternal characteristics. Age seems to be a moderator, with children older than 16 months demonstrating the strongest association between bottle use and iron depletion. Daily volume of milk consumed may act as a mediator, with bottle-fed children consuming larger volumes of milk per day and having a higher probability of iron depletion at all volumes of milk, compared with cup-fed children.

Healthy children were enrolled from an urban community primary care practice and demonstrated socioeconomic diversity. Eligibility criteria ensured that children with conditions or variables known to be strongly associated with the exposure or outcome were excluded. Accuracy of the outcome measurement was ensured by performing a standardized biochemical laboratory test (measuring serum ferritin level) at enrollment and using an accepted cutoff of less than 10 µg/L. Con-

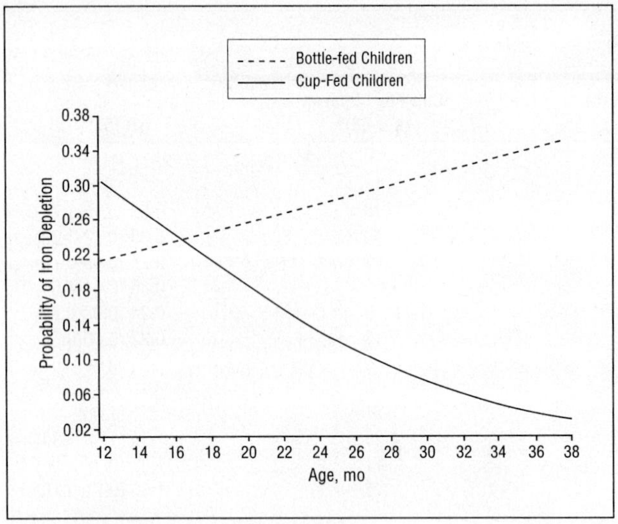


**Figure 1.** Probability of iron depletion in bottle- vs cup-fed children, by age.

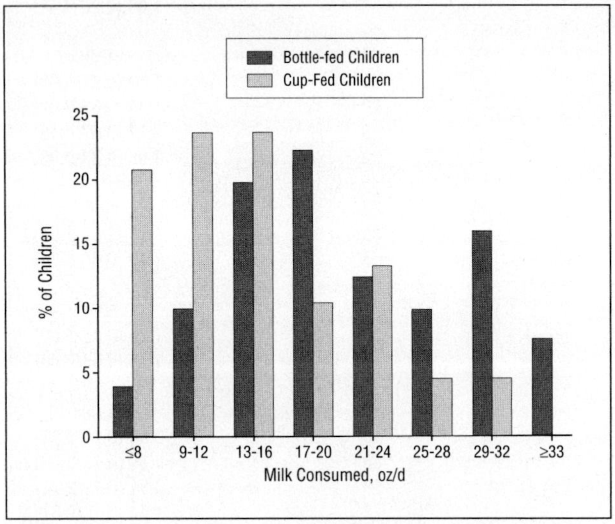


**Figure 2.** Daily milk volume consumed in bottle- vs cup-fed children.

current measurement of exposure and the primary outcome decreased the potential for recall bias. To balance covariates in the bottle and cup groups, a score measuring the child's propensity for bottle use was developed and entered into the final regression model, thus minimizing confounding bias.

Study limitations include recruitment from a single primary care practice, assessment of iron depletion rather than IDA (which required a larger sample size) as the primary outcome, and use of parental report of diet variables. Diet questions, individually or in combination, do not have adequate sensitivity and specificity to identify IDA.[25,26] The question used to classify exposure status did not allow us to examine the role of mixed bottle-feeding and cup feeding. However, the question was designed to avoid misclassification of children who were predominately bottle users.

The findings in the present study share some similarities with several studies conducted in urban US centers. Graham et al[16] found that children of Southeast Asian ethnicity were more likely to be iron deficient than chil-

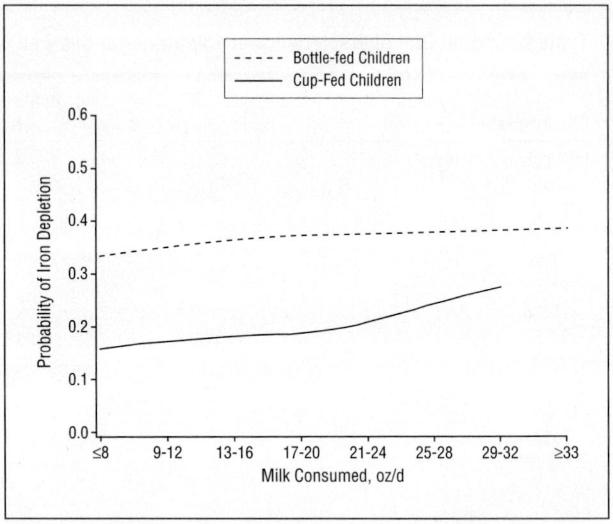


**Figure 3.** Probability of iron depletion in bottle- vs cup-fed children, by daily milk volume consumed.

dren of other ethnicities (12 of 17 vs 2 of 21 children), and were more likely to be bottle-fed at the age of 2 years (17 of 17 vs 10 of 21 children). These researchers used the zinc protoporphyrin–heme ratio as a measure of iron deficiency (identified to be altered by other causes, such as lead poisoning, febrile illness, or some hemoglobinopathies). Lampe and Velez[17] found that, among thirty-four 18-month-old children from a primary care practice, bottle-feeding was associated with significantly greater daily milk consumption (24 vs 16 oz; $P<.001$) and a lower ferritin concentration (18.6 vs 16.4 µg/L; $P$ value not significant). The small sample size may have precluded a finding of significance. Bonuck and Kahn[18] found that, among 95 inner-city Hispanic and African American low-income children aged 18 months to 5 years, bottle-feeding, compared with not bottle-feeding, was associated with anemia (15 of 61 vs 5 of 34 children; $P<.05$). The researchers defined IDA using hemoglobin level and hematocrit alone, without measures of iron stores. Brotanek et al,[19] using cross-sectional data from a US national health survey, found that bottle-feeding to the age of 24 to 48 months and Mexican ethnicity were associated with iron deficiency (odds ratio, 2.8 and 2.9, respectively). In all of these studies, the contributions of milk volume and other diet variables were not available or analyzed.

Other investigators have identified an association between volume of milk consumed and iron status. Cowin et al[27] found that ferritin levels were negatively associated with the amount of cow's milk consumed in 18-month-old children. Lozoff et al[28] found that children with IDA, aged 12 to 23 months, consumed more milk per day and took more bottles. This supports the concept that milk volume consumed may be a mediator in the causal pathway, causing variation in iron status (outcome) and itself caused to vary by bottle use (exposure).

Risk factors and mechanisms for iron depletion in the second and third years of life may differ from those in the first year of life. James et al[29] found poor correlation between children with IDA at the end of the first year (14 months) and children with IDA at the end of the second year (24 months). Lind et al[30] have suggested that dietary iron may be channeled to erythropoiesis in the first year of life and to storage in the second year of life. In developed countries, promotion of breastfeeding and iron-fortified cereals and formula and delayed introduction of whole cow's milk have contributed to the primary prevention of iron depletion in the first year of life. Less is known about the primary prevention of iron depletion in the second and third years of life.

Secondary prevention through population screening of children in the second year of life has been controversial because of lack of clear evidence of the benefits of iron therapy in reversing the developmental outcomes of children with IDA,[5] the changing patterns of IDA from the first to the second year of life,[29] and the lack of evidence regarding the feasibility of screening.[31] Identifying risk factors for iron depletion for children in the second and third years of life might lead to the development of secondary prevention strategies for high-risk groups and primary prevention strategies for the population.

There are several possible mechanisms by which bottle-feeding in 1- to 3-year-old children might lead to iron depletion. The bottle may act as a vehicle for excessive milk consumption, which may compromise iron absorption or the intake of iron-rich foods or juices. In this study, bottle-fed children consumed larger volumes of milk and smaller amounts of pure juice compared with cup-fed children.

The bottle may interfere with the development of age-appropriate feeding practices or may be associated with behavioral and developmental feeding difficulties. Previous research[29] has shown that children described as difficult to feed at the age of 2 years had a risk ratio of 3.5 (95% CI, 1.9-6.7) for anemia. The interaction between diet and developmentally appropriate feeding practices, and their association with iron depletion, is likely to be complex.

Results from this and other studies suggest that prolonged bottle-feeding may be a risk factor for iron depletion in children in the second and third years of life. Children using a bottle beyond the age of 12 to 16 months may be selected for screening and counseling. Bottle use is a potentially modifiable practice. The promotion of bottle weaning before the age of 12 months, or weaning directly from the breast to the cup, may be a potentially simple primary prevention strategy. These hypotheses must be tested in prospective trials.

**Accepted for Publication:** June 5, 2006.

**Correspondence:** Patricia C. Parkin, MD, FRCPC, Division of Pediatric Medicine and Pediatric Outcomes Research Team, Hospital for Sick Children, 555 University Ave, Toronto, Ontario, Canada M5G 1X8 (patricia.parkin@sickkids.ca).

**Author Contributions:** The authors completed all aspects of the study (design, conduct, data collection, management, analysis, interpretation, manuscript preparation, and approval) independent of the funding organization. *Study concept and design:* Sutcliffe, Khambalia, Jacobson, Peer, and Parkin. *Acquisition of data:* Sutcliffe, Khambalia, Westergard, Jacobson, Peer, and Parkin. *Analysis and interpretation of data:* Sutcliffe, Khambalia, and Parkin. *Drafting of the manuscript:* Sutcliffe, Khambalia, and Parkin. *Critical revision of the manuscript for important intellectual content:* Sutcliffe, Khambalia, Jacobson, Peer, and Parkin. *Statistical analysis:* Khambalia and Parkin. *Obtained funding:* Sutcliffe, Khambalia, and Parkin. *Administrative, technical, and material support:* Khambalia, Jacobson, Peer, and Parkin. *Study supervision:* Khambalia and Parkin.

**Financial Disclosure:** None reported.

**Funding/Support:** This study was supported by grant-in-aid-01 from Danone Institute of Canada. The Pediatric Outcomes Research Team is supported by a grant from the Hospital for Sick Children Foundation.

**Role of the Sponsor:** The funding bodies had no role in data extraction and analyses, in the writing of the manuscript, or in the decision to submit the manuscript for publication.

**Acknowledgments:** We thank Derek Stephens, MSc, and Cristina Goia, MSc, biostatisticians who helped in the analysis and interpretation of data; Gurvinder Dohl for patient recruitment in the first part of the study; and Nike Onabajo for assistance in the preparation of the manuscript.

## REFERENCES


1. Oski FA. Iron deficiency in infancy and childhood. *N Engl J Med.* 1993;329:190-193.
2. Grantham-McGregor S, Ani C. A review of studies on the effect of iron deficiency on cognitive development in children. *J Nutr.* 2001;131(2) (suppl 2):649S-668S.
3. Lozoff B, Jimenez E, Wolf AW. Long-term developmental outcome of infants with iron deficiency. *N Engl J Med.* 1991;325:687-694.
4. Lozoff B, Jimenez E, Hagen J, Mollen E, Wolf AW. Poorer behavioral and developmental outcome more than 10 years after treatment for iron deficiency in infancy. *Pediatrics.* 2000;105:e51 http://pediatrics.aappublications.org/cgi/content/full/105/4/e51. Accessed April 28, 2006.
5. Logan S, Martins S, Gilbert R. Iron therapy for improving psychomotor development and cognitive function in children under the age of three with iron deficiency anaemia. *Cochrane Database Syst Rev.* 2001;(2):CD001444.
6. Eden AN, Mir MA. Iron deficiency in 1- to 3-year-old children: a pediatric failure? *Arch Pediatr Adolesc Med.* 1997;151:986-988.
7. Booth IW, Aukett MA. Iron deficiency anaemia in infancy and early childhood. *Arch Dis Child.* 1997;76:549-554.
8. Zlotkin SH, Ste-Marie M, Kopelman H, Jones A, Adam J. The prevalence of iron depletion and iron-deficiency anemia in a randomly selected group of infants from four Canadian cities. *Nutr Res.* 1996;16:729-733.
9. Kaste LM, Gift HC. Inappropriate infant bottle feeding: status of the Healthy People 2000 objective. *Arch Pediatr Adolesc Med.* 1995;149:786-791.
10. American Academy of Pediatrics. *Guidelines for Health Supervision III.* Elk Grove Village, Ill: American Academy of Pediatrics; 1997:197.
11. Early childhood: 1-4 years. http://www.brightfutures.org/nutrition/pdf/ec.pdf. Accessed April 28, 2006.
12. Hammer LD, Bryson S, Agras WS. Development of feeding practices during the first 5 years of life. *Arch Pediatr Adolesc Med.* 1999;153:189-194.
13. Frazier JP, Countie D, Elerian L. Parental barriers to weaning infants from the bottle. *Arch Pediatr Adolesc Med.* 1998;152:889-892.
14. Sutcliffe T, Parkin PC. Anticipatory guidelines for bottle weaning: a survey of pediatricians [abstract]. *Paediatr Child Health.* 2002;7:43A.
15. Safer DL, Bryson S, Agras WS, Hammer LD. Prolonged bottle feeding in a cohort of children: does it affect caloric intake and dietary composition? *Clin Pediatr (Phila).* 2001;40:481-487.
16. Graham EA, Carlson TH, Sodergren KK, Detter JC, Labbe RF. Delayed bottle weaning and iron deficiency in Southeast Asian toddlers. *West J Med.* 1997;167:10-14.
17. Lampe JB, Velez N. The effect of prolonged bottle feeding on cow's milk intake and iron stores at 18 months of age. *Clin Pediatr (Phila).* 1997;36:569-572.

18. Bonuck KA, Kahn R. Prolonged bottle use and its association with iron deficiency anemia and overweight: a preliminary study [published correction appears in *Clin Pediatr (Phila).* 2003;42:280]. *Clin Pediatr (Phila).* 2002;41:603-607.
19. Brotanek JM, Halterman JS, Auinger P, Flores G, Weitzman M. Iron deficiency, prolonged bottle-feeding and racial/ethnic disparities in young children. *Arch Pediatr Adolesc Med.* 2005;159:1038-1042.
20. Canadian Paediatric Society, Dietitians of Canada and Health Canada. Nutrition for healthy term infants—statement of the joint working group: Canadian Paediatric Society, Dietitians of Canada and Health Canada. http://www.hc-sc.gc.ca/fn-an/pubs/infant-nourrisson/nut_infant_nourrisson_term_e.html. Accessed April 28, 2006.
21. Expert Scientific Working Group. Summary of a report on assessment of the iron nutritional status of the United States population. *Am J Clin Nutr.* 1985;42:1318-1330.
22. Looker AC, Dallman PR, Carroll MD, Gunter EW, Johnson CL. Prevalence of iron deficiency in the United States. *JAMA.* 1997;277:973-976.
23. D'Agostino RB. Tutorial in biostatistics: propensity score methods for bias reduction in the comparison of a treatment to a non-randomized control group. *Stat Med.* 1998;17:2265-2281.
24. Kraemer HC, Stice E, Kazdin A, Offord D, Kupfer D. How do risk factors work together? mediators, moderators, and independent, overlapping, and proxy risk factors. *Am J Psychiatry.* 2001;158:848-856.
25. Boutry M, Needlman R. Use of diet history in the screening of iron deficiency. *Pediatrics.* 1996;98(pt 1):1138-1142.
26. Bogen DL, Duggan AK, Dover GJ, Wilson MH. Screening for iron deficiency anemia by dietary history in a high-risk population. *Pediatrics.* 2000;105:1254-1259.
27. Cowin I, Emond A, Emmett P; ALSPAC Study Group. Association between composition of the diet and haemoglobin and ferritin levels in 18-month-old children. *Eur J Clin Nutr.* 2001;55:278-286.
28. Lozoff B, Brittenham GM, Wolf AW, et al. Iron deficiency anemia and iron therapy effects on infant developmental test performance [published correction appears in *Pediatrics.* 1988;81:683]. *Pediatrics.* 1987;79:981-995.
29. James JA, Laing GJ, Logan S. Changing patterns of iron deficiency anaemia in the second year of life [published correction appears in *BMJ.* 1995;311:545]. *BMJ.* 1995;311:230.
30. Lind T, Hernell O, Lonnerdal B, Stenlund H, Domellof M, Persson LA. Dietary iron intake is positively associated with hemoglobin concentration during infancy but not during the second year of life. *J Nutr.* 2004;134:1064-1070.
31. James JA, Laing GJ, Logan S, Rossdale M. Feasibility of screening toddlers for iron deficiency anaemia in general practice. *BMJ.* 1997;315:102-103.


"Was animal instinct a compelling force that enabled humans to find food, plants, substances, and procedures to nurture themselves? If so, it may have been the beginning of healing methods. The almost reflex rubbing of an injured part, using heat to relieve discomfort, and applying cold to deaden pain may all parallel the similar activities of animals who wallow in cool water and apply mud to irritated areas."

—From *Medicine: An Illustrated History* by Albert S. Lyons, MD, and R. Joseph Petrucelli, MD, 1987

Now:

**The Purple Pill™ is FDA-approved for use in kids 12 to 17 years old with GERD**

# NEXIUM for the NEXT GENERATION

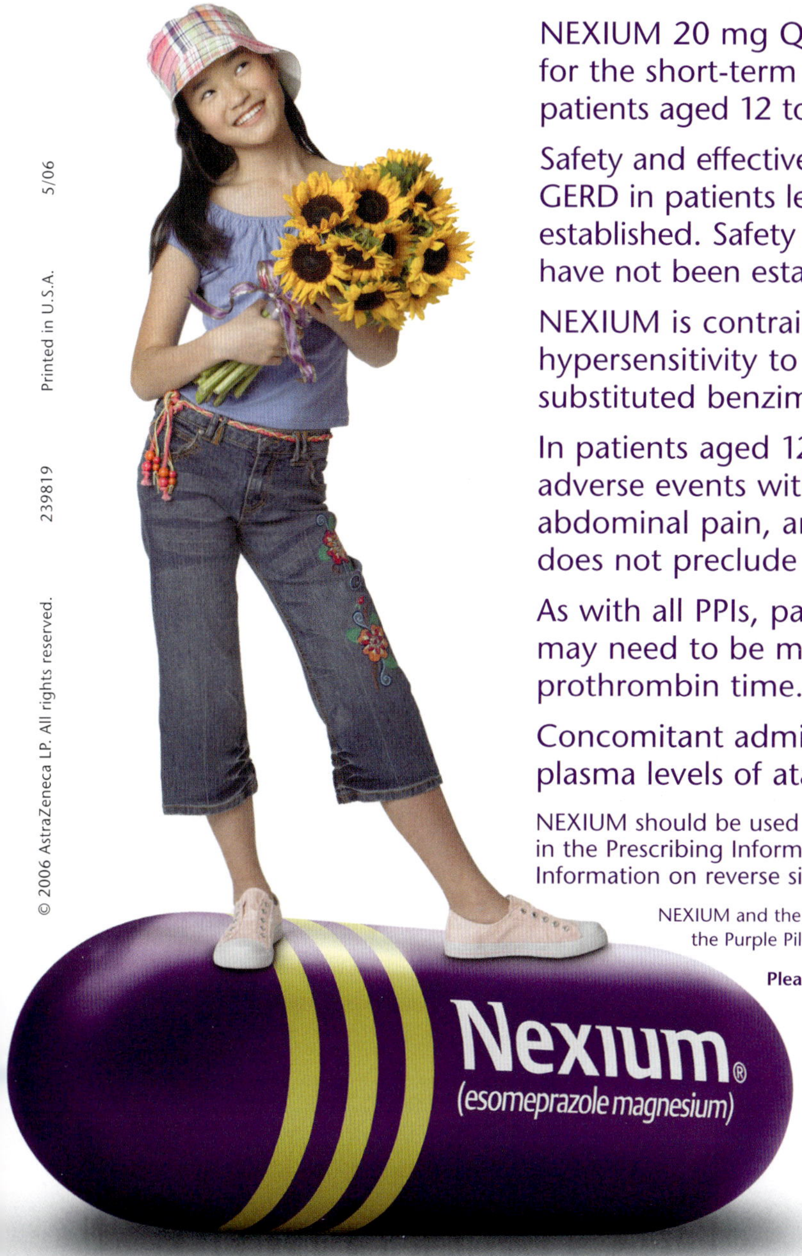


NEXIUM 20 mg QD and NEXIUM 40 mg QD are approved for the short-term treatment (up to 8 weeks) of GERD in patients aged 12 to 17 years.

Safety and effectiveness for the treatment of symptomatic GERD in patients less than 12 years of age have not been established. Safety and effectiveness for other pediatric uses have not been established.

NEXIUM is contraindicated in patients with known hypersensitivity to any component of the formulation or to substituted benzimidazoles.

In patients aged 12 to 17 years, the most frequently reported adverse events with NEXIUM include headache, diarrhea, abdominal pain, and nausea. Symptomatic response to therapy does not preclude the presence of gastric malignancy.

As with all PPIs, patients treated concomitantly with warfarin may need to be monitored for increases in INR and prothrombin time.

Concomitant administration of esomeprazole may reduce the plasma levels of atazanavir.

NEXIUM should be used only for the conditions, dosages, and durations specified in the Prescribing Information. Please see the brief summary of full Prescribing Information on reverse side.

NEXIUM and the color purple as applied to the capsule are registered trademarks and the Purple Pill is a trademark of the AstraZeneca group of companies.

**Please visit our Web site at www.Nexium-us.com**

**Nexium®**
(esomeprazole magnesium)

AstraZeneca

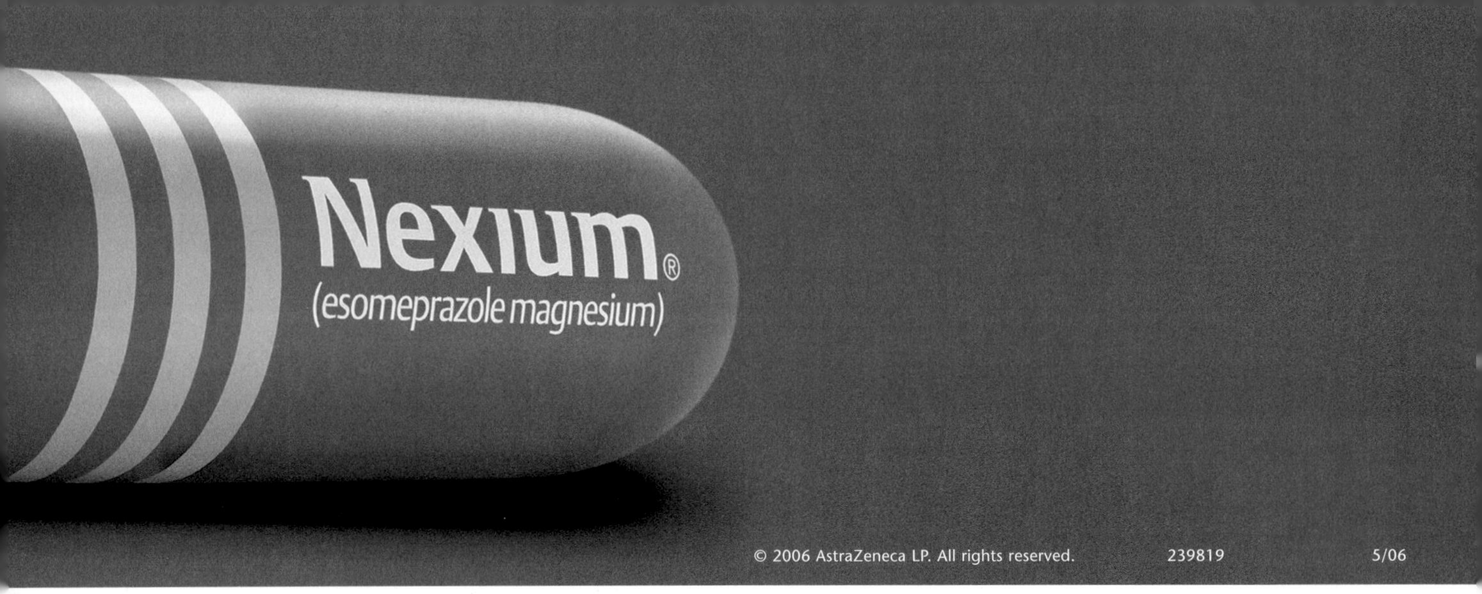


# NEXIUM® *(esomeprazole magnesium)*

## 20-mg, 40-mg Delayed-Release Capsules

**BRIEF SUMMARY** of Prescribing Information.

**INDICATIONS AND USAGE Treatment of GERD** NEXIUM is indicated for the short-term treatment (4 to 8 weeks) in the healing and symptomatic resolution of diagnostically confirmed erosive esophagitis; the maintenance of symptom resolution and healing of erosive esophagitis (controlled studies do not extend beyond 6 months); the treatment of heartburn and other symptoms associated with GERD; **Risk Reduction of NSAID-Associated Gastric Ulcer; *H.pylori* Eradication to Reduce the Risk of Duodenal Ulcer Recurrence.**

**CONTRAINDICATIONS** NEXIUM is contraindicated in patients with known hypersensitivity to any component of the formulation or to substituted benzimidazoles.

**PRECAUTIONS General** Symptomatic response to therapy with NEXIUM does not preclude the presence of gastric malignancy. Atrophic gastritis has been noted occasionally in gastric corpus biopsies from patients treated long-term with omeprazole, of which NEXIUM is an enantiomer. **Information for Patients** NEXIUM Delayed-Release Capsules should be swallowed whole and taken at least one hour before meals. For patients who have difficulty swallowing capsules, one tablespoon of applesauce can be added to an empty bowl and the NEXIUM Delayed-Release Capsule can be opened, and the pellets carefully emptied onto the applesauce. The pellets should be mixed with the applesauce and then swallowed immediately. The applesauce used should not be hot and should be soft enough to be swallowed without chewing. The pellets should not be chewed or crushed. The pellet/applesauce mixture should not be stored for future use. Antacids may be used while taking NEXIUM. **Drug Interactions** Esomeprazole is extensively metabolized in the liver by CYP2C19 and CYP3A4. *In vitro* and *in vivo* studies have shown that esomeprazole is not likely to inhibit CYPs 1A2, 2A6, 2C9, 2D6, 2E1 and 3A4. No clinically relevant interactions with drugs metabolized by these CYP enzymes would be expected. Drug interaction studies have shown that esomeprazole does not have any clinically significant interactions with phenytoin, warfarin, quinidine, clarithromycin or amoxicillin. Post-marketing reports of changes in prothrombin measures have been received among patients on concomitant warfarin and esomeprazole therapy. Increases in INR and prothrombin time may lead to abnormal bleeding and even death. Patients treated with proton pump inhibitors and warfarin concomitantly may need to be monitored for increases in INR and prothrombin time. Esomeprazole may potentially interfere with CYP2C19, the major esomeprazole metabolizing enzyme. Coadministration of esomeprazole 30 mg and diazepam, a CYP2C19 substrate, resulted in a 45% decrease in clearance of diazepam. Increased plasma levels of diazepam were observed 12 hours after dosing and onwards. However, at that time, the plasma levels of diazepam were below the therapeutic interval, and thus this interaction is unlikely to be of clinical relevance. Coadministration of oral contraceptives, diazepam, phenytoin, or quinidine did not seem to change the pharmacokinetic profile of esomeprazole. Concomitant administration of esomeprazole may reduce the plasma levels of atazanavir. Studies evaluating concomitant administration of esomeprazole and either naproxen (non-selective NSAID) or rofecoxib (COX-2 selective NSAID) did not identify any clinically relevant changes in the pharmacokinetic profiles of esomeprazole or these NSAIDs. Esomeprazole inhibits gastric acid secretion. Therefore, esomeprazole may interfere with the absorption of drugs where gastric pH is an important determinant of bioavailability (eg, ketoconazole, iron salts and digoxin). **Carcinogenesis, Mutagenesis, Impairment of Fertility** The carcinogenic potential of esomeprazole was assessed using omeprazole studies. In two 24-month oral carcinogenicity studies in rats, omeprazole at daily doses of 1.7, 3.4, 13.8, 44.0 and 140.8 mg/kg/day (about 0.7 to 57 times the human dose of 20 mg/day expressed on a body surface area basis) produced gastric ECL cell carcinoids in a dose-related manner in both male and female rats; the incidence of this effect was markedly higher in female rats, which had higher blood levels of omeprazole. Gastric carcinoids seldom occur in the untreated rat. In addition, ECL cell hyperplasia was present in all treated groups of both sexes. In one of these studies, female rats were treated with 13.8 mg omeprazole/kg/day (about 5.6 times the human dose on a body surface area basis) for 1 year, then followed for an additional year without the drug. No carcinoids were seen in these rats. An increased incidence of treatment-related ECL cell hyperplasia was observed at the end of 1 year (94% treated vs 10% controls). By the second year the difference between treated and control rats was much smaller (46% vs 26%) but still showed more hyperplasia in the treated group. Gastric adenocarcinoma was seen in one rat (2%). No similar tumor was seen in male or female rats treated for 2 years. For this strain of rat no similar tumor has been noted historically, but a finding involving only one tumor is difficult to interpret. A 78-week mouse carcinogenicity study of omeprazole did not show increased tumor occurrence, but the study was not conclusive. Esomeprazole was negative in the Ames mutation test, in the *in vivo* rat bone marrow cell chromosome aberration test, and the *in vivo* mouse micronucleus test. Esomeprazole, however, was positive in the *in vitro* human lymphocyte chromosome aberration test. Omeprazole was positive in the *in vitro* human lymphocyte chromosome aberration test, the *in vivo* mouse bone marrow cell chromosome aberration test, and the *in vivo* mouse micronucleus test. The potential effects of esomeprazole on fertility and reproductive performance were assessed using omeprazole studies. Omeprazole at oral doses up to 138 mg/kg/day in rats (about 56 times the human dose on a body surface area basis) was found to have no effect on reproductive performance of parental animals. **Pregnancy** *Teratogenic Effects. Pregnancy Category B* Teratology studies have been performed in rats at oral doses up to 280 mg/kg/day (about 57 times the human dose on a body surface area basis) and in rabbits at oral doses up to 86 mg/kg/day (about 35 times the human dose on a body surface area basis) and have revealed no evidence of impaired fertility or harm to the fetus due to esomeprazole. There are, however, no adequate and well-controlled studies in pregnant women. Because animal reproduction studies are not always predictive of human response, this drug should be used during pregnancy only if clearly needed. Teratology studies conducted with omeprazole in rats at oral doses up to 138 mg/kg/day (about 56 times the human dose on a body surface area basis) and in rabbits at doses up to 69 mg/kg/day (about 56 times the human dose on a body surface area basis) did not disclose any evidence for a teratogenic potential of omeprazole. In rabbits, omeprazole in a dose range of 6.9 to 69.1 mg/kg/day (about 5.5 to 56 times the human dose on a body surface area basis) produced dose-related increases in embryo-lethality, fetal resorptions, and pregnancy disruptions. In rats, dose-related embryo/ fetal toxicity and postnatal developmental toxicity were observed in offspring resulting from parents treated with omeprazole at 13.8 to 138.0 mg/kg/day (about 5.6 to 56 times the human doses on a body surface area basis). There are no adequate and well-controlled studies in pregnant women. Sporadic reports have been received of congenital abnormalities occurring in infants born to women who have received omeprazole during pregnancy. **Nursing Mothers** The excretion of esomeprazole in milk has not been studied. However, omeprazole concentrations have been measured in breast milk of a woman following oral administration of 20 mg. Because esomeprazole is likely to be excreted in human milk, because of the potential for serious adverse reactions in nursing infants from esomeprazole, and because of the potential for tumorigenicity shown for omeprazole in rat carcinogenicity studies, a decision should be made whether to discontinue nursing or to discontinue the drug, taking into account the importance of the drug to the mother. **Pediatric Use** Use of NEXIUM in adolescent patients 12 to 17 years of age for short-term treatment of GERD is supported by a) extrapolation of results, already included in the currently approved labeling, from adequate and well-controlled studies that supported the approval of NEXIUM for adults, and b) safety and pharmacokinetic studies performed in adolescent patients. (See **CLINICAL PHARMACOLOGY, Pharmacokinetics,** *Pediatric* for pharmacokinetic information.) The safety and effectiveness of NEXIUM for the treatment of symptomatic GERD in patients <12 years of age have not been established. The safety and effectiveness of NEXIUM for other pediatric uses have not been established. **12 to 17 Years of Age GERD** In a multi-center, randomized, double-blind, parallel-group study, 149 adolescent patients (12 to 17 years of age; 89 female; 124 Caucasian, 15 Black, 10 Other) with clinically diagnosed GERD were treated with either NEXIUM 20 mg or NEXIUM 40 mg once daily for up to 8 weeks to evaluate safety and tolerability. Patients were not endoscopically characterized as to the presence or absence of erosive esophagitis. The most frequently reported (at least 2%) treatment related adverse events in these patients were headache (8.1%), abdominal pain (2.7%), diarrhea (2%) and nausea (2%). No new safety concerns were identified. **Geriatric Use** Of the total number of patients who received NEXIUM in clinical trials, 1459 were 65 to 74 years of age and 354 patients were ≥75 years of age. No overall differences in safety and efficacy were observed between the elderly and younger individuals, and other reported clinical experience has not identified differences in responses between the elderly and younger patients, but greater sensitivity of some older individuals cannot be ruled out.

**ADVERSE REACTIONS** The safety of NEXIUM was evaluated in over 15,000 patients (aged 18-84 years) in clinical trials worldwide including over 8,500 patients in the United States and over 6,500 patients in Europe and Canada. Over 2,900 patients were treated in long-term studies for up to 6-12 months. In general, NEXIUM was well tolerated in both short and long-term clinical trials. A study was performed evaluating the safety of NEXIUM in pediatric patients aged 12-17 for the treatment of symptomatic GERD (see **PRECAUTIONS – Pediatric Use**). The safety in the treatment of healing of erosive esophagitis was assessed in four randomized comparative clinical trials, which included 1,240 patients on NEXIUM 20 mg, 2,434 patients on NEXIUM 40 mg, and 3,008 patients on omeprazole 20 mg daily. The most frequently occurring adverse events (≥1%) in all three groups was headache (5.5, 5.0, and 3.8, respectively) and diarrhea (no difference among the three groups). Nausea, flatulence, abdominal pain, constipation, and dry mouth occurred at similar rates among patients taking NEXIUM or omeprazole. Additional adverse events that were reported as possibly or probably related to NEXIUM with an incidence <1% are listed below by body system: ***Body as a Whole:*** abdomen enlarged, allergic reaction, asthenia, back pain, chest pain, chest pain substernal, facial edema, peripheral edema, hot flushes, fatigue, fever, flu-like disorder, generalized edema, leg edema, malaise, pain, rigors; ***Cardiovascular:*** flushing, hypertension, tachycardia; ***Endocrine:*** goiter; ***Gastrointestinal:*** bowel irregularity, constipation aggravated, dyspepsia, dysphagia, dysplasia GI, epigastric pain, eructation, esophageal disorder, frequent stools, gastroenteritis, GI hemorrhage, GI symptoms not otherwise specified, hiccup, melena, mouth disorder, pharynx disorder, rectal disorder, serum gastrin increased, tongue disorder, tongue edema, ulcerative stomatitis, vomiting; ***Hearing:*** earache, tinnitus; ***Hematologic:*** anemia, anemia hypochromic, cervical lymphoadenopathy, epistaxis, leukocytosis, leukopenia, thrombocytopenia; ***Hepatic:*** bilirubinemia, hepatic function abnormal, SGOT increased, SGPT increased; ***Metabolic/Nutritional:*** glycosuria, hyperuricemia, hyponatremia, increased alkaline phosphatase, thirst, vitamin B12 deficiency, weight increase, weight decrease; ***Musculoskeletal:*** arthralgia, arthritis aggravated, arthropathy, cramps, fibromyalgia syndrome, hernia, polymyalgia rheumatica; ***Nervous System/Psychiatric:*** anorexia, apathy, appetite increased, confusion, depression aggravated, dizziness, hypertonia, nervousness, hypoesthesia, impotence, insomnia, migraine, migraine aggravated, paresthesia, sleep disorder, somnolence, tremor, vertigo, visual field defect; ***Reproductive:*** dysmenorrhea, menstrual disorder, vaginitis; ***Respiratory:*** asthma aggravated, coughing, dyspnea, larynx edema, pharyngitis, rhinitis, sinusitis; ***Skin and Appendages:*** acne, angioedema, dermatitis, pruritus, pruritus ani, rash, rash erythematous, rash maculo-papular, skin inflammation, sweating increased, urticaria; ***Special Senses:*** otitis media, parosmia, taste loss, taste perversion; ***Urogenital:*** abnormal urine, albuminuria, cystitis, dysuria, fungal infection, hematuria, micturition frequency, moniliasis, genital moniliasis, polyuria; ***Visual:*** conjunctivitis, vision abnormal. Endoscopic findings that were reported as adverse events include: duodenitis, esophagitis, esophageal stricture, esophageal ulceration, esophageal varices, gastric ulcer, gastritis, hernia, benign polyps or nodules, Barrett's esophagus, and mucosal discoloration. Two placebo-controlled studies were conducted in 710 patients for the treatment of symptomatic gastroesophageal reflux disease. The most common adverse events that were reported as possibly or probably related to NEXIUM were diarrhea (4.3%), headache (3.8%), and abdominal pain (3.8%). Postmarketing Reports – There have been spontaneous reports of adverse events with postmarketing use of esomeprazole. These reports occurred rarely and are listed below by body system: ***Blood And Lymphatic System Disorders:*** agranulocytosis, pancytopenia; ***Eye Disorders:*** blurred vision; ***Gastrointestinal Disorders:*** pancreatitis; ***Hepatobiliary Disorders:*** hepatitis with or without jaundice; ***Immune System Disorders:*** anaphylactic reaction/shock; ***Musculoskeletal And Connective Tissue Disorders:*** myalgia; ***Psychiatric Disorders:*** depression; ***Skin and Subcutaneous Tissue Disorders:*** alopecia, erythema multiforme, Stevens-Johnson syndrome, toxic epidermal necrolysis (TEN, some fatal). Other adverse events not observed with NEXIUM, but occurring with omeprazole can be found in the omeprazole package insert, **ADVERSE REACTIONS** section.

**OVERDOSAGE** A single oral dose of esomeprazole at 510 mg/kg (about 103 times the human dose on a body surface area basis), was lethal to rats. The major signs of acute toxicity were reduced motor activity, changes in respiratory frequency, tremor, ataxia, and intermittent clonic convulsions. There have been some reports of overdosage with esomeprazole. Reports have been received of overdosage with omeprazole in humans. Doses ranged up to 2,400 mg (120 times the usual recommended clinical dose). Manifestations were variable, but included confusion, drowsiness, blurred vision, tachycardia, nausea, diaphoresis, flushing, headache, dry mouth, and other adverse reactions similar to those seen in normal clinical experience (see omeprazole package insert-**ADVERSE REACTIONS**). No specific antidote for esomeprazole is known. Since esomeprazole is extensively protein bound, it is not expected to be removed by dialysis. In the event of overdosage, treatment should be symptomatic and supportive. As with the management of any overdose, the possibility of multiple drug ingestion should be considered. For current information on treatment of any drug overdose, a certified Regional Poison Control Center should be contacted. Telephone numbers are listed in the Physicians' Desk Reference (PDR) or local telephone book. **DOSAGE AND ADMINISTRATION** Please see full Prescribing Information for recommended dosages and dosage adjustments for **Special Populations** for NEXIUM.

NEXIUM and the color purple as applied to the capsule are registered trademarks of the AstraZeneca group of companies.



Distributed by: AstraZeneca LP, Wilmington, DE 19850
Product of France 31026-02 Rev. 04/06 240260

AstraZeneca

# Efficacy of Duct Tape vs Placebo in the Treatment of Verruca Vulgaris (Warts) in Primary School Children

*Marloes de Haen, MD; Marcus G. Spigt, PhD; Caro J. T. van Uden, PhD; Pierre van Neer, MD; Frans J. M. Feron, MD; André Knottnerus, PhD*

**Objective:** To determine the efficacy of duct tape compared with placebo in the treatment of verruca vulgaris.

**Design and Setting:** A randomized placebo-controlled trial in 3 primary schools in Maastricht, the Netherlands.

**Participants:** One hundred three children aged 4 to 12 years with verruca vulgaris.

**Interventions:** Duct tape applied to the wart or placebo, a corn pad (protection ring for clavi), applied around the wart for 1 night a week. Both treatments were applied for a period of 6 weeks. Patients were blinded to the hypothesis of the study.

**Main Outcome Measurement:** Complete resolution of the treated wart.

**Results:** After 6 weeks, the wart had disappeared in 16% of the children in the duct tape group compared with 6% in the placebo group ($P=.12$). The estimated effect of duct tape compared with placebo on diameter reduction of the treated wart was 1.0 mm ($P=.02$, 95% confidence interval, −1.7 to −0.1). After 6 weeks, in 7 children (21%) in the duct tape group, a surrounding wart had disappeared compared with 9 children (27%) in the placebo group ($P=.79$). Fifteen percent of the children in the duct tape group reported adverse effects such as erythema, eczema, and wounds compared with 0 in the placebo group ($P=.14$).

**Conclusion:** In a 6-week trial, duct tape had a modest but nonsignificant effect on wart resolution and diameter reduction when compared with placebo in a cohort of primary school children.

*Arch Pediatr Adolesc Med. 2006;160:1121-1125*

THREE PERCENT TO 20% OF school-aged children have warts.[1] Warts (verruca vulgaris) are skin infections caused by the human papillomavirus. Although they are harmless and usually self-limiting, they can stigmatize a child or cause physical discomfort, for example, in the case of plantar warts.[2] Many therapies have been developed for the treatment of warts, but most of these treatments have adverse effects such as pain and irritation or need to be applied for a long time. In a Cochrane review of 50 wart therapy trials, sufficient evidence was found only for the efficacy of salicylic acid.[3]

In the department of general practice at Maastricht University, general practitioners can propose new topics for research by using the "idea box." In January 2005, a proposal was submitted about researching the effects of duct tape on warts. Duct tape is a strong sticking tape normally used by do-it-yourselfers for small industrial applications. To our knowledge, only 1 study has been published on duct tape treatment for warts. In this study, Focht et al[4] treated warts with either cryotherapy or duct tape occlusion therapy. After 2 months, 85% in the duct tape arm vs 60% in the cryotherapy arm had complete resolution of their warts. However, this result has been debated because of the small number of subjects (n=61), the large loss to follow-up (16%), the method of application of the cryotherapy, and the lack of a placebo arm.[5]

*See also page 1126*

Considering the serious discomfort of cryotherapy and the awkwardness of applying salicylic acid for a long time, simply applying tape would be a cheap and helpful alternative, especially in children. However, according to the critics on Focht et al,[4] a blinded randomized control trial comparison of duct tape with placebo and/or salicylate is first indicated.

## METHODS

We performed a randomized controlled trial in which we treated warts in primary school children with either duct tape or placebo for a

Author Affiliations: Departments of General Practice (Drs de Haen, Spigt, and Knottnerus) and Dermatology (Dr van Neer), Maastricht University, Maastricht, the Netherlands; Department of Integrated Care, University Hospital Maastricht, Maastricht (Dr van Uden); and Youth Health Care Division, Regional Public Health Institute, Maastricht (Dr Feron).

period of 6 weeks. Children treated their warts at home, and 1 researcher (M.D.) performed the outcome measurements at school. At the baseline measurement, she counted the total number of warts and measured the diameter of the warts. She also decided which wart would be treated. Only 1 wart (usually the largest; otherwise, 1 surrounded by other warts) was treated in each child. To evaluate the effect of the tape on the primary and surrounding warts, the diameters of a maximum of 5 warts were measured. To blind the assessor, a second researcher (M.S.), who was not involved in the follow-up measurements, applied the first treatment. He telephoned the central randomization office that assigned the intervention and kept the randomization key. Randomization was performed in blocks of 10 stratified in 2 groups (single or multiple warts).

## POWER CALCULATION

In a review about wart therapies, it was estimated that approximately 30% of warts disappear after 10 weeks of placebo therapy.[3] To provide evidence for a minimal difference of 30% against placebo with a power of 80%, an $\alpha$ of .05, and 2-tailed statistical testing, we calculated that we would need 39 children in each group. Taking into account probable loss to follow-up, the aimed study population was set at 100 children.

## PARTICIPANTS

In cooperation with the Youth Health Care Division of the Regional Public Health Institute (Maastricht, the Netherlands), we approached children of 3 primary schools to take part in this study. Every child in these 3 schools received a letter to inform the parents about the trial. A special "child folder" was added with information about the study written at a child's reading level. Children aged 4 to 12 years with verruca vulgaris were included. Exclusion criteria were immune suppression, bandage allergy, skin diseases in the area surrounding the wart, and warts on the face or anogenital region. Parents were asked to fill in a written questionnaire about the history of the wart and the inclusion and exclusion criteria. The informed consent form had to be signed by both parents. If a child showed any resistance to the measurements or treatments during the study, no further investigations were performed. The ethical review board of the University Hospital Maastricht and Maastricht University approved the research protocol and the informed consent procedure.

## INTERVENTIONS

Children treated their warts at home. They received written instruction, including pictures, on how to apply the duct tape or the placebo. Both interventions had to be applied for their respective periods for 6 weeks. The intervention group received a duct tape that was fabricated by 3M (Leiden, the Netherlands). To minimize the risk that people would recognize the duct tape, we used the transparent version. In addition, we figured that the transparent version would be more cosmetic. The tape was removed from the original roll and pasted on sticker paper. The duct tape group received 10 strips of duct tape, which the participants had to cut to the size of the wart. The tape had to remain on the wart for 7 days. If the tape fell off, the parents had to apply a new piece of tape on the wart. In accordance with the study by Focht et al[4], at the evening of the seventh day, the parents had to remove the tape, soak the wart for 5 minutes in warm water, and rub the wart gently with a pumice stone. On that night, the wart was left untreated, and the next day the participants started the duct tape application again.

The placebo group received 10 pieces of placebo, a protection ring for clavi, which they had to apply around the wart. The clavi rings were also pasted on sticker paper so that the brand name was unknown. Because this ring had an open center, the wart itself was left clear. To avoid any influence of the glue in the ring, the children were instructed to apply the placebo only 1 night per week. As in the duct tape group, they were asked to soak and rub the wart with a pumice stone once a week.

Because it is unknown how duct tape achieves its possible effect, it was impossible to fabricate a placebo copy. Therefore, participants were not informed about the specific treatment investigated in this study. We mentioned that they would be allocated in a random fashion to 2 interventions and that they would receive "some kind of tape" for their wart. They were also informed that it was possible that they would receive an ineffective intervention for a period of 6 weeks. All participants were fully informed about the study aim after study termination.

## MEASUREMENTS AND OUTCOME PARAMETERS

Outcome measurements were performed at school at 0, 2, 4, and 6 weeks of treatment. One assessor (M.D.), who was aware of the study hypothesis, examined all children. To blind the assessor, parents were asked to remove the tape before each measurement. The location of the wart was defined by a picture and written description. At each measurement, the total number of warts was counted and the presence of the treated wart was checked. In addition, the sizes of the primary wart and a maximum of 4 surrounding warts were measured. The diameters of the warts were measured in tenth of millimeters using a sliding caliper. The primary outcome measurement of this study was complete resolution of the treated wart. Secondary outcome measurements were disappearance of other warts and reduction in diameter of the treated wart and surrounding warts.

In addition to these outcome measurements, we assessed the success of blinding. First, to check the success of our attempt to blind them for the hypothesis for this study, we asked parents about their expectations about the efficacy of the tape in the first week. Second, the assessor noted at each effect measurement whether she was blinded to the treatment that was used. Finally, to monitor the applicability, adverse effects, use of additional therapies, and discontinuation of the treatment, parents were asked to fill in a short questionnaire at the end of the treatment period before they were unblinded to the study goals.

## STATISTICAL ANALYSIS

Differences between the 2 groups in wart disappearance were analyzed using a $\chi^2$ test. Diameter reduction was analyzed by linear regression in which the treatment was the independent variable and the baseline diameter the covariable. A *P* value of $<.05$ was considered statistically significant. Differences in adverse effects and differences in blinding of the patients and researcher were analyzed using $\chi^2$ tests.

# RESULTS

## PATIENTS

Fourteen hundred forty children of 3 primary schools received the information about the trial (**Figure**). One hundred twenty-one children were scheduled for a baseline assessment. Two children were excluded because they were absent on the day of measurement; 16 others were excluded for reasons shown in the Figure. Finally, 103

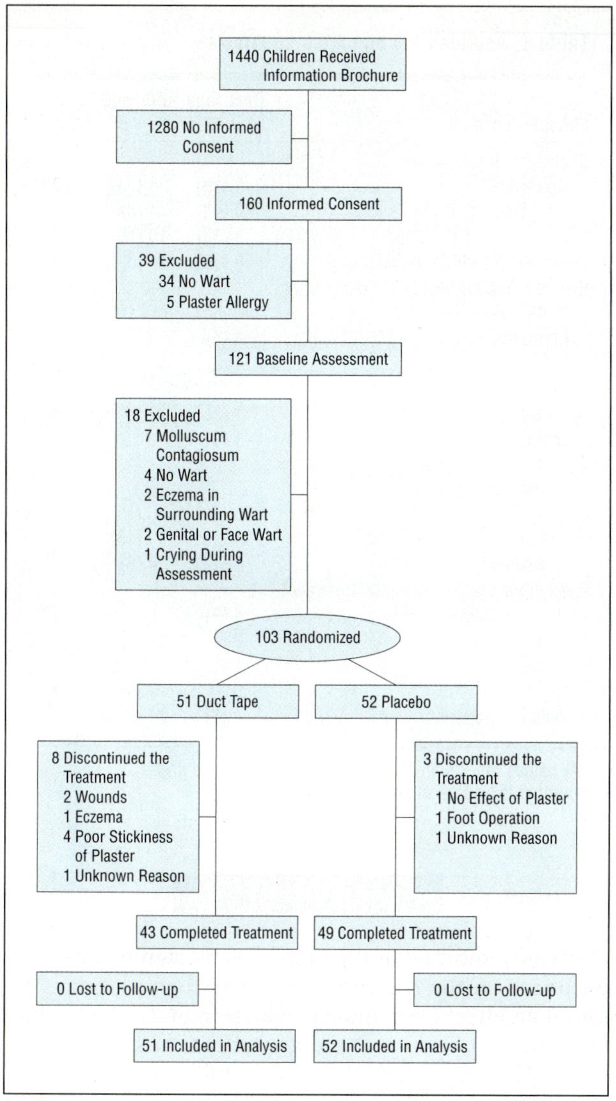


**Figure.** Trial profile.

children were randomized of whom 51 were assigned to the duct tape group and 52 to the placebo group. During the study, 8 children (17%) in the duct tape group stopped applying the duct tape, most of them in the first 2 weeks. One stopped for unknown reasons, 4 stopped because of the poor stickiness of the tape (eg, less than 1 hour), and 3 were advised to stop because of wounds or eczema caused by the tape. The reasons for discontinuation for 3 children in the placebo group were as follows: 1 was in the hospital because of an operation, 1 child stopped because he did not experience any effect of the treatment, and for 1 child the reason was unknown. These children stopped in the last 2 weeks. Parents of children who discontinued the treatment were asked for the reason of discontinuing and were instructed about the necessity of follow-up. These outcome measurements were included in the analysis.

## BASELINE CHARACTERISTICS

**Table 1** shows the baseline characteristics of the 2 treatment groups. The mean number of warts as well as

**Table 1. Baseline Characteristics**

| Characteristic | Duct Tape (n = 51) | Placebo (n = 52) |
|---|---|---|
| Sex, % | | |
| Male | 45 | 52 |
| Age, mean ± SD (range), y | 8.2 ± 2.0 (5-12) | 8.3 ± 2.0 (5-12) |
| Single/multiple warts, No. (%) | | |
| Single | 18 (35) | 19 (37) |
| Multiple | 33 (65) | 33 (64) |
| Warts, mean ± SD (range), No. | 3.4 ± 3.4 (1-16) | 3.7 ± 4.1 (1-17) |
| Location of treated wart, No. (%) | | |
| Finger/dorsum of hand | 11 (22) | 18 (35) |
| Palm of hand | 3 (6) | 2 (4) |
| Toe/dorsum of foot | 15 (29) | 13 (25) |
| Plantar part of foot | 10 (20) | 10 (19) |
| Back of heel | 1 (2) | 0 |
| Other | 11 (22) | 9 (17) |
| Duration of wart, mean ± SD (range), wk | 34.2 ± 33.9 (4-156) | 38.5 ± 34.7 (2-156) |
| Prior treatment, No. (%) | | |
| None | 27 (53) | 19 (37) |
| Cryotherapy | 8 (16) | 14 (27) |
| Salicylic acid | 15 (29) | 16 (31) |
| Other | 1 (2) | 2 (4) |
| Baseline size of treated wart mean ± SD (range), mm | 4.6 ± 2.3 (1.8-13.5) | 4.4 ± 1.7 (2.1-10.0) |

the baseline size of the treated wart was comparable between the 2 groups. In the duct tape group, fewer warts were located on the finger or dorsum of the hand (22% vs 35%) and more warts were located at the toe or foot (29% vs 25%). The warts had existed longer in the duct tape group than in the placebo group (34.2 vs 38.5 weeks). Forty-seven percent in the duct tape group vs 62% in the placebo group had received prior treatment for their warts.

## TREATMENT OUTCOME

Complete resolution of the treated wart was seen in only a few children. The first resolution in both the duct tape and placebo groups was noted after 4 weeks. At the end of the study, after 6 weeks, the warts of 8 children (16%) in the duct tape group and the warts of 3 children (6%) in the placebo group had disappeared (**Table 2**), resulting in a number needed to treat of 10 (95% confidence interval, 5 to ∞). This difference was not statistically significant.

In the duct tape group, there was a diameter reduction of 27% (from a mean of 4.6 mm to 3.4 mm) after 6 weeks. In the placebo group, this was 9% (from 4.4 mm to 4.0 mm). When adjusted for the baseline diameter, this resulted in a statistically significant difference in diameter reduction of 1.0 mm between the 2 groups ($P = .008$).

The duct tape did not seem to have any effect on surrounding warts. After 6 weeks, in only 7 children (21%) in the duct tape group a surrounding wart had disappeared compared with 9 children (27%) in the placebo group ($P = .79$) (Table 2), resulting in a number needed

**Table 2. Outcomes From 6 Weeks of Treatment With Duct Tape**

| Effect Parameter | Duct Tape | Placebo | *P* Value |
|---|---|---|---|
| **Effects on Treated Wart** | | | |
| Patients, No. | 51 | 52 | |
| Complete resolution | | | |
| 2 wk, No. | 0 | 0 | |
| 4 wk, No. | 5 | 3 | |
| 6 wk, No. (%) | 8 (16) | 3 (6) | .12 |
| Diameter of wart (range), mm | | | |
| 0 wk | 4.6 (1.8-13.5) | 4.4 (2.1-10.0) | |
| 2 wk | 4.3 (1.6-15.7) | 4.2 (1.4-9.1) | |
| 4 wk | 3.8 (0-22.2) | 3.9 (0-10.4) | |
| 6 wk | 3.4 (0-18.4) | 4.0 (0-11.2) | |
| Diameter reduction after 6 wk, %† | −27 | −9 | .02 |
| **Effect on Surrounding Warts*** | | | |
| Patients, No. | 33 | 33 | |
| Complete resolution of at least 1 surrounding wart | | | |
| 2 wk, No. | 4 | 2 | |
| 4 wk, No. | 8 | 7 | |
| 6 wk, No. (%) | 7 (21) | 9 (27) | .79 |
| Diameter of warts (range), mm | | | |
| 0 wk | 3.2 (1.7-5.8) | 3.0 (1.7-6.0) | |
| 2 wk | 3.2 (0-10.8) | 3.0 (1.0-6.6) | |
| 4 wk | 2.9 (0-6.2) | 2.7 (0-6.2) | |
| 6 wk | 3.0 (0-5.6) | 2.6 (0-6.8) | |
| Diameter reduction after 6 wk, %‡ | −21 | −27 | .22 |

*Only children with multiple warts are included in this analysis.
†The calculated difference between the 2 groups adjusted for baseline size, location of the wart, previous treatment, and duration of the wart was −1.0 mm (95% confidence interval, −1.7 to −0.1).
‡The calculated difference between the 2 groups adjusted for baseline size, previous treatment, and duration of the wart was 0.4 mm (95% confidence interval, −0.2 to 1.0).

**Table 3. Applicability and Adverse Effects***

| Effect Parameter | Duct Tape (n = 47)† | Placebo (n = 52) | *P* Value |
|---|---|---|---|
| Stickiness of the plaster | | | |
| Good | 9 (19) | 38 (73) | <.001 |
| Moderate | 20 (43) | 4 (8) | |
| Bad | 18 (38) | 10 (19) | |
| Use of extra fixation material | 15 (32) | 17 (33) | .93 |
| Skin reaction caused by the tape | | | |
| None | 40 (85) | 52 (100) | .14 |
| Erythema | 3 (6) | | |
| Itching | 1 (2) | | |
| Eczema | 1 (2) | | |
| Bleeding | 1 (2) | | |
| Other | 1 (2) | | |
| Skin reaction caused by the pumice stone | | | |
| None | 28 (60) | 38 (75) | .24 |
| Pain | 11 (23) | 9 (18) | |
| Bleeding | 8 (17) | 4 (8) | |
| Reason for discontinuing the treatment | | | |
| Poor stickiness | 4 (9) | | .75 |
| Wounds | 2 (4) | | |
| Eczema | 1 (2) | | |
| Other | 0 | 2 (4) | |
| Unknown reason | 1 (2) | 1 (2) | |

*All values other than *P* values are numbers (percentages).
†Number is less because of missing values.

to harm of 17 (95% confidence interval, 4 to ∞). There was no difference in diameter reduction of surrounding warts between the 2 groups.

Only 19% of the duct tape group judged the stickiness of the tape as good (**Table 3**). Both groups used additional fixation material (32% vs 33%). Seven children (15%) in the duct tape group showed a skin reaction caused by the duct tape, mostly erythema ($P=.14$) None of the participants in the placebo group showed any skin reaction. Both groups reported pain and/or bleeding caused by the pumice stone. None of the participants used other wart therapies during the study.

The prior expectations of the participants toward the efficacy of their treatment was rather low but comparable between the 2 study groups ($P=.38$). The duct tape scored 5.6 on a scale from 0 to 10 and the placebo scored 5.1 (**Table 4**). During the measurements, the assessor recorded whether she knew which kind of treatment had been applied when she performed the measurements. It turned out that she was blinded in 69% of the measurements in the duct tape group. In the placebo group, this was significantly higher: 83% ($P=.03$) (Table 4).

## COMMENT

Our study shows that duct tape has no significantly better effect on the resolution of warts than placebo. We found an effect on diameter reduction of 27%. The duct tape did not seem to have any effect on surrounding warts. The majority (81%) of the children reported that the duct tape would not stick and 15% reported adverse effects such as erythema. This is inconsistent with the previously reported positive results observed by Focht et al.[4]

An important finding in our study was the applicability and adverse effects of the duct tape. In the study by Focht et al, only "a minimal amount of local irritation and erythema and difficulty for some patients in keeping the tape on" was mentioned. In our study, the latter turned out to be highly important. Only 19% of the duct tape group judged the stickiness of the tape as good; 32% used extra fixation material. In our view, this is crucial because it makes the treatment a bothersome rather than a feasible alternative for other wart therapies. In addition, 15% of the children in the duct tape group showed adverse effects varying from erythema to eczema and small wounds.

### DIFFERENCES BETWEEN THE 2 STUDIES

How can we explain the differences in effects between our study and that of Focht et al?[4] Maybe the high efficacy of duct tape in the study by Focht et al could be explained by their follow-up. Part of the follow-up in that study was performed by telephone. This can result in a more positive judgment about wart resolution by the parents, especially if the parents were not blinded to the objective of the study (ie, to investigate the effects of duct tape).

The poor stickiness of the duct tape may have negatively influenced our observed effects. However, we emphasized to parents the importance of keeping the tape on, and parents said they tried their utmost to comply with this instruction. For that reason, we do not think that the short periods the wart was uncovered can explain the low efficacy of the duct tape. In addition, we analyzed whether children who had complete resolution of the treated wart judged the tape as sticking well. If the effect of the duct tape would be so low because of the bad stickiness, one would expect that the children who had complete resolution of their wart had a better sticking tape, which turned out not to be the case. Only 1 of 8 children in the duct tape group who had complete resolution judged the tape as sticking well. However, it is possible that Focht et al[4] used a different and maybe more effective kind of duct tape. We do not know which kind of duct tape was used in their study. We used the transparent version of duct tape produced by 3M. The producer of the tape guaranteed this tape had the same stickiness as the well-known silver variant.

Finally, the overall low effectiveness of both interventions in our study is surprising.

Considering the estimated placebo effect of 30% in 10 weeks, the observed 6% effect in our placebo group was small. One explanation could be that in both groups, a part of the children had already used other wart therapies, which could result in more resistant warts. Besides that, the effects in a placebo group are the result of many variables, such as natural course of the disease, regression to the mean, cointerventions, placebo effects, and probably many other unknown variables. All these different variables can sum up to a large effect in the placebo group or, in our case, can explain a small effect. Hence, both the duct tape and the placebo could do better in other studies, but it is crucial that in our study the duct tape was not more effective than placebo although it did have more adverse effects. Therefore, we do not think that, when subjected to firm investigation, the duct tape would do much better than placebo or better than other effective interventions.

## FUTURE RESEARCH

The effect on diameter reduction could be a reason for further investigation, although we do not think that this is of clinical importance. Nevertheless, we advise taking the following suggestions into account when studying duct tape any further. First, it is important to use a very sticky tape. Second, a longer follow-up period is needed to observe any effect of the duct tape. Finally, we suggest not using a pumice stone. We used the pumice stone to make our study comparable with that of Focht et al[4], but the reasons to use the pumice stone besides the duct tape are unclear. Many children in our study experienced scrubbing with the pumice stone as very unpleasant, and bleeding of the wart (caused by the pumice stone) could lead to spreading of the wart virus.

**Table 4. Success of Blinding Patients and Researcher**

| Measure | Duct Tape (n = 51) | Placebo (n = 52) | *P* Value |
|---|---|---|---|
| Expectation rating by the patient about the efficacy of the treatment after 1 week of treatment, mean ± SD (range, 1-10)* | 5.6 ± 2.3 | 5.1 ± 2.8 | .38 |
| Blinding of the researcher during the outcome measurements, % | 69 | 83 | .03 |

*A score of 10 is the most favorable score.

## CONCLUSION

In this 6-week study, duct tape was no more effective than placebo. The duct tape was difficult to use because of poor stickiness, and it caused a skin reaction in 15% of the children. Further research with longer follow-up would only be useful with a tape that is better sticking.

**Accepted for Publication:** July 4, 2006.

**Correspondence:** Marcus G. Spigt, PhD, Department of General Practice, Maastricht University, PO Box 616, 6200 MD Maastricht, the Netherlands (m.spigt@hag.unimaas.nl).

**Author Contributions:** All authors had full access to all the data in the study and take responsibility for the integrity of the data and the accuracy of the data analysis. *Study concept and design:* de Haen, Spigt, van Uden, van Neer, and Knottnerus. *Acquisition of data:* de Haen, Spigt, and Feron. *Analysis and interpretation of data:* de Haen and Spigt. *Drafting of the manuscript:* de Haen and Spigt. *Critical revision of the manuscript for important intellectual content*: Spigt, van Uden, van Neer, Feron, and Knottnerus. *Statistical analysis:* de Haen. *Administrative, technical, and material support:* de Haen, Spigt, Feron, and Knottnerus. *Study supervision:* Spigt, van Uden, van Neer, and Knottnerus.

**Financial Disclosure:** None reported.

## REFERENCES

1. Burns DA, Breathnach SM, Cox N, Griffiths CE. *Rook's Textbook of Dermatology.* 7th ed. Oxford, England: Blackwell Publishers; 2004.
2. van de Lisdonk EH, van den Bosch WJHM, Lagro-Janssen ALM. *Ziekten in de Huisartspraktijk.* Maarssen, the Netherlands: Elsevier; 2003.
3. Gibbs S, Harvey I, Sterling J, Stark R. Local treatments for cutaneous warts: systematic review. *BMJ.* 2002;325:461.
4. Focht DR III, Spicer C, Fairchok MP. The efficacy of duct tape vs cryotherapy in the treatment of verruca vulgaris (the common wart). *Arch Pediatr Adolesc Med.* 2002;156:971-974.
5. Ringold S, Mendoza JA, Tarini BA, Sox C. Is duct tape occlusion therapy as effective as cryotherapy for the treatment of the common wart? *Arch Pediatr Adolesc Med.* 2002;156:975-977.

SECTION EDITORS: DIMITRI A. CHRISTAKIS, MD, MPH

# Interpreting Negative Results From an Underpowered Clinical Trial

## Warts and All

In the randomized, placebo-controlled trial by de Haen et al[1] that appears in this issue of the Archives, the application of duct tape is compared with placebo as a treatment for common warts. The investigators recruited 103 children in the Netherlands from primary schools and assessed them for warts. Those with warts were randomized to 1 of 2 groups. One group received duct tape to apply to a designated wart, and the other group received a placebo in the form of a corn pad to apply around the wart. The primary outcome of the study was resolution of the designated wart 6 weeks after initiation of therapy. Other outcomes included change in the size of the designated wart and resolution of surrounding warts. Differences in complete resolution of the designated wart were not statistically significant. However, the investigators did find a statistically significant difference in the change in wart diameter: those treated with duct tape had a greater reduction in size compared with the placebo group. Importantly, 15% of the duct tape group stopped treatment early either because of a skin reaction to the treatment or because the tape did not stick well. Given the problems with the duct tape treatment as well as its lack of efficacy, de Haen and colleagues concluded that duct tape has a modest, nonsignificant effect as a therapy for warts.

*See also page 1121*

This study merits a detailed examination for several reasons. Warts are common, and a quick, effective, and inexpensive treatment is not available. Although warts are medically benign, they are unsightly and may cause a child to feel self-conscious. A recent review[2] concluded that the only treatment shown consistently to be effective is salicylic acid, but the treatment time is long and application is tedious. A randomized, controlled trial by Focht et al[3] published in the Archives in 2002 comparing duct tape with cryotherapy showed a benefit to using duct tape. Although primary care physicians and persons with warts welcomed this news, further studies were needed to verify these results. We critiqued this study using the framework suggested by the *Users' Guide to the Medical Literature: A Manual for Evidence-Based Clinical Practice*[4] for therapeutic trials.

### WERE THE STUDY PATIENTS SIMILAR TO ACTUAL PATIENTS?

A randomized, controlled trial ideally recruits participants who would most accurately reflect the population to whom the treatment would be applied in reality. For a common condition like warts, to test a treatment (duct tape) that can be purchased over the counter presents challenges to subject recruitment. Recruiting from a physician's office may not result in a representative sample, as many persons who develop warts do not seek medical attention but try other treatments at home first. Therefore, clinic-setting study participants would likely include those with warts that are more difficult to treat.

de Haen and colleagues attempted to address this limitation by recruiting from schools, which would be expected to yield a more representative, community-based sample. However, considering epidemiologic data showing that 30% of warts resolve without treatment by 32 weeks,[5] the mean length of time that the subjects had had their warts was quite long—34.2 weeks for the experimental group and 38.5 weeks for the control group. In addition, many subjects had already tried another treatment. Therefore, the warts in the participants may be particularly resistant not only to spontaneous resolution but also to any treatment. Thus, we are doubtful that this study population is optimally representative of those who would likely consider the treatment in question. There also may have been a selection bias in recruiting, as those who were particularly motivated to enroll in the study may have been those most frustrated by warts refractory to other over-the-counter therapies. These factors may also partially explain the surprisingly low rate of spontaneous resolution within the 6-week study period as compared with the rate in other studies.[2]

*See the enhanced version at http://www.archpediatrics.com*

## WERE PATIENTS RANDOMIZED? WERE THE PATIENTS IN THE TREATMENT AND CONTROL GROUPS SIMILAR WITH RESPECT TO KNOWN PROGNOSTIC FACTORS?

All of the 103 children were randomized to duct tape or a placebo clavi ring. Despite randomization, there were differences between the 2 groups: patients in the duct tape group reported longer wart duration on average. If we assume, in general, that older warts are more likely to spontaneously resolve, this difference in wart "age" would likely bias away from the study's null hypothesis that treatment with duct tape for 6 weeks is no different from placebo in wart resolution. However, more patients in the placebo group had already tried another treatment, which would likely bias toward null findings because such refractory warts in the placebo group would be less likely to resolve spontaneously.

## WERE PATIENTS AWARE OF GROUP ALLOCATION? WAS THE OBSERVER AWARE OF GROUP ALLOCATION?

Although participants could not practically be blinded to the kind of tape they received, they were blinded to the hypothesis of the study. Randomization was blinded to the observer (wart size assessor) by having the subjects remove the tape or clavi ring prior to each assessment. The CONSORT statement[6] recommends reporting the method used to assess blinding; however, this is often not done.[7] To their credit, de Haen and colleagues assessed blinding in this study using 2 methods. First, the investigators asked how well the parents of participants (subject proxies) expected the treatment to work. The assumption is that those who believe they are in the experimental group will have higher expectations of treatment success. In this study, parents in both groups had similar expectations. Second, the investigators asked the observer whether she knew which kind of tape the subjects received. The observer reported that she knew the assigned group in 31% of the duct tape group compared with 17% of the placebo group, a statistically significant difference. Although the observer was incorrect about assignment more than half of the time overall, the presence of incomplete, asymmetric blinding of the observer would theoretically bias the results toward finding that duct tape was more effective. The investigators did mention that the observer was aware of the study hypothesis. Even if she were blinded to the study hypothesis, the observer could still have subconsciously formed hypotheses of her own, which could potentially bias the results.

## WAS FOLLOW-UP COMPLETE? WERE PATIENTS ANALYZED IN THE GROUPS TO WHICH THEY WERE RANDOMIZED?

In contrast to the prior randomized, controlled trial of duct tape for warts by Focht et al,[3] follow-up by de Haen and colleagues was complete, which improves the validity of these results. All of the patients were accounted for at the end of the study, and follow-up was conducted in person rather than by telephone for all of the subjects. Furthermore, all of the participants were analyzed in the groups to which they were randomized, and this even included those who did not complete treatment. This intention-to-treat analysis included everyone regardless of adherence to treatment and was designed to produce conclusions that are more applicable to real-life situations.

An intention-to-treat analysis reflects the potential real-world experience in which not all of the patients adhere to treatment recommendations. However, including in the analysis those who did not finish the course of treatment could dilute a positive effect of the treatment. For example, if all of the 8 subjects in the duct tape group whose warts resolved had completed treatment, analyzing treatment completers as a subgroup may have yielded a different result and led to different conclusions. If duct tape for warts was effective for this subgroup, improving the stickiness of the tape and treating concomitant eczema more aggressively may be more appropriate than entirely dismissing duct tape as a potentially beneficial treatment. Although such post hoc analyses are methodologically less appealing than approaches chosen by investigators prior to a study, they can potentially inform future studies as well as clinical management.

## STATISTICAL POWER AND TYPE II ERROR

de Haen and colleagues found no statistical difference in wart resolution between duct tape and placebo. As these were negative results, it is essential to consider the likelihood of a type II error, or that the investigators erroneously concluded that duct tape was ineffective. Did the study have enough power to detect a clinically meaningful difference between the 2 groups, and how did the investigators decide how big that difference should be?

The primary outcome in this study was binary, meaning that there were 2 possible and distinct outcomes: either the wart resolved or it did not. To calculate how many subjects are needed to detect a difference in a binary outcome, one must estimate how many subjects in each group will have the desired outcome. Previous studies[8] have suggested that 30% of warts resolve after 10 weeks with no treatment, and de Haen and colleagues decided that an acceptable treatment alternative should be 30 percentage points better than the natural history of warts.[1] Thus, they calculated how many subjects were needed to detect a significant difference if 30% of warts in the placebo group resolved and 60% of warts in the duct tape group resolved.

However, de Haen and colleagues misjudged 2 critical pieces of information in calculating their desired sample size. First, for a 6-week—rather than 10-week—follow-up, they should have anticipated a lower rate of wart resolution because of the shorter time frame. Second, they should have elaborated more on how they concluded that a 30-percentage-point difference was clinically meaningful, especially because many persons with warts may consider a smaller effect size beneficial enough—and the treatment accessible enough—to try the duct tape treatment on their own.

If de Haen and colleagues had recruited a larger sample to detect a smaller but still clinically relevant effect, they may have reached different conclusions with the very same

**Table. Precision of Estimates of the Effect of Duct Tape vs Placebo for Wart Therapy**

| Treatment | Patients, No. | Treated Warts That Resolved, % | 95% CI* |
|---|---|---|---|
| Duct tape | 51 | 16 | 7.0-28.6 |
| Placebo | 52 | 6 | 1.2-15.9 |

Abbreviation: CI, confidence interval.
*The CIs were calculated from data provided by de Haen et al.[1]

effect size they described. With 6% spontaneous resolution in the placebo group and a difference of only 10 percentage points between duct tape and placebo, de Haen and colleagues had insufficient power (only 26%) to reject their null hypothesis of no difference between duct tape and placebo. In contrast, if they assumed a priori 30% spontaneous resolution in placebo and a 20-percentage-point meaningful difference, they would have needed to recruit 184 patients evenly split between the groups to achieve 90% power to reject the null hypothesis. If they had such a sample and had identical findings to what they described (ie, lower spontaneous resolution rate and smaller treatment effect than anticipated),[1] they would have had 53% power to reject the null hypothesis. If instead they had assumed a priori 30% resolution and a 15-percentage-point difference, their target sample size would have been about 350 children. A sample of this size would have given them more than 80% statistical power; importantly, the same results they described would have led them to *reject* the null hypothesis at $P<.05$. Although such a study would have been more expensive, it would have provided a better test of the null hypothesis.

## HOW PRECISE WAS THE ESTIMATE OF THE TREATMENT EFFECT?

In a randomized, controlled trial, the measured effect on the subjects is an estimate of what the true effect would be if the treatment were applied to a larger population. The precision of the estimate is important in interpreting these results. Precision is estimated by confidence intervals. The 95% confidence intervals give us parameters with which we can say that if we repeat the same study 100 times, the result would fall within these parameters 95% of the time. Although de Haen and colleagues did not report confidence intervals, we calculated them to provide insights into the reported data (**Table**).

These confidence intervals are somewhat wide, largely attributable to the small sample noted earlier. There is considerable overlap with these confidence intervals, consistent with the failure by de Haen and colleagues to reject the null hypothesis of no difference between 6 weeks of treatment vs placebo.

## WERE ALL CLINICALLY IMPORTANT OUTCOMES CONSIDERED?

As a secondary outcome, de Haen and colleagues measured the change in the diameter of the wart over the 6-week study period and found significant differences between the groups. This is an important finding, especially given the short observation period. The warts treated with duct tape were improving more rapidly. It is reasonable to speculate that if the study continued, the warts treated with duct tape would be likely to resolve more quickly than the placebo-treated warts, and at some point, meaningful differences in resolution rates that de Haen and colleagues anticipated would be achieved.

## CONCLUSIONS

The negative study published by de Haen and colleagues is illustrative for several reasons. First, it allows us to examine the potential effect of selection bias in recruiting subjects for a study of a common condition. Second, de Haen and colleagues assessed how well the subjects and observers were blinded, which provides the opportunity to discuss this very important but often underreported component of randomized, controlled trials. Third, this study shows possible limitations of intention-to-treat analyses and the potential benefit of as-treated subgroup analyses in randomized, controlled trials to assess the treatment effects when the sample is heterogeneous with respect to treatment exposure. Fourth and perhaps most importantly, the study illustrates the perils of study design with respect to sample size. Although investigators must always balance scientific goals with fiscal and logistic constraints, the assumptions by de Haen and colleagues regarding the spontaneous wart resolution rate and a meaningful clinical difference were so substantively different from what they actually found that they were left underpowered to assess their study hypotheses.

In summary, this study tests an inexpensive treatment for a common condition, and the results contradict an earlier randomized, controlled trial that had flaws of its own.[3] However, several methodological limitations in the study by de Haen and colleagues lead us to question the investigators' conclusions that the effects of duct tape were not significant. Further studies that address the limitations of these extant studies are needed before such definitive conclusions can be drawn.

*Jeanne Van Cleave, MD*
*Alex R. Kemper, MD, MPH, MS*
*Matthew M. Davis, MD, MAPP*

**Correspondence**: Dr Davis, Division of General Pediatrics, University of Michigan, 300 N Ingalls Bldg, Room 6C23, Ann Arbor, MI 48109-0456 (mattdav@med.umich.edu).

**Author Contributions**: *Study concept and design:* Davis and Van Cleave. *Analysis and interpretation of data:* Davis and Kemper. *Drafting of the manuscript:* Davis and Van Cleave. *Critical revision of the manuscript for important intellectual content*: Davis and Kemper. *Statistical analysis:* Davis and Van Cleave. *Administrative, technical, and material support:* Davis. *Study supervision:* Davis.
**Financial Disclosure**: None reported.

## REFERENCES

1. de Haen M, Spigt MG, van Uden CJT, van Neer P, Feron FJM, Knottnerus A. Efficacy of duct tape vs placebo in the treatment of verruca vulgaris (warts) in primary school children. *Arch Pediatr Adolesc Med.* 2006;160:1121-1125.
2. Gibbs S, Harvey I, Sterling JC, Stark R. Local treatments for cutaneous warts [update of *Cochrane Database Syst Rev.* 2001;(2):CD001781]. *Cochrane Database Syst Rev.* 2003;(3):CD001781. doi:10.1002/14651858.CD001781. Processed June 29, 2006.
3. Focht DR, Spicer C, Fairchok MP. The efficacy of duct tape vs cryotherapy in the treatment of verruca vulgaris (the common wart). *Arch Pediatr Adolesc Med.* 2002; 156:971-974.
4. Guyatt G, Rennie D. *Users' Guide to the Medical Literature: A Manual for Evidence-Based Clinical Practice.* Chicago, Ill: American Medical Association; 2002.
5. Massing AM, Epstein WL. Natural history of warts: a two-year study. *Arch Dermatol.* 1963;87:306-310.
6. Altman DG, Schulz KF, Moher D, et al. The revised CONSORT statement for reporting randomized trials: explanation and elaboration. *Ann Intern Med.* 2001; 134:663-694.
7. Boutron I, Estellat C, Ravaud P. A review of blinding in randomized controlled trials found results inconsistent and questionable. *J Clin Epidemiol.* 2005;58:1220-1226.
8. Gibbs S, Harvey I, Sterling J, Stark R, Altman DG. Local treatments for cutaneous warts: systematic review. *BMJ.* 2002;325:461.

### *Announcement*

**Topic Collections**. The *Archives* offers collections of articles in specific topic areas to make it easier for physicians to find the most recent publications in a field. These are available by subspecialty, study type, disease, or problem. In addition, you can sign up to receive a Collection E-Mail Alert when new articles on specific topics are published. Go to http://archpedi.ama-assn.org/collections to see these collections of articles.

ARTICLE

# Parental Reactions to Information About Increased Genetic Risk of Type 1 Diabetes Mellitus in Infants

*Paula Simonen, PhLic; Tapio Korhonen, PhD; Tuula Simell, MPH, PhD; Päivi Keskinen, MD, PhD; Maarit Kärkkäinen, MHSci; Mikael Knip, MD, PhD; Jorma Ilonen, MD, PhD; Olli Simell, MD, PhD*

**Objective:** To assess the anxiety, emotions, thoughts, and coping behaviors of parents 1 week after they receive the results of screening of their infant's genetic risk of type 1 diabetes mellitus.

**Design:** Survey.

**Setting:** The population-based Type 1 Diabetes Prediction and Prevention project conducted in Turku.

**Participants:** Parents of 443 consecutive high-risk infants and 506 next-born low-risk infants.

**Interventions:** An infant's genetic risk of type 1 diabetes mellitus was measured from cord blood. High-risk information was delivered by telephone and low-risk information by mail 4 weeks later.

**Main Outcome Measures:** Anxiety measured using the state anxiety scale of the State-Trait Anxiety Inventory, and feelings, thoughts, and coping behaviors extracted from the questionnaire.

**Results:** One week after obtaining the results, 67% of mothers and 63% of fathers of high-risk children and 58% of mothers and 54% of fathers of low-risk children had returned the questionnaire. Anxiety levels of parents of high-risk infants were similar to those of parents of low-risk infants ($P = .86$). More than 90% of the parents thought that it was good to know about the risk. Fifty-five percent of mothers and 37% of fathers of high-risk infants expressed modest worry. Increased anxiety was connected with other stressful life events, catastrophizing thoughts of diabetes mellitus risk, and emotion-focused or avoiding coping attitudes.

**Conclusions:** Learning about their infant's genetic diabetes mellitus risk induces only mild anxiety in most parents. Identifying the few parents with stronger anxiety helps focus intensified counseling.

*Arch Pediatr Adolesc Med. 2006;160:1131-1136*

ADVANCED BIOTECHNOLOGY has made population-based genetic screening of several diseases possible. Although the prevention of type 1 diabetes mellitus (T1DM), a multifactorial, polygenic disease, remains a dream, screening for genetic risk combined with follow-up of high-risk individuals has been accepted to enhance our understanding of the etiopathogenesis of diabetes mellitus and to expedite the discovery of preventive measures. By nature, T1DM differs markedly from the single-gene disorders commonly searched for in conventional infant screening. Information of increased T1DM risk received soon after a child's birth may have a strong psychological impact on the family and the child. Most parents first react with anxiety or worry, but the intensity and duration of the psychological sequelae are likely to vary markedly.

Johnson and coworkers[1,2] studied individuals at risk for T1DM because they had islet cell antibodies, which are regarded as immune markers of the disease. Such knowledge induced anxiety that dissipated to normal levels across time in islet cell autoantibody–positive individuals and their families. The impact of risk screening probably depends on the disease and its genetic features, the velocity of progression, the prognosis, the availability of prevention or treatment, the background of the family, and other factors.

In population-based genetic T1DM risk screening, at best, only approximately 75% of future cases are detected. Most individuals at risk never develop T1DM, and the family has to wait years to learn whether their child will develop β-cell autoimmunity as a marker of prediabetes. We have been conducting a population-based infant screening study for 11½ years to recognize children with genetic T1DM risk. We hypothesized that the parents will accept the risk information with tolerable anxiety and that high anxiety scores indicate recent exposure also to other stressful events. To test these hypotheses

Author Affiliations: Departments of Psychology (Ms Simonen and Dr Korhonen), Child Psychiatry (Dr Korhonen), Pediatrics (Drs T. Simell and O. Simell and Ms Kärkkäinen), and Virology (Dr Ilonen), University of Turku, Turku; Hospital District of Satakunta, Pori (Ms Simonen); Department of Pediatrics, Tampere University School of Medicine, Tampere (Dr Keskinen); and Hospital for Children and Adolescents, University of Helsinki, Helsinki (Dr Knip), Finland.

and explore the impact of screening, we assessed the anxiety, psychosocial reactions, and coping behaviors of parents who had just learned that their infant is at genetic risk and compared these findings with those from families who had just learned that their infant has no increased risk.

## METHODS

### PROCEDURE

The population-based Type 1 Diabetes Prediction and Prevention project was launched in Turku on November 7, 1994, and was soon expanded to Oulu and Tampere.[3-5] The risk and protective *HLA-DQ* gene alleles of newborns are analyzed in cord blood, and children at genetic risk are observed for islet-specific autoimmunity and T1DM. The project is expected to identify 70% of the children who will develop T1DM before 15 years of age. Although the T1DM risk before this age in Finland is 0.75%, the risk in at-risk children varies from 3% to 7% according to the genotype. This project comprises a double-blind, placebo-controlled trial evaluating the efficacy of nasal insulin therapy in T1DM prevention.[3-5]

The ethics committee of Turku University Hospital approved the study. The parents were asked before postpartum hospital discharge whether they wanted their infant's genetic T1DM risk assessed. The sample was analyzed only after the parents had received information about T1DM and the study and had consented to the screening. Only 1.4% of the families refused.

Parents of infants at genetic risk ("high-risk parents") received the risk information by telephone 4 weeks after the child's birth. The parents were offered a counseling appointment with a study physician to discuss the risk and potential follow-up within a few days of the telephone call. The "low-risk parents" were informed of the result by mail. The letter also reminded the parents that not all children who will develop T1DM are found by screening, and it described the symptoms and signs of T1DM. The physician delivered the questionnaire to the mother and father of the high-risk infant and asked them to return it by mail within a week. The questionnaires were completed when the infant was aged 1 to 1½ months, and the parents had been aware of the risk for 1 to 2 weeks. In most families, the mother and father both attended the counseling. For each high-risk infant, the parents of the next-born infant without T1DM risk were approached via mail requesting that they also complete similar questionnaires and return them within a week.

### PARTICIPANTS

The study group comprised the parents of infants born at Turku University Hospital between April 13, 1995, and June 12, 1996, who had defined *HLA-DQ* risk alleles.[3-5] Altogether, 523 high-risk infants were identified; 88.5% of the families with a high-risk infant attended the counseling session, and 84.7% (n=443) continued in follow-up. They were the high-risk parents of the present study, whereas the low-risk parents were those whose infant was born in the same hospital, was screened next after the high-risk child, but was found not to be at high risk for T1DM (n=506).

### MEASUREMENTS

#### Social Readjustment Scale

Ten events from the Social Readjustment Scale of Holmes and Rahe[6] were selected to establish a stress sum variable for rating parents' stressful life events in the preceding year. Although widely used, this shortened scale remains to be validated.

#### State-Trait Anxiety Inventory

This standardized measure was used to collect information on the parents' anxiety level.[7,8] The State-Trait Anxiety Inventory (STAI) comprises self-report scales for 2 anxiety concepts in healthy adults: state anxiety (A-State) and trait anxiety. We used the A-State scale, which refers to a transitory emotional state or condition characterized by subjective, consciously perceived feelings of tension and apprehension and increased autonomic nervous system activity. It consists of 20 statements that indicate how the individual feels at a particular moment. The scales were scored as directed in the manual. The reliability coefficients for the A-State scale have ranged from 0.83 to 0.92 and are typically higher under psychological stress.[7] Our data led to a Cronbach coefficient of 0.94 for high-risk parents and 0.92 for low-risk parents. The validity of the STAI A-State scale has been previously documented.[8]

#### Parents' Feelings, Thoughts, and Behaviors

The emotional reactions, thoughts, and coping strategies of parents of high-risk children were assessed using questions designed for this study within the framework of the Lazarus and Folkman stress theory.[9,10] Low-risk parents were asked what they thought about screening for genetic illnesses and how they supposed such information would affect parents. Questions concerning emotions were based on the 15 different emotions identified by Lazarus.[11] Questions about coping behavior were drawn from a standardized measure, the Ways of Coping checklist,[12,13] but they were formulated to fit the situation of the study. The questions represented the 8 factors found in a previous factor analytic study[10]: confrontational coping, distancing, self-control, seeking social support, accepting responsibility, escape-avoidance, planned problem solving, and positive reappraisal. The participants indicated on a 4-point Likert scale the extent to which each stake was involved. A possibility to answer "I don't know" was also included.

### STATISTICAL ANALYSIS

The data were analyzed using a software program (SAS; SAS Institute Inc, Cary, NC). Unanswered items and "I don't know" answers were removed and analyzed separately, resulting in a slight variation in the number of observations. Analysis of variance was applied to compare data between the groups. The $\chi^2$ test was used to compare the distributions of classified variables between the 2 groups, and the 2-tailed *t* test was used to compare the group means.

## RESULTS

A total of 67.3% of mothers and 63.0% of fathers of high-risk infants and 57.5% of mothers and 54.0% of fathers of low-risk infants returned the questionnaires. The ages of the parents and the incidence of diabetes mellitus in the family in the 2 groups did not differ between those who returned or did not return the questionnaire. Those who did not return the questionnaire had a lower education level and more children than those who returned the questionnaire ($P<.01$ for both). The number of children in the family, the sex of the infant, and the age, ba-

**Table. Characteristics of Families of Infants at Increased Genetic Risk for Type 1 Diabetes Mellitus (High-Risk Infants) and of Infants Without Such Increased Risk (Low-Risk Infants)***

| | Families | |
|---|---|---|
| | With High-Risk Infants | With Low-Risk Infants |
| Families, No. | 519-554† | 513-552† |
| Parental age, mean (SD), y | | |
| Mother | 29.0 (4.6) | 29.3 (4.6) |
| Father | 30.9 (6.4) | 31.6 (5.5) |
| Basic education, %‡ | | |
| 1 | 1.1 | 0.6 |
| 2 | 38.7 | 40.8 |
| 3 | 6.1 | 5.2 |
| 4 | 54.1 | 53.4 |
| Vocational education, %§ | | |
| 1 | 7.9 | 7.2 |
| 2 | 27.6 | 28.5 |
| 3 | 14.8 | 14.0 |
| 4 | 24.6 | 21.8 |
| 5 | 9.4 | 8.5 |
| 6 | 15.4 | 18.8 |
| Sex of the infant, % | | |
| M | 52.8 | 53.3 |
| F | 47.2 | 46.7 |
| No. of children in the family, % | | |
| 1 | 43.5 | 44.0 |
| 2 | 36.2 | 36.2 |
| 3 | 16.2 | 14.0 |
| 4 | 4.2 | 5.8 |
| Stress sum score, mean (SD)‖ | | |
| Mother | 9.3 (5.6) | 8.9 (4.6) |
| Father | 7.9 (4.6) | 7.9 (4.8) |

*All differences in means and distributions are nonsignificant.

†The number varies because the background information of 35 families was incomplete.

‡Scale: 1 = less than comprehensive school, 2 = comprehensive school, 3 = part of upper secondary school, and 4 = upper secondary school.

§Scale: 1 = no vocational education, 2 = vocational school or course, 3 = upper secondary-level vocational qualification, 4 = postsecondary-level vocational qualification, 5 = academic studies without degree, and 6 = academic degree.

‖Stress index: the sum of experienced stress caused by the birth of the infant, divorce, unemployment, illness or accident, death of a loved one, or any problems with social relations, alcohol, mental health, economy, or something else.

sic education, or vocational education of the parents did not differ between high- and low-risk families (**Table**).

## PARENTS OF AT-RISK INFANTS IN FOLLOW-UP VS THOSE WHO LEFT THE STUDY

Eighteen families attended the counseling and returned the questionnaires but did not join the follow-up. The STAI A-State measure showed no difference in the anxiety scores between parents who continued in the study and those who did not ($P = .14$). The mean (SD) anxiety score of mothers of high-risk children who did not continue in the study was 36.4 (11.8), and that of fathers was 36.1 (9.6). However, parents of high-risk children who did not continue in the study had higher stress sum scores than those who continued ($P < .001$), and they were also younger ($P = .04$).

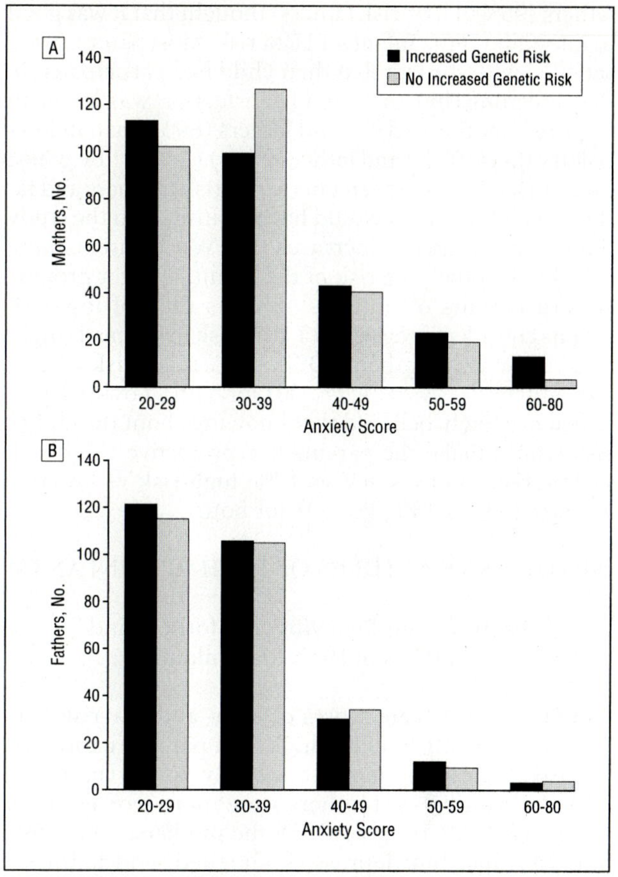


**Figure.** Distribution of the anxiety scores of mothers (A) and fathers (B) of infants with vs without increased genetic risk of type 1 diabetes mellitus.

## PARENTS OF HIGH-RISK INFANTS VS PARENTS OF LOW-RISK INFANTS

### Social Readjustment Rating Scale

The stress sum score did not differ between high- and low-risk parents ($P = .61$ by analysis of variance).

### A-State Scale

The standardized STAI A-State measure showed no difference in the scores between high- and low-risk parents 1 to 2 weeks after they had learned about their infant's screening results. The mean (SD) anxiety scores of mothers ($n = 291$) and fathers ($n = 272$) of high-risk infants were 34.9 (11.4) and 32.1 (9.0), respectively, and those of mothers ($n = 290$) and fathers ($n = 266$) of low-risk children were 33.9 (9.0) and 32.3 (8.9), respectively ($P = .86$ by analysis of variance). Similarly, no difference was observed when high-risk mothers were compared with low-risk mothers and high-risk fathers with low-risk fathers (**Figure**). However, high-risk mothers showed higher anxiety than high-risk fathers ($P < .001$), and the same sex difference was seen when low-risk mothers and fathers were compared ($P < .01$).

### Parents' Thoughts

Ninety-two percent of high-risk mothers (96% of low-risk mothers; $P < .001$ by $\chi^2$ test) and 95% of high-risk fathers (95% of low-risk fathers) thought that it was good to know about the infant's T1DM risk. Most parents were satisfied with the fact that their child had participated in the screening, but the rate of satisfaction was lower in high-risk mothers (88%) and fathers (89%) than in low-risk mothers (98%) and fathers (96%) ($P<.001$ by $\chi^2$ test for both). Ninety-six percent of low-risk mothers and fathers stated that they would have continued in the study if their infant had had increased risk. When parents were asked to estimate the risk of the infant, a larger proportion of parents of high-risk infants than of low-risk infants considered the actual T1DM risk to be small (high-risk vs low-risk mothers: 83% vs 66%; high-risk vs low-risk fathers: 87% vs 64%; $P<.001$ for both). Low-risk parents more likely believed that knowing about the child's risk would make the parents overprotective (high-risk vs low-risk mothers: 8% vs 17%; high-risk vs low-risk fathers: 14% vs 28%; $P<.001$ for both).

## MOTHERS VS FATHERS OF HIGH-RISK INFANTS

### Feelings and Behaviors of Mothers and Fathers of High-Risk Infants

Although the A-State scores of high- and low-risk parents did not differ, many high-risk parents expressed negative emotions, most commonly worry (mothers, 55%; fathers, 37%). Mothers were more worried than fathers ($P<.001$ by $\chi^2$ test). Of the mothers, 30%, 25%, and 24% had felt depressed, shocked, and helpless, respectively, and the respective percentages of fathers were 12%, 12%, and 12% ($P<.001$ for the difference between the sexes in all tests). However, 64% of the mothers (64% of the fathers) reported that they were happy because the study offered hope that T1DM can be prevented some day.

The most common way for high-risk parents to cope with the news about their infant's risk status was to seek social support from the spouse. More than 90% of the parents had discussed the infant's risk with the spouse. Mothers (85%) discussed the matter with other relatives or friends more often than fathers (59%) ($P<.001$). Most mothers (64%) and fathers (61%) had also been thinking about how the risk is going to affect the future life of their child, and more than half of the mothers and fathers (56% and 52%, respectively) decided to do everything they can to prevent T1DM. Mothers had cried more often than fathers (10% vs 1%), and fathers had decided to keep feelings to themselves more often than mothers (14% vs 10%) ($P<.001$ for both).

### Anxious vs Nonanxious Parents of High-Risk Infants

Mothers and fathers of high-risk children were then classified as anxious or nonanxious. Owing to the lack of STAI norms for Finland, the parents were classified using the mean + 1.5 SD STAI A-State score as the lower limit for the anxious group (score $\geq$47 for 17% of the mothers; score $\geq$46 for 8% of the fathers). Parents with scores below these values were considered nonanxious. The mean (SD) anxiety score of anxious mothers was 55.3 (7.7) and of anxious fathers was 53.5 (5.8).

Scores of anxious and nonanxious parents of high-risk infants showed an association with the amount of stress they reported having experienced lately. The higher stress sum score of anxious vs nonanxious parents was not explained by differences in age, education or vocational education of the parents, number of children in the family, prevalence of T1DM among family members, or the infant's sex ($P<.001$). When anxious and nonanxious parents of low-risk infants were compared, the findings were similar, and anxiety scores showed an association with stress sum scores ($P<.001$).

The thoughts of anxious parents could be defined as catastrophizing. They felt more often than nonanxious parents that they were losing control of their life, that their infant already had T1DM, and that the chances of the infant getting T1DM were very high ($P<.001$ for the difference between the 2 groups of mothers and the 2 groups of fathers). Anxious parents also thought more often than nonanxious parents that the information they had received makes parents overprotective ($P<.01$ for mothers and for fathers). The coping behavior of anxious parents was more emotion-focused or avoiding than that of nonanxious parents, and they also cried and felt angry more often ($P<.001$ for both features in mothers and fathers). Furthermore, they more often developed substitute activities and hoped that the screening result would be incorrect ($P<.001$ for mothers and for fathers). A larger proportion of anxious than nonanxious parents also began to look after their infant more carefully once they had heard of the risk ($P<.01$ for mothers and $P<.001$ and for fathers). Anxious fathers reported more often than nonanxious fathers that they did not tell others about their feelings ($P<.001$).

## COMMENT

These data suggest that learning about increased T1DM risk of the infant through a telephone call and in a subsequent counseling session does not induce serious parental anxiety according to a standardized anxiety questionnaire when studied at the child's age of 1 to 1½ months, 1 to 2 weeks after the parents had heard of the risk and discussed its implications with a physician. However, more than half of the mothers and a third of the fathers of high-risk children felt worried, and one quarter of the mothers reported depressive feelings, shock, or helplessness. Mothers of high-risk children reported more positive and negative feelings than fathers.

In studies regarding single-gene disorders, such as cystic fibrosis, anxiety in pregnant women associated with information of being a carrier disappeared when their male partners had negative test results,[14] and the carriers reported no anxiety 6 months later.[15] Also, screening for Tay-Sachs disease carriers among high school students resulted in anxiety among the carriers, but 1 year later anxiety levels of carriers and noncarriers showed no difference.[16] After genetic testing for Huntington chorea, most people experienced major emotional distress, but no severe psychiatric responses were observed.[17] However, in Sweden, neonatal screening for $\alpha_1$-antitrypsin deficiency was discontinued because of negative psychological consequences. The parents reported immediate and long-lasting worrying, anxiety, and fear, which were still recognizable after 5 to 7 years.[18-21] Prenatal detection of a serious fetal defect always induced traumatic reactions in parents,[22] but parents coped with the news using similar strategies as parents in the present study.

The impact of information concerning the genetic risk of Huntington chorea,[17] Tay-Sachs disease,[16] or cystic fibrosis[14,15] differs from this study because the risk can be expressed accurately, in some cases with 100% certainty. In contrast to studies of carriers of some monogenic diseases, information regarding the T1DM risk of the infant induced no more than modest anxiety in parents. Because data on parental anxiety after testing for genetic T1DM risk in infants are scanty, the present findings are important for T1DM prediction and prevention programs. Bennett Johnson and Tercyak[2] interviewed by telephone older children and adults soon after they had been told that they were islet cell autoantibody positive but had not met with a physician to discuss the implications of the results in detail. The participants also completed the A-State questionnaire, and they were asked to respond to the questions about diabetes mellitus risk. In the present study, parents returned the questionnaire by mail after they had met with the study physician and learned that the child's absolute risk of developing T1DM before age 15 years was 3% to 7%, a risk 4 to 10 times higher than that in the background population but still rather small.

Almost all the parents of children with or without increased T1DM risk thought that it was good to be aware of the child's risk and were happy that they took part in the study. These data support the findings suggesting that the attitude of the general population in Finland is favorable toward genetic screening.[23]

Parents of high-risk children believed that the child's actual risk of getting T1DM was smaller than what parents of low-risk children thought of the risk of high-risk children. Parents of low-risk children also more commonly believed that the infant's risk of T1DM would increase parental overprotectiveness. However, parents of high- and low-risk children had received risk information and counseling to a different extent. Furthermore, low-risk parents were asked to answer the questions as they believed they would answer if they had an infant at risk.

Parents of diabetic children regard T1DM as a less serious disease than parents of unaffected children.[24] Close acquaintance with a disease changes one's view of its severity, suggesting that proper information about the risk of multifactorial diseases may alleviate the overly pessimistic opinion of the risk.

Mothers of high-risk children used more emotion-focused coping than fathers, who used more avoiding. These sex-associated strategies may partly explain the higher anxiety scores of mothers, as mothers probably more readily reveal their emotions. The most common coping behavior of parents was to seek social support from the spouse, and more than half of the parents decided to do everything they can to prevent T1DM. This tendency to try some means of T1DM prevention has to be taken into account in T1DM prediction and prevention trials.

High anxiety scores were linked with existing life stresses rather than with the information of the infant's T1DM risk per se. Anxiety was also associated with catastrophizing thoughts of the infant's T1DM risk and emotion-focused coping strategies. According to the stress theory of Lazarus,[9-12] the outcome of the evaluative first phase of coping, the appraisal phase, makes the person respond to stress with certain coping strategies and also affects the emotions evoked in that situation. Individuals who thought that the new situation was a catastrophe mainly used emotion-focused coping strategies and were prone to high anxiety scores. Because the anxiety levels of the parents, including symptoms of postpartum depression, remain unknown from the time before they learned about the child's risk, the possibility exists that parents who were more anxious beforehand were more prone to find the situation catastrophic, leading often to passive coping strategies.

A brief anxiety assessment when a pediatrician or a nurse meets with the parents of a child with increased disease risk is likely to help identify those most in need of assistance in coping with the risk information. Cognitive behavioral therapy has also shown long-term promise in such circumstances.[25-27] The different ways mothers and fathers react should also be remembered, and fathers should probably be encouraged to accompany mothers to the appointments.

Although we think that the key findings of this study are generalizable, some limitations may exist. Among others, the participating families may not entirely represent the general population, although the number of families recruited was reasonably large and the enrollment rate was excellent. The participating families were all from Finland, with a closely similar cultural background, living circumstances, and features of mentality, which differ from those in other countries. Finally, the T1DM incidence is markedly higher in Finland than in other countries, suggesting that the disease may be better known in Finland than elsewhere. Because screening for genetic T1DM risk has recently been initiated in many countries, we should soon know whether the findings of this study are valid in other populations as well.

In conclusion, the results of this study suggest that the infant's genetic T1DM risk information does not lead to differences in anxiety levels between parents of high- and low-risk infants. However, reactions such as worrying and depressive feelings do occur, and they have to be assessed when the long-term impact of screening on the families is evaluated. As the at-risk children in this study grow older, it also becomes possible to analyze the children's own views and feelings about having been screened as a newborn. The general population also needs to be informed about the nature of screening of genetic risk for multifactorial diseases to prevent unnecessary labeling of individuals at risk and to decrease information-induced unnecessary worries in the family.

**Accepted for Publication:** July 4, 2006.

**Correspondence:** Olli Simell, MD, PhD, Department of Pediatrics, University of Turku, Kiinamyllynkatu 4-8, FI-20520 Turku, Finland (olli.simell@utu.fi).

**Author Contributions:** *Study concept and design:* Simonen, Korhonen, T. Simell, Keskinen, Knip, and O. Simell. *Acquisition of data:* Simonen, Korhonen, T. Simell,

Keskinen, Ilonen, and O. Simell. *Analysis and interpretation of data:* Simonen. *Drafting of the manuscript:* Simonen, Korhonen, Ilonen, and O. Simell. *Critical revision of the manuscript for important intellectual content:* Korhonen, T. Simell, Keskinen, Kärkkäinen, Knip, and O. Simell. *Statistical analysis:* Simonen. *Obtained funding:* Simonen, T. Simell, Knip, Ilonen, and O. Simell. *Administrative, technical, and material support:* Korhonen, T. Simell, Keskinen, Knip, Ilonen, and O. Simell. *Study supervision:* Korhonen and O. Simell.

**Financial Disclosure:** None reported.

**Funding/Support:** This study was supported in part by grants from the Signe and Ane Gyllenberg Foundation, the Oskar Öflund Foundation, the Finnish Cultural Foundation's Satakunta Fund, Special Federal Funds for Health Care Research of Turku University Central Hospital, and grant 4-1999-731 from the Juvenile Diabetes Research Foundation International (Dr O. Simell).

**Acknowledgment:** We thank all the families in the study and the entire Type 1 Diabetes Prediction and Prevention project study group.

## REFERENCES

1. Johnson SB, Riley WJ, Hansen CA, Nurick MA. Psychological impact of islet-cell antibody screening: preliminary results. *Diabetes Care.* 1990;13:93-97.
2. Bennett Johnson S, Tercyak KP Jr. Psychological impact of islet cell antibody screening for IDDM on children, adults, and their family members. *Diabetes Care.* 1995;18:1370-1372.
3. Hahl J, Simell T, Ilonen J, Knip M, Simell O. Costs of predicting IDDM. *Diabetologia.* 1998;41:79-85.
4. Kupila A, Muona P, Simell T, et al. Feasibility of genetic and immunological prediction of type I diabetes in a population-based birth cohort. *Diabetologia.* 2001;44:290-297.
5. Kukko M, Kimpimäki T, Korhonen S, et al. Dynamics of diabetes-associated autoantibodies in young children with human leukocyte antigen–conferred risk of type 1 diabetes recruited from the general population. *J Clin Endocrinol Metab.* 2005;90:2712-2717.
6. Holmes TH, Rahe RH. The Social Readjustment Rating Scale. *J Psychosom Res.* 1967;11:213-218.
7. Spielberger C, Gorsuch RL, Lushene R. *Manual for the State-Trait Anxiety Inventory.* Palo Alto, Calif: Consulting Psychologists Press; 1970.
8. Knight RG, Waal-Manning HJ, Spears GF. Some norms and reliability data for the State-Trait Anxiety Inventory and the Zung Self-Rating Depression Scale. *Br J Clin Psychol.* 1983;22:245-249.
9. Lazarus RS. *Patterns of Adjustment.* New York, NY: McGraw-Hill; 1976.
10. Folkman S, Lazarus RS, Dunkel-Schetter C, DeLongis A, Gruen RJ. Dynamics of a stressful encounter: cognitive appraisal, coping, and encounter outcomes. *J Pers Soc Psychol.* 1986;50:992-1003.
11. Lazarus RS. From psychological stress to the emotions: a history of changing outlooks. *Annu Rev Psychol.* 1993;44:1-21.
12. Lazarus RS, Folkman S. *Stress, Appraisal and Coping.* New York, NY: Springer Publishing Co; 1984.
13. Folkman S, Lazarus RS. An analysis of coping in a middle-aged community sample. *J Health Soc Behav.* 1980;21:219-239.
14. Mennie ME, Gilfillan A, Compton M, et al. Prenatal screening for cystic fibrosis. *Lancet.* 1992;340:214-216.
15. Watson EK, Myall ES, Lamb J, Chapple J, Williamson R. Psychological and social consequences of community carriers screening programme for cystic fibrosis. *Lancet.* 1992;340:217-220.
16. Clow CL, Scriver CR. Knowledge about and attitudes toward genetic screening among high-school students: the Tay-Sachs experience. *Pediatrics.* 1977;59:86-90.
17. Blomhoff S, Malt U, Weisaeth L. Psychosocial aspects in presymptomatic testing for genetic diseases: experiences after 2 years of counseling in Huntington disease [in Norwegian]. *Tidsskr Nor Laegeforen.* 1995;115:27-29.
18. McNeil TF, Thelin T, Aspegren-Jansson E, Sveger T. Identifying children at high somatic risk: possible long-term effects on parental conceptualizations of the children's personality and behavior. *Acta Psychiatr Scand.* 1985;72:498-504.
19. Thelin T, McNeil TF, Aspegren-Jansson E, Sveger T. Psychological consequences of neonatal screening for $\alpha$1-antitrypsin deficiency: parental reactions to the first news of their infants' deficiency. *Acta Paediatr Scand.* 1985;74:787-793.
20. Thelin T, McNeil TF, Aspegren-Jansson E, Sveger T. Psychological consequences of neonatal screening for $\alpha$1-antitrypsin deficiency (ATD): parental attitudes toward "ATD-check-ups" and parental recommendations regarding future screening. *Acta Paediatr Scand.* 1985;74:841-847.
21. Thelin T, McNeil TF, Aspegren-Jansson E, Sveger T. Identifying children at high somatic risk: parents' long-term emotional adjustment to their children's $\alpha$1-antitrypsin deficiency. *Acta Psychiatr Scand.* 1985;72:323-330.
22. Posa T. *Ultrasono-graphically Detected Fetal Defect as a Parental Crisis* [PhD thesis]. Oulu, Finland: Oulu University; 1998.
23. Hietala M, Hakonen A, Aro AR, Niemelä P, Peltonen L, Aula P. Attitudes toward genetic testing among the general population and relatives of patients with severe genetic disease: a survey from Finland. *Am J Hum Genet.* 1995;56:1493-1500.
24. Marteau TM, Johnston M. Determinants of beliefs about illness: a study of parents of children with diabetes, asthma, epilepsy, and no chronic illness. *J Psychosom Res.* 1986;30:673-683.
25. Abramowitz JS, Schwartz SA, Moore KM, Luenzmann KR. Obsessive-compulsive symptoms in pregnancy and the puerperium: a review of the literature. *J Anxiety Disord.* 2003;17:461-478.
26. Wenzel A, Haugen EN, Jackson LC, Brendle JR. Anxiety symptoms and disorders at eight weeks postpartum. *J Anxiety Disord.* 2005;19:295-311.
27. Otto MW, Smits JA, Reese HE. Cognitive-behavioral therapy for the treatment of anxiety disorders. *J Clin Psychiatry.* 2004;65(suppl 5):34-41.

> "I was 1 of 6 children, and when you travel in a pack like that, your early memories of your father all involve discipline. For the longest time, my dad was simply a black-haired arm reaching into the backseat of the car to grab one of us."
>
> —Conan O'Brien discussing fatherhood

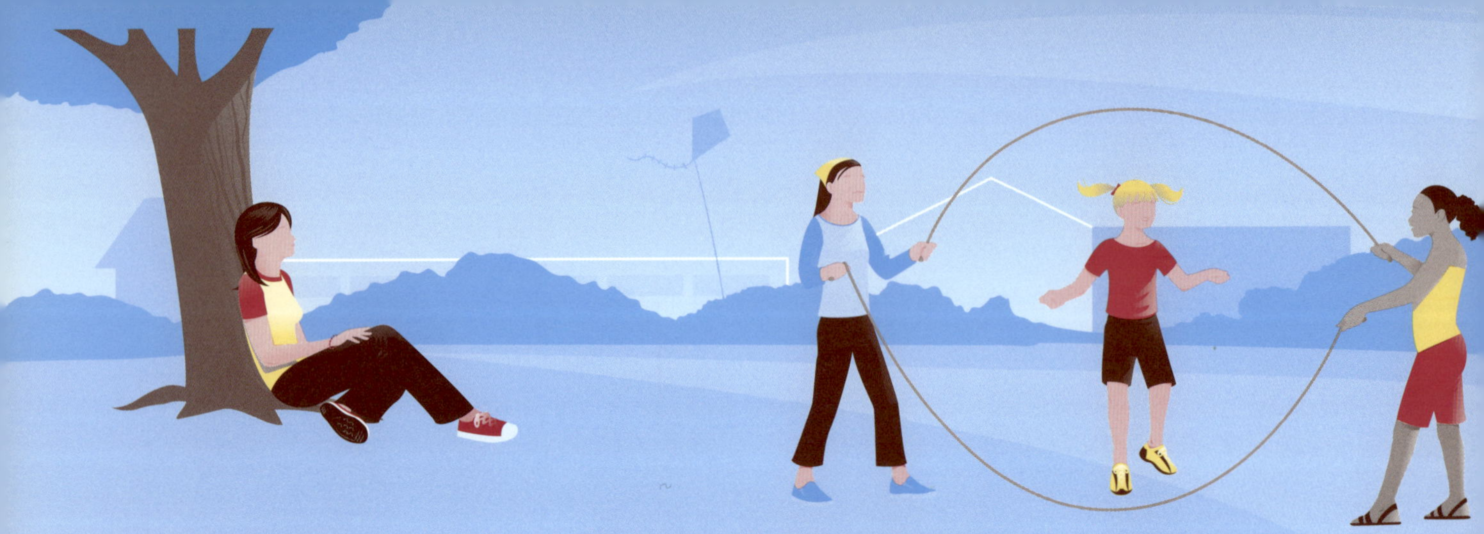

# Introducing GARDASIL—helping you

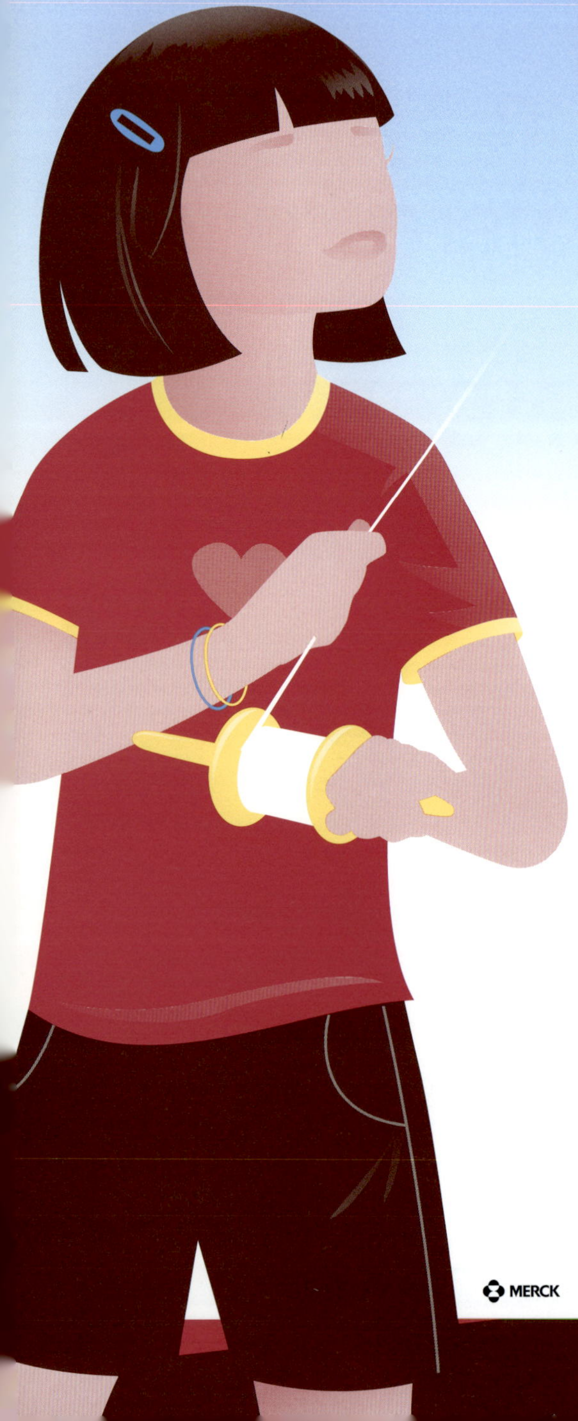

- **GARDASIL is a vaccine indicated in girls and women 9 to 26 years of age for the prevention of cervical cancer, precancerous or dysplastic lesions, and genital warts caused by human papillomavirus (HPV) Types 6, 11, 16, and 18.**
- **A complete vaccination regimen of GARDASIL consists of a 3-dose schedule.**

## Select safety information

GARDASIL is contraindicated in individuals who are hypersensitive to the active substances or to any of the excipients of the vaccine.

GARDASIL does not substitute for routine cervical cancer screening, and women who receive GARDASIL should continue to undergo screening per standard of care.

Vaccination with GARDASIL may not result in protection in all vaccine recipients.

GARDASIL is not intended to be used for treatment of active genital warts; cervical cancer; cervical intraepithelial neoplasia, vulvar intraepithelial neoplasia, or vaginal intraepithelial neoplasia.

To place an order, call **1-800-MERCK-RX,** or visit **www.MerckVaccines.com.**

MERCK

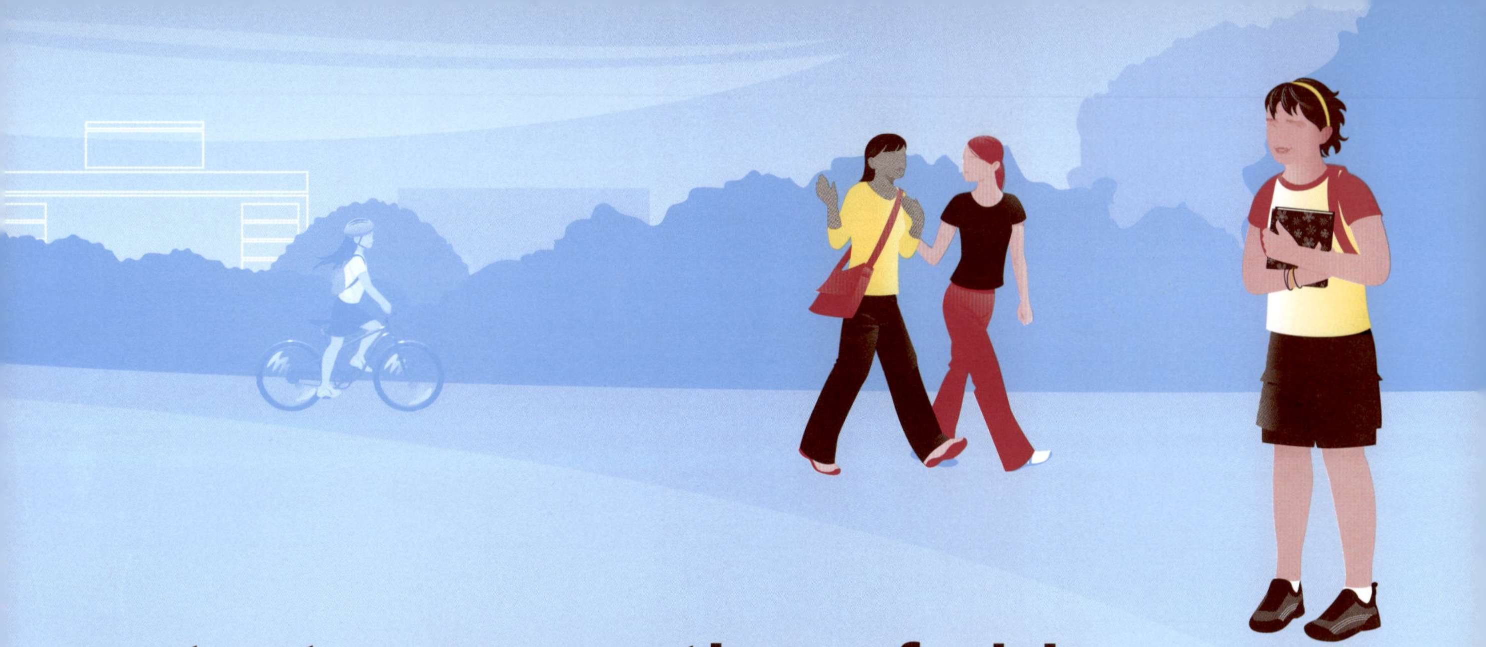

# GARDASIL®

## [Quadrivalent Human Papillomavirus (Types 6,11,16,18) Recombinant Vaccine]



**BRIEF SUMMARY OF PRESCRIBING INFORMATION**

**CONTRAINDICATIONS:** Hypersensitivity to the active substances or to any of the excipients of the vaccine.

Individuals who develop symptoms indicative of hypersensitivity after receiving a dose of GARDASIL should not receive further doses of GARDASIL.

**PRECAUTIONS:** *General:* As for any vaccine, vaccination with GARDASIL may not result in protection in all vaccine recipients.

This vaccine is not intended to be used for treatment of active genital warts; cervical cancer; cervical intraepithelial neoplasia (CIN), vulvar intraepithelial neoplasia (VIN), or vaginal intraepithelial neoplasia (VaIN).

This vaccine will not protect against diseases that are not caused by human papillomavirus (HPV).

GARDASIL has not been shown to protect against diseases due to non-vaccine HPV types.

As with all injectable vaccines, appropriate medical treatment should always be readily available in case of rare anaphylactic reactions following the administration of the vaccine.

The decision to administer or delay vaccination because of a current or recent febrile illness depends largely on the severity of the symptoms and their etiology. Low-grade fever itself and mild upper respiratory infection are not generally contraindications to vaccination.

Individuals with impaired immune responsiveness, whether due to the use of immunosuppressive therapy, a genetic defect, Human Immunodeficiency Virus (HIV) infection, or other causes, may have reduced antibody response to active immunization (see PRECAUTIONS, ***Drug Interactions***).

As with other intramuscular injections, GARDASIL should not be given to individuals with bleeding disorders such as hemophilia or thrombocytopenia, or to persons on anticoagulant therapy unless the potential benefits clearly outweigh the risk of administration. If the decision is made to administer GARDASIL to such persons, it should be given with steps to avoid the risk of hematoma following the injection.

*Information for the Patient, Parent, or Guardian:* The health care provider should inform the patient, parent, or guardian that vaccination does not substitute for routine cervical cancer screening. Women who receive GARDASIL should continue to undergo cervical cancer screening per standard of care.

The health care provider should provide the vaccine information required to be given with each vaccination to the patient, parent, or guardian.

The health care provider should inform the patient, parent, or guardian of the benefits and risks associated with vaccination. For risks associated with vaccination, see PRECAUTIONS and ADVERSE REACTIONS.

GARDASIL is not recommended for use in pregnant women.

The health care provider should inform the patient, parent, or guardian of the importance of completing the immunization series unless contraindicated.

Patients, parents, or guardians should be instructed to report any adverse reactions to their health care provider.

***Drug Interactions:*** *Use with Other Vaccines:* Results from clinical studies indicate that GARDASIL may be administered concomitantly (at a separate injection site) with hepatitis B vaccine (recombinant) (see CLINICAL PHARMACOLOGY, *Studies with Other Vaccines*). Co-administration of GARDASIL with other vaccines has not been studied.

*Use with Hormonal Contraceptives:* In clinical studies, 13,293 subjects (vaccine = 6644; placebo = 6649) who had post-Month 7 follow-up used hormonal contraceptives for a total of 17,597 person-years (65.1% of the total follow-up time in the study for these subjects). Use of hormonal contraceptives or lack of use of hormonal contraceptives among study participants did not alter vaccine efficacy in the per-protocol efficacy (PPE) population.

*Use with Systemic Immunosuppressive Medications:* Immunosuppressive therapies, including irradiation, antimetabolites, alkylating agents, cytotoxic drugs, and corticosteroids (used in greater than physiologic doses), may reduce the immune responses to vaccines (see PRECAUTIONS, ***General***).

*Carcinogenesis, Mutagenesis, Impairment of Fertility:* GARDASIL has not been evaluated for the potential to cause carcinogenicity or genotoxicity.

GARDASIL administered to female rats at a dose of 120 mcg total protein, which corresponds to approximately 300-fold excess relative to the projected human dose, had no effects on mating performance, fertility, or embryonic/fetal survival.

*Pregnancy: Pregnancy Category B:* Reproduction studies have been performed in female rats at doses up to 300 times the human dose (on a mg/kg basis) and have revealed no evidence of impaired female fertility or harm to the fetus due to GARDASIL. However, it is not known whether GARDASIL can cause fetal harm when administered to a pregnant woman or if it can affect reproductive capacity. GARDASIL should be given to a pregnant woman only if clearly needed. An evaluation of the effect of GARDASIL on embryo-fetal, pre- and postweaning development was conducted using rats. One group of rats was administered GARDASIL twice prior to gestation, during the period of organogenesis (gestation day 6) and on lactation day 7. A second group of pregnant rats was administered GARDASIL during the period of organogenesis (gestation day 6) and on lactation day 7 only. GARDASIL was administered at 0.5 mL/rat/occasion (approximately 300-fold excess relative to the projected human dose on a mg/kg basis) by intramuscular injection. No adverse effects on mating, fertility, pregnancy, parturition, lactation, embryo-fetal or pre- and postweaning development were observed. There were no vaccine-related fetal malformations or other evidence of teratogenesis noted in this study. In addition, there were no treatment-related effects on developmental signs, behavior, reproductive performance, or fertility of the offspring. The effect of GARDASIL on male fertility has not been studied.

In clinical studies, women underwent urine pregnancy testing prior to administration of each dose of GARDASIL. Women who were found to be pregnant before completion of a 3-dose regimen of GARDASIL were instructed to defer completion of their vaccination regimen until resolution of the pregnancy.

During clinical trials, 2266 women (vaccine = 1115 vs. placebo = 1151) reported at least 1 pregnancy each. Overall, the proportions of pregnancies with an adverse outcome were comparable in subjects who received GARDASIL and subjects who received placebo. Overall, 40 and 41 subjects in the group that received GARDASIL or placebo, respectively (3.6% and 3.6% of all subjects who reported a pregnancy in the respective vaccination groups), experienced a serious adverse experience during pregnancy. The most common events reported were conditions that can result in Caesarean section (e.g., failure of labor, malpresentation, cephalopelvic disproportion), premature onset of labor (e.g., threatened abortions, premature rupture of membranes), and pregnancy-related medical problems (e.g., pre-eclampsia, hyperemesis). The proportions of pregnant subjects who experienced such events were comparable between the vaccination groups.

There were 15 cases of congenital anomaly in pregnancies that occurred in subjects who received GARDASIL and 16 cases of congenital anomaly in pregnancies that occurred in subjects who received placebo.

Further sub-analyses were conducted to evaluate pregnancies with estimated onset within 30 days or more than 30 days from administration of a dose of GARDASIL or placebo. For pregnancies with estimated onset within 30 days of vaccination, 5 cases of congenital anomaly were observed in the group that received GARDASIL compared to 0 cases of congenital anomaly in the group that received placebo. The congenital anomalies seen in pregnancies with estimated onset within 30 days of vaccination included pyloric stenosis, congenital megacolon, congenital hydronephrosis, hip dysplasia and club foot. Conversely, in pregnancies with onset more than 30 days following vaccination, 10 cases of congenital anomaly were observed in the group that received GARDASIL compared with 16 cases of congenital anomaly in the group that received placebo. The types of anomalies observed were consistent (regardless of when pregnancy occurred in relation to vaccination) with those generally observed in pregnancies in women aged 16 to 26 years.

*Pregnancy Registry for GARDASIL:* Merck & Co., Inc. maintains a Pregnancy Registry to monitor fetal outcomes of pregnant women exposed to GARDASIL. Patients and health care providers are encouraged to report any exposure to GARDASIL during pregnancy by calling (800) 986-8999.

*Lactation:* It is not known whether vaccine antigens or antibodies induced by the vaccine are excreted in human milk.

Because many drugs are excreted in human milk, caution should be exercised when GARDASIL is administered to a nursing woman.

A total of 995 nursing mothers (vaccine = 500, placebo = 495) were given GARDASIL or placebo during the vaccination period of the clinical trials. Geometric mean titers (GMTs) in nursing and non-nursing mothers were as follows:

The GMTs in nursing mothers were 595.9 (95% CI: 522.5, 679.5) for anti-HPV 6, 864.3 (95% CI: 754.0, 990.8) for anti-HPV 11, 3056.9 (95% CI: 2594.4, 3601.8) for anti-HPV 16, and 527.2 (95% CI: 450.9, 616.5) for anti-HPV 18. The GMTs for women who did not nurse during vaccine administration were 540.1 (95% CI: 523.5, 557.2) for anti-HPV 6, 746.3 (95% CI: 720.4, 773.3) for anti-HPV 11, 2290.8 (95% CI: 2180.7, 2406.3) for anti-HPV 16, and 456.0 (95% CI: 438.4, 474.3) for anti-HPV 18.

Overall, 17 and 9 infants of subjects who received GARDASIL or placebo, respectively (representing 3.4% and 1.8% of the total number of subjects who were breast-feeding during the period in which they received GARDASIL or placebo, respectively), experienced a serious adverse experience. None was judged by the investigator to be vaccine related.

In clinical studies, a higher number of breast-feeding infants (n = 6) whose mothers received GARDASIL had acute respiratory illnesses within 30 days post-vaccination of the mother as compared to infants (n = 2) whose mothers received placebo. In these studies, the rates of other adverse experiences in the mother and the nursing infant were comparable between vaccination groups.

*Pediatric Use:* The safety and efficacy of GARDASIL have not been evaluated in children younger than 9 years.

*Geriatric Use:* The safety and efficacy of GARDASIL have not been evaluated in adults above the age of 26 years.

**ADVERSE REACTIONS:** In 5 clinical trials (4 placebo-controlled), subjects were administered GARDASIL or placebo on the day of enrollment, and approximately 2 and 6 months thereafter. Few subjects (0.1%) discontinued due to adverse experiences. In all except 1 of the clinical trials, safety was evaluated using vaccination report card (VRC)-aided surveillance for 14 days after each injection of GARDASIL or placebo. The subjects who were monitored using VRC-aided surveillance included 5088 girls and women 9 through 26 years of age at enrollment who received GARDASIL and 3790 girls and women who received placebo.

*Common Adverse Experiences: Vaccine-related Common Adverse Experiences:* The vaccine-related adverse experiences that were observed among female recipients of GARDASIL at a frequency of at least 1.0% and also at a greater frequency than that observed among placebo recipients are shown in Table 1.

**Table 1. Vaccine-related Injection-site and Systemic Adverse Experiences***

| Adverse Experience (1 to 5 Days Postvaccination) | GARDASIL (N = 5088) % | Aluminum-Containing Placebo (N = 3470) % | Saline Placebo (N = 320) % |
|---|---|---|---|
| *Injection Site* | | | |
| Pain | 83.9 | 75.4 | 48.6 |
| Swelling | 25.4 | 15.8 | 7.3 |
| Erythema | 24.6 | 18.4 | 12.1 |
| Pruritus | 3.1 | 2.8 | 0.6 |

| Adverse Experience (1 to 15 Days Postvaccination) | GARDASIL (N = 5088) % | Placebo (N = 3790) % |
|---|---|---|
| *Systemic* | | |
| Fever | 10.3 | 8.6 |

*The vaccine-related adverse experiences that were observed among recipients of GARDASIL were at a frequency of at least 1.0% and also at a greater frequency than that observed among placebo recipients.

*All-cause Common Systemic Adverse Experiences:* All-cause systemic adverse experiences for female subjects reported 1 to 15 days postvaccination and observed at a frequency of ≥1% with incidence in the GARDASIL group (N = 5088) ≥ that of the placebo group (N = 3790), respectively, were: pyrexia (13.0% vs. 11.2%), nausea (6.7% vs. 6.6%), nasopharyngitis (6.4% vs. 6.4%), dizziness (4.0% vs. 3.7%), diarrhea (3.6% vs. 3.5%), vomiting (2.4% vs. 1.9%), myalgia (2.0% vs. 2.0%), cough (2.0% vs. 1.5%), toothache (1.5% vs. 1.4%), upper respiratory tract infection (1.5% vs. 1.5%), malaise (1.4% vs. 1.2%), arthralgia (1.2% vs. 0.9%), insomnia (1.2% vs. 0.9%), and nasal congestion (1.1% vs. 0.9%).

*Evaluation of Injection-site Adverse Experiences by Dose:* An analysis of injection-site adverse experiences in female subjects by dose is shown in Table 2. Overall, 94.3% of subjects who received GARDASIL judged their injection-site adverse experience to be mild or moderate in intensity.

**Table 2. Postdose Evaluation of Injection-site Adverse Experiences**

| | Vaccine (% occurrence) | | | |
|---|---|---|---|---|
| **Adverse Experience** | Post-dose 1 | Post-dose 2 | Post-dose 3 | Post Any Dose |
| **Pain** | 63.4 | 60.7 | 62.7 | 83.9 |
| Mild/Moderate | 62.5 | 59.7 | 61.2 | 81.1 |
| Severe | 0.9 | 1.0 | 1.5 | 2.8 |
| **Swelling*** | 10.2 | 12.8 | 15.1 | 25.4 |
| Mild/Moderate | 9.6 | 11.9 | 14.3 | 23.3 |
| Severe | 0.6 | 0.8 | 0.8 | 2.0 |
| **Erythema*** | 9.2 | 12.1 | 14.7 | 24.7 |
| Mild/Moderate | 9.0 | 11.7 | 14.3 | 23.7 |
| Severe | 0.2 | 0.3 | 0.4 | 0.9 |

*Intensity of swelling and erythema was measured by size (inches): Mild = 0 to ≤1; Moderate = >1 to ≤2; Severe = >2.

| | Aluminum-Containing Placebo (% occurrence) | | | | Saline Placebo (% occurrence) | | | |
|---|---|---|---|---|---|---|---|---|
| **Adverse Experience** | Post-dose 1 | Post-dose 2 | Post-dose 3 | Post Any Dose | Post-dose 1 | Post-dose 2 | Post-dose 3 | Post Any Dose |
| **Pain** | 57.0 | 47.8 | 49.5 | 75.4 | 33.7 | 20.3 | 27.3 | 48.6 |
| Mild/Moderate | 56.6 | 47.3 | 48.9 | 74.1 | 33.3 | 20.3 | 27.0 | 48.0 |
| Severe | 0.4 | 0.5 | 0.6 | 1.3 | 0.3 | 0.0 | 0.3 | 0.6 |
| **Swelling*** | 8.2 | 7.5 | 7.6 | 15.8 | 4.4 | 3.0 | 3.3 | 7.3 |
| Mild/Moderate | 8.0 | 7.2 | 7.3 | 15.2 | 4.4 | 3.0 | 3.3 | 7.3 |
| Severe | 0.2 | 0.3 | 0.2 | 0.6 | 0.0 | 0.0 | 0.0 | 0.0 |
| **Erythema*** | 9.8 | 8.4 | 8.9 | 18.4 | 7.3 | 5.3 | 5.7 | 12.1 |
| Mild/Moderate | 9.5 | 8.3 | 8.8 | 18.0 | 7.3 | 5.3 | 5.7 | 12.1 |
| Severe | 0.3 | 0.1 | 0.1 | 0.4 | 0.0 | 0.0 | 0.0 | 0.0 |

*Evaluation of Fever by Dose:* An analysis of fever in girls and women by dose is shown in Table 3.

**Table 3. Postdose Evaluation of Fever**

| | Vaccine (% occurrence) | | | Placebo (% occurrence) | | |
|---|---|---|---|---|---|---|
| **Temperature (°F)** | Post-dose 1 | Post-dose 2 | Post-dose 3 | Post-dose 1 | Post-dose 2 | Post-dose 3 |
| ≥100 to <102 | 3.7 | 4.1 | 4.4 | 3.1 | 3.8 | 3.6 |
| ≥102 | 0.3 | 0.5 | 0.5 | 0.3 | 0.4 | 0.6 |

*Serious Adverse Experiences:* A total of 102 subjects out of 21,464 total subjects (9- to 26-year-old girls and women and 9- to 15-year-old boys) who received both GARDASIL and placebo reported a serious adverse experience on Day 1-15 following any vaccination visit during the clinical trials for GARDASIL. The most frequently reported serious adverse experiences regardless of causality for GARDASIL compared to placebo, respectively, were: headache (0.03% vs. 0.02%), gastroenteritis (0.03% vs. 0.01%), appendicitis (0.02% vs. 0.01%), and pelvic inflammatory disease (0.02% vs. 0.01%).

One case of bronchospasm and 2 cases of asthma were reported as serious adverse experiences that occurred during Day 1-15 of any vaccination visit.

*Deaths:* Across the clinical studies, 17 deaths were reported in 21,464 male and female subjects. The events reported were consistent with events expected in healthy adolescent and adult populations. The most common cause of death was motor vehicle accident (4 subjects who received GARDASIL and 3 placebo subjects), followed by overdose/suicide (1 subject who received GARDASIL and 2 subjects who received placebo), and pulmonary embolus/deep vein thrombosis (1 subject who received GARDASIL and 1 placebo subject). In addition, there were 2 cases of sepsis, 1 case of pancreatic cancer, and 1 case of arrhythmia in the group that received GARDASIL, and 1 case of asphyxia in the placebo group.

*Systemic Autoimmune Disorders:* In the clinical studies, subjects were evaluated for new medical conditions that occurred over the course of up to 4 years of follow up. The number of subjects who received both GARDASIL and placebo and developed a new medical condition potentially indicative of a systemic immune disorder is shown in Table 4.

**Table 4. Summary of Subjects Who Reported an Incident Condition Potentially Indicative of Systemic Autoimmune Disorder After Enrollment in Clinical Trials of GARDASIL**

| Potential Autoimmune Disorder | GARDASIL (N = 11,813) | Placebo (N = 9701) |
|---|---|---|
| Specific Terms | 3 (0.025%) | 1 (0.010%) |
| Juvenile arthritis | 1 | 0 |
| Rheumatoid arthritis | 2 | 0 |
| Systemic lupus erythematosus | 0 | 1 |
| Other Terms | 6 (0.051%) | 2 (0.021%) |
| Arthritis | 5 | 2 |
| Reactive Arthritis | 1 | 0 |

N = Number of subjects enrolled

*Safety in Concomitant Use with Other Vaccines:* The safety of GARDASIL when administered concomitantly with hepatitis B vaccine (recombinant) was evaluated in a placebo-controlled study. There were no statistically significant higher rates in systemic or injection-site adverse experiences among subjects who received concomitant vaccination compared with those who received GARDASIL or hepatitis B vaccine alone.

*Reporting of Adverse Events:* The US Department of Health and Human Services has established a Vaccine Adverse Event Reporting System (VAERS) to accept all reports of suspected adverse events after the administration of any vaccine, including but not limited to the reporting of events required by the National Childhood Vaccine Injury Act of 1986. For information or a copy of the vaccine reporting form, call the VAERS toll-free number at 1-800-822-7967 or report on line to www.vaers.hhs.gov.

For more detailed information, please read the Prescribing Information.
GARDASIL is a registered trademark of Merck & Co., Inc.

MERCK



20650343(2)(300)-GRD

ARTICLE

# The Association Between Parents' Past Agricultural Injuries and Their Children's Risk of Injury

## *Analyses From the Regional Rural Injury Study–II*

*Kathleen Ferguson Carlson, PhD; Deborah Langner, MS; Bruce H. Alexander, PhD; James G. Gurney, PhD; Susan G. Gerberich, PhD; Andrew D. Ryan, MS; Colleen M. Renier, BS; Steven J. Mongin, MS*

**Objective:** To examine associations between parents' and children's agricultural injuries in a cohort of farming and ranching households.

**Design:** Analyses from a population-based, nested case-control study.

**Setting:** The 1999 Regional Rural Injury Study–II, involving a cohort of 3765 agricultural households. Demographic, injury, and exposure data were collected for household members for 1 year.

**Participants:** A total of 203 injured children (cases) and 755 randomly selected control children were identified for the study.

**Main Exposure:** Children's risk of injury was estimated in reference to individual and combined parental injury experience. Two periods were evaluated, separately and in combination.

**Main Outcome Measures:** Odds ratios (ORs) and 95% confidence intervals (CIs) were calculated by using logistic regression; directed acyclic graphs guided selection of potential confounders.

**Results:** When controlling for potential confounders, children whose fathers were injured before the study year had twice the risk of injury of those whose fathers were not injured (OR, 2.1; 95% CI, 1.5-3.0). Children had increased risk of injury if their mothers were injured before the study (OR, 2.5; 95% CI, 1.7-3.8) or during the study (OR, 2.0; 95% CI, 0.9-4.2). Children whose parents both reported agricultural injuries before the study had a 4-fold increase in injury risk over those with neither parent injured (OR, 4.2; 95% CI, 2.6-6.9).

**Conclusions:** Positive associations between parents' and children's injuries were observed, with a potential additive effect if both parents were injured. These results indicate a need for further research into the social and/or physical environments driving these associations so that appropriate interventions for pediatric injury can be determined.

*Arch Pediatr Adolesc Med. 2006;160:1137-1142*

**Author Affiliations:** Regional Injury Prevention Research Center, Division of Environmental Health Sciences, School of Public Health, University of Minnesota, Minneapolis (Drs Carlson, Alexander, and Gerberich; Ms Langner; and Messrs Ryan and Mongin); Child Health Evaluation and Research Unit, Department of Pediatrics, University of Michigan, Ann Arbor (Dr Gurney); and Division of Education and Research, St Mary's Duluth Clinic Health System, Duluth, Minn (Ms Renier).

INJURY, THE LEADING CAUSE OF death among children,[1] results in substantial costs in terms of disability, rehabilitation, and lost productivity.[2] Children working on farming and ranching operations are at a particularly high risk of fatal and nonfatal injury.[3,4] Injury-related mortality and morbidity rates for the agricultural trade are among the highest of all US industries.[5,6] For farming and ranching families, the proximity between the household and the operation makes hazardous exposures nearly unavoidable, even for children not actively engaged in operation-related tasks.[7] In response to this issue, a national initiative for the reduction of agricultural injury among children was established.[8]

*For editorial comment see page 1180*

Injuries are not distributed randomly among populations at risk. Positive associations between one's prior injuries and risk of subsequent injury have been observed in studies of sports,[9,10] occupational,[11] and agricultural[12,13] injuries and for medically attended injuries among adults and children.[14-16] Risk also appears to be associated within families; sibling injury was shown to be associated with at least a short-term increase in children's risk of injury.[17,18] Individuals' past injuries may increase their vulnerability to future injuries,[12] and the association between sibling injuries could be related to periods of heightened familial stress after initial injuries.[17,18] Another likely explanation is that certain environments are inherently more hazardous than others and continue to be so even after an injury occurs.

An area that remains to be examined is the association between parents' and children's injuries. A positive association might be expected, given the theories that increased familial stress or sustained hazardous environments or both lead to multiple injuries within households. However, parents' injuries might lead to implementation of preventive measures for their children. Improved understanding of the effect of parents' injury experiences on children's risk may help practitioners identify high-risk populations and exposures as well as effective interventions. The objective of this study was to determine whether an association exists between parents' agricultural injuries and children's risk of injury among farm and ranch households.

## METHODS

### STUDY DESIGN

This study was based on data from the 1999 Regional Rural Injury Study–II,[19] a prospective, population-based cohort study of agricultural households in Minnesota, North Dakota, South Dakota, Nebraska, and Wisconsin. We conducted a nested case-control study of agricultural injuries involving children younger than 20 years. The University of Minnesota Institutional Review Board Human Subjects Committee approved the protocol for this study.

### STUDY POPULATION

A random sample of 16 000 agricultural operations was generated (n=3200 from each state) by using the US Department of Agriculture's National Agricultural Statistics Service Master ListFrame of Farming Operations.[20] Eligible operations had to have produced $1000 or more of agricultural goods during 1998 and/or have land enrolled in a Conservation Reserve Program, and they had to be actively engaged in farming or ranching as of January 1, 1999. In addition, the operator's household had to be associated with the farm or ranch and include children younger than 20 years in residence as of January 1, 1999.

Of the 16 000 sampled operations, 12 677 were screened successfully, of which 8288 (51.8%) were found ineligible. Of the 4402 (27.5%) households identified as eligible, 3765 (85.5%) participated in the first 6-month interview, and 3677 (83.5%) participated in both full interviews. Demographic and injury data were collected for 16 538 household members, including 8488 children. An agricultural injury was defined as any event resulting from activities or objects associated with the family agricultural operation leading to restriction of normal activities for 4 hours or more, loss of consciousness or awareness or amnesia for any length of time, and/or treatment by a health professional.

### DATA COLLECTION

Subsequent to introductory mailings, computer-assisted telephone interviews were conducted to obtain informed consent, establish eligibility, and enroll households. As an incentive to participate, all sampled operations were eligible for a drawing that provided at least a 1 in 32 probability of receiving a $100 US savings bond.

Participating households received packets containing study details and materials to facilitate collection of information during each of 2 full-length interviews. The interviews occurred in July 1999 and January 2000, and information was collected about each 6-month recall period of 1999 (January through June and July through December). Nonrespondents for whom eligibility status was not established were sent a 1-page survey to ascertain eligibility of the household. Copies of the materials used, including interview instruments, are available on a Web site.[21]

The female head of household was the primary respondent for demographic and injury data, whereas the male head of household was preferred for operation exposure information. With parents' permission, children 12 years and older were requested to be their own respondents. The proxy for those who refused, and children younger than 12 years, was the female head of household.

### IDENTIFICATION OF CASES AND CONTROLS

Cases were all agricultural injury events sustained by children younger than 20 years on their own operation during the reporting periods. The control population came from households randomly sampled to achieve a minimum ratio of 3 controls per case on the basis of injury rates from a previous study.[3] An incidence-density sampling scheme was used to sample from the agricultural injury-free person-time experience (months) of children younger than 20 years in residence on the operation. One child with at least 1 agricultural injury–free month was selected randomly from each control household. The exposure experience was collected for the month before the month of injury for cases and the month before an agricultural injury–free month for controls, sampled to reflect expected monthly incidence rates.[3] This method allowed cases to be sampled as controls for months in which they did not sustain an agricultural injury. The final population included 203 (91.0%) of 223 eligible case events and 755 (97.0%) of 778 sampled eligible controls.

### PARENTAL INJURY

Agricultural injury data also were collected for respondents identified as the children's mothers and fathers. Parents were asked whether they had incurred an agricultural injury before or during the study year. Use of the 6-month recall periods is key for validity of injury reporting;[22,23] in this study, this method also was expected to decrease the potential for exposure (parents' injuries) misclassification.

Children were categorized as having a father, a mother, or both parents injured any time before or during the study period. For the analyses to address the temporal nature of the study question, parents' injuries had to have occurred before the case injury month. For controls, parents' injuries had to have occurred before a randomly selected target month. In addition, each parent's injury experiences were combined to reflect their overall injury history through both periods.

### DATA ANALYSIS

Multivariable logistic regression was used to estimate risk of agricultural injury to children, subsequent to parental agricultural injury, while controlling for potentially confounding covariates.[24] To determine potential confounders, we used a causal model[21] to guide the design and use of directed acyclic graphs, according to the methods in Greenland et al[25] and Hernan et al.[26] These methods facilitated identification of covariates that may introduce bias if included in the statistical models and reduced potential of overfitting the models. For parent-related covariates, data specific to fathers or mothers were used for the respective analyses of fathers' and mothers' injuries. For analyses of combined parental injury history, mothers' data were included, assuming these factors have a greater effect on children's risk.

**Table 1. Characteristics of Case and Control Subjects Younger Than 20 Years: 1999 Regional Rural Injury Study–II**

| Characteristic | Cases (n = 203) No. (%) | Controls (n = 755) No. (%) |
| --- | --- | --- |
| Sex | | |
| Male | 136 (67.0) | 429 (56.8) |
| Female | 67 (33.0) | 326 (43.2) |
| Age, y | | |
| <5 | 13 (6.4) | 95 (12.6) |
| 5-9 | 33 (16.3) | 160 (21.2) |
| 10-14 | 88 (43.3) | 222 (29.4) |
| 15-19 | 69 (34.0) | 276 (36.6) |
| Missing/unknown/refused | 0 | 2 (0.3) |
| Type of agricultural operation requiring most work time | | |
| Beef cattle | 56 (27.6) | 178 (23.6) |
| Dairy cattle | 47 (23.2) | 97 (12.8) |
| Other animals | 25 (12.3) | 67 (8.9) |
| Field, forage, or specialty crops or Conservation Reserve Program | 71 (35.0) | 384 (50.9) |
| Nothing during month of inquiry, or missing/unknown/refused | 4 (2.0) | 29 (3.8) |
| Household hours worked per week on agricultural operation | | |
| ≤40 | 11 (5.4) | 100 (13.2) |
| 41-80 | 41 (20.2) | 242 (32.1) |
| 81-120 | 66 (32.5) | 205 (27.2) |
| 121-160 | 33 (16.3) | 124 (16.4) |
| >160 | 52 (25.6) | 84 (11.1) |
| No. of children in household | | |
| 1 | 34 (16.7) | 208 (27.5) |
| 2 | 73 (36.0) | 288 (38.1) |
| 3 | 50 (24.6) | 163 (21.6) |
| ≥4 | 46 (22.7) | 94 (12.5) |
| Unknown/missing/refused | 0 | 2 (0.3) |

Results were adjusted for within-household correlation by using generalized estimating equations.[27] To account partially for selection bias, we addressed nonresponse at the household level by weighting observed responses with inverse probabilities of response[28] on the basis of characteristics from the Master ListFrame (operation state, operation type, annual revenue by quintile). To account for unknown eligibility for nonrespondents, we estimated probability of eligibility for these same characteristics and used them to adjust weights.[29] Parents' injury status was unknown for 4% to 6% of children in each analysis; a separate exposure level was evaluated for these missing data in each model.

## RESULTS

Among the 203 cases and 755 controls, agricultural injuries before the study period were reported for 118 (58.1%) and 306 (40.5%) fathers and 63 (31.0%) and 112 (14.8%) mothers, respectively. During the study period, injuries were identified for 18 (8.9%) and 59 (7.8%) fathers and 15 (7.4%) and 29 (3.8%) mothers, respectively.

### PARTICIPANT CHARACTERISTICS

Case vs control children more often resided in households affiliated with dairy operations (23.2% and 12.8%); controls were more often associated with field, forage, or specialty crop operations or Conservation Reserve Programs (50.9% and 35.0%, respectively) (**Table 1**). Compared with control households, case households worked more hours per week on their operations: 25.6% vs 11.1% worked 160 hours or more. Nearly 23% of case households had 4 or more children in residence, compared with 12.7% of control households. Control households more often had only 1 child in residence (27.6% vs 16.8%). There were no differences between cases and controls in parents' age or educational status.

**Table 2. Risk of Children's Agricultural Injury According to Fathers' and Mothers' Injury Histories: 1999 Regional Rural Injury Study–II**

| Parent Injury Status | Cases (n = 203) No. (%) | Controls (n = 755) No. (%) | Multivariable Analyses Odds Ratio* (95% Confidence Interval) |
| --- | --- | --- | --- |
| Father's injury status† | | | |
| Injured before study | | | |
| Yes | 118 (58.1) | 306 (40.5) | 2.1 (1.5-3.0) |
| No | 74 (36.5) | 419 (55.5) | 1.0 |
| Missing | 11 (5.4) | 30 (4.0) | 1.3 (0.5-3.3) |
| Injured during study | | | |
| Yes | 18 (8.9) | 59 (7.8) | 1.0 (0.5-1.9) |
| No | 175 (86.2) | 667 (88.3) | 1.0 |
| Missing | 10 (4.9) | 29 (3.8) | 0.8 (0.3-2.0) |
| Ever injured | | | |
| One time period | 108 (53.2) | 298 (39.5) | 2.0 (1.4-2.9) |
| Both time periods | 14 (6.9) | 33 (4.4) | 1.8 (0.8-4.1) |
| Neither time period | 70 (34.5) | 394 (52.2) | 1.0 |
| Missing | 11 (5.4) | 30 (4.0) | 1.3 (0.5-3.3) |
| Mother's injury status‡ | | | |
| Injured before study | | | |
| Yes | 63 (31.0) | 112 (14.8) | 2.5 (1.7-3.8) |
| No | 131 (64.5) | 600 (79.5) | 1.0 |
| Missing | 9 (4.4) | 43 (5.7) | 1.2 (0.5-3.1) |
| Injured during study | | | |
| Yes | 15 (7.4) | 29 (3.8) | 2.0 (0.9-4.2) |
| No | 178 (87.7) | 683 (90.5) | 1.0 |
| Missing | 10 (4.9) | 43 (5.7) | 1.3 (0.5-1) |
| Ever injured | | | |
| One time period | 58 (28.6) | 125 (16.6) | 2.0 (1.3-3.0) |
| Both time periods | 10 (4.9) | 8 (1.1) | 8.0 (2.5-25.4) |
| Neither time period | 125 (61.6) | 579 (76.7) | 1.0 |
| Missing | 10 (4.9) | 43 (5.7) | 1.4 (0.6-3.4) |

*Adjusted for within-household correlation by using generalized estimating equations[27] and weighted for nonresponse.[28,29]

†Models included state, enterprise, number of children in the household, father's age and education level, and total household hours worked on the operation.

‡Models included state, enterprise, number of children in the household, mother's age and education level, and total household hours worked on the operation.

### MULTIVARIABLE ANALYSES

When controlling for potential confounders, children of fathers who sustained an agricultural injury before the study period had twice the risk of injury as those whose fathers did not report an injury (odds ratio [OR], 2.1; 95% confidence interval [CI], 1.5-3.0) (**Table 2**). Children whose fathers were injured during the study were no more or less likely to be injured (OR, 1.0; 95% CI, 0.5-1.9) than children whose fathers were not injured. Children whose

**Table 3. Risk of Children's Agricultural Injury According to Parents' Combined Injury History: 1999 Regional Rural Injury Study–II**

| Parent Injury Status* | No. (%) Cases (n = 203) | No. (%) Controls (n = 755) | Multivariable Analyses Odds Ratio† (95% Confidence Interval) |
|---|---|---|---|
| Before study | | | |
| Both injured | 55 (27.1) | 71 (9.4) | 4.2 (2.6-6.9) |
| One injured | 71 (35.0) | 268 (36.0) | 1.5 (1.0-2.2) |
| Neither injured | 65 (32.0) | 369 (48.9) | 1.0 |
| Missing | 12 (5.9) | 47 (6.2) | 2.0 (0.8-4.8) |
| During study | | | |
| Both injured | 1 (0.5) | 9 (1.2) | 0.4 (0.04-4.4) |
| One injured | 30 (14.8) | 68 (9.0) | 1.5 (0.8-2.5) |
| Neither injured | 160 (78.8) | 632 (83.7) | 1.0 |
| Missing | 12 (5.9) | 46 (6.1) | 1.5 (0.7-3.5) |
| Either time period | | | |
| Both injured | 60 (29.6) | 87 (11.5) | 3.5 (2.2-5.7) |
| One injured | 69 (34.0) | 281 (37.2) | 1.4 (0.9-2.0) |
| Neither injured | 61 (30.0) | 340 (45.0) | 1.0 |
| Missing | 13 (6.4) | 47 (6.2) | 2.3 (1.0-5.2) |

*Models included state, type of agricultural operation, number of children in the household, mother's age and education level, and total household hours worked on the operation.

†Adjusted for within-household correlation by using generalized estimating equations[27] and weighted for nonresponse.[28,29]

fathers were injured during both periods had a greater, albeit imprecise, risk of injury than children whose fathers were never injured (OR, 1.8; 95% CI, 0.8-4.1).

The risk of injury among children whose mothers were injured before the study period was more than twice that for children whose mothers did not sustain an injury (OR, 2.5; 95% CI, 1.7-3.8) (Table 2). A more modest association was observed for mothers' agricultural injuries during the study (OR, 2.0; 95% CI, 0.9-4.2). The highest risk was observed among children whose mothers reported injuries both before and during the study year (OR, 8.0; 95% CI, 2.5-25.4).

Compared with those with neither parent injured before the study period, increased risks of agricultural injury were observed for children with one (OR, 1.5; 95% CI, 1.0-2.2) or both (OR, 4.2; 95% CI, 2.6-6.9) parents injured (**Table 3**). Similarly, if both parents were injured during either time period analyzed, the children's risk was also increased (OR, 3.5; 95% CI, 2.2-5.7) compared with children with neither parent ever injured.

Although data were too sparse to evaluate all exposures of interest, the effect of parents' injuries on children varied slightly according to sex. For example, the relative risks of injury for boys and girls whose fathers reported an injury before the study period were 1.9 (95% CI, 1.2-3.0) and 2.5 (95% CI, 1.3-4.7), respectively. For those whose mothers reported injuries before the study period, relative risks were 2.4 (95% CI, 1.3-4.2) and 3.2 (95% CI, 1.7-6.0).

## COMMENT

Results of this study showed a positive association between parents' history of agricultural injury and children's risk of subsequent injury. Although the underlying reasons for this association cannot be identified from the data, 2 explanations are plausible: (1) certain agricultural environments may be inherently more hazardous than others, regardless of operation type, and (2) behavioral characteristics of some families may lead to increased high-risk exposure. No matter the cause, this association indicates that interventions to prevent childhood injury can be targeted specifically to families with injured parents (ie, parents treated by health professionals can be sentinel events for prevention efforts).

Although it is postulated that prior injury is associated with risk perception[30] and that risk perception may lead to improved preventive practices and reduced likelihood of injuries,[31] results of this study indicate that parents' experiences with agricultural injuries, alone, do not convey a lower risk to children. Results of studies conducted with other populations support these findings. A recent analysis of self-reported hospital emergency department visits indicated that increased parental emergency department use was associated with increased child emergency department use.[32] Further studies showed that parents rarely alter the environment or change safety behaviors to prevent reinjury among children,[33,34] and relatively few parents who perceive their agricultural operations as high risk make safety-related changes to mediate this risk.[35] These findings may be partly due to parents' beliefs that children's injuries are unpreventable or a normative part of child development.[34,36-39]

Although fathers and mothers may perceive injuries as a normal part of childhood, mothers relay more conservative perceptions of injury,[39] which may explain the greater awareness and focus on safety-related behaviors among mothers.[40,41] In the current study, mothers' injuries appeared to be associated more strongly with children's risk than fathers' injuries were. It is unknown whether this is influenced by the divergence between mothers' and fathers' perceptions of injury or by distinct gender roles among parents on agricultural operations. The latter could explain the strength of association between mothers' and children's injuries. For example, mothers may have been working on their operation while also caring for children. Supervision by a caregiver engaged in farmwork, compared with that in the home, is associated with increased risk of injury among children.[42] The associations observed in the current study could result from the tendency of mothers and children to share environments that potentiate injury risk.

A unique finding was the apparent additive effect of parents' agricultural injuries on children's risk of injury. Children whose parents were both injured before the study were 4 times more likely to be injured, and children whose parents both had a lifetime history of injury (either before or during the study) were 3.5 times more likely to be injured. This finding may be attributable to inherent hazard levels of certain operations. The type of operation, however, was controlled in the multivariable analyses to address this problem, although residual confounding cannot be ruled out. A second rationale for this finding is the possible modeling of parental behaviors by children, particularly pertaining to risk awareness. For example, children are more likely to practice safety precautions, such as using personal protective equipment, when such precautions are modeled by their parents.[43] The current finding emphasizes the potential benefit of clinic-based injury prevention measures targeted to parents treated for agricultural injuries.

Limitations of this study should be considered when interpreting the results. For example, some families may be better reporters of injuries than others, which could lead to misinterpretation of the observed associations. Furthermore, because of the self-reported nature of the data, the results are susceptible to information bias. However, the use of 6-month recall periods, which improves injury reporting validity,[22,23] was expected to minimize reporting bias for the injuries occurring in the study year. Also, a particular strength of this study was the large number of participating households (3765 [85.5%] of 4402 eligible). Although the high participation rate should reduce the potential for selection bias to affect study results, an attempt to control such bias also was made through adjustments for nonresponse and within-household correlation.

The complexity of agricultural operations limits our ability to fully account for environmental characteristics in multivariable analyses. Agricultural injuries result from multiple and complex causal pathways. Although this study is one of the largest of its kind and contains a substantial amount of detailed data, we could not identify single pathways or circumstances that may explain intrafamilial risk of injury. Despite this limitation, these findings are useful in the context of identifying families at higher risk to whom interventions might be targeted, particularly in a clinical setting. Future studies of the shared physical and social environments contributing to such risk may lead to more effective population-based injury prevention measures.

**Accepted for Publication:** June 15, 2006.
**Correspondence**: Susan G. Gerberich, PhD, Regional Injury Prevention Research Center, Division of Environmental Health Sciences, School of Public Health, University of Minnesota, MMC 807, 420 Delaware St SE, Minneapolis, MN 55455 (gerbe001@umn.edu).
**Author Contributions:** Dr Gerberich had full access to all of the data in the study and takes responsibility for the integrity of the data and the accuracy of these data analyses. *Study concept and design:* Carlson, Langner, Alexander, Gurney, Gerberich, Ryan, and Renier. *Acquisition of data:* Ryan, Renier, and Mongin. *Analysis and interpretation of data:* Carlson, Langner, Alexander, Gurney, Gerberich, Ryan, Renier, and Mongin. *Drafting of the manuscript:* Carlson, Langner, Gerberich, and Ryan. *Critical revision of the manuscript for important intellectual content*: Carlson, Alexander, Gurney, Gerberich, Renier, and Mongin. *Statistical analysis:* Carlson, Alexander, Gerberich, Ryan, Renier, and Mongin. *Obtained funding:* Gerberich. *Administrative, technical, and material support:* Carlson, Gerberich, Ryan, and Renier. *Study supervision:* Alexander and Gurney.
**Financial Disclosure:** None reported.
**Funding/Support:** This study was supported by grant R01 CCR514375 from the National Institute for Occupational Safety and Health, Centers for Disease Control and Prevention, US Department of Health and Human Services; a National Institute for Occupational Safety and Health grant T42/CCT510-422 for the Occupational Injury Prevention Research Training Program; the National Occupational Research Agenda Program, Midwest Center for Occupational Health and Safety, University of Minnesota; and the Regional Injury Prevention Research Center and Center for Violence Prevention and Control, Division of Environmental Health Sciences, School of Public Health, University of Minnesota.
**Acknowledgment:** We thank the US Department of Agriculture's National Agricultural Statistics Service for collaboration on this project and are indebted to the farm and ranch families who shared their time and personal information during participation in the Regional Rural Injury Study–II.

## REFERENCES

1. Anderson RN, Smith BL. Deaths: leading causes for 2001. *Natl Vital Stat Rep.* 2003;52(9):1-85.
2. Baker SP. *The Injury Fact Book.* New York, NY: Oxford University Press; 1992: 11-15.
3. Gerberich SG, Gibson RW, French LR, et al. *The Regional Rural Injury Study–I (RRIS-I): A Population-Based Effort. A Report to the Centers for Disease Control and Prevention.* Minneapolis: Regional Injury Prevention Center, University of Minnesota; 1993.
4. Hard D, Myers J, Snyder K, et al. Young workers at risk when working in agricultural production. *Am J Ind Med.* 1999(suppl 1):31-33.
5. National Safety Council. *Injury Facts, 2005-2006 Edition.* Itasca, Ill: National Safety Council; 2006:68.
6. 2004 Census of Fatal Occupational Injuries: fatal occupational injuries by industry and event or exposure, all United States, 2004. US Department of Labor, Bureau of Labor Statistics Web site. http://www.bls.gov/iif/oshwc/cfoi/cftb0196.pdf. Accessed April 11, 2006.
7. Pickett W, Brison RJ, Berg RL, Zentner J, Linneman J, Marlenga B. Pediatric farm injuries involving non-working children injured by a farm work hazard: five priorities for primary prevention. *Inj Prev.* 2005;11:6-11.
8. Castillo D, Hard D, Myers J, Pizatella T, Stout N. A national childhood agricultural injury prevention initiative. *J Agric Saf Health.* 1998;1(special issue):183-191. http://asae.frymulti.com/abstract.asp?aid=15368&t=2. Accessed November 15, 2005.
9. Emery CA, Meeuwisse WH. Risk factors for groin injuries in hockey. *Med Sci Sports Exerc.* 2001;33:1423-1433.
10. Hagel BE, Fick GH, Meeuwisse WH. Injury risk in men's Canada West University football. *Am J Epidemiol.* 2003;157:825-833.
11. Schneider GA, Bigelow C, Amoroso PJ. Evaluating risk of re-injury among 1214 army airborne soldiers using a stratified survival model. *Am J Prev Med.* 2000; 18(3)(suppl):156-163.
12. Browning SR, Truszczynska H, Reed D, McKnight RH. Agricultural injuries among older Kentucky farmers: the Farm Family Health and Hazard Surveillance Study. *Am J Ind Med.* 1998;33:341-353.
13. Low JM, Griffith GR, Alston CL. Australian farm work injuries: incidence, diversity and personal risk factors. *Aust J Rural Health.* 1996;4:179-189.
14. Kendrick D, Marsh P. Injury prevention programmes in primary care: a high risk group or a whole population approach? *Inj Prev.* 1997;3:170-175.
15. Madden C, Garrett JM, Cole TB, Runge JW, Porter CQ. The urban epidemiology of recurrent injury: beyond age, race, and gender stereotypes. *Acad Emerg Med.* 1997;4:772-775.
16. Spady DW, Saunders DL, Schopflocher DP, Svenson LW. Patterns of injury in children: a population-based approach. *Pediatrics.* 2004;113:522-529.
17. Johnston BD, Grossman DC, Connell FA, Koepsell TD. High-risk periods for childhood injury among siblings. *Pediatrics.* 2000;105:562-568.
18. Johnston BD, Grossman DC, Thompson RS. Transient elevation in risk of injury in siblings following injury encounters. *J Pediatr.* 2003;142:79-83.
19. Gerberich SG, Gibson RW, French LR, et al. *Etiology and Consequences of Injuries Among Children in Farm Households: A Regional Rural Injury Study: Technical Report to the Centers for Disease Control and Prevention.* Minneapolis: Regional Injury Prevention Center, University of Minnesota; 2003.
20. National Agricultural Statistics Service. US Department of Agriculture Web site. http://www.nass.usda.gov/Data_and_Statistics/Quick_Stats/index.asp. Accessed August 17, 2006.
21. Regional Injury Prevention Research Center Web site. http://enhs.umn.edu/riprc/riprc.html. Accessed October 15, 2005.

22. Braun BL, Gerberich SG, Sidney S. Injury events: utility of self-report in retrospective identification in the USA. *J Epidemiol Community Health.* 1994;48:604-605.
23. Gerberich SG, Gibson RW, Gunderson PD, et al. *The Olmsted Agricultural Trauma Study (OATS): A Population-Based Effort: A Report to the Centers for Disease Control.* Minneapolis: Regional Injury Prevention Center, University of Minnesota; 1991.
24. Breslow NE, Day NE. Statistical methods in cancer research: volume II—the design and analysis of cohort studies. *IARC Sci Publ.* 1987;(82):1-406.
25. Greenland S, Pearl J, Robins J. Causal diagrams for epidemiologic research. *Epidemiology.* 1999;10:37-48.
26. Hernan MA, Hernandez-Diaz S, Werler MM, Mitchell AA. Causal knowledge as a prerequisite for confounding evaluation: an application to birth defects epidemiology. *Am J Epidemiol.* 2002;155:176-184.
27. Liang KY, Zeger SL. Longitudinal data analysis using generalized linear models. *Biometrika.* 1986;73:13-22.
28. Horvitz DG, Thompson DJ. A generalization of sampling without replacement from a finite universe. *J Am Stat Assoc.* 1952;47:663-685.
29. Mongin SJ. Adjustment for non-response in the Minnesota Nurses Study. Division of Environmental and Occupational Health, University of Minnesota Web site. http://www1.umn.edu/eoh/NewFiles/researchpdffiles/response.adjustment.1.pdf. Accessed October 15, 2005.
30. Glik D, Kronenfeld J, Jackson K. Predictors of risk perception of childhood injury among parents of preschoolers. *Health Educ Q.* 1991;18:285-301.
31. Conrad P, Bradshaw YS, Lamsudin R, Kasniyah N, Costello C. Helmets, injuries, and cultural definitions: motorcycle injury in urban Indonesia. *Accid Anal Prev.* 1996;28:193-200.
32. Mistry RD, Hoffmann RG, Yauck JS, Brousseau DC. Association between parental and childhood emergency department utilization. *Pediatrics.* 2005;115:e147-e151.
33. Peterson L, Bartelstone J, Kern T, Gillies R. Parents' socialization of children's injury prevention: description and some initial parameters. *Child Dev.* 1995;66:224-235.
34. Langley J, Silva P. Childhood accidents: parents' attitudes to prevention. *Aust Paediatr J.* 1982;18:247-249.
35. Zentner J, Berg RL, Pickett W, Marlenga B. Do parents' perceptions of risks protect children engaged in farm work? *Prev Med.* 2005;40:860-866.
36. Morrongiello BA, Dayler L. A community-based study of parents' knowledge, attitudes and beliefs related to childhood injuries. *Can J Public Health.* 1996;87:383-388.
37. Coffman S, Martin V, Prill N, Langley B. Perceptions, safety behaviors, and learning needs of parents of children brought to an emergency department. *J Emerg Nurs.* 1998;24:133-139.
38. Bennett Murphy LM. Adolescent mothers' beliefs about parenting and injury prevention: results of a focus group. *J Pediatr Health Care.* 2001;15:194-199.
39. Lewis T, DiLillo D, Peterson L. Parental beliefs regarding developmental benefits of childhood injuries. *Am J Health Behav.* 2004;28(suppl 1):S61-S68.
40. Garling A, Garling T. Mothers' anticipation and prevention of unintentional injury to young children in the home. *J Pediatr Psychol.* 1995;20:23-36.
41. Garling A, Garling T. Mothers' supervision and perception of young children's risk of unintentional injury in the home. *J Pediatr Psychol.* 1993;18:105-114.
42. Pryor SK, Caruth AK, McCoy CA. Children's injuries in agriculture related events: the effect of supervision on the injury experience. *Issues Compr Pediatr Nurs.* 2002;25:189-205.
43. Hu X, Wesson DF, Parlin PC, Chipman ML, Spence LJ. Current bicycle helmet ownership, use, and related factors among school-aged children in metropolitan Toronto. *Can J Public Health.* 1994;85:121-124.

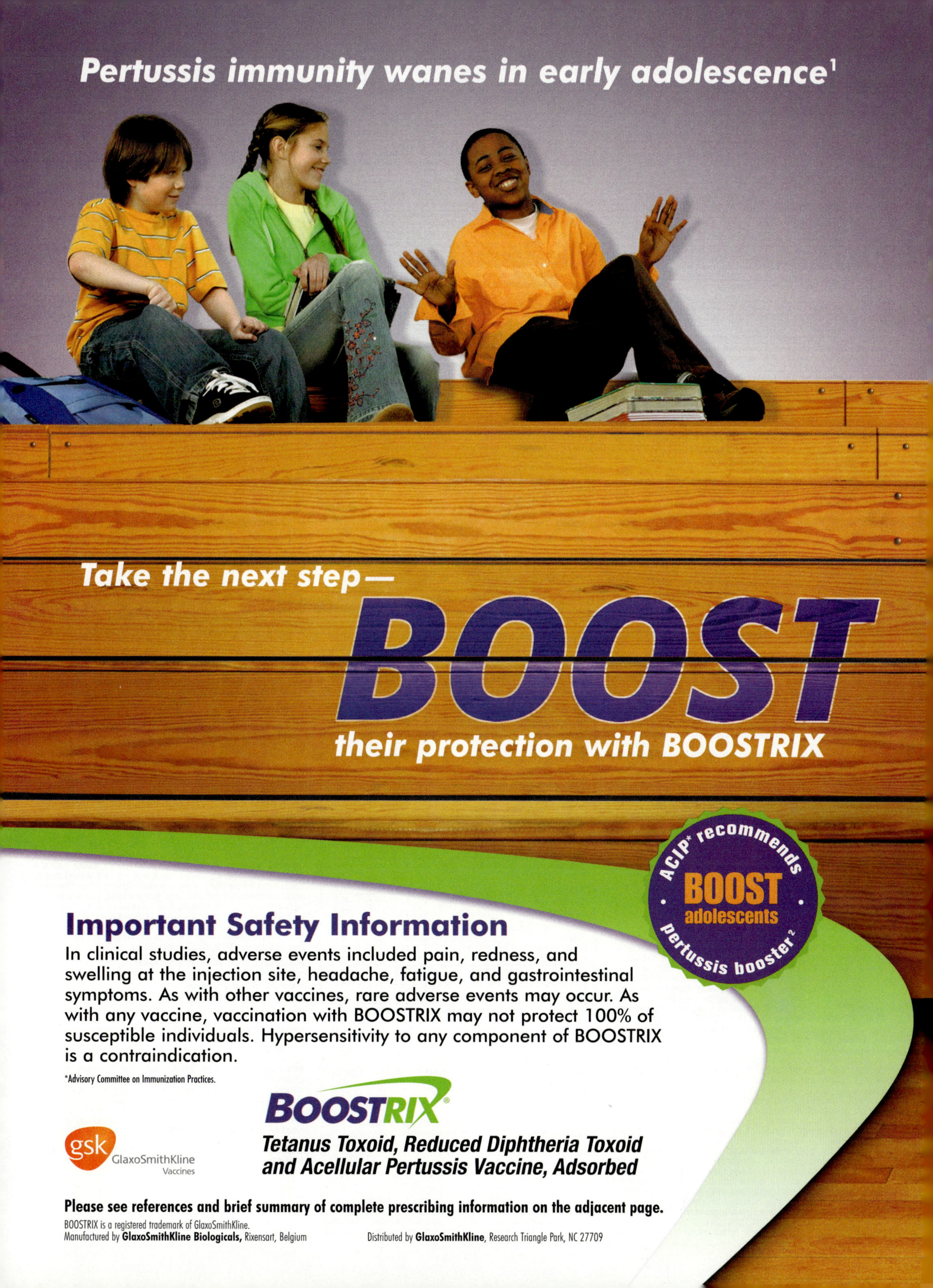
Pertussis immunity wanes in early adolescence[1]
Take the next step—
BOOST
their protection with BOOSTRIX
ACIP* recommends
BOOST
adolescents
pertussis booster[2]
Important Safety Information
In clinical studies, adverse events included pain, redness, and swelling at the injection site, headache, fatigue, and gastrointestinal symptoms. As with other vaccines, rare adverse events may occur. As with any vaccine, vaccination with BOOSTRIX may not protect 100% of susceptible individuals. Hypersensitivity to any component of BOOSTRIX is a contraindication.
*Advisory Committee on Immunization Practices.
BOOSTRIX®
Tetanus Toxoid, Reduced Diphtheria Toxoid and Acellular Pertussis Vaccine, Adsorbed
gsk GlaxoSmithKline Vaccines
Please see references and brief summary of complete prescribing information on the adjacent page.
BOOSTRIX is a registered trademark of GlaxoSmithKline.
Manufactured by GlaxoSmithKline Biologicals, Rixensart, Belgium
Distributed by GlaxoSmithKline, Research Triangle Park, NC 27709

# BOOSTRIX®

## (Tetanus Toxoid, Reduced Diphtheria Toxoid and Acellular Pertussis Vaccine, Adsorbed) (Tdap)

The following is a brief summary only; see full prescribing information for complete product information.

**INDICATIONS AND USAGE:** BOOSTRIX is indicated for active booster immunization against tetanus, diphtheria, and pertussis as a single dose in individuals 10 through 18 years of age. The use of BOOSTRIX as a primary series or to complete the primary series has not been studied. As with any vaccine, BOOSTRIX may not protect 100% of individuals receiving the vaccine.

**CONTRAINDICATIONS:** Hypersensitivity to any component of the vaccine is a contraindication (see DESCRIPTION in full prescribing information). Do not use BOOSTRIX after a serious allergic reaction (e.g., anaphylaxis) following any other tetanus toxoid, diphtheria toxoid or pertussis-containing vaccine, or any component of this vaccine (see DESCRIPTION in full prescribing information). Because of the uncertainty as to which component of the vaccine might be responsible, do not give further vaccination with any of these components; or, refer such individuals to an allergist for evaluation. The following events are contraindications to administration of BOOSTRIX: encephalopathy (e.g., coma, decreased level of consciousness, prolonged seizures) within 7 days of administration of a previous dose of a pertussis-containing vaccine that is not attributable to another identifiable cause; progressive neurologic disorder, uncontrolled epilepsy, or progressive encephalopathy. Do not vaccinate individuals with these conditions until a treatment regimen has been established and the condition has stabilized.

**WARNINGS:** The tip cap and the rubber plunger of the needleless prefilled syringes contain dry natural latex rubber that may cause allergic reactions in latex sensitive individuals. The vial stopper is latex-free. If any of the following events occurred in temporal relation to previous receipt of a Diphtheria and Tetanus Toxoids and Pertussis Vaccine Adsorbed (DTwP) vaccine or a vaccine containing an acellular pertussis component, consider carefully whether to give subsequent doses of BOOSTRIX: temperature of ≥40.5°C (105°F) within 48 hours not due to another identifiable cause; collapse or shock-like state (hypotonic-hyporesponsive episode) within 48 hours; persistent, inconsolable crying lasting ≥3 hours, occurring within 48 hours; seizures with or without fever occurring within 3 days. Persons who experienced serious Arthus-type hypersensitivity reactions following a prior dose of tetanus toxoid usually have high serum tetanus antitoxin levels and should not be given Tetanus and Diphtheria Toxoids Adsorbed For Adult Use (Td) or Tdap vaccines or even emergency doses of Td more frequently than every 10 years, even if the wound is neither clean nor minor. If Guillain-Barré syndrome has occurred within 6 weeks of receipt of prior vaccine containing tetanus toxoid, the decision to give BOOSTRIX or any vaccine containing tetanus toxoid should be based on careful consideration of the potential benefits and possible risks. The decision to administer a pertussis-containing vaccine to individuals with stable central nervous system (CNS) disorders must be made by the physician on an individual basis, with consideration of all relevant factors, and assessment of potential risks and benefits for that individual. Advise the patient, parent, or guardian of the potential increased risk involved (see PRECAUTIONS). A family history of seizures or other CNS disorders is not a contraindication to pertussis vaccine. The Advisory Committee on Immunization Practices (ACIP) has published guidelines for vaccination of persons with recent or acute illness (www.cdc.gov). Do not give BOOSTRIX to individuals with bleeding disorders such as hemophilia or thrombocytopenia, or to persons on anticoagulant therapy unless the potential benefit clearly outweighs the risk of administration. If the decision is made to administer BOOSTRIX to such persons, it should be given with caution with steps taken to avoid the risk of hematoma following the injection.

**PRECAUTIONS: General:** Before the injection of any biological, the physician should take all reasonable precautions to prevent allergic or other adverse reactions. Epinephrine injection (1:1,000) and other appropriate agents used for the control of immediate allergic reactions must be immediately available should an acute anaphylactic reaction occur. Immunosuppressed persons, including individuals receiving immunosuppressive therapy, may not develop the expected immune response. **Drug Interactions:** Do not mix BOOSTRIX with any other vaccine in the same syringe or vial. **Carcinogenesis, Mutagenesis, Impairment of Fertility:** BOOSTRIX has not been evaluated for carcinogenic or mutagenic potential, or for impairment of fertility. **Pregnancy:** Pregnancy Category C. Animal reproduction studies have not been conducted with BOOSTRIX. It is also not known whether BOOSTRIX can cause fetal harm when administered to a pregnant woman or can affect reproductive capacity. BOOSTRIX should be given to a pregnant woman only if clearly needed. Animal fertility studies have not been conducted with BOOSTRIX. In a developmental toxicity study, the effect of BOOSTRIX on embryo-fetal and pre-weaning development was evaluated in pregnant rats. Animals were administered INFANRIX® (Diphtheria and Tetanus Toxoids and Acellular Pertussis Vaccine Adsorbed) prior to gestation and BOOSTRIX during the period of organogenesis (gestation days 6, 8, 11) and later in pregnancy (gestation day 15), 0.1 mL/rat/occasion (a 45-fold increase compared to the human dose of BOOSTRIX on a body weight basis), by intramuscular injection. No adverse affect on pregnancy and lactation parameters, embryo-fetal or pre-weaning development was observed. There were no fetal malformations or other evidence of teratogenesis noted in this study. **Nursing Mothers:** It is not known whether BOOSTRIX is excreted in human milk. Because many drugs are excreted in human milk, caution should be exercised when BOOSTRIX is administered to a nursing woman. **Pregnancy Exposure Registry:** Healthcare providers are encouraged to register pregnant women who receive BOOSTRIX in the GlaxoSmithKline vaccination pregnancy registry by calling 1-888-825-5249. **Geriatric Use:** BOOSTRIX is not indicated for use in individuals older than 18 years. **Pediatric Use:** BOOSTRIX is not indicated for use in individuals younger than 10 years (see DOSAGE AND ADMINISTRATION in full prescribing information). For immunization of infants and children younger than 7 years against diphtheria, tetanus, and pertussis, refer to the manufacturers' package inserts for Diphtheria and Tetanus Toxoids and Acellular Pertussis Vaccine Adsorbed (DTaP) vaccines.

**ADVERSE REACTIONS:** A total of 3,608 adolescents were vaccinated with a single dose of BOOSTRIX during clinical trials. An additional 1,092 adolescents 10 to 18 years of age received a non-US formulation of BOOSTRIX (formulated to contain 0.5 mg aluminum per dose) in non-US clinical studies.

The primary safety study, conducted in the United States, was a randomized, observer-blinded, controlled study in which 3,080 adolescents 10 to 18 years of age received a single dose of BOOSTRIX and 1,034 received the control Td vaccine manufactured by Massachusetts Public Health Biologic Laboratories. There were no substantive differences in demographic characteristics between the vaccine groups. Among BOOSTRIX and control vaccine recipients approximately 75% were 10 to 14 years of age and approximately 25% were 15 to 18 years of age. Approximately 98% of participants in this study had received the recommended series of 4 or 5 doses of either DTwP or a combination of DTwP and DTaP in childhood. Data on adverse events were collected by the subjects, parents and/or guardians using standardized diaries for 15 consecutive days following the vaccine dose (i.e., day of vaccination and the next 14 days). Subjects were monitored for unsolicited adverse events that occurred within 31 days of vaccination (day 0-30) using diary cards (day 0-14) supplemented by spontaneous reports and a medical history as reported by subjects, parents, and/or guardians. Subjects were also monitored for 6 months post-vaccination for non-routine medical visits, visits to an emergency room, onset of new chronic illness, and serious adverse events. Information regarding late onset adverse events was obtained via a telephone call 6 months following vaccination. At least 97% of subjects completed the 6-month follow-up evaluation.

In a study conducted in Germany, BOOSTRIX was administered to 319 children 10 to 12 years of age previously vaccinated with 5 doses of acellular pertussis-containing vaccines, 193 of these subjects had previously received 5 doses of INFANRIX. Adverse events were recorded on diary cards during the 15 days following vaccination. Unsolicited adverse events that occurred within 31 days of vaccination (day 0-30) were recorded on the diary card or verbally reported to the investigator. Subjects were monitored for 6 months post-vaccination for physician office visits, emergency room visits, onset of new chronic illness, and serious adverse events. The 6-month follow-up evaluation, conducted via telephone interview, was completed by 90% of subjects.

The adverse event information from clinical trials provides a basis for identifying adverse events that appear to be related to vaccine use and for approximating rates. However, because clinical trials are conducted under widely varying conditions, adverse event rates observed in the clinical trials of a vaccine cannot be directly compared to rates in the clinical trials of another vaccine, and may not reflect the rates observed in practice.

**Serious Adverse Events in All Safety Studies:** In the US-safety study and German-safety study, no serious adverse events were reported to occur within 31 days of vaccination. During the 6-month extended safety evaluation period, no serious adverse events that were of potential autoimmune origin or new onset and chronic in nature were reported to occur. In non-US studies in which serious adverse events were monitored for up to 37 days, one subject was diagnosed with insulin dependent diabetes 20 days following administration of BOOSTRIX. No other serious adverse events of potential autoimmune origin or that were new onset and chronic in nature were reported to occur in these studies.

**Solicited Adverse Events in the US-Safety Study:** In a US study, the most common local adverse events following administration of BOOSTRIX were pain, redness, and swelling at the injection site. The most common general adverse events were headache and fatigue. Most of these events were reported at a similar frequency in recipients of both BOOSTRIX and Td. Any pain, grade 2 or 3 pain (but not grade 3 alone), and grade 2 or 3 headache (but not grade 3 alone) were reported at a higher rate in recipients of BOOSTRIX. The primary safety endpoint of the US study was the incidence of grade 3 pain (spontaneously painful and/or prevented normal activity) at the injection site within 15 days of vaccination. Grade 3 pain was reported in 4.6% of those who received BOOSTRIX compared with 4.0% of those who received the Td vaccine. The difference in rate of grade 3 pain was within the pre-defined clinical limit for non-inferiority (upper limit of the 95% CI for the difference ≤4%). These were the rates for solicited local and general adverse events within 15 days of vaccination with BOOSTRIX or Td vaccine for the total vaccinated cohort (all enrolled, vaccinated subjects with safety data available analyzed by vaccine received):

**Percentage of Individuals 10 to 18 Years of Age Reporting Solicited Local Adverse Events or Solicited General Adverse Events Within the 15-day* Post-Vaccination Period**

| | BOOSTRIX (N = 3,032) % | Td (N =1,013) % |
|---|---|---|
| **Local** | | |
| Pain,† any | 75.3 | 71.7 |
| Pain,† grade 2 or 3 | 51.2 | 42.5 |
| Pain,‡ grade 3 | 4.6 | 4.0 |
| Redness, any | 22.5 | 19.8 |
| Redness, >20 mm | 4.1 | 3.9 |
| Redness, ≥50 mm | 1.7 | 1.6 |
| Swelling, any | 21.1 | 20.1 |
| Swelling, >20 mm | 5.3 | 4.9 |
| Swelling, ≥50 mm | 2.5 | 3.2 |
| Arm circumference increase,§ >5 mm | 28.3 | 29.5 |
| Arm circumference increase,§ >20 mm | 2.0 | 2.2 |
| Arm circumference increase,§ >40 mm | 0.5 | 0.3 |
| **General** | | |
| Fever,‖ ≥99.5°F | 13.5 | 13.1 |
| Fever,‖ >100.4°F | 5.0 | 4.7 |
| Fever,‖ >102.2°F | 1.4 | 1.0 |
| Headache, any | 43.1 | 41.5 |
| Headache,† grade 2 or 3 | 15.7 | 12.7 |
| Headache, grade 3 | 3.7 | 2.7 |
| Fatigue, any | 37.0 | 36.7 |
| Fatigue, grade 2 or 3 | 14.4 | 12.9 |
| Fatigue, grade 3 | 3.7 | 3.2 |
| Gastrointestinal symptoms,¶ any | 26.0 | 25.8 |
| Gastrointestinal symptoms,¶ grade 2 or 3 | 9.8 | 9.7 |
| Gastrointestinal symptoms,¶ grade 3 | 3.0 | 3.2 |

Td = Tetanus and Diphtheria Toxoids Adsorbed For Adult Use manufactured by Massachusetts Public Health Biologic Laboratories.
N = number of subjects in the total vaccinated cohort with local/general symptoms sheets completed.
Grade 2 = Local: painful when the limb was moved; General: interfered with normal activity.
Grade 3 = Local: spontaneously painful and/or prevented normal activity; General: prevented normal activity.
*Day of vaccination and the next 14 days.
†Statistically significantly higher (P<0.05) following BOOSTRIX as compared to Td vaccine.
‡Grade 3 injection site pain following BOOSTRIX was not inferior to Td (upper limit of two-sided 95% CI for the difference in the percentage of subjects ≤4%).
§Mid-upper region of the vaccinated arm.
‖Oral temperatures or axillary temperatures.
¶Gastrointestinal symptoms included nausea, vomiting, diarrhea and/or abdominal pain.

Mid-upper arm circumference was measured by the adolescent or their parent/guardian prior to injection and daily for 15 days following vaccination. There was no significant difference between BOOSTRIX recipients and Td recipients in the proportion of subjects reporting an increase in mid-upper arm circumference in the vaccinated arm. The incidence of unsolicited adverse events reported in the 31 days after vaccination was comparable between the 2 groups.

**Solicited Adverse Events in the German Safety Study:** No cases of whole arm swelling were spontaneously reported. Two individuals (2/193) reported large injection site swelling (range 110 to 200 mm diameter), in one case associated with grade 3 pain. Neither individual sought medical attention. These episodes were reported to resolve without sequelae within 5 days. These were the rates of solicited local adverse events and fever within 15 days of vaccination for those subjects who had previously been vaccinated with 5 doses of INFANRIX:

**Rates of Solicited Adverse Events Reported Within the 15-day* Post-Vaccination Period Following Administration of BOOSTRIX in Individuals 10 to 12 Years of Age Who Had Previously Received 5 Doses of INFANRIX**

| Adverse Event | BOOSTRIX (N = 193) % (95% CI) |
|---|---|
| Pain, any | 62.2 (54.9-69.0) |
| Pain, grade 2 or 3 | 33.2 (26.6-40.3) |
| Pain, grade 3 | 5.7 (2.9-10.0) |
| Redness, any | 47.7 (40.4-55.0) |
| Redness, >20 mm | 15.0 (10.3-20.9) |
| Redness, ≥50 mm | 10.9 (6.9-16.2) |
| Swelling, any | 38.9 (31.9-46.1) |
| Swelling, >20 mm | 17.6 (12.5-23.7) |
| Swelling, ≥50 mm | 14.0 (9.4-19.7) |
| Fever, ≥99.5 | 8.8 (5.2-13.7) |
| Fever, >100.4 | 4.1 (1.8-8.0) |
| Fever, >102.2 | 1.0 (0.1-3.7) |

N = number of subjects with local/general symptoms sheets completed.
Grade 2 = Painful when the limb was moved.
Grade 3 = Spontaneously painful and/or prevented normal activity.
*Day of vaccination and the next 14 days.

As with any vaccine, there is the possibility that broad use of BOOSTRIX could reveal adverse events not observed in clinical trials.

**Postmarketing Reports:** Worldwide voluntary reports of adverse events received for BOOSTRIX in persons 10 to 18 years of age since market introduction of this vaccine are listed below. This list includes serious events or events which have causal connection to components of this or other vaccines or drugs. Because these events are reported voluntarily from a population of uncertain size, it is not possible to reliably estimate their frequency or establish a causal relationship to vaccine exposure. *Blood and lymphatic system disorders:* Lymphadenitis, lymphadenopathy. *Cardiac disorders:* Myocarditis. *Injection site reactions:* Induration, inflammation, mass, nodule, warmth, local reaction. *Metabolism and nutrition disorders:* Diabetes mellitus insulin-dependent. *Musculoskeletal and connective tissue disorders:* Arthralgia, back pain, myalgia. *Nervous system disorders:* Convulsion, encephalitis, facial palsy, paraesthesia. *Skin and subcutaneous tissue disorders:* Exanthem, Henoch-Schönlein purpura, rash. In addition, extensive swelling of the injected limb has been reported following administration of BOOSTRIX.

**Reporting Adverse Events:** Report the occurrence following immunization of any event set forth in the Vaccine Injury Table from the National Childhood Vaccine Injury Act including: Anaphylaxis or anaphylactic shock within 7 days, encephalopathy or encephalitis within 7 days, brachial neuritis within 28 days, or an acute complication or sequelae (including death) of an illness, disability, injury, or condition referred to above, or any events that would contraindicate further doses of vaccine, according to this prescribing information. These events should be reported to VAERS. The VAERS toll-free number is 1-800-822-7967. Reporting forms may also be obtained at the VAERS website at www.vaers.hhs.gov.

**DOSAGE AND ADMINISTRATION: Recommended Dose:** BOOSTRIX should be administered as a single 0.5 mL injection by the intramuscular route into the deltoid muscle of the upper arm in individuals 10 through 18 years of age. Do not administer this product subcutaneously or intravenously. There are no data to support repeat administration of BOOSTRIX. Five years should elapse between the subject's last dose of the recommended series of childhood DTwP and/or DTaP vaccine and the administration of BOOSTRIX. Limited data are available on the use of BOOSTRIX following Tetanus and Diphtheria Toxoids Adsorbed For Adult Use (Td) vaccine. **Additional Dosing Information:** ***Wound Management:*** Clinicians should refer to guidelines for tetanus prophylaxis in routine wound management. Adolescents 10 to 18 years of age who have completed a primary series against tetanus and who sustain wounds which are minor and uncomplicated, should receive a booster dose of a tetanus toxoid-containing vaccine only if they have not received tetanus toxoid within the preceding 10 years. In case of tetanus-prone injury (e.g., wounds contaminated with dirt, feces, soil, and saliva; puncture wounds; avulsions; and wounds resulting from missles, crushing, burns, and frostbite) in an adolescent who is in need of tetanus toxoid, BOOSTRIX can be used as an alternative to Tetanus and Diphtheria Toxoids Adsorbed For Adult Use (Td) vaccine in patients for whom the pertussis component is also indicated (see INDICATIONS AND USAGE).

Manufactured by **GlaxoSmithKline Biologicals**
Rixensart, Belgium, US License 1617

Distributed by **GlaxoSmithKline**
Research Triangle Park, NC 27709

BOOSTRIX and INFANRIX are registered trademarks of GlaxoSmithKline.

Full prescribing information for BOOSTRIX is available at www.BOOSTRIX.com.
BRS-BO:L3

**References: 1.** Centers for Disease Control and Prevention. Preventing tetanus, diphtheria, and pertussis among adolescents: use of tetanus toxoid, reduced diphtheria toxoid and acellular pertussis vaccines: recommendations of the Advisory Committee on Immunization Practices (ACIP). Early Release 2006;55(February 23, 2006):1–43. **2.** Centers for Disease Control and Prevention. Recommended childhood and adolescent immunization schedule—United States, 2006. *MMWR.* 2006;54(51&52):Q1–Q4.

ARTICLE

# The Interpreter as Cultural Educator of Residents

## *Improving Communication for Latino Parents*

*Ann Chen Wu, MD; John M. Leventhal, MD; Jacqueline Ortiz, MPhil; Ernesto E. Gonzalez, BS; Brian Forsyth, MBChB*

**Objective:** To determine whether augmentation of the Spanish interpreter's role to include cultural education of residents can improve the satisfaction of Latino patients.

**Design:** We assessed parent satisfaction during 4 sequential 2-month periods between June 1, 2004, and February 11, 2005, using different interpretation methods: telephone interpretation (n=91 patient encounters), trained in-person interpretation (n=49), in-person interpretation with cultural education of residents (n=65), and postprogram telephone interpretation (n=45).

**Setting:** General pediatric practice at a large teaching hospital.

**Participants:** A total of 250 Spanish-speaking parents who were limited in English proficiency.

**Interventions:** The cultural education program included 3 brief preclinic conferences taught by an interpreter and one-on-one teaching of residents about language and cultural issues after each clinical encounter.

**Main Outcome Measures:** Parent satisfaction was assessed using 8 questions that have previously been validated in Spanish. Lower scores indicated more satisfaction.

**Results:** Because they were limited in English proficiency, our Spanish-speaking patients were significantly more satisfied when an in-person interpreter was used compared with a telephone interpreter (mean total satisfaction score of 14.5 [in-person] vs 17.4 [telephone]; $P=.006$) but were even more satisfied when the interpreter educated residents in cultural and language issues (mean, 11.5 [in-person with education] vs 17.4 [telephone]; $P<.001$).

**Conclusion:** Although use of an in-person interpreter can increase Latino parents' satisfaction, a program using an interpreter to educate residents in cultural and language issues can increase satisfaction further.

*Arch Pediatr Adolesc Med. 2006;160:1145-1150*

COMMUNICATION BETWEEN patient and physician is a fundamental aspect of patient care, but unfortunately in the United States, physicians often do not share the same language and culture as their patients, making communication difficult. Latino individuals are currently the largest racial/ethnic minority group of US children, and language issues are one of the major barriers to accessing health care encountered by such children.[1] Communication gaps due to language differences compromise medical care in many different ways. Studies have documented that language barriers lead to a decreased likelihood of follow-up appointments being made after a visit to an emergency department[2]; a higher rate of resource utilization for diagnostic tests[3]; less satisfaction with medical care when seen in the emergency department or by primary care physicians[4,5]; a decreased likelihood of having had a health care visit, mental health visit, or influenza vaccination[6]; decreased explanation of adverse effects; decreased compliance with medications[7]; an increased incidence of medical errors during hospitalizations[8]; and a decreased likelihood of receiving all preventive health visits in the first year of life.[9] The ability for physicians to communicate effectively either in Spanish or with the use of interpreters is an important desire expressed by Latino patients.[10] Case studies demonstrate that in addition to addressing language barriers, it is important to understand normative cultural values, folk illnesses, and parent and patient beliefs in pediatric health care.[11] Pachter[12] describes a system of culturally sensitive health care that respects ethnic and cultural values along with linguistic considerations to enhance the quality of the interaction between the patient and the health care system. Similarly, Kleinman et al[13] suggest that the negotiation of a shared explanatory

Author Affiliations:
Department of Pediatrics, Yale University School of Medicine (Drs Wu, Leventhal, and Forsyth and Mr Gonzalez), Office of Interpreter Services, Yale-New Haven Hospital (Ms Ortiz), and Department of Sociology, Yale University (Ms Ortiz), New Haven, Conn. Dr Wu is currently with the Department of Ambulatory Care and Prevention, Harvard Medical School, and Children's Hospital, Boston, Mass.

model between patient and physician may be a crucial step in developing trust, encouraging adherence to medical regimens, and improving patient satisfaction.

Studies[14] demonstrate that bilingual health care professionals and trained professional interpreters result in the best patient satisfaction, outcomes, and quality of care compared with untrained or ad hoc interpreters. For example, Mazor et al[15] taught pediatric emergency department physicians a 10-week intensive medical Spanish course and demonstrated that at the end of the course physicians were able to care for Spanish-speaking patients without the use of interpreters more frequently than before the course. Furthermore, families had greater satisfaction with the care they received.[15] Unfortunately, teaching physicians Spanish can lead to problems with false fluency because physicians are less likely to use interpreters and instead rely on their own inadequate Spanish-speaking skills.[16]

Medical interpreters are crucial to effective communication between patients limited in English proficiency (LEP) and health care professionals, yet Spanish-speaking Latino persons are less satisfied than their English-proficient counterparts even when interpreters are used.[17] When language barriers are present, cultural barriers are present as well.[18] Therefore, the medical system needs further interventions beyond that of the trained, professional interpreter to help bridge cultural barriers with LEP patients.

Effectively using interpreters to communicate with LEP patients is not traditionally part of medical training. In a study of pediatric residents, Burbano O'Leary et al[19] found that non–Spanish-fluent residents rarely used professional interpreters.

Common methods to help overcome language barriers include the use of a telephone interpreter, an in-person interpreter, or an ad hoc interpreter (untrained individuals such as a family member, friend, nonclinical health care worker, or stranger from the waiting room). Studies[20,21] disagree on whether telephone interpretation or trained in-person interpretation is best; significant shortcomings exist with both methods of interpretation. We sought to examine the effects of a novel method using an in-person interpreter as a cultural educator of residents.

The goal of the study was to evaluate an intervention aimed at improving communication between pediatric residents and Spanish-speaking parents who are LEP. We hypothesized that by understanding Latino cultural values and home remedies, learning to use interpreters, and mastering Spanish phrases that helped establish rapport, pediatric resident physicians would be able to communicate more effectively with their Latino patients, resulting in improved satisfaction among the patients.

## METHODS

### STUDY DESIGN

The study was conducted in a general pediatric practice of a large teaching hospital that serves a predominantly Medicaid population and has approximately 22 000 visits per year. The study was approved by the Yale University School of Medicine's institutional review board. The study involved 4 sequential 2-month phases using different interpretation methods: telephone interpretation (phase A), in-person interpretation (phase B), in-person interpretation with resident education (phase C), and postprogram telephone interpretation (phase D). The study began on June 1, 2004, and ended February 11, 2005. The same individual (J.O.) served as in-person interpreter (phase B) and resident educator (phase C).

Eligible study participants included all parents who were Spanish-speaking, who were LEP, and whose children were being seen for either a well or sick visit by a pediatric resident who was not fluent in Spanish. We defined LEP as self-rated ability to speak English as fair or poor. The age range of the children was 2 days to 12 years; adolescent patients are seen in a separate clinic. Triage nurses who were blinded to the purpose of the study identified parents who needed an interpreter; a nurse evaluated parents by asking basic questions about the child. If the mother could not understand or respond properly, an interpreter was called. In the cases in which the mother spoke some English, she was asked if she wished to have an interpreter. After patient visits, a bilingual research assistant (E.E.G.) approached every LEP, Spanish-speaking parent who used an interpreter (telephone or in person). The research assistant presented the study as one of parent satisfaction in the clinic and did not mention that it was a study of interpretation method. After written informed consent was obtained, a patient satisfaction questionnaire was administered orally in Spanish by the research assistant.

One of the 50 pediatric residents at our hospital described herself as a native Spanish speaker and was excluded from the study. The remaining 49 residents participated in the study and completed written questionnaires describing their experiences with Spanish interpreters before and after the program. Each resident in our program has a weekly continuity clinic in our hospital; thus, all 49 residents in the program participated in the study. No resident was involved with more than 3 of the encounters in this study.

Both the telephone and in-person interpreters at the study hospital receive more than 60 hours of extensive training in proper interpreting technique, professional ethics, interpreter roles, medical terms, and cultural brokerage. Interpreter training specifically emphasizes the use of appropriate interventions to clarify possible misunderstandings caused by educational or cultural issues. Although the in-person interpreter in this study was from a South American background, she had extensive experience with many Latino groups in the United States. Telephone interpretation was conducted with telephones that were placed in patient rooms at the time of the visit, and interpretation was performed with speaker telephones.

### INTERVENTION

The trained in-person interpreter served as a cultural educator for a 2-month period. The teaching occurred in (1) 30-minute group sessions during preclinic seminars in a conference room and (2) individual sessions related to specific clinical encounters with patients.

The goals of the group didactic sessions were to introduce Latino cultural values and home remedies that could contribute to a physician's history taking, to optimize the use of interpreters in improving communication, to teach residents a few Spanish expressions to help establish rapport with Spanish-speaking patients, and to teach techniques for using interpreters.

The individual sessions between interpreter and resident occurred at the end of a patient visit when the patient was not present or when the resident stepped out of the room. The interpreter reviewed language or cultural issues that emerged during the visit. For example, in Latino culture, parents commonly place bracelets with amulets on a baby's wrist to ward off the "evil eye" or simply to protect the child. The interpreter observed that residents frequently cautioned parents against using jewelry on infants, and once even removed the bracelet from a child's wrist, causing embarrassment and offense. Once the residents understood the traditional use of these amulets, their teaching with parents was modified. Instead of cautioning parents to remove the amulets, they asked parents to check if the bracelets were cutting off circulation or suggested that they secure the amulets to clothing, thus ensuring safety while respecting the parents' beliefs.

Furthermore, the interpreter reminded the residents to introduce themselves to parents because the initial greeting is particularly important in Latino culture. The resident educator taught the residents to say to their patients, "Hello, my name is Dr ____" in Spanish to demonstrate an attempt to communicate in the parent's native language. In addition, the resident educator taught the residents proper technique when using interpreters. For example, she reminded the residents to maintain eye contact with the patient and/or parent and to avoid speaking directly to the interpreter. With each topic covered in both group sessions and individual teaching, the interpreter was careful to point out differences in customs from each national group. Despite general cultural commonalities among the Latino population as a whole, important variations in cultural practices also exist among Latino individuals from various countries.

## MAIN OUTCOME MEASURES

Parent satisfaction was measured using a patient satisfaction instrument that has been validated in both Spanish and English.[15] The instrument uses a 5-point Likert scale (with 1 meaning excellent and 5 meaning poor) for each of 8 questions about the respondent's satisfaction with the physician. These 8 questions are given in **Table 1**. The range of total satisfaction scores was 8 to 40, with 8 indicating excellent.

Residents completed questionnaires before and after the program about their experiences with treating LEP, Spanish-speaking patients in the clinic. The questionnaires asked for the resident's self-reported race/ethnicity. In addition, using a 5-point Likert scale, residents were asked to rank their abilities to speak Spanish; to take care of LEP, Spanish-speaking patients; and to use telephone interpreters or in-person interpreters. Residents were asked how often they used interpreters, and they were asked to rank a list of potential benefits of an in-person interpreter providing cultural education.

## STATISTICAL ANALYSIS

Analyses were performed using SAS statistical software, version 8.02 (SAS Institute Inc, Cary, NC). We present mean scores of satisfaction for each question and total summed scores in all 4 interpretation groups. To take into account that the satisfaction scores are nonparametric, we used the Kruskal-Wallis test to compare the scores among groups. To adjust for multiple comparisons, we applied the Bonferroni correction.

# RESULTS

## PARENT SATISFACTION

Of 460 parents approached, 83 (18.0%) were ineligible because their health care professionals for the visits were nurse practitioners or medical students, the families were in the clinic for nurse encounters only, or the parents had already participated in the study. A total of 250 (66.3%) of the 377 eligible parents participated in the study, and the proportion who participated in the study was similar in the 4 phases. Ninety-one LEP, Spanish-speaking parents were enrolled in the telephone interpretation phase (A), 49 in the in-person interpretation phase (B), 65 during in-person interpretation with cultural education of residents (C), and 45 in the telephone interpretation phase that followed the interpretation with cultural education (D). More parents were enrolled in phase A, since it was possible to have 2 simultaneous telephone interpretations because multiple telephone interpreters were available, whereas only 1 in-person interpreter was present.

**Table 1. Patient Satisfaction Questionnaire***

| |
|---|
| How was the doctor at listening to you? |
| How was the doctor at answering your questions? |
| How was the examiner at using words that you could understand, instead of confusing medical words? |
| How was the doctor at being friendly to you? |
| How was the doctor at spending enough time with you? |
| How was the doctor at treating you with respect? |
| How was the doctor at showing concern for you as a person? |
| How was the doctor at making you feel comfortable? |

*1 Indicates excellent; 2, very good; 3, good; 4, fair; and 5, poor.

The mean age of the children was 27.9 months, and 50.3% were female. There were no statistically significant differences among the 4 groups with respect to the child's age or sex. The most common countries of origin of the LEP, Spanish-speaking parents were Mexico (44.0%), Puerto Rico (15.7%), Ecuador (15.7%), Guatemala (8.5%), Peru (4.8%), and Colombia (3.2%). The remaining 8.1% were from Chile, El Salvador, the Dominican Republic, Argentina, Cuba, the United States (excluding Puerto Rico), Honduras, and Nicaragua. There were no statistically significant differences among patients in the 4 phases of the study with respect to the country of origin. During the telephone interpretation phases before and after the cultural education of residents, a significantly lower proportion of patients was seen by first-year residents ($P<.001$). First-year residents saw 14 patients (15.4%) in the initial telephone interpretation phase, 19 patients (38.8%) in the in-person interpretation phase, 27 patients (41.5%) in the cultural education of residents phase, and 10 patients (22.2%) in the postprogram telephone interpretation phase. No significant variability was found in the Spanish-speaking ability of the residents across the phases.

**Table 2** gives the means for the total satisfaction scores and individual item scores for the 4 phases of the study. The mean total satisfaction score during the initial telephone interpretation phase was 17.4. During the in-person interpretation phase, the mean total satisfaction score was significantly improved at 14.5 ($P=.006$), and during the cultural education of residents phase, the score was significantly better than both the telephone interpretation and in-person interpretation phases at 11.5 (vs telephone: $P<.001$; vs in-person interpreter: $P<.001$). The mean total satisfaction score was 17.2 during the post-

**Table 2. Comparison of Mean Satisfaction Scores Among Interpretation Methods***

| Satisfaction Item | Telephone (A) | In Person (B) | Cultural Education (C) | Telephone (D) | *P* Value B vs A | C vs B | D vs C |
|---|---|---|---|---|---|---|---|
| Total score | 17.4 | 14.5 | 11.5 | 17.2 | .006 | <.001 | <.001 |
| Listening | 2.2 | 1.8 | 1.5 | 2.0 | .01 | .02† | .02 |
| Answering | 2.4 | 2.1 | 1.7 | 2.4 | .14 | .01 | <.001 |
| Words | 2.4 | 2.0 | 1.3 | 2.3 | .02 | <.001 | <.001 |
| Friendly | 2.1 | 1.7 | 1.4 | 2.0 | .02 | .03† | <.001 |
| Time | 2.1 | 1.8 | 1.4 | 2.2 | .11 | .005 | <.001 |
| Respect | 1.9 | 1.7 | 1.4 | 1.8 | .11 | .004 | .003 |
| Concern | 2.0 | 1.7 | 1.4 | 2.2 | .07 | .01 | <.001 |
| Comfortable | 2.1 | 1.6 | 1.4 | 2.1 | .003 | .07 | <.001 |

*Phase A was telephone interpretation (n = 91); B, trained in-person interpretation (n = 49); C, in-person interpretation with cultural education of residents (n = 65); and D, postprogram telephone interpretation (n = 45). Lower scores indicate more satisfaction.
†No longer significant when using a cutoff of .017 for significance when applying the Bonferroni correction for multiple comparisons.

**Table 3. Results of Resident Preintervention Survey**

| Variable | Excellent, % | Very Good, % | Good, % | Fair, % | Poor, % |
|---|---|---|---|---|---|
| Self-rated Spanish-speaking ability (n = 50) | 2.0 | 4.0 | 40.0 | 20.0 | 34.0 |
| Overall ability to take care of Spanish-speaking patients in clinic (n = 50) | 8.0 | 38.0 | 40.0 | 12.0 | 2.0 |
| Ability to take care of Spanish-speaking patients with use of telephone interpreter (n = 49) | 18.4 | 40.8 | 26.5 | 12.2 | 2.0 |
| Ability to take care of Spanish-speaking patients with use of in-person interpreter (n = 49) | 30.6 | 32.7 | 18.4 | 18.4 | 0 |

program telephone interpretation phase, which was similar to that in the initial telephone interpretation phase.

For the 8 individual questions, the differences among groups in the mean scores were similar to the differences in total satisfaction scores. Compared with the telephone interpretation phase, the individual scores of each satisfaction item were significantly improved at $P<.001$ during the resident education phase, similar to the total satisfaction score. When telephone interpretation was reintroduced, scores for each of the satisfaction items worsened and were not significantly different from the scores in the initial telephone interpretation phase, although "spending enough time" was slightly worse when telephone interpretation was reintroduced ($P=.02$).

## RESIDENT ASSESSMENT OF IN-PERSON INTERPRETER AS RESIDENT EDUCATOR

For the description of residents at baseline, all 50 residents completed the preprogram questionnaire; of these, 6% reported their ethnicity/race as Latino or part Latino, 74% as white, 10% as Asian, 8% as black, and 6% as other. The results of the survey that was completed by all of the residents before implementation of the program are presented in **Table 3**. Before implementation of the program, 18.4% of the residents rated use of the telephone interpreter as excellent, a figure that was unchanged at the end of the program. Although 30.6% of residents rated use of an in-person interpreter as an excellent preprogram, 71.4% rated use of an in-person interpreter as an excellent postprogram ($P=.02$).

At the conclusion of the resident education phase, potential benefits of the program were listed in the postprogram questionnaire, and residents were asked to rank the benefits. For the 49 residents responding, the most important benefits of an in-person interpreter were efficiency, convenience, and the ability to make patients feel comfortable, and 10.2% felt that the ability to elaborate on cultural values and home remedies was also important. Examples of statements supporting these benefits are listed in **Table 4**.

## COMMENT

This study demonstrates that an educational program that includes an interpreter with an interactive role in educating and providing feedback to residents improves satisfaction of Latino parents with LEP. To our knowledge, this is the first study that uses an interpreter as a resident educator and the first study to measure parent satisfaction after educating health care professionals about culture and the use of interpreters. As language barriers between patient and physician become more common in the United States, it is even more critical to develop ways beyond the traditional use of a trained professional interpreter to overcome the negative clinical consequences of these barriers.

This study shows that LEP, Spanish-speaking parents are most satisfied with medical care when an interpreter acts not only to translate words from one language to another but also to interpret cultural meanings for both the physician and the patient. This improvement in parent satisfaction is possibly a marker for improvement in communication between non–Spanish-speaking physicians and LEP, Spanish-speaking patients. Our results also suggest that patients are more satisfied with in-person interpretation compared with telephone interpretation. To our knowledge, no previous study has compared the use of in-person interpretation with telephone interpretation. Lee et al[20] have suggested that Spanish-speaking patients using telephone interpretation are more satisfied than patients who use ad hoc interpreters, possibly because telephone interpreters are unbiased third parties. In our study, LEP, Spanish-speaking patients who experienced an in-person interpreter who educated residents were even more satisfied with the physician than Latino patients who experienced a standard in-person interpreter, likely because health care professionals were better able to understand the patient and to treat the specific problem by eliminating cultural misunderstanding.

Our program attempts to eliminate problems associated with language barriers by teaching health care professionals how to work most effectively with interpreters and to use select Spanish phrases to establish rapport with their patients. In addition, the program teaches health care professionals about Latino cultural values to diminish cultural barriers. Our study suggests that a physician's ability to use an interpreter effectively and understand a parent's culture are important factors in parent satisfaction. An alternative explanation for the improvement in parent satisfaction when the interpreter acted as an educator is that the residents knew that they would be critiqued at the end of the visit and therefore spent more time with the parents. However, residents stated that they were unaware that the interpreter was evaluating them but thought that she was only acting in a helpful manner.

This program, which uses the interpreter as a resident educator, was well received by the residents. Interacting with the interpreter during educational sessions clarified common misunderstandings that occur between Latino patients and non–Spanish-speaking physicians and provided physicians with tools to communicate better with their patients. We also demonstrated that residents rated the use of in-person interpretation better after the program, likely because they learned skills that helped them use an in-person interpreter and because many residents had not previously used in-person interpretation.

This intervention is simple and effective at improving parent satisfaction. One other study demonstrated an improvement in patient satisfaction after a more extensive intervention. In a study by Mazor et al,[15] 9 pediatric emergency department physicians took an intensive 10-week Spanish course. Although patient satisfaction improved, problems with false fluency arise when physicians provide medical care in Spanish after a short language course.

Despite the strengths of the study, several limitations deserve mention. This was a small, single-site study with 1 Spanish interpreter, which may limit generalizability. The intervention conducted by the in-person interpreter, however, was relatively simple and could be taught to other interpreters. Because the same interpreter was used during the in-person interpretation phase and the cultural education of residents phase, the satisfaction scores could have been higher when she was also serving as cultural educator because of altered behavior toward the patients by the interpreter. To address this, the interpreter was instructed not to alter her behavior toward the patients and to strictly translate what the health care professional said. We believe that using the same interpreter is a strength of the study because we do not have to account for different interpreters being the source of differing satisfaction scores.

In addition, this study occurred sequentially during an 8-month period, and residents likely gained experience as physicians and in using interpreters. It is possible that parents in the resident education phase were more satisfied with care than parents in the standard in-person interpretation phase because the residents were 2 months further along in their training. On the other hand, in the subsequent telephone interpretation phase after the program, parents were less satisfied than either of the 2 phases in which in-person interpretation was used, suggesting that the presence of the in-person interpreter explained the improvement in parent satisfaction. Seasonal variation could also explain variations in satisfaction, since parent satisfaction may decrease during the busier months; however, the highest satisfaction scores occurred when the interpreter served as cultural

**Table 4. Most Important Benefits of In-Person Interpreter**

| Benefit | Residents Reporting Benefit as Most Important, % | Statement by Resident Explaining Quality |
|---|---|---|
| Efficiency and convenience | 42.9 | "It's really difficult when you're on the phone and there are so many delays and you feel like you have a finite amount of time because you're on the phone. So you basically have to run through everything in your mind immediately. And then, you get off the phone and all of a sudden you remember, Oh, yeah, I have this to ask and great, I don't have an interpreter anymore." |
| Makes patients comfortable | 26.5 | "For the patients,. . .culturally, I think they like having somebody who they can relate to in their own language and who kind of understands some of where they're coming from better than any of us would." |
| Ability to elaborate on cultural values and home remedies | 10.2 | One resident stated that the interpreter was helpful when she said, "Well, they went to a healer. Sometimes in this country, that means a curandero who provides herbal remedies." |

educator during October and November, which are typically busy months. The parent satisfaction scores for the 2 telephone interpretation phases, which occurred from May to June and then from December to February, were not significantly different, suggesting that the satisfaction scores were not affected by the season.

A further potential bias may be that the proportion of LEP, Spanish-speaking patients seeing second- or third-year residents was significantly greater in the 2 telephone interpretation phases compared with the 2 in-person interpretation phases. During the 2 telephone interpretation phases, the satisfaction scores were worse than for the in-person interpretation phases even though the residents were more experienced. Although it may seem to be a limitation that the residents' level of training was not the same among groups, no studies to our knowledge have demonstrated a difference in patient satisfaction based on the year of the resident. In addition, although the mean satisfaction scores were significantly highest when the in-person interpreter was a resident educator, further studies are needed to determine the clinical significance of these results.

In summary, we have demonstrated that a unique intervention in which an interpreter also provides education on cultural and language issues to residents improves the satisfaction of LEP, Spanish-speaking parents. Native Spanish-speaking interpreters not only have the linguistic resources to make communication possible but also possess insights into cultural subtleties that can be taught to health care professionals as they interact with their patients. Wider application of this intervention has the potential to contribute to improvements in health care of LEP, Spanish-speaking patients.

**Accepted for Publication:** July 14, 2006.
**Correspondence:** Ann Chen Wu, MD, Department of Ambulatory Care and Prevention, 133 Brookline Ave, Sixth Floor, Boston, MA 02215-5301 (ann.wu@childrens.harvard.edu).

**Author Contributions:** Dr Wu, the principal investigator, had full access to all of the data in the study and takes responsibility for the integrity of the data and the accuracy of the data analysis. *Study concept and design:* Wu, Leventhal, and Forsyth. *Acquisition of data:* Wu, Ortiz, and Gonzalez. *Analysis and interpretation of data:* Wu and Forsyth. *Drafting of the manuscript:* Wu. *Critical revision of the manuscript for important intellectual content:* Wu, Leventhal, Ortiz, Gonzalez, and Forsyth. *Statistical analysis:* Wu. *Obtained funding:* Wu. *Administrative, technical, and material support:* Ortiz and Gonzalez. *Study supervision:* Wu, Leventhal, and Forsyth.

**Financial Disclosure:** None reported.

**Funding/Support:** This study was supported by the Connecticut Health Foundation, Friends of the Yale-New Haven Children's Hospital, American Medical Association, United Illuminating, and Swindells Charitable Foundation.

**Acknowledgment:** We thank Cathi Kroon, MS, from the Office of Interpreter Services at Yale-New Haven Hospital, for technical advice and providing trained interpreters for the study and Diana Edmonds for administrative support.

## REFERENCES

1. Flores G, Fuentes-Afflick E, Barbot O, et al. The health of Latino children: urgent priorities, unanswered questions, and a research agenda. *JAMA.* 2002;288:82-90.
2. Sarver J, Baker DW. Effect of language barriers on follow-up appointments after an emergency department visit. *J Gen Intern Med.* 2000;15:256-264.
3. Hampers LC, Cha S, Gutglass DJ, Binns HJ, Krug SE. Language barriers and resource utilization in a pediatric emergency department. *Pediatrics.* 1999;103:1253-1256.
4. Carrasquillo O, Orav EJ, Brennan TA, Burstin HR. Impact of language barriers on patient satisfaction in an emergency department. *J Gen Intern Med.* 1999;14:82-87.
5. Mosen DM, Carlson MJ, Morales LS, Hanes PP. Satisfaction with provider communication among Spanish-speaking Medicaid enrollees. *Ambul Pediatr.* 2004;4:500-504.
6. Fiscella K, Franks P, Doescher MP, Saver BG. Disparities in health care by race, ethnicity, and language among the insured. *Med Care.* 2002;40:52-59.
7. David RA, Rhee M. The impact of language as a barrier to effective health care in an underserved urban Hispanic community. *Mt Sinai J Med.* 1998;65:393-397.
8. Cohen AL, Rivara F, Marcuse EK, McPhillips H, Davis R. Are language barriers associated with serious medical events in hospitalized pediatric patients? *Pediatrics.* 2005;116:575-579.
9. Cohen AL, Christakis DA. Primary language of parent is associated with disparities in pediatric preventive care. *J Pediatr.* 2006;148:254-258.
10. Tucker CM, Herman KC, Pedersen TR, et al. Cultural sensitivity in physician-patient relationships. *Med Care.* 2003;41:859-870.
11. Flores G, Abreu M, Schwartz I, Hill M. The importance of language and culture in pediatric care: case studies from the Latino community. *J Pediatr.* 2000;137:842-848.
12. Pachter LM. Culture and clinical care: folk illness beliefs and behaviors and their implications for health care delivery. *JAMA.* 1994;271:690-694.
13. Kleinman A, Eisenberg L, Good B. Culture, illness, and care: clinical lessons from anthropologic and cross-cultural research. *Ann Intern Med.* 1978;88:251-258.
14. Flores G. The impact of medical interpreter services on the quality of health care: a systematic review. *Med Care Res Rev.* 2005;62:255-299.
15. Mazor SS, Hampers LC, Chande VT, Krug SE. Teaching Spanish to pediatric emergency physicians: effects on patient satisfaction. *Arch Pediatr Adolesc Med.* 2002;156:693-695.
16. Flores G. Dolor aqui? fiebre?: a little knowledge requires caution. *Arch Pediatr Adolesc Med.* 2002;156:638-640.
17. Baker DW, Hayes R, Fortier JP. Interpreter use and satisfaction with interpersonal aspects of care for Spanish-speaking patients. *Med Care.* 1998;36:1461-1470.
18. Haffner L. Translation is not enough: interpreting in a medical setting. *West J Med.* 1992;157:255-259.
19. Burbano O'Leary SC, Federico S, Hampers LC. The truth about language barriers: one residency program's experience. *Pediatrics.* 2003;111:e569-e573.
20. Lee LJ, Bata HA, Maselli JH. Effect of Spanish interpretation method on patient satisfaction in an urban walk-in clinic. *J Gen Intern Med.* 2002;17:640-645.
21. Kuo D, Fagan MJ. Satisfaction with methods of Spanish interpretation in an ambulatory care clinic. *J Gen Intern Med.* 1999;14:547-550.

# Public Opinion on Sex Education in US Schools

*Amy Bleakley, PhD, MPH; Michael Hennessy, PhD, MPH; Martin Fishbein, PhD*

**Objective:** To examine US public opinion on sex education in schools to determine how the public's preferences align with those of policymakers and research scientists.

**Design:** Cross-sectional survey.

**Setting:** July 2005 through January 2006.

**Participants:** Randomly selected nationally representative sample of US adults aged 18 to 83 years (N = 1096).

**Main Outcome Measures:** Support for 3 different types of sex education in schools: abstinence only, comprehensive sex education, and condom instruction.

**Results:** Approximately 82% of respondents indicated support for programs that teach students about both abstinence and other methods of preventing pregnancy and sexually transmitted diseases. Similarly, 68.5% supported teaching how to properly use condoms. Abstinence-only education programs, in contrast, received the lowest levels of support (36%) and the highest level of opposition (about 50%) across the 3 program options. Self-identified conservative, liberal, and moderate respondents all supported abstinence-plus programs, although the extent of support varied significantly.

**Conclusions:** Our results indicate that US adults, regardless of political ideology, favor a more balanced approach to sex education compared with the abstinence-only programs funded by the federal government. In summary, abstinence-only programs, while a priority of the federal government, are supported by neither a majority of the public nor the scientific community.

*Arch Pediatr Adolesc Med. 2006;160:1151-1156*

THE SOCIAL MERITS AND PRACtical efficacy of sex education in schools generate considerable debate among public health professionals and government officials. The choice of appropriate and effective sex education policies is critical, as human immunodeficiency virus (HIV) infection and AIDS increased by 10% from 2000 to 2003 among 15- to 24-year-olds in the United States.[1] In addition, this age group acquires half of all new sexually transmitted disease (STD) infections, but represents only about 25% of the sexually active population.[2] Direct medical costs associated with the 9 million STD infections, including HIV, among this age group in 2000 were estimated at \$6.5 billion, which is likely an underestimate.[3] Although teen pregnancy, birth, and abortion rates declined in recent years, rates in the United States are persistently higher compared with other developed countries.[1,4,5] Epidemiological data suggest that by 15 years of age, 25.1% of youth have had vaginal sex, and this figure increases to 37.5% at 16 years of age, and 46.9% by 17 years of age.[1] These data underscore the relevance of timely and informative sex education in middle and high schools as an important component to the public health goal of promoting safe behaviors and preventing additional infections and unintended pregnancies.

*For editorial comment see page 1182*

At the core of the federal government's response to sexual activity and STD and HIV rates among youth is abstinence-only education. Federal requirements for abstinence-only education programs focus on the promotion of abstinence until marriage (ie, postponing sexual intercourse) as a lifestyle choice (ie, "a mutually monogamous relationship in the context of marriage is the expected standard").[6] Abstinence is endorsed as "the only certain way to avoid out-of-wedlock pregnancy, sexually transmitted diseases, and other associated health problems."[6] Implementation of federally funded programs precludes mentioning contraception and other forms of birth control or protection, such as condoms, unless it is to mention their limitations (eg, failure rates).

For abstinence-only education, the federal government identified 8 requirements or central program components.

**Author Affiliations:** Annenberg Public Policy Center, Annenberg School for Communication, University of Pennsylvania, Philadelphia.

Originally articulated in Section 510 of Title V of the Social Security Act of 1996,[6] and highlighted in a recent review of abstinence policies by Santelli and colleagues,[7] abstinence education is a program which:

1. as its exclusive purpose, teaches the social, psychological, and health gains to be realized by abstaining from sexual activity;
2. teaches abstinence from sexual activity outside marriage as the expected standard for all school-age children;
3. teaches that abstinence from sexual activity is the only certain way to avoid out-of-wedlock pregnancy, STDs, and other associated health problems;
4. teaches that a mutually faithful monogamous relationship in the context of marriage is the expected standard of human sexual activity;
5. teaches that sexual activity outside of the context of marriage is likely to have harmful psychological and physical effects;
6. teaches that bearing children out of wedlock is likely to have harmful consequences for the child, the child's parents, and society;
7. teaches young people how to reject sexual advances and how alcohol and drug use increases vulnerability to sexual advances; and
8. teaches the importance of attaining self-sufficiency before engaging in sexual activity.

There are 3 federal funding sources for abstinence-only education: the Adolescent and Family Life Act (AFLA), Section 510 of the Welfare Reform Act in 1996, and Community-Based Abstinence Education through Special Programs of Regional and National Significance (SPRANS). Support for abstinence-only education began in 1981 through AFLA; in fiscal year 2005, AFLA dollars represented only 7.8% of the total dollars spent ($167 million) on abstinence funding. Section 510 funding started in 1996 and gives (since 1998) $50 million a year to states. It requires states to match $3 for every $4 of federal funding, and the act explicitly identifies the 8 requirements of abstinence-only education funded under Section 510, AFLA, and SPRANS. If a state accepts federal funds, nonfederal funds are also subject to the federal restrictions on providing information on contraception. Funding through SPRANS, created in 2001, goes directly to community-based organizations and other agencies, including faith-based organizations. In contrast to Section 510 funds that originally allowed for more flexibility in content, programs that receive SPRANS funding are obligated to teach all 8 of the aforementioned components. The SPRANS dollars for abstinence-only education increased from $20 million in fiscal year 2001 to $104 million in fiscal year 2005.

The number of studies evaluating abstinence-only education is few compared with those assessing more comprehensive approaches. A recent review of abstinence-only programs concluded "there do not currently exist any abstinence-only programs with strong evidence that they either delay sex or reduce teen pregnancy."[8] Reasons often cited for the lack of more rigorous evaluations of abstinence-only education, as well as school-based education programs in general, include cost, a social environment in which research on sex is often seen as controversial, and a "prejudice" against messages that only emphasize abstinence.[9-11] However, a randomized controlled trial of an abstinence intervention demonstrated promising effects for delaying sex in the short-term (ie, 3 months postintervention), but those effects disappeared by 6 months.[12] Another recent study found that adolescents who took virginity pledges—public commitments to remain abstinent until marriage—experienced a delayed sexual debut but reported lower frequency of condom use at first intercourse. Pledgers were more likely to substitute oral and/or anal sex for vaginal sex, and had the same rates of STDs as nonpledgers.[13]

Abstinence-plus programs (also referred to as comprehensive sex education) emphasize abstinence and a delay of sexual debut but also offer information on contraception and protection against STDs. These programs may or may not include instruction on how to properly use a condom. Systematic reviews of empirical studies on sex education efficacy provide evidence that support a more balanced approach (ie, comprehensive sex education). These reviews suggest that comprehensive programs may delay initiation of sexual intercourse, reduce frequency of sex, reduce frequency of unprotected sex, and reduce the number of sexual partners.[8,11,14,15] Based on this evidence, an Institute of Medicine report in 2001 recommended "eliminating congressional, federal, state, and local requirements that public funds be used for abstinence-only education, and that states and local school districts implement and continue to support age-appropriate comprehensive sex education and condom availability programs in schools."[10]

Public opinion on sex education in schools is, however, largely absent from discourse on this issue, as few studies report on what types of sex education the public supports.[16-18] This study examines public opinion on sex education in schools to determine how the public's preferences align with those of policymakers and research scientists. Using a nationally representative sample of adults, this study describes levels of support among the public for the different sex education approaches.

## METHODS

The Annenberg National Health Communication Survey is a nationally representative, repeated cross-sectional survey with a sample universe of all people aged 18 years and older living in the United States.[19] The online survey is administered by a survey research firm that uses a list-assisted random-digit-dialing telephone method to provide a probability-based starting sample of US telephone-accessible households. The recruited panel members are provided with free Web access and a WebTV set-top box that uses a telephone line to connect to the Internet and the television as a monitor to enable their participation in Internet surveys. The provision of identical hardware to all participating households allows for consistent delivery of the survey content and does not bias the sample in favor of current Internet users or computer owners. The Web-enabled panel closely tracks the US population on age, race, Hispanic ethnicity, geographical region, employment status, and other demographic elements. The differences that do exist are small and are corrected statistically in survey data (ie, by nonresponse adjustments).

Each month a sample for the Annenberg National Health Communication Survey is drawn from the firm's participating households. The current study used data collected from July

**Table 1. Frequencies and Means for Beliefs About Sex Education Programs***

| Beliefs About Sex Education Programs | Strongly Disagree, % | Somewhat Disagree, % | No Opinion, % | Somewhat Agree, % | Strongly Agree, % | Mean ± SD |
|---|---|---|---|---|---|---|
| Abstinence-only education is an effective way to prevent unplanned pregnancy and sexually transmitted diseases. | 29.8 | 24.7 | 6.4 | 22.9 | 16.2 | −.292 ± 1.49 |
| Sex education that teaches about abstinence and other methods of preventing pregnancy is an effective way to prevent unplanned pregnancy and sexually transmitted diseases. | 6.3 | 8.7 | 4.6 | 43.6 | 36.9 | .961 ± 1.15 |
| Teaching teens how to properly use a condom encourages them to have sex. | 23.8 | 33.1 | 6.0 | 23.5 | 13.5 | −.302 ± 1.40 |

*N = 1096.

2005 through January 2006. Rates of completion of the Annenberg National Health Communication Survey range from 73% to 76%. The survey features a core set of items answered by the entire sample as well as modules randomly assigned to half the sample. The variables used in this analysis were part of the noncore modules and resulted in a total sample of 1096 respondents. Data were collected on sex education policy preferences, beliefs regarding sex education programs, political ideology, and frequency of attendance at religious services. The primary variables of interest were the beliefs and policy preferences about sex education; ideology and attendance at religious services were treated as background characteristics.

To justify pooling the data across months, we conducted equivalency tests on the means, variances, and covariances of the belief and policy preference variables. Fit statistics, assuming no difference between months, were consistent with the assumption of no change over time: $\chi^2=26.143$, $P=.35$; root-mean-squared error of approximation = 0.009; and Tucker-Lewis Index = 0.996. For information on these types of goodness-of-fit indices, see Kline.[20]

## POLICY PREFERENCES

Three measures assessed policy preferences for sex education in schools by using a 5-point scale (from −2 to 2) from strongly oppose to strongly support. The measures each represented a different type of sex education: abstinence only, abstinence plus (ie, comprehensive sex education), and comprehensive sex education that includes condom instruction. The survey items were as follows: "Do you support or oppose sex education programs in schools in your community that teach abstinence only? Abstinence-only education promotes abstinence until marriage and does not teach students about other methods of preventing pregnancy and sexually transmitted diseases," "Do you support or oppose sex education programs in schools in your community that teach students about other methods of preventing pregnancy and sexually transmitted diseases in addition to teaching about abstinence?", and "Do you support or oppose sex education programs in schools in your community that include instruction on how to use condoms properly to prevent pregnancy and sexually transmitted diseases?"

## BELIEFS

Respondents were also asked about their beliefs or expectations about the educational efficacy of different sex education approaches. They answered 3 items regarding their beliefs on sex education (disagree to agree, −2 to 2): "Abstinence-only education is an effective way of preventing teens from having unplanned pregnancies," "Sex education that teaches about abstinence and other methods of preventing pregnancy is an effective way of preventing teens from having unplanned pregnancies," and "Teaching teens how to properly use a condom encourages them to have sex."

## BACKGROUND CHARACTERISTICS

Self-reported political ideology was measured on a 7-point scale from "extremely liberal" to "extremely conservative," with moderates at the midpoint. For the purposes of analysis, it was collapsed into 3 groups: liberals, moderates, and conservatives. Attendance at religious services, often used as an indicator of religiosity, was a 6-level ordinal estimate of attending religious services ranging from "never" to "more than once a week."

## SAMPLE DESCRIPTION

The mean age of the sample was 46.8 years (±15.94; range, 18-83 years) and 46% of the sample were male adults. The race/ethnicity distribution was consistent with other nationally representative surveys. According to the 2000 Census, 72.0% of adults aged 18 years or older were white, non-Hispanic; 11.2% were African American, non-Hispanic; 11.0% were Hispanic (all races); and 4.5% were classified as other, non-Hispanic (1.3% were classified as 2 or more races).[21] Race and ethnicity estimates from our survey were as follows: 78.7% white, non-Hispanic; 9.6% black, non-Hispanic; 7.6% Hispanic; and 4.1% other, non-Hispanic. Politically, 39.5% of the sample identified themselves as moderate, 35.5% as conservative, and 25% as liberal. This distribution is also consistent with self-reported ideological identification in several national surveys.[22,23] Respondents attended religious services with the following frequency: 20.4% never, 16.5% once a year or less, 20.6% a few times a year, 10.6% once or twice a month, 21.4% once a week, and 10.6% more than once a week.

# RESULTS

## BELIEFS REGARDING SEX EDUCATION PROGRAMS

**Table 1** shows the distribution of beliefs regarding sex education programs. In general, the majority of respondents disagreed with the beliefs that abstinence-only programs were effective in preventing unplanned pregnancies and that teaching condom instruction encourages teens to have sex. Thirty-nine percent of respondents agreed that abstinence only was an effective way to prevent unplanned pregnancies, whereas 80.4% believed a

**Table 2. Frequencies and Means for Policy Preferences for Sex Education Programs***

| Sex Education Policy Preferences | Strongly Oppose, % | Somewhat Oppose, % | No Opinion, % | Somewhat Support, % | Strongly Support, % | Mean ± SD |
|---|---|---|---|---|---|---|
| Support or oppose abstinence only? | 18.8 | 31.9 | 13.1 | 20.9 | 15.3 | -.180 ± 1.36 |
| Support or oppose teaching other methods of preventing pregnancy and sexually transmitted diseases in addition to teaching about abstinence? | 3.3 | 6.5 | 8.1 | 43.6 | 38.5 | 1.08 ± 1.01 |
| Support or oppose instruction on how to use condoms properly? | 7.7 | 13.2 | 10.8 | 41.3 | 27.0 | .668 ± 1.22 |

*N = 1096.

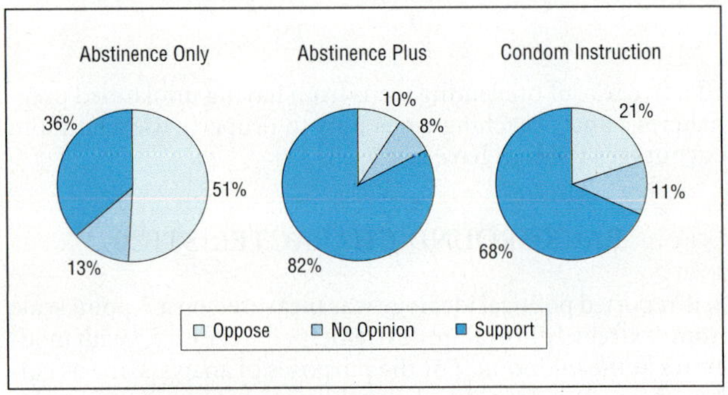

**Figure 1.** Policy preferences for sex education approaches.

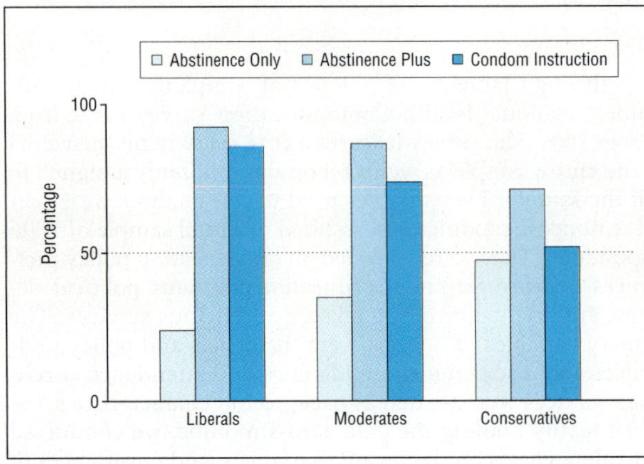

**Figure 2.** Percentage of support for sex education programs by political ideology.

combination of abstinence and other methods was effective. Fifty-seven percent disagreed that teaching teens how to use a condom encourages them to have sex. There were no differences between men and women on 2 of the 3 belief measures. Women reported significantly stronger disagreement with the belief that abstinence-only education is an effective way of preventing unplanned pregnancies (female mean: −0.400 ± 1.50; male mean: −0.167 ± 1.47; $t = -2.585$; $P < .01$).

## POLICY PREFERENCES FOR SEX EDUCATION PROGRAMS

The distribution for policy preferences is similar to that of the corresponding beliefs (**Table 2**). **Figure 1** depicts support and opposition for abstinence-only education, abstinence-plus education, and condom instruction. As shown, approximately 82% of respondents indicated support for programs that teach students about both abstinence and other methods of preventing pregnancy and STDs. Similarly, about 68% supported teaching how to properly use condoms. Abstinence-only education programs, in contrast, received the lowest levels of support (36%) and the highest level of opposition (about 50%) across the 3 program options. Only about 10% of the sample opposed comprehensive sex education, and 21% opposed condom instruction. Women also showed more opposition to abstinence-only policies (female mean: −0.233 ± 1.38; male mean: −0.118 ± 1.34; $t = 2.018$; $P < .05$).

## POLICY PREFERENCES FOR SEX EDUCATION PROGRAMS BY IDEOLOGY AND RELIGION

**Figure 2** presents support for sex education programs by political ideology. Support for abstinence-plus programs and condom instruction is greater than 50% across all ideologies. Self-identified conservative, liberal, and moderate respondents all supported abstinence-plus programs, although the extent of support varied significantly. Seventy percent of conservatives supported abstinence plus, compared with 86.4% of moderates and 91.6% of liberals ($F2 = 78.86$; $P < .01$). More conservatives supported condom instruction in schools (51.2%) than supported abstinence-only education (47%), and conservatives opposed abstinence-only programs (39.9%) at approximately the same rate as they opposed condom instruction (37.5%). Opposition to condom instruction among liberals (9.1%) and moderates (13.4%) was much lower than opposition among conservatives. Nineteen percent of conservatives opposed abstinence-plus education, compared with 5.3% of moderates and 3.7% of liberals. Sixty-seven percent of liberals and 50.4% of moderates opposed abstinence only.

Differences in policy support by attendance at religious services were also assessed (**Figure 3**). Abstinence plus was supported by all religious attendance groups, with levels of support ranging from 87.4% among those who reported never attending religious services to 60.3% among those who attend more than once a week ($F5 = 16.46$; $P < .01$). Condom instruction was also supported by a majority across all groups, with the exception of those who attend services more than once a week (37.9%); opposition to condom instruction in this group was 52.6% ($F5 = 35.19$; $P < .01$). It is interesting to note that among the most religious respondents (ie, those who attend services more than once a week), abstinence only and abstinence plus received equivalent levels of support (60.3%). Opposition to abstinence-only programs was lowest for those who attended services more than once a week (31.3%) and at its highest (57.9%) among those who never attend religious services.

## COMMENT

It appears that current investments in abstinence-only sex education programs do not correspond with either public opinion or scientific consensus on how sex education should be taught in schools. Our results demonstrated that American adults, regardless of political ideology, favor a more balanced approach to sex education compared with the abstinence-only programs funded by the federal government. Abstinence-only education received the lowest levels of public support and the highest levels of public opposition; more respondents supported teaching adolescents how to properly use a condom than teaching only about abstinence. This finding is consistent with respondents' beliefs about the efficacy of different sex education approaches: 39% agreed that abstinence only was an effective way to reduce unplanned teenage pregnancies.

The federal government's support of abstinence-only education is in contrast to the broad public and scientific support for comprehensive sex education demonstrated by our research review and study results. This discrepancy in the realm of sex education highlights a gap between science and policy.[24] Sex education in schools is clearly a politically charged issue, but public opinion in this instance offers an opportunity to diffuse some of the inherent tension between science and policymaking. Our data indicated that among politically conservative respondents, support for comprehensive sex education was at 70%, compared with 47% support for abstinence-only education. With such high support for comprehensive sex education among the public from liberals, conservatives, and moderates alike, political leaders could capitalize on this rare occasion to enact public policy that is supported by both sound scientific evidence as well as public opinion.

Moving beyond the politics of sex education might also require reframing the issues. For example, Santelli and colleagues[7] discussed abstinence-only programs in a human-rights context, citing the deprivation of scientifically accurate information as unethical. Their position, supported by the Society for Adolescent Medicine and the American College Health Association,[25] is provocative insofar as it shifts the debate to focus on the more compelling theme of the strategic provision and withholding of information.

There are several limitations to this analysis. The sample universe is landline telephone subscribers and therefore does not include those who rely solely on cellular telephones. Telephone subscribership in the United States penetrated 92.4% of households as of March 2005; about 6% of households, mostly younger and single Americans, rely only on wireless service.[26] It is also possible that, because of question wording, respondents did not fully appreciate the extent of differences between abstinence-only and abstinence-plus education. The results however are consistent with the assumption that citizens have a basic understanding of the sex education options: liberals and conservatives differ significantly in the extent of their support. In addition, study findings of overall support for comprehensive sex education are also consistent with results from similar studies.[16-18]

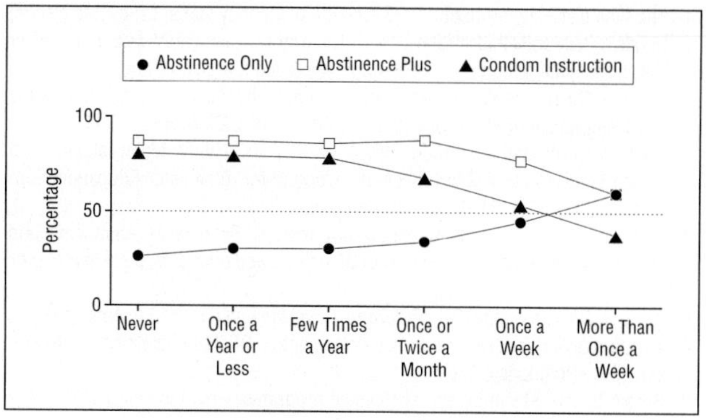


**Figure 3.** Percentage of support for sex education programs by attendance at religious services.

In summary, public opinion favors comprehensive sex education. Abstinence-only programs, while a priority of the federal government, are supported by neither a majority of the public nor the scientific community. The public at large, across the ideological spectrum, supports programs that teach a combination of abstinence and other methods to prevent unplanned pregnancies and STDs.

**Accepted for Publication:** May 28, 2006.

**Correspondence:** Amy Bleakley, PhD, MPH, Annenberg Public Policy Center, Annenberg School for Communication, University of Pennsylvania, 3620 Walnut St, Philadelphia, PA 19104 (ableakley@asc.upenn.edu).

**Author Contributions:** *Study concept and design:* Bleakley, Hennessy, and Fishbein. *Analysis and interpretation of data:* Bleakley and Hennessy. *Drafting of the manuscript:* Bleakley and Hennessy. *Critical revision of the manuscript for important intellectual content:* Bleakley, Hennessy, and Fishbein. *Statistical analysis:* Bleakley and Hennessy. *Study supervision:* Fishbein.

**Financial Disclosure:** None reported.

**Acknowledgment:** The authors would like to thank the Annenberg School for Communication and the Annenberg Foundation Trust at Sunnylands for their generous support of the Annenberg National Health Communication Survey.

## REFERENCES


1. Centers for Disease Control and Prevention. *HIV/AIDS Surveillance Report, 2003.* Vol 15. Atlanta, Ga: US Dept of Health and Human Services, Centers for Disease Control and Prevention; 2004.
2. Mosher W, Chandra A, Jones J. *Sexual Behavior and Selected Health Measures: Men and Women 15-44 Years of Age, United States, 2002. Advance Data From Vital and Health Statistics; No. 362.* Hyattsville, Md: National Center for Health Statistics; 2005.
3. Chesson HW, Blandford J, Gift T, Tao G, Irwin K. The estimated direct medical costs of sexually transmitted diseases among American youth, 2000. *Perspect Sex Reprod Health.* 2004;36:11-19.

4. The Alan Guttmacher Institute. US teenage pregnancy statistics: overall trends, trends by race and ethnicity and state-by-state information. http://www.guttmacher.org/pubs/state_pregnancy_trends.pdf. Accessed March 8, 2005.
5. Singh S, Darroch J. Adolescent pregnancy and childbearing: levels and trends in developed countries. *Fam Plann Perspect.* 2000;32:14-23.
6. Social Security Administration. Social Security Act: Title V: Maternal and Child Health Services Black Grant. Separate Program for Abstinence Education, Section 510 [42 U.S.C. 710].
7. Santelli J, Ott M, Lyon M, Rogers J, Summers D, Schleifer R. Abstinence and abstinence-only education: a review of US policies and programs. *J Adolesc Health.* 2006;38:72-81.
8. Kirby D. *Do Abstinence-Only Programs Delay the Initiation of Sex Among Young People and Reduce Teen Pregnancy?* Washington, DC: National Campaign to Prevent Teen Pregnancy; 2002.
9. Brown S. Sex education and abstinence programs: why don't we know more? *Child Youth Serv Rev.* 1997;19:455-463.
10. Institute of Medicine. *No Time to Lose: Getting More From HIV Prevention.* Washington, DC: National Academy Press; 2001.
11. Eng TR, Butler WT, eds. *The Hidden Epidemic: Confronting Sexually Transmitted Diseases.* Washington, DC: National Academy Press; 1997.
12. Jemmott JB III, Jemmott LS, Fong GT. Abstinence and safer sex HIV risk-reduction interventions for African American adolescents: a randomized controlled trial. *JAMA.* 1998;279:1529-1536.
13. Bruckner H, Bearman P. After the promise: the STD consequences of adolescent virginity pledges. *J Adolesc Health.* 2005;36:271-278.
14. Kirby D. *Emerging Answers: Research Findings on Programs to Reduce Teen Pregnancy (Summary).* Washington, DC: National Campaign to Prevent Teen Pregnancy; 2001.
15. Manlove J, Papillio A, Ikramullah E. *Not Yet: Programs to Delay First Sex Among Teens.* Washington, DC: National Campaign to Prevent Tenn Pregnancy; 2004.
16. Albert B. *American Opinion on Teen Pregnancy and Related Issues 2003.* Washington, DC: National Campaign to Prevent Teen Pregnancy; 2004.
17. Harris Interactive Inc. Majorities of US adults do not believe abstinence programs are effective in preventing or reducing HIV/AIDS, unwanted pregnancies or extra-marital sex. *The Harris Poll #2.* http://www.harrisinteractive.com/news/allnewsbydate.asp?NewsID=1013. Accessed March 8, 2006.
18. NPR/Kaiser/Kennedy School Poll. Sex education in America. http://www.kff.org/newsmedia/upload/Sex-Education-in-America-Summary.pdf. Accessed March 8, 2005.
19. Knowledge Networks. *Field Report: Annenberg National Health Communication Survey 2005.* Prepared for the Annenberg School for Communication. Menlo Park, Calif; 2006.
20. Kline R. *Principles and Practice of Structural Equation Modeling.* New York, NY: Guilford; 2004.
21. Census Bureau. Population by race and Hispanic or Latino origin for the United States: 1990 and 2000. http://www.census.gov/population/cen2000/phc-t1/tab01.pdf. Accessed March 28, 2006.
22. Romer D, Kenski K, Winneg K, Adasiewicz C, Jamieson K. *Capturing Campaign Dynamics, 2000 and 2004: The National Annenberg Election Survey.* Philadelphia: University of Pennsylvania Press; 2006.
23. The ANES guide to public opinion and electoral behavior. The American National Election Studies. http://www.umich.edu/~nes/nesguide/text/tab3_1.txt. Accessed February 22, 2006.
24. Brownson RC, Royer C, Ewing R, McBride TD. Researchers and policymakers: travelers in parallel universes. *Am J Prev Med.* 2006;30:164-172.
25. Santelli J, Ott M. Abstinence-only education policies and programs: a position paper of the Society for Adolescent Medicine. *J Adolesc Health.* 2006;38:83-87.
26. Belinfante A. Telephone subscribership in the United States. Federal Communications Commission. http://www.fcc.gov/Bureaus/Common_Carrier/Reports/FCC-State_Link/IAD/subs0305.pdf. Accessed May 8, 2006.

### *Announcement*

**Trial Registration Required.** In concert with the International Committee of Medical Journal Editors (ICMJE), *Archives of Pediatrics and Adolescent Medicine* will require, as a condition of consideration for publication, registration of all trials in a public trials registry (such as http://ClinicalTrials.gov). Trials must be registered at or before the onset of patient enrollment. This policy applies to any clinical trial starting enrollment after July 1, 2005. For trials that began enrollment before this date, registration will be required by September 13, 2005, before considering the trial for publication. The trial registration number should be supplied at the time of submission.

For details about this new policy, and for information on how the ICMJE defines a clinical trial, see the editorials by DeAngelis et al in the September 8, 2004 (2004;292:1363-1364) and June 15, 2005 (2005;293:2927-2929) issues of *JAMA*. Also see the Instructions to Authors on our Web site: www.archpediatrics.com.

**PEDIARIX® [Diphtheria and Tetanus Toxoids and Acellular Pertussis Adsorbed, Hepatitis B (Recombinant) and Inactivated Poliovirus Vaccine Combined]**

The following is a brief summary only; see full prescribing information for complete product information.

**CONTRAINDICATIONS:** Hypersensitivity to any component of the vaccine, including yeast, neomycin, and polymyxin B, is a contraindication (see DESCRIPTION in complete prescribing information). Do not use PEDIARIX after a serious allergic reaction (e.g., anaphylaxis) temporally associated with a previous dose of this vaccine or with any components of this vaccine. Because of the uncertainty as to which component of the vaccine might be responsible, do not give further vaccination with any of these components; or, refer such individuals to an allergist for evaluation. The following events are contraindications to administration of PEDIARIX: encephalopathy (e.g., coma, decreased level of consciousness, prolonged seizures) within 7 days of administration of a previous dose of a pertussis-containing vaccine that is not attributable to another identifiable cause; progressive neurologic disorder, including infantile spasms, uncontrolled epilepsy, or progressive encephalopathy. Do not vaccinate individuals with these conditions until a treatment regimen has been established and the condition has stabilized.

**WARNINGS:** Administration of PEDIARIX is associated with higher rates of fever relative to separately administered vaccines. In a safety study that evaluated medically attended fever after PEDIARIX or separately administered vaccines when coadministered with 7-valent pneumococcal and Hib conjugate vaccines, infants who received PEDIARIX had a higher rate of medical encounters for fever within the first 4 days following the first vaccination. In some infants, these encounters included the performance of diagnostic studies to evaluate other causes of fever (see ADVERSE REACTIONS). The tip cap and the rubber plunger of the needleless prefilled syringes contain dry natural latex rubber that may cause allergic reactions in latex sensitive individuals. The vial stopper is latex-free. If any of the following events occur in temporal relation to receipt of DTwP or a vaccine containing an acellular pertussis component, consider carefully whether to give any pertussis vaccine, including PEDIARIX: temperature of ≥40.5°C (105°F) within 48 hours not due to another identifiable cause; collapse or shock-like state (hypotonic-hyporesponsive episode) within 48 hours; persistent, inconsolable crying lasting ≥3 hours, occurring within 48 hours; seizures with or without fever occurring within 3 days. If Guillain-Barré syndrome occurs within 6 weeks of receipt of prior vaccine containing tetanus toxoid, the decision to give any tetanus toxoid-containing vaccine, including PEDIARIX, should be based on careful consideration of the potential benefits and possible risks. If tetanus toxoid is withheld, other available vaccines should be given, as indicated. The decision to administer a pertussis-containing vaccine to individuals with stable central nervous system (CNS) disorders must be made by the physician on an individual basis, with consideration of all relevant factors, and assessment of potential risks and benefits for that individual. Advise the parent or guardian of the potential increased risk involved (see PRECAUTIONS). For children at higher risk for seizures than the general population, an appropriate antipyretic may be administered at the time of vaccination and for the ensuing 24 hours according to the respective prescribing information recommended dosage to reduce the possibility of post-vaccination fever. The ACIP has published guidelines for vaccination of persons with recent or acute illness (www.cdc.gov/nip).

**PRECAUTIONS:** PEDIARIX should be given with caution in children with bleeding disorders such as hemophilia or thrombocytopenia and in children on anticoagulant therapy, with steps taken to avoid the risk of hematoma following the injection. Before the injection of any biological, the physician should take all reasonable precautions to prevent allergic or other adverse reactions. Epinephrine injection (1:1,000) and other appropriate agents used for the control of immediate allergic reactions must be immediately available should an acute anaphylactic reaction occur. Immunosuppressed individuals, including those receiving immunosuppressive therapy, may not develop the expected immune response. The ACIP has published guidelines for vaccination of persons on such therapies (www.cdc.gov/nip). **Drug Interactions:** For information regarding concomitant administration with other vaccines, refer to DOSAGE AND ADMINISTRATION in complete prescribing information. Do not mix PEDIARIX with any other vaccine in the same syringe or vial. **Carcinogenesis, Mutagenesis, Impairment of Fertility:** PEDIARIX has not been evaluated for carcinogenic or mutagenic potential, or for impairment of fertility. **Pregnancy:** Pregnancy Category C: PEDIARIX is not indicated for women of child-bearing age. Animal reproduction studies have not been conducted with PEDIARIX. It is not known whether PEDIARIX can cause fetal harm when administered to a pregnant woman or if PEDIARIX can affect reproductive capacity. **Geriatric Use:** PEDIARIX is not indicated for use in adult populations. **Pediatric Use:** Safety and effectiveness of PEDIARIX in infants younger than 6 weeks of age have not been evaluated. PEDIARIX is not recommended for persons 7 years of age or older.

**ADVERSE REACTIONS:** A total of 23,849 doses of PEDIARIX have been administered to 8,088 infants who received one or more doses as part of a 3-dose primary series during 14 clinical studies. The most common adverse reactions observed in clinical trials were local injection site reactions (pain, redness, or swelling), fever, and fussiness. In comparative studies, administration of PEDIARIX was associated with higher rates of fever relative to separately administered vaccines (see WARNINGS and ADVERSE REACTIONS Table 1). The prevalence of fever was highest on the day of vaccination and the day following vaccination. More than 96% of episodes of fever resolved within the 4-day period following vaccination (i.e., the period including the day of vaccination and the next 3 days). In the largest of the 14 studies, conducted in Germany, safety data were available for 4,666 infants who received PEDIARIX administered concomitantly at separate sites with 1 of 4 *Haemophilus influenzae* type b (Hib) vaccines at 3, 4, and 5 months of age and for 768 infants in the control group that received INFANRIX® (Diphtheria and Tetanus Toxoids and Acellular Pertussis Vaccine Adsorbed), Hib conjugate vaccine, and oral poliovirus vaccine (OPV) separately. Data on adverse events were collected by parents using standardized diary cards for 4 consecutive days following each vaccine dose (i.e., day of vaccination and the next 3 days). Infants were also monitored for unsolicited adverse events that occurred within 30 days following vaccination using diaries which were returned at subsequent visits and were supplemented by spontaneous reports and a medical history as reported by parents. More than 95% of study participants were white.

In a US study, the safety of PEDIARIX administered to 673 infants was compared to the safety of separately administered INFANRIX, ENGERIX-B® [Hepatitis B Vaccine (Recombinant)], inactivated poliovirus vaccine (IPV) in 335 infants. In both groups, infants received Hib and 7-valent pneumococcal conjugate vaccines concomitantly at separate sites. All vaccines were administered at 2, 4, and 6 months of age. The study was powered to evaluate fever >101.3° F following dose 1. Data on solicited adverse events were collected by parents using standardized diary cards for 4 consecutive days following each vaccine dose (i.e., day of vaccination and the next 3 days) and are presented in Table 1. Telephone follow-up was conducted 1 month and 6 months after the third vaccination to inquire about serious adverse events. At the 6-month follow-up, information also was collected on new onset of chronic illnesses. 638 subjects who received PEDIARIX and 313 subjects who received INFANRIX, ENGERIX-B, and IPV completed the 6-month follow-up. Among subjects in both study groups combined, 69% were white, 18% were Hispanic, 7% were black, 3% were Oriental, and 3% were of other racial/ethnic groups.

The adverse event information from clinical trials provides a basis for identifying adverse events that appear to be related to vaccine use and for approximating rates. However, because clinical trials are conducted under widely varying conditions, adverse event rates observed in the clinical trials of a vaccine cannot be directly compared to rates in the clinical trials of another vaccine, and may not reflect the rates observed in practice. As with any vaccine, there is the possibility that broad use of PEDIARIX could reveal adverse events not observed in clinical trials.

**Deaths:** In 14 clinical trials, 5 deaths were reported among 8,088 (0.06%) recipients of PEDIARIX and 1 death was reported among 2,287 (0.04%) recipients of comparator vaccines. Causes of death in the group that received PEDIARIX included 2 cases of Sudden Infant Death Syndrome (SIDS) and one case of each of the following: Convulsive disorder, congenital immunodeficiency with sepsis, and neuroblastoma. One case of SIDS was reported in the comparator group. The rate of SIDS among all recipients of PEDIARIX across the 14 trials was 0.25/1,000. The rate of SIDS observed for recipients of PEDIARIX in the German safety study was 0.2/1,000 infants (reported rate of SIDS in Germany in the latter part of the 1990s was 0.7/1,000 newborns). The reported rate of SIDS in the United States from 1990 to 1994 was 1.2/1,000 live births. By chance alone, some cases of SIDS can be expected to follow receipt of pertussis-containing vaccines.

**Serious Adverse Events:** Within 30 days following any dose of vaccine in the US safety study in which all subjects received concomitant pneumococcal and Hib conjugate vaccines, 7 serious adverse events were reported in 7 subjects (1% [7/673]) who received PEDIARIX (1 case each of pyrexia, gastroenteritis, and culture negative clinical sepsis and 4 cases of bronchiolitis) and 5 serious adverse events were reported in 4 subjects (1% [4/335]) who received INFANRIX, ENGERIX-B, and IPV (uteropelvic junction obstruction and testicular atrophy in one subject and 3 cases of bronchiolitis).

**Onset of Chronic Illnesses:** In the US safety study in which all subjects received concomitant pneumococcal and Hib conjugate vaccines, 21 subjects (3%) who received PEDIARIX and 14 subjects (4%) who received INFANRIX, ENGERIX-B, and IPV reported new onset of a chronic illness during the period from 1 to 6 months following the last dose of study vaccines. Among the chronic illnesses reported in the subjects who received PEDIARIX, there were 4 cases of asthma and 1 case each of diabetes mellitus and chronic neutropenia. There were 4 cases of asthma in subjects who received INFANRIX, ENGERIX-B, and IPV.

**Seizures:** In the German safety study over the entire study period, 6 subjects in the group that received PEDIARIX reported seizures. Two of these subjects had a febrile seizure, 1 of whom also developed afebrile seizures. The remaining 4 subjects had afebrile seizures, including 2 with infantile spasms. Two subjects reported seizures within 7 days following vaccination (1 subject had both febrile and afebrile seizures, and 1 subject had afebrile seizures), corresponding to a rate of 0.22 seizures per 1,000 doses (febrile seizures 0.07 per 1,000 doses, afebrile seizures 0.14 per 1,000 doses). No subject who received concomitant INFANRIX, Hib vaccine, and OPV reported seizures. In a separate German study that evaluated the safety of INFANRIX in 22,505 infants who received 66,867 doses of INFANRIX administered as a 3-dose primary series, the rate of seizures within 7 days of vaccination with INFANRIX was 0.13 per 1,000 doses (febrile seizures 0.0 per 1,000 doses, afebrile seizures 0.13 per 1,000 doses). Over the entire study period in the US safety study in which all subjects received concomitant pneumococcal and Hib conjugate vaccines, 4 subjects in the group that received PEDIARIX reported seizures. Three of these subjects had a febrile seizure and 1 had an afebrile seizure. Over the entire study period, 2 subjects in the group that received INFANRIX, ENGERIX-B, and IPV reported febrile seizures. There were no afebrile seizures in this group. No subject in either study group had seizures within 7 days following vaccination.

**Other Neurological Events of Interest:** No cases of hypotonic-hyporesponsiveness or encephalopathy were reported in either the German safety study or the US safety study.

**Solicited Adverse Events:** Table 1 presents data from the US safety study on solicited local and systemic adverse events within 4 days of vaccination with PEDIARIX or INFANRIX, ENGERIX-B, and IPV, administered concomitantly with Hib and 7-valent pneumococcal conjugate vaccines. In this study, medical attention (a visit to or from medical personnel) for fever within 4 days following vaccination was sought in the group who received PEDIARIX for 8 infants after the first dose (1.2%), 1 infant following the second dose (0.2%), and 5 infants following the third dose (0.8%) (Table 1). Following dose 2, medical attention for fever was sought for 2 infants (0.6%) who received separately administered vaccines (Table 1). Among infants who had a medical visit for fever within 4 days following vaccination, 9 of 14 who received PEDIARIX and 1 of 2 who received separately administered vaccines, had one or more diagnostic studies performed to evaluate the cause of fever.

**Safety of PEDIARIX after a previous dose of hepatitis B vaccine:** Limited data are available on the safety of administering PEDIARIX after a previous dose of hepatitis B vaccine. In 2 separate studies, 160 Moldovan infants and 96 US infants, respectively, received 3 doses of PEDIARIX following 1 previous dose of hepatitis B vaccine. Neither study was designed to detect significant differences in rates of adverse events associated with PEDIARIX administered after a previous dose of hepatitis B vaccine compared to PEDIARIX administered without a previous dose of hepatitis B vaccine.

**Table 1. Percentage of US Infants With Solicited Local Reactions or Systemic Adverse Events Within 4 Days of Vaccination* at 2, 4, and 6 Months of Age With PEDIARIX Administered Concomitantly With Hib Conjugate Vaccine and 7-valent Pneumococcal Conjugate Vaccine (PCV7) or With Separate Concomitant Administration of INFANRIX, ENGERIX-B, IPV, Hib Conjugate Vaccine, and PCV7 (Modified ITT cohort)**

| | PEDIARIX, Hib Vaccine, & PCV7 | | | INFANRIX, ENGERIX-B, IPV, Hib Vaccine, & PCV7 | | |
|---|---|---|---|---|---|---|
| | **Dose 1** | **Dose 2** | **Dose 3** | **Dose 1** | **Dose 2** | **Dose 3** |
| **Local[†]** | | | | | | |
| **N** | **671** | **653** | **648** | **335** | **323** | **315** |
| Pain, any | 36.1 | 36.1 | 31.2 | 31.9 | 30.0 | 29.8 |
| Pain, grade 2 or 3 | 11.5 | 10.9 | 10.6 | 9.0 | 8.7 | 8.9 |
| Pain, grade 3 | 2.4 | 2.5 | 1.7 | 2.7 | 1.5 | 1.3 |
| Redness, any | 29.9[§] | 37.2 | 40.1 | 18.2 | 32.8 | 39.0 |
| Redness, >5 mm | 6.0[§] | 9.6[§] | 12.7[§] | 1.8 | 5.9 | 7.3 |
| Redness, >20 mm | 0.9 | 1.2[§] | 2.8 | 0.3 | 0.0 | 1.9 |
| Swelling, any | 17.3[§] | 26.5[§] | 28.7 | 9.6 | 20.4 | 24.8 |
| Swelling, >5 mm | 5.8[§] | 9.6[§] | 9.3[§] | 1.8 | 5.0 | 4.1 |
| Swelling, >20 mm | 1.9 | 2.5[§] | 3.1 | 0.6 | 0.0 | 1.3 |
| **Systemic** | | | | | | |
| **N** | **667** | **644** | **645** | **333** | **321** | **311** |
| Fever[‡], ≥100.4°F | 27.9[§] | 38.8[§] | 33.5[§] | 19.8 | 30.2 | 23.8 |
| Fever[‡], >101.3°F | 7.0 | 14.1[§] | 8.8 | 4.5 | 9.7 | 5.8 |
| Fever[‡], >102.2°F | 2.2[§] | 3.6 | 3.4 | 0.3 | 3.1 | 2.3 |
| Fever[‡], >103.1°F | 0.4 | 1.4 | 1.1 | 0.0 | 0.3 | 0.3 |
| Fever[‡], M.A. | 1.2[§] | 0.2 | 0.8 | 0.0 | 0.6 | 0.0 |
| **N** | **671** | **653** | **648** | **335** | **323** | **315** |
| Drowsiness, any | 57.2 | 51.6 | 40.9 | 54.0 | 48.3 | 38.4 |
| Drowsiness, grade 2 or 3 | 15.8 | 13.8 | 11.4 | 17.6 | 12.4 | 11.1 |
| Drowsiness, grade 3 | 2.5 | 1.2 | 0.9 | 3.6 | 0.6 | 1.9 |
| Irritability/Fussiness, any | 60.5 | 64.9 | 61.1 | 61.5 | 61.6 | 56.5 |
| Irritability/Fussiness, grade 2 or 3 | 19.8 | 27.9[§] | 25.2[§] | 19.4 | 21.1 | 19.4 |
| Irritability/Fussiness, grade 3 | 3.4 | 4.4 | 3.5 | 3.9 | 3.4 | 3.2 |
| Loss of appetite, any | 30.4 | 30.6 | 26.2 | 27.8 | 26.6 | 23.8 |
| Loss of appetite, grade 2 or 3 | 6.6 | 7.8[§] | 5.9 | 5.1 | 3.4 | 5.4 |
| Loss of appetite, grade 3 | 0.7 | 0.3 | 0.2 | 0.6 | 0.3 | 0.0 |

Modified ITT cohort = all vaccinated subjects for whom safety data were available

N = number of infants for whom at least one symptom sheet was completed; for fever, numbers exclude missing temperature recordings or tympanic measurements.

M.A. = Medically attended (a visit to or from medical personnel).

Grade 2 defined as sufficiently discomforting to interfere with daily activities.

Grade 3 defined as preventing normal daily activities.

[*] Within 4 days of vaccination defined as day of vaccination and the next 3 days.

[†] Local reactions at the injection site for PEDIARIX or INFANRIX.

[‡] Rectal temperatures or axillary temperatures increased by 1°C to derive equivalent rectal temperature.

[§] Rate significantly higher in the group that received PEDIARIX compared to separately administered vaccines [p value < 0.05 (2-sided Fisher Exact test) or the 95% CI on the difference between groups (Separate minus PEDIARIX) does not include 0].

**Postmarketing Reports With PEDIARIX:** Worldwide voluntary reports of adverse events received for PEDIARIX since market introduction of this vaccine are listed below. This list includes serious adverse events or events which have a suspected causal connection to components of PEDIARIX or other vaccines or drugs. Because these events are reported voluntarily from a population of uncertain size, it is not always possible to reliably estimate their frequency or establish a causal relationship to vaccine exposure. *Cardiac Disorders:* Cyanosis. *Gastrointestinal Disorders:* Diarrhea, vomiting. *General Disorders and Administrative Site Conditions:* Fatigue, injection site cellulitis, injection site induration, injection site itching, injection site nodule/lump, injection site pain, injection site reactions, injection site redness, injection site swelling, injection site warmth, irritability, limb pain, limb swelling, pyrexia, Sudden Infant Death Syndrome. *Immune System Disorders:* Anaphylactic reaction, anaphylactoid reaction, hypersensitivity. *Infections and Infestations:* Upper respiratory tract infection. *Investigations:* Abnormal liver function tests. *Metabolism and Nutrition Disorders:* Anorexia. *Nervous System Disorders:* Bulging fontanelle, convulsions, depressed level of consciousness, febrile convulsion, hypotonia, hypotonic-hyporesponsive episode, lethargy, somnolence. *Psychiatric Disorders:* Crying, insomnia, irritability, nervousness, restlessness, screaming, unusual crying. *Respiratory, Thoracic and Mediastinal Disorders:* Apnea, dyspnea. *Skin and Subcutaneous Tissue Disorders:* Angioedema, erythema, rash, urticaria. *Vascular Disorders:* Pallor, petechiae.

**Postmarketing Reports With INFANRIX and/or ENGERIX-B:** Worldwide voluntary reports of adverse events received for INFANRIX and/or ENGERIX-B in children younger than 7 years of age but not already reported for PEDIARIX are listed below. This list includes serious adverse events or events which have a suspected causal connection to components of INFANRIX and/or ENGERIX-B or other vaccines or drugs. Because these events are reported voluntarily from a population of uncertain size, it is not always possible to reliably estimate their frequency or establish a causal relationship to vaccine exposure. *Blood and Lymphatic System Disorders:* Idiopathic thrombocytopenic purpura[a,b], lymphadenopathy[a], thrombocytopeni[a,b]. *Gastrointestinal Disorders:* Abdominal pain[b], intussusception[a,b], nausea[b]. *General Disorders and Administrative Site Conditions:* Asthenia[b], malaise[b]. *Hepatobiliary Disorders:* Jaundice[b]. *Immune System Disorders:* Anaphylactic shock[a], serum sickness–like disease[b]. *Musculoskeletal and Connective Tissue Disorders:* Arthralgia[b], myalgia[b]. *Nervous System Disorders:* Encephalopathy[a], headache[b]. *Skin and Subcutaneous Tissue Disorders:* Alopecia[b], erythema multiforme[b], pruritus[a,b], Stevens-Johnson syndrome[a]. [[a] Following INFANRIX; [b] Following ENGERIX-B]

**Reporting Adverse Events:** Report the occurrence following immunization of any event set forth in the Vaccine Injury Table from the National Childhood Vaccine Injury Act including: Anaphylaxis or anaphylactic shock within 7 days, encephalopathy or encephalitis within 7 days, brachial neuritis within 28 days, or an acute complication or sequelae (including death) of an illness, disability, injury, or condition referred to above, or any events that would contraindicate further doses of PEDIARIX. These events should be reported to VAERS. The VAERS toll-free number is 1-800-822-7967. Reporting forms may also be obtained at the VAERS website at www.vaers.hhs.gov.

Manufactured by **GlaxoSmithKline Biologicals**, Rixensart, Belgium, US License 1617

Distributed by **GlaxoSmithKline,** Research Triangle Park, NC 27709



Full prescribing information for PEDIARIX is available at www.GSKVaccines.com/Pediarix.

BRS-PE:L3

 PED644R0 May 2006

ARTICLE

# Adolescent and Parent Perceptions on Youth Participation in Risk Behavior Research

*Ryan H. Pasternak, MD, MPH; Gail Geller, ScD; Catherine Parrish, MD; Tina L. Cheng, MD*

**Objectives:** To assess and compare parent and adolescent views on the importance of risk behavior research and the need for parental consent and to identify predictors of views.

**Design:** Confidential survey.

**Setting:** Adolescent, general pediatrics clinics.

**Participants:** Adolescents aged 14 to 17 years presenting alone (solo) or with a parent or guardian (paired) and parents or guardians. Of 265 eligible pairs (199 solo adolescents), 134 (93) had useable surveys. The proportion of females in the parent or guardian, paired adolescent, and solo adolescent groups was 92%, 59%, and 75%, respectively; and the proportion of African Americans in these groups was 67%, 69%, and 91%, respectively.

**Main Outcome Measures:** Views on the importance of and requirement of parental consent for confidential risk behavior research.

**Results:** Most parents (98%), paired adolescents (99%), and solo adolescents (100%) believed confidential risk behavior research surveys with teenagers were important; greater than 90% of all groups believed surveys should be conducted. The proportion of parents, paired adolescents, and solo adolescents that endorsed requiring parental permission was 84%, 53%, and 19%, respectively. Parents were less likely to endorse requiring permission if they had confidential health concerns as teenagers and were more likely to endorse requiring permission if their child was younger or female, if they believed their child had sex, and if they were a parent vs a guardian. Adolescents were more likely to endorse requiring permission if they were younger, not African American, and had more educated parents. Adolescents presenting with parents were more likely to endorse requiring permission.

**Conclusions:** Parents and adolescents believed risk behavior research with adolescents was important. Most parents believed parental permission is needed for participation. Compared with parents, fewer adolescents believed parental consent was necessary. It is not clear what effect requirement of parental permission would have on participation or validity. Further research is needed to elucidate views on adolescent risk behavior research.

*Arch Pediatr Adolesc Med. 2006;160:1159-1166*

Adolescent risk behaviors, such as tobacco use, alcohol and other drug use, unprotected sexual intercourse, and weapon carrying, account for significant morbidity and mortality. Research on these risk behaviors, including the perspectives of adolescents, is essential to address these issues and improve adolescent health.[1] Information on adolescent risk behaviors has frequently been obtained from confidential research surveys conducted without parental consent. Considerable uncertainty and controversy exist regarding the ethical guidelines and legal statutes that relate to adolescents' involvement in research.[2,3] Legal and legislative challenges have led to increased scrutiny of such research.[4,5] Including adolescents as research subjects has resulted in debate among parents and schools,[6] in research review boards,[7] in regulatory and legislative bodies,[8-10] and in the existence of conflicting guidelines.[11-14]

Recent legal decisions have also questioned the involvement of minors in research[4,15] and the need for parental knowledge regarding their children's participation in the research.[6,8,16] This has directly impacted research with adolescents. *CN v Ridgewood Board of Education*[6] challenged schools' ability to conduct confidential risk behavior surveys and led to the cancellation of subsequent surveys.[17] This case was framed as an issue of "parents' rights" and, while struck down by the Supreme Court, led to legislative change in New Jersey, limiting adolescent research and increasing requirements for parental consent. Because of difficulty in interpreting federal regulations on adolescent involvement in research, adolescents have been excluded from participation in clinical trials, studies in public health prevention, and other critical research efforts.[13,18,19] These surveys are con-

Author Affiliations:
Department of Pediatrics, Louisiana State University, New Orleans (Dr Pasternak); The Phoebe R. Berman Bioethics Institute (Dr Geller) and Department of Pediatrics (Dr Cheng), The Johns Hopkins University, Baltimore, Md; and The Johns Hopkins Community Physicians, The Johns Hopkins Medical Institutions, Baltimore (Dr Parrish).

sidered minimal-risk research. Recent studies[20,21] have shown increased parent and adolescent acceptance of adolescent participation in minimal-risk clinical research. Amid this discussion, there has been little systematic research exploring parent and adolescent perspectives on this important issue of parental consent for risk behavior survey research involving adolescents.

The primary objectives of this study were to assess parent and adolescent (1) perceptions regarding the importance and need for research on adolescent risk behaviors and (2) attitudes regarding a requirement for parental consent for adolescent involvement in confidential risk behavior survey research. Our secondary objectives were to compare parents'/guardians' attitudes and views with those of their adolescents, to compare the views of adolescents receiving care with parents present vs those of adolescents receiving care alone, and to identify predictors of these views.

## METHODS

### STUDY DESIGN AND SAMPLE

The study sample was drawn from a population of adolescents and parents or guardians at 2 clinical sites: an urban academic adolescent medicine clinic and a community general pediatrics clinic. Between November 23, 2003, and August 19, 2004, participants were recruited in waiting rooms during a clinic visit. Adolescents were eligible for enrollment if they spoke English and were aged between 14 and 17 years. Adolescent participants were either "solo," if they presented without a parent or guardian; or "paired," if they presented with a parent or guardian, both spoke English, and both completed the informed consent process. The selected age range for adolescents was based on prior studies[22] suggesting that teenagers of this age had the capacity for informed consent/assent. Persons without the physical or mental capacity to participate (eg, hearing loss in one grandmother) were excluded.

An audiotaped questionnaire was used to improve confidentiality, lessen literacy concerns, and allow participation of multiple pairs at once. This modality has been shown to increase survey completion and accuracy when sensitive data are being gathered.[23] The study was approved by The Johns Hopkins University institutional review board and the research review board for the community pediatric clinic.

### MEASURES

Survey items were initially drawn from other confidentiality questionnaires on adolescent research.[24,25] Focus groups and in-depth interviews with talk-aloud pretesting were conducted with 25 adolescents and 19 parents or guardians to assess relevance and comprehension. The recorded surveys and consent process were also tested to evaluate understanding of specific items, audio quality of the recorded survey, and timing of the enrollment process.

Questions included Likert-scaled, true or false, multiple choice, short fill-in, and yes or no responses. The surveys consisted of questions on demographics, perceptions of the importance of and need for adolescent risk behavior research surveys, perceived need for a requirement for parental permission to participate in this research for various topics (smoking, alcohol use, other drug use, having sex or using birth control, abortion, depression, carrying a weapon, and physical or sexual abuse), and past experience with giving informed consent for relevant research. Predictor variables assessed included relationship to the adolescent (parent vs guardian), parent or guardian and adolescent gender, adolescent age, race/ethnicity, and parental educational level; parent or guardian personal history of a confidential health issue as a teenager and parent or guardian belief that the adolescent had experienced or been involved in risk-taking behaviors and belief that the adolescent has a current confidential health concern; and adolescent report of a current confidential health concern. Race/ethnicity was included as a self-selected demographic variable because prior studies[24] have indicated differences in perceptions regarding the confidentiality of risk behavior issues. Research surveys were described as "surveys . . . used to gather information about teens' behaviors and attitudes on sex, drugs and violence. Research surveys help develop programs for teenagers as a group, but NOT for each person answering the survey." The study focused on confidential survey research, with questions specifying research in which "no names are used."

### SURVEY PROCEDURE

Participants were recruited in clinic waiting rooms at each site on randomly chosen clinic days by one of us (R.H.P.) or a trained research assistant. Potential participants were identified via clinic flyers or approached directly by research staff. Written informed consent was obtained from parents or guardians and solo adolescents, and written assent was also obtained from paired adolescents. Each participant then received an audiocassette player containing the recorded survey and a written answer sheet. Participants were instructed on proper survey completion and use of the equipment and completed surveys independently.

Separate color-coded answer sheets were provided to adolescents and parents. Answer sheets contained no questions but only response options, contained no personal identifiers, and were coded to link parent-adolescent pairs. Research staff were available during survey completion to answer questions and ensure that participants worked independently. Each adolescent completing the survey received a $5 gift card, and parents received a brochure on parenting adolescents.

### STATISTICAL ANALYSIS

Data were entered into a Microsoft Access 2000 Version 9.0 database (Microsoft Corp, Redmond, Wash). Double data entry was performed, with less than 1.0% data error. For analysis, data were exported to Microsoft Excel, version 9.0 (Microsoft Corp), for use with Stata 8.0 (Stata Corp, College Station, Tex) and SAS statistical software. Responses to questions on perceived need for adolescent risk behavior research, perceived need for a requirement for parental permission, and predictors were tabulated as frequencies. The McNemar test for paired data was used to test the statistical significance of differences in proportions for parent and adolescent attitudes toward research. $\chi^2$ Tests were used to test the differences in proportions for solo and paired adolescent attitudes toward research and the associations between predictors and outcome variables on endorsement of parental permission for adolescent involvement in risk behavior research. Outcome variables included endorsement of a requirement for parental permission for adolescent involvement in research generally and on each research topic. An additional variable was generated for endorsement of parental permission for all 8 research topics combined vs endorsement of fewer than 8 topics. Initial logistic regression models were developed using predictors with $P \leq .10$ in bivariate analyses controlling for adolescent age, gender, current confidential health concern, or participation in risk behavior.

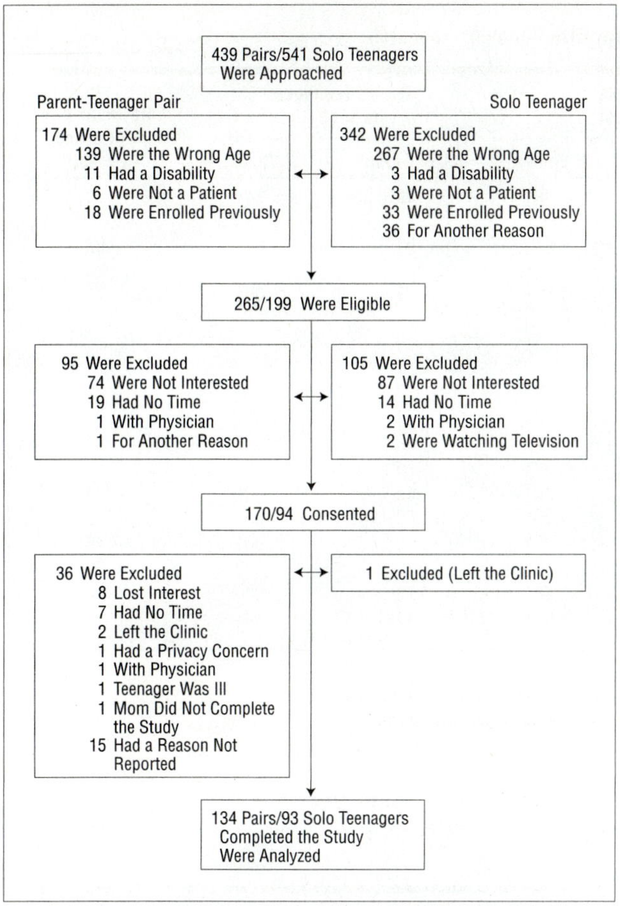


**Figure.** Flow diagram of enrollment for parent-teenager pairs and solo teenagers.

**Table 1. Demographic Characteristics of Participants***

| Characteristic | Parents (n = 134) | Paired Teenagers (n = 134) | Solo Teenagers (n = 93) |
|---|---|---|---|
| Age, y | | | |
| Mean (SD) | 41.0 (9.7) | 15.0 (1.1) | 15.9 (1.0) |
| Range | 22-77 | 14-17 | 14-17 |
| Female sex | 92 | 59 | 75 |
| Race/ethnicity | | | |
| African American | 67 | 69 | 91 |
| White | 25 | 21 | 3 |
| Asian/Pacific Islander | 2 | 3 | 0 |
| Hispanic | 1 | 2 | 1 |
| Native American | 2 | 1 | 0 |
| Not answered | 4 | 4 | 4 |
| Relation to teenager | | | |
| Parent | 64 | NA | NA |
| Other | 36 | NA | NA |
| Educational level of parents | | | |
| <High school | 15 | NA | NA |
| High school or GED | 52 | NA | NA |
| College | 26 | NA | NA |
| Graduate school | 7 | NA | NA |
| Last grade of teenager | | | |
| 6-8 | NA | 37 | 8 |
| 9-12 | NA | 63 | 92 |

Abbreviations: GED, general equivalency diploma; NA, data not applicable.
*Data are given as percentage of each group unless otherwise indicated. Percentages may not total 100 because of rounding.

## RESULTS

### SAMPLE CHARACTERISTICS

Of the 439 parent or guardian–adolescent pairs approached at the 2 sites, 265 were eligible. Of those eligible, 74 were not interested and 19 noted a time constraint; 170 (64.2%) of those eligible gave consent, and there were 134 useable surveys (**Figure**). Of the 541 solo adolescents approached, 199 were eligible. Of those adolescents, 87 were not interested and 14 noted a time constraint; 94 (47.2%) gave consent. There were 93 useable surveys (Figure). **Table 1** presents participant characteristics. Nearly all of the parents or guardians were female, and most of all 3 groups described themselves as African American.

### ATTITUDES REGARDING ADOLESCENT RISK BEHAVIOR RESEARCH

Virtually all parents or guardians and adolescents believed that research surveys involving teenagers aged 14 to 17 years were important; 95% of parents, 94% of paired teenagers, and 92% of solo teenagers believed these surveys should be done (**Table 2**). When asked if a teenager should "be REQUIRED to have written parent or guardian permission to do a research survey," in which no names are used, 84% of parents, 53% of paired teenagers, and 19% of solo teenagers said yes. There was little variability in parental views on parental permission by risk behavior topic; 75% of parents or guardians endorsed a requirement for consent for all 8 topics. Adolescents demonstrated more variability in their views, with only 37% of paired teenagers and only 16% of solo teenagers endorsing a requirement for consent for all 8 topics.

There was a significant difference in paired parent or guardian and adolescent responses for all questions on parental permission, with fewer adolescents than parents or guardians endorsing required parental permission (Table 2). Parent-adolescent differences in proportions were greatest for research involving sexual activity or use of birth control, depression, and abortion. Of parents or guardians, 83% and 81%, compared with 63% and 66% of paired adolescents, endorsed a requirement for parental permission for research involving sexual activity and depression, respectively.

There was a significant difference in paired and solo adolescent responses for all questions on parental permission, with fewer solo adolescents than paired adolescents endorsing required parental permission (Table 2).

Participants were asked about prior experience with research consent and assent forms. Of parents or guardians, 53%, and 45% and 49% of paired and solo adolescents, respectively, reported having signed a consent or assent form in the past; and 27% of parents or guardians and 26% and 27% of paired and solo adolescents, respectively, had previously refused to sign a consent form. Of parents or guardians, 31% had previously been asked to sign research consent for their child. Parent refusal to sign

**Table 2. Parent or Guardian and Adolescent Attitudes Toward Adolescent Risk Behavior Research**

| Question | Parents (n = 134) | | Paired Teenagers (n = 134) | | Solo Teenagers, % of Group (n = 93)* |
|---|---|---|---|---|---|
| | % of Group* | *P* Value† | % of Group* | *P* Value‡ | |
| "Research surveys with teenagers ages 14-17 are important." | 98 | >.99 | 99 | .24 | 100 |
| "If no names are used, do you believe that research surveys should be done with teenagers ages 14-17?" | 95 | .27 | 94 | .61 | 92 |
| "If no names are used, do you feel that a teenager 14 to 17 years old should be REQUIRED to have written parent or guardian permission to do a research survey?" | 84 | <.001 | 53 | <.001 | 19 |
| "Should teens be required to have written permission for research involving:" | | | | | |
| Smoking cigarettes | 86 | <.001 | 74 | <.001 | 35 |
| Alcohol use | 84 | <.001 | 70 | <.001 | 44 |
| Drug use | 84 | <.001 | 76 | <.001 | 42 |
| Having sex or using birth control | 83 | <.001 | 63 | .004 | 44 |
| Having an abortion | 85 | <.001 | 66 | .02 | 52 |
| Depression | 81 | <.001 | 66 | .001 | 45 |
| Carrying a weapon | 83 | .005 | 72 | .009 | 56 |
| Physical or sexual abuse | 83 | <.001 | 76 | .04 | 64 |
| All topics | 75 | <.001 | 37 | .001 | 16 |

*Data indicate those who agreed with the item.
†The McNemar test was used to determine the difference in proportions between parent and paired teenager responses.
‡The Pearson $\chi^2$ test was used to determine the difference between paired teenager and solo teenager responses.

**Table 3. Parent Bivariate Associations: Endorsement of a Requirement for Parental Permission for Adolescent Involvement in Risk Behavior Research***

| Research Topic | Adolescent Gender | | Adolescent Age, y | | Relation to Adolescent | | Parent or Guardian History of Confidential Issue as a Teenager | | Parent or Guardian Believes Adolescent Has Had Sex | |
|---|---|---|---|---|---|---|---|---|---|---|
| | Male | Female | 14-15 | 16-17 | Parent | Guardian | Yes | No | Yes | No |
| General risk behavior | 84 | 85 | 87 | 79 | 86 | 83 | 78† | 88 | 86 | 82 |
| Smoking | 84 | 89 | 89 | 89 | 92 | 83 | 81† | 91 | 96‡ | 79 |
| Alcohol use | 80† | 90 | 86 | 85 | 93‡ | 70 | 82 | 88 | 93§ | 79 |
| Sex | 82 | 87 | 86 | 83 | 89 | 79 | 81 | 87 | 89 | 81 |
| Other drug use | 81 | 89 | 87 | 85 | 93† | 79 | 81 | 89 | 95§ | 79 |
| All topics | 69 | 79 | 75 | 75 | 80 | 67 | 72 | 77 | 79 | 73 |

*Data are given as percentage of each group. n = 134 for each group.
†*P*=.10 to *P*=.005, using the 2-sided α for the Pearson $\chi^2$ test.
‡*P*<.01, using the 2-sided α for the Pearson $\chi^2$ test.
§*P*<.05 to *P*=.01, using the 2-sided α for the Pearson $\chi^2$ test.

consent or history of signing consent for a child was not related to parental attitudes on parental permission.

**Table 3** presents bivariate analyses of factors associated with parents' or guardians' views on requirements for parental permission. Compared with parents of female adolescents, parents of male adolescents were less likely to endorse a requirement for parental permission for adolescent involvement in research on alcohol (odds ratio, 0.4 and 0.5, respectively; *P*<.10). Parents who had had a confidential health concern were not significantly different from parents without history of a confidential health concern with respect to race or ethnicity (*P*=.62) or level of education (*P*=.90).

**Table 4** presents logistic regression analyses of parents' views regarding requirement for parental permission of adolescent involvement in risk behavior research. Being a parent, compared with being a guardian, was predictive of an increased need for permission for research involving alcohol use. Parents of younger teenagers (aged 14-15 vs 16-17 years) were more likely to endorse a requirement for parental permission for research generally, and parents of female vs male adolescents endorsed parental permission for research involving alcohol and all topics combined. Parents who believed their adolescents had had sex were much more likely to believe permission was needed for research involving smoking, alcohol use, and other drug use.

**Table 4. Parent Logistic Regression Data Predicting Endorsement of a Requirement for Parental Permission for Adolescent Involvement in Risk Behavior Research***

| Research Topic | Adolescents: Male vs Female Gender | Adolescents: Aged 14-15 vs 16-17 y | Relation to Adolescent: Parent vs Guardian | Parent or Guardian History of Confidential Issue as a Teenager: Yes vs No | Parent or Guardian Believes Adolescent Has Had Sex: Yes vs No |
|---|---|---|---|---|---|
| General risk behavior | 0.5 (0.2-1.7) | 4.5 (1.4-14.7) | 1.3 (0.3-4.8) | 0.5 (0.2-1.7) | 1.5 (0.5-4.7) |
| Smoking | 0.6 (0.2-2.6) | 1.7 (0.4-6.9) | 3.4 (0.8-15.0) | 0.7 (0.2-2.7) | 11.9 (1.7-102.6) |
| Alcohol use | 0.3 (0.1-1.3) | 2.7 (0.7-10.8) | 8.7 (2.1-35.3) | 1.1 (0.3-4.2) | 4.4 (1.0-20.2) |
| Sex | 0.7 (0.2-2.2) | 2.2 (0.6-7.2) | 2.7 (0.7-9.7) | 0.7 (0.2-2.5) | 2.6 (0.7-9.4) |
| Other drug use | 0.6 (0.1-2.5) | 2.6 (0.6-11.4) | 5.5 (1.2-24.7) | 0.6 (0.1-2.6) | 14.1 (1.6-127.1) |
| All topics | 0.4 (0.2-1.1) | 2.0 (0.7-5.3) | 1.8 (0.6-5.4) | 1.1 (0.4-3.0) | 1.2 (0.5-3.1) |

*Data are given as odds ratio (95% confidence interval). Data are controlled for adolescent gender, adolescent age, relation to adolescent, parental history of confidential health concern as a teenager, and parental belief that the adolescent has had sex.

**Table 5. Paired Adolescent Bivariate Associations: Endorsement of a Requirement for Parental Permission for Adolescent Involvement in Risk Behavior Research***

| Research Topic | Adolescent Gender | | Adolescent Age, y | | Confidential Health Concern | | Adolescent Race/Ethnicity | | Parental Education | |
|---|---|---|---|---|---|---|---|---|---|---|
| | Male | Female | 14-15 | 16-17 | Yes | No | African American | Other Ethnicity | High School or Less | More Than High School |
| General risk behavior | 56 | 52 | 55 | 51 | 47 | 57 | 100 | 59 | 49 | 62 |
| Smoking | 71 | 78 | 72 | 81 | 70 | 71 | 73 | 78 | 70 | 84 |
| Alcohol use | 68 | 72 | 67 | 77 | 70 | 71 | 66† | 81 | 68 | 76 |
| Sex | 57 | 68 | 60 | 70 | 60 | 65 | 58‡ | 76 | 58† | 73 |
| Other drug use | 75 | 79 | 75 | 81 | 77 | 77 | 72† | 86 | 77 | 78 |
| All topics | 30 | 42 | 34 | 43 | 33 | 39 | 36 | 41 | 33 | 44 |

*Data are given as percentage of each group. n = 134 for each group.
†$P$=.10 to $P$=.05, using the 2-sided $\alpha$ for the Pearson $\chi^2$ test.
‡$P$<.01.

**Table 6. Paired Adolescent Logistic Regression Data Predicting Endorsement of a Requirement for Parental Permission for Adolescent Involvement in Risk Behavior Research***

| Research Topic | Adolescents: Male vs Female Gender | Adolescents: Aged 14-15 vs 16-17 y | Confidential Health Concern: Yes vs No | Adolescent Race or Ethnicity: African American vs Other Ethnicity | Parental Education: High School or Less vs More Than High School |
|---|---|---|---|---|---|
| General risk behavior | 1.6 (0.8-3.4) | 1.4 (0.6-3.1) | 0.8 (0.4-1.8) | 0.5 (0.2-1.2) | 0.5 (0.2-1.0) |
| Smoking | 0.8 (0.3-1.7) | 0.6 (0.3-1.6) | 1.0 (0.3-2.5) | 0.7 (0.3-1.8) | 0.5 (0.2-1.2) |
| Alcohol use | 0.9 (0.4-1.9) | 0.7 (0.3-1.7) | 1.0 (0.4-2.5) | 0.4 (0.2-1.1) | 0.6 (0.3-1.5) |
| Sex | 0.7 (0.4-1.5) | 0.8 (0.3-1.7) | 1.0 (0.5-2.4) | 0.4 (0.1-0.9) | 0.4 (0.2-1.0) |
| Other drug use | 0.9 (0.4-2.1) | 0.9 (0.4-2.2) | 1.2 (0.4-2.1) | 0.4 (0.1-1.1) | 0.8 (0.3-1.9) |
| All topics | 0.7 (0.3-1.5) | 0.7 (0.3-1.4) | 0.8 (0.4-1.9) | 0.8 (0.4-1.9) | 0.7 (0.3-1.6) |

*Data are given as odds ratio (95% confidence interval). Data are controlled for adolescent gender, adolescent age, current confidential health concern, adolescent race, and parental educational level.

**Table 5** presents the bivariate associations for paired adolescents regarding the outcome variables with significant differences only, noted by race/ethnicity and level of parental education. In the multivariable analyses presented in **Table 6**, we found that African American race and lower parental education were independently predictive of decreased odds for endorsing a requirement for parental permission for research on general and specific topics, controlling for adolescent gender, age, and history of current confidential health concern.

**Table 7** presents bivariate associations for solo adolescents, and **Table 8** presents the logistic regression analyses. Because parental education was not known for this group, this variable and race/ethnicity were not included in the logistic regression analyses. Younger adolescents were much more likely to believe permission should be required for research. Current confidential

**Table 7. Solo Adolescent Bivariate Associations: Endorsement of a Requirement for Parental Permission for Adolescent Involvement in Risk Behavior Research***

| | Adolescent Gender | | Adolescent Age, y | | Confidential Health Concern | |
|---|---|---|---|---|---|---|
| Research Topic | Male | Female | 14-15 | 16-17 | Yes | No |
| General risk behavior | 0† | 25 | 23 | 16 | 25‡ | 10 |
| Smoking | 40 | 34 | 63† | 21 | 32 | 35 |
| Alcohol use | 35 | 47 | 80† | 26 | 48 | 39 |
| Sex | 35 | 47 | 63† | 34 | 38 | 47 |
| Other drug use | 36 | 44 | 73† | 27 | 40 | 42 |
| All topics | 9 | 19 | 33† | 8 | 10 | 18 |

*Data are given as percentage of each group. n = 93 for each group.
†$P<.01$, by 2-sided $\alpha$ for the Pearson $\chi^2$ test.
‡$P=.10$ to $P=.05$, by 2-sided $\alpha$ for the Pearson $\chi^2$ test.

**Table 8. Solo Adolescent Logistic Regression Data Predicting Endorsement of a Requirement for Parental Permission for Adolescent Involvement in Risk Behavior Research***

| Research Topic | Adolescents: Male vs Female Gender | Adolescents: Aged 14-15 vs 16-17 y | Confidential Health Concern: Yes vs No |
|---|---|---|---|
| General risk behavior | NA | 1.2 (0.4-4.0) | 2.1 (0.6-7.1) |
| Smoking | 8.0 (1.6-40.3)† | 20.1 (5.0-81.7) | 1.4 (0.4-4.5) |
| Alcohol use | 2.7 (0.7-9.8) | 19.6 (5.6-68.7) | 2.0 (0.7-6.0) |
| Sex | 0.9 (0.3-2.8) | 3.6 (1.3-10.0) | 0.6 (0.2-1.6) |
| Other drug use | 2.3 (0.7-8.0) | 11.9 (3.8-37.4) | 1.1 (0.4-2.9) |
| All topics | 1.4 (0.2-10.6) | 11.4 (2.1-60.8) | 0.4 (0.1-1.7) |

Abbreviation: NA, data not applicable (removed from the model because of no variability).
*Data are given as odds ratio (95% confidence interval). Data are controlled for adolescent gender, adolescent age, and current confidential health concern.
†$P<.01$.

health concern was not predictive of views on permission for solo adolescents.

## COMMENT

Information from research on youth risk behavior is important to understand health issues among adolescents and to determine the appropriate distribution of funds for education and health care services for adolescents. As research and controversy have grown, the need to develop guidelines for adolescent research and clinical care has become increasingly apparent. Professional society and legal and ethical guidelines[26-32] have been developed for the inclusion of adolescents in research, and the challenges regarding confidentiality and consent have been discussed. The Society for Adolescent Medicine[13(p407)] has suggested in its policy statements that adolescents be allowed to participate in minimal-risk research, including confidential surveys, with a waiver of parental consent stating "for research of low risk (eg, confidential or anonymous survey research) . . . informed consent of the adolescent can be substituted for parental permission." This recommendation has been debated in the research community and within research review boards because of misunderstandings about the legal statutes regarding adolescent consent, fear of litigation, state variability, or a perception that adolescents are not as capable as adults of giving consent.[22] To our knowledge, there has been little systematic study of parental and adolescent perspectives on this important issue.

In the present study, we focused on risk behavior survey research involving adolescent minors and found that virtually all parents and adolescents believed that this research is important and should be done. Our research also revealed variability in attitudes regarding the need for parental consent by research topic, substantial differences between adolescents and parents, and substantial differences between adolescents presenting to the clinic with parents and adolescents presenting to the clinic without parents.

Most parents believed parental consent or permission is needed for adolescent participation in risk behavior research. Prior research[33] has demonstrated parents' complex and sometimes conflicting responses related to confidentiality in clinical care for adolescents, particularly regarding contraception and reproductive health care. In our study, parents of male adolescents felt less need for permission than parents of female adolescents. However, parents vs other guardians were more likely to believe permission should be required. Parents who believed their adolescent was involved in risk behavior, like "had sex," were more likely to endorse a requirement for parental consent. This may represent efforts by parents to monitor the behavior of an at-risk adolescent.

Adolescents were less likely than parents to endorse a requirement for parental consent on all topics. There was variability in adolescent attitudes depending on the topic, suggesting recognition of the differential impact of some of the issues. Only 37% and 16% of paired and solo adolescents, respectively, endorsed requirements for parental consent for all topics. Parent-adolescent differences were significant for research involving sexual activity or birth control. This difference in opinion on reproductive health care issues is consistent with the literature and supports research and clinical guidelines that protect adolescent confidentiality regarding these issues.[13]

The attitudes of teenagers presenting to the clinic were significantly different based on whether they presented to the clinic with (paired) or without (solo) their parent or guardian. Compared with paired teenagers, solo teenagers were less likely to endorse a requirement for parental permission. This may reflect the fact that solo teenagers were more likely to have a confidential health concern because they likely had a chief complaint regarding a medically emancipated condition. Participation of solo teenagers in research is a controversial issue on many institutional review boards.[7] This study demonstrates that these solo teenagers had different views from those presenting with parents and underscores the potential bias introduced if they were not included in adolescent research.

For adolescents presenting to clinics with parents, African American race was associated with a decreased perceived need for permission for research after controlling for parental educational level. "Closeness to parent" was included in the survey and was not significantly associated with adolescent race or gender. This finding may be related to a more open relationship between African American adolescents and their parents in discussing these risk behaviors and, therefore, less concern regarding loss of confidentiality with required parental consent. Past studies[24,34] have shown that African American adolescents are less concerned with disclosure of risk behaviors than their peers of other ethnicities.

Our study findings on parental and youth attitudes regarding parental permission for research are similar to those of other studies. Like Sikand et al,[25] we found that most parents endorsed parental consent for surveys of adolescents involving sexual behavior and found differences in attitudes between parents and adolescents (parents, 83%; paired adolescents, 63%; and solo adolescents, 44%). The proportions of paired parents and adolescents endorsing a requirement for parental permission for research on the various risk behavior research topics were higher in this study than in previous studies.[25] This may reflect differences between studies, with this survey's focus on risk behaviors and confidential surveys compared with previous work that addressed a broad array of research topics and methods.

There are limitations to our study. Most parents in our sample were female, most were African American, and all were recruited from clinic settings. Most solo adolescents were African American. These sampling characteristics may affect generalizability. Also, our study was conducted amid a time of much public debate regarding parental consent in pediatric and adolescent health care and pediatric research, including the case of *CN v Ridgewood Board of Education*[6] and the cancelled risk behavior survey in northern Virginia public schools.[17] Local and national media, lawmakers, and politicians have addressed these controversies. In addition, the study prompting *Grimes v Kennedy Krieger Institute, Inc*[15] was conducted within the metropolitan area of the study sample. This may have biased results toward greater endorsement requiring parental permission. Another potential limitation may have been respondent confusion regarding clinical research vs confidential survey research. This may have biased results toward greater endorsement of parental permission; however, the study clearly defined survey research and emphasized confidential risk behavior surveys with no names used. Finally, the fact that parent-adolescent pairs were sampled concurrently could affect perceived confidentiality, although headsets were used and safeguards were developed to address this issue.

It is not clear what effect requirement of parental permission for adolescent involvement in risk behavior research would have on external research validity. It is probable that participation in this research would decrease because of logistic issues in contacting parents, parental refusal of participation, and adolescent refusal of participation related to confidentiality concerns. This could increase selection bias and decrease generalizability. In addition, it is possible that the truthfulness of adolescent responses could be influenced by knowledge that their parents are aware of their participation and concerns about disclosure of their responses. This study adds the adolescent and parent perspective on the issue of adolescent risk behavior research importance and parental permission, although further study is needed on the impact of parental consent on research participation and validity.

Parents and adolescents agree that risk behavior research is important and should be done. Policy decisions on whether parental consent should be required for adolescent risk behavior research must consider parental and adolescent views, the impact of required consent on the validity of research, the risk and benefits of the research, and the importance of this research for public health. Clearly, requirement of parental consent for confidential adolescent research would exclude some of the solo adolescents in this study who had different attitudes compared with adolescents presenting with their parents. This study contributes to our understanding of parental and adolescent views that may foster improved communication regarding research and consent. Better communication among parents, researchers, study subjects, and governing bodies is essential to improving adolescent risk behavior research and participation. Agreement on guidelines is needed for research that all agree is important for adolescent health.

**Accepted for Publication:** June 14, 2006.
**Correspondence:** Ryan H. Pasternak, MD, MPH, Department of Pediatrics, Louisiana State University, School of Medicine, 1542 Tulane Ave, Campus Box T8-1, New Orleans, LA 70112 (rpaste@lsuhsc.edu).
**Author Contributions:** Dr Pasternak had full access to all of the data in the study and takes full responsibility for the integrity of the data and the accuracy of the data analysis. *Study concept and design:* Pasternak, Geller, and Cheng. *Acquisition of data:* Pasternak and Parrish. *Drafting of the manuscript:* Pasternak, Geller, and Cheng. *Critical revision of the manuscript for important intellectual content:* Pasternak, Geller, Parrish, and Cheng. *Statistical analysis:* Pasternak, Geller, and Cheng. *Obtained funding:* Pasternak, Geller, and Cheng. *Administrative, technical, and material support:* Pasternak, Geller, Parrish, and Cheng. *Study supervision:* Cheng.
**Financial Disclosure:** None reported.
**Funding/Support:** This study was supported by grant U48/CCU309674 through the Prevention Research Centers, Centers for Disease Control and Prevention; and by a Pri-

mary Care Faculty Development training grant from the Health Resources and Services Administration.
**Role of the Sponsor:** The funding bodies had no role in data extraction and analyses, in the writing of the manuscript, or in the decision to submit the manuscript for publication.
**Disclaimer:** The opinions expressed in this article do not necessarily reflect those of the Centers for Disease Control and Prevention or the Health Resources and Services Administration.
**Previous Presentation:** This study was presented in part as a platform presentation at the annual meeting of the Society for Adolescent Medicine; April 2, 2005; Los Angeles, Calif.
**Acknowledgments:** We thank Anne Duggan, ScD, Department of Pediatrics, The Johns Hopkins University, for her support and contributions toward this study; Kristen Ehrenberger, now with the University of Illinois School of Medicine, for her dedication to the early development of this project; Diane Markakis, MS, Department of Pediatrics, The Johns Hopkins University, for her assistance with data entry and analysis; Merisa Aranas Pasternak, MPH, Department of Medicine, Tulane University Health Sciences Center, for her critique and for providing a voice for the survey; and the research assistants, for their indispensable and appreciated work.

## REFERENCES

1. Reif CJ, Elster AB. Adolescent preventive services. *Prim Care.* 1998;25:1-21.
2. Scarr S. Ethical problems in research on risky behaviors and risky populations. *Ethics Behav.* 1994;4:147-155.
3. Wilfond BS, Geller G, Lerman C, Audrain-McGovern J, Shields AE. Ethical issues in conducting behavioral genetics research: the case of smoking prevention trials among adolescents. *J Health Care Law Policy.* 2002;6:73-88.
4. Glantz LH. Nontherapeutic research with children: *Grimes v Kennedy Krieger Institute. Am J Public Health.* 2002;92:1070-1073.
5. Gardner W, Wilcox BL. Political intervention in scientific peer review: research on adolescent sexual behavior. *Am Psychol.* 1993;48:972-983.
6. *CN v Ridgewood Board of Education*, 319 F2d 483 (NJ 2004).
7. Mammel KA, Kaplan DW. Research consent by adolescent minors and institutional review boards. *J Adolesc Health.* 1995;17:323-330.
8. Kopelman LM. Pediatric research regulations under legal scrutiny: Grimes narrows their interpretation. *J Law Med Ethics.* 2002;30:38-49.
9. Mastroianni AC, Kahn JP. Risk and responsibility: ethics, *Grimes v Kennedy Krieger*, and public health research involving children. *Am J Public Health.* 2002;92:1073-1076.
10. Pearce M. Children as subjects in nontherapeutic research: *Grimes v Kennedy Krieger Institute, Inc. J Leg Med.* 2002;23:421-436.
11. McHale JV. Guidelines for medical research: some ethical and legal problems. *Med Law Rev.* 1993;1:160-185.
12. The National Commission for the Protection of Human Subjects of Biomedical and Behavioral Research. *The Belmont Report: Ethical Principles and Guidelines for the Protection of Human Subjects of Research.* Washington, DC: US Government Printing Office; 1978. DHEW publication (OS) 78-0012.
13. Santelli JS, Smith Rogers A, Rosenfeld WD, et al; Society for Adolescent Medicine. Guidelines for adolescent health research: a position paper of the Society for Adolescent Medicine. *J Adolesc Health.* 2003;33:396-409.
14. Office for Human Research Protections, Department of Health and Human Services. Special protections for children as research subjects: children involved as subjects in research: guidance on the HHS 45 CFR 46.407 ("407") review process. http://www.hhs.gov/ohrp/children/guidance_407process.html. Accessed June 7, 2005.
15. *Grimes v Kennedy Krieger Institute, Inc*, 782 A2d 807 (Md 2001).
16. Roeder KH, Martin SH, Rees JS. Maryland Court ruling sets precedent on research involving minors: Grimes v Kennedy Krieger Institute, Inc. *GHA Today.* 2001;45:3, 8.
17. Kalita SM. Fairfax cancels student survey on sex, drugs company distributing the questionnaire feared angry parents might file lawsuits. *Washington Post.* April 23, 2003;§B:B1.
18. Select Committee on Children, Youth, and Families, US House of Representatives. *A Decade of Denial: Teens and AIDS in America.* Washington, DC: US Government Printing Office; 1992.
19. Rogers AS, D'Angelo L, Futterman D. Guidelines for adolescent participation in research: current realities and possible resolutions. *IRB.* 1994;16:1-6.
20. Geller G, Tambor ES, Bernhardt BA, Fraser G, Wissow LS. Informed consent for enrolling minors in genetic susceptibility research: a qualitative study of at-risk children's and parents' views about children's role in decision-making. *J Adolesc Health.* 2003;32:260-271.
21. Brody JL, Annett RD, Scherer DG, Perryman DL, Cofrin KM. Comparisons of adolescent and parent willingness to participate in minimal and above-minimal risk pediatric asthma research protocols. *J Adolesc Health.* 2005;37:229-235.
22. Petersen AC, Leffert N. Developmental issues influencing guidelines for adolescent health research: a review. *J Adolesc Health.* 1995;17:298-305.
23. Boekeloo BO, Schiavo L, Rabin DL, Conlon RT, Jordan CS, Mundt DJ. Self-reports of HIV risk factors by patients at a sexually transmitted disease clinic: audio vs written questionnaires. *Am J Public Health.* 1994;84:754-760.
24. Cheng TL, Savageau JA, Sattler AL, DeWitt TG. Confidentiality in health care: a survey of knowledge, perceptions, and attitudes among high school students. *JAMA.* 1993;269:1404-1407.
25. Sikand A, Schubiner H, Simpson PM. Parent and adolescent perceived need for parental consent involving research with minors. *Arch Pediatr Adolesc Med.* 1997;151:603-607.
26. Sigman G, Silber TJ, English A, Epner JE. Confidential health care for adolescents: position paper of the Society for Adolescent Medicine. *J Adolesc Health.* 1997;21:408-415.
27. English A. Treating adolescents: legal and ethical considerations. *Med Clin North Am.* 1990;74:1097-1112.
28. English A. Guidelines for adolescent health research: legal perspectives. *J Adolesc Health.* 1995;17:277-286.
29. Santelli J. Human subjects protection and parental permission in adolescent health research. *J Adolesc Health.* 1997;21:384-387.
30. Santelli J, Rogers AS. Parental permission, passive consent, and "children" in research. *J Adolesc Health.* 2002;31:303-304.
31. Santelli JS, Rosenfeld WD, DuRant RH, et al. Guidelines for adolescent health research: a position paper of the Society for Adolescent Medicine. *J Adolesc Health.* 1995;17:270-276.
32. Levine RJ. Adolescents as research subjects without permission of their parents or guardians: ethical considerations. *J Adolesc Health.* 1995;17:287-297.
33. Eisenberg ME, Swain C, Bearinger LH, Sieving RE, Resnick MD. Parental notification laws for minors' access to contraception: what do parents say? *Arch Pediatr Adolesc Med.* 2005;159:120-125.
34. Jones RK, Purcell A, Singh S, Finer LB. Adolescents' reports of parental knowledge of adolescents' use of sexual health services and their reactions to mandated parental notification for prescription contraception. *JAMA.* 2005;293:340-348.

# Autism

## A Review of the State of the Science for Pediatric Primary Health Care Clinicians

William J. Barbaresi, MD; Slavica K. Katusic, MD; Robert G. Voigt, MD

Autism is a complex neurodevelopmental disorder characterized by impaired reciprocal social interaction, impaired communication, and restricted, repetitive, or stereotyped behaviors. Autism seems to affect more children than was previously believed, although this phenomenon may be due to broadening of the diagnostic criteria and increased awareness of the condition. Recent research has clearly indicated the importance of early identification, since early intensive treatment is associated with better long-term outcome. There are many controversies and competing theories about the etiology and treatment of autism, often leaving families confused about the best course of treatment and intervention. Pediatric primary health care clinicians have an important role in both the early identification and ongoing management of children with autism. It is, therefore, essential that primary care clinicians have up-to-date information about the science of autism. *Arch Pediatr Adolesc Med. 2006;160:1167-1175*

### WHY A REVIEW ON AUTISM?

Autism and related conditions in the autism spectrum have become the focus of intense interest fueled by concerns about the apparent increase in the number of children with these developmental disorders.[1,2] Pediatricians have an important role in the identification and ongoing management of children with autism. This article provides pediatric clinicians with a contemporary understanding of autism, including definitions, epidemiology, initial identification, formal diagnostic approaches, medical evaluation, treatment, controversies, and caregiver support.

### WHAT IS AUTISM?

Autism, first described in 1943, is a complex developmental disorder characterized by severe impairment in reciprocal social interaction and communication and by a pattern of repetitive or stereotyped behavior.[3,4] The *Diagnostic and Statistical Manual of Mental Disorders, Fourth Edition, Text Revision* (*DSM-IV, TR*) includes autistic disorder in the broader category of pervasive developmental disorders, along with pervasive developmental disorder, not otherwise specified (PDD-NOS), Asperger's disorder, Rett's disorder, and childhood disintegrative disorder.[3] Autistic disorder, PDD-NOS, and Asperger's disorder are often collectively referred to as the autism spectrum disorders (ASDs), while the term autism is used interchangeably with the *DSM-IV, TR* term autistic disorder. The term ASDs reflects the notion that these conditions are related and may be difficult to differentiate with current diagnostic tools.[5-8] Pervasive developmental disorder, not otherwise specified is a somewhat ill-defined diagnosis of exclusion reserved for children with problems similar to those seen in autistic disorder but insufficient to meet the criteria for autistic disorder in number, severity, or age at onset.[3,6,7]

The diagnostic criteria for autism require the presence of 6 symptoms from 3 categories: impaired reciprocal social in-

**Author Affiliations:** Departments of Pediatric and Adolescent Medicine, Division of Developmental and Behavioral Pediatrics (Drs Barbaresi and Voigt), and Health Sciences Research, Division of Epidemiology (Dr Katusic), and Mayo Clinic–Dana Child Development and Learning Disorders Program (Drs Barbaresi, Katusic, and Voigt), Mayo Clinic College of Medicine, Rochester, Minn.

**Table 1. Diagnostic Criteria for Autistic Disorder***

A. A total of ≥6 items from the following criteria 1, 2, and 3, with at least 2 from criterion 1 and 1 each from criteria 2 and 3
  1. Qualitative impairment in social interaction as manifested by at least 2 of the following:
    a. Marked impairment in the use of multiple nonverbal behaviors such as eye-to-eye gaze, facial expression, body posture, and gestures to regulate social interaction
    b. Failure to develop peer relationships appropriate to developmental level
    c. Lack of spontaneous seeking to share enjoyment, interests, or achievements with other people (eg, lack of showing, bringing, or pointing out objects of interest)
    d. Lack of social or emotional reciprocity
  2. Qualitative impairments in communication as manifested by at least 1 of the following:
    a. Delay in or total lack of development of spoken language (not accompanied by an attempt to compensate through alternative modes of communication such as gesture or mime)
    b. In individuals with adequate speech, marked impairment in the ability to initiate or sustain a conversation
    c. Stereotyped and repetitive use of language or idiosyncratic language
    d. Lack of varied, spontaneous make-believe play or social imitative play appropriate to developmental level
  3. Restricted, repetitive, and stereotyped patterns of behavior, interests, and activities as manifested by at least 1 of the following:
    a. Encompassing preoccupation with 1 or more stereotyped and restricted patterns of interest that is abnormal either in intensity or focus
    b. Apparently inflexible adherence to specific, nonfunctional routines or rituals
    c. Stereotyped and repetitive motor mannerisms (eg, hand or finger flapping or twisting, or complex whole-body movements
    d. Persistent preoccupation with parts of objects

B. Delay or abnormal functioning in at least 1 of the following areas, with onset before age 3 years:
  1. Social interaction
  2. Language as used in social communication
  3. Symbolic or imaginative play

C. Disturbance not better accounted for by Rett's disorder or childhood disintegrative disorder

*Reprinted with permission from the *Diagnostic and Statistical Manual of Mental Disorders, Fourth Edition, Text Revision*.[3]

**Table 2. Autism-Specific Screening Tools**

| Screening Tool | Characteristics |
|---|---|
| Checklist for Autism in Toddlers (CHAT) | For use in children aged 18 mo; 14 items, 9 derived from parent history and 5 from direct observation; specificity 98%, sensitivity 38%; does not discriminate well between children with autism and children with mental retardation |
| Social Communication Questionnaire (formerly called Autism Screening Questionnaire) | For use in children aged ≥4 y |
| Modified Checklist for Autism in Toddlers (M-CHAT) | For use in children aged 24 mo; 23 items, all based on parental report; specificity 87%, sensitivity 99%; efficient for use in a primary care setting |

teraction (at least 2 symptoms), impaired communication, and restricted, repetitive, or stereotyped behaviors (**Table 1**). These criteria reflect the central role of deficits in social behavior in children with ASDs.[3,9,10] One of the earliest and most important indicators of autism is the failure to develop joint attention,[7,11,12] which refers to the child's ability to share interests, pleasurable experiences, or requests by using gestures or verbal communication in combination with eye contact with another person.

## EPIDEMIOLOGY

There is widespread public concern about the apparent increase in autism, based on prevalence studies during the last 20 years.[1,13-17] Studies from the 1980s and early 1990s reported a prevalence of 4 to 10 per 10 000 children, whereas recent studies have reported prevalences of 30 to 50 per 10 000 children.[1,13-18] Studies that rely on administrative data for children who receive special education services have reported significant increases in prevalence from 1992 to 2001.[19] A recent study in a single US county demonstrated an apparent increase in the incidence of research-identified autism among individuals 21 years of age or younger, from 5.5 per 100 000 in the 1980-1983 period to 44.9 per 100 000 in the 1995-1997 period.[1] The advantage this incidence study had over previous prevalence studies was in its reporting rates of newly identified cases in the same community over many years with the use of consistent *DSM-IV, TR*–based research criteria for case identification. The timing of this apparent increase coincided with the introduction of broader diagnostic criteria, increased availability of educational services, and increased awareness of autism. These findings were not consistent with the hypotheses that immunization policy or the vaccine preservative thimerosal have contributed to this epidemiologic phenomenon.[1,20] A recent review also noted the absence of published literature that demonstrates increased rates of autism in children who have been immunized with vaccines containing thimerosal.[20] A study from the United Kingdom also concluded that the observed increase in the rate of diagnosis of pervasive developmental disorder is likely the result of better case ascertainment rather than a true increase in autism.[21]

## IDENTIFICATION OF AUTISM BY PEDIATRIC PRIMARY HEALTH CARE CLINICIANS

Early identification of autism is important because early intervention services may be more effective in children with autism than in children with other developmental disabilities.[22] Pediatric clinicians are ideally positioned to assume this role, aided by practice guidelines for the diagnosis and management of ASDs in children.[7,23,24] A 2-level approach to autism screening and diagnosis is recommended.[7] In children who fail routine developmental screening, specific screening for autism should be performed[25-28] (**Table 2**). In children who fail specific autism screening, referral for a formal evaluation by an experienced clinician is recommended. Referral is also recommended for any child who does not babble or point or use other gestures by the age of 12 months, who uses no single words by 16 months or no spontaneous (nonecholalic) 2-word phrases by 24 months, or who experiences any loss of any language or social skills at any age.[7]

Deficits in joint attention differentiate infants with autism from those with mental retardation or typical development.[29-32] These behaviors include deficits in the following areas: eye contact, orientation to name being called, pointing, and showing. In the toddler age group, a lack of pretend play and imitation, deficits in nonverbal communication, and disproportionate language delays differentiate autism from other developmental disorders.[7] Although repetitive behaviors, stereotypic motor mannerisms, atypical sensory responses, and behavioral outbursts are generally observed in children with autism, these behaviors do not consistently differentiate autism from other developmental disorders at early ages.[7]

The Modified Checklist for Autism in Toddlers (M-CHAT) has been developed as an autism-specific screening tool for use in 24-month-old children (Table 2).[33-36] It consists of 23 items based on parental report, which makes this checklist efficient for use in primary care settings. Other promising screening instruments include the Pervasive Developmental Disorders Screening Test–II[37] and the Screening Tool for Autism in Two-Year Olds.[38] For children who are 4 years or older, the Social Communication Questionnaire may be used as an autism screening instrument.[7,27,28]

Children with autism can also be identified by a characteristic early developmental profile, with relative strengths in visuomotor problem solving and discrepant and disproportionate weaknesses in language.[39-50] The Cognitive Adaptive Test/Clinical Linguistic and Auditory Milestone Scale (Capute Scales) provides quantitative information about a child's development in the domains of language and visuomotor problem solving and can be used efficiently for this purpose in primary care settings.[51]

## DIAGNOSING AUTISM

A comprehensive, multidisciplinary assessment is required to evaluate a child for an ASD and to differentiate ASDs from other developmental disorders.[5-7,12,52] Since there are no definitive diagnostic tests, a clinical diagnosis by an expert, based on *DSM-IV, TR* criteria, remains the gold standard of ASD diagnosis.[6,7,12,52] The *DSM-IV, TR* criteria consist of a list of behaviors that are not described in detail, leaving considerable latitude for clinical judgment.[3,7,12] Children who have been evaluated exclusively by school or early intervention staff should not be considered to have undergone a thorough diagnostic assessment. This can be confusing to both parents and pediatricians, given the existence of the explicit special education category "Autism Spectrum Disorders" (Individuals with Disabilities Education Act [IDEA] 97, Pub L No. 105-17).[53] An ASD designation for special education purposes may be obtained without a clinical diagnosis of an ASD. Furthermore, children with autism or PDD-NOS often have severe cognitive, communicative, and behavioral problems that can only be assessed by a team of professionals (**Table 3**). The clinical diagnosis of an ASD is facilitated by the use of rating scales and direct assessment tools specifically developed for this purpose (**Table 4**).[54-59]

**Table 3. Professionals Who May Be Included in Multidisciplinary Assessment for Autism**

| Discipline | Role |
|---|---|
| Developmental and behavioral pediatrician, child psychiatrist, child neurologist or neurodevelopmental disabilities pediatrician | Clinical diagnostic assessment based on *DSM-IV, TR* criteria, case coordination for medical workup and treatment |
| Child psychologist | Psychometric testing, administration of Autism Diagnostic Observation Schedule if indicated |
| Speech pathologist | Formal speech, language, and communication assessment |
| Medical geneticist | Clinical dysmorphology examination, coordination of genetic and metabolic testing |
| Physiatrist, occupational therapist, physical therapist | Assessment of fine and gross motor disorders and development of treatment recommendations |
| Medical social worker | Assessment of family resources, coordination of services, family support |

Abbreviation: *DSM-IV, TR, Diagnostic and Statistical Manual of Mental Disorders, Fourth Edition, Text Revision.*

**Table 4. Autism-Specific Diagnostic Tools**

| Instrument | Characteristics |
|---|---|
| Autism Diagnostic Interview-Revised (ADI-R)* | Semistructured interview that is reliable, valid, and differentiates autism from other developmental disorders; takes 1½ h to administer, limiting clinical use |
| Autism Diagnostic Observation Schedule-Generic (ADOS-G)* | Reliable, valid, direct assessment that helps to differentiate ASDs from other developmental disorders; requires specific training; takes 30 min to administer, making it practical for clinical use |
| Gilliam Autism Rating Scale | Checklist that may be used by parents and teachers and other professionals to quantify autism symptoms |
| Childhood Autism Rating Scale | Structured interview and observational tool designed to be used by experienced clinicians or other professionals to identify symptoms consistent with ASDs |

Abbreviation: ASDs, autistic spectrum disorders.
*Neither the ADI-R nor the ADOS-G is sufficient to enable a diagnosis of autism. The diagnosis depends on assessment by an experienced clinician.

Approximately 60% to 75% of children with autistic disorder or PDD-NOS have cognitive skills in the mentally retarded range (standard scores $<70$ on formal cognitive tests).[1,3] Fewer children with PDD-NOS are likely to function in the mentally retarded range.[52] Children with autism or PDD-NOS often demonstrate relative strength in visual problem-solving skills and relative weakness in language-based cognitive skills; this discrepant cogni-

**Table 5. Cognitive Assessment Tools**

| |
|---|
| Bayley Scales of Infant Development |
| Mullen Scales of Early Learning |
| Differential Abilities Scales |
| Stanford-Binet IV |
| Wechsler Scales of Intelligence for Children, Fourth Edition |
| Leiter International Performance Scale–Revised* |
| Merrill-Palmer Scale* |

*May be more appropriate for use in nonverbal children.

**Table 6. Medical and Genetic Evaluation of Children With Autism**

| |
|---|
| Required evaluations |
| Careful examination to identify dysmorphic physical features |
| Wood's lamp examination for tuberous sclerosis |
| Formal audiologic evaluation |
| Lead test; repeat periodically in children with pica |
| High-resolution karyotype |
| Molecular DNA testing for fragile X syndrome |
| Consider if results of above evaluations are normal, and in children with comorbid mental retardation |
| FISH test for region 15q11q13 to rule out duplications in Prader-Willi/Angelman syndrome region |
| FISH test for telomeric abnormalities |
| Test for mutations in *MECP2* gene (Rett syndrome) |
| Metabolic testing to consider based on other clinical features |
| Fasting blood glucose |
| Plasma amino acids |
| Ammonia and lactate |
| Fatty acid profile, paroxysmal |
| Carnitine |
| Acylcarnitine, quantitative |
| Homocysteine |
| Plasma 7-dehydrocholesterol (Smith-Lemli-Opitz disease screening) |
| Urine amino acids |
| Urine organic acids |
| Urine testing for purines and pyrimidines |
| Urine acylglycine, random |
| Other testing to consider based on clinical features |
| Liver enzymes |
| Thyroxine, thyroid-stimulating hormone |
| Biotinidase |
| Complete blood cell count |
| Ceruloplasmin and serum copper |
| Electroencephalography if the following clinical features are noted |
| Clinically observable seizures |
| History of significant regression in social or communication functioning |

Abbreviation: FISH, fluorescent in situ hybridization.

tive profile may be reflected in a significant discrepancy between verbal and performance IQ scores.[3,7,39-50,52] Formal cognitive assessment should be completed using instruments that have been demonstrated to be appropriate[60-67] (**Table 5**).

Similarly, formal speech and language assessment is essential because communication deficits of varying severity are always present in children with ASD.[3,7,12] Children with ASD may have specific deficits in the social use of language, often referred to as pragmatic language.[3,7,12] For example, a child may be able to recite long segments of dialogue from a favorite video yet not be able to use a 3-word sentence to ask for something to eat. Problems with pragmatic language are often identified only by a careful history or direct observation of the child in his or her natural environment.[3,7,12]

Social-adaptive behavioral assessments should include assessment of functional skills such as sleeping, eating, and toileting and problem behaviors such as aggression, oppositionality, and self-injury. This assessment is facilitated by the use of formal questionnaires and rating scales including, among others, the Vineland Adaptive Behavior Scales and the Scales of Independent Behavior.[68,69] Formal assessments of fine and gross motor skills may be incorporated into the evaluation as indicated. Parent resources should be carefully assessed to enable the team to understand the context of the child's developmental problems and to ensure that plans are made to provide appropriate support to the family.

## MEDICAL EVALUATION OF CHILDREN WITH AUTISM

Every child with autism should undergo a formal audiologic evaluation, whether or not the child passed a newborn hearing screening test. In addition, children with autism are at risk of lead toxicity, given their high prevalence of putting objects in their mouths.[70] Thus, periodic lead screening should be performed until pica resolves.[7]

Although a recognizable etiologic disorder is found in fewer than 25% of individuals with autism, attempts to establish an etiologic diagnosis to account for this clinical syndrome are important to identify diagnoses that may affect prognosis, risk of recurrence, and associated medical morbidity. A thorough history and physical examination should guide the medical diagnostic workup[71-77] (**Table 6**). Since tuberous sclerosis accounts for up to 3% to 4% of autism cases, Wood's lamp examinations should be performed in every child with autism to detect the hypopigmented macules associated with this syndrome, especially if the child has an intercurrent seizure disorder.[78] While routine head imaging (computed tomography or magnetic resonance imaging) is not recommended, recent studies have reported abnormal patterns of brain growth in individuals with autism.[79] Functional imaging techniques are currently used as research tools but are not indicated in routine clinical practice.[7,80,81]

Autism has been associated with many genetic syndromes, including Down syndrome, Angelman syndrome, de Lange syndrome, Smith-Magenis syndrome, and Smith-Lemli-Opitz syndrome.[82,83] Seven percent to 8% of individuals with autism have fragile X syndrome.[84] In addition, anomalies in almost every chromosome have been reported in individuals with autism, although more consistent linkage findings have been associated with chromosomes 2q, 7q, and 15q.[85] Thus, DNA testing for fragile X syndrome and high-resolution chromosome analyses are recommended in the laboratory workup in children with autism, especially those with mental retardation, dysmorphic features, congenital anomalies, or a family history of autism or mental retardation.[7,84] Fluorescent in situ hybridization testing for specific chromosome deletions, duplications, or inversions should be considered if initial investigations produce negative results[84-87] (Table 6). Even in the absence of a specific genetic diagnosis, the recurrence rate in siblings of children with autism is between 2% and 8%, increasing the risk of having a second child with autism nearly 50-fold over that in the general population.[84]

Although a wide range of inborn errors of metabolism have been associated with autistic behavior, less than 5% of children with autism have identifiable metabolic disorders.[88-93] Thus, metabolic testing is particularly indicated when the autistic behaviors are accompanied by a history of developmental plateauing or regression; decompensation with mild illness, unusual odors, or food intolerance; failure to thrive; episodic lethargy; cyclic vomiting; seizures; coarse features; mental retardation; questionable newborn screening results; or birth outside the United States[7] (Table 6).

By adulthood, about one third of individuals with autism will have at least 2 unprovoked epileptic seizures.[82] Onset of seizures in individuals with autism follows a bimodal age distribution, with peaks in early childhood and adolescence.[7,94] All seizure types, including infantile spasms, can be associated with autism, but partial complex seizures, with electroencephalographic abnormalities occurring most often over the temporal lobes, appear to be most prevalent.[95] About one third of parents of children with autism report regression of language in their children, most commonly the loss of their toddler's first few words, between age 18 and 24 months.[94,96] Approximately 10% of children with autism also have a paroxysmal electroencephalographic pattern similar to that seen in Landau-Kleffner syndrome (acquired epileptic aphasia) or electrical status epilepticus during slow-wave sleep.[94] While there have been reports of the use of anticonvulsant therapy and even epilepsy surgery, there is insufficient evidence to recommend routine electroencephalography in all children with autism.[97-99] Indications for prolonged sleep-deprived electroencephalography with adequate sampling of slow-wave sleep are listed in Table 6.[7]

## EDUCATIONAL AND BEHAVIORAL INTERVENTIONS

Pediatricians have an important role in helping to guide families toward intervention approaches that have been empirically demonstrated as effective.[5,52,100] In the Internet era, families have access to virtually limitless information about treatments and interventions for autism. Since family resources of time, energy, and finances are limited, it is essential to ensure that these resources are directed toward interventions that offer the best hope for improved outcome.

The Individuals with Disabilities Education Act mandates educational services for children in the special education category of Autism Spectrum Disorders.[52] The provisions of the Individuals with Disabilities Education Act do not, however, ensure that children will receive empirically validated interventions of appropriate intensity. There is, therefore, considerable variability in the quality of educational interventions for children with ASD. This is an additional important reason for pediatricians to understand and advocate for optimal services.

Decades-worth of scientific research provide clear and convincing support for the technique referred to as Applied Behavior Analysis (ABA).[5,100] This technique uses the principles of operant conditioning to teach specific social, communicative, and behavioral skills to children with ASD.[5,100] It involves teaching new behaviors by explicit reinforcement of these behaviors; problem behaviors are often addressed by carefully analyzing triggers or antecedents of the problem behavior in order to change the factors in the environment that are contributing to the problem behavior. Applied Behavior Analysis also uses careful collection of data to demonstrate the efficacy of treatment in the individual child; the data are used to assess progress and to continually modify the intervention as the child progresses toward specific learning objectives.[101]

Interest in ABA as a primary, comprehensive treatment approach in children with ASD was sparked by the research of Lovaas,[102,103] who reported that 9 (47%) of 19 young children with autism who received intensive, early ABA (40 hours per week for ≥2 years) had outcomes that were indistinguishable from their normally developing peers.[103] Subsequent studies have led many experts in the field to conclude that intensive ABA is an effective intervention but that it is unlikely that 50% of children who receive early, intensive ABA will achieve completely normal developmental outcomes.[100,104-107] Practice guidelines have used these and other research findings to formulate recommendations on the key features of appropriate intervention for children with autism.[5,52,100] Characteristics of effective intervention are believed to include a minimum of 20 hours per week of carefully organized services initiated at an early age (preferably younger than 4 years) and involving direct adult attention in individual or very small group instruction.[5,7,52,100] Recent studies have concluded that intensity of intervention is important (ie, a minimum of 20 hours per week) and that ABA is superior to other intervention strategies.[100,108]

Another intervention model with a long history and well-defined instructional methods is TEACCH (Treatment and Education of Autistic and Related Communication Handicapped Children).[109] The TEACCH approach takes advantage of relative strengths in visual information processing, characteristic of many children with ASD, using strategies such as visual schedules, clearly structured and organized classrooms, and highly structured learning activities that are broken down into manageable, visually organized steps. Published reports demonstrate improvement in behaviors and functional skills and parent satisfaction with the TEACCH approach.[52,109,110] However, there appear to be no direct studies of treatment outcomes attributable to TEACCH interventions.

While other intervention strategies are often recommended, there do not appear to be approaches that have the empirical support of ABA or the long history and well-developed curricula of TEACCH. The weight of currently available scientific evidence, however, indicates that ABA should be viewed as the optimal, comprehensive treatment approach in young children with ASD.

Pediatricians should also be aware of sensory integration therapy because this approach is often used in special education programs. Interest in sensory integration is related to the observation that children with ASD often exhibit unusual sensory responses, such as hypersensitivity to certain noises. Techniques used in this therapy include "brushing" of the skin, "swinging" to stimulate vestibular responses, and deep-pressure massage applied in an effort to calm the child.[52] There is no available empirical support for sensory integration therapy, and it should, therefore, neither be routinely recommended nor viewed as a primary intervention strategy in children with ASD.[5,52]

Many other unproved nonmedical therapies have been recommended for use in children with autism. There is no evidence to support the use of facilitated communication, auditory integration training, or music therapy.[5,111-115]

## MEDICAL INTERVENTIONS FOR CHILDREN WITH AUTISM

Although psychopharmacologic therapies have been studied for more than 50 years, there are no Food and Drug Administration–approved indications for the treatment of autism with any agent and there is no medication available for treatment of the core deficits in communication and social interaction.[116] In addition, when used to treat similar target behaviors, psychotropic medications tend to be less effective and result in more adverse effects when used in children with autism compared with children without autism because of similar target behavioral symptoms. However, there is an evidence base for prescribing risperidone to assist in managing tantrums, aggression, and self-injurious and stereotypic behaviors and for prescribing methylphenidate to manage inattentive, impulsive, and hyperactive behaviors in children with autism.[117,118] To date, there is insufficient evidence to support the use of selective serotonin reuptake inhibitors, $\alpha_2$-adrenergic agonists, or mood stabilizers, despite reports of their effectiveness in managing target behavioral symptoms in some children with autism in short-term open-label trials with small sample sizes.[119-121] Psychotropic medications should never be used in isolation but used only in conjunction with behavioral, educational, and habilitative therapies.[122] If psychotropic medications are used, initial dosage should be low, with gradual increases in dosage until optimal positive effects, without significant adverse effects, are achieved.

## UNPROVED THEORIES OF CAUSATION AND UNPROVED OR INEFFECTIVE TREATMENTS IN CHILDREN WITH AUTISM

Traditional medicine does not offer a cure for autism. As a result, unproved complementary and alternative treatments are often provided to children with autism by parents who are seeking effective biomedical interventions.[123] Patients with chronic conditions with unclear pathophysiologic features, fluctuating courses, highly subjective symptoms, and few effective evidence-based treatments are most vulnerable to the placebo effect.[124] Such is clearly the case in autism, and unproved explanations of causation and unproved therapies abound.

One example is the controversy about whether the mercury-containing compound thimerosal, which has been included in certain vaccines to protect multiple-dose vials from bacterial and fungal contamination, is related to the increased prevalence of autism.[125] However, no children with autism have been reported to have an abnormal body burden of mercury or an excess of mercury in hair, urine, or blood.[126] Neither the clinical signs and symptoms of mercury-induced neurologic damage nor the neuropathologic changes associated with mercury exposure parallel the clinical signs and symptoms of autism.[20] Population-based studies have also shown that the risk of autism in children given thimerosal-containing vaccines is no different from that in children given thimerosal-free vaccines.[20,127] Further, since thimerosal was removed from childhood vaccines in Denmark in 1992, the incidence of autism in that country has continued to rise.[128] Despite this overwhelming scientific evidence, some children with autism are receiving treatment with chelating agents.[129] However, even if exposure to mercury or other heavy metals was causative of autism, chelation therapy has not been found to improve the neurodevelopmental sequelae of heavy metal toxicity.[130] Also, children being treated with chelating agents are at risk of renal and hepatic toxic adverse effects.[129]

There have been concerns about the potential role of the measles-mumps-rubella (MMR) vaccine in the causation of autism, based on findings that have been partially retracted.[131] This theory hypothesizes that the MMR vaccine produces enterocolitis, causing "leaky gut," which then leads to increased absorption of peptides with bioactive properties of endogenous opioids that produce the symptoms of autism.[123] However, large-scale epidemiologic studies have failed to show an association between the MMR vaccine and autism.[1,132-135] Furthermore, a dramatically increased incidence of autism has been associated with the withdrawal of the MMR vaccine in Japan.[135] Despite strong evidence against an association between either thimerosal or MMR vaccines and autism, fear generated by these scientifically disproved theories may be leading more parents to decline to have their children immunized.[136]

The leaky gut hypothesis has also led to unproved claims that variants of celiac disease, yeast overgrowth, and immunologic abnormalities can cause autism.[123,129] Many children with autism have been given very restrictive gluten- and casein-free diets because of unfounded fears that opioidlike peptides derived from gluten and casein are absorbed through their leaky guts and can be detected in their urine. However, children with autism have not been found to have an increased rate of celiac disease and do not have excessive amounts of opioidlike compounds in their urine.[137-142]

Although hypothesized as another cause of leaky gut, fungal overgrowth in the intestines has not been documented at endoscopy in children with autism.[143] While there is no evidence that systemic antifungal medications improve autistic behavior, these medications are associated with liver toxicity, anemia, diarrhea, and exfoliative dermatitis.[123,129]

It has been hypothesized that autism is an autoimmune disorder; however, treatment with intravenous immunoglobulin has not proved effective.[144] The pancreatic hormone secretin has also been proposed as a treatment of autism. However, more than a dozen published, peer-reviewed, randomized, double-blind, placebo-controlled trials have failed to show secretin to be effective in treating the symptoms of autism.[129] Other medical therapies that have been recommended but that do not have sufficient evidence to support their effectiveness or safety include vitamin and mineral supplements (vitamin $B_6$ and magnesium, vitamin C, vitamin $B_{12}$, and folic acid), amino acid and peptide supplements (dimethyl glycine and carnosine), and ω-3 long-chain polyunsaturated fatty acids.[129]

Clinicians should counsel parents of children with autism to be sure that any treatment they may consider is supported by evidence from randomized, double-blind, placebo-controlled clinical trials published in the peer-reviewed medical literature. Families should be informed about potential health risks associated with unproved therapies. Finally, parents should be reminded that such treatments may take time, effort, and financial resources away from effective, evidence-based interventions.

## FAMILY AND CAREGIVER SUPPORT

Families that include a child with one of the ASDs experience considerable stress as they are confronted with extraordinary demands on their time, energy, and financial resources. It is essential to offer clear explanations of diagnostic findings and treatment recommendations and to guide families toward effective treatment approaches. This requires the combined effort of experts in the ASD field working collaboratively with primary care clinicians.

Parents need reliable sources of information about ASDs. This is particularly important in an era when the Internet makes misinformation as easily available as accurate information. The Web sites sponsored by the Autism Society of America (www.autism-society.org/site/PageServer), TEACCH (www.teacch.com), and the National Institute of Child Health and Human Development (www.nichd.nih.gov/publications/pubs/autismfacts.pdf) are particularly useful sources of reliable information. However, even accurate information about ASDs is subject to misinterpretation because of the inherent complexity of the topic and the many unanswered questions in the field. There is no substitute for knowledgeable professionals who provide ongoing advice in the context of regular primary care management of children with ASDs.

**Accepted for Publication:** May 5, 2006.
**Correspondence:** William J. Barbaresi, MD, Departments of Pediatric and Adolescent Medicine, Division of Developmental and Behavioral Pediatrics, Mayo Clinic College of Medicine, 200 First St SW, Rochester, MN 55905 (barbaresi.william@mayo.edu).
**Author Contributions:** *Study concept and design:* Barbaresi, Katusic, and Voigt. *Drafting of the manuscript:* Barbaresi, Katusic, and Voigt. *Critical revision of the manuscript for important intellectual content:* Barbaresi, Katusic, and Voigt. *Administrative, technical, and material support:* Barbaresi, Katusic, and Voigt. *Study supervision:* Barbaresi.
**Financial Disclosure:** None reported.

## REFERENCES

1. Barbaresi WJ, Katusic SK, Colligan RC, Weaver AL, Jacobsen SJ. The incidence of autism in Olmsted County, Minnesota, 1976-1997: results from a population-based study. *Arch Pediatr Adolesc Med.* 2005;159:37-44.
2. Stratton K, Gable A, Shetty P, McCormich M, eds. *Immunization Safety Review: Measles-Mumps-Rubella Vaccine and Autism.* Washington, DC: National Academy Press; 2001.
3. American Psychiatric Association. *Diagnostic and Statistical Manual of Mental Disorders, Fourth Edition, Text Revision.* Washington, DC: American Psychiatric Association; 2000.
4. Kanner L. Autistic disturbances of affective contact. *Nervous Child.* 1943;2:217-250.
5. New York State Department of Health Early Intervention Program. *Clinical Practice Guideline: Report of the Recommendations, Autism/Pervasive Developmental Disorders.* Albany: New York State Dept of Health, Health Education Services; 1999.
6. Lord C, Risi S. Frameworks and methods in diagnosing autism spectrum disorders. *Ment Retard Dev Disabil Res Rev.* 1998;4:90-96.
7. Filipek PA, Accardo PJ, Baranek GT, et al. The screening and diagnosis of autistic spectrum disorders [published correction appears in *J Autism Dev Disord.* 2000;30:81]. *J Autism Dev Disord.* 1999;29:439-484.
8. Lord C, Volkmar F. Genetics of childhood disorders, XLII: autism, part 1: diagnosis and assessment in autistic spectrum disorders. *J Am Acad Child Adolesc Psychiatry.* 2002;41:1134-1136.
9. Wing L, Gould J. Severe impairments of social interaction and associated abnormalities in children: epidemiology and classification. *J Autism Dev Disord.* 1979;9:11-29.
10. Beglinger L, Smith T. Concurrent validity of social subtype and IQ after early intensive behavioral intervention in children with autism: a preliminary investigation. *J Autism Dev Disord.* 2005;35:295-303.
11. Volkmar F, Chawarska K, Klin A. Autism in infancy and early childhood. *Annu Rev Psychol.* 2005;56:315-336.
12. Volkmar FR, Lord C, Bailey A, Schultz RT, Klin A. Autism and pervasive developmental disorders. *J Child Psychol Psychiatry.* 2004;45:135-170.
13. Wing L, Potter D. The epidemiology of autistic spectrum disorders: is the prevalence rising? *Mental Retard Dev Dis Res Rev.* 2002;8:151-161.
14. Fombonne E, Simmons H, Ford T, Meltzer H, Goodman R. Prevalence of pervasive developmental disorder in the British nationwide survey of child mental health. *J Am Acad Child Adolesc Psychiatry.* 2001;40:820-827.
15. Fombonne E. The prevalence of autism. *JAMA.* 2003;289:87-89.
16. Yeargin-Allsopp M, Rice C, Karapurkar T, Doernberg N, Boyle C, Murphy C. Prevalence of autism in a US metropolitan area. *JAMA.* 2003;289:49-55.
17. Bertrand J, Mars A, Boyle C, Bove F, Yeargin-Allsopp M, Decoufle P. Prevalence of autism in a United States population: the Brick Township, New Jersey, investigation. *Pediatrics.* 2001;108:1155-1161.
18. Gernsbacher M, Dawson M, Goldsmith H. Three reasons not to believe in an autism epidemic. *Curr Dir Psychol Sci.* 2005;14:55-58.
19. Newschaffer CJ, Falb MD, Gurney JG. National autism prevalence trends from United States special education data. *Pediatrics.* 2005;115:e277-e282.
20. Nelson KB, Bauman ML. Thimerosal and autism? *Pediatrics.* 2003;111:674-679.
21. Smeeth L, Cook C, Fombonne PE, et al. Rate of first recorded diagnosis of autism and other pervasive developmental disorders in United Kingdom general practice, 1988 to 2001. *BMC Med.* 2004;2:39.
22. Lipkin PH, Schertz M. An assessment of the efficacy of early intervention programs. In: Capute AJ, Accardo PJ, eds. *Developmental Disabilities in Infancy and Childhood.* 2nd ed. Baltimore, Md: Brookes Publishing Co; 1996:525-547.
23. American Academy of Pediatrics, Council on Children with Disabilities. Identifying infants and young children with developmental disorders in the medical home: an algorithm for developmental surveillance and screening. *Pediatrics.* 2006;118:405-420.
24. American Academy of Pediatrics, Committee on Children with Disabilities. The pediatrician's role in the diagnosis and management of autistic spectrum disorder in children. *Pediatrics.* 2001;107:1221-1226.
25. Baron-Cohen S, Allen J, Gillberg C. Can autism be detected at 18 months? the needle, the haystack, and the CHAT. *Br J Psychiatry.* 1992;161:839-843.
26. Baron-Cohen S, Wheelwright S, Cox A, et al. Early identification of autism by the CHecklist for Autism in Toddlers (CHAT). *J R Soc Med.* 2000;93:521-525.
27. Berument SK, Rutter M, Lord C, Pickles A, Bailey A. Autism screening questionnaire: diagnostic validity. *Br J Psychiatry.* 1999;175:444-451.
28. Rutter M, Bailey A, Lord C. *SCQ: Social Communication Questionnaire.* Los Angeles, Calif: Western Psychological Services; 2003.
29. Osterling J, Dawson G. Early recognition of children with autism: a study of first birthday home videotapes. *J Autism Dev Disord.* 1994;24:247-257.

30. Mars AE, Mauk JE, Dowrick P. Symptoms of pervasive developmental disorders as observed in prediagnostic home videos of infants and toddlers. *J Pediatr.* 1998;132:500-504.
31. Werner E, Dawson G, Osterling J, Dinno N. Brief report: recognition of autism spectrum disorder before one year of age: a retrospective study based on home videotapes. *J Autism Dev Disord.* 2000;30:157-162.
32. Baranek GT. Autism during infancy: a retrospective video analysis of sensory-motor and social behaviors at 9-12 months of age. *J Autism Dev Disord.* 1999; 29:213-224.
33. Baird G, Charman T, Baron-Cohen S, et al. A screening instrument for autism at 18 months of age: a 6-year follow-up study. *J Am Acad Child Adolesc Psychiatry.* 2000;39:694-702.
34. Chouieri R, Bridgemohan C. To make the biggest difference, screen early for autism spectrum disorders. *Contemp Pediatr.* 2005;22:54-64.
35. Robins DL, Fein D, Barton ML, Green JA. The modified checklist for autism in toddlers: an initial study investigating the early detection of autism and pervasive developmental disorders. *J Autism Dev Disord.* 2001;31:131-144.
36. Dumont-Mathieu T, Fein D. Screening for autism in young children: the Modified Checklist for Autism in Toddlers (M-CHAT) and other measures. *Ment Retard Dev Disabil Res Rev.* 2005;11:253-262.
37. Siegel B. *Pervasive Developmental Disorders Screening Test—II.* San Antonio, Tex: Harcourt Assessment Inc; 2004.
38. Stone WL, Coonrod EE, Turner LM, Pozdol SL. Psychometric properties of the STAT for early autism screening. *J Autism Dev Disord.* 2004;34:691-701.
39. Lockyer L, Rutter M. A five- to fifteen-year follow-up study of infantile psychosis, IV: Patterns of cognitive ability. *Br J Soc Clin Psychol.* 1970;9:152-163.
40. Happe FGE. Wechsler IQ profile and theory of mind in autism: a research note. *J Child Psychol Psychiatry.* 1994;35:1461-1471.
41. Dennis M, Lockyer L, Lazenby AL, Donnelly RE, Wilkinson M, Schoonheyt W. Intelligence patterns among children with high-functioning autism, phenylketonuria, and childhood head injury. *J Autism Dev Disord.* 1999;29:5-17.
42. Joseph RM, Tager-Flusberg H, Lord C. Cognitive profiles and social-communicative functioning in children with autism spectrum disorder. *J Child Psychol Psychiatry.* 2002;43:807-821.
43. Ehlers S, Nyden A, Gillberg C, et al. Asperger syndrome, autism, and attention disorders: a comparative study of the cognitive profiles of 120 children. *J Child Psychol Psychiatry.* 1997;38:207-217.
44. Klin A, Volkmar FR, Sparrow SS, Cicchetti DV, Rourke BP. Validity and neuropsychological characterization of Asperger syndrome: convergence with nonverbal learning disabilities syndrome. *J Child Psychol Psychiatry.* 1995;36: 1127-1140.
45. Mayes SD, Calhoun SL. Similarities and differences in Wechsler intelligence Scale for Children, third edition (WISC-III) profiles: support for subtest analysis in clinical referrals. *Clin Neuropsychol.* 2004;18:559-572.
46. Mayes SD, Calhoun SL. Ability profiles in children with autism: influence of age and IQ. *Autism.* 2003;7:65-80.
47. Mayes SD, Calhoun SL. Analysis of WISC-II, Stanford–Binet IV, and academic achievement test scores in children with autism. *J Autism Dev Disord.* 2003; 33:329-341.
48. Shah A, Frith U. Why do autistic individuals show superior performance on the block design task? *J Child Psychol Psychiatry.* 1993;34:1351-1364.
49. Voigt RG, Childers DO, Dickerson CL, et al. Early pediatric neurodevelopmental profile of children with autistic spectrum disorders. *Clin Pediatr (Phila).* 2000; 39:663-668.
50. Voigt RG. The Capute Scales in research. In: Accardo PJ, Capute AJ, eds. *The Capute Scales.* Baltimore, Md: Brookes Publishing Co; 2005:41-46.
51. Accardo PJ, Capute AJ, eds. *The Capute Scales.* Baltimore, Md: Brookes Publishing Co; 2005.
52. Lord C, McGee JP, eds, for the Committee on Educational Interventions for Children with Autism, Division of Behavioral and Social Sciences and Education, National Research Council. *Educating Children With Autism.* Washington, DC: National Academy Press; 2001.
53. Individuals with Education Disabilities Act, Public Law 105-117 (1997).
54. Lord C, Rutter M, Le Couteur A. Autism Diagnostic Interview–Revised: a revised version of a diagnostic interview for caregivers of individuals with possible pervasive developmental disorders. *J Autism Dev Disord.* 1994;24: 659-685.
55. Klinger LG, Renner P. Performance-based measures in autism: implications for diagnosis, early detection, and identification of cognitive profiles. *J Clin Child Psychol.* 2000;29:479-492.
56. Lord C, Pickles A, McLennan J, et al. Diagnosing autism: analyses of data from the Autism Diagnostic Interview. *J Autism Dev Disord.* 1997;27:501-517.
57. Lord C, Risi S, Lambrecht L, et al. The Autism Diagnostic Observation Schedule–Generic: a standard measure of social and communication deficits associated with the spectrum of autism. *J Autism Dev Disord.* 2000;30:205-223.
58. Gilliam J. *Gilliam Autism Rating Scale (GARS).* Austin, Tex: PRO-ED, Inc; 1995.
59. Schopler E, Reichler R, Rochen-Renner B. *The Childhood Autism Rating Scale (CARS).* Los Angeles, Calif: Western Psychological Services; 1988.
60. Bayley N. *Bayley Scale of Infant Development.* 2nd ed. San Antonio, Tex: Psychological Corp; 1993.
61. Mullen E. *Mullen Scales of Early Learning.* Los Angeles, Calif: Western Psychological Services; 1997.
62. Elliot C. *Differential Abilities Scale (DAS).* New York, NY: Psychological Corp; 1990.
63. Thorndike R, Hagen E, Sattler J. *The Stanford-Binet Intelligence Scale: Guide for Administering and Scoring.* 4th ed. Chicago, Ill: Riverside Publishing Co; 1986.
64. Wechsler D. *Wechsler Intelligence Scale for Children.* 4th ed. San Antonio, Tex: Psychological Corp; 2003.
65. Wechsler D. *Wechsler Adult Intelligence Scale* . 3rd ed. San Antonio, Tex: Psychological Corp; 1997.
66. Roid G, Miller L. *Leiter International Performance Scale-Revised.* Wood Dale, Ill: Stoelting Co; 1997.
67. Stutsman R. *The Merrill-Palmer Scale of Mental Tests.* Chicago, Ill: Stoelting Co; 1948.
68. Sparrow S, Balla D, Cicchetti D. *Vineland Adaptive Behavior Scales, Expanded Edition.* Circle Pines, Minn: American Guidance Service; 1984.
69. Bruininks R, Woodcock R, Weatherman R, Hill B. *Scales of Independent Behavior–Revised (SIB-R).* Chicago, Ill: Riverside Publishing Co; 1996.
70. Shannon M, Graef J. Lead intoxication in children with pervasive developmental disorders. *J Toxicol Clin Toxicol.* 1997;34:177-182.
71. Gillberg C, Coleman M. Autism and medical disorders: a review of the literature. *Dev Med Child Neurol.* 1996;38:191-202.
72. Challman TD, Barbaresi WJ, Katusic SK, Weaver A. The yield of the medical evaluation of children with pervasive developmental disorders. *J Autism Dev Disord.* 2003;33:187-192.
73. Voigt RG, Dickerson CL, Reynolds AM, Childers DO, Rodriguez DL, Brown FR. Laboratory evaluation of children with autistic spectrum disorders: a guide for primary care pediatricians. *Clin Pediatr (Phila).* 2000;39:669-671.
74. Shevell MI, Majnemer A, Rosenbaum P, Abrahamowicz M. Etiologic yield of autistic spectrum disorder: a prospective study. *J Child Neurol.* 2001;16: 509-512.
75. Chudley AE, Gutierrez E, Jocelyn LJ, Chodirker BN. Outcomes of genetic evaluation in children with pervasive developmental disorder. *J Dev Behav Pediatr.* 1998;19:321-325.
76. Kielinen M, Rantala H, Timonen E, Linna SL, Moilanen I. Associated medical disorders and disabilities in children with autistic disorder: a population-based study. *Autism.* 2004;8:49-60.
77. Kosinovsky B, Hermon S, Yoran-Hegesh R, et al. The yield of laboratory investigations in children with infantile autism. *J Neural Transm.* 2005;112:587-596.
78. Curatolo P, Porfirio MC, Manzi B, Seri S. Autism in tuberous sclerosis. *Eur J Paediatr Neurol.* 2004;8:327-332.
79. Redcay E, Courchesne E. When is the brain enlarged in autism? a meta-analysis of all brain size reports. *Biol Psychiatry.* 2005;58:1-9.
80. Boddaert N, Zilbovicius M. Functional neuroimaging and childhood autism. *Pediatr Radiol.* 2002;32:1-7.
81. Herbert MR, Ziegler DA, Deutsch CK, et al. Brain asymmetries in autism and developmental language disorder: a nested whole-brain analysis. *Brain.* 2005; 128:213-226.
82. Rapin I. Autism. *N Engl J Med.* 1997;337:97-104.
83. Cohen D, Pichard N, Tordjman S, et al. Specific genetic disorders and autism: clinical contribution towards their identification. *J Autism Dev Disord.* 2005; 35:103-116.
84. Muhle R, Trentacoste SV, Rapin I. The genetics of autism. *Pediatrics.* 2004;113: e472-e486.
85. Wassink TH, Brzustowicz LM, Bartlett CW, Szatmari P. The search for autism disease genes. *Ment Retard Dev Disabil Res Rev.* 2004;10:272-283.
86. Dykens EM, Sutcliffe JS, Levitt P. Autism and 15Q11-Q13 disorders: behavioral, genetic, and pathophysiological issues. *Ment Retard Dev Disabil Res Rev.* 2004;10:284-291.
87. Carney RM, Wolpert CM, Ravan SA, et al. Identification of MeCP2 mutations in a series of females with autistic disorder. *Pediatr Neurol.* 2003;28:205-211.
88. Rutter M, Bailey A, Bolton P, Le Couteur A. Autism and known medical conditions: myth and substance. *J Child Psychol Psychiatry.* 1994;35:311-322.
89. Baieli S, Pavone L, Meli C, Fiumara A, Coleman M. Autism and phenylketonuria. *J Autism Dev Disord.* 2003;33:201-204.
90. Gorker I, Tuzun U. Autistic-like findings associated with a urea cycle disorder in a 4-year-old girl. *J Psychiatry Neurosci.* 2005;30:133-135.
91. Kohler M, Assmann B, Brautigam C, et al. Adenylosuccinase deficiency: pos-

sibly under diagnosed encephalopathy with variable clinical features. *Eur J Paediatr Neurol.* 1999;3:3-6.
92. Tierney E, Nwokoro NA, Kelley RI. Behavioral phenotype of RSH/Smith-Lemli-Opitz syndrome. *Ment Retard Dev Disabil Res Rev.* 2000;6:131-134.
93. Oliveira G, Diogo L, Grazina M, et al. Mitochondrial dysfunction in autism spectrum disorders: a population-based study. *Dev Med Child Neurol.* 2005; 47:185-189.
94. Tuchman R, Rapin I. Epilepsy in autism. *Lancet Neurol.* 2002;1:352-358.
95. Olsson I, Steffenburg S, Gillberg C. Epilepsy in autism and autistic-like conditions: a population-based study. *Arch Neurol.* 1988;45:666-668.
96. Tuchman RF, Rapin I. Regression in pervasive developmental disorders: seizures and epileptiform electroencephalogram correlates. *Pediatrics.* 1997; 99:560-566.
97. Scott RC, Neville BG. Developmental perspectives on epilepsy. *Curr Opin Neurol.* 1998;11:115-118.
98. Nass R, Petrucha D. Acquired aphasia with convulsive disorder: a pervasive developmental disorder variant. *J Child Neurol.* 1990;5:327-328.
99. Lewine JD, Andrews R, Chez M, et al. Magnetoencephalographic patterns of epileptiform activity in children with regressive autism spectrum disorders. *Pediatrics.* 1999;104:405-418.
100. Rogers SJ. Empirically supported comprehensive treatments for young children with autism. *J Clin Child Psychol.* 1998;27:168-179.
101. Lovaas OI. *Teaching Individuals With Developmental Delays: Basic Intervention Techniques.* Austin, Tex: PRO-ED, Inc; 2003.
102. Lovaas OI. Behavioral treatment and normal educational and intellectual functioning in young autistic children. *J Consult Clin Psychol.* 1987;55:3-9.
103. McEachin JJ, Smith T, Lovaas OI. Long-term outcome for children with autism who received early intensive behavioral treatment. *Am J Ment Retard.* 1993; 97:359-372.
104. Schopler E, Short A, Mesibov G. Relation of behavioral treatment to "normal functioning": comment on Lovaas. *J Consult Clin Psychol.* 1989;57:162-164.
105. Smith T, Eikeseth S, Klevstrand M, Lovaas O. Intensive behavioral treatment for preschoolers with severe mental retardations and pervasive developmental disorder. *Am J Ment Retard.* 1997;102:238-249.
106. Sheinkopf SJ, Siegel B. Home-based behavioral treatment of young children with autism. *J Autism Dev Disord.* 1998;28:15-23.
107. Eikeseth S, Smith T, Jahr E, Eldevik S. Intensive behavioral treatment at school for 4- to 7-year-old children with autism: a 1-year comparison controlled study. *Behav Modif.* 2002;26:49-68.
108. Howard JS, Sparkman CR, Cohen HG, Green G, Stanislaw H. A comparison of intensive behavior analytic and eclectic treatments for young children with autism. *Res Dev Disabil.* 2005;26:359-383.
109. Mesibov G, Shea V, Schopler E. *The TEACCH Approach to Autism Spectrum Disorders.* New York, NY: Springer; 2005.
110. Mesibov G. Formal and informal measures on the effectiveness of the TEACCH programme. *Autism.* 1997;1:25-35.
111. Mostert MP. Facilitated communication since 1995: a review of published studies. *J Autism Dev Disord.* 2001;31:287-313.
112. American Academy of Pediatrics, Committee on Children With Disabilities. Auditory integration training and facilitated communication for autism. *Pediatrics.* 1998;102:431-433.
113. Mudford OC, Cross BA, Breen S, et al. Auditory integration training for children with autism: no behavioral benefits detected. *Am J Ment Retard.* 2000;105: 118-129.
114. Sinha Y, Silove N, Wheeler D, Williams K. Auditory integration training and other sound therapies for autism spectrum disorders. *Cochrane Database Syst Rev.* 2004;1:CD003681.
115. Dawson G, Watling R. Interventions to facilitate auditory, visual, and motor integration in autism: a review of the evidence. *J Autism Dev Disord.* 2000; 30:415-421.
116. Aman MG, Novotny S, Samango-Sprouse C, et al. Outcome measures for clinical drug trials in autism. *CNS Spectr.* 2004;9:36-47.
117. McCracken JT, McGough J, Shah B, et al; Research Units on Pediatric Psychopharmacology Autism Network. Risperidone in children with autism and serious behavioral problems. *N Engl J Med.* 2002;347:314-321.
118. Research Units on Pediatric Psychopharmacology (RUPP) Autism Network. Randomized, controlled, crossover trial of methylphenidate in pervasive developmental disorders with hyperactivity. *Arch Gen Psychiatry.* 2005;62:1266-1274.
119. DeLong GR, Teague LA, McSwain Kamran M. Effects of fluoxetine treatment in young children with idiopathic autism. *Dev Med Child Neurol.* 1998;40:551-562.
120. Jaselskis CA, Cook EH Jr, Fletcher KE, Leventhal BL. Clonidine treatment of hyperactive and impulsive children with autistic disorder. *J Clin Psychopharmacol.* 1992;12:322-327.
121. Steingard R, Biederman J. Lithium responsive manic-like symptoms in two individuals with autism and mental retardation. *J Am Acad Child Adolesc Psychiatry.* 1987;26:932-935.
122. American Academy of Pediatrics, Committee on Children With Disabilities. Technical report: the pediatrician's role in diagnosis and management of autistic spectrum disorder in children. *Pediatrics.* 2001;107:1221-1226. http://www.pediatrics.org/cgi/content/full/107/5/e85. Accessed October 1, 2005.
123. Hyman SL, Levy SE. Autistic spectrum disorders: when traditional medicine is not enough. *Contemp Pediatr.* 2000;17:101-116.
124. Kaptchuk TJ, Eisenberg DM. The persuasive appeal of alternative medicine. *Ann Intern Med.* 1998;129:1061-1065.
125. Bernard S, Enayati A, Redwood L, Roger H, Binstock T. Autism: a novel form of mercury poisoning. *Med Hypotheses.* 2001;56:462-471.
126. Aschner M, Walker SJ. The neuropathogenesis of mercury toxicity. *Mol Psychiatry.* 2002;7(suppl 2):S40-S41.
127. Hviid A, Stellfeld M, Wohlfahrt J, Melbye M. Association between thimerosal-containing vaccine and autism. *JAMA.* 2003;290:1763-1766.
128. Madsen KM, Lauritsen MB, Pedersen CB, et al. Thimerosal and the occurrence of autism: negative ecological evidence from Danish population-based data. *Pediatrics.* 2003;112:604-606.
129. Levy SE, Hyman SL. Novel treatments for autistic spectrum disorders. *Ment Retard Dev Disabil Res Rev.* 2005;11:131-142.
130. Dietrich KN, Ware HH, Salganik M, et al. Effect of chelation therapy on the neuropsychological and behavioral development of lead-exposed children after school entry. *Pediatrics.* 2004;114:19-24.
131. Wakefield AJ, Murch SH, Anthony A. Ileal lymphoid nodular hyperplasia, nonspecific colitis, and pervasive developmental disorder. *Lancet.* 1998;351: 637-641.
132. Dales L, Hammer SJ, Smith NJ. Time trends in autism and in MMR immunization coverage in California. *JAMA.* 2001;285:1183-1185.
133. Madsen KM, Hviid A, Vestergaard M, et al. A population-based study of measles, mumps, and rubella vaccination and autism. *N Engl J Med.* 2002;347:1477-1482.
134. Taylor B, Lingam R, Simmons A, Stowe J, Miller E, Andrews N. Autism and MMR vaccination in North London: no causal relationship. *Mol Psychiatry.* 2002; 7(suppl 2):S7-S8.
135. Honda H, Shimizu Y, Rutter M. No effect of MMR withdrawal on the incidence of autism: a total population study. *J Child Psychol Psychiatry.* 2005;46: 572-579.
136. Paterson R. MMR debate fall-out continues. *Lancet Infect Dis.* 2004;4:653.
137. Pavone L, Fiumara A, Bottaro G, Mazzone D, Coleman M. Autism and celiac disease: failure to validate the hypothesis that a link might exist. *Biol Psychiatry.* 1997;42:72-75.
138. Kuddo T, Nelson KB. How common are gastrointestinal disorders in children with autism? *Curr Opin Pediatr.* 2003;15:339-343.
139. Black C, Kaye JA, Jick H. Relation of childhood gastrointestinal disorders to autism: nested case-control study using data from the UK General Practice Research Database. *BMJ.* 2002;325:419-421.
140. Hunter LC, O'Hare A, Herron WJ, Fisher LA, Jones GE. Opioid peptides and dipeptidyl peptidase in autism. *Dev Med Child Neurol.* 2003;45:121-128.
141. Williams KM, Marshall T. Urinary protein patterns in autism as revealed by high resolution two-dimensional electrophoresis. *Biochem Soc Trans.* 1992;20: 189S.
142. Le Couteur A, Trygstad O, Evered C, Gillberg C, Rutter M. Infantile autism and urinary excretion of peptides and protein-associated peptide complexes. *J Autism Dev Disord.* 1988;18:181-190.
143. Horvath K, Papadimitriou JC, Rabsztyn A, Drachenberg C, Tildon JT. Gastrointestinal abnormalities in children with autistic disorder. *J Pediatr.* 1999; 135:559-563.
144. DelGiudice-Asch G, Simon L, Schmeidler J, Cunningham-Rundles C, Hollander E. A pilot open clinical trial of intravenous immunoglobulin in childhood autism. *J Autism Dev Disord.* 1999;29:157-160.

SECTION EDITOR: ALBERT C. YAN, MD; ASSISTANT SECTION EDITOR: SAMIR S. SHAH, MD

# Picture of the Month

*Jon M. Burnham, MD; Portia A. Kreiger, MD; Michele Paessler, DO; Leslie S. Kersun, MD; Randy Q. Cron, MD, PhD*

AN 11-YEAR-OLD BOY DEVELOPED A GENERALized erythematous macular rash 5 weeks prior to hospitalization. The rash resolved in 3 weeks but he then developed fevers and a sore on his inner left arm (**Figure 1**). The lesion was painful and red. One week prior to hospital admission, a complete blood cell count revealed a low white blood cell count of $3.6 \times 10^3/\mu L$ with a normal hemoglobin concentration and platelet count. A sore throat was present and he complained of oral ulcers.

On hospital admission, he was ill appearing and febrile (40°C), with marked oral ulceration. In addition to an eschar measuring 1.5 cm on his left upper arm with underlying induration (Figure 1), he had a tender lymph node in the nearby axilla. His laboratory test results showed a white blood cell count of $1.6 \times 10^3/\mu L$ (12% band forms, 67% segmented neutrophils, 20% lymphocytes), a hemoglobin concentration of 9.4 g/dL, and a platelet count of $71 \times 10^3/\mu L$. His fibrin split products were elevated and the fibrinogen level was falling. His serum ferritin level was 18 070 ng/mL (40 603 pmol/L). His C-reactive protein level was elevated at greater than 20 mg/dL, but surprisingly, his erythrocyte sedimentation rate was normal at 5 mm/h. His serum and urine electrolyte levels were consistent with syndrome-inappropriate antidiuretic hormone, and his uric acid and lactate dehydrogenase levels were elevated. Epstein-Barr virus testing was consistent with prior infection.

Biopsy specimens of the rash (**Figure 2** and **Figure 3**) and a bone marrow aspirate (**Figure 4**) were diagnostic. Despite therapy for his underlying condition, the patient subsequently died of fungal sepsis.

**Author Affiliations:** Divisions of Rheumatology (Drs Burnham and Cron) and Oncology (Dr Kersun), Department of Pediatrics, and Department of Anatomic Pathology (Drs Kreiger and Paessler), Children's Hospital of Philadelphia, Philadelphia, Pa.

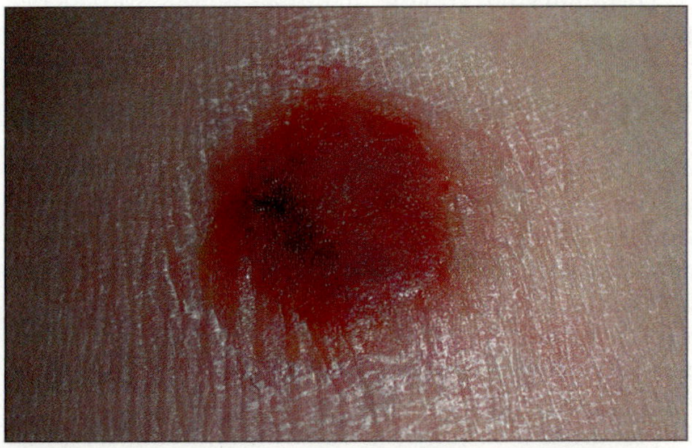

**Figure 1.** Painful, indurated left upper arm eschar with surrounding erythema.

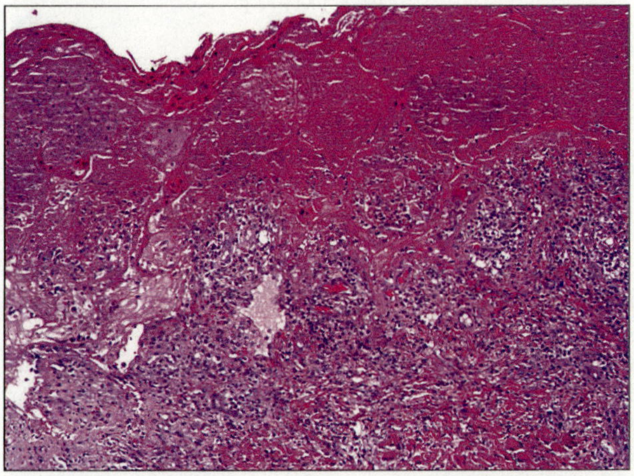

**Figure 2.** Skin biopsy specimen revealing superficial necrosis and underlying atypical lymphoid infiltrate (hematoxylin-eosin, original magnification ×10).

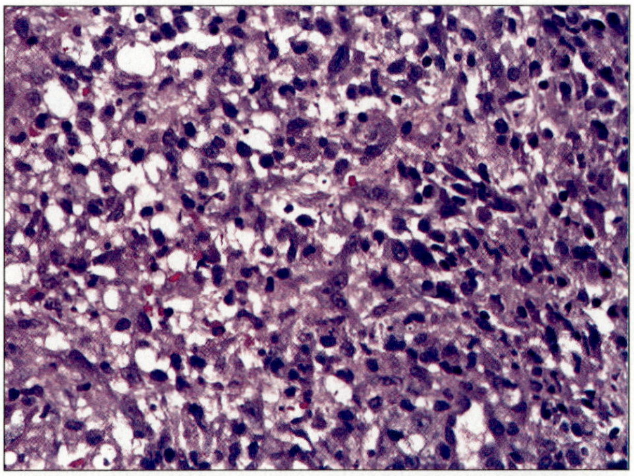

**Figure 3.** Higher-power view of skin biopsy specimen revealing atypical lymphoid infiltrate (hematoxylin-eosin, original magnification ×80).

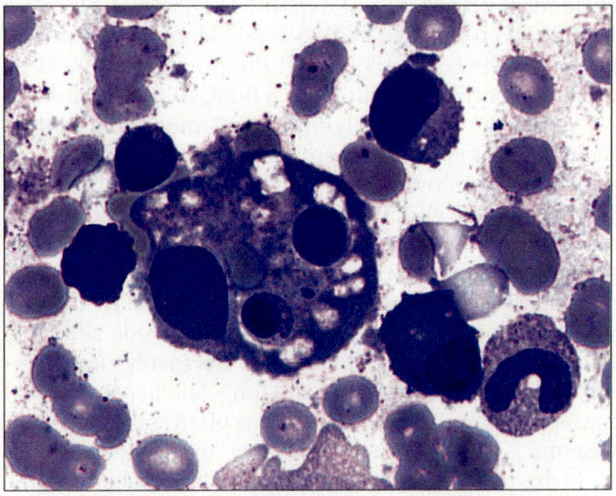

**Figure 4.** Bone marrow aspirate revealing hemophagocytosis.

# Denouement and Discussion

## *Anaplastic Large Cell Lymphoma With Hemophagocytic Lymphohistiocytosis*

Hemophagocytic lymphohistiocytosis (HLH) may occur in a primary form, often associated with mutations in the perforin gene responsible for natural killer cell cytotoxic activity,[1] or secondary to underlying rheumatic disease (most commonly systemic-onset juvenile rheumatoid arthritis), infection (usually herpesvirus infections such as Epstein-Barr virus or virtually any bacteria, fungus, or parasite), immunodeficiency (Griscelli syndrome), lysinuric protein intolerance, and malignancies. Lymphomas are the most common malignancies associated with HLH, and although HLH is frequently associated with subcutaneous T-cell lymphomas,[2] it is exceedingly rare as part of anaplastic large cell lymphoma (ALCL), as was observed in this case.[3]

Lymphomas, including Hodgkin and non-Hodgkin (NHL), account for 10% to 15% of childhood cancer in developed countries, and ALCL accounts for 10% of NHL in childhood. Anaplastic large cell lymphoma is a mature T-cell or null-cell lymphoma that has been recognized as a distinct entity in the classification of NHL.[4] The 2 subtypes of ALCL include systemic or cutaneous; however, the primary cutaneous form is rare in children.[5] In 80% of cases, the systemic form of ALCL is associated with a chromosomal translocation, t(2;5)(p23; q35), specific to this disease. This translocation results in a chimeric protein whose expression has oncogenic properties and may contribute to malignant transformation in these lymphomas.[6]

### CLINICAL MANIFESTATIONS

The clinical presentation of HLH is a direct result of the underlying hyperinflammatory syndrome and uncontrolled activation of T lymphocytes and macrophages. Diagnostic criteria include familial disease or known genetic defect and 5 of the following clinical or laboratory criteria: fever, splenomegaly, cytopenias, hypertriglyceridemia with or without hypofibrinogenemia, elevated ferritin level, elevated sCD25 level, decreased or absent natural killer cell activity, and the presence of HLH in the bone marrow, cerebrospinal fluid, or lymph nodes.[7]

Anaplastic large cell lymphoma is more common in males and the clinical presentation is unusual since it can present with a slowly progressive course and patients often have peripheral, intrathoracic, and intra-abdominal nodal involvement instead of the typical extranodal involvement seen in other types of NHL. Other common sites of disease characteristic of patients with ALCL and not often seen in other forms of NHL include skin and bone. Furthermore, this lymphoma can involve less common sites such as soft tissue and lung, and hepatosplenomegaly is common. Finally, ALCL is often associated with systemic symptoms including fever and weight loss.

In this patient, fevers may have been attributable to either HLH or lymphoma, while the significant oral ulceration was likely a manifestation of his neutropenia. The progressive pancytopenia with elevated lactate dehydrogenase and uric acid concentrations were suspicious for either HLH or hematologic malignancy, but the eschar with underlying induration (Figure 1) was suspicious for an infiltrative lesion, such as lymphoma, and necessitated the bone marrow examination and skin biopsies.

### DIAGNOSIS

Diagnosis of both ALCL and HLH are made by biopsy of the skin and bone marrow or other involved organs (eg, lymph node). In this case, a biopsy specimen of the skin revealed superficial epidermal ulceration with necrosis and an underlying atypical lymphoid infiltrate within the dermis. The atypical cells were large and contained eosinophilic cytoplasm and convoluted nuclei, suggesting a diagnosis of ALCL. The diagnosis was confirmed by immunohistochemical evaluation, which revealed staining for T-cell antigens and both the epithelial membrane antigen and the anaplastic lymphoma kinase (ALK-1) protein. Thus, the combined histologic and immunohistochemical findings were most consistent with ALCL.

Histologically, HLH is identified by the presence of histiocytes containing engulfed cells and cellular fragments from red and white blood cells, as well as platelets.[8] This can be seen within the skin, the bone marrow, or other involved organs. In the clinical setting, evaluation of a patient for HLH involves obtaining a complete blood cell count to test for cytopenias, hepatic function test results to check for hepatitis, prothrombin and activated partial thromboplastin times, D-dimers levels, and fibrinogen levels to test for coagulopathy. Hyperferritinemia and hypertriglyceridemia are also characteristic of HLH. Once the diagnosis of HLH is made, an evaluation of natural killer cell numbers and function should be performed to distinguish primary from secondary forms of the disease.

### TREATMENT

The goals of treatment for HLH are to suppress the significant inflammation responsible for the symptoms and to kill pathogen-infected antigen-presenting cells in order to decrease natural killer cell and T-suppressor cell activation.[7] The pathogenesis of HLH is thought to be due to an uncontrolled cytokine storm from T-lymphocyte activation. Cytokines such as interferon-$\gamma$, IL-12, IL-18, and tumor necrosis factor $\alpha$ are believed to contribute to the macrophage activation and cytophagocytosis.[9] To counteract this cytokine storm, high-dose corticosteroids and cyclosporine A are often used to combat the T-cell activation.[8] For severe familial forms, or those refractory to highly immunosuppressive therapy, a protocol using etoposide and dexamethasone is available.[8] If the HLH is eventually controlled, then the underlying associated illness needs to be treated.

Recent advances in the treatment for children with NHL have resulted in a significant improvement in cure rates. Combination chemotherapy protocols are based on the tumor cell immunophenotype, whereas early regimens were based on the histologic features of the tumor.[10-12] With any of the protocols, the long-term survival is estimated to be approximately 60% to 70%; however, newer combinations of chemotherapeutic agents, increasing dose intensity of some medications, and targeted immunotherapy are currently under investigation. For patients with relapse of ALCL after combination chemotherapy, intensive combinations of other drugs have induced remission in a small proportion of patients. Those children would be candidates for high-dose chemotherapy with stem cell rescue.[13] Few patients, late recurrences, disparate staging systems, and treatment by different groups prevent generalizations from being made about optimal treatment, and the approach to this condition continues to evolve.[10-14]

**Accepted for Publication:** December 8, 2005.
**Correspondence:** Randy Q. Cron, MD, PhD, Division of Rheumatology, Department of Pediatrics, Children's Hospital of Philadelphia, 3615 Civic Center Blvd, ARC 1102B, Philadelphia, PA 19104-4318 (cron@email.chop.edu).
**Author Contributions:** *Study concept and design:* Burnham, Kersun, and Cron. *Acquisition of data:* Burnham and Kreiger. *Analysis and interpretation of data:* Burnham and Paessler. *Drafting of the manuscript:* Burnham, Kersun, and Cron. *Critical revision of the manuscript for important intellectual content:* Burnham, Kreiger, Paessler, Kersun, and Cron. *Administrative, technical, and material support:* Burnham. *Study supervision:* Cron.
**Financial Disclosure:** None reported.

## REFERENCES

1. Grom AA. Natural killer cell dysfunction: a common pathway in systemic-onset juvenile rheumatoid arthritis, macrophage activation syndrome, and hemophagocytic lymphohistiocytosis? *Arthritis Rheum.* 2004;50:689-698.
2. Yung A, Snow J, Jarrett P. Subcutaneous panniculitic T-cell lymphoma and cytophagic histiocytic panniculitis. *Australas J Dermatol.* 2001;42:183-187.
3. Chen GS, Chang YF, Chang MC, Tsan KW. Response of Epstein-Barr virus-associated Ki-1+ anaplastic large cell lymphoma to 13-cis retinoic acid and interferon alpha. *J Formos Med Assoc.* 1998;97:420-424.
4. Harris NL, Jaffe ES, Diebold J, et al. World Health Organization classification of neoplastic diseases of the hematopoietic and lymphoid tissues: report of the Clinical Advisory Committee meeting—Airlie House, Virginia, November 1997. *J Clin Oncol.* 1999;17:3835-3849.
5. Tomaszewski MM, Moad JC, Lupton GP. Primary cutaneous Ki-1(CD30) positive anaplastic large cell lymphoma in childhood. *J Am Acad Dermatol.* 1999;40:857-861.
6. Hinshaw M, Towers AB, Kodish E, Kuerbitz S, Shurin S, Wood GS. Three children with CD30 cutaneous anaplastic large cell lymphomas bearing the t(2;5)(p23;q35) translocation. *Pediatr Dermatol.* 2004;21:212-217.
7. Janka GE, Schneider EM. Modern management of children with haemophagocytic lymphohistiocytosis. *Br J Haematol.* 2004;124:4-14.
8. Fisman DN. Hemophagocytic syndromes and infection. *Emerg Infect Dis.* 2000;6:601-608.
9. Larroche C, Mouthon L. Pathogenesis of hemophagocytic syndrome (HPS). *Autoimmun Rev.* 2004;3:69-75.
10. Seidemann K, Tiemann M, Schrappe M, et al. Short-pulse B-non-Hodgkin lymphoma-type chemotherapy is efficacious treatment for pediatric anaplastic large cell lymphoma: a report of the Berlin-Frankfurt-Munster Group Trial NHL-BFM 90. *Blood.* 2001;97:3699-3706.
11. Zinzani PL, Martelli M, Magagnoli M, et al. Anaplastic large cell lymphoma Hodgkin's-like: a randomized trial of ABVD versus MACOP-B with and without radiation therapy. *Blood.* 1998;92:790-794.
12. Brugieres L, Deley MC, Pacquement H, et al. CD30(+) anaplastic large-cell lymphoma in children: analysis of 82 patients enrolled in two consecutive studies of the French Society of Pediatric Oncology. *Blood.* 1998;92:3591-3598.
13. Kobrinsky NL, Sposto R, Shah NR, et al. Outcomes of treatment of children and adolescents with recurrent non-Hodgkin's lymphoma and Hodgkin's disease with dexamethasone, etoposide, cisplatin, cytarabine, and l-asparaginase, maintenance chemotherapy, and transplantation: Children's Cancer Group Study CCG-5912. *J Clin Oncol.* 2001;19:2390-2396.
14. Sandlund JT, Downing JR, Crist WM. Non-Hodgkin's lymphoma in childhood. *N Engl J Med.* 1996;334:1238-1248.

"Mankind owes to the child the best it has to give."
—United Nations Declaration

# Understanding Shared Injury Risk on the Family Farm

Although unintentional injury remains a major cause of morbidity and mortality among children, significant progress has been made toward reducing the burden of trauma over the past 30 years.[1] An important factor in this success has been the application of an epidemiological approach to injury as a disease, most famously advanced by William Haddon, Jr.[2] Epidemiologists studying the determinants and distribution of injury consider factors in the host (the child at risk for injury), the vehicles or vectors that cause injury, and the environments in which child injury occurs. Because injury risk and outcome are so often behaviorally determined, the salient "environment" in injury epidemiology includes both the physical context of injury and the child's sociocultural milieu.

*See also page 1137*

Children in farming families are known to bear a disproportionately high risk of morbidity, disability, and mortality due to injury.[3-5] Their increased risk is typically attributed to prolonged or repeated exposure to agricultural hazards in their home environment, often collocated with their parents' occupational setting. Many children in farming families also work, at least informally and often from an early age, in this agricultural environment, engaged in activities, exposed to animals, and using tools, vehicles, or products that can cause injury. However, not all children in farm families are injured. The factors that place some children at greater risk than others in a similar environment have not been well studied.

In this issue of the Archives, Carlson and colleagues[6] suggest that injury risk in farming families is, at least in part, the result of vulnerabilities shared by parents and children within a household. They studied 203 injured children and 755 uninjured control subjects drawn from a sample of 3765 farming households participating in the Regional Rural Injury Study–II in 1999. This population-based longitudinal study was designed to determine the etiology and consequences of injury in agricultural operations in the upper Midwest of the United States. The authors report that the odds of agricultural injury in 1999 was more than doubled among children whose mother or father was injured before 1999 and increased more than 4-fold if both parents reported a previous agricultural injury.

Some caution is warranted in interpreting these findings. Although the study was prospective in design, injury history was based on respondent recall, a method that is commonly used but prone to some inaccuracy.[7] If parents who were better able to recall and report their child's injury were also more likely to recall their own injury experience, the strength of the reported association could be artificially inflated. In addition, the propensity to seek medical care for an injury is driven by appraisal of severity, beliefs about the need for professional attention, and access to health care resources.[8-10] All of these factors would be held in common within a family group and could influence patterns of injury care and the apparent association between parent and child experiences.

Although there is insufficient detail in the data available from the study by Carlson et al, it is interesting to speculate about mechanisms of shared vulnerability to injury within a family. Again, an epidemiologic approach is instructive.

At the level of the individual (or host), one could postulate the existence of heritable genetic factors contributing to injury risk in parents and their biological children. Some behavioral risk factors for injury, such as impulsivity, aggression, and sensation seeking, may have a neurochemical or genetic basis that permits clustering of these risk factors in families.[11,12] Other vaguer concepts such as "injury proneness" are sometimes used to retrospectively describe an individual's injury experience but are not sufficiently specific to allow their use in an explanatory model for intergenerational transmission of injury risk.[13] It is not helpful to note that some people have more injuries than others unless the factors that underlie this vulnerability can be identified.[14]

The vehicles or vectors that cause injury in an agricultural environment may also be sources of shared injury risk among family members. Not all agricultural operations are equally hazardous.[15] Family members living on the same farm share exposure to the same hazardous animals or machinery and, as a consequence, a common level of injury risk. Although Carlson and colleagues attempted to control for the type of agricultural operation, the ability to model salient characteristics of individual farms is inherently limited.

Finally, parents and children in farming families share exposure to the same physical and sociocultural environments. While the contribution of static physical hazards to shared injury risk is obvious, the role of the family as the most important social environment for children is often overlooked. The perception of injury risk, the relative valuation of children's exposure to potentially hazardous environments while working, and the patterns of adult supervision that ensue are all family-level factors that will influence child injury risk in agricultural settings. The extent to which each of these factors is also associated with adult injury liability is unclear but could be an important mediator in any association between parent and child injury risk.

Family structure, defined as the number of children and adults in the household and the roles that each plays, is an important mediator of child injury.[16-18] Family function is a more dynamic concept that may also play a role in shared injury risk.[19-21] Families have processes in place for identifying, appraising, and accommodating to both normal and extraordinary stresses and transitions. The success and facility with which these transitions and adaptations are achieved may influence injury risk within the family because patterns of behavior and supervision change in response to new stresses and requirements. Indeed, sibling groups have been shown to share a transient increase in injury risk when any one of the children in the home is injured.[22,23] This clustering of injuries within families over short periods suggests a dynamic perturbation in risk and protection but does not explain the more prolonged association of parent and child injury risk described in the study by Carlson et al.

Can clinicians use these observations to help children living and working on family farms? Unfortunately, there is a paucity of experimental data to identify interventions that reduce agricultural injury and even fewer that apply specifically to children.[24] Most farming families place a high value on the participation of their children in farm-related chores.[25] Even those who do not require children to participate in farm tasks may find it difficult to limit their children's exposure to agricultural hazards because their residence and place of occupation are one and the same.

The North American Guidelines for Children's Agricultural Tasks (NAGCAT) were developed in 1999 as a resource for parents to help identify developmentally appropriate agricultural work, its associated injury hazards, and recommended countermeasures.[26] The guidelines match farming tasks to children's developmental abilities and thus account for variation in skills and abilities among the 7- to 16-year-olds targeted.

Gadomski and colleagues[27] recently reported a randomized trial involving almost 900 farm families. Their results suggest that the NAGCAT guidelines, when delivered with a single introductory educational session and boosted by periodic mailings, could significantly reduce the risk of injuries related to work covered by the guidelines.[27] In addition, intervention families were noted to delay child use of all-terrain vehicles, an important and growing injury problem in rural areas.[28,29] These positive results suggest that a prevention message promoting gradual and individualized attainment of work responsibility may be both acceptable to farm families and useful in the prevention of children's occupational farm injuries.

Although these results are encouraging, only about 30% of child agricultural injuries are work-related.[30] Additional harm-reduction strategies to reduce injury risk to children on farms thus might include the provision of developmentally appropriate nonoccupational safety advice, advocacy for product design and policy to protect all farm workers and their family members, and promotion of resources for child care or alternate supervision, especially during times of intense agricultural activity.[31]

The reported association between parent injury and subsequent child injury risk might also prompt clinicians who see adults to use a parent's agricultural injury visit as a "teachable moment"; safety advice or behavior-change interventions could be offered when the parent may be most receptive to this information.[32] The results of the study by Carlson et al do not suggest that parent injury is, in itself, a sufficient intervention to mitigate the risk to children in the family; however, with a nudge at the appropriate time, clinicians might open the door to discussion of the social and environmental context of injury, a realistic reframing of the risks involved, and a shared understanding of the possible consequences for that family. An intervention based on these principles, with content modeled after the NAGCAT guidelines, could be tested in an experimental trial that would be of great interest to farming families and the clinicians who help them care for their children.

More broadly, the results reported by Carlson et al suggest that injury control efforts might be directed productively toward the familial context of child injury. Targeting the middle ground between broad modification of products or environments and individual interventions to change child behavior, family-focused injury control would address the child's most intimate and influential sociocultural milieu. Families, through patterns of interaction and shared exposure, shape the safety of everyday life. Moreover, they are the forge and crucible of health, health beliefs, health behaviors, and the consequent risk or resilience that mediate a child's interaction with the broader environment. Timely intervention with families at risk and the creation of programs or policies to support the health-promoting functions of resilient families could prove to be an efficient and effective strategy for reducing the toll of injury among children and parents alike.

*Brian D. Johnston, MD, MPH*

**Correspondence:** Dr Johnston, Department of Pediatrics, University of Washington, 325 Ninth Ave, Campus Box 359774, Seattle, WA 98104 (bdj@u.washington.edu).

**Financial Disclosure:** None reported.

## REFERENCES

1. Rivara FP, Grossman DC, Cummings P. Injury prevention—second of two parts. *N Engl J Med.* 1997;337:613-618.
2. Haddon W Jr. The changing approach to the epidemiology, prevention, and amelioration of trauma: the transition to approaches etiologically rather than descriptively based. *Am J Public Health Nations Health.* 1968;58:1431-1438.
3. Browning SR, Westneat SC, Donnelly C, Reed D. Agricultural tasks and injuries among Kentucky farm children: results of the Farm Family Health and Hazard Surveillance Project. *South Med J.* 2003;96:1203-1212.
4. Rivara FP. Fatal and non-fatal farm injuries to children and adolescents in the United States, 1990-3. *Inj Prev.* 1997;3:190-194.
5. Reed DB, Claunch DT. Nonfatal farm injury incidence and disability to children: a systematic review. *Am J Prev Med.* 2000;18(4)(suppl):70-79.

6. Carlson KF, Langner D, Alexander BH, et al. The association between parents' past agricultural injuries and their children's risk of injury: analyses from the Regional Rural Injury Study–II. *Arch Pediatr Adol Med.* 2006;160:1137-1142.
7. Cummings P, Rivara FP, Thompson RS, Reid RJ. Ability of parents to recall the injuries of their young children. *Inj Prev.* 2005;11:43-47.
8. Schor EL. Unintentional injuries: patterns within families. *AJDC.* 1987;141:1280-1284.
9. Riley AW, Finney JW, Mellits ED, et al. Determinants of children's health care use: an investigation of psychosocial factors. *Med Care.* 1993;31:767-783.
10. Newacheck PW, Halfon N. The association between mother's and children's use of physician services. *Med Care.* 1986;24:30-38.
11. Kluger AN, Siegfried Z, Ebstein RP. A meta-analysis of the association between DRD4 polymorphism and novelty seeking. *Mol Psychiatry.* 2002;7:712-717.
12. Lynn DE, Lubke G, Yang M, et al. Temperament and character profiles and the dopamine D4 receptor gene in ADHD. *Am J Psychiatry.* 2005;162:906-913.
13. Wazana A. Are there injury-prone children? a critical review of the literature. *Can J Psychiatry.* 1997;42:602-610.
14. Sass R, Crook G. Accident proneness: science or non-science? *Int J Health Serv.* 1981;11:175-190.
15. *National Census of Fatal Occupational Injuries in 2004.* Washington, DC: Bureau of Labor Statistics, US Dept of Labor; August 25, 2005. http://www.bls.gov/news.release/pdf/cfoi.pdf. Accessed April 20, 2006.
16. Kendrick D, Mulvaney C, Burton P, Watson M. Relationships between child, family and neighbourhood characteristics and childhood injury: a cohort study. *Soc Sci Med.* 2005;61:1905-1915.
17. O'Connor TG, Davies L, Dunn J, Golding J; ALSPAC Study Team. Distribution of accidents, injuries, and illnesses by family type: Avon Longitudinal Study of Pregnancy and Childhood. *Pediatrics.* 2000;106:E68 http://pediatrics.aappublications.org/cgi/content/full/106/5/e68. Accessed April 20, 2006.
18. Roberts I. Sole parenthood and the risk of child pedestrian injury. *J Paediatr Child Health.* 1994;30:530-532.
19. Beautrais AL, Fergusson DM, Shannon FT. Life events and childhood morbidity: a prospective study. *Pediatrics.* 1982;70:935-940.
20. Christoffel KK, Donovan M, Schofer J, Wills K, Lavigne JV; Kids 'n' Cars Team. Psychosocial factors in childhood pedestrian injury: a matched case-control study. *Pediatrics.* 1996;97:33-42.
21. Schor EL. Use of health care services by children and diagnoses received during presumably stressful life transitions. *Pediatrics.* 1986;77:834-841.
22. Johnston BD, Grossman DC, Connell FA, Koepsell TD. High-risk periods for childhood injury among siblings. *Pediatrics.* 2000;105(3)(pt 1):562-568.
23. Johnston BD, Grossman DC, Thompson RS. Transient elevation in risk of injury in siblings following injury encounters. *J Pediatr.* 2003;142:79-83.
24. DeRoo LA, Rautiainen RH. A systematic review of farm safety interventions. *Am J Prev Med.* 2000;18(4)(suppl 1):51-62.
25. Neufeld S, Wright SM, Gaut J. Not raising a "bubble kid": farm parents' attitudes and practices regarding the employment, training and supervision of their children. *J Rural Health.* 2002;18:57-66.
26. Lee B, Marlenga B, eds. *Professional Resource Manual: North American Guidelines for Children's Agricultural Tasks.* Marshfield, Wis: Marshfield Clinic; 1999.
27. Gadomski A, Ackerman S, Burdick P, Jenkins P. Efficacy of the North American Guidelines for Children's Agricultural Tasks in reducing childhood agricultural injuries. *Am J Public Health.* 2006;96:722-727.
28. Shults RA, Wiles SD, Vajani M, Helmkamp JC. All-terrain vehicle–related nonfatal injuries among young riders: United States, 2001-2003. *Pediatrics.* 2005;116:e608-e612. Accessed April 18, 2006. doi:10.1542/peds.2005-0937.
29. Killingsworth JB, Tilford JM, Parker JG, Graham JJ, Dick RM, Aitken ME. National hospitalization impact of pediatric all-terrain vehicle injuries. *Pediatrics.* 2005;115:e316-e321. Accessed April 18, 2006. doi:10.1542/peds.2004-1585.
30. Marlenga B, Brison RJ, Berg RL, Zentner J, Linneman J, Pickett W. Evaluation of the North American Guidelines for Children's Agricultural Tasks using a case series of injuries. *Inj Prev.* 2004;10:350-357.
31. Committee on Injury and Poison Prevention and Committee on Community Health Services, American Academy of Pediatrics. Prevention of agricultural injuries among children and adolescents. *Pediatrics.* 2001;108:1016-1019.
32. Rollnick S, Mason P, Butler C. *Health Behavior Change: A Guide for Practitioners.* Edinburgh, Scotland: Churchill Livingstone; 1999.

# Comprehensive Sex Education

## *Strong Public Support and Persuasive Evidence of Impact, but Little Funding*

THE ARTICLE BY BLEAKLEY ET AL[1] PROVIDES strong evidence that a very large majority of adults in this country supports comprehensive sex education programs that teach about abstinence and also other methods of preventing pregnancy and sexually transmitted disease, whereas only a minority of adults supports the teaching of only abstinence.

*See also page 1151*

These results build on numerous somewhat similar surveys that have been conducted for decades demonstrating such support. Indeed, as long ago as 1943, the Gallup Poll found that 68% of adults approved of sex education in schools.[2] By 1985, that support had increased to 85%.[3] Furthermore, for decades these polls have demonstrated that adults want the instruction to include both abstinence and condoms and other methods of contraception.[4] Notably, this support is not limited to only certain parts of the country; similar polls in more conservative southern states, such as North Carolina, South Carolina, and Texas, have demonstrated strong support for programs that encourage abstinence but also encourage the use of condoms and other contraceptives among those who do have sex.

The article by Bleakley et al provides additional evidence that not only does a large majority of American adults support comprehensive sex education but about half actually oppose abstinence-only programs and more than half believe it is not an effective way to prevent unintended teen pregnancy.

As the article by Bleakley et al summarizes, few abstinence-only programs have been well evaluated and found to be effective. There have been very few studies conducted of abstinence-only programs and even fewer studies of programs that meet all the federal Title V guidelines. These studies of abstinence-only programs have produced mixed results. Several had no significant impact on sexual behavior, 2 had positive effects in helping youth return to abstinence, 1 reduced the number of sexual partners, and 1 even appeared to increase the frequency of sex. This mixture of results does not mean that abstinence-only programs cannot work, but it does mean that (1) given the great diversity of abstinence-only programs, we cannot judge their effectiveness as a whole and (2) there are few abstinence-only programs with sufficiently strong evidence of success to recommend their widespread dissemination and implementation.

This is in contrast to comprehensive sex and human immunodeficiency virus (HIV) education programs, which have been evaluated more than 50 times and frequently found to be effective.[5] Some of these programs have been demonstrated to delay sex, reduce the frequency of sex, reduce the number of sexual partners, increase condom use, or increase contraceptive use more generally. Some reduce sexual risk, both by delaying sex and increasing condom and overall contraceptive use. A few even have evidence that they reduce teen pregnancy or sexually transmitted disease (STD) rates. Notably, the evidence is very strong that these programs do not increase sexual behavior, even when they do encourage condom or other contraceptive use. What is particularly encouraging about the evidence from these studies of comprehensive sex and HIV education programs is that when some curricula found to be effective in 1 study were implemented by other educators in other states and evaluated by independent research teams, they remained effective if they were implemented with fidelity in the same type of setting.

Given high teen pregnancy[6] and STD rates,[7] persuasive evidence that comprehensive sex and HIV education programs can reduce sexual risk,[5] and solid public support for these programs,[1] one might guess that federal and state programs would provide strong support for their dissemination and replication. However, this is not the case.

As the article by Bleakley et al demonstrates, the federal government is spending instead a large amount of money on abstinence-only programs. By the end of this year, the federal government, with mandatory matching grants from the states, will have spent roughly a billion dollars on abstinence-only programs. In this field in particular, this is a very large amount of money, and it has dramatically changed the landscape. There are now many large, well-funded organizations focusing solely on the promotion of abstinence and opposing programs that cover both abstinence and condom or contraceptive use. Some of these organizations encourage school districts to teach only abstinence-only programs and offer free abstinence-only instruction in the classroom. Partially as a result of this funding and these efforts, the proportion of sexuality educators in schools that teach abstinence as the only method of preventing pregnancy and STDs increased markedly during the 1990s as did the percentage of teachers who cited abstinence as the most important message they wanted to convey.[8] Furthermore, according to a 1999 nationally representative sample of school district superintendents or their representatives, 23% of all school districts require that "abstinence be taught as the only option outside of marriage, with discussion of contraception either prohibited entirely or permitted only to emphasize its short-comings.[9(p280)]

To the extent that unproven abstinence-only programs have displaced effective comprehensive programs, the abstinence-only funding may have had much less effect on the behavior of youth than its supporters have hoped. In fact, it is even possible that by making the funds so restrictive, they had the opposite effect intended.

Personally, I do not oppose abstinence-only programs for some grade levels. In every school district, there is some grade level where very few, if any, students are having sex, but some students are considering sex or being pressured to have sex by other, often older, potential sexual partners. At this grade level, emphasizing only abstinence, without denigrating condoms or other forms of contraception, may be appropriate.

However, I do oppose only abstinence-only programs in schools, especially in grades where some teens are having sex. Once 10% to 20% of the students are beginning to have sex, I believe they have the right to accurate and balanced information about abstinence, condoms, and other forms of contraception. Furthermore, from a public health standpoint, they should be given such information, as well as the skills, and access to condoms and contraception so that they are more likely to use protection if they do have sex.

Given the solid evidence of public support for comprehensive programs, the paucity of studies of abstinence-only programs, and the strong evidence of effectiveness for some comprehensive sex education programs, what should be done?

I believe we should devote more funds to evaluating the impact of abstinence-only programs using rigorous research designs (ideally randomized controlled trials). Abstinence-only programs are extremely diverse and we know far too little about the impact of different kinds of programs. Until we have strong evidence that particular abstinence-only programs are effective, we certainly should relax the funding restrictions and fund programs (including comprehensive programs) that effectively delay sex among young people. (After all, it makes no practical sense to fund programs that may not work and to legally prevent the funding of comprehensive programs that actually delay sex.) And, of course, we should always appropriately balance the funding for programs that effectively increase abstinence with funding for programs that increase condom and contraceptive use. Given that some programs both delay sex and increase condom and other contraceptive use, implementing these programs especially makes sense.

If we can agree to focus on programs with strong evidence that they effectively reduce sexual risk, regardless of whether they are abstinence-only or comprehensive programs, there still remain important questions to resolve. These include: How can we make programs even more effective? What other approaches are effective at addressing the risk and protective factors of youth? How can we generate the political support needed to disseminate effective programs widely? How can we best disseminate evidence-based programs so that they are replicated broadly with fidelity? To what extent can or should programs be implemented exactly as designed as opposed to being adapted for individual communities and groups of youth? How can we secure the resources needed to replicate and evaluate these programs (eg, financial resources, educator training, and adequate time in classrooms or other youth-serving agencies)? The more quickly we can resolve these issues, the more rapidly we can reduce teen pregnancy and STD rates in this country.

*Douglas Kirby, PhD*

**Correspondence:** Dr Kirby, ETR Associates, 4 Carbonero Way, Scotts Valley, CA 95066-4200 (dougk@etr.org).
**Financial Disclosure:** None reported.

## REFERENCES

1. Bleakley A, Hennessy M, Fishbein M. Public opinion on sex education in US schools. *Arch Pediatr Adolesc Med.* 2006;160:1151-1156.
2. Gallup G. *Gallup Poll Public Opinion 1935-1971.* New York, NY: Random House; 1972.
3. Louis Harris and Associates Inc. *Public Attitudes About Sex Education, Family Planning, and Abortion in the United States.* New York, NY: Louis Harris & Associates Inc; 1985.
4. National Public Radio; Kaiser Family Foundation; Kennedy School of Government. Sex Education in America: general public/parents survey. January 2004. http://www.kff.org/newsmedia/upload/Sex-Education-in-America-General-Public-Parents-Survey-Toplines.pdf.
5. Kirby D, Laris B, Rolleri L. *Impact of Sex and HIV Curriculum-Based Education Programs on Sexual Behaviors of Youth in Developing and Developed Countries.* Washington, DC: Family Health International; 2005.
6. Alan Guttmacher Institute. *US Teenage Pregnancy Statistics: Overall Trends, Trends by Race and Ethnicity and State-By-State Information.* New York, NY: Alan Guttmacher Institute; 2004.
7. Weinstock H, Berman S, Cates W. Sexually transmitted diseases among American youth: incidence and prevalence estimates. *Perspect Sex Reprod Health.* 2004;36:6-10.
8. Darroch JE, Landry DJ, Singh S. Changing emphases in sexuality education in US public secondary schools, 1988-1999. *Fam Plann Perspect.* 2000;32:204-211, 265.
9. Landry DJ, Kaeser L, Richards CL. Abstinence promotion and the provision of information about contraception in public school district sexuality education policies. *Fam Plann Perspect.* 1999;31:280-286.

## *Announcement*

**Submissions.** The Editors welcome contributions to Picture of the Month. Submissions should describe common problems presenting uncommonly, rather than total zebras. Cases should be of interest to practicing pediatricians, highlighting problems that they are likely to at least occasionally encounter in the office or hospital setting. High-quality clinical images (in either 35-mm slide or electronic format) along with parent or patient permission to use these images must accompany the submission. The entire discussion should comprise no more than 750 words. Articles and photographs accepted for publication will bear the contributor's name. There is no charge for reproduction and printing of color illustrations. For details regarding electronic submission, please see: http://archpedi.ama-assn.org.

## Primum Non Nocere

Kim et al[1] demonstrated that in the practice of pediatric oncology, computerized physician order entry (CPOE) reduced improper dosing, missing cumulative doses, and incomplete nursing checklists. In contrast to these benefits, however, CPOE also resulted in a 5-fold increase in "not matching medication orders to treatment plans." Although little detail was provided on the nature of these medication order/treatment plan "mismatches," it implies that chemotherapy ordered through CPOE deviated more often from intended protocol therapy as compared with paper-ordered chemotherapy. While CPOE ostensibly led to more precise chemotherapy dosing, it increased the risk of that chemotherapy being the wrong chemotherapy.

Increasing the risk of protocol deviation in pediatric oncology has both individual patient and nationwide/study ramifications. For the individual patient, receiving protocol therapy in an unintended way has the potential to cause harm either by overtreament or undertreatment. For patients having data submitted for national study purposes, variability in protocol delivery has the potential to create misleading or unevaluable data.

Kim et al appropriately took on the responsibility of systematically evaluating the implementation of CPOE at their institution. In doing so, they were able to identify process steps contributing to errors, their likelihood of occurrence, and recommendations to reduce those errors. Regarding protocol deviations, a recommendation for limited menus and order sets was made. In our experience with an industry leader in medical informatics, such order sets do not yet exist. We encountered significant difficulty in modifying available informatics coding to support the complexities of pediatric chemotherapy protocols. In particular, timed chemotherapy, whose initiation is dependant on patients meeting certain clinical criteria, could not be supported by existing programs.

The sheer number of pediatric chemotherapy protocols, the continued deployment of new protocols, and the routine use of nonprotocol therapy would make the creation of computerized order sets a full-time undertaking and therefore remain out of reach for many institutions. One solution could be to organize a cooperative group effort to standardize order sets nationally. However, electronic compatibility issues between different treatment centers would likely limit the utility of such efforts. Unless these problems are solved first, CPOE for pediatric oncology has risks of greater concern than their reported benefit. As statistician John Tukey warns, "Far better an approximate answer to the right question, which is often wrong, than an exact answer to the wrong question, which can always be made precise."[2(pp13-14)]

*David Dickens, MD*
*Dianne Sinsabaugh, RPh*
*Brenda Winger, PharmD*

**Correspondence:** Dr Dickens, Pediatric Hematology/Oncology, DeVos Children's Hospital, 100 Michigan St, NE Mail Code 85, Grand Rapids, MI 49503 (david.dickens@spectrum-health.org).
**Financial Disclosure:** None reported.

1. Kim GR, Chen AR, Arceci RJ, et al. Error reduction in pediatric chemotherapy: computerized order entry and failure modes and effects analysis. *Arch Pediatr Adolesc Med*. 2006;160:495-498.
2. Tukey JW. The future of data analysis. *Ann Math Stat*. 1962;33:13-14.

*In reply*

*We appreciate the comments by Drs Dickens, Sinsabaugh, and Winger as an opportunity to continue the discussion on improving safety in pediatric chemotherapy.*

*First, to clarify the type of error classified as medication order/treatment plan mismatches: our divisional policy requires that each chemotherapy order identify precisely the therapy that is due (including protocol, treatment arm, course, cycle, week, and day). If any of this information was missing or did not match the treatment plan verbatim, pharmacists and nurses were expected to reject the order as potentially incorrect or unclear, and prescribers were expected to generate a corrected order to ensure accurate delivery of the intended therapy. In our study, it was these mismatches in the specification of the point in therapy that increased. The wrong agent, dose, route, or schedule was never prescribed.*

*Second, the failure modes analysis and CPOE features targeted process errors in the prescribing/ordering, dispensing, and administration steps of the medication process[1] (primarily prescribing/ordering for CPOE). The complexity of chemotherapy may increase failure modes outside of these steps. In addition, interfaces may introduce new errors. The CPOE interface design (the data entry field was too narrow to display the full required text) may have contributed to the rate of the error described in the evaluation.*

*We concur that order sets and clinical decision support in pediatric oncology are still in development by vendors and not yet standardized. Collective experience shows that CPOE systems "out of the box" are a far cry from the vision of point-of-care clinical decision support that prevents all medication errors. Nevertheless, we believe that commercially available CPOE software includes order set tools that can at least match the degree of decision support provided by paper-based order sets, as long as it is recognized that human intelligence is still required to write orders, dispense medica-*

*tions, and (particularly) administer therapy. For chemotherapy schedules, the initiation of which depends on patients meeting certain clinical criteria, with paper, a nurse must manually calculate the time each medication is due on the medication administration record, when the criteria are met; with CPOE (and a bidirectional pharmacy interface), without (event-triggered) decision support for scheduling medications, at worst, the nurse would similarly need to retime all chemotherapy on an electronic medication administration record.*

*Even with standards, meeting organizational, technical, and resource needs (in different hospital environments) to optimize pediatric chemotherapy can become progressively multidisciplinary (and complex). Our institutional goal is to develop order set templates and practices that require no more multidisciplinary effort than for paper-based order sets. We suggest that the first step to developing and sharing standardized order sets is to define collectively the best and safest practices for chemotherapy ordering, dispensing, and administration that the standards will facilitate.*

*George R. Kim, MD*
*Allen R. Chen, MD, PhD*
*Robert J. Arceci, MD, PhD*
*Christoph U. Lehmann, MD*

**Correspondence**: Dr Kim, Division of Health Sciences Informatics, Johns Hopkins University School of Medicine, 600 N Wolfe St, Nelson 2-133, Baltimore, MD 21287-3200 (georkim@pol.net).
**Financial Disclosure**: None reported.

1. Robinson DL, Heigham M, Clark J. Using failure mode and effects analysis for safe administration of chemotherapy to hospitalized children with cancer. *Jt Comm J Qual Patient Saf.* 2006;32:161-166.

## Correction

**Errors in Figures.** In the Article by Villarruel et al titled "A Randomized Controlled Trial Testing an HIV Prevention Intervention for Latino Youth," published in the August issue of the ARCHIVES (2006;160: 772-777), errors occurred in the symbol keys of **Figures 2**, **3**, and **4** on page 775. The keys should have indicated that the squares represent the health-promotion group and the diamonds represent the human immunodeficiency virus (HIV) risk-reduction group. The corrected figures are reprinted here with their legends.

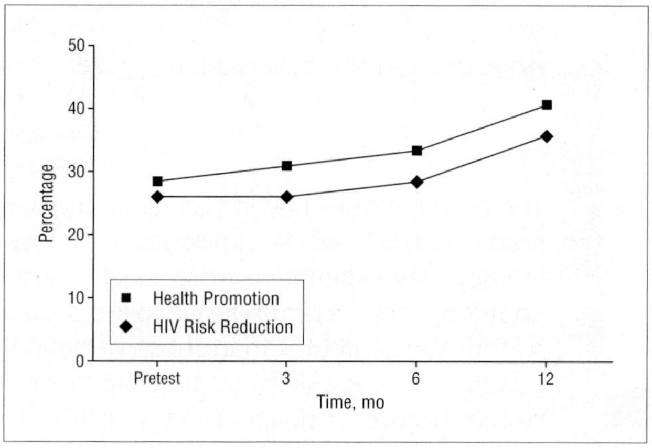


**Figure 2.** Self-report of sexual intercourse in the past 3 months. This graph does not represent results of generalized estimation equation analyses. The percentage (SE) was calculated for the outcome variable; unadjusted scores are presented for each time period. Values for the human immunodeficiency virus (HIV) risk-reduction group are as follows: pretest, 25.9% (0.44%); 3 mo, 26.0% (0.44%); 6 mo, 28.4% (0.45%); and 12 mo, 35.7% (0.48%). Values for the health-promotion group are as follows: pretest, 28.4% (0.45%); 3 mo, 31.0% (0.46%); 6 mo, 33.3% (0.47%); and 12 mo, 40.7% (0.49%).

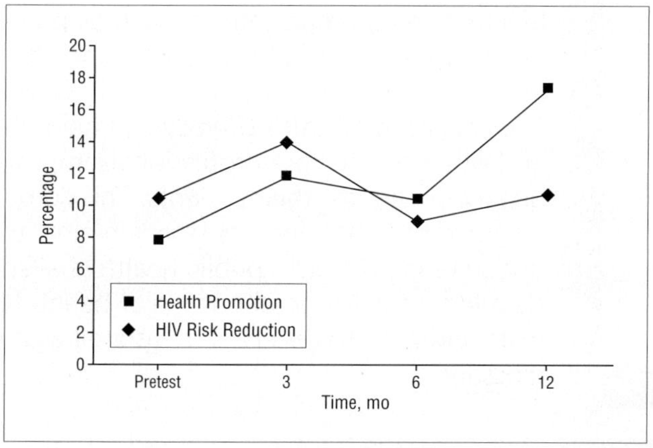


**Figure 3.** Self-report of multiple partners in the past 3 months. This graph does not represent results of generalized estimation equation analyses. The percentage (SE) was calculated for the outcome variable; unadjusted scores are presented for each time period. Values for the human immunodeficiency virus (HIV) risk-reduction group are as follows: pretest, 10.4% (0.31%); 3 mo, 14.0% (0.35%); 6 mo, 9.0% (0.29%); and 12 mo, 10.7% (0.31%). Values for the health-promotion group are as follows: pretest, 7.8% (0.27%); 3 mo, 11.7% (0.32%); 6 mo, 10.3% (0.30%); and 12 mo, 17.3% (0.38%).

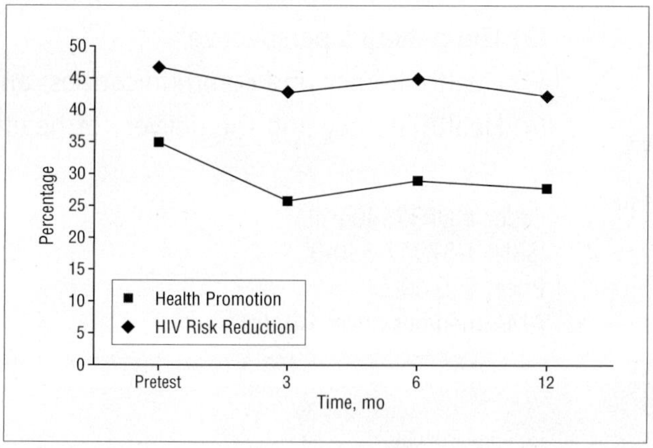


**Figure 4.** Consistent condom use in the past 3 months. This graph does not represent results of generalized estimation equation analyses. The percentage (SE) was calculated for the outcome variable; unadjusted scores are presented for each time period. Scores were calculated only for participants who were sexually active at baseline (human immunodeficiency virus [HIV] risk-reduction group [n=106], health-promotion group [n=127]). Values for the HIV risk-reduction group are as follows: pretest, 46.8% (0.50%); 3 mo, 42.6% (0.50%); 6 mo, 44.8% (0.50%); and 12 mo, 42.2% (0.50%). Values for the health-promotion group are as follows: pretest, 34.8% (0.48%); 3 mo, 25.7% (0.44%); 6 mo, 28.8% (0.46%); and 12 mo, 27.6% (0.45%).

United States Postal Service

## Statement of Ownership, Management, and Circulation

| 1. Publication Title | 2. Publication Number | 3. Filing Date |
|---|---|---|
| Archives of Pediatrics & Adolescent Medicine | 0 0 1 9 – 6 8 0 | 9/29/06 |
| **4. Issue Frequency** | **5. Number of Issues Published Annually** | **6. Annual Subscription Price** |
| Monthly | 12 | $185 |

7. Complete Mailing Address of Known Office of Publication (Not printer) (Street, city, county, state, and ZIP+4)
515 N. State Street, Chicago, Cook, Illinois 60610-4325

Contact Person: Michael McGraw
Telephone: 312-464-2570

8. Complete Mailing Address of Headquarters or General Business Office of Publisher (Not printer)
515 N. State Street, Chicago, Cook, Illinois 60610-4325

9. Full Names and Complete Mailing Addresses of Publisher, Editor, and Managing Editor (Do not leave blank)

Publisher (Name and complete mailing address)
American Medical Association
515 N. State Street, Chicago, Illinois 60610-4325

Editor (Name and complete mailing address)
Frederick P. Rivara, MD, MPH
515 N. State Street, Chicago, Illinois 60610-4325

Managing Editor (Name and complete mailing address)
Cheryl Iverson
515 N. State Street, Chicago, Illinois 60610-4325

10. Owner (Do not leave blank. If the publication is owned by a corporation, give the name and address of the corporation immediately followed by the names and addresses of all stockholders owning or holding 1 percent or more of the total amount of stock. If not owned by a corporation, give the names and addresses of the individual owners. If owned by a partnership or other unincorporated firm, give its name and address as well as those of each individual owner. If the publication is published by a nonprofit organization, give its name and address.)

| Full Name | Complete Mailing Address |
|---|---|
| American Medical Association | 515 N. State Street, Chicago, Illinois 60610-4325 |

11. Known Bondholders, Mortgagees, and Other Security Holders Owning or Holding 1 Percent or More of Total Amount of Bonds, Mortgages, or Other Securities. If none, check box → XX None

| Full Name | Complete Mailing Address |
|---|---|
| None | |

12. Tax Status (For completion by nonprofit organizations authorized to mail at nonprofit rates) (Check one)
The purpose, function, and nonprofit status of this organization and the exempt status for federal income tax purposes:
☒ Has Not Changed During Preceding 12 Months
☐ Has Changed During Preceding 12 Months (Publisher must submit explanation of change with this statement)

PS Form **3526,** October 1999 (See Instructions on Reverse)

13. Publication Title: Archives of Pediatrics & Adolescent Medicine
14. Issue Date for Circulation Data Below: September 2006

| 15. Extent and Nature of Circulation | | | Average No. Copies Each Issue During Preceding 12 Months | No. Copies of Single Issue Published Nearest to Filing Date |
|---|---|---|---|---|
| a. Total Number of Copies (Net press run) | | | 23039 | 23651 |
| b. Paid and/or Requested Circulation | (1) | Paid/Requested Outside-County Mail Subscriptions Stated on Form 3541. (Include advertiser's proof and exchange copies) | 15639 | 14130 |
| | (2) | Paid In-County Subscriptions Stated on Form 3541 (Include advertiser's proof and exchange copies) | 0 | 0 |
| | (3) | Sales Through Dealers and Carriers, Street Vendors, Counter Sales, and Other Non-USPS Paid Distribution | 589 | 567 |
| | (4) | Other Classes Mailed Through the USPS | 0 | 0 |
| c. Total Paid and/or Requested Circulation [Sum of 15b. (1), (2),(3),and (4)] | | | 16227 | 14697 |
| d. Free Distribution by Mail (Samples, compliment ary, and other free) | (1) | Outside-County as Stated on Form 3541 | 5190 | 7430 |
| | (2) | In-County as Stated on Form 3541 | 0 | 0 |
| | (3) | Other Classes Mailed Through the USPS | 0 | 0 |
| e. Free Distribution Outside the Mail (Carriers or other means) | | | 395 | 294 |
| f. Total Free Distribution (Sum of 15d. and 15e.) | | | 5585 | 7724 |
| g. Total Distribution (Sum of 15c. and 15f) | | | 21812 | 22421 |
| h. Copies not Distributed | | | 1227 | 1230 |
| i. Total (Sum of 15g. and h.) | | | 23039 | 23651 |
| j. Percent Paid and/or Requested Circulation (15c. divided by 15g. times 100) | | | 74% | 66% |

16. Publication of Statement of Ownership
XX Publication required. Will be printed in the 11/01/06 issue of this publication. ☐ Publication not required.

17. Signature and Title of Editor, Publisher, Business Manager, or Owner — Date 9/29/06

I certify that all information furnished on this form is true and complete. I understand that anyone who furnishes false or misleading information on this form or who omits material or information requested on the form may be subject to criminal sanctions (including fines and imprisonment) and/or civil sanctions (including civil penalties).

### Instructions to Publishers

1. Complete and file one copy of this form with your postmaster annually on or before October 1. Keep a copy of the completed form for your records.
2. In cases where the stockholder or security holder is a trustee, include in items 10 and 11 the name of the person or corporation for whom the trustee is acting. Also include the names and addresses of individuals who are stockholders who own or hold 1 percent or more of the total amount of bonds, mortgages, or other securities of the publishing corporation. In item 11, if none, check the box. Use blank sheets if more space is required.
3. Be sure to furnish all circulation information called for in item 15. Free circulation must be shown in items 15d, e, and f.
4. Item 15h., Copies not Distributed, must include (1) newsstand copies originally stated on Form 3541, and returned to the publisher, (2) estimated returns from news agents, and (3), copies for office use, leftovers, spoiled, and all other copies not distributed.
5. If the publication had Periodicals authorization as a general or requester publication, this Statement of Ownership, Management, and Circulation must be published; it must be printed in any issue in October or, if the publication is not published during October, the first issue printed after October.
6. In item 16, indicate the date of the issue in which this Statement of Ownership will be published.
7. Item 17 must be signed.

***Failure to file or publish a statement of ownership may lead to suspension of Periodicals authorization.***

PS Form **3526,** October 1999 *(Reverse)*

JAMACAREERNET NetWorking for Physicians

www.jamacareernet.com

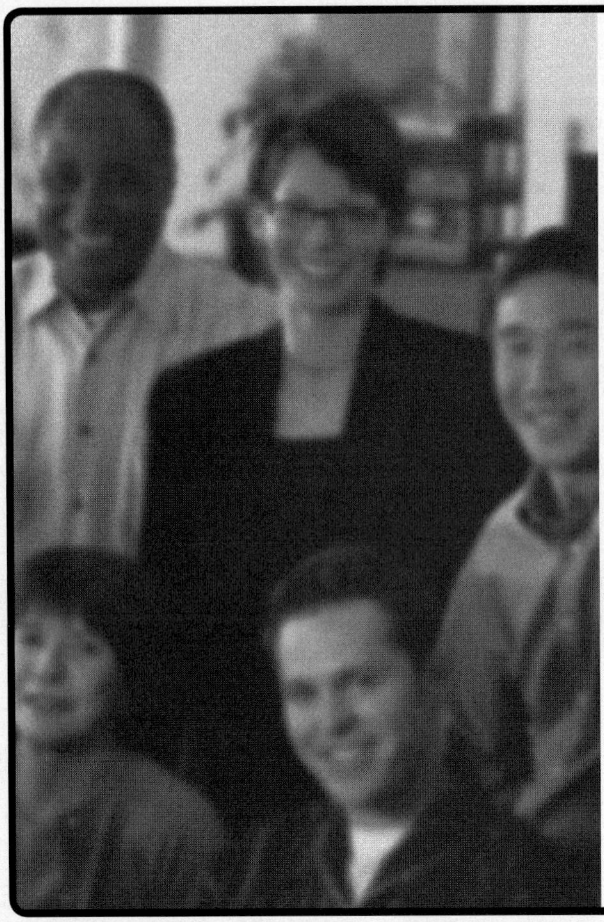

# *Simplify* Your Search.

**JAMACAREERNET**
*NetWorking for Physicians*

Are you a physician seeking a new position?
Each week, JAMA CareerNet brings you a wide array of clinical and academic career opportunities from every part of the nation.

As the most widely circulated medical journal in the world, *JAMA* is read by physicians in virtually every specialty and practice setting. So whether you want a career move that takes you across the country or across the hall, make JAMA CareerNet your resource.

## MEDICAL DIRECTOR
### CHILD ADVOCACY & PROTECTION PROGRAM

Children's Hospital at Dartmouth seeks a full-time medical director for its Child Advocacy and Protection Program. The successful candidate must be Board certified in Pediatrics, have additional fellowship training in child abuse or the equivalent, and should have at least five years of post-residency clinical experience in evaluations of cases of child maltreatment. Additionally, candidates should have prior experience in program development and a record of academic achievement. Support is available for academic and program development. The chosen candidate will lead an experienced team consisting of an NP, a child advocacy center coordinator, a social worker, and an administrative assistant. Faculty appointment at Dartmouth Medical School commensurate with experience.

Please direct inquiries and CVs to:

**Richard P. Morse, M.D.,**
**Department of Pediatrics,**
**Dartmouth-Hitchcock Medical Center,**
**Lebanon, NH 03756.**
**E mail: Richard.P.Morse@hitchcock.org**

DARTMOUTH–HITCHCOCK MEDICAL CENTER

Dartmouth-Hitchcock Medical Center is an affirmative action/equal opportunity employer and is especially interested in identifying female and minority candidates.

**www.dhmc.org**

BrownMed BROWN MEDICAL SCHOOL

MH MEMORIAL HOSPITAL OF RHODE ISLAND

## General Pediatrician

The Department of Pediatrics is seeking a General Pediatrician to join its growing academic faculty. The successful candidate will have opportunities for family-centered care, teaching and clinical research. Memorial Hospital is a major teaching hospital for Brown Medical School. The Division of General Pediatrics provides clinical care and medical homes for community children as well as medical support to community schools. The Division pursues excellence in clinical care and in the teaching and mentoring of medical students, resident and fellows. The successful candidate will have a unique opportunity for professional growth and will be encouraged to develop innovative forward-looking healthcare programs or resident educational programs that will be needed by Pediatric training programs in the future.

Candidates must be BC/BE in Pediatrics and eligible for a faculty appointment at the assistant or associate professor level at Brown Medical school. Research experience is valued but not required.

Interested candidates should forward correspondence and curriculum vitae to: **Joseph J Hallett, M.D., c/o Rose Tremblay, Department of Pediatrics, Memorial Hospital, 111 Brewster Street, Pawtucket, RI 02860 or email Rose_Tremblay@mhri.org.**

We are an equal opportunity employer M/F/D/V.

## JOURNAL ADVERTISER INDEX


**ABBOTT LABS**
Omnicef OS .......... 1097-1099

**ALLIANT PHARMACEUTICALS**
Orapred Odt .......... 1091-1092

**ASTRAZENECA**
http://www.astrazeneca.com
Nexium .......... 1120A-B

**CLASSIFIED ADVERTISING** .......... 1190-1191
http://www.amapublications.com

**GLAXOSMITHKLINE**
Boostrix .......... 1143-1144, COVER 3-4
Pediarix .......... 1157-1158, COVER 2-1089

**MERCK & COMPANY**
Gardasil .......... 1136A-D


*Demographic and "Mini" inserts and/or ROB ad pages

While every precaution is taken to ensure accuracy, we cannot guarantee against the possibility of an occasional change or omission in the preparation of this index.

ARCHIVES OF PEDIATRICS & ADOLESCENT MEDICINE

# CONTACT INFORMATION

## EDITORIAL OFFICE

**Editorial Office Information:** *Archives of Pediatrics & Adolescent Medicine*, Department of Pediatrics, Child Health Institute, University of Washington, 6200 NE 74th St, Suite 210, Seattle, WA 98115-8160, USA; phone: (206) 685-3573; fax: (206) 685-3572; e-mail: archpediatrics@jama-archives.org.

**Electronic Submission:** Manuscripts should be submitted via our online manuscript submission and review system (http://manuscripts.archpediatrics.com). Manuscripts submitted through our online system should not also be submitted by mail or fax. Signed authorship forms should be sent by regular mail or fax with the assigned manuscript number noted on each page in the upper right-hand corner. See the Instructions for Authors (www.archpediatrics.com) for more details.

## CONSORTIUM OF *JAMA* & *ARCHIVES* JOURNALS

The *Archives of Pediatrics & Adolescent Medicine* is a member of the consortium of AMA journals listed below.

The Journal of the American Medical Association (JAMA)
Archives of Dermatology
Archives of Facial Plastic Surgery
Archives of General Psychiatry
Archives of Internal Medicine
Archives of Neurology
Archives of Ophthalmology
Archives of Otolaryngology–Head & Neck Surgery
Archives of Pediatrics & Adolescent Medicine
Archives of Surgery

## *JAMA/ARCHIVES* MEDIA RELATIONS

Jann Ingmire; phone: (312) 464-5262; e-mail: mediarelations@jama-archives.org.

## *ARCHIVES OF PEDIATRICS* ONLINE

*Archives of Pediatrics & Adolescent Medicine* is available online at www.archpediatrics.com.

## *JAMA/ARCHIVES* REPRINTS

**Author/Educational Institution Reprints:** Anna Goins at (312) 464-2477; fax: (312) 464-5843; e-mail: anna.goins@ama-assn.org. Minimum order: 100 reprints.

**Commercial Reprints:** Phone: (312) 464-0776; fax: (312) 464-0708; e-mail: reprints@ama-assn.org. Minimum order: 100 reprints.

## PERMISSIONS

Information about obtaining permission to republish, reprint, or adapt material published in *Archives of Pediatrics & Adolescent Medicine* is available from Rhonda Bailey Brown; phone: (312) 464-2513; fax: (312) 464-5843; e-mail: permissions@ama-assn.org.

## DOCUMENT DELIVERY

Copies of individual articles are available online at www.archpediatrics.com and from the following: Infotrieve, phone: (800) 422-4633; fax: (310) 208-5971; URL: www.infotrieve.com; e-mail: orders@infotrieve.com; Institute for Scientific Information (ISI), phone: (800) 603-4367; fax: (856) 787-1679; URL: http://www.isidoc.com; e-mail: service@isidoc.com.

## ADVERTISING

Information about advertising is available from the following sales representatives and online at www.archpediatrics.com.

**Account Manager:** Tim Melroy (nationally); phone: (973) 263-9191 ext 213.

**Manager, Marketing Services:** Nancy Bell; phone: (973) 263-9191 ext 216.

**Advertising Office:** 119 Cherry Hill Rd, Suite 330, Parsippany, NJ 07054-1114; phone: (973) 263-9191.

**Classified Advertising:** Thalia Moss, Shana Brown, Kim Jenkins, Sophie Levandoski, 515 N State St, Chicago, IL 60610; phone: (800) 262-2260; e-mail: classifieds@jama-archives.org.

## ADVERTISING PRINCIPLES

Advertisements in this issue have been reviewed to comply with the principles governing advertising in AMA publications. A copy of these principles is available on request and online at www.archpediatrics.com. The appearance of advertising in AMA publications is not an AMA guarantee or endorsement of the product or the claims made for the product by the manufacturer.

## ADDRESS CHANGES

Send all address changes to *Archives of Pediatrics & Adolescent Medicine*, c/o the AMA Unified Service Center, American Medical Association, 515 N State St, Chicago, IL 60610. Notification of address changes must be made at least 6 weeks in advance; include both old and new addresses and a recent mailing label if sending via mail.

## SUBSCRIPTION RATES AND SERVICE

Subscription rates are shown in the table below. For service in the US and Americas, inquiries on pricing, address changes, missing issues, subscription billing, subscription renewal, and back issues, contact the AMA Unified Service Center, 24 hours a day, 7 days a week.

**AMA members:** phone: (800) 262-3211; e-mail: msc@ama-assn.org. **Other physicians and nonphysician customers, including subscription agents:** phone: (800) 262-2350 or (312) 670-7827; fax: (312) 464-5831; e-mail: ama-subs@ama-assn.org. **Inquiries:** Unified Service Center, American Medical Association, PO Box 10946, Chicago, IL 60610-0946. For subscribers with mailing addresses outside the United States & Americas: Contact *JAMA* & *Archives* Journals, c/o EMD GmbH, Birkenstr.67, 10559 Berlin, Germany. Phone: +49 (30) 33099828; fax: +49 (30) 33099829; e-mail: ama@emd-germany.de.

**Annual Subscription Rates**

| | United States | Americas | UK | Rest of World |
|---|---|---|---|---|
| INDIVIDUAL | | | | |
| Print and Online | $185 | $240 | £165 | €250 |
| INSTITUTION | | | | |
| Print and Online | $400 | $485 | £315 | €470 |

In Canada, US rate plus GST. Rates for residents and medical students available at pubs.ama-assn.org, or from the AMA Unified Service Center.

The ARCHIVES OF PEDIATRICS & ADOLESCENT MEDICINE (ISSN 01072–4710) is published monthly by the American Medical Association, 515 N State St, Chicago, IL 60610–0946, and is an official publication of the Association. The ARCHIVES OF PEDIATRICS & ADOLESCENT MEDICINE reaches more than 30 900 readers in over 83 countries each month. Periodicals postage paid at Chicago, Ill, and at additional mailing offices. GST registration number 12622 5556 RT. Canada Post International Publications Mail (Canadian Distribution) Sales Agreement No. 318728. POSTMASTER, send all address changes to *Archives of Pediatrics & Adolescent Medicine,* c/o the AMA Unified Service Center, American Medical Association, 515 N State St, Chicago, IL 60610. Printed in the USA.

# ARCHIVES OF PEDIATRICS & ADOLESCENT MEDICINE

WWW.ARCHPEDIATRICS.COM

DECEMBER 2006

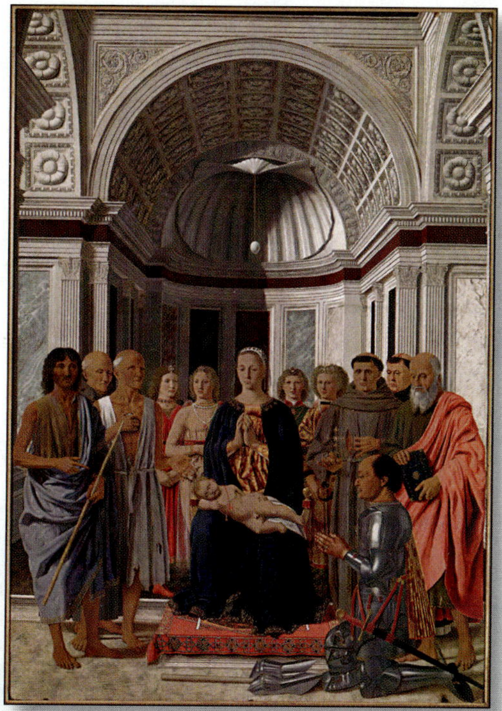

Piero della Francesca (ca 1415-1492), *Madonna and Child With Saints*. See page 1204.

TOBACCO MARKETING AND USE IN FILMS AND CHILDREN'S USE OF TOBACCO

IMPACT OF INFLUENZA VACCINATION DURING PREGNANCY ON RESPIRATORY ILLNESS IN INFANTS

RISKY ALCOHOL USE, AGE OF DRINKING ONSET, AND ADVERSE CHILDHOOD EXPERIENCES

DEXTROMETHORPHAN ABUSE IN ADOLESCENCE, 1999-2004

COMPLETE TABLE OF CONTENTS ON PAGE 1195



JAMA & ARCHIVES JOURNALS
American Medical Association

In the treatment or prevention of bronchospasm

# Expect Xopenex

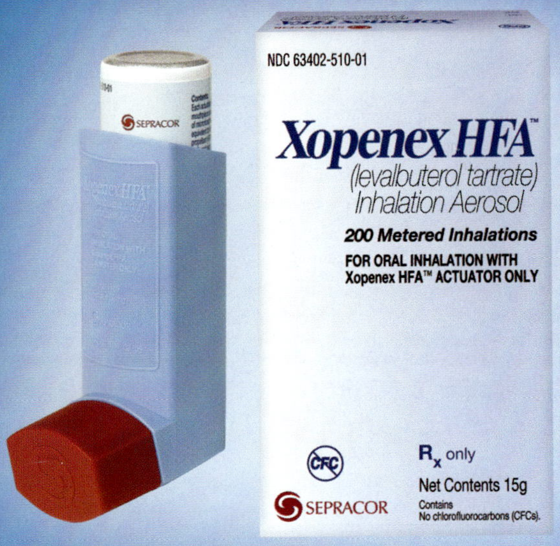


## ...in an MDI

**Same trusted single-isomer technology**

**Does not contain (S)-albuterol[1]**

# Xopenex HFA™

(levalbuterol tartrate) Inhalation Aerosol

XOPENEX HFA™ (levalbuterol tartrate) Inhalation Aerosol is indicated for the treatment or prevention of bronchospasm in adults, adolescents, and children 4 years of age and older with reversible obstructive airway disease.

**Important Safety Information**

Xopenex HFA™ (levalbuterol tartrate) Inhalation Aerosol is contraindicated in patients with a history of hypersensitivity to levalbuterol, racemic albuterol, or any other component of Xopenex HFA. Xopenex HFA and other β-agonists can produce paradoxical bronchospasm, which may be life threatening. If additional adrenergic drugs, including other short-acting sympathomimetic bronchodilators or epinephrine, are to be administered by any route, they should be used with caution to avoid deleterious cardiovascular effects. Due to the cardiovascular side effects associated with β-agonists, caution is generally recommended for patients with cardiovascular disorders (especially coronary insufficiency, cardiac arrhythmias, and hypertension), diabetes, hyperthyroidism, or convulsive disorders. Do not exceed the recommended dose. Fatalities have been reported in association with excessive use of inhaled sympathomimetic drugs in patients with asthma. Please refer to the complete prescribing information for further information and in regard to potential drug interactions with β-blockers, diuretics, digoxin, or MAOI and tricyclic antidepressants.

**In patients aged 4 to 11 years,** the most common adverse events (occurring in greater than 2% of patients and more frequently than patients receiving placebo) were (90 mcg Xopenex HFA and placebo, respectively): accidental injury (9.2%; 5.7%), vomiting (10.5%; 5.7%), bronchitis (2.6%; 0%), and pharyngitis (6.6%; 5.7%).

**In patients aged 12 years and older,** the most common adverse events (occurring in greater than 2% of patients and more frequently than patients receiving placebo) were (90 mcg Xopenex HFA and placebo, respectively): pain (4.0%; 3.6%), dizziness (2.7%; 1.8%), asthma (9.4%; 6.0%), pharyngitis (7.9%; 2.4%), and rhinitis (7.4%; 3.0%).


**Reference:** 1. Xopenex HFA Prescribing Information.


Please see brief summary of prescribing information.

# BOOSTRIX®

## (Tetanus Toxoid, Reduced Diphtheria Toxoid and Acellular Pertussis Vaccine, Adsorbed) (Tdap)

The following is a brief summary only; see full prescribing information for complete product information.

**INDICATIONS AND USAGE:** BOOSTRIX is indicated for active booster immunization against tetanus, diphtheria, and pertussis as a single dose in individuals 10 through 18 years of age. The use of BOOSTRIX as a primary series or to complete the primary series has not been studied. As with any vaccine, BOOSTRIX may not protect 100% of individuals receiving the vaccine.

**CONTRAINDICATIONS:** Hypersensitivity to any component of the vaccine is a contraindication (see DESCRIPTION in full prescribing information). Do not use BOOSTRIX after a serious allergic reaction (e.g., anaphylaxis) following any other tetanus toxoid, diphtheria toxoid or pertussis-containing vaccine, or any component of this vaccine (see DESCRIPTION in full prescribing information). Because of the uncertainty as to which component of the vaccine might be responsible, do not give further vaccination with any of these components; or, refer such individuals to an allergist for evaluation. The following events are contraindications to administration of BOOSTRIX: encephalopathy (e.g., coma, decreased level of consciousness, prolonged seizures) within 7 days of administration of a previous dose of a pertussis-containing vaccine that is not attributable to another identifiable cause; progressive neurologic disorder, uncontrolled epilepsy, or progressive encephalopathy. Do not vaccinate individuals with these conditions until a treatment regimen has been established and the condition has stabilized.

**WARNINGS:** The tip cap and the rubber plunger of the needleless prefilled syringes contain dry natural latex rubber that may cause allergic reactions in latex sensitive individuals. The vial stopper is latex-free. If any of the following events occurred in temporal relation to previous receipt of a Diphtheria and Tetanus Toxoids and Pertussis Vaccine Adsorbed (DTwP) vaccine or a vaccine containing an acellular pertussis component, consider carefully whether to give subsequent doses of BOOSTRIX: temperature of ≥40.5°C (105°F) within 48 hours not due to another identifiable cause; collapse or shock-like state (hypotonic-hyporesponsive episode) within 48 hours; persistent, inconsolable crying lasting ≥3 hours, occurring within 48 hours; seizures with or without fever occurring within 3 days. Persons who experienced serious Arthus-type hypersensitivity reactions following a prior dose of tetanus toxoid usually have high serum tetanus antitoxin levels and should not be given Tetanus and Diphtheria Toxoids Adsorbed For Adult Use (Td) or Tdap vaccines or even emergency doses of Td more frequently than every 10 years, even if the wound is neither clean nor minor. If Guillain-Barré syndrome has occurred within 6 weeks of receipt of prior vaccine containing tetanus toxoid, the decision to give BOOSTRIX or any vaccine containing tetanus toxoid should be based on careful consideration of the potential benefits and possible risks. The decision to administer a pertussis-containing vaccine to individuals with stable central nervous system (CNS) disorders must be made by the physician on an individual basis, with consideration of all relevant factors, and assessment of potential risks and benefits for that individual. Advise the patient, parent, or guardian of the potential increased risk involved (see PRECAUTIONS). A family history of seizures or other CNS disorders is not a contraindication to pertussis vaccine. The Advisory Committee on Immunization Practices (ACIP) has published guidelines for vaccination of persons with recent or acute illness (www.cdc.gov). Do not give BOOSTRIX to individuals with bleeding disorders such as hemophilia or thrombocytopenia, or to persons on anticoagulant therapy unless the potential benefit clearly outweighs the risk of administration. If the decision is made to administer BOOSTRIX to such persons, it should be given with caution with steps taken to avoid the risk of hematoma following the injection.

**PRECAUTIONS: General:** Before the injection of any biological, the physician should take all reasonable precautions to prevent allergic or other adverse reactions. Epinephrine injection (1:1,000) and other appropriate agents used for the control of immediate allergic reactions must be immediately available should an acute anaphylactic reaction occur. Immunosuppressed persons, including individuals receiving immunosuppressive therapy, may not develop the expected immune response. **Drug Interactions:** Do not mix BOOSTRIX with any other vaccine in the same syringe or vial. **Carcinogenesis, Mutagenesis, Impairment of Fertility:** BOOSTRIX has not been evaluated for carcinogenic or mutagenic potential, or for impairment of fertility. **Pregnancy:** Pregnancy Category C. Animal reproduction studies have not been conducted with BOOSTRIX. It is also not known whether BOOSTRIX can cause fetal harm when administered to a pregnant woman or can affect reproductive capacity. BOOSTRIX should be given to a pregnant woman only if clearly needed. Animal fertility studies have not been conducted with BOOSTRIX. In a developmental toxicity study, the effect of BOOSTRIX on embryo-fetal and pre-weaning development was evaluated in pregnant rats. Animals were administered INFANRIX® (Diphtheria and Tetanus Toxoids and Acellular Pertussis Vaccine Adsorbed) prior to gestation and BOOSTRIX during the period of organogenesis (gestation days 6, 8, 11) and later in pregnancy (gestation day 15), 0.1 mL/rat/occasion (a 45-fold increase compared to the human dose of BOOSTRIX on a body weight basis), by intramuscular injection. No adverse affect on pregnancy and lactation parameters, embryo-fetal or pre-weaning development was observed. There were no fetal malformations or other evidence of teratogenesis noted in this study. **Nursing Mothers:** It is not known whether BOOSTRIX is excreted in human milk. Because many drugs are excreted in human milk, caution should be exercised when BOOSTRIX is administered to a nursing woman. **Pregnancy Exposure Registry:** Healthcare providers are encouraged to register pregnant women who receive BOOSTRIX in the GlaxoSmithKline vaccination pregnancy registry by calling 1-888-825-5249. **Geriatric Use:** BOOSTRIX is not indicated for use in individuals older than 18 years. **Pediatric Use:** BOOSTRIX is not indicated for use in individuals younger than 10 years (see DOSAGE AND ADMINISTRATION in full prescribing information). For immunization of infants and children younger than 7 years against diphtheria, tetanus, and pertussis, refer to the manufacturers' package inserts for Diphtheria and Tetanus Toxoids and Acellular Pertussis Vaccine Adsorbed (DTaP) vaccines.

**ADVERSE REACTIONS:** A total of 3,608 adolescents were vaccinated with a single dose of BOOSTRIX during clinical trials. An additional 1,092 adolescents 10 to 18 years of age received a non-US formulation of BOOSTRIX (formulated to contain 0.5 mg aluminum per dose) in non-US clinical studies.

The primary safety study, conducted in the United States, was a randomized, observer-blinded, controlled study in which 3,080 adolescents 10 to 18 years of age received a single dose of BOOSTRIX and 1,034 received the control Td vaccine manufactured by Massachusetts Public Health Biologic Laboratories. There were no substantive differences in demographic characteristics between the vaccine groups. Among BOOSTRIX and control vaccine recipients approximately 75% were 10 to 14 years of age and approximately 25% were 15 to 18 years of age. Approximately 98% of participants in this study had received the recommended series of 4 or 5 doses of either DTwP or a combination of DTwP and DTaP in childhood. Data on adverse events were collected by the subjects, parents and/or guardians using standardized diaries for 15 consecutive days following the vaccine dose (i.e., day of vaccination and the next 14 days). Subjects were monitored for unsolicited adverse events that occurred within 31 days of vaccination (day 0-30) using diary cards (day 0-14) supplemented by spontaneous reports and a medical history as reported by subjects, parents, and/or guardians. Subjects were also monitored for 6 months post-vaccination for non-routine medical visits, visits to an emergency room, onset of new chronic illness, and serious adverse events. Information regarding late onset adverse events was obtained via a telephone call 6 months following vaccination. At least 97% of subjects completed the 6-month follow-up evaluation.

In a study conducted in Germany, BOOSTRIX was administered to 319 children 10 to 12 years of age previously vaccinated with 5 doses of acellular pertussis-containing vaccines, 193 of these subjects had previously received 5 doses of INFANRIX. Adverse events were recorded on diary cards during the 15 days following vaccination. Unsolicited adverse events that occurred within 31 days of vaccination (day 0-30) were recorded on the diary card or verbally reported to the investigator. Subjects were monitored for 6 months post-vaccination for physician office visits, emergency room visits, onset of new chronic illness, and serious adverse events. The 6-month follow-up evaluation, conducted via telephone interview, was completed by 90% of subjects.

The adverse event information from clinical trials provides a basis for identifying adverse events that appear to be related to vaccine use and for approximating rates. However, because clinical trials are conducted under widely varying conditions, adverse event rates observed in the clinical trials of a vaccine cannot be directly compared to rates in the clinical trials of another vaccine, and may not reflect the rates observed in practice.

**Serious Adverse Events in All Safety Studies:** In the US-safety study and German-safety study, no serious adverse events were reported to occur within 31 days of vaccination. During the 6-month extended safety evaluation period, no serious adverse events that were of potential autoimmune origin or new onset and chronic in nature were reported to occur. In non-US studies in which serious adverse events were monitored for up to 37 days, one subject was diagnosed with insulin dependent diabetes 20 days following administration of BOOSTRIX. No other serious adverse events of potential autoimmune origin or that were new onset and chronic in nature were reported to occur in these studies.

**Solicited Adverse Events in the US-Safety Study:** In a US study, the most common local adverse events following administration of BOOSTRIX were pain, redness, and swelling at the injection site. The most common general adverse events were headache and fatigue. Most of these events were reported at a similar frequency in recipients of both BOOSTRIX and Td. Any pain, grade 2 or 3 pain (but not grade 3 alone), and grade 2 or 3 headache (but not grade 3 alone) were reported at a higher rate in recipients of BOOSTRIX. The primary safety endpoint of the US study was the incidence of grade 3 pain (spontaneously painful and/or prevented normal activity) at the injection site within 15 days of vaccination. Grade 3 pain was reported in 4.6% of those who received BOOSTRIX compared with 4.0% of those who received the Td vaccine. The difference in rate of grade 3 pain was within the pre-defined clinical limit for non-inferiority (upper limit of the 95% CI for the difference ≤4%). These were the rates for solicited local and general adverse events within 15 days of vaccination with BOOSTRIX or Td vaccine for the total vaccinated cohort (all enrolled, vaccinated subjects with safety data available analyzed by vaccine received):

**Percentage of Individuals 10 to 18 Years of Age Reporting Solicited Local Adverse Events or Solicited General Adverse Events Within the 15-day* Post-Vaccination Period**

| | BOOSTRIX (N = 3,032) % | Td (N =1,013) % |
|---|---|---|
| **Local** | | |
| Pain,† any | 75.3 | 71.7 |
| Pain,† grade 2 or 3 | 51.2 | 42.5 |
| Pain,‡ grade 3 | 4.6 | 4.0 |
| Redness, any | 22.5 | 19.8 |
| Redness, >20 mm | 4.1 | 3.9 |
| Redness, ≥50 mm | 1.7 | 1.6 |
| Swelling, any | 21.1 | 20.1 |
| Swelling, >20 mm | 5.3 | 4.9 |
| Swelling, ≥50 mm | 2.5 | 3.2 |
| Arm circumference increase,§ >5 mm | 28.3 | 29.5 |
| Arm circumference increase,§ >20 mm | 2.0 | 2.2 |
| Arm circumference increase,§ >40 mm | 0.5 | 0.3 |
| **General** | | |
| Fever,‖ ≥99.5°F | 13.5 | 13.1 |
| Fever,‖ >100.4°F | 5.0 | 4.7 |
| Fever,‖ >102.2°F | 1.4 | 1.0 |
| Headache, any | 43.1 | 41.5 |
| Headache,† grade 2 or 3 | 15.7 | 12.7 |
| Headache, grade 3 | 3.7 | 2.7 |
| Fatigue, any | 37.0 | 36.7 |
| Fatigue, grade 2 or 3 | 14.4 | 12.9 |
| Fatigue, grade 3 | 3.7 | 3.2 |
| Gastrointestinal symptoms,¶ any | 26.0 | 25.8 |
| Gastrointestinal symptoms,¶ grade 2 or 3 | 9.8 | 9.7 |
| Gastrointestinal symptoms,¶ grade 3 | 3.0 | 3.2 |

Td = Tetanus and Diphtheria Toxoids Adsorbed For Adult Use manufactured by Massachusetts Public Health Biologic Laboratories.
N = number of subjects in the total vaccinated cohort with local/general symptoms sheets completed.
Grade 2 = Local: painful when the limb was moved; General: interfered with normal activity.
Grade 3 = Local: spontaneously painful and/or prevented normal activity; General: prevented normal activity.
*Day of vaccination and the next 14 days.
†Statistically significantly higher (P<0.05) following BOOSTRIX as compared to Td vaccine.
‡Grade 3 injection site pain following BOOSTRIX was not inferior to Td (upper limit of two-sided 95% CI for the difference in the percentage of subjects ≤4%).
§Mid-upper region of the vaccinated arm.
‖Oral temperatures or axillary temperatures.
¶Gastrointestinal symptoms included nausea, vomiting, diarrhea and/or abdominal pain.

Mid-upper arm circumference was measured by the adolescent or their parent/guardian prior to injection and daily for 15 days following vaccination. There was no significant difference between BOOSTRIX recipients and Td recipients in the proportion of subjects reporting an increase in mid-upper arm circumference in the vaccinated arm. The incidence of unsolicited adverse events reported in the 31 days after vaccination was comparable between the 2 groups.

**Solicited Adverse Events in the German Safety Study:** No cases of whole arm swelling were spontaneously reported. Two individuals (2/193) reported large injection site swelling (range 110 to 200 mm diameter), in one case associated with grade 3 pain. Neither individual sought medical attention. These episodes were reported to resolve without sequelae within 5 days. These were the rates of solicited local adverse events and fever within 15 days of vaccination for those subjects who had previously been vaccinated with 5 doses of INFANRIX:

**Rates of Solicited Adverse Events Reported Within the 15-day* Post-Vaccination Period Following Administration of BOOSTRIX in Individuals 10 to 12 Years of Age Who Had Previously Received 5 Doses of INFANRIX**

| Adverse Event | BOOSTRIX (N = 193) % (95% CI) |
|---|---|
| Pain, any | 62.2 (54.9-69.0) |
| Pain, grade 2 or 3 | 33.2 (26.6-40.3) |
| Pain, grade 3 | 5.7 (2.9-10.0) |
| Redness, any | 47.7 (40.4-55.0) |
| Redness, >20 mm | 15.0 (10.3-20.9) |
| Redness, ≥50 mm | 10.9 (6.9-16.2) |
| Swelling, any | 38.9 (31.9-46.1) |
| Swelling, >20 mm | 17.6 (12.5-23.7) |
| Swelling, ≥50 mm | 14.0 (9.4-19.7) |
| Fever, ≥99.5 | 8.8 (5.2-13.7) |
| Fever, >100.4 | 4.1 (1.8-8.0) |
| Fever, >102.2 | 1.0 (0.1-3.7) |

N = number of subjects with local/general symptoms sheets completed.
Grade 2 = Painful when the limb was moved.
Grade 3 = Spontaneously painful and/or prevented normal activity.
*Day of vaccination and the next 14 days.

As with any vaccine, there is the possibility that broad use of BOOSTRIX could reveal adverse events not observed in clinical trials.

**Postmarketing Reports:** Worldwide voluntary reports of adverse events received for BOOSTRIX in persons 10 to 18 years of age since market introduction of this vaccine are listed below. This list includes serious events or events which have causal connection to components of this or other vaccines or drugs. Because these events are reported voluntarily from a population of uncertain size, it is not possible to reliably estimate their frequency or establish a causal relationship to vaccine exposure. *Blood and lymphatic system disorders:* Lymphadenitis, lymphadenopathy. *Cardiac disorders:* Myocarditis. *Injection site reactions:* Induration, inflammation, mass, nodule, warmth, local reaction. *Metabolism and nutrition disorders:* Diabetes mellitus insulin-dependent. *Musculoskeletal and connective tissue disorders:* Arthralgia, back pain, myalgia. *Nervous system disorders:* Convulsion, encephalitis, facial palsy, paraesthesia. *Skin and subcutaneous tissue disorders:* Exanthem, Henoch-Schönlein purpura, rash. In addition, extensive swelling of the injected limb has been reported following administration of BOOSTRIX.

**Reporting Adverse Events:** Report the occurrence following immunization of any event set forth in the Vaccine Injury Table from the National Childhood Vaccine Injury Act including: Anaphylaxis or anaphylactic shock within 7 days, encephalopathy or encephalitis within 7 days, brachial neuritis within 28 days, or an acute complication or sequelae (including death) of an illness, disability, injury, or condition referred to above, or any events that would contraindicate further doses of vaccine, according to this prescribing information. These events should be reported to VAERS. The VAERS toll-free number is 1-800-822-7967. Reporting forms may also be obtained at the VAERS website at www.vaers.hhs.gov.

**DOSAGE AND ADMINISTRATION: Recommended Dose:** BOOSTRIX should be administered as a single 0.5 mL injection by the intramuscular route into the deltoid muscle of the upper arm in individuals 10 through 18 years of age. Do not administer this product subcutaneously or intravenously. There are no data to support repeat administration of BOOSTRIX. Five years should elapse between the subject's last dose of the recommended series of childhood DTwP and/or DTaP vaccine and the administration of BOOSTRIX. Limited data are available on the use of BOOSTRIX following Tetanus and Diphtheria Toxoids Adsorbed For Adult Use (Td) vaccine. **Additional Dosing Information:** ***Wound Management:*** Clinicians should refer to guidelines for tetanus prophylaxis in routine wound management. Adolescents 10 to 18 years of age who have completed a primary series against tetanus and who sustain wounds which are minor and uncomplicated, should receive a booster dose of a tetanus toxoid-containing vaccine only if they have not received tetanus toxoid within the preceding 10 years. In case of tetanus-prone injury (e.g., wounds contaminated with dirt, feces, soil, and saliva; puncture wounds; avulsions; and wounds resulting from missles, crushing, burns, and frostbite) in an adolescent who is in need of tetanus toxoid, BOOSTRIX can be used as an alternative to Tetanus and Diphtheria Toxoids Adsorbed For Adult Use (Td) vaccine in patients for whom the pertussis component is also indicated (see INDICATIONS AND USAGE).

Manufactured by **GlaxoSmithKline Biologicals**
Rixensart, Belgium, US License 1617

Distributed by **GlaxoSmithKline**
Research Triangle Park, NC 27709



Full prescribing information for BOOSTRIX is available at www.BOOSTRIX.com.
BRS-BO:L3

**References: 1.** Centers for Disease Control and Prevention. Preventing tetanus, diphtheria, and pertussis among adolescents: use of tetanus toxoid, reduced diphtheria toxoid and acellular pertussis vaccines: recommendations of the Advisory Committee on Immunization Practices (ACIP). Early Release 2006;55(February 23, 2006):1–43. **2.** Centers for Disease Control and Prevention. Recommended childhood and adolescent immunization schedule—United States, 2006. *MMWR.* 2006;54(51&52):Q1–Q4.

# Xopenex HFA™
(levalbuterol tartrate) Inhalation Aerosol

FOR ORAL INHALATION ONLY

## BRIEF SUMMARY

### INDICATIONS AND USAGE

XOPENEX HFA (levalbuterol tartrate) Inhalation Aerosol is indicated for the treatment or prevention of bronchospasm in adults, adolescents, and children 4 years of age and older with reversible obstructive airway disease.

### CONTRAINDICATIONS

XOPENEX HFA (levalbuterol tartrate) Inhalation Aerosol is contraindicated in patients with a history of hypersensitivity to levalbuterol, racemic albuterol, or any other component of XOPENEX HFA Inhalation Aerosol.

### WARNINGS

1. Paradoxical Bronchospasm: Like other inhaled beta-adrenergic agonists, XOPENEX HFA Inhalation Aerosol can produce paradoxical bronchospasm, which may be life-threatening. If paradoxical bronchospasm occurs, XOPENEX HFA (levalbuterol tartrate) Inhalation Aerosol should be discontinued immediately and alternative therapy instituted. It should be recognized that paradoxical bronchospasm, when associated with inhaled formulations, frequently occurs with the first use of a new canister. 2. Deterioration of Asthma: Asthma may deteriorate acutely over a period of hours or chronically over several days or longer. If the patient needs more doses of XOPENEX HFA Inhalation Aerosol than usual, this may be a marker of destabilization of asthma and requires reevaluation of the patient and treatment regimen, giving special consideration to the possible need for anti-inflammatory treatment, e.g., corticosteroids.
3. Use of Anti-Inflammatory Agents: The use of a beta-adrenergic agonist alone may not be adequate to control asthma in many patients. Early consideration should be given to adding anti-inflammatory agents, e.g., corticosteroids, to the therapeutic regimen. 4. Cardiovascular Effects: XOPENEX HFA Inhalation Aerosol, like other beta-adrenergic agonists, can produce clinically significant cardiovascular effects in some patients, as measured by heart rate, blood pressure, and/or symptoms. Although such effects are uncommon after administration of XOPENEX HFA Inhalation Aerosol at recommended doses, if they occur, the drug may need to be discontinued. In addition, beta-agonists have been reported to produce electrocardiogram (ECG) changes, such as flattening of the T wave, prolongation of the QTc interval, and ST segment depression. The clinical significance of these findings is unknown. Therefore, XOPENEX HFA Inhalation Aerosol, like all sympathomimetic amines, should be used with caution in patients with cardiovascular disorders, especially coronary insufficiency, cardiac arrhythmias, and hypertension. 5. Do Not Exceed Recommended Dose: Fatalities have been reported in association with excessive use of inhaled sympathomimetic drugs in patients with asthma. The exact cause of death is unknown, but cardiac arrest following an unexpected development of a severe acute asthmatic crisis and subsequent hypoxia is suspected.
6. Immediate Hypersensitivity Reactions: Immediate hypersensitivity reactions may occur after administration of racemic albuterol, as demonstrated by rare cases of urticaria, angioedema, rash, bronchospasm, anaphylaxis, and oropharyngeal edema. The potential for hypersensitivity must be considered in the clinical evaluation of patients who experience immediate hypersensitivity reactions while receiving XOPENEX HFA Inhalation Aerosol.

### PRECAUTIONS

#### General

XOPENEX HFA (levalbuterol tartrate) Inhalation Aerosol, like all sympathomimetic amines, should be used with caution in patients with cardiovascular disorders, especially coronary insufficiency, hypertension, and cardiac arrhythmias; in patients with convulsive disorders, hyperthyroidism, or diabetes mellitus; and in patients who are unusually responsive to sympathomimetic amines. Clinically significant changes in systolic and diastolic blood pressure have been seen in individual patients and could be expected to occur in some patients after the use of any beta-adrenergic bronchodilator.

Large doses of intravenous racemic albuterol have been reported to aggravate preexisting diabetes mellitus and ketoacidosis. As with other beta-adrenergic agonist medications, XOPENEX HFA Inhalation Aerosol may produce significant hypokalemia in some patients, possibly through intracellular shunting, which has the potential to produce adverse cardiovascular effects. The decrease is usually transient, not requiring supplementation.

#### Information for Patients

The action of XOPENEX HFA Inhalation Aerosol should last for 4 to 6 hours. XOPENEX HFA Inhalation Aerosol should not be used more frequently than recommended. Do not increase the dose or frequency of doses of XOPENEX HFA Inhalation Aerosol without consulting your physician. If you find that treatment with XOPENEX HFA Inhalation Aerosol becomes less effective for symptomatic relief, your symptoms become worse, and/or you need to use the product more frequently than usual, you should seek medical attention immediately. While you are using XOPENEX HFA Inhalation Aerosol, other inhaled drugs and asthma medications should be taken only as directed by your physician.

Common adverse effects of treatment with inhaled beta-agonists include palpitations, chest pain, rapid heart rate, tremor, and nervousness. If you are pregnant or nursing, contact your physician about use of XOPENEX HFA Inhalation Aerosol. Effective and safe use of XOPENEX HFA Inhalation Aerosol includes an understanding of the way that it should be administered.

Use XOPENEX HFA Inhalation Aerosol only with the actuator supplied with the product. Discard the canister after 200 sprays have been used. Never immerse the canister in water to determine how full the canister is ("float test").

In general, the technique for administering XOPENEX HFA Inhalation Aerosol to children is similar to that for adults. Children should use XOPENEX HFA Inhalation Aerosol under adult supervision, as instructed by the patient's physician.

#### Drug Interactions

Other short-acting sympathomimetic aerosol bronchodilators or epinephrine should be used with caution with XOPENEX HFA Inhalation Aerosol. If additional adrenergic drugs are to be administered by any route, they should be used with caution to avoid deleterious cardiovascular effects.

1. Beta-blockers: Beta-adrenergic receptor-blocking agents not only block the pulmonary effect of beta-adrenergic agonists, such as XOPENEX HFA Inhalation Aerosol, but may produce severe bronchospasm in asthmatic patients. Therefore, patients with asthma should not normally be treated with beta-blockers. However, under certain circumstances, e.g., as prophylaxis after myocardial infarction, there may be no acceptable alternatives to the use of beta-adrenergic blocking agents in patients with asthma. In this setting, cardioselective beta-blockers should be considered, although they should be administered with caution. 2. Diuretics: The ECG changes and/or hypokalemia that may result from the administration of non–potassium-sparing diuretics (such as loop and thiazide diuretics) can be acutely worsened by beta-agonists, especially when the recommended dose of the beta-agonist is exceeded. Although the clinical significance of these effects is not known, caution is advised in the coadministration of beta-agonists with non–potassium-sparing diuretics. 3. Digoxin: Mean decreases of 16% to 22% in serum digoxin levels were demonstrated after single-dose intravenous and oral administration of racemic albuterol, respectively, to normal volunteers who had received digoxin for 10 days. The clinical significance of these findings for patients with obstructive airway disease who are receiving XOPENEX HFA Inhalation Aerosol and digoxin on a chronic basis is unclear. Nevertheless, it would be prudent to carefully evaluate the serum digoxin levels in patients who are currently receiving digoxin and XOPENEX HFA Inhalation Aerosol. 4. Monoamine Oxidase Inhibitors or Tricyclic Antidepressants: XOPENEX HFA Inhalation Aerosol should be administered with extreme caution to patients being treated with monoamine oxidase inhibitors or tricyclic antidepressants, or within 2 weeks of discontinuation of such agents, because the action of albuterol on the vascular system may be potentiated.

**Carcinogenesis, Mutagenesis, and Impairment of Fertility** No carcinogenesis or impairment of fertility studies have been carried out with levalbuterol tartrate. However, racemic albuterol sulfate has been evaluated for its carcinogenic potential and ability to impair fertility.

In a 2-year study in Sprague-Dawley rats, racemic albuterol sulfate caused a significant dose-related increase in the incidence of benign leiomyomas of the mesovarium at, and above, dietary doses of 2 mg/kg/day (approximately 30 times the maximum recommended daily inhalation dose of levalbuterol tartrate for adults on a $mg/m^2$ basis and approximately 15 times the maximum recommended daily inhalation dose of levalbuterol tartrate for children on a $mg/m^2$ basis). In another study, this effect was blocked by the coadministration of propranolol, a non-selective beta-adrenergic antagonist. In an 18-month study in CD-1 mice, racemic albuterol sulfate showed no evidence of tumorigenicity at dietary doses up to 500 mg/kg/day (approximately 3800 times the maximum recommended daily inhalation dose of levalbuterol tartrate for adults on a $mg/m^2$ basis and approximately 1800 times the maximum recommended daily inhalation dose of levalbuterol tartrate for children on a $mg/m^2$ basis). In a 22-month study in the Golden hamster, racemic albuterol sulfate showed no evidence of tumorigenicity at dietary doses up to 50 mg/kg/day (approximately 500 times the maximum recommended daily inhalation dose of levalbuterol tartrate for adults on a $mg/m^2$ basis and approximately 240 times the maximum recommended daily inhalation dose of levalbuterol tartrate for children on a $mg/m^2$ basis).

Levalbuterol HCl was not mutagenic in the Ames test or the CHO/HPRT Mammalian Forward Gene Mutation Assay.

Levalbuterol HCl was not clastogenic in the in vivo micronucleus test in mouse bone marrow. Racemic albuterol sulfate was negative in an in vitro chromosomal aberration assay in CHO cell cultures.

Reproduction studies in rats using racemic albuterol sulfate demonstrated no evidence of impaired fertility at oral doses up to 50 mg/kg/day (approximately 750 times the maximum recommended daily inhalation dose of levalbuterol tartrate for adults on a $mg/m^2$ basis).

**Teratogenic Effects - Pregnancy Category C** A reproduction study in New Zealand White rabbits demonstrated that levalbuterol HCl was not teratogenic when administered orally at doses up to 25 mg/kg/day (approximately 750 times the maximum recommended daily inhalation dose of levalbuterol tartrate for adults on a $mg/m^2$ basis).

However, racemic albuterol sulfate has been shown to be teratogenic in mice and rabbits. A study in CD-1 mice given racemic albuterol sulfate subcutaneously showed cleft palate formation in 5 of 111 (4.5%) fetuses at 0.25 mg/kg/day (approximately 2 times the maximum recommended daily inhalation dose of levalbuterol tartrate for adults on a $mg/m^2$ basis) and in 10 of 108 (9.3%) fetuses at 2.5 mg/kg/day (approximately 20 times the maximum recommended daily inhalation dose of levalbuterol tartrate for adults on a $mg/m^2$ basis). The drug did not induce cleft palate formation when administered subcutaneously at a dose of 0.025 mg/kg/day (less than the maximum recommended daily inhalation dose of levalbuterol tartrate for adults on a $mg/m^2$ basis). Cleft palate also occurred in 22 of 72 (30.5%) fetuses from females treated subcutaneously with 2.5 mg/kg/day of isoproterenol (positive control).

A reproduction study in Stride Dutch rabbits revealed cranioschisis in 7 of 19 (37%) fetuses when racemic albuterol sulfate was administered orally at a dose of 50 mg/kg/day (approximately 1500 times the maximum recommended daily inhalation dose of levalbuterol tartrate for adults on a $mg/m^2$ basis).

A study in which pregnant rats were dosed with radiolabeled racemic albuterol sulfate demonstrated that drug-related material is transferred from the maternal circulation to the fetus.

There are no adequate and well-controlled studies of XOPENEX HFA Inhalation Aerosol in pregnant women. Because animal reproduction studies are not always predictive of human response, XOPENEX HFA Inhalation Aerosol should be used during pregnancy only if the potential benefit justifies the potential risk to the fetus.

During marketing experience of racemic albuterol, various congenital anomalies, including cleft palate and limb defects, have been rarely reported in the offspring of patients being treated with racemic albuterol. Some of the mothers were taking multiple medications during their pregnancies. No consistent pattern of defects can be discerned, and a relationship between racemic albuterol use and congenital anomalies has not been established.

**Use in Labor and Delivery** Because of the potential for beta-adrenergic agonists to interfere with uterine contractility, the use of XOPENEX HFA Inhalation Aerosol for the treatment of bronchospasm during labor should be restricted to those patients in whom the benefits clearly outweigh the risk.

**Tocolysis** XOPENEX HFA Inhalation Aerosol has not been approved for the management of preterm labor. The benefit:risk ratio when levalbuterol tartrate is administered for tocolysis has not been established. Serious adverse reactions, including maternal pulmonary edema, have been reported during or following treatment of premature labor with beta2-agonists, including racemic albuterol.

**Nursing Mothers** Plasma concentrations of levalbuterol after inhalation of therapeutic doses are very low in humans. It is not known whether levalbuterol is excreted in human milk.

Because of the potential for tumorigenicity shown for racemic albuterol in animal studies and the lack of experience with the use of XOPENEX HFA Inhalation Aerosol by nursing mothers, a decision should be made whether to discontinue nursing or to discontinue the drug, taking into account the importance of the drug to the mother. Caution should be exercised when XOPENEX HFA Inhalation Aerosol is administered to a nursing woman.

**Pediatrics** The safety and efficacy of XOPENEX HFA Inhalation Aerosol have been established in pediatric patients 4 years of age and older in an adequate and well-controlled clinical trial. Use of XOPENEX HFA Inhalation Aerosol in children is also supported by evidence from adequate and well-controlled studies of XOPENEX HFA Inhalation Aerosol in adults, considering that the pathophysiology, systemic exposure of the drug, and clinical profile in pediatric and adult patients are substantially similar. Safety and effectiveness of XOPENEX HFA Inhalation Aerosol in pediatric patients below the age of 4 years have not been established.

**Geriatrics** Clinical studies of XOPENEX HFA Inhalation Aerosol did not include sufficient numbers of subjects aged 65 and older to determine whether they respond differently from younger subjects. Other reported clinical experience has not identified differences in responses between the elderly and younger patients. In general, dose selection for an elderly patient should be cautious, usually starting at the low end of the dosing range, reflecting the greater frequency of decreased hepatic, renal, or cardiac function, and of concomitant diseases or other drug therapy.

Albuterol is known to be substantially excreted by the kidney, and the risk of toxic reactions may be greater in patients with impaired renal function. Because elderly patients are more likely to have decreased renal function, care should be taken in dose selection, and it may be useful to monitor renal function.

**ADVERSE REACTIONS** Adverse event information concerning XOPENEX HFA (levalbuterol tartrate) Inhalation Aerosol in adults and adolescents is derived from two 8-week, multicenter, randomized, double-blind, active- and placebo-controlled trials in 748 adult and adolescent patients with asthma that compared XOPENEX HFA Inhalation Aerosol, a marketed albuterol HFA inhaler, and an HFA-134a placebo inhaler. The following lists the incidence (% XOPENEX HFA 90 mcg, marketed albuterol HFA inhaler 180 mcg, placebo, respectively) of all adverse events (whether considered by the investigator to be related or unrelated to drug) from these trials that occurred at a rate of 2% or greater in the group treated with XOPENEX HFA Inhalation Aerosol and more frequently than in the HFA-134a placebo inhaler group. Body as a whole: pain (4.0%, 3.4%, 3.6%). Central nervous system: dizziness (2.7%, 0.6%, 1.8%). Respiratory system: asthma (9.4%, 7.3%, 6.0%), pharyngitis (7.9%, 2.2%, 2.4%), rhinitis (7.4%, 2.2%, 3.0%).

Adverse events reported by less than 2% and at least 2 or more of the adolescent and adult patients receiving XOPENEX HFA Inhalation Aerosol and by a greater proportion than receiving HFA-134a placebo inhaler include cyst, flu syndrome, viral infection, constipation, gastroenteritis, myalgia, hypertension, epistaxis, lung disorder, acne, herpes simplex, conjunctivitis, ear pain, dysmenorrhea, hematuria, and vaginal moniliasis. There were no significant laboratory abnormalities observed in these studies.

Adverse event information concerning XOPENEX HFA Inhalation Aerosol in children is derived from a 4-week, randomized, double-blind trial of XOPENEX HFA Inhalation Aerosol, a marketed albuterol HFA inhaler, and an HFA-134a placebo inhaler in 150 children aged 4 to 11 years with asthma. The following lists the adverse events (% XOPENEX HFA 90 mcg, marketed albuterol HFA inhaler 180 mcg, placebo, respectively) reported for XOPENEX HFA Inhalation Aerosol in children at a rate of 2% or greater and more frequently than for placebo. Body as a whole: accidental injury (9.2%, 10.3%, 5.7%). Digestive system: vomiting (10.5%, 7.7%, 5.7%). Respiratory system: bronchitis (2.6%, 0%, 0%), pharyngitis (6.6%, 12.8%, 5.7%).

The incidence of systemic beta-adrenergic adverse effects (e.g., tremor, nervousness) was low and comparable across all treatment groups, including placebo.

**Postmarketing** In addition to the adverse events reported in clinical trials, the following adverse events have been observed in postapproval use of levalbuterol inhalation solution. These events have been chosen for inclusion due to their seriousness, their frequency of reporting, or their likely beta-mediated mechanism: angioedema, anaphylaxis, arrhythmias (including atrial fibrillation, supraventricular tachycardia, extrasystoles), asthma, chest pain, cough increased, dyspnea, nausea, nervousness, rash, tachycardia, tremor, urticaria. Because these events have been reported spontaneously from a population of unknown size, estimates of frequency cannot be made.

In addition, XOPENEX HFA Inhalation Aerosol, like other sympathomimetic agents, can cause adverse reactions such as hypertension, angina, vertigo, central nervous system stimulation, sleeplessness, headache, and drying or irritation of the oropharynx.

Rx only.

SEPRACOR 12/05

# ARCHIVES OF PEDIATRICS & ADOLESCENT MEDICINE

DECEMBER 2006 VOLUME 160, NUMBER 12 PAGES 1193-1312


## COVER ART


**Piero della Francesca (circa 1415-1492): *Madonna and Child With Saints*, circa 1474** 1204
*Thomas D. Koepsell, MD, MPH*


## ARTICLES


**Risky Alcohol Use, Age at Onset of Drinking, and Adverse Childhood Experiences in Young Men Entering the US Marine Corps** 1207
*Sylvia Y. N. Young, MD, MPH; Christian J. Hansen, BS; Roger L. Gibson, PhD, DVM, MPH; Margaret A. K. Ryan, MD, MPH*

**Dextromethorphan Abuse in Adolescence: An Increasing Trend: 1999-2004** 1217
*Jodi K. Bryner, PharmD; Uerica K. Wang, PharmD; Jenny W. Hui, PharmD; Merilin Bedodo, PharmD; Conan MacDougall, PharmD; Ilene B. Anderson, PharmD*

**Reduction in Newborns With Discharge Coding of In Utero Alcohol Effects in the United States, 1993 to 2002** 1224
*James M. Robbins, PhD; T. M. Bird, MS; John M. Tilford, PhD; J. Alex Reading, MS; Mario A. Cleves, PhD; Mary E. Aitken, MD, MPH; Charlotte M. Druschel, MD, MPH; Charlotte A. Hobbs, MD, PhD*

**Effect of Early Childhood Adversity on Child Health** 1232
*Emalee G. Flaherty, MD; Richard Thompson, PhD; Alan J. Litrownik, PhD; Adrea Theodore, MD, MPH; Diana J. English, PhD; Maureen M. Black, PhD; Traci Wike, MSW; Lakecia Whimper, MA; Desmond K. Runyan, MD, PhD; Howard Dubowitz, MD, MS*

**The Other Children: A Survey of Child Abuse Physicians on the Medical Evaluation of Children Living With a Physically Abused Child** 1241
*Kristine A. Campbell, MD, MSc; Debra L. Bogen, MD; Rachel P. Berger, MD, MPH*

**Nondisclosure of Sexual Orientation to a Physician Among a Sample of Gay, Lesbian, and Bisexual Youth** 1248
*Garth D. Meckler, MD, MSHS; Marc N. Elliott, PhD; David E. Kanouse, PhD; Kristin P. Beals, PhD; Mark A. Schuster, MD, PhD*

**Effects of a Life Skills Intervention for Increasing Physical Activity in Adolescent Girls** 1255
*Deborah Rohm Young, PhD; Jennie A. Phillips, MS; Tao Yu, MS; Jennifer A. Haythornthwaite, PhD*

**Objectively Measured Physical Activity in Sixth-Grade Girls** 1262
*Russell R. Pate, PhD; June Stevens, PhD; Charlotte Pratt, PhD; James F. Sallis, PhD; Kathryn H. Schmitz, PhD, MPH; Larry S. Webber, PhD; Gregory Welk, PhD; Deborah R. Young, PhD*

**YOUTH: A Health Plan–Based Lifestyle Intervention Increases Bone Mineral Density in Adolescent Girls** 1269
*Lynn L. DeBar, PhD, MPH; Cheryl Ritenbaugh, PhD, MPH; Mikel Aickin, PhD; Eric Orwoll, MD; Diane Elliot, MD; John Dickerson, MS; Nancy Vuckovic, PhD; Victor J. Stevens, PhD; Esther Moe, PhD; Lori M. Irving, PhD*

**Impact of Maternal Influenza Vaccination During Pregnancy on the Incidence of Acute Respiratory Illness Visits Among Infants** 1277
*Eric K. France, MD, MSPH; Renae Smith-Ray, MA; David McClure, PhD; Simon Hambidge, MD, PhD; Stanley Xu, PhD; Kristi Yamasaki, PharmD; David Shay, MD, MPH; Eric Weintraub, MPH; Alicia M. Fry, MD, MPH; Steve B. Black, MD; Henry R. Shinefield, MD; John P. Mullooly, PhD; Lisa A. Jackson, MD, MPH; for the Vaccine Safety Datalink Team*


## REVIEW ARTICLE


**The Extent to Which Tobacco Marketing and Tobacco Use in Films Contribute to Children's Use of Tobacco: A Meta-analysis** 1285
*Robert J. Wellman, PhD; David B. Sugarman, PhD; Joseph R. DiFranza, MD; Jonathan P. Winickoff, MD, MPH*

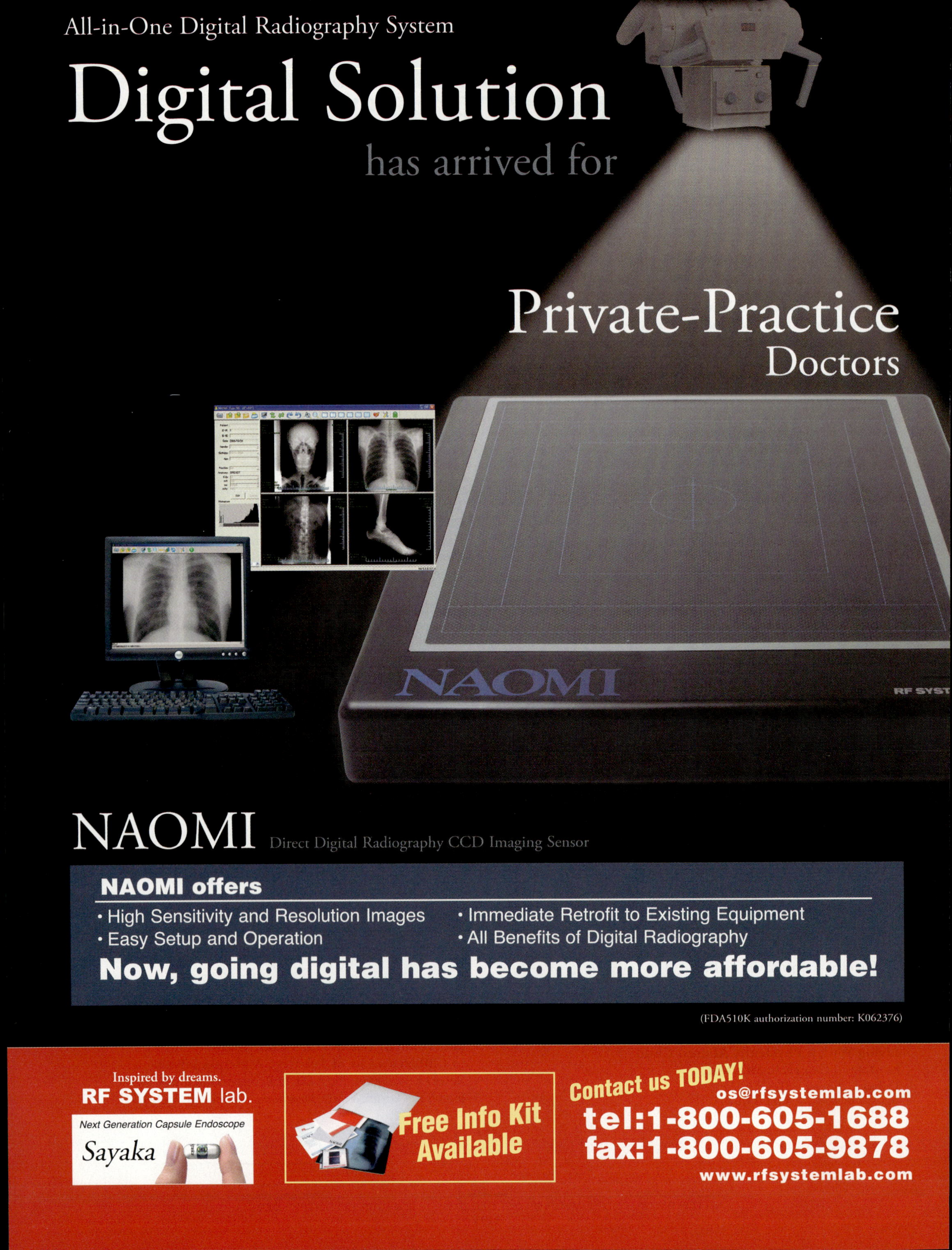
All-in-One Digital Radiography System
Digital Solution
has arrived for
Private-Practice
Doctors
NAOMI
RF SYST
NAOMI
Direct Digital Radiography CCD Imaging Sensor
NAOMI offers
• High Sensitivity and Resolution Images
• Easy Setup and Operation
• Immediate Retrofit to Existing Equipment
• All Benefits of Digital Radiography
Now, going digital has become more affordable!
(FDA510K authorization number: K062376)
Inspired by dreams.
RF SYSTEM lab.
Next Generation Capsule Endoscope
Sayaka
Free Info Kit
Available
Contact us TODAY!
os@rfsystemlab.com
tel:1-800-605-1688
fax:1-800-605-9878
www.rfsystemlab.com

ARCHIVES OF PEDIATRICS & ADOLESCENT MEDICINE

## SPECIAL FEATURE

**Picture of the Month** 1297
*Hossam Al-Tatari, MD; Nahed Abdel-Haq, MD; Basim Asmar, MD; Michael Haupert, DO; Raja Rabah, MD*

## EDITORIALS

**The Role of Early Stressors in Child Health and Mental Health Outcomes** 1300
*Mary Dozier, PhD; Elizabeth Peloso, MS*

**Adolescent Homosexuality: Dare We Ask the Question?** 1303
*Gary Remafedi, MD, MPH*

## THE PEDIATRIC FORUM

**The Association Between Caregiver Knowledge of Antiretroviral Therapy Regimens and Disease Parameters Among Perinatally Human Immunodeficiency Virus–Infected Children** 1307
*Ouzama Nicholson, MD, MS; Claude Mellins, PhD; Curtis Dolezal, PhD; E. Karina Santamaria, BA; Elizabeth Brackis-Cott, PhD; Elaine J. Abrams, MD*

## REGULAR DEPARTMENTS

**This Month in *Archives of Pediatrics & Adolescent Medicine*** 1202

**Announcements** 1222, 1231, 1254, 1261

**Classified Advertising** 1311

**Journal Advertiser Index** 1311

**Contact Information** 1312

**Instructions for authors and the author and subject indexes are available on our Web site: http://www.archpediatrics.com. If you do not have access to the Web, contact Suzanne Shuey at (206) 685-3573.**

### About the Cover

Piero della Francesca (circa 1415-1492), Italian. *Madonna and Child With Saints*, circa 1474. Photo credit: Scala/Art Resource, New York, NY.

# ARCHIVES OF PEDIATRICS & ADOLESCENT MEDICINE


**Mission Statement:** *The Archives of Pediatrics & Adolescent Medicine* is a monthly, peer-reviewed journal for physicians and other health care professionals who contribute to the health of children and adolescents. The *Archives* provides an open forum for dialogue on a full range of clinical, scientific, advocacy, and humanistic issues relevant to the care of pediatric patients from infancy through young adulthood. The *Archives* is a vehicle for increased attention to adolescent health, the education of pediatric health care professionals, and disease prevention and health promotion. The *Archives* publishes original studies, editorials, reviews by experts, practice commentaries, case quizzes, and updates on clinical science and practice management. The Pediatric Forum provides our readers with opportunities to express their views. *Archives* incorporates *AJDC*, the oldest journal in US pediatric literature, which originated in 1911.




JAMA & ARCHIVES JOURNALS
American Medical Association

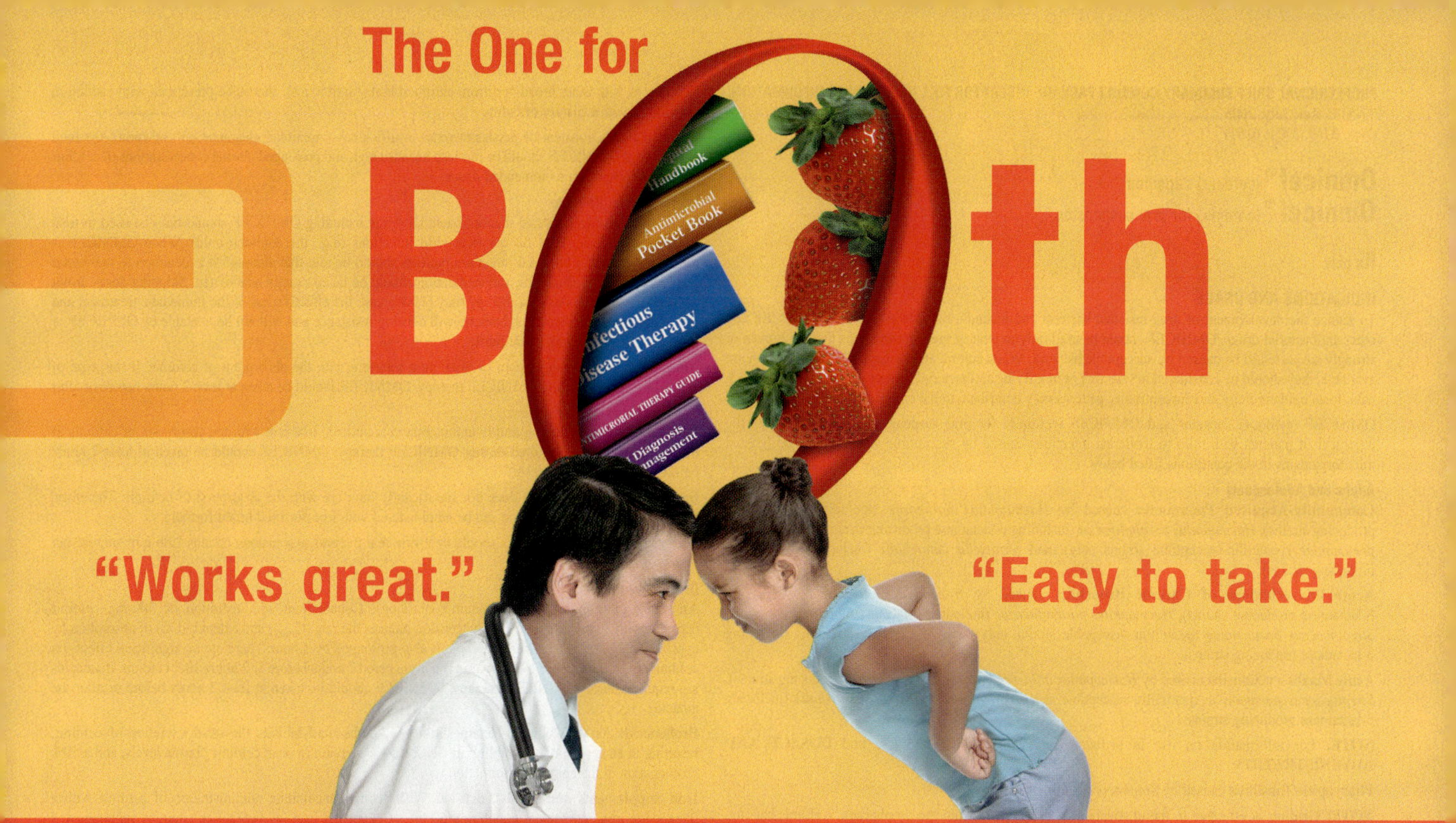


# 250 mg/5 mL* — Half the Volume†

**According to published peer-reviewed literature,[1-3] compliance factors that make an antibiotic easy to take include:**

- **Taste (palatability)**
- **Tolerability**
- **Short duration of treatment**
- **Number of daily doses**

**Indications** OMNICEF (cefdinir) for Oral Suspension is indicated in patients 6 months through 12 years for mild to moderate **Acute Bacterial Otitis Media** caused by susceptible strains of *H influenzae* (including ß-lactamase producing strains), *S pneumoniae* (penicillin-susceptible strains only), and *M catarrhalis* (including ß-lactamase producing strains).[4]

**Important Safety Information**[4]

- To reduce the development of drug-resistant bacteria and maintain the effectiveness of OMNICEF and other antibacterial drugs, OMNICEF should be used only to treat or prevent infections that are proven or strongly suspected to be caused by bacteria
- OMNICEF is contraindicated in patients with known allergy to the cephalosporin class of antibiotics
- For patients with previous hypersensitivity reaction to penicillins, caution should be exercised because cross-hypersensitivity among ß-lactam antibiotics has been clearly documented. If an allergic reaction to cefdinir occurs, the drug should be discontinued
- Safety and efficacy in neonates and infants less than 6 months of age have not been established
- 2% of 2,289 pediatric patients discontinued medication due to adverse events in US and non-US clinical trials. Discontinuations were primarily for gastrointestinal disturbance, usually diarrhea
- The most common reported adverse events occurring in ≥1% of pediatric patients in US clinical trials (N=1,783) were diarrhea (8%), rash (3%), and vomiting (1%)
- Maximum dose of OMNICEF for pediatric patients weighing ≥43 kg is 600 mg/day. For pediatric patients with a creatinine clearance of <30 mL/min/1.73 $m^2$ and not requiring hemodialysis, the dose of cefdinir should be 7 mg/kg (up to 300 mg) given once daily
- Antacids that contain magnesium or aluminum and iron supplements, including multivitamins that contain iron, should be taken at least 2 hours before or 2 hours after taking OMNICEF

***For pediatric patients weighing 20 lbs, use the 125 mg/5 mL product.[4]**
**†Of the 125 mg/5 mL formulation.**

**References: 1.** Brixner DI. Improving acute otitis media outcomes through proper antibiotic use and adherence. *Am J Manag Care.* 2005;11:S202-S210. **2.** Kardas P. Patient compliance with antibiotic treatment for respiratory tract infections. *J Antimicrob Chemother.* 2002;49:897-903. **3.** Ramgoolam A, Steele R. Formulations of antibiotics for children in primary care. *Pediatr Drugs.* 2002;4:323-333. **4.** OMNICEF (cefdinir) Capsules and for Oral Suspension Prescribing Information, Abbott Laboratories.

**Please see adjacent brief summary of full prescribing information.**

OMNICEF®
(cefdinir) for oral suspension
*125 mg/5 mL and 250 mg/5 mL*
"Works great." "Easy to take."

astellas
Under License of **Astellas Pharma Inc.** Japan

**Abbott**
A Promise for Life

**PROFESSIONAL BRIEF SUMMARY-CONSULT PACKAGE INSERT FOR FULL PRESCRIBING INFORMATION.**
03-5435-Rev. July, 2005
(Nos. 3769, 3771, 6151)

# Omnicef® (cefdinir) capsules
# Omnicef® (cefdinir) for oral suspension

## Rx only

### INDICATIONS AND USAGE

To reduce the development of drug-resistant bacteria and maintain the effectiveness of OMNICEF and other antibacterial drugs, OMNICEF should be used only to treat or prevent infections that are proven or strongly suspected to be caused by susceptible bacteria. When culture and susceptibility information are available, they should be considered in selecting or modifying antibacterial therapy. In the absence of such data, local epidemiology and susceptibility patterns may contribute to the empiric selection of therapy.

OMNICEF (cefdinir) capsules and OMNICEF (cefdinir) for oral suspension are indicated for the treatment of patients with mild to moderate infections caused by susceptible strains of the designated microorganisms in the conditions listed below.

**Adults and Adolescents**

**Community-Acquired Pneumonia** caused by *Haemophilus influenzae* (including β-lactamase producing strains), *Haemophilus parainfluenzae* (including β-lactamase producing strains), *Streptococcus pneumoniae* (penicillin-susceptible strains only), and *Moraxella catarrhalis* (including β-lactamase producing strains).

**Acute Exacerbations of Chronic Bronchitis** caused by *Haemophilus influenzae* (including β-lactamase producing strains), *Haemophilus parainfluenzae* (including β-lactamase producing strains), *Streptococcus pneumoniae* (penicillin-susceptible strains only), and *Moraxella catarrhalis* (including β-lactamase producing strains).

**Acute Maxillary Sinusitis** caused by *Haemophilus influenzae* (including β-lactamase producing strains), *Streptococcus pneumoniae* (penicillin-susceptible strains only), and *Moraxella catarrhalis* (including β-lactamase producing strains).

**NOTE:** For information on use in pediatric patients, see **Pediatric Use** and **DOSAGE AND ADMINISTRATION**.

**Pharyngitis/Tonsillitis** caused by *Streptococcus pyogenes*.

**NOTE:** Cefdinir is effective in the eradication of *S. pyogenes* from the oropharynx. Cefdinir has not, however, been studied for the prevention of rheumatic fever following *S. pyogenes* pharyngitis/tonsillitis. Only intramuscular penicillin has been demonstrated to be effective for the prevention of rheumatic fever.

**Uncomplicated Skin and Skin Structure Infections** caused by *Staphylococcus aureus* (including β-lactamase producing strains) and *Streptococcus pyogenes*.

**Pediatric Patients**

**Acute Bacterial Otitis Media** caused by *Haemophilus influenzae* (including β-lactamase producing strains), *Streptococcus pneumoniae* (penicillin-susceptible strains only), and *Moraxella catarrhalis* (including β-lactamase producing strains).

**Pharyngitis/Tonsillitis** caused by *Streptococcus pyogenes*.

**NOTE:** Cefdinir is effective in the eradication of *S. pyogenes* from the oropharynx. Cefdinir has not, however, been studied for the prevention of rheumatic fever following *S. pyogenes* pharyngitis/tonsillitis. Only intramuscular penicillin has been demonstrated to be effective for the prevention of rheumatic fever.

**Uncomplicated Skin and Skin Structure Infections** caused by *Staphylococcus aureus* (including β-lactamase producing strains) and *Streptococcus pyogenes*.

### CONTRAINDICATIONS

OMNICEF (cefdinir) is contraindicated in patients with known allergy to the cephalosporin class of antibiotics.

### WARNINGS

**BEFORE THERAPY WITH OMNICEF (CEFDINIR) IS INSTITUTED, CAREFUL INQUIRY SHOULD BE MADE TO DETERMINE WHETHER THE PATIENT HAS HAD PREVIOUS HYPERSENSITIVITY REACTIONS TO CEFDINIR, OTHER CEPHALOSPORINS, PENICILLINS, OR OTHER DRUGS. IF CEFDINIR IS TO BE GIVEN TO PENICILLIN-SENSITIVE PATIENTS, CAUTION SHOULD BE EXERCISED BECAUSE CROSS-HYPERSENSITIVITY AMONG β-LACTAM ANTIBIOTICS HAS BEEN CLEARLY DOCUMENTED AND MAY OCCUR IN UP TO 10% OF PATIENTS WITH A HISTORY OF PENICILLIN ALLERGY. IF AN ALLERGIC REACTION TO CEFDINIR OCCURS, THE DRUG SHOULD BE DISCONTINUED. SERIOUS ACUTE HYPERSENSITIVITY REACTIONS MAY REQUIRE TREATMENT WITH EPINEPHRINE AND OTHER EMERGENCY MEASURES, INCLUDING OXYGEN, INTRAVENOUS FLUIDS, INTRAVENOUS ANTIHISTAMINES, CORTICOSTEROIDS, PRESSOR AMINES, AND AIRWAY MANAGEMENT, AS CLINICALLY INDICATED.**

**Pseudomembranous colitis has been reported with nearly all antibacterial agents, including cefdinir, and may range in severity from mild- to life-threatening. Therefore, it is important to consider this diagnosis in patients who present with diarrhea subsequent to the administration of antibacterial agents.**

Treatment with antibacterial agents alters the normal flora of the colon and may permit overgrowth of clostridia. Studies indicate that a toxin produced by *Clostridium difficile* is a primary cause of "antibiotic-associated colitis."

After the diagnosis of pseudomembranous colitis has been established, appropriate therapeutic measures should be initiated. Mild cases of pseudomembranous colitis usually respond to drug discontinuation alone. In moderate to severe cases, consideration should be given to management with fluids and electrolytes, protein supplementation, and treatment with an antibacterial drug clinically effective against *Clostridium difficile*.

### PRECAUTIONS

**General**

Prescribing OMNICEF in the absence of a proven or strongly suspected bacterial infection or a prophylactic indication is unlikely to provide benefit to the patient and increases the risk of the development of drug-resistant bacteria.

As with other broad-spectrum antibiotics, prolonged treatment may result in the possible emergence and overgrowth of resistant organisms. Careful observation of the patient is essential. If superinfection occurs during therapy, appropriate alternative therapy should be administered.

Cefdinir, as with other broad-spectrum antimicrobials (antibiotics), should be prescribed with caution in individuals with a history of colitis.

In patients with transient or persistent renal insufficiency (creatinine clearance <30 mL/min), the total daily dose of OMNICEF should be reduced because high and prolonged plasma concentrations of cefdinir can result following recommended doses.

**Information for Patients**

Patients should be counseled that antibacterial drugs including OMNICEF should only be used to treat bacterial infections. They do not treat viral infections (e.g., the common cold). When OMNICEF is prescribed to treat a bacterial infection, patients should be told that although it is common to feel better early in the course of therapy, the medication should be taken exactly as directed. Skipping doses or not completing the full course of therapy may (1) decrease the effectiveness of the immediate treatment and (2) increase the likelihood that bacteria will develop resistance and will not be treatable by OMNICEF or other antibacterial drugs in the future.

Antacids containing magnesium or aluminum interfere with the absorption of cefdinir. If this type of antacid is required during OMNICEF therapy, OMNICEF should be taken at least 2 hours before or after the antacid.

Iron supplements, including multivitamins that contain iron, interfere with the absorption of cefdinir. If iron supplements are required during OMNICEF therapy, OMNICEF should be taken at least 2 hours before or after the supplement.

Iron-fortified infant formula does not significantly interfere with the absorption of cefdinir. Therefore, OMNICEF for Oral Suspension can be administered with iron-fortified infant formula.

Diabetic patients and caregivers should be aware that the oral suspension contains 2.86 g of sucrose per teaspoon.

**Drug Interactions**

**Antacids:** (aluminum- or magnesium-containing): Concomitant administration of 300-mg cefdinir capsules with 30 mL Maalox® TC suspension reduces the rate ($C_{max}$) and extent (AUC) of absorption by approximately 40%. Time to reach $C_{max}$ is also prolonged by 1 hour. There are no significant effects on cefdinir pharmacokinetics if the antacid is administered 2 hours before or 2 hours after cefdinir. If antacids are required during OMNICEF therapy, OMNICEF should be taken at least 2 hours before or after the antacid.

**Probenecid:** As with other β-lactam antibiotics, probenecid inhibits the renal excretion of cefdinir, resulting in an approximate doubling in AUC, a 54% increase in peak cefdinir plasma levels, and a 50% prolongation in the apparent elimination $t_{1/2}$.

**Iron Supplements and Foods Fortified With Iron:** Concomitant administration of cefdinir with a therapeutic iron supplement containing 60 mg of elemental iron (as $FeSO_4$) or vitamins supplemented with 10 mg of elemental iron reduced extent of absorption by 80% and 31%, respectively. If iron supplements are required during OMNICEF therapy, OMNICEF should be taken at least 2 hours before or after the supplement.

The effect of foods highly fortified with elemental iron (primarily iron-fortified breakfast cereals) on cefdinir absorption has not been studied.

Concomitantly administered iron-fortified infant formula (2.2 mg elemental iron/6 oz) has no significant effect on cefdinir pharmacokinetics. Therefore, OMNICEF for Oral Suspension can be administered with iron-fortified infant formula.

There have been reports of reddish stools in patients receiving cefdinir. In many cases, patients were also receiving iron-containing products. The reddish color is due to the formation of a nonabsorbable complex between cefdinir or its breakdown products and iron in the gastrointestinal tract.

**Drug/Laboratory Test Interactions**

A false-positive reaction for ketones in the urine may occur with tests using nitroprusside, but not with those using nitroferricyanide. The administration of cefdinir may result in a false-positive reaction for glucose in urine using Clinitest®, Benedict's solution, or Fehling's solution. It is recommended that glucose tests based on enzymatic glucose oxidase reactions (such as Clinistix® or Tes-Tape®) be used. Cephalosporins are known to occasionally induce a positive direct Coombs' test.

**Carcinogenesis, Mutagenesis, Impairment of Fertility**

The carcinogenic potential of cefdinir has not been evaluated. No mutagenic effects were seen in the bacterial reverse mutation assay (Ames) or point mutation assay at the hypoxanthine-guanine phosphoribosyltransferase locus (HGPRT) in V79 Chinese hamster lung cells. No clastogenic effects were observed *in vitro* in the structural chromosome aberration assay in V79 Chinese hamster lung cells or *in vivo* in the micronucleus assay in mouse bone marrow. In rats, fertility and reproductive performance were not affected by cefdinir at oral doses up to 1000 mg/kg/day (70 times the human dose based on mg/kg/day, 11 times based on mg/m²/day).

**Pregnancy - Teratogenic Effects**

**Pregnancy Category B:** Cefdinir was not teratogenic in rats at oral doses up to 1000 mg/kg/day (70 times the human dose based on mg/kg/day, 11 times based on $mg/m^2$/day) or in rabbits at oral doses up to 10 mg/kg/day (0.7 times the human dose based on mg/kg/day, 0.23 times based on $mg/m^2$/day). Maternal toxicity (decreased body weight gain) was observed in rabbits at the maximum tolerated dose of 10 mg/kg/day without adverse effects on offspring. Decreased body weight occurred in rat fetuses at ≥ 100 mg/kg/day, and in rat offspring at ≥ 32 mg/kg/day. No effects were observed on maternal reproductive parameters or offspring survival, development, behavior, or reproductive function.

There are, however, no adequate and well-controlled studies in pregnant women. Because animal reproduction studies are not always predictive of human response, this drug should be used during pregnancy only if clearly needed.

**Labor and Delivery**

Cefdinir has not been studied for use during labor and delivery.

**Nursing Mothers**

Following administration of single 600-mg doses, cefdinir was not detected in human breast milk.

**Pediatric Use**

Safety and efficacy in neonates and infants less than 6 months of age have not been established. Use of cefdinir for the treatment of acute maxillary sinusitis in pediatric patients (age 6 months through 12 years) is supported by evidence from adequate and well-controlled studies in adults and adolescents, the similar pathophysiology of acute sinusitis in adult and pediatric patients, and comparative pharmacokinetic data in the pediatric population.

**Geriatric Use**

Efficacy is comparable in geriatric patients and younger adults. While cefdinir has been well-tolerated in all age groups, in clinical trials geriatric patients experienced a lower rate of adverse events, including diarrhea, than younger adults. Dose adjustment in elderly patients is not necessary unless renal function is markedly compromised.

## ADVERSE EVENTS

**Clinical Trials - OMNICEF Capsules (Adult and Adolescent Patients):**

In clinical trials, 5093 adult and adolescent patients (3841 US and 1252 non-US) were treated with the recommended dose of cefdinir capsules (600 mg/day). Most adverse events were mild and self-limiting. No deaths or permanent disabilities were attributed to cefdinir. One hundred forty-seven of 5093 (3%) patients discontinued medication due to adverse events thought by the investigators to be possibly, probably, or definitely associated with cefdinir therapy. The discontinuations were primarily for gastrointestinal disturbances, usually diarrhea or nausea. Nineteen of 5093 (0.4%) patients were discontinued due to rash thought related to cefdinir administration.

In the US, the following adverse events were thought by investigators to be possibly, probably, or definitely related to cefdinir capsules in multiple-dose clinical trials (N = 3841 cefdinir-treated patients):

**ADVERSE EVENTS ASSOCIATED WITH CEFDINIR CAPSULES US TRIALS IN ADULT AND ADOLESCENT PATIENTS (N=3841)[a]**

| | | |
|---|---|---|
| Incidence ≥ 1% | Diarrhea | 15% |
| | Vaginal moniliasis | 4% of women |
| | Nausea | 3% |
| | Headache | 2% |
| | Abdominal pain | 1% |
| | Vaginitis | 1% of women |
| Incidence <1% but >0.1% | Rash | 0.9% |
| | Dyspepsia | 0.7% |
| | Flatulence | 0.7% |
| | Vomiting | 0.7% |
| | Abnormal stools | 0.3% |
| | Anorexia | 0.3% |
| | Constipation | 0.3% |
| | Dizziness | 0.3% |
| | Dry mouth | 0.3% |
| | Asthenia | 0.2% |
| | Insomnia | 0.2% |
| | Leukorrhea | 0.2% of women |
| | Moniliasis | 0.2% |
| | Pruritus | 0.2% |
| | Somnolence | 0.2% |

[a] 1733 males, 2108 females

The following laboratory value changes of possible clinical significance, irrespective of relationship to therapy with cefdinir, were seen during clinical trials conducted in the US:

**LABORATORY VALUE CHANGES OBSERVED WITH CEFDINIR CAPSULES US TRIALS IN ADULT AND ADOLESCENT PATIENTS (N=3841)**

| | | |
|---|---|---|
| Incidence ≥ 1% | ↑ Urine leukocytes | 2% |
| | ↑ Urine protein | 2% |
| | ↑ Gamma-glutamyltransferase[a] | 1% |
| | ↓ Lymphocytes, ↑ Lymphocytes | 1%, 0.2% |
| | ↑ Microhematuria | 1% |
| Incidence <1% but >0.1% | ↑ Glucose[a] | 0.9% |
| | ↑ Urine glucose | 0.9% |
| | ↑ White blood cells, ↓ White blood cells | 0.9%, 0.7% |
| | ↑ Alanine aminotransferase (ALT) | 0.7% |
| | ↑ Eosinophils | 0.7% |
| | ↑ Urine specific gravity, ↓ Urine specific gravity[a] | 0.6%, 0.2% |
| | ↓ Bicarbonate[a] | 0.6% |
| | ↑ Phosphorus, ↓ Phosphorus[a] | 0.6%, 0.3% |
| | ↑ Aspartate aminotransferase (AST) | 0.4% |
| | ↑ Alkaline phosphatase | 0.3% |
| | ↑ Blood urea nitrogen (BUN) | 0.3% |
| | ↓ Hemoglobin | 0.3% |
| | ↑ Polymorphonuclear neutrophils (PMNs), ↓ PMNs | 0.3%, 0.2% |
| | ↑ Bilirubin | 0.2% |
| | ↑ Lactate dehydrogenase[a] | 0.2% |
| | ↑ Platelets | 0.2% |
| | ↑ Potassium[a] | 0.2% |
| | ↑ Urine pH[a] | 0.2% |

[a] N<3841 for these parameters

**Clinical Trials - OMNICEF for Oral Suspension (Pediatric Patients):**

In clinical trials, 2289 pediatric patients (1783 US and 506 non-US) were treated with the recommended dose of cefdinir suspension (14 mg/kg/day). Most adverse events were mild and self-limiting. No deaths or permanent disabilities were attributed to cefdinir. Forty of 2289 (2%) patients discontinued medication due to adverse events considered by the investigators to be possibly, probably, or definitely associated with cefdinir therapy. Discontinuations were primarily for gastrointestinal disturbances, usually diarrhea. Five of 2289 (0.2%) patients were discontinued due to rash thought related to cefdinir administration.

In the US, the following adverse events were thought by investigators to be possibly, probably, or definitely related to cefdinir suspension in multiple-dose clinical trials (N=1783 cefdinir-treated patients):

**ADVERSE EVENTS ASSOCIATED WITH CEFDINIR SUSPENSION US TRIALS IN PEDIATRIC PATIENTS (N=1783)[a]**

| | | |
|---|---|---|
| Incidence ≥ 1% | Diarrhea | 8% |
| | Rash | 3% |
| | Vomiting | 1% |
| Incidence <1% but >0.1% | Cutaneous moniliasis | 0.9% |
| | Abdominal pain | 0.8% |
| | Leukopenia[b] | 0.3% |
| | Vaginal moniliasis | 0.3% of girls |
| | Vaginitis | 0.3% of girls |
| | Abnormal stools | 0.2% |
| | Dyspepsia | 0.2% |
| | Hyperkinesia | 0.2% |
| | Increased AST[b] | 0.2% |
| | Maculopapular rash | 0.2% |
| | Nausea | 0.2% |

[a] 977 males, 806 females

[b] Laboratory changes were occasionally reported as adverse events.

NOTE: In both cefdinir- and control-treated patients, rates of diarrhea and rash were higher in the youngest pediatric patients. The incidence of diarrhea in cefdinir-treated patients ≤2 years of age was 17% (95/557) compared with 4% (51/1226) in those >2 years old. The incidence of rash (primarily diaper rash in the younger patients) was 8% (43/557) in patients ≤2 years of age compared with 1% (8/1226) in those >2 years old.

The following laboratory value changes of possible clinical significance, irrespective of relationship to therapy with cefdinir, were seen during clinical trials conducted in the US:

**LABORATORY VALUE CHANGES OF POSSIBLE CLINICAL SIGNIFICANCE OBSERVED WITH CEFDINIR SUSPENSION US TRIALS IN PEDIATRIC PATIENTS (N=1783)**

| | | |
|---|---|---|
| Incidence ≥ 1% | ↑ Lymphocytes, ↓ Lymphocytes | 2%, 0.8% |
| | ↑ Alkaline phosphatase | 1% |
| | ↓ Bicarbonate[a] | 1% |
| | ↑ Eosinophils | 1% |
| | ↑ Lactate dehydrogenase | 1% |
| | ↑ Platelets | 1% |
| | ↑ PMNs, ↓ PMNs | 1%, 1% |
| | ↑ Urine protein | 1% |
| Incidence <1% but >0.1% | ↑ Phosphorus, ↓ Phosphorus | 0.9%, 0.4% |
| | ↑ Urine pH | 0.8% |
| | ↓ White blood cells, ↑ White blood cells | 0.7%, 0.3% |
| | ↓ Calcium[a] | 0.5% |
| | ↓ Hemoglobin | 0.5% |
| | ↑ Urine leukocytes | 0.5% |
| | ↑ Monocytes | 0.4% |
| | ↑ AST | 0.3% |
| | ↑ Potassium[a] | 0.3% |
| | ↑ Urine specific gravity, ↓ Urine specific gravity | 0.3%, 0.1% |
| | ↓ Hematocrit[a] | 0.2% |

[a] N=1387 for these parameters

**Postmarketing Experience**

The following adverse experiences and altered laboratory tests, regardless of their relationship to cefdinir, have been reported during extensive postmarketing experience, beginning with approval in Japan in 1991: Stevens-Johnson syndrome, toxic epidermal necrolysis, exfoliative dermatitis, erythema multiforme, erythema nodosum, serum sickness-like reactions, conjunctivitis, stomatitis, acute hepatitis, cholestasis, fulminant hepatitis, hepatic failure, jaundice, increased amylase, shock, anaphylaxis, facial and laryngeal edema, feeling of suffocation, acute enterocolitis, bloody diarrhea, hemorrhagic colitis, melena, pseudomembranous colitis, pancytopenia, granulocytopenia, leukopenia, thrombocytopenia, idiopathic thrombocytopenic purpura, hemolytic anemia, acute respiratory failure, asthmatic attack, drug-induced pneumonia, eosinophilic pneumonia, idiopathic interstitial pneumonia, fever, acute renal failure, nephropathy, bleeding tendency, coagulation disorder, disseminated intravascular coagulation, upper GI bleed, peptic ulcer, ileus, loss of consciousness, allergic vasculitis, possible cefdinir-diclofenac interaction, cardiac failure, chest pain, myocardial infarction, hypertension, involuntary movements, and rhabdomyolysis.

**Cephalosporin Class Adverse Events**

The following adverse events and altered laboratory tests have been reported for cephalosporin-class antibiotics in general:

Allergic reactions, anaphylaxis, Stevens-Johnson syndrome, erythema multiforme, toxic epidermal necrolysis, renal dysfunction, toxic nephropathy, hepatic dysfunction including cholestasis, aplastic anemia, hemolytic anemia, hemorrhage, false-positive test for urinary glucose, neutropenia, pancytopenia, and agranulocytosis. Pseudomembranous colitis symptoms may begin during or after antibiotic treatment (see **WARNINGS**).

Several cephalosporins have been implicated in triggering seizures, particularly in patients with renal impairment when the dosage was not reduced (see **OVERDOSAGE**). If seizures associated with drug therapy occur, the drug should be discontinued. Anticonvulsant therapy can be given if clinically indicated.

## OVERDOSAGE

Information on cefdinir overdosage in humans is not available. In acute rodent toxicity studies, a single oral 5600-mg/kg dose produced no adverse effects. Toxic signs and symptoms following overdosage with other β-lactam antibiotics have included nausea, vomiting, epigastric distress, diarrhea, and convulsions. Hemodialysis removes cefdinir from the body. This may be useful in the event of a serious toxic reaction from overdosage, particularly if renal function is compromised.

**Rx only**

Ref: 03-5435-Rev. July, 2005
(Nos. 3769, 3771, 6151)



05J-034-L150-2 **MASTER**

Manufactured by:
**CEPH** International Corporation
Carolina, Puerto Rico 00986

Under License of:
astellas Astellas Pharma Inc.
Tokyo, Japan

For:
**Abbott Laboratories**
North Chicago, IL 60064, U.S.A.

06F-034-Q068-1
Printed in U.S.A.

## The Extent to Which Tobacco Marketing and Tobacco Use in Films Contribute to Children's Use of Tobacco: A Meta-analysis

More than 80% of adults who smoke begin to do so before age 18 years. The authors examined the relationship between exposure to tobacco in marketing materials and media and changes in adolescents' attitudes and use of tobacco. The 51 studies examined in this meta-analysis demonstrated that exposure to pro-tobacco marketing and media significantly increased the chance that youth would hold positive attitudes toward tobacco and that they would initiate tobacco use. These effects were observed over time, in different countries, and with different study designs. The results indicate that restriction exposure of adolescents to tobacco marketing materials and use of tobacco in the media may have an effect on smoking rates in both adolescents and adults.

See page 1285

## Impact of Maternal Influenza Vaccination During Pregnancy on the Incidence of Acute Respiratory Illness Visits Among Infants

Infants in their first 6 months of life have high susceptibility to respiratory infections, but have poor immunogenic response to some respiratory vaccines, such as influenza. One strategy is to immunize the mother during pregnancy to both boost passive protection of the infant as well as decrease the risk of infection in the mother. In this cohort study of 41 129 infants studied during a 6-year period, maternal influenza vaccination did not reduce the risk of an emergency department, physician, or inpatient respiratory illness visit for their infants, nor did it delay the onset of the first respiratory illness.

See page 1277

## Risky Alcohol Use, Age at Onset of Drinking, and Adverse Childhood Experiences in Young Men Entering the US Marine Corps

Nearly 90% of new users of alcohol are younger than age 21 years at initiation of alcohol use. Young and colleagues screened 41 482 males aged 18 to 20 years and identified 15% as risky drinkers. Risk of problem drinking increased as age of first alcohol use decreased, with those who started drinking by age 13 years at 5.5-fold increased odds of having risky drinking at age 18 to 20 years compared with those who began drinking after age 17 years. Individuals who were abused as a child or who grew up with a problem drinker in the home were also at increased risk of problem drinking. This study indicates a group at high risk of later alcohol problems, who potentially should be targeted with intervention even at earlier ages.

See page 1207

## Dextromethorphan Abuse in Adolescence, An Increasing Trend: 1999-2004

High doses of dextromethorphan may produce dissociative hallucinations, and its potential for abuse has been recognized for decades. This study examined the trends in dextromethorphan abuse in California and compares those trends with national data (**Figure**). There was a 10-fold increase in cases of dextromethorphan abuse between 1999 and 2004. Three fourths of these cases were among adolescents, with the highest frequency of abuse among 15- and 16-year-olds. The source of dextromethorphan was usually inexpensive, over-the-counter cough and cold medications. Measures to prevent abuse of this drug, such as requiring dispensing by a pharmacist, may be needed.

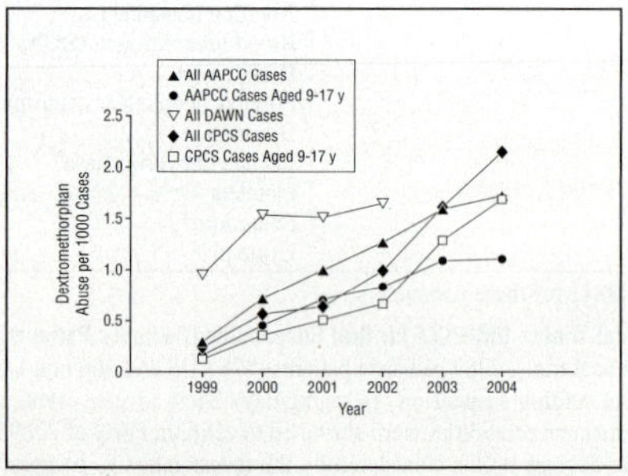


**Figure.** The proportion of California Poison Control System (CPCS), American Association of Poison Control Centers (AAPCC), and Drug Abuse Warning Network (DAWN) dextromethorphan abuse cases compared with the total exposures reported to each database. Dextromethorphan DAWN data are unavailable for 2003 and 2004.

See page 1217

# Piero della Francesca (circa 1415-1492)

## Madonna and Child With Saints, *circa 1474*

Once upon a time in the town of Urbino, Italy, there lived a man named Federico da Montefeltro, the Duke of Urbino. By profession, he was a *condottiere*—a soldier for hire who led recruits from his hometown into battle on behalf of well-to-do clients, including the city of Florence and the pope, who in those days had his own army. Federico was a clever strategist and an effective leader, and he usually won his battles. Over the years, he and his men were much in demand and well compensated for their efforts, and little Urbino became a prosperous center of culture and the arts.

"It is a truth universally acknowledged that a single man in possession of a good fortune must be in want of a wife."[1] Federico's true love was Battista Sforza, his beautiful young bride from a prominent family in Milan. Theirs proved to be a happy marriage, with Battista managing the affairs of state capably when Federico was away at war. She knew full well that her responsibility was to produce a male heir, and she got right to work. Their first child was a daughter. So was their second. And their third, fourth, fifth, sixth, seventh, and eighth. After 8 daughters in a row, the increasingly desperate Federico and Battista prayed to Saint Guido Ubaldo, patron saint of the nearby town of Gubbio, for divine intercession. Battista was said to have offered up her own life in return for the birth of a son. Early the next year, she did bear a son whom the happy parents named Guidobaldo. Six months later, Battista was dead at age 26 years, leaving behind 9 children and their grieving father.[2]

Soon afterward, Federico commissioned *Madonna and Child With Saints* from Piero della Francesca for the altar of a small church in his beloved Urbino. In the painting, Federico himself kneels before the Virgin Mary and the infant Jesus, who are flanked by 6 saints and 4 angels in a scene of timeless stillness. The ostrich egg suspended over Mary's head symbolizes new life. By one interpretation, the painting is a traditional portrayal of a donor affirming his devotion to Mary and Jesus. However, Federico also had deep personal reasons for celebrating the birth of a baby boy, and the sleeping infant before whom he kneels with hands raised in thanks can also be viewed as representing his own long-awaited son Guidobaldo. Yet another interpretation is suggested by noting that the painting's otherwise near-perfect symmetry is disturbed by an empty space in the left foreground opposite Federico. Had Battista survived, she would almost certainly have been shown there in front of her own name saint, John the Baptist. Like an empty chair at the banquet table, the open space in Piero della Francesca's painting honors someone not seen—the departed wife and mother, Battista.

Guidobaldo led a pampered boyhood, being tutored by a doting father. When Federico's luck finally ran out and he died in battle, the 10-year-old Guidobaldo succeeded him as Duke of Urbino. He grew up to continue the family's prowess in military affairs and patronage of the arts. During Guidobaldo's lifetime, the great Renaissance painter Raphael was born and raised in Urbino, receiving his first serious exposure to fine art in the ducal palace collection. Like his father before him, Guidobaldo married well; however, the union produced no children. When Guidobaldo died of gout at age 36 years, the Montefeltro line and the golden era of Urbino came to an end.

*Thomas D. Koepsell, MD, MPH*

**Correspondence**: Dr Koepsell, Department of Epidemiology, University of Washington, F-261F Health Sciences, Box 357236, Seattle, WA 98195-7236 (koepsell@u.washington.edu).

**Financial Disclosure:** None reported.

## REFERENCES

1. Austen J. *Pride and Prejudice.* London, England: Penguin Books; 1813.
2. Meiss M. *The Painter's Choice: Problems in the Interpretation of Renaissance Art.* New York, NY: Harper & Row; 1976.

# Pertussis immunity wanes in early adolescence[1]

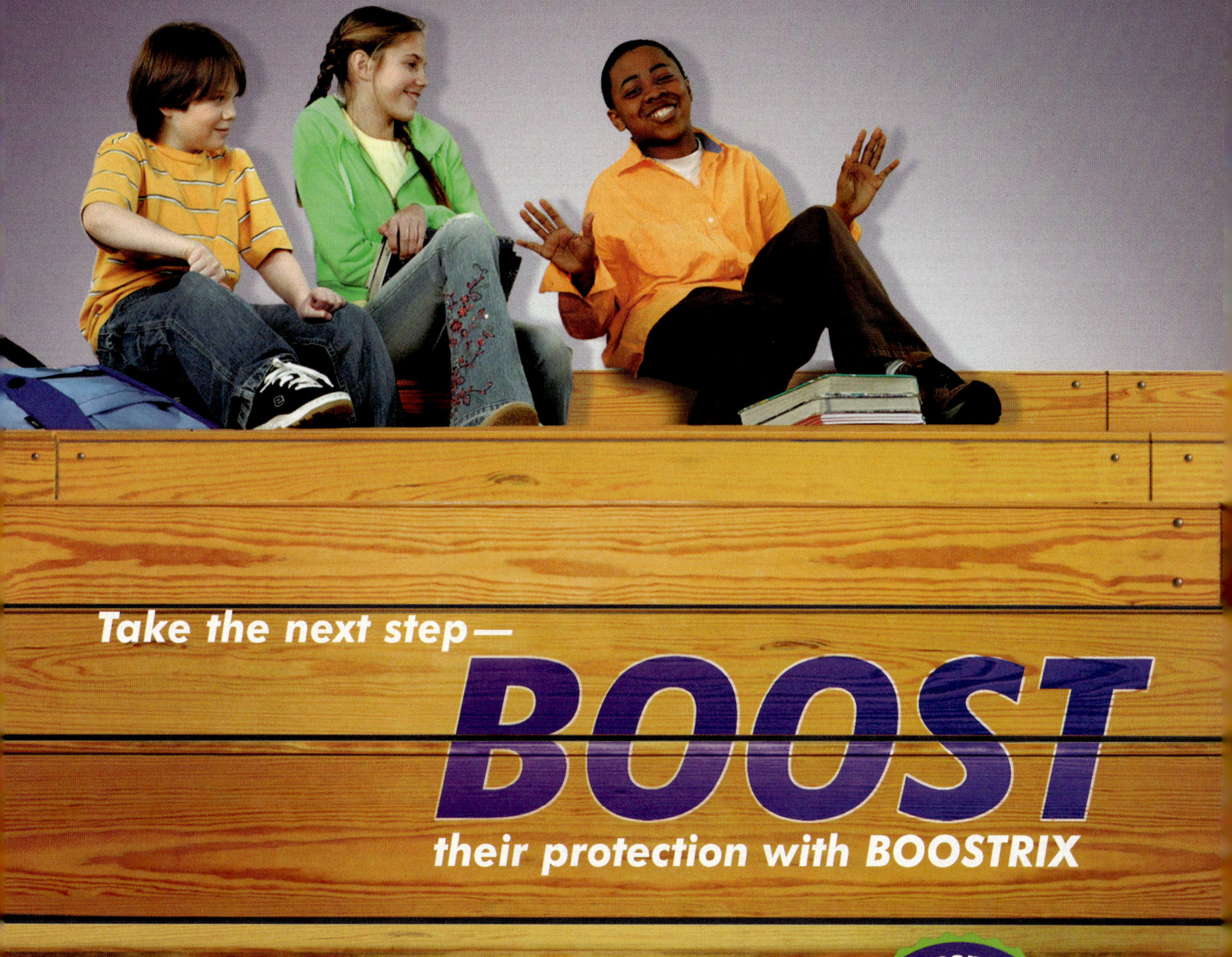

**Take the next step—**

# BOOST

**their protection with BOOSTRIX**

ACIP* recommends · BOOST adolescents · pertussis booster[2]

## Important Safety Information

In clinical studies, adverse events included pain, redness, and swelling at the injection site, headache, fatigue, and gastrointestinal symptoms. As with other vaccines, rare adverse events may occur. As with any vaccine, vaccination with BOOSTRIX may not protect 100% of susceptible individuals. Hypersensitivity to any component of BOOSTRIX is a contraindication.

*Advisory Committee on Immunization Practices.

**BOOSTRIX®**

***Tetanus Toxoid, Reduced Diphtheria Toxoid and Acellular Pertussis Vaccine, Adsorbed***

gsk GlaxoSmithKline Vaccines

**Please see references and brief summary of complete prescribing information on the adjacent page.**



Manufactured by **GlaxoSmithKline Biologicals,** Rixensart, Belgium

Distributed by **GlaxoSmithKline,** Research Triangle Park, NC 27709

# BOOSTRIX®

## (Tetanus Toxoid, Reduced Diphtheria Toxoid and Acellular Pertussis Vaccine, Adsorbed) (Tdap)

The following is a brief summary only; see full prescribing information for complete product information.

**INDICATIONS AND USAGE:** BOOSTRIX is indicated for active booster immunization against tetanus, diphtheria, and pertussis as a single dose in individuals 10 through 18 years of age. The use of BOOSTRIX as a primary series or to complete the primary series has not been studied. As with any vaccine, BOOSTRIX may not protect 100% of individuals receiving the vaccine.

**CONTRAINDICATIONS:** Hypersensitivity to any component of the vaccine is a contraindication (see DESCRIPTION in full prescribing information). Do not use BOOSTRIX after a serious allergic reaction (e.g., anaphylaxis) following any other tetanus toxoid, diphtheria toxoid or pertussis-containing vaccine, or any component of this vaccine (see DESCRIPTION in full prescribing information). Because of the uncertainty as to which component of the vaccine might be responsible, do not give further vaccination with any of these components; or, refer such individuals to an allergist for evaluation. The following events are contraindications to administration of BOOSTRIX: encephalopathy (e.g., coma, decreased level of consciousness, prolonged seizures) within 7 days of administration of a previous dose of a pertussis-containing vaccine that is not attributable to another identifiable cause; progressive neurologic disorder, uncontrolled epilepsy, or progressive encephalopathy. Do not vaccinate individuals with these conditions until a treatment regimen has been established and the condition has stabilized.

**WARNINGS:** The tip cap and the rubber plunger of the needleless prefilled syringes contain dry natural latex rubber that may cause allergic reactions in latex sensitive individuals. The vial stopper is latex-free. If any of the following events occurred in temporal relation to previous receipt of a Diphtheria and Tetanus Toxoids and Pertussis Vaccine Adsorbed (DTwP) vaccine or a vaccine containing an acellular pertussis component, consider carefully whether to give subsequent doses of BOOSTRIX: temperature of ≥40.5°C (105°F) within 48 hours not due to another identifiable cause; collapse or shock-like state (hypotonic-hyporesponsive episode) within 48 hours; persistent, inconsolable crying lasting ≥3 hours, occurring within 48 hours; seizures with or without fever occurring within 3 days. Persons who experienced serious Arthus-type hypersensitivity reactions following a prior dose of tetanus toxoid usually have high serum tetanus antitoxin levels and should not be given Tetanus and Diphtheria Toxoids Adsorbed For Adult Use (Td) or Tdap vaccines or even emergency doses of Td more frequently than every 10 years, even if the wound is neither clean nor minor. If Guillain-Barré syndrome has occurred within 6 weeks of receipt of prior vaccine containing tetanus toxoid, the decision to give BOOSTRIX or any vaccine containing tetanus toxoid should be based on careful consideration of the potential benefits and possible risks. The decision to administer a pertussis-containing vaccine to individuals with stable central nervous system (CNS) disorders must be made by the physician on an individual basis, with consideration of all relevant factors, and assessment of potential risks and benefits for that individual. Advise the patient, parent, or guardian of the potential increased risk involved (see PRECAUTIONS). A family history of seizures or other CNS disorders is not a contraindication to pertussis vaccine. The Advisory Committee on Immunization Practices (ACIP) has published guidelines for vaccination of persons with recent or acute illness (www.cdc.gov). Do not give BOOSTRIX to individuals with bleeding disorders such as hemophilia or thrombocytopenia, or to persons on anticoagulant therapy unless the potential benefit clearly outweighs the risk of administration. If the decision is made to administer BOOSTRIX to such persons, it should be given with caution with steps taken to avoid the risk of hematoma following the injection.

**PRECAUTIONS: General:** Before the injection of any biological, the physician should take all reasonable precautions to prevent allergic or other adverse reactions. Epinephrine injection (1:1,000) and other appropriate agents used for the control of immediate allergic reactions must be immediately available should an acute anaphylactic reaction occur. Immunosuppressed persons, including individuals receiving immunosuppressive therapy, may not develop the expected immune response. **Drug Interactions:** Do not mix BOOSTRIX with any other vaccine in the same syringe or vial. **Carcinogenesis, Mutagenesis, Impairment of Fertility:** BOOSTRIX has not been evaluated for carcinogenic or mutagenic potential, or for impairment of fertility. **Pregnancy:** Pregnancy Category C. Animal reproduction studies have not been conducted with BOOSTRIX. It is also not known whether BOOSTRIX can cause fetal harm when administered to a pregnant woman or can affect reproductive capacity. BOOSTRIX should be given to a pregnant woman only if clearly needed. Animal fertility studies have not been conducted with BOOSTRIX. In a developmental toxicity study, the effect of BOOSTRIX on embryo-fetal and pre-weaning development was evaluated in pregnant rats. Animals were administered INFANRIX® (Diphtheria and Tetanus Toxoids and Acellular Pertussis Vaccine Adsorbed) prior to gestation and BOOSTRIX during the period of organogenesis (gestation days 6, 8, 11) and later in pregnancy (gestation day 15), 0.1 mL/rat/occasion (a 45-fold increase compared to the human dose of BOOSTRIX on a body weight basis), by intramuscular injection. No adverse affect on pregnancy and lactation parameters, embryo-fetal or pre-weaning development was observed. There were no fetal malformations or other evidence of teratogenesis noted in this study. **Nursing Mothers:** It is not known whether BOOSTRIX is excreted in human milk. Because many drugs are excreted in human milk, caution should be exercised when BOOSTRIX is administered to a nursing woman. **Pregnancy Exposure Registry:** Healthcare providers are encouraged to register pregnant women who receive BOOSTRIX in the GlaxoSmithKline vaccination pregnancy registry by calling 1-888-825-5249. **Geriatric Use:** BOOSTRIX is not indicated for use in individuals older than 18 years. **Pediatric Use:** BOOSTRIX is not indicated for use in individuals younger than 10 years (see DOSAGE AND ADMINISTRATION in full prescribing information). For immunization of infants and children younger than 7 years against diphtheria, tetanus, and pertussis, refer to the manufacturers' package inserts for Diphtheria and Tetanus Toxoids and Acellular Pertussis Vaccine Adsorbed (DTaP) vaccines.

**ADVERSE REACTIONS:** A total of 3,608 adolescents were vaccinated with a single dose of BOOSTRIX during clinical trials. An additional 1,092 adolescents 10 to 18 years of age received a non-US formulation of BOOSTRIX (formulated to contain 0.5 mg aluminum per dose) in non-US clinical studies.

The primary safety study, conducted in the United States, was a randomized, observer-blinded, controlled study in which 3,080 adolescents 10 to 18 years of age received a single dose of BOOSTRIX and 1,034 received the control Td vaccine manufactured by Massachusetts Public Health Biologic Laboratories. There were no substantive differences in demographic characteristics between the vaccine groups. Among BOOSTRIX and control vaccine recipients approximately 75% were 10 to 14 years of age and approximately 25% were 15 to 18 years of age. Approximately 98% of participants in this study had received the recommended series of 4 or 5 doses of either DTwP or a combination of DTwP and DTaP in childhood. Data on adverse events were collected by the subjects, parents and/or guardians using standardized diaries for 15 consecutive days following the vaccine dose (i.e., day of vaccination and the next 14 days). Subjects were monitored for unsolicited adverse events that occurred within 31 days of vaccination (day 0-30) using diary cards (day 0-14) supplemented by spontaneous reports and a medical history as reported by subjects, parents, and/or guardians. Subjects were also monitored for 6 months post-vaccination for non-routine medical visits, visits to an emergency room, onset of new chronic illness, and serious adverse events. Information regarding late onset adverse events was obtained via a telephone call 6 months following vaccination. At least 97% of subjects completed the 6-month follow-up evaluation.

In a study conducted in Germany, BOOSTRIX was administered to 319 children 10 to 12 years of age previously vaccinated with 5 doses of acellular pertussis-containing vaccines, 193 of these subjects had previously received 5 doses of INFANRIX. Adverse events were recorded on diary cards during the 15 days following vaccination. Unsolicited adverse events that occurred within 31 days of vaccination (day 0-30) were recorded on the diary card or verbally reported to the investigator. Subjects were monitored for 6 months post-vaccination for physician office visits, emergency room visits, onset of new chronic illness, and serious adverse events. The 6-month follow-up evaluation, conducted via telephone interview, was completed by 90% of subjects.

The adverse event information from clinical trials provides a basis for identifying adverse events that appear to be related to vaccine use and for approximating rates. However, because clinical trials are conducted under widely varying conditions, adverse event rates observed in the clinical trials of a vaccine cannot be directly compared to rates in the clinical trials of another vaccine, and may not reflect the rates observed in practice.

**Serious Adverse Events in All Safety Studies:** In the US-safety study and German-safety study, no serious adverse events were reported to occur within 31 days of vaccination. During the 6-month extended safety evaluation period, no serious adverse events that were of potential autoimmune origin or new onset and chronic in nature were reported to occur. In non-US studies in which serious adverse events were monitored for up to 37 days, one subject was diagnosed with insulin dependent diabetes 20 days following administration of BOOSTRIX. No other serious adverse events of potential autoimmune origin or that were new onset and chronic in nature were reported to occur in these studies.

**Solicited Adverse Events in the US-Safety Study:** In a US study, the most common local adverse events following administration of BOOSTRIX were pain, redness, and swelling at the injection site. The most common general adverse events were headache and fatigue. Most of these events were reported at a similar frequency in recipients of both BOOSTRIX and Td. Any pain, grade 2 or 3 pain (but not grade 3 alone), and grade 2 or 3 headache (but not grade 3 alone) were reported at a higher rate in recipients of BOOSTRIX. The primary safety endpoint of the US study was the incidence of grade 3 pain (spontaneously painful and/or prevented normal activity) at the injection site within 15 days of vaccination. Grade 3 pain was reported in 4.6% of those who received BOOSTRIX compared with 4.0% of those who received the Td vaccine. The difference in rate of grade 3 pain was within the pre-defined clinical limit for non-inferiority (upper limit of the 95% CI for the difference ≤4%). These were the rates for solicited local and general adverse events within 15 days of vaccination with BOOSTRIX or Td vaccine for the total vaccinated cohort (all enrolled, vaccinated subjects with safety data available analyzed by vaccine received):

**Percentage of Individuals 10 to 18 Years of Age Reporting Solicited Local Adverse Events or Solicited General Adverse Events Within the 15-day* Post-Vaccination Period**

| | BOOSTRIX (N = 3,032) % | Td (N =1,013) % |
|---|---|---|
| **Local** | | |
| Pain,† any | 75.3 | 71.7 |
| Pain,† grade 2 or 3 | 51.2 | 42.5 |
| Pain,‡ grade 3 | 4.6 | 4.0 |
| Redness, any | 22.5 | 19.8 |
| Redness, >20 mm | 4.1 | 3.9 |
| Redness, ≥50 mm | 1.7 | 1.6 |
| Swelling, any | 21.1 | 20.1 |
| Swelling, >20 mm | 5.3 | 4.9 |
| Swelling, ≥50 mm | 2.5 | 3.2 |
| Arm circumference increase,§ >5 mm | 28.3 | 29.5 |
| Arm circumference increase,§ >20 mm | 2.0 | 2.2 |
| Arm circumference increase,§ >40 mm | 0.5 | 0.3 |
| **General** | | |
| Fever,‖ ≥99.5°F | 13.5 | 13.1 |
| Fever,‖ >100.4°F | 5.0 | 4.7 |
| Fever,‖ >102.2°F | 1.4 | 1.0 |
| Headache, any | 43.1 | 41.5 |
| Headache,† grade 2 or 3 | 15.7 | 12.7 |
| Headache, grade 3 | 3.7 | 2.7 |
| Fatigue, any | 37.0 | 36.7 |
| Fatigue, grade 2 or 3 | 14.4 | 12.9 |
| Fatigue, grade 3 | 3.7 | 3.2 |
| Gastrointestinal symptoms,¶ any | 26.0 | 25.8 |
| Gastrointestinal symptoms,¶ grade 2 or 3 | 9.8 | 9.7 |
| Gastrointestinal symptoms,¶ grade 3 | 3.0 | 3.2 |

Td = Tetanus and Diphtheria Toxoids Adsorbed For Adult Use manufactured by Massachusetts Public Health Biologic Laboratories.
N = number of subjects in the total vaccinated cohort with local/general symptoms sheets completed.
Grade 2 = Local: painful when the limb was moved; General: interfered with normal activity.
Grade 3 = Local: spontaneously painful and/or prevented normal activity; General: prevented normal activity.
*Day of vaccination and the next 14 days.
†Statistically significantly higher (P<0.05) following BOOSTRIX as compared to Td vaccine.
‡Grade 3 injection site pain following BOOSTRIX was not inferior to Td (upper limit of two-sided 95% CI for the difference in the percentage of subjects ≤4%).
§Mid-upper region of the vaccinated arm.
‖Oral temperatures or axillary temperatures.
¶Gastrointestinal symptoms included nausea, vomiting, diarrhea and/or abdominal pain.

Mid-upper arm circumference was measured by the adolescent or their parent/guardian prior to injection and daily for 15 days following vaccination. There was no significant difference between BOOSTRIX recipients and Td recipients in the proportion of subjects reporting an increase in mid-upper arm circumference in the vaccinated arm. The incidence of unsolicited adverse events reported in the 31 days after vaccination was comparable between the 2 groups.

**Solicited Adverse Events in the German Safety Study:** No cases of whole arm swelling were spontaneously reported. Two individuals (2/193) reported large injection site swelling (range 110 to 200 mm diameter), in one case associated with grade 3 pain. Neither individual sought medical attention. These episodes were reported to resolve without sequelae within 5 days. These were the rates of solicited local adverse events and fever within 15 days of vaccination for those subjects who had previously been vaccinated with 5 doses of INFANRIX:

**Rates of Solicited Adverse Events Reported Within the 15-day* Post-Vaccination Period Following Administration of BOOSTRIX in Individuals 10 to 12 Years of Age Who Had Previously Received 5 Doses of INFANRIX**

| Adverse Event | BOOSTRIX (N = 193) % (95% CI) |
|---|---|
| Pain, any | 62.2 (54.9-69.0) |
| Pain, grade 2 or 3 | 33.2 (26.6-40.3) |
| Pain, grade 3 | 5.7 (2.9-10.0) |
| Redness, any | 47.7 (40.4-55.0) |
| Redness, >20 mm | 15.0 (10.3-20.9) |
| Redness, ≥50 mm | 10.9 (6.9-16.2) |
| Swelling, any | 38.9 (31.9-46.1) |
| Swelling, >20 mm | 17.6 (12.5-23.7) |
| Swelling, ≥50 mm | 14.0 (9.4-19.7) |
| Fever, ≥99.5 | 8.8 (5.2-13.7) |
| Fever, >100.4 | 4.1 (1.8-8.0) |
| Fever, >102.2 | 1.0 (0.1-3.7) |

N = number of subjects with local/general symptoms sheets completed.
Grade 2 = Painful when the limb was moved.
Grade 3 = Spontaneously painful and/or prevented normal activity.
*Day of vaccination and the next 14 days.

As with any vaccine, there is the possibility that broad use of BOOSTRIX could reveal adverse events not observed in clinical trials.

**Postmarketing Reports:** Worldwide voluntary reports of adverse events received for BOOSTRIX in persons 10 to 18 years of age since market introduction of this vaccine are listed below. This list includes serious events or events which have causal connection to components of this or other vaccines or drugs. Because these events are reported voluntarily from a population of uncertain size, it is not possible to reliably estimate their frequency or establish a causal relationship to vaccine exposure. *Blood and lymphatic system disorders:* Lymphadenitis, lymphadenopathy. *Cardiac disorders:* Myocarditis. *Injection site reactions:* Induration, inflammation, mass, nodule, warmth, local reaction. *Metabolism and nutrition disorders:* Diabetes mellitus insulin-dependent. *Musculoskeletal and connective tissue disorders:* Arthralgia, back pain, myalgia. *Nervous system disorders:* Convulsion, encephalitis, facial palsy, paraesthesia. *Skin and subcutaneous tissue disorders:* Exanthem, Henoch-Schönlein purpura, rash. In addition, extensive swelling of the injected limb has been reported following administration of BOOSTRIX.

**Reporting Adverse Events:** Report the occurrence following immunization of any event set forth in the Vaccine Injury Table from the National Childhood Vaccine Injury Act including: Anaphylaxis or anaphylactic shock within 7 days, encephalopathy or encephalitis within 7 days, brachial neuritis within 28 days, or an acute complication or sequelae (including death) of an illness, disability, injury, or condition referred to above, or any events that would contraindicate further doses of vaccine, according to this prescribing information. These events should be reported to VAERS. The VAERS toll-free number is 1-800-822-7967. Reporting forms may also be obtained at the VAERS website at www.vaers.hhs.gov.

**DOSAGE AND ADMINISTRATION: Recommended Dose:** BOOSTRIX should be administered as a single 0.5 mL injection by the intramuscular route into the deltoid muscle of the upper arm in individuals 10 through 18 years of age. Do not administer this product subcutaneously or intravenously. There are no data to support repeat administration of BOOSTRIX. Five years should elapse between the subject's last dose of the recommended series of childhood DTwP and/or DTaP vaccine and the administration of BOOSTRIX. Limited data are available on the use of BOOSTRIX following Tetanus and Diphtheria Toxoids Adsorbed For Adult Use (Td) vaccine. **Additional Dosing Information:** ***Wound Management:*** Clinicians should refer to guidelines for tetanus prophylaxis in routine wound management. Adolescents 10 to 18 years of age who have completed a primary series against tetanus and who sustain wounds which are minor and uncomplicated, should receive a booster dose of a tetanus toxoid-containing vaccine only if they have not received tetanus toxoid within the preceding 10 years. In case of tetanus-prone injury (e.g., wounds contaminated with dirt, feces, soil, and saliva; puncture wounds; avulsions; and wounds resulting from missles, crushing, burns, and frostbite) in an adolescent who is in need of tetanus toxoid, BOOSTRIX can be used as an alternative to Tetanus and Diphtheria Toxoids Adsorbed For Adult Use (Td) vaccine in patients for whom the pertussis component is also indicated (see INDICATIONS AND USAGE).

Manufactured by **GlaxoSmithKline Biologicals**
Rixensart, Belgium, US License 1617

Distributed by **GlaxoSmithKline**
Research Triangle Park, NC 27709



Full prescribing information for BOOSTRIX is available at www.BOOSTRIX.com.
BRS-BO:L3

**References: 1.** Centers for Disease Control and Prevention. Preventing tetanus, diphtheria, and pertussis among adolescents: use of tetanus toxoid, reduced diphtheria toxoid and acellular pertussis vaccines: recommendations of the Advisory Committee on Immunization Practices (ACIP). Early Release 2006;55(February 23, 2006):1–43. **2.** Centers for Disease Control and Prevention. Recommended childhood and adolescent immunization schedule—United States, 2006. *MMWR.* 2006;54(51&52):Q1–Q4.

ARTICLE

# Risky Alcohol Use, Age at Onset of Drinking, and Adverse Childhood Experiences in Young Men Entering the US Marine Corps

*Sylvia Y. N. Young, MD, MPH; Christian J. Hansen, BS; Roger L. Gibson, PhD, DVM, MPH; Margaret A. K. Ryan, MD, MPH*

**Objective:** To examine how childhood experiences relate to risky underage drinking.

**Design:** A survey study of men starting military training between June 11, 2002, and April 5, 2006. Multivariate logistic regression models compared risky drinkers with "all others" or with nonrisky drinkers; excluding nondrinkers.

**Setting:** Marine Corps Recruit Depot, San Diego, Calif.

**Participants:** Forty-one thousand four hundred eighty-two men aged 18 to 20 years.

**Main Exposures:** Age at drinking onset; childhood emotional, physical, and sexual abuse; childhood emotional and physical neglect; and household alcohol abuse, mental illness, domestic violence, or divorce.

**Main Outcome Measures:** Risky drinking identified by scoring responses to 3 questions about alcohol consumption.

**Results:** Of 41 482 young men, 6128 (14.8%) were identified as risky drinkers, 18 693 (45.1%) as nonrisky drinkers, and 16 661 (40.2%) as nondrinkers. Among drinkers, early initiation of alcohol use was strongly associated with risky drinking, with a 5.5-fold risk if age at onset of drinking was 13 years or younger. Other associated factors included tobacco use, rural or small hometown, higher education, motivation to join the military for travel or adventure or to leave problems at home, numerous close friends and relatives, household alcohol abuse or mental illness, and childhood sexual or emotional abuse. When the comparison group included nondrinkers, additional associated factors included childhood physical abuse and domestic violence.

**Conclusions:** These analyses confirm previous findings on risks for alcohol misuse in young adults and quantify these risks in new, large, multivariable models, adding unique perspective from a population of young Marines. Public health efforts to decrease alcohol misuse may be effectively targeted by prevention of underage alcohol use, tobacco use, and childhood abuse.

*Arch Pediatr Adolesc Med. 2006;160:1207-1214*

**Author Affiliations:** Department of Defense Center for Deployment Health Research, Naval Health Research Center, San Diego, Calif (Drs Young and Ryan and Mr Hansen); and the Armed Forces Epidemiological Board, Falls Church, Va (Dr Gibson).

IN 2004, HALF OF PERSONS LIVING in the United States aged 12 years or older (121 million persons) reported current alcohol use, with prevalence ranging from 2.3% in 12-year-old children to 69.8% in persons aged 21 years.[1] Approximately 4.4 million persons in the United States used alcohol for the first time in 2004, and most new users (86.9%) were younger than 21 years at first use of alcohol.[1] Heavy alcohol use among male Marines aged 18 to 25 years occurs at twice the civilian rate for the same age group (38.6% vs 17.8%, respectively).[2]

Many studies have shown a relationship between adverse childhood experiences, and alcohol misuse and abuse as an adult,[3-8] with the largest study including 13 494 participants.[5] Additional studies have found that early first use of alcohol increases the risk of developing alcohol disorders and alcohol-related injuries.[9-14] To our knowledge, no studies have examined both adverse childhood experiences and age at first use of alcohol in relation to alcohol misuse.

The Recruit Assessment Program (RAP) study was begun at the Marine Corps Recruit Depot, San Diego, Calif (MCRD San Diego), on June 12, 2001, to collect computerized comprehensive baseline health data from new military personnel.[15,16] The RAP questionnaire is administered to recruits in the first days of 12-week recruit training. Most recruits (>80%) have not reached legal drinking age when they begin their Marine training; thus, our objective was to examine the relationship between factors including adverse childhood

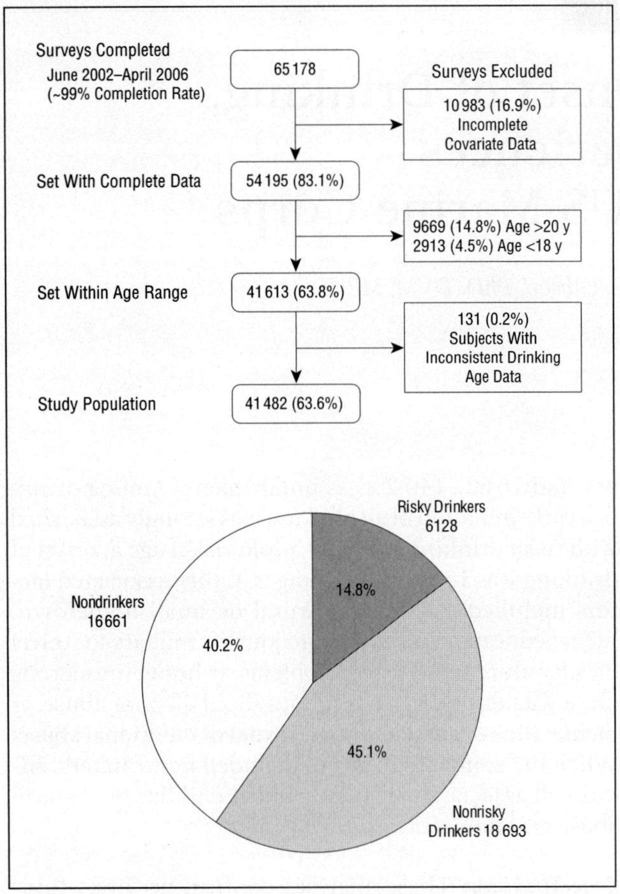


**Figure.** Schematic diagram illustrating exclusions for analysis of risky drinking in male recruits at onset of training at the Marine Corps Recruit Depot, San Diego, Calif.

experiences and age at onset of drinking with risky drinking in an underage military population, using self-reported RAP data.

## METHODS

### STUDY POPULATION AND DESIGN

The RAP study was approved by institutional review boards of the Naval Health Research Center and the Naval Medical Center, San Diego. The MCRD San Diego trains between 17 000 and 18 000 recruits per year. Because only men are trained in San Diego, our evaluation excluded women. All recruits were invited to complete an RAP questionnaire; participation rates were approximately 99% during the study period. Recruits were told that their answers would not disqualify them for military service, and informed consent was obtained before recruits completed the questionnaire. Between June 11, 2002, and April 5, 2006, 65 178 surveys were collected from male Marine recruits at MCRD San Diego. Selected self-reported characteristics were evaluated to include demographic data (age, race, hometown, marital status, educational achievement, and reasons for joining the military), family background (parental educational achievement and number of close relatives and friends for support), general history (frequency of attendance at a religious gathering and tobacco use), and childhood experiences (whether grew up with 2 parents, a mentally ill or depressed person, or a problem drinker or alcoholic; parental divorce; domestic violence; physical or emotional neglect; and emotional, physical, or sexual abuse). In addition to sexual abuse, a related question regarding history of rape was included.

Of 65 178 surveys, 54 195 (83.1%) contained complete outcome and covariate data for this analysis. Because our focus was underage drinking behavior among those aged 18 to 20 years, we excluded 9669 recruits (14.8%) aged 21 years or older and 2913 recruits (4.5%) younger than 18 years. In addition, we excluded 117 inconsistent recruits (0.2%) who gave a positive response about alcohol use but a contradictory response ("I have never had a drink") when asked at what age they first used alcohol, and 14 recruits (0.02%) who were aged 18 to 20 years but responded that they first used alcohol at age 21 years or older. For the remaining 41 482 respondents (63.6%), self-reported exposures in this survey study were examined (**Figure**).

### MEASURES

The RAP questionnaire was developed by public health officials, clinicians, and researchers from the Department of Defense, Department of Veterans Affairs, and Department of Health and Human Services. Questions were derived from standardized survey instruments, including the Alcohol Use Disorders Identification Test (AUDIT),[17-22] National Comorbidity Study,[23,24] Adverse Childhood Experiences Study,[5,6,25-27] Childhood Trauma Questionnaire,[28,29] and Conflict Tactics Scales.[30] The Adverse Childhood Experiences Study questions were first added to the RAP survey instrument in June 2002.

Because of time limitation, not all items of the 10-item AUDIT are asked on the RAP questionnaire. Focus group testing of the questionnaire in small groups of recruits led to inclusion of 3 questions derived from the AUDIT–Alcohol Consumption Questions (AUDIT-C)[18-22] questionnaire, with possible scores ranging from 0 to 12 points (**Table 1**).

Our primary outcome, risky drinking, was defined using the 3 questions derived from AUDIT-C. To meet the outcome definition, a score of 4 points or more, of the maximum of 12 points, was required. A score of 4 points has been shown to be an optimal cutoff in screening for risky drinking.[18,21,22] It is possible that men could drink 1 or 2 drinks daily and score 4 points, but since the men in our analyses were all younger than the legal drinking age, we considered 4 points to be a fair cutoff to screen for risky drinking. Nonrisky drinkers were recruits who scored 1 to 3 points of the maximum of 12 points. Nondrinkers consistently marked negative responses to the 3 questions (Table 1), although they may have responded positively to another question about age at onset of drinking, as may be expected for many nondrinkers who experimented with tasting alcohol. The "all other" group comprised both nonrisky drinkers and nondrinkers.

Our exposures of interest included age at onset of drinking. This was initially defined as, "How old were you when you first had a drink containing alcohol?" In July 2005, this question was revised as, "Not counting sips, how old were you when you first had a drink containing alcohol?" With either question, the response options were, "I have never had a drink of alcohol," "13 years or younger," "14 to 15 years old," 16 to 17 years old," "18 to 20 years old," and "21 years or older."

To assess adverse childhood experiences, we used questions from the Adverse Childhood Experiences Study,[5,6,25-27] the Childhood Trauma Questionnaire,[28,29] and the Conflict Tactics Scales,[30] prefacing them with, "The following are statements about you when you were growing up, before you were 17 years old. Please choose the one answer that comes closest to the way you felt."

Physical neglect was defined by the responses "never true," "rarely true," or "sometimes true" to the statement, "There was someone to take care of you and protect you." Emotional neglect was defined by the responses, "never true," "rarely true," or "sometimes true" to the statement "You felt loved."

**Table 1. Risky Drinking Scoring for the Recruit Assessment Program Survey Derived From the AUDIT-C**

| Question | Score 0 | 1 | 2 | 3 | 4 |
|---|---|---|---|---|---|
| During the year (12 mo) before entering the military, how often did you have a drink containing alcohol?* | Never | Once or twice, a few times, or monthly | Weekly | | Daily |
| During the past year, how many drinks containing alcohol did you have on a typical day of drinking? | None, 1, or 2 | 3 or 4 | 5 or 6 | 7-9 | ≥10 |
| During the past year, how often did you have ≥6 drinks at one sitting? | Never | Once or twice, or a few times | Monthly | Weekly | Daily |

Abbreviation: AUDIT-C, Alcohol Use Disorders Identification Test–Alcohol Consumption Questions.
*One drink equals 1 bottle or can of beer, 1 glass of wine, 1 wine cooler, or 1 shot of hard liquor.

To assess emotional abuse, we asked, "How often did a parent or adult living in your home swear at you, insult you, or put you down?" Emotional abuse was defined as present if the response was "often" or "very often."

Domestic violence was assessed with the question "How often did a parent or other adult living in your home push, grab, shove, slap, or throw something at each other?" Domestic violence was defined as present if the response was "sometimes," "often," or "very often."

To assess childhood physical abuse, we asked, "How often did a parent or other adult living in your home push, grab, shove, slap, or throw something at you?" Childhood physical abuse was defined as present if the response was "often" or "very often."

Childhood sexual abuse was assessed with the question, "How often did an adult ever touch you sexually or try to make you touch them sexually?" Childhood sexual abuse was defined as present if the response was "once or twice," "sometimes," "often," or "very often."

Tobacco use was assessed by asking the following 4 questions: "Have you smoked more than 100 cigarettes (5 packs) in your entire life?" "How many years did you smoke more than 3 cigarettes on most days?" "When you were smoking regularly, how many packs did you smoke each day?" "When did you last smoke a cigarette?" The never smoked group included those who consistently answered, "I have never smoked" to these questions; past smokers were those who had positive responses to the first 3 questions and last smoked a cigarette more than 1 year ago; current smokers, less than 2 pack-years, were those with a positive response to the first question and a history of smoking less than 2 pack-years for the second and third questions, and last smoked a cigarette within the past year; and current smokers, 2 or more pack-years, were similar to current light smokers except they had a history of smoking at least 2 pack-years.

## DATA ANALYSIS

Descriptive investigations of population characteristics were completed. Univariate analyses, including $\chi^2$ and measures of association, were performed to assess the significance of associations between exposures of interest and risky drinking. An exploratory model analysis was performed to assess regression diagnostics, significant associations, and possible confounding while simultaneously adjusting for all other variables in the model. These analyses yielded a consistent set of influential covariates, with $P \leq .15$, that were then included in subsequent model analyses. Multivariate logistic regression analysis using SAS software (version 9.1; SAS Institute Inc, Cary, NC) was used to determine the odds of an outcome of risky drinking using 2 comparisons: with "all other" recruits to include nonrisky drinkers and nondrinkers, and with nonrisky drinkers excluding nondrinkers. Odds ratios and 95% confidence intervals were calculated for Marine recruits with complete covariate data.

## RESULTS

Of 41 482 recruits in our analysis, 6128 (14.8%) were identified as risky drinkers, 18 693 (45.1%) as nonrisky drinkers, and 16 661 (40.2%) as nondrinkers. **Table 2** summarizes frequency and percentage distribution of risky drinking scores by exposures of interest. Univariate analyses suggested significant associations between higher risky drinking scores and many covariates, particularly early age when having a first alcohol drink, tobacco use, and adverse childhood events.

To simultaneously control for many covariates, we used all covariates from Table 2 in multivariable logistic regression analyses for 6128 risky drinkers and 35 354 other recruits (**Table 3**). Risky drinkers were more likely to be smokers, from a rural or small hometown background, to have grown up with someone who was a problem drinker or alcoholic or who was depressed or mentally ill, and to have experienced childhood sexual or emotional abuse. They were more likely to report educational achievement beyond high school, having more close family members or friends available for personal support, and motivation to join the military for travel or adventure or to leave problems at home. Risky drinkers were slightly more likely to report childhood physical abuse and a history of witnessing domestic violence and to be 19 or 20 years of age at survey completion, rather than 18 years of age.

Factors inversely associated with risky drinking were being married, attending religious services weekly or more often, neither parent having completed high school, not knowing parental educational achievement, and motivation to join the military "to serve my country," for education and new job skills, or for a 20-year military career. A history of emotional neglect was also inversely associated.

Further analyses compared the 6128 risky drinkers and 18 693 nonrisky drinkers, excluding nondrinkers, from the comparison group (Table 3). Compared with those recruits who first used alcohol at age 18 to 20 years, drinkers who started younger were more likely to be identified as risky drinkers; those who started drinking at age 13 years were 5.5-fold more likely to be identified as risky

**Table 2. Selected Characteristics of Male Marine Recruits at Onset of Training in San Diego, Calif***

| Characteristic | Nondrinkers (Score, 0) (n = 16 661) | Nonrisky Drinkers (Score, 1-3) (n = 18 693) | Risky Drinkers (Score, 4-12) (n = 6128) |
|---|---|---|---|
| Age at first alcohol use, y | | | |
| Never | 11 507 (69.1) | 0 | 0 |
| 18-20 | 778 (4.7) | 4749 (25.4) | 541 (8.8) |
| 16-17 | 2399 (14.4) | 8642 (46.2) | 2304 (37.6) |
| 14-15 | 1149 (6.9) | 3425 (18.3) | 1978 (32.3) |
| ≤13 | 828 (5.0) | 1877 (10.0) | 1305 (21.3) |
| Age at survey completion, y | | | |
| 18 | 10 095 (60.6) | 9998 (53.5) | 2976 (48.6) |
| 19 | 4762 (28.6) | 5794 (31.0) | 2032 (33.2) |
| 20 | 1804 (10.8) | 2901 (15.5) | 1120 (18.3) |
| Race/ethnic group | | | |
| White | 10 397 (62.4) | 12 475 (66.7) | 4539 (74.1) |
| African American | 742 (4.5) | 555 (3.0) | 77 (1.3) |
| Hispanic | 3770 (22.6) | 3954 (21.2) | 1054 (17.2) |
| Other | 1752 (10.5) | 1709 (9.1) | 458 (7.5) |
| Hometown | | | |
| City with >100 000 persons | 4997 (30.0) | 5492 (29.4) | 1468 (24.0) |
| Town or city with <100 000 persons | 8308 (49.9) | 9442 (50.5) | 3220 (52.6) |
| Rural (eg, farm or ranch) | 1611 (9.7) | 2049 (11.0) | 948 (15.5) |
| Moved a lot to different cities | 1415 (8.5) | 1446 (7.7) | 422 (6.9) |
| Not sure | 330 (2.0) | 264 (1.4) | 70 (1.1) |
| Marital status | | | |
| Married | 258 (1.6) | 319 (1.7) | 81 (1.3) |
| Single, separated, divorced, or widowed | 16 403 (98.5) | 18 374 (98.3) | 6047 (98.7) |
| Highest educational achievement | | | |
| Some high school but did not graduate | 143 (0.9) | 140 (0.8) | 55 (0.9) |
| High school graduate or GED | 14 129 (84.8) | 15 129 (80.9) | 4762 (77.7) |
| Some college or trade school, or higher | 2389 (14.3) | 3424 (18.3) | 1311 (21.4) |
| Reason for joining the military† | | | |
| Education and new job skills | 9445 (56.7) | 10 873 (58.2) | 3410 (55.7) |
| Travel or adventure | 6106 (36.7) | 7399 (39.6) | 2650 (43.2) |
| Job to earn money | 4448 (26.7) | 5105 (27.3) | 1746 (28.5) |
| Leave problems at home | 764 (4.6) | 959 (5.1) | 459 (7.5) |
| Family member was in the military | 1829 (11.0) | 2206 (11.8) | 767 (12.5) |
| 20-Year career in the military | 2544 (15.3) | 2726 (14.6) | 864 (14.1) |
| "To serve my country" | 10 264 (61.6) | 11 686 (62.5) | 3805 (62.1) |
| Other reason | 4838 (29.0) | 5543 (29.7) | 1835 (29.9) |
| Highest level of parental education | | | |
| Neither parent completed high school | 1640 (9.8) | 1688 (9.0) | 424 (6.9) |
| At least 1 parent was a high school graduate or had a GED | 9078 (54.5) | 10 557 (56.5) | 3595 (58.7) |
| At least 1 parent was a college graduate | 4704 (28.2) | 5287 (28.3) | 1846 (30.1) |
| Unknown | 1239 (7.4) | 1161 (6.2) | 263 (4.3) |
| No. of close friends or relatives for support | | | |
| None | 1661 (10.0) | 1036 (5.5) | 308 (5.0) |
| 1 or 2 | 4553 (27.3) | 4848 (25.9) | 1405 (22.9) |
| ≥3 | 10 447 (62.7) | 12 809 (68.5) | 4415 (72.1) |
| Attendance at religious gathering (eg, church) | | | |
| Weekly or more often | 6514 (39.1) | 5893 (31.5) | 1521 (24.8) |
| Less than weekly | 10 147 (60.9) | 12 800 (68.5) | 4607 (75.2) |
| Tobacco use‡ | | | |
| Never smoked | 14 529 (87.2) | 12 931 (69.2) | 2909 (47.5) |
| Past smoker | 232 (1.4) | 420 (2.3) | 156 (2.6) |
| Current smoker, <2 pack-years | 1492 (9.0) | 4112 (22.0) | 2035 (33.2) |
| Current smoker, ≥2 pack-years | 408 (2.5) | 1230 (6.6) | 1028 (16.8) |
| Raised by 2 parents | | | |
| No | 4714 (28.3) | 5314 (28.4) | 1662 (27.1) |
| Yes | 11 947 (71.7) | 13 379 (71.6) | 4466 (72.9) |
| Parents divorced | | | |
| No | 10 574 (63.5) | 11 183 (59.8) | 3543 (57.8) |
| Yes, when respondent <10 y | 4280 (25.7) | 5336 (28.6) | 1814 (29.6) |
| Yes, when respondent >10 y | 1807 (10.9) | 2174 (11.6) | 771 (12.6) |
| Physically neglected as a child | 2901 (17.4) | 3050 (16.3) | 1080 (17.6) |
| Emotionally neglected as a child | 2665 (16.0) | 2767 (14.8) | 970 (15.8) |
| Emotionally abused as a child | 1942 (11.7) | 2289 (12.3) | 951 (15.5) |
| Physically abused as a child | 360 (2.2) | 489 (2.6) | 214 (3.5) |
| Sexually abused as a child | 254 (1.5) | 286 (1.5) | 137 (2.2) |
| Witnessed domestic violence as a child | 1081 (6.5) | 1480 (7.9) | 595 (9.7) |
| Grew up with mentally ill or depressed person | 863 (5.2) | 1161 (6.2) | 550 (9.0) |
| Grew up with problem drinker or alcoholic | 1459 (8.8) | 2021 (10.8) | 902 (14.7) |
| Ever raped | 37 (0.2) | 80 (0.4) | 38 (0.6) |

Abbreviation: GED, general equivalency diploma.
*Data are given as number (percentage), unless otherwise indicated.
†More than 1 reason could be selected.
‡For assessment of tobacco use, see the "Measures" subsection of the "Methods" section.

**Table 3. Final Multivariate Regression Models for 6128 Risky Drinkers vs "All Others" (35 354)* and Nonrisky Drinkers (18 693)†**

| Characteristic | Risky Drinkers vs All Others‡ | Risky Drinkers vs Nonrisky Drinkers‡ |
|---|---|---|
| Age at first alcohol use, y | | |
| 18-20 | NA | 1.0 |
| 16-17 | NA | 2.3 (2.1-2.6) |
| 14-15 | NA | 4.7 (4.2-5.2) |
| ≤13 | NA | 5.5 (4.9-6.2) |
| Age at survey completion, y | | |
| 18 | 1.0 | 1.0 |
| 19 | 1.1 (1.0-1.2) | 1.2 (1.1-1.3) |
| 20 | 1.2 (1.1-1.3) | 1.4 (1.3-1.5) |
| Race/ethnic group | | |
| White | 1.0 | 1.0 |
| African American | 0.5 (0.4-0.6) | 0.5 (0.4-0.7) |
| Hispanic | 1.1 (1.0-1.2) | 1.1 (1.0-1.2) |
| Other | 0.8 (0.7-0.9) | 0.9 (0.8-1.0) |
| Hometown | | |
| City with >100 000 persons | 1.0 | 1.0 |
| Town or city with <100 000 persons | 1.3 (1.2-1.3) | 1.2 (1.1-1.3) |
| Rural (eg, farm or ranch) | 1.7 (1.5-1.9) | 1.5 (1.4-1.7) |
| Moved a lot to different cities | 0.9 (0.8-1.0) | 0.9 (0.8-1.1) |
| Not sure | 1.0 (0.8-1.3) | 1.1 (0.8-1.4) |
| Marital status | | |
| Single, separated, divorced, or widowed | 1.0 | 1.0 |
| Married | 0.7 (0.5-0.9) | 0.7 (0.5-0.8) |
| Highest educational achievement | | |
| High school graduate or GED | 1.0 | 1.0 |
| Some high school but did not graduate | 1.0 (0.7-1.3) | 1.0 (0.7-1.4) |
| Some college or trade school, or higher | 1.3 (1.2-1.5) | 1.2 (1.1-1.3) |
| Reason for joining the military | | |
| Education and new job skills§ | 0.9 (0.8-0.9) | 0.9 (0.8-1.0) |
| Travel or adventure§ | 1.3 (1.2-1.3) | 1.2 (1.1-1.3) |
| Leave problems at home§ | 1.3 (1.2-1.5) | 1.3 (1.1-1.4) |
| 20-Year career in the military§ | 0.9 (0.8-1.0) | 0.9 (0.8-1.0) |
| "To serve my country"§ | 0.9 (0.8-1.0) | 0.9 (0.9-1.0) |
| Other reason§ | 1.0 (0.9-1.0) | 0.9 (0.9-1.0) |
| Highest level of parental education | | |
| At least 1 parent was a high school graduate or had a GED | 1.0 | 1.0 |
| Neither parent completed high school | 0.8 (0.7-0.9) | 0.8 (0.7-0.9) |
| At least 1 parent was a college graduate | 1.0 (0.9-1.1) | 1.0 (1.0-1.1) |
| Unknown | 0.7 (0.6-0.8) | 0.7 (0.6-0.9) |
| No. of close friends or relatives for support | | |
| None | 1.0 | 1.0 |
| 1-2 | 1.3 (1.1-1.4) | 1.0 (0.9-1.2) |
| ≥3 | 1.6 (1.4-1.9) | 1.2 (1.0-1.4) |
| Attendance at religious gathering (eg, church) | | |
| Less than weekly | 1.0 | 1.0 |
| Weekly or more often | 0.7 (0.6-0.7) | 0.8 (0.7-0.8) |
| Tobacco use‖ | | |
| Never smoked | 1.0 | 1.0 |
| Past smoker | 2.1 (1.8-2.5) | 1.3 (1.1-1.6) |
| Current smoker, <2 pack-years | 3.2 (3.0-3.4) | 2.0 (1.8-2.1) |
| Current smoker, ≥2 pack-years | 5.3 (4.8-5.8) | 2.7 (2.5-3.0) |
| Raised by 2 parents§ | 1.1 (1.0-1.2) | 1.1 (1.0-1.2) |
| Emotionally neglected as a child§ | 0.9 (0.9-1.0) | 0.9 (0.8-1.0) |
| Emotionally abused as a child§ | 1.2 (1.1-1.3) | 1.1 (1.0-1.2) |
| Physically abused as a child§ | 1.1 (1.0-1.4) | |
| Sexually abused as a child§ | 1.3 (1.0-1.6) | 1.3 (1.1-1.7) |
| Witnessed domestic violence as a child§ | 1.1 (1.0-1.2) | |
| Grew up with mentally ill or depressed person§ | 1.3 (1.2-1.4) | 1.2 (1.1-1.3) |
| Grew up with problem drinker or alcoholic§ | 1.3 (1.2-1.5) | 1.2 (1.1-1.3) |

Abbreviations: GED, general equivalency diploma; NA, not applicable.
*Nondrinkers and nonrisky drinkers are combined in the "all others" classification.
†Nonrisky drinkers excludes nondrinkers.
‡Data are given as adjusted odds ratio (95% confidence interval). Risk estimates are adjusted for all other factors in the table.
§Dichotomous variable.
‖For assessment of tobacco use, see the "Measures" subsection of the "Methods" section.

drinkers. Age at first use of alcohol was excluded from the previous analysis with "all other" recruits because this question did not apply to nondrinkers in this group.

In addition to age at first alcohol use, factors associated with risky drinking were the same as in the previous analysis, in which nondrinkers were included in the comparison group, except that the covariates for having experienced childhood physical abuse and for reporting household domestic violence were not found to be significant in the final multivariate logistic regression model. Factors inversely associated with risky drinking were identical to those in the previous analysis with the "all others" comparison group.

## COMMENT

Several points are highlighted in this large survey study examining age at onset of drinking and adverse childhood experiences in relation to alcohol use in 18- to 20-year-old male Marine recruits. Our risky drinking scores were based on the AUDIT-C instrument, in which scores of 4 points or more have been demonstrated to have sensitivity ranging from 83.7% to 92.6% and specificity ranging from 69.0% to 92.0% in identifying patients with heavy drinking or active alcohol abuse or dependence.[18,22] This led to the identification of 14.8% of 18- to 20-year-old recruits as risky drinkers, consistent with previous large community surveys using detailed interviews where prevalence of alcohol abuse and dependence in the previous year among men who were 18 to 29 years old was 14% to 26%.[1,24,31]

While previous studies tend to look separately at associations between adverse childhood experiences with alcohol abuse and tobacco abuse,[3-6,25,26] our study was large enough that we were able to evaluate risky drinking, simultaneously controlling for tobacco use and adverse childhood experiences, in addition to other covariates, including age at onset of drinking. Early age at first alcohol use, adverse childhood experiences, and tobacco use are each independently associated with risky drinking behavior.

Among drinkers, the strongest correlate of a high risky drinking score was early age at first alcohol use, with a 5.5-fold risk if age at onset of drinking was 13 years or younger. This is consistent with previous studies that found that early alcohol use increases risk of developing alcohol disorders and experiencing alcohol-related injuries.[9-14] However, to our knowledge, this is the first time that the relationship between age at onset of drinking and risky drinking has been quantified in multivariable models of a large Marine Corps cohort.

Our findings underscore the need for programs and policies to reduce underage drinking, such as the minimum legal drinking age of 21 years. The American Medical Association recommends the following actions to address underage drinking[32]:

- Expand physician involvement by educating physicians about alcohol screening and intervention, especially for adolescents.
- Examine alcohol advertising and marketing practices and develop mandatory standards to prevent the targeting of young people.
- Increase alcohol excise taxes.
- Develop and fund counteradvertising and public awareness campaigns.
- Expand research on the harmful effects of alcohol on adolescents.
- Improve product labeling to warn people of the dangers and negative health effects of alcohol.
- Implement comprehensive school health programs to provide our children with decision-making skills and age-appropriate information to counter the impact of alcohol advertisements.
- Step up enforcement of existing regulations and underage drinking laws.

Our study results also reinforce the need for public health efforts to prevent tobacco use and child abuse. After early age at first alcohol use, the factor most strongly associated with risky drinking was tobacco use. Whether reducing smoking will reduce risky drinking among youth is an important but unexplored question.

The magnitude of the associations between individual adverse childhood experiences and risky drinking was smaller but still significant in our large sample. Langeland and Hartgers[4] concluded in their review of child abuse and alcoholism that there is insufficient evidence on which to base conclusions about relationships between childhood sexual abuse or childhood physical abuse and alcoholism in male subjects. The largest study in their review included 802 participants, which may not have been a large enough sample to show these relationships. Our data showed an increased association between childhood sexual, physical, and emotional abuse and risky drinkers when compared with all other recruits and an increased risk of childhood sexual and emotional abuse when compared with other drinkers. Our findings that growing up with a problem drinker or with someone who is mentally ill and that childhood emotional or sexual abuse were all independently associated with risky drinking are consistent with previous studies that concluded that adverse childhood events may contribute to negative consequences in adulthood, including adult alcohol abuse.[3-8,25-27]

Finding that being married is inversely associated with risky drinking is supported by studies noting that married men show lower levels of alcohol consumption.[33-35] Finding that weekly attendance at religious gatherings is inversely associated with risky drinking is also supported by literature noting that existential well-being is inversely associated with alcohol abuse or dependence.[36,37]

In many studies, older and better-educated subjects generally report healthier behaviors, but in this study focusing on 18- to 20-year-old male recruits, higher education increased risk of risky drinking behavior. A plausible explanation may be that 20-year-old recruits with some college education have drinking experience related to college, compared with younger men who enlisted right after high school. Binge drinking and heavy alcohol use rates are known to be significantly higher in full-time college students compared with other persons aged 18 to 22 years.[1]

It was unexpected to find that risky drinkers were more likely to report having many close friends or relatives for support, but this may indicate that young men are more likely to indulge in risky drinking behavior for reasons of conviviality and peer group pressure.[38,39] It was also unexpected to find that a history of emotional neglect was inversely associated with risky drinking and that risky drinkers were slightly more likely to report being raised by 2 parents. While it is possible that multiple statistical comparisons may have resulted in spurious results, another explanation may be that risky underage drinking is such an enormous problem in the United States that not only youth from families with household dysfunction are susceptible to alcohol misuse but that this is a problem that also affects youth from intact and loving homes. Thus, it is plausible that many young men identified in our study as risky drinkers were raised in 2-parent families and felt loved and supported while growing up. Further research is needed to confirm these unexpected findings.

Finally, a novel finding of these analyses was the association between motivation to join the military and risky drinking. Those who joined to escape problems at home or for travel and adventure were more likely to report risky drinking behavior. Motivation to join for travel and adventure is perhaps not surprising if considered a surrogate for risk-taking behavior. In contrast, those who joined to have a 20-year career in the military or "to serve my country" were slightly less likely to report risky drinking behavior.

Our study was restricted to male Marine recruits who had passed initial screening for military entrance, and the findings can only be generalized to other similar populations. Our study was limited to self-reported data, which may have led to underreporting of adverse childhood experiences, risky drinking behavior, early age at first alcohol use, and misclassification of identified risky drinkers, nonrisky drinkers, and nondrinkers. Based on κ statistics to measure reproducibility,[40] recruits are generally candid in filling out these questionnaires. However, the sensitive nature of the questions evaluated in this study may have resulted in underreporting and, thus, underestimation of both predictor and outcome variables. Nevertheless, with our large sample size, we were able to simultaneously control for many potential confounders and detect many significant associations.

Similar to other studies, our findings do not show causality, but they support other work suggesting the importance of adverse childhood experiences on adult behavior and that the prevention of childhood abuse is of public health importance. Further studies are needed to examine how early age at onset of drinking and adverse childhood events relate to alcohol misuse in new female military members. Studies in Navy recruits suggest that a high percentage of female recruits had been raped and that many had experienced childhood physical or sexual abuse at much higher frequency than noted in male Marine recruits with the RAP questionnaire.[41,42]

Although the RAP was implemented at MCRD San Diego as a pilot study, the Department of Defense is taking steps to implement routine collection of computerized baseline health data from each person entering the armed forces. Recruit assessment health data will not be used to screen out candidates for the armed forces, but collection of accurate baseline health data is essential to evaluate health risks and behaviors before entrance into military service, to understand the potential effects of deployments and other exposures of military concern throughout the service member's military career and thereafter, and to develop and assess intervention and prevention programs for force health protection.

Our RAP database represents vital baseline health information from many US Marines who have been, are, or will be deployed overseas. A separate study, the United States Marine Corps Health Assessment Project, is presently resurveying Marines who are previous RAP participants to assess later health status in a large cohort of Marines several years after boot camp, with additional questions about deployment and exposure information; and to determine whether baseline health data were associated with subsequent postdeployment mental and physical health problems identifiable from surveys and inpatient or outpatient encounters. Future plans include studies to follow health and career outcomes of Marines identified from RAP as risky drinkers. Future studies may determine whether adverse childhood experiences help build resiliency and coping skills so that Marines subsequently involved in combat are less susceptible to developing mental health problems or whether they contribute to increased susceptibility to problems such as posttraumatic stress disorder and problems related to alcohol misuse. These kinds of studies enhance efforts for intervention and prevention programs to protect health and readiness, add to research in chronic multisymptom illnesses and mental health challenges, and should be considered important to the health of military personnel in future deployments.

**Accepted for Publication:** July 8, 2006.
**Correspondence:** Margaret A. K. Ryan, MD, MPH, Department of Defense Center for Deployment Health Research, Naval Health Research Center, PO Box 85122, San Diego, CA 92186-5122 (ryan@nhrc.navy.mil).
**Author Contributions:** *Study concept and design:* Young and Ryan. *Acquisition of data:* Young, Hansen, and Ryan. *Analysis and interpretation of data:* Young, Gibson, and Ryan. *Drafting of the manuscript:* Young, Hansen, Gibson, and Ryan. *Critical revision of the manuscript for important intellectual content:* Young, Gibson, and Ryan. *Statistical analysis:* Young, Hansen, Gibson, and Ryan. *Obtained funding:* Young and Ryan. *Administrative, technical, and material support:* Young, Gibson, and Ryan. *Study supervision:* Young and Ryan.
**Financial Disclosure:** None reported.
**Funding/Support:** This study (report 05-12) was supported by the Department of Defense under work unit 60002.
**Disclaimer:** The views expressed in this article are those of the authors and do not reflect the official policy or position of the Department of the Navy, Department of the Army, Department of Defense, or the US Government. Approved for public release; distribution is unlimited.
**Additional Information:** This research was conducted in compliance with all applicable federal regulations governing the protection of human subjects in research (protocol NHRC.2000.0003).
**Acknowledgment:** We thank Christina Brocco, BA; Christina Corpuz, BA; William Honner, BA; Suzanne Lane,

BA; Chrislee Leyco, BS; Meghan Morris, BS; Annie Wang, BS; Steven Speigle, and Jim Whitmer, Department of Defense Center for Deployment Health Research, Naval Health Research Center, for data collection and database management; and Col Rick Riddle, USAF, BSC, Air Force Research Laboratory; COL Charles Engel, MC, USA, Department of Defense Deployment Health Clinical Center; Lt Col Bruce Ruscio, USAF, BSC, Office of the Assistant Secretary of Defense for Health Affairs; Greg Gray, MD, MPH, University of Iowa; Keith Hauret, MSPH, MPT, US Army Center for Health Promotion; COL Brian Lukey, MS, USA, US Army Medical Research and Materiel Command; COL Karl Friedl, MS, USA, US Army Research Institute of Environmental Medicine; and COL Charles Hoge, MC, USA, and Stephen Messer, PhD, Walter Reed Army Institute of Research, for support with development of the Recruit Assessment Program instrument and protocol, and review of the manuscript. We also thank LCDR Janet Whitney-Spira, MC, USNR, who worked on a related analysis on the relationship of personal lifestyle choices to underage drinking for her Master of Public Health thesis.

## REFERENCES


1. Substance Abuse and Mental Health Services Administration. *Results From the 2004 National Survey on Drug Use and Health: National Findings.* Rockville, Md: Substance Abuse and Mental Health Services Administration; 2005. Office of Applied Studies, NSDUH Series H-28, US Dept of Health and Human Services Publication No. SMA 05-0462.
2. Bray RM, Hourani LL, Rae KL, et al. *2002 Department of Defense Survey of Health Related Behaviors Among Military Personnel.* Research Triangle Park, NC: Research Triangle Institute; 2003. Report No. RTI/7841/006-FR.
3. Kunitz SJ, Levy JE, McCloskey J, Gabriel KR. Alcohol dependence and domestic violence as sequelae of abuse and conduct disorder in childhood. *Child Abuse Negl.* 1998;22:1079-1091.
4. Langeland W, Hartgers C. Child sexual and physical abuse and alcoholism: a review. *J Stud Alcohol.* 1998;59:336-348.
5. Dube SR, Anda RF, Felitti VJ, Edwards VJ, Croft JB. Adverse childhood experiences and personal alcohol abuse as an adult. *Addict Behav.* 2002;27:713-725.
6. Anda RF, Whitfield CL, Felitti VJ, et al. Adverse childhood experiences, alcoholic parents, and later risk of alcoholism and depression. *Psychiatr Serv.* 2002; 53:1001-1009.
7. Tam TW, Zlotnick C, Robertson MJ. Longitudinal perspective: adverse childhood events, substance use, and labor force participation among homeless adults. *Am J Drug Alcohol Abuse.* 2003;29:829-846.
8. Moran PB, Vuchinich S, Hall NK. Associations between types of maltreatment and substance use during adolescence. *Child Abuse Negl.* 2004;28:565-574.
9. Clapper RL, Buka SL, Goldfield EC, Lipsitt LP, Tsuang MT. Adolescent problem behaviors as predictors of adult alcohol diagnoses. *Int J Addict.* 1995;30:507-523.
10. DeWit DJ, Adlaf EM, Offord DR, Ogborne AC. Age at first alcohol use: a risk factor for the development of alcohol disorders. *Am J Psychiatry.* 2000;157:745-750.
11. Hingson RW, Heeren T, Jamanka A, Howland J. Age of drinking onset and unintentional injury involvement after drinking. *JAMA.* 2000;284:1527-1533.
12. Hingson R, Heeren T, Zakocs R, Winter M, Wechsler H. Age of first intoxication, heavy drinking, driving after drinking, and risk of unintentional injury among US college students. *J Stud Alcohol.* 2003;64:23-31.
13. McCarty CA, Ebel BE, Garrison MM, DiGiuseppe DL, Christakis DA, Rivara FP. Continuity of binge and harmful drinking from late adolescence to early adulthood. *Pediatrics.* 2004;114:714-719.
14. Hingson RW, Heeren T, Winter MR. Age of drinking onset and alcohol dependence. *Arch Pediatr Adolesc Med.* 2006;160:739-746.
15. Hyams KC, Barrett DH, Duque D, et al. The Recruit Assessment Program: a program to collect comprehensive baseline health data from U.S. military personnel. *Mil Med.* 2002;167:44-47.
16. Lane SE, Young SYN, Bayer L, Hogan B, Hyams KC, Ryan MAK. *Recruit Assessment Program: Implementation at Marine Corps Recruit Depot, San Diego.* San Diego, Calif: Naval Health Research Center; 2002. NHRC Report 02-17.
17. Babor TF, Higgins-Biddle JC, Saunders JB, Monteiro MG. *AUDIT: The Alcohol Use Disorders Identification Test.* 2nd ed. Geneva, Switzerland: World Health Organization; 2001.
18. Bush K, Kivlahan DR, McDonell MB, Fihn SD, Bradley KA. The AUDIT alcohol consumption questions (AUDIT-C): an effective brief screening test for problem drinking. Ambulatory Care Quality Improvement Project (ACQUIP). Alcohol Use Disorders Identification Test. *Arch Intern Med.* 1998;158:1789-1795.
19. Gordon AJ, Maisto SA, McNeil M, et al. Three questions can detect hazardous drinkers. *J Fam Pract.* 2001;50:313-320.
20. Reinert DF, Allen JP. The Alcohol Use Disorders Identification Test (AUDIT): a review of recent research. *Alcohol Clin Exp Res.* 2002;26:272-279.
21. Bradley KA, Bush KR, Epler AJ, et al. Two brief alcohol-screening tests from the Alcohol Use Disorders Identification Test (AUDIT): validation in a female Veterans Affairs patient population. *Arch Intern Med.* 2003;163:821-829.
22. Dawson DA, Grant BF, Stinson FS, Zhou Y. Effectiveness of the derived Alcohol Use Disorders Identification Test (AUDIT-C) in screening for alcohol use disorders and risk drinking in the US general population. *Alcohol Clin Exp Res.* 2005; 29:844-854.
23. Kessler RC. The U.S. National Comorbidity Survey: onset, chronicity and comorbidity patterns of mood disorders in the general population. In: Langer SZ, Brunello N, Racagni G, Mendlewicz J, eds. *Critical Issues in the Treatment of Affective Disorders.* Basel, Switzerland: S Karger AG; 1994:154-157.
24. Kessler RC, McGonagle KA, Zhao S, et al. Lifetime and 12-month prevalence of *DSM-III-R* psychiatric disorders in the United States: results from the National Comorbidity Survey. *Arch Gen Psychiatry.* 1994;51:8-19.
25. Felitti VJ, Anda RF, Nordenberg D, et al. Relationship of childhood abuse and household dysfunction to many of the leading causes of death in adults: the Adverse Childhood Experiences (ACE) Study. *Am J Prev Med.* 1998;14:245-258.
26. Anda RF, Croft JB, Felitti VJ, et al. Adverse childhood experiences and smoking during adolescence and adulthood. *JAMA.* 1999;282:1652-1658.
27. Dube SR, Anda RF, Felitti VJ, Chapman DP, Williamson DF, Giles WH. Childhood abuse, household dysfunction, and the risk of attempted suicide throughout the life span: findings from the Adverse Childhood Experiences Study. *JAMA.* 2001;286:3089-3096.
28. Bernstein DP, Fink L, Handelsman L, et al. Initial reliability and validity of a new retrospective measure of child abuse and neglect. *Am J Psychiatry.* 1994;151: 1132-1136.
29. Bernstein DP, Stein JA, Newcomb MD, et al. Development and validation of a brief screening version of the Childhood Trauma Questionnaire. *Child Abuse Negl.* 2003;27:169-190.
30. Straus M, Gelles RJ. *Physical Violence in American Families: Risk Factors and Adaptations to Violence in 8,145 Families.* New Brunswick, NJ: Transaction Press; 1990.
31. Grant BF. Alcohol consumption, alcohol abuse and alcohol dependence: the United States as an example. *Addiction.* 1994;89:1357-1365.
32. Fleming M, Towey K, eds. *Educational Forum on Adolescent Health: Youth Drinking Patterns and Alcohol Advertising.* Chicago, Ill: American Medical Association; 2004.
33. Rosengren A, Wedel H, Wilhelmsen L. Marital status and mortality in middle-aged Swedish men. *Am J Epidemiol.* 1989;129:54-64.
34. Lillard LA, Waite LJ. 'Til death do us part: marital disruption and mortality. *Am J Sociol.* 1995;100:1131-1156.
35. Hill EM, Chow K. Life-history theory and risky drinking. *Addiction.* 2002;97:401-413.
36. Baetz M, Larson DB, Marcoux G, Bowen R, Griffin R. Canadian psychiatric inpatient religious commitment: an association with mental health. *Can J Psychiatry.* 2002;47:159-166.
37. Tsuang MT, Williams WM, Simpson JC, Lyons MJ. Pilot study of spirituality and mental health in twins. *Am J Psychiatry.* 2002;159:486-488.
38. Kilty KM. Drinking styles of adolescents and young adults. *J Stud Alcohol.* 1990; 51:556-564.
39. Hawkins JD, Catalano RF, Miller JY. Risk and protective factors for alcohol and other drug problems in adolescence and early adulthood: implications for substance abuse prevention. *Psychol Bull.* 1992;112:64-105.
40. Young SYN, Leard CA, Hansen CJ, et al . The Recruit Assessment Program (RAP) Experience With Adverse Childhood Experiences (ACE) Questions. San Diego, Calif: Naval Health Research Center; 2006. Publication NHRC report 06-04.
41. Merrill LL, Newell CE, Milner JS, et al. Prevalence of premilitary adult sexual victimization and aggression in a Navy recruit sample. *Mil Med.* 1998;163:209-212.
42. Merrill LL, Newell CE, Thomsen CJ, et al. Childhood abuse and sexual revictimization in a female Navy recruit sample. *J Trauma Stress.* 1999;12:211-225.

**PEDIARIX® [Diphtheria and Tetanus Toxoids and Acellular Pertussis Adsorbed, Hepatitis B (Recombinant) and Inactivated Poliovirus Vaccine Combined]**

The following is a brief summary only; see full prescribing information for complete product information.

**CONTRAINDICATIONS:** Hypersensitivity to any component of the vaccine, including yeast, neomycin, and polymyxin B, is a contraindication (see DESCRIPTION in complete prescribing information). Do not use PEDIARIX after a serious allergic reaction (e.g., anaphylaxis) temporally associated with a previous dose of this vaccine or with any components of this vaccine. Because of the uncertainty as to which component of the vaccine might be responsible, do not give further vaccination with any of these components; or, refer such individuals to an allergist for evaluation. The following events are contraindications to administration of PEDIARIX: encephalopathy (e.g., coma, decreased level of consciousness, prolonged seizures) within 7 days of administration of a previous dose of a pertussis-containing vaccine that is not attributable to another identifiable cause; progressive neurologic disorder, including infantile spasms, uncontrolled epilepsy, or progressive encephalopathy. Do not vaccinate individuals with these conditions until a treatment regimen has been established and the condition has stabilized.

**WARNINGS:** Administration of PEDIARIX is associated with higher rates of fever relative to separately administered vaccines. In a safety study that evaluated medically attended fever after PEDIARIX or separately administered vaccines when coadministered with 7-valent pneumococcal and Hib conjugate vaccines, infants who received PEDIARIX had a higher rate of medical encounters for fever within the first 4 days following the first vaccination. In some infants, these encounters included the performance of diagnostic studies to evaluate other causes of fever (see ADVERSE REACTIONS). The tip cap and the rubber plunger of the needleless prefilled syringes contain dry natural latex rubber that may cause allergic reactions in latex sensitive individuals. The vial stopper is latex-free. If any of the following events occur in temporal relation to receipt of DTwP or a vaccine containing an acellular pertussis component, consider carefully whether to give any pertussis vaccine, including PEDIARIX: temperature of ≥40.5°C (105°F) within 48 hours not due to another identifiable cause; collapse or shock-like state (hypotonic-hyporesponsive episode) within 48 hours; persistent, inconsolable crying lasting ≥3 hours, occurring within 48 hours; seizures with or without fever occurring within 3 days. If Guillain-Barré syndrome occurs within 6 weeks of receipt of prior vaccine containing tetanus toxoid, the decision to give any tetanus toxoid-containing vaccine, including PEDIARIX, should be based on careful consideration of the potential benefits and possible risks. If tetanus toxoid is withheld, other available vaccines should be given, as indicated. The decision to administer a pertussis-containing vaccine to individuals with stable central nervous system (CNS) disorders must be made by the physician on an individual basis, with consideration of all relevant factors, and assessment of potential risks and benefits for that individual. Advise the parent or guardian of the potential increased risk involved (see PRECAUTIONS). For children at higher risk for seizures than the general population, an appropriate antipyretic may be administered at the time of vaccination and for the ensuing 24 hours according to the respective prescribing information recommended dosage to reduce the possibility of post-vaccination fever. The ACIP has published guidelines for vaccination of persons with recent or acute illness (www.cdc.gov/nip).

**PRECAUTIONS:** PEDIARIX should be given with caution in children with bleeding disorders such as hemophilia or thrombocytopenia and in children on anticoagulant therapy, with steps taken to avoid the risk of hematoma following the injection. Before the injection of any biological, the physician should take all reasonable precautions to prevent allergic or other adverse reactions. Epinephrine injection (1:1,000) and other appropriate agents used for the control of immediate allergic reactions must be immediately available should an acute anaphylactic reaction occur. Immunosuppressed individuals, including those receiving immunosuppressive therapy, may not develop the expected immune response. The ACIP has published guidelines for vaccination of persons on such therapies (www.cdc.gov/nip). **Drug Interactions:** For information regarding concomitant administration with other vaccines, refer to DOSAGE AND ADMINISTRATION in complete prescribing information. Do not mix PEDIARIX with any other vaccine in the same syringe or vial. **Carcinogenesis, Mutagenesis, Impairment of Fertility:** PEDIARIX has not been evaluated for carcinogenic or mutagenic potential, or for impairment of fertility. **Pregnancy:** Pregnancy Category C: PEDIARIX is not indicated for women of child-bearing age. Animal reproduction studies have not been conducted with PEDIARIX. It is not known whether PEDIARIX can cause fetal harm when administered to a pregnant woman or if PEDIARIX can affect reproductive capacity. **Geriatric Use:** PEDIARIX is not indicated for use in adult populations. **Pediatric Use:** Safety and effectiveness of PEDIARIX in infants younger than 6 weeks of age have not been evaluated. PEDIARIX is not recommended for persons 7 years of age or older.

**ADVERSE REACTIONS:** A total of 23,849 doses of PEDIARIX have been administered to 8,088 infants who received one or more doses as part of a 3-dose primary series during 14 clinical studies. The most common adverse reactions observed in clinical trials were local injection site reactions (pain, redness, or swelling), fever, and fussiness. In comparative studies, administration of PEDIARIX was associated with higher rates of fever relative to separately administered vaccines (see WARNINGS and ADVERSE REACTIONS Table 1). The prevalence of fever was highest on the day of vaccination and the day following vaccination. More than 96% of episodes of fever resolved within the 4-day period following vaccination (i.e., the period including the day of vaccination and the next 3 days). In the largest of the 14 studies, conducted in Germany, safety data were available for 4,666 infants who received PEDIARIX administered concomitantly at separate sites with 1 of 4 *Haemophilus influenzae* type b (Hib) vaccines at 3, 4, and 5 months of age and for 768 infants in the control group that received INFANRIX® (Diphtheria and Tetanus Toxoids and Acellular Pertussis Vaccine Adsorbed), Hib conjugate vaccine, and oral poliovirus vaccine (OPV) separately. Data on adverse events were collected by parents using standardized diary cards for 4 consecutive days following each vaccine dose (i.e., day of vaccination and the next 3 days). Infants were also monitored for unsolicited adverse events that occurred within 30 days following vaccination using diaries which were returned at subsequent visits and were supplemented by spontaneous reports and a medical history as reported by parents. More than 95% of study participants were white.

In a US study, the safety of PEDIARIX administered to 673 infants was compared to the safety of separately administered INFANRIX, ENGERIX-B® [Hepatitis B Vaccine (Recombinant)], inactivated poliovirus vaccine (IPV) in 335 infants. In both groups, infants received Hib and 7-valent pneumococcal conjugate vaccines concomitantly at separate sites. All vaccines were administered at 2, 4, and 6 months of age. The study was powered to evaluate fever >101.3° F following dose 1. Data on solicited adverse events were collected by parents using standardized diary cards for 4 consecutive days following each vaccine dose (i.e., day of vaccination and the next 3 days) and are presented in Table 1. Telephone follow-up was conducted 1 month and 6 months after the third vaccination to inquire about serious adverse events. At the 6-month follow-up, information also was collected on new onset of chronic illnesses. 638 subjects who received PEDIARIX and 313 subjects who received INFANRIX, ENGERIX-B, and IPV completed the 6-month follow-up. Among subjects in both study groups combined, 69% were white, 18% were Hispanic, 7% were black, 3% were Oriental, and 3% were of other racial/ethnic groups.

The adverse event information from clinical trials provides a basis for identifying adverse events that appear to be related to vaccine use and for approximating rates. However, because clinical trials are conducted under widely varying conditions, adverse event rates observed in the clinical trials of a vaccine cannot be directly compared to rates in the clinical trials of another vaccine, and may not reflect the rates observed in practice. As with any vaccine, there is the possibility that broad use of PEDIARIX could reveal adverse events not observed in clinical trials.

**Deaths:** In 14 clinical trials, 5 deaths were reported among 8,088 (0.06%) recipients of PEDIARIX and 1 death was reported among 2,287 (0.04%) recipients of comparator vaccines. Causes of death in the group that received PEDIARIX included 2 cases of Sudden Infant Death Syndrome (SIDS) and one case of each of the following: Convulsive disorder, congenital immunodeficiency with sepsis, and neuroblastoma. One case of SIDS was reported in the comparator group. The rate of SIDS among all recipients of PEDIARIX across the 14 trials was 0.25/1,000. The rate of SIDS observed for recipients of PEDIARIX in the German safety study was 0.2/1,000 infants (reported rate of SIDS in Germany in the latter part of the 1990s was 0.7/1,000 newborns). The reported rate of SIDS in the United States from 1990 to 1994 was 1.2/1,000 live births. By chance alone, some cases of SIDS can be expected to follow receipt of pertussis-containing vaccines.

**Serious Adverse Events:** Within 30 days following any dose of vaccine in the US safety study in which all subjects received concomitant pneumococcal and Hib conjugate vaccines, 7 serious adverse events were reported in 7 subjects (1% [7/673]) who received PEDIARIX (1 case each of pyrexia, gastroenteritis, and culture negative clinical sepsis and 4 cases of bronchiolitis) and 5 serious adverse events were reported in 4 subjects (1% [4/335]) who received INFANRIX, ENGERIX-B, and IPV (uteropelvic junction obstruction and testicular atrophy in one subject and 3 cases of bronchiolitis).

**Onset of Chronic Illnesses:** In the US safety study in which all subjects received concomitant pneumococcal and Hib conjugate vaccines, 21 subjects (3%) who received PEDIARIX and 14 subjects (4%) who received INFANRIX, ENGERIX-B, and IPV reported new onset of a chronic illness during the period from 1 to 6 months following the last dose of study vaccines. Among the chronic illnesses reported in the subjects who received PEDIARIX, there were 4 cases of asthma and 1 case each of diabetes mellitus and chronic neutropenia. There were 4 cases of asthma in subjects who received INFANRIX, ENGERIX-B, and IPV.

**Seizures:** In the German safety study over the entire study period, 6 subjects in the group that received PEDIARIX reported seizures. Two of these subjects had a febrile seizure, 1 of whom also developed afebrile seizures. The remaining 4 subjects had afebrile seizures, including 2 with infantile spasms. Two subjects reported seizures within 7 days following vaccination (1 subject had both febrile and afebrile seizures, and 1 subject had afebrile seizures), corresponding to a rate of 0.22 seizures per 1,000 doses (febrile seizures 0.07 per 1,000 doses, afebrile seizures 0.14 per 1,000 doses). No subject who received concomitant INFANRIX, Hib vaccine, and OPV reported seizures. In a separate German study that evaluated the safety of INFANRIX in 22,505 infants who received 66,867 doses of INFANRIX administered as a 3-dose primary series, the rate of seizures within 7 days of vaccination with INFANRIX was 0.13 per 1,000 doses (febrile seizures 0.0 per 1,000 doses, afebrile seizures 0.13 per 1,000 doses). Over the entire study period in the US safety study in which all subjects received concomitant pneumococcal and Hib conjugate vaccines, 4 subjects in the group that received PEDIARIX reported seizures. Three of these subjects had a febrile seizure and 1 had an afebrile seizure. Over the entire study period, 2 subjects in the group that received INFANRIX, ENGERIX-B, and IPV reported febrile seizures. There were no afebrile seizures in this group. No subject in either study group had seizures within 7 days following vaccination.

**Other Neurological Events of Interest:** No cases of hypotonic-hyporesponsiveness or encephalopathy were reported in either the German safety study or the US safety study.

**Solicited Adverse Events:** Table 1 presents data from the US safety study on solicited local and systemic adverse events within 4 days of vaccination with PEDIARIX or INFANRIX, ENGERIX-B, and IPV, administered concomitantly with Hib and 7-valent pneumococcal conjugate vaccines. In this study, medical attention (a visit to or from medical personnel) for fever within 4 days following vaccination was sought in the group who received PEDIARIX for 8 infants after the first dose (1.2%), 1 infant following the second dose (0.2%), and 5 infants following the third dose (0.8%) (Table 1). Following dose 2, medical attention for fever was sought for 2 infants (0.6%) who received separately administered vaccines (Table 1). Among infants who had a medical visit for fever within 4 days following vaccination, 9 of 14 who received PEDIARIX and 1 of 2 who received separately administered vaccines, had one or more diagnostic studies performed to evaluate the cause of fever.

**Safety of PEDIARIX after a previous dose of hepatitis B vaccine:** Limited data are available on the safety of administering PEDIARIX after a previous dose of hepatitis B vaccine. In 2 separate studies, 160 Moldovan infants and 96 US infants, respectively, received 3 doses of PEDIARIX following 1 previous dose of hepatitis B vaccine. Neither study was designed to detect significant differences in rates of adverse events associated with PEDIARIX administered after a previous dose of hepatitis B vaccine compared to PEDIARIX administered without a previous dose of hepatitis B vaccine.

**Table 1. Percentage of US Infants With Solicited Local Reactions or Systemic Adverse Events Within 4 Days of Vaccination* at 2, 4, and 6 Months of Age With PEDIARIX Administered Concomitantly With Hib Conjugate Vaccine and 7-valent Pneumococcal Conjugate Vaccine (PCV7) or With Separate Concomitant Administration of INFANRIX, ENGERIX-B, IPV, Hib Conjugate Vaccine, and PCV7 (Modified ITT cohort)**

| | PEDIARIX, Hib Vaccine, & PCV7 | | | INFANRIX, ENGERIX-B, IPV, Hib Vaccine, & PCV7 | | |
|---|---|---|---|---|---|---|
| | Dose 1 | Dose 2 | Dose 3 | Dose 1 | Dose 2 | Dose 3 |
| **Local†** | | | | | | |
| **N** | **671** | **653** | **648** | **335** | **323** | **315** |
| Pain, any | 36.1 | 36.1 | 31.2 | 31.9 | 30.0 | 29.8 |
| Pain, grade 2 or 3 | 11.5 | 10.9 | 10.6 | 9.0 | 8.7 | 8.9 |
| Pain, grade 3 | 2.4 | 2.5 | 1.7 | 2.7 | 1.5 | 1.3 |
| Redness, any | 29.9§ | 37.2 | 40.1 | 18.2 | 32.8 | 39.0 |
| Redness, >5 mm | 6.0§ | 9.6§ | 12.7§ | 1.8 | 5.9 | 7.3 |
| Redness, >20 mm | 0.9 | 1.2§ | 2.8 | 0.3 | 0.0 | 1.9 |
| Swelling, any | 17.3§ | 26.5§ | 28.7 | 9.6 | 20.4 | 24.8 |
| Swelling, >5 mm | 5.8§ | 9.6§ | 9.3§ | 1.8 | 5.0 | 4.1 |
| Swelling, >20 mm | 1.9 | 2.5§ | 3.1 | 0.6 | 0.0 | 1.3 |
| **Systemic** | | | | | | |
| **N** | **667** | **644** | **645** | **333** | **321** | **311** |
| Fever‡, ≥100.4°F | 27.9§ | 38.8§ | 33.5§ | 19.8 | 30.2 | 23.8 |
| Fever‡, >101.3°F | 7.0 | 14.1§ | 8.8 | 4.5 | 9.7 | 5.8 |
| Fever‡, >102.2°F | 2.2§ | 3.6 | 3.4 | 0.3 | 3.1 | 2.3 |
| Fever‡, >103.1°F | 0.4 | 1.4 | 1.1 | 0.0 | 0.3 | 0.3 |
| Fever‡, M.A. | 1.2§ | 0.2 | 0.8 | 0.0 | 0.6 | 0.0 |
| **N** | **671** | **653** | **648** | **335** | **323** | **315** |
| Drowsiness, any | 57.2 | 51.6 | 40.9 | 54.0 | 48.3 | 38.4 |
| Drowsiness, grade 2 or 3 | 15.8 | 13.8 | 11.4 | 17.6 | 12.4 | 11.1 |
| Drowsiness, grade 3 | 2.5 | 1.2 | 0.9 | 3.6 | 0.6 | 1.9 |
| Irritability/Fussiness, any | 60.5 | 64.9 | 61.1 | 61.5 | 61.6 | 56.5 |
| Irritability/Fussiness, grade 2 or 3 | 19.8 | 27.9§ | 25.2§ | 19.4 | 21.1 | 19.4 |
| Irritability/Fussiness, grade 3 | 3.4 | 4.4 | 3.5 | 3.9 | 3.4 | 3.2 |
| Loss of appetite, any | 30.4 | 30.6 | 26.2 | 27.8 | 26.6 | 23.8 |
| Loss of appetite, grade 2 or 3 | 6.6 | 7.8§ | 5.9 | 5.1 | 3.4 | 5.4 |
| Loss of appetite, grade 3 | 0.7 | 0.3 | 0.2 | 0.6 | 0.3 | 0.0 |

Modified ITT cohort = all vaccinated subjects for whom safety data were available

N = number of infants for whom at least one symptom sheet was completed; for fever, numbers exclude missing temperature recordings or tympanic measurements.

M.A. = Medically attended (a visit to or from medical personnel).

Grade 2 defined as sufficiently discomforting to interfere with daily activities.

Grade 3 defined as preventing normal daily activities.

* Within 4 days of vaccination defined as day of vaccination and the next 3 days.

† Local reactions at the injection site for PEDIARIX or INFANRIX.

‡ Rectal temperatures or axillary temperatures increased by 1°C to derive equivalent rectal temperature.

§ Rate significantly higher in the group that received PEDIARIX compared to separately administered vaccines [p value < 0.05 (2-sided Fisher Exact test) or the 95% CI on the difference between groups (Separate minus PEDIARIX) does not include 0].

**Postmarketing Reports With PEDIARIX:** Worldwide voluntary reports of adverse events received for PEDIARIX since market introduction of this vaccine are listed below. This list includes serious adverse events or events which have a suspected causal connection to components of PEDIARIX or other vaccines or drugs. Because these events are reported voluntarily from a population of uncertain size, it is not always possible to reliably estimate their frequency or establish a causal relationship to vaccine exposure. *Cardiac Disorders:* Cyanosis. *Gastrointestinal Disorders:* Diarrhea, vomiting. *General Disorders and Administrative Site Conditions:* Fatigue, injection site cellulitis, injection site induration, injection site itching, injection site nodule/lump, injection site pain, injection site reactions, injection site redness, injection site swelling, injection site warmth, irritability, limb pain, limb swelling, pyrexia, Sudden Infant Death Syndrome. *Immune System Disorders:* Anaphylactic reaction, anaphylactoid reaction, hypersensitivity. *Infections and Infestations:* Upper respiratory tract infection. *Investigations:* Abnormal liver function tests. *Metabolism and Nutrition Disorders:* Anorexia. *Nervous System Disorders:* Bulging fontanelle, convulsions, depressed level of consciousness, febrile convulsion, hypotonia, hypotonic-hyporesponsive episode, lethargy, somnolence. *Psychiatric Disorders:* Crying, insomnia, irritability, nervousness, restlessness, screaming, unusual crying. *Respiratory, Thoracic and Mediastinal Disorders:* Apnea, dyspnea. *Skin and Subcutaneous Tissue Disorders:* Angioedema, erythema, rash, urticaria. *Vascular Disorders:* Pallor, petechiae.

**Postmarketing Reports With INFANRIX and/or ENGERIX-B:** Worldwide voluntary reports of adverse events received for INFANRIX and/or ENGERIX-B in children younger than 7 years of age but not already reported for PEDIARIX are listed below. This list includes serious adverse events or events which have a suspected causal connection to components of INFANRIX and/or ENGERIX-B or other vaccines or drugs. Because these events are reported voluntarily from a population of uncertain size, it is not always possible to reliably estimate their frequency or establish a causal relationship to vaccine exposure. *Blood and Lymphatic System Disorders:* Idiopathic thrombocytopenic purpura[a,b], lymphadenopathy[a], thrombocytopenia[a,b]. *Gastrointestinal Disorders:* Abdominal pain[b], intussusception[a,b], nausea[b]. *General Disorders and Administrative Site Conditions:* Asthenia[b], malaise[b]. *Hepatobiliary Disorders:* Jaundice[b]. *Immune System Disorders:* Anaphylactic shock[a], serum sickness–like disease[b]. *Musculoskeletal and Connective Tissue Disorders:* Arthralgia[b], myalgia[b]. *Nervous System Disorders:* Encephalopathy[a], headache[b]. *Skin and Subcutaneous Tissue Disorders:* Alopecia[b], erythema multiforme[b], pruritus[a,b], Stevens-Johnson syndrome[a]. [[a] Following INFANRIX; [b] Following ENGERIX-B]

**Reporting Adverse Events:** Report the occurrence following immunization of any event set forth in the Vaccine Injury Table from the National Childhood Vaccine Injury Act including: Anaphylaxis or anaphylactic shock within 7 days, encephalopathy or encephalitis within 7 days, brachial neuritis within 28 days, or an acute complication or sequelae (including death) of an illness, disability, injury, or condition referred to above, or any events that would contraindicate further doses of PEDIARIX. These events should be reported to VAERS. The VAERS toll-free number is 1-800-822-7967. Reporting forms may also be obtained at the VAERS website at www.vaers.hhs.gov.

Manufactured by **GlaxoSmithKline Biologicals**, Rixensart, Belgium, US License 1617

Distributed by **GlaxoSmithKline**, Research Triangle Park, NC 27709



Full prescribing information for PEDIARIX is available at www.GSKVaccines.com/Pediarix.

BRS-PE:L3

Now:
The Purple Pill™ is FDA-approved for use in kids 12 to 17 years old with GERD

# NEXIUM for the NEXT GENERATION

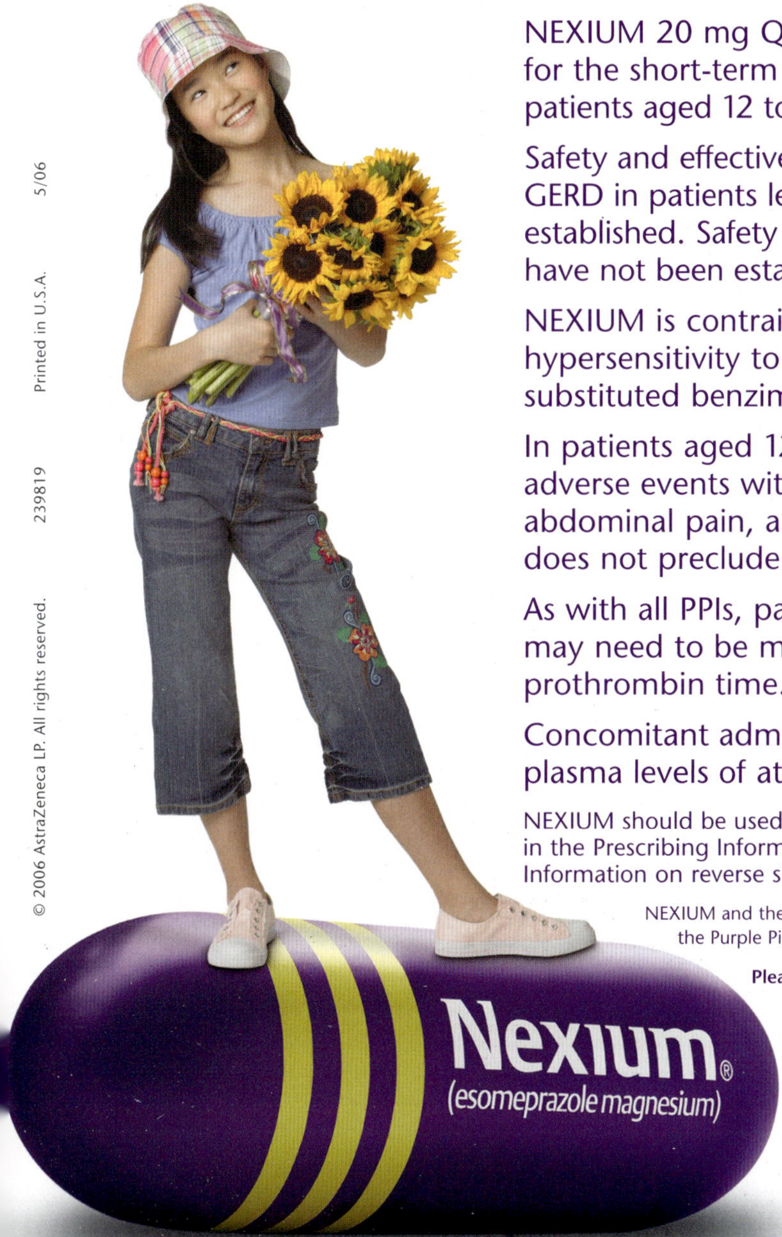


NEXIUM 20 mg QD and NEXIUM 40 mg QD are approved for the short-term treatment (up to 8 weeks) of GERD in patients aged 12 to 17 years.

Safety and effectiveness for the treatment of symptomatic GERD in patients less than 12 years of age have not been established. Safety and effectiveness for other pediatric uses have not been established.

NEXIUM is contraindicated in patients with known hypersensitivity to any component of the formulation or to substituted benzimidazoles.

In patients aged 12 to 17 years, the most frequently reported adverse events with NEXIUM include headache, diarrhea, abdominal pain, and nausea. Symptomatic response to therapy does not preclude the presence of gastric malignancy.

As with all PPIs, patients treated concomitantly with warfarin may need to be monitored for increases in INR and prothrombin time.

Concomitant administration of esomeprazole may reduce the plasma levels of atazanavir.

NEXIUM should be used only for the conditions, dosages, and durations specified in the Prescribing Information. Please see the brief summary of full Prescribing Information on reverse side.

NEXIUM and the color purple as applied to the capsule are registered trademarks and the Purple Pill is a trademark of the AstraZeneca group of companies.

**Please visit our Web site at www.Nexium-us.com**

**Nexium®**
(esomeprazole magnesium)

AstraZeneca

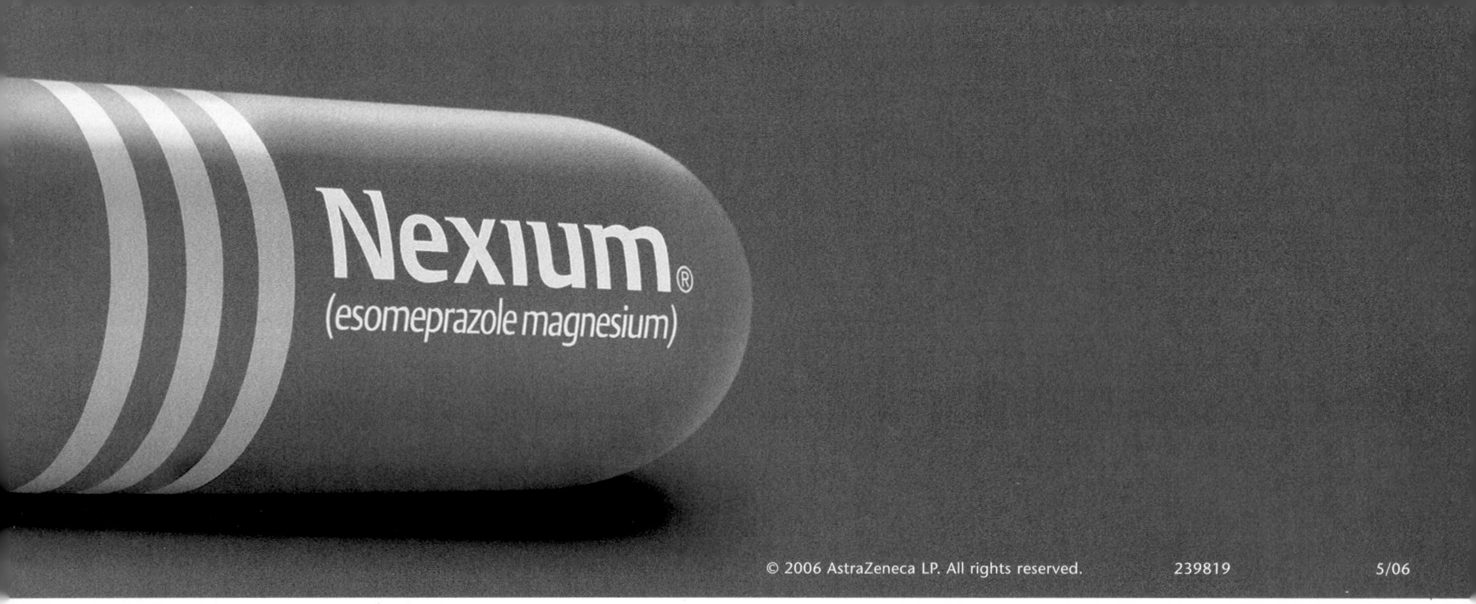


# NEXIUM® *(esomeprazole magnesium)*

## 20-mg, 40-mg Delayed-Release Capsules

**BRIEF SUMMARY** of Prescribing Information.

**INDICATIONS AND USAGE Treatment of GERD** NEXIUM is indicated for the short-term treatment (4 to 8 weeks) in the healing and symptomatic resolution of diagnostically confirmed erosive esophagitis; the maintenance of symptom resolution and healing of erosive esophagitis (controlled studies do not extend beyond 6 months); the treatment of heartburn and other symptoms associated with GERD; **Risk Reduction of NSAID-Associated Gastric Ulcer; *H.pylori* Eradication to Reduce the Risk of Duodenal Ulcer Recurrence.**

**CONTRAINDICATIONS** NEXIUM is contraindicated in patients with known hypersensitivity to any component of the formulation or to substituted benzimidazoles.

**PRECAUTIONS General** Symptomatic response to therapy with NEXIUM does not preclude the presence of gastric malignancy. Atrophic gastritis has been noted occasionally in gastric corpus biopsies from patients treated long-term with omeprazole, of which NEXIUM is an enantiomer. **Information for Patients** NEXIUM Delayed-Release Capsules should be swallowed whole and taken at least one hour before meals. For patients who have difficulty swallowing capsules, one tablespoon of applesauce can be added to an empty bowl and the NEXIUM Delayed-Release Capsule can be opened, and the pellets carefully emptied onto the applesauce. The pellets should be mixed with the applesauce and then swallowed immediately. The applesauce used should not be hot and should be soft enough to be swallowed without chewing. The pellets should not be chewed or crushed. The pellet/applesauce mixture should not be stored for future use. Antacids may be used while taking NEXIUM. **Drug Interactions** Esomeprazole is extensively metabolized in the liver by CYP2C19 and CYP3A4. *In vitro* and *in vivo* studies have shown that esomeprazole is not likely to inhibit CYPs 1A2, 2A6, 2C9, 2D6, 2E1 and 3A4. No clinically relevant interactions with drugs metabolized by these CYP enzymes would be expected. Drug interaction studies have shown that esomeprazole does not have any clinically significant interactions with phenytoin, warfarin, quinidine, clarithromycin or amoxicillin. Post-marketing reports of changes in prothrombin measures have been received among patients on concomitant warfarin and esomeprazole therapy. Increases in INR and prothrombin time may lead to abnormal bleeding and even death. Patients treated with proton pump inhibitors and warfarin concomitantly may need to be monitored for increases in INR and prothrombin time. Esomeprazole may potentially interfere with CYP2C19, the major esomeprazole metabolizing enzyme. Coadministration of esomeprazole 30 mg and diazepam, a CYP2C19 substrate, resulted in a 45% decrease in clearance of diazepam. Increased plasma levels of diazepam were observed 12 hours after dosing and onwards. However, at that time, the plasma levels of diazepam were below the therapeutic interval, and thus this interaction is unlikely to be of clinical relevance. Coadministration of oral contraceptives, diazepam, phenytoin, or quinidine did not seem to change the pharmacokinetic profile of esomeprazole. Concomitant administration of esomeprazole may reduce the plasma levels of atazanavir. Studies evaluating concomitant administration of esomeprazole and either naproxen (non-selective NSAID) or rofecoxib (COX-2 selective NSAID) did not identify any clinically relevant changes in the pharmacokinetic profiles of esomeprazole or these NSAIDs. Esomeprazole inhibits gastric acid secretion. Therefore, esomeprazole may interfere with the absorption of drugs where gastric pH is an important determinant of bioavailability (eg, ketoconazole, iron salts and digoxin). **Carcinogenesis, Mutagenesis, Impairment of Fertility** The carcinogenic potential of esomeprazole was assessed using omeprazole studies. In two 24-month oral carcinogenicity studies in rats, omeprazole at daily doses of 1.7, 3.4, 13.8, 44.0 and 140.8 mg/kg/day (about 0.7 to 57 times the human dose of 20 mg/day expressed on a body surface area basis) produced gastric ECL cell carcinoids in a dose-related manner in both male and female rats; the incidence of this effect was markedly higher in female rats, which had higher blood levels of omeprazole. Gastric carcinoids seldom occur in the untreated rat. In addition, ECL cell hyperplasia was present in all treated groups of both sexes. In one of these studies, female rats were treated with 13.8 mg omeprazole/kg/day (about 5.6 times the human dose on a body surface area basis) for 1 year, then followed for an additional year without the drug. No carcinoids were seen in these rats. An increased incidence of treatment-related ECL cell hyperplasia was observed at the end of 1 year (94% treated vs 10% controls). By the second year the difference between treated and control rats was much smaller (46% vs 26%) but still showed more hyperplasia in the treated group. Gastric adenocarcinoma was seen in one rat (2%). No similar tumor was seen in male or female rats treated for 2 years. For this strain of rat no similar tumor has been noted historically, but a finding involving only one tumor is difficult to interpret. A 78-week mouse carcinogenicity study of omeprazole did not show increased tumor occurrence, but the study was not conclusive. Esomeprazole was negative in the Ames mutation test, in the *in vivo* rat bone marrow cell chromosome aberration test, and the *in vivo* mouse micronucleus test. Esomeprazole, however, was positive in the *in vitro* human lymphocyte chromosome aberration test. Omeprazole was positive in the *in vitro* human lymphocyte chromosome aberration test, the *in vivo* mouse bone marrow cell chromosome aberration test, and the *in vivo* mouse micronucleus test. The potential effects of esomeprazole on fertility and reproductive performance were assessed using omeprazole studies. Omeprazole at oral doses up to 138 mg/kg/day in rats (about 56 times the human dose on a body surface area basis) was found to have no effect on reproductive performance of parental animals. **Pregnancy** *Teratogenic Effects. Pregnancy Category B* Teratology studies have been performed in rats at oral doses up to 280 mg/kg/day (about 57 times the human dose on a body surface area basis) and in rabbits at oral doses up to 86 mg/kg/day (about 35 times the human dose on a body surface area basis) and have revealed no evidence of impaired fertility or harm to the fetus due to esomeprazole. There are, however, no adequate and well-controlled studies in pregnant women. Because animal reproduction studies are not always predictive of human response, this drug should be used during pregnancy only if clearly needed. Teratology studies conducted with omeprazole in rats at oral doses up to 138 mg/kg/day (about 56 times the human dose on a body surface area basis) and in rabbits at doses up to 69 mg/kg/day (about 56 times the human dose on a body surface area basis) did not disclose any evidence for a teratogenic potential of omeprazole. In rabbits, omeprazole in a dose range of 6.9 to 69.1 mg/kg/day (about 5.5 to 56 times the human dose on a body surface area basis) produced dose-related increases in embryo-lethality, fetal resorptions, and pregnancy disruptions. In rats, dose-related embryo/ fetal toxicity and postnatal developmental toxicity were observed in offspring resulting from parents treated with omeprazole at 13.8 to 138.0 mg/kg/day (about 5.6 to 56 times the human doses on a body surface area basis). There are no adequate and well-controlled studies in pregnant women. Sporadic reports have been received of congenital abnormalities occurring in infants born to women who have received omeprazole during pregnancy. **Nursing Mothers** The excretion of esomeprazole in milk has not been studied. However, omeprazole concentrations have been measured in breast milk of a woman following oral administration of 20 mg. Because esomeprazole is likely to be excreted in human milk, because of the potential for serious adverse reactions in nursing infants from esomeprazole, and because of the potential for tumorigenicity shown for omeprazole in rat carcinogenicity studies, a decision should be made whether to discontinue nursing or to discontinue the drug, taking into account the importance of the drug to the mother. **Pediatric Use** Use of NEXIUM in adolescent patients 12 to 17 years of age for short-term treatment of GERD is supported by a) extrapolation of results, already included in the currently approved labeling, from adequate and well-controlled studies that supported the approval of NEXIUM for adults, and b) safety and pharmacokinetic studies performed in adolescent patients. (See **CLINICAL PHARMACOLOGY, Pharmacokinetics,** *Pediatric* for pharmacokinetic information.) The safety and effectiveness of NEXIUM for the treatment of symptomatic GERD in patients <12 years of age have not been established. The safety and effectiveness of NEXIUM for other pediatric uses have not been established. **12 to 17 Years of Age GERD** In a multi-center, randomized, double-blind, parallel-group study, 149 adolescent patients (12 to 17 years of age; 89 female; 124 Caucasian, 15 Black, 10 Other) with clinically diagnosed GERD were treated with either NEXIUM 20 mg or NEXIUM 40 mg once daily for up to 8 weeks to evaluate safety and tolerability. Patients were not endoscopically characterized as to the presence or absence of erosive esophagitis. The most frequently reported (at least 2%) treatment related adverse events in these patients were headache (8.1%), abdominal pain (2.7%), diarrhea (2%) and nausea (2%). No new safety concerns were identified. **Geriatric Use** Of the total number of patients who received NEXIUM in clinical trials, 1459 were 65 to 74 years of age and 354 patients were ≥75 years of age. No overall differences in safety and efficacy were observed between the elderly and younger individuals, and other reported clinical experience has not identified differences in responses between the elderly and younger patients, but greater sensitivity of some older individuals cannot be ruled out.

**ADVERSE REACTIONS** The safety of NEXIUM was evaluated in over 15,000 patients (aged 18-84 years) in clinical trials worldwide including over 8,500 patients in the United States and over 6,500 patients in Europe and Canada. Over 2,900 patients were treated in long-term studies for up to 6-12 months. In general, NEXIUM was well tolerated in both short and long-term clinical trials. A study was performed evaluating the safety of NEXIUM in pediatric patients aged 12-17 for the treatment of symptomatic GERD (see **PRECAUTIONS – Pediatric Use**). The safety in the treatment of healing of erosive esophagitis was assessed in four randomized comparative clinical trials, which included 1,240 patients on NEXIUM 20 mg, 2,434 patients on NEXIUM 40 mg, and 3,008 patients on omeprazole 20 mg daily. The most frequently occurring adverse events (≥1%) in all three groups was headache (5.5, 5.0, and 3.8, respectively) and diarrhea (no difference among the three groups). Nausea, flatulence, abdominal pain, constipation, and dry mouth occurred at similar rates among patients taking NEXIUM or omeprazole. Additional adverse events that were reported as possibly or probably related to NEXIUM with an incidence <1% are listed below by body system: ***Body as a Whole:*** abdomen enlarged, allergic reaction, asthenia, back pain, chest pain, chest pain substernal, facial edema, peripheral edema, hot flushes, fatigue, fever, flu-like disorder, generalized edema, leg edema, malaise, pain, rigors; ***Cardiovascular:*** flushing, hypertension, tachycardia; ***Endocrine:*** goiter; ***Gastrointestinal:*** bowel irregularity, constipation aggravated, dyspepsia, dysphagia, dysplasia GI, epigastric pain, eructation, esophageal disorder, frequent stools, gastroenteritis, GI hemorrhage, GI symptoms not otherwise specified, hiccup, melena, mouth disorder, pharynx disorder, rectal disorder, serum gastrin increased, tongue disorder, tongue edema, ulcerative stomatitis, vomiting; ***Hearing:*** earache, tinnitus; ***Hematologic:*** anemia, anemia hypochromic, cervical lymphoadenopathy, epistaxis, leukocytosis, leukopenia, thrombocytopenia; ***Hepatic:*** bilirubinemia, hepatic function abnormal, SGOT increased, SGPT increased; ***Metabolic/Nutritional:*** glycosuria, hyperuricemia, hyponatremia, increased alkaline phosphatase, thirst, vitamin B12 deficiency, weight increase, weight decrease; ***Musculoskeletal:*** arthralgia, arthritis aggravated, arthropathy, cramps, fibromyalgia syndrome, hernia, polymyalgia rheumatica; ***Nervous System/Psychiatric:*** anorexia, apathy, appetite increased, confusion, depression aggravated, dizziness, hypertonia, nervousness, hypoesthesia, impotence, insomnia, migraine, migraine aggravated, paresthesia, sleep disorder, somnolence, tremor, vertigo, visual field defect; ***Reproductive:*** dysmenorrhea, menstrual disorder, vaginitis; ***Respiratory:*** asthma aggravated, coughing, dyspnea, larynx edema, pharyngitis, rhinitis, sinusitis; ***Skin and Appendages:*** acne, angioedema, dermatitis, pruritus, pruritus ani, rash, rash erythematous, rash maculo-papular, skin inflammation, sweating increased, urticaria; ***Special Senses:*** otitis media, parosmia, taste loss, taste perversion; ***Urogenital:*** abnormal urine, albuminuria, cystitis, dysuria, fungal infection, hematuria, micturition frequency, moniliasis, genital moniliasis, polyuria; ***Visual:*** conjunctivitis, vision abnormal. Endoscopic findings that were reported as adverse events include: duodenitis, esophagitis, esophageal stricture, esophageal ulceration, esophageal varices, gastric ulcer, gastritis, hernia, benign polyps or nodules, Barrett's esophagus, and mucosal discoloration. Two placebo-controlled studies were conducted in 710 patients for the treatment of symptomatic gastroesophageal reflux disease. The most common adverse events that were reported as possibly or probably related to NEXIUM were diarrhea (4.3%), headache (3.8%), and abdominal pain (3.8%). Postmarketing Reports – There have been spontaneous reports of adverse events with postmarketing use of esomeprazole. These reports occurred rarely and are listed below by body system: ***Blood And Lymphatic System Disorders:*** agranulocytosis, pancytopenia; ***Eye Disorders:*** blurred vision; ***Gastrointestinal Disorders:*** pancreatitis; ***Hepatobiliary Disorders:*** hepatitis with or without jaundice; ***Immune System Disorders:*** anaphylactic reaction/shock; ***Musculoskeletal And Connective Tissue Disorders:*** myalgia; ***Psychiatric Disorders:*** depression; ***Skin and Subcutaneous Tissue Disorders:*** alopecia, erythema multiforme, Stevens-Johnson syndrome, toxic epidermal necrolysis (TEN, some fatal). Other adverse events not observed with NEXIUM, but occurring with omeprazole can be found in the omeprazole package insert, **ADVERSE REACTIONS** section.

**OVERDOSAGE** A single oral dose of esomeprazole at 510 mg/kg (about 103 times the human dose on a body surface area basis), was lethal to rats. The major signs of acute toxicity were reduced motor activity, changes in respiratory frequency, tremor, ataxia, and intermittent clonic convulsions. There have been some reports of overdosage with esomeprazole. Reports have been received of overdosage with omeprazole in humans. Doses ranged up to 2,400 mg (120 times the usual recommended clinical dose). Manifestations were variable, but included confusion, drowsiness, blurred vision, tachycardia, nausea, diaphoresis, flushing, headache, dry mouth, and other adverse reactions similar to those seen in normal clinical experience (see omeprazole package insert-**ADVERSE REACTIONS**). No specific antidote for esomeprazole is known. Since esomeprazole is extensively protein bound, it is not expected to be removed by dialysis. In the event of overdosage, treatment should be symptomatic and supportive. As with the management of any overdose, the possibility of multiple drug ingestion should be considered. For current information on treatment of any drug overdose, a certified Regional Poison Control Center should be contacted. Telephone numbers are listed in the Physicians' Desk Reference (PDR) or local telephone book. **DOSAGE AND ADMINISTRATION** Please see full Prescribing Information for recommended dosages and dosage adjustments for **Special Populations** for NEXIUM.


Distributed by: AstraZeneca LP, Wilmington, DE 19850
Product of France 31026-02 Rev. 04/06 240260

AstraZeneca

ARTICLE

# Dextromethorphan Abuse in Adolescence

## An Increasing Trend: 1999-2004

*Jodi K. Bryner, PharmD; Uerica K. Wang, PharmD; Jenny W. Hui, PharmD; Merilin Bedodo, PharmD; Conan MacDougall, PharmD; Ilene B. Anderson, PharmD*

**Objectives:** To analyze the trend of dextromethorphan abuse in California and to compare these findings with national trends.

**Design:** A 6-year retrospective review.

**Setting:** California Poison Control System (CPCS), American Association of Poison Control Centers (AAPCC), and Drug Abuse Warning Network (DAWN) databases from January 1, 1999, to December 31, 2004.

**Participants:** All dextromethorphan abuse cases reported to the CPCS, AAPCC, and DAWN. The main exposures of dextromethorphan abuse cases included date of exposure, age, acute vs long-term use, coingestants, product formulation, and clinical outcome.

**Main Outcome Measure:** The annual proportion of dextromethorphan abuse cases among all exposures reported to the CPCS, AAPCC, and DAWN databases.

**Results:** A total of 1382 CPCS cases were included in the study. A 10-fold increase in CPCS dextromethorphan abuse cases from 1999 (0.23 cases per 1000 calls) to 2004 (2.15 cases per 1000 calls) (odds ratio, 1.48; 95% confidence interval, 1.43-1.54) was identified. Of all CPCS dextromethorphan abuse cases, 74.5% were aged 9 to 17 years; the frequency of cases among this age group increased more than 15-fold during the study (from 0.11 to 1.68 cases per 1000 calls). Similar trends were seen in the AAPCC and DAWN databases. The highest frequency of dextromethorphan abuse occurred among adolescents aged 15 and 16 years. The most commonly abused product was Coricidin HBP Cough & Cold Tablets.

**Conclusions:** Our study revealed an increasing trend of dextromethorphan abuse cases reported to the CPCS that is paralleled nationally as reported to the AAPCC and DAWN. This increase was most evident in the adolescent population.

*Arch Pediatr Adolesc Med. 2006;160:1217-1222*

DEXTROMETHORPHAN HAS been used safely for years as a cough suppressant and is available in many over-the-counter (OTC) cough and cold preparations. Whereas therapeutic doses of dextromethorphan act at the sigma receptor to produce its antitussive effects, high doses are metabolized to dextrorphan, an active metabolite that antagonizes *N*-methyl-D-aspartate receptors.[1] Because of its similar pharmacology to phencyclidine and ketamine, dextrorphan and, to a lesser degree, dextromethorphan may produce dissociative hallucinations at high doses.[2,3] In addition, tachycardia, hypertension, agitation, ataxia, and psychosis also have been reported following high-dose dextromethorphan.[4-7]

Dextromethorphan abuse was recognized as early as the 1960s when it was marketed as the sole active ingredient in Romilar, an OTC product that was voluntarily removed from the market because of abuse.[8] Since the late 1990s, adolescents have been increasingly abusing OTC dextromethorphan products because of their easy accessibility and false perception of safety. Several states, such as California, North Dakota, Texas, and New York, have even proposed legislation to control the sale of dextromethorphan-containing products to minors. There are numerous slang names for dextromethorphan, such as CCC, Triple C, DXM, Dex, Poor Man's PCP, Skittles, and Robo.[9] Many of these slang terms refer to particular brand name products containing dextromethorphan. Two previously reported studies, one in California[6] and another in Texas,[10] identified Coricidin products (Schering-Plough HealthCare Products Inc, Kenilworth, NJ) as agents of abuse with a high prevalence in the ado-

Author Affiliations: Department of Clinical Pharmacy, School of Pharmacy, University of California, San Francisco (Drs Bryner, Wang, Hui, Bedodo, MacDougall, and Anderson), and San Francisco Division, California Poison Control System (Dr Anderson).

lescent population. The Texas Poison Center study identified a possible increasing trend of Coricidin abuse from 1998 to 1999.

The goals of this retrospective review were to analyze the trend of dextromethorphan abuse in California and to compare the findings with national trends. We also hoped to gain insight into the particular products involved and the most common age groups abusing dextromethorphan, and the effect on health care facilities. Evaluating patterns of dextromethorphan abuse may help health care practitioners target interventions, such as prevention and treatment.

## METHODS

We conducted a retrospective case record review analyzing all suspected dextromethorphan abuse cases reported to the California Poison Control System (CPCS) from January 1, 1999, through December 31, 2004. The CPCS is a 24-hour emergency telephone consultation service that offers treatment advice to the public and health care professionals regarding poisonings and overdoses. The CPCS database consists of case records documenting all consultations. All data in the case records are collected by the CPCS staff in accordance with American Association of Poison Control Centers (AAPCC) guidelines.[11] This study was approved by the Committee on Human Research, University of California, San Francisco. Subject consent was not required because the study involved a retrospective review of case records, in which all patient identifiers were removed before evaluation.

Case records were identified for evaluation by electronically searching the CPCS database for all cases coded as abuse and containing any of the AAPCC dextromethorphan-containing generic or product codes. Cases were excluded if they involved any of the following: (1) drug information, (2) unintentional misuse, (3) duplicate cases, (4) product miscoded as dextromethorphan abuse, and (5) symptoms unrelated to dextromethorphan ingestion. Cases were reviewed by 1 of 4 data reviewers (J.K.B., U.K.W., J.W.H., or M.B.), with 183 (13.2%) of the 1382 cases undergoing a second review to ensure consistency. All major outcome cases underwent a second review. Data collected included age, sex, caller site, disposition, product ingested, dose form, coingestants, clinical symptoms, short- vs long-term use, ethanol level, and acetaminophen level. Outcomes were coded according to the AAPCC definitions.[11] Examples of each category include the following: (1) no effect; (2) minor effect (self-limiting minimal symptoms that generally resolve rapidly, including drowsiness, gastrointestinal symptoms, and/or sinus tachycardia); (3) moderate effect (more pronounced, prolonged, or systemic symptoms that are not life threatening, including agitation, disorientation, hallucinations, brief hypotension, and/or a single brief seizure); and (4) major effect (life-threatening symptoms or symptoms that resulted in significant residual disability, including cardiovascular and respiratory compromise and/or prolonged or multiple seizures).

The primary outcome measured was the proportion of dextromethorphan abuse cases among all cases reported to the CPCS yearly from 1999 to 2004. Secondary outcomes analyzed included the proportion of dextromethorphan abuse cases in patients aged 9 to 17 years, the proportion of users classified as long-term abusers, the proportion of solid vs other dose forms, the frequency of individual product exposures, and the frequency of clinical outcomes (classified as no effect, minor, moderate, or major). Changes in primary and secondary outcomes over the study years were analyzed using logistic regression. A multivariate logistic regression model was constructed to determine the effect of age, sex, year, presence of coingestants, and product on clinical outcome.

Data were analyzed from 2 additional sources reporting nationwide drug abuse. The first was composed of dextromethorphan abuse cases reported to the AAPCC from January 1, 1999, through December 31, 2004. The AAPCC data were derived from a written report generated from the Toxic Exposure Surveillance System involving human exposures to dextromethorphan reported as intentional abuse to US Poison Control Centers from 1999 to 2004 (AAPCC, Washington, DC, Report 27, unpublished data, December 16, 2005).[11] The second was composed of dextromethorphan abuse cases reported to the Substance Abuse and Mental Health Services Administration program, Drug Abuse Warning Network (DAWN), from January 1, 1999, through December 31, 2002.[12] Dextromethorphan-related exposures reported to DAWN are not currently available after 2002. The following data from CPCS were compared with data from the DAWN and AAPCC databases: (1) age distribution (for AAPCC only, not available through DAWN) and (2) total number of dextromethorphan abuse cases reported annually. Only the AAPCC cases for which the exact age was known and the age was at least 9 years were included in the analysis. The AAPCC and DAWN databases were analyzed for temporal trends in dextromethorphan reporting by logistic regression, and the proportion of dextromethorphan cases reported in adolescents was investigated in the AAPCC database. The general approach we used in this study of combining detailed analysis of CPCS data juxtaposed with general surveillance data from other sources parallels the methods previously used to study γ-hydroxybutyrate, another drug of abuse.[13]

## RESULTS

During the 6-year study period, the CPCS had 1411 reports coded as dextromethorphan abuse and all underwent manual case record review. Ultimately, 1382 dextromethorphan abuse cases were included in the final analysis. On review, 29 cases were excluded because of the following reasons: drug information cases (n=10), duplicate cases (n=2), product reported did not contain dextromethorphan (n=1), misclassified as abuse (n=14), and reported symptoms were unrelated to dextromethorphan ingestion (n=2). During the study, the CPCS received 1 336 475 human exposure calls.

From 1999 through 2004, the frequency of all dextromethorphan abuse cases reported to the CPCS increased 10-fold (**Table**). The average effect was an almost 50% increase in the frequency of reported cases each year compared with the previous year (odds ratio, 1.48; 95% confidence interval, 1.43-1.54). This increase in the number of dextromethorphan abuse cases (**Figure 1**) and the proportion of dextromethorphan cases among all exposures reported (**Figure 2**) was also seen in the data collected by the AAPCC (odds ratio, 1.31; 95% confidence interval, 1.29-1.33) and DAWN (through 2002) (odds ratio, 1.15; 95% confidence interval, 1.13-1.18). The CPCS dextromethorphan abuse reports are included in the cases reported to the AAPCC, but these alone would not account for the national AAPCC trend.

The overall increase in the frequency of dextromethorphan abuse cases was paralleled by an increase in the frequency of dextromethorphan abuse cases reported in

**Table. Dextromethorphan Abuse Cases Reported to the CPCS From 1999 Through 2004***

| Case Characteristics | 1999 | 2000 | 2001 | 2002 | 2003 | 2004 | All Years |
|---|---|---|---|---|---|---|---|
| CPCS data | | | | | | | |
| Dextromethorphan cases | | | | | | | |
| Total | 48 | 125 | 149 | 226 | 356 | 478 | 1382 |
| Those aged 9-17 y† | 23 (47.9) | 79 (63.2) | 114 (76.5) | 152 (67.3) | 286 (80.3) | 375 (78.5) | 1029 (74.5) |
| Total CPCS human exposure cases | 209 991 | 220 418 | 230 819 | 231 716 | 220 867 | 222 664 | 1 336 475 |
| Dextromethorphan cases/1000 calls | | | | | | | |
| All | 0.23 | 0.57 | 0.65 | 0.97 | 1.61 | 2.15 | 1.03 |
| Those aged 9-17 y | 0.11 | 0.36 | 0.49 | 0.66 | 1.30 | 1.68 | 0.77 |
| Case characteristics of CPCS data | | | | | | | |
| Males† | 30 (62.5) | 75 (60.0) | 105 (70.5) | 145 (64.2) | 184 (51.7) | 289 (60.5) | 828 (59.9) |
| Mean age, y | 21.5 | 18.8 | 17.9 | 17.4 | 16.6 | 16.6 | 18.1 |
| Median age, y | 18.0 | 16.0 | 16.0 | 16.0 | 15.0 | 16.0 | 16.0 |
| Disposition† | | | | | | | |
| HCF | 31 (64.6) | 78 (62.4) | 102 (68.5) | 132 (58.4) | 235 (66.0) | 303 (63.4) | 881 (63.7) |
| NHCF | 17 (35.4) | 47 (37.6) | 47 (31.5) | 94 (41.6) | 121 (34.0) | 175 (36.6) | 501 (36.3) |
| Long-term abusers† | 7 (14.6) | 8 (6.4) | 4 (2.7) | 8 (3.5) | 3 (0.8) | 2 (0.4) | 32 (2.3) |
| Outcome† | | | | | | | |
| Minor or no effect | 26 (54.2) | 80 (64.0) | 75 (50.3) | 137 (60.6) | 185 (52.0) | 227 (47.5) | 730 (52.8) |
| Moderate effect | 19 (39.6) | 42 (33.6) | 73 (49.0) | 83 (36.7) | 142 (39.9) | 219 (45.8) | 578 (41.8) |
| Major effect | 1 (2.1) | 0 | 1 (0.7) | 1 (0.4) | 2 (0.6) | 2 (0.4) | 7 (0.5) |
| Unknown | 2 (4.2) | 3 (2.4) | 0 | 5 (2.2) | 27 (7.6) | 30 (6.3) | 67 (4.8) |
| Most common products abused†‡ | | | | | | | |
| Coricidin HBP Cough & Cold Tablets | 9 (18.8) | 72 (57.6) | 106 (71.1) | 144 (63.7) | 248 (69.7) | 330 (69.0) | 909 (65.8) |
| Robitussin formulations with dextromethorphan | 11 (22.9) | 24 (19.2) | 27 (18.1) | 41 (18.1) | 38 (10.7) | 50 (10.5) | 191 (13.8) |
| Coricidin, other dextromethorphan-containing formulations | 3 (6.2) | 3 (2.4) | 0 | 7 (3.1) | 23 (6.5) | 26 (5.4) | 62 (4.5) |
| Nyquil formulations with dextromethorphan | 10 (20.8) | 9 (7.2) | 4 (2.7) | 5 (2.2) | 10 (2.8) | 10 (2.1) | 48 (3.5) |
| Slang term used to identify dextromethorphan | 0 | 3 (2.4) | 2 (1.3) | 14 (6.2) | 8 (2.2) | 17 (3.6) | 44 (3.2) |
| Tussin DM liquid | 1 (2.1) | 0 | 0 | 5 (2.2) | 3 (0.8) | 6 (1.3) | 15 (1.1) |
| Vicks formulations with dextromethorphan | 2 (4.2) | 3 (2.4) | 2 (1.3) | 1 (0.4) | 4 (1.1) | 2 (0.4) | 14 (1.0) |
| Other§ | 0 | 5 (4.0) | 1 (0.7) | 1 (0.4) | 8 (2.2) | 16 (3.3) | 31 (2.2) |
| Unknown dextromethorphan-containing product | 12 (25.0) | 6 (4.8) | 7 (4.7) | 8 (3.5) | 14 (3.9) | 21 (4.4) | 68 (4.9) |

Abbreviations: CPCS, California Poison Control System; HCF, health care facility; NHCF, non-HCF (home or other site).

*The age was unknown for 22 subjects; the sex was known for all subjects. The exact dates of the study were from January 1, 1999, through December 31, 2004.

†Data are given as number (percentage) of total for each year. Percentages may not total 100 because of rounding.

‡Coricidin HBP Cough & Cold Tablets are a combination of chlorpheniramine maleate and dextromethorphan hydrobromide and are manufactured by Schering-Plough HealthCare Products Inc, Kenilworth, NJ; Robitussin formulations are manufactured by Wyeth, Madison, NJ; Nyquil formulations are manufactured by Proctor & Gamble, Cincinnati, Ohio; Tussin DM is a combination of guaifenesin and dextromethorphan hydrobromide and is manufactured by various manufacturers; and Vicks formulations are manufactured by Proctor & Gamble.

§Individual brand name products each had a frequency of 10 or fewer.

adolescents (defined as those aged 9-17 years). During the 6-year study period, 74.5% of all reported CPCS dextromethorphan abuse cases involved adolescents. The overall median age was 16 years. The proportion of all dextromethorphan abuse cases that occurred in adolescents increased over the duration of the study according to the CPCS (odds ratio, 1.25; 95% confidence interval, 1.15-1.36) and AAPCC (odds ratio, 1.03; 95% confidence interval, 1.01-1.05) databases. The largest proportional increase in adolescent abuse was seen from 1999 to 2000 (Table). The highest frequency of dextromethorphan abuse in the CPCS and AAPCC databases was among adolescents aged 15 and 16 years (**Figure 3**). The younger adolescent age distribution is further underscored by the observation that in CPCS reporting the combined frequency among 12- to 13-year-old subjects exceeded that of 18-year-old subjects.

Of the 1382 cases of dextromethorphan abuse included in our study, the most commonly abused product was Coricidin HBP Cough & Cold Tablets. This was followed by dextromethorphan-containing Robitussin products (Wyeth, Madison, NJ) (Table). The proportion of abused dextromethorphan products represented by Coricidin HBP Cough & Cold Tablets increased over the study period (odds ratio, 1.23; 95% confidence interval, 1.13-1.26). This increasing trend in abuse of Coricidin HBP Cough & Cold Tablets corresponded to an increase in the number of exposures that involved a solid dose form of dextromethorphan (odds ratio, 1.43; 95% confidence interval, 1.31-1.56). In contrast to the increase in acute cases of dextromethorphan abuse, long-term abuse reports to the CPCS were uncommon (n=32) and declined over the study period (odds ratio, 0.51; 95% confidence interval, 0.40-0.64).

Most dextromethorphan cases resulted in minor (636 cases [46.0%]) or moderate (578 cases [41.8%]) outcomes. Seven cases (0.5%) had major outcomes. For the remaining cases, either no symptoms were reported (94 cases [6.8%]) or the outcome was unknown (67 cases [4.8%]) (Table). There were no fatalities reported. All 7 major outcome cases involved serious pulmonary complications, such as respiratory depression or aspiration requiring intubation. Five of the major outcome cases involved coingestants, 3 of which involved ethanol. Among

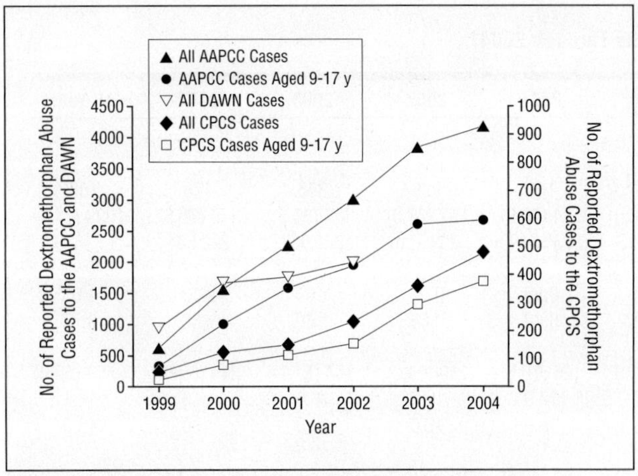


**Figure 1.** A comparison of California Poison Control System (CPCS), American Association of Poison Control Centers (AAPCC), and Drug Abuse Warning Network (DAWN)[12] dextromethorphan abuse cases. Dextromethorphan DAWN data were unavailable for 2003 and 2004. Dextromethorphan abuse reported to the AAPCC represents 15 543 cases; and to DAWN, 6447 cases.

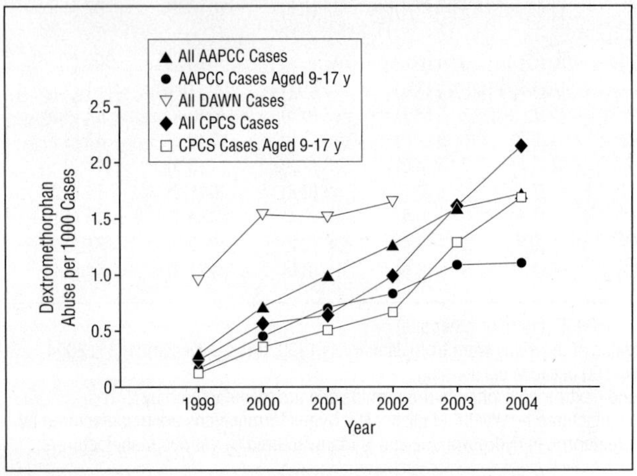


**Figure 2.** The proportion of California Poison Control System (CPCS), American Association of Poison Control Centers (AAPCC), and Drug Abuse Warning Network (DAWN)[12] dextromethorphan abuse cases compared with the total exposures reported to each database. Dextromethorphan DAWN data are unavailable for 2003 and 2004.

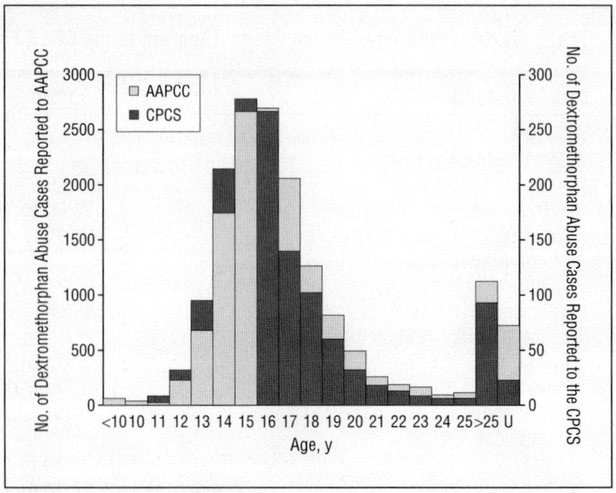


**Figure 3.** A comparison of the trends in abuse according to age for cases reported to the California Poison Control System (CPCS) and the American Association of Poison Control Centers (AAPCC) during the study. The age was not reported in 22 of the CPCS cases and in 733 of the AAPCC cases. U indicates unknown.

the major outcome cases, only 2 involved minors. There was an increase in combined moderate and major outcomes during the study (odds ratio, 1.09; 95% confidence interval, 1.01-1.17). A multivariate model incorporating study year, age, sex, presence of coingestants, and exposure to Coricidin HBP Cough & Cold Tablets showed an increased incidence of moderate and major outcomes among patients in later years (odds ratio, 1.09; 95% confidence interval, 1.01-1.18) and among male adolescents (odds ratio, 1.22; 95% confidence interval, 1.09-1.37).

Polysubstance use was reported by history in 278 (20.1%) of all subjects. The most common agents reported were ethanol (n=93), marijuana (n=40), opiates (n=23), acetaminophen (n=17), amphetamines (n=14), selective serotonin reuptake inhibitors (n=10), pseudoephedrine (n=10), and benzodiazepines (n=9). Self-reported ethanol coingestion was documented among 93 (6.7%) subjects; however, only 23 cases had laboratory confirmation. Three cases were coded as having major outcomes (levels ranged from 230-373 mg/dL), and 11 were coded as having moderate outcomes. Only 17 patients reported ingesting acetaminophen by history; however, there were 26 patients with confirmed laboratory acetaminophen levels (range, 9.1-111.0 μg/mL). More important, 8 patients had a delayed presentation to the hospital (range, 8 hours–4 days), and in 4 additional patients the time of ingestion was unknown. Sixteen patients received *N*-acetylcysteine therapy, of whom 7 experienced elevated transaminase levels. Of these 7 patients, 1 was a long-term alcohol user. Of the 26 subjects with acetaminophen involvement, 14 were coded as having a moderate outcome and 0 were coded as having a major outcome. There was no significant difference in the occurrence of the combined major and moderate outcomes between patients who did or did not have any coingestant (odds ratio, 0.96; 95% confidence interval, 0.83-1.14).

The most common adverse effects reported were tachycardia (n=593), lethargy (n=481), hypertension (n=289), confusion or altered mental status (n=277), mydriasis (n=251), agitation (n=171), gastrointestinal effects (n=159), dizziness (n=94), ataxia (n=83), hallucinations (n=80), slurred speech (n=77), nystagmus (n=75), fever (n=54), loss of consciousness (n=26), tachypnea (n=20), seizure (n=12), and hypotension (n=12).

## COMMENT

Our study reveals a 10-fold increase in all dextromethorphan abuse cases reported to the CPCS from 1999 through 2004. This increasing trend of dextromethorphan abuse is consistent with the national trend documented by the AAPCC, whose data revealed a 7-fold increase during the same time frame. In addition, DAWN also reported an overall increase in dextromethorphan abuse from 1999 to 2002, although the increase was not as pronounced. The highest frequency of abuse was in adolescents aged 15 and 16 years, as reported to the CPCS and the AAPCC. Abuse of solid dose forms increased more dramatically during the study, compared with the liquid formulations. According to CPCS reports, Coricidin HBP Cough & Cold Tablets was the most commonly reported dextromethorphan-containing product abused, followed by dextromethorphan-containing Robitussin formulations (Table). There may be multiple explanations for the apparent preference of Coricidin HBP Cough & Cold Tablets abuse, including widespread OTC availability, high dextromethorphan content, palatability of the tablet formulation, and, most important, its frequent promotion as a product of abuse on many Internet Web sites. An increase in combined moderate and major outcomes was also identified during the study. The explanation for this trend is likely multifactorial; however, it may be because of the increased abuse of Coricidin HBP Cough & Cold Tablets and the contribution of chlorpheniramine in the formulation following high doses. However, a detailed examination of the actual cause of this particular trend is beyond the scope of this study.

The increasing trend of teenage dextromethorphan abuse is multifactorial. Dextromethorphan is available in multiple OTC cough and cold products legally sold at pharmacies and most grocery stores. As little as 1 package may contain enough dextromethorphan to produce euphoric and hallucinatory effects.[14] Adolescents are increasingly abusing OTC medications because they are easily available and relatively inexpensive, and many have a false perception that even high doses of dextromethorphan are not dangerous. In contrast, other drugs of abuse, such as γ-hydroxybutyrate, methylenedioxymethamphetamine (Ecstasy), and lysergic acid diethylamide, which are not as easily accessible to minors, have shown an annual decline in use among adolescents and all age groups over the past few years.[13,15] Considering ease of availability as a reason for teenage abuse, it is not surprising that abuse of a readily available OTC medication like dextromethorphan, with its euphoric effects, is increasing. Another factor is that it is easy to fool parents because these OTC products are commonly kept in the household. Because dextromethorphan is an OTC medication, it lacks the stigma of a drug of abuse and there are numerous Web sites promoting dextromethorphan abuse and even providing instructions on how to abuse and manufacture the drug.[16,17] More and more children younger than 18 years have unsupervised access to the World Wide Web, including dextromethorphan abuse Web sites. The peer pressure that commonly plagues adolescents could certainly play an important role in the increasing abuse.

Another serious concern with taking large amounts of OTC cough and cold products for the dextromethorphan content involves toxicity from the hidden ingredients, such as pseudoephedrine, acetaminophen, and antihistamines. For example, high doses of acetaminophen may result in delayed liver failure.[18] Typically, the intoxication from the dextromethorphan resolves within 6 to 8 hours; however, acetaminophen may not even start to show signs of toxicity for 10 hours and, even then, the first signs may be gastrointestinal upset only. Unless these patients seek medical care, acetaminophen-induced hepatotoxicity may ensue. Our study revealed that of the 26 patients who had elevated serum acetaminophen levels, only 17 reported acetaminophen use by history. It is highly likely that some of these patients were unaware of their acetaminophen exposure because it is a common "hidden" ingredient in many OTC cough and cold products. Sixteen patients received the antidote, *N*-acetylcysteine, and 7 had elevated transaminase levels.

The major limitation of our study was the retrospective design, primarily because of incomplete documentation of clinical data on some of the poison center charts. Because the poison center reporting is a passive reporting system, calls to the poison center regarding drugs of abuse are usually secondary to an adverse reaction. To our knowledge, there is no study that correlates the true incidence of abuse in the general population to the incidence of poison center reports. Therefore, dextromethorphan abuse may be far higher than the cases reported in our study. Another limitation of our study is that laboratory testing of dextromethorphan is not routinely available at hospital laboratories. Consequently, our patients' dextromethorphan exposure was based on history rather than urine or blood test confirmation. In addition, dextromethorphan may trigger a false positive on the phencyclidine laboratory drug screen, resulting in some patients being falsely diagnosed as having phencyclidine intoxication when in actuality dextromethorphan was the agent responsible for the intoxication, further lowering the dextromethorphan incidence reported.[6] Moreover, dextromethorphan abuse is likely underreported to DAWN for 2 reasons. First, dextromethorphan was not a drug that was specifically listed on the DAWN data collection form during the early years of this study, but rather would only be documented in the "other" category. Second, dextromethorphan is a hidden ingredient in OTC cough and cold preparations and, therefore, may have been missed by the DAWN hospital medical record evaluator during the medical record review process. Last, another limitation of our study is our inability to attribute case-specific symptoms to dextromethorphan as opposed to other ingredients found in combination products. For example, in some cases, tachycardia, a common finding, could have been due, at least in part, to the antihistamine (eg, chlorpheniramine) or the decongestant (eg, pseudoephedrine) components in the OTC cough and cold products.

In conclusion, this study showed an increasing trend of dextromethorphan abuse over a 6-year period, particularly in adolescents younger than 18 years. The data from the CPCS showed a 10-fold increase in dextromethorphan abuse in all ages and a 15-fold increase in adolescents from 1999 through 2004. This increase in dextromethorphan abuse in adolescents is most likely due to the hallucinogenic effects of these easily accessible inexpensive OTC products and the false perception that high-dose dextromethorphan is safe. It is important for health care practitioners, manufacturers, and retail establishments selling dextromethorphan-containing products to be aware of increasing dextromethorphan abuse to educate and hopefully prevent dextromethorphan abuse and the ensuing toxicity from occurring. Preventive measures, such as placing dextromethorphan-containing products behind pharmacy counters, may be an effective action to limit this increasing trend of abuse in adolescents.

**Accepted for Publication:** July 20, 2006.
**Correspondence:** Ilene B. Anderson, PharmD, San Francisco Division, California Poison Control System, UCSF Box 1369, San Francisco, CA 94143-1369 (iba@calpoison.org).
**Author Contributions:** Dr Anderson had full access to all the data in the study and takes responsibility for the integrity of the data and the accuracy of the data analysis. *Study concept and design:* Bryner, Wang, Hui, Bedodo, and Anderson. *Acquisition of data:* Bryner, Wang, Hui, Bedodo, and Anderson. *Analysis and interpretation of data:* Bryner, Wang, Hui, Bedodo, MacDougall, and Anderson. *Drafting of the manuscript:* Bryner, Wang, Hui, Bedodo, and MacDougall. *Critical revision of the manuscript for important intellectual content:* Bryner, Wang, Hui, MacDougall, and Anderson. *Statistical analysis:* MacDougall. *Obtained funding:* Anderson. *Administrative, technical, and material support:* Bryner, Hui, and Bedodo. *Study supervision:* Anderson. *Background data search:* Bedodo.
**Financial Disclosure:** None reported.
**Funding/Support:** This study was supported in part by grant R01 DA 14935 from the National Institute on Drug Abuse.
**Role of the Sponsor:** The funding body had no role in data extraction and analyses, in the writing of the manuscript, or in the decision to submit the manuscript for publication.
**Additional Information:** This study was conducted as a partial requirement to earn a doctor of pharmacy degree from the School of Pharmacy, University of California, San Francisco, for the following authors: Bryner, Wang, Hui, and Bedodo.
**Acknowledgment:** We thank Terry S. Carlson, PharmD, at the CPCS, for his invaluable assistance as a computer systems analyst in extracting the poison center case records.

## REFERENCES

1. Ramachander G, Williams FD, Emele JF. Determination of dextrorphan in plasma and evaluation of bioavailability of dextromethorphan hydrobromide in humans. *J Pharm Sci.* 1977;66:1047-1048.
2. Ginski MJ, Witkin JM. Sensitive and rapid behavioral differentiation of *N*-methyl-D-aspartate receptor antagonists. *Psychopharmacology (Berl).* 1994;114:573-582.
3. Bobo WV, Fulton RB. Commentary on: severe manifestations of Coricidin intoxication. *Am J Emerg Med.* 2004;22:624-625.
4. Price LH, Lebel J. Dextromethorphan-induced psychosis [letter]. *Am J Psychiatry.* 2000;157:304.
5. Sharma A, Dewan V, Petty F. Acute psychosis with Coricidin cold medicine. *Ann Pharmacother.* 2005;39:1577-1578.
6. Banerji S, Anderson IB. Abuse of Coricidin HBP Cough & Cold Tablets: episodes recorded by a poison center. *Am J Health Syst Pharm.* 2001;58:1811-1814.
7. Kirages TJ, Sule HP, Mycyk MB. Severe manifestations of Coricidin intoxication. *Am J Emerg Med.* 2003;21:473-475.
8. Wolfe TR, Caravati EM. Massive dextromethorphan ingestion and abuse. *Am J Emerg Med.* 1995;13:174-176.
9. Dextromethorphan (DXM). [*www.streetdrugs.org* Web site.] http://www.streetdrugs.org/dxm.htm. Accessed March 18, 2006.
10. Baker SD, Borys DJ. A possible trend suggesting increased abuse of Coricidin exposures reported to the Texas Poison Network: comparing 1998 to 1999. *Vet Hum Toxicol.* 2002;44:169-171.
11. Watson WA, Litovitz TL, Rodgers GC Jr, et al. 2004 Annual report of the American Association of Poison Control Centers Toxic Exposure Surveillance System. *Am J Emerg Med.* 2005;23:589-666.
12. Drug Abuse Warning Network. ED mentions for respiratory agents by drug category: estimates for the coterminous US by half year: trends from the Drug Abuse Warning Network, final estimates 1995-2002: 2003 [report 2.9.0 and 2.10.0]. http://dawninfo.samhsa.gov/old_dawn/pubs_94_02/pickatable/drugtable1.asp. Accessed January 10, 2006.
13. Anderson IB, Kim SY, Dyer JE, et al. Trends in γ-hydroxybutyrate (GHB) and related drug intoxication: 1999 to 2003. *Ann Emerg Med.* 2006;47:177-183. doi:10.1016/j.annemergmed.2005.10.012.
14. The vaults of Erowid. [The Vaults of Erowid Web site.] http://www.erowid.org/chemicals/dxm/. Accessed March 18, 2006.
15. National Institute on Drug Abuse. Monitoring the Future Survey: overview of key findings, 2005. http://www.monitoringthefuture.org/. Accessed March 22, 2006.
16. The third plateau: beginner's guide to DXM. [The Third Plateau: Beginner's Guide to DXM Web site.] http://www.third-plateau.org/knowledgebase/beginners.shtml. Accessed April 24, 2006.
17. Dextroverse. [Dextroverse Web site.] http://www.dextroverse.org. Accessed February 19, 2006.
18. Rumack BH, Peterson RC, Koch GG, Amara IA. Acetaminophen overdose: 662 cases with evaluation of oral acetylcysteine treatment. *Arch Intern Med.* 1981;141:380-385.

# From Underdog

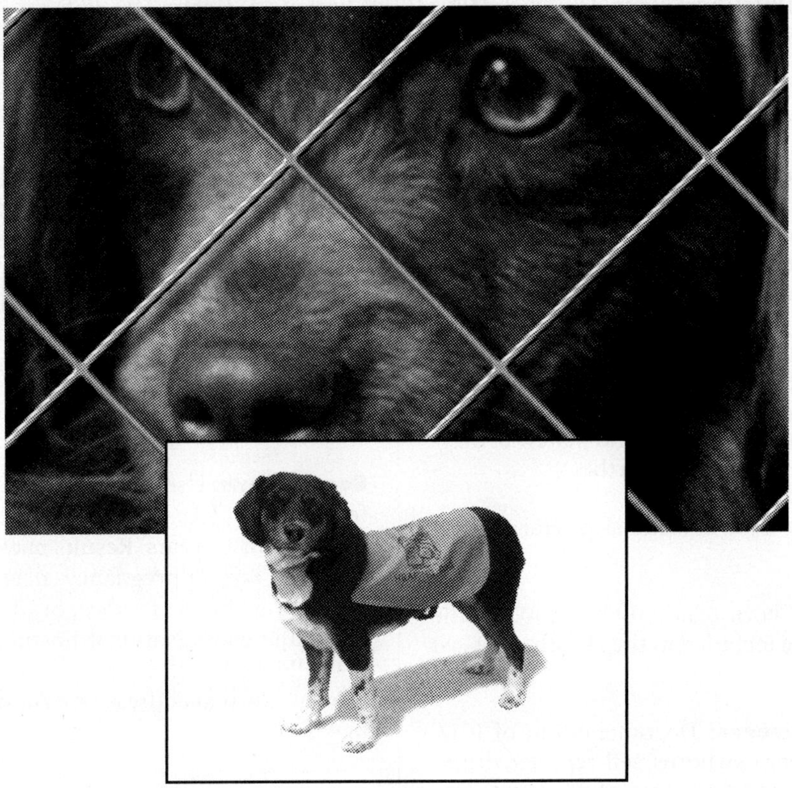

# to Wonder Dog!

For nearly a quarter of a century, Dogs for the Deaf has changed the destiny of hundreds of shelter dogs while enhancing the lives of people who are deaf or hearing impared. We've been able to do this because of people like you, people who support our efforts to rescue these lovable pups and train them to become the "ears" of those who need them.

We place these specially trained dogs nationwide at no cost to the recipient. Your contribution is the lifeblood of this special program, and we need your help to continue to make a difference.

Call us at **1-800-990-DOGS (3647)** or visit our website: www.dogsforthedeaf.org

**DOGS FOR THE DEAF, INC.**

10175 Wheeler Road • Central Point, Oregon 97502

**www.dogsforthedeaf.org**

ARTICLE

# Reduction in Newborns With Discharge Coding of In Utero Alcohol Effects in the United States, 1993 to 2002

*James M. Robbins, PhD; T. M. Bird, MS; John M. Tilford, PhD; J. Alex Reading, MS; Mario A. Cleves, PhD; Mary E. Aitken, MD, MPH; Charlotte M. Druschel, MD, MPH; Charlotte A. Hobbs, MD, PhD*

**Objective:** To determine whether use of the *International Classification of Diseases, Ninth Revision, Clinical Modification* (*ICD-9-CM*) code for fetal alcohol effects has declined during the past 10 years among hospitalized newborns in the United States.

**Design:** Trends in use of the *ICD-9-CM* code 760.71, "alcohol affecting the fetus," among newborns from 1993 through 2002 were compared with trends in self-reported drinking during pregnancy and maternal diagnoses of alcohol abuse during childbirth.

**Setting:** Sampled short-term, nonfederal general and specialty hospitals.

**Participants:** Infants born from 1993 to 2002 in the United States who were included in the Healthcare Cost and Utilization Project databases.

**Main Outcome Measures:** Documentation of *ICD-9-CM* code 760.71 among newborns, self-reported drinking during pregnancy, and diagnoses of maternal alcohol abuse during childbirth from 1993 through 2002.

**Results:** The prevalence of the *ICD-9-CM* code 760.71 for alcohol affecting the fetus, as documented in the discharge record of newborns, declined from 0.73 (95% confidence interval, 0.56-0.92) per 1000 live births in 1993 to 0.17 (95% confidence interval, 0.13-0.20) per 1000 live births in 2002. Rates declined concurrently with those of self-reported alcohol consumption during pregnancy and diagnoses of maternal alcohol abuse during childbirth.

**Conclusions:** Use of the *ICD-9-CM* code for alcohol affecting the fetus among newborns declined 75% throughout 10 years. Results may be due to decreases in drinking during pregnancy, decreases in disclosure of alcohol use by the mother, or more selective use of the discharge code. National hospital discharge databases may allow cost-effective monitoring of public health interventions that address rare conditions of the fetus and newborn.

*Arch Pediatr Adolesc Med. 2006;160:1224-1231*

SELF-REPORTED ALCOHOL USE during pregnancy has declined during the past 10 years.[1,2] Comparable longitudinal data on rates of newborns diagnosed as having in utero alcohol effects are not available. Newly developed national hospital discharge databases may allow effective monitoring of fetal alcohol diagnoses. Alcohol affecting the fetus is documented in the newborn medical record as *International Classification of Diseases, Ninth Revision, Clinical Modification* (*ICD-9-CM*) code 760.71. This code is intended to identify "noxious influences affecting fetus or newborn via the placenta or breast milk, specifically alcohol."[3(p485)] The newborn *ICD-9-CM* code may be viewed as a marker for problems associated with in utero exposure to alcohol.[4]

Alcohol effects on the fetus represent a spectrum of structural anomalies and behavioral and neurocognitive disabilities termed *fetal alcohol spectrum disorders*.[5] Children with fetal alcohol spectrum disorder often experience learning disabilities, mental retardation, and behavioral problems throughout life.[6,7] Children at the severe end of the spectrum will meet diagnostic criteria for fetal alcohol syndrome (FAS). Conclusive diagnosis of FAS is often not made until the child is 6 years or older.[8] Fetal alcohol spectrum disorder results directly from maternal alcohol consumption during pregnancy and is completely preventable if a woman does not drink alcohol when she is pregnant. The *ICD-9-CM* code 760.71 applied to the newborn is predictive of later identification of fetal alcohol spectrum disorder.[9,10]

**Author Affiliations:** Arkansas Center for Birth Defects Research and Prevention (Drs Robbins, Tilford, Cleves, and Hobbs), Department of Pediatrics, College of Medicine, University of Arkansas for Medical Sciences, and Arkansas Children's Hospital, Little Rock (Drs Robbins, Tilford, Cleves, Aitken, and Hobbs, Mr Bird, and Ms Reading); and Congenital Malformations Registry, New York State Department of Health, New York (Dr Druschel).

Because earlier identification of infants and children affected by in utero alcohol exposure facilitates earlier referral for needed care, prevention of secondary disabilities, and reduced risk of a subsequent pregnancy affected by alcohol,[11-13] it is important to monitor newborns suspected of alcohol effects or exposure. In this study, we used the Healthcare Cost and Utilization Project (HCUP) series of databases to examine *ICD-9-CM* diagnoses of 760.71, alcohol affecting the fetus, among hospitalized newborns during a 10-year period from 1993 through 2002. We determined whether changes in estimated rates of these diagnoses differed for white, black, and Hispanic newborns and whether changes were associated with household income. To offer evidence of the concurrent validity of changes in documentation of alcohol affecting the fetus, we assessed co-occurring changes in self-reported drinking during pregnancy based on a national sample and changes in diagnoses of alcohol abuse or dependency documented in the maternal medical record during childbirth.

## METHODS

### DATABASES

Data for this study came from 2 large national hospital discharge databases developed for the HCUP of the Agency for Healthcare Research and Quality (AHRQ) and the Behavioral Risk Factor Surveillance System (BRFSS), a national survey of self-reported behaviors and health risks. The HCUP Nationwide Inpatient Sample (NIS)[14] was used to examine yearly trends in newborn hospitalizations with documented *ICD-9-CM* code 760.71 for 10 years from 1993 through 2002. The NIS is designed to approximate a 20% stratified random sample of all US community hospitals from states that contribute their State Inpatient Databases to the HCUP. The NIS includes discharge information for all age groups and all payers from each sampled hospital. In 1993, 17 states contributed their data to NIS. In 2002, 35 states contributed data.

Because the NIS samples 20% of hospitals from participating states, some rare conditions of infancy and childhood might not be adequately represented. To guarantee proper sampling of a large number of discharges of infants and children, the AHRQ generated the Kids' Inpatient Database (KID)[15] for discharge years 1997 and 2000. For each year, the KID includes a 10% sample of all healthy newborn hospitalizations and an 80% sample of all other pediatric hospitalizations from short-term, nonfederal general and specialty hospitals. In 1997, 22 states participated in the KID, representing 2521 hospitals and 1.9 million discharge records from children aged 0 to 18 years. In 2000, 27 states participated, representing 2784 hospitals and 2.5 million discharge records from children aged 0 to 20 years. Only newborns (668 956 in 1997 and 784 191 in 2000) were included in this analysis.

The AHRQ has developed discharge weights to generate national estimates of hospitalizations from the NIS and the KID. With these weights, national estimates of hospitalizations and hospitalization rates are comparable across years despite the differing sampling designs of the NIS and KID and the varying number of states participating each year in the HCUP.[14,15] The HCUP databases have been used to generate national rates of newborns with birth defects,[16] study the impact of fortification of grains with folic acid on neural tube defects,[17] study the epidemiologic features of Kawasaki disease,[18] and investigate the hospital management of other rare conditions of infancy and childhood.[19]

Infants in the NIS and KID with the *ICD-9-CM* newborn discharge code 760.71, "noxious influences affecting fetus or newborn via the placenta or breast milk, specifically alcohol; including fetal alcohol syndrome,"[3(p485)] were identified. The *ICD-9-CM* code has been used to represent adverse effects on the newborn of maternal alcohol consumption during pregnancy.[20,21] It has been our experience that newborns are given the presumptive diagnosis when long-term alcohol use is documented or strongly suspected in the obstetric record and the newborn is observed to have intrauterine growth retardation, small head circumference, and/or abnormal facial features.[22]

The NIS was also used to determine the number of women with a documented diagnosis of alcohol abuse or dependence during childbirth. Alcohol abuse or dependence was measured by *ICD-9-CM* diagnosis codes 303.00 to 303.93 or 305.00 to 305.03. Childbirth was identified by diagnosis-related group codes 370 to 375[23,24] or *ICD-9-CM* V-codes V27.0 to V27.9. The combination of an alcohol-related diagnosis and childbirth-related diagnosis was used to measure changes over time in alcohol abuse diagnoses of the mother during childbirth.

Rates of drinking alcohol during pregnancy were estimated from the BRFSS data. The BRFSS is a national survey conducted yearly and coordinated by the Centers for Disease Control and Prevention (CDC).[25] The BRFSS sampling frame of adults 18 years and older has remained constant during the 10 years of study, thereby allowing comparison of rates over time. Questions are asked about any drinking and binge drinking (≥5 drinks at one time) in the past month and current pregnancy. Because no safe threshold of alcohol use during pregnancy has been established[11] and because women are known to underreport the amount of alcohol use during pregnancy,[26] reports of any drinking should be taken seriously.

### STATISTICAL ANALYSIS

Newborn hospitalization rates were calculated per 1000 newborns. Numbers of observed cases with a discharge *ICD-9-CM* diagnosis of 760.71 (alcohol affecting the fetus) were first computed from the NIS and the KID. Weights were then applied to the observed cases to derive national estimates. Similarly, numbers of all newborns were computed from the NIS and the KID, then weighted up to represent all hospital births in the United States. This value forms the denominator in the calculation of *ICD-9-CM* diagnosis rates per 1000 newborns. Statistical analyses were completed with Stata statistical software, version 8.0 (StataCorp, College Station, Tex), to take into account the complex sampling designs and sample weights of the NIS and the KID. The SVYRATIO command was used to calculate the proportion of newborn hospital births with *ICD-9-CM* documentation of alcohol affecting the fetus and associated 95% confidence intervals for both overall yearly rates and subpopulation rates. Differences in rates across years were compared using the LINCOM command. Ten-year trends toward decreasing (or increasing) rates were tested for significance with the Cochran-Armitage trend test.

Income is defined in the NIS and the KID as the median income of households in the census tract of residence of the patient. Income was classified for our analyses into 3 categories roughly corresponding to the top, middle, and bottom third of the income distribution each year. For example, in 2000 the top third of the distribution included households from census tracts with a yearly income of $45 000 or more. The middle third included households from tracts with a yearly income of $35 000 to $44 999. The bottom third included households from census tracts with a yearly income of less than $35 000.

Three mutually exclusive racial/ethnic codes (white, black, and Hispanic) are available in the NIS and the KID with suffi-

**Table 1. Rates of Documentation of Discharge Code 760.71 (Alcohol Affecting the Fetus) Among Hospitalized Newborns by Ethnicity, 1993-2002***

| | Rate (95% Confidence Interval) | | | | |
|---|---|---|---|---|---|
| Ethnicity | 1993 | 1994 | 1995 | 1996 | 1997 |
| All | 0.73 (0.56-0.92) | 0.62 (0.51-0.73) | 0.56 (0.47-0.66) | 0.53 (0.44-0.63) | 0.48 (0.40-0.56) |
| White | 0.53 (0.34-0.71) | 0.38 (0.29-0.46) | 0.41 (0.33-0.48) | 0.41 (0.31-0.51) | 0.36 (0.28-0.43) |
| Black | 2.03 (1.34-2.72) | 1.93 (1.39-2.47) | 1.65 (1.15-2.15) | 1.44 (1.10-1.78) | 1.23 (0.95-1.51) |
| Hispanic | 0.25 (0.11-0.39) | 0.25 (0.11-0.39) | 0.32 (0.21-0.43) | 0.29 (0.11-0.36) | 0.19 (0.10-0.28) |

(*continued*)

cient numbers of cases to allow for meaningful stratified analyses. Race-specific rates of alcohol affecting the fetus were calculated per 1000 newborn hospitalizations.

Some newborns require more intensive medical management owing to a variety of conditions and thus may be transferred from the birthing hospital to another acute care inpatient facility. To avoid double-counting these newborn cases, age of admission was limited to a maximum of 10 days, and those whose hospital disposition was listed as transferred to another short-term, acute care hospital were excluded from computation of rates.[27] These patients would likely be included (a single time) based on the discharge diagnosis from the hospital to which the newborn was transferred.

Numbers of maternal alcohol-related diagnoses were identified from the NIS. Weights were applied to the observed cases to derive national estimates and 95% confidence intervals per 1000 hospital births. The BRFSS databases for the years 1993 to 2002 were accessed to compute the percentage and 95% confidence intervals of pregnant women who reported any alcohol consumption during the past month.

## RESULTS

Estimated rates of *ICD-9-CM* code 760.71 documentation per 1000 live hospital births are presented in **Table 1**. In 1993, 2746 of 3 741 144 live births in the United States (0.73 per 1000 live births) received the discharge diagnosis. In 2002, 684 of 4 148 092 live births (0.17 per 1000 live births) received the diagnosis. This finding represents more than a 75% reduction in the rate of documentation of the 760.71 code during the study period. Documentation of code 760.71 among black newborns is approximately 4 times the rate for white newborns across 10 years of births. Hispanic newborns consistently have lower rates than black or white newborns. Cochran-Armitage trend tests confirm statistically significantly ($P<.001$) decreasing rates for the total and for each racial group.

Declines in estimated rates of documentation of alcohol affecting the fetus across time are depicted in **Figure 1** separately for white, black, and Hispanic newborns. The decline is most apparent among black newborns, although rates for all groups have decreased substantially during the decade examined.

In **Figure 2**, rates are presented separately for high, middle, and low income categories of infants. Across years, rates of documentation of alcohol affecting the fetus are highest for the lowest income category and lowest for the highest income category. Rates have declined consistently across each income category, most precipitously among those from areas with lower income. Cochran-Armitage trend tests confirm statistically significant ($P<.001$) decreases for each income category.

In **Table 2**, estimated rates of *ICD-9-CM* code 760.71 documented in the newborn medical record are presented for years 1997 and 2000 and are stratified by race and income. Absolute rates of the diagnosis have decreased most strikingly for lower-income black newborns (from 1.82 to 0.93 per 1000 live births; $P=.02$). Significant relative reductions in rates are also seen for middle- and higher-income white newborns. Rates for lower-income white newborns and middle- or higher-income black newborns were not significantly lower in 2000 than in 1997. Rates did not change significantly during this 4-year period for Hispanic newborns in any income category.

**Figure 3** presents estimated rates of diagnosis of alcohol affecting the fetus among hospitalized newborns superimposed on rates of drinking during pregnancy derived from the BRFSS[25] and rates of maternal alcohol abuse or dependence diagnoses during childbirth computed from the NIS. Rates of documentation of the *ICD-9-CM* code for alcohol affecting the fetus have declined concurrently with trends in drinking during pregnancy and trends in alcohol abuse or dependence diagnoses of the mother during childbirth. Cochran-Armitage trend tests confirm statistically significant ($P<.001$) decreases in drinking and alcohol diagnoses.

In **Figure 4**, estimated rates of documentation of alcohol affecting the fetus among hospitalized newborns derived from the NIS are presented along with comparable rates among hospitalized newborns generated from the CDC Birth Defects Monitoring Program (BDMP).[28-30] The BDMP, active from 1979 through 1993, relied on hospital discharge data contributed on a voluntary basis by participating hospitals. As seen from this figure, rates of documentation of code 760.71, as reported by the BDMP, were 0.10 per 1000 live births in 1979 and increased to 0.67 per 1000 live births by 1993.[20,21] By comparison, NIS-based rates begin at 0.36 per 1000 live births in 1988, peaking at 0.73 in 1993, then declining to 0.17 by 2002.

## COMMENT

Our study demonstrated a decline in the number of newborns with a discharge *ICD-9-CM* diagnosis of 760.71 (alcohol affecting the fetus) during the past decade: a 75%

**Table 1. Rates of Documentation of Discharge Code 760.71 (Alcohol Affecting the Fetus) Among Hospitalized Newborns by Ethnicity, 1993-2002 (cont)***

| | Rate (95% Confidence Interval) | | | | |
|---|---|---|---|---|---|
| Ethnicity | 1998 | 1999 | 2000 | 2001 | 2002 |
| All | 0.34 (0.27-0.41) | 0.25 (0.20-0.31) | 0.21 (0.17-0.24) | 0.18 (0.14-0.22) | 0.17 (0.13-0.20) |
| White | 0.21 (0.15-0.27) | 0.15 (0.10-0.19) | 0.11 (0.08-0.14) | 0.18 (0.11-0.24) | 0.08 (0.05-0.11) |
| Black | 0.90 (0.56-1.23) | 0.87 (0.48-1.26) | 0.73 (0.52-0.93) | 0.41 (0.22-0.60) | 0.56 (0.39-0.74) |
| Hispanic | 0.18 (0.09-0.26) | 0.09 (0.03-0.14) | 0.16 (0.10-0.22) | 0.13 (0.07-0.19) | 0.08 (0.03-0.13) |

*Data are from the Healthcare Cost and Utilization Project, Nationwide Inpatient Sample, 1993-2002. Rates are per 1000 live hospital births. Code 760.71 is from the *International Classification of Diseases, Ninth Revision, Clinical Modifications.*

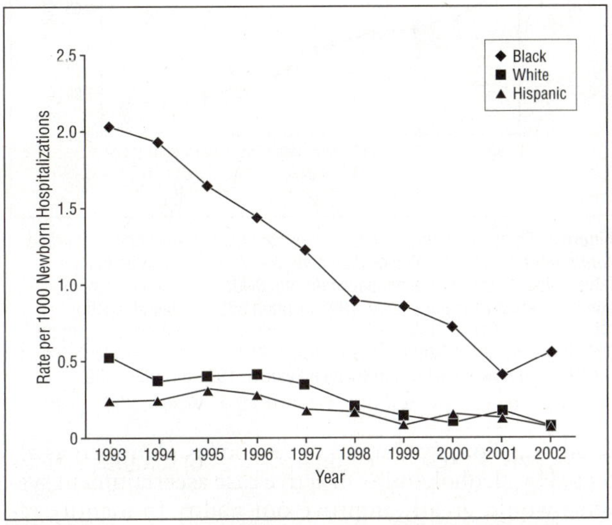


**Figure 1.** Rates of documentation of *International Classification of Diseases, Ninth Revision, Clinical Modification* code 760.71 (alcohol affecting the fetus) among hospitalized newborns by ethnicity, 1993 through 2002. Data are from the Healthcare Cost and Utilization Project, Nationwide Inpatient Sample.

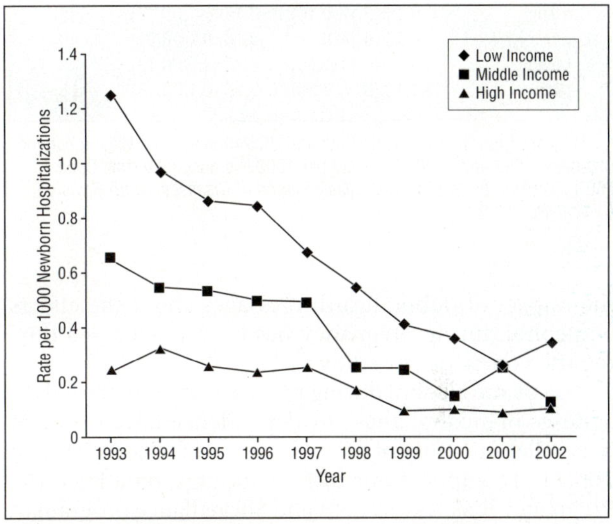


**Figure 2.** Rates of documentation of *International Classification of Diseases, Ninth Revision, Clinical Modification* code 760.71 (alcohol affecting the fetus) among hospitalized newborns by income, 1993 through 2002. Data are from the Healthcare Cost and Utilization Project, Nationwide Inpatient Sample.

reduction was observed from 1993 to 2002. Our results are consistent with a prior study[31] of infants born at Albert Einstein College of Medicine–affiliated hospitals from 1985 through 1996 and a study[2] documenting a declining prevalence of FAS in Washington state from 1993 to 1998. Our findings are also consistent with longitudinal data from the BDMP that measured earlier trends in diagnosis of alcohol affecting the fetus.[20,21]

Declines in use of the diagnosis for alcohol affecting the fetus were seen among white, black, and Hispanic newborns, but a far greater absolute decline was seen among black newborns. Within racial categories, rates declined significantly among lower-income black newborns and middle- and higher-income white newborns. Reductions in rates of documentation of alcohol affecting the fetus in the medical record paralleled reduced drinking during pregnancy and reduced maternal diagnosis of alcohol abuse and dependence during childbirth.[1,25]

Several explanations for these findings should be considered: (1) changes in preference for the discharge diagnosis code among health care professionals or coders, (2) changes in mothers' disclosure of alcohol use during pregnancy, and (3) changes in exposure to alcohol during pregnancy. The newborn diagnosis code 760.71 specifies only that an infant has been affected by alcohol. It is possible that health care professionals and coders have come to avoid this code. Public health campaigns and professional education may have altered the attitudes of health care professionals, making them increasingly less likely to apply a diagnosis that may be somewhat uncertain and potentially stigmatizing. Similarly, coders may have discontinued use of the code if insurers increasingly refused to pay for fetal alcohol–related hospital care.[22] We are not aware of evidence supporting this selective coding explanation.

The results we observed may be due to increased underreporting of alcohol use during pregnancy. Documentation of alcohol effects in the newborn medical record often depends on maternal self-report of drinking or documentation of alcohol use during pregnancy in the obstetric medical record. Underreporting of alcohol use during pregnancy is known to occur.[26] Maternal knowledge of the potential harmful effects of alcohol on the infant and potential loss of custody of the child if alcohol use is discovered may result in nondisclosure of drinking during pregnancy. It is not known whether nondisclosure has increased sufficiently during the study period to explain our findings. Related evidence suggests that

**Table 2. Rates of Documentation of Discharge Code 760.71 (Alcohol Affecting the Fetus) Among Hospitalized Newborns by Ethnicity and Income, 1997 and 2000***

| Ethnicity and Income Category | Rate (95% Confidence Interval) 1997 | 2000 | *P* Value |
|---|---|---|---|
| White | 0.22 (0.18-0.26) | 0.15 (0.13-0.17) | .007 |
| Low | 0.23 (0.16-0.29) | 0.25 (0.20-0.30) | .57 |
| Middle | 0.30 (0.19-0.40) | 0.17 (0.12-0.21) | .02 |
| High | 0.16 (0.12-0.20) | 0.08 (0.06-0.11) | .003 |
| Black | 1.22 (0.81-1.62) | 0.80 (0.66-0.94) | .06 |
| Low | 1.82 (1.07-2.58) | 0.93 (0.72-1.13) | .02 |
| Middle | 0.78 (0.60-0.96) | 0.74 (0.47-1.00) | .80 |
| High | 0.42 (0.28-0.56) | 0.45 (0.35-0.55) | .73 |
| Hispanic | 0.14 (0.12-0.16) | 0.15 (0.13-0.17) | .48 |
| Low | 0.16 (0.14-0.19) | 0.18 (0.14-0.21) | .49 |
| Middle | 0.15 (0.11-0.19) | 0.11 (0.08-0.13) | .08 |
| High | 0.12 (0.08-0.16) | 0.15 (0.13-0.18) | .18 |

*Data are from the Healthcare Cost and Utilization Project, Kids' Inpatient Database, 1997 and 2000. Rates are per 1000 live hospital births. Code 760.71 is from the *International Classification of Diseases, Ninth Revision, Clinical Modification.*

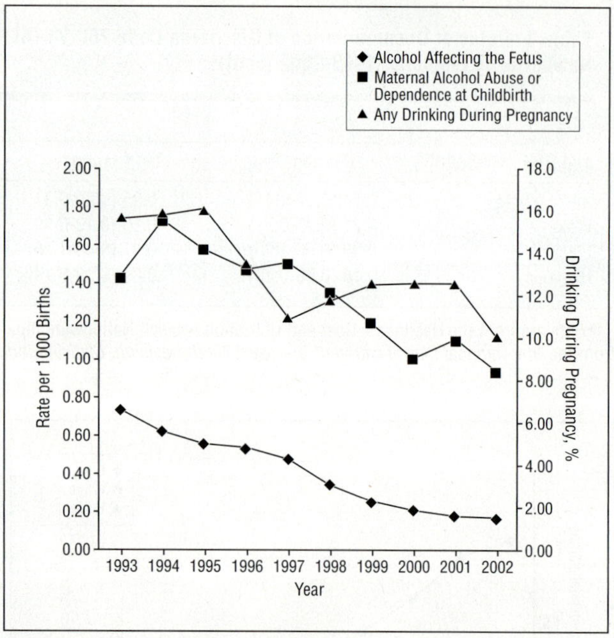


**Figure 3.** Rates of documentation of *International Classification of Diseases, Ninth Revision, Clinical Modification* code 760.71 (alcohol affecting the fetus), alcohol abuse or dependence during childbirth, and any alcohol consumption during pregnancy, 1993 through 2002. Rates of alcohol affecting the fetus and maternal alcohol abuse or dependence are from the Nationwide Inpatient Sample, 1993 through 2002; alcohol use rates are from the Behavioral Risk Factor Surveillance System, 1993 through 2002.

the impact of public health messages about the effects of alcohol during pregnancy has been unchanged during the course of our study.[32,33]

Use of any alcohol during pregnancy and maternal diagnoses of alcohol abuse or dependence have declined in parallel with rates of documentation of *ICD-9-CM* code 760.71. To support our BRFSS findings, data from the Pregnancy Risk Assessment and Surveillance program in 12 states with longitudinal data show that rates of self-reported drinking during the last 3 months of pregnancy declined significantly from 1993 to 1999 in 7 states. Drinking declined, although not significantly, in the remaining 5 states.[1] Drinking during the 3 months before conception, perhaps most representative of behavior during the early weeks of pregnancy before a woman is aware she is pregnant, declined significantly only in Washington state.[1] Public health campaigns, prenatal screening for drinking during pregnancy, and warning labels on bottles have had significant effects on drinking during pregnancy[33-37] and may partly explain our results.

Data on heavy or risky drinking patterns during pregnancy from the BRFSS show that self-reported binge drinking during pregnancy has not declined during the past 10 years.[25] These data are not consistent with our findings.

Our results point to the need for better surveillance of the effects of alcohol on the fetus in the United States. Currently, cases of FAS are reported to the National Birth Defects Prevention Network by participating states on a voluntary basis. State surveillance systems vary greatly in how aggressively cases of FAS are ascertained. As of 2004, 23 states did not collect data on FAS and 10 states relied exclusively on discharge data provided by hospitals.[38] Although fetal alcohol spectrum disorder continues to have a great impact on families, the health care system, and the educational system, we are currently without a comprehensive, well-funded program to monitor our prevention efforts in this regard. If rates of FAS are declining along with rates of newborns identified as affected by alcohol, uniform active case ascertainment systems would greatly improve our ability to identify responsible protective factors. A program in place in Washington state since 1997 uses facial photographic software and a 4-digit diagnostic code to ascertain cases of FAS among birth cohorts entering foster care. Findings from this model program have shown decreases in rates of FAS from 1993 to 1998 that parallel decreases in maternal alcohol use during pregnancy as reported to the Pregnancy Risk Assessment and Surveillance program.[2] As an alternative to this labor-intensive state ascertainment program, hospital discharge databases may represent a cost-effective method of monitoring national changes in the number of infants affected by maternal alcohol use over time.

The limitations of our study should be acknowledged. Because we have used an ecological design, we have no direct evidence in our analysis that cases of newborn hospitalizations with a documentation of *ICD-9-CM* 760.71 (alcohol affecting the fetus) were exposed to alcohol. We are unable to state that women who over time delivered fewer infants affected by alcohol were those who consumed less alcohol during pregnancy.

We are also limited by the use of the *ICD-9-CM* code. Dysmorphic features typical of older children with fetal alcohol spectrum disorders are not required for this code. The Institute of Medicine–based case definition of FAS used by many fetal alcohol spectrum disorders researchers[39-42] and the more recent CDC definition[8] require documentation by a physician of abnormal facial features consistent with FAS (including short palpebral fissures, abnormal philtrum, and thin upper lip), central ner-

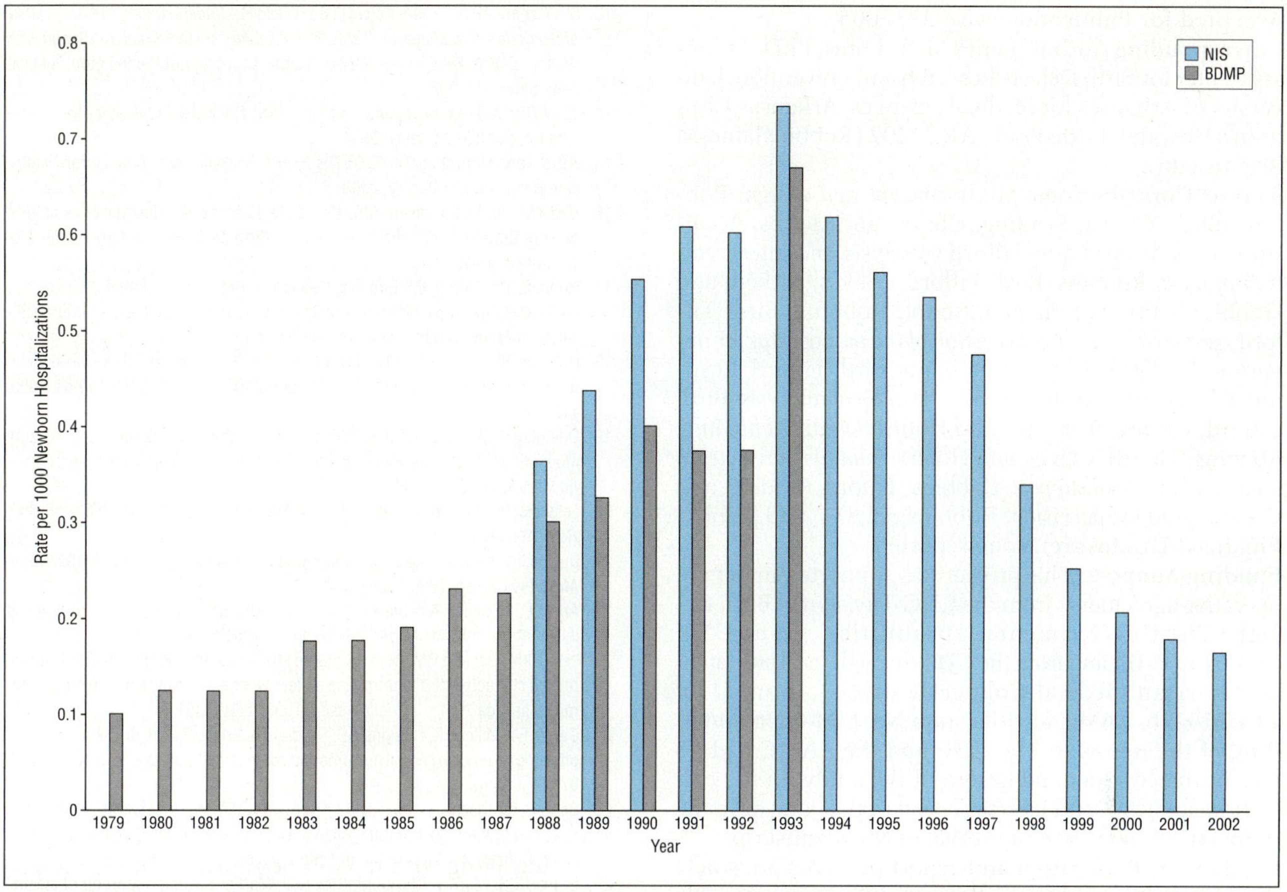


**Figure 4.** Rates of documentation of *International Classification of Diseases, Ninth Revision, Clinical Modification* code 760.71 (alcohol affecting the fetus) among hospitalized newborns, 1979 through 2002. Data from 1979 through 1993 are from the Centers for Disease Control and Prevention Birth Defects Monitoring Program (BDMP); data from 1988 through 2002 are from the Nationwide Inpatient Sample (NIS).

vous system abnormalities (including small head circumference, developmental delay, and mental retardation), and growth retardation (including low birth weight and delayed postnatal growth). Most of these criteria cannot be assessed reliably in the newborn period.[43-47] Typically, FAS is identified and diagnosed in the preschool or early school years.[8] Fox and Druschel[9] found that only 44% of cases identified by the *ICD-9-CM* newborn code were confirmed as cases of FAS by the age of 2 years and that only 56% of confirmed cases of FAS based on Institute of Medicine criteria were first recognized at birth. Although not meeting syndrome criteria, most neonates with the discharge code of alcohol affecting the fetus have growth deficiencies, central nervous system impairment, and documented maternal alcohol consumption during pregnancy, suggesting that the diagnosis might best be viewed as a marker for problems associated with in utero exposure to alcohol.[4]

The newborn *ICD-9-CM* code can also be the basis of referral for needed early intervention. The *ICD-9-CM* code of alcohol affecting the fetus is considered a "presumptive eligibility" diagnosis in Part C of the federal Individuals With Disabilities Education Act. This diagnosis allows children from birth to 3 years of age who are "at risk" of later developmental delay to receive early intervention services without meeting more stringent eligibility criteria of significant developmental delay.[8]

Rates of alcohol affecting the fetus at birth are known to miss many cases of FAS identified as the child ages.[9] Estimates of the number of infants and children who meet full criteria for FAS have proved elusive even with the best of surveillance methods. Rates vary between and within types of state surveillance systems and between clinic-based studies and surveillance studies.[48] Rates per 1000 live births vary across existing studies by a factor of 10 or more.[48] The NIS- and KID-based rates of alcohol affecting the fetus, although limited to the newborn period, have the advantage of a standardized collection method across millions of hospital discharges per year mandated by state participation in the federal Medicaid program. Yearly rates generated from the NIS may be the most accurate current means of monitoring the rate of fetal alcohol effects over time.

In conclusion, the coded diagnosis of alcohol effects among newborns has decreased significantly during the past 10 years. Further research is required to determine the importance of decreases in risky drinking behavior, changes in maternal disclosure of drinking to health care professionals, and changes in hospital coding tendencies as explanations for this finding. Large-scale discharge databases such as the NIS and KID may provide a cost-effective method of monitoring the success of public health interventions that address rare conditions that affect the newborn.

**Accepted for Publication:** May 27, 2005.
**Corresponding Author:** James M. Robbins, PhD, Arkansas Center for Birth Defects Research and Prevention, University of Arkansas for Medical Sciences, Arkansas Children's Hospital, Little Rock, AR 72202 (RobbinsJamesM@uams.edu).
**Author Contributions:** *Study concept and design:* Robbins, Bird, Tilford, Reading, Cleves, and Hobbs. *Acquisition of data:* Bird and Tilford. *Analysis and interpretation of data:* Robbins, Bird, Tilford, Cleves, Aitken, and Hobbs. *Drafting of the manuscript:* Robbins, Bird, Tilford, and Hobbs. *Critical revision of the manuscript for important intellectual content:* Robbins, Bird, Tilford, Reading, Cleves, Aitken, and Hobbs. *Statistical analysis:* Bird, Tilford, Cleves, Druschel, and Hobbs. *Obtained funding:* Robbins, Tilford, Cleves, and Hobbs. *Administrative, technical, and material support:* Robbins, Tilford, Reading, and Cleves. *Study supervision:* Robbins, Cleves, and Hobbs.
**Financial Disclosure:** None reported.
**Funding/Support:** This project was supported under cooperative agreements from the CDC, Division of Birth Defects and Developmental Disabilities, grant U50/CCU613236-02; and from the CDC through the Association of American Medical Colleges (AAMC), grant U36/CCU319276, AAMC identification No. MM-0636-04/04.
**Role of the Sponsor:** The CDC and the AAMC had no role in the conduct and design of the study; in the collection, analysis, and interpretation of the data; or in the preparation, review, or approval of the manuscript.
**Disclaimer:** Publication and report contents are solely the responsibility of the authors and do not necessarily represent the official views of the CDC or the AAMC.

## REFERENCES

1. Beck LF, Johnson CH, Morrow B, et al. *PRAMS 1999 Surveillance Report.* Atlanta, Ga: Division of Reproductive Health, National Center for Chronic Disease Prevention and Health Promotion, Centers for Disease Control and Prevention; 2003.
2. Astley SJ. Fetal alcohol syndrome prevention in Washington State: evidence of success. *Paediatr Perinat Epidemiol.* 2004;18:344-351.
3. *International Classification of Diseases, Ninth Revision, Clinical Modification.* Washington, DC: Public Health Service, US Dept of Health and Human Services; 1988.
4. Use of. *International Classification of Diseases* coding to identify fetal alcohol syndrome–Indian Health Service facilities, 1981-1992. *MMWR Morb Mortal Wkly Rep.* 1995;44:253-255, 261.
5. Hoyme HE. A practical clinical approach to diagnosis of fetal alcohol spectrum disorders: clarification of the 1996 Institute of Medicine criteria: in reply. *Pediatrics.* 2005;115:1787.
6. O'Leary CM. Fetal alcohol syndrome: diagnosis, epidemiology, and developmental outcomes. *J Paediatr Child Health.* 2004;40:2-7.
7. Institute of Medicine. *Fetal Alcohol Syndrome: Diagnosis, Epidemiology, Prevention, and Treatment.* Washington, DC: National Academy Press; 1996.
8. Bertrand J, Floyd RL, Weber MK, et al. *Fetal Alcohol Syndrome: Guidelines for Referral and Diagnosis, 1-50.* Atlanta, Ga: Centers for Disease Control and Prevention; 2004.
9. Fox DJ, Druschel CM. Estimating prevalence of fetal alcohol syndrome (FAS): effectiveness of a passive birth defects registry system. *Birth Defects Res Part A Clin Mol Teratol.* 2003;67:604-608.
10. Miller LA, Shaikh T, Stanton C, et al. Surveillance for fetal alcohol syndrome in Colorado. *Public Health Rep.* 1995;110:690-696.
11. Bertrand J, Floyd LL, Weber MK. Guidelines for identifying and referring persons with fetal alcohol syndrome. *MMWR Recomm Rep.* 2005;54:1-14.
12. Coles CD, Kable JA, Drews-Botsch C, Falek A. Early identification of risk for effects of prenatal alcohol exposure. *J Stud Alcohol.* 2000;61:607-616.
13. Streissguth AP, Barr HM, Kogan J, Bookstein FL. *Understanding the Occurrence of Secondary Disabilities in Clients With Fetal Alcohol Syndrome (FAS) and Fetal Alcohol Effects (FAE): Final Report.* Seattle: University of Washington Publications Services; 1996.
14. *The HCUP Nationwide Inpatient Sample (NIS).* Rockville, Md: Agency for Healthcare Research and Quality; 2004.
15. *KIDS' Inpatient Database (KID):The HCUP.* Rockville, Md: Agency for Healthcare Research and Quality; 2003.
16. Bird TM, Hobbs CA, Cleves MA, Tilford JM, Robbins JM. National rates of birth defects among hospitalized newborns. *Birth Defects Res Part A Clin Mol Teratol.* In press.
17. Robbins JM, Tilford JM, Bird TM, Cleves MA, Reading JA, Hobbs CA. Hospitalizations of newborns with folate-sensitive birth defects before and after fortification of foods with folic acid. *Pediatrics.* In press.
18. Holman RC, Curns AT, Belay ED, Steiner CA, Schonberger LB. Kawasaki syndrome hospitalizations in the United States, 1997 and 2000. *Pediatrics.* 2003;112:495-501.
19. Odetola FO, Tilford JM, Davis MM. Variation in the use of intracranial pressure monitoring and mortality in critically ill children with meningitis in the United States. *Pediatrics.* 2006;117:1893-1900.
20. Fetal alcohol syndrome–United States, 1979-1992. *MMWR Morb Mortal Wkly Rep.* 1993;42:339-341.
21. Update: trends in fetal alcohol syndrome–United States, 1979-1993. *MMWR Morb Mortal Wkly Rep.* 1995;44:249-251.
22. Abel EL, Sokol RJ. A revised conservative estimate of the incidence of FAS and its economic impact. *Alcohol Clin Exp Res.* 1991;15:514-524.
23. Leung KM, Elashoff RM, Rees KS, Hasan MM, Legorreta AP. Hospital- and patient-related characteristics determining maternity length of stay: a hierarchical linear model approach. *Am J Public Health.* 1998;88:377-381.
24. Garcia FA, Miller HB, Huggins GR, Gordon TA. Effect of academic affiliation and obstetric volume on clinical outcome and cost of childbirth. *Obstet Gynecol.* 2001;97:567-576.
25. Centers for Disease Control and Prevention (CDC). *Behavioral Risk Factor Surveillance System Survey Data.* Atlanta, Ga: US Dept of Health and Human Services, Centers for Disease Control and Prevention; 2004:1993-2002.
26. Ernhart CB, Morrow-Tlucak M, Sokol RJ, Martier S. Underreporting of alcohol use in pregnancy. *Alcohol Clin Exp Res.* 1988;12:506-511.
27. Westfall JM, McGloin J. Impact of double counting and transfer bias on estimated rates and outcomes of acute myocardial infarction. *Med Care.* 2001;39:459-468.
28. Edmonds LD, Layde PM, James LM, Flynt JW, Erickson JD, Oakley GP Jr. Congenital malformations surveillance: two American systems. *Int J Epidemiol.* 1981;10:247-252.
29. Windham GC, Edmonds LD. Current trends in the incidence of neural tube defects. *Pediatrics.* 1982;70:333-337.
30. Lynberg MC, Chavez GF, Edmonds LD, Mulinare J. Evaluation of the birth defects monitoring program, 1982-1985. *Teratology.* 1993;48:650-657.
31. Hoffman JD, Shanske A. Trends in fetal alcohol syndrome. *Int Pediatr.* 2003;18:114-118.
32. Greenfield TK, Kaskutas LA. Five years exposure to the alcohol warning label messages and their impacts: evidence from diffusion analysis. *Appl Behav Sci Rev.* 1998;6:39-68.
33. Hankin JR, Sloan JJ, Firestone IJ, Ager JW, Sokol RJ, Martier SS. Has awareness of the alcohol warning label reached its upper limit? *Alcohol Clin Exp Res.* 1996;20:440-444.
34. Kaskutas LA, Graves K. Relationship between cumulative exposure to health messages and awareness and behavior-related drinking during pregnancy. *Am J Health Promot.* 1994;9:115-124.
35. Kaskutas LA. Understanding drinking during pregnancy among urban American Indians and African Americans: health messages, risk beliefs, and how we measure consumption. *Alcohol Clin Exp Res.* 2000;24:1241-1250.
36. Sokol RJ, Martier SS, Ager JW. The T-ACE questions: practical prenatal detection of risk-drinking. *Am J Obstet Gynecol.* 1989;160:863-868.
37. Hankin JR, Sloan JJ, Sokol RJ. The modest impact of the alcohol beverage warning label on drinking during pregnancy among a sample of African American women. *J Public Policy Marketing.* 1998;17:61-69.
38. National Birth Defects Prevention Network. State birth defects surveillance program directory. *Birth Defects Res Part A Clin Mol Teratol.* 2005;73:700-757.
39. Sampson PD, Streissguth AP, Bookstein FL, et al. Incidence of fetal alcohol syndrome and prevalence of alcohol-related neurodevelopmental disorder. *Teratology.* 1997;56:317-326.
40. Burd L, Martsolf JT, Klug MG, Kerbeshian J. Diagnosis of FAS: a comparison

of the fetal alcohol syndrome diagnostic checklist and the Institute of Medicine Criteria for fetal alcohol syndrome. *Neurotoxicol Teratol.* 2003;25:719-724.
41. Hymbaugh K, Miller LA, Druschel CM, Podvin DW, Meaney FJ, Boyle CA. A multiple source methodology for the surveillance of fetal alcohol syndrome–The Fetal Alcohol Syndrome Surveillance Network (FASSNet). *Teratology.* 2002;66 (suppl 1):S41-S49.
42. Meaney FJ, Miller LA. A comparison of fetal alcohol syndrome surveillance network and birth defects surveillance methodology in determining prevalence rates of fetal alcohol syndrome. *Birth Defects Res Part A Clin Mol Teratol.* 2003; 67:819-822.
43. Jones KL. From recognition to responsibility: Josef Warkany, David Smith, and the fetal alcohol syndrome in the 21st century. *Birth Defects Res Part A Clin Mol Teratol.* 2003;67:13-20.
44. Lyons Jones K. Early recognition of prenatal alcohol effects: a pediatrician responsibility. *J Pediatr.* 1999;135:405.
45. Aase JM. Clinical recognition of FAS: difficulties of detection and diagnosis. *Alcohol Res Health.* 1994;18:5-9.
46. Little BB, Snell LM, Rosenfeld CR, Gilstrap LC III, Gant NF. Failure to recognize fetal alcohol syndrome in newborn infants. *AJDC.* 1990;144:1142-1146.
47. Streissguth AP, Aase JM, Clarren SK, Randels SP, LaDue RA, Smith DF. Fetal alcohol syndrome in adolescents and adults. *JAMA.* 1991;265:1961-1967.
48. May PA, Gossage JP. Estimating the prevalence of fetal alcohol syndrome: a summary. *Alcohol Res Health.* 2001;25:159-167.

## *Trial Registration Required*

In concert with the International Committee of Medical Journal Editors (ICMJE), *Archives of Pediatrics and Adolescent Medicine* will require, as a condition of consideration for publication, registration of all trials in a public trials registry (such as http://ClinicalTrials.gov). Trials must be registered at or before the onset of patient enrollment. This policy applies to any clinical trial starting enrollment after July 1, 2005. For trials that began enrollment before this date, registration will be required by September 13, 2005, before considering the trial for publication. The trial registration number should be supplied at the time of submission.

For details about this new policy, and for information on how the ICMJE defines a clinical trial, see the editorials by DeAngelis et al in the September 8, 2004 (2004;292:1363-1364) and June 15, 2005 (2005;293: 2927-2929) issues of *JAMA*. Also see the Instructions to Authors on our Web site: www.archpediatrics.com.

# Effect of Early Childhood Adversity on Child Health

*Emalee G. Flaherty, MD; Richard Thompson, PhD; Alan J. Litrownik, PhD; Adrea Theodore, MD, MPH; Diana J. English, PhD; Maureen M. Black, PhD; Traci Wike, MSW; Lakecia Whimper, MA; Desmond K. Runyan, MD, PhD; Howard Dubowitz, MD, MS*

**Objective:** To examine the effect of child abuse and other household dysfunction on child health outcomes.

**Design:** Data from the Longitudinal Studies of Child Abuse and Neglect collected through interviews and questionnaires administered when target children were 4 years old and 6 years old.

**Setting:** Children in the South, East, Midwest, Northwest, and Southwest United States.

**Participants:** One thousand forty-one children at high risk for child abuse and neglect (3 cohorts derived primarily from among children recruited through social service mechanisms, 1 cohort recruited at birth from among high-risk infants, and 1 cohort recruited from a medical setting).

**Main Outcome Measures:** (1) Association of 7 adverse exposures (3 categories of child abuse [physical abuse, sexual abuse, and psychological maltreatment] and 4 categories of household dysfunction [caregiver problem drinking, caregiver depression, caregiver treated violently, and criminal behavior in the household]) derived from data collected when the child was 4 years old. (2) Indexes of child physical health at age 6 years (caregiver overall assessment of child health and reports of illness requiring medical attention).

**Results:** Two thirds of the sample had experienced at least 1 adverse exposure. One adverse exposure almost doubled the risk of overall poor health (odds ratio, 1.89; 95% confidence interval, 1.02-3.48), and 4 adverse exposures or more almost tripled the risk of illness requiring medical attention (odds ratio, 2.83; 95% confidence interval, 1.10-7.31).

**Conclusion:** Adverse environmental exposures, including child abuse and other household dysfunction, are associated with poor child health even at an early age, although our data do not support a dose-response relationship.

*Arch Pediatr Adolesc Med. 2006;160:1232-1238*

**Author Affiliations:** Department of Pediatrics, Children's Memorial Hospital, Chicago, Ill (Dr Flaherty) Department of Research, Juvenile Protective Association (Dr Thompson), and Department of Psychology, San Diego State University, and Joint Doctoral Program in Clinical Psychology, San Diego State University and University of California at San Diego (Dr Litrownik); Departments of Social Medicine and Pediatrics, School of Medicine (Drs Theodore and Runyan), Department of Maternal and Child Health, School of Public Health (Ms Wike), and Department of Pediatrics, Children's Memorial Hospital (Ms Whimper), University of North Carolina at Chapel Hill; School of Social Work, University of Washington, Seattle (Dr English); and Department of Pediatrics, University of Maryland School of Medicine, Baltimore (Drs Black and Dubowitz).

CHILDHOOD EXPOSURE TO household dysfunction and abuse correlates with adverse health outcomes in adulthood.[1] The Adverse Childhood Experiences (ACE) Study[1] found a relationship between childhood exposure to abuse and household dysfunction and medical disorders in adulthood, including cancer, liver disease, skeletal fractures, chronic lung disease, and ischemic heart disease . In addition, the ACE Study investigators found relationships between early adverse life events and other health problems such as smoking, suicide, depression, obesity, illicit drug use, alcoholism, teen pregnancy, sexual risk behaviors, and sexually transmitted disease.[2-13]

The initial ACE Study[1] considered an index of 7 adverse childhood exposures (psychological abuse, physical abuse, sexual abuse, violence against the mother, living with household members who abused drugs, household members who were mentally ill or suicidal, and household members who were imprisoned). In later analyses, the ACE Study investigators included emotional neglect, physical neglect, and parental marital discord.[11,14-16] These later analyses focused more attention on psychosocial outcomes rather than physical outcomes.

The importance of childhood adversities to adult health outcomes has been corroborated by smaller investigations examining the long-term consequences of child

***For editorial comment see page 1300***

abuse. A study[17] of middle-class women in a gynecologic practice included an assessment of childhood abuse. Women who reported a history of abuse (approximately half the subjects) also reported more hospitalizations and more physical and psychological problems and rated their overall health as poorer than women who did not report a history of childhood abuse. In a study[18] of undergraduate students in the United Kingdom, a history of childhood physical or sexual abuse was associated with more hospital admissions and surgical procedures. Others have simi-

**Table 1. Description of Sampling at 5 Consortium for LONGSCAN Sites**

| Site | No. (% of Study Sample) | Sampling Criteria |
|---|---|---|
| East | 203 (19.5) | Children at high risk for abuse (failure-to-thrive children, children at high risk for HIV infection, or low-income families) |
| Midwest | 189 (18.2) | Family reported to CPS, with neighborhood control subjects |
| South | 194 (18.6) | Children at high risk for abuse (young mothers, single parents, low birth weight, poverty, or reported to CPS for abuse or neglect), with matched control subjects |
| Southwest | 230 (22.1) | Maltreated children placed in foster care |
| Northwest | 225 (21.6) | Maltreated children identified by CPS |

Abbreviations: CPS, Child Protective Services; HIV, human immunodeficiency virus; LONGSCAN, Longitudinal Studies of Child Abuse and Neglect.

larly linked childhood abuse to adult physical and emotional problems.[19-21]

Other investigations have examined the effects of childhood abuse on health in adolescents, typically focusing on heath-related behavior or emotional health.[22] A US national survey found that adolescent girls reporting both physical and sexual abuse were at risk for having depressive symptoms, smoking tobacco, using illicit drugs, and drinking alcohol regularly.[23] Several studies[11,24,25] confirmed these findings and showed that abused adolescents are more likely to engage in risky behaviors, including running away and having unprotected sex that results in teen pregnancy.

The effect of household dysfunction or child abuse on the physical health of children has rarely been investigated. Most research (including past research involving the sample used for this study) has examined the behavioral and developmental consequences of child abuse.[25-27] A recently published review of articles about childhood exposure to intimate partner violence found no data that established a clear link between intimate partner violence exposure and child physical health.[28]

The primary strength of the ACE Study[1] is that it included a comprehensive and sophisticated assessment of health outcomes through medical examinations and medical record reviews of the adult subjects. However, information regarding childhood experiences came only from recall, the value of which has come under question.[29] In addition, many chronic diseases begin in childhood, suggesting that it would be useful to evaluate the more immediate effect of household dysfunction and child abuse on children's health.

We hypothesized that exposure to child abuse and other household dysfunction would result in poor health or illness even in early childhood and that these exposures would have a dose-response effect. Using the ACE Study[1] as a model, we prospectively examined the same 7 categories of adverse childhood experiences (based on Child Protective Services [CPS] data and caregiver reports) and general health outcomes in a sample of 6-year-old children. We included demographic variables similar to those used in the ACE Study (child's sex and race/ethnicity, caregiver's marital status, and family income).

## METHODS

### PARTICIPANTS AND STUDY DESIGN

The Consortium for Longitudinal Studies of Child Abuse and Neglect (LONGSCAN)[30] is a consortium of 5 study sites that are investigating prospectively the antecedents and consequences of child maltreatment. The study sites, located in different regions of the United States (South, East, Midwest, Northwest, and Southwest), operate under common protocols. The present analysis uses pooled data. At each site, a sample of children who had been maltreated or who were at risk of maltreatment was recruited when children were 4 years old or younger. The samples were distinct and were meant to include children in several categories, including those at risk before any reports of child maltreatment, those reported but whose investigations were not yet complete, those reported and substantiated and left in their homes with or without intervention, and those placed in foster care. The sampling criteria used at each site are given in **Table 1**.

We collected data at the ages of 4 years and 6 years, using 2-hour interviews conducted face to face with primary female caregivers (mothers or foster mothers). For each child, we reviewed CPS records and coded for official reports of child maltreatment from birth through age 4 years. Of the 1354 caregivers who completed interviews at age 4 years or age 6 years, 1041 (76.9%) had complete data (ie, caregivers completed both interviews and CPS records were reviewed) and were included in the analyses. For 26.7% of the children, someone other than the biological mother was interviewed when the child was 6 years old; in most of these cases, the respondent was another relative (eg, grandmother or aunt), although some respondents were nonrelative foster parents. $\chi^2$ Analyses revealed no significant demographic differences between those included and those excluded ($P>.20$ for all).

### VARIABLES AND THEIR MEASUREMENT

The LONGSCAN consortium shared common interview procedures and measures across the 5 sites. Data were entered locally and were processed at the LONGSCAN coordinating center at the University of North Carolina at Chapel Hill. A random 10% of the interviews were reentered to verify data entry procedures and coding. Measures were selected, as far as possible, from among available standard instruments previously published in the child abuse literature, as discussed herein. Data periods varied by measure, but each instrument referred to contemporaneous exposures; some measures asked caregivers about events in the prior year or in the prior 6 months. Unless otherwise specified, we dichotomized each predictor and outcome variable to construct a risk profile.

### DEMOGRAPHIC CONTROL VARIABLES

The caregiver interview at age 4 years recorded the child's sex, child's race/ethnicity (white, African American, or other), caregiver's marital status (married, never married, or formerly married), and family income. Family income was dichotomized into above the federal poverty level or at or below the federal poverty level, based on the total annual household income and the number of people dependent on that income.

## CHILD ABUSE AND HOUSEHOLD DYSFUNCTION

We examined the pool of variables from the interviews at age 4 years to identify indicators of adverse childhood experiences. Mirroring the ACE Study,[1] we studied 7 categories of abuse and household dysfunction, including 3 categories of child abuse and 4 categories of exposure to household dysfunction.

### Child Abuse

Each site reviewed their local CPS records for alleged and substantiated reports of child abuse. Based on prior research suggesting that distinctions between allegations and substantiations are not useful,[31,32] official reports of alleged child abuse were coded using a slightly modified version[33] of the maltreatment classification scheme developed by Barnett et al.[34] Three general indicators of child abuse were created, each dichotomized as present or not, based on the coding of the following records: (1) physical abuse (any blows or injury to the head, torso, buttocks, or limbs; and violent handling, choking, burning, shaking, or nondescript injury); (2) sexual abuse (any sexual exposure, exploitation, molestation, or penetration); and (3) psychological maltreatment (threats to psychological safety and security, lack of acceptance and threats to self-esteem, or failure to allow age-appropriate autonomy). Domestic violence exposure was not considered psychological maltreatment in the LONGSCAN version of the maltreatment classification scheme but was examined separately.

### Household Dysfunction

The indicators of household dysfunction use the following 4 standardized measures:

**Caregiver Problem Drinking.** The CAGE (acronym for cut down on drinking, annoyed by people criticizing, guilty about drinking, and eye-opener or drink first thing in the morning) questionnaire is a widely used alcoholism screening tool.[35] It was administered if the caregiver responded that she had ever drunk alcoholic beverages. The following 4 questions comprising the CAGE alcoholism screening test were asked: Have you ever felt you ought to cut down on your drinking? Have you ever felt annoyed by people criticizing your drinking? Have you ever felt bad or guilty about your drinking? Have you ever had a drink first thing in the morning to steady your nerves or get rid of a hangover? Problem drinking was coded as present if the caregiver endorsed more than 1 of the 4 items on the CAGE.

**Caregiver Depression.** Caregiver depressive symptoms were assessed using the Center for Epidemiological Studies Depression Scale (CES-D).[36] The CES-D questionnaire includes 20 items about symptoms commonly associated with depression. Consistent with typical clinical cutoff points for the CES-D, marked depressive symptoms were coded as present if the CES-D scores exceeded 16. The CES-D is a reliable and valid measure of the number, types, and duration of depressive symptoms.[36]

**Caregiver Treated Violently.** A widely used and validated measure (partner-to-partner Conflict Tactics Scales[37]) was used to assess the type and level of domestic violence between the caregiver and a partner. Caregivers were asked how many times in the past 3 months a spouse or partner had engaged in violent behavior, including kicking, biting, choking, hitting with a fist or object, threatening with a knife or gun, using a knife or gun, or beating her up. The caregiver was coded as having been treated violently if she indicated that any of these behaviors was directed at her more than once or if her partner engaged in more than 1 type of specific violent behavior.

**Criminal Behavior in the Household.** The child life-events report[38] assessed events in the child's life during the past year. Criminal behavior was coded as present if the caregiver responded yes to the question "Was anyone in the family or household jailed or imprisoned?"

### Development of the Adversity Index

The child abuse and household dysfunction variables were dichotomized into 7 indicators of adverse childhood experience, yielding a score of 0 vs 1 (absent vs present) for each indicator. The 7 dichotomous scores on the indexes of child abuse and household dysfunction were summed to produce an overall adversity index, with scores ranging from 0 (best) to 7 (worse). This adversity index was based on the methods used in the ACE Study.[1]

## ASSESSMENT OF HEALTH AND SERIOUS ILLNESS

The caregiver's overall assessment of the child's health and serious illness in the past year at the interview at age 6 years was used to assess the outcome variables. Primary outcome variables were dichotomized. The following 2 variables were measured—child health and serious illness.

### Child Health

The caregivers described the child's health using a child health assessment form.[39] Caregivers were asked "How would you describe [your child's] health compared to other children his/her age? Would you say that his/her health is: excellent, good, fair, or poor?" Using the same approach as that used by Felitti et al[1] to obtain global ratings of health, ratings of poor or fair overall health were coded as indicators of poor health, and ratings of good or excellent health were coded as indicators of good health. Extensive prior work has demonstrated the utility of the global health ratings in predicting hospitalization and mortality.[40]

### Serious Illness

Caregivers were also asked "Did [your child] have a serious illness in the past year?" If the response was yes, the caregiver was asked if the child saw a physician. An illness that received professional attention was coded as present if the caretaker selected this response on the child life-events report.[38]

## STATISTICAL ANALYSIS

The analyses were conducted using Statistical Package for the Social Sciences (SPSS 12.0.1; SPSS Inc, Chicago, Ill) software. Preliminary descriptive analyses were conducted for each of the control, predictor, and outcome variables. In addition, bivariate relationships between the control and predictor variables were examined. Similar to the ACE Study analyses, for each outcome variable, a binary logistic regression was applied to test the relationship of the adversity index score (0, 1, 2, 3, or ≥4) to the outcome, after entering the control variables (child's sex, child's race/ethnicity, caregiver's marital status, and family income). Subsequently, the adversity index score was entered as a categorical predictor. This allowed for examination not only

**Table 2. Prevalence of Early Exposure to Child Abuse and Household Dysfunction Among 1041 Children**

| Variable | Prevalence, % |
|---|---|
| Indicator of child abuse | |
| Psychological maltreatment | 25.3 |
| Physical abuse | 23.2 |
| Sexual abuse | 10.8 |
| Indicator of household dysfunction | |
| Caregiver problem drinking | 16.9 |
| Caregiver depression | 32.3 |
| Caregiver treated violently | 7.9 |
| Criminal behavior in the household | 13.4 |
| No. of adverse exposures | |
| 0 | 33.2 |
| 1 | 29.2 |
| 2 | 20.5 |
| 3 | 10.8 |
| ≥4 | 6.3 |

of the possibility of a simple linear relationship but also of the possibility that particular levels of adversity were especially harmful. The adjusted odds ratios and 95% confidence intervals reported for these logistic regression analyses represent the increased likelihood of the outcome of interest, compared with having experienced no adversities.

### ASSESSING THE POSSIBLE EFFECT OF EXCLUSIONS

We examined whether the results were affected by excluding those with incomplete data on childhood exposure. We performed separate analyses that included those participants with missing data (n = 313), but we assumed that those with missing data on a given childhood exposure did not have that category of childhood exposure. In these reanalyses, there were no significant differences from the results reported herein. The direction and strength of the associations between the number of childhood exposures and the outcomes were almost identical (data not shown). Therefore, the results appear to be unaffected by the exclusion of those with missing data on childhood exposure.

### HUMAN SUBJECTS

Each site followed informed consent procedures approved by their institutional or local human subjects review committee. The coordinating center data handling and analysis procedures were approved by the School of Medicine, University of North Carolina at Chapel Hill, committee for the protection of human subjects. The primary caregiver gave informed consent to participate. Caregivers were reimbursed for their time and effort.

## RESULTS

### ADVERSE CHILDHOOD EXPOSURES

The prevalence of adverse exposures at age 4 years is given in **Table 2**. Two thirds of the children had at least 1 adverse exposure. Caregiver depression was the most prevalent household dysfunction, present in about one third of the maternal caregivers. Twenty-five percent of the children had experienced psychological maltreatment, while 7.9% of caregivers had a history of domestic violence in the past 3 months (which represented the lowest prevalence among the 7 indicators of adverse childhood experience in our sample).

**Table 3. Prevalence of Adverse Exposures by Demographic Characteristics***

| Characteristic | No. of Adverse Exposures 0 | 1 | 2 | 3 | ≥4 |
|---|---|---|---|---|---|
| Sex | | | | | |
| Male | 29.2 | 28.2 | 21.5 | 12.0 | 9.1 |
| Female | 27.0 | 27.2 | 20.6 | 15.0 | 10.3 |
| Site | | | | | |
| East | 37.9 | 32.5 | 20.2 | 6.9 | 2.5 |
| South | 45.9 | 26.3 | 16.5 | 7.7 | 3.6 |
| Midwest | 38.1 | 35.4 | 18.0 | 5.3 | 3.2 |
| Northwest | 7.6 | 20.0 | 26.2 | 25.8 | 20.4 |
| Southwest | 16.1 | 25.7 | 23.0 | 19.1 | 16.1 |
| Race/ethnicity | | | | | |
| White | 26.5 | 25.4 | 18.3 | 16.5 | 13.3 |
| African American | 32.7 | 29.7 | 21.8 | 10.0 | 5.7 |
| Other | 17.2 | 25.1 | 22.7 | 19.2 | 15.8 |
| Poverty | | | | | |
| Yes | 28.0 | 26.5 | 21.1 | 13.9 | 10.6 |
| No | 28.6 | 30.5 | 20.2 | 12.9 | 7.8 |
| Marital status | | | | | |
| Married | 32.5 | 27.1 | 18.2 | 14.0 | 8.2 |
| Never married | 31.1 | 27.8 | 20.0 | 12.1 | 9.0 |
| Formerly married | 17.1 | 28.3 | 16.4 | 15.5 | 12.8 |
| Total with No. of adverse exposures | 28.0 | 27.7 | 21.0 | 13.5 | 9.7 |

*Data are given as percentages.

The prevalence of adverse exposures varied as a function of some demographic characteristics (**Table 3**). Children whose race/ethnicity was other than white or African American were less likely to have had no adverse exposures; African American children were less likely than other children to have had at least 3 adverse exposures ($\chi^2_8$=45.62, $P<.05$). Children whose mothers had previously been married were more likely than other children to have had at least 1 adversity ($\chi^2_8$=21.20, $P<.05$). Child sex and economic status were not associated with adverse exposures.

There were some significant site differences (Table 3). Almost half of the southern participants had no adverse exposures, while 92.4% of the northwest participants had 1 or more adverse exposures ($\chi^2_{16}$=174.04, $P<.05$). These differences were expected given the differences in the sampling frame; the southern sample consisted of children considered at high risk for abuse, while the northwest sample consisted of children who had been identified by CPS as maltreated (Table 1).

### RELATIONSHIP BETWEEN CHILDHOOD EXPOSURES AND HEALTH

The relationship between adverse exposures and negative health outcomes is summarized in **Table 4**. The relationship between numbers of adverse exposures and adjusted odds ratios of health outcomes is summarized in **Table 5**. Two significant relationships emerged. The odds ratio for general health to be rated as poor was 1.89 (95% confidence interval, 1.02-3.48) when there was 1 vs 0 adverse childhood experiences, and the odds ratio was 2.83 (95% confidence interval, 1.10-7.31) that a child

**Table 4. Relationship Between Adverse Exposures and Negative Health Outcomes**

| | Health Outcome | | |
|---|---|---|---|
| Variable, % | Poor Health | Illness Requiring Professional Care | Poor Health or Illness Requiring Professional |
| Overall rate | 7.2 | 6.7 | 12.1 |
| Indicator of child abuse | | | |
| Psychological maltreatment | 4.2 | 8.0 | 10.6 |
| Physical abuse | 5.0 | 9.6 | 12.5 |
| Sexual abuse | 4.5 | 7.1 | 9.8 |
| Indicator of household dysfunction | | | |
| Caregiver problem drinking | 8.5 | 6.3 | 14.2 |
| Caregiver depression | 11.9 | 10.4 | 19.0 |
| Caregiver treated violently | 4.9 | 6.1 | 11.0 |
| Criminal behavior in the household | 4.3 | 6.4 | 12.1 |

**Table 5. Relationship Between Numbers of Adverse Exposures and Adjusted Odds Ratios (OR) of Negative Health Outcomes**

| Health Outcome | No. of Adverse Exposures | Prevalence, % | Adjusted OR (95% Confidence Interval)* |
|---|---|---|---|
| Poor health | 0 | 5.5 | 1.00 |
| | 1 | 9.9 | 1.89 (1.02-3.48) |
| | 2 | 8.5 | 1.84 (0.90-3.73) |
| | 3 | 4.5 | 0.96 (0.30-3.00) |
| | ≥4 | 4.5 | 1.38 (0.38-5.10) |
| Illness requiring professional care | 0 | 4.7 | 1.00 |
| | 1 | 7.9 | 1.72 (0.88-3.35) |
| | 2 | 6.6 | 1.36 (0.62-2.96) |
| | 3 | 6.3 | 1.20 (0.45-3.20) |
| | ≥4 | 13.6 | 2.83 (1.10-7.31) |
| Poor health or illness requiring professional care | 0 | 9.0 | 1.00 |
| | 1 | 14.9 | 1.79 (1.09-2.95) |
| | 2 | 13.1 | 1.64 (0.92-2.90) |
| | 3 | 10.7 | 1.33 (0.62-2.88) |
| | ≥4 | 15.2 | 2.31 (1.01-5.28) |

*Adjusted for site, child's sex, child's race/ethnicity, caregiver's marital status, and family income.

would have an illness that required medical attention when there were 4 or more adverse exposures. Several relationships between the number of adverse exposures and health approached significance, including 2 vs 0 adversities on overall health and 1 vs 0 adversities on illness requiring medical attention. Based on the overall pattern of odds ratios for poor health and illness, there was some support for the hypothesized relationship between the extent of exposure to adverse factors and negative health outcomes (ie, odds ratios tended to increase relative to 1 vs 0 to ≥4 vs 0 adversities).

## COMMENT

Adverse childhood exposures seem to already begin to affect a child's health early in childhood. Our results suggest a relationship between adverse childhood exposures and negative health indicators by age 6 years. In our sample, having 1 adverse exposure almost doubled the odds that these children would have overall poor health compared with children who had no early adverse exposures. Furthermore, the presence of 4 adverse exposures or more almost tripled the likelihood of childhood illness for exposed children compared with children who did not experience adversities.

The presence of a single adverse environmental exposure early in life affected children's health. Very young children may be more susceptible to poor health or illness because of their almost complete dependence on the presence, attentiveness, and reasonable actions of their caregivers. Measurable household dysfunction, including child abuse, likely affects the ability of the caregiver to parent a child well. Parents' inability to respond quickly and adequately to emerging health problems may lead to complications. In addition, stressed parents may be less able to carefully supervise young children, jeopardizing their safety.[41] Some aspects of household dysfunction (eg, problem drinking) may have predated the birth of the child. The vulnerability of children in these families to early poor health speaks to the need for timely help for young families.

The baseline prevalence of adverse exposures in our sample deserves comment. Two thirds of the sample of 6-year-old children had at least 1 adverse environmental exposure, and almost one third of families had evidence of caregiver depression. This is not surprising, given the LONGSCAN consortium's selection criteria; children in the study had been maltreated or were considered at risk for child abuse.

This high prevalence of exposures may help explain why our study did not find a dose-response relationship between the number of adverse exposures and overall child health. Although the presence of 1 adversity and of 4 or more adversities was associated with poor child health, this effect did not hold in cases in which there were 2 or 3 adverse exposures.

There are other possible explanations why we did not find a significant relationship between different levels of adversity compared with no adversity. Our subjects were only 6 years old when we assessed their health. Larger or dose-related effects may become clearer over time. Our global measurement of health outcomes may not have been sensitive enough to detect important differences. The effect of adverse exposures at this early age may manifest as psychosocial problems rather than physical health problems,[42] or the model of adverse exposures may not be the most useful construct in younger age groups. It is also possible that children in our sample with more adversities were more likely to receive interventions to ameliorate the effects of these adversities. A high number of adversities (ie, $\geq$4) may have negated the helpful effects of the intervention.

Some of these children may have had congenital disorders or other medical conditions that predisposed them to poor health and illness. Certain disabilities, chronic health problems, and prematurity increase the risk that a child will be maltreated.[43-45] Although we might postulate that these health problems would be evenly distributed among families with and without adverse exposures, we have no information that supports that hypothesis.

Only 7.9% of the caregivers described domestic violence as occurring in the prior 3 months. Although this number may appear somewhat low, most caregivers had no partner at the time of the interview, resulting in a lack of opportunity for domestic violence to occur during that 3-month period. Other adversities were assessed during a longer period (ie, during the past year), and the use of different measurement periods constitutes a weakness of our data.

A strength of our study is that we prospectively documented the presence of the adverse exposures. This may explain some of the differences between the ACE Study[1] findings and our results. The ACE Study subjects may not have accurately recalled early childhood experiences, and those with later problems may have been more inclined to recall childhood adversity. Our prospective design minimizes such recall bias. On the other hand, we relied on the parent or full-time caregiver for information about the child's health, whereas the health of ACE Study participants was ascertained from medical records or self-reports. Negligent or abusive caregivers may not accurately assess their children's health or seek medical care for illnesses needing medical treatment. Our dependence on the caregiver's assessment of the child's health and health care may not clearly reflect childhood health status. This population of caregivers may deny that children living in their homes experience adverse effects of their behaviors, or they may have less capacity to empathize with the children and to assess child health. Illness data may more accurately depict child health status than caregiver assessment in these households. We were unable to review medical records or conduct independent assessments of the health of the children in this study. Using caregivers' assessments of child health is supported by studies[46,47] showing that adults fairly accurately rate their health, although the use of such ratings in dysfunctional households may require further examination.

## CONCLUSIONS

Findings from this study suggest that a relationship between adverse childhood experiences and negative health indicators begins early in childhood. Because the effect on the child's health becomes evident early in childhood, physicians may have a window of opportunity to intervene and prevent the long-term medical complications described in the ACE Study.[1] We speculate that, as children age, the negative health effects of these adverse childhood experiences and child maltreatment will increase. These negative childhood exposures may play a role in the development or exacerbation of certain childhood diseases such as asthma, diabetes mellitus, and obesity. Family, environment, and community intervention may have a mediating effect on these adverse childhood experiences. Further research is needed to examine a link between adverse childhood experiences and specific childhood illnesses, to understand the mechanisms underlying such a link, and to identify interventions that mediate or ameliorate negative health consequences.

**Accepted for Publication:** June 15, 2006.
**Correspondence:** Emalee G. Flaherty, MD, Department of Pediatrics, Children's Memorial Hospital, 2300 Children's Plaza, Box 16, Chicago, IL 60614 (e-flaherty@northwestern.edu).
**Author Contributions:** *Study concept and design:* Flaherty, Thompson, Litrownik, and Wike. *Acquisition of data:* Thompson, Litrownik, English, Runyan, and Dubowitz. *Analysis and interpretation of data:* Flaherty, Thompson, Litrownik, Theodore, English, Whimper, and Dubowitz. *Drafting of the manuscript:* Flaherty, Thompson, English, and Whimper. *Critical revision of the manuscript for important intellectual content:* Flaherty, Thompson, Litrownik, Theodore, Black, Wike, Runyan, and Dubowitz. *Statistical analysis:* Thompson, Whimper, and Runyan. *Obtained funding:* Litrownik, Runyan, and Dubowitz. *Administrative, technical, and material support:* Theodore, Whimper, Runyan, and Dubowitz. *Study supervision:* Flaherty and Runyan.
**Financial Disclosure:** None reported.
**Funding/Support:** This research was supported by grants to the LONGSCAN consortium from the National Center on Child Abuse and Neglect, the Children's Bureau, the Office on Child Abuse and Neglect, the National Institute of Child Health and Human Development, and the Administration for Children, Youth, and Families.

## REFERENCES


1. Felitti VJ, Anda RF, Nordenberg D, et al. Relationship of childhood abuse and household dysfunction to many of the leading causes of death in adults: the Adverse Childhood Experiences (ACE) Study. *Am J Prev Med.* 1998;14:245-258.
2. Dube SR, Anda RF, Felitti VJ, Chapman DP, Williamson DF, Giles WH. Childhood abuse, household dysfunction, and the risk of attempted suicide throughout the life span: findings from the Adverse Childhood Experiences Study. *JAMA.* 2001;286:3089-3096.
3. Dube SR, Felitti VJ, Dong M, Chapman DP, Giles WH, Anda RF. Childhood abuse, neglect, and household dysfunction and the risk of illicit drug use: the adverse childhood experiences study. *Pediatrics.* 2003;111:564-572.
4. Anda RF, Chapman DP, Felitti VJ, et al. Adverse childhood experiences and risk of paternity in teen pregnancy. *Obstet Gynecol.* 2002;100:37-45.
5. Anda RF, Felitti VJ, Chapman DP, et al. Abused boys, battered mothers, and male involvement in teen pregnancy. *Pediatrics.* 2001;107:e19.
6. Chapman DP, Whitfield CL, Felitti VJ, Dube SR, Edwards VJ, Anda RF. Adverse childhood experiences and the risk of depressive disorders in adulthood. *J Affect Disord.* 2004;82:217-225.
7. Dietz PM, Spitz AM, Anda RF, et al. Unintended pregnancy among adult women exposed to abuse or household dysfunction during their childhood. *JAMA.* 1999; 282:1359-1364.
8. Dube SR, Anda RF, Felitti VJ, Edwards VJ, Croft JB. Adverse childhood experiences and personal alcohol abuse as an adult. *Addict Behav.* 2002;27:713-725.
9. Felitti VJ. Childhood sexual abuse, depression, and family dysfunction in adult obese patients: a case control study. *South Med J.* 1993;86:732-736.
10. Felitti VJ. Long-term medical consequences of incest, rape, and molestation. *South Med J.* 1991;84:328-331.
11. Hillis SD, Anda RF, Dube SR, Felitti VJ, Marchbanks PA, Marks JS. The association between adverse childhood experiences and adolescent pregnancy, long-term psychosocial consequences, and fetal death. *Pediatrics.* 2004;113:320-327.
12. Hillis SD, Anda RF, Felitti VJ, Nordenberg D, Marchbanks PA. Adverse childhood experiences and sexually transmitted diseases in men and women: a retrospective study. *Pediatrics.* 2000;106:e11.
13. Williamson DF, Thompson TJ, Anda RF, Dietz WH, Felitti V. Body weight and obesity in adults and self-reported abuse in childhood. *Int J Obes Relat Metab Disord.* 2002;26:1075-1082.
14. Dong M, Anda RF, Felitti VJ, et al. The interrelatedness of multiple forms of childhood abuse, neglect, and household dysfunction. *Child Abuse Negl.* 2004;28: 771-784.
15. Dube SR, Anda RF, Whitfield CL, et al. Long-term consequences of childhood sexual abuse by gender of victim. *Am J Prev Med.* 2005;28:430-438.
16. Whitfield CL, Dube SR, Felitti VJ, Anda RF. Adverse childhood experiences and hallucinations. *Child Abuse Negl.* 2005;29:797-810.
17. Moeller TP, Bachmann GA, Moeller JR. The combined effects of physical, sexual, and emotional abuse during childhood: long-term health consequences for women. *Child Abuse Negl.* 1993;17:623-640.
18. Salmon P, Calderbank S. The relationship of childhood physical and sexual abuse to adult illness behavior. *J Psychosom Res.* 1996;40:329-336.
19. Katon W, Sullivan M, Walker E. Medical symptoms without identified pathology: relationship to psychiatric disorders, childhood and adult trauma, and personality traits. *Ann Intern Med.* 2001;134:917-925.
20. Reilly J, Baker GA, Rhodes J, Salmon P. The association of sexual and physical abuse with somatization: characteristics of patients presenting with irritable bowel syndrome and non-epileptic attack disorder. *Psychol Med.* 1999;29:399-406.
21. Morse DS, Suchman AL, Frankel RM. The meaning of symptoms in 10 women with somatization disorder and a history of childhood abuse. *Arch Fam Med.* 1997; 6:468-476.
22. DiClemente RJ, Wingood GM, Lang DL, et al. Adverse health consequences that co-occur with depression: a longitudinal study of black adolescent females. *Pediatrics.* 2005;116:78-81.
23. Diaz A, Simantov E, Rickert VI. Effect of abuse on health: results of a national survey. *Arch Pediatr Adolesc Med.* 2002;156:811-817.
24. Hibbard RA, Brack CJ, Rauch S, Orr DP. Abuse, feelings, and health behaviors in a student population. *AJDC.* 1988;142:326-330.
25. Johnson RM, Kotch JB, Catellier DJ, et al. Adverse behavioral and emotional outcomes from child abuse and witnessed violence. *Child Maltreat.* 2002;7:179-186.
26. Kerr MA, Black MM, Krishnakumar A. Failure-to-thrive, maltreatment and the behavior and development of 6-year-old children from low-income, urban families: a cumulative risk model. *Child Abuse Negl.* 2000;24:587-598.
27. Thompson R, Briggs E, English DJ, et al. Suicidal ideation among 8-year-olds who are maltreated and at risk: findings from the LONGSCAN studies. *Child Maltreat.* 2005;10:26-36.
28. Bair-Merritt MH, Blackstone M, Feudtner C. Physical health outcomes of childhood exposure to intimate partner violence: a systematic review. *Pediatrics.* 2006 117:e278.
29. Widom CS, Raphael KG, DuMont KA. The case for prospective longitudinal studies in child maltreatment research: commentary on Dube, Williamson, Thompson, Felitti, and Anda (2004). *Child Abuse Negl.* 2004;28:715-722.
30. Runyan DK, Curtis PA, Hunter WM, et al. LONGSCAN: a consortium for longitudinal studies of maltreatment and the life course of children. *Aggress Violent Behav.* 1998;3:275-285.
31. English DJ, Upadhyaya MP, Litrownik AJ, et al. Maltreatment's wake: the relationship of maltreatment dimensions to child outcomes. *Child Abuse Negl.* 2005; 29:597-619.
32. Hussey JM, Marshall JM, English DJ, et al. Defining maltreatment according to substantiation: distinction without a difference? *Child Abuse Negl.* 2005;29: 479-492.
33. English DJ, Bangdiwala SI, Runyan D. The dimensions of maltreatment: introduction. *Child Abuse Negl.* 2005;29:441-460.
34. Barnett D, Manly JT, Cicchetti D. *Defining Child Maltreatment: The Interface Between Policy and Research.* Norwood, NJ: Ablex Publishing; 1993.
35. Mayfield D, McLeod G, Hall P. The CAGE questionnaire: validation of a new alcoholism screening instrument. *Am J Psychiatry.* 1974;131:1121-1123.
36. Radloff LS. The CES-D Scale: a self-report depression scale for research in the general population. *Appl Psychol Meas.* 1977;1:385-401.
37. Straus MA. *New Scoring Methods for Violence and New Norms for the Conflict Tactics Scales.* New Brunswick, NJ: Transaction Books; 1990.
38. Coddington RD. The significance of life-events as etiologic factors in the diseases of children, II: a study of a normal population. *J Psychosom Res.* 1972; 16:205-213.
39. Krause NM, Jay GM. What do global self-rated health items measure? *Med Care.* 1994;32:930-942.
40. Runyan DK. *Monitoring Child Health and Well-being in Large Population Surveys.* Ann Arbor: University of Michigan Press; 2001.
41. Morrongiello BA, Ondejko L, Littlejohn A. Understanding toddlers' in-home injuries, I: context, correlates, and determinants. *J Pediatr Psychol.* 2004;29: 415-431.
42. Egeland B, Sroufe LA, Erickson M. The developmental consequence of different patterns of maltreatment. *Child Abuse Negl.* 1983;7:459-469.
43. Wu SS, Ma CX, Carter RL, et al. Risk factors for infant maltreatment: a population-based study. *Child Abuse Negl.* 2004;28:1253-1264.
44. Spencer N, Devereux E, Wallace A, et al. Disabling conditions and registration for child abuse and neglect: a population-based study. *Pediatrics.* 2005;116: 609-613.
45. Sidebotham P, Heron J, Team AS. Child maltreatment in the "children of the nineties": the role of the child. *Child Abuse Negl.* 2003;27:337-352.
46. LaRue A, Bank L, Jarvik L, Hetland M. Health in old age: how do physicians' ratings and self-ratings compare? *J Gerontol.* 1979;34:687-691.
47. Garrity TF, Somes GW, Marx MB. Factors influencing self-assessment of health. *Soc Sci Med.* 1978;12:77-81.

# New Orapred ODT™

(prednisolone sodium phosphate orally disintegrating tablets)

## Grape Taste That's Good to Go

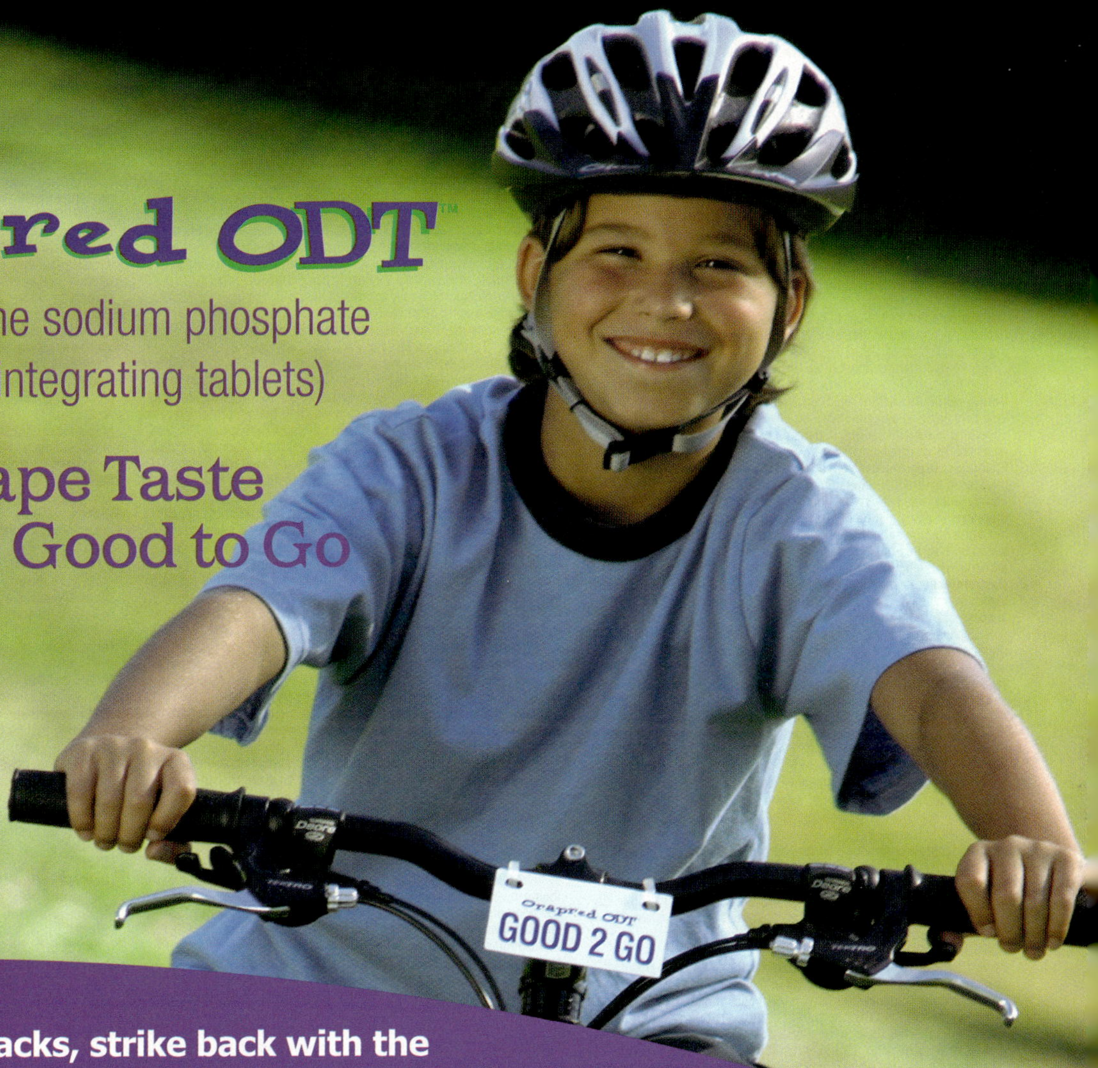


**When asthma attacks, strike back with the kid-friendly tablet that melts in the mouth.**

**The first and only orally disintegrating prednisolone tablet**
**Disintegrates on the tongue without water or messy spoons**
**Kid-preferred grape taste[1]**
**Natural flavors and sweeteners help mask prednisolone's unpleasant taste**

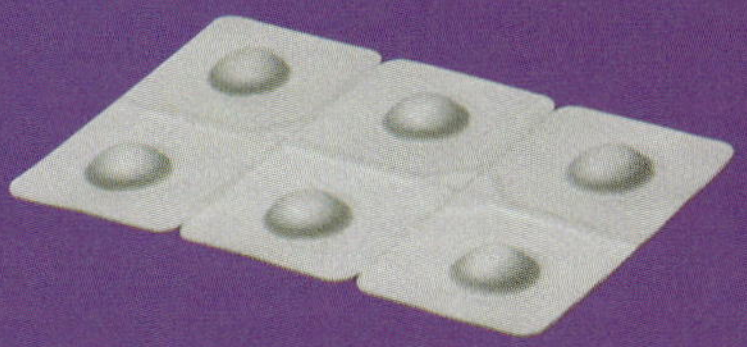

**Orapred ODT™**

(prednisolone sodium phosphate orally disintegrating tablets)
Equivalent to prednisolone 15mg

Important Safety Information.

Orapred ODT™ (prednisolone sodium phosphate orally disintegrating tablets) is a prescription drug product indicated for the control of severe or incapacitating allergic conditions intractable to adequate trials of conventional treatment in adult and pediatric populations with asthma or asthma caused by respiratory disorders. Orapred is contraindicated in patients with systemic fungal infections. **Administration of live or live, attenuated vaccines is contraindicated in patients receiving immunosuppressive doses of corticosteroids. Killed or inactivated vaccines may be administered, however, the response to such vaccines cannot be predicted. Immunization procedures may be undertaken in patients who are receiving corticosteroids as replacement therapy, e.g., for Addison's disease.** Orapred may cause mood swings. Adverse effects of Orapred include the following: endocrine (including development of cushingoid state, increased requirements for insulin or oral hypoglycemic agents in diabetic patients, manifestations of latent diabetes mellitus); fluid and electrolyte disturbances (including fluid retention, hypertension); gastrointestinal (including peptic ulcer with possible perforation and hemorrhage); increased appetite; and weight gain.

For additional safety information, please see brief summary prescribing information on the following page.

Reference: 1. Prednisolone 12 Study. Data on file. Alliant Pharmaceuticals.

**Orapred ODT™**

(prednisolone sodium phosphate orally disintegrating tablets)

**BRIEF SUMMARY:** Please see full prescribing information.

**DESCRIPTION:**
Orapred ODT orally disintegrating tablets are available in strengths containing 13.4 mg, 20.2 mg, and 40.3 mg prednisolone sodium phosphate (equivalent to 10 mg, 15 mg, or 30 mg prednisolone base, respectively).

**PRECAUTIONS: General: Do not break or use partial Orapred ODT tablets.** The lowest possible dose of corticosteroid should be used to control the condition under treatment, and when reduction in dosage is possible, the reduction should be gradual.
Since complications of treatment with glucocorticoids are dependent on the size of the dose and the duration of treatment, a risk/benefit decision must be made in each individual case as to dose and duration of treatment and as to whether daily or intermittent therapy should be used.
There is an enhanced effect of corticosteroids in patients with hypothyroidism and in those with cirrhosis
Kaposi's sarcoma has been reported to occur in patients receiving corticosteroid therapy, most often for chronic conditions. Discontinuation of corticosteroids may result in clinical improvement.
**Cardio-renal:** As sodium retention with resultant edema and potassium loss may occur in patients receiving corticosteroids, these agents should be used with caution in patients with hypertension, congestive heart failure, or renal insufficiency.
**Endocrine:** Drug-induced secondary adrenocortical insufficiency may be minimized by gradual reduction of dosage. This type of relative insufficiency may persist for months after discontinuation of therapy; therefore, in any situation of stress occurring during that period, hormone therapy should be reinstituted. Since mineralocorticoid secretion may be impaired, salt and/or a mineralocorticoid should be administered concurrently.
**Gastrointestinal:** Steroids should be used with caution in nonspecific ulcerative colitis, if there is a probability of impending perforation, abscess or other pyogenic infection;
diverticulitis; fresh intestinal anastomoses; active or latent peptic ulcer. Signs of peritoneal irritation following gastrointestinal perforation in patients receiving corticosteroids may be minimal or absent.
**Musculoskeletal:** Corticosteroids decrease bone formation and increase bone resorption both through their effect on calcium regulation (i.e., decreasing absorption and increasing excretion) and inhibition of osteoblast function. This, together with a decrease in the protein matrix of the bone secondary to an increase in protein catabolism, and reduced sex hormone production, may lead to inhibition of bone growth in children and adolescents and the development of osteoporosis at any age. Special consideration should be given to patients at increased risk of osteoporosis (i.e., postmenopausal women) before initiating corticosteroid therapy.
**Neuro-psychiatric:** Although controlled clinical trials have shown corticosteroids to be effective in speeding the resolution of acute exacerbations of multiple sclerosis, they do not show that they affect the ultimate outcome or natural history of the disease. The studies do show that relatively high doses of corticosteroids are necessary to demonstrate a significant effect. (See DOSAGE AND ADMINISTRATION.)
An acute myopathy has been observed with the use of high doses of corticosteroids, most often occurring in patients with disorders of neuromuscular transmission (e.g., myasthenia gravis), or in patients receiving concomitant therapy with neuromuscular blocking drugs (e.g., pancuronium). This acute myopathy is generalized, may involve ocular and respiratory muscles, and may result in quadriparesis. Elevation of creatinine kinase may occur. Clinical improvement or recovery after stopping corticosteroids may require weeks to years.
Psychic derangements may appear when corticosteroids are used, ranging from euphoria, insomnia, mood swings, personality changes, and severe depression, to frank psychotic manifestations. Also, existing emotional instability or psychotic tendencies may be aggravated by corticosteroids.
**Ophthalmic:** Intraocular pressure may become elevated in some individuals. If steroid therapy is continued for more than 6 weeks, intraocular pressure should be monitored.
**Information For Patients:** Patients should be warned not to discontinue the use of Orapred abruptly or without medical supervision, to advise any medical attendants that they are taking it, and to seek medical advice at once should they develop fever or other signs of infection. Persons who are on immunosuppressant doses of corticosteroids should be warned to avoid exposure to chickenpox or measles. Patients should also be advised that if they are exposed, medical advice should be sought without delay.
**Drug Interactions:** Drugs such as barbiturates, phenytoin, ephedrine, and rifampin, which induce hepatic microsomal drug metabolizing enzyme activity may enhance metabolism of prednisolone and require that the dosage of Orapred be increased.
Increased activity of both cyclosporin and corticosteroids may occur when the two are used concurrently. Convulsions have been reported with this concurrent use.
Estrogens may decrease the hepatic metabolism of certain corticosteroids thereby increasing their effect.
Ketoconazole has been reported to decrease the metabolism of certain corticosteroids by up to 60% leading to an increased risk of corticosteroid side effects.
Coadministration of corticosteroids and warfarin usually results in inhibition of response to warfarin, although there have been some conflicting reports. Therefore, coagulation indices should be monitored frequently to maintain the desired anticoagulant effect.
Concomitant use of aspirin (or other non-steroidal anti-inflammatory agents) and corticosteroids increases the risk of gastrointestinal side effects. Aspirin should be used cautiously in conjunction with corticosteroids in hypoprothrombinemia. The clearance of salicylates may be increased with concurrent use of corticosteroids. When corticosteroids are administered concomitantly with potassium-depleting agents (i.e., diuretics, amphotericin-B), patients should be observed closely for development of
hypokalemia. Patients on digitalis glycosides may be at increased risk of arrhythmias due to hypokalemia.
Concomitant use of anticholinesterase agents and corticosteroids may produce severe weakness in patients with myasthenia gravis. If possible, anticholinesterase agents should be withdrawn at least 24 hours before initiating corticosteroid therapy.
Due to inhibition of antibody response, patients on prolonged corticosteroid therapy may exhibit a diminished response to toxoids and live or inactivated vaccines. Corticosteroids may also potentiate the replication of some organisms contained in live attenuated vaccines. If possible, routine administration of vaccines or toxoids should be deferred until corticosteroid therapy is discontinued.
Because corticosteroids may increase blood glucose concentrations, dosage adjustments of antidiabetic agents may be required.
Corticosteroids may suppress reactions to skin tests.
**Pregnancy: Teratogenic Effects:** *Pregnancy Category C.*
Prednisolone has been shown to be teratogenic in many species when given in doses equivalent to the human dose. Animal studies in which prednisolone has been given to pregnant mice, rats, and rabbits have yielded an increased incidence of cleft palate in the offspring. There are no adequate and well-controlled studies in pregnant women. Orapred should be used during pregnancy only if the potential benefit justifies the potential risk to the fetus. Infants born to mothers who have received corticosteroids during pregnancy should be carefully observed for signs of hypoadrenalism.
**Nursing Mothers:** Systemically administered corticosteroids appear in human milk and could suppress growth, interfere with endogenous corticosteroid production, or cause other untoward effects. Caution should be exercised when Orapred is administered to a nursing woman.
**Pediatric Use:** The efficacy and safety of prednisolone in the pediatric population are based on the well-established course of effect of corticosteroids, which is similar in pediatric and adult populations. Published studies provide evidence of efficacy and safety in pediatric patients for the treatment of nephrotic syndrome (>2 years of age), and aggressive lymphomas and leukemias (>1 month of age). However, some of these conclusions and other indications for pediatric use of corticosteroid, e.g., severe asthma and wheezing, are based on adequate and well-controlled trials conducted in adults, on the premises that the course of the diseases and their pathophysiology are considered to be substantially similar in both populations.
The adverse effects of prednisolone in pediatric patients are similar to those in adults (see ADVERSE REACTIONS). Like adults, pediatric patients should be carefully observed with frequent measurements of blood pressure, weight, height, intraocular pressure, and clinical evaluation for the presence of infection, psychosocial disturbances, thromboembolism, peptic ulcers, cataracts, and osteoporosis. Children, who are treated with corticosteroids by any route, including systemically administered corticosteroids, may experience a decrease in their growth velocity. This negative impact of corticosteroids on growth has been observed at low systemic doses and in the absence of laboratory evidence of HPA axis suppression (i.e., cosyntropin stimulation and basal cortisol plasma levels). Growth velocity may therefore be a more sensitive indicator of systemic corticosteroid exposure in children than some commonly used tests of HPA axis function. The linear growth of children treated with corticosteroids by any route should be monitored, and the potential growth effects of prolonged treatment should be weighed against clinical benefits obtained and the availability of other treatment alternatives. In order to minimize the potential growth effects of corticosteroids, children should be *titrated* to the lowest effective dose.
**Geriatric Use:** Clinical studies of prednisolone sodium phosphate oral solution did not include sufficient numbers of subjects aged 65 and over to determine whether they respond differently from younger subjects. Other reported clinical experience with prednisolone sodium phosphate has not identified differences in responses between the elderly and younger patients. However, the incidence of corticosteroid-induced side effects may be increased in geriatric patients and appear to be dose-related. Osteoporosis is the most frequently encountered complication, which occurs at a higher incidence rate in corticosteroid-treated geriatric patients as compared to younger populations and in agematched controls. Losses of bone mineral density appear to be greatest early on in the course of treatment and may recover over time after steroid withdrawal or use of lower doses (i.e., 5 mg/day). Prednisolone doses of 7.5 mg/day or higher, have been associated with an increased relative risk of both vertebral and nonvertebral fractures, even in the presence of higher bone density compared to patients with involutional osteoporosis.
Routine screening of geriatric patients, including regular assessments of bone mineral density and institution of fracture prevention strategies, along with regular review of Orapred indication should be undertaken to minimize complications and keep the Orapred dose at the lowest acceptable level. Co-administration of bisphosphonates has been shown to retard the rate of bone loss in corticosteroid-treated males and postmenopausal females, and these agents are recommended in the prevention and treatment of corticosteroid-induced osteoporosis.
It has been reported that equivalent weight-based doses yield higher total and unbound prednisolone plasma concentrations and reduced renal and non-renal clearance in elderly patients compared to younger populations. However, it is not clear whether dosing reductions would be necessary in elderly patients, since these pharmacokinetic alterations may be offset by age-related differences in responsiveness of target organs and/or less pronounced suppression of adrenal release of cortisol. Dose selection for an elderly patient should be cautious, usually starting at the low end of the dosing range, reflecting the greater frequency of decreased hepatic, renal, or cardiac function, and of concomitant disease or other drug therapy.
This drug is known to be substantially excreted by the kidney, and the risk of toxic reactions to this drug may be greater in patients with impaired renal function. Because elderly patients are more likely to have decreased renal function, care should be taken in dose selection, and it may be useful to monitor renal function (see CLINICAL PHARMACOLOGY).

**ADVERSE REACTIONS: (listed alphabetically under each subsection):**
**Cardiovascular:** Hypertrophic cardiomyopathy in premature infants.
**Dermatologic:** Facial erythema; increased sweating; impaired wound healing; may suppress reactions to skin tests; petechiae and ecchymoses; thin fragile skin; urticaria; edema.
**Endocrine:** Decreased carbohydrate tolerance; development of cushingoid state; hirsutism; increased requirements for insulin or oral hypoglycemic agents in diabetic patients; manifestations of latent diabetes mellitus; menstrual irregularities; secondary adrenocortical and pituitary unresponsiveness, particularly in times of stress, as in trauma, surgery or illness; suppression of growth in children.
**Fluid and Electrolyte Disturbances:** Congestive heart failure in susceptible patients; fluid retention; hypertension; hypokalemic alkalosis; potassium loss; sodium retention.
**Gastrointestinal:** Abdominal distention; elevation in serum liver enzyme levels (usually reversible upon discontinuation); pancreatitis; peptic ulcer with possible perforation and hemorrhage; ulcerative esophagitis.
**Metabolic:** Negative nitrogen balance due to protein catabolism.
**Musculoskeletal:** Aseptic necrosis of femoral and humeral heads; loss of muscle mass; muscle weakness; osteoporosis; pathologic fracture of long bones; steroid myopathy; tendon rupture; vertebral compression fractures.
**Neurological:** Convulsions; headache; increased intracranial pressure with papilledema
(pseudotumor cerebri) usually following discontinuation of treatment; psychic disorders; vertigo.
**Ophthalmic:** Exophthalmos; glaucoma; increased intraocular pressure; posterior subcapsular cataracts.
**Other:** Increased appetite; malaise; nausea; weight gain.
In clinical trials with ORAPRED ODT, the following adverse reactions were seen.
Facial edema, pharyngolaryngeal pain, blood in stool, eye irritation, eyelid edema.

**OVERDOSAGE:** The effects of accidental ingestion of large quantities of prednisolone over a very short period of time have not been reported, but prolonged use of the drug can produce mental symptoms, moon face, abnormal fat deposits, fluid retention, excessive appetite, weight gain, hypertrichosis, acne, striae, ecchymosis, increased sweating, pigmentation, dry scaly skin, thinning scalp hair, increased blood pressure, tachycardia, thrombophlebitis, decreased resistance to infection, negative nitrogen balance with delayed bone and wound healing, headache, weakness, menstrual disorders, accentuated menopausal symptoms, neuropathy, fractures, osteoporosis, peptic ulcer, decreased glucose tolerance, hypokalemia, and adrenal insufficiency. Hepatomegaly and abdominal distention have been observed in children.

Treatment of acute overdosage is by immediate gastric lavage or emesis followed by supportive and symptomatic therapy. For chronic overdosage in the face of severe disease requiring continuous steroid therapy, the dosage of prednisolone may be reduced only temporarily, or alternate day treatment may be introduced.

**Do not break or use partial Orapred ODT tablets.** Keep out of the reach of children.

**Rx only**
Revised May 2006.

Manufactured for Alliant Pharmaceuticals, Inc.
Alpharetta, GA 30022

by CIMA LABS INC., Eden Prairie, MN 55344 (Orapred ODT)

# The Other Children

## *A Survey of Child Abuse Physicians on the Medical Evaluation of Children Living With a Physically Abused Child*

*Kristine A. Campbell, MD, MSc; Debra L. Bogen, MD; Rachel P. Berger, MD, MPH*

**Objective:** To explore the practice and attitudes of child abuse physicians regarding the evaluation of "contact children" identified in the home of a physically abused index child.

**Design:** A self-administered survey.

**Setting:** E-mail and postal mailings from May 10 through September 30, 2005.

**Participants:** Physicians in the United States recognized as experts in child abuse medicine based on membership in the Helfer Society.

**Main Outcome Measures:** Descriptive measures of recommended medical evaluations of contact children in 3 clinical settings, estimates of association between these recommendations, and respondent experiences.

**Results:** There was a 61% (93/153) response rate. Respondents uniformly endorsed medical evaluation for contact children, although there was substantial variability in the extent of evaluation recommended. Recommended diagnostic testing varied by age of contact child and by type of abuse in the index child. Recommendations were influenced by anecdotal recall of abused contact children "missed" during the initial evaluation of another child in the household. Of our 93 respondents, 37 (40%) reported routine disagreement with child protection workers about the need for medical evaluation of contact children.

**Conclusions:** Child abuse physicians perceive that findings of abuse in contact children are sufficiently frequent to warrant medical examination of most contact children, but there is no consensus on the extent of evaluation needed for contact children. A better understanding of risk of abuse in contact children and improved collaboration between physicians and child protection workers are needed to improve evidence-based care of this high-risk population.

*Arch Pediatr Adolesc Med. 2006;160:1241-1246*

**Author Affiliations:** General Academic Pediatrics (Drs Campbell and Bogen) and Child Advocacy Center (Dr Berger), Children's Hospital of Pittsburgh, Pittsburgh, Pa. Dr Campbell is now with the Division of Safe and Healthy Families, Department of Pediatrics, Primary Children's Medical Center, Salt Lake City, Utah.

IN 2004, MORE THAN 2 PER 1000 US children were documented as experiencing physical abuse.[1] Many of these children were living with siblings, stepsiblings, cousins, and other children. In a medical model for communicable disease, these household children would be identified as at-risk contacts and would receive medical care for exposure to pertussis or meningococcus. In the field of child abuse, however, there are little data describing (1) the risk of abuse for "contact children" living in a physically abusive household, (2) the role of the medical evaluation in assessing this risk, or (3) the extent of medical evaluation needed to detect abusive injury in these children.

Public concern for these contact children of abuse has earned national media attention in recent months.[2,3] Contrary to popular theories that families tend to scapegoat a single child,[4-7] experience suggests that all children identified in a violent home are at a high risk of experiencing abuse. Limited observations drawn from several case series[5,8-12] describe reports of suspected abuse in 30% to 60% of siblings of abused children over the years following an initial report of abuse in the home. A larger review[7] documented concern for abuse in siblings in 175 (56%) of 310 British families in which a single child was reported as being abused. Unfortunately, none of these studies provides descriptions of the pattern or timing of abuse found in contact children. We do not know how often contact children have findings of abuse coincident with the recognition of physical abuse in an index child, and cannot say whether a medical evaluation is likely to reveal abusive injury not already suspected by the child protection worker.

We recently evaluated 2 children for abusive injuries in the days and months following recognition of physical abuse in another child in their households. In each

**Table. Characteristics of Survey Respondents**

| Characteristic | No. (%) of the 93 Respondents* |
|---|---|
| Female sex | 48 (52) |
| Sees >50 physical abuse cases annually | 42 (45) |
| Spends at least 50% of professional time in clinical child abuse medicine | 49 (53) |
| Routinely participates in MDT meetings | 68 (73) |
| Time spent in child abuse medicine, y | |
| <10 | 26 (28) |
| 10-20 | 33 (35) |
| >20 | 31 (33) |
| No response | 3 (3) |
| Recalls a contact child who experienced further abuse attributed to incomplete evaluation following an earlier index report | |
| Yes | 48 (52) |
| No | 31 (33) |
| Not sure | 13 (14) |
| No response | 1 (1) |

Abbreviation: MDT, multidisciplinary team.
*Percentages do not sum to 100 because of rounding.

case, there was discussion within our medical team regarding the urgency and extent of evaluation needed for the contact child at the time of the index report. Given the lack of evidence regarding the medical evaluation of children living in the home of a physically abused child, we decided to explore practices and attitudes of other child abuse physicians in the evaluation of these children.

We designed a survey instrument to elicit perceptions of child abuse physicians regarding risk of abuse in contact children and to gather recommendations of child abuse physicians regarding appropriate medical evaluation of these children. We hypothesized that respondents would recommend medical evaluations of contact children and that the extent of the recommended evaluation would relate to the age of the contact child and to the severity of abuse in the index child. We conducted analyses to determine whether there was expert consensus regarding the evaluation of contact children and to highlight areas in the care of contact children that may require future investigation.

## METHODS

### STUDY DESIGN

We surveyed members of the Helfer Society (http://helfersociety.org/), an honorary society of physicians elected for leadership in diagnosis, treatment, and research related to child abuse and neglect. We distributed surveys through the Helfer Society membership Internet listserv in May 2005. Eligible nonresponders subsequently received surveys via US mail and personal e-mail accounts through September 30, 2005. Our administrative assistant received completed surveys and removed all identifying information before responses were entered into a database for analysis. The Helfer Society received a donation of $2 for each completed survey. The study was approved by the institutional review board of the University of Pittsburgh.

### PARTICIPANTS

We chose to survey members of the Helfer Society because we wanted to describe the practice and perceptions of physicians who had substantial experience in the field of child abuse medicine. Helfer Society officers provided us with access to the 175 members for the study. We excluded non-US members (n = 12), members with ties to the Children's Hospital of Pittsburgh (n = 3), and pathologists not directly involved in clinical care (n = 7).

### SURVEY

The survey was designed to elicit perceptions, experiences, and medical recommendations of respondents in relation to risk of abuse in children identified in the home of a child diagnosed as being physically abused. Eight items surveyed perceptions and experiences of participants regarding abuse in contact children using yes, no, or unknown or 5-point Likert scale response options. Three case scenarios presented choices for the evaluation of index and contact children of varying ages and abuse exposures. The survey was designed by one of us (K.A.C.) with assistance from a measurements expert at the University of Pittsburgh. Two of us (D.L.B. and R.P.B.) and 6 others in child abuse medicine (not members of the Helfer Society) graded the instrument for clarity and relevance. We examined these responses and revised and retested the instrument before distribution.

### STATISTICAL ANALYSIS

We calculated frequencies to describe the perceptions and experiences of respondents and the medical evaluations recommended for case scenarios. To account for ordinal response data, we examined associations between perceptions and experiences using Spearman rank correlation and Wilcoxon rank sum statistics. We compared medical recommendations for contact children of different ages and abuse exposures using Fisher exact test statistics. Significance was defined as $P < .05$. All analyses were conducted using Stata statistics software, version 9.0 (StataCorp LP, College Station, Tex).

## RESULTS

### SURVEY RESPONDENTS

We received 93 completed surveys from 153 eligible members, for a response rate of 61%. Respondents did not differ from nonrespondents by sex or geographic region. Of the respondents, 49 (53%) spent more than half of their professional time in child abuse clinical practice; 42 (45%) evaluated at least 1 case of physical abuse per week. Most respondents reported routine participation in multidisciplinary team meetings with community child protection teams (**Table**). Of the respondents, 48 (52%) recalled a contact child who experienced abuse that the respondent attributed to incomplete evaluation at the time of report of physical abuse in an index child.

### PERCEPTIONS AND EXPERIENCES REGARDING RISK OF ABUSE IN CONTACT CHILDREN

#### Need for Medical Evaluations in Contact Children

All respondents believed that physicians diagnosing physical abuse in an index child should make recommenda-

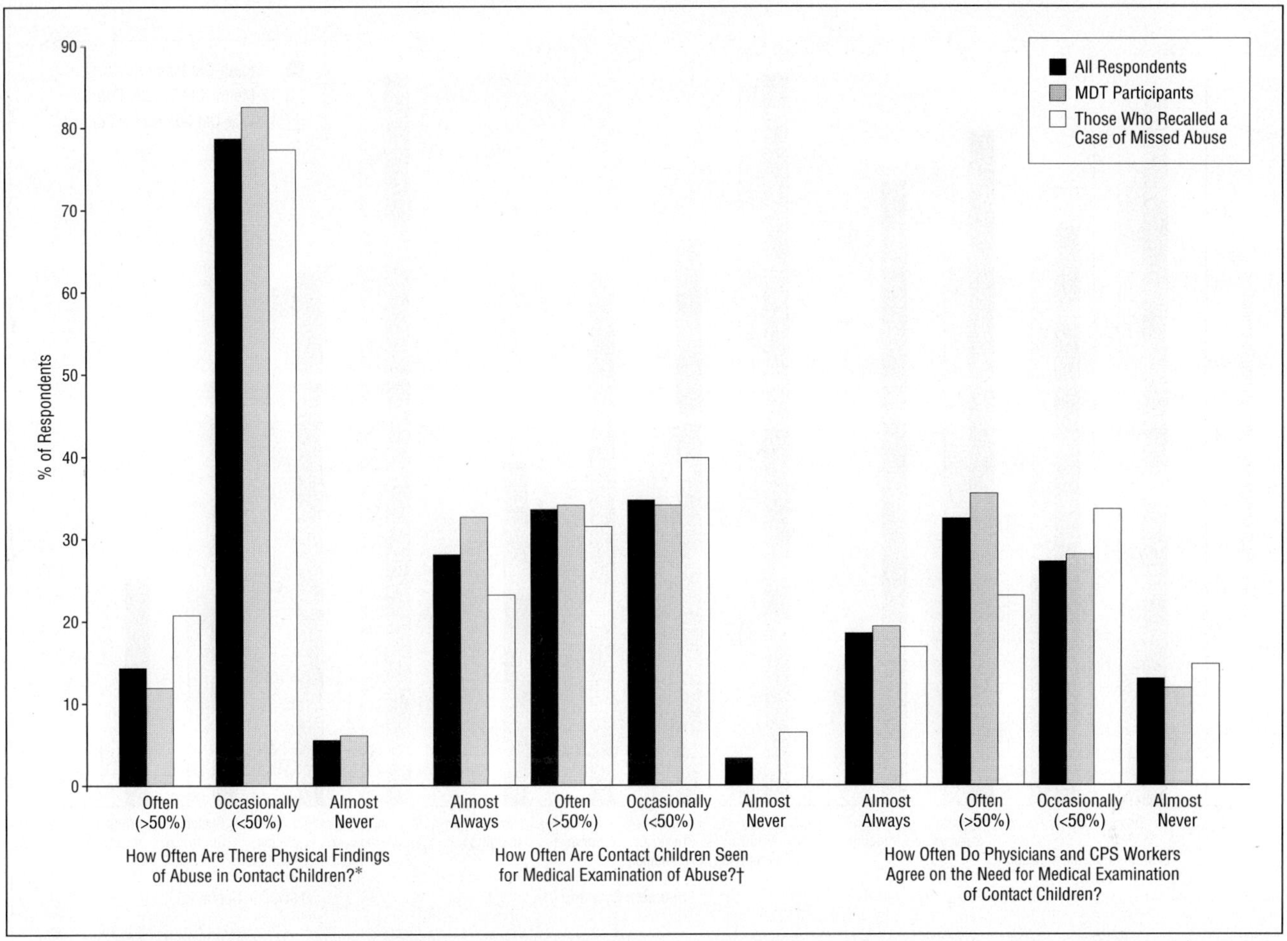


**Figure 1.** Experiences and perceptions of respondents regarding the need and the frequency of medical evaluations of contact children and agreement with child protective service (CPS) workers regarding medical evaluations of contact children. The asterisk indicates that respondents who recalled a case of "missed abuse" in a contact child reported findings of abuse in contact children more frequently than those who did not recall a case of missed abuse (*P* = .009, Wilcoxon rank sum test) and the dagger that respondents who served on a multidisciplinary team (MDT) perceived that contact children were seen more frequently than respondents who did not serve on an MDT (*P* = .049, Wilcoxon rank sum test).

tions regarding the need for medical evaluations of other children in the home. Respondents rated severity of injury to the index child, age of the contact child, and history of prior abuse in the home as the most important factors in determining the need for medical evaluation of contact children. Most respondents (73 [78%]) believed that contact children occasionally had findings of physical abuse on examination (**Figure 1**).

### Frequency of Medical Evaluations in Contact Children

Although respondents favored medical evaluations for contact children, there was wide variability in the frequency that experts reported seeing contact children in practice. Of the respondents, 3 (3%) indicated that contact children were "almost never" seen for medical evaluations; the remainder reported that contacts were "occasionally" (32 [34%]), "often" (31 [33%]), or "almost always" (26 [28%]) seen (Figure 1). One respondent (1%) was unsure of the frequency of contact evaluations. Respondents participating in multidisciplinary team meetings with child protective service (CPS) workers reported a higher frequency of medical evaluations among contact children compared with respondents who were not multidisciplinary team meeting participants (Wilcoxon rank sum test, *P*=.049).

### Agreement With CPS Workers

Of our respondents, 37 (40%) reported disagreement with CPS workers on indications for medical evaluation of contact children in at least half of all abuse cases. There was a positive correlation between the frequency of contact evaluation and the frequency of agreement with CPS workers (Spearman $\rho$=0.74, *P*<.005). Multidisciplinary team participation did not influence agreement with CPS workers (Wilcoxon rank sum test, *P*=.90).

## MEDICAL EVALUATIONS OF CONTACT CHILDREN

Three case scenarios were used to elicit medical recommendations for the evaluation of contact children. Each scenario involved a family composed of a mother, a father, 1-month-old twins, a 19-month-old boy, and a 12-year-old girl. In each case, a different child was identified as the index child. Participants were asked about their

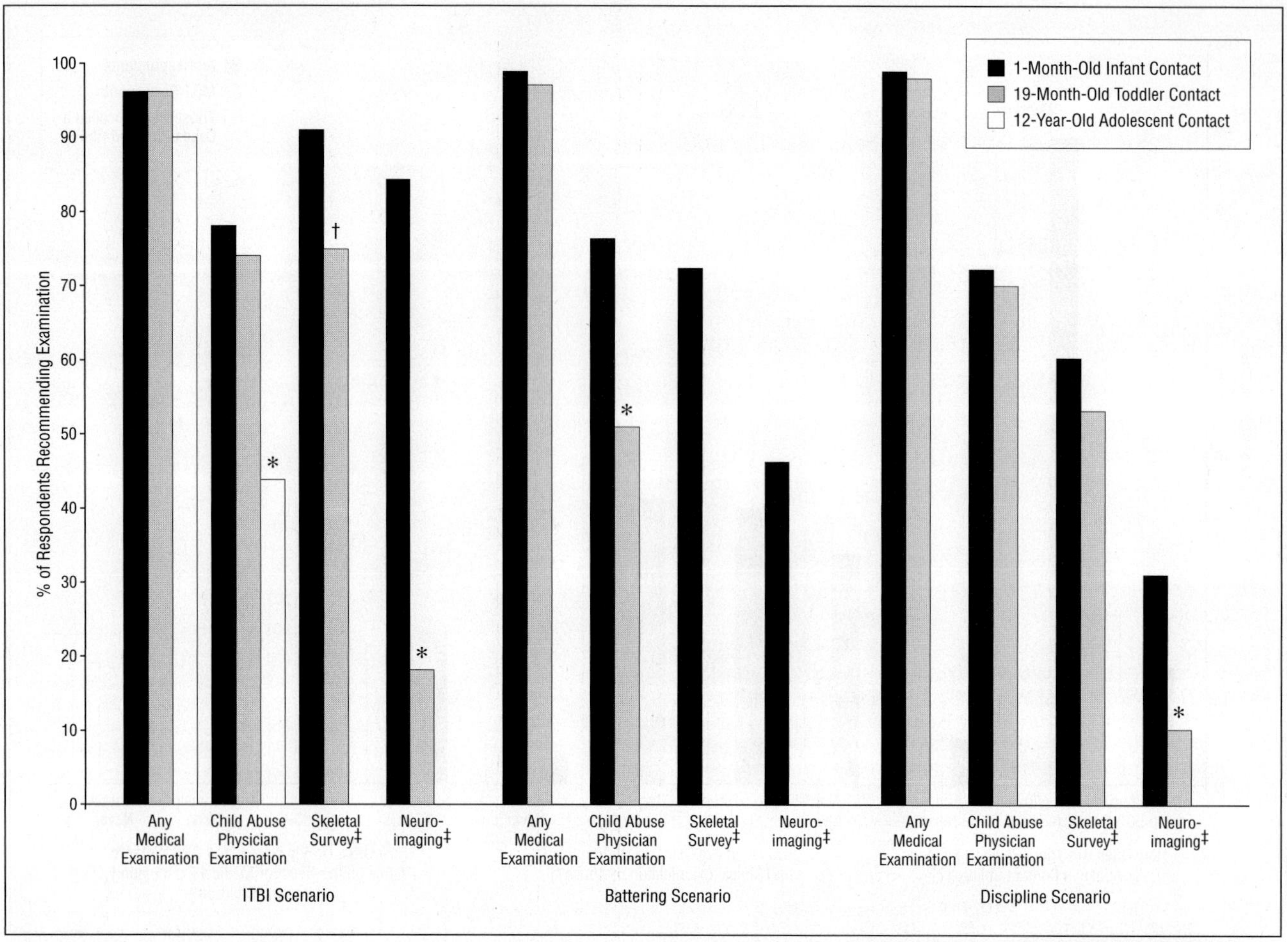


**Figure 2.** Medical evaluations recommended for contact children. Detailed descriptions of case scenarios are given in the "Medical Evaluations of Contact Children" subsection of the "Results" section. ITBI indicates inflicted traumatic brain injury. The asterisk ($P<.001$) and dagger ($P=.003$) indicate that this value differs from the same evaluation in the next youngest contact child. The double dagger indicates that participants were not asked about imaging recommendations for teen contacts.

recommended evaluations for each contact child (**Figure 2**).

### Inflicted Traumatic Brain Injury Scenario

In this scenario, one of the 1-month-old twins presents with scalp bruising. The twin has a subdural hemorrhage and is diagnosed as having inflicted traumatic brain injury (ITBI). All contacts are well, with unremarkable "foster placement evaluations" in the emergency department. Of the respondents, 93 (100%) recommended further medical evaluation of the twin and toddler; 84 (90%) recommended further evaluation of the 12-year-old girl. Respondents believed that the younger siblings should be seen by a child abuse physician; most believed that the adolescent could be seen by a primary care physician. Of the respondents, 78 (84%) recommended imaging for possible ITBI in the twin; 85 respondents (91%) and 70 respondents (75%) recommended imaging for skeletal injury in the twin and toddler, respectively.

### Battering Scenario

In this scenario, the 19-month-old boy presents with facial bruising. The boy has extensive bruising and adult bite marks, and he is diagnosed as being physically abused. All contacts are healthy according to CPS workers. Almost all respondents (90-93 [97%-100%]) recommended medical evaluation of the contacts. Recommendations for brain and skeletal imaging of the twins were made by 46 (49%) and 67 (72%) of the respondents, respectively. Write-in recommendations for forensic interviews (8 [9%] respondents) and counseling referrals (2 [2%] respondents) were made for the adolescent contact child.

### Discipline Scenario

In this scenario, the 12-year-old girl presents with bruises. She has patterned skin injuries and discloses "whippings." She is diagnosed as being physically abused. All contacts are well according to CPS workers. Respondents recommended medical evaluation of the infant and toddler siblings, but fewer indicated a preference for a child abuse physician evaluation over a primary care physician evaluation. Brain imaging for the twins was recommended by 29 (31%) of the respondents, while skeletal surveys were recommended by 56 (60%) of the respondents.

## Influence of Index Case on Recommended Evaluation

While respondents consistently supported medical evaluations for contact infants, the recommended diagnostic evaluation varied according to characteristics of the index case (**Figure 3**). Of the respondents, 78 (84%) believed that neuroimaging was indicated for the infant contact of a twin with ITBI, but only 29 (31%) would seek neuroimaging for the infant contact of a physically abused adolescent ($P<.001$). Similarly, skeletal surveys were recommended by 85 respondents (91%) in the case of ITBI in a twin but only by 56 respondents (60%) if living with an abused adolescent ($P<.001$).

## Influence of Recall of "Missed Abuse" in a Contact Child on Recommended Evaluation

Participants reporting recall of a case of missed abuse in a contact child were significantly more likely to recommend computed tomography of the head (Fisher exact test, $P=.02$). These respondents also favored skeletal surveys in toddler contacts compared with respondents who did not recall a case of missed abuse (Fisher exact test, $P=.09$).

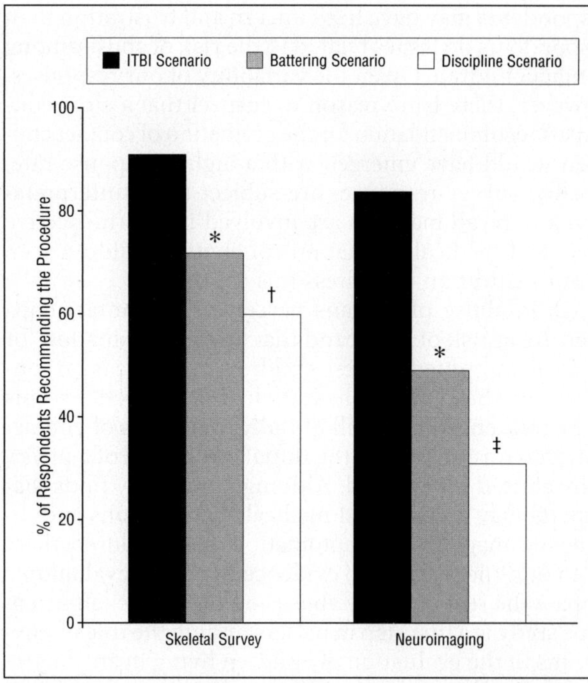


**Figure 3.** Diagnostic evaluations recommended for the infant contact, by index case. Detailed descriptions of case scenarios are given in the "Medical Evaluations of Contact Children" subsection of the "Results" section. ITBI indicates inflicted traumatic brain injury; $^*P<.001$; †, $P=.09$; and ‡, $P=.01$.

## COMMENT

To our knowledge, this is the first study to address the medical evaluation of children sharing a home with a physically abused child. The results support our initial hypotheses on the perceived need for medical evaluations of abuse and the extent of diagnostic evaluations recommended for contact children. Respondents believed that contact children should undergo medical evaluations following a report of physical abuse of an index child in the home. Respondents recommended more extensive diagnostic evaluations for younger contacts and for contacts of more severely injured index children.

Except in the ITBI scenario, no clear pattern of recommendations for the medical evaluation of contact children emerged from our study results. We observed wide variability in recommended diagnostic evaluations even among this small and expert respondent set. The consistency in recommendations for skeletal and neurologic imaging of the twin of an infant with ITBI was expected and supported by a small but intuitive set of literature on the increased risk of abuse among twin sets.[13-15] This consistency disappeared when respondents were asked about the diagnostic evaluations of contact toddlers or the need for child abuse physician evaluations in older contact children. Anecdotal experience with abused contact children seemed to inform diagnostic recommendations, particularly for toddler contacts.

Recommendations for imaging of well-appearing contacts reflect a valid concern for missed opportunities to diagnose inflicted injuries.[16-18] Hesitation to recommend imaging in asymptomatic children demonstrates recognition of long-term health risks and short-term economic costs associated with such evaluations. Without improved understanding of the probability of abusive injury in contact children, it is difficult to know whether diagnostic imaging for occult injury is "worth" the associated short- and long-term costs. We conclude that there is no consensus on the diagnostic evaluations needed to evaluate possible abuse in contact children. Our study supports the need for further research on risks and patterns of abuse in this high-risk population.

The decision to seek medical evaluation for abuse in contact children generally falls to local CPS workers, so it is not surprising that the rate of medical evaluations for contacts varies between respondents. More concerning is the frequency with which child abuse physicians disagree with local CPS workers on the need for medical evaluations of contact children. Frustration with CPS has been recognized as a barrier to appropriate reporting of suspected child maltreatment by general pediatricians.[19-21] It is disheartening to find that even experts working with multidisciplinary teams report frequent disagreement. As child abuse medicine grows as a discipline, efforts to create and sustain ties between medical and social service teams are needed to improve care of children evaluated for abuse.

The interpretation of our results must be made in the context of study limitations. We chose a limited sample to define expert practice in this area. The experiences and practices of these physicians may not reflect general pediatric practice. Similarly, we did not attempt to survey social work colleagues in this study. Understanding the experiences and practices of CPS workers would contribute to the interdisciplinary cooperation we believe is necessary in this field. Future studies should consider the experiences and attitudes of a wider range of respondents toward risk of abuse in contact children. As with all surveys, there is the potential for response bias. Nonrespondents may have less concern and frustration than respondents on issues related to the risk of abuse among contact children. Given the variability of our responses, however, there is no reason to suspect that a clear consensus recommendation for the evaluation of contact children would have emerged with a higher response rate. Finally, survey responses are subject to misinterpretation and recall bias. We are involved in a retrospective review of medical evaluations of contact children seen at our institution to address this concern.

Child abuse physicians perceive that contact children are at risk of abuse and that medical evaluation for abuse is warranted in these children, but there is no consensus on the extent of these evaluations. Practice seems to be influenced by recall of individual cases of contact children missed during the initial evaluation of a physically abused index child. Although our study finds that experts may recommend medical examinations and diagnostic imaging in asymptomatic contact children, there is, to our knowledge, no evidence that such evaluations impact the risk of future abuse among contact children. This study is a first step in understanding the role of physicians in the evaluation of children living in an abusive home. Further research is needed to provide an evidence base to guide the multidisciplinary care of this at-risk population.

**Accepted for Publication:** July 5, 2006.
**Correspondence:** Kristine A. Campbell, MD, MSc, Department of Pediatrics, The University of Utah, Intermountain Injury Control Research Center and Primary Children's Medical Center, Safe and Healthy Families Team, 295 Chipeta Way, PO Box 581289, Salt Lake City, UT 84158 (kristine.campbell@hsc.utah.edu).
**Author Contributions:** *Study concept and design:* Campbell, Bogen, and Berger. *Acquisition of data:* Campbell. *Analysis and interpretation of data:* Campbell and Bogen. *Drafting of the manuscript:* Campbell, Bogen, and Berger. *Critical revision of the manuscript for important intellectual content:* Campbell and Bogen. *Statistical analysis:* Campbell and Bogen. *Obtained funding:* Campbell. *Study supervision:* Berger.
**Financial Disclosure:** None reported.
**Funding/Support:** This study was funded by grant D55HP05156-01-00 from Health Resources and Services Administration (Dr Campbell).
**Acknowledgment:** We thank Galen Switzer, PhD, and Janet Squires, MD, for their assistance with survey design and development; Dianna Ploof, EdD, for her expert assistance with manuscript preparation; and the Helfer Society members for their thoughtful participation.

## REFERENCES

1. *Child Maltreatment 2004.* Washington, DC: US Government Printing Office; 2006.
2. Kaufman L, Baker A. Bronx boy, 4, is dead: family was investigated. *New York Times.* January 31, 2006:A1.
3. Bernstein N. A tough road for siblings who survived abuse. *New York Times.* January 15, 2006:§1:27.
4. Halperin SM. Family perceptions of abused children and their siblings. *Child Abuse Negl.* 1983;7:107-115.
5. Herrenkohl EC, Herrenkohl RC. A comparison of abused children and their nonabused siblings. *J Am Acad Child Psychiatry.* 1979;18:260-269.
6. Nakou S, Adam H, Stathacopoulou N, Agathonos H. Health status of abused and neglected children and their siblings. *Child Abuse Negl.* 1982;6:279-284.
7. Hamilton-Giachritsis CE, Browne KD. A retrospective study of risk to siblings in abusing families. *J Fam Psychol.* 2005;19:619-624.
8. Doueck HJ, Bronson DE, Levine M. Evaluating risk assessment implementation in child protection: issues for consideration. *Child Abuse Negl.* 1992;16:637-646.
9. Rivara FP. Physical abuse in children under two: a study of therapeutic outcomes. *Child Abuse Negl.* 1985;9:81-87.
10. Jean-Gilles M, Crittenden PM. Maltreating families: a look at siblings. *Fam Relations J Appl Fam Child Stud.* 1990;39:323-329.
11. Hicks RA, Gaughan DC. Understanding fatal child abuse. *Child Abuse Negl.* 1995; 19:855-863.
12. Alexander R, Crabbe L, Sato Y, Smith W, Bennett T. Serial abuse in children who are shaken. *AJDC.* 1990;144:58-60.
13. Groothuis JR, Altemeier WA, Robarge JP, et al. Increased child abuse in families with twins. *Pediatrics.* 1982;70:769-773.
14. Nelson HB, Martin CA. Increased child abuse in twins. *Child Abuse Negl.* 1985; 9:501-505.
15. Hansen KK. Twins and child abuse. *Arch Pediatr Adolesc Med.* 1994;148:1345-1346.
16. Jenny C, Hymel KP, Ritzen A, Reinert SE, Hay TC. Analysis of missed cases of abusive head trauma [published correction appears in *JAMA.* 1999;282:29]. *JAMA.* 1999;281:621-626.
17. Laskey AL, Holsti M, Runyan DK, Socolar RR. Occult head trauma in young suspected victims of physical abuse. *J Pediatr.* 2004;144:719-722.
18. Rubin DM, Christian CW, Bilaniuk LT, Zazyczny KA, Durbin DR. Occult head injury in high-risk abused children. *Pediatrics.* 2003;111:1382-1386.
19. Theodore AD, Runyan DK. A medical research agenda for child maltreatment: negotiating the next steps. *Pediatrics.* 1999;104:168-177.
20. Flaherty EG, Sege R, Binns HJ, Mattson CL, Christoffel KK; Pediatric Practice Research Group. Health care providers' experience reporting child abuse in the primary care setting. *Arch Pediatr Adolesc Med.* 2000;154:489-493.
21. Flaherty EG, Jones R, Sege R; Child Abuse Recognition Experience Study Research Group. Telling their stories: primary care practitioners' experience evaluating and reporting injuries caused by child abuse. *Child Abuse Negl.* 2004; 28:939-945.

ARTICLE

# Nondisclosure of Sexual Orientation to a Physician Among a Sample of Gay, Lesbian, and Bisexual Youth

*Garth D. Meckler, MD, MSHS; Marc N. Elliott, PhD; David E. Kanouse, PhD; Kristin P. Beals, PhD; Mark A. Schuster, MD, PhD*

**Background:** The American Medical Association, the American Academy of Pediatrics, and the Society for Adolescent Medicine recommend discussing sexual orientation as part of the health supervision of all adolescents. Little is known about whether lesbian, gay, and bisexual (LGB) youth hide their orientation from health care providers, which can potentially lead to missed opportunities in identifying individual health risks and provide appropriate screening and counseling.

**Objectives:** To describe the health care experiences of a nonclinical sample of LGB youth and identify factors associated with disclosure and nondisclosure of orientation to physicians.

**Design:** Community-based participatory study using a self-administered questionnaire.

**Setting:** Los Angeles youth empowerment conference held in October 2003 targeting high school–aged LGB youth.

**Participants:** One hundred thirty-one youth aged 14 to 18 years who identified themselves as LGB.

**Main Outcome Measure:** Physician's knowledge of participant's sexual orientation.

**Results:** Thirty-five percent of the sample reported that their physician knew they were LGB. Bisexual youth were less likely than gay and lesbian youth to have disclosed. The strongest predictor of disclosure was having discussed sex or sexual health of any kind with a physician (odds ratio, 15.47; 95% confidence interval, 4.34-55.18). When asked what a physician could do to make talking about being LGB more comfortable, 64% of participants chose the survey response, "Just ask me."

**Conclusions:** Even among a nonclinical sample of LGB youth who were open enough about their orientation to attend a conference on the subject, only 35% reported that their physician knew their orientation. The results indicate that physicians had not discussed sexuality with most LGB youth in the study and that most youth would welcome such a discussion.

*Arch Pediatr Adolesc Med. 2006;160:1248-1254*

THE DEVELOPMENT OF A healthy sexual identity during adolescence is often fraught with stress.[1,2] The process may be particularly difficult for lesbian, gay, and bisexual (LGB) youth, who not only face challenges and health risks in common with their heterosexual peers, but who also must confront stigma while struggling to reconcile emerging sexual feelings with social norms.[2-4] Some LGB youth are at heightened risk for depression, suicide, substance abuse, rejection by family, violence, school failure, and sexually transmitted infections, including human immunodeficiency virus.[3,5-21] Although particular sexual behaviors, rather than sexual orientation itself, determine a youth's risk for sexually transmitted infection, self-identification as LGB may be associated with feelings of isolation and stigma, which contribute to the risk for psychosocial problems. Therefore, guidelines from the American Academy of Pediatrics (AAP), the American Medical Association, and the Society for Adolescent Medicine recommend that health care providers discuss sexuality with all adolescents and provide nonjudgmental communication about sexual orientation.[22-28]

Despite these recommendations, several studies report low rates of disclosure of sexual orientation to health care providers by LGB adolescents and adults.[29-33] Obstacles to disclosure include homophobia among health care providers; a lack of

*For editorial comment see page 1303*

**Author Affiliations:** UCLA/RAND Center for Adolescent Health Promotion, Los Angeles, Calif (Drs Meckler, Elliott, Kanouse, and Schuster); RAND, Santa Monica, Calif (Drs Kanouse and Schuster); Department of Psychology, California State University, Fullerton (Dr Beals); Department of Pediatrics, School of Medicine, University of California, Los Angeles (Dr Schuster); and Department of Health Services, School of Public Health, University of California, Los Angeles (Dr Schuster). Dr. Meckler is now with Oregon Health and Sciences University, Portland.

provider training, knowledge, and comfort about LGB issues; and patient concerns about confidentiality.[2,7,29,34-44] Nondisclosure may result in missed opportunities for health care providers to offer appropriate health education and counseling, perform targeted screening and treatment, and identify individual risks. Disclosure of sexual orientation to a provider has been associated with increased levels of patient satisfaction[2,29,30,33,34,36,45] and quality of care.[46] Although many studies have described the health care experiences of LGB adults, few have included LGB youth.[47-49] One study that surveyed 18- to 23-year-olds about their experiences at ages 14 to 18 years found that only 13% of self-identified LGB youth had disclosed their orientation to a provider.[47] Little is known about the health care experiences of nonclinical samples of LGB youth, or how growing public awareness and increasing societal acceptance of homosexuality in recent years[50] may have affected their experiences discussing sexual orientation with a provider.

We examined the health care experiences of LGB youth using a nonclinical sample from a 2003 LGB conference. We aimed to (1) describe access to and use of health services among LGB youth, (2) determine rates of disclosure of LGB sexual orientation, as perceived by LGB youth, (3) identify potential barriers to disclosure and elicit suggestions for how to make discussing sexual orientation more comfortable, and (4) identify factors that were associated with disclosure.

## METHODS

### HUMAN SUBJECTS APPROVAL

This study was reviewed and approved by the institutional review board at the University of California, Los Angeles.

### PARTICIPANTS

Participants were invited to take part during the Models of Pride Youth Conference held in October 2003 on a southern California college campus. This privately funded conference is an annual full-day youth empowerment event that is open to all LGB high school–aged youth from Los Angeles County. Among 192 conference participants, aged 14 to 18 years, 179 (93%) completed the questionnaire. Analyses presented here do not include 25 respondents self-identified as heterosexual, 9 who were identified as transgender (because survey items analyzed for this article focused on orientation rather than gender identity), 5 who were missing data (>90% of items missing), and 9 who had not visited a physician since realizing their sexual orientation. The analytic sample size was 131.

### COMMUNITY-BASED PARTICIPATORY RESEARCH

The study was conducted using a Community-Based Participatory Research framework.[51-53] The head of Project 10 (Los Angeles Unified School District's LGB anti-discrimination office) partnered with the research team in developing and implementing this study. In addition, the Models of Pride conference planning committee (which included youth) provided input on the study design and questionnaire content. The UCLA/RAND Center for Adolescent Health Promotion's Community Advisory Board also participated in developing the study.

### DATA COLLECTION

On arrival, conference participants received a packet containing a cover letter, information sheet, and anonymous questionnaire. Participants received a pair of movie passes for returning a packet, even if the questionnaire was not completed.

### QUESTIONNAIRE AND MEASURES

The self-administered questionnaire was mostly multiple-choice and included the following topics:

*Primary Outcome Variable*: Disclosure of sexual orientation to a physician was measured with the question: "Does your doctor know that you are LGB?" This item was analyzed as a dichotomous variable.

*Demographics*: Age, gender, race/ethnicity, and maternal education were included.

*Orientation and Disclosure:* Sexual orientation was assessed on a 5-point continuum from "100% lesbian or gay" to "100% straight/heterosexual." Youth who responded "100% straight/heterosexual" were omitted from analysis, and the remaining 4 categories were dichotomized into "100% or mostly lesbian/gay" and "bisexual or mostly straight." Disclosure of orientation to others was measured by 5 ordered responses to the question "How 'out' are you overall?" (out to everyone, out to most, out to some, out to a few, not out to anyone), which were treated linearly as a predictor of disclosure. In addition, participants were asked to identify from a list everyone who knew that they were LGB (mother/stepmother, father/stepfather, sister/brother, gay friend(s), straight friend(s), teacher, counselor/psychologist, doctor).

*Health Care Variables:* Usual setting of care was measured by the question: "What kind of place do you usually go to for your health care?" Responses were coded into 1 of 3 categories: doctor's office, no usual source of care ("I don't have a place where I go for health care"), or other setting (eg, school clinic or teen health center). Length of time since the most recent visit for routine or preventive care was measured in 12-month increments from "within the past 12 months" to "more than 4 years ago"; these categories were treated as linear. Communication with a physician about sexual issues was assessed by asking, "Has a doctor ever talked to you about sex (gay or straight) or sexual health?"

*Attitudes and Expectations*: Attitude toward disclosure of patient orientation was assessed with: "How important do you think it is for a doctor to know that you are LGB in order to give you the best health care possible?" Answers ranged on a 4-point scale from "very important" to "not at all important." The questions, "How do you think your care would change if your doctor knew that you were LGB?" and "If your doctor does know that you are LGB, how has your care changed as a result?" used a 5-point scale. Possible responses ranged from "my care would be/is a lot better" to "my care would be/is a lot worse." We analyzed respondents separately by whether they had disclosed to their physician.

*Reasons for Nondisclosure and Suggestions to Make Disclosure More Comfortable*: All participants were asked, "What could your doctor do to make you more comfortable talking about being LGB?" and were instructed to indicate which of 6 listed items applied. Participants who had not disclosed their orientation to their physician chose from a list of 7 reasons for nondisclosure (**Table 1**). Items for both lists were derived from previously published qualitative work with LGB youth.[46]

### DATA ANALYSIS

Data were analyzed using SPSS 11.0. All hypothesis tests were 2-sided. We calculated descriptive statistics for health

**Table 1. Perceived Barriers and Recommendations to Improve Disclosure of Sexual Orientation**

| | Percentage |
|---|---|
| Reasons for not disclosing* | |
| I don't think it's important | 46 |
| He/she hasn't asked me | 33 |
| My parents are always in the room | 30 |
| I'm scared my doctor will tell my parents | 14 |
| I don't know how to bring it up | 11 |
| I'm embarrassed | 6 |
| I think my doctor would disapprove | 0 |
| Suggestions to make disclosure more comfortable† | |
| Just ask me | 64 |
| Talk to me without my parents in the room | 25 |
| Put LGB materials in waiting/exam rooms | 21 |
| Post a nondiscrimination sign | 17 |
| Assure me he/she won't write it in my chart | 17 |
| Assure me he/she won't tell my parents | 25 |

Abbreviation: LGB, lesbian, gay, or bisexual.
*n = 86.
†n = 117.

**Table 2. Sexual Orientation and Patterns of Disclosure**

| Variable | Percentage |
|---|---|
| "Do you consider yourself. . ."* | |
| 100% lesbian or gay | 55 |
| Mostly lesbian or gay | 14 |
| Bisexual | 27 |
| Mostly straight | 4 |
| "How out are you overall?"† | |
| Out to everyone | 33 |
| Out to most | 37 |
| Out to some | 21 |
| Out to a few | 9 |
| Out to no one | 0 |
| "Who knows that you are LGB?"† | |
| Mother | 57 |
| Father | 45 |
| Sibling | 54 |
| Gay friend | 85 |
| Straight friend | 83 |
| Teacher | 52 |
| Counselor/psychologist | 41 |

Abbreviation: LGB, lesbian, gay, or bisexual.
*n = 131.
†n = 128.

care utilization, attitudes, barriers to disclosing sexual orientation to a physician, and suggestions for increasing the likelihood of disclosure. Missing values for specific items were less than 5% for all variables except maternal education (13%). Missing values were replaced using mean imputation. Bivariate analyses ($\chi^2$ tests and simple logistic regression) and multivariate logistic regression were used to evaluate associations between disclosure of respondent's sexual orientation to a physician, and demographics, sexual orientation, health care experiences, and attitudes toward disclosure. Variables were included in the multivariate regression if they had at least marginal bivariate significance in our data ($P<.10$) or had been identified as relevant in previously published research.

**Table 3. Disclosure of Sexual Orientation to a Provider: Attitudes and Experiences**

| | Percentage |
|---|---|
| "How important is it for a doctor to know that you are LGB in order to give you the best health care possible?"* | |
| Very important | 33 |
| Somewhat important | 33 |
| Not very important | 19 |
| Not at all important | 15 |
| "Does your doctor know that you are LGB?"* | |
| Yes | 35 |
| No | 65 |
| "How did your doctor find out you are LGB?"† | |
| He/she brought it up | 21 |
| I brought it up | 62 |
| Someone else told him/her | 15 |
| He/she read it in my chart | 2 |
| "How helpful has your doctor been at providing information and advice about being LGB?"‡ | |
| Very helpful | 39 |
| Somewhat helpful | 19 |
| Not very helpful | 12 |
| Not at all helpful | 30 |

Abbreviation: LGB, lesbian, gay, or bisexual.
*n = 131.
†n = 47.
‡n = 57.

## RESULTS

### SAMPLE CHARACTERISTICS

The sample was 57% female, 52% Latino, 21% white, 8% African American, and 19% "other." Primary languages spoken at home were English (64%), Spanish (19%), and other (13%). The median age was 17 years (range, 14-18 years).

Most respondents (69%) identified themselves as either 100% or mostly lesbian or gay (**Table 2**). Respondents reported high levels of disclosure of their sexual orientation to others: 70% said they were "out to everyone" or to "most people," specifically, to their friends (85%), mother (57%), father (45%), and teacher (52%).

### HEALTH CARE EXPERIENCES

Ninety percent of survey respondents had been to a physician for preventive health care within the past 2 years, and 66% had been within the past 12 months. Most participants (76%) received their health care in a physician's office, while 11% had no usual source of health care. Forty-nine percent said that a physician had ever discussed sex or sexual health with them.

### DISCLOSURE OF SEXUAL ORIENTATION TO A PHYSICIAN

Sixty-six percent of study participants thought that it was very or somewhat important that a physician know their sexual orientation to provide the best health care possible (**Table 3**). However, only 35% reported that their physician knew their orientation, and only 21% of respondents whose physician knew their orientation said that their physician had raised the topic.

Among youth who had not disclosed their orientation to their physician, 27% thought their care would be better if their physician knew that they were LGB, 65% thought it would have no impact on care, and 8% feared that their care would be worse. In contrast, 57% of those who had disclosed thought their care had improved as a result, 39% thought it had remained the same, and 4% felt it had become worse.

Although 17% to 23% of participants whose physician did not know their orientation cited concerns about privacy and confidentiality as barriers to disclosure, 37% stated that their physician simply had not asked about their orientation, and almost half (46%) did not think it was important (Table 1). Females were more likely than males to say that they did not know how to raise the topic (23% vs 7%, $P=.05$) and to report that they had not disclosed because a parent was in the examination room (34% vs 12%, $P=.02$). Older respondents (aged 17 to 18 years) were more likely to report that they were too embarrassed to bring up the topic of sexual orientation with a provider (22% vs 6%, $P=.04$). To make disclosure more comfortable, 64% of respondents thought that their physicians should "just ask" them.

In a multivariate model (**Table 4**), the strongest predictor of disclosure was having discussed sex or sexual health of any kind with a physician; 58% of youth who had discussed sex with their physician reported that the physician knew their orientation, compared with 9.7% who had not discussed sex (odds ratio [OR], 15.47; 95% confidence interval [CI], 4.34-55.18). The more important it was to participants that their physicians know their sexual orientation, the more likely it was that they did know (OR, 1.96 per level; 95% CI, 1.16-3.32). Youth who were more out overall were more likely to report having physicians who were aware of their orientation (OR, 2.66 per level; 95% CI, 1.28-5.57). Participants who had seen a physician for a routine physical examination more recently were more likely to have physicians who knew they were LGB (OR, 2.14; 95% CI, 1.05-4.35). The usual setting of care was no longer independently associated with disclosure after adjusting for covariates.

**Table 4. Multivariate Predictors of Disclosure of Sexual Orientation to Provider**

| Variable | OR (95% CI) |
|---|---|
| Physician talked about sex* | 15.47 (4.34-55.18) |
| It is important for a doctor to know† | 1.96 (1.16-3.32) |
| Sexual orientation | |
| 100%/mostly lesbian or gay | 1.00 |
| Bisexual/mostly heterosexual | 0.41 (0.12-1.39) |
| How out, per level†‡ | 2.66 (1.28-5.57) |
| Age, per y | 0.91 (0.55-1.49) |
| Female | 0.87 (0.29-2.55) |
| Race/ethnicity | |
| White | 1.00 |
| Latino | 1.12 (0.21-5.94) |
| Other | 0.97 (0.24-3.84) |
| Usual setting of care | |
| Physician's Office | 1.00 |
| Other | 0.38 (0.03-4.71) |
| No USOC§ | 1.01 (0.23-4.43) |
| Years since last preventive care visit‖ | 2.14 (1.05-4.35) |
| Maternal education, per level¶ | 1.31 (0.90-1.89) |

Abbreviations: CI, confidence interval; OR, odds ratio; USOC, usual source of care.

*$P<.001$.

†$P=.001$.

‡Analyzed as linear from 1 to 5 ("out to everyone" to "not out to anyone").

§Includes teen health center; lesbian, gay, and bisexual clinic; school clinic; and hospital emergency department.

‖$P=.04$.

¶Analyzed as linear from 1 to 6 ("less than high school" to "attended professional school").

## COMMENT

Although 70% of lesbian, gay, and bisexual youth in this study described themselves as out to everyone or most people, only 35% reported that their physician knew of their orientation. Respondents' perceptions that their physician knew their orientation was significantly less common among those who identified themselves as bisexual or mostly heterosexual than among gay and lesbian youth. Physician knowledge of patients' sexual orientation is important in identifying both the infectious risks associated with some sexual behaviors and the psychosocial issues that some LGB youth experience. Nondisclosure of sexual orientation to health care providers may lead to missed opportunities for providers to explore individual sexual risks; provide appropriate screening; and offer guidance, information, and support to LGB youth. Specific recommendations for addressing sexual orientation have been published by the AAP and others.[23,28,54]

Although access to health care in this sample was generally good, with 89% of the overall sample identifying a regular place where they received health care, about half (49%) of youth recall their physician as ever having discussed sex or sexual health with them. This finding is consistent with earlier studies of general samples. A survey of providers in a large health maintenance organization found that although 68% of pediatricians asked their patients about sexual intercourse, only 17% asked about sexual orientation.[55] Similarly, in a study of more than 2000 southern California high school students, 49% reported having discussed at least 1 sexual topic with a physician, but only 8% had talked about sexual orientation.[56]

The importance of discussing sex and sexual health with all adolescents has been stressed in guidelines for adolescent preventive services published by several professional organizations.[23-27,35,44,54,57-59] In "Sexual Orientation and Adolescents," the AAP states: "Most nonheterosexual youths are 'invisible' and will pass through pediatricians' offices without raising the issue of sexual orientation on their own. Therefore, health care professionals should raise issues of sexual orientation and sexual behavior with all adolescent patients."[28] Suggestions for discussing sexual behavior and sexual orientation have been published elsewhere.[23,44,48,60-63]

In our multivariate analysis, having discussed sex or sexual health with a physician was the strongest predictor of disclosure of the respondent's sexual orientation, lending support to the AAP's assertion that discussion of sexual behavior with adolescent patients may help identify nonheterosexual youth who might otherwise remain unrecognized. Moreover, the second most common reason for nondisclosure cited by youth in our sample was that a physician had not asked about sexual orientation. Nearly two thirds of youth selected "just ask me" from a list of actions their physician could take to make talking about being LGB more comfortable. Because general discussions of sex with a provider were included in the multivariate model, the effects of other predictor variables in the model should be interpreted as specific to disclosure of sexual orientation after these more general discussions have been taken into account.

Earlier research suggested that many gay and lesbian adults do not disclose their sexual orientation to providers because they fear their provider will not support them or that they will receive worse care.[7,30,64,65] Such fears were consistent with findings from a study in which 67% of LGB physicians surveyed said they had witnessed colleagues giving "substandard" care to patients whom those colleagues knew to be LGB.[42,43,66] These historically important barriers to disclosure of orientation to a provider appear to be less salient to our study population; only 8% of youth feared that their care would be worse if their physician knew they were LGB, and only 7% worried that their physician would not approve of their orientation. It is unclear whether this difference reflects improving provider acceptance of nonheterosexual patients, as some, more recent studies suggest[38]; developmental differences between youth and adults; or characteristics of the current study population.

Privacy and confidentiality are important concerns for many adolescent patients and may influence decisions to seek care or disclose sensitive information to providers.[40,41,44,48,56,67-70] Lesbian and gay youth in 1 study identified these concerns as among the most important barriers to disclosure of sexual orientation to their provider: 75% said they had not disclosed because they did not want to discuss sexual orientation in front of a parent, 57% were afraid that their provider would tell a parent, and 26% said that a parent was always in the examination room with them.[47,48] In our study, issues of privacy and confidentiality were cited by some respondents as reasons for not disclosing to a physician: 23% said that a parent was always in the room and 17% were afraid that their physician would tell a parent. Eighteen percent said reassurance that their physician would not write their orientation in their medical record would make talking about orientation more comfortable.

Some respondents also indicated that placing LGB materials in waiting or examination rooms or posting a nondiscrimination policy in the office would help them feel more comfortable. However, previous studies have reported mixed attitudes from LGB youth with regard to this approach. Although some youth reported that they would appreciate these gestures, others felt that they were unnecessary and might even make them uncomfortable.[47,48,66] Most of the research in this area has focused on self-identified LGB youth, but those who are unsure of their orientation or who have disclosed their orientation to fewer people may find such indirect displays of openness more helpful. Additional suggestions for creating a safe clinical environment for sexual minority youth have been published and include staff sensitivity training and the use of gender- and orientation-neutral intake forms.*

Studies have shown various effects of disclosing sexual orientation to providers. Early studies found that many LGB adults had a negative experience when they told their physician about their sexual orientation.[7,30,66] Other studies have found higher rates of satisfaction with care among those who disclosed.[30,33] In a recent study that suggested that disclosure might be associated with higher quality of care, disclosure was independently associated with receipt of recommended Papanicolaou screenings among lesbian adults.[46]

Because we used self-reports, some respondents may have forgotten prior discussions with providers; however, we believe that discussions about orientation would usually be salient and well remembered by youth. Although our results provide an indication of the prevalence of discussions between LGB youth and their physicians about sexuality, they do not provide information on the content or quality of those discussions. Future research addressing those aspects of communication is needed for a more complete picture of the quality of care received by LGB youth.

As with all cross-sectional studies, temporal ambiguity complicates causal interpretation in this study. The directionality of the observed association between talking with a physician about sex and disclosure of sexual orientation to a physician, for instance, cannot be determined from our study. Although some youth may have disclosed their orientation because their physician initiated a conversation about sexuality, other youth may have disclosed their orientation first, leading their physician to then discuss sexuality or sexual health. In addition, it is possible that youth who said that their physician knew their sexual orientation had not disclosed directly, but rather that their physician had become aware of their orientation indirectly, through a parent or another source.

Our sample of LGB respondents is probably not representative of most LGB youth. Most participants in this study described themselves as being out to everyone or most people, and a high degree of initiative was required for them to arrange transportation to the conference at which the study was conducted. These characteristics are of most concern for prevalence estimates, and may bias our results toward higher estimates of disclosure of orientation. Nonetheless, it is not necessarily the case that the overrepresentation of highly motivated out youth biases relationship estimates of predictors with disclosure presented here. Our findings, therefore, likely fall near the upper end of the range of disclosure to providers of LGB youth.

Despite these limitations, it is striking that even among this sample of highly motivated youth who have shared their sexual orientation with most people in their lives, only about one third had physicians who were aware of their orientation. This study is one of the first to exam-

*References 2, 7, 16, 26, 35, 40, 57, 58, 61, 69, 70.

ine the health care experiences of a nonclinical sample of high school–aged LGB youth, and the results reinforce the AAP's assertion that primary care providers do not recognize the orientation or sexual experiences of many nonheterosexual youth. Nearly two thirds of our sample reported that they would be more comfortable discussing their sexual orientation if their physician would "just ask." Further research is needed to explore the effect of disclosure or nondisclosure of sexual orientation to all types of health care providers on the quality of health care they deliver and on subsequent health outcomes.

**Accepted for Publication:** June 7, 2006.
**Correspondence:** Garth D. Meckler, MD, MSHS, Oregon Health and Sciences University, 3181 SW Sam Jackson Park Rd, CDW-EM, Portland, OR 97201-3098 (meckler g@ohsu.edu).
**Author Contributions:** *Study concept and design:* Meckler, Elliott, Kanouse, Beals, and Schuster. *Acquisition of data:* Meckler, Beals, and Schuster. *Drafting of the manuscript:* Meckler, Elliott, Kanouse, Beals, and Schuster. *Critical revision of the manuscript for important intellectual content:* Meckler, Elliott, Kanouse, Beals, and Schuster. *Statistical analysis:* Meckler, Elliott, Kanouse, Beals, and Schuster. *Obtained funding:* Meckler and Schuster. *Administrative, technical, and material support:* Meckler and Schuster. *Study supervision:* Schuster.
**Financial Disclosure:** None reported.
**Funding/Support:** Funding for this study was provided by the National Research Scientist Award Training Grant (PE1-9001) and grants from the Centers for Disease Control and Prevention (U48-CCU915773 and U48-DP000056).
**Acknowledgment:** We would like to acknowledge Gail Rolf, Project 10 advisor to the Los Angeles Unified School District, for partnering with us in developing, designing, and implementing the study. We would also like to thank the planning committee for Models of Pride Youth Conference and the Community Advisory Board of the UCLA/RAND Center for Adolescent Health Promotion for their participation in the study.

## REFERENCES


1. Futterman D, Ryan C. *Lesbian and Gay Youth: Care and Counseling.* New York, NY: Columbia University Press; 1998.
2. Perrin E. *Sexual Orientation in Child and Adolescent Health Care.* New York, NY: Kluwer Academic; 2002.
3. Stronski Huwiler SM, Remafedi G. Adolescent homosexuality. *Adv Pediatr.* 1998; 45:107-144.
4. Taylor BA, Remafedi G. Youth coping with sexual orientation issues. J Sch Nurs. 1993;9:26-27, 30-39.
5. Gay teens at risk for injection drug use. *AIDS Patient Care STDS.* 2004;18:553-554.
6. Bontempo DE, D'Augelli AR. Effects of at-school victimization and sexual orientation on lesbian, gay, or bisexual youths' health risk behavior. *J Adolesc Health.* 2002;30:364-374.
7. Dean L. Lesbian, gay, bisexual, and transgender health: findings and concerns. *J Gay Lesbian Med Assoc.* 2000;4:101-151.
8. DuRant RH, Krowchuk DP, Sinal SH. Victimization, use of violence, and drug use at school among male adolescents who engage in same-sex sexual behavior. *J Pediatr.* 1998;133:113-118.
9. Eisenberg M. Differences in sexual risk behaviors between college students with same-sex and opposite-sex experience: results from a national survey. *Arch Sex Behav.* 2001;30:575-589.
10. Garofalo R, Wolf RC, Kessel S, Palfrey SJ, DuRant RH. The association between health risk behaviors and sexual orientation among a school-based sample of adolescents. *Pediatrics.* 1998;101:895-902.
11. Igartua KJ, Gill K, Montoro R. Internalized homophobia: a factor in depression, anxiety, and suicide in the gay and lesbian population. *Can J Commun Ment Health.* 2003;22:15-30.
12. Kreiss JL, Patterson DL. Psychosocial issues in primary care of lesbian, gay, bisexual, and transgender youth. *J Pediatr Health Care.* 1997;11:266-274.
13. Noell JW, Ochs LM. Relationship of sexual orientation to substance use, suicidal ideation, suicide attempts, and other factors in a population of homeless adolescents. *J Adolesc Health.* 2001;29:31-36.
14. Remafedi G. Sexual orientation and youth suicide. *JAMA.* 1999;282:1291-1292.
15. Remafedi G, French S, Story M, Resnick MD, Blum R. The relationship between suicide risk and sexual orientation: results of a population-based study. *Am J Public Health.* 1998;88:57-60.
16. Ryan C, Futterman D. Lesbian and gay youth: care and counseling. *Adolesc Med.* 1997;8:207-374.
17. Saewyc EM, Bearinger LH, Heinz PA, Blum RW, Resnick MD. Gender differences in health and risk behaviors among bisexual and homosexual adolescents. *J Adolesc Health.* 1998;23:181-188.
18. Udry JR, Chantala K. Risk assessment of adolescents with same-sex relationships. *J Adolesc Health.* 2002;31:84-92.
19. Valleroy LA, MacKellar DA, Karon JM, et al. HIV prevalence and associated risks in young men who have sex with men. Young Men's Survey Study Group. *JAMA.* 2000;284:198-204.
20. Wainright JL, Russell ST, Patterson CJ. Psychosocial adjustment, school outcomes, and romantic relationships of adolescents with same-sex parents. *Child Dev.* 2004;75:1886-1898.
21. Williams T, Connolly J, Pepler D, Craig W. Questioning and sexual minority adolescents: high school experiences of bullying, sexual harassment and physical abuse. *Can J Commun Ment Health.* 2003;22:47-58.
22. SAM. Society for Adolescent Medicine position paper on reproductive health care for adolescents. *J Adolesc Health.* 1991;12:649-661.
23. AAP. American Academy of Pediatrics Committee on Adolescence: homosexuality and adolescence. *Pediatrics.* 1993;92:631-634.
24. AAP. Nondiscrimination in pediatric health care. Committee on Pediatric Workforce. *Pediatrics.* 2001;108:1215.
25. AAP. Nondiscrimination in the care of pediatric patients. *Pediatrics.* 1996;97:596.
26. Health care needs of gay men and lesbians in the United States. *JAMA.* 1996;275: 1354-1359.
27. APA; Commission on Psychotherapy by Psychiatrists. Position statement on therapies focused on attempts to change sexual orientation (reparative or conversion therapies). *Am J Psychiatry.* 2000;157:1719-1721.
28. Frankowski BL. Sexual orientation and adolescents. *Pediatrics.* 2004;113:1827-1832.
29. Cochran SD, Mays VM. Disclosure of sexual preference to physicians by black lesbian and bisexual women. *West J Med.* 1988;149:616-619.
30. Dardick L, Grady KE. Openness between gay persons and health professionals. *Ann Intern Med.* 1980;93:115-119.
31. Elford J, Bolding G, Maguire M, Sherr L. Do gay men discuss HIV risk reduction with their GP? *AIDS Care.* 2000;12:287-290.
32. Fitzpatrick R, Dawson J, Boulton M, McLean J, Hart G, Brookes M. Perceptions of general practice among homosexual men. *Br J Gen Pract.* 1994;44: 80-82.
33. Klitzman RL, Greenberg JD. Patterns of communication between gay and lesbian patients and their health care providers. *J Homosex.* 2002;42:65-75.
34. Diamant AL, Wold C, Spritzer K, Gelberg L. Health behaviors, health status, and access to and use of health care: a population-based study of lesbian, bisexual, and heterosexual women. *Arch Fam Med.* 2000;9:1043-1051.
35. East JA, El Rayess F. Pediatricians' approach to the health care of lesbian, gay, and bisexual youth. *J Adolesc Health.* 1998;23:191-193.
36. Koh AS. Use of preventive health behaviors by lesbian, bisexual, and heterosexual women: questionnaire survey. *West J Med.* 2000;172:379-384.
37. Price JH, Telljohann SK. School counselors' perceptions of adolescent homosexuals. *J Sch Health.* 1991;61:433-438.
38. Ramos MM, Tellez CM, Palley TB, Umland BE, Skipper BJ. Attitudes of physicians practicing in New Mexico toward gay men and lesbians in the profession. *Acad Med.* 1998;73:436-438.
39. Tesar CM, Rovi SL. Survey of curriculum on homosexuality/bisexuality in departments of family medicine. *Fam Med.* 1998;30:283-287.
40. Ford CA, Millstein SG. Delivery of confidentiality assurances to adolescents by primary care physicians. *Arch Pediatr Adolesc Med.* 1997;151:505-509.
41. Ginsburg KR, Slap GB, Cnaan A, Forke CM, Balsley CM, Rouselle DM. Adolescents' perceptions of factors affecting their decisions to seek health care. *JAMA.* 1995;273:1913-1918.

42. Mathews WC, Booth MW, Turner JD, Kessler L. Physicians' attitudes toward homosexuality: survey of a California County Medical Society. *West J Med.* 1986;144:106-110.
43. Morrissey M. Attitudes of practitioners to lesbian, gay and bisexual clients. *Br J Nurs.* 1996;5:980-982.
44. Sankar P, Merz JF. Assuring adolescents about medical confidentiality. *JAMA.* 1998;279:116-117.
45. Mays VM, Yancey AK, Cochran SD, Weber M, Fielding JE. Heterogeneity of health disparities among African American, Hispanic, and Asian American women: unrecognized influences of sexual orientation. *Am J Public Health.* 2002;92:632-639.
46. Diamant AL, Schuster MA, Lever J. Receipt of preventive health care services by lesbians. *Am J Prev Med.* 2000;19:141-148.
47. Allen LB, Glicken AD, Beach RK, Naylor KE. Adolescent health care experience of gay, lesbian, and bisexual young adults. *J Adolesc Health.* 1998;23:212-220.
48. Ginsburg KR, Winn RJ, Rudy BJ, Crawford J, Zhao H, Schwarz DF. How to reach sexual minority youth in the health care setting: the teens offer guidance. *J Adolesc Health.* 2002;31:407-416.
49. Paroski PA Jr. Health care delivery and the concerns of gay and lesbian adolescents. *J Adolesc Health Care.* 1987;8:188-192.
50. Brewer PR. The shifting foundations of public opinion about gay rights. *J Polit.* 2003;65:1208-1220.
51. Minkler M, Wallerstein N, eds. *Community Based Participatory Research for Health.* San Francisco, Calif: Jossey-Bass; 2003.
52. McAllister CL, Green BL, Terry M, Herman V, Mulvey L. Parents, practitioners, and researchers: community based participatory research with early head start. *Am J Public Health.* 2003;93:1672-1679.
53. Gebbie K, Rosenstock L, Hernandez L, eds. *Who Will Keep the Public Healthy: Educating Public Health Professionals for the 21st Century.* Washington, DC: National Academies Press; 2002.
54. National Association of Pedatric Nurse Associates & Practitioners. Position statement on health risks and needs of gay, lesbian, bisexual, and transgender adolescents. *J Pediatr Health Care.* 2000;14:28A.
55. Halpern-Felsher BL, Ozer EM, Millstein SG, et al. Preventive services in a health maintenance organization: how well do pediatricians screen and educate adolescent patients? *Arch Pediatr Adolesc Med.* 2000;154:173-179.
56. Schuster MA, Bell RM, Petersen LP, Kanouse DE. Communication between adolescents and physicians about sexual behavior and risk prevention. *Arch Pediatr Adolesc Med.* 1996;150:906-913.
57. Arnold LM. Promoting culturally competent care for the lesbian, gay, bisexual, and transgender population. *Am J Public Health.* 2001;91:1731.
58. Perrin EC. Pediatricians and gay and lesbian youth. *Pediatr Rev.* 1996;17:311-318.
59. Perrin EC, Cohen KM, Gold M, Ryan C, Savin-Williams RC, Schorzman CM. Gay and lesbian issues in pediatric health care. *Curr Probl Pediatr Adolesc Health Care.* 2004;34:355-398.
60. Young F. How to take a sexual history. *J Fam Health Care.* 2005;15:149-151.
61. Association GLMA. MSM: Clinician's Guide to Incorporating Sexual Risk Assessment in Routine Visits. http://www.glma.org/_data/n_0001/resources/live/msm_assessment.pdf. Accessed June 10, 2004.
62. Andrews WC. Approaches to taking a sexual history. *J Womens Health Gend Based Med.* 2000;9(suppl 1):S21-S24.
63. Tomlinson J. ABC of sexual health: taking a sexual history. *BMJ.* 1998;317:1573-1576.
64. Kass NE, Faden RR, Fox R, Dudley J. Homosexual and bisexual men's perceptions of discrimination in health services. *Am J Public Health.* 1992;82:1277-1279.
65. Smith EM, Johnson SR, Guenther SM. Health care attitudes and experiences during gynecologic care among lesbians and bisexuals. *Am J Public Health.* 1985;75:1085-1087.
66. Schatz B, O'Hanlan K. Anti-gay discrimination in medicine: results of a national survey of lesbian, gay and bisexual physicians. Paper presented at: American Association of Physicians for Human Rights/Gay Lesbian Medical Association; May 1994; San Francisco, Calif.
67. Burack R. Young teenagers' attitudes towards general practitioners and their provision of sexual health care. *Br J Gen Pract.* 2000;50:550-554.
68. Cheng TL, Savageau JA, Sattler AL, DeWitt TG. Confidentiality in health care: a survey of knowledge, perceptions, and attitudes among high school students. *JAMA.* 1993;269:1404-1407.
69. Ford CA, Millstein SG, Halpern-Felsher BL, Irwin CE Jr. Influence of physician confidentiality assurances on adolescents' willingness to disclose information and seek future health care: a randomized controlled trial. *JAMA.* 1997;278:1029-1034.
70. Moon MW, O'Briant A, Friedland M. Caring for sexual minority youths: a guide for nurses. *Nurs Clin North Am.* 2002;37:405-422.

## *Announcement*

**Submissions.** The Editors welcome contributions to Picture of the Month. Submissions should describe common problems presenting uncommonly, rather than total zebras. Cases should be of interest to practicing pediatricians, highlighting problems that they are likely to at least occasionally encounter in the office or hospital setting. High-quality clinical images (in either 35-mm slide or electronic format) along with parent or patient permission to use these images must accompany the submission. The entire discussion should comprise no more than 750 words. Articles and photographs accepted for publication will bear the contributor's name. There is no charge for reproduction and printing of color illustrations. For details regarding electronic submission, please see: http://archpedi.ama-assn.org.

# Effects of a Life Skills Intervention for Increasing Physical Activity in Adolescent Girls

*Deborah Rohm Young, PhD; Jennie A. Phillips, MS; Tao Yu, MS; Jennifer A. Haythornthwaite, PhD*

**Background:** Although adolescence is a time when physical activity levels decline, few interventions have targeted high school–aged girls in the school setting.

**Objective:** To evaluate the effects of a life skills–oriented physical activity intervention for increasing overall physical activity in high school–aged girls.

**Design:** Randomized controlled trial.

**Setting:** Baltimore magnet high school.

**Participants:** A total of 221 ninth-grade girls, 83.0% of whom were African American.

**Intervention:** Participants were randomized to an 8-month physical intervention conducted in physical education class or to a standard physical education class (control).

**Main Outcome Measures:** Self-reported estimated daily energy expenditure (physical activity), self-reported sedentary activities (television viewing and computer or Internet use), cardiorespiratory fitness, and selected cardiovascular disease risk factors.

**Results:** Intervention classes spent 46.9% of physical education class time in moderate to vigorous activity compared with 30.5% of time for control classes ($P<.001$). There were no significant between-treatment group differences for mean daily energy expenditure ($P=.93$), moderate-intensity energy expenditure ($P=.77$), or hard to very hard energy expenditure ($P=.69$). The proportion of participants who spent 3 or more hours viewing television during school days declined from 22.3% to 17.0% in the intervention group, but remained at 26.7% for the control group ($P=.03$). Both groups improved their cardiorespiratory fitness ($P<.001$).

**Conclusion:** A life skills–oriented physical education curriculum may need to be combined with other approaches to increase the magnitude of effects on physical activity behavior in predominantly African American high school–aged girls.

*Arch Pediatr Adolesc Med. 2006;160:1255-1261*

PHYSICAL ACTIVITY PARTICIPATION in the United States is insufficient to provide protection from adverse health consequences; hence, national recommendations were formulated to increase awareness and to encourage people of all ages to increase physical activity.[1-3] Healthy People 2010 guidelines recommend that adolescents participate in moderate physical activity for at least 30 minutes on 5 or more days per week and engage in at least 20 minutes of vigorous activity at least 3 times per week.[4] The 2003 National Youth Risk Behavior Survey indicated that 40% of high school girls and 27% of high school boys had insufficient physical activity to meet these recommendations.[5] Participation was even lower for African American girls.[5] Thus, the high school years represent a life stage in which girls, particularly African American girls, are not engaging in sufficient physical activity.

Physical education (PE) class provides an opportunity to participate in physical activity and learn relevant skills to be physically active.[6] Progressing from traditional PE, which emphasizes team sports–related skills, to a model in which lifestyle-oriented physical activity skills are taught is feasible.[7] In recent years, the Centers for Disease Control and Prevention[6] and the American Heart Association[8] recommended that PE instruction emphasize enjoyable participation in physical activity to help students develop knowledge, skills, and confidence needed to adopt and maintain active lifestyles.

While physical activity interventions have been previously conducted in PE class, most worked with elementary school–aged children,[9-11] with less focus on middle and high school students. Few school-based interventions were tested with high school students,[12-17] and fewer still solely focused on promoting physical activity.[16,17] This stage of adolescence

**Author Affiliations:** Department of Kinesiology, University of Maryland, College Park (Dr Young and Mss Phillips and Yu); and Department of Psychiatry, The Johns Hopkins School of Medicine, Baltimore, Md (Dr Haythornthwaite).

is critical to establish health attitudes and behaviors that are likely to be carried into adulthood. Interventions focused at this age group can reduce the burden of physical inactivity–related chronic diseases that begin in adolescence and typically present in adulthood.

This trial tests the effectiveness of a life skills–oriented physical activity intervention, conducted in PE class by a teacher hired by the project, for increasing physical activity and fitness in ninth-grade girls. We hypothesized that participants in the intervention would increase physical activity and fitness compared with control subjects. The trial extends previous work[17] by providing an intervention that targeted all students regardless of risk factor status.

## METHODS

### PARTICIPANTS

Ninth-grade girls enrolled in an all-girl public magnet high school and who were also enrolled in 2 consecutive semesters of required PE were eligible to participate. Of the entering ninth-grade class, approximately two thirds were eligible based on their PE class schedules. Exclusion criteria were as follows: (1) being excused from meeting Maryland state PE requirements, (2) being pregnant or breastfeeding, (3) planning to leave the geographic area, and (4) having a sister enrolled in the trial. Participants were recruited using multiple strategies, such as presentations at parent and student orientation meetings, mass mailings to parents, and classroom presentations to students. Students were recruited over 3 successive years. Informed consent was obtained from a parent or legal guardian, and child assent was provided. The study was approved by the institutional review boards at The Johns Hopkins University and the University of Maryland.

### MEASURES

Assessments were made by trained study staff over a 4- to 5-week period before randomization in a dedicated classroom that was refitted as a project office. Measurements were obtained primarily during PE class, although assessments were also made before and after school and during lunch. Measurements were obtained in September (baseline) and, for follow-up, during the last 2 months of the spring semester (April and May). Self-report physical activity, clinical assessments, submaximal fitness, and questionnaires composed the measurement protocol. After baseline data collection was completed, participants were randomized into intervention or control PE classes. This required some participants to transfer from their current PE class to the alternate one occurring at the same time.

#### Estimated Daily Energy Expenditure

Daily energy expenditure, the trial's primary outcome, was determined from the 7-day Physical Activity Recall.[18,19] The instrument is widely used to determine change in physical activity interventions.[18,20-22] The 7-day Physical Activity Recall is an interviewer-administered instrument that estimates daily expenditure by asking participants to estimate the amount of time spent sleeping and doing physical activities of moderate (eg, brisk walk), hard, and very hard (eg, run) intensity over the previous 7 days. The survey was designed for adults, but it has been validated and used with children.[23] Test-retest reliability was 0.59 for a sample of eighth graders and 0.81 for eleventh-grade students, and it correlated with another self-report instrument ($r = 0.76$ for girls), time spent with a heart rate of at least a moderate intensity, and skinfold thicknesses.[23] The daily time frame in which physical activity was recalled was modified to allow for recall to be prompted by the school-day schedule. Weekend days were separated by meals, as suggested by the instrument developers.[24]

#### Cardiorespiratory Fitness

Cardiorespiratory fitness was assessed with a submaximal 3-stage step test designed for adolescents.[25] The protocol was designed for participants to exercise successively at 50%, 59%, and 70% of estimated maximal heart rate reserve by stepping up and down on 3 steps whose heights were calculated to meet the required energy expenditure.[25] Participants stepped up and down at progressive step heights until the test was completed or until the participant reached the target heart rate (70% of estimated heart rate reserve).

Participants' exercise heart rate was recorded at 2:30, 2:45, and 3:00 of each 3-minute stage. If a student's average heart rate did not exceed the target heart rate, she proceeded to the next stage. If the target heart rate was achieved, the test was terminated.

A decrease in average heart rate from baseline to follow-up at a given stage was used to assess fitness improvement. A 1- to 2-week test-retest reliability of 21 participants indicated that heart rate was 1 to 3 beats/min lower at the end of a stage during the second administration of the test (difference not significant). Thus, a significant decrease in heart rate indicated fitness improvement rather than familiarity with testing procedures.

#### Sedentary Activities

Time spent in sedentary activities was assessed using selected items from a questionnaire.[26] Participants were asked to estimate how much time they spent (1) watching television, movies, or videotapes (ie, television time); and (2) playing video games, surfing the Internet, e-mailing, or participating in chat rooms (ie, computer time). School days and weekends were queried. Response options were 0 minutes, less than 30 minutes, 30 minutes to less than 1 hour, 1 to 3 hours, and more than 3 hours.

#### Anthropometric and Clinical Variables

Height, weight, and waist and hip circumferences were determined using standard methods. Height was measured to the nearest 0.1 cm and weight to the nearest 0.11 kg. Waist circumference was measured from the horizontal plane at 1 cm above the navel. Hip circumference was measured in a horizontal plane at the site of maximum extension of the buttocks. Four waist and hip circumferences were measured in consecutive order and averaged. Body mass index was calculated as weight in kilograms divided by the square of height in meters. Waist-hip ratio was calculated by dividing the mean waist circumference by the mean hip circumference. Adolescent body mass index,[27,28] waist circumference,[27,28] and waist-hip ratio[29-31] are associated with childhood cardiovascular risk factors and adult overweight or obesity and risk factor status.[32]

Resting blood pressure was measured in the nondominant arm using an automated blood pressure monitor (Dinamap) in a seated position after 5 minutes of rest. Three blood pressure measurements were made, with a 1-minute interval between measures. Three 30-second peripheral pulse rates were also obtained. Measures were averaged.

Plasma total cholesterol, high-density lipoprotein cholesterol, and low-density lipoprotein cholesterol levels were obtained from a venous blood sample drawn after a 12-hour fast. Blood samples were analyzed by a local commercial laboratory (Quest Diagnostics, Lyndhurst, NJ).

## ALTERNATIVE PE INTERVENTION

The intervention was designed to be congruent with the Social Action Theory, which emphasizes social interdependence, environmental factors, and problem-solving skills.[33] It was taught by a teacher hired by the project. Intervention content included information to make an informed decision about the personal benefits of a physically active lifestyle, develop problem-solving skills, and obtain support from others. Specific strategies that were taught and reinforced included goal setting, problem-solving barriers, communication skills, reinforcement of goal achievement through internal and external rewards, and learning from relevant role models. Skills were taught using class lectures and discussions, small-group discussions, and homework activities. Physical activity self-monitoring was given a strong focus. Students were encouraged to keep weekly exercise logs from which the teacher provided feedback on progress toward goal attainment and reward strategies. All students in class received the intervention, irrespective of whether they were trial participants.

The intervention was also designed to maximize physical activity during PE class. The format was congruent with the school's PE curriculum—1 semester of individual sports and 1 semester of team sports—taught 5 days per week. Classes were optimized for physical activity by teaching units that were active in nature (eg, soccer instead of softball [personal fitness unit]), breaking skills training into small-group activities, and playing games in small groups (eg, 3-on-3 basketball). Skills training was limited to that needed for competency rather than proficiency. Written tests focused on health-related physical activity and fitness concepts and behavioral skills.

The family support component consisted of a family workshop, monthly newsletters, and adult-child homework assignments. A 2-hour family workshop, scheduled shortly after randomization, featured tips on how parents could provide support to their daughters. As an in-class activity, students worked on skits illustrating support strategies that were videotaped and viewed at the workshop. Families who did not attend were mailed copies. Families also received a 2-page family support newsletter each month that contained an article on ways families can support physical activity with their daughter.

## STANDARD PE (CONTROL)

Standard PE class was a curriculum in which students were taught skills in individual and team sports. For example, during the basketball unit, students were taught how to dribble, shoot, and pass, and were tested on concepts such as game rules and defense strategies. Similar to the intervention structure, 1 semester focused on individual sports and the other on team sports. Classes were taught by certified PE teachers employed by the school.

Parents of participants in the standard PE class also received monthly newsletters. Topics were of general health interests and included an article about PE class content that month.

## INTERVENTION FIDELITY

The percentage of PE class time spent in physical activity was assessed in intervention and control classes using a modification of the System for Observing Fitness Instruction Time.[34] This was used to determine fidelity to the intervention goal of optimizing physical activity in class. Trained assessors determined physical activity levels of selected students in all quadrants of the activity area at 5-minute intervals. Physical activity level was recorded as (1) lying down, (2) sitting, (3) standing, (4) walking, and (5) active. At the class start time, observers mentally divided the activity area into quadrants, identified a student in the northeast quadrant, observed for 10 seconds, then identified another student in the northwest quadrant, observed for 10 seconds, and so on. The process was repeated every 5 minutes. In a 45-minute class period, there were 36 student observations recorded. Thus, there was an opportunity for each student to be observed. The percentage of time in class spent in physical activity was calculated as the number of observations of the categories "walking" and "active" relative to the total number of observations.[34]

## STATISTICAL ANALYSES

Means and standard deviations were calculated at baseline and follow-up for continuous physical activity, fitness, and secondary outcome variables. Baseline means were examined for comparability between intervention and control groups using unpaired *t* tests. Mean change and standard errors from baseline to follow-up were calculated after controlling for baseline values and race (African American vs other). To determine the effects of the intervention, an analysis of covariance was used, with change in physical activity as the dependent variable, intervention group as the independent variable, and baseline physical activity and race as the covariates. The same approach was used for secondary outcome variables. Initial models tested for treatment × race interactions; none were significant, so they were not included in the final models. Race was a significant covariate and, thus, was retained. Within-treatment group change was assessed by paired *t* tests, after controlling for baseline values and race.

For the sedentary activities' variables, the proportion of participants who reported 3 or more hours per day of television viewing or video game or Internet use during school days and weekends was computed. To test for intervention effects, between-group differences in the reduction of high prevalence of sedentary activities (≥3 hours) were tested using the Fisher exact test. Within-intervention group differences were assessed using the McNemar test. Initial analyses indicated no differences by race, so data were not stratified to test for race differences.

All analyses were conducted using SAS statistical software, version 9.1 (SAS Institute Inc, Cary, NC). Significance was set at a 2-tailed α of .05.

# RESULTS

The study flow is displayed in the **Figure**. Of the 442 students eligible to participate across 3 successive school years, 221 (50.0%) agreed to participate and were randomized. There was greater than 90% power to detect a 1.7-kcal/kg per day treatment group difference (5% change) in daily energy expenditure at follow-up. Common reasons for nonparticipation were the following: did not want to miss PE class to undergo baseline measurements, did not want to provide a blood sample, and did not want to be randomized and risk moving to the alternate class. The sample was a mean ± SD age of 13.8 ± 0.5 years. Most (83.0%) were African American, with the remainder predominantly white, consistent with the demographics of the school. More than half of the participants' mothers (56.3%) had greater than a high school education. We report mother's education because of the many participants (29.2%) who did not know their father's educational level. Follow-up data were obtained for 210 (95.0%) of the participants.

Observations occurred in 81 (40 intervention and 41 control) PE classes. Interrater reliability of physical activity level (active [walking or active categories] vs inactive) was κ=0.83. Intervention PE classes spent significantly more time (46.9%) walking or active than control PE classes (30.5%) (*P*<.001). Most of this difference was for the walking category (28.1% vs 18.8%, respectively), with less difference for the active category (16.6% vs 13.9%, respectively).

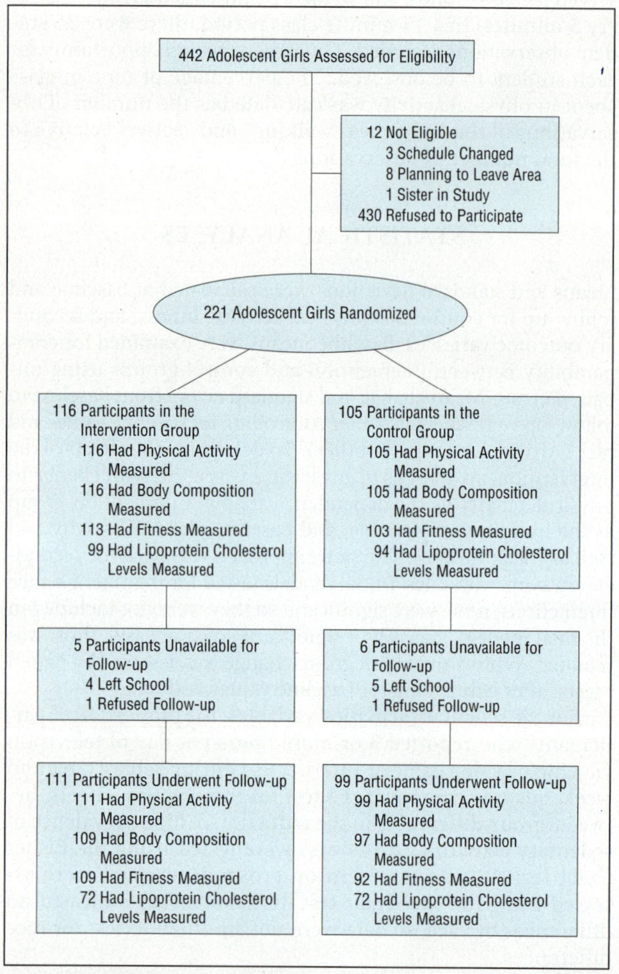


**Figure.** Participant study flow diagram.

The results of the physical activity and sedentary activity measures are displayed in **Table 1** and **Table 2**. At baseline, groups were comparable for mean daily energy expenditure. Based on the previously established cut point for sedentary behavior of 35 kcal/kg per day,[22] most participants were sedentary, although daily energy expenditure ranged from 30.2 to 50.7 kcal/kg per day. Baseline sedentary activity prevalence did not differ between treatment groups.

There were no significant between-treatment group differences for mean daily energy expenditure, moderate energy expenditure, or hard to very hard energy expenditure (Table 1). The results of additional analyses' testing for possible treatment group differences for those who increased (n=92) or decreased (n=113) their physical activity also were not statistically significant.

Both treatment groups significantly increased in fitness, as assessed by reduction in submaximal heart rate (Table 1).

The proportion of participants who reported 3 or more hours per day of television viewing or video game or Internet use declined in the intervention group, with minimal change in the control group (Table 2). For high television viewing during school days, the intervention group declined by 5.3%, with no change in the controls (*P*=.03). The proportion of participants who reported 3 or more hours per day in at least 1 of the sedentary variables of interest declined from 44.1% to 36.0% in the intervention group, but remained at 45.5% in the control group (*P*=.06).

Mean body mass index, waist-hip ratio, waist circumference, blood pressure, total cholesterol level, or lipoprotein level did not differ from baseline to follow-up by treatment status (**Table 3**). However, there were improvements in waist-hip ratio, blood pressure, and high-density lipoprotein cholesterol level in both groups that either were statistically significant or approached significance.

**Table 1. Baseline, Follow-up, and Change in Estimated Daily Energy Expenditure, Its Subcomponents, and Submaximal Heart Rate by Randomized Treatment Group***

| | Intervention Group | | | | Control Group | | | | |
|---|---|---|---|---|---|---|---|---|---|
| Variable | Baseline† | Follow-up† | Within-Group Change‡ | *P* Value* | Baseline† | Follow-up† | Within-Group Change‡ | *P* Value* | Between-Group *P* Value* |
| Estimated daily energy expenditure, kcal/kg | | | | | | | | | |
| Total | 34.6 (3.2) | 34.2 (2.9) | −0.1 (0.3) | .79 | 34.9 (2.7) | 34.2 (2.1) | −0.1 (0.3) | .72 | .93 |
| Moderate | 2.0 (1.9) | 1.8 (3.0) | 0.0 (0.3) | .94 | 2.4 (2.1) | 2.0 (1.4) | 0.1 (0.3) | .68 | .77 |
| Hard or very hard | 1.9 (3.6) | 1.5 (2.7) | −0.1 (0.3) | .70 | 2.0 (3.0) | 1.4 (2.4) | −0.0 (0.3) | .92 | .69 |
| Change in submaximal heart rate (fitness) | NA | −6.2 (16.4) | −7.1 (1.8) | <.001 | NA | −3.5 (18.3) | −7.4 (2.0) | <.001 | .91 |

Abbreviation: NA, data not applicable.
*Values are given for analysis of covariance testing for within-group change and difference of change between treatment groups for a given variable, with baseline physical activity and race as covariates.
†Data are given as unadjusted mean (SD).
‡Data are given as mean change (SE), adjusted for baseline value and race.

**Table 2. Baseline, Follow-up, and Change in Prevalence of Sedentary Activities**

| Variable | Intervention Group Baseline* | Intervention Group Follow-up* | Intervention Group Within-Group Change | Intervention Group P Value† | Control Group Baseline* | Control Group Follow-up* | Control Group Within-Group Change | Control Group P Value† | Between-Group P Value‡ |
|---|---|---|---|---|---|---|---|---|---|
| ≥3 h of watching television | | | | | | | | | |
| School day | 22.3 | 17.0 | −5.3 | .27 | 26.7 | 26.7 | 0 | .99 | .03 |
| Weekend | 34.2 | 27.0 | −7.2 | .16 | 35.6 | 35.6 | 0 | .99 | .25 |
| ≥3 h of playing video games or using the Internet | | | | | | | | | |
| School day | 4.4 | 1.8 | −2.6 | .18 | 7.6 | 5.0 | −2.6 | .32 | .99 |
| Weekend | 11.4 | 9.9 | −1.5 | .62 | 13.2 | 16.8 | 3.6 | .47 | .44 |

*Data are given as percentage of the group.
†Value for the McNemar test comparing baseline with follow-up change of prevalence of sedentary activities.
‡Value for the Fisher exact test determining the treatment group difference in change of prevalence of sedentary activities.

**Table 3. Baseline, Follow-up, and Change in Anthropometric and Cardiovascular Risk Factors by Randomized Treatment Group**

| Risk Factor | Intervention Group Baseline* | Intervention Group Follow-up* | Intervention Group Within-Group Change† | Intervention Group P Value‡ | Control Group Baseline* | Control Group Follow-up* | Control Group Within-Group Change† | Control Group P Value‡ | Between-Group P Value‡ |
|---|---|---|---|---|---|---|---|---|---|
| Body mass index§ | 25.0 (6.9) | 25.3 (7.1) | 0.3 (0.2) | .20 | 25.2 (6.7) | 25.6 (6.5) | 0.2 (0.2) | .34 | .81 |
| Waist-hip ratio | 0.79 (0.08) | 0.77 (0.06) | −0.02 (0.006) | .001 | 0.78 (0.07) | 0.77 (0.06) | −0.01 (0.006) | .05 | .20 |
| Waist circumference, cm | 77.6 (14.9) | 77.9 (15.0) | −0.1 (0.5) | .83 | 77.6 (14.3) | 78.6 (14.5) | 0.2 (0.5) | .77 | .67 |
| Blood pressure, mm Hg | | | | | | | | | |
| Systolic | 109.4 (10.4) | 108.3 (11.1) | −1.6 (0.9) | .09 | 110.3 (12.0) | 106.8 (10.0) | −3.7 (1.0) | .001 | .06 |
| Diastolic | 59.5 (5.9) | 57.7 (7.2) | −1.4 (0.7) | .05 | 58.8 (7.4) | 56.8 (5.8) | −2.0 (0.8) | .008 | .49 |
| Cholesterol level, mg/dL | | | | | | | | | |
| Total | 154.9 (27.6) | 155.4 (28.3) | −0.3 (2.2) | .91 | 161.0 (25.5) | 162.8 (29.0) | 1.8 (2.2) | .42 | .43 |
| LDL | 90.3 (23.8) | 88.7 (22.4) | −2.6 (1.9) | .18 | 95.2 (23.7) | 94.4 (27.4) | −2.3 (1.9) | .24 | .90 |
| HDL | 52.2 (12.0) | 54.0 (12.4) | 2.3 (1.0) | .02 | 52.7 (10.7) | 55.7 (10.3) | 4.2 (1.0) | <.001 | .10 |

Abbreviations: HDL, high-density lipoprotein; LDL, low-density lipoprotein.
SI conversion factor: To convert HDL, LDL, and total cholesterol to millimoles per liter, multiply by 0.0259.
*Data are given as unadjusted mean (SD).
†Data are given as mean change (SE), adjusted for baseline value and race.
‡Values are given for analysis of covariance testing for within-group change and difference of change between groups for a given variable, with baseline physical activity and race as covariates.
§Calculated as weight in kilograms divided by height in meters squared.

## COMMENT

Study results indicate that the life skills physical activity intervention, while successful in increasing physical activity in PE class, did not result in total increased physical activity. That is, there was no change in overall daily, moderate, or hard to very hard mean energy expenditure in either the intervention or the control group. The intervention did demonstrate, however, a decline in prevalence of high participation in sedentary activities, particularly school-day television viewing. Thus, to our knowledge, it is the first to report a reduction in sedentary activities among high school girls.

The prevalence of 3 or more hours per day of television viewing on school days declined in the intervention group, but did not change in controls. Although the intervention targeted moderate to vigorous physical activity, it did include inferences as to how sedentary activities could be replaced with more active pursuits. The reduction in television viewing may have resulted in an increase in light physical activity, which the 7-day Physical Activity Recall is not designed to assess. Previous school-based interventions aimed at reducing the prevalence of sedentary activities among elementary and middle school–aged children did not find a concomitant increase in physical activity,[26,35] confirming our findings.

Most previous work[12-15,17] with high school–aged adolescents separated study participants into specialized targeted PE and/or health education classes. While interventions targeting students with particular characteristics have greater potential for positive results, they are limited in generalizability. We reduced this limitation by conducting a trial with generous eligibility criteria and implemented an intervention that was applied within the school's existing PE curriculum. Pate et al[16] used the same approach, but augmented the intervention by promoting physical activity schoolwide. Their results demonstrated an increase in vigorous physical activity.[16] Thus, while integrating physical activity promotion in PE class enhances reach and generalizability, efforts may need to extend beyond PE class for sufficient potency to increase out-of-class physical activity.

To our knowledge, our study is the first to report results of participants who were overwhelmingly minority (83.0%), which may have contributed to our mixed results. While intervention materials and discussions were designed to be appropriate for African American and white students, there may not have been sufficient cultural targeting to result in substantial out-of-class physical activity participation.

We hypothesized that the intervention would result in an increase in physical activity relative to the control group, a hypothesis that was optimistic in retrospect. Cross-sectional and longitudinal studies document a decline in physical activity in girls throughout adolescence. From a recent longitudinal cohort study of black and white girls, Kimm et al[36] found an annual mean decline of 4.1 metabolic equivalent times per week for black girls and 3.5 metabolic equivalent times per week for white girls at similar ages as our participants. In contrast, the predominantly African American participants reported no change in physical activity over an 8-month period, irrespective of treatment assignment. Although PE class did not result in increased daily energy expenditure, perhaps it provided sufficient stimulus to blunt the age-expected decline.

Fitness, assessed by reduction in submaximal heart rate, improved in both groups. While the intervention PE classes resulted in greater physical activity compared with the control classes, the difference was largely because of more class time spent walking, rather than more active (vigorous), activity. The vigorous physical activity that occurred in PE class may have been sufficient to improve fitness. These results provide additional evidence for national groups that advocate PE requirements for all ages.[6,8]

We found improvements in waist-hip ratio, blood pressure, and high-density lipoprotein cholesterol level in both groups, without a decline in weight, waist circumference, or body mass index or an improvement in overall physical activity. These improvements are important, given the high risk of hypertension and cardiovascular disease that African American women carry.[37] In another report,[38] we found that, at baseline, almost 20% of our sample met the criteria for metabolic syndrome. Thus, these adolescent girls are at high risk for future cardiovascular and metabolic diseases. Perhaps the combination of vigorous activity in PE class and improved fitness resulted in favorable physiologic variables. Future work should continue to explore public health strategies to improve cardiovascular risk factors in adolescents.

The trial had several limitations, most of which limit generalizability. The study was conducted in 1 high school, although the high school was a magnet that enrolls students from most Baltimore neighborhoods. Only about 50% of eligible participants chose to enroll. The intervention was delivered by a teacher who was hired by the project. While this approach maximizes the intervention fidelity, it is less generalizable than if the school's PE teachers were the implementers. And finally, our primary outcome, physical activity, was assessed by self-report. Although the instrument we used is valid for high school–aged populations, it may not have been sensitive enough to detect the change in physical activity we were able to produce.

In conclusion, a physical activity intervention conducted in PE class targeting ninth-grade girls increased in-class physical activity and reduced high prevalence of school-day television viewing, but did not result in an increase in overall daily energy expenditure. Given the alarming decline in physical activity during adolescence and the associated increase in prevalence of adolescent obesity, future work should continue to identify potentially effective intervention strategies.

**Accepted for Publication:** July 5, 2006.
**Correspondence:** Deborah Rohm Young, PhD, Department of Kinesiology, University of Maryland, 2312 Health and Human Performance Building, College Park, MD 20742 (dryoung@umd.edu).
**Author Contributions:** All authors had full access to all the data in the study and take responsibility for the integrity of the data and the accuracy of the data analysis. *Study concept and design:* Young, Phillips, and Haythornthwaite. *Acquisition of data:* Young, Phillips, and Haythornthwaite. *Analysis and interpretation of data:* Young, Yu, and Haythornthwaite. *Drafting of the manuscript:* Young. *Critical revision of the manuscript for important intellectual content*: Phillips, Yu, and Haythornthwaite. *Statistical analysis:* Yu. *Obtained funding:* Young and Haythornthwaite. *Administrative, technical, and material support:* Phillips. *Study supervision:* Young and Haythornthwaite.
**Financial Disclosure:** None reported.
**Funding/Support:** This study was supported by grant RO1 HL063861 from the National Heart, Lung, and Blood Institute, National Institutes of Health.
**Role of the Sponsor:** The funding body had no role in data extraction and analyses, in the writing of the manuscript, or in the decision to submit the manuscript for publication.
**Acknowledgment:** We thank Jeanette Harris, Sue Shang, MS, Tavon English, Jie Li, PhD, and Marcella Sapun, MS, for their contributions to this study; and the administration of the high school for allowing us to conduct the trial.

## REFERENCES


1. US Department of Health and Human Services. *Physical Activity and Health: A Report of the Surgeon General.* Atlanta, Ga: Centers for Disease Control and Prevention; 1996.
2. Pate RR, Pratt M, Blair SN, et al. Physical activity and public health: a recommendation from the Centers for Disease Control and Prevention and the American College of Sports Medicine. *JAMA.* 1995;273:402-407.
3. NIH Consensus Development Panel on Physical Activity and Cardiovascular Health. Physical activity and cardiovascular health. *JAMA.* 1996;276:241-246.
4. US Department of Health and Human Services. *Healthy People 2010: Understanding and Improving Health.* 2nd ed. Washington, DC: US Dept of Health and Human Services; 2000.
5. Grunbaum JA, Kann L, Kinchen S, et al. Youth risk behavior surveillance: United States, 2003. *MMWR Surveill Summ.* 2004;53:1-96.
6. National Center for Chronic Disease Prevention and Health Promotion; Centers for Disease Control and Prevention. Guidelines for school and community programs to promote lifelong physical activity among young people. *J Sch Health.* 1997;67:202-219.

7. Sallis JF, McKenzie TL. Physical education's role in public health. *Res Q Exerc Sport.* 1991;62:124-137.
8. Gidding SS, Deckelbaum RJ, Strong W, Moller JH. Improving children's heart health: a report from the American Heart Association's Children's Heart Health Conference. *J Sch Health.* 1995;65:129-132.
9. Sallis JF, McKenzie TL, Alcaraz JE, Kolody B, Faucette N, Hovell MF. The effects of a 2-year physical education program (SPARK) on physical activity and fitness in elementary school students: Sports, Play and Active Recreation for Kids. *Am J Public Health.* 1997;87:1328-1334.
10. McKenzie TL, Nader PR, Strikmiller PK, et al. School physical education: effect of the Child and Adolescent Trial for Cardiovascular Health. *Prev Med.* 1996; 25:423-431.
11. Caballero B, Clay T, Davis SM, et al; Pathways Study Research Group. Pathways: a school-based, randomized controlled trial for the prevention of obesity in American Indian schoolchildren. *Am J Clin Nutr.* 2003;78:1030-1038.
12. Bayne-Smith M, Fardy PS, Azzollini A, Magel J, Schmitz KH, Agin D. Improvements in heart health behaviors and reduction in coronary artery disease risk factors in urban teenaged girls through a school-based intervention: the PATH program. *Am J Public Health.* 2004;94:1538-1543.
13. Killen JD, Telch MJ, Robinson TN, Maccoby N, Taylor CB, Farquhar JW. Cardiovascular disease risk reduction for tenth graders: a multiple-factor school-based approach. *JAMA.* 1988;260:1728-1733.
14. Fardy PS, White RE, Clark LT, et al. Health promotion in minority adolescents: a Healthy People 2000 pilot study. *J Cardiopulm Rehabil.* 1995;15:65-72.
15. Neumark-Sztainer D, Story M, Hannan PJ, Rex J. New Moves: a school-based obesity prevention program for adolescent girls. *Prev Med.* 2003;37:41-51.
16. Pate RR, Ward DS, Saunders RP, Felton G, Dishman RK, Dowda M. Promotion of physical activity among high-school girls: a randomized controlled trial. *Am J Public Health.* 2005;95:1582-1587.
17. Ewart CK, Young DR, Hagberg JM. Effects of school-based aerobic exercise on blood pressure in adolescent girls at risk for hypertension. *Am J Public Health.* 1998;88:949-951.
18. Blair SN, Haskell WL, Ho P, et al. Assessment of habitual physical activity by a seven-day recall in a community survey and controlled experiments. *Am J Epidemiol.* 1985;122:794-804.
19. Sallis JF, Haskell WL, Wood PD, et al. Physical activity assessment methodology in the Five-City Project. *Am J Epidemiol.* 1985;121:91-106.
20. Dunn AL, Marcus BH, Kampert JB, Garcia ME, Kohl HW III, Blair SN. Comparison of lifestyle and structured interventions to increase physical activity and cardiorespiratory fitness: a randomized trial. *JAMA.* 1999;281:327-334.
21. Albright CL, Pruitt L, Castro C, Gonzalez A, Woo S, King AC. Modifying physical activity in a multiethnic sample of low-income women: one-year results from the IMPACT (Increasing Motivation for Physical ACTivity) project. *Ann Behav Med.* 2005;30:191-200.
22. Writing Group for the Activity Counseling Trial Research Group. Effects of physical activity counseling in primary care: the Activity Counseling Trial: a randomized controlled trial. *JAMA.* 2001;286:677-687.
23. Sallis JF, Buono MJ, Roby JJ, Micale FG, Nelson JA. Seven-day recall and other physical activity self-reports in children and adolescents. *Med Sci Sports Exerc.* 1993;25:99-108.
24. Pereira MA, FitzerGerald SJ, Gregg EW, et al. A collection of Physical Activity Questionnaires for health-related research. *Med Sci Sports Exerc.* 1997;29 (suppl):S1-S205.
25. Ewart CK. School-based exercise to lower blood pressure in high-risk African-American girls: project design and baseline findings. *J Health Educ.* 1995;26 (suppl):S99-S105.
26. Robinson TN. Reducing children's television viewing to prevent obesity: a randomized controlled trial. *JAMA.* 1999;282:1561-1567.
27. Duncan GE, Li SM, Zhou XH. Prevalence and trends of a metabolic syndrome phenotype among US adolescents, 1999-2000. *Diabetes Care.* 2004;27:2438-2443.
28. Katzmarzyk PT, Srinivasan SR, Chen W, Malina RM, Bouchard C, Berenson GS. Body mass index, waist circumference, and clustering of cardiovascular disease risk factors in a biracial sample of children and adolescents. *Pediatrics.* 2004; 114:e198-e205. http://pediatrics.aappublications.org/cgi/content/full/114/2/e198. Accessed September 7, 2006.
29. Freedman DS, Serdula MK, Srinivasan SR, Berenson GS. Relation of circumferences and skinfold thicknesses to lipid and insulin concentrations in children and adolescents: the Bogalusa Heart Study. *Am J Clin Nutr.* 1999;69:308-317.
30. Gillum RF. Distribution of waist-to-hip ratio, other indices of body fat distribution and obesity and associations with HDL cholesterol in children and young adults aged 4-19 years: the Third National Health and Nutrition Examination Survey. *Int J Obes Relat Metab Disord.* 1999;23:556-563.
31. Huang KC, Lin RC, Kormas N, et al. Plasma leptin is associated with insulin resistance independent of age, body mass index, fat mass, lipids, and pubertal development in nondiabetic adolescents. *Int J Obes Relat Metab Disord.* 2004; 28:470-475.
32. Janssen I, Katzmarzyk PT, Srinivasan SR, et al. Utility of childhood BMI in the prediction of adulthood disease: comparison of national and international references. *Obes Res.* 2005;13:1106-1115.
33. Ewart CK. Social action theory for a public health psychology. *Am Psychol.* 1991; 46:931-946.
34. McKenzie TL, Sallis JF, Nader PR. SOFIT: System for Observing Fitness Instruction Time. *J Teach Phys Educ.* 1991;11:195-205.
35. Gortmaker SL, Peterson K, Wiecha J, et al. Reducing obesity via a school-based interdisciplinary intervention among youth: Planet Health. *Arch Pediatr Adolesc Med.* 1999;153:409-418.
36. Kimm SY, Glynn NW, Kriska AM, et al. Decline in physical activity in black girls and white girls during adolescence. *N Engl J Med.* 2002;347:709-715.
37. Centers for Disease Control and Prevention. Public health focus: physical activity and the prevention of coronary heart disease. *MMWR Morb Mortal Wkly Rep.* 1993;42:669-672.
38. Camhi S, Kuo J, Young DR. Evaluating BMI and waist circumference cutpoints to identify urban female adolescents at risk for metabolic syndrome [abstract]. *Med Sci Sports Exerc.* 2005;37(suppl):S69.

# Objectively Measured Physical Activity in Sixth-Grade Girls

*Russell R. Pate, PhD; June Stevens, PhD; Charlotte Pratt, PhD; James F. Sallis, PhD; Kathryn H. Schmitz, PhD, MPH; Larry S. Webber, PhD; Gregory Welk, PhD; Deborah R. Young, PhD*

**Objectives:** To describe the objectively measured physical activity characteristics of a diverse sample of sixth-grade girls, to examine influences on physical activity, and to report compliance with physical activity guidelines.

**Design:** Cross-sectional study.

**Setting:** Six locations across the United States.

**Participants:** A total of 1578 sixth-grade girls. Accelerometers were worn for 7 days, and data for 6 days were included in the analyses.

**Main Exposures:** Race/ethnicity, free or reduced-price lunch, and geographic region.

**Main Outcome Measures:** Six operational definitions of adequate activity (60 or 30 minutes of daily moderate to vigorous physical activity at or above 4.6, 3.8, or 3.0 metabolic equivalents) were used to examine whether girls met physical activity guidelines.

**Results:** Average times spent in sedentary, light, moderate, and vigorous activities were 460, 342, 18, and 6 min/d, respectively. White girls were more active than girls in other race/ethnic groups, and girls who did not receive free or reduced-price lunch were more active than girls who did. Girls in western states were most active. Percentages of girls in compliance with the 6 thresholds for adequate activity varied widely and ranged from 0.6% to 100.0%.

**Conclusions:** When physical activity is measured objectively and a 4.6–metabolic equivalents cut point for moderate to vigorous physical activity is used, most sixth-grade girls do not meet guidelines for adequate physical activity. One notable finding was the effect of different accelerometer scoring protocols on estimates of compliance. Conceptual and empirical work is needed to define appropriate physical activity for youth using objective physical activity measures.

*Arch Pediatr Adolesc Med. 2006;160:1262-1268*

Author Affiliations: Department of Exercise Science, University of South Carolina, Columbia (Dr Pate); Departments of Nutrition and Epidemiology, The University of North Carolina at Chapel Hill (Dr Stevens); National Heart, Lung, and Blood Institute, Bethesda, Md (Dr Pratt); Department of Psychology, San Diego State University, San Diego, Calif (Dr Sallis); Center for Clinical Epidemiology and Biostatistics, University of Pennsylvania, Philadelphia (Dr Schmitz); Department of Biostatistics, Tulane University, New Orleans, La (Dr Webber); Department of Health and Human Performance, Iowa State University, Ames (Dr Welk); and Department of Kinesiology, University of Maryland, College Park (Dr Young).

NUMEROUS GOVERNMENT health agencies and private organizations have emphasized the importance of physical activity to public health.[1-4] Among children and adolescents, higher levels of physical activity are associated with reduced risk of obesity, more favorable cardiovascular risk profiles, greater lean weight and bone mass, and enhanced psychological well-being.[5-9] Because of the immediate and likely long-term benefits of physical activity for young people, several organizations have issued guidelines on participation in physical activity for children and adolescents. The consensus recommendation is that young people should participate in moderate to vigorous physical activity (MVPA) for at least 60 minutes on most days.[10-13]

The significance of physical activity to the health of children and adolescents has led to increased interest in developing surveillance systems to monitor compliance with physical activity guidelines in young people.[14,15] Most large-scale studies of physical activity behavior have relied on self-report measures, but this approach has clear limitations for use with children.[16] Because accelerometers have not yet been used in a surveillance capacity to evaluate large samples of youth in the United States, there is uncertainty regarding activity levels of youth and the percentage who meet current physical activity recommendations.[17] Although accelerometers are objective measures, there are challenges in using them in studies of children and youth.[18] For example, there is no consensus on the methods of converting accelerometer output to minutes of physical activity,[19] so it is important to explore the effect of different accelerometer scoring protocols on the interpretation of results.

Results of previous studies in young people consistently have shown that physical activity decreases with increasing age and that girls tend to be less active than boys.[14,15,17,20-22] Furthermore, there is some evidence that physical activity is associated with demographic factors such as socioeconomic status,[23,24] race/ethnicity,[20,25] and geographic location.[1] However, accelerometers have not been used in previous studies to examine the associations with these demographic factors in population-based samples of youth.

To respond to the need to increase physical activity in girls, the National Heart, Lung, and Blood Institute is sponsoring the Trial of Activity for Adolescent Girls (TAAG), a multicenter study designed to promote physical activity in middle-school girls. The primary goal of TAAG is to determine if a physical activity intervention that links schools to community organizations reduces the age-related decrease in MVPA in girls in sixth through eighth grades. The purposes of this article are to describe the baseline physical activity characteristics of a diverse sample of sixth-grade girls by using an objective measure of physical activity and to examine the relation of race/ethnicity, socioeconomic status, and geographic region to physical activity levels in those girls. The percentage of girls meeting physical activity guidelines and the influence of varying accelerometer scoring protocols also are reported.

## METHODS

### SUBJECTS

This is a cross-sectional examination of sixth-grade girls recruited from 6 communities in the United States. University-based field centers were located in and around the cities of Tucson, Arizona; San Diego, California; New Orleans, Louisiana; Washington, DC, and Baltimore, Maryland; Minneapolis, Minnesota; and Columbia, South Carolina. Six middle schools in each community were recruited for the study. To be eligible, schools had to have a minimum of 90 girls in the eighth grade and offer physical education at all grade levels. Schools were selected for convenience but with ethnic diversity as a goal. Within each school, girls were selected by means of random sampling of all eligible sixth-grade girls. Girls were considered eligible unless they had a health problem that contraindicated physical activity or if a school administrator requested that the girl not be included in the study. Study coordination was provided by The University of North Carolina at Chapel Hill and the National Heart, Lung, and Blood Institute Project Office.

The study was approved by the participating universities' institutional review boards. Each participant's parent or guardian provided written informed consent, and all subjects assented to participation. Consent for measurement was obtained for 1721 girls. Differences in measurement rates across racial and ethnic groups were not significant. For the analyses described in this article, girls who were missing data for ethnicity (n=6), free or reduced-price lunch (n=27), or physical activity (n=110) were excluded. Thus, 1578 (91.7%) of 1721 girls with consent were included in the analysis sample.

### MEASURES

Girls classified themselves in 1 of 5 race/ethnicity categories: Asian American, African American, Hispanic, white, or other. Girls were categorized as Hispanic if they indicated Hispanic ethnicity on the questionnaire. Otherwise, girls who indicated more than one race group or who selected "Native Hawaiian or other Pacific Islanders" were classified as "other." Socioeconomic status was assessed by asking each girl if she received free or reduced-price school lunch. The answer set included the options "yes," "no," and "don't know." The investigators found that reported school lunch eligibility associated well with US Census figures for neighborhood income among TAAG subjects. Date of birth was self-reported. Weight and height were measured by using standard protocols.

Physical activity was measured by using accelerometers (MTI model 7164; Actigraph, Ft Walton Beach, Fla). Participating girls wore an accelerometer during most waking hours for 7 consecutive days. Accelerometers were initialized before data collection and were set to begin collecting data at 5:00 AM on the day after they were distributed to participants; thus, data for 6 complete days were available for analysis. Data were collected and stored in 30-second intervals. Trained and certified staff members provided detailed oral and written instruction on how and when to wear the monitors. Girls wore the accelerometer on their right hip, attached to a belt. They were asked to wear it all the time, except at night while sleeping and while bathing or swimming.

Measurement coordinators from each field site were trained and certified at a centralized training event. The TAAG Measurement Committee provided oversight for all measures. On the basis of the recommendations of a TAAG preliminary study, all data were collected during at least 2 separate calendar weeks in each participating school to minimize the school-level intraclass correlation between girls within a school.[26]

### DATA REDUCTION

Data from the accelerometers were downloaded to the same laptop computer that was used to initialize them. Accelerometer data were reduced by using methods previously described by Treuth et al.[19] Briefly, missing accelerometry data within a girl's 6-day record were replaced via imputation based on the Expectation Maximization algorithm; details on the imputation methods are provided elsewhere.[27] On average, approximately 12 hours of data per girl were imputed across the 6 days of data collection. The count thresholds (counts $\times$ 30 seconds$^{-1}$) established by Treuth and colleagues[19] in a study of eighth-grade girls were used for the activity intensities of interest: sedentary ($\leq$50), light physical activity (51-1499), moderate physical activity (1500-2600), and vigorous physical activity (>2600).

The primary analyses performed in this study were conducted by using an accelerometry count cut point for moderate-intensity physical activity (1500 counts per 30 seconds) corresponding to 4.6 metabolic equivalents (METs; 1 MET=3.5 mL $O_2 \times kg^{-1} \times min^{-1}$). Thirty-second increments with counts at or above that level were summed across the period between 6:00 AM and midnight to determine minutes of MVPA. Also, for each time increment above the 4.6-MET cut point, METs were estimated by using a regression equation.[19] The MET-weighted minutes of MVPA were calculated as the sum of the MET values for all time increments above the 4.6-MET cut point. As previously reported, the 4.6-MET cut point was selected as the intensity that best discriminated between slow and brisk walking in eighth-grade girls.[19] Two additional cut points for defining MVPA were used in some analyses. A 3.0-MET cut point (579 counts per 30 seconds) was used because it has been taken as the threshold for moderate-intensity physical activity in some studies of youth[17,28,29] and is typically used in studies of adults.[1,30] A 3.8-MET cut point (1047 counts per 30 seconds) was used because it is the intensity midway between the means for slow and brisk walking in the accelerometry calibration study.[19]

Because accelerometry is a recent innovation in public health surveillance of physical activity, there is no broad consensus as to how physical activity guidelines should be defined in terms of accelerometry data. Accordingly, compliance with physical

**Table 1. Descriptive Characteristics of Girls According to State**

| Characteristic | California (n = 291) | Arizona (n = 229) | Minnesota (n = 269) | Louisiana (n = 286) | South Carolina (n = 274) | Maryland (n = 229) |
|---|---|---|---|---|---|---|
| Age, y, mean (SD) | 11.8 (0.4) | 12.0 (0.3) | 12.0 (0.4) | 12.3 (0.7) | 12.1 (0.5) | 11.7 (0.4) |
| Weight, kg, mean (SD) | 47.1 (12.7) | 46.6 (12.8) | 47.5 (11.3) | 51.7 (14.4) | 52.0 (16.6) | 48.5 (14.8) |
| Height, cm, mean (SD) | 150.8 (7.0) | 151.9 (7.7) | 153.9 (7.3) | 153.4 (7.7) | 153.5 (7.7) | 150.8 (7.4) |
| Ethnicity, No. (%) | | | | | | |
| Asian American | 14 (4.8) | 6 (2.6) | 10 (3.7) | 10 (3.5) | 7 (2.6) | 14 (6.1) |
| African American | 18 (6.2) | 7 (3.1) | 5 (1.9) | 154 (53.8) | 102 (37.2) | 58 (25.3) |
| Hispanic | 122 (41.9) | 86 (37.6) | 27 (10.0) | 56 (19.6) | 18 (6.6) | 34 (14.8) |
| White | 104 (35.7) | 122 (53.3) | 210 (78.1) | 44 (15.4) | 121 (44.2) | 105 (45.9) |
| Other | 33 (11.3) | 8 (3.5) | 17 (6.3) | 22 (7.7) | 26 (9.5) | 18 (7.9) |
| School lunch subsidy, No. (%) | | | | | | |
| No | 143 (49.1) | 122 (53.3) | 136 (50.6) | 56 (19.6) | 137 (50.0) | 126 (55.0) |
| Yes | 115 (39.5) | 80 (34.9) | 64 (23.8) | 218 (76.2) | 111 (40.5) | 73 (31.9) |
| Don't know | 33 (11.3) | 27 (11.8) | 69 (25.7) | 12 (4.2) | 26 (9.5) | 30 (13.1) |

activity guidelines was calculated by using 6 different operational definitions. In the first definition, a girl was considered compliant if she had accumulated 60 or more minutes of physical activity at or above a cut point of 4.6 METs on 4 or more of the 6 days on which the accelerometer recorded physical activity data. The second definition was similar but used the 3.8-MET cut point. A third definition used a cut point of 3.0 METs, a standard often used with adults.[1] We also examined compliance by using 30 min/d of physical activity as the standard instead of 60 minutes because 30 minutes of daily activity is the consensus guideline for adults.[1]

## STATISTICAL METHODS

Data were analyzed by using commercially available software (Statistical Analysis System, version 8.2, PROC MIXED and PROC GLIMMIX; SAS Institute, Inc, Cary, NC). Unadjusted means and frequencies were calculated. Mixed models were used to test for group differences in mean levels of activity, and generalized linear models with a logit link function were used to test for group differences in the percentage of girls who met physical activity guidelines. By treating "school" as a random effect, these models account for the correlation in responses resulting from clustering of girls within schools. Means, adjusted for clustering of girls nested within schools, and percentages were estimated by using least squares means based on the observed marginal (the OM option in SAS) distributions of categorical variables . Three-way and 2-way interactions between location, ethnicity, and lunch subsidy were tested.

## RESULTS

**Table 1** describes characteristics of the girls according to state, arbitrarily listed from west to east. The mean (SD) age of the girls ranged from 11.7 (0.4) years to 12.3 (0.7) years across the 6 sites. Each of 4 ethnic groups was represented at each of the 6 study sites, although distributions varied considerably. In Arizona, Maryland, Minnesota, and South Carolina, the highest percentage of girls was white; in California, the highest percentage was Hispanic; and in Louisiana, the highest percentage was African American. Fewer than 10 Asian American girls participated at the Arizona and South Carolina sites, and fewer than 10 African American girls participated at the Arizona and Minnesota sites. Overall, 706 white girls, 344 African American girls, 343 Hispanic girls, and 61 Asian American girls participated. The percentage of girls who reported receiving subsidized school lunch ranged from 23.8% in Minnesota to 76.2% in Louisiana. Across the sites, 4.2% to 25.7% of girls did not know if they received a subsidy for school lunch.

**Table 2** shows the adjusted mean minutes and unadjusted overall mean minutes of sedentary, light, moderate, and vigorous physical activity according to location, ethnicity, and school lunch subsidy status. Overall, on a daily basis, girls spent 459.9 minutes in sedentary activity, 341.6 minutes in light activity, 18.1 minutes in moderate activity, and 5.6 minutes in vigorous activity. Girls in Arizona and California had the smallest number of sedentary minutes and the largest number of moderate and vigorous minutes. Examination of adjusted means showed that Asian American girls had the largest number of sedentary minutes and the smallest number of moderate and vigorous minutes compared with the other racial/ethnic groups. White girls were more active than girls in other race/ethnic groups. Girls who reported they did not receive subsidized school lunch had the largest number of moderate and vigorous minutes.

As a first step in the examination of the independent effects of location, race/ethnicity, and subsidized school lunch, we tested the 3-way interaction and found that it was not statistically significant for any of the physical activity variables. We then tested 2-way interactions. Two-way interactions with school lunch subsidy were not significant, but the interaction between location and race/ethnicity was significant ($P<.05$) for sedentary and vigorous activity, moderate and vigorous activity, and MET-weighted MVPA with the 4.6-MET cut point. Visual examination of plots of residuals indicated that African American girls in Arizona were likely responsible for the interaction between location and race/ethnicity. African American girls living in Arizona were more active than African American girls in other locations.

**Table 3** shows the percentage of girls meeting a physical activity guideline, which differed markedly depending on the operational definition used. Using the guideline of 60 min/d at or above the 4.6-MET cut point, we found that less than 1% of girls met the guideline. However, when the lower cut points of 3.8 and 3.0 METs were used with the same requirement of 60 minutes, the per-

**Table 2. Minutes of Physical Activity and MET-Weighted Minutes of Physical Activity According to Geographic Location, Ethnicity, and Receipt of Subsidy for School Lunch***

| Characteristic | Sedentary | Light | Moderate | Vigorous | MVPA (≥4.6 METs) | MET-Weighted MVPA (≥4.6 METs) |
|---|---|---|---|---|---|---|
| Location | | | | | | |
| *P* value | .003 | .009 | <.001 | .002 | <.001 | <.001 |
| California | 453.3 (5.6) | 347.0 (5.8) | 20.5 (0.7) | 6.7 (0.4) | 27.1 (1.0) | 166.7 (7.1) |
| Arizona | 438.9 (6.0) | 346.8 (6.0) | 20.8 (0.8) | 6.9 (0.4) | 27.7 (1.1) | 173.5 (7.5) |
| Minnesota | 456.0 (5.8) | 351.2 (5.9) | 18.1 (0.7) | 4.8 (0.4) | 22.9 (1.1) | 136.7 (7.2) |
| Louisiana | 465.4 (5.7) | 349.1 (5.8) | 16.3 (0.7) | 5.2 (0.4) | 21.5 (1.1) | 134.2 (7.1) |
| South Carolina | 473.6 (5.7) | 321.7 (5.8) | 15.7 (0.7) | 5.1 (0.4) | 20.8 (1.1) | 130.1 (7.2) |
| Maryland | 470.4 (6.0) | 334.2 (6.0) | 17.4 (0.8) | 5.1 (0.4) | 22.5 (1.1) | 137.8 (7.5) |
| Ethnicity | | | | | | |
| *P* value | .09 | .99 | .004 | .001 | .001 | .001 |
| Asian American | 478.8 (9.0) | 340.0 (7.5) | 14.6 (1.1) | 3.9 (0.6) | 18.5 (1.6) | 110.8 (10.8) |
| African American | 465.2 (4.6) | 342.8 (4.2) | 18.0 (0.6) | 5.7 (0.3) | 23.7 (0.9) | 146.6 (6.0) |
| Hispanic | 456.5 (4.5) | 340.8 (4.1) | 17.7 (0.6) | 4.9 (0.3) | 22.6 (0.9) | 137.3 (5.8) |
| White | 457.0 (3.5) | 341.7 (3.3) | 18.6 (0.5) | 5.9 (0.3) | 24.6 (0.7) | 152.7 (4.8) |
| Other | 459.3 (6.5) | 342.4 (5.6) | 18.4 (0.8) | 6.1 (0.4) | 24.5 (1.2) | 152.2 (8.0) |
| School lunch subsidy | | | | | | |
| *P* value | .49 | .59 | .23 | .01 | .07 | .03 |
| No | 458.8 (3.5) | 341.8 (3.3) | 18.5 (0.5) | 6.0 (0.2) | 24.5 (0.7) | 152.5 (4.5) |
| Yes | 458.9 (3.7) | 342.8 (3.4) | 17.8 (0.5) | 5.3 (0.3) | 23.1 (0.7) | 140.9 (4.7) |
| Don't know | 465.1 (5.5) | 338.0 (4.7) | 17.8 (0.7) | 5.3 (0.4) | 23.1 (1.0) | 142.0 (6.7) |
| Overall | 459.9 (1.7) | 341.6 (1.4) | 18.1 (0.2) | 5.6 (0.1) | 23.7 (0.3) | 146.1 (2.1) |

Abbreviations: METs, metabolic equivalents; MVPA, moderate to vigorous physical activity.

*Data are given as adjusted mean (SE). Data are adjusted for clustering of girls nested within schools; overall means are unadjusted. The first row of *P* values refers to tests of the equality of mean activity across site; the second row, tests of the equality of mean activity across race groups; and the third row, tests of the equality of mean activity between girls who did or did not receive free or reduced-price school lunches.

centage increased to 11.8% and 87.7%, respectively. Reducing the amount of time of MVPA from 60 to 30 minutes resulted in 16.1% of girls meeting the standard when the 4.6-MET cut point was used. When the 3.8- and 3.0-MET cut points were used, 73.3% and 100.0% of girls met the standard. The differences were highly significant for all pairwise comparisons.

## COMMENT

This study is the first to use an objective measure of physical activity to describe the physical activity levels of a large and diverse sample of American youth. Accelerometers were worn by more than 1500 sixth-grade girls in 6 widely separated geographic locations. Intensity-weighted time spent in MVPA was higher in girls residing in western states compared with those living in other regions. Activity was higher in white girls than in ethnic minority groups. Also, when we used school lunch subsidy as an indicator of socioeconomic status, girls in the higher socioeconomic stratum were more active than girls in the lower socioeconomic status group.

The overall sample of sixth-grade girls engaged in an average of 24 minutes of MVPA per day. Of this total, less than 6 min/d were of vigorous intensity. Several expert panels have recommended that youth participate in at least 60 minutes of MVPA per day, and this recommendation was recently reaffirmed by a panel convened by the US Centers for Disease Control and Prevention.[13] The findings of this study suggest that most sixth-grade girls are well below the prevailing public health guideline for physical activity. However, it should be noted that, in the present study as in previous studies, physical activity showed high interindividual variability. With a standard deviation for daily minutes of MVPA of 11.8 minutes, we could expect 95% of girls to accumulate approximately 0 to 50 minutes of MVPA (±2 SD of the mean).The observation that physical activity levels differed across geographic areas is consistent with previous surveys based on self-report measures. In the 2003 Youth Risk Behavior Survey, high school girls in the western states reported participating in more vigorous physical activity than did girls in other regions.[15] Girls in the southern states reported the lowest level of vigorous physical activity, and those in the eastern and midwestern states reported activity levels between those of girls in the western and southern regions. A similar pattern was observed in the present study. Activity levels were lowest in South Carolina and Louisiana, slightly higher in Maryland and Minnesota, and highest in Arizona and California. The geographic pattern for time spent being sedentary was, in general, inversely related to the time spent in MVPA, with girls in Arizona and California spending less time being sedentary than girls at the other sites.

Results of previous studies showed that white adolescents were more physically active than adolescents from other race/ethnic groups,[20,25] and results of a national survey showed white youth reported more vigorous physical activity than African American or Hispanic youth.[15] In TAAG, white girls had slightly higher minutes of moderate and vigorous physical activity than girls in the other race/ethnic groups and had the highest MET-weighted MVPA. White girls had a higher prevalence than African American or Hispanic girls of meeting the 60-

**Table 3. Adjusted Percentage of Girls Meeting Guidelines for MVPA According to Geographic Location, Ethnicity, and Receipt of Subsidy for School Lunch***

| Characteristic | ≥60 min/d† | | | ≥30 min/d† | | |
|---|---|---|---|---|---|---|
| | ≥4.6 METs | ≥3.8 METs | ≥3.0 METs | ≥4.6 METs | ≥3.8 METs | ≥3.0 METs |
| Location | | | | | | |
| *P* value | .53 | .008 | .01 | <.001 | .004 | .99 |
| California | 0.3 | 15.4 | 95.1 | 24.0 | 85.7 | 99.8 |
| Arizona | 1.3 | 19.5 | 91.9 | 25.3 | 75.5 | 100 |
| Minnesota | 0 | 7.3 | 91.4 | 12.6 | 80.0 | 100 |
| Louisiana | 1.4 | 12.6 | 87.2 | 11.9 | 70.1 | 100 |
| South Carolina | 0.4 | 5.2 | 79.4 | 8.4 | 61.5 | 100 |
| Maryland | 0.4 | 12.1 | 84.2 | 15.2 | 68.4 | 100 |
| Ethnicity | | | | | | |
| *P* value | .66 | .09 | .19 | .03 | .007 | .99 |
| Asian American | 0 | 1.7 | 82.3 | 4.8 | 55.5 | 100 |
| African American | 1.2 | 13.9 | 90.6 | 20.2 | 74.8 | 100 |
| Hispanic | 0 | 12.0 | 87.1 | 13.0 | 70.5 | 99.9 |
| White | 0.6 | 10.1 | 80.0 | 15.0 | 76.7 | 100 |
| Other | 1.6 | 14.6 | 87.9 | 17.8 | 77.4 | 100 |
| School lunch subsidy | | | | | | |
| *P* value | .87 | .01 | .84 | .55 | .64 | .88 |
| No | 0.6 | 12.8 | 89.2 | 16.6 | 73.0 | 99.9 |
| Yes | 0.8 | 11.5 | 88.5 | 14.7 | 74.9 | 99.9 |
| Don't know | 0.5 | 5.3 | 89.9 | 14.3 | 76.0 | 100 |
| Overall | 0.6 | 11.8 | 87.7 | 16.1 | 73.3 | 100 |

Abbreviations: METs, metabolic equivalents; MVPA, moderate to vigorous physical activity.

*Adjusted for clustering of girls nested within schools; overall proportions are unadjusted. The first row of *P* values refers to tests of the equality of the proportion of girls who meet the guidelines for MVPA across site; the second row, tests of the equality of the proportion of girls who meet the guidelines for MVPA across race groups; and the third row, tests of the equality of the proportion of girls who meet the guidelines for MVPA between girls who did or did not receive free or reduced-price school lunches.

†Number of minutes per day of MVPA 4 or more days per week.

minute MVPA guidelines. However, the differences among white, African American, and Hispanic girls were small for minutes of moderate and vigorous physical activity considered separately. Few investigators have evaluated the physical activity behavior of Asian American girls. Although the present sample was relatively small, Asian American girls consistently had the lowest levels of physical activity and highest levels of sedentary behavior. These findings of race/ethnic differences in large samples of adolescents by using an objective measure of physical activity confirm the disparities reported in studies that used self-report measures.[31-33] These disparities appear to increase as minority youth move from adolescence to adulthood,[31] so interventions to promote physical activity in minority adolescents should be designated a public health priority. Research to improve understanding of the reasons for these disparities in physical activity also is needed.

Findings on the relationship between socioeconomic status and physical activity in adolescents have been inconsistent,[20] possibly because a wide range of indicators of socioeconomic status have been used. Results of a large national survey, however, showed that vigorous physical activity was directly related to family income and educational level, after adjusting for other variables.[31] In TAAG, reported free or reduced-price lunch was used as an indicator of family income, although approximately 12% of girls did not know their free or reduced-price lunch status. We found no variation in physical activity according to lunch subsidy status for sedentary, light, and moderate physical activity. However, girls who received no lunch subsidy engaged in significantly ($P = .01$) more vigorous physical activity than those who received a subsidy, similar to the findings in a national survey.[31] This finding suggests that lower income adolescent girls may be less physically active, but the mean difference in the present study was small. A prudent interpretation is that adolescent-reported lunch subsidy status did not permit an adequate test of the relationship of socioeconomic status to physical activity.

One of the most notable findings of the present study was the effect of different accelerometer scoring protocols on estimates of physical activity. Although there is reasonable consensus that 3.0 METs is an appropriate cut point for moderate-intensity physical activity in adults,[1] there is no such consensus in youth. Resting energy expenditure in children is higher than the assumed value of 3.5 mL/kg per minute for adults, so a value of 3.0 METs represents a lower relative activity level for youth. Differences in metabolic and biomechanical efficiency because of growth and maturation[34] also alter the relationship between accelerometer counts and energy expenditure. A detailed calibration study conducted by the TAAG investigators determined that a value of 4.6 METs provides an appropriate cut point for moderate-intensity physical activity in adolescent girls.[19] Operationally, this cut point was established by using accelerometer values that distinguished between a slow and a brisk walk. The activity levels reported with this cut point are considerably lower than those reported in other studies,[17,35] but this result is because of the differences in cut points used in the different studies.

By definition, cut points impart a somewhat artificial categorization to continuous data. To provide an indication of how the cut point can influence the results, the data were analyzed by using 3.0- and 3.8-MET cut points, the former being a value commonly used in other studies.[17] The percentage of girls meeting the current physical activity standard for youth (ie, 60 minutes of MVPA per day) varied dramatically, depending on the accelerometry cut point for moderate-intensity physical activity. With the 4.6-MET cut point, almost no girls met the standard. However, if a 3.0-MET cut point was used, 87.7% of girls met the standard. If the adult guideline (30 min/d) was used, all the girls met the standard with a 3.0-MET cut point, but only 16.1% met the 30-minute goal with the 4.6-MET cut point. Using the 3.8-MET cut point yielded compliance rates that were intermediate to those obtained with 4.6 and 3.0 METs but with a different pattern for the 60- and 30-minute standards. Only 11.8% of girls met the 60-minute 3.8-MET standard, but most of them met the 30-minute 3.8-MET standard (73.3%). The difference in compliance estimates because of choice of cut points makes it difficult to draw definitive conclusions about the activity patterns in these youth. The cut point of 3.0 provides a liberal estimate of activity patterns and favors sensitivity over specificity, whereas the 3.8 and 4.6 cut points provide more conservative estimates and favor specificity over sensitivity. Misclassification is always a concern when attempting to determine compliance with public health recommendations, and the dramatic differences demonstrate the need to develop consensus guidelines for reducing and reporting accelerometer data. In addition, conceptual and empirical work are likely to be needed to define health-related physical activity for youth. At present, physical activity guidelines for youth are based on a body of knowledge that experts agree is too limited.[13] Hence, there is a need to strengthen the basis for physical activity guidelines and adopt improved methods for monitoring compliance with those guidelines.

Although absolute determinations of activity levels must be made with caution, this study demonstrates the potential for large-scale surveillance of activity patterns with accelerometers. Data from large and ethnically diverse samples were collected in a standardized way from 6 different regions throughout the United States. Obtaining objective physical activity information for 6 days is a major strength because this time frame is sufficient to capture reliable patterns.[36] Sophisticated data reduction procedures and imputation methods were used to improve the accuracy and stability of the reported values. Using cut points for MVPA that were empirically determined specifically for adolescent girls is another strength. As the data suggest, the proportion of girls meeting national recommendations varies substantially on the basis of the MET cut point used. Given the increasing epidemic of obesity in adolescents,[37,38] it is likely that the percentage of girls achieving sufficient physical activity is reflective of the data reported by using the 4.6-MET cut point. Without having conducted this prior work and being able to use this cut point, the data would suggest almost 90% of sixth-grade girls met recommendations.

Some limitations in the design should be noted. First, the data cannot be considered representative of youth in these regions. The participating TAAG sites were from predominantly urban settings, so the participating schools tended to be from the densely populated metropolitan areas. Second, subtle differences in population profiles, community characteristics, and seasonality could explain the interaction observed between location and ethnicity, but additional research will be needed to understand these influences and to capture possible differences between rural and urban youth. Designs that permit linkages with geographic information system and census data may be particularly helpful in examining the influence of social, environmental, and policy variables on physical activity. The results are limited in that not all geographic regions of the country were represented. Nevertheless, an ethnic/racially diverse sample was obtained. Although the schools were not randomly selected, the girls within the schools were randomly selected. Because girls were sampled from middle schools that met eligibility criteria for participation in the TAAG trial, there is a loss of generalizability. The TAAG schools offered physical education at all grade levels, and girls who participate in physical education may be more active than girls who do not.

The present study demonstrated the feasibility of using accelerometers to collect objective physical activity data in a large number of adolescents. Race/ethnic disparities in physical activity levels were documented, with white girls having slightly higher activity levels than girls of ethnic minority groups. On average, girls living in the West were more physically active than those in other parts of the United States. The difficulty of estimating the prevalence of meeting physical activity guidelines was demonstrated by the dramatic effect of different accelerometer protocols on prevalence rates. Because there is no consensus on the most suitable protocols, a high priority should be given to research to guide the development of accelerometer scoring protocols that can be applied across all ages.

**Accepted for Publication:** August 3, 2006.
**Correspondence:** Russell R. Pate, PhD, Department of Exercise Science, University of South Carolina, 921 Assembly St, Columbia, SC 29208 (rpate@gwm.sc.edu).
**Author Contributions:** Dr Pate had full access to all the data in the study and takes responsibility for the integrity of the data and the accuracy of the data analysis. *Study concept and design:* Pate, Pratt, Sallis, Schmitz, Webber, and Young. *Acquisition of data:* Stevens, Schmitz, and Webber. *Analysis and interpretation of data:* Welk. *Drafting of the manuscript:* Pate, Stevens, Pratt, Sallis, Schmitz, and Welk. *Critical revision of the manuscript for important intellectual content*: Pratt, Schmitz, Webber, Welk, and Young. *Statistical analysis:* Stevens and Webber. *Obtained funding:* Pate, Stevens, Sallis, Webber, and Young. *Administrative, technical, and material support:* Pate, Pratt, Sallis, Webber, and Welk. *Study supervision:* Pate.
**Financial Disclosure:** None reported.
**Funding/Support:** The study was supported by grant 5U01HL066852 from the National Institutes of Health.
**Acknowledgment:** We thank Leslie Lytle, PhD, Univer-

sity of Minnesota, Minneapolis, and Timothy Lohman, PhD, University of Arizona, Tucson, for their leadership of the TAAG field centers in Minnesota and Arizona and Gaye Groover Christmus, MPH, University of South Carolina, Columbia, for assistance in developing and editing the manuscript.

## REFERENCES

1. US Department of Health and Human Services. *Physical Activity and Health: A Report of the Surgeon General.* Atlanta, Ga: US Dept of Health and Human Services/Centers for Disease Control; 1996.
2. Physical activity and cardiovascular health: NIH Consensus Development Panel on Physical Activity and Cardiovascular Health. *JAMA.* 1996;276:241-246.
3. Williams CL, Hayman LL, Daniels SR, et al. Cardiovascular health in childhood: a statement for health professionals from the Committee on Atherosclerosis, Hypertension, and Obesity in the Young (AHOY) of the Council on Cardiovascular Disease in the Young, American Heart Association [published correction appears in *Circulation.* 2002;106:1178]. *Circulation.* 2002;106:143-160.
4. US Department of Health and Human Services. *Healthy People 2010.* 2nd ed. Washington, DC: US Dept of Health and Human Services; 2000.
5. Rowland TW. The role of physical activity and fitness in children in the prevention of adult cardiovascular disease. *Prog Pediatr Cardiol.* 2001;12:199-203.
6. Hager RL, Tucker LA, Seljaas GT. Aerobic fitness, blood lipids, and body fat in children. *Am J Public Health.* 1995;85:1702-1706.
7. Hagberg JM, Goldring D, Ehsani AA, et al. Effect of exercise training on the blood pressure and hemodynamic features of hypertensive adolescents. *Am J Cardiol.* 1983;52:763-768.
8. Armstrong N, Simons-Morton B. Physical activity and blood lipids in adolescents. *Pediatric Exerc Sci.* 1994;6:381-405.
9. Calfas KJ, Taylor WC. Effects of physical activity on psychological variables in adolescents. *Pediatric Exerc Sci.* 1994;6:406-423.
10. Corbin CB, Pangrazzi RP. *Physical Activity for Children: A Statement of Guidelines.* Reston, Va: National Association for Sport and Physical Education; 1998.
11. Sallis JF, Patrick K. Physical activity guidelines for adolescents: consensus statement. *Pediatric Exerc Sci.* 1994;6:302-314.
12. Health Education Authority. Policy framework for young people and health-enhancing physical activity. In: Biddle S, Sallis JF, Cavill NA, eds. *Young and Active? Young People and Health-Enhancing Physical Activity—Evidence and Implications.* London, England: Health Education Authority; 1998:3.
13. Strong WB, Malina RM, Blimkie CJ, et al. Evidence based physical activity for school-age youth. *J Pediatr.* 2005;146:732-737.
14. Grunbaum JA, Kann L, Kinchen SA, et al. Youth risk behavior surveillance—United States, 2001. *MMWR Surveill Summ.* 2002;51:1-62.
15. Grunbaum JA, Kann L, Kinchen SA, et al. Youth risk behavior surveillance—United States, 2003 [published corrections appear in *MMWR Surveill Summ.* 2004;53:536 and 2005;54:608]. *MMWR Surveill Summ.* 2004;53:1-96.
16. Sallis JF, Saelens BE. Assessment of physical activity by self-report: status, limitations, and future directions [published correction appears in *Res Q Exerc Sport.* 2000;71:409]. *Res Q Exerc Sport.* 2000;71(2 suppl):S1-S14.
17. Pate RR, Freedson PS, Sallis JF, et al. Compliance with physical activity guidelines: prevalence in a population of children and youth. *Ann Epidemiol.* 2002;12:303-308.
18. Welk GJ. Use of accelerometry-based activity monitors to assess physical activity. In: Welk GJ, ed. *Physical Activity Assessments for Health-related Research.* Champaign, Ill: Human Kinetics; 2002.
19. Treuth MS, Schmitz K, Catellier DJ, et al. Defining accelerometer thresholds for activity intensities in adolescent girls. *Med Sci Sports Exerc.* 2004;36:1259-1266.
20. Sallis JF, Prochaska JJ, Taylor WC. A review of correlates of physical activity of children and adolescents. *Med Sci Sports Exerc.* 2000;32:963-975.
21. Sallis JF, Zakarian JM, Hovell MF, Hofstetter CR. Ethnic, socioeconomic, and sex differences in physical activity among adolescents. *J Clin Epidemiol.* 1996;49:125-134.
22. Aaron DJ, Kriska AM, Dearwater SR, et al. The epidemiology of leisure physical activity in an adolescent population. *Med Sci Sports Exerc.* 1993;25:847-853.
23. Pate RR, Heath GW, Dowda M, Trost SG. Associations between physical activity and other health behaviors in a representative sample of US adolescents. *Am J Public Health.* 1996;86:1577-1581.
24. Gordon-Larsen P, McMurray RG, Popkin BM. Determinants of adolescent physical activity and inactivity patterns. *Pediatrics.* 2000;105:e83 http://pediatrics.aappublications.org/cgi/content/full/105/6/e83. Accessed September 8, 2006.
25. Kimm SY, Glynn NW, Kriska AM, et al. Decline in physical activity in black girls and white girls during adolescence. *N Engl J Med.* 2002;347:709-715.
26. Murray DM, Catellier DJ, Hannan PJ, et al. School-level intraclass correlation for physical activity in adolescent girls. *Med Sci Sports Exerc.* 2004;36:876-882.
27. Catellier DJ, Hannan PJ, Murray DM, et al. Imputation of missing data when measuring physical activity by accelerometry. *Med Sci Sports Exerc.* 2005;37(suppl 11):S555-S562.
28. Trost SG, Kerr LM, Ward DS, Pate RR. Physical activity and determinants of physical activity in obese and non-obese children. *Int J Obes Relat Metab Disord.* 2001;25:822-829.
29. Thompson AM, Campagna PD, Rehman LA, Murphy RJ, Rasmussen RL, Ness GW. Physical activity and body mass index in grade 3, 7, and 11 Nova Scotia students. *Med Sci Sports Exerc.* 2005;37:1902-1908.
30. Pate RR, Pratt M, Blair SN, et al. Physical activity and public health: a recommendation from the Centers for Disease Control and Prevention and the American College of Sports Medicine. *JAMA.* 1995;273:402-407.
31. Pratt M, Macera CA, Blanton C. Levels of physical activity and inactivity in children and adults in the United States: current evidence and research issues. *Med Sci Sports Exerc.* 1999;31(suppl 11):S526-S533.
32. Dowda M, Pate RR, Felton GM, et al. Physical activities and sedentary pursuits in African American and Caucasian girls. *Res Q Exerc Sport.* 2004;75:352-360.
33. Felton GM, Dowda M, Ward DS, et al. Differences in physical activity between black and white girls living in rural and urban areas. *J Sch Health.* 2002;72:250-255.
34. Sallis JF, Buono MJ, Freedson PS. Bias in estimating caloric expenditure from physical activity in children: implications for epidemiological studies. *Sports Med.* 1991;11:203-209.
35. Riddoch CJ, Bo Andersen L, Wedderkopp N, et al. Physical activity levels and patterns of 9- and 15-yr-old European children. *Med Sci Sports Exerc.* 2004;36:86-92.
36. Trost SG, Pate RR, Freedson PS, Sallis JF, Taylor WC. Using objective physical activity measures with youth: how many days of monitoring are needed? *Med Sci Sports Exerc.* 2000;32:426-431.
37. Hedley AA, Ogden CL, Johnson CL, Carroll MD, Curtin LR, Flegal KM. Prevalence of overweight and obesity among US children, adolescents, and adults, 1999-2002. *JAMA.* 2004;291:2847-2850.
38. Ogden CL, Flegal KM, Carroll MD, Johnson CL. Prevalence and trends in overweight among US children and adolescents, 1999-2000. *JAMA.* 2002;288:1728-1732.

"Another father might tell you to put that coat on and zip it up."

"Just tell me then! Pretend you're the kind of father who tells his kid to put on her coat so she won't catch a cold."

"We don't tell you what to do. If you want to get chilled, it's really none of our business."

"Since when did reverse psychology work on me?"

"Do you want to talk about it?"

—From *My Latest Grievance* by Elinor Lippman, 2006

# YOUTH

## A Health Plan–Based Lifestyle Intervention Increases Bone Mineral Density in Adolescent Girls

*Lynn L. DeBar, PhD, MPH; Cheryl Ritenbaugh, PhD, MPH; Mikel Aickin, PhD; Eric Orwoll, MD; Diane Elliot, MD; John Dickerson, MS; Nancy Vuckovic, PhD; Victor J. Stevens, PhD; Esther Moe, PhD; Lori M. Irving, PhD†*

**Objective:** To test the efficacy of a health plan–based lifestyle intervention to increase bone mineral density in adolescent girls.

**Design:** Two-year randomized, controlled trial.

**Setting:** Large health maintenance organization.

**Participants:** Girls 14 to 16 years old with body mass index below the national median.

**Intervention:** Behavioral intervention (bimonthly group meetings, quarterly coaching telephone calls, and weekly self-monitoring) designed to improve diet and increase physical activity.

**Main Outcome Measures:** Total bone mineral density was measured by dual-energy x-ray absorptiometry. Behavioral outcomes included intake of calcium, vitamin D, soda, and fruits and vegetables; high-impact and strength-training physical activity; measures of strength and fitness; and biomarkers (osteocalcin and naltrexone).

**Results:** Compared with control subjects, girls in the intervention group had significantly higher bone mineral density in the spine and trochanter regions during the first study year, which was maintained during the second study year. The naltrexone biomarker demonstrated a greater relative decrease in the intervention group compared with the control group, with nonsignificant changes in osteocalcin consistent with more bone building in the intervention group. Participants in the intervention group reported significantly greater consumption of calcium in both study years, vitamin D in the first year, and fruits and vegetables in both years. We found no effect on soda consumption or target exercise rates.

**Conclusions:** A comprehensive health care–based lifestyle intervention can effectively improve dietary intake and increase bone mineral gains in adolescent girls. To our knowledge, this study is the first to significantly improve bone mass in adolescent girls in a non–school-based intervention.

**Trial Registration:** Clinicaltrials.gov Identifier: NCT67600.

*Arch Pediatr Adolesc Med. 2006;160:1269-1276*

THE PRIMARY PREVENTION OF osteoporosis is an important public health target. Almost half of all women in the United States older than 50 years demonstrate low bone density (osteopenia).[1] An estimated 1.3 million osteoporosis-related fractures occur each year in the United States, with annual costs of approximately $13.8 billion.[2] One determinant of lifetime osteopenia and osteoporosis risk is low bone mineral density (BMD). Because 90% of peak bone mass is acquired by age 18 years,[3-5] interventions to maximize BMD in youth may decrease the incidence of osteopenia later in life. For this reason, the National Institute of Child Health and Health Development recently requested applications (RFA: HD-97-006) for the prevention of adult osteoporosis by targeting BMD in youth.

Although a substantial component of osteoporosis risk is genetic,[6,7] both diet and physical activity are important modifiers of bone accrual.[3] Several controlled trials have found that increasing calcium intake increases BMD in youth.[8-10] Other dietary factors also may maximize the retention of calcium in bones, but few randomized trials have examined these factors in adolescents. Studies suggest that greater fruit and vegetable intake is important for bone health[11,12] and is associated with higher BMD.[13,14] In addition, studies[15,16] suggest that achievement of peak bone mass in adolescent girls is contingent on adequate vitamin D intake. Further, consuming caffeinated beverages, particularly colas, increases risk of bone fracture.[17,18] Finally, many studies have suggested that increasing weight-bearing activity increases BMD in children and adolescents.[19-24]

**Author Affiliations:** Center for Health Research, Kaiser Permanente Northwest, Portland, Ore (Drs DeBar, Vuckovic, and Stevens, and Mr Dickerson); University of Arizona College of Medicine, Tucson (Drs Ritenbaugh and Aickin); Oregon Health & Science University, Portland (Drs Orwoll, Elliot, and Moe); Washington State University, Vancouver (Dr Irving).
†Deceased.

**Table 1. Study Intervention and Adherence Components**

| Component | Enhanced Fitness (Intervention) | Total Health (Comparison) |
|---|---|---|
| **Intervention** | | |
| Re-treat, to create group cohesion among study participants and orient to study* | 1 Time at study beginning | 1 Time at study beginning |
| Annual individual visits to provide individualized feedback and motivation* | Annually | Annually |
| Coaching calls to address individual adherence issues | 4 Times per year | NA |
| Team meetings: information and group support | Bimonthly | NA |
| Self-monitoring postcards with behavioral targets shifting weekly | Weekly | NA |
| **Adherence and retention** | | |
| Study Web site: information and monitoring own point accumulation* | Ongoing | Ongoing |
| Team meetings: social interaction and parental involvement | Quarterly | Quarterly |
| Study incentives/points | Ongoing | Ongoing |
| Youth and parent newsletter* | Twice yearly | Twice yearly |
| Participant membership in fitness center | Ongoing | Ongoing |

Abbreviation: NA, not available.
*Content differs for intervention and comparison conditions; intervention focused on diet and exercise, whereas comparison focused on other health issues.

Although much of the research on building healthy bones in youth has targeted younger children,[19,21,23,25,26] adolescents may be an equally important target population. Eating and exercise patterns established in adolescence may be more likely to be sustained into adulthood than similar efforts aimed at younger children.[27,28] Gains in bone mass are most rapid during adolescence, with as much as 51% of peak bone mass accumulated during pubertal growth.[29,30] Interventions to prevent osteoporosis are particularly important in adolescent girls, because they are at a higher risk of developing osteoporosis in adulthood than males.[31] Recent reports suggest that vigorous exercise declines in adolescents,[32] which makes this time key for intervention.

Preventive interventions conducted in youth generally have involved calcium supplementation, controlled feeding trials, or prescribed exercise in a controlled setting; that is, they have not emphasized sustainable behavioral practices and, thus, not represented community trials. Further, existing youth interventions are mainly school based,[33-36] largely overlooking the opportunities in other settings such as health care. Inasmuch as most children and adolescents (about 80%) visit a medical provider at least annually (76 million annual contacts with physicians[37]), such visits are a largely untapped setting in which to offer primary prevention programs. Pediatric patients are influenced by physician advice and are receptive to health behavior recommendations.[38] Thus, adolescents may comply with targeted lifestyle interventions offered through health care settings more than with those offered in schools.

## METHODS

### OVERVIEW

This randomized controlled trial (YOUTH) tested the efficacy of a lifestyle intervention for increasing BMD in adolescent girls initially 14 to 16 years old. The goal of the intervention was to improve diet and increase physical activity. The 3 dietary targets were increasing dairy consumption, eating 8 servings of fruits and vegetables daily, and decreasing soft drink intake. The 2 primary physical activity targets were high-impact exercise and strength training.

### SETTING

Kaiser Permanente Northwest is a nonprofit, group-model health maintenance organization (HMO) in the Portland, Ore, metropolitan region that provides comprehensive medical care to more than 440 000 members, including 15 768 female adolescents between 14 and 16 years of age. The research center is located within the HMO but conducts independent, public domain research. The HMO Human Subjects Protection Committee monitored and approved all study procedures.

### STUDY POPULATION AND RECRUITMENT, SCREENING, AND RANDOMIZATION

We selected adolescent girls with body mass index below the national median to enrich our sample with girls at risk of low peak BMD.[39,40] We also targeted potential participants by selecting for characteristics we expected would enhance adherence to the study (ie, younger girls [freshmen and sophomores], parent or guardian willing to participate in the study, and no indication of psychiatric or psychosocial disorders). We excluded potential participants with any apparent contraindication to the dietary or exercise portions of the intervention, including current or past disordered eating behavior. Potential participants were identified through the HMO's electronic medical record. Health plan member contracts with the HMO provide consent for use of their data in research. Members who met the selection criteria were mailed study invitations, followed by telephone calls from research staff. An informational meeting for interested families meeting study criteria preceded randomization. Eligible adolescent girls were randomized by a computer program developed by one of us (M.A.) into either the lifestyle intervention group or an attentional control group after baseline data collection (between September 1, 2000, and August 31, 2001). The project manager informed participants of group assignment to keep assessors blinded. Treatment group assignment was made by a design-adaptive randomization to minimize group imbalance on physical activity, calcium intake, age, and other factors.[41,42] Design-adaptive randomization sequentially assigned girls to the control or intervention groups to achieve, at each step, the maximum balance of factors predictive of bone measurements, such as menarcheal age and participation in organized sports. To conceal allocation, the project biostatistician (M.A.) made allocations in response to project staff requests.

### INTERVENTION

The YOUTH intervention emphasized adolescents actively developing strategies for healthy dietary and exercise practices that they could maintain in adulthood. Participants attended group and individual meetings, participated in activities, and received coaching telephone calls (**Table 1**). They also received psychoeducational information, recorded their diet and exercise goals and achievements, and kept in touch with their cohort through a Web-based study site. We combined elements especially for adolescents (peer-oriented, community-building activities) with those widely recognized as important in lifestyle interventions (individual tailoring). Further, our intervention drew heavily from both mentoring models and motivational interviewing or enhancement techniques.[43] Because this trial involved a 2-year intervention and follow-up, we incorporated several adherence and retention components (Table 1). The intervention has been extensively described elsewhere.[39]

## ASSESSMENT

Staff who performed clinical and dietary and physical activity assessments were masked to the experimental condition of the participants. These assessors had no additional contact with participants.

## BONE MINERAL DENSITY

Bone mineral density was measured using dual-energy x-ray absorptiometry (DEXA; QDR 2000, Hologic Inc, Waltham, Mass) at baseline and at 1- and 2-year follow-up. We assessed BMD and bone mineral content (BMC) for the total body and at specific sites: lumbar spine (L2 through L4), trochanter, femoral neck, and total hip. Independently determined in vivo precision (coefficient of variation) for total hip and lumbar spine in our laboratory were 1.4% and 1.7%, respectively. Phantom scans performed daily during the observation period revealed no change in DEXA machine performance. Our adolescent girls had mostly completed linear growth, and we anticipated little change in bone dimensions during follow-up. Thus, BMD was the primary outcome measure. Nevertheless, we also measured BMC, bone mineral apparent density (BMAD), and bone area. Because volumetric density (BMAD) is difficult to estimate using DEXA, we limited BMAD results to L2 through L4, for which there are established reference ranges for teenagers.[44]

## BODY COMPOSITION AND PHYSICAL DEVELOPMENT

Certified technicians measured weight and height using a standardized protocol.[45] Body mass index was calculated as weight in kilograms divided by height in meters squared. The total-body scan (DEXA) was used to measure lean and fat masses. We used years since menarche at baseline as our measure of sexual maturation because[46] our minimum age requirement (14 years) meant that most subjects (97%) had reached menarche. Month and year of menarche was updated at every diet recall for those who had not reached menarche at baseline.

## BIOMARKERS

We collected blood samples from participants at the beginning and end of the study to examine biochemical markers of bone formation (osteocalcin; Diagnostic Products Corp, Los Angeles, Calif) and bone resorption (*N*-terminal telopeptides; Ostex International, Inc, Seattle, Wash). Blood samples were drawn in the morning after overnight fasting and handled and assayed according to the manufacturer's specifications.

## DIETARY INTAKE

Certified dietary interviewers used unannounced 24-hour telephone diet recalls to obtain data on all foods consumed, preparation method, and portion sizes. Participants were trained to estimate portion size using real food and food models at the screening visit, and received visual aids for estimating portion size of various foods. At baseline, we obtained data from 3 unannounced diet recalls for a 2-week period. Postrandomization, 1 recall was obtained every other month, targeting 4 weekdays and 2 weekend days per year to cover seasonal effects. The 6 dietary recalls in each year were averaged for analysis. Data were directly entered into the ESHA database (ESHA Food Processor, version 8.1, 2003; ESHA Research Inc, Salem, Ore). We limited the nutrient variables to the food group–based nutrition categories potentially relevant for bone mineral accrual: total calcium intake, in milligrams per day; total vitamin D, in international units per day; and fruits and vegetables, in servings per day. In addition, we adapted the ESHA program to output soda intake, in ounces per day, and vitamin supplementation.

## WEIGHT-BEARING PHYSICAL ACTIVITY, STRENGTH, AND FITNESS

We used both laboratory and self-reported measures to assess weight-bearing physical activity, strength, and fitness. To determine weight-bearing physical activity, we adapted a 72-hour physical activity recall from the Previous Day Physical Activity Recall form[47,48] and administered it like the dietary recalls. Because we examined activity most relevant for bone mineral accrual (high impact, spinal motion, and weight-loading activities), physical activity recall focused on exercise rather than usual daily activities or sedentary behaviors. We defined "high impact" as movement in which both feet were simultaneously off the ground (eg, jumping or running) and "strength training" as any activity that provided muscular resistance (eg, weight training and resistance band use).

Strength and fitness were assessed at the 3 annual clinic visits using standardized protocols and trained assessors. Assessments included hand grip (overall strength), Roman chair and sit-ups (lower back strength), and vertical jump (hip and upper thigh strength). We used sit-ups and vertical jump as representative strength measures.

## OTHER STUDY MEASURES

At baseline and follow-up visits, girls completed questionnaires about potential moderators and mediators of outcomes. Only the demographic characteristics and the participant's osteoporosis risk are included here. We defined "adult osteoporosis risk" as the proportion of first- and second-degree relatives of the participant's parents (eg, their parents, aunts, and uncles) whom the parents identified as having hip fractures or osteoporosis. Teen participants also reported their self-perceived risk of osteoporosis later in life.

## ANALYSIS

Statistical analyses were conducted using SAS Release 8.2 (SAS Institute Inc, Cary, NC) and STATA version 6.0 (StataCorp, College Station, Tex). Bone mineral density was our primary dependent variable, and the intervention effect was estimated as the adjusted (for baseline values) mean difference between the intervention and control conditions after years 1 and 2. We used a conditional change model and the Zellner seemingly unrelated regression models.[49-51] This approach uses joint estimates of several regression models. Baseline and change equations were estimated simultaneously because we expected that the 2 equations were not independent. Adjusting for the correlated errors generally leads to more efficient estimates of the coefficients and reduced standard errors in both equations than would result from the use of separate equation estimations. Treat-

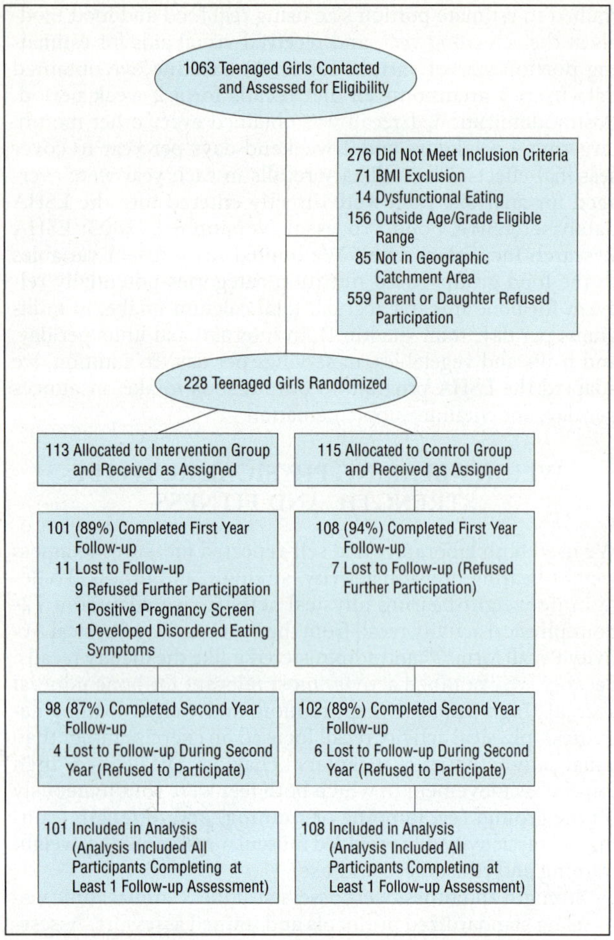


**Figure 1.** Consolidated Standards of Reporting Trials (CONSORT) diagram. Participant flow through the clinical trial. BMI, body mass index (calculated as weight in kilograms divided by height in meters squared).

ment condition was the primary independent variable. All analyses were adjusted for baseline age, years since menarche, risk of adult osteoporosis, height, body mass index, and the respective bone mass variable. We analyzed the intervention's effects on bone mineral over the initial year of the intervention and across the entire 2-year period. All significance tests were 2-sided.

We used the same regression approach for secondary outcomes: changes in diet and physical activity. In addition, we examined behavioral (overall energy intake and overall physical activity) and anthropometric factors (weight, height, body mass index, and lean and fat masses) that were not targeted for behavioral change.

Of the 1063 girls originally contacted, 228 met the inclusion criteria, agreed to participate, and were randomized to either the intervention or the control group (**Figure 1**). Of those randomized, 210 (92%) underwent at least 1 bone mineral follow-up test. For those with missing values for the first-year follow-up DEXA measurement (n=8), the data were imputed by averaging baseline and second-year DEXA values. One girl was excluded after a positive pregnancy screening, bringing the 1-year outcome analysis sample to 209. Two hundred girls had DEXA data at the 2-year follow-up; the sustainability analysis was limited to these girls. Blood was drawn in all girls for biomarker analyses. In a laboratory error, a box of samples was lost; all remaining paired samples (n=130) were analyzed. We repeated all nonblood analyses with this biomarker subsample; patterns (direction and significance of results) were comparable to those of the entire sample (data not shown).

## RESULTS

### DESCRIPTIVE CHARACTERISTICS

Baseline values for study participants (**Table 2**) showed they were mainly white (81%) and from middle- to upper-middle-income working homes. The participants were in the lower half of the body mass index distribution (20.6) per the selection criteria, and 97% had reached menarche at enrollment. At baseline, average consumption included 986 mg/d of calcium, 161 IU of vitamin D, 3.6 servings of fruits and vegetables, and less than 6 oz per day of soda. At baseline, total physical activity was 61.9 min/d (including 13.9 min/d of high-impact activity and 6.9 min/d of strength training), with 68.9% of participants reporting participation in organized team sports. No statistically significant differences were found for these variables between the intervention and control groups at baseline.

### INTERVENTION EFFECTS ON MAIN DIET AND EXERCISE TARGETS

The intervention had a substantial effect on the 3 main dietary targets but not on exercise (Table 2). Participants in the intervention group reported significantly higher consumption compared with those in the control group for calcium in both study years (adjusted mean difference [AMD], 216.6 and 241.3 mg, respectively; $P<.001$), vitamin D in the first year of the study (AMD, 34.3 IU; $P=.02$), and fruit and vegetable servings in both study years (AMD, 0.74 and 0.79 servings, respectively; $P\leq.01$). We found no effect of the intervention on soda consumption or significant differences between the conditions in target exercise rates during either year.

### INTERVENTION EFFECTS ON BONE MINERAL VARIABLES AND MARKERS OF BONE TURNOVER

Significantly higher BMD was found in the intervention group compared with the control group in the spine (AMD, 0.01; $P<.001$) and trochanter region (AMD, 0.007; $P=.05$) and a trend toward higher density in the total hip (AMD, 0.006; $P=.08$) after 1 year of intervention (**Table 3** and **Figure 2**). We found no significant differences between the groups for BMD for the total body or the femoral neck region or for bone area or BMC for any of the bone regions. The 2 groups differed in spinal BMAD at the year 1 follow-up (AMD, 0.01; $P=.001$).

Data in Table 3 and Figure 2 suggest that the intervention effects on BMD in the spine (AMD, 0.01; $P=.007$) and trochanter region (AMD, 0.01; $P=.03$) were maintained during the second study year. During the second year, we observed no differences in bone areas in the 2 groups but significantly higher levels of BMC for the total body (AMD, 19.78; $P=.43$) and spine (AMD, 7.09; $P=.03$) in the intervention group compared with the control group. Also, the 2 groups differed in spinal BMAD at the year 2 follow-up (AMD, 0.01; $P=.02$). In addition, the *N*-terminal telopeptides biomarker demonstrated a larger relative decrease in the intervention group compared with the control group (AMD, 2.05; $P=.02$), with nonsignifi-

**Table 2. Baseline to Year 1 and Year 2 Intervention Outcomes: Behavioral and Other Intermediary Factors***

| | Control Group (n = 108) | | | Intervention Group (n = 101) | | | *P* Value | |
|---|---|---|---|---|---|---|---|---|
| Factor | Baseline Value | Adjusted Change to Year 1† | Adjusted Change to Year 2† | Baseline Value | Adjusted Change to Year 1† | Adjusted Change to Year 2† | Baseline to Year 1† | Baseline to Year 2† |
| Diet | | | | | | | | |
| Energy, kcal | 1 724.35 (41.39) | -83.86 (36.65) | -22.60 (31.34) | 1733.09 (43.91) | 42.29 (37.90) | 91.57 (33.00) | .02 | 0.01 |
| Total calcium level, mg/d | 977.43 (38.78) | -64.41 (38.41) | −13.72 (39.27) | 994.37 (46.70) | 152.21 (39.72) | 227.56 (41.35) | <.001 | <.001 |
| Vitamin D level, IU/d | 157.01 (11.28) | 2.95 (10.33) | 54.03 (13.76) | 166.42 (14.13) | 37.27 (10.68) | 86.13 (14.49) | .02 | 0.11 |
| Fruits and vegetables, servings/d | 3.53 (0.21) | 0.01 (0.18) | 0.16 (0.21) | 3.68 (0.24) | 0.74 (0.19) | 0.95 (0.22) | .005 | .01 |
| Soda, oz/d | 5.20 (0.69) | −0.05 (0.47) | −0.98 (0.38) | 5.13 (0.69) | −0.95 (0.48) | −1.24 (0.40) | .18 | .65 |
| Strength and physical activity | | | | | | | | |
| High-impact activity, min/d | 14.44 (1.77) | −0.14 (1.19) | −2.98 (0.96) | 13.23 (1.44) | −2.63 (1.23) | −4.07 (1.01) | .15 | .43 |
| Strength training, min/d | 8.05 (2.58) | −3.36 (0.97) | −0.94 (0.66) | 5.74 (1.05) | −0.83 (1.00) | −0.70 (0.70) | .07 | .80 |
| Total activity, min/d | 61.43 (5.32) | −7.98 (3.22) | −10.01 (3.21) | 62.45 (4.29) | −11.24 (3.33) | −14.51 (3.38) | .48 | .34 |
| Sit-ups, No./min‡ | 34.21 (0.92) | 0.64 (0.61) | 1.57 (0.67) | 32.91 (0.82) | 0.96 (0.63) | 2.57 (0.69) | .71 | .30 |
| Vertical jump, in‡ | 12.62 (0.28) | 0.92 (0.23) | 0.84 (0.23) | 12.67 (0.23) | 0.86 (0.23) | 0.65 (0.23) | .86 | .55 |
| Anthropometry | | | | | | | | |
| Height, in‡ | 64.69 (0.25) | 0.20 (0.07) | 0.37 (0.07) | 64.34 (0.29) | 0.30 (0.07) | 0.48 (0.07) | .29 | .29 |
| Weight, lb‡ | 123.79 (1.52) | 3.00 (0.54) | 4.73 (0.78) | 120.83 (1.40) | 1.71 (0.56) | 4.38 (0.80) | .10 | .75 |
| BMI‡ | 20.75 (0.19) | 0.38 (0.09) | 0.55 (0.13) | 20.51 (0.19) | 0.10 (0.09) | 0.42 (0.13) | .03 | .46 |

Abbreviation: BMI, body mass index (calculated as weight in kilograms divided by height in meters squared).

SI conversion factors: To convert calcium to millimoles per liter, multiply by 0.25; ounces to grams, multiply by 28; inches to centimeters, multiply by 2.54; and pounds to kilograms, multiply by 0.45.

*Data are given as mean (standard error), unless otherwise indicated.

†Adjusted for baseline values.

‡Missing values for both control and intervention groups were imputed by matching the participant with missing data with a similar participant in the control group based on menarcheal age, baseline BMI, and baseline height. Missing data were as follows: height, weight, and BMI in 7 girls in the control group and 1 girl in the intervention group; vertical jump, 7 girls in the control group and 3 girls in the intervention group; and sit-ups, 8 girls in the control group and 3 girls in the intervention group.

cant changes in osteocalcin. This combination is consistent with more net bone formation in participants in the intervention group.

## COMMENT

The YOUTH health care–based lifestyle intervention increased BMD gains and improved dietary intake during a 2-year period. The intervention resulted in significant increases in BMD in the spine and femoral trochanter and increases in dietary calcium, vitamin D, and fruit and vegetable consumption. As expected, in adolescents who had essentially finished growing, we observed no changes in bone size, and the greater increase in BMD seemed to come from a greater accrual of BMC in the intervention group. Further, the biomarkers collected in the baseline and second-year follow-up visits were consistent with the observed bone mineral changes. Changes achieved in BMD and dietary behavior were achieved largely during the first year of the intervention. In the second year, the difference between groups was maintained and BMD and dietary behavior were not further improved in the intervention group. Finally, our retention rate for participants was 88% for the 2 years of the study.

Although we did not directly examine the cellular basis for the BMD changes, the maintenance of serum osteocalcin levels (a marker of osteoblastic function) with a relative reduction in *N*-terminal telopeptides levels (a marker of osteoclast activity) in the intervention group suggests that the intervention reduced bone resorption while allowing bone formation to continue. We would expect increases in fruit and vegetable intake to reduce dietary acid load, and fruits and vegetables have been associated with reduced bone resorption, maintained bone formation, and higher BMD.[13] Similarly, increased calcium and vitamin D intake has been shown to reduce bone resorption. These findings suggest that the skeletal changes induced by the intervention are biologically credible and are likely to enhance bone strength.

The significant increase in BMD in the intervention group was associated with targeted dietary behaviors. This increase in BMD is especially significant because the dietary changes occurred in a community setting. The researchers had no control over the physical environment, and the individually targeted intervention did not affect the girls' peer groups. Other studies with calcium-related bone mineral changes have relied on supplementation rather than influence of adolescents' dietary behavior.[52,53] One recent study targeting dietary calcium showed significant increases in dietary calcium but not associated bone mineral changes.[54] In addition, studies targeting bone mineral changes have not emphasized other

**Table 3. Baseline to Year 1 and Year 2 Bone Marker and Body Composition Outcomes***

| | Control Group (n = 108) | | | Intervention Group (n = 101) | | | *P* Value | |
|---|---|---|---|---|---|---|---|---|
| Outcome | Baseline Value | Adjusted Change to Year 1† | Adjusted Change to Year 2† | Baseline Value | Adjusted Change to Year 1† | Adjusted Change to Year 2† | Baseline Year 1† | Baseline Year 2† |
| Bone mineral density | | | | | | | | |
| Total body, g/cm² | 1.114 (0.008) | 0.024 (0.002) | 0.025 (0.002) | 1.114 (0.008) | 0.027 (0.002) | 0.029 (0.003) | .27 | .19 |
| Spine, g/cm² | 0.973 (0.009) | 0.017 (0.002) | 0.033 (0.003) | 0.962 (0.010) | 0.029 (0.002) | 0.045 (0.003) | <.001 | 0.007 |
| Trochanter, cm² | 0.775 (0.010) | 0.003 (0.002) | 0.003 (0.003) | 0.763 (0.011) | 0.010 (0.002) | 0.013 (0.003) | .03 | .03 |
| Femoral neck, cm² | 0.894 (0.010) | 0.009 (0.003) | 0.015 (0.004) | 0.891 (0.012) | 0.010 (0.003) | 0.020 (0.004) | .70 | .44 |
| Total hip, cm² | 0.974 (0.010) | 0.009 (0.002) | 0.017 (0.003) | 0.966 (0.011) | 0.015 (0.002) | 0.021 (0.003) | .06 | .36 |
| Bone mineral apparent density‡ | | | | | | | | |
| Spine | 0.148 (0.001) | 0.002 (0.000) | 0.005 (0.000) | 0.148 (0.001) | 0.004 (0.000) | 0.006 (0.000) | 0.003 | 0.02 |
| Bone mineral content | | | | | | | | |
| Total body, g | 2087.951 (28.515) | 74.499 (4.943) | 91.847 (6.408) | 2059.446 (26.311) | 85.134 (5.113) | 110.629 (6.561) | .14 | .04 |
| Spine, g | 54.602 (1.101) | 1.369 (0.314) | 2.554 (0.229) | 53.643 (0.998) | 2.001 (0.324) | 3.263 (0.235) | .17 | .03 |
| Trochanter, g | 7.561 (0.185) | 0.124 (0.061) | 0.169 (0.066) | 7.274 (0.141) | 0.189 (0.063) | 0.334 (0.067) | .47 | .08 |
| Femoral neck, g | 4.152 (0.058) | 0.103 (0.016) | 0.113 (0.022) | 4.117 (0.059) | 0.078 (0.017) | 0.095 (0.023) | .30 | .59 |
| Total hip, g | 30.648 (0.489) | 0.505 (0.121) | 1.077 (0.120) | 29.818 (0.438) | 0.667 (0.125) | 1.203 (1.203) | .36 | .46 |
| Bone area | | | | | | | | |
| Total body, cm² | 1867.373 (15.757) | 25.966 (3.224) | 41.651 (3.468) | 1844.583 (15.056) | 30.560 (3.335) | 49.348 (3.551) | .33 | .12 |
| Spine, cm² | 55.787 (0.842) | 0.530 (0.280) | 0.769 (0.099) | 55.546 (0.680) | 0.403 (0.289) | 0.770 (0.102) | .75 | .997 |
| Trochanter, cm² | 9.696 (0.160) | 0.119 (0.062) | 0.178 (0.064) | 9.532 (0.126) | 0.096 (0.064) | 0.269 (0.066) | .80 | .33 |
| Femoral neck, cm² | 4.642 (0.037) | 0.069 (0.016) | 0.050 (0.019) | 4.629 (0.034) | 0.037 (0.016) | 0.008 (0.019) | .16 | .13 |
| Total hip, cm² | 31.412 (0.323) | 0.247 (0.084) | 0.574 (0.072) | 30.888 (0.277) | 0.182 (0.087) | 0.541 (0.073) | .60 | .75 |
| Body composition | | | | | | | | |
| Fat mass, % of weight | 24.353 (0.512) | 0.582 (0.204) | 0.673 (0.275) | 24.106 (0.443) | 0.285 (0.211) | 0.482 (0.282) | .32 | .63 |
| Lean mass, % of weight | 67.147 (.488) | −0.002 (0.194) | −0.188 (0.266) | 67.446 (0.428) | −0.079 (0.200) | −0.223 (0.272) | .72 | .93 |
| Biomarkers | | | | | | | | |
| Osteocalcin, ng/mL§ | 17.932 (0.715) | | −5.597 (0.438) | 19.214 (1.006) | | −5.557 (0.420) | | .95 |
| Naltrexone, nM BCE‖ | 36.462 (2.024) | | −11.163 (0.618) | 37.024 (1.825) | | −13.211 (0.610) | | .02 |

Abbreviation: BCE, bone collagen equivalents.
*Data are given as mean (standard error), unless otherwise indicated.
†Adjusted for baseline values age, menarche, risk of osteoporosis, height, and BMI.
‡Intervention group, n = 90; control group, n = 94.
§Intervention group, n = 69; control group, n = 65.
‖Intervention group, n = 66; control group, n = 66.

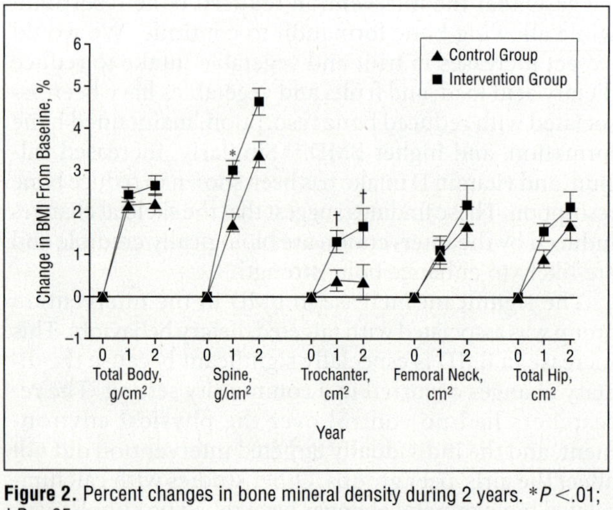


**Figure 2.** Percent changes in bone mineral density during 2 years. *$P<.01$; †$P<.05$.

dietary factors that may contribute to BMD.[11-13] In this study, baseline calcium intake was already close to recommendations, whereas vitamin D and fruit and vegetable intake was below recommendations; this suggests the importance of vitamin D and fruits and vegetables in the outcomes. The improvements achieved in the intervention group in fruit and vegetable consumption (about 20% increase in year 1 and 26% overall increase by year 2; from 3.68 servings at baseline to 4.42 and 4.62 for follow-up years 1 and 2, respectively) exceeded changes achieved in school-based adolescent studies that have specifically examined fruit and vegetable consumption.[55,56] The intervention did not significantly affect soda consumption; however, study participants reported drinking little soda.

Despite significant improvements in BMD and dietary targets, reported levels of physical activity and physiologic strength measures did not differ between the intervention and comparison groups. Although levels in individual girls varied substantially, overall trends suggested that physical activity declined in both study conditions. This finding mirrors reports of overall decline in physical activity during adolescence[32,57,58] and a recent community trial that attempted to increase weight-bearing physical activity to promote bone mass gains in younger girls.[54] Studies that have positively affected adolescent girls' physical activity were school-based interventions that enrolled girls in structured physical education classes[53,59-61] rather than relying on self-directed changes. In addition to this study's component of self-directed change, our study population reported an initially high level of physical activity: 69% of the girls participated in team sports. Since they were already active, this group may have been a particularly difficult population in which to increase or even shift physical activity. Finally, despite the decline in physical activity, we did not observe a commensurate decline in physical strength or fitness measures.

Although this study uniquely contributes to the previous research, this medical setting has some limitations. Our population was largely white, from middle- to upper-middle-income working families, and had relatively high levels of reported calcium consumption and physical activity at baseline. Therefore, the intervention might need adjustments in different populations. Further, some intervention elements, such as events for participant motivation and retention, may not be easily replicated in all medical settings. Another limitation is that health plans might have less participant contact than schools do. We addressed this limitation by providing a wide range of intervention components with both in-person and remote study contact to maximize participant exposure to the intervention. The effect on participants' dietary habits was more substantial than that achieved in most school-based interventions targeting these factors, although possible differences in participant socioeconomic status may have influenced the ease of achieving the dietary targets. Our results suggest that the dietary intervention designed to empower high school–aged girls to take charge of their health was reasonably successful. Conversely, we had more difficulty in achieving our physical activity targets than school-based interventions do. Health care settings may be best suited to helping adolescents achieve change in domains in which individual tailoring is important and the behavior is more individual; conversely, substantially increasing physical activity may be maximized with the built-in community and structure that school interventions provide.

In summary, the YOUTH project is one of very few preventive research interventions in adolescents conducted in a health plan setting. Information available to medical providers may provide ways of targeting such interventions (eg, a family history of hip fracture or osteoporosis). Our results suggest that a comprehensive health care–based lifestyle intervention can effectively increase bone mineral gains and improve dietary intake. Future research should examine what this magnitude of BMD gain means for adult osteoporosis risk. To our knowledge, this study is the first to significantly improve bone mass in adolescents in a non–school-based intervention emphasizing self-directed behavioral change.

**Accepted for Publication:** July 7, 2006.
**Correspondence:** Lynn L. DeBar, PhD, MPH, Center for Health Research, Kaiser Permanente Northwest, 3800 N Interstate Ave, Portland, OR 97227 (lynn.debar@kpchr.org).

**Author Contributions:** Dr DeBar had full access to all of the data in the study and takes responsibility for the integrity of the data and the accuracy of the data analysis. *Study concept and design:* DeBar, Ritenbaugh, Aicken, Orwoll, Elliot, Vuckovic, Stevens, and Moe. *Intervention design:* Stevens. *Acquisition of data:* DeBar, Ritenbaugh, and Dickerson. *Analysis and interpretation of data:* Ritenbaugh, Aicken, Orwoll, Dickerson, Vuckovic, and Stevens. *Drafting of the manuscript:* DeBar, Ritenbaugh, and Aicken. *Critical revision of the manuscript for important intellectual content:* Ritenbaugh, Aicken, Orwoll, Elliot, Dickerson, Vuckovic, Stevens, and Moe. *Statistical analysis:* Aicken. *Obtained funding:* Ritenbaugh, Aicken, and Stevens. *Administrative, technical, and material support:* DeBar, Ritenbaugh, Orwoll, Elliot, Dickerson, Stevens, and Moe. *Study supervision:* DeBar and Ritenbaugh. *Qualitative research:* Vuckovic.

**Financial Disclosure:** None reported.

**Funding/Support:** This study was supported by grant R01-HD037744 to Dr DeBar from the National Institute of Child Health and Human Development.

**Trial Registration:** ClinicalTrials.gov Identifier: NCT67600

**Acknowledgment:** We thank Jen Coury, MA (Center for Health Research, Kaiser Permanente Northwest, Portland, Ore), for helpful comments about previous versions of this article and for editorial assistance; and Gina Keppel, BS, Chris Catlin, BS, Patty LeGarda, BS, Colleen Flattum, RD, Megan Porter, RD, Cynthia Roh, RD, Amanda Petrik, BS, and Pat Elmer, PhD, for assistance with this study.

**Dedication:** We dedicate this article to the memory of Dr Irving, who was an essential part of the conceptualization and realization of the project.

## REFERENCES


1. Siris ES, Miller PD, Barrett-Connor E, et al. Identification and fracture outcomes of undiagnosed low bone mineral density in postmenopausal women: results from the National Osteoporosis Risk Assessment. *JAMA.* 2001;286:2815-2822.
2. US Preventive Services Task Force. *Guide to Clinical Preventive Services.* Alexandria, Va: International Medical Publishing; 1996.
3. Teegarden D, Proulx WR, Martin BR, et al. Peak bone mass in young women. *J Bone Miner Res.* 1995;10:711-715.
4. Bailey DA, McKay HA, Mirwald RL, Crocker PR, Faulkner RA. A six-year longitudinal study of the relationship of physical activity to bone mineral accrual in growing children: the University of Saskatchewan bone mineral accrual study. *J Bone Miner Res.* 1999;14:1672-1679.
5. Bonjour JP, Theintz G, Buchs B, Slosman D, Rizzoli R. Critical years and stages of puberty for spinal and femoral bone mass accumulation during adolescence. *J Clin Endocrinol Metab.* 1991;73:555-563.
6. Slemenda CW, Christian JC, Williams CJ, Norton JA, Johnston CC Jr. Genetic determinants of bone mass in adult women: a reevaluation of the twin model and the potential importance of gene interaction on heritability estimates. *J Bone Miner Res.* 1991;6:561-567.
7. Smith DM, Nance WE, Kang KW, Christian JC, Johnston CC Jr. Genetic factors in determining bone mass. *J Clin Invest.* 1973;52:2800-2808.
8. Chan GM, Hoffman K, McMurry M. Effects of dairy products on bone and body composition in pubertal girls. *J Pediatr.* 1995;126:551-556.
9. Lloyd T, Andon MB, Rollings N, et al. Calcium supplementation and bone mineral density in adolescent girls. *JAMA.* 1993;270:841-844.
10. Jackman LA, Millane SS, Martin BR, et al. Calcium retention in relation to calcium intake and postmenarcheal age in adolescent females. *Am J Clin Nutr.* 1997;66:327-333.
11. Lemann J Jr, Litzow JR, Lennon EJ. The effects of chronic acid loads in normal man: further evidence for the participation of bone mineral in the defense against chronic metabolic acidosis. *J Clin Invest.* 1966;45:1608-1614.

12. Wachman A, Bernstein DS. Diet and osteoporosis. *Lancet.* 1968;1:958-959.
13. New SA, Robins SP, Campbell MK, et al. Dietary influences on bone mass and bone metabolism: further evidence of a positive link between fruit and vegetable consumption and bone health? *Am J Clin Nutr.* 2000;71:142-151.
14. Tucker KL, Hannan MT, Chen H, Cupples LA, Wilson PW, Kiel DP. Potassium, magnesium, and fruit and vegetable intakes are associated with greater bone mineral density in elderly men and women. *Am J Clin Nutr.* 1999;69:727-736.
15. Lehtonen-Veromaa MK, Mottonen TT, Nuotio IO, Irjala KM, Leino AE, Viikari JS. Vitamin D and attainment of peak bone mass among peripubertal Finnish girls: a 3-y prospective study. *Am J Clin Nutr.* 2002;76:1446-1453.
16. Du X, Zhu K, Trube A, et al. School-milk intervention trial enhances growth and bone mineral accretion in Chinese girls aged 10-12 years in Beijing [published correction appears in *Br J Nutr.* 2005;93:571-572]. *Br J Nutr.* 2004;92:159-168.
17. Draper HH, Scythes CA. Calcium, phosphorus, and osteoporosis. *Fed Proc.* 1981; 40:2434-2438.
18. Wyshak G. Teenaged girls, carbonated beverage consumption, and bone fractures. *Arch Pediatr Adolesc Med.* 2000;154:610-613.
19. Fuchs RK, Bauer JJ, Snow CM. Jumping improves hip and lumbar spine bone mass in prepubescent children: a randomized controlled trial. *J Bone Miner Res.* 2001;16:148-156.
20. Gutin B, Owens S, Okuyama T, Riggs S, Ferguson M, Litaker M. Effect of physical training and its cessation on percent fat and bone density of children with obesity. *Obes Res.* 1999;7:208-214.
21. Heinonen A, Sievanen H, Kannus P, Oja P, Pasanen M, Vuori I. High-impact exercise and bones of growing girls: a 9-month controlled trial. *Osteoporos Int.* 2000;11:1010-1017.
22. McKay HA, Petit MA, Schutz RW, Prior JC, Barr SI, Khan KM. Augmented trochanteric bone mineral density after modified physical education classes: a randomized school-based exercise intervention study in prepubescent and early pubescent children. *J Pediatr.* 2000;136:156-162.
23. Morris FL, Naughton GA, Gibbs JL, Carlson JS, Wark JD. Prospective ten-month exercise intervention in premenarcheal girls: positive effects on bone and lean mass. *J Bone Miner Res.* 1997;12:1453-1462.
24. Snow-Harter C, Bouxsein ML, Lewis BT, Carter DR, Marcus R. Effects of resistance and endurance exercise on bone mineral status of young women: a randomized exercise intervention trial. *J Bone Miner Res.* 1992;7:761-769.
25. Bradney M, Pearce G, Naughton G, et al. Moderate exercise during growth in prepubertal boys: changes in bone mass, size, volumetric density, and bone strength; a controlled prospective study. *J Bone Miner Res.* 1998;13:1814-1821.
26. McKay HA, Petit MA, Khan KM, Schutz RW. Lifestyle determinants of bone mineral: a comparison between prepubertal Asian- and Caucasian-Canadian boys and girls. *Calcif Tissue Int.* 2000;66:320-324.
27. Petersen AC, Leffert N. Developmental issues influencing guidelines for adolescent health research: a review. *J Adolesc Health.* 1995;17:298-305.
28. Steinberg L, Silverberg SB. The vicissitudes of autonomy in early adolescence. *Child Dev.* 1986;57:841-851.
29. Gordon CL, Halton JM, Atkinson SA, Webber CE. The contributions of growth and puberty to peak bone mass. *Growth Dev Aging.* 1991;55:257-262.
30. MacKelvie KJ, Khan KM, McKay HA. Is there a critical period for bone response to weight-bearing exercise in children and adolescents? a systematic review. *Br J Sports Med.* 2002;36:250-257.
31. Campion JM, Maricic MJ. Osteoporosis in men. *Am Fam Physician.* 2003;67:1521-1526.
32. Kimm SY, Glynn NW, Kriska AM, et al. Decline in physical activity in black girls and white girls during adolescence. *N Engl J Med.* 2002;347:709-715.
33. MacKelvie KJ, McKay HA, Petit MA, Moran O, Khan KM. Bone mineral response to a 7-month randomized controlled, school-based jumping intervention in 121 prepubertal boys: associations with ethnicity and body mass index. *J Bone Miner Res.* 2002;17:834-844.
34. Perry CL, Bishop DB, Taylor G, et al. Changing fruit and vegetable consumption among children: the 5-a-Day Power Plus program in St. Paul, Minnesota. *Am J Public Health.* 1998;88:603-609.
35. Petit MA, McKay HA, MacKelvie KJ, Heinonen A, Khan KM, Beck TJ. A randomized school-based jumping intervention confers site and maturity-specific benefits on bone structural properties in girls: a hip structural analysis study. *J Bone Miner Res.* 2002;17:363-372.
36. Reynolds KD, Franklin FA, Binkley D, et al. Increasing the fruit and vegetable consumption of fourth-graders: results from the High 5 Project. *Prev Med.* 2000; 30:309-319.
37. Sallis JF, Patrick K, Frank E, Pratt M, Wechsler H, Galuska DA. Interventions in health care settings to promote healthful eating and physical activity in children and adolescents. *Prev Med.* 2000;31(suppl 2):S112-S121.
38. Fleming GV. Pediatricians and health promotion practitioner goals for the year 2000. *Patient Educ Counsel.* 1993;21:143-154.
39. Rollins D, Imrhan V, Czajka-Narins DM, Nichols DL. Lower bone mass detected at femoral neck and lumbar spine in lower-weight vs normal-weight small-boned women. *J Am Diet Assoc.* 2003;103:742-744.
40. Blum M, Harris SS, Must A, Phillips SM, Rand WM, Dawson-Hughes B. Weight and body mass index at menarche are associated with premenopausal bone mass. *Osteoporos Int.* 2001;12:588-594.
41. Taves DR. Minimization: a new method of assigning patients to treatment and control groups. *Clin Pharmacol Ther.* 1974;15:443-453.
42. Aickin M. Randomization, balance, and the validity and efficiency of design-adaptive allocation methods. *J Stat Plan Inference.* 2001;94:97-119.
43. Miller WR, Rollnick S. *Motivational Interviewing: Preparing People for Change.* 2nd ed. New York, NY: Guilford Press; 2002.
44. Bachrach LK. Dual energy X-ray absorptiometry (DEXA) measurements of bone density and body composition: promise and pitfalls. *J Pediatr Endocrinol Metab.* 2000;13(suppl 2):983-988.
45. Lohman TG, Roche AF, Martorell R, eds. *Anthropometric Standardization Reference Manual.* Champaign, Ill: Human Kinetics Books; 1998.
46. Slemenda CW, Reister TK, Hui SL, Miller JZ, Christian JC, Johnston CC Jr. Influences on skeletal mineralization in children and adolescents: evidence for varying effects of sexual maturation and physical activity. *J Pediatr.* 1994;125: 201-207.
47. Weston AT, Petosa R, Pate RR. Validation of an instrument for measurement of physical activity in youth. *Med Sci Sports Exerc.* 1997;29:138-143.
48. Lee KS, Trost SG. Validity and reliability of the 3-day physical activity recall in Singaporean adolescents. *Res Q Exerc Sport.* 2005;76:101-106.
49. Zellner A. An efficient method of estimating seemingly unrelated regressions and tests for aggregation bias. *J Am Stat Assoc.* 1962;57:348-368.
50. Zellner A, Huang DS. Further properties of efficient estimators for seemingly unrelated regression equations. *Int Econ Rev.* 1962;3:300-313.
51. Zellner A. Estimators for seemingly unrelated regression equations: some exact finite sample results. *J Am Stat Assoc.* 1963;58:977-992.
52. Matkovic V, Goel PK, Badenhop-Stevens NE, et al. Calcium supplementation and bone mineral density in females from childhood to young adulthood: a randomized controlled trial. *Am J Clin Nutr.* 2005;81:175-188.
53. Stear SJ, Prentice A, Jones SC, Cole TJ. Effect of a calcium and exercise intervention on the bone mineral status of 16-18-y-old adolescent girls. *Am J Clin Nutr.* 2003;77:985-992.
54. French SA, Story M, Fulkerson JA, et al. Increasing weight-bearing physical activity and calcium-rich foods to promote bone mass gains among 9-11-year-old girls: outcomes of the Cal-Girls study. *Int J Behav Nutr Phys Act.* 2005;2:8.
55. Lytle LA, Murray DM, Perry CL, et al. School-based approaches to affect adolescents' diets: results from the TEENS study. *Health Educ Behav.* 2004;31: 270-287.
56. Nicklas TA, Johnson CC, Myers L, Farris RP, Cunningham A. Outcomes of a high school program to increase fruit and vegetable consumption: Gimme 5, a fresh nutrition concept for students. *J Sch Health.* 1998;68:248-253.
57. Heath GW, Pratt M, Warren CW, Kann L. Physical activity patterns in American high school students: results from the 1990 Youth Risk Behavior Survey. *Arch Pediatr Adolesc Med.* 1994;148:1131-1136.
58. Aaron DJ, Kriska AM, Dearwater SR, et al. The epidemiology of leisure physical activity in an adolescent population. *Med Sci Sports Exerc.* 1993;25:847-853.
59. Jamner MS, Spruijt-Metz D, Bassin S, Cooper DM. A controlled evaluation of a school-based intervention to promote physical activity among sedentary adolescent females: project FAB. *J Adolesc Health.* 2004;34:279-289.
60. Mcmurray RG, Harrell JS, Bangdiwala SI, Bradley CB, Deng S, Levine A. A school-based intervention can reduce body fat and blood pressure in young adolescents. *J Adolesc Health.* 2002;31:125-132.
61. Pate RR, Ward DS, Saunders RP, Felton G, Dishman RK, Dowda M. Promotion of physical activity among high-school girls: a randomized controlled trial. *Am J Public Health.* 2005;95:1582-1587.

# Impact of Maternal Influenza Vaccination During Pregnancy on the Incidence of Acute Respiratory Illness Visits Among Infants

*Eric K. France, MD, MSPH; Renae Smith-Ray, MA; David McClure, PhD; Simon Hambidge, MD, PhD; Stanley Xu, PhD; Kristi Yamasaki, PharmD; David Shay, MD, MPH; Eric Weintraub, MPH; Alicia M. Fry, MD, MPH; Steve B. Black, MD; Henry R. Shinefield, MD; John P. Mullooly, PhD; Lisa A. Jackson, MD, MPH; for the Vaccine Safety Datalink Team*

**Objective:** To determine whether influenza vaccination of pregnant women prevents visits for respiratory illness in their infants born during the influenza season.

**Design:** Retrospective matched cohort study.

**Setting:** Four managed care organizations in the United States.

**Patients:** A total of 41 129 infants (3160 and 37 969 born to vaccinated and unvaccinated mothers, respectively) born between 1995 and 2001.

**Main Exposure:** Maternal influenza vaccination. Infants were considered exposed if their gestational age at birth was at least 30 weeks, if the time from maternal vaccination to birth was at least 28 days, and if they were exposed to at least 14 days of the influenza season.

**Main Outcome Measures:** Incidence of acute respiratory illnesses (outpatient, emergency department, and inpatient settings combined) and incident rate ratios (IRRs) for infants exposed and unexposed to maternal vaccination during the following 4 periods: peak influenza, respiratory syncytial virus predominant, periseasonal, and summer weeks. The time to the first acute respiratory illness during peak influenza weeks was also assessed.

**Results:** During the peak influenza weeks, infant visit rates were 15.4 and 17.1 per 100 person-months for exposed and unexposed infants, respectively (IRR, 0.90; 95% confidence interval, 0.80-1.02). Adjusted IRRs for the 4 periods found a protective effect of infant female sex, whereas Medicaid status and maternal high-risk status increased infant visit rates. Maternal influenza vaccination did not reduce visit rates during any of the 4 time periods (IRR for peak influenza season, 0.96; 95% confidence interval, 0.86-1.07) and did not delay the onset of first respiratory illness.

**Conclusion:** We were unable to demonstrate that maternal influenza vaccination reduces respiratory illness visit rates among their infants.

*Arch Pediatr Adolesc Med. 2006;160:1277-1283*

**Author Affiliations** are listed at the end of this article.
**Group Information:** The Vaccine Safety Datalink Team members are listed at the end of this article.

BEGINNING IN 2004, THE ADvisory Committee on Immunization Practices has recommended universal influenza vaccination of children aged 6 to 23 months.[1] This recommendation was based primarily on studies that found high hospitalization rates for infants attributable to influenza illness,[2,3] particularly for infants younger than 6 months.[3] Influenza vaccination of infants younger than 6 months has not succeeded owing to the poor immunogenic response elicited by vaccination in this age group[4,5]; also, the immature immune system of neonates has posed a challenge to the efforts of vaccinating newborns.[6] Tetanus immunization of women during pregnancy has been very successful in reducing the incidence of neonatal tetanus worldwide.[7] Experts have proposed that influenza vaccination of the mother during pregnancy could protect infants during the first few months of life through transplacentally acquired antibodies or by reducing exposure to a mother with influenza infection.[8-10]

To date, 2 small studies have explored the effect of maternally acquired antibodies on influenza illness in infants. Puck et al[11] found a direct correlation between the level of cord blood antibody to influenza A and the time of culture-documented influenza A infection in 26 infants younger than 4 months: infants with high levels of antibody to influenza A had a delay in influenza A infection. Reuman et al[12] followed up 39 families in Houston, Tex, and found no difference in the rate of influenza virus infection between infants based on levels of cord blood antibodies to influenza A (H1N1). The onset of illness from the beginning of the influenza season was significantly later for infants with high antibody levels in cord blood (27.0 vs 8.2 days), and the duration of respiratory symptoms (cough and rapid breathing) was shorter. In both of these studies, cord blood antibodies to influenza A were from naturally acquired infections in the mothers rather than from influenza vaccination during pregnancy. A third study by Englund et al[13] assessed the effect of maternal influenza vaccination on infant cord blood antibodies to influenza virus and found significantly increased levels of IgG specific to influenza virus in the cord blood of infants born to vaccinated mothers compared with those born to unvaccinated mothers.

We undertook this study to determine whether infants born to mothers who received influenza vaccination during their pregnancy had lower incidence rates of medically attended acute respiratory illnesses (MAARIs) (combined outpatient, inpatient, and emergency department settings) during peak influenza weeks compared with infants born to unvaccinated mothers. A study performed in 2003 at Northern California Kaiser Permanente that assessed the effectiveness and safety of the influenza vaccine among pregnant women and their infants found no impact of the mother's vaccination on the rates of infant health care visits during the influenza season.[14] Our current study expands on this work by using viral surveillance data to define peak influenza weeks, by requiring 4 weeks from vaccination to birth to ensure maternal antibody transfer, and by measuring incidence of acute respiratory illness across 4 periods (peak influenza, respiratory syncytial virus [RSV]–predominant, periseasonal, and summer weeks). We hypothesized that the incidence rate ratio (IRR) would be less than 1 (ie, protective) during peak influenza weeks, whereas the IRRs during the RSV-predominant and summer weeks would equal 1 (ie, no protective effect). Our secondary objectives were to determine whether infants born during the peak influenza weeks to vaccinated mothers had a delay in their first acute respiratory illness compared with infants born to unvaccinated mothers and to determine whether the proportion of infants with severe MAARIs (eg, pneumonia and hospitalization) differed between these 2 groups.

## METHODS

### STUDY POPULATION

Infants who were born before or during the influenza season at 4 managed care organizations (MCOs) (Kaiser Permanente Colorado, Denver; Kaiser Permanente Northern California, Oakland; Kaiser Permanente Northwest, Portland, Ore; and Group Health Cooperative, Seattle, Wash) between October 1, 1995, and September 30, 2001, were eligible for study inclusion. Mother-infant pairs were included in the final study population if (1) the mothers were aged 18 to 45 years and enrolled in the MCO for longer than 1 year; (2) the infants' gestational age was at least 30 weeks at birth; (3) the infants were continuous MCO members for at least 14 days during the influenza season; and (4) the infants had a least 1 outpatient visit during the first 3 months of life. To ensure adequate maternal transfer of IgG, an infant was considered exposed if the mother was vaccinated against influenza during the pregnancy and there were at least 28 days from the vaccination date of the mother to the birth date of the infant.[15] Infants of mothers vaccinated within 27 days of birth were excluded from the primary analysis. Infants born during the influenza season began contributing person-time on the day after their birth hospitalization discharge; if the date of discharge from the birth hospitalization was unavailable, person-time began after the first outpatient visit.

In comparing acute respiratory illness rates between exposed and unexposed infants, important potential confounders include age, MCO site, and season. Unexposed infants were therefore matched by birth week and MCO to exposed infants, and thus also matched for influenza season.

### HEALTH SERVICES DATA

We used data sets created for the Vaccine Safety Datalink (VSD) Study to perform all analyses. The VSD is a large, linked database project that is funded by the Centers for Disease Control and Prevention (CDC).[16] Member enrollment dates, vaccination histories, and inpatient, outpatient, and emergency department visits are included in these data sets. During the study period (1995-2001), a specific MCO site would contribute data only for those years in which reliable data were available. For example, outpatient data were available from Kaiser Permanente Northwest from 1997 through 2001. The study was approved by the institutional review boards at each of the 4 MCOs and the CDC.

Comorbid conditions in the mother were defined by the codes from the *International Classification of Diseases, Ninth Revision* (*ICD-9*) assigned to medical encounters in the year before delivery. Mothers were considered at high risk for complications of influenza if, in the year before delivery, they had an *ICD-9* diagnosis code for a high-risk condition (cardiac, pulmonary, renal, or hematologic disease; diabetes or metabolic disorders; neoplasm or immunodeficiencies; or hepatic or neurological disorders[1]). A total of 1617 *ICD-9* codes across the 10 conditions were used; this list was developed for a CDC-sponsored study of the impact of influenza on adult health care services utilization (available from the authors on request). In addition to high-risk status, other maternal variables used in the analyses include influenza vaccination status (current and preceding season), age, high-risk status, and Medicaid insurance coverage. Other variables used include infant gestational age at birth, MCO site, and influenza season.

Influenza illness in young children is not often coded as influenza, per se, but as a number of illnesses that can be caused by the influenza virus (eg, upper respiratory infection, febrile illness, sepsis, and pneumonia). A visit was defined as a MAARI if any of the following *ICD-9* codes were used: 460, 462, 463, 464.0, 464.10, 464.11, 464.20, 464.21, 464.4, 465.0, 465.8, 465.9, 478.9, 487.1, 487.8, 490, 078.89, 079.99, or 786.2 for viral or upper respiratory infection; 466, 480.8, 480.9, 481.0, 482.2, 482.3, 482.4, 482.41, 482.49, 484.0, 484.1, 485, 486, 487.0, or 511.9 for lower respiratory infection or pneumonia; 038 for sepsis; 780.31 or 779.0 for febrile seizure; or 780.6 for fever. To maximize power, we combined outpatient, emergency department, and inpatient visits for acute respiratory illnesses in the primary analysis.

### VIRAL SURVEILLANCE DATA AND STUDY PERIODS

For each influenza season, peak influenza and RSV-predominant weeks were defined using viral surveillance data from each of the MCO sites. Influenza surveillance data for each MCO's area were provided by the CDC and were collected as part of the World Health Organization Influenza Surveillance system.[17] Annual RSV data were collected by the National Respiratory and Enteric Virus Surveillance System at the Respiratory Enteric Viruses Branch of the CDC.[18] Laboratories participating in these 2 national surveillance systems are in state or local health departments, universities, and hospitals. Because the surveillance data for the Portland area were unreliable for the 1999-2001 influenza seasons, we used the Northern California Kaiser Permanente laboratory viral surveillance data to define the peak influenza and RSV-predominant seasons in the Portland area. The 1997-1999 influenza surveillance data for Northern California Kaiser Permanente have a sensitivity of 69% and a specificity of 97% in matching peak influenza weeks to the 1997-1999 influenza surveillance data for Kaiser Permanente Northwest.

For this study, we defined 4 seasonal study periods:

1. *Peak influenza weeks* as any week from October 1 to April 30 in which influenza accounted for at least 5% of the season's total number of influenza virus isolates. Other viruses such as RSV could have been circulating during these weeks.

2. *RSV-predominant weeks* as any week from October 1 to April 30 in which RSV accounted for at least 5% of the season's total number of RSV virus isolates and influenza accounted for less than 5% of the season's total influenza virus isolates.

3. *Periseasonal weeks* as any week from October 1 to April 30 in which each week accounted for less than 3% of total RSV isolates and less than 3% of influenza virus isolates.

4. *Summer weeks* as the period each year from July 1 to September 30.

## STATISTICAL ANALYSIS OF THE STUDY HYPOTHESES

The primary hypothesis of this study was that the incidence of MAARI visits during peak influenza weeks would be lower for infants born to mothers vaccinated against influenza compared with infants born to unvaccinated mothers and that the MAARI incidence rates during the RSV-predominant and summer weeks would be equal between the exposed and unexposed groups. We estimated a priori that there would be 4500 exposed and 40 000 unexposed infants in the VSD cohort based on an observed 2% annual maternal influenza vaccination rate at Kaiser Permanente Colorado and on the pregnancy rate across the MCOs. We assessed the power of this sample size by 2 methods. First, we determined our ability to see a reduction of a rare event, pneumonia, among exposed infants. Given a background incidence of 2.4 per 100 person-months, we would have 80% power to see a 20% reduction in the incidence of visits for pneumonia. Second, we determined that 1900 exposed infants during the peak influenza weeks would be needed to detect a 20% reduction in febrile illness, a common event, based on an assumed risk of 0.11 for developing this diagnosis during an 8-week period (estimate based on Kaiser Permanente Colorado data). Planned secondary analyses included the time to first illness, limited to infants born during the peak influenza weeks, and the severity of MAARI, assessed by comparing the proportion of MAARI coded as upper respiratory infection, pneumonia, and hospitalization.

Bivariate comparisons between exposed and unexposed infants were evaluated with the 2-tailed, unpaired $t$ (or if not normally distributed, Wilcoxon signed rank) and $\chi^2$ tests for continuous and discrete variables, respectively. We calculated crude IRRs of exposed to unexposed infants during the 4 study periods for MAARI outcomes in all settings while ignoring matching by MCO site and infant birth week. We generated adjusted IRRs by Poisson regression, accounting for the matching by MCO site and infant birth week while controlling for other covariates. We obtained coefficients and their standard errors using generalized estimating equations that take into account the dependence of the data introduced by matching.[19] Cox proportional hazards regression modeling was also performed to evaluate the time to the first MAARI outcome between exposed and unexposed infants while controlling for other covariates. For all regression models, customary residual and influential statistics were examined to assess model fit and to evaluate influential outliers. All analyses were conducted using commercially available software (SAS version 8.2; SAS Institute Inc, Cary, NC).

## RESULTS

Before matching, a total of 54 385 women meeting all other inclusion criteria gave birth at the 4 MCOs between October 1 and April 30 of the included study years (1995-2001). The proportion of mothers vaccinated against influenza during a given season ranged from 0.7% to 20.8% across the 4 MCOs. Diagnoses for a condition that increased maternal risk for a complication from influenza infection were present in 11.5% of mothers (range across MCOs, 9.2%-12%); almost two thirds of these were for a pulmonary condition (primarily asthma). Combined data were available from 21 site-specific influenza seasons (6 seasons from 2 sites; 5 seasons from the third site, and 4 seasons from the fourth site). There were 124 peak influenza weeks, 97 RSV-predominant weeks, 310 periseasonal weeks, and 336 summer weeks among the 4 MCOs. Only 1 of the influenza seasons (1997-1998) had a notable mismatch between circulating influenza strains and the strains used in the seasonal vaccine.

In all, 3815 infants were born to vaccinated mothers during the study period. The mean number of days between maternal influenza vaccination and birth of the infant was 68 (range, 1-172), and the mean gestational age of the infant at the time of maternal vaccination was 29.4 (range, 9.8-41.6) weeks. Six hundred fifty-five infants were exposed less than 28 days in utero and were excluded. A total of 37 969 infants born to unvaccinated mothers were matched by birth week and MCO to the 3160 infants exposed at least 28 days in utero, yielding 41 129 infants in the matched cohort (**Figure**).

**Table 1** compares exposed and unexposed mothers and infants across study variables. Vaccinated mothers were more likely to have a high-risk condition than were unvaccinated mothers ($P<.001$). The mean age of the exposed infants at the end of the influenza season was 65 (range, 14-177) days; of unexposed infants, 75 (range, 14-180) days. There were no meaningful differences in gestational age or birth weight between the groups. Hospital discharge dates were present in 98.4% of infants.

**Table 2** lists the crude incidence rates for acute respiratory illnesses across the 4 study periods in exposed and unexposed populations matched by infant age, MCO site, and influenza season. The IRRs across the 4 study periods were all similar: 0.90 (95% confidence interval [CI], 0.80-1.02) for the peak influenza weeks; 0.93 (95% CI, 0.84-1.02) for the RSV-predominant weeks; 1.12 (95%

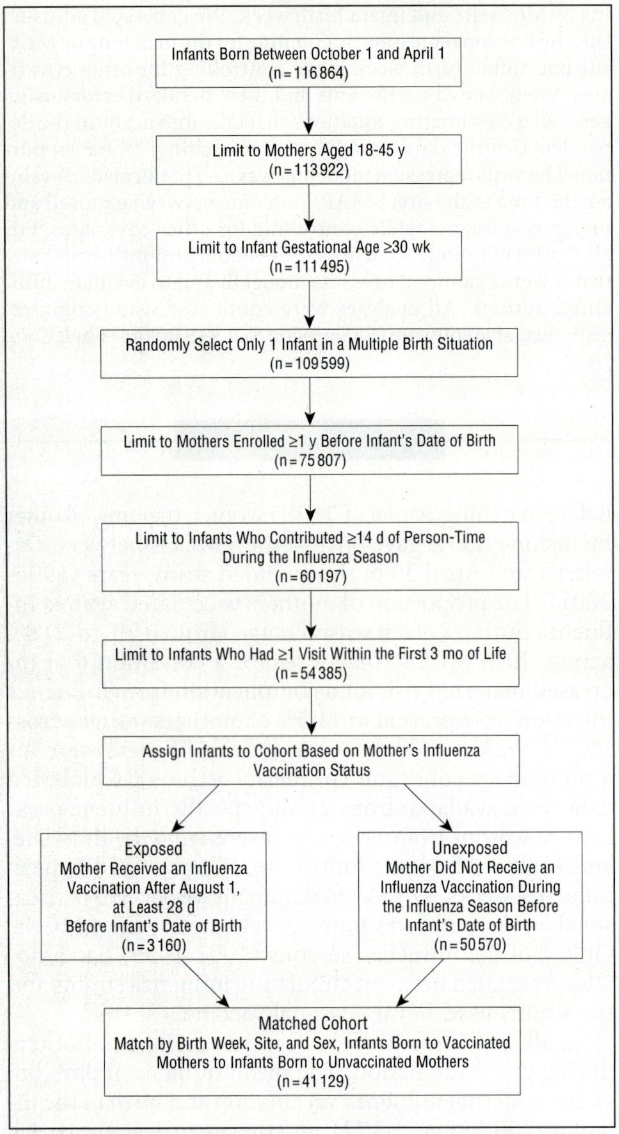


**Figure.** Medically attended acute respiratory illness cohort development based on study exclusion criteria.

CI, 0.94-1.34) for the periseasonal weeks; and 1.04 (95% CI, 0.99-1.10) for the summer weeks. The MAARI incidence during the summer weeks, when the mean age of the exposed infants was 210 days, was similar to the MAARI incidence during the peak influenza weeks, when the mean age of the infants was 65 days.

Models using generalized estimating equations included the following independent variables: maternal vaccination status, infant gestational age at birth, infant sex, maternal age, Medicaid coverage, maternal history of prior influenza vaccination, and maternal high-risk status. Exposed infants were matched to unexposed infants by MCO site and birth week. Female sex was significantly associated with reduced infant MAARI incidence, whereas maternal high-risk status and infant Medicaid coverage were significantly associated with increased MAARI incidence (**Table 3**). Maternal influenza vaccination did not reduce MAARI incidence: the adjusted IRRs (95% CIs) for the peak influenza, RSV-predominant, periseasonal, and summer periods were

**Table 1. Comparison of Mother-Infant Pairs by Maternal Influenza Vaccination Status***

| Cohort Characteristic | Maternal Influenza Vaccination | No Maternal Influenza Vaccination |
|---|---|---|
| No. of birth mothers | 3160 | 37 969 |
| Mothers | | |
| High-risk status, %† | 14.9‡ | 11.3 |
| Age, y | 30.8 (5.5)‡ | 29.7 (5.5) |
| Medicaid insurance, % | 2.2‡ | 3.1 |
| Influenza vaccination in preceding season, % | 25.4‡ | 4.5 |
| Infants | | |
| Gestational age at birth, wk | 39.1 (1.6)‡ | 39.2 (1.6) |
| Birth weight, g | 3425 (550)‡ | 3442 (539) |
| Female, % | 49.0 | 49.0 |
| Length of stay for birth hospitalization, d | 2.3 (1.7)‡ | 2.1 (1.6) |
| Age at end of influenza season, d | 65 (34)‡ | 75 (36) |

*Unless otherwise indicated, data are expressed as mean (SD).
†Maternal high-risk status is explained in the "Health Services Data" subsection of the "Methods" section.
‡Indicates $P<.05$ compared with the group with no maternal influenza vaccination.

**Table 2. Incidence Rates for Acute Respiratory Illnesses Among Infants Exposed and Unexposed to Maternal Influenza Vaccination, 1995-2001**

| Acute Respiratory Illness by Study Period | MAARI Incidence* Among Exposed Infants | MAARI Incidence* Among Unexposed Infants | IRR (95% CI) |
|---|---|---|---|
| Peak influenza weeks† | 15.4 | 17.1 | 0.90 (0.80-1.02) |
| RSV-predominant weeks‡ | 19.0 | 20.5 | 0.93 (0.84-1.02) |
| Periseasonal weeks§ | 15.5 | 13.8 | 1.12 (0.94-1.34) |
| Summer weeks‖ | 17.6 | 16.9 | 1.04 (0.99-1.10) |

Abbreviations: CI, confidence interval; IRR, incident rate ratio; MAARI, medically attended acute respiratory illness; RSV, respiratory syncytial virus.
*Calculated as number of visits per 100 person-months, with outpatient, emergency department, and inpatient visits combined.
†Indicates any week during influenza season (October 1 to April 30) in which influenza accounted for 5% or more of the season's total number of influenza virus isolates.
‡Indicates any week during influenza season in which RSV accounted for 5% or more of the season's total number of RSV virus isolates and less than 5% of the season's total influenza virus isolates.
§Indicates any week during influenza season in which each week accounted for less than 3% of total RSV isolates and less than 3% of influenza virus isolates.
‖Indicates any week from July 1 to September 30.

0.96 (0.86-1.07), 0.95 (0.84-1.06), 1.12 (0.91-1.37), and 1.04 (0.98-1.10), respectively.

For infants born during the peak influenza weeks, the mean time in days from birth to the first MAARI did not vary by exposure status: exposed and unexposed infants' mean times to first acute respiratory illness were 49 and 53 days, respectively ($P=.84$). A Cox proportional hazards model comparing the time to the first

**Table 3. Adjusted IRRs for Acute Respiratory Illnesses Among Matched Infants Exposed and Unexposed to Maternal Influenza Vaccination, 1995-2001***

| Independent Variable | IRR (95% CI) by Study Period† Peak Influenza Weeks | RSV-Predominant Weeks | Periseasonal Weeks | Summer Weeks |
|---|---|---|---|---|
| Exposed infants | 0.96 (0.86-1.07) | 0.95 (0.84-1.06) | 1.12 (0.91-1.37) | 1.04 (0.98-1.10) |
| Gestation age | 0.96 (0.94-0.98) | 0.98 (0.96-1.00) | 0.96 (0.93-0.98) | 0.99 (0.98-1.00) |
| Maternal high-risk status‡ | 1.14 (1.01-1.27) | 1.14 (1.03-1.27) | 1.26 (1.10-1.44) | 1.22 (1.15-1.29) |
| Infant female sex | 0.88 (0.82-0.94) | 0.85 (0.80-0.91) | 0.95 (0.89-1.02) | 0.89 (0.86-0.92) |
| Medicaid coverage | 1.03 (0.85-1.25) | 1.29 (1.05-1.58) | 1.41 (1.08-1.85) | 1.21 (1.11-1.33) |
| Maternal age at infant birth | 0.98 (0.97-0.98) | 0.98 (0.97-0.99) | 0.98 (0.97-0.99) | 0.99 (0.99-0.99) |
| Maternal influenza vaccination in the preceding season | 1.06 (0.90-1.23) | 1.06 (0.94-1.20) | 0.87 (0.68-1.10) | 1.08 (1.01-1.16) |

Abbreviations: CI, confidence interval; IRR, incident rate ratio; RSV, respiratory syncytial virus.

*Calculated as outpatient, emergency department, and inpatient visits combined, and matched by managed care organization site and infant birth date within the same week.

†Study periods are described in the footnotes to Table 2.

‡Maternal high-risk status is explained in the "Health Services Data" subsection of the "Methods" section.

MAARI between exposed and unexposed infants born during the peak influenza weeks, controlling for maternal risk status, maternal age, gestational age, MCO site, and season, found no difference between exposed and unexposed infants (hazard ratio, 1.02; 95% CI, 0.83-1.25).

During peak influenza weeks, of all acute respiratory illnesses experienced by exposed infants, 59 (89.4%) were an upper respiratory infection, 4 (6.1%) were pneumonia, and 3 (4.5%) were hospitalizations. Similarly, in 851 (92.9%), 39 (4.3%), and 26 (2.8%) of the unexposed infants, acute respiratory illnesses were upper respiratory infections, pneumonia, and hospitalizations, respectively. The proportions between exposed and unexposed infants were not statistically significant (*P*=.32).

## COMMENT

Our study found no reduction in the incidence rate of MAARIs during peak influenza weeks among infants born to mothers vaccinated against influenza during their pregnancy. This finding is consistent with the work by Black et al[14] performed at Kaiser Permanente Northern California. The presence of other circulating respiratory viruses during the peak influenza weeks could mask any potential reduction in MAARI visits associated with maternal influenza vaccination. Similarly, we did not see any evidence that maternal influenza vaccination delayed the onset or reduced the severity of MAARI illness among infants born during the peak influenza weeks. This study was designed to maximize the possibility of seeing an effect on infant MAARI visits of maternal influenza vaccination, and therefore the analysis was limited to infants who had at least 28 days in utero for development and transfer of maternal antibodies, focused on peak influenza weeks, required infants to contribute person-time during the influenza season, and used data from a large linked database to maximize the number of study subjects. Although our study confirmed known predictors of acute respiratory illness visits in infants (sex and Medicaid coverage), we did not see an effect of maternal vaccination on rates of infant MAARI health care visits. Although it may be that maternal influenza vaccination reduces the risk of serious influenza illness among infants during their first months of life, this does not translate to a decrease in the number of visits to the physician's office or hospitalizations for acute respiratory illnesses.

We overestimated the maternal vaccination rate across our MCOs, which ranged from 0.7% to 20.8% during the 6 seasons, and thus had a smaller-than-expected number of infants exposed to maternal influenza vaccination. Because of the smaller sample size, our study is limited in its power to detect a reduced visit rate among exposed infants. Although we did not have the power to look at the effect of maternal vaccination on rare events such as infant pneumonia, our power to assess our primary outcome, MAARI incidence during peak influenza weeks, was good: We had the power to detect a 15% or greater reduction in MAARI visits (IRR, 0.85) during the peak influenza weeks ($\beta = .80$; $\alpha = .05$; unexposed background incidence, 17 per 100 person-months).

Although we had information on important variables that predict infant health care services utilization (eg, sex, gestational age, and Medicaid coverage), some variables predicting the incidence of acute respiratory illness in infants are not available in the VSD data. These include the number of siblings in the home, parental smoking status, breastfeeding, and attendance at day care. Glezen et al[20] studied influenza illness during the first year of life and found that having at least 3 siblings constituted a significant risk for infant influenza infection. More data from another database are available on the 5530 Colorado infants in this study, which suggest that there may not be great differences between families of exposed and unexposed infants, because the numbers of first-time mothers (45% exposed vs 43% unexposed), mothers intending to breastfeed (83% exposed vs 78% unexposed), and mothers who smoked (8.4% exposed vs 10% unexposed) are all similar.

Influenza illness in the first 6 months of life is more likely to present as an afebrile upper respiratory infection compared with the second 6 months of life. Glezen et al[20] reported that 58% of influenza illness among infants younger than 6 months were afebrile, compared with 28% among infants aged 6 to 11 months. Parents of afebrile infants with an upper respiratory infection may be less likely to seek medical care, and these infants would be missed in our study. Higher MAARI incidence rates among infants aged 6 to 11 months compared with 0 to 5 months could explain our finding of similar incidence rates of MAARIs for infants during the peak influenza (mean age, 2½ months) and the summer weeks (mean age, 7 months). Work by the New Vaccine Surveillance Network Group[21] confirms this lower rate of influenza illness among infants younger than 6 months. Outpatient surveillance of all children younger than 5 years at 2 study sites, in which viral culture or reverse transcriptase polymerase chain reaction testing for influenza virus was performed on nasal and throat swabs, found low rates of influenza infection—that is, less than 10% of acute respiratory infections occurring among infants aged 0 to 5 months during the 2002-2003 and 2003-2004 influenza seasons were due to influenza virus.[21]

Any study of the effect of maternal influenza vaccination on acute respiratory tract infection in infants faces a number of challenges. A randomized placebo-controlled trial would best control for unknown imbalances in confounders; however, given the current national recommendation that all pregnant women be vaccinated against influenza, it would be unethical to randomly assign women to vaccination or placebo. Any controlled trial allowing mothers to select vaccination could potentially suffer from confounding. The restrictive period studied reduces the number of mother-infant pairs available to study: the VSD files have more than 200 000 newborns during the study years, yet only 40 000 contributed to this work. The small number of peak influenza weeks during the winter months (average, 9.5 weeks per influenza season) means that even with large numbers of children, there will be limited person-time experience for analysis. A mismatch between the circulating strains of wild influenza virus and the strains used for vaccine development could explain the absence of an effect of maternal vaccination on MAARI visits. However, only 1 of the 6 seasons (1997-1998) was considered a fair rather than a good match. Finally, influenza cohort studies are challenged by the vagaries of the influenza season: the 2 influenza seasons after our study (2001-2002 and 2002-2003) were both unusually mild, whereas the 2003-2004 season was early (November to January), eliminating much opportunity for maternal influenza to protect infants born during that season against moderate to severe influenza infection. Future work should include multiple influenza seasons, use accurate tools such as viral culture and reverse transcriptase polymerase chain reaction to diagnose influenza, and focus on hospitalization as the outcome of interest. Small effect sizes, such as a reduction in hospitalization of 10% to 30%, will require large numbers of subjects to detect. Although this vaccination did not appear to have an effect on the rates of infant health care visits, vaccination is still important and is primarily recommended to protect the health of the mother.

**Accepted for Publication:** July 14, 2006.

**Author Affiliations:** Department of Preventive Medicine (Dr France) and Clinical Research Unit (Ms Smith-Ray and Drs McClure, Hambidge, Xu, and Yamasaki), Kaiser Permanente Colorado, Denver; The National Immunization Program, Influenza Branch (Dr Shay), Vaccine Safety Branch (Mr Weintraub), and Respiratory and Enteric Viruses Branch (Dr Fry), Division of Viral and Rickettsial Diseases, National Center for Infectious Diseases, Centers for Disease Control and Prevention, Atlanta, Ga; Kaiser Permanente Vaccine Study Center, Oakland, Calif (Drs Black and Shinefield); Center for Health Research, Kaiser Permanente Northwest, Portland, Ore (Dr Mullooly); and The Center for Health Studies, Group Health Cooperative, Seattle, Wash (Dr Jackson). The Vaccine Safety Branch has been transferred to the Office of the Chief Science Officer, Office of the Director, Centers for Disease Control and Prevention. Ms Smith-Ray is now with Human Cognitive Neuroscience at the University of Edinburgh, Edinburgh, Scotland.

**Correspondence:** Eric K. France, MD, MSPH, Kaiser Permanente Colorado, 10065 E Harvard Ave, Suite 250, Denver, CO 80231 (eric.k.france@kp.org).

**Author Contributions:** *Study concept and design:* France, Smith-Ray, McClure, Hambidge, Xu, Yamasaki, Shay, Weintraub, and Black. *Acquisition of data:* France, Smith-Ray, McClure, Weintraub, Shinefield, and Mullooly. *Analysis and interpretation of data:* France, Smith-Ray, McClure, Hambidge, Xu, Fry, Mullooly, and Jackson. *Drafting of the manuscript:* France, Smith-Ray, McClure, Hambidge, Yamasaki, and Fry. *Critical revision of the manuscript for important intellectual content*: France, Smith-Ray, McClure, Hambidge, Xu, Shay, Weintraub, Shinefield, and Jackson. *Statistical analysis:* McClure, Xu, Weintraub, Black, and Mullooly. *Obtained funding:* France. *Administrative, technical, and material support:* Smith-Ray, McClure, Yamasaki, Shay, and Fry. *Study supervision:* France, Hambidge, and Mullooly.

**Group Members:** The following are VSD investigators: Frank DeStefano, MD, MPH, William W. Thompson, PhD, James Baggs, PhD, and Robert L. Davis, MD, MPH (Immunization Safety Office, Office of the Chief Science Officer, Office of the Director, CDC, Atlanta, Ga); Lisa A. Jackson, MD, MPH, Karl Bohlke, ScD, and William E. Barlow, PhD (Center for Health Studies, Group Health Cooperative, Seattle, Wash); Steve B. Black, MD, and Henry R. Shinefield, MD (Kaiser Vaccine Study Center, Oakland, Calif); John P. Mullooly, PhD (Center for Health Research, Northwest Kaiser Permanente, Portland, Ore); Richard Platt, MD, MSc, and Tracy A. Lieu, MD, MPH (Harvard Pilgrim Health Care, Boston, Mass); Joel I. Ward, MD, Ken Zangwill, MD, and S. Michael Marcy, MD (Center for Vaccine Research, Harbor University of California–Los Angeles Medical Center, Torrance); Eric K. France, MD, MSPH, Simon Hambidge, MD, PhD, and Jason M. Glanz, PhD (Clinical Research Unit, Kaiser Permanente of Colorado, Denver); Mike Goodman, PhD (Health Partners Research Foundation, Minneapolis, Minn); and Edward A. Belongia, MD (Marshfield Clinic, Marshfield, Wis).

**Financial Disclosure:** Drs France and Yamasaki have received research funding from Sanofi-Aventis,

MedImmune, Inc, and Chiron Corp. Dr Jackson has received speakers bureau funding from Sanofi-Aventis and research funding from GlaxoSmithKline Vaccines and Chiron Corp.
**Funding/Support:** This study was supported by the CDC through an agreement with America's Health Insurance Plans.
**Previous Presentation:** This study was presented in part at the European Society for Paediatric Infectious Disease Meeting; May 19, 2005; Valencia, Spain.
**Acknowledgment:** The manuscript was approved through the clearance process of the CDC prior to submission. We thank the data management staff at the participating managed care organizations for their work in putting together the VSD files and the staff at America's Health Insurance Plans for their assistance.

## REFERENCES

1. Harper SA, Fukuda K, Uyeki TM, Cox NJ, Bridges CB; Centers for Disease Control and Prevention (CDC) Advisory Committee on Immunization Practices (ACIP). Prevention and control of influenza: recommendations of the Advisory Committee on Immunization Practices [ACIP] [published correction appears in *MMWR Recomm Rep.* 2004;53:743]. *MMWR Recomm Rep.* 2004;53:1-40.
2. Izurieta HS, Thompson WW, Kramarz P, et al. Influenza and the rates of hospitalization for respiratory disease among infants and young children. *N Engl J Med.* 2000;342:232-239.
3. Neuzil KM, Mellen BG, Wright PF, Mitchel EF, Griffin MR . The effect of influenza on hospitalizations, outpatient visits, and courses of antibiotics in children. *N Engl J Med.* 2000;342:225-231.
4. Groothuis JR, Levin MR, Rabalais GP, Meiklejohn G, Lauer BA. Immunization of high-risk infants younger than 18 months of age with split-product influenza vaccine. *Pediatrics.* 1991;87:823-828.
5. Piedra PA, Glezen WP, Mbawuike I, et al. Studies on reactogenicity and immunogenicity of attenuated bivalent cold recombinant influenza type A (CRA) and inactivated trivalent influenza virus (TI) vaccines in infants and young children. *Vaccine.* 1993;11:718-724.
6. Siegrist CA. Neonatal and early life vaccinology. *Vaccine.* 2001;19:3331-3346.
7. Global Programme for Vaccines and Immunization. *Programme Report 1995: WHO/GPV/96.01.* Geneva, Switzerland: World Health Organization; 1996.
8. Stephenson M. Protecting kids against influenza begins with maternal immunization. *Infect Dis Child.* September 2001. http://www.idinchildren.com/200109/frameset.asp?article=flu.asp. Accessed June 2002.
9. Englund JA. Maternal immunization with inactivated influenza vaccine: rationale and experience. *Vaccine.* 2003;21:3460-3464.
10. Terebuh P, Uyeki T, Fukuda K. Impact of influenza on young children and the shaping of United States influenza vaccine policy [published correction appears in *Pediatr Infect Dis J.* 2004;23:294]. *Pediatr Infect Dis J.* 2003;22:S231-S235.
11. Puck JM, Glezen WP, Frank AL, Six HR. Protection of infants from infection with influenza A virus by transplacentally acquired antibody. *J Infect Dis.* 1980;142:844-849.
12. Reuman PD, Ayoub EM, Small PA. Effect of passive maternal antibody on influenza illness in children: a prospective study of influenza A in mother-infant pairs. *Pediatr Infect Dis J.* 1987;6:398-403.
13. Englund JA, Mbawuike IN, Hammill H, Holleman MC, Baxter BD, Glezen WP. Maternal immunization with influenza or tetanus toxoid vaccine for passive antibody protection in young infants. *J Infect Dis.* 1993;168:647-656.
14. Black SB, Shinefield HR, France EK, Fireman BH, Platt ST, Shay D. Effectiveness of influenza vaccine during pregnancy in preventing hospitalizations and outpatient visits for respiratory illness in pregnant women and their infants. *Am J Perinatol.* 2004;21:333-339.
15. Kohler PF, Farr RS. Elevation of cord over maternal IgG immunoglobulin: evidence for an active placental IgG transport. *Nature.* 1966;210:1070-1071.
16. Chen RT, Glasser JW, Rhodes PH, et al; Vaccine Safety Datalink Team. Vaccine Safety Datalink Project: a new tool for improving vaccine safety monitoring in the United States. *Pediatrics.* 1997;99:765-773.
17. Centers for Disease Control and Prevention. Flu activity: reports and surveillance methods in the United States. http://www.cdc.gov/flu/weekly/fluactivity.htm. Accessed September 8, 2005.
18. Centers for Disease Control and Prevention. Respiratory syncytial virus trends. http://www.cdc.gov/ncidod/dvrd/revb/nrevss/rsvtre1.htm. Accessed September 8 2005.
19. Zeger SL, Liang KY. Longitudinal data analysis for discrete and continuous outcomes. *Biometrics.* 1986;42:121-130.
20. Glezen WP, Taber LH, Frank AL, Gruber WC, Piedra PA. Influenza virus infections in infants. *Pediatr Infect Dis J.* 1997;16:1065-1068.
21. National Immunization Program, Centers for Disease Control and Prevention. Morbidity from influenza infections in infants (and children). http://cdc.confex.com/cdc/nic2005/techprogram/paper_8719.htm. Accessed August 9, 2005.

### *When Is the Right Time for Toilet Training?*

Only a child can decide when the time for toilet training has come. Any pressure parents may feel from grandparents, nursery schools, or helpful friends had better be disregarded. It's got to be his achievement, not theirs.
—From *Touchpoints* by Dr T. Berry Brazelton, 2004

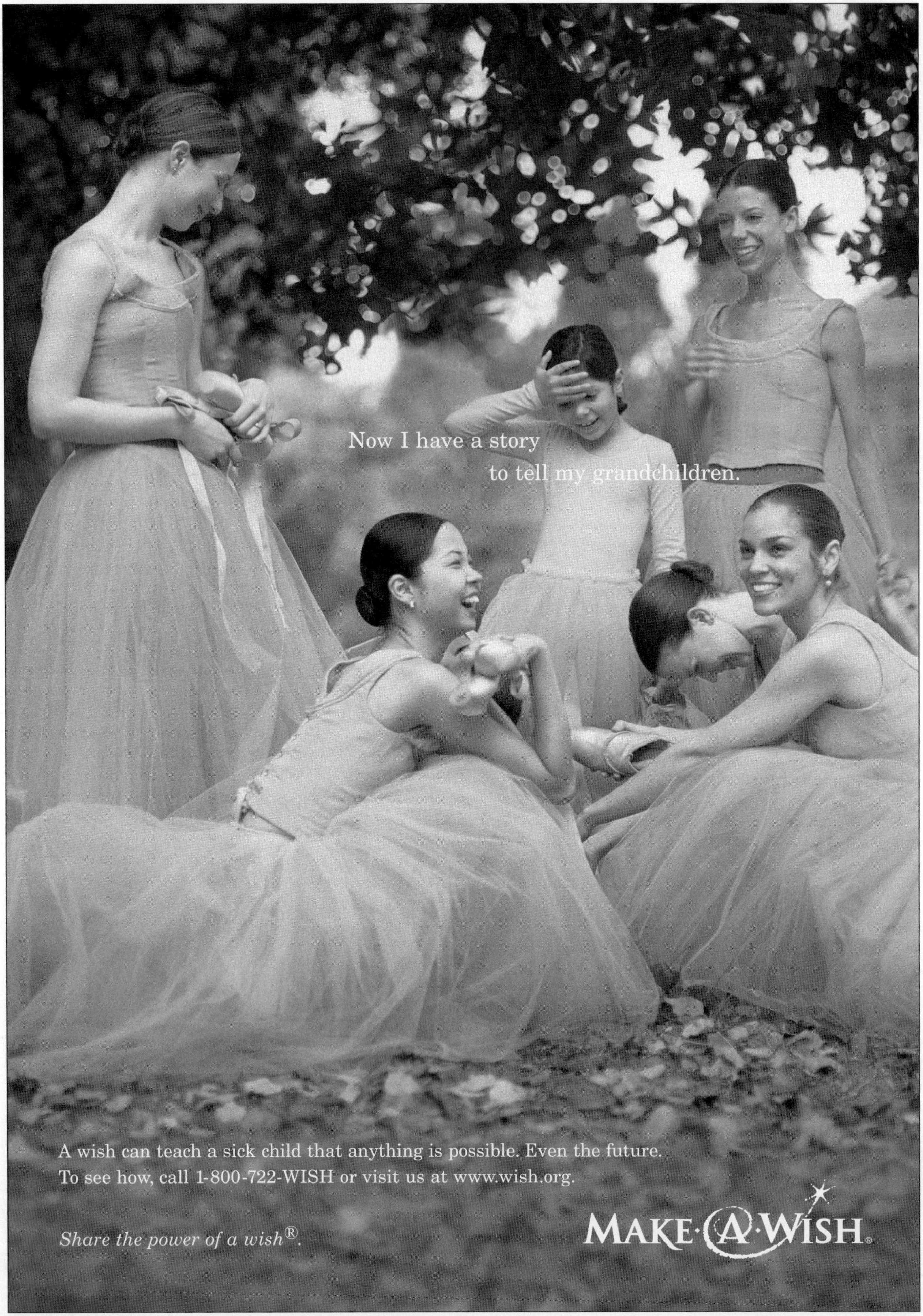
Now I have a story
to tell my grandchildren.
A wish can teach a sick child that anything is possible. Even the future.
To see how, call 1-800-722-WISH or visit us at www.wish.org.
Share the power of a wish®.
MAKE·A·WISH

# The Extent to Which Tobacco Marketing and Tobacco Use in Films Contribute to Children's Use of Tobacco

## *A Meta-analysis*

*Robert J. Wellman, PhD; David B. Sugarman, PhD; Joseph R. DiFranza, MD; Jonathan P. Winickoff, MD, MPH*

**Objective:** To quantify the effect of exposure on initiation of tobacco use among adolescents.

**Data Sources:** A systematic literature search of MEDLINE, PsychINFO, ABI/INFORM, and Business Source Premier through October/November 2005 was conducted. Unpublished studies were solicited from researchers.

**Study Selection:** Of 401 citations initially identified, 51 (n = 141 949 participants) met the inclusion criteria: reporting on exposure and tobacco use outcomes and participants younger than 18 years. Included studies reported 146 effects; 89 were conceptually independent effects. Data were extracted independently by 3 of us using a standardized tool. Weighted averages were calculated using a linear mixed-effects model. Heterogeneity and publication bias were assessed.

**Main Exposures:** Exposures (tobacco advertising, promotions, and samples and pro-tobacco depictions in films, television, and videos) were categorized as low or high engagement based on the degree of psychological involvement required.

**Main Outcome Measures:** Outcomes were categorized as cognitive (attitudes or intentions) or behavioral (initiation, tobacco use status, or progression of use).

**Results:** Exposure to pro-tobacco marketing and media increases the odds of youth holding positive attitudes toward tobacco use (odds ratio, 1.51; 95% confidence interval, 1.08-2.13) and more than doubles the odds of initiating tobacco use (odds ratio, 2.23; 95% confidence interval, 1.79-2.77). Highly engaging marketing and media are more effective at promoting use (odds ratio, 2.67; 95% confidence interval, 2.19-3.25). These effects are observed across time, in different countries, with different study designs and measures of exposure and outcome.

**Conclusions:** Pro-tobacco marketing and media stimulate tobacco use among youth. A ban on all tobacco promotions is warranted to protect children.

*Arch Pediatr Adolesc Med. 2006;160:1285-1296*

**Author Affiliations:** Department of Family Medicine and Community Health, University of Massachusetts Medical School, Worcester (Drs Wellman and DiFranza); Department of Behavioral Sciences, Fitchburg State College, Fitchburg, Mass (Dr Wellman); Department of Psychology, Rhode Island College, Providence (Dr Sugarman); and Center for Child and Adolescent Health Policy, Massachusetts General Hospital, Boston (Dr Winickoff).

APPROXIMATELY 1.4 MILLION children younger than 18 years in the United States begin smoking cigarettes each year.[1] Addiction to tobacco begins quickly, and the earlier a person initiates use the more likely he or she is to develop a severe and persistent addiction.[2-4] Therefore, factors that influence children to start using tobacco represent a significant public health risk.

DiFranza et al[5] applied the criteria of Hill[6] for assessing causality in epidemiologic studies to examine the marketing of tobacco products and children's initiation of tobacco use. Youth exposed to marketing develop positive attitudes, beliefs, and expectations about tobacco use, which foster the intention to use, and intention leads to initiation. They concluded that the evidence strongly supported a causal inference. Other reviews[7-9] have concluded that children's risk of using tobacco is increased by industry-sponsored tobacco promotion and the depiction of tobacco use in films. This meta-analysis assesses the magnitude of the risk and the stability of the effect across study design characteristics. We use the terms *pro-tobacco marketing* and *media* to refer to tobacco advertising, promotions, and samples and to pro-tobacco depictions in films, television, and videos, respectively. A quantified measure of risk will help resolve the tobacco industry–driven controversy about whether their marketing efforts are harmful[10-14] and, if the risk is substantial, will provide evidence to policy makers supporting measures to restrict children's exposure.

## METHODS

### STUDY SELECTION

Following the Meta-analysis of Observational Studies in Epidemiology standards for reporting meta-analyses,[15] we conducted a systematic search of MEDLINE (January 1966 to October 2005), PsychINFO (January 1985 to October 2005), Business Source Premier (January 1965 to October 2005), and ABI/INFORM Global (January 1971 to November 2005) to identify studies that assessed a link between any of 5 tobacco use outcomes (attitudes toward use, intention to use, initiation of use, tobacco use status, and progression to heavier use) and tobacco marketing (advertising, promotions, and samples) and media (depictions of tobacco use in films, television, and videos). We searched using Medical Subject Headings and the text key words *advertising* or *tobacco advertising* coupled with *adolescent* or *adolescence* and *smoking* or *smoking initiation* (or related headings appropriate to the database). Separate searches were conducted using the headings/key words *motion pictures* or *television* coupled with *adolescent* or *adolescence* and *smoking* or *smoking initiation*, or appropriate terms. Searches were limited to studies of humans published in English in peer-reviewed journals. We then searched the reference lists of review articles and all potentially relevant articles to identify additional candidates, and we solicited unpublished studies via a posting on the Society for Research on Nicotine and Tobacco Listserv and by talking with colleagues.

All potentially relevant articles were independently assessed for inclusion by 2 evaluators (R.J.W. and J.R.D.); in cases of disagreement, a third evaluator (D.B.S.) assessed the study and a consensus was reached.[16] To be included, a study had to measure both a tobacco use outcome and exposure to marketing or media. Measures of exposure included asking participants to recognize a brand name or logo, recall a brand, identify a favorite brand, express appreciation of advertisements, report whether they had received a sample of tobacco or had received or would use a tobacco promotional item, or report how many actors they had seen smoking in movies or which movies they had seen. Measures of tobacco use outcome included attitudes toward or expectations about the act of using (rather than attitudes about users), intention to use among youths who had never done so, initiation of use, status as a nonuser or user, and progression to heavier use. We excluded articles without original data and those where the primary focus was on (1) tobacco in the context of disease, (2) adult tobacco use, (3) law or policy, (4) anti-tobacco campaigns, (5) effects of advertising on adult tobacco consumption, (6) comparison of smoking rates across nations without controlling for any factor other than advertising, or (7) marketing practices.

### DATA EXTRACTION

Data were extracted independently by 3 of us (R.J.W., J.R.D., and D.B.S.) using a standardized tool. In the rare instances when coding did not match, mismatches were resolved by consensus.[16] We noted the first author's affiliation (medicine/public health, behavioral sciences, business/marketing, communications, government, or private industry); year of publication; year of data collection (first year for prospective studies); country and sample breadth (national, regional, single state, or local); sampling strategy (representative or convenience); final sample size; age, sex, and ethnicity of the sample; research design (cross-sectional, prospective, or experimental); and the number of effect size estimates (ESs) (which are unadjusted odds ratios [ORs] with accompanying 95% confidence intervals [CIs]).

Before the resolution of mismatches, raters coded categorical study characteristics identically 98.0% of the time on average (range, 93.9%-100%). For continuous variables, the mean correlation was 0.98 (range, 0.95-1.00). Before the resolution of mismatches, the raters coded exposure measures identically 97.3% of the time and outcome measures 97.9% of the time. Because of a high proportion of missing data, several variables (year of data collection, age, sex, and ethnicity) could not be included in analyses of moderator variables.

For each ES we determined the operational definition of the exposure variable and classified it within a conceptual category: awareness (eg, recognition of a brand name or logo, ability to name a brand, or expressed awareness of tobacco promotions), advertising exposure (eg, having seen advertisements or the number of advertisements seen), movie exposure (eg, the number of smoking scenes viewed in movies), appreciation of advertisements (eg, naming a favorite advertisement or rating advertisements as appealing), receipt of a tobacco promotional item or a sample of tobacco, participation in a promotional campaign (eg, willingness to use or actual use of a promotional item), or a scale of receptivity to marketing and media that combined aspects of the other measures. Likewise, we determined the operational definition of the outcome variable and classified it as follows: attitudes toward use, intention to use (typically measured either by a yes answer to a question about intention or by a score on the standardized susceptibility measure of Pierce et al[17,18]), initiation of use, status as a user or nonuser, or progression of use (ie, heavier use or earlier age at initiation).

In cases in which multiple studies used the same data to investigate conceptually equivalent exposure measures and outcomes, we used the study that most clearly showed the relationship. For example, if one study reported a dichotomous effect[19] and a second reported a dose-response relationship,[20] we chose the dichotomous effect. In cases in which a single article reported data derived from separate samples (eg, 2 different age groups[21] or data collected in different years[22]) or from separate designs (eg, cross-sectional and longitudinal[23]), the sets of data were treated as separate studies.

### STATISTICAL ANALYSIS

To avoid overweighting of individual studies, when multiple ESs in a single study addressed the same conceptual categories of exposure and outcome (eg, comparing smokers' and nonsmokers' recognition of 6 brand names and logos, all of which would address awareness[24]), we averaged the ESs using DSTAT version 1.11.[25]

The primary analyses were conducted using Comprehensive Meta-analysis version 2.2.023.[26] Exposures and outcomes were treated as dichotomous variables. Weighted averages are reported as ORs and 95% CIs; study weights were assigned by means of inverse variance weighting. The overall ES and ESs for the analyses of moderator variables were calculated using a linear mixed-effects model to account for differences between studies.[27,28] The consistency of effects across studies is reported as $I^2$, the percentage of total variance attributable to heterogeneity among studies rather than to chance.[29] Values of $I^2$ less than 25% are considered low, those around 50% are moderate, and those greater than 75% indicate high heterogeneity.

We assessed the potential for publication bias in 6 ways. We calculated Begg and Mazumdar rank correlations[30] and the regression intercept of Egger et al.[31] Because the Egger et al regression test can yield false-positive results when ESs are reported as ORs, we also performed the alternative regression test of Peters et al.[32] We calculated fail-safe *N*s to determine how many additional null findings would be needed to render the results nonsignificant at $\alpha = .05$, using the Rosenthal methods,[33,34] or to yield a "trivial" OR of 1.05, using the Orwin method.[35] Rosenthal suggested that meta-analysts calculate a tolerance level around a fail-safe *N* equal to 5 times the number of effects included in the meta-analysis (symbolized by $k$) plus 10 (the "$5k + 10$" benchmark)[34,36,37]; we used this benchmark to assess the observed fail-safe *N*s. Finally, to assess whether smaller studies distorted the overall ES we conducted a cumulative meta-analysis, adding studies sequentially from largest to smallest sample size.[38]

To assess the relationship between design quality and ES, we analyzed differences in ES between 5 subgroups created to represent a continuum of increasing design quality: cross-sectional design/convenience sample, cross-sectional/representative, experimental/convenience, prospective/convenience, and prospective/representative. Ordinarily, an experimental design would be considered strongest for demonstrating causality, but because of ethical considerations, experimental studies in this field are limited to assessments of attitudes. Prospective studies, which can track the change from nonuse to use, were, therefore, ranked highest.

Long ago, the Federal Trade Commission raised concerns that tobacco industry marketing was targeted at young people.[39] Similar concerns have been raised about depictions of tobacco use in movies.[40] In 1998, the Master Settlement Agreement between the industry and 46 US states banned advertising on billboards and in youth-oriented magazines.[41] To determine whether there was a decrease in ESs across time that might be attributed to changes in marketing and media, we conducted a second cumulative meta-analysis in which studies were sorted from oldest to most recent.

## RESULTS

### STUDY CHARACTERISTICS

The initial search yielded 331 nonduplicated citations addressing marketing and 70 addressing media (**Figure 1**). After reviewing the abstracts we excluded 317 articles and retained 84 full-text articles for detailed evaluation; review of their reference lists yielded 9 additional published studies, and data from 2 unpublished studies were provided by colleagues. Via e-mail we requested additional data from the authors of 20 studies with insufficient published data. Up to 3 requests were made at monthly intervals; 8 authors met the request, providing data from 10 studies.[12,17,19,80-84] Full review of the 95 studies resulted in excluding 44 for the following reasons: unavailable data (n=10),[42-51] no outcome measure (n=8),[52-59] no exposure measure (n=8),[18,60-66] duplicated another article (n=6),[20,67-71] no original data (n=7),[8,10,11,13,72-74] only time series data from which an ES could not be calculated (n=2),[75,76] included only tobacco users (n=2),[77,78] and studied only antismoking campaigns (n=1).[79] The 51 studies retained for the meta-analysis included 141 949 participants (**Table 1**) and presented 146 ESs, 89 of which were included in the analysis after averaging those estimates that were conceptually equivalent. **Figures 2**, **3**, and **4** present

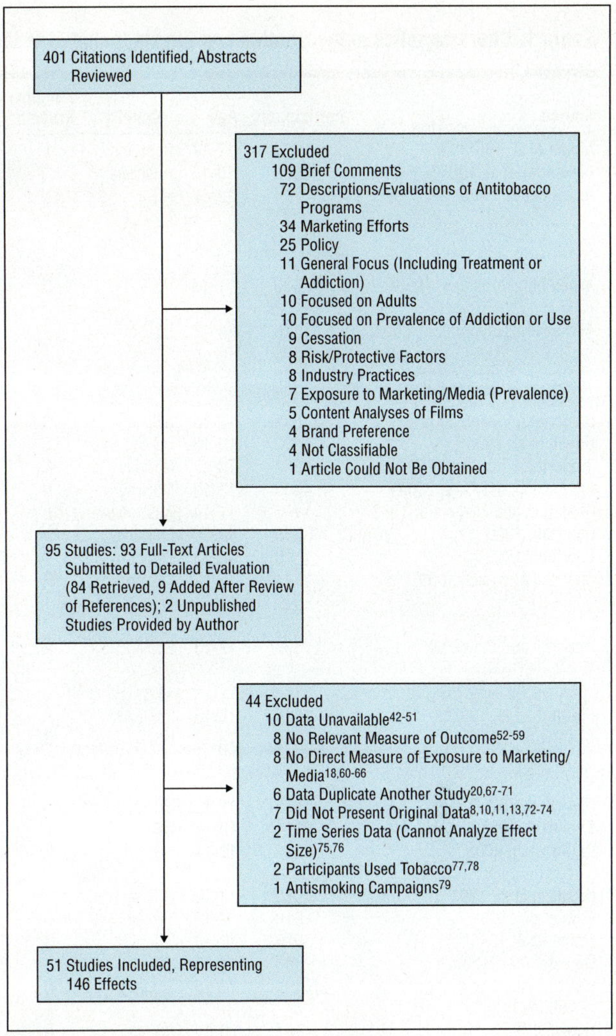


**Figure 1.** Study selection, inclusion, and exclusion.

the ESs and 95% CIs for all the studies, divided by decade of publication.

### QUANTITATIVE DATA SYNTHESIS

The overall ESs from the fixed- and mixed-effects models did not differ (fixed-effects: OR, 2.17; 95% CI, 2.12-2.22; mixed-effects: OR, 2.19; 95% CI, 1.93-2.47; $P < .001$ for both), and there was considerable heterogeneity among studies ($I^2 = 96.9$). Evidence of publication bias was not observed with either the Begg and Mazumdar[30] rank correlation ($P = .89$, 2-tailed) or the Egger et al[31] regression intercept ($P = .57$, 2-tailed), although the Peters et al[32] alternative regression method yielded a significant result (slope=−67.34; $P < .001$). The Rosenthal fail-safe *N* indicated that 86 514 additional null effects would be needed to render the overall ES nonsignificant at $P = .05$; the Orwin fail-safe *N* indicated that 1324 null effects would be needed to yield an OR of 1.05 or less. Both fail-safe *N*s greatly exceed the 455 ESs representing the $5k + 10$ threshold. Together, these tests suggest little likelihood of publication bias and, given the strength of the effect, little likelihood that the exclusion of studies with negative results (due to a file

**Table 1. Characteristics of the Studies and Effects Included in the Meta-analysis**

| Source | Participants | Age, y | Country | Sample Breadth | Sampling Strategy | Design | Exposure Measure | Outcome Measure | OR (SE) | Comment | Exposure/ Outcome |
|---|---|---|---|---|---|---|---|---|---|---|---|
| Aitken et al, 1987[24] | 359 | 12-17 | Scotland | L | Rep | CS | Awa | Att | 1.66 (0.19) | Mean of 12 ESs | LC |
| Alexander et al, 1983[85] | 4082 | 10-12 | Australia | R | NA | P | App | Sta | 2.69 (0.13) | None | HB |
| Altman et al, 1996[86] | 874 | 12-17 | US | N | Rep | CS | Awa | Int | 2.72 (0.30) | None | LC |
| | | | | | | | RP | Int | 0.05 (0.46) | | LC |
| | | | | | | | PP | Int | 2.64 (0.18) | | HC |
| | | | | | | | RT | Int | 0.11 (0.43) | | LC |
| Arnett and Terhanian, 1998[87] | 532 | 11-18 | US | R | C | CS | AE | Sta | 1.30 (0.16) | Mean of 5 ESs | LB |
| | | | | | | | App | Sta | 1.80 (0.16) | Mean of 10 ESs | HB |
| Audrain-McGovern et al, 2004[81] | 1115 | 14-17 | US | S | C | P | RS | Sta | 2.17 (0.17) | 9th grade | HB |
| | 1065 | | | | | | RS | Ini | 2.42 (0.17) | 10th grade | HB |
| | 1042 | | | | | | RS | Ini | 3.18 (0.16) | 11th grade | HB |
| | 1007 | | | | | | RS | Ini | 2.60 (0.16) | 12th grade | HB |
| Biener and Siegel, 2000[88] | 529 | 12-15 | US | S | Rep | P | RS | Prg | 1.78 (0.29) | None | HB |
| Botvin et al, 1993[89] | 602 | 12-13 | US | L | C | CS | AE | Sta | 2.93 (0.17) | None | LB |
| Braverman and Aaro, 2004[22] | 4292 | 13-15 | Norway | N | Rep | CS | AE | Sta | 1.98 (0.08) | None | LB |
| Braverman and Aaro, 2004[22] | 4065 | 13-15 | Norway | N | Rep | CS | AE | Sta | 2.01 (0.07) | None | LB |
| Chapman and Fitzgerald, 1982[90] | 1195 | 11-14 | Australia | L | C | CS | Awa | Sta | 2.72 (0.11) | Mean of 16 ESs | HB |
| Charlton, 1986[21] | 833 | 9-10 | England | R | Rep | CS | App | Sta | 3.50 (0.21) | None | HB |
| Charlton, 1986[21] | 1119 | 12-13 | England | R | Rep | CS | App | Sta | 2.51 (0.16) | None | HB |
| Charlton and Blair, 1989[23] | 2321 | 12-13 | England | R | Rep | CS | Awa | Sta | 4.79 (0.17) | None | LB |
| | | | | | | | App | Sta | 2.09 (0.11) | | HB |
| | | | | | | | AE | Sta | 0.95 (0.09) | | LB |
| Charlton and Blair, 1989[23] | 1390 | 12-13 | England | R | Rep | P | Awa | Ini | 1.77 (0.21) | None | LB |
| | | | | | | | App | Ini | 1.43 (0.19) | | HB |
| | | | | | | | AE | Ini | 0.88 (0.15) | | LB |
| Charlton et al, 1997[91] | 1029 | 12-13 | England | R | NA | P | AE | Prg | 1.96 (0.30) | None | LB |
| Chen et al, 2002[92] | 20,332 | 12-17 | US | S | Rep | CS | App | Sta | 1.87 (0.03) | Mean of 2 ESs | HB |
| | | | | | | | RP | Sta | 3.79 (0.07) | | LB |
| | | | | | | | PP | Sta | 3.30 (0.05) | | HB |
| Choi et al, 2002[93] | 965 | 12-17 | US | S | Rep | P | RS | Prg | 1.61 (0.19) | None | HB |
| Choi et al, 1995[80] | 2814 | 12-17 | US | S | Rep | CS | Awa | Sta | 8.83 (0.10) | None | LB |
| Dalton et al, 2003[94] | 2603 | 10-14 | US | R | C | P | PP | Ini | 2.45 (0.15) | None | HB |
| | | | | | | | ME | Ini | 3.95 (0.23) | | LB |
| DiFranza et al, 1991[95] | 1055 | 12-19 | US | R | C | CS | App | Int | 2.69 (0.32) | None | LC |
| Emri et al, 1998[96] | 918 | 7-13 | Turkey | L | C | CS | Awa | Sta | 0.96 (0.12) | Mean of 6 ESs | LB |
| Evans et al, 1995[17] | 3536 | 12-17 | US | S | Rep | CS | RS | Int | 3.81 (0.27) | None | LC |
| Goldstein et al, 1987[97] | 306 | 14-17 | US | L | C | CS | Awa | Sta | 8.12 (0.24) | None | LB |
| Health Education Authority, 1993[98] | 5,451 | 11-15 | England | N | Rep | CS | AE | Sta | 1.43 (0.09) | None | LB |
| Henke, 1995[99] | 81 | 3-8 | US | L | C | CS | Awa | Att | 2.49 (0.56) | None | LC |
| Henriksen et al, 2004[82] | 2,125 | 11-13 | US | L | C | CS | PP | Sta | 6.03 (0.13) | None | HB |
| | | | | | | | AE | Sta | 1.94 (0.08) | Mean of 2 ESs | LB |
| | | | | | | | ME | Sta | 2.17 (0.13) | | LB |
| Klein et al, 1992[100] | 195 | 13 | US | L | C | CS | PP | Sta | 2.25 (0.48) | Average age | HB |
| Lam et al, 1998[101] | 6,304 | 14 | Hong Kong | L | Rep | CS | PP | Sta | 1.69 (0.06) | None | HB |
| | | | | | | | AE | Sta | 1.35 (0.06) | | LB |
| | | | | | | | App | Sta | 4.72 (0.06) | | HB |
| Lopez et al, 2004[83] | 3,664 | 13-14 | Spain | R | C | P | Awa | Sta | 3.82 (0.29) | Baseline | LB |
| | 2743 | | | | | | Awa | Sta | 1.05 (0.23) | 6 mo | LB |
| | 2631 | | | | | | Awa | Sta | 1.24 (0.22) | 12 mo | LB |
| | 2149 | | | | | | Awa | Sta | 1.23 (0.20) | 18 mo | LB |
| Maassen et al, 2004[102] | 282 | 14-18 | Gambia | N | Rep | CS | ME | Sta | 0.51 (0.22) | None | LB |
| | | | | | | | AE | Sta | 0.77 (0.13) | Mean of 3 ESs | LB |
| | | | | | | | RT | Sta | 8.44 (0.29) | | LB |
| MacFadyen et al, 2001[113] | 618 | 15 | England | R | Rep | CS | Awa | Sta | 1.68 (0.16) | Average age | LB |
| | | | | | | | PP | Sta | 2.16 (0.20) | | HB |
| Maziak et al, 2003[114] | 3,489 | 12-15 | Germany | L | Rep | CS | App | Sta | 16.18 (0.09) | None | HB |
| Mizerski, 1995[12] | 790 | 3-6 | US | R | Rep | CS | Awa | Att | 0.83 (0.26) | Mean of 4 ESs | LC |
| Otake and Shimai, 2002[115] | 757 | – | Japan | L | C | CS | App | Sta | 5.95 (0.35) | None | HB |
| Pechmann and Knight, 2002[116] | 718 | 14 | US | L | C | E | AE | Int | 2.67 (0.28) | Average age | LC |
| Pechmann and Shih, 1999[104] | 113 | 14-15 | US | L | C | E | ME | Int | 1.56 (0.24) | None | LC |
| Peters et al, 1995[105] | 9,591 | 8-14 | Hong Kong | L | Rep | CS | Awa | Sta | 2.34 (0.07) | None | LB |
| Pierce et al, 1998[106] | 1,752 | 12-17 | US | S | Rep | P | RS | Ini | 1.85 (0.20) | None | HB |
| Pierce et al, 2005[117] | 2,119 | 12-15 | US | S | Rep | P | RS | Ini | 2.04 (0.20) | None | HB |

(continued)

drawer effect[34] or unavailability of data) could have led to this outcome. The cumulative meta-analysis revealed no shift in ES as smaller studies were included. The ES after addition of the 2 largest studies,[92,103] which accounted for 6 ESs, was 1.92 (95% CI, 1.28-2.88), and the ES after all the studies were included was 2.19. Because the overall ES is well within the 95% CI for that of the largest studies, there is no evidence of a "small study effect."[38] There was no correlation between sample size and ES (slope=0.00; *P*=.29).

**Table 1. Characteristics of the Studies and Effects Included in the Meta-analysis (cont)**

| Source | Participants | Age, y | Country | Sample Breadth | Sampling Strategy | Design | Exposure Measure | Outcome Measure | OR (SE) | Comment | Exposure/Outcome |
|---|---|---|---|---|---|---|---|---|---|---|---|
| Santana et al, 2003[84] | 1,732 | 12-14 | Spain | R | Rep | CS | App | Sta | 3.79 (0.09) | None | HB |
| J. D. Sargent, unpublished data, 1999 | 5,389 | 10-13 | US | R | Rep | CS | PP | Sta | 3.60 (0.08) | None | HB |
| J. D. Sargent, unpublished data, 2002 | 2603 | 10-13 | US | R | Rep | P | PP | Ini | 2.45 (0.15) | None | HB |
| Sargent et al, 2005[112] | 6,522 | 10-14 | US | N | Rep | CS | ME | Sta | 6.64 (0.17) | None | LB |
| Sargent et al, 2001[118] | 4,919 | 9-15 | US | R | Rep | CS | ME | Sta | 5.43 (0.13) | None | LB |
| | | | | | | | PP | Sta | 3.02 (0.08) | | HB |
| Sargent et al, 2000[107] | 480 | 8-17 | US | L | C | P | PP | Int | 3.25 (0.21) | None | HC |
| Sargent et al, 1997[19] | 1,008 | 10-19 | US | L | C | CS | PP | Sta | 1.79 (0.15) | None | HB |
| Sargent et al, 2002[119] | 3,702 | 9-15 | US | R | Rep | CS | ME | Int | 2.29 (0.10) | None | LC |
| | | | | | | | ME | Att | 1.72 (0.07) | | LC |
| Schooler et al, 1996[108] | 571 | 14 | US | L | Rep | CS | AE | Sta | 1.92 (0.16) | Mean of 4 ESs | LB |
| | | | | | | | RP | Sta | 3.66 (0.24) | | LB |
| | | | | | | | PP | Sta | 3.83 (0.20) | | HB |
| Tickle et al, 2001[120] | 632 | 10-19 | US | L | C | CS | ME | Sta | 1.15 (0.16) | None | LB |
| Turco, 1997[109] | 178 | 10-14 | US | L | C | E | AE | Att | 1.39 (0.84) | None | LC |
| Unger and Chen, 1999[103] | 10,030 | 12-18 | US | S | Rep | CS | App | Prg | 0.87 (0.06) | None | HB |
| | | | | | | | RP | Prg | 1.68 (0.14) | | LB |
| | | | | | | | PP | Prg | 1.46 (0.10) | | HB |
| Unger et al, 2001[121] | 5,821 | 11-16 | US | S | Rep | CS | AE | Sta | 1.11 (0.05) | None | LB |
| | | | | | | | ME | Sta | 1.27 (0.05) | | LB |
| | | | | | | | App | Sta | 5.46 (0.06) | | HB |
| | | | | | | | RP | Sta | 2.50 (0.06) | | LB |
| | | | | | | | PP | Sta | 4.04 (0.09) | | HB |
| Vaidya et al, 1996[110] | 1948 | 13-16 | India | L | Rep | CS | AE | Sta | 1.69 (0.22) | None | LB |
| | | | | | | | AE | Att | 1.92 (0.28) | | LC |
| While et al, 1996[111] | 1450 | 11-12 | England | R | Rep | P | Awa | Ini | 3.26 (0.20) | None | LB |
| **Grand Mean ES (95% Confidence Interval)** | | | | | | | | | | | |
| Fixed-effects model | | | | | | | | | 2.17 (2.12-2.22), *P*<.001, n = 89 | | |
| Mixed-effects model | | | | | | | | | 2.19 (1.93-2.47), *P*<.001 | | |

Abbreviations: AE, advertising exposure; App, appreciation of advertisements; Att, attitudes toward smoking; Awa, awareness of marketing; C, convenience; CS, cross-sectional; E, experimental; ESs, effect sizes; HB, high-engagement exposure/behavioral outcome; HC, high-engagement exposure/cognitive outcome; Ini, initiation of use; Int, intention to use; L, local; LB, low-engagement exposure/behavioral outcome; LC, low-engagement exposure/cognitive outcome; ME, movie exposure; N, national; NA, not applicable; OR, odds ratio; P, prospective; PP, participated in promotional campaign; Prg, progression of use; R, regional; Rep, representative; RP, received promotional item; RT, received tobacco sample; RS, receptivity scale; S, state; Sta, user vs nonuser; US, United States.

| Source | OR (95% CI) | *Z* Value | *P* Value |
|---|---|---|---|
| Chapman and Fitzgerald[90] | 2.72 (2.19-3.36) | 9.17 | <.001 |
| Alexander et al[85] | 2.69 (2.10-3.46) | 7.77 | <.001 |
| Charlton[21a] | 3.50 (2.31-5.29) | 5.94 | <.001 |
| Charlton[21b] | 2.51 (1.85-3.40) | 5.91 | <.001 |
| Aitken et al[24] | 1.66 (1.14-2.43) | 2.62 | .009 |
| Goldstein et al[97] | 8.12 (5.07-13.01) | 8.70 | <.001 |
| Charlton and Blair[23a] | 4.79 (3.40-6.74) | 8.98 | <.001 |
| Charlton and Blair[23b] | 2.09 (1.70-2.58) | 6.94 | <.001 |
| Charlton and Blair[23c] | 0.95 (0.80-1.13) | −0.58 | .57 |
| Charlton and Blair[23d] | 1.77 (1.17-2.68) | 2.69 | .007 |
| Charlton and Blair[23e] | 1.43 (0.99-2.07) | 1.89 | .06 |
| Charlton and Blair[23f] | 0.88 (0.66-1.18) | −0.86 | .39 |
| **Total** | 2.24 (1.59-3.15) | 4.64 | <.001 |

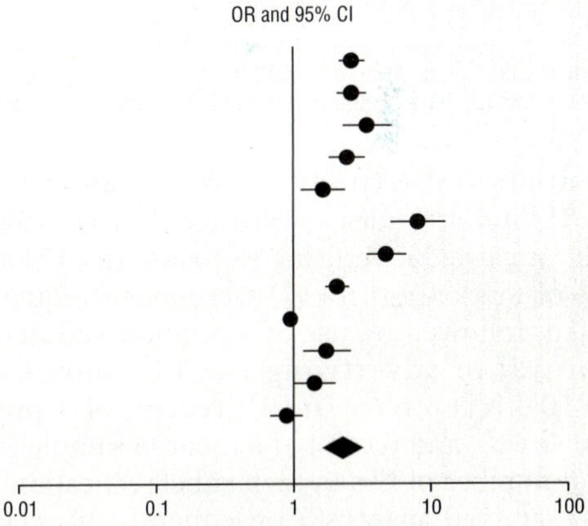


**Figure 2.** Odds ratios (ORs) and 95% confidence intervals (CIs) for studies conducted in the 1980s. The total represents the average OR derived from a mixed-effects model analysis. Lowercase letters after a reference number indicate different effects from the same study.

We next examined the effects of design quality and sampling breadth (**Table 2**). Overall, quality of design was unrelated to ES. In the initial analysis, studies with national samples tended to yield lower ESs than those with regional, state, or local samples (*P*=.06). However, 2 ESs from 1 study[86] were significantly different from the other ESs in that study and from those derived from the other 5 studies with national samples.[22,98,102,112] When the 2 outlying ESs were removed from the analysis there was no difference among studies on the basis of sampling breadth (*P*=.67).

A preliminary analysis revealed that 56 of the 89 ESs had tobacco use status (nonuser vs user) as the outcome variable, followed by initiation of use (n=13),

| Source | OR (95% CI) | *Z* Value | *P* Value |
|---|---|---|---|
| DiFranza et al[95] | 2.69 (1.44-5.03) | 3.09 | .002 |
| Klein et al[100] | 2.25 (0.88-5.72) | 1.70 | .09 |
| Botvin et al[89] | 2.93 (2.10-4.09) | 6.32 | <.001 |
| Health Education Authority[98] | 1.43 1.20-1.69) | 4.12 | <.001 |
| Choi et al[80] | 8.83 (7.27-10.72) | 21.96 | <.001 |
| Evans et al[17] | 3.81 (2.25-6.45) | 4.98 | <.001 |
| Henke[99] | 2.49 (0.84-7.40) | 1.65 | .10 |
| Mizerski[12] | 0.83 (0.50-1.38) | −0.71 | .48 |
| Peters et al[105] | 2.34 (2.05-2.68) | 12.60 | <.001 |
| Altman et al[86a] | 2.72 (1.53-4.85) | 3.40 | .001 |
| Altman et al[86b] | 0.05 (0.02-0.13) | −6.33 | <.001 |
| Altman et al[86c] | 2.64 (1.85-3.78) | 5.32 | <.001 |
| Altman et al[86d] | 0.11 (0.05-0.25) | −5.24 | <.001 |
| Schooler et al[108a] | 1.92 (1.42-2.61) | 4.24 | <.001 |
| Schooler et al[108b] | 3.66 (2.28-5.85) | 5.40 | <.001 |
| Schooler et al[108c] | 3.83 (2.59-5.67) | 6.74 | <.001 |
| Vaidya et al[110a] | 1.69 (1.10-2.59) | 2.42 | .02 |
| Vaidya et al[110b] | 1.92 (1.10-3.35) | 2.31 | .02 |
| While et al[111] | 3.26 (2.20-4.83) | 5.90 | <.001 |
| Charlton et al[91] | 1.96 (1.09-3.51) | 2.26 | .02 |
| Sargent et al[19] | 1.79 (1.34-2.40) | 3.93 | <.001 |
| Turco[109] | 1.39 (0.27-7.22) | 0.39 | .70 |
| Arnett and Terhanian[87a] | 1.30 (0.95-1.77) | 1.64 | .10 |
| Arnett and Terhanian[87b] | 1.80 (1.31-2.46) | 3.67 | <.001 |
| Emri et al[96] | 0.96 (0.76-1.22) | −0.31 | .76 |
| Lam et al[101a] | 1.69 (1.51-1.90) | 8.99 | <.001 |
| Lam et al[101b] | 1.35 (1.20-1.51) | 4.97 | <.001 |
| Lam et al[101c] | 4.72 (4.20-5.30) | 26.22 | <.001 |
| Pierce et al[106] | 1.85 (1.25-2.74) | 3.06 | .002 |
| Pechmann and Shih[104] | 1.56 (0.98-2.50) | 1.87 | .06 |
| Unger and Chen[103a] | 0.87 (0.77-0.98) | −2.28 | .02 |
| Unger and Chen[103b] | 1.68 (1.28-2.20) | 3.72 | <.001 |
| Unger and Chen[103c] | 1.46 (1.21-1.76) | 4.00 | <.001 |
| Biener and Siegel[88] | 1.78 (1.01-3.13) | 2.01 | .04 |
| Sargent et al[107] | 3.25 (2.16-4.89) | 5.66 | <.001 |
| Chen et al[92b] | 3.79 (3.29-4.37) | 18.50 | <.001 |
| J. D. Sargent, unpublished data, 1999 | 3.60 (3.08-4.21) | 16.12 | <.001 |
| **Total** | 1.89 (1.52-2.35) | 5.66 | <.001 |

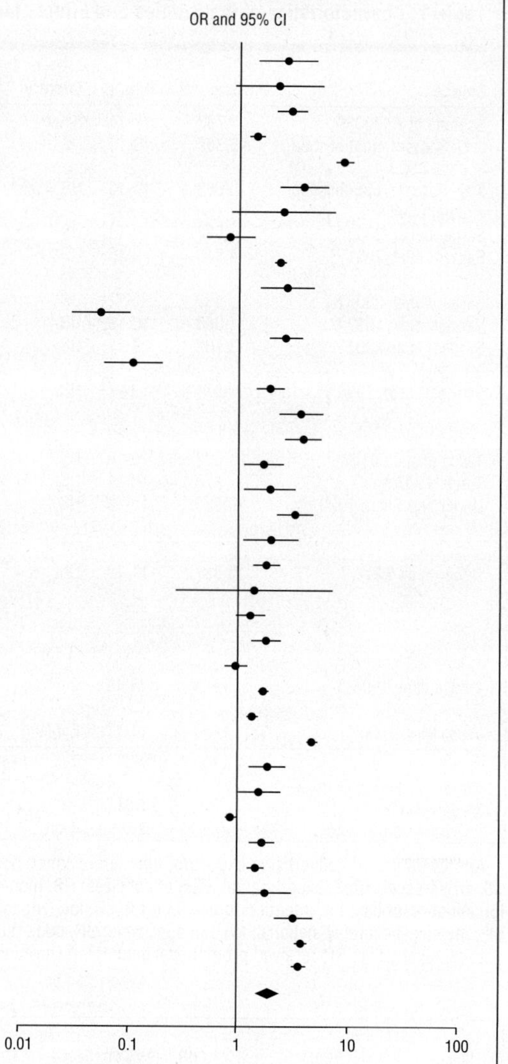


**Figure 3.** Odds ratios (ORs) and 95% confidence intervals (CIs) for studies conducted in the 1990s. The total represents the average OR derived from a mixed-effects model analysis. Lowercase letters after a reference number indicate different effects from the same study.

intention to use (n=10), progression to heavier use (n=5), and attitudes toward use (n=5). Among exposure measures, advertising exposure (n=17) and awareness of marketing (n=17) were most frequently represented, followed by use of a promotional item (n=14), approval of advertising (n=14), movie exposure (n=10), receptivity (n=9), receipt of a promotional item (n=6), and receipt of a tobacco sample (n=2). The small number of ESs in each subclassification precluded a fine-grained analysis. Consequently, we classified exposure measures by the degree of psychological involvement required: low engagement (awareness of marketing, advertising exposure, movie exposure, and receipt of a promotional item or tobacco sample) or high engagement (appreciation of advertising, willingness to use a promotional item, and receptivity). We classified outcome measures as either cognitive (attitudes toward use and intention to use) or behavioral (initiation of use, status, and progression). Overall, high-engagement exposures produced higher ESs than did low-engagement exposures, and ESs for behavioral outcomes were greater than those for cognitive outcomes (**Table 3**). The ES for progression to heavier use (OR, 1.42) was significantly lower than those for initiation of use (OR, 2.23) and tobacco use status (OR, 2.46).

The classification scheme gave us 4 possible combinations of exposure and outcome (see Table 1 for the classification of each ES). The overall ES for studies using a cognitive outcome was 1.51 (95% CI, 1.08-2.13; $P=.02$); the ES for low-engagement exposure was smaller than for high-engagement exposure with a cognitive outcome (**Table 4**). Because of the small number of included studies, we assessed the potential for publication bias in studies with a cognitive outcome. The Rosenthal fail-safe *N* indicated that 340 null effects would be needed to render the ES nonsignificant at $P<.05$. The Orwin fail-safe *N* indicated that 179 null effects would be necessary to yield a trivial OR of 1.05. These fail-safe *N*s greatly exceed the $5k+10$ threshold of 85 null effects. Given that the ratio of excluded null effects to included effects is greater than 5:1, there is little likelihood that the exclusion of studies led to the observed

| Source | OR (95% CI) | *Z* Value | *P* Value |
|---|---|---|---|
| MacFadyen et al[113a] | 1.68 (1.24-2.28) | 3.30 | .001 |
| MacFadyen et al[113b] | 2.16 (1.47-3.17) | 3.90 | <.001 |
| Sargent et al[118a] | 5.43 (4.17-7.06) | 12.59 | <.001 |
| Sargent et al[118b] | 3.02 (2.58-3.54) | 13.81 | <.001 |
| Tickle et al[120] | 1.15 (0.84-1.58) | 0.87 | .38 |
| Unger et al[121a] | 1.11 (1.01-1.22) | 2.18 | .03 |
| Unger et al[121b] | 1.27 (1.14-1.41) | 4.44 | <.001 |
| Unger et al[121c] | 5.46 (4.87-6.11) | 29.35 | <.001 |
| Unger et al[121d] | 2.50 (2.25-2.79) | 16.59 | <.001 |
| Unger et al[121e] | 4.04 (3.37-4.84) | 15.08 | <.001 |
| Chen et al[92a] | 1.87 (1.78-1.97) | 23.65 | <.001 |
| Chen et al[92c] | 3.30 (2.97-3.67) | 22.21 | <.001 |
| Choi et al[93] | 1.61 (1.12-2.33) | 2.55 | .01 |
| Otake and Shimai[115] | 5.95 (2.99-11.85) | 5.07 | <.001 |
| Pechmann and Knight[116] | 2.67 (1.55-4.59) | 3.56 | <.001 |
| Sargent et al[119a] | 2.29 (1.90-2.76) | 8.63 | <.001 |
| Sargent et al[119b] | 1.72 (1.52-1.96) | 8.35 | <.001 |
| Dalton et al[94a] | 2.45 (1.84-3.26) | 6.12 | <.001 |
| Dalton et al[94b] | 3.95 (2.53-6.17) | 6.03 | <.001 |
| Maziak et al[114] | 16.18 (13.57-19.30) | 30.99 | <.001 |
| Santana et al[84] | 3.79 (3.17-4.53) | 14.57 | <.001 |
| Audrain-McGovern et al[81a] | 2.17 (1.55-3.04) | 4.52 | <.001 |
| Audrain-McGovern et al[81b] | 2.42 (1.75-3.35) | 5.34 | <.001 |
| Audrain-McGovern et al[81c] | 3.18 (2.32-4.34) | 7.26 | <.001 |
| Audrain-McGovern et al[81d] | 2.60 (1.92-3.53) | 6.13 | <.001 |
| Braverman and Aaro[22a] | 1.98 (1.71-2.30) | 9.04 | <.001 |
| Braverman and Aaro[22b] | 2.01 (1.74-2.32) | 9.43 | <.001 |
| Henriksen et al[82a] | 6.03 (4.68-7.77) | 13.86 | <.001 |
| Henriksen et al[82b] | 1.94 (1.65-2.26) | 8.25 | <.001 |
| Henriksen et al[82c] | 2.17 (1.68-2.80) | 5.91 | <.001 |
| Lopez et al[83a] | 3.82 (2.18-6.72) | 4.67 | <.001 |
| Lopez et al[83b] | 1.05 (0.68-1.63) | 0.22 | .82 |
| Lopez et al[83c] | 1.24 (0.81-1.90) | 1.00 | .32 |
| Lopez et al[83d] | 1.23 (0.83-1.82) | 1.03 | .30 |
| Maassen et al[102a] | 0.51 (0.33-0.78) | −3.11 | .002 |
| Maassen et al[102b] | 0.77 (0.60-0.98) | −2.09 | .04 |
| Maassen et al[102c] | 8.44 (4.78-14.93) | 7.34 | <.001 |
| Pierce et al[117] | 2.04 (1.39-3.00) | 3.64 | <.001 |
| Sargent et al[112] | 6.64 (4.72-9.34) | 10.89 | <.001 |
| J. D. Sargent, unpublished data, 2002 | 2.45 (1.84-3.26) | 6.12 | <.001 |
| **Total** | 2.46 (2.05-2.96) | 9.61 | <.001 |

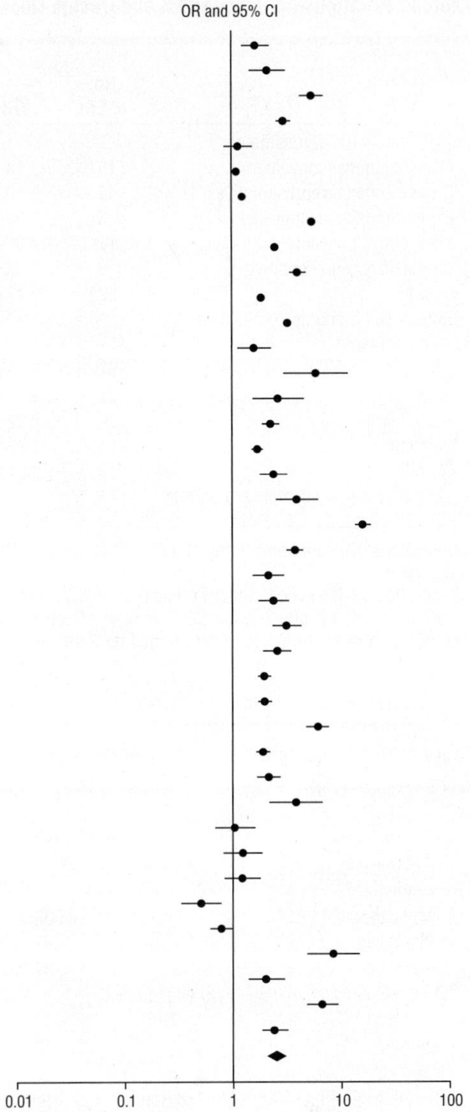


**Figure 4.** Odds ratios (ORs) and 95% confidence intervals (CIs) for studies conducted in the 2000s. The total represents the average OR derived from a mixed-effects model analysis. Lowercase letters after a reference number indicate different effects from the same study.

outcome. The overall ES for studies using a behavioral outcome was 2.33 (95% CI, 2.03-2.67; *P*<.001); low- and high-engagement exposures with behavioral outcomes produced equivalent ESs (Table 4).

The cumulative meta-analysis by publication date did not reveal a trend toward decreasing ESs across time. There was no overall difference in ESs derived from studies conducted between 1981 and 1990 (8 studies and 12 ESs), 1991 and 2000 (26 studies and 37 ESs), or 2001 and 2005 (21 studies and 40 ESs) (*P*=.15). However, studies conducted since 2001 tended to yield larger ESs (overall ES, 2.45; 95% CI, 2.05-2.95) than did those conducted in the 1990s (overall ES, 1.89; 95% CI, 1.52-2.35; *P*=.07).

## COMMENT

DiFranza et al[5] concluded that exposure to marketing causes children to initiate tobacco use. We quantified this risk; the odds of becoming a tobacco user are more than doubled by exposure to marketing and media. This relationship is robust, with similar effects observed across time in different countries, in cross-sectional and prospective designs using a variety of measures of exposure, and whether the outcome is initiation or tobacco use status.

Exposure that does not actively engage the recipient has a substantial impact, increasing the odds of tobacco use by approximately 90%. This suggests that youth are highly susceptible to the pervasive presence of marketing and media. Once a recipient is psychologically involved, the odds increase almost 3-fold, suggesting that the interaction between exposure and an individual's psychological processes is powerful. The impact of marketing and media remains powerful even after the initiation of use; exposure increased the odds of progression to heavier use by 42%.

A variety of psychosocial factors (eg, age, ethnicity, family structure, parental socioeconomic status, per-

**Table 2. Relationship Between ES and Design Quality and Sampling Breadth**

| | No. of ESs | Fixed-Effects Analysis | | | | | Mixed-Effects Analysis* | |
|---|---|---|---|---|---|---|---|---|
| | | OR (95% CI) | *P* Value | Cochran *Q* | *P* Value | $I^2$ | OR (95% CI) | *P* Value |
| Design quality (design/sample) | | | | | | | | |
| Cross-sectional/convenience | 15 | 2.13 (1.98-2.30) | <.001 | 184.72 | <.001 | 92.42 | 2.39 (1.78-3.21) | <.001 |
| Cross-sectional/representative | 49 | 2.16 (2.11-2.21) | <.001 | 2542.01 | <.001 | 98.11 | 2.19 (1.83-2.61) | <.001 |
| Experimental/convenience | 3 | 1.94 (1.37-2.74) | <.001 | 2.30 | .32 | 13.19 | 1.95 (1.32-2.87) | .001 |
| Prospective/convenience | 11 | 2.31 (2.07-2.58) | <.001 | 46.55 | <.001 | 78.52 | 2.27 (1.78-2.89) | <.001 |
| Prospective/representative | 9 | 2.27 (2.05-2.51) | <.001 | 91.13 | <.001 | 91.22 | 1.88 (1.29-2.73) | .001 |
| Overall | 87† | 2.17 (2.12-2.21) | <.001 | | | | 2.18 (1.94-2.45) | <.001 |
| Difference among design qualities | | | | | | | | .84 |
| Sampling breadth | | | | | | | | |
| Local | 27 | 2.53 (2.42-2.65) | <.001 | 904.43 | <.001 | 97.13 | 2.60 (1.97-3.43) | <.001 |
| State | 21 | 2.08 (2.02-2.14) | <.001 | 1207.68 | <.001 | 98.34 | 2.35 (1.83-3.02) | <.001 |
| Regional | 30 | 2.22 (2.11-2.32) | <.001 | 385.88 | <.001 | 92.49 | 2.14 (1.79-2.57) | <.001 |
| National | 11 | 1.72 (1.60-1.86) | <.001 | 282.27 | <.001 | 96.46 | 1.29 (0.83-2.01) | .26 |
| Overall | 89 | 2.17 (2.12-2.22) | <.001 | | | | 2.19 (1.93-2.47) | <.001 |
| Difference among sampling breadths | | | | | | | | .06 |

Abbreviations: CI, confidence interval; ESs, effect sizes; $I^2$, the percentage of total variance attributable to heterogeneity among studies rather than to chance; OR, odds ratio.

*Mixed-effects (also called random-effects) models assume that true differences exist among studies and so estimate within-study and between-study variance. Mixed-effects models produce wider CIs than fixed-effects models and so are more conservative.

†The design quality could not be determined for 2 studies.

**Table 3. Relationship Between ES and Exposure Type and Outcome Type**

| | No. of ESs | Fixed-Effects Analysis | | | | | Mixed-Effects Analysis* | |
|---|---|---|---|---|---|---|---|---|
| | | OR (95% CI) | *P* Value | Cochran *Q* | *P* Value | $I^2$ | OR (95% CI) | *P* Value |
| Exposure type | | | | | | | | |
| Low engagement | 52 | 1.85 (1.79-1.91) | <.001 | 1295.72 | <.001 | 96.06 | 1.90 (1.62-2.24) | <.001 |
| High engagement | 37 | 2.51 (2.44-2.59) | <.001 | 1373.91 | <.001 | 97.38 | 2.67 (2.19-3.25) | <.001 |
| Overall | 89 | 2.17 (2.12-2.22) | <.001 | | | | 2.19 (1.93-2.47) | <.001 |
| Difference between low and high engagement | | | | | | | | .009 |
| Outcome type | | | | | | | | |
| Cognitive | 15 | 1.88 (1.72-2.05) | <.001 | 143.06 | <.001 | 90.21 | 1.51 (1.08-2.13) | .02 |
| Behavioral | 74 | 2.19 (2.14-2.24) | <.001 | 2717.94 | <.001 | 97.31 | 2.33 (2.03-2.67) | <.001 |
| Difference between cognitive and behavioral | | | | | | | | .02 |
| Outcome | | | | | | | | |
| Initiation | 13 | 2.21 (2.02-2.43) | <.001 | 66.68 | <.001 | 82.00 | 2.23 (1.79-2.77) | <.001 |
| Tobacco use status | 56 | 2.28 (2.23-2.34) | <.001 | 2389.20 | <.001 | 97.70 | 2.46 (2.10-2.89) | <.001 |
| Progression | 5 | 1.12 (1.02-1.23) | .01 | 40.57 | <.001 | 90.14 | 1.42 (1.00-2.00) | .049 |
| Difference among outcomes | | | | | | | | .02 |

Abbreviations: CI, confidence interval; ESs, effect sizes; $I^2$, the percentage of total variance attributable to heterogeneity among studies rather than to chance; OR, odds ratio.

*Mixed-effects (also called random-effects) models assume that true differences exist among studies and so estimate within-study and between-study variance. Mixed-effects models produce wider confidence intervals than fixed-effects models and so are more conservative.

sonal income, parental attitudes and tobacco use, sibling and peer tobacco use, peer attitudes and norms, family environment, engagement in other risky behaviors, stress, depression, and self-esteem) raise the odds of initiation.[122-124] The appearance of symptoms of addiction seems to be the primary factor driving progression to heavier use.[125] Thus, it is not surprising that marketing and media have a greater impact on initiation of use than on progression to heavier use.

Compared with unexposed youth, exposed youth had approximately 50% greater odds of holding positive attitudes toward tobacco use or expressing an intention to use in the future and more than twice the odds of initiating use. For years the tobacco industry has claimed that a cross-sectional association between exposure to marketing and tobacco use is found because users are more likely than nonusers to attend to marketing.[13] If use causes exposure rather than vice versa, ESs in cross-sectional studies should exceed those in prospective studies of nonusers, in which assessment of exposure precedes the onset of use. The present findings refute the industry's argument; the ESs in prospective studies are equivalent to those in cross-sectional studies.

**Table 4. Subgroup Analysis (Exposure Type by Outcome Type)**

| | No. of ESs | Fixed-Effects Analysis: OR (95% CI) | P Value | Cochran Q | P Value | $I^2$ | Mixed-Effects Analysis*: OR (95% CI) | P Value |
|---|---|---|---|---|---|---|---|---|
| Low-engagement cognitive | 11 | 1.72 (1.57-1.90) | <.001 | 121.30 | <.001 | 91.76 | 1.12 (0.73-1.72) | .61 |
| Low-engagement behavioral | 41 | 1.86 (1.81-1.93) | <.001 | 1172.05 | <.001 | 96.59 | 2.12 (1.77-2.54) | <.001 |
| High-engagement cognitive | 4 | 3.01 (2.41-3.77) | <.001 | 1.55 | .67 | 0.00 | 3.01 (2.41-3.77) | <.001 |
| High-engagement behavioral | 33 | 2.51 (2.43-2.58) | <.001 | 1369.82 | <.001 | 97.66 | 2.63 (2.13-3.24) | <.001 |
| Overall | 89 | 2.17 (2.12-2.22) | <.001 | | | | 2.19 (1.93-2.47) | <.001 |
| Difference among subgroups | | | | | | | | <.001 |
| Difference between exposures with cognitive outcome | | | | | | | | <.001 |
| Difference between exposures with behavioral outcome | | | | | | | | .13 |

Abbreviation: CI, confidence interval; ESs, effect sizes; $I^2$, the percentage of total variance attributable to heterogeneity among studies rather than to chance; OR, odds ratio.

*Mixed-effects (also called random-effects) models assume that true differences exist among studies and so estimate within-study and between-study variance. Mixed-effects models produce wider confidence intervals than fixed-effects models and so are more conservative.

If attempts to mitigate the harm posed by marketing and media, embodied in voluntary and mandatory restrictions instituted during the past 2 decades, were effective, we would expect to observe a decrease in ESs across time. We did not. Indeed, the ES shows a trend toward increasing since 2001, suggesting that the risk to youth has increased. These measures have not had an evident effect on exposure. The tobacco industry has been remarkably adept at shifting strategies to avoid the restrictions imposed by the Master Settlement Agreement by preferentially placing their advertisements in magazines whose youth readership exceeds 20%,[126,127] and tobacco use in current movies is comparable with that seen in the 1950s, when it was rampant.[128]

The strengths of this meta-analysis include the large number of ESs available for analysis, lack of evidence for publication bias, large overall sample size, the time during which data were collected, and diversity among studies in design, geographic distribution, and exposure and outcome measures. Potential limitations include the inability to assess possible moderation by demographic or psychosocial factors because of a lack of data or to conduct a fine-grained analysis of the interaction between exposure and outcome measures because of a paucity of studies in particular categories.

Despite the industry-fueled controversy surrounding the relationship between exposure to pro-tobacco marketing and media and initiation of use,[10-14] the present findings offer considerable evidence for a causal link. First, the overall ES is strong and robust, showing consistency between cross-sectional and prospective studies. Second, the 3 experimental studies reviewed demonstrated that greater exposure led to more positive attitudes toward use. Third, the failure of design-related moderator variables to impact the ES suggests that such alternative explanations are limited. Most important, in 13 prospective studies, exposure more than doubled the odds of initiating tobacco use.

Ethical considerations preclude experimental studies that would expose youth to marketing and media to see whether they would initiate tobacco use. However, laboratory and field-based experiments have shown that media portrayals of violence in films (low engagement) and video games (high engagement) produce subsequent violent attitudes and behaviors in children and adolescents.[129,130] The causal relationship between violent media and behavior makes it plausible that tobacco marketing and media also affect behavior.

Given the money spent by the tobacco industry on worldwide marketing and the global distribution of American movies, it is unlikely that many children escape exposure. Our findings suggest that half of all children who initiate tobacco use do so because of exposure to marketing and media. Half the youth who initiate smoking will likely continue for more than 15 years,[3] making themselves vulnerable to serious harm. Smoking causes 36 diseases,[131] which kill almost half of all smokers.[132] Current and future schemes that expose children to pro-tobacco messages, products, or images are a public health menace. More definitive measures to curtail exposure, such as a ban on all tobacco promotional activities, as called for in the World Health Organization Framework Convention on Tobacco Control,[133] are needed and warranted.

**Accepted for Publication:** June 27, 2006.

**Correspondence:** Robert J. Wellman, PhD, Department of Family Medicine and Community Health, University of Massachusetts Medical School, 55 Lake Ave N, Worcester, MA 01655 (Robert.Wellman@umassmed.edu).

**Author Contributions:** Dr Wellman had full access to all the data presented in this study and takes responsibility for the integrity of the data and the accuracy of the data analysis. *Study concept and design:* Wellman, Sugarman, and DiFranza. *Acquisition of data:* Wellman, Sugarman, DiFranza, and Winickoff. *Analysis and interpretation of data:* Wellman, Sugarman, DiFranza,and Winickoff. *Drafting of the manuscript:* Wellman, Sugarman, and DiFranza. *Critical revision of the manuscript for important intellectual content*: Wellman, Sugarman, DiFranza, and Winickoff. *Statistical analysis:* Wellman and Sugarman. *Obtained funding:* Wellman and DiFranza. *Administrative, technical, and material support:* Wellman, Sugarman, DiFranza, and Winickoff. *Study supervision:* Wellman and Winickoff.

**Financial Disclosure:** None reported.
**Funding/Support:** This study was supported by grant 53081 from the Robert Wood Johnson Foundation (Dr Wellman).
**Role of the Sponsor:** The funding agency played no role in designing or conducting the study; in collecting, managing, analyzing, or interpreting the data; or in preparing, reviewing, or approving the manuscript.
**Disclaimer:** The ideas expressed herein are those of the authors and not necessarily those of the funding agency.
**Acknowledgment:** We thank Bethany J. Hipple, MPH (Center for Child and Adolescent Health Policy, Massachusetts General Hospital), for assistance in searching the business literature and for reviewing the first draft of the manuscript and William Shadel, PhD (Rand Corp) for reviewing the first draft.

## REFERENCES

1. Substance Abuse and Mental Health Services Administration. Overview of findings from the 2004 national survey on drug use and health. http://www.oas.samhsa.gov/NSDUH/2k4NSDUH/2k4Overview/2k4Overview.pdf. Accessed December 8, 2005.
2. DiFranza JR, Savageau JA, Rigotti NA, et al. Development of symptoms of tobacco dependence in youths: 30 month follow up data from the DANDY study. *Tob Control.* 2002;11:228-235.
3. Pierce JP, Gilpin E. How long will today's new adolescent smoker be addicted to cigarettes? *Am J Public Health.* 1996;86:253-256.
4. Chen J, Millar WJ. Age of smoking initiation: implications for quitting. *Health Rep.* 1998;9:39-46.
5. DiFranza JR, Wellman RJ, Sargent JD, Weitzman M, Hipple BJ, Winickoff JP. Tobacco promotion and the initiation of tobacco use: assessing the evidence for causality. *Pediatrics.* 2006;117:e1237-e1248.
6. Hill AB. The environment and disease: association or causation? *Proc R Soc Med.* 1965;58:295-300.
7. Charlesworth A, Glantz SA. Smoking in the movies increases adolescent smoking: a review. *Pediatrics.* 2005;116:1516-1528.
8. Lovato C, Linn G, Stead LF, Best A. Impact of tobacco advertising and promotion on increasing adolescent smoking behaviours. *Cochrane Database Syst Rev.* 2003;(4):CD003439.
9. Sargent JD. Smoking in movies: impact on adolescent smoking. *Adolesc Med Clin.* 2005;16:345-370.
10. Boddewyn JJ. Cigarette advertising bans and smoking: the flawed policy connection. *Int J Advertising.* 1994;13:311-332.
11. Jenkins J. Tobacco advertising and children: some Canadian findings. *Int J Advertising.* 1988;7:357-367.
12. Mizerski R. The relationship between cartoon trade character recognition and attitude toward product category in young children. *J Mark.* 1995;59:58-70.
13. Moschis GP. Cigarette advertising and young smokers. *J Advertising Res.* April/May: 1989:51-60.
14. Sullum J. Unclear link between cigarette ads and adolescent smoking. *Health Aff (Millwood).* 2002;21:280-281.
15. Stroup DF, Berlin JA, Morton SC, et al; Meta-analysis of Observational Studies in Epidemiology (MOOSE) Group. Meta-analysis of observational studies in epidemiology: a proposal for reporting. *JAMA.* 2000;283:2008-2012.
16. Deeks JJ, Higgins JPT, Altman DG. Analysing and presenting results. In: Higgins JPT, Green S, eds. *Cochrane Handbook for Systematic Reviews of Interventions 4.2.5* [updated May 2005]. http://www.cochrane.org/resources/handbook/hbook.htm. Accessed March 30, 2006.
17. Evans N, Farkas A, Gilpin E, Berry C, Pierce JP. Influence of tobacco marketing and exposure to smokers on adolescent susceptibility to smoking. *J Natl Cancer Inst.* 1995;87:1538-1545.
18. Pierce JP, Choi WS, Gilpin EA, Farkas AJ, Merritt RK. Validation of susceptibility as a predictor of which adolescents take up smoking in the United States. *Health Psychol.* 1996;15:355-361.
19. Sargent JD, Dalton MA, Beach M, Bernhardt A, Pullin D, Stevens M. Cigarette promotional items in public schools. *Arch Pediatr Adolesc Med.* 1997;151:1189-1196.
20. Sargent JD, Dalton M, Beach M. Exposure to cigarette promotions and smoking uptake in adolescents: evidence of a dose-response relation. *Tob Control.* 2000;9:163-168.
21. Charlton A. Children's advertisement awareness related to their views on smoking. *Health Educ J.* 1986;45:75-78.
22. Braverman MT, Aaro LE. Adolescent smoking and exposure to tobacco marketing under a tobacco advertising ban: findings from 2 Norwegian national samples. *Am J Public Health.* 2004;94:1230-1238.
23. Charlton A, Blair V. Predicting the onset of smoking in boys and girls. *Soc Sci Med.* 1989;29:813-818.
24. Aitken PP, Leathar DS, O'Hagan FJ, Squair SI. Children's awareness of cigarette advertisements and brand imagery. *Br J Addict.* 1987;82:615-622.
25. DSTAT Software for the Meta-analytic Review of Research Literature. *Version 1.11.* Mahwah, NJ: Lawrence Earlbaum Associates; 1995.
26. Comprehensive Meta-analysis. *A Computer Program for Research Synthesis: Version 2.2.023.* Englewood, NJ: Biostat; 2005.
27. Overton RC. A comparison of fixed-effects and mixed (random-effects) models for meta-analysis tests of moderator variable effects. *Psychol Methods.* 1998;3:354-379.
28. Stram DO. Meta-analysis of published data using a linear mixed-effects model. *Biometrics.* 1996;52:536-544.
29. Higgins JP, Thompson SG, Deeks JJ, Altman DG. Measuring inconsistency in meta-analyses. *BMJ.* 2003;327:557-560.
30. Begg CB, Mazumdar M. Operating characteristics of a rank correlation test for publication bias. *Biometrics.* 1994;50:1088-1101.
31. Egger M, Davey Smith G, Schneider M, Minder C. Bias in meta-analysis detected by a simple, graphical test. *BMJ.* 1997;315:629-634.
32. Peters JL, Sutton AJ, Jones DR, Abrams KR, Rushton L. Comparison of two methods to detect publication bias in meta-analysis. *JAMA.* 2006;295:676-680.
33. Rosenthal R. Combining results of independent studies. *Psychol Bull.* 1978;85:185-193.
34. Rosenthal R. The file drawer problem and tolerance for null results. *Psychol Bull.* 1979;86:638-641.
35. Orwin RG. A fail-safe *N* for effect size in meta-analysis. *J Educ Stat.* 1983;8:157-159.
36. Mullen B, Muellerleile P, Bryant B. Cumulative meta-analysis: a consideration of indicators of sufficiency and stability. *Pers Soc Psychol Bull.* 2001;27:1450-1462.
37. Muellerleile P, Mullen B. Sufficiency and stability of evidence for public health interventions using cumulative meta-analysis. *Am J Public Health.* 2006;96:515-522.
38. Borenstein M. Software for publication bias. In: Rothstein HR, Sutton AJ, Borenstein M, eds. *Publication Bias in Meta-analysis: Prevention, Assessment and Adjustments.* Chichester, England: John Wiley & Sons Ltd; 2005:193-220.
39. *Report to Congress Pursuant to the Cigarette Smoking Act 1978: An Action Oriented Research Program for Discovering and Creating the Best Possible Image for Viceroy Cigarettes, Ted Bates Advertising, 1975.* Washington, DC: Federal Trade Commission; 1975. Document AD11345.
40. Tye JB. Cigarette ads in kids' movies. *Tob Youth Rep.* 1989;4:1-2.
41. National Association of Attorneys General. *Master Settlement Agreement.* Washington, DC: National Association of Attorneys General; 1998.
42. Aitken PP, Eadie DR, Hastings GB, Haywood AJ. Predisposing effects of cigarette advertising on children's intentions to smoke when older. *Br J Addict.* 1991;86:383-390.
43. Armstrong BK, de Klerk NH, Shean RE, Dunn DA, Dolin PJ. Influence of education and advertising on the uptake of smoking by children. *Med J Aust.* 1990;152:117-124.
44. Arnett JJ. Adolescents' responses to cigarette advertisements for five "youth brands" and one "adult brand." *J Res Adolesc.* 2001;11:425-443.
45. Borzekowski DL, Flora JA, Feighery E, Schooler C. The perceived influence of cigarette advertisements and smoking susceptibility among seventh graders. *J Health Commun.* 1999;4:105-118.
46. Goldberg ME. American media and the smoking-related behaviors of Asian adolescents. *J Advertising Res.* 2003;43:2-11.
47. Hawkins K, Hane AC. Adolescents' perceptions of print cigarette advertising: a case for counteradvertising. *J Health Commun.* 2000;5:83-96.
48. Kaufman NJ, Castrucci BC, Mowery PD, Gerlach KK, Emont S, Orleans CT. Predictors of change on the smoking uptake continuum among adolescents. *Arch Pediatr Adolesc Med.* 2002;156:581-587.
49. Klitzner M, Gruenewald PJ, Bamberger E. Cigarette advertising and adolescent experimentation with smoking. *Br J Addict.* 1991;86:287-298.
50. Straub DM, Hills NK, Thompson PJ, Moscicki AB. Effects of pro- and anti-tobacco advertising on nonsmoking adolescents' intentions to smoke. *J Adolesc Health.* 2003;32:36-43.
51. Unger JB, Johnson CA, Rohrbach LA. Recognition and liking of tobacco and alcohol advertisements among adolescents: relationships with susceptibility to substance use. *Prev Med.* 1995;24:461-466.
52. Aitken PP, Leathar DS, Squair SI. Children's awareness of cigarette brand sponsorship of sports and games in the UK. *Health Educ Res.* 1986;1:203-211.

53. Donovan RJ, Jancey J, Jones S. Tobacco point of sale advertising increases positive brand user imagery. *Tob Control.* 2002;11:191-194.
54. Fischer PM, Schwartz MP, Richards JW, et al. Brand logo recognition by children aged 3 to 6 years. *JAMA.* 1991;266:3145-3148.
55. McCool JP, Cameron LD, Petrie KJ. Adolescent perceptions of smoking imagery in film. *Soc Sci Med.* 2001;52:1577-1587.
56. Pechmann C, Ratneshwar S. The effects of antismoking and cigarette advertising on young adolescents' perceptions of peers who smoke. *J Consum Res.* 1994;21:236-251.
57. Shadel WG, Niaura R, Abrams DB. Who am I? the role of self-conflict in adolescents' responses to cigarette advertising. *J Behav Med.* 2004;27:463-475.
58. Shadel WG, Niaura R, Abrams DB. Adolescents' responses to the gender valence of cigarette advertising imagery: the role of affect and the self-concept. *Addict Behav.* 2004;29:1735-1744.
59. Sun D, Anderson M, Shah A, Julliard K. Early adolescents' perceptions of cigarette smoking: a cross-sectional survey in a junior high school. *Adolescence.* 1998;33:805-810.
60. Charlton A. Children's opinions about smoking. *J R Coll Gen Pract.* 1984;34:483-487.
61. Distefan JM, Gilpin EA, Sargent JD, Pierce JP. Do movie stars encourage adolescents to start smoking? evidence from California. *Prev Med.* 1999;28:1-11.
62. Gidwani PP, Sobol A, DeJong W, Perrin JM, Gortmaker SL. Television viewing and initiation of smoking among youth. *Pediatrics.* 2002;110:505-508.
63. Goldberg ME, Baumgartner H. Cross-country attraction as a motivation for product consumption. *J Bus Res.* 2002;55:901-906.
64. Hunter SM, Croft JB, Burke GL, Parker FC, Webber LS, Berenson GS. Longitudinal patterns of cigarette smoking and smokeless tobacco use in youth: the Bogalusa Heart Study. *Am J Public Health.* 1986;76:193-195.
65. Unger JB, Johnson CA, Stoddard JL, Nezami E, Chou CP. Identification of adolescents at risk for smoking initiation: validation of a measure of susceptibility. *Addict Behav.* 1997;22:81-91.
66. Vaidya SG, Vaidya JS, Naik UD. Sports sponsorship by cigarette companies influences the adolescent children's mind and helps initiate smoking: results of a national study in India. *J Indian Med Assoc.* 1999;97:354-356, 359.
67. Albers AB, Biener L. Adolescent participation in tobacco promotions: the role of psychosocial factors. *Pediatrics.* 2003;111:402-406.
68. Biener L, Siegel M. The role of tobacco advertising and promotion in smoking initiation. In: National Cancer Institute, ed. *Changing Adolescent Smoking Prevalence.* Bethesda, Md: US Dept of Health and Human Services, National Institutes of Health, National Cancer Institute; 2001. NIH publication 02-5086.
69. Feighery E, Borzekowski DL, Schooler C, Flora J. Seeing, wanting, owning: the relationship between receptivity to tobacco marketing and smoking susceptibility in young people. *Tob Control.* 1998;7:123-128.
70. Gilpin EA, Pierce JP, Rosbrook B. Are adolescents receptive to current sales promotion practices of the tobacco industry? *Prev Med.* 1997;26:14-21.
71. Pierce JP, Distefan JM, Jackson C, White MM, Gilpin EA. Does tobacco marketing undermine the influence of recommended parenting in discouraging adolescents from smoking? *Am J Prev Med.* 2002;23:73-81.
72. Hastings GB, Ryan H, Teer P, MacKintosh AM. Cigarette advertising and children's smoking: why Reg was withdrawn. *BMJ.* 1994;309:933-937.
73. Wakefield M, Flay B, Nichter M, Giovino G. Role of the media in influencing trajectories of youth smoking. *Addiction.* 2003;98(suppl 1):79-103.
74. Young EC, Moschis GP. *Review of Eye Tracking and Recall Study of Adolescents Viewing Tobacco Advertisements.* Fort Lee, NJ: Perception Research Services, American Tobacco Document Collection; January 5, 1989. Bates No. 980108834/8845.
75. Pierce JP, Gilpin EA. A historical analysis of tobacco marketing and the uptake of smoking by youth in the United States: 1890-1977. *Health Psychol.* 1995;14:500-508.
76. Pierce JP, Lee L, Gilpin EA. Smoking initiation by adolescent girls, 1944 through 1988: an association with targeted advertising. *JAMA.* 1994;271:608-611.
77. Wakefield MA, Ruel EE, Chaloupka FJ, Slater SJ, Kaufman NJ. Association of point-of-purchase tobacco advertising and promotions with choice of usual brand among teenage smokers. *J Health Commun.* 2002;7:113-121.
78. Pucci LG, Siegel M. Exposure to brand-specific cigarette advertising in magazines and its impact on youth smoking. *Prev Med.* 1999;29:313-320.
79. Andrews J, Netemeyer RG, Burton S, Moberg D, Christiansen A. Understanding adolescent intentions to smoke: an examination of relationships among social influence, prior trial behavior, and antitobacco campaign advertising. *J Mark.* 2004;68:110-123.
80. Choi WS, Farkas AJ, Rosbrook B, Elder JP, Pierce JP. Does advertising promote smokeless tobacco use among adolescent boys? evidence from California. *Tob Control.* 1995;4(suppl 1):S57-S63.
81. Audrain-McGovern J, Rodriguez D, Tercyak KP, Cuevas J, Rodgers K, Patterson F. Identifying and characterizing adolescent smoking trajectories. *Cancer Epidemiol Biomarkers Prev.* 2004;13:2023-2034.
82. Henriksen L, Feighery EC, Wang Y, Fortmann SP. Association of retail tobacco marketing with adolescent smoking. *Am J Public Health.* 2004;94:2081-2083.
83. Lopez ML, Herrero P, Comas A, et al. Impact of cigarette advertising on smoking behaviour in Spanish adolescents as measured using recognition of billboard advertising. *Eur J Public Health.* 2004;14:428-432.
84. Santana Y, Gonzalez B, Pinilla J, Calvo JR, Barber P. Young adolescents, tobacco advertising, and smoking. *J Drug Educ.* 2003;33:427-444.
85. Alexander HM, Callcott R, Dobson AJ, et al. Cigarette smoking and drug use in schoolchildren, IV: factors associated with changes in smoking behaviour. *Int J Epidemiol.* 1983;12:59-66.
86. Altman DG, Levine DW, Coeytaux R, Slade J, Jaffe R. Tobacco promotion and susceptibility to tobacco use among adolescents aged 12 through 17 years in a nationally representative sample. *Am J Public Health.* 1996;86:1590-1593.
87. Arnett JJ, Terhanian G. Adolescents' responses to cigarette advertisements: links between exposure, liking, and the appeal of smoking. *Tob Control.* 1998;7:129-133.
88. Biener L, Siegel M. Tobacco marketing and adolescent smoking: more support for a causal inference. *Am J Public Health.* 2000;90:407-411.
89. Botvin GJ, Goldberg CJ, Botvin EM, Dusenbury L. Smoking behavior of adolescents exposed to cigarette advertising. *Public Health Rep.* 1993;108:217-224.
90. Chapman S, Fitzgerald B. Brand preference and advertising recall in adolescent smokers: some implications for health promotion. *Am J Public Health.* 1982;72:491-494.
91. Charlton A, While D, Kelly S. Boys' smoking and cigarette-brand-sponsored motor racing [letter]. *Lancet.* 1997;350:1474.
92. Chen X, Cruz TB, Schuster DV, Unger JB, Johnson CA. Receptivity to protobacco media and its impact on cigarette smoking among ethnic minority youth in California. *J Health Commun.* 2002;7:95-111.
93. Choi WS, Ahluwalia JS, Harris KJ, Okuyemi K. Progression to established smoking: the influence of tobacco marketing. *Am J Prev Med.* 2002;22:228-233.
94. Dalton MA, Sargent JD, Beach ML, et al. Effect of viewing smoking in movies on adolescent smoking initiation: a cohort study. *Lancet.* 2003;362:281-285.
95. DiFranza JR, Richards JW, Paulman PM, et al. RJR Nabisco's cartoon camel promotes Camel cigarettes to children [published correction appears in *JAMA.* 1992;268:2034]. *JAMA.* 1991;266:3149-3153.
96. Emri S, Bagci T, Karakoca Y, Baris E. Recognition of cigarette brand names and logos by primary schoolchildren in Ankara, Turkey. *Tob Control.* 1998;7:386-392.
97. Goldstein AO, Fischer PM, Richards JW Jr, Creten D. Relationship between high school student smoking and recognition of cigarette advertisements. *J Pediatr.* 1987;110:488-491.
98. Health Education Authority. *An Investigation of the Appeal and Impact of the Embassy Regal "Reg" Campaign on Young People.* London, England: Health Education Authority; 1993.
99. Henke LL. Young children's perceptions of cigarette brand advertising symbols: awareness, affect, and target market identification. *J Advertising.* 1995;4:13-28.
100. Klein JD, Forehand B, Oliveri J, Patterson CJ, Kupersmidt JB, Strecher V. Candy cigarettes: do they encourage children's smoking? *Pediatrics.* 1992;89:27-31.
101. Lam TH, Chung SF, Betson CL, Wong CM, Hedley AJ. Tobacco advertisements: one of the strongest risk factors for smoking in Hong Kong students. *Am J Prev Med.* 1998;14:217-223.
102. Maassen IT, Kremers SP, Mudde AN, Joof BM. Smoking initiation among Gambian adolescents: social cognitive influences and the effect of cigarette sampling. *Health Educ Res.* 2004;19:551-560.
103. Unger JB, Chen X. The role of social networks and media receptivity in predicting age of smoking initiation: a proportional hazards model of risk and protective factors. *Addict Behav.* 1999;24:371-381.
104. Pechmann C, Shih C-F. Smoking scenes in movies and antismoking advertisements before movies: effects on youth. *J Mark.* 1999;63:1-13.
105. Peters J, Betson CL, Hedley AJ, et al. Recognition of cigarette brand names and logos by young children in Hong Kong. *Tob Control.* 1995;4:150-155.
106. Pierce JP, Choi WS, Gilpin EA, Farkas AJ, Berry CC. Tobacco industry promotion of cigarettes and adolescent smoking. *JAMA.* 1998;279:511-515.
107. Sargent JD, Dalton M, Beach M, Bernhardt A, Heatherton T, Stevens M. Effect of cigarette promotions on smoking uptake among adolescents. *Prev Med.* 2000;30:320-327.
108. Schooler C, Feighery E, Flora JA. Seventh graders' self-reported exposure to cigarette marketing and its relationship to their smoking behavior. *Am J Public Health.* 1996;86:1216-1221.
109. Turco RM. Effects of exposure to cigarette advertisements on adolescents' attitudes toward smoking. *J Appl Soc Psychol.* 1997;27:1115-1130.
110. Vaidya SG, Naik UD, Vaidya JS. Effect of sports sponsorship by tobacco companies on children's experimentation with tobacco. *BMJ.* 1996;313:400.
111. While D, Kelly S, Huang W, Charlton A. Cigarette advertising and onset of smoking in children: questionnaire survey. *BMJ.* 1996;313:398-399.

112. Sargent JD, Beach ML, Adachi-Mejia AM, et al. Exposure to movie smoking: its relation to smoking initiation among US adolescents. *Pediatrics.* 2005;116:1183-1191.
113. MacFadyen L, Hastings G, MacKintosh AM. Cross sectional study of young people's awareness of and involvement with tobacco marketing. *BMJ.* 2001;322:513-517.
114. Maziak W, Rzehak P, Keil U, Weiland SK. Smoking among adolescents in Muenster, Germany: increase in prevalence (1995-2000) and relation to tobacco advertising. *Prev Med.* 2003;36:172-176.
115. Otake K, Shimai S. Relationship between stages of smoking acquisition and environmental factors among junior high school students. *Psychol Rep.* 2002;90:257-261.
116. Pechmann C, Knight SJ. An experimental investigation of the joint effects of advertising and peers on adolescents' beliefs and intentions about cigarette consumption. *J Consum Res.* 2002;29:5-19.
117. Pierce JP, Distefan JM, Kaplan RM, Gilpin EA. The role of curiosity in smoking initiation. *Addict Behav.* 2005;30:685-696.
118. Sargent JD, Beach ML, Dalton MA, et al. Effect of seeing tobacco use in films on trying smoking among adolescents: cross sectional study. *BMJ.* 2001;323:1394-1397.
119. Sargent JD, Dalton MA, Beach ML, et al. Viewing tobacco use in movies: does it shape attitudes that mediate adolescent smoking? *Am J Prev Med.* 2002;22:137-145.
120. Tickle JJ, Sargent JD, Dalton MA, Beach ML, Heatherton TF. Favourite movie stars, their tobacco use in contemporary movies, and its association with adolescent smoking. *Tob Control.* 2001;10:16-22.
121. Unger JB, Cruz TB, Schuster D, Flora JA, Johnson CA. Measuring exposure to pro- and anti-tobacco marketing among adolescents: intercorrelations among measures and associations with smoking status. *J Health Commun.* 2001;6:11-29.
122. Conrad KM, Flay BR, Hill D. Why children start smoking cigarettes: predictors of onset. *Br J Addict.* 1992;87:1711-1724.
123. de Vries H, Engels R, Kremers S, Wetzels J, Mudde A. Parents' and friends' smoking status as predictors of smoking onset: findings from six European countries. *Health Educ Res.* 2003;18:627-636.
124. Tyas SL, Pederson LL. Psychosocial factors related to adolescent smoking: a critical review of the literature. *Tob Control.* 1998;7:409-420.
125. Wellman RJ, DiFranza JR, Savageau JA, Dussault GF. Short term patterns of early smoking acquisition. *Tob Control.* 2004;13:251-257.
126. Chung PJ, Garfield CF, Rathouz PJ, Lauderdale DB, Lantos J. Youth targeting by tobacco manufacturers since the Master Settlement Agreement: the first study to document violations of the youth-targeting ban in magazine ads by the three top U.S. tobacco companies. *Health Aff (Millwood).* 2001;21:254-263.
127. Hamilton WL, Turner-Bowker DM, Celebucki CC, Connolly GN. Cigarette advertising in magazines: the tobacco industry's response to the Master Settlement Agreement and to public pressure. *Tob Control.* 2002;11(suppl 2):ii54-ii58.
128. Glantz SA, Kacirk KW, McCulloch C. Back to the future: smoking in movies in 2002 compared with 1950 levels. *Am J Public Health.* 2004;94:261-263.
129. Anderson CA, Bushman BJ. Effects of violent video games on aggressive behavior, aggressive cognition, aggressive affect, physiological arousal, and prosocial behavior: a meta-analytic review of the scientific literature. *Psychol Sci.* 2001;12:353-359.
130. Paik H, Comstock G. The effects of television violence on antisocial behavior: a meta-analysis. *Communication Res.* 1994;21:516-546.
131. US Department of Health and Human Services. *The Health Consequences of Smoking: A Report of the Surgeon General.* Rockville, Md: US Dept of Health and Human Services, Public Health Service, Centers for Disease Control and Prevention, Office on Smoking and Health; 2004. DHHS publication 0-16-051576-2.
132. Burns DM, Garfinkel G, Samet JM. Introduction, summary and conclusions. In: *Changes in Cigarette-Related Disease Risks and Their Implication for Prevention and Control: Smoking and Tobacco Control Monograph 8.* Bethesda, Md: US Dept of Health and Human Services, Public Health Service, National Institute of Health, National Cancer Institute; 1997. NIH publication 97-4213.
133. World Health Organization. WHO Framework Convention on Tobacco Control (World Health Assembly resolution 56.1). http://www.who.int/tobacco/framework/final_text/en/index5.html. Accessed June 1, 2006.


The battle against infectious diseases and other dread killers of the early twentieth century has been spectacularly successful. But there is another dread killer, against which our efforts have proved not nearly so effective. This, indeed, has become the leading cause of children's death, and its name is 'accident.'

—From *A Parent's Guide to Children's Illnesses* by Dr John Henderson, 1957

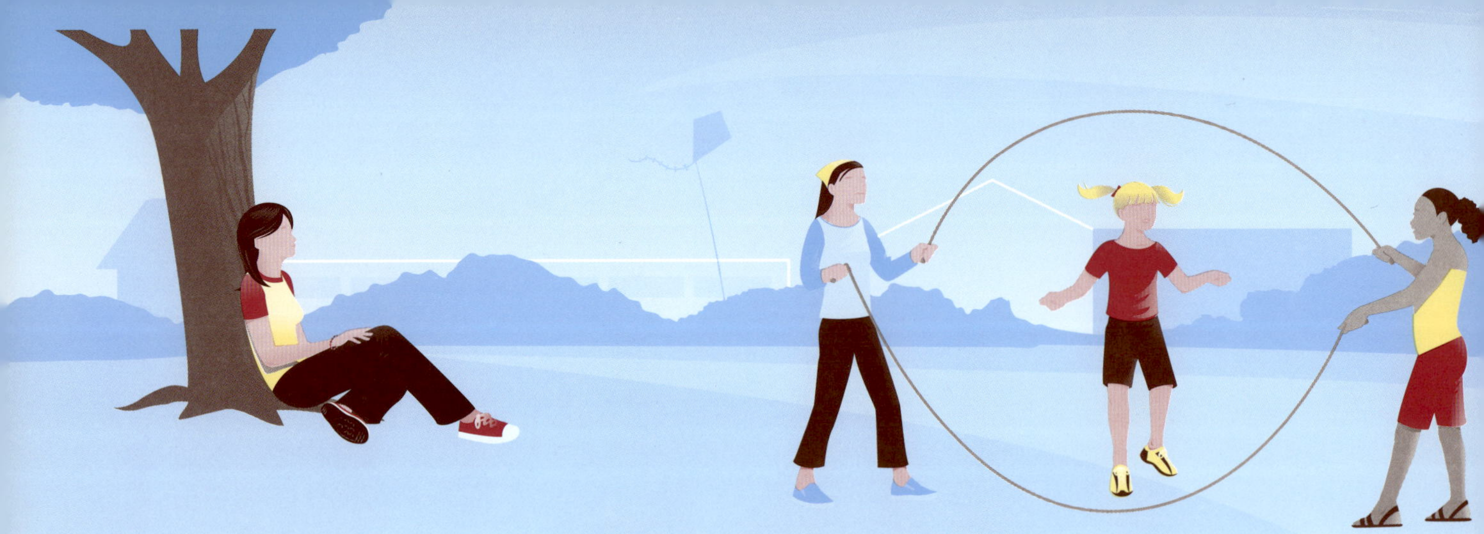

# Introducing GARDASIL—helping you

- **GARDASIL is a vaccine indicated in girls and women 9 to 26 years of age for the prevention of cervical cancer, precancerous or dysplastic lesions, and genital warts caused by human papillomavirus (HPV) Types 6, 11, 16, and 18.**
- **A complete vaccination regimen of GARDASIL consists of a 3-dose schedule.**

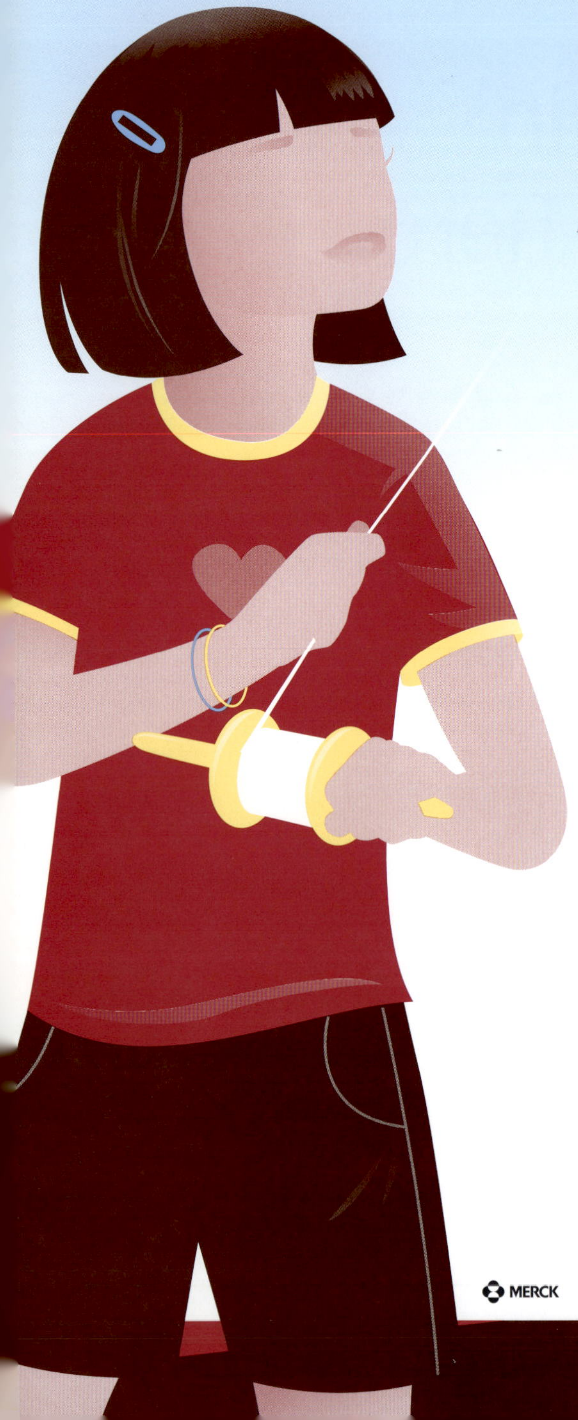

## Select safety information

GARDASIL is contraindicated in individuals who are hypersensitive to the active substances or to any of the excipients of the vaccine.

GARDASIL does not substitute for routine cervical cancer screening, and women who receive GARDASIL should continue to undergo screening per standard of care.

Vaccination with GARDASIL may not result in protection in all vaccine recipients.

GARDASIL is not intended to be used for treatment of active genital warts; cervical cancer; cervical intraepithelial neoplasia, vulvar intraepithelial neoplasia, or vaginal intraepithelial neoplasia.

To place an order, call **1-800-MERCK-RX,** or visit **www.MerckVaccines.com.**

MERCK

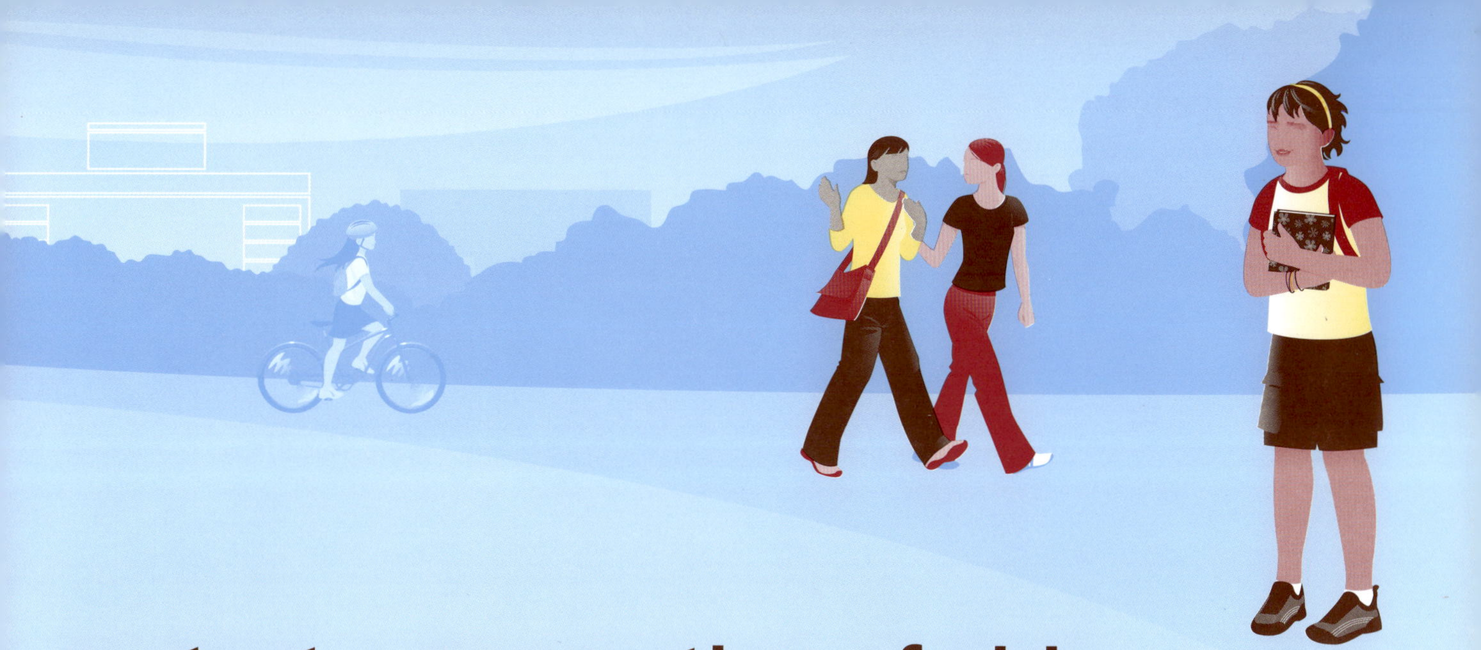

# protect a generation of girls

**The only quadrivalent vaccine that prevents disease caused by significant human papillomavirus (HPV) types: 6, 11, 16, and 18**

- **CERVICAL CANCER**
- **CERVICAL DYSPLASIA**
- **GENITAL WARTS**

- **Now is the time to vaccinate girls and young women 9 to 26 years of age.**

The vaccine-related adverse experiences that were observed among recipients of GARDASIL at a frequency of at least 1.0% and greater than placebo were pain, swelling, erythema, fever, nausea, pruritus, and dizziness.

Please see Brief Summary of Prescribing Information on adjacent page.

GARDASIL®

**[Quadrivalent Human Papillomavirus (Types 6,11,16,18) Recombinant Vaccine]**

# GARDASIL®

## [Quadrivalent Human Papillomavirus (Types 6,11,16,18) Recombinant Vaccine]



**BRIEF SUMMARY OF PRESCRIBING INFORMATION**

**CONTRAINDICATIONS:** Hypersensitivity to the active substances or to any of the excipients of the vaccine.

Individuals who develop symptoms indicative of hypersensitivity after receiving a dose of GARDASIL should not receive further doses of GARDASIL.

**PRECAUTIONS:** *General:* As for any vaccine, vaccination with GARDASIL may not result in protection in all vaccine recipients.

This vaccine is not intended to be used for treatment of active genital warts; cervical cancer; cervical intraepithelial neoplasia (CIN), vulvar intraepithelial neoplasia (VIN), or vaginal intraepithelial neoplasia (VaIN).

This vaccine will not protect against diseases that are not caused by human papillomavirus (HPV).

GARDASIL has not been shown to protect against diseases due to non-vaccine HPV types.

As with all injectable vaccines, appropriate medical treatment should always be readily available in case of rare anaphylactic reactions following the administration of the vaccine.

The decision to administer or delay vaccination because of a current or recent febrile illness depends largely on the severity of the symptoms and their etiology. Low-grade fever itself and mild upper respiratory infection are not generally contraindications to vaccination.

Individuals with impaired immune responsiveness, whether due to the use of immunosuppressive therapy, a genetic defect, Human Immunodeficiency Virus (HIV) infection, or other causes, may have reduced antibody response to active immunization (see PRECAUTIONS, ***Drug Interactions***).

As with other intramuscular injections, GARDASIL should not be given to individuals with bleeding disorders such as hemophilia or thrombocytopenia, or to persons on anticoagulant therapy unless the potential benefits clearly outweigh the risk of administration. If the decision is made to administer GARDASIL to such persons, it should be given with steps to avoid the risk of hematoma following the injection.

*Information for the Patient, Parent, or Guardian:* The health care provider should inform the patient, parent, or guardian that vaccination does not substitute for routine cervical cancer screening. Women who receive GARDASIL should continue to undergo cervical cancer screening per standard of care.

The health care provider should provide the vaccine information required to be given with each vaccination to the patient, parent, or guardian.

The health care provider should inform the patient, parent, or guardian of the benefits and risks associated with vaccination. For risks associated with vaccination, see PRECAUTIONS and ADVERSE REACTIONS.

GARDASIL is not recommended for use in pregnant women.

The health care provider should inform the patient, parent, or guardian of the importance of completing the immunization series unless contraindicated.

Patients, parents, or guardians should be instructed to report any adverse reactions to their health care provider.

***Drug Interactions:*** *Use with Other Vaccines:* Results from clinical studies indicate that GARDASIL may be administered concomitantly (at a separate injection site) with hepatitis B vaccine (recombinant) (see CLINICAL PHARMACOLOGY, *Studies with Other Vaccines*). Co-administration of GARDASIL with other vaccines has not been studied.

*Use with Hormonal Contraceptives:* In clinical studies, 13,293 subjects (vaccine = 6644; placebo = 6649) who had post-Month 7 follow-up used hormonal contraceptives for a total of 17,597 person-years (65.1% of the total follow-up time in the study for these subjects). Use of hormonal contraceptives or lack of use of hormonal contraceptives among study participants did not alter vaccine efficacy in the per-protocol efficacy (PPE) population.

*Use with Systemic Immunosuppressive Medications:* Immunosuppressive therapies, including irradiation, antimetabolites, alkylating agents, cytotoxic drugs, and corticosteroids (used in greater than physiologic doses), may reduce the immune responses to vaccines (see PRECAUTIONS, ***General***).

*Carcinogenesis, Mutagenesis, Impairment of Fertility:* GARDASIL has not been evaluated for the potential to cause carcinogenicity or genotoxicity.

GARDASIL administered to female rats at a dose of 120 mcg total protein, which corresponds to approximately 300-fold excess relative to the projected human dose, had no effects on mating performance, fertility, or embryonic/fetal survival.

***Pregnancy:*** *Pregnancy Category B:* Reproduction studies have been performed in female rats at doses up to 300 times the human dose (on a mg/kg basis) and have revealed no evidence of impaired female fertility or harm to the fetus due to GARDASIL. However, it is not known whether GARDASIL can cause fetal harm when administered to a pregnant woman or if it can affect reproductive capacity. GARDASIL should be given to a pregnant woman only if clearly needed. An evaluation of the effect of GARDASIL on embryo-fetal, pre- and postweaning development was conducted using rats. One group of rats was administered GARDASIL twice prior to gestation, during the period of organogenesis (gestation day 6) and on lactation day 7. A second group of pregnant rats was administered GARDASIL during the period of organogenesis (gestation day 6) and on lactation day 7 only. GARDASIL was administered at 0.5 mL/rat/occasion (approximately 300-fold excess relative to the projected human dose on a mg/kg basis) by intramuscular injection. No adverse effects on mating, fertility, pregnancy, parturition, lactation, embryo-fetal or pre- and postweaning development were observed. There were no vaccine-related fetal malformations or other evidence of teratogenesis noted in this study. In addition, there were no treatment-related effects on developmental signs, behavior, reproductive performance, or fertility of the offspring. The effect of GARDASIL on male fertility has not been studied.

In clinical studies, women underwent urine pregnancy testing prior to administration of each dose of GARDASIL. Women who were found to be pregnant before completion of a 3-dose regimen of GARDASIL were instructed to defer completion of their vaccination regimen until resolution of the pregnancy.

During clinical trials, 2266 women (vaccine = 1115 vs. placebo = 1151) reported at least 1 pregnancy each. Overall, the proportions of pregnancies with an adverse outcome were comparable in subjects who received GARDASIL and subjects who received placebo. Overall, 40 and 41 subjects in the group that received GARDASIL or placebo, respectively (3.6% and 3.6% of all subjects who reported a pregnancy in the respective vaccination groups), experienced a serious adverse experience during pregnancy. The most common events reported were conditions that can result in Caesarean section (e.g., failure of labor, malpresentation, cephalopelvic disproportion), premature onset of labor (e.g., threatened abortions, premature rupture of membranes), and pregnancy-related medical problems (e.g., pre-eclampsia, hyperemesis). The proportions of pregnant subjects who experienced such events were comparable between the vaccination groups.

There were 15 cases of congenital anomaly in pregnancies that occurred in subjects who received GARDASIL and 16 cases of congenital anomaly in pregnancies that occurred in subjects who received placebo.

Further sub-analyses were conducted to evaluate pregnancies with estimated onset within 30 days or more than 30 days from administration of a dose of GARDASIL or placebo. For pregnancies with estimated onset within 30 days of vaccination, 5 cases of congenital anomaly were observed in the group that received GARDASIL compared to 0 cases of congenital anomaly in the group that received placebo. The congenital anomalies seen in pregnancies with estimated onset within 30 days of vaccination included pyloric stenosis, congenital megacolon, congenital hydronephrosis, hip dysplasia and club foot. Conversely, in pregnancies with onset more than 30 days following vaccination, 10 cases of congenital anomaly were observed in the group that received GARDASIL compared with 16 cases of congenital anomaly in the group that received placebo. The types of anomalies observed were consistent (regardless of when pregnancy occurred in relation to vaccination) with those generally observed in pregnancies in women aged 16 to 26 years.

*Pregnancy Registry for GARDASIL:* Merck & Co., Inc. maintains a Pregnancy Registry to monitor fetal outcomes of pregnant women exposed to GARDASIL. Patients and health care providers are encouraged to report any exposure to GARDASIL during pregnancy by calling (800) 986-8999.

*Lactation:* It is not known whether vaccine antigens or antibodies induced by the vaccine are excreted in human milk.

Because many drugs are excreted in human milk, caution should be exercised when GARDASIL is administered to a nursing woman.

A total of 995 nursing mothers (vaccine = 500, placebo = 495) were given GARDASIL or placebo during the vaccination period of the clinical trials. Geometric mean titers (GMTs) in nursing and non-nursing mothers were as follows:

The GMTs in nursing mothers were 595.9 (95% CI: 522.5, 679.5) for anti-HPV 6, 864.3 (95% CI: 754.0, 990.8) for anti-HPV 11, 3056.9 (95% CI: 2594.4, 3601.8) for anti-HPV 16, and 527.2 (95% CI: 450.9, 616.5) for anti-HPV 18. The GMTs for women who did not nurse during vaccine administration were 540.1 (95% CI: 523.5, 557.2) for anti-HPV 6, 746.3 (95% CI: 720.4, 773.3) for anti-HPV 11, 2290.8 (95% CI: 2180.7, 2406.3) for anti-HPV 16, and 456.0 (95% CI: 438.4, 474.3) for anti-HPV 18.

Overall, 17 and 9 infants of subjects who received GARDASIL or placebo, respectively (representing 3.4% and 1.8% of the total number of subjects who were breast-feeding during the period in which they received GARDASIL or placebo, respectively), experienced a serious adverse experience. None was judged by the investigator to be vaccine related.

In clinical studies, a higher number of breast-feeding infants (n = 6) whose mothers received GARDASIL had acute respiratory illnesses within 30 days post-vaccination of the mother as compared to infants (n = 2) whose mothers received placebo. In these studies, the rates of other adverse experiences in the mother and the nursing infant were comparable between vaccination groups.

*Pediatric Use:* The safety and efficacy of GARDASIL have not been evaluated in children younger than 9 years.

*Geriatric Use:* The safety and efficacy of GARDASIL have not been evaluated in adults above the age of 26 years.

**ADVERSE REACTIONS:** In 5 clinical trials (4 placebo-controlled), subjects were administered GARDASIL or placebo on the day of enrollment, and approximately 2 and 6 months thereafter. Few subjects (0.1%) discontinued due to adverse experiences. In all except 1 of the clinical trials, safety was evaluated using vaccination report card (VRC)-aided surveillance for 14 days after each injection of GARDASIL or placebo. The subjects who were monitored using VRC-aided surveillance included 5088 girls and women 9 through 26 years of age at enrollment who received GARDASIL and 3790 girls and women who received placebo.

*Common Adverse Experiences: Vaccine-related Common Adverse Experiences:* The vaccine-related adverse experiences that were observed among female recipients of GARDASIL at a frequency of at least 1.0% and also at a greater frequency than that observed among placebo recipients are shown in Table 1.

**Table 1. Vaccine-related Injection-site and Systemic Adverse Experiences***

| Adverse Experience (1 to 5 Days Postvaccination) | GARDASIL (N = 5088) % | Aluminum-Containing Placebo (N = 3470) % | Saline Placebo (N = 320) % |
|---|---|---|---|
| *Injection Site* | | | |
| Pain | 83.9 | 75.4 | 48.6 |
| Swelling | 25.4 | 15.8 | 7.3 |
| Erythema | 24.6 | 18.4 | 12.1 |
| Pruritus | 3.1 | 2.8 | 0.6 |

| Adverse Experience (1 to 15 Days Postvaccination) | GARDASIL (N = 5088) % | Placebo (N = 3790) % |
|---|---|---|
| *Systemic* | | |
| Fever | 10.3 | 8.6 |

*The vaccine-related adverse experiences that were observed among recipients of GARDASIL were at a frequency of at least 1.0% and also at a greater frequency than that observed among placebo recipients.

*All-cause Common Systemic Adverse Experiences:* All-cause systemic adverse experiences for female subjects reported 1 to 15 days postvaccination and observed at a frequency of ≥1% with incidence in the GARDASIL group (N = 5088) ≥ that of the placebo group (N = 3790), respectively, were: pyrexia (13.0% vs. 11.2%), nausea (6.7% vs. 6.6%), nasopharyngitis (6.4% vs. 6.4%), dizziness (4.0% vs. 3.7%), diarrhea (3.6% vs. 3.5%), vomiting (2.4% vs. 1.9%), myalgia (2.0% vs. 2.0%), cough (2.0% vs. 1.5%), toothache (1.5% vs. 1.4%), upper respiratory tract infection (1.5% vs. 1.5%), malaise (1.4% vs. 1.2%), arthralgia (1.2% vs. 0.9%), insomnia (1.2% vs. 0.9%), and nasal congestion (1.1% vs. 0.9%).

*Evaluation of Injection-site Adverse Experiences by Dose:* An analysis of injection-site adverse experiences in female subjects by dose is shown in Table 2. Overall, 94.3% of subjects who received GARDASIL judged their injection-site adverse experience to be mild or moderate in intensity.

**Table 2. Postdose Evaluation of Injection-site Adverse Experiences**

| Adverse Experience | Vaccine (% occurrence) Post-dose 1 | Post-dose 2 | Post-dose 3 | Post Any Dose |
|---|---|---|---|---|
| **Pain** | 63.4 | 60.7 | 62.7 | 83.9 |
| Mild/Moderate | 62.5 | 59.7 | 61.2 | 81.1 |
| Severe | 0.9 | 1.0 | 1.5 | 2.8 |
| **Swelling*** | 10.2 | 12.8 | 15.1 | 25.4 |
| Mild/Moderate | 9.6 | 11.9 | 14.3 | 23.3 |
| Severe | 0.6 | 0.8 | 0.8 | 2.0 |
| **Erythema*** | 9.2 | 12.1 | 14.7 | 24.7 |
| Mild/Moderate | 9.0 | 11.7 | 14.3 | 23.7 |
| Severe | 0.2 | 0.3 | 0.4 | 0.9 |

*Intensity of swelling and erythema was measured by size (inches): Mild = 0 to ≤1; Moderate = >1 to ≤2; Severe = >2.

| Adverse Experience | Aluminum-Containing Placebo (% occurrence) Post-dose 1 | Post-dose 2 | Post-dose 3 | Post Any Dose | Saline Placebo (% occurrence) Post-dose 1 | Post-dose 2 | Post-dose 3 | Post Any Dose |
|---|---|---|---|---|---|---|---|---|
| **Pain** | 57.0 | 47.8 | 49.5 | 75.4 | 33.7 | 20.3 | 27.3 | 48.6 |
| Mild/Moderate | 56.6 | 47.3 | 48.9 | 74.1 | 33.3 | 20.3 | 27.0 | 48.0 |
| Severe | 0.4 | 0.5 | 0.6 | 1.3 | 0.3 | 0.0 | 0.3 | 0.6 |
| **Swelling*** | 8.2 | 7.5 | 7.6 | 15.8 | 4.4 | 3.0 | 3.3 | 7.3 |
| Mild/Moderate | 8.0 | 7.2 | 7.3 | 15.2 | 4.4 | 3.0 | 3.3 | 7.3 |
| Severe | 0.2 | 0.3 | 0.2 | 0.6 | 0.0 | 0.0 | 0.0 | 0.0 |
| **Erythema*** | 9.8 | 8.4 | 8.9 | 18.4 | 7.3 | 5.3 | 5.7 | 12.1 |
| Mild/Moderate | 9.5 | 8.3 | 8.8 | 18.0 | 7.3 | 5.3 | 5.7 | 12.1 |
| Severe | 0.3 | 0.1 | 0.1 | 0.4 | 0.0 | 0.0 | 0.0 | 0.0 |

*Evaluation of Fever by Dose:* An analysis of fever in girls and women by dose is shown in Table 3.

**Table 3. Postdose Evaluation of Fever**

| Temperature (°F) | Vaccine (% occurrence) Post-dose 1 | Post-dose 2 | Post-dose 3 | Placebo (% occurrence) Post-dose 1 | Post-dose 2 | Post-dose 3 |
|---|---|---|---|---|---|---|
| ≥100 to <102 | 3.7 | 4.1 | 4.4 | 3.1 | 3.8 | 3.6 |
| ≥102 | 0.3 | 0.5 | 0.5 | 0.3 | 0.4 | 0.6 |

*Serious Adverse Experiences:* A total of 102 subjects out of 21,464 total subjects (9- to 26-year-old girls and women and 9- to 15-year-old boys) who received both GARDASIL and placebo reported a serious adverse experience on Day 1-15 following any vaccination visit during the clinical trials for GARDASIL. The most frequently reported serious adverse experiences regardless of causality for GARDASIL compared to placebo, respectively, were: headache (0.03% vs. 0.02%), gastroenteritis (0.03% vs. 0.01%), appendicitis (0.02% vs. 0.01%), and pelvic inflammatory disease (0.02% vs. 0.01%).

One case of bronchospasm and 2 cases of asthma were reported as serious adverse experiences that occurred during Day 1-15 of any vaccination visit.

*Deaths:* Across the clinical studies, 17 deaths were reported in 21,464 male and female subjects. The events reported were consistent with events expected in healthy adolescent and adult populations. The most common cause of death was motor vehicle accident (4 subjects who received GARDASIL and 3 placebo subjects), followed by overdose/suicide (1 subject who received GARDASIL and 2 subjects who received placebo), and pulmonary embolus/deep vein thrombosis (1 subject who received GARDASIL and 1 placebo subject). In addition, there were 2 cases of sepsis, 1 case of pancreatic cancer, and 1 case of arrhythmia in the group that received GARDASIL, and 1 case of asphyxia in the placebo group.

*Systemic Autoimmune Disorders:* In the clinical studies, subjects were evaluated for new medical conditions that occurred over the course of up to 4 years of follow up. The number of subjects who received both GARDASIL and placebo and developed a new medical condition potentially indicative of a systemic immune disorder is shown in Table 4.

**Table 4. Summary of Subjects Who Reported an Incident Condition Potentially Indicative of Systemic Autoimmune Disorder After Enrollment in Clinical Trials of GARDASIL**

| Potential Autoimmune Disorder | GARDASIL (N = 11,813) | Placebo (N = 9701) |
|---|---|---|
| Specific Terms | 3 (0.025%) | 1 (0.010%) |
| Juvenile arthritis | 1 | 0 |
| Rheumatoid arthritis | 2 | 0 |
| Systemic lupus erythematosus | 0 | 1 |
| Other Terms | 6 (0.051%) | 2 (0.021%) |
| Arthritis | 5 | 2 |
| Reactive Arthritis | 1 | 0 |

N = Number of subjects enrolled

*Safety in Concomitant Use with Other Vaccines:* The safety of GARDASIL when administered concomitantly with hepatitis B vaccine (recombinant) was evaluated in a placebo-controlled study. There were no statistically significant higher rates in systemic or injection-site adverse experiences among subjects who received concomitant vaccination compared with those who received GARDASIL or hepatitis B vaccine alone.

*Reporting of Adverse Events:* The US Department of Health and Human Services has established a Vaccine Adverse Event Reporting System (VAERS) to accept all reports of suspected adverse events after the administration of any vaccine, including but not limited to the reporting of events required by the National Childhood Vaccine Injury Act of 1986. For information or a copy of the vaccine reporting form, call the VAERS toll-free number at 1-800-822-7967 or report on line to www.vaers.hhs.gov.

For more detailed information, please read the Prescribing Information.
GARDASIL is a registered trademark of Merck & Co., Inc.

MERCK



20650343(2)(300)-GRD

SECTION EDITOR: ALBERT C. YAN, MD; ASSISTANT SECTION EDITOR: SAMIR S. SHAH, MD

# Picture of the Month

*Hossam Al-Tatari, MD; Nahed Abdel-Haq, MD; Basim Asmar, MD; Michael Haupert, DO; Raja Rabah, MD*

A 16-YEAR-OLD, PREVIOUSLY HEALTHY Hispanic American female complained of coughing up small, round "brainlike" structures for the last 6 weeks. The cough was always preceded by a foreign body sensation or "something stuck" in the throat. The episodes occurred 3 to 4 times a week and were often associated with choking. Examination of the oral cavity revealed slightly enlarged tonsils without exudates. The rest of the examination results were normal. During her first visit to our clinic, she handed over 2 small, lobulated masses of white-gray material, which she had expectorated during the last few days (**Figure 1**). The material was sent for histopathologic examination (**Figure 2**).

**Author Affiliations:** Divisions of Pediatric Infectious Diseases (Drs Al-Tatari, Abdel-Haq, and Asmar) and Pediatric ENT (Dr Haupert) and Department of Pathology (Dr Rabah), Children's Hospital of Michigan, Detroit.

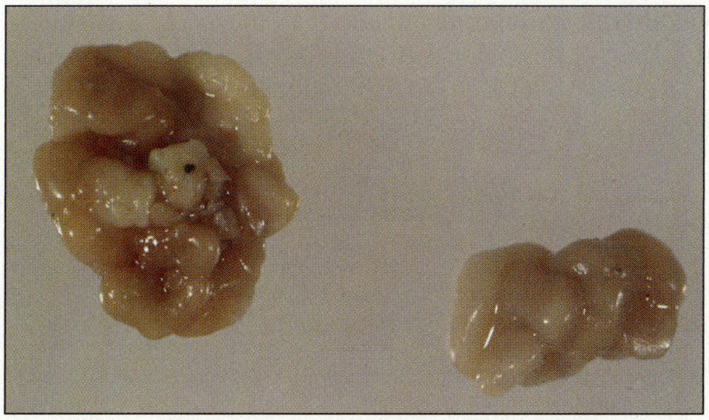

**Figure 1.** Two masses that the patient expectorated. Both consisted of lobulated, soft, white-gray material that measured 10 mm × 12 mm and 5 mm × 8 mm.

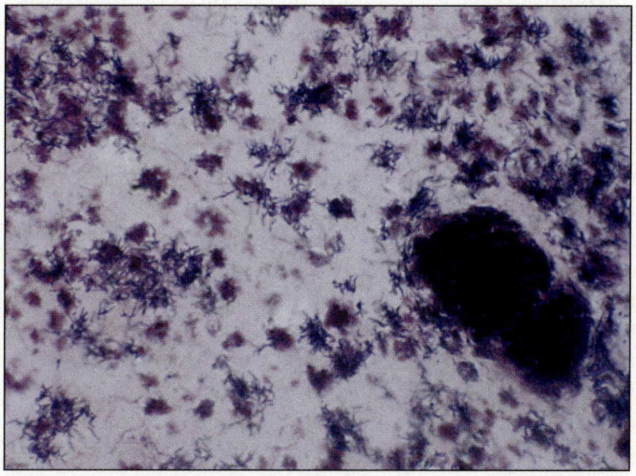

**Figure 2.** Gram stain highlights coccoid and filamentous structures.

# Denouement and Discussion

## *Tonsillar Actinomycosis*

Tonsillar actinomycosis was diagnosed in an otherwise healthy adolescent girl. Tissue histopathologic examination revealed amorphous fragments composed of slender filaments. Gram stain and Gomori methamine silver fungal stain confirmed the presence of gram-positive bacilli and granules compatible with actinomycosis. Staining for acid-fast bacilli was negative. Diagnostic evaluation was performed to locate the source of the granules. Neck and chest radiographs were normal and sputum cytologic results were negative. Direct laryngobronchoscopy revealed enlarged tonsils with copious amounts of thick particulate material in the crypts of the right tonsil.

She remained symptomatic despite 6 weeks of oral amoxicillin therapy. Subsequently, tonsillectomy was performed, and postoperatively, she stopped coughing up debris and had no further choking spells. She completed 6 months of amoxicillin therapy. She has remained well and has not expectorated any further masses.

*Actinomyces* species are strictly anaerobic, gram-positive, nonsporulating bacteria that are considered part of the normal flora of the mouth and gastrointestinal tract. Actinomycosis can involve virtually any anatomical site.[1,2] Infections are typically indolent and spread contiguously, crossing soft-tissue planes and organs with ultimate formation of draining sinus tracts. Cervicofacial infections, otherwise known as "lumpy jaw," are the most common and frequently follow tooth extraction, oral surgery, or facial trauma.[2,3]

Actinomycosis of the tonsils is a rare and poorly defined clinical entity. The presence of *Actinomyces* species in both inflamed and uninflamed tonsils has been recognized.[4] Pransky et al[5] reviewed histologic preparations from 460 patients undergoing tonsillectomy or adenotonsillectomy for recurrent tonsillitis or obstructive tonsillar hypertrophy. Actinomycetes were more prevalent in the tissues of patients with obstructive tonsillar hypertrophy. Actinomycosis was diagnosed in a 12-year-old girl who presented with difficulty swallowing for 3 months and had a tonsillar mass suggestive of a tumor.[6] Cervicofacial actinomycosis may rarely present as acute upper respiratory tract obstruction requiring urgent airway management.[7] To our knowledge, only 1 previous case of tonsillar actinomycosis presenting with a history of expectorating debris has been reported.[8] That was of an adult who complained of chronic productive cough for 3 months. He had 1 episode of expectorating a small whitish mass. Histologic examination revealed *Actinomyces* species. The patient was treated with a course of oral phenoxymethylpenicillin with no further episodes. The symptoms in our patient were more pronounced since she was producing larger masses and more often and some of her coughing episodes were associated with significant choking. The coughing episodes and foreign body sensation were probably induced by aspirating or swallowing the masses that were formed in the right tonsil.

The optimal treatment of tonsillar actinomycosis is not clear. Although a patient may respond to antibiotic treatment,[8] it is not clear if antibiotic treatment alone without surgical intervention is adequate. Our patient did not respond to antibiotic therapy alone and required tonsillectomy to clear the infection. Other forms of actinomycosis are usually treated with high-dose intravenous penicillin G or ampicillin for 4 to 6 weeks followed by high doses of oral penicillin, amoxicillin, erythromycin, clindamycin, minocycline, or tetracycline for a total of 6 to 12 months. However, surgical resection of the lesions and debridement of surrounding tissues and draining sinuses is necessary in most cases.[2,3,9,10]

Tonsillar actinomycosis should be considered in patients presenting with coughing associated with expectoration of particulate material. Tonsillectomy may be required in those patients who fail to respond to antibiotic treatment.

**Accepted for Publication:** February 7, 2006.
**Correspondence:** Hossam Al-Tatari, MD, Division of Pediatric Infectious Diseases, Children's Hospital of Michigan, 3901 Beaubien Blvd, Detroit, MI 48201 (haltatari@dmc.org).
**Author Contributions:** *Study concept and design:* Al-Tatari. *Acquisition of data:* Al-Tatari, Abdel-Haq, Asmar, Haupert, and Rabah. *Analysis and interpretation of data:* Al-Tatari, Abdel-Haq, and Asmar. *Drafting of the manuscript:* Al-Tatari, Abdel-Haq, and Asmar. *Critical revision of the manuscript for important intellectual content*: Al-Tatari, Abdel-Haq, Asmar, Haupert, and Rabah. *Study supervision:* Al-Tatari, Abdel-Haq, Asmar, Haupert, and Rabah.
**Financial Disclosure:** None reported.

## REFERENCES

1. Bhargava D, Bhusnurmath B, Sundaram KR, et al. Tonsillar actinomycosis: a clinicopathological study. *Acta Trop.* 2001;80:163-168.
2. Richtsmeier WJ, Johns ME. Actinomycosis of the head and neck. *CRC Crit Rev Clin Lab Sci.* 1979;11:175-202.
3. Miller M, Haddad AJ. Cervicofacial actinomycosis. *Oral Surg Oral Med Oral Pathol Oral Radiol Endod.* 1998;85:496-508.
4. Gaffney R, Harrison M, Walsh M, Sweeney E, Cafferkey M. The incidence and role of actinomyces in recurrent acute tonsillitis. *Clin Otolaryngol.* 1993;18:268-271.
5. Pransky SM, Feldman JI, Kearns DB, Seid AB, Billman GF. Actinomycosis in obstructive tonsillar hypertrophy and recurrent tonsillitis. *Arch Otolaryngol Head Neck Surg.* 1991;117:883-885.
6. Yadav SP, Chanda R, Gathwala G, Yadav RK. Actinomycosis of tonsil masquerading as tumour in a 12-year old child. *Int J Pediatr Otorhinolaryngol.* 2002;63:73-75.
7. Balatsouras DG, Kaberos AK, Eliopoulos PN, Kandiloros D, Economou CN. Cervicofacial actinomycosis presenting as acute upper respiratory tract obstruction. *J Laryngol Otol.* 1994;108:801-803.
8. Blackburn LM, Green ST. Tonsillar actinomycosis presenting as expectorated debris. *J Infect.* 1997;34:283-284.
9. Lockhart GR, Williams GP, Gilbert-Barness E. Pathological case of the month: thoracic and abdominal actinomycosis. *AJDC.* 1993;147:317-318.
10. Lippes J. Pelvic actinomycosis: a review and preliminary look at prevalence. *Am J Obstet Gynecol.* 1999;180:265-269.

EDITORIAL

# The Role of Early Stressors in Child Health and Mental Health Outcomes

STARTING OUT LIFE WITH A DEPRESSED OR AN abusive parent appears to make a number of issues challenging for children. Infants are dependent on caregivers for help with regulating behavior, physiological state, and emotions. With development, children increasingly take over these functions themselves. When a caregiver is unresponsive (as often happens with a depressed caregiver) or frightening (as often happens with a maltreating caregiver), children may not receive the help they need in taking over these regulatory functions. There has been strong evidence that these and other early environmental risk factors place children at increased risk for a host of psychological and social problems.[1-3] Flaherty et al[4] found that early adversity is also associated with problematic child health outcomes.

A number of studies have linked early adversity with later problematic mental health outcomes,[1-3] as Flaherty et al discuss. When considering mental health outcomes, these effects typically show a linear (ie, dose-response) relation. The preponderance of evidence suggests that the effects of risk are additive, with each additional factor increasing the odds of problematic outcomes.[2,3] Some investigations, on the other hand, have found evidence that the effects of risk factors are multiplicative, with 3 or 4 risk factors, for example, showing a much stronger effect than fewer risk factors.[1,4,5] Although neither an additive nor a multiplicative model is clearly supported by the findings of Flaherty et al,[4] an association nonetheless emerges between early adversity and risk for health problems. These results suggest that the association between risk and adverse outcomes extends to health outcomes as well as mental health outcomes.

*See also page 1232*

What are the mechanisms by which early adversity affects mental health and physical health? The experience of chronic stress appears to affect the developing brain in ways that make coping with both immune and psychological challenges difficult. Infants and children are equipped to deal with minor, transient stressors effectively. One of the systems central to the body's response to stress is the hypothalamic-pituitary-adrenal (HPA) axis. When stressors are experienced, the HPA axis is activated, with glucocorticoids (cortisol in humans and nonhuman primates and corticosterone in rodents) released as one of the system's products. There is a negative feedback loop such that the production of glucocorticoids signals the system to shut down. Under conditions for which the organism was evolutionarily prepared, this system functions well in mounting a response to the threat and then terminating the response.

When stressors are experienced that are beyond what the organism can cope with (in scope, duration, concomitant conditions), the HPA system may adapt in ways that are problematic in the long-term. Several different patterns have been observed in the functioning of this system among children who have experienced chronic or traumatic stress. High levels of circulating glucocorticoids are sometimes seen even after the stressful conditions have apparently ended.[6-8] Given that the system evolved to deal with high levels of circulating glucocorticoids for brief periods only, high levels for extended periods have deleterious consequences. On the other hand, very low basal levels of glucocorticoids are sometimes seen among those who have experienced early adversity.[6,7] This "hypocortisolism" is thought to be the result of down-regulation of the HPA system in response to initially high levels of circulating glucocorticoids.[9,10]

In our research with young children in foster care,[6] and in the Pears and Fisher[7] work with preschoolers in foster care, some children showed atypically high patterns of diurnal cortisol production and some children showed atypically low levels of cortisol production. Several researchers have suggested that high levels are likely to be seen when stress is first experienced, followed by low levels later as the system is down-regulated.[9-11] Although such changes in patterns over time make intuitive sense, a strong case for this cannot yet be made. Longitudinal studies that carefully track children following removal from stressful living conditions will be important in developing a fuller picture of the course of change over time. In addition to time since adversity, temperamental differences and developmental differences may well be important in predicting whether children who have experienced early adversity show low or high patterns of cortisol production.[6,7]

Both high and low patterns of cortisol production have important consequences for immune functioning. High levels of cortisol production are designed to affect immune functioning under emergency conditions. The effects are somewhat complex, involving both suppression and activation of various aspects of the immune system. Whereas the system is efficient when stressors are short-lived, long-term recovery from illness is problematic under such conditions. Low patterns of cortisol production are generally associated with overactivity of the immune system and increased inflammatory response.[10] Among adults, a number of problematic conditions, such as chronic fatigue syndrome and fibromyalgia, are characterized by high levels of stress and low levels of cortisol production.[10-12]

The results of the Flaherty et al study suggest that associations between stressors and illness may well emerge for children as has been seen for adults. We expect that the link between stress and problematic outcomes is mediated by an emerging neurobiological mechanism that predisposes to later disorder.[13,14] This study, as well as studies linking early adversity with psychological problems,[1-3] have important implications for policy. Most especially, it seems critical to interrupt the pattern whereby stressors accumulate, leading to a neurobiological mechanism that makes children vulnerable to psychological and physical disorders. Second, interventions that target existing regulatory deficits directly appear to have effects on both neurobiological and behavioral outcomes[15] (P. Fisher, PhD, M. Gunnar, PhD, M.D., J. Burns, PhD, K. Pears, PhD, unpublished data, 2005). Early intervention is likely most effective because brain and behavior become increasingly less plastic with development. Nonetheless, even later social support appears important in moderating the effects of early life stressors.[16]

The associations between exposure to stressors and physical health have practical implications for the practice of pediatric medicine. Routine pediatrician visits give the physician the opportunity to assess risk for the child and to be a first line of defense in recommending services for the family to lessen that risk. Taking the time to assess family stressors when children are very young may be a valuable investment in ensuring good child health outcomes.

*Mary Dozier, PhD*
*Elizabeth Peloso, MS*

**Correspondence:** Dr Dozier, Department of Psychology, University of Delaware, Newark, DE 19716 (mdozier@udel.edu).
**Financial Disclosure:** None reported.

## REFERENCES

1. Rutter M. Protective factors in children's responses to stress and disadvantage. In: Kent MW, Rolf JE, eds. *Primary Prevention of Psychopathology, Vol 3: Social Competence in Children.* Hanover, NJ: University Press of New England; 1979:49-74.
2. Sameroff A, Seifer R, Zax M, Barocas R. Early indicators of developmental risk: the Rochester Longitudinal Study. *Schizophr Bull.* 1987;13:383-394.
3. Appleyard K, Egeland B, van Dulmen HM, Sroufe LA. When more is not better: the role of cumulative risk in child behavior outcomes. *J Child Psychol Psychiatry.* 2005;46:235-245.
4. Flaherty EG, Thompson R, Litrownik AJ, et al. Effect of early childhood adversity on child health. *Arch Pediatr Adolesc Med.* 2006;160:1232-1238.
5. Biederman J, Milberger S, Farasone SV, et al. Family-environment risk factors for attention deficit hyperactivity disorder: a test of Rutter's indicators of adversity. *Arch Gen Psychiatry.* 1995;52:464-470.
6. Dozier M, Manni M, Gordon MK, et al. Foster children's diurnal production of cortisol: an exploratory study. *Child Maltreat.* 2006;11:189-197.
7. Pears K, Fisher P. Developmental, cognitive, and neuropsychological functioning in preschool-aged foster children: associations with prior maltreatment and placement history. *J Dev Behav Pediatr.* 2005;26:112-122.
8. Gunnar MR, Morison SJ, Chisholm K, Schuder M. Salivary cortisol levels in children adopted from Romanian orphanages. *Dev Psychopathol.* 2001;13:611-628.
9. Gunnar MR, Vazquez DM. Low cortisol and a flattening of expected daytime rhythm: potential indices of risk in human development. *Dev Psychopathol.* 2001;13:515-538.
10. Fries E, Hesse J, Hellhammer J, Hellhammer DH. A new view on hypocortisolism. *Psychoneuroendocrinology.* 2005;30:1010-1016.
11. Heim C, Ehlert U, Hellhammer DK. The potential role of hypocortisolism in the pathophysiology of stress-related bodily disorders. *Psychoneuroendocrinology.* 2000;25:1-35.
12. De Bellis MD. Developmental traumatology: a contributory mechanism for alcohol and substance use disorders. *Psychoneuroendocrinology.* 2002;27:155-170.
13. Levine S, Weiner SG, Coe CL. Temporal and social factors influencing behavioral and hormonal responses to separation in mother and infant squirrel monkeys. *Psychoneuroendocrinology.* 1993;18:297-306.
14. Sanchez MM, Ladd CO, Plotsky PM. Early adverse experience as a developmental risk factor for later psychopathology: evidence from rodent and primate models. *Dev Psychopathol.* 2001;13:419-449.
15. Dozier M, Peloso E, Lindhiem O, et al. Developing evidence-based interventions for foster children: an example of a randomized clinical trial with infants and toddlers. *J Soc Issues.* 2006;62:765-783.
16. Kaufman J, Yang B, Douglas-Palumberi H, et al. Social supports and serotonin transporter gene moderate depression in maltreated children. *Proc Natl Acad Sci U S A.* 2004;101:17316-17321.

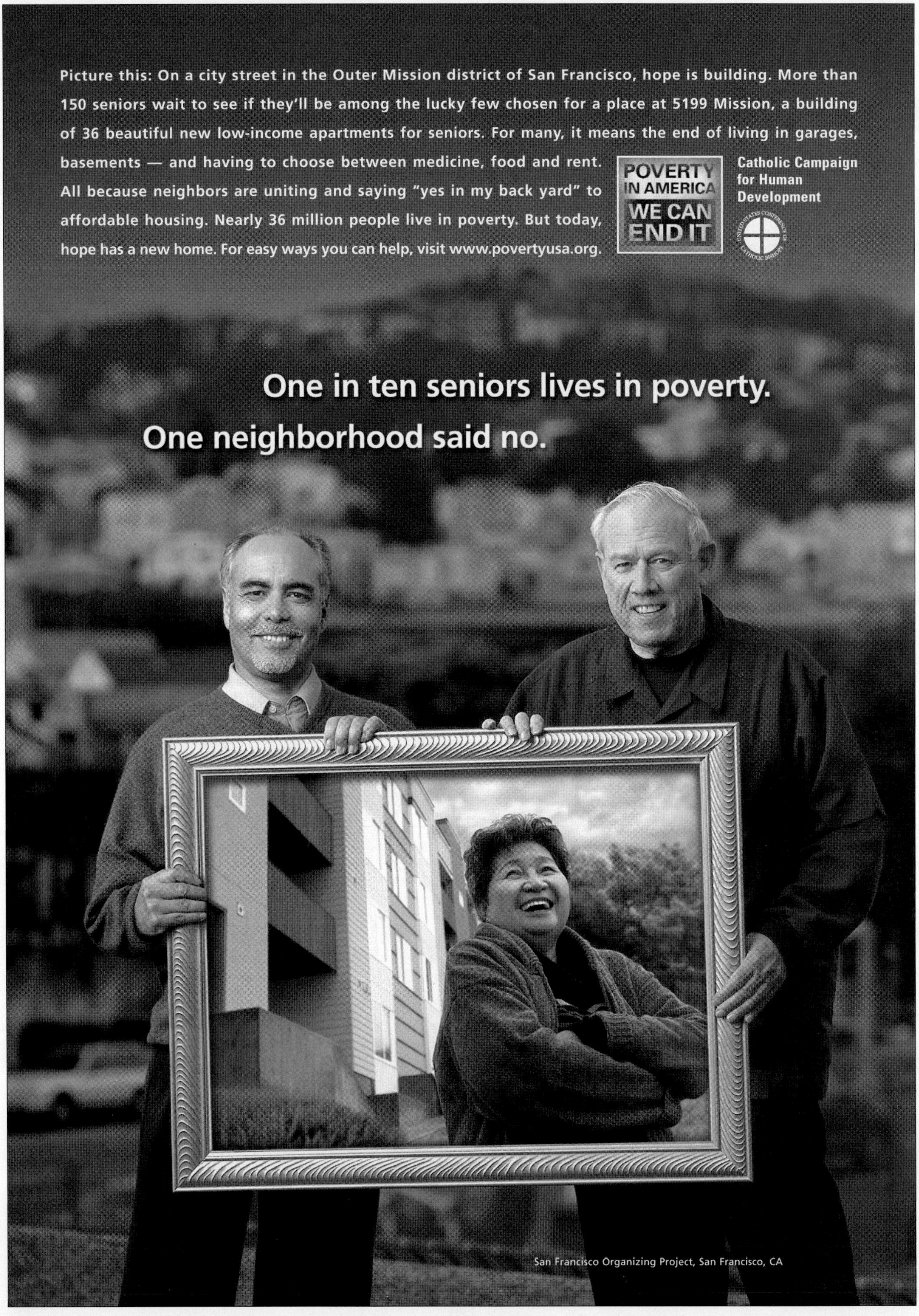
Picture this: On a city street in the Outer Mission district of San Francisco, hope is building. More than 150 seniors wait to see if they'll be among the lucky few chosen for a place at 5199 Mission, a building of 36 beautiful new low-income apartments for seniors. For many, it means the end of living in garages, basements — and having to choose between medicine, food and rent. All because neighbors are uniting and saying "yes in my back yard" to affordable housing. Nearly 36 million people live in poverty. But today, hope has a new home. For easy ways you can help, visit www.povertyusa.org.
POVERTY IN AMERICA WE CAN END IT
Catholic Campaign for Human Development
One in ten seniors lives in poverty.
One neighborhood said no.
San Francisco Organizing Project, San Francisco, CA

# Adolescent Homosexuality

## *Dare We Ask the Question?*

SERIOUS DISPARITIES RELATED TO SEXUAL ORIentation adversely affect the health and well-being of lesbian, gay, bisexual, and transgender (LGBT) youth.[1] Running away, homelessness, difficulties in school, tobacco and other substance use, suicidality, eating disorders, and human immunodeficiency virus (HIV)/AIDS and other sexually transmitted diseases are among the many medical and psychosocial challenges they face.[2] Existing data suggest that rates of these problems have not abetted over time in LGBT populations.[3,4]

On the recent 25th anniversary of the first reported cases in the United States, HIV/AIDS provides a stunning example of persistent and devastating health disparities. Although fewer than 3% of high school–aged students report same sex experiences,[5] young men (13-24 years of age) who have sex with men account for 57% of all reported HIV/AIDS cases in adolescents and young adults in the US.[6] A large percentage of HIV-seropositive gay and bisexual youth have not been tested and are unaware of their serostatus.[7]

*See also page 1248*

One of the best ways to bridge gaps in health outcomes is to reach affected individuals with preventive services. This approach has long been espoused by the American Academy of Pediatrics. The American Academy of Pediatrics issued its first statement of policy on adolescent homosexuality in 1983, recognizing pediatricians' responsibility to care for "homosexual youth and other young people struggling with the problem of sexual expression."[8] In the most recent version,[9] the academy recommended that pediatricians:

- "discuss emerging sexuality with all adolescents,"
- "carefully identify all risky behaviors (sexual behaviors; use of tobacco, alcohol, and drugs; etc) and offer advice and treatment if indicated," and
- "explore the adolescent's understanding and concerns about sexual orientation, dispel any misconceptions, provide appropriate medical care and anticipatory guidance, and connect the adolescent to appropriate supportive community resources."

In this issue of ARCHIVES, Meckler and colleagues[10] described the health care experiences of lesbian, gay, and bisexual youth and factors associated with disclosure of orientation to physicians. The participants were 140 teens at a youth empowerment conference. Only 35% of them reported that their physician knew they were lesbian, gay, or bisexual. The strongest predictor of disclosure was discussing sex or sexual health with a provider. When asked what a physician could do to make talking about being lesbian, gay, or bisexual more comfortable, 64% advised, "Just ask me."

This is the latest of only a few available studies that capture the experiences of LGBT youth in health care systems. Although most of the participants had "come out" (ie, revealed their sexual orientation) to others, surprisingly few had talked about it with health care providers. Their advice to physicians was simply to ask directly. This sentiment is quite new and different from popular opinion in the day when LGBT people feared discrimination and went without basic health services like HIV and Papanicolaou tests.[11,12]

Even today, the advice of the "out" respondents in this study must be tempered with an understanding that some young people are uncertain about their feelings or afraid to disclose their orientation. "Just ask" just might not work. Rarely, however, is there an urgency to classify sexual orientation in a medical setting. Most of the participants in the study had regular health care providers, and their familiarity might have helped them share personal information. Building a trusting relationship with a vulnerable adolescent often takes repeated interaction in safe surroundings.

Yet the findings still give us reason to wonder why more physicians are not broaching the topic of sexual orientation. The argument has been made that following the Guidelines for Adolescent Preventive Services (which include recommendations for the care of young men who have sex with men) takes time without evidence of improving health outcomes.[13] Lack of provider know-how is another barrier to inquiry. A Canadian study found that pediatricians felt unprepared to address the health care needs of gay adolescents, despite being interested in learning more about homosexuality.[14] In another study of physicians in the United Kingdom, non-LGBT providers expressed unfamiliarity with cultural and sexual practices, uncertainty about the correct use of language, and incorrect assumptions about gay relationships.[15] Conversely, research in the US has shown that providing training, resource materials, patient questionnaires, and clinician manuals can improve providers' use of Guidelines for Adolescent Preventive Services and increase discussion of sexual orientation from 13% to 27% of patient encounters.[16]

The current study cites evidence from prior research that pediatricians are more reluctant to discuss sexual orientation than other sexual topics. Some physicians might fear offending non-LGBT young people or parents, although it has not been my experience that patients are upset by sensitively delivered questions. Perhaps other factors are influencing physicians' practices, such as the negative attitudes toward homosexual patients and providers that medical students, residents, practitioners, and patients have reported in prior research.[14,17-20] Fueled by fears of contagion, discrimination against homosexual patients and providers reportedly peaked in the early years of the HIV/AIDS pandemic and subsided with the advent of highly active retroviral treatment.[21]

While inquiring about sexual orientation per se is not enough, it is one in a series of necessary steps to correct health disparities for LGBT people. The serious and complex problems previously mentioned can only be addressed with multifaceted and comprehensive approaches aimed at protecting children from maltreatment in homes, schools, and institutional settings; encouraging public policies that guarantee equal treatment; sponsoring research to understand the scope of health problems and disparities, resiliencies, and strategies to prevent the problems discussed; building community awareness of LGBT needs; implementing programs known to be successful, such as evidenced-based approaches to HIV prevention[22]; and fostering inclusive clinical service systems.

Working effectively with LGBT youth and other diverse populations are teachable skills[23] that entail creating a private and inclusive professional environment, highlighting parameters of confidentiality, asking open and nonjudgmental questions, and encouraging honest answers. Even if some young people aren't ready to answer openly, our sensitive questions and language speak volumes about who we are as supportive and trustworthy professionals. By asking about sexuality and other sensitive topics, pediatricians begin to dispel isolation and stigma, help young people clarify their feelings, acknowledge their struggles, provide potentially life-saving services, and narrow the gaps in health disparities within larger communities and societies.

*Gary Remafedi, MD, MPH*

**Correspondence:** Dr Remafedi, University of Minnesota Youth and AIDS Projects, 428 Oak Grove St, Minneapolis, Minn 55403 (remaf001@umn.edu).
**Financial Disclosure:** None reported.

## REFERENCES

1. Sell RL, Becker JB. Sexual orientation data collection and progress toward Healthy People 2010. *Am J Public Health.* 2001;91:876-882.
2. Stronski Huwiler SM, Remafedi G. Adolescent homosexuality. *Adv Pediatr.* 1998; 45:107-144.
3. Herrell R, Goldberg J, True WR, et al. Sexual orientation and suicidality: a co-twin control study in adult men. *Arch Gen Psychiatry.* 1999;56:867-874.
4. Wolitski RJ, Valdiserri RO, Denning PH, Levine WC. Are we headed for a resurgence of the HIV epidemic among men who have sex with men? *Am J Public Health.* 2001;91:883-888.
5. Garofalo R, Wolf RC, Kessel S, Palfrey SJ, DuRant RH. The association between health risk behaviors and sexual orientation among a school-based sample of adolescents. *Pediatrics.* 1998;101:895-902.
6. Centers for Disease Control and Prevention. Estimated AIDS incidence in adolescents and adults under age 25, by sex and exposure category, diagnosed in 2001, and cumulative totals though 2001, United States [Table 24]. HIV/AIDS Surveillance Report. 2002;13:1-44.
7. MacKellar DA, Valleroy LA, Secura GM, et al. Unrecognized HIV infection, risk behaviors, and perceptions of risk among young men who have sex with men: opportunities for advancing HIV prevention in the third decade of HIV/AIDS. *J Acquir Immune Defic Syndr.* 2005;38:603-614.
8. American Academy of Pediatrics' Committee on Adolescence LWC. Homosexuality and adolescence. *Pediatrics.* 1983;72:249-250.
9. Frankowski BL; Committee on Adolescence. Sexual orientation and adolescents. *Pediatrics.* 2004;113:1827-1832.
10. Meckler GD, Elliott MN, Kanouse DE, Beals KP, Schuster MA. Nondisclosure of sexual orientation to a physician among a sample of gay, lesbian, and bisexual youth. *Arch Pediatrics Adolesc Med.* 2006;160:1248-1254.
11. Rankow EJ, Tessaro I. Cervical cancer risk and Papanicolaou screening in a sample of lesbian and bisexual women. *J Fam Pract.* 1998;47:139-143.
12. Fitzpatrick R, Dawson J, Boulton M, McLean J, Hart G, Brookes M. Perceptions of general practice among homosexual men. *Br J Gen Pract.* 1994;44:80-82.
13. Stevens M. Adolescent guidelines: should we use them? *Am Fam Physician.* 1998; 57:2060, 2066.
14. Druzin P, Shrier I, Yacowar M, Rossignol M. Discrimination against gay, lesbian and bisexual family physicians by patients. *CMAJ.* 1998;158:593-597.
15. Hinchliff S, Gott M, Galena E. 'I daresay I might find it embarrassing': general practitioners' perspectives on discussing sexual health issues with lesbian and gay patients. *Health Soc Care Community.* 2005;13:345-353.
16. Klein JD, Allan MJ, Elster AB, et al. Improving adolescent preventive care in community health centers. *Pediatrics.* 2001;107:318-327.
17. Ramos MM, Tellez CM, Palley TB, Umland BE, Skipper BJ. Attitudes of physicians practicing in New Mexico toward gay men and lesbians in the profession. *Acad Med.* 1998;73:436-438.
18. Rose L. Homophobia among doctors. *BMJ.* 1994;308:586-587.
19. Oriel KA, Madlon-Kay DJ, Govaker D, Mersy DJ. Gay and lesbian physicians in training: family practice program directors' attitudes and students' perceptions of bias. *Fam Med.* 1996;28:720-725.
20. Andersson D, Westerstahl A. Gynecologists about lesbian women—an interview study:there is a risk that lesbian women receive worse treatment [in Swedish]. *Lakartidningen.* 2000;97:5796-5800.
21. Hayward RA, Weissfeld JL. Coming to terms with the era of AIDS: attitudes of physicians in U.S. residency programs. *J Gen Intern Med.* 1993;8:10-18.
22. Centers for Disease Control and Prevention. Diffusion of effective behavioral interventions. http://www.effectiveinterventions.org/. 2005. Accessed on June 15, 2006.
23. Taylor M, Prescott L, Brown J, et al. Activities to increase provider awareness of early syphilis in men who have sex with men in 8 cities, 2000-2004. *Sex Transm Dis.* 2005;32(suppl 10):S24-S29.

# BOOSTRIX®

## (Tetanus Toxoid, Reduced Diphtheria Toxoid and Acellular Pertussis Vaccine, Adsorbed) (Tdap)

The following is a brief summary only; see full prescribing information for complete product information.

**INDICATIONS AND USAGE:** BOOSTRIX is indicated for active booster immunization against tetanus, diphtheria, and pertussis as a single dose in individuals 10 through 18 years of age. The use of BOOSTRIX as a primary series or to complete the primary series has not been studied. As with any vaccine, BOOSTRIX may not protect 100% of individuals receiving the vaccine.

**CONTRAINDICATIONS:** Hypersensitivity to any component of the vaccine is a contraindication (see DESCRIPTION in full prescribing information). Do not use BOOSTRIX after a serious allergic reaction (e.g., anaphylaxis) following any other tetanus toxoid, diphtheria toxoid or pertussis-containing vaccine, or any component of this vaccine (see DESCRIPTION in full prescribing information). Because of the uncertainty as to which component of the vaccine might be responsible, do not give further vaccination with any of these components; or, refer such individuals to an allergist for evaluation. The following events are contraindications to administration of BOOSTRIX: encephalopathy (e.g., coma, decreased level of consciousness, prolonged seizures) within 7 days of administration of a previous dose of a pertussis-containing vaccine that is not attributable to another identifiable cause; progressive neurologic disorder, uncontrolled epilepsy, or progressive encephalopathy. Do not vaccinate individuals with these conditions until a treatment regimen has been established and the condition has stabilized.

**WARNINGS:** The tip cap and the rubber plunger of the needleless prefilled syringes contain dry natural latex rubber that may cause allergic reactions in latex sensitive individuals. The vial stopper is latex-free. If any of the following events occurred in temporal relation to previous receipt of a Diphtheria and Tetanus Toxoids and Pertussis Vaccine Adsorbed (DTwP) vaccine or a vaccine containing an acellular pertussis component, consider carefully whether to give subsequent doses of BOOSTRIX: temperature of ≥40.5°C (105°F) within 48 hours not due to another identifiable cause; collapse or shock-like state (hypotonic-hyporesponsive episode) within 48 hours; persistent, inconsolable crying lasting ≥3 hours, occurring within 48 hours; seizures with or without fever occurring within 3 days. Persons who experienced serious Arthus-type hypersensitivity reactions following a prior dose of tetanus toxoid usually have high serum tetanus antitoxin levels and should not be given Tetanus and Diphtheria Toxoids Adsorbed For Adult Use (Td) or Tdap vaccines or even emergency doses of Td more frequently than every 10 years, even if the wound is neither clean nor minor. If Guillain-Barré syndrome has occurred within 6 weeks of receipt of prior vaccine containing tetanus toxoid, the decision to give BOOSTRIX or any vaccine containing tetanus toxoid should be based on careful consideration of the potential benefits and possible risks. The decision to administer a pertussis-containing vaccine to individuals with stable central nervous system (CNS) disorders must be made by the physician on an individual basis, with consideration of all relevant factors, and assessment of potential risks and benefits for that individual. Advise the patient, parent, or guardian of the potential increased risk involved (see PRECAUTIONS). A family history of seizures or other CNS disorders is not a contraindication to pertussis vaccine. The Advisory Committee on Immunization Practices (ACIP) has published guidelines for vaccination of persons with recent or acute illness (www.cdc.gov). Do not give BOOSTRIX to individuals with bleeding disorders such as hemophilia or thrombocytopenia, or to persons on anticoagulant therapy unless the potential benefit clearly outweighs the risk of administration. If the decision is made to administer BOOSTRIX to such persons, it should be given with caution with steps taken to avoid the risk of hematoma following the injection.

**PRECAUTIONS: General:** Before the injection of any biological, the physician should take all reasonable precautions to prevent allergic or other adverse reactions. Epinephrine injection (1:1,000) and other appropriate agents used for the control of immediate allergic reactions must be immediately available should an acute anaphylactic reaction occur. Immunosuppressed persons, including individuals receiving immunosuppressive therapy, may not develop the expected immune response. **Drug Interactions:** Do not mix BOOSTRIX with any other vaccine in the same syringe or vial. **Carcinogenesis, Mutagenesis, Impairment of Fertility:** BOOSTRIX has not been evaluated for carcinogenic or mutagenic potential, or for impairment of fertility. **Pregnancy:** Pregnancy Category C. Animal reproduction studies have not been conducted with BOOSTRIX. It is also not known whether BOOSTRIX can cause fetal harm when administered to a pregnant woman or can affect reproductive capacity. BOOSTRIX should be given to a pregnant woman only if clearly needed. Animal fertility studies have not been conducted with BOOSTRIX. In a developmental toxicity study, the effect of BOOSTRIX on embryo-fetal and pre-weaning development was evaluated in pregnant rats. Animals were administered INFANRIX® (Diphtheria and Tetanus Toxoids and Acellular Pertussis Vaccine Adsorbed) prior to gestation and BOOSTRIX during the period of organogenesis (gestation days 6, 8, 11) and later in pregnancy (gestation day 15), 0.1 mL/rat/occasion (a 45-fold increase compared to the human dose of BOOSTRIX on a body weight basis), by intramuscular injection. No adverse affect on pregnancy and lactation parameters, embryo-fetal or pre-weaning development was observed. There were no fetal malformations or other evidence of teratogenesis noted in this study. **Nursing Mothers:** It is not known whether BOOSTRIX is excreted in human milk. Because many drugs are excreted in human milk, caution should be exercised when BOOSTRIX is administered to a nursing woman. **Pregnancy Exposure Registry:** Healthcare providers are encouraged to register pregnant women who receive BOOSTRIX in the GlaxoSmithKline vaccination pregnancy registry by calling 1-888-825-5249. **Geriatric Use:** BOOSTRIX is not indicated for use in individuals older than 18 years. **Pediatric Use:** BOOSTRIX is not indicated for use in individuals younger than 10 years (see DOSAGE AND ADMINISTRATION in full prescribing information). For immunization of infants and children younger than 7 years against diphtheria, tetanus, and pertussis, refer to the manufacturers' package inserts for Diphtheria and Tetanus Toxoids and Acellular Pertussis Vaccine Adsorbed (DTaP) vaccines.

**ADVERSE REACTIONS:** A total of 3,608 adolescents were vaccinated with a single dose of BOOSTRIX during clinical trials. An additional 1,092 adolescents 10 to 18 years of age received a non-US formulation of BOOSTRIX (formulated to contain 0.5 mg aluminum per dose) in non-US clinical studies.

The primary safety study, conducted in the United States, was a randomized, observer-blinded, controlled study in which 3,080 adolescents 10 to 18 years of age received a single dose of BOOSTRIX and 1,034 received the control Td vaccine manufactured by Massachusetts Public Health Biologic Laboratories. There were no substantive differences in demographic characteristics between the vaccine groups. Among BOOSTRIX and control vaccine recipients approximately 75% were 10 to 14 years of age and approximately 25% were 15 to 18 years of age. Approximately 98% of participants in this study had received the recommended series of 4 or 5 doses of either DTwP or a combination of DTwP and DTaP in childhood. Data on adverse events were collected by the subjects, parents and/or guardians using standardized diaries for 15 consecutive days following the vaccine dose (i.e., day of vaccination and the next 14 days). Subjects were monitored for unsolicited adverse events that occurred within 31 days of vaccination (day 0-30) using diary cards (day 0-14) supplemented by spontaneous reports and a medical history as reported by subjects, parents, and/or guardians. Subjects were also monitored for 6 months post-vaccination for non-routine medical visits, visits to an emergency room, onset of new chronic illness, and serious adverse events. Information regarding late onset adverse events was obtained via a telephone call 6 months following vaccination. At least 97% of subjects completed the 6-month follow-up evaluation.

In a study conducted in Germany, BOOSTRIX was administered to 319 children 10 to 12 years of age previously vaccinated with 5 doses of acellular pertussis-containing vaccines, 193 of these subjects had previously received 5 doses of INFANRIX. Adverse events were recorded on diary cards during the 15 days following vaccination. Unsolicited adverse events that occurred within 31 days of vaccination (day 0-30) were recorded on the diary card or verbally reported to the investigator. Subjects were monitored for 6 months post-vaccination for physician office visits, emergency room visits, onset of new chronic illness, and serious adverse events. The 6-month follow-up evaluation, conducted via telephone interview, was completed by 90% of subjects.

The adverse event information from clinical trials provides a basis for identifying adverse events that appear to be related to vaccine use and for approximating rates. However, because clinical trials are conducted under widely varying conditions, adverse event rates observed in the clinical trials of a vaccine cannot be directly compared to rates in the clinical trials of another vaccine, and may not reflect the rates observed in practice.

**Serious Adverse Events in All Safety Studies:** In the US-safety study and German-safety study, no serious adverse events were reported to occur within 31 days of vaccination. During the 6-month extended safety evaluation period, no serious adverse events that were of potential autoimmune origin or new onset and chronic in nature were reported to occur. In non-US studies in which serious adverse events were monitored for up to 37 days, one subject was diagnosed with insulin dependent diabetes 20 days following administration of BOOSTRIX. No other serious adverse events of potential autoimmune origin or that were new onset and chronic in nature were reported to occur in these studies.

**Solicited Adverse Events in the US-Safety Study:** In a US study, the most common local adverse events following administration of BOOSTRIX were pain, redness, and swelling at the injection site. The most common general adverse events were headache and fatigue. Most of these events were reported at a similar frequency in recipients of both BOOSTRIX and Td. Any pain, grade 2 or 3 pain (but not grade 3 alone), and grade 2 or 3 headache (but not grade 3 alone) were reported at a higher rate in recipients of BOOSTRIX. The primary safety endpoint of the US study was the incidence of grade 3 pain (spontaneously painful and/or prevented normal activity) at the injection site within 15 days of vaccination. Grade 3 pain was reported in 4.6% of those who received BOOSTRIX compared with 4.0% of those who received the Td vaccine. The difference in rate of grade 3 pain was within the pre-defined clinical limit for non-inferiority (upper limit of the 95% CI for the difference ≤4%). These were the rates for solicited local and general adverse events within 15 days of vaccination with BOOSTRIX or Td vaccine for the total vaccinated cohort (all enrolled, vaccinated subjects with safety data available analyzed by vaccine received):

**Percentage of Individuals 10 to 18 Years of Age Reporting Solicited Local Adverse Events or Solicited General Adverse Events Within the 15-day* Post-Vaccination Period**

| | BOOSTRIX (N = 3,032) % | Td (N =1,013) % |
|---|---|---|
| **Local** | | |
| Pain,† any | 75.3 | 71.7 |
| Pain,† grade 2 or 3 | 51.2 | 42.5 |
| Pain,‡ grade 3 | 4.6 | 4.0 |
| Redness, any | 22.5 | 19.8 |
| Redness, >20 mm | 4.1 | 3.9 |
| Redness, ≥50 mm | 1.7 | 1.6 |
| Swelling, any | 21.1 | 20.1 |
| Swelling, >20 mm | 5.3 | 4.9 |
| Swelling, ≥50 mm | 2.5 | 3.2 |
| Arm circumference increase,§ >5 mm | 28.3 | 29.5 |
| Arm circumference increase,§ >20 mm | 2.0 | 2.2 |
| Arm circumference increase,§ >40 mm | 0.5 | 0.3 |
| **General** | | |
| Fever,‖ ≥99.5°F | 13.5 | 13.1 |
| Fever,‖ >100.4°F | 5.0 | 4.7 |
| Fever,‖ >102.2°F | 1.4 | 1.0 |
| Headache, any | 43.1 | 41.5 |
| Headache,† grade 2 or 3 | 15.7 | 12.7 |
| Headache, grade 3 | 3.7 | 2.7 |
| Fatigue, any | 37.0 | 36.7 |
| Fatigue, grade 2 or 3 | 14.4 | 12.9 |
| Fatigue, grade 3 | 3.7 | 3.2 |
| Gastrointestinal symptoms,¶ any | 26.0 | 25.8 |
| Gastrointestinal symptoms,¶ grade 2 or 3 | 9.8 | 9.7 |
| Gastrointestinal symptoms,¶ grade 3 | 3.0 | 3.2 |

Td = Tetanus and Diphtheria Toxoids Adsorbed For Adult Use manufactured by Massachusetts Public Health Biologic Laboratories.
N = number of subjects in the total vaccinated cohort with local/general symptoms sheets completed.
Grade 2 = Local: painful when the limb was moved; General: interfered with normal activity.
Grade 3 = Local: spontaneously painful and/or prevented normal activity; General: prevented normal activity.
*Day of vaccination and the next 14 days.
†Statistically significantly higher (P<0.05) following BOOSTRIX as compared to Td vaccine.
‡Grade 3 injection site pain following BOOSTRIX was not inferior to Td (upper limit of two-sided 95% CI for the difference in the percentage of subjects ≤4%).
§Mid-upper region of the vaccinated arm.
‖Oral temperatures or axillary temperatures.
¶Gastrointestinal symptoms included nausea, vomiting, diarrhea and/or abdominal pain.

Mid-upper arm circumference was measured by the adolescent or their parent/guardian prior to injection and daily for 15 days following vaccination. There was no significant difference between BOOSTRIX recipients and Td recipients in the proportion of subjects reporting an increase in mid-upper arm circumference in the vaccinated arm. The incidence of unsolicited adverse events reported in the 31 days after vaccination was comparable between the 2 groups.

**Solicited Adverse Events in the German Safety Study:** No cases of whole arm swelling were spontaneously reported. Two individuals (2/193) reported large injection site swelling (range 110 to 200 mm diameter), in one case associated with grade 3 pain. Neither individual sought medical attention. These episodes were reported to resolve without sequelae within 5 days. These were the rates of solicited local adverse events and fever within 15 days of vaccination for those subjects who had previously been vaccinated with 5 doses of INFANRIX:

**Rates of Solicited Adverse Events Reported Within the 15-day* Post-Vaccination Period Following Administration of BOOSTRIX in Individuals 10 to 12 Years of Age Who Had Previously Received 5 Doses of INFANRIX**

| Adverse Event | BOOSTRIX (N = 193) % (95% CI) |
|---|---|
| Pain, any | 62.2 (54.9-69.0) |
| Pain, grade 2 or 3 | 33.2 (26.6-40.3) |
| Pain, grade 3 | 5.7 (2.9-10.0) |
| Redness, any | 47.7 (40.4-55.0) |
| Redness, >20 mm | 15.0 (10.3-20.9) |
| Redness, ≥50 mm | 10.9 (6.9-16.2) |
| Swelling, any | 38.9 (31.9-46.1) |
| Swelling, >20 mm | 17.6 (12.5-23.7) |
| Swelling, ≥50 mm | 14.0 (9.4-19.7) |
| Fever, ≥99.5 | 8.8 (5.2-13.7) |
| Fever, >100.4 | 4.1 (1.8-8.0) |
| Fever, >102.2 | 1.0 (0.1-3.7) |

N = number of subjects with local/general symptoms sheets completed.
Grade 2 = Painful when the limb was moved.
Grade 3 = Spontaneously painful and/or prevented normal activity.
*Day of vaccination and the next 14 days.

As with any vaccine, there is the possibility that broad use of BOOSTRIX could reveal adverse events not observed in clinical trials.

**Postmarketing Reports:** Worldwide voluntary reports of adverse events received for BOOSTRIX in persons 10 to 18 years of age since market introduction of this vaccine are listed below. This list includes serious events or events which have causal connection to components of this or other vaccines or drugs. Because these events are reported voluntarily from a population of uncertain size, it is not possible to reliably estimate their frequency or establish a causal relationship to vaccine exposure. *Blood and lymphatic system disorders:* Lymphadenitis, lymphadenopathy. *Cardiac disorders:* Myocarditis. *Injection site reactions:* Induration, inflammation, mass, nodule, warmth, local reaction. *Metabolism and nutrition disorders:* Diabetes mellitus insulin-dependent. *Musculoskeletal and connective tissue disorders:* Arthralgia, back pain, myalgia. *Nervous system disorders:* Convulsion, encephalitis, facial palsy, paraesthesia. *Skin and subcutaneous tissue disorders:* Exanthem, Henoch-Schönlein purpura, rash. In addition, extensive swelling of the injected limb has been reported following administration of BOOSTRIX.

**Reporting Adverse Events:** Report the occurrence following immunization of any event set forth in the Vaccine Injury Table from the National Childhood Vaccine Injury Act including: Anaphylaxis or anaphylactic shock within 7 days, encephalopathy or encephalitis within 7 days, brachial neuritis within 28 days, or an acute complication or sequelae (including death) of an illness, disability, injury, or condition referred to above, or any events that would contraindicate further doses of vaccine, according to this prescribing information. These events should be reported to VAERS. The VAERS toll-free number is 1-800-822-7967. Reporting forms may also be obtained at the VAERS website at www.vaers.hhs.gov.

**DOSAGE AND ADMINISTRATION: Recommended Dose:** BOOSTRIX should be administered as a single 0.5 mL injection by the intramuscular route into the deltoid muscle of the upper arm in individuals 10 through 18 years of age. Do not administer this product subcutaneously or intravenously. There are no data to support repeat administration of BOOSTRIX. Five years should elapse between the subject's last dose of the recommended series of childhood DTwP and/or DTaP vaccine and the administration of BOOSTRIX. Limited data are available on the use of BOOSTRIX following Tetanus and Diphtheria Toxoids Adsorbed For Adult Use (Td) vaccine. **Additional Dosing Information:** ***Wound Management:*** Clinicians should refer to guidelines for tetanus prophylaxis in routine wound management. Adolescents 10 to 18 years of age who have completed a primary series against tetanus and who sustain wounds which are minor and uncomplicated, should receive a booster dose of a tetanus toxoid-containing vaccine only if they have not received tetanus toxoid within the preceding 10 years. In case of tetanus-prone injury (e.g., wounds contaminated with dirt, feces, soil, and saliva; puncture wounds; avulsions; and wounds resulting from missles, crushing, burns, and frostbite) in an adolescent who is in need of tetanus toxoid, BOOSTRIX can be used as an alternative to Tetanus and Diphtheria Toxoids Adsorbed For Adult Use (Td) vaccine in patients for whom the pertussis component is also indicated (see INDICATIONS AND USAGE).

Manufactured by **GlaxoSmithKline Biologicals**
Rixensart, Belgium, US License 1617

Distributed by **GlaxoSmithKline**
Research Triangle Park, NC 27709

BOOSTRIX and INFANRIX are registered trademarks of GlaxoSmithKline.

Full prescribing information for BOOSTRIX is available at www.BOOSTRIX.com.
BRS-BO:L3

**References: 1.** Centers for Disease Control and Prevention. Preventing tetanus, diphtheria, and pertussis among adolescents: use of tetanus toxoid, reduced diphtheria toxoid and acellular pertussis vaccines: recommendations of the Advisory Committee on Immunization Practices (ACIP). Early Release 2006;55(February 23, 2006):1–43. **2.** Centers for Disease Control and Prevention. Recommended childhood and adolescent immunization schedule—United States, 2006. *MMWR.* 2006;54(51&52):Q1–Q4.

## The Association Between Caregiver Knowledge of Antiretroviral Therapy Regimens and Disease Parameters Among Perinatally Human Immunodeficiency Virus–Infected Children

The ability of caregivers of human immunodeficiency virus (HIV)–infected children to correctly identify or describe their child's antiretroviral therapy (ART) regimen has been associated with higher levels of ART adherence.[1,2] We hypothesized that children whose caregivers could correctly describe their ART regimens would also have better HIV disease parameters as measured by CD4 percentage and HIV viral load.

**Methods.** Children (aged 3-13 years) and their caregivers were recruited for a cross-sectional study examining factors associated with child ART medication adherence.[3,4] During a 90-minute interview, caregivers were asked to describe their child's ART regimen and comparisons were made with the medical and/or pharmacy records. Knowledge of medication regimens was defined as the percentage of antiretroviral medications reported in the medical or pharmacy record that was correctly named or whose appearance was correctly described by the child's caregiver, dichotomized as 100% vs less than 100%. We examined the association between knowledge of medication regimens and several covariates, including caregiver/child race, caregiver HIV status, caregiver primary language, number of antiretroviral medications prescribed, and the degree to which the child was responsible for medication administration. Viral load and CD4 percentage were obtained from medical records and dichotomized as undetectable (<400 copies/mL) vs detectable and severe (CD4<15%) vs moderate or no immunosuppression.

We examined the degree to which knowledge of medication regimens was associated with viral load and CD4 percentage both before and after controlling for other covariates significant at the $P \leq .05$ level in the bivariate analysis using SAS software for Windows version 9.0 (SAS Institute Inc, Cary, NC).

**Results.** Of the 77 children, 75 were taking ART and 72 had complete medical record information. Seventy-five percent (54 to 72) of caregivers were able to name or accurately describe the appearance of all of their child's antiretroviral medications and scored 100% on the knowledge of medication regimens variable. The **Table** provides a summary of the frequency and type of medication errors made. Knowledge of medication regimens was not related to any demographic or medication-related covariates (data not shown). Caregivers who were unable to identify their child's medications were 4.8 times more likely to have a child with severe immunosuppression when compared with those who could name their child's antiretroviral medications (odds ratio, 4.8 [95% confidence interval, 1.1-20.5]; $P = .04$). Caregivers' knowledge of medication regimens was not significantly associated with HIV RNA viral load, either before or after controlling for the number of antiretroviral medications prescribed.

**Table. Frequency and Type of Medication Errors Made by Caregivers**

| Type of Medication Error | No. (%) |
|---|---|
| Any medication error | 43 (31) |
| Incorrectly identifying number of pills or volume per dose | 32 (23) |
| Incorrectly identifying number of doses per day | 8 (6) |
| Identifying antiretroviral medications not prescribed | 7 (5) |
| Failing to identify prescribed antiretroviral medication | 22 (16) |

**Comment.** Our results indicate that caregiver knowledge of antiretroviral medication regimens is strongly associated with better immunologic status in HIV-infected children. Our study provides valuable information on the degree to which caregivers are knowledgeable about ART regimens. Also, 25% of caregivers could not completely identify their children's regimen. Studies of HIV-positive adults have shown similar levels of regimen misunderstanding.[5] Our study has several limitations, including a relatively small sample and a cross-sectional design that prevents us from establishing a causal relationship between study variables. In addition, caregivers with more severely immunocompromised children may have experienced recent changes in medication regimens that might account for their lower knowledge. Finally, because adherence was overreported in this sample, we were unable to adequately evaluate its impact on the variables in question.[3]

Despite these limitations, our study provides valuable information on the degree to which caregivers are knowledgeable about ART regimens and their importance in disease management. Caregivers who can correctly name or identify medications are more likely to administer medications as prescribed, thereby avoiding suboptimal response to therapy or undue toxic effects. Assessing caregiver knowledge of regimens may help to identify children who are taking medications incorrectly and may help health care professionals target families for educational interventions to improve disease outcomes.

*Ouzama Nicholson, MD, MS*
*Claude Mellins, PhD*
*Curtis Dolezal, PhD*
*E. Karina Santamaria, BA*
*Elizabeth Brackis-Cott, PhD*
*Elaine J. Abrams, MD*

**Correspondence:** Dr Nicholson, Partners AIDS Research Center, Charlestown Navy Yard, 149 13th St, Fifth Floor, Charlestown, MA 02129 (onicholson1@partners.org).

**Author Contributions:** Dr Mellins, the principal investigator, had full access to all the data in the study and takes responsibility for the integrity of the data and the accuracy of the data analysis. *Study concept and design:* Mellins. *Acquisition of data:* Mellins, Santamaria, Brackis-Cott, and Abrams. *Analysis and interpretation of data:* Nicholson, Mellins, Dolezal, and Abrams. *Drafting of the manuscript:* Nicholson. *Critical revision of the manuscript for important intellectual content:* Nicholson, Mellins, Dolezal, Santamaria, Brackis-Cott, and Abrams. *Statistical analysis:* Nicholson and Dolezal. *Obtained funding:* Mellins and Brackis-Cott. *Administrative, technical, and material support:* Santamaria and Abrams. *Study supervision:* Mellins, Brackis-Cott, and Abrams.

**Financial Disclosure:** None reported.

**Funding/Support:** This research was supported by pilot grant P30 AI42848 from the Columbia-Rockefeller Center for AIDS Research (Dr Mellins [principal investigator, David Ho, MD]) and center grant P30-MH43520 from the National Institute of Mental Health (NIMH) to the HIV Center for Clinical and Behavioral Studies at New York State Psychiatric Institute and Columbia University (principal investigator, Anke A. Ehrhardt, PhD). Dr Nicholson is supported by NIMH training grant T-32 MH19139 to the HIV Center.

1. Marhefka SL, Farley JJ, Rodrigue JR, Sandrik LL, Sleasman JW, Tepper VJ. Clinical assessment of medication adherence among HIV-infected children: examination of the Treatment Interview Protocol (TIP). *AIDS Care.* 2004;16:323-338.
2. Katko E, Johnson GM, Fowler SL, Turner RB. Assessment of adherence with medications in human immunodeficiency virus-infected children. *Pediatr Infect Dis J.* 2001;20:1174-1176.
3. Mellins CA, Brackis-Cott E, Dolezal C, Abrams EJ. The role of psychosocial and family factors in adherence to antiretroviral treatment in human immunodeficiency virus-infected children. *Pediatr Infect Dis J.* 2004;23:1035-1041.
4. Dolezal C, Mellins C, Brackis-Cott E, Abrams EJ. The reliability of reports of medical adherence from children with HIV and their adult caregivers. *J Pediatr Psychol.* 2003;28:355-361.
5. Bangsberg DR, Bronstone A, Hofmann R. A computer-based assessment detects regimen misunderstandings and nonadherence for patients on HIV antiretroviral therapy. *AIDS Care.* 2002;14:3-15.

If a growing object is both fresh and spoiled at the same time, chances are it is a child.
—Morris Goldfischer

## PRACTICE FOR SALE

WESTERN CONNECTICUT PEDIATRIC PRACTICE FOR SALE. Established 50 years. Near excellent community Hospital. One hour to New York City, New Haven, Hartford. Reply to Box 2860, c/o ADC, 515 N State St, 11th Fl, Chicago, IL 60610.

## ACKNOWLEDGMENT SERVICE

Acknowledgments in confirmation of advertising orders are sent each week. Upon receipt, please verify that your ad will be running under the appropriate heading and that your scheduling is correct. Changes to the schedule, cancellations or corrections must be communicated in writing by fax, e-mail, or regular mail prior to the published closing date of the scheduled issue.

## Fondation Jérôme Lejeune

The main target of the Fondation Jerome Lejeune, a state-recommended foundation, is research into Intelligence Disability.

"Searching, Healing, Defending"

### Grants

The Fondation Jerome Lejeune invites interested teams and researchers to submit fundamental or clinical research projects to its Scientific Committee (neurosciences, behaviour, genetics, molecular biology, therapeutics, adult or cord blood stem cells, etc), aimed at leading to the discovery of treatments for genetic intelligence disabilities, especially the trisomy 21 (Down syndrome). The Fondation also considers support for congresses or courses organization.

### Practical Information

Please fill in the "on-line" application form on **www.fondationlejeune.org** (validation deadline: 30/03/2007).

For any further information, please contact:

**Conseil Scientifique**
**Fondation Jerome Lejeune**
**48 rue Galande - 75005 PARIS - France**
**Tel: +33 1 5310 0830 Fax: +33 1 5310 8598**

Fondation Jérôme LEJEUNE

## JOURNAL ADVERTISER INDEX


**ABBOTT LABS**
Omnicef OS ........ 1199-1201

**ALLIANT PHARMACEUTICALS**
Orapred Odt ........ 1239-1240

**ASTRAZENECA**
http://www.astrazeneca.com
Nexium ........ 1216A-B

**CLASSIFIED ADVERTISING** ........ 1311
http://www.amapublications.com

**GLAXOSMITHKLINE**
Boostrix ........ 1205-1206, 1305-1306
Pediarix ........ 1215-1216, COVER 3-COVER 4

**MERCK & COMPANY**
Gardasil ........ 1296A-D

**RF COMPANY LTD** ........ 1196

**SCHERING-PLOUGH**
Claritin Grape Chewables ........ 1194, 1247

**SEPRACOR**
Xopenex ........ COVER 2-1193


*Demographic and "Mini" inserts and/or ROB ad pages

While every precaution is taken to ensure accuracy, we cannot guarantee against the possibility of an occasional change or omission in the preparation of this index.

## UT SOUTHWESTERN MEDICAL CENTER

University of Texas Southwestern Medical Center at Dallas and Children's Medical Center of Dallas

### FACULTY POSITIONS IN GENERAL ACADEMIC PEDIATRICS

The University of Texas Southwestern Medical Center at Dallas invites applications for faculty positions in the Division of General Academic Pediatrics. Applicants can expect an opportunity for a well-balanced career in teaching, research, and clinical medicine. The medical campus, which houses the medical school and its affiliated hospitals, offers all the resources that are necessary for a productive academic career.

We specifically seek physicians with expertise in the following areas: Adolescent Medicine, Child Abuse, and General Pediatric Medicine. The Division of General Academic Pediatrics is located in Children's Medical Center of Dallas, a state-of-the art 406 bed free-standing facility that provides comprehensive care to the children of Dallas and surrounding areas. Members of the Division attend both on in-patient and ambulatory services, where they supervise and teach residents from the categorical pediatric residency training program and students from UTSW School of Medicine.

Candidates must be trained in and Board eligible or certified in Pediatrics, and have a dedication to academic excellence. Positions are available at the Assistant or Associate Professor level, commensurate with experience. Applications from minority and female candidates are encouraged. A letter of interest and curriculum vitae should be sent to:

M. Douglas Baker, MD
Director of Medical Services
Professor, Department of Pediatrics
University of Texas Southwestern Medical Center at Dallas
5323 Harry Hines Blvd
Dallas, TX 75390-9063
Phone: (214) 456-4472
Fax: (214) 456-2397
E-mail: douglas.baker@utsouthwestern.edu

*The University of Texas Southwestern Medical Center is an Equal Opportunity/Affirmative Action Employer.*

## MEDICAL DIRECTOR
## CHILD ADVOCACY & PROTECTION PROGRAM

Children's Hospital at Dartmouth seeks a full-time medical director for its Child Advocacy and Protection Program. The successful candidate must be Board certified in Pediatrics, have additional fellowship training in child abuse or the equivalent, and should have at least five years of post-residency clinical experience in evaluations of cases of child maltreatment. Additionally, candidates should have prior experience in program development and a record of academic achievement. Support is available for academic and program development. The chosen candidate will lead an experienced team consisting of an NP, a child advocacy center coordinator, a social worker, and an administrative assistant. Faculty appointment at Dartmouth Medical School commensurate with experience.

Please direct inquiries and CVs to:

**Richard P. Morse, MD**
**Department of Pediatrics**
**Dartmouth-Hitchcock Medical Center**
**Lebanon, NH 03756**
**E-mail: Richard.P.Morse@hitchcock.org**

DARTMOUTH-HITCHCOCK MEDICAL CENTER

Dartmouth-Hitchcock Medical Center is an affirmative action/equal opportunity employer and is especially interested in identifying female and minority candidates.

**www.dhmc.org**

ARCHIVES OF PEDIATRICS & ADOLESCENT MEDICINE

# CONTACT INFORMATION

## EDITORIAL OFFICE

**Editorial Office Information:** *Archives of Pediatrics & Adolescent Medicine*, Department of Pediatrics, Child Health Institute, University of Washington, 6200 NE 74th St, Suite 210, Seattle, WA 98115-8160, USA; phone: (206) 685-3573; fax: (206) 685-3572; e-mail: archpediatrics@jama-archives.org.

**Electronic Submission:** Manuscripts should be submitted via our online manuscript submission and review system (http://manuscripts.archpediatrics.com). Manuscripts submitted through our online system should not also be submitted by mail or fax. Signed authorship forms should be sent by regular mail or fax with the assigned manuscript number noted on each page in the upper right-hand corner. See the Instructions for Authors (www.archpediatrics.com) for more details.

## CONSORTIUM OF *JAMA* & *ARCHIVES* JOURNALS

The *Archives of Pediatrics & Adolescent Medicine* is a member of the consortium of AMA journals listed below.

The Journal of the American Medical Association (JAMA)
Archives of Dermatology
Archives of Facial Plastic Surgery
Archives of General Psychiatry
Archives of Internal Medicine
Archives of Neurology
Archives of Ophthalmology
Archives of Otolaryngology–Head & Neck Surgery
Archives of Pediatrics & Adolescent Medicine
Archives of Surgery

## *JAMA/ARCHIVES* MEDIA RELATIONS

Jann Ingmire; phone: (312) 464-5262; e-mail: mediarelations@jama-archives.org.

## *ARCHIVES OF PEDIATRICS* ONLINE

*Archives of Pediatrics & Adolescent Medicine* is available online at www.archpediatrics.com.

## *JAMA/ARCHIVES* REPRINTS

**Author/Educational Institution Reprints:** Anna Goins at (312) 464-2477; fax: (312) 464-5843; e-mail: anna.goins@ama-assn.org. Minimum order: 100 reprints.

**Commercial Reprints:** Phone: (312) 464-0776; fax: (312) 464-0708; e-mail: reprints@ama-assn.org. Minimum order: 100 reprints.

## PERMISSIONS

Information about obtaining permission to republish, reprint, or adapt material published in *Archives of Pediatrics & Adolescent Medicine* is available from Rhonda Bailey Brown; phone: (312) 464-2513; fax: (312) 464-5843; e-mail: permissions@ama-assn.org.

## DOCUMENT DELIVERY

Copies of individual articles are available online at www.archpediatrics.com and from the following: Infotrieve, phone: (800) 422-4633; fax: (310) 208-5971; URL: www.infotrieve.com; e-mail: orders@infotrieve.com; Institute for Scientific Information (ISI), phone: (800) 603-4367; fax: (856) 787-1679; URL: http://www.isidoc.com; e-mail: service@isidoc.com.

The ARCHIVES OF PEDIATRICS & ADOLESCENT MEDICINE (ISSN 01072–4710) is published monthly by the American Medical Association, 515 N State St, Chicago, IL 60610–0946, and is an official publication of the Association. The ARCHIVES OF PEDIATRICS & ADOLESCENT MEDICINE reaches more than 30 900 readers in over 83 countries each month. Periodicals postage paid at Chicago, Ill, and at additional mailing offices. GST registration number 12622 5556 RT. Canada Post International Publications Mail (Canadian Distribution) Sales Agreement No. 318728. POSTMASTER, send all address changes to *Archives of Pediatrics & Adolescent Medicine,* c/o the AMA Unified Service Center, American Medical Association, 515 N State St, Chicago, IL 60610. Printed in the USA.

## ADVERTISING

Information about advertising is available from the following sales representatives and online at www.archpediatrics.com.

**Account Manager:** Tim Melroy (nationally); phone: (973) 263-9191 ext 213.

**Manager, Marketing Services:** Nancy Bell; phone: (973) 263-9191 ext 216.

**Advertising Office:** 119 Cherry Hill Rd, Suite 330, Parsippany, NJ 07054-1114; phone: (973) 263-9191.

**Classified Advertising:** Thalia Moss, Shana Brown, Kim Jenkins, Sophie Levandoski, 515 N State St, Chicago, IL 60610; phone: (800) 262-2260; e-mail: classifieds@jama-archives.org.

## ADVERTISING PRINCIPLES

Advertisements in this issue have been reviewed to comply with the principles governing advertising in AMA publications. A copy of these principles is available on request and online at www.archpediatrics.com. The appearance of advertising in AMA publications is not an AMA guarantee or endorsement of the product or the claims made for the product by the manufacturer.

## ADDRESS CHANGES

Send all address changes to *Archives of Pediatrics & Adolescent Medicine*, c/o the AMA Unified Service Center, American Medical Association, 515 N State St, Chicago, IL 60610. Notification of address changes must be made at least 6 weeks in advance; include both old and new addresses and a recent mailing label if sending via mail.

## SUBSCRIPTION RATES AND SERVICE

Subscription rates are shown in the table below. For service in the US and Americas, inquiries on pricing, address changes, missing issues, subscription billing, subscription renewal, and back issues, contact the AMA Unified Service Center, 24 hours a day, 7 days a week.

**AMA members:** phone: (800) 262-3211; e-mail: msc@ama-assn.org. **Other physicians and nonphysician customers, including subscription agents:** phone: (800) 262-2350 or (312) 670-7827; fax: (312) 464-5831; e-mail: ama-subs@ama-assn.org. **Inquiries:** Unified Service Center, American Medical Association, PO Box 10946, Chicago, IL 60610-0946. For subscribers with mailing addresses outside the United States & Americas: Contact *JAMA* & *Archives* Journals, c/o EMD GmbH, Birkenstr.67, 10559 Berlin, Germany. Phone: +49 (30) 33099828; fax: +49 (30) 33099829; e-mail: ama@emd-germany.de.

**Annual Subscription Rates**

| | United States | Americas | UK | Rest of World |
|---|---|---|---|---|
| INDIVIDUAL | | | | |
| Print and Online | $185 | $240 | £165 | €250 |
| INSTITUTION | | | | |
| Print and Online | $400 | $485 | £315 | €470 |

In Canada, US rate plus GST. Rates for residents and medical students available at pubs.ama-assn.org, or from the AMA Unified Service Center.

**PEDIARIX® [Diphtheria and Tetanus Toxoids and Acellular Pertussis Adsorbed, Hepatitis B (Recombinant) and Inactivated Poliovirus Vaccine Combined]**

The following is a brief summary only; see full prescribing information for complete product information.

**CONTRAINDICATIONS:** Hypersensitivity to any component of the vaccine, including yeast, neomycin, and polymyxin B, is a contraindication (see DESCRIPTION in complete prescribing information). Do not use PEDIARIX after a serious allergic reaction (e.g., anaphylaxis) temporally associated with a previous dose of this vaccine or with any components of this vaccine. Because of the uncertainty as to which component of the vaccine might be responsible, do not give further vaccination with any of these components; or, refer such individuals to an allergist for evaluation. The following events are contraindications to administration of PEDIARIX: encephalopathy (e.g., coma, decreased level of consciousness, prolonged seizures) within 7 days of administration of a previous dose of a pertussis-containing vaccine that is not attributable to another identifiable cause; progressive neurologic disorder, including infantile spasms, uncontrolled epilepsy, or progressive encephalopathy. Do not vaccinate individuals with these conditions until a treatment regimen has been established and the condition has stabilized.

**WARNINGS:** Administration of PEDIARIX is associated with higher rates of fever relative to separately administered vaccines. In a safety study that evaluated medically attended fever after PEDIARIX or separately administered vaccines when coadministered with 7-valent pneumococcal and Hib conjugate vaccines, infants who received PEDIARIX had a higher rate of medical encounters for fever within the first 4 days following the first vaccination. In some infants, these encounters included the performance of diagnostic studies to evaluate other causes of fever (see ADVERSE REACTIONS). The tip cap and the rubber plunger of the needleless prefilled syringes contain dry natural latex rubber that may cause allergic reactions in latex sensitive individuals. The vial stopper is latex-free. If any of the following events occur in temporal relation to receipt of DTwP or a vaccine containing an acellular pertussis component, consider carefully whether to give any pertussis vaccine, including PEDIARIX: temperature of ≥40.5°C (105°F) within 48 hours not due to another identifiable cause; collapse or shock-like state (hypotonic-hyporesponsive episode) within 48 hours; persistent, inconsolable crying lasting ≥3 hours, occurring within 48 hours; seizures with or without fever occurring within 3 days. If Guillain-Barré syndrome occurs within 6 weeks of receipt of prior vaccine containing tetanus toxoid, the decision to give any tetanus toxoid-containing vaccine, including PEDIARIX, should be based on careful consideration of the potential benefits and possible risks. If tetanus toxoid is withheld, other available vaccines should be given, as indicated. The decision to administer a pertussis-containing vaccine to individuals with stable central nervous system (CNS) disorders must be made by the physician on an individual basis, with consideration of all relevant factors, and assessment of potential risks and benefits for that individual. Advise the parent or guardian of the potential increased risk involved (see PRECAUTIONS). For children at higher risk for seizures than the general population, an appropriate antipyretic may be administered at the time of vaccination and for the ensuing 24 hours according to the respective prescribing information recommended dosage to reduce the possibility of post-vaccination fever. The ACIP has published guidelines for vaccination of persons with recent or acute illness (www.cdc.gov/nip).

**PRECAUTIONS:** PEDIARIX should be given with caution in children with bleeding disorders such as hemophilia or thrombocytopenia and in children on anticoagulant therapy, with steps taken to avoid the risk of hematoma following the injection. Before the injection of any biological, the physician should take all reasonable precautions to prevent allergic or other adverse reactions. Epinephrine injection (1:1,000) and other appropriate agents used for the control of immediate allergic reactions must be immediately available should an acute anaphylactic reaction occur. Immunosuppressed individuals, including those receiving immunosuppressive therapy, may not develop the expected immune response. The ACIP has published guidelines for vaccination of persons on such therapies (www.cdc.gov/nip). **Drug Interactions:** For information regarding concomitant administration with other vaccines, refer to DOSAGE AND ADMINISTRATION in complete prescribing information. Do not mix PEDIARIX with any other vaccine in the same syringe or vial. **Carcinogenesis, Mutagenesis, Impairment of Fertility:** PEDIARIX has not been evaluated for carcinogenic or mutagenic potential, or for impairment of fertility. **Pregnancy:** Pregnancy Category C: PEDIARIX is not indicated for women of child-bearing age. Animal reproduction studies have not been conducted with PEDIARIX. It is not known whether PEDIARIX can cause fetal harm when administered to a pregnant woman or if PEDIARIX can affect reproductive capacity. **Geriatric Use:** PEDIARIX is not indicated for use in adult populations. **Pediatric Use:** Safety and effectiveness of PEDIARIX in infants younger than 6 weeks of age have not been evaluated. PEDIARIX is not recommended for persons 7 years of age or older.

**ADVERSE REACTIONS:** A total of 23,849 doses of PEDIARIX have been administered to 8,088 infants who received one or more doses as part of a 3-dose primary series during 14 clinical studies. The most common adverse reactions observed in clinical trials were local injection site reactions (pain, redness, or swelling), fever, and fussiness. In comparative studies, administration of PEDIARIX was associated with higher rates of fever relative to separately administered vaccines (see WARNINGS and ADVERSE REACTIONS Table 1). The prevalence of fever was highest on the day of vaccination and the day following vaccination. More than 96% of episodes of fever resolved within the 4-day period following vaccination (i.e., the period including the day of vaccination and the next 3 days). In the largest of the 14 studies, conducted in Germany, safety data were available for 4,666 infants who received PEDIARIX administered concomitantly at separate sites with 1 of 4 *Haemophilus influenzae* type b (Hib) vaccines at 3, 4, and 5 months of age and for 768 infants in the control group that received INFANRIX® (Diphtheria and Tetanus Toxoids and Acellular Pertussis Vaccine Adsorbed), Hib conjugate vaccine, and oral poliovirus vaccine (OPV) separately. Data on adverse events were collected by parents using standardized diary cards for 4 consecutive days following each vaccine dose (i.e., day of vaccination and the next 3 days). Infants were also monitored for unsolicited adverse events that occurred within 30 days following vaccination using diaries which were returned at subsequent visits and were supplemented by spontaneous reports and a medical history as reported by parents. More than 95% of study participants were white.

In a US study, the safety of PEDIARIX administered to 673 infants was compared to the safety of separately administered INFANRIX, ENGERIX-B® [Hepatitis B Vaccine (Recombinant)], inactivated poliovirus vaccine (IPV) in 335 infants. In both groups, infants received Hib and 7-valent pneumococcal conjugate vaccines concomitantly at separate sites. All vaccines were administered at 2, 4, and 6 months of age. The study was powered to evaluate fever >101.3° F following dose 1. Data on solicited adverse events were collected by parents using standardized diary cards for 4 consecutive days following each vaccine dose (i.e., day of vaccination and the next 3 days) and are presented in Table 1. Telephone follow-up was conducted 1 month and 6 months after the third vaccination to inquire about serious adverse events. At the 6-month follow-up, information also was collected on new onset of chronic illnesses. 638 subjects who received PEDIARIX and 313 subjects who received INFANRIX, ENGERIX-B, and IPV completed the 6-month follow-up. Among subjects in both study groups combined, 69% were white, 18% were Hispanic, 7% were black, 3% were Oriental, and 3% were of other racial/ethnic groups.

The adverse event information from clinical trials provides a basis for identifying adverse events that appear to be related to vaccine use and for approximating rates. However, because clinical trials are conducted under widely varying conditions, adverse event rates observed in the clinical trials of a vaccine cannot be directly compared to rates in the clinical trials of another vaccine, and may not reflect the rates observed in practice. As with any vaccine, there is the possibility that broad use of PEDIARIX could reveal adverse events not observed in clinical trials.

**Deaths:** In 14 clinical trials, 5 deaths were reported among 8,088 (0.06%) recipients of PEDIARIX and 1 death was reported among 2,287 (0.04%) recipients of comparator vaccines. Causes of death in the group that received PEDIARIX included 2 cases of Sudden Infant Death Syndrome (SIDS) and one case of each of the following: Convulsive disorder, congenital immunodeficiency with sepsis, and neuroblastoma. One case of SIDS was reported in the comparator group. The rate of SIDS among all recipients of PEDIARIX across the 14 trials was 0.25/1,000. The rate of SIDS observed for recipients of PEDIARIX in the German safety study was 0.2/1,000 infants (reported rate of SIDS in Germany in the latter part of the 1990s was 0.7/1,000 newborns). The reported rate of SIDS in the United States from 1990 to 1994 was 1.2/1,000 live births. By chance alone, some cases of SIDS can be expected to follow receipt of pertussis-containing vaccines.

**Serious Adverse Events:** Within 30 days following any dose of vaccine in the US safety study in which all subjects received concomitant pneumococcal and Hib conjugate vaccines, 7 serious adverse events were reported in 7 subjects (1% [7/673]) who received PEDIARIX (1 case each of pyrexia, gastroenteritis, and culture negative clinical sepsis and 4 cases of bronchiolitis) and 5 serious adverse events were reported in 4 subjects (1% [4/335]) who received INFANRIX, ENGERIX-B, and IPV (uteropelvic junction obstruction and testicular atrophy in one subject and 3 cases of bronchiolitis).

**Onset of Chronic Illnesses:** In the US safety study in which all subjects received concomitant pneumococcal and Hib conjugate vaccines, 21 subjects (3%) who received PEDIARIX and 14 subjects (4%) who received INFANRIX, ENGERIX-B, and IPV reported new onset of a chronic illness during the period from 1 to 6 months following the last dose of study vaccines. Among the chronic illnesses reported in the subjects who received PEDIARIX, there were 4 cases of asthma and 1 case each of diabetes mellitus and chronic neutropenia. There were 4 cases of asthma in subjects who received INFANRIX, ENGERIX-B, and IPV.

**Seizures:** In the German safety study over the entire study period, 6 subjects in the group that received PEDIARIX reported seizures. Two of these subjects had a febrile seizure, 1 of whom also developed afebrile seizures. The remaining 4 subjects had afebrile seizures, including 2 with infantile spasms. Two subjects reported seizures within 7 days following vaccination (1 subject had both febrile and afebrile seizures, and 1 subject had afebrile seizures), corresponding to a rate of 0.22 seizures per 1,000 doses (febrile seizures 0.07 per 1,000 doses, afebrile seizures 0.14 per 1,000 doses). No subject who received concomitant INFANRIX, Hib vaccine, and OPV reported seizures. In a separate German study that evaluated the safety of INFANRIX in 22,505 infants who received 66,867 doses of INFANRIX administered as a 3-dose primary series, the rate of seizures within 7 days of vaccination with INFANRIX was 0.13 per 1,000 doses (febrile seizures 0.0 per 1,000 doses, afebrile seizures 0.13 per 1,000 doses). Over the entire study period in the US safety study in which all subjects received concomitant pneumococcal and Hib conjugate vaccines, 4 subjects in the group that received PEDIARIX reported seizures. Three of these subjects had a febrile seizure and 1 had an afebrile seizure. Over the entire study period, 2 subjects in the group that received INFANRIX, ENGERIX-B, and IPV reported febrile seizures. There were no afebrile seizures in this group. No subject in either study group had seizures within 7 days following vaccination.

**Other Neurological Events of Interest:** No cases of hypotonic-hyporesponsiveness or encephalopathy were reported in either the German safety study or the US safety study.

**Solicited Adverse Events:** Table 1 presents data from the US safety study on solicited local and systemic adverse events within 4 days of vaccination with PEDIARIX or INFANRIX, ENGERIX-B, and IPV, administered concomitantly with Hib and 7-valent pneumococcal conjugate vaccines. In this study, medical attention (a visit to or from medical personnel) for fever within 4 days following vaccination was sought in the group who received PEDIARIX for 8 infants after the first dose (1.2%), 1 infant following the second dose (0.2%), and 5 infants following the third dose (0.8%) (Table 1). Following dose 2, medical attention for fever was sought for 2 infants (0.6%) who received separately administered vaccines (Table 1). Among infants who had a medical visit for fever within 4 days following vaccination, 9 of 14 who received PEDIARIX and 1 of 2 who received separately administered vaccines, had one or more diagnostic studies performed to evaluate the cause of fever.

**Safety of PEDIARIX after a previous dose of hepatitis B vaccine:** Limited data are available on the safety of administering PEDIARIX after a previous dose of hepatitis B vaccine. In 2 separate studies, 160 Moldovan infants and 96 US infants, respectively, received 3 doses of PEDIARIX following 1 previous dose of hepatitis B vaccine. Neither study was designed to detect significant differences in rates of adverse events associated with PEDIARIX administered after a previous dose of hepatitis B vaccine compared to PEDIARIX administered without a previous dose of hepatitis B vaccine.

**Table 1. Percentage of US Infants With Solicited Local Reactions or Systemic Adverse Events Within 4 Days of Vaccination* at 2, 4, and 6 Months of Age With PEDIARIX Administered Concomitantly With Hib Conjugate Vaccine and 7-vaient Pneumococcal Conjugate Vaccine (PCV7) or With Separate Concomitant Administration of INFANRIX, ENGERIX-B, IPV, Hib Conjugate Vaccine, and PCV7 (Modified ITT cohort)**

| | PEDIARIX, Hib Vaccine, & PCV7 | | | INFANRIX, ENGERIX-B, IPV, Hib Vaccine, & PCV7 | | |
|---|---|---|---|---|---|---|
| | **Dose 1** | **Dose 2** | **Dose 3** | **Dose 1** | **Dose 2** | **Dose 3** |
| **Local[†]** | | | | | | |
| **N** | **671** | **653** | **648** | **335** | **323** | **315** |
| Pain, any | 36.1 | 36.1 | 31.2 | 31.9 | 30.0 | 29.8 |
| Pain, grade 2 or 3 | 11.5 | 10.9 | 10.6 | 9.0 | 8.7 | 8.9 |
| Pain, grade 3 | 2.4 | 2.5 | 1.7 | 2.7 | 1.5 | 1.3 |
| Redness, any | 29.9[§] | 37.2 | 40.1 | 18.2 | 32.8 | 39.0 |
| Redness, >5 mm | 6.0[§] | 9.6[§] | 12.7[§] | 1.8 | 5.9 | 7.3 |
| Redness, >20 mm | 0.9 | 1.2[§] | 2.8 | 0.3 | 0.0 | 1.9 |
| Swelling, any | 17.3[§] | 26.5[§] | 28.7 | 9.6 | 20.4 | 24.8 |
| Swelling, >5 mm | 5.8[§] | 9.6[§] | 9.3[§] | 1.8 | 5.0 | 4.1 |
| Swelling, >20 mm | 1.9 | 2.5[§] | 3.1 | 0.6 | 0.0 | 1.3 |
| **Systemic** | | | | | | |
| **N** | **667** | **644** | **645** | **333** | **321** | **311** |
| Fever[‡], ≥100.4ºF | 27.9[§] | 38.8[§] | 33.5[§] | 19.8 | 30.2 | 23.8 |
| Fever[‡], >101.3ºF | 7.0 | 14.1[§] | 8.8 | 4.5 | 9.7 | 5.8 |
| Fever[‡], >102.2ºF | 2.2[§] | 3.6 | 3.4 | 0.3 | 3.1 | 2.3 |
| Fever[‡], >103.1ºF | 0.4 | 1.4 | 1.1 | 0.0 | 0.3 | 0.3 |
| Fever[‡], M.A. | 1.2[§] | 0.2 | 0.8 | 0.0 | 0.6 | 0.0 |
| **N** | **671** | **653** | **648** | **335** | **323** | **315** |
| Drowsiness, any | 57.2 | 51.6 | 40.9 | 54.0 | 48.3 | 38.4 |
| Drowsiness, grade 2 or 3 | 15.8 | 13.8 | 11.4 | 17.6 | 12.4 | 11.1 |
| Drowsiness, grade 3 | 2.5 | 1.2 | 0.9 | 3.6 | 0.6 | 1.9 |
| Irritability/Fussiness, any | 60.5 | 64.9 | 61.1 | 61.5 | 61.6 | 56.5 |
| Irritability/Fussiness, grade 2 or 3 | 19.8 | 27.9[§] | 25.2[§] | 19.4 | 21.1 | 19.4 |
| Irritability/Fussiness, grade 3 | 3.4 | 4.4 | 3.5 | 3.9 | 3.4 | 3.2 |
| Loss of appetite, any | 30.4 | 30.6 | 26.2 | 27.8 | 26.6 | 23.8 |
| Loss of appetite, grade 2 or 3 | 6.6 | 7.8[§] | 5.9 | 5.1 | 3.4 | 5.4 |
| Loss of appetite, grade 3 | 0.7 | 0.3 | 0.2 | 0.6 | 0.3 | 0.0 |

Modified ITT cohort = all vaccinated subjects for whom safety data were available

N = number of infants for whom at least one symptom sheet was completed; for fever, numbers exclude missing temperature recordings or tympanic measurements.

M.A. = Medically attended (a visit to or from medical personnel).

Grade 2 defined as sufficiently discomforting to interfere with daily activities.

Grade 3 defined as preventing normal daily activities.

* Within 4 days of vaccination defined as day of vaccination and the next 3 days.

† Local reactions at the injection site for PEDIARIX or INFANRIX.

‡ Rectal temperatures or axillary temperatures increased by 1°C to derive equivalent rectal temperature.

§ Rate significantly higher in the group that received PEDIARIX compared to separately administered vaccines [p value < 0.05 (2-sided Fisher Exact test) or the 95% CI on the difference between groups (Separate minus PEDIARIX) does not include 0].

**Postmarketing Reports With PEDIARIX:** Worldwide voluntary reports of adverse events received for PEDIARIX since market introduction of this vaccine are listed below. This list includes serious adverse events or events which have a suspected causal connection to components of PEDIARIX or other vaccines or drugs. Because these events are reported voluntarily from a population of uncertain size, it is not always possible to reliably estimate their frequency or establish a causal relationship to vaccine exposure. *Cardiac Disorders:* Cyanosis. *Gastrointestinal Disorders:* Diarrhea, vomiting. *General Disorders and Administrative Site Conditions:* Fatigue, injection site cellulitis, injection site induration, injection site itching, injection site nodule/lump, injection site pain, injection site reactions, injection site redness, injection site swelling, injection site warmth, irritability, limb pain, limb swelling, pyrexia, Sudden Infant Death Syndrome. *Immune System Disorders:* Anaphylactic reaction, anaphylactoid reaction, hypersensitivity. *Infections and Infestations:* Upper respiratory tract infection. *Investigations:* Abnormal liver function tests. *Metabolism and Nutrition Disorders:* Anorexia. *Nervous System Disorders:* Bulging fontanelle, convulsions, depressed level of consciousness, febrile convulsion, hypotonia, hypotonic-hyporesponsive episode, lethargy, somnolence. *Psychiatric Disorders:* Crying, insomnia, irritability, nervousness, restlessness, screaming, unusual crying. *Respiratory, Thoracic and Mediastinal Disorders:* Apnea, dyspnea. *Skin and Subcutaneous Tissue Disorders:* Angioedema, erythema, rash, urticaria. *Vascular Disorders:* Pallor, petechiae.

**Postmarketing Reports With INFANRIX and/or ENGERIX-B:** Worldwide voluntary reports of adverse events received for INFANRIX and/or ENGERIX-B in children younger than 7 years of age but not already reported for PEDIARIX are listed below. This list includes serious adverse events or events which have a suspected causal connection to components of INFANRIX and/or ENGERIX-B or other vaccines or drugs. Because these events are reported voluntarily from a population of uncertain size, it is not always possible to reliably estimate their frequency or establish a causal relationship to vaccine exposure. *Blood and Lymphatic System Disorders:* Idiopathic thrombocytopenic purpura[a,b], lymphadenopathy[a], thrombocytopenia[b]. *Gastrointestinal Disorders:* Abdominal pain[b], intussusception[a,b], nausea[b]. *General Disorders and Administrative Site Conditions:* Asthenia[b], malaise[b]. *Hepatobiliary Disorders:* Jaundice[b]. *Immune System Disorders:* Anaphylactic shock[a], serum sickness–like disease[b]. *Musculoskeletal and Connective Tissue Disorders:* Arthralgia[b], myalgia[b]. *Nervous System Disorders:* Encephalopathy[a], headache[b]. *Skin and Subcutaneous Tissue Disorders:* Alopecia[b], erythema multiforme[b], pruritus[a,b], Stevens-Johnson syndrome[a]. [[a] Following INFANRIX; [b] Following ENGERIX-B]

**Reporting Adverse Events:** Report the occurrence following immunization of any event set forth in the Vaccine Injury Table from the National Childhood Vaccine Injury Act including: Anaphylaxis or anaphylactic shock within 7 days, encephalopathy or encephalitis within 7 days, brachial neuritis within 28 days, or an acute complication or sequelae (including death) of an illness, disability, injury, or condition referred to above, or any events that would contraindicate further doses of PEDIARIX. These events should be reported to VAERS. The VAERS toll-free number is 1-800-822-7967. Reporting forms may also be obtained at the VAERS website at www.vaers.hhs.gov.

Manufactured by **GlaxoSmithKline Biologicals**, Rixensart, Belgium, US License 1617

Distributed by **GlaxoSmithKline**, Research Triangle Park, NC 27709

PEDIARIX, TIP-LOK, INFANRIX, and ENGERIX-B are registered trademarks of GlaxoSmithKline.

Full prescribing information for PEDIARIX is available at www.GSKVaccines.com/Pediarix.

BRS-PE:L3

## Pertussis is on the rise[1,2]...

*Infants may be at risk when they are not vaccinated on time*[3]

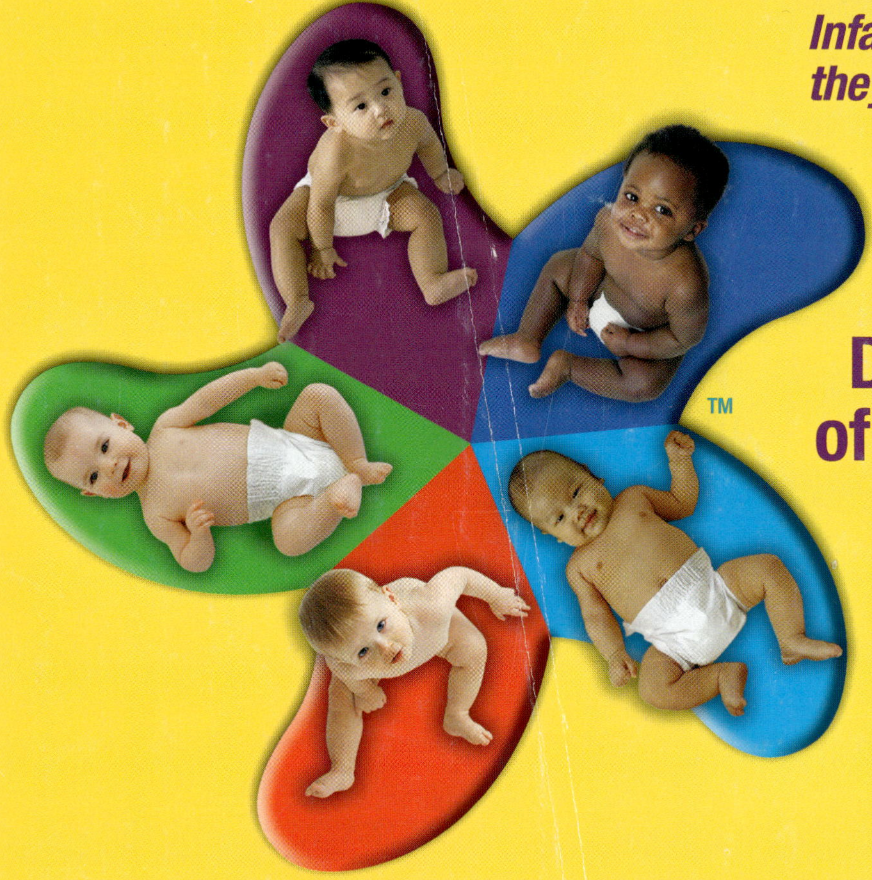


# Don't run the risk of letting one child get away

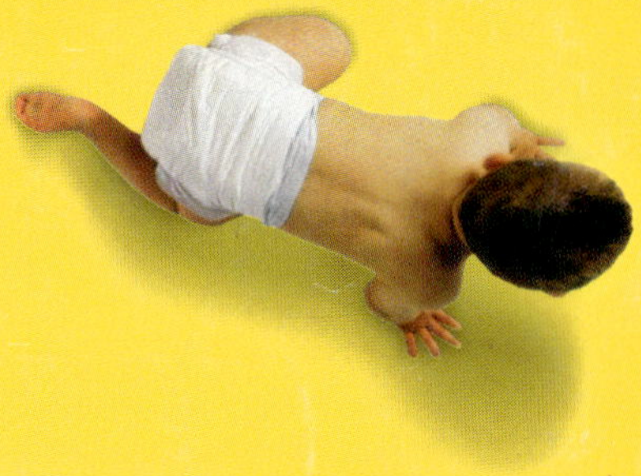

## PEDIARIX may help ensure timely vaccination with fewer injections

- 5 serious childhood diseases—1 combination vaccine*[4]
- With just 1 dose at 2, 4, and 6 months of age (in infants born of HBsAg-negative mothers)

## Important Safety information

In clinical studies, adverse events in infants receiving PEDIARIX included injection-site reactions (pain, redness, or swelling), fever, and fussiness. Administration of PEDIARIX was associated with higher rates of fever relative to separately administered vaccines (see Adverse Reactions section of the Brief Summary). PEDIARIX is contraindicated in infants with known hypersensitivity to any component of the vaccine including yeast, neomycin, and polymyxin B. As with any vaccine, vaccination with PEDIARIX may not protect 100% of susceptible individuals.

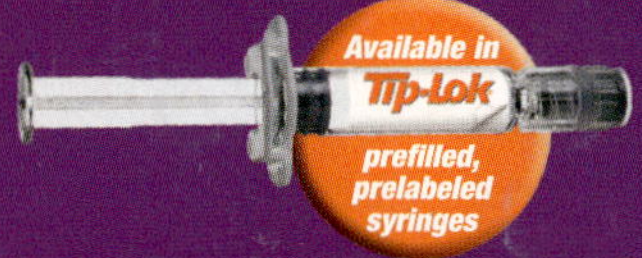


**Please see brief summary for PEDIARIX on adjacent page.**

**References: 1.** Centers for Disease Control and Prevention. Pertussis Surveillance Report—2004 (final data). Issued 8/12/05. **2.** Centers for Disease Control and Prevention. *Epidemiology and Prevention of Vaccine-Preventable Diseases.* Reported Cases and Deaths from Vaccine Preventable Diseases, United States, 1950-2003. Available at http://www.cdc.gov/nip/publications/pink/appendices/G/cases&deaths.pdf. Accessed May 10, 2006. **3.** Centers for Disease Control and Prevention. *Epidemiology and Prevention of Vaccine-Preventable Diseases.* Atkinson W, Hamborsky J, McIntyre L, Wolfe S, eds. 9th ed. Washington, DC: Public Health Foundation;2006: 84. **4.** PEDIARIX Prescribing Information.

*Does not require reconstitution.



Manufactured by **GlaxoSmithKline Biologicals,** Rixensart, Belgium
Distributed by **GlaxoSmithKline,** Research Triangle Park, NC 27709

**Pediarix**

**Diphtheria and Tetanus Toxoids and Acellular Pertussis Adsorbed, Hepatitis B (Recombinant) and Inactivated Poliovirus Vaccine Combined**

gsk GlaxoSmithKline Vaccines